TOPICAL TABLE OF CONTENTS

CLINICAL DISORDERS

TOPIC	CHAPTER	PAGE
Congenital heart disease		
Echocardiography	24	479
Ultrafast CT	37	714
MRI	48	886
Valvular heart disease		
Basic physiology	5	56
Echocardiography	21	419
Intraoperative echocardiography	31	618
Ultrafast CT	33	669
MRI	49	896
Ischemic heart disease		
Basic physiology	2	8
Myocardial metabolism	4	39
Coronary angiography	12	182
Quantitative coronary angiography	13	211
Digital angiography	16	310
Stress echocardiography	28	575
Echocardiography	29	594
Ultrafast CT and bypass grafts	34	682
Perfusion assessment with CT	35	688
MRI in ischemic heart disease	50	911
Thallium-201 imaging	58	1047
Infarct avid imaging	59	1074
Tc-99m perfusion imaging	61	1097
Monoclonal antibody imaging	62	1110
PET and perfusion	66	1169
PET and metabolism	67	1196
Cardiomyopathy		
Echocardiography	22	449
MRI	51	929
PET	68	1244
Pericardial disease		
Echocardiography	23	460
Ultrafast CT	36	703
MRI	52	936
Cardiac masses		
Echocardiography	25	511
Ultrafast CT	36	703
Indium-111 thrombus imaging	63	1121

CARDIAC IMAGING

A Companion to Braunwald's HEART DISEASE

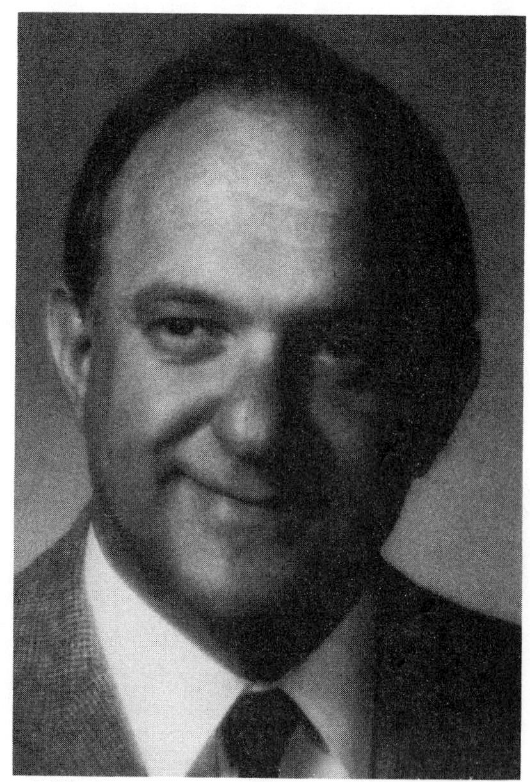

In memoriam:
Melvin L. Marcus, M.D.
1940–1989
scholar, educator, humanitarian, and friend.

H. R. Schelbert
D. J. Skorton
G. L. Wolf

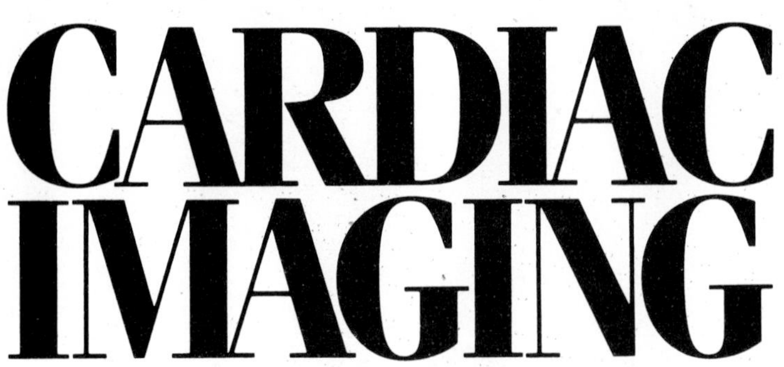

CARDIAC IMAGING

A Companion to Braunwald's HEART DISEASE

EDITED BY

Melvin L. Marcus, M.D.
Professor, Department of Internal Medicine;
Director, Coronary Physiology Laboratory,
Director, Specialized Center of Research in Ischemic Heart Disease,
College of Medicine,
The University of Iowa;
Consultant Physician,
Department of Veterans Affairs Medical Center,
Iowa City, Iowa

Heinrich R. Schelbert, M.D.
Professor of Radiological Sciences
Division of Nuclear Medicine and Biophysics
Department of Radiological Sciences
UCLA School of Medicine
Principal Investigator
The Laboratory of Nuclear Medicine
The Laboratory of Biomedical and Environmental Sciences
University of California at Los Angeles
Los Angeles, California

David J. Skorton, M.D.
Professor and Associate Chair for Clinical Programs,
Department of Internal Medicine,
College of Medicine;
Professor, Department of Electrical and Computer Engineering,
College of Engineering,
The University of Iowa;
Consultant Physician,
Department of Veterans Affairs Medical Center,
Iowa City, Iowa

Gerald L. Wolf, Ph.D., M.D.
Professor of Radiology
Harvard Medical School
Director, Center for Imaging and Pharmaceutical Research
Massachusetts General Hospital
Boston, Massachusetts

CONSULTING EDITOR

Eugene Braunwald, M.D.
Hersey Professor of the Theory and Practice of Medicine
Harvard Medical School
Chairman, Department of Medicine
Brigham and Women's Hospital
Boston, Massachusetts

W.B. SAUNDERS COMPANY
Harcourt Brace Jovanovich, Inc.
Philadelphia London Toronto Montreal Sydney Tokyo

W. B. SAUNDERS COMPANY
Harcourt Brace Jovanovich, Inc.

The Curtis Center
Independence Square West
Philadelphia, PA 19106

Library of Congress Cataloging-in-Publication Data

Cardiac imaging: a companion to Braunwald's Heart disease / edited by Melvin L. Marcus . . . [et al.]. ; consulting editor, Eugene Braunwald.

p. cm.

Companion to: Heart disease / edited by Eugene Braunwald. 3rd ed. 1988.

1. Heart—Imaging. 2. Heart—Diseases—Diagnosis. I. Marcus, Melvin L. II. Braunwald, Eugene. III. Heart disease. [DNLM: 1. Diagnostic Imaging. 2. Heart Diseases—diagnosis. WG 141 C2648]

RC683.5.I42C37 1990 616.1'2075—dc20

DNLM/DLC 90-8928

ISBN 0-7216-5862-8

Editor: Richard Zorab
Developmental Editor: Rosanne Hallowell
Designer: Joan Wendt
Production Manager: Peter Faber
Manuscript Editor: W. B. Saunders Staff
Illustration Coordinator: Walt Verbitski
Indexer: Linda Van Pelt

Cardiac Imaging:
A Companion to Braunwald's Heart Disease ISBN 0-7216-5862-8

Printed in the United States of America.

Last digit is the print number: 9 8 7 6 5 4 3 2

To my wife, Rita,
for being the primary source
encouraging me to pursue completion of this book,
to the Marcus children,
Daniel, Cheryl, Bethany, and David,
to the Schnoll children,
Marc, Danna, Jason, and Leslie,
and to my brother, Jack, and my sister-in-law, Susan,
for their continuing support.

M.L.M.

To Barbara, Kristina, and Mark,
for their patience and encouragement.

H.R.S.

To my son, Joshua,
and my wife, Judith Cooper Skorton,
for constant inspiration and support.

D.J.S.

To the memory of my mentor, Bill Wilson,
and his boundless enthusiasm for cardiac imaging, sailing, and Sue.

G.L.W.

Contributors

NICOLE AEBISCHER, M.D.
Assistant Professor, Brown University Program-in-Medicine; Director of Echocardiography, Division of Cardiology, Roger Williams General Hospital, Providence, Rhode Island
Echocardiographic Assessment of Ventricular Function

LEON AXEL, M.D., Ph.D.
Associate Professor of Radiology, University of Pennsylvania; Medical Staff, Hospital of the University of Pennsylvania, Philadelphia, Pennsylvania
Flow Phenomena in MRI; Dynamic Imaging: Principles of Cine Magnetic Resonance Imaging

RAMESH C. BANSAL, M.D.
Associate Professor of Medicine, and Director, Echocardiography Laboratory, Loma Linda University Medical Center, Loma Linda, California
Echocardiography in Cardiomyopathies

JACQUES D. BARTH, M.D., Ph.D.
Assistant Professor of Medicine, University of Southern California, Los Angeles, California; Assistant Professor of Cardiology, University of Nijmegen, The Netherlands; Director, Outpatient Clinic, Radboud University Hospital, Nijmegen, The Netherlands
Quantitative Coronary Angiography

BENICO BARZILAI, M.D.
Assistant Professor of Medicine, Washington University; Assistant Physician, Barnes Hospital, St. Louis, Missouri
Ultrasonic Characterization of Cardiovascular Tissue

THOMAS BEHRENBECK, M.D., Ph.D.
Assistant Professor of Medicine, Mayo Graduate School of Medicine and Mayo Clinic and Hospitals, Rochester, Minnesota
Measurement of Myocardial Perfusion Using Fast Computed Tomography

MALCOLM R. BELL, M.B.B.S.
Research Associate, Cardiovascular Disease, Mayo Graduate School of Medicine and Mayo Clinic and Hospitals, Rochester, Minnesota
Measurement of Myocardial Perfusion Using Fast Computed Tomography

GEORGE A. BELLER, M.D.
Professor of Medicine and Head, Division of Cardiology, Department of Internal Medicine, University of Virginia Medical School and Health Sciences Center, Charlottesville, Virginia
Myocardial Perfusion Imaging with Thallium-201

A. RESAI BENGUR, M.D.
Assistant Professor of Pediatrics (Cardiology), University of Texas Southwestern Medical Center at Dallas, Dallas, Texas
Two-Dimensional and Doppler Echocardiography in the Evaluation of Congenital Heart Disease

KEVIN S. BERBAUM, Ph.D.
Associate Professor of Radiology, The University of Iowa College of Medicine, Iowa City, Iowa
Perceptual Aspects of Cardiac Imaging

DANIEL S. BERMAN, M.D.
Professor of Medicine, UCLA School of Medicine; Director, Nuclear Cardiology, Cedars-Sinai Medical Center, Los Angeles, California
Technetium-99m Myocardial Perfusion Imaging Agents

DAVID A. BLUEMKE, M.D., Ph.D.
Resident, Department of Radiology, Johns Hopkins Hospital, Baltimore, Maryland
Nuclear Magnetic Resonance Assessment of Pericardial Disease

FREDERICK J. BONTE, M.D.
Professor of Radiology; Effie and Wofford Caine Distinguished Chair in Diagnostic Imaging; Director, Nuclear Medicine Center, The University of Texas Southwestern Medical Center at Dallas, Dallas, Texas
Infarct Avid Imaging

ELIAS H. BOTVINICK, M.D.
Professor of Medicine and Radiology, School of Medicine, Department of Radiology, University of California, San Francisco; Associate Director, Adult Cardiac Noninvasive Laboratory, Medical Center at University of California, San Francisco, California
Imaging Cardiac Neurons and Receptors

JEROME F. BREEN, M.D.
Instructor, Mayo Medical School, Mayo Graduate School; Senior Associate Consultant at Mayo Clinic, Rochester, Minnesota
Clinical Aspects of Chest Roentgenology

GARY M. BROCKINGTON, M.D.
Assistant Professor of Medicine, Tufts University School of Medicine, Boston, Massachusetts; Physician, The Faulkner Hospital, Jamaica Plain, Massachusetts
Echocardiography in Pericardial Diseases

RICHARD C. BRUNKEN, M.D.
Assistant Professor of Radiological Sciences, University of California, School of Medicine; Attending Physician, UCLA Center for the Health Sciences, Los Angeles, California
Evaluation of Myocardial Substrate Metabolism in Ischemic Heart Disease

L. MAXIMILIAN BUJA, M.D.
Professor and Chairman, Department of Pathology and Laboratory Medicine, The University of Texas Medical School at Houston; Chief of Service, Clinical Pathology Laboratory, Hermann Hospital; Chief of Service, Clinical Pathology Laboratory, Lyndon Baines Johnson Hospital; Director of Cardiovascular Pathology Research, Texas Heart Institute at St. Luke's Episcopal Hospital, Houston, Texas
Infarct Avid Imaging

PETER T. BUSER, M.D.
Director of Cardiac Magnetic Resonance Imaging, Division of Cardiology, Department of Internal Medicine, University Hospital Basel, Basel, Switzerland
Cardiomyopathy; Assessment by Magnetic Resonance

DENIS B. BUXTON, Ph.D.
Assistant Professor of Radiological Sciences, UCLA School of Medicine, Los Angeles, California
Myocardial Metabolism

PAUL J. CANNON, M.D.
Professor of Medicine, Columbia University, College of Physicians and Surgeons; Attending in Medicine, Columbia-Presbyterian Medical Center, New York, New York
Use of Sodium-23 for Cardiac Magnetic Resonance Imaging and Spectroscopy

SCOTT R. CANNON, Ph.D.
Associate Professor of Computer Science, Utah State University, Logan, Utah; Consultant, Veterans and University of New Mexico Hospitals, Albuquerque, New Mexico
Physiologic Basis for the Evaluation of Valvular Function; Principles and Physics of Doppler

STEVE M. COLLINS, Ph.D.
Professor of Electrical and Computer Engineering, and Radiology, The University of Iowa, Iowa City, Iowa
Ultrasonic Characterization of Cardiovascular Tissue

JAMES R. CORBETT, M.D.
Associate Professor of Radiology and Director of Nuclear Cardiology, The University of Texas Southwestern Medical Center at Dallas, Dallas, Texas
Infarct Avid Imaging

MICHAEL H. CRAWFORD, M.D.
Robert S. Flinn Professor of Cardiology, and Chief, Division of Cardiology, University of New Mexico School of Medicine, Albuquerque, New Mexico
Stress Echocardiography

JOHANNES CZERNIN, M.D.
Postdoctoral Scholar, Division of Nuclear Medicine and Biophysics, UCLA School of Medicine, Los Angeles, California
Metabolic Imaging with Single Photon–Emitting Tracers

MICHAEL W. DAE, M.D.
Associate Professor of Radiology and Medicine, School of Medicine, Department of Radiology, University of California, San Francisco; Associate Director, Adult Cardiac Noninvasive Laboratory, Medical Center at University of California, San Francisco, California
Imaging Cardiac Neurons and Receptors

KEVIN C. DELLSPERGER, M.D., Ph.D.
Assistant Professor, Department of Internal Medicine and the Cardiovascular Center, University of Iowa, College of Medicine; Assistant Professor, Department of Internal Medicine and the Cardiovascular Division, University of Iowa Hospitals and Clinics, Iowa City, Iowa
Determinants of Systolic and Diastolic Ventricular Function

LINDA L. DEMER, M.D., Ph.D.
Assistant Professor of Medicine, University of California, Los Angeles School of Medicine; Attending Physician, UCLA Medical Center, Los Angeles, California
Evaluation of Myocardial Blood Flow in Cardiac Disease

W. JAY ELDREDGE, M.D.
Associate Clinical Professor of Pediatrics, Robert Wood Johnson Medical School, Piscataway, N.J.; Director, Section of Cardiac Imaging; Attending Pediatric Cardiologist, Deborah Heart and Lung Center, Browns Mills, New Jersey
Comprehensive Evaluation of Congenital Heart Disease Using Ultrafast Computed Tomography

STEVEN B. FEINSTEIN, M.D.
Assistant Professor of Medicine, Division of Cardiology, University of Chicago; Director, Noninvasive Cardiology Department, University of Chicago Hospitals/Louis A. Weiss Memorial Hospital, Chicago, Illinois
Contrast Echocardiography

ANDREW J. FEIRING, M.D.
Associate Professor of Medicine, Medical College of Wisconsin; Director, Cardiac Catheterization Laboratory, Milwaukee Regional Medical Complex, Milwaukee, Wisconsin
Measurement of Myocardial Perfusion Using Fast Computed Tomography

STEVEN R. FLEAGLE, B.S.E.E.
Technical Director, Cardiovascular Image Processing Laboratory, University of Iowa, Iowa City, Iowa
Quantitative Methods in Cardiac Imaging: An Introduction to Digital Image Processing

EDWARD D. FOLLAND, M.D.
Associate Professor of Medicine, University of Massachusetts Medical School; Director, Cardiac Catheterization Laboratory, Medical Center of Central Massachusetts/Memorial, Worcester, Massachusetts
Echocardiographic Assessment of Ventricular Function

THOMAS L. FORCE, M.D.
Assistant Professor of Medicine, Harvard University; Medical Director, Cardiovascular Health Center, Massachusetts General Hospital, Boston, Massachusetts
Echocardiographic Assessment of Ventricular Function

E. A. FRANKEN, Jr., M.D.
Professor and Head, Department of Radiology, University of Iowa, College of Medicine; Director of Radiology, University of Iowa Hospitals and Clinics, Iowa City, Iowa
Perceptual Aspects of Cardiac Imaging

JEFFREY R. GALVIN, M.D.
Assistant Professor, Chief of Thoracic Radiology, The University of Iowa, Iowa City, Iowa
Assessment of Intracardiac Masses and Extracardiac Abnormalities by Ultrafast Computed Tomography

ERNEST V. GARCIA, Ph.D.
Professor of Radiology and Director of Nuclear Medicine Physics, Emory University School of Medicine, Atlanta, Georgia
Physics and Instrumentation of Radionuclide Imaging

EDWARD A. GEISER, M.D.
Professor of Medicine, University of Florida College of Medicine; Associate Director, Clinical Research Center, Shands Hospital at the University of Florida, Gainesville, Florida
Echocardiography: Physics and Instrumentation

EDWARD M. GELTMAN, M.D.
Associate Professor of Medicine, Washington University School of Medicine; Medical Director, Cardiac Diagnostic Laboratory, Barnes Hospital, St. Louis, Missouri
Metabolic Findings in Cardiomyopathies

RAYMOND J. GIBBONS, M.D.
Associate Professor of Medicine, Mayo Medical School; Co-Director, Nuclear Cardiology Laboratory; Consultant in Cardiovascular Diseases and Internal Medicine, Mayo Clinic, Rochester, Minnesota
Equilibrium Radionuclide Angiography

ANTOINETTE S. GOMES, M.D.
Associate Professor of Radiology and Medicine, UCLA School of Medicine, UCLA Medical Center, Los Angeles, California
Pulmonary Angiography

DIANA F. GUTHANER, M.D., M.B.B.S. (Syd.), M.R.C.P. (U.K.), F.R.C.R.
Clinical Associate Professor, Department of Radiology and Nuclear Medicine, Stanford University Medical Center, Stanford, California
Clinical Aspects of Chest Roentgenology

PAUL V. HARPER, M.D.
Professor (Emeritus), Surgery and Radiology, University of Chicago, Chicago, Illinois
Contrast Echocardiography

DAVID G. HARRISON, M.D.
Professor of Medicine, Emory University, Atlanta, Georgia
Physiologic Basis for Myocardial Perfusion Imaging

WALTER L. HENRY, M.D.
Professor of Medicine/Cardiology, University of California, Irvine, California College of Medicine; Vice Chancellor, Health Sciences, UCI Medical Center; Dean, California College of Medicine, University of California at Irvine, Irvine, California
Ventricular Function Assessed with Digital Subtraction Angiography

ROBERT J. HERFKENS, M.D.
Associate Professor, Department of Diagnostic Cardiology, Stanford University Medical School, Stanford University Hospital, Stanford, California
Nuclear Magnetic Resonance Assessment of Valvular Disease

CHARLES B. HIGGINS, M.D.
Professor of Radiology, University of California; Chief, Magnetic Resonance Imaging, University of California Medical Center, San Francisco, California
Cardiomyopathy: Assessment by Magnetic Resonance

JOHN W. HIRSHFELD, Jr., M.D.
Professor of Medicine, University of Pennsylvania School of Medicine; Director, Cardiac Catheterization Laboratory, Hospital of the University of Pennsylvania, Philadelphia, Pennsylvania
Radiographic Contrast Agents

MARYL R. JOHNSON, M.D.
Assistant Professor of Medicine and Associate Medical Director, Cardiac Transplant Program, Loyola University Medical Center, Maywood, Illinois
Clinical Aspects of Data Acquisition in Coronary Angiography

ROBERT H. JONES, M.D.
Mary and Deryl Hart Professor of Surgery, Associate Professor of Radiology, Duke University School of Medicine and Duke University Medical Center, Durham, North Carolina
Radionuclide Angiography

JOSE KATZ, Ph.D., M.D.
Assistant Professor of Medicine and Radiology, Columbia University College of Physicians and Surgeons; Co-director of Cardiovascular MR; Assistant Attending in Medicine, Columbia-Presbyterian Medical Center, New York, New York
Use of Sodium-23 for Cardiac Magnetic Resonance Imaging and Spectroscopy

RICHARD E. KERBER, M.D.
Professor of Medicine, University of Iowa College of Medicine; Associate Director of Cardiovascular Division, Department of Medicine, University of Iowa Hospitals and Clinics, Iowa City, Iowa
Echocardiography in Coronary Artery Disease: Myocardial Ischemia and Infarction; Intraoperative Echocardiography

BAN AN KHAW, Ph.D.
Associate Professor, Department of Radiology, Harvard Medical School; Associate Radiochemist, Associate Biochemist, Massachusetts General Hospital, Boston, Massachusetts
Monoclonal Antibody Imaging

HOSEN KIAT, M.D.
Staff Specialist, Division of Cardiology, Department of Medicine and Department of Nuclear Medicine, Cedars-Sinai Medical Center, Los Angeles, California
Technetium-99m Myocardial Perfusion Imaging Agents

EDMOND LEE, M.D.
Director of Noninvasive Cardiology, Sutter Heart Institute, Sacramento, California; Formerly, Clinical Instructor and Co-Director, Adult Echocardiography Laboratory, Medical Center at University of California, San Francisco, California
Transesophageal Echocardiography in Clinical Cardiology

JEFFREY A. LEPPO, M.D.
Associate Professor, Medicine and Nuclear Medicine, University of Massachusetts Medical Center; Associate Professor, Medicine and Nuclear Medicine; Director, Nuclear Cardiology, University of Massachusetts Medical Center, Boston, Massachusetts
Technetium-99m Myocardial Perfusion Imaging Agents

MARTIN J. LIPTON, M.D.
Chairman, Department of Radiology, University of Chicago, Chicago, Illinois
Nuclear Magnetic Resonance Assessment of Pericardial Disease

JEFFREY T. LUND, M.D.
Northern Wyoming Diagnostic Radiology, Sheridan, Wyoming
Nuclear Magnetic Resonance Assessment of Pericardial Disease

JAMSHID MADDAHI, M.D.
Associate Professor, UCLA School of Medicine; Director, Nuclear Cardiology Research, Cedars-Sinai Medical Center, Los Angeles, California
Technetium-99m Myocardial Perfusion Imaging Agents

G. B. JOHN MANCINI, M.D.
Associate Professor of Internal Medicine, University of Michigan; Director, Digital Cardiac

Angiography, University of Michigan Medical Center; Chief, Cardiology at Ann Arbor VA Medical Center, Ann Arbor, Michigan
Applications of Digital Angiography to the Coronary Circulation

MELVIN L. MARCUS, M.D.*
Professor, Department of Internal Medicine; Director, Coronary Physiology Laboratory; Director, Specialized Center of Research in Ischemic Heart Disease, College of Medicine, The University of Iowa; Consultant Physician, Department of Veterans Affairs Medical Center, Iowa City, Iowa
*Deceased.
Goals of Cardiac Imaging; Physiologic Basis for Myocardial Perfusion Imaging; Determinants of Systolic and Diastolic Ventricular Function; Evaluation of Cardiac Structure and Function with Ultrafast Computed Tomography; Determination of Bypass Graft Patency with Ultrafast Computed Tomography; Measurement of Myocardial Perfusion Using Fast Computed Tomography

BARRY M. MASSIE, M.D.
Professor of Medicine, University of California, San Francisco; Associate Staff Member, Cardiovascular Research Institute; Director, Coronary Care Unit and Hypertension Unit, San Francisco Veterans Administration Medical Center, San Francisco, California
Clinical Applications of Spectroscopy

A. IAIN McGHIE, M.B., M.R.C.R.
Registrar in General Internal Medicine and Cardiology, Stobhill General Hospital, Glasgow, United Kingdom
Infarct Avid Imaging

JAMES G. MILLER, Ph.D.
Professor of Physics, Research Professor of Medicine, Washington University, St. Louis, Missouri
Ultrasonic Characterization of Cardiovascular Tissue

MATTHEW D. MITCHELL, B.A.
Research Fellow, Department of Biochemistry and Biophysics, University of Pennsylvania, Philadelphia, Pennsylvania
Magnetic Resonance Spectroscopy to Study Myocardial Metabolism and Cellular Function

RICHARD L. MORIN, Ph.D.
Associate Professor of Physics of Diagnostic Radiology, Mayo Medical School, Rochester, Minnesota
Principles and Instrumentation for Dynamic X-ray Computed Tomography

ORHAN NALCIOGLU, Ph.D.
Professor, Radiological Sciences; Head, Division of Physics and Engineering, University of California at Irvine, Irvine, California
Ventricular Function Assessed with Digital Subtraction Angiography

PHILIP D. NICOL, M.D.
Assistant Professor, University of Toronto; Assistant Professor, The Wellesley Hospital, Division of Cardiology, Toronto, Ontario, Canada
Monoclonal Antibody Imaging

LYLE J. OLSON, M.D.
Assistant Professor of Medicine, Mayo Medical School; Senior Associate Consultant, Division of Cardiovascular Diseases and Internal Medicine, Mayo Clinic and Mayo Foundation, Rochester, Minnesota
Echocardiographic Evaluation of Valvular Heart Disease

MARY D. OSBAKKEN, M.D., Ph.D.
Assistant Professor of Medicine (Cardiology), Department of Anesthesia, Biochemistry/Biophysics, University of Pennsylvania; Staff Physician, Hospital of University of Pennsylvania, Philadelphia, Pennsylvania
Magnetic Resonance Spectroscopy to Study Myocardial Metabolism and Cellular Function

NATESA G. PANDIAN, M.D.
Associate Professor of Medicine and Radiology, Tufts University School of Medicine, Staff Physician, Director, Non-Invasive Cardiac Laboratory, Tufts–New England Medical Center Hospital, Boston, MA
Echocardiography in Pericardial Diseases

ALFRED F. PARISI, M.D.
Professor of Medicine and Director, Division of Cardiology, Brown University Program in Medicine; Chief, Cardiology, The Miriam Hospital and Roger Williams General Hospital, Providence, Rhode Island
Echocardiographic Assessment of Ventricular Function

ROBERT W. PARKEY, M.D.
Professor and Chairman, University of Texas Southwestern Medical School; Parkland Memorial Hospital, Children's Medical Center, Veterans Administration Medical Center Dallas, St. Paul Hospital, Zale-Lipshy University Hospital, Baylor Hospital, Dallas Rehabilitation Center, Dallas, Texas
Infarct Avid Imaging

ALAN S. PEARLMAN, M.D.
Professor of Medicine, University of Washington School of Medicine; Director, Echocardiography, University of Washington Medical Center, Seattle, Washington
Evaluation of Cardiac Function by Doppler Echocardiographic Techniques

JULIO E. PEREZ, M.D.
Associate Professor of Medicine, Washington University; Director of Echocardiography, Associate Physician, Barnes Hospital, St. Louis, Missouri
Ultrasonic Characterization of Cardiovascular Tissue

RONALD M. PESHOCK, M.D.
Associate Professor of Internal Medicine and Radiology; Clinical Director, Mary Nell and Ralph B. Rogers Magnetic Resonance Center; University of Texas Southwestern Medical Center; Staff Cardiologist, Zale-Lipshy University Hospital; Staff Cardiologist, Parkland Memorial Hospital, Dallas, Texas
Magnetic Resonance Imaging of the Heart: Quantitation; NMR Imaging of the Great Vessels

RONALD PETCHENY, R.T.(R.)
Clinical MRI Applications Specialist, General Electric Medical Systems, Milwaukee, Wisconsin
Optimizing MR Image Quality: Artifact Causes and Cures

CHARLES F. PRESTI, M.D.
Assistant Professor of Medicine, University of Texas Health Sciences Center, San Antonio, Texas
Stress Echocardiography

RICHARD PROROK, R.T.
MR Clinical Applications Specialist, General Electric Medical Systems, Milwaukee, Wisconsin
Optimizing MR Image Quality: Artifact Causes and Cures

JOHAN H. C. REIBER, Ph.D.
Director, Laboratory for Clinical and Experimental Image Processing, Thoraxcenter, Erasmus University and University Hospital Rotterdam-Dijkzigt, Rotterdam, The Netherlands
Quantitative Coronary Angiography

NATHANIEL REICHEK, M.D.
Professor of Medicine, University of Pennsylvania; Director, Noninvasive Laboratory, Hospital of the University of Pennsylvania, Philadelphia, Pennsylvania
Dynamic Imaging; Principles of Cine Magnetic Resonance Imaging

KENT L. RICHARDS, M.D.
Professor of Medicine, University of New Mexico; Chief of Cardiology, VA Hospital, Albuquerque, New Mexico
Physiologic Basis for the Evaluation of Valvular Function; Principles and Physics of Doppler

ERIK L. RITMAN, M.D., Ph.D.
Professor of Biophysics, Department of Physiology and Biophysics, Mayo Graduate School of Medicine, Rochester, Minnesota
Measurement of Myocardial Perfusion Using Fast Computed Tomography

RICHARD A. ROBB, Ph.D.
Professor of Biophysics, Mayo Graduate School of Medicine, Rochester, Minnesota
Principles and Instrumentation for Dynamic X-ray Computed Tomography

SEYED A. ROOHOLAMINI, M.D.
Clinical Professor, Radiological Sciences, UCLA School of Medicine, Los Angeles, California
Assessment of Intracardiac Masses and Extracardiac Abnormalities by Ultrafast Computed Tomography

JOHN A. RUMBERGER, Ph.D., M.D.
Assistant Professor of Medicine, Department of Cardiovascular Diseases and Internal Medicine, Mayo Graduate School of Medicine; Associate Professor of Internal Medicine, Mayo Clinic and Hospitals, Rochester, Minnesota
Measurement of Myocardial Perfusion Using Fast Computed Tomography

SAUL SCHAEFER, M.D.
Assistant Professor of Medicine and Radiology, University of California, San Francisco; Cardiology Staff, VA Medical Center, San Francisco, California
Clinical Applications of Cardiac Spectroscopy

HEINRICH R. SCHELBERT, M.D.
Professor of Radiological Sciences, Division of Nuclear Medicine and Biophysics, Department of Radiological Sciences, UCLA School of Medicine; Principal Investigator, The Laboratory of Nuclear Medicine, The Laboratory of Biomedical and Environmental Sciences, University of California at Los Angeles, Los Angeles, California
Goals of Cardiac Imaging; Metabolic Imaging with Single Photon-Emitting Tracers; Principles of Positron Emission Tomography; Evaluation of Myocardial Substrate Metabolism in Ischemic Heart Disease

NELSON B. SCHILLER, M.D.
Professor of Medicine, University of California, San Francisco; Director of Adult Echocardiography Laboratory, University of California, San Francisco, Medical Center, Moffitt Hospital, San Francisco, California
Transesophageal Echocardiography in Clinical Cardiology

INGELA SCHNITTGER, M.D.
Assistant Professor of Medicine (Cardiology), Co-director Non-Invasive Laboratory, Stanford University Medical Center, Stanford, California
Cardiac and Extracardiac Masses: Echocardiographic Evaluation

STEVEN L. SCHWARTZ, M.D.
Assistant Professor of Medicine, Tufts University School of Medicine; Physician, Associate Director, Non-Invasive Cardiac Laboratory, Tufts–New England Medical Center Hospital, Boston, Massachusetts
Echocardiography in Pericardial Diseases

LAWRENCE J. SEGIL, M.D.
Clinical Assistant Professor, Department of Anesthesia and Critical Care Medicine, Michael Reese Hospital and Medical Center, Chicago, Illinois
Contrast Echocardiography

PATRICK W. SERRUYS, M.D.
Professor of Interventional Cardiology, and Research Director, Catheterisations Laboratory, Erasmus University, Rotterdam, The Netherlands
Quantitative Coronary Angiography

PRAVIN M. SHAH, M.D.
Professor of Medicine and Director of Academic Programs, Loma Linda University Medical Center, Loma Linda, California
Echocardiography in Cardiomyopathies

SATISH SHARMA, M.D.
Associate Professor, Brown University Program in Medicine; Chief of Cardiology, VA Medical Center, Davis Park, Providence, Rhode Island
Echocardiographic Assessment of Ventricular Function

FLORENCE H. SHEEHAN, M.D.
Research Associate Professor, University of Washington, Seattle, Washington
Cardiac Angiography

DAVID J. SKORTON, M.D.
Professor and Associate Chair for Clinical Programs, Department of Internal Medicine, College of Medicine; Professor, Department of Electrical and Computer Engineering, College of Engineering, The University of Iowa; Consultant Physician, Department of Veterans Affairs Medical Center, Iowa City, Iowa
Goals of Cardiac Imaging; Quantitative Methods in Cardiac Imaging: An Introduction to Digital Image Processing; Ultrasonic Characterization of Cardiovascular Tissue; Assessment of Congenital Heart Disease by Nuclear Magnetic Resonance Imaging

WILBUR L. SMITH, Jr., M.D.
Professor of Radiology, Vice-Chairman, Department of Radiology, The University of Iowa, College of Medicine, Iowa City, Iowa
Assessment of Congenital Heart Disease by Nuclear Magnetic Resonance Imaging

A. REBECCA SNIDER, M.D.
Professor of Pediatrics and Communicable Diseases, C.S. Mott Children's Hospital, University of Michigan Medical Centers, Ann Arbor, Michigan
Two-Dimensional and Doppler Echocardiography in the Evaluation of Congenital Heart Disease

HEINZ SOCHOR, M.D.
Universitätsdozent, Kardiologische Universitätsklinik, Wien, Austria
Metabolic Imaging with Single Photon–Emitting Tracers

WILLIAM STANFORD, M.D.
Associate Professor, Department of Radiology, University of Iowa College of Medicine; Director, Cardiovascular Radiology, University of Iowa Hospitals, Iowa City, Iowa
Determination of Bypass Graft Patency with Ultrafast Computed Tomography; Assessment of Intracardiac Masses and Extracardiac Abnormalities by Ultrafast Computed Tomography; Assessment of Congenital Heart Disease by Nuclear Magnetic Resonance Imaging

WILLIAM J. STEWART, M.D.
Staff Cardiologist, The Cleveland Clinic Foundation, Cleveland, Ohio
Intraoperative Echocardiography

JOHN R. STRATTON, M.D.
Associate Professor of Medicine; Director, Echocardiography Laboratory; Staff Cardiologist, University of Washington, Seattle, Washington
Thrombosis Imaging with Indium-111–Labeled Platelets

ANDRÉ SYROTA, M.D., Ph.D.
Professor of Biophysics and Nuclear Medicine, Head of Service Hospitalier Frédéric Joliot, Commissariat à l'Energie Atomique; Service Hospitalier Frédéric Joliot, Orsay, France
Positron Emission Tomography: Evaluation of Cardiac Receptors

A. JAMIL TAJIK, M.D., F.A.C.C.
Professor of Medicine and Pediatrics, Mayo Medical School; Consultant, Cardiovascular Diseases, Internal Medicine, and Pediatric Cardiology, Director, Cardiovascular Ultrasound Imaging and Hemodynamic Laboratory, Mayo Clinic and Mayo Foundation, Rochester, Minnesota
Echocardiographic Evaluation of Valvular Heart Disease

S. L. TALAGALA, Ph.D.
Magnetic Resonance Physicist, Pittsburgh NMR Institute, Pittsburgh, Pennsylvania
Principles of Nuclear Magnetic Resonance; Principles of Magnetic Resonance Imaging

JONATHAN M. TOBIS, M.D.
Associate Professor, Medicine/Cardiology, University of California at Irvine, California College of Medicine, Irvine, California; Acting Chief, Division of Cardiology, Director, Cardiac Catheterization Laboratory, University of California, Irvine Medical Center, Orange, California
Ventricular Function Assessed with Digital Subtraction Angiography

JOSEPH A. UTZ, M.D.
Clinical Associate Professor of Radiology, Uniformed Services University of the Health Sciences, Bethesda, Maryland; Attending Radiologist, Baptist Medical Center, Memorial Medical Center, Jacksonville, Florida
Nuclear Magnetic Resonance Assessment of Valvular Disease

PAOLO VOCI, M.D.
Assistant Professor of Cardiology, University of Rome "La Sapienza," Rome, Italy
Contrast Echocardiography

MICHAEL W. WEINER, M.D.
Scientific Director, Magnetic Resonance Unit, Professor of Medicine and Radiology, University of California, San Francisco, California
Clinical Applications of Cardiac Spectroscopy

ROBERT M. WEISS, M.D.
Assistant Professor of Medicine, Department of Internal Medicine, University of Iowa College of Medicine, Iowa City, Iowa
Evaluation of Cardiac Structure and Function with Ultrafast Computed Tomography

JAMES S. WHITING, Ph.D.
Assistant Professor, Department of Radiological Sciences, University of California, Los Angeles; Director, Medical Physics and Imaging, Cedars-Sinai Medical Center, Los Angeles, California
Physical Principles and Instrumentation in Digital Angiography

SAMUEL A. WICKLINE, M.D.
Assistant Professor of Medicine, Washington University; Assistant Physician, Barnes Hospital, St. Louis, Missouri
Ultrasonic Characterization of Cardiovascular Tissue

JAMES T. WILLERSON, M.D.
Professor and Chairman, Department of Internal Medicine, University of Texas Medical School at Houston, Texas; Director of Cardiology Research, Texas Heart Institute; Chief of Internal Medicine Services at Hermann Hospital and Lyndon Baines Johnson Hospital, Houston, Texas
Infarct Avid Imaging

GERALD WISENBERG, M.D., F.R.C.P.
Associate Professor, Department of Medicine, University of Western Ontario; Chief, Division of Cardiology, St. Joseph's Hospital, London, Ontario, Canada
Evaluation of Ischemic Heart Disease by Nuclear Magnetic Resonance

GERALD L. WOLF, Ph.D., M.D.
Professor of Radiology, Harvard Medical School; Director, Center for Imaging and Pharmaceutical Research, Massachusetts General Hospital, Boston, Massachusetts
Goals of Cardiac Imaging; Principles of Nuclear Magnetic Resonance; Principles of Magnetic Resonance Imaging; Biologic Basis of Proton Relaxation; Contrast Agents for Cardiac MRI; Assessment of Congenital Heart Disease by Nuclear Magnetic Resonance Imaging; Glossary

PAUL WOZNEY, M.D.
Assistant Clinical Professor, University of Miami, Miami, Florida; Staff Radiologist, Medical Center Hospital of Punta Gorda, Florida; Staff Radiologist, Southwest Florida Regional MRI Center, Port Charlotte, Florida
Optimizing MR Image Quality: Artifact Causes and Cures

Foreword

It is a special honor to have been invited to write this foreword to the first edition of what I predict will be an important new text—*Cardiac Imaging.*

Since the days of William Harvey, clinicians and basic scientists alike have marveled at both the simplicity of the heart's pumping function and the complexity of its structure. The intimacy of the reciprocal relations between cardiac structure and function—each simultaneously and profoundly influencing the other—is one of the wonders of biology. However, until the end of the nineteenth century physiologists and physicians could correlate the structure and function of the heart only by visual inspection, an approach that had little if any implication for clinical medicine. The first approaches to cardiac imaging (i.e., roentgenography and fluoroscopy, followed by peripheral angiocardiography and then selective angiocardiography) have allowed extensive simultaneous assessment of cardiac structure and function in intact subjects. During the past 25 years, clinical cardiovascular investigators, specialists in imaging techniques, nuclear physicists, and engineers have devoted enormous effort to the development of noninvasive imaging techniques. As a consequence, we now have available, in addition to conventional radiology, a broad array of such techniques, including cardiac and vascular angiography, various modes of echocardiography, computed tomography, magnetic resonance imaging and spectroscopy, several forms of radionuclide imaging, and positron emission tomography.

Consider, for example, how the care of a patient with aortic stenosis and regurgitation may be facilitated by these techniques. Ultimately, this valvular deformity leads to hemodynamic overload, cardiac hypertrophy and dilatation, and an increase in myocardial wall tension, which in turn, is somehow sensed by the cardiac cell and leads to changes in gene expression, which result in enhanced myocardial protein synthesis and ventricular hypertrophy. The heart's total oxygen consumption rises while the aortic valvular abnormality interferes with myocardial perfusion. Thus, the left ventricle may become ischemic when acute stress is superimposed, and ultimately cardiac dysfunction and failure develop. Persistence of the latter leads to "down-regulation" of myocardial beta receptors and the loss of adrenergic support of the failing myocardium. As the heart dilates further, mitral regurgitation develops, followed in turn by pulmonary hypertension, right ventricular enlargement, and tricuspid regurgitation. It is possible, of course, to interrupt this vicious circle by surgical treatment, but selecting the optimal time for operation can be very difficult.

The modern cardiologist, by judicious application of a number of noninvasive imaging techniques, can now assess the valvular deformity and determine its impact on ventricular function. The configuration and severity of obstruction of the aortic valve, the transvalvular pressure gradient, the magnitude of regurgitant flow, the ventricular volume throughout the cardiac cycle, the thickness of the ventricular wall at rest and during stress, its ability to shorten, its diastolic properties, the height of the pulmonary artery pressure, the presence and severity of secondary mitral and tricuspid regurgitation, the regional perfusion of the myocardium, its metabolism of glucose and of fatty acids, and even the density of beta-adrenergic receptors can now all be assessed at appropriate intervals by application of the modern imaging techniques described in this book. Thus, these methods, many of which are noninvasive or only minimally invasive, can provide all of the information required for developing a rational therapeutic plan for such a patient and for assessing the effects on cardiac structure and function of pharmacologic or surgical intervention, or simply of the passage of time. Similar analyses are now possible in patients presenting with a wide variety of cardiovascular disorders.

In this splendid new book, the editors—Drs. Marcus, Schelbert, Skorton and Wolf—working with a group of talented authors, have provided an elegant analysis of the most important cardiovascular diagnostic imaging techniques currently available. This interdisciplinary book will be of enormous aid to those involved in the care of patients with heart disease—whether they are adult or pediatric cardiologists, cardiovascular surgeons, radiologists, echocardiographers, or specialists in nuclear medicine. It will provide them with information on the theoretical background, clinical utility, and relative values and limitations of each of these techniques. The first section of the book is particularly useful. It includes clear presentations of the goals and quantitative and perceptual aspects of cardiac imaging as well as the physiologic bases for the evaluation of ventricular performance, myocardial perfusion, myocardial metabolism, and valvular function.

We now have an embarrassment of riches insofar as available imaging techniques are concerned. If all were applied in a single patient, an enormous amount of redundant information would be obtained. Some techniques have special advantages—the equipment is relatively inexpensive and portable; it can be used in a physician's office or an emergency room, or it can be easily wheeled into an intensive care unit. Other types of equipment provide unique information, but they are quite large and require expensive fixed installations. *Cardiac Imaging* presents not only detailed descriptions of these various techniques and their strengths and limitations but also the bases for comparing them. In this era of cost-conscious medical practice, this book will be equally useful to the individual physician who is deciding on which technique to employ in a given patient as well as to the department head faced with the decision of whether and how to upgrade the institution's cardiac imaging facilities.

The untimely death of Dr. Marcus, the founding editor of *Cardiac Imaging*, just as the finishing touches were put on this book, represents a serious loss to cardiovascular science. Dr. Marcus' enthusiasm, creativity, and overall positive influence on this field will live on in his trainees, his many seminal research contributions, and certainly in *Cardiac Imaging*, an effort that I know occupied his devoted attention during his final illness.

The editors deserve congratulations for preparing this very scholarly, yet quite readable and useful text. I am delighted to acknowledge its association with *Heart Disease: A Textbook of Cardiovascular Medicine* with which it will share readership, i.e., the physician, regardless of specialty, who bears responsibility for and who has a deep interest in patients with heart disease as well as the serious student who seeks to acquire the most accurate current understanding and information that will allow assumption of that responsibility. It is my hope that the current and future editions of these two books will complement one another in benefiting the many patients with disorders of the heart and circulatory system.

EUGENE BRAUNWALD, M.D.
BOSTON, MA

Preface

The field of cardiac imaging is of great importance to the care of patients with cardiovascular disease. Virtually all patients with suspected or known cardiovascular disease undergo one and frequently several different cardiac imaging procedures as part of their initial evaluation. Often these diagnostic tests are repeated at variable intervals during the course of the illness. The information gleaned from the interpretation of these imaging procedures is often crucial to establishing a precise diagnosis, assessing the severity of the disease and its likely course, and evaluating the efficacy of various therapeutic approaches.

In the past two decades, there has been explosive development in the field of cardiac imaging. Prior to 1970, chest roentgenography and invasive angiography were the only widely used cardiac imaging modalities. In the 1970's, four new technologies were introduced (M-mode, two-dimensional and Doppler echocardiography, conventional nuclear medicine studies, digital subtraction angiography, and positron emission tomography) and in the 1980's another four were launched (single-photon emission computed tomography, magnetic resonance imaging and spectroscopy, color flow Doppler ultrasound, and ultrafast computed tomography). At present, most of these individual modalities are in an accelerated phase of development.

As a consequence of the rapid introduction and impressive progress in the development of complex imaging methods, it has become very difficult for a single practicing cardiologist, radiologist, or academician to completely master this vast array of new diagnostic technology. As a result of economic considerations, overlapping applications and lack of sufficient expertise in various imaging areas, very few hospitals have access to all of these diagnostic methods. At the same time, in this era, it is no longer acceptable for a cardiologist or radiologist to have a knowledge base that is limited to only a few of these imaging methods. Studying only texts that focus on a single modality can lead to a very restricted frame of reference. Optimal utilization of these disparate diagnostic methods requires a broad appreciation of the relative strengths and weaknesses of the various modalities.

Dr. Eugene Braunwald's book, *Heart Disease*, contains several chapters that relate to cardiac imaging. However, this vast subject area cannot be comprehensively addressed in a general cardiology textbook. The present volume is intended to be a companion to Dr. Braunwald's book, providing an in-depth review of cardiac imaging to those who have a particular interest in this area.

In planning this textbook, several guiding principles were followed. First, editors were selected who had complementary areas of expertise, the sum of which would encompass the entire field of cardiac imaging. Second, the introductory chapters in the book provide the physiologic and biochemical bases for cardiac imaging that transcend any of the individual modalities. Third, all of the individual cardiac imaging modalities are comprehensively reviewed, and at the beginning of each section there is at least one chapter that reviews the basic principles of the techniques. In general, the information content in these sections is greater than that found in many of the monographs available in a similar area. Finally, a large portion of the entire text was written by the editors and the contributed chapters were carefully reviewed and almost always extensively revised at the suggestion of the editors.

This textbook has a number of other features that we hope will be helpful to the reader. Two tables of contents are provided. One, following this preface, lists the chapters in the sequence in which they appear in the book, while the other, located inside the book's cover, regroups the chapters under topical headings. Thus, the reader can quickly find all the information that pertains to imaging a given clinical entity such as congenital or valvular heart disease. Each chapter begins with a detailed outline that should facilitate finding information on specific subtopics. The book contains a large number of carefully selected and reproduced black and white and color images. Extensive references to both classic articles and recent studies are provided. Finally, since the senior editor (MLM) reviewed the entire volume, duplication between chapters was minimized and diverse opinions on specific points among contributors and editors were adjudicated in an effort to present a balanced view in controversial areas.

Major textbooks invariably represent the efforts of many individuals in addition to the editors and contributors. We want to particularly thank Dr. Eugene Braunwald for encouraging us to undertake this project and for advising us on many aspects of the book.

We gratefully acknowledge Cindy Evans, Carolyn Frisbie, Rita Griffin, Maureen Kent, Ruth Lillie, Tina Schrunk, and Lea Williams at The University of Iowa for their efforts in many organizational aspects of the project and for expert preparation of the manuscripts. We have been fortunate to work with William Lamsback (former acquisitions editor at W. B. Saunders), Richard Zorab, Rosanne Hallowell, Peter Faber, Carol DiBerardino, Betty Barth, and Jody Murphy at W. B. Saunders; these professionals gave invaluable advice and constructive criticism, generously sharing their experience in the publishing arts.

If this textbook provides a vehicle that will enable cardiology fellows, cardiologists, radiology residents, radiologists, and cardiac surgeons to substantially increase the breadth and depth of their knowledge in cardiac imaging, then it will have accomplished its primary purpose.

MELVIN L. MARCUS
HEINRICH R. SCHELBERT
DAVID J. SKORTON
GERALD L. WOLF

Contents

PART I

INTRODUCTION 1

CHAPTER 1

Goals of Cardiac Imaging 1
David J. Skorton, M.D. ■ Melvin L. Marcus, M.D. ■ Heinrich R. Schelbert, M.D. ■ Gerald L. Wolf, Ph.D., M.D.

CHAPTER 2

Physiologic Basis for Myocardial Perfusion Imaging 8
Melvin L. Marcus, M.D. ■ David G. Harrison, M.D.

CHAPTER 3

Determinants of Systolic and Diastolic Ventricular Function 24
Melvin L. Marcus, M.D. ■ Kevin C. Dellsperger, M.D., Ph.D.

CHAPTER 4

Myocardial Metabolism 39
Denis B. Buxton, Ph.D.

CHAPTER 5

Physiologic Basis for the Evaluation of Valvular Function 56
Kent L. Richards, M.D. ■ Scott R. Cannon, Ph.D.

CHAPTER 6

Quantitative Methods in Cardiac Imaging: An Introduction to Digital Image Processing 72
Steven R. Fleagle, B.S.E.E. ■ David J. Skorton, M.D.

CHAPTER 7

Perceptual Aspects of Cardiac Imaging 87
E. A. Franken, Jr., M.D. ■ Kevin S. Berbaum, Ph.D.

PART II

CONVENTIONAL RADIOGRAPHY 93

CHAPTER 8

Clinical Aspects of Chest Roentgenology 93
Diana F. Guthaner, M.D. ■ Jerome F. Breen, M.D.

CHAPTER 9

Cardiac Angiography 109
Florence H. Sheehan, M.D.

CHAPTER 10

Pulmonary Angiography 149
Antoinette S. Gomes, M.D.

CHAPTER 11

Radiographic Contrast Agents 162
John W. Hirshfeld, Jr., M.D.

PART III

CORONARY ANGIOGRAPHY 182

CHAPTER 12

Clinical Aspects of Data Acquisition in Coronary Angiography 182
Maryl R. Johnson, M.D.

CHAPTER 13

Quantitative Coronary Angiography 211
Johan H. C. Reiber, Ph.D. ■ Patrick W. Serruys, M.D., Ph.D. ■ Jacques D. Barth, M.D., Ph.D.

PART IV

DIGITAL ANGIOGRAPHY 281

CHAPTER 14

Physical Principles and Instrumentation in Digital Angiography 281
James S. Whiting, Ph.D.

CHAPTER 15

Ventricular Function Assessed with Digital Subtraction Angiography 295
Jonathan M. Tobis, M.D. ■ Orhan Nalcioglu, Ph.D. ■ Walter L. Henry, M.D.

CHAPTER 16

Applications of Digital Angiography to the Coronary Circulation 310
G. B. John Mancini, M.D.

PART V

ECHOCARDIOGRAPHY 348

CHAPTER 17

Echocardiography: Physics and Instrumentation 348
Edward A. Geiser, M.D.

CHAPTER 18

Principles and Physics of Doppler 365
Scott R. Cannon, Ph.D. ■ Kent L. Richards, M.D.

CHAPTER 19

Echocardiographic Assessment of Ventricular Function 374
Thomas L. Force, M.D. ■ Edward D. Folland, M.D. ■ Nicole Aebischer, M.D. ■ Satish Sharma, M.D. ■ Alfred F. Parisi, M.D.

CHAPTER 20

Evaluation of Cardiac Function by Doppler Echocardiographic Techniques 402
Alan S. Pearlman, M.D.

CHAPTER 21

Echocardiographic Evaluation of Valvular Heart Disease .. 419
Lyle J. Olson, M.D. ■ A. Jamil Tajik, M.D.

CHAPTER 22

Echocardiography in Cardiomyopathies 449
Pravin M. Shah, M.D. ■ Ramesh C. Bansal, M.D.

CHAPTER 23

Echocardiography in Pericardial Diseases 460
Gary M. Brockington, M.D. ■ Steven L. Schwartz, M.D. ■ Natesa G. Pandian, M.D.

CHAPTER 24

Two-Dimensional and Doppler Echocardiography in the Evaluation of Congenital Heart Disease 479
A. Rebecca Snider, M.D. ■ A. Resai Bengur, M.D.

CHAPTER 25

Cardiac and Extracardiac Masses: Echocardiographic Evaluation 511
Ingela Schnittger, M.D.

CHAPTER 26

Ultrasonic Characterization of Cardiovascular Tissue 538
David J. Skorton, M.D. ■ James G. Miller, Ph.D. ■ Samuel A. Wickline, M.D. ■ Benico Barzilai, M.D. ■ Steve M. Collins, Ph.D. ■ Julio E. Perez, M.D.

CHAPTER 27

Contrast Echocardiography 557
Steven B. Feinstein, M.D. ■ Paolo Voci, M.D. ■ Lawrence J. Segil, M.D. ■ Paul V. Harper, M.D.

CHAPTER 28

Stress Echocardiography 575
Charles F. Presti, M.D. ■ Michael H. Crawford, M.D.

CHAPTER 29

Echocardiography in Coronary Artery Disease: Myocardial Ischemia and Infarction 594
Richard E. Kerber, M.D.

CHAPTER 30

Transesophageal Echocardiography in Clinical Cardiology 605
Edmond Lee, M.D. ■ Nelson B. Schiller, M.D.

CHAPTER 31

Intraoperative Echocardiography 618
William J. Stewart, M.D. ■ Richard E. Kerber, M.D.

PART VI

ULTRAFAST COMPUTED TOMOGRAPHY 634

CHAPTER 32

Principles and Instrumentation for Dynamic X-ray Computed Tomography 634
Richard A. Robb, Ph.D. ■ Richard L. Morin, Ph.D.

CHAPTER 33

Evaluation of Cardiac Structure and Function with Ultrafast Computed Tomography 669
Melvin L. Marcus, M.D. ■ Robert M. Weiss, M.D.

CHAPTER 34

Determination of Bypass Graft Patency with Ultrafast Computed Tomography 682
William Stanford, M.D. ■ Melvin L. Marcus, M.D.

CHAPTER 35

Measurement of Myocardial Perfusion Using Fast Computed Tomography 688
John A. Rumberger, M.D., Ph.D. ■ Malcolm R. Bell, M.B.B.S. ■ Andrew J. Feiring, M.D. ■ Thomas Behrenbeck, M.D., Ph.D. ■ Melvin L. Marcus, M.D. ■ Erik L. Ritman, M.D., Ph.D.

CHAPTER 36

Assessment of Intracardiac Masses and Extracardiac Abnormalities by Ultrafast Computed Tomography 703
William Stanford, M.D. ■ Seyed A. Rooholamini, M.D. ■ Jeffrey R. Galvin, M.D.

CHAPTER 37

Comprehensive Evaluation of Congenital Heart Disease Using Ultrafast Computed Tomography 714
W. Jay Eldredge, M.D.

PART VII

CARDIAC NUCLEAR MAGNETIC RESONANCE IMAGING 732

CHAPTER 38

Principles of Nuclear Magnetic Resonance 732
S. L. Talagala, M.D., Ph.D. ■ Gerald L. Wolf, Ph.D., M.D.

Chapter 39

Principles of Magnetic Resonance Imaging 744
S. L. Talagala, M.D., Ph.D. ■ Gerald L. Wolf, Ph.D., M.D.

Chapter 40

Biologic Basis of Proton Relaxation 759
Gerald L. Wolf, Ph.D., M.D.

Chapter 41

Flow Phenomena in MRI 769
Leon Axel, M.D., Ph.D.

Chapter 42

Optimizing MR Image Quality: Artifact Causes and Cures 776
Paul Wozney, M.D. ■ Richard Prorok, R.T. ■ Ronald Petcheny, R.T.(R.)

Chapter 43

Contrast Agents for Cardiac MRI 794
Gerald L. Wolf, Ph.D., M.D.

Chapter 44

Magnetic Resonance Imaging of the Heart: Quantitation 811
Ronald M. Peshock, M.D.

Chapter 45

Use of Sodium-23 for Cardiac Magnetic Resonance Imaging and Spectroscopy 828
Jose Katz, M.D., Ph.D. ■ Paul J. Cannon, M.D.

Chapter 46

Magnetic Resonance Spectroscopy to Study Myocardial Metabolism and Cellular Function 841
Mary D. Osbakken, M.D., Ph.D. ■ Matthew D. Mitchell, B.A.

Chapter 47

NMR Imaging of the Great Vessels 864
Ronald M. Peshock, M.D.

Chapter 48

Assessment of Congenital Heart Disease by Nuclear Magnetic Resonance Imaging 886
Wilbur L. Smith, Jr., M.D. ■ William Stanford, M.D. ■ David J. Skorton, M.D. ■ Gerald L. Wolf, Ph.D., M.D.

Chapter 49

Nuclear Magnetic Resonance Assessment of Valvular Disease 896
Robert J. Herfkens, M.D. ■ Joseph A. Utz, M.D.

Chapter 50

Evaluation of Ischemic Heart Disease by Nuclear Magnetic Resonance 911
Gerald Wisenberg, M.D., F.R.C.P.C

Chapter 51

Cardiomyopathy: Assessment by Magnetic Resonance 929
Peter T. Buser, M.D. ■ Charles B. Higgins, M.D.

Chapter 52

Nuclear Magnetic Resonance Assessment of Pericardial Disease 936
David A. Bluemke, M.D., Ph.D. ■ Jeffrey T. Lund, M.D. ■ Martin J. Lipton, M.D.

Chapter 53

Dynamic Imaging: Principles of Cine Magnetic Resonance Imaging 948
Nathaniel Reichek, M.D. ■ Leon Axel, M.D., Ph.D.

Chapter 54

Clinical Applications of Cardiac Spectroscopy 967
Saul Schaefer, M.D. ■ Michael W. Weiner, M.D. ■ Barry M. Massie, M.D.

PART VIII

CONVENTIONAL RADIONUCLIDE IMAGING 977

Chapter 55

Physics and Instrumentation of Radionuclide Imaging 977
Ernest V. Garcia, Ph.D.

Chapter 56

Radionuclide Angiocardiography 1006
Robert H. Jones, M.D.

Chapter 57

Equilibrium Radionuclide Angiography 1027
Raymond J. Gibbons, M.D.

Chapter 58

Myocardial Perfusion Imaging with Thallium-201 1047
George A. Beller, M.D.

Chapter 59

Infarct Avid Imaging 1074
James T. Willerson, M.D. ■ Iain McGhie, M.D. ■ Robert W. Parkey, M.D. ■ Frederick J. Bonte, M.D. ■ L. Maximilian Buja, M.D. ■ James R. Corbett, M.D.

Chapter 60

Metabolic Imaging with Single-Photon Emitting Tracers 1085
Heinz Sochor, M.D. ■ Johannes Czernin, M.D. ■ Heinrich R. Schelbert, M.D.

PART IX

NEW DEVELOPMENTS IN CARDIAC RADIONUCLIDE IMAGING 1097

CHAPTER 61

Technetium–99m Myocardial Perfusion Imaging Agents 1097
Daniel S. Berman, M.D. ■ Hosen Kiat, M.D. ■ Jeffrey A. Leppo, M.D. ■ Jamshid Maddahi, M.D.

CHAPTER 62

Monoclonal Antibody Imaging 1110
Philip D. Nicol, M.D. ■ Ban An Khaw, Ph.D.

CHAPTER 63

Thrombosis Imaging with Indium-111–Labeled Platelets 1121
John R. Stratton, M.D.

CHAPTER 64

Imaging Cardiac Neurons and Receptors 1135
Michael W. Dae, M.D. ■ Elias H. Botvinick, M.D.

PART X

POSITRON EMISSION TOMOGRAPHY 1140

CHAPTER 65

Principles of Positron Emission Tomography 1140
Heinrich R. Schelbert, M.D.

CHAPTER 66

Evaluation of Myocardial Blood Flow in Cardiac Disease 1169
Linda L. Demer, M.D., Ph.D.

CHAPTER 67

Evaluation of Myocardial Substrate Metabolism in Ischemic Heart Disease 1196
Richard C. Brunken, M.D. ■ Heinrich R. Schelbert, M.D.

CHAPTER 68

Metabolic Findings in Cardiomyopathies 1244
Edward M. Geltman, M.D.

CHAPTER 69

Positron Emission Tomography: Evaluation of Cardiac Receptors 1256
André Syrota, M.D., Ph.D.

NMR GLOSSARY 1271

INDEX 1279

The color plates are located between pages 648 and 649.

Part I

Introduction

Chapter 1

Goals of Cardiac Imaging

- *DAVID J. SKORTON, M.D.* ▪ *MELVIN L. MARCUS, M.D.*
- *HEINRICH R. SCHELBERT, M.D.*
- *GERALD L. WOLF, M.D., Ph.D.*

CURRENT CAPABILITIES AND NEEDS IN DIAGNOSTIC CARDIAC IMAGING 1
Anatomy 1
Chamber Function 2
Valvular Function 3
Myocardial Perfusion 4
Myocardial Metabolism 4
Tissue Characterization 5
CONCLUSIONS 5

The twentieth century has witnessed an astounding increase in our knowledge concerning the normal and abnormal cardiovascular system. This change has been intimately linked to developments in cardiac diagnosis. At present, the cardiac diagnostic process is complex. Current diagnostic aims are not merely oriented toward placing a patient into a broad category of disease. Instead, the modern diagnostician aims for a comprehensive evaluation of anatomy, physiology, prognosis, and treatment planning.

The diagnostic process still begins with obtaining the bedside history and performing the physical examination, usually followed by obtaining the resting electrocardiogram and chest roentgenogram. Based on this initial information, tentative diagnostic hypotheses are formed. Confirmation and extension of these initial hypotheses are possible through an array of diagnostic tools that include biochemical analyses of blood and urine; electrocardiographic recordings at rest, with graded exercise, during everyday activities, and within the heart chambers; and several sophisticated methods of imaging the heart and vasculature. With the exception of electrocardiographic and electrophysiologic testing, the most commonly used laboratory diagnostic procedures in current practice are the imaging techniques. Thus, cardiac imaging has become a dominant force in modern cardiovascular diagnosis.

This chapter prepares the reader for the remainder of this book by briefly reviewing the goals of cardiac imaging as part of the comprehensive approach to diagnostic evaluation. Through cardiac imaging methods, a clinician first attempts to visualize cardiac *anatomy* and to derive quantitative descriptors. Anatomic assessment includes determination of the size, shape, and structure of the cardiac chambers, the valve annuli and leaflets, and the coronary arteries. Next, chamber and valvular *function* are addressed, which includes evaluation of systolic and diastolic functions and assessment of the severity of valvular stenosis or regurgitation.

Until recently, cardiac imaging methods offered information chiefly restricted to these two areas of anatomy and function. In the last decade, however, rapid progress in the laboratory and at the bedside have placed three further goals within the realm of clinical utility: assessment of myocardial *perfusion, metabolism,* and *tissue characteristics.*[S1] Particularly in the present era of aggressive intervention to minimize the deleterious effects of acute myocardial ischemia,[G1, T1] the clinician desires accurate information concerning myocardial perfusion. Ideally, this information would include regional and transmural estimates of cardiac perfusion at rest, with pharmacologic or physical exercise stress, and during acute ischemia.[M1] At a more basic level, investigators and clinicians seek further insights into myocardial metabolism under normal and abnormal conditions,[G2] including details of myocardial substrate uptake, of certain aspects of intermediary metabolism, and of myocardial bioenergetics, especially of the kinetics of high-energy phosphate metabolism. Finally, the clinician seeks information regarding myocardial tissue composition,[S2] including identification of abnormal deposition of collagen, iron, amyloid, or other substances, delineation of the nature of intracardiac masses, and identification of acute and chronically ischemic myocardium.

Thus, the goals of cardiac imaging are broad. How do current, widely available techniques measure up to these goals, and what needs are still to be met in cardiac imaging? Answers to these questions are attempted briefly in this chapter and in greater detail throughout this book.

CURRENT CAPABILITIES AND NEEDS IN DIAGNOSTIC CARDIAC IMAGING

Anatomy

Chest roentgenography, echocardiography, radionuclide ventriculography, and selective left heart angiography are commonly used to assess the anatomy of the heart and great vessels. Properly performed and interpreted, chest roentgenography permits qualitative identification of enlargement of each cardiac chamber and gives important information on the physiologic state of the pulmonary vasculature, especially in chronic disorders. Echocardiography,[G3] radionuclide imaging,[S3] and angiography[W1] permit quantitative assessment of volumes of the left and right ventricles.

Echocardiography and angiography also permit estimates of

left ventricular mass.[D1, R1] Because it provides clear delineation of wall thickness, echocardiography has been the method most widely used for estimation of left ventricular mass, especially in patients with left ventricular hypertrophy related to hypertensive and valvular heart disease.[L1] Because contrast angiography depicts only the intracardiac blood pool, assessment of ventricular mass is less precise and usually requires assumptions concerning the distribution of wall thickness in the normal and abnormal heart. Shortcomings of standard, transthoracic echocardiography include difficulties of the examination in some patients and the need to approximate the shapes of the left and right ventricles by the use of simple geometric models.[D1, L1] Even methods that utilize "Simpson's rule" and are based on echocardiographic data suffer from an important theoretic limitation: The various echocardiographic images used to integrate mass or volume across the entire left or right ventricle are not truly mutually parallel; they are obtained at somewhat arbitrary orientations based in part on the patient's thoracic habitus and on the availability of acoustic "windows" at particular anatomic sites.

Increased accuracy in determination of mass and volume requires methods that can delineate endocardial and epicardial interfaces in multiple, mutually parallel sections, preferably within the same cardiac cycle, or within only a few cardiac cycles. This type of information for both ventricles appears to be available through the use of rapid-acquisition computed tomographic (CT) methods.[I1, R2] Although currently requiring many cardiac cycles for acquisition, cine- and standard techniques of nuclear magnetic resonance imaging (MRI) also permit accurate anatomic assessment.[C1, D2, F1] The problems of acoustic access and the varying orientation of images produced by transthoracic echocardiography may be alleviated with the use of transesophageal echocardiography, a promising and important extension of ultrasound examination of the heart.[S4]

In addition to the determination of global left ventricular mass, the assessment of regional ventricular wall thickness in selected patients is important, as in the subject with suspected left ventricular aneurysm or localized scar from prior myocardial infarction. Echocardiography provides excellent information on regional wall thickness and systolic thickening[P1] in patients in whom good-quality studies are obtained. Computed tomography and MRI appear to provide data of at least equal accuracy in this application.[L2, P2]

Clinicians are often interested in determining the size and shape of the thoracic aorta to evaluate the patient with suspected aneurysm, coarctation, or dissection. Both echocardiography and angiography permit excellent delineation of aortic root size and anatomic characteristics. Transthoracic echocardiography is less consistently useful than is aortography in the definition of proximal aortic dissection.[K1] Angiography fulfills this goal but requires an invasive left heart study. Again, the newer tomographic methods of transesophageal echocardiography,[E1] ultrafast CT,[D3] and MRI[D4] appear to permit better noninvasive assessment of the size and shape of the thoracic aorta. Furthermore, MRI permits acquisition of images along many arbitrarily oriented planes, potentially permitting the entire thoracic aorta to be viewed in a single image.

Delineation of the detailed anatomy of the coronary arteries has remained the exclusive domain of selective coronary angiography. Unfortunately, although some assessment of coronary arterial size may be made by subjective evaluation of standard cineangiograms, studies have identified a large degree of interobserver and intraobserver variability in the assessment of percent coronary arterial narrowing,[Z1] the parameter most commonly derived from angiograms. Furthermore, in patients with multivessel coronary disease, the physiologic significance of a particular coronary stenosis may not be defined by the standard arteriographic technique of visually estimating percent diameter stenosis.[W2] Improved determination of the absolute size of the arterial lumen in normal and atherosclerotic areas, and of the physiologic significance of individual stenosis, is offered by techniques of quantitative, computer-based angiographic analysis.[B1, F2, R3] These techniques are being applied to both digital and film-based cineangiographic data with extremely promising results.

An additional capability recently offered by modern cardiac imaging techniques is that of three-dimensional (3D) reconstruction of cardiac anatomy.[C2] The clinician usually assesses the 3D characteristics of the heart by mentally reassembling data from multiple echocardiographic or angiographic images. Three-dimensional computer-based reconstructive techniques seek to replace this process of mental reassembly with a computer-generated model of the heart capable of showing regional changes in chamber size, shape, and function. These advanced methods are now possible by the application of techniques involving digital processing of cardiac images. Promising results have been obtained by applying techniques of 3D reconstruction to data acquired from echocardiograms,[C4, M2] CT scans,[S5] magnetic resonance images,[L3] and tomographic radionuclide scans.[M3] Further application of 3D reconstruction and display technology should offer the clinician more precise assessment of cardiac anatomy from noninvasive imaging data.

Chamber Function

Ventricular systolic performance is an important determinant of prognosis in ischemic and valvular heart disease.[M4] The choice of medical versus surgical therapy in coronary artery disease or in chronic valvular disease often depends partly on measurements of global left ventricular function, at rest and with exercise. Several procedures that permit assessment of global and regional left ventricular function have been developed. Current approaches focus largely on systolic performance of the left ventricle. Ejection phase indices,[B2] such as ejection fraction, give estimates of ventricular performance based on data from echocardiograms, angiograms, radionuclide ventriculograms, CT scans, and MRI studies. Although clinically useful, ejection phase indices are highly dependent on afterload. Isovolumic phase indices,[B2] such as dP/dt, are directly obtainable only by high-fidelity intraventricular pressure measurements and are affected by ventricular preload. Recent advances in Doppler echocardiography have permitted the accurate measurement of aortic outflow velocity patterns, which also offer insight into ventricular function, particularly in serial studies.[L4] Finally, *regional* systolic ventricular performance (whether assessed by wall motion or by wall thickening) offers important insights into the extent of acute and chronic myocardial ischemic injury.[C3]

Despite the widespread clinical use of standard global and regional systolic functional indices, many important problems remain in their application. First is the aforementioned load dependence of most of these measures, which often makes comparisons of studies between patients, and even comparisons of serial studies in the same patient, difficult to interpret. The second problem is that measures of global ventricular function that depend on geometric assumptions in their calculation (such as angiographic and echocardiographic ejection fractions) may be inaccurate in patients whose ventricles do not conform to these ideal geometric figures. Finally, regional left ventricular contraction patterns are heterogeneous in the normal heart,[P3] and this heterogeneity of the pattern of contraction may be affected by loading conditions.[S6]

Because of these and other difficulties, research continues at a brisk pace toward improvements in the assessment of left ventricular systolic function. Substantial recent work has been directed toward developing relatively load-independent indices of function. The left ventricular pressure-volume relationship has been used to generate end-systolic indices of ventricular function that appear to give information on left ventricular inherent contractility that is somewhat less load-dependent than that given by standard isovolumic or ejection phase indices.[C4] Similarly, the increased geometric accuracy of left ventricular anatomic analysis by CT and MRI promises more accurate estimation of absolute left ventricular volumes as well as of ejection fractions. Finally, 3D reconstruction techniques performed throughout the cardiac cycle may offer additional information in the assessment of left ventricular systolic function.

Assessment of right ventricular performance is even more complex, partly because of the unusual shape of the right ventricle, which precludes the use of simple geometric models for volumetric or ejection fraction analyses. Currently, gated first-pass radionuclide scintigraphy, using a region of interest of variable size, appears to be the most widely available and reliable method of determining right ventricular ejection fraction.[R4] Echocardiography may supplement this information, and ultrafast CT appears to be an accurate,[R2] though expensive, alternative to radionuclide imaging for determining right ventricular ejection fraction.

Although the largest body of work concerning left ventricular function has focused on systolic performance, the importance of diastolic function in cardiac symptoms and in therapeutic considerations has become increasingly clear.[G5] For example, pulmonary congestion and resultant dyspnea may occur as a result of impaired left ventricular filling function, even in cases of normal or super-normal systolic performance.[D5] Often, the constellation of normal systolic and abnormal diastolic function is related to myocardial hypertrophy,[L5] as in hypertrophic cardiomyopathy.

Diastolic function has proved to be a difficult parameter to evaluate quantitatively in the clinical setting. Diastole comprises a complex series of events, not merely a passive phase of ventricular filling.[G5] Isovolumic relaxation and early diastolic filling occur largely because of active muscular relaxation with active transport of calcium into the sarcoplasmic reticulum. Following the active phases of isovolumic relaxation and rapid ventricular filling, a period of diastasis occurs, with a small volume of filling depending mainly on passive (elastic) properties of the left ventricular myocardium. Finally, in patients in sinus rhythm, atrial systole completes ventricular filling with the rapid addition of a variable bolus of blood, depending on atrial size and function as well as on left ventricular compliance. Because of these various diastolic phases, each with its own mechanism of ventricular filling, the literature of diastolic ventricular performance has been somewhat confusing. High-fidelity pressure measurement in the catheterization laboratory yields indices of isovolumic relaxation such as $-dP/dt$. On the other hand, the measurement of left ventricular end-diastolic (or pulmonary artery wedge) pressure provides information on average or late diastolic filling. Finally, Doppler echocardiographic indices of diastolic function provide information on early versus late relative filling.[O1] The various mechanisms of ventricular filling responsible for the phases of diastolic function make it difficult to compare functional parameters derived from different portions of diastole.

Current research in diastolic ventricular function is focusing more extensively on measurement of intrinsic muscle properties by the use of finite element analysis methods and other techniques for assessing global and regional stress-strain characteristics of the myocardium. Finite element analysis techniques have been used with echocardiographic,[M5] CT,[P4] and angiographic[R5] image data. The finite element method and other stress-strain analyses are complex and not available for routine clinical use. Thus, continuing attention is being directed to interpretation of global filling curves such as those generated by echocardiographic, radionuclide,[B3] and CT techniques.

Like global systolic function, diastolic ventricular muscle function is load-dependent.[B4] Furthermore, the regional pattern of left ventricular filling appears to be heterogeneous,[F3] as is the pattern of regional systolic contractile performance. Thus, the assessment of diastolic function is a complex process and remains a challenging task for imaging or pressure-based techniques.

Valvular Function

The study and treatment of valvular heart disease account for a significant portion of modern cardiovascular practice. The etiology of valvular disease is progressively changing, involving less chronic rheumatic heart disease and a greater prevalence of degenerative and congenital disorders. Despite the change in etiology, however, the physiologic principles related to the assessment of valvular disorders remain similar to those that have been clarified over the past several decades. Clinical and physiologic assessment of stenotic valve lesions focuses on the estimation of transvalvular pressure drop (gradient) and, ultimately, of stenotic orifice area. The evaluation of valvular regurgitation is oriented toward determination of the amount of regurgitation and its subsequent physiologic effects on ventricular function.

The laboratory evaluation of patients with stenotic valve lesions changed substantially with the development of accurate quantitative methods of Doppler echocardiography.[H1] Pulsed, continuous-wave, and color Doppler echocardiography have had an important impact on the diagnostic process in patients with stenotic valve lesions. Echocardiography can be used to accurately identify abnormal valvular morphology, to measure transvalvular gradient,[S7] and to identify other physiologic sequelae of the valve disorder, such as left ventricular hypertrophy related to aortic valve stenosis. Because the transvalvular gradient for any given stenotic orifice size is directly related to transvalvular flow, estimation of the blood flow passing through the orifice of interest is additional information required for fully assessing the severity of valvular stenosis. Echocardiographic techniques have been developed to assess aortic valve orifice area based on the measurement of transvalvular flow and gradient.[R6] A variation on this approach, employing the so-called "continuity equation," has also been explored for the diagnosis of the severity of aortic stenosis.[O2] Mitral valve stenotic orifice area may be derived by direct imaging of the flow-limiting orifice in two-dimensional echocardiographic images of adequate quality,[M6] as well as by estimation of valve area from mitral pressure half-time data.[H2]

These echocardiographic methods of assessing stenotic valve areas and gradients are sufficiently accurate for routine distinction of trivial from significant valvular stenosis. Especially in intermediate degrees of stenosis, however, technical limitations of echocardiography may sometimes add enough variability to the measurements to make clinical decisions more difficult. For example, methods of assessing valve stenosis by echocardiography that depend on measurements of chamber or annular dimensions suffer from variability in these measurements that is introduced by the sometimes inadequate image quality of echocardiograms. This difficulty in measuring left ventricular outflow tract dimension, for example, probably explains some of the variability found in estimates of aortic valve areas by the continuity equation as compared with invasive hemodynamic data.[O2] Further improvements in the technology of echocardiography are likely to continue to improve the precision and accuracy of assessment of stenotic valve severity. Despite the current drawback, however, ultrasound continues to be the method of choice in the initial assessment of stenotic lesions. Furthermore, in expert hands, echocardiographic assessment permits decisions regarding the need for valve surgery to be made without additional invasive hemodynamic or angiographic studies.

The assessment of valvular regurgitation is more complex. The degree of regurgitation through a particular valve depends on several factors, including the size of the regurgitant orifice, cardiac function, the resistance of the downstream vascular bed, and the compliance of the chamber receiving the regurgitant flow. The most widely used laboratory technique for identification of valvular regurgitation is echocardiography. Doppler techniques may be used to identify regurgitation and to offer a semiquantitative assessment of its severity.[P5] The advent of color Doppler flow mapping techniques has added to the semiquantitative assessment of valvular regurgitation.[Y1] Doppler estimates compare favorably with angiographic parameters of valvular regurgitation.[P5, Y1] Angiographic estimates, however, which are commonly used as an independent standard, are themselves subjective, imprecise,[C5] and likely to depend on loading conditions and other factors. Thus, an important goal of current research in assessing valvular regurgitation is to develop more quantitative indices of regurgitation based on noninvasive measurements of regurgitant fraction,[R7] regurgitant orifice size, and other parameters. The precise geometric measurements necessary for calculation of biventricular stroke volumes, which are needed to estimate regurgitant fraction, may be achieved through the use of echocardiographic, CT, or MRI techniques. Improving the assessment of valvular regurgitation remains an important diagnostic goal for cardiac imaging.

Myocardial Perfusion

The present emphasis on interventional maneuvers in acute myocardial ischemia has intensified the desire to obtain accurate and reproducible estimates of regional myocardial perfusion. Currently available imaging techniques give no information on absolute regional perfusion. Semiquantitative estimates of perfusion may be obtained through use of inert gas washout methods as well as coronary sinus thermodilution techniques.[M7] Although both inert gas washout and selective cardiac vein sampling have been used to estimate regional ventricular perfusion, these methods are beset by a variety of difficulties, which discourage their common clinical use.[M7] Thallium-201 (^{201}Tl) scintigraphy is the only commonly available method used to identify relative regional deficits in perfusion, but it gives no information on absolute regional perfusion. Furthermore, delineation of only relative perfusion abnormalities may be limited by the suboptimal physical characteristics of ^{201}Tl as a radionuclide for external imaging, leading to inaccuracies due to Compton scatter and other problems.

The assessment of epicardial coronary arterial anatomy using angiographic techniques is a commonly employed, indirect method of detecting abnormalities in regional coronary flow reserve. In other words, clinicians often interpret severe coronary artery stenosis (such as a greater than 50 per cent reduction in luminal diameter) as indicating a hydraulically significant obstruction likely to lead to perfusion deficits under conditions of stress. As alluded to previously, however, visual assessment of percent diameter arterial stenosis is not always an accurate indication of the physiologic significance of individual coronary stenoses, particularly in the setting of diffuse, multivessel coronary disease.[M8]

Several new approaches are currently being investigated as means of estimating regional myocardial perfusion. These approaches may be divided into those that evaluate the kinetics of an indicator traversing the cardiac microvasculature and those that evaluate myocyte uptake of an indicator. Several different substances can be used as indicators for the study of regional perfusion via analysis of tracer transit through the coronary circulation. These indicators include iodinated contrast material studied with radiographic or CT imaging systems,[R8, W3] ultrasonic contrast material studied with echocardiographic imaging techniques,[F4, K2] and magnetic resonance contrast agents, studied with MRI.[B5, M9] Whether the imaging sensor is an image intensifier, a CT detector, or an echocardiographic transducer, the resulting data frequently consist of indicator appearance and washout curves, which may be evaluated using indicator-dilution mathematical techniques.[Z2] Thus, to yield accurate estimates of perfusion, the indicator and subsequent imaging procedure must follow the assumptions of indicator-dilution theory. These assumptions are satisfied to varying degrees by the different imaging methods. For example, some early attempts at CT-based perfusion measurements were hampered by the prolonged duration of initial indicator appearance (the so-called input function) after intravenous infusion.[R8] This prolonged input function may be shortened, and the resulting perfusion estimate rendered more precise, by aortic root injection of a contrast agent.[W4]

The other major category of perfusion measurement techniques consists of those based on myocyte uptake of a radiotracer. Several radionuclide techniques are being developed toward the goal of perfusion measurements in clinical practice. Through the use of single-photon emission computed tomography (SPECT) methods, technetium-99m (^{99m}Tc)–based radionuclides are being studied as perfusion imaging tracers.[S8, W5] Because of higher photon energies, these tracers provide images of improved diagnostic quality. Like ^{201}Tl, however, the myocardial uptake of these tracers correlates with myocardial blood flow in a nonlinear fashion, tending toward a plateau at higher flows. Therefore, identification of mild-to-moderate relative perfusion abnormalities in the high-flow range may remain difficult. On the other hand, positron-emitting tracers, employed with positron emission tomography (PET), show substantial promise for estimating regional myocardial perfusion.[B6, G6, S9] Partially extracted tracers (^{13}N ammonia, ^{82}Rb rubidium) and freely diffusible tracers (^{15}O water) have been used to assess myocardial perfusion. Although not yet widely available, PET methods are of potential value for assessing regional perfusion in the clinical setting. Nuclear magnetic resonance techniques may also supply data on myocardial perfusion through the use of contrast agents. These substances shorten proton magnetic resonance relaxation time in areas of normal perfusion and may be useful as methods of assessing myocardial perfusion in a quantitative, noninvasive fashion.[B5, M9]

Myocardial Metabolism

One of the ultimate goals of cardiac diagnosis is the study of the biochemistry of myocardium in patients with heart disease. Cardiac metabolism represents the link between perfusion and mechanical function and is of obvious importance in many cardiac disorders, including ischemic, valvular, myopathic, traumatic, and congenital diseases. Until recently, virtually no information on myocardial metabolism was available except for the calculation of lactate extraction via coronary sinus sampling methods.

Again, the recent emphasis on interventional techniques in acute myocardial ischemia has intensified the search for methods of noninvasive evaluation of salient aspects of myocardial metabolism. The reason for this intensified effort may be demonstrated by consideration of a clinical scenario. Consider the evaluation of a patient with severe chest discomfort and a history of known coronary heart disease. An abnormal electrocardiogram may be the result of prior ischemic injury; electrocardiographic conduction abnormalities may make even this determination difficult. Assessment of regional myocardial contraction may reveal regional wall motion disturbances. These wall motion abnormalities are nonspecific, however, and may be found in acute ischemia as well as in acute and chronic myocardial infarction. Abnormal levels of serum cardiac enzymes indicate injury but do not localize its site. Finally, even if measurements of myocardial perfusion were widely available, an area of decreased perfusion could represent acute injury or prior infarction in an area now replaced with scar. Only the assessment of regional myocardial metabolism or direct evaluation of tissue characteristics (discussed later) would differentiate chronic from acute injury in this setting. The addition of a measure of substrate uptake to the determination of perfusion has helped to differentiate irreversibly damaged from potentially viable myocardium in the acute and chronic ischemic settings.[B7, S10, T2]

Various aspects of myocardial metabolism are evaluated by different investigative techniques. Both SPECT and PET methods may be used to assess the uptake and turnover of myocardial fuel substrates, including fatty acids and glucose. Other aspects of intermediary metabolism may also be studied using PET techniques.[B8, S11] Nuclear magnetic resonance (NMR) technology, especially that employing phosphorus-31 (^{31}P) spectroscopy, offers important insights into myocardial bioenergetics, specifically the metabolism of high-energy phosphate compounds.[K3, M10, R9] Proton and carbon spectroscopy also offer data on aspects of intermediary metabolism and on other myocardial biochemical features of clinical interest.

These evolving technologies are likely to provide new insights into disease-specific abnormalities of myocardial substrate and energy metabolism. They offer the possibility of demonstrating, localizing, and measuring metabolic consequences of structural abnormalities as well as the effects of treatment. Conversely, they offer the possibility of identifying metabolic abnormalities that ultimately result in structural changes; thus, they may permit early detection of disease. At the same time, they may offer new and important insights into the physiology of the human heart.

At present, none of the emerging methods of myocardial metabolic imaging is widely available, and no consensus exists on the relative merits of radionuclide versus NMR approaches to studying cardiac biochemistry. Recent research in both of these directions, however, has brought the clinician far closer to the goal of assessing the biochemistry of the myocardium in health and disease.

Tissue Characterization

Just as assessment of perfusion and metabolism represents the ultimate analysis of myocardial vascular and cellular function, research into "tissue characterization" may supply definitive data on the physical status or composition of the myocardium. In other words, the goal of tissue characterization is to identify abnormalities in myocardial architecture (as in hypertrophic cardiomyopathy), the deposition of abnormal substances (as in amyloidosis), and the replacement of myocardium with collagen (as in chronic infarction).

Currently, information on regional myocardial tissue characteristics is inferred by indirect means, such as the observation of abnormalities in regional wall motion or the lack of uptake of ^{201}Tl. Abnormalities in wall motion not related to acute myocardial ischemia may be attributed to previous injury and subsequent scar formation. Similarly, a deficit in regional ^{201}Tl uptake that is not reversible after a period of rest is commonly assumed to represent scar. Unfortunately, both of these findings are nonspecific. For example, investigators have estimated that as many as 50 percent of regions demonstrating "fixed" defects of thallium uptake may, in fact, represent chronically ischemic, but potentially viable, tissue.[G7, L6] The only currently available method of directly identifying myocardial tissue abnormalities in vivo is endomyocardial biopsy. This technique is useful but is limited by the shallowness of the biopsy and by obvious sampling problems. Thus, the goal of tissue characterization research is to identify directly, in a noninvasive fashion, abnormalities in the composition or physical state of myocardium.

The two methods that appear most promising for noninvasive tissue characterization are ultrasound and NMR. Ultrasound appears to interact differently with abnormal versus normal myocardium. For example, ultrasound is reflected more strongly by acutely ischemic and infarcted tissue as compared with normal tissue; it is strongly reflected by scar from infarction as well.[F5, M11, S12, S13, V1] Similarly, changes in the two-dimensional pattern or "texture" of tissue echoes imaged on standard two-dimensional echocardiograms may indicate the presence of infarction, or of specific cardiomyopathies such as amyloidosis or hypertrophic cardiomyopathy.[C6, S14] Based on these and other promising data, investigative effort continues into methods of ultrasound tissue characterization.

Nuclear magnetic resonance methods offer a great wealth of information on cardiac anatomy and function as a result of high-resolution imaging techniques. In addition, as mentioned previously, spectroscopic methods may provide unique information on myocardial perfusion and metabolism. In addition to these two lines of information, nuclear magnetic resonance techniques may also be useful in tissue characterization through the study of proton relaxation times. Spin-lattice (T_1) or spin-spin (T_2) relaxation times are altered by a variety of changes in tissue structure, including ischemia[J1] and infarction.[B9, M12, W6] Although the precise mechanisms of alteration of magnetic resonance relaxation in ischemic disease are not yet fully elucidated, NMR techniques used for tissue characterization appear promising.

CONCLUSIONS

Modern cardiac imaging techniques represent the predominant laboratory methods of diagnosis in 1990. The field of cardiac imaging currently resides at the threshold between structural and functional imaging and perfusion, metabolic, and tissue characterization capabilities. The extremely promising results of current research into all of these areas strongly suggest that all five goals of cardiac imaging will soon be realized for both investigative and clinical use. Throughout this book, we attempt to introduce the reader to the details and physiologic and physical principles relevant to cardiac imaging as it is now practiced and as it moves into the future.

References

B

1. Brown, B. G., Bolson, E., Frimer, M., and Dodge, H. T.: Quantitative coronary arteriography: Estimation of dimensions, hemodynamic resistance, and atheroma mass of coronary artery lesions using the arteriogram and digital computation. Circulation 55:329, 1977.
2. Braunwald, E.: Assessment of cardiac function. *In* Braunwald, E. (ed.): Heart Disease: A Textbook of Cardiovascular Medicine. 3rd ed. W. B. Saunders, Philadelphia, 1988, p. 449.
3. Bonow, R. O., Bacharach, S. L., Green, M. V., et al.: Impaired left ventricular diastolic filling in patients with coronary artery disease: Assessment with radionuclide angiography. Circulation•64:315, 1981.
4. Braunwald, E., Ross, J., Jr., and Sonnenblick, E. H.: Mechanisms governing contraction of the whole heart. *In* Braunwald, E., et al.: (eds.): Mechanisms of Contraction of the Normal and Failing Heart. 2nd ed. Little, Brown, Boston, 1976, p. 92.
5. Brown, J. J., and Higgins, C. B.: Myocardial paramagnetic contrast agents for MR imaging. AJR 151:865, 1988.
6. Bergmann, S. R., Fox, K. A. A., Rand, A. L., et al.: Quantification of regional myocardial blood flow in vivo with $H_2{}^{15}O$. Circulation 70:724, 1984.
7. Brunken, R., Schwaiger, M., Grover-McKay, M., et al.: Positron emission tomography detects tissue metabolic activity in myocardial segments with persistent thallium perfusion defects. J. Am. Coll. Cardiol. 10:557, 1987.
8. Bergmann, S. R., Fox, K. A. A., Geltman, E. M., and Sobel, B. E.: Positron emission tomography of the heart. Prog. Cardiovasc. Dis. 28:165, 1985.
9. Been, M., Smith, M. A., Ridgway, J. P., et al.: Serial changes in the T_1 magnetic relaxation parameter after myocardial infarction in man. Br. Heart J. 59:1, 1988.

C

1. Caputo, G. R., Tscholakoff, D., Sechtem, U., and Higgins, C. B.: Measurement of canine left ventricular mass using MR imaging. AJR 148:33, 1987.
2. Collins, S. M., Chandran, K. B., and Skorton, D. J.: Three-dimensional cardiac imaging. Echocardiography 5:311, 1988.
3. Collins, S. M., Kerber, R. E., and Skorton, D. J.: Quantitative analysis of left ventricular regional function by imaging methods. *In* Miller, D. D. (ed.): Clinical Cardiac Imaging. McGraw-Hill, New York, 1988, p. 223.
4. Carabello, B. A., and Spann, J. F.: The uses and limitations of end-systolic indexes of left ventricular function. Circulation 69:1058, 1984.
5. Croft, C. H., Lipscomb, K., Matthis, K., et al.: Limitations of qualitative grading in aortic or mitral regurgitation. Am. J. Cardiol. 53:1593, 1984.
6. Chandrasekaran, K., Aylward, P. E., Fleagle, S. R., et al.: Feasibility of identifying amyloid and hypertrophic cardiomyopathy with the use of computerized quantitative texture analysis of clinical echocardiographic data. J. Am. Coll. Cardiol. 13:832, 1989.

D

1. Devereux, R. B., and Reichek, N.: Echocardiographic determinants of LV mass in man: Anatomic validation of the method. Circulation 55:613, 1977.
2. Dilworth, L. R., Aisen, A. M., Mancinci, J., et al.: Determination of left ventricular volumes and ejection fraction by nuclear magnetic resonance imaging. Am. Heart J. 113:24, 1987.
3. Drucker, E. A., Miller, S. W., Shepard, J. O., and Waltman, A. C.: The great vessels: Acquired diseases of the thoracic aorta. *In* Miller, D. D., et al. (eds.): Clinical Cardiac Imaging. McGraw-Hill, New York, 1988, p. 591.
4. Dinsmore, R. E., Wedeen, V. J., Miller, S. W., et al.: MRI of dissection of the aorta: Recognition of the intimal tear and differential flow velocities. AJR 143:1135, 1984.
5. Dougherty, A. H., Naccarelli, G. V., Gray, E. L., et al.: Congestive heart failure with normal systolic function. Am. J. Cardiol. 54:778, 1984.

E

1. Engberding, R., Bender, E., Grosse-Heitmeyer, W., et al.: Identification of dissection or aneurysm of the descending thoracic aorta by conventional and transesophageal two-dimensional echocardiography. Am. J. Cardiol. 59:717, 1987.

F

1. Florentine, M. S., Grosskreutz, C. L., Chang, W., et al.: Measurement of left ventricular mass in vivo using gated nuclear magnetic resonance imaging. J. Am. Coll. Cardiol. 8:107, 1986.
2. Fleagle, S. R., Johnson, M. R., Wilbricht, C. J., et al.: Automated analysis of coronary arterial morphology in cineangiograms: Geometric and physiologic validation in humans. IEEE Trans. Med. Imag. 8:387, 1989.
3. Funai, J. T., Pandian, N. G., Salem, D. N., and Levine, H. J.: Heterogeneity of regional diastolic filling dynamics in normal left ventricle: Experimental two-dimensional echocardiographic studies. (Abstract.) J. Am. Coll. Cardiol. 5:426A, 1985.
4. Feinstein, S. B., Lang, R. M., Dick, C. D., et al.: Contrast echocardiography during coronary arteriography in humans: Perfusion and anatomic studies. J. Am. Coll. Cardiol. 11:59, 1988.

5. Fitzgerald, P. J., McDaniel, M. D., Rolett, E. L., et al.: Two-dimensional ultrasonic tissue characterization: Backscatter power, endocardial wall motion, and their relationship for normal, ischemic and infarcted myocardium. Circulation 76:850, 1987.

G

1. Gruppo Italiano per lo Studio della Streptochinasi Nell'Infarto Miocardico (GISSI). Effectiveness of intravenous thrombolytic treatment in acute myocardial infarction. Lancet 2:349, 1986.
2. Grover-McKay, M., Schelbert, H. R., Schwaiger, M., et al.: Identification of impaired metabolic reserve in patients with significant coronary artery stenosis by atrial pacing. Circulation 74:281, 1986.
3. Gueret, P., Meerbaum, S., Wyatt, H. L., et al.: Two-dimensional echocardiographic quantitation of left ventricular volumes and ejection fraction: Importance of accounting for dyssynergy in short-axis reconstruction mode. Circulation 62:1308, 1980.
4. Geiser, E. A., Lupkiewicz, S. M., Christie, L. G., et al.: A framework for three-dimensional time-varying reconstruction of the human left ventricle: Sources of error and estimation of their magnitude. Comput. Biomed. Res. 13:225, 1980.
5. Gilbert, J. C., and Glantz, S. A.: Determinants of left ventricular filling and of the diastolic pressure-volume relation. Circ. Res. 64:827, 1989.
6. Gould, K. L.: Identifying and measuring severity of coronary artery stenosis: Quantitative coronary arteriography and positron emission tomography. Circulation 78:237, 1988.
7. Gibson, R. S., Watson, D. D., Taylor, G. J., et al.: Prospective assessment of regional myocardial perfusion before and after coronary revascularization surgery by quantitative thallium-201 scintigraphy. J. Am. Coll. Cardiol. 1:804, 1983.

H

1. Hatle, L., and Angelsen, B. (eds.): Doppler Ultrasound in Cardiology: Physical Principles and Clinical Applications. 2nd ed. Lea & Febiger, Philadelphia, 1985.
2. Hatle, L., Angelsen, B., and Tromsdal, A.: Noninvasive assessment of atrioventricular pressure half-time by Doppler ultrasound. Circulation 60:1096, 1979.

I

1. Iwasaki, T., Sinak, L. J., Hoffman, E. A., et al.: Mass of left ventricular myocardium estimated with dynamic spatial reconstructor. Am. J. Physiol. 15:H138, 1984.

J

1. Johnston, D. L., Brady, T. J., Ratner, A. V., et al.: Assessment of myocardial ischemia with proton magnetic resonance: Effects of a three hour coronary occlusion with and without reperfusion. Circulation 71:595, 1985.

K

1. Khandheria, B. K., Tajik, A. J., Taylor, C. L., et al.: Aortic dissection: Review of value and limitations of two-dimensional echocardiography in a six-year experience. J. Am. Soc. Echo. 2:17, 1989.
2. Kaul, S., Kelly, P., Oliner, J. D., et al.: Assessment of regional myocardial blood flow with myocardial contrast two-dimensional echocardiography. J. Am. Coll. Cardiol. 13:468, 1989.
3. Kavanaugh, K. M., Aisen, A. M., Fechner, K. P., et al.: Regional metabolism during coronary occlusion, reperfusion, and reocclusion using ^{31}phosphorus nuclear magnetic resonance spectroscopy in the intact rabbit. Am. Heart J. 117:53, 1989.

L

1. Liebson, P. R., Devereux, R. B., and Horan, M. J.: Hypertension research: Echocardiography in the measurement of LV wall mass. Hypertension 9(Suppl. II):2, 1987.
2. Lanzer, P., Garrett, J. S., Lipton, M. J., et al.: Quantitation of regional myocardial function by cine-computed tomography: Pharmacological changes in wall thickening dynamics. J. Am. Coll. Cardiol. 8:682, 1986.
3. Laschinger, J. C., Vannier, M. W., Gronemeyer, S., et al.: Noninvasive three-dimensional reconstruction of the heart and great vessels by ECG-gated magnetic resonance imaging: A new diagnostic modality. Ann. Thorac. Surg. 45:505, 1988.
4. Labovitz, A. J., Lewen, M. K., Kern, M., et al.: Evaluation of left ventricular systolic and diastolic dysfunction during transient myocardial ischemia produced by angioplasty. J. Am. Coll. Cardiol. 10:748, 1987.
5. Lorell, B. H., and Grossman, W.: Cardiac hypertrophy: The consequences for diastole. J. Am. Coll. Cardiol. 9:1189, 1987.
6. Liu, P., Kiess, M. C., Okada, R. D., et al.: The persistent defect on exercise thallium imaging and its fate after myocardial revascularization: Does it represent scar or ischemia? Am. Heart J. 110:996, 1985.

M

1. Marcus, M. L., Wilson, R. F., and White, C. W.: Methods of measurement of myocardial blood flow in patients: A critical review. Circulation 76:245, 1987.
2. Moritz, W. E., Pearlman, A. S., McCabe, D. H., et al.: An ultrasonic technique for imaging the ventricle in three dimensions and calculating its volume. IEEE Trans. Biomed. Eng., 30:482, 1983.
3. Miller, T. R., Starren, J. B., and Grothe, R. A., Jr.: Three-dimensional display of positron emission tomography of the heart. J. Nucl. Med. 29:530, 1988.
4. Mock, M. B., Ringvist, I., Fisher, L. D., et al.: Survival of medically treated patients in the Coronary Artery Surgery Study (CASS) Registry. Circulation 66:562, 1982.
5. McPherson, D. D., Skorton, D. J., Kodiyalam, S., et al.: Finite element analysis of myocardial diastolic function using three-dimensional echocardiographic reconstructions: Application of a new method for study of acute ischemia in dogs. Circ. Res. 60:674, 1987.
6. Martin, R. P., Rakowski, H., Kleiman, J. H., et al.: Reliability and reproducibility of two-dimensional echocardiographic measurement of the stenotic mitral valve orifice area. Am. J. Cardiol. 43:560, 1979.
7. Marcus, M. L.: Methods of measuring coronary blood flow. *In* Marcus, M. L. (ed.): The Coronary Circulation in Health and Disease. McGraw-Hill, New York, 1983, p. 25.
8. Marcus, M. L., Skorton, D. J., Johnson, M. R., et al.: Visual estimates of percent diameter coronary stenosis: A battered gold standard. J. Am. Coll. Cardiol. 11:882, 1988.
9. Miller, D. D., Holmuang, G., Gill, J. B., et al.: MRI detection of myocardial perfusion changes by gadolinium-DTPA infusion during dipyridamole hyperemia. Magn. Reson. Med. 10:246, 1989.
10. Massie, B., and Weiner, M. W.: Response of myocardial metabolites to graded regional ischemia: ^{31}P NMR spectroscopy of porcine myocardium in vivo. Circ. Res. 64:968, 1989.
11. Miller, J. G., Perez, J. E., and Sobel, B. E.: Ultrasonic characterization of myocardium. Prog. Cardiovasc. Dis. 28:85, 1985.
12. McNamara, M. T., Higgins, C. B., Schechtmann, N., et al.: Detection and characterization of acute myocardial infarction in man with use of gated magnetic resonance. Circulation 71:717, 1985.

O

1. Otto, C. M., Pearlman, A. S., and Amsler, L. C.: Doppler echocardiographic evaluation of left ventricular diastolic filling in isolated valvular aortic stenosis. Am. J. Cardiol. 63:313, 1989.
2. Otto, C. M., and Pearlman, A. S.: Doppler echocardiography in adults with symptomatic aortic stenosis: Diagnostic utility and cost-effectiveness. Arch. Intern. Med. 148:2553, 1988.

P

1. Pandian, N. G., and Kerber, R. E.: Two-dimensional echocardiography in experimental coronary stenosis. I. Sensitivity and specificity in detecting transient myocardial dyskinesis: Comparison with sonomicrometers. Circulation 66:597, 1982.
2. Peshock, R. M., Rokey, R., Malloy, C. M., et al.: Assessment of myocardial systolic wall thickening using nuclear magnetic resonance imaging. J. Am. Coll. Cardiol. 14:653, 1989.
3. Pandian, N. G., Skorton, D. J., Collins, S. M., et al.: Heterogeneity of left ventricular segmental wall thickening and excursion in 2-dimensional echocardiograms of normal humans. Am. J. Cardiol. 51:1667, 1983.
4. Pao, Y. C., and Ritman, E. L.: Estimation of passive and active muscle properties of working heart. Proc. Intl. Conf. on Finite Elements in Biomechanics. Tucson, AZ, 1980. Vol. 2. 1980, p. 657.
5. Pearlman, A. S., and Otto, C. M.: The use of Doppler techniques for quantitative evaluation of valvular regurgitation. Eur. Heart J., 8(Suppl. C):35, 1987.

R

1. Rackley, C. E., Dodge, H. T., Coble, Y. D., Jr., and Hay, R. E.: A method for determining left ventricular mass in man. Circulation 29:666, 1964.
2. Reiter, S. J., Rumberger, J. A., Feiring, A. J., et al.: Precision of measurements of right and left ventricular volume by cine computed tomography. 74:890, 1986.
3. Reiber, J. H. C.: Morphologic and densitometric quantitation of coronary stenoses: An overview of existing quantitation techniques. *In* Reiber, J. H. C., and Serruys, P. W. (eds.): New Developments in Quantitative Coronary Arteriography. Kluwer Academic, Dordrecht, 1988, p. 34.
4. Rezai, K., Weiss, R., Preslar, J., et al.: ECG gating improves the accuracy of radionuclide right ventricular ejection fraction determinations. (Abstract.) J. Am. Coll. Cardiol. 11:215A, 1988.
5. Ray, G., Chandran, K. B., Nikravesh, P. E., et al.: Estimation of local elastic modulus of the normal and infarcted left ventricle from angiographic data. *In* Saha, S. (ed.): Proceedings of the 4th New England Bioengineering Conference. Pergamon Press, Elmsford, NY, 1976, p. 173.
6. Richards, K. L.: Doppler echocardiography in the diagnosis and quantification of valvular disease. Mod. Concepts Cardiovasc. Dis. 56:43, 1987.
7. Reiter, S. J., Rumberger, J. A., Stanford, W., and Marcus, M. L.: Quantitative determination of aortic regurgitant volumes in dogs by ultrafast computed tomography. Circulation 76:728, 1987.
8. Rumberger, J. A., Feiring, A. J., Lipton, M. J., et al.: Use of ultrafast CT to quantitate regional myocardial perfusion. A preliminary report. J. Am. Coll. Cardiol. 9:59, 1987.
9. Robitaille, P. M., Merkle, H., Sublett, E., et al.: Spectroscopic imaging and spatial localization using adiabatic pulses and applications to detect transmural metabolite distribution in the canine heart. Magn. Reson. Med. 10:14, 1989.

S

1. Skorton, D. J., and Collins, S. M.: New directions in cardiac imaging. Ann. Intern. Med. 102:795, 1985.
2. Skorton, D. J., and Collins, S. M.: Characterization of myocardial structure with ultrasound. *In* Greenleaf, J. (ed.): Tissue Characterization With Ultrasound. Vol. II. Results and Applications. CRC Press, Boca Raton, FL, 1986, p. 123.
3. Stadius, M. L., Williams, D. L., Harp, G., et al. Left ventricular volume determination using single-photon emission computed tomography. Am. J. Cardiol. 55:1185, 1985.
4. Seward, J. B., Khandheria, B. K., Oh, J. K., et al.: Transesophageal echocardiography: Technique, anatomic correlations, implementation and clinical applications. Mayo Clin. Proc. 63:649, 1988.
5. Sinak, L. J., Hoffman, E. A., Julsrud, P. R., et al.: The dynamic spatial reconstructor: Investigating congenital heart disease in four dimensions. Cardiovasc. Intervent. Radiol. 7:124, 1984.
6. Stark, C. A., Rumberger, J. A., Stanford, W., and Marcus, M. L.: Dobutamine stress with cine CT. (Abstract.) Circulation 74(Suppl. II):II-122, 1987.
7. Stamm, R. B., and Martin, R. P.: Quantification of pressure gradients across stenotic valves by Doppler ultrasound. J. Am. Coll. Cardiol. 2:707, 1983.
8. Seldin, D. W., Johnson, L. L., Blood, D. K., et al.: Myocardial perfusion imaging with technetium-99m SQ 30217: Comparison with thallium-201 and coronary anatomy. J. Nucl. Med. 30:312, 1989.
9. Shah, A., Schelbert, H. R., Schwaiger, M., et al.: Measurement of regional myocardial blood flow with N-13-ammonia and positron emission tomography in intact dogs. J. Am. Coll. Cardiol. 5:92, 1985.
10. Schelbert, H. R., and Buxton, D.: Insights into coronary artery disease gained from metabolic imaging. Circulation 78:496, 1988.
11. Schelbert, H. R., and Schwaiger, M.: PET studies of the heart. *In* Phelps, M., et al. (eds.): Positron Emission Tomography and Autoradiography: Principles and Applications for the Brain and Heart. Raven Press, New York, 1986, p. 581.
12. Skorton, D. J., Melton, H. E., Jr., Pandian, N. G., et al.: Detection of acute myocardial infarction in closed-chest dogs by analysis of regional two-dimensional echocardiographic gray-level distributions. Circ. Res. 52:36, 1983.
13. Sagar, K. B., Rhyne, T. L., Warltier, D. C., et al.: Intramyocardial variability in integrated backscatter: Effects of coronary occlusion and reperfusion. Circulation 75:436, 1987.
14. Siqueira-Filho, A. G., Cunha, C. L. P., Tajik, A. J., et al.: M-mode and two-dimensional echocardiographic features in cardiac amyloidosis. Circulation 63:188, 1981.

T

1. TIMI Study Group: Comparison of invasive and conservative strategies after treatment with intravenous tissue plasminogen activator in acute myocardial infarction: Results of the thrombolysis in myocardial infarction (TIMI) Phase II trial. N. Engl. J. Med. 320:618, 1989.
2. Tillisch, J., Brunken, R., Marshall, R., et al.: Reversibility of cardiac wall-motion abnormalities predicted by positron tomography. N. Engl. J. Med. 314:884, 1986.

V

1. Vered, Z., Mohr, G. A., Barzilai, B., et al.: Ultrasonic integrated backscatter tissue characterization of remote myocardial infarction in human subjects. J. Am. Coll. Cardiol. 13:84, 1989.

W

1. Wynne, J., Green, L. H., Mann, T., et al.: Estimation of left ventricular volumes in man from biplane cineangiograms filmed in oblique projections. Am. J. Cardiol. 41:726, 1978.
2. White, C. W., Wright, C. B., Doty, D. B., et al.: Does the visual interpretation of the coronary arteriogram predict the physiological significance of a coronary stenosis? N. Engl. J. Med. 310:819, 1984.
3. Wolfkiel, C., Ferguson, J. L., Chomka, E. V., et al.: Measurement of myocardial blood flow by ultrafast computed tomography. Circulation 76:1262, 1987.
4. Weiss, R. M., Hajduczok, Z. D., and Marcus, M. L.: A new cine CT algorithm for quantitation of myocardial perfusion. (Abstract.) Circulation 78:II-398, 1988.
5. Wackers, F. J. T., Berman, D. S., Maddahi, J., et al.: Technetium 99m hexakis 2-methoxyisobutyl isonitrile: Human biodistribution, dosimetry, safety, and preliminary comparison to thallium-201 for myocardial perfusion imaging. J. Nucl. Med. 30:301, 1989.
6. Wisenberg, G., Prato, F. S., Carroll, S. E., et al.: Serial nuclear magnetic resonance imaging of acute myocardial infarction with and without reperfusion. Am. Heart J. 115:510, 1988.

Y

1. Yoshikawa, J., Yoshida, K., Akasaka, T., et al.: Value and limitations of color Doppler flow mapping in the detection and semi-quantification of valvular regurgitation. Int. J. Cardiac Imag. 2:85, 1987.

Z

1. Zir, L. M., Miller, S. W., Dinsmore, R. E., et al.: Interobserver variability in coronary angiography. Circulation 53:627, 1976.
2. Zierler, K. L.: Theoretical basis of indicator-dilution methods for measuring flow and volume. Circ. Res. 10:393, 1962.

Chapter 2

Physiologic Basis for Myocardial Perfusion Imaging

MELVIN L. MARCUS, M.D. ▪ *DAVID G. HARRISON, M.D.*

MAJOR DETERMINANTS OF MYOCARDIAL PERFUSION 8
Metabolic Control 8
Autoregulation 9
Compressive Forces 10
Neural Control 10
Humoral Control 11
Myogenic Control 11
SPECIAL CONSIDERATIONS RELATED TO THE REGULATION OF THE CORONARY CIRCULATION 11
Regulation of Transmural Perfusion 11
Heterogeneity of Perfusion to Small Segments of the Myocardium 12
Endothelial Relaxing Factor 12
Differences in Flow to Various Cardiac Chambers 12
CORONARY VASODILATOR RESERVE 13
Nonhemodynamic Conditions That Influence Coronary Reserve 13
Effects of Hemodynamics on Coronary Reserve 14
Drug Effects on Coronary Flow Reserve 14
Effects of Disease on Coronary Flow Reserve 14
Absolute Versus Relative Assessment of Coronary Flow Reserve 14
Summary 14
CLINICAL USE OF CORONARY VASODILATORS 15
Submaximal Coronary Dilator Stimuli 15
Maximal Coronary Dilators 15
CORONARY COLLATERAL CIRCULATION 16
Native Collaterals 16
Mature Collaterals 17
CORONARY STENOSIS 18
Hydraulic Principles 18
Intra- and Interobserver Variability 18
Diffuse Coronary Disease 18
Correlations with Direct Measurements of Flow Reserve 18
Coexisting Factors That Influence Coronary Reserve 18
CORONARY OCCLUSION AND INFARCTION 19
Infarct/Risk Relationship 19
EFFECTS OF HYPERTROPHY ON MYOCARDIAL PERFUSION 19
EFFECTS OF CORONARY VASODILATION ON CORONARY VASCULAR VOLUME 20
CONCLUSION 20

Almost all cardiovascular imaging techniques have measurement of regional myocardial perfusion as one of their goals. Interest in achieving this aim is intense at present. Many groups of investigators using newer imaging modalities (magnetic resonance imaging, positron emission tomography, ultrafast computed tomography, digital angiography, single photon emission computed tomography, and contrast echocardiography) are devoting an enormous amount of time and energy in pursuit of a clinically useful approach for the precise measurement of regional myocardial perfusion over a broad range of flow rates. The current status of these investigations will be reviewed in many of the chapters in this volume.

Precise measurement of regional myocardial perfusion in humans would have immense clinical applicability. Such measurements could be employed to measure coronary reserve, the physiologic significance of a coronary obstructive lesion, the functional capacity of coronary collateral vessels, or the physiologic effectiveness of a treatment procedure such as coronary bypass surgery or angioplasty.

Knowledge of the physiologic basis for perfusion imaging is essential to understanding and placing in proper perspective the progress made in this area by the various imaging modalities. In this chapter, we will address general issues regarding perfusion imaging that transcend any specific approach to the problem.

MAJOR DETERMINANTS OF MYOCARDIAL PERFUSION

The coronary circulation is regulated by three major and three minor control mechanisms. The dominant regulatory factors are cardiac metabolism or oxygen consumption, autoregulation, and effects of compressive forces. The factors of lesser importance are neural, humoral, and myogenic control. The relative importance of these individual control mechanisms has been reasonably well defined in normal hearts.[B1, 2, C2, K1, M1–6, R1, S1, V1] In pathophysiologic states, however, the importance of these control mechanisms can be shifted dramatically. For example, neurohumoral stimuli may become more important if the endothelium is removed or dysfunctional[C3] in vessels distal to a critical stenosis,[H1] or in hearts with regions of myocardium perfused by collaterals.[H2, S2]

In this section, the six major component factors that modulate myocardial perfusion are reviewed.

Metabolic Control

Myocardial oxygen consumption and coronary vascular resistance are tightly coupled in normal hearts.[B3, H3, R2] The minimal time interval between a change in oxygen consumption and a directionally appropriate change in coronary vascular resistance is only a few hundred milliseconds.[S3] In addition, the gain of this control system is very high. An intense metabolic stimulus can produce maximal coronary dilation (500 to 600 percent increase in coronary flow) in 10 to 15 seconds.[V2] Also, changes in metabolic demand result in an appropriate change in coronary vascular resistance that is precisely limited to the area involved.[W1] The close association between changes in myocardial oxygen consumption and in coronary vascular resistance has not only been demonstrated in the left ventricle but also in the right ventricle[D1, F1] and the atria.[W1] Thus, the coupling of myocardial metabolism to coronary vascular resistance has high gain and impressive temporal and spatial characteristics. Potential mechanisms responsible for this coupling include adenosine,[B4] tissue oxygen tension,[C4] tissue carbon dioxide tension,[C5, 6] prostaglandins,[D2] and hydrogen ion concentration.[M7]

Myocardial oxygen consumption is determined by a combination of six known factors: contractility, chamber wall stress, heart rate, electrical activation, fiber shortening, and basal metabolic demand.[B5] Selective increases in each of these factors produce an increment in myocardial oxygen consumption. However, a fixed percent increase in each factor produces a very different percent increase in myocardial oxygen consumption. This critically important point is often ignored. An example of this problem relates to the frequent use of an increase in heart rate to augment myocardial oxygen consumption and, thereby, decrease coronary vascular resistance or provoke myocardial ischemia. An increase in heart rate is not a potent metabolic stress to the heart. In the dog, for example, an increase in heart rate from 90 beats per minute to 200 beats per minute only increases coronary blood flow about twofold.[B6, M8] Thus, it is not surprising that the moderate tachycardia utilized in clinical studies (resting heart rate of 70, stimulated heart rate with atrial pacing of 120 to 150 beats per minute) produces only a modest increase in coronary flow (typically less than twofold).[G1] This represents a very small stress to the normal coronary circulation, which can increase flow 500 or 600 percent in response to an intense stimulus.

One reason that tachycardia is a relatively impotent coronary dilator stimulus is that in association with tachycardia there is a decrease in intracardiac volume, myocardial shortening, and frequently aortic pressure. This combination leads to a substantial decline in chamber wall stress. These factors in concert decrease myocardial oxygen consumption and, thereby, attenuate any direct increase in myocardial oxygen consumption secondary to the tachycardia alone.

Many protocols in cardiac imaging procedures employ a metabolic stress such as pacing, treadmill or bicycle exercise, handgrip, or infusion of a vasopressor or inotropic agent to increase myocardial oxygen consumption and, thereby, increase coronary flow or precipitate myocardial ischemia. Although this approach is widely accepted, it should be appreciated that these maneuvers seldom produce maximal coronary dilation. When the stress employed simultaneously increases some determinants of myocardial consumption and decreases other factors, then the stimulus produces only moderate coronary dilation. Examples of such stresses on the coronary circulation include tachycardia and infusion of a vasopressor that will usually engender baroreflex-related bradycardia. Only one form of stress—treadmill or bicycle exercise—is associated with simultaneous increases in all the individual factors that augment myocardial oxygen consumption and, thereby, produce moderately intense coronary dilation. Maximal coronary dilation, however, seldom can be achieved by exercise in the typical patient with suspected heart disease. Furthermore, commonly used antianginal drugs, such as beta-adrenergic receptor antagonists or calcium channel blockers, may attenuate increases in oxygen consumption with exercise, owing to blunted heart rate and blood pressure responses. In theory, the sensitivity of detecting perfusion abnormalities or evidence of myocardial ischemia in patients with obstructive coronary disease will decline in proportion to the inadequacy of the coronary dilator employed.

Autoregulation

The ability to maintain myocardial perfusion constant or nearly constant in the face of large changes in perfusion pressure is termed *autoregulation*. This phenomenon can be demonstrated in many vascular beds and is particularly well developed in the heart[B7, G2, M3] and the brain.[S4] In the awake, normal adult dog, autoregulation is extraordinarily powerful.[F2, H4, K7] Decreases in mean coronary perfusion pressure from 100 to 40 mmHg are unassociated with any change in myocardial perfusion (Fig. 2–1). In general, autoregulation is less effective in anesthetized open-chest animal preparations. Although autoregulation has not been formally studied in detail in patients, a wealth of clinical information strongly suggests that autoregulation is very effective in clinical situations. For example, many patients with severe stenosis in a proximal coronary artery have a marked reduction in distal coronary perfusion pressure at rest and no evidence of myocardial ischemia or inadequate perfusion in the field of the obstructed vessel. This could occur only if autoregulation were remarkably effective.

Three regional aspects of autoregulation are of special note. First, there is controversy about the effectiveness of autoregulation in the right ventricle.[M9, U1] This is of little current concern to the field of cardiac imaging, because present techniques for assessing myocardial perfusion cannot quantitatively or qualitatively determine perfusion in the free wall of the normal right ventricle.

Second, the gain of autoregulation is substantially less in the subendocardium than in the subepicardium of the left ventricle (Fig. 2–2). This well-accepted aspect of coronary physiology has very important implications for the field of cardiac imaging. If a technique became available that could separate subendocardial from subepicardial perfusion, it would significantly enhance the sensitivity of perfusion imaging for detecting physiologically significant coronary obstructive lesions. Only ultrafast computed tomography and magnetic resonance imaging are likely to accomplish this goal in the next several years. If one employs a method for perfusion imaging that has poor transmural spatial resolution, such as thallium-201 or positron emission tomography with currently available cameras—a priori, one must accept the notion that for the most part, perfusion abnormalities limited to the subendocardium will not be detectable unless they are extremely

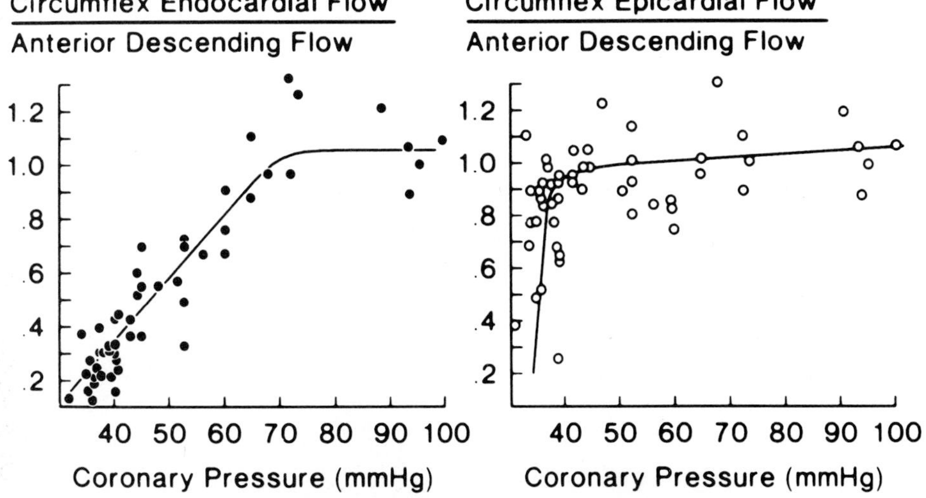

Figure 2–1. Pressure flow relationships in the endocardial (left) and epicardial (right) thirds of the left ventricular myocardium. The ability of epicardial vessels to autoregulate is substantially greater than that of endocardial vessels. (Redrawn from data originally presented by Guyton, R. A., McClenathan, J. H., Newman, G. E., and Michaelis, L. L.: Significance of subendocardial S-T segment elevation caused by coronary stenosis in the dog. Am. J. Cardiol. 40:373, 1977.)

severe. In effect, this implies that only relatively severe coronary obstructive lesions will be detectable.

The third aspect of regional autoregulation of special note is that chronic hypertension and left ventricular hypertrophy seriously decrease the gain of autoregulation in the subendocardium.[H4] This effect amplifies the adverse consequences of coronary obstructive lesions and under some circumstances could decrease subendocardial perfusion significantly even in the absence of an obstructive coronary lesion if sufficient stress were applied to the myocardium. Abnormalities in autoregulation of hypertrophied ventricles should be considered when employing any imaging modality for detecting coronary obstructive disease in patients with cardiac hypertrophy. This is especially true if the imaging procedure assesses relative, as opposed to absolute, myocardial perfusion.

It is critical to separate the effects of "autoregulation" from the effects of a change in coronary driving pressure in a clinical setting. Autoregulation can be demonstrated only if other factors that regulate coronary flow, such as cardiac metabolism and compressive forces, are held constant. This can be achieved only in an animal research laboratory. This is typically accomplished by perfusing a coronary vessel at a constant predetermined pressure that is controlled independently from aortic or left ventricular pressure. In a clinical situation, except under very rare circumstances, a change in aortic pressure is associated with a similar change in coronary driving pressure and left ventricular pressure. Therefore, if aortic pressure is increased, there will be an increase in left ventricular wall stress, baroreflex-mediated bradycardia, a decrease in shortening, and an increase in compressive forces. In addition, other neural, humoral, and myogenic mechanisms may be activated. The usual net effect of an increase in aortic pressure is an increase in coronary flow secondary to the net increase in myocardial oxygen consumption. This increase in coronary flow will be attenuated by autoregulation and reflex bradycardia. A decrease in aortic pressure produces the opposite effect.

The most important aspect of autoregulation relevant to the field of cardiac imaging is the observation that autoregulation is less effective in the subendocardium, as opposed to the subepicardium, of the left ventricle,[G2] and this difference is further exaggerated by the presence of pressure-induced left ventricular hypertrophy.[H4] As a consequence, the first detectable effect of a proximal coronary stenosis on myocardial perfusion is a decrement in subendocardial perfusion.

Compressive Forces

Skeletal muscle and heart muscle are the only two tissues that compress their own blood supply under normal physiologic conditions. When the heart contracts, two compressive forces limit myocardial perfusion. The most obvious one is an increase in intracavitary pressure and tension in the chamber wall, which compresses intramural coronary vessels. The second is the twisting of cardiac fibers. In the left ventricle, the "twisting component" is of greater importance than the increase in intracavitary pressure.[D3] This becomes vividly clear if one observes the phasic waveform of coronary flow in the left anterior descending coronary artery in a contracting left ventricle generating normal pressure and compares it with the phasic waveform of coronary flow in a contracting left ventricle that is empty and vented to the atmosphere so that intracavitary pressure is zero. In both situations, the phasic coronary flow waveforms are remarkably similar.[D3] The only explanation for this observation is that the "twisting component" must importantly contribute to compressive forces that act on the coronary vasculature. A third compressive force is left ventricular diastolic pressure.

From the point of view of a physiologist, compressive forces modulate several aspects of coronary function, including the phasic nature of myocardial perfusion and, to a lesser extent, the transmural distribution of left ventricular perfusion. In the normal heart, the abolition of compressive forces leads to a prompt but relatively small increase in coronary flow.[D3] In pathologic states during the presence of maximal coronary dilation, the effects of compressive forces are strikingly exaggerated.[K2] In addition, compressive forces can play an important role in modulating collateral perfusion.

From the point of view of cardiac imaging methods, compressive forces are of limited importance, because phasic coronary flow cannot be accurately assessed with current imaging modalities, and collateral flow can be only crudely estimated.

Neural Control

The coronary vessels are densely innervated by sympathetic and parasympathetic nerves. Numerous studies have shown that neural mechanisms can alter myocardial perfusion.[B1, C1, F3, 4, M1, 2, 10, S1] These mechanisms are complex, because activation of the nerves produces a direct effect on coronary vessels and many indirect effects that under normal circumstances are dominant.

Activation of sympathetic nerves produces certain effects that indirectly alter coronary flow by modulating myocardial oxygen consumption: increase in aortic pressure, increase in heart rate, and increase in contractility. Direct coronary vascular actions of sympathetic nerve activation may include (1) beta-adrenergic dilation of both large conduit coronary arteries[V3] and small microarterial vessels less than 100 μm in diameter;[C8] (2) α_2-adrenergic release of the endothelium-derived relaxing factor;[C3] and (3) α-adrenergic constriction of large coronary arteries[V1, 4] and arterioles greater than 100 μm in diameter.[C8] The net effect of

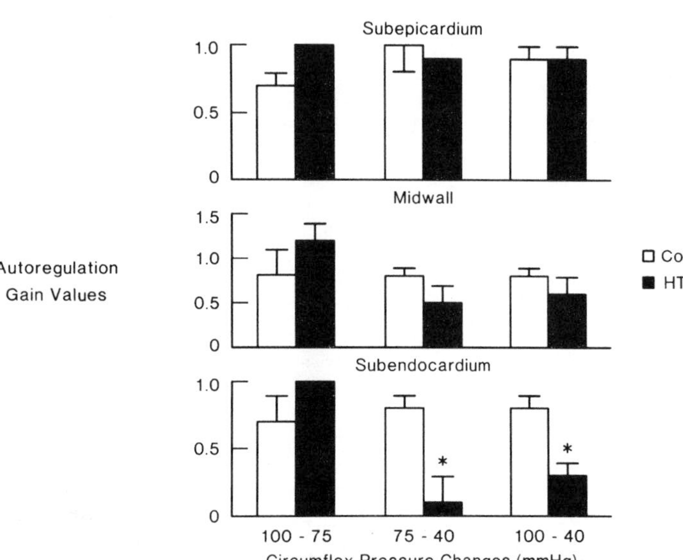

Figure 2–2. Autoregulation gain values for the subepicardium, midwall, and subendocardium of the left ventricle obtained during decreases of circumflex perfusion pressure from 100 to 75 and from 75 to 40 mmHg. Data are shown for control dogs and for dogs with chronic hypertension and left ventricular hypertrophy. Values of one indicate perfect autoregulation, whereas values approaching zero indicate absence of autoregulation. For pressure changes of 100 to 75 mmHg, autoregulation is excellent both in controls and in dogs with hypertension and left ventricular hypertrophy. In contrast, autoregulation is virtually absent in the subendocardium of dogs with hypertension and left ventricular hypertrophy during pressure changes of 75 to 40 mmHg. * = $p < .05$ versus controls. (From Harrison, D. G., Florentine, M. S., Brooks, L. A., et al.: The effect of hypertension and left ventricular hypertrophy on the lower range of coronary autoregulation. Circulation 77:1108, 1988. Used with permission from the American Heart Association.)

sympathetic activation in the normal heart is to increase coronary flow. However, under pathologic conditions such as in the presence of a severe coronary obstructive lesion, sympathetic activation can decrease flow markedly by selectively constricting the coronary vessel at the site of the stenotic lesion.[H1] Further, after α-adrenergic blockade, α-adrenergic constriction may be unmasked.[M1]

Activation of parasympathetic nerves engenders hemodynamic alterations that indirectly modify coronary flow. Parasympathetic activation decreases heart rate, increases atrial contractility, decreases ventricular contractility, and can produce generalized vasodilation.[B8, L2] The direct action of parasympathetic stimulation of coronary vessels is to produce a generalized but modest coronary dilation.[B8, L1] The net effect of an increase in parasympathetic activity is a striking decrease in coronary flow, because the intense bradycardia has such a dominant effect on decreasing myocardial oxygen consumption.

Although the effects of neural activation on the coronary circulation are very complex, most of them are too small to influence the outcome of cardiac imaging procedures. Only two of these effects are large enough to be of clinical importance, given the current sensitivity of imaging modalities. They are (1) indirect effects of sympathetic activation; and (2) directly mediated constriction of severely stenotic coronary segments. If the action of the sympathetic nerves is partially blocked, for example, by beta-blockade, the effects of exercise on myocardial oxygen consumption will be strikingly attenuated. This will limit increases in coronary flow and make it more difficult to detect moderate coronary obstructive lesions. If the alpha-adrenergic effects of the sympathetic nerves are blocked, then coronary obstructive lesions may not be constricted with exercise; this may prevent exaggeration of the hydraulic effects of the obstruction and, thereby, decrease the likelihood of detecting the presence of an obstructive lesion.

Humoral Control

Both circulating and noncirculating humoral agents can influence coronary vascular resistance. Some of the potent circulating substances include norepinephrine, epinephrine,[B2, M5, 6, V1] vasopressin,[N1, 2] and angiotensin.[B9, C9, D4, 5, F5, M11] Prostacyclin,[D2, H5, N3] thromboxane,[K3, R3] and endothelial relaxing factors are examples of noncirculating humoral agents that can modulate coronary tone. In addition, a host of substances can influence coronary resistance when injected in pharmacologic amounts but have little demonstrated effect on the coronary circulation under physiologic conditions. Examples of substances in this class include glucagon,[M12] substance P,[L2] endogenous dopamine,[B10, C10, N4] many of the prostaglandins,[H5] and vasoactive intestinal peptide.[S5]

This is a particularly complex area of coronary physiology, because the number of humoral substances that have some vasoactive effects on coronary vessels under experimental conditions is legion. Furthermore, the action of any one humoral substance is often complex and frequently not fully understood. An example that illustrates this point relates to the effects of vasopressin on the coronary circulation. At low concentrations (less than 10 μU/ml), which are present normally, vasopressin has no effect on coronary tone.[P1] At higher concentrations (over 100 μU/ml), which are present during pathologic states such as hemorrhage, vasopressin can increase systolic pressure and reflexly decrease heart rate.[N1, 2] These higher concentrations of vasopressin have no effect or dilate coronary arterial vessels greater than 100 μm in diameter, while constricting coronary arterial vessels less than 100 μm in diameter.

It is interesting that modest elevations of vasopressin (more than 100 μU/ml) can constrict mature collaterals markedly and decrease coronary collateral perfusion in dogs with mature collaterals developed by chronic ameroid coronary occlusion.[P1] This pronounced effect of vasopressin appears related to a marked sensitivity of well-developed collaterals to vasopressin and endothelial dysfunction of microvessels within the collateral-dependent myocardium.[S2] Why the endothelium is dysfunctional in microvessels chronically perfused by mature collaterals is an interesting but so far unanswered question.

Other humoral substances, such as histamine and serotonin, may have enhanced effects on diseased coronary segments. Histamine and platelet-derived products may cause enhanced constriction of diseased coronary artery segments.[K4, S6–8] It is unlikely that these enhanced effects of humoral substances will influence the results of any cardiac imaging procedures under normal circumstances. It is quite possible that if procedures are performed during physiologic stresses that elevate the circulating levels of vasopressin or histamine, or enhance the release of serotonin from platelets, these substances may predispose to the development of myocardial ischemia and influence the outcome of the study.

Myogenic Control

Many blood vessels exhibit a characteristic referred to as "myogenic tone." In response to an increase in intraluminal pressure, the vessel constricts, and in response to a decrease in intraluminal pressure, it dilates. This regulatory mechanism has been well documented in several peripheral vascular beds.[B11, J1] The importance of the myogenic response in the coronary circulation remains debatable. Recently, it has been shown that the myogenic response is at least in part modulated by the endothelium.[H6, K5]

SPECIAL CONSIDERATIONS RELATED TO THE REGULATION OF THE CORONARY CIRCULATION

In addition to the aforementioned six factors that primarily regulate coronary tone, four areas deserve special consideration: regional and transmural distribution of perfusion to the right and left ventricles, heterogeneity of perfusion to small ventricular segments, endothelial relaxing factor, and differences in flow to the various cardiac chambers.

Regulation of Transmural Perfusion

The development of the labeled microsphere technique[R13] has made it possible to explore in detail the regulation of perfusion to different zones and different transmural layers of the left and right ventricles. It was soon demonstrated that, in the absence of disease, perfusion around the circumference of the left ventricle, including the septum and from apex to base of the left ventricle, was essentially uniform[D6, M13, U2] (Fig. 2–3), with the exception of minor variations of perfusion that are likely related to the accuracy of the measurement technique.

In normal awake animals, subendocardial flow per gram is 10 to 30 percent greater than subepicardial flow.[C11, F6, M14] In several situations, the ratio of subendocardial to subepicardial flow decreases and in a few it increases. Situations often associated with decreases in the subendocardial to subepicardial flow ratio include a striking decrease in the systolic-pressure-time:diastolic-pressure-time index ratio;[B12] severe coronary stenosis with a distal coronary perfusion pressure of less than 40 mmHg;[G2] severe pressure-induced left ventricular hypertrophy;[V5] coronary occlusion, especially if subepicardial collaterals are present, as occurs in the dog;[F7] a marked increase in left ventricular pressure;[M15, W2] and maximal coronary dilation.[R4] Conditions in which the subendocardial:subepicardial flow ratio may increase primarily involve infusion of vasodilators such as the endothelium-dependent dilator substances, including acetylcholine, histamine, and moderate doses of adenosine.[G3, R4] Although the normal subendocardial:subepicardial flow ratio is 1.2:1, this ratio can decrease to as low as 0:2 with severe ischemia and increase to as high as 3:0 during adenosine infusion.

Even though current imaging techniques cannot measure perfusion in the subendocardium of the left ventricle accurately, understanding the factors that modulate transmural perfusion is critical to an in-depth appreciation of the major factors that determine the eventual outcome of perfusion imaging studies.

Heterogeneity of Perfusion to Small Segments of the Myocardium

The ability accurately to measure perfusion to segments of myocardium that weigh less than 250 mg has enabled investigators to quantify the pattern of blood flow in the myocardium under various conditions. Many studies[F8, M16] have confirmed that, under control conditions, perfusion to various tiny regions of the cardiac chamber walls at any one time is strikingly heterogeneous. Under control conditions, perfusion between adjacent segments of normal myocardium may vary by ± 50 percent of mean perfusion to the chamber wall (Fig. 2–4). Furthermore, over a period of seconds to minutes, perfusion in any single tiny myocardial segment may vary tremendously even though average flow to the chamber wall and hemodynamics remain constant.[M16] Meticulously designed studies have excluded experimental error as a significant component of the observed variability of perfusion. This "transient heterogeneity of perfusion" is sometimes referred to as "twinkling." Mechanisms responsible for the heterogeneity remain unknown. It should be emphasized that when perfusion in very large segments of myocardium is examined (entire septum, anterior wall, lateral wall, inferior wall), the pattern of perfusion to segments of myocardium then appears to be relatively uniform.[D6, M13, U2]

The substantial heterogeneity that exists in the perfusion of small segments of left ventricular wall has important ramifications for the interpretation and validation of perfusion imaging procedures. If a given perfusion agent is extracted almost entirely in one pass through the myocardium (such as albumin macroaggregates labeled with a radionuclide), the heterogeneity of perfusion will likely be apparent if the spatial resolution of the technique is sufficiently fine. If the perfusion agent accumulates over many cardiac cycles, such as ^{15}O-labeled H_2O, then the heterogeneity will average out over time. In either case, because validation studies almost always utilize radiolabeled microspheres that are almost fully extracted in one pass, perfusion to tiny zones of myocardium cannot be compared quantitatively unless the myocardial zones in the two techniques (positron emission tomography and radiolabeled spheres) are matched within a few square millimeters. In practice, this is impossible. As a consequence of these considerations for the present and the near future, it will be possible to validate perfusion measurements only with imaging techniques to relatively large zones of myocardium (3- to 10-gram segments). In addition, the occasional detection of a "tiny isolated hypoperfused zone" in an imaging examination may not reflect the presence of disease but simply be an example of "the twinkling phenomenon."

Endothelial Relaxing Factor

When the endothelium is physically removed from a vessel or is dysfunctional because of disease, the vasoactive response of the vessel to various stimuli changes dramatically.[F9, G4, K6] This observation, originally described by Furchgott and Zawadski,[F9] is related to the release of an endothelial relaxing factor. It is now suspected that there are several endothelial relaxing factors and one or more endothelial constricting factors.[F10, R5] The exact nature of these factors remains unknown. It is appreciated, however, that the dominant endothelial relaxing factor has a low molecular weight, a half-life in vivo of less than 15 seconds, and contains or can give rise to nitric oxide.[P2]

There are a host of substances, including acetylcholine, thrombin, adenosine diphosphate, norepinephrine, and vasopressin, whose vascular effects are modulated by the release of an endothelial relaxing factor.[C3, D7, F11, M17] Other substances, including adenosine, nitroglycerin, and nitroprusside, do not depend on the endothelium. It has also been shown that several common disease states, including diabetes,[M18] hypertension,[W3] and atherosclerosis[F11, H7, L3, V6] can impair the release of endothelial relaxing factor. Ascending dilation is also probably related to the release of endothelial relaxing factor.[P3, R6] Finally, situations associated with physical disruption of the endothelium, such as angioplasty or plaque rupture associated with unstable angina or acute myocardial infarction, obviously can interfere with release of endothelial relaxing factors. The effect of atherosclerosis on this process has been extensively reviewed recently.[H8]

Endothelial relaxing factors significantly influence the tone of several segments in the coronary vasculature and thereby can influence myocardial perfusion. It remains unclear under what clinical conditions coronary tone related to the release of endothelial relaxing factor will influence the outcome of cardiac imaging studies.

Differences in Flow to Various Cardiac Chambers

Total flow to a given cardiac chamber wall is obviously equal to flow per gram times the mass of the chamber wall. In the normal heart, flow per gram is greatest in the left ventricle and least in the atria.[W1] These differences are further exaggerated because the weight of the normal left ventricle (free wall and septum) is 3.5 times more than that of the right ventricular free wall and also substantially greater than that of the right atrial or left atrial wall. As a consequence, the left ventricle receives about 80 percent of total flow to the heart. It is also known that certain regulatory mechanisms concerning perfusion of the chamber walls are not uniform in the four chambers. In particular, for example, flow reserve in the atria is only about 2.5-fold, whereas it is five- or sixfold in both the right and left ventricles.[W1]

Because current perfusion imaging techniques are relatively

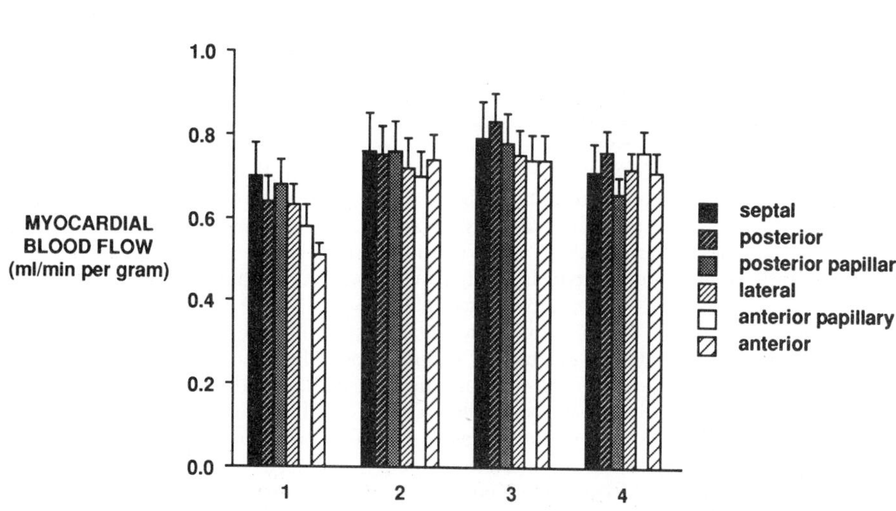

Figure 2–3. Myocardial blood flow measurements obtained from four transmural layers and multiple circumferential regions of the left ventricular myocardium. Although there is some random variability, the circumferential distribution of perfusion is essentially uniform. (Redrawn from data originally presented by Murdock, R. H., Jr., and Cobb, F. R.: Effects of infarcted myocardium on regional blood flow measurements to ischemic regions in canine heart. Circ. Res. 47(5):701, 1980 by permission of the American Heart Association, Inc., and the authors.)

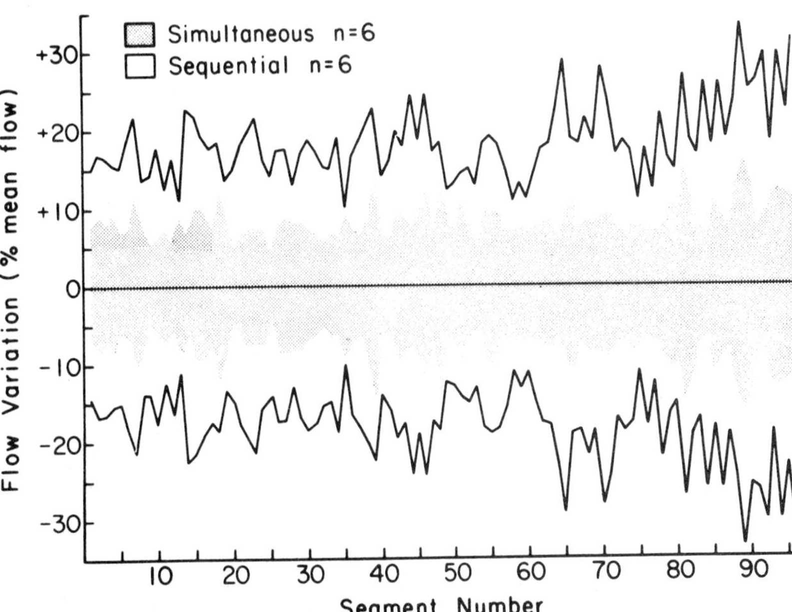

Figure 2–4. Distribution of segmental flow variations for simultaneous and sequential injections of microspheres in conscious dogs. The middle band indicates the average range of perfusion variability in simultaneously injected dogs. The larger outside band indicates the average range of perfusion for sequentially injected dogs. All data were normalized to eliminate the effect of spatial heterogeneity and variance in the intra-animal mean left ventricular perfusion. (Redrawn from data originally presented by Marcus, M. L., Kerber, R. E., Erhardt, J. C., et al.: Spatial and temporal heterogeneity of left ventricular perfusion in awake dogs. Am. Heart J. 94:748, 1977. Used with permission of the publisher.)

insensitive, in the normal heart only the left ventricle is imaged with sufficient clarity to derive diagnostic information. The walls of the atria are almost never seen, and the right ventricle is usually visualized only if it is hypertrophied and has increased flow per gram secondary to a pressure load. If the entire right ventricular free wall cannot be visualized well with perfusion imaging techniques, it is no wonder that small perfusion defects in the left ventricle are often not detected.

CORONARY VASODILATOR RESERVE

As noted earlier, in large mammals, including humans, coronary flow under resting conditions is only a small fraction of maximal coronary flow. The ratio between resting and maximal flow is about 5:1 or 6:1 under normal conditions. Katz and Linder described coronary reserve in 1939,[K7] and this was further explored by Coffman and Gregg in 1960.[C12] The concept of coronary reserve was popularized and further refined as a consequence of the work of Gould and his associates.[G5–7] The first accurate measurements of coronary reserve in anesthetized patients were obtained by Marcus and associates[M19] and in awake patients by Wilson and associates.[W4]

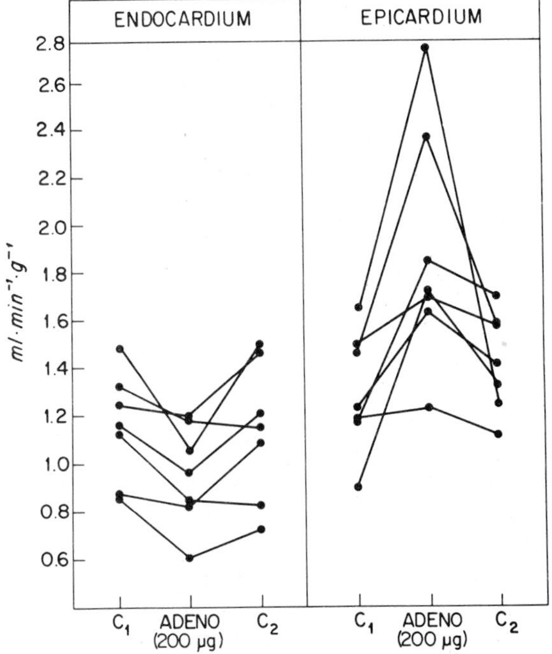

Figure 2–5. Changes in myocardial blood flow distal to a flow-limiting coronary stenosis during adenosine infusion. Vasodilator reserve is abolished in the endocardium but persists in the epicardium. (From Gewirtz, H., Williams, D. O., Ohley, W. H., and Most, A. S.: Influence of coronary vasodilatation on the transmural distribution of myocardial blood flow distal to a severe fixed coronary artery stenosis. Am Heart J. 106:674, 1983. Used with permission of the publisher, the author and the editor.)

The difference between resting and maximal coronary flow is usually elicited by three types of stimuli: transient coronary occlusion to produce coronary reactive hyperemia;[C12, K7, M19] intense metabolic stress usually secondary to bicycle or treadmill exercise;[K1] or intense pharmacologic coronary dilation.[G5, 6, T1] In both animals and humans, coronary reserve values obtained with any of these approaches are very similar.

Several specific aspects of coronary reserve should be emphasized:

- Coronary reserve can be altered by disease processes,[M8, 20, 21, T1] nonhemodynamic conditions,[G4–6, W5] hemodynamic alterations,[B13, 14] and drug effects.[B15, E1] All the factors that can modify coronary reserve must be considered whenever coronary reserve measurements are being interpreted.
- Coronary reserve is not altered by age or gender.[E2, M19]
- Coronary reserve is not equal in all cardiac chambers. It is 5:1 to 6:1 in both the right and left ventricles and only 2:1 to 3:1 in the right or left atria.[W1]
- Coronary reserve is not uniform in different transmural layers of the left ventricle under all conditions.[B16, D8] When a coronary obstruction is present, reserve can be strikingly decreased in the subendocardial layer and relatively normal in the subepicardial layer of the left ventricle[G8] (Fig. 2–5).

Because coronary reserve is of enormous importance to the field of perfusion imaging, several of the factors that can modify this phenomenon will be discussed in greater detail.

Nonhemodynamic Conditions That Influence Coronary Reserve

Many nonhemodynamic factors that may directly influence the major hemodynamic determinants of myocardial oxygen consumption (heart rate, wall stress, and contractility) can modulate coronary reserve. In the broad sense, these factors: changes in body temperature,[B5] hypoxia,[M4] carbon monoxide,[E3] abnormal hemoglobin,[R7] and hematocrit do have "hemodynamic effects," such as altering blood viscosity, but, in a more conventional sense, these factors can be classified as nonhemodynamic because they may not alter the traditional hemodynamic parameters that are measured routinely.

Temperature changes are rarely of concern except during cardiac surgical procedures that include cold potassium cardioplegia.[A1, C13, B17, 18, G9] Likewise, noncellular causes of increased blood viscosity, such as myeloma and macroglobulinemia, are rarely of sufficient severity to affect minimal coronary vascular resistance materially. Hypoxia[M4] or carbon monoxide poisoning[E3] can increase resting coronary flow strikingly and, hence, decrease coronary flow reserve if it is measured as a ratio to maximal flow, as opposed to absolute minimal coronary vascular resistance. Polycythemia decreases perfusion to the subendocardium of the left ventricle,[R7] and anemia decreases minimal coronary vascular resistance.[V7] Polycythemia, therefore, decreases flow under control conditions, and anemia does the opposite. If coronary reserve is assessed as a ratio of resting-to-peak flow, as opposed to absolute minimal coronary vascular resistance, then polycythemia may produce little or no change in coronary reserve, whereas severe anemia will reduce coronary reserve strikingly, since resting flow is markedly increased.

It should be emphasized that these "nonhemodynamic factors" can influence coronary reserve profoundly and must be considered whenever measurements of coronary reserve are interpreted.

Effects of Hemodynamics on Coronary Reserve

Perturbations of routinely measured hemodynamics can modify coronary reserve in several ways. If a given hemodynamic change, such as an increase in heart rate, alters resting coronary flow, even if minimal coronary resistance is not modified, coronary reserve will change, particularly if it is assessed as a ratio between control and maximal flow. Hemodynamic perturbations also can modulate coronary reserve by altering compressive forces or coronary driving pressure or activating reflex mechanisms.

In the animal laboratory, it has been shown that tachycardia decreases, and augmentation of myocardial contractility increases, coronary flow reserve.[H3] As expected, marked decreases in coronary driving pressure severely decrease coronary reserve.[D9]

Studies in humans by Winniford and associates indicate that a 40 beat per minute increase in heart rate from a resting heart rate of 80 beats per minute results in an increase in resting coronary blood flow velocity and about a one third decrease in coronary flow reserve.[W6] Moderate increases in aortic pressure in patients do not change coronary flow reserve. In light of these observations, it is clear that the interpretation of measurements of coronary flow reserve requires that the hemodynamic conditions during the examination be carefully considered. This is particularly critical when repeated measurements are compared in one patient or groups of measurements are compared between patients.

Drug Effects on Coronary Flow Reserve

Any pharmacologic agent that can influence hemodynamics will indirectly modulate coronary flow reserve. Cardiac drugs that often influence hemodynamics at rest include beta-blockers, calcium channel blockers, inotropic agents, vasodilators, vasoconstrictors, and atropine-like drugs.

In addition, drugs may have a direct effect on coronary vascular resistance and can modify coronary reserve. In dogs, the calcium channel blocker diltiazem markedly decreases coronary flow reserve even after the hemodynamic effects of the drug have dissipated.[B15] In humans, Rossen and associates have shown that the decrease in flow reserve secondary to intravenous or intracoronary diltiazem is negligible.[R8] Simonetti and associates have shown that nitroglycerin does not alter coronary flow reserve after its transient effects on overall coronary vascular resistance have abated.[S9] The effects of beta-blockade on flow reserve have not been studied in detail.

At present, evidence of a direct pharmacologic action of drugs on coronary flow reserve, particularly in humans, is lacking. In contrast, numerous drugs can modify coronary flow reserve indirectly by influencing systemic hemodynamics. As a consequence, whenever measurements of coronary reserve are evaluated, concomitant drug effects must be taken into account.

Effects of Disease on Coronary Flow Reserve

Both noncardiac and cardiac diseases can influence coronary flow reserve. Noncardiac diseases exert their influence on coronary flow reserve primarily by affecting hemodynamics or the oxygen-carrying or oxygen-delivering capacity of the blood. Classic examples include febrile illnesses associated with tachycardia, changes in arterial pressure and myocardial contractility, diseases associated with severe hypoxia such as emphysema, and anemia secondary to chronic blood loss.

Cardiac diseases that typically influence coronary reserve include pathologic problems of the conduit coronary vessels, such as congenital coronary anomalies,[E4, V8] or coronary obstructive disease.[G2, G5, G7] Diffuse diseases of the coronary vasculature also can decrease coronary reserve. These may include collagen vascular diseases,[S10] syndrome X,[C14, G10] or the diffuse atherosclerosis that frequently occurs in cardiac transplant patients.

Pathologic types of cardiac hypertrophy—volume-induced[D10] and pressure-induced[M21] hypertrophy of either the right or left ventricles—profoundly decrease flow reserve in humans. It is not known whether the hypertrophy associated with various types of athletic conditioning or thyrotoxicosis is associated with a decrease in coronary flow reserve. Finally, large coronary collaterals may influence coronary flow reserve by increasing baseline flow in the vessels supplying the collaterals, allowing only limited perfusion of collateral-dependent myocardium or permitting coronary steal to develop.

Absolute Versus Relative Assessment of Coronary Flow Reserve

When coronary flow reserve is measured, the clinician is usually attempting to estimate minimal coronary vascular resistance. In the animal laboratory, this is measured by determining absolute as opposed to relative flow and calculating minimal resistance with one of the conventional formulations,[M22] which takes coronary driving pressure and perhaps other forces into account. Most of the factors that modulate coronary reserve when it is measured as a ratio of resting to maximal flow would have either no effect or a lesser effect on absolute minimal vascular resistance. Tachycardia, for example, which decreases coronary flow reserve substantially when it is measured as a ratio of resting to maximal flow,[W6] has only minor effects on absolute minimal coronary vascular resistance measurements. A few factors do modestly increase (cardiac hypertrophy) or decrease (profound anemia and thyrotoxicosis) minimal coronary vascular resistance.

At present, there is no clinically acceptable method of measuring absolute coronary flow in a single coronary vessel, hence minimal vascular resistance cannot be calculated in humans. Therefore, at present, we must rely on relative measurements of flow reserve—the ratio of resting to maximal flow—and accept the numerous limitations this imposes.

Summary

Coronary flow reserve can be modulated enormously by four major categories of effects, including cardiac disease, specific hemodynamic perturbations, drug effects, and a variety of cardiac diseases. Therefore, it is critical to consider all these factors whenever coronary reserve measurements are interpreted. This is of overwhelming importance to the field of perfusion imaging, because all current imaging approaches attempt to assess regional or global coronary flow reserve in relative terms, as opposed to absolute minimal coronary resistance, which would be less affected by many of these factors.

CLINICAL USE OF CORONARY VASODILATORS

Clinicians employing perfusion imaging techniques must either be content to assess perfusion under control conditions only or to employ a stimulus to produce coronary vasodilation. In certain clinical settings, such as patients with acute myocardial infarction, unstable angina, or coronary spasm, regions of myocardium may be underperfused at rest, and imaging techniques that reflect regional myocardial perfusion may yield valuable clinical information. In most clinical settings, however, it is essential to measure regional myocardial perfusion in the presence of coronary vasodilation. This substantially enhances the likelihood of detecting obstructive coronary disease, because only the most severe coronary obstructive lesions decrease perfusion under control conditions (Fig. 2–6).

Cardiac perfusion imaging techniques have utilized a broad range of interventions intended to produce coronary dilation. These can be categorized into those that usually produce submaximal coronary dilation and those that usually produce maximal coronary dilation. It should be noted that several potent coronary dilators that are useful in animal experiments, such as carbocromen[G11, N5, R9] and large intracoronary doses of acetylcholine,[B8, L1] are not utilized in imaging studies because they are either not approved for human use (carbocromen) or they are not thought to be clinically safe (large intracoronary doses of acetylcholine).

Submaximal Coronary Dilator Stimuli

This category includes interventions that indirectly produce coronary dilation by increasing myocardial oxygen consumption. Examples of such interventions include pacing,[G1] intravenous atropine,[M11] handgrip,[B19] the cold pressor test,[M10] infusion of inotropic agents such as norepinephrine,[B2, V1, 4] isoproterenol,[B2] or dopamine,[B10, N4] or vasoconstrictors such as angiotensin.[F5] Several drugs also produce submaximal coronary dilation, such as intracoronary infusion of contrast media[G4, 5] or oral administration of submaximal doses of dipyridamole.[T2]

The most popular intervention in this category of stimuli that usually produce submaximal coronary dilation is moderate treadmill or bicycle exercise. When exercise is performed by patients taking drugs such as beta-blockers that limit the hemodynamic response to exercise, maximal coronary dilation is never achieved. The approaches that produce submaximal coronary dilation have been employed in the overwhelming majority of cardiac imaging procedures. These interventions are readily available to practicing physicians, are relatively safe, and are well accepted by patients. Furthermore, they provide four types of valuable clinical information in addition to producing coronary dilation: electrocardiographic or hemodynamic evidence of stress-induced myocardial ischemia, angina pectoris, stress-induced arrhythmias, and an assessment of exercise capacity. For these reasons, there is no doubt that these interventions for producing coronary dilation will continue to be extremely popular.

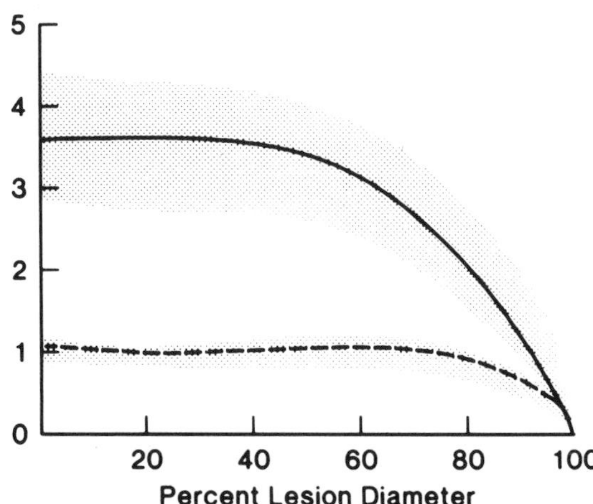

Figure 2–6. Relationship between resting (dashed line) and maximal coronary blood flow (solid line) and percent diameter stenosis in a dog. Increasing severity of coronary stenosis was achieved by progressively narrowing a short segment of a proximal coronary artery. Resting coronary blood flow did not change until coronary diameter stenosis exceeded 90 percent. Maximal coronary blood flow began to decrease when percent diameter stenosis exceeded 50 percent. (Modified from data originally presented by Gould, K. L., Lipscomb, K., and Hamilton, G. W.: Physiologic basis for assessing critical coronary stenosis. Am. J. Cardiol. 33:87, 1974. Used with permission of the publisher.)

Unfortunately, none of these agents produces maximal coronary dilation, and many of them are associated with less than a twofold increase in coronary flow. If a cardiac imaging procedure is capable of measuring maximal coronary flow (five to six times control) and a relatively impotent coronary dilator is utilized, sensitivity will inevitably suffer. However, if the imaging procedure can assess only moderate increases in coronary flow, utilizing an intense coronary dilator will not necessarily enhance the sensitivity of the procedure for detecting an obstructive coronary lesion. Most conventional techniques that employ diffusable indicators cannot accurately track high coronary flow rates under clinical conditions. However, other newer approaches of assessing coronary reserve, such as digital angiographic assessments of coronary transient time or the intracoronary Doppler catheter, can accurately measure maximal coronary flow rates. If physicians employ coronary vasodilators that produce submaximal coronary dilation in association with a cardiac imaging procedure, it is a foregone conclusion that the sensitivity of detecting hemodynamically significant coronary obstructions will decline in proportion to the impotence of the dilator employed.

Maximal Coronary Dilators

There are four clinically acceptable approaches to producing maximal coronary dilation: intravenous dipyridamole, intracoronary papaverine, intracoronary adenosine, and intense exercise. In addition, under special conditions (balloon angioplasty, open heart surgery), transient coronary occlusion can produce maximal coronary dilation by eliciting the reactive hyperemia response.

Exhaustive exercise in animals and humans[V2, 9] can produce near-maximal coronary dilation. Maximal increases in coronary flow do not occur during intense exercise, because the sympathetic nervous system is activated and alpha-adrenergic–mediated coronary constriction modestly limits coronary flow.[M23] However, the main reason that exercise does not produce intense coronary dilation clinically is that patients suspected of having heart disease can rarely achieve the intense exercise level required to produce near-maximal coronary dilation. Ordinarily, such levels of exercise can be achieved only by trained athletes.

The three pharmacologic agents that can produce maximal coronary dilation differ in a variety of ways. Two of them, papaverine and adenosine, traditionally have been administered only intracoronary. Therefore, these agents have not been used for imaging procedures such as ultrafast computed tomography, standard nuclear imaging, positron emission tomography, or magnetic resonance imaging, that are "relatively noninvasive." However, for invasive procedures such as digital angiographic estimates of coronary transit time or use of the Doppler catheter, intracoronary papaverine and adenosine have been extremely valuable.[W4, 7, 8] Although intracoronary administration of papaverine or adenosine has minimal effects on systemic hemodynamics, both drugs have potentially serious side effects. In about 0.1 to 0.5 percent of patients, intracoronary papaverine can produce transient or sustained ventricular tachycardia, which occasionally requires cardioversion. In experimental animals, adenosine impairs the function of the sinus[W9] and atrioventricular[C15] nodes and, thereby, may produce profound bradycardia, primarily when it is injected into the vascular supply of these structures (usually the right coronary artery). Both papaverine[W9] and adenosine have a brief duration of action—less than 2 minutes—and can be administered repeatedly during a study. This facilitates the determination of dose-response curves and allows a great deal of flexibility in protocol design. Neither agent exhibits tachyphylaxis.

Recently, Wilson and associates examined the utility of intravenous adenosine as a coronary vasodilator in 30 patients.[W10] These investigators found that 140 μg/kg/min produced maximal coronary flow (measured with intracoronary Doppler) in 83 percent of patients. This dose was well tolerated, producing an average decrease in blood pressure of 5 ± 1 mmHg and increasing heart rate by 19 beats per minute.

Dipyridamole is a clinically useful dilator that has many favorable characteristics. The drug's mechanism of action involves inhibition of cellular uptake and metabolism of the endogenous release of adenosine.[K8, W11] Although this agent is not currently approved for use intravenously in the United States, it is likely to reach the commercial market in a relatively short time. Dipyridamole is relatively simple to administer and can produce maximal coronary dilation. Unfortunately, a small percentage of patients (10 to 25 percent) given the drug do not achieve maximal coronary dilation if the conventional dose (0.56 mg/kg intravenously over 4 minutes) is administered. These submaximal responses cannot be predicted on the basis of either the patient's clinical characteristics or hemodynamic response to drug infusion and are not always overcome by infusing a 50 percent increase in the dose of intravenous dipyridamole. The drug achieves its maximal coronary dilator effect 9 minutes after the onset of infusion. The physiologic half-life of dipyridamole is 30 to 45 minutes.[W11] Hence, for practical reasons, dipyridamole can be administered only once during a study in the cardiac catheterization laboratory. Although one study suggested that handgrip would increase the coronary dilator response associated with dipyridamole infusion,[B19] subsequent studies by Rossen and associates[R10] with more accurate measurement of coronary blood flow velocity suggest that handgrip does not significantly increase the coronary dilator response to dipyridamole.

Dipyridamole infusion is associated with a small increase in cardiac output, and, furthermore, the distribution of cardiac output in various organs is much different with dipyridamole than with intense treadmill exercise. With dipyridamole, the relative blood flow to abdominal viscera increases, whereas with exercise, it decreases. Thus, a perfusion agent such as thallium-201 will accumulate in the liver and spleen to a greater extent when coronary dilation is achieved with dipyridamole versus exercise. This can interfere with assessing perfusion of the inferior wall of the left ventricle, which is immediately adjacent to these abdominal viscera.

Many minor side effects of dipyridamole administration occur frequently: nausea, dizziness, vomiting, mild chest discomfort, perspiration, and headache.[L4] In addition, typically the drug increases heart rate by 5 to 20 beats per minute and decreases mean aortic pressure by 5 to 15 mmHg. The more serious side effects occur less frequently. These are severe chest pain (18 to 42 percent of patients) and a striking decrease in systemic pressure (6 to 10 percent of patients). These effects almost always are quickly ameliorated immediately following intravenous infusion of aminophylline (125 to 250 mg intravenously). Also, a few patients develop ST segment depression or ventricular wall motion abnormalities,[L4, P4] suggesting the presence of myocardial ischemia secondary to coronary steal.

In addition to these mild and moderate side effects of dipyridamole, a study conducted by the drug's manufacturer indicates that 2 of 5000 patients given intravenous dipyridamole died and 2 patients suffered a myocardial infarction thought to be related to drug infusion. All four of the patients had a clinical history suggesting unstable angina pectoris. Hence, in this patient group, dipyridamole infusion is contraindicated.

Despite these various limitations, intravenous dipyridamole is the most clinically useful potent coronary dilator available. The side effects of the drug in patients without unstable angina can be easily managed. Furthermore, there is no other potent safe coronary dilator on the horizon that can be administered intravenously. The newer sophisticated perfusion imaging techniques, such as magnetic resonance imaging, positron emission tomography, contrast echocardiography, and ultrafast computed tomography, all depend entirely on an effective pharmacologic coronary dilator, and dipyridamole is the only choice likely to be available in the next several years. Dipyridamole is probably as safe as intense level exercise in patients who do not have unstable pectoris or acute myocardial infarction, and it produces more intense coronary dilation than the exercise usually achieved by patients suspected of having coronary heart disease.

CORONARY COLLATERAL CIRCULATION

Coronary collaterals are arteriovascular channels that connect large arterial systems, such as the left anterior descending and circumflex coronary beds. A basic concept in understanding the collateral circulation relates to the differences between native, immature, or unstimulated collaterals and mature coronary collaterals. These two main classes of coronary collaterals will be discussed separately.

Native Collaterals

Native collaterals are tiny vascular channels typically ranging in size from 40 to 200 μm that exist from birth.[F12, S11] The density and distribution of these pre-existing or native collaterals are genetically determined. There are vast differences between species and also within a single species. In mongrel dogs, the density of native collaterals varies over at least a hundredfold range.[S12] Furthermore, the distribution of collaterals within the left ventricular wall is also genetically determined. In dogs, epicardial collaterals constitute at least 50 percent of the native collaterals, whereas, in pigs, the few collaterals that exist are primarily subendocardial.[S11] This difference in the transmural distribution of collaterals explains in part why experimentally induced infarcts in dogs are predominantly subendocardial and transmural in pigs. The flow that can be delivered by native collaterals in dogs is roughly 5 to 10 percent of resting myocardial perfusion.[M24, S12, 13] Typically, the distribution of coronary collateral perfusion by native collaterals is such that the ratio of subendocardial to subepicardial perfusion in myocardium served by native collaterals is typically 0:5 or less.[S13]

In animals, the native collaterals are normally closed, because no pressure gradient exists between the two bridged vascular systems. However, if the pressure in one of the vessels connected to a collateral drops strikingly due to a severe upstream stenosis or occlusion, then the native collaterals can open quickly. In response to sudden occlusion, the native collaterals immediately open, but the opening is only partial. Over a period of 10 to 30 minutes, the vessel opens maximally.[M24] Typically, in the dog, flow via native collaterals increases about twofold in the first 10 to 30 minutes following coronary occlusion.[M24]

A number of additional characteristics of native collaterals are of importance. In the dog, the collaterals are more abundant per gram of tissue in the atria and right ventricle, compared with the left ventricle.[S14] This may explain why atrial and right ventricular infarctions are more difficult to produce in dogs than left ventricular infarction. Also, the density and functional capacity of mature collaterals in dogs are inversely proportional to the perfusion field served by the vessel receiving collateral perfusion[G12] (Fig. 2–7). This probably explains why occlusion of coronary vessels with small perfusion fields may not be associated with infarction. Collateral density is not altered in pressure-induced hypertrophy in either dogs or humans.[H9] Finally, the functional capacity of the native collaterals is very sensitive to extravascular compressive forces, coronary driving pressure,[S11] and the vasomotor tone of the vascular bed downstream of the collaterals.

Although a great deal is known about the characteristics of the collateral circulation in animals, little is known about the native coronary collateral circulation in humans, other than its existence. The topography of infarcts (subendocardial greater than subepi-

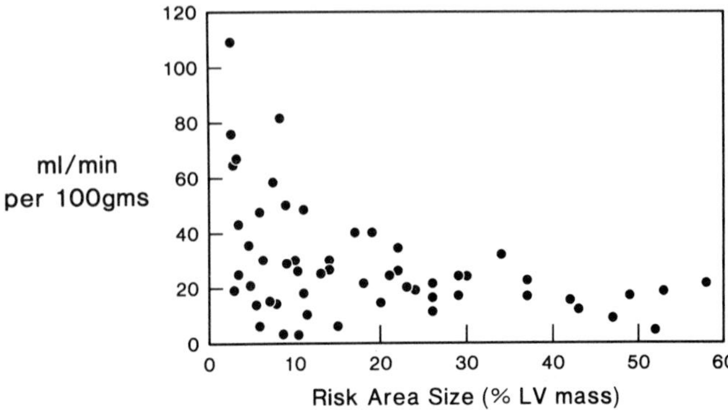

Figure 2–7. Relationship between coronary collateral blood flow and the size of an ischemic region (risk area as a percent of left ventricular mass). Although there is a great deal of variability in coronary collateral flow, it is apparent that absolute collateral flow is inversely proportional to the size of the region of myocardium at risk. (From Gumm, D. C., Thompson, S. B., Marcus, M. L., and Harrison, D. G.: The influence of risk area on native collateral resistance and ischemic zone perfusion. Am. J. Physiol. 254:H473, 1988. Used with permission of the American Physiological Society.)

cardial) in patients suggests that collaterals are more abundant in the subepicardial layers in patients. Also, the rare occurrence of atrial infarction and the relatively small size of right ventricular infarctions in humans suggest that these chambers have more abundant collaterals than the left ventricle. A limited number of measurements of distal pressure in normal coronaries of patients subjected to transient occlusion at surgery suggest that the overall density of collaterals in humans is roughly equivalent to that observed in the dog.[G13] Obviously, what is needed is more direct measurements of coronary collateral function in humans. These will be done when an appropriate method becomes available.

Mature Collaterals

Either gradual, progressive occlusion with an ameroid constrictor or intermittent brief occlusions in dogs will cause the native coronary collaterals to develop to vascular channels that are fiftyfold their original size.[S15] This remarkable transformation occurs because of growth of all constituents of the vessel wall. In dogs, mature collaterals can maintain normal perfusion to a collateral-dependent bed during intense exercise (Fig. 2–8).[B20] However, minimal coronary vascular resistance in collateral-dependent myocardium served by mature collaterals is significantly greater than that in the normal coronary circulation of the dog.[H10]

Although mature coronary collaterals histologically appear remarkably similar to conduit coronary vessels of similar size, their functional characteristics in dogs are different from normal conduit coronary vessels. Mature coronary collaterals have no functional alpha-receptors,[H10] have normal beta-receptors,[F13] and are hyperresponsive to vasopressin.[P1] The absence of alpha-receptors is probably beneficial, because it prevents sympathetically mediated constriction of mature collaterals during stress. The hyperresponse of mature collaterals to vasopressin may explain why patients with coronary disease occasionally have catastrophic responses to vasopressin infusion or high endogenous levels of vasopressin that may develop in certain stressful situations such as hemorrhage. Because some mature collaterals arise distal to a source of resistance in the vessel giving rise to the collaterals, increasing flow in the normal vessel can produce "steal" or decrease perfusion to the collateral-dependent region.[S16]

Mature coronary collaterals can have a profound effect on the perfusion of collateral-dependent myocardium in the dog. In humans, the importance of mature collaterals is less certain, primarily because there is no acceptable method of directly measuring coronary collateral flow in patients.

In humans, mature coronary collaterals can be demonstrated angiographically.[L5] Usually, these vessels are not angiographically demonstrable unless they perfuse an area served by a vessel that is either occluded or severely (greater than 90 percent diameter narrowing) obstructed.[C16] Large mature collaterals can produce an increase in distal coronary pressure that indicates that these collateral vessels provide a significant amount of perfusion to the collateral-dependent myocardium.[B11] Although there is much evidence that mature collaterals can maintain normal resting

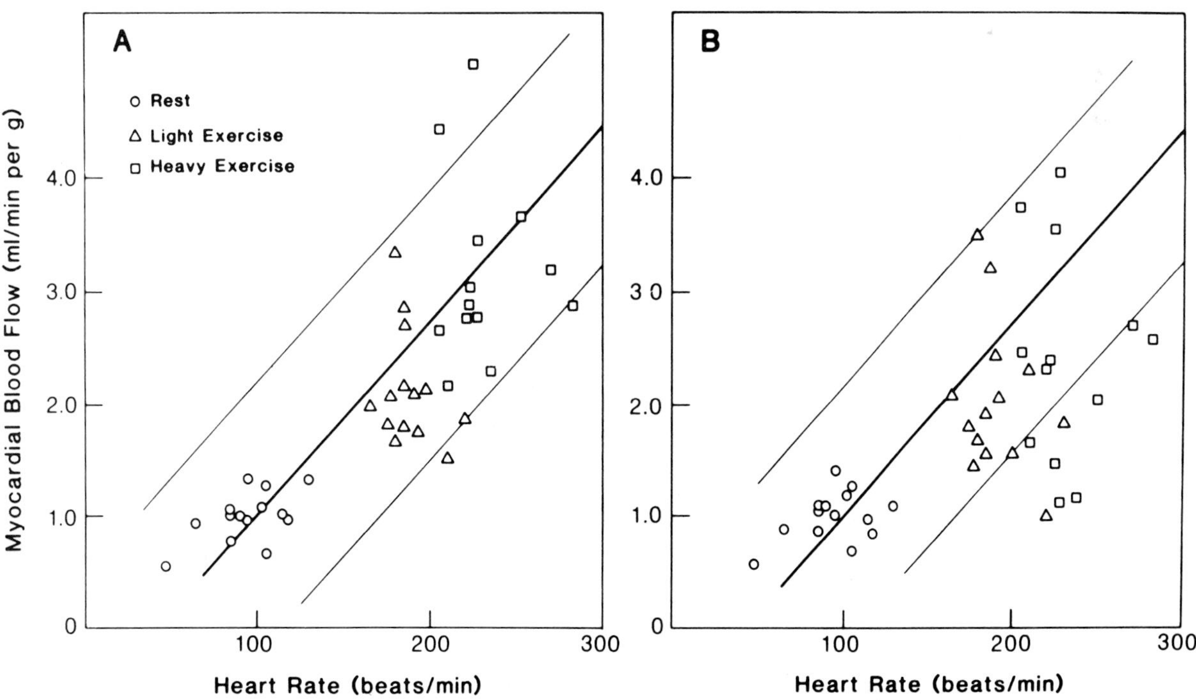

Figure 2–8. Mean blood flow at rest and during two levels of treadmill exercise in normally perfused (*A*) and collateral-dependent myocardium (*B*) plotted as a function of heart rate for 14 dogs with mature coronary collaterals. Mature collaterals were stimulated to develop by ameroid occlusion of the circumflex coronary artery for one month. Under most circumstances, collateral blood-flow increased proportionately with heart rate. During heavy exercise there was a tendency for subnormal increase in blood flow in the collateral-dependent areas. (From Bache, R. J., and Schwartz, J. S.: Myocardial blood flow during exercise after gradual coronary occlusion in the dog. Am. J. Physiol. 245(Heart Circ. Physiol. 14):H131, 1983. Used with permission of the American Physiological Society.)

perfusion in humans, it is less certain that normal perfusion during stress can be maintained in collateral-dependent myocardium. Utilizing ultrafast computed tomography, we have observed normal wall motion during dobutamine infusion in two patients with totally collateral-dependent myocardium. This suggests that the collateral-dependent myocardium could increase its perfusion with this type of stress.

The status of the coronary collateral circulation has a significant impact on the outcome of many types of cardiac imaging studies. In general, the presence of collaterals will decrease wall motion abnormalities during stress and improve perfusion when assessed with an exercise thallium perfusion scintigram. In one study, 50 percent of patients with an occluded coronary vessel served by mature collaterals had normal thallium distribution in the collateral-dependent zones.[E5] When imaging studies employ maximal coronary dilators such as dipyridamole, the presence of collaterals sets the stage for "collateral steal." This can result in wall motion abnormalities and decreases in perfusion in collateral-dependent myocardium.[P4] Finally, mature collaterals permit the development of ischemia at a distance.[S17] This occurs when the parent vessel supplying collaterals to an adjacent bed becomes compromised, and as a consequence the adjacent bed is suddenly underperfused.

The results of current imaging procedures are confounded by the existence of mature collaterals, because patients with total coronary occlusion can demonstrate normal wall motion and perfusion in the collateral-dependent zone. Whether this implies that the myocardium served by the collaterals is normally perfused and functions normally, or that currently available tests are too insensitive to detect the abnormalities that exist, remains unanswered.

CORONARY STENOSIS

The hydraulic effects of an obstruction in a pulsatile vascular bed have been exhaustively explored both in vitro[Y1–4] and in vivo,[G5, 6] and detailed equations that precisely predict energy losses across the obstruction have been presented.[Y1–4] In summary, the key factors that determine the functional significance of an obstruction are the blood velocity and viscosity, the entrance and exit angles of the obstruction, and the length, shape, and relative and absolute narrowing produced by the obstruction. The effects of obstructions in series have also been accurately described.[F14] Although these hydraulic principles are soundly established, for decades they have been ignored by physicians caring for patients with coronary obstructive disease. Instead of paying attention to the fund of knowledge available, clinicians have chosen to assess the severity of a coronary stenosis by visual estimates of percent diameter narrowing. This approach became widely accepted by both clinicians and clinical investigators for two reasons: (1) it was quick and simple to apply; and (2) studies in normal dogs with short, relatively round obstructions demonstrated an orderly relationship between percent diameter stenosis and decrements in maximal and resting coronary flow (see Fig. 2–6).

It has now been convincingly demonstrated in studies performed primarily in patients with coronary disease that visual estimates of percent diameter narrowing are no longer acceptable as a means of predicting the physiologic significance of a coronary obstruction. Because this is a critical issue in cardiac imaging, the reasons why percent diameter stenosis is a poor predictor of the functional significance of a coronary obstruction will be reviewed (Table 2–1).

Hydraulic Principles

As mentioned, many geometric factors and blood flow characteristics determine the hemodynamic effects of a given obstruction, and most of them are ignored if one focuses only on percent diameter narrowing as the sole predictor of the physiologic significance of a coronary obstructive lesion.

Table 2–1. REASONS WHY VISUAL ESTIMATES OF PERCENT DIAMETER NARROWING ARE NO LONGER ACCEPTABLE FOR ESTIMATING THE PHYSIOLOGIC SIGNIFICANCE OF AN OBSTRUCTIVE LESION

Ignore important hydraulic principles
Large intra- and interobserver variability
Ignore the ubiquitous presence of angiographically undetectable diffuse disease
Correlate poorly with direct measurements of flow reserve in individual diseased vessels
Disregard other coexistent factors that may influence coronary reserve in patients with coronary obstructions, such as hypertrophy, microvascular disease, and myocardial infarction, in the perfusion field of the obstructed vessel

Intra- and Interobserver Variability

Numerous studies have now demonstrated that the inter- and intraobserver variability associated with the determination of the percent diameter stenosis by visual interpretation of coronary arteriograms is enormous.[D12, 13, Z1] Although errors are less severe at the ends of the spectrum (normal coronary arteries versus coronary vessels with greater than 90 percent diameter obstruction), the magnitude of the error is very significant, with coronary obstructions in the midrange (20 to 80 percent diameter narrowing).[W12]

Diffuse Coronary Disease

Whenever percent diameter narrowing is used as a predictor of the physiologic significance of an obstructive lesion in the coronary tree, one accepts the notion that the reference segment ("adjacent normal vascular segment") is free of atherosclerotic disease. Both pathologic studies[A2, S18] and in vivo cross-sectional images of coronary vessels obtained with high-frequency echocardiography[M25] have now demonstrated very conclusively that focal disease in the coronary tree is infrequent, and diffuse disease is ubiquitous. Furthermore, the severity of diffuse disease is quite variable and can be angiographically undetectable. The presence of diffuse disease is likely more prevalent in patients with multivessel disease than in patients with single-vessel disease. Thus, in patients with single-vessel disease, the use of quantitative coronary angiography to determine percent area stenosis does provide a reasonable index of the physiologic significance of the obstructive lesion.[W7]

Correlations with Direct Measurements of Flow Reserve

Studies with Doppler systems[W4, 7] and digital angiography[M26] have now made it possible to measure coronary reserve in either individual vessels or the perfusion field of individual coronary vessels in humans. These studies have regularly demonstrated a very poor relationship between percent diameter stenosis and coronary reserve, particularly in patients with multivessel coronary disease. These observations from direct physiologic measurement severely undermine the usefulness of percent diameter narrowing as a precise predictor of the physiologic significance of a coronary obstructive lesion.

Coexisting Factors That Influence Coronary Reserve

In addition to a coronary obstructive lesion, coronary reserve can be impaired because of other coexisting factors that are known to influence coronary vasodilator capacity. These include cardiac hypertrophy secondary to either pressure or volume overload,[B6, D10, M8, 21] microvascular disease,[C14, G10] or infarction of the myocardium served by the diseased vessel. As a consequence of these problems, a relatively minor coronary obstructive lesion in the pressure-hypertrophied ventricle can have profound physiologic effects, and this would be totally overlooked if the physiologic significance of the coronary obstruction were based solely on a visual estimate of percent diameter stenosis.

In the aggregate, an impressive body of evidence has now been presented that provides a convincing argument that percent diameter narrowing determined by visual inspection of the coronary arteriogram is no longer acceptable for estimating the physiologic significance of coronary obstructive lesions. Although investigators studying cardiac imaging procedures and the coronary circulation in general are beginning to accept this dictum, many cardiologists continue to use percent diameter stenosis as the primary means of detecting the physiologic significance of a coronary obstructive lesion. It is hoped that as the availability of more sophisticated methods for determining the physiologic significance of coronary obstructions is improved, all cardiologists will begin to assess the significance of coronary obstructions, utilizing far more sophisticated approaches than visual estimates of percent diameter stenosis.

CORONARY OCCLUSION AND INFARCTION

When a coronary vessel is totally occluded, the perfusion to the involved territory is primarily dependent on the coronary collateral circulation. If the coronary collaterals are well developed, coronary occlusion may not be associated with any decrease in resting perfusion. In contrast, if the collaterals are poorly developed, the perfusion will decrease usually to less than 10 percent of flow.[M24, S13] Furthermore, the subendocardium in the involved zone receives less than half the flow that goes to the subepicardium.[M24]

The border that separates normally perfused and hypoperfused myocardium in the perfusion field of an occluded vessel is extremely narrow and very irregular. In the dog, this "border zone" is well below 0.5 mm in width.[F15, H11, O1] Studies that suggest that this border zone is much wider than 0.5 mm are usually plagued by methodologic artifacts. Although the border zone in dogs is very narrow, it is less certain how wide this zone is in humans.

Perfusion of a zone of recent infarction is typically very low, less than 10 percent of control flow. For reasons that are obscure, perfusion to infarcted myocardium increases over a period of hours quite significantly.[R11]

Imaging studies of perfusion or metabolism frequently demonstrate a relatively broad border zone between areas supplied by the occluded vessel and adjacent normal vessels. Although this may occasionally reflect relatively good collateral perfusion to the border zone, in most instances, this "broad-based border zone" simply implies that the imaging technique has poor spatial resolution. Imaging studies of hearts with an occluded vessel frequently demonstrate wall motion abnormalities that correlate poorly with the size of the perfusion deficit. This is best explained by four factors: (1) poor spatial resolution of the imaging technique; (2) tethering; (3) effects of loading conditions on wall motion of ischemic myocardium; and (4) variable extent of collateral flow.

Infarct/Risk Relationship

Many studies in patients[F16] and animals[K9] have demonstrated a linear relationship between the size of a perfusion field of an occluded vessel and the size of the resulting infarction. Furthermore, the rate at which the infarct progresses across the risk zone from subendocardium to subepicardium is variable. The slope of the infarct/risk relationship and the rate at which the infarct progresses across the risk zone depend on the extent of collateral flow.[L6, M27] Since both parameters are quite different between species, it follows that the infarct/risk relationship is variable from species to species.

Several other factors that influence the infarct/risk relationship deserve emphasis. In many animal species, small-risk zones are not associated with any infarction. This is probably because collateral density is inversely related to risk area size.[G12] Thus, small-risk areas receive sufficient collateral perfusion to maintain viability. Furthermore, large-risk zones are associated with the most adverse complications of infarction, i.e., markedly impaired left ventricular function and death. This has been shown to be true in both animals and humans.

The infarct/risk relationship can be shifted in a favorable direction by reperfusion.[R12] The risk area of individual coronary vessels in both humans[F16] and animals[K9] is quite variable. Although in most patients the size of the perfusion field of the right coronary artery is smaller than the perfusion field of the left anterior descending (LAD) artery, this can be variable. This difference in the perfusion field sizes of the right coronary artery and the LAD explains in part why right coronary artery occlusions have less dire consequences than LAD occlusions in most patients.

EFFECTS OF HYPERTROPHY ON MYOCARDIAL PERFUSION

Many investigations in animals and humans have shown that most types of cardiac hypertrophy are associated with decrements in coronary flow reserve[B6, D10, M8, 21] (Fig. 2–9). Furthermore, pressure-induced left ventricular hypertrophy limits autoregulation in the subendocardium of the left ventricle.[H4] Because cardiac hypertrophy is common, the effects of hypertrophy on perfusion have important implications for many imaging procedures. Most important, with our present relatively insensitive techniques, it is almost impossible to assess the physiologic significance of coronary obstructions in hypertrophied ventricles, because both hypertrophy and coronary obstruction can severely impair coronary reserve and, thereby, engender myocardial ischemia. Hence, interpretation of the results of imaging tests designed to assess perfusion metabolism or wall motion in hypertrophied ventricles with superimposed coronary obstructive disease must be very guarded.

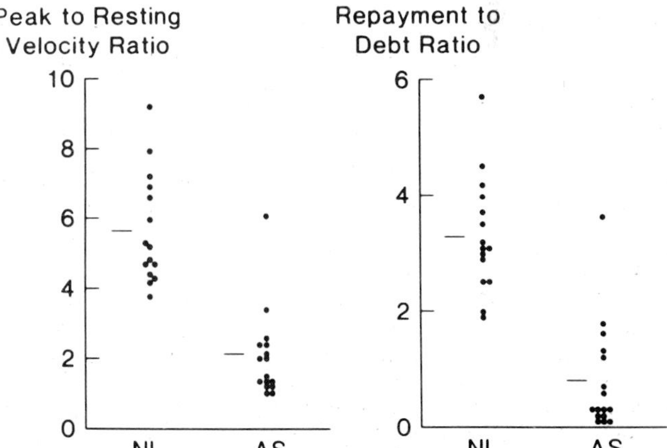

Figure 2–9. Characteristics of coronary reactive hyperemia in the left anterior descending coronary artery of patients with aortic stenosis (AS) and controls (NL). All studies were obtained at the time of open heart surgery prior to cardiopulmonary bypass. The left ventricles in the normal group were not enlarged and were functionally normal; the left ventricles in patients with aortic stenosis were markedly hypertrophied. All coronary arteries were angiographically normal. Following release of a 20-second occlusion of the left anterior descending coronary artery, the peak to resting velocity ratios and the repayment/debt ratios were markedly decreased in patients with aortic stenosis. (Based on data originally presented by Marcus, M. L., Thurman, J. C., Tranquili, W. J., et al.: Regional myocardial blood flow and coronary vascular reserve in unanesthetized young calves with severe concentric right ventricular hypertrophy. Circ. Res. 48:785, 1981. Used with permission from the editor.)

EFFECTS OF CORONARY VASODILATION ON CORONARY VASCULAR VOLUME

The left ventricular myocardium is an extremely vascular organ. Capillary density is about 2000 to 3000 capillaries per square mm. Several studies suggest that the total volume of all vessels in the left ventricular myocardium is equivalent to 10 to 13 percent of total left ventricular mass.

In the past several years, it has been demonstrated that the vascular volume of the left ventricle is not fixed but can increase quite significantly during various conditions independent of flow. This is particularly apparent during hypoxia.[D14] This property of the volume of the vasculature to change has important implications for perfusion imaging techniques that employ intravascular indicators. Such techniques include digital subtraction angiography, contrast echocardiography, and ultrafast computed tomography. When these techniques are utilized, failure to quantitatively assess changes in vascular volume that may concomitantly occur with changes in flow may lead to errors in estimates of myocardial perfusion rates.

CONCLUSION

Understanding basic mechanisms that regulate various aspects of myocardial perfusion is critical to the interpretation of all cardiac imaging procedures and particularly to cardiac imaging procedures directed toward estimating myocardial perfusion. Those interested in developing expertise in cardiac imaging will be well advised to master these basic concepts prior to examining the detailed aspects of a particular cardiac imaging modality.

References

A

1. Archie, J.P., and Kirklin, J.W.: Effect of hypothermic perfusion on myocardial oxygen consumption and coronary resistance. Surg. Forum 24:186, 1973.
2. Arnett, E.N., Isner, J.M., Redwood, D.R., et al.: Coronary artery narrowing in coronary heart disease: Comparison of cineangiographic and necropsy findings. Ann. Intern. Med. 91:350, 1979.

B

1. Berne, R.M., DeGeest, H., and Levy, M.N.: Influence of the cardiac nerves on coronary resistance. Am. J. Physiol. 208:763, 1965.
2. Berne, R.M.: Effect of epinephrine and norepinephrine on coronary circulation. Circ. Res. 6:644, 1958.
3. Berne, R.M., and Rubio, R.: Coronary circulation. In Berne, R.M. (ed.): Handbook of Physiology. Vol. 1, Sect. 2, The Cardiovascular System. Bethesda, Md., American Physiological Society, 1979, p. 873.
4. Berne, R.M.: The role of adenosine in the regulation of coronary blood flow. Circ. Res. 47:807, 1980.
5. Braunwald, E.: Control of myocardial oxygen consumption: Physiologic and clinical considerations. Am. J. Cardiol. 27:416, 1971.
6. Bache, R.J., Vrobel, T.R., Arentzen, C.E., and Ring, W.S.: Effect of maximal coronary vasodilation on transmural myocardial perfusion during tachycardia in dogs with left ventricular hypertrophy. Circ. Res. 49:742, 1981.
7. Boatwright, R.B., Downey, H.F., Bashour, F.A., and Crystal, G.J.: Transmural variation in autoregulation of coronary blood flow in hyperperfused canine myocardium. Circ. Res. 47:599, 1980.
8. Blesa, M.I., and Ross, G.: Cholinergic mechanisms on the heart and coronary circulation. Br. J. Pharm. 38:93, 1970.
9. Britton, S., and DiSalvo, J.: Effects of angiotensin I and angiotensin II on hindlimb and coronary vascular resistance. Am. J. Physiol. 225:1226, 1973.
10. Brooks, H.L., Stein, P.D., Matson, J.L., and Hyland, J.W.: Dopamine-induced alterations in coronary hemodynamics in dogs. Circ. Res. 24:699, 1969.
11. Bayless, W.M.: On the local reaction of the arterial wall to changes of internal pressure. J. Physiol. (Lond.) 28:220, 1902.
12. Brazier, J., Cooper, N., and Buckberg, G.D.: The adequacy of subendocardial oxygen delivery: The interaction of determinants of flow, arterial oxygen content and myocardial oxygen need. Circulation 49:968, 1974.
13. Barnard, R.J., Duncan, H.W., Levesay, J.J., and Buckberg, G.D.: Coronary vasodilator reserve and flow distribution during near-maximal exercise in dogs. J. Appl. Physiol. Resp. Environ. Exer. Physiol. 43:988, 1977.
14. Bache, R.J., Cobb, F.R., and Greenfield, J.C., Jr.: Effect of increased myocardial oxygen consumption on coronary reactive hyperemia in the awake dog. Circ. Res. 33:588, 1973.
15. Bache, R.J., and Dymek, D.J.: Effect of diltiazem on myocardial blood flow. Circulation 65:I–19, 1982.
16. Bache, R.J., and Lambert, P.R.: Transmural myocardial blood flow during coronary reactive hyperemia in the dog. Circulation 55/56(Suppl. 3):III-37, 1977.
17. Badeer, H.S.: Influence of cooling the heart on reactive hyperemia of the coronary bed in the heart-lung preparation. Circ. Res. 16:19, 1965.
18. Buckberg, G.D., Brazier, J.R., Nelson, R.H., et al.: Studies on the effects of hypothermia on regional myocardial blood flow and metabolism during cardiopulmonary bypass. I. The adequately perfused beating, fibrillating, and arrested heart. J. Thorac. Cardiovasc. Surg. 73:87, 1977.
19. Brown, B.G., Josephson, M.A., Petersen, R.B., et al.: Intravenous dipyridamole combined with isometric handgrip for near maximal acute increase in coronary flow in patients with coronary artery disease. Am. J. Cardiol. 48:1077, 1981.
20. Bache, R.J., and Schwartz, J.S.: Myocardial blood flow during exercise after gradual coronary occlusion in the dog. Am. J. Physiol. 245(Heart Circ. Physiol. 14):H131, 1983.

C

1. Chilian, W.M., Boatwright, R.B., Shoji, T., and Griggs, D.M.: Evidence against significant resting sympathetic coronary vasoconstrictor tone in the conscious dog. Circ. Res. 49:866, 1981.
2. Cross, C.E., Rieben, P.A., and Salisbury, P.F.: Coronary driving pressure and vasomotor tonus as determinants of coronary blood flow. Circ. Res. 9:589, 1961.
3. Carrier, G.O., and White, R.E.: Enhancement of alpha-1 and alpha-2 adrenergic agonist-induced vasoconstriction by removal of endothelium in rat aorta. J. Pharmacol. Exp. Ther. 232(3):682, 1985.
4. Case, R.B., Greenberg, H., and Moskowitz, R.: Alterations in coronary sinus pO_2 and O_2 saturation resulting from pCO_2 changes. Cardiovasc. Res. 9:167, 1975.
5. Case, R.B., Felix, A., Wachter, M., et al.: Relative effect of CO_2 on canine coronary vascular resistance. Circ. Res. 42:410, 1978.
6. Case, R.B., and Greenberg, H.: The response of canine coronary vascular resistance to local alterations in coronary arterial PCO_2. Circ. Res. 39:558, 1976.
7. Canty, J.M., Jr.: Coronary pressure-function and steady-state pressure-flow relations during autoregulation in the unanesthetized dog. Circ. Res. 63:821, 1988.
8. Chilian, W.M., Layne, S.M., Eastham, C.L., and Marcus, M.L.: Heterogeneous microvascular coronary α-adrenergic vasoconstriction. Circ. Res. 64:376, 1989.
9. Cohen, M.V., and Kirk, E.S.: Differential response of large and small coronary arteries to nitroglycerin and angiotensin. Circ. Res. 33:445, 1973.
10. Cobb, F.R., McHale, P.A., Bache, R.J., and Greenfield, J.C., Jr.: Coronary and systemic hemodynamic effects of dopamine in the awake dog. Am. J. Physiol. 222:1355, 1972.
11. Cobb, F.R., Bache, R.J., and Greenfield, J.C., Jr.: Regional myocardial blood flow in awake dogs. J. Clin. Invest. 53:H1618, 1974.
12. Coffman, J.D., and Gregg, D.E.: Reactive hyperemia characteristics of the myocardium. Am. J. Physiol. 199:1143, 1960.
13. Chitwood, W.R., Sink, J.D., Hill, R.C., et al.: The effects of hypothermia on myocardial oxygen consumption and transmural coronary blood flow in the potassium-arrested heart. Ann. Surg. 190:106, 1979.
14. Cannon, R.O. III, Watson, R.M., Rosing, D.R., and Epstein, S.E.: Angina caused by reduced vasodilator reserve of the small coronary arteries. J. Am. Coll. Cardiol. 1:1359, 1983.
15. Clemo, H.F., and Belardinelli, L.: Effect of adenosine on atrioventricular conduction. I. Site and characterization of adenosine action in the guinea pig atrioventricular node. Circ. Res. 59:427, 1986.
16. Cohen, M., Sherman, W., Rentrop, K.P., and Gorlin, R.: Determinants of collateral filling observed during sudden controlled coronary artery occlusion in human subjects. J. Am. Coll. Cardiol. 13(2):297, 1989.

D

1. Domenech, R.J., and Ayuy, A.H.: Total and regional coronary blood flow during acute right ventricular pressure overload. Cardiovasc. Res. 8:611, 1974.
2. Dusting, G.J., Moncada, S., and Vane, J.R.: Prostaglandins, their intermediates and precursors: Cardiovascular actions and regulatory roles in normal and abnormal circulatory systems. Prog. Cardiovasc. Dis. 21:405, 1979.
3. Downey, J.M., Downey, H.F., and Kirk, E.S.: Effects of myocardial strains on coronary blood flow. Circ. Res. 34:286, 1974.
4. Douglas, C.R., Ponce/Zumino, A., Ruiz-Petrich, E., et al.: Effect of angiotensin upon coronary flow and oxygen consumption of the isolated heart of the cat. Acta Physiol. Lat. Am. 14:161, 1967.
5. Drimal, J., Pavek, K., and Selecky, F.V.: Primary and secondary effects of angiotensin on the coronary circulation. Cardiologia 54:1, 1969.
6. Domenech, R.J., Hoffman, J.I.E., Noble, M.I.M., et al.: Total and regional coronary blood flow measured by radioactive microspheres in conscious and anesthetized dogs. Circ. Res. 25:581, 1969.
7. DeMay, J.G., Claeys, M., and Vanhoutte, P.M.: Endothelium dependent inhibitory effects of acetylcholine, adenosine triphosphate, thrombin, and arachidonic acid in the canine femoral artery. J. Pharmacol. Exp. Ther. 222:166, 1982.
8. Downey, H.F., Crystal, G.J., and Bashour, F.A.: Transmural variations in myocardial blood flow during reactive hyperemia. Physiologist 24:26, 1981.
9. Dole, W.P., Montville, W.J., and Bishop, V.S.: Dependence of myocardial reactive hyperemia on coronary artery pressure in the dog. Am. J. Physiol. 240:H709, 1981.

10. Doty, D.B., Wright, C.B., Hiratzka, L.F., et al.: Coronary reserve in volume-induced right ventricular hypertrophy from atrial septal defect. Am. J. Cardiol. 54:1059, 1984.
11. de Bruyne, B., Meier, B., Finci, L., et al.: Potential protective effect of high coronary wedge pressure on left ventricular function after coronary occlusion. Circulation 78:455, 1988.
12. Detre, K.M., Wright, E., Murphy, M.L., and Takaro, T.: Observer agreement in evaluating coronary angiograms. Circulation 52:979, 1975.
13. DeRouen, T.A., Murray, J.A., and Owen, W.: Variability in the analysis of coronary arteriograms. Circulation 55:2, 1977.
14. Downey, H.F., Crystal, G.J., Bockman, E.L., and Bashour, F.A.: Nonischemic myocardial hypoxia: Coronary dilation without increased tissue adenosine. Am. J. Physiol. 12(6):H512, 1982.

E

1. Eikens, E., and Wilcken, D.E.L.: Myocardial reactive hyperaemia in conscious dogs: Effect of dipyridamole and aminophylline on responses to four- and eight-second coronary artery occlusions. Aust. J. Exp. Biol. Med. Sci. 51:617, 1973.
2. Eastham, C., Doty, D., Wright, C., and Marcus, M.: Effects of age on coronary reserve in man. Circulation 62(Suppl. 3):III-64, 1980.
3. Ehrich, W.E., Bellet, S., and Lewey, F.H.: Cardiac changes from CO poisoning. Am. J. Med. 208:511, 1944.
4. Engel, H.J., Torres, C., and Page, H.L.: Major variations in anatomical origin of the coronary arteries: Angiographic observations in 4250 patients without associated congenital heart disease. Cath. Cardiovasc. Diagn. 1:157, 1975.
5. Eng, C., Patterson, R.E., Horowitz, S.F., et al.: Coronary collateral function during exercise. Circulation 66(2):309, 1982.

F

1. Fixler, D.E., Archie, J.P., Ullyot, D.J., et al.: Effect of acute right ventricular systolic hypertension on regional myocardial blood flow in anesthetized dogs. Am. Heart J. 85:491, 1973.
2. Farhi, E.R., Canty, J.M., Jr., and Klocke, F.J.: Effects of graded reductions in coronary perfusion pressure on the diastolic pressure-segment length relation and the rate of isovolumic relaxation in the resting conscious dog. Circulation 80:1458, 1989.
3. Feigl, E.O.: Parasympathetic control of coronary blood flow in dogs. Circ. Res. 25:509, 1969.
4. Feigl, E.O.: Reflex parasympathetic coronary vasodilation elicited from cardiac receptors in the dog. Circ. Res. 37:175, 1975.
5. Fowler, N.O., and Holmes, J.C.: Coronary and myocardial actions of angiotensin. Circ. Res. 14:191, 1964.
6. Fedor, M., McIntosh, D.M., Rembert, J.C., and Greenfield, J.C., Jr.: Coronary and transmural myocardial blood flow responses in awake domestic pigs. Am. J. Physiol. 235:H435, 1978.
7. Flameng, W., Wusten, B., Winkler, B., et al.: Influence of perfusion pressure and heart rate on local myocardial flow in the collateralized heart with chronic coronary occlusion. Am. Heart J. 89:51, 1975.
8. Falsetti, H.L., Carroll, R.J., and Marcus, M.L.: Temporal heterogeneity of myocardial blood flow in anesthetized dogs. Circulation 52:848, 1975.
9. Furchgott, R.F., and Zawadski, J.V.: The obligatory role of endothelial cells in the relaxation of arterial smooth muscle by acetylcholine. Nature 288:373, 1980.
10. Forstermann, U., Trogisch, G., and Busse, R.: Species-dependent differences in the nature of endothelium-derived vascular relaxing factor. Eur. J. Pharm. 106:639, 1984.
11. Freiman, P.C., Mitchell, G.G., Heistad, D.D., et al.: Atherosclerosis impairs endothelium-dependent vascular relaxation to acetylcholine and thrombin in primates. Circ. Res. 58:783, 1986.
12. Fulton, W.F.M.: The Coronary Arteries. Charles C Thomas, Springfield, Ill., 1965.
13. Feldman, R.D., Christy, J.P., Paul, S.T., and Harrison, D.G.: β-Adrenergic receptors on canine coronary collateral vessels: Characterization and function. Am. J. Physiol. 257(Heart Circ. Physiol. 26):H1634, 1989.
14. Feldman, R.L., Nichols, W.W., Pepine, C.J., and Conti, C.R.: Hemodynamic effects of long and multiple coronary arterial narrowings. Chest 74:280, 1978.
15. Factor, S.M., Okun, E.M., and Kirk, E.S.: The histological lateral border of acute canine myocardial infarction. Circ. Res. 48:640, 1981.
16. Feiring, A.J., Johnson, M.R., Kioschos, J.M., et al.: The importance of determining the myocardial area at risk when evaluating the outcome of acute myocardial infarction in patients. Circulation 75(5):980, 1987.

G

1. Ganz, W., Yoshida, S., and Swan, H.J.C.: Coronary hemodynamics during progressive elevation of heart rate by pacing in subjects with normal coronary arteries and coronary artery disease. *In* Maseri, A. (ed.): Myocardial Blood Flow in Man. Turin, Minerva Medica, 1972, p. 509.
2. Guyton, R.A., McClenathan, J.H., Newman, G.E., and Michaelis, L.L.: Significance of subendocardial S-T segment elevation caused by coronary stenosis in the dog. Am. J. Cardiol. 40:373, 1977.
3. Gross, G.J., Buck, J.D., and Warltier, D.C.: Transmural distribution of blood flow during activation of coronary muscarinic receptors. Am. J. Physiol. 240:H941, 1981.
4. Griffith, T.M., Edwards, D.H., Lewis, M.J., et al.: The nature of endothelium-derived relaxant factor. Nature 308:645, 1984.
5. Gould, K.L., Lipscomb, K., and Hamilton, G.W.: Physiologic basis for assessing critical coronary stenosis. Am. J. Cardiol. 33:87, 1974.
6. Gould, K.L., and Lipscomb, K.: Effects of coronary stenoses on coronary flow reserve and resistance. Am. J. Cardiol. 34:48, 1974.
7. Gould, K.L.: Pressure-flow characteristics of coronary stenoses in unsedated dogs at rest and during coronary vasodilation. Circ. Res. 43:245, 1978.
8. Gewirtz, H., Williams, D.O., Ohley, W.H., and Most, A.S.: Influence of coronary vasodilatation on the transmural distribution of myocardial blood flow distal to a severe fixed coronary artery stenosis. Am. Heart J. 106:674, 1983.
9. Greenberg, J.J., Edmunds, H., Jr., and Brown, R.B.: Myocardial metabolism and postarrest function in the cold and chemically arrested heart. Surgery 48:31, 1960.
10. Greenberg, M.A., Neuburger, N., Grose, R., et al.: Decreased coronary reserve in syndrome X. Circulation 64(Suppl. IV):305, 1981.
11. Grayson, J., Irvine, M., and Parratt, R.: Effects of carbocromen and dipyridamole on blood flow and heat production in the normal and ischemic canine myocardium. Cardiovasc. Res. 5:41, 1971.
12. Gumm, D.C., Thompson, S.B., Marcus, M.L., and Harrison, D.G.: The influence of risk area on native collateral resistance and ischemic zone perfusion. Am. J. Physiol. 254:H473, 1988.
13. Goldstein, R.E., Michaelis, L.L., Morrow, A.G., and Epstein, S.E.: Coronary collateral function in patients without occlusive coronary artery disease. Circulation 51:118, 1975.

H

1. Heusch, G., and Deussen, A.: The effects of cardiac sympathetic nerve stimulation on perfusion of stenotic coronary arteries in the dog. Circ. Res. 53:8, 1983.
2. Hautamaa, P.V., Dai, X.Z., Homans, D.C., and Bache, R.J.: Vasomotor activity of moderately well-developed canine coronary collateral circulation. Am. J. Physiol. (Heart Circ. Physiol.) 25(3):H890, 1989.
3. Hoffman, J.I.E.: Determinants and prediction of transmural myocardial perfusion. Circulation 58:381, 1978.
4. Harrison, D.G., Florentine, M.S., Brooks, L.A., et al.: The effect of hypertension and left ventricular hypertrophy on the lower range of coronary autoregulation. Circulation 77(5):1108, 1988.
5. Hintze, T.H., and Kaley, G.: Prostaglandins in the control of blood flow in the canine myocardium. Circ. Res. 40:313, 1977.
6. Harder, D.R.: Pressure-induced myogenic activation of cat cerebral arteries is dependent on intact endothelium. Circ. Res. 60:102, 1987.
7. Habib, J.B., Bossaler, C., Wells, S., et al.: Preservation of endothelium-dependent vascular relaxation in cholesterol-fed rabbit by treatment with the calcium blocker PN 200110. Circ. Res. 58:305, 1986.
8. Harrison, D.G., Minor, R.L., Guerra, R., et al.: Endothelial dysfunction in atherosclerosis. *In* Rubanyi, G. (ed.): Cardiovascular Significance of Endothelium-Derived Vasoactive Factors. Futura Publishing, New York, 1990.
9. Harrison, D.G., Barnes, D.H., Hiratzka, L.F., et al.: The effect of cardiac hypertrophy on the coronary collateral circulation. Circulation 71:1135, 1985.
10. Harrison, D.G., Chilian, W.M., and Marcus, M.L.: Absence of functioning α-adrenergic receptors in mature canine coronary collaterals. Circ. Res. 59:133, 1986.
11. Hirzel, H.O., Sonnenblock, E.H., and Kirk, E.S.: Absence of a lateral border zone of intermediate creatine phosphokinase depletion surrounding a central infarct 24 hours after acute coronary occlusion in the dog. Circ. Res. 41(5):673, 1977.

J

1. Johnson, P.C.: The myogenic response. *In* Bohr, D.F., Somlyo, A.P., and Sparks, H.V., Jr. (eds.): Handbook of Physiology. Vol. II, Sec. 2, The Cardiovascular System. American Physiological Society, Bethesda, Md., 1980, p. 409.

K

1. Khouri, E.M., Gregg, D.E., and Rayford, C.R.: Effect of exercise on cardiac output, left coronary flow and myocardial metabolism in the anesthetized dog. Circ. Res. 17:427, 1965.
2. Kjekshus, J.K.: Mechanism for flow distribution in normal and ischemic myocardium during increased ventricular preload in the dog. Circ. Res. 23:489, 1973.
3. Kuzuya, T., Tada, M., Inoue, M., et al.: Increased levels of thromboxane A_2 in peripheral and coronary circulation in patients with angina pectoris. Am. J. Cardiol. 45:454, 1980.
4. Kawachi, Y., Tomoike, H., Maruoka, Y., et al.: Selective hypercontraction caused by ergonovine in the canine coronary artery under conditions of induced atherosclerosis. Circulation 69:441, 1984.
5. Katusic, Z.S., Shepherd, J.T., and Vanhoutte, P.M.: Endothelium-dependent contraction to stretch in canine basilar arteries. Am. J. Physiol. (Heart Circ. Physiol.) 21:H671, 1987.
6. Ku, D.: Coronary vascular reactivity after acute myocardial ischemia. Science 218:576, 1982.
7. Katz, L.N., and Linder, E.: Quantitative relation between reactive hyperemia and the myocardial ischemia which it follows. Am. J. Physiol. 126:283, 1939.
8. Kinsella, D., Troup, W., and McGregor, M.: Studies with a new coronary vasodilator drug: Persantin. Am. Heart J. 63:146, 1963.
9. Koyanagi, S., Eastham, C.L., Harrison, D.G., and Marcus, M.L.: Transmural variation in the relationship between myocardial infarct size and risk area. Am. J. Physiol. 242:H867, 1982.

L

1. Levy, M.N., and Zieske, H.: Comparison of the cardiac effects of vagus nerve stimulation and of acetylcholine infusions. Am. J. Physiol. 216:890, 1969.
2. Losay, J., Mroz, E.A., Treagear, G.W., et al.: Action of substance P on the coronary blood flow in the isolated dog heart. *In* von Euler, U.S., Pernow, B. (eds.): Substance P. Raven Press, New York, 1976.
3. Ludmer, P.L., Selwyn, A.P., Shook, T.L., et al.: Paradoxical vasoconstriction induced by acetylcholine in atherosclerotic coronary arteries. N. Engl. J. Med. 315:1046, 1986.
4. Levin, D.C.: Pathways and functional significance of the coronary collateral circulation. Circulation 50:831, 1974.
5. Leppo, J.A.: Dipyridamole-thallium imaging: The lazy man's stress test. J. Nucl. Med. 30:281, 1989.
6. Lubbe, W.F., Perach, M., Pretorius, R., et al.: Distribution of myocardial blood flow before and after coronary artery ligation in the baboon: Relation to early ventricular fibrillation. Cardiovasc. Res. 8:478, 1974.

M

1. Mohrman, D.E., and Feigl, E.O.: Competition between sympathetic vasoconstriction and metabolic vasodilation in the canine coronary circulation. Circ. Res. 42:79, 1978.
2. Mudge, G.H., Jr., Goldberg, S., Gunther, S., et al.: Comparison of metabolic and vasoconstrictor stimuli on coronary vascular resistance in man. Circulation 59:544, 1979.
3. Mosher, P., Ross, J., Jr., McFate, P.A., and Shaw, R.F.: Control of coronary blood flow by an autoregulatory mechanism. Circ. Res. 14:250, 1964.
4. Markwalder, J., and Starling, E.H.: Note on some factors which determine blood flow through coronary circulation. J. Physiol. 47:275, 1914.
5. McRaven, D.R., Mark, A.L., Abboud, F.M., and Mayer, H.E.: Responses of coronary vessels to adrenergic stimuli. J. Clin. Invest. 50:773, 1971.
6. Mark, A.L., Abboud, R.M., Schmid, P.G., et al.: Differences in direct effects of adrenergic stimuli on coronary, cutaneous, and muscular vessels. J. Clin. Invest. 51:279, 1972.
7. Merrill, G.J., Haddy, F.J., and Dabney, J.M.: Adenosine, theophylline and perfusate pH in the isolated, perfused guinea pig heart. Circ. Res. 42:225, 1978.
8. Mueller, T.M., Marcus, M.L., Kerber, R.E., et al.: Effect of renal hypertension and left ventricular hypertrophy on the coronary circulation in dogs. Circ. Res. 42:543, 1978.
9. Murray, P.A., and Vatner, S.F.: Carotid sinus baroreceptor control of right coronary circulation in normal, hypertrophied, and failing right ventricles of conscious dogs. Circ. Res. 49:1339, 1981.
10. Mudge, G.H., Jr., Grossman, W., Mills, R.M., Jr., et al.: Reflex increase in coronary vascular resistance in patients with ischemic heart disease. N. Engl. J. Med. 295:1333, 1976.
11. Meier, M., Wirz, E., Brunner, H., and Stamm, W.: Effects of norepinephrine and angiotensin II-amide on coronary flow and myocardial oxygen consumption in the cat. Cardiologia 47:127, 1965.
12. Moir, T.W., and Nayler, W.G.: Coronary vascular effects of glucagon in the isolated dog heart. Circ. Res. 26:29, 1970.
13. Murdock, R.H., Jr., and Cobb, F.R.: Effects of infarcted myocardium on regional blood flow measurements to ischemic regions in canine heart. Circ. Res. 47(5):701, 1980.
14. Manohar, M., Bisgard, G.E., Bullard, V., et al.: Myocardial perfusion and function during acute right ventricular systolic hypertension. Am. J. Physiol. 235:H628, 1978.
15. Monroe, R.G., Gamble, W.G., LaFarge, C.G., et al.: The Anrep effect reconsidered. J. Clin. Invest. 51:2573, 1972.
16. Marcus, M.L., Kerber, R.E., Erhardt, J.C., et al.: Spatial and temporal heterogeneity of left ventricular perfusion in awake dogs. Am. Heart J. 94(6):748, 1977.
17. Myers, P.R., Banitt, P.F., Guerra, R., Jr., and Harrison, D.G.: Characteristics of canine coronary resistance arteries: Importance of endothelium. Am. J. Physiol. 256H603–H610, 1989.
18. Mayhan, W.G.: Impairment of endothelium-dependent dilatation of cerebral arterioles during diabetes mellitus. Am. J. Physiol. 256:H621, 1989.
19. Marcus, M., Wright, C., Doty, D., et al.: Measurements of coronary velocity and reactive hyperemia in the coronary circulation of humans. Circ. Res. 49:877, 1981.
20. Manohar, M., Thurmon, J.C., Tranquili, W.J., et al.: Regional myocardial blood flow and coronary vascular reserve in unanesthetized young calves with severe concentric right ventricular hypertrophy. Circ. Res. 48:785, 1981.
21. Marcus, M.L., Doty, D.B., Hiratzka, L.F., et al.: Decreased coronary reserve—a mechanism for angina pectoris in patients with aortic stenosis and normal coronary arteries. N. Engl. J. Med. 307:1362, 1982.
22. Marcus, M.L.: The Coronary Circulation in Health and Disease. McGraw-Hill Book Company, New York, 1983, p. 108.
23. Murray, P.A., and Vatner, S.F.: Alpha-adrenoceptor attenuation of the coronary vascular response to severe exercise in the conscious dog. Circ. Res. 45:654, 1979.
24. Marcus, M.L., Kerber, R.E., Ehrhardt, J., and Abboud, F.M.: Effects of time on volume and distribution of coronary collateral flow. Am. J. Physiol. 230:279, 1976.
25. McPherson, D.D., Hiratzka, L.F., Lamberth, W.C., et al.: Delineation of the extent of coronary atherosclerosis by high frequency epicardial echocardiography. N. Engl. J. Med. 316:304, 1987.
26. Mancini, G.B.J., Simon, S.B., McGillem, M.J., et al.: Automated quantitative coronary arteriography: Morphologic and physiologic validation in vivo of a rapid digital angiographic method. Circulation 75:452, 1987.
27. Most, A.S., Williams, D.O., and Millard, R.W.: Acute coronary occlusion in the pig: Effect of nitroglycerin on regional myocardial blood flow. Am. J. Cardiol. 42:947, 1978.

N

1. Nakano, J.: Cardiovascular actions of vasopressin. Jap. Circ. J., 37:363, 1973.
2. Nakano, J.: Cardiovascular responses to neurohypophysial hormones. *In* Greep, R.O., and Astwood, E.B. (eds.): Handbook of Physiology. Vol. 4, Sec. 7, Endocrinology. American Physiological Society, Washington, D.C., 1974, p. 395.
3. Needleman, P., and Kaley, G.: Cardiac and coronary prostaglandin synthesis and function. N. Engl. J. Med. 298:1122, 1978.
4. Nayler, W.G., McInnes, J.S., Carson, V., and Lowe, T.E.: Effect of dopamine on coronary vascular resistance and myocardial function. Cardiovasc. Res. 5:161, 1971.
5. Nitz, R.E., and Poetzch, E.: 3(β-diethylaminoethyl)4-methyl-7-carbethoxymethoxy-2-oxo-(1,2-chromen)—a specific, long acting coronary dilator. Arzneim Forsch 13:243, 1963.

O

1. Okun, E.M., Factor, S.M., and Kirk, E.S.: End-capillary loops in the heart: An explanation for discrete myocardial infarctions without border zones. Science 206(2):565, 1979.

P

1. Peters, K.G., Marcus, M.L., and Harrison, D.G.: Vasopressin and the mature coronary collateral circulation. Circulation 79(6):1324, 1989.
2. Palmer, R.M.J., Rerrige, A.G., and Moncada, S.: Nitric oxide release accounts for the biological activity of the endothelium-derived relaxing factor. Nature 327:524, 1987.
3. Pohl, U., Holtz, J., Busse, R., and Bassenge, E.: Crucial role of the endothelium in the vasodilator response to increased flow in vivo. Hypertension 8:37, 1986.
4. Picano, E., Simonetti, I., Masini, M., et al.: Transient myocardial dysfunction during pharmacologic vasodilation as an index of reduced coronary reserve: A coronary hemodynamic and echocardiographic study. J. Am. Coll. Cardiol. 8:84, 1986.

R

1. Rouleau, J., Boerboom, L.E., Surjadhana, A., and Hoffman, J.I.E.: The role of autoregulation and tissue diastolic pressures in the transmural distribution of left ventricular blood flow in anesthetized dogs. Circ. Res. 45:804, 1979.
2. Rubio, R., and Berne, R.M.: Regulation of coronary blood flow. Prog. Cardiovasc. Dis. 18:105, 1975.
3. Robertson, R.M., Robertson, D., Roberts, L.J., et al.: Thromboxane A_2 in vasotonic angina pectoris. N. Engl. J. Med. 304:998, 1981.
4. Rembert, J.C., Boyd, L.M., Watkinson, W.P., and Greenfield, J.C., Jr.: Effect of adenosine on transmural myocardial blood flow distribution in the awake dog. Am. J. Physiol. 239:H7, 1980.
5. Rubanyi, G.M., and Vanhoutte, P.M.: Nature of endothelium-derived relaxing factor: Are there two relaxing mediators? Circ. Res. 61(Suppl. II):II61, 1987.
6. Rubanyi, G.M., Romero, J.C., and Vanhoutte, P.F.: Flow-induced release of endothelium-derived relaxing factor. Am. J. Physiol. 250:H145, 1986.
7. Rosenthall, D.S., and Braunwald, E.: Hematologic-oncologic disorders and heart disease. *In* Braunwald, E. (ed.): Heart Disease: A Textbook of Cardiovascular Medicine. Vol. 2. W.B. Saunders, Philadelphia, 1980, p. 1771.
8. Rossen, J.D., Simonetti, I., Marcus, M.L., et al.: The effect of diltiazem on coronary flow reserve in humans. Circulation 80:1240, 1989.
9. Rowe, G.G., Terry, W., Stenlund, R.R., et al.: Systemic and coronary hemodynamic effects of 3-(β-diethylaminoethyl)4-methyl-7-carbethyoxymethoxy-2-oxo-(1,2-chromen) hydrochloride (Intensain, A-27053). Arch. Int. Pharmacodyn. Ther. 178:99, 1969.
10. Rossen, J.D., Simonetti, I., Marcus, M.L., and Winniford, M.D.: Coronary dilation with standard dose dipyridamole and dipyridamole combined with handgrip. Circulation 79:566, 1989.
11. Rivas, F., Cobb, F.R., Bache, R.J., and Greenfield, J.C., Jr.: Relationship between blood flow to ischemic regions and extent of myocardial infarction. Circ. Res. 38(5):439, 1976.
12. Reimer, K.A., and Jennings, R.B.: The "wave front phenomenon" of myocardial ischemic cell death. II. Transmural progression of necrosis within the framework of ischemic bed size (myocardium at risk) and collateral flow. Lab. Invest. 40:633, 1979.
13. Rudolph, A.M., and Heymann, M.A.: The circulation of the fetus in utero: Methods for studying distribution of blood flow, cardiac output, and organ blood flow. Circ. Res. 21:163, 1967.

S

1. Schwartz, P.J., and Stone, H.L.: Tonic influence on the sympathetic nervous system on myocardial reactive hyperemia and on coronary blood flow distribution in dogs. Circ. Res. 41:51, 1977.
2. Sellke, F.W., Quillen, J.E., Brooks, L.A., and Harrison, D.G.: Endothelial modulation of the coronary vasculature in vessels perfused via mature collaterals. Circulation (in press).
3. Schwartz, G.C., McHale, P.A., and Greenfield, J.C., Jr.: Coronary vasodilation

after a single ventricular extra-activation in the conscious dog. Circ. Res. 50:28, 1982.

4. Strandgaard, S., Jones, J.V., MacKenzie, E.T., and Harper, A.M.: Upper limit of cerebral blood flow autoregulation in experimental renovascular hypertension in the baboon. Circ. Res. 37:164, 1975.
5. Said, S.I.: Vasoactive intestinal polypeptide (VIP) as a neural peptide. *In* Miyoshi, A. (ed.): Gut Peptides: Secretion, Function and Clinical Aspects. Kodansha Ltd., Tokyo, 1979.
6. Shimokawa, H., Tomoike, H., Nabeyama, S., et al.: Coronary artery spasm induced in miniature swine: Angiographic evidence and relation to coronary atherosclerosis. Am. Heart J. 110:300, 1985.
7. Shimokawa, H., Tomoike, H., Nabeyama, S., et al.: Coronary artery spasm induced in atherosclerotic miniature swine. Science 221:560, 1983.
8. Shimokawa, H., and Vanhoutte, P.M.: Impaired endothelium-dependent relaxation to aggregating platelets and related vasoactive substances in porcine coronary arteries in hypercholesterolemia and atherosclerosis. Circ. Res. 64:900, 1989.
9. Simonetti, I., Rossen, J.D., Winniford, M.D., and Marcus, M.L.: Biphasic effect of nitroglycerin on coronary hemodynamics in normal subjects. Cardiology 78(Suppl. II):52, 1989.
10. Strauer, B.E.: Personal communication. Department of Medicine, University of Munich, July 1981.
11. Schaper, W.: The Collateral Circulation of the Heart. North-Holland Publishing Company (American Elsevier), New York, 1971.
12. Scheel, K.W., Banet, M., Ott, C., and Lehan, P.H.: A quantitative approach to collateral and antegrade flows after coronary occlusion. Am. J. Physiol. 222:687, 1972.
13. Schaper, W., Flameng, W., Winkler, B., et al.: Quantification of collateral resistance in acute and chronic experimental coronary occlusion in the dog. Circ. Res. 39:371, 1976.
14. Salmon, D., Holida, M., Dole, W., et al.: Reduced incidence of infarction in the right heart may be explained by a low native collateral resistance. (Abstract.) Clin. Res. 33(4):816A, 1985.
15. Schaper, W., Schaper, J., Xhonneux, R., and Vandesteene, R.: Morphology of intercoronary anastomoses in chronic coronary artery occlusion. Cardiovasc. Res. 3:315, 1969.
16. Simonetti, I., Cooper, S.M., and Harrison, D.G.: Dependence of native coronary collateral perfusion on normal zone resistance. Circulation 76(Suppl. IV):1301, 1987.
17. Schuster, E.H., and Bulkley, B.H.: Early post-infarction angina. Ischemia at a distance and ischemia in the infarct zone. N. Engl. J. Med. 305(19):1101, 1981.
18. Schwartz, J.N., Kong, Y., Hackell, D.B., et al.: Comparison of angiographic and postmortem findings in patients with coronary artery disease. Am. J. Cardiol. 36:174, 1975.

T

1. Tauchert, M., and Hilger, H.H.: Application of the coronary reserve concept to the study of myocardial perfusion. *In* Schaper, W. (ed.): The Patho-Physiology of Myocardial Perfusion. Amsterdam Elsevier/North-Holland Biomedical Press, Amsterdam, 1979, p. 141.
2. Taillefer, R., Lette, J., Phaneuf, D.-C., et al.: Thallium-201 myocardial imaging during pharmacologic coronary vasodilation: Comparison of oral and intravenous administration of dipyridamole. J. Am. Coll. Cardiol. 8:76, 1986.

U

1. Urabe, Y., Tomoike, H., Ohzono, K., et al.: Role of afterload in determining regional right ventricular performance during coronary underperfusion in dogs. Circ. Res. 57:96, 1985.
2. Utley, J., Carlson, E.L., Hoffman, J.I.E., et al.: Total and regional myocardial blood flow measurements with 25μ, 15μ, 9μ, and filtered 1-10μ diameter microspheres and antipyrine in dogs and sheep. Circ. Res. 34:391, 1974.

V

1. Vatner, S.F., Higgins, C.B., and Braunwald, E.: Effects of norepinephrine on coronary circulation and left ventricular dynamics in the conscious dog. Circ. Res. 34:812, 1974.
2. Vatner, S.F., Higgins, C.B., Franklin, D., and Braunwald, E.: Role of tachycardia in mediating the coronary hemodynamic response to severe exercise. J. Appl. Physiol. 32:380, 1972.
3. Vatner, S.F., and Hintze, T.H.: Regulation of large coronary arteries by beta-adrenergic mechanisms in the conscious dog. Circ. Res. 51:56, 1983.
4. Vatner, S.F., McRitchie, R.J., Maroko, P.R., et al.: Effects of catecholamines, exercise and nitroglycerin on the normal and ischemic myocardium in conscious dogs. J. Clin. Invest. 54:563, 1974.
5. Vincent, W.R., Buckberg, G.D., and Hoffman, J.I.E.: Left ventricular subendocardial ischemia in severe valvular and supravalvular aortic stenosis: A common mechanism. Circulation 49:326, 1974.
6. Verbeuren, T.J., Jordaens, F.H., Zonnekeyn, L.L., et al.: Effect of hypercholesterolemia on vascular reactivity in the rabbit. Circ. Res. 58:552, 1986.
7. von Restorff, W., Hofling, B., Holtz, J., and Bassenge, E.: Effect of increased blood fluidity through hemodilution on coronary circulation at rest and during exercise in dogs. Pflugers Arch. 357:15, 1975.
8. Verani, M., Marcus, M., Ehrhardt, J., and Doty, D.: Demonstration of improved myocardial perfusion following aortic implantation of anomalous left coronary artery. J. Nucl. Med. 19:1032, 1978.
9. Van Citters, R.L., and Franklin, D.L.: Cardiovascular performance of Alaska sled dogs during exercise. Circ. Res. 24:33, 1969.

W

1. White, C.W., Kerber, R., Weiss, H.R., and Marcus, M.L.: Effect of atrial fibrillation on wall stress, oxygen consumption and perfusion of the left atrium. Circulation (Suppl. 2)64:IV-65, 1981.
2. Walston, A., Rembert, J.C., Fedor, J.M., and Greenfield, J.C.: Regional myocardial blood flow after sudden aortic constriction in awake dogs. Circ. Res. 42:419, 1978.
3. Wei, E.P., Kontos, H.A., Christman, C.W., et al.: Superoxide generation and reversal of acetylcholine-induced cerebral arteriolar dilation after acute hypertension. Circ. Res. 57:781, 1985.
4. Wilson, R.F., Laughlin, D.E., Ackell, P.H., et al.: Transluminal subselective measurement of coronary artery blood flow velocity and vasodilator reserve in man. Circulation 72:82, 1985.
5. Wangler, R.D., Peters, K.G., Marcus, M.L., and Tomanek, R.J.: Effects of duration and severity of arterial hypertension on cardiac hypertrophy and coronary vasodilator reserve. Circ. Res. 51:10, 1982.
6. Winniford, M.D., Rossen, J.D., Simonetti, I., and Stark, C.A.: Effect of changes in myocardial metabolism on coronary flow reserve in patients. (Abstract.) Circulation (Suppl. II)78(4):II-256, 1988.
7. Wilson, R.F., Marcus, M.L., Drews, T.A., and White, C.W.: Prediction of the physiologic significance of coronary arterial lesions by quantitative lesion geometry in patients with limited coronary artery disease. Circulation 75(4):723, 1987.
8. Wilson, R.F., and White, C.W.: Intracoronary papaverine: An ideal coronary vasodilator for studies of the coronary circulation in conscious humans. Circulation 73:444, 1986.
9. West, G.A., and Belardinelli, L.: Sinus slowing and pacemaker shift caused by adenosine in rabbit SA node. Pflugers Arch. 403:66, 1985.
10. Wilson, R.F., Wyche, K., Christensen, B.V., et al.: The effects of adenosine on the human coronary circulation. Circulation (in press).
11. West, J.W., Bellet, S., Monzoli, V.C., and Muller, O.F.: Effects of persantin (RA8), a new coronary vasodilator, on coronary blood flow and cardiac dynamics in the dog. Circ. Res. 10:35, 1962.
12. White, C.W., Wright, C.B., Doty, D.B., et al.: Does visual interpretation of the coronary arteriogram predict the physiologic importance of a coronary stenosis? N. Engl. J. Med. 310:819, 1984.

Y

1. Young, D.R., Cholvin, N.R., Kirkeeide, R.L., and Roth, A.C.: Hemodynamics of arterial stenoses at elevated flow rates. Circ. Res. 41:99, 1977.
2. Young, D.F., Cholvin, N.R., Roth, A.C.: Pressure drop across artificially induced stenoses in the femoral arteries of dogs. Circ. Res. 36:735, 1975.
3. Young, D.F., and Tsai, F.Y.: Flow characteristics in models of arterial stenoses. I. Steady flow. J. Biomech. 6:395, 1973.
4. Young, D.F., and Tsai, F.Y.: Flow characteristics in models of arterial stenoses. II. Unsteady flow. J. Biomech. 6:547, 1973.

Z

1. Zir, L.M., Miller, S.W., Dinsmore, R.E., et al.: Interobserver variability in coronary angiography. Circulation 53:4, 1976.

Chapter 3

Determinants of Systolic and Diastolic Ventricular Function

MELVIN L. MARCUS, M.D.
KEVIN C. DELLSPERGER, M.D., Ph.D.

COMPLEXITIES OF CARDIAC SHAPE 25
COMPLEXITIES OF LEFT VENTRICULAR MOTION 25
HOW IMPORTANT ARE THE VARIOUS COMPONENTS OF LEFT VENTRICULAR MOTION? 25
COMPLEXITIES OF RIGHT VENTRICULAR MOTION 25
GLOBAL LEFT AND RIGHT VENTRICULAR ANATOMY AND FUNCTION 26
FACTORS OTHER THAN DISEASE STATES THAT MODULATE LEFT VENTRICULAR FUNCTION AND VOLUME 26
Preload 26
Afterload 26
Contractility 26
Heart Rate 27
DIFFERENCES BETWEEN EFFECTS OF SUPINE AND UPRIGHT EXERCISE ON LEFT VENTRICULAR HEMODYNAMICS 27
FORMS OF STRESS OTHER THAN EXERCISE USED TO EVALUATE VENTRICULAR FUNCTION 27
PRESSURE-VOLUME MEASUREMENTS OF VENTRICULAR FUNCTION 27
FACTORS OTHER THAN DISEASES THAT MODULATE RIGHT VENTRICULAR FUNCTION AND VOLUME 28
VENTRICULAR INTERDEPENDENCE 28
REGIONAL LEFT VENTRICULAR FUNCTION 28
INHERENT HETEROGENEITY OF LEFT VENTRICULAR FUNCTION 30
Implications of Heterogeneity for Acquisition and Interpretation in Cardiac Imaging Procedures 30
PATHOLOGIC STATES THAT MODIFY REGIONAL VENTRICULAR FUNCTION 31
Transient Ischemia 31
Stunned Myocardium 31
Clinical Implications 32
Hibernating Myocardium 32
Clinical Implications 32
Infarcted Myocardium 32
Infarct Expansion 33
Reactive Hypertrophy 33
Compensatory Hyperfunction 33
DIASTOLIC VENTRICULAR FUNCTION 33
Basic Factors That Modulate Diastolic Left Ventricular Function 34
Triphasic Nature of Diastolic Left Ventricular Filling 34
Heterogeneity of Diastolic Left Ventricular Function 34
Clinical Parameters That Influence the Practical Assessment of Diastolic Left Ventricular Function 34
Cardiac Rhythm 34
Heart Rate 34
End-Diastolic Left Ventricular Volume 35
Systolic Left Ventricular Performance 35
Age 35
Clinical Implications 35

Accurate information concerning ventricular function is essential in the evaluation of patients with heart disease. Not surprisingly, most of the major imaging techniques in current use have as one objective the assessment of structure, and of systolic and/or diastolic function, of the right and left ventricles.

The functional status and anatomic characteristics of the ventricles are important in many respects. First, the prognosis for a patient with almost any type of heart disease (coronary disease, valvular disease, cardiomyopathy, hypertensive heart disease) is profoundly influenced by the status of ventricular performance. For example, annual expected mortality rates of patients with three-vessel coronary disease with normal or with severely impaired left ventricular function are approximately 5 and 20 per cent, respectively.[M1] Second, the mechanism responsible for clinical symptoms and signs of congestive heart failure may be dysfunction—systolic, diastolic, or both—of either or both ventricles. Although in adults in the United States, heart failure is usually related to an impairment of systolic left ventricular function,[B1] several recent studies suggest that up to 30 per cent of adults with clinical heart failure have isolated diastolic dysfunction of the left ventricle.[B1, D1, T1] Finally, certain specific anatomic or functional features of the left or right ventricles are often essential to precise definition of a patient's cardiac disease. Examples include left ventricular aneurysm, idiopathic hypertrophic subaortic stenosis, and infundibular pulmonic stenosis.

Thus, accurate information about the structure and function of the left and right ventricles is useful in estimating prognosis, defining the mechanism responsible for the clinical syndrome, and sometimes, identifying the precise cause of the patient's problem. Although this concept is widely acknowledged by physicians involved in the care of cardiac patients, debate is substantial regarding how precise the diagnostic information needs to be. The controversy includes concerns about the cost-effectiveness, and the relative risks and merits, of multiple techniques that can provide clinically relevant and somewhat overlapping data.

This chapter reviews general aspects of global and regional function of the right and left ventricles that are essential to an understanding of the basic problems in this diagnostic area. The material covered applies to all technologies that seek to define structure and function of the left and right ventricles.

COMPLEXITIES OF CARDIAC SHAPE

If the three-dimensional shapes of the right and left ventricles were simple spheres, and if the shapes remained unchanged by disease processes or during the sequence of cardiac contraction, most of the problems that have plagued attempts to define cardiac structure and function by imaging techniques would not exist. The shapes of the left and right ventricle cannot be precisely defined, however, by simple three-dimensional geometric figures. Ventricular shape changes throughout the cardiac cycle, and disease processes may severely distort the shapes of the ventricular chambers. The normal left ventricle at end-diastole has a shape that is similar to a prolate ellipsoid.[H1] The right ventricular shape at end-diastole is far more complex.[F1, F2, H1, M2, R1, R2] In addition, the inner walls of the ventricles are trabeculated (more so in the right than in the left ventricle), and the trabeculation is greatly accentuated during systole. This characteristic imparts an irregular shape to the inner wall. In both ventricles, the size and shape of the papillary muscles and other muscle bands further complicate the overall shape.

Because of the complexity of the shapes of the left and right ventricles, projection imaging techniques (e.g., contrast and radionuclide ventriculography, and digital angiography) are not able to measure ventricular size and shape precisely. These techniques give particularly poor information regarding ventricular wall thickness. Objects that have complex shapes are best imaged by techniques that have a tomographic format, especially if multiple, thin, parallel tomographic images can be obtained throughout the entire structure at frequent intervals in the cardiac cycle. At present, only two-dimensional echocardiography, ultrafast computed tomography, single-photon emission computed tomography and nuclear magnetic resonance imaging provide tomographic images of the cardiac chambers.

COMPLEXITIES OF LEFT VENTRICULAR MOTION

Left ventricular motion during systole involves five specific movements: (1) translation, (2) rotation, (3) wringing, (4) accordion-like motion, and (5) movement of the endocardial circumference toward the center of the ventricular chamber. Each of these primary movements is not uniform throughout the left ventricle. For example, the accordion-like motion is strikingly asymmetric. During systole, the mitral valve plane in adults with normal cardiac function descends 1 to 2 cm toward the apex, but the apex barely moves up toward the base of the heart.[F3] In addition, disease processes can sometimes disproportionately augment one or more of the components of left ventricular motion. Finally, changes in the inotropic state or loading conditions have been shown to alter various components and the heterogeneity of left ventricular motion.[F3, M3, P1, S1]

Of the five cardiac movements, motion of the endocardial surface toward the center of the ventricle is by far the dominant motion for both the right and left ventricles. The second most important motion of the left ventricle is the accordion-like movement. Studies using several techniques (two-dimensional echocardiography, ventriculography with contrast media or implanted tantalum clips, ultrafast computed tomography, or magnetic resonance imaging) indicate that this type of motion is of sufficient magnitude to influence significantly measurements of regional ventricular function.[B2, C1, F3, G1, G2, H1, I1, K1, L1, L2, M4–M6, P1, P2, R3, S2, S3, T2, Z1] The other three cardiac movements (translation, rotation, and wringing) are of minor importance if the pericardium is normal. In the absence of the pericardium, however, or in the presence of a large pericardial effusion, these movements become significant.[B3]

None of the existing methods of assessing left ventricular geometry can measure the specific contribution of each of the five primary sources of motion to overall ventricular function. All existing methods ignore one of the five components—the wringing motion. Several relatively crude approximations to provide correction for some of the remaining primary movements—translation and rotation—have been suggested, but they are seldom used in routine clinical practice. The accordion-like motion of the base of the left ventricle is ignored by radionuclide ventriculography, but it appears as a prominent component in studies involving ultrafast computed tomography, magnetic resonance imaging, two-dimensional echocardiography, and contrast ventriculography. All methods in current use place most emphasis on movement of the endocardial circumference toward the center of the ventricular cavity.

Recently, several investigators using magnetic resonance imaging technology have succeeded in placing "reference markers" at multiple positions on the ventricle by altering the protocol used to obtain the magnetic resonance images. This ingenious method coupled with three-dimensional reconstruction techniques should allow careful examination of all five cardiac movements, because the "reference markers" fully compensate for out-of-plane imaging. Unfortunately, this method can be applied only to "gated" magnetic resonance images. Therefore, the distortion in gated images may possibly limit the precision of this approach. Any imaging method in which "reference markers" cannot be used, either placed with magnetic resonance imaging technology or implanted externally on the ventricle, is plagued by the problem of "out-of-plane" motion. For example, if a fixed tomographic location is imaged, the accordion motion of the left ventricle causes segments imaged in end-diastole and end-systole to be nonidentical in a given tomographic slice. This problem causes artifactual augmentation of the apparent heterogeneity of left ventricular contraction and becomes an enormous problem when one attempts to measure changes in wall thickness during the cardiac cycle in small ventricular segments.[F3, P1, Z1]

HOW IMPORTANT ARE THE VARIOUS COMPONENTS OF LEFT VENTRICULAR MOTION?

Because endocardial movement toward the center of the cardiac chamber is so dominant, estimates of some parameters of global left ventricular function remain relatively accurate and sufficient for clinical purposes, even if all other types of motion are ignored. Radionuclide ventriculography ignores four of the five components of left ventricular motion; nevertheless, left ventricular ejection fraction measured with this technique is reasonably accurate. The accuracy of stroke volume measurements of the left ventricle, and particularly of the right ventricle, is severely impaired when only endocardial motion toward the center of the ventricular chamber is considered. For accurate measurements of regional ventricular function, particularly during attempts to examine small segments, consideration of many of the five components of cardiac motion is essential.

In general, projection imaging techniques (digital angiography, standard ventriculography, and isotope ventriculography) involve difficulty in completely measuring or compensating for the five movements of the left ventricle. Hence, measurements of regional function with these methods are always imprecise. The tomographic imaging techniques (two-dimensional echocardiography, ultrafast computed tomography, and magnetic resonance imaging) could potentially measure all five cardiac movements throughout the left ventricle if the following three conditions were met: (1) parallel and relatively thin tomographic slices were obtained, (2) a reference marker system was used, and (3) other potential imaging artifacts, such as those associated with gated studies, were eliminated. At present, no imaging technique can satisfy all of these conditions.

COMPLEXITIES OF RIGHT VENTRICULAR MOTION

Less is known about various primary movements of the right ventricle in comparison with those of the left ventricle. Three major components of right ventricular motion clearly exist, however: (1) translation, (2) motion of the tricuspid valve plane in a counterclockwise fashion toward the lateral wall of the right ventricle, and (3) contraction of the endocardial circumference toward the center of the chamber. Failure to account properly for movement of the tricuspid valve plane during cardiac contraction has led to large errors in attempts to measure right ventricular ejection fraction with the radionuclide technique.[K2, M7] The extent of rotation and of wringing motion of the right ventricle has not been defined.

Consideration of the various primary movements of the right ventricle is at least as important as for the left ventricle.

GLOBAL LEFT AND RIGHT VENTRICULAR ANATOMY AND FUNCTION

Studies of global left and right ventricular structure and function in normal adults have been performed through the use of many imaging techniques, including digital angiography, standard ventriculography, isotope ventriculography, M-mode and two-dimensional echocardiography, magnetic resonance imaging, single-photon emission tomography, and ultrafast computed tomography. All of these methods have led to similar general conclusions about most aspects of global left and right ventricular structure and function. At present, data obtained with ultrafast computed tomography probably provide the most precise information and can be used to compare measurements of the structure and function of the left and right ventricles in normal humans.

Studies using ultrafast computed tomography indicate that the mass of the free wall of the right ventricle is slightly less than one third the mass of the left ventricular walls, including the septum.[H2] Wall thickness in the right ventricle is about 3 to 4 mm whereas left ventricular wall thickness is 9 to 13 mm. These measurements agree closely with data obtained from pathologic specimens. The end-diastolic volume of the right ventricle is about 18 percent larger than that of the left ventricle. At end-systole, the volume of the right ventricle is 76 percent larger than that of the ventricle. Consequently, right ventricular ejection fraction is lower than left ventricular ejection fraction in normal adults. In the absence of respiratory movement, right and left ventricular stroke volumes are nearly identical.[R2] A small volume of bronchial flow is responsible for left ventricular stroke volume being slightly in excess of right ventricular stroke volume.

Although these anatomic and structural features of the right and left ventricles are well established, the precision of most imaging techniques is not sufficient to demonstrate all of these parameters. All of the available techniques can reasonably approximate left ventricular ejection fraction and, to a lesser extent, right ventricular ejection fraction. Several techniques allow accurate volume measurements of the left ventricle, but such measurements are far more difficult in the right ventricle. Only ultrafast computed tomography has been demonstrated to measure right ventricular mass accurately. Several techniques (echocardiography, single and biplane ventriculography, digital angiography, ultrafast computed tomography, magnetic resonance imaging, and single-photon emission computed tomography) can be used to estimate left ventricular mass.

FACTORS OTHER THAN DISEASE STATES THAT MODULATE LEFT VENTRICULAR FUNCTION AND VOLUME

The left ventricle is extremely sensitive to many factors constantly modulating its function. Not only can the volume of the left ventricular chamber in various phases of the cardiac cycle be modified, but even the mass of the left ventricle can be changed within narrow limits. Acute changes in mass of the left ventricular wall can occur, because in the presence of various stimuli that promote coronary vasodilation, the volume of blood in the coronary vasculature increases,[K3, K4, M8] and during ischemia, it decreases.[K4, S4] In addition, effects of systolic compression on coronary blood volume can slightly alter left ventricular mass within a single cardiac cycle.

Table 3–1 lists most of the common factors that have been shown to alter left ventricular function and volume. Under clinical conditions, alteration by more than one factor is not unusual. With exercise, for example, the heart rate, afterload, preload, and inotropic state of the cardiac muscle are augmented simultaneously. In addition to the physiologic and anatomic factors listed in Table 3–1, drugs, toxins, and various disease states can also significantly modify left ventricular function and volume. Although the purpose of this chapter is not the exhaustive and precise description of how each of the factors listed in Table 3–1 influence the function or volume of the left ventricle, several factors of particular importance are briefly described. They are preload, afterload, contractility, and heart rate. The information presented summarizes the response of the normal left ventricle to an isolated change in one of these parameters.

Preload

If other hemodynamic parameters remain constant, an increase in preload, by definition, increases end-diastolic volume in accordance with the diastolic compliance of the ventricular chamber. This increase in end-diastolic volume is associated with a decrease in end-systolic volume, and increase in stroke volume, and an increase in ejection fraction. Decreases in preload have the opposite effects.[S5]

Afterload

An isolated increase in afterload produces an increase in end-diastolic volume, an increase in end-systolic volume, a decrease in stroke volume, and a decrease in ejection fraction. The decrease in ejection fraction associated with increases in afterload can be prominent. Decreases in afterload usually decrease left ventricular end-diastolic volume and end-systolic volume, and they increase left ventricular ejection fraction and stroke volume.[R4]

Contractility

An augmentation in contractility leads to a decrease in end-diastolic volume, a greater decrease in end-systolic volume, an

Table 3–1. FACTORS THAT MODULATE LEFT VENTRICULAR FUNCTION AND VOLUME

Hemodynamic Factors
Preload
Afterload
Heart rate
Intrinsic Functional Factors
Systolic contractility
Diastolic function
Compressive Forces
Thoracic deformities
Shifts in lung volumes
Pericardial abnormalities (congenital absence of the pericardium, effusion, constriction)
Pharmacologic Factors
Positive and negative inotropic agents
Drugs that alter hemodynamics
Drugs that alter diastolic function
Disease States
Volume overload
Pressure overload
Hypertrophy
Atrophy
Infarction

increase in stroke volume, and an increase in ejection fraction.[K5] Acute administration of negative inotropic agents has the opposite effects.[R5]

Heart Rate

When heart rate increases to greater than 160 beats per minute, end-diastolic volume, end-systolic volume, ejection fraction, and stroke volume all decrease. Cardiac output remains unchanged because the increase in heart rate offsets the decrement in stroke volume.[M9]

The previous information makes clear that whenever measurements of ventricular size and function are interpreted, consideration of the prevailing conditions under which the data were obtained is critically important.

DIFFERENCES BETWEEN EFFECTS OF SUPINE AND UPRIGHT EXERCISE ON LEFT VENTRICULAR HEMODYNAMICS

With the exception of magnetic resonance imaging and single-photon emission computed tomography, the other cardiac imaging techniques (contrast ventriculography, echocardiography, radionuclide angiography, digital angiography, and ultrafast computed tomography) have been employed to assess left ventricular function, both at rest and during exercise. For technical reasons, upright exercise cannot be easily used in contrast angiography or digital angiography. These methods almost always employ recumbent bicycle exercise with the legs elevated. Echocardiography, radionuclide angiography, and ultrafast computed tomography can use either recumbent or upright exercise. These techniques often assess effects of exercise on ventricular performance by allowing measurements to be obtained immediately after exercise rather than during peak exertion. Posture and the phase of exercise examined significantly influence the effects of exercise on ventricular performance, and these factors affect the interpretation of the results of various imaging procedures. A brief review of this topic follows.

Left ventricular volume is posture-dependent. It is maximal in Trendelenburg's position and minimal when the patient is upright. In adults with normal ventricular function, end-diastolic left ventricular volume in Trendelenburg's position is approximately 15 percent greater than it is in an upright position.[G3]

If end-diastolic left ventricular volume is maximal in Trendelenburg's position, then exercise does not appreciably increase it.[P3, R6] In contrast, with upright exercise, end-diastolic left ventricular volume starts at a much lower value and can appreciably increase during exercise.[P3] Because part of the exercise-induced change in stroke volume is related to an increase in end-diastolic volume and a decrease in end-systolic volume, recumbent exercise is accompanied by smaller changes in stroke volume than is upright exercise.[I2, P3] In most patients, the intensity of exercise stress achieved is greater with upright than with supine exercise, because with the former, patient participation is more intense. This greater intensity probably occurs because this type of exertion is more familiar to most patients. Also, recumbent exercise that is performed with the legs elevated adds a component of isometric stress, which can increase arterial pressure.[P3] As a consequence of these factors, the effects of upright exercise on left ventricular performance are quite different from those of recumbent exercise.

Immediately following exercise, particularly when it has been performed in the recumbent position with legs up, arterial pressure and heart rate begin to decline rapidly, but high circulating levels of catecholamines cause the inotropic state to remain intense for a short time. This combination of factors (intense inotropic stimulation and falling afterload) can produce a transient post-exercise increase in left ventricular ejection fraction.[I2, P3]

The rate at which the hemodynamic stress of exercise declines following cessation of exertion is related primarily to cardiac function and conditioning. In highly trained individuals with normal cardiac function, hemodynamics return toward normal levels quickly (i.e., within a few minutes) following cessation of exercise. In poorly trained individuals or patients with impaired left ventricular function, hemodynamics return toward control levels very slowly following completion of exercise. Finally, regional wall motion abnormalities produced by ischemia that occurs as a consequence of exertional stress can persist for many minutes following completion of exercise, particularly if the ischemia has been severe and persisted for several minutes during exercise.[I2] This prolongation of regional wall motion abnormalities in patients with intense ischemia allows echocardiographers to detect exercise-induced wall motion abnormalities a few minutes after treadmill exercise through use of ultrasound examinations with the patient in the recumbent position.

FORMS OF STRESS OTHER THAN EXERCISE USED TO EVALUATE VENTRICULAR FUNCTION

In many ways, exercise is an ideal form of stress for ventricular function studies, but in some patients with coexistent noncardiac disease, adequate exercise may not be possible. In addition, exercise stress may limit ideal patient positioning for a particular type of imaging study and is associated with marked chest motion mainly related to hyperpnea. These limitations of exercise stress have encouraged investigators to develop many other approaches to enhancing ventricular performance. These interventions are listed in Table 3–2. One of the problems with many of these approaches is that they provoke hemodynamic responses that may simultaneously increase or decrease ventricular performance. For example, infusion of a pressor substance such as phenylephrine or angiotensin increases afterload, but by activating the baroreceptor mechanism, it promotes sympathetic withdrawal and vagal stimulation. The end result is significant bradycardia. Another problem with non-exercise forms of stress is that the intensity of the hemodynamic stress achieved is often much less than the hemodynamics achievable through intense upright exertion. For example, a dobutamine infusion (10 μg/kg/min IV) increases the product of heart rate and systolic arterial pressure by less than twofold in young healthy men, whereas with intense upright exercise, the rate-pressure product can increase threefold or fourfold.[G4]

PRESSURE-VOLUME MEASUREMENTS OF VENTRICULAR FUNCTION

To obtain detailed studies of left ventricular function, chamber volume or dimensions and intraventricular pressure must be

Table 3–2. NON-ISOTONIC EXERCISE APPROACHES TO ALTERING VENTRICULAR FUNCTION

Pharmacologic Agents
- Positive inotropic agents—dobutamine, dopamine, isoproterenol, norepinephrine
- Negative inotropic agents—calcium blockers, beta blockers
- Increases in afterload—phenylephrine, angiotensin
- Decreases in afterload—nitroprusside, nitroglycerine
- Increases in heart rate—isoproterenol, atropine

Electrical Stimulation
- Pacing
- Paired extrasystolic potentiation

Isometric Exercise
- Hand grip

Neural Activation
- Neck suction
- Lower body negative suction
- Cold pressor test

Intensive Coronary Dilation
- Intravenous dipyridamole

Respiratory Maneuvers
- Valsalva's maneuver
- Müller's maneuver

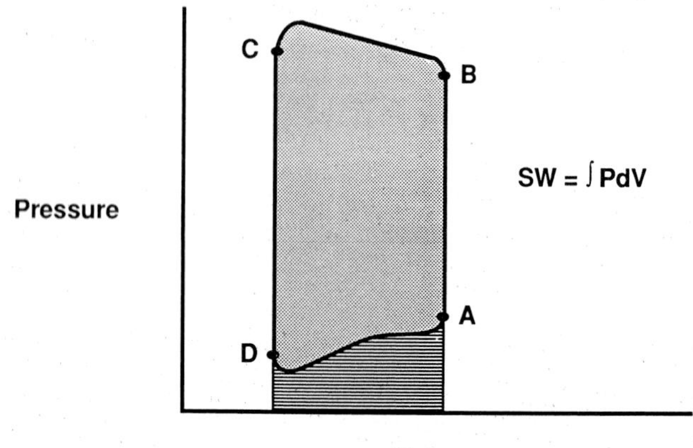

Figure 3–1. Schematic diagram of left ventricular pressure (P) versus simultaneous left ventricular volume (V) for a single cardiac cycle. Point A represents end diastole; the segment AB represents isovolumic contraction. Aortic valve opening is shown by point B, and left ventricular ejection by segment BC. Point C represents aortic valve closure and the end of ejection. Segment CD represents isovolumic relaxation, and point D the mitral valve opening. The segment DA represents left ventricular filling. The left ventricular stroke work (SW), the area within the pressure-volume loop, is designated by stippling. The striped area represents the diastolic work performed on the left ventricle by the right ventricle and the left atrium.

measured simultaneously. The chamber dimensions are assessed with an imaging technique such as M-mode or two-dimensional echocardiography, single-plane or biplane ventriculography, or ultrafast computed tomography.

Pressure-volume data are often presented in one of two formats: the classic pressure-volume loop (Fig. 3–1)[G5] or the end-systolic pressure-volume relationship (Fig. 3–2).[S6] With either approach, the accuracy of the information obviously depends on the precision of the input data. Pressure measurements are most accurate when obtained with manometer-tipped pressure catheters. The

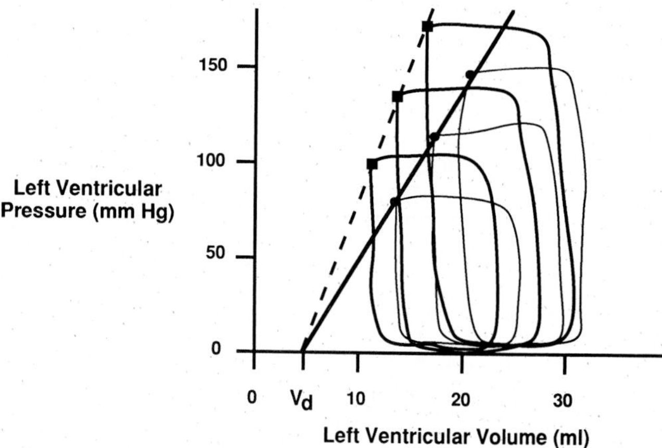

Figure 3–2. Schematic diagram of several pressure-volume loops. The control loading conditions *(solid line)* differ from those produced during an epinephrine infusion *(dashed line)*. The premise of the end-systolic pressure-volume index is that left ventricular chamber pressure is related to volume at the end of end-systole by a single line that is independent of various loading conditions. This line is characterized by a slope and an x intercept that is called V_d (the extrapolated end-systolic volume when end-systolic pressure is zero). This diagram illustrates that when an infusion of epinephrine is given to experimental animals to increase contractility, the slope of this line is steeper, whereas when an agent that depresses cardiac contractility is given, the slope of the line is shallower (i.e., to the right of the solid line). Although uncertainty exists regarding the usefulness of the end-systolic volume at zero pressure, the slope of the line is generally considered to be of some use in the clinical evaluation of contractility.

most accurate volume measurements are obtained when tomographic imaging techniques are employed. Although pressure-volume data are extremely useful in understanding ventricular mechanics,[B4] they are seldom obtained outside of research laboratories, for practical reasons.

FACTORS OTHER THAN DISEASES THAT MODULATE RIGHT VENTRICULAR FUNCTION AND VOLUME

Most of the factors that have been shown to modulate end-diastolic volume, end-systolic volume, stroke volume, and ejection fraction of the left ventricle also affect the volume and function of the right ventricle. Changes in systemic pressure have lesser effects on right ventricular performance than on left ventricular performance, just as perturbations in pulmonary arterial pressure mainly influence right ventricular size and function and have only minimal effects on the left ventricle. Ventilation has a greater effect on the right ventricular volume than on left ventricular volume because of the buffering effect of the pulmonary reservoir. Similarly, other ventilatory maneuvers (e.g., Valsalva's maneuver, Müller's maneuver) have greater effects on right ventricular performance than on left ventricular performance. Studies of right ventricular function based on pressure measurements or on assessment of right ventricular ejection fraction have been performed for many years. Accurate measurements of right ventricular volume and regional right ventricular function, however, have only recently become possible with the introduction of sophisticated tomographic imaging techniques (Fig. 3–3).

VENTRICULAR INTERDEPENDENCE

Profound dysfunction of one of the ventricular chambers may coexist with normal function or hyperfunction of the other chamber. Also, a reasonably normal life may be possible even for patients in whom the right ventricle has been surgically excluded.[F4] These observations, however, do not totally undermine the concept of ventricular interdependence.[O1] Many situations exist in which the function, shape, or size of one ventricle can influence the other ventricle.[B5, G6, P1, R7] A good example of ventricular interdependence is marked right ventricular volume overload, which occurs in patients with large atrial septal defects. In this condition, the dilated right ventricle, with increased end-diastolic pressure, bows the interventricular septum toward the left. This action in turn decreases left ventricular volume and unfavorably alters the pressure-volume characteristics of the left ventricular chamber.[B5] Septal hypertrophy secondary to idiopathic hypertropic subaortic stenosis can sometimes be severe enough to cause partial obstruction of the outflow tract of the right ventricle.

Because the function of one ventricle is not a reliable predictor of the performance of the other pumping chamber, and because ventricular interdependence is occasionally clinically relevant, assessment of the function of both ventricles is always wise in patients suspected of heart disease. With the use of several imaging techniques, this assessment requires little or no change in the routine procedure (magnetic resonance imaging, ultrafast computed tomography, echocardiography, and radionuclide angiography). With two of the commonly used procedures, however—digital angiography and standard ventriculography—accurate assessment of both ventricles requires more extensive equipment (biplane as opposed to single-plane x-ray imaging), which prolongs and slightly increases the risk of the diagnostic procedure. In practice, when digital angiography or standard ventriculography is employed to assess ventricular function, only the left ventricle is usually examined.

REGIONAL LEFT VENTRICULAR FUNCTION

Although measurements of global left ventricular function are clinically valuable, many cardiac conditions primarily produce

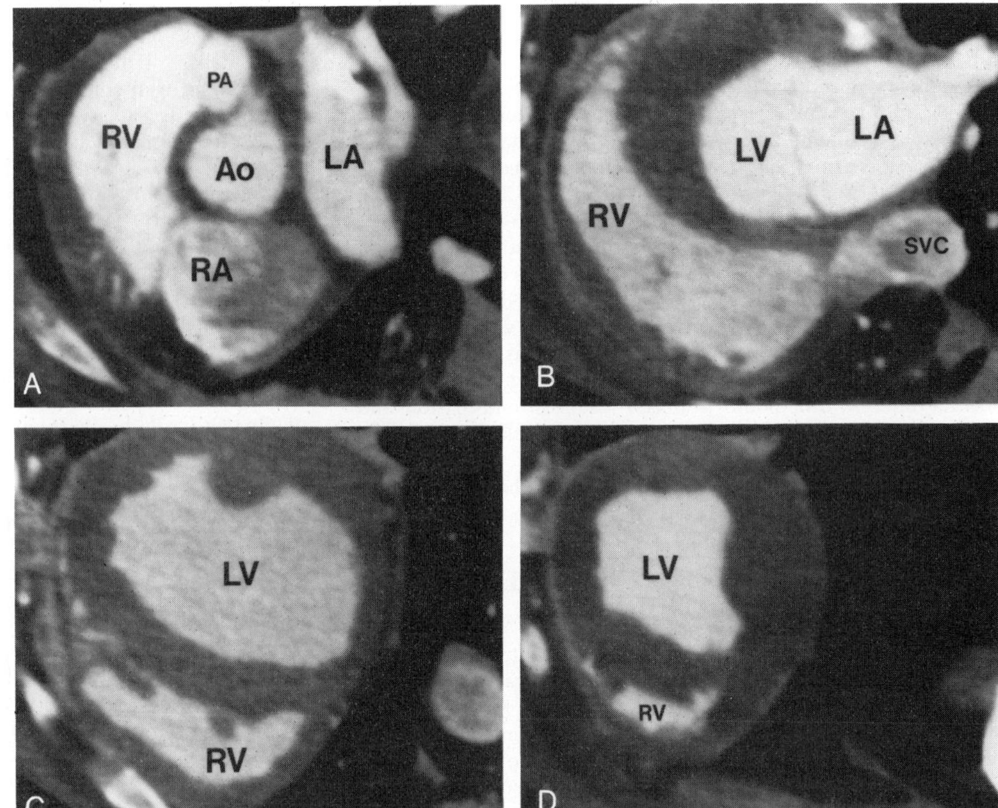

Figure 3–3. The right ventricle (RV) of a dog is imaged during end-diastole, using ultrafast computed tomography at four levels and a 3-mm slice thickness. An image of the base of the heart *(A)*, an image toward the apex *(B)*, a midventricular image *(C)*, and a tomographic image near the apex *(D)* are shown. The anterior aspect of the animal's chest is to the left of each image. Note the marked anatomic diversity of the right ventricular shape in comparison with that of the left ventricle (LV). Border recognition is sharp, and accurate measurements of both end-diastolic volume and end-diastolic mass of the right ventricle can be easily obtained. Ao—aorta; LA—left atrium; PA—pulmonary artery; RA—right atrium; SVC—superior vena cava. (Courtesy of Zina Hajduczok, M.D., University of Iowa, Department of Internal Medicine.)

regional disturbances in ventricular function. Measurement of regional function is essential in many cardiac conditions, such as ischemia, infarction, ventricular aneurysm, and idiopathic hypertrophic subaortic stenosis.

Precise evaluation of regional left ventricular function is much more difficult than assessment of global function. Reasons for this difficulty can be grouped into two general categories: technologic and physiologic (Table 3–3). The technologic problems are several. *First*, as one attempts to study smaller and smaller regions of the left ventricle, examination of all surfaces of the ventricular chambers becomes increasingly important. Over- and undersampling of various regions can occur because the imaging system employed does not provide parallel images. This problem occurs, for example, in standard echocardiography and contributes to suboptimal assessment of regional ventricular performance. With transesophageal echocardiography, however, the entire surface of the left ventricle can be examined in detail.[L3]

Second, superimposition of various segments of the left ventricular wall, an inherent characteristic of radionuclide angiography, digital angiography, and standard ventriculography, also undermines attempts to define regional ventricular performance accurately. *Third*, as progressively smaller regions are examined, the spatial resolution of the imaging technique must improve appropriately. Techniques with inherently modest spatial resolution, such as planar radionuclide angiography, are consequently limited in their ability to perform detailed measurements of regional ventricular function.

Fourth, even with high-resolution tomographic imaging systems—such as ultrafast computed tomography, magnetic resonance imaging, and transesophageal echocardiography—out-of-plane motion of the cardiac structures confounds accurate measurements of regional ventricular function if a "reference marker system" is not employed. *Finally*, an ideal examination of regional ventricular function would include measurements of left ventricular wall thickness in multiple segments. At present, only three imaging techniques—echocardiography, magnetic resonance imaging, and ultrafast computed tomography—can measure left ventricular wall thickness in multiple regions.

The physiologic problems that limit accurate assessment of regional wall motion are even more formidable and less surmountable than the technical barriers. They are related to the complex motion of the left ventricle, the inherent spatial heterogeneity of regional performance of the normal left ventricle, and the temporal heterogeneity of left ventricular contraction.

In a previous section of this chapter, the five primary components of left ventricular motion were emphasized: rotation, wringing, translation, accordion-like motion, and movement of the endocardial surface toward the center of the left ventricular chamber. Although most of these components can be ignored without jeopardizing accurate assessment of global left ventricular ejection fraction, the accurate measurement of regional function requires that many of these components be considered.

As noted earlier, the contraction of the normal left ventricle is heterogeneous, both from apex to base and around the circumference of individual tomographic slices. Because different segments contribute variably to overall ventricular performance, dysfunction of different areas of the left ventricle should be expected to have varying effects on global left ventricular function. Studies have shown that anterior and posterior infarcts of similar size have different effects on global ventricular performance. Anterior infarcts produce greater decrements in global left ventricular ejection fraction than do posterior infarcts.[F5]

Table 3–3. REQUIREMENTS OF IMAGING METHODS FOR ACCURATE ASSESSMENT OF REGIONAL VENTRICULAR FUNCTION

Technologic Requirements
Examination of entire surface of left ventricle
Lack of superimposition of left ventricular segments
Optimum spatial resolution
"Reference marker" system to identify specific segments
Measurements of wall thickness in multiple segments
Physiologic Considerations
Complex motion of the heart
Rotation
Wringing
Translation
Accordion-like movement
Endocardial movement
Spatial heterogeneity of contraction
Temporal heterogeneity of contraction

Another factor that contributes to the heterogeneity of contraction is temporal variability. Even in the normal heart, all ventricular segments are not depolarized simultaneously. Excitation of the normal left ventricle generally proceeds from apex to base.[F6] Such disease processes as infarction and conduction disturbances can substantially augment the extent of temporal heterogeneity. Most analytic protocols for evaluating systolic and diastolic function tacitly assume that all segments in the ventricle reach peak contraction or relaxation simultaneously. Such simultaneity does not occur, however, even in normal ventricles; thus, this assumption contributes to the apparent measured heterogeneity of performance. This problem can be managed by analyzing several different time points near end-systole or end-diastole and selecting peak systolic contraction or diastolic relaxation of individual segments at the optimal point in time. When such a procedure is performed, the magnitude of the heterogeneity of regional function decreases modestly.[F3, R8]

INHERENT HETEROGENEITY OF LEFT VENTRICULAR FUNCTION

Many methods of evaluating regional left ventricular function have tacitly assumed that the left ventricle contracts and relaxes in a homogeneous manner. This assumption is fundamental to predictions of global left ventricular function when only a limited area of the left ventricle is imaged (as in M-mode and early two-dimensional echocardiographic studies). This assumption is also fundamental to estimates of left ventricular wall stress obtained from measurement of left ventricular wall thicknesss and diameter from one site in the chamber. Tomographic imaging techniques have provided convincing data that establish the concept that the normal left ventricle contracts in a heterogeneous manner (Fig. 3–4).[F3]

The heterogeneity of contraction of the left ventricle has been described from three perspectives: apex-to-base function, circumferential variability within a single tomographic plane, and accordion-like motion. Studies performed with several imaging techniques including ultrafast computed tomography[F3] have shown that the contraction of the basal area of the left ventricle differs greatly from the apical sections. At the base of the heart, the overall regional ejection fraction is lower than at the apex, but the end-diastolic volume and stroke volume are greater at the base. Furthermore, a nearly continuous apex-to-base gradation of these parameters (regional sectional ejection fraction, sectional end-diastolic volume, sectional volume/mass ratio, and sectional stroke volume) has been noted.[F3] Although problems with out-of-plane motion may augment the magnitude of this apex-to-base heterogeneity, the heterogeneity is clearly of considerable importance. Circumferentially, studies with two-dimensional echocardiography[P1] and ultrafast computed tomography[F3] have shown striking heterogeneity of regional cavity ejection fraction and regional wall thickening. The accordion-like motion of the left ventricle is also asymmetric. The mitral valve plane descends 1 to 2 cm toward the apex in systole, but the apex hardly moves toward the base in systole. Thus far, no studies have described heterogeneity of rotation (apex to base) or the twisting movement of the left ventricle.

A further complication of this matter is the demonstration by investigators using ultrafast computed tomography that inotropic stimulation with dobutamine decreases circumferential heterogeneity of left ventricular contraction.[S1] In addition, increases in afterload decrease both apex-to-base and circumferential heterogeneity of left ventricular performance.[M4] Together, these investigations suggest that when a stress is imposed, the left ventricle adapts to it partly by contracting in a more homogeneous manner.

Implications of Heterogeneity for Acquisition and Interpretation in Cardiac Imaging Procedures

Many clinical examinations of left ventricular function using imaging techniques have either ignored or attempted to account crudely for the problem of heterogeneity of contraction of the normal human left ventricle. As a consequence, several approaches to regional analysis of left ventricular function are relatively insensitive and nonspecific in detecting subtle localized cardiac contraction abnormalities, such as those occurring with regional myocardial ischemia of intermediate severity. This problem is obviously minimized if abnormalities in regional ventricular function are more severe (i.e., dyskinetic as opposed to hypokinetic). Furthermore, a myriad of methods have been proposed, including various placements of a "centroid" and corrections for rotation, that are intended to compensate for unmeasured components of left ventricular motion.[P1] None of these methods has achieved wide-scale acceptance either within one imaging approach (e.g., two-dimensional echocardiography) or across several approaches.

If quantitative analysis of left ventricular function in multiple small regions (40 to 100 segments) of the left ventricle is to be successful, either for research or for clinical care, at least three criteria must be satisfied: (1) the technique employed must provide images of high spatial and temporal resolution of the entire left ventricular surface; (2) most or all of the five primary movements of the left ventricle must be directly measured, which requires an appropriate reference marker system; and (3) the "normal" range for each segment or cluster of segments must be defined under a given set of conditions. Only three of the available cardiac imaging techniques (ultrafast computed tomography, magnetic resonance imaging, and echocardiography)—if they can develop an internal reference marker system—are likely to satisfy these stringent criteria. A marker system is currently available

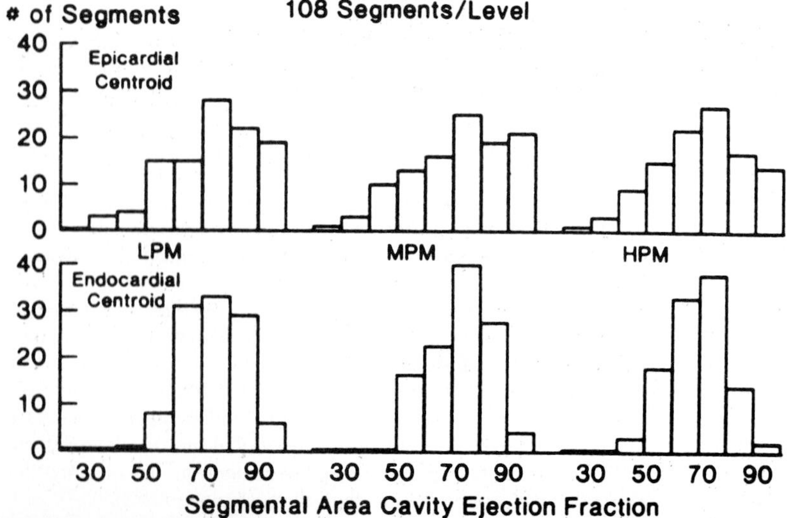

Figure 3–4. Graphic representation of the heterogeneity of regional left ventricular ejection fraction using ultrafast cine–computed tomography. These data are from 11 volunteers and reflect the regional segmental cavity ejection fractions obtained using an epicardial centroid *(top panel)* and an endocardial centroid *(bottom panel)* at the low, middle, and high papillary muscle levels (LPM, MPM, and HPM, respectively). Marked heterogeneity of segmental area cavity ejection fraction can be seen at each level using either centroid. (From Feiring, A. J., Rumberger, J. A., Reiter, S. J., et al.: Sectional and segmental variability of left ventricular function: Experimental and clinical studies using ultrafast computed tomography. J. Am. Coll. Cardiol. 12:415, 1988. Reprinted with permission from the American College of Cardiology.)

only for magnetic resonance imaging. *The experience of the last two decades suggests that the use of simpler approaches that ignore the aforementioned criteria are likely to limit the success of further attempts at quantitative analysis of regional left ventricular function.*

PATHOLOGIC STATES THAT MODIFY REGIONAL VENTRICULAR FUNCTION

In this section, several of the most important pathologic states that have major effects on regional left ventricular function are described. These include transient ischemia, stunned myocardium, hibernating myocardium, and infarcted myocardium.

Transient Ischemia

Transmural myocardial ischemia profoundly decreases regional wall motion within a few cardiac cycles. This observation, first made in 1935 by Tennant and Wiggers in their study of dogs,[T3] has been repeatedly confirmed in numerous animal investigations and in humans. Studies in humans have been performed using two approaches. In the first approach, during open-heart surgery and a proximal coronary artery occlusion, the regional wall thickening distal to the site of occlusion is measured with an M-mode echocardiographic miniature 5- to 7-MHz transducer held on the cardiac surface with a suction cup.[H3] The second approach involves coronary artery occlusion with a balloon during angioplasty in awake patients, during which regional left ventricular wall motion in the perfusion field of the occluded vessel is assessed with transthoracic two-dimensional echocardiography.[H4] Both types of studies have confirmed that in humans, transient coronary occlusion is associated with a prompt alteration of regional ventricular function. If the occlusion is released in seconds, regional wall function is fully restored in less than 1 minute. Interestingly, following coronary occlusion, regional wall motion abnormalities occurred more quickly in anesthetized dogs than in anesthetized humans (5 versus 20 cardiac cycles), and wall motion abnormalities were less intense (thinning versus a marked decrease in thickening) in humans.[H4, P4] The explanation for this quantitative difference in the response to coronary occlusion is unknown.

The introduction of sophisticated experimental techniques such as sonomicrometers and radiolabeled microspheres has allowed detailed exploration of the relationship between the extent and site of myocardial ischemia and the associated changes in regional mechanical function of the myocardium. These elegant investigations have uncovered several new aspects of the relationship between regional perfusion and function. In normal and hypertrophied ventricles, a somewhat linear relationship has been shown between the percentage of decrease in regional myocardial perfusion and percentage of decrease in regional wall thickening or fiber shortening.[C2, K6, K7, P4] When perfusion is decreased to 20 percent of control values in dogs, no thickening or shortening of ischemic myocardium occurs. If blood flow is reduced to 5 percent of control values, one observes dyskinesis or wall thinning.[V1] Also, changes in wall thickening are slightly more sensitive to decreases in myocardial perfusion than to alterations in segment shortening.[C2, K6, P4, V1] Transmural ischemia is associated with a decrease in diastolic left ventricular wall thickness because the "blood volume" in the ischemic zone of the left ventricular wall decreases.[C2, P4]

Studies have also been performed to evaluate the perfusion/function relationship in different transmural layers of the left ventricular wall. These studies have demonstrated that the subepicardial thickening/perfusion relationship is quite different from the subendocardial thickening/perfusion relationship.[L4, P4] The decline in subendocardial wall thickening is clearly coupled to a subendocardial perfusion deficit, as opposed to a subepicardial perfusion deficit. As a corollary of this observation, studies have shown that when 40 percent of left ventricular wall (subendocardium-to-midwall) thickness is ischemic, thickening of the entire left ventricular wall segment ceases.[G7] As a consequence, measurements of regional wall thickening often overestimate the extent of transmural myocardial ischemia.

Since the seminal studies of Kerber and associates,[K7] investigators have established that the extent of regional wall dysfunction extends laterally beyond the borders of the ischemic zone. The "width" of this lateral border of dysfunctional, normally perfused myocardium is narrow (1 to 3 mm) in anesthetized and awake dogs studied under control hemodynamic conditions.[C2, P4] The width of this border of normally perfused but mechanically dysfunctional myocardium, however, is highly load-dependent and can be significantly expanded with a moderate increase in afterload.

Taken together, these observations indicate that both the transmural extent and lateral extent of mechanical dysfunction extend well beyond the size of a regional perfusion deficit, and that the magnitude of the discrepancy is highly sensitive to hemodynamic loading. This conclusion has important implications for the interpretation of regional wall motion abnormalities in the presence of regional ischemia. Clearly, the size of the wall motion abnormality exaggerates the magnitude of the perfusion deficit. Hence, the practice of estimating the size of an ischemic zone from the size of a wall motion abnormality or a change in global left ventricular ejection fraction leads to variable errors. *Physicians involved in the care of cardiac patients should be cautious about predicting ischemic zone or infarct size from the extent of a regional wall motion abnormality. This relationship is crude at best and can often be misleading.* At the same time, extensive abnormalities in regional wall motion in patients who sustain a myocardial infarction do reliably indicate a bleak long-term prognosis.

Although the response of myocardial function to sudden severe myocardial ischemia has been exhaustively described, the mechanisms responsible for this phenomenon remain unclear. The decrement in mechanical function occurs earlier than a profound decrease in tissue glycogen or adenosine triphosphate content.[B6, F7, J1, P5] Tissue creatine phosphate, however, decreases significantly within seconds of sudden coronary occlusion.[F7, P5] The development of tissue acidosis or an increase in tissue P_{CO_2} occurs more slowly than does the decline in regional mechanical functioning. Also, perfusion of a coronary vessel with blood in which the hemoglobin has been converted to methemoglobin, and thus carries no oxygen, produces a similar but slightly more delayed effect on regional mechanical functioning in the perfusion field of the perfused coronary vessel.[P5] Thus, washout of a toxic metabolite is not the crucial factor, and investigators therefore remain uncertain regarding the proximate cause of the response of regional wall motion to sudden severe myocardial ischemia.

Stunned Myocardium

When severe regional myocardial ischemia occurs for less than 1 minute, regional ventricular function returns to control levels within 60 seconds if reperfusion is adequate. When the duration of the severe ischemia is longer, that is, 5 minutes or greater, reperfusion is associated with a marked delay in the return of normal mechanical function of the ischemic myocardium to control levels. Reperfused, viable myocardium that displays prolonged mechanical dysfunction was called "stunned myocardium" by Braunwald and Kloner in 1982.[B7] This phenomenon was also described by Heyndrickx and colleagues in 1975 and 1978.[H5, H6]

The concept of stunned myocardium has ignited a major research effort to explore two aspects of this phenomenon: detailed description of its occurrence under variable conditions and its potential mechanisms.

The time course of the delayed return of function of reperfused, viable, dysfunctional myocardium is related to the duration of occlusion, the severity of the perfusion deficit, and the extent of superimposed transmural infarction.[B8, P6] In addition, a transient occlusion has been demonstrated to sensitize the myocardium to subsequent brief occlusions if the repeat occlusion occurs within less than 30 minutes of the sensitizing stimulus.[S7] If a 20-minute occlusion is used in dogs, no necrosis occurs,[R9] but the reperfused myocardium may not function normally for as long as 48 hours.[B8] The delay in the return of function of reperfused, previously ischemic myocardium is approximately 50 times longer if regional collateral perfusion is less than 25 percent, as opposed to greater than 50 percent, of normal zone flow, when occlusion time is held constant.[B8]

Although most studies of stunned myocardium have employed an experimental model that involves transient total occlusion, Homans and co-workers sought evidence of prolonged dysfunction in dogs that were exercised in the presence of a critical coronary stenosis. In this clinically relevant model, evidence of prolonged dysfunction following cessation of exercise and restoration of normal perfusion was noted.[H7] Thus, the "stunning phenomenon" can occur with either coronary stenosis or coronary occlusion when the duration of severe ischemia is several minutes or longer.

When coronary occlusion duration is greater than 20 minutes in the dog, some degree of myocardial necrosis usually occurs. Therefore, in this setting, the return of mechanical function is complicated by the presence of superimposed infarction. As a consequence, function of the reperfused myocardium after an occlusion that is 20 minutes or longer in duration may never be restored to its normal level. Studies in dogs have shown that with occlusions of 1 to 6 hours, return of mechanical function may occur over a period of many days (3 to 15 days)[K8, L5] and is generally slower if the ischemia is more intense or if the extent of transmural infarction is substantial.

In general, studies of the stunning phenomenon in humans have confirmed the concepts resulting from animal investigations.[B8, H5–H7, P6] Numerous investigators have documented that in humans, prolonged periods of ischemia followed by reperfusion are associated with a significant delay in the return of regional myocardial function toward normal levels. This delay can sometimes extend from a period of days to weeks.

A second aspect of the stunning phenomenon that has been the subject of extensive investigation is its mechanism. The most promising theory suggested that the prolonged decrease in regional function after reperfusion was related to a prolonged delay in the replenishment of high-energy phosphate stores (adenosine triphosphate). Restoration to control levels can require many hours or days following reperfusion.[C3] This theory has been challenged by two experiments. In the first experiment, the stunned myocardium responds well to a variety of inotropic stimuli, including paired pacing, dopamine, and norepinephrine infusion.[A1, B9, E1] Because inotropic stimulation does not increase high-energy phosphate stores, this result implies that sufficient amounts of high-energy phosphates are present to allow more vigorous cardiac contraction. In the second experiment, more rapid restoration of adenosine triphosphate stores, accomplished by manipulating metabolic pathways, did not diminish the extent or severity of the stunning phenomenon.[K9, P7, P8] Thus, the theory that depressed levels of high-energy phosphate stores are responsible for the stunning phenomenon is no longer held in high regard by many investigators.

Clinical Implications

The stunning phenomenon has broad implications for the interpretation of cardiac imaging studies of regional wall motion abnormalities produced by ischemia. From a negative perspective, the stunning phenomenon severely undermines the usefulness of the extent of wall motion abnormalities as a predictor of the magnitude of necrosis in acute or subacte ischemic syndromes. After a 1- to 4-hour coronary occlusion, mechanical function in the reperfused myocardium may not be maximally restored for many days, or possibly weeks. During this long interval, other simultaneous processes—edema, cellular infiltration, fibrosis, reactive hypertrophy, infarct expansion, and hemodynamic perturbations—further complicate the relationship between the size of the wall motion abnormality and the size of the eventual infarction. From a positive perspective, the stunning phenomenon allows studies of exercise-induced ischemia to be performed soon after exercise is completed.[B2, N1, R10] Such timing minimizes imaging artifacts related to excessive respiratory motion that would occur during exercise and permits optimal positioning of the patient. This procedure has been used in echocardiograpahic and radionuclide examination of exercise-induced ischemic dysfunction.

Hibernating Myocardium

The amount of blood flow needed to prevent necrosis of myocardial cells is only about 15 to 20 percent of the perfusion required to maintain normal contraction.[K7] Hence, theoretically in chronically ischemic myocardium, a "twilight zone" exists, in which cellular viability can be maintained with limited perfusion if mechanical function is attenuated. Myocardium that exists in the twilight zone for a prolonged period has been termed "hibernating myocardium."[B10, R11] The designation implies that mechanical function returns toward normal levels when adequate perfusion is restored. Substantial data now support the concept of hibernating myocardium. When flow is limited, the myocardium quickly reduces its contractile activity. This response limits oxygen requirements and permits cellular viability in the presence of limited perfusion.

In patients with severe obstructive coronary disease, studies using positron emission tomography have identified myocardial segments with markedly decreased perfusion and decreased function, but with active metabolic activity as evidenced by studies of glucose utilization.[M10, S8, T4] Reperfusion of such segments with coronary bypass surgery or potentially percutaneous transluminal coronary angioplasty can restore normal or near normal mechanical function to these hibernating segments.[A2, S9, S10, T5] Studies of patients with unstable angina have identified myocardial segments, with decreased thallium uptake at rest and decreased mechanical function, in which flow and function can be restored with coronary bypass surgery.[B11]

Hibernating myocardium undoubtedly exists in some patients with chronic obstructive coronary disease. The extent to which this entity contributes to the clinical picture of coronary heart disease has not been well defined. More importantly, the short- or long-term stability of the hibernating state remains to be defined.

Clinical Implications

From the standpoint of interpreting cardiac imaging studies of regional wall motion of the left ventricle, hibernating myocardium is one of many potential mechanisms responsible for reversible severe regional dysfunction.

Infarcted Myocardium

Wall motion abnormalities associated with infarcted myocardium have many characteristics in common with ischemic, stunned, and hibernating myocardium. All segments of infarcted myocardium were ischemic at one point in their evolution, and many infarcted segments may have previously exhibited the stunning phenomenon or hibernation. Once infarction occurs, however, manifestation of several new features begins.

Over a short interval (hours to days), infarcted myocardial segments change their wall thickness and mechanical properties. Severe ischemia or infarction is associated with damage to the microvasculature, which allows leakage of fluid and cellular elements into the abnormal interstitium. This leakage produces swelling or edema in the involved segments. Studies using sonomicrometers,[S11, T6] computed tomography,[H8, P9] and echocardiography[L6, P10] indicate that during this acute phase, the diastolic thickness of the infarcted myocardial segments can increase by 5 to 41 percent. In the ensuing days, the edema and cellular elements recede, and the necrotic myocardium is gradually replaced by fibrous tissue, which frequently contains small islands of viable myocytes. The fibrous tissue contracts, which leads to diastolic thinning of the infarcted segments.[P10, S11, T6] The diastolic thickness of infarcted myocardium may decrease from 9 to 12 mm (normal myocardium) to the point of rupture, with sealing by the pericardium. Under these circumstances, a pseudoaneurysm develops.

The eventual diastolic thickness of infarcted myocardium depends on the interplay of six factors: (1) the original wall thickness, (2) the transmural and, to a lesser extent, lateral dimensions of the infarct, (3) the collateral flow, (4) the emergence of reactive hypertrophy, (5) the development of infarct expansion, and (6) the presence of a mural thrombus, which can falsely exaggerate the true thickness of the wall and may slightly influence mechanical properties of the involved wall. Small subendocardial infarctions may not perceptibly change regional diastolic wall thickness. Extensive infarctions typically decrease the diastolic wall thickness of the most involved segments to 3 to 4 mm.[P9, T6]

During the evolution of infarction, the mechanical properties of the involved region undergo vast alterations. Initially, when ischemia is severe, the region behaves almost passively, and during systole, dyskinesis and wall thinning characterize the behavior of the abnormal region. During diastole, the segments augment the stiffness of the left ventricular chamber. Over a period of weeks, dyskinesis and wall thinning in systole may persist or gradually give way to akinesis or even hypokinesis. The mechanisms responsible for this transition include gradual improvement in function of viable areas of stunned or hibernating myocardium, increased coronary flow from reperfusion due to coronary bypass surgery or percutaneous transluminal coronary angioplasty, development of reactive hypertrophy, and an increase in the tensile strength of the developing scar tissue.

Three components of the evolutionary process of infarction require special emphasis: infarct expansion, reactive hypertrophy, and compensatory hyperfunction.

Infarct Expansion

Bulkley and others, in studies of both animals and humans, have described delayed diastolic thinning or stretching of infarcted regions, accompanied by some lateral expansion of the abnormal zone.[B12, E2, F8, H9–H11, M11, N2, P11, R12, W1, W2] This phenomenon is observed only in association with extensive infarcts and never occurs in small subendocardial infarctions. Infarct expansion is more common in patients with hypertension[P11, P12, W3] and in those with minimal evidence of coronary collaterals.[H11, P12, P13] Both situations predispose the patient to extensive transmural infarction.

Infarct expansion has several deleterious consequences. First, the incidence of ventricular rupture is increased in patients with infarct expansion.[P13, S12] Whether infarct expansion contributes directly to the rupture or simply represents extensive transmural infarction is not known. Second, infarct expansion is mechanically disadvantageous because it augments the size of the dysfunctional zone and may exaggerate the severity or retard the recovery, if any occurs, of the wall motion disorder.[E2, F8] Third, infarct expansion undoubtedly contributes to development of chronic ventricular aneurysms.[H9, H11, P13, R12, S12, W3] Finally, infarct expansion is yet another factor that undermines the relationship between size of wall motion abnormality and true infarct size.

Reactive Hypertrophy

The infarcted ventricle can compensate for muscle loss associated with the infarction by developing hypertrophy of the remaining, normally perfused myocytes. This process—hypertrophy secondary to muscle loss—is called reactive hypertrophy.[A3, A4, C8, P14, R13] Reactive hypertrophy has been documented well in experimental studies of rats, and to a lesser extent in studies of dogs[G9, H12] and humans.[H7, H13, M12, S13] The hypertrophy is usually greatest in the areas adjacent to the infarct zone.[A3, A4, H12, P14] The net effect of reactive hypertrophy in smaller infarcts is the return of left ventricular mass to the pre-infarct level. In larger infarcts, this mechanism is not sufficient to compensate fully for all the muscle loss, and the final left ventricular mass is less than pre-infarct mass.

Many questions concerning the effects of reactive hypertrophy remain unanswered at present. These questions include the degree to which reactive hypertrophy contributes to the gradual improvement in ventricular function that is often seen following acute myocardial infarction. Furthermore, the adequacy of the vascular supply to cardiac muscle that undergoes reactive hypertrophy needs definition.

From an imaging standpoint, reactive hypertrophy has two implications: (1) It contributes to the complex ventricular remodeling process that ensues following an acute myocardial infarction. (2) It may be a contributing factor to the gradual improvement of ventricular function that occurs following completion of a myocardial infarction.

Compensatory Hyperfunction

When a segment of the left ventricular myocardium ceases to function as a result of trauma, ischemia, or infarction, the remaining myocardium almost immediately undergoes hyperfunction and thereby compensates, in part, for the loss. Compensatory hyperfunction has been documented through use of various imaging techniques, including M-mode and two-dimensional echocardiography,[P10] contrast ventriculography, and ultrafast computed tomography.[G10, H8, S14] This response is not primarily neurally mediated; rather, it occurs as a consequence of "internal unloading," which is conceptually similar to the development of a low impedance leak such as mitral regurgitation. The dyskinetic, ventricular segment no longer restrains the contraction of the normal myocardium. Although compensatory hyperfunction of the myocardium can be demonstrated within a few cardiac cycles of the onset of profound dysfunction in a remote myocardial segment, this hyperfunction does not persist for long. Most studies suggest that the hyperfunction recedes over a period of days to weeks toward the control level. In a few instances, cardiac hyperfunction may persist for a much longer period.

Compensatory hyperfunction is one of many factors that make measurements of global left ventricular function an unreliable and imprecise approach to estimating infarct or risk area size. In addition, compensatory hyperfunction extends the already broad range of what constitutes the normal function of a given ventricular segment. This problem further complicates any approach to developing criteria for identifying abnormally contracting segments.

DIASTOLIC VENTRICULAR FUNCTION

For many decades, physicians involved in cardiovascular medicine have focused their attention on systolic function of the left and right ventricles and, to a large extent, ignored diastolic function. At least three reasons can be found for their doing so. First, many investigators believed that the relationship between diastolic pressure and volume could not change acutely and could only be altered by chronic changes in the material properties of cardiac muscle, such as scarring related to infarction or significant hypertrophy. Second, few, if any, therapeutic approaches were available to modify diastolic ventricular function. Third, because diastolic function is a triphasic process, it is far more difficult to characterize than peak systolic ejection.

Now that the ability of ventricular diastolic function to change acutely is well established, therapeutic approaches to modifying diastolic function have been introduced, and sophisticated semi-automated methods of characterizing diastolic function have become commercially available. Furthermore, evidence is increasing that isolated left ventricular dysfunction is responsible for a significant percentage of cases of cardiac failure.[B1, D1, T1] Therefore, in the 1990's, evaluation of diastolic left ventricular and eventually right ventricular function will become progressively more important in the routine practice of cardiovascular medicine. At present, diastolic left ventricular function can be evaluated through use of several imaging techniques—conventional radionuclide ventriculography, digital angiography, standard contrast ventriculography, echocardiography, magnetic resonance imaging, and ultrafast computed tomography.

Basic Factors That Modulate Diastolic Left Ventricular Function

Diastolic left ventricular function is modulated primarily by diastolic left ventricular pressure and the material properties of the left ventricular myocardium. In the past two decades, however, several other important factors have been emphasized. These include active relaxation of the myocardium, mechanical ventricular interaction, the pericardium, diastolic suction, pulmonary-cardiac contact pressure, myocardial viscoelasticity, and engorgement of the coronary vasculature. Each of these factors affects specific segments of the diastolic function curve (Fig. 3–5). A detailed discussion of each of these factors is beyond the scope of this text. The interested reader is referred to a recent review.[G11]

Triphasic Nature of Diastolic Left Ventricular Filling

When heart rate in a normal heart is relatively slow during sinus rhythm (i.e., less than 120 beats per minute), the diastolic filling curve is triphasic. The initial phase is rapid diastolic filling, the second phase is diastasis or very slow diastolic filling, and the third phase is atrial contraction (Fig. 3–6). When heart rate increases, the diastasis phase becomes progressively abbreviated, and eventually, the rapid filling phase and the atrial contraction phase merge and cannot be easily separated.

Several imaging techniques—particularly, conventional radionuclide ventriculography—have focused on the rapid filling phase of diastole. Many other parameters, however, are used to characterize diastolic left ventricular function (Table 3–4). Parameters that require measurements of left ventricular pressure obviously cannot be studied using imaging techniques alone and instead require simultaneous acquisition of both pressure and volume data.

Heterogeneity of Diastolic Left Ventricular Function

Like systolic function, diastolic function of the normal left ventricle is heterogeneous. The filling rate of the apical segments of the left ventricle proceed more rapidly than do the basal segments of the left ventricle.[F9, R14, R15] Although this question has been subject to intensive investigation, the disease processes—particularly ischemia and infarction—most likely augment the heterogeneity of diastolic left ventricular function.

Table 3–4. PARAMETERS OF DIASTOLIC FUNCTION

Peak filling rate
Peak filling rate referenced to end-diastolic volume
Time to peak filling rate
Echocardiographic pulsed Doppler mitral valve velocimetry
Pressure-volume loops
Rate of reduction of left ventricular pressure (−dP/dt)

Clinical Parameters That Influence the Practical Assessment of Diastolic Left Ventricular Function

In addition to fundamental disease proceses, five parameters significantly influence the practical assessment of diastolic left ventricular function. These factors are (1) cardiac rhythm, (2) heart rate, (3) end-diastolic volume, (4) left ventricular systolic performance, and (5) patient age.

Cardiac Rhythm

Several methods of assessing diastolic left ventricular function can be employed only in hearts with regular cardiac rhythm, and the atrial contribution phase is obviously affected by both the timing and the vigor of atrial contraction. The imaging methods that require regular cardiac rhythm include equilibrium, radionuclide ventriculography, magnetic resonance imaging, and ultrafast computed tomography. Although other imaging methods can evaluate left ventricular diastolic function based on a single cardiac cycle (first-pass radionuclide ventriculography, Doppler echocardiography, digital angiography, and conventional contrast ventriculography), the interpretation of such data is complicated by irregular cardiac rhythm because of variation in end-diastolic volume and contractile state.

Heart Rate

The triphasic character of diastolic filling is demonstrable only at heart rates less than about 120 beats per minute. Hence, tachycardia complicates some approaches to assessing diastolic left ventricular function. In addition, extreme tachycardia may not permit complete relaxation of ventricular muscle, which would also modify diastolic left ventricular function.

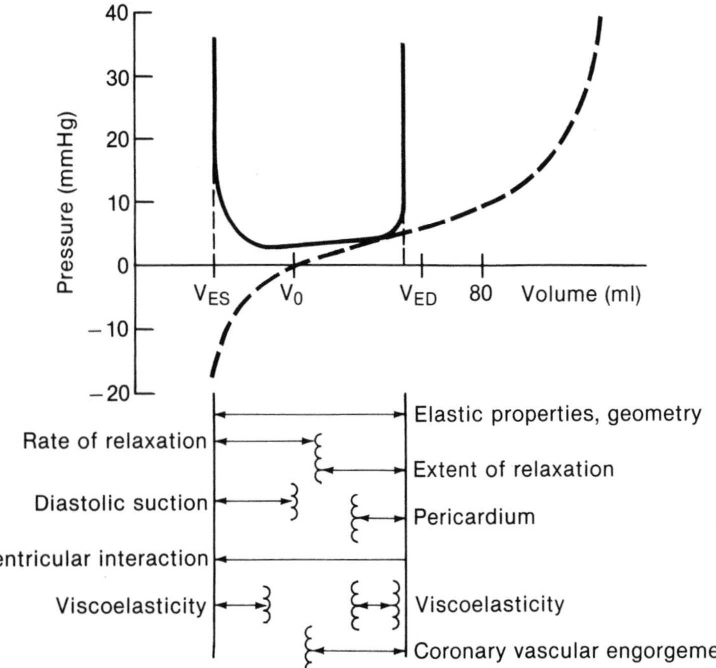

Figure 3–5. Many factors affect diastolic pressure during diastole, with different factors exerting their importance at different times. The elasticity and geometry (size and wall thickness) of the myocardium are important throughout diastole; the other factors are superimposed on the pressure because of the myocardial elasticity. During early diastole, active relaxation and the recoiling effect of elastic energy stored in the myocardium from the previous systole ("diastolic suction") determine the atrial-ventricular pressure gradient and the ventricular filling rate. The *dashed line* in the graph represents the purely elastic pressure volume curve of the myocardial shell and the absence of the component due to active relaxation from the previous beat. Late in diastole, ventricular interaction and the pericardium become important. Viscoelastic properties of the myocardium play a small role in rapid filling and atrial contraction. Coronary vascular engorgement has a small effect late in diastole. These various factors are listed below the curve, and the time course of their significance is indicated by the lines. V_{ES}—end-systolic volume; V_{ED}—end-diastolic volume; V_0—equilibrium volume. (From Gilbert, J. C., and Glantz, S. A.: Determinants of left ventricular filling and of the diastolic pressure-volume relation. Circ. Res. 64:827, 1989, with permission by the American Heart Association, Inc.)

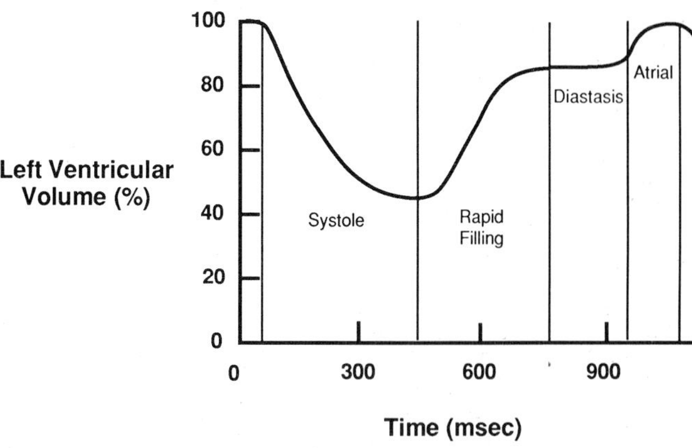

Figure 3–6. A diagrammatic representation of left ventricular volume versus time for a single cardiac cycle, illustrating the three major components of diastole. The initial rapid filling phase of diastolic filling is demonstrated by a marked rise in left ventricular volume over time. The second phase of diastole is diastasis, which is demonstrated by the short period of minimal change in volume. The third phase of diastolic filling is due to atrial contraction. Following atrial contraction, left ventricular volume decreases rapidly in association with systole.

End-Diastolic Left Ventricular Volume

The rapid filling segment of the diastolic filling curve is sensitive to alterations in end-diastolic left ventricular volume. Because end-diastolic volume can change significantly from the upright to the recumbent position, it must be considered in the interpretation of data. In addition, some approaches to assessing early diastolic left ventricular filling, particularly equilibrium radionuclide ventriculography, normalize the filling rate by dividing it by end-diastolic volume and report filling rates in units of end-diastolic volume per second.[R15] Obviously, with this approach, chronically dilated ventricles nearly always appear to have decreased filling rates, even when the absolute rate of left ventricular filling as expressed in milliliters per minute is significantly increased.

Systolic Left Ventricular Performance

Although investigators have noted several clinical states in which chronically slow diastolic filling of the left ventricle can be associated with normal systolic left ventricular function,[A5, D2, L7] the opposite is almost never the case. As systolic left ventricular function deteriorates, rapid diastolic filling declines in a parallel fashion. Because measurement of diastolic function is, with most techniques, more difficult and more expensive than assessment of systolic function, detailed measurements of diastolic left ventricular function do not provide useful diagnostic information in patients with impaired systolic function of the left ventricle. In this setting, evaluation of diastolic function can often be eliminated.

Age

The rapid diastolic filling phase of the left ventricle undergoes a progressive decline with age.[T1] This situation poses a major problem for the interpretation of rapid filling rates in older patients, because age-adjusted normal values are not well established and may vary depending on the precise method used to measure rapid diastolic filling.

Clinical Implications

When measurements of diastolic left ventricular function are interpreted, proper consideration of the patient's cardiac rhythm, heart rate, end-diastolic left ventricular volume, systolic left ventricular performance, and age is essential. In addition, pharmacologic, neural, and humoral factors undoubtedly can influence diastolic left ventricular function. If these factors are ignored, measurement of diastolic left ventricular filling may be of limited clinical value.

The systolic and diastolic functions of the left and right ventricles are complex and modulated by many potent influences. In addition, many of the currently available imaging techniques cannot precisely characterize the movements of the cardiac chambers in three-dimensional space. Therefore, physicians involved in the performance and interpretation of cardiac imaging procedures designed to assess left ventricular size and function must first be thoroughly familiar with the basic concepts in this area. Time and effort devoted to mastering these basic concepts result in improved application of any of the existing imaging technologies.

References

A

1. Arnold, J. M. O., Braunwald, E., Sandor, T., and Kloner, R. A.: Inotropic stimulation of reperfused myocardium with dopamine: Effects on infarct size and myocardial function. J. Am. Coll. Cardiol. 6:1026, 1985.
2. Akins, C. W., Pohost, G. M., DeSanctis, R. W., and Block, P. C.: Selection of angina-free patients with severe left ventricular dysfunction for myocardial revascularization. Am. J. Cardiol. 46:695, 1980.
3. Anversa, P., Beghi, C., Kikkawa, Y., and Olivetti, G.: Myocardial infarction in rats: Infarct size, myocyte hypertrophy and capillary growth. Circ. Res. 58:26, 1986.
4. Anversa, P., Lond, A. V., Levicky, V., and Guiden, G.: Left ventricular failure induced by myocardial infarction. I. Myocyte hypertrophy. Am. J. Physiol. 248:H876, 1985.
5. Abelmann, W. H., and Lorell, B. H.: The challenge of cardiomyopathy. J. Am. Coll. Cardiol. 13:1219, 1989.

B

1. Braunwald, E.: Clinical manifestations of heart failure. *In* Braunwald, E. (ed.): Heart Disease: A Textbook of Cardiovascular Medicine. 3rd ed. W.B. Saunders, Philadelphia, 1988, p. 471.
2. Borer, J. S., Bacharach, S. L., Green, M. V., et al.: Real-time radionuclide cine angiography in the non-invasive evaluation of global and regional left ventricular function at rest and during exercise in patients with coronary artery disease. N. Engl. J. Med. 296:839, 1977.
3. Bhargava, V., Shahetai, R., Ross, J., Jr., et al.: Influence of the pericardium on left ventricular diastolic pressure volume curves in dogs with sustained volume overload. Am. Heart J. 105:995, 1983.
4. Borow, K. M., Lang, R. M., Neumann, A., et al.: Physiologic mechanisms governing hemodynamic responses to positive inotropic therapy in patients with dilated cardiomyopathy. Circulation 77:625, 1988.
5. Bemis, L. E., Serur, J. R., Korkenhagen, D., et al.: Influence of right ventricular filling pressure on left ventricular pressure and dimension. Circ. Res. 34:498, 1974.
6. Barrett, E. J., Alger, J. R., and Zaret, B. L.: Nuclear magnetic resonance spectroscopy: Its evolving role in the study of myocardial metabolism. J. Am. Coll. Cardiol. 6:497, 1985.
7. Braunwald, E., and Kloner, R. A.: The stunned myocardium: Prolonged, postischemic ventricular dysfunction. Circulation 66:1146, 1982.
8. Bolli, R., Zhu, W.-X., Thornby, J. I., et al.: Time course and determinants of recovery of function after reversible ischemia in conscious dogs. Am. J. Physiol. 254:H102, 1988.
9. Bolli, R., Zhu, W.-X., Myers, H. L., et al.: Beta-adrenergic stimulation reverses postischemic myocardial dysfunction with producing subsequent functional deterioration. Am. J. Cardiol. 56:964, 1985.
10. Braunwald, E., and Rutherford, J. D.: Reversible ischemic left ventricular dysfunction: Evidence for "hibernating myocardium." J. Am. Coll. Cardiol. 8:1467, 1986.
11. Bodenheimer, M. M., Banka, V. S., Fooskee, C., et al.: Relationship between regional myocardial perfusion and the presence, severity and reversibility of asynergy in patients with coronary heart disease. Circulation 58:789, 1978.
12. Bulkley, B. H.: Site and sequelae of myocardial infarction. N. Engl. J. Med. 305:337, 1981.

C

1. Chaitman, B. R., Bristow, J. D., and Rahimtoola, S. A.: Left ventricular wall motion assessed by using a fixed external reference system. Circulation 48:1043, 1973.
2. Cox, D. A., and Vatner, S. F.: Myocardial function in areas of heterogeneous perfusion after coronary artery occlusion in conscious dogs. Circulation 66:1154, 1982.
3. Carmeliet, E.: Myocardial ischemia: Reversible and irreversible changes. Circulation 70:149, 1984.

D

1. Dougherty, A. H., Naccarelli, G. V., Gray, E. L., et al.: Congestive heart failure with normal systolic function. Am. J. Cardiol. 54:778, 1984.
2. Diver, D. J., Royal, H. D., Aroesty, J. M., et al.: Diastolic function in patients with aortic stenosis: Influence of left ventricular load reduction. J. Am. Coll. Cardiol. 12:642, 1988.

DETERMINANTS OF SYSTOLIC AND DIASTOLIC VENTRICULAR FUNCTION

E

1. Ellis, S. G., Wysone, J., Braunwald, E., et al.: Response of the reperfusion-salvaged, stunned myocardium to inotropic stimulation. Am. Heart J., 107:13, 1984.
2. Eaton, L. W., and Bulkley, B. H.: Expansion of acute myocardial infarction: Its relationship to infarct morphology in a canine model. Circ. Res. 49:80, 1981.

F

1. Fisher, E. A., DuBrow, I. W., and Hastreiter, A. R.: Right ventricular volume in congenital heart disease. Am. J. Cardiol. 36:67, 1975.
2. Ferlinz, J., Gorlin, R., Cohn, P. F., and Herman, M. V.: Right ventricular performance in patients with coronary artery disease. Circulation 52:608, 1975.
3. Feiring, A. J., Rumberger, J. A., Reiter, S. J., et al.: Sectional and segmental variability of left ventricular function: Experimental and clinical studies using ultrafast computed tomography. J. Am. Coll. Cardiol. 12:415, 1988.
4. Furey III, S. A., Zieske, H. A., and Levy, M. N.: The essential function of the right ventricle. Am. Heart J. 107:404, 1984.
5. Feiring, A. J., Johnson, M. R., Kioschos, J. M., et al.: The importance of the determination of the myocardial area at risk in the evaluation of the outcome of acute myocardial infarction in patients. Circulation 75:980, 1987.
6. Fisch, C.: Electrocardiography and vector cardiography. *In* Braunwald, E. (ed.): Heart Disease: A Textbook of Cardiovascular Medicine, 3rd ed. W.B. Saunders, Philadelphia, 1988, p. 180.
7. Flaherty, J. T., Weisfeldt, M. L., Bulkley, B. H., et al.: Mechanisms of ischemic myocardial cell damage assessed by phosphorus-31 nuclear magnetic resonance. Circulation 65:561, 1982.
8. Fletcher, P. J., Pfeffer, J. M., Pfeffer, M. A., and Braunwald, E.: Left ventricular diastolic pressure-volume relations in rats with healed myocardial infarction: Effects on systolic function. Circ. Res. 49:618, 1981.
9. Funai, J. T., Pandian, N. G., Salem, D. N., and Levine, H. J.: Heterogeneity of regional diastolic filling dynamics in normal left ventricle: Experimental two-dimensional echocardiographic studies. (Abstract.) J. Am. Coll. Cardiol. 5:426A, 1985.

G

1. Greenbaum, R. A., and Gibson, D. G.: Regional non-uniformity of left ventricular movement in man. Br. Heart J. 45:29, 1981.
2. Gibson, D. G., Brown, D. J., and Logan-Sinclair, R. B.: Analysis of regional left ventricular wall movement by phased array echocardiography. Br. Heart J. 40:1334, 1978.
3. Guyton, A. C., Jones, C. E., and Coleman, T. G.: Graphical analysis of cardiac output regulation. *In* Circulatory Physiology: Cardiac Output and Its Regulation. 2nd ed. W.B. Saunders, Philadelphia, 1973, p. 237.
4. Gobel, F. L., Nordstrom, L. A., Nelson, R. R., et al.: The rate-pressure product as an index of myocardial oxygen consumption during exercise in patients with angina pectoris. Circulation 57:549, 1978.
5. Grossman, W.: Evaluation of systolic and diastolic function of the myocardium. *In* Grossman, W. (ed.): Cardiac Catheterization and Angiography. 3rd ed. Lea & Febiger, Philadelphia, 1986, p. 301.
6. Glantz, S. A., and Parmley, W. W.: Factors which affect the diastolic pressure volume curve. Circ. Res. 42:171, 1978.
7. Gallagher, K. P., Osakada, G., Hess, O. M., et al.: Subepicardial segmental function during coronary stenosis and the role of myocardial fiber orientation. Circ. Res. 50:352, 1982.
8. Gerdes, A. M., Locket, S., and Zimmer, H.-G.: Function and cellular responses of the rat left heart to severe myocardial infarction. (Abstract.) Circulation 78(Suppl. II):II-648, 1988.
9. Ginzton, L. E., Thigpen, T., Garner, D., and Laks, M. M.: Post-infarction hypertrophy of the non-infarcted myocardium: A compensatory response? (Abstract.) Circulation 72(Suppl. III):III-66, 1985.
10. Gribier, A., Berland, J., Champond, O., et al.: Intracoronary thrombolysis in evolving myocardial infarction: Sequential angiographic analysis of left ventricular performance. Br. Heart J. 50:401, 1983.
11. Gilbert, J. C., and Glantz, S. A.: Determinants of left ventricular filling and of the diastolic pressure-volume relation. Circ. Res. 64:827, 1989.

H

1. Hoffman, E. A., and Ritman, E. L.: Body computed tomography: Shape and dimensions of cardiac chambers; importance of CT section thickness and orientation. Radiology 155:739, 1985.
2. Hajduczok, Z. D., Weiss, R. M., and Marcus, M. L.: Right ventricular mass can be accurately assessed by ultrafast computed tomography. (Abstract.) J. Am. Coll. Cardiol. 13:8A, 1989.
3. Hiratzka, L. F., Eastham, C., Doty, D., et al.: Directly measured coronary flow velocity/left ventricular wall thickening relationship in patients. (Abstract.) Circulation 68(Suppl. III):III–157, 1983.
4. Hansen, A. M., Gangadharan, V., Ramos, R. G., et al.: Sequence of mechanical, electrocardiographic and clinical effects of repeated coronary artery occlusion in human beings: Echocardiographic observations during coronary angioplasty. J. Am. Coll. Cardiol. 5:193, 1985.
5. Heyndrickx, G. R., Millard, R. W., McRitchie, R. J., et al.: Regional myocardial functional and electrophysiological alterations after a brief coronary artery occlusion in conscious dogs. J. Clin. Invest. 56:978, 1975.
6. Heyndrickx, G. R., Baig, H., Nellers, P., et al.: Depression of regional myocardial blood flow and wall thickening after brief coronary occlusions. Am. J. Physiol. 234:H653, 1978.
7. Homans, D. C., Sublett, E., Dai, X.-Z., and Bache, R. J.: Persistence of regional left ventricular dysfunction after exercise-induced myocardial ischemia. J. Clin. Invest. 77:66, 1986.
8. Hajduczok, Z., Weiss, R. M., Stanford, W., and Marcus, M. L.: Ventricular remodeling following infarction. (Abstract.) Circulation 78(Suppl. II):II-400, 1988.
9. Hodiman, J. S., and Bulkley, B. H.: Pathogenesis of left ventricular aneurysms: An experimental study in the rat model. Am. J. Cardiol. 50:83, 1982.
10. Hutchins, G. M., and Bulkley, B. H.: Infarct expansion vs. extension: Two different complications of acute myocardial infarction. Am. J. Cardiol. 41:1127, 1978.
11. Hirai, T., Fujita, M., Nakajima, H., et al.: Importance of collateral circulation for prevention of left ventricular aneurysm formation in acute myocardial infarction. Circulation 79:791, 1989.
12. Hood, W. B., Jr.: Experimental myocardial infarction. III. Recovery of left ventricular function in the healing phase: Contribution of increased fiber shortening in noninfarcted myocardium. Am. Heart J. 79:531, 1970.
13. Henning, H., O'Rourke, R. A., Crawford, M. H., et al.: Inferior myocardial infarction as a cause of asymmetric septal hypertrophy. Am. J. Cardiol. 41:817, 1978.

I

1. Ingels, N. B., Jr., Daughters II, G. T., Stinson, E. B., and Alderman, E. L.: Measurement of midwall myocardial dynamics in intact man by radiography of surgically implanted markers. Circulation 52:859, 1975.
2. Iskandrian, A. S., Hakki, A. H., DePace, N. L., et al.: Evaluation of left ventricular function by radionuclide angiography during exercise in normal subjects and in patients with chronic coronary heart disease. J. Am. Coll. Cardiol. 1:1518, 1983.

J

1. Jennings, R. B., and Reimer, K. A.: Lethal myocardial ischemic injury. Am. J. Pathol. 102:241, 1981.

K

1. Kong, Y., Morris, J. J., Jr., and McIntosh, H. D.: Assessment of regional myocardial performance from biplane cine angiograms. Am. J. Cardiol. 27:529, 1971.
2. Kaul, S., Boucher, C. A., Okada, R. D., et al.: Sources of variability in the radionuclide angiographic assessment of ejection fraction: A comparison of first pass and gated equilibration techniques. Am. J. Cardiol. 53:823, 1984.
3. Kajiya, F., Tsujiokak, H., Goto, M., et al.: Functional characteristics of intramyocardial capacitance vessels during diastole in the dog. Circ. Res. 58:476, 1986.
4. Klocke, F. J., Mates, R. E., Canty, J. M., Jr., and Ellis, A. K.: Coronary pressure flow relationships—controversial issues and probable implications. Circ. Res. 56:310, 1985.
5. Katz, A. M.: Regulation of myocardial contractility 1958–1983: An odyssey. J. Am. Coll. Cardiol. 1:42, 1983.
6. Kanaide, H., Yashimura, R., Makio, N., and Nakamura, M.: Regional myocardial function and metabolism during acute coronary artery occlusion. Am. J. Physiol. 242:H980, 1982.
7. Kerber, R. E., Marcus, M. L., Erhardt, J., et al.: Correlation between echocardiographically demonstrated segmental dyskinesis and regional myocardial perfusion. Circulation 52:1097, 1975.
8. Kloner, R. A., DeBoer, L. W. V., Darsee, J. R., et al.: Recovery from prolonged abnormalities of canine myocardium salvaged from ischemic necrosis by coronary reperfusion. Proc. Natl. Acad. Sci. USA 78:7152, 1981.
9. Krause, S. M., Jacobus, W. E., and Becker, L. C.: Alterations in sarcoplasmic reticulum Ca^{2+} transport in the postischemic "stunned" myocardium. (Abstract.) Circulation 74(Suppl II):II-67, 1986.

L

1. LeWinter, M. M., Kent, R. S., Kroener, J. M., et al.: Regional differences in myocardial performance in the left ventricle of the dog. Circ. Res. 37:191, 1975.
2. Lynch, P. R., and Bove, A. A.: Geometry of the left ventricle as studied by high-speed cine radiographic technique. Fed. Proc. 28:1330, 1969.
3. Lee, E., and Schiller, N. B.: Ambulatory and intraoperative transesophageal echocardiography. Cardiol. Clin. 7:511, 1989.
4. LeWinter, M. M., Kent, R. S., Kroener, J. M., et al.: Regional differences in myocardial performance in the left ventricle of the dog. Circ. Res. 37:191, 1975.
5. Lavallee, M., Cox, D., and Vatner, S. F.: Time required for myocardial function salvaged by coronary artery reperfusion to respond appropriately to stress. (Abstract.) Clin. Res. 30:483A, 1982.
6. Lieberman, A. N., Weiss, J. L., Jugdutt, B. I., et al.: Two-dimensional echocardiography and infarct size: Relationship of regional wall motion and thickening to the extent of myocardial infarction in the dog. Circulation 63:739, 1981.
7. Lorell, B. H., and Grossman, W.: Cardiac hypertrophy: The consequences for diastole. J. Am. Coll. Cardiol. 9:1189, 1987.

M

1. Mock, M. B., Ringvist, I., Fisher, L. D., et al.: Survival of medically treated patients in the coronary artery surgery study (CASS) registry. Circulation 66:562, 1982.
2. Mahoney, L. T., Smith, W., Noel, M. P., et al.: Measurement of right ventricular volume using cine computed tomography. Invest. Radiol. 22:451, 1987.
3. Marcus, M. L., Stanford, W., Hajduczok, Z., and Weiss, R. M.: Ultrafast computed tomography in the diagnosis of cardiac disease. Am. J. Cardiol. 64:54E, 1989.
4. McDonald, I. G.: The shape and movements of the human left ventricle during systole. Am. J. Cardiol. 26:221, 1970.
5. Mitchell, J. H., Wildenthal, K., and Mullins, C. B.: Geometrical studies of the left ventricle utilizing biplane cine fluorography. Fed. Proc. 28:1334, 1969.
6. Moynihan, P. F., Parisi, A. F., and Feldman, C. L.: Quantitative detection of regional left ventricular contraction abnormalities by two-dimensional echocardiography. I. Analysis of methods. Circulation 63:752, 1981.
7. Manno, B. V., Iskandrian, A. S., and Hakki, A.: Right ventricular function: Methodologic and clinical considerations in non-invasive scintigraphic assessment. J. Am. Coll. Cardiol. 3:1072, 1984.
8. Moe, G. K., Wood, E. H., and Visscher, M. B.: Aortic pressure and the diastolic volume loss of energy output in cardiac contraction. Proc. Soc. Exp. Biol. Med. 40:460, 1939.
9. Mitchell, J. H., Wallace, A. G., and Skinner, N. S., Jr.: Intrinsic effects of heart rate on left ventricular performance. Am. J. Physiol. 205:41, 1963.
10. Marshall, R. C., Tillisch, J. H., Phelps, M. E., et al.: Identification and differentiation of resting myocardial ischemia and infarction in man with positron computed tomography ^{18}F-labeled fluorodeoxyglucose and N-13 ammonia. Circulation 67:766, 1983.
11. Mehta, P. M., Alker, K. J., and Kloner, R. A.: Functional infarct expansion, left ventricular dilation and isovolumic relaxation time after coronary occlusion: A two-dimensional echocardiographic study. J. Am. Coll. Cardiol. 11:630, 1988.
12. McKay, R. G., Pfeffer, M. A., Pasternack, R. C., et al.: Left ventricular remodeling after myocardial infarction: A corollary to infarct expansion. Circulation 74:693, 1986.

N

1. Nixon, J. V., Brown, C. N., and Smitherman, T. C.: Identification of transient and persistent segmental wall abnormalities in patients with unstable angina by two-dimensional echocardiography. Circulation 65:1497, 1982.
2. Nicklas, J. M., Maughan, W. L., Ciuffo, A., et al.: The effect of varied systolic load on acute infarct expansion. (Abstract.) Clin. Res. 31:208A, 1983.

O

1. Olsen, G. O., Tyson, G. S., Maier, G. W., et al.: Dynamic ventricular interaction in the conscious dog. Circ. Res. 52:85, 1983.

P

1. Pandian, N. G., Skorton, D. J., Collins, S. M., et al.: Heterogeneity of left ventricular segmental wall thickening and excursion in 2-dimensional echocardiograms of normal human subjects. Am. J. Cardiol. 51:1667, 1983.
2. Pflugfelder, P. N., Sechtem, U. P., White, R. D., et al.: Quantification of regional myocardial function by rapid cine MR imaging. Am. J. Radiol. 150:523, 1988.
3. Poliner, L. R., Dehmr, G. J., Lewis, S. E., et al.: Left ventricular performance in normal subjects: A comparison of the responses to exercise in the upright and supine positions. Circulation 62:528, 1980.
4. Pagani, M., Vatner, S. F., Baig, H., and Braunwald, E.: Initial myocardial adjustments to brief periods of ischemia and reperfusion in the conscious dog. Circ. Res. 43:83, 1978.
5. Pernot, A.-C., Ingwall, J. S., Menasche, P., et al.: Evaluation of high-energy phosphate metabolism during cardioplegic arrest and reperfusion: A phosphorus-31 nuclear magnetic resonance study. Circulation 67:1296, 1983.
6. Przyklenk, K., and Kloner, R. A.: What factors predict recovery of contractile function in the canine model of the stunned myocardium? Am. J. Cardiol. 64:18F, 1989.
7. Przyklenk, K., and Kloner, R. A.: Superoxide dismutase plus catalase improve contractile function in the canine model of the "stunned myocardium." Circ. Res. 58:148, 1986.
8. Przyklenk, K., and Kloner, R. A.: Effect of verapamil on postischemic "stunned" myocardium: Importance of the timing of treatment. J. Am. Coll. Cardiol. 11:614, 1988.
9. Peck, W. W., Mancini, G. B. J., Slutsky, R. A., et al.: In vivo assessment by computed tomography of the natural progression of infarct size, left ventricular muscle mass and function after acute myocardial infarction in the dog. Am. J. Cardiol. 53:929, 1984.
10. Pandian, N. G., Koyanagi, S., Skorton, D. J., et al.: Relations between 2-dimensional echocardiographic wall thickening abnormalities, myocardial infarct size and coronary risk area in normal and hypertrophied myocardium. Am. J. Cardiol. 52:1318, 1983.
11. Pfeffer, M. A., and Pfeffer, J. M.: Ventricular enlargement and reduced survival after myocardial infarction. Circulation 75(Suppl. IV):IV93, 1987.
12. Pfeffer, M. A., Lamas, G. A., Vaughan, D. E., et al.: Effect of captopril on progressive ventricular dilation after anterior myocardial infarction. N. Engl. J. Med. 319:80, 1988.
13. Pirolo, J. S., Hutchins, G. M., and Moore, G. W.: Infarct expansion: Pathologic analysis of 204 patients with a single myocardial infarct. J. Am. Coll. Cardiol. 7:349, 1986.
14. Pfeffer, M. A., Pfeffer, J. M., Fishbein, M. C., et al.: Myocardial infarct size and ventricular function in rats. Circ. Res. 44:503, 1979.

R

1. Rappaport, E., Wong, M., Ferguson, R. E., et al.: Right ventricular volumes in patients with and without heart failure. Circulation 31:531, 1965.
2. Reiter, S. J., Rumberger, J. A., Feiring, A. J., et al.: Precision of measurements of right and left ventricular volume by cine computed tomography. Circulation 74:890, 1986.
3. Rankin, J. S., McHale, P. A., Arentzen, C. E., et al.: The three-dimensional dynamic geometry of the left ventricle in the conscious dog. Circ. Res. 39:304, 1976.
4. Ross, J., Jr., and Braunwald, E.: The study of left ventricular function in man by increasing resistance to ventricular ejection with angiotensin. Circulation 29:739, 1965.
5. Ross, J., Jr., Covell, J. W., and Sonnenblick, E. H.: The mechanics of left ventricular contraction in acute experimental cardiac failure. J. Clin. Invest. 46:299, 1967.
6. Ross, J., Jr., Gault, J. H., Mason, O. T., et al.: Left ventricular performance during muscular exercise in patients with and without cardiac dysfunction. Circulation 34:597, 1966.
7. Ross, J., Jr.: Acute displacement of the diastolic pressure volume curve of the left ventricle: Role of the pericardium and right ventricle. Circulation 59:32, 1979.
8. Rumberger, J. A., Feiring, A. J., Skorton, D. J., and Marcus, M. L.: Patterns of segmental ejection fraction in normal adults within ventricular levels. (Abstract.) Circulation 72(Suppl. II):II-721, 1985.
9. Reimer, K. A., Lowe, J. E., Rusmussen, M. M., and Jennings, R. B.: The wavefront phenomenon of ischemic cell death. I. Myocardial infarct size vs. duration of coronary occlusion in dogs. Circulation 56:786, 1977.
10. Robertson, W. S., Feigenbaum, H. S., Armstrong, W. F., et al.: Exercise echocardiography: A clinically practical addition in the evaluation of coronary artery disease. J. Am. Coll. Cardiol. 2:1085, 1983.
11. Rahimtoola, S. H.: The hibernating myocardium. Am. Heart J. 117:211, 1989.
12. Roberts, C. S., Maclean, D., Maroko, P. R., and Kloner, R. A.: Early and late remodeling of the left ventricle after acute myocardial infarction. Am. J. Cardiol. 54:407, 1984.
13. Rubin, S. A., Fishbein, M. C., and Swan, H. J. C.: Compensatory hypertrophy in the heart after myocardial infarction in the rat. J. Am. Coll. Cardiol. 1:1435, 1983.
14. Rumberger, J. A., Stark, C. A., Stanford, W., and Marcus, M. L.: Heterogeneity of diastolic filling in normal patients as assessed by cine computed tomography. (Abstract.) J. Am. Coll. Cardiol. 9:159A, 1987.
15. Rumberger, J. A., Weiss, R. M., Feiring, A. J., et al.: Patterns of regional diastolic function in the normal human ventricle: An ultrafast computed tomographic study. J. Am. Coll. Cardiol. 14:119, 1989.

S

1. Stark, C. A., Rumberger, J. A., Stanford, W., and Marcus, M. L.: Dobutamine stress with cine CT. (Abstract.) Circulation 74(Supp-II):II-122, 1987.
2. Shapiro, E., Marier, D. L., St. John Sutton, M. G., and Gibson, D. G.: Regional non-uniformity of wall dynamics in normal left ventricle. Br. Heart J. 45:264, 1981.
3. Sechtem, U., Sommerhoff, B. A., Markiewicz, W., et al.: Regional left ventricular wall thickening by magnetic resonance imaging: Evaluation in normal persons and patients with global and regional dysfunction. Am. J. Cardiol. 59:145, 1987.
4. Scharf, S. M., and Brumberger-Barnea, B.: Influence of coronary flow and pressure on cardiac function and coronary vascular volume. Am. J. Physiol. 224:918, 1973.
5. Starling, E. H.: Linacre Lecture on the Law of the Heart. Langmans Green and Co., London, 1915, p. 1918.
6. Suga, H., Katabatake, A., and Sagawa, K.: End-systolic pressure determines stroke volume from fixed end-diastolic volume in the isolated canine left ventricle under a constant contractile state. Circ. Res. 44:238, 1979.
7. Schroder, E., Kieso, R. A., Laughlin, D., et al.: Altered response of reperfused myocardium to repeated coronary occlusions in dogs. J. Am. Coll. Cardiol. 10:898, 1987.
8. Schelbert, H. R.: Myocardial ischemia and clinical applications of positron emission tomography. Am. J. Cardiol. 64:46E, 1989.
9. Shanes, J. G., Kondos, G. T., Levitsky, S., et al.: Coronary artery obstruction: A potentially reversible cause of dilated cardiomyopathy. Am. Heart J. 110:173, 1985.
10. Shearn, D. L., and Brent, B. N.: Coronary artery bypass surgery in patients with left ventricular dysfunction. Am. J. Med. 80:405, 1986.
11. Sasayama, S., Tomoika, H., Crozatier, B., et al.: Wall thickness and endocardial segment dynamics during chronic myocardial infarction in conscious dogs. (Abstract.) Am. J. Cardiol. 37:169, 1976.
12. Schuster, E. H., and Bulkley, B. H.: Expansion of transmural myocardial infarction: A pathophysiologic factor in cardiac rupture. Circulation 60:1532, 1979.
13. Stern, A., Kessler, K. M., Hammer, W. J., et al.: Septal-free wall disproportion in inferior infarction: The echocardiographic differentiation from hypertrophic cardiomyopathy. Circulation 58:700, 1978.
14. Serruys, P. W., Simoons, M. L., Soryapranata, H., et al.: Preservation of global and regional left ventricular function after early thrombolysis in acute myocardial infarction. J. Am. Coll. Cardiol. 7:729, 1986.

38
DETERMINANTS OF SYSTOLIC AND DIASTOLIC VENTRICULAR FUNCTION

T

1. Topol, E. J., Traill, T. A., and Fortuin, N. J.: Hypertensive hypertrophic cardiomyopathy of the elderly. N. Engl. J. Med. 312:277, 1985.
2. Tsakiris, A. G., Donald, D. E., Sturm, R. E., and Wood, E. H.: Volume ejection fraction and internal dimensions of left ventricle determined by biplane videometry. Fed. Proc. 28:1358, 1969.
3. Tennant, R., and Wiggers, C. J.: The effect of coronary occlusion on myocardial contraction. Am. J. Physiol. 112:351, 1935.
4. Tillisch, J. H., Bunken, R., Marshall, R., et al.: Predication of cardiac wall motion abnormalities predicted by using positron tomography. N. Engl. J. Med. 314:884, 1986.
5. Topol, E. J., Weiss, J. L., and Guzman, P. A.: Immediate improvement of dysfunctional myocardial segments after coronary revascularization: Detection by intraoperative transesophageal echocardiography. J. Am. Coll. Cardiol. 4:1123, 1984.
6. Theroux, P., Ross, J., Jr., Franklin, D., et al.: Regional myocardial function and dimensions early and late after myocardial infarction in the unanesthetized dog. Circ. Res. 40:158, 1977.

V

1. Vatner, S. F.: Correlation between acute reductions in myocardial blood flow and function in conscious dogs. Circ. Res. 47:201, 1980.

W

1. Weisman, H. F., Bush, D. E., Mannisi, J. A., and Bulkley, B. H.: Effect of extent of transmurality on infarct expansion. (Abstract.) Clin. Res. 32:447A, 1984.
2. Weisman, H. F., Bush, D. E., Mannisi, J. A., et al.: Early reperfusion reduces the severity of infarct expansion. (Abstract.) Circulation 70(Suppl. II):II-261, 1984.
3. Weisman, H. F., and Healy, B.: Myocardial infarct expansion, infarct extension and reinfarction: Pathophysiological concepts. Prog. Cardiovasc. Dis. 30:73, 1987.

Z

1. Zerhouni, E. A., Parish, D. M., Rogers, W. J., et al.: Human heart: Tagging with MR imaging—a method for noninvasive assessment of myocardial motion. Radiology 169:59, 1988.

■ Chapter 4

Myocardial Metabolism

■ *DENIS B. BUXTON, Ph.D.*

GENERAL CONSIDERATIONS 39
ENERGY PRODUCTION IN MYOCARDIUM 39
CARBOHYDRATE METABOLISM 39
Glucose Uptake and Phosphorylation 39
Glycogen Metabolism 40
Glycolysis 42
Pyruvate Metabolism 42
Pyruvate Dehydrogenase 42
Lactate Metabolism 44
Malate-Aspartate Shuttle 44
LIPID METABOLISM 44
Fatty Acid Metabolism 44
Uptake and Activation 44
Transport of Acyl Coenzyme A into Mitochondria 45
β-Oxidation 46
Ketone Metabolism 46
TRICARBOXYLIC ACID CYCLE ACTIVITY 46
Respiratory Control in Myocardium 47
MYOCARDIAL SUBSTRATE INTERACTIONS 48
Fasting 49
Diabetes and Insulin 49
Increased Work and Exercise 49
Catecholamines 49
Ischemia 49
Reperfusion 50
COMPARTMENTATION OF ENERGY UTILIZATION 50
PROTEIN TURNOVER 50
Protein Synthesis 50
Amino Acid Transport and Aminoacyl-tRNA Synthesis 50
Peptide Chain Initiation 50
Peptide Elongation and Termination 52
Protein Degradation 52
Regulation of Protein Turnover 52
Insulin and Diabetes 52
Starvation 52
Hypertrophy 52
Ischemia 53
SUMMARY 53

The myocardium displays eclectic substrate tastes and modifies its fuel selection in response to a wide range of influences, including nutritional status, hormonal signals, cardiac innervation, myocardial demand, and pathophysiologic status. The rate of energy production is closely linked to myocardial workload, allowing the heart to maintain its stores of high-energy phosphates—adenosine triphosphate (ATP) and phosphocreatine—at relatively constant levels during changes in workload or substrate utilization. This chapter summarizes the major myocardial energy-producing metabolic pathways and discusses the regulation of these pathways under different physiologic and pathophysiologic conditions. Regulation of the protein synthetic and degradative pathways under varying metabolic conditions is also addressed. For additional information on cardiac muscle metabolism, the reader is referred to several excellent reviews.[L1, N1, R1]

GENERAL CONSIDERATIONS

Regulation of biochemical pathways has traditionally been considered in terms of rate-limiting steps that control the flux through the pathway. The elegant studies of Kacser and Burns have demonstrated that this concept is an oversimplification, and that limitation of flux through a pathway cannot be attributed solely to a single step.[K1, K2] For the purposes of this general overview of myocardial metabolism, however, the less rigorous approach of considering rate-limiting steps is used, because most experimental work on myocardial metabolism is based on this approach.

ENERGY PRODUCTION IN MYOCARDIUM

Under normoxic conditions, the vast majority of myocardial energy production takes place via the complete oxidation of fuels to carbon dioxide and water. The pathways of oxidative myocardial energy production can be divided into three sections (Fig. 4–1). In the first section, the many fuels that can contribute to myocardial energy production are broken down to acetyl coenzyme A (acetyl-CoA) and other tricarboxylic acid cycle intermediates. In the second section, oxidation of acetyl-CoA via the tricarboxylic acid (TCA) cycle, yielding carbon dioxide and water, is coupled to reduction of the oxidized form of nicotinamide-adenine dinucleotide (NAD^+) and flavin adenine dinucleotide (FAD) to NADH and $FADH_2$, respectively. Finally, NADH and $FADH_2$ are reoxidized by transfer of electrons to molecular oxygen via the electron transport chain. Movement of electrons through the electron transport chain is coupled to the vectorial pumping of protons out of the mitochondrion to form a proton gradient, and ATP synthesis is in turn coupled to return of protons down the gradient via adenosine triphosphatase (ATPase).

The pathways for production of acetyl-CoA from the various myocardial substrates are now considered.

CARBOHYDRATE METABOLISM

Glucose Uptake and Phosphorylation

Entry of glucose into myocardial cells occurs via carrier-mediated facilitated diffusion, which requires no energy or counter-ion. Transport of glucose in myocardium is acutely regulated by insulin and other hormones. Insulin stimulation of glucose transport activity in myocardium occurs primarily through increased maximum transport velocity rather than through changes in the apparent affinity (K_m) of the carrier for glucose.[C1] This effect is believed to be achieved at least in part by the reversible, stoichiometric, energy-dependent translocation of glucose transporters from an intracellular pool to the surface of the sarcolemma.[S1] Glucose transport is accelerated by anoxia, increased cardiac work in the absence of insulin, and epinephrine and is inhibited by oxidation of fatty acids, ketone bodies, and pyruvate.[R2] Transport of glucose is not limiting in the presence of adequate glucose levels with high insulin levels, at high workloads, or in hypoxia, but glucose metabolism is limited in the absence of insulin and at low workloads in normoxia.

Once inside the cell, glucose is phosphorylated by the ATP-dependent hexokinase reaction. When glucose transport is activated, phosphorylation of glucose becomes rate-limiting. Hexokinase is present as three isozymes in muscle and is also found in both soluble and particulate forms.[N1] Both forms are inhibited noncompetitively by glucose-6-phosphate, and this inhibition appears to be the major regulatory factor in vivo.[E1] Adenosine diphosphate (ADP) and adenosine monophosphate (AMP) also inhibit competitively with magnesium (Mg) ATP^{2-}. Rates of glucose phosphorylation in vivo were found to correlate well with those predicted from the kinetic properties of the enzyme and intracellular concentrations of substrates and effectors.[E1] Dephosphorylation of the glucose-6-phosphate analog fluorodeoxyglucose-6-phosphate has been demonstrated to occur at a low but significant rate,[K3] which raises the possibility of futile cycling between glucose and glucose-6-phosphate.

Glucose-6-phosphate can now enter one of three alternative pathways in myocardium: storage as glycogen, glycolytic breakdown to pyruvate, or the pentose phosphate pathway (Fig. 4–2). The pentose phosphate pathway yields ribose and the reduced form of nicotinamide-adenine dinucleotide phosphate (NADPH) primarily for biosynthetic purposes and is quantitatively of little importance in glucose oxidation.[G1]

Glycogen Metabolism

Glycogen is synthesized and degraded by two separate pathways. Synthesis of glycogen proceeds via isomerization of glucose-6-phosphate to glucose-1-phosphate, followed by the uridine triphosphate (UTP)–dependent formation of uridine diphosphate glucose (UDPG) by UDPG pyrophosphorylase. Uridine diphosphate glucose is then transferred to the glycogen chain. The transfer of the α-glucosyl residue to the 4-glucosyl position of the

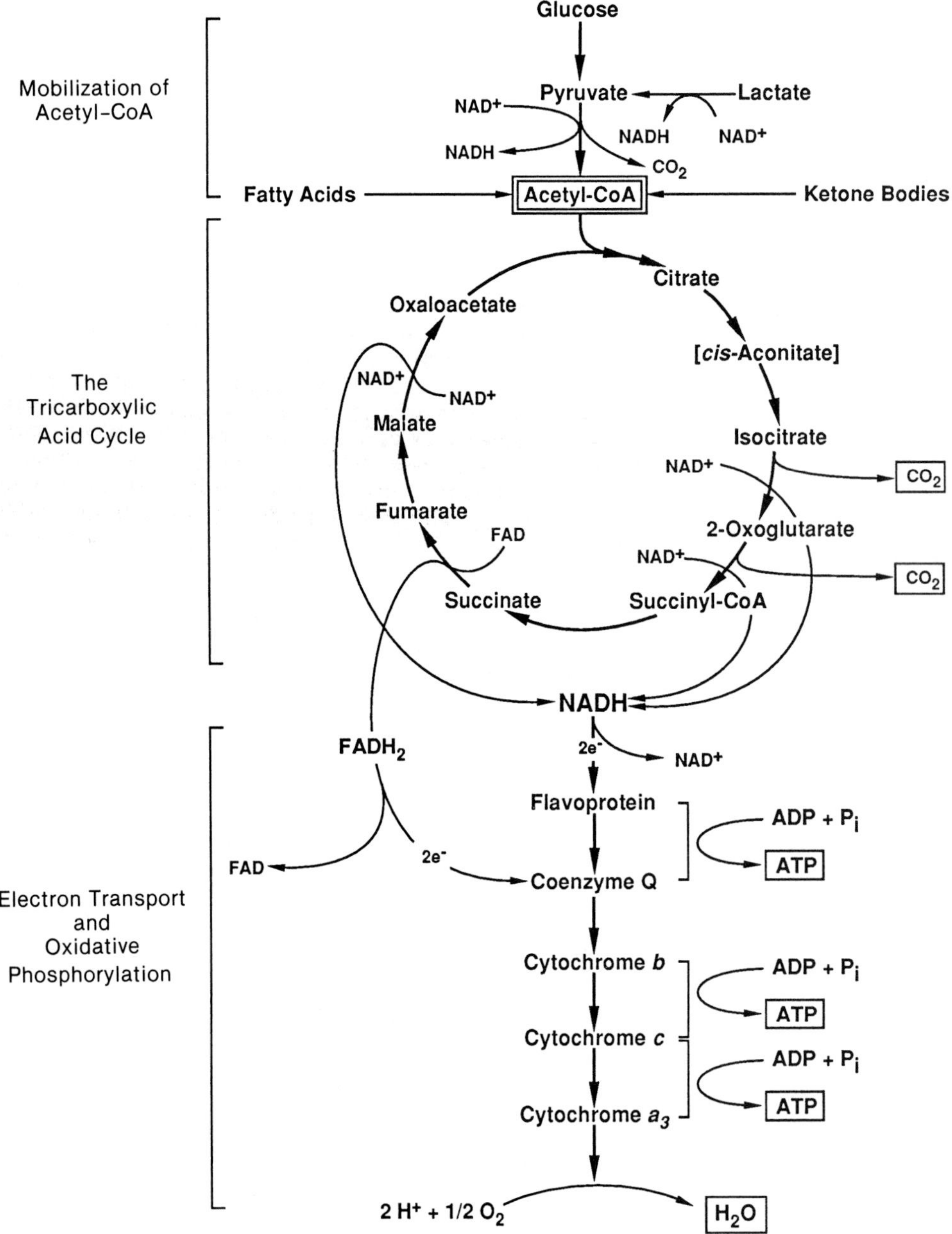

Figure 4–1. Catabolic breakdown of substrates. In the first stage, fuels are broken down to acetyl-CoA by the individual catabolic pathways. In the second stage, acetyl-CoA is oxidized to carbon dioxide by the tricarboxylic acid cycle, producing reducing equivalents (reduced coenzymes). In the third stage, electrons flow from the reduced coenzymes to molecular oxygen via the electron transport chain, leading to ATP synthesis via oxidative phosphorylation. (Modified from Lehninger, A. L.: Biochemistry. Worth, New York, 1975, p. 465.)

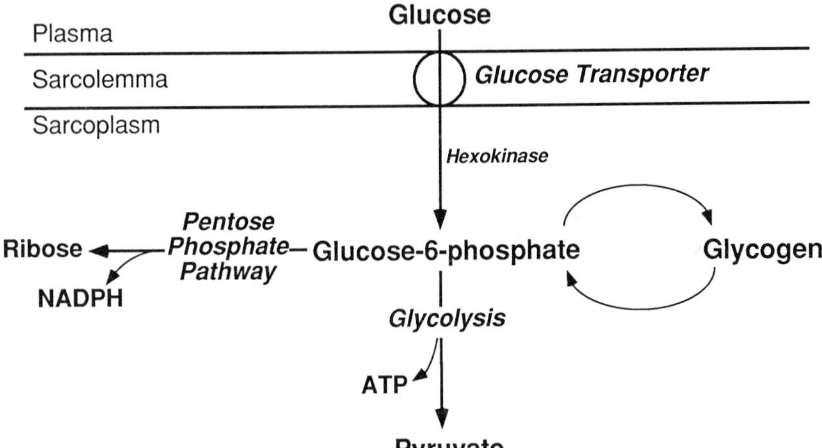

Figure 4–2. Pathways of glucose utilization.

chain is catalyzed by glycogen synthetase, which requires a primer of at least four glucose residues, formed by an additional enzyme and carrier protein.[K4] A further enzyme, 1,4-α-glucan branching enzyme, inserts branch points in the growing chain by transferring six or seven glucosyl residues from the end of the chain to form an α(1→6) linkage with the 6-hydroxyl group of a glucosyl residue. The branched structure of glycogen allows more rapid mobilization of glucosyl residues, because degradation of glycogen can occur simultaneously on the multiple branches.

Degradation of glycogen requires glycogen phosphorylase, which cleaves the terminal α(1→4) glycosidic linkage at the nonreducing end of the glycogen chain by phosphorolytic introduction of orthophosphate. The products are glucose-1-phosphate and a glycogen chain with one less glucose unit. This is followed by isomerization of glucose-1-phosphate to glucose-6-phosphate by phosphoglucomutase. Because glycogen phosphorylase cannot cleave α(1→6) glycosidic linkages, a debranching enzyme, hydrolytic amylo-1,6-glucosidase, removes branch points, allowing glycogen phosphorylase to continue progressive cleavage of the glycogen chain.

Regulation of glycogen metabolism for skeletal muscle has been studied in detail, and cardiac muscle is generally assumed to follow a similar pattern.[R1] In skeletal muscle, glycogen phosphorylase and glycogen synthetase are regulated in a coordinated fashion, thus limiting futile cycling and producing a large amplification of the stimulus by the enzymatic cascade systems (Fig. 4–3). Glycogen phosphorylase exists in phosphorylated and dephosphorylated forms: The phosphorylated enzyme is termed *a*, and the dephosphorylated enzyme is termed *b*. Phosphorylation of the *b* form is catalyzed by phosphorylase kinase, and dephosphorylation of *a* is catalyzed by the same protein phosphatase involved in activation of glycogen synthetase. Glycogen phosphorylase *a* is active in the absence of AMP at high concentrations of the substrates glycogen and inorganic phosphate, and it requires AMP only at low substrate concentrations. In contrast,

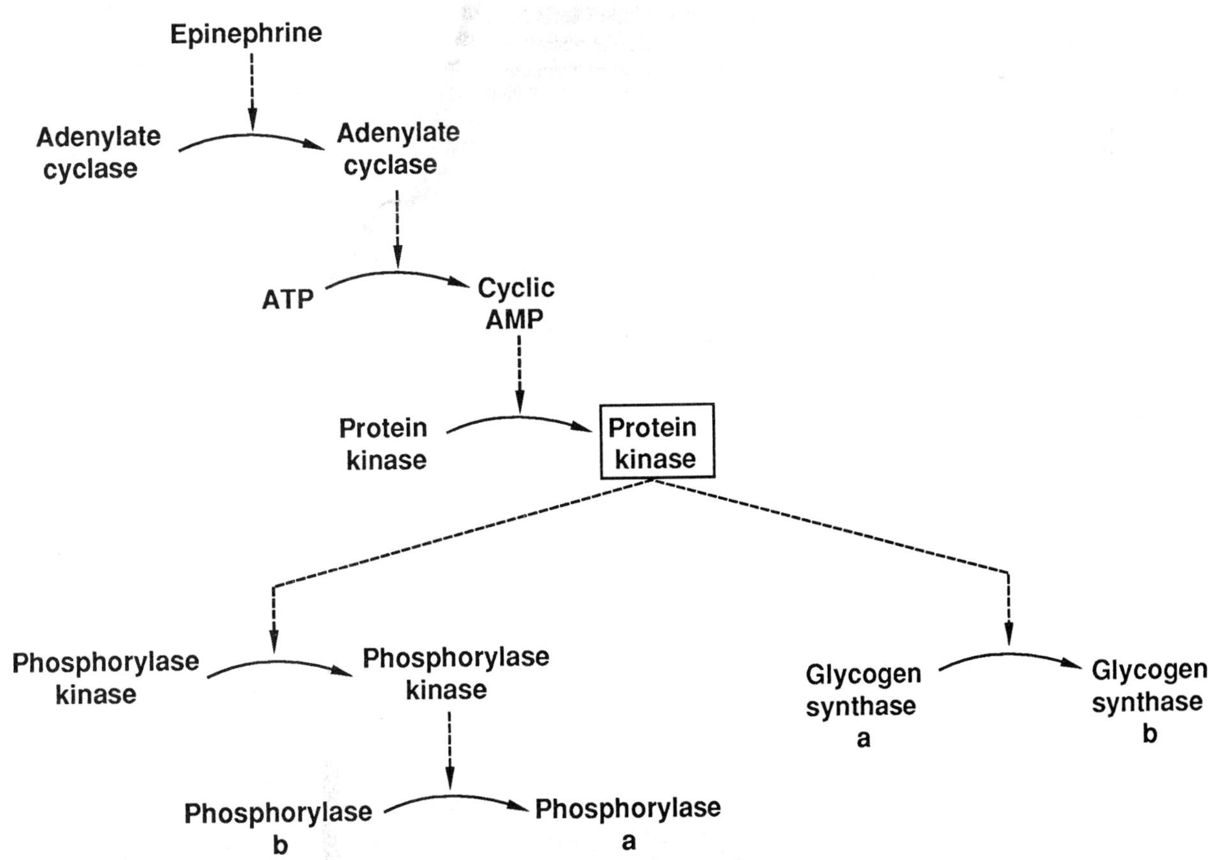

Figure 4–3. Regulation of glycogen phosphorylase and synthetase by covalent modification.

phosphorylase *b* requires AMP for activity; the activation by AMP is antagonized by ATP and glucose-6-phosphate.

The enzyme responsible for covalent activation of phosphorylase, phosphorylase kinase, is also regulated in turn by phosphorylation and dephosphorylation. Activation by phosphorylation is catalyzed by cyclic adenosine monophosphate (cAMP)–dependent protein kinase, while protein phosphatase again carries out the dephosphorylation reaction. Activity of phosphorylase kinase is Ca^{2+}-dependent, which allows glycogen breakdown to be coordinated with contractility on a beat-to-beat basis by the transient increase in cytosolic calcium concentration.

Glycogen synthetase also exists in dephosphorylated and phosphorylated forms, termed *a* and *b* respectively. Cyclic AMP–dependent protein kinase and protein phosphatase catalyze interconversion of the two forms of glycogen synthetase. Glycogen synthetase *a* is active in the absence of glucose-6-phosphate and only weakly inhibited by ATP, ADP, and inorganic phosphate. Glucose-6-phosphate lowers the K_m for UDPG, but has no effect on maximum transport velocity. In contrast, glycogen synthetase *b* requires a glucose-6-phosphate–mediated increase in maximum transport velocity for full activation, because it has only low activity in the absence of the effector. Adenosine triphosphate, ADP, and inorganic phosphate strongly inhibit glycogen synthetase *b* competitively with glucose-6-phosphate. Under normal in vivo conditions, the *a* form is active, whereas the *b* form is inactive.

In myocardium, the importance of inactivation of glycogen synthetase during activation of phosphorylase is less apparent than in skeletal muscle, because the synthetase appears to be 80 to 90 percent in the *b* form under basal conditions, and most studies show no further inactivation of glycogen synthetase in response to catecholamines under conditions in which glycogen phosphorylase is activated.[G2, M1]

Glycolysis

The reactions involved in the breakdown of glucose to pyruvate by glycolysis are shown in Figure 4–4. The pathway can be divided into two halves. In the first half, from glucose to the triose phosphates dihydroxyacetone phosphate and glyceraldehyde-3-phosphate, ATP is utilized in two priming steps. In the second half, from the triose phosphates to pyruvate, two ATP molecules are produced from each of the two triose phosphates, producing a net gain of two ATP molecules per glucose molecule. In addition, two molecules of NADH are produced for production of ATP via the electron transport chain after transfer of the reducing equivalents to the mitochondria via the malate-aspartate shuttle.

Regulation of glycolysis under most conditions is believed to reside at the level of phosphofructokinase, an enzyme whose activity can be regulated in vivo by a large number of allosteric effectors.[U1] The precise physiologic roles of the various effectors of phosphofructokinase are not fully understood. Phosphofructokinase is inhibited by ATP, phosphocreatine, and citrate and is activated by ADP, AMP, inorganic phosphate and the end product, fructose-1,6-bisphosphate. Allosteric control of phosphofructokinase is sensitive to pH, showing decreased allosteric sensitivity as the pH is increased from 6.8 to 7.3.[M2]

Increased citrate levels are believed to be important in inhibiting phosphofructokinase when fatty acid oxidation rates are high,[M2] but they cannot explain increased glycolysis observed in hearts perfused with insulin and glucose, in which citrate levels also rise.[O1] The recent discovery of fructose-2,6-bisphosphate as a potent stimulator of phosphofructokinase,[H1, U2] and demonstration that fructose-2,6-bisphosphate is required for in vitro activity of phosphofructokinase purified from perfused rat hearts,[N2] indicate an additional potential control mechanism. Fructose-2,6-bisphosphate is synthesized from fructose-6-phosphate by phosphofructokinase-2 and is broken down by fructose-2,6-bisphosphatase. Further experiments in perfused rat hearts demonstrated that changes in glycolytic rate induced by insulin or increased work correlated well with changes in the substrate, fructose-6-phosphate, and the activator fructose-2,6-bisphosphate, but not with other effectors.[L3] An additional level of control of phosphofructokinase may consist of covalent modification. Epinephrine activation appears to activate phosphofructokinase via covalent modification, possibly phosphorylation, in addition to changes in effector concentrations.[C2, N2] Also, evidence has been found for covalent activation of myocardial phosphofructokinase-2 in response to insulin[R3] and epinephrine.[N2]

When phosphofructokinase is activated, glyceraldehyde-3-phosphate dehydrogenase may become rate-limiting for glycolysis under certain conditions, including ischemia[R4] and extremely high workloads.[K5] Regulation of glyceraldehyde-3-phosphate dehydrogenase occurs via product inhibition by NADH and 1,3-diphosphoglycerate. Glycolysis is probably limited by the rate of disposal of cytosolic NADH, which must be reoxidized either by the malate aspartate shuttle or by lactate dehydrogenase.[K5]

Pyruvate Metabolism

Pyruvate generated in the cytosol by glycolysis can undergo one of several processes. Lactate dehydrogenase, a near-equilibrium cytosolic enzyme, converts pyruvate to lactate, regenerating NAD^+ from NADH simultaneously. In normoxia this pathway is less important, but in hypoxia it is increased, and the NAD^+ formed in this manner is important for maintenance of glycolysis. Similarly, formation of alanine by alanine aminotransferase, in which glutamate is used as an amino-group donor, occurs primarily in the cytosol by a near-equilibrium reaction and is accelerated by hypoxia. Oxidation of pyruvate by pyruvate dehydrogenase and carboxylation to oxaloacetate by pyruvate carboxylase take place in the mitochondrial matrix and thus require transport of pyruvate across the inner mitochondrial membrane. This transport is achieved by the monocarboxylate carrier.[M3] Pyruvate carboxylation to oxaloacetate represents a method by which the levels of tricarboxylic acid cycle intermediates can be increased, a process termed anaplerosis.

Pyruvate Dehydrogenase

Under normoxic conditions, the main route for pyruvate disposition is oxidation to acetyl-CoA by pyruvate dehydrogenase. Pyruvate dehydrogenase consists of a high-molecular-weight complex containing multiple copies of three polypeptides that catalyze a series of reactions: pyruvate decarboxylase, dihydrolipoyl acetyltransferase, and dihydrolipoyl dehydrogenase.[R5, W1] The pyruvate decarboxylase reaction is essentially irreversible under physiologic conditions, so the enzyme represents a vital committed step in breakdown of carbohydrate and hence in myocardial fuel selection. Not surprisingly, therefore, the pyruvate dehydrogenase complex is tightly regulated. Two interrelated regulatory mechanisms—allosteric regulation and covalent modification by a cycle of phosphorylation and dephosphorylation—operate to control the activity of pyruvate dehydrogenase (Fig. 4–5).[O2, R5, W1]

Allosteric control is mediated by feedback inhibition by the reaction products NADH and acetyl-CoA, which compete with NAD^+ and CoA respectively. Phosphorylation and inactivation of the pyruvate decarboxylase subunit of pyruvate dehydrogenase are mediated by an intrinsic kinase activity tightly bound to the pyruvate dehydrogenase complex. Pyruvate dehydrogenase kinase activity is stimulated by high ratios of [ATP]/[ADP], [acetyl/CoA]/[CoA], and [NADH]/[NAD^+] and inhibited by pyruvate, Ca^{2+}, and Mg^{2+}. The products of the pyruvate dehydrogenase reaction, acetyl-CoA and NADH, thus regulate activity of the complex both directly by allosterism and indirectly via kinase-mediated covalent inhibition. Reactivation by removal of the phosphate is accomplished by a phosphatase, pyruvate dehydrogenase phosphatase, which is not tightly bound to the pyruvate dehydrogenase complex. The phosphatase is stimulated by Ca^{2+} and dependent on Mg^{2+}.

In diabetes and starvation, myocardial pyruvate dehydrogenase

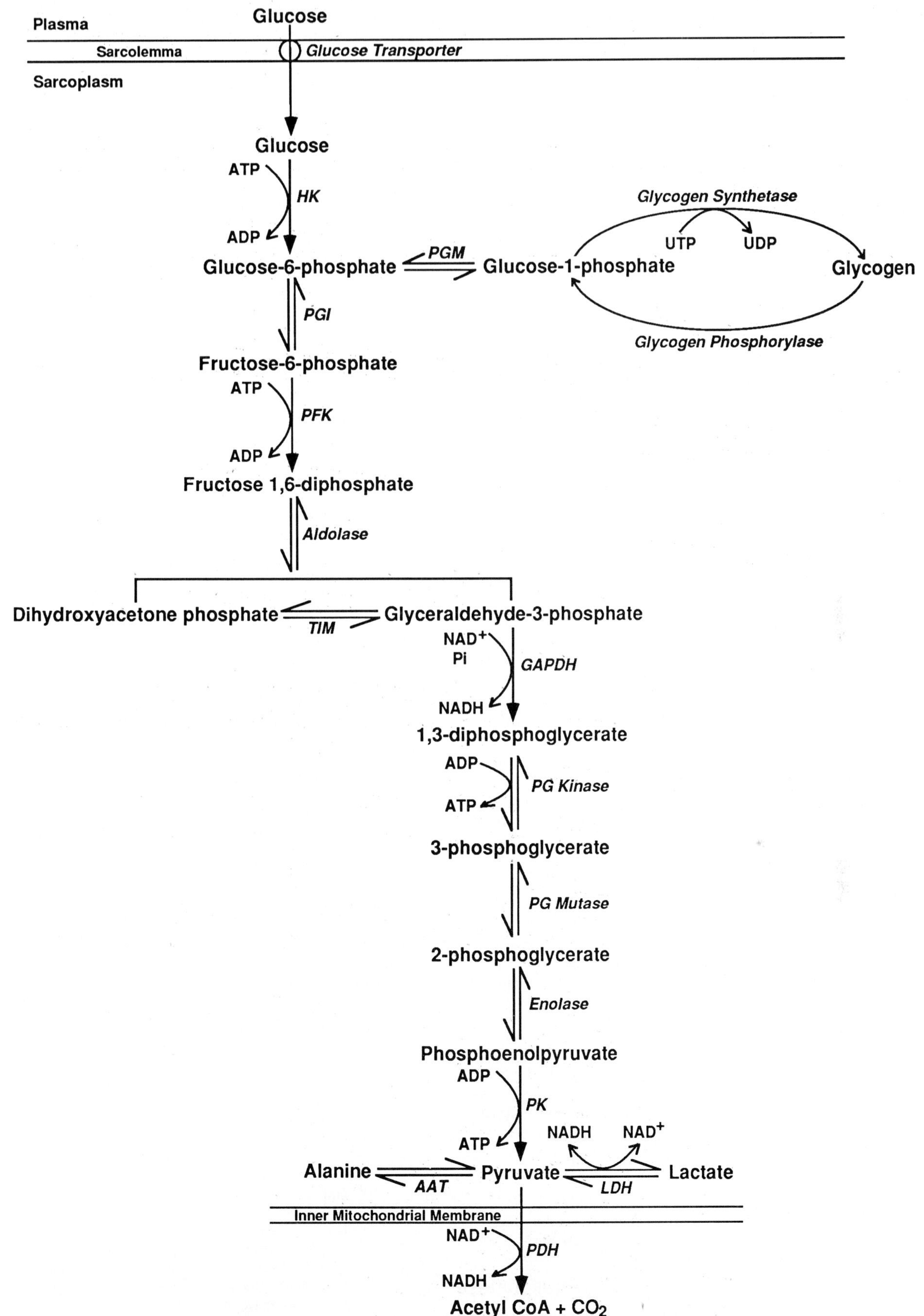

Figure 4–4. Glucose metabolism in myocardium. Under aerobic conditions, most glucose taken up is broken down to pyruvate and ultimately to carbon dioxide and water via the tricarboxylic acid cycle. In hypoxia and ischemia, release of lactate and alanine is increased. HK—hexokinase; PGM—phosphoglucomutase; PGI—phosphoglucoisomerase; PFK—phosphofructokinase; TIM—triosephosphate isomerase; GAPDH—glyceraldehyde-3-phosphate dehydrogenase; PG kinase—phosphoglycerate kinase; PG mutase—phosphoglycerate mutase; PK—pyruvate kinase; AAT—alanine aminotransferase; LDH—lactate dehydrogenase; PDH—pyruvate dehydrogenase. (Modified from Taegtmeyer, H.: Myocardial metabolism. *In* Phelps, M. E., et al. (eds.): Positron Emission Tomography and Autoradiography: Principles and Applications for the Brain and Heart. Raven Press, New York, 1986, p. 149.)

is present almost entirely in the inactive phosphorylated form, and reactivation of the enzyme by pyruvate or dichloroacetate, inhibitors of the kinase reaction, is decreased.[R1]

Lactate Metabolism

Exogenous lactate is readily taken up and metabolized by myocardium,[D1] and evidence exists for a stereospecific transporter.[M4] Lactate is then converted to pyruvate by lactate dehydrogenase, and the pyruvate enters the tricarboxylic acid cycle as acetyl-CoA produced by the pyruvate dehydrogenase reaction. Under normoxic conditions, lactate utilization in dogs was proportional to the arterial lactate concentration up to about 4.5 mM lactate. At this concentration, approximately 90 percent of myocardial oxygen consumption was supplied by lactate.[D2] In hypoxia, lactate utilization is limited by high cytosolic NADH levels, which push the lactate dehydrogenase equilibrium toward lactate. Decreased pyruvate utilization by pyruvate dehydrogenase also increases net lactate formation through the glycolytic pathway. In humans, recent experiments using dual carbon-labeled substrates have demonstrated that even during net chemical extraction of lactate, release of lactate from myocardium occurs.[G3, W2] In patients with coronary artery disease, lactate derived from exogenous glucose constitutes about 25 percent of lactate release at rest in the absence of clinical evidence for ischemia.[W2]

Malate-Aspartate Shuttle

The inner mitochondrial membrane is impermeable to NAD^+ and NADH, which means that NADH formed in the cytosol by glycolysis must be transported into the mitochondrion by an indirect mechanism. In cardiac muscle, this mechanism is the malate-aspartate shuttle (Fig. 4–6), in which oxaloacetate, generated by transamination of aspartate, is reduced to malate in the cytosol, thereby regenerating NAD^+. Cytosolic malate undergoes electroneutral exchange with mitochondrial 2-oxoglutarate and, in the mitochondrion, is reoxidized to oxaloacetate by malate dehydrogenase. In this latter reaction, mitochondrial NAD^+ is converted to NADH, completing the transfer of reducing equivalents from cytosolic to mitochondrial NADH. Transamination of oxaloacetate forms aspartate, which exchanges with glutamate across the mitochondrial membrane to complete the shuttle. Aspartate efflux in exchange for glutamate entry is accompanied by uptake of a proton; thus, the exchange is driven by the mitochondrial membrane potential.[R1] When glucose is used as the myocardial fuel, flux through the malate dehydrogenase reaction is approximately double the flux through the other reactions of the TCA cycle, because malate is also being delivered to the enzyme from the cytosol, bringing in the reducing equivalents from glycolysis.[R1]

LIPID METABOLISM

Fatty Acid Metabolism

Uptake and Activation

Investigators have long recognized that under most conditions fatty acids constitute the preferred fuel for myocardial energy supply.[B1] Nevertheless, the metabolism of fatty acids, the main pathways of which are shown in Figure 4–7, is less understood than carbohydrate metabolism. The heart is able to use both nonesterified fatty acids, which are largely bound to albumin in the circulation, and circulating triglycerides, which can be broken down by the lipoprotein lipase found at the extracellular surface in myocardium and other extrahepatic cells.[R1] The relative importance of these two sources of fatty acid has not been well characterized. The uptake of fatty acids into cells is also poorly understood. Most investigators believe that uptake occurs through a simple process of diffusion,[D3] although others have argued for the existence of a specific carrier in addition to the process of diffusion.[S2, S3] Recent studies have demonstrated a protein in myocyte membranes with high binding affinity for long-chain fatty acids; a specific antibody against this protein was able to reduce both binding and uptake of long-chain fatty acids by myocytes. In general, fatty acid uptake is governed by the circulating nonesterified fatty acid levels and the rate of intracellular fatty acid utilization.[R1]

On entering the cell, fatty acids are bound to a soluble protein, termed fatty acid binding protein.[G4, S4] The physiologic significance of fatty acid binding protein has not been clarified.[S4] Subsequent metabolism of fatty acids requires activation by formation of a coenzyme A thioester. Acyl coenzyme A synthesis requires hydrolysis of ATP to produce AMP and inorganic pyrophosphate. The location of the acyl-CoA synthetases responsible for this reaction depend on the chain length of the fatty acid; short-chain acyl-CoA synthetases, which activate fatty acids of C_8 or shorter, are present in the mitochondrion.[G5] Thus, short-chain fatty acids can be oxidized by heart mitochondria in the absence of external carnitine or coenzyme A. In contrast, the long-chain fatty acids, which in general are of much greater physiologic importance, are activated to their coenzyme A derivatives via extramitochondrial acyl-CoA synthetases, for which the majority of the activity is bound to the mitochondrial outer membrane.[D4]

Following activation, long-chain acyl-CoA can be either esterified to form triglyceride, a process taking place in the cytosol, or oxidized to acetyl-CoA, which takes place intramitochondrially. The regulation of partitioning between these two pathways has also not been clarified; increased net esterification of fatty acids

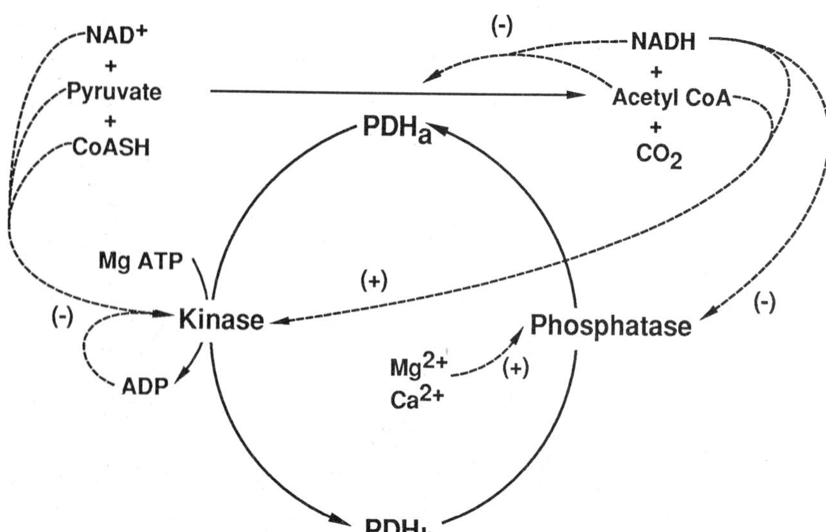

Figure 4–5. Regulation of pyruvate dehydrogenase by allosteric and covalent mechanisms. In addition to direct feedback product inhibition of the active pyruvate dehydrogenase (PDH_a), substrates, products, and metal ions modulate the reversible covalent inactivation to the phosphorylated PDH_b by allosteric effects on the kinase/phosphatase system.

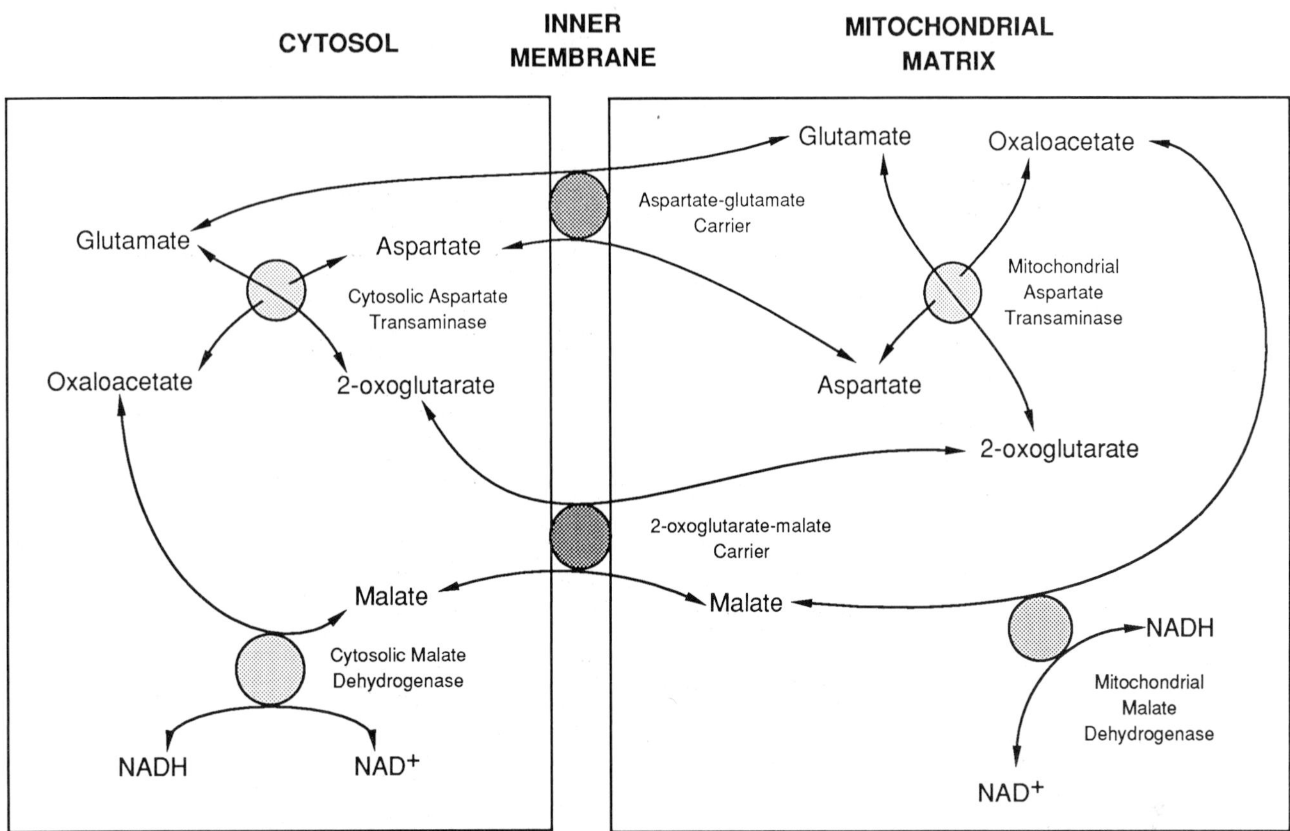

Figure 4–6. The malate-aspartate shuttle. The shuttle allows the reversible transfer of reducing equivalents, which are produced in the cytosol during breakdown of glucose to pyruvate, to the mitochondrial electron transport chain. Three molecules of ATP are produced from ADP for each cytosolic NADH transferred to the mitochondrion. (Modified from Lehninger, A. L.: Biochemistry. Worth, New York, 1975, p. 535.)

into triglyceride occurs in ischemia, when fatty acid oxidation is inhibited, as well as in starvation and diabetes, when fatty acid levels are elevated in the plasma. Triglyceride synthesis rates may thus reflect, in part, the relative rates of fatty acid uptake from the plasma, and the disposition via mitochondrial oxidation.

Transport of Acyl Coenzyme A into Mitochondria

Because activation of long-chain fatty acids takes place extramitochondrially and β-oxidation occurs in the mitochondrial matrix, the long-chain acyl-CoA moieties must be transported into the mitochondrion before being oxidized (Fig. 4–8). Transport of long-chain acyl-CoA across the inner mitochondrial membrane occurs via a carnitine-dependent system involving two carnitine palmitoyltransferase enzymes, one present on each surface of the inner mitochondrial membrane, and carnitine translocase, which catalyzes the stoichiometric exchange of carnitine and acylcarnitine across the inner mitochondrial membrane.[B2] The outer carnitine palmitoyltransferase, CPT I, which

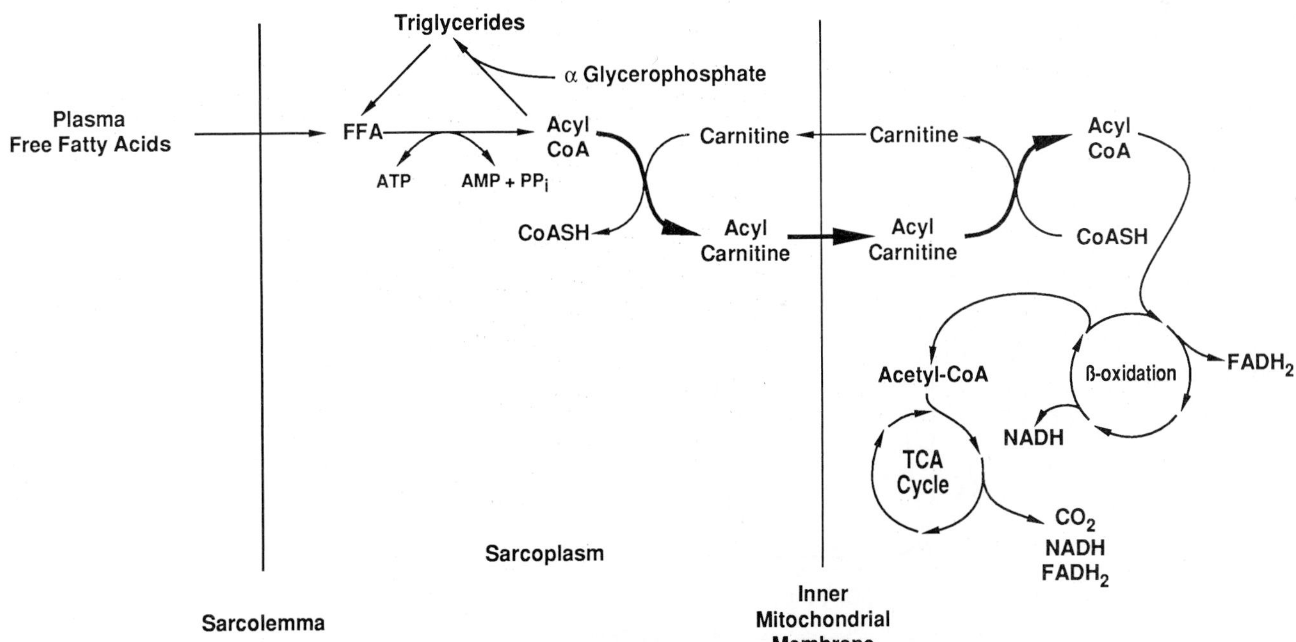

Figure 4–7. Metabolism of long-chain fatty acid in myocardium. Following entry into the cell, the fatty acid must first be activated to form an acyl-CoA derivative. The acyl-CoA can then be transported into the mitochondrion, via a carnitine-dependent shuttle, to undergo β-oxidation to acetyl-CoA for entry into the tricarboxylic acid cycle, or it can be esterified in the cytosol to form triglyceride.

catalyzes the freely reversible formation of acylcarnitine and coenzyme A from acyl-CoA and carnitine, is inhibited by malonyl-CoA. Malonyl coenzyme A inhibition of CPT I is thought to represent an important regulatory mechanism in fatty acid oxidation,[M5] and CPT I of cardiac mitochondria is more sensitive than that of liver mitochondria to malonyl-CoA.[S6] Following translocation of the acylcarnitine across the inner mitochondrial membrane, acyl-CoA is reformed by the inner carnitine palmitoyltransferase, CPT II.

β-*Oxidation*

Oxidation of intramitochondrial acyl-CoA requires the repetitive sequential action of four enzymes: acyl-CoA dehydrogenase, enoyl-CoA hydratase, 3-hydroxyacyl-CoA dehydrogenase and 3-oxoacyl-CoA thiolase (Fig. 4–9). Each passage through the enzyme sequence results in the liberation of acetyl-CoA, with concomitant shortening of the acyl-CoA by two carbons. Additional mitochondrial enzymes are responsible for the conversion of intermediates that are formed during oxidation of unsaturated fatty acids to normal β-oxidation intermediates.[B2] Under normal conditions, intermediates of β-oxidation are present only at low concentrations in mitochondria. The intermediates also display anomalous turnover kinetics, leading to the suggestion that the β-oxidation enzymes are arranged in a loose complex that breaks apart during isolation of the enzymes, thus channeling the intermediates from enzyme to enzyme.[S7] The free intermediates would thus represent leakage from the complex. Acetyl coenzyme A formed by β-oxidation appears to enter the general mitochondrial acetyl-CoA pool.[L4]

Because ketogenesis is absent in myocardium, β-oxidation is tightly coupled to disposition of acetyl-CoA via the tricarboxylic acid cycle, and accumulation of acetyl-CoA has been proposed to regulate β-oxidation.[O3] Approximately 85 percent of myocardial coenzyme A is found in the mitochondria. Carnitine is predominantly cytosolic; only 9 percent of carnitine is associated with the mitochondria.[O4] This arrangement is believed to assist in directing fatty acids primarily toward oxidation in myocardium.

Ketone Metabolism

Myocardial tissue has the highest rate of ketone body utilization, reflecting the continuous high-energy requirements of cardiac muscle.[R5] Uptake of ketones at the plasma membrane is believed to occur by diffusion of the undissociated acids,[R6] whereas entry into the mitochondria can take place as anions via the monocarboxylate carrier used by pyruvate,[L5, P1] in addition to diffusion. Inside the mitochondrion, 3-hydroxybutyrate is converted to acetoacetate by 3-hydroxybutyrate dehydrogenase, an enzyme tightly bound to the inner mitochondrial membrane. The reaction, which also generates NADH from NAD^+, is reversible. Acetoacetate is then activated to acetoacetyl-CoA in an unusual reaction catalyzed by 3-oxoacid-CoA transferase (Fig. 4–10), in which succinyl-CoA acts as coenzyme donor with formation of succinate. Thus, in effect, acetoacetyl-CoA synthesis bypasses the succinate thiokinase reaction of the tricarboxylic acid cycle and hence, the substrate-level phosphorylation of guanosine diphosphate (GDP) to guanosine triphosphate (GTP).[T1] Acetoacetyl-CoA is then cleaved by acetoacetyl-CoA thiolase, with the net reaction of formation of two molecules of acetyl-CoA from acetoacetyl-CoA and coenzyme A.[R5] No evidence has been found for regulation of ketone body metabolism at any particular step.[T1] Utilization of ketone bodies in heart is linearly related to the plasma concentration at low concentrations and reaches a plateau at higher plasma concentrations.[R7, W3]

Experimental studies in isolated hearts have demonstrated an inability of ketone bodies to act as sole myocardial substrates at high workloads, which is due to a relative inhibition of the tricarboxylic acid cycle at the 2-oxoglutarate dehydrogenase step.[T2] This phenomenon has been proposed to reflect sequestration of coenzyme A in the form of acetyl-CoA and acetoacetyl-CoA, and it is overcome by glucose.[T1]

TRICARBOXYLIC ACID CYCLE ACTIVITY

The tricarboxylic acid cycle represents the means by which acetyl-CoA derived from the breakdown of glucose, fatty acid, ketone bodies, lactate, and pyruvate, in addition to other cycle intermediates derived from the metabolism of amino acids, are catabolized to carbon dioxide and water, with the production of reduced coenzymes (NADH and $FADH_2$) and GTP. The reduced coenzymes can then donate electrons to the electron transport chain, leading to synthesis of ATP and the reduction of molecular oxygen. Because the tricarboxylic acid cycle is responsible for approximately two thirds of the energy production from the major myocardial fuels under normoxic conditions, flux through the

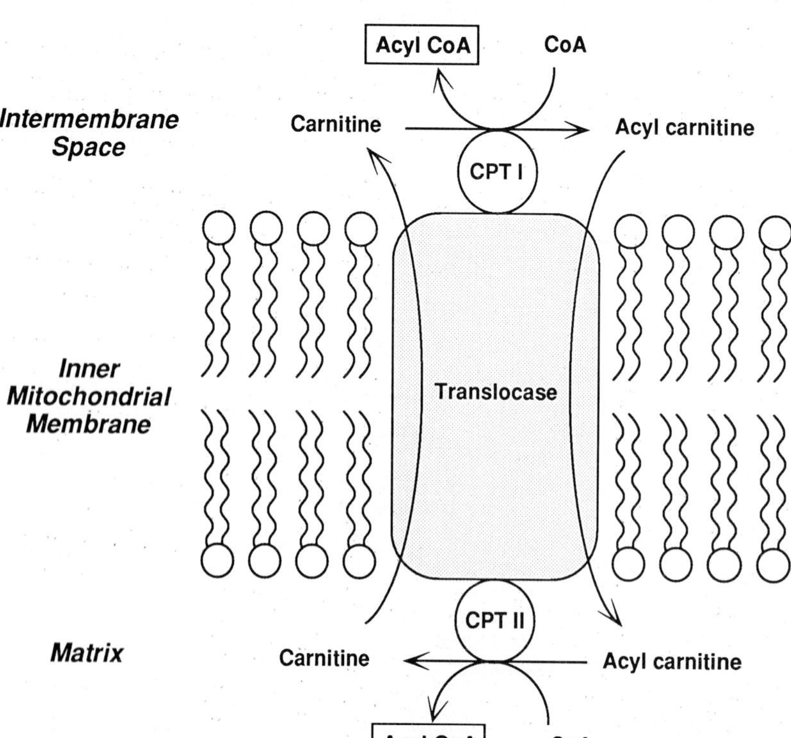

Figure 4–8. The carnitine shuttle. Acyl coenzyme A crosses the inner mitochondrial membrane via a carnitine-dependent shuttle system. The acyl group is first transferred to carnitine by the action of carnitine palmitoyltransferase I (CPT I) on the cytosolic face of the inner mitochondrial membrane. Acylcarnitine then exchanges via a translocase with free carnitine across the inner mitochondrial membrane, and the acyl group is transferred back to form intramitochondrial acyl-CoA by a second transferase, CPT II, situated on the matrix side. (Modified from Stryer, L.: Biochemistry. W. H. Freeman, New York, 1988, p. 474.)

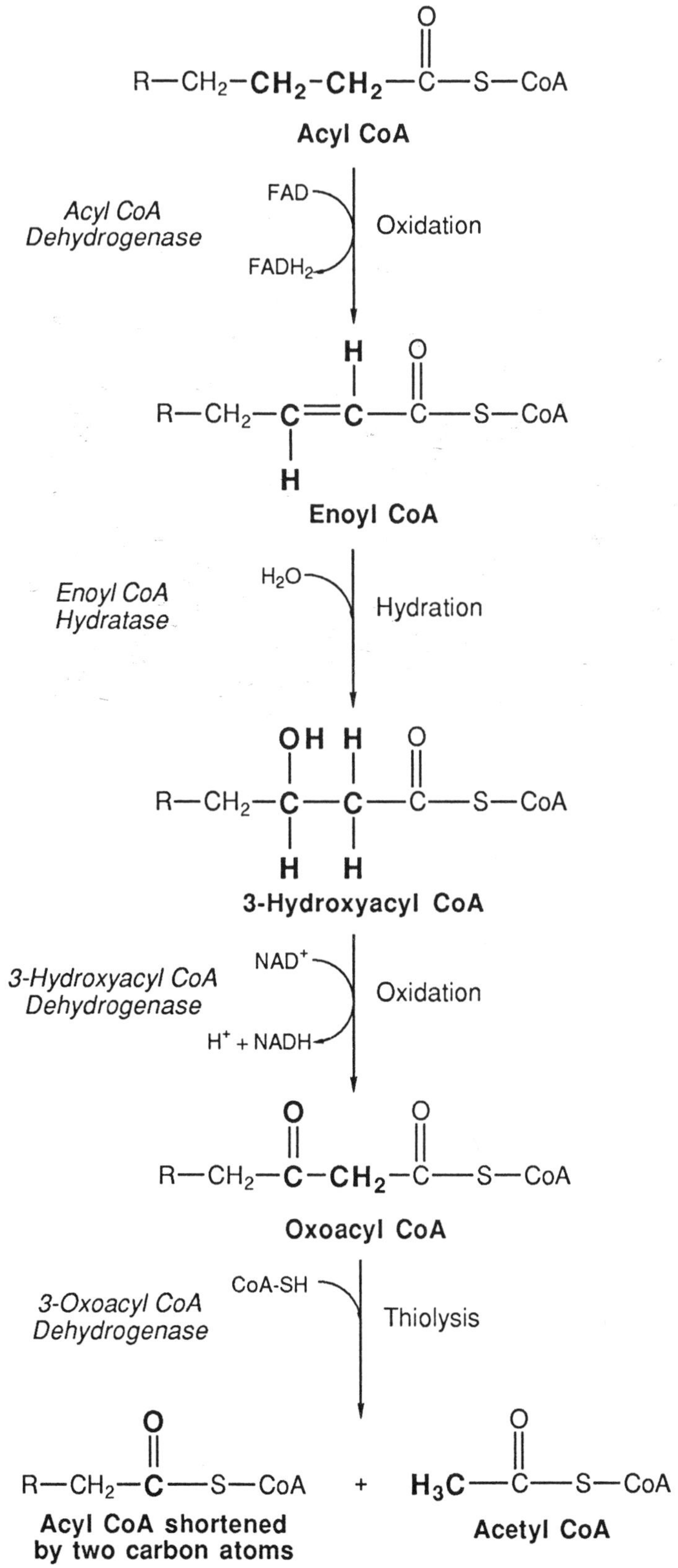

$R-CH_2-CH_2-CH_2-C(=O)-S-CoA$

Acyl CoA

Acyl CoA Dehydrogenase — $FAD \rightarrow FADH_2$ — Oxidation

$R-CH_2-CH=CH-C(=O)-S-CoA$

Enoyl CoA

Enoyl CoA Hydratase — H_2O — Hydration

$R-CH_2-CH(OH)-CH_2-C(=O)-S-CoA$

3-Hydroxyacyl CoA

3-Hydroxyacyl CoA Dehydrogenase — $NAD^+ \rightarrow H^+ + NADH$ — Oxidation

$R-CH_2-C(=O)-CH_2-C(=O)-S-CoA$

Oxoacyl CoA

3-Oxoacyl CoA Dehydrogenase — CoA-SH — Thiolysis

$R-CH_2-C(=O)-S-CoA \quad + \quad H_3C-C(=O)-S-CoA$

Acyl CoA shortened by two carbon atoms — **Acetyl CoA**

Figure 4–9. β-Oxidation of fatty acids.

tricarboxylic acid cycle must be closely coupled to myocardial energy demand. Determination of the mechanisms of regulation of the tricarboxylic acid cycle is complicated by the cyclical nature of the process, which makes interpretation of data more difficult than in a linear system.[W4] The current state of knowledge on the regulatory mechanisms linking flux through the tricarboxylic acid cycle to myocardial energy demand has been reviewed extensively.[H2, R1, T3, W4] The main points are summarized in the following discussion.

The main role of the tricarboxylic acid cycle is the efficient oxidation of the acetyl group of acetyl-CoA to carbon dioxide and water, with the concomitant production of reducing equivalents for energy production. A secondary function of the tricarboxylic acid cycle is the coordinated regulation of fatty acid metabolism and glycolysis.[R1] Thus, increased β-oxidation and, hence, increased flux of acetyl-CoA from fatty acid into the tricarboxylic acid cycle elevates citrate levels, leading to inhibition of phosphofructokinase and glycolysis.[R1]

The main candidates for regulation of activity of the tricarboxylic acid cycle, based on identification of disequilibrium enzymes,[W4] are citrate synthetase and the tricarboxylic acid cycle dehydrogenases—NAD-linked isocitrate dehydrogenase and 2-oxoglutarate dehydrogenase—which are linked directly to reduction of coenzymes. Citrate synthetase has been assumed to be a rate-limiting enzyme because of its position in committing acetyl-CoA to oxidation.[R8] Although citrate synthetase is inhibited by NADH, ATP, and succinyl-CoA in vitro, thus providing possible feedback regulation of the enzyme, the significance of these factors in vivo has been questioned.[T1, T3] The possible functional and structural linkage of citrate synthetase and malate dehydrogenase[S8] has been proposed as a means by which citrate synthetase is linked to the mitochondrial redox state.[T3] The equilibrium of citrate synthetase favors citrate synthesis, and the equilibrium of malate dehydrogenase favors malate formation. Therefore, due to the competition of the two enzymes for oxaloacetate, consideration of the two reactions as a unit demonstrates that purely on the basis of thermodynamic equilibria, NADH inhibits flux through citrate synthetase whereas NAD^+ promotes it.[T3] The importance of citrate synthesis as a regulatory step in myocardial regulation of tricarboxylic acid cycle flux is still unclear, however.[T3]

NAD-linked isocitrate dehydrogenase is strongly inhibited by NADH and stimulated by ADP, and it appears to be the site most sensitive to changes in the [NADH]/[NAD^+] ratio.[W4] Results obtained in isolated heart mitochondria have demonstrated increased flux througth isocitrate dehydrogenase in uncoupled mitochondria treated with oligomycin. These mitochondria have a high [ATP]/[ADP] ratio but a low [NADH]/[NAD^+] ratio, which suggests that the redox state of the mitochondrial nicotinamide adenine nucleotides may be of greater importance than the phosphorylation state of the adenine nucleotides in regulating NAD^+-linked isocitrate dehydrogenase.[H3, L6]

The 2-oxoglutarate dehydrogenase reaction commits 2-oxoglutarate to oxidation, in contrast to the alternative fates of efflux from the mitochondrion as part of the malate-aspartate shuttle, or transamination.[H2] In addition, 2-oxoglutarate dehydrogenase is inhibited by increases in the [NADH]/[NAD^+] ratio and is strongly inhibited by the product succinyl-CoA. The [succinyl-CoA]/[CoA] ratio is increased in high mitochondrial energy states by the actions of succinate thiokinase and nucleoside diphosphate kinase, which tend to decrease flux through 2-oxoglutarate dehydrogenase.[L7] The inhibitory effects of succinyl-CoA depend on the relative concentrations of the substrate 2-oxoglutarate and the inhibitor succinyl-CoA.

An additional level of control of tricarboxylic acid cycle flux may result from the Ca^{2+} sensitivity of the NAD-linked isocitrate dehydrogenase and 2-oxoglutarate dehydrogenase reactions, as well as of the pyruvate dehydrogenase reaction that feeds in acetyl-CoA from glycolysis.[D5] This mechanism may be of particular importance in catecholamine stimulation and is discussed in more detail in the later section on the role of catecholamines in myocardial substrate interactions.

Thus, there are multiple mechanisms by which tricarboxylic acid cycle flux can be linked to the energy state of the mitochondrion, as reflected by the [ATP]/[ADP] ratio and, probably of primary importance, by the [NADH]/[NAD^+] ratio. As a result, energy utilization is tightly coupled to the provision of reducing equivalents via the tricarboxylic acid cycle and energy production through the electron transport chain.

Respiratory Control in Myocardium

Under normal conditions, the healthy myocardium has the ability to match energy production closely to the rate of myocardial energy utilization, but the regulatory mechanisms involved in this coordination are incompletely understood. A number of models have been offered to explain the control of myocardial respiration. These include (1) limitation of respiration by the availability of ADP and inorganic phosphate,[C3, J1, L8] (2) regulation of the translocation of ATP and ADP through kinetic control by the substrates and electrophoretic control by the membrane potential,[K6] and (3) the near-equilibrium hypothesis, in which a near equilibrium exists between the extramitochondrial adenylate system and the respiratory chain reactions across the first two energy-conserving sites. According to this hypothesis, the rate of oxygen consumption is determined by the redox state of the mitochondrial free [NADH]/[NAD] couple.[N3] This topic has been discussed in several reviews.[E2, H4, H5, W4] The mechanism, or mechanisms, of respiratory control thus remain a controversial area at present.

MYOCARDIAL SUBSTRATE INTERACTIONS

The selection of fuels by myocardium is governed by several factors.[R1, T1] The utilization of a substrate first depends on its plasma concentration. Whereas plasma glucose levels remain relatively constant, the concentrations of fatty acids, ketone bodies, and lactate in blood can vary widely with changes in nutritional status and with exercise. Increases in plasma concentrations of any of these substrates tend to lead to increased myocardial utilization of that substrate.[R1] The presence and nature of alternate substrates also have a profound effect on utilization of a particular substrate. Taegtmeyer has pointed out that the ease of access of a substrate to the tricarboxylic acid cycle is an important factor in substrate selection.[T1] Thus, ketone bodies[R2, W3] and lactate,[I1, D1] which have few control steps in their metabolic pathways, tend to be used preferentially in proportion to their plasma concentrations, while glucose and fatty acid oxidation pathways have more potential for regulation and are thus more affected by alternate substrates. Plasma levels of hormones can control the provision of substrates in the circulation as well as myocardial uptake and oxidation of substrates.

The importance of fatty acids as the primary substrate for myocardium under normal conditions, and the "glucose-sparing" effects of lipid substrates in myocardium, have long been recognized.[B3, R2] Fatty acids and ketone bodies inhibit glucose utilization at multiple sites, the most important of which involves inhibition of phosphofructokinase. Metabolism of fatty acids and ketone bodies increases mitochondrial citrate levels as a result of increased mitochondrial acetyl-CoA production and, hence, substrate effects on citrate synthetase.[N4, R8] Transport of citrate to the cytosol resulting in inhibition of phosphofructokinase occurs by citrate-malate exchange or by efflux of 2-oxoglutarate and synthesis of citrate by cytosolic isocitrate dehydrogenase.[R1] Inhibition of phosphofructokinase causes accumulation of glucose-6-phosphate, with resultant inhibition of hexokinase.[N4] Transport of glucose into myocardium is inhibited by oxidation of fatty acids and ketone bodies, although the mechanism remains unclarified at present.[R2] Lastly, oxidation of fatty acids or ketones inhibits pyruvate dehydrogenase activity by increasing mitochondrial [acetyl CoA]/[CoA] and [NADH]/[NAD$^+$], with resultant allosteric inhibition of pyruvate dehydrogenase in addition to covalent inactivation by stimulation of pyruvate dehydrogenase kinase.[O1, R1, W1]

The regulation of fatty acid metabolism by alternate substrates has also been demonstrated, although the mechanisms are not well understood. Carbohydrate feeding of animals, with resultant increases in plasma glucose and insulin, decreases myocardial fatty acid uptake, in part by decreasing plasma free fatty acid levels.[G6] Additional regulation at the level of the myocardium, however, has been demonstrated both in vivo and in vitro.

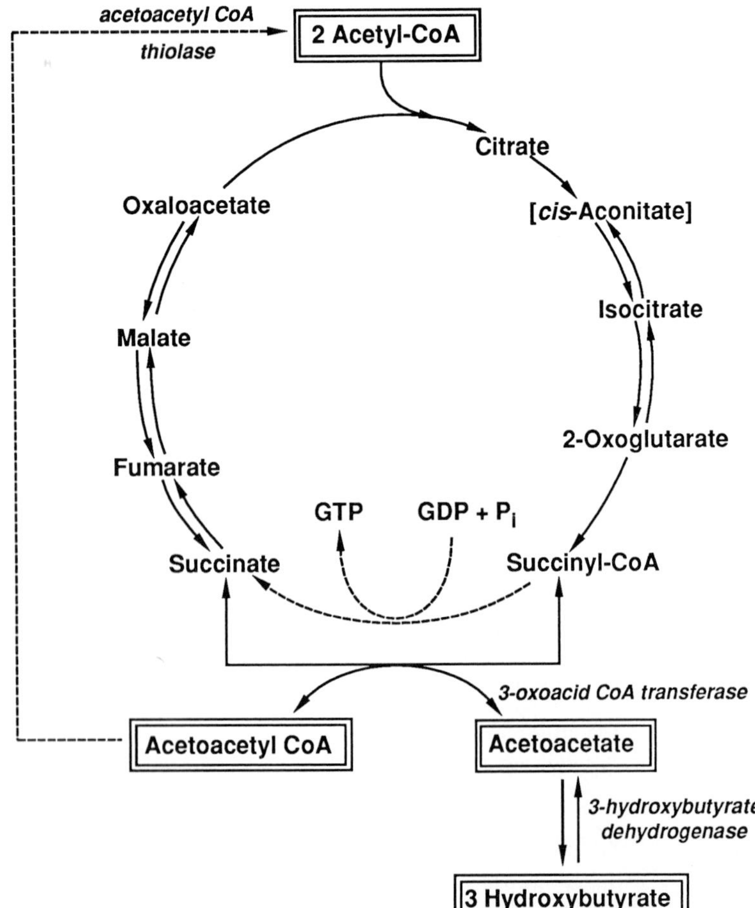

Figure 4–10. Mechanism of entry of ketone bodies into the tricarboxylic acid cycle. Acetoacetyl-coenzyme A is synthesized using succinyl-CoA as a CoA donor, thus bypassing the GTP-yielding substrate-level phosphorylation step catalyzed by succinyl-CoA synthetase. Cleavage of acetoacetyl-CoA yields two acetyl-CoA units. (Modified from Taegtmeyer, H.: Myocardial metabolism. *In* Phelps, M. E., et al. (eds.) Positron Emission Tomography and Autoradiography: Principles and Applications for the Brain and Heart. Raven Press, New York, 1986, p. 149.)

Inhibition of fatty acid oxidation by glucose and insulin,[S9] lactate, [D2, I1] and ketone bodies[B4, L9] has been demonstrated in vivo. Similar results have been obtained in vitro.[B5, F1, T2] Interestingly, lactate, pyruvate, and glucose inhibited oxidation of long-chain, but not medium-chain, fatty acids in perfused hearts,[B5, F1] which is consistent with an effect at the level of the transport of long-chain fatty acids into the mitochondrion. In contrast, ketones inhibited both oleate and octanoate oxidation, which suggests an intramitochondrial site of action.[F1]

Fasting

Fasting leads to elevated plasma concentrations of free fatty acids and to low levels of circulating insulin. Myocardial triglyceride and glycogen stores are increased, reflecting increased esterification of free fatty acid to triglyceride, and inhibition of glycolysis in response to increased β-oxidation.[R1] Perfused hearts from starved rats demonstrate decreased glucose transport, glycolysis, and pyruvate dehydrogenase activity.[N4, R1] Accumulation of citrate is observed in vivo and in vitro and is believed to be responsible for the inhibition of phosphofructokinase, with consequent accumulation of glucose-6-phosphate and inhibition of hexokinase.[N4, R1] Pyruvate dehydrogenase inhibition probably reflects increases in [acetyl CoA]/[CoA] and [NADH]/[NAD] in response to increased β-oxidation of fatty acids.[W1]

Diabetes and Insulin

Myocardial metabolism in diabetes is markedly similar to the situation produced by fasting. Rats made diabetic by administration of alloxan are characterized by high plasma levels of free fatty acids, elevated blood glucose concentrations, ketonemia, and undetectable levels of circulating insulin.[R1] As observed in fasting, increased β-oxidation of fatty acids leads to accumulation of citrate with concomitant inhibition of phosphofructokinase and glycolysis.[N4] Despite the presence of high plasma glucose levels, transport of glucose into myocardium is limited, owing to the absence of insulin; treatment with insulin in vivo (but not in vitro) restores glucose transport, although the sensitivity of the glucose transport system to insulin is decreased.[D1, N4, R1] The percentage of active pyruvate dehydrogenase is decreased by phosphorylation of the enzyme in diabetes, which is mediated at least in part by increases in [acetyl CoA]/[CoA] and [NADH]/[NAD]. Some evidence has been found for additional, as yet incompletely defined, inhibition of the reactivation of the enzyme by multi-site phosphorylation.[S10]

Increased Work and Exercise

Increased myocardial work leads to an increased rate of ATP utilization, with a consequent increase in tricarboxylic acid cycle flux and oxygen consumption. Experiments in vitro have shown that free fatty acid consumption is increased preferentially over glucose metabolism at higher workloads.[N1, R1, W5] As a sole substrate, glucose was found to be unable to support maximal rates of cardiac work, owing to the inability to dispose of cytosolic NADH and consequent inhibition of glyceraldehyde-3-phosphate dehydrogenase.[K5]

In exercise in vivo, changes in plasma substrate concentrations are an additional factor. Exercise leads to increases in arterial plasma lactate concentrations from the low levels of approximately 1 mmol/L found at rest to 5 to 12 mmol/L occurring with moderate or heavy exercise, respectively.[D2] Exercise has been shown to lead to an increase in lactate oxidation,[K7, S11] which is consistent with the increased plasma availability of lactate. In addition, myocardial glucose uptake and oxidation have been shown to increase with exercise.[S11]

Catecholamines

Stimulation of myocardium with catecholamines affects cardiac metabolism in a number of ways. Myocardial oxygen consumption increases, providing additional energy to fuel the chronotropic and inotropic actions of catecholamines on heart. Experimental evidence suggests that the catecholamine-mediated stimulation of cardiac respiration may have both α- and β-adrenergic mechanisms. α-Adrenergic stimulation has been shown to activate Ca^{2+} influx into mitochondria via the Ca^{2+} uniporter,[K8] while β-adrenergic stimulation increases cytoplasmic [Ca^{2+}], leading to enhanced mitochondrial Ca^{2+} uptake.[M6] Increased mitochondrial [Ca^{2+}] is then believed to activate key Ca^{2+}-dependent intramitochondrial dehydrogenases, NAD-linked isocitrate dehydrogenase, 2-oxoglutarate dehydrogenase, and pyruvate dehydrogenase phosphatase. Stimulation of pyruvate dehydrogenase phosphatase by Ca^{2+} leads to dephosphorylation (and hence activation) of pyruvate dehydrogenase, while Ca^{2+} lowers the K_m of the two tricarboxylic acid cycle dehydrogenases for their respective substrates, stimulating tricarboxylic acid cycle fluxes.[D5]

Glucose metabolism is stimulated at several steps by catecholamines. α-Adrenergic activity stimulates glucose uptake[C4] and activates phosphofructokinase.[C2] β-Adrenergic activity also stimulates glucose uptake,[C4] and activates glycogen phosphorylase, which in turn stimulates glycogen breakdown.[W6] Activation of glycogen phosphorylase occurs via the cyclic adenosine monophosphate (cAMP)–dependent phosphorylation cascade (see Fig. 4–3).

Ischemia

The alterations in substrate metabolism occurring in ischemia have been discussed in detail in extensive review articles.[L1, O5] A summary of the main points follows, with a focus on ischemia (reduction in blood flow) rather than anoxia (removal of oxygen from perfusate) because of the former's greater relevance to clinical heart disease.

Reduction of blood flow resulting in decreased delivery of oxygen to myocardium leads to a reduction in tricarboxylic acid cycle flux approximately in proportion to flow,[O6] which reflects the limited capacity of myocardium to increase oxygen extraction. Tricarboxylic acid cycle flux is limited by elevated mitochondrial [NADH]/[NAD^+] as a consequence of the oxygen limitation of the respiratory chain, with resultant inhibition of the key dehydrogenase steps in the tricarboxylic acid cycle. Pyruvate dehydrogenase flux is also limited by elevated [NADH]; the relative contributions of allosteric and covalent control to the inhibition of flux have not been clarified.[K9, P2] Ischemia is accompanied by a rapid decline in contractile function and thus a decrease in myocardial energy demand.[A1]

In ischemia, glucose metabolism accounts for an increased percentage of the residual oxygen consumption, with a concomitant decrease in fatty acid oxidation.[O6] Metabolism of glucose is accelerated in oxygen deficiency at a number of steps. Utilization of both exogenous and endogenous glucose supplies is increased in ischemia. Transport of glucose is increased,[M7] although the mechanism has not been defined, and activation of glycogen phosphorylase leads to increased glycogen breakdown. Phosphofructokinase activity is increased because of decreased inhibition resulting from decreased tissue ATP levels, together with stimulation through elevation of AMP and inorganic phosphate.[M8] Increased flux through phosphofructokinase decreases glucose-6-phosphate levels, relieving inhibition of hexokinase, which is also stimulated by elevated inorganic phosphate levels.[M8, W7] Overall, glycolytic flux is increased in ischemia, but the degree of stimulation depends on the extent of residual flow; in severe ischemia, glycolysis falls below control heart levels.[N5] Because pyruvate dehydrogenase flux is limited, pyruvate is converted to lactate, with concomitant regeneration of NAD from NADH. Increased alanine production is also observed;[P3, T4] the probable source of the alanine is disposal of tricarboxylic acid cycle metabolites rather than glycolysis.[P3]

As flow decreases, washout of tissue lactate produced by glycolysis, and of H^+ produced by breakdown of ATP, is inhibited. Accumulation of lactate prevents regeneration of NAD^+ via the lactate dehydrogenase reaction. The resulting increase in cytosolic NADH produced by triose phosphate dehydrogenation, in conjunction with lactate itself, inhibits glyceraldehyde-3-phosphate dehydrogenase.[M9] The accumulation of metabolites in ischemia thus prevents glycolysis from reaching the maximum levels observed in anoxia with normal flows. Anaerobic glycolysis may account for greater than 50 percent of the glycolytic flux in ischemic myocardium. However, because of the low yield of ATP from anaerobic glycolysis (2 moles of ATP per mole of glucose) compared with that from aerobic glycolysis (36 moles of ATP per mole of glucose), aerobic metabolism still contributes greater than 90 percent of ATP production in ischemia in canine myocardium, with 7 percent residual flow from collaterals. The possibility of compartmentation of ATP production exists, however.

Unlike glucose metabolism, no anaerobic alternative exists for energy-producing metabolism of fatty acids. Increases in mitochondrial [NADH]/[NAD$^+$] rapidly inhibit β-oxidation; production of β-hydroxy fatty acid by ischemic heart suggests that the NAD$^+$-dependent β-hydroxyacyl-CoA dehydrogenase may be the most sensitive locus.[M10] Fatty acid uptake is decreased,[V1, W8] fatty acid activation is decreased by product inhibition, and transport of long-chain acyl-CoA into mitochondria is decreased.[W9] Free fatty acids,[V1] acylcarnitine, and acyl-CoA[W8] accumulate in ischemia. The possible deleterious effects of accumulation of intermediates of fatty acid metabolism on cardiac function in ischemia have been reviewed elsewhere.[L1]

Studies in humans in vivo have demonstrated similar metabolic patterns in ischemia. Increased glucose metabolism in relation to blood flow has been demonstrated in ischemic myocardial segments compared with normal myocardial segments in patients with abnormal wall motion.[M11, T5] Pacing-induced stress increases glucose extraction and lactate production in patients with coronary artery disease[M12, W2] and decreases oxidation of long-chain fatty acids.[G7] Thus, clinical studies have demonstrated a switch to glucose from fatty acid metabolism and increased anaerobic glucose utilization during ischemia.

Reperfusion

The prolonged functional abnormalities following brief periods of regional myocardial ischemia, often referred to as stunned myocardium, are well established.[B6] Reperfused myocardium also demonstrates profound metabolic disturbances. Myocardial ATP levels remain depressed following reperfusion,[D6] but these decreased ATP levels are not thought to be the cause of the contractile dysfunction.[T4] Glycogen levels also show prolonged depletion in reperfused myocardium.[S12] The changes in substrate metabolism observed in reperfusion have proved to be rather variable, which probably reflects differences in the experimental models used. In general, uptake and oxidation of fatty acids have been found to be decreased immediately following reperfusion,[M13, S13, S14] with the return of fatty acid oxidation paralleling the return of function;[S14] however, increased oxidation of fatty acids has also been reported immediately following reperfusion.[L10] In dogs, glucose uptake immediately following reperfusion has been found to be decreased compared with glucose uptake in normal myocardium,[S14] but 24 hours following reperfusion, glucose uptake is enhanced in the reperfused tissue.[S14, S15] Increased anaerobic glucose utilization contributes to the enhanced glucose utilization observed 24 hours following reperfusion.[S12] In patients with coronary artery disease, increased glucose metabolism was demonstrated after exercise-induced angina in the presence of normal flow.[S5]

Oxygen consumption is generally lower in the reperfused area compared with that in control myocardium,[B7, L10, M13, S15] although whether this change is secondary to the decreased contractile work is not clear. Some studies have demonstrated increased oxygen consumption in reperfused myocardium and have proposed a decreased efficiency of energy utilization in reperfused tissue.[S16]

COMPARTMENTATION OF ENERGY UTILIZATION

Studies in a number of laboratories have suggested that ATP derived directly from glycolysis via substrate level phosphorylation at the phosphoglycerate kinase and pyruvate kinase steps may be used preferentially in the maintenance of membrane integrity in ischemia, while energy derived from oxidative metabolism is used for support of contractile function. Inhibition of glycolysis has been shown to lead to increased enzyme leakage,[B8, H6] shortening of the action potential,[M14] accelerated onset of contracture,[B9] and increased extracellular K$^+$ accumulation,[H7, W10] and to have little effect on contractility, whereas inhibition of oxidative metabolism has a much greater effect on contractility than on membrane function.[H7, W10] Preferential inhibition of ATP-sensitive K$^+$ channels in isolated guinea pig cardiomyocytes by glycolysis has also been demonstrated.[W11]

On the basis of these and other experimental results, investigators have proposed that the glycolytic enzymes are positioned close to the sarcolemma, which allows glycolytically generated ATP to be readily used at the ATP-sensitive K$^+$ channels and to be used for other energy-dependent membrane processes. Conversely, the close proximity of the mitochondria to the myofibrils would allow ready utilization of ATP derived from oxidative metabolism for contractility. A phosphocreatine shuttle has been proposed by which ATP from the mitochondria is transferred to the contractile apparatus in the form of phosphocreatine, which is then converted to ATP by myosin-bound creatine kinase.[B10]

PROTEIN TURNOVER

Myocardial protein turnover reflects a balance between the rates of protein synthesis and degradation, a balance that can be disturbed by several physiologic variations.[M15] Myocardium shows an overall fractional protein synthesis rate of 8 to 9 percent per day in rabbits and rats,[P4, S17] while individual proteins display markedly heterogeneous turnover rates.[Z1] The pathways of protein synthesis and degradation, and the factors controlling the balance between these two pathways, are discussed in the following sections.

Protein Synthesis

The pathway for protein synthesis can conveniently be divided into three sections: (1) amino acid transport and aminoacyl–transfer ribonucleic acid (tRNA) synthesis, (2) peptide chain initiation, and (3) elongation and termination of peptide chains.

Amino Acid Transport and Aminoacyl-tRNA Synthesis

Transport of amino acids into cells takes place via a number of transport systems with overlapping substrate specificities.[C6] Availability of amino acids does not appear to limit cardiac protein synthetic rate when amino acids are available at physiologic concentrations.[M15] Synthesis of aminoacyl-tRNA derivatives takes place by the enzymatic action of aminoacyl-tRNA synthetases specific for each amino acid and its corresponding tRNA. Interestingly, many of the tRNA synthetases are found as a loose complex in the cell.[S18] Measurement of the specific activity of the aminoacyl-tRNA pools using radiolabeled amino acids has demonstrated it to be generally greater than that of the intracellular amino acid pool, but less than that of the extracellular pool, suggesting that extracellular amino acids are used for synthesis of aminoacyl-tRNA prior to mixing with the bulk intracellular amino acid pool.[M15]

Peptide Chain Initiation

Initiation of protein synthesis in mammalian cells has been reviewed recently[P5] and is summarized in Figure 4–11. Initiation of protein synthesis utilizes a specific initiator tRNA, methionyl-tRNA$_f$, which donates methionine exclusively into the N-terminal

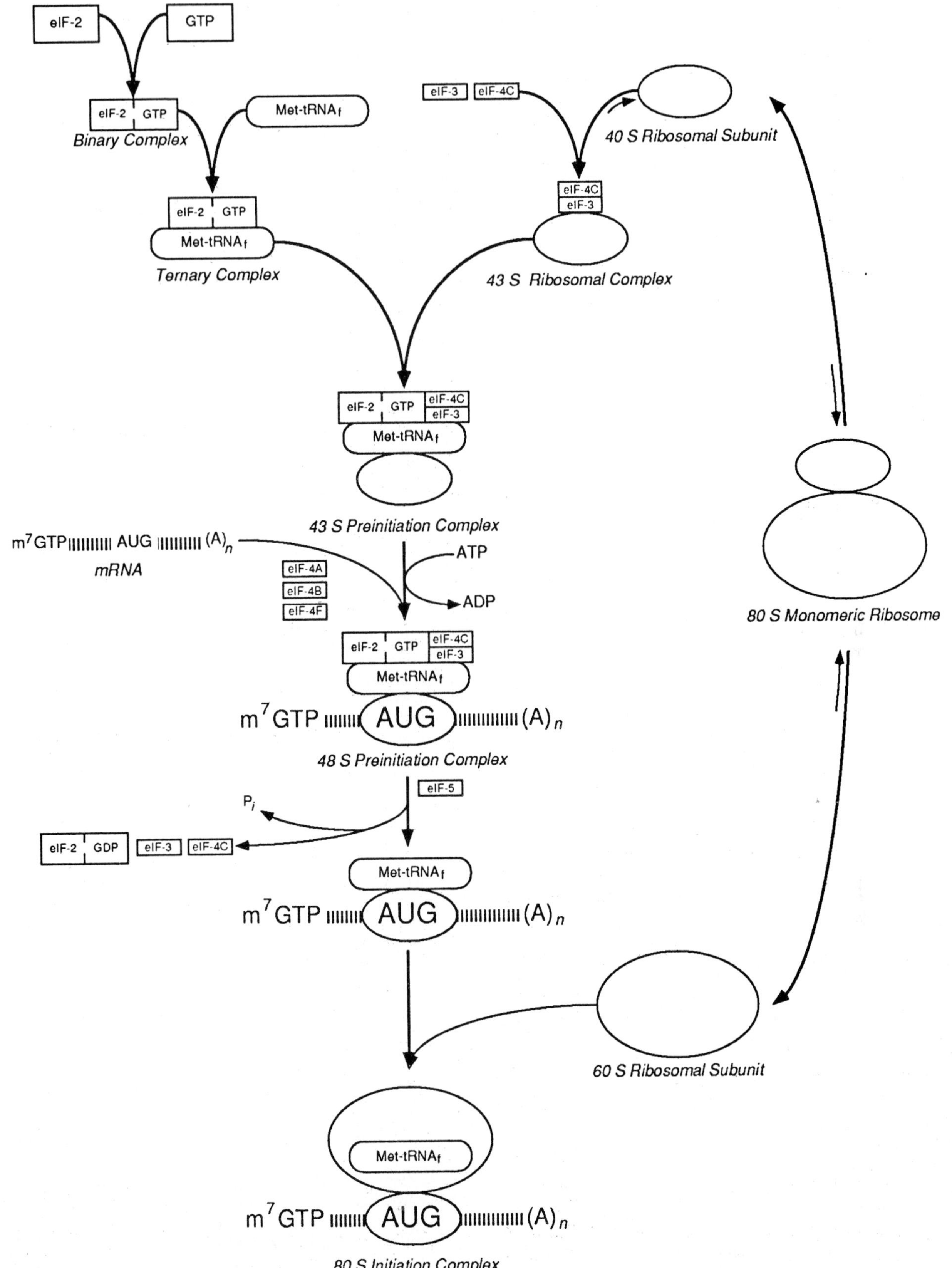

Figure 4–11. Initiation of protein synthesis in mammalian cells. (Modified from Pain, V. M.: Initiation of protein synthesis in mammalian cells. Biochem. J. 235:625, 1986.)

position of newly synthesized peptides. A separate methionine-accepting tRNA is used for incorporation of methionine into internal positions. Methionyl-tRNA$_f$ binds to eukaryotic initiation factor 2 (eIF-2) in a GTP-dependent reaction to form a ternary complex. The ternary complex binds to a 43S ribosomal complex consisting of the 40S ribosomal subunit, eIF-3, and eIF-4C, and forms a 43S preinitiation complex. The 43S preinitiation complex then binds to the 5′ end of messenger ribonucleic acid (mRNA) and migrates to the initiation codon, AUG. Eukaryotic initiation factors 4A, 4B, and 4F are required, as well as ATP hydrolysis. Eukaryotic initiation factor 5 then promotes dissociation of the other initiation factors bound to the 40S subunit and hydrolysis of the GTP that entered as part of the ternary complex. Finally, the 60S ribosomal subunit joins to form an 80S initiation complex on the mRNA.

Regulation of protein synthesis initiation has been studied in most detail in the reticulocyte lysate, where protein synthesis depends on the continued presence of hemin. Inhibition of protein synthesis in the absence of hemin involves decreased 43S preinitiation complex formation, which is accompanied by an increase in the phosphorylation of one of the subunits of eIF-2 by a cAMP-independent protein kinase. The mechanism by which eIF-2 phosphorylation inhibits 43S complex formation is not fully understood, however.[P5] Decreased formation of 43S preinitiation complexes has also been demonstrated in skeletal muscle from starved or diabetic rats,[H8, K10] suggesting that a similar regulatory mechanism may be operative.

Peptide Elongation and Termination

Elongation of peptides requires two elongation factors: EF-1 and EF-2.[M16] EF-1 forms a ternary complex with GTP and charged aminoacyl-tRNA,[S19] which binds to the acceptor site of the ribosomes, with hydrolysis of GTP. Peptide bond formation, catalyzed by a peptidyltransferase activity located on the 60S ribosomal subunit, is then followed by translocation of the peptidyl-tRNA from the acceptor (A) site to the donor (P) site, and translocation of the ribosome one codon along the mRNA. This reaction probably requires EF-2–mediated GTP hydrolysis.[H9]

Termination occurs when a termination codon is reached by the A site, and it requires binding of GTP and a specific release factor RF.[T6] In the presence of a termination codon in the A site and binding of RF and GTP, peptidyltransferase catalyzes the hydrolysis of the peptidyl-tRNA ester, releasing the completed polypeptide chain from the tRNA. Release of RF, the terminal tRNA, and the ribosomal subunits from the mRNA requires GTP hydrolysis; the released ribosomal subunits then enter the ribosomal subunit pool and are available for another round of protein synthesis, starting with the initiation process. A detailed account of the elongation and termination processes is available in a recent review.[M16]

Protein Degradation

Protein degradation occurs via two pathways: lysosomal and nonlysosomal.[M17] Lysosomal protein degradation has been proposed to have two components: the first is macroautophagy, which is responsible for acceleration of protein degradation under various stimuli; the second is microautophagy or basal autophagy, in which proteins are sequestered through smaller vacuoles with high surface-to-volume ratios via invaginative or single-walled vesicular mechanisms, and which is responsible for basal levels of protein degradation. In muscle, macroautophagic protein degradation appears to be limited to nonmyofibrillar proteins, while myofibrillar protein degradation probably involves nonlysosomal calcium-activated disassembly of myofibrils into separate contractile proteins,[Z2] at least for the initial steps in myofibrillar degradation. The macroautophagic pathway appears to be the component of total protein breakdown suppressed by insulin and amino acids in perfused hearts, and by food intake in vivo.[M17]

Regulation of Protein Turnover

Net protein turnover is determined by the relative rates of protein synthesis and degradation, which can be modified by many physiologic stimuli.

Insulin and Diabetes

Perfusion of isolated hearts in the absence of insulin leads to dissociation of polyribosomal complexes and increased levels of ribosomal subunits, which indicate decreased polypeptide initiation.[M15] A negative nitrogen balance is also observed in such hearts: protein degradation rates are double the protein synthesis rates.[M15, P4] Addition of insulin was found to decrease protein degradation rates and to increase protein synthesis rates, restoring a positive nitrogen balance.[M15, P4] Addition of insulin to the perfusate increased latency of lysosomal enzymes, possibly indicating stabilization of the lysosomes.[R9]

Diabetes was not found to lead to decreases in polyribosomal content or increases in levels of ribosomal subunits, indicating that initiation of protein synthesis remained rapid in relation to peptide elongation.[R10] Increased plasma fatty acid levels in diabetes have been proposed to maintain peptide chain initiation, because addition of fatty acids to perfused hearts mimicked the effect of insulin of maintaining peptide initiation and thus preserving polyribosomal profiles.[R10, R11] A reduced level of protein synthesis in diabetic rat hearts in vivo was found to reflect both a decreased number of ribosomes and a decreased efficiency of protein synthesis per ribosome.[P5] The effect of diabetes on protein degradation has not been investigated in detail, but preliminary results indicate that protein degradation may be increased in diabetes.[M15]

Starvation

Starvation leads to decreases in myocardial mass and protein content, which indicate a negative myocardial nitrogen balance.[C7, P4] Prolonged starvation inhibits protein synthesis.[C7, P4, S17] While starvation caused the RNA content of cardiac muscle to decrease, its major effect was to decrease the efficiency of protein synthesis (the rate of protein synthesis relative to RNA content).[P4] Polyribosomal profiles were maintained without breakdown to ribosomal subunits, again indicating maintenance of peptide initiation in relation to elongation.[R11] Elevated fatty acid levels in serum produced by fasting may also contribute to the relative maintenance of peptide initiation, in contrast to such levels in skeletal muscle, where inhibition of protein synthesis initiation is observed in fasting.[R10, R11] Starvation has been shown to have different effects on the synthesis rates for different myocardial proteins. A disproportionate reduction of actin synthesis relative to myosin heavy-chain and total protein synthesis has been demonstrated;[C7, S17] this effect is readily reversible on refeeding.[C7] The decrease in actin synthesis could be explained at least in part by a disproportionately large decrease in actin mRNA.[C7] Also of interest was the finding that a similar disproportionate decrease in actin synthesis did not occur in skeletal muscle.[C7]

The effects of starvation on protein degradation are less clear, which probably reflects the greater methodologic difficulties involved in estimation of protein degradation rates.[M15] Although in vivo studies have shown increased fractional rates of protein degradation in starvation,[P4, S17] in vitro studies have shown decreased degradation rates in cardiac tissue from fasted animals.[C8, C9, P4] These results are likely to reflect the involvement of systemic factors in the regulation of protein degradation in vivo during starvation.

Hypertrophy

Cardiac hypertrophy is characterized by increases in flux through both the protein synthetic and protein degradative pathways. Aortic banding leads to rapid increases in cardiac muscle protein content.[W12] Studies from several laboratories have demonstrated protein synthetic rates in hypertrophy ranging from 165 to 400 percent of initial rates, and in each case the increase in the protein synthetic rate was greater than the increase in myocardial growth, indicating that protein degradative rates must also increase.[W12] Similarly, in left ventricular hypertrophy that was induced in rabbits by thyroxine treatment, the rate of protein synthesis increased in excess of the rate of total protein accumulation, again indicating an increase in left ventricular protein degradative rates.[P6] An increased protein synthetic rate was observed prior to significant changes in left ventricular RNA content, which suggests that an increase in the efficiency of protein synthesis per ribosome is responsible, at least in part, for the increase in protein synthesis.[P6]

Imposition of acute pressure overload in isolated perfused hearts has also been demonstrated to lead to increased rates of myocardial protein synthesis, and some evidence suggests that peptide chain initiation was increased.[M15] Protein degradation was not increased by acute pressure overload.[M15]

Ischemia

The effects of oxygen deprivation on the rates of protein synthesis and degradation have been studied both in vitro and in vivo. In vitro inhibition of both protein synthesis and degradation was observed in perfused rat hearts made ischemic by reduction of coronary flow.[M15] Anoxia, induced by perfusion with buffer equilibrated with N_2/CO_2 instead of O_2/CO_2, caused a more profound inhibition of protein synthesis, but a lesser inhibition of protein degradation, compared with that caused by ischemia. Energy deprivation was more severe in the anoxic hearts than in the ischemic hearts, as indicated by a greater decline in myocardial creatine phosphate levels.[M15]

Exposure of rats to mild hypoxia in vivo (10 per cent O_2 atmosphere) for 6 hours led to a modest decrease (20 per cent) in the myocardial protein synthesis rate, which was attributable to decreased efficiency of protein synthesis.[P7] After 24 hours of mild hypoxia, protein synthesis rates were found to be normal, however.[P8] Short-term exposure to severe hypoxia (5 per cent O_2 atmosphere) for as little as 1 hour caused approximately a 50 percent inhibition of myocardial protein synthesis; decreased efficiency was again the cause.[P8]

SUMMARY

This chapter has focused on the major metabolic pathways in myocardium and on their regulation under various physiologic and pathophysiologic conditions. The current understanding of the regulation of these pathways is by no means complete, particularly with respect to regulatory mechanisms in vivo. Investigators hope that cardiac imaging will play an increasing role in furthering the understanding of these complex pathways in health and sickness.

References

A

1. Allen, D. G., and Orchard, C. H.: Myocardial contractile function during ischemia and hypoxia. Circ. Res. 60:153, 1987.

B

1. Bing, R. J.: The metabolism of the heart. Harvey Lect. 50:27, 1955.
2. Bremer, J., and Osmundsen, H.: Fatty acid oxidation and its regulation. *In* Numa, S. (ed.): Fatty Acid Metabolism and Its Regulation. Elsevier, Amsterdam, 1984, p. 113.
3. Bing, R. J.: Cardiac metabolism. Physiol. Rev. 45:171, 1965.
4. Bassenge, E., Wendt, V. E., Schollmeyer, P., et al.: Effects of ketone bodies on cardiac metabolism. Am. J. Physiol. 208:162, 1965.
5. Bielefeld, D. R., Vary, T. C., and Neely, J. R.: Inhibition of carnitine palmitoyl-CoA transferase activity and fatty acid oxidation by lactate and oxfenicine in cardiac muscle. J. Mol. Cell. Cardiol. 17:619, 1985.
6. Braunwald, E., and Kloner, R. A.: The stunned myocardium: Prolonged, postischemic ventricular dysfunction. Circulation 66:1146, 1982.
7. Buxton, D. B., Schwaiger, M., Vaghaiwalla Mody, F., et al.: Regional abnormality of oxygen consumption in reperfused myocardium assessed with [1-^{11}C]acetate and positron emission tomography. Am. J. Cardiac Imag. 3:276, 1989.
8. Bricknell, O. L., and Opie, L. H.: Effects of substrates on tissue metabolic changes in the isolated rat heart during underperfusion and on release of lactate dehydrogenase and arrhythmias during reperfusion. Circ. Res. 43:102, 1978.
9. Bricknell, O. L., Davies, P. S., and Opie, L. H.: A relationship between adenosine triphosphate, glycolysis and ischemic contracture in the isolated rat heart. J. Mol. Cell. Cardiol. 13:941, 1981.
10. Bessman, S. P., and Geiger, P. J.: Transport of energy in muscle: The phosphorylcreatine shuttle. Science 211:448, 1981.

C

1. Cheung, J. Y., Conover, C., Regen, D. M., et al.: Effects of insulin on kinetics of sugar transport in heart muscle. Am. J. Physiol. 234:E70, 1978.
2. Clark, M. G., and Patten, G. S.: Adrenaline activation of phosphofructokinase in rat heart mediated by α-receptor mechanism independent of cyclic AMP. Nature 292:461, 1981.
3. Chance, B., and Williams, G. R.: Respiratory enzymes in oxidative phosphorylation. 1. Kinetics of oxygen utilization. J. Biol. Chem. 217:383, 1955.
4. Clark, M. G., and Patten, G. S.: Adrenergic regulation of glucose metabolism in rat heart. J. Biol. Chem. 259:15204, 1984.
5. Camici, P., Araujo, L. I., Spinks, T., et al.: Increased uptake of ^{18}F-fluorodeoxyglucose in postischemic myocardium of patients with exercise-induced angina. Circulation 74:81, 1986.
6. Collarini, E. J., and Oxender, D. L.: Mechanisms of transport of amino acids across membranes. Annu. Rev. Nutr. 7:75, 1987.
7. Clark, A. F., and Wildenthal, K.: Disproportionate reduction of actin synthesis in hearts of starved rats. J. Biol. Chem. 261:13168, 1986.
8. Crie, J. S., Sanford, C. F., and Wildenthal, K.: Influence of starvation and refeeding on cardiac protein degradation in rats. J. Nutr. 108:22, 1980.
9. Curfman, G. D., O'Hara, D. S., Hopkins, B. E., and Smith, T. W.: Suppression of myocardial protein degradation in the rat during fasting: Effects of insulin, glucose and leucine. Circ. Res. 46:581, 1980.

D

1. Drake, A. J., Haines, J. R., and Noble, M. I. M.: Preferential uptake of lactate by normal myocardium in dogs. Cardiovasc. Res. 14:65, 1980.
2. Drake-Holland, A. J.: Substrate utilization. *In* Drake, A. J., and Noble, M. I. (eds.): Cardiac Metabolism. John Wiley & Sons, New York, 1983, p. 195.
3. DeGrella, R. F., and Light, R. J.: Uptake and metabolism of fatty acids by dispersed adult rat heart myocytes. J. Biol. Chem. 255:9731, 1980.
4. De Jong, J. W., and Hülsmann, W. C.: A comparative study of palmitoyl-CoA synthetase activity in rat liver, heart and gut mitochondrial and microsomal preparations. Biochim. Biophys. Acta 197:127, 1970.
5. Denton, R. M., and McCormack, J. G.: On the role of the calcium transport cycle in heart and other mammalian mitochondria. FEBS Lett. 119:1, 1980.
6. DeBoer, L. W. V., Ingwall, J. S., Kloner, R. A., and Braunwald, E.: Prolonged derangement of canine myocardial purine metabolism after a brief coronary artery occlusion not associated with anatomical evidence of necrosis. Proc. Natl. Acad. Sci. USA 77:5471, 1980.

E

1. England, P. J., and Randle, P. J.: Effectors of rat heart hexokinases and the control of rates of glucose phosphorylation in the perfused rat. Biochem. J. 105:907, 1967.
2. Erecinska, M., and Wilson, D. F.: Regulation of cellular energy metabolism. J. Membr. Biol. 70:1, 1982.

F

1. Forsey, R. G. P., Reid, K., and Brosnan, J. T.: Competition between fatty acids and carbohydrate or ketone bodies as metabolic fuels for the isolated perfused heart. Can. J. Physiol. Pharmacol. 65:401, 1987.

G

1. Green, M. H., and Landau, B. R.: Contribution of the pentose cycle to glucose metabolism in muscle. Arch. Biochem. Biophys. 1111:569, 1965.
2. Grably, S., and Rossi, A.: Changes in cardiac glycogen synthase and phosphorylase activities following stimulation of beta-adrenergic receptors in rats. Basic Res. Cardiol. 80:175, 1985.
3. Gertz, E. W., Wisneski, J. A., Neese, R., et al.: Myocardial lactate metabolism: Evidence of lactate release during net chemical extraction in man. Circulation 63:1273, 1981.
4. Glatz, J. F. C., Janssen, A. M., Baerwaldt, C. C. F., and Veerkamp, J. H.: Purification and characterization of fatty acid–binding proteins from rat heart and liver. Biochim. Biophys. Acta 837:57, 1985.
5. Groot, P. G. E., Scholte, H. R., and Hulsmann, W. C.: Fatty acid activation: Specificity, localization and function. Adv. Lipid. Res. 14:75, 1976.
6. Goodale, W. T., Olson, R. E., and Hackel, D. B.: The effects of fasting and diabetes mellitus on myocardial metabolism in man. Am. J. Med. 27:212, 1959.
7. Grover-McKay, M., Schelbert, H. R., Schwaiger, M., et al.: Identification of impaired metabolic reserve by atrial pacing in patients with impaired coronary reserve. Circulation 74:281, 1986.

H

1. Hers, H. G., and Van Schaftigen, E.: Fructose 2,6-bisphosphate 2 years after its discovery. Biochem J. 206:1, 1982.
2. Hansford, R. G.: Control of mitochondrial substrate oxidation. Curr. Top. Cell. Regul. 10:217, 1980.
3. Hansford, R. G., and Johnson, R. N.: Steady state concentrations of coenzyme A-SH, coenzyme A thioester, citrate and isocitrate during tricarboxylate cycle oxidation in rabbit heart mitochondria. J. Biol. Chem. 250:8361, 1975.
4. Hansford, R. G.: Relation between mitochondrial Ca^{2+} transport and control of energy metabolism. Rev. Physiol. Biochem. Pharmacol. 102:1, 1985.
5. Hassinen, I. E.: Mitochondrial respiratory control in the myocardium. Biochim. Biophys. Acta 853:135, 1986.
6. Higgins, T. J. C., and Bailey, P. J.: The effects of cyanide and iodoacetate intoxication and ischaemia on enzyme release from the perfused rat heart. Biochim. Biophys. Acta 762:67, 1983.
7. Hasin, Y., and Barry, W. H.: Myocardial metabolic inhibition and membrane potential, contraction and potassium uptake. Am. J. Physiol. 247:H322, 1984.
8. Harmon, C. S., Proud, C. G., and Pain, V. M.: Effects of starvation, diabetes and acute insulin treatment on the regulation of polypeptide initiation in rat skeletal muscle. Biochem. J. 223:687, 1984.
9. Henriksen, O., Robinson, E. A., and Maxwell, E. S.: Interaction of guanine nucleotides with elongation factor-2. 1. Equilibrium dialysis studies. J. Biol. Chem. 250:720, 1975.

I

1. Issekutz, B., Jr., Miller, H. I., Paul, P., et al.: Effect of lactic acid on free fatty acids and glucose oxidation in dogs. Am. J. Physiol. 209:1137, 1965.

J

1. Jacobus, W. E., Moreadith, R. W., and Vandegaer, K. M.: Mitochondrial respiratory control. J. Biol. Chem. 257:2377, 1982.

K

1. Kacser, H., and Burns, J. A.: The control of flux. Symp. Soc. Exp. Biol. 32:65, 1973.
2. Kacser, H.: The control of enzyme systems in vivo—elasticity analysis of the steady state. Biochem. Soc. Trans. 11:35, 1983.
3. Krivokapich, J., Huang, S.-C., Phelps, M. E., et al.: Estimation of rabbit myocardial metabolic rate for glucose using fluorodeoxyglucose. Am. J. Physiol. 243:H884, 1982.
4. Krisman, C. R., and Barengo, R.: A precursor of glycogen biosynthesis: Alpha-1,4-glucan-protein. Eur. J. Biochem. 52:117, 1975.
5. Kobayashi, K., and Neely, J. R.: Control of maximum rates of glycolysis in rat cardiac muscle. Circ. Res. 44:166, 1979.
6. Klingenberg, M.: The ADP-ATP translocation in mitochondria: A membrane potential controlled transport. J. Membr. Biol. 56:97, 1980.
7. Keul, J., Doll, E., Steim, H., et al.: Uber den Stoffwechsel des menschlichen Herzens III: Der oxydative Stoffwechsel des menschlichen Herzens under vershiedenen Arbeitsbedigungen. Pflügers Arch. 282:43, 1965.
8. Kessar, P., Crompton, M.: The α-adrenergic–mediated activation of Ca^{2+} influx into cardiac mitochondria. Biochem. J. 200:379, 1981.
9. Kobayashi, K., and Neely, J. R.: Effects of ischemia and reperfusion on pyruvate dehydrogenase activity in isolated rat hearts. J. Mol. Cell. Cardiol. 15:359, 1983.
10. Kelly, F. J., and Jefferson, L. S.: Control of peptide-chain initiation in rat skeletal muscle: Development of methods for preparation of native ribosomal subunits and analysis of the effects of insulin on formation of 40 S initiation complexes. J. Biol. Chem. 260:6677, 1985.

L

1. Liedtke, A. J.: Alterations of carbohydrate and lipid metabolism in the acutely ischemic heart. Prog. Cardiovasc. Dis. 23:321, 1981.
2. Lehninger, A. L.: Biochemistry. Worth, New York, 1975.
3. Lawson, J. W. R., and Uyeda, K.: Effects of insulin and work on fructose 2,6-bisphosphate content and phosphofructokinase activity in perfused rat hearts. J. Biol. Chem. 262:3165, 1987.
4. Lopes-Cardozo, M., Klazinga, W., and van den Bergh, S. G.: Evidence for a homogeneous pool of acetyl CoA in rat liver mitochondria. Eur. J. Biochem. 83:635, 1978.
5. Land, J. M., Mowbray, J., and Clark, J. B.: Control of pyruvate and β-hydroxybutyrate utilization in rat brain mitochondria and its relevance to phenylketonuria and maple syrup urine disease. J. Neurochem. 26:823, 1976.
6. LaNoue, K. F., Bryla, J., and Williamson, J. R.: Feedback interactions in the control of citric acid cycle activity in rat heart mitochondria. J. Biol. Chem. 247:667, 1972.
7. LaNoue, K. F., Walajtys, E. I., and Williamson, J. R.: Regulation of glutamate metabolism and interactions with the citric acid cycle in rat heart mitochondria. J. Biol. Chem. 248:7171, 1973.
8. Lowenstein, J. M.: Oxygen in the Animal Organism. Pergamon Press, London, 1963, p. 163.
9. Little, J. R., Goto, M., and Spitzer, J. J.: Effects of ketones on metabolism of free fatty acids by dog myocardium and skeletal muscle in vivo. Am. J. Physiol. 219:1458, 1971.
10. Liedtke, A. J., DeMaison, L., Eggleston, A. M., et al.: Changes in substrate metabolism and effects of excess fatty acids in reperfused myocardium. Circ. Res. 62:535, 1988.

M

1. McCollough, T. E., and Walsh, D. A.: Phosphorylation of glycogen synthase in the perfused rat heart. J. Biol. Chem. 254:7336, 1979.
2. Mansour, T. E.: Phosphofructokinase. Curr. Top. Cell. Regul. 5:1, 1972.
3. Mowbray, J.: A mitochondrial monocarboxylate transporter in rat liver and heart and its possible function in cell control. Biochem. J. 148:41, 1975.
4. Mann, G. E., Zlokovic, B. V., and Yudilevich, D. L.: Evidence for a lactate transport system in the sarcolemmal membrane of the perfused rabbit heart: Kinetics of unidirectional influx, carrier specificity and effects of glucagon. Biochim. Biophys. Acta 819:241, 1985.
5. McGarry, J. D., Mills, S. E., Long, C. S., and Foster, D. W.: Observations on the affinity for carnitine, and malonyl-CoA sensitivity, of carnitine, palmitoyl-transferase I in animal and human tissues. Biochem. J. 214:21, 1983.
6. McCormack, J. G., and Denton, R. M.: The activation of pyruvate dehydrogenase in the perfused rat heart by adrenaline and other inotropic agents. Biochem. J. 194:639, 1981.
7. Morgan, H. E., Randle, P. J., and Regen, D. M.: Regulation of glucose uptake by muscle. III. Effects of insulin, anoxia, salicylate and 2:4-dinitrophenol on membrane transport and intracellular phosphorylation of glucose in the isolated rat heart. Biochem. J. 73:573, 1959.
8. Morgan, H. E., Henderson, M. J., Regen, D. M., and Park, C. R.: Regulation of glucose uptake in muscle. 1. The effects of insulin and anoxia on glucose transport and phosphorylation in the isolated perfused heart of the normal rat. J. Biol. Chem. 236:253, 1961.
9. Mochizuki, S., and Neely, J. R.: Control of glyceraldehyde-3-phosphate dehydrogenase in cardiac muscle. J. Mol. Cell. Cardiol. 11:221, 1979.
10. Moore, K. H., Radloff, J. F., Hull, F. E., and Sweeley, C. C.: Incomplete fatty acid oxidation by ischemic heart: β-hydroxy fatty acid production. Am. J. Physiol. 239:H257, 1980.
11. Marshall, R. C., Tillisch, J. H., Phelps, M. E., et al.: Identification and differentiation of resting myocardial ischemia and infarction in man with positron computed tomography, ^{18}F-labeled fluorodeoxyglucose and N-13 ammonia. Circulation 67:766, 1983.
12. Most, A. S., Gorlin, R., and Soeldner, J. S.: Glucose extraction by the human myocardium during pacing stress. Circulation 45:92, 1972.
13. Myears, D. W., Sobel, B. E., and Bergmann, S. R.: Substrate use in ischemic and reperfused canine myocardium: Quantitative considerations. Am. J. Physiol. 253:H107, 1987.
14. McDonald, T. F., Hayahi, H., Ponnambalam, C., and Watanabe, T.: Cardiac Function Under Ischemia and Hypoxia. University of Nagoya Press, Nagoya, Japan, 1986.
15. Morgan, H. E., Rannels, D. E., and McKee, E. E.: Protein metabolism of the heart. *In* Berne, R., and Sperelakis, N. (eds.): Handbook of Physiology: Circulation. Section 1, The Cardiovascular System. Vol. 1. Am. Physiological Society. Williams & Wilkins, Baltimore, 1979, p. 845.
16. Moldave, K.: Eukaryotic protein synthesis. Annu. Rev. Biochem. 54:1109, 1985.
17. Mortimore, G. E., Pösö, A. R.: Intracellular protein catabolism and its control during nutrient deprivation and supply. Annu. Rev. Nutr. 7:539, 1987.

N

1. Neely, J. R., and Morgan, H. E.: Relationship between carbohydrate and lipid metabolism and the energy balance of heart muscle. Ann. Rev. Physiol. 36:414, 1974.
2. Narabayashi, H., Lawson, J. W. R., and Uyeda, K.: Regulation of phosphofructokinase in perfused rat heart. J. Biol. Chem. 260:9750, 1985.
3. Nishiki, K., Erecinska, M., and Wilson, D.: Energy relationships between cytosolic metabolism and mitochondrial respiration in rat heart. Am. J. Physiol. 234:C73, 1978.
4. Newsholme, E. A., and Randle, P. J.: Regulation of glucose uptake by muscle. 7. Effects of fatty acids, ketone bodies and pyruvate, and of alloxan diabetes, starvation hypophysectomy and adrenalectomy, on the concentrations of hexose phosphates, nucleotides and inorganic phosphate in perfused rat heart. Biochem. J. 93:641, 1964.
5. Neely, J. R., Whitmer, J. T., and Rovetto, M. J.: Effect of coronary blood flow on glycolytic flux and intracellular pH in isolated rat hearts. Circ. Res. 37:733, 1975.

O

1. Opie, L. H., Mansford, K. R. L., and Owen, P.: Effects of increased heart work on glycolysis and adenine nucleotides in the perfused hearts of normal and diabetic rats. Biochem. J. 124:475, 1971.
2. Olson, M. S., Scholz, R., Buffington, C., et al.: Regulation of α-keto acid dehydrogenase multienzyme complexes in isolated perfused organs. *In* Veneziale, C. M. (ed.): The Regulation of Carbohydrate Formation and Utilization in Mammals. Baltimore, University Park Press, 1981, p. 153.
3. Oram, J. F., Bennetch, S. L., and Neely, J. R.: Regulation of fatty acid utilization in isolated perfused rat hearts. J. Biol. Chem. 248:5299, 1973.
4. Oram, J. F., Wenger, J. J., and Neely, J. R.: Regulation of long chain fatty acid activation in heart muscle. J. Biol. Chem. 250:73, 1975.
5. Opie, L. H.: Effects of regional ischemia on metabolism of glucose and fatty acids: Relative rates of aerobic and anaerobic energy production during myocardial infarction and comparison with effects of anoxia. Circulation 38(Suppl. I):52, 1976.
6. Opie, L. H., Owen, P., and Riemersma, R. A.: Relative rates of oxidation of glucose and free fatty acids by ischaemic and non-ischaemic myocardium after coronary artery ligation in the dog. Eur. J. Clin. Invest. 3:419, 1973.

P

1. Pande, S. V., and Parvin, R.: Pyruvate and acetoacetate transport in mitochondria: A reappraisal. J. Biol. Chem. 253:1565, 1978.
2. Patel, T. B., and Olson, M. S.: Regulation of pyruvate dehydrogenase complex in ischemic rat heart. Am. J. Physiol. 246:H858, 1984.
3. Peuhkurinen, K. J., Takala, T. E. S., Nuutinen, E. M., and Hassinen, I. E.: Tricarboxylic acid cycle metabolites during ischemia in isolated perfused rat heart. Am. J. Physiol. 244:H281, 1983.
4. Preedy, V. R., Smith, D. M., Kearney, N. F., and Sugden, P. H.: Rates of protein turnover in vivo and in vitro in ventricular muscle of hearts from fed and starved rats. Biochem. J. 222:395, 1984.
5. Pain, V. M.: Initiation of protein synthesis in mammalian cells. Biochem. J. 235:625, 1986.
6. Parmacek, M. S., Magid, N. M., Lesch, M., et al.: Cardiac protein synthesis and degradation during thyroxine-induced left ventricular hypertrophy. Am. J. Physiol. 251:C727, 1986.
7. Preedy, V. R., Smith, D. M., and Sugden, P. H.: The effects of 6 hours of hypoxia on protein synthesis in rat tissues in vivo and in vitro. Biochem. J. 228:179, 1985.
8. Preedy, V. R., and Sugden, P. H.: The effects of fasting or hypoxia on rates of protein synthesis in vivo in subcellular fractions of rat heart and gastrocnemius muscle. Biochem. J. 257:519, 1989.

R

1. Randle, P. J., and Tubbs, P. K.: Carbohydrate and fatty acid metabolism. *In* Berne, R., and Sperelakis, N. (eds.): Handbook of Physiology: Circulation. Section 2, The Cardiovascular System. Vol. 1. American Physiological Society. Williams & Wilkins, Baltimore, 1979, p. 805.
2. Randle, P. J., Newsholme, E. A., and Garland, P. B.: Regulation of glucose uptake by muscle. 8. Effects of fatty acids, ketone bodies, and pyruvate, and of alloxan diabetes and starvation, on the uptake and metabolic fate of glucose in rat heart and diaphragm muscle. Biochem. J. 93:652, 1964.
3. Rider, M. H., and Hue, L.: Activation of rat heart phosphofructokinase-2 by insulin in vivo. FEBS Lett. 176:484, 1984.
4. Rovetto, M. J., Lamerton, W. F., and Neely, J. R.: Mechanisms of glycolytic inhibition in ischemic rat hearts. Circ. Res. 37:742, 1975.
5. Reed, L. J.: Regulation of mammalian pyruvate dehydrogenase complex by a phosphorylation-dephosphorylation cycle. Curr. Top. Cell. Regul. 18:95, 1981.
6. Robinson, A. M., and Williamson, D. H.: Physiological roles of ketone bodies as substrates and signals in mammalian tissues. Physiol. Rev. 60:143, 1980.
7. Rudolph, W., Maas, D., Richter, J., et al.: Über die Bedeutung von Acetoacetat und β-Hydroxybutyrat im Stoffwechsel der menschlichen Herzens. Klin. Wochenschr. 43:445, 1965.
8. Randle, P. J., England, P. J., and Denton, R. M.: Control of the tricarboxylate cycle and its interactions with glycolysis during acetate utilization in the rat heart. Biochem. J. 117:677, 1970.
9. Rannels, D. E., Kao, R., and Morgan, H. E.: Effect of insulin on protein turnover in heart muscle. J. Biol. Chem. 250:1694, 1975.
10. Rannels, D. E., Jefferson, L. S., Hjalmarson, A. C., et al.: Maintenance of protein synthesis in hearts of diabetic animals. Biochem. Biophys. Res. Commun. 40:1110, 1970.
11. Rannels, D. E., Hjalmarson, A. C., and Morgan, H. E.: Effects of non-carbohydrate substrates on protein synthesis in muscle. Am. J. Physiol. 226:528, 1974.

S

1. Simpson, I. A., and Cushman, S. W.: Hormonal regulation of mammalian glucose transport. Annu. Rev. Biochem. 55:1059, 1986.
2. Samuel, D., Paris, S., and Ailhaud, G.: Uptake and metabolism of fatty acids and analogues by cultured cardiac cells from chick embryo. Eur. J. Biochem. 64:583, 1976.
3. Stremmel, W.: Fatty acid uptake by isolated rat heart myocytes represents a carrier-mediated transport process. J. Clin. Invest. 81:844, 1988.
4. Sweetser, D. A., Heuckeroth, R. O., and Gordon, J. I.: The metabolic significance of mammalian fatty-acid-binding proteins: Abundant proteins in search of a function. Annu. Rev. Nutr. 7:337, 1987.
5. Stryer, L.: Biochemistry, W.H. Freeman, New York, 1988.
6. Saggerson, E. D., and Carpenter, C. A.: Carnitine palamitoyltransferase and carnitine octanoyltransferase activities in liver, kidney cortex, adipocyte, lactating mammary gland, skeletal muscle and heart—relative activities, latency and effect of malonyl CoA. FEBS Lett. 129:229, 1981.
7. Stanley, K. K., and Tubbs, P. K.: The role of intermediates in fatty acid oxidation. Biochem. J. 150:77, 1975.
8. Srere, P. A., Halper, L. A., and Finkelstein, M. B.: Interaction of citrate synthase and malate dehydrogenase. *In* Srere, P. A., and Estabrook, R. W. (eds.): Microenvironments and Metabolic Compartmentation. Academic Press, New York, 1978, p. 419.
9. Schelbert, H. R., Henze, E., Schon, H. R., et al.: C-11 palmitate for the non-invasive evaluation of regional myocardial fatty acid metabolism with positron computed tomography. III. In vivo demonstration of the effects of substrate availability on myocardial metabolism. Am. Heart. J. 105:492, 1983.
10. Sale, G. J., and Randle, P. J.: Occupancy of sites of phosphorylation in inactive rat heart pyruvate dehydrogenase phosphate in vivo. Biochem. J. 193:935, 1981.
11. Stanley, W. C., Wisneski, J. A., Gertz, E. W., and Neese, R. A.: Enhanced carbohydrate utilization by the myocardium during exercise. Circulation 78(Suppl. II):54, 1988.
12. Schwaiger, M., Neese, R., Araujo, L., et al.: Sustained nonoxidative glucose utilization and depletion of glycogen in reperfused canine myocardium. J. Am. Coll. Cardiol. 13:745, 1989.
13. Schwaiger, M., Schelbert, H. R., Keen, R., et al.: Retention and clearance of C-11 palmitate in ischemic and reperfused myocardium. J. Am. Coll. Cardiol. 6:311, 1985.
14. Schwaiger, M., Schelbert, H. R., Ellison, D., et al.: Sustained regional abnormalities in cardiac metabolism after transient ischemia in the chronic dog model. J. Am. Coll. Cardiol. 6:336, 1985.
15. Schwaiger, M., Hansen, H. W., Sochor, W., et al.: Delayed recovery of regional glucose metabolism in reperfused canine myocardium demonstrated by positron-CT (PCT). J. Am. Coll. Cardiol. 3:574, 1984.
16. Stahl, L. D., Weiss, H. R., and Becker, L. C.: Myocardial oxygen consumption, oxygen supply/demand heterogeneity, and microvascular patency in regionally stunned myocardium. Circulation 77:865, 1988.
17. Samarel, A. M., Parmacek, M. S., Magid, N. M., et al.: Protein synthesis and degradation during starvation-induced cardiac atrophy in rabbits. Circ. Res. 60:933, 1987.
18. Schimmel, P. R., and Söll, D.: Aminoacyl t-RNA synthetases: General features and recognition of transfer RNAs. Annu Rev. Biochem. 48:601, 1979.
19. Slobin, L. I.: Eukaryotic initiation factor Ts is an integral component of rabbit reticulocyte elongation factor-1. Eur. J. Biochem. 96:287, 1979.

T

1. Taegtmeyer, H.: Myocardial metabolism. *In* Phelps, M. E., et al. (eds.): Positron Emission Tomography and Autoradiography: Principles and Applications for the Brain and Heart. Raven Press, New York, 1986, p. 149.
2. Taegtmeyer, H., Hems, R., and Krebs, H. A.: Utilization of energy providing substrates in the isolated working rat heart. Biochem. J. 186:701, 1980.
3. Taegtmeyer, H.: Six blind men explore an elephant: Aspects of fuel metabolism and the control of tricarboxylic acid cycle activity in heart muscle. Basic Res. Cardiol. 79:322, 1984.
4. Taegtmeyer, H., Roberts, A. F. C., and Raine, A. E. G.: Energy metabolism in reperfused heart muscle: Metabolic correlates to return of function. J. Am. Coll. Cardiol. 6:864, 1985.
5. Tillisch, J., Brunken, R., Marshall, R., et al.: Reversibility of cardiac wall–motion abnormalities predicted by positron tomography. N. Engl. J. Med. 314:884, 1986.
6. Tate, W. P., and Caskey, C. T.: The mechanism of peptide chain termination. Mol. Cell. Biochem. 5:115, 1974.

U

1. Uyeda, K.: Phosphofructokinase. Adv. Enzymol. 48:193, 1979.
2. Uyeda, K., Furuya, E., Richards, C. S., and Yokoyama, M.: Fructose 2,6-P2: Chemistry and biological function. Mol. Cell. Biochem. 48:97, 1982.

V

1. van der Vusse, G. J., Roemen, T. H., Prinzen, F. W., et al.: Uptake and tissue content of fatty acids in dog myocardium under normoxic and ischemic conditions. Circ. Res. 50:538, 1982.

W

1. Wieland, O. H.: The mammalian pyruvate dehydrogenase complex: Structure and regulation. Rev. Physiol. Biochem. Pharmacola. 96:123, 1983.
2. Wisneski, J. A., Gertz, E. W., Neese, R. A., et al.: Dual carbon-labeled isotope experiments using D-[6-^{14}C] glucose and L-[1,2,3-^{13}C]lactate: A new approach for investigating human myocardial metabolism during ischemia. J. Am. Coll. Cardiol. 5:1138, 1985.
3. Wick, A. N., and Drury, D. R.: The effect of concentration on the rate of utilization of β-hydroxybutyric acid by the rabbit. J. Biol. Chem. 138:129, 1951.
4. Williamson, J. R.: Mitochondrial function in the heart. Ann. Rev. Physiol. 41:485, 1979.
5. Williamson, J. R., Ford, C., Illingworth, J., and Safer, B.: Coordination of citric acid cycle activity with electron transport flux. Circ. Res. 38(Suppl. I):I39, 1976.
6. Williamson, J. R.: Metabolic effects of epinephrine in the isolated perfused rat heart. J. Biol. Chem. 239:2721, 1964.
7. Williamson, J. R.: Glycolytic control mechanisms: II. Kinetics of intermediate changes during the aerobic-anoxic transition in perfused rat heart. J. Biol. Chem. 2411:5026, 1966.
8. Whitmer, J. T., Idell-Wenger, J. A., Rovetto, M. J., and Neely, J. R.: Control of fatty acid metabolism in ischemic and hypoxic hearts. J. Biol. Chem. 253:4305, 1978.
9. Wood, J. M., Hanley, H. G., Entman, M. L., et al.: Biochemical and morphological correlates of acute experimental ischemia in the dog. IV. Energy mechanisms during very early ischemia. Circ. Res. 44:52, 1979.
10. Weiss, J. N., and Hiltbrand, B.: Functional compartmentation of glycolytic versus oxidative metabolism in isolated rabbit heart. J. Clin. Invest. 75:436, 1985.
11. Weiss, J. N., and Lamp, S. T.: Glycolysis preferentially inhibits ATP-sensitive K^+ channels in isolated guinea pig myocytes. Science 238:67, 1987.
12. Waterlow, J. C., Garlick, P. J., and Millward, D. J.: Protein Turnover in Mammalian Tissues and in the Whole Body. North-Holland, Amsterdam, 1978, p. 580.

Z

1. Zak, R., Martin, A. F., Prior, G., and Rabinowitz, M.: Comparison of turnover of several myofibrillar proteins and critical evaluation of double isotope method. J. Biol. Chem. 252:3430, 1977.
2. Zeman, R. J., Kameyama, T., Matsumoto, K., et al.: Regulation of protein degradation in muscle by calcium. J. Biol. Chem. 260:13619, 1985.

Chapter 5

Physiologic Basis for the Evaluation of Valvular Function

▪ *KENT L. RICHARDS, M.D.* ▪ *SCOTT R. CANNON, Ph.D.*

HEMODYNAMIC EQUATIONS USEFUL IN QUANTIFYING VALVULAR HEART DISEASE 56
Quantification of Cardiac Output 56
Invasive Standards for Measuring Cardiac Output 56
Velocity-Based Flow Measurements 57
Relationship Among Velocity, Cross-Sectional Area, and Flow Rate Using the Continuity Equation 58
VALVE STENOSIS 59
Velocity Patterns Near Stenotic Valves 59
Quantification of Pressure Gradients 60
Relationship Between Velocity and Pressure Gradient Using the Bernoulli Equation 60
Calculation of Blood Velocity Using the Doppler Equation 61
Invasive Standards for Measuring Pressure Gradients 62
Calculation of "Flow-Independent" Measures of Stenosis 63
Valve Area 63
Valve Resistance 64
Variable-Orifice Stenotic Valves 64
Clinical Comparisons of Valve Stenoses 64
VALVULAR REGURGITATION 64
Velocity Patterns Near a Regurgitant Valve 65
Proximal Velocity Patterns and the Concepts of Regurgitant Orifice Cross-Sectional Area and Pressure Gradient 66
Distal Velocity Patterns and the Concept of Regurgitant Fraction 66
Invasive Standards for Quantifying Regurgitation 67
Regurgitant Fraction 67
Angiographic Severity 67
Other Hemodynamic Indicators of Severity of Regurgitation 68
Blood Pressure and Pressure Gradients 68
Pulmonary Artery Pressure 68
Regurgitant Orifice Cross-Sectional Area 68
Comparison of Regurgitant Valves 69
SUMMARY 69

The goal of this chapter is to familiarize the reader with the hemodynamics of common valvular lesions. Blood velocity is used to contrast normal with abnormal valve hemodynamics, because it best facilitates an understanding of the relationships among volume flow rate, cross-sectional area, and pressure gradient. In each section, parameters derived from catheterization, imaging, and Doppler echocardiography are emphasized because these are the techniques most widely available. For ease of discussion, this chapter first discusses equations that are useful in quantifying both stenotic and regurgitant lesions, and then discusses valvular stenosis and regurgitation in separate sections.

HEMODYNAMIC EQUATIONS USEFUL IN QUANTIFYING VALVULAR HEART DISEASE

The severity of valve stenosis is quantified clinically by measuring the transvalvular pressure gradient and valve cross-sectional area; valve resistance can also be calculated by combining pressure gradient and flow data. Because the physiology of pressure gradients is most easily understood as a function of velocity changes produced as blood flows through a reduced cross-sectional area, our discussion starts with quantification of blood flow rates and applications of the continuity equation, moves to measurement of pressure gradients, and ends with calculation of valve area and resistance.

Quantification of Cardiac Output

Invasive Standards for Measuring Cardiac Output

Two invasive techniques are used as the diagnostic standards for quantifying cardiac output. Both the Fick technique and the indicator dilution techniques (using green dye or thermodilution) are based on the principle proposed by Adolph Fick, which states that the total uptake of a substance by an organ is the product of the rate of blood flow through the organ multiplied by the difference between the arterial and the venous concentrations of that substance.[G1] If oxygen is the indicator substance, then determination of the oxygen consumption (Vo_2) and the arterial minus the venous oxygen concentration, that is, the arteriovenous oxygen difference (AV O_2 difference), allows calculation of pulmonary blood flow (Q_p) and systemic flow (Q_s) using Fick's principle (CO_f).

$$\text{If } Q_p = Q_s = CO_f, \text{ therefore, } CO_f = (Vo_2)/(\text{AV } O_2 \text{ difference})$$

In practice, oxygen consumption is estimated by quantifying the difference between the oxygen content of room air and that of expired air and measuring the volume of expired air. Because systemic arterial blood allows good approximation of pulmonary venous oxygen content, and pulmonary arterial blood allows approximation of mixed venous oxygen content, these samples are used to calculate the arteriovenous oxygen difference.

Major sources of error in the Fick method include incomplete collection or improper timing of the expired air samples, and contamination of the blood samples by room air or saturated blood (from the pulmonary artery wedge position). The error in the Fick method, when it is performed carefully, is about 10 percent.[V1] Although the Fick method is least accurate in cases of high cardiac output, in which a narrow arteriovenous oxygen difference is detected, it is more accurate than indicator dilution techniques when net forward cardiac output is low.

The indicator dilution techniques commonly used in intensive care units or catheterization laboratories involve injection of a bolus of a substance that is assumed to pass through a central part of the circulation (usually the lungs), where it mixes completely with the blood in that portion of the circulation before passing completely through the site at which its concentration (C) is determined with respect to time. Under these conditions, the amount of the substance injected (I) is the product of the flow rate (Q) and the integral of the concentration with respect to time [C(t)dt]:

$$I = Q \int C(t)dt$$

$$\text{therefore, } Q = I / \int C(t)dt$$

When indocyanine green dye is used as the indicator, it is usually injected into the pulmonary artery and sampled in the brachial or femoral artery. Because recirculation may occur before the first circulation has been completed, replotting of the downslope of the green dye concentration curve is required. If recirculation occurs during the early part of the downslope, significant errors result. Thus, in the presence of low cardiac output or severe valvular regurgitation, the green dye technique may be inaccurate. In the thermodilution technique, a bolus of cold saline or dextrose solution is injected into the vena cava, and a sample is obtained from the pulmonary artery with a sensitive thermistor. Inaccurate results are noted in the presence of significant tricuspid regurgitation or low cardiac output. In both of the indicator dilution techniques, samples are obtained over a relatively short period of flow (about 12 to 30 seconds in the green dye technique and about 1 to 3 seconds in the thermodilution technique). Because of the short sampling time, cardiac output determined by the dilution technique is more likely to be influenced by transient factors such as arrhythmias than is cardiac output determined by the Fick method, which averages flow over several minutes (usually 2 to 5 minutes). Arrhythmias that occur during the beats used to replot the downslope of the indicator dilution curves may cause significant errors. Indicator dilution techniques are widely used and usually produce accurate results (5 to 10 percent error) in moderate to high flow rates but less accurate results when flow rates are low.[G1]

Velocity-Based Flow Measurements

Figure 5–1 illustrates the Doppler echocardiographic equation, which is used to calculate the rate at which blood flows through a cylindric vessel. The volume flow rate (Q), is the product of the mean velocity of blood across the vessel (V_{mean}) and the mean cross-sectional area (A_{mean}) of the flowing blood:

$$Q = (V_{mean})(A_{mean})$$

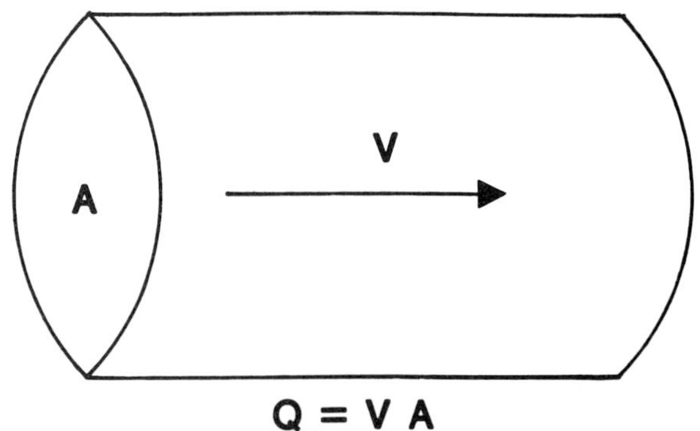

Figure 5–1. The flow rate (Q) of blood through the cylinder is the product of the cross-sectional area of flow (A) and the mean velocity (V) across that cross section. The velocity vector, shown as an arrow, denotes the anatomic site at which velocity is sampled at its tail, the speed of blood by the length of the shaft, and the direction of flow by the direction of the shaft and head.

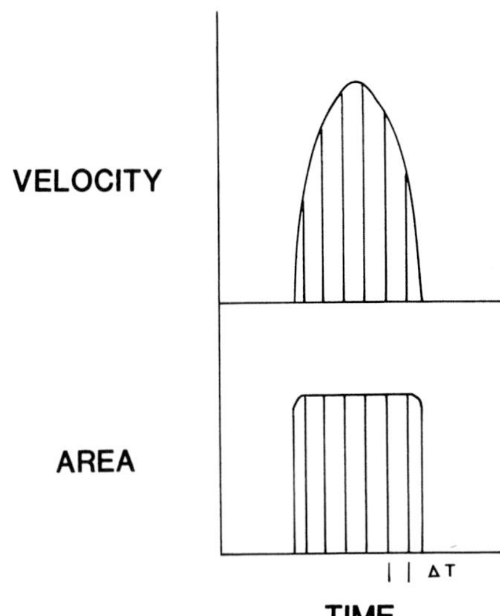

Figure 5–2. Blood velocity and cross-sectional area of pulsatile flow are plotted against the same time axis so that simultaneous, instantaneous velocities and cross-sectional areas can be measured at multiple, small time-intervals (ΔT). Multiple instantaneous volume flow rates are calculated as the product of instantaneous velocities and cross-sectional areas.

The concept that both the velocity and the cross-sectional area are averaged in time and space is important in the application of this equation to the heart.

Pulsatile flow produced by the heart introduces complexity into measurement of volume flow rate because both cross-sectional area and velocity change with time. Figure 5–2 shows graphs of hypothetic velocity and cross-sectional area versus time that might be expected near the aortic valve or in the ascending aorta. Velocity and time have been measured at a large number (n) of equally spaced times (Δt) throughout the cardiac cycle. The flow rate (Q_i) at each of these times is:

$$Q_i = (V_i)(A_i)$$

where (V_i) and (A_i) are the instantaneous velocities and cross-sectional areas.

The mean velocity and the mean cross-sectional area with respect to time are simply the averages of these individual measurements over the time of observation (usually a cardiac cycle):

$$V_{mean} = 1/n \sum_{i=1}^{n} V_i \qquad A_{mean} = 1/n \sum_{i=1}^{n} A_i$$

In a pulsatile system, in which area and velocity are in phase (that is, they start and end simultaneously and become larger or smaller to the same degree and at the same time), the mean flow rate is the product of the mean velocity and mean cross-sectional area:

$$Q_{mean} = (V_{mean})(A_{mean})$$

If differences in the phase relationship exist between instantaneous velocities and cross-sectional areas, then the products of multiple synchronous instantaneous velocities and instantaneous cross-sectional areas must be averaged to calculate accurate mean flow rate:

$$Q_{mean} = 1/n \sum_{i=1}^{n} (V_i)(A_i)$$

The observation that velocity is not the same across the cross section of the vessel complicates the calculation of mean velocity with respect to space. Determining the average velocity in space is usually accomplished by either sampling a portion of the vessel cross section, which is representative of velocity across the entire vessel, or by sampling all velocities across its cross section simultaneously. Examination of velocities recorded from vessels, such as the aorta, shows that a family of velocities is present at all times. The average spatial velocity at any time is usually approximated by the most common or modal velocity. The velocity-time envelope, used to estimate mean velocity, is drawn using the modal portion of the velocity tracing, as shown in Figure 5–3.

Measurement of the cross-sectional area of flow is simplified in most clinical situations by assuming (1) that flow cross-sectional area and anatomic cross-sectional area of the conduit that contains that flow are equal, and (2) that flow cross-sectional area remains constant throughout the part of the cardiac cycle in which blood is flowing through the vessel. These assumptions are reasonable when flow rates and pressures are normal and when the ascending aorta or aortic valve is used as a site for flow and area measurements. If flow rate is less than normal, blood velocities along the vessel wall slow because of the viscosity of blood. In this situation, the cross-sectional area of flow is smaller than that of the vessel; flow rates calculated using anatomic rather than flow cross-sectional area overestimate actual flow rates. Similarly, both anatomic and flow cross-sectional area can change significantly if blood pressure varies widely over the period of flow measurement. Under such circumstances, actual calculation of the mean cross-sectional area over the time of flow is required. Because mitral and tricuspid valve annulus and leaflet cross-sectional areas change greatly during diastolic flow time,[F1] mean cross-sectional area must be either calculated or estimated using a constant.[F1]

An early application of combined Doppler and imaging echocardiography was calculation of stroke volume through use of cross-sectional area and velocity data obtained from the aortic root.[H1] As shown in Figure 5–3, the velocity waveform from the aortic root exhibits a pulsatile contour. Because the phase of the velocity and cross-sectional area events is similar with respect to time, mean systolic cross-sectional area and velocity can be used. Stroke volume (SV) is the product of mean systolic cross-sectional area (A) and the area under the systolic velocity-time curve (VT):

$$SV = (A)\,(VT)$$

The two components of the equation are cross-sectional area (A) and the stroke distance (VT). The stroke distance is the distance that the cross section of blood moves in one cardiac cycle:

$$[(VT)] = [(\text{cm/sec})\,(\text{sec})] = [\text{cm}]$$

Stroke volume is converted to cardiac output by multiplying by the heart rate (HR = beats/min) and the constant (1 L/1000 cm^3) to produce units in familiar L/min from velocity-time integral (cm/beat) and vessel cross-sectional area (cm^2):

$$CO = (A)\,(VT)\,(HR)\,(\text{L}/1000\ \text{cm}^3)$$

Although Doppler echocardiographic measurements of cardiac flow have been made at all four heart valves,[F1, G2, L1, S1] their accuracy at sites other than the aorta, aortic valve, and mitral annulus has not been well established in adults. Because changes in both velocity and cross-sectional area usually accompany large changes in hemodynamics, both area and velocity measurements should be made when large changes in flow are anticipated or large changes in pressure are detected.

Relationship Among Velocity, Cross-Sectional Area, and Flow Rate Using the Continuity Equation

The continuity equation is based on concepts illustrated in Figure 5–4, in which blood flows steadily from left to right in a cylindrical vessel that tapers at its middle. Because there are no branches in the system, the rate at which volume flows into the vessel (Q_1) through cross-sectional area A_1 at velocity V_1 is the same as that at which blood flows out of the vessel (Q_2). Flow rates Q_1 and Q_2 are thus calculated:

$$Q_1 = (V_1)\,(A_1) = (V_2)\,(A_2) = Q_2$$

Rearrangement of the equation to calculate the stenotic cross-sectional area (A_2) yields the following:

$$(A_2) = (V_1)\,(A_1)/(V_2)$$

This approach can be applied directly to calculation of cross-sectional areas of stenotic aortic valves.[O1, S2, Z1] The valve area (A_a) is calculated as the product of the velocity in the left ventricular outflow tract (V_{lvot}) and the cross-sectional area of the outflow tract (A_{lvot}) divided by the velocity in the aortic valve orifice (V_a):

$$(A_a) = (V_{lvot})\,(A_{lvot})/(V_a)$$

This approach works well clinically despite the approximations used to obtain cross-sectional area and velocity measurements. The method used to calculate cross-sectional area of the left ventricular outflow tract is based on a single systolic diameter rather than an average of the cross-sectional areas measured throughout systole. Significant error can be introduced by this approach because the cross-sectional area of the outflow tract is not circular and because both cross-sectional area and shape change throughout systole. The exact site at which diameter of the left ventricular outflow tract should be measured is not clearly defined. In addition, blood velocities increase continuously, not discretely, as blood moves from the large cross-sectional area of

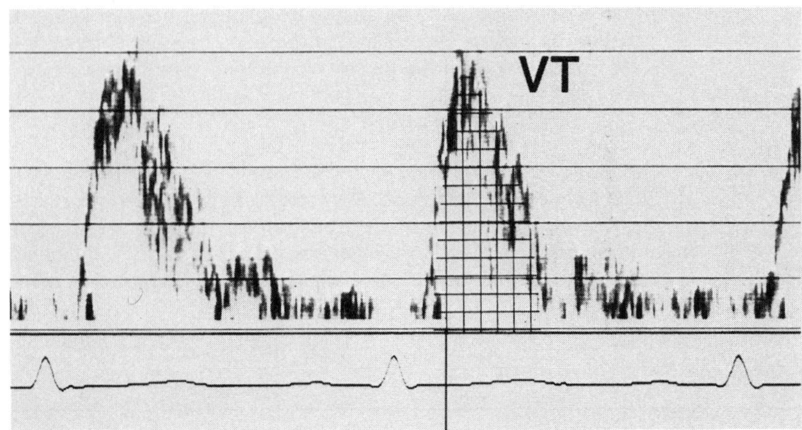

Figure 5–3. In this Doppler spectral tracing of velocities within the ascending aorta, time is plotted in the *x* axis (using 50-msec time lines) with the electrocardiogram for timing within the cardiac cycle. Velocity is plotted in the *y* axis using 20-cm/sec velocity lines; the double horizontal line represents zero. The velocity-time integral (VT) is shown as a cross-hatched region between the modal velocity (most prevalent velocity as indicated by the darkest shade of gray) and the zero baseline.

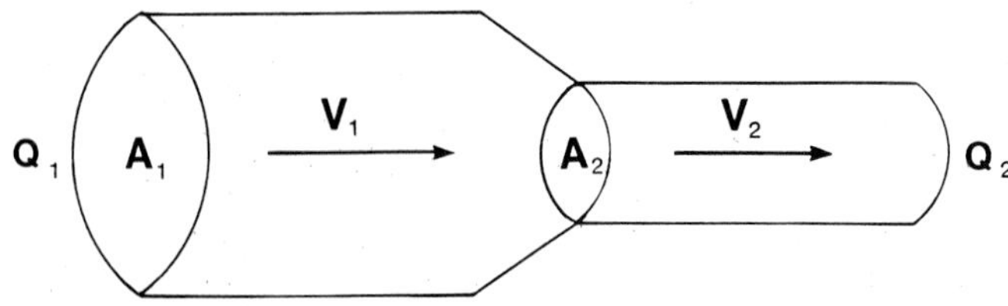

$$Q_1 = (A_1)(V_1) = (A_2)(V_2) = Q_2$$
$$(A_2) = (A_1)(V_1)/(V_2)$$

Figure 5–4. Blood flows from a widely patent cylinder with cross-sectional area (A_1) and velocity (V_1) through a constricted cylinder with cross-sectional area (A_2) and velocity (V_2). Because no branches occur in the system, the flow rate entering the cylinder (Q_1) equals that exiting the cylinder (Q_2). The stenotic cross-sectional area can be determined by measuring both velocities and the cross-sectional area in the wide portion of the vessel.

the left ventricle into the left ventricular outflow tract and through the stenotic valve orifice. Care must be taken to obtain the velocity sample of the left ventricular outflow tract at a site proximal to the site at which velocities begin to increase abruptly, and at the same site at which cross-sectional area is measured. Likewise, the valve orifice velocities must be obtained from the orifice rather than at a proximal site.

A simplified application of the same concept is illustrated in Figure 5–5. The heart is modeled as if it were a conduit in which, during each cardiac cycle, flow into the mitral valve (Q_m) equals flow out of the aortic valve (Q_a):

$$Q_m = (A_m)(V_m) = (A_a)(V_a) = Q_a$$

Rearrangement of the equation to calculate the ratio of cross-sectional area yields the following:

$$(A_a)/(A_m) = (V_m)/(V_a)$$

If the ratio of valve cross-sectional areas in normal subjects is assumed to be nearly constant, a direct relationship should exist

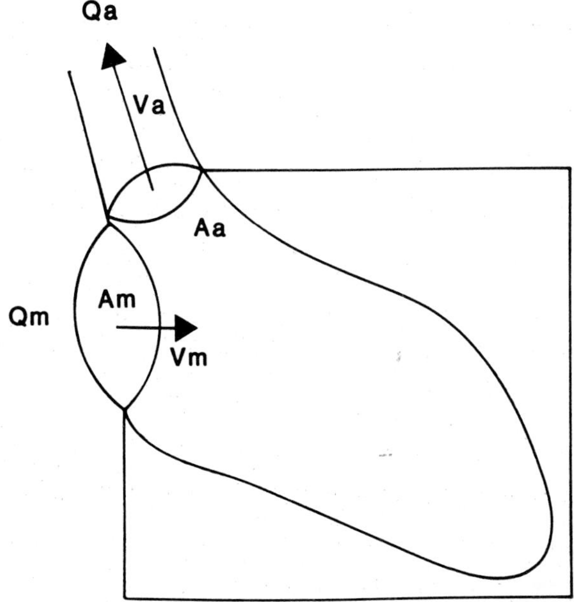

$$Qm = (Am)(Vm) = (Aa)(Va) = Qa$$

Figure 5–5. If an entire cardiac cycle is considered, the left atrium, left ventricle, and aortic valve can be modeled as a conduit in which blood enters at the mitral valve with cross-sectional area A_m at velocity V_m and exits at the aortic valve with cross-sectional area A_a at velocity V_a. If regurgitation and shunting are absent, the flow into the mitral valve (Q_m) equals that exiting the aortic valve (Q_a).

between the ratio of velocities in these valves $[(V_m)/(V_a)]$ and aortic valve area:[R1]

$$(A_a) \sim (V_m)/(V_a) \qquad \text{(Aortic)}$$

The inverse of this ratio has been shown to be directly proportional to mitral valve area in the presence of mitral stenosis:[R2, N1]

$$(A_m) \sim (V_a)/(V_m) \qquad \text{(Mitral)}$$

These abbreviated approaches have the advantage of requiring no imaging data. They are applicable only when mitral and aortic stroke volumes are equal; they are inaccurate when more than mild mitral or aortic regurgitation is present, or when intracardiac shunts are present.

In addition to the applications in valvular disease, the continuity equation should allow accurate calculation of cross-sectional area reduction in peripheral and central arteries.

VALVE STENOSIS

Velocity Patterns Near Stenotic Valves

Knowledge of the velocity patterns near stenotic cardiac valves is helpful in understanding the basis by which catheterization and echocardiography identify valve stenosis. Quantification of the lesions requires knowledge of the spatial distribution of velocities as well as use of the preceding concepts from the flow and continuity equations. The universal presence of subvalvular, valvular, and postvalvular pressure gradients is easily understood by employing these concepts.

Blood velocity patterns near a stenotic orifice are illustrated in Figure 5–6. The model consists of a straight cylinder in which blood flows steadily from left to right. A long, tapered, stenotic region exists in the middle of the cylinder. Blood velocities are shown by arrows, which represent blood velocity vectors. The anatomic sites sampled are shown by the beginning of each arrow. The direction of each velocity vector is shown by its arrowhead. The speed represented by a velocity vector is proportional to the length of the arrow shaft. Curved arrows are drawn to imply circular motion of blood.

Proximal to the stenotic region, the speed of the blood is moderate and nearly uniform across the vessel; the velocity vectors are parallel to each other.[C1, M1] This type of blood flow is referred to as laminar flow, meaning that small adjacent units of flowing blood have nearly the same speeds and directions. As the anatomic cross-sectional area of the tube is reduced in the region proximal to the stenosis, the blood velocities increase, because the same volume of blood must now pass through progressively smaller cross-sectional areas of the vessel. Blood velocities are further elevated within the stenosis but reach a peak in a region called the vena contracta, which is usually just distal to the most severe anatomic narrowing. A high-velocity jet, formed within the stenosis, extends distally 2 to 5 valve orifice diameters in relation to the stenotic region.[C2] As the equal lengths of the blood velocity vectors within the jet suggest, the velocities across the jet are frequently similar to each other. If the stenotic orifice is asymmetric, however, the velocities can be skewed, and the orientation of the jet may not parallel the conduit into which it flows.

As the high-velocity jet enters the vessel at a site that is distal to the stenosis, it interacts with blood moving at much lower velocities. Because blood is viscous, this interaction causes a flow disturbance that produces multidirectional velocity patterns, which appear as small whirlpools and are frequently referred to as eddies.[C2, C3] At sites more distal from the jet, blood velocity vectors again become parallel and resume near-equal distribution across the cross section of the vessel. If the cross-sectional areas of the proximal and distal portions of the vessel are the same, the slight loss in blood velocity that is distal to the stenosis is proportional to the energy loss caused by the stenosis.

In this and subsequent discussions, the clinical term "disturbed flow" refers to a blood velocity pattern in which velocity vectors within a small volume of blood have an abnormally wide range of velocities and directions when observed over a short period. Disturbed flow is manifested clinically as the simultaneous presence of an abnormally wide range of velocities within the volume of blood sampled by pulsed Doppler echocardiography.

Two important concepts are illustrated by the model of the stenotic valve. The first is that velocities that are extremely high or disturbed in relation to velocities measured at other sites in the same vessel are useful indicators of stenosis. Furthermore, the site of stenosis is indicated by the anatomic location of these regions of high velocity or disturbed flow, and by their timing with respect to the cardiac cycle. These two simple concepts form the basis by which stenotic vascular or valvular lesions are detected in patients by color flow imaging or standard duplex pulsed and continuous-wave Doppler echocardiography.[B1, D1, R3]

Stenoses that involve heart valves are more accurately represented by short, abrupt stenotic regions, as shown in Figure 5–7, rather than the long, tapering stenotic regions shown in Figure 5–6. Although the walls of the heart and great vessels that are proximal and distal to the stenosis may not taper anatomically, the streamlines used to depict the boundaries of the flowing blood taper as the column of blood narrows to flow through the stenotic orifice. As illustrated by the streamlines in Figure 5–7, the flow cross-sectional area proximal to the stenosis is continuously reduced as blood moves closer to the valve orifice. Velocity increases inversely with this reduction in cross-sectional area.

The relationship among velocity (V), cross-sectional area (A), and flow rate (Q) is described by the volume flow rate equation [$Q = (V)(A)$]. Because the volume of blood flowing into the proximal end of the vessel across the large proximal flow cross-sectional area (A_1) is the same as that flowing across the pre-stenotic area (A_2), the stenotic area (A_3), and the vena contracta (A_4), one can apply the continuity equation:

$$Q_1 = Q_2 = Q_3 = Q_4 = (V_1)(A_1) = (V_2)(A_2) = (V_3)(A_3) = (V_4)(A_4)$$

If, as the illustration suggests, the cross-sectional areas of flow are different at each of these sites ($A_1 > A_2 > A_3 > A_4$), then the velocities must increase in a continuous manner within the pre-stenotic region ($V_1 < V_2 < V_3 < V_4$) and reach a maximum within the vena contracta.

Figure 5–8 extends the information presented in Figures 5–6 and 5–7 by graphing changes in pressure with respect to the anatomy of the stenosis. As shown in the lower panel, pressure is highest proximal to the stenosis prior to convergence of the streamlines. Pressure decreases in the pre-stenotic region as flow cross-sectional areas decrease and blood velocities increase. The sites of minimum pressure and maximum velocity are immediately distal to the region of maximum anatomic stenosis at the vena contracta. As velocities return to a more uniform distribution across the cross section of the tube, pressure recovery occurs. If the cross-sectional areas of the pre-stenotic and post-stenotic regions of the cylinder are identical, the difference in proximal and distal pressures is due to the energy lost because of the stenosis.[N2]

The observations concerning subvalvular gradients have implications in the catheterization lab because subvalvular pressure gradients are present in many normal individuals and in all adults who have valvular aortic stenosis.[P1] In the normal subjects, the gradients are confined to early and late systole and thus are largely of inertial origin. Pasipoularides and associates noted that in the presence of valvular aortic stenosis, such gradients were located in the subvalvular region starting at a site that is 1 cm proximal to the valve.[P1] Because these pathologic subvalvular gradients are largest in early systole and persist throughout systole, they have significant inertial and convective components.

Subvalvular gradients have clinical importance in the Doppler lab,[S2] because the subvalvular region (left ventricular outflow tract) is commonly used as a site for measuring velocity and cross-sectional area, which in turn can be used in conjunction with velocities from the valve orifice (V_a) to calculate aortic valve area (A_a):

$$(A_a) = (V_{lvot})(A_{lvot})/(V_a)$$

Both the left ventricular outflow tract velocity (V_{lvot}) and area (A_{lvot}) must be measured at a site that is proximal to the pre-stenotic region where velocities increase rapidly over the 1 cm that is proximal to the valve orifice. Likewise, the valve orifice velocity (V_a) should be measured in the vena contracta near the valve orifice, and the true velocity should not be underestimated by substitution of velocities from the pre-stenotic region. Either error can result in significant overestimation of the aortic valve orifice area.

Quantification of Pressure Gradients

Relationship Between Velocity and Pressure Gradient Using the Bernoulli Equation

The key to understanding the hemodynamic principles governing flow through a stenotic valve is the realization that steady-state flow entering a vessel possesses a given amount of energy in terms of pressure (potential energy) and velocity or momentum (kinetic energy). The relationship between these two energy values is expressed by the Bernoulli equation:[H1, H2, V1]

$$P_1 - P_2 = \rho/2[(V_2)^2 - (V_1)^2] + \rho\int_1^2 \frac{dv}{dt}\,ds + R(V)$$

Convective acceleration + Inertial acceleration + Viscous friction

P_1, P_2, V_1, and V_2 represent pressure and velocity values at two positions along the vessel; ρ is a physical constant, the density of blood, which equals 1.06×10^3 kg/m^3. The left side of the equation represents potential energy in terms of a pressure gradient ($P_1 - P_2$), and the right side represents kinetic energy in terms of its convective, inertial, and viscous components.

Several assumptions are made to simplify the Bernoulli equation for clinical applications.[H2, H3, H4, V1] First, because viscous frictional losses [R(V)] are small with respect to the two other

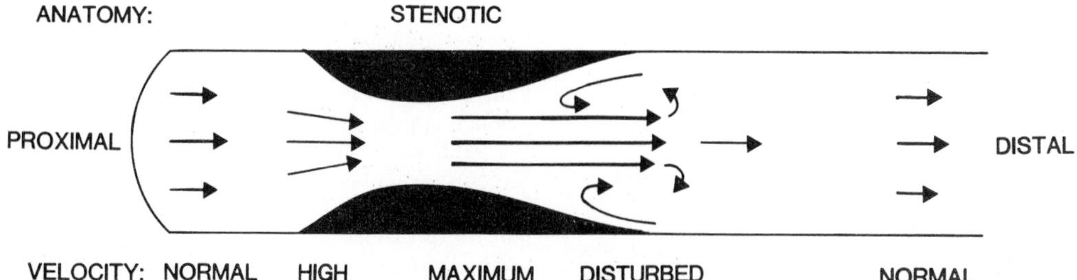

Figure 5–6. The blood velocity patterns are shown by vectors as blood flows from a proximal site at which velocities are normal through a long, tapered stenotic valve at which high velocities are noted. A region of disturbed flow that is distal to the stenosis and is characterized by velocity vectors that have a wide range of speeds and directions is observed. Velocities return to normal at a more distal site.

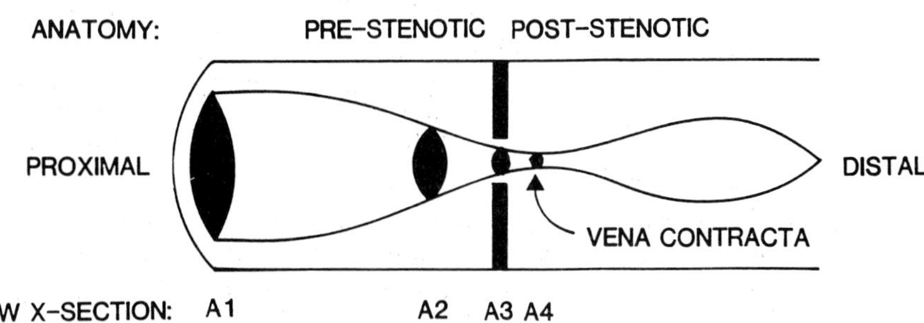

Figure 5–7. Blood flowing from left to right through a discrete stenotic region in a cylinder tapers from a wide cross-sectional area proximal to the stenosis (A_1) to progressively narrower areas ($A_1 > A_2 > A_3 > A_4$) until minimum cross-sectional area is noted within the vena contracta, where velocity is maximal.

kinetic terms, they are assumed to be zero. Second, because acceleration and deceleration are confined to brief periods in early and late portions of valve flow, the acceleration component is also neglected. The simplified Bernoulli equation for estimating pressure gradients across severe, abrupt stenoses is:

$$P_1 - P_2 = 4\,[(V_2)^2 - (V_1)^2]$$

According to this simplified equation, any changes in velocity between two points are accounted for as changes in pressure. If the flow across the stenosis illustrated in Figure 5–8 is reconsidered, velocity increases and a subvalvular gradient are produced as flow is constricted in the pre-stenotic region. Further reduction of cross-sectional area in the anatomic stenosis and vena contracta increases velocity; a decrease in the pressure and increase in the pressure gradient between the proximal site and the vena contracta result. In the pressure recovery region, velocity approaches its original value, and pressure returns to its original value except for its frictional losses.

As velocity increases and decreases in a pulsatile system like the heart, blood flow must accelerate—a factor ignored by the simplified Bernoulli equation. The acceleration term in the complete Bernoulli equation is nondissipative when it is considered over the entire flow cycle; that is, it does not result in any energy loss. If actual velocities shown in the top panel of Figure 5–9 are used to calculate the pressure gradient using only their convective component and neglecting their inertial component, the mean gradient is accurate, but the timing of the calculated gradient and its exact shape are inaccurate. As shown in the bottom panel of Figure 5–9, the calculated gradient *(solid line)* lags behind the actual pressure gradient *(dashed line)* when the acceleration component is not considered. Furthermore, the magnitude of the actual pressure drop is slightly greater during positive acceleration and slightly smaller during negative acceleration than would be indicated using the simplified Bernoulli equation.

In most clinical situations, further simplification of the equation is possible. If the stenosis is severe and a single lesion is present, the proximal velocity (V_1) is ignored, and the pressure gradient (PG) is calculated using only the orifice velocity (V_2):

$$PG = 4(V_2)^2$$

Figure 5–10 illustrates a situation in which serial lesions, such as subvalvular and valvular pulmonic stenoses, are present in the same patient. In such a case, calculation of the pressure gradient at each lesion is helpful so that the need to surgically correct one or both of the lesions can be determined.

$$PG_a = 4[(V_2)^2 - (V_1)^2]$$
and
$$PG_b = 4[(V_4)^2 - (V_3)^2]$$

If numbers are substituted into both equations, one can see that when velocities in the region that is proximal to the stenosis are small (usually less than 1.5 m/sec), then the proximal velocities can be neglected and only the orifice velocities need to be used in calculating the pressure gradient. If, however, the proximal velocities are greater than 2 m/sec, then proximal velocities must be used in the calculation.

Calculation of Blood Velocity using the Doppler Equation

The Doppler equation allows calculation of blood velocity (V) if the variables Doppler frequency shift (F_d) and the cosine of the Doppler angle (cos θ) are measured, and if the speed of ultrasound in tissue (C_t = 1.6×10^3 m/sec) and the carrier frequency (F_c), both of which are constants, are known:

$$V = (F_d)/(\cos\theta) \times (C_t)/2(F_c)$$
$$\text{Variables} \times \text{Constants}$$

The Doppler angle, as shown in Figure 5–11, is the angle between the ultrasound beam and the blood velocity vectors, shown as arrows. In most clinical examinations, the Doppler angle is not actually measured. Multiple ultrasound windows are used in order to provide the smallest Doppler angle possible. It is usually indicated by the window in which the largest Doppler frequency shift is detected for the sampling site to be evaluated.[H3, H4] The Doppler angle is then assumed to be zero and thus the cosine θ becomes 1:

$$V = (F_d)/1 \times (C_t)/2(F_c)$$

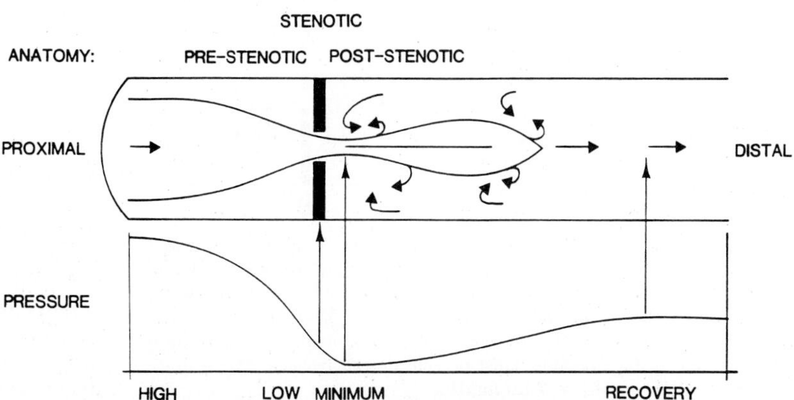

Figure 5–8. Diagram combines concepts from the velocity model and the pressures recorded from the model. The characteristics of velocity are shown in the upper panel, and the corresponding pressures are shown in the lower panel. Pressure proximal to the stenosis is highest, but it decreases progressively to a minimum at the vena contracta. Pressure is at least partially recovered at a site distal to the stenosis, as convective velocities are converted back into pressure (recovery region).

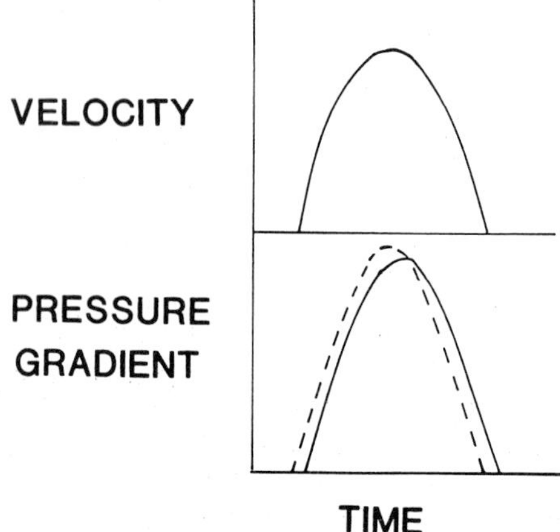

Figure 5–9. Actual velocity and the pressure gradient—calculated using the simplified Bernoulli equation, which considers only the convective components of the pressure gradient—are graphed as solid lines versus the same horizontal time base. The dashed line shows the actual pressure gradient present and illustrates that failure to consider the inertial components of the pressure gradient may lead to errors in timing, especially during times of rapid acceleration and deceleration.

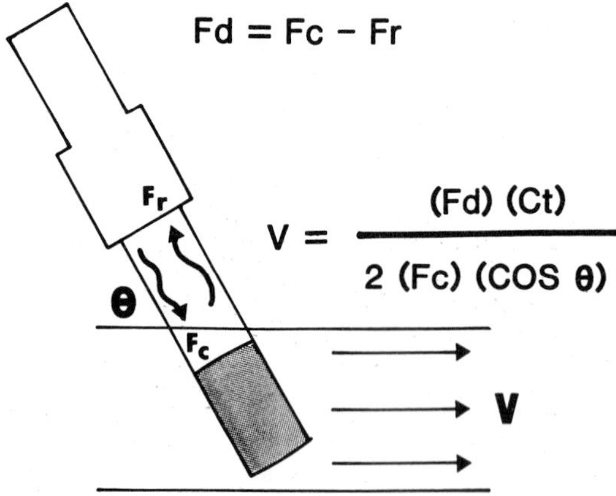

Figure 5–11. Blood flowing through the cylinder in the bottom of the figure at a given velocity (V) causes the ultrasound carrier frequency broadcast by the transducer to change such that the reflected frequency differs from the broadcast frequency. The difference between carrier (F_c) and reflected (F_r) ultrasound frequency is the Doppler frequency shift (F_d). Blood velocity can be calculated with the Doppler equation if the Doppler frequency shift (F_d), the speed of ultrasound in tissue (C_t = 1.6 × 10^3 m/sec), the carrier frequency (F_c), and the cosine of the Doppler angle (cos θ = the cosine of the angle between the ultrasound beam and the velocity vectors) are known.

The assumption of a Doppler angle of zero is accurate when the actual angle is 25 degrees or less, because the cosine function changes from 1.00 at zero degrees to 0.91 at 25 degrees. If the angle is larger than 30 degrees, significant underestimation of the true velocity results from application of the Doppler equation.

Invasive Standards for Measuring Pressure Gradients

Although the concept of transvalvular pressure gradients is simple, the different methods used to acquire and analyze them have led to considerable confusion. To illustrate the dilemmas created, our discussion focuses on the following three problems encountered in patients with aortic stenosis:

1. Different pressure gradients can be measured from different sites within the left ventricle and the systemic arterial circulation.
2. Three different kinds of gradients can be calculated for each gradient measured.
3. Gradients can be measured under different hemodynamic conditions.

As discussed previously, the velocity abnormalities produced by valvular stenoses result in subvalvular and valvular pressure drops and partial post-valvular pressure recovery. Waves reflected from branch points in the peripheral circulation produce marked differences between central aortic pressure waves and those encountered in the radial or femoral artery. For this reason, the locations from which pressure data are acquired can greatly affect the timing, shape, and magnitude of pressure gradients.

The maximum pressure gradient is present between the body of the left ventricle and the vena contracta. Gradients acquired from the left ventricular outflow tract or distal to the vena contracta underestimate the actual gradient.[P1] Because of the marked differences in pressure waveforms and systolic pressures between the ascending aorta and more distal arterial sites, such as the femoral or brachial artery, substitution of such pressures for those from the ascending aorta produces further degradation of the magnitude of the gradient and its timing.[M2] The low-fidelity recordings obtained by most fluid-filled catheter and transducer systems add additional degradation to the pressure waveforms, which could be obtained with high-fidelity catheter-tip manometers.[M3] Errors in timing, contour, and magnitude of the pressure gradients are most marked when peak-to-peak and peak instantaneous gradients are measured but are usually less severe when mean gradients are calculated. Thus, pressure records should be made with transducers sensing pressure in the body of the left ventricle and in the vena contracta. Simultaneous recordings increase the chance of recording pressures under identical flow conditions. High-fidelity recordings are vital for research applications, especially when peak gradients are to be quantified.

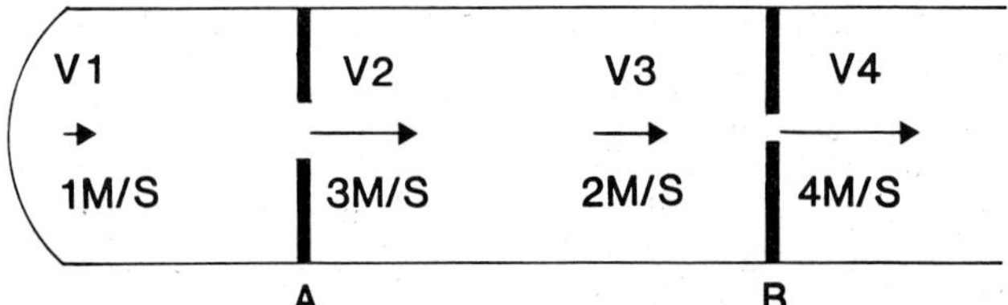

Figure 5–10. The serial stenoses cause blood velocity to increase from 1 meter per second (m/sec) to 3 m/sec proximally and distally to *A* and from 2 m/sec to 4 m/sec at *B*. On application of the Bernoulli equation, the convective pressure gradient at $A = 4[(3)^2 - (1)^2] = 4[(9) - (1)] \sim 4(9)$ mmHg; thus, the proximal velocity (V_1) can be neglected. At *B*, both proximal and distal velocities must be considered, because $PG = 4[(4)^2 - (2)^2] = 4[(16) - (4)] = 4(12)$ mmHg.

Three different pressure gradients can be calculated from left ventricular and aortic pressure waveforms in patients with aortic stenosis (Fig. 5–12). The peak-to-peak gradient is the difference between the peak left ventricular pressure and the peak aortic pressure. Close examination of the tracings shows that peak left ventricular and aortic pressures do not occur at the same time in the cardiac cycle. Because the peak-to-peak gradient does not really occur, it lacks a physiologic basis and should not be used.

The peak instantaneous gradient is the maximum gradient noted any time during systole; by definition, it is the largest gradient measured and may exceed the mean or peak-to-peak gradient by as much as 200 percent. Although it was not commonly measured at catheterization prior to development of Doppler echocardiography, it can be accurately measured from high-fidelity pressure tracings. Its current clinical importance is that it can be easily calculated by use of the Bernoulli equation and the peak aortic valve orifice velocity obtained by Doppler echocardiography. Clinical use of the peak instantaneous gradient is complicated because it tends to provide poor differentiation of the severity of aortic stenosis in the presence of high-flow states (high cardiac output or aortic regurgitation) or of systemic hypertension.

In addition, high peak instantaneous gradients early in systole are calculated in many normally functioning prosthetic aortic valves. The mean systolic gradient (MSG), the average of multiple instantaneous gradients, allows easier categorization of the severity of stenosis. In addition, it can be accurately measured at

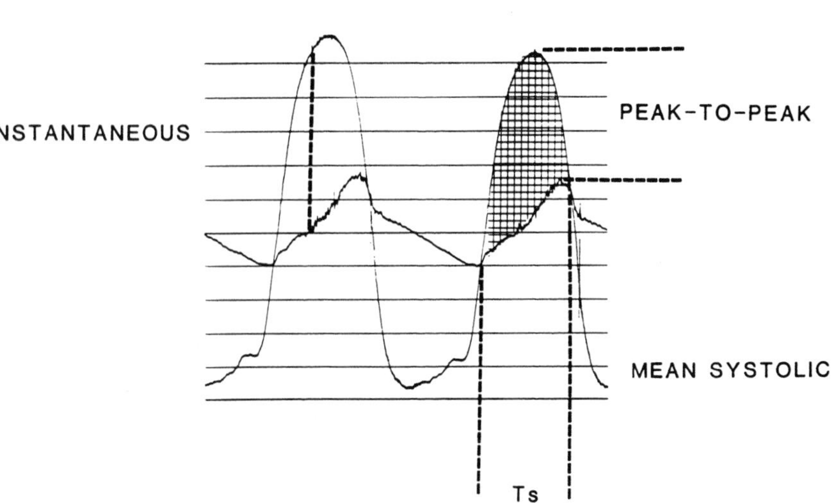

Figure 5–12. From the left ventricular and aortic pressures noted in this patient with severe aortic stenosis, three different pressure gradients are commonly measured. Peak instantaneous is the maximum pressure measured at any time during systole. Peak-to-peak is the difference between the nonsimultaneous peaks of left ventricular and aortic pressures. Mean systolic is the average of the systolic pressure gradients and is commonly determined by dividing the systolic gradient-time area *(cross-hatched)* by systolic ejection period (Ts).

catheterization or from Doppler velocity records.[H3, H4, C4] It should be the pressure gradient used for comparison of Doppler and catheterization data. It is calculated from catheterization data by integrating the pressure gradient-time area and dividing by the systolic ejection period. It is calculated from Doppler velocity data by measuring multiple, equally spaced velocities during systole (V_i), squaring these velocities, dividing by the number of observations (n), and multiplying by the constant 4:

$$MSG = 4\left[\Sigma\frac{(V_i)^2}{n}\right]$$

When estimating pressure gradients from Doppler data, one should remember that the velocity used to calculate the gradient is usually determined with the assumption that the Doppler angle is less than 25 degrees; if the actual Doppler angle is larger, significant underestimation of the velocity and the pressure gradient is possible.

Because the pressure gradient is affected by both the cross-sectional area of the valve orifice and the flow rate of blood across the valve, the pressure gradient may be significantly affected by changes in flow induced by physical or mental stress, medications, or changes in heart rhythm. This consideration is particularly important when serial tracings are acquired for comparison in the same patient, or when comparisons between Doppler and catheterization are made using data acquired at different times. Although these effects may not be marked in most adult patients, they can be marked in children and young adults, who are usually not sedated in the echocardiographic lab but are universally sedated in the catheterization lab. Realization of this problem has led to the practice of sedating pediatric patients prior to Doppler examinations in which pressure gradients are to be quantified.[S3]

Calculation of "Flow-Independent" Measures of Stenosis

Valve Area

Evaluation of valve stenosis based solely on the pressure gradient is difficult because pressure gradient is a function of both the size of the valve orifice and the flow rate across that orifice. Therefore, calculation of valve area from other hemodynamic parameters is an attractive approach, because it is thought to provide an indication of severity, which remains constant despite changes in valve flow rates in the same patient, and to allow comparison of severity despite differences in flow rates among patients. As discussed previously, use of the continuity equation and of parameters derived from Doppler and imaging echocardiography is promising, but may be inaccurate in patients in whom data quality is low because of associated disease.

The Gorlin equation, which has been used for nearly four decades to provide an estimate of anatomic valve area,[G3] remains the clinical standard of reference. Because the Gorlin equation is designed for use in nonpulsatile flow, pulsatile parameters (flow rates and pressure gradients) must be expressed as steady flow parameters averaged over the time of flow. For aortic stenosis, flow rate or aortic valve flow (AVF) is expressed as if the cardiac output was distributed only in systole:

$$AVF = CO/SEP$$

where SEP is the number of seconds of systolic flow per minute of cardiac cycle. Because systole occupies about 25 percent to 50 percent of the cardiac cycle, aortic valve flow exceeds cardiac output by a factor of approximately two to four. Pressure gradients are the average or mean systolic gradients across the aortic valve (PG_a). To calculate valve area (A_g), the Gorlin equation requires an empiric constant (K), which has been validated for mitral but not for aortic stenosis:[G3]

$$A_g = (AVF)/K\sqrt{PG_a}$$

Derivation of the Gorlin equation is based on a combination of the volume flow rate equation and the Bernoulli equation. If aortic valve flow rate (Q_a) is proportional to mean blood velocity (V_a) multiplied by mean cross-sectional area of the stenotic aortic valve (A_a), then the flow rate equation can be rearranged in terms of aortic valve area (A_a):

$$\text{If } Q_a = (V_a)(A_a), \text{ then } (A_a) = (Q_a)/(V_a)$$

In the 1950's, valve flow rates could be measured, but velocity within the aortic valve orifice could not be reliably quantified. Therefore, the simplified Bernoulli equation was used to allow the unknown variables in the Gorlin equation to become pressure gradient (PG_a) and aortic valve flow rate:

$$\text{If } (PG_a) \sim (V_a)^2$$
$$\text{then } (V_a) \sim \sqrt{PG_a}$$
$$\text{Therefore, } (A_a) = (Q_a)/K\sqrt{PG_a}$$

Although the constant (K) in the equation was never validated experimentally for aortic stenosis, it was derived for mitral stenosis from 13 patients for whom catheterization and surgical anatomic valve area measurements were available. Interestingly, all the unknown variables in the Gorlin equation can be provided by data determined at catheterization or with combined Doppler and imaging echocardiography.

Despite our clinical dependence on the Gorlin equation, numerous studies suggest that such valve area estimates are either inaccurate or may change with differences in hemodynamic conditions. Richter reported a single patient in whom severe mitral stenosis was documented at catheterization but in whom anatomic valve areas were 1.4 to 2.3 cm^2 at autopsy.[R4] Significant discrepancies have been documented between anatomic and calculated valve areas for normal aortic and mitral prosthetic valves.[C5] Bache and associates noted a 16 percent increase in valve areas of native stenotic aortic valves in patients undergoing mild supine exercise at cardiac catheterization.[B1] Ubago and colleagues noted that the valve area of prosthetic porcine valves increases as flow and pressure gradients increase.[U1]

Both experimental and clinical studies suggest that inaccuracy in the Gorlin equation itself may at least partially account for the discrepancies between calculated and anatomic valve area.[C6] In a pulsatile flow tank model in which fixed, stenotic valve orifices of known cross-sectional area were used, an excellent correlation was noted between the Gorlin equation "constant" and the square root of the mean systolic pressure gradient. If the Gorlin equation is used to calculate the Gorlin constant (K_g):

$$K_g = (Q_a)/(A_a)\sqrt{(PG_a)}$$

If one considers the observation that the Gorlin constant is not a constant, but is proportional to the square root of the mean pressure gradient, then K_g is proportional to a new constant (K_c) multiplied by the square root of the mean gradient:

$$K_g\sqrt{(PG_a)} = [K_c\sqrt{(PG_a)}]\sqrt{(PG_a)} = K_c\,(PG_a)$$

The new constant (K_c) was independent of both flow and pressure gradients in the flow tank as well as in clinical studies.[C6] Interestingly, the study suggests that a more flow-independent indicator of the severity of valve stenosis would use an equation in the form:

$$(A_a) = (Q_a)/K_c\,(PG_a)$$

where the denominator is a new and as yet undetermined constant multiplied by the mean systolic pressure gradient.

Valve Resistance

The use of valve resistance as an indicator of severity of valve stenosis is based on an old concept that was debated heavily when the Gorlin equation was adopted as an indicator of severity of mitral stenosis.[G3] Aortic valve resistance (R_a) is calculated as:

$$(R_a) = (PG_a)/(Q_a)$$

Upon closer consideration of the equation derived in the flow tank experiments discussed earlier, one can see that it allows calculation of aortic valve conductance (C_a); the reciprocal of the equation allows calculation of aortic valve resistance (R_a):

$$(R_a) = 1/(C_a) = (PG_a)/(Q_a)$$

Because of the stability of aortic valve conductance and resistance despite changes in hemodynamics, this method deserves further investigation as a clinically important indicator of the severity of valve stenosis.

An additional attractive feature of the use of resistance as an indicator of severity of valve stenosis is that it allows assessment of the workload imposed on the heart by the valve disease as well as of the peripheral circulation. For aortic stenosis, the total resistive load (R_t) imposed by a stenotic valve (R_a) plus that imposed by the systemic circulation (R_c) is:

$$(R_t) = (R_a) + (R_c)$$

Thus, the total resistive load, as well as its components, can be assessed using similar parameters. Perhaps such an approach will provide more accurate evaluation of the complications of aortic stenosis, such as development of left ventricular dysfunction, and will allow more accurate clinical intervention with medical as opposed to surgical therapy.

Variable-Orifice Stenotic Valves

The dilemma concerning discrepancies between anatomic valve area and valve area calculated by the Gorlin equation is only partially explained by the equation's flow-dependent "constant." When rest and exercise data are examined for patients with aortic stenosis assessed by the Gorlin equation, a 26 percent increase in valve area is noted to occur with exercise; in the same patients, a 10 percent increase in aortic valve resistance suggests that anatomic valve area actually increases with mild changes in mean systolic gradient.[H4]

As shown in Figure 5–13, direct measurement of anatomic aortic valve area at the time of aortic valve surgery[R5] demonstrates that aortic valve area increases as force distending the valve is increased. Pulsatile flow tank experiments on unfixed, intact severely stenotic aortic valves demonstrate the same linear relationship between pressure gradient and aortic valve orifice cross-sectional area.[R6]

Interestingly, the compliance of the aortic valves evaluated at surgery is inversely related to the severity of their stenoses. Thus, severe stenosis is indicated not only by a small valve cross-sectional area but also by little change in that cross-sectional area with increases in pressure gradient.[R5]

Clinical Comparisons of Valve Stenoses

Although the discussion has focused on the dynamics of aortic valve stenosis, the same concepts can be applied to mitral stenosis. In contrast to the high pressure gradients that characterize aortic stenosis, those of mitral stenosis are in the range of 5 to 15 mmHg. Mean diastolic gradients are clinically useful and can be determined using catheterization or Doppler echocardiography. Valve area can be quantified by direct echocardiographic imaging techniques. Although Doppler echocardiography allows estimation of mitral valve area using the pressure half-time technique,[H6, S4] application of the continuity equation is more accurate, especially in the presence of aortic regurgitation.[N1] In addition to accurate quantification of pressure gradient and valve area, detection of pulmonary hypertension and quantification of pulmonary artery pressure[H4, K1] are important in the assessment of mitral stenosis.

Clinical evaluation of the severity of pulmonic stenosis can be easily accomplished by Doppler echocardiographic quantification of the mean systolic pressure gradient.[H4] Evaluation of the severity of tricuspid stenosis is based on both two-dimensional echocardiographic imaging and Doppler determination of the transvalvular pressure gradient. Because the pressure gradients are low, simultaneous right atrial and right ventricular pressures are required to quantify the severity of tricuspid stenosis at catheterization. Valve area determinations have not been validated for pulmonic or tricuspid stenosis.

VALVULAR REGURGITATION

The approaches used to detect valvular regurgitation and assess its severity are best understood by studying the abnormal velocity patterns near regurgitant valves. These hemodynamic abnormalities are used to help in understanding the concept of regurgitant fraction and other hemodynamic indicators of severity. Difficulties encountered in using angiography to assess severity of regurgi-

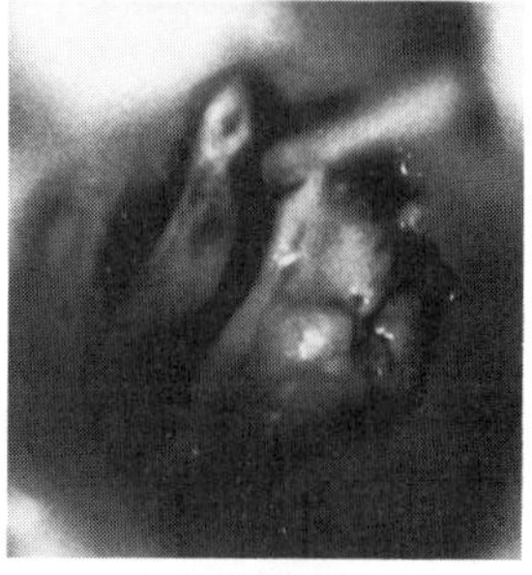
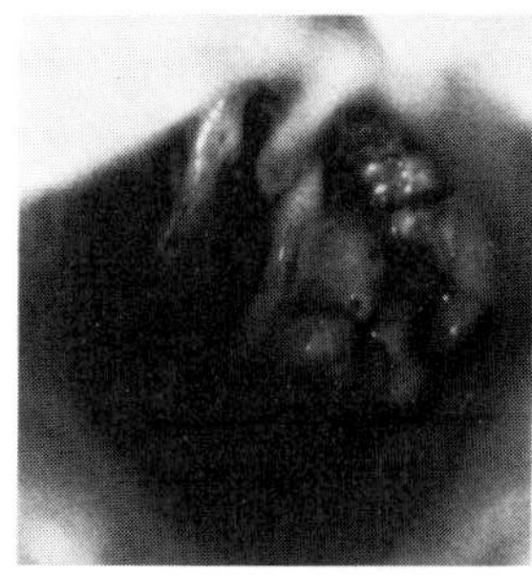
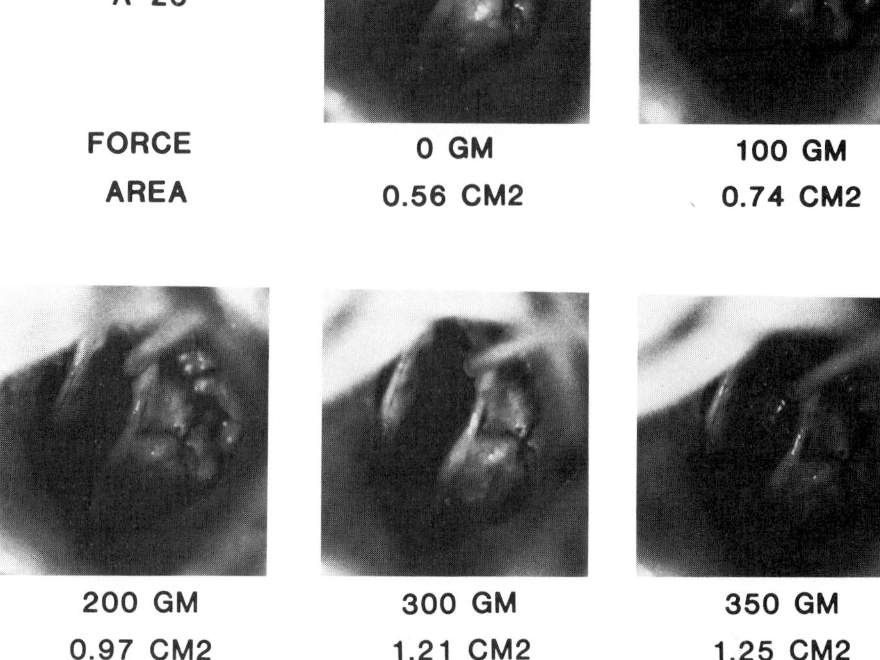

Figure 5–13. The anatomic aortic valve area in this patient with severe aortic stenosis varies from 0.56 cm² to 1.25 cm² as a No. 7 French Fogarty balloon is pulled against the left ventricular surface of the valve with 0 to 350 g of force.

tation are discussed. As in the preceding section, catheterization and echocardiographic techniques are stressed. Although aortic regurgitation is used to illustrate hemodynamic concepts, application of these concepts to mitral, tricuspid, and pulmonic regurgitation is discussed at the end of the section.

Velocity Patterns Near a Regurgitant Valve

Figure 5–14 contrasts the velocity patterns found in the normal valve *(left panels)* with those noted in the regurgitant valve *(right panels)*. For simplicity, the valve illustrated is the aortic; the left ventricular outflow tract is to the left and the aorta to the right in each of the four panels. The systolic panel (T_1) in the normal valve shows moderate velocities in contrast to the slightly elevated forward velocities that are characteristic of many regurgitant valves. Forward systolic flow is elevated in the presence of aortic regurgitation because total forward flow (Q_t) includes the net forward volume, which is delivered to the systemic circulation (Q_n) as well as the regurgitant diastolic flow (Q_r):

$$Q_t = Q_n + Q_r$$

Because values for normal forward flow velocity and stroke volume frequently overlap those detected in mild to moderate regurgitation, the diagnosis of valvular regurgitation is based on detection of abnormal regurgitant velocity patterns.[A1, B2, C7, D3, Q1] Unlike the normal aortic valve, which has little blood motion adjacent to it during diastole (T_2), the regurgitant aortic valve exhibits abnormal diastolic flow patterns on both of its sides. Proximal to the regurgitant lesion is a retrograde, high-velocity jet surrounded by a region of disturbed flow. The velocity patterns that are proximal to regurgitant lesions are noted to be similar to those whose production is distal to stenotic valves, except that the regurgitant jets are (1) on the side of the valve opposite that of normal blood flow, (2) directed opposite the direction of forward flow, and (3) produced at a time in the cardiac cycle when flow is normally absent.

Accurate diagnosis of a specific lesion by Doppler echocardiography depends on identifying the abnormal regurgitant jet and defining its anatomic location, direction, and timing. The regurgitant velocities distal to the valve in the ascending aorta are less

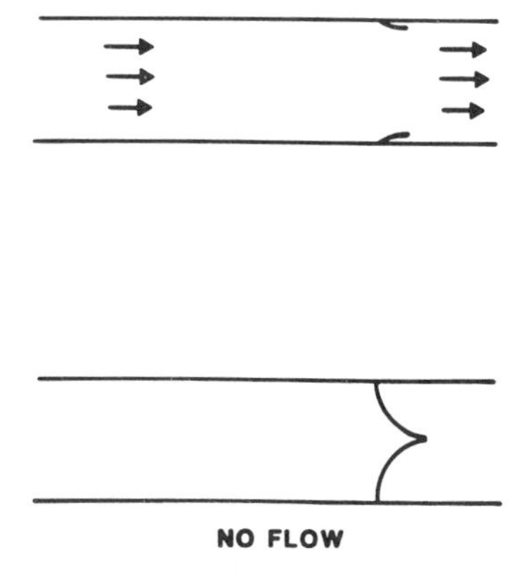

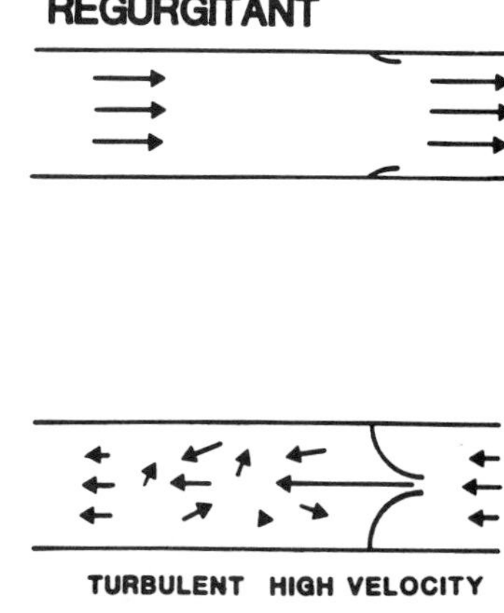

Figure 5–14. Velocity vectors are shown at two opposite times in the cardiac cycle (T_1 & T_2) to allow comparison of the velocity patterns near normal valves *(left panels)* and regurgitant valves *(right panels)*. During T_2, when no flow across the normal valve occurs, reversed high velocity and disturbed (or turbulent) flow through the regurgitant valve occur.

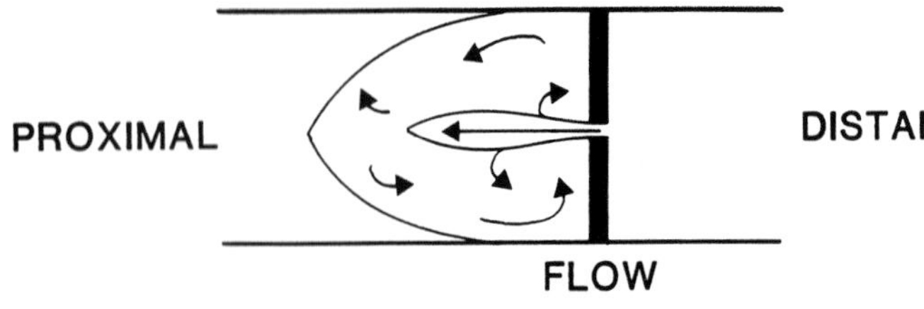

Figure 5–15. The velocity patterns on the proximal side of a regurgitant lesion are the result of a relatively small regurgitant orifice that produces a small cross-sectional area, high-velocity jet extending 2 to 5 jet diameters distance from the orifice. The high-velocity jet is surrounded by a larger region of disturbed flow characterized by velocity vectors that have a wide range of directions and speeds.

helpful in identifying aortic regurgitation because they are frequently of low velocity and may not be detected by Doppler echocardiographic techniques. To understand the parameters useful in quantifying the severity of the lesion, we will examine regurgitant flow patterns that are proximal and distal to the regurgitant valve.

Proximal Velocity Patterns and the Concepts of Regurgitant Orifice Cross-Sectional Area and Pressure Gradient

The high-velocity jet and the parajet region of disturbed flow proximal to a regurgitant valve provide three sets of parameters that are used to estimate the severity of regurgitation: (1) volume and dimensions of the parajet region of disturbed velocities, (2) jet cross-sectional area or diameter, or both, at its origin from the regurgitant orifice, and (3) pressure gradient across the regurgitant orifice.

As shown in Figure 5–15, the region of disturbed flow is large in relation to the regurgitant orifice and thus was easily detected by early duplex pulsed Doppler instruments. Initial studies revealed a correlation between the severity of regurgitation and the length, width, or area of the region of disturbed flow.[A1, C7, J1, Q1] More recent studies have demonstrated that the dimensions of the region of disturbed flow displayed by color flow imagers are greatly influenced by individual instruments and instrument settings,[S6] as well as by the duration of regurgitation, driving pressure producing the regurgitation, and the cross-sectional area of the valve orifice.[W1] Because of the multiple factors responsible for the dimensions of the region of disturbed flow, it remains an important site for detection of regurgitation but serves as only an approximate indicator of the severity of the regurgitation.

The high-velocity region within and immediately proximal to the regurgitant orifice provides a more reproducible and promising area for quantification of regurgitant lesions. Color flow imaging studies have focused on determining the diameter or cross-sectional area of the regurgitant orifice by indirectly imaging the abnormal velocities within that orifice.[P2, P3, H7] The ability of color flow to image the orifice when standard two-dimensional imaging techniques have failed is probably due to the high-velocity gradients between the jet and the adjacent blood pool or the tissue at the regurgitant orifice, or both. This approach allows estimation of the regurgitant orifice cross-sectional area but neglects measurement of the pressure gradient across and the regurgitant volume passing through that orifice.[D2]

The Bernoulli equation has been helpful in estimating pressure gradients across regurgitant orifices. In the presence of aortic regurgitation, the magnitude of the pressure gradient at end-diastole and the slope of the pressure gradient or velocity decay are helpful indicators of the severity of the lesion.[B3, G4, T1]

Distal Velocity Patterns and the Concept of Regurgitant Fraction

As shown in Figure 5–16, the velocity patterns distal to a regurgitant aortic valve are slightly elevated during forward flow but are considerably lower during regurgitant flow. Regurgitant fraction (RF) is an indicator of severity of regurgitation that compares regurgitant volume (Q_r) with total forward flow (Q_t):

$$RF = (Q_r)/(Q_t)$$

Regurgitant fraction becomes larger as regurgitation becomes more severe.

Use of the volume flow rate equation [Q = (V) (A)] to calculate regurgitant and total forward flow rates requires quantification of mean velocity (V) and mean cross-sectional area of flow (A) during regurgitant flow (r) and total forward flow (t):

$$RF = (Q_r)/(Q_t) = [(V_r)\,(A_r)/(V_t)\,(A_t)]$$

As shown in Figure 5–17, abnormal regurgitant velocities are detectable in the presence of severe aortic regurgitation during diastole in the descending aorta. Note that during systole (s), velocities are negative because blood moves away from the suprasternal notch where the transducer is located; during diastole (d), regurgitant velocities are observed toward the transducer in a positive direction. Because flow is pulsatile, calculation of regurgitant and total forward flows is based on stroke volume (SV); stroke volume is the product of the velocity-time integral (VT) multiplied by the cross-sectional area. Regurgitant fraction becomes:

$$RF = (Q_r)/(Q_t) = (SV_d)/(SV_s) = [(VT_d)\,(A_d)/(VT_s)(A_s)]$$

This approach is helpful in the assessment of aortic regurgitation because both the forward and regurgitant stroke volumes affect aortic blood velocities.[B4, T2]

Quantification of mitral, tricuspid, and pulmonic regurgitation by direct calculation of regurgitant fraction from Doppler and echocardiographic data is much more complex, because unlike the aorta, these valves do not deliver both volumes into a cylindric conduit. Mean mitral diastolic velocity-time integral (VT_m) and mean mitral cross-sectional area (A_m) can be used to calculate total forward mitral valve stroke volume (SV_t):

$$(SV_t) = (VT_m)\,(A_m) = (SV_n) + (SV_r)$$

The total forward stroke volume includes both net forward (SV_n) and regurgitant stroke volume (SV_r). Because the flow measurements are made at the mitral valve, which has a variable cross-sectional area during diastolic flow, the mean cross-sectional area must be calculated either by using a constant[S1, L1] or by obtaining

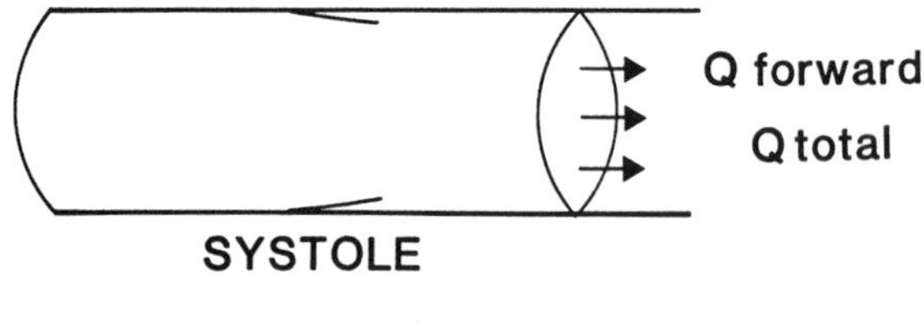

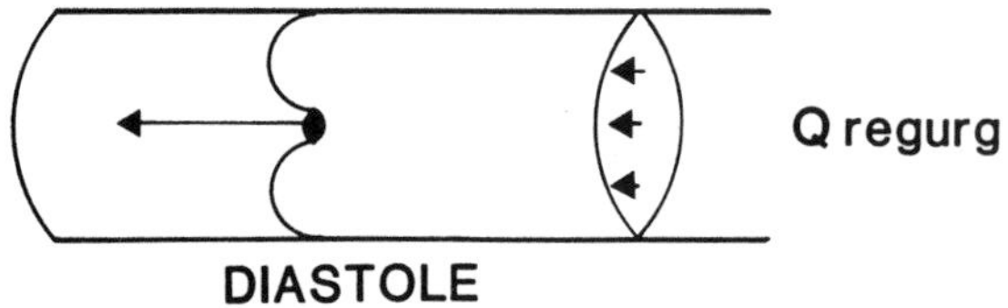

Figure 5–16. The velocity patterns distal to a regurgitant lesion *(toward right)* are characterized by lower, more evenly distributed velocities than those that are proximal to the lesion *(toward left)*. For aortic regurgitation, forward or total flow (Q forward or Q total) is noted during systole, and regurgitant flow (Q regurg) is noted during diastole.

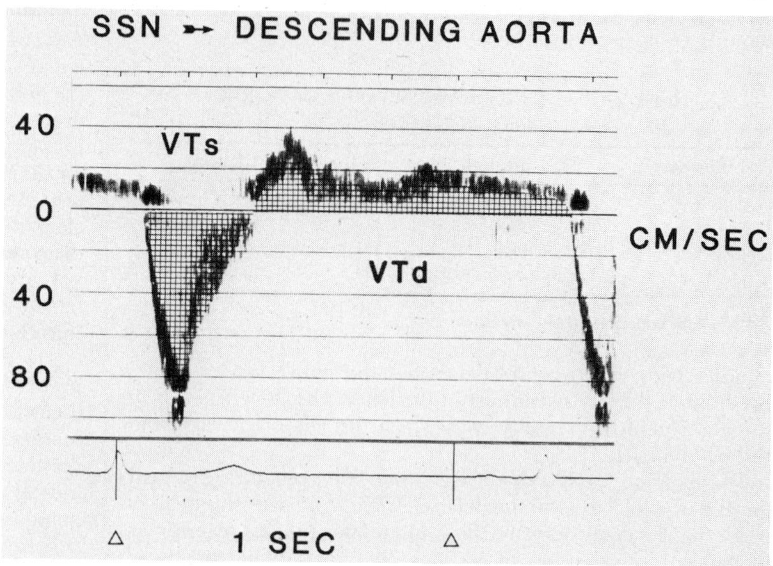

Figure 5–17. In this Doppler spectral tracing of velocities from the descending aorta, regurgitant fraction can be calculated as the ratio of the product of the diastolic velocity-time integral (VT_d) and the aortic diastolic cross-sectional area divided by the product of the systolic velocity-time integral (VT_s) and the aortic systolic cross-sectional area. Cross-hatching denotes the velocity-time integral.

indirect measurements through use of M-mode echocardiographic imaging.[F1] The velocity-time integral is usually determined using an apical four-chamber view, because it allows parallel alignment of the ultrasound beam and the velocity vectors from the mitral valve diastolic orifice. Satisfactory results have been reported by sampling at either the mitral valve orifice[F1] or the mitral valve annulus.[L1]

To calculate the unknown variables in the equation, the net forward stroke volume is measured at the aortic annulus[L1] or the proximal ascending aorta.[H1] The difference between total forward and net forward stroke volumes is used to calculate regurgitant stroke volume, which is required to calculate regurgitant fraction:

$$(SV_r) = (SV_t) - (SV_n)$$

$$RF = (SV_r)/(SV_t) = [(SV_t) - (SV_n)]/(SV_t)$$

Because this approach requires tedious data acquisition from two different sites, and calculation of two different velocity-time integrals and orifice cross-sectional areas, it is seldom performed. In addition, the multiple measurements allow introduction of error, especially when lesions in addition to mitral regurgitation are present. For these reasons, other techniques, which depend on assessment of the characteristics of the regurgitant jet, have been more popular.

Invasive Standards for Quantifying Regurgitation

The severity of aortic and mitral regurgitation is judged clinically by the angiographic severity and the size of the regurgitant fraction.[G1] Secondary indicators of the severity of aortic regurgitation include aortic pulse pressure and end-diastolic pressure; large, early V waves are frequently seen on the left atrial or pulmonary artery wedge pressure recordings in severe mitral regurgitation, especially if it is acute. Because patients with severe aortic or mitral regurgitation may remain asymptomatic for long periods, valve replacement is frequently deferred until symptoms are noted or until left ventricular dysfunction is evident. If left ventricular dysfunction becomes advanced prior to valve replacement, complete recovery is uncommon. For these reasons, assessment of ventricular function as well as of the severity of the lesion is an important task in patients with left-sided regurgitant lesions. Physical or pharmacologic stress is frequently used to detect ventricular dysfunction before it becomes apparent at rest.

Evaluation of the severity of right-sided regurgitant lesions is much more difficult because the catheter required to perform angiography must cross the regurgitant valve. Because pressures within the right side of the heart are generally lower than those within the left side of the heart, the catheter across the affected valve may actually produce at least a portion of the regurgitation. In addition, because the angiographic techniques by which right ventricular stroke volume is quantified are less accurate than those for left ventricular stroke volume, calculation of regurgitant fraction is infrequently used.

Regurgitant Fraction

Regurgitant fraction allows more accurate quantification of valvular regurgitation than is possible with angiography alone.[A2, G1] Also, because it can be calculated from both catheterization and Doppler echocardiographic data, it provides a common means of comparing the accuracy of both. As shown previously, regurgitant fraction is the ratio of regurgitant over total forward flow rates:

$$RF = (Q_r)/(Q_t)$$

At cardiac catheterization, total ventricular cardiac output is determined by performing left ventricular angiography and subtracting end-systolic from end-diastolic volumes. New forward cardiac output (CO_n) is calculated from the cardiac output measurements obtained from indicator dilution (thermodilution or green dye) techniques or from the Fick method. Regurgitant cardiac output is the difference between total forward output (CO_t) and net forward output (CO_n). Therefore, at catheterization, regurgitant fraction (RF_c) is calculated as:

$$RF_c = (CO_r)/(CO_t) = [(CO_t) - (CO_n)]/(CO_t)$$

Although determination of regurgitant fraction at catheterization is the most accurate standard of reference, it commonly results in 10 to 20 percent differences between sequential measurements. For this reason, normal individuals who have no valvular regurgitation can have calculated regurgitant fractions that differ as much as 10 to 20 percentage points. Accuracy is impaired because ventriculographic and net forward output measurements are not simultaneous and because of the difficulties involved in accurate determination of ventriculographic output. Ultrafast computed tomography is proving to be extremely accurate in calculating regurgitant volumes.[R8]

Angiographic Severity

Quantification of severity of regurgitation by angiography provides a less exact indication of severity than is possible with regurgitant fraction. With aortic regurgitation used as an example, the angiographic severity depends on subjective characterization of the movement of contrast material retrograde into the left ventricle from the aorta, where it is injected.[C8] The division of severity into its four grades (Table 5–1) is based on observing the

Table 5–1. ANGIOGRAPHIC SEVERITY OF AORTIC REGURGITATION

Grade	Opacification	Density	Clearing
+	Incomplete in LV	AO >> LV	Each beat
+ +	Complete but faint	AO > LV	Incomplete
+ + +	Rapid into LV	AO = LV	Slow
+ + + +	Complete in first beat	AO < LV	Slow

LV—left ventricle; AO—aorta.

rapidity with which contrast opacifies the entire left ventricle, the relative density of contrast in the left ventricle versus that in the aorta, and the rapidity with which the contrast clears from the left ventricle.[G1]

The volume of blood regurgitating, the pressure gradient driving the blood into the left ventricle, and the duration of regurgitant versus forward flow all influence the severity as judged by angiography. In addition, the volume and timing of contrast injection, the plane in which the left ventricle is visualized, the configuration of the valve orifice, and the relative volumes of the ventricle and aorta influence the timing and density of opacification and thus the apparent severity of the regurgitation. Because of the multiple factors that are unrelated to the severity of regurgitation, angiography remains a crude, although commonly used, method of estimating the severity of regurgitation. No echocardiographic technique that is similar to aortic angiography for quantification of aortic regurgitation has been found.

Other Hemodynamic Indicators of Severity of Regurgitation

Useful information about the severity of valvular regurgitation is based on parameters other than regurgitant fraction. These parameters include (1) blood pressure and pressure gradients; (2) pulmonary artery pressure; and (3) regurgitant orifice cross-sectional area.

Blood Pressure and Pressure Gradients

Aortic regurgitation can be quantified by hemodynamic parameters other than regurgitant fraction because it modifies aortic blood pressure in two different ways: (1) Peak systolic pressure is elevated because total forward systolic stroke volume includes normal net forward flow plus regurgitant flow; and (2) end-diastolic pressure is subnormal because blood flows from the aorta into the systemic circulation as well as through the regurgitant valve into the left ventricle.

Low aortic end-diastolic pressure (<55 mmHg) and abnormally wide pulse pressure are thus hemodynamic markers of severe aortic regurgitation.[G1] Both parameters can be detected directly from aortic pressure recordings or by using Doppler echocardiographic measurements of the high regurgitant velocities detected in the left ventricular outflow tract.[B3, T1]

Figure 5–18 contrasts the hemodynamic pressure and Doppler velocity findings in a patient with mild aortic regurgitation *(left)* and a patient with severe aortic regurgitation *(right)*. In the patient with mild aortic regurgitation, the forward stroke volume is normal, and the systolic aortic and left ventricular pressures are normal. Because only a small volume of blood leaks across the aortic valve in diastole, the pressure gradient between the aorta and the left ventricle is well maintained throughout diastole; the end-diastolic pressure in the aorta is normal. The velocity pattern produced by the mild regurgitant jet is pandiastolic; velocity remains high at end-diastole. The slope of the diastolic velocities in the left ventricular outflow tract is shallow; the time required for the pressure gradient to drop from its diastolic maximum to half of that maximum is long in the presence of mild aortic regurgitation.

In contrast, the patient with severe aortic regurgitation frequently has elevation of aortic peak systolic pressure, which leads to a slightly elevated early diastolic pressure gradient and velocity. As a large volume of blood flows rapidly from the aorta into the left ventricle, the diastolic pressure gradient and velocity drop rapidly to subnormal values. The time required for the pressure gradient to drop from its maximum to half of that maximum is short. Thus, the Doppler velocity records in the presence of severe aortic regurgitation are characterized by (1) a steep diastolic slope and short pressure half-time and (2) low end-diastolic velocity. The slope, pressure half-time, and end-diastolic velocity, derived from Doppler echocardiographic records obtained in the regurgitant jet, contain information useful in quantification of the severity of aortic regurgitation.[B3, G4, T1]

An interesting consequence of severe aortic regurgitation is premature closure of the mitral valve leaflets. Hemodynamically, if aortic regurgitation is severe, the pressure in the left ventricle increases rapidly, so that it exceeds left atrial pressure before diastole is completed. In such a case, diastolic closure of the mitral leaflets may occur. Upon imaging, premature closure is noted in severe, usually acute, aortic regurgitation. With Doppler echocardiography, premature cessation of mitral diastolic flow is detected. Interestingly, angiography or Doppler echocardiography can occasionally reveal diastolic mitral regurgitation in such patients.

Pulmonary Artery Pressure

Although quantification of the pulmonary artery systolic pressure is helpful in assessing all valvular lesions, it is of particular importance in assessing mitral valve disease. Doppler echocardiography can be used to assess the presence of pulmonary hypertension by two different techniques. The first technique is based on the observation that reaching peak velocity across the pulmonary valve takes longer when the pressure is elevated.[K1] Thus, the time from onset of flow to time of peak pulmonary artery velocity (T to V_{max}) is proportional to the peak systolic pulmonary artery pressure (P_{pa-s}):

$$P_{pa-s} \sim T \text{ to } V_{max}$$

In practice, small differences in the time to peak pulmonary velocity and the difficulty in identifying the onset of flow accurately significantly affect the calculated pulmonary artery systolic pressure.

A more exact method of estimating pulmonary systolic pressure involves assessment of the peak systolic velocity present across regurgitant tricuspid valves (V_{tr}), which are frequently associated with mitral valve disease. The Bernoulli equation is used to calculate the peak systolic pressure gradient[S5] between the right ventricle and the right atrium (PG_{rv-ra}):

$$(PG_{rv-ra}) = 4(V_{tr})^2$$

The pulmonary artery systolic pressure can be calculated by estimating right atrial mean pressure (P_{ra}) and adding that to the pressure gradient estimated from the tricuspid regurgitation:

$$(P_{pa-s}) = (P_{ra}) + 4(V_{tr})^2$$

Similar calculations can be performed with patients in whom pulmonary regurgitation is noted with Doppler echocardiography. Pulmonary artery diastolic pressure is estimated in that manner.

Regurgitant Orifice Cross-Sectional Area

One of the first observations made in attempting to assess the severity of valvular regurgitation by pulsed Doppler techniques was that the region of disturbed flow in the chamber proximal to the regurgitant valve seemed to be larger in the presence of more severe regurgitation. Early duplex pulsed Doppler techniques were used to map the width and the depth of the region of disturbed flow, and an approximate correlation was found between the dimensions of the disturbed flow region and the angiographic severity of regurgitation.[A1, C7, J1] Later studies with

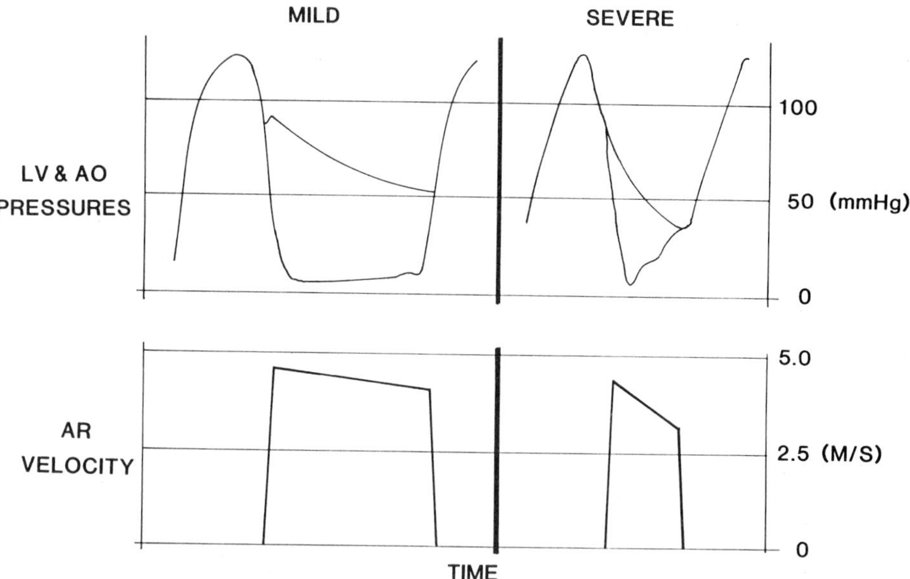

Figure 5–18. Diastolic pressure gradients between the left ventricle (LV) and the aorta (AO) and the corresponding diastolic peak velocity recordings from the regurgitant orifice, are shown in mild *(left)* and severe *(right)* aortic regurgitation (AR). Note that in mild aortic regurgitation, the pressure gradient remains high at the end of diastole; therefore, the velocity-time slope falls slowly, and end-diastolic velocity is high. In severe aortic regurgitation, the pressure gradient may be eliminated before diastole ends; therefore, the velocity-time slope falls steeply and the end-diastolic velocity is low.

color flow imaging instruments led to an enthusiastic series of reports, because the ease of examination and the accuracy with which the region of disturbed flow could be measured were increased. Planar area measurements and actual volume measurements were additional improvements.

Many factors are responsible for the dimensions of the apparent region of flow disturbance:[S6, W1]

1. Pressure gradient driving the jet
2. Regurgitant orifice cross-sectional area
3. Duration of regurgitation
4. Characteristics of the individual instrument
5. Settings of the instrument at the time of use
6. Physical characteristics of the tissue through which the ultrasound was transmitted
7. Configuration of the jet

Consideration of these factors makes accurate prediction of the severity of regurgitation based on measurement of the region of disturbed flow very unlikely, whether measurements are based on standard duplex pulsed Doppler or color flow instruments.

More recent studies have used two-dimensional color Doppler imaging to assess velocity patterns produced by the regurgitant jet at its origin in the left ventricular outflow tract and the left atrium. When the dimensions and the cross-sectional area of the color flow image are measured, they are found to be accurate indicators of the severity of regurgitation.[P2, P3] Slight improvement in performance is noted when the dimension or area is indexed for the size of the outflow tract by dividing by its anatomic diameter or cross-sectional area. Confirmation of the accuracy of two-dimensional color Doppler imaging in quantifying regurgitant orifice dimensions or cross-sectional area has not been accomplished, but it is suggested by the good correlation between these dimensions and the severity of valvular regurgitation.

Calculation of the regurgitant orifice cross-sectional area is cumbersome but possible at catheterization. It requires use of the Gorlin equation and measurement of regurgitant orifice flow rate and mean pressure gradient. The continuity equation, although its use seems promising, has not been directly applied to assess the severity of aortic or mitral regurgitation.

Comparison of Regurgitant Valves

Although the previous discussion has focused on quantification of aortic regurgitation, the concepts presented can be applied to mitral, pulmonic, and tricuspid regurgitation. Quantification of the severity of mitral regurgitation at catheterization is based on measurement of its angiographic severity as well as the regurgitant fraction.[G1] Because calculation of regurgitant fraction from Doppler echocardiographic data is difficult in patients with mitral regurgitation, estimation of regurgitant orifice dimension using two-dimensional color Doppler echocardiography is more widely performed. Assessment of left and right ventricular function as well as detection of pulmonary artery pressure is important in the evaluation of mitral regurgitation.

Tricuspid regurgitation occurs in two different forms. The usual secondary form is associated with marked dilatation of the right atrium and right ventricle and is secondary to annulus dilatation combined with displacement of the tricuspid papillary muscles. It is usually secondary to elevation of pulmonary arteriolar resistance but may also be caused by pulmonary stenosis, right ventricular dysfunction, or left ventricular dysfunction. Cardiac output is usually subnormal; significant elevation of right atrial pressure usually occurs. Because the tricuspid regurgitation is secondary to elevation of right ventricular systolic pressure, a significant right ventricular–right atrial pressure gradient is present. Systolic tricuspid regurgitant orifice velocities are therefore elevated. Usually, when tricuspid regurgitation occurs because of a structural defect of the tricuspid valve, only a slight elevation of right ventricular or pulmonary artery systolic pressures occurs. The transvalvular regurgitant velocities are usually low.

Angiographic evaluation of the severity of pulmonic and tricuspid regurgitation is difficult because the catheter must cross the regurgitant valve. Despite the tendency of the catheter to induce mild regurgitation, which distorts the valve cusps, differentiation of mild from severe regurgitation is frequently based on angiography. Doppler echocardiographic techniques have the advantage of not distorting the valve when measurements are made and thus provide a theoretically more accurate approach to detection and quantification. Assessment is usually based on the dimensions of the region of disturbed flow as noted with two-dimensional color Doppler imaging.

An interesting controversy has arisen because of the ability of standard continuous-wave and pulsed Doppler echocardiography and two-dimensional color Doppler imaging to detect tricuspid and pulmonic regurgitation in a large number of otherwise normal individuals in whom pulmonary hypertension and cardiac disease are absent by other examinations.[H4] If the pulmonic regurgitant velocities are confined to the right ventricular outflow tract within 1 cm of the pulmonic valve, the finding is thought to be within normal limits even though it represents actual (but trivial) valvular regurgitation.

SUMMARY

The concepts presented should provide the clinician with a knowledge of the abnormal hemodynamics of valvular disease. We hope that this knowledge base will be used to select appropriate invasive and noninvasive tests more wisely to answer specific questions regarding patients with valvular lesions. Although the discussions have used catheterization, Doppler techniques, and echocardiographic imaging to illustrate hemodynamic points, radionuclide angiography, magnetic resonance imaging, and other techniques such as ultrafast computed tomography can provide high-quality imaging and flow data that are useful in answering diagnostic questions concerning these patients.

References

A

1. Abbasi, A., Allen, M., DeCristofaro, D., and Ungar, I.: Detection and estimation of the degree of mitral regurgitation by range-gated pulsed Doppler echocardiography. Circulation 61:143, 1980.
2. Arvidsson, H., and Karnell, J.: Quantitative assessment of mitral and aortic insufficiency by angiography. Acta Radiol. 2:105, 1964.

B

1. Bache, R. J., Wang, Y., and Jorgensen, C. R.: Hemodynamic effects of exercise in isolated aortic stenosis. Circulation 44:1003, 1971.
2. Brubakk, A. O., Angelsen, B. A. J., and Hatle, L.: Diagnosis of valvular disease using transcutaneous Doppler ultrasound. Cardiovasc. Res. 11:461, 1977.
3. Beyer, R. W., Rameriz, M., Josephson, M. A., and Shan, P. M.: Correlation of continuous wave Doppler assessment of chronic aortic regurgitation with hemodynamics and angiography. Am. J. Cardiol. 60:852, 1987.
4. Boughner, D. R.: Assessment of aortic insufficiency by transcutaneous Doppler ultrasound. Circulation 52:874, 1975.

C

1. Clark, C., and Schultz, D. L.: Velocity distribution in aortic flow. Cardiovasc. Res. 7:601, 1973.
2. Clark, C.: Relationship between pressure differences across the aortic valve and left ventricular outflow. Cardiovasc. Res. 12:276, 1978.
3. Clark, C.: The propagation of turbulence produced by a stenosis. J. Biomech. 13:591, 1980.
4. Currie, P. J., Seward, J. B., Reeder, G. S., et al.: Continuous wave Doppler echocardiographic assessment of the severity of calcific aortic stenosis. Circulation 71:1162, 1985.
5. Cannon, S. R., Richards, K. L., Crawford, M. H., et al.: Inadequacy of the Grolin formula for predicting prosthetic valve area. Am. J. Cardiol. 62:113, 1988.
6. Cannon, S. R., Richards, K. L., and Crawford, M. H.: Hydraulic estimation of stenotic orifice area: A correction of the Gorlin formula. Circulation 71:1170, 1985.
7. Ciobanu, M., Abbasi, A. S., Allen, M., et al.: Pulsed Doppler echocardiography in the diagnosis and estimation of severity of aortic insufficiency. Am. J. Cardiol. 49:339, 1982.
8. Cohn, L. H., Mason, D. T., Ross, J., et al.: Preoperative assessment of aortic regurgitation in patients with mitral valve disease. Am. J. Cardiol. 19:177, 1967.

D

1. DeMaria, A. N.: Two-dimensional Doppler (color) flow imaging: State of the art. Echocardiography 3:459, 1986.
2. Dennig, K., Heneke, K. H., Dacian, S., and Rudolph, W.: Combined use of continuous wave and color flow Doppler for the estimation of the regurgitant volume in aortic regurgitation. J. Am. Coll. Cardiol. 11:176a, 1988.
3. Diebold, B., Peronneau, P., Blanchard, D., et al.: Noninvasive quantification of aortic regurgitation by Doppler echocardiography. Br. Heart J. 49:167, 1983.

F

1. Fisher, D. C., Sahn, D. J., Friedman, M. J., et al.: The mitral valve orifice method for noninvasive two-dimensional echo Doppler determination of cardiac output. Circulation 67:872, 1983.

G

1. Grossman, W. (ed.): Cardiac Catheterization and Angiography. Lea & Febiger, Philadelphia, 1986.
2. Goldberg, S. J., Sahn, D. J., Allen, H., and Valdes-Cruz, L. M.: Evaluation of pulmonary and systemic flow by two-dimensional echo Doppler fast Fourier transform spectral analysis. Am. J. Cardiol. 50:1394, 1982.
3. Gorlin, R., and Gorlin, S. G.: Hydraulic formula for the calculation of the area of the stenotic mitral valve, other cardiac valves, and central circulatory shunts. Am. Heart J. 41:1, 1951.
4. Grayburn, P. A., Handshoe, R., Smith, M. D., et al.: Quantitative assessment of the hemodynamic consequences of aortic regurgitation by means of continuous wave Doppler recordings. J. Am. Coll. Cardiol. 10:135, 1987.

H

1. Huntsman, L. L., Stewart, D. K., Barnes, S. R., et al.: Noninvasive Doppler determination of cardiac output in man: Clinical validation. Circulation 67:593, 1983.
2. Holen, J., and Simonsen, S.: Determination of pressure gradient in mitral stenosis with Doppler echocardiography. Br. Heart J. 41:529, 1979.
3. Hatle, L.: Noninvasive assessment and differentiation of left ventricular outflow obstruction by Doppler ultrasound. Circulation 64:381, 1981.
4. Hatle, L., and Angelsen, B.: Doppler Ultrasound in Cardiology. Lea & Febiger, Philadelphia, 1984.
5. Hart, T. T., Richards, K. L., Cannon S. R., et al.: Exercise induced changes in cardiac output and calculated valve area in adults with severe aortic stenosis. Circulation 74:314, 1986.
6. Hatle, L., Angelson, B., and Tromsdal, A.: Noninvasive assessment of atrioventricular pressure half-time by Doppler ultrasound. Circulation 60:1096, 1979.
7. Helmcke, F., Nanda, N. C., Hsiung, M. C., et al.: Color Doppler assessment of mitral regurgitation with orthogonal planes. Circulation 75:175, 1987.

J

1. Johnson, S. L., Baker, D. W., Lute, A. R., and Murray, J. A.: Detection of mitral regurgitation by Doppler echocardiography. Am. J. Cardiol. 33:146, 1974.

K

1. Kitabatake, A., Inoue, M., Asao, M., et al.: Noninvasive estimation of pulmonary hypertension by a pulsed Doppler technique. Circulation 68:302, 1983.

L

1. Lewis, J. F., Kuo, L. C., Nelson, J. G., et al.: Pulsed Doppler echocardiographic determination of stroke volume in cardiac output: Clinical validation of two methods using the apical window. Circulation 70:425, 1984.
2. Lima, C., Sahn, D. J., Valdes-Cruz, L. M., et al.: Noninvasive prediction of transvalvular pressure gradient in patients with pulmonary stenosis by quantitative two-dimensional echo Doppler studies. Circulation 67:866, 1983.

M

1. McDonald, D. A.: Blood Flow in Arteries. Williams & Wilkins, Baltimore, 1974.
2. Murgo, J. P., Westerhof, N., Giolma, J. P., and Altobelli, S. A.: Aortic input impedance in normal man: Relationship to pressure wave forms. Circulation 62:105, 1980.
3. Murgo, J. P., Giolma, J. P., and Altobelli, S. A.: Signal acquisition and processing for human hemodynamic research. Proc. IEEE 65:696, 1977.

N

1. Nakatani, S., Kodama, K., and Fujii, K.: Value and limitation of Doppler echocardiography in quantitating stenotic mitral valve area: Comparison of pressure half-time and continuity equation methods. Circulation 77:78, 1988.
2. Nerem, R. M., and Seed, W. A.: An in vivo study of aortic flow disturbances. Cardiovasc. Res. 6:1, 1972.

O

1. Otto, C. M., Pearlman, A. S., Comess, K. A., et al.: Determination of the stenotic aortic valve area in adults using Doppler echocardiography. J. Am. Coll. Cardiol. 7:509, 1986.

P

1. Pasipoularides, A., Murgo, J. P., Bird, J. J., and Craig, W. E.: Fluid dynamics of aortic stenosis: Mechanisms for the presence of subvalvular pressure gradients. Am. J. Physiol. 264:H542, 1984.
2. Perry, G. J., Nanda, N. C.: Diagnosis and quantitation of valvular regurgitation by color Doppler flow mapping. Echocardiography 3:493, 1986.
3. Perry, G. J., Helmcke, F., Nanda, N. C., et al.: Evaluation of aortic insufficiency by Doppler color flow mapping. J. Am. Coll. Cardiol. 9:952, 1987.

Q

1. Quinones, M. A., Young, J. B., Waggoner, A. S., et al.: Assessment of pulsed Doppler echocardiography in detection and quantification of aortic and mitral regurgitation. Br. Heart J. 44:612, 1980.

R

1. Richards, K. L., Cannon, S. R., Miller, J. F., and Crawford, M. H.: Calculation of aortic valve area by Doppler echocardiography: A direct application of the continuity equation. Circulation 73:964, 1986.
2. Richards, K. L., Cannon, S. R., and Crawford, M. H.: Noninvasive quantification of mitral valve area using high PRF Doppler. J. Am. Coll. Cardiol. 3:493, 1984.
3. Richards, K. L., Cannon, S. R., Crawford, M. H., and Sorensen, S. G.: Noninvasive diagnosis of aortic and mitral valve disease with pulsed-Doppler spectral analysis. Am. J. Cardiol. 51:1122, 1983.

4. Richter, H. S.: Mitral valve area: Measurement soon after catheterization. Circulation 28:451, 1963.
5. Richards, K. L., Hart, T. T., Cannon, S. R., et al.: Confirmation of variable orifice native valves in adults with severe aortic stenosis. Circulation 74:314, 1986.
6. Richards, K. L., Cannon, S. R., Lujan, M., et al.: Anatomical valve area varies with pressure gradient and flow rate in severe aortic stenosis. Circulation 78:209, 1988.
7. Rodrigo, F. A., and Snellen, H. A.: Estimation of valve area and valvular resistance. Am. Heart J. 45:1, 1953.
8. Reiter, S. J., Rumberger, J. A., Stanford, W. W., and Marcus, M. L.: Quantitative determination of aortic regurgitant volumes in dogs by ultrafast computed tomography. Circulation 76:728, 1987.

S

1. Stewart, W. J., Jiang, L., Mich, R., et al.: Variable effects of changes in flow rate through the aortic, pulmonary and mitral valves on valve area and flow velocity: Impact on quantitative Doppler flow calculations. J. Am. Coll. Cardiol. 6:653, 1985.
2. Skjaerpe, T., Hegrenaes, L., and Hatle, L.: Noninvasive estimation of valve area in patients with aortic stenosis by Doppler ultrasound and 2-D echocardiography. Circulation 72:810, 1985.
3. Stevenson, J. G., and Kawabori, I.: Noninvasive determination of pressure gradients in children: Two methods employing pulsed Doppler echocardiography. J. Am. Coll. Cardiol. 3:179, 1984.
4. Smith, M. D., Handshoe, B., Handshoe, S., et al.: Comparative accuracy of two-dimensional echocardiography and Doppler pressure half-time methods in assessing severity of mitral stenosis in patients with and without prior commissurotomy. Circulation 73:100, 1986.
5. Skjaerpe, T., and Hatle, L.: Noninvasive estimation of pulmonary artery pressure by Doppler ultrasound. *In* Spencer, M. (ed.): Cardiac Doppler Diagnosis. Martinus Nijhoff, The Hague, 1983, p. 247.
6. Stevenson, J. G.: Two-dimensional color Doppler estimation of the severity of atrioventricular valve regurgitation: Important effects of instrument gain setting, pulse repetition frequency and carrier frequency. J. Am. Soc. Echo. 2:1, 1989.

T

1. Teague, S. M., Heinsimer, J. A., Anderson, J. L., et al.: Quantification of aortic regurgitation utilizing continuous wave Doppler ultrasound. J. Am. Coll. Cardiol. 8:592, 1986.
2. Touche, T., Prasquier, R., Nitenberg, A., et al.: Assessment of follow-up patients with aortic regurgitation by an updated Doppler echocardiographic measurement of the regurgitant fraction in the aortic arch. Circulation 72:819, 1985.

U

1. Ubago, J. L., Figueroa, A., Colman, T., et al.: Hemodynamic factors that affect calculated areas in the mitral Hancock xenograft valve. Circulation 61:388, 1980.

V

1. Visscher, M. B., and John, J. A.: The Fick principle: Analysis of potential errors in its conventional application. J. Appl. Physiol. 5:635, 1953.
2. Valdes-Cruz, L. M., Yoganathan, A. P., Tamura, T., et al.: Studies in vitro of the relationship between ultrasound and Doppler velocimetry and the applicability of the simplified Bernoulli relationship. Circulation 73:300, 1986.

W

1. Wranne, B., Ask, P., and Loyd, D.: Quantification of heart valve regurgitation: A critical analysis from a theoretical and experimental point of view. Clin. Physiol. 5:81, 1985.

Z

1. Zohgbi, W. A., Farmer, K. L., Soto, J. G., et al.: Accurate noninvasive quantification of stenotic aortic valve area by Doppler echocardiography. Circulation 73:452, 1986.

Chapter 6

Quantitative Methods in Cardiac Imaging: An Introduction to Digital Image Processing

■ STEVEN R. FLEAGLE, B.S.E.E. ■ DAVID J. SKORTON, M.D.

QUANTITATION IN CARDIAC IMAGING: ASSESSMENT OF ANATOMY AND FUNCTION 72
General Considerations 72
Three-Dimensional Reconstruction of the Heart .. 73
DIGITAL IMAGE PROCESSING: A PRIMER 74
Introduction 74
Digital Images and Their Characteristics 74
Image Enhancement 77
Point Operations 77
Geometric Operations 79
Filtering Operations 82
Segmentation 82
Future Directions of Quantitative Image Processing 83

Modern cardiac imaging encompasses an extremely broad variety of methods in which several energy forms are used to create diagnostically useful pictures of the cardiovascular system. Although many basic differences distinguish the various imaging techniques and, thus, the information offered, at least two similarities are shared by all methods. First, modern modalities are based to an increasing degree on digital computer processing technology for creation, display, storage, and analysis or image data.[B1, C1] Second, the current clinical practice of cardiac imaging is making increased use of image quantitation. For example, the subjective, visual assessment of coronary arterial narrowing due to atherosclerosis may now be complemented by computer-based quantitative coronary arteriographic techniques that permit reproducible, precise delineation of minimal coronary lumen area and other important parameters of stenosis severity.[B2, F1, K1] Similarly, qualitative analysis of planar thallium-201 scintigrams is giving way to computer-based quantitation of single photon emission computed tomograms (SPECT).[G1, G2] Many other examples may be considered as evidence of the trend toward image quantitation and its importance in cardiac diagnosis, therapy, and prognosis.

The orientation toward quantitation in imaging is due in turn to at least two evolutionary factors. First, the clinician caring for the patient with heart disease is becoming increasingly sophisticated in the assessment of cardiovascular physiology. For example, investigators and clinicians are demanding quantitative capabilities in the assessment of ventricular function and myocardial perfusion. Second, the increasing sophistication and decreasing costs of digital computing systems have permitted sophisticated computational devices to be integrated into modern imaging systems. From relatively simple measures such as left ventricular ejection fraction to more complex assessment of regional myocardial glucose uptake by positron emission tomography (PET) scanning, most modern imaging systems contain sufficient computing power for many forms of sophisticated analysis. In addition, off-line computer systems can be used to supplement the capability of the main imaging system (e.g., in radionuclide scanning) or as an added capability offered by the original equipment vendor or other manufacturers (e.g., of echocardiography and coronary angiography equipment). These two factors—the *need* for quantitation and the *capability* for quantitation—are combining to make cardiovascular imaging an increasingly quantitative science.

In this chapter we present some of the principles common to quantitation of cardiac images based on digital image processing methods. We begin by briefly reviewing an example of the evolution of quantitation in imaging: assessment of left ventricular anatomy throughout the heart cycle. This example demonstrates the progression from qualitative estimates of ventricular size and shape to a precise, dynamic three-dimensional representation of ventricular morphology. These advances in the assessment of ventricular anatomy and function occurred in part due to progress in the science of digital image processing. Thus, the major portion of this chapter constitutes a brief primer on digital image processing. Because the orientation of this book is toward the clinician, detailed and mathematically rigorous descriptions of image processing techniques are not within the scope of this chapter. However, we hope to introduce the reader to enough of the basic concepts of image processing that new ideas and their implementation in clinical practice may be viewed in their proper perspective. The orientation of the chapter is toward general principles of digital processing. Detailed descriptions of specific quantitative analyses are presented in the chapter dealing with each particular imaging technique.

QUANTITATION IN CARDIAC IMAGING: ASSESSMENT OF ANATOMY AND FUNCTION

General Considerations

Cardiac anatomy and function are assessed by ascertaining the size and shape of the cardiac chambers throughout the heart cycle. Although quantitative analysis of all four cardiac chambers is of physiologic and diagnostic importance, the vast majority of investigative and clinical work has gone into evaluating the size, shape, and function of the left ventricle because of its predominant role in many cardiac disorders. Left ventricular anatomy and function are generally evaluated by assuming an idealized geometric model, commonly a prolate ellipsoid,[B3] to represent the shape of this chamber. Area-length angiographic methods as well as some echocardiographic and radionuclide techniques depend on this assumed prolate ellipsoid geometry to assess left ventricular volume, mass, and ejection fraction. However, the normal shape of the left ventricle does not precisely match that of a prolate ellipsoid. Because of this and because wide variations in shape (causing an even poorer match) occur with disease, especially ischemic disorders, methods of quantitation not based on the assumption of a limited geometric model will be more generally applicable. Since the advent of tomographic or "slice-like" imaging methods, various approaches have been used with an approximation technique based on Simpson's rule to delineate left ventricular volume and mass throughout the heart cycle. In the current context, the term "Simpson's rule" is used to refer to the summation of the volumes of several tomographic slices through a part of the heart, such as the left ventricle, to obtain a total volume for the left ventricular cavity and for myocardial mass. The ideal Simpson's rule-based approximation would require many mutually parallel slices through the left ventricle; the volume encompassed by the endocardium and epicardium in each slice, multiplied by the distance between slices, would then yield an estimate of left ventricular cavity and muscle volume. Multiplication of the myocardial volume by the specific gravity of muscle (generally taken to be 1.05) would yield left ventricular mass. Simpson's rule-based approximations of left ventricular volume or mass from echocardiographic,[S1] computed tomographic (CT),[F2] or magnetic resonance image (MRI) data[F3] have supplied accurate and precise delineation of these variables. It should be appreciated that three important requirements form the basis for Simpson's rule-based approximations of left ventricular volume and mass. First, endocardial and epicardial contours must be accurately delineated in each tomographic slice. Second, the location of the imaging plane and of the patient during all slice acquisitions must be known precisely. Third, for techniques in which the slices are not all obtained within a single cardiac cycle (including echocardiography, CT, and MRI), stability of the cardiac cycle length and hemodynamics is required, since the calculated volume and mass will be "average" values across the several cardiac cycles required for image data acquisition.

Three-Dimensional Reconstruction of the Heart

Ultimately, complete evaluation of cardiac anatomy and function will require appreciation of cardiac size and *shape* throughout the heart cycle. The shape of the heart is complex and, as mentioned, does not precisely fit any simple geometric model. This is particularly true for the right ventricle and the atria. Thus, in the evaluation of cardiac shape, clinicians often utilize the information from several individual images to conceptualize mentally the three-dimensional (3D) shape of the portion of the heart under study. Particularly in disorders of complex morphology, such as congenital heart disease, this 3D conceptualization of cardiac shape may be quite difficult, even for the experienced observer. Thus, there has been growing interest in 3D modeling of the heart. Based on 3D reconstruction techniques originally developed for industrial and engineering applications, especially computer-aided design and manufacturing,[R1] these techniques permit visualization of an object without the need for a physical model. Precise information of geometry and information concerning the physical load to which a structure may be subjected (such as the weight expected on a bridge) may be combined through a variety of mathematical techniques to estimate the stresses and strains that will occur in the actual structure.[C2]

Three-dimensional image processing methods applied to biomedical images have already shown utility in planning maxillofacial surgery[H1] and in imaging the spine and other bony structures.[T1] Cardiovascular applications of 3D reconstructions are recent but appear capable of accurately calculating chamber volume and mass[L1] as well as analyzing regional stress-strain characteristics of the heart. For example, 3D reconstruction of the left ventricle, combined with high-fidelity intracavitary pressure information, may be used to evaluate regional stress-strain characteristics of the normal left ventricle and alteration of these characteristics in the setting of acute ischemia.[M1] It is clear that the great potential of sophisticated 3D reconstruction techniques is just beginning to be appreciated in cardiovascular image processing.

The basic requirements for 3D cardiac reconstruction include several steps (Table 6–1).[C3, G3, S2] First, individual images must be acquired, along with information about the position and orientation of each image relative to other images or to a common reference system. This process of acquiring information on the relative orientation and position of various images may be referred to as "spatial registration." The important structural contours (such as endocardium and epicardium) in each image must then be identified and their location entered into the computer system. When the contours in each image have been spatially registered, they may be reconstructed into a 3D data structure. Data "missing" between actual image slices must be interpolated, usually by use of polynomial curves or other similar procedures.

Display of the 3D reconstructions has included two basic approaches: wire-frame displays and shaded-surface displays. Wire-frame displays depict the important image contours (such as endocardium and epicardium), along with lines interpolated between individual image slices (Fig. 6–1*A*). Calculations of volume, mass, and ejection fraction and stress-strain analysis may be expedited by the use of wire-frame structures. For structures of relatively simple shape, such as the left ventricle, wire-frame displays allow the structure to be represented with an amount of data small enough to be easily manipulated. On the other hand, the multiplicity of lines of a wire-frame model of a complex structure make the display less appealing than solid, shaded-surface displays.

The shaded-surface display procedure produces a more visually pleasing rendering of the 3D reconstruction. The display appears as a solid object with shading effects calculated by the computer program (Fig. 6–1*B*).[H2] Qualitative visual evaluation of these structures is easier than that of wire-frame displays because the shaded-surface displays more closely resemble actual anatomic structures. However, these shaded-surface displays involve manipulation and storage of substantially more data than the wire-frame displays.

Once the 3D reconstruction information is available throughout the heart cycle (or for selected portions of the cycle), these images may be combined sequentially to produce cine loop animated displays of cardiac motion that may closely resemble the actual cardiac appearance.

Three-dimensional reconstruction techniques have been applied to echocardiographic,[A1, G3, L1, M1, M2, S3] angiographic,[R2, S4] CT,[H2, I1, R3] radionuclide,[G1, M3] and MRI image data.[A2, L2] Static cardiac geometry (such as left ventricular mass), left ventricular function, and complex stress-strain characteristics of the heart have all been assessed by use of 3D reconstruction techniques. Continuing improvements in digital display and reconstruction technology

Table 6–1. REQUIREMENTS FOR THREE-DIMENSIONAL CARDIAC RECONSTRUCTION

1. Acquisition of several tomographic images encompassing the entire structure of interest.
2. Registration of spatial position and orientation of each image.
3. Identification and digitization of important image contours (e.g., endocardium).
4. Reconstruction of individual digitized image contours into a three-dimensional data structure.
5. Display of three-dimensional reconstruction.
6. Extraction of quantitative data.

and the increasing emphasis on digital picture archiving and communications systems (PACS) in departments of radiology will probably lead to increased utilization of cardiac 3D reconstructions.

As a general conclusion, it can be appreciated that newer imaging methods, coupled with the trend toward quantitation in cardiac imaging, are improving the assessment of left ventricular function. Part of the improved capability of modern imaging modalities must be credited to advances in the physics and engineering of imaging energy sources and sensors, demonstrated so dramatically in the development of PET scanning, ultrafast CT, and MRI. A great deal of the progress must also be credited to the ingenious use of digital computational techniques—methods that permit rapid image reconstruction, flexible display, and unique data analysis. We will now provide an overview of this fascinating science that is so integral to modern imaging—digital image processing.

DIGITAL IMAGE PROCESSING: A PRIMER

Introduction

Digital image processing is a type of computerized data processing in which an image is stored in a numerical format that can easily be manipulated and analyzed by a computer. Using the computational abilities of modern computers, quantitative analyses that were formerly impossible are now routine.

Computers have been used to analyze digital images for many years. Much of the early work in digital image processing was done at the Jet Propulsion Laboratory.[C4] The early technological advances were achieved in the process of maximizing the information extractable from images transmitted from unmanned exploration spacecraft; this work was done in the early 1960s and continues today. Over this period, many advances in the science of digital image processing have occurred, primarily due to the decreased cost and increased availability of the imaging equipment needed by researchers. One of the major applications of digital image processing has been the field of medical imaging. Medical image processing has benefited tremendously from other nonbiological applications of image processing and has also served to advance the general science of digital image processing.

Digital image processing has many important advantages over other techniques such as optical or analog image processing. These advantages include ease of implementing new algorithms, relative immunity to noise generated during the application, and an abundance of available techniques. In contrast, the nondigital techniques are usually faster (most optical and analog operations are performed at video frame rates) and are occasionally more desirable in special, dedicated applications.[S5]

Digital Images and Their Characteristics

Since computers work with numerical data, images must be represented in numerical form prior to computer manipulation and analysis. The process of transforming an image into numerical form is called *digitization* or analog-to-digital conversion. There are many ways of digitizing images, largely because there are many sources of images. For instance, the method of choice for digitizing echocardiographic images stored on videotape is not applicable to images stored on radiographic films. Images from videotape are available as a video signal (a time-varying voltage) when the tape is played back. The voltage of the video signal at a particular point in time corresponds directly to the brightness of a portion of the image. The film, however, is a static, two-dimensional distribution (pattern) of film densities. In each case the signal (voltage or density) at a particular portion of the image represents the feature of interest (e.g., backscattered ultrasound amplitude or x-ray exposure). It is common to have the image converted from its natural state of energy into a voltage by use of some sort of transducer. A video camera is an example of a transducer that converts energy in the form of light into a voltage signal that varies in proportion to the amount of light received. The video camera accomplishes this much in the same way as we read text from a printed page. Just as we scan the page and turn

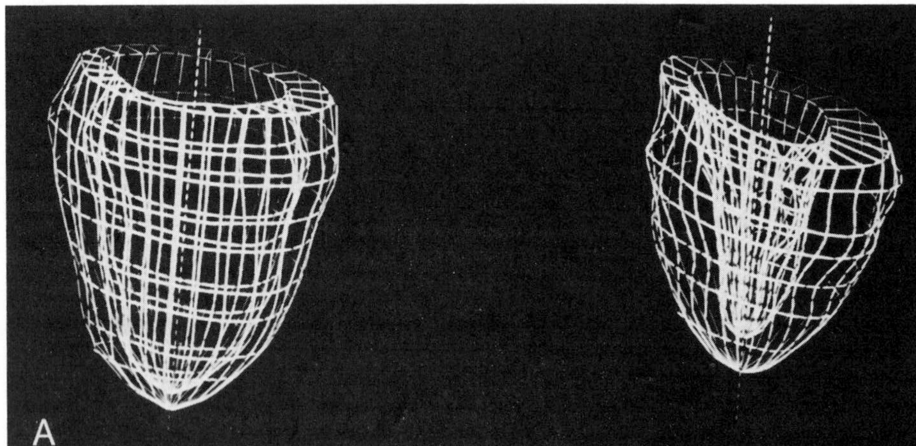

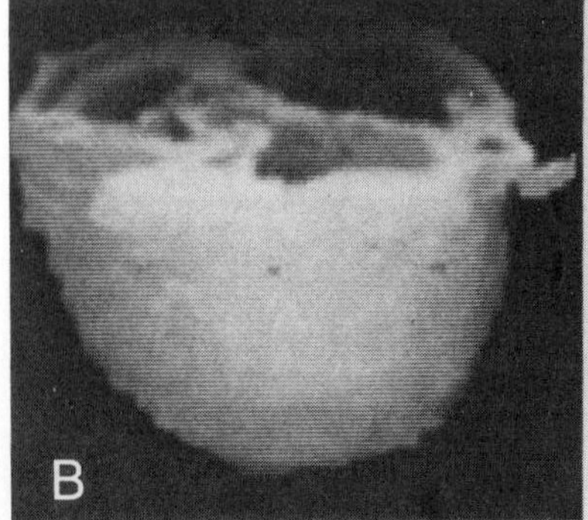

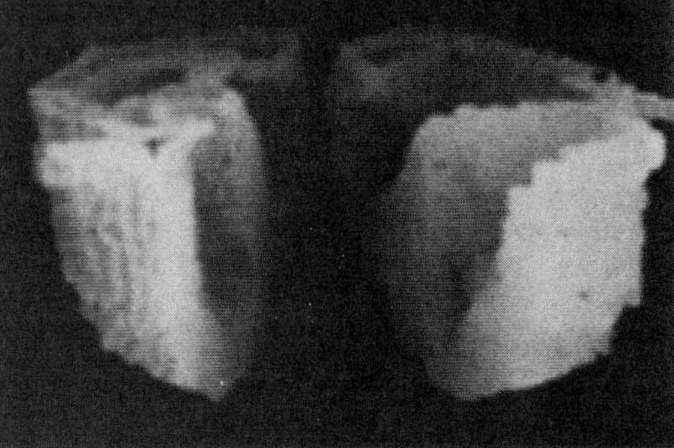

Figure 6–1. Three-dimensional reconstructions of the heart based on noninvasive imaging methods. *A*, Wire-frame display of reconstruction of the left ventricle from ultrafast computed tomographic images. At the left is an end-diastolic reconstruction, and at the right is an end-systolic reconstruction. *B*, Shaded-surface display of reconstruction produced from CT data. At the left is a reconstruction of the entire heart, and at the right the three-dimensional data structure has been "sectioned" mathematically, revealing details of internal anatomy. (*A*, From Collins, S. M., Chandran, K. B., and Skorton, D. J.: Three-dimensional cardiac imaging. Echocardiography 5:311, 1988, with permission; *B*, from Herman, G. T., and Liu, H. K.: Display of three-dimensional information in computed tomography. J. Comput. Assist. Tomogr. 1:155, 1977, with permission.)

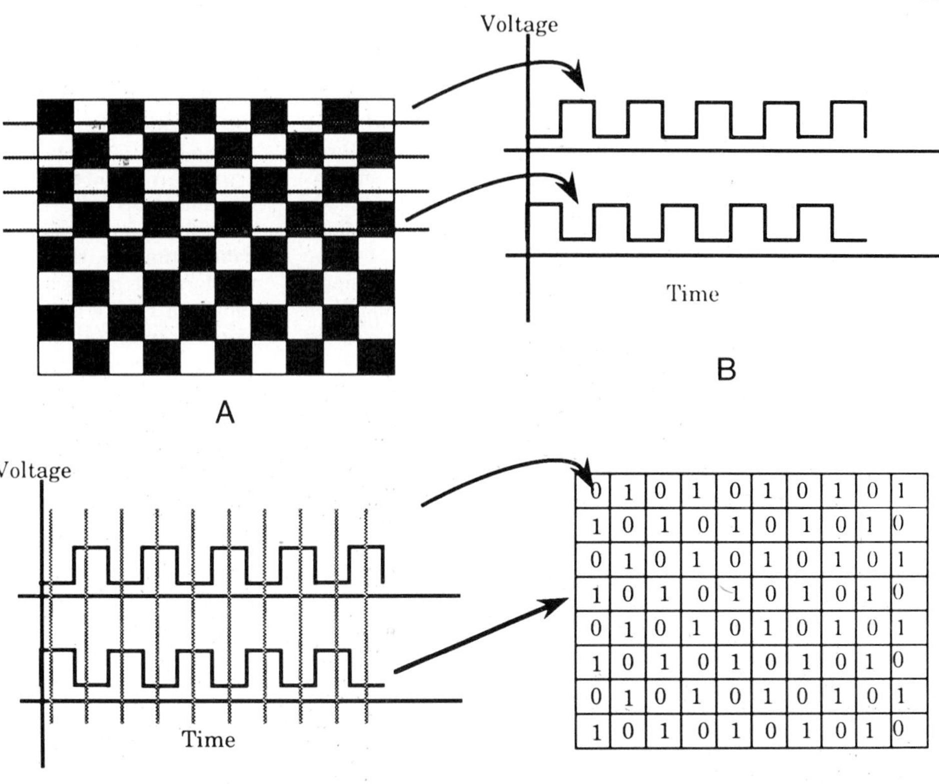

Figure 6–2. The concept of image digitization as implemented with a video camera. *A*, An "image" representing a checkerboard pattern. The horizontal lines drawn through the first four rows of the image indicate scan lines for a video camera. *B*, The resulting voltage signals from two of the scan lines. The voltage signals are then sampled at points in time indicated by vertical lines in *C*. The value of the voltage at each of these times is then quantized (in this case as 0 or 1) and stored as a rectangular grid of numbers, as shown in *D*.

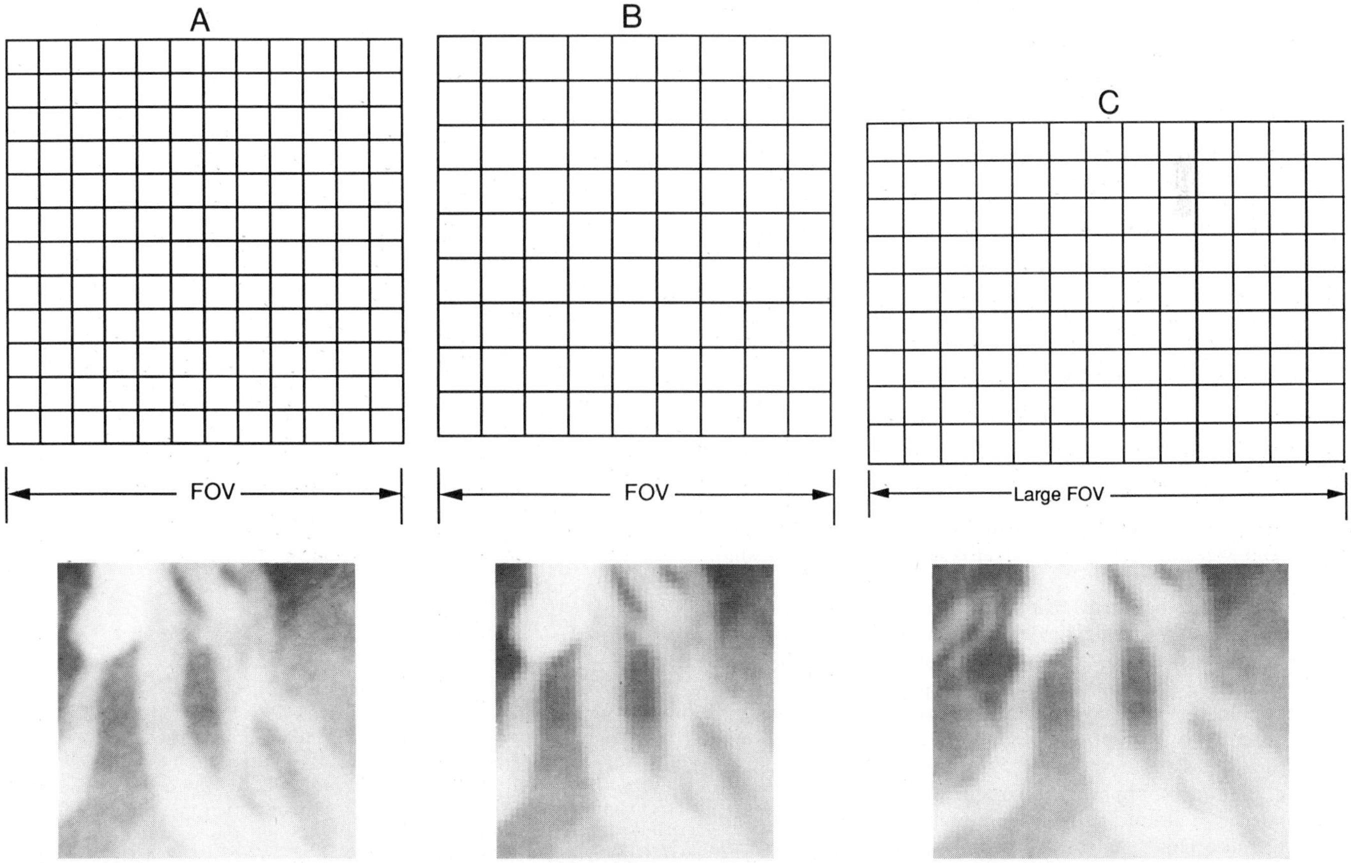

A B C

FOV FOV Large FOV

Figure 6–3. Relationship between matrix size and spatial resolution. Panels *A*, *B*, and *C* each have a schematic image matrix (above) and an example image (below). If *A* is considered the standard spatial resolution and matrix size, then *B* has a lower spatial resolution because it has the same field of view (FOV) but a smaller matrix size. Panel *C*, on the other hand, shows the same matrix size but a lower spatial resolution than *A* because the field of view has increased. Note that *B* and *C* have the same spatial resolution even though the matrix size and field of view are different in each.

characters into words, the video camera scans across the image, line by line, and converts the brightness at each point in the line into a voltage. The most common method of scanning is from upper left to lower right, transversing in nearly horizontal rows from top to bottom. The scanning process is quite rapid, usually being completed in less than 30 msec. The resulting voltage signal, in turn, must be converted into a signal that can be processed by a computer. Converting the voltage signals representing an image into digital form involves two steps: *sampling* (dividing the image into small areas) and *quantizing* (converting the intensity of each small area into a number). In the case of the video voltage that results from scanning with the video camera, the image is divided into small areas by measuring the voltage at frequent time intervals. Each time interval is therefore related to a particular image region. This process of digitization results in a digital image composed of an ordered array of *pixels* (picture elements). With each pixel is associated a gray level, which describes the intensity of that region, and a unique location. Figure 6–2 shows some of the steps taken in digitizing an image. In cases in which the location is described by three dimensions, the elements of the array are termed *voxels* (volume elements). For example, if the pixel dimensions in a CT image are 2 × 2 mm and the image "slice" thickness is 3 mm, each voxel will be a rectangular volume element of 2 × 2 × 3 mm.

When referring to the characteristics of digital images, the term *resolution* is often used. *Spatial resolution,* which is most commonly used, refers to how much detail can be represented in the image. The higher the spatial resolution, the finer the detail that can be represented in the image or the closer together two objects can be and still be resolved as separate objects. *Temporal resolution* is determined by the number of images per unit time and defines how well a series of images can represent changes that occur over time; imaging techniques with higher temporal resolution are able to represent events that occur more rapidly. Finally, *contrast resolution* describes how well an image can discriminate various intensity attributes, such as displaying differing tissues as separate shades (levels) of gray.

The number of pixels into which an image is divided (the matrix size), the size of each pixel (the spatial resolution), and the number and range of intensity levels each pixel can represent have important effects on the characteristics of digital images.

The matrix size and spatial resolution are closely related but not identical and are often confused. The matrix size is simply the number of pixels used to represent an image and has no effect on spatial resolution. Confusion arises because the region to be digitized, or the "field of view," is usually assumed to be of constant size. If the field of view is held constant, the matrix size and spatial resolution are directly related, as shown in Figure 6–3. Adding more pixels by making the matrix larger requires that each pixel be smaller in order to maintain the same field of view. As each pixel becomes smaller, the spatial resolution increases. Conversely, if the matrix size is decreased each pixel must be larger in order to maintain the field of view, and the spatial resolution decreases. Figure 6–3 also shows how the matrix size can increase while spatial resolution stays the same. To accomplish this, the field of view must also be increased. Thus, one must take great care when comparing matrix sizes between different imaging devices to ascertain the relationship between matrix size and actual spatial resolution.

The lower the spatial resolution of a digital image, the poorer the approximation to the original data. But how do we know if we have sufficient spatial resolution? The answer can be found in the Nyquist sampling theorem,[R4, J1] which states that to preserve all information found in the original image, the image must be sampled at a minimum of twice the highest *spatial frequency* found in the original image. We define spatial frequency as the number of gray level fluctuations over a given region of the image. High spatial frequencies are found at points in the image where there are rapid gray level transitions, such as object borders. The "sharper" the border, the higher the spatial frequency. Thus, if the image contains high spatial frequencies, we need high spatial resolution to represent it. What happens if the sampling rate is less than twice the highest spatial frequency? In this situation, known as undersampling, we not only lose some information but also introduce image artifacts known as *aliasing* errors.[R5] Aliasing errors occur when a signal is undersampled and information is lost. As shown in Figure 6–4, the sampled points seem to form a signal of lower frequency than that of the original data. In images, these artifacts of lower frequency may appear in the form of moiré patterns. An example of such a pattern is shown in Figure 6–5. If the image is undersampled, any aliasing errors introduced are permanent, so care should be taken to avoid undersampling the image data. When digitizing an image it can be difficult to determine the proper sampling frequency unless some information is available about the range of spatial frequencies contained in the data.

Errors introduced by representing pixels with too few gray levels are called quantization errors. Some quantization error usually occurs with digitization because the pixel can rarely assume as many values as the original, continuous data. To use a familiar analogy, the column of mercury in a common thermometer may assume an infinite variety of lengths and thus represent an infinite variety of temperatures, but a digital thermometer may yield the temperature only in discrete units of, for example, 0.1 degree. In the case of image data, if a signal actually has a value of 104.63 and the nearest allowable pixel values are 100 and 110, the pixel is assigned a value of 100 and the difference of 4.63 is the quantization error. The effects of quantization error can appear to be just as dramatic as those of undersampling errors. The most common error is the appearance of false contours as edges in an area of an image that should exhibit a smoothly varying gray level. This effect can be seen in Figure 6–6.

The number of gray levels represented in a digital system is usually expressed as a power of two. This is a result of the binary representation of numbers by computers. The gray scale data are stored in binary digits or "bits" (0's or 1's). Each bit available in a binary number doubles the number of values (gray levels) that may be represented. Thus, an 8-bit system can represent four times more gray levels ($2^8 = 256$) than a 6-bit system ($2^6 = 64$). The number of bits available depends on the image storage or display device. Storage and display of 6- to 8-bit images are currently most common, although technology is making 10- to 12-bit devices (1024 to 4096 gray levels) increasingly popular.

If spatial resolution and pixel quantization can introduce errors, why not always sample at the highest possible rate and represent

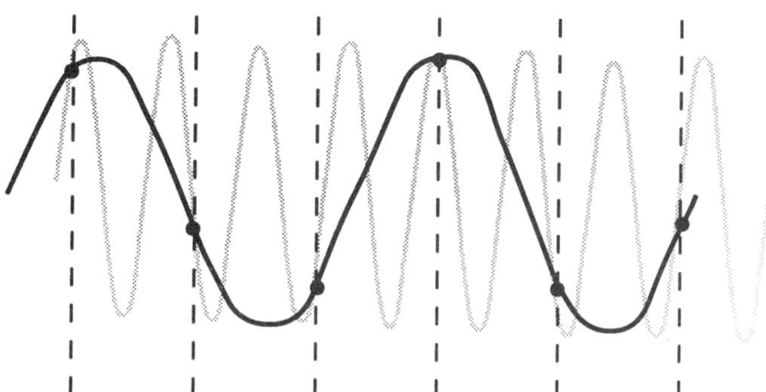

Figure 6–4. Effect of undersampling during the process of digitization. A time-varying voltage signal is represented as a sinusoidal wave pattern (gray line). The vertical, dashed lines indicate times at which the voltage values are sampled in the digitization process. The intersections of the vertical lines and the original sinusoid, indicated here by dots, are the voltage values measured at these times. The darker line through the dots indicates a signal that might be fit through the sampled points. The sampled signal differs from the original sinusoidal signal because the original signal was sampled at too low a frequency (not enough samples per unit time). The distortion of the original signal because of undersampling is often referred to as aliasing.

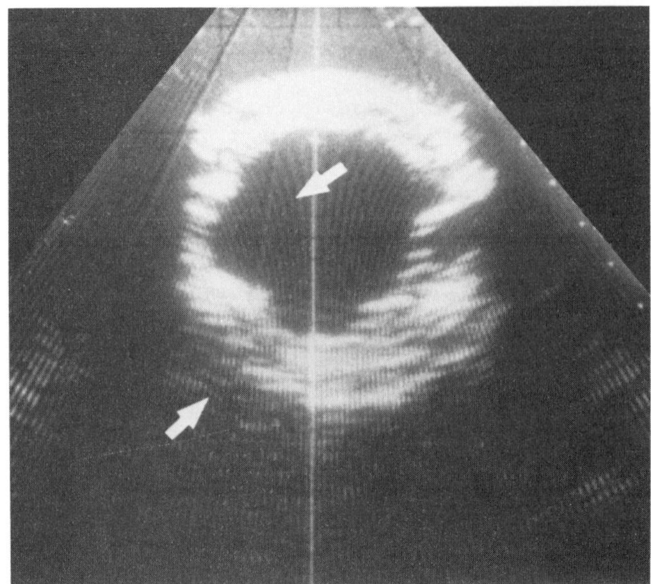

Figure 6–5. Illustration of a moiré pattern. The lines identified by the arrows are another undersampling artifact sometimes noted in digital images. (From Collins, S. M., and Skorton, D. J. [eds.]: Cardiac Imaging and Image Processing. McGraw-Hill Book Company, New York, 1986, p. 128, with permission.)

pixels with the largest possible number of gray levels? Increasing the spatial resolution or the number of allowable gray levels increases digital data storage requirements and potentially increases the time required to analyze the image. In many cases, improvements in image quality (either in spatial resolution or in the number of allowable gray levels) require a much larger investment in both image acquisition time and equipment expenses.

After manipulation by the computer, the digital image must be converted back into a form easily viewed by the human eye. This reverse process is ditital-to-analog conversion or digital image display. Displays may be temporary (as on video monitors) or permanent (film recorders). Just as there are important considerations regarding image digitization, there are many factors that influence the proper display of digital images.[C5] It is frequently not possible to display all the information available in the digital image. If the range of data (either spatially or in gray levels) exceeds the range of the available display, some transformation must be done. This may mean compressing the image data or omitting some information from the display. For example, with echocardiographic data only a fraction of the broad dynamic range of the echo transducer can be accommodated by common video displays. Most commercial echocardiographic systems thus allow the user to adjust the compression of the data before display. Some common forms of data compression are shown in Figure 6–7. One should always keep in mind that the computer may be processing more information than can be seen on the display.

Image Enhancement

One major application of digital image processing is enhancement of images. Enhancement operations may be performed to improve the appearance of the image or to make quantitation easier or more accurate. Examples of such enhancement would be accentuating an important feature (e.g., the endocardial border) or removing some undesirable feature of the image such as noise.

Point Operations

Among the most common forms of image enhancement are gray level histogram modification techniques. These operations are also called *point operations* because the operators (calculations) have no spatial dependences. In other words, the output (processed) pixel gray level value depends only on the input (original) image pixel value at the same image location or "point." Point operators are, in general, easy to implement, and most modern image processing systems support point operations as part of their basic operation at or near video rates (that is, the calculations can be performed at the rate of 30 frames per second). Point operators are most efficiently implemented in either hardware or software, through the use of a *lookup table*. A lookup table is simply a list of gray levels used to map the input (original) pixel values to the output (processed) pixel values. The length of the list is equal to the number of possible input (original) gray levels. At each place or address on the list, the desired output or processed value for that particular input pixel is placed. To determine the output for a particular input, the input value is used to "look up" the corresponding element of the list. As shown in Figure 6–8, if the third element of the list has a value of 18, then whenever an input pixel has a value of 3, the output pixel will be assigned a value of 18. The advantage of using

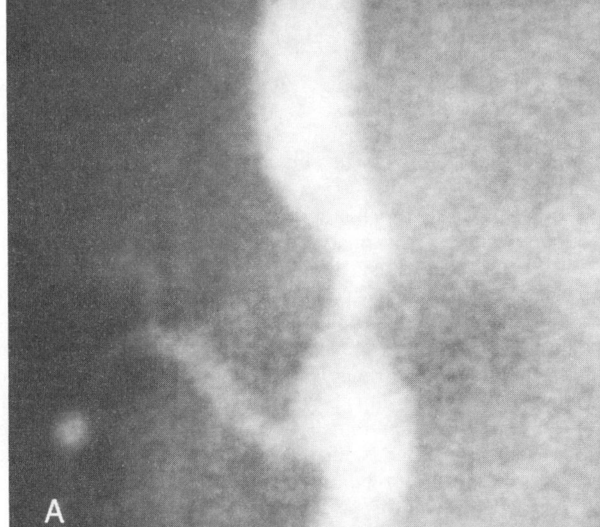

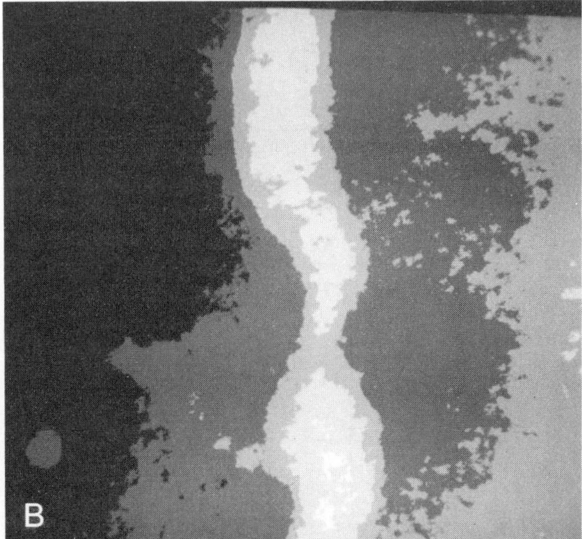

Figure 6–6. Effect of variable gray scale quantization on digital image appearance. *A*, Magnified image of a coronary arteriogram digitized using a large number of gray levels. *B*, The same image data, digitized using a smaller number of gray levels. The image quantized with fewer gray levels shows so-called false contours in which artifactual edges are produced because of inadequate gray level sampling.

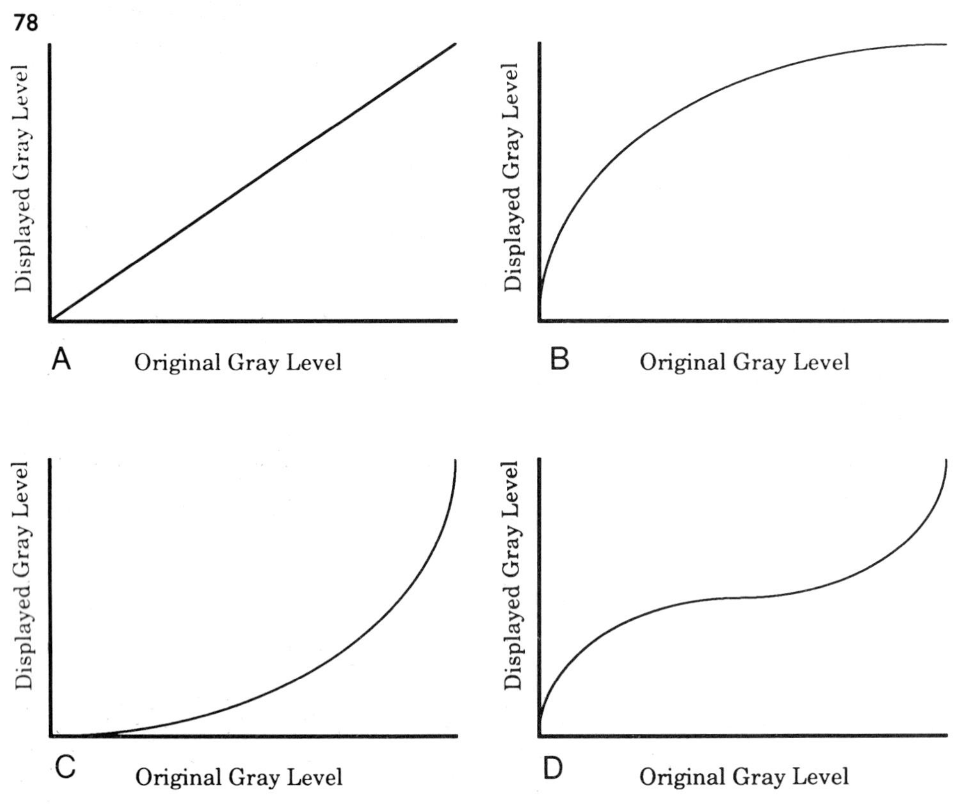

Figure 6–7. Four functions commonly used for gray scale compression in digital imaging. Each graph shows the displayed gray level plotted against the original gray level; notice that the original gray level range is wider than the displayed gray level range, necessitating compression. *A*, The data are compressed in a linear fashion. *B*, The function compresses higher gray levels more than middle gray levels. *C*, The function compresses lower gray levels more than higher ones. *D*, Middle level gray levels are compressed most.

lookup tables is that there are usually many fewer elements in the lookup table than there are pixels in the image. In the previous example, it might have been difficult to compute an output value of 18 for the input value of 3, but once this has been computed, it need not be done again, even if there are many pixels in the input image with a value of 3. The input and output lookup table do not necessarily have the same ranges of values. An important example of this is related to the pseudocolor display found in some medical imaging systems.[C6, G4] In this sort of display, the input values are image intensities, but the output values are color hues or intensities instead of gray levels. The pseudocolor lookup table thus converts a gray scale image to a color image. The human eye is much more sensitive to variations in color than it is to small changes in gray scale.[G5] Thus, by assigning color values that change quickly in the gray level range of interest, the pseudocolor display can amplify small differences in gray scale of the original image.

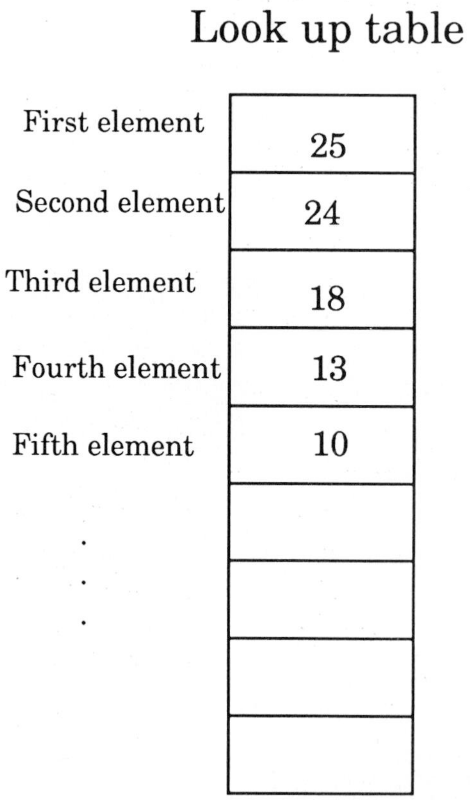

Look up table

First element	25
Second element	24
Third element	18
Fourth element	13
Fifth element	10
.	
.	
.	

Figure 6–8. The structure of a lookup table. The value of each pixel is used as an address to "look up" a value in the table. This value is then used as the output value for the pixel.

Lookup tables can be used to implement many different point operations, as shown in Figure 6–9. One special operation, histogram equalization, deserves special attention because of its important properties. Histogram equalization attempts to produce an image with a uniform gray level distribution or histogram. The *gray level histogram* is simply the number of occurrences of each particular gray level in an image (this is also the *probability density function* for gray levels in the image). In an image with a uniform histogram, all gray levels occur with the same frequency, which has the effect of spreading out the gray scale and increasing image contrast. If the image does not occupy the complete range of available gray levels, histogram equalization can be a powerful image enhancement technique, as shown in Figure 6–10.

In contrast to the histogram equalization techniques, which depend only on the image gray level values, another common point operation adjusts the image "window" and "level." This operation is found in virtually all MRI and CT scanners. Implemented as interactive processes, the window and level operations allow the user to isolate part of the gray scale and expand this part to fill the full range of display gray levels available. The range of input gray level values mapped to the entire range of the display is the *window*. The center of the window is the *level*. Increasing the window size or "width" decreases contrast but displays a wider range of gray levels from the input image. Window and level displays are most common when the available range of gray scales is high and exceeds the display capability of a standard monitor. The window can then be adjusted so that only a desired portion of the entire range of gray levels is

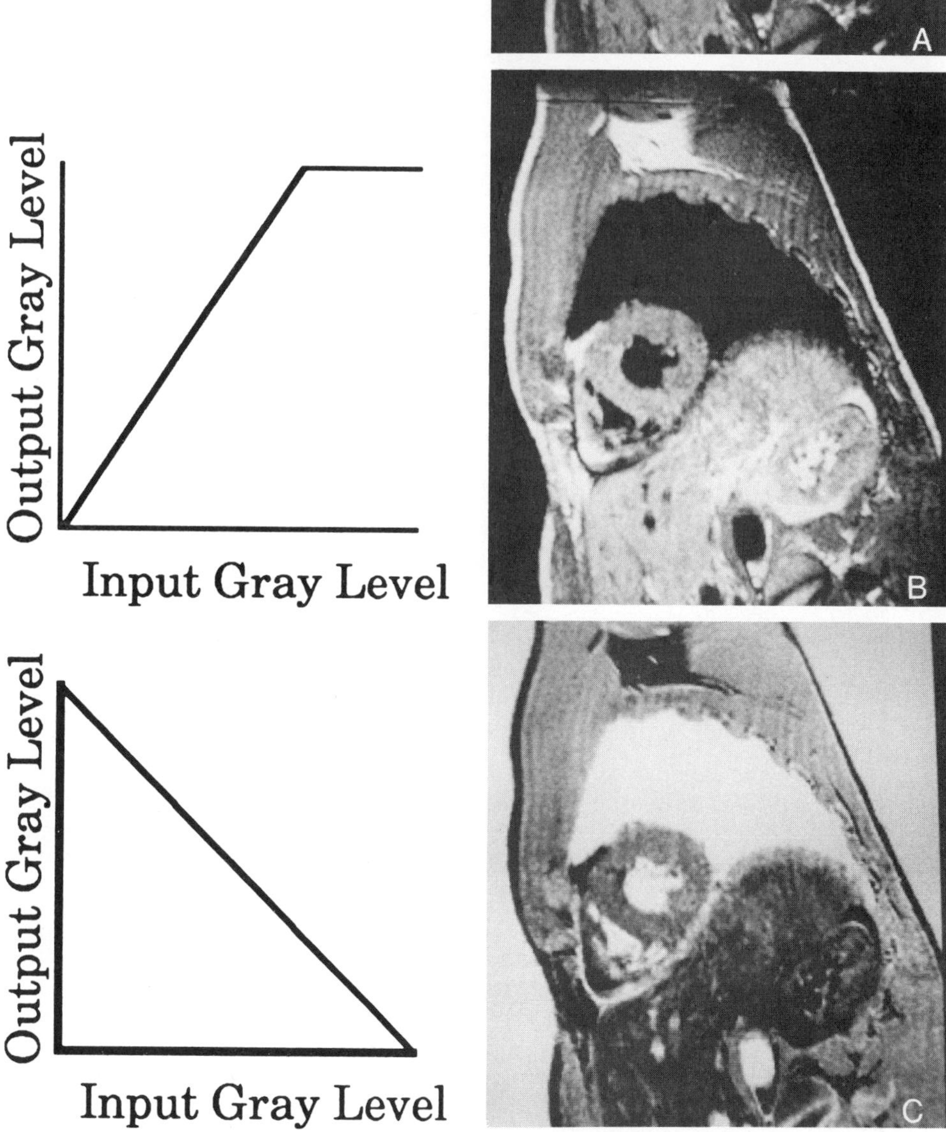

Figure 6–9. Effect of two lookup tables on magnetic resonance images. *A*, The original image. *B* and *C*, The lookup tables and resulting images for white stretching and gray level inversion, respectively.

displayed. A CT image at different window and level settings is shown in Figure 6–11.

Geometric Operations

Rotating, magnifying, and translating images are all examples of *geometric transformations*. Geometric transformations can all be considered special cases of a polynomial or "rubber sheet" warping.[C7] The basic idea is to map the input image into the output image as described by the warping function. In this context, "warping" refers to changing some geometric characteristic of the image. Correcting an angiographic image for pincushion distortion is an example of corrective warping. Problems arise in polynomial warping because the locations of pixels in a digital image must have discrete integral coordinates. A pixel in the input image may be mapped to a location between integral locations in the output image, two pixels may map to the same location, or the output pixels may have "holes" because no pixels were mapped there.

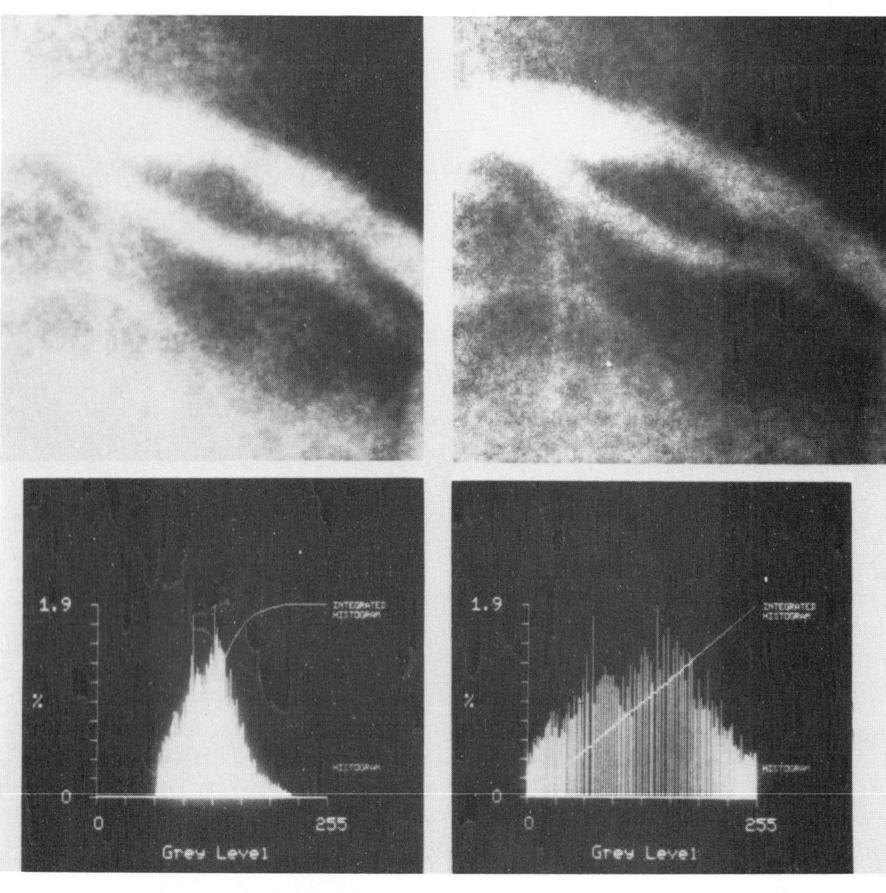

Figure 6–10. Illustration of the effect of histogram equalization. At the top are shown two images of a coronary arteriogram. The image at the left is the original digitized image; its gray level histogram (display of the frequency of occurrence of all gray levels in the image) is shown below. On the right, the alteration of image quality is shown after histogram equalization, a process that spreads the gray levels in the image over the entire available display range. Notice the improved contrast in the image. (From Collins, S. M., and Skorton, D. J. (eds.): Cardiac Imaging and Image Processing. McGraw-Hill Book Company, New York, 1986, p. 128, with permission.)

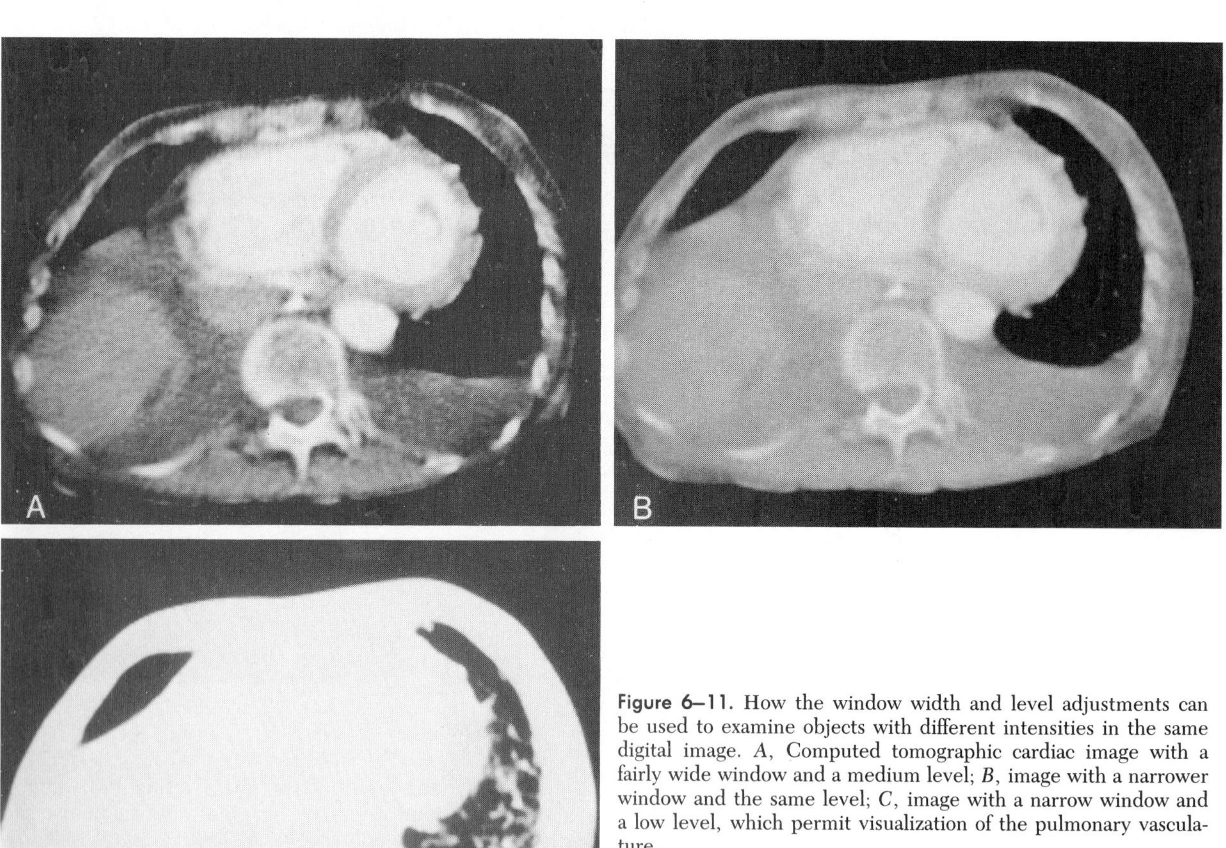

Figure 6–11. How the window width and level adjustments can be used to examine objects with different intensities in the same digital image. *A*, Computed tomographic cardiac image with a fairly wide window and a medium level; *B*, image with a narrower window and the same level; *C*, image with a narrow window and a low level, which permit visualization of the pulmonary vasculature.

Two methods exist for mapping the input image pixel to the output image pixel. The first method starts by calculating the output location for a particular input pixel. If the output location falls between the integral positions in the output image, the pixel is divided up between the nearest neighbors. The input pixel need not be equally divided among the neighboring output pixels. Instead, the closer output locations receive a proportionally larger share of the input pixel. This method is usually termed the "forward mapping" method.[C7]

In the second method, known as the "reverse mapping" method,[C7] calculations are made in the opposite direction. Starting at an integral output location, the location of the input pixel is calculated. When this location falls between pixels in the input image, the pixel value is interpolated from the four nearest neighbors in the input image. This method ensures that each pixel in the output image is assigned a value. However, sometimes an input pixel location may fall entirely outside the input image location, and thus no data will be available to map into the output image. The usual procedure is to set the output image value to zero when this occurs.

In both methods, pixel values must be interpolated because of the discrete nature of the image matrix. The two most popular interpolation schemes are *nearest-neighbor* interpolation and *bilinear* interpolation. The nearest-neighbor method is a simple technique in which the pixel is interpolated by using the value of the closest pixel in the image matrix. This method, although fast and simple, can produce images that appear "blocky." The more complicated method of bilinear interpolation fits a complex surface (a hyperbolic paraboloid) to the four pixels surrounding the nonintegral location. Once the coefficients describing this surface are known, any point between those four neighbors may be found. Bilinear interpolation produces images that have no abrupt intensity transitions and thus do not appear blocky. It is, however, a computationally intensive task because a surface must be fit to each set of four neighboring pixels.

Geometric operations in general can be computationally very intensive. Some cases may be implemented in standard image processing hardware to reduce the burden on the image processing system, but more complex operations usually require dedicated hardware for this process.

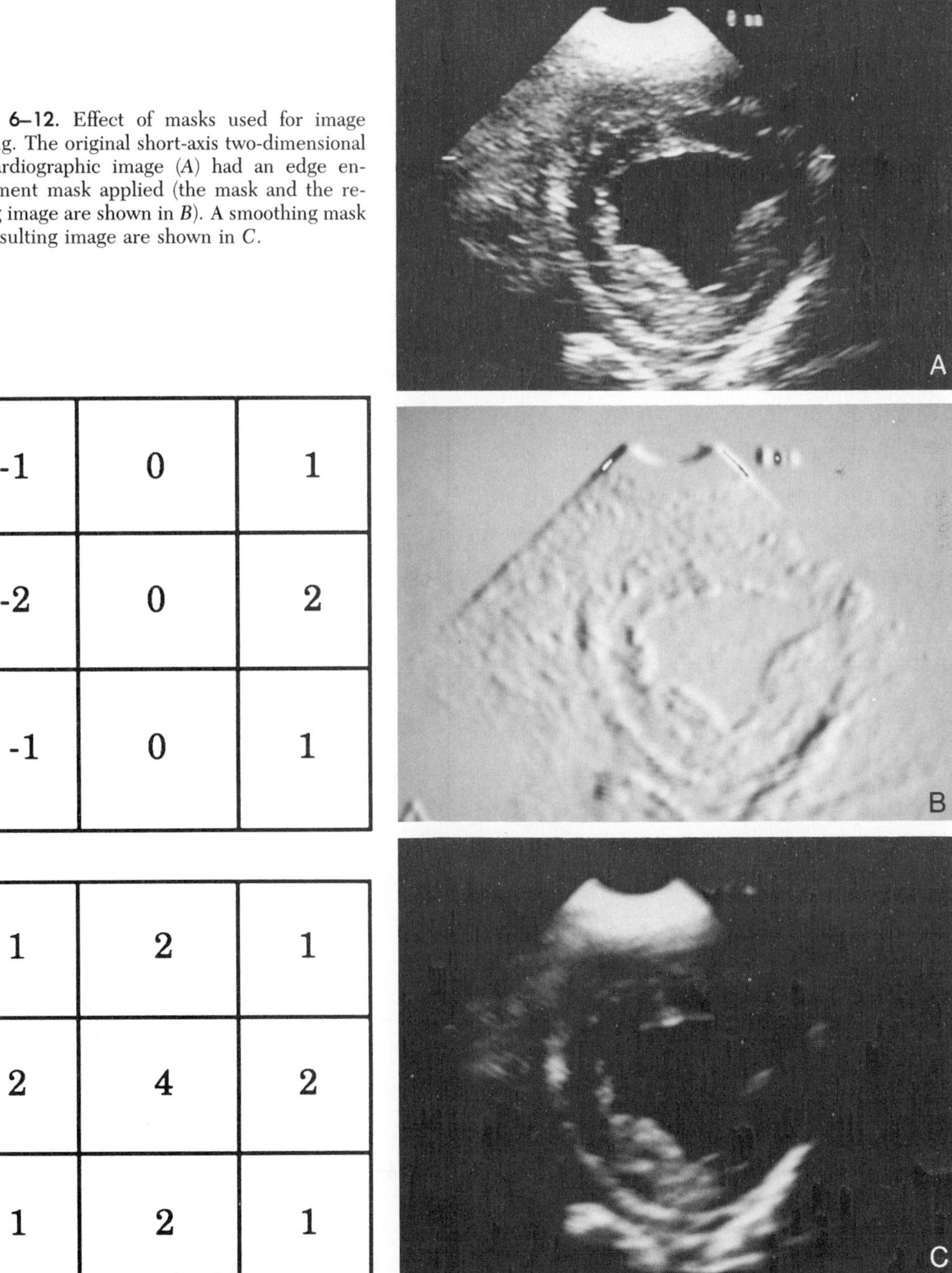

Figure 6–12. Effect of masks used for image filtering. The original short-axis two-dimensional echocardiographic image (*A*) had an edge enhancement mask applied (the mask and the resulting image are shown in *B*). A smoothing mask and resulting image are shown in *C*.

Filtering Operations

Some of the most powerful image enhancement techniques are often grouped together in the general category of *filtering* operations. Filtering operations are image enhancement techniques that either accentuate or de-emphasize some feature of the image. Originally, image filtering received more attention than other forms of image enhancement, so there is a large body of literature on the subject.[P1] We will introduce a few of the basic concepts illustrated with some examples and refer the interested reader to more in-depth reviews.[C8, G4, J2, P2, R6]

For our purposes, filtering can be thought of as having two major functions: to remove noise from the image or to enhance edges. Most filtering operations can be described in two ways, in the spatial domain and in the frequency domain. As will be shown, there is a direct mathematical relationship between these two domains that allows filters to be transformed from one domain to the other. Because of this direct mathematical relationship, filtering operators can be expressed in either the spatial or the frequency domain. Most filters, however, are more easily expressed in one domain or the other.

Spatial domain filters are described by an operation that is performed on a group of pixels called the "neighborhood." For example, a filter that removes noise from images might be an averaging operator. In this case the spatial operator replaces each pixel value with the average value of that pixel and its neighbors. The more neighbors that are included, the more averaging, or smoothing, is performed. If the image noise is random, it will be reduced by averaging. The image data, which are not random, will not be removed by averaging. Spatial operations of this type are usually easy to implement and are often done through *mask operators*, which define a neighborhood size and a weighting function for each pixel in the neighborhood. The pixel in the center of the mask is replaced by the sum of all the pixel values, each multiplied by the respective weight of the mask. Figure 6–12 shows examples of some common mask operators and their effects on an image. As can be seen, mask operators can produce widely varying results depending on their size and the particular weighting scheme employed.

Before describing the frequency domain operators, it is appropriate to describe exactly what is meant by the frequency domain. The direct relationship between the spatial domain and the frequency domain is known as the *Fourier transform*. The basis for the Fourier transform is that all images may be represented by a unique set of sinusoidal functions that vary in both frequency and phase (Fig. 6–13). The Fourier transform changes the representation of an image from spatial locations of gray scales to frequency amplitudes and phases. The Fourier transform is invertible (reversible), no information is lost in the transform, and if the process is reversed, the original data may be recovered. The motivation for using the frequency domain is that some operations are much easier to define in terms of frequencies and phases. High frequencies in images correspond to areas of rapidly changing gray levels (such as edges). Images with many edges contain more high frequencies than images without a large complement of edges.

Frequency domain filters usually fall into one of three classes: high pass, low pass, or bandpass. *High-pass* filters allow only relatively high frequencies to pass through, *low-pass* filters allow only relatively high frequencies to pass through, and *bandpass* filters allows some bandwidth (range) of frequencies to pass through (Fig. 6–14). Frequency domain filters are most easily applied after the image has been transformed into the frequency domain. The filtering may then be accomplished by multiplying each of the frequency components by the filter functions and then transforming the image back into the spatial domain.

The choice between a spatial and a frequency domain filter is usually based on implementation. Some filters, such as the averaging filter in the example above, are easily represented in the spatial domain, whereas others, such as a high-pass filter, are more easily represented in the frequency domain.

Segmentation

Medical image processing problems often contain a step that involves isolating a particular object or region of interest within an image. This process, known as *segmentation*, is sometimes the goal in itself, but more often it is a preprocessing step before further measurements of the object region can be made.[R7, S6] For example, the left ventricular cavity area in an echocardiographic image must be separated or segmented from the remainder of the image before the area can be measured. Segmentation procedures can be divided into five categories: (1) thresholding techniques, (2) region-growing techniques, (3) region-partitioning techniques, (4) split-and-merge techniques, and (5) border detection.

The simplest method of segmenting an image is through the use of *gray level thresholds*.[B4] In this method, all pixels with values falling above a particular gray level (the threshold) are said to belong to one region; those whose values fall below the threshold belong to the other region. The difficulty in this method is that of finding the proper threshold. For images that have

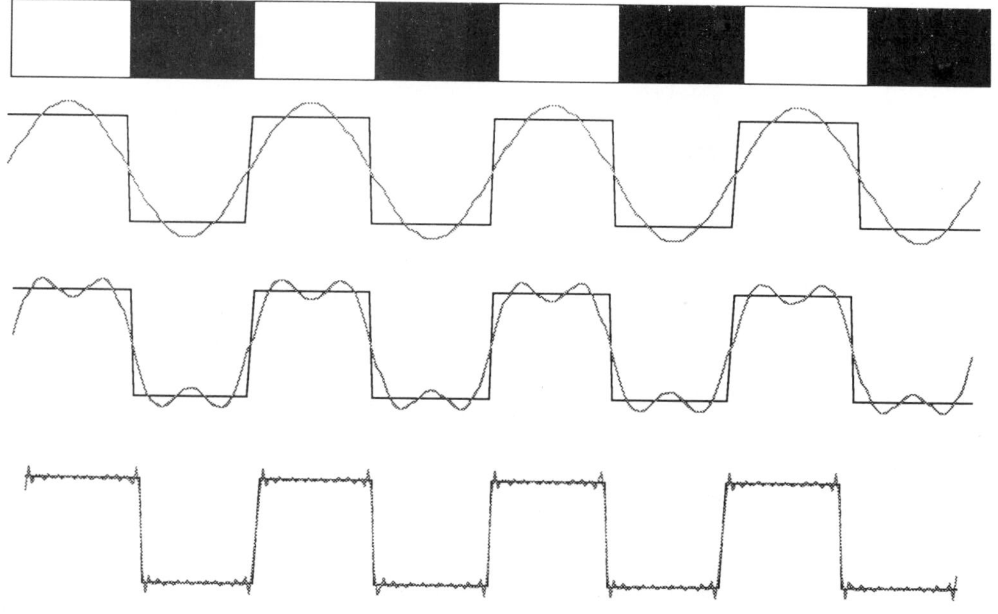

Figure 6–13. Illustration of the concept of Fourier transformation. The upper panel shows a digital "image" consisting of alternating black and white pixels. The second panel shows the representation of this image as alternating high and low values. Superimposed on the values (square waves) is a single sine wave that may be used to approximate roughly this pattern of image intensities. The bottom two panels show increasingly accurate representation of the square-wave pattern by the addition of multiple sinusoids of varying phase and amplitude to represent the data more accurately.

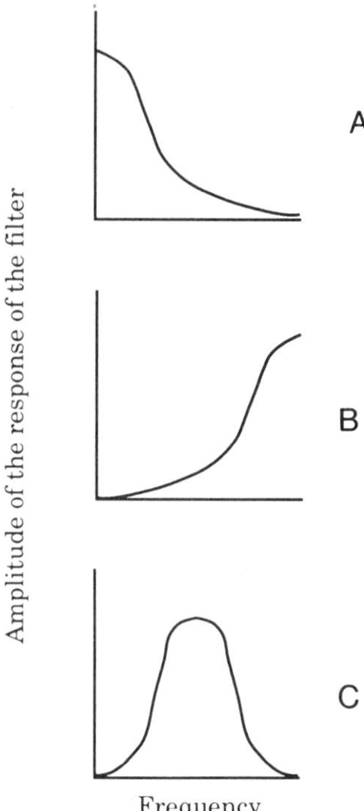

Figure 6–14. Effect of various frequency domain filters. Each graph shows how much each of the frequency components in the image is attenuated by the filter. *A*, Low-pass filter; lower frequencies are allowed to pass at relatively high amplitude while higher frequencies are reduced to a great extent. *B*, High-pass filter; higher frequencies are permitted to pass at a high amplitude while lower-frequency components of the signal are removed. *C*, Bandpass filter; both lowest and highest frequencies are filtered and middle-level frequencies are allowed to pass.

bimodal histograms, the "valley" or local minimum of the histogram can be used as the threshold value,[B4] as shown in Figure 6–15. Alternatively, the distributions expected from the image can be fit to the histograms to determine the proper threshold.[C9] Simple thresholding techniques are not useful in all cases. For example, using a gray level threshold to identify an object placed on a slowly varying background (which could be caused by camera shading) will fail because the threshold remains constant but the background and object intensities do not. A possible solution in this case is to perform the analysis adaptively on a regional basis, using a separate threshold for each region, to compensate for the slowly varying background. A related technique is to use a multidimensional threshold. In this method, thresholds are picked for several image features. With color images one could pick a separate threshold for each color.

For many kinds of segmentation, thresholding techniques prove inadequate. A second type of segmentation technique is known as *region growing*. Region-growing techniques start with a "seed" location. The seed is a pixel or group of pixels known to be within the region, as indicated by an observer or perhaps determined automatically. From this seed the region is "grown" by adding neighboring pixels that fit some criterion (e.g., their gray level is similar). The procedure stops when no neighboring pixels can be added to the region. An advanced form of this method starts with many seed locations and grows as many regions as needed until each pixel in the image belongs to a region.[Z1]

Region-partitioning techniques approach the segmentation problem in a related manner. These techniques start with the entire image as a region. The region is then divided or partitioned into smaller subregions, and the characteristics of the subregions are calculated and examined. If these characteristics meet a homogeneity requirement, the region is not partitioned further. If the homogeneity requirement is not met, the subregions are further partitioned until the sub-subregions meet the requirement. When no regions can be partitioned further, the procedure stops. By combining region-growing and region-partitioning techniques a class of powerful *split-and-merge* techniques can be defined. Split-and-merge techniques first split the entire image into subregions. For each subregion the neighboring subregions are examined to see if they are similar. Similar neighboring subregions are merged to form larger regions, and dissimilar subregions are split to form smaller subregions. When no more subregions can be split or merged, the procedure stops (Fig. 6–16).

A completely different approach to segmentation is not to identify regions but instead to find the boundaries between the regions. *Border detection* has been extensively studied in many applications of medical imaging[A3, F1, L3] with varying degrees of success. Traditionally, border detection consists of two steps. First, all pixels in the image or region of interest are evaluated for their potential to be points on the boundary. Second, the list of these candidate points is reduced by using the information contained in the first step. An example would be to find the spatial gradient (change in gray level) across each point in the image and then select border points as those points with a gradient greater than some threshold value. There are many ways to implement both steps in border detection. A particularly interesting approach to the second procedure (that of selecting the boundaries) involves the use of graph-searching techniques to implement a minimum-cost search. The problem is restated so that a "cost" is assigned to each pixel such that the higher the probability that the particular pixel is a part of the border, the lower is the assigned cost. Paths through the image may be found by connecting locations. Each path has an overall cost that is defined as the sum of the costs of all the locations along the path. The goal is to find the minimum-cost path. An exhaustive search of all paths through the image would always find this optimum path, but the large number of possible paths available precludes such a search in all but the simplest cases. Fortunately, intelligent heuristic search algorithms or dynamic programming techniques may be used to produce globally optimal borders with a reasonable amount of computation.

Future Directions of Quantitative Image Processing

The disciplines of image processing, computer graphics, signal processing, and artificial intelligence have all existed for more than 20 years, and each has made contributions to quantitation in medical imaging. In the past several years the traditional distinction between these disciplines has become blurred as techniques from the various disciplines have been combined to solve specific problems. An interesting illustration of this is the

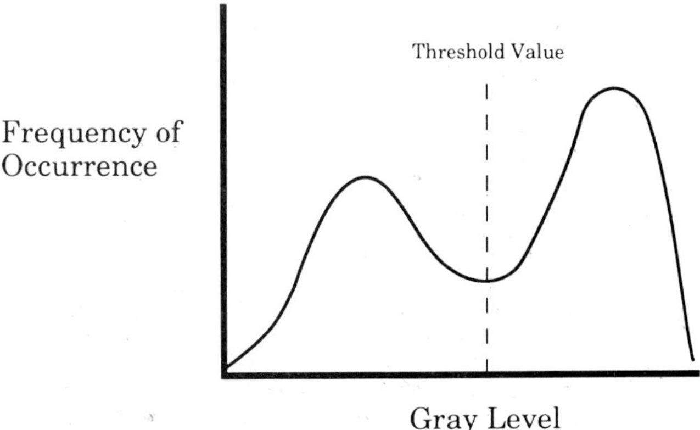

Figure 6–15. Concept of simple gray level thresholding. The gray level histogram displays the frequency of occurrence of all gray levels in an image. In the example shown, the histogram is bimodal; that is, two distinct populations of gray levels are present. The image may be divided into segments of high and low gray level by choosing a threshold level at the local minimum ("valley") of the histogram (vertical line).

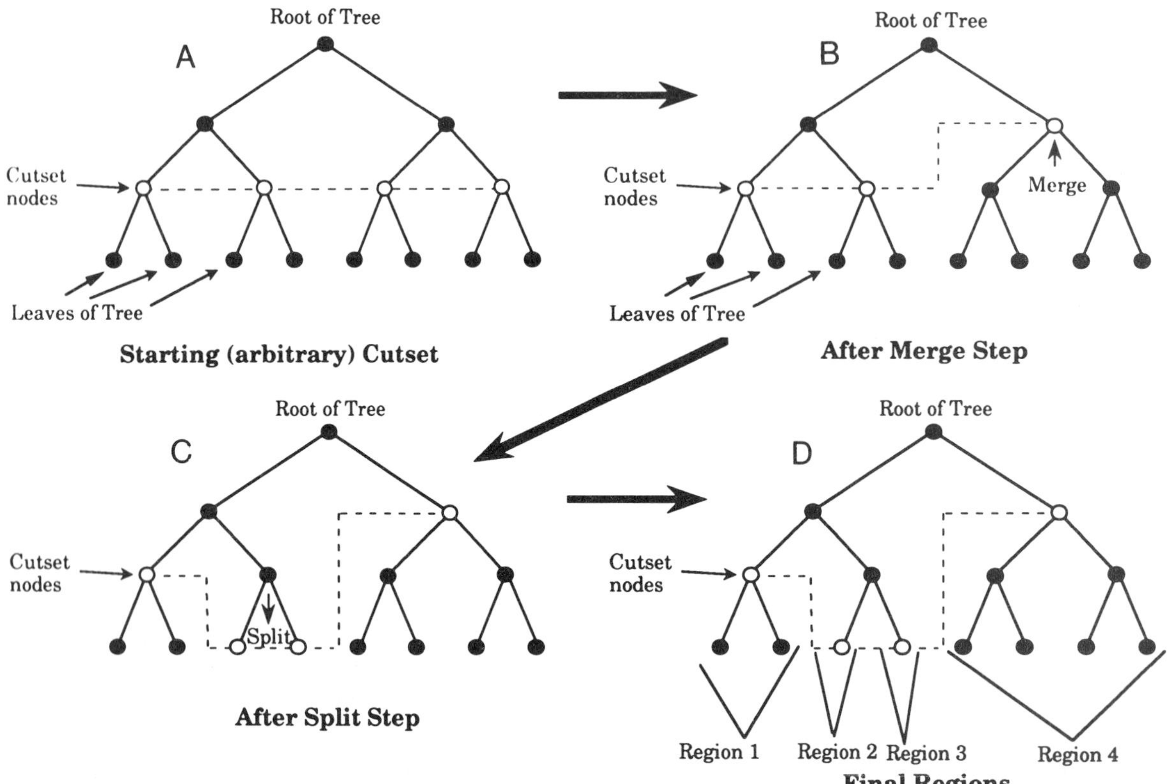

Figure 6–16. A split-and-merge procedure as applied to a binary tree. (Binary trees and the two-dimensional extension, the quad tree, can be used to organize the image data.) *A*, The tree is segmented into four regions along the dashed lines. *B*, The result of a merge operation resulting in three regions. *C*, The resulting four regions after a split operation. *D*, The final region.

dual representation of information as either the image data or a higher-level description. An example of such duality is the information contained in the geometry of the left ventricle, which can be represented as either a set of echocardiographic images or a three-dimensional mathematical model such as a prolate ellipsoid. Techniques from each of the disciplines can be used to provide methods for transforming the image data into a description and vice versa. Specifically, computer graphic techniques transform the description into the image data, image and signal processing techniques enhance or modify the data, and pattern recognition/image processing/artificial intelligence techniques transform image data and objects into descriptions (Fig. 6–17). In addition, image processing techniques can modify image data so that descriptions can be generated more easily. An example of the combination of these disciplines may be found in quantitative coronary angiography. A typical processing sequence involves some sort of preprocessing, such as with a smoothing filter (an image processing technique) followed by an edge operator (another image processing technique). A graph-searching technique (from the artificial intelligence discipline) is then applied to generate the borders of the coronary artery. These borders form the quantitative description of the part of the image data in which the researcher is interested. If multiple views of the coronary artery are obtained, the descriptions can be used to generate a three-dimensional model (from computer graphics) so that complex lesions may be easily visualized. As awareness of these various disciplines and their interrelationships increases, more researchers will combine techniques from the various disciplines to solve specific problems.

Not only will separate techniques be combined to solve the

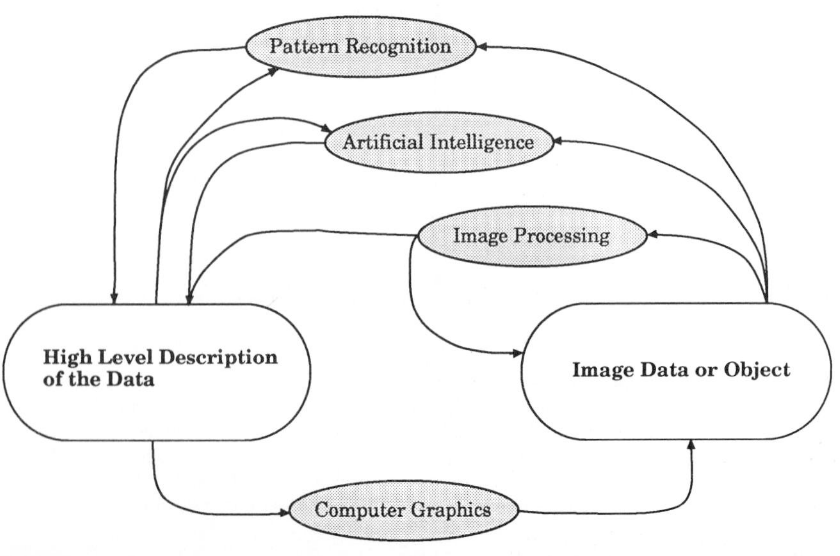

Figure 6–17. The concept of transformation of data using the various image quantitation techniques available.

intricate problems in cardiac imaging but also the disciplines will evolve and provide better individual tools to help solve these problems. An example is the development of three-dimensional analysis techniques. Much of three-dimensional analysis is a natural extension of two-dimensional image analysis. The three-dimensional techniques have, however, been limited by the computational abilities and display methods currently available. An example of an extension from two- to three-dimensional image processing is surface detection, which is related to the two-dimensional edge detection problem.[M4] Because most cardiac analysis problems are inherently three-dimensional (or four-dimensional, if time is included), many of the two-dimensional techniques will be replaced by higher-dimensional extensions.

The capabilities of modern digital computers are being increasingly applied to cardiovascular image data for the purposes of image enhancement, extraction of features of interest, derivation of quantitative data more objectively than is possible with visual interpretation, and extraction of information not easily extractable by simple visual means. The recent advances in rapid CT scanning, color Doppler flow imaging, and nuclear magnetic resonance scanning have been possible because of the application of digital computer techniques for rapid image reconstruction and analysis. The ubiquitous presence of computers in modern imaging departments as well as the need for quantitation will increase the prevalence of computer image processing techniques, and of image quantitation in general, in modern cardiac imaging practice.

Acknowledgments

The authors acknowledge Johathan Elion, M.D., Edward Geiser, M.D., Christopher Wilbricht, M.S.E.E., Thomas Scholz, M.D., and Michael Noel, M.S.E.E., for thoughtful review of the chapter and Rita Griffin and Carolyn Frisbie for expert preparation of the manuscript.

References

A

1. Ariet, M., Geiser, E. A., Lupkiewicz, S. M., et al.: Evaluation of a three-dimensional reconstruction to compute left ventricular volume and mass. Am. J. Cardiol. 54:415, 1984.
2. Axel, L., Herman, G. T., Udupa, J. K., et al.: Three-dimensional display of nuclear magnetic resonance (NMR) cardiovascular images. J. Comput. Assist. Tomogr. 7:172, 1983.
3. Ashkar, G. P., and Modestino, J. W.: The contour extraction problem with biomedical application. Comput. Graph. Image Process. 7:331, 1978.

B

1. Buda, A. J., and Delp, E. J. (eds.): Digital cardiac imaging. Martinus Nijhoff, Boston, 1985.
2. Brown, B. G., Bolson, E., Frimer, M., and Dodge, H. T.: Quantitative coronary arteriography. Estimation of dimensions, hemodynamic resistance, and atheroma mass of coronary artery lesions using the arteriogram and digital computation. Circulation 55:329, 1977.
3. Braunwald, E.: Assessment of cardiac function. *In* Braunwald, E. (ed.): Heart Disease, 3rd ed. W. B. Saunders Co., Philadelphia, 1988, p. 449.
4. Ballard, D. H., and Brown, C. M.: Computer vision. Prentice-Hall, Englewood Cliffs, NJ, 1982, p. 152.

C

1. Collins, S. M., and Skorton, D. J. (eds.): Cardiac Imaging and Image Processing. McGraw-Hill Book Company, New York, 1986.
2. Cook, R. D.: Concepts and Applications of Finite Element Analysis, 2nd ed. John Wiley & Sons, New York, 1981.
3. Collins, S. M., Chandran, K. B., and Skorton, D. J.: Three-dimensional cardiac imaging. Echocardiography 5:311, 1988.
4. Castleman, K. R.: Digital Image Processing. Prentice-Hall, Englewood Cliffs, NJ, 1979, p. 383.
5. Castleman, K. R.: Digital Image Processing. Prentice-Hall, Englewood Cliffs, NJ, 1979, p. 39.
6. Collins, S. M., and Skorton, D. J. (eds.): Cardiac Imaging and Image Processing. McGraw-Hill Book Company, New York, 1986, p. 128.
7. Castleman, K. R.: Digital Image Processing. Prentice-Hall, Englewood Cliffs, NJ, 1979, p. 110.
8. Castleman, K. R.: Digital Image Processing. Prentice-Hall, Englewood Cliffs, NJ, 1979, p. 190.
9. Chow, C. K., and Kaneko, T.: Automatic boundary detection of the left ventricle from cineangiograms. Comput. Biomed. Res. 5(4):388, 1972.

F

1. Fleagle, S. R., Johnson, M. R., Wilbricht, C. J., et al.: Automated analysis of coronary arterial morphology in cineangiograms: Geometric and physiologic validation in humans. IEEE Trans. Med. Imag. 8:387, 1989.
2. Feiring, A. J., Rumberger, J. A., Reiter, S. J., et al.: Determination of left ventricular mass in dogs with rapid-acquisition cardiac computed tomographic scanning. Circulation 72:1355, 1985.
3. Florentine, M. S., Grosskreutz, C. L., Chang, W., et al.: Measurement of left ventricular mass in vivo using gated nuclear magnetic resonance imaging. J. Am. Coll. Cardiol. 8:107, 1986.

G

1. Garcia, E. V., Ezquerra, N. F., DePuey, E. G., et al.: An artificial intelligence approach to interpreting thallium-201 3-dimensional myocardial distributions (Abstract). J. Nucl. Med. 27:1005, 1986.
2. Garcia, E. V., DePuey, E. G., and DePasquale, E. E.: Quantitative planar and tomographic thallium-201 myocardial perfusion imaging. Cardiovasc. Intervent. Radiol. 10:374, 1987.
3. Geiser, E. A., Lupkiewicz, S. M., Christie, L. G., et al.: A framework for three-dimensional time-varying reconstruction of the human left ventricle: Sources of error and estimation of their magnitude. Comput. Biomed. Res. 13:225, 1980.
4. Gonzalez, R. C., and Wintz, P.: Digital Image Processing. Addison-Wesley Publishing Co. Reading, MA, 1987.
5. Gonzalez, R. C., and Wintz, P.: Digital Image Processing. Addison-Wesley Publishing Co. Reading, MA, 1987, p. 13.

H

1. Hemmy, D. C., David, D. J., and Herman, G. T.: Three-dimensional reconstruction of craniofacial deformity using computed tomography. Neurosurgery 13:534, 1983.
2. Herman, G. T., and Liu, H. K.: Display of three-dimensional information in computed tomography. J. Comput. Assist. Tomogr. 1:155, 1977.

I

1. Iwasaki, T., Sinak, L. J., Hoffman, E. A., et al.: Mass of left ventricular myocardium estimated with dynamic spatial reconstructor. Am. J. Physiol. 246:H138, 1984.

J

1. Jain, A. K.: Fundamentals of Digital Image Processing. Prentice-Hall, Englewood Cliffs, NJ, 1989, p. 80.
2. Jain, A. K.: Fundamentals of Digital Image Processing. Prentice-Hall, Englewood Cliffs, NJ, 1989, p. 267.

K

1. Kirkeeide, R. L., Gould, K. L., and Parsel, L.: Assessment of coronary stenoses by myocardial perfusion imaging during pharmacologic coronary vasodilation. VII. Validation of coronary flow reserve as a single integrated functional measure of stenosis severity reflecting all its geometric dimensions. J. Am. Coll. Cardiol. 7:103, 1986.

L

1. Linker, D. T., Moritz, W. E., and Pearlman, A. S.: A new three-dimensional echocardiographic method of right ventricular volume measurements: In vitro validation. J. Am. Coll. Cardiol. 8:101, 1986.
2. Laschinger, J. C., Vannier, M. W., Gronemeyer, S., et al.: Noninvasive three-dimensional reconstruction of the heart and great vessels by ECG-gated magnetic resonance imaging: A new diagnostic modality. Ann. Thorac. Surg. 45:505, 1988.
3. Lester, J. M., Williams, H. A., Weintraub, B. A., and Brenner, J. F.: Two graph searching techniques for boundary finding in white blood cell images. Comput. Biol. Med. 8:293, 1978.

M

1. McPherson, D. D., Skorton, D. J., Kodiyalam, S., et al.: Finite element analysis of myocardial diastolic function using three-dimensional echocardiographic reconstructions: Application of a new method for study of acute ischemia in dogs. Circ. Res. 60:674, 1987.
2. Moritz, W. E., Pearlman, A. S., McCabe, D. H., et al.: An ultrasonic technique for imaging the ventricle in three dimensions and calculating its volume. IEEE Trans. Biomed. Eng. 30:482, 1983.
3. Miller, T. R., Starren, J. B., and Grothe, R. A., Jr.: Three-dimensional display of positron emission tomography of the heart. J. Nucl. Med. 29:530, 1988.
4. Monga, O., and Deriche, R.: 3D edge detection using recursive filtering: Application to scanner images. Proceedings of the IEEE Computer Society, Washington, D.C. Vision and Pattern Recognition 1989, p. 28.

QUANTITATIVE METHODS IN CARDIAC IMAGING: AN INTRODUCTION TO DIGITAL IMAGE PROCESSING

P

1. Pratt, W. K.: Digital Image Processing. John Wiley & Sons, New York, 1978, p. 279.
2. Pratt, W. K.: Digital Image Processing. John Wiley & Sons, New York, 1978, p. 291.

R

1. Ranky, P. G.: Computer Integrated Manufacturing. Prentice-Hall International, Englewood Cliffs, NJ, 1986.
2. Ray, G., Chandran, K. B., Nikravesh, P. E., et al.: Estimation of the local elastic modulus of the normal and infarcted left ventricle from angiographic data. *In* Saha, S. (ed.): Proceedings of the 4th New England Bioengineering Conference. 1976, 173–176.
3. Ritman, E. L., Kinsey, J. H., Robb, R. A., et al.: Three-dimensional imaging of heart, lungs, and circulation. Science 210:273, 1980.
4. Rosenfeld, A., and Kak, A.: Digital Picture Processing. Academic Press, New York, 1976, p. 65.
5. Rosenfeld, A., and Kak, A.: Digital Picture Processing. Academic Press, New York, 1976, p. 75.
6. Rosenfeld, A., and Kak, A.: Digital Picture Processing. Academic Press, New York, 1976, p. 179.
7. Rosenfeld, A., and Kak, A.: Digital Picture Processing. Academic Press, New York, 1976, p. 256.

S

1. Schiller, N. B., Acquatella, H., Ports, T. A., et al.: Left ventricular volume from paired biplane two-dimensional echocardiography. Circulation 60:547, 1979.
2. Skorton, D. J., and Geiser, E. A.: Three-dimensional echocardiography: A geometric reconstruction. *In* Talano, J. V., and Gardin, J. M. (eds.): Textbook of Two-Dimensional Echocardiography. Grune & Stratton, New York, 1983, p. 357.
3. Sawada, H., Fujii, J., Kato, K., et al.: Three-dimensional reconstruction of the left ventricle from multiple cross-sectional echocardiograms. Value for measuring left ventricular volume. Br. Heart J. 50:438, 1983.
4. Sasayama, S., Nonogi, H., Fujita, M., et al.: Three-dimensional analysis of regional myocardial function in response to nitroglycerin in patients with coronary artery disease. J. Am. Coll. Cardiol. 3:1187, 1984.
5. Stark, H. (ed): Applications of Optical Fourier Transforms. Academic Press, New York, 1982.
6. Sklansky, J.: Image segmentation and feature extraction. IEEE Trans. Syst. Man Cybern. SMC-8:237, 1978.

T

1. Tessier, P., and Hemmy, D.: Three-dimensional imaging in medicine. A critique by surgeons. Scand. J. Plast. Reconstr. Surg. 20:3, 1986.

Z

1. Zucker, S.: Region growing: Childhood and adolescence. Comput. Graph. Image Process. 5(3):382, 1976.

Chapter 7

Perceptual Aspects of Cardiac Imaging

■ *E. A. FRANKEN, JR., M.D.* ■ *KEVIN S. BERBAUM, Ph.D.*

MOTION AND PERCEPTION 88
IMAGE SEARCH 88
SOME COMMON PERCEPTUAL ERRORS AND STRATEGIES TO HELP 89
JUDGMENT CALLS AND THEIR EVALUATION 90
PERCEPTION AND EVALUATION OF HEART DISEASE 90
SUMMARY 91

Image evaluation has three dimensions: image quality, perception and recognition, and interpretation of findings. The body of knowledge on factors of importance in producing an image is substantial. Similarly, there is a considerable literature on the interpretation of recognized findings, as evidenced by the multitude of publications on descriptive aspects of images. The perceptual process, wherein the information implicit in the image is transferred explicitly to the level of consciousness and decision making, is less well studied. Understanding the perceptual process requires study of human brain activity with its acknowledged imperfections. Most errors of image interpretation occur in this category and are the subject of this chapter.

Clinical medicine, being an imperfect science, is universally associated with error. In almost all clinically ambiguous situations, disagreement among competent practitioners occurs in up to one-third of cases.[S1, S2] Such disagreements or errors may be noted among physicians (interobserver error) or within the same individual (intraobserver error). Examples abound in therapeutics, in which yesterday's dogma frequently mutates into today's nonsense. Similarly, what previously seemed an ejection murmur is on repeat examination unequivocally mitral regurgitation. Factors producing such errors can generally be attributed to three mechanisms: (1) biologic variability of the patient, (2) fallibility of the physician/observer, and (3) variation in clinical judgment. In this chapter we attempt to raise awareness of error in diagnostic imaging, to familiarize the reader with sources of error, and to illustrate methods of evaluating error. Finally, we discuss some strategies for minimizing such error.

Errors in diagnostic imaging are in the same general range as elsewhere in clinical medicine, occurring in about one-third of ambiguous situations. Although our understanding of the nature of such errors has improved considerably, the error rate in diagnostic radiology has not changed substantially in the past 50 years. The inherent tendency of the radiologist (and presumably other physicians) is to under-read a positive case (false-negative interpretation); this type of error accounts for about 80 percent of all mistakes.[S1, S2] The highest rate of disagreement will be found between individual observers, especially those with different backgrounds. But in a blind situation the competent physician observer will disagree with his or her own interpretations in up to one-fifth of cases.

Sources of imaging error are multiple. Obviously, more mistakes are made with a poor image than with an image in which pathologic anatomy is well demonstrated. Environmental factors can be of considerable importance. For instance, minimizing indirect light sources around an image produces substantial improvement in contrast resolution,[B1] but it is the infrequent physician who maximizes viewing conditions. Similarly, fine detail is best detected at short viewing distances (sometimes with a magnifying glass), whereas minimal contrast differences may be best noted several meters away (or with a minifying lens), but physicians seldom utilize such devices.

Image factors involved in perception are fairly well understood and can be measured. High spatial resolution is needed for fine structures (e.g., Kerley's B lines). Contrast sensitivity allows recognition of minimal differences in density (e.g., mitral insufficiency on a left ventriculogram). Motion can be of critical importance in recognizing abnormality but has been minimally investigated in clinical angiocardiography.

Knowledge and experience would seem of importance in minimizing clinical errors in imaging, but in fact lack of knowledge accounts for less than 5 percent of imaging mistakes in clinical practice.[S1] Mind-set (clinical prejudice) and physiologic state (boredom, distraction) are important.[K1, S2] We must recognize that the human perceptual system is imperfect, and error occurs because of inherent limitations in human perception and cognition in addition to any limitations in an individual's visual acuity.[C1]

The most frequent cause of error in imaging is the faulty judgment call. In the imperfect world of clinical medicine, distinction from black and white goes through several shades of gray, and individuals vary in judging the point(s) of separation. By "judgment call" we mean that, although an image feature may always be observed (repeatedly fixated), different observers (or the same observer at different times) may require different levels of apparent abnormality to report a finding as positive. Such judgment calls may be quite deliberate—for instance, spending a great deal of time and worry about whether to raise a question of cardiac calcification after noting an ambiguous shadow on the chest radiograph. Conversely, based on individual previous training, knowledge, and experience (or on characteristics of the image), such a decision may be automatic, never rising to the level of conscious deliberation. For example, the pulmonary artery segment of the normal adolescent female is known to be prominent on the chest radiograph. When an observer views the radiograph of such a person, the possibility that the patient has valvar pulmonic stenosis may never be logically deliberated—based on previous experience, the observer tends to discard this observation automatically in the appropriate situation.

Distraction may prevent potential observations. For example, mitral valve calcification would be much more likely to be detected with routine fluoroscopy of the heart than on a cineangiocardiogram of the pulmonary arterial tree. With the latter, the observer's perceptual attention is directed to opacified vessels rather than other cardiac structures.

The perceptual processes of the observer can be considered as a hardware and software system.[J1] By hardware we mean aspects of registration of the visual stimulus. Software refers to aspects of how the observer knows and perceives the stimulus. Hardware factors include visual acuity, edge gradients of abnormalities, retinal illusions such as Mach bands, and the "limited channel" carrying retinal information to the brain. The hardware aspect of the system has been extensively studied and can be reasonably well quantified. The software processing of images is more obscure and complex.[K2] Study of the software, the science of psychophysics, is introduced below.

Most of the studies involving interaction of the physician observer and the diagnostic image have utilized radiologists as the experimental subjects. Our own investigations involving orthopedic physicians[B2] indicate that the same mechanisms apply but are of varying importance when the experienced clinician evaluates images.

There are two general theories regarding perception of images: top-down theory (concept- and context-driven processing) and bottom-up theory (data-driven processing).[K3] Bottom-up theory suggests that the image data occurring at the senses are sufficient to form a coherent percept. Experience with radiologists indicates that top-down theory better explains image perception in this group; that is, there is rapid processing of the entire image to give a global percept. This step is followed by entry of new data into the percept, as the observer uses foveal vision to fill in specific details. The influence of context on perception also helps explain the role of experience. Radiologists are no better than laypersons in discovering simple objects in a camouflaged environment.[R1] But for a medical image, which the physician is trained to recognize, vast differences between radiologist and layperson are demonstrated. An example to illustrate this phenomenon is the typical chest radiograph in tetralogy of Fallot, in which overall heart size is usually normal. The experienced observer immediately recognizes the unusual cardiac contour on a top-down basis (according to a learned set of features) and, after confirming the observation with further gathering of information from the radiograph, gives a confident diagnosis. Unless one were trained to recognize a boot-shaped heart (couer en sabot) as indicative of abnormality, the diagnosis would not be made.

For an observer to recognize a radiographic abnormality, the abnormality must be recognizable and separable from normal structures. To use the terminology of signal detection theory, the signal (abnormality) must be distinguishable from noise (background), or, put another way, there must be a favorable signal-to-noise ratio. A simple example: gross cardiomegaly is easily recognized on an otherwise normal chest radiograph, as the heart is surrounded by aerated lung. In a neonate with primary failure to inflate the lungs, heart size cannot be evaluated because heart and lungs are of the same radiographic density. In the latter situation the signal is indistinguishable from the noise. An everyday example is radiographic recognition of increased pulmonary vascularity in those with left-to-right shunts. Unless pulmonary flow is greater than twice normal, the signal is not sufficient to be deciphered from the noise of normal pulmonary vascularity.

MOTION AND PERCEPTION

Motion can be a powerfully informative diagnostic cue because motion perception influences the perception of structure (form). There are several clear demonstrations of this in the literature on perception. For example, a number of researchers[A1, B3–B5, J2, L1–L2] have demonstrated that apparent motion can readily be seen when random-dot cinematograms are used as stimuli (see Fig. 67–1). Each half of the cinematogram pair in Figure 7–1 consists of a matrix of black and white squares or dots (e.g., 100 × 100 or 250 × 250). The sequence of black and white squares is random. When either half is viewed alone, the observer may see only a random pattern of squares but no global form. A central region depicting a square or some other form is identical in the two halves but displaced horizontally in one half relative to the other. Since global form cues become available only when the information from the two cinematograms is integrated, perception of motion must logically precede the perception of form. The practical implication of this research is that elements of structure may be perceived on the basis of motion even where the static images alternated to generate the motion do not themselves contain the information. In images with diagnostic structures of low contrast, the structures may not be apparent in the static views but readily apparent in a cinematographic presentation.

A number of authors[B6, B7, G1, J3] have suggested that dynamic visual information is of greatest importance to the survival of organism and therefore the most important determinant of perception. The most informative type of visual motion is believed to be relative motion (motion of an element relative to another element) rather than absolute motion (motion of an element relative to the observer). A number of experiments indicate that relative motion is perceptually antecedent to object quality. Thus, it would hardly be surprising if relative motion in diagnostic images (e.g., motion of the heart wall) were informative with regard to structural qualities (e.g., dyskinesia).

Another way in which the motion of image elements may contribute to diagnosis derives from the influence of visual motion on visual search and attention. Selection of locations for subsequent fixation depends on data acquired in the peripheral visual field. Initial analysis of peripherally imaged objects may depend partly on their motion. The peripheral mechanisms may act as an early warning system of attention for control of eye movement, signaling the locations of unusual, unexpected, or informative events.[B8] Temporal modulation in diagnostic images demonstrates changes or differences between images that may be particularly informative and directs attention toward these aspects.

In dynamic environments in which many stimulus elements are in motion, visual search may depend on specific characteristics of target motion that are known in advance.[B9] When the stimulus elements move in various directions, prior knowledge of the target's direction of motion reduces search time. Because direction of motion is available at relatively early stages of visual processing, attention and eye movements can be voluntarily attuned to this information. Thus, even particular types of motion may be influential in guiding visual search.

IMAGE SEARCH

Visual search is one of the most common of human activities: searching for the appropriate entry in a phone book, attempting to locate a friend in a crowd, or looking for a book in the library. Evidence[B10, H1, N1–N2] suggests that when human beings search the visual field for some target item (a word, object, form), two types of cognitive activities are involved: an identification of the part of the visual field centered on the fovea, and a decision as to where in the peripheral visual field to move the eyes next. These two activities taken together are often referred to as "focal attention." Identification seems to require the allotment of analyzing mechanisms to a limited area of the visual field. Attentional mechanisms cannot work on the whole visual field simultaneously. Because of this spatial limitation in identification, any task that requires analysis of a large part of the visual field will require successive fixation(s). A visual search task will be serial in nature, with steps in the search corresponding to eye movements. The decision as to where to move the eyes next is of great importance for the effectiveness of visual search. In order to explain visual search it has proved necessary to postulate an intermediate stage of analysis between the mechanisms responsible for stimulus registration and the sequential analysis of parts of the visual field referred to as focal attention. This is a preattentive stage of analysis in which the visual field is segmented into (meaningful) parts. According to this postulate, guidance of eye movement and focal attention depends on more complex aspects of the stimulus than are available in a receptor-level description. Other elements such as perceptual tasks given to the observer modify subsequent search.

Not surprisingly, search patterns of physicians looking at images are similar to those observed in picture search experiments. For example, there is a strong tendency to fixate on edges and exclude broad uniform areas.[K4, L3, L4] There appears to be preattentive segmentation that provides the perceptual system with information needed to carry out search. Tachistoscopic presen-

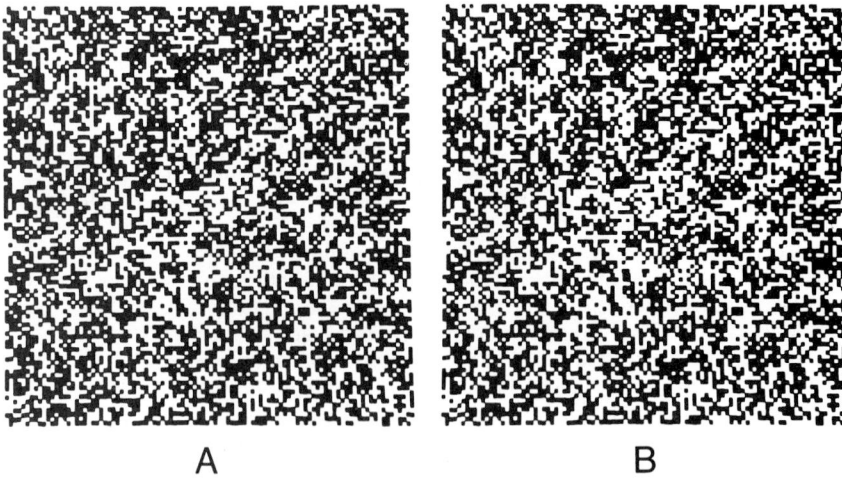

Figure 7–1. A pair of random-dot cinematograms of the type introduced by Julesz,[J2] which, when viewed alone, permit no global form to be seen. When *A* and *B* are spatially superimposed and temporally alternated, a form is seen in the center (in this case a small square) because elements in the region of the square have been displaced horizontally in *A* relative to *B*. This effect demonstrates that the perception of a structure may depend on prior perception of its motion.

tation of radiographs at an interval sufficiently brief to preclude eye movements (0.2 second) allows 70 percent true-positives.[K5] Thus visual search begins with a global response that establishes context and organizes subsequent fixations. Another finding common to both picture and radiograph search experiments is that the eye movement pattern is influenced by the search tasks. Kundel and Wright[K4] showed that there is a difference between the eye movement pattern of subjects searching for nodules and the pattern exhibited in a more general search task. There is a definite evolution of the pattern of fixation from that of an untrained observer to that of a mature radiologist.[K6] Such learned behavior is not that of a step-by-step organized search. The untrained observer tends to exhibit a localized central pattern of search, whereas the radiologist tends to exhibit a circumferential pattern that requires fewer fixations to sample the radiograph with the fovea.

Visual search and eye movement pattern are not synonymous. Attention can be directed sequentially at different organ systems without eye movements. Eye movements are ordinarily superimposed on the attentional pattern but do not follow it exactly.[K4] Search may be quantitated by time. In one experiment, experienced readers concluded their visual search while they were still making a significant number of true-positive observations and while the true-positive rate was higher than the false-positive rate.[C2] Less experienced readers, on the other hand, observed the radiographs for half again as long and found only 70 percent of the lesions found by more experienced observers. In fact, with neophyte observers, late observations may be more likely to be false-positive.

Visual search experiments in which eye movements were recorded during inspection of radiographs have been used to determine particular sources of diagnostic error.[K7, N3] Scanning or sampling errors occur when locations containing lesions are not covered by foveal fixation. Recognition error occurs when the viewer spends no more time attending to an unreported target than is spent attending to a normal anatomic structure. Decision-making error occurs when more time is spent attending to an unreported target than to a normal anatomic structure (three to four fixations in a cluster). Here elements of the abnormality have been segmented, allowing increased interrogation with eye movements and fixation. However, the observer's criterion for apparent abnormality has not been met, so the lesion is not reported. A study of lung nodule detection showed that 10 percent of the misses were due to sampling, 30 percent to recognition, and 60 percent to decision making.[K5]

Another area of research relevant to visual search of images concerns the effect of clinical history on detection of lesions. Numerous studies involving radiologists indicate a powerful positive effect of clinical information. Subsequent experiments with orthopedic surgeons[B2] suggest that nonradiologists exhibit an even greater dependence on localizing clues to direct visual search. A true increase in perceptual ability can be demonstrated here.

SOME COMMON PERCEPTUAL ERRORS AND STRATEGIES TO HELP

Some situations are particularly apt to induce perceptual error. If there are two or more separate abnormalities on a radiograph (e.g., cardiomegaly and bronchogenic carcinoma), observers are considerably less likely to recognize both abnormalities than to find either of the abnormalities singly. This error, known as satisfaction of search, is presumed to occur because the observer ceases the search after discovering one abnormality. Undetermined perceptual mechanisms in the brain may subtract certain aspects of an image before the percept reaches the level of consciousness. Common foreign bodies such as safety pins are often overlooked for this reason, particularly if the perceptual task is related to a different end. The observer frequently fails to recognize visible abnormalities outside the area of clinical interest. Examples include abnormalities of the shoulder and abdomen unrecognized on chest radiographs of patients with heart disease.

Certain strategies minimize perceptual error in evaluating images. Appropriate image quality and optimal viewing conditions are obvious aids. Experience in viewing images is of utmost importance. A neophyte in cardiology may easily learn the differential diagnosis and imaging characteristics of the various types of atrial septal defects. However, the same individual would not usually recognize a subtle puff of contrast material entering the right atrium after pulmonary arteriography until he or she had had experience with many similar studies. Minimum length of time to gain the experience necessary for a good "eye" for cardiac studies has, to our knowledge, not been determined. Experience with plain-film radiography[H2] suggests that a year or less may be quite sufficient.

Having a directed perceptual task is of enormous benefit to a radiologist.[B11] This translates clinically into having an appropriate clinical history so that the radiographic search is directed toward abnormality. This direction may raise the number of false-positive observations slightly, but there is a much greater increase in true-positive findings. This effect may be even more powerful for clinical physicians.[B2]

Although one might anticipate that increasing the time spent in viewing an image would improve perception, this is not the case for chest radiographs.[C2] Most observations are made after a short period of viewing. Although more positive diagnoses occur with prolonged viewing, many of these late diagnoses are false-positive. In some circumstances the rate of false-positive observation increases more rapidly than the rate of true-positive observation, so prolonged viewing of images actually decreases observer accuracy.

Use of comparison radiographs facilitates interpretation by radiologists. We would assume the same for nonphysician observers. Although the mechanisms of this facilitation are not entirely understood, it is recognized that length of previous training changes the way in which observers utilize comparison films.[B11]

Effects of motion are considerable in the interpretation of clinical images such as cineangiograms, but the mechanisms and nature of these effects are not well determined. Additional experimental work is necessary to evaluate the beneficial (or detrimental) effects of motion on perception in cardiovascular diagnosis.

Interpretation of images by more than one observer increases the accuracy of diagnosis. Probabilities of true- and false-positives are summated for the observers,[H2] so the numbers of both true- and false-positives increase. This approach is of value in studies where sensitivity is of greatest importance. There are various mechanisms for arriving at a consensus diagnosis when multiple observers are involved. Such evaluations are necessary for formal investigations but are seldom needed in clinical practice.

JUDGMENT CALLS AND THEIR EVALUATION

A traditional method for evaluating a diagnostic system involves analysis of a two-by-two decision matrix in which truth is crossed with the system's judgment of positive (abnormal) and negative (normal). With this characterization, difficulties arise in comparing two diagnostic systems. One system may yield not only more true-positives (disease-present judged abnormal) but also more false-positives (disease-absent judged abnormal). The fundamental probem with the decision matrix description of diagnostic systems is that it assumes a fixed threshold of abnormality for deciding whether to judge a case normal or abnormal. In fact, when human beings are the decision makers, they can change the criterion of abnormality on which the normal-abnormal decision is based, depending on costs of various kinds of errors. In other words, increases or decreases in true-positive rate can be traded for increases or decreases in false-positive rate. Thus, a family of decision matrices is needed to describe the performance of a diagnostic system. This is exactly what receiver operating characteristic (ROC) analysis involves. Probability of true-positive is plotted as a function of probability of false-positive. Each diagnostic system is forced to adopt several different criteria of abnormality in judging whether cases are abnormal or normal. Each criterion leads to a decision matrix and thus becomes an ROC point relating probability of true-positive to probability of false-positive response. The ROC curve can be extrapolated from the points to describe the potential behavior of the system—every potential true-positive rate is related to its corresponding false-positive rate. True-positive rates of different systems can thus be compared at the same false positive rate. Figure 7–2 illustrates these points. Figure 7–2*A* presents three ROC points for one hypothetical diagnostic system (black) and three ROC points for another diagnostic system (white). In practice, each system would tend to operate at a single point; however, that point may be anywhere on the curve. If black operates at the highest point shown in Figure 7–2*A* and white operates at the lowest, there would be no adequate way to tell if the points for black and white lie on the same curve. To establish the underlying curve, both systems are forced to operate at several *criterion* levels. The chief benefit of this kind of analysis is that a difference in true-positive rates between systems can be attributed either to simple changes in willingness to call a case normal or abnormal, so-called response bias *(as in Fig. 7–2B)*, or to an actual difference in the systems' ability to discriminate normal and abnormal, their relative accuracies *(as in Fig. 7–2A)*. Note that for both Figure 7–2*A* and 7–2*B* the true-positive rate for black points is always higher than that for corresponding white points. In Figure 7–2*B*, however, differences in true-positive rates are completely compensated by differences in false-positive rates. In one case, the ROC points for two diagnostic systems lie along the same fitted curve with the points for one system being higher along the curve (see Fig. 7–2*B*). In the other case, the ROC points for the two diagnostic systems lie along different curves (see Fig. 7–2*A*). Rigorous curve-fitting methods for deriving separate parameters of ROC curves that describe detection accuracy and response

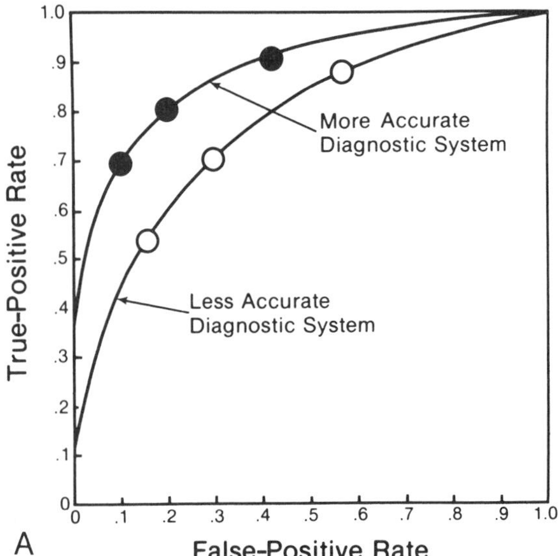

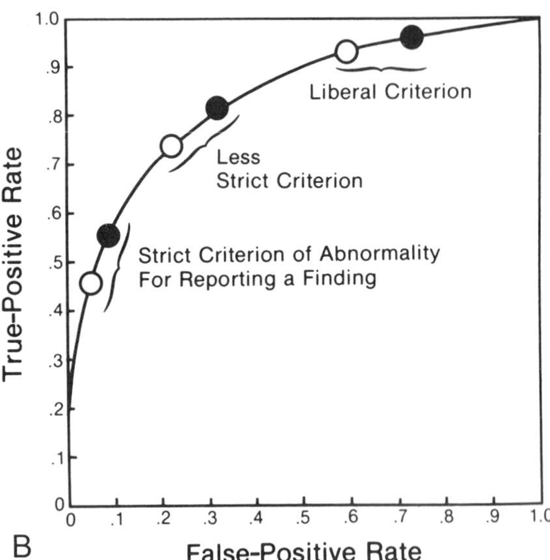

Figure 7–2. Receiver operating characteristic (ROC) points and curves for two hypothetical diagnostic systems (black and white) where black has either *(A)* greater accuracy or *(B)* simply a less stringent decision criterion of abnormality. Without relating true-positive rates to corresponding false-positive rates and forcing each system to operate at several criterion levels of apparent abnormality by which cases are called normal or abnormal, there would be no way to determine whether one system was more accurate than the other.

bias have been developed,[D1, D2, M1] and statistics may be used to analyze these parameters to generalize to case and observer populations.[B11, H3]

PERCEPTION AND EVALUATION OF HEART DISEASE

Disagreement and error in detecting heart disease have been known for years. In the early days of roentgenology many elaborate attempts were made to quantitate heart size on the chest radiograph, and both simple and complex measurement techniques were developed to separate the normal from the abnormal heart. It is now recognized that the chest radiograph cannot be utilized to recognize all patients with abnormal hearts; the sensitivity of the x-ray for this task is considerably less than 100 percent. Current studies[M2] indicate that the predictive value of the chest radiograph for cardiomegaly or normal-sized heart is about 70 percent, and there is wide observer variability in such an evaluation. Attempts to extend these judgments to determine enlargement of specific chambers are much less successful, with sensitivity values of 30 to 40 percent, depending on the chamber being evaluated.

Recognition of increased vascularity in left-to-right shunts on chest radiographs is limited to situations in which pulmonary flow is twice normal. Unless the increased flow is of this magnitude, the signal of engorged vascular structures cannot be recognized within the noise of the normal pulmonary vessels. In contrast, trained observers are quite accurate in diagnosis of congestive heart failure on plain film of the chest,[B12] with a correlation above 0.8 in estimating measured pulmonary capillary wedge pressure. Accuracy can be further increased by using consensus results from several observers. This is accomplished by assessing the degree of pulmonary blood flow redistribution and other specific signs of pulmonary venous hypertension.

Plain-film diagnosis of the type of congenital heart disease was attempted (with variable success) even before the development of palliative and curative surgery for such patients. The subject has been a popular one for books, as well as many descriptive reports. However, the sensitivity of diagnosis is suboptimal. There are marked differences in physicians' capabilities in this area, which range from very poor to fair in recognition of type and/or nature of disease present.[S3]

Although nuclear medicine studies are relied on for many clinical judgments in cardiology, studies of the performance of observers in such cases are limited in number. One group[T2] noted overall agreement in the interpretation of myocardial images using thallium in about 80 percent of cases. Acero and coworkers[C1] noted such inconsistency among observers of images utilizing ^{99m}Tc-labeled phosphates that the authors suggested "that uncorrected visual defects could play an important role in the reading of nuclear medicine images." Variation in interpretation can be reduced by reliance on quantitative data.[F3]

With the notable exception of coronary arteriography (see below), there have been few investigations of the reliability and reproducibility of diagnosis in angiocardiography. Motion effects are of obvious importance in evaluation of cine studies, but formal perceptual investigations of these effects have been minimal. Cinecardiography is best for situations in which minimal changes in contrast are necessary for diagnosis or in which motion of structures is important. An example is the puff of contrast entering the left atrium from the left ventricle with minimal mitral insufficiency. Conversely, serial standard films from a film changer are of greatest benefit in situations in which spatial resolution must be optimal, such as determining the thickness of the pulmonary valve. Overall agreement between cine and cut film is 84 percent,[B13] which indicates that the experience of observers and the nature of the abnormality are of considerably greater importance than the mechanism of image recording.

Interpretation of individual structures within the heart has about the same variation as interpretation of structures elsewhere in the body. Assessment of ventricular volumes by angiocardiography is inexact compared with the assessment in autopsy material.[R2] Although consistency of angiographic diagnoses of ventricular aneurysm is good,[D3] correlation with pathologic material is inconsistent. Variability in "softer" diagnoses is considerable—one observer's definite wall dyskinesia is another's normal finding.[Z1]

Studies of observer performance in coronary artery examinations are more numerous than in other aspects of cardiac imaging. A significant problem in such investigation is determining a "gold standard," that is, knowing the truth in assessing degree of coronary artery narrowing. Interpretation of pathologic material, even with injection of resin into arteries of a specimen, has variation in quantitation of up to 45 percent.[R3] Except in cases of severe stenosis, consensus panels evaluating angiograms are not reliable indicators of truth.[G2] And measured degree of arterial narrowing does not correlate well with actual perfusion through the vessel.[H4]

Except for one study[T1] that indicated high agreement among observers, investigations of observer agreement in assessing coronary artery narrowing have shown wide interpretive variation.[B14, D3, D4, F1, R3] Factors of particular importance in error included[B4] experience of the observer, disease of distal segments, poor opacification, inadequate technical quality, and more severe disease. Left circumflex and distal left anterior descending arteries are the most common locations for disagreements.[D3]

For imaging studies, variability of both intraobserver and interobserver nature is so high that it makes the recording method of minimal importance. For instance, one study[B14] compared 16-mm cinecardiography with 70-mm serial images—two systems with substantial differences in resolution and image contrast. The two techniques were similar in accuracy, but there were large interobserver differences in estimates of degree of narrowing.

Because of the recognized difficulties in using human observers for reproducible and reliable measurements of arterial stenosis, various machine-based techniques have been advocated.[L5, S4, S5, V1] In the authors' opinion, the common results with such techniques indicate that measurements of structures by machines can be much more consistent than measurements by human observers. However, the "validity" of such techniques—that is, whether they give consistent results regarding arterial stenosis that accurately reflect dynamics of flow in the coronary arteries—has yet to be demonstrated.

In contrast to the considerable disagreement rate in assessment of arterial stenosis, assessment of extent of collateral in circulation shows little variability.

There is minimal information on the accuracy of cardiac diagnosis with the newer imaging modalities. Fast CT has been evaluated for accuracy in several dimensions—ventricular volumes, left ventricular mass, ejection fractions, and patency of coronary artery grafts—and found to be comparable to or better than other clinical studies.[M3] Magnetic resonance imaging is emerging as a diagnostic tool in cardiac imaging, and the sensitivity and specificity of diagnosis of atrial septal defect are over 90 percent with this technique.[D5]

SUMMARY

In summary, errors of a perceptual and judgmental nature occur in evaluating cardiac images in the same fashion (and probably at the same rate) as in other imaging categories. Awareness of error allows a realistic approach to image interpretation and avoidance of some of the common pitfalls. Such avoidance is facilitated by familiarity with the clinical history of individual patients, utilizing previous examinations for comparison, using readings by multiple observers, maximizing physical circumstances for interpretation sessions, and, where appropriate, using motion to improve perception.

References

A

1. Anstis, S. M.: Phi movement as a subtraction process. Vision Res. 10:1411, 1970.

B

1. Baxter, B., Ravindra, H., and Normann, R. A.: Changes in lesion detectability caused by light adaptation in retinal photoreceptors. Invest. Radiol. 17:394, 1982.
2. Berbaum, K. S., El-Khoury, G. Y., and Franken, E. A., Jr.: Impact of clinical history on radiographic detection of fractures: A comparison of radiologists and orthopedists. AJR 153:1221, 1989.
3. Bell, H. H., and Lappin, J. S.: Sufficient conditions for discrimination of motion. Percept. Psychophys. 14:45, 1973.
4. Braddick, O.: The masking of apparent motion in random-dot patterns. Vision Res. 13:355, 1973.
5. Braddick, O.: A short-range process in apparent motion. Vision Res. 14:519, 1974.
6. Boynton, R. M., and Boss, D. E.: The effect of background luminance and contrast upon visual search performance. Illum. Eng. 66:173, 1971.
7. Boynton, R. M., Elworth, C., and Palmer, R. M.: Laboratory Studies Pertaining to Visual Air Reconnaissance. Wright Air Development Center, Technical Report 55–304, part 3, 1958.
8. Breitmeyer, B. G., and Ganz, L.: Implications of sustained and transient channels for theories of visual pattern masking, saccadic suppression, and information processing. Psychol. Rev. 83:1, 1976.
9. Berbaum, K. S., Chung, C. S., and Loke, W. H.: Improved localization of moving targets with prior knowledge of direction of target motion. Am. J. Psychol. 99:509, 1986.

10. Beck, J.: Similarity grouping and peripheral discriminability under uncertainty. Am. J. Psychol. 85:1, 1972.
11. Berbaum, K. S., Franken, E. A., Jr., Dorfman, D. D., and Barloon, T. J.: Influence of clinical history upon detection of nodules and other lesions. Radiology 23:48, 1988.
12. Baumstark, A., Swensson, R. G., Hessel, S. J., et al.: Evaluating the radiographic assessment of pulmonary venous hypertension in chronic heart disease. AJR 141:877, 1984.
13. Bjork, L.: Cineangiocardiography or full-size angiocardiography? Radiology 86:663, 1966.
14. Bjork, L., Spindola-Franco, H., Van Houten, F. X., et al.: Comparison of observer performance with 16 mm cinefluorography and 70 mm camera fluorography in coronary arteriography. Am. J. Cardiol. 36:474, 1975.

C

1. Cuaron, A., Acero, A. P., Cardenas, M., et al.: Interobserver variability in the interpretation of myocardial images with Tc-99m-labeled diphosphonate and pyrophosphate. J. Nucl. Med. 21:1, 1980.
2. Christiansen, E. E., Murry, R. C., Holland, K., et al.: The effect of search time on perception. Radiology 138:361, 1981.

D

1. Dorfman, D. D., and Alf, E.: Maximum likelihood estimation of parameters of signal-detection theory and determination of confidence intervals—rating method data. J. Math. Psychol. 6:487, 1969.
2. Dorfman, D. D., and Berbaum, K.: RSCORE-J: Pooled rating method data: A computer program for analyzing pooled ROC curves. Behav. Res. Methods Instrum. Comput. 18:452, 1986.
3. Detre, K. M., Wright, E., Murphy, M. L., and Takaro, T.: Observer agreement in evaluating coronary angiograms. Circulation 52:979, 1975.
4. DeRouen, T. A., Murray, J. A., and Owen, W.: Variability in the analysis of coronary arteriograms. Circulation 55(2):324, 1977.
5. Diethelm, L., Dery, R., Lipton, M. J., and Higgins, C. B.: Atrial-level shunts: Sensitivity and specificity of MR in diagnosis. Radiology 162:181, 1987.

F

1. Fisher, L. D., Judkins, M. P., Lespernce, J., et al.: Reproducibility of coronary arteriographic reading in the coronary artery surgery study (CASS). Catheterization Cardiovasc. Diagn. 8:565, 1982.
2. Froehlich, R. T., Falsetti, H. L., Doty, D. B., and Marcus, M. L.: Prospective study of surgery for left ventricular aneurysm. Am. J. Cardiol. 45(5):923, 1980.
3. Francisco, D. A., Collins, S. M., Go, R. T., et al.: Tomographic thallium-201 myocardial perfusion scintigrams after maximal coronary artery vasodilation with intravenous dipyridamole: Comparison of qualitative and quantitative approaches. Circulation 66(2):370, 1982.

G

1. Gibson, J. J.: The Perception of the Visual World. Houghton Mifflin, Boston, 1950.
2. Galbraith, J. E., Murphy, M. L., and de Soyza, N.: Coronary angiogram interpretation. JAMA 240:2053, 1978.

H

1. Haber, R. N., and Hershenson, M.: The Psychology of Visual Perception, 2nd ed. Holt, Rinehart and Winston, Chicago, 1980.
2. Hessel, S. J., Herman, P. G., and Swensson, R. G.: Improving performance by multiple interpretations of chest radiographs: Effectiveness and cost. Radiology 127:589, 1978.
3. Hanley, J. A.: Alternative approaches to receiver operating characteristic analysis. Radiology 168:568, 1988.
4. Harrison, D. G., White, C. W., Hiratzka, L. F., et al.: The value of lesion cross-sectional area determined by quantitative coronary angiography in assessing the physiologic significance of proximal left anterior descending coronary arterial stenoses. Circulation 69:1111, 1984.

J

1. Jaffe, C. C.: Medical imaging, vision, and visual psychophysics. Med. Radiogr. Photogr. 60:1, 1984.
2. Julesz, B.: Foundations of Cyclopean Perception. University of Chicago Press, Chicago, 1971.
3. Johannson, G.: Spatial temporal differentiation and integration in visual motor perception. Psychol. Rev. 35:379, 1976.

K

1. Kundel, H. L., and Hendee, W. R.: The perception of radiologic image information. Invest. Radiol. 20:874, 1985.
2. Kundel, H. L.: Images, image quality and observer performance. Radiology 132:265, 1979.
3. Kundel, H. L., and Nodine, C. F.: A visual concept shapes image perception. Radiology 146:363, 1983.
4. Kundel, H. L., and Wright, D. J.: The influence of prior knowledge on visual search strategies during the viewing of chest radiographs. Radiology 93:315, 1969.
5. Kundel, H. L., and Nodine, C. F.: Interpreting chest radiographs without visual search. Radiology 116:527, 1975.
6. Kundel, H. L., and LaFollette, P. S., Jr.: Visual search patterns and experience with radiological images. Radiology 103:523, 1972.
7. Kundel, H. L., Nodine, C. F., and Carmody, D.: Visual scanning, pattern recognition and decision making in pulmonary nodule detection. Invest. Radiol. 13:175, 1978.

L

1. Lappin, J. S., and Bell, H. H.: The detection of coherence in moving random-dot patterns. Vision Res. 16:161, 1976.
2. Lenel, J. C., and Berbaum, K. S.: Measurements of displacement and type of background in apparent motion with random-dot cinematograms. Am. J. Psychol. 97:563, 1984.
3. Lewellyn-Thomas, E., and Lansdowne, E. L.: Visual search patterns of radiologists in training. Radiology 81:288, 1963.
4. Lewellyn-Thomas, E.: Search behavior. Radiol. Clin. North Am. 7:403, 1969.
5. LeFree, M. T., Simon, S. B., Mancini, G. B. J., et al.: A comparison of 35 mm cine film and digital radiographic image recording: Implications for quantitative coronary arteriography: Film vs. digital coronary quantification. Invest. Radiol. 23:176, 1988.

M

1. Metz, C. E., Wang, P., and Kronman, H. B.: A new approach for testing the significance of differences between ROC curves measured from correlated data. *In* Deconick, F. (ed.): Information Processing in Medical Imaging. Martinus Nijhoff, Rotterdam, 1984, p. 432.
2. Murphy, M. L., Blue, L. R., Thenabadu, N., et al.: The reliability of the routine chest roentgenogram for determination of heart size based on specific ventricular chamber evaluation at postmortem. Invest. Radiol. 20:21, 1985.
3. Marcus, M. L., Rumberger, J. A., Start, C. A., et al.: Cardiac applications of ultrafast computed tomography. Am. J. Cardiac Imag. 2:116, 1988.

N

1. Neisser, U.: Decision-time without reaction-time: Experiments in visual scanning. Am. J. Psychol. 76:376, 1963.
2. Neisser, U.: Cognitive Psychology. Appleton-Century-Crofts, New York, 1967.
3. Nodine, C. F., and Kundel, H. L.: Using eye movements to study visual search and to improve tumor detection. Radiographics 7:1241, 1987.

R

1. Rackow, P. L., Spitzer, V. M., and Hendee, W. R.: Detection of low-contrast signals: a comparison of observers with and without radiology training. Invest. Radiol. 22:311, 1987.
2. Ringertz, H. G., Rodgers, B., Lipton, M. J., et al.: Assessment of human right ventricular cast volume by CT and angiocardiography. Invest. Radiol. 20:29, 1985.
3. Robbins, S. L., Rodriguez, F. L., Wragg, A. L., and Fish, S. J.: Problems in the quantitation of coronary arteriosclerosis. Am. J. Cardiol. 18:153, 1966.

S

1. Smith, M. C.: Error and Variation in Diagnostic Radiology. Springfield, IL, Charles C Thomas, 1967.
2. Spodick, D. H.: On experts and expertise: the effect of variability in observer performance. Am. J. Cardiol. 36:592, 1975.
3. Steinbach, W. R., and Richter, K.: Multiple classification and receiver operating characteristic (ROC) analysis. Med. Decision Making 7:234, 1987.
4. Simons, M. A., Bastian, B. V., Bray, B. E., and Dedrickson, D. R.: Comparison of observer and videodensitometric measurements of simulated coronary artery stenoses. Invest. Radiol. 22:562, 1987.
5. Sandor, T., and Swensson, R. G.: Evaluation of observer performance in detecting blood vessels on simulated angiographic images. Med. Phys. 5:380, 1978.

T

1. Trask, N., Califf, R. M., Conley, M. J., et al.: Accuracy and interobserver variability of coronary cineangiography: A comparison with postmortem evaluation. J. Am. Coll. Cardiol. 3:1145, 1984.
2. Trobaugh, G. B., Wackers, F. J. Th., Sokole, E. B., et al.: Thallium-201 myocardial imaging: An interinstitutional study of observer variability. J. Nucl. Med. 19:359, 1977.

V

1. Vas, R., Eigler, N., Miyazono, C., et al.: Digital quantification eliminates intraobserver and interobserver variability in the evaluation of coronary artery stenosis. Am. J. Cardiol. 56:718, 1985.

Z

1. Zir, L. M., Miller, S. W., Dinsmore, R. E., et al.: Interobserver variability in coronary angiography. Circulation 53:627, 1976.

Part II

Conventional Radiography

Chapter 8

Clinical Aspects of Chest Roentgenology

▪ *DIANA F. GUTHANER, M.D.* ▪ *JEROME F. BREEN, M.D.*

TECHNIQUES ... 93
INTERPRETATION ... 93
Pulmonary Vasculature ... 93
Cardiac Silhouette ... 98
ACQUIRED HEART DISEASE ... 103
Ischemic Heart Disease ... 103
Valvular Disease ... 104
Cardiomyopathy ... 105
Pericardial Disease ... 106
Cardiac Masses ... 106
Aortic Disease ... 107

Imaging of the heart has undergone dramatic advances with the development and refinement of new imaging modalities such as echocardiography, ultrafast computed tomography, magnetic resonance imaging, and radionuclide emission tomography. However, the plain chest roentgenogram remains the foundation of clinical cardiac imaging, having provided useful, readily available information for the clinical care of patients for nearly a century. A basic but thorough understanding of the anatomic and physiologic information provided by this "low-tech" but highly informative examination provides the key to interpreting the plain chest film.

TECHNIQUES

The standard upright posteroanterior and lateral projections of the chest are obtained with high kilovoltage (120–140 kVp) and high milliamperage (1000 mA) technique at maximum inspiration to permit short exposure times, which stop cardiac motion, and sufficient penetration to visualize retrocardiac structures and pleural reflections. Interstitial markings are accentuated on an expiratory film and mislead the interpreter. A tube-to-film distance of at least 6 feet minimizes distortion and magnification.

It is often necessary to obtain chest films of severely ill, bedridden patients using a portable apparatus, which necessitates a compromise between the desired and the allowable technical factors. Technicians should routinely record the technical factors (kVp and mA) as well as respirator settings to provide some degree of standardization and basis for serial comparisons. Typically, a distance of 40 inches is used, which will keep magnification and distortion of the anterior structures such as the heart within acceptable limits. The position of the patient (supine, semiupright, or upright) should be noted to facilitate appropriate interpretation of the pulmonary vasculature and the size of cardiac and central vascular structures.

The "standard" roentgenologic examination varies in different institutions. The traditional four-projection cardiac film series—posteroanterior (PA), lateral, left anterior oblique (LAO), and right anterior oblique (RAO)—with barium in the esophagus is rarely obtained and has been replaced with two views, PA and lateral, of the chest. Although fluoroscopy remains an inexpensive and simple tool for evaluating the dynamics of cardiac contraction, it, too, has been replaced by two-dimensional echocardiography with its improved accuracy. The ability to detect coronary artery calcification has renewed interest in high-definition image-intensified fluoroscopy as an inexpensive means of screening for asymptomatic coronary disease. However, the major use of cardiac fluoroscopy today is simply for guidance during catheterization and other instrumentation of the heart.[M1]

INTERPRETATION

Pulmonary Vasculature

Interpretation of the chest radiograph requires a systematic approach and comprehensive analysis of the entire film. In assessing cardiac disease, the most important and often the most difficult step in this analysis is the evaluation of the pulmonary vasculature, which will reflect the basic physiologic effects of a cardiac lesion and, therefore, provides important clues to the diagnosis. Roentgenographic abnormalities are primarily the result of an increase in pulmonary blood flow or an obstruction to flow somewhere in the pulmonary circuit.[M2, S1]

NORMAL PULMONARY FLOW. The pulmonary arteries and veins branch outward from each hilum in an orderly arborizing fashion with gradual tapering peripherally (Fig. 8–1). The hilar density is composed of the proximal pulmonary arteries with the left hilum normally projecting more cranially than the right owing to the course of the left pulmonary artery over the left

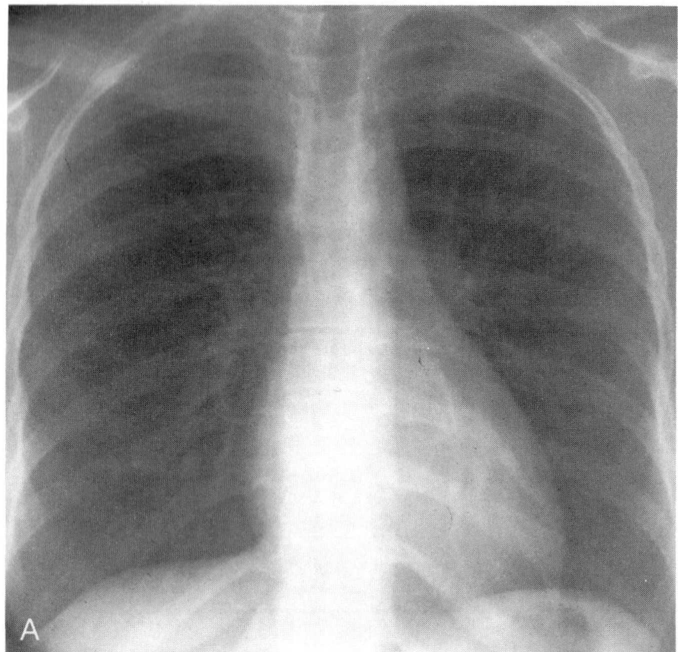

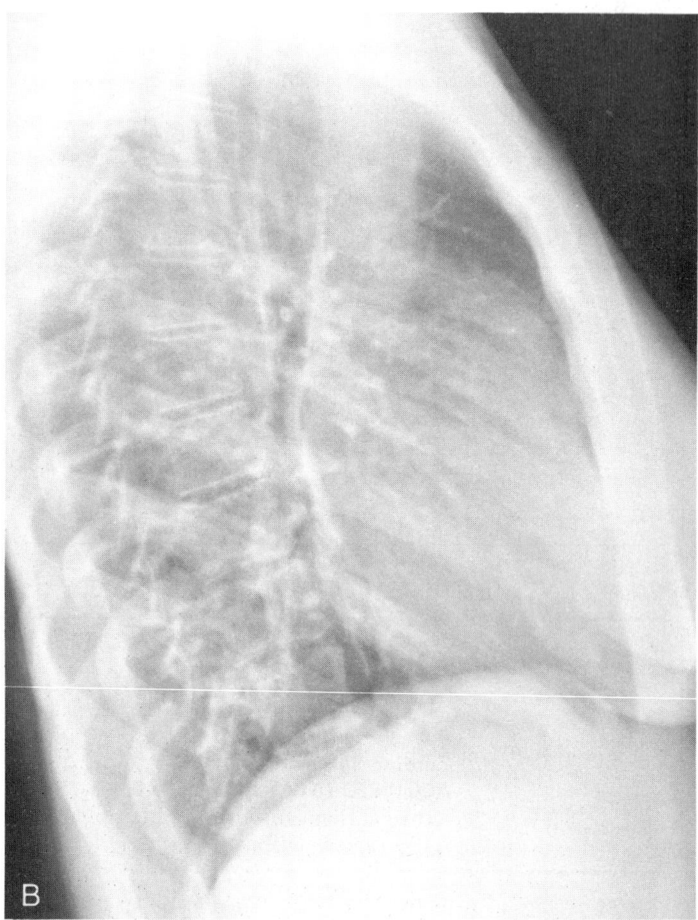

Figure 8–1. *A*, Posteroanterior and *B*, lateral chest radiographs with normal pulmonary vasculature and cardiac silhouette.

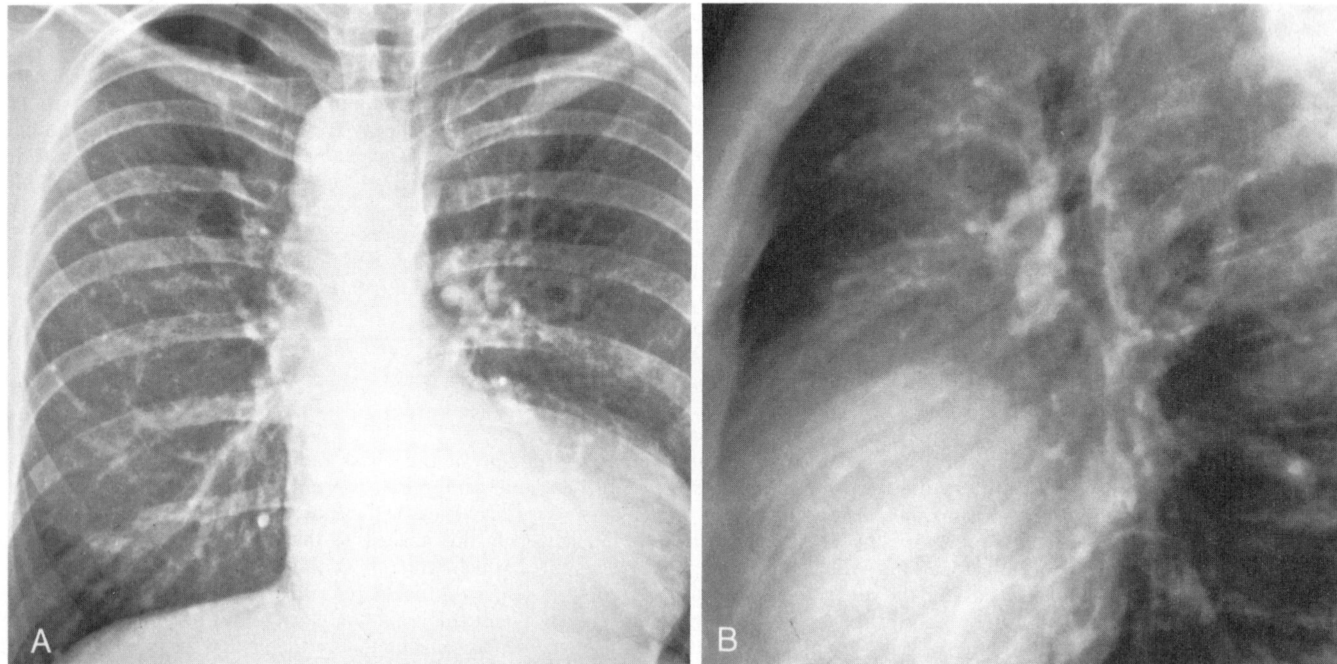

Figure 8–2. *A*, Posteroanterior and *B*, lateral chest radiographs of a patient with pseudotruncus, showing an upturned apex seen in right ventricular enlargement, a right-sided aortic arch as commonly seen in association with truncus arteriosus, and absence of hilar structures. A tangle of vessels in the hilar regions, well seen on the left side, is due to bronchial arterial supply to the lung fields.

main bronchus. In the upper lobes, the veins and arteries are essentially parallel with the veins lying lateral to their corresponding arteries. The major arteries and veins in the lower lung fields cross each other with the veins taking a more horizontal course toward the left atrium. In the upright position there is increased flow to the lung bases, largely due to the effects of gravity, which causes the lower-lobe vessels to increase in size. It may be difficult to identify the apical vessels clearly because pulmonary flow to the apices is negligible in the upright position.[M3] Therefore, position has a marked effect on flow distribution. For example, in the supine position the pulmonary blood flow is greatest to the dependent or posterior portions of the lungs, so pulmonary vasculature as seen from the front appears evenly distributed across the upper, middle, and lower lung zones. It must be remembered that the lung has a dual blood supply and receives oxygenated blood from the bronchial circulation. These bronchial arteries are not ordinarily visible except in pathologic conditions (Fig. 8–2).

INCREASED PULMONARY FLOW. As pulmonary flow increases, the pulmonary vessels, both arteries and veins, become enlarged and prominent. These enlarged vessels become apparent when pulmonary flow is approximately twice normal. The overcirculation pattern may be symmetric or asymmetric. High-output states with increased circulating blood volume, such as anemia, pregnancy, thyrotoxicosis, overhydration, and fever, result in a symmetric increase in vascularity, as do various congenital defects characterized by left-to-right shunts, such as ventricular and atrial septal defects (Fig. 8–3), patent ductus arteriosus, various admixture lesions such as truncus arteriosus, transposition (Fig. 8–4*B*), and anomalous pulmonary venous return. An asymmetric increase in pulmonary flow may be congenital in origin (e.g., pulmonary arteriovenous malformation, anomalous origin of a pulmonary artery) but is more commonly the result of surgical intervention to create a systemic-to-pulmonary shunt to improve pulmonary blood flow in the presence of severe pulmonary stenosis or atresia (e.g., a Blalock-Taussig shunt).

DECREASED PULMONARY FLOW. Since all the linear shadows in normal lung fields are due to pulmonary vasculature, when flow and, therefore, vessel size are diminished, the lung fields appear abnormally radiolucent. Both symmetric and asymmetric patterns of abnormal vascularity can be observed. Generalized undercirculation can be secondary to an obstructive lesion in the right heart, as in tetralogy of Fallot, pulmonary atresia (Fig. 8–5), right ventricular tumor, or tricuspid valve atresia. Small-caliber pulmonary vessels with relatively hyperlucent lungs and a small heart are evidence of a marked decrease in the circulating blood volume (e.g., in Addison's disease, hemorrhage). Chronic obstructive pulmonary disease (COPD) may result in generalized lung destruction or, more commonly, a patchy distribution of decreased vascularity. Segmental and asymmetric decreases in pulmonary vascularity are seen with pulmonary embolic disease (Westermark's sign), segmental COPD, partial pneumonectomy, and branch pulmonary artery stenoses. Rarely, postinflammatory changes (e.g., granulomatous mediastinitis), extrinsic compression (e.g., aortic aneurysm), and congenital hypoplasia as seen in the scimitar syndrome result in areas of decreased pulmonary flow. Bronchial collateral circulation may become prominent with a somewhat disordered pattern when there is a decrease in pulmonary artery blood flow and occasionally gives the illusion that the overall vascularity is actually normal or even increased. Small hila in tetralogy of Fallot or pulmonary atresia and loss of the normal branching pattern of pulmonary vasculature should be evident on the chest radiograph (see Fig. 8–2).

INCREASED RESISTANCE TO PULMONARY FLOW. Pulmonary hypertension with redistribution of flow is the result of increased resistance in the pulmonary circuit. Recognition of the various redistribution patterns shown by chest radiographs often allows one to determine the level of the increased resistance and the possible underlying pathology.

Pulmonary Venous Hypertension. Lesions acting beyond the pulmonary capillary level result in elevation of the pulmonary venous pressure. Left ventricular dysfunction (Figs. 8–6, 8–7, and 8–8) and mitral valve disease (Fig. 8–9) are the most common causes of pulmonary venous hypertension; other obstructive lesions at the left atrial level (e.g., atrial myxoma, cor triatriatum, thrombus) or pulmonary vein (see Fig. 8–4*C*) level (e.g., stenosis, veno-occlusive disease, or thrombosis) are relatively rare.

Initially, because of the increase in venous pressure, venous dilatation takes place throughout the lungs. However, the roentgenographic pattern typically seen is that of prominent upper lung vessels, both arteries and veins. This phenomenon is thought to be secondary to a localized segmental reflex initiated by the elevation of pulmonary venous pressure above a critical level of about 10 to 15 mmHg. An additional factor is fluid accumulation around compressible small vessels when plasma oncotic pressure

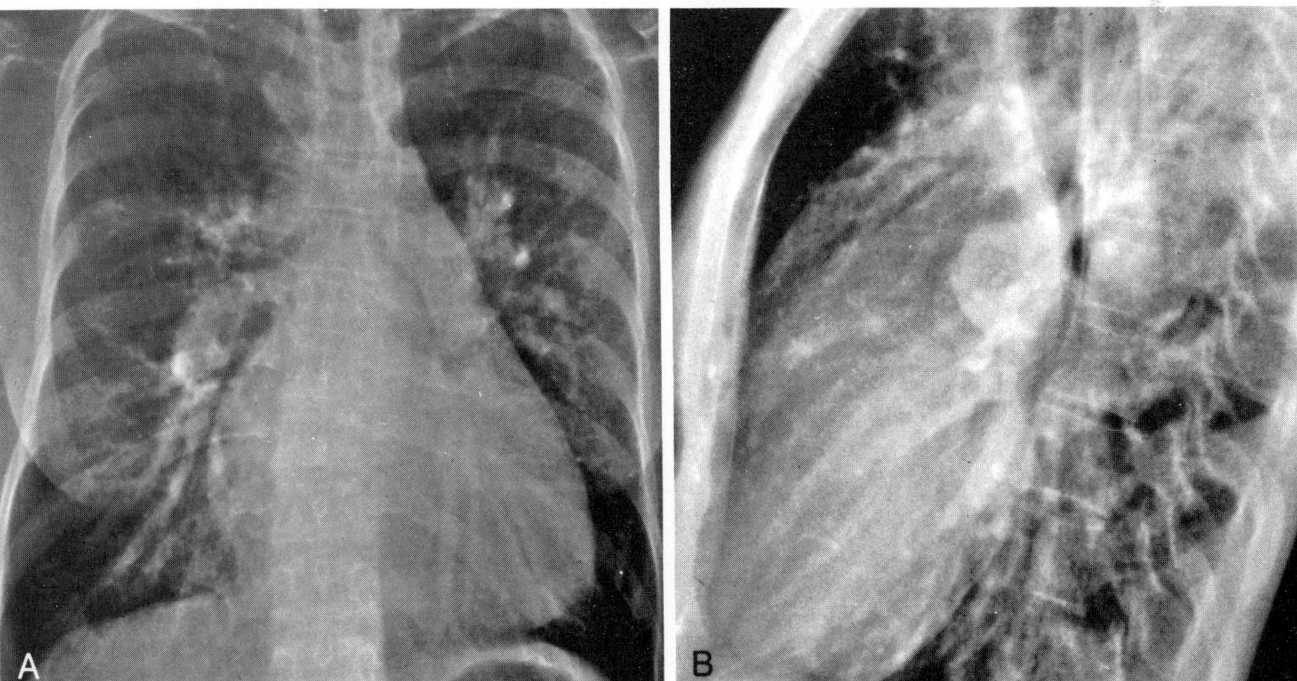

Figure 8–3. Chest films of a 32-year-old woman with an atrial septal defect. There is diffuse overall increase in the size of the pulmonary vessels (*A*) with evidence of right heart enlargement (*B*) and enlargement of the main pulmonary artery, manifest by straightening of the pulmonary artery segment (*A*) and the proximal pulmonary arteries.

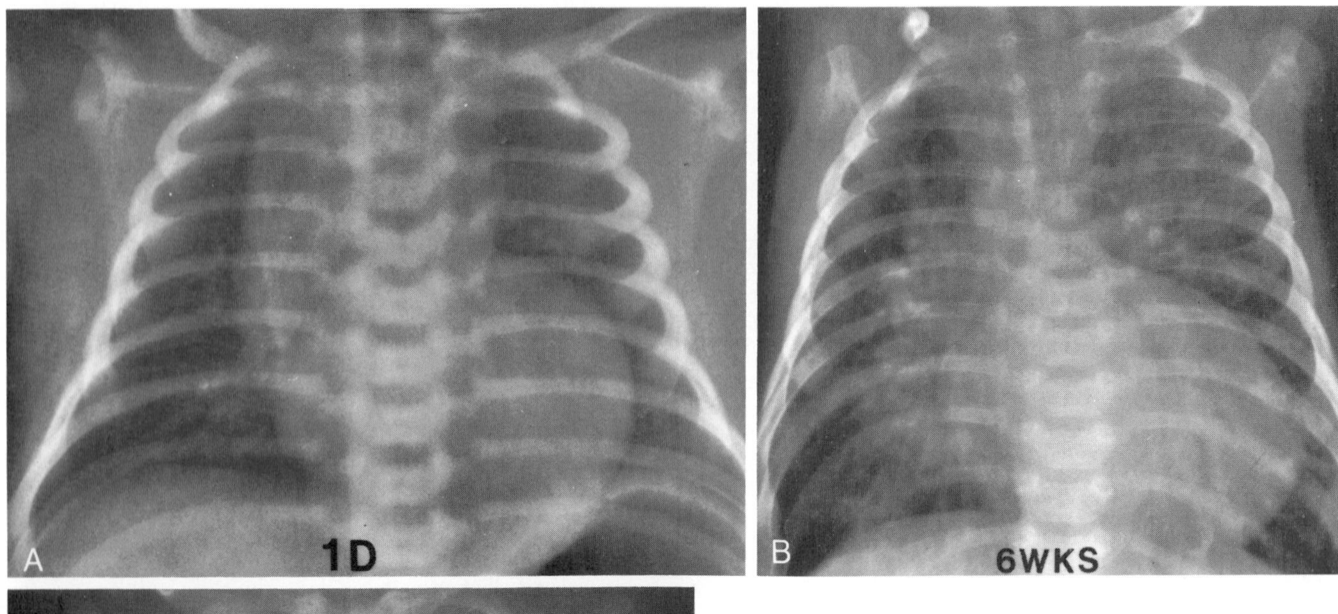

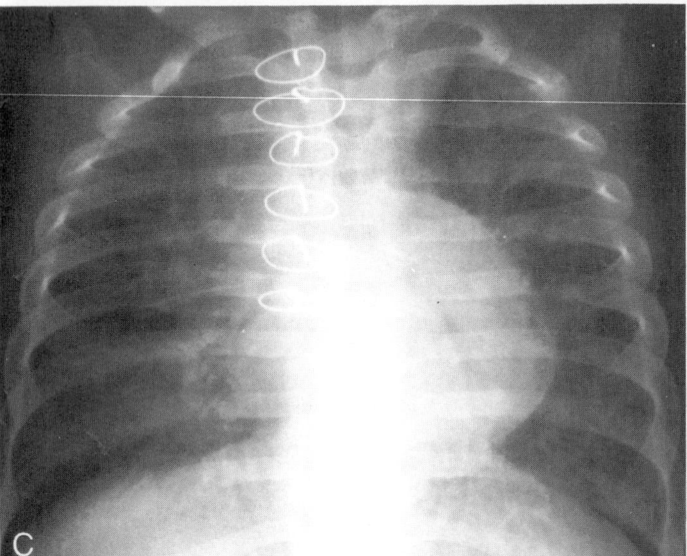

Figure 8–4. Chest films of a child with complete 1D transposition *A*, in the newborn period and *B*, at 6 weeks of age, when the more classic signs of an enlarged heart with the configuration of an "egg on side" together with the narrow waist of the vascular pedicle is seen. With the fall in pulmonary hypertension there has been an increase in the pulmonary vascularity. *C*, Following the Mustard operation, a change occurred in the appearances of the lung fields, which now demonstrate marked interstitial edema due to pulmonary venous obstruction.

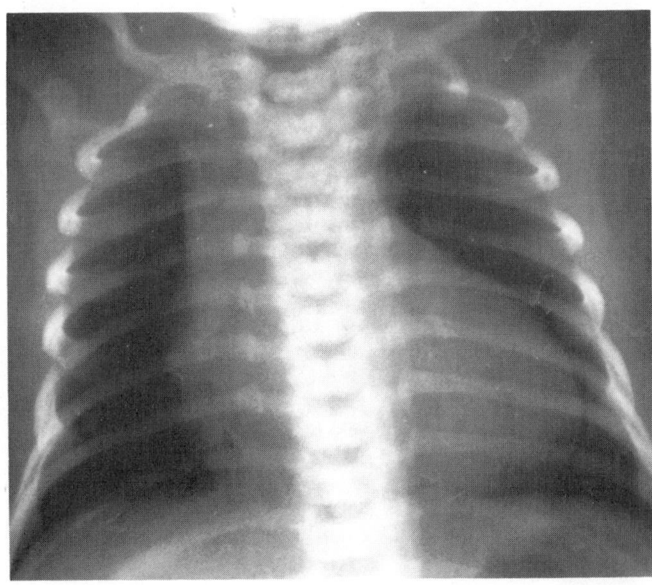

Figure 8–5. Chest film of a newborn with an atrial septal defect, patent ductus arteriosus, and pulmonary atresia. Diffusely oligemic lung fields due to decreased pulmonary flow are seen.

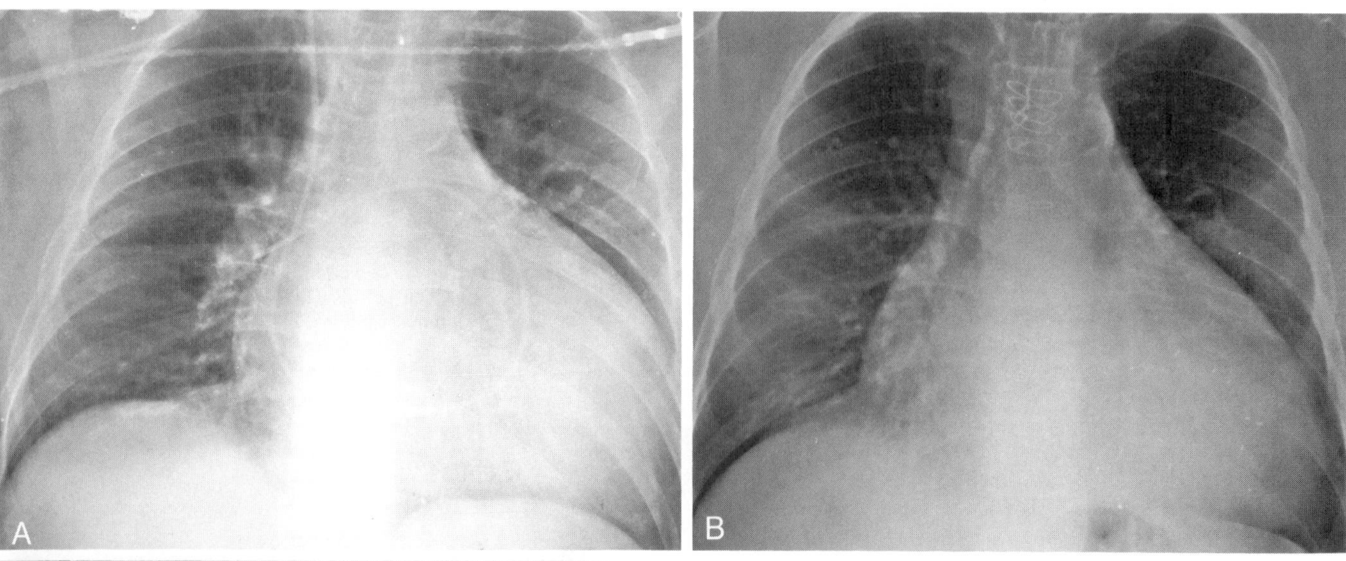

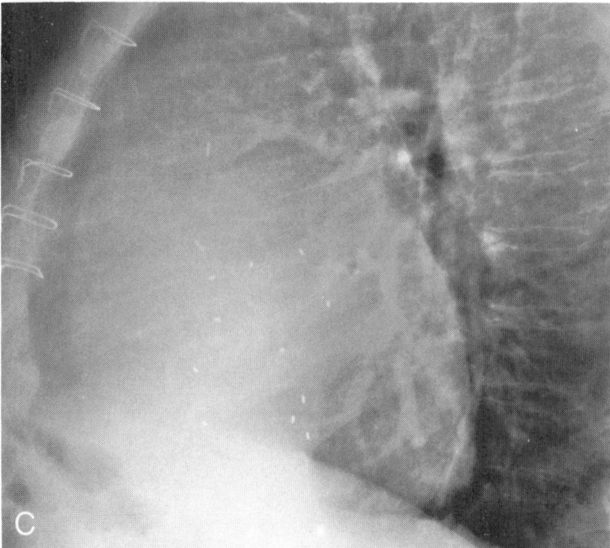

Figure 8–6. *A*, Chest film of a patient with dilated cardiomyopathy preoperatively, showing evidence of interstitial changes and pulmonary venous hypertension. *B* and *C*, Following transplantation the heart remains enlarged. The marked disparity between the metallic markers indicating the endocardium and the cardiac silhouette is consistent with the presence of a pericardial effusion.

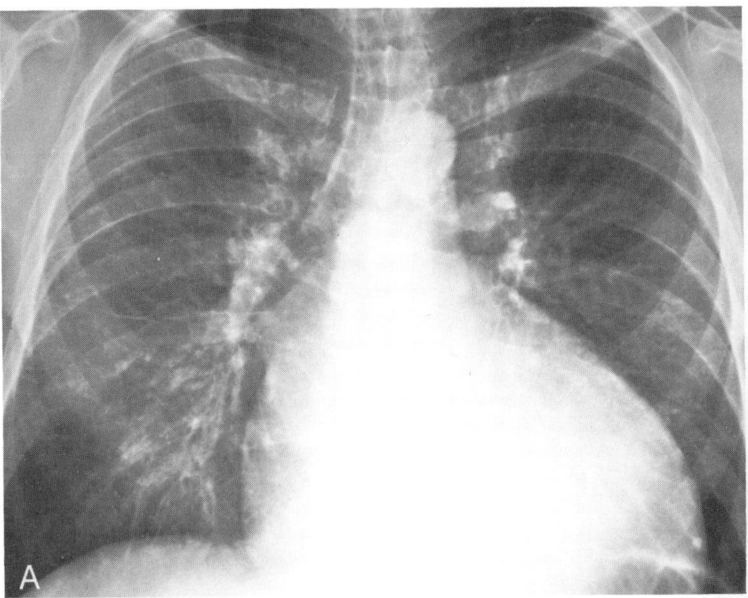

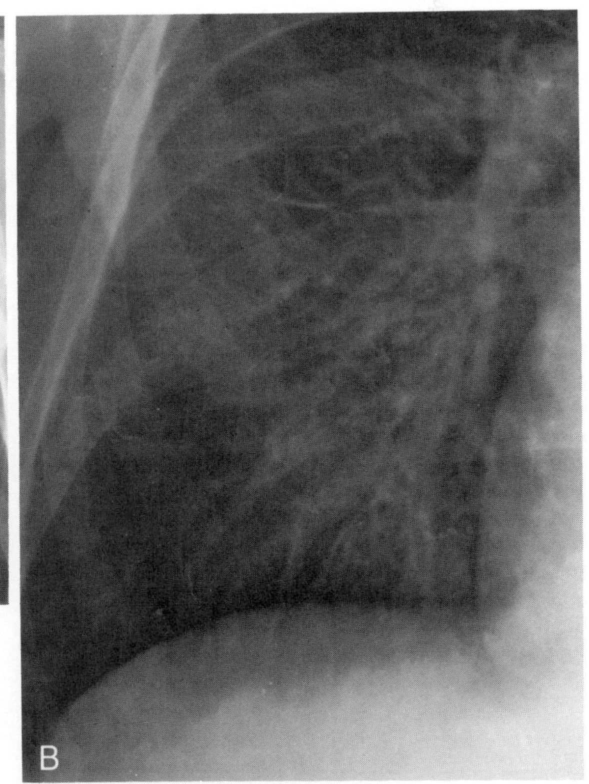

Figure 8–7. *A*, Chest film of a 43-year-old with dilated cardiomyopathy, showing an enlarged cardiac silhouette and evidence of pulmonary venous hypertension and interstitial pulmonary edema. *B*, Detailed image in which the findings of interstitial changes in the lung fields including Kerley's B lines are well seen.

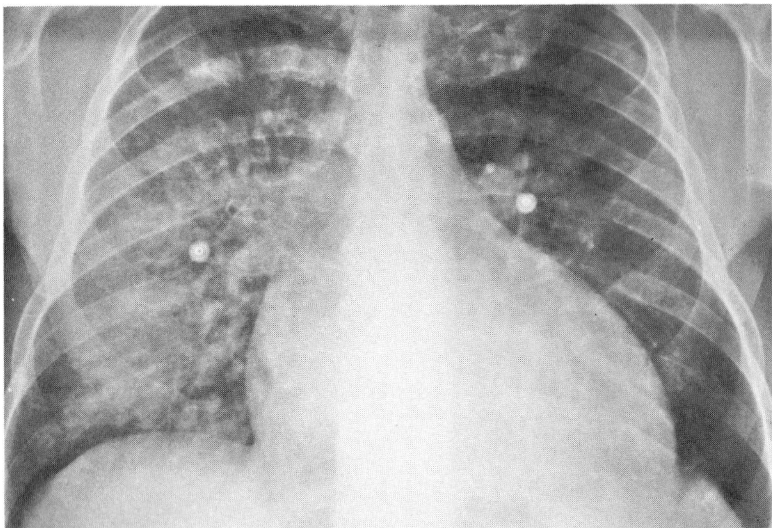

Figure 8–8. Chest film of a 50-year-old with dilated cardiomyopathy and left ventricular failure, showing an enlarged heart, a relatively small aortic knob, and a patchy infiltrate particularly seen perihilar in distribution on the right due to alveolar pulmonary edema.

is exceeded by the pulmonary venous pressure. Since the pressure in the lower lung is greater in the upright position because of hydrostatic forces, vasoconstriction of both arteries and veins occurs here first and increases resistance to flow, thereby reducing the circulatory volume through these vessels. To overcome the increased resistance and maintain a gradient in the presence of increased pulmonary venous pressure, the pulmonary artery pressure must rise, resulting in increased flow to the apices. The diverted pulmonary flow increases the size and visibility of the upper-lobe vessels. As pulmonary venous hypertension increases to the order of 25 mmHg, there is increased transudation of plasma from the lower lung capillaries that results in interstitial edema. In addition to further obscuring the now smaller and crowded lower-lobe vessels, this transudation results in the radiographic appearance of septal lines (Kerley's lines) owing to fluid within the interlobular septa. Still further elevation of the pulmonary venous pressure results in transudation of plasma into the alveoli, producing classic alveolar edema when the pressure exceeds 30 mmHg.[81]

Pulmonary Arterial Hypertension. Increased resistance at the pulmonary capillary level or in the pulmonary arterioles produces elevation of the pulmonary artery pressure. The causes of pulmonary arterial hypertension include (1) obstructive processes (e.g., chronic pulmonary emboli, idiopathic or primary pulmonary arterial hypertension, pulmonary schistosomiasis), (2) obliterative processes (e.g., pulmonary fibrosis, COPD), (3) constrictive processes (e.g., chronic hypoxia), and (4) increased flow as seen in large left-to-right shunts with development of Eisenmenger's syndrome (Fig. 8–10). Radiographically, pulmonary arteries are dilated centrally with an abrupt disparity in the caliber of the central and intrapulmonary arteries or "pruning" of the intrapulmonary branches. This uneven response is thought to be due to constriction of the muscular intrapulmonary branches in response to the increased intraluminal pressures with dilatation of the more elastic central arteries.

Cardiac Silhouette

The image of the heart and great vessels on the chest radiograph is a two-dimensional display of dynamic three-dimensional struc-

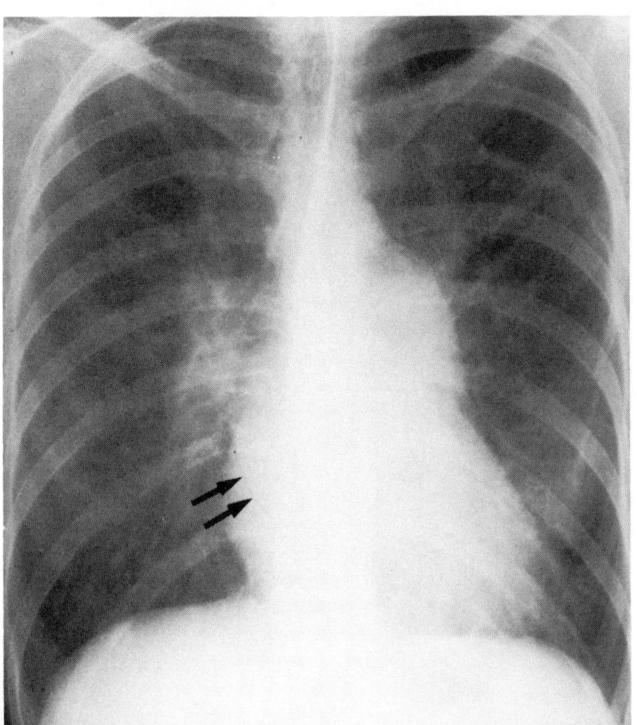

Figure 8–9. Chest film of a 28-year-old woman with mitral stenosis status post mitral valve commissurotomy via a left lateral thoracotomy. The heart is not enlarged, but there is evidence of enlarged proximal pulmonary vessels due to pulmonary venous hypertension and marked interstitial changes in the lung fields. Left atrium is seen to be enlarged with splaying of the bronchus, and a double density is seen *(arrows)*. There is evidence of secondary pulmonary arterial hypertension with enlarged main pulmonary artery and proximal pulmonary arteries.

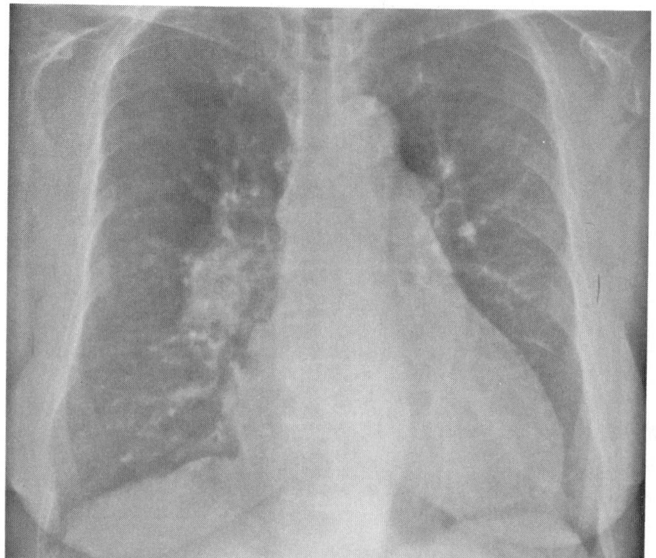

Figure 8–10. Chest film of a 65-year-old woman with atrial septal defect and Eisenmenger complex. Marked enlargement of the proximal pulmonary arteries is seen with a pruned appearance of the peripheral pulmonary vessels as seen in pulmonary arterial hypertension. The left atrium does not appear enlarged.

tures (see Fig. 8–1). The appearance of the cardiovascular silhouette varies not only with pathology but also with body habitus, age, respiratory depth, cardiac cycle, and position of the patient.

POSTEROANTERIOR PROJECTION. The right mediastinal contour comprises a straight superior vertical border owing to the superior vena cava and a smooth convex lower cardiac contour owing to the right atrium. The junction of the superior vena cava and right atrium often shows a shallow notch. Occasionally, where the right atrium meets the diaphragm, a short segment of inferior vena cava is interposed as a border-forming structure.

The normal left mediastinal contour is formed by a series of convexities due, in order, to the aortic knob superiorly, the pulmonary trunk, the left atrial appendage, and the left ventricle abutting the diaphragm. The pulmonary trunk segment varies in shape with age and body habitus. Most frequently, this segment is only slightly convex; however, it can be prominent in women in their twenties and thirties and straight or even concave in older patients and still be within normal limits. Occasionally, the cardiophrenic junction of the cardiac silhouette is not formed by the left ventricle but by a fat pad. Less common, but not rare, is a border-forming fat pad in the right cardiophrenic angle.

LATERAL PROJECTION. Typically, the patient's left side is positioned against the film cassette to minimize distortion of the heart due to geometric magnification. Superiorly, the anterior border is formed by the ascending aorta posterior to the retrosternal air space; inferiorly, the right ventricle and right ventricular outflow tract abut the sternum and blend imperceptibly into the main pulmonary artery, which then courses posteriorly to its bifurcation. The posterior cardiac contour is formed by the left atrium superiorly beneath the carina and the left ventricle curving inferiorly to the diaphragm, where the straight vertical edge of the inferior vena cava is apparent within the thorax as it enters the right atrium.

HEART SIZE. Cardiac enlargement always suggests underlying cardiac pathophysiology. The experienced observer evaluates cardiac size by visual inspection and subjectively grades any degree of cardiac enlargement. A more objective method of assessment may be desirable. All objective methods of determining cardiac size on the chest radiograph are subject to considerable error due to the wide variation in the appearance of the heart with body habitus, age, sex, depth of respiration, position of the patient, and radiographic technique. The cardiothoracic (CT) ratio—the ratio of the transverse cardiac diameter to the maximum internal diameter of the thorax at the level of the diaphragm on an upright posteroanterior chest radiograph—corrects for body build variables and magnification produced by slight differences in radiographic techniques. In adults, a CT ratio greater than 0.5 is considered to represent cardiomegaly (see Figs. 8–6, 8–7, and 8–8); however, rigid adherence to this value will result in both false-positives and false-negatives.[G1] Often, in aortic regurgitation the left ventricle is enlarged primarily downward rather than horizontally. The CT ratio may be less than 0.5 in the presence of cardiac enlargement. A high diaphragm position, as seen with obesity, expiration, or shallow inspiration, will produce an erroneous CT ratio greater than 0.5. Chest wall deformity, as in pectus excavatum, displaces the heart posteriorly and rotates the apex laterally, again resulting in a CT ratio greater than 0.5 in the presence of a normal-sized heart. Large pericardial fat pads give a falsely increased CT ratio. These factors, together with the performance of nonstandard radiographic techniques, make reliance on the CT ratio alone in diagnosing cardiomegaly often misleading except to serve as a baseline for future comparisons. Calculation of total cardiac silhouette volume, based on both PA and lateral projections, provides a closer correlation with angiographically determined cardiomegaly. Since it is not clinically very useful and the calculation itself is cumbersome, cardiac volume is not routinely calculated.[K1]

Generalized Cardiac Enlargement. Symmetric global enlargement, with maintenance of an otherwise normal cardiac contour, is usually due to a diffuse disturbance of structure or function with enlargement of all chambers of the heart. Hypertrophy or dilatation due to myocardial disease (see Figs. 8–6*A*, 8–7, and 8–8), increased stress secondary to abnormal volume or pressure loads, increased work as in hyperthyroidism, and decreased work capacity as in anemia or hypothyroidism all result in an enlarged cardiac silhouette. Pericardial effusions similarly produce enlargement of the cardiac silhouette (see Fig. 8–6*B*, *C*). Asymmetric generalized enlargement with left ventricular prominence can be seen in the late stages of essential hypertension and other left-sided obstructive lesions with secondary left ventricular failure, or in left-sided regurgitant valvular lesions with secondary increase in pulmonary pressures and subsequent right-sided hypertrophy and dilatation.

Specific Cardiac Chamber Enlargement. Unlike generalized cardiomegaly, enlargement of a specific cardiac chamber on the plain films often suggests the nature of the underlying pathology.

Left Atrium. Enlargement of the left atrium is the chamber enlargement most reliably demonstrated on the chest radiograph (Figs. 8–9, 8–11, and 8–12). The left atrium nestles just below the angle of the carina, in close proximity to the left bronchus and esophagus, so its enlargement is readily reflected in displacement of these neighboring structures. Enlargement usually produces a double density behind the right atrial margin on a PA projection as the left atrium bulges out from the mediastinum into the right lung. Occasionally, a double density can be seen in the presence of a normal-sized left atrium in young patients or patients in whom a prominent right pulmonary venous confluence has a tongue of lung between it and the right atrium.

Other signs of left atrial enlargement on the PA projection include upward and posterior displacement of the left main bronchus, resulting in a less acute carinal angle. Massive enlargement of the left atrium may cause leftward displacement of the descending aorta. Enlargement of the left atrial appendage causes first straightening, and later a convexity, in the upper left cardiac contour. In the presence of a giant left atrium, the left atrium itself may project beyond the right atrium and form a portion of the right cardiac contour. On the lateral projection, left atrial enlargement can be recognized by posterior and upward displacement of the left main stem bronchus. The left atrium itself enlarges upward and posteriorly to form an increasing convex density (Fig. 8–13). If the esophagus is opacified with barium, posterior displacement by the enlarged left atrium is demonstrated.[G1, H1]

Isolated left atrial enlargement (Fig. 8–14) is most commonly due to mitral valve stenosis secondary to rheumatic heart disease. Left atrial myxoma can also cause isolated enlargement. Isolated enlargement of the left atrial appendage or apparent enlargement

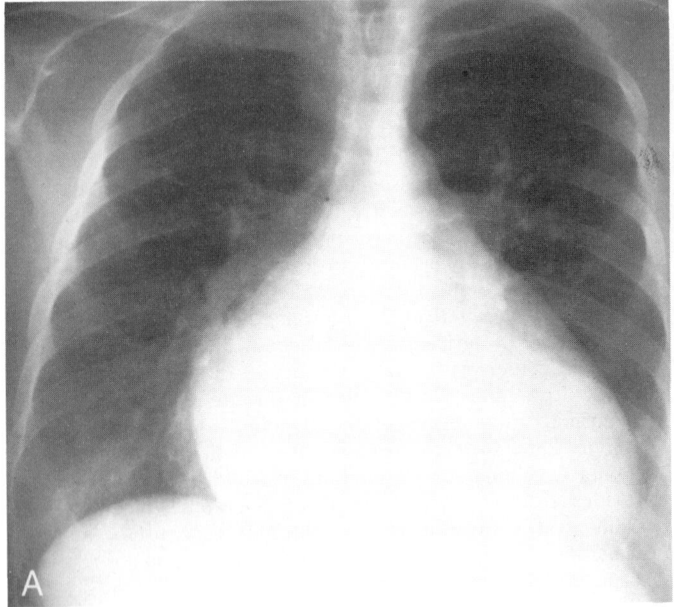

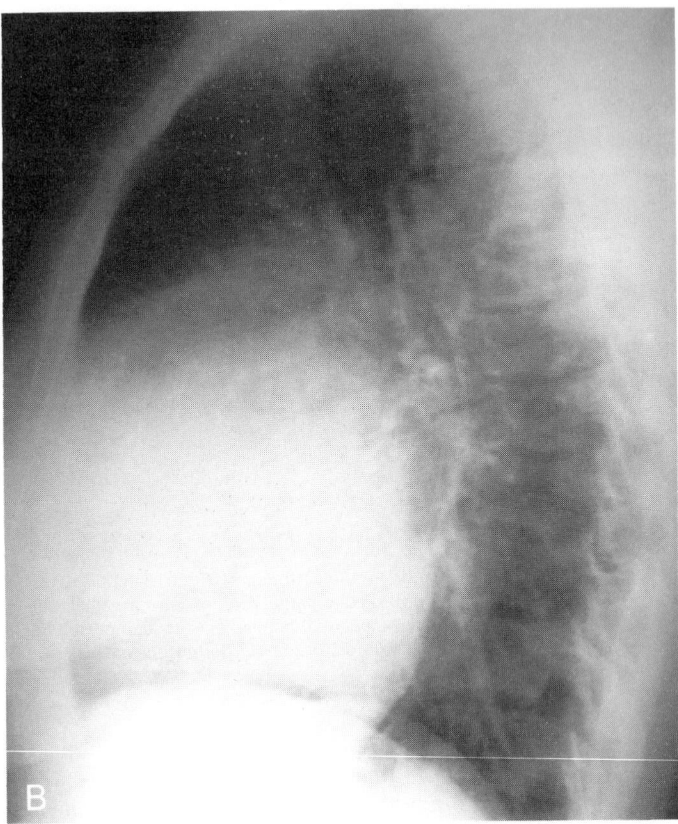

Figure 8–11. *A*, Posteroanterior and *B*, lateral chest radiographs demonstrating cardiac enlargement with evidence of a giant left atrium elevating and narrowing the left main stem bronchus. The left atrium extends almost to reach the right cardiac border *(A)*. There is also evidence of left ventricular enlargement and right heart enlargement *(B)*. The lung fields demonstrate interstitial changes and findings consistent with pulmonary venous hypertension in this patient with mitral regurgitation.

due to pericardial defect and focal herniation of the appendage may cause a localized bulge in the upper left cardiac contour without other signs of left atrial dilatation. Left atrial enlargement combined with additional chamber involvement may be produced by various conditions, such as left ventricular failure, left-sided obstructive lesions, or certain shunts (e.g., ventricular septal defects, patent ductus arteriosus, and aortopulmonary window). Left atrial enlargement is not seen, however, with simple atrial septal defects. When left atrial enlargement is marked, it is most often secondary to rheumatic valvular disease.

Left Ventricle. Left ventricular enlargement can be secondary to hypertrophy, dilatation, or both. Considerable hypertrophy must be present to enlarge the cardiac shadow appreciably. The classic appearance of left ventricular hypertrophy on the PA projection is rounding of the cardiac apex with downward and lateral displacement without cardiac enlargement (Fig. 8–15). Left ventricular dilatation causes an increase in the transverse diameter of the heart and the cardiothoracic ratio together with an apparent increase in the length of the left heart border. The cardiac apex may be displaced to such an extent that it projects

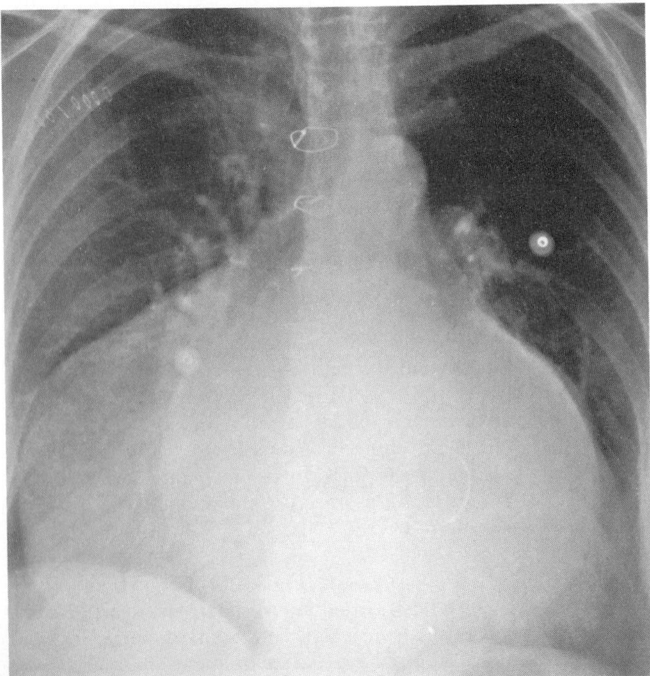

Figure 8–12. Frontal chest radiograph of a patient with rheumatic heart disease and significant tricuspid and mitral regurgitation. Marked right atrial enlargement is seen, with the right atrium enlarged almost to the right chest wall. There is also evidence of marked left atrial enlargement with splaying of the carina and a prominent double density. The patient has a mitral valve prosthesis in place.

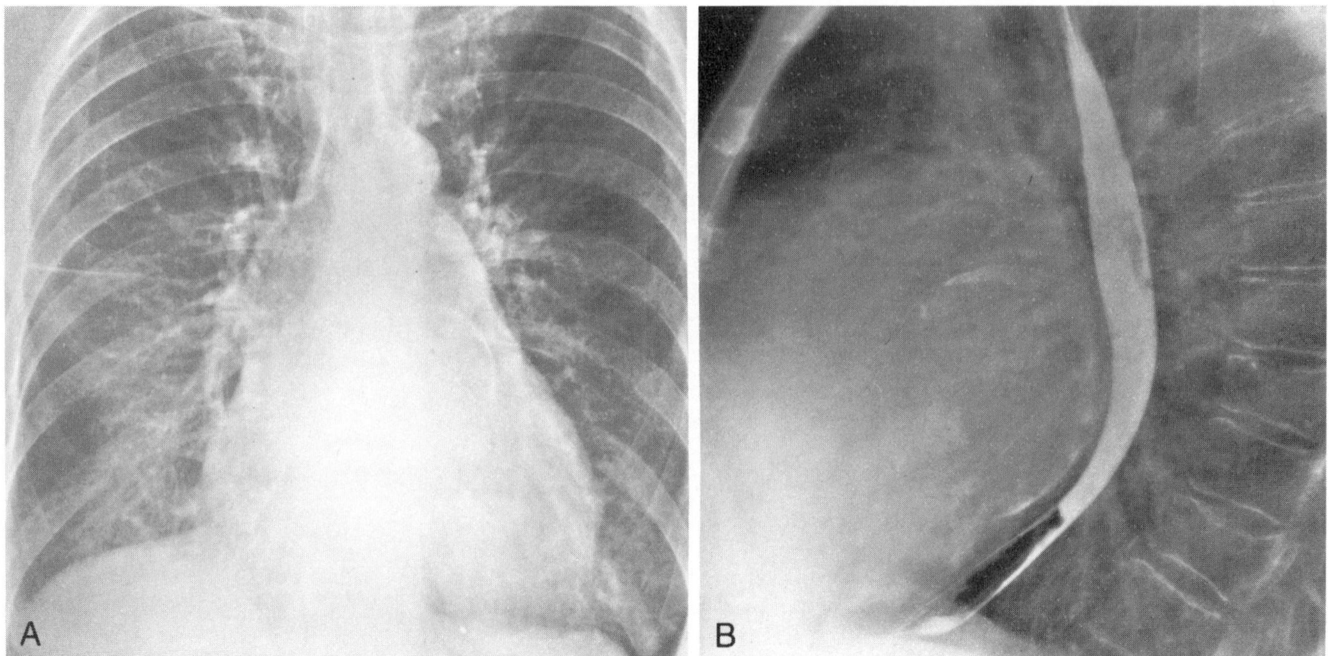

Figure 8–13. *A*, Frontal and *B*, lateral chest radiographs of a patient with mitral stenosis, showing extensive calcification outlining the left atrium and calcification in the mitral valve.

below the diaphragm. On the lateral projection, dilatation increases the posterior convexity of the left ventricular contour, which will project behind the edge of the vertical inferior vena cava (Rigler's sign) (see Fig. 8–15).[H2] Obstruction to left ventricular emptying, or increased afterload, as caused by systemic hypertension, aortic coarctation, or aortic valve stenosis, leads to hypertrophy initially, with rounding of the cardiac apex. Left ventricular dilatation with cardiac failure may follow.

Congestive or dilated cardiomyopathy, especially ischemic cardiomyopathy, primarily enlarges the left ventricle (see Figs. 8–6, 8–7, and 8–8). Aortic valve regurgitation and mitral valve regurgitation enlarge the left ventricle and are associated with dilatation of the aorta (Fig. 8–16) and left atrium, respectively. Volume overload secondary to left-to-right shunt, as in ventricular septal defects or aortopulmonary window, may also lead to left ventricular enlargement. More likely, right ventricular enlargement causes posterior displacement of the left atrium and ventricle with exaggeration of any true left ventricular enlargement. Left ventricular aneurysms, usually the result of a previous myocardial infarction, occasionally result in a localized bulge projecting beyond the normal ventricular contour[B1] or an angulation to the left ventricular contour (Fig. 8–17). A large apical aneurysm can appear similar to simple left ventricular chamber dilatation. Sometimes the heart appears normal in size and contour with true aneurysms of the left ventricle. False aneurysms often are paracardiac in location, posterior and inferior to the left ventricle. Aneurysms can also be secondary to trauma, surgery, or infection. All cardiac chambers have been reported to be involved with aneurysm formation, although atrial aneurysms are very rare.

Right Atrium. Isolated right atrial enlargement is best detected on the frontal chest film. Enlargement is to the right and causes increased fullness and convexity of the right cardiac contour and angulation of the junction of the superior vena cava and right

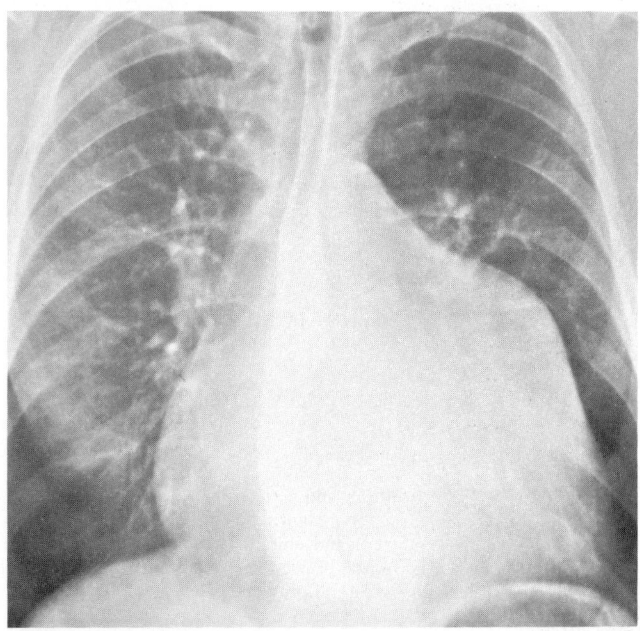

Figure 8–14. Frontal chest radiograph of a patient with mitral stenosis and marked left atrial enlargement. A convexity in the left cardiac contour below the left main stem bronchus is due to the enlarged left atrial appendage in this patient, who has other signs of left atrial enlargement and pulmonary venous hypertension.

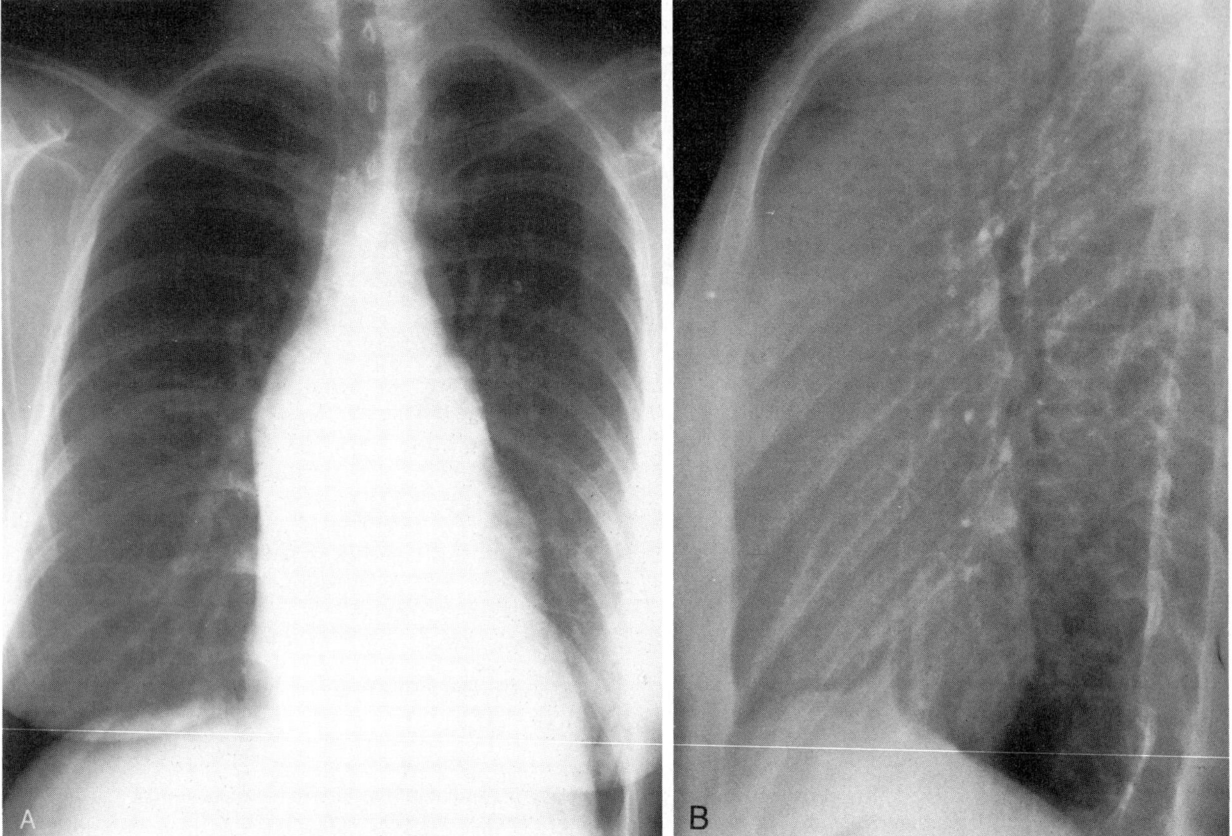

Figure 8–15. *A*, Posteroanterior and *B*, lateral chest radiographs of a patient with Marfan's syndrome. The patient has aortic stenosis with aortic root aneurysm. The enlargement of the aortic sinus extends to become border forming in the midportion of the left cardiac contour *(A)*. The aneurysm of the ascending aorta fills in the retrosternal air space on the lateral projection *(B)* and produces a convexity in the superior cardiac contour on the frontal projection *(A)*. There is evidence of left ventricular enlargement.

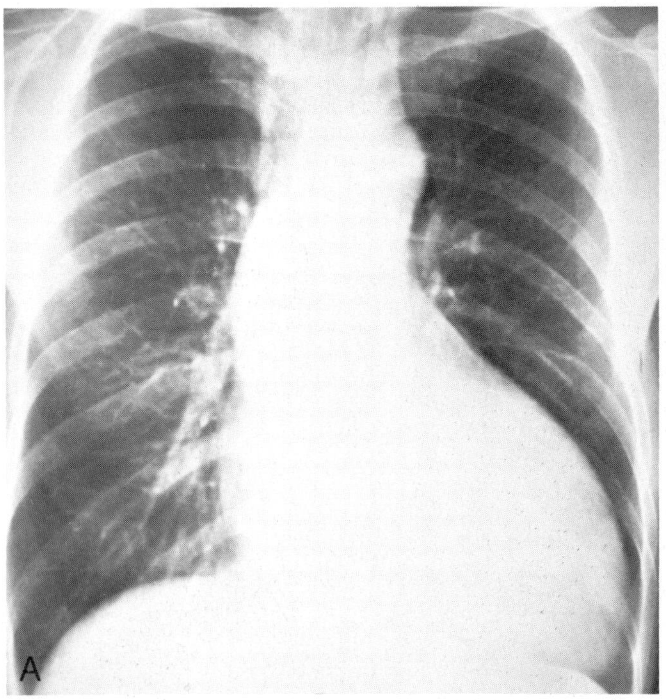

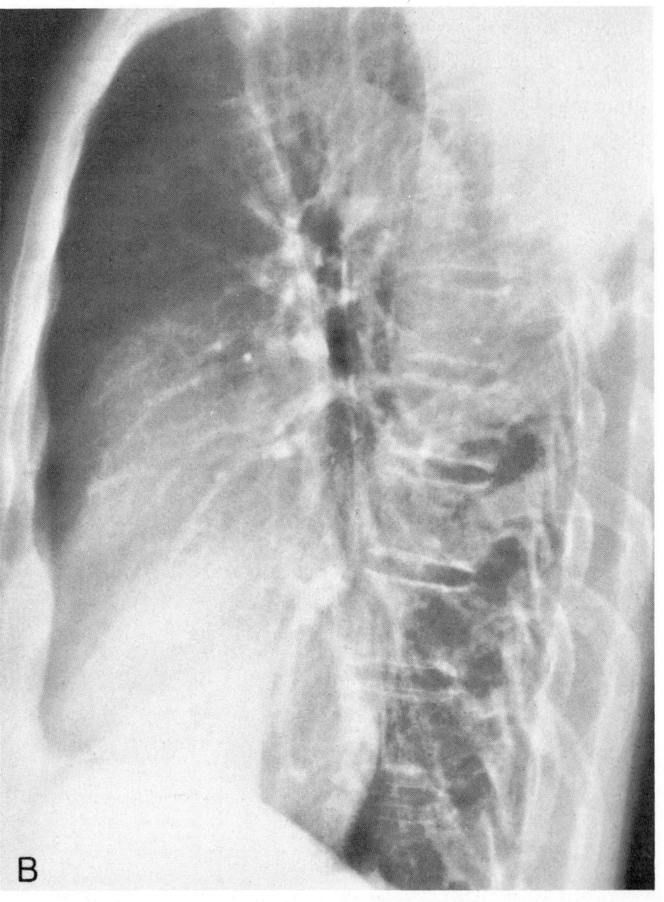

Figure 8–16. *A*, Posteroanterior and *B*, lateral chest radiographs of a 28-year-old with aortic regurgitation, showing an enlarged cardiac silhouette with an enlarged left ventricle and unfolded aorta. The ascending aorta shows a convexity on the frontal projection *(A)* and encroachment on the retrosternal air space on the lateral projection *(B)*.

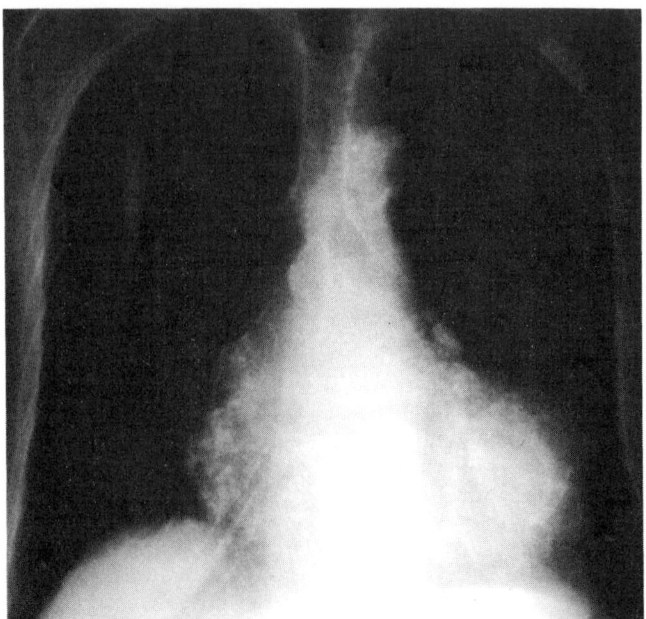

Figure 8–17. Frontal chest radiograph of an 83-year-old woman with a left ventricular aneurysm following a prior myocardial infarction. The angulation of the left cardiac contour is consistent with a left ventricular aneurysm. Calcification is seen in the left ventricular aneurysm.

atrium. There may be associated dilatation of the superior and inferior venae cavae that causes widening of the right superior mediastinum and an additional border in the right cardiophrenic angle. On the lateral projection, right atrial dilatation causes a filling-in of the retrosternal clear space anteriorly and superiorly, with the cardiac silhouette extending behind the sternum more than one-third above the cardiophrenic angle, similar to that seen with right ventricular enlargement. There may be a double density that merges with the inferior vena caval shadow, which now may be a slightly convex structure. Left atrial enlargement can be simulated by marked right atrial dilatation.

Isolated right atrial enlargement is uncommon and is usually secondary to tricuspid stenosis or right atrial tumor. Right atrial dilatation associated with other chamber enlargement, primarily right ventricular enlargement, can be seen in multiple conditions, such as tricuspid regurgitation (see Fig. 8–12), pulmonary arterial hypertension, shunts to the right atrium, and cardiomyopathies. Marked isolated right atrial enlargement resulting in a "box-shaped" heart is seen in Ebstein's malformation of the tricuspid valve. This configuration of the heart is the result of marked angulation at the superior vena caval–right atrial junction as the right atrium enlarges.

Right Ventricle. The right ventricle enlarges by broadening its triangular shape primarily in the superior and leftward direction. With increasing right ventricular enlargement, the whole heart rotates to the left around its long axis and displaces the left ventricle posteriorly. This displacement causes increased convexity of the left upper heart border and elevation of the cardiac apex (see Fig. 8–2). The rotation also makes the pulmonary trunk appear prominent (it often will be dilated as well) and the aorta appear relatively small. With marked dilatation, the right ventricle may form the left heart border on the PA projection.

On the lateral projection one sees the right ventricle extending cranially behind the sternum with increased bulk anteriorly (Fig. 8–18). Normally, the heart does not extend more than one-third of the distance from the cardiophrenic angle to the angle of Louis or the level of the carina; however, the normal extension can vary with body habitus. Isolated right ventricular enlargement is very unusual. More typically there is associated prominence of the right atrium and pulmonary trunk.

ACQUIRED HEART DISEASE

Ischemic Heart Disease

Radiographs of the heart can be very useful in the evaluation of patients with coronary artery disease, although occasionally

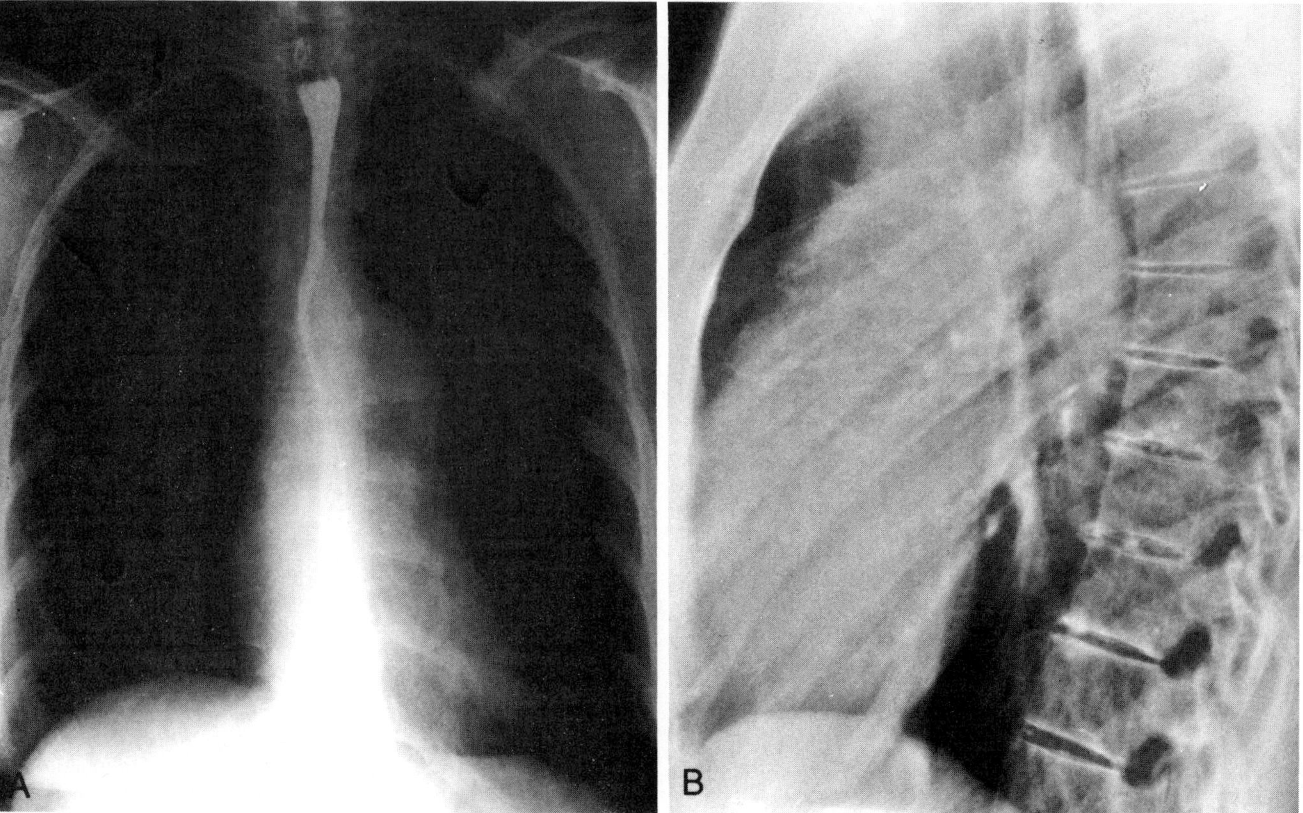

Figure 8–18. *A*, Posteroanterior and *B*, lateral chest radiographs of a 28-year-old woman with pulmonary stenosis. Classic findings of an enlarged right heart are seen on the lateral projection *(B)* with post-stenotic dilatation of the main pulmonary artery extending to enlarge the left pulmonary artery *(A, B)*.

the patient with severe symptomatic coronary disease may have a normal chest x-ray.[S2] When myocardial function is significantly impaired, radiologic manifestations of left ventricular failure will be present on the chest film. Commonly, left ventricular enlargement is seen when there is impairment of left ventricular contractility. Cardiac decompensation results in secondary ventricular dilatation, decreased ventricular compliance, increased left ventricular end-diastolic pressure, and increased pulmonary venous pressure leading to pulmonary vascular redistribution. The left atrium will also be enlarged as a result of the increase in ventricular filling pressure or concomitant mitral regurgitation. All four chambers dilate when there is progression to right ventricular failure, and the appearance of the ischemic cardiomyopathic heart resembles that of the heart in other congestive cardiomyopathies (see Figs. 8–6, 8–7, and 8–8). Differentiation from the enlarged cardiac silhouette of pericardial effusion may be impossible if diuretic therapy has been effective in decreasing pulmonary interstitial and alveolar edema and the overt signs of congestive failure are not evident.

Acute or recent myocardial infarction may be indicated by several findings on the chest radiograph. Acute, often transient, left ventricular failure associated with infarction may be seen as pulmonary vascular congestion and pulmonary edema with normal heart size. Papillary muscle rupture or dysfunction secondary to infarction may also produce acute pulmonary venous hypertension. Postinfarction ventricular septal defect may result in the abrupt appearance of shunt vascularity, usually superimposed on a pattern of overt pulmonary edema. Postmyocardial infarction syndrome (Dressler's syndrome) is characterized by enlargement of the cardiac silhouette secondary to pericardial effusion, together with pleural effusions and pulmonary infiltrates, often without signs of left ventricular failure.[A1, D1] Left ventricular aneurysms seldom form until several months after infarction (see Fig. 8–17), and the incidence of formation is estimated to be 12 to 14 percent.[A2] Calcification in an aneurysm occasionally is seen as a focal linear or curvilinear density, which can mimic pericardial calcification. Occasionally, a simple infarction can necrose and develop an area of smudgy calcification many years after the infarction. This is most commonly seen in the ventricular septum.

Valvular Disease

The clinical and radiologic manifestations of valvular disease result from obstruction of flow across a stenotic valve, regurgitation of flow across an incompetent valve, or a combination of both. Obstruction results in pressure overload with resultant proximal chamber hypertrophy. Regurgitation causes volume overload, which results primarily in chamber dilatation on both sides of the diseased valve.

AORTIC VALVE STENOSIS. Isolated aortic stenosis is usually due to either a congenitally bicuspid valve or a degenerative calcific process producing commissural fusion. Congenital bicuspid aortic valve occurs in about 2 percent of the population. Typically, the older adult patient with a bicuspid valve becomes symptomatic in the fifth to seventh decade due to stenosis resulting from calcification and limited mobility of valve leaflets. Occasionally, a bicuspid valve that is severely dysplastic is seen in childhood or even infancy.

Calcification of a bicuspid aortic valve is common over the age of 40 years. It is best seen on the lateral projection, where it is located above a line drawn from the junction of the sternum and diaphragm to the hilum. On the frontal projection the calcification often projects over the spine. Congenitally bicuspid aortic valve occasionally may be differentiated on plain films from acquired aortic stenosis. Three calcified curved lines representing the lines of insertion of the three cusps of the aortic valve suggest the diagnosis of acquired aortic stenosis. A characteristic bulbous appearance of a calcified raphe of a congenital bicuspid valve has been described.[S3]

Radiographically, the obstruction to the left ventricular outflow results in concentric left ventricular hypertrophy, initially without ventricular dilatation, and produces little change in the overall size of the cardiac silhouette. Slight rounding of the left ventricular apex is seen on the PA projection (see Fig. 8–15). Long-standing aortic stenosis often results in post-stenotic dilatation of the ascending aorta, seen as a localized bulge of the right contour of the superior mediastinum above the right atrium on the frontal projection and prominence of the ascending aorta protruding into the retrosternal air space on the lateral projection.[A3, K2] Left ventricular dilatation without associated aortic regurgitation indicates left ventricular decompensation and onset of end-stage disease. There will also be other radiographic signs of left ventricular failure.

AORTIC REGURGITATION. Rheumatic heart disease commonly involves the aortic valve. However, many other causes of aortic regurgitation must be considered, especially in the presence of isolated regurgitation. Lesions affecting the aortic cusps include infectious endocarditis, traumatic rupture, connective tissue diseases such as ankylosing spondylitis or Reiter's syndrome, congenitally bicuspid valve, and prolapse of a valve leaflet in the presence of a subaortic ventricular septal defect. Aortic root pathology such as seen in Marfan's syndrome (see Fig. 8–15), ascending aortic dissection (type A, Stanford classification), luetic aortitis, atherosclerotic aneurysms of the aortic root, and aorto–left ventricular fistulas can result in aortic regurgitation.

The chest radiograph may appear normal in mild regurgitation. Increasing enlargement of the left ventricle is seen as the severity of regurgitation progresses. The ventricle elongates and dilates and the apex is displaced downward, laterally, and posteriorly. Mild to moderate enlargement of the ascending aorta may be present, but classically there is diffuse unfolding of the thoracic aorta as a result of the increasingly wide pulse pressure (see Fig. 8–16). The pulmonary vasculature is often normal. The appearance of pulmonary venous hypertension heralds left ventricular decompensation.

MITRAL STENOSIS. Mitral valve stenosis in the adult is almost always secondary to rheumatic heart disease. Thickened, immobile, and often calcified valve leaflets form many years after the episode of rheumatic fever, which may not even have been recognized clinically. Radiographic features of mitral valve stenosis (see Figs. 8–9 and 8–14) reflect the physiology of pressure overload of the left atrium and pulmonary veins and ultimately the right ventricle. Although overall heart size may appear normal, discrete left atrial enlargement develops with significant obstruction. Prominence of the left atrial appendage on the PA view may be the only sign of atrial enlargement.

There is poor correlation between the degree of left atrial enlargement and the severity of stenosis. Changes in the pulmonary vasculature more accurately reflect the severity of obstruction. Pulmonary venous hypertension with interstitial edema and septal lines indicates severe disease, and these are the classic features of mitral valve disease. Prominent proximal pulmonary arteries combined with right ventricular hypertrophy and dilatation are features of long-standing mitral valve stenosis, pulmonary venous hypertension, and the development of pulmonary arterial hypertension.[C1] Valvular calcifications associated with rheumatic mitral stenosis are located to the left of the spine in the frontal projection and below a line drawn from the junction of the diaphragm and sternum to the hilum on the lateral projection. Curvilinear calcifications outlining the left atrial wall are associated with long-standing atrial mural thrombus, and tiny calcified nodules in the lung bases are seen in association with hemosiderosis secondary to chronic pulmonary hypertension.[S4] The plain-film findings resulting from left atrial myxoma that obstructs the mitral valve are often indistinguishable from those seen in rheumatic mitral stenosis.

MITRAL REGURGITATION. Causes of mitral regurgitation are multiple and include structural or functional disturbances in the mitral valve apparatus including the leaflets, the papillary muscles, the chordae, and the valve annulus. Rheumatic endocarditis is a common cause of mitral regurgitation, which is due to shortening and scarring of the valve leaflets. Leaflet or chordal destruction is also commonly seen with infective endocarditis. Mitral valve prolapse, as seen in Marfan's syndrome, may also result from stretching and rupture of chordae. Ischemic heart disease causes papillary muscle dysfunction and/or left ventricular enlargement with dilatation of the mitral valve annulus, which can cause mitral regurgitation. Papillary muscle rupture, often secondary to myocardial infarction, is a well-recognized cause of acute mitral regurgitation.

Plain films are typically normal with mild mitral valve regurgitation. As the regurgitant volume increases, the left ventricle enlarges to maintain cardiac output. The presence of left ventricular enlargement differentiates mitral regurgitation from mitral stenosis in which the left ventricle remains normal in size. The left atrium enlarges in mitral regurgitation, usually to a greater degree than in mitral stenosis. As the left atrium enlarges, it becomes border-forming along the right cardiac margin. When the left atrium becomes enormous, it can approach the right chest wall (see Fig. 8–11). The left atrial appendage classically is dilated if the mitral regurgitation is of rheumatic etiology. The pulmonary vascular changes resulting from pulmonary venous hypertension are usually less marked in mitral regurgitation than in mitral stenosis. Interstitial edema and alveolar edema are quite uncommon except in acute mitral valve regurgitation, as occurs with papillary muscle rupture or acute myocardial infarction. As mitral regurgitation secondary to rheumatic heart disease is often combined with some degree of mitral stenosis, it may be difficult to determine the dominant lesion. However, in general, if the heart is small relative to the degree of pulmonary vascular and interstitial changes, mitral stenosis is the dominant lesion, whereas a large heart and left atrium are seen with only mild changes of pulmonary venous hypertension when regurgitation is the dominant lesion.

PULMONARY STENOSIS. Isolated valvular pulmonary stenosis is nearly always congenital in etiology but symptoms may not develop until adulthood (see Fig. 8–18). Rheumatic heart disease may rarely result in stenosis but typically other valves are involved as well. Carcinoid plaques may result in fusion of pulmonary valve cusps.

Radiographically, pulmonary stenosis has a classic appearance caused by post-stenotic dilatation of the pulmonary trunk and the left pulmonary artery due to the jet phenomenon across the stenosis. The right pulmonary artery is normal in size where it is visible in the right hilum (see Fig. 8–18).[C2] Rarely, calcification of a stenotic pulmonary valve is seen. Heart size and contour are typically normal, but mild enlargement can be seen due predominantly to hypertrophy and dilatation of the right ventricle. Right atrial enlargement may follow secondary to stretching of the tricuspid valve annulus and regurgitation. The plain-film appearance of idiopathic dilatation of the pulmonary artery, a rarer condition, is indistinguishable from that of mild pulmonary valve stenosis.

PULMONARY REGURGITATION. Pulmonary regurgitation may be secondary to dilatation of the valve ring as seen in pulmonary hypertension (of any etiology), connective tissue disorders, and idiopathic dilatation of the pulmonary artery. Regurgitation can also be due to a variety of lesions involving the leaflets, such as a congenitally dysplastic valve, infectious endocarditis, or rheumatic disease. A not uncommon cause is surgical removal of the dysplastic or atretic pulmonary valve.

There are no specific radiologic signs of pulmonary regurgitation. Plain chest films are usually normal or demonstrate changes due to the underlying cause of the regurgitation, e.g., pulmonary arterial hypertension.

TRICUSPID STENOSIS. Rheumatic tricuspid stenosis is rare and is usually associated with mitral valve stenosis. Rare causes of acquired obstruction to right atrial emptying include carcinoid syndrome and right atrial myxoma. Congenital tricuspid stenosis is also rare.

The chest radiograph demonstrates a dilated right atrium, often with a prominent superior vena cava and azygous vein. Associated changes of mitral stenosis are often present, although the pulmonary vascular prominence may be less evident.

TRICUSPID REGURGITATION. Acquired tricuspid regurgitation is often functional, resulting from right ventricular hypertension of any cause with right ventricular dilatation and stretching of the tricuspid annulus. Organic tricuspid regurgitation can result from multiple causes including rheumatic endocarditis, infectious endocarditis, carcinoid syndrome, and trauma that causes acute rupture of the tricuspid valve.

Plain films often show considerable cardiomegaly in cases of functional regurgitation with right ventricular dilatation in addition to right atrial dilatation. In rheumatic valvular disease, tricuspid regurgitation may be functional, owing to associated pulmonary arterial hypertension and dilatation of the tricuspid annulus, or organic, owing to tricuspid rheumatic endocarditis. Whether it is functional or organic, the findings of tricuspid regurgitation on the chest radiograph are similar; however, signs of pulmonary arterial hypertension are present in functional regurgitation. Right atrial enlargement may be difficult to appreciate in the presence of left atrial enlargement, as the two borders can overlap on the frontal and lateral projections.

A special cause of tricuspid regurgitation is Ebstein's anomaly of the tricuspid valve, in which the leaflets are malformed and attached abnormally in the right ventricle. A spectrum of functional changes result, including tricuspid regurgitation; thinning of the portion of the right ventricle between the tricuspid annulus and the abnormally attached tricuspid leaflets (atrialization of the right ventricular inflow tract); right ventricular obstruction between the inflow and outflow portions of the ventricle due to an enlarged, sail-like anterior tricuspid leaflet; and a small functional segment, the residual infundibular or outflow portion of the right ventricle. Cardiac enlargement, particularly right atrial enlargement, results, with decreased pulmonary flow and a prominent, hyperdynamic pulmonary infundibulum in the most severe cases.

Cardiomyopathy

Cardiomyopathies are diseases of the myocardium of diverse etiology and may be classified pathophysiologically into three groups: dilated (congestive), restrictive, and hypertrophic. Often the specific etiology is unknown or at best inferred. The three groups are not always distinct, and some cardiomyopathies show a combination of impaired contraction with congestive heart failure together with restrictive diastolic filling. Hypertrophic cardiomyopathy may eventually develop impaired contractility.

DILATED CARDIOMYOPATHY. This group is the largest and most diverse of the cardiomyopathies, and the majority in this group are idiopathic in origin. The chest radiograph appearances are quite similar.[H3, S5] There is usually diffuse cardiac enlargement (see Figs. 8–6, 8–7, 8–8). There may be left ventricular prominence, but often the cardiac contour is globular and resembles that of a large pericardial effusion. The degree of enlargement varies considerably depending on the severity and duration of the illness. The aorta is usually of normal size but the vascular pedicle may appear relatively small, in part because of the decreased cardiac output. Oligemic lungs reflect involvement of the right cardiac chambers with low pulmonary pressures and low cardiac output. Pulmonary venous hypertension with interstitial edema is indicative of predominant left heart failure and adequate right ventricular function. Vigorous diuresis and vasodilator therapy also result in small but sharply defined pulmonary vessels. The circulating blood volume can be monitored by observing the prominence of the superior vena cava and azygous vein.

RESTRICTIVE CARDIOMYOPATHY. Unlike dilated cardiomyopathies, many restrictive cardiomyopathies have identifiable causes. They are the result of impaired diastolic function with relatively unimpaired contractile function. Infiltrating processes such as amyloid deposition, sarcoidosis, or hemochromatosis result in rigid ventricular walls that fail to relax and contract fully. Fibrotic processes such as endocardial fibroelastosis or endomyocardial fibrosis are relatively rare causes of restrictive cardiomyopathies. Neoplastic involvement by metastases or direct invasion can result in a restrictive pattern. Radiation therapy delivered to the heart and some antineoplastic drugs such as doxorubicin (Adriamycin) are cardiotoxic and result in permanent restrictive cardiomyopathy. The plain-film appearance is quite nonspecific. The heart may be normal or enlarged and indistinguishable from that in a dilated cardiomyopathy. The atria may be disproportionately enlarged secondary to functional regurgitation with dilatation of the mitral and tricuspid valve rings. Normal or congested and enlarged pulmonary vascularity may be present. An important finding on the chest radiograph is absence of calcification within the pericardium, since clinical differentiation of constrictive pericarditis from restrictive cardiomyopathy may be very difficult.[H3, S5]

HYPERTROPHIC CARDIOMYOPATHY. Hypertrophic cardiomyopathy can have both an obstructive and a nonobstructive clinical and radiographic presentation. The presence of a systolic gradient across the left ventricular outflow tract determines the degree of obstructive component. The plain-film appearance is classically very similar to that in other left ventricular outflow obstructions such as aortic or subaortic stenosis; however, the aorta is normal in size. The heart may be enlarged in about 50 percent of symptomatic patients, with the frontal projection demonstrating a rounded left heart border produced by the left ventricular hypertrophy.[M4] There can be left atrial enlargement and changes of pulmonary venous hypertension due to the presence of associated mitral valve regurgitation; the appearance is then more suggestive of primary mitral disease. Findings of left heart failure can occur when the obstruction becomes severe.

Pericardial Disease

The normal pericardium is seldom identified on plain chest radiographs. It may be visible as a sharp line at the cardiac apex outlined by epicardial and mediastinal fat.

PERICARDIAL EFFUSION. A pericardial stripe wider than 2 mm paralleling the lower heart border, usually in the lateral projection, and best identified in the sternophrenic angle is diagnostic of a pericardial effusion (see Fig. 8–6*B*, *C*).[K3, L1] This sign is easily overlooked but has been reported to be positive in up to 53 percent of adults and 83 percent of children with pericardial effusions.[C3, S6] The only clue to a relatively small effusion may be a noticeable change in heart size compared with that on prior films. The classic "water flask" configuration of a large effusion may not be present, and the appearance of the cardiac silhouette may be identical to that in a dilated cardiomyopathy with no significant distortion other than enlargement. A large heart with a prominent superior vena cava and azygous vein combined with decreased pulmonary vasculature should raise the question of cardiac tamponade. Acutely, a relatively small effusion can cause tamponade with minimal enlargement of the cardiac shadow.

PERICARDIAL CALCIFICATION. Constrictive pericarditis may occur as the end result of pericarditis and pericardial effusion of any etiology. Calcification of the pericardium is highly suggestive but not pathognomonic of constrictive pericarditis. Approximately 50 percent of patients with constrictive pericarditis do not show calcifications on the plain chest film or fluoroscopy.[C4] Calcifications are frequently found on the anterior and diaphragmatic surfaces but may be over any part of the heart (Fig. 8–19). Often best seen on the lateral view, linear or plaque-like calcifications are typically projected over the right ventricle or the atrioventricular groove. The entire heart may appear encased in a shell. The calcification may be quite dense and thick.

PERICARDIAL DEFECTS. Congenital or surgical absence of the pericardium may result in changes in the cardiac contours. Congenital absence is more commonly left sided and rarely right sided. Partial defects may allow a portion of the heart (usually the left atrial appendage in congenital defects) to herniate outside the pericardial sac with the herniated portion producing a bulge in the contour of the heart.[C5, C6] "Complete" absence of the pericardium is actually a unilateral defect and nearly always left sided. The heart appears shifted to the left without tracheal shift. The left cardiac contour has an elongated appearance. The pulmonary artery often appears prominent and sharply defined. A somewhat similar appearance is seen on the frontal projection when the heart is rotated secondary to chest wall compression in patients with pectus excavatum deformity.

Cardiac Masses

The role of the plain chest radiograph in the identification of cardiac masses is often limited. Radiologic manifestations are dependent on tumor size and location as well as type. With many intracavitary and intramural tumors of even moderate size, no changes are seen on plain films unless hemodynamic alterations are produced, such as the mimicking of mitral stenosis by a left atrial myxoma.[A4] Left ventricular aneurysms, pericardial cysts, extracardiac mediastinal masses, and loculated pericardial effusions are all common causes of abnormal contours that can be indistinguishable from neoplasms (Fig. 8–20). The presence of calcification may help in the detection of a mass, but calcification patterns are not specific and differentiation from calcification of thrombus or normal structures usually requires additional imaging modalities.

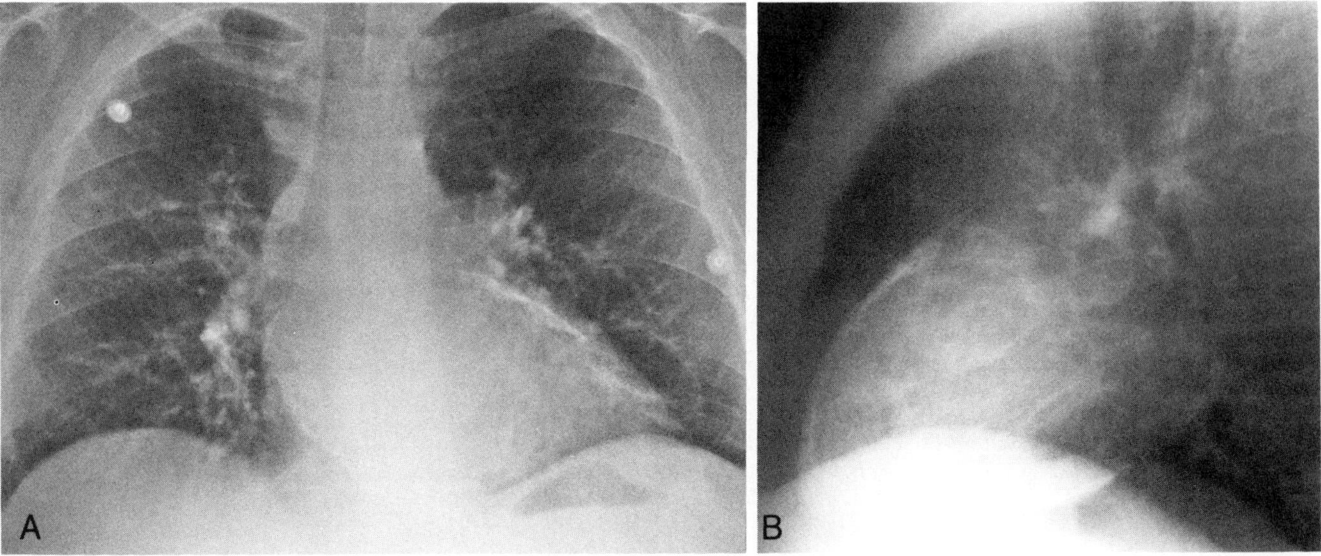

Figure 8–19. *A*, Posteroanterior and *B*, lateral chest radiographs of a patient with secondary hyperparathyroidism and renal failure with calcific pericarditis. Calcification is seen outlining the heart but without specific signs of pericardial constriction on the chest radiograph.

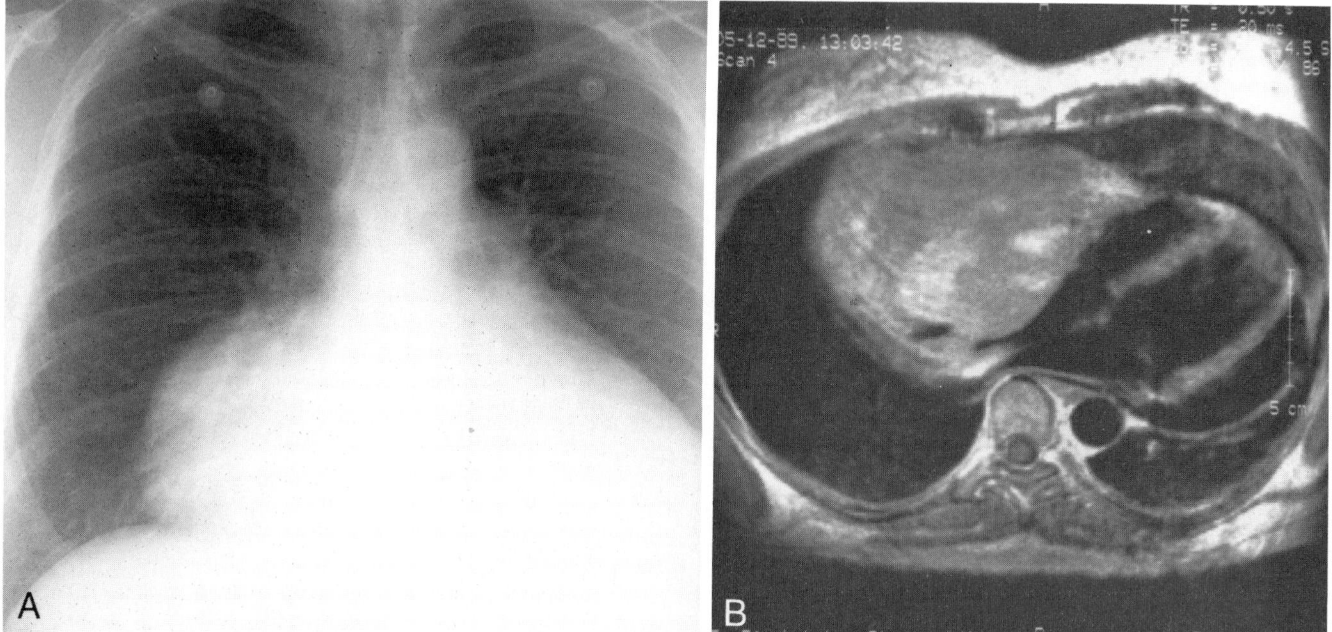

Figure 8–20. *A*, Posteroanterior chest radiograph and *B*, spin-echo image from an ECG-gated magnetic resonance image of a 40-year-old woman with a history of palpitations and a large angiosarcoma invading the free wall of the right atrium. The chest radiograph demonstrates a markedly enlarged cardiac contour with an abnormal configuration of the enlarged right heart. The overall enlarged heart is due in part to the pericardial effusion confirmed on the magnetic resonance image. A large infiltrating mass arising from the lateral wall of the right atrium and right ventricle and extending to encase the inferior vena cava is demonstrated on the magnetic resonance image.

Aortic Disease

The aortic knob, representing the foreshortened transverse aortic arch, is the only border-forming portion of the normal thoracic aorta that is otherwise hidden within the mediastinum.[G2] The descending thoracic aorta parallels the thoracic spine on the left and is delineated on a plain chest radiograph by the pleural reflection from the left side of the spine over the descending aorta. With the development of atherosclerotic aortic disease, unfolding and ectasia (dilatation and elongation) of the aorta occur. The left paraspinal line becomes displaced to the left. As the descending aorta swings into the left chest, more and more of the contour becomes silhouetted by lung; on the lateral projection a portion of the descending aorta may be demon-

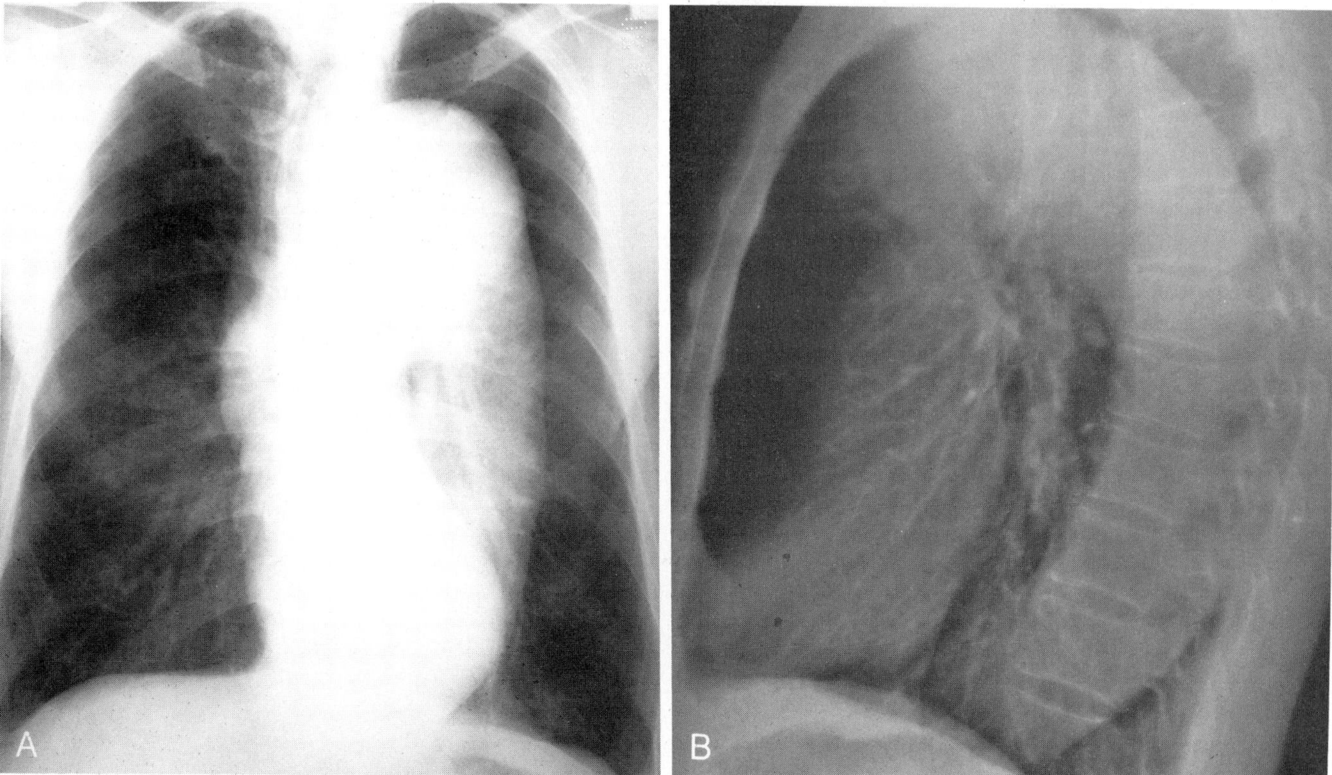

Figure 8–21. *A*, Posteroanterior and *B*, lateral chest radiographs of a 50-year-old with a chronic type B aortic dissection demonstrating widening of the superior mediastinum with displacement of the trachea and marked enlargement of the aortic knob *(A)*. The aneurysm extends to involve the descending thoracic aorta with marked displacement of the left paraspinal line *(B)*.

strated, and only then is a clue to the presence of an aneurysm obtained. Unfolding or ectasia of the ascending aorta produces a convexity of the right superior mediastinum. These findings may be indistinguishable from those present with an aortic aneurysm (Fig. 8–21). The most common finding of an aortic aneurysm on a frontal chest radiograph is widening of the superior mediastinum. Other chest film findings suggestive of a thoracic aortic aneurysm, whether atherosclerotic, luetic, dissecting, or traumatic, include displacement and/or compression of the trachea and esophagus either to the left and posteriorly by an ascending aortic aneurysm or to the right and anteriorly by an aneurysm of the descending aorta. Calcification in the aorta is a common finding in atherosclerotic aortic disease. Displacement of intimal calcification from the outer aortic contour by more than 4 to 10 mm, as seen on the frontal chest radiograph, can be a useful sign of a dissecting hematoma.[E1] Since the aorta is largely hidden within the mediastinal silhouette, the cross-sectional modalities, such as computed tomography and magnetic resonance imaging, are complementary in the evaluation and follow-up of aortic disease.

References

A

1. Arnold, H.R.: Postmyocardial infarction syndrome. AJR 90:628, 1963.
2. Abrams, D.L., Edelist, A., Luria, M.H., et al.: Ventricular aneurysm: A reappraisal based on a study of sixty-five consecutive autopsied cases. Circulation 27:164, 1963.
3. Amplatz, K.: The roentgenographic diagnosis of mitral and aortic valvular disease. Am. Heart J. 64:556, 1962.
4. Abrams, H.L., Adams, D.F., and Grant, H.A.: The radiology of tumors of the heart. Radiol. Clin. North Am. 9:299, 1971.

B

1. Baron, M.G.: Postinfarction aneurysm of the left ventricle. Circulation 43:762, 1971.

C

1. Chen, J.T.T., Behar, V.S., Morris, J.J., et al.: Correlation of roentgen findings with hemodynamic data in pure mitral stenosis. AJR 102:280, 1968.
2. Chen, J.T.T., Robinson, A.E., Goodrich, J.K., et al.: Uneven distribution of pulmonary blood flow between left and right lungs in isolated valvular pulmonary stenosis. AJR 107:343, 1969.
3. Carsky, E.W., Mauceri, R.A., and Azimi, F.: The epicardial fat pad sign. Radiology 137:303, 1980.
4. Cornell, S.H., and Rossi, N.P.: Roentgenographic findings in constrictive pericarditis. AJR 102:301, 1968.
5. Chang, C.H., and Leigh, T.F.: Congenital partial defect of the pericardium associated with herniation of the left atrial appendage. AJR 86:517, 1961.
6. Chang, C.H., and Amory, H.I.: Congenital partial right pericardial defect associated with herniation of the right atrial appendage. Radiology 84:660, 1965.

D

1. Dressler, W.: Postmyocardial infarction syndrome. JAMA 160:1379, 1956.

E

1. Eyler, W.R., and Clark, M.D.: Dissecting aneurysm of the aorta: Roentgen manifestations including a comparison with other types. Radiology 85:1047, 1965.

G

1. Glover, L., Baxley, W.A., and Dodge, H.T.: A quantitative evaluation of heart size measurements from chest roentgenograms. Circulation 47:1289, 1973.
2. Guthaner, D.F.: The plain chest film in assessing aneurysms and dissecting hematomas of the thoracic aorta. Radiology 2:1, 1986.

H

1. Higgins, C.B., Reinke, R.T., Jones, N.E., et al.: Left atrial dimension on the frontal thoracic radiograph: A method for assessing left atrial enlargement. AJR 130:251, 1978.
2. Hoffman, R.B., and Rigler, L.G.: Evaluation of left ventricular enlargement in the lateral projection of the chest. Radiology 85:93, 1965.
3. Hill, C.A., Harle, T.S., and Gaston, W.: Cardiomyopathy: A review of 59 patients with emphasis on the plain chest roentgenogram. AJR 104:433, 1968.

K

1. Keats, T.E., and Enge, I.P.: Cardiac mensuration by the cardiac volume method. Radiology 85:850, 1965.
2. Klatte, E.C., Tampas, J.P., Campbell, J.A., et al.: The roentgenographic manifestations of aortic stenosis and aortic valvular insufficiency. AJR 88:57, 1962.
3. Kremens, V.: Demonstration of the pericardial shadow on the routine chest roentgenogram: A new roentgen finding: preliminary report. Radiology 64:72, 1955.

L

1. Lane, E.J., and Carsky, E.W.: Epicardial fat: Lateral plain film analysis in normals and in pericardial effusion. Radiology 91(1):1, 1968.

M

1. Margolis, J.R., Chen, J.T.T., Kong, Y., et al.: The diagnostic and prognostic significance of coronary artery calcification. Radiology 137:609, 1980.
2. Milne, E.N.C.: Some new concepts of pulmonary blood flow and volume. Radiol. Clin. North Am. 16:515, 1978.
3. Milne, E.N.C.: Correlation of physiologic findings with chest roentgenology. Radiol. Clin. North Am. 11:17, 1973.
4. Morrow, A.G., Lambrew, C.T., and Braunwald, E.: Idiopathic hypertrophic subaortic stenosis: Operative treatment and the results of pre- and postoperative hemodynamic evaluations. Circulation 29:120, 1964.

S

1. Simon, M.: The pulmonary vessels: Their hemodynamic evaluation using routine radiographs. Radiol. Clin. North Am. 11:363, 1963.
2. Soulen, R.L., and Freeman, E.: Radiologic evaluation of myocardial infarction. Radiol. Clin. North Am. 9:567, 1971.
3. Spindola-Franco, H., Fish, B.G., Dachman, A., et al.: Recognition of bicuspid aortic valve by plain film calcification. AJR 139:867, 1982.
4. Shaw, D.R., Chen, J.T.T., and Lester, R.G.: X-ray appearance and clinical significance of left atrial wall calcification. Invest. Radiol. 11:501, 1976.
5. Steiner, R.E.: The roentgen features of the cardiomyopathies. Semin. Roentgenol. 4:311, 1969.
6. Spooner, E.W., Kuhns, L.R., and Stern, A.M.: Diagnosis of pericardial effusion in children: A new radiographic sign. AJR 128:23, 1977.

Chapter 9

Cardiac Angiography

FLORENCE H. SHEEHAN, M.D.

ANGIOGRAPHIC TECHNIQUE 109
QUALITATIVE ASSESSMENT OF THE CONTRAST LEFT VENTRICULOGRAM 110
QUANTITATIVE ANALYSIS OF THE CONTRAST LEFT VENTRICULOGRAM: VOLUME DETERMINATION 110
Volume Determination in Theory 110
Volume Determination in Practice 118
Parameters Derived from Volume Measurements 122
Volumes, Indices, and Output 122
Ejection Fraction 122
Regurgitant Flow and Valve Areas 122
Left Ventricular Mass and Stress 123
QUANTITATIVE ANALYSIS OF REGIONAL LEFT VENTRICULAR WALL MOTION 124
Wall Motion Analysis in Theory 124
Methods of Wall Motion Analysis 124
Assumptions in Methods of Wall Motion Analysis 127
Parameters of Regional Function 129
Definition of Abnormal Motion 131
Variability 132
Measuring Wall Motion in the Region of Interest 132
Method Selection: Theoretical, Empirical, and Clinical Considerations 134
APPLICATIONS OF QUANTITATIVE ANALYSIS .. 134
Normal Values 134
Ventricular Function in Coronary Artery Disease 135
Measurement of Left Ventricular Function as a Diagnostic Tool: Relationship Between Coronary Artery Stenosis Severity and Function 135
Stress Ventriculography: Assessment of Cardiac Reserve and Viability 135
Assessment of Myocardial Viability 135
Left Ventricular Function in Acute Myocardial Infarction: Abnormalities in the Infarct Region 135
Wall Motion Remote From an Infarction 137
Time Course of Functional Recovery After Infarction 137
Ventricular Function as a Predictor of Survival 138
Evaluating Response to Therapeutic Intervention 138
Theoretical Considerations 138
Timing of Measurements 138
Parameter Selection 138
FURTHER APPLICATIONS OF ANGIOGRAPHIC ANALYSIS 139
Right Ventriculography 139
Analysis of Left Ventricular Function Throughout the Cardiac Cycle 139
Global Function 139
Regional Function 140

Contrast cineangiography provides visualization of the projected image of a cardiac chamber, from which assessment can be made of its dimensions and shape through the phases of the cardiac cycle. Left ventriculography is performed routinely; right ventriculography may be added if necessary. Angiographic studies of the atria can be performed, and methods have been developed for calculation of right or left atrial volume and function, but these are outside the scope of clinical practice.

From subjective evaluation of the angiogram, a trained observer can estimate chamber size and function, grade the severity of valvular regurgitation, and search for pathognomonic findings. Beginning in the late 1950's, quantitative techniques have been developed for measurement of chamber volume, ejection fraction, and wall motion and of regurgitation valve flow. The advent and accessibility of high-speed computers made it possible to combine angiographic dimension data with high-fidelity pressure measurement for analysis of stroke work and diastolic function. The results derived from ventriculographic analysis are useful in determining the functional status of the patient's heart and the degree of compensation, gauging response to therapy, and assessing prognosis. Furthermore, quantitative analysis of ventricular function provides a reproducible, prognosis-related end point for clinical trials.

ANGIOGRAPHIC TECHNIQUE

The goal is to obtain images of the chamber, contracting in normal sinus rhythm, of adequate contrast quality to allow confident identification of the endocardial contour throughout the cardiac cycle.

The left ventricle is most commonly imaged by injecting contrast agent directly into that chamber. Alternative routes are injection into the right side of the heart with filming of the levo phase when contrast agent has passed through the pulmonary vessels, the left atrium, and into the left ventricle; injection directly into the left atrium via transseptal catheterization; and injection into the ascending aorta in patients with aortic regurgitation.

A pigtail catheter is usually preferred, as the unwinding of the catheter tip absorbs and distributes the force of injection and prevents inadvertent damage by intramyocardial injection of contrast agent. Placing the catheter in the inflow tract or reducing the acceleration in the flow of contrast agent from the injector will minimize ectopy.[H1] In some patients, particularly those studied during acute myocardial infarction, it may be helpful to perform a small test injection of 5 to 10 ml to evaluate chamber opacification as well as irritability.

The volume and rate of injection needed for adequate opacification of the left ventricle depend on the size of the chamber, the heart rate, and the function of the heart and valves. Patients with hypercontractile hearts, tachycardia, or mitral or aortic regurgitation require a higher volume and rate of injection. Conversely, in patients with poor ventricular function or low forward cardiac output, circulation is poor and contrast agent is slowly cleared, so less is required. Hildner and associates have shown that good-quality ventriculograms can be achieved in cases in which the tolerable contrast volume is reduced by injecting at low flow rates through a six-hole catheter in the apex.[H1]

Images are usually acquired on 35-mm cine film at a rate of 30 or 60 frames per second. The higher rate allows more precise selection of the end-diastolic and end-systolic frames and is particularly desirable if the heart rate is high or if frame-by-frame analysis of function throughout the cardiac cycle will be performed. The projection or view is most commonly 30 degrees right anterior oblique (RAO), which allows visualization of the left ventricle at full length without foreshortening or overlap of the heart with the spine, as occurs with the anteroposterior (AP) view. Views orthogonal to these provide additional information about regional function, which may be of use in evaluating patients with ischemic heart disease. For instance, hypokinesis due to stenosis of the circumflex coronary artery is better appreciated in the 60-degree left anterior oblique (LAO) view than in the 30-degree RAO view.[S1]

QUALITATIVE ASSESSMENT OF THE CONTRAST LEFT VENTRICULOGRAM

Visual inspection of the cineventriculogram provides an impression of chamber dimension and performance and of valvular function and may reveal structural pathology.

The shape of the normal left ventricle in diastole is elliptical (Fig. 9–1) and has been likened to the shape of an avocado. Following atrial systole, which is evident from the abrupt final expansion of the contour, contraction begins. There is normally some asynchrony[R1] with the anterior and inferior walls moving inward before the apex, but the difference in timing is barely perceptible. With systole, the papillary muscles thicken and may become prominent. Normality in regional function is assessed from the uniform inward motion of all the walls in systole (Fig. 9–2) and their uniform outward motion in diastole. With experience, one develops a mental composite image of the "normal" ventriculogram.

Abnormality in ventricular volume can be appreciated from the extent to which the chamber filled with contrast agent fills the image field and from the shape of the ventricle. In ventricular dilatation associated with depressed ventricular performance, the ventricle assumes a more spherical shape as wall stresses become more evenly distributed (Fig. 9–3).[D1] In patients with hyperkinesis due to hypertrophic cardiomyopathy, the diastolic volume is normal or small but the end-systolic volume may be reduced nearly to the point of "cavity obliteration" at the apex (Fig. 9–4).

Abnormality in ventricular function may be either diffuse or regional, affecting only part of the ventricular contour. Diffuse dysfunction can result from ischemic heart disease, valvular dysfunction, or cardiomyopathy. Depression of regional wall motion usually indicates the presence of coronary artery disease, occurring in the ischemic region, although it has been reported in valvular disease of rheumatic origin.[T1] For the purpose of semiquantitative assessment, the ventricular contour is commonly divided into segments whose motion is graded individually. Based on the original definitions by Herman and associates, motion is classified as normal, hypokinetic if wall motion is reduced, akinetic if the wall is motionless, or dyskinetic if the segment displays paradoxic outward motion during systole.[H2] If numeric values are assigned to each grade, their sum over all the segments provides a so-called wall motion score, which indicates the circumferential extent of dysfunction. Such visual assessment of the size and function of the left ventricle can be used to gauge surgical risk and prognosis in patients with coronary artery disease.[K1]

Asynchrony or abnormal timing of wall motion can also be appreciated from a visual inspection of the ventriculogram.[H2] Patients with ischemia or infarction may have a discoordinate contraction pattern if the inward motion of the affected region is delayed into early diastole, when normally perfused regions are relaxing.[H3]

Although contrast ventriculography is not the primary tool for diagnosing mitral regurgitation, the retrograde filling of the left atrium by contrast agent from the left ventricle has been used for many years to grade the severity of mitral regurgitation. Thus, a jet of contrast agent that enters the left atrium but clears immediately is assigned grade 1, light atrial opacification as grade 2, atrial opacification equal to that of the ventricle as grade 3, and denser opacification of the atrium than of the ventricle as grade 4 (Fig. 9–5). In patients with left atrial dilatation, the subjective grade may be underestimated because of dilution of contrast. The artifactual appearance of mitral regurgitation may result from poor catheter placement near or even across the valve or from arrhythmia. In mitral valve prolapse, the valve can be seen to balloon into the atrium during systole (Fig. 9–6).

Other valve disease entities may also result in ventriculographic abnormalities, but of a less specific or diagnostic nature. Mitral stenosis is associated with a small but normally functioning ventricle. In patients with aortic stenosis, the severity of hypertrophy may be appreciable from the thickness of the anterior wall, where the epicardium is most visible.[H4] Limitation of aortic valve motion or calcification or thickening of the leaflets may also be appreciable. Aortic regurgitation is, of course, evident from the reflux across the valve (Fig. 9–7) but also results in left ventricular dilatation and hypertrophy.

On inspection of the ventriculogram, other pathology may be visible. Filling defects due to intraventricular thrombi are not uncommon in patients with a large contraction defect or aneurysm due to myocardial infarction. In a patient in whom ventricular septal defect is suspected, ventriculography in the 45-degree LAO view may show a systolic passage of contrast agent into the right heart. Transmural myocardial infarction involving the anteroapical wall is the most frequent cause of left ventricular aneurysm (Fig. 9–8), a condition in which part of the ventricle is dyskinetic. The paradoxic motion of the aneurysm reduces the efficiency of the heart because blood is sequestered in the aneurysm instead of being ejected.

QUANTITATIVE ANALYSIS OF THE CONTRAST LEFT VENTRICULOGRAM: VOLUME DETERMINATION

Although much information can be gleaned from a subjective assessment of the ventriculogram, quantitative analysis is recommended for its accuracy and reproducibility as well as for the increased information content. When the end-diastolic and end-systolic endocardial contours have been delineated, it is possible to calculate rapidly the end-diastolic, end-systolic, and stroke volumes; cardiac output; ejection fraction; and wall motion. The only adjustment to the cardiac catheterization routine needed is either filming of a grid at the end of the procedure or performance of biplane ventriculography with a banded catheter to correct for magnification.

Because of its accuracy, volume determination by contrast ventriculography is the gold standard by which other imaging modalities are judged. The agreement between volumes calculated from ventriculographic images by the area-length method,[D2] and the true volumes of postmortem hearts filled with barium paste was close: $r = 0.995$, standard error of the estimate $= 8.2$ ml (Fig. 9–9). The accuracy of angiographic stroke volume determination in vivo was demonstrated by comparison with volumes measured by Fick's method or the indicator dilution technique (Fig. 9–10).[H5]

Whether this level of accuracy is achieved outside the research laboratory depends on both theoretic and practical considerations. First, the method used to calculate volume contains inherent assumptions about the geometry of the ventricle. Second, corrections must be made for the volume of the papillary muscles and trabeculae and for magnification and distortion in the imaging chain. Finally, the element of human error must be taken into consideration.

Volume Determination in Theory

In the area-length method, volume is calculated as if the left ventricle were an ellipsoid of revolution (see Fig. 9–1). The

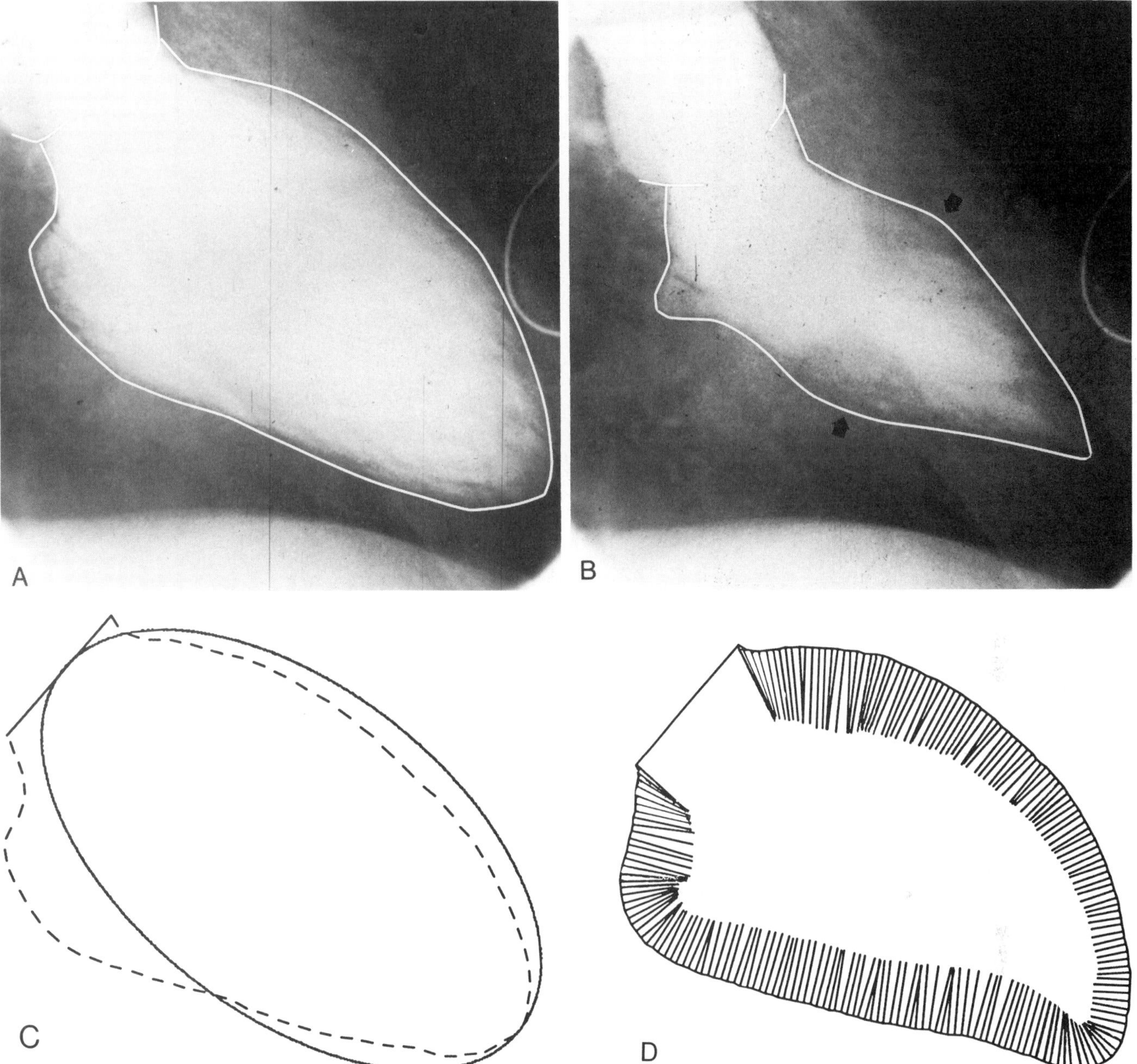

Figure 9–1. Contrast ventriculogram (30 degrees RAO) of a patient with normal cardiac function and anatomy at end-diastole *(A)* and end-systole *(B)*. The papillary muscles, visible only at end-systole *(arrows)* are included in the chamber volume when tracing the endocardial contour. Chamber volume is calculated by comparing the contour to an ellipse of equivalent area and long axis length (*C*, end-diastole only). Normal wall motion was calculated as the mean motion for 52 patients with normal cardiac anatomy and function *(D)*.

diameter (D) of the contour is calculated from the area (A) and the long axis length (L):

$$D = \frac{4A}{\pi L}$$

Volume (V) is calculated as

$$V = \frac{\pi}{6} LD_aD_b$$

where D_a and D_b are the diameters of two orthogonal projections and L is the length of the longer long axis.

Biplane ventriculography is most commonly performed in the 30-degree RAO and 60-degree LAO projections. Because the long axis is frequently foreshortened in the straight LAO view (Fig. 9–11), however, addition of 15 to 30 degrees cranial angulation has been advocated.[A1, R2] The diameters D_a and D_b are similar in orthogonal projections, so volume can be accurately determined from single-plane ventriculograms in 30-degree RAO or AP projections.[K2, S2]

Most of the other methods proposed for determining left ventricular volume have proved to be less accurate. The exception employs Simpson's rule, whose accuracy is comparable to that of the area-length method, despite the more complex computation required. The accuracy or validity of the area-length method may

Text continued on page 118

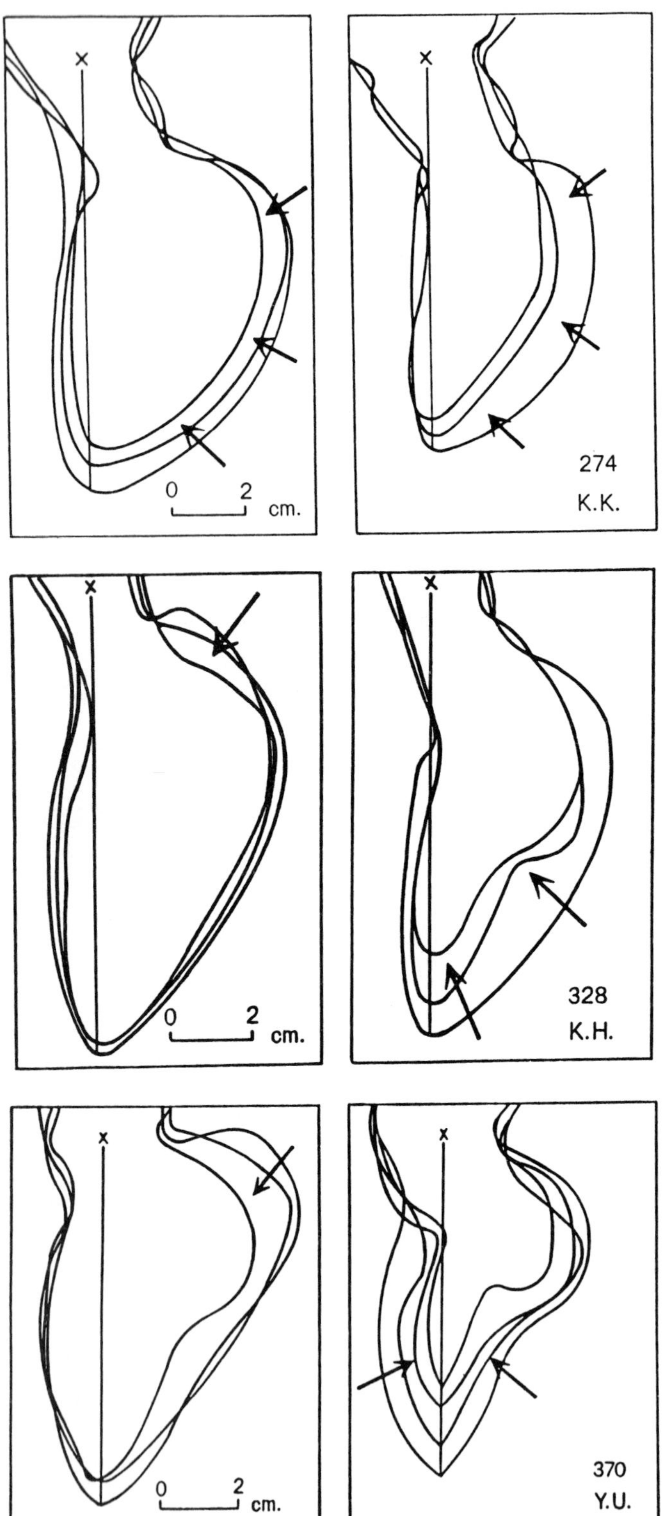

Figure 9–2. Left ventricular endocardial contours in the 60-degree left anterior oblique view in subjects with a normal heart *(top)*, mitral regurgitation *(middle)*, or hypertrophic cardiomyopathy *(bottom)*. Panels at the left display the contours at end-diastole and 50 msec and 100 msec later. Panels at the right display contours from the second 100 msec after end-diastole. The normal subject has uniform inward motion. In the two patients with heart disease, motion begins at the base and apical contraction is delayed. (From Ueda, H., Ueda, K., Morooka, S., et al.: A cineangiocardiographic study of the regional contraction sequence of the normal and diseased left ventricle in man. Jap. Heart J. 10:95, 1969, with permission.)

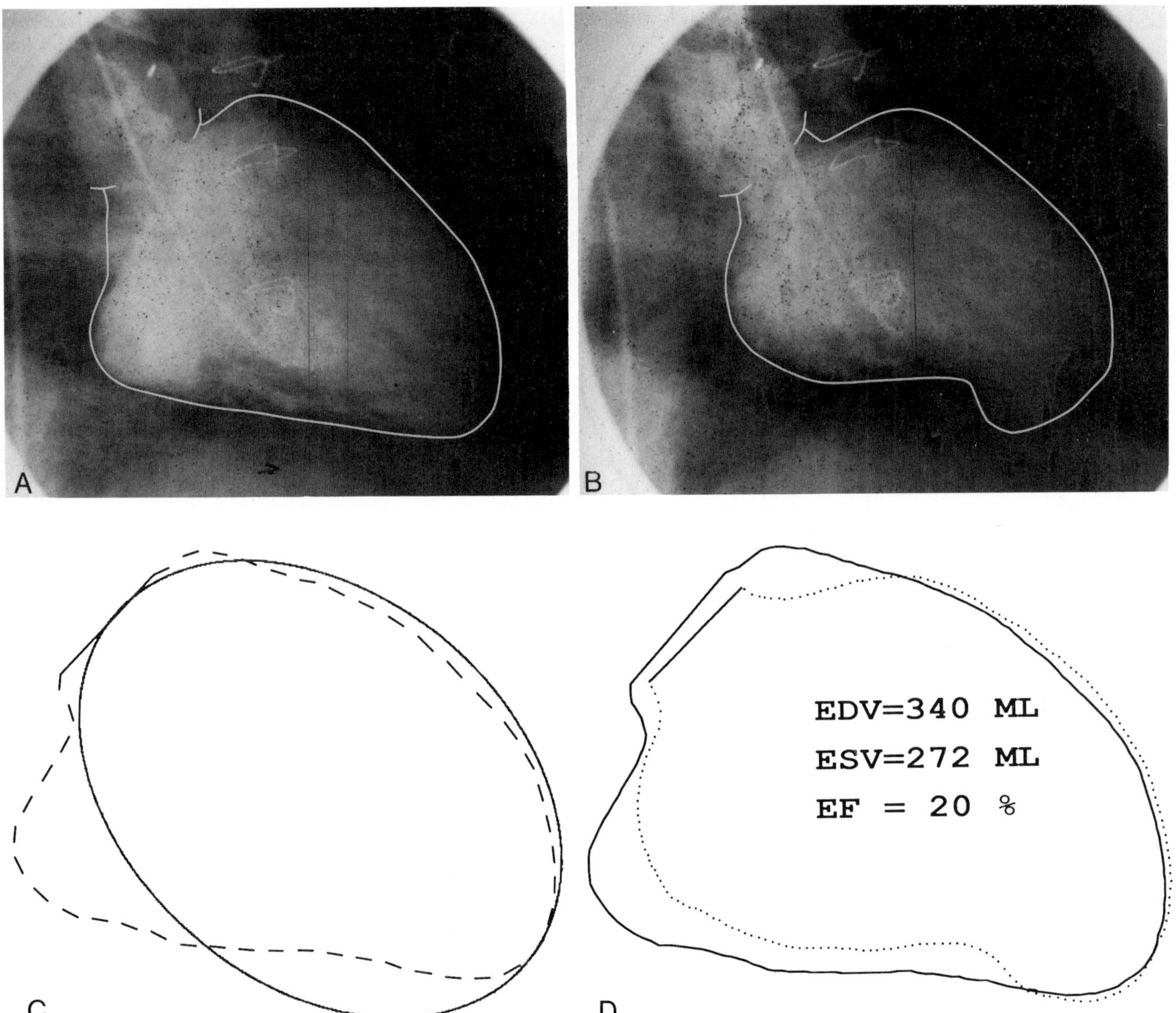

Figure 9–3. Ventriculogram (30 degrees RAO) at end-diastole *(A)* and end-systole *(B)* of a patient with left ventricular dilatation and congestive heart failure due to acute myocardial infarction and three-vessel coronary artery disease. The ventricle is more spherical than normal *(C)*, the ejection fraction is reduced, and there is anteroapical akinesis *(D)*.

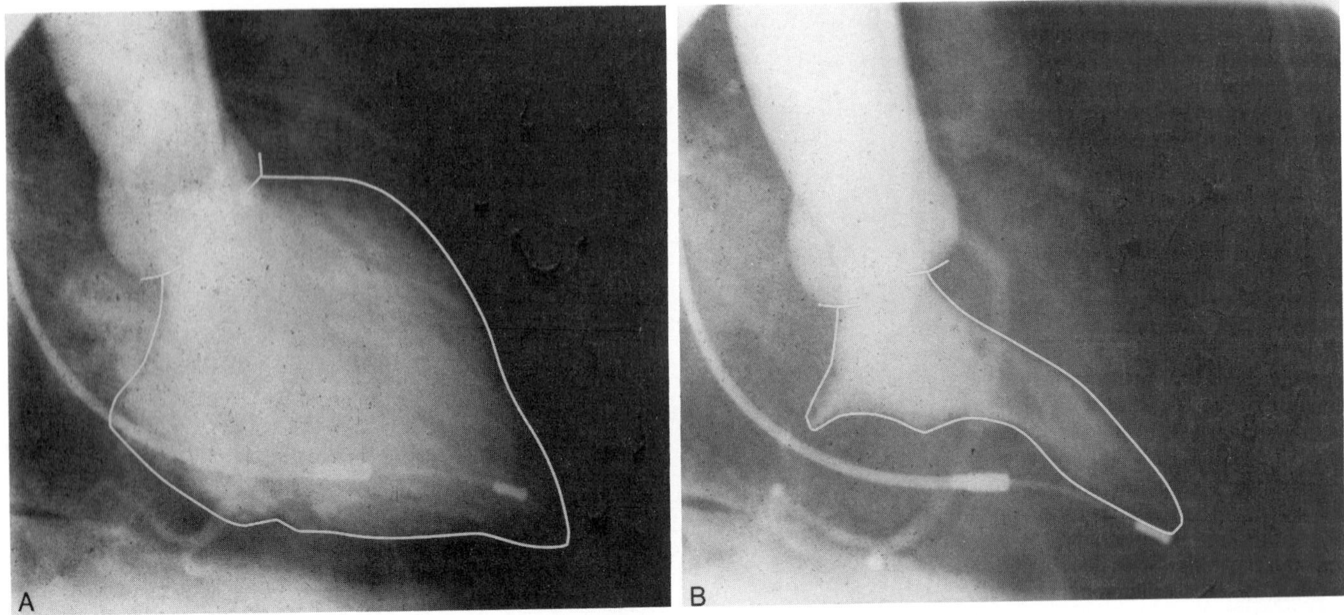

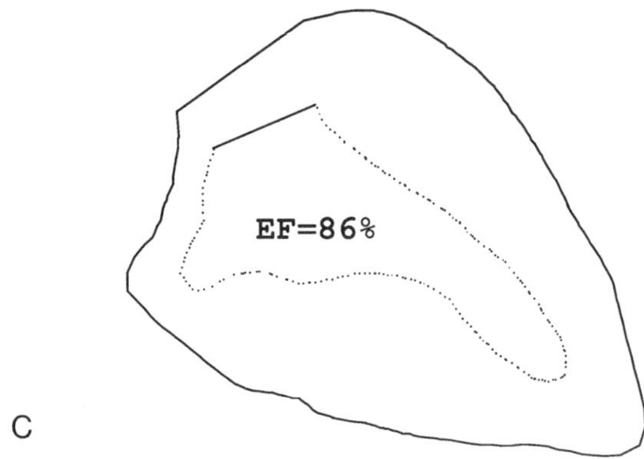

Figure 9–4. *A*, Ventriculogram (30 degrees RAO) of a patient with hypertrophic cardiomyopathy at end-diastole. *B*, At end-systole, there is "cavity obliteration." *C*, The ejection fraction is elevated.

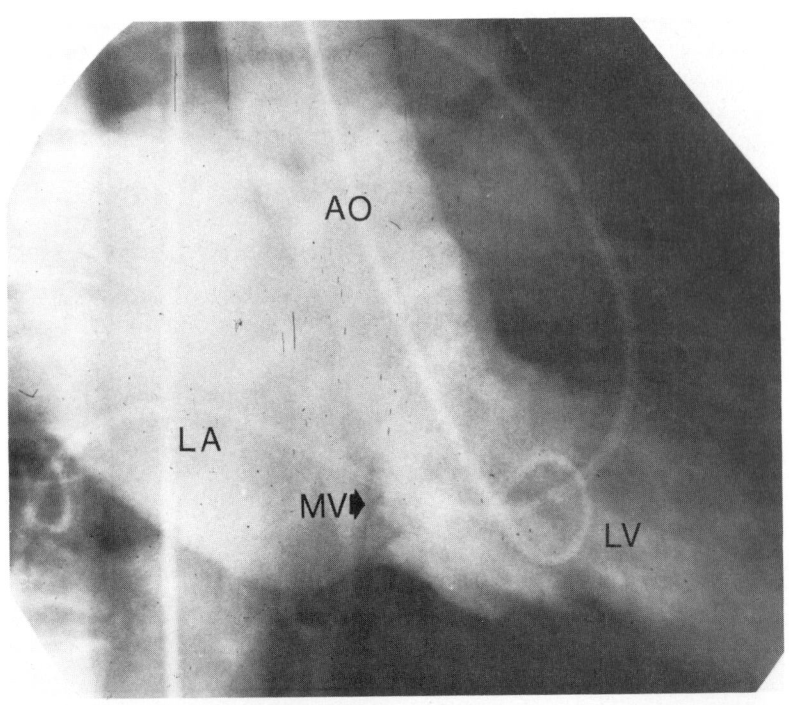

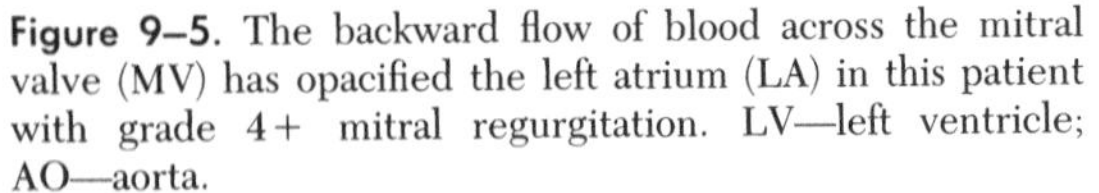

Figure 9–5. The backward flow of blood across the mitral valve (MV) has opacified the left atrium (LA) in this patient with grade 4+ mitral regurgitation. LV—left ventricle; AO—aorta.

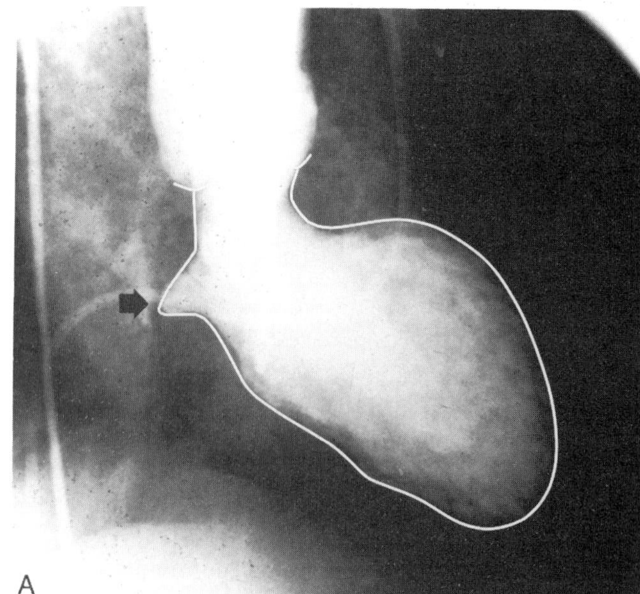

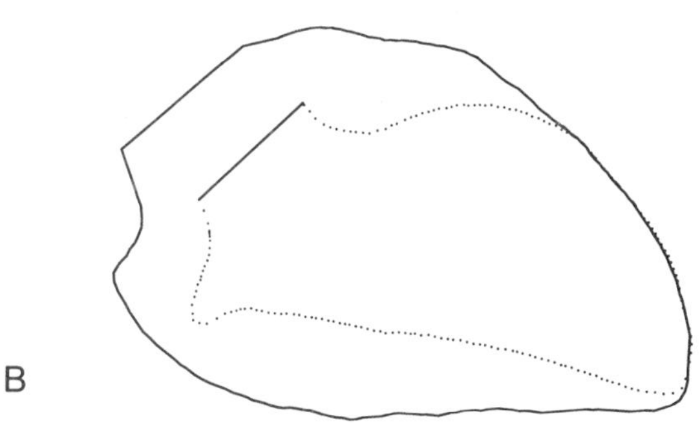

Figure 9–6. *A*, Mitral valve prolapse is evident at end-systole *(arrow)*. *B*, The end-diastolic contour is normal. The view is 30 degrees RAO.

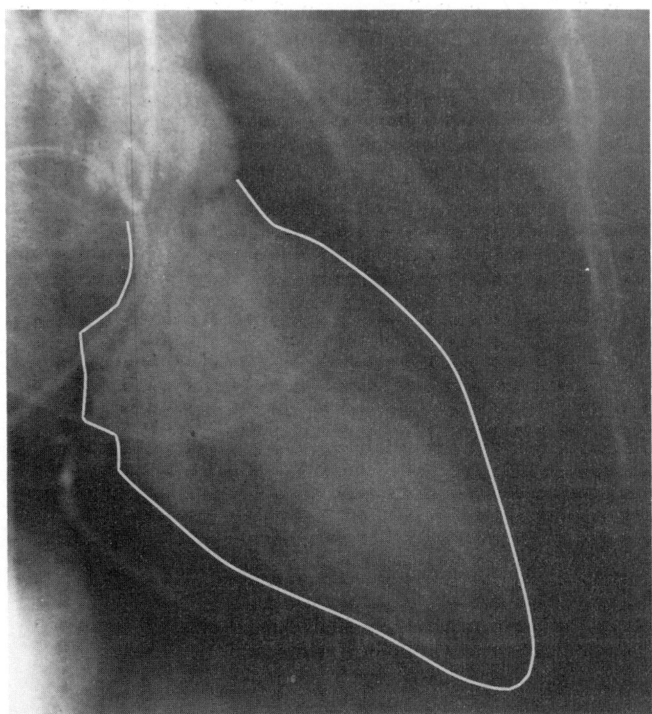

Figure 9–7. In aortic valvular regurgitation, contrast agent injected into the aortic root opacifies the left ventricle.

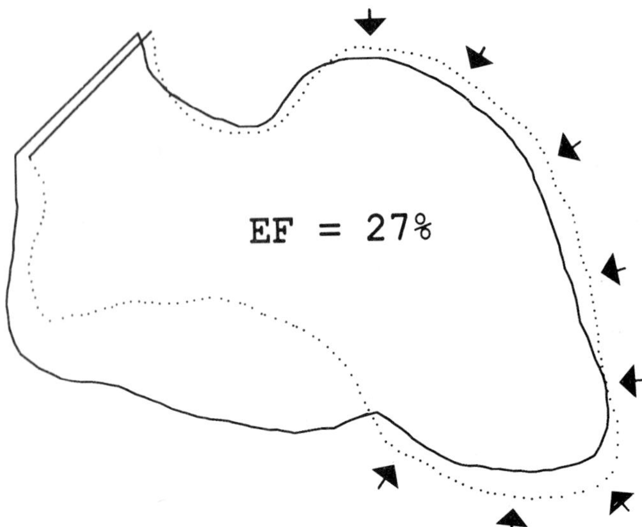

Figure 9–8. End-diastolic and end-systolic contours (30 degrees RAO) of a patient with aneurysm due to recent anterior myocardial infarction. There is dyskinesis around the anteroapical region *(arrows)*.

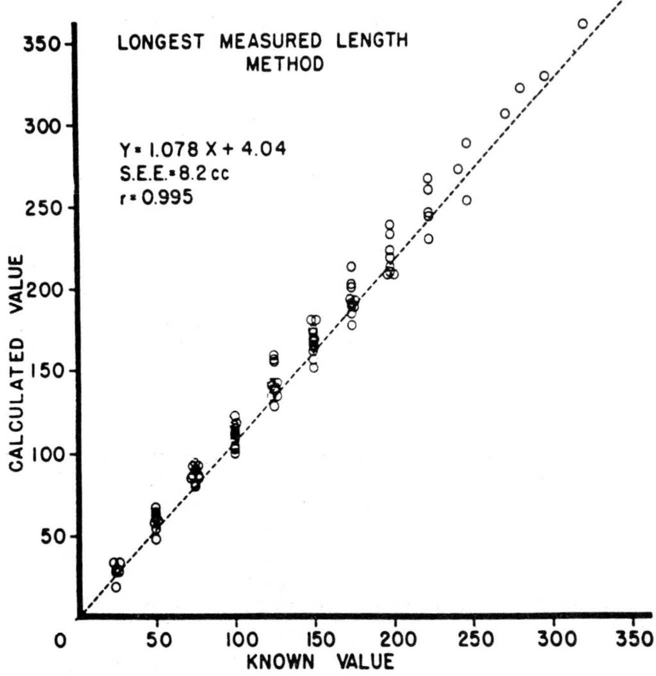

Figure 9–9. The area-length method of measuring left ventricular chamber volume was validated by comparing the volume calculated from angiograms of barium-filled heart casts with the true volume of these hearts. (From Dodge, H.T., Sandler, H., Balew, D.W., Lord, J.D., Jr.: The use of biplane angiocardiography for the measurement of left ventricular volume in man. Am. Heart J. 60:762, 1960, with permission.)

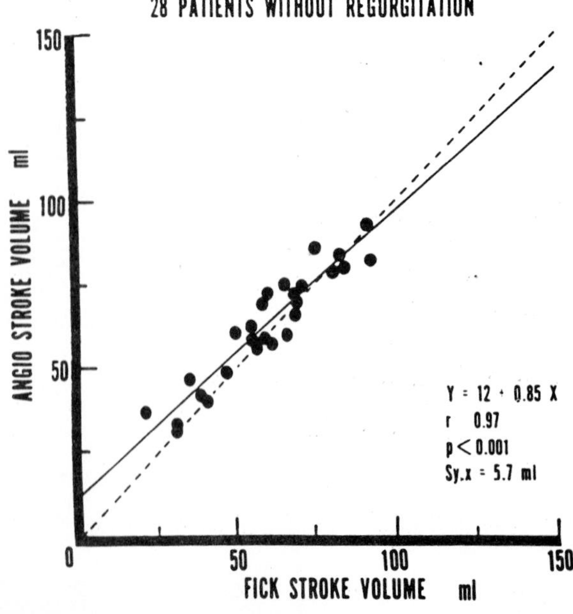

Figure 9–10. The area-length method of volume determination has been further validated in vivo by comparing the angiographic stroke volume against that measured by the Fick technique. (From Hunt, D., Baxley, W.A., Kennedy, J.W., et al.: Quantitative evaluation of cineaortography in the assessment of aortic regurgitation. Am. J. Cardiol. 31:696, 1973, with permission.)

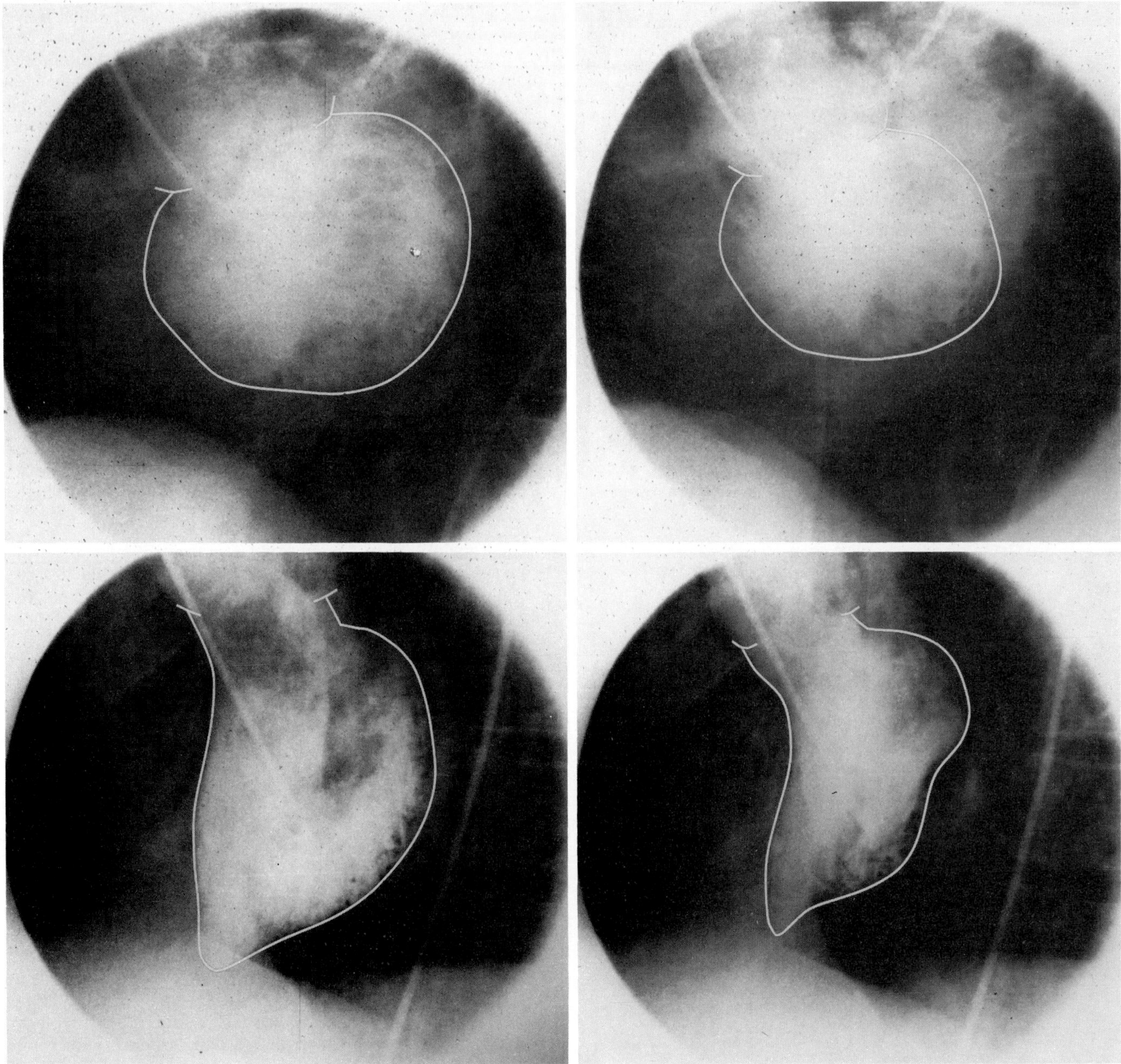

Figure 9–11. End-diastolic *(left)* and end-systolic *(right)* contours in the 60-degree LAO view of two patients. When the left ventricle is foreshortened *(top)*, the motion of the apex cannot be assessed. In order to visualize the full length of the ventricle *(bottom)*, some angiographers advocate addition of cranial angulation.

appear questionable for grossly abnormal ventricles such as those with aneurysms. However, despite its inherent assumption of an ellipsoidal chamber, the area-length method has proved accurate for determining the volume of the right ventricle, right atrium, and left atrium.[C1, L1, S3]

The papillary muscles, trabeculae carneae, and chordae tendineae occupy a volume that is not calculable. Instead, correction is made by using regression equations.[D2, K2, W1] Correction must also be made for magnification in the imaging chain, which includes magnification when projecting the cine film for tracing, and for pincushion distortion. This correction is most easily accomplished by filming a grid of known dimension placed at the level of the patient's heart with the imaging equipment positioned and set as it was during ventriculography (Fig. 9–12). Such grids are commercially available but can be made by embedding fine wires at 1-cm intervals in a 10 × 10 cm Plexiglas plate. The heart may be assumed to be at midchest level. When the cineventriculogram is projected for tracing, the size of the grid is measured and compared with the true grid size. The correction factor is calculated as the ratio of the number of grid squares to the measured span of grid squares.[K3] As magnification increases, the correction factor decreases. Since this factor is applied to diameter and long axis lengths, the correction is cubed.[D2] If volume is calculated from a biplane ventriculogram, a grid must be filmed for each projection and correction factors calculated and applied to the dimensions measured in each projection. Alternatively, a pigtail catheter with metallic bands at known spacing can be employed and a correction factor determined trigonometrically.[C1] Variations in the procedure used to determine the correction factor affect the volume calculation in proportion to the magnification made and the size of the left ventricle.[S4]

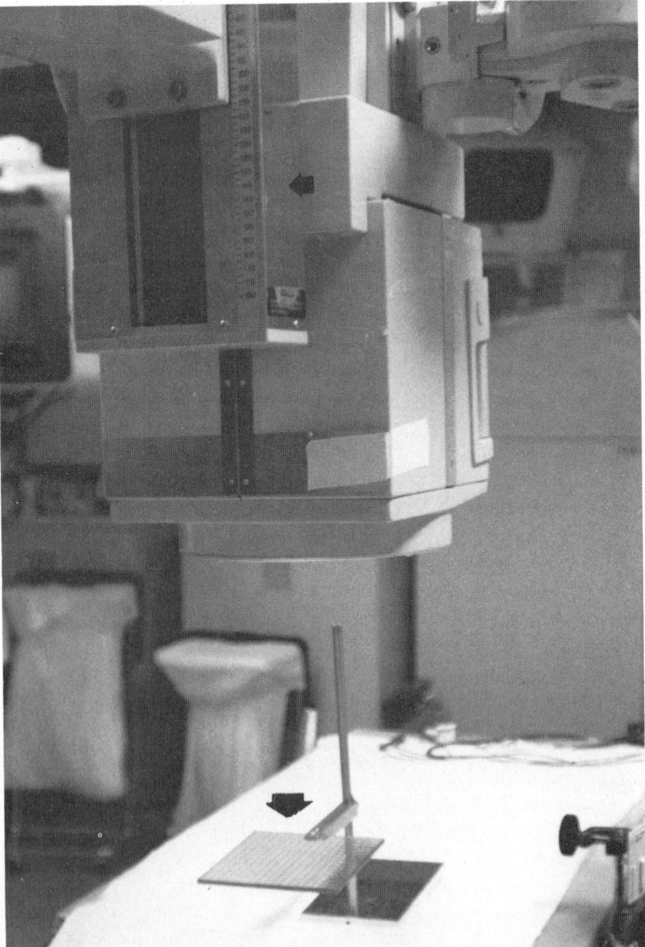

Figure 9–12. The calibration grid is filmed at the level of the patient's midchest *(large arrow)*. The height of the image intensifier is recorded at the time ventriculography is performed *(small arrow)* so that the equipment can be returned to this position to film the grid.

Volume Determination in Practice

In practice, the accuracy of volume determination is influenced by technical factors such as image quality and the care with which the endocardial contours are traced. The combined influence of these factors is usually assessed in terms of the variability or reproducibility of volume determination.

Studies have shown that interobserver variability—that is, the mean absolute difference in volume determination when two people analyze the same ventriculogram—ranges from 6.6 to 20 ml for end-diastolic volume, 5.7 to 10 ml for end-systolic volume (Fig. 9–13), and 4 to 5 percent for ejection fraction.[C2, C3, D3, R3] Both beat-to-beat variability and intraobserver variability, which is measured between repeated analyses by the same observer, are similarly low.[C2, D3] However, study-to-study variability is considerably greater, even when measured from serial ventriculograms of clinically stable patients.[C2] This variability may be due to differences in hemodynamic state in addition to variability in tracing the ventricular contours; for example, pacing to different heart rates alters volume and ejection fraction.[R4] It is probably advisable to have the same observer trace serial ventriculograms to avoid worsening study-to-study variability by the addition of interobserver variability.

Quantitative analysis requires higher-quality images than qualitative assessment, simply because the projector must be stopped for tracing. Visual assessment is performed with the projector running and thus is aided by the visual integration of motion. The ability to track the motion of the endocardial contour allows the observer to estimate ventricular dimensions and function even from poor-quality images in which the contour is unidentifiable when the images are viewed singly.

The capabilities of the imaging system are, of course, the primary determinant of image quality. The most skilled angiographic technique cannot compensate for an x-ray system that has too little power to penetrate the patient or magnification modes so high that the ventricle does not fit into the imaging field.

With adequate equipment, angiographic technique can make the difference between an accurate ejection fraction determined with confidence and ease and a pseudoquantitative, poorly reproducible value created after a struggle from a patchwork of guesses. As for visual assessment, the goal is to opacify the entire ventricle throughout the cardiac cycle. Care must be taken to avoid ectopy, which is undesirable for several reasons. First, contrast is wasted. Second, the normal beat following it is usually not analyzed because function is potentiated and therefore nonrepresentative. Finally, this potentiated beat empties the ventricle of much of its remaining contrast, so the ensuing normal sinus beats are poorly opacified.

It is helpful to record the electrocardiogram simultaneously with the ventriculogram, particularly in a mode that allows correlation of the two. The timing of ventriculographic frames may be printed with the electrocardiogram on a strip-chart recorder (Fig. 9–14), or the electrocardiogram may be displayed as a "cine trace" in a corner of the cine image. Having such a timing strip makes it easier to check the regularity of the rhythm, to select a normal sinus beat of representative cycle length, and to determine the R-R interval. If such a recording is unavailable, the length of each cardiac cycle is estimated by counting the number of frames from one end-diastole to the next. The process must be repeated over several successive cycles to check on the regularity of the rhythm: The R-R interval and heart rate are calculated as follows:

$$\text{R-R interval (sec)} = \frac{\text{number of frames/cardiac cycle}}{\text{filming rate (frames/sec)}}$$

$$\text{Heart rate (beats/min)} = \frac{60}{\text{R-R interval (sec/beat)}}$$

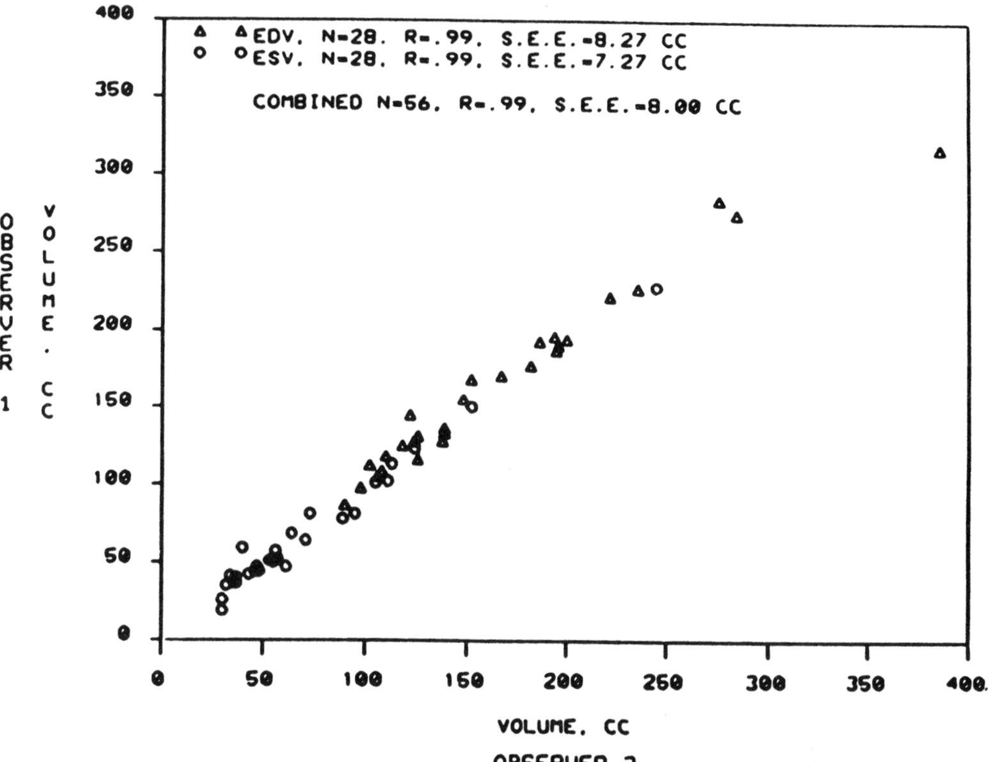

Figure 9–13. Variability in left ventricular volume between measurements made independently by different observers. (From Dodge, H.T., Sheehan, F.H., and Stewart, D.K.: Estimation of ventricular volume, fractional ejected volumes, and stroke volume and quantitation of regurgitant flow. *In* Just, H., and Heintzen, P.H. (eds.): Angiocardiography: Current Status and Future Developments. Springer-Verlag, Berlin, 1986, p. 99, with permission.)

Because of the cardiodepressive effect of the contrast agent, analysis should be performed on the earliest possible beat following contrast injection. Using epicardial clips to track serial ventricular functional changes (Fig. 9–15), Vine and associates found that the contrast-related changes in end-systolic volume and ejection fraction from their preinjection values are small but become significant seven cardiac cycles after contrast agent injection.[V1] Usually, the ventricle has emptied of contrast agent by then, but in occasional studies with early ectopy and low contractile function, the tracing of a relatively late beat incurs

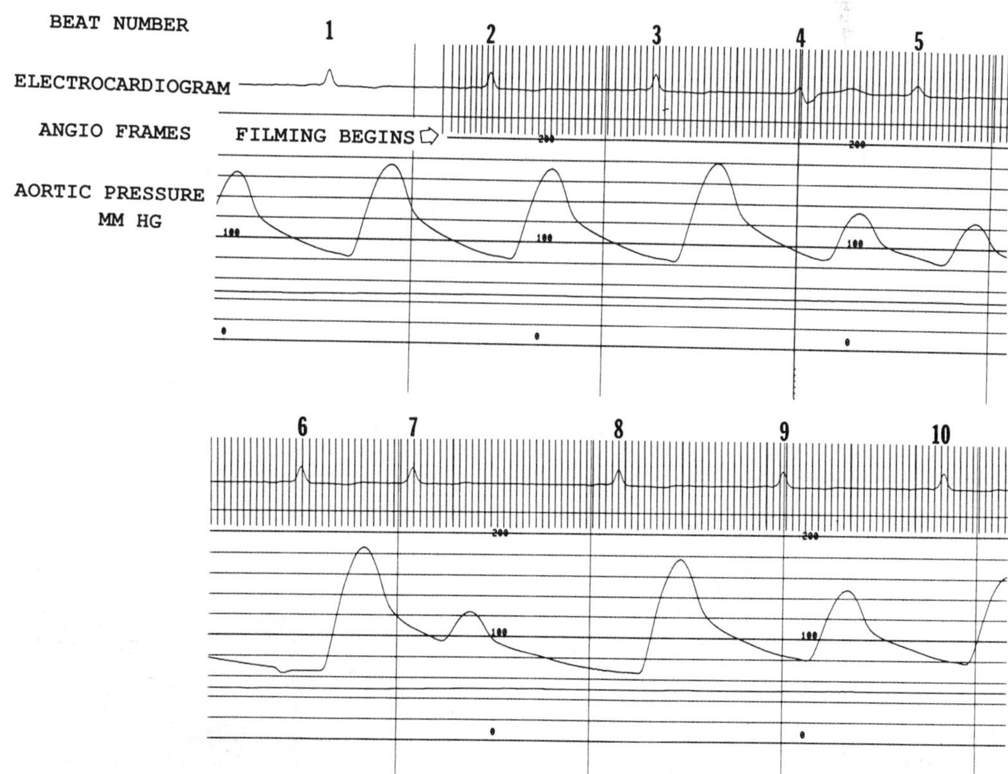

Figure 9–14. Continuous recording of the electrocardiogram (ECG) during contrast ventriculography allows accurate selection of a non-postpremature normal sinus beat for analysis. In this tracing, recorded at 100 mm/sec, the timing of angiographic (angio) frames is indicated by the vertical lines for comparison with the ECG. The R-R interval preceding beat number 4 is nearly normal and approaches the interval preceding beats 2 and 3. Nevertheless, beat 4 is a slightly premature ventricular contraction, with a wide QRS interval, and is associated with reduced pressure. If this angiogram were evaluated without the ECG, the slight prematurity of beat 4 might be overlooked; it could then be identified only by the lack of an atrial kick.

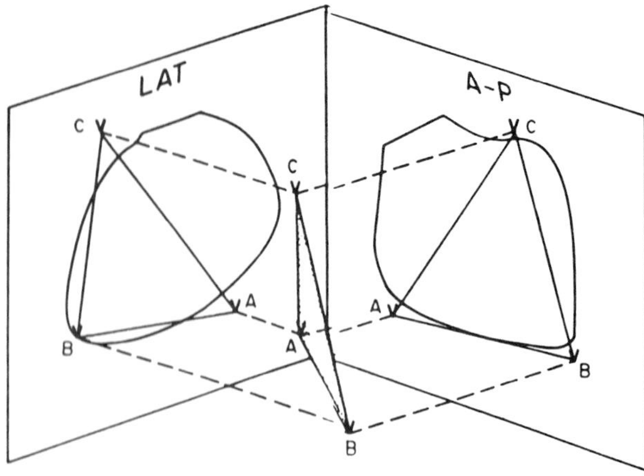

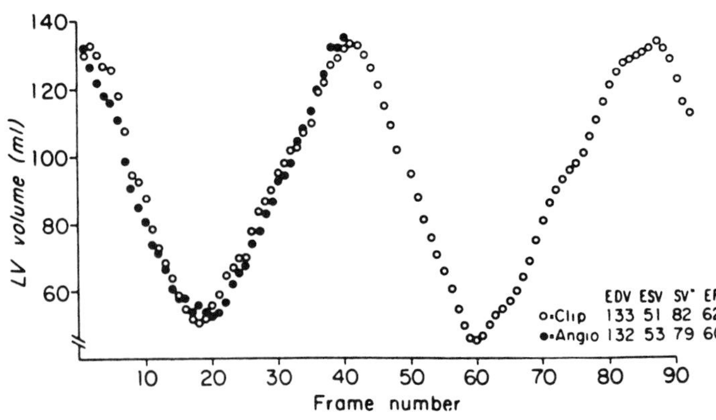

Figure 9–15. To measure the effect of contrast material on left ventricular volume and ejection fraction, volume was determined continuously beginning before contrast injection from the motion of epicardial clips *(left)*. There was close agreement between clip-derived volume and angiographic volume *(right)*. (From Vine, D.L., Dodge, H.T., Frimer, M.J., et al.: Quantitative measurement of left ventricular volumes in man from radio-opaque epicardial markers. Circulation 54:391, 1976, with permission from the American Heart Association, Inc.)

less error than tracing a postectopic beat, in which the ejection fraction is about 12 percent higher than normal. Alternatively, ventriculography may be performed with one of the nonionic contrast media. These nonionic media cause less hypotension, fewer arrhythmias, or less fluctuation in ventricular function than Renografin[G2, H6] and may be safer for patients with congestive heart failure or acute myocardial infarction.

For clinical studies, only the end-diastolic and end-systolic endocardial contours are traced. End-diastole is the frame at which ventricular volume appears to be largest. If the electrocardiogram is recorded, the choice of the end-diastolic frame can be facilitated by looking for the peak of the R wave (see Fig. 9–14). The end-systolic contour is traced from the frame of minimum chamber volume. End injection has been proposed as a more appropriate marker of end-systole.[M1] In practice, however, the closure of the aortic valve is visible angiographically in only 20 to 35 percent of studies and requires a measurable period of time so that the leaflets do not coapt until several frames after the time of minimum volume.[S5] It may be difficult to select the end-systolic frame in patients with asynchronous motion, in whom contraction is proceeding in one wall while relaxation has already begun elsewhere. In such cases, it is helpful to trace several frames and calculate the volume in each to find the frame of minimum volume.

One of the most important factors influencing the accuracy of quantitative analysis is the care with which the endocardial contours are identified, traced, and digitized. It is a common misconception that the number of decimal places in the answer is proportional to the accuracy of the measurement. Instead, the old saying "garbage in, garbage out" more appropriately fits the situation. It makes good common sense to design the physical layout of the laboratory with the needs of the tracer in mind. Such an atmosphere is more conducive to attention to frame selection, checking of traced contours, and patience in analyzing "difficult" films, that is, those with poor image quality, arrhythmias, heavy trabeculation, asynchrony, or other problems that may hinder delineation of the endocardial contour.

Tracing is best performed on a horizontal or slightly sloped table down to which the cine images are displayed from a projector mounted overhead (Fig. 9–16). It is much more awkward and fatiguing to trace on a wall or vertical projector screen. Often the projector must be played back and forth to track endocardial motion in the process of tracing or for error checking and editing. This procedure is an important step for accurate measurements and is comfortably performed with an overhead projector. If the contours of the projected images are traced on paper, editing is a simple matter of erasing the pencil line and redrawing (Fig. 9–17). The *x-y* coordinates of the final endocardial contours are then entered into the computer by using a digitizing tablet (Fig. 9–18).

With a digital analysis system, the tracer views the image on a vertical screen while tracing onto a digitizing tablet on the table; the traced contour appears on the screen as an overlay. Advanced digital systems offer capabilities comparable to those of cine analysis. For example, endocardial motion can be tracked by playing a "cine loop" of images under the traced border. Editing is also performed as with cine: the errant border section is identified with the cursor, deleted, and then redrawn. Such

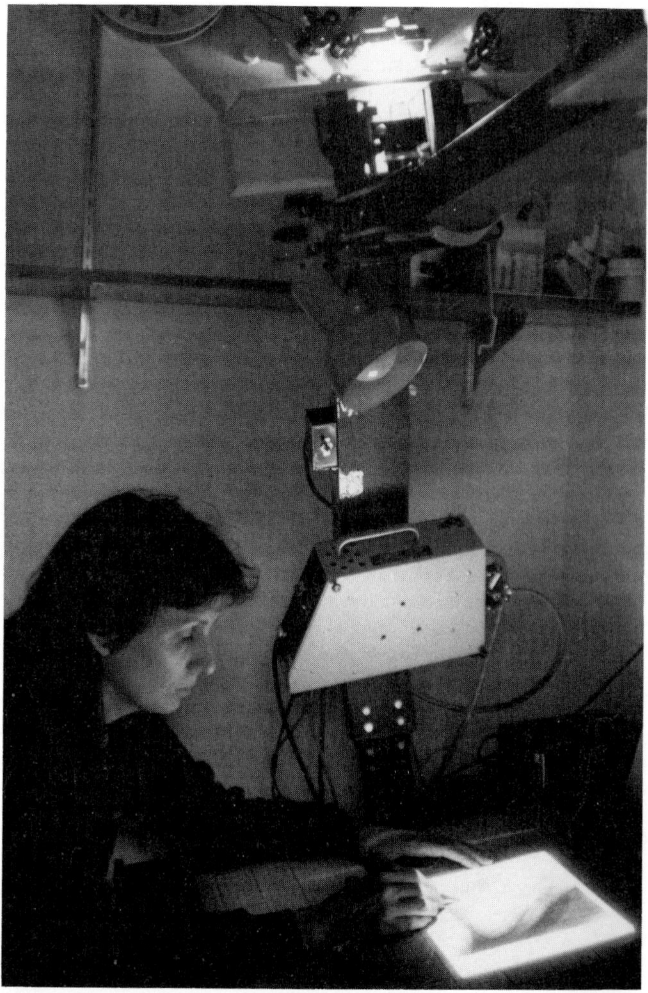

Figure 9–16. With a projector mounted overhead, the image is projected onto the table, where it can be traced more comfortably.

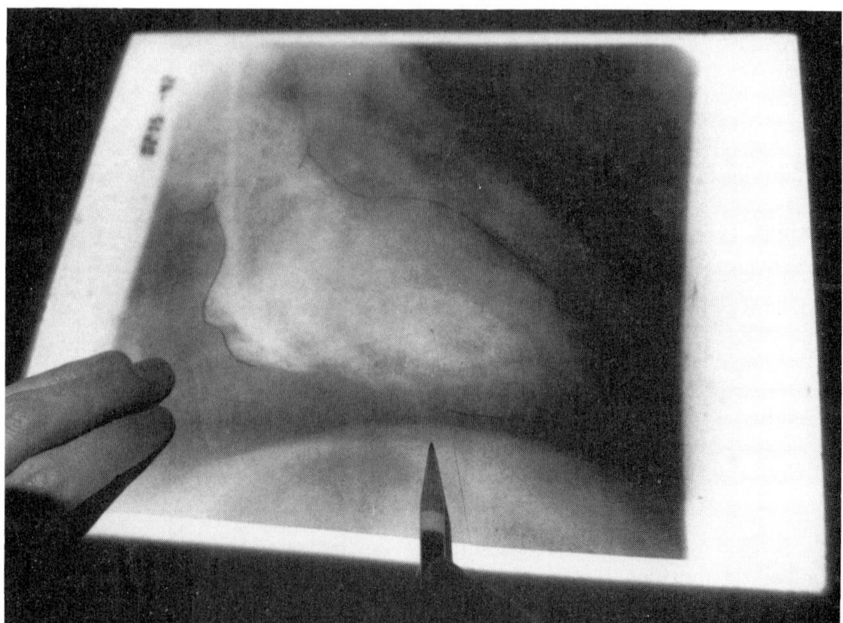

Figure 9–17. The endocardial contour of this end-diastolic frame has been traced. The operator covers the tracing with a blank sheet of paper, mentally retraces the endocardial contour, slides off the blank paper, and checks to see whether the new impression of the contour agrees with the penciled tracing.

systems are to be preferred to more primitive arrangements, such as projecting the image directly onto a tablet and attempting to trace and digitize in one step. One disadvantage of such one-step processing is that the contour must be traced in a single sweep from the stopped frame, unaided by visual tracking of the motion of the walls. Another disadvantage is that the entire contour must be redrawn to alter any segment, which inhibits the tracer from correcting errors. It is naive to assume that all digitally acquired or processed images will have such superior image quality that the contours will be easily traceable from the stopped frame alone. This may be true if a standard volume of contrast agent is injected and the rhythm is normal. However, angiographers may wish to perform a low-volume contrast injection and then rely on digital processing to enhance the images up to the quality of a routine cineventriculogram. In such cases, having the features detailed above would facilitate accurate angiographic analysis.

By convention, the endocardial contours begin and end where they intersect the aortic valve. The papillary muscles and trabeculae carneae are not traced (see Fig. 9–1). The volume they

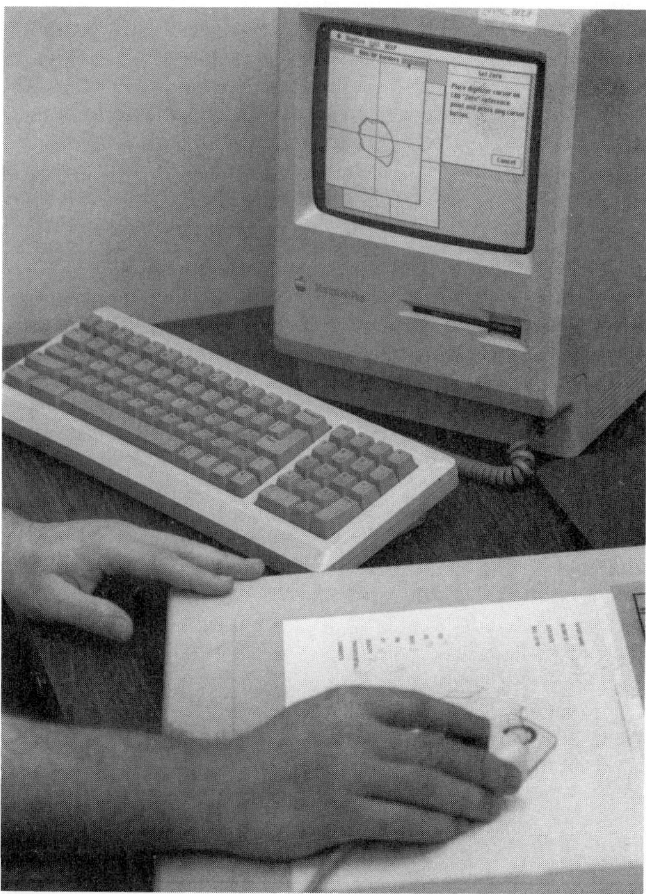

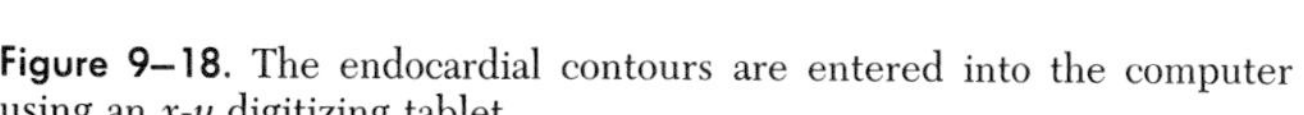

Figure 9–18. The endocardial contours are entered into the computer using an *x-y* digitizing tablet.

occupy is included with the ventricular chamber. As a result, the calculated volume is elevated and must be corrected back by using regression equations (see earlier). Tracing the contour is most difficult in the anterobasal region, where a faintly opacified left anterior descending artery may be mistaken for the ventricular contour, and in the apex, because it is often less well opacified.[S6] The tracing room should be darkened; otherwise function is overestimated because the faintly opacified fingers of contrast between trabeculae at end-systole are hard to see and the contour is mistakenly traced at the tips of the trabeculae rather than at their roots.

Training is obviously a factor influencing the accuracy of volume determination. At the University of Washington, interobserver variability is minimized by requiring that new tracers pass a variability test after their training. The test consists of a standard set of 20 ventriculograms whose measurements are known.

For monitoring quality and performance, it is useful to assign a grade to the image quality of each ventriculogram. This grade is recorded together with the identity of the tracer and the numbers of the frames from which the end-diastolic and end-systolic contours were traced. If the imaging system does not print frame numbers on the cine film, the numbers can be read from the frame counter on the projector after zeroing at the beginning of the ventriculogram.

Parameters Derived from Volume Measurements

Volumes, Indices, and Output

The end-diastolic volume is that measured when the ventricle has reached peak dilatation for a given cardiac cycle. The end-systolic volume is a measure of the residual volume of blood remaining in the ventricle at the end of contraction. The difference between them is the stroke volume. The product of stroke volume and heart rate yields the cardiac output, the volume of blood ejected from the ventricle per minute. These measurements are commonly normalized for differences in size of patients[M2] by dividing by the body surface area, and expressed as a volume or cardiac index. The body surface area is easily calculated from the patient's height and weight using a nomogram.[D4]

Ejection Fraction

The ratio of the stroke volume to the end-diastolic volume is the ejection fraction. This parameter expresses the mechanical performance of the left ventricle in a variety of cardiac conditions. It correlates with other parameters of ventricular performance such as the peak rate of pressure rise (dP/dt),[M3] can be measured with a high degree of reproducibility, and is useful as an index of prognosis (Fig. 9–19).[R5, S7] The ejection fraction, however, is not a measure of contractility and is influenced by acute changes in preload, afterload, or heart rate and by drugs that alter contractility. Under chronically altered loading conditions, as in valvular regurgitation or stenosis, the ejection fraction remains normal as long as there is adequate compensation by dilatation and/or hypertrophy.[K4, M3] In mitral regurgitation, however, ventricular performance may be poorer than the ejection fraction indicates because of reduced afterload.[B1, V2]

Regurgitant Flow and Valve Areas

The close correlation between angiographic stroke volume and the stroke volume measured with Fick's or the indicator dilution method[D5, G3] in patients without arrhythmias, shunts, or valvular regurgitation makes it possible to measure the volume of regurgitant flow across the mitral or aortic valve.[S8] Since the angiographic stroke volume is the volume output from the left ventricle, but the Fick or dilution stroke volume is the forward output, the difference between them is the regurgitant flow per beat. The severity of regurgitation may be expressed as a percentage of the angiographic stroke volume. Although the quantitative measurements correlate significantly with the grades of aortic

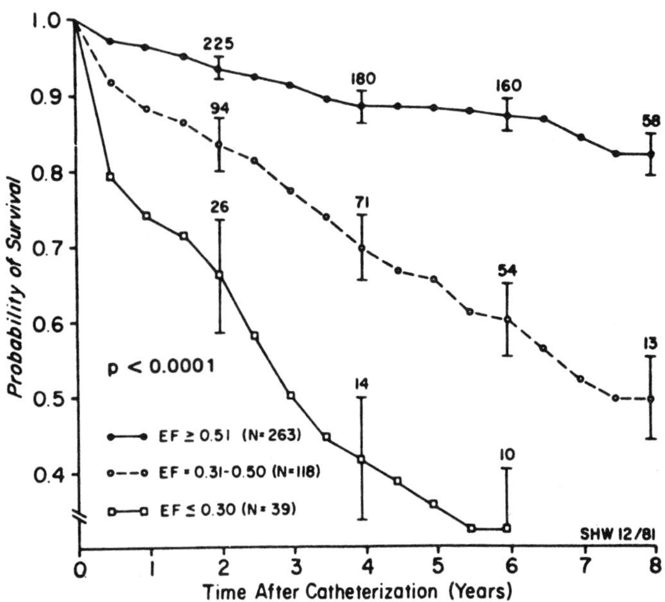

Figure 9–19. Left ventricular ejection fraction was found to be one of the strongest prognostic indicators in the Seattle Heart Watch Study. This figure displays survival in patients randomized to medical therapy, subgrouped according to initial ejection fraction. (From Hammermeister, K.E., DeRouen, T.A., Zia, M.S., and Dodge, H.T.: Survival of medically treated coronary artery disease patients in the Seattle Heart Watch Angiography Registry. *In* Hammermeister, K.E. (ed.): Coronary Bypass Surgery, the Late Results. Praeger Publishers, New York, 1983, p. 167. Copyright © 1983 by Praeger Publishers. Reprinted with permission.)

regurgitation assessed visually from the aortogram ($r = 0.56$, $P < 0.001$, $N = 69$) (Fig. 9–20),[H7] there is considerable overlap because the appearance of regurgitation is affected by the size and function of the left ventricle and the presence of valvular stenosis. For example, the severity of regurgitation may be overestimated from the aortogram in patients with a normal heart size because there is less dilution of contrast agent.

From the cardiac output and pressure gradient across a valve, the cross-sectional area of a stenotic valve can be calculated using a hydraulic formula[G4] as

$$\text{Valve orifice area} = \frac{\text{valve flow}}{K\sqrt{\text{pressure gradient}}}$$

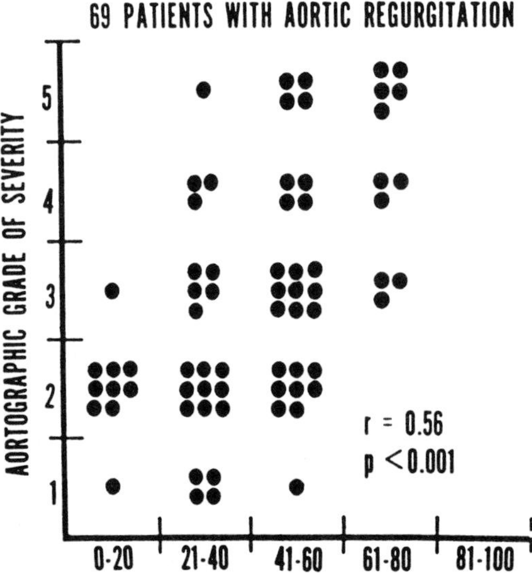

Figure 9–20. Correlation between visual assessment and quantitative measurement of aortic regurgitation expressed as a percentage of stroke volume. (From Hunt, D., Baxley, W.A., Kennedy, J.W., et al.: Quantitative evaluation of cineaortography in the assessment of aortic regurgitation. Am. J. Cardiol. 31:696, 1973, with permission.)

where K = 31.0 for the mitral valve and K = 44.5 for the aortic valve, and valve flow is measured during diastole for the mitral valve and during systole for the aortic valve. The accuracy of this approach has been established by comparing the calculated area with the valve area measured at surgery or autopsy.

Left Ventricular Mass and Stress

By delineating the epicardial border of the left ventricle, it is possible to measure the thickness of the wall and to calculate the mass of the left ventricular myocardium (Fig. 9–21).[R6] The epicardium is visible only along the anterior wall, and wall thickness is assumed to be homogeneous. The equation for mass in grams is

$$\text{Mass (g)} = \left(\frac{4}{3}\pi\left[\frac{D_{AP}}{2} + h\right]\left[\frac{D_{lat}}{2} + h\right]\left[\frac{L}{2} + h\right] - V\right) \cdot 1.050$$

where L is the longest long-axis length measured in the two views, in centimeters; D_{AP} and D_{lat} are the minor axes in the AP and lateral views, respectively, in centimeters; h is left ventricular wall thickness in centimeters; V is corrected left ventricular chamber volume in milliliters; and 1.050 is the specific gravity of heart muscle. Comparison of calculated mass with postmortem weight has revealed close agreement (r = 0.97, standard error of the estimate = 32.7 g) over a range of 99 to 609 g (Fig. 9–22),[K5] except in patients with right ventricular hypertrophy or pericardial disease.

Left ventricular stress can be calculated throughout the cardiac cycle from measurements of dimensions, wall thickness, and pressure.[S9] Because of trabecular thickening, the mass calculated from direct measurement of wall thickness in late systole exceeds mass at end-diastole. To avoid this artifactual increase in mass, wall thickness in systole and diastole is calculated by assuming that mass is constant at the end-diastolic value and spread homogeneously over a changing chamber volume.[H4] With this approach, stress can be calculated by using the Laplace relationship:

$$\frac{P}{h} = \frac{\sigma_1}{R_1} + \frac{\sigma_2}{R_2}$$

where σ_1 and σ_2 are the stresses along the principal radii of curvature in dynes/cm², R_1 and R_2 are the radii of curvature, P is

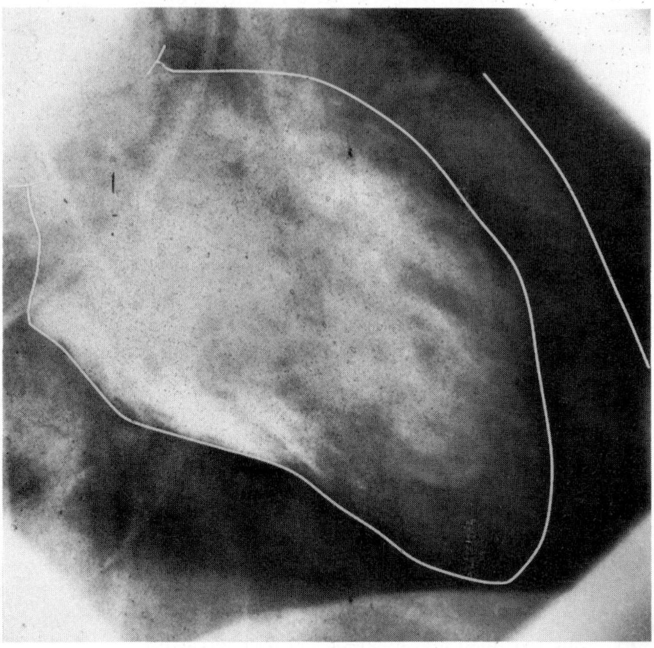

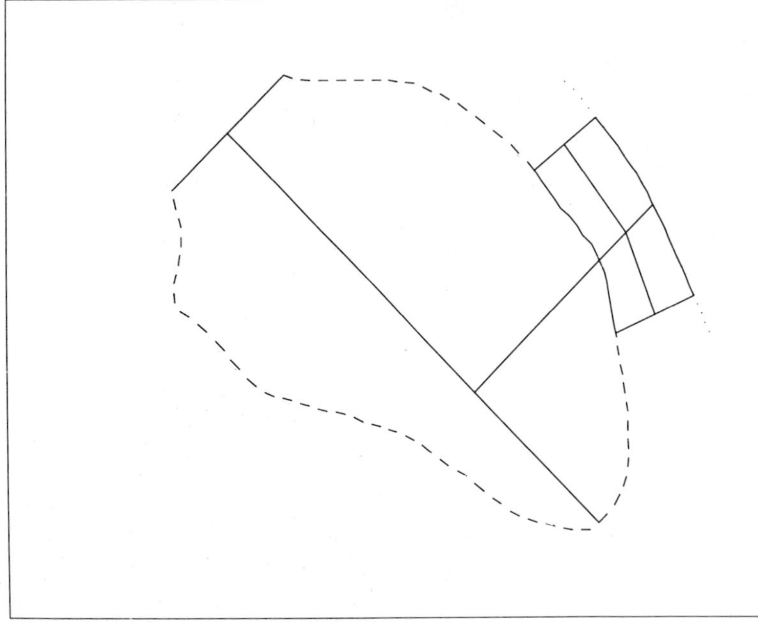

Figure 9–21. The thickness of the myocardium is measured along the anterior wall, in the neighborhood of the hemiaxis between the middle and distal third of the long axis, where the epicardium is visible.

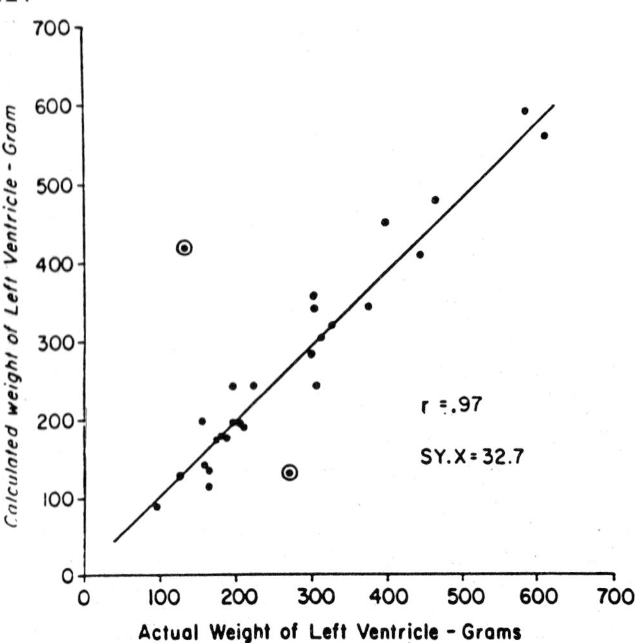

Figure 9–22. Validation of the method for measuring left ventricular mass. The two outliers represent patients with right ventricular hypertrophy and were excluded from statistical analysis. (From Kennedy, J.W., Reichenbach, D.D., Baxley, W.A., and Dodge, H.T.: Left ventricular mass: A comparison of angiocardiographic measurements with autopsy weight. Am. J. Cardiol. 19:221, 1967, with permission.)

left ventricular chamber pressure in dynes/cm^2, and h is wall thickness in centimeters.

The capability of measuring wall thickness and stress has led to increased understanding of the effect of pressure or volume overload on left ventricular function and the mechanism underlying the compensatory hypertrophy and dilatation that develop in response (Fig. 9–23). In pressure overload, the myocardium thickens without dilating; in volume overload, on the other hand, wall thickness remains normal but total mass increases with the increase in volume. In both conditions, the result of the change is reduction in wall stress.[H8] Examination of changes in ventricular shape as well as size has shown that the two types of load cause different patterns of hypertrophy.[G5] In decompensated patients with impaired ventricular performance, the ventricle becomes more spherical and stresses redistribute.[D1, G6, L2] The adaptations to volume overload are analogous to normal cardiac growth.[G7]

Although of great value in understanding the mechanisms of myocardial hypertrophy, measurement of wall stress is not useful for evaluating the functional status of individual patients.[G6]

QUANTITATIVE ANALYSIS OF REGIONAL LEFT VENTRICULAR WALL MOTION

It has long been recognized that coronary artery occlusion causes dysfunction in the ischemic region.[T2] Wall motion abnormalities in the normal region in patients with chronic or acute ischemia have also been identified and their relationship to the ejection fraction has been measured.[F1, S10, S11] More recently, the effect of reperfusion therapy on the function of the peripheral infarct region was analyzed and shown to affect global function significantly early after myocardial infarction.[S12] The ejection fraction reflects the net effect of abnormalities in the various regions of the left ventricle. The value of wall motion analysis derives from its greater sensitivity to the function of the region of interest and its usefulness for interpreting observed changes in the ejection fraction. The illustrative examples have been prepared using the centerline method developed at the University of Washington, to allow a more uniform presentation (Fig. 9–24).

Wall Motion Analysis in Theory

The accuracy of volume determination by each proposed method was established by postmortem heart studies. However, no such gold standard exists for verifying the accuracy of wall motion measurements. It is possible to implant metallic markers in the epicardium, midwall, or even endocardium and to track their motion. Such studies have been performed in attempts to validate one or another approach to wall motion analysis.[D6, I1, K6, M4, S13] None of these marker methods has won universal acceptance. The fact that wall thickening contributes half of the perceived endocardial wall motion implies that epicardial or midwall marker motion underestimates the extent of endocardial motion. Even endocardial marker motion does not correspond to the motion measured from a contrast ventriculogram because the markers become embedded in the trabeculae as the latter thicken in systole. Thus, a one-to-one correspondence cannot be established between points on the end-diastolic contour and points on the end-systolic contour.[H4]

The lack of a gold standard for wall motion has led to a proliferation of methods, founded on hypotheses that can be neither proved nor disproved. These methods were then accepted or discarded on the basis of purely empirical criteria such as the accuracy with which the resulting wall motion measurements distinguished normal subjects from patients with ischemic heart disease or how homogeneous the motion in the normal group appeared. These criteria are influenced by the size and selection of the normal subjects and populations of patients used for testing and by the statistical approach.[K7, L3, L4, R7]

The problem is further complicated by the translational motion of the heart within the chest, which cannot be distinguished angiographically from the perceived inward motion of the projected endocardial contours. To correct for translational motion, a number of approaches have been proposed in which the end-systolic contour is realigned relative to the end-diastolic contour (Fig. 9–25). Like the wall motion analysis methods, the approaches to realignment were founded and validated empirically. All three approaches developed on the basis of marker motion analysis eschew realignment. They rely instead on external referencing, in which the *x-y* coordinates of the endocardial contours are related to their location in the angiographic frame. Of course, the positions of the patient and of the imaging equipment must remain constant during ventriculography; panning is not allowed. The validity of performing realignment is being questioned on theoretical grounds, and more recent studies indicate that realignment worsens variability in wall motion measurement and may artifactually give the appearance of motion in patients with akinesis.[C4, L5, S6] Thus, the problem of distinguishing wall motion from the heart's translational motion has not been solved to date.

The problem can be bypassed by measuring wall thickening, which is independent of translational motion, as a parameter of regional function. However, it is difficult to delineate the epicardial border from contrast ventriculograms. The wall thickness measurements used to calculate the mass of the left ventricle are made on the anterior wall alone. In patients with ischemia the wall thickness may not be homogeneous. Methods have been proposed for measuring wall thickness around the entire contour, but they require digital processing.[B2]

In addition to the translational motion of the heart, the rotational motion of the left ventricle about its long axis should be considered when performing wall motion analysis. This rotation has been attributed to the spiral orientation of endocardial and epicardial muscle fibers.[M4] The magnitude of this rotation is small. Nevertheless, in view of its presence and the other factors described earlier, it is more appropriate to consider the various methods that purport to measure wall motion as models of regional function.

Methods of Wall Motion Analysis

In the absence of a gold standard by which to gauge the accuracy of the methods of wall motion analysis, it is necessary to consider other criteria in selecting a method. All the methods

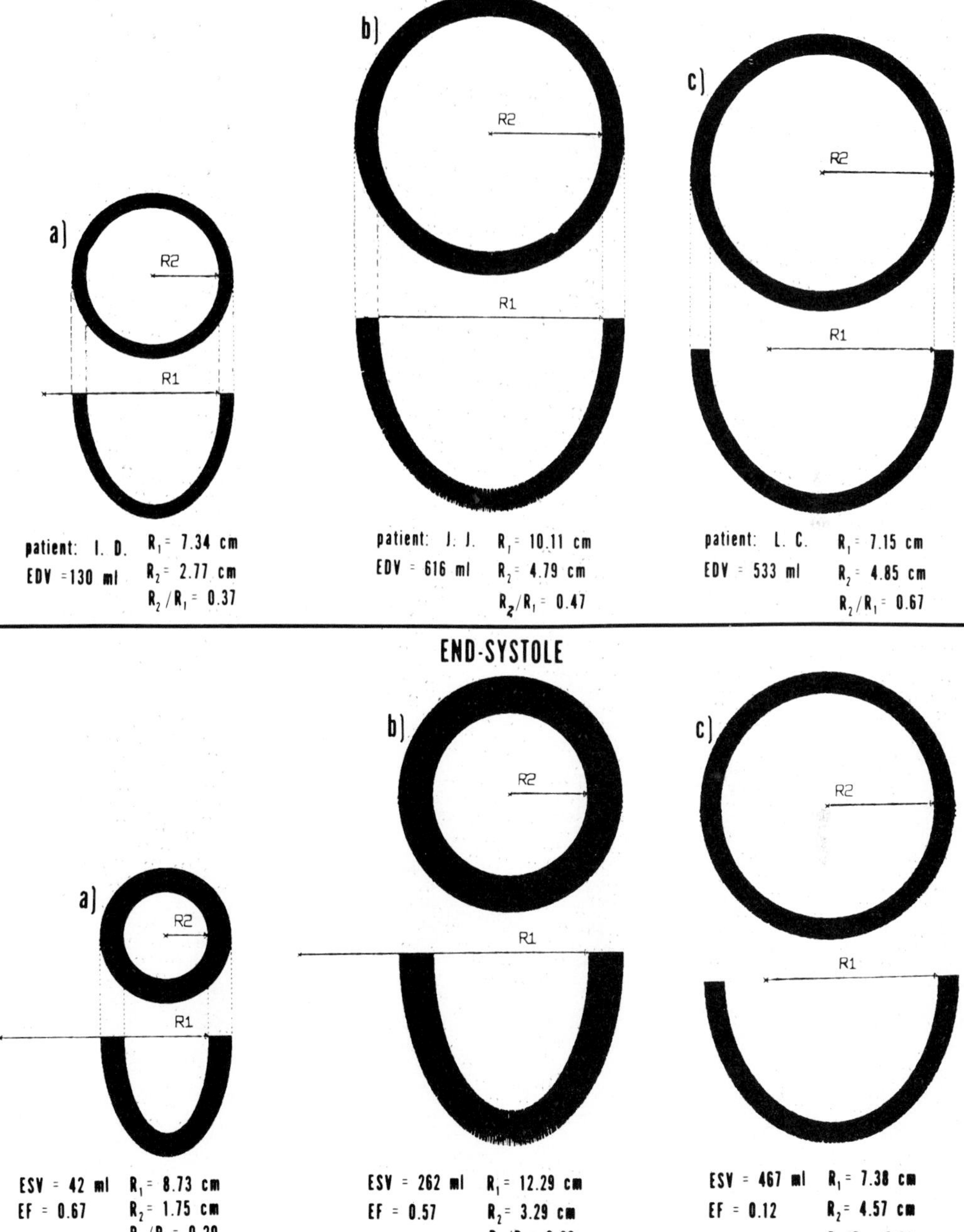

Figure 9–23. Schematic drawings for three subjects: *a*, normal; *b*, volume overload with hypertrophy and intact left ventricular function; *c*, dilated hypertrophied ventricle with depressed function. In *c*, the ventricle is rounder, as evident from the elevated ratio of the principal radii of curvature, R_2/R_1, calculated by comparing the ventricle to an ellipsoid of revolution. In the more spherical ventricle, wall stress in the meridional direction increases relative to stress in the equatorial direction. (From Dodge, H.T., Frimer, M., and Stewart, D.K.: Functional evaluation of the hypertrophied heart in man. Circ. Res. 34–35(Suppl. II):II-122, 1974, with permission from the American Heart Association, Inc.)

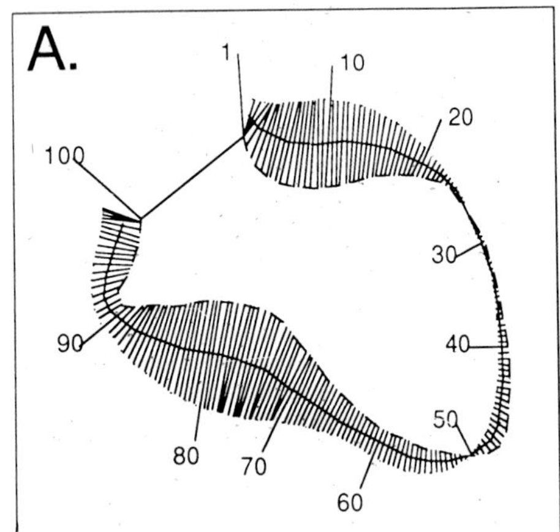

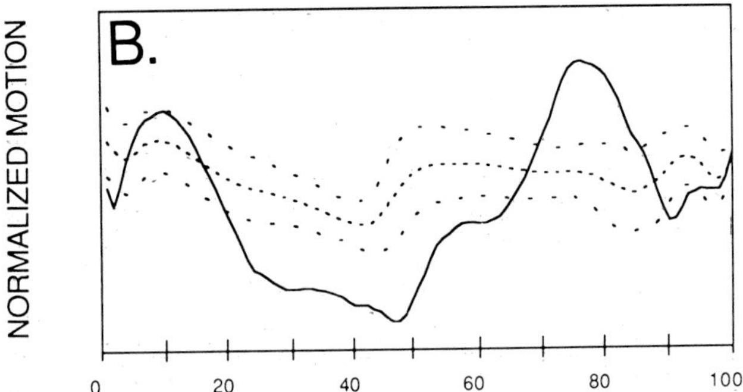

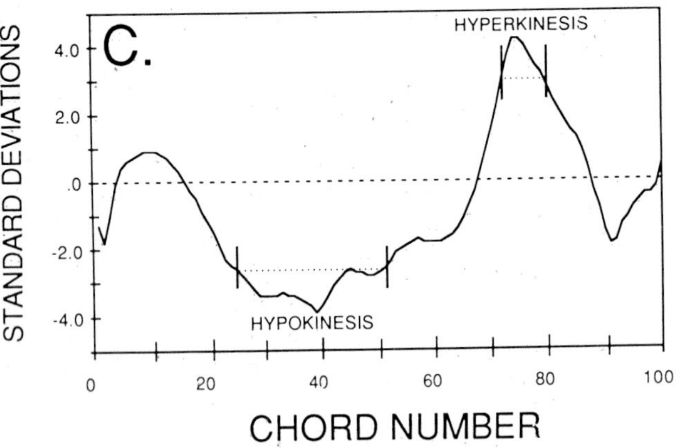

Figure 9–24. Wall motion measured by the centerline method. A centerline is constructed midway between the end-diastolic and end-systolic endocardial contours. Motion is measured along 100 chords perpendicular to the centerline *(A)*. To adjust for heart size, the motion of each chord is normalized by the length of the end-diastolic perimeter. When comparing the patient's motion *(solid curve)* to the normal range (mean ± 1 standard deviation, *dotted curves*), the regional variability of normal motion is apparent *(B)*. Therefore motion is converted to units of standard deviations from the normal mean *(horizontal axis)* *(C)*. Abnormality in a region of interest is calculated as the mean motion of chords lying in the most abnormally contracting part of the respective coronary artery territory. (From Sheehan, F.H., Mathey, D.G., Schofer, J., et al.: Limitations in the interpretation of rest-exercise ejection fraction changes after early thrombolytic therapy during myocardial infarction. Am. J. Cardiol. 61:743, 1988.)

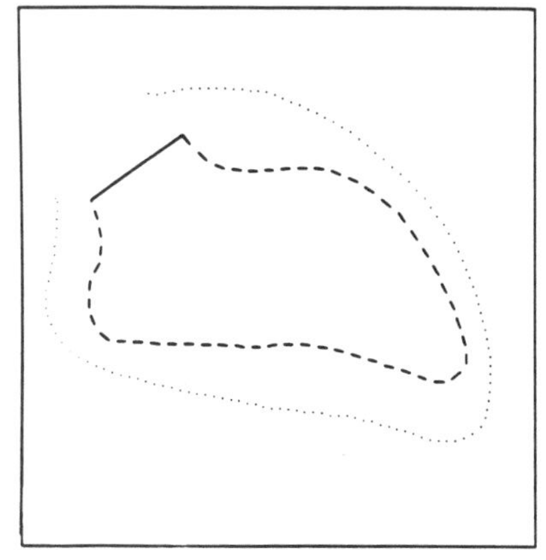
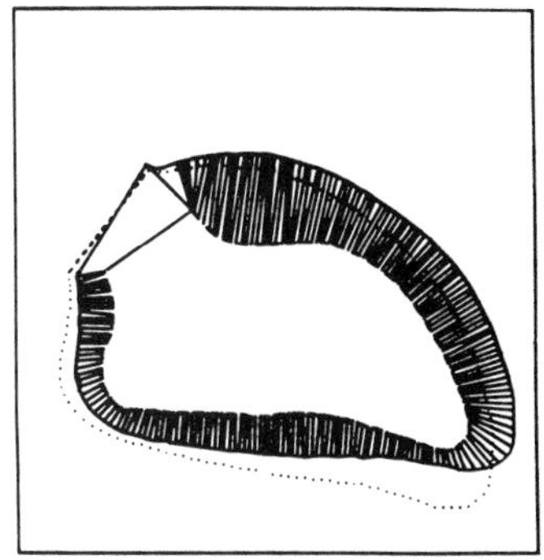
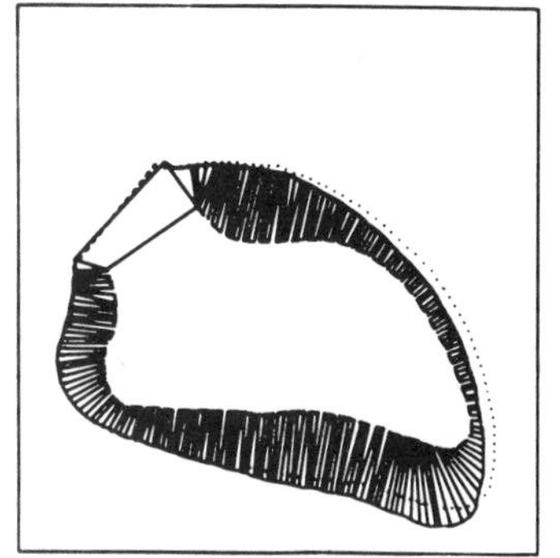
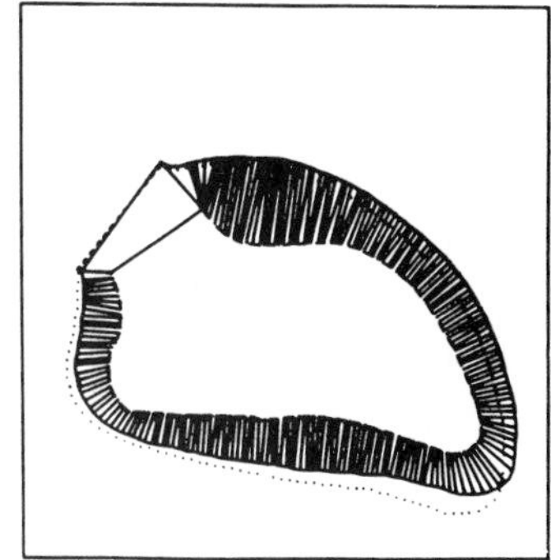

Figure 9–25. The displacement of the endocardial contour between end-diastole and end-systole measures the net effect of inward wall motion and translational motion of the heart in the chest. When the contours are realigned in an attempt to correct for translational motion, the apparent inward wall motion is altered. Here the contours traced under external referencing *(upper left)* have been realigned to give the appearance of anterior hypokinesis, normal motion, and inferior hypokinesis *(proceeding clockwise)*. It is evident that if realignment is performed, the method must be carefully chosen and tested to avoid artifact in wall motion analysis.

have inherent assumptions about the directionality of wall motion. It is important to identify the assumption implicit in each method under consideration and to evaluate the validity of the assumption in the light of available experimental data. However, the selection of a method implies more than the definition of motion vectors. Additional considerations include the parameter used to express regional function and the way in which abnormality will be defined and measured. Having a clear understanding of the method assists in interpreting the results of the empirical studies used to validate it, since the method's performance is the second criterion. Practically, performance is assessed by four empirical criteria. First, the measurements made should be reproducible; variability should be minimal to increase accuracy in detecting abnormalities and changes. Having low variability in the measurement itself helps to lower the variability observed in a study population. The importance of enhancing the "signal-to-noise ratio" becomes evident from the equation used to estimate sample size in a clinical trial:

$$N = 2\left[\frac{(Z_\alpha - Z_\beta)\sigma}{\mu_T - \mu_c}\right]^2$$

that is, the number, N, of patients needed in each treatment group is proportional to the second power of α, the variability in the measurement in the study population.[C5] In this equation, Z_α and Z_β are cut-off values on the standard normal distribution for the specified α and β errors, μ_T is the sample mean for a treatment group, μ_C is the sample mean for the control group and σ is the standard deviation. Second, the motion of normal subjects should have a narrow standard deviation to enhance sensitivity for abnormality (Fig. 9–26). Third, although wall motion analysis is most often performed on patients with ischemic heart disease, it has provided useful information about patients with valvular disease and cardiomyopathy. Hypokinesis in these conditions can occur anywhere in the left ventricle. For this reason, the method used to measure wall motion should be able to focus on the region of interest, wherever it is located. Any method that meets these three criteria will probably meet the fourth: it will demonstrate sensitivity and specificity in distinguishing the function of normal subjects from that of patients with hypokinesis or hyperkinesis.

Assumptions in Methods of Wall Motion Analysis

There are almost as many methods as there are laboratories interested in performing wall motion analysis. The methods fall into two broad categories, depending on whether they are based on a coordinate system. Most methods utilize either a rectangular or radial coordinate system (Fig. 9–27). Motion is measured along hemiaxes or radii from the end-diastolic to the end-systolic contour. To adjust for patient-to-patient differences in heart size, the measured motion is normalized by the end-diastolic length of the hemiaxis or radius to calculate a shortening fraction, a linear version of the volume ejection fraction. If the coordinate system is used to divide the ventricle into regions, the area change in each region can similarly be normalized by the end-diastolic area to express regional function as an area ejection fraction.

Two of the methods developed on the basis of metallic marker studies utilize a coordinate system. The method of Ingels and associates measures motion along radii to an origin located 69 percent down the long axis, drawn from the anterior aspect of the aortic valve to the apex. This approach yielded the closest agreement with the motion of markers surgically implanted in the midwall of patients undergoing coronary artery bypass surgery. However, the authors noted that the location of the origin was not critical and small changes in its position incurred little additional error.[12] Slager and associates developed their method on the basis of motion of endocardial markers implanted in pigs. They subsequently extended their studies to normal human ventriculograms and used an automated border recognition system to identify and track the motion of individual irregularities on the endocardial contour. The mean motion of irregularities proceeding from each of 20 points on the end-diastolic contour was used to define 20 pathways along which wall motion could be measured.[S13] They then related the intersection of the 20 pathways with the end-diastolic and end-systolic contours to a rectangular coordinate system and calculated 20 regional contributions to the global ejection fraction.

There are several problems associated with coordinate system methods. Foremost, the apex is not an anatomic landmark. It is often poorly visualized because of (1) its distance from the catheter, (2) the presence of aneurysms or intraluminal thrombus, or (3) the disfiguring effect of apical venting during surgery. The highest variability in delineating the contour occurs at the apex.[S6, S13]

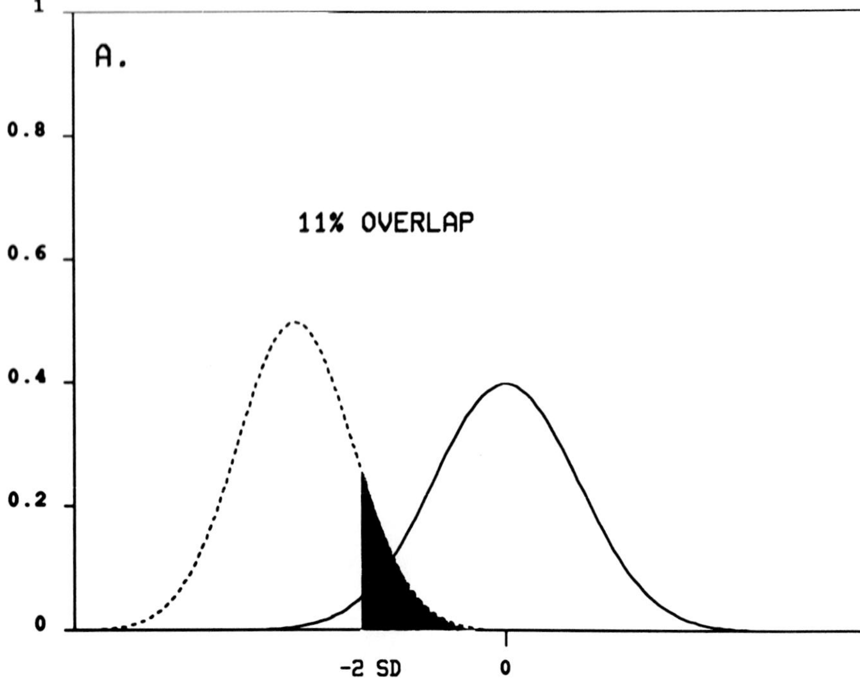

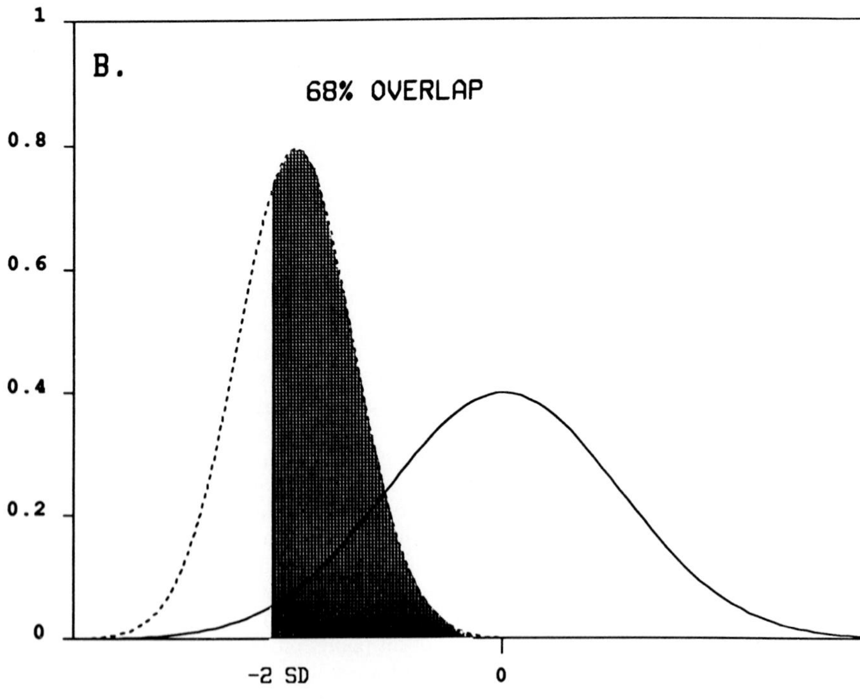

Figure 9–26. Distribution of wall motion in normal subjects and in patients with recent myocardial infarction by different imaging modalities. *A,* In this method there is relatively little variability in the normal group's motion, and the standard deviation is low. Consequently, separation of normal individuals from diseased patients is much greater than for the method in *B,* indicating that the method in *A* can more accurately distinguish between these two populations. (Reproduced from Comparative Cardiac Imaging by B. Brundage [ed.], with permission of Aspen Publishers, Inc., © 1990.)

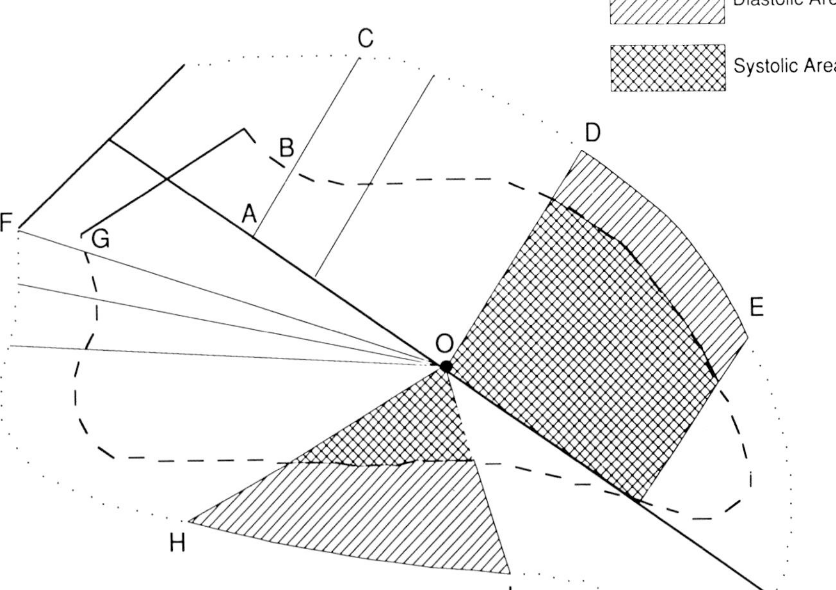

Figure 9–27. Most methods of wall motion analysis utilize a rectangular or radial coordinate system. In a rectangular system, motion is measured along a hemiaxis such as AC; fractional shortening is calculated as BC/AC. Similarly, a fractional shortening can be determined from motion along radius FO as FG/FO. Alternatively, the area ejection fraction may be determined from the areas spanned by two hemiaxes or two radii. For the border segments DE and HI, this is calculated as (diastolic area − systolic area)/diastolic area.

For these reasons, the reliance of coordinate system methods on identification of the apex introduces a source of error and inconsistency. Second, methods based on coordinate systems assume that the motion of the walls proceeds toward the long axis or a central origin. This assumption, while convenient, has been challenged by more recent studies indicating that the direction of wall motion is multicentric.[G8] The motion pattern depicted in the various marker studies consistently shows systolic descent of the base toward the apex;[I2, M5, S13] this observation invalidates methods using a rectangular coordinate system to measure motion at the base because the vectors run perpendicular to the long axis. It has been suggested that the center of mass be used as the origin of a radial system.[P1] However, implementation of this approach is difficult because only the center of the chamber can be calculated from the endocardial contour; delineation of the epicardium would be required to determine the center of mass of the myocardium. This may explain why the center of mass approach has proved to be less sensitive than other methods on empirical testing.[C6, K7, S15] A third problem is a practical one—the ability of the method to handle contours of varying shapes. All of the methods were developed for analysis of the AP or RAO view of the left ventricle. Neither of the marker-based methods has been validated for analysis of left ventriculograms filmed in the LAO view. The rectangular coordinate methods are not suitable for the LAO view in cases where the contour is foreshortened and appears nearly circular (see Fig. 9–11). Radial methods may function well in this circumstance, if the coordinate system does not require identification of an apex, and radial methods can be used to measure wall motion in the RAO view of the right ventricle as well. However, radial methods cannot be used to analyze wall motion in the LAO view of the right ventricle because of its indented shape (Fig. 9–28).

There are a few methods that do not rely on construction of a coordinate system. One approach is to divide the end-diastolic and end-systolic contours evenly into the same number of points and then measure motion between the two contours at parallel points.[D6] The method assumes that the ventricular contour shortens homogeneously around its circumference. Unfortunately, this assumption might be invalid in patients with ischemic heart disease because the local hypokinesis may cause the end-systolic borders of an akinetic region to be related to normally contracting sections of the end-diastolic contour, giving the artifactual appearance of motion.

Two methods minimize the assumptions concerning wall motion by measuring motion in the direction of locally determined vectors. Gibson and associates connected points on the end-diastolic contour to the nearest point on the end-systolic contour.[G9] This method is free of serious theoretical drawbacks, although it occasionally creates undesirable motion vectors in tightly curved sections of the contour.[B3] The centerline method (see Fig. 9–24) measures wall motion along perpendiculars to a centerline drawn midway between the end-diastolic and end-systolic contours.[S16] The measured motion is normalized by the end-diastolic perimeter length to generate a shortening fraction. Abnormality in motion is expressed in units of standard deviations from the mean of a reference population with normal findings on cardiac catheterization.

There are two alternatives to wall motion as a measure of regional ventricular function. Studies have shown that regional wall thickening is more accurate than wall motion in discriminating normal from infarcted tissue.[L6] Unfortunately, it is difficult to visualize the epicardial contour from contrast ventriculograms, and the need to trace four contours—the epicardial and endocardial contours at end-diastole and end-systole—tends to increase variability. The second alternative is to measure the curvature of the endocardial contour. Abnormalities in regional curvature correlate with reduced wall motion in patients with coronary artery disease.[G10, M6] Measurements of wall thickening and curvature are independent of the translational motion of the heart within the chest.

Parameters of Regional Function

There are many methods for measuring wall motion but only two ways to express the results: in terms of the magnitude of inward motion or in terms of the circumferential extent of wall motion abnormality (Fig. 9–29). The latter, usually referred to as the hypokinetic segment length, is determined as the number of points on the contour with motion depressed below a specified threshold. For example, the akinetic segment length is the percentage of the contour with motion less than or equal to zero and is easily determined from tracings of the end-diastolic and end-systolic contours with a planimeter. Measurements of hypokinetic or akinetic segment length indicate the percentage of the contour suffering decreased function, but they are uninformative concerning the magnitude of dysfunction in any specific region. Measurements of inward motion express the level of function of a point or region on the ventricular contour but indicate nothing about the function of surrounding regions.

Which parameter is preferable depends on the question being addressed. For example, the effect of thrombolytic therapy in salvaging myocardium is most sensitively detected by measuring inward motion in the infarct region;[S17] measuring hypokinetic segment length would introduce variability because the intervention cannot be expected to affect function in regions outside the

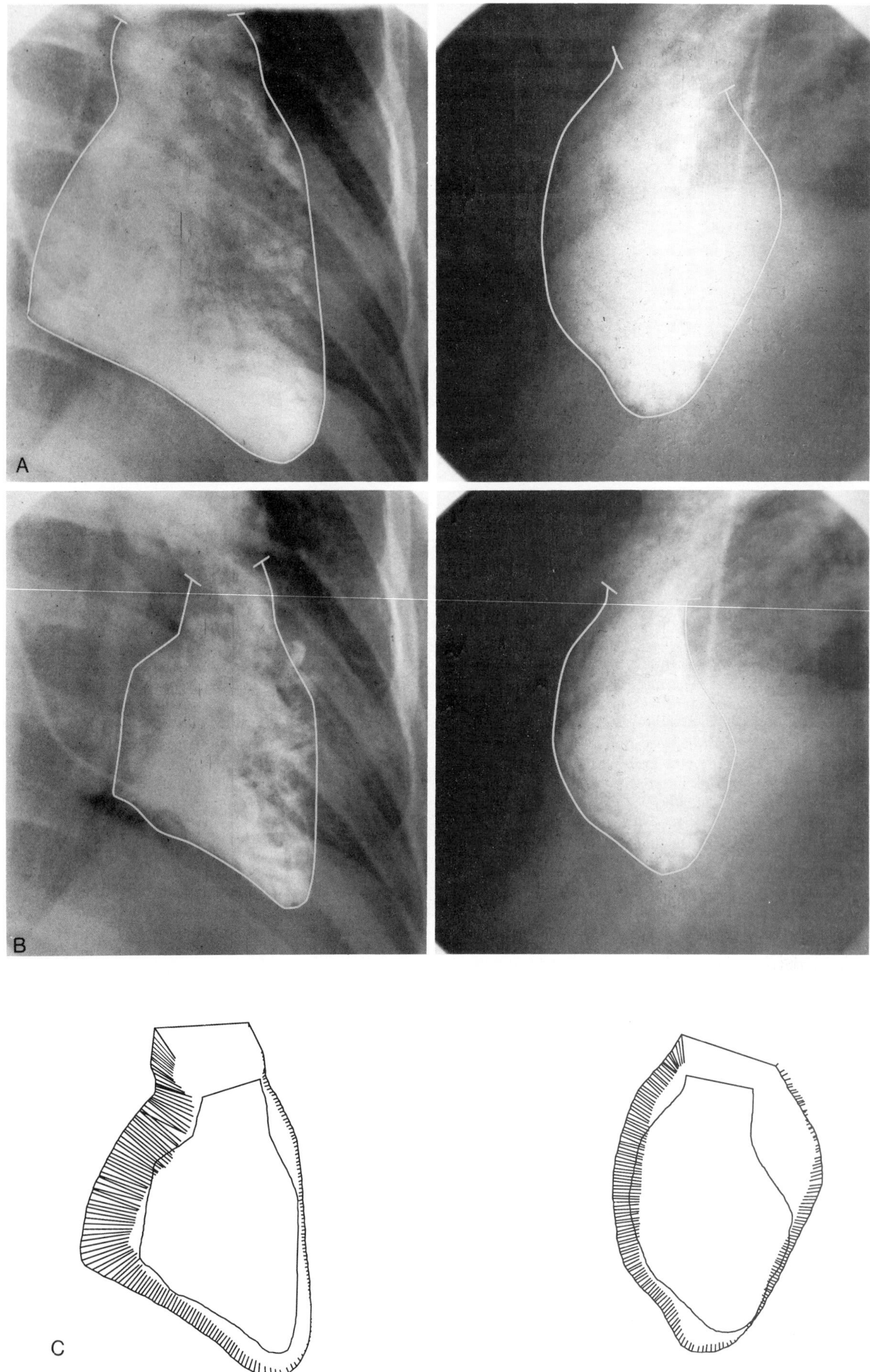

Figure 9–28. Analysis of chamber volume, ejection fraction, and wall motion can be performed for the right ventricle as well as for the left. The end-diastolic *(A)* and end-systolic *(B)* images, contours, and wall motion analysis *(C)* are displayed in the 30-degree RAO *(left)* and 60-degree LAO *(right)* projections. This patient, a survivor of sudden cardiac death, has normal left ventricular function and normal cardiac anatomy. The right ventricular ejection fraction (by Simpson's rule) is 61 percent and wall motion is hyperkinetic (contours) compared to normal (chords).

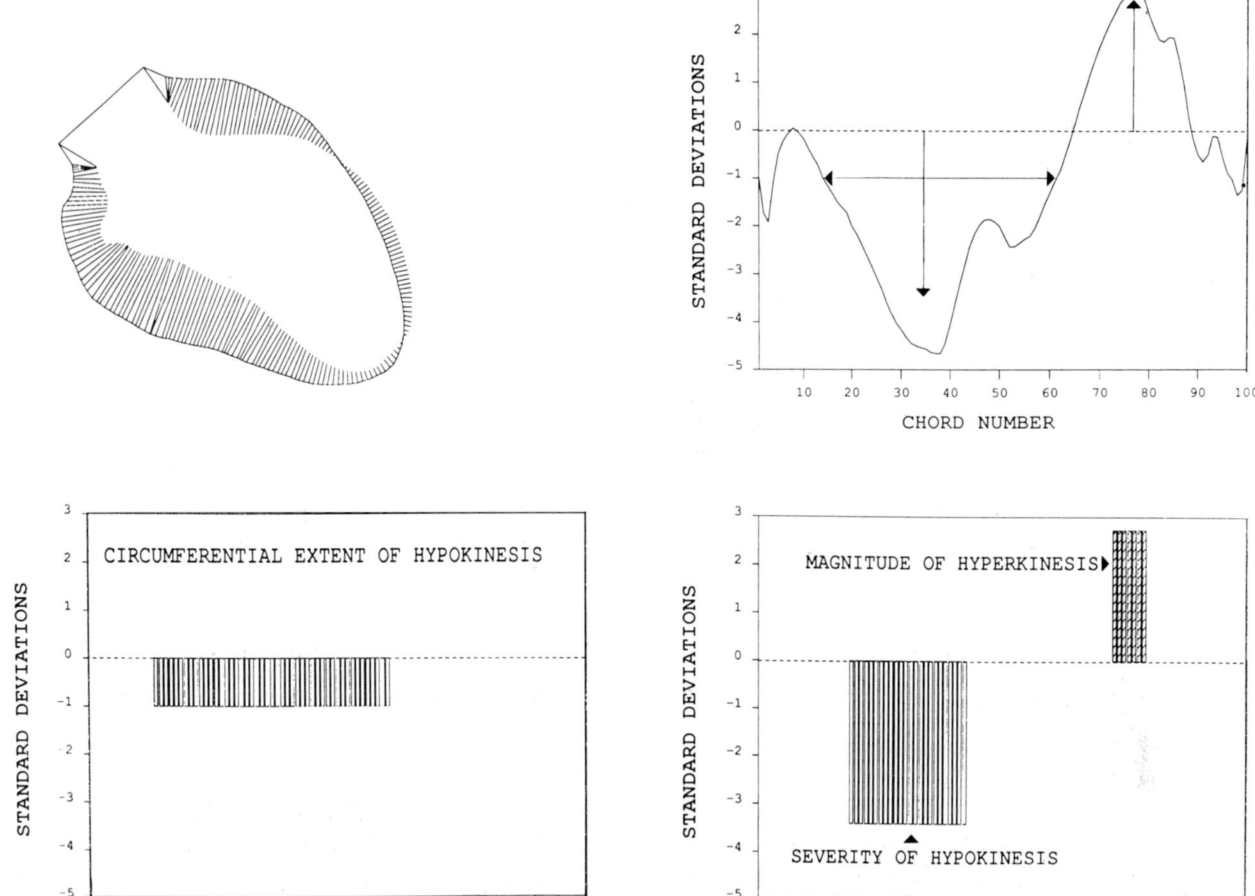

Figure 9–29. Wall motion abnormality is commonly expressed in terms of its severity within a region of interest *(lower right)* or its circumferential extent *(lower left)*. The two parameters give quite different impressions of the heart's function. The original contours and full wall motion analysis are above.

acute infarct, such as in the site of previous infarction. On the other hand, comparison of function in patients with stenosis of the left anterior descending versus the right coronary artery would be more appropriately done with a parameter of hypokinetic segment length, to demonstrate that the former affects a larger segment of the ventricle.

Definition of Abnormal Motion

In order to identify and measure abnormality, it is first necessary to define the limits of normal wall motion by determining the mean and standard deviation for motion in a normal reference population. Because of the small but measurable risk of cardiac catheterization, it is difficult to obtain contrast ventriculograms of truly normal subjects. Instead, data for patients who underwent diagnostic cardiac catheterization and in whom no cardiac pathology was discovered are commonly used. Although Bayesian normals, asymptomatic subjects who by age, sex, or other criteria have a low probability of cardiac disease, may have more normal exercise tolerance,[R8] one can argue that "cath normals" are (1) closer in age to the patients with ischemic heart disease who are the most likely subjects of a wall motion analysis and (2) angiographically proven rather than statistically likely to have normal coronary arteries.

Since one of the empiric criteria used to evaluate methods of wall motion is the homogeneity of function measured in normal subjects, there have been several studies of normal wall motion. Regardless of the method, these studies agree in showing that the normal extent of inward motion varies by region around the ventricle (see Fig. 9–24).[G11, H9, I1] As for wall motion, there are regional differences in the normal curvature of the ventricle as well. This regional variability can be related to the local architecture of the muscle fibers as they spiral around the ventricle.[B4, G10, H10] As a result of the nonuniformity of normal regional function, the definition of abnormality is necessarily also nonuniform. That is, no matter what threshold for wall motion is selected, it will indicate different severities of abnormality in different regions of the ventricle. For example, in the anterior or inferior walls, akinesis represents a grave dysfunction, but at the apex it lies within two standard deviations of the normal mean for motion (see Fig. 9–24).[L5]

Due to the variation in normal mean, abnormality must be assessed in the context of the normal range for motion in each vector. This was a simple matter for the ejection fraction, whose threshold value of 55 percent represents two standard deviations below the mean of a normal population,[K8] but becomes unwieldy if there are many wall motion measurements. Gelberg and associates have suggested that motion be expressed as a Z score, in terms of the number of standard deviations by which it differs from the normal mean.[G11] By this simple conversion, the motion of all regions is expressed in equivalent units, so the function of different regions can be summed, averaged, or compared (see Fig. 9–24). The standard deviation units indicate not only the magnitude but also the significance of the abnormality. Even the sign is informative: positive values indicate hyperkinesis, negative values hypokinesis, and zero motion means that function is normal.

In general, the application of a threshold to a continuous variable such as function acts to dichotomize it into two values, "normal" and "abnormal." This process is undesirable because it reduces the data and may alter the outcome of an analysis depending on what cutoff value is selected.[J1] Accordingly, statistical power is sacrificed if the threshold yielding the "best results" is selected. These considerations argue against measuring the circumferential extent of abnormality as the parameter of regional function, because it requires selection of a threshold. If, despite these drawbacks, dichotomization is desired, the threshold selected should exceed the variability of the measurement. For example, an improvement of one standard deviation in wall motion exceeds even study-to-study variability,[S6] and a change in ejection fraction greater than 5 percent would exceed the highest reported interobserver variability for this parameter.[B3]

There are actually two reasons why a wall motion method should portray the results with reference to the normal values. The practical reason is, of course, that it facilitates the interpretation of the data. The more important reason is that mortality in ischemic heart disease is related to the absolute level of ventricular dysfunction, not to the change in function after an intervention.[S12]

Variability

As for volume, measurements of wall motion are subject to variability. The greatest variability arises from differences between repeated studies, but there is also variability between different beats of the same angiogram, between observers tracing the same beat, or even between repeated tracings by the same observer.[C3, C7, S6, S18] In addition, these sources of variability vary by region around the ventricle. Variability affects the measurement of volume less than that of wall motion for two reasons. First, volume and ejection fraction measurements, unlike wall motion measurements, are unaffected by the translational motion of the heart within the chest. The effect of translation on study-to-study variability can be appreciated from a study in which the end-systolic contour was realigned relative to the end-diastolic contour in an attempt at correction; the procedure increased rather than decreased variability, particularly at the apex.[S6] Second, wall motion measurements are subject to point-to-point variability. This is less of a problem when motion is measured over regions rather than at discrete points on the contour,[G11] perhaps because the point-to-point differences between measurements are "averaged out." In a larger sense, the global ejection fraction is an average of the motion of all regions of the ventricle. Variability can be substantially reduced by averaging the motion of points lying within the region of interest (Fig. 9–30).[S6] Indeed, it is the capability provided by wall motion analysis to focus on a particular region that compensates for its greater variability compared with ejection fraction analysis.

Measuring Wall Motion in the Region of Interest

In spite of the methodologic difficulties detailed above, wall motion analysis has increasingly proved to be a useful adjunct to ejection fraction analysis because of its ability to focus on a specified region of interest. There are several ways in which this can be done. One approach is to divide the ventricle into a number of areas and measure area ejection fractions. Unfortunately, the region of dysfunction in a particular patient may not fall exactly into one of these areas (Fig. 9–31). The American Heart Association has prepared guidelines for the assessment of contrast ventriculograms that divide the contour seen in the 30-degree RAO view into five areas.[A2] However, in a study of patients with acute myocardial infarction due to isolated stenosis of the left anterior descending artery, the dysfunctional segment spanned two adjacent areas in about half of the patients. In such cases, the severity of dysfunction will be underestimated by either segment's function because each segment contains only part of the infarct region and partly normal myocardium (see Fig. 9–31). The problem arises because of the variable length, and consequently perfusion territory, of the coronary arteries and because the location of coronary stenosis in an artery varies from patient to patient.

One could, of course, measure motion in all of the vectors spanning the perfusion bed of the artery of interest and present these data together with the respective normal values for comparison. This approach is straightforward but is relatively insensitive because the dysfunctional segment has a variable location. Consequently, no single vector captures the wall motion of the dysfunctional segment in all patients.

To address this problem, the centerline method measures wall motion in the region of interest, which in coronary disease is the perfusion territory of that artery (Fig. 9–32). To maximize diagnostic accuracy, only the most abnormally contracting 50 percent of the artery territory is sought and the motion of its chords is averaged.[S19, S20] In validation studies, this approach yielded a greater correlation between wall motion and severity of coronary stenosis than the mean motion of larger or smaller proportions of the artery territory. Each artery's territory is defined simply as the set of chords whose motion, when measured in patients with isolated stenosis of that artery, is significantly depressed compared to normal.[S21] The centerline method thus yields a single

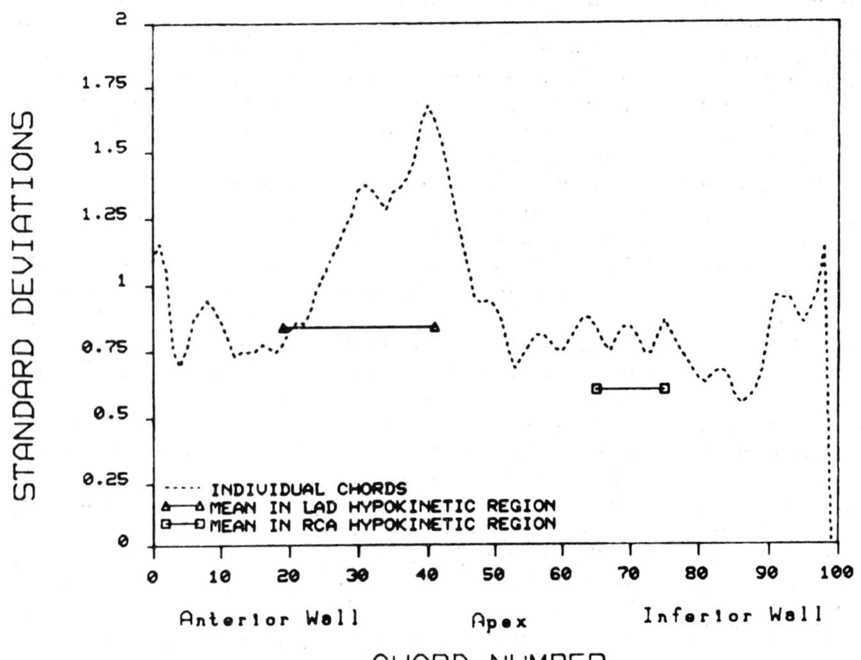

Figure 9–30. Variability in the motion of individual chords between repeated angiographic studies is relatively high, even in stable patients. This variability is reduced by averaging the motion of chords lying in the region of interest. (From Sheehan, F.H., Stewart, D.K., Dodge, H.T., et al.: Variability in the measurement of regional ventricular wall motion from contrast angiograms. Circulation 68:550, 1983, with permission from the American Heart Association, Inc.)

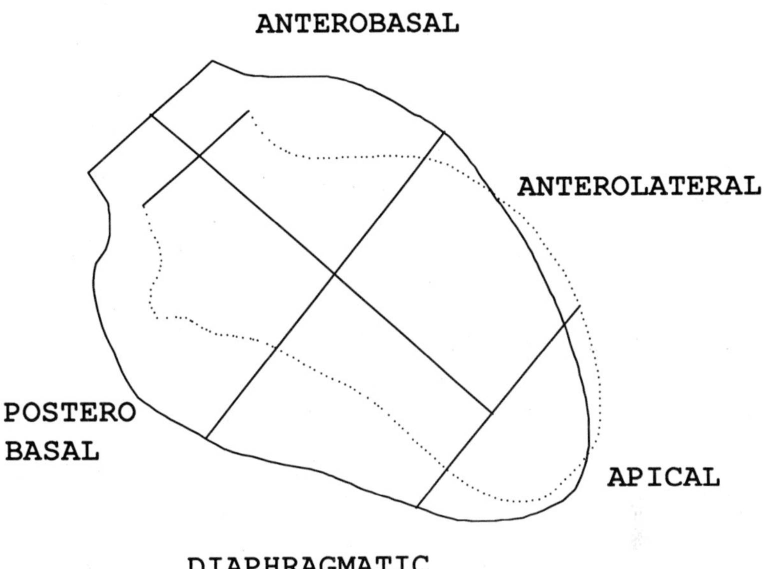

Figure 9–31. Segmentation of the ventricular contour into fixed regions results in underestimation of the severity of wall motion because the location of the hypokinetic segment often spans adjacent segments.

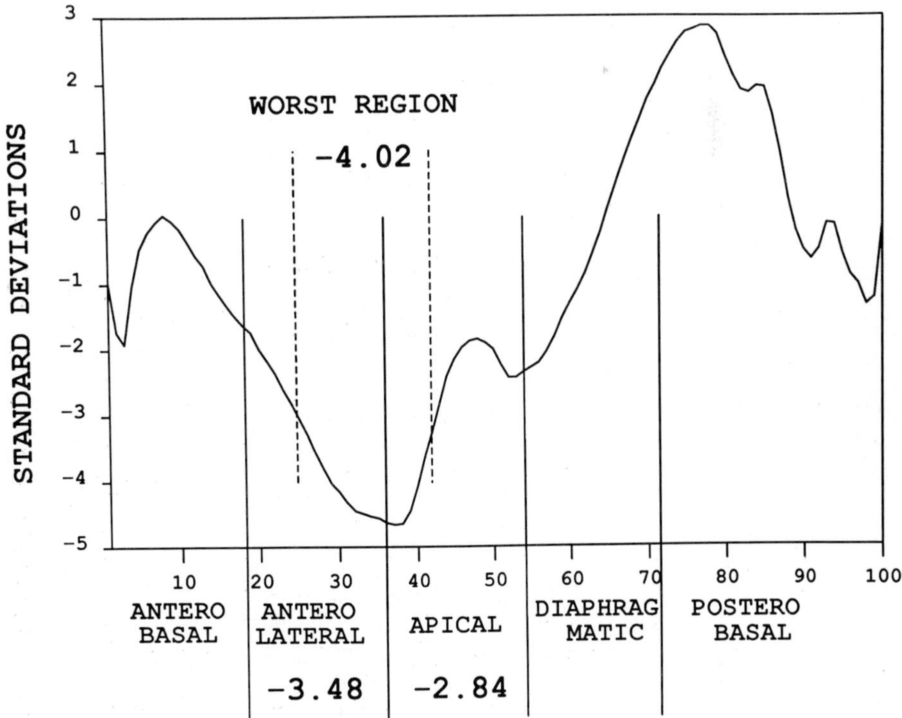

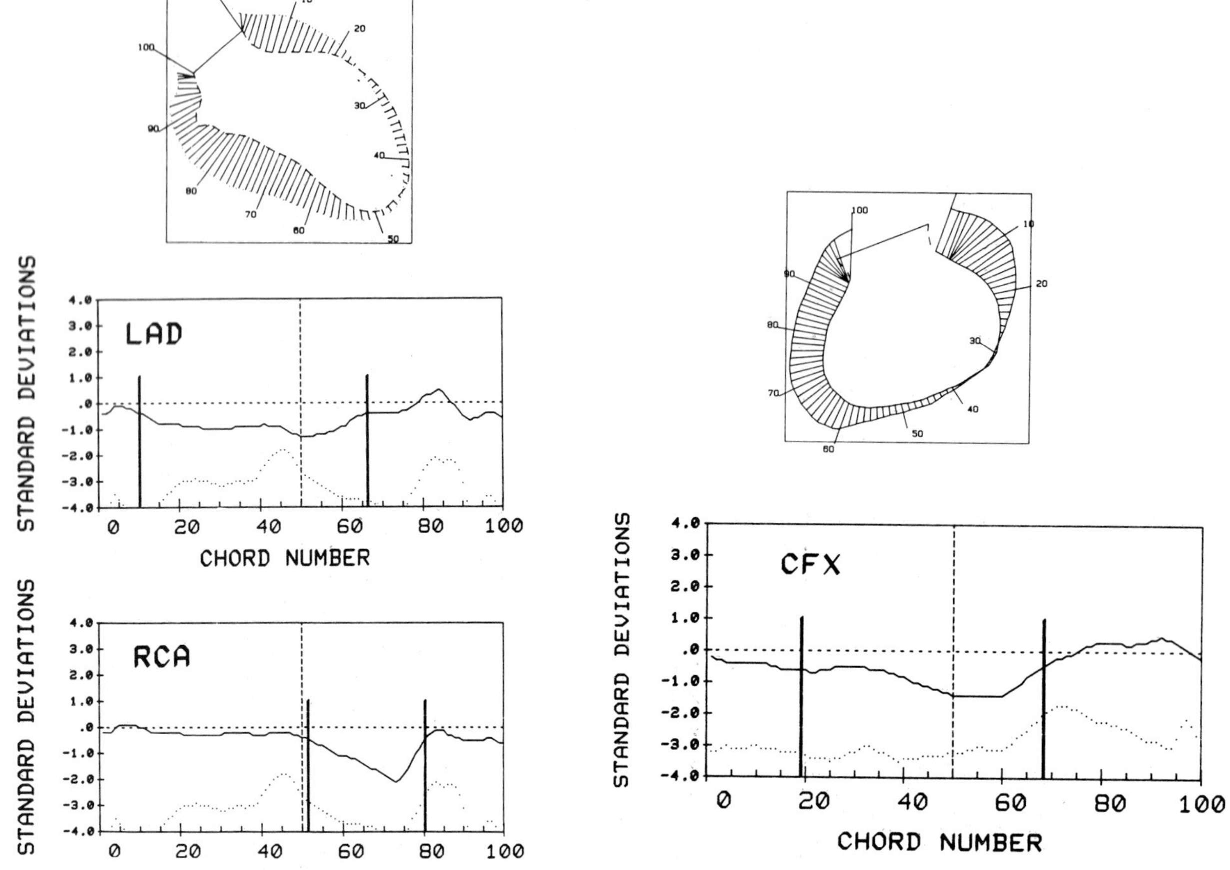

Figure 9–32. The territories of the left anterior descending artery (LAD), right coronary artery (RCA), and circumflex artery (CFX) were defined as the sequence of contiguous chords having significantly depressed wall motion in patients with isolated stenosis of the respective artery. The LAD and RCA territories are well visualized in the 30-degree RAO projection *(left)* and the CFX in the 60-degree LAO projection *(right)*. (From Sheehan, S. H., Schofer, J., Mathey, D. G., et al.: Measurement of regional wall motion from biplane contrast ventriculograms: A comparison of the 30 degree RAO and 60 degree LAO projections in patients with acute myocardial infarction. Circulation 74:796, 1986 with permission of the American Heart Association, Inc.)

parameter that expresses the severity of wall motion abnormality within a region of interest, in units of standard deviations to indicate the significance of that abnormality. Either hypokinesis or hyperkinesis can be measured by this approach.

A similar approach can be used with other methods of wall motion analysis, provided that (1) there are enough measurement vectors to avoid sampling error and (2) the abnormality in motion at each vector is expressed in equivalent and comparable units such as the Z score.

Method Selection: Theoretical, Empirical, and Clinical Considerations

The foregoing discussion reviewed the theoretical basis, or lack thereof, of many of the methods for wall motion analysis. It can be seen that many methods incorporate implicit assumptions, whether intentionally or not. The very lack of assumption concerning the direction of motion is an assumption. The types of empirical criteria used to evaluate and compare the methods have also been described and their validity criticized. In the absence of a gold standard, the facility with which a regional analysis can be performed and interpreted naturally becomes one of the criteria by which the various methods are compared and judged.

Several comparisons have been made in which 2 to 19 methods were tested for diagnostic accuracy in the same patient population. These studies have had somewhat variable results, but in general radial methods and the centerline method perform better than methods based on a rectangular coordinate system.[C6, G12, I2, K7] The methods of Gibson and associates[G9] and Slager and associates[S13] have not been compared extensively to other methods.

A final test of a method's usefulness may be more clinically oriented criteria such as which method is flexible enough to answer all of the practitioner's analysis needs, or which method produces results that are easy to interpret or to correlate with the results of other diagnostic tests ordered for the patients. Nebulous as these criteria may be, they represent the element of practicality that influences acceptance.

APPLICATIONS OF QUANTITATIVE ANALYSIS

Normal Values

Normal ranges for end-diastolic volume, end-systolic volume, and stroke volume, the volume indices after normalization for body surface area, and the ejection fraction have been determined for children and adults (Table 9–1).[B5, G13, K8, M2, W1] The normal ranges for wall motion are more variable from study to study because they are dependent on the method used to measure wall motion and whether realignment is performed to attempt correction for the translational motion of the heart within the chest.

Table 9–1. NORMAL VALUES FOR LEFT VENTRICULAR VOLUME AND MASS IN ADULTS

End-diastolic volume	70 ± 20 ml/m^2
End-systolic volume	24 ± 10 ml/m^2
Ejection fraction	0.67 ± 0.08
Mass	92 ± 16 g/m^2
Wall thickness	10.9 ± 2.0 mm

Reprinted with permission from the American College of Cardiology (Journal of the American College of Cardiology, Vol. 1, 1983, pp. 73–81).

Ventricular Function in Coronary Artery Disease

Quantitative ventriculography may be used to (1) assist in the diagnosis of ischemic heart disease or infarction, (2) assess the impact of coronary artery stenosis on resting function and functional reserve, (3) measure the compensatory response, (4) gauge the patient's prognosis for survival, or (5) evaluate the effect of therapeutic interventions. The ejection fraction is the most commonly measured parameter of function and has been consistently a strong index of prognosis. However, the ejection fraction measures global function and thus expresses the net effect of function in the various regions. Analysis of wall motion provides information that assists in the interpretation of observed abnormalities or changes in the ejection fraction, particularly in a situation where a disease process or therapy may have different effects in involved and normal regions.

Measurement of Left Ventricular Function as a Diagnostic Tool: Relationship Between Coronary Artery Stenosis Severity and Function

Patients with chronic stable angina have a normal ejection fraction. Resting hypokinesis, which occurs in the ischemic region,[H2, T2] is unusual unless the artery stenosis exceeds a critical threshold.[S19] This relationship confirms experimental data showing that during progressive coronary artery stenosis, left ventricular function remains normal until compensatory mechanisms maintaining coronary blood flow fail and resting coronary flow falls below normal.[S22] At that point, function declines exponentially. Studies to determine the threshold for a critical stenosis using quantitative coronary artery analysis have reported a minimum cross-sectional area $\leq 0.88 \pm 0.14$ mm^2 in patients with unstable angina, $\leq 0.64 \pm 0.08$ mm^2 in those who developed subendocardial infarction, and ≤ 0.6 mm^2 in patients with significant hypokinesis.[M7, S19]

Thus, function is relatively insensitive to reductions in coronary artery lumen size until stenosis has reached a critical level and resting coronary flow is impaired. Therefore, the measurement of resting ventricular function is not useful for the diagnosis of coronary artery stenosis. Furthermore, the finding of regional hypokinesis, although most probably due to myocardial infarction, is nondiagnostic of myocardial infarction because regional hypokinesis may be seen in other diseases such as valvular regurgitation and cardiomyopathy.[B6, O1, W2]

Stress Ventriculography: Assessment of Cardiac Reserve and Viability

Because ischemia results from a mismatch between coronary perfusion and myocardial metabolic demands, application of a stress that worsens the mismatch will exacerbate the ischemia and produce electrocardiographic changes and/or reduction in ventricular function.[S23] This effect is the basis for exercise electrocardiography and radionuclide ventriculography and can be applied as well to contrast ventriculography, using either supine exercise or pacing as the ischemia-inducing stress. The noninvasive stress tests are performed to diagnose the presence of coronary artery disease in lieu of performing cardiac catheterization. After diagnosis is made by coronary angiography, ventriculography may be performed to determine cardiac reserve in those with normal resting function or viability in patients with resting hypokinesis or akinesis.

The advantage of contrast ventriculography for this purpose is its greater image resolution compared with radionuclide ventriculography. This is important because the ejection fraction response to exercise, like the resting ejection fraction, measures the net effect of regional contributions. The exercise response in nonischemic regions may differ from, compensate for, or oppose exercise-induced changes in an ischemic region. In such cases, motion analysis may be more sensitive in measuring functional response of the ischemic region.[S24] The disadvantage is the discomfort of peddling a bicycle supine with a catheter in the femoral artery, which is only partially relieved by using the Sones technique.

Various alternatives have been tried, such as performance of handgrip, arm ergometry, cold pressor testing, or atrial pacing. However, each of these alternatives has a drawback that limits its usefulness.[D7] Pharmacologic and metabolic stresses have also been tested. Infusion of bioactive amines, isoproterenol, norepinephrine, epinephrine, dopamine, dobutamine, methoramine, phenylephrine, and angiotensin increases myocardial oxygen consumption[H11] and thereby induces ischemia. Ischemia may also be elicited by dipyridamole infusion, which increases coronary flow to normally perfused regions and decreases flow to underperfused regions, the "coronary steal" phenomenon.

These modes of stress testing have been developed primarily for the detection of ischemia and the diagnosis of coronary artery disease. Not surprisingly, there has been a concerted move to combine the stress test with noninvasive imaging. Stress ventriculography is now performed only as the gold standard for evaluation and validation of the various test protocols, in the context of a research protocol, or semi-invasively with digital processing of the levo phase of a right ventricular injection.

Assessment of Myocardial Viability

A determination of viability is sometimes desirable when weighing the chances for functional recovery after a revascularization procedure. For example, the advisability of bypass graft surgery to an artery supplying an akinetic and possibly infarcted region may be debatable. If the myocardium is viable, despite its hypocontractility, wall motion should improve in response to an infusion of epinephrine or nitroglycerin or to postextrasystolic potentiation. In patients with a positive response to such tests, the chances are better for resting function to recover following coronary artery bypass graft surgery.[B7, C8, H12] More recently, the response to postextrasystolic potentiation during acute myocardial infarction has been found to predict later function in patients who do or do not undergo thrombolytic therapy.[A3, H12]

Practical limitations that tend to inhibit viability testing are the need to perform two ventriculograms and the time required to assess response. These may be alleviated by the capabilities of digital angiography.

Left Ventricular Function in Acute Myocardial Infarction: Abnormalities in the Infarct Region

Coronary artery occlusion causes hypokinesis in the ischemic region. Hypokinesis due to occlusion of the left anterior descending and right coronary arteries is similar in severity, averaging -2.7 standard deviations by the centerline method. The circumferential extent of hypokinesis is smaller after right coronary artery occlusion. It is the greater size of the infarcted and dysfunctional segment in patients with occlusion of the left anterior descending artery that is responsible for their lower ejection fraction.[M8] The size of the dysfunctional segment is related to the coronary anatomy;[C9, S25] in humans the left anterior descending artery supplies 42 percent of the left ventricle.[K9] Dysfunction due to circumflex artery occlusion is slightly better appreciated in the LAO view (see Fig. 9–32), which allows visualization of the posterior wall, although the RAO view gives an adequate measure of the severity of hypokinesis.[S1, S26] When the circumflex gives rise to the posterior descending artery, the circulation is said to be left dominant and dysfunction is greatest along the inferior wall, which is usually perfused by the right coronary artery.

Many studies have shown that the dysfunction due to myocardial infarction occurs over a larger area of the myocardium than hypoperfusion. This phenomenon has been attributed to several mechanisms. Hypofunction in the normally perfused "border zone" may be due to tethering of normal muscle fibers to adjacent infarcted, akinetic fibers.[K10] Alternatively, the border region may be a zone in which infarction is restricted to a thin layer of the subendocardium, since regional hypokinesis occurs after fibrosis of as little as 6 percent of the wall and akinesis after fibrosis of only 14 percent.[I3] The dysfunction of the border zone has also been attributed to amplification of local stress in the border zone.[B8] Methodologically, the apparent overestimation of infarct size by measurement of the hypokinetic segment length is related to the threshold used to define hypokinesis; the error can be

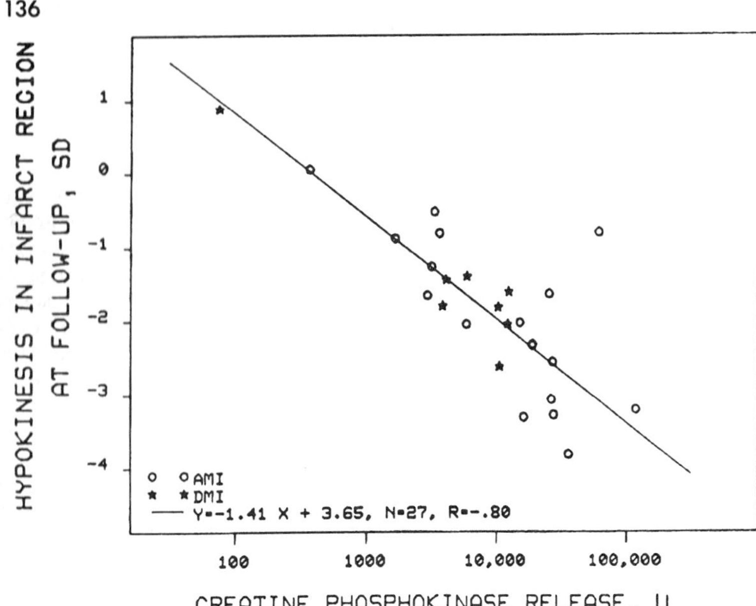

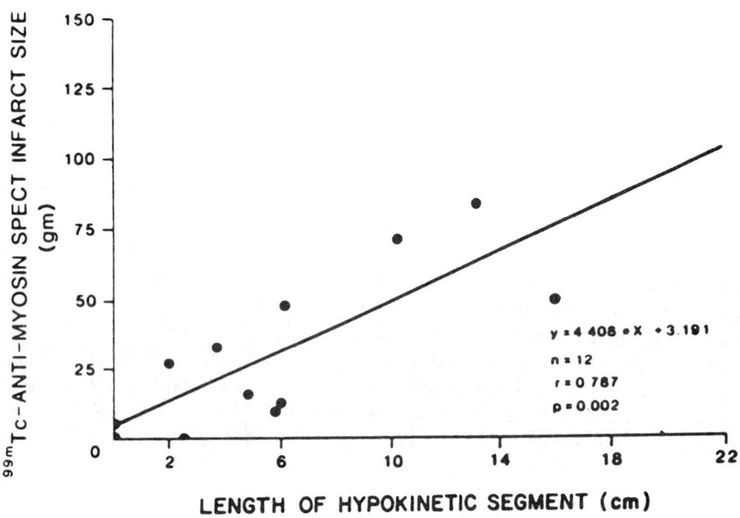

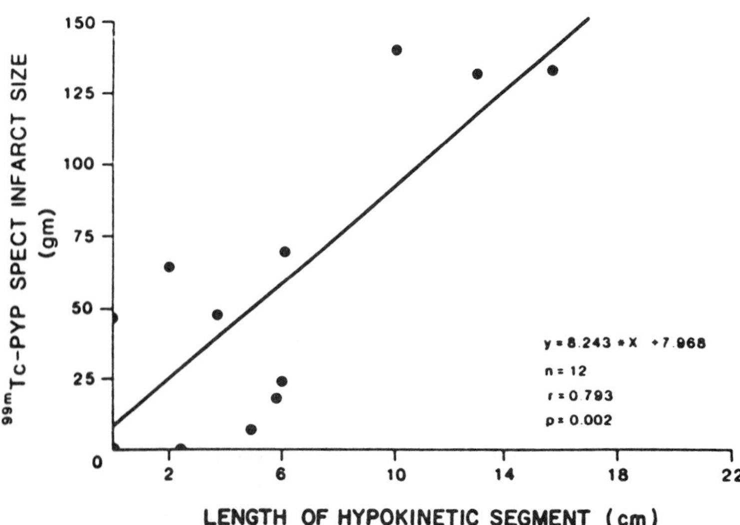

Figure 9–33. The severity of hypokinesis in left ventricular wall motion correlates significantly with infarct size estimated from release of creatine phosphokinase *(top)*, technetium pyrophosphate imaging *(center)*, or antimyosin antibody scintigraphy *(bottom)*. (Top: from Sheehan, F.H., Bolson, E.L., Dodge, H.T., et al.: Advantages and applications of the centerline method for characterizing regional ventricular function. Circulation 74:293, 1986, with permission from the American Heart Association, Inc. Middle and bottom: from Ban An Khaw, Gold, H.K., Yasuda, T., et al.: Scintigraphic quantification of myocardial necrosis in patients after intravenous injection of myosin-specific antibody. Circulation 74:501, 1986, with permission of the American Heart Association, Inc.)

reduced if severe reduction in motion is used to define the infarcted region.[G14] Also, measurement of function immediately after infarction may overestimate infarct size because the apparent border zone at this time probably represents a region that is ischemic but salvageable; by 48 hours this region has either infarcted or recovered, and measurements of hypokinetic segment length correlate better with pathologic infarct size.[N1]

Although it is tempting to assess infarct size from measurements of wall motion, there are several complicating factors, such as the nonlinear relationship between function and fibrosis[L6] and the presence of a border zone. In addition, left ventricular wall motion is naturally asynergic; this is exacerbated by ischemia and infarction. Frame-by-frame analysis of function throughout the cardiac cycle to determine the full extent of akinesis or dyskinesis yields a closer correlation with infarct size.[K11] Finally, experimental studies suggest that measurements of regional function are insensitive to small (≤ 6 percent of left ventricular mass) infarcts.[P2]

Nevertheless, significant correlation with infarct size was found with measurements of either the severity of hypokinesis or the length of the hypokinetic segment, using the centerline method. The strength of the correlation is, of course, influenced by the accuracy of the infarct size determination, since it is difficult to measure infarct size in vivo, as well as the accuracy of the wall motion measurement, and ranged from $r = 0.69$ for thallium scintigraphy, $r = 0.78$ for creatine phosphokinase release, and $r = 0.79$ for antimyosin antibody scintigraphy or technetium pyrophosphate imaging to $r = 0.85$ for nuclear magnetic resonance imaging (Fig. 9–33).[J2, K12, S16, S27]

Wall Motion Remote From an Infarction

Motion in the wall opposite the site of acute infarction is frequently increased (Fig. 9–34). Although hyperkinesis may be seen in experimental animals, function measured in the noninfarct region may be normal or even reduced.[C10, T3] The reason for the variability in response is unclear. In man, the incidence of hyperkinesis in acute infarction ranges from 16 to 67 percent[J3, S25, S28] and is higher in patients with single-vessel disease than in those with multivessel disease.[J3, S28] It is not surprising, therefore, that patients with hyperkinesis have a higher ejection fraction and a better prognosis: they also have less severe hypokinesis.[J3, M9, S25] The presence of hyperkinesis has been shown to benefit global function independent of the severity of hypokinesis in the infarct site.[S11]

The appearance of compensatory hyperkinesis during acute myocardial infarction often results in a normal (≥ 55 percent) ejection fraction. Conversely, patients with hypokinesis in the noninfarct region may have an ejection fraction lower than expected from the severity of hypokinesis in the infarct region.[S11]

Time Course of Functional Recovery After Infarction

The influence of regional function on the ejection fraction is best seen from serial studies in the postinfarct period because of the differing time course over which function recovers in the infarct and noninfarct regions.[S29] Contraction ceases immediately

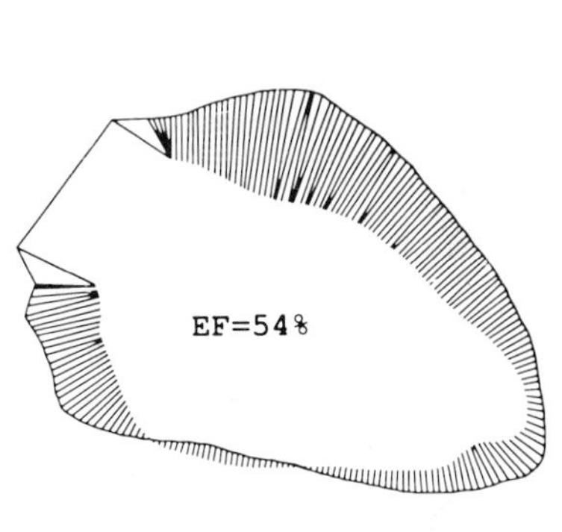

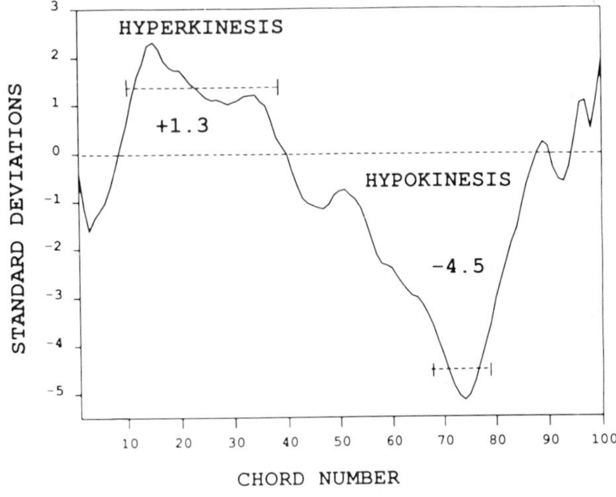

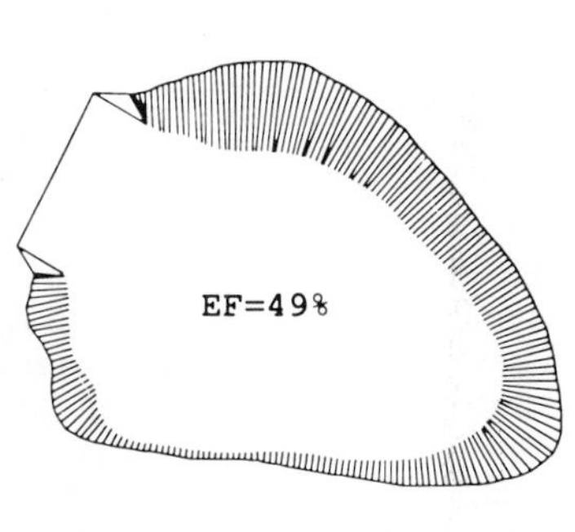

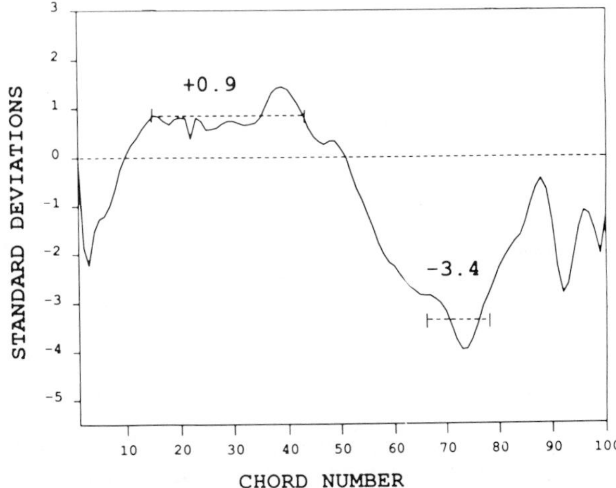

Figure 9–34. The development of compensatory hyperkinesis during acute myocardial infarction improves global function *(top)*. However, the effect of thrombolytic therapy on functional recovery in the infarct region may be underestimated by measurement of the ejection fraction because of concomitant regression of hyperkinesis following infarction *(bottom)*.

following coronary artery occlusion. However, following reperfusion, even in myocardium that is reversibly ischemic, there is a delay before function recovers to baseline levels or reaches a plateau. This delay ranges from 15 minutes after a 5-minute occlusion to 4 weeks after a permanent occlusion.[H14, L7, P3] Both the magnitude of recovery and the rate are related to the severity of the ischemic result. Thus, recovery is more rapid in the peripheral than in the central infarct region.[E1, L7, R9] In humans, function begins to recover between 3 and 5 days following thrombolysis.[S12, W3] This phenomenon of the "stunned" myocardium has been attributed to the need to repair damaged metabolic processes.[B9] In the noninfarct region, regression of compensatory hyperkinesis is largely complete by 3 days after infarction, before function in the infarct region recovers.[S29] In response, the ejection fraction declines the first few days and improves later.

Ventricular Function as a Predictor of Survival

The left ventricular ejection fraction was consistently proved to be one of the most powerful predictors of survival in patients with coronary artery disease. In the Seattle Heart Watch Study, which surveyed over 2000 patients with angina, the ejection fraction was one of the best correlates of survival in both medically and surgically treated groups (see Fig. 9–19).[H15] In patients with myocardial infarction, the ejection fraction is a strong predictor of survival regardless of whether it is measured acutely, after 3 days, before hospital discharge, or later.[M10, N2, S12, S30]

Measurements of wall motion are also useful prognostic indicators. In the Coronary Artery Surgery Study, the wall motion score measured preoperatively correlated well with the patient's subsequent surgical risk.[K1] However, measurements of regional function also correlate significantly with the ejection fraction and therefore closely parallel the ejection fraction as a prognostic indicator. For example, in the Western Washington Intracoronary Streptokinase Study, the hypokinetic segment length was slightly more predictive of 6-month survival than the ejection fraction, but the opposite was true for 1-year survival.[S30, S31] Similarly, hyperkinesis in the noninfarct region was more predictive of hospital mortality than the ejection fraction in one study but less predictive of survival in another study.[G15, S12] Therefore, the usefulness of a wall motion parameter in predicting survival should be evaluated in comparison with the ejection fraction and with consideration of possible covarying factors such as the function of other regions of the ventricle. For example, the higher mortality reported in patients lacking compensatory hyperkinesis in the noninfarct region could have been related to their higher wall motion score.[J3] The end-systolic volume has also been reported to be a powerful prognostic indicator in patients with myocardial infarction.[W4]

Measurement of left ventricular function can be used to identify subsets of patients who are likely to benefit from a therapeutic intervention. The results of two recent multicenter trials comparing coronary artery bypass graft surgery with medical therapy for angina patients with three-vessel disease showed better survival with surgery if the patients had an ejection fraction less than 50 percent,[C11, V3] despite their higher operative mortality.[K1] In patients with three-vessel disease and ejection fraction greater than or equal to 50 percent, trial results were conflicting as to the benefit of surgery[E2] and indicated the need for a more sensitive prognostic indicator to assist in decision making. One possibility is stress ventriculography to identify patients with borderline cardiac reserve, whose function falls under stress.

Another application of ventricular function analysis is in preoperative evaluation of patients with aneurysms. Aneurysms most frequently arise as a complication of myocardial infarction. When they cause arrhythmias, angina, or congestive heart failure, aneurysmectomy may provide relief. Studies have shown that the ejection fraction of the nonaneurysmal part of the ventricle correlates with survival, even though the studies differed in how the calculation was made.[K13, K14]

Evaluating Response to Therapeutic Intervention

Theoretical Considerations

There are several advantages of ventricular function as an end point for clinical trials of interventions that reduce ischemia and/or salvage myocardium. The use of quantitative techniques improves accuracy, reduces variability, and thereby enhances the study's power to detect a treatment effect. Also, the measurement of function, especially regional function, provides a very specific end point compared with death, which may occur from noncardiac causes. Ventricular function is objective, uninfluenced by either the patient's or the physician's perspective, in contrast to parameters such as return to work or angina class.

In selecting ventricular function to be the end point for a clinical trial, however, several aspects must be considered. Naturally, the underlying hypothesis should be that the proposed intervention benefits the patient by its effect on ventricular function. In addition, parameters of function such as the ejection fraction and wall motion are influenced by preload, afterload, and heart rate. White and associates reported the end-systolic volume to be a parameter of function that correlated with survival after infarction better than the ejection fraction, perhaps because of its independence from preload.[C12, W4] The time-varying elastance is a parameter of contractility that is independent of both preload and afterload.[S32] However, elastance is difficult to measure clinically because it requires that volume and pressure be determined under at least three loading conditions.

Timing of Measurements

The effect of therapy on function may be assessed either from the change observed between the baseline and follow-up studies or from the level of function achieved by the time of follow-up. Measurement of function prior to treatment allows (1) comparison of treatment groups to be sure they were similar at baseline, (2) measurement of the change in function after the intervention, and (3) adjustment for the influence of patient-to-patient variability in baseline function.

On the other hand, it is the absolute level of function achieved, not the change in function, that correlates with survival. Thus, the measurement of both function and the severity of residual dysfunction at follow-up may be more pertinent to outcome.

In studies of acute myocardial infarction, the time at which ventricular function is measured has critical importance because of the time course of changes. Consequently, the extent of recovery may be incorrect if measured too soon, either because it is incomplete in the infarct region or because hyperkinesis in the noninfarct region is still evolving.

Parameter Selection

The ejection fraction is generally the parameter of ventricular function that is selected as the end point of a therapeutic trial. However, for studies of thrombolytic therapy the change in wall motion in the site of acute myocardial infarction proved to be more sensitive than the ejection fraction to the effect of reperfusion, because the ejection fraction was influenced by the sometimes opposing changes in the noninfarct region.[S10, S21] As a result, wall motion analysis was very useful in pinpointing factors that influence functional recovery.[S33] Even if the ejection fraction is the main end point, the analysis of wall motion may provide information that aids in the interpretation of the trial results. For example, streptokinase therapy was associated with a higher predischarge ejection fraction than was seen in placebo-treated patients in the Western Washington Intravenous Streptokinase Trial. Wall motion analysis revealed that streptokinase improved function in the noninfarct region, which suggested that the drug may benefit function via mechanisms other than reperfusion of the infarct-related artery.[M11]

When evaluating change in regional function, for example, between serial studies, attention must be paid to the method used for wall motion analysis, to avoid regression toward the mean. That is, if follow-up function is measured from the wall motion vectors that demonstrated severe abnormality at baseline, there is a statistical likelihood for function to be less abnormal on repeated study.[J1] The centerline method avoids this bias by searching for the most abnormally contracting segment independently in each study.

FURTHER APPLICATIONS OF ANGIOGRAPHIC ANALYSIS

Right Ventriculography

Until recently, interest in evaluating right ventricular function was restricted to pediatric cardiologists for management of patients with congenital heart disease. Experimental studies had suggested that the right ventricle was a superfluous structure.[S34, S35] The clinical consequences of right ventricular infarction were first recognized in 1974.[C13] Subsequently, methods for measurement of right ventricular volume and ejection fraction were developed and applied to study patients with myocardial infarction.

The right ventricle has an irregular three-dimensional shape and curves concavely over the right anterolateral aspect of the left ventricle. Nevertheless, studies have shown that the techniques developed to measure left ventricular volume can be applied to the right ventricle. Thus, even though the right ventricle bears no resemblance to an ellipsoid of revolution, its volume can be calculated using the area-length method from biplane angiograms with an accuracy (range of standard error of the estimate is 7.8 to 13.6 ml, depending on the orientation of the right ventricle) comparable to that of the measurements of the left ventricle and to that of calculations by the multiple-slice method.[L1]

Other investigators have compared the right ventricle to other geometric structures such as a parallelogram[A4] or a prism.[F2] In an analysis of 21 methods for right ventricular volume determination, the pyramid method of Ferlinz yielded the greatest accuracy.[D8, F3] Measurement of right ventricular volume from single-plane angiograms increases the standard error of the estimate by 2.7 ml and results in systematic underestimation of stroke volume and ejection fraction; the error can be reduced by applying phase-specific correction factors at end-diastole and end-systole. Others have reported that the single-plane and biplane volumes correlate with $r = 0.93$.[F4] Accuracy is not increased by calculating the volumes of the apex and inflow and outflow tracts with separate correction factors.[L1] The high incidence of ectopy during right ventriculography can be reduced by using a balloon-tipped catheter.[U1]

There have been few studies of regional right ventricular wall motion. These studies have utilized either a rectangular coordinate system or the centerline method (see Fig. 9–28).[F5, S16] The elongated shape of the LAO view makes radial coordinate methods unsuitable.

Studies of normal subjects indicate that right ventricular is lower than left ventricular ejection fraction.[G16] This finding has not been universally confirmed[F3, S36] but is consistently supported by studies employing radionuclide ventriculography.[M12] Since stroke volumes of the two ventricles are equal in the absence of a shunt, right ventricular end-diastolic and end-systolic volumes and volume indices are greater than the left ventricular values. The normal ranges for these parameters cannot be stated reliably because none of the angiographic studies has included more than 10 adult normal subjects and all have used different methods for calculating right ventricular volume.[F3, G16, S36] Similarly, the normal extent of inward wall motion is lower in the right ventricle.[S36] Consequently, it is more difficult to identify abnormalities in wall motion, unless the disease process results in frank dyskinesis.

In contrast to the plethora of reports on left ventricular function in coronary artery disease, studies of right ventricular involvement have been recent and few. These studies have shown that right ventricular infarction occurs much less frequently than, and is virtually always associated with, left ventricular infarction.[R10] As is the case for the left ventricle, dysfunction of the right ventricle occurs in the hypoperfused region.[F5] The right and left anterior descending coronary arteries have diminished wall motion in the free wall or septum, respectively,[F5, M13] but the circumferential extent of hypokinesis is small.

Analysis of Left Ventricular Function Throughout the Cardiac Cycle

Global Function

VOLUME CURVE. Most studies of ventricular function are made from only two points in the cardiac cycle, end-diastole and end-systole. From calculations of volume at each frame through the cardiac cycle, a volume curve can be constructed relating volume to time (Fig. 9–35). Rapid filming at 30 to 60 frames per second allows accurate determination of the rate of ejection or filling from the slopes of the systolic and diastolic portions of the volume-time curve. The peak ejection rate is a parameter of ventricular performance but offers no advantage over the ejection fraction.[H16]

Because the ejection fraction is normal in patients with coronary disease without infarction, there has been a search for a functional parameter that is more sensitive to ischemia. The partial ejection fraction, or volume ejected in early systole, was not consistently found to be reduced in patients with a normal holosystolic ejection fraction.[D9, J4] The opposite is true for diastole. Hammermeister and Warbasse first reported that diastolic filling rates are reduced in patients with coronary artery disease.[H17] Studies using radionuclide techniques for their ease and noninvasive nature have shown that the peak filling rate and time to peak filling rate are abnormal in the majority of patients with coronary artery disease and normal systolic function.[B10]

PRESSURE-VOLUME RELATIONSHIP. Integration of volume and ventricular pressure data allows measurement of stroke work.[A5, B11, D10, R11] Systolic stroke work is calculated from the area under the systolic portion of the curve, and the work of filling is calculated from the diastolic portion:

$$\text{Systolic stroke work} = \int_{V_d}^{V_s} PdV$$

where V_d and V_s are the end-diastolic and end-systolic volumes, respectively, and P is the ventricular systolic pressure. Systolic stroke work increases when the ventricle dilates or afterload increases, as with aortic stenosis.

$$\text{Diastolic stroke work} = \int_{V_d}^{V_s} PdV$$

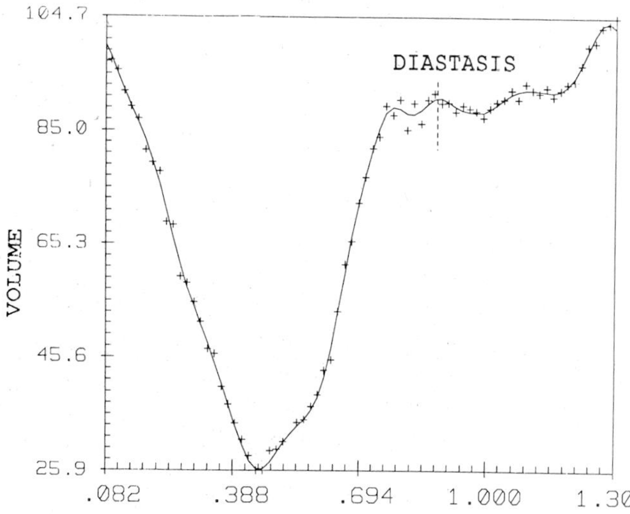

Figure 9–35. From frame-by-frame analysis of left ventricular chamber volume, the volume-time curve can be plotted. At low heart rates (heart rate = 46 in this study), the diastasis period is prolonged.

The work of filling the ventricle in diastole is related to its distensibility. In patients with increased wall thickness, compliance is chronically reduced: more work must be performed by the left atrium and perhaps by the right ventricle to fill the left ventricle. This is manifested by an elevation in end-diastolic pressure, shifting the diastolic portion of the pressure-volume curve upward. Acute myocardial ischemia can also decrease compliance by increasing muscle stiffness without changing the volume/mass ratio.[B12, G17] This effect has been attributed to impaired relaxation or to sustained contraction. Even without performing further quantitative analysis, the effect of heart disease on stroke work can be appreciated from the shape and location of the pressure-volume loop (Fig. 9–36).

The time-varying volume elastance of the left ventricle can be determined from repeated measurements of the pressure-volume relationship under varying loading conditions.[S32, S37] The elastance is calculated as

$$E(t) = P(t)/V(t) - V_0(t)$$

where E(t) is the elastance in mmHg/ml at time t after onset of contraction, P(t) and V(t) are the instantaneous pressure and volume at time t, and $V_0(t)$ is the ventricular volume at zero pressure during systole. The maximum elastance, E_{max}, has been used as a load-independent measure of contractility. In clinical studies, E_{max} is generally approximated by calculating the elastance at end-systole, E_{ES}.[G18] More recent studies report that the end-systolic pressure-volume relationship is curvilinear under conditions of regional myocardial ischemia and is not adequately described by a simple slope and intercept.[S38]

The preload recruitable stroke work is another parameter of contractility that is load independent. It can be determined from the same set of pressure-volume loops as elastance.[G19]

In humans, it is difficult to perform more than three ventriculograms to determine E_{ES} with confidence. Nevertheless, even visual examination of the pressure-volume relationship may provide clinically useful information on the performance of a patient's heart throughout the cardiac cycle and apart from load considerations.[K15]

Regional Function

As for analysis of left ventricular function at end-diastole and end-systole, assessment of regional wall motion throughout the cardiac cycle is useful for interpreting observed abnormalities in global function (Fig. 9–37).

METHODS. As for two-frame studies, many different methods have been used for frame-by-frame analysis of wall motion. The advantages and drawbacks of these various methods are the same as those of two-frame studies, and the question remains of how to adjust for translation. In addition, a method is needed to adjust for heart rate and to express the wall motion results so that they are clearly understandable (Fig. 9–38).

The duration of systole is fairly constant, varying within narrow limits of 0.36 ± 0.04 second over the clinical spectrum of heart rates.[H17] It is the duration of diastole that adjusts to changes in heart rate. At rates below 80 beats per minute, diastasis becomes clearly visible and progressively prolonged. The duration of diastasis correlates highly with the length of the cardiac cycle (r = 0.87) in normal subjects.[H17] Consequently, systolic wall motion can be analyzed by fractionating the duration of systole (Fig. 9–39). The extent of motion at each fraction of systole is then measured and compared between patients.[L8] Alternatively, the linearity of the correlation between wall motion and time through systole can be used as an index of function.[C14, H9] The strength of the correlation indicates the linearity of motion with time; the slope of the regression and its direction indicate whether motion is hyperkinetic or hypokinetic. The situation is more difficult for diastole. If the duration of diastole is fractionated, measurements of function made at a given fraction will correspond to different parts of diastole in patients with different heart rates (Fig. 9–40). In experimental animals, of course, this problem is eliminated by pacing all study subjects to the same heart rate.

An alternative for clinical studies is measurement of asynchrony. For example, asynchrony may be defined as the difference between the time of end-systole and the time at which each region around the ventricular contour reaches maximum contraction and calculated as the mean absolute value or as the standard deviation of the differences. Or, asynchrony may be defined as the time each region reaches peak rate of contraction or peak rate of relaxation and measured from the first derivative of the motion-time curve.[M14] As for global function, diastolic indices of regional function are more sensitive than systolic indices in separating patients with coronary artery disease from normal subjects.

The parameters of asynchrony measure the timing of wall motion but provide no information about the magnitude of wall motion. Conversely, methods that measure motion at a particular time point do not indicate whether the wall is moving in synchrony or not. The correlation of motion with time is more informative, if the correlation coefficient is high, provided that akinetic regions are distinguished from regions contracting with normal synchrony. Both have linear motion-time curves, but the slope of the regression is zero for the akinetic region. However, when the correlation is poor, neither the coefficient of correlation nor the slope indicates when in the cardiac cycle asynchrony is occurring. As can be seen from Figure 9–39, a single patient may have a variety of motion-time patterns.

Regardless of the method or approach used, the motion pattern of normal subjects must be determined in order to define abnormality. There is regional variability in the timing of the phases of diastole,[L9] in the timing of the onset of systolic inward motion,[C15, H10] in the extent and velocity of outward motion during

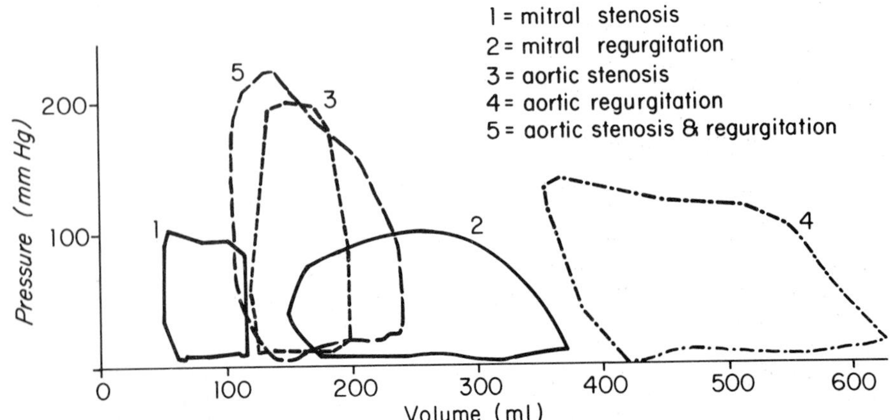

Figure 9–36. Examples of left ventricular pressure-volume curves from patients with different types of heart diseases.[D12] The curve from the patient with mitral stenosis (1) shows well-defined isovolumic contraction and relaxation periods, a normal stroke volume, and relatively normal stroke work. The other patients have large stroke work values, as estimated by the areas under the systolic limb of the curves. The patients with aortic (4) or mitral (2) regurgitation and aortic stenosis and regurgitation (5) have elevated stroke work values with large stroke volumes, as shown by the excursion of the curves along the horizontal or volume axis. Patients with valvular insufficiency have shortening or absence of isovolumic contraction and relaxation periods. Patients with aortic valve stenosis (3) have elevated systolic pressures. Patients with large stroke volumes have elevated end-diastolic volumes.

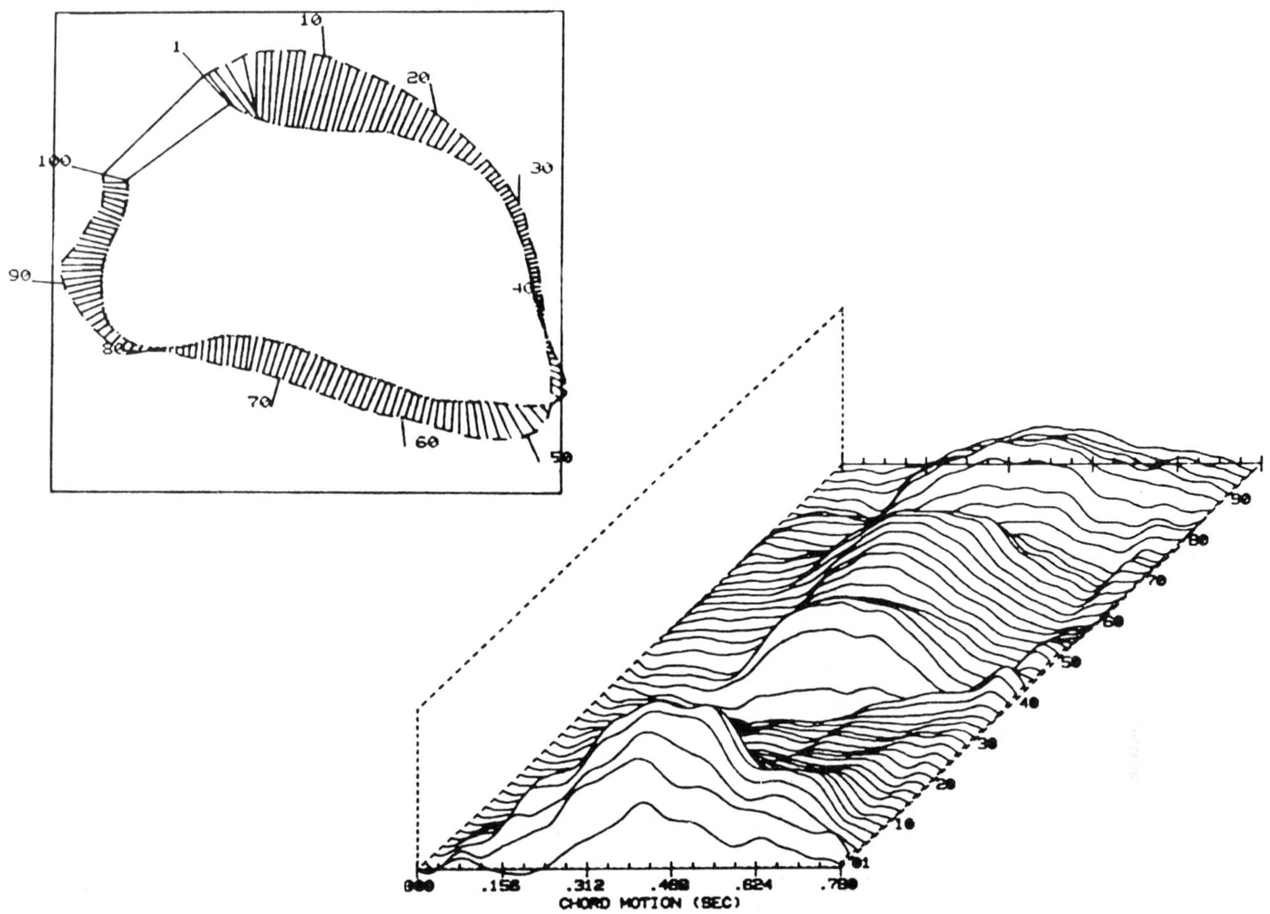

Figure 9–37. Wall motion throughout the cardiac cycle can be plotted as a three-dimensional plot, with chord number, time, and motion on the x, y, and z axes. Normal motion is a "mountain range" extending the length of the y axis. Akinesis is depicted as a flat "plain." The patient was studied during acute anterior myocardial infarction.

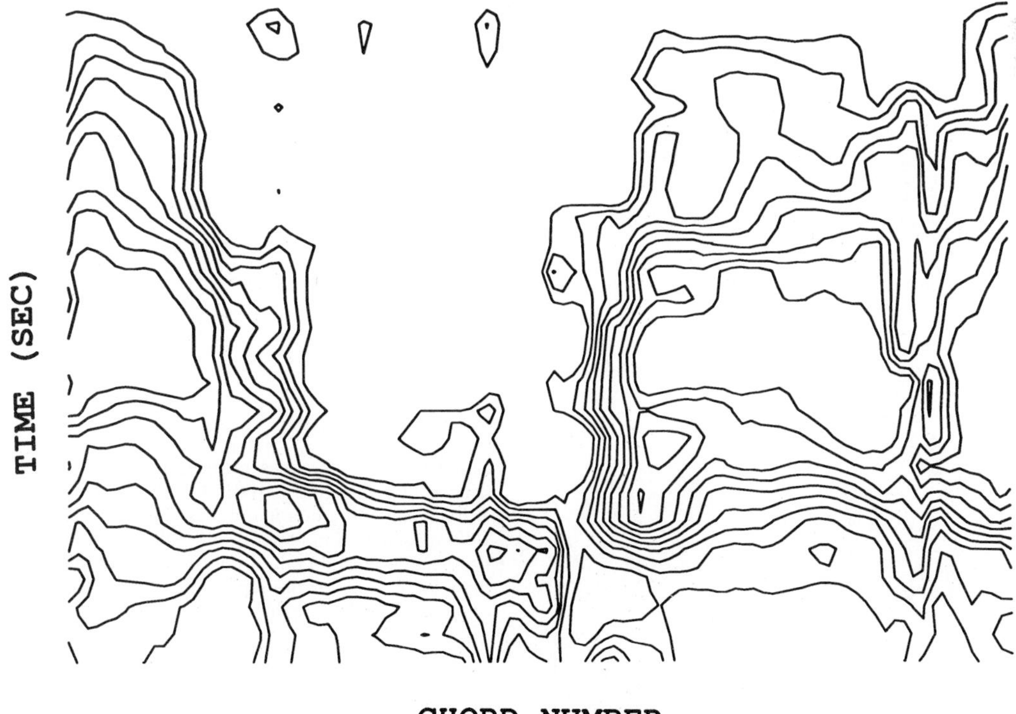

Figure 9–38. The timing of motion depicted with a contour plot[G22] for the same patient as in Figure 9–37.

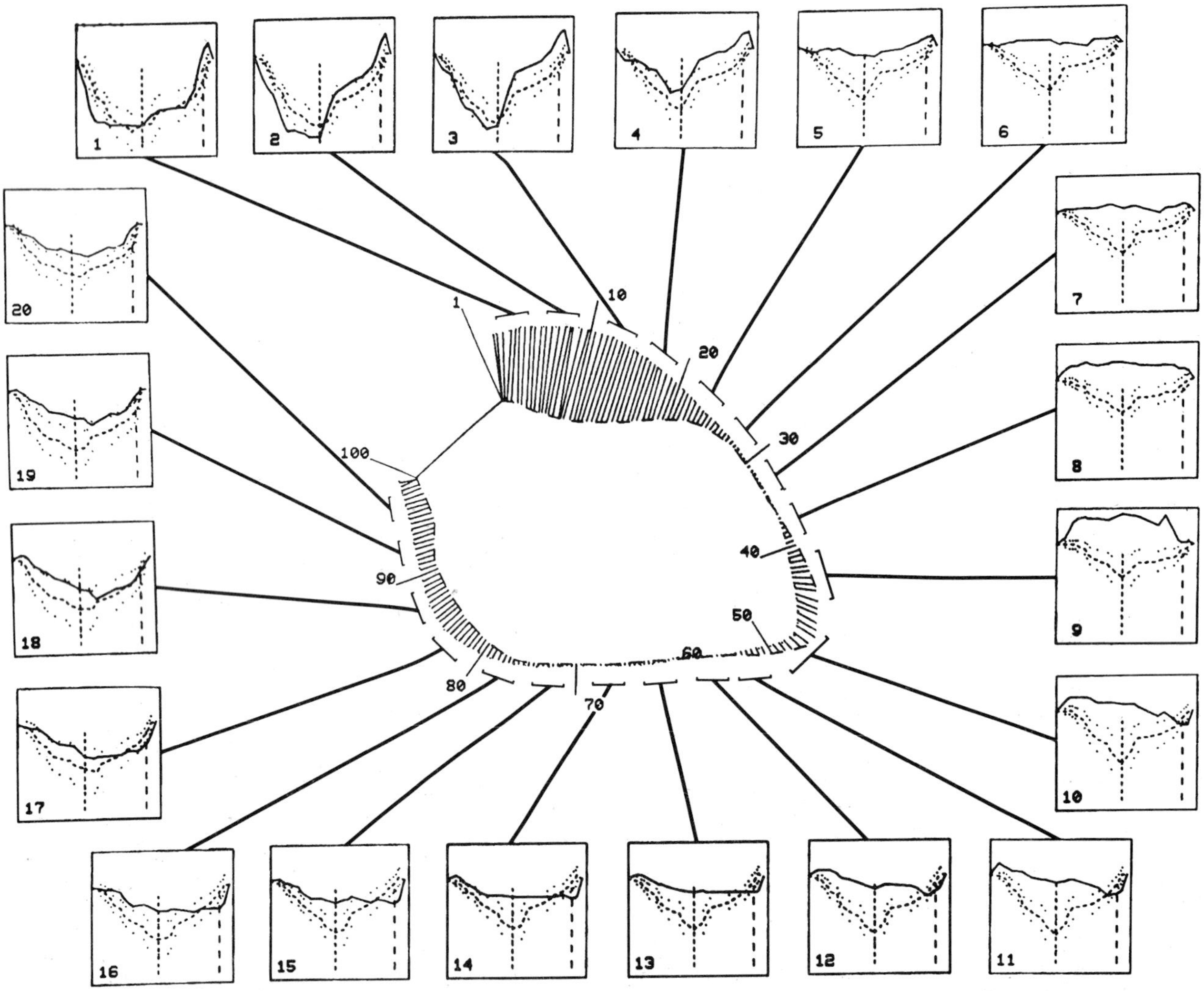

Figure 9–39. Wall motion *(vertical axis)* in 20 regions around the left ventricle plotted against time *(horizontal axis)* through the cardiac cycle from end-diastole to end-diastole. End-systole is marked by the finely dashed vertical line. The time in diastole at which inward motion ceases is marked by the coarsely dashed vertical line. The solid curve is the patient's motion. The dotted curves indicate the mean ± 1 standard deviation for motion in 31 normal patients. Motion is akinetic along the anterior wall (regions 6–8) in this patient with acute thrombosis of the left anterior descending artery. There is apical dyskinesis. Along the inferior wall, postsystolic shortening can be seen. In segments with normal, synchronous motion *(segment 3)* or akinesis *(segment 6 or 7)*, the correlation of motion with time is linear, differing only in slope. In some regions, motion is asynchronous. For example, segment 14 displays slight paradoxic motion at the onset of systole, contraction at a normal rate in early systole, and then near-akinesis through mid-diastole.

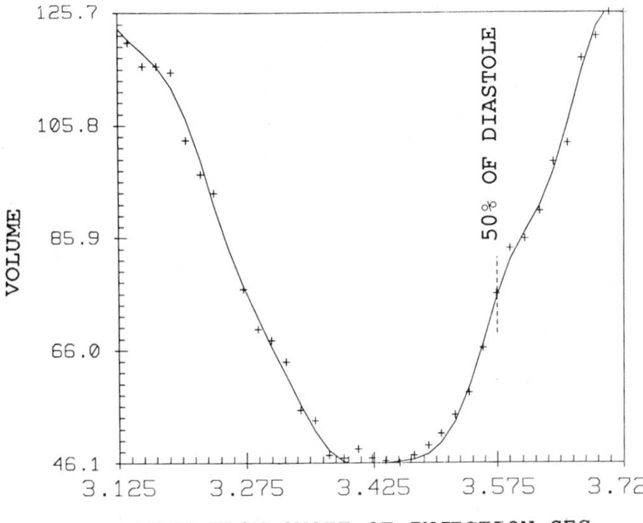

Figure 9–40. Differences in heart rate primarily affect the duration of diastole by prolonging diastasis. Consequently, when function is measured at fractions of the duration of diastole, different parts of the cardiac cycle will be compared in patients with different heart rates. In this study, the heart rate is 96 and mid-diastole occurs near mid-filling. In contrast, mid-diastole occurs after the rapid filling period has ended, at the beginning of diastasis, at a heart rate of 54, as seen in Figure 9–35.

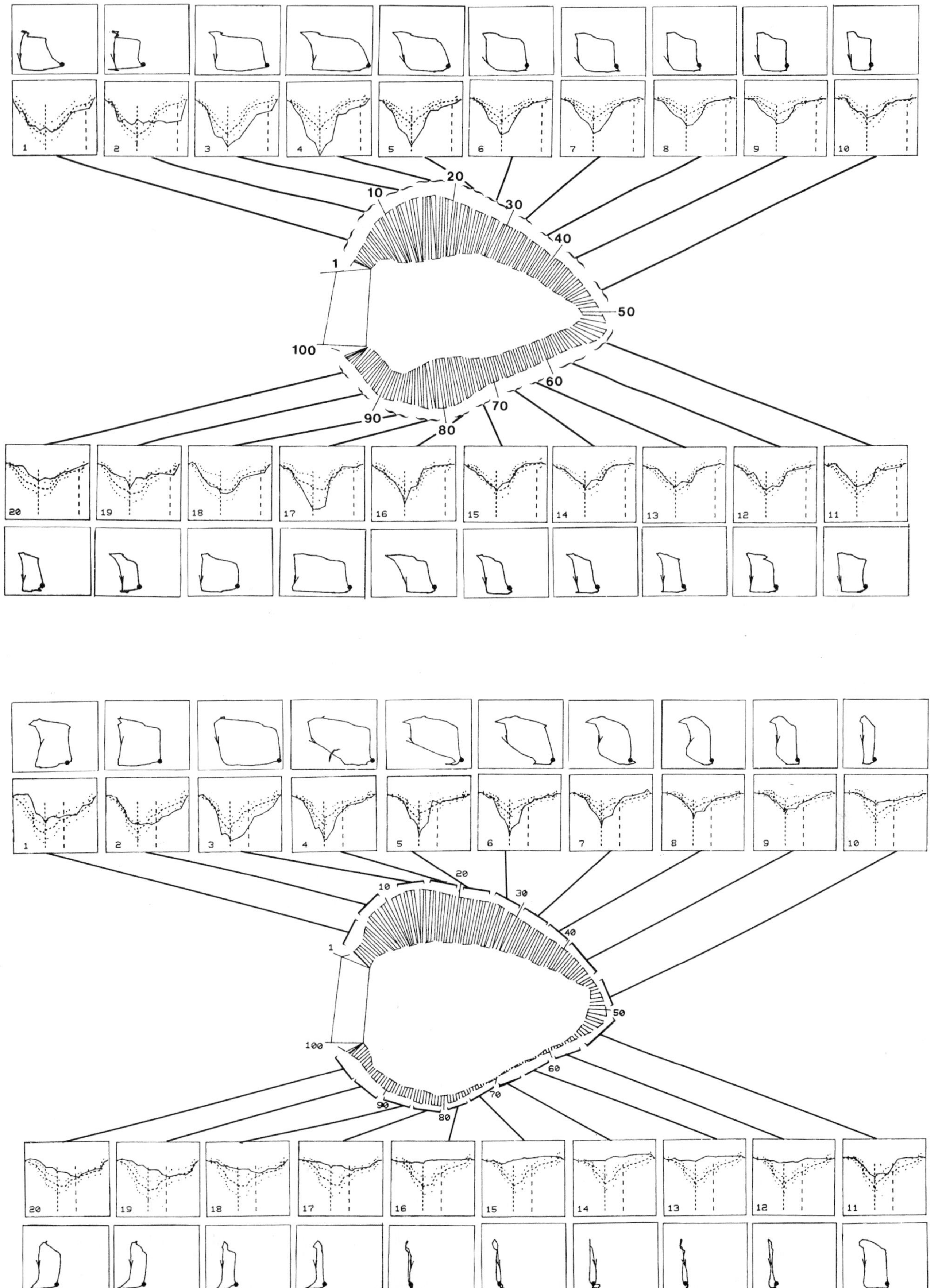

Figure 9–41. Pressure-motion loops relate the motion measured throughout the cardiac cycle with changes in intraventricular pressure. These studies were performed before *(top)* and during *(bottom)* occlusion of the left anterior descending coronary artery in a patient undergoing angioplasty. The motion-time curves of the same regions are presented for comparison.

isovolumic relaxation,[G20] and in the peak velocity of systolic inward motion,[G9] as well as in the extent of motion at end-systole.[G11, H9, I1] Some of this regional, temporal variability is due to the sequence of activation[K16] and to loading conditions.[G21, L10]

In patients with coronary artery disease, the extent of wall motion in the ischemic region is not accurately reflected by the measurement at end-systole.[L8, W5] The onset of contraction may be delayed, or there may be paradoxic outward motion during isovolumic contraction.[G22, L8] These abnormalities are associated with abnormal inward motion during isovolumic relaxation.[G22] It has been suggested that inward motion occurring in diastole represents residual contractile activity in patients with acute myocardial infarction.[T4] These patterns of asynchrony can be classified into a progression of abnormality with increasing severity of coronary artery disease.[H3]

Examination of asynchrony has not proved useful in studies attempting to correlate function with infarct size, the clinical status of the patient, or the presence of surgical aneurysm.[D11, L11] On the other hand, analysis of regional diastolic function has been helpful in elucidating observed abnormalities in global diastolic function. For example, prolongation of the time constant of pressure delay and decrease in the diastolic filling rate at rest and during acute ischemia have been related to reduced regional outward wall motion in the ischemic region.[S39, T5, Y1] The abnormalities in diastolic wall motion are reversible after coronary angioplasty in patients with normal systolic function.[B13]

Measurements of the displacement of the ventricular wall with time can be combined with intraventricular pressure data in a manner analogous to pressure-volume curves (Fig. 9–41). The area enclosed within the loop provides an index of regional stroke work, and the shape of the loop graphically displays the effect of disease processes on regional contraction.[F6, G23] Sasayama and associates have demonstrated the different effects of pacing-induced ischemia on diastolic pressure-length relationships in normal and ischemic regions and their contribution to the global pressure-volume relation.[S40] In pressure-dimension analyses, as in two-frame wall motion studies, it must be remembered that the translational motion of the heart within the chest cannot be distinguished from endocardial motion.

In summary, angiographic measurements of various parameters of the size and function of the right and left ventricles have been employed for decades and an enormous body of experience has established the value of this type of diagnostic procedure. The measurements have been extensively validated, are readily performed in community hospitals, and continue to be one of the dominant cardiac imaging approaches in use today.

References

A

1. Als, A.V., Paulin, S., and Aroesty, J.M.: Biplane angiographic volumetry using the right anterior oblique and half-axial left anterior oblique technique. Radiology 126:511, 1978.
2. Austen, W.G., Edwards, J.E., Frye, R.L., et al.: A reporting system on patients evaluated for coronary artery disease. Circulation 51:6, 1975.
3. Azancot, I., Beaufils, P., Masquet, C., et al.: Detection of residual myocardial function in acute transmural infarction using postextrasystolic potentiation. Circulation 64:46, 1981.
4. Arcilla, R.A., Tsai, P., Thilenius, O., and Ranniger, K.: Angiographic method for volume estimation of right and left ventricles. Chest 60:446, 1971.
5. Arvidsson, H.: Angiocardiographic determination of left ventricular volume. Acta Radiol. 56:321, 1961.

B

1. Braunwald, E.: Mitral regurgitation: Physiologic, clinical and surgical considerations. N. Engl. J. Med. 281:425, 1969.
2. Bursch, J.H., and Heintzen, P.H.: Endocardial and epicardial contour detection of the left ventricle by digital angiocardiography. *In* Ventricular Wall Motion: International Symposium Lausanne 1982. Georg Thieme Verlag, Stuttgart, 1984.
3. Bolson, E.L., Kliman, S., Sheehan, E., and Dodge, H.T.: Left ventricular segmental wall motion—a new method using local direction information. *In:* Computers in Cardiology. IEEE Computer Society, Long Beach, CA, 1980, p. 245.
4. Brutsaert, D.L.: Nonuniformity: A physiologic modulator of contraction and relaxation of the normal heart. J. Am. Coll. Cardiol. 9:341, 1987.
5. Bartle, S. H., and Sanmarco, M. E.: Comparison of angiographic and thermal washout techniques for left ventricular volume measurement. Am. J. Cardiol. 18:235, 1966.
6. Bottcher, D., Holper, H., Meindl, S., et al.: Muster der regionalen Wandbewegungsstorung bei primarer dilatativer Kardiomyopathie. Z. Kardiol. 75:37, 1986.
7. Banka, V.S., Bodenheimer, M.M., Shah, R., and Helfant, R.H.: Intervention ventriculography. Comparative value of nitroglycerin, post-extrasystolic potentiation and nitroglycerin plus post-extrasystolic potentiation. Circulation 53:632, 1976.
8. Bogen, D.K., Rabinowitz, S.A., Needleman, A., et al.: An analysis of the mechanical disadvantage of myocardial infarction in the canine left ventricle. Circ. Res. 47:728, 1980.
9. Braunwald, E., and Kloner, R.A.: The stunned myocardium: Prolonged, postischemic ventricular dysfunction. Circulation 66:1146, 1982.
10. Bonow, R.O., Bacharach, S.L., Green, M.V., et al.: Impaired left ventricular diastolic filling in patients with coronary artery disease: Assessment with radionuclide angiography. Circulation 64:315, 1981.
11. Bunnell, I.L., Grant, C., and Greene, D.G.: Left ventricular function derived from the pressure-volume diagram. Am. J. Med. 39:881, 1965.
12. Barry, W.H., Brooker, J.Z., Alderman, E.L., and Harrison, D.C.: Changes in diastolic stiffness and tone of the left ventricle during angina pectoris. Circulation 49:255, 1974.
13. Bonow, R.O., Vitale, D.F., Bacharach, S.L., et al.: Asynchronous left ventricular regional function and impaired global diastolic filling in patients with coronary artery disease: Reversal after coronary angioplasty. Circulation 71:297, 1985.

C

1. Cha, S.D., Incarvito, J., and Maranhao, V.: Calculation of magnification factor from an intracardiac marker. Cathet. Cardiovasc. Diagn. 9:79, 1983.
2. Cohn, P.F., Levine, J.A., Bergeron, G.A., and Gorlin, R.: Reproducibility of the angiographic left ventricular ejection fraction in patients with coronary artery disease. Am. Heart J. 88:713, 1974.
3. Chaitman, B.R., DeMots, H., Bristow, J.D., et al.: Objective and subjective analysis of left ventricular angiograms. Circulation 52:420, 1975.
4. Clayton, P.D., Jeppson, G.M., and Klausner, S.C.: Should a fixed external reference system be used to analyze left ventricular wall motion? Circulation 65:1518, 1982.
5. Colton, T.: Statistics in medicine. Little, Brown and Company, Boston, 1974, p. 145.
6. Colle, J.P., LeGoff, G., Page, A., and Besse, P.: Validité de la méthode de Stanford dans l'évaluation des dyskinesies segmentaires du ventricule gauche. Arch. Mal. Coeur 75:395, 1982.
7. Clayton, P.D., Klausner, S.C., Blair, T.L., et al.: Sources and magnitude of variability in measurements of regional left ventricular function. *In* Sigwart, U., and Heintzen, P.H. (eds.): Ventricular Wall Motion. Georg Thieme Verlag, Stuttgart, 1984, p. 90.
8. Cohn, P.F., Gorlin, R., Herman, M.V., et al.: Relation between contractile reserve and prognosis in patients with coronary artery disease and a depressed ejection fraction. Circulation 51:414, 1975.
9. Cortina, A., Ambrose, J.A., Prieto-Granada, J., et al.: Left ventricular function after myocardial infarction: Clinical and angiographic correlations. J. Am. Coll. Cardiol. 5:619, 1985.
10. Corday, E., Kaplan, L., Meerbaum, S., et al.: Consequences of coronary arterial occlusion on remote myocardium: Effects of occlusion and reperfusion. Am. J. Cardiol. 36:385, 1975.
11. CASS Principal Investigators and Their Associates: Myocardial infarction and mortality in the coronary artery surgery study (CASS randomized trial). N. Engl. J. Med. 310:750, 1984.
12. Carabello, B.A., and Spann, J.F.: The uses and limitations of end-systolic indexes of left ventricular function. Circulation 69:1058, 1984.
13. Cohn, J.N., Guiha, N.H., Broder, M.I., and Limas, C.J.: Right ventricular infarction: Clinical and hemodynamic features. Am. J. Cardiol. 33:209, 1974.
14. Chen, C., Bonzel, T., Just, H., et al.: Quantitative assessment of temporal and spatial ventricular wall motion in normal and infarcted human left ventricles. Am. Heart J. 112:712, 1986.
15. Clayton, P.D., Bulawa, W.F., Klausner, S.C., et al.: The characteristic sequence for the onset of contraction in the normal human left ventricle. Circulation 59:671, 1979.

D

1. Dodge, H.T., Frimer, M., and Stewart, D.K.: Functional evaluation of the hypertrophied heart in man. Circ. Res. (Suppl. II) 34–35:II-122, 1974.
2. Dodge, H.T., Sandler, H., Ballew, D.W., and Lord, J.D., Jr.: The use of biplane angiocardiography for the measurement of left ventricular volume in man. Am. Heart J. 60:762, 1960.
3. Dodge, H.T., Sheehan, F.H., and Stewart, D.K.: Estimation of ventricular volume, fractional ejected volumes, stroke volume, and quantitation of regurgitant flow. *In* Just, H., and Heintzen, P.H. (eds.): Angiocardiography: Current Status and Future Developments. Springer-Verlag, Berlin, 1986, p. 99.
4. DuBois, D., and DuBois, E.: A formula to estimate the approximate surface area if height and weight be known. Arch. Intern. Med. 17:863, 1916.
5. Dodge, H.T., Hay, R.E., and Sandler, H.: An angiocardiographic method for determining left ventricular stroke volume in man. Circ. Res. 11:739, 1962.
6. Doss, J.K., Hillis, L.D., Curry, G., et al.: A new model for the assessment of regional ventricular wall motion. Radiology 143:763, 1982.
7. David, D., Lang, R.M., and Borow, K.M.: Clinical utility of exercise, pacing, and pharmacologic stress testing for the noninvasive determination of myocardial contractility and reserve. Am. Heart J. 116:235, 1988.

8. Dubel, H.P., Romaniuk, P., and Tschapek, A.: Investigation of human right ventricular cast specimens. Cardiovasc. Intervent. Radiol. 5:296, 1982.
9. Denenberg, B.S., Makler, P.T., Bove, A.A., and Spann, J.F.: Normal left ventricular emptying in coronary artery disease at rest: Analysis by radiographic and equilibrium radionuclide ventriculography. Am. J. Cardiol. 48:311, 1981.
10. Dodge, H.T., Sandler, H., Baxley, W.A., and Hawley, R.R.: Usefulness and limitations of radiographic methods for determining left ventricular volume. Am. J. Cardiol. 18:10, 1966.
11. Dawson, J.R., and Sutton, G.C.: Incoordinate left ventricular wall motion after acute myocardial infarction. Br. Heart J. 51:545, 1984.
12. Dodge, H.T., and Kennedy, J.W.: Cardiac output, cardiac performance, hypertrophy, dilation, valvular disease, ischemic heart disease and pericardial disease. *In* Sodeman, W.A., Jr., and Sodeman, W.A. (eds.): Pathologic Physiology: Mechanisms of Disease, 7th ed. W.B. Saunders Co., Philadelphia, 1985, p. 292.

E

1. Ellis, S.G., Henschke, C.I., Sandor, T., et al.: Time course of functional and biochemical recovery of myocardium salvaged by reperfusion. J. Am. Coll. Cardiol. 1:1047, 1983.
2. European Coronary Surgery Study Group: Long-term results of prospective randomised study of coronary artery bypass surgery in stable angina pectoris. Lancet 2:1172, 1982.

F

1. Feild, B.J., Russel, O., Dowling, J.T., and Rackley, C.E.: Regional left ventricular performance in the year following myocardial infarction. Circulation 46:679, 1972.
2. Fisher, E.A., DuBrow, I.W., and Hastreiter, A.R.: Right ventricular volume in congenital heart disease. Am. J. Cardiol. 36:67, 1975.
3. Ferlinz, J., Gorlin, R., Cohn, P.F., and Herman, M.W.: Right ventricular performance in patients with coronary artery disease. Circulation 52:608, 1975.
4. Ferlinz, J.: Measurements of right ventricular volumes in man from single plane cineangiograms. Am. Heart J. 94:87, 1977.
5. Ferlinz, J., Delvicario, M., and Gorlin, R.: Incidence of right ventricular asynergy in patients with coronary artery disease. Am. J. Cardiol. 38:557, 1976.
6. Forrester, J.S., Wyatt, H.L., Da Luz, P.L., et al.: Functional significance of regional ischemic contraction abnormalities. Circulation 54:64, 1976.

G

1. Graham, T.P., Jr., Atwood, G.F., Faulkner, S.L., and Nelson, J.H.: Right atrial volume measurements from biplane cineangiocardiography. Circulation 49:709, 1974.
2. Gertz, E.W., Wisneski, J.A., Chiu, D., et al.: Clinical superiority of a new nonionic contrast agent (Iopamidol) for cardiac angiography. J. Am. Coll. Cardiol. 5:250, 1985.
3. Gribbe, P.: Comparison of the angiocardiographic and direct Fick methods in determining cardiac output. Cardiologia 36:20, 1960.
4. Gorlin, R., and Gorlin, S.G.: Hydraulic formula for calculation of the area of the stenotic mitral valve, other cardiac valves and central circulatory shunts. Am. Heart J. 41:1, 1951.
5. Grossman, W., Jones, D., and McLaurin, L.P.: Wall stress and patterns of hypertrophy in the human left ventricle. J. Clin. Invest. 56:56, 1975.
6. Gould, K.L., Lipscomb, K., Hamilton, G.W., and Kennedy, J.W.: Relation of left ventricular shape, function and wall stress in man. Am. J. Cardiol. 34:627, 1974.
7. Grossman, W., Carabello, B.A., Gunther, S., and Fifer, M.A.: Ventricular wall stress and the development of cardiac hypertrophy and failure. Perspect. Cardiovasc. Res. 7:1, 1983.
8. Goodyer, A.V.N., and Langou, R.A.: The multicentric character of normal left ventricular wall motion. Implications for the evaluation of regional wall motion abnormalities by contrast angiography. Cathet. Cardiovasc. Diagn. 8:225, 1982.
9. Gibson, D.G., Sanderson, J.E., Traill, T.A., et al.: Regional left ventricular wall movement in hypertrophic cardiomyopathy. Br. Heart J. 40:1327, 1978.
10. Greenbaum, R.A., and Gibson, D.G.: Regional non-uniformity of left ventricular wall movement in man. Br. Heart J. 45:29, 1981.
11. Gelberg, H.J., Brundage, B.H., Glantz, S., and Parmley, W.W.: Quantitative left ventricular wall motion analysis: A comparison of area, chord and radial methods. Circulation 59:991, 1979.
12. Ginzton, L.E., Berntzen, R., Lobodzinski, S., et al.: Computerized quantitative segmental wall motion analysis during exercise: Radial vs. centerline left ventricular segmentation. *In* Computers in Cardiology. IEEE Computer Society, Long Beach, CA, 1985, p. 157.
13. Graham, T.P., Jr., Jarmakani, J.M., Canent, R.V., and Morrow, M.N.: Left heart volume estimation in infancy and childhood: Reevaluation of methodology and normal values. Circulation 43:895, 1971.
14. Gallagher, K.P., Gerren, R.A., Stirling, M.C., et al.: The distribution of functional impairment across the lateral border of acutely ischemic myocardium. Circ. Res. 58:570, 1986.
15. Grines, C.L., Topol, E.J., Califf, R.M., et al.: Prognostic implications and predictors of enhanced wall motion of the noninfarct zone after thrombolysis and angioplasty therapy of acute myocardial infarction. Circulation 80:245, 1989.
16. Gentzler, R.D., Briselli, M.F., and Gault, J.H.: Angiographic estimation of right ventricular volume in man. Circulation 50:324, 1974.
17. Gaasch, W.H., Levine, H.J., Quinones, M.A., and Alexander, J.K.: Left ventricular compliance: Mechanisms and clinical implications. Am. J. Cardiol. 38:645, 1976.
18. Grossman, W., Braunwald, E., Mann, T., et al.: Contractile state of the left ventricle in man as evaluated from end-systolic pressure-volume relations. Circulation 56:845, 1977.
19. Glower, D.D., Spratt, J.A., Snow, N.D., et al.: Linearity of the Frank-Starling relationship in the intact heart: The concept of preload recruitable stroke work. Circulation 71:994, 1985.
20. Gibson, D.G., Prewitt, T.A., and Brown, D.J.: Analysis of left ventricular wall movement during isovolumic relaxation and its relation to coronary artery disease. Br. Heart J. 38:1010, 1976.
21. Gaasch, W.H., Blaustein, A.S., and Bing, O.H.L.: Asynchronous (segmental early) relaxation of the left ventricle. J. Am. Coll. Cardiol. 5:891, 1985.
22. Gibson, D.G., Doran, J.H., Traill, T.A., and Brown, D.J.: Abnormal left ventricular wall movement during early systole in patients with angina pectoris. Br. Heart J. 40:758, 1978.
23. Gibson, D.G., and Brown, D.J.: Assessment of left ventricular systolic function in man from simultaneous echocardiographic and pressure measurements. Br. Heart J. 38:8, 1976.

H

1. Hildner, F.J., Furst, A., Krieger, R., et al.: New principles for optimum left ventriculography. Cathet. Cardiovasc. Diagn. 12:266, 1986.
2. Herman, M.V., Heinle, R.A., Klein, M.D., and Gorlin, R.: Localized disorders in myocardial contraction: Asynergy and its role in congestive heart failure. N. Engl. J. Med. 277:222, 1967.
3. Holman, B.L., Wynne, J., Idoine, J., and Neill, J.: Disruption in the temporal sequence of regional ventricular contraction. Circulation 61:1075, 1980.
4. Hugenholtz, P.G., Kaplan, E., and Hull, E.: Determination of left ventricular wall thickness by angiocardiography. Am. Heart J. 78:513, 1969.
5. Hugenholtz, P.G., Wagner, H.R., and Sandler, H.: The in vivo determination of left ventricular volume: Comparison of the fiberoptic-indicator dilution and the angiocardiographic methods. Circulation 37:489, 1968.
6. Higgins, C.B., Gerber, K.H., Mattrey, R.F., and Slutsky, R.A.: Evaluation of the hemodynamic effects of intravenous administration of ionic and nonionic contrast materials. Radiology 143:681, 1982.
7. Hunt, D., Baxley, W.A., Kennedy, J.W., et al.: Quantitative evaluation of cineaortography in the assessment of aortic regurgitation. Am. J. Cardiol. 31:696, 1973.
8. Hood, W.P., Rackley, C.E., and Rolett, E.L.: Wall stress in the normal and hypertrophied human left ventricle. Am. J. Cardiol. 22:550, 1968.
9. Harris, L.D., Clayton, P.D., Marshall, H.W., and Warner, H.R.: A technique for the detection of asynergic motion in the left ventricle. Comput. Biomed. Res. 7:380, 1974.
10. Hammermeister, K.E., Gibson, D.G., and Hughes, D.: Regional variation in the timing and extent of left ventricular wall motion in normal subjects. Br. Heart J. 56:226, 1986.
11. Horn, H.R., Teichholz, L.E., Cohn, P.F., et al.: Augmentation of left ventricular contraction pattern in coronary artery disease by an inotropic catecholamine. Circulation 49:1063, 1974.
12. Hamby, R.I., Aintablian, A., Wisoff, B.G., and Hartstein, M.L.: Response of the left ventricle in coronary artery disease to postextrasystolic potentiation. Circulation 51:428, 1975.
13. Hodgson, J.M., O'Neill, L.W.W., Laufer, N., et al.: Assessment of potentially salvageable myocardium during acute myocardial infarction: Use of postextrasystolic potentiation. Am. J. Cardiol. 54:1237, 1984.
14. Heyndrickx, G.R., Millard, R.W., McRitchie, R.J., et al.: Regional myocardial functional and electrophysiological alterations after brief coronary artery occlusion in conscious dogs. J. Clin. Invest. 56:978, 1975.
15. Hammermeister, K.E., DeRouen, T.A., and Dodge, H.T.: Variables predictive of survival in patients with coronary disease. Circulation 59:421, 1979.
16. Hammermeister, K.E., Brooks, R.C., and Warbasse, J.R.: Rate of change of left ventricular volume in man. I. Validation and peak systolic ejection rate in health and disease. Circulation 49:729, 1974.
17. Hammermeister, K.E., and Warbasse, J.R.: The rate of change of left ventricular volume in man. II. Diastolic events in health and disease. Circulation 49:739, 1974.
18. Hammermeister, K.E., DeRouen, T.A., Zia, M.S., and Dodge, H.T.: Survival of medically treated coronary artery disease patients in the Seattle Heart Watch Angiography Registry. *In* Late Results of Coronary Bypass Surgery. Praeger, New York, 1983, p. 167.

I

1. Ingels, N.B., Jr., Daughters, G.T., II, Stinson, E.B., and Alderman, E.L.: Measurement of midwall myocardial dynamics in intact man by radiography of surgically implanted markers. Circulation 52:859, 1975.
2. Ingels, N.B., Jr., Daughters, G.T., II, Stinson, E.B., and Alderman, E.L.: Evaluation of methods for quantitating left ventricular segmental wall motion in man using myocardial markers as a standard. Circulation 61:966, 1980.
3. Ideker, R.E., Behar, V.S., Wagner, G.S., et al.: Evaluation of asynergy as an indicator of myocardial fibrosis. Circulation 57:715, 1978.

J

1. Jeppson, G.M., Clayton, P.D., Blair, T.J., et al.: Changes in left ventricular wall motion after coronary artery bypass surgery: Signal or noise. Circulation 64:945, 1981.
2. Johns, J.A., Leavitt, M.B., Newell, J.B., et al.: Quantitation of acute myocardial

infarct size by nuclear magnetic resonance imaging. J. Am. Coll. Cardiol. 15:143, 1990.
3. Jaarsma, W., Visser, C.A., Van, M.J.E., et al.: Prognostic implications of regional hyperkinesia and remote asynergy of noninfarcted myocardium. Am. J. Cardiol. 58:394, 1986.
4. Johnson, L.L., Ellis, K., Schmidt, D., et al.: Volume ejected in early systole: A sensitive index of left ventricular performance in coronary artery disease. Circulation 52:378, 1975.

K

1. Kennedy, J.W., Kaiser, G.C., Fisher, L.D., et al.: Clinical and angiographic predictors of operative mortality from the Collaborative Study in Coronary Artery Stenosis (CASS). Circulation 63:793, 1981.
2. Kennedy, J.W., Trenholme, S.E., and Kasser, I.S.: Left ventricular volume and mass from single-plane cineangiocardiogram: A comparison of anteroposterior and right anterior oblique methods. Am. Heart J. 80:343, 1970.
3. Kasser, I.S., and Kennedy, J.W.: Measurement of left ventricular volumes in man by single-plane cineangiocardiography. Invest. Radiol. 4:83, 1969.
4. Kennedy, J.W., Twiss, R.D., Blackmon, J.R., and Dodge, H.T.: Quantitative angiocardiography. III. Relationships of left ventricular pressure, volume, and mass in aortic valve disease. Circulation 38:838, 1968.
5. Kennedy, J.W., Reichenbach, D.D., Baxley, W.A., and Dodge, H.T.: Left ventricular mass: A comparison of angiocardiographic measurements with autopsy weight. Am. J. Cardiol. 19:221, 1967.
6. Kong, Y., Morris, J.J., Jr., and McIntosh, H.D.: Assessment of regional myocardial performance from biplane coronary cineangiograms. Am. J. Cardiol. 27:529, 1971.
7. Karsch, K.R., Lamm, U., Blanke, H., and Rentrop, K.P.: Comparison of nineteen quantitative models for assessment of localized left ventricular wall motion abnormalities. Clin. Cardiol. 3:123, 1980.
8. Kennedy, J.W., Baxley, W.A., Figley, M.M., et al.: Quantitative angiography. I. The normal left ventricle in man. Circulation 34:272, 1966.
9. Kalbfleisch, H., and Hort, W.: Quantitative study on the size of coronary artery supplying areas postmortem. Am. Heart J. 94:183, 1977.
10. Kerber, R.E., Marcus, M.L., Ehrhardt, J., et al.: Correlation between echocardiographically demonstrated segmental dyskinesis and regional myocardial perfusion. Circulation 52:1097, 1975.
11. Kaul, S., Pandian, N.G., Gillam, L.D., et al.: Contrast echocardiography in acute myocardial ischemia. III. An in vivo comparison of the extent of abnormal wall motion with the area at risk for necrosis. J. Am. Coll. Cardiol. 7:383, 1986.
12. Khaw, B.A., Gold, H.K., Yasuda, T., et al.: Scintigraphic quantification of myocardial necrosis in patients after intravenous injection of myosin-specific antibody. Circulation 74:501, 1986.
13. Kiefer, S.K., Flaker, G.C., Martin, R.H., and Curtis, J.J.: Clinical improvement after ventricular aneurysm repair: Prediction by angiographic and hemodynamic variables. J. Am. Coll. Cardiol. 2:30, 1983.
14. Kapelanski, D.P., Al-Sadir, J., Lamberti, J.J., and Angnostopoulos, C.E.: Ventriculographic features predictive of surgical outcome for left ventricular aneurysm. Circulation 58:1167, 1978.
15. Kass, D.A., and Maughan, W.L.: From "E_{max}" to pressure-volume relations: A broader view. Circulation 77:1203, 1988.
16. Klausner, S.C., Blair, T.J., Bulawa, W.F., et al.: Quantitative analysis of segmental wall motion throughout systole and diastole in the normal human left ventricle. Circulation 65:580, 1982.

L

1. Lange, P.E., Onnasch, D., Farr, F.L., and Heintzen, P.H.: Angiocardiographic right ventricular volume determination. Accuracy, as determined from human casts, and clinical application. Eur. J. Cardiol. 8:477, 1978.
2. Lewis, R.P., and Sandler, H.: Relationship between changes in left ventricular dimensions and the ejection fraction in man. Circulation 44:548, 1971.
3. Lorente, P., Azancot, I., Masquet, C., et al.: Comparison of decision rules in assessing regional wall motion. *In* Computers in Cardiology. IEEE Computer Society, Long Beach, CA, 1984, p. 83.
4. Lorente, P., Azancot, I., Masquet, C., et al.: Relationships between single-vessel coronary artery obstructions and wall motion dysfunction analyzed by four computer-based methods. Int. J. Cardiol. 7:361, 1985.
5. Leighton, R.F., Drobinski, G., Fontaine, G.H., et al.: Effects of correcting apical displacement on regional wall motion in severely damaged ventricles. *In* Computers in Cardiology. IEEE Computer Society, Long Beach, CA, 1983, p. 173.
6. Lieberman, A.N., Weiss, J.L., Jugdutt, B.I., et al.: Two-dimensional echocardiography and infarct size: Relationship of regional wall motion and thickening to the extent of myocardial infarction in the dog. Circulation 63:739, 1981.
7. Lavallee, M., Cox, D., Patrick, T.A., and Vatner, S.F.: Salvage of myocardial function by coronary artery reperfusion 1, 2, and 3 hours after occlusion in conscious dogs. Circ. Res. 53:235, 1983.
8. Leighton, R.F., Pollack, M.E.M., and Welch, T.G.: Abnormal left ventricular wall motion at mid-ejection in patients with coronary heart disease. Circulation 52:238, 1975.
9. Lew, W.Y., and LeWinter, M.M.: Regional circumferential lengthening patterns in canine left ventricle. Am. J. Physiol. 245:H741, 1983.
10. Ludbrook, P.A., Byrne, J.D., and Tiefenbrunn, A.J.: Association of asynchronous protodiastolic segmental wall motion. Circulation 64:1201, 1981.
11. Leighton, R.F., Drobinski, G., Eugene, M., et al.: The timing of paradoxical wall motion in ventricular aneurysms and in asynergic ventricles. Int. J. Cardiol. 12:321, 1986.

M

1. Marier, D.L., and Gibson, D.G.: Limitations of two frame method for displaying regional left ventricular wall motion in man. Br. Heart J. 44:555, 1980.
2. Miller, G.A.H., and Swan, H.J.C.: Effect of chronic pressure and volume overload on left heart volumes in subjects with congenital heart disease. Circulation 30:205, 1964.
3. Miller, G.A.H., Kirklin, J.W., and Swan, H.J.C.: Myocardial function and left ventricular volumes in acquired valvular insufficiency. Circulation 31:374, 1965.
4. McDonald, I.G.: The shape and movements of the human left ventricle during systole. Am. J. Cardiol. 26:221, 1970.
5. McDonald, I.G.: Echocardiographic demonstration of abnormal motion of the interventricular septum in left bundle branch block. Circulation 48:272, 1973.
6. Mancini, G.B.J., DeBoe, S.F., Anselmo, E., and LeFree, M.T.: A comparison of traditional wall motion assessment and quantitative shape analysis: A new method for characterizing left ventricular function in humans. Am. Heart J. 114:1183, 1987.
7. McMahon, M.M., Brown, B.G., Cukingnan, R., et al.: Quantitative coronary angiography: Quantitation of the critical stenosis in patients with unstable angina and single-vessel disease without collaterals. Circulation 60:106, 1979.
8. Miller, R.R., Olson, H.G., Vismara, L.A., et al.: Pump dysfunction after myocardial infarction: Importance of location, extent and pattern of abnormal left ventricular segmental contraction. Am. J. Cardiol. 37:340, 1976.
9. Mathes, P., Baxley, W.A., Neiss, A., et al.: Ventrikelfunktion nach abgelaufenem Herzinfarkt in Abhangigkeit vom Kontraktionsverhalten des Uberlebenden Herzmuskels. Dtsch. Med. Wochenschr. 104:175, 1979.
10. Multicenter Postinfarction Research Group: Risk stratification and survival after myocardial infarction. N. Engl. J. Med. 309:321, 1983.
11. Martin, G.V., Sheehan, F.H., Stadius, M., et al.: Intravenous streptokinase for acute myocardial infarction: Effects on global and regional systolic function. Circulation 78:258, 1988.
12. Maddahi, J., Berman, D., Matsuoka, D.T., et al.: A new technique for assessing right ventricular ejection fraction using rapid multiple-gated equilibrium cardiac blood pool scintigraphy. Circulation 60:581, 1979.
13. Morrison, D.A., Hartnett, S.D., and Adcock, K.: Radionuclide and angiographic assessment of the right heart. Cardiovasc. Clin. 17:19, 1987.
14. Melchior, J.P., Doriot, P.A., Chatelain, P., et al.: Improvement of left ventricular contraction and relaxation synchronism after recanalization of chronic total coronary occlusion by angioplasty. J. Am. Coll. Cardiol. 9:763, 1987.

N

1. Nieminen, M., Parisi, A.F., O'Boyle, J.E., et al.: Serial evaluation of myocardial thickening and thinning in acute experimental infarction: Identification and quantification using two-dimensional echocardiography. Circulation 66:174, 1982.
2. Norris, R.M., Barnaby, P.F., Brandt, P.W.T., et al.: Prognosis after recovery from first acute myocardial infarction: Determinants of reinfarction and sudden death. Am. J. Cardiol. 53:408, 1984.

O

1. Osbakken, M.D., Bove, A.A., and Spann, J.F.: Left ventricular regional wall motion and velocity of shortening in chronic mitral and aortic regurgitation. Am. J. Cardiol. 47:1005, 1981.

P

1. Papapietro, S.E., Smith, L.R., Hood, W.P., Jr., et al.: An optimal method for angiographic definition and quantification of regional left ventricular contraction. *In* Computers in Cardiology. IEEE Computer Society, Long Beach, CA, 1978, p. 293.
2. Pandian, N.G., Skorton, D.J., Collins, S.M., et al.: Myocardial infarct size threshold for two-dimensional echocardiographic detection: Sensitivity of systolic wall thickening and endocardial motion abnormalities in small versus large infarcts. Am. J. Cardiol. 55:551, 1985.
3. Pairolero, P., Hallermann, F.J., and Ellis, F., Jr.: Left ventriculogram in experimental myocardial infarction. Radiology 95:311, 1970.

R

1. Rushmer, R.F.: Initial phase of ventricular systole: Asynchronous contraction. Am. J. Physiol. 184:188, 1956.
2. Rogers, W.J., Smith, L.R., Bream, P.R., et al.: Quantitative axial oblique contrast left ventriculography: Validation of the method by demonstrating improved visualization of regional wall motion and mitral valve function with accurate volume determinations. Am. Heart J. 103:185, 1982.
3. Rogers, W.J., Smith, L.R., Hood, W.P., Jr., et al.: Effect of filming projection and interobserver variability on angiographic biplane left ventricular volume determination. Circulation 59:96, 1979.
4. Ricci, D.R., Orlick, A.E., Alderman, E.L., et al.: Influence of heart rate on left ventricular ejection fraction in human beings. Am. J. Cardiol. 44:447, 1979.
5. Rackley, C.E.: Quantitative evaluation of left ventricular function by radiographic techniques. Circulation 54:862, 1976.
6. Rackley, C.E., Dodge, H.T., Coble, Y.D., Jr., and Hay, R.E.: A method for determining left ventricular mass in man. Circulation 29:666, 1964.
7. Ransohoff, D.F., and Feinstein, A.R.: Problems of spectrum and bias in evaluating the efficacy of diagnostic tests. N. Engl. J. Med. 299:926, 1978.

8. Rozanski, A., Diamond, G.A., Forrester, J.S., et al.: Alternative referent standards for cardiac normality. Ann. Intern. Med. 101:164, 1984.
9. Roan, P.G., Buja, M., Izquierdo, C., et al.: Interrelationships between regional left ventricular function, coronary blood flow, and myocellular necrosis during the initial 24 hours and 1 week after experimental coronary occlusion in awake, unsedated dogs. Circ. Res. 49:31, 1981.
10. Rackley, C.E., Russell, R.O., Jr., Mantle, J.A., et al.: Right ventricular infarction and function. Am. Heart J. 101:215, 1981.
11. Rackley, C.E., Behar, V.S., Whalen, R.E., and McIntosh, H.D.: Biplane cineangiographic determinations of left ventricular function: Pressure-volume relationships. Am. Heart J. 74:766, 1967.

S

1. Sheehan, F.H., Schofer, J., Mathey, D.G., et al.: Measurement of regional wall motion from biplane contrast ventriculograms: A comparison of the 30 degree RAO and 60 degree LAO projections in patients with acute myocardial infarction. Circulation 74:796, 1986.
2. Sandler, H., and Dodge, H.T.: The use of single plane angiocardiograms for the calculation of left ventricular volume in man. Am. Heart J. 75:325, 1968.
3. Sauter, H.J., Dodge, H.T., Johnston, R.R., and Graham, T.P.: The relationship of left atrial pressure and volume in patients with heart disease. Am. Heart J. 67:635, 1964.
4. Sheehan, F.H., and Mitten-Lewis, S.: Factors influencing accuracy in left ventricular volume determination. Am. J. Cardiol. 64:661, 1989.
5. Sheehan, F.H., Dodge, H.T., Mathey, D.G., et al.: Measurement of abnormalities in the timing and extent of motion from frame-by-frame analysis of contrast left ventriculograms. *In* Computers in Cardiology. IEEE Computer Society, Long Beach, CA, 1983, p. 35.
6. Sheehan, F.H., Stewart, D.K., Dodge, H.T., et al.: Variability in the measurement of regional ventricular wall motion from contrast angiograms. Circulation 68:550, 1983.
7. Sonnenblick, E.H., and Strobeck, J.E.: Derived indexes of ventricular and myocardial function. N. Engl. J. Med. 296:978, 1977.
8. Sandler, H., Dodge, H.T., Hay, R.E., and Rackley, C.E.: Quantitation of valvular insufficiency in man by angiocardiography. Am. Heart J. 65:501, 1963.
9. Sandler, H., and Dodge, H.T.: Left ventricular tension and stress in man. Circ. Res. 13:91, 1963.
10. Stack, R.S., Phillips, H.R., III, Grierson, D.S., et al.: Functional improvement of jeopardized myocardium following intracoronary streptokinase infusion in acute myocardial infarction. J. Clin. Invest. 72:34, 1983.
11. Sheehan, F.H., Szente, A., Mathey, D.G., and Dodge, H.T.: Assessment of left ventricular function in acute myocardial infarction: The relationship between global ejection fraction and regional wall motion. Eur. Heart J. 6(Suppl. E):117, 1985.
12. Sheehan, F.H., Doerr, R., Schmidt, W.G., et al.: Early recovery of left ventricular function after thrombolytic therapy for acute myocardial infarction: An important determinant of survival. J. Am. Coll. Cardiol. 12:289, 1988.
13. Slager, C.J., Hooghoudt, T.E.H., Serruys, P.W., et al.: Quantitative assessment of regional left ventricular motion using endocardial landmarks. J. Am. Coll. Cardiol. 7:317, 1986.
14. Sandor, T., Paulin, S., and Hanlon, W.B.: Left ventricular wall motion analysis using operator-independent contour positioning. Comput. Biomed. Res. 17:129, 1984.
15. Skorton, D.J., Collins, S.M., and Kerber, R.E.: Digital image processing and analysis in echocardiography. *In* Collins, S.M., and Skorton, D.J. (eds.): Cardiac Imaging and Image Processing. McGraw-Hill, New York, 1986, p. 171.
16. Sheehan, F.H., Bolson, E.L., Dodge, H.T., et al.: Advantages and applications of the centerline method for characterizing regional ventricular function. Circulation 74:293, 1986.
17. Sheehan, F.H., Braunwald, E., Canner, P., et al.: The effect of intravenous thrombolytic therapy on left ventricular function: A report on tissue plasminogen activator and streptokinase from the thrombolysis in myocardial infarction (TIMI Phase I) trial. Circulation 75:817, 1987.
18. Sigel, H., Nechwatal, W., and Stauch, M.: Quantitative evaluation of regional and global parameters of left ventriculography with different methods in an intra- and interobserver test. Z. Kardiol. 70:742, 1981.
19. Sheehan, F.H., Brown, B.G., Dodge, H.T., et al.: Quantitative analysis of the relationship between coronary artery stenosis and regional left ventricular wall motion. *In* Sigwart, U., and Heintzen, P.H. (eds.): Ventricular Wall Motion. Georg Thieme Verlag, Stuttgart, 1984, p. 198.
20. Sheehan, F.H., Dodge, H.T., Mathey, D.G., et al.: Application of the centerline method: Analysis of change in regional left ventricular wall motion in serial studies. *In* Computers in Cardiology. IEEE Computer Society, Long Beach, CA, 1982, p. 97.
21. Sheehan, F.H., Mathey, D.G., Schofer, J., et al.: Effect of interventions in salvaging left ventricular function in acute myocardial infarction: A study of intracoronary streptokinase. Am. J. Cardiol. 52:431, 1983.
22. Schwarz, F., Flameng, W., Thiedemann, K.-U., et al.: Effect of coronary stenosis on myocardial function, ultrastructure and aortocoronary bypass graft hemodynamics. Am. J. Cardiol. 42:193, 1978.
23. Sharma, B., Goodwin, J.F., Raphael, M.J., et al.: Left ventricular angiography on exercise. A new method of assessing left ventricular function in ischaemic heart disease. Br. Heart J. 38:59, 1976.
24. Sheehan, F.H., Mathey, D.G., Schofer, J., et al.: Limitations in the interpretation of rest-exercise ejection fraction changes after early thrombolytic therapy during acute myocardial infarction. Am. J. Cardiol. 61:743, 1988.
25. Stadius, M.L., Maynard, C., Fritz, J.K., et al.: Coronary anatomy and left ventricular function in the first 12 hours of acute myocardial infarction: The Western Washington Randomized Intracoronary Streptokinase Trial. Circulation 72:292, 1985.
26. Sheehan, F.H.: Left ventricular dysfunction in acute myocardial infarction due to isolated left circumflex coronary artery disease. Am. J. Cardiol. 64:440, 1989.
27. Schofer, J., Sheehan, F.H., Spielmann, R., et al.: Early intracoronary thallium/technetium-pyrophosphate scintigraphy is a reliable method to predict myocardial salvage (Abstract). Circulation 74(Suppl. II):II-273, 1986.
28. Stamm, R.B., Gibson, R.S., Bishop, H.L., et al.: Echocardiographic detection of infarct-localized asynergy and remote asynergy during acute myocardial infarction: Correlation with the extent of angiographic coronary disease. Circulation 67:233, 1983.
29. Schmidt, W.G., Sheehan, F.H., von Essen, R., et al.: Evolution of left ventricular function after intracoronary thrombolysis for acute myocardial infarction. Am. J. Cardiol. 63:497, 1989.
30. Stadius, M.L., Davis, K., Maynard, C., et al.: Risk stratification for 1 year survival based on characteristics identified in the early hours of acute myocardial infarction. The Western Washington Intracoronary Streptokinase Trial. Circulation 74:703, 1986.
31. Stadius, M.L., Maynard, C., Sheehan, F.H., et al.: Six month prognosis after acute MI based on clinical and acute angiographic variables from streptokinase trial (WWIST) (Abstract). Circulation 70(Suppl. II):II-257, 1984.
32. Sagawa, K.: Editorial: The end-systolic pressure-volume relationship of the ventricle: Definition, modifications and clinical use. Circulation 63:1223, 1981.
33. Sheehan, F.H., Mathey, D.G., Schofer, J., et al.: Factors determining recovery of left ventricular function following thrombolysis in acute myocardial infarction. Circulation 71:1121, 1985.
34. Starr, I., Jeffers, W.A., and Meade, R.H., Jr.: The absence of conspicuous increments of venous pressure after severe damage to the right ventricle of the dog, with a discussion of the relation between clinical congestive failure and heart disease. Am. Heart J. 26:291, 1943.
35. Sade, R.M., and Castaneda, A.R.: The dispensable right ventricle. Surgery 77:624, 1975.
36. Sheehan, F.H., Mathey, D.G., Wygant, J., et al.: Measurement of regional right ventricular wall motion from biplane contrast angiograms using the centerline method. *In* Computers in Cardiology. IEEE Computer Society, Long Beach, CA, 1985, p. 149.
37. Sagawa, K.: The ventricular pressure-volume diagram revisited. Circ. Res. 43:677, 1978.
38. Sunagawa, K., Maughan, W.L., and Sagawa, K.: Effect of regional ischemia on the left ventricular end-systolic pressure-volume relationship of isolated canine hearts. Circ. Res. 52:170, 1983.
39. Serruys, P.W., Wijns, W., Van den Brand, M., et al.: Left ventricular performance, regional blood flow, wall motion, and lactate metabolism during transluminal angioplasty. Circulation 70:25, 1984.
40. Sasayama, S., Nonogi, H., Miyazaki, S., et al.: Changes in diastolic properties of the regional myocardium during pacing-induced ischemia in human subjects. J. Am. Coll. Cardiol. 5:599, 1985.
41. Sheehan, F.H.: Measurement of left ventricular function from contrast angiograms in patients with coronary artery disease. *In* Brundage, B. (ed.): Comparative Cardiac Imaging—Function, Flow, Anatomy, Quantitation. Rockville, MD, Aspen (In Press).

T

1. Thompson, R., Ahmed, M., Seabra-Gomes, R., et al.: Influence of preoperative left ventricular function on results of homograft replacement of the aortic valve for aortic regurgitation. J. Thorac. Cardiovasc. Surg. 77:411, 1979.
2. Tennant, R., and Wiggers, C.J.: Effect of coronary occlusion on myocardial contraction. Am. J. Physiol. 112:351, 1935.
3. Theroux, P., Franklin, D., Ross, J., Jr., and Kemper, W.S.: Regional myocardial function during acute coronary artery occlusion and its modification by pharmacologic agents in the dog. Circ. Res. 35:896, 1974.
4. Takayama, M., Norris, R.M., Brown, M.A., et al.: Post-systolic shortening of acutely ischemic canine myocardium predicts early and late recovery of function following coronary artery reperfusion. Circulation 78:994, 1988.
5. Takeuchi, M., Fujitani, K., and Fukuzaki, H.: The relation between left ventricular asynchrony, relaxation, outward wall motion and filling characteristics during control period and pacing-induced myocardial ischemia in coronary artery disease. Int. J. Cardiol. 9:45, 1985.

U

1. Ubago, J.L., Figueroa, A., Colman, T., et al.: Right ventriculography as a valid method for the diagnosis of tricuspid insufficiency. Cathet. Cardiovasc. Diagn. 7:433, 1981.
2. Ueda, H., Ueda, K., Morooka, S., et al.: A cineangiocardiographic study of the regional contraction sequence of the normal and diseased left ventricle in man. Jap. Heart J. 10:95, 1969.

V

1. Vine, D.L., Hegg, T.D., Dodge, H.T., et al.: Immediate effect of contrast medium injection on left ventricular volumes and ejection fraction: A study using metallic epicardial markers. Circulation 56:379, 1977.
2. Vokonas, P.S., Gorlin, R., Cohn, P.F., et al.: Dynamic geometry of the left ventricle in mitral regurgitation. Circulation 48:786, 1973.
3. The Veterans Administration Coronary Artery Bypass Surgery Cooperative Study Group: Eleven-year survival in the Veterans Administration randomized trial of coronary bypass surgery for stable angina. N. Engl. J. Med. 21:1333, 1984.
4. Vine, D.L., Dodge, H.T., Frimer, M.J., et al.: Quantitative measurement of left ventricular volumes in man from radio-opaque epicardial markers. Circulation 54:391, 1976.

W

1. Wynne, J., Green, L.H., Mann, T., et al.: Estimation of left ventricular volumes in man from biplane cineangiograms filmed in oblique projections. Am. J. Cardiol. 41:726, 1978.
2. Wallis, D.E., O'Connell, J.B., Henkin, R.E., et al.: Segmental wall motion abnormalities in dilated cardiomyopathy: A common finding and good prognostic sign. J. Am. Coll. Cardiol. 4:674, 1984.
3. Widimsky, P., Cervenka, V., Gregor, P., et al.: First month course of left ventricular asynergy after intracoronary thrombolysis in acute myocardial infarction. A longitudinal echocardiographic study. Eur. Heart J. 6:759, 1985.
4. White, H.D., Norris, R.M., Brown, M.A., et al.: Left ventricular end-systolic volume as the major determinant of survival after recovery from myocardial infarction. Circulation 76:44, 1987.
5. Weyman, A.E., Hogan, T.D., Jr., Gilliam, L.D., et al.: Importance of temporal heterogeneity in assessing the contraction abnormalities associated with acute myocardial ischemia. Circulation 70:102, 1984.

Y

1. Yamagishi, T., Ozaki, M., Kumada, T., et al.: Asynchronous left ventricular diastolic filling in patients with isolated disease of the left anterior descending coronary artery: Assessment with radionuclide ventriculography. Circulation 69:933, 1984.

Chapter 10

Pulmonary Angiography

ANTOINETTE S. GOMES, M.D.

INDICATIONS 149
CONTRAINDICATIONS 149
TECHNIQUE 149
NORMAL ANATOMY OF PULMONARY VASCULATURE 151
PULMONARY ANGIOGRAPHY IN PULMONARY EMBOLISM 151
Timing 152
Interpretation 153
Complications 154
Therapeutic Maneuvers at Time of Angiography 154
PULMONARY ANGIOGRAPHY FOR OTHER PULMONARY VASCULAR LESIONS 155
Pulmonary Arteriovenous Fistulae 155
Pulmonary Artery Stenosis 156
Pulmonary Artery Aneurysms 156
Pulmonary Varix 157
Neoplasms 157
Pulmonary Sequestration 157
Congenital Dysplasia of the Lung 157
Anomalous Pulmonary Venous Connection 159

INDICATIONS

Pulmonary arteriography is the most reliable technique for evaluation of the status of the pulmonary vessels. It is indicated in the diagnosis of suspected pulmonary embolism and in the evaluation of other vascular abnormalities of the pulmonary arteries. Other vascular lesions diagnosed with angiography include pulmonary arteriovenous fistulae; pulmonary artery stenoses, aneurysms, neoplasms, and sequestration; and congenital lesions of both the pulmonary arteries and the pulmonary veins. By far, the most frequent clinical indication is in the diagnosis of suspected pulmonary embolism.

CONTRAINDICATIONS

In the past, the only absolute contraindication to pulmonary angiography was a known allergy to contrast media.[D1] Because medication prior to angiography has been shown effective, a history of contrast allergy is a relative contraindication. Other relative contraindications to angiography are severe pulmonary hypertension, recent myocardial infarction, ventricular irritability, left bundle branch block, and severe bleeding diathesis. In patients with a previous documented reaction to contrast material, premedication with corticosteroids is necessary. Several regimens have been employed. Prednisone given orally 50 mg for three doses beginning 18 hours before the study with the intramuscular administration of 50 mg of benadryl just prior to angiography has been found to be an effective means of blocking allergic reactions to contrast agents.[K1] Use of the new nonionic contrast agents is also recommended because these agents have been suggested to reduce the overall incidence of reactions to contrast agents.

Pulmonary hypertension and right ventricular dysfunction have been found to be associated with a higher incidence of sudden death at angiography. In a large series, Mills and associates noted a similar incidence of major nonfatal complications in patients with pulmonary hypertension compared with those having normal right ventricular and pulmonary artery pressures.[M1] Mortality, however, was higher in patients with severe pulmonary hypertension (pulmonary artery systolic pressure greater than 70 mmHg) and moderate right ventricular dysfunction (right ventricular end-diastolic pressure greater than 20 mmHg). The degree to which pulmonary angiography contributed to the death of these patients has not been clarified, because they were all gravely ill. Nonetheless, others have observed that patients with systemic pulmonary artery pressures tolerate large injections of contrast material poorly,[D1] and in these patients, low-volume subselective injection of contrast agents into high probability areas is recommended. The use of the new nonionic or low osmolar contrast agents may also be beneficial in this patient subgroup.

Patients with a left bundle branch block are at risk for developing complete heart block as the pulmonary angiography catheter is passed along the right ventricular wall into the pulmonary artery. Complete heart block can result in acute decompensation with hypotension. Patients with left bundle branch block who require pulmonary angiography should have a temporary pacemaker placed before angiography.

TECHNIQUE

Pulmonary angiography should be performed in a well-functioning angiographic fluoroscopic radiographic suite with, at minimum, single-plane rapid serial filming capability. The focal spot of the x-ray tube should be adequate for obtaining magnification film. Often, spot filming capability may also be of value. The availability of biplane filming capability, U or C arms, and cineangiography may in certain selected instances allow the use of reduced volumes of contrast medium and facilitate the study. Because the pulmonary embolism does not require a dynamic display, the use of cineangiography, with its attendant higher radiation dose, is not recommended. Digital subtraction angiography is not routinely employed in pulmonary angiography in the adult patient. It may be of value in the diagnosis of large congenital lesions in children. In the older patient, although the main pulmonary artery may be well visualized, severe problems due to motion artifact and poor resolution make digital subtraction angiography unreliable for the diagnosis of pulmonary embolism or evaluation of abnormalities of smaller pulmonary artery branches. The angiography suite must be equipped with an electrocardiographic (ECG) monitor, a blood pressure monitor, and a physiologic monitor for measurement of right ventricular and pulmonary artery pressures. The physiologic monitor should allow collection of a printed record of these pressures. In certain instances, pulse oximetry may be important. A life support cart should be readily available, and the angiographers should be knowledgeable in its use.

When a pulmonary angiogram is requested, the indications for the study and the patient's overall condition should be discussed with the referring physician. All of the patient's pertinent studies should be reviewed, in particular the chest x-ray and, in patients being studied for pulmonary embolism, the lung scan. A radionuclide lung scan prior to the arteriogram is strongly recommended, because it may obviate the need for the angiogram, and if the angiogram is indicated, the lung scan directs the angiographer to the most suspicious areas of the lung. Baseline serum creatinine and coagulation studies should be obtained. Severe bleeding abnormalities should be corrected, if possible, before the study. If the patient is receiving heparin therapy, however, such therapy needs to be stopped 1 to 2 hours before the study. The ECG should be examined to rule out acute myocardial infarction, a conduction defect, or a cardiac arrhythmia.

As before any type of arteriography, informed consent should be obtained. Patients with renal insufficiency should be well hydrated, and patients on dialysis should have provisions made for dialysis following arteriography.

The patient should be sedated before the angiogram, with the selection of sedation and dosage adjusted appropriately for the patient's degree of hypoxia.

Pulmonary angiography can be performed from the arm, the groin, or through a jugular vein approach. The femoral vein approach is the most frequently used. When such access is not possible because of occlusion of the femoral vein or inferior vena cava, an antecubital vein approach via the basilic vein may be performed. Percutaneous puncture using Seldinger's technique is used at both sites. Infrequently, a cutdown may be required when performing the study through an arm vein. If a Swan-Ganz catheter has been passed through a sheath positioned in the internal jugular vein, the Swan-Ganz catheter may be exchanged for the angiographic catheter if the sheath size is at least 6 Fr. When the study is completed, a new Swan-Ganz catheter is passed through the sheath. The catheter most frequently used for pulmonary angiography is the 7 to 8 French Grollman pigtail catheter with multiple side holes.[G1] Patients with a dilated heart may be more easily catheterized using a pigtail catheter.[G2]

Stiff, straight 8 French multi-sidehole catheters of the National Institutes of Health (NIH) type are not recommended, because of the increased risk of myocardial perforation attendant with their use.[A1]

After administration of local anesthetic, the femoral vein is punctured below the inguinal ligament, using either a single-wall or double-wall puncture needle. The position of the vein is medial to the femoral artery, and the femoral artery passes diagonally across the medial one third of the femoral head. Once the vein is entered and the needle stylet is removed, a syringe or connecting tubing is attached to the needle, and suction is applied as the needle is slowly withdrawn. When freely aspirated venous blood is obtained, the tubing is removed from the needle hub, and a guidewire is passed into the vein and advanced up the vena cava to the right side of the heart under fluoroscopic guidance. Failure to pass the guidewire freely is due to (1) passage of the wire up into the ipsilateral ascending lumbar vein, in which case the wire tip should be reoriented, or (2) the occlusion of the vein or inferior vena cava, in which case the procedure should be performed from the arm.

Once the guidewire has entered the inferior vena cava, the catheter is passed over the guidewire and advanced into the inferior vena cava. Often, a test injection of contrast agent into the inferior vena cava is made to document free flow within it. A theoretic possibility is that a catheter could dislodge a caval thrombus; however, the likelihood of this occurring is low, and for complete evaluation of the cava, a separate cavogram is necessary. In most instances, the catheter is passed directly up into the right side of the heart.

The guidewire is then exchanged for a Cook deflecting wire, (Cook Inc., Bloomington IN) and the deflecting wire is used to facilitate passage of the Grollman catheter across the tricuspid valve and into the right ventricle. Using clockwise torque, the catheter is pushed across the pulmonic valve. The catheter is then manipulated into the right or left pulmonary artery. The left pulmonary artery is entered most frequently. Fluoroscopically, if the tip of the catheter lies above the left mainstem bronchus, the catheter is committed to the left pulmonary artery. Deflection of the catheter when it is just below the left mainstem bronchus results in its passage into the right pulmonary artery. The deflecting wire is usually removed at this point and exchanged for a J guidewire or soft-tip Bentson wire to assist in passage of the catheter out into the distal right or left pulmonary artery for injection. Pulmonary artery pressures are then recorded. In the interests of reducing overall study time and particularly in those cases in which difficulty was encountered in reaching the pulmonary artery, pullback pressures of the right side of the heart are not usually recorded before the angiogram. Pulmonary artery pressures however, are always recorded, and if pulmonary artery pressures are markedly elevated, it may be useful to pull the catheter back and record right ventricular pressures, because patients with high right ventricular pressures are at greater risk. If pulmonary artery pressures are elevated, subselective angiography is preferred. In patients with normal or near-normal pressures, the catheter is positioned in the proximal portion of the descending pulmonary artery on the selected side. In patients with suspected pulmonary embolism, the area of highest probability on the lung scan should be the site of the first injection. In selected instances, main pulmonary artery injections may be performed.

A test injection is made to determine catheter position and to assess the pulmonary flow rate. A standard injection is 40 ml of contrast medium injected at a rate of 20 to 25 ml/sec with the flow rate dependent on the rate of pulmonary blood flow and the patient's heart rate. In general, patients with a higher heart rate require a higher injection rate. Rapid serial filming is performed at a rate of 3 films per second for 3 seconds and 1 film per second for 3 seconds. The initial position for filming is the anteroposterior projection. If the thrombi are suspected in the lower lobes, oblique filming is performed in the ipsilateral posterior oblique projection. If the suspected thrombus is in the upper lobe, the ipsilateral anterior oblique projection is used.[G3] The lateral view may be helpful in difficult cases. Each lung should be visualized in two projections. Magnification is recommended although full two-to-one magnification is not necessary. When filming is complete, the patient is allowed to stabilize after the final injection, and pullback pressures of the right side of the heart are performed with recording of pulmonary artery, right ventricular, and right atrial pressures. After the study, the patient is given bedrest for 2 to 4 hours with frequent monitoring of vital signs.

The antecubital approach is performed via puncture of a basilic vein or through a cutdown. Entry via the cephalic vein is not desirable, because it may be difficult to pass a catheter from the cephalic vein into the subclavian vein. A short 2-inch, 18-gauge needle may be used for the venous puncture, after which a guidewire is passed. If an 18-gauge needle is too large for the size of the vein, a smaller gauge needle and guidewire may be used for entry and exchanged for a small dilator through which a guidewire with a larger bore may then be passed. Once a suitable size guidewire has been passed into the right atrium, a pigtail catheter is then advanced over the wire. A straight pigtail catheter may be used, or alternatively, a gentle 6-cm curve is steamed into the distal portion of the catheter at a site that is proximal to that of the pigtail. This procedure facilitates passage of the catheter out into the right ventricular outflow tract. A Cook deflecting wire is used to manipulate the catheter out into the pulmonary artery. The pulmonary angiogram is then performed with the same technique as with the femoral vein approach.

In certain instances, balloon occlusion pulmonary arteriography may be performed. This technique is occasionally used in patients with severe pulmonary hypertension and suspected pulmonary embolism in whom standard arteriography is precluded, or in cases of suspected small pulmonary emboli and equivocal cut-film arteriography.[B1] Under fluoroscopic guidance, a 7 French pulmonary wedge balloon catheter is passed into the pulmonary artery and the appropriate branch subselectively catheterized. The balloon is inflated to obstruct flow, and 5 to 10 ml of contrast is then injected slowly until the entire vessel is opacified and 3 to 4 films are obtained (preferably 105-mm spot films). The balloon is deflated immediately after filming. Overinflation of the balloon should be avoided, as this may cause vessel injury or rupture.

Another angiographic technique used in pulmonary arteriography is the pulmonary vein wedge angiogram. This technique is used for evaluating the patency and drainage pattern of pulmonary arteries and is used most often in patients with congenital heart disease.[N1] An end-hole catheter is wedged into a pulmonary vein branch and 7 to 10 ml of contrast medium is hand injected over 2 to 4 seconds. Cine, spot film, or cut film recording is then done.

Pulmonary angiography can be performed using either the new low osmolar ionic or nonionic agents or conventional Renografin 76. The nonionic agents have been shown to be associated with less patient discomfort, diminished incidence of coughing, and consequently less motion artifact.[S1] Similar findings were observed in a comparison study of ioxaglate 320, a low osmolar ionic agent, and diatrizoate meglumine and diatrizoate sodium.[S2] The new agents have not yet been determined to result in fewer allergic reactions or significantly less nephrotoxicity.

NORMAL ANATOMY OF PULMONARY VASCULATURE

The main pulmonary artery arises from the right ventricle, is anterior to the aorta, and is within the pericardium. It passes to the left of the aorta and divides into the right and left pulmonary arteries. The left pulmonary artery is shorter than the right, courses higher and more posteriorly than the right, and is foreshortened in the frontal angiogram. In the left hilus, the left pulmonary artery divides into ascending and descending branches that supply the left upper and lower lobe, respectively. The right pulmonary artery passes behind the ascending aorta, superior vena cava, and right upper lobe pulmonary vein. Its position is anterior to the esophagus and the right upper lobe bronchus. At the level of the hilus of the right lung, it divides into superior and inferior branches. The ascending branch supplies the right upper lobe, and the descending branch supplies the middle and lower segments of the right lobe. The pulmonary artery branches to both lungs usually follow the segmental bronchi; however, variations occur frequently, usually in the upper lobes.

The pulmonary veins drain into the left atrium. On the right side, the middle lobe vein joins the upper lobe vein to form the right superior pulmonary vein. The inferior pulmonary vein drains the lower lobe. On the left, the three segmental upper lobe veins form the superior pulmonary vein. The two lower lobe veins join to form the inferior pulmonary vein. In general, filming during pulmonary angiography should be carried out to the levophase so that previously unsuspected venous disease is not missed.

PULMONARY ANGIOGRAPHY IN PULMONARY EMBOLISM

The clinical diagnosis of pulmonary embolism can be difficult because the signs and symptoms of pulmonary embolism are nonspecific and can mimic a variety of other disease processes. Because of difficulties in diagnosis, the precise incidence of pulmonary embolism is unknown. In 1975, Dalen and Alpert estimated that a total of 630,000 symptomatic cases of pulmonary embolism occur per year.[D2] Pulmonary embolism is the direct cause of death or a major contributor to death in approximately 200,000 cases. Of the 630,000 cases, 11 percent of the patients died within the first hour. The diagnosis was not made in 71 percent of the 563,000 patients who survived beyond the first hour, and 30 percent of these patients died. In the 163,000 patients in whom the diagnosis was made and therapy was instituted, however, only 8 percent died. The diagnosis and treatment of pulmonary embolism are therefore imperative. Similarly, Barker observed that postoperative patients who suffered an episode of pulmonary embolism and were not treated with anticoagulants had a 33 percent chance of recurrence and an 18 percent chance of fatal recurrence.[B2]

An autopsy study by Smith and associates demonstrated that most pulmonary emboli (46 percent) arise from thrombosis in the veins of the leg.[S3] Other sites of origin in that study were the right atrium (23 percent), the inferior vena cava (19 percent), and the pelvic veins (16 percent). Clinical studies indicate that 35 to 71 percent of patients with documented pulmonary emboli have deep vein thrombosis.[H1, S4]

Usually, the symptoms of pulmonary embolism are misinterpreted as those of primary respiratory disease or ischemic heart disease. Pulmonary embolism may mimic myocardial infarction, arrhythmia, pneumonia, pneumothorax, and other systemic diseases. These disease processes should be excluded prior to performance of pulmonary angiography. The typical clinical workup of a patient with suspected pulmonary embolism should include an electrocardiogram, chest radiograph, complete blood count, arterial blood gases, and a ventilation perfusion (V/Q) scan. This initial workup helps to exclude other causes of the patient's symptoms. It also provides valuable information regarding the patient's ability to tolerate angiography. Ventilation perfusion scanning is recommended in the initial evaluation of suspected pulmonary embolism because it helps to establish the relative probability of a pulmonary embolus and serves as a useful guide should the patient undergo angiography.

As with clinical findings, the laboratory findings in pulmonary embolism are nonspecific. Although a chest radiograph should be obtained in all patients with suspected pulmonary embolus, the absence of specific findings on the chest radiograph makes it unreliable for diagnosis.[G4] The chest radiograph is often most

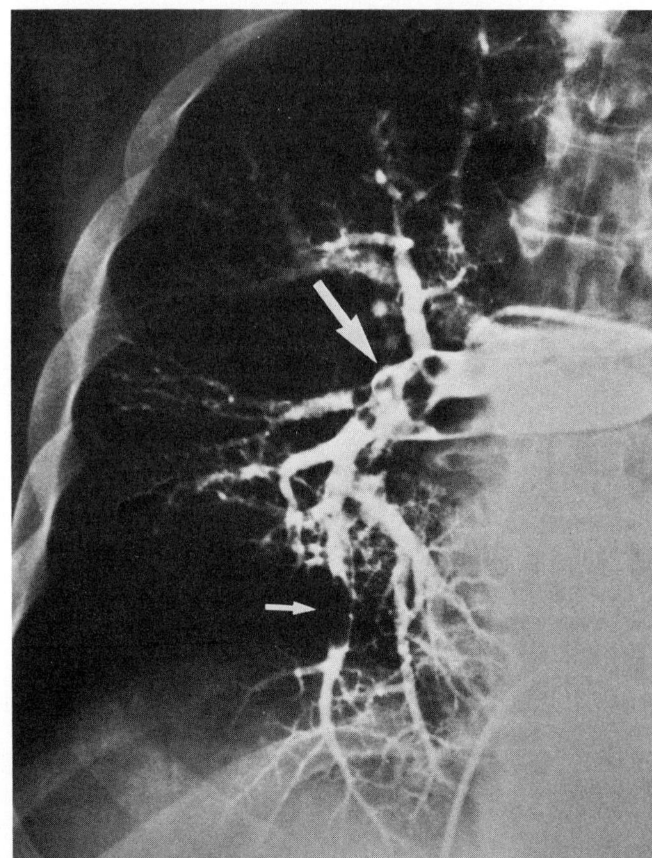

Figure 10–1. Selective right pulmonary artery injection angiogram shows typical appearance of multiple pulmonary emboli involving right main pulmonary artery and multiple right lower lobe segmental pulmonary arteries. Pulmonary emboli appear as radiolucent filling defects surrounded by contrast medium *(arrows)*.

helpful in excluding other conditions that can mimic pulmonary embolism and is essential for interpretation of the radionuclide lung scan. The radionuclide lung scan is the only currently available noninvasive imaging mode with documented sensitivity and specificity in the diagnosis of pulmonary embolism.[A1, S5, W1] Unfortunately, ventilation perfusion imaging has limitations. The most reliable criterion for pulmonary embolus in ventilation perfusion imaging is lack of perfusion with persistent ventilation. Although the ventilation perfusion scan is sensitive to changes in pulmonary perfusion, perfusion abnormalities can occur from causes other than pulmonary emboli. In addition, the technique for performing ventilation perfusion imaging, as well as the sensitivity and specificity of the various criteria used in interpretation of the scan criteria, has been the subject of controversy.[B3, M2, S6, S7]

Pulmonary angiography is indicated in those instances in which the diagnosis of pulmonary embolism must be made with certainty. The most frequent indication is an indeterminate ventilation perfusion scan. This situation often occurs in the presence of pulmonary parenchymal disease and congestive heart failure. Pulmonary angiography is indicated in the presence of a high-probability ventilation perfusion study when anticoagulation is contraindicated, and in patients with a low-probability ventilation perfusion scan when the clinical suspicion of pulmonary embolism is strong. It is also indicated when the patient has an underlying disease process that may cause a perfusion defect. Angiography should be performed prior to caval filter placement and prior to treatment with thrombolytic therapy.

Timing

Both clinical and experimental evidence indicate considerable variability in the resolution rate of pulmonary emboli.[B4, C1, F1, M3] The rate of resolution may be adversely affected by the presence of concomitant cardiac or lung disease.[F1] Angiographic evidence of complete resolution has been reported at 25 and 128 days,[S8] and at 6 weeks after embolism.[S9] Dalen and colleagues reported the results of follow-up arteriography in 15 patients with previous angiographically documented bilateral pulmonary emboli.[D3] The follow-up arteriograms were performed 1 to 7 days after the initial study in seven patients, from 10 to 21 days in 10 patients, and at 34 days in two patients. Only minimal angiographic and hemodynamic signs of resolution were present at 7 days. By 10 to 21 days, pressures in the right side of the heart had returned to almost normal levels, and unmistakable angiographic evidence of resolution was noted. Complete resolution of emboli with normal arteriographic results and hemodynamic data was noted in three patients at 14, 15, and 34 days, respectively. In other patients, hemodynamic abnormalities persisted for weeks. In another series of nine patients with major pulmonary embolism, who were free of cardiopulmonary disease, follow-up angiography that was performed an average of 26.5 hours after heparin therapy showed that little resolution of major pulmonary embolism occurs during the first 24 to 48 hours of heparin therapy.[M4]

The rate of early resolution of pulmonary embolus was also assessed in the Urokinase Pulmonary Embolism Trial.[U1] Lung scans and pulmonary angiograms were repeated 18 hours after a 12-hour heparin infusion in 78 patients with documented emboli. The follow-up angiograms documented slight improvement at 24 hours with a 20 percent decrease in the degree of embolic

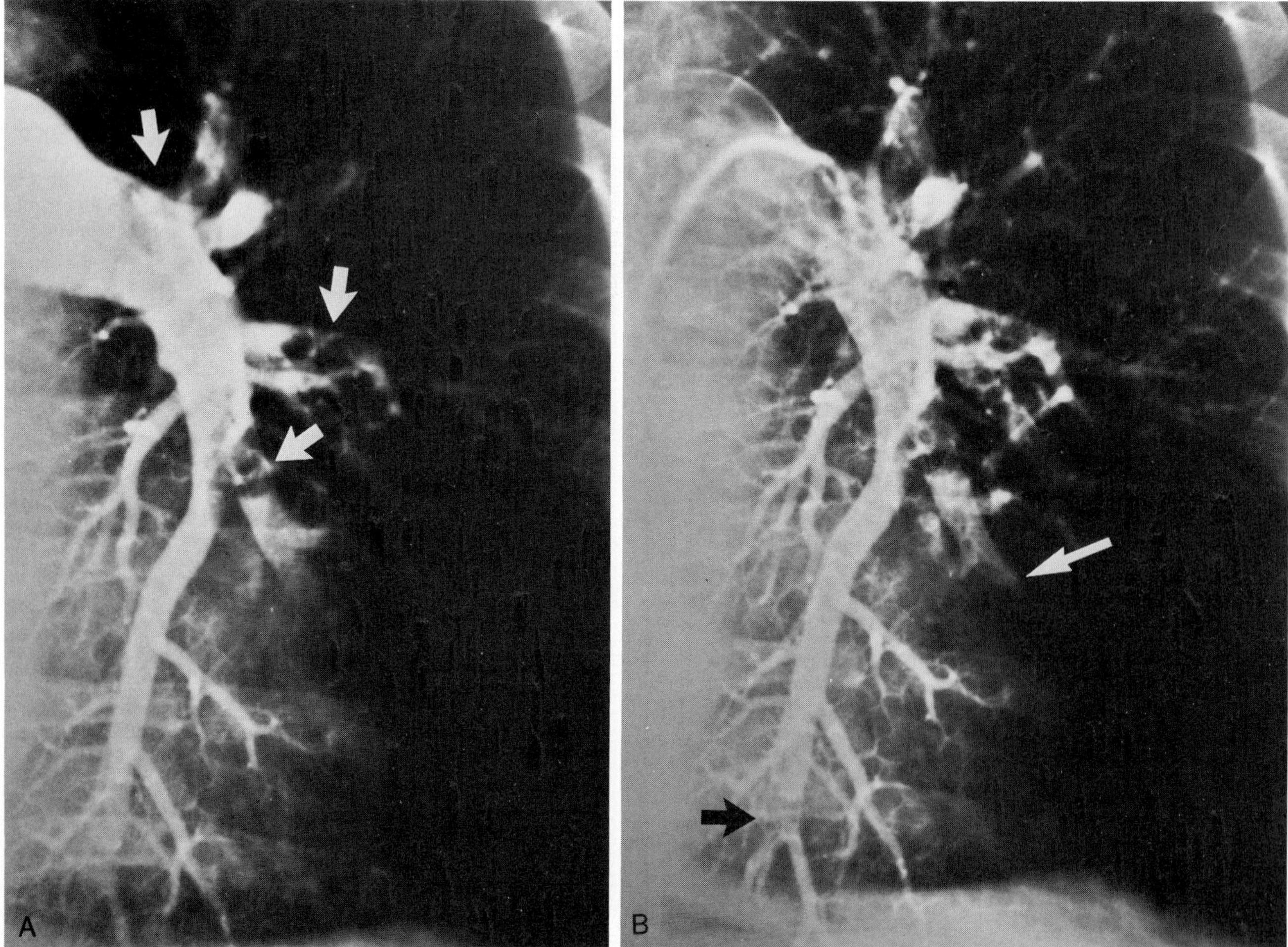

Figure 10–2. *A*, Left pulmonary artery injection angiogram shows multiple filling defects consistent with multiple pulmonary emboli in distal left pulmonary artery and in the lobar branches to the right upper lobe, middle lobe, and lower lobe *(arrows)*. *B*, Next film from the angiographic series shows a vessel cutoff *(white arrow)* and an additional embolus in the segmental pulmonary artery to the left lower lobe *(black arrow)*. Intravascular filling defects and vessel cutoffs are the two most reliable angiographic signs of pulmonary embolism.

obstruction. Repeat lung scans demonstrated an 8 percent resolution at 24 hours. These studies indicate that pulmonary embolism is not likely to be missed if arteriography is performed within 24 to 48 hours of the event. Studies performed within 7 days of the embolic event should also not result in a significant incidence of misdiagnosis.

The overall condition of the patient should be taken into consideration in the determination of the optimal time for performance of arteriography. In acutely ill patients who are in shock and under consideration for emergency embolectomy or thrombolytic therapy, the study may need to be performed on an emergency basis. In other patients, delay of the arteriography until heparin therapy has been instituted and the patient's condition has stabilized may be more appropriate. Many patients, shortly after embolism, are acutely ill and dyspneic and are unable to lie flat or cooperate for angiography. These same patients, if brought to arteriography 12 to 14 hours after institution of heparin, are typically more stable and tolerate angiography better. This improved tolerance may reflect several hemodynamic factors. Early improvement may be due to in vivo fibrinolysis or decrease in pulmonary vascular obstruction due to subtle changes in the locations of the pulmonary emboli.[D2]

Miller and associates evaluated right atrial, right ventricular, and pulmonary artery hemodynamics in two groups of patients with massive pulmonary embolism.[M5] Hemodynamics were measured within 24 hours of the embolus in one group, and 24 to 48 hours after the clinical event in the other group. All but 2 of the 23 patients studied were free of pre-existing cardiorespiratory disease. Right atrial, right ventricular, and pulmonary artery hemodynamics were found to be significantly more abnormal in those patients studied within 24 hours. Patients studied more than 24 hours after the event no longer showed evidence of right ventricular failure. Because massive pulmonary embolism was still present, this finding suggests an adaptation of the right ventricle to the stress. The hypotension sometimes seen following pulmonary angiography may be due to the vasodilative effect of contrast in patients with right ventricular failure and a fixed cardiac output. This finding suggests that the acutely stressed right ventricle is unable to increase pulmonary artery pressures to a degree adequate to maintain pulmonary artery pressure and systemic output. Adaptation of the right ventricle most likely explains the improved ability of patients to tolerate angiography after a delay of some hours.

Other important considerations are the vasoconstriction and bronchoconstriction that frequently accompany pulmonary embolism.[S10] When an embolus is examined within a few minutes of the event, degranulation of platelets is evident, with release of serotonin, adenine nucleotides, histamine, catecholamines, prostaglandins, thromboxanes, and other substances, which results in smooth muscle constriction of the pulmonary arteries and bronchi.[S11] Acute bronchoconstriction that occurs with pulmonary embolism involves the small peripheral airways (terminal bronchioles and alveolar ducts), which are perfused by the pulmonary artery. Thrombin stimulates the degranulation of platelets. Heparin, by its inhibitory effect on thrombin, blocks this vasoconstrictive response.

Given that angiographic studies indicate only minimal resolution of pulmonary emboli occurring within 24 hours of the embolic event, and hemodynamic responses in most patients improve with therapy during this period, the indications for emergency pulmonary arteriography would appear to be limited to extreme situations.

Interpretation

The two most reliable signs of pulmonary embolism are an intraluminal filling defect and a vessel cutoff, which may occur singly or in combination.[D4] Intraluminal filling defects appear as negative defects outlined by surrounding radiopaque contrast medium (Figs. 10–1 through 10–3). Oligemia and asymmetry of blood flow are frequently observed in pulmonary embolism but are not specific findings. These abnormalities may occur in

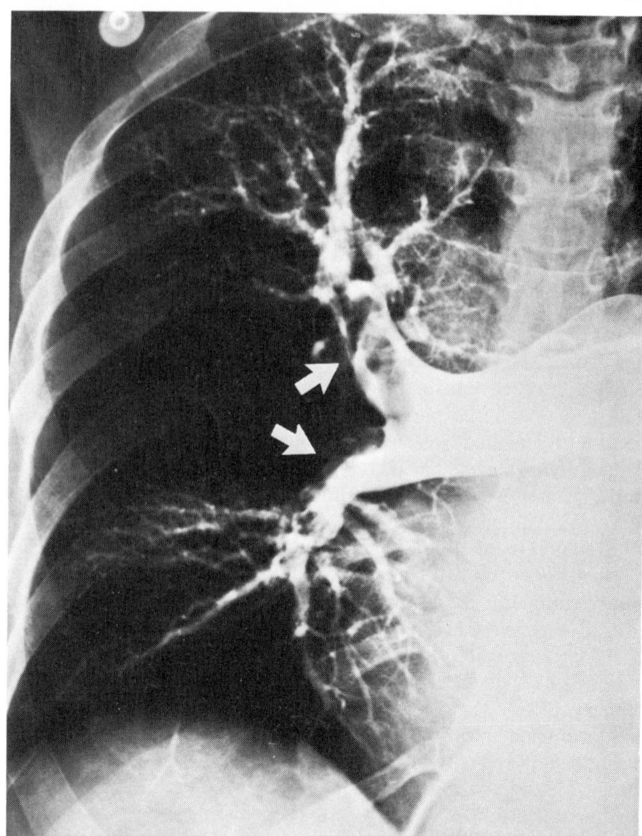

Figure 10–3. Acute and chronic pulmonary embolism. Right pulmonary artery injection angiogram shows a large acute saddle embolus involving right upper lobe artery, right middle lobe artery, and right lower lobe pulmonary artery *(arrows)*. Note the severe oligemia in right middle lobe distribution. Although observed with pulmonary embolism, oligemia can occur with other pulmonary disorders. The paucity of vessels and the stringy appearance in the right lower lobe segmental arteries suggest chronic recurrent emboli.

chronic lung disease or congestive heart failure without pulmonary embolism.[D4] When the strict criterion of intraluminal filling defects or vessel cutoff is used for the diagnosis of pulmonary embolism, interobserver variation is low (less than 3 percent).[U1]

Novelline and co-workers followed the clinical course of 180 patients with clinically suspected pulmonary embolization and a negative pulmonary arteriogram.[N2] The arteriograms were performed with selective injections and subselective magnification views of areas of lung scan abnormality within 24 to 48 hours after the onset of symptoms. None of the untreated 167 patients died as a result of thromboembolic disease during their acute illness. During a follow-up period of 6 months or more, 20 patients died from unrelated causes, and none of the 147 patients who survived suffered from "recurrent" pulmonary embolism. These findings indicate that a negative pulmonary arteriogram of good quality can effectively exclude the presence of clinically significant pulmonary emboli.

In cases of chronic pulmonary emboli, organization of the thrombus occurs if the emboli do not lyse and fragment. Organization may result in little or no persistent recognizable abnormality, total occlusion of the vessel, transverse webs, eccentric plaques, or longitudinal strands. Multiple small recurrent peripheral pulmonary emboli may occur over time, causing pulmonary hypertension and right ventricular failure. Angiographically, these tend to appear as a lacy network of vessels and may be associated with bronchial arterial dilatation and pleural collateral flow, especially if infarction has occurred.[B5] These changes are not specific, and neoplastic, postinflammatory, and other fibrotic obliterations may have a similar appearance. A variety of nonembolic disorders may be seen on pulmonary angiography during evaluation for pulmonary embolus. These disorders include arteritis, primary and metastatic pulmonary artery neoplasms, extrinsic compression of the pulmonary arteries by granulomatous or neoplastic hilar lymph nodes, and pulmonary arteriovenous malformations.[C2]

Complications

The complications of pulmonary arteriography fall into three broad categories: those related to the angiographic technique, those due to altered hemodynamics resulting from contrast injections, and those arising from adverse reactions to contrast material. Two large series, one involving 367 patients[D4] and the other involving 298 patients,[M6] reported a total of three deaths as a consequence of pulmonary arteriography. Two of the patients had greater than 90 percent occlusion of the pulmonary vascular bed, and one had severe pulmonary hypertension. Dalen and colleagues reported an overall 3 percent incidence of complications.[D4] In the Urokinase Pulmonary Embolism Trial, five cases of ventricular tachycardia and one cardiac perforation occurred, all of which were treated successfully.[U1]

More recently, Mills and associates evaluated the incidence of complications in 1350 pulmonary arteriograms.[M1] He reported an overall 4 percent incidence of complications. Three deaths (0.2 percent) were directly attributable to the procedure. All three patients had severe pulmonary hypertension with systolic pulmonary artery pressures greater than 75 mmHg and diastolic right ventricular pressures greater than 20 mmHg. The precipitating event was the injection of contrast medium, which produced a sudden drop in systemic pressure. In the same series, cardiac perforation occurred in 1 percent of patients, and endocardial stain in 0.04 percent. These latter complications occurred exclusively in catheterizations performed with the NIH or Gensini catheter. No perforations occurred when the pigtail configuration catheter was used. Other complications included cardiac arrhythmias in 0.08 percent of patients, cardiac arrest in 0.03 percent, and contrast reaction in 0.08 percent. This study confirmed the general experience regarding the safety of pulmonary arteriography when performed by experienced personnel using appropriate techniques and precautions.

Therapeutic Maneuvers at Time of Angiography

Traditional therapy for pulmonary embolism consists of anticoagulant therapy with intravenous heparin followed by anticoagulation with oral sodium warfarin (Coumadin). Heparin limits the propagation of existing thrombi while the body's endogenous fibrinolytic system lyses the clot. Heparin interferes with the activation of factor IX by activated factor XI (intrinsic pathway) and by acting as a potent antithrombin (common pathway) to inhibit the conversion of fibrinogen to fibrin. Its effectiveness is measured by the activated partial thromboplastin time (APTT) test. Heparin is not a benign drug. Its administration is the most common cause of drug-related complications in hospitalized patients. Serious bleeding complications have been reported in 10 to 15 percent of patients who were being treated with appropriately adjusted doses.[M7, U2]

Systemic heparinization is accomplished through administration of an intravenous loading dose of 5000 units per hour followed by 800 to 1000 intravenous units per hour with the dose adjusted to maintain the APTT at 1.5 to 2.5 times the control value. Oral anticoagulation with sodium warfarin is usually instituted several days after institution of heparin therapy. Sodium warfarin inhibits hepatic synthesis of vitamin K–dependent factors and interferes with fibrin formation and growth of thrombi. Warfarin is administered orally, and its effectiveness is monitored by the prothrombin time.

Another form of treatment is thrombolytic therapy. Suitable candidates for thrombolytic therapy are patients with large pulmonary emboli that produce an obstruction of two or more segmental arteries or of one lobar artery, or patients with multiple

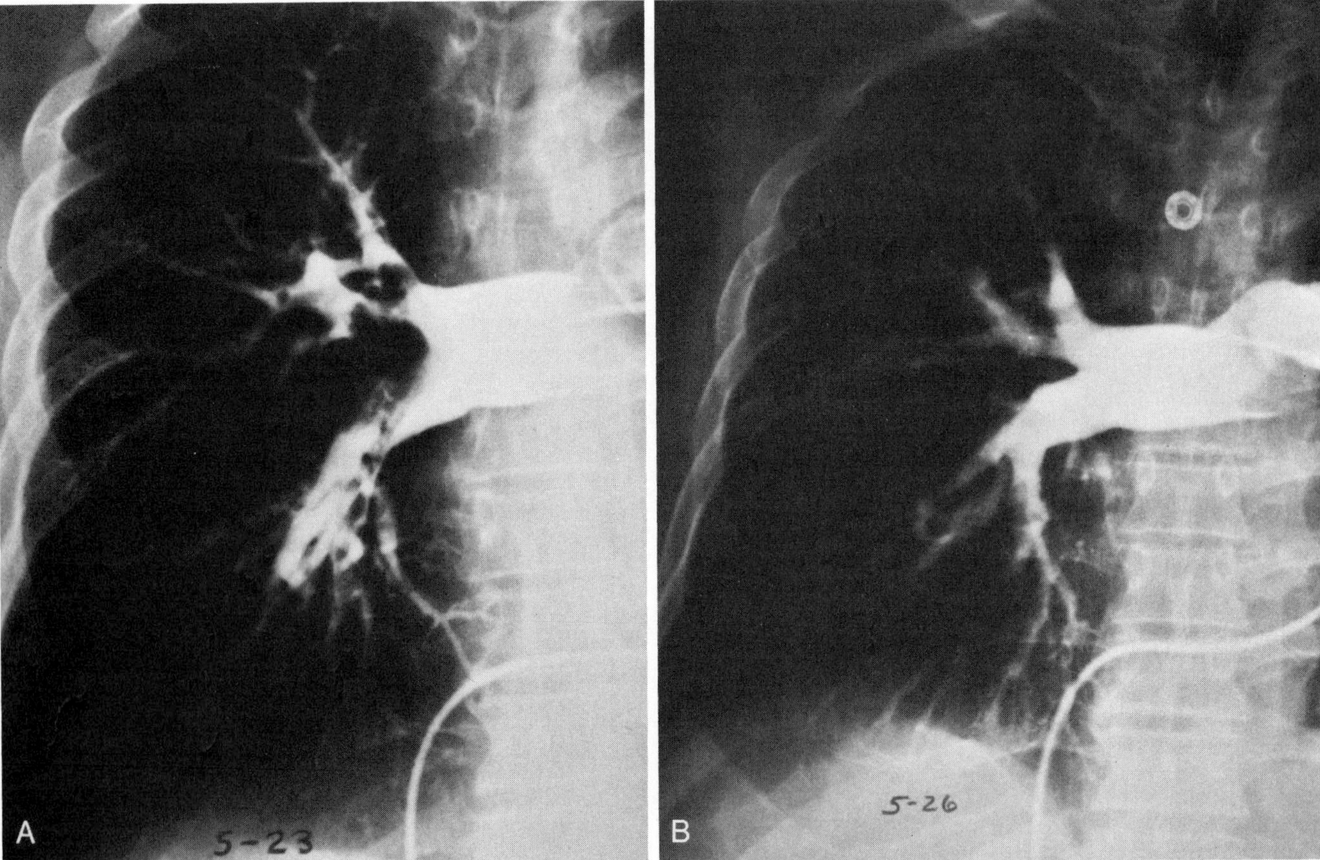

Figure 10–4. *A*, Patient with large saddle embolus to right upper and lower lobe pulmonary artery. This patient was treated with systemic doses of a thrombolytic agent infused into the right pulmonary artery. *B*, Repeat pulmonary arteriogram at 72 hours shows lysis of the thrombus with improved pulmonary perfusion.

smaller pulmonary emboli that produce hemodynamic compromise in the presence of severe left ventricular dysfunction (Fig. 10–4). Patients should be screened to exclude those with a contraindication to thrombolytic therapy. Contraindications include active or recent internal bleeding, recent cerebrovascular accident, recent major surgery, serious trauma, or severe arterial hypertension.[C3]

Both the Urokinase Pulmonary Embolism Trial (UPET)[U2] and the Urokinase/Streptokinase Pulmonary Embolism Trial (USPET)[U3] documented the value of thrombolytic therapy. The Phase I study established that urokinase increased the resolution rate of pulmonary emboli, especially massive emboli as judged by arteriography, hemodynamics testing, and lung scanning. The trial was not designed to demonstrate a difference in mortality, and none was found. Patients selected at random for lytic therapy had the best hemodynamic response, with a significantly greater reduction in their pulmonary artery pressure and right atrial pressure than in patients treated with heparin.

The Phase II trial was organized to determine if 24 hours of urokinase therapy further increased clot resolution, compared with 12 hours of urokinase therapy. Another goal was to compare 24 hours of streptokinase therapy with 24 hours of urokinase therapy. All three Phase II dosage regimens were found to be superior to heparin alone in accelerating the rate of resolution of acute pulmonary embolism. Patients treated with urokinase achieved the best angiographic and hemodynamic response, although the difference between the response to urokinase and the response to streptokinase was not statistically significant. Mortality did not differ significantly. Two-week follow-up of participants in the UPET and USPET showed significant improvement in both diffusing capacity and pulmonary capillary blood flow for patients treated with lytic agents compared with those receiving heparin therapy. Long-term studies show that patients who receive lytic therapy for massive pulmonary embolism have improved capillary blood volume at 2 weeks and at 1 year, compared with heparin-treated patients, who have demonstrated decreased capillary blood volume at 1 year.[S12] In these studies, however, these drugs show no difference in recurrence rates of pulmonary embolism, and the use of thrombolytic agents is associated with a significantly higher rate of bleeding complications.

Forty-five percent of patients receiving urokinase had bleeding complications compared with 27 percent of those given heparin alone. Both of these bleeding rates were considered unacceptable for clinical practice, and this issue has been readdressed on several occasions.[C3, M8] The 45 percent incidence of bleeding with use of urokinase included both moderate and severe bleeding, and superficial oozing from a venous cutdown site was considered in the same manner as a retroperitoneal or other major hemorrhage. The incidence of clinically meaningful bleeding episodes (i.e., those that occurred during the infusion and required transfusion or discontinuation of therapy, as opposed to those that could be easily prevented or managed) was 9 percent for patients treated with urokinase and 4 percent for patients treated with heparin.[U2] In these trials, both the heparin and the thrombolytic agent were administered through a peripheral intravenous line. Systemic doses of lytic therapy were used.

More recently, a newer thrombolytic agent, recombinant human tissue–type plasminogen activator (rt-TPA) has undergone evaluation in the treatment of acute pulmonary embolism. This agent has greater affinity for fibrin-bound plasminogen than for circulating unbound plasminogen and therefore should allow effective lysis of fibrin clots with minimal systemic fibrinogenolysis, which should reduce the risk of hemorrhagic complications.

The effectiveness of this agent as compared with that of urokinase was tested in a randomized controlled trial.[G5] The principal end points of the study were clot lysis at 2 hours, as assessed by angiography, and pulmonary reperfusion at 24 hours, as assessed by lung scanning. By 2 hours, a significantly greater number of patients treated with rt-TPA demonstrated clot lysis as compared with the patients treated with urokinase (82 percent versus 48 percent). A significantly lower incidence of hemorrhagic complications occurred in the patients treated with rt-TPA. The results indicated that in the dosage regimens employed (100 mg rt-TPA delivered at 50 mg/hr, or 2000-U/lb body-weight urokinase bolus followed by 2000 U/lb/hr for 24 hours), rt-TPA acted more rapidly and was safer than urokinase in the treatment of acute pulmonary embolism.[G5] In a small series of patients, Verstraete and associates were unable to show that the intrapulmonary infusion of rt-TPA offered significant benefit over the intravenous route.[V1] Their results suggested that a prolonged infusion of 100 mg of rt-TPA over 7 hours was superior to a single infusion of 50 mg delivered over 2 hours. Nonetheless, the administration of rt-TPA or other thrombolytic agent via the pulmonary angiographic catheter has the theoretic advantages of obviating the need for repeat venipuncture when follow-up arteriography is performed and of permitting a higher concentration of the agent to be delivered to the thrombus.

Other therapeutic maneuvers that can be performed at angiography are percutaneous embolectomy and percutaneous placement of an inferior vena cava filter. Transvenous percutaneous embolectomy was first proposed by Greenfield in the early 1970's.[G6] This technique involves the passing of a specially designed catheter with a suction tip through the right ventricle out into the pulmonary artery and aspiration of the clots. The technique has never gained widespread popularity.

The placement of an inferior vena cava filter, however, is often effective therapy. Placement of a filter is indicated in patients with an absolute contraindication to anticoagulant therapy, acute bleeding in the presence of anticoagulant therapy, or recurrent emboli occurring in the presence of appropriately managed full anticoagulation. The first caval filter was the Mobin-Uddin filter.[M9] It was placed through a jugular vein cutdown. Its use was limited by its tendency to generate caval thrombosis and its tendency to migrate to the right ventricle. The Kimray-Greenfield filter is associated with a lower incidence of complications.[G7] Initially, it was placed through either a jugular or femoral vein cutdown. More recently, the system has been modified to permit percutaneous placement via a femoral vein or jugular vein puncture using a 24-gauge sheath. This procedure is now typically performed in the angiographic suite following an inferior venacavogram to identify the location of the renal veins (Fig. 10–5). The filter is placed below the renal veins. Femoral vein thrombosis has been described as a complication of the procedure, but it occurs in less than 10 percent of patients.[D5, T1] Another filter now available is the bird's nest filter. This filter is designed for percutaneous placement through a 10 Fr. sheath. Lund and colleagues have described early experience with a filter that may be placed prophylactically and may be removed when the risk of embolism has been resolved.[L1] Gunther and associates are evaluating another percutaneous filter that may be placed through a 10 Fr. sheath.[G8]

PULMONARY ANGIOGRAPHY FOR OTHER PULMONARY VASCULAR LESIONS

Pulmonary arteriography is essential for accurate diagnosis of other pulmonary vascular lesions. Among these are pulmonary artery stenosis, pulmonary arteriovenous fistulae, arteritis, and pulmonary artery aneurysms.

The technique of pulmonary angiography applied in cases of these suspected lesions is the same as that employed in the evaluation of suspected pulmonary embolism. Indeed, a pulmonary vascular abnormality is often found in a patient initially suspected of having a pulmonary embolus. The preangiographic workup should include routine laboratory admission studies, chest radiography, and ECG and should be tailored to the patient's suspected underlying disease process. The risks of pulmonary arteriography are similar to those previously described.

Pulmonary Arteriovenous Fistulae

Pulmonary arteriovenous fistulae are abnormal communications between pulmonary arteries and veins, the majority of which are congenital. They may occur as an isolated anomaly, but they occur most frequently in cases of hereditary hemorrhagic telangiectasia in which 30 to 40 percent of the patient's family members may be affected.[D6] Acquired fistulae are rare and are often secondary to pulmonary arterial hypertension resulting from mitral stenosis and to hepatic cirrhosis with portal hypertension. Other acquired causes include schistosomiasis, trauma, and metastatic disease to the lung, especially thyroid carcinoma.

Pulmonary arteriovenous fistulae may often be suspected from the chest radiograph. At angiography, selective injections into the area of corresponding radiographic abnormality disclose the typical angiographic findings of a fistula. These fistulae may be simple or complex.[M10, W2] The simple type are characterized by a single feeding artery draining into a bulbous, nonseptated aneurysmal part with two or more draining veins. Complex fistulae have two or more pulmonary arterial branches communicating with a bulbous, septated, cirsoid, aneurysmal part with two or more draining veins. In both types, the feeding artery may also give rise to branches to the uninvolved adjacent lung. Both types may occur in the same patient, and diffuse involvement can occur with evidence of multiple large or small lesions (Fig. 10–6). The size of fistulae may vary from microscopic to large bulbous structures.

In the past, surgical excision of single or several of the largest pulmonary arteriovenous malformations was the therapy of choice. With time, however, symptoms recurred as smaller malformations grew. Currently, the preferred treatment of these fistulae involves transcatheter embolization therapy. Particular skill is required in the transcatheter embolization of these lesions, because faulty technique can result in inadvertent passage of the embolic agent to the pulmonary veins and subsequent systemic embolization.[W2]

Pulmonary Artery Stenosis

Pulmonary artery stenosis is characterized by narrowing of the pulmonary artery or of its branches. The stenoses may be central, peripheral, or combined. The condition exists as an isolated anomaly in approximately 40 percent of cases, and in the remaining 60 percent, it is associated with valvular pulmonic stenosis or other congenital heart disease, usually tetralogy of Fallot or ventricular septal defect.[G9] Acquired stenosis of a main branch pulmonary artery may be secondary to a hilar mass, such as an aortic aneurysm, thymoma, or bronchogenic carcinoma. Peripheral branch pulmonary artery stenosis may be a part of the congenital rubella syndrome, the supravalvular aortic stenosis syndrome, or Takayasu's arteritis.

Takayasu's arteritis primarily involves the aortic arch and great vessels, but it may involve the pulmonary arteries in as many as 50 percent of patients.[K2, L2] Usually, the main pulmonary arterial branches are involved. Segmental stenoses, vessel irregularities and occlusions are usually seen on the angiogram (Fig. 10–7). Pulmonary hypertension is common, and most patients have exertional dyspnea. If pulmonary hypertension is severe, subselective injections should be performed during arteriography. Because the disease often occurs in young patients, the disease process should be considered so that early angiography may be performed.

Pulmonary Artery Aneurysms

Almost 90 percent of pulmonary artery aneurysms involve the main pulmonary artery and are asymptomatic.[T2] They may occur

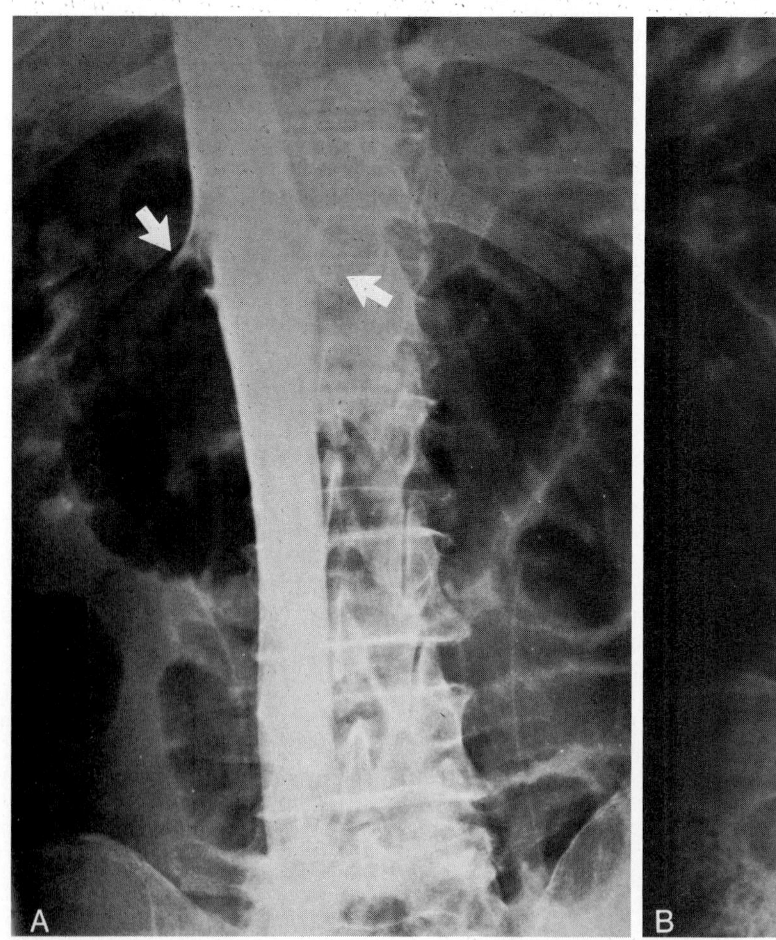

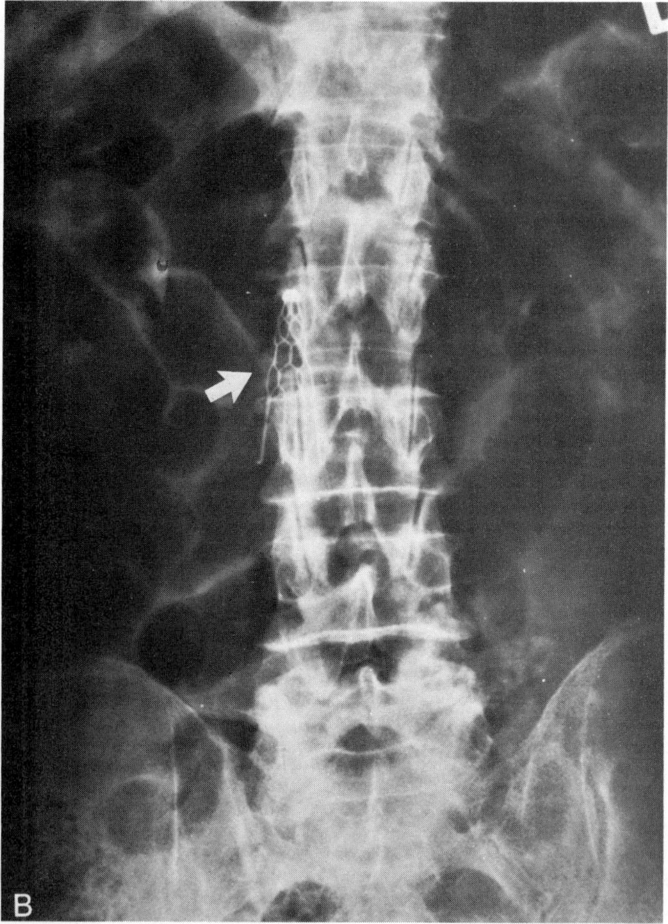

Figure 10–5. *A*, Inferior venacavogram shows a patent inferior vena cava. Radiolucent defects in upper vena cava indicate site of drainage of the right and left renal veins *(arrows)*. The location of the renal veins should be determined prior to filter placement, as the filter should be placed below their site of entrance into the vena cava. *B*, A Kimray-Greenfield filter has been percutaneously placed in the inferior vena cava. Note the upright position of the filter. If the filters are placed incorrectly and tilted, they are less effective in trapping thrombi.

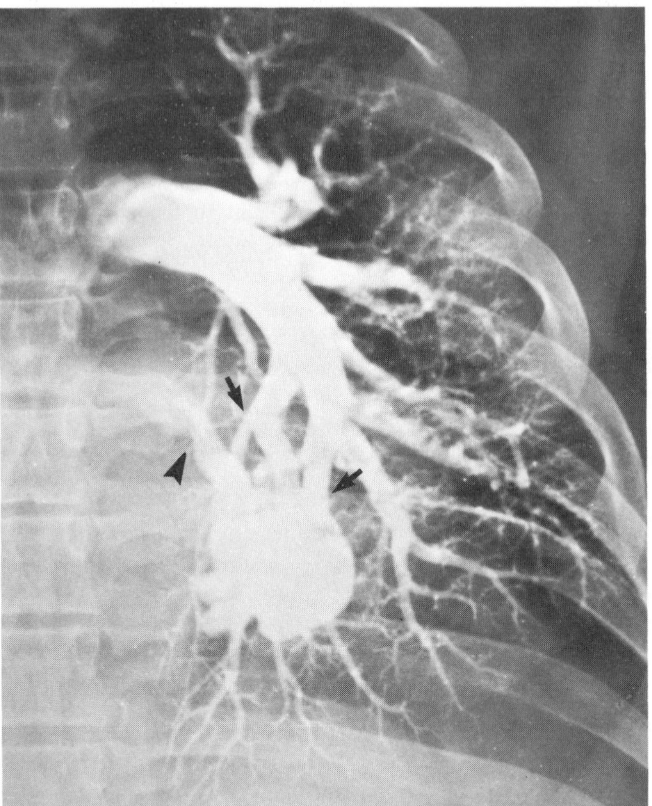

Figure 10–6. Left pulmonary arterial injection angiogram shows a large pulmonary arteriovenous fistula involving the left lower lobe in a patient with hereditary hemorrhagic telangiectasia. This fistula is complex and supplied by two lower lobe segmental pulmonary arteries *(arrows)*, which communicate with a bulbous aneurysm. The draining pulmonary vein opacifies *(arrowhead)*.

in Marfan's syndrome. Most peripheral pulmonary artery aneurysms are multiple, are of mycotic origin, and are associated with a high incidence of rupture (Fig. 10–8). They may also occur following trauma. Solitary peripheral aneurysms are usually tuberculous in origin. Rasmussen's aneurysms, as they are called, are false aneurysms of the pulmonary arteries resulting from arterial erosion in chronic cavitary tuberculosis. They are most often found in the upper lobe. They usually present with hemoptysis and are associated with a high incidence of fatal rupture.[A2]

Pulmonary Varix

On the chest radiograph, pulmonary varices appear as cylindric or oval-shaped densities that are centrally located. They may be unilateral or bilateral, and congenital or acquired in origin. The acquired lesions are usually secondary to venous hypertension or mitral insufficiency. They may bleed, but such bleeding is rare. They are usually asymptomatic, and their diagnosis is important to prevent unnecessary operation. They are identified on the venous phase of pulmonary arteriography.

Neoplasms

Malignant lesions involving the pulmonary arteries can also be identified at arteriography (Fig. 10–9). Arterial narrowing and occlusion have been documented in patients with bronchogenic carcinoma and large mass lesions.[B6] Primary pulmonary artery sarcoma can mimic pulmonary embolism. It is rare and typically arises from the main pulmonary artery. Pulmonary infarcts due to tumor emboli or small thrombi arising on the mass may produce symptoms similar to pulmonary emboli. The clinical symptoms of this tumor more typically simulate chronic or recurrent embolism. Pulmonary carcinosarcoma is an uncommon pulmonary neoplasm. Two varieties occur. The central type is a pedunculated endobronchial lesion producing bronchial obstruction. The peripheral type grows rapidly and has a propensity to invade the chest wall, mediastinum, and vascular structures. Symptoms may be indistinguishable from pulmonary embolism, and neoplasia should be included in the differential diagnosis of acute pulmonary embolism in patients in whom perfusion scan defects do not change with appropriate anticoagulation or who show a progression of perfusion defects on lung scanning despite adequate anticoagulation.[O1]

Pulmonary Sequestration

Pulmonary sequestration is a condition in which part of a lung is not connected with the pulmonary artery, and sometimes is not connected with the bronchial tree. The abnormal lung segment receives its blood supply from an artery arising from the thoracic or abdominal aorta. In intralobar sequestration, the nonfunctional segment of lung is enclosed within the visceral pleura. The posterobasilar segment is usually involved, and the majority of cases occur on the left side.[T3] In intralobar sequestration, venous drainage to pulmonary veins occurs. In extralobar sequestration, the abnormal lung segment is contained within its own visceral pleura outside the pleural space either above or below the diaphragm. The blood is supplied from a systemic source, typically the thoracic aorta, but venous drainage involves a systemic vein such as the inferior vena cava, the azygos vein, or the hemiazygos system. These abnormalities usually occur on the left side.

Congenital Dysplasia of the Lung

Embryologically, the aorta and the main pulmonary artery arise from a common trunk that septates to form the ascending

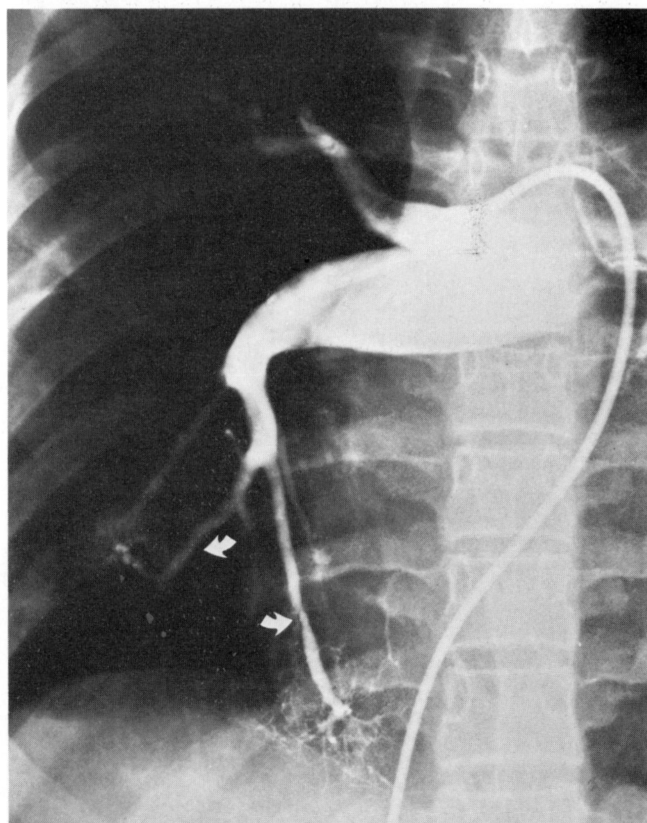

Figure 10–7. Takayasu's arteritis involving pulmonary artery. Right pulmonary arterial injection angiogram shows rapid tapering of distal vessels, with occlusion of several segmental branches and areas of irregular stenosis typical of vasculitis *(arrows)*. This patient had severe pulmonary hypertension. (From Cassling, R.J., et al.: Unusual pulmonary angiographic findings in suspected pulmonary embolism. AJR 145:995, 1985, with permission. © by American Roentgen Ray Society.)

aorta and the main pulmonary artery. The main right and left pulmonary arteries arise from the ventral portions of the sixth primitive arches; dorsal portions form the ductus on the side that retains its fourth arch, the forerunner of the descending aorta. The lung buds develop as a ventral outgrowth from the foregut and transiently receive blood from small systemic vessels arising from the paired dorsal aortae. Pulmonary parenchymal vessels then develop and join on each side with the corresponding sixth arch.

Abnormalities of the pulmonary arteries are seen in conjunction with congenital dysplasia of the lung. Hypoplasia, interruption, agenesis, or anomalous origin of the pulmonary vessels may be evident. Chest radiographs may show a unilaterally small hemithorax, decreased or absent pulmonary vascular markings, a small or absent hilus, and a mediastinal shift to the affected side. Hypogenetic lung syndrome causes lobar or segmental absence

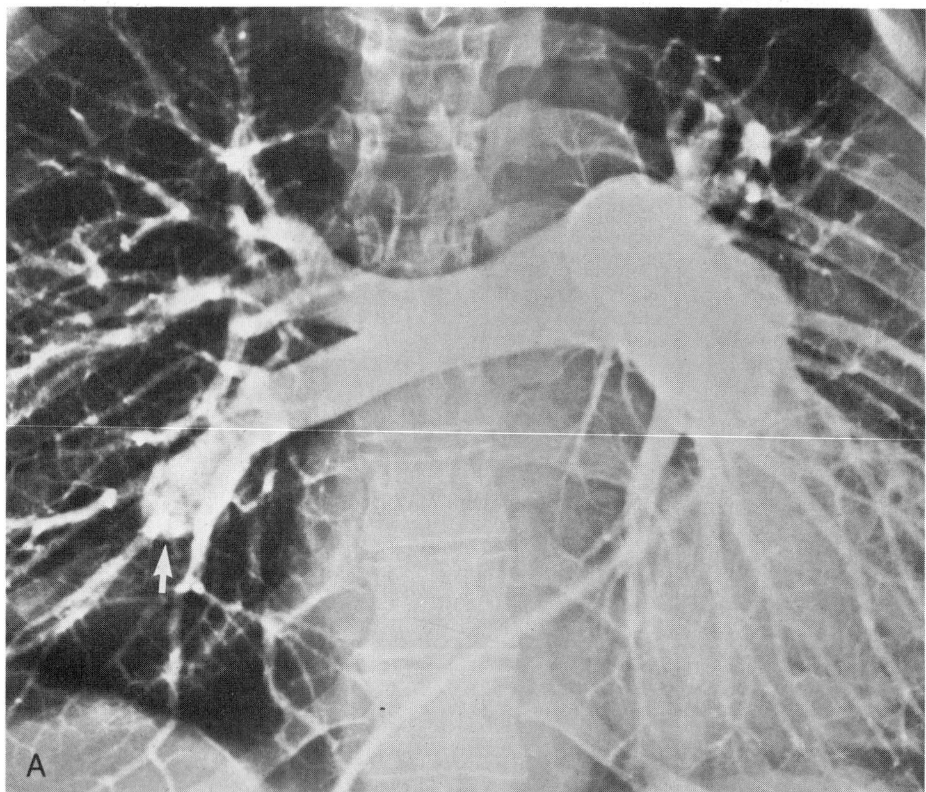

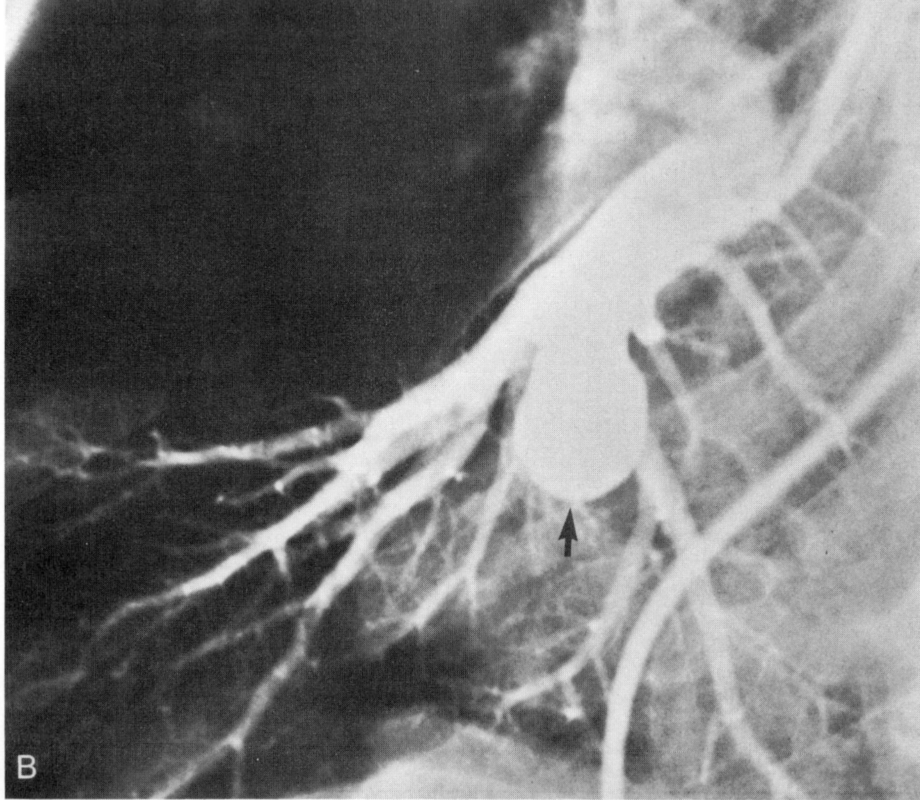

Figure 10–8. *A*, Peripheral pulmonary artery aneurysm. Pulmonary arteriogram in a patient with a history of intravenous drug abuse shows an aneurysm of the right lower lobe pulmonary artery *(arrow)*. *B*, Selective pulmonary artery injection angiogram shows this mycotic aneurysm arising from the anterior basal segmental artery *(arrow)*.

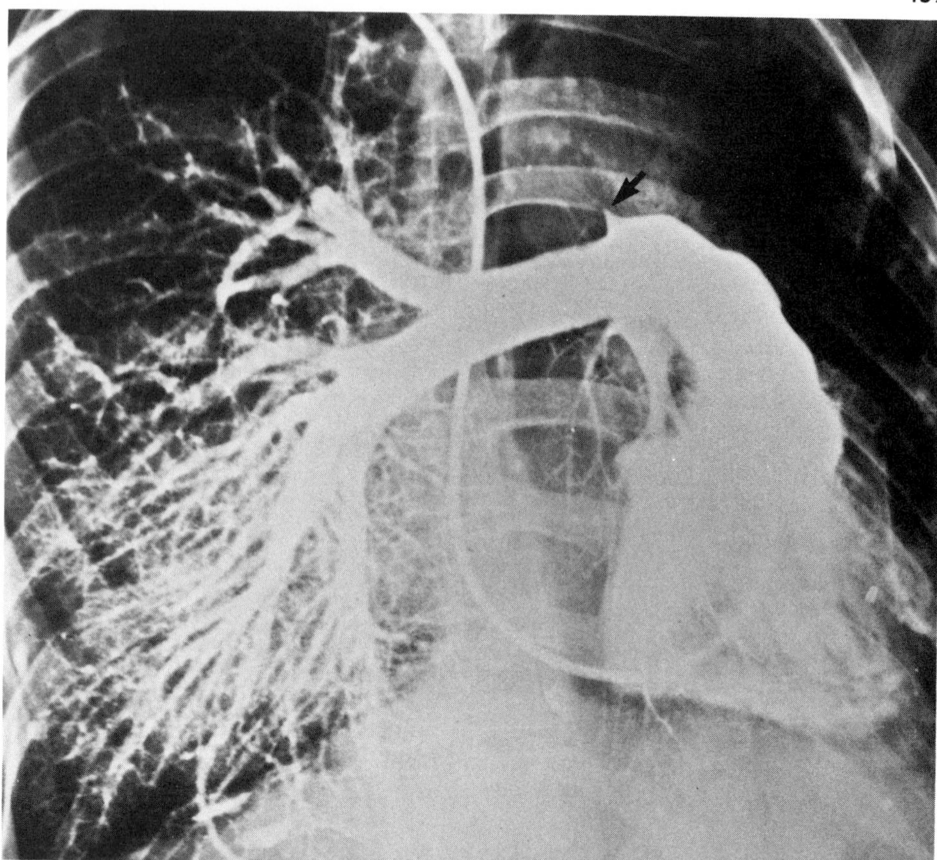

Figure 10–9. Metastatic rectal carcinoma to lung. Main pulmonary artery injection angiogram shows oblique view of left upper lobe lung infiltrate. The left upper lobe pulmonary artery is occluded by tumor encasement *(arrow)*.

of pulmonary tissue, bronchi, and vessels. Occasionally, it may involve anomalous systemic arterial supply and partially or totally anomalous venous drainage from the right lung into systemic veins, usually the inferior vena cava or the right atrium ("scimitar syndrome").[R1]

Interruption of the right or left pulmonary artery occurs when the ventral portion of the sixth arch does not communicate with its corresponding pulmonary parenchymal plexus. Usually, a left-sided arch is present when the right pulmonary artery is interrupted, and a right-sided arch is present when the left pulmonary artery is interrupted. In agenesis of the lung, no pulmonary vessels or parenchymal tissue is present.

The pulmonary artery can also arise anomalously from the aorta. This phenomenon is explained embrologically by persistence of the dorsal portion of the sixth arch (ductus) with agenesis of its ventral portion. Typically, anomalous origin of the right pulmonary artery is associated with a left aortic arch, and anomalous origin of the left pulmonary artery is associated with a right aortic arch. The left pulmonary artery may also arise anomalously from the right pulmonary artery "sling," or rarely, from the abdominal aorta. The pulmonary artery sling can produce obstruction of the distal trachea or right bronchus, or of both.[E1]

Anomalous Pulmonary Venous Connection

Anomalous pulmonary venous return can be diagnosed on the venous phase or levophase of a pulmonary arteriogram. The anomalous drainage may be partial or complete. When partial, it most frequently consists of drainage of the right upper lobe pulmonary vein to the right superior vena cava. In total anomalous pulmonary venous connection, the anomalous return, in order of frequency, is to the left superior vena cava, to the coronary sinus, to the right atrium, to the right superior vena cava, and finally, to below the diaphragm. Less frequently, the connection may be mixed with one or more veins draining into a different site. These anomalies are typically associated with an atrial septal defect that allows oxygenated blood to reach the systemic circulation. These anomalies are best identified with selective pulmonary arterial injections and delayed filming.

Pulmonary arteriography is currently the most reliable test for the diagnosis of abnormalities of the pulmonary vessels. The most frequent indication is for diagnosis of pulmonary embolism. When performed by experienced physicians, pulmonary angiography can be performed with little morbidity. The procedure should be performed in a well-equipped angiographic suite with ECG and pressure monitoring. Selective right and left pulmonary arterial injections should be performed. Particular care should be taken when studying patients with pulmonary hypertension. In these patients, subselective injections of contrast should be made into the area of highest probability. In patients with pulmonary embolism, heparin therapy followed by oral anticoagulation is usually sufficient to prevent recurrence. Patients with massive pulmonary embolism should be considered for treatment with thrombolytic therapy if no contraindications exist. When heparin therapy fails or the patient's medical condition precludes anticoagulation, vena caval filter placement can be performed. Filter placement should not be undertaken in the absence of angiographically documented pulmonary embolism. These filters can now be placed percutaneously, avoiding the need for operative placement. Pulmonary angiography is also indicated in the diagnosis of other pulmonary vascular lesions, such as pulmonary arteriovenous fistulae, vasculitis, and pulmonary artery stenosis.

References

A

1. Alderson, P.O., and Martin, E.C.: Pulmonary embolism: Diagnosis with multiple imaging modalities. Radiology 164:297, 1987.
2. Auerbach, O.: Pathology and pathogenesis of pulmonary arterial aneurysm in tuberculous cavities. Am. Rev. Tuberc. 39:99, 1939.

B

1. Bynum, L.J., Wilson, J.E., III, Christenson, E.E., and Sorensen, C.: Radiographic techniques for balloon occlusion pulmonary angiography. Radiology 133:518, 1979.
2. Barker, N.W.: The diagnosis and treatment of pulmonary embolism. Med. Clin. North Am. 42:1053, 1958.
3. Biello, D.R., Mattar, A.G., McKnight, R.C., and Siegel, B.A.: Ventilation-perfusion studies in suspected pulmonary embolism. AJR 133:1033, 1979.
4. Bjork, L., and Ansusinha, T.: Angiographic diagnosis of acute pulmonary embolism. Acta Radiol. (Diagn.) 3:129, 1965.

5. Bookstein, J.J., and Silver, T.M.: The angiographic differential diagnosis of acute pulmonary embolism. Radiology 110:25, 1974.
6. Ballantyne, A.J., Clagett, O.T., and McDonald, J.R.: Vascular involvement in bronchogenic carcinoma. Thorax 12:294, 1957.

C

1. Chait, A., Summers, D., Krasnow, N., and Wechsler, B.M.: Observations on the fate of large pulmonary emboli. AJR 100:364, 1967.
2. Cassling, R.J., Lois, J.F., and Gomes, A.S.: Unusual pulmonary angiographic findings in suspected pulmonary embolism. AJR 145:995, 1985.
3. Consensus Developmental Panel: Thrombolytic therapy in thrombosis: A National Institutes of Health Consensus Development Conference. Ann. Intern. Med. 93:141, 1980.

D

1. Dalen, J.E.: Pulmonary angiography in pulmonary embolism. Bull. Physiopathol. Resp. 6:45, 1970.
2. Dalen, J.E., and Alpert, J.S.: Natural history of pulmonary embolism. Prog. Cardiovasc. Dis. 17:259, 1975.
3. Dalen, J.E., Banas, J.S., Brooks, H.L., et al.: Resolution rate of acute pulmonary embolism in man. N. Engl. J. Med. 280:1194, 1969.
4. Dalen, J.E., Brooks, H.L., Johnson, L.W., et al.: Pulmonary angiography in acute pulmonary embolism: Indications, techniques, and results in 367 patients. Am. Heart J. 81:175, 1971.
5. Denny, D.F., Cronan, J.J., Dorfman, G.S., and Esplin, C.: Percutaneous Kimray-Greenfield filter placement by femoral vein puncture. AJR 145:827, 1985.
6. Dines, D.E., Arms, R.A., Bernatz, P., and Gomes, M.R.: Pulmonary arteriovenous fistulas. Mayo Clin. Proc. 49:460, 1974.

E

1. Ellis, K., Seamen, W.B., Griffiths, S.P., et al.: Some congenital anomalies of the pulmonary arteries. Semin. Roentgenol. 2:325, 1967.

F

1. Fred, H.L., Axelrad, M.A., Lewis, J.M., and Alexander, J.K.: Rapid resolution of pulmonary thromboemboli in man: An angiographic study. JAMA 196:1137, 1966.

G

1. Grollman, J.H., Jr., Gypes, M.T., and Helmer, E.: Transfemoral selective bilateral pulmonary arteriography with a pulmonary-artery–seeking catheter. Radiology 96:202, 1970.
2. Green, G.S.: Use of the pigtail catheter for pulmonary angiography (L). Radiology 138:744, 1981.
3. Gomes, A.S., Grollman, J.H., Jr., and Mink, J.: Pulmonary angiography for pulmonary emboli: Rational selection of oblique views. AJR 129:1019, 1977.
4. Greenspan, R.H., Ravin, C.E., Polansky, S.M., and McLoud, T.C.: Accuracy of the chest radiograph in diagnosis of pulmonary embolism. Invest. Radiol. 17:539, 1982.
5. Goldhaber, S.Z., Heit, J., Sharma, G.V., et al.: Randomised controlled trial of recombinant tissue plasminogen activator versus urokinase in the treatment of acute pulmonary embolism. Lancet 2:293, 1988.
6. Greenfield, L.J.: Pulmonary embolism: Diagnosis and management. Curr. Probl. Cardiol. 13:1, 1976.
7. Greenfield, L.J., Peyton, R., Crute, S., and Barnes, R.: Greenfield vena caval filter experience: Late results in 156 patients. Arch. Surg. 116:1451, 1981.
8. Gunther, R.W., Schild, H., Fries, A., and Storkel, S.: Vena cava filter to prevent pulmonary embolism: Experimental study. Radiology 156:315, 1985.
9. Gay, B.B., Jr., French, R.H., and Shuford, W.H., et al.: The roentgenologic features of single and multiple coarctations of the pulmonary artery and branches. AJR 90:599, 1963.

H

1. Hull, R.D., Hirsh, J., Carter, C.J., et al.: Pulmonary angiography, ventilation lung scanning and venography for clinically suspected pulmonary embolism with abnormal perfusion scan. Ann. Intern. Med. 98:891, 1983.

K

1. Kelly, J.F., Patterson, R., Lieberman, P., et al.: Radiographic contrast media studies in high-risk patients. J. Allergy Clin. Immunol. 62:181, 1978.
2. Kawai, C., Ishikawa, K., Kato, M., et al.: Pulmonary pulseless disease: Clinical Conference in Cardiology from the Third Medical Division, Kyoto University Hospital, Kyoto, Japan. Chest 73:651, 1978.

L

1. Lund, G., Rysavy, J.A., Hunter, D.W., et al.: Retrievable vena caval filter percutaneously introduced. Radiology 155:831, 1985.
2. Lupi-Herrera, E., Sanchez-Torres, G., Marcushamer, J., et al.: Takayasu's arteritis: Clinical study of 107 cases. Am. Heart J. 93:94, 1977.

M

1. Mills, S.R., Jackson, D.C., Older, R.A., et al.: The incidence, etiologies, and avoidance of complications of pulmonary angiography in a large series. Radiology 136:295, 1980.
2. McNeil, B.J.: A diagnostic strategy using ventilation perfusion studies in patients suspected for pulmonary embolism. J. Nucl. Med. 17:613, 1976.
3. Murphy, M.L., and Bulloch, R.T.: Factors influencing the restoration of blood flow following pulmonary embolization as determined by angiography and scanning. Circulation 38:1116, 1968.
4. McDonald, I.G., Hirsh, J., and Hale, G.S.: Early rate of resolution of major pulmonary embolism: A study of angiographic and hemodynamic changes occurring in the first 24–48 hours. Br. Heart J. 33:432, 1971.
5. Miller, G.A.H., and Sutton, G.C.: Acute massive pulmonary embolism: Clinical and hemodynamic findings in 23 patients studied by cardiac catheterization and pulmonary arteriography. Br. Heart J. 32:518, 1970.
6. Moses, D.L., Silver, T.M., and Bookstein, J.J.: The complementary roles of chest radiography lung scanning and selective pulmonary arteriography in the diagnosis of pulmonary embolism. Circulation 49:179, 1974.
7. Mant, M.J., Thong, K.L., Kirtwhistle, R.V., et al.: Fibrinolytic therapy. Radiology 159:619, 1986.
8. Marder, V.J.: Are we using fibrinolytic agents often enough? [Editorial.] Ann. Intern. Med. 93:136, 1980.
9. Mobin-Uddin, K., McLean, R., and Jude, J.R.: A new catheter technique of interruption of inferior vena cava for prevention of pulmonary embolism. Am. J. Surg. 35:889, 1969.
10. Moyer, J.H., Glentz, G., and Brest, A.N.: Pulmonary arteriovenous fistulas. Am. J. Med. 32:417, 1962.

N

1. Nihill, M.R., Mullins, C.E., and McNamara, D.G.: Visualization of the pulmonary arteries in pseudotruncus by pulmonary vein wedge angiography. Circulation 58:140, 1978.
2. Novelline, R.A., Baltarowich, O.H., Athanasoulis, C.A., et al.: The clinical course of patients with suspected pulmonary embolism and a negative pulmonary arteriogram. Radiology 126:561, 1978.

O

1. Olsson, H.E., Spitzer, R.M., and Erston, W.F.: Primary and secondary pulmonary artery neoplasia mimicking acute pulmonary embolus. Radiology 118:49, 1976.

R

1. Roehm, J., Jue, K., and Amplatz, K.: Radiographic features of the scimitar syndrome. Radiology 86:856, 1966.

S

1. Saeed, M., Braun, S.D., Cohan, R.H., et al.: Pulmonary angiography with iopamidol: Patient comfort, image quality, and hemodynamics. Radiology 165:345, 1987.
2. Smith, D.C., Lois, J.F., Gomes, A.S., et al.: Pulmonary arteriography: Comparison of cough stimulation effects of diatrizoate and ioxaglate. Radiology 162:617, 1987.
3. Smith, G.T., Dexter, L., and Dammin, G.J.: Postmortem quantitative studies in pulmonary embolism. *In* Sasahara, A.A., and Stein, M. (eds.): Pulmonary Embolic Disease. Grune & Stratton, New York, 1965, p. 120.
4. Sasahara, A.: Clinical studies in pulmonary thromboembolism. *In* Sasahara, A.A., and Stein, M. (eds.): Pulmonary Embolic Disease. Grune & Stratton, New York, 1965, p. 256.
5. Sostman, H.D., Rapoport, S., Gottschalk, A., and Greenspan, R.H.: Imaging of pulmonary embolism. Invest. Radiol. 21:443, 1986.
6. Sostman, H.D., Ravin, C.E., and Sullivan, D.C.: Use of pulmonary angiography for suspected pulmonary embolism: Influence of scintigraphic diagnosis. AJR 139:673, 1982.
7. Sullivan, D.C., Coleman, R.E., and Mills, S.R.: Lung scan interpretation: Effect of different observers and different criteria. Radiology 149:803, 1983.
8. Sautter, R.D., Fletcher, F.W., Emmanuel, D.A., et al.: Clinical notes: Complete resolution of massive pulmonary thromboembolism. JAMA 189:948, 1964.
9. Simon, M., and Sasahara, A.A.: Observations on the angiographic changes in pulmonary thrombolism. *In* Sasahara, A.A., and Stein, M. (eds.): Pulmonary Embolic Disease. Grune & Stratton, New York, 1965, p. 214.
10. Sasahara, A.A., Sidd, J.J., Tremblay, G., and Leland, O.S.: Cardiopulmonary consequences of acute pulmonary embolic disease. Prog. Cardiovasc. Dis. 9:259, 1966.
11. Stein, M., Hirose, T., Yasutake, T., and Tarabeith, A.: Airway responses to pulmonary embolism—pharmacologic aspects. *In* Moser, K.M., and Stein, M. (eds.): Pulmonary Thromboembolism. Yearbook, Chicago, 1973, p. 166.
12. Sharma, G.V., Burleson, V.A., and Sasahara, A.A.: Effect of thrombolytic therapy on pulmonary capillary blood volume in patients with pulmonary embolism. N. Engl. J. Med. 303:842, 1980.

T

1. Tadavarthy, S.M., Castaneda-Zuniga, W.R., Salomowitz, E., et al.: Kimray-Greenfield vena cava filter: Percutaneous introduction. Radiology 151:525, 1984.

2. Trell, E.: Pulmonary arterial aneurysm. Thorax 28:644, 1973.
3. Turk, L.N., III, and Lindskog, G.E.: The importance of angiographic diagnosis in intralobar pulmonary sequestration. J. Thorac. Cardiovasc. Surg. 41:299, 1961.

U

1. Urokinase Pulmonary Embolism Trial: A national cooperative study. Circulation 47 and 48 (Suppl. 2):1, 1973.
2. Urokinase Pulmonary Embolism Trial Phase I Results: A cooperative study. JAMA 214:2163, 1970.
3. Urokinase-Streptokinase Pulmonary Embolism Trial Phase II Results: A cooperative study. JAMA 229:1606, 1974.

V

1. Verstraete, M., Miller, G.A.H., Bounameaux, H., et al.: Intravenous and intrapulmonary recombinant tissue type plasminogen activator in the treatment of acute massive pulmonary embolism. Circulation 77:353, 1988.

W

1. Wellman, H.N.: Pulmonary thromboembolism: Current status report on the role of nuclear medicine. Semin. Nucl. Med. 6:236, 1986.
2. White, R.I., Jr., Mitchell, S.E., Barth, K.H., et al.: Angioarchitecture of pulmonary arteriovenous malformations: An important consideration before embolotherapy. AJR 140:681, 1983.

Chapter 11

Radiographic Contrast Agents

JOHN W. HIRSHFELD, JR., M.D.

THE PHYSICS OF DIAGNOSTIC X-RAY IMAGING 162
PERFORMANCE CRITERIA FOR INTRAVASCULAR RADIOGRAPHIC CONTRAST AGENTS 162
HISTORICAL BACKGROUND 162
ANGIOGRAPHIC CONTRAST AGENTS CURRENTLY MARKETED IN THE UNITED STATES 165
Importance of Iodine Concentration 165
1.5 Ratio Ionic Agents 166
3.0 Ratio Ionic Agent 166
3.0 Ratio Nonionic Agents 166
PHARMACOLOGIC EFFECTS OF ANGIOGRAPHIC CONTRAST AGENTS 166
Acute Toxicity 166
Effects of Intravascular Bolus Injection 168
Effect on Intravascular Volume 168
Effect on Systemic Vascular Resistance 168
Effect on Systemic Arterial Pressure 169
Effect on Ventricular Filling Pressure 169
Effect on Cardiac Output 169
Effects of Selective Intracoronary Injection 170
Effect of Myocardial Performance and Systemic Arterial Pressure 170
Cardiac Electrophysiologic Effects 171
Other Noncardiovascular Effects 174
Immediate Generalized or Anaphylactoid Reaction 174
Effects on Renal Function 176
Effects on Pulmonary Function 176
Gastrointestinal Effects 176
Hematologic Effects 176
Effects on Blood Vessels 176
CRITERIA FOR SELECTION OF CONTRAST AGENTS FOR CARDIAC ANGIOGRAPHY 177

THE PHYSICS OF DIAGNOSTIC X-RAY IMAGING

All imaging techniques in which diagnostic x-ray methods are used rely on regional differences in the absorbance of x-ray photons. The conventional radiographic image is a two-dimensional analog display of the spatial variations in x-ray absorbance of the three-dimensional structure being imaged. In the display, a large signal (black on a conventional x-ray film) represents a comparatively small x-ray absorbance or radiographic density, and a small signal (white on a conventional x-ray film) represents a greater density. For a structure to be imaged, its x-ray absorbance must be either greater or less than that of the surrounding tissues. The amount of difference, or image contrast, required is related inversely to the size of the structure.

Conventional radiographic imaging employs x-ray photon energies in the so-called diagnostic range of 60 to 125 kilovolts peak (kVp). The ability of a material to absorb these photons is determined predominantly by two properties: (1) the *atomic number* of the elements in the material and (2) the *elemental density* of the atoms in the material. Most tissues of the body are solid- or fluid-phase structures composed predominantly of hydrogen, carbon, and oxygen, which have atomic numbers of 1, 6, and 8, respectively. Bones are solid-phase structures that are easily resolved from surrounding structures because they contain large quantities of calcium (atomic number 20). Lungs contain predominantly gases that are composed of nitrogen (atomic number 7), oxygen, hydrogen, and carbon. These gases are distinguished from surrounding fluid and solid structures by the smaller elemental densities of the atoms.

Diagnostic x-ray techniques cannot resolve internal cardiac structure and blood vessels because the x-ray absorbance of these structures is identical to that of the blood contained within them. Thus, they have no "radiographic contrast" and cannot be imaged by conventional radiographic techniques. Radiographic contrast can be created, however, by transiently replacing the blood inside these structures with a contrast agent.

PERFORMANCE CRITERIA FOR INTRAVASCULAR RADIOGRAPHIC CONTRAST AGENTS

Intravascular radiographic contrast agents make cardiac and vascular structures visible by increasing the x-ray absorbance of the fluid inside them, thus increasing the radiographic density of the structure's lumen. Theoretically, cardiovascular structures could also be imaged by decreasing their x-ray density. This approach has been tried to a limited extent by using gases such as carbon dioxide as contrast agents. All currently used techniques employ fluids to increase x-ray absorbance.

To resolve an object 1 mm in diameter (the diameter of small coronary branches), image contrast that is roughly 10 percent greater than the surrounding structures is required.[M6] Larger structures require less of a percentage of image contrast. Accordingly, the x-ray absorbance of an intravascular contrast agent must be sufficiently greater than that of blood to increase the vessel's radiographic density to a value 10 percent greater than that of the entire thickness of the tissues traversed by the x-ray beam.

Therefore, a suitable angiographic contrast agent must meet several criteria:

1. It must be a liquid at body temperature, with a viscosity similar to that of blood. To be suitable for intravascular injection, it probably should be an aqueous solution, like blood plasma.
2. It must contain an element with a sufficiently high atomic number in a concentration adequate to provide an x-ray absorbance that is at least 10 percent greater than that of blood.
3. Its constituents must be biocompatible, have minimal deleterious effects in the required concentrations, and be easily eliminated from the body.

HISTORICAL BACKGROUND

Roentgen discovered x-rays in 1895.[R5] Excited endeavors to image internal body structures ensued rapidly thereafter. The need for contrast agents to image blood vessels promptly became apparent but most of the elements with high atomic number proved to be too toxic for intravascular administration in the concentrations needed to generate sufficient image contrast. Many workers investigated potential contrast agent preparations. The first vascular images of diagnostic quality in a living human were obtained in 1923 by Berberich and Hirsch, who used injection of a 20 percent solution of strontium bromide (atomic numbers 38 and 35, respectively).[B2]

Iodine (atomic number 53) soon emerged as the element with the optimum combination of physical, chemical, and pharmacologic properties for intravascular imaging. In 1924, Brooks reported vascular imaging with intra-arterial injection of sodium iodide.[B8] Taking advantage of sodium iodide's high aqueous solubility, he prepared a solution that was approximately 40 percent iodine by weight (and that had a sodium concentration of approximately 5 mol/L) by dissolving 100 g of sodium iodide in 100 ml of water. His description of the angiographic procedure makes clear that this preparation was less than ideal as an arteriographic agent:

> The entire thigh is prepared for operation. A sterile tourniquet is placed around the thigh as high as possible, but is not tightened. With a local anesthetic of 0.5 percent procain, the femoral artery is exposed in the proximal end of Hunter's canal. Only enough of the artery is exposed to permit the application of a Crile artery clamp, which is not tightened. The roentgen-ray tube is placed over the knee region, and a large photographic film with a screen is placed under the knee and leg. The patient is now given nitrous oxid gas. It has been found that there is pain during the period the solution is in the artery, and the patient cannot be kept still enough to get a good roentgenogram unless a general anesthetic is used. The tourniquet proximal to the exposed artery is tightened enough to produce a filling of the veins. When the veins are full, the clamp on the artery is tightened enough to occlude the artery completely. A short interval is then allowed to elapse for the artery distal to the clamp to empty its blood. A medium sized needle is introduced into the lumen of the artery, and 10 c.c. of the sodium iodid solution is injected. The roentgen-ray tube is then operated for the briefest period possible to secure a good plate. A second plate may be taken of the distal third of the leg and foot. The tourniquet is released, the clamp removed from the artery, and the gas anesthetic discontinued. The wound is then closed.[B8]

Brooks's experience demonstrated the feasibility of arteriography using iodine as the contrast agent element. It also demonstrated that the iodide ion itself was unacceptable in this role because of absolute physiochemical limitations. The molar concentrations of iodide ion required to achieve adequate image contrast are 20 times greater than the molar concentration of ions in body fluids, and the quantities of iodine needed to perform the typical angiographic examination are enormous compared with either total body stores or the normal daily intake (Fig. 11–1). An improved method of delivering the large quantities of highly concentrated iodine was needed.

Fortunately, iodine is readily incorporated into organic molecules. The history of the molecular evolution of iodinated radiographic contrast agents is illustrated in Figure 11–2. The first attempt to use organified iodine as a contrast agent employed a complex of sodium iodide and urea.[R6] This complex, however, also proved to be unacceptably toxic. Selectan, the first iodinated organic molecule that was successfully administered to humans, was introduced in 1928. It had been synthesized originally as a potential antibiotic by Binz and Rath.[B4] It was studied and found to be effective as a urographic contrast agent by Swick.[S9] It also proved to be unacceptably toxic, however (the maximum tolerated human dose was 18 g), and not adequately soluble in water. Two years later, in 1930, the substitution of the methyl moiety with a carboxyl group produced Uroselectan. Development of this compound represented a true breakthrough. Its toxicity was one tenth that of Selectan, and it was substantially more water-soluble.[S10] Although Swick studied it primarily as a urographic agent, other investigators, including Forssmann, who used it to opacify the right heart in animals,[F2] recognized its potential as a vascular and cardiac contrast agent.

Once organified iodine was established as a successful intravascular contrast agent, work was directed to develop improved molecules. Investigators rapidly realized that a satisfactory intravascular contrast agent formulation required an iodine content of at least 20 percent by weight, and that better opacification and detail resolution required even greater concentrations. This fundamental physical problem required that the formulations of intravascular contrast agent molecules be highly concentrated in comparison with the solute concentrations of body fluids. The problem was to design molecules that had physical and biochemical properties compatible with intravascular administration and that incorporated an adequate elemental density of iodine into solution.

A molecule's ability to deliver iodine is characterized by its *iodine ratio*, the ratio of the number of iodine atoms in a molecule to the number of osmotically active particles that the molecule produces in solution. Uroselectan contains one iodine atom per two osmotically active particles. Thus, it has an iodine ratio of 0.5. Since 1930, the contrast agent molecule "horsepower race" has been directed at increasing the iodine ratio and correspondingly reducing the toxicity of contrast agent molecules.

Development focused initially on increasing the iodine content of the contrast agent molecule. If a molecule contained more iodine atoms, a lower molar concentration would be required to achieve a given iodine density. The first major improvement occurred in 1931 with the synthesis of iodopyracet (Diodrast) and neo-iopax (Uroselectan B), which have two iodine atoms per molecule and, accordingly, are 1.0 ratio agents.[C1] These molecules were used actively for 20 years, and considerable work that laid the groundwork for cardiac angiography was performed with these molecules. The next significant advance was the synthesis

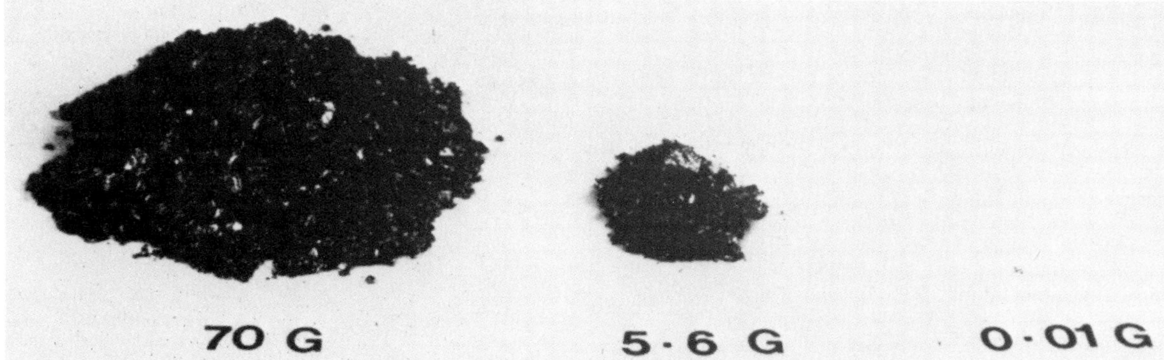

Figure 11–1. Illustration demonstrating the relationship between the quantities of iodine employed in angiographic examinations and total body stores. The 70-g pile of crystalline iodine on the left represents the amount of iodine in 200 ml (a representative total patient dose for a complex procedure) of a contrast agent containing 350 mg/ml iodine. The 5.6-g pile in the center represents the amount of iodine contained in 16 ml of contrast agent. The 0.01-g pile on the right represents the normal total body content of iodine. (From Grainger, R.G.: Osmolalities of intravascular radiological contrast media. Brit. J. Radiol. 53:739, 1980, with permission.)

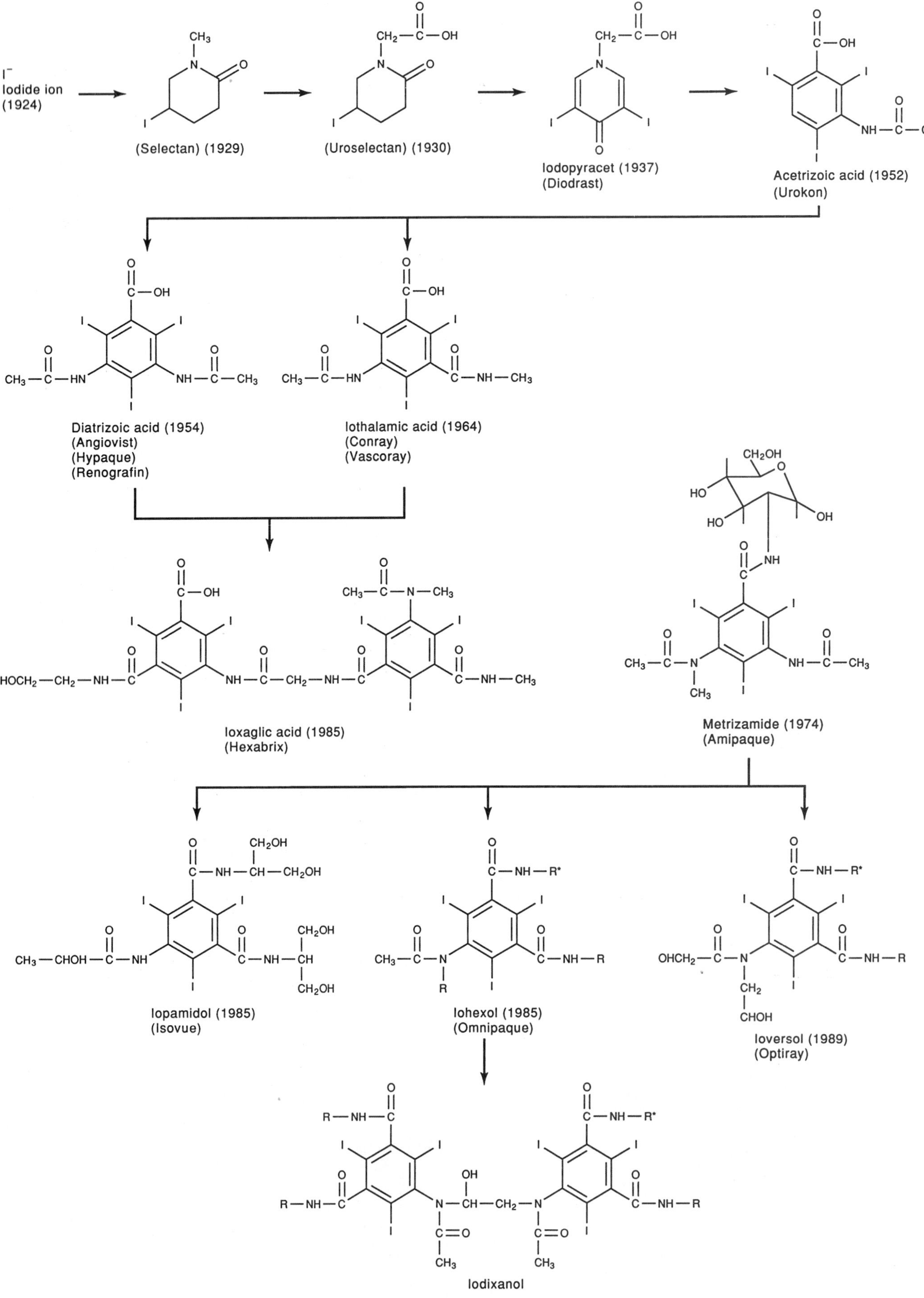

Figure 11–2. The molecular history of the evolution of iodine-based angiographic contrast agents. For each compound, the generic name is listed along with common trade names and the year of introduction into clinical use.

of acetrizoic acid by Wallingford (Urokon), which was introduced into clinical radiology in 1952. This material added a third iodine atom, producing a 1.5 ratio agent, which carried the halogen-substituted benzene ring to its maximum achievable iodine content.[H11] This accomplishment was the culmination of 20 years of work (slowed somewhat by World War II) to overcome the organic synthetic problems of creating 2,4,6-tri-iodinated aromatic molecules and to reduce the substantial toxicity of the first molecules synthesized in this class.

The acetrizoic acid class of contrast agents was further refined by substituting the 5 position with an amide. The first and prototypical member of this class is diatrizoic acid (Angiovist, Hypaque, MD-76, Renografin), which was introduced into clinical use in 1954 and until recently has been the most widely used of all intravascular contrast agent molecules.[H10] Iothalamic acid (Conray) was subsequently developed as a derivative of diatrizoic acid and was found to have similar properties.

By 1960, investigators established that despite substantial improvements in radiographic equipment, an angiographic contrast agent required at least 30 percent iodine by weight to produce satisfactory opacification of small vessels. Even the tri-iodinated molecules required very large molar concentrations to achieve iodine contents in this range.

To maintain the required high degree of aqueous solubility, all of the previously synthesized contrast agent molecules relied on an ionizing functional group at the 1 position. These ionic characteristics caused two problems. The first problem was that the cation associated with the contrast agent molecule was present in such large concentrations that its pharmacologic, electrophysiologic, and physiochemical properties became an important determinant of the properties of the contrast agent formulation. The simplest formulation of an ionic contrast agent would use an inorganic biocompatible cation such as sodium. Achieving a satisfactory concentration of the iodine containing anion, however, requires a cation concentration of approximately 1000 mEq/L (over six times the normal concentration of sodium in plasma). A solution with this large a sodium concentration is electrophysiologically unacceptable for direct injection into coronary arteries. Consequently, a cation that is not electrophysiologically active needs to be furnished.

Methylglucamine (Meglumine) has such properties and is used as the cation in most currently used ionic contrast agent formulations. A shortcoming of methylglucamine, however, is that compared with sodium, it increases the solution viscosity, making extremely concentrated solutions difficult to inject through catheters. The currently used formulations therefore represent a compromise; they contain a concentration of sodium that is approximately isotonic, and the remaining cation space is filled with methylglucamine. Thus, a typical diatrizoate-based contrast agent formulation contains 10 percent sodium diatrizoate and 66 percent methylglucamine diatrizoate by weight. The sodium concentration of such a formulation is 160 mEq/L.[H6]

The second problem of the previously synthesized contrast agent molecules was that the ionic nature of the compound required that the associated cation be in solution, which doubled the number of osmotically active particles associated with the contrast agent molecule.

The tri-iodinated ionic contrast agents, although substantially improved over the molecules used earlier, still have toxicities that limit the volume that can be administered, particularly to hemodynamically fragile patients (see later discussion). In 1969, Almen reasoned that a major component of the toxicity was not the contrast agent molecule itself, but the high osmolality of the solution of the contrast agent formulation (five to six times that of plasma).[A2]

Almen identified several potential approaches to reducing contrast agent osmolality (and increasing the iodine ratio). One approach was the replacement of the ionizable functional group with a polar nonionizing functional group that would maintain aqueous solubility, but because of the absence of an associated cation, would reduce the osmolality of a formulation by a factor of two.[A2] This reasoning led to the synthesis of metrizamide, a tri-iodinated aromatic molecule in which the carboxyl group is replaced by a sugar.[A1]

Metrizamide, the first 3.0 ratio agent, was introduced into clinical radiology in 1974. Because of aggregation of contrast agent molecules in solution, it proved to have a measured osmolality that is actually lower than that predicted from theoretic calculations.[G3] Experimental and clinical studies showed that compared with the ionic acetrizoic acid derivatives, it was remarkably less toxic, and that it caused fewer hemodynamic and electrophysiologic changes.[T4] Unfortunately, metrizamide is extremely expensive to synthesize and lacks thermostability. These problems make it cumbersome to use and have limited its usefulness in procedures that require large amounts of contrast agent, such as cardiac angiography. It proved to be extremely successful, however, as a myelographic agent and clearly demonstrated the value of reducing contrast agent osmolality to improve tolerance.

Subsequent research focused on compounds that would achieve osmolality reduction and that were practical to use. Two of the approaches proposed by Almen were used. The first approach was the synthesis of other 3.0 ratio nonionic compounds. This led to the introduction of iohexol[L5] and iopamidol[M4, T2] in 1985, and of ioversol[H7] in 1989. All three of these compounds are 3.0 ratio agents that are thermostable and less expensive to synthesize than metrizamide. Their pharmacologic properties and toxicities are similar to metrizamide. The second approach was the synthesis of an ionic agent with six iodine atoms per molecule, which was accomplished by linking two 1.5 ratio ionic molecules together and converting one of the carboxyl groups to an amide. This class of molecules (termed monoacid dimers), which also have a 3.0 iodine ratio, is represented by ioxaglate, which was introduced in 1984.[H8] Ioxaglate proved to have hemodynamic performance comparable to the 3.0 ratio nonionic agents, but a frequency of minor adverse reactions (chiefly, nausea) that was intermediate between the 1.5 ratio ionic agents and the 3.0 ratio nonionic agents.[W2]

Radiographic contrast agent design is currently developing in two directions. The first involves identification of nonionic 3.0 ratio molecules that are either more economical to produce than other available compounds or that have improved physical properties. One such molecule under current consideration is Iopentol.[B6] The second direction involves further reduction of the osmolality of nonionic molecules by synthesis of a nonionic dimer to create a 6.0 ratio molecule. One such molecule under evaluation is iodixanol, which appears to cause even less hemodynamic disturbance than do the 3.0 ratio nonionic agents.[A3, R3]

The iodixanol molecule applies the dimer strategy to nonionic molecules. Because it is a 6.0 ratio agent, it offers the promise of even lower osmolality for any given iodine concentration than that of the 3.0 ratio nonionic agents. In fact, the osmolality of an iodixanol solution containing 300 mg/ml of iodine is 200 mosm/kg, which is less than that of blood plasma. Correspondingly, the mouse intravenous median lethal dose (LD_{50}) of iodixanol is reported to be greater than that of the 3.0 ratio nonionic agents. Solutions of iodixanol are considerably more viscous (18.9 mPa • sec at 20°C for 300 mg of iodine per ml), however, than comparably concentrated solutions of 3.0 ratio nonionic agents (iohexol viscosity is 11.6 mPa • sec at 20°C for 300 mg of iodine per ml).[A8] This viscosity may preclude the use of iodixanol as an angiographic agent. In addition, iodixanol is likely to be even more costly to produce than the 3.0 ratio nonionic agents that are already substantially more expensive than the 1.5 ratio ionic agents. Thus, although iodixanol represents a potential advance in contrast agent design, its clinical and commercial viability remains to be determined. At this time, it is of theoretic interest because it represents the logical next step in increasing the iodine ratio of radiographic intravascular contrast agents.

ANGIOGRAPHIC CONTRAST AGENTS CURRENTLY MARKETED IN THE UNITED STATES

Importance of Iodine Concentration

As discussed earlier, an angiographic contrast agent must deliver to the vascular structure being imaged an elemental density of iodine that is adequate to resolve that structure. The lowest iodine concentration that is adequate for the resolution of small vessels such as coronary arteries in large, heavy patients is 300 mg/ml. All of the contrast agents marketed in the United States for cardiac angiography meet this criterion, with iodine concentrations ranging from 320 to 400 mg/ml. All of these agents provide acceptable opacification. In fact, differences between the levels of opacification provided by the different marketed iodine concentrations are essentially imperceptible in clinical use (Fig. 11–3). Thus, a preparation with an iodine concentration of 370 mg/ml does not provide vascular opacification that is clinically superior to that provided by a preparation with an iodine concentration of 320 mg/ml.

Some of the relevant properties of contrast agents that are currently marketed for cardiac angiography are compiled in Table 11–1.

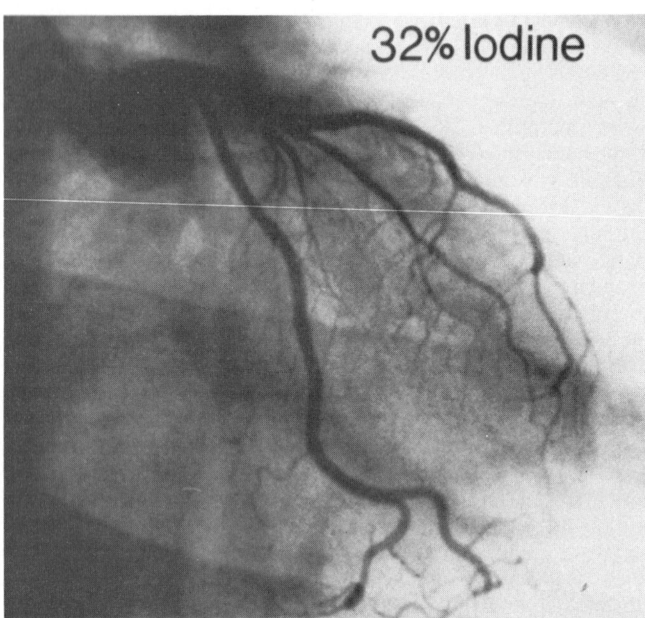

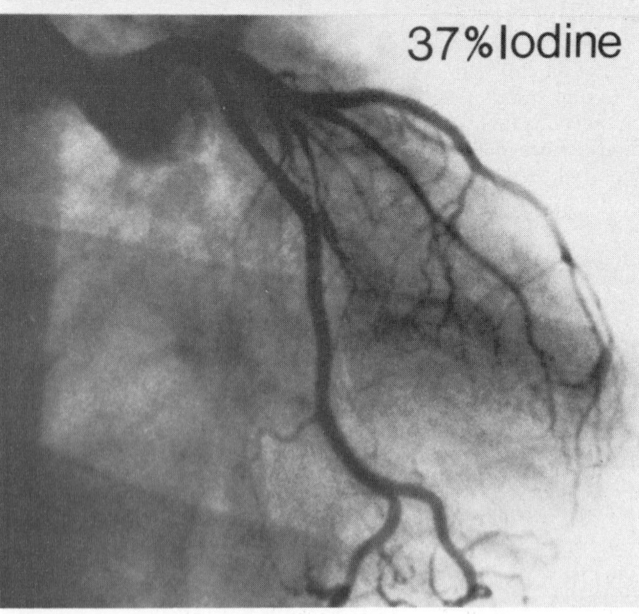

Figure 11–3. Frames from two left coronary cineangiograms from the same patient (height, 70 inches; weight, 225 lb) exposed in the same radiographic projection. The upper frame was obtained with a contrast agent containing 320 mg/ml iodine, and the lower frame was obtained with an agent continuing 370 mg/ml iodine.

1.5 Ratio Ionic Agents

The diatrizoate anion is the basis of virtually all of the 1.5 ratio ionic agents used for cardiac angiography in the United States. An iothalamate-based agent is also marketed and is widely used in cerebral angiography but has been of limited use in cardiac angiography. Diatrizoate is available in many formulations and concentrations for different intravascular applications and is marketed in the United States under four different trade names. All preparations used for cardiac angiography contain 76 percent contrast agent by weight with a ratio of methylglucamine cation to sodium cation of 6.6:1.0. Because of differences in other additives, the sodium concentration of the different formulations varies from 160 to 190 mEq/L. This range of sodium concentration has been found to be optimum in terms of minimizing cardiac electrophysiologic effects during selective coronary injection.[A4, H6, S5, S7] Higher or lower sodium concentrations cause a greater frequency of ventricular fibrillation during selective intracoronary injection.

The diatrizoate formulations also differ from each other in their calcium-binding properties. All of the formulations contain ethylenediaminetetraacetic acid (EDTA), but in two of the formulations (Angiovist and Hypaque-76), the EDTA is enriched with calcium. The other two formulations (M.D.-76 and Renografin-76) contain EDTA that is not calcium-enriched. In addition, these latter two formulations contain citrate ion (for the purpose of chelating trace quantities of heavy metals to enhance shelf life). The significance of the differences in calcium-binding properties and sodium concentration is examined in the discussion of cardiac electrophysiologic effects of selective intracoronary injection, which is found later in this chapter.

The iothalamate anion is marketed in the United States for cardiac use under the trade name of Vascoray. Its formulation by weight contains 26 percent sodium salt and 52 percent methylglucamine salt, and it has an iodine content of 400 mg/ml. Its formulation also contains calcium-enriched EDTA, and it does not contain citrate.

3.0 Ratio Ionic Agent

Ioxaglate is marketed in the United States as Hexabrix. Unlike the other agents, its formulation is somewhat less concentrated, containing 32 percent iodine. This lower concentration is a consequence of the molecule's physical properties. A concentration that would contain 37 percent iodine would have an unacceptably high viscosity. Its formulation by weight includes 39.3 percent methylglucamine salt and 19.6 percent sodium salt. It contains calcium-enriched EDTA and does not contain citrate.

3.0 Ratio Nonionic Agents

Three 3.0 ratio nonionic agents are currently marketed in the United States: iohexol (Omnipaque), iopamidol (Isovue), and ioversol (Optiray). These three molecules have similar structures. The formulations are also similar, except for the concentrations of the contrast agent molecule: iohexol, 35 percent iodine; iopamidol, 37 percent iodine; and ioversol, 32 percent iodine. Only trace quantities of sodium are present in the formulations of the nonionic agents. A comparison of the performance of these agents with the performance of the 1.5 ratio ionic agents and with that of the 3.0 ratio ionic agent is discussed in detail in the next section.

PHARMACOLOGIC EFFECTS OF ANGIOGRAPHIC CONTRAST AGENTS

An overall summary of the cardiovascular and noncardiovascular actions of radiographic contrast agents is provided by Tables 11–2 and 11–3.

Acute Toxicity

The ideal contrast agent would be biologically inert. The agents currently used are not inert but have remarkably little toxicity.

Table 11–1. CHEMICAL COMPOSITIONS AND SELECTED PHYSICAL AND PHARMACOLOGIC PROPERTIES OF ANGIOCARDIOGRAPHIC CONTRAST AGENTS

	Angiovist	Hypaque-76	Renografin-76	M.D.-76	Vascoray	Isovue	Omnipaque	Optiray	Hexabrix
Iodine concentration (mg/ml)	370	370	370	370	400	370	350	320	320
Iodine-containing molecule	Diatrizoate	Diatrizoate	Diatrizoate	Diatrizoate	Iothalamate	Iopamidol	Iohexol	Ioversol	Ioxaglate
Cations	Methylglucamine, Sodium	Methylglucamine, Sodium	Methylglucamine, Sodium	Methylglucamine, Sodium	Methylglucamine, Sodium	None	None	None	Methylglucamine, Sodium
Intravenous LD_{50} (g iodine/kg)	7.5	7.5	7.5		6.2	21.8	24.2	17.0	11.2
Measured osmolality (mosm/kg)	2076	2016	1940	2140	2400	796	844	702	600
Viscosity (37°C)	8.4	8.32	8.4	9.1	9.0	9.4	10.4	5.8	7.5
Sodium concentration (mEq/L)	160	160	190	190	408	Trace	Trace	Trace	150
Other additives	.01% Sodium calcium EDTA	.01% Sodium calcium EDTA	.32% Sodium citrate .04% Sodium EDTA	.32% Sodium citrate .04% Sodium EDTA	.0125% NaH_2PO_4 .011% Sodium calcium EDTA	.05% Disodium calcium EDTA 0.02% Tromethamine	.01% Disodium calcium EDTA 0.02% Tromethamine	.02% Disodium calcium EDTA 0.02% Tromethamine	.01% Disodium calcium EDTA

Table 11–2. CARDIOVASCULAR ACTIONS OF RADIOGRAPHIC CONTRAST AGENTS*

Action	1.5 Ratio Ionic Agents†	3.0 Ratio Ionic Agents	3.0 Ratio Nonionic Agents
Acute expansion of intravascular volume	+ + +	+	+
Transient systemic arteriolar vasodilation	+ + +	+	+
Transient depression of myocardial contractile function	+ +	+	0
Alteration of myocardial metabolism	+ +	?	+
Transient increase in cardiac filling pressure	+ + +	+	+
Transient increase in cardiac output	+ + +	+	+
Transient decrease in arterial pressure	+ + (Ca^{2+} binding) + (Non-Ca^{2+} binding)	+	0
Bradycardia following intracoronary injection	+ + + (Ca^{2+} binding) + (Non-Ca^{2+} binding)	+	0
Prolongation of ventricular repolarization	+ + + + (Ca^{2+} binding) + + (Non-Ca^{2+} binding)	+ +	+
Decrease in ventricular fibrillation threshold	+ + + (Ca^{2+} binding) + (Non-Ca^{2+} binding)	+	+

*Administered via intravascular bolus or intracoronary injection.
†Where appropriate, the effects of these agents are subdivided into formulations with and without calcium-binding properties.

Table 11–3. NONCARDIOVASCULAR ACTIONS OF RADIOGRAPHIC CONTRAST AGENTS*

Action	1.5 Ratio Ionic Agents	3.0 Ratio Ionic Agents	3.0 Ratio Nonionic Agents
Frequency of immediate generalized (anaphylactoid) reaction. (Severe form is rare with all agents.)	+ +	Inadequate data	+
Frequency of nephrotoxicity			
Low-risk patients	Rare	Inadequate data	Rare
High-risk patients (renal disease, diabetes, myeloma)	Related to volume administered	Inadequate data	Inadequate data
Effects on lung airway dynamics. (Effect is greater in asthmatics.)	+	0	0
Effect on vascular endothelium (disruption by large concentrations)	+ + +	+	+
Anticoagulant activity	+ + + +	+ + + +	+ +
Effect on red blood cell morphology (RBC crenation)	+ + +	Inadequate data	+
Frequency of nausea and vomiting	+ + +	+ +	Rare
Severity of pain during extracardiac selective intra-arterial injection	+ + +	+	+

*Administered via intravascular bolus or intracoronary injection.

This characteristic results in part from their lack of affinity for protein binding, high water solubility, large molecular size, and lack of transport mechanisms, all of which prevent them from entering the intracellular space when cell membrane structure is intact.

Because the purpose of these molecules is delivery of iodine, their toxicity is most meaningfully expressed as the LD_{50} in terms of grams of iodine delivered per kilogram of body weight. This value expresses the pharmacologic toxicity in terms of the molecule's medical role.

Published LD_{50} values vary somewhat from study to study, because the actual value is highly influenced by the conditions of the particular experiment (e.g., the injection rate), and not all LD_{50} determinations are made using the same experimental protocol. For example, published LD_{50} values for diatrizoate vary from 4.6 to 8.0 g iodine per kg.[S3, W12] The data cited here and in Table 11–1 are taken from the manufacturers' published data as approved by the United States Food and Drug Administration. Thus, they may be considered to represent roughly comparable experimental protocols and provide an approximate basis for comparing the toxicities of the different agents. The intravenous mouse LD_{50} for bolus injection varies from 8.0 g iodine per kg for diatrizoate to 24.2 g iodine per kg for iohexol.[S3] For a solution containing 37 percent iodine, this range represents an injection volume range of 21.6 to 65.4 ml/kg. Because total blood volume is approximately 70 ml/kg, the LD_{50} for an intravenous bolus dose of these agents ranges from 31 to 93 percent of total blood volume.

Animals that are given lethal intravenous boluses of contrast agents die in respiratory distress because of pulmonary edema. This phenomenon is not surprising when one considers the total quantity of agent injected. The LD_{50} of each of the currently used agents, when expressed in terms of the quantity of osmotically active solute, is comparable to the total intravascular volume.

Generalization of these data to humans indicates that in a 70-kg subject, the intravenous bolus LD_{50} for these agents ranges from 1400 ml for diatrizoate to 4500 ml for 3.0 ratio nonionic agents. The typical contrast agent dose for a cardiac angiographic procedure is 145 ml.[H8] Thus, the therapeutic index in healthy subjects for these compounds probably ranges from 10 to 31. Obviously, in seriously ill patients, particularly those with severe and unstable cardiac disease, the therapeutic index may be smaller.

Effects of Intravascular Bolus Injection

Cardiac angiography involves intravascular bolus injection of contrast agents. Typical injection volumes vary from 3 to 9 ml for selective coronary opacification and from 45 to 60 ml for cardiac and great vessel opacification. The effects of bolus injection may be separated into three groups: (1) effects on intravascular volume, (2) effects on the systemic vasculature, and (3) direct myocardial effects. The direct myocardial effects are discussed in detail in the later sections on selective intracoronary injection and myocardial performance.

Effect on Intravascular Volume

In the rapid intravascular injection of 50 ml of a contrast agent, the same quantity of osmotically active solute is administered as is present in 100 to 250 ml of plasma (depending on which contrast agent is used). The large quantity of osmotically active solute rapidly draws water into the intravascular volume. Some of this water is drawn from red blood cells, but the majority comes from the extravascular compartment. The magnitude of this effect is directly related to the osmolality of the particular contrast agent molecule and to the volume injected. The effect is reflected in a transient decrease in blood hemoglobin concentration (Fig. 11–4), which is caused by red blood cell dilution from the acute expansion of intravascular plasma volume.

The contrast agent molecule is initially confined to the intravascular compartment, but it gains access to the entire extracellular fluid compartment fairly rapidly.[D3, N3] The typical elimination half-life from the intravascular compartment is 24.4 ± 6.3 minutes.[A8] This elimination is a combination of movement out of the intravascular compartment into the extracellular fluid and excretion (predominantly renal). Little, if any, of the contrast agent molecule enters the intracellular compartment when cell membrane structure is intact.

Effect on Systemic Vascular Resistance

Contrast agents all produce acute vasodilation activity, causing an acute transient reduction in systemic vascular resistance shortly after injection. The onset of the vasodilation coincides with the arrival of the contrast agent molecule at the systemic arterioles, and the magnitude is related to the concentration of the agent as it reaches the systemic arterioles. This vasodilation is mediated by a physiochemical rather than a pharmacologic process and is related predominantly to the osmolality of the solution that reaches the systemic vasculature. Similar responses to the injection of other hypertonic solutions have been observed, and the magnitude of the response is related to the osmolality of the solution (Fig. 11–5).[M3, R2] Possibly, the transient vasodilation is caused by the osmotically driven extraction of water from the cells of the systemic microvasculature.[H5]

Thus, the magnitude of the effect is related to three variables:

1. The injection volume. (The larger the volume, the greater the vasodilation.)

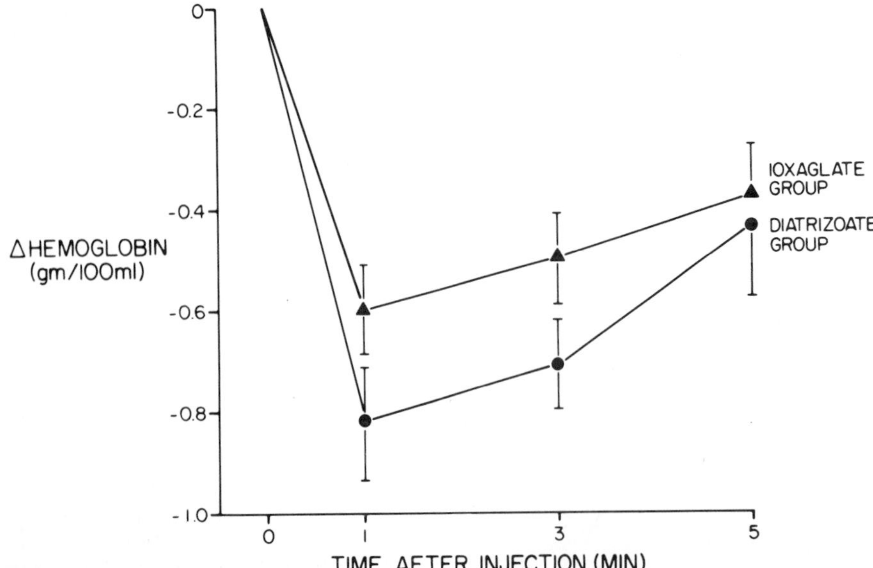

Figure 11–4. The time-related change in whole-blood hemoglobin concentration that occurs after bolus injection of 45 ml of a 1.5 ratio ionic agent (diatrizoate, 370 mg/ml iodine concentration) compared with the changes caused by a 3.0 ratio ionic agent (ioxaglate, 320 mg/ml iodine concentration). The decrease in hemoglobin concentration reflects the degree of the acute expansion of plasma volume caused by the contrast agent. The magnitude of the change is less with the 3.0 ratio agent. (From Hirshfeld, J.W., Jr., et al.: Hemodynamic changes induced by cardiac angiography with ioxaglate: Comparison with diatrizoate. J. Am. Coll. Cardiol. 2:954, 1983. Reprinted with permission from the American College of Cardiology.)

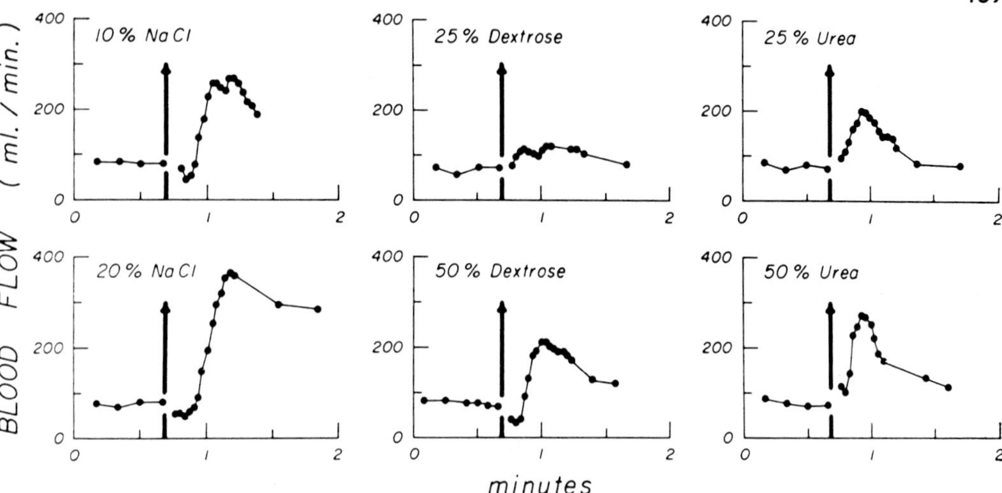

Figure 11–5. The vasodilative response to the injection of several solutions of different solute concentrations into the femoral artery of the dog. Note that all of the solutions produce vasodilation and that the magnitude of vasodilation is related to the concentration of the solution. (From Marshall, R.J., and Shepherd, J.T.: Effects of injections of hypertonic solutions on blood flow throughout the femoral artery of the dog. Am. J. Physiol. 197:951, 1959, with permission.)

2. The osmolality of the injected agent. (High osmolar agents cause a greater vasodilation than low osmolar agents.)

3. The site of injection. (Injections on the arterial side of the circulation produce greater effects than injections on the venous side.)

Effect on Systemic Arterial Pressure

The vasodilation caused by contrast agents causes a transient reduction in arterial pressure, which begins within 10 seconds after injection. The arterial pressure usually reaches its nadir by 30 to 45 seconds after injection and returns to the baseline value within 60 to 90 seconds after injection (Fig. 11–6).[H7, H8] Overshooting to a level above the pre-injection pressure occurs frequently. Because the drop in arterial pressure is mediated principally by the osmotically induced systemic vasodilation, the magnitude and duration of the decrease are related to the osmolality of the injected contrast agent. The 3.0 ratio agents cause less change than the 1.5 ratio agents.

Effect on Ventricular Filling Pressure

Contrast agents cause acute expansion of intravascular volume and a late increase in arterial pressure; some contrast agents also depress myocardial contractile performance (see later discussion). These effects combine to produce a transient elevation of cardiac filling pressures.[H3] This phenomenon occurs on both the left and the right sides of the heart, but because most cardiac disease predominantly affects the left side of the heart, and because elevation of filling pressure of the left side of the heart has greater immediate clinical consequences than does the same pressure increase in the right side of the heart, the immediate clinical consequences of elevation of filling pressure of the left side are greater than those of the elevation of the right side (Figs. 11–7 and 11–8).

For a typical bolus injection, such as 45 ml for ventriculography, the magnitude of the increase in left ventricular end-diastolic pressure varies with the osmolality of the contrast agent injected and with the nature of the particular patient's heart disease. The increases are the smallest in healthy individuals and are greater in individuals whose ventricular compliance is reduced by hypertrophy and in individuals with impaired left ventricular function who are on the steep portion of the diastolic pressure-volume relationship. An early report suggested that the degree of increase in left ventricular end-diastolic pressure was related to the presence and severity of coronary artery disease,[G1] but more recent studies have shown no such relationship.[W10] The average increase in left ventricular end-diastolic pressure after injection of a 1.5 ratio ionic agent is 9 mmHg, whereas the average increase after injection of a 3.0 ratio ionic or nonionic agent is 4 mmHg (Fig. 11–9; see Fig. 11–8).[H7, H8]

The clinical significance of an increase in left ventricular filling pressure is determined by the magnitude of the increase and the level from which it began. Obviously, an increase of 9 mmHg in a healthy individual with a baseline value of 12 mmHg is of no clinical consequence; however, a comparable (or possibly greater) increase from a baseline value of 35 mmHg in a precariously ill patient with severe aortic stenosis and coronary disease is of much greater significance.

Effect on Cardiac Output

In most patients, the increased intravascular volume and the systemic arteriolar vasodilation increase cardiac output transiently (Fig. 11–10). The magnitude of the increase in cardiac output is determined by the nature of the patient's heart disease and by the osmolality of the injected contrast agent. Because the 3.0 ratio agents increase intravascular volume less than the 1.5 ratio agents, they cause less of a change in cardiac output. The cardiac output peaks approximately 2 minutes after injection, and cardiac output usually returns to the preinjection value within 5 minutes after the injection.[H7, H8]

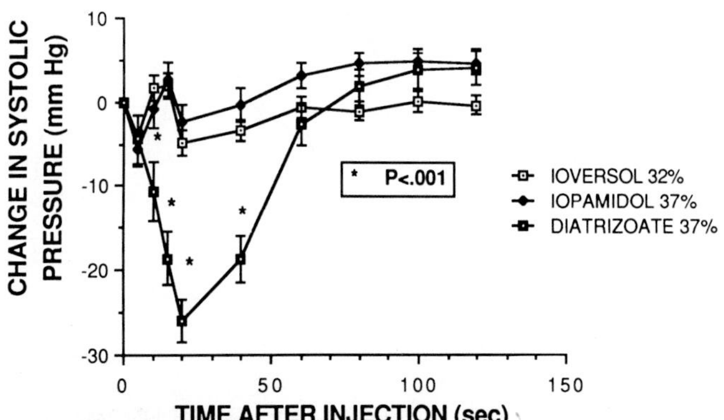

Figure 11–6. The time-related change in systemic arterial pressure following left ventriculography with 45 ml of 1.5 ratio ionic contrast agent (diatrizoate, 370 mg/ml iodine concentration) and two 3.0 ratio nonionic contrast agents (ioversol, 320 mg/ml iodine concentration, and iopamidol, 370 mg/ml iodine concentration). The magnitude of the decrease is greater with the 1.5-ratio ionic contrast agent. (From Hirshfeld, J.W., Jr., et al.: Hemodynamic and electrocardiographic effects of ioversol during cardiac angiography comparison with diatrizoate. Invest. Radiol. 24:138, 1989, with permission.)

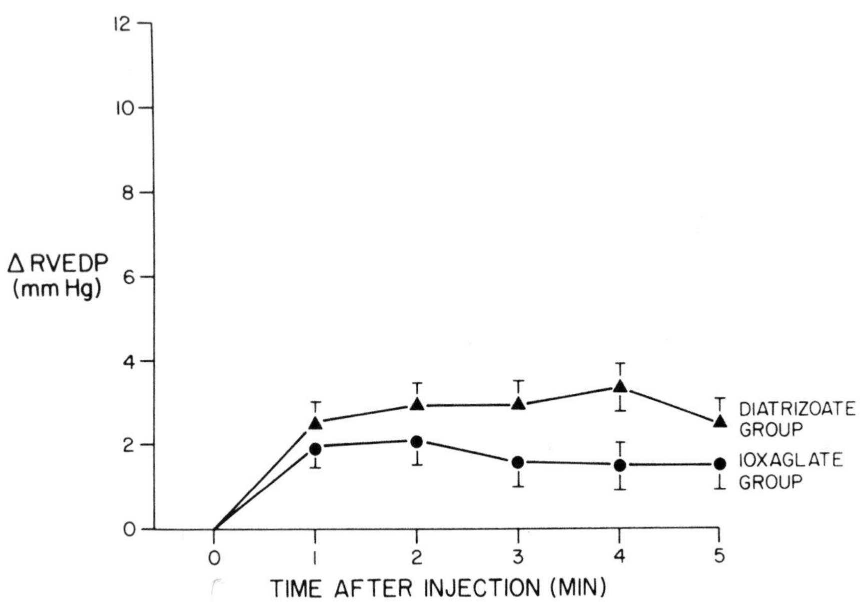

Figure 11–7. The time-related change in right ventricular end-diastolic pressure (RVEDP) after left ventriculography with 1.5 ratio ionic and 3.0 ratio ionic contrast agents. The increase caused by the 3.0 ratio agent is less than that caused by the 1.5 ratio agent. (From Hirshfeld, J.W., Jr., et al.: Hemodynamic changes induced by cardiac angiography with ioxaglate: Comparison with diatrizoate. J. Am. Coll. Cardiol. 2:954, 1983, with permission.)

Effects of Selective Intracoronary Injection

Coronary arteriography involves the selective intracoronary injection of 3 to 9 ml of contrast agent. During each injection, the blood passing through the coronary vascular bed is replaced for approximately 5 seconds with nearly undiluted contrast agent. The effects of this intervention are attributable to the properties of the contrast agent molecule and of the other constituents of the contrast agent formulation, and to the osmolality of the formulation. Most experimental studies of the response to selective intracoronary injection attempt to replicate clinical coronary arteriography. They use bolus intracoronary injections of contrast agent in volumes and durations that are comparable to those achieved in clinical coronary arteriography.

Effect on Myocardial Performance and Systemic Arterial Pressure

Investigators have noted substantial differences in the response to intracoronary injection of the different classes of clinically available contrast agents (Fig. 11–11). Injection of 1.5 ratio ionic agents transiently depresses left ventricular contractile function. A transient decrease in left ventricular peak systolic pressure occurs in association with a decrease in the maximum rate of increase of left ventricular pressure (peak dP/dt) and with an increase in left ventricular end-systolic and end-diastolic diameter. These changes are maximal 10 seconds after the onset of the injection and resolve within 45 to 60 seconds.[H4, T3] The magnitude of the evoked changes is modest (see Fig. 11–11) and of no clinical significance in an individual with normal or moderately impaired cardiac function.

Intracoronary injection of ioxaglate (a 3.0 ratio ionic agent) causes changes that are qualitatively similar but smaller in magnitude than those of the 1.5 ratio ionic agents.[H4] The response to injection of a 3.0 ratio nonionic agent is quite different, however. Instead of depressing left ventricular systolic performance, a 3.0 ratio nonionic agent actually transiently enhances contractile performance and increases left ventricular systolic shortening. This phenomenon, rather than being due to an intrinsic positive ionotropic property of the 3.0 ratio nonionic agents, is probably caused by the absence of sodium in their formulations.[K3]

These changes in myocardial contractile performance are not merely due to the transient replacement of blood by a fluid that does not transport oxygen. Injection of a solution that has a physiologic ionic composition but does not transport oxygen (such

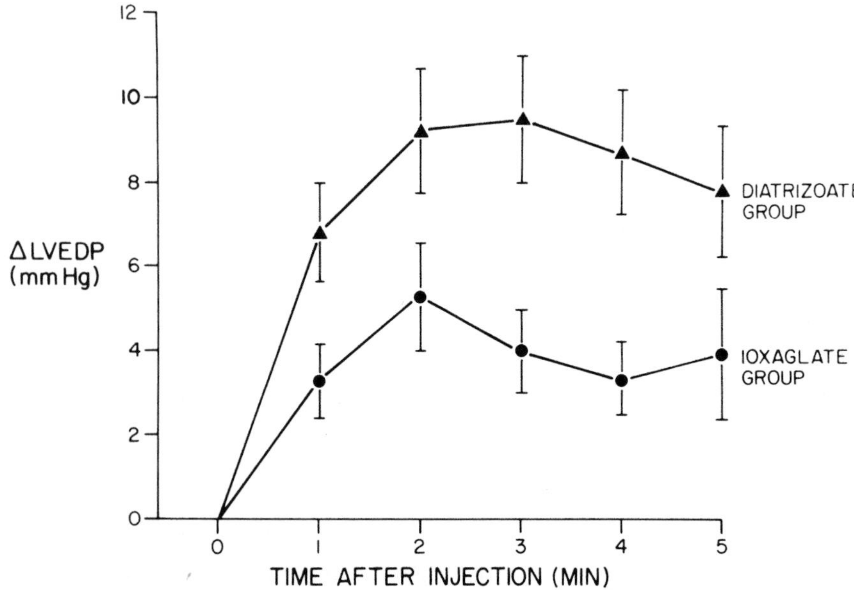

Figure 11–8. The time-related change in left ventricular end-diastolic pressure (LVEDP) after left ventriculography with 1.5 ratio ionic and 3.0 ratio ionic contrast agents. The format of this figure is identical to that of Figure 11–7. The change caused by the 1.5 ratio agent is greater. (From Hirshfeld, J.W., Jr., et al.: Hemodynamic changes induced by cardiac angiography with ioxaglate: Comparison with diatrizoate. J. Am. Coll. Cardiol. 2:954, 1983, with permission.)

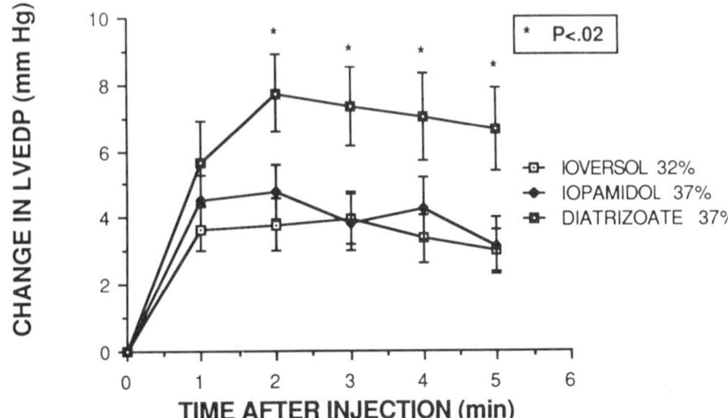

Figure 11–9. The time-related change in left ventricular end-diastolic pressure after left ventriculography with 1.5 ratio ionic and two 3.0 ratio nonionic contrast agents. The format of this figure is identical to that of Figure 11–6. The increase caused by the 1.5 ratio ionic agent is greater. (From Hirshfeld, J.W., Jr., et al.: Hemodynamic and electrocardiographic effects of ioversol during cardiac angiography comparison with diatrizoate. Invest. Radiol. 24:138, 1989, with permission.)

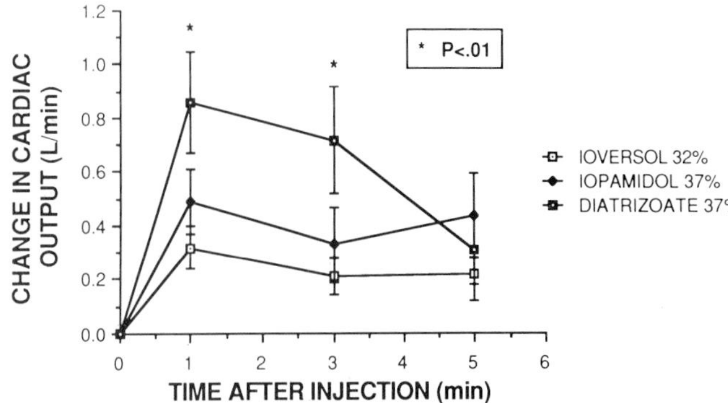

Figure 11–10. The time-related change in cardiac output after left ventriculography with a 1.5 ratio ionic and two 3.0 ratio nonionic contrast agents. The increase caused by the 1.5 ratio ionic agent is greater. (From Hirshfeld, J.W., Jr., et al.: Hemodynamic and electrocardiographic effects of ioversol during cardiac angiography comparison with diatrizoate. Invest. Radiol. 24:138, 1989, with permission.)

as Hartman's solution) produces little change in left ventricular systolic performance.[T2] Rather, the changes are attributable to actual metabolic actions of the formulations.

A major contributor to the effect on myocardial contractile performance is the calcium-binding property of the formulations of some of the 1.5 ratio ionic agents. Those with calcium-binding activity reduce the concentration of ionized calcium in the effluent from vascular beds into which the contrast agent has been injected.[C2, M2, M7] Calcium binding would be expected to decrease myocardial contractile force transiently until the contrast agent washes out of the vascular bed and normal myocardial concentrations of calcium are restored. The reduction in left ventricular contractile performance correlates temporally with the reduction in calcium ion concentration in the coronary sinus effluent (Fig. 11–12).[B7]

The magnitude of myocardial contractile depression caused by the ionic agents is related to the osmolality of the solution.[P7] The 1.5 ratio ionic agents also cause longer-lasting effects on myocardial metabolism. After injection, myocardial uptake of free fatty acids increases, and uptake of lactate and of glucose decreases. The clinical and functional significance of this observation has not been defined.[W3]

The integrated clinical consequence of all of these effects is that selective coronary arteriography with ionic 1.5 ratio agents causes a transient decrease in systemic arterial pressure, whereas injections of 3.0 ratio nonionic agents produce little or no change. The overall magnitude of the effect of any particular contrast agent on arterial pressure, however, is modest and of little clinical importance. The effect of the contrast agent itself is, in general, greatly overshadowed by the effect of the voluntary held inspiration that the patient performs during the injection (Fig. 11–13).

Cardiac Electrophysiologic Effects

Not surprisingly, contrast agents affect several cardiac electrophysiologic properties. Many contrast agent–induced adverse

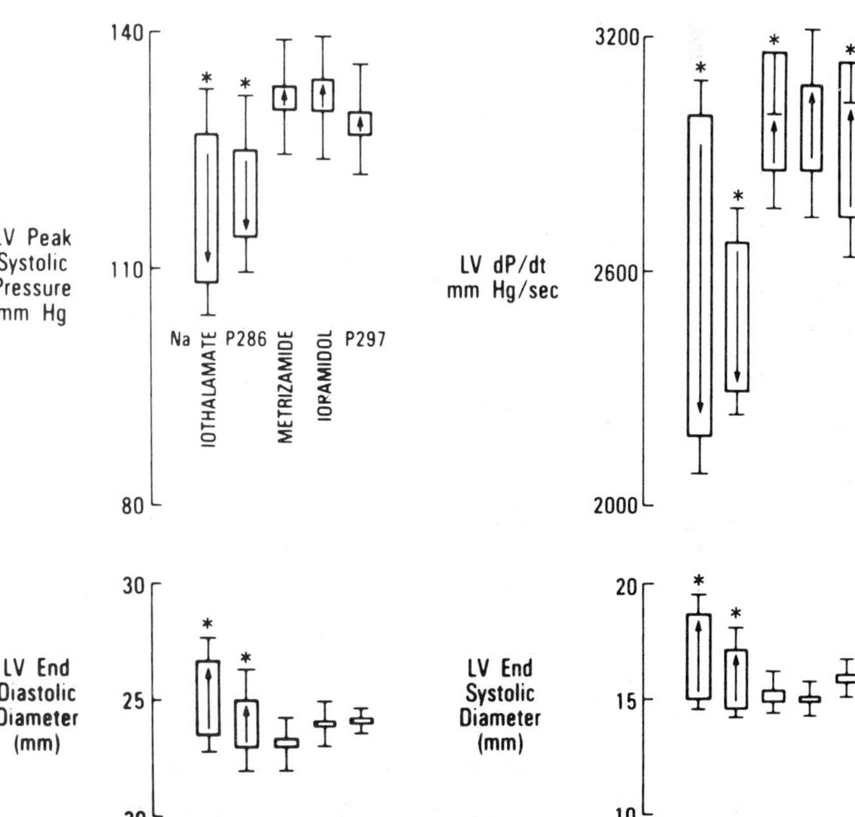

Figure 11–11. Block diagrams illustrating the effects of selective intracoronary injection of 1.5 ratio ionic (iothalamate), 3.0 ratio ionic (P-286 = ioxaglate), and 3.0 ratio nonionic contrast agents (metrizamide, iopamidol, and P-297) in volumes comparable to those used in clinical coronary arteriography. The data presented are for left ventricular peak systolic pressure, peak systolic dP/dt, and end-diastolic and end-systolic diameters. One end of each block indicates the average value and the standard error of the mean (SEM) during the control period, and the other end indicates the average value and SEM at the peak of the response. The direction of the change is indicated by the arrow in each block. The ionic agents depress left ventricular myocardial performance, whereas the nonionic agents enhance it. (From Higgins, C.B., et al.: Direct myocardial effects of intracoronary administration of new contrast materials with low osmolality. Invest. Radiol. 15:39, 1980, with permission.)

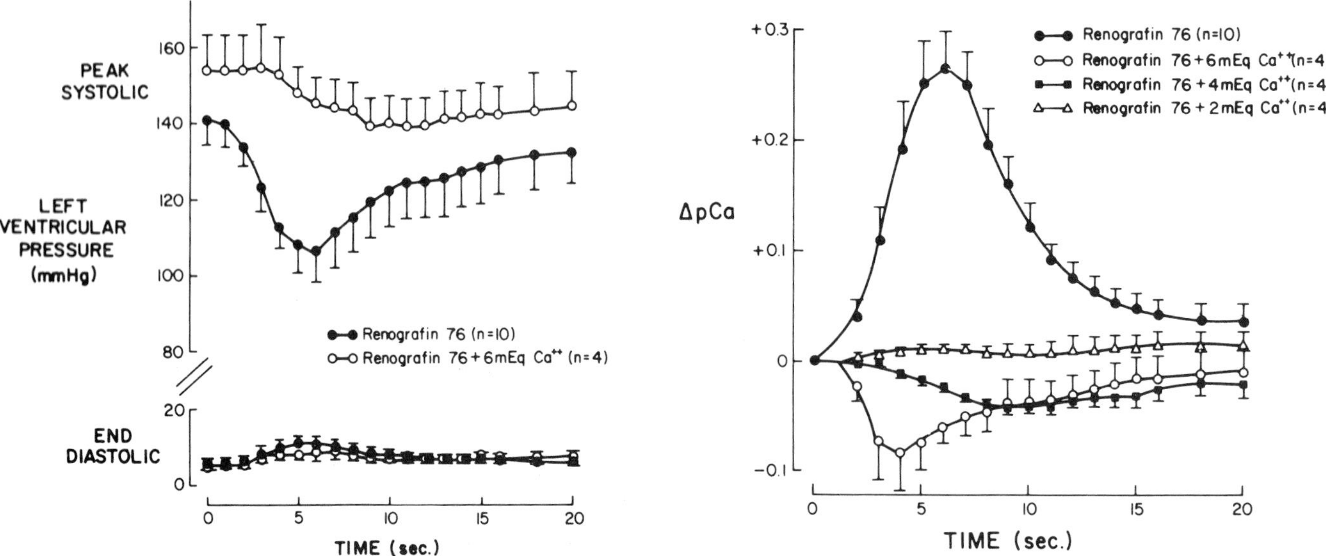

Figure 11–12. The time-related changes in left ventricular pressure *(left panel)* and the negative log of coronary sinus ionized calcium pCa *(right panel)* following selective left coronary injection of Renografin-76 with and without calcium enrichment. (An increase in pCa represents a decrease in calcium ion concentration.) Note that calcium enrichment increases coronary sinus calcium ion concentration and attenuates the contrast agent–induced depression of myocardial contractile performance. (From Boundillion, P.D., et al.: Effects of a new nonionic and a conventional ionic contrast agent on coronary sinus ionized calcium and left ventricular hemodynamics in dogs. J. Am. Coll. Cardiol. 6:845, 1985. Reprinted with permission from the American College of Cardiology.)

reactions are due to alterations in these properties. Indeed, until Sones serendipitously observed that inadvertent selective coronary injection of a diatrizoate contrast agent did not cause cardiac arrest, the prevailing belief was that the heart would not tolerate selective coronary arteriography.

The cardiac electrophysiologic effects of contrast agents may be divided into those of impulse formation and conduction, repolarization, and arrhythmias.

Impulse Formation and Conduction

A transient reduction in sinus heart rate accompanies selective coronary injection of 1.5 ratio ionic contrast agents. Typically, the reduction in heart rate is greatest 10 to 15 seconds after injection, and the heart rate returns to baseline values within 30 seconds (Fig. 11–14). The degree of slowing evoked by right coronary injection is greater than that caused by left coronary

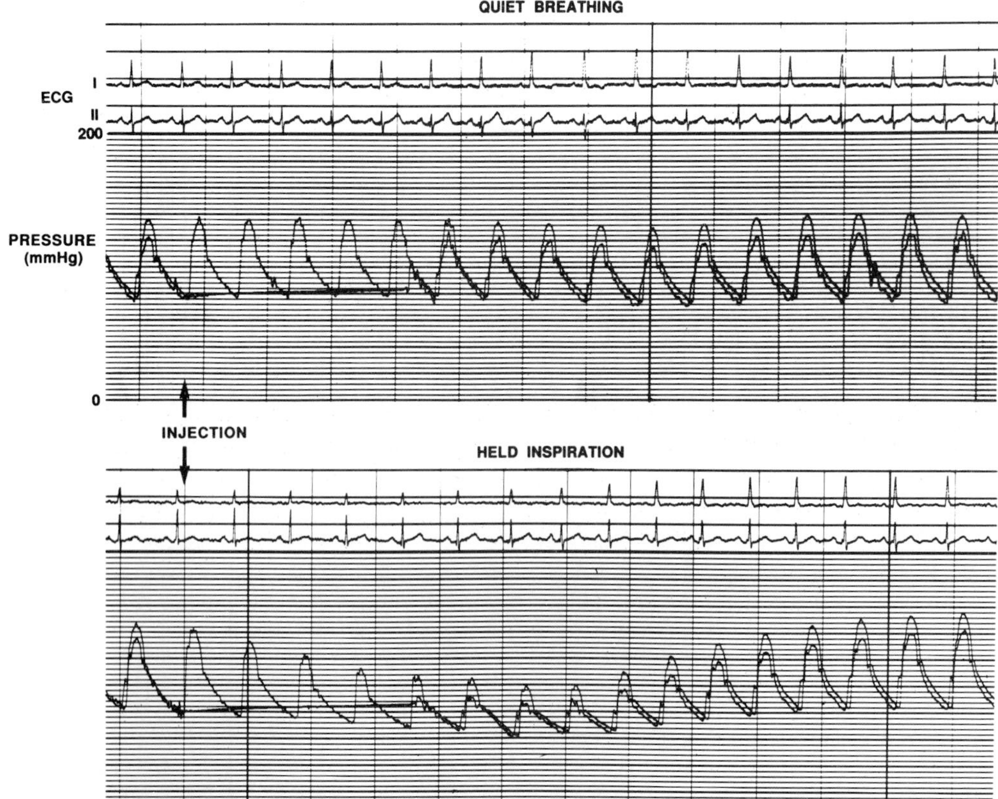

Figure 11–13. Comparison of the time-related change in arterial pressure during clinical coronary arteriography with a 1.5 ratio ionic contrast agent during quiet breathing and during the customary held inspiration. The majority of the decrease in arterial pressure is caused by the hemodynamic effect of breath holding.

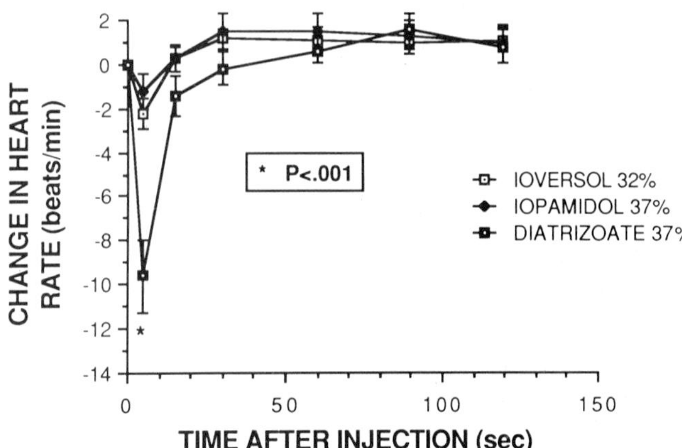

Figure 11–14. The time-related change in heart rate after left coronary arteriography with 1.5 ratio ionic and two 3.0 ratio nonionic contrast agents. The decrease caused by the 1.5 ratio ionic agent is greater. (From Hirshfeld, J.W., Jr., et al.: Hemodynamic and electrocardiographic effects of ioversol during cardiac angiography comparison with diatrizoate. Invest. Radiol. 19:563, 1984, with permission.)

injection, presumably because the arterial supply to the sinoatrial and atrioventricular nodes is most commonly derived from the right coronary artery.[M1] Because bradycardia also follows selective left coronary injection, however, the mechanism is clearly more complex than simply a direct effect on the sinoatrial node. The response may be evoked by superselective infusion of contrast agents into the sinoatrial nodal artery. It is attenuated but not abolished by pharmacologic autonomic blockade.[H2] On the other hand, the bradycardia caused by injection into an artery that does not supply the sinoatrial node is completely blocked by atropine.[F3] These observations show that the bradycardia is due to a combination of a direct depression of impulse formation in the sinoatrial node and an autonomically mediated reflex. The degree of slowing caused by 3.0 ratio nonionic and ionic agents is less than that evoked by 1.5 ratio ionic agents.[P3, S8]

In general, this slowing is of little clinical significance because it may be minimized by proper operator technique. The slowing may be more pronounced if the impulse-forming cells are allowed to remain in contact with the contrast agent for too long. Such circumstances occur when duration of the injection is excessive, when the injection is made after a period of obstruction of coronary flow by a catheter tip wedged in the coronary orifice, or when a wedged catheter tip is not promptly removed from a coronary orifice to allow washout of the contrast agent.[W9]

Selective intracoronary injection of contrast agents also prolongs atrioventricular conduction by slowing conduction through the atrioventricular node without affecting infranodal conduction.[N1] In contrast to the effect on the sinoatrial node, the effect on the atrioventricular node has no autonomic component, and the degree of impairment of its conduction is not influenced by pharmacologic autonomic blockade.[H2] The degree of impairment of atrioventricular nodal conduction evoked by 3.0 ratio nonionic agents is less than that evoked by 1.5 ratio ionic agents.[H2]

Repolarization

Prolongation of ventricular myocardial repolarization occurs in response to selective intracoronary injection of all contrast agents and is reflected in a prolongation of the Q-T interval on the body surface electrocardiogram.[S2] This effect is the result of three properties of a contrast agent formulation, which combine to delay repolarization. These properties are:

1. The specific contrast agent molecule
2. The osmolality of the contrast agent formulation
3. The ionic composition (including calcium-binding properties) of the contrast agent formulation

The 1.5 ratio ionic agents evoke a greater prolongation of the Q-T interval than either the 3.0 ratio ionic agent (which is intermediate) or the 3.0 ratio nonionic agents (which prolong it the least).[B5, H7, T5, W2, W11] The maximum prolongation of the Q-T interval after selective intracoronary injection of a 3.0 ratio nonionic agent is approximately 20 msec, as opposed to 30 msec for the 3.0 ratio ionic agent. The prolongation evoked by 1.5 ratio ionic agents, however, not only is considerably greater, but varies substantially in relation to the calcium-binding properties of the different formulations. Formulations that are not enriched with calcium, such as MD-76 and Renografin 76, prolong the Q-T interval by as much as 160 msec. On the other hand, calcium-enriched formulations such as Angiovist and Hypaque-76 prolong the Q-T interval by only 50 msec,[W5] a longer duration than that of the nonionic 3.0 ratio agents, but similar to that of the 3.0 ratio ionic agent (Fig. 11–15).

Ventricular Fibrillation Threshold

Ventricular fibrillation is a dramatic adverse reaction to selective coronary arteriography. It occurs as a consequence of both the inherent properties of the contrast agent and the operator technique.

All contrast agents decrease the heart's resistance to ventricular fibrillation as measured by the ventricular fibrillation threshold (the square-wave current required to induce ventricular fibrillation); this effect occurs for approximately 60 seconds after selective coronary injection (Fig. 11–16). The degree of reduction of ventricular fibrillation threshold by contrast agents is influenced by the quantity of contrast agent injected, the duration of injection, and the properties and formulation of the particular contrast agent molecule.[W9] The ventricular fibrillation threshold is also reduced by myocardial ischemia.[L3] The combination of ischemia and contrast agent injection reduces the threshold even further.[W9] Both the 3.0 ratio nonionic agents and the 3.0 ratio ionic agent cause less reduction of ventricular fibrillation threshold than do the 1.5 ratio ionic agents.[W7]

Also, significant differences among the ionic compositions of the different formulations of the 1.5 ratio ionic agents affect their fibrillatory propensity. These differences are in the content of two important ions—sodium and calcium.

Early experience with coronary angiography, in which ionic diatrizoate-based contrast agents were used, involved considerable work to determine the optimal composition of the cationic component of the agent. If sodium was used to fill the entire cation space, the resulting agent would have a sodium concentration of 1000 mEq/L, a concentration that would certainly have detrimental electrophysiologic effects when injected selectively into the coronary arteries. Consequently, a portion of the cation space was filled with methylglucamine, a cation that is not electrophysiologically active. Reducing the sodium concentration below 118 mEq/L, however, was found to increase the fibrillatory propensity of an ionic contrast agent formulation.[A4] A sodium concentration between 150 and 190 mEq/L was found to cause the least ventricular fibrillation in experimental and clinical studies.[H6, P5, S5, S7] Thus, although diatrizoate is marketed in many formulations with different sodium concentrations, the formulations that are appropriate for use in coronary arteriography have a sodium concentration between 160 and 190 mEq/L.

The other important property of a contrast agent formulation that influences its electrophysiologic activity is its calcium-binding activity. The formulations of all contrast agents contain ethylenediaminetetra-acetic acid (EDTA) as a chelating agent to sequester any trace quantities of heavy metal contaminants left in the preparation from manufacturing. EDTA is an avid calcium chelator. In two of the diatrizoate preparations (Angiovist and Hypaque-76), the EDTA is enriched with calcium to reduce its calcium-binding potential. In the other two preparations (MD-76 and Renografin-76), the EDTA is not calcium-enriched, and in addition, sodium citrate (another calcium chelating agent) is added to the formulation. Thus, the latter two formulations have considerably greater calcium-binding activity than the former two.

The difference between the calcium-enriched and the calcium-binding formulations is clearly detectable clinically and is probably clinically important. Hypocalcemia delays ventricular repo-

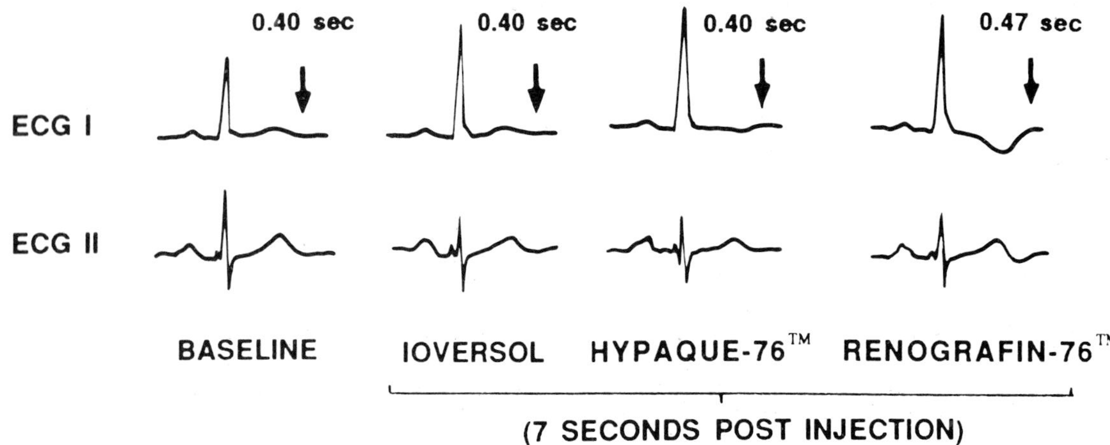

Figure 11–15. A comparison of the electrocardiographic changes caused by left coronary arteriography with 1.5 ratio ionic contrast agents with (Renografin-76) and without (Hypaque-76) calcium-binding activity and a 3.0 ratio nonionic agent (ioversol). Representative complexes from ECG leads I and II are shown. The pre-injection complexes are shown on the left. The corresponding complexes recorded at the peak effect (7 seconds after injection) are shown to the right. The changes are most marked after the injection of a calcium-binding 1.5 ratio ionic contrast agent.

larization, which prolongs the Q-T interval. Also, because myocardial contractile force depends on calcium-mediated actin-myosin interaction, hypocalcemia can reduce myocardial contractile force. Ionic contrast agent formulations with calcium-binding activity cause a greater prolongation of the Q-T interval than do otherwise identical formulations that do not bind calcium (see Fig. 11–15).[W5] In addition, they cause a greater decrease in arterial pressure following intracoronary injection (Fig. 11–17; see Fig. 11–12).

In 1978, Thompson and colleagues, and Violante and associates, showed that the frequency of ventricular fibrillation caused by experimental intracoronary injection of Renografin-76 in dogs was reduced by the addition of calcium ions.[T3, V1] Subsequently, Wolf found that the reduction in ventricular fibrillation threshold caused by Renografin-76 was attenuated by the addition of 5 mEq/L calcium chloride.[W9] Wolf and colleagues also found that under identical experimental conditions, Hypaque-76 caused less reduction in ventricular fibrillation threshold than did Renografin-76.[W6] In subsequent clinical studies, investigators have observed a reduction in the frequency of episodes of ventricular fibrillation during clinical coronary arteriography, from 0.5 to 2.4 percent in patients studied with Renografin-76 to zero to 0.1 percent in patients studied with Angiovist—a non–calcium-binding diatrizoate agent.[B1, M8, Z1]

The 3.0 ratio nonionic agents and the 3.0 ratio ionic agent have been shown experimentally to have less fibrillatory propensity than calcium-binding formulations of 1.5 ratio ionic agents.[W9] Differences in fibrillatory propensity between the 3.0 ratio agents and the non–calcium-binding formulations of 1.5 ratio ionic agents have not been demonstrated, however.

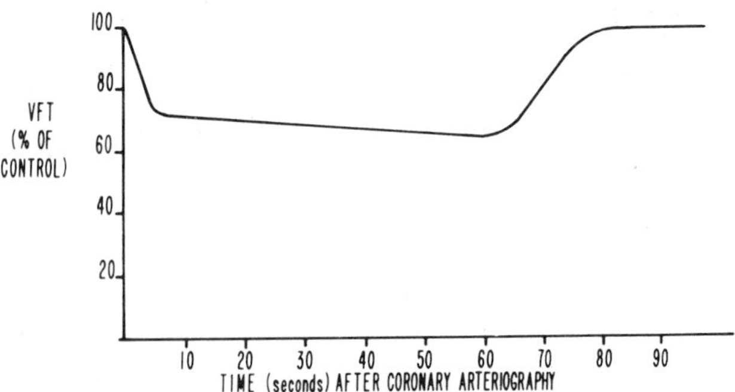

Figure 11–16. The time-related change in ventricular fibrillation threshold after left coronary injection of a 1.5 ratio ionic contrast agent. The curve is a smoothed compilation of many determinations. The heart's vulnerability to ventricular fibrillation increases after injection. The increased vulnerability persists for nearly a minute after injection. (From Wolf, G.L.: The fibrillatory properties of contrast agents. Invest. Radiol. 15:S208, 1980, with permission.)

Because ventricular fibrillation is such a rare event in cardiac angiography,[D4, K2, M8] demonstration of a statistically significant difference in the frequency of ventricular fibrillation between two contrast agents would require a large study population (greater than 1000 patients per group). One study compared the frequency of ventricular fibrillation in patients randomized to receive either Renografin-76 or iopamidol during coronary angioplasty (a circumstance in which myocardial ischemia is often provoked). In this study, the Renografin-76 group had a 2.3 percent frequency of ventricular fibrillation, while the iopamidol group had a 0.7 percent frequency.[L4] If a non–calcium-binding formulation of diatrizoate had been used instead of Renografin-76, the frequency of ventricular fibrillation in the diatrizoate group would probably have been lower. Because the frequency of ventricular fibrillation caused by non–calcium-binding formulations of 1.5 ratio agents is so low in clinical use, the 3.0 ratio agents would be unlikely to offer any clinically significant advantage regarding arrhythmia generation.

Other Noncardiovascular Effects

Most studies of the noncardiovascular effects of angiographic contrast agents have been performed using intravenous injections for other radiographic procedures such as intravenous urography and computed tomography. Thus, they may not be strictly comparable to circumstances occurring in cardiac angiography. Nevertheless, they do provide some useful information concerning other effects of these agents.

Immediate Generalized or Anaphylactoid Reaction

The immediate generalized reaction has been termed the *anaphylactoid reaction* because it mimics gamma E immunoglobulin (IgE)–mediated anaphylaxis. This reaction is perhaps the most feared of all reactions because it can be life-threatening. The fully developed reaction is caused by the release of large quantities of histamine. It typically occurs following the initial injection of contrast agent and is not related to the volume of contrast agent injected. Such reactions include varying severities of urticaria, angioedema (including laryngeal edema), bronchospasm, vasodilation, and increased capillary permeability. Severe immediate generalized reactions can produce life-threatening circulatory collapse or airway obstruction.

These reactions do not appear to be immunologically mediated. No IgE antibody to any contrast agent has ever been identified, and the reactions can occur during a patient's initial exposure to a contrast agent.[G6] The final common pathway of the immediate generalized reaction is the activation of the complement pathway

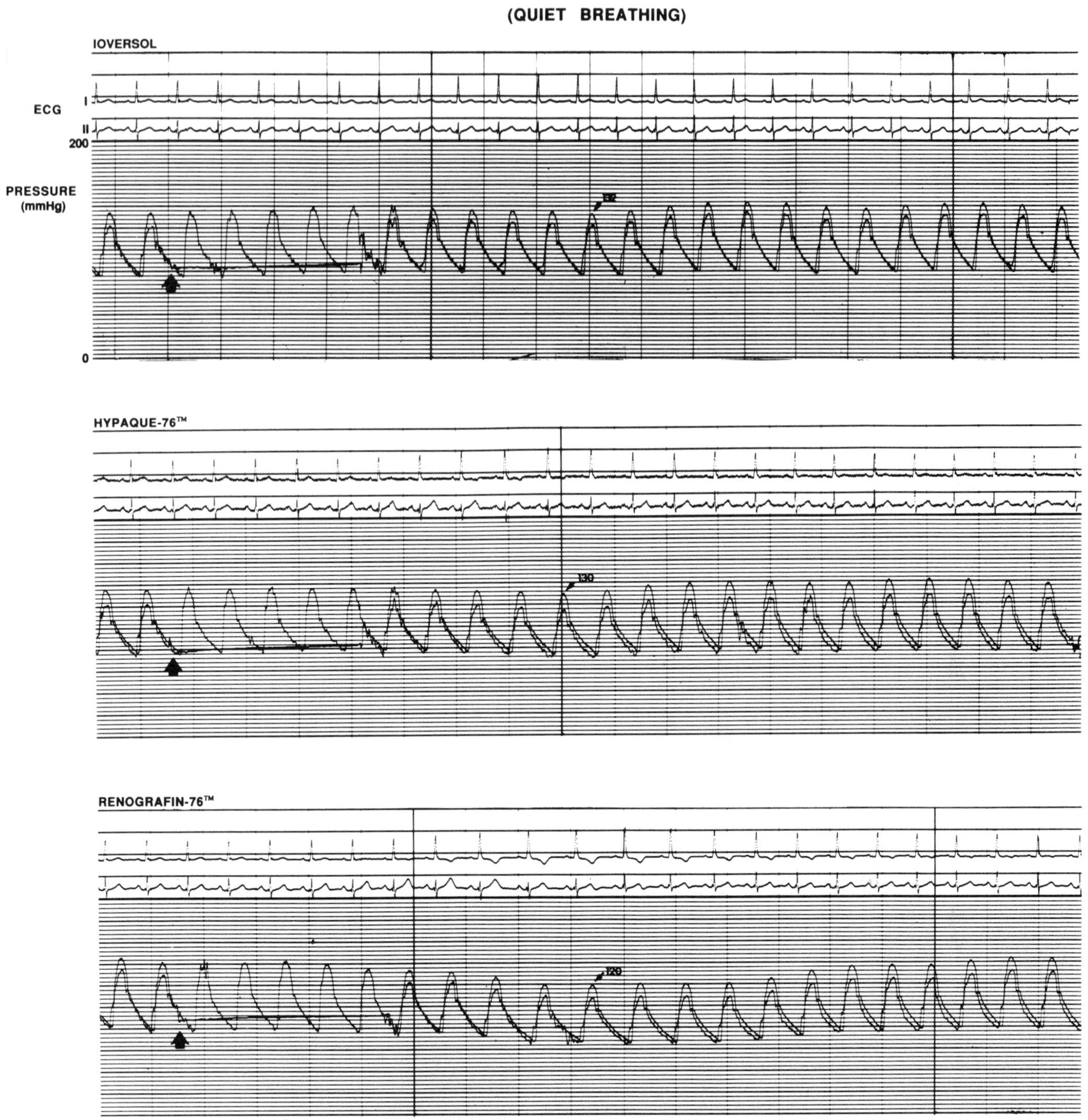

Figure 11–17. The time-related changes in systolic arterial pressure and electrocardiography caused by left coronary arteriography with 1.5 ratio ionic contrast agents with (Renografin-76) and without (Hypaque-76) calcium-binding activity and a 3.0 ratio nonionic agent (ioversol). The recordings were made during quiet breathing to isolate the effect of the contrast agent. Note that the decrease in arterial pressure is greatest with the calcium-binding 1.5 ratio ionic agent and is least with the nonionic agent.

leading to mast cell degranulation. The mechanism by which the reaction is initiated is not known.[G5]

The frequency of all immediate generalized reactions (including minor urticaria) to 1.5 ratio ionic agents is approximately 5 percent.[G4] The frequency of life-threatening immediate generalized reactions to 1.5 ratio ionic agents is approximately 0.1 percent.[S4] No diagnostic test is available to detect patients at risk of an immediate generalized reaction.

The severe immediate generalized reaction has long been known to occur after injection of 1.5 ratio ionic agents. Severe immediate generalized reactions to 3.0 ratio nonionic agents have also been reported.[G5] Investigators believe, but have not yet proved, that the frequency of *severe* immediate generalized reactions to 3.0 ratio nonionic contrast agents is less than the frequency of such severe reactions to 1.5 ratio ionic agents. Data that support this idea include a reduced overall fatality rate following contrast agent exposure[B3] and a small frequency of repeat reactions when 3.0 ratio nonionic agents are used in patients who have previously had an immediate generalized reaction to 1.5 ratio ionic agents.[H9, L1] Also, the frequency of cutaneous reactions to the 3.0 ratio nonionic contrast agents is less than the frequency of such reactions to the 1.5 ratio agents.

The conclusion that the frequency of severe immediate generalized reactions to the 3.0 ratio nonionic agents is reduced must be drawn with caution, however, because the frequency of *repeat* immediate generalized reactions to contrast agents is small (approximately 15 percent).[S3, S4]

On the other hand, Lasser and associates have reported that pretreatment with two doses of 32 mg methylprednisolone, 12 hours and 2 hours prior to contrast agent administration, causes a substantial reduction in the frequency of all adverse reactions to 1.5 ratio ionic contrast agents (9.5 to 6.4 percent), including severe, life-threatening reactions (0.7 to 0.2 percent).[L2] Investigators have not compared the clinical efficacy of corticosteroid pretreatment with that of substitution of a 3.0 ratio nonionic contrast agent for prevention of immediate generalized reactions in patients who have had a previous reaction.

Effects on Renal Function

Renal excretion is essentially the sole means of elimination of contrast agents. The quantity of contrast agent molecule administered is often quite large—over 100 g. This material functions as an osmotic diuretic and probably also causes transient mild renal dysfunction. This dysfunction is not detectable with routine screening tests in individuals with normal renal function because it is obscured by reserve capacity. In individuals with pre-existing renal disease, diabetes mellitus, or reduced cardiac output, however, the risk and severity of renal injury increase substantially.[C3, D1, P8]

Clinically important renal failure is extremely rare in patients who undergo cardiac angiography with 1.5 ratio ionic agents, who have no diabetes or pre-existing renal disease, and who receive a total contrast agent dose less than 125 ml. On the other hand, patients with the combination of pre-existing renal insufficiency and low cardiac output, or pre-existing renal insufficiency and diabetes mellitus, have approximately a 40 percent chance of developing a detectable increase in serum creatinine after exposure to 1.5 ratio ionic contrast agents. In less than 10 percent of those high-risk patients who develop measurable changes in renal function, however, is the renal failure severe enough to require dialysis.[T1]

The mechanism of contrast agent–induced renal injury is probably a combination of medullary ischemia, which is due to vasoconstriction caused by the contrast agent, and a direct toxic effect of high concentrations of contrast agent on renal tubular cells.[S1] Currently, no information is available to distinguish between 1.5 ratio ionic agents and 3.0 ratio agents in terms of the hazard of renal injury. The comparative studies that have been reported have shown no difference between the two classes of contrast agents, in terms of either measurable changes in renal function following contrast agent exposure or clinically important renal injury.[H1] This lack of data may result from inadequate statistical power. At present, this question is being examined in trials of greater statistical power.

Investigators believe that the frequency and severity of contrast agent–induced renal injury can be minimized in susceptible patients by careful attention to maintenance of optimal hydration and cardiac output, concurrent furosemide diuresis, and, perhaps, concurrent administration of mannitol.[M5]

The frequency of contrast agent–induced renal failure seems to have decreased in recent years. Parfrey and associates recently reported an experience of administering large volumes of contrast agent (both 1.5 ratio and 3.0 ratio agents) to 135 patients with renal insufficiency. The patients had serum creatinine levels between 2 and 5 mg per 100 ml, and some had coexisting diabetes. The frequency of clinically significant renal injury (defined as an increase in serum creatinine greater than 50 percent) was 7 percent, whereas a comparable control group of hospitalized patients who did not receive contrast agents exhibited a 1.5 percent frequency of deterioration of renal function.[P2] No difference in the frequency of renal injury was observed between patients studied with 1.5 ratio agents and those studied with 3.0 ratio agents. The average volume of contrast agent administered was 110 ml. Such experience suggests that careful attention to the patient's hydrational status and limitation of the quantity of contrast agent administered enhance the safety of the use of both 1.5 and 3.0 ratio contrast agents in patients with previously existing renal disease.

Effects on Pulmonary Function

All contrast agents affect airway dynamics, causing a decrease in the 1-second forced expiratory volume.[L6] In healthy individuals, this change is modest (0.21 L/sec or 7.5 percent) and is not clinically apparent unless direct measurements are made. In patients with underlying airway obstruction such as asthma, however, the decrease could be clinically significant. The decrease in 1-second forced expiratory volume caused by the 3.0 ratio nonionic agents (0.03 L/sec or 0.8 percent) is less than that caused by the 1.5 ratio ionic agents.[D2]

Coughing frequently accompanies injections of contrast agents into the right side of the heart and into the pulmonary artery. Not only is this side effect unpleasant for the patient, but it can also compromise the quality of the examination. Presumably, the coughing results from irritation of the lungs by the contrast agent as it passes through the pulmonary microcirculation. It occurs in two thirds of studies with 1.5 ratio agents. In one study comparing 1.5 ratio agents with ioxaglate, the frequency of cough evoked by ioxaglate during selective pulmonary angiography was only 0.4 percent.[S6]

Gastrointestinal Effects

The most frequent adverse reactions to 1.5 ratio ionic contrast agents are nausea and vomiting, which occur in 10 to 20 percent of patients. This response typically occurs only during the first injection of contrast agent and does not recur with subsequent injections. The frequency of nausea is somewhat less with the 3.0 ratio ionic agent[H8] and is virtually eliminated by the 3.0 ratio nonionic agents.[G2, P6, W2]

Hematologic Effects

Contrast agents have several measurable effects on blood cells and blood coagulation that are of potential clinical importance.

In clinically used concentrations, all contrast agent molecules cause red blood cell deformation. This deformation occurs both through a direct toxic effect on the cell membrane, which produces a crenated "echinocyte,"[B9] and through osmotic extraction of water from the interior of the red cell, which produces a "desiccocyte."[N2] Of the two effects, the osmotic effect is more important; as a result, the effect of the 3.0 ratio agents is less than the effect of the 1.5 ratio ionic agents.[A6] Although such actions can potentially affect blood viscosity and the rheology of flow through the microcirculation, the clinical significance of these effects has not been established. Nor has the clinical importance of the measurable differences between the 1.5 ratio agents and the 3.0 ratio agents been established.

All intravascular contrast agents have inherent anticoagulant properties. If blood is mixed with clinically used concentrations of contrast agents, its clotting time is markedly prolonged. The magnitude of this effect is greatest for the 1.5 ratio ionic agents, particularly for those containing citrate in their formulations, and for ioxaglate, the 3.0 ratio ionic agent. (Both citrate and ioxaglate prolong the whole blood clotting time from 15 minutes to more than 330 minutes.) The 3.0 ratio nonionic agents also prolong the clotting time, but to a lesser degree (from 15 minutes to 160 minutes).[E1, R1]

This property of contrast agents has provided a margin of safety that could partially compensate for inadequacies in technique, such as allowing blood to mingle with contrast agent in catheters and syringes. Clearly, the reduced anticoagulant effect of the nonionic 3.0 ratio agents provides less margin for safety in this regard. Several reports of thrombus formation and embolization during use of nonionic contrast agents have appeared.[G7, R4] These differences should be clinically unimportant, however, if operators adhere to proper technique. Systemic heparinization, which is employed in many cardiac angiographic studies, should further reduce the risk of thrombus formation. Arterial embolization has occurred, however, during coronary angiography in heparinized patients studied with 3.0 ratio nonionic agents.[G7]

Effects on Blood Vessels

All contrast agents exert toxic effects on endothelium. Ultrastructural changes are visible in the aortic endothelium for up to 4 hours after the 1-ml/kg intravenous injection of 1.5 ratio agents having an iodine concentration of 370 mg/ml.[P4] The significance of these observations has not been determined, however. Similar evidence of endothelial damage by contrast agents has been derived from silver staining studies of the aorta after contrast agent exposure.[N4] This damage appears to be predominantly an osmotically mediated effect, with the effects of the 1.5 ratio ionic agents being most pronounced and the effects of the 3.0 ratio ionic and nonionic agents being equivalent to each other and less than those of the 1.5 ratio ionic agents. The significance of these observations for cardiac angiography is also undetermined. The silver staining studies involve 5-minute applications of undiluted contrast agent to isolated aorta, a condition considerably harsher than that occurring in arterial and cardiac angiography in vivo. These observations may be relevant for phlebography, in which undiluted contrast agent remains in contact with the veins for a longer period of time.

CRITERIA FOR SELECTION OF CONTRAST AGENTS FOR CARDIAC ANGIOGRAPHY

The creation of the 3.0 ratio contrast agents has presented cardiac angiographers with both an opportunity and a dilemma. The opportunity derives from the clear-cut hemodynamic and electrophysiologic superiority and from the reduced adverse reaction rate offered by the low-osmolality agents. The dilemma derives from the substantial disparity in price between the 1.5 ratio agents and the 3.0 ratio agents. In the United States, the price disparity varies between 12- and 25-fold, depending on locally negotiated prices. (In Europe, the price disparity is smaller, because 1.5 ratio agents are more expensive than in the United States, and the 3.0 ratio agents are cheaper.) The problem is particularly magnified in cardiac angiography because of the large volumes of contrast agent used in a typical procedure. The price disparity compels physicians to consider the clinical importance of the superior properties of the 3.0 ratio agents and to confront the issue of assigning a monetary value to the difference.

A priori, one would expect that the superior hemodynamic and cardiac electrophysiologic properties of the 3.0 ratio agents would render them safer and, as a consequence, more efficacious than the 1.5 ratio ionic agents. This assumption appears to be correct, but the increment of safety offered by the 3.0 ratio agents appears to be modest and not pragmatically relevant in all classes of patients.

Two large trials have recently been published that support the concept of decreased adverse reaction rates with 3.0 ratio nonionic agents; however, these trials were not blinded or randomized, and they involved predominantly intravenous administration in noncardiac procedures. In Japan, 119,621 procedures were evaluated. Of these, 77,040 procedures were performed with 1.5 ratio agents, which resulted in a "severe" adverse reaction frequency of 0.45 percent and one death. In the 42,581 procedures performed with 3.0 ratio agents, a 0.10 percent frequency of severe adverse reactions and one death resulted.[K1] In Australia, 61,000 procedures were evaluated. Of these, 46,262 procedures were performed with 1.5 ratio ionic agents, resulting in a severe adverse reaction rate of 0.10 percent and two deaths. The 3.0 ratio nonionic agents were used in 14,738 procedures, which resulted in a severe adverse reaction rate of 0.01 percent and no deaths.[P1] The differences in overall frequencies of severe adverse reactions between the two studies probably reflect differences in definitions. Nevertheless, in both studies, the lower rates of severe adverse reactions in procedures performed with 3.0 ratio nonionic agents are statistically significant. The fatality rates are so low in both studies, however, that no statistically significant difference between the two classes of agents is detectable.

In a study of the adverse reactions to contrast agent administration, Wolf and colleagues surveyed a large group of patients who had received either 1.5 ratio ionic agents or 3.0 ratio nonionic agents for intravenous examinations.[W4] They observed the expected differences in the frequency of minor adverse reactions (2.5 percent in the 1.5 ratio ionic agent group and 0.6 percent in the 3.0 ratio nonionic agent group) and in the frequency of reactions requiring treatment (1.3 percent in the 1.5 ratio ionic agent group and 0.2 percent in the 3.0 ratio nonionic agent group). No deaths were reported in more than 13,000 examinations, which were equally divided between the two classes of contrast agents. The authors of the study also observed a slightly greater frequency of aftereffects in patients who received the 1.5 ratio ionic agents. Forty percent of patients who received a 1.5 ratio agent reported not feeling completely well for at least 24 hours after the study. In contrast, 32 percent of patients who received a 3.0 ratio nonionic agent reported such aftereffects.[W4] Thus, the frequency of aftereffects caused by the 3.0 ratio nonionic agents is modestly lower than the frequency of aftereffects caused by the 1.5 ratio ionic agents.

The magnitude of the financial impact of the choice between 1.5 and 3.0 ratio agents is substantial—at the levels of both the individual laboratory and society. If a laboratory were to switch completely from 1.5 ratio to 3.0 ratio agents, the increment in expense would most likely exceed the laboratory's total expense for technical personnel. The aggregate increment in expense over 2 years for a moderately large-volume laboratory (performing 2000 procedures per year) would be equivalent to the price of a complete cineradiographic x-ray unit.

At the societal level, Jacobson and Rosenquist estimate that universal adoption of 3.0 ratio contrast agents for all radiologic examinations requiring intravascular contrast agents would cost the United States health care system $1.1 billion.[J1] This calculation includes the incremental saving derived from the reduced cost of treating the expected smaller number of severe contrast agent reactions that would occur if only 3.0 ratio agents were used. The authors calculate that the universal use of 3.0 ratio contrast agents in the United States would avert 293 contrast agent–related fatalities per year, at a cost of $3.4 million per death averted or $106,000 per year of life saved. This monetary value is large compared with prices that society is willing to pay for other life-prolonging procedures.[J1]

The problem of selecting the most appropriate contrast agent has stimulated considerable debate. Some individuals believe that the benefits of the 3.0 ratio agents outweigh their financial cost and that, accordingly, they should be universally adopted.[W8] Others feel that the 3.0 agents should be reserved for certain subsets of patients, but they have difficulty identifying criteria for separating high-risk from low-risk patients.[F1, W1]

The issue is brought to a particular focus in cardiac angiography, an expensive, widely used procedure that requires large volumes of contrast agent and is performed in patients with severe heart disease—the type of patient who might benefit the most from the advantages of 3.0 ratio agents. On the other hand, cardiac angiography is carried out in a highly controlled and monitored environment and is performed by physicians who are specifically trained to recognize and treat cardiovascular problems.

Accumulated experience shows that cardiac angiography performed with 1.5 ratio contrast agents can have an excellent safety record in terms of clinically important outcome. In a study of cardiac angiography involving 4630 procedures, using 1.5 ratio agents, the overall frequency of minor adverse reactions to contrast agents was 14 percent, and the frequency of major adverse reactions was 1.3 percent.[D4] The frequency of major adverse reactions increased with increasing severity of heart disease (Fig. 11–18). In this study, however, no deaths resulted, and all of the major adverse reactions were successfully managed without any sequelae. Nevertheless, 6 percent of the procedures were abbreviated either because of an adverse reaction or because of concern that the patient could not tolerate further contrast agent injections.

These data indicate that physicians achieve safety in cardiac angiography with 1.5 ratio agents by tailoring the procedure to the patient's condition. Because some of the studies were abbreviated in the interest of patient safety, 0.8 percent of all studies yielded partially inadequate diagnostic data.[D4] Possibly, in certain patients, the superior properties of the 3.0 ratio agents might allow the safe performance of a more complete examination than can be performed with a 1.5 ratio agent. The use of a 3.0 ratio agent would be clearly justified in this circumstance. In almost all patients, however, a diagnostically complete study can be obtained safely, without adverse reactions, with a 1.5 ratio agent.

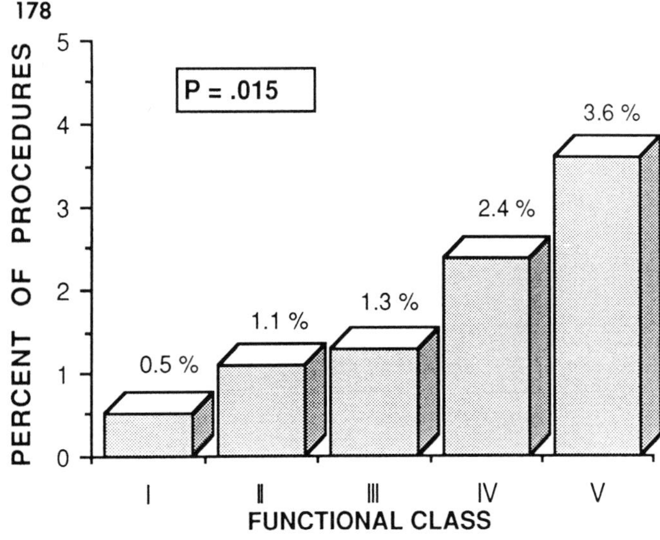

Figure 11–18. The relationship of the frequency of major contrast agent–related adverse reactions during cardiac angiography to New York Heart Association clinical functional class. (Class V represents patients who were in extreme circulatory failure at the time of the procedure.) Note that the frequency of adverse reactions is increased in the more seriously ill patients. (From DiBattiste, P.M., et al.: The safety of cardiac angiography with conventional contrast agents. Circulation 78(Suppl. II):II-377, 1988, by permission of the American Heart Association, Inc.)

Despite the current lack of rigorous data to guide the choice of the most appropriate contrast agent, physicians performing cardiac angiography must make reasonable decisions based on the information currently available. The most reasonable approach appears to be one in which the physician recognizes that certain "high-risk" patients probably derive clinically important benefit from the superior pharmacologic properties of the 3.0 ratio agents, whereas other patients can be safely and effectively studied with 1.5 ratio agents.

A framework for identifying patients who may benefit from the use of 3.0 ratio agents is outlined in Table 11–4. The documentation of the validity of the indication (if available) is also listed in the table.

Indications for the use of 3.0 ratio agents are divided into three groups. *Strong* indications are those in which the physiologic rationale for the importance of the benefit of a 3.0 ratio agent is strong. These include patients who have had a documented previous severe anaphylactoid reaction and patients in severe

Table 11–4. INDICATIONS FOR SELECTING 3.0 RATIO CONTRAST AGENTS OVER 1.5 RATIO CONTRAST AGENTS FOR CARDIAC ANGIOGRAPHY

Indication	Rationale	Documentation of Effectiveness
Strong Indications		
Previous severe anaphylactoid reaction	Reduced frequency of first reactions and possible reduced frequency of repeat reactions in patients with a previous reaction.	Reports of a small number of cases, indicating a lower likelihood of repeat reactions. No comparison with corticosteroid pretreatment.
Severe hemodynamic disturbance. (Left atrial pressure >25 mmHg; cardiac index <2.0 L/min; mean arterial pressure <60 mmHg; requirement for intravenous pressors; requirement for mechanical circulatory assistance)	Reduced expansion of intravascular volume and less pronounced myocardial depression of low osmolality agents should cause less hemodynamic perturbation.	No documentation of increased safety in such patients exists currently.
Severely impaired left ventricular contractile function. (Left ventricular ejection fraction <20%)	Reduced expansion of intravascular volume and less pronounced myocardial depression of low-osmolality agents should affect left ventricular performance less.	No documentation of increased safety in such patients exists currently.
Moderately Strong Indications		
Acute myocardial infarction and severe unstable cardiac ischemic syndromes	Less hemodynamic and electrophysiologic disturbance should improve tolerance of both ventricular and coronary injections.	No documentation of increased safety in such situations exists currently. The degree of safety enhancement should be related to the severity of the myocardial infarction and the total volume of contrast agent used.
Severe aortic stenosis with impaired left ventricular contractile function. (Aortic valve area <0.7 cm²; left ventricular end-diastolic pressure >30 mmHg)	Less hemodynamic disturbance and myocardial depression should improve tolerance.	No documentation of increased safety exists currently. The degree of safety enhancement is probably related to the total volume of contrast agent used.
Internal mammary artery angiography	Less pain during injections.	Well documented. The discomfort caused by such angiography is minimal if the internal mammary orifice is selectively engaged.
Possible Indications		
Complex coronary angioplasty	Improved tolerance may enhance safety—particularly if large volumes of contrast agent are required.	Not documented. The reduced anticoagulant properties of nonionic agents may increase the likelihood of thrombi forming within a catheter.
Renal disease	Reduced likelihood of renal injury.	No clinical documentation currently exists. Studies in low-risk patients have shown negative results. Animal studies suggest possible mechanisms for reducing renal injury.
Diabetes mellitus	Reduced likelihood of renal injury.	Same as for renal disease (above).

hemodynamic distress. Despite the fact that these situations are considered strong indications, one should recognize that even such severely ill patients can frequently be studied safely with 1.5 ratio agents, and that corticosteroid pretreatment reduces the likelihood of a repeat anaphylactoid reaction to 1.5 ratio agents.

Moderately strong indications are circumstances in which potentially fragile patients might stand to benefit significantly from 3.0 ratio agents. This category also includes angiography of the internal mammary and of other peripheral arteries—procedures that may be painful when conducted with 1.5 ratio agents.

Possible indications include circumstances in which large volumes of contrast agent may be administered to potentially fragile patients and patients with underlying systemic disorders that may predispose them to contrast agent–induced injury. These indications are only theoretic, as all currently available clinical trials have failed to demonstrate differences between the 1.5 ratio and the 3.0 ratio agents in these settings.

Universal adoption of 3.0 ratio agents appears to be unwarranted for cardiac angiography. As yet, however, the criteria for identifying those patients in whom the benefits of 3.0 ratio agents offer a safer, higher-quality study have not been developed. This problem represents an important area for future clinical research in radiographic contrast agents.

References

A

1. Anonymous: Metrizamide—a non-ionic water-soluble contrast medium. Acta Radiol. [Suppl.] (Stockh.) 1973.
2. Almen, T.: Contrast agent design. J. Theor. Biol. 24:216, 1969.
3. Almen, T.: Effects of iodixanol, iopentol, and metrizoate on femoral blood flow after injection into the femoral artery of the dog. Acta Radiol. [Suppl.] (Stockh.) 370:69, 1987.
4. Almen, T.: Effects of metrizamide and other contrast media on the isolated rabbit heart. Acta Radiol. [Suppl. 335] (Stockh.) vol. 216, 1973.
5. Almen, T.: Effects of metrizamide and other contrast media on the isolated rabbit heart. Acta Radiol. [Suppl.] (Stockh.) 335:216, 1973.
6. Aspelin, P.: Effect of ionic and non-ionic contrast media on morphology of human erythrocytes. Acta Radiol. (Diagn.) 19:675, 1978.
7. Aulie, Michelet, A., and Skinnemoen, K.: Pharmacokinetics of iopentol in the rat. Acta Radiol. [Suppl.] (Stockh.) 370:101, 1987.
8. Aulie Michelet, A.: Effects of intravascular contrast media on blood-brain barrier: Comparison between iothalamate, iohexol, iopentol, and iodixanol. Acta Radiol. 28:329, 1987.

B

1. Bashore, T.M., Davidson, C.J., Mark, D.B., et al.: Iopamidol use in the cardiac catheterization laboratory: A retrospective analysis of 3313 patients. Cardio 5:6, 1988.
2. Berberich, J., and Hirsch, S.: Die rontgenographische darstellun der arterien und venen am lebenden. Muench. Klin. Wschr. 49:2226, 1923.
3. Bettmann, M.A., and Morris, T.W.: Recent advances in contrast agents. Radiol. Clin. North Am. 24:347, 1986.
4. Binz, A., and Rath, C.: Uber Biochemische eigenschaften von derivaten des pyridins und chinolins. Biochem. Z. 203:218, 1928.
5. Bjork, L., Eldh, P., and Paulin, S.: Non-ionic and dimeric contrast media in coronary angiography. Acta Radiol. (Diagn.) 18:235, 1976.
6. Boijsen, E., and Kormano, M. (eds.): Iopentol: Chemistry, toxicology and pharmacology of a non-ionic contrast medium. Acta Radiol. [Suppl.] (Stockh.) vol. 370, 1987.
7. Bourdillion, P.D., Bettmann, M.A., McCracken, S., et al.: Effects of a new nonionic and a conventional ionic contrast agent on coronary sinus ionized calcium and left ventricular hemodynamics in dogs. J. Am. Coll. Cardiol. 6:845, 1985.
8. Brooks, B.: Intraarterial injection of sodium iodid. JAMA 82:1016, 1924.
9. Bessis, M., Weed, R.J., and LeBlond, P.F.: Red cell shape: Physiology, pathology, and ultrastructure. Springer-Verlag, New York, 1973.

C

1. Castellanos, A., Pereiras, R., and Garcia, A.: La angiocardiografica radio-opaca. Arch. Soc. Estud. Clin. Habana 31:523, 1937.
2. Caulfield, J.B., Zir, L., and Hawthorne, J.W.: Blood calcium levels in the presence of arteriographic contrast material. Circulation 52:119, 1975.
3. Cochran, S.T., Wong, W.S., and Roe, D.J.: Predicting angiography induced acute renal impairment: Clinical risk model. AJR 141:1027, 1983.

D

1. D'Elia, J.A., Gleason, R.E., Alday, M., et al.: Nephrotoxicity from angiographic contrast material. Am. J. Med. 72:719, 1982.
2. Dawson, P., Pitfield, J., and Britton, J.: Contrast media and bronchospasm: A study with iopamidol. Clin. Radiol. 34:227, 1982.
3. Dean, P.B., Kivisaari, L., and Kormano, M.: The diagnostic potential of contrast enhancement pharmacokinetics. Invest. Radiol., 13:533, 1978.
4. DiBattiste, P.M., Kussmaul, W.G., and Hirshfeld, J.W., Jr.: The safety of cardiac angiography with conventional contrast agents. Circulation 78 (Suppl. II):II-377, 1988.

E

1. Engelhart, J.A., Smith, D.C., Maloney, M.D., et al.: A technique for estimating the probability of clots in blood/contrast agent mixtures. Invest. Radiol. 23:923, 1988.

F

1. Fischer, H.W.: Cost vs safety: The use of low-osmolar contrast media. JAMA 260:1614, 1988.
2. Forssmann, W.: Uber kontrastdarstellun der hohlen des levenden rechten herzens und der lungenschlagader. Muench. Med. Wschr. Wochenschr. 78:489, 1931.
3. Frink, R.J., Merrick, B., and Lowe, H.M.: Mechanism of the bradycardia during coronary angiography. Am. J. Cardiol. 35:17, 1975.

G

1. Gensini, G.G., Dubiel, J., Huntington, P.P., and Kelly, A.E.: Left ventricular end-diastolic pressure before and after coronary arteriography. Am. J. Cardiol. 27:453, 1971.
2. Gertz, E.W., Wisneski, J.A., Chiu, D., et al.: Clinical superiority of a new nonionic contrast agent (iopamidol) for cardiac angiography. J. Am. Coll. Cardiol. 5:250, 1985.
3. Grainger, R.G.: Osmolalities of intravascular radiological contrast media. Br. J. Radiol. 53:739, 1980.
4. Greenberger, P.A., Meyers, S.N., Kramer, B.L., and Kramer, B.L.: Effects of beta-adrenergic and calcium antagonists on development of anaphylactoid reactions from radiographic contrast media during cardiac angiography. J. Allergy Clin. Immunol. 80:698, 1987.
5. Greenberger, P.A., and Patterson, R.: Adverse reactions to radiocontrast media. Prog. Cardiovasc. Dis. 31:239, 1988.
6. Greenberger, P.A.: Contrast media reactions. J. Allergy Clin. Immunol. 74:600, 1984.
7. Grollman, J.H., Jr., Liu, C.K., Astone, R.A., and Lurie, M.D.: Thromboembolic complication in coronary angiography associated with the use of nonionic contrast medium. Cathet. Cardiovasc. Diagn. 14:159, 1988.

H

1. Heyman, S., Brezis, M., Greenfield, Z., and Rosen, S.: Protective role of furosemide and saline in radiocontrast-induced acute renal failure. (Abstract.) Clin. Res. 36:520A, 1988.
2. Higgins, C.B., and Feld, G.K.: Direct chronotropic and dromotropic actions of contrast media: Ineffectiveness of atropine in the prevention of bradyarrhythmias and conduction disturbances. Radiology 212:205, 1976.
3. Higgins, C.B., Gerber, K.H., Mattrey, R.F., et al.: Evaluation of the hemodynamic effects of intravenous administration of ionic and nonionic contrast materials. Radiology 142:681, 1983.
4. Higgins, C.B., Sovak, M., Schmidt, W.S., et al.: Direct myocardial effects of intracoronary administration of new contrast materials with low osmolality. Invest. Radiol. 15:39, 1980.
5. Hilal, S.: Hemodynamic changes associated with intra-arterial injection of contrast media. Radiology 86:615, 1966.
6. Hildner, F.J., Scherlag, B.J., and Samet, P.: Evaluation of Renografin M76 as a contrast agent for angiocardiography. Radiology 100:329, 1971.
7. Hirshfeld, J.W., Jr., Wieland, J., Davis, C.A., et al.: Hemodynamic and electrocardiographic effects of ioversol during cardiac angiography comparison with diatrizoate. Invest. Radiol. 24:138, 1989.
8. Hirshfeld, J.W., Jr., Laskey, W.K., Martin, J.L., et al.: Hemodynamic changes induced by cardiac angiography with ioxaglate: Comparison with diatrizoate. J. Am. Coll. Cardiol. 2:954, 1983.
9. Holtas, S.: Iohexol in patients with previous adverse reactions to contrast media. Invest. Radiol. 19:563, 1984.
10. Hoppe, J.O., Larsen, H.A., and Coulston, F.J.: Observations on the toxicity of a new urographic contrast medium, sodium 3,5-diacetamido-2,4,6 triiodobenzoate (Hypaque sodium) and related compounds. J. Pharmacol. Exp. Ther. 116:394, 1956.
11. Hoppe, J.O.: Some pharmacological aspects of radiopaque compounds. Ann. N.Y. Acad. Sci. 78:727, 1959.

J

1. Jacobson, P.D., and Rosenquist, C.J.: The introduction of low-osmolar contrast agents in radiology: Medical, economic, legal and public policy issues. JAMA 260:1586, 1988.

K

1. Katayama, H.: Clinical survey on adverse reactions of iodinated contrast media. *In* Matsuura, K., et al. (eds.): Advance and Future Trends of Contrast Media. Japan Convention Services, Tokyo, 1988, p. 145.

2. Kennedy, J.W.: Complications associated with cardiac catheterization and angiography. Cathet. Cardiovasc. Diagn. 8:5, 1982.
3. Kozeny, G.A., Murdock, D.K., Euler, D.E., et al.: In vivo effects of acute changes in osmolality and sodium concentration in myocardial contractility. Am. J. Heart 109:290, 1985.

L

1. Lalli, A.F.: Urography, shock reaction, and repeat urography. (Editorial.) AJR 125:264, 1975.
2. Lasser, E.C., Berry, C.C., Talner, L.B., et al.: Pretreatment with corticosteroids to alleviate reactions to intravenous contrast material. N. Engl. J. Med. 317:845, 1987.
3. Lazarra, R., El-Sherif, N., Hope, R.R., et al.: Ventricular arrhythmias and electrophysiological consequences of myocardial ischemia and infarction. Circ. Res. 35:391, 1974.
4. Lembo, N.J., Roubin, G.S., Chin, H.K., et al.: Does non-ionic contrast media decrease the incidence of PTCA related complications? Circulation 78(Suppl. II):II-378, 1978.
5. Lindgren, E. (ed.): Iohexol: A non-ionic contrast medium: Pharmacology and toxicology. Acta Radiol. [Suppl.] (Stockh.) vol. 362, 1980.
6. Littner, M.R., Rosenfield, A.T., Ulreich, S., and Puttman, C.E.: Evaluation of bronchospasm during excretory urography. Radiology 124:17, 1977.

M

1. MacAlpin, R.N., Weidner, W.A., Kattus, A.A., Jr., and Hanafee, W.N.: Electrocardiographic changes during selective coronary cinearteriography. Circulation 34:627, 1966.
2. Mallette, L.E., and Gomez, L.S.: Systemic hypocalcemia after clinical injections of radiographic contrast media: Amelioration by omission of calcium chelating agents. Radiology 147:677, 1983.
3. Marshall, R.J., and Shepherd, J.T.: Effects of injections of hypertonic solutions on blood flow throughout the femoral artery of the dog. Am. J. Physiol. 197:951, 1959.
4. McKinstry, D.N., Rommel, A.J., and Sugarman, A.: Pharmacokinetics, metabolism, and excretion of iopamidol in healthy subjects. Invest. Radiol. 19:S171, 1984.
5. Messina, J.M., Cieslinski, D.A., Nguyen, V.D., and Holmes, H.D.: Comparison of the toxicity of the radiocontrast agents iopamidol and diatrizoate to rabbit renal proximal tubule cells in vitro. J. Pharmacol. Exp. Ther. 244:1139, 1988.
6. Morgan, R.H.: Physics of diagnostic radiology. *In* Goodwin, P.N., et al. (eds.): Physical Foundations of Radiology. 4th ed. Harper & Row, New York, 1970.
7. Morris, T.W., Sahler, L.G., and Fischer, H.W.: Calcium binding by radiopaque media. Invest. Radiol 17:501, 1982.
8. Murdock, D.K., Johnson, S.A., Loeb, H.S., and Scanlon, P.J.: Ventricular fibrillation during coronary angiography: Reduced incidence in man with contrast media lacking calcium binding additives. Cathet. Cardiovasc. Diagn. 11:153, 1985.

N

1. Nakjavan, F.K.: Continuous recording of His bundle electrogram during selective coronary cineangiography in man. J. Electrocardiol. 5:233, 1972.
2. Nathan, D.G., and Shohet, S.B.: Erythrocyte ion transport and hemolytic anemia: Hydrocytosis and desiccocytosis. Semin. Hematol. 7:381, 1970.
3. Newhouse, J.H.: Fluid compartment distribution of intravenous iothalamate in the dog. Invest. Radiol. 12:364, 1977.
4. Nyman, U., and Almen, T.: Effects of contrast media on aortic endothelium. Acta Radiol. [Suppl.] (Stockh.) 362:65, 1980.

P

1. Palmer, F.J.: The R.C.A.R. survey of intravenous contrast media reactions: A preliminary report. Australas. Radiol. 32:8, 1988.
2. Parfrey, P.S., Griffiths, S.M., Barrett, B.J., et al.: Contrast material–induced renal failure in patients with diabetes mellitus, renal insufficiency, or both. N. Engl. J. Med. 320:143, 1989.
3. Partridge, J.B., Robinson, P.J., Turnbull, C.M., et al.: Clinical cardiovascular experiences with iopamidol: A new non-ionic contrast medium. Clin. Radiol. 32:451, 1981.
4. Parvez, Z., Kahn, T., and Moncada, R.: Ultrastructural changes in rat aortic endothelium during contrast media infusion. Invest. Radiol. 20:407, 1985.
5. Paulin, S., and Adams, D.F.: Increased ventricular fibrillation during coronary arteriography with a new contrast medium preparation. Radiology 101:45, 1971.
6. Peck, R.J., Bull, M.J., and Cumberland, D.C.: Comparison of low-osmolar contrast media in cardiac angiography. Br. J. Radiol. 58:1177, 1985.
7. Popio, K.A., Ross, A.M., Oravec, J.M., and Ingram, J.T.: Identification and description of separate mechanisms for two components of Renografin cardiotoxicity. Circulation 58:520, 1978.
8. Port, F.K., Wagoner, R.D., and Fulton, R.E.: Acute renal failure after arteriography. AJR 121:544, 1974.

R

1. Rasuli, P., McLeish, W.A., and Hammond, D.T.: Anticoagulant effects of contrast materials: In vitro study of iohexol, ioxaglate, and diatrizoate. AJR 152:309, 1989.
2. Read, R.C., Johnson, J.A., Vick, J.A., and Meyer, M.W.: Vascular effects of hypertonic solutions. Circ. Res. 8:538, 1960.
3. Renaa, T., and Jacobsen, T.: Contrast media research: An investment for the future. Acta Radiol. [Suppl.] (Stockh.) 370:9, 1987.
4. Robertson, H.J.F.: Blood clot formation in angiographic syringes containing nonionic contrast media. Radiology 163:621, 1987.
5. Roentgen, W.C.: On a new kind of rays. Erst Mitt. Sitzber. Phys.-Med. Ges. (Wurzburg) 137, 1895.
6. Roseno, A.: Die intravenose pyelographie: II Mitteilung klinische ergebnisse. Klin. Wochenschr. 8:1165, 1929.

S

1. Schwab, S.J., Hlatky, M.A., Pieper, K.S., et al.: Contrast nephrotoxicity: A randomized controlled trial of a nonionic and an ionic radiographic contrast agent. N. Engl. J. Med. 320:149, 1989.
2. Shabetai, R., Surawicz, B., and Hammill, W.: Monophasic action potential in man. Circulation 38:341, 1968.
3. Shaw, D.D., and Potts, D.G.: Toxicity of iohexol. Invest. Radiol. 20:S10, 1984.
4. Shehadi, W.H.: Contrast media adverse reactions: Occurrence, recurrence, and distribution patterns. Radiology 143:11, 1982.
5. Simon, A.L., Shabetai, R., Lang, J.H., and Lasser, E.C.: The mechanism of production of ventricular fibrillation in coronary angiography. AJR 114:810, 1972.
6. Smith, D.C., Luis, J.F., Gomes, A.S., et al.: Pulmonary arteriography: Comparison of cough stimulation effects of diatrizoate and ioxaglate. Radiology 162:617, 1987.
7. Snyder, C.F., Formanek, A., Frech, R.S., and Amplatz, K.: The role of sodium in promoting ventricular arrhythmia during selective coronary arteriography. AJR 113:567, 1971.
8. Sullivan, I.D., Wainwright, R.J., Freidy, J.F., and Sowton, E.: Comparative trial of iohexol 350, a non-ionic contrast medium with diatrizoate (Urografin 370) in left ventriculography and coronary arteriography. Br. Heart J. 51:643, 1984.
9. Swick, M.: Darstellum der niere und harnwefe in rontenbild durch intravenose einbringung eines neuen kontraststoffes des uroselectans. Klin. Wochenschr. 8:2087, 1929.
10. Swick, M.: Intravenous urography by means of Uroselectan. Am. J. Surg. 8:405, 1930.

T

1. Talierco, C.P., Vlietstra, R.E., Fisher, L.D., and Burnett, J.D.: Risks for renal dysfunction with cardiac angiography. Ann. Intern. Med. 104:501, 1986.
2. Thompson, K.R., Evill, C.A., Fritzche, J., et al.: Comparison of iopamidol, ioxaglate, and diatrizoate during coronary angiography in dogs. Invest. Radiol. 15:234, 1980.
3. Thompson, K.R., Violante, M.R., Kenyon, T., and Fischer, H.W.: Reduction of ventricular fibrillation using calcium-enriched Renografin-76. Invest. Radiol. 13:238, 1978.
4. Tragardh, B., Lynch, P.R., and Vinciguerra, T.: Effects of metrizamide, a new non-ionic contrast medium, on cardiac function during coronary arteriography in the dog. Radiology 115:59, 1976.
5. Tragardh, B., and Lynch, P.R.: ECG changes and arrhythmias induced by ionic and non-ionic contrast media during coronary arteriography in dogs. Invest. Radiol. 13:223, 1978.

V

1. Violante, M.R., Thompson, K.R., Fischer, H.W., and Kenyon, T.: Ventricular fibrillation from diatrizoate with and without chelating agents. Radiology 128:497, 1978.

W

1. White, R.I., Jr., and Holden, W.J., Jr.: Liquid gold: Low osmolarity contrast media. Radiology 159:559, 1986.
2. Wisneski, J.A., Gertz, E.W., Dahlgren, M., and Muslin, A.: Double-blind comparison of low osmolality ionic (ioxaglate) versus nonionic (iopamidol) contrast media in cardiac angiography. Am. J. Cardiol. 63:489, 1989.
3. Wisneski, J.A., Gertz, E.W., Reese, R., et al.: Myocardial metabolic alterations after contrast angiography. Am. J. Cardiol. 50:239, 1982.
4. Wolf, G.L., Arenson, R.L., and Cross, A.P.: A prospective trial of ionic versus nonionic contrast agents in routine clinical practice: Comparison of adverse effects. AJR 152:939, 1989.
5. Wolf, G.L., and Hirshfeld, J.W., Jr.: Changes in QTc interval with Renografin-76 and Hypaque-76 during coronary arteriography. J. Am. Coll. Cardiol. 1:1489, 1983.

6. Wolf, G.L., LeVeen, R.F., Mulry, C., and Kilzer, K.: The influence of contrast media additives upon ventricular fibrillation threshold during coronary angiography in ischemic and normal canine hearts. Cardiovasc. Intervent. Radiol. 4:145, 1981.
7. Wolf, G.L., Mulry, C.C., Kilzer, K., and Laski, P.A.: New angiographic agents with less fibrillatory propensity. Invest. Radiol. 16:320, 1981.
8. Wolf, G.L.: Safer, more expensive iodinated contrast agents: How do we decide? Radiology 159:557, 1986.
9. Wolf, G.L.: The fibrillatory properties of contrast agents. Invest. Radiol. 15:S208, 1980.
10. Wolfe, C.L., Winniford, M.D., Wheelan, K.R., et al.: Relation of coronary artery disease and left ventricular systolic dysfunction to left ventricular end-diastolic pressure after left ventriculography. Am. J. Cardiol. 55:1622, 1985.
11. Wolpers, H.G., Boller, D., Hoeft, A., et al.: The effect of ion composition on cellular membrane potentials during selective coronary arteriography. Invest. Radiol. 19:291, 1984.
12. Winthrop Pharmaceuticals Inc.: Upper range of mouse intravenous L.D.$_{50}$ for Hypaque-76.™ (Published in package insert.)

Z

1. Zuckerman, L.S., Friehling, T.D., Wolf, N.M., et al.: Effect of calcium-binding additives on ventricular fibrillation and repolarization changes during coronary arteriography. J. Am. Coll. Cardiol. 10:1249, 1987.

Part III

Coronary Angiography

Chapter 12

Clinical Aspects of Data Acquisition in Coronary Angiography

MARYL R. JOHNSON, M.D.

HISTORIC EVENTS IN THE DEVELOPMENT OF CORONARY ANGIOGRAPHY 183
INDICATIONS 183
CONTRAINDICATIONS 184
COMPLICATIONS 185
CONTRAST MEDIA AND THEIR EFFECTS IN CORONARY ANGIOGRAPHY 187
Arrhythmias 187
Bradycardias 187
Ventricular Arrhythmias 187
Electrocardiographic Changes 187
Hemodynamic Changes 187
Nephrotoxicity 188
"Allergic" Reactions 188
PREPARATION AND MANAGEMENT OF PATIENTS 189
CORONARY ANGIOGRAPHIC TECHNIQUES 190
Sones Technique 190
Judkins Technique 191
Amplatz Technique 191
Schoonmaker Technique 192
Other Techniques 192
Bypass Graft and Internal Mammary Artery Angiography 193
IMPORTANCE OF ADEQUATE ANGIOGRAPHIC VIEWS 193
NORMAL CORONARY ANATOMY 194
CONGENITAL ANOMALIES OF THE CORONARY ARTERIES 196
Coronary Anomalies That Alter Myocardial Perfusion 197
Coronary Artery Fistulas 197
Origin of the Left Coronary Artery from the Pulmonary Artery 197
Congenital Stenosis or Atresia of the Coronary Arteries 198
Origin of the Left or the Right Coronary Artery from the Opposite Coronary Sinus with Passage of the Vessel Between the Aorta and the Right Ventricular Outflow Tract 198
Coronary Anomalies That Do Not Alter Myocardial Perfusion 198
Origin of the Circumflex Coronary Artery from the Right Coronary Sinus or the Right Coronary Artery 198
Origin of the Left Anterior Descending Artery from the Right Coronary Artery or Right Coronary Sinus 198
Single Coronary Artery 198
Multiple Ostia of the Coronary Arteries 199
High Origin of the Coronary Arteries 199
Horseshoe Coronary Artery (with Two Ostia to the Aorta): Origin of the First Septal Perforator from the Right Coronary Artery or RightCoronary Sinus 199
CORONARY COLLATERALS 199
Collateral Pathways to the Left Anterior Descending Artery 199
Collateral Pathways to the Right Coronary Artery 199
Collateral Pathways to the Circumflex Coronary Artery 200
CORONARY BRIDGING 200
VALIDITY OF CORONARY ANGIOGRAMS 200
Postmortem/Angiographic Comparisons 200
Intraobserver and Interobserver Variability 201
EVALUATION/INTERPRETATION/IMPLICATIONS OF THE CORONARY ANGIOGRAM 201
TRAPS TO AVOID IN THE PERFORMANCE AND INTERPRETATION OF CORONARY ANGIOGRAMS 206
OUTPATIENT CARDIAC CATHETERIZATION 206
GENERAL RECOMMENDATIONS 207

Coronary artery disease remains the major cause of morbidity and mortality in the United States. It is estimated that 1.2 million myocardial infarctions occur each year and nearly 600,000 deaths per year are related to coronary artery disease.[A1] Over the past several years there has been increased use of coronary angiography to define the coronary arterial narrowings responsible for the morbidity and mortality caused by ischemic heart disease. In contrast to the situation of years ago, when coronary angiography was performed only when coronary bypass or valvular surgery was clearly indicated, coronary angiography is currently used to define coronary anatomy whenever the information obtained will be beneficial in management of the patient. Although numerous attempts have been made with other imaging modalities to define the presence, extent, and functional significance of coronary artery disease, coronary angiography remains the only method of defining coronary vascular anatomy in closed-chest humans in vivo, and coronary angiography remains the "gold standard" for determining the presence, extent, localization, and severity of coronary artery disease. Coronary angiography also allows visualization of coronary collaterals, intracoronary thrombus, coronary artery spasm, and congenital anomalies of the coronary arteries. If coronary stenoses are present, coronary angiography permits analysis of the distal coronary vessels and also provides a rough index of the area "at risk" distal to a coronary stenosis.

Because over 300,000 coronary angiograms are performed each year in the United States, it is important to review the techniques of coronary angiography and the implications of the information found on coronary angiograms. Numerous authors have written about coronary angiography. It is the goal of this chapter to review previously reported data, stressing aspects of the clinical performance and interpretation of coronary angiograms that should be useful to the clinical cardiologist, to scientists interested in improving the safety and validity of coronary angiography, and to clinicians interested in using angiographic information to define the prognostic significance of coronary artery stenoses and thus define appropriate means of therapy. Although this chapter cannot reiterate all the details presented elsewhere, it is hoped that the references provided will allow the interested reader to more fully explore selected areas.

HISTORIC EVENTS IN THE DEVELOPMENT OF CORONARY ANGIOGRAPHY

We will begin by recalling some historic events important in the development of coronary angiography. The history actually begins over a century ago when catheters were placed into the arteries and veins of horses by Claude Bernard.[S1] Subsequently, Chauveau and Marey reported recording pressures from such catheters.[S1] Catheterization in humans began in 1929 when Werner Forssman, a 25-year-old surgical resident, inserted a ureteral catheter into his left antecubital vein, advanced it to the right atrium, and climbed several flights of stairs to radiology to document the intracardiac position of the catheter.[S1] In 1937 Castellanos injected iodine into the antecubital vein of humans to better define the anatomy of patients with congenital heart disease. In 1938 Robb and Steinberg placed catheters into the right atrium and right ventricle and performed contrast injections.[C1]

Although these reports served as the background for the development of coronary angiography, it was not until 1945 that human coronary arteries were first seen in vivo at the time of retrograde aortography (performed following direct needle puncture through the sternum into the aorta).[R1] Similar observations were reported by Jonsson in 1948.[L1] In 1952 DiGuglielmo and Guttadauro published diagrams of the x-ray appearance of the coronary arteries based on thoracic aortograms. However, visualization was adequate in only 112 of 159 cases.[L1] Attempts were subsequently made to increase opacification of the coronary arteries during thoracic aortography by using balloon occlusion, as reported for a dog model by Dotter and Frische,[D1] or acetylcholine-induced circulatory arrest, as reported by Lehman and associates.[L1] Injections were also attempted in late systole or early diastole or with Valsalva's maneuver to decrease contrast dilution.[A2] In 1960, Bellman and associates reported the injection of contrast medium into the aortic root with a loop catheter containing side holes such that a larger volume of contrast medium was injected into the region of the coronary ostia.[B1, W1] They also suggested that carotid compression during contrast injection would decrease the cerebral flow of the contrast agent. By using the loop catheter and carotid compression, the coronary arteries were seen in 27 of 32 males.[W1] The development of angiography in general, and the pursuit of adequate coronary visualization in particular, was facilitated in 1952 when Seldinger reported his technique of obtaining vascular access.[S2] Despite all of these advances, however, visualization of the coronary arteries was still inadequate in most cases.

In 1959, Sones and associates reported a brachial approach in which better coronary opacification was produced by injecting 20 to 30 ml of contrast agent directly into the coronary sinuses.[S3] With this technique, coronary collaterals were seen angiographically for the first time. In April 1959, Sones began the era of selective coronary angiography with selective catheter entry of the right and left coronary arteries.[S4] Both coronary arteries were entered in 954 of 1020 cases, and at least one artery was entered in every patient. Selective coronary injection decreased the interference arising from contrast agent in the aortic root, decreased the volume of contrast agent needed for each injection, and made possible the use of additional projections to better define coronary anatomy. Ricketts and Abrams reported the use of selective catheters from the femoral approach in 1962.[R2] Judkins reported the use of preformed catheters from the femoral approach in 1967,[J1] and Amplatz and associates, in the same year, pioneered the use of selective catheters from the femoral approach with catheter tips designed to arise perpendicular to the wall of the aorta and thus more easily enter the coronary ostia, which are funnel shaped and arise perpendicular to the sinuses.[A3]

Thus, we have come a long way from the time when Werner Forssman showed that intravascular placement of catheters in humans was possible. Although many of these developmental techniques seem far-fetched, archaic, and dangerous today, they serve as the background on which our current techniques of coronary angiography are based and still provide lessons concerning selective coronary angiography.

INDICATIONS

The purpose of coronary angiography is to define the presence or absence of significant narrowings of the coronary arteries. This information is then used to define the patient's prognosis and determine appropriate therapy. Although complications can arise during coronary angiography, as will subsequently be discussed, the risk of coronary angiography may be small compared to that of undertaking therapy with incomplete or inaccurate diagnostic information. Although in the past angiography was performed only in patients with symptoms significant enough to warrant surgical therapy, improved angiographic techniques, advances in cardiac surgery, and the development of new methods of therapy (particularly thrombolysis and angioplasty) have expanded indications for cardiac catheterization. General guidelines concerning patients for whom coronary angiography should be considered can be presented, but it is impossible to provide absolute indications or contraindications; the appropriateness of coronary angiography depends not only on the patient's cardiac status but also on his age (in particular, his physiologic age), overall health, occupation, and desired level of activity. Factors such as the availability of experienced angiographers, the physician's philosophy concerning appropriate therapy for coronary disease, and local results from angioplasty and surgery also play a role. Thus, although coronary angiography requires specialized technical skills for safe and adequate studies to be performed, it is essential that angiographers retain the clinical acumen necessary to individualize the use of angiography for each patient in whom it is considered.

An excellent review of the indications for coronary angiography can be found in reference G1. Following is a list of indications for coronary angiography as proposed by several authors.[A1, B2, C2–C4, G1, G2]

1. History of angina
   - A. Angina unresponsive to medical management. This is perhaps the most uniformly accepted indication for coronary angiography, as long as the patient is otherwise healthy enough for anatomic correction by coronary artery bypass grafting or angioplasty to be considered.
   - B. Unstable angina. This syndrome refers to anginal chest pain that is new in onset, is crescendo in character (increased in frequency or duration or occurring with lesser degrees of exertion), or occurs at rest.
   - C. Stable angina, with high-risk noninvasive tests. High-risk treadmill results would include a positive test at a heart rate of less than 120 or a work load of less than 6.5 mets, a test with greater than 2.0 mm or greater than 6 minutes of ST depression, or a test with electrocardiographic (ECG) changes in multiple leads or a decrease in blood pressure with exercise. A thallium scan with multiple areas of abnormal thallium uptake or a decrease in ejection fraction of greater than 10 percent with exercise as shown on radionuclide ventriculography is also considered indicative of high risk.
   - D. Angina following myocardial infarction.
   - E. Recurrent angina following coronary artery bypass surgery or angioplasty, particularly if it is not readily responsive to medical management.
   - F. Angina and planned major vascular surgery.
2. History of myocardial infarction.
   - A. Patients with recurrent angina following myocardial infarction, particularly if the angina occurs close to the time of the infarct.
   - B. Patients with non-Q-wave myocardial infarction.
   - C. Patients with myocardial infarction at a "young" age.
   - D. Patients with severe heart failure following myocardial infarction that may be due to infarct complications (mitral regurgitation, ventricular septal defect, or ventricular aneurysm).
   - E. Patients with high-risk noninvasive studies.
3. Asymptomatic patients for whom there is a high suspicion of significant coronary artery disease.
   - A. Patients with abnormal ECGs or positive treadmill tests, particularly if they are involved in public safety-related occupations, such as airline pilots, truck drivers, and air traffic controllers.
   - B. Patients with numerous coronary risk factors.
   - C. Patients who have sustained a myocardial infarction, particularly if they are young.
   - D. Patients in whom noninvasive tests suggest the high likelihood of significant silent ischemia.
4. Chest pain of uncertain cardiac etiology. This indication is one of the more controversial. However, for patients with atypical chest pain in whom the coronary arteries are found to be normal, subsequent therapy may be significantly aided. If the patient's coronary arteries are normal but the suspicion of a cardiac etiology for chest pain remains high, ergonovine testing to diagnose coronary artery spasm[H1] or testing to evaluate for "microvascular angina"[C5] should be considered.
5. Patients who require surgery for valvular heart disease. If patients undergoing surgery for valvular heart disease have significant coronary disease, their long-term prognosis may be better if the coronary lesions are bypassed.[R3] Thus, preoperative coronary angiography is indicated when valvular surgery is planned if the patient's age and/or risk factor profile suggests a significant likelihood of coronary disease. Noninvasive tests may be used to define the patients at the highest risk of having associated coronary disease; however, many of these patients have left ventricular hypertrophy, which makes an exercise test difficult to interpret. It has been said that if patients with isolated aortic stenosis do not have angina, coronary angiography is not necessary; however, in a study of 103 patients with isolated aortic stenosis, Green and associates found that 25 percent of the patients with no history of angina had significant coronary disease that would have been missed had coronary angiograms not been performed.[G3]
6. Left ventricular dysfunction of uncertain etiology. Coronary angiography in this setting determines whether ischemia is the cause of left ventricular dysfunction. This determination has become more important as improved surgical techniques allow coronary bypass grafting to be performed more safely in patients with ventricular dysfunction. Data from the Coronary Artery Surgery Study (CASS) have revealed prolongation of life in patients with three-vessel coronary disease and left ventricular dysfunction who are treated surgically.[P1]
7. To identify coronary anomalies. Coronary anomalies can be of functional significance (as will be discussed) or might complicate surgical repair in patients with congenital heart disease.
8. Intractable ventricular arrhythmias, particularly following cardiac arrest.
9. Patients for whom interventional therapy, such as angioplasty or intracoronary thrombolysis, is being considered.
10. Patients who have received intravenous thrombolytic therapy.
11. Potential donors for cardiac transplantation whose age or history suggests a possibility of coronary disease. This indication will likely become more common as attempts are made to expand the pool of cardiac donors.
12. Patients following cardiac transplantation, who must have yearly surveillance catheterizations to evaluate for graft atherosclerosis, which does not result in angina as the heart is denervated.[G4] This disease tends to be diffuse and is thought to have an immune etiology. (See Fig. 12–1.)
13. Patients in whom noninvasive tests cannot be performed (i.e., amputees, patients with peripheral vascular disease) and coronary risk must be defined.

CONTRAINDICATIONS

Just as the indications for coronary angiography must be individualized, most of the contraindications are also relative, and the risks versus benefits of proceeding to coronary angiography in an individual patient must be considered carefully. There are situations in which angiography may be of such clinical benefit as to outweigh the presence of factors that would generally be strong contraindications. Indeed, perhaps the only absolute contraindication to coronary angiography is the lack of experienced angiographers and suitable laboratory facilities. However, in patients with any of the following problems the risk/benefit ratio of proceeding to coronary angiography, particularly prior to stabilizing the problematic clinical condition, must be evaluated thoroughly.[C2, C3, G1, G2]

- Bleeding diatheses, whether due to underlying illness or anticoagulation therapy.
- Advanced physiologic age.
- Uncontrolled hypertension.
- Significant electrolyte abnormalities or digitalis toxicity.
- Fever, particularly with documented infection.
- Decompensated congestive heart failure (which might prevent the patient from assuming a supine enough posture to allow a complete study).
- Severe anemia.
- Active gastrointestinal bleeding.
- A mental or physical condition that precludes the patient's cooperation.
- A significant cerebrovascular accident within the previous few months.
- The presence of noncardiac disease that precludes long-term survival.
- Previous history of a contrast reaction (although pretreatment may decrease the incidence of recurrence, as will be discussed).

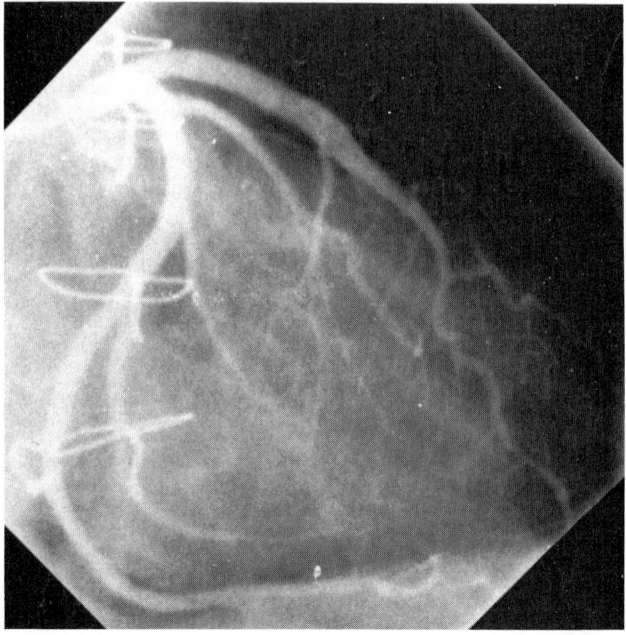
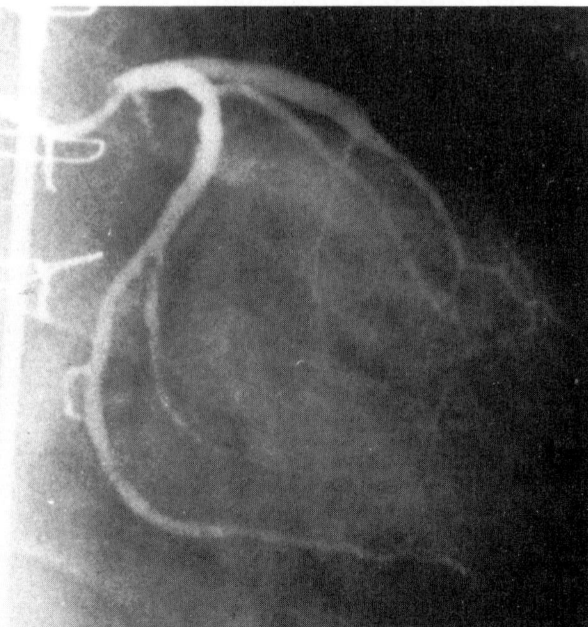

Figure 12–1. Serial coronary angiograms of a patient following cardiac transplantation, demonstrating the diffuse coronary disease that can develop in the transplanted coronary arteries. *Left,* The left coronary angiogram (right anterior oblique projection) 2 years following transplantation. Only minimal irregularities were noted. *Right,* The same vessel 3 years following transplantation reveals severe diffuse disease with pruning of the distal vessels. The patient was asymptomatic at the time the 3-year angiogram was taken but died suddenly 2 months later, before a suitable donor heart for retransplantation was obtained.

- Significant renal insufficiency or anuria.
- Refusal to undergo any interventional therapy, regardless of the outcome of the coronary angiogram.

COMPLICATIONS

In evaluating the risk/benefit ratio of coronary angiography, the angiographer must be aware of the risk of complications from the procedure. As coronary angiography is invasive and is generally performed in patients with cardiovascular disease, it is associated with complications. The complications may be cardiovascular in origin (myocardial infarction, cerebrovascular accident, arrhythmia, death) or may be related to the vascular access site (local arterial damage, clot formation, embolism, or infection). Although the "forefathers" of coronary angiography each reported complication rates, Adams and associates reported the first large series in which complications that occurred during or within the 24 hours following cardiac catheterization and coronary angiography were tabulated.[A4] They reported a survey of 46,904 patients studied in 173 centers during 1970 and 1971. The mortality rate was 0.45 percent. Cardiovascular complications were significantly higher with the femoral than with the brachial approach, with a death rate of 0.78 percent versus 0.13 percent. The overall cardiovascular complication rate (death, myocardial infarction, or cerebrovascular accident) was 2.2 percent for the femoral approach and 0.38 percent for the brachial approach. However, arterial clot formation was higher with the brachial approach (1.67 percent) than the femoral approach (1.19 percent). A significant contributor to the cardiovascular complication rate for angiograms obtained by the femoral approach, however, was that in 55 percent of these cases the technique was performed in laboratories that did fewer than 50 cardiac catheterizations per year. The complication rate was higher in laboratories performing fewer than 200 cardiac catheterizations per year than in laboratories performing more than 800. The risk of complications also increased with longer procedures and with sicker patients.

In 1976 Bourassa and Noble reported complication rates in 5250 patients in whom angiograms were obtained using the femoral approach (without heparin) from 1970 to 1974.[B3] In patients with normal coronary arteries, no serious complications resulted. The mortality rate was 0.23 percent, and all 12 patients who died had left main disease. The five patients who suffered myocardial infarction (0.09 percent) also had severe coronary artery disease. The incidence of significant arrhythmias (ventricular fibrillation, ventricular tachycardia, or transient asystole) was 0.80 percent. Femoral site complications occurred in 0.85 percent (with a higher incidence in females), cerebral ischemia in 0.13 percent, and impending pulmonary edema in 0.1 percent. The study concluded that complications were related mainly to disease severity.

In 1979 Davis and associates reported the complications occurring in the CASS.[D2] In this study 7553 patients were evaluated prospectively at 13 centers in 1975 and 1976. Eighty-four percent of the cardiac catheterizations were performed by the femoral approach. The death rate was 0.20 percent and the myocardial infarction rate 0.25 percent. Similar to the results of Bourassa et al., the complications all occurred in patients with left main or three-vessel disease. In 657 patients with significant left main disease, there were 5 deaths and 3 myocardial infarctions, a complication rate 6.8 times that of the remainder of the group. In contrast to the earlier study of Adams and associates,[A4] cardiovascular complications were more frequent in patients undergoing the procedure from the brachial approach. However, this was not true in centers that performed more than 80 percent of their procedures by the brachial route. Thus, complications appeared to be related to the familiarity of the operators with the technique used. In the CASS survey, the mortality was higher among patients with congestive heart failure, hypertension, significant premature ventricular contractions (PVCs), greater than 50 percent left main disease, or a left ventricular ejection fraction less than 30 percent. There was also an increased risk of myocardial infarction in patients with unstable angina. There were two cerebrovascular accidents (0.03 percent), seven arterial emboli, 56 vascular injuries, and 48 episodes of ventricular fibrillation without myocardial infarction (0.63 percent). The authors found that heparin did not significantly alter any of the risks. As in the study of Adams et al.,[A4] local complications were higher in patients catheterized by the brachial approach.

The most recent large series reporting complications is from the Registry of the Society for Cardiac Angiography.[K1] In this study data were obtained for 53,581 patients in 66 laboratories over a 14-month period in 1979 and 1980. Forty-three percent of procedures were brachial and 54 percent femoral; the arterial access site was not reported in 3 percent. Heparin was used in 71 percent. The overall complication rate was 1.8 percent and mortality was 0.14 percent. Mortality was equal for males and females and for patients catheterized from the brachial and the femoral approach. However, mortality was increased for patients less than 1 year of age or more than 60 years of age, for patients who were functional Class IV versus those who were functional Class I and II, for patients with left ventricular dysfunction, and for patients with left main coronary artery disease. Nonfatal myocardial infarctions occurred in 0.07 percent and significant arrhythmias in 0.56 percent (including ventricular fibrillation, ventricular tachycardia, and bradycardias). Vascular complications occurred in 0.57 percent, with local complications significantly higher when procedures were performed via the brachial rather than the femoral approach.

Wyman and his colleagues reported data on complications of 1609 diagnostic cardiac catheterizations performed from July 1986 through December 1987 at Beth Israel Hospital.[W13] In these diagnostic studies (performed primarily via the femoral approach), the rates for mortality (0.12 percent), myocardial infarction (0.00 percent), and significant arrhythmias (0.30 percent) were the same as or less than those in previous studies, despite the fact that the patients included in this study were older and had more severe coronary disease. Vascular complications occurred in 1.6 percent of the procedures, but approximately one-third of the vascular problems arose in patients who required intra-aortic balloon counterpulsation. The incidence of cerebrovascular events was 0.20 percent.

Table 12–1 summarizes the complications of coronary angiography reported in the five series described above. Although there has been a gradually decreasing risk of cardiac complications since 1970, the incidence of cerebrovascular events and vascular complications has not shown much change.

In 1984 Nishimura and associates reported the arrhythmic complications that occurred in 7915 patients who had coronary angiography between 1978 and 1983.[N1] Thirty-nine significant ventricular arrhythmias occurred (0.5 percent), with 12 patients developing ventricular tachycardia, 23 ventricular fibrillation, and 4 ventricular tachycardia that degenerated into ventricular fibrillation. All of the patients had successful cardioversion. Sixty-seven percent of the arrhythmias occurred with injections to normal or minimally diseased coronary arteries. In these patients the arrhythmias were preceded by bradycardia and widening of the QRS complex and Q-T interval. On the other hand, arrhythmias that occurred with injection into diseased coronary arteries began with a PVC on the T wave. Twenty-four of the arrhythmias occurred with right coronary injection. Seven arrhythmias were preceded by ventricularization of the pressure waveform monitored at the tip of the coronary catheter. These authors concluded that the incidence of ventricular arrhythmias could be decreased by allowing time between injections, as many of the arrhythmias occurred late in the study (77 percent occurred with the last or next to last coronary injection). They also emphasized that close attention should be paid to the arterial pressure waveform. They hypothesized that atropine might prevent some arrhythmias, particularly those that followed bradycardia.

Franch and associates reported on 23,000 patients who underwent coronary arteriography from the femoral approach.[F1] Thromboembolic risk in this series increased with the use of increased numbers of catheters and wire changes. They suggested that heparinization and careful aspiration and flushing of the catheter might decrease the risk of thromboemboli. In 1987 Gordon and associates reported on angiographic complications in 107 patients with left main disease.[G5] There were three deaths, three myocardial infarctions, three patients with angina requiring intra-aortic balloon pumping and/or coronary artery bypass grafting, two episodes of ventricular fibrillation, and one episode of hypotension requiring intra-aortic balloon pump support. The risk of complications was greater if angina occurred within the 24 hours prior to catheterization and if there was a short distance from the catheter tip to the left main lesion. No significant differences in complication rates were related to New York Heart Association functional class, femoral versus brachial artery approach, number of coronary injections, amount of contrast agent used, severity of left main disease, number of diseased vessels, or the patient's blood pressure, left ventricular end-diastolic pressure, or ejection fraction.

The most recent data from the Society for Cardiac Angiography Registry, on 271,586 diagnostic procedures performed from July 1984 through June 1988, reveal a mortality rate of 0.11 percent, a myocardial infarction rate of 0.06 percent, a cerebrovascular accident rate of 0.07 percent, and a vascular complication rate of 0.42 percent. Complication rates for outpatient catheterization have also been reported and are detailed in a subsequent section on outpatient coronary angiography.

For catheterization-related cardiovascular complications, it is of interest to know whether the complications result from the catheterization or from the underlying coronary disease. Hildner and associates in 1973 reported on what they called "pseudo-complications" occurring within the 48 hours prior to or more than 24 hours following catheterization.[H2] The pseudo-complication rate was 2.3 percent, with a 1.2 percent mortality rate during this time period. In the 24 hours immediately following catheterization, there was a 2.6 percent complication rate and a 0.56 percent mortality. Thus, many complications resulted from the coronary disease itself rather than the catheterization. Hildner and associates followed up on these data in 1982 and reported a 0.81 percent incidence of complications with no catheterization-related deaths compared to a 0.81 percent incidence of pseudo-complications including four deaths (0.24 percent).[H3] Seven of the 13 pseudo-complications occurred within 2 hours prior to the scheduled procedure, which suggests that the patients' anxiety might have contributed to their occurrence.

Vagal responses characterized by nausea, hypotension, and bradycardia also occur during and following angiography. Particularly in elderly patients, a vasodepressor response can occur without bradycardia; this response generally responds to discontinuation of catheter maneuvering, intravenous atropine, elevation of the legs, and/or intravenous fluids. Pyrogen reactions due

Table 12–1. COMPLICATIONS OF CORONARY ANGIOGRAPHY

	Adams et al.[A4]	Bourassa and Noble[B3]	Davis et al.[D2]	Kennedy et al.[K1]	Wyman et al.[W13]
Number of angiograms	46,904	5250	7553	53,581	1609
Years of study	1970–1971	1970–1974	1975–1976	1979–1980	1986–1987
Vascular approach (% femoral/% brachial)	49/51	100/0	84/16	54/43*	95/5
Deaths (%)	0.45	0.23	0.20	0.14	0.12
Myocardial infarctions (%)	0.61	0.09	0.25	0.07	0.00
Arrhythmias (%)†	1.28	0.80	0.63	0.56	0.30
Cerebrovascular events (%)	0.23	0.13	0.03	0.07	0.20
Vascular complications (%)	1.62	0.85	0.74	0.57	1.60

*Site of vascular access was not reported in 3%.

†Generally includes ventricular fibrillation or prolonged ventricular tachycardia requiring countershock or bradyarrhythmias significant enough to require medical or pacemaker therapy. Davis and colleagues[D2] reported only ventricular fibrillation data.

to contamination by foreign proteins can also occur and generally respond to morphine sulfate, antihistamines, and/or antipyretics, The radiation exposure during coronary angiography varies from 20 to 45 rads and presents little risk to the patient unless multiple procedures are performed.[F1]

In summary, complications can and do occur during and following coronary angiography. The incidence is related to the patient's disease and to the experience of the angiographer and the laboratory. Therefore, Judkins and Gander suggested that each angiographer select a particular approach (brachial or femoral) and become proficient at it.[J2] It has been suggested that if a laboratory has a mortality rate greater than 0.1 percent, the selection of the patients and the skills of the angiographers should be re-evaluated; if the mortality rate is greater than 0.3 percent, procedures should be terminated.[G6] Although randomized studies have not defined specific means of decreasing angiographic complications, there are commonsense things that can be done to minimize complication rates. The angiographer must carefully examine and evaluate each patient prior to the angiographic study. Any electrolyte or hemodynamic instability should be corrected, unless the catheterization is an emergency procedure and must be performed without further stabilization of the patient. Dehydration should be avoided and premedication used to decrease the patient's anxiety. A temporary pacemaker should be available and in some cases should be inserted prior to the procedure. The amount of contrast agent used should be minimized, as greater than 3 ml/kg has been said to increase complication rates. If patients are unstable, filling pressures should be monitored (using a Swan-Ganz catheter), and if abnormalities are found they should be treated prior to coronary angiography. If the patient is extremely unstable, an intra-aortic balloon pump can be used to stabilize the patient during catheterization.[G7, W2] In techniques in which exchange wires are used, anticoagulation may be of benefit, but even more important are careful aspiration and flushing of the catheters, wiping of the wires, and limiting the time that the wire remains in the vascular system to 3 minutes. During the procedure the electrocardiogram should be monitored constantly and careful attention should be paid to the catheter tip pressure. Minimal time should be spent in the coronary arteries (no longer than 2½ to 4 minutes), and contrast agent should not be injected during episodes of ECG changes or significant chest pain until therapy has been given. For patients with small or diseased arteries, the use of 7 Fr. rather than 8 Fr. catheters might decrease local complications. However, the most important factors in reducing complication rates are the skill of the operator (particularly in the technique he has chosen), meticulous attention to details, and expediency in obtaining the necessary information in the least amount of time possible.

CONTRAST MEDIA AND THEIR EFFECTS IN CORONARY ANGIOGRAPHY

As contrast media are discussed in detail elsewhere in this book, the purpose here is not to review the different contrast media comprehensively but to provide an overview of the effects of intracoronary injection of contrast media on the electrocardiogram and hemodynamics and to review some of the adverse reactions that occur with such injections and possible ways to prevent these reactions. Such information is important as the angiographer considers the risk/benefit ratio of coronary angiography for a patient and plans the protocol for the study to minimize the adverse effects of contrast media on the patient.

Organic contrast agents were introduced in Germany by Dr. Moses Swick in the 1920's.[M1] Contrast media are generally substituted benzene rings that contain iodine. The most commonly used contrast media have been Renografin 76 (370 mg of iodine per ml in the form of 66 percent methylglucamine diatrizoate and 10 percent sodium diatrizoate) and Angiovist (also 370 mg of iodine per ml but formulated to cause less calcium binding). The commonly available contrast media have been of high osmolarity, and as some of the adverse effects of contrast media are due to the high osmolarity, newer agents have been developed with lower osmolarity. Low-osmolarity agents have been produced that are either nonionic (that is, do not form particles in solution) or dimers (such that the iodine content is twice as high for the number of particles in solution). Although low-osmolarity contrast agents have less effect on hemodynamics, the electrocardiogram, coronary blood flow, and renal blood flow than conventional contrast agents, their appropriate use is still in question, mainly because of their high cost. Contrast agents are excreted by glomerular filtration with a half-life of approximately 20 minutes. Less important routes of excretion are the biliary tract, the small bowel, sweat, tears, and saliva.

Some of the effects of the contrast agents used in coronary angiography are summarized in the following paragraphs.[F2, H4, M2]

Arrhythmias

Bradycardias

MacAlpin and associates reported that 58 percent of 107 patients showed an increase in the P-P interval of at least 0.10 second with intracoronary injection of a contrast agent.[M2] Sinus slowing is greater with injection into the right coronary artery than the left,[F2] and on occasion transient sinus arrest occurs. Reynolds found that in 50 of 75 patients sinus slowing occurred 20 to 30 seconds after contrast agent injection associated with an increase in the P-R interval, an increase in the QRS duration, and ST-T changes.[R4] Sinus slowing is related to the hypertonicity of the contrast agent. Studies by White and Eckberg and their associates have shown that the bradycardia is due to both a direct effect of the contrast medium on the sinus node and a reflex arising in the proximal coronary artery.[E1, W3] The bradycardia is attenuated but not prevented by atropine.

Ventricular Arrhythmias

Ventricular tachycardia and ventricular fibrillation occur in 0.1 to 1.28 percent of patients who have intracoronary contrast injections.[N1] Wolf found that injection of contrast media in dogs decreased the ventricular fibrillation threshold, and in vitro studies showed that this was due to activation of the slow response potential with initiation of reentry.[W4] The risk of ventricular fibrillation increases when an increased volume of contrast agent is injected and with injection into the right coronary artery. The incidence is also related to the sodium, calcium, and magnesium content of the contrast media.

Electrocardiographic Changes

MacAlpin and associates reported on the ECG changes in lead III in 107 patients during coronary angiography.[M2] With injection into the left coronary artery there was a decrease in R-wave amplitude in lead III with or without an increase in S-wave amplitude; there was also an increase in T-wave amplitude. Injection into the right coronary artery resulted in an increased R-wave amplitude in lead III with or without a decrease in the S wave; there was concomitant inversion of the T wave. (See Fig. 12–2.) The QRS axis rotated toward the site of the injection, and the T-wave axis rotated in the opposite direction.[F2, M2] Thus, injections in the right coronary artery generally result in inverted T waves in leads II, III, and aVF, whereas injections in the left coronary artery result in peaked T waves in leads II, III, and aVF.

Hemodynamic Changes

Following intracoronary injection of contrast medium, coronary blood flow increases up to 3.5 times the normal value. This increase was shown in dogs[L2] and has been confirmed in humans by measuring coronary sinus flow by the thermodilution technique.[B4] The increase in coronary blood flow may be protective, as it decreases the time during which contrast agent is present in the coronary arteries.

Injection of a contrast agent also produces vasodilatation, with a decrease in blood pressure, a 50 percent increase in cardiac

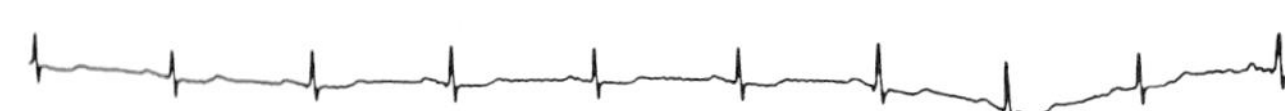

LEFT CORONARY ARTERY INJECTION

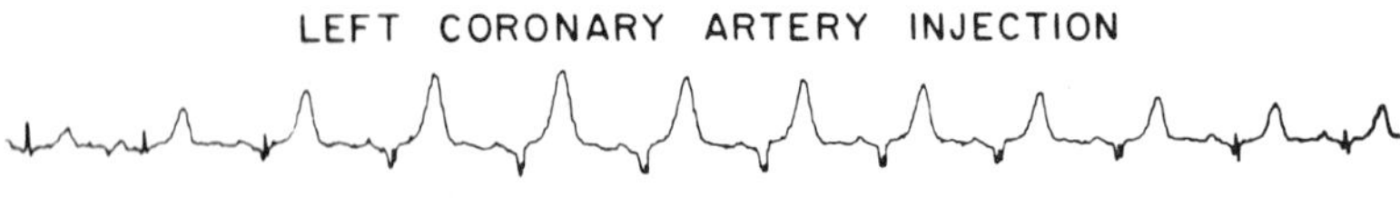

RIGHT CORONARY ARTERY INJECTION

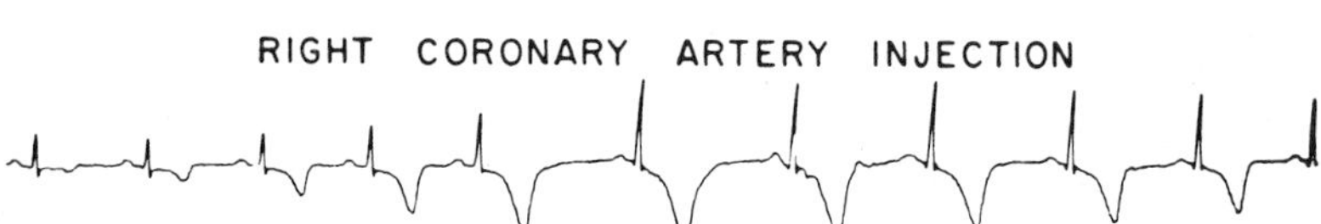

Figure 12–2. Lead III recording of an electrocardiogram taken before and after selective injections of contrast media into the left and right coronary arteries. With left coronary artery injection there are a decrease in R-wave amplitude and an increase in T-wave amplitude. Following right coronary artery injection, the lead III electrocardiogram shows an increase in R-wave amplitude and inverted T waves. (From MacAlpin, R.N., Weidner, W.A., Kattus, A.A., Jr., and Harafu, W.N.: Electrocardiographic changes during selective coronary cineangiography. Circulation 34:627, 1966, by permission of the American Heart Association, Inc.)

output, a decrease in systemic vascular resistance, and an increase in vascular volume. This induced vasodilatation is due to a direct effect of the contrast agent on the endothelium and a cholinergic reflex. Contrast agent injection increases left ventricular end-diastolic pressure and decreases left ventricular dP/dt. These hemodynamic changes are produced by either direct toxicity, the hypertonicity of the contrast medium, a decrease in O_2 delivery, or calcium chelation.[B2] If significant bradycardia and hypotension occur, aortic pressure and pulse can be increased by having the patient cough, which speeds washout of the contrast agent from the coronary arteries. Atropine and a pacemaker can also be used to decrease or treat bradycardia. It may also be helpful to remove the catheter from the coronary ostium to allow faster return of blood to the coronary circulation.

Nephrotoxicity

In a random population, the risk of nephropathy induced by contrast medium is 0 to 0.5 percent. However, a decrease in renal function occurs in up to 90 percent of patients in high-risk groups. Contrast nephropathy is defined as an acute impairment of renal function that occurs after the injection of contrast medium and for which other causes have been ruled out. Contrast nephropathy is due to acute tubular necrosis with an increase in creatinine level (and sometimes a decrease in urine volume) occurring within 24 hours. The creatinine level peaks in 2 to 5 days, and recovery occurs in 75 percent of affected patients in 4 to 14 days.[B5, H4]

Although several risk factors for the development of contrast-induced nephropathy have been proposed, the most important is baseline renal dysfunction. If the creatinine level is greater than 2.5 mg/dl prior to injection of the contrast agent, more than one-third of patients will have a creatinine rise greater than or equal to 1 mg/dl. Patients with diabetes mellitus have been said to have an increased risk of contrast agent-induced renal insufficiency, but whether this is due to the diabetes itself or underlying diabetic renal insufficiency is unclear. Other potential risk factors include age (greater than 60 years), dehydration, recent exposure to large volumes of contrast media, advanced atherosclerotic vascular disease, congestive heart failure with low cardiac output, impaired hepatic function, and multiple myeloma.[H4, W5] The risks of hyperuricemia and hypertension are most likely related to underlying renal insufficiency.

Of 139 patients with a creatinine level greater than 2 mg/dl who underwent 141 cardiac procedures at the Mayo Clinic, 23 percent developed contrast nephropathy.[T1] If there was no congestive heart failure, use of other contrast media, or insulin-dependent diabetes mellitus, the incidence of contrast nephropathy was 2 percent if less than 125 ml of contrast agent was used but 19 percent if more than 125 ml was used.[T1] In a study of 13 juvenile-onset diabetics with a mean creatinine level of 6.8 mg/dl, 12 (92 percent) developed some degree of progressive renal insufficiency following contrast agent injection, including 6 who required dialysis and 2 who required a potassium exchange resin.[W5] In 378 patients undergoing peripheral nonrenal angiography, the risk of renal failure was related only to underlying renal disease and not to the volume of contrast agent, the injection site, or a history of cardiac disease or diabetes mellitus.[D3] However, a positive renal nephrogram at 24 hours was a sensitive indicator of renal insufficiency. The authors stated that up to 50 percent of patients with a creatinine level of 4 to 5 mg/dl may require at least temporary dialysis.

The mechanism of contrast nephropathy has not been determined, but possibilities include renal hemodynamic changes (a transient increase in blood flow followed by a decrease due to contrast agent hyperosmolarity), a shift of renal blood flow from the cortex to the medulla, direct tubular toxicity, toxic effects on the red blood corpuscles and the microcirculation, tubular obstruction by protein or uric acid, and immune mechanisms (which have been seen in two cases, but probably do not play a role in the majority).[B6]

Although renal insufficiency induced by contrast agent injection is uncommon in patients without risk factors, in patients who do have risk factors and for whom coronary angiography is essential, it is important to try to prevent or minimize renal insult. It has been suggested that patients whose creatinine level is greater than 2 mg/dl should be treated with 500 ml of 20 percent mannitol to which furosemide has been added at a dose of 100 mg for each 1 mg/dl creatinine, beginning at a rate of 20 ml/hr 1 hour prior to the procedure and continuing for 6 hours following the procedure. Although no randomized studies have shown the benefit of this treatment, in small groups of patients it has appeared to be beneficial.[B5]

"Allergic" Reactions

"Allergic" reactions to contrast media occur in 3 percent of patients who undergo cardiac angiography and in 5 percent of all patients who receive contrast media. The incidence of reactions is higher in patients who have a history of an allergy to shellfish and can be as high as 17 to 60 percent in patients who have had a prior contrast reaction.[G8, G9] The allergic reactions consist of urticaria, pruritis, angioedema, bronchospasm, shock, vasodilatation, and/or true anaphylaxis. Reactions related to contrast media cause 500 deaths per year in the United States.[L3] Risk factors for contrast reactions in addition to those mentioned above include age greater than 50 years or less than 1 year, cardiac dysfunction, and coronary artery disease.[M1] The etiology of contrast reactions is not clear, but suggested mechanisms include anaphylactoid processes, endothelial damage (resulting in the release of serotonin, histamine, and prekallikrein with complement activation, activation of the coagulation pathway, and platelet aggregation), and direct cardiovascular effects (producing hypotension and changes in heart rate, contractility, and intravascular volume). The contrast agent may also cross the blood-brain barrier and produce direct chemotoxic effects on the central nervous system.[L4, M1] The stabilizer and preservatives in contrast agents may also play a role in the reactions.[H4]

Skin testing or small-dose testing is not predictive of the development of severe contrast reactions. Several pretreatment regimens have been suggested to decrease the incidence of contrast reactions, but their benefit has not been proved.[B2, G8, G9, L3, L5, M3, Z1] Suggested premedications include steroids (prednisone or methylprednisolone beginning 1 to 4 days prior to the procedure), antihistamines (diphenhydramine 25 mg q 6 hrs × 18 to 24 hours), and possibly H_2 blockers (cimetidine 300 mg q 6 hrs). Although studies have shown a decreased incidence of contrast reactions compared to historical controls when prednisone and diphenhydramine with or without ephedrine were used,[G8, G9] no documented benefit of cimetidine was seen. A decreased incidence of expected reactions was also seen when patients were given only prednisone (150 mg 18 hours before and 12 hours following angiography).[Z1] However, pretreatment does not prevent severe contrast reactions.[M3] Although the benefit of preangiographic cimetidine is unproved, a patient who developed a reaction despite pretreatment with steroids and antihistamines responded promptly to intravenous cimetidine.[M4] Severe reactions that occur with the use of contrast media, with or without premedication, should be treated like any anaphylactic reaction, with intravenous epinephrine, corticosteroids, and antihistamines and with appropriate resuscitative measures.

Other reactions related to contrast media include nausea and vomiting (perhaps related to a direct central nervous system effect), transient elevation of thyroxine, abnormal platelet and coagulation factor function, sickle-cell crisis, hemolysis, parotid swelling, tetany, and red cell aggregation.

The nonionic and low-osmolarity contrast media result in fewer side effects than traditional contrast media; however, major systemic reactions have been reported. These agents cause little or no change in left ventricular end-diastolic pressure or dP/dt and cause only minor changes in the electrocardiogram and heart rate. They also produce fewer osmotic changes in red blood cells and cause less endothelial damage. In animals, they produced a smaller increase in renal blood flow and less proteinuria, which suggests that the incidence of renal dysfunction might be decreased with use of these agents.[B7] Low-osmolarity contrast media also result in less nausea, vomiting, and anxiety. Overall, although experience is limited, low-osmolarity contrast media produce fewer than one-half of the reactions that occur with traditional contrast agents. The incidence of death with the low-osmolarity agents has been reported to be 0.0004 percent.[M1] However, the increase in comfort and safety with low-osmolarity agents carries a high price tag, as these agents cost 12 to 15 times more than conventional agents. Low-osmolarity contrast agents are currently being used in 15 to 25 percent of all angiographic studies. However, the exact situations in which these agents are indicated remain unclear. It is reasonable to suggest that low-osmolarity agents be used for high-risk patients, high-risk procedures, or procedures in which large volumes of contrast agent are needed.[J3, M1]

PREPARATION AND MANAGEMENT OF PATIENTS

Although each laboratory develops its own protocols for precatheterization management, use of medications during catheterization, and postcatheterization care, several guidelines have been proposed.[B2, C2, C3, F1, F3, G2, G6] Some of these recommendations are summarized here.

One of the most important factors in determining the safety and usefulness of coronary angiography is the precatheterization evaluation of the patient by the angiographer. Complete review of the patient's history and physical examination, laboratory data, chest x-ray, ECG, and past angiograms is essential to define the questions that need to be answered during the procedure as well as to evaluate the risk of the procedure to the patient. A baseline ECG in the 24 hours prior to catheterization is essential. After careful evaluation of the patient, the angiographer should define the catheterization protocol (access site, sequence of studies, contrast medium to use) for the patient. Although contrast medium affects hemodynamic measurements and can depress left ventricular function, it is better to obtain the most critical pieces of information first rather than state that left ventricular angiography should always be performed prior to coronary angiography. For example, if it has been decided on the basis of noninvasive testing that the patient has adequate left ventricular function to undergo coronary bypass surgery, perhaps the coronary angiogram should be performed prior to the left ventricular angiogram, for if any untoward events occur that require emergency surgical intervention, it would be more likely that the essential pieces of information have been obtained. If the patient's ventricular function is in question, performing the left ventricular angiogram first is prudent, because this sequence allows the most accurate assessment of left ventricular function. When hemodynamic measurements are important (i.e., in valvular heart disease), measurement of intracardiac pressures and cardiac output should generally be completed prior to any contrast agent injection. Potential exceptions would be cases of aortic stenosis in which the critical nature of the aortic stenosis has been defined by noninvasive testing (Doppler echocardiography) and the most important piece of information is whether the patient has concomitant coronary artery disease. In such cases, perhaps coronary angiograms should be performed first, followed by hemodynamic measurements and the other required angiograms.

In addition to allowing for careful evaluation of the patient and planning of the catheterization protocol, the precatheterization meeting should be the time when the patient is informed about the procedure, the reasons for the procedure, the potential risks of the procedure, and the reasons why the risk/benefit ratio is in favor of proceeding. It is important that a family member is also present for this discussion. Telling the patient what to expect during the procedure, and the things that will be expected of him, can decrease his anxiety. The patient should be informed of the potential need to cough on request and to take deep breaths and hold them during coronary injections. (It is particularly important that the patient not perform Valsalva's maneuver, as this elevates the diaphragm and makes coronary visualization more difficult.)

Following the precatheterization meeting, precatheterization orders should be written. Although formerly there was concern about continuing antianginals, particularly β-blockers, until the time of catheterization, all antianginal medications should generally be continued to prevent the development of increased angina due to medication withdrawal. The patient should take nothing by mouth for 6 to 8 hours prior to the catheterization; however, if the study is to be performed in the afternoon a light breakfast should be ordered. To prevent dehydration prior to the procedure, intravenous hydration should be given during the time when the patient is receiving nothing by mouth; this may decrease the incidence of vasovagal reactions and contrast-induced renal insufficiency. Antibiotics are not required. Prophylactic antiarrhythmic therapy, unless otherwise clinically indicated, is not necessary.

Premedication regimens vary; however, a sedative is generally used to decrease the patient's anxiety. The sedative may be diazepam (5–10 mg PO or IV) or secobarbital (50–100 mg PO). An antihistamine is also frequently included, either diphenhydramine (25–50 mg PO or IV) or promethazine (25–50 mg PO or IV). The use of atropine is variable; but unless the patient is unstable, tachycardic, to undergo an ergonovine study, or in atrial fibrillation, atropine (0.4–0.6 mg SC) can decrease vasovagal reactions and the sinus bradycardia that follow contrast agent injection. However, it must be realized that atropine can also increase heart rate and thus myocardial oxygen consumption; the resulting increased coronary flow may also decrease coronary opacification. Many physicians avoid intramuscular injections because they cause elevations of creatine phosphokinase (CPK) levels from skeletal muscle, which can complicate the interpretation of CPK levels following catheterization. However, the group at Emory reports use of a premedication regimen of 6.25 mg of promethazine, 6.25 mg of chlorpromazine, and 25 mg of meperidine IM.[F1] They use additional intravenous meperidine or diazepam as needed and also give 0.6 mg of atropine IV in many of their patients.

Medication protocols during angiography also vary. Many laboratories use full-dose heparin (5000 units IV at the beginning of the case, after the lines have been inserted) in an attempt to decrease thromboembolic phenomena; this was not shown to be beneficial in the CASS Registry.[D2] (If heparin is used and the femoral approach is taken, protamine is frequently given to reverse the anticoagulation at the end of the case.) Nitroglycerin (either sublingual or intracoronary) is commonly given to decrease coronary artery spasm, to decrease coronary vascular tone and allow better visualization of coronary lesions, and to allow better visualization of coronary collaterals. I prefer to perform the first left coronary angiogram prior to giving nitroglycerin. In the absence of left main coronary disease or hemodynamic instability, I routinely give sublingual or intracoronary nitroglycerin after the first left coronary angiogram. If a significant left main lesion is present or the patient is at all hemodynamically unstable, possibly nitroglycerin should be withheld as it could result in hypotension and decreased coronary perfusion, which might lead to complications. In cases of left main coronary stenosis or hemodynamic instability in which nitroglycerin is considered essential for better visualization of distal coronary vessels, a Swan-Ganz catheter should be placed prior to nitroglycerin therapy so that filling pressures can be monitored and treated appropriately. Several additional medications should be available for emergency use, including atropine, lidocaine, furosemide (or a similar diuretic), steroids, antihistamines, epinephrine, pressor agents (dopamine, norepinephrine), morphine, and nifedipine.

During the catheterization, the ECG and arterial pressure should be monitored continuously. Time should be allowed for the ECG and arterial pressure to return to the baseline state before the next injection of contrast agent. In cases of prolonged bradycardia or asystole with hypotension, having the patient cough can speed resolution of the hemodynamic and electrocardiographic changes by clearing contrast agent from the coronary vessels and providing a mechanical stimulus to the heart. The ability to place a temporary transvenous pacemaker and an intra-aortic balloon pump, if indicated, is also important.[G7, W2] Multiple projections of each coronary artery should be imaged with a 6-inch or higher-magnification image intensifier. The angiographic study should be recorded on videotape for immediate review.

Care of the patient following cardiac catheterization depends on the approach used. When the brachial approach is used, the patient can sit up and, if stable, can be out of bed almost immediately. When the procedure is performed by the femoral route, at least 4 to 8 hours of bed rest is important to achieve adequate hemostasis. The patient's vital signs should be monitored frequently (for example, every 15 minutes × 4, every 30 minutes × 4, every hour × 4, and every 4 hours until the following day). The arterial entry site and pulses distal to the site should be examined with each vital sign check. Unless the patient has had nausea and vomiting with the procedure, resumption of fluid intake and gradual resumption of full diet can occur very soon after catheterization. It is essential that the patient remain well hydrated, so if the patient is not taking sufficient oral fluids (1–2 liters over the 8 hours following catheterization) intravenous hydration should be continued. (Maintaining good hydration appears to decrease the incidence of vasovagal episodes following catheterization. If such episodes still occur they can be treated with atropine 1–3 mg IV and additional intravenous fluids.) Patients may be uncomfortable following the procedure, particularly when the femoral approach is used, and sedatives and analgesics should be given as necessary. Postcatheterization care should also include palpating the vascular site for an aneurysm and listening for a bruit, which might indicate the presence of an arteriovenous fistula. Previously ordered medications should be resumed as soon as possible.

If complications occur in the angiography laboratory, there are techniques that can be used to stabilize the patient. If congestive heart failure is aggravated, it can be treated with nitroglycerin and diuretics, with monitoring of right heart pressures if necessary. Angina can be treated with nitroglycerin (sublingual, intravenous, or intracoronary) or nifedipine. Elevation of left ventricular end-diastolic pressure frequently responds to nitrates and/or oxygen. Hypertension and tachycardia respond to intravenous β-blockers; hypertension can also be treated with nifedipine.

CORONARY ANGIOGRAPHIC TECHNIQUES

Prior to performing coronary angiography, one must decide about the arterial access site (brachial, femoral, or axillary), the access technique (cutdown and arteriotomy or the Seldinger technique with either wire exchanges or a vascular sheath), and the specific catheters to be used. Brachial access might be advantageous in patients with peripheral vascular disease, abdominal aortic aneurysms, or indwelling femoral clots. Brachial access may also be advantageous in patients with coarctation of the aorta or in obese patients in whom hemostasis following femoral access may be difficult. The major disadvantages of the brachial approach are an increased incidence of local arterial complications and the fact that tortuous subclavian vessels may make access difficult. The femoral technique is advantageous for patients with subclavian arterial disease, and, because preformed catheters are available for use in the femoral approach, direct catheter entry into the coronary artery may be easier. (However, this may actually be disadvantageous because less-skilled operators may perform the procedure and complication rates may increase.) Disadvantages of the femoral approach are that access may be difficult in the presence of aorto-iliac disease and that the use of multiple catheters may increase the embolic risk. The transaxillary approach as reported by Weidner and associates[W6] has been less commonly used than either the brachial or the femoral approach. Its advantage is that it allows vascular access closer to the coronary arteries and in an artery large enough so that reexamination via the same artery can be performed. A cutdown procedure on the brachial artery might be the least risky approach in patients who are anticoagulated, have defective hemostasis, are hypertensive, or have significant aortic regurgitation (in whom bleeding complications following percutaneous access, particularly from the femoral approach, may be increased).

Thorough reviews of the techniques of arterial entry and coronary angiography are provided elsewhere.[A1, B2, C3, C4, C6, F1, G2, G6, H5, J4, K2, K3, L6] Prior to summarizing four of the most commonly used techniques of coronary angiography, some general points deserve emphasis. First, if arterial spasm develops during cutdown or percutaneous entry into the brachial artery, it can be treated with morphine sulfate or decreased by using a smaller catheter. If a clot produces loss of distal pulses when the brachial or femoral approach is used, a Fogarty catheter can be used to remove the clot and restore distal perfusion. During brachial approaches, particularly cutdowns, proximal and distal heparin is recommended. For femoral approaches the use of heparin is more variable. When femoral access is used, the level of arterial puncture is important. To decrease bleeding complications the arterial entry site must be below the inguinal ligament; however, if vascular access is attempted too far distally, it may be difficult as the artery and vein separate. Almost all techniques of coronary angiography involve the use of a coronary manifold in which three different ports are used for contrast medium, waste, and monitoring of arterial pressure. Such a setup allows rapid return to monitoring of intracoronary pressure following injection of contrast medium through the coronary catheter.

Sones Technique

The Sones technique of brachial artery cutdown and use of a single catheter (with an end hole and four side holes) for left coronary angiography, right coronary angiography, and left ventriculography has the advantage of requiring only a single catheter. However, because of the presence of side holes as well as an end hole, obstruction at the distal tip may not damp catheter pressure. With the Sones technique it is necessary to learn the catheter manipulations involved in engaging the coronary arteries, but because the catheter tip is closer to the manipulating hand, the operator has a better "feel" for the catheter than in many of the femoral techniques.

Selective coronary artery entry is performed with the patient in a left anterior oblique position. Although several maneuvers can be used to perform selective coronary artery cannulation with the Sones catheter,[B2, H5] for left coronary artery cannulation the catheter tip is generally placed in the left coronary sinus and a shallow loop is formed. With gradual rotation and advancement of the catheter tip, the left coronary ostium is entered. (See Fig. 12–3.) For right coronary artery entry, a shallow loop toward the left coronary artery is rotated clockwise, with slight withdrawal, and the catheter is manipulated toward the right sinus of Valsalva until the right coronary artery is engaged. If ostial engagement is difficult, a deep breath may allow easier catheter entry into the coronary artery.[C3, C4]

Judkins Technique

Judkins catheters are preformed catheters with different designs for the right and left coronary arteries and with different sizes appropriate for different-sized aortic arches. The key to success with the Judkins technique is proper catheter selection. Judkins catheters come in sizes 3.5, 4, 5, and 6, where the size refers to the distance between the primary and secondary curvatures of the catheter. A size 4 catheter is for standard aortas; size 5 for older patients or those with unfolded aortas, hypertension, or medial disease; and size 6 for patients with aortic dilatation distal to a stenotic aortic valve. If a Judkins left coronary catheter is too small, it will double back on itself as it reaches the coronary ostium; if it is too long, it will be positioned vertically and rest on the tip of the sinus rather than in the coronary ostium.[J1]

The Judkins technique of selective coronary catheterization is illustrated in Figure 12–4. The left coronary artery is entered with the patient in a shallow left anterior oblique position. In this orientation, the left coronary catheter is placed en face (i.e., in profile) and slowly advanced with continuous tip pressure monitoring. After the catheter has apparently entered the coronary ostium, contrast agent is gently injected. If ventricularization or damping of the pressure occurs, the catheter is pulled back. If damping recurs on repositioning the catheter in the artery, nonselective injections may be used to rule out ostial disease. For right coronary artery entry, a shallow left anterior oblique position is again used. The right coronary catheter is positioned one-half to one rib interspace cephalad to the aortic valve and rotated clockwise until the catheter enters the right coronary ostium. If damping occurs, it may imply stenosis, subselective entry into the conus branch, or spasm around the catheter (which is much more common in the right coronary artery than in the left). Whether spasm or a significant lesion exists can be determined in many cases by repeating angiograms after nitroglycerin treatment or by performing sinus injections of contrast agent. (The Judkins technique of coronary angiography has been reviewed in detail elsewhere.)[J4, L6]

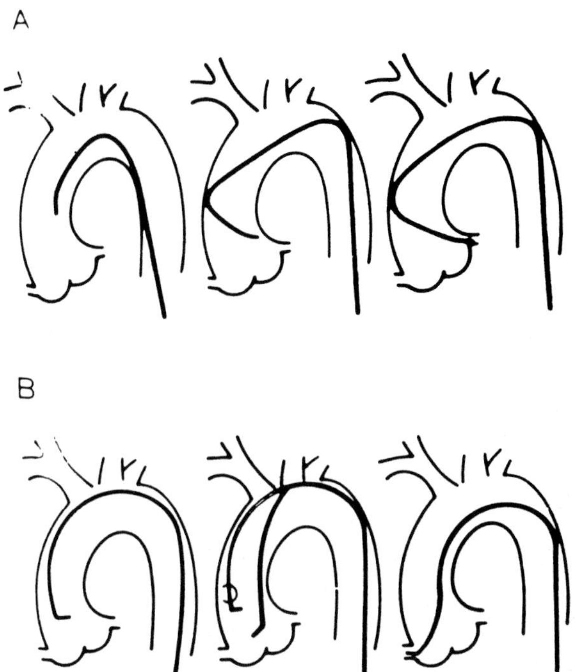

Figure 12–4. Selective catheterization of the left (*A*) and right (*B*) coronary arteries by the Judkins technique. Additional details concerning the Judkins technique can be found in the text. (From Conti, C.R.: Coronary arteriography. Circulation 55:227, 1977, by permission of the American Heart Association, Inc.)

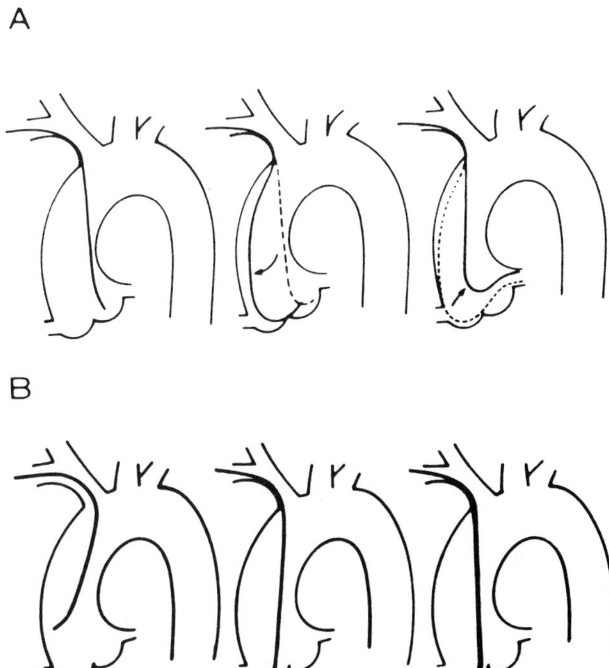

Figure 12–3. Illustration of the Sones technique for selective catheterization of the left (*A*) and right (*B*) coronary arteries. See text for additional details. (From Conti, C.R.: Coronary arteriography. Circulation 55:227, 1977, by permission of the American Heart Association, Inc.)

Amplatz Technique

Amplatz coronary catheters are preformed catheters and have the advantage that they can be used from either the brachial or the femoral approach. The disadvantages are that from the femoral approach, and on many occasions from the brachial approach, multiple catheter changes may be necessary, and if the angle of takeoff of the coronary artery from the aorta is unusual, selective coronary entry may be difficult.

To position the left Amplatz catheter in the left coronary ostium, the curve of the catheter is stabilized in the noncoronary cusp; to position the right Amplatz catheter, the curve of the catheter is placed in the left coronary cusp. The left catheter is advanced until its tip points upward and enters the coronary ostium; then with gradual, slight withdrawal the catheter is locked in place. (See Fig. 12–5.) Maneuvering of the right Amplatz catheter is similar to that previously described for the right Judkins catheter. If the catheter is too small it may slip through the valve or recoil from the ostium with injection or valve motion, or the tip may be unable to reach the coronary ostium. If the

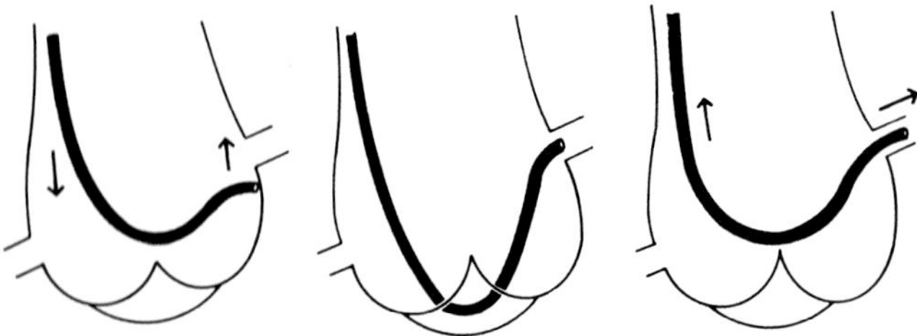

Figure 12–5. The technique of selective catheterization of the left coronary artery with an Amplatz catheter. (From Baim, D.S., and Grossman, W.: Coronary angiography. *In* Grossman, W. [ed.]: Cardiac Catheterization and Angiography. Lea & Febiger, Philadelphia, 1986, p. 179, with permission.)

Amplatz catheter is too large, the catheter may buckle so that the tip does not ascend to the level of the ostium or the tip may extend beyond the ostium itself.

Zir reported on 500 catheterizations performed by the brachial approach with preformed catheters (Amplatz catheters modified for the brachial approach in that they had a smaller curve and less hook on the end).[Z2] In many cases the right coronary artery was difficult to cannulate because of its sharp angle of origin. The use of the preformed catheters rather than Sones catheters was thought to be advantageous, however, because it allowed easier arterial entry, resulted in excellent opacification, allowed stable catheter position during contrast agent injection, and required minimal manipulation of the catheters.

Schoonmaker Technique

An additional catheter technique reported by Schoonmaker in 1974 is illustrated in Figure 12–6. In this technique a single catheter is used from the femoral approach.[S5] The single-catheter technique requires a bit more training than the use of preformed catheters from the femoral route; however, with experience, angiography can be performed in approximately 15 minutes by most operators.

The catheter is an 8 French 100-cm catheter with a 45-degree angle at its tip. To position the Schoonmaker catheter in the left coronary artery, a 30-degree right anterior oblique projection is used and the catheter tip is placed in the noncoronary cusp. In this position a loop of the tip of the catheter is formed, after which clockwise rotation results in the tip being positioned at the mouth of the coronary orifice. To enter the right coronary artery a 45- to 60-degree left anterior oblique projection is used. The catheter body is placed in the left coronary cusp, and with withdrawal and clockwise rotation the tip of the catheter is rotated into the right coronary ostium. Thus, the maneuvering of this catheter is very much like that described by Sones for his brachial technique. (Details of the Schoonmaker, multipurpose technique of coronary angiography may be found elsewhere.[K3, S5]) In a series of 6800 cases over 7 years, only 10 patients required use of a second catheter for selective coronary angiography. Embolic complications occurred in this series only if catheter exchanges were necessary, so proponents of this technique suggest that use of a single catheter decreases embolic complications.[S5]

Other Techniques

Many authors have proposed changes in the methods used to obtain arterial access. In 1979 Barry and associates reported the use of a sheath with a side arm and a hemostasis valve.[B8] The sheath made catheter changes easier and decreased the patient's discomfort during catheter changes. Side-arm pressure could be monitored during coronary injection, and, as a wire was not essential for catheter insertion, catheters without an endhole could be placed. The investigators reported that the arterial puncture had to occur at an angle of 45 degrees or less or the sheath would become kinked, and they routinely used heparin. Of 562 patients, two had local complications that required surgical repair and 10 percent required groin compression for longer than 10 minutes to achieve hemostasis. It was proposed that the sheath might decrease the incidence of thromboemboli by decreasing

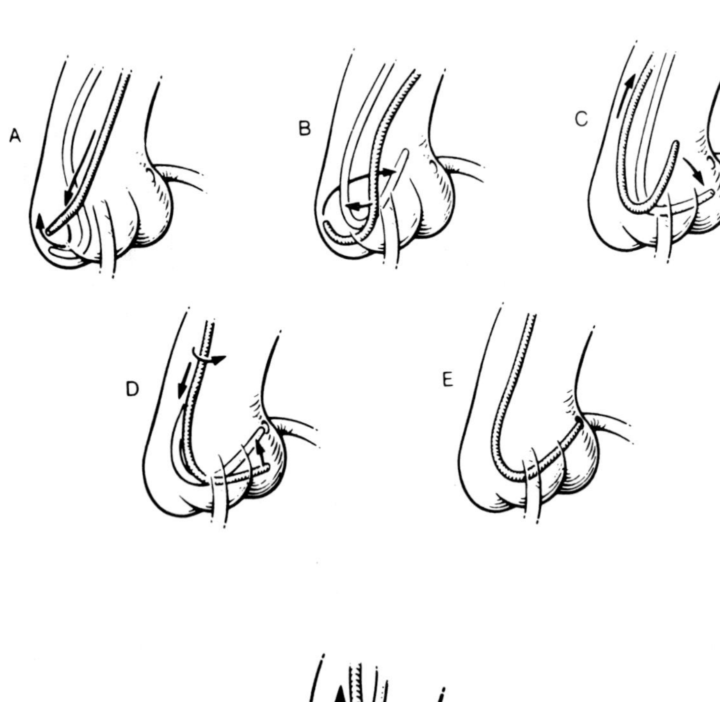

Figure 12–6. The Schoonmaker technique of selectively catheterizing the left coronary artery in the right anterior oblique projection (*top, A–E*) and the right coronary artery in the left anterior oblique projection (*bottom*). For entry into the left coronary artery the catheter tip is positioned in the noncoronary cusp, and clockwise rotation and slight withdrawal followed by gradual catheter advancement result in selective entry into the artery. For selective catheterization of the right coronary artery the catheter body is placed in the left coronary cusp. Withdrawal and clockwise rotation of the catheter are required to accomplish selective entry into the artery. (From King, S.B., III, and Douglas, J.S., Jr.: Coronary arteriography and left ventriculography: Multipurpose technique. *In* King, S.B., III, and Douglas, J.S., Jr. [eds.]: Coronary Arteriography and Angioplasty. McGraw-Hill, New York, 1985, pp. 252 and 256, with permission.)

the arterial trauma that occurs with catheter changes, by allowing aspiration and flushing between catheters, by requiring the guide wire to be present for shorter periods, and by decreasing the duration of the procedure.

In 1981 Fergusson and Kamada described percutaneous access via the brachial artery by use of a sheath without a hemostasis valve or side port,[F4] and in 1986 they reported results with this technique for 1783 patients.[F5] Ninety-six percent of attempts were successful with a 1.3 percent incidence of brachial occlusion, which in general was easily repaired. Three arteriovenous fistulas occurred. During catheter changes a blood pressure cuff and not a hemostasis valve was used for hemostasis, as it was thought that the catheter was easier to maneuver without a hemostasis valve. In the 62 cases in which percutaneous brachial entry was unsuccessful, the procedure was completed with either brachial cutdown or the femoral technique. The authors proposed this technique for use in the outpatient setting because of the easier achievement of hemostasis than with other techniques.

In 1984 Pepine and associates reported a slightly different percutaneous brachial technique in which a 7 French side-arm sheath with a hemostasis valve was used.[P2] One hundred patients underwent the procedure without failure or serious complications. Twelve of the patients had had at least one previous brachial cutdown. One patient with loss of a radial pulse was treated with cutdown and thrombectomy. The only other significant complications were 11 ecchymoses and 4 small hematomas. These authors suggested that sheaths protected the artery from the trauma of catheter motion. Cohen and associates reported on a series of brachial catheterizations performed by two angiographers at Mount Sinai between 1982 and 1984.[C7] The brachial catheterizations were done percutaneously in 254 patients and via cutdown in 184 patients. The complication rates were 3.1 percent and 2.1 percent, respectively. In four patients in whom the percutaneous route failed, successful cutdown was performed. The average duration of the procedure was 39 ± 10 minutes for the percutaneous route and 44 ± 13 minutes for cutdown.

In addition to the specific observations on each technique above, there are some pointers that are applicable to all techniques of coronary angiography. These are as follows:

- Damping or ventricularization of the pressure recorded at the catheter tip is indicative of restriction of inflow to the coronary artery. The restriction can be due to proximal stenosis, adverse catheter position, catheter-induced spasm, or subselective entry into a branch vessel.
- A vessel must be studied perpendicular to its course and in orthogonal views to allow adequate evaluation. (This is discussed further in a later section concerning the importance of angulated views in coronary angiography.)
- If resistance is met or the catheter tip pressure damps, do not advance the catheter.
- If one waits for ECG changes to identify catheter obstruction of the coronary artery, it is too late!
- Perform cineangiography during deep inspiration to clear the liver from the field of view.
- Inject the contrast agent in such a manner as to replace blood in the coronary artery for a period of 3 to 4 seconds (generally 3–9 ml in the left coronary artery and 2–4 ml in the right coronary artery).
- Failure of contrast to clear following coronary injection may be an indication of catheter obstruction of the coronary ostium. The catheter should be withdrawn.
- Tortuous arteries can impede torque control and may necessitate the use of catheters that require less manipulation.
- Be cautious if the catheter tip does not rotate when the catheter is being rotated outside the body. Evaluate the entire course of the catheter using fluoroscopy to rule out "kink" formation in tortuous iliac or abdominal vessels.
- If no lesions are seen on the angiograms and the patient's history strongly suggests coronary disease, take additional views to be certain no lesions have been missed.
- When lining up views for cineangiography, position the left coronary artery with the catheter tip near the top of the screen. The right coronary artery should be positioned with the catheter tip in the upper quadrant and not at the top of the screen, as the conus and sinus node branches frequently course cephalad.
- Allow hemodynamic and ECG changes to normalize before the next injection of contrast agent.

Instability of the patient was formerly considered a contraindication to cardiac catheterization. However, the possibility of acute interventions for patients with unstable angina or myocardial infarction has resulted in clinical circumstances in which angiography is indicated even though the patient is unstable. In addition to the use of medical therapy to stabilize these patients as much as possible prior to catheterization, it has been suggested that an intra-aortic balloon pump can produce resolution of ischemia and stabilization of the patient.[G7, W2] In a study by Gold and associates,[G7] all 11 patients with rest angina had significant relief of angina following intra-aortic balloon pumping, and recurrent angina occurred in 5 of the 11 when balloon pumping was interrupted. Weintraub and associates studied 16 similar patients and found that balloon counterpulsation produced significant resolution of chest pain and ECG changes in 15 patients.[W2] The mechanism of stabilization with balloon pumping is not clear, but theories include decreased oxygen demand due to decreased afterload, increased coronary perfusion pressure and thus increased coronary blood flow, augmentation of collateral blood flow, and redistribution of coronary blood flow.

Bypass Graft and Internal Mammary Artery Angiography

The location of coronary artery bypass grafts is less predictable than that of native coronary arteries; however, in general, right coronary grafts are placed on the right anterolateral aorta and left anterior descending and circumflex grafts are placed anteriorly. If the bypass graft itself or the stump of a graft cannot be defined by using selective bypass graft catheters or right coronary catheters, an aortogram may define a graft stump or a patent graft that could not be selectively cannulated. Internal mammary arteries are frequently studied in patients with previous vein bypass graft surgery (to confirm the integrity of these arteries should subsequent surgery be indicated) or in patients with recurrent angina following internal mammary artery grafting. An internal mammary artery catheter is guided into the subclavian artery over a wire, and the catheter is then gradually withdrawn until the internal mammary artery is selectively entered. Conventional high-osmolarity contrast agents produce significant chest pain when injected undiluted into the internal mammary arteries, so low-osmolarity contrast agents or contrast agents diluted with sterile saline should be used. In performing bypass graft or internal mammary artery graft angiograms, not only should vessel patency be analyzed but also the anastomosis to the native vessel and the distal vessel beyond the site of anastomosis should be evaluated.[L6]

IMPORTANCE OF ADEQUATE ANGIOGRAPHIC VIEWS

Despite the best efforts of the angiographer to obtain safe and correct catheter position and optimum opacification of the coronary vessels, lesions will be missed if angiographic views are not selected properly. For complete evaluation of a vessel for lesions, the entire vessel must be evaluated perpendicular to the x-ray beam and without foreshortening or overlap. Left anterior oblique (LAO) and right anterior oblique (RAO) views are routinely used; however, because of the oblique orientation of the heart in the thorax and the fact that the vessels curve around the epicardial surface of the heart, angles in the cranial-to-caudal plane are also required for adequate visualization of all portions of the coronary tree. The recent widespread use of C-arm angiographic systems has greatly facilitated the acquisition of such cranial and caudal angulated views.

Because of confusion about the terminology for angulated views, Paulin proposed in 1981 that projections should be described as if the observer was seeing the object transluminated by the x-ray source on the opposite side.[P3] The projections referred to as caudocranial and craniocaudal are illustrated in Figure 12–7. The view is considered caudocranial (subsequently referred to as cranial) if the observer's view appears to be downward from the patient's head and craniocaudal (subsequently referred to as caudal) if the observer's view appears to be upward from the patient's feet. Although angulated views increase the demand on the x-ray generator and also increase radiation scatter, they are essential in some cases for adequate visualization of the coronary arteries. Because of the increased demand and scatter, however, it is recommended that screening LAO and RAO views be done first, followed by angulated projections to bring out areas in question.[B2] For the left coronary artery, standard LAO and RAO views result in foreshortening and overlap of the proximal vessels; for the right coronary artery, the LAO projection foreshortens the posterior descending and right ventricular branches and the RAO projection foreshortens the proximal and distal right coronary artery. Thus, the major problem areas that may require specific evaluation are the left main coronary artery, the proximal circumflex and left anterior descending coronary arteries, the diagonal branches of the left anterior descending artery, and the distal right coronary artery plus the proximal portions of the posterior descending and posterolateral branches.[G6]

Numerous investigators have extolled the benefits of angulated projections.[A5–A8, B9, E2, E3, G10, S6] Many have found that in up to 50 percent of cases angulated views result in improved visualization of lesions, if not the uncovering of lesions not previously seen. Bunnell and associates suggested that the angle most helpful for bringing out the proximal left coronary artery and its branches is a shallow LAO or RAO with cranial angulation.[B9] Diagnosis was improved in 33 of 72 cases by using this view. In 1974, using a cut-film technique, Sos and associates confirmed that the use of lordotic views assisted in the evaluation of left main disease, of proximal left anterior descending and circumflex disease, and of left anterior descending and diagonal disease.[S6] Also in 1974, Eldh and Silverman proposed elevation of the patient on a wedge to obtain cranial angulation.[E2] In 1975 Arani and associates stated that LAO angulation with caudal projection was helpful in 47 percent of cases.[A5] Aldridge and co-workers found that in 20 percent of 100 consecutive coronary angiograms additional views unmasked lesions and in 34 percent analysis was improved.[A6] In 4 of 12 patients whose coronary arteries had been considered normal, angulated views unmasked lesions. Gomes and associates reported that shallow LAO projections of the right coronary artery with cranial angulation of 15 to 25 degrees allowed avoidance of errors at the takeoff of the posterior descending coronary artery in 12 of 20 cases.[G10] RAO projections with 15 degrees of either cranial or caudal angulation also improved separation of the distal right coronary artery and the posterior descending coronary artery. In 1981 Elliott and associates reported on 300 patients in whom cranial angulation in the RAO projection improved visualization of 80 percent of left anterior descending lesions and uncovered lesions in 70 percent.[E3] Similar projections improved the diagnosis of diagonal lesions in 75 percent. For 15 right coronary arteries, a cranial RAO projection improved separation of the posterior descending and posterolateral coronary arteries in over 80 percent. Aldridge reported that angled projections improved lesion visualization in 54 to 93 percent of patients.[A7] However, such angulation was problematic if patients were obese or had dense diaphragms, as adequate x-ray penetration was not always possible.

It is difficult to predict which angiographic view might be helpful for an individual patient because of variability in the lie of the heart and in each patient's coronary anatomy. However, there are views that are considered helpful for bringing out specific problem areas. The left main artery can generally be best visualized in a shallow LAO or RAO projection (such that the vessel is just off the spine) with 20 to 25 degrees of caudal angulation; the proximal left anterior descending artery can be brought out at 45 to 60 degrees LAO with 25 to 45 degrees of cranial angulation; and the proximal circumflex artery is frequently best seen in a 60 to 75 degree LAO projection with 20 to 45 degrees of caudal angulation. An RAO angle of 30 to 45 degrees with caudal angulation can also be used to bring out the proximal circumflex artery. To better evaluate the portion of the right coronary artery adjacent to the crux or the posterior descending and posterolateral coronary arteries, a shallow LAO or RAO view with a small amount of either cranial or caudal angulation, variable from patient to patient, can be useful. It is important for the angiographer to be experienced enough to determine the areas that are not adequately seen on routine views and then, beginning with these general guidelines, obtain the additional views that are necessary. Some of the more commonly used angulated angiographic projections are shown in Figure 12–8.

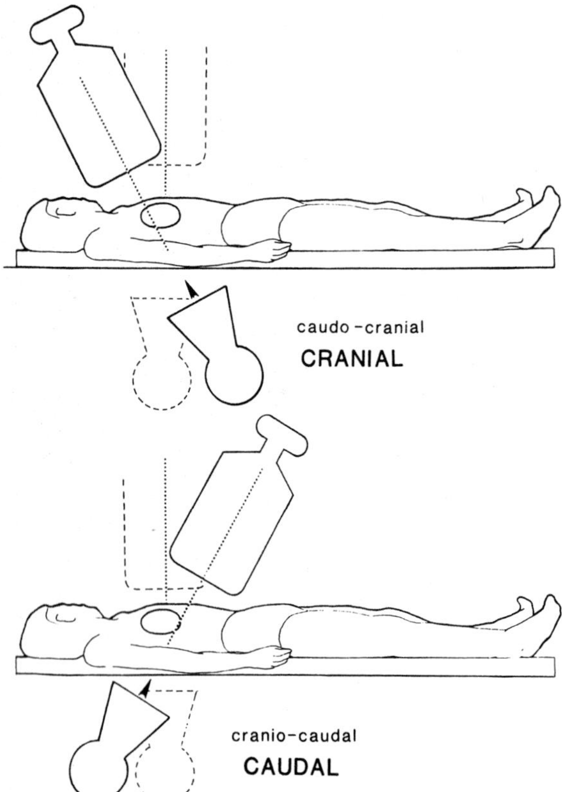

Figure 12–7. Illustration of the terminology used for describing angulations in the cranial/caudal plane. The arrowheads indicate the direction of travel of x-ray photons. The view is described as caudocranial or simply cranial (*top*) if the view is as if the observer is looking down from the patient's head; the craniocaudal or caudal view (*bottom*) is the projection as if the observer is looking upward from the patient's feet. (From Paulin, S.: Terminology for radiographic projections in cardiac angiography. Cathet. Cardiovasc. Diagn. 7:341, 1981, with permission.)

NORMAL CORONARY ANATOMY

The coronary arteries run in the atrioventricular and interventricular grooves along the epicardial surface. (See Fig. 12–9.) Although this description is straightforward, analyzing the coronary arteries on angiograms is somewhat difficult, and angulated views are necessary for adequate visualization, because the planes of the atrioventricular groove and the interventricular septum are set at 45-degree angles to the major planes of the body. The interventricular septum runs from right posterior to left anterior at 45 degrees from the frontal and sagittal planes. The atrioventricular groove runs from right anterior to left posterior and is also tilted 45 degrees to the horizontal and sagittal planes, running from right inferior to left superior. In addition, it is tilted 45 degrees to the horizontal and frontal planes, running from anteroinferior to posterosuperior. Thus, although the coronary arteries

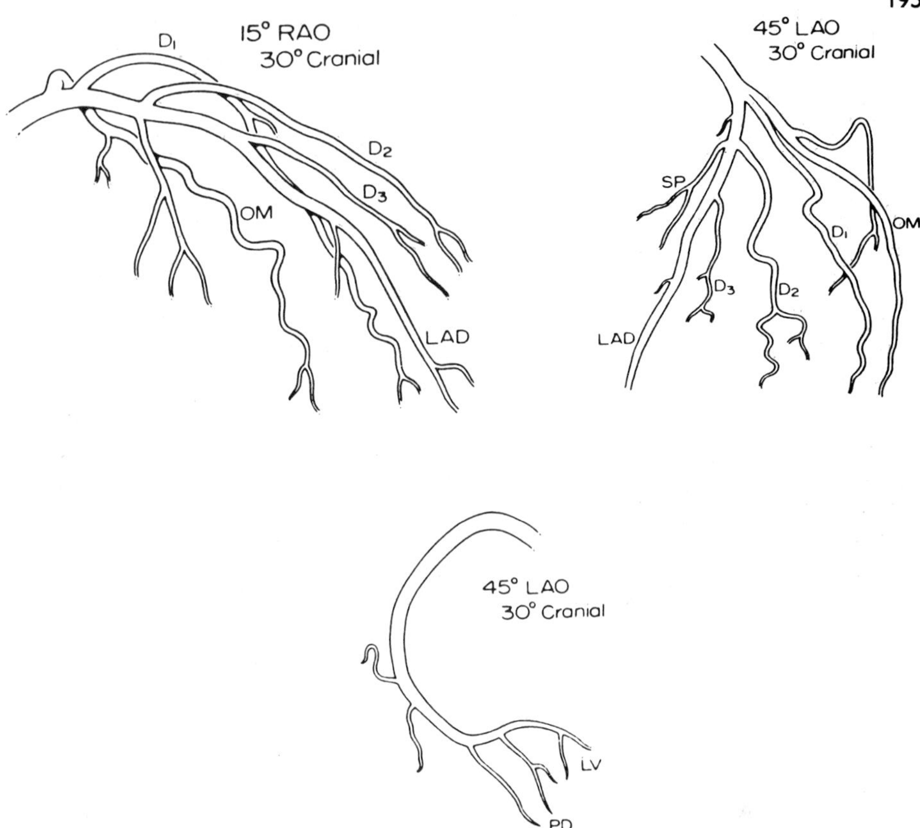

Figure 12–8. Specially angulated views of the coronary arteries designed to show areas that are frequently masked in conventional angiographic projections. (*Upper left*) A shallow right anterior oblique-cranial view of the left coronary artery that is helpful for evaluating the proximal left anterior descending coronary artery and its diagonal branches. (*Upper right*) A left anterior oblique view of the left coronary artery with cranial angulation; this view is useful for evaluating the proximal left anterior descending and circumflex coronary arteries in the left anterior oblique projection because it decreases the foreshortening of the proximal left coronary artery. (*Bottom*) A cranially angulated left anterior oblique projection of the right coronary artery better defines the takeoff of the posterior descending coronary artery from the distal right coronary artery. RAO—right anterior oblique; LAD—left anterior descending coronary artery; OM—obtuse marginal coronary artery; D1, D2, D3—diagonal branches of the left anterior descending coronary artery; LAO—left anterior oblique; SP—septal artery; PD—posterior descending coronary artery; LV—left ventricular branch. (From King, S.B., III, Douglas, J.S., Jr., and Morris, D.C.: New angiographic views for coronary arteriography. *In* Hurst, J.W. [ed.]: Update IV: The Heart. McGraw-Hill, New York, 1981, pp. 206, 208, and 210, with permission.)

follow the atrioventricular and interventricular grooves, the oblique positioning of the heart makes description and analysis of their course more difficult. The anterior descending and posterior descending arteries course along the anterior and posterior aspects of the interventricular septum, respectively, and the right and circumflex coronary arteries course in the atrioventricular groove.

Terms that describe certain borders of the heart will help in understanding the descriptions of the course of the coronary arteries. The obtuse margin of the heart is the superior (i.e., left)

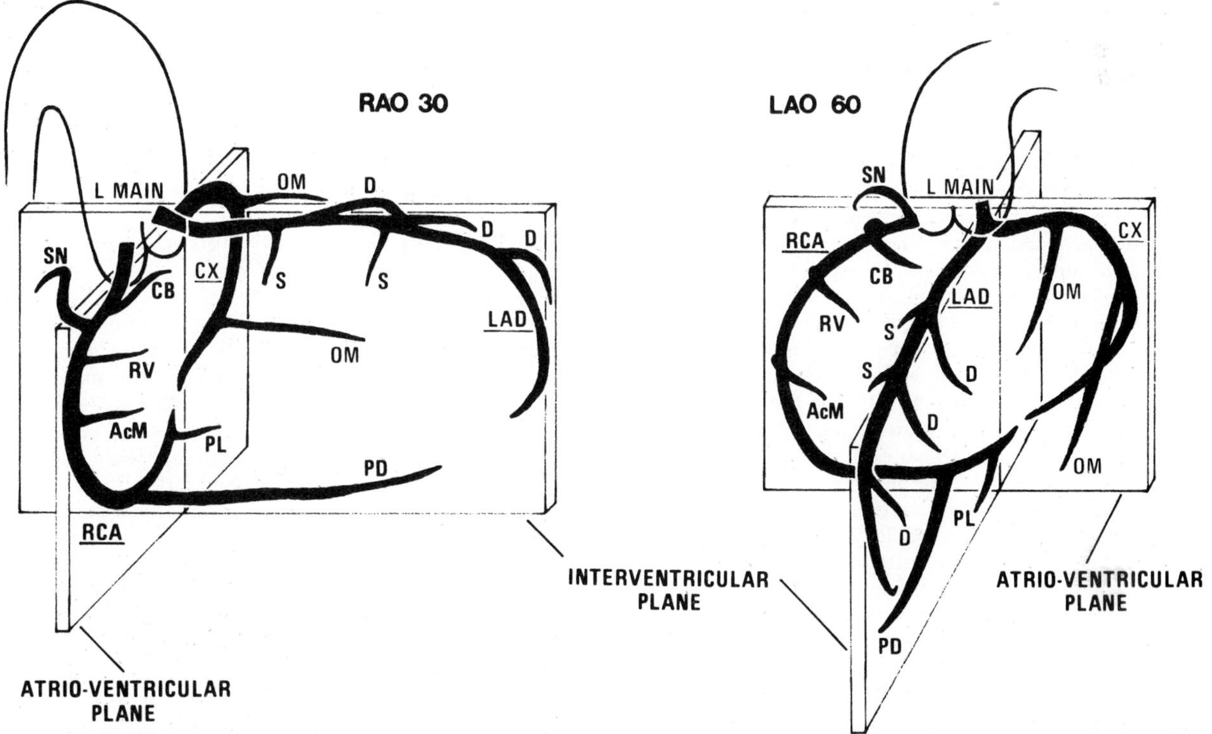

Figure 12–9. Relationship of the right and left coronary arteries to the interventricular and atrioventricular planes of the heart. RAO—right anterior oblique; LAO—left anterior oblique; L Main—left main; LAD—left anterior descending; D—diagonal; S—septal; CX—circumflex; OM—obtuse marginal; RCA—right coronary artery; CB—conus branch; SN—sinus node artery; RV—right ventricular branch; AcM—acute marginal; PD—posterior descending; PL—posterolateral left ventricular branch. (From Baim, D.S., and Grossman, W.: Coronary angiography. *In* Grossman, W. [ed.]: Cardiac Catheterization and Angiography. 3rd ed. Lea & Febiger, Philadelphia, 1986, p. 185, with permission.)

border of the heart, and the acute margin is the inferior (i.e., right) border of the heart. Other authors have described the course of the coronary arteries,[A1, B2, F1, G6, L6] and the following description of coronary anatomy is based on a compilation of previous descriptions supplemented by personal experience. The important thing to remember is that coronary anatomy is variable from person to person. This variability contributes to the challenge of correct interpretation of coronary angiograms, whether the coronary arteries are normal or abnormal.

The right coronary artery arises from the right or anterior sinus of Valsalva; the left coronary artery arises from the left sinus of Valsalva, which is to the left and posterior; and the noncoronary cusp, which is slightly larger than either of the two coronary cusps, lies to the right and posterior, between the two coronary cusps. The left coronary ostium tends to arise higher in the aorta than the right coronary ostium.

The concept of coronary dominance was described by Schlesinger in 1940.[S7] (The classification refers to the relative dominance of the right and left circumflex coronary arteries, for in humans the left coronary artery nearly always supplies the greatest portion of the left ventricular myocardium.) The dominant coronary artery was described by Schlesinger as that which supplies the inferior portion of the septum and the diaphragmatic wall of the left ventricle. In Schlesinger's original series, coronary circulations were right dominant in 45 percent, balanced in 34 percent, and left dominant in 18 percent. However, subsequent series have shown the right coronary artery to be dominant in 77 to 90 percent of cases. Of the remaining patients, one-half to two-thirds have left-dominant coronary systems (that is, the inferior wall of the left ventricle and the atrioventricular nodal artery arise from the circumflex coronary artery, and thus the entire septum is supplied by the left coronary system) and one-third to one-half have codominant coronary artery systems (in which both the right and circumflex coronary arteries provide blood to the inferior septum and diaphragmatic wall of the left ventricle).

The left coronary artery arises from the left sinus of Valsalva, has an initial diameter of approximately 4.5 mm, and courses behind the right ventricular outflow tract for 0 to 10 mm before dividing into the left anterior descending and cirumflex coronary arteries. (If difficulty is noted in distinguishing the left anterior descending and circumflex coronary arteries, note that they move in opposite directions, with the left anterior descending showing less motion than the circumflex.[G6]) In 20 to 37 percent of patients, the division of the left main artery is actually a trifurcation with a ramus medianus (ramus intermedius) branch arising between the left anterior descending and circumflex coronary arteries. The left anterior descending artery continues along the anterior interventricular groove and in 70 to 80 percent of patients courses around the apex to supply a portion of the apical inferior septum. In the RAO projection the left anterior descending coronary artery follows the anterior border of the heart, whereas in the LAO projection it is located in the midline of the heart. The left anterior descending artery gives off septal branches and a variable number of diagonal branches, which course to the anterolateral wall of the heart. In 90 percent of patients one to three diagonal branches are present. Thus, the left anterior descending coronary artery and its branches supply the anterior left ventricle, the anterolateral wall (the left ventricular free wall), and the interventricular septum. Although terminology varies, the proximal left anterior descending artery generally includes that portion of the vessel proximal to the origin of the first septal perforator and the mid left anterior descending artery includes that portion of the vessel between the first septal and second diagonal branches.

The circumflex coronary artery runs in the left atrioventricular groove, with its more distal course paralleling that of the coronary sinus. The circumflex artery supplies the lateral and posterior left ventricle, giving off one to three obtuse marginal branches. (These marginal branches are variable and the terminology concerning them is among the most variable in coronary angiography. In some centers the largest branch that courses to the actual obtuse margin of the heart is called the obtuse marginal and all the other branches are called lateral branches; in other centers the marginals are simply numbered first marginal, second marginal, third marginal, etc., similar to the system for numbering the diagonal branches of the left anterior descending coronary artery; others refer to the branches of the circumflex coronary artery that go to the posterolateral wall as lateral branches and number them sequentially. Thus, in describing coronary anatomy among various angiographers, the terminology used needs to be clarified.) The circumflex artery also gives off atrial branches. In 40 to 50 percent of patients the sinus node artery arises from the circumflex, and in 8 to 10 percent of patients the atrioventricular nodal artery and the posterior descending artery arise from the circumflex coronary artery, making the circumflex the "dominant" coronary artery.

The right coronary artery has an initial diameter of approximately 2.5 mm. It follows the right atrioventricular groove to the crux of the heart (the portion of the heart where the right atrioventricular groove, the left atrioventricular groove, and the posterior interventricular groove join). In 50 percent of cases the conus branch is the first branch of the right coronary artery; otherwise it arises from a separate ostium in the right coronary sinus. (This is an important anatomic variation, for the conus branch frequently supplies collaterals to the left anterior descending system.) The sinus node artery arises from the right coronary artery in 50 to 60 percent of cases. (It can be helpful in trying to distinguish the conus and the sinus node arteries to recall that their initial courses are in opposite directions.) The right coronary artery provides right ventricular branches, and in patients with a right-dominant coronary circulation it gives off the posterior descending coronary artery, which provides branches to the inferior portion of the ventricular septum. Following the posterior descending takeoff, the dominant right coronary artery continues in the atrioventricular groove to give off posterolateral left ventricular branches. The distal portion of the right coronary artery is extremely variable; two posterior descending arteries can be present, or in some cases one of the right ventricular branches actually provides a portion of the blood supply to the inferior ventricular wall. The acute marginal branches of the right coronary artery arise below the right atrium and just before or at the acute margin of the heart. These branches run toward the apex of the heart and in some cases also reach the inferior ventricular wall and provide a portion of the blood supply to the interventricular septum.

In coronary angiograms, only large to medium-sized coronary arteries (at least 100–200 μm in size) are seen; thus, only a small part of the entire coronary tree is actually visualized (the epicardial coronary arteries and some second-, third-, and fourth-order branches).

CONGENITAL ANOMALIES OF THE CORONARY ARTERIES

Congenital anomalies of the coronary arteries occur in 1 to 2 percent of patients. They frequently occur in association with other forms of congenital heart disease, but in many cases they are of no clinical significance. In angiographic series the incidence of anomalous origin of the coronary arteries was reported as 0.83 percent of 3750 patients at the Montreal Heart Institute,[C8] 1.2 percent of 4250 patients at St. Thomas Hospital in Nashville,[E4] and 0.64 percent of 7000 angiograms at Hahneman in Philadelphia.[K4] (See Table 12–2.) In the Hahneman series, associated valvular heart disease was present in 31 percent of patients. Variations in origin from the right coronary sinus are more frequent than variations from the left, and origin of the coronary arteries from the noncoronary sinus is rare.

Since coronary anomalies are infrequent and most are not clinically significant, it might be questioned why it is important to consider them at all. Knowledge of coronary anomalies is important for coronary angiographers for three reasons. First, if an anomalous coronary origin is not realized, a totally occluded coronary artery may be mistakenly diagnosed. Second, some coronary anomalies can result in myocardial ischemia. Third, it is important for surgeons to be aware of anomalous coronary

Table 12–2. ANOMALOUS AORTIC ORIGINS OF THE CORONARY ARTERIES

	Chaitman et al.[C8]	Engel et al.[E4*]	Kimbiris et al.[K4†]
Number of patients	3750	4250	7000
Incidence of anomalous coronary arteries (%)			
Total	0.83	1.20	0.64
Origin of Cx‡ from right sinus of Valsalva	0.45	0.71	0.37
Origin of both coronary arteries from left sinus of Valsalva	0.19	0.07	0.17
Origin of both coronary arteries from right sinus of Valsalva	0.19	0.11	0.06
Origin of LAD‡ from right sinus of Valsalva	NR‡	0.07	0.03
Origin of first septal artery from right sinus of Valsalva	NR	0.09	0.04

*The series reported by Engel and associates[E4] also included one case of left main origin from the pulmonary artery, one case of LAD origin from the pulmonary artery and Cx origin from the right coronary sinus, and eight cases of separate ostia for the LAD and Cx in the left coronary sinus.

†In the series of Kimbiris and colleagues[K4] two patients had a combination of the listed coronary anomalies.

‡Cx—circumflex coronary artery; LAD—left anterior descending coronary artery; NR—not reported.

arteries as they can be damaged during open-heart surgery. For convenience, coronary artery anomalies can be divided into those that affect perfusion and those that have no effect on perfusion.[G6, L6, L7] We will first describe coronary anomalies that can result in perfusion abnormalities.

Coronary Anomalies That Alter Myocardial Perfusion

Coronary Artery Fistulas

These are the most common anomalies that can affect coronary perfusion. In half of patients, coronary fistulas are totally asymptomatic; in the other half they may be detected because of a heart murmur or may present with complications such as congestive heart failure, myocardial ischemia or infarction (due to a coronary steal phenomenon), endocarditis, or rupture of the aneurysmal segments of the coronary arteries. About 50 percent of fistulas arise from the right coronary artery, 42 percent from the left coronary artery, and 5 percent from both.[L7] Coronary fistulas drain into the right side of the heart more commonly than the left, and in one series the right ventricle was the site of drainage in 41 percent, the right atrium in 26 percent, the pulmonary artery in 17 percent, the coronary sinus in 7 percent, the left atrium in 5 percent, the left ventricle in 3 percent, and the superior vena cava in 1 percent.[L7] An example of a fistula from the right coronary artery that drains into the coronary sinus is shown in Figure 12–10. If patients have symptoms due to coronary artery fistulas, the treatment is to obliterate the fistula but preserve forward coronary flow, usually by means of coronary artery bypass grafting.

Coronary fistulas can be acquired as well as congenital. They can occur following myocardial infarction,[R5] and recently an increased incidence of coronary artery fistulas has been described in patients following cardiac transplantation.[S8] An incidence of coronary fistulas of 8 percent was found in 176 heart transplant patients, compared to an incidence of 0.2 percent in 1000 control patients. In the transplant population the fistulas were single in nine patients and multiple in five. Fifty-two percent arose from the right coronary artery, 43 percent from the left anterior descending coronary artery, and 5 percent from the circumflex coronary artery. All drained into the right ventricle, none were symptomatic, and no shunts were detected by oxygen saturation. However, the transplant patients with coronary fistulas had a slightly higher cardiac index and pulmonary arterial oxygen saturation than those without coronary fistulas. On follow-up angiograms, three of the fistulas increased in size, three remained the same, two decreased in size, and three disappeared. Fitchett and associates also reported coronary arterial–right ventricular fistulas in five post-transplantation patients. Two of these fistulas were not seen on the first yearly angiogram, so they were not congenital anomalies present in the donor heart.[F6] Although the etiology of the increased incidence of coronary fistulas in the cardiac transplant population is uncertain, one hypothesis is that they are related to the biopsies of right ventricular endomyocardium that are performed for the diagnosis of rejection.

Origin of the Left Coronary Artery from the Pulmonary Artery[L7, W7, W8]

Origin of the left coronary artery from the pulmonary artery generally produces early myocardial ischemia that results in an infant syndrome of failure to thrive, tachypnea, wheezing, and angina. In 75 to 90 percent of reported cases, the patients die as infants or children. Those who survive to adulthood present with mitral regurgitation, angina, and congestive heart failure. There is also a high incidence of sudden death in adults with this syndrome. Origin of the left coronary artery from the pulmonary artery results in low coronary perfusion pressure and low oxygen saturation in the blood perfusing the left coronary artery. Survival depends on the development of collaterals from the right coronary artery; however, a steal syndrome can develop in which flow proceeds from the right coronary system to the left coronary artery and on into the pulmonary artery. In patients in whom the anomaly is diagnosed, treatment consists of ligation of the left coronary artery at its origin from the pulmonary artery, either

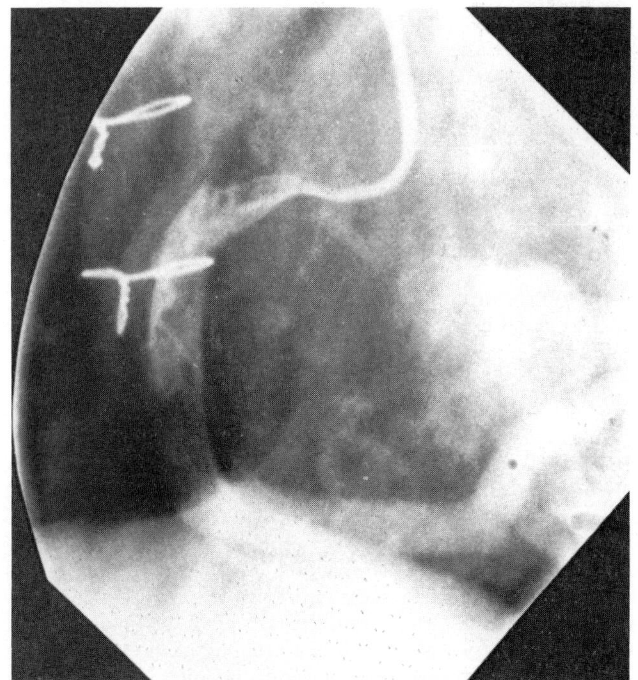

Figure 12–10. A fistula from the right coronary artery to the coronary sinus is shown here (left anterior oblique projection). The right coronary artery is markedly dilated, possibly because of the increased right coronary flow caused by the fistula.

alone or associated with coronary artery bypass grafting or reimplantation of the left coronary artery into the aorta.

Congenital Stenosis or Atresia of the Coronary Arteries

This rare anomaly usually occurs in association with other congenital heart diseases, including calcific coronary sclerosis, supravalvular aortic stenosis, homocystinuria, Hurler's syndrome, progeria, or the congenital rubella syndrome.[L7]

Origin of the Left or the Right Coronary Artery from the Opposite Coronary Sinus with Passage of the Vessel Between the Aorta and the Right Ventricular Outflow Tract[C8, C9, K4] (See Fig. 12–11.)

Origin of the left coronary artery from the right coronary sinus or the right coronary artery with passage of the left main coronary trunk between the aorta and pulmonary artery was seen in 33 of 475,000 autopsies.[C9] It has been associated with sudden death in 27 to 33 percent of patients. The mechanism of sudden death is not known but may be related to "squeezing" of the left main coronary artery between the two vessels (although this is unlikely due to the low pulmonary artery pressure involved), to a congenitally small left coronary artery, to kinking or spasm of the artery as it passes between the other vascular structures, or to the slitlike orifice of the left main artery or the acute angle of its takeoff when it arises in this position.

Origin of the right coronary artery from the left coronary sinus with passage of this vessel between the aorta and the right ventricular outflow tract was initially thought to be benign; however, angina, myocardial infarction, syncope, and sudden death (associated with left ventricular scarring in the absence of coronary artery disease) have been reported. Brandt and associates described a patient in whom the right coronary artery arose from the left coronary sinus and passed between the great vessels. They found that coronary flow reserve (evaluated with an epicardial Doppler probe in the operating room) was decreased by 50 percent in this anomalously originating right coronary artery. The abnormality in flow reserve was corrected by coronary artery bypass grafting.[B10] Thus, origin of the right coronary artery from the left sinus or left coronary artery can have pathophysiologic significance. Again, the reason for the physiologic significance of this anomaly is unclear but may involve the slitlike origin of the right coronary artery or compression of the vessel between the aorta and pulmonary outflow tract. Kragel and Roberts have recently suggested that the dominance of the coronary system may be the most important factor in determining whether anomalous vessels coursing between the aorta and pulmonary outflow tract are of clinical significance.[K5]

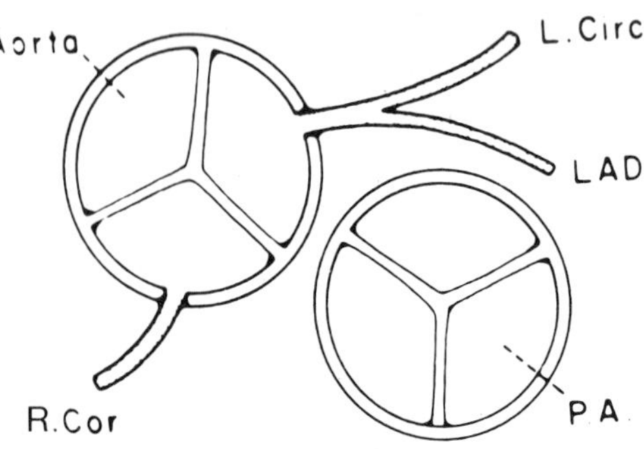

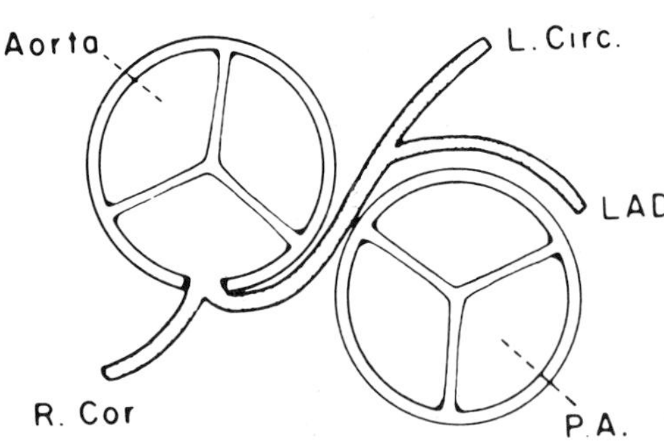

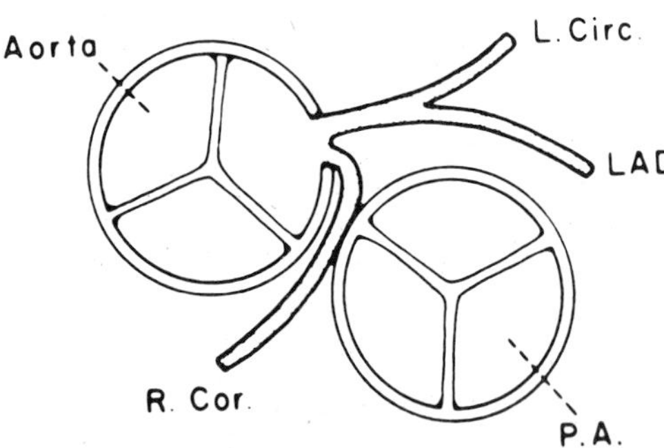

Figure 12–11. (*Top*) Normal relationship of the aorta, the pulmonary artery (P.A.), and the origins of the right (R. Cor.), left circumflex (L. Circ.), and left anterior descending (LAD) coronary arteries. (*Middle*) Anomalous origin of the left main coronary artery from the right sinus of Valsalva and (*bottom*) anomalous origin of the right coronary artery from the left sinus of Valsalva. For the anomalous coronary origins illustrated here, the anomalous coronary artery passes between the aorta and the pulmonary artery; such anomalies may be of physiologic significance. (From Cheitlin, M.D., DeCastro, C.M., and McAllister, H.A.: Sudden death as a complication of anomalous left coronary origin from the anterior sinus of Valsalva. A not-so-minor congenital anomaly. Circulation 50:780, 1974, by permission of the American Heart Association, Inc.)

Coronary Anomalies That Do Not Alter Myocardial Perfusion

Origin of the Circumflex Coronary Artery from the Right Coronary Sinus or the Right Coronary Artery

This anomaly occurs in 0.67 percent of cases[C8] and is the most common of all congenital coronary anomalies.[V1] In one-half of patients it is found in association with other cardiac anomalies. The vessel courses posterior to the aortic root and the noncoronary sinus to enter the left atrioventricular groove and supply its usual territory of the posterolateral left ventricle. Two angiographic signs have been suggested for anticipating origin of the circumflex coronary artery from the right coronary sinus.[P4] These are the aortic root sign, which is a profiling of the vessel across the aortic root during right anterior oblique left ventricular angiography, and the presence of a nonperfused region of the heart in the left circumflex territory after completion of left and right coronary angiography.

Origin of the Left Anterior Descending Artery from the Right Coronary Artery or Right Coronary Sinus

This anomalous vessel generally courses anterior to the pulmonary artery and is thought to be of no physiologic significance. If difficulty is noted in determining the course of the left anterior descending coronary artery—that is, whether it passes anterior or posterior to the pulmonary artery—positioning a catheter in the pulmonary artery during coronary angiography may be helpful.

Single Coronary Artery

A single coronary artery was reported in 0.04 percent of cases at Hahneman[K4] and in 0.024 percent of cases in another series;[L8] in the latter series, 40 percent of the cases were associated with other congenital cardiac anomalies. A single coronary artery is of potential importance only if the artery passes between the aorta and the pulmonary artery. Three types of single coronary artery have been described. In the first, the single artery initially follows the course of one of the normal coronary arteries and then swings around the heart to supply the distribution of the second coronary artery. In the second, the ostium is in the position of one of the normal coronary ostia, but branches come off proximally to supply the other coronary territory. In the third type, totally irregular coronary perfusion is seen. As the corrected cross-sectional area of the single coronary artery is less than that of a left coronary artery plus a right coronary artery, it has been suggested that the anomaly may be of clinical significance. Accelerated atherosclerosis may also occur due to the irregular course and bending of the artery. Congestive heart failure and sudden death have been reported.[L8]

Multiple Ostia of the Coronary Arteries

In a pathologic series, 50 percent of patients had a separate origin for the conus artery in the right coronary sinus. This is important, as the conus artery can be a major source of collaterals in cases of left anterior descending stenosis or occlusion. Separate origin of the anterior descending and circumflex coronary arteries was observed in 1 percent of 2000 autopsy cases.[V1]

High Origin of the Coronary Arteries

In a pathologic series, Vlodaver and associates found that in 30 percent of patients the left coronary ostium arose above the junction of the coronary sinuses and the tubular aorta, in 8 percent the right coronary artery arose above this junction, and in 6 percent both coronary arteries arose from the tubular aorta.[V1]

Horseshoe Coronary Artery (with Two Ostia to the Aorta): Origin of the First Septal Perforator from the Right Coronary Artery or Right Coronary Sinus

Thus, although coronary anomalies are uncommon, they can be of clinical significance, and the presence of an anomalous coronary artery should be considered in a young person with chest pain or sudden death.

CORONARY COLLATERALS

Coronary collaterals are said to be present when a coronary artery is seen beyond the site of an occlusion or a stenosis so severe that it prevents significant antegrade flow. In normal hearts at postmortem examination small anastomotic vessels are seen, and it is suggested that in the presence of coronary artery disease these vessels actually increase in size to form collaterals, probably due to the pressure gradients that develop between normally perfused portions of the heart and the small nonfunctioning collaterals distal to sites of coronary occlusion. Collateral vessels are generally not seen until the stenosis reaches 75 to 90 percent severity. One hundred angiograms were reviewed by Gensini and DaCosta.[G11] Fifty-three angiograms with no evidence of significant coronary artery disease showed no collateral vessels. Of 47 angiograms with evidence of significant coronary disease, 37 showed collateral vessels and all but 1 of 67 vessels with collaterals contained greater than 90 percent stenoses.

Since collaterals were first seen, there has been controversy concerning their clinical importance. Initially it was thought that collaterals indicated severe disease but that they were of no functional significance. Helfant and associates reported in 1970 that in 111 patients with coronary artery disease, there was no difference in wall motion abnormalities, left ventricular end-diastolic pressure, or cardiac index between patients with collaterals and those without collaterals.[H6] Helfant and Gorlin reported in 1972 that postobstructive coronary flow was not changed in the presence of collateral vessels, that ECGs were not different whether collaterals were present or absent, and that treadmill tests were more commonly positive in patients with collaterals than in patients without collaterals.[H7] In 1976 Hamby and associates reported that collaterals appeared to be of benefit in patients with left anterior descending coronary artery occlusions but of no benefit in patients with right coronary artery occlusions.[H8] In 1981 Tubau and associates reported on 37 patients with one-vessel coronary artery disease, 16 of whom had collaterals.[T2] Some protective effect of collaterals was suggested, as exercise thallium perfusion scans showed defects in only 40 percent of patients with collaterals versus 100 percent of patients without collaterals. However, ST segment depression and work capacity on the treadmill were not affected by collaterals.

The most convincing evidence for functional significance of collaterals in humans is that angiographic total occlusions are seen in patients without pathologic evidence of myocardial infarction. Furthermore, several studies suggest that coronary collateral vessels are functionally important. In 1975 Hecht and associates reported that in 43 patients with coronary artery disease, normal wall motion was more common if good collateral filling was present than if no collateral filling was present.[H9] They suggested that it was the size rather than the presence or absence of collaterals that was important in determining their functional significance. In 1976 Williams and associates reported on 20 patients with acute myocardial infarction, 6 of whom were considered to have "adequate" collateral vessels.[W9] In this series, patients with adequate collaterals had lower left ventricular end-diastolic pressure, less dyssynergy, higher cardiac index, higher stroke work index, higher ejection fraction, and greater survival than patients without collaterals. In 1978 Schwarz and associates reported that ejection fraction and wall motion were better in patients with coronary collaterals and that these patients had fewer myocardial infarctions.[S9] However, rapid pacing resulted in wall motion abnormalities in 12 patients with left anterior descending coronary occlusions and collaterals. This study suggested that although collateral vessels may preserve myocardial viability at rest, they are not adequate to prevent myocardial ischemia during stress. In 1982 it was reported that patients with collateral-dependent beds could have normal exercise thallium scans.[E5] Patients who, in angiographic studies, had shorter times to the appearance of contrast agent in the collaterals were more likely to have normal thallium perfusion scans. Finally, Probst and co-workers reported that in 63 patients with single-vessel coronary artery disease who underwent angioplasty, there was a significant positive relationship between distal coronary occlusion pressure and the extent of angiographic collaterals.[P5] There was also less difference in the distal coronary pressure before and during balloon occlusion in the presence of collaterals.

The pathways most commonly taken by coronary collaterals have been described in detail by other authors.[A1, L9] Collaterals can arise from the artery in which the occlusive stenosis is seen (homocoronary or intracoronary collaterals) or from other coronary vessels (intercoronary collaterals). Some of the most common coronary collateral pathways are listed in the following section.

Collateral Pathways to the Left Anterior Descending Artery

1. From the posterior descending via septal branches.
2. From the posterior descending around the apex.
3. From the acute marginal branch of the right coronary artery.
4. From the conus branch of the right coronary artery via Vieussen's circle.
5. From the obtuse marginal branch of the circumflex artery.
6. From diagonal branches of the left anterior descending artery.
7. From left anterior descending septal to septal collaterals.

Collateral Pathways to the Right Coronary Artery

1. From the left anterior descending via septal branches.
2. From the left anterior descending around the apex.

3. From the distal circumflex to the right coronary artery or the atrioventricular nodal artery.
4. From the obtuse marginal via posterior left ventricular branches.
5. From the right ventricular branch of the left anterior descending artery to the marginal branch of the right coronary artery.
6. From Kugel's artery along the anterior atrial septum to the atrioventricular nodal artery.
7. From the sinus node artery to the left atrial circumflex artery and subsequently to the right coronary artery.
8. From the conus branch or the acute marginal branch of the right coronary artery to more distal branches.
9. From the distal or left atrial circumflex artery to the atrioventricular nodal artery.

Collateral Pathways to the Circumflex Coronary Artery

1. From the left atrial circumflex to the more distal circumflex.
2. From a proximal marginal branch to a more distal marginal branch.
3. From a diagonal branch of the left anterior descending artery to a marginal branch.
4. From the distal right coronary artery to the distal circumflex artery.
5. From a posterior left ventricular branch of the right coronary artery to the obtuse marginal branch.

CORONARY BRIDGING

Bridging of myocardial vessels was first described by Block in 1796. Bridging refers to the intramural location of a coronary artery that appears on an angiogram as a systolic narrowing. Although autopsy reports show a widely variable incidence of bridging (5–86 percent), angiographic studies show an incidence of 0.5 to 12 percent. The functional significance of coronary bridging remains controversial. Generally, bridging is not thought to result in symptoms, as the coronary narrowing occurs during systole and most coronary flow occurs during diastole. This was confirmed by Kramer and associates, who reported a 12 percent incidence of bridging in 658 otherwise normal cineangiograms.[K6] In this series all of the bridges occurred in the left anterior descending distribution. The 5-year survival was 97 percent, and no myocardial infarctions occurred in the survivors.[K6] Marcus has reported that the flow reserve of a human coronary artery with a prominent myocardial bridge studied intraoperatively was nearly normal and diastolic inflow to the vessel was not delayed.[R6]

In 1976 Noble and associates reported a 0.51 percent incidence of intramyocardial left anterior descending coronary arteries on 5250 coronary angiograms.[N2] A more extensive study of 11 of these patients showed that if the systolic narrowing resulted in greater than 75 percent obstruction of the vessel, there was ST segment depression and lactate production with pacing. At 50 to 75 percent systolic narrowing, two of four patients developed angina and ECG changes but no changes in lactate metabolism; less than 50 percent systolic narrowing resulted in no angina, ECG changes, or metabolic changes. It has also been suggested that the duration of coronary obstruction due to myocardial bridging (i.e., whether obstruction is purely systolic or extends into diastole) is a determinant of the physiologic consequences of bridging. Krawczyk and co-workers found in a dog model of coronary bridging that the duration of occlusion did influence myocardial flow.[K9] For systolic occlusion alone, mean flow decreased 8 ± 5 percent, whereas occlusions extending into diastole reduced mean flow 20 ± 14 percent. However, the delay in diastolic opening required to produce significant ischemia was equal to one-quarter to one-half of the diastolic interval at heart rates of 60 to 120 beats per minute, and the frequency with which this duration of occlusion occurs in humans in vivo is unknown. Faruqui and associates reported on two patients with symptomatic coronary arterial bridging who responded to therapy with debridging and coronary artery bypass surgery.[F7]

Thus, although coronary bridging is generally not of physiologic or pathologic significance, cases of documented abnormalities have been reported. Indeed, bridges may be important when they are prominent, when vascular occlusion extends into diastole, or when there is concomitant left ventricular hypertrophy or a hypercontractile state. One of the major questions concerning bridges is why patients develop symptoms later, if the bridges are present from birth. Possibilities include tachycardia resulting in decreased diastolic flow, changes in vascular beds and flow that occur with aging, changes in oxygen requirements, or increases in systolic wall tension that occur with the development of hypertrophy.

VALIDITY OF CORONARY ANGIOGRAMS

Postmortem/Angiographic Comparisons

It is important to consider how well the coronary angiogram defines the disease present in the coronary arteries. (In evaluating studies of angiographic-pathologic correlation, it must be remembered that an angiographic 50 percent diameter stenosis is equivalent to a histologic 75 percent cross-sectional area stenosis; likewise, an angiographic 75 percent diameter stenosis correlates with a histologic 90 percent cross-sectional area stenosis.) One of the first studies to address this point was reported by Eusterman and associates in 1962.[E6] At postmortem examination, 75 percent of adults had significant coronary disease. Of 479 coronary segments from 50 postmortem hearts, 19 percent contained focal as well as nonfocal disease. For areas with nonfocal disease, postmortem angiograms agreed with the pathologic diagnosis in 61 percent of cases, underestimated disease in 22 percent of cases, and overestimated disease in 17 percent of cases. For areas with focal disease, however, agreement was present in only 11 percent of cases, with angiographic underestimation occurring in 76 percent and overestimation in 3 percent. Agreement was best if less than 50 percent stenosis was present.[E6] In 1967 Kemp and associates compared the postmortem diagnosis of disease with premortem angiographic findings in 145 coronary segments from 29 patients.[K7] In these 145 segments, 23 "errors," only 3 of which were considered functionally significant, were noted. The greatest errors involved angiographic underestimation of disease severity. Problems were particularly noted in segments with crescentic lumens or in areas of vessel overlap on angiography. Errors were also common when the diagonal and circumflex branches were small but were erroneously interpreted as showing diffuse disease. These authors stressed the importance of high-quality angiograms and expert observers for obtaining accurate angiographic diagnoses.[K7]

In 1972 Vlodaver and co-workers reported the pathologic distribution of disease in 50 adult hearts.[V1] Coronary disease was most common in the right coronary artery between the acute margin and the posterior descending branch; the next most common areas of disease were the proximal left anterior descending artery and the proximal right coronary artery. In the left anterior descending and circumflex systems, proximal disease was more common than distal disease. There was a strong tendency for disease to be present in more than one artery. Pathologically, most atherosclerotic plaques were distributed in an arc around the periphery of the lumen, with few lesions showing circumferential distribution. The angiographic significance of diseased segments with a slitlike lumen was frequently misinterpreted. In patients with a false-negative angiogram, 68 percent of the lesions whose significance was underestimated had slitlike lumens.

In a follow-up study, Vlodaver and co-workers compared premortem angiograms with necropsy findings in 10 cases.[V2] For 135 coronary segments, the angiograms were falsely negative in 44 (33 percent). Many of the angiographic false-negative segments were diffusely diseased pathologically and contained slitlike lumens. Only five coronary segments (3.5 percent) had false-positive angiograms. For only five of 10 left main segments was agreement noted between angiographic and postmortem diagnoses. Angiographic underestimation of disease was especially common in the mid right coronary artery, the left main artery, and the proximal circumflex coronary artery.[V2]

Grondin and associates evaluated the hearts of 23 patients who died following coronary bypass grafting and for whom angiograms were available within 30 days of postmortem evaluation.[G12] In nine cases there was an appreciable difference between the severity of coronary disease defined angiographically and that defined at postmortem evaluation, and in four of these nine cases incomplete revascularization had occurred because of angiographic underestimation of disease. Eleven of 145 lesions (7.5 percent) were underestimated angiographically. Hutchins and co-workers compared clinical angiograms and pathologic findings for 28 patients who died within 3 months of angiography.[H10] For 21 (7 percent) of 315 segments with greater than 50 percent diameter narrowing on the angiogram, discrepancies were noted between angiographic and postmortem findings. In six segments the angiogram overestimated the disease, but in 3 segments spasm was clearly present. In 15 segments the angiogram underestimated the coronary disease, and in 12 the discrepancy was due to overlap of the left anterior descending and diagonal coronary arteries.

Several subsequent studies also evaluated the correlation between the angiographic and histologic diagnoses of coronary disease. Isner and co-workers studied 29 patients postmortem who had angiograms less than 6 weeks prior to death.[I1] Of 15 patients with histologic evidence of a greater than 75-percent decrease in luminal cross-sectional area, seven (47 percent) had normal angiographic findings; of 14 patients with histologic evidence of less than 75 percent narrowing, six (or 43 percent) were thought to have severe narrowing on the angiogram. Thus, in nearly 50-percent of cases angiographic underestimation or overestimation of disease occurred. Arnett and associates compared premortem angiograms and postmortem findings for 10 patients.[A9] For 61 coronary segments there was no angiographic overestimation of disease. For 11 segments with 0- to 50-percent narrowing, there was perfect angiographic and pathologic correlation. Of eight segments with 51- to 75-percent cross-sectional narrowing, seven were underestimated angiographically, and of 42 segments with 76- to 100-percent pathologic narrowing, 17 were underestimated on angiograms. Diffuse plaque formation rather than focal disease was noted pathologically in 90 percent of 467 5-mm segments. Seventeen of 24 segments with eccentric lumens were underestimated angiographically. Murphy and associates compared pathologic and angiographic findings for 20 patients.[M5] They evaluated 313 coronary segments on LAO and 311 on RAO angiograms. For single-plane views, angiographic sensitivity was 72 to 78 percent and specificity was 85 to 87 percent. When both angiographic views were evaluated, the stenosis was seen in both views for only 61 percent of the segments; however, if narrowing was seen in both views, 93 percent specificity was noted. Left main disease was overestimated in 10 percent of cases. The most common area of false-positive diagnosis was the proximal right coronary artery, possibly due to catheter-induced spasm.[M5] Ganz and associates found that of 15 stenoses with severity graded as 25 to 75 percent on angiograms, seven had significant pressure gradients at rest with an increase in the gradient following contrast agent injection.[G13]

Thus, comparative studies of the angiographic and postmortem definition of coronary artery disease suggest that angiograms frequently underestimate the severity of coronary disease. However, this interpretation must be made with some caution, as many of the pathologic studies were not performed on pressure-perfusion-fixed arteries. Although pathologic studies show a significant incidence of crescentic or slitlike residual coronary lumens, such lumens are rarely seen in vivo.

Intraobserver and Interobserver Variability

An additional problem concerning the clinical validity of the coronary angiogram is the high degree of intra- and interobserver variability in interpreting the degree and significance of coronary stenoses. In 1975 Detre and associates reported on a subset of 13 angiograms from the Veterans Administration Cooperative Study that were reviewed by 22 physicians on two different occasions.[D4] The individuals who showed the highest intraobserver variability also had the highest interobserver variability, and more experienced angiographers tended to show less variability in angiographic interpretation. Highest agreement was noted for lesions in the right coronary artery, the proximal left anterior descending artery, and the left main artery; the most disagreement was seen for distal left anterior descending and circumflex lesions.

In a more quantitative study, Zir and associates reported on the variability observed when four experienced angiographers (two radiologists and two cardiologists) independently assessed 20 coronary angiograms.[Z3] In only 65 percent of cases did all the angiographers agree about the significance of stenoses in the proximal or mid left anterior descending coronary artery. Agreement about the presence or absence of significant disease in the left main occurred in 85 percent of cases, in the circumflex coronary artery in 75 percent of cases, and in the proximal right coronary artery in 65 percent of cases.[Z3]

DeRouen and associates reported on 11 readers evaluating 10 angiograms.[D5] The standard deviation for diagnosis of coronary disease per segment was 18 percent. Disagreement about which vessels contained 70 percent or greater stenosis occurred in 31 percent of cases, especially those involving distal vessels, non-opacified segments, diffusely diseased segments, or angiograms of poor technical quality. Best agreement occurred for the proximal right coronary artery, the proximal left anterior descending artery, and the left main coronary artery. Least agreement was seen for diagonal lesions, distal right coronary lesions, and distal left anterior descending lesions.[D5]

Galbraith and co-workers reported a study in which interpretation of premortem coronary angiograms was compared with postmortem histology.[G14] When 624 angiographic segments were evaluated by three cardiologists, there was actually a higher incidence of false-positive than false-negative angiograms. For slightly more than 50 percent of the misinterpreted segments, at least two of the three interpreters made the same misdiagnosis. Thus, use of a consensus opinion might not improve the validity of angiographic interpretation. In 82 to 84 percent of cases, the angiographic definition correlated with pathologic findings.

In 1982 Fisher and associates reported on the reproducibility between two readers analyzing 870 coronary angiograms from participants in the CASS.[F8] Interpretation of left main coronary lesions was least reproducible and that of proximal right coronary artery lesions was most reproducible. If one reader read 50 percent or greater left main stenosis, the second reader read no left main disease 18.6 percent of the time. (See Fig. 12–12.) However, in only 5.3 percent of cases did the numbers of vessels considered diseased differ by more than one vessel. It was found that good quality and complete studies resulted in less interobserver variability.

Thus, the standard method of interpreting coronary angiograms, that of visually estimating stenosis as percent diameter reduction, frequently underestimates the severity of coronary artery disease[A9] and also results in substantial intraobserver and interobserver variability.[D4, D5, F8, G14, Z3] Underestimation of the severity of coronary stenoses may be related to the presence of eccentric lesions that cannot be evaluated adequately unless several perpendicular views are seen, and of diffuse disease such that the "normal" segment used as a denominator in defining percent stenosis frequently is not normal.[A9, M6]

EVALUATION/INTERPRETATION/ IMPLICATIONS OF THE CORONARY ANGIOGRAM

Eighty-one percent of patients referred for catheterization with the diagnosis of coronary artery disease are found to have coronary disease, and in 77 percent the disease is significant (defined as greater than 50 percent narrowing of the diameter of the left main coronary artery or greater than 75 percent narrowing of the

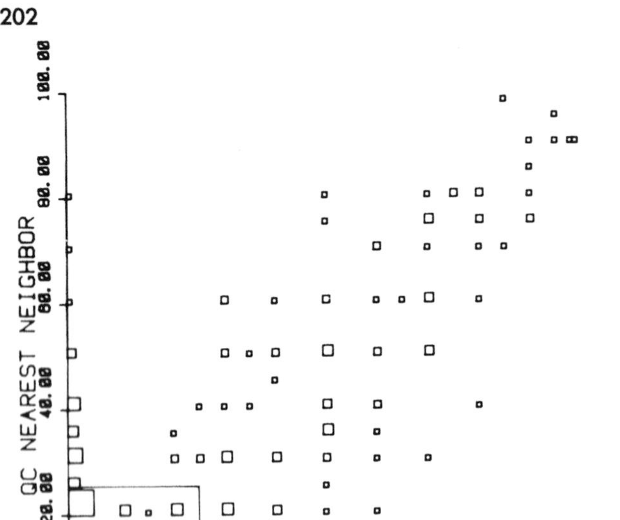

Figure 12–12. The variability noted between the quality control (QC) site (vertical axis) and the clinical site (horizontal axis) for readings of percent stenosis of the left main coronary artery in the Coronary Artery Surgery Study. The area of each square is proportional to the number of cases with that reading. The large square at the lower left represents cases for which both readers considered the segment nonstenotic. The marked variability in interpretation of the degree of disease in the left main coronary artery is readily apparent. (From Fisher, L.D., Judkins, M.P., Lesperance, J., et al.: Reproducibility of coronary arteriographic reading in the Coronary Artery Surgery Study (CASS). Cathet. Cardiovasc. Diagn. 8:565, 1982, with permission.)

other vessels).[G6] One-vessel disease is found in 24 percent of cases, two-vessel disease in 27 percent, three-vessel disease in 49 percent, and left main disease in 10 percent. Seventy-five percent of patients have complete or nearly complete occlusions, usually in association with disease elsewhere. It is important to evaluate the coronary angiogram systematically to define the extent and severity of disease present. The course and caliber of each vessel should be carefully traced. The number of diseased vessels, number of lesions in each vessel, and severity of the lesions also must be evaluated. It is important to consider the area of myocardium supplied by each diseased vessel and whether the diseased vessel supplies viable or necrotic myocardium. The status of the distal vessel should also be considered. Lesion length and proximal versus distal location of the stenosis are also clinically important. The coronary angiogram should not be evaluated in isolation, but in conjunction with information about the function of each left ventricular region. Collateral vessels should be looked for, time to filling of the collaterals evaluated, and the presence of coronary artery spasm or bridging considered.[A1, G6] It should be remembered that assessment of collaterally filled vessels is unreliable in determining the status of the vessel. Also remember that slow distal filling of vessels may imply proximal disease.

It is relevant at this time to review some of the studies on which definitions of the significance of coronary stenoses are based. These definitions are based mainly on studies by Gould and his colleagues in which the effects of varying degrees of stenosis on resting and hyperemic coronary blood flow were evaluated in a dog model.[G15–G17] (These studies are illustrated in Fig. 12–13.) Resting coronary blood flow was found to be an insensitive indicator of the significance of coronary disease, as resting flow was unaffected until 85 percent stenosis was reached. However, hyperemic flow began to decrease at 30 to 45 percent stenosis, and no hyperemia was noted when stenoses reached 88 to 93 percent in diameter.[G16] Gould and Lipscomb also found that the resistance to flow produced by stenoses in series was additive, and thus each of the stenoses in the vessel was important, not only the most severe one.[G15] In a follow-up study, it was found that distal vasodilatation could maintain near-normal resting flow to between 60 to 85 percent stenosis, but resting flow decreased beyond this point.[G17] On the basis of results such as these, clinical studies have generally used 50 or 75 percent diameter narrowing to define significant coronary artery disease. That the length of stenoses as well as their number and severity had to be considered was confirmed in a study in dogs by Feldman and associates.[F9] They noted that a pressure gradient and change in resting coronary flow occurred only with greater

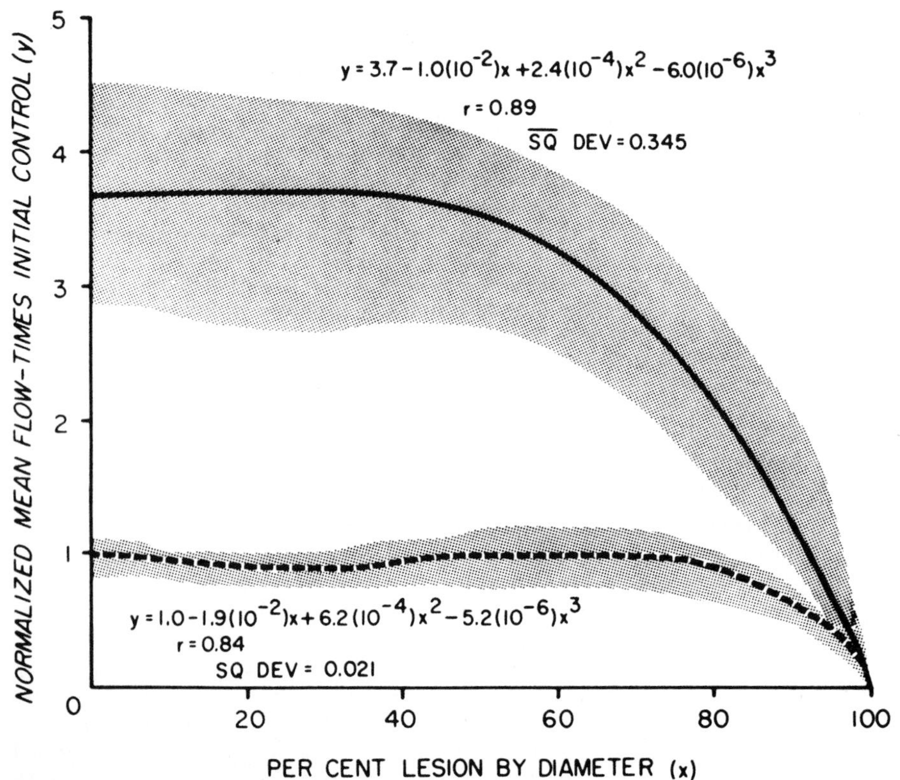

Figure 12–13. These data from a study by Gould and his colleagues illustrate the effects of varying degrees of coronary stenosis on resting and hyperemic coronary blood flow as evaluated in a dog model. Resting mean flow is shown by the dashed line and hyperemic flow after the intracoronary injection of Hypaque is shown by the solid line. Flows are expressed as ratios to control flow. The shaded area indicates the limits of the data when plotted for the individual dogs. SQ DEV—mean square of deviations. (From Gould, K.L., Lipscomb, K., and Hamilton, G.W.: Physiologic basis for assessing critical coronary stenosis. Instantaneous flow response and regional distribution during coronary hyperemia as measures of coronary flow reserve. Am. J. Cardiol. 33:87, 1974, with permission.)

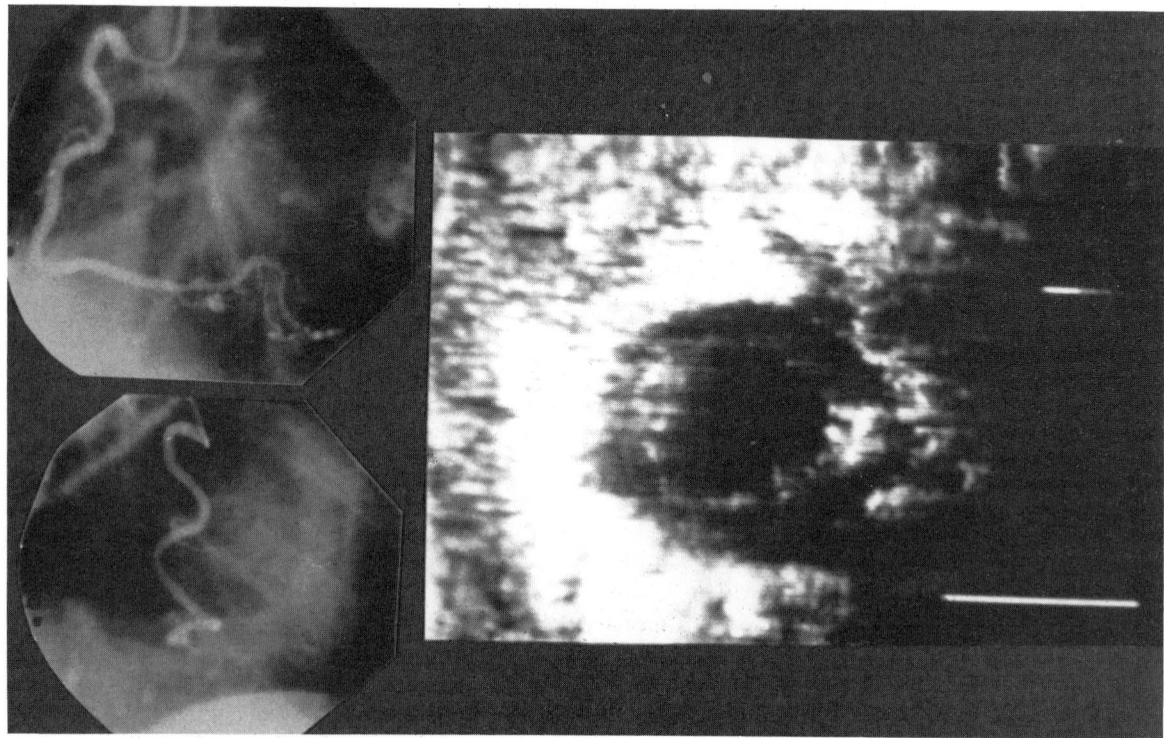

Figure 12–14. The left anterior oblique (*top left*) and right anterior oblique (*bottom left*) angiograms of this right coronary artery show only mild irregularities. However, the high-frequency echocardiographic image of the mid right coronary artery (*right*) shows diffuse thickening of the arterial wall. This confirms that vessels that are nearly normal in angiographic appearance may be diffusely diseased. (From McPherson, D.D., Hiratzka, L.F., Lamberth, W.C., et al.: Delineation of the extent of coronary atherosclerosis by high-frequency epicardial echocardiography. Reprinted with permission from The New England Journal of Medicine 316:306, 1987.)

than 80 percent stenosis when the stenosis was short; however, when stenosis length was increased to 10 to 15 mm, a 40 to 60 percent stenosis resulted in a pressure gradient and a decrease in resting flow.

Subsequent studies have suggested that these indicators of the significance of coronary disease may not apply in humans, who often have diffuse coronary disease (originally seen in pathologic studies[A9] and confirmed in vivo by high-frequency epicardial echocardiography, as shown in Fig. 12–14[M6]). The problem with using percent diameter stenosis to reflect the significance of coronary lesions in the presence of diffuse coronary artery disease is shown graphically in Figure 12–15. Particularly in patients with multivessel coronary artery disease, percent stenosis does not correlate with coronary flow reserve.[W10] (See Fig. 12–16.) It has been shown that minimum lesion luminal area is one of the major determinants of the physiologic significance of coronary lesions.[M7] In fact, minimum luminal area defined by quantitative coronary arteriography (Fig. 12–17)[H11] or videodensitometry (Fig. 12–18)[J5] does predict the physiologic significance of coronary lesions. The minimal diameter of coronary lesions defined by other geometric methods has also been correlated with physiologic significance.[J6] Quantitation of absolute luminal dimensions may substantially decrease intra- and interobserver variability in angiographic interpretation. As the next chapter in this book is devoted to the quantitative analysis of coronary angiograms, neither the individual methods nor their validity and application are discussed in detail here. Suffice it to say that problems do exist with the conventional means of defining the clinical importance of coronary stenoses in terms of percent diameter stenosis, and physicians who use angiographic data for clinical decision making should be aware of these problems and of potential approaches for improving the clinical significance of the information obtained by coronary angiography.

In spite of the controversy concerning the use of percent

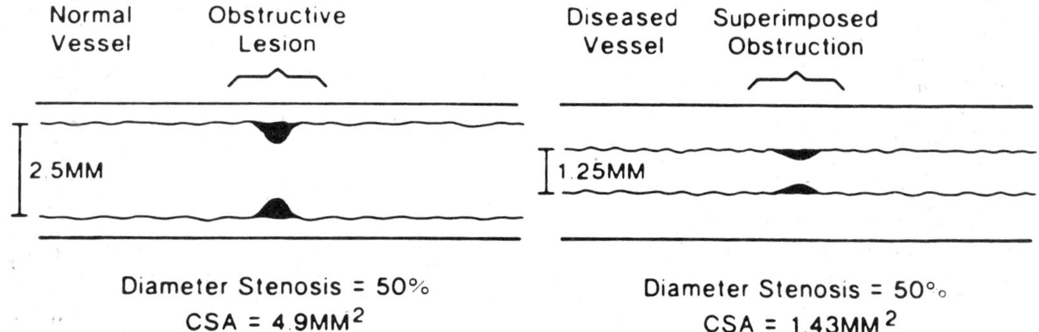

Figure 12–15. The markedly different effects of a 50 percent diameter stenosis depending on whether the vessel is normal (*left*) or diffusely diseased (*right*) are illustrated. In a normal vessel of 2.5 mm diameter, a 50 percent diameter lesion results in a luminal cross-sectional area (CSA) of 4.9 mm^2, whereas if the same vessel is diffusely diseased with a luminal diameter of 1.25 mm, a 50 percent stenosis results in a markedly decreased luminal area of 1.43 mm^2. As coronary disease frequently is a diffuse process, percent stenosis alone is an inadequate means of assessing the severity of coronary artery disease. (From Harrison, D.G., White, C.W., Hiratzka, L.F., et al.: The value of lesion cross-sectional area determined by quantitative coronary arteriography in assessing the physiologic significance of proximal left anterior descending coronary arterial stenoses. Circulation 69:1111, 1984, by permission of the American Heart Association, Inc.)

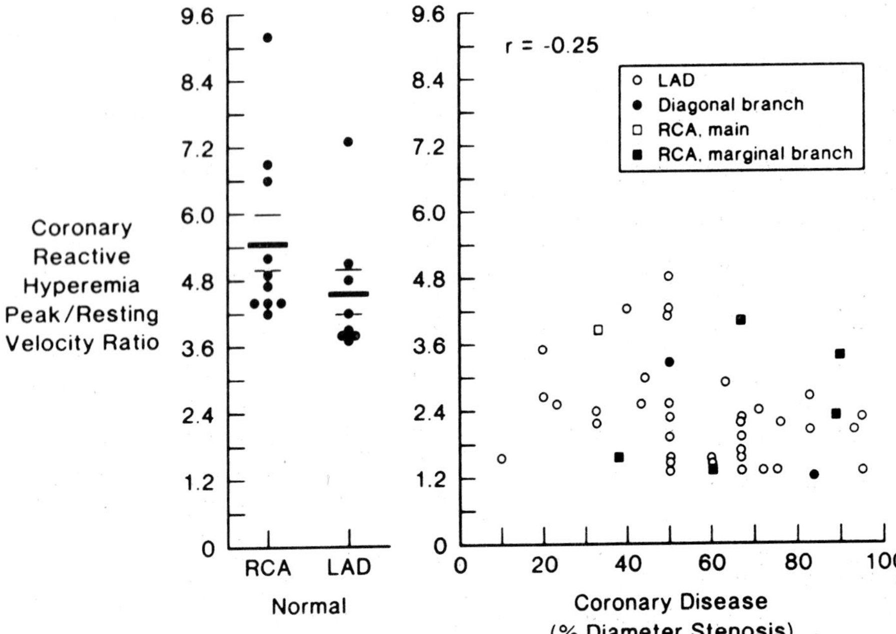

Figure 12–16. Relationship between the coronary hyperemic response obtained during intraoperative Doppler studies (vertical axis) and percent diameter stenosis (horizontal axis) for normal coronary vessels (*left*) and diseased coronary arteries (*right*). The normal peak/resting velocity ratio is greater than 3.6 to 1. The right panel clearly shows that percent diameter stenosis does not adequately predict the coronary reactive hyperemic response and thus does not accurately reflect the physiologic significance of coronary lesions. RCA—right coronary artery; LAD—left anterior descending coronary artery. (From White, C.W., Wright, C.B., Doty, D.B., et al.: Does visual interpretation of the coronary arteriogram predict the physiologic importance of a coronary stenosis? Reprinted with permission from The New England Journal of Medicine 310:821, 1984.)

Figure 12–17. Relationship between the peak/resting velocity ratio and coronary luminal minimal cross-sectional area defined by the Brown-Dodge method of quantitative coronary arteriography. (From Harrison, D.G., White, C.W., Hiratzka, L.F., et al.: The value of lesion cross-sectional area determined by quantitative coronary arteriography in assessing the physiologic significance of proximal left anterior descending coronary arterial stenoses. Circulation 69:1111, 1984, by permission of the American Heart Association, Inc.)

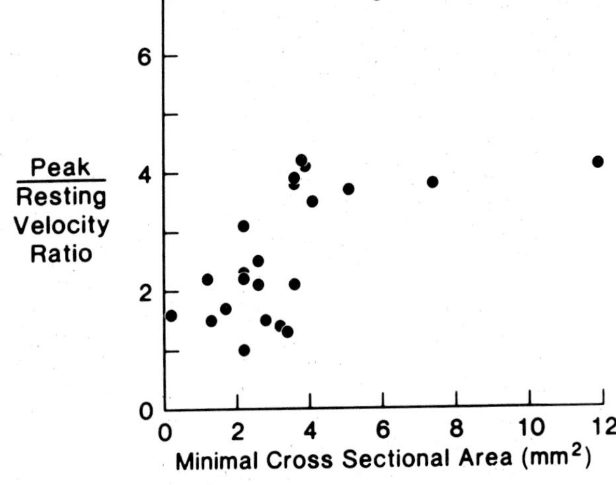

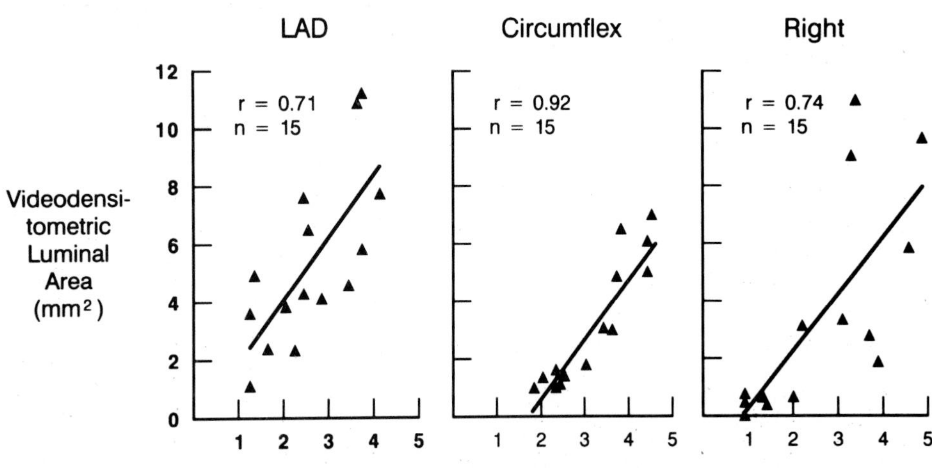

Figure 12–18. Absolute coronary luminal areas defined by videodensitometric techniques also correlate with the coronary reactive hyperemic response as defined by studies of the peak-to-resting velocity ratio in the left anterior descending (LAD), circumflex, and right coronary arteries. (From Johnson, M.R., Skorton, D.J., Ericksen, E.E., et al.: Videodensitometric analysis of coronary stenoses: In vivo geometric and physiologic validation in humans. Invest. Radiol. 23:891, 1988, with permission.)

diameter stenosis to define the significance of coronary artery disease,[G18, M8] definition of significant coronary artery disease in terms of the classic 50 percent or 75 percent diameter stenosis does predict coronary risk. In 1970 Friesinger and associates reported on 244 patients with chest pain who were followed for a mean of 53 months.[F10] Five-year survival was 97 percent for patients with normal coronary arteries and 73 percent for patients with coronary artery disease. Survival decreased with increasing severity of coronary disease as defined by a coronary artery disease score. Bruschke and co-workers confirmed the effect of the presence or absence of coronary artery disease on the risk of cardiac mortality.[B11] In 342 patients with normal coronary arteries, 5-year cardiac mortality was 0.6 percent and the incidence of myocardial infarction was 0.9 percent, compared to 5.3 percent and 3.5 percent, respectively, in patients with minimal (30–50 percent) coronary narrowings. In 1974 Webster and associates reported on 469 patients with 80 to 100 percent proximal coronary lesions.[W11] Yearly attrition was 4 percent with left anterior descending coronary artery disease, 2.3 percent with right coronary artery disease, 6.6 percent with two-vessel disease, and 10 percent with three-vessel disease. Six-year mortality was 25.5, 14, 41.5, and 63 percent, respectively, in these groups of patients confirming the influence of coronary artery disease on mortality. Harris and associates reported that the 5-year survival of patients with coronary disease who were treated medically was related inversely to the number of vessels with 75 percent or greater stenosis but was also related to left ventricular function.[H12] Burggraf and Parker, in a review of 259 patients, found that survival was related to the number of vessels with greater than 50 percent or greater than 75 percent stenosis but was also affected by hypertension, congestive heart failure, abnormal hemodynamics, and left ventricular asynergy.[B12]

The CASS Registry data for patients treated medically show that 4-year survival was inversely related to the number of vessels with greater than 70 percent stenosis; 4-year survival was 92 percent with one-vessel disease, 84 percent with two-vessel disease, and 68 percent with three-vessel disease.[M9] (See Fig. 12–19.) Three-year survival was only 41 percent in those with greater than 70 percent left main stenosis, which confirms the high risk of left main disease. Others have looked more specifically at the effect of left main stenoses. Conley and associates reported that 3-year survival was only 50 percent in patients with 50 percent or greater left main stenosis and decreased to 41 percent in patients with greater than 70 percent left main stenosis.[C10] Congestive heart failure, resting chest pain, cardiomegaly on chest x-ray, ST-T changes, abnormal left ventricular function, and elevated left ventricular end-diastolic pressure were also predictive of mortality. Campeau and associates reported in 1978 that the medical survival of patients with greater than 50 percent left main stenosis was 48.5 percent in the early portion of the study but improved to 60.4 percent in patients entered after 1972.[C11]

Thus, although there are problems in interpretation of the coronary angiogram relative to pathologic specimens, in variability in angiographic interpretation, and in the definition of a significant coronary stenosis, the presence of coronary disease on coronary angiograms does have prognostic significance.

It has been suggested that the angiographic characteristics of coronary stenoses may also be predictive of the clinical state. In their classic paper on the high incidence of total thrombotic arterial occlusion in the early hours following myocardial infarction, DeWood and colleagues reported that in 59 patients with angiographic features suggestive of clots, a Fogarty catheter retrieved clots in 88 percent, which suggested that clots could be defined angiographically.[D6] In only 5 patients was a clot found intraoperatively that was not seen angiographically. Others have determined the presence of coronary thrombi angiographically and correlated it with the patient's clinical status. Capone and associates evaluated the angiograms of 119 patients with unstable angina and 35 patients with stable angina.[C12] Intracoronary thrombi, defined as intravascular filling defects, were present in 37 percent of patients with unstable angina but in no patients with stable angina. If the patients with unstable angina had rest pain within 24 hours of catheterization the incidence of intracoronary thrombi was 52 percent, compared to 28 percent in those whose rest pain occurred 1 to 14 days prior to the angiogram. In a similar study, Bresnahan and associates evaluated 286 angiograms and in 86 of them found intracoronary thrombus, defined as contrast staining or an intravascular filling defect without associated calcification.[B13] Eighty-three percent of patients with intracoronary thrombi had unstable angina. Likewise, thrombus was found in 36 percent of patients with unstable angina and 2.5 percent of those with stable angina. No clot was found in patients with stable angina unless they had a prior history of myocardial infarction. Thus, it appears that thrombus is commonly seen on the angiograms of patients with unstable angina; however, whether the thrombus progresses to result in total occlusion and myocardial infarction requires further study.

Others have evaluated the morphology of a coronary stenosis and related it to the patient's clinical status. Levin and Fallon evaluated 73 coronary stenoses by postmortem angiography and histology.[L10] When stenoses had a smooth or hourglass angiographic appearance without associated intracoronary lucency, only 11.4 percent were histologically complicated by plaque rupture, hemorrhage, or clot. On the other hand, if angiographically the stenoses were irregular or there was intracoronary

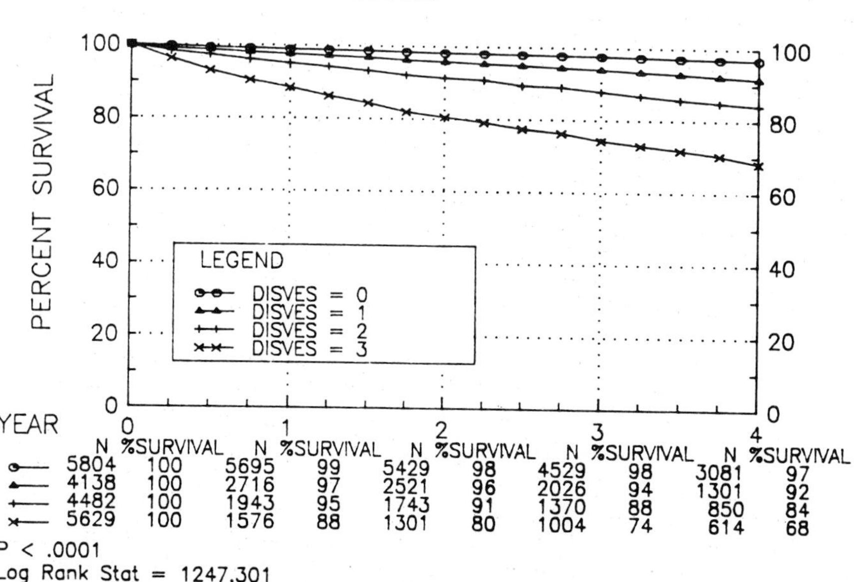

	Year 0 N	%SURVIVAL	Year 1 N	%SURVIVAL	Year 2 N	%SURVIVAL	Year 3 N	%SURVIVAL	Year 4 N	%SURVIVAL
DISVES = 0	5804	100	5695	99	5429	98	4529	98	3081	97
DISVES = 1	4138	100	2716	97	2521	96	2026	94	1301	92
DISVES = 2	4482	100	1943	95	1743	91	1370	88	850	84
DISVES = 3	5629	100	1576	88	1301	80	1004	74	614	68

Figure 12–19. Despite our difficulties in interpreting the data on coronary angiograms, survival is indeed related to the number of coronary arteries containing significant disease (here defined as greater than 70 percent stenosis). DISVES—diseased vessels. (From Mock, M.B., Ringquist, I., Fisher, L.D., et al.: Survival of medically treated patients in the Coronary Artery Surgery Study (CASS) Registry. Circulation 66:562, 1982, by permission of the American Heart Association, Inc.)

lucency, 78.9 percent were histologically complicated plaques. The angiogram was 88 percent sensitive and 79 percent specific for defining histologically complicated plaques. Ambrose and coworkers reported that eccentric stenoses with a narrow neck or totally irregular stenoses were seen in 71 percent of patients with unstable angina but in only 16 percent of patients with stable angina.[A10, A11] They found no difference in the number of vessels diseased or the degree of coronary obstruction between the groups of patients. In 41 patients with recent myocardial infarction and subtotal occlusions, 66 percent of infarct vessel stenoses were eccentric with a narrow neck or irregular; this type of stenosis was found in only 11 percent of noninfarct vessels. There was also a high incidence (61 percent) of eccentric stenoses with narrow necks or irregular stenoses in infarct vessels following streptokinase therapy.

Wilson and associates described a quantitative definition of luminal irregularity, the ulceration index, and found that luminal irregularity was significantly greater in patients with unstable angina or following myocardial infarction than in patients with stable angina or in the noninfarct vessels of patients following myocardial infarction.[W12] Quantitative angiography indicated that the lesions in the patients with unstable angina were somewhat more severe than those in the other clinical classes.

Although these studies suggest that more precise characterization of the angiographic appearance of coronary stenoses may be of prognostic importance, the overall clinical significance of these findings awaits further study.

TRAPS TO AVOID IN THE PERFORMANCE AND INTERPRETATION OF CORONARY ANGIOGRAMS

Accurate diagnosis of coronary artery disease depends on performing a complete angiographic study and correctly interpreting the study. Several authors have described problems that commonly arise in coronary angiography.[B2, C4, G6, L6, L11, L12] Potential errors in the performance or interpretation of the coronary angiogram that can result in an incomplete or misinterpreted study include the following:

1. Use of a fixed number of projections or only specific projections, particularly without cranially or caudally angulated projections. Unless each vascular segment is viewed perpendicular to the plane of the x-ray beam (i.e., without foreshortening), it cannot be adequately analyzed. In addition, adequate views and angles are needed so that no superimposition of vessels masks lesions. For the evaluation of eccentric stenoses, angiograms in two views at least 90 degrees apart are essential.
2. Inadequate force of injection or pulsatile injection of contrast media. Unless the contrast medium is injected to produce nearly complete opacification of the vessel (with some reflux of contrast medium into the coronary sinus), pockets of nonopacified blood may be interpreted as stenoses or ostial lesions may be missed.
3. Iatrogenically induced coronary artery spasm. Such spasm, which could be misinterpreted as a proximal coronary lesion, is much more common in the right coronary artery than the left. If a proximal lesion must be differentiated from spasm, refilming the vessel after nitroglycerin or nifedipine administration or performing sinus flush shots may help resolve the question. Spasm is also suggested when the narrowing occurs at or within a few millimeters of the catheter tip without any alteration in coronary flow, chest pain, or ST-T changes.
4. Superselective coronary injections. Superselective injections can result in the angiographer misinterpreting a branch vessel as being totally occluded and, in the case of injection into a right coronary artery beyond the conal branch, missing collaterals to the left anterior descending circulation. Superselective injection can also produce ventricular fibrillation. Reflux of contrast agent into the coronary sinus should be seen, and the proximal segment of the vessel should be carefully analyzed.
5. Performing angiograms in projections where the vessels overlie dense structures such as the spine or the diaphragm. This technique makes adequate visualization of the coronary arteries difficult. For good visualization of the distal right coronary artery to be achieved, the patient must inspire during injections to move the diaphragm out of the way. Similarly, it is critical to obtain views in which the segment of interest is not obscured by the spine.
6. Missing left main lesions. To avoid this, the left main artery should be filmed in the frontal projection and with the vessel off the spine. Catheter damping and absence of reflux into the coronary sinus suggest an ostial lesion.
7. Absent blood supply to a portion of the heart. This may be produced by a flush coronary occlusion or by an anomalous coronary vessel that has not yet been visualized. Collaterals suggest an occlusion or severe disease in a vessel proximal to the collateral-dependent bed.
8. Re-canalized vessels. In one-third of cases, vessels that have been totally occluded subsequently re-canalize.
9. Coronary bridging. Bridging must be distinguished from a coronary lesion, as the implications of bridging, as discussed elsewhere, are different from those of atherosclerotic coronary disease.
10. Coronary veins mistaken for arteries.
11. "Artifactual" collaterals. These may appear if contrast agent is injected too vigorously.

OUTPATIENT CARDIAC CATHETERIZATION

Although outpatient cardiac catheterization is considered relatively new, Fierens reported that 12,719 outpatient angiograms were performed using the Sones technique between 1968 and 1982 at Butterworth Hospital in Detroit.[F11] Fierens reviewed the most recent 5107 cases, in which there were no deaths or myocardial infarctions and a 2.2 percent incidence of complications. Specific protocols were followed. The patients were seen 1 to 2 weeks prior to the planned procedure, at which time the procedure was explained and they were given a brochure to review. Chest x-ray, electrocardiogram, hematocrit/hemoglobin level, white blood cell count, blood chemistries and electrolytes, and prothrombin time were obtained and treadmill tests, thallium scans, or radionuclide ventriculograms were performed as indicated. On the day of the procedure the patient fasted for 4 hours and reported to the catheterization facility 30 minutes prior to the scheduled procedure. Informed consent was obtained, and the patient underwent coronary angiography by the Sones technique. Following the procedure, patients were allowed to leave the area but required to remain in the hospital, and they returned in 30 to 60 minutes for evaluation of the radial pulse, the catheterization site, blood pressure, and any complications. On the following day, the patients were seen again and their angiograms were reviewed. Ventricular fibrillation occurred in 0.14 percent of patients; most of the patients were discharged without hospital admission. Cerebrovascular complications occurred in 0.02 percent, anaphylactic complications in 0.02 percent, brachial artery lacerations in 0.04 percent, and decreased radial pulses in 2 percent. Twenty-four patients (0.5 percent) were hospitalized because of chest pain, angiographic findings, hypotension, malaise, nausea, or oozing at the catheterization site. Subsequently, two patients died (one had critical aortic stenosis and the other had a stroke following carotid and coronary angiography).

Mahrer and Eshoo reported on 288 patients who underwent outpatient coronary angiography, 95 percent by the percutaneous Judkins technique and 5 percent by the Sones technique.[M10] There were six complications (one death, two myocardial infarctions, one embolism, and two hematomas). Three of the six complications occurred in patients with left main disease, and only two of the complications were thought to be related to the outpatient nature of the procedure. However, these authors emphasized careful selection of patients and excluded patients with unstable angina, recent heart failure, severe arrhythmias, severe valvular heart disease, concomitant insulin-dependent diabetes mellitus, chronic obstructive pulmonary disease, or steroid dependence. In patients studied with the Judkins technique, the arterial site was treated with pressure for 6 to 10 minutes following catheter removal and with a pressure dressing for 4 hours. If there was no bleeding at this time, ambulation and discharge were allowed. The patients were to rest at home for 1 day and then resume normal activity. Ninety-one percent of patients were discharged at 4 hours. Eleven (3.6 percent) were hospitalized for chest pain or hypotension but were subsequently discharged without complications. Ten (3.2 percent) were hospitalized for emergency coronary artery bypass surgery, mainly because of left main disease.

Klinke and associates reported that for 3071 outpatient catheterizations performed by the femoral approach there was 0.13 percent mortality, 0.07 percent myocardial infarction, 0.42 percent arrhythmias, 0.14 percent cerebrovascular complications, and 0.35 percent local vascular complications.[K8] Recently, Block and associates reported a prospective randomized trial of outpatient versus inpatient cardiac catheterization.[B14] Because of the careful selection of patients, only 20 percent of patients were eligible for study. There were no deaths and no cerebrovascular accidents. Although there were no significant differences between the two groups in hematomas, number of weak, cold, or blue extremities, or acute myocardial infarctions, the incidence of hematomas, vascular insufficiency, and myocardial infarcts was slightly higher in the outpatients. Twelve percent of outpatients were hospitalized because of disease severity or complications. As expected, costs were lower for the outpatients.

Thus, coronary angiography, whether by the Judkins or the Sones technique, can be performed safely and cost-efficiently on an outpatient basis in selected cases. However, selection of patients is critical, and the status of the patient as well as his suspected pathology must be evaluated to determine whether inpatient or outpatient catheterization is appropriate.

GENERAL RECOMMENDATIONS

The safest and most complete coronary angiographic study requires an expert and skilled angiographer, a competent and dedicated catheterization laboratory team, and a good imaging system; it should be the briefest possible complete study. A catheterization laboratory should generally be operated only in conjunction with surgical facilities. Performance of safe and adequate coronary angiography requires not only technical skills but also good clinical judgment and attention to detail. Less than 25 percent of angiograms performed for chest pain in a catheterization laboratory should have no significant coronary artery disease.[G1]

The Intersociety Commission on Heart Disease Resources recommended in 1983 that no fewer than 150 cases per year be performed by each physician to obtain the best-quality studies at the least risk to the patient.[F3] A laboratory minimum of 300 cases per year was also suggested. In addition, not more than 1 percent of studies should be considered inadequate or have to be repeated for diagnosis, unless the initial study had become prolonged for some reason. Deaths among stable patients undergoing elective angiography should be less than 0.1 percent.

References

A

1. Assessment of coronary artery disease. *In* Yang, S.S., Bentivoglio, L.G., Maranhao, V., and Goldberg, H. (eds.): From Cardiac Catheterization Data to Hemodynamic Parameters. 3rd ed. F.A. Davis, Philadelphia, 1988, p. 256.
2. Amplatz, K.: Techniques of coronary arteriography. Circulation 27:101, 1963.
3. Amplatz, K., Formanek, G., Stanger, P., and Wilson, W.: Mechanics of selective coronary artery catheterization via femoral approach. Radiology 89:1040, 1967.
4. Adams, D.F., Fraser, D.B., and Abrams, H.L.: The complications of coronary arteriography. Circulation 48:609, 1973.
5. Arani, D.T., Bunnell, I.L., and Greene, D.G.: Lordotic right posterior oblique projection of the left coronary artery. A special view for special anatomy. Circulation 52:504, 1975.
6. Aldridge, H.E., McLoughlin, M.J., and Taylor, K.W.: Improved diagnosis in coronary cinearteriography with routine use of 110° oblique views and cranial and caudal angulations. Comparison with standard transverse oblique views in 100 patients. Am. J. Cardiol. 36:468, 1975.
7. Aldridge, H.E.: A decade or more of cranial and caudal angled projections in coronary arteriography—another look (Editorial.) Cathet. Cardiovasc. Diagn. 10:539, 1984.
8. Aldridge, H.E.: Better visualization of the asymmetric lesion in coronary arteriography using cranial and caudal angulated projections. Chest 71:502, 1977.
9. Arnett, E.N., Isner, J.M., Redwood, D.R., et al.: Coronary artery narrowing in coronary heart disease: Comparison of cineangiographic and necropsy findings. Ann. Intern. Med. 91:350, 1979.
10. Ambrose, J.A., Winters, S.L., Arora, R.R., et al.: Coronary angiographic morphology in myocardial infarction: A link between the pathogenesis of unstable angina and myocardial infarction. J. Am. Coll. Cardiol. 6:1223, 1985.
11. Ambrose, J.A., Winters, S.L., Stern, A., et al.: Angiographic morphology and the pathogenesis of unstable angina pectoris. J. Am. Coll. Cardiol. 5:609, 1985.

B

1. Bellman, S., Frank, H.A., Lambert, P.B., et al.: Coronary arteriography. I. Differential opacification of the aortic stream by catheters of special design—experimental development. N. Engl. J. Med. 262:325, 1960.
2. Baim, D.S., and Grossman, W.: Coronary angiography. *In* Grossman, W. (ed.): Cardiac Catheterization and Angiography. Lea & Febiger, Philadelphia, 1986, p. 173.
3. Bourassa, M.C., and Noble, J.: Complication rate of coronary arteriography. A review of 5250 cases studied by a percutaneous femoral technique. Circulation 53:106, 1976.
4. Bassan, M., Ganz, W., Marcus, H.S., and Swan, H.J.C.: The effect of intracoronary injections of contrast medium upon coronary blood flow. Circulation 51:442, 1975.
5. Berkseth, R.O., and Kjellstrand, C.M.: Radiologic contrast-induced nephropathy. Med. Clin. North Am. 68:351, 1984.
6. Byrd, L., and Sherman, R.: Radiocontrast-induced acute renal failure. A clinical and pathophysiologic review. Medicine 58:270, 1979.
7. Bettman, M.A.: Angiographic contrast agents: Conventional and new media compared. AJR 139:787, 1982.
8. Barry, W.H., Levin, D.C., Green, L.H., et al.: Left heart catheterization and angiography via the percutaneous femoral approach using an arterial sheath. Cathet. Cardiovasc. Diagn. 5:401, 1979.
9. Bunnell, I.L., Greene, D.G., Tandon, R.N., and Arani, D.T.: The half-axial projection. A new look at the proximal left coronary artery. Circulation 48:1151, 1973.
10. Brandt, B., III, Martins, J.B., and Marcus, M.L.: Anomalous origin of the right coronary artery from the left sinus of Valsalva. N. Engl. J. Med. 10:596, 1983.
11. Bruschke, A.V.G., Proudfit, W.L., and Sones, F.M., Jr.: Clinical course of patients with normal and slightly or moderately abnormal coronary arteriograms. A follow-up study on 500 patients. Circulation 47:936, 1973.
12. Burggraf, G.W., and Parker, J.O.: Prognosis in coronary artery disease. Angiographic, hemodynamic, and clinical factors. Circulation 51:146, 1975.
13. Bresnahan, D.R., Davis, J.L., Holmes, D.R., Jr., and Smith, H.C.: Angiographic occurrence and clinical correlates of intraluminal coronary artery thrombus: Role of unstable angina. J. Am. Coll. Cardiol. 6:285, 1985.
14. Block, P.C., Ockene, I., Goldberg, R.J., et al.: A prospective randomized trial of outpatient versus inpatient cardiac catheterization. N. Engl. J. Med. 319:1251, 1988.

C

1. Chavez, I., Dorbecker, N., and Celis, A.: Direct intracardiac angiography—its diagnostic value. Am. Heart J. 33:560, 1947.
2. Carabello, B.A., and Grossman, W.: Bedside hemodynamic monitoring, cardiac catheterization, and pulmonary angiography. *In* Cohn, P.F., and Wynne, J. (eds.): Diagnostic Methods in Clinical Cardiology. Little, Brown, Boston, 1982, p. 235.
3. Cohn, P.F., and Goldberg, S.: Cardiac catheterization and coronary arteriography. *In* Cohn, P.F. (ed.): Diagnosis and Therapy of Coronary Artery Disease. Martinus Nijhoff, Boston, 1985, p. 219.
4. Conti, C.R.: Coronary arteriography. Circulation 55:227, 1977.
5. Cannon, R.O., III, Watson, R.M., Rosing, D.R., and Epstein, S.E.: Angina caused by reduced vasodilator reserve of the small coronary arteries. J. Am. Coll. Cardiol. 1:1359, 1983.
6. Coronary Arteriography. *In* Verel, D., and Grainger, R.G. (eds.): Cardiac Catheterization and Angiocardiography. Churchill Livingstone, Edinburgh, 1978, p. 107.
7. Cohen, M., Rentrop, K.P., Cohen, B.M., and Holt, J.: Safety and efficacy of percutaneous entry of the brachial artery versus cutdown and arteriotomy for left-sided cardiac catheterization. Am. J. Cardiol. 57:682, 1986.
8. Chaitman, B.R., Lesperance, J., Saltiel, J., and Bourassa, M.G.: Clinical, angiographic, and hemodynamic findings in patients with anomalous origin of the coronary arteries. Circulation 53:122, 1976.
9. Cheitlin, M.D., DeCastro, C.M., and McAllister, H.A.: Sudden death as a complication of anomalous left coronary origin from the anterior sinus of Valsalva. A not-so-minor congenital anomaly. Circulation 50:780, 1974.
10. Conley, M.J., Ely, R.L., Kisslo, J., et al.: The prognostic spectrum of left main stenosis. Circulation 57:947, 1978.
11. Campeau, L., Corbara, F., Crochet, D., and Petitclerc, R.: Left main coronary

artery stenosis. The influence of aortocoronary bypass surgery on survival. Circulation 57:1111, 1978.
12. Capone, G., Wolf, N.M., Meyer, B., and Meister, S.G.: Frequency of intracoronary filling defects by angiography in angina pectoris at rest. Am. J. Cardiol. 56:403, 1985.

D

1. Dotter, C.T., and Frische, L.H.: Visualization of the coronary circulation by occlusion aortography: A practical method. Radiology 71:502, 1958.
2. Davis, K., Kennedy, J.W., Kemp, H.G., et al.: Complications of coronary arteriography from the Collaborative Study of Coronary Artery Surgery (CASS). Circulation 59:1105, 1979.
3. D'Elia, J.A., Gleason, R.E., Alday, M., et al.: Nephrotoxicity from angiographic contrast media. A prospective study. Am. J. Med. 72:719, 1982.
4. Detre, K.M., Wright, P.H.E., Murphy, M.L., and Takaro, T.: Observer agreement in evaluating coronary angiograms. Circulation 52:979, 1975.
5. DeRouen, T.A., Murray, J.A., and Owen, W.: Variability in the analysis of coronary arteriograms. Circulation 55:324, 1977.
6. DeWood, M.A., Spore, J., Notske, R., et al.: Prevalence of total coronary occlusion during the early hours of transmural myocardial infarction. N. Engl. J. Med. 303:897, 1980.

E

1. Eckberg, D.L., White, C.W., Kioschos, J.M., and Abboud, F.M.: Mechanisms mediating bradycardia during coronary arteriography. J. Clin. Invest. 54:1455, 1974.
2. Eldh, P., and Silverman, J.F.: Methods of studying the proximal left anterior descending coronary artery. Radiology 113:738, 1974.
3. Elliott, L.P., Green, C.E., Rogers, W.J., et al.: Advantage of the cranial-right anterior oblique view in diagnosing mid left anterior descending and distal right coronary artery disease. Am. J. Cardiol. 48:754, 1981.
4. Engel, H.J., Torres, C., and Page, H.L.: Major variations in anatomical origin of the coronary arteries: Angiographic observations in 4,250 patients without associated congenital heart disease. Cathet. Cardiovasc. Diagn. 1:157, 1975.
5. Eng, C., Patterson, R.E., Horowitz, S.F., et al.: Coronary collateral function during exercise. Circulation 66:309, 1982.
6. Eusterman, J.H., Achor, R.W.P., Kincaid, O.W., and Brown, A.L., Jr.: Atherosclerotic disease of the coronary arteries. A pathologic-radiologic correlative study. Circulation 26:1288, 1962.

F

1. Franch, R.H., King, S.B., III, and Douglas, J.S., Jr.: Techniques of cardiac catheterization including coronary arteriography. *In* Hurst, J.W. (ed): The Heart, 6th ed. McGraw-Hill, New York, 1986, p. 1768.
2. Fischer, H.W., and Thomson, K.R.: Contrast media in coronary arteriography: A review. Invest. Radiol. 13:450, 1978.
3. Friesinger, G.C., Adams, D.F., Bourassa, M.G., et al.: Optimal resources for examination of the heart and lung: Cardiac catheterization and radiographic facilities. Circulation 68:893A, 1983.
4. Fergusson, D.J.G., and Kamada, R.O.: Percutaneous entry of the brachial artery for left heart catheterization using a sheath. Cathet. Cardiovasc. Diagn. 7:111, 1981.
5. Fergusson, D.J.G., and Kamada, R.O.: Percutaneous entry of the brachial artery for left heart catheterization using a sheath: Further experience. Cathet. Cardiovasc. Diagn. 12:209, 1986.
6. Fitchett, D.H., Forbes, C., and Guerraty, A.J.: Repeated endomyocardial biopsy causing coronary arterial-right ventricular fistula after cardiac transplantation. Am. J. Cardiol. 62:829, 1988.
7. Faruqui, A.M.A., Maloy, W.C., Felner, J.M., et al.: Symptomatic myocardial bridging of coronary artery. Am. J. Cardiol. 41:1305, 1978.
8. Fisher, L.D., Judkins, M.P., Lesperance, J., et al.: Reproducibility of coronary arteriographic reading in the Coronary Artery Surgery Study (CASS). Cathet. Cardiovasc. Diagn. 8:565, 1982.
9. Feldman, R.L., Nichols, W.W., Pepine, C.J., and Conti, C.R.: Hemodynamic significance of the length of a coronary arterial narrowing. Am. J. Cardiol. 41:865, 1978.
10. Friesinger, G.C., Page, E.E., and Ross, R.S.: Prognostic significance of coronary arteriography. Trans. Assoc. Am. Physicians 83:78, 1970.
11. Fierens, E.: Outpatient coronary arteriography. Cathet. Cardiovasc. Diagn. 10:27, 1984.

G

1. Guidelines for coronary angiography. A report of the American College of Cardiology/American Heart Association Task Force on Assessment of Diagnostic and Therapeutic Cardiovascular Procedures (Subcommittee on Coronary Angiography). Circulation 76:963A, 1987.
2. Grossman, W., and Barry, W.H.: Cardiac catheterization. *In* Braunwald, E. (ed.): Heart Disease. 3rd ed. W.B. Saunders, Philadelphia, 1988, p. 242.
3. Green, S.J., Pizzarello, R.A., Padmanabhan, V.T., et al.: Relation of angina pectoris to coronary artery disease in aortic valve stenosis. Am. J. Cardiol. 55:1063, 1985.
4. Gao, S.Z., Schroeder, J.S., Hunt, S., and Stinson, E.B.: Retransplantation for severe accelerated coronary artery disease in heart transplant recipients. Am. J. Cardiol. 62:876, 1988.
5. Gordon, P.R., Abrams, C., Gash, A.K., and Carabello, B.A.: Pericatheterization risk factors in left main coronary artery stenosis. Am. J. Cardiol. 59:1080, 1987.
6. Gensini, G.G.: Coronary arteriography. *In* Braunwald, E. (ed.): Heart Disease. 2nd ed. W.B. Saunders, Philadelphia, 1984, p. 304.
7. Gold, H.K., Leinbach, R.C., Sanders, C.A., et al.: Intraaortic balloon pumping for control of recurrent myocardial ischemia. Circulation 47:1197, 1973.
8. Greenberger, P.A., Patterson, R., and Tapio, C.M.: Prophylaxis against repeated radiocontrast media reactions in 857 cases. Adverse experience with cimetidine and safety of β-adrenergic antagonists. Arch. Intern. Med. 145:2197, 1985.
9. Greenberger, P.A., Patterson, R., and Radin, R.C.: Two pretreatment regimens for high-risk patients receiving radiographic contrast media. J. Allergy Clin. Immunol. 74:540, 1984.
10. Gomes, A.S., Esposito, V.A., Grollman, J.H., Jr., and O'Reilly, R.J.: Angled views in the evaluation of the right coronary artery. (Abstract.) Circulation 59, 60:II-161, 1979.
11. Gensini, G.G., and DaCosta, B.C.B.: The coronary collateral circulation in living man. Am. J. Cardiol. 24:393, 1969.
12. Grondin, C.M., Dyrda, I., Pasternac, A., et al.: Discrepancies between cineangiographic and postmortem findings in patients with coronary artery disease and recent myocardial revascularization. Circulation 49:703, 1974.
13. Ganz, P., Abben, R., Friedman, P.L., et al.: Usefulness of transstenotic coronary pressure gradient measurements during diagnostic catheterization. Am. J. Cardiol. 55:910, 1985.
14. Galbraith, J.E., Murphy, M.L., and deSoyza, N.: Coronary angiogram interpretation. Interobserver variability. JAMA 240:2053, 1978.
15. Gould, K.L., and Lipscomb, K.: Effects of coronary stenoses on coronary flow reserve and resistance. Am. J. Cardiol. 34:48, 1974.
16. Gould, K.L., Lipscomb, K., and Hamilton, G.W.: Physiologic basis for assessing critical coronary stenosis. Instantaneous flow response and regional distribution during coronary hyperemia as measures of coronary flow reserve. Am. J. Cardiol. 33:87, 1974.
17. Gould, K.L., Lipscomb, K., and Calvert, C.: Compensatory changes of the distal coronary vascular bed during progressive coronary constriction. Circulation 51:1085, 1975.
18. Gould, K.L.: Percent coronary stenosis: Battered gold standard, pernicious relic, or clinical practicality? (Editorial.) J. Am. Coll. Cardiol. 11:886, 1988.

H

1. Heupler, F.A., Proudfit, S.L., and Razavi, M.: Ergonovine maleate provocative test for coronary arterial spasm. Am. J. Cardiol. 41:631, 1978.
2. Hildner, F.J., Javier, R.P., Ramaswamy, K., and Samet, P.: Pseudo complications of cardiac catheterization. Chest 63:15, 1973.
3. Hildner, F.J., Javier, R.P., Tolentino, A., and Samet, P.: Pseudo complications of cardiac catheterization: Update. Cathet. Cardiovasc. Diagn. 8:43, 1982.
4. Hanley, P.C., Holmes, D.R., Jr., Julsrud, P.R., and Smith, H.C.: Use of conventional and newer radiographic contrast agents in cardiac angiography. Prog. Cardiovasc. Dis. 28:435, 1986.
5. Heupler, F., Jr.: Coronary arteriography and left ventriculography: Sones technique. *In* King, S.B., III, and Douglas, J.S. (eds.): Coronary Arteriography and Angioplasty. McGraw-Hill, New York, 1985, p. 137.
6. Helfant, R.H., Kemp, H.G., and Gorlin, R.: Coronary atherosclerosis, coronary collaterals, and their relation to cardiac function. Ann. Intern. Med. 73:189, 1970.
7. Helfant, R.H., and Gorlin, R.: The coronary collateral circulation. (Editorial.) Ann. Intern. Med. 77:995, 1972.
8. Hamby, R.I., Aintablian, A., and Schwartz, A.: Appraisal of the functional significance of the coronary collateral circulation. Am. J. Cardiol. 38:305, 1976.
9. Hecht, H., Aroesty, J.M., Morkin, E., et al.: Role of the coronary collateral circulation in the preservation of left ventricular function. Radiology 114:305, 1975.
10. Hutchins, G.M., Bulkley, B.H., Ridolfi, R.L., et al.: Correlation of coronary arteriograms and left ventriculograms with postmortem studies. Circulation 56:32, 1977.
11. Harrison, D.G., White, C.W., Hiratzka, L.F., et al.: The value of lesion cross-sectional area determined by quantitative coronary arteriography in assessing the physiologic significance of proximal left anterior descending coronary arterial stenoses. Circulation 69:1111, 1984.
12. Harris, P.J., Harrell, F.E., Jr., Lee, K.L., et al.: Survival in medically treated coronary artery disease. Circulation 60:1259, 1978.

I

1. Isner, J.M., Kishel, J., Kent, K.M., et al.: Inaccuracy of angiographic determination of left main coronary arterial narrowing. (Abstract.) Circulation 59,60:II, 1979.

J

1. Judkins, M.P.: Selective coronary arteriography. Part 1: A percutaneous transfemoral technic. Radiology 89:815, 1967.
2. Judkins, M.P., and Gander, M.P.: Prevention of complications of coronary arteriography. (Editorial.) Circulation 49:599, 1974.
3. Jacobson, P.D., and Rosenquist, C.J.: The introduction of low-osmolar contrast agents in radiology. Medical, economic, legal, and public policy issues. JAMA 260:1586, 1988.
4. Judkins, M.P., and Judkins, E.: Coronary arteriography and left ventriculography: Judkins technique. Part I: The Judkins technique. *In* King, S.B., III,

and Douglas, J.S. (eds.): Coronary arteriography and angioplasty. McGraw-Hill, New York, 1985, p. 182.
5. Johnson, M.R., Skorton, D.J., Ericksen, E.E., et al.: Videodensitometric analysis of coronary stenoses: In vivo geometric and physiologic validation in humans. Invest. Radiol. 23:891, 1988.
6. Johnson, M.R., Fleagle, S.R., Aylward, P.E., et al.: Digital processing and analysis of coronary cineangiograms: Geometric and physiological assessment of coronary stenosis. (Abstract.) Circulation 70:II-324, 1984.

K

1. Kennedy, J.W., and the Registry Committee of the Society for Cardiac Angiography: Complications associated with cardiac catheterization and angiography. Cathet. Cardiovasc. Diagn. 8:5, 1982.
2. King, S.B., III, and Douglas, J.S.: Indications, limitations, and risks of coronary arteriography and left ventriculography. *In* King, S.B., III, and Douglas, J.S. (eds.): Coronary Arteriography and Angioplasty. McGraw-Hill, New York, 1985, p. 122.
3. King, S.B., III, and Douglas, J.S., Jr.: Coronary arteriography and left ventriculography: Multipurpose technique. *In* King, S.B., III, and Douglas, J.S. (eds.): Coronary Arteriography and Angioplasty. McGraw-Hill, New York, 1985, p. 239.
4. Kimbiris, D., Iskandrian, A.S., Segal, B.L., and Bemis, C.E.: Anomalous aortic origin of coronary arteries. Circulation 58:606, 1978.
5. Kragel, A.H., and Roberts, W.C.: Anomalous origin of either the right or left main coronary artery from the aorta with subsequent coursing between aorta and pulmonary trunk: Analysis of 32 necropsy cases. Am. J. Cardiol. 62:771, 1988.
6. Kramer, J.R., Kitazume, H., Proudfit, W.L., and Sones, F.M., Jr.: Clinical significance of isolated coronary bridges: Benign and frequent condition involving the left anterior descending artery. Am. Heart J. 103:283, 1982.
7. Kemp, H.G., Evans, H., Elliott, W.C., and Gorlin, R.: Diagnostic accuracy of selective coronary cinearteriography. Circulation 36:526, 1967.
8. Klinke, W.P., Kubac, G., Talibi, T., and Lee, S.J.K.: Safety of outpatient catheterizations. Am. J. Cardiol. 56:639, 1985.
9. Krawczyk, J.A., Dashkoff, N., Mays, A., and Klocke, F.J.: Reduced coronary flow in a canine model of "muscle bridge" with inflow occlusion extending into diastole; possible role of downstream vascular closure. Trans. Assoc. Am. Physicians 93:100, 1980.

L

1. Lehman, J.S., Boyer, R.A., and Winter, F.S.: Coronary Arteriography. AJR 81:749, 1959.
2. Levin, D.C., Phillips, D.A., Lee-son, S., and Maroko, P.R.: Hemodynamic changes distal to selective arterial injections. Invest. Radiol. 12:116, 1977.
3. Lieberman, P., Siegle, R.L., and Taylor, W.W., Jr.: Anaphylactoid reactions to iodinated contrast material. J. Allergy Clin. Immunol. 62:174, 1980.
4. Lalli, A.F.: Contrast media reactions: Data analysis and hypothesis. Radiology 134:1, 1980.
5. Lasser, E.C., Berry, C.C., Talner, L.B., et al.: Pretreatment with corticosteroids to alleviate reactions to intravenous contrast material. N. Engl. J. Med. 317:845, 1987.
6. Levin, D.C., and Gardiner, G.A., Jr.: Coronary arteriography. *In* Braunwald, E. (ed.): Heart Disease. 3rd ed. W.B. Saunders, Philadelphia, 1988, p. 268.
7. Levin, D.C., Fellow, K.E., and Abrams, H.L.: Hemodynamically significant primary anomalies of the coronary arteries. Circulation 58:25, 1978.
8. Lipton, M.J., Barry, W.H., Obrez, I., et al.: Isolated single coronary artery: Diagnosis, angiographic classification, and clinical significance. Radiology 130:39, 1979.
9. Levin, D.C.: Pathways and functional significance of the coronary collateral circulation. Circulation 50:831, 1974.
10. Levin, D.C., and Fallon, J.T.: Significance of the angiographic morphology of localized coronary stenoses: Histopathologic correlations. Circulation 66:316, 1982.
11. Levin, D.C., Baltaxe, H.A., Lee, J.G., and Sos, T.A.: Potential sources of error in coronary arteriography. I. In performance of the study. AJR 124:378, 1975.
12. Levin, D.C., Baltaxe, H.A., and Sos, T.A.: Potential sources of error in coronary arteriography. II. In interpretation of the study. AJR 124:386, 1975.

M

1. McClennan, B.L.: Low-osmolality contrast media: Premises and promise. Radiology 162:1, 1987.
2. MacAlpin, R.N., Weidner, W.A., Kattus, A.A., Jr., and Hanafee, W.N.: Electrocardiographic changes during selective coronary cineangiography. Circulation 34:627, 1966.
3. Madowitz, J.S., and Schweiger, M.J.: Severe anaphylactioid reaction to radiographic contrast media. Recurrence despite premedication with diphenhydramine and prednisone. JAMA 241:813, 1979.
4. Myers, G.E., and Bloom, F.L.: Cimetidine (Tagamet) combined with steroids and H_1 antihistamines for the prevention of serious radiographic contrast material reactions. Cathet. Cardiovasc. Diagn. 7:65, 1981.
5. Murphy, M.L., Galbraith, J.E., and deSoyza, N.: The reliability of coronary angiogram interpretation: An angiographic-pathologic correlation with a comparison of radiographic views. Am. Heart J. 97:578, 1979.
6. McPherson, D.D., Hiratzka, L.F., Lamberth, W.C., et al.: Delineation of the extent of coronary atherosclerosis by high-frequency epicardial echocardiography. N. Engl. J. Med. 316:304, 1987.
7. Mates, R.E., Gupta, R.L., Bell, A.C., and Klocke, F.J.: Fluid dynamics of coronary artery stenosis. Circ. Res. 42:152, 1978.
8. Marcus, M.L., Skorton, D.J., Johnson, M.R., et al.: Visual estimates of percent diameter coronary stenosis: "A battered gold standard." (Editorial.) J. Am. Coll. Cardiol. 11:882, 1988.
9. Mock, M.B., Ringquist, I., Fisher, L.D., et al.: Survival of medically treated patients in the Coronary Artery Surgery Study (CASS) Registry. Circulation 66:562, 1982.
10. Mahrer, P.R., and Eshoo, N.: Outpatient cardiac catheterization and coronary angiography. Cathet. Cardiovasc. Diagn. 7:355, 1981.

N

1. Nishimura, R.A., Holmes, D.R., Jr., McFarland, T.M., et al.: Ventricular arrhythmias during coronary angiography in patients with angina pectoris or chest pain syndrome. Am. J. Cardiol. 53:1496, 1984.
2. Noble, J., Bourassa, M.G., Petitclerc, R. and Dyrda, I.: Bridging and milking effect of the left anterior descending coronary artery: Normal variant or obstruction? Am. J. Cardiol. 37:993, 1976.

P

1. Passamani, E., Davis, K.B., Gillespie, M.J., et al.: A randomized trial of coronary artery bypass surgery. Survival of patients with a low ejection fraction. N. Engl. J. Med. 312: 1665, 1985.
2. Pepine, C.J., VonGunten, C., Hill, J.A., et al.: Percutaneous brachial catheterization using a modified sheath and new catheter system. Cathet. Cardiovasc. Diagn. 10:637, 1984.
3. Paulin, S.: Terminology for radiographic projections in cardiac angiography. (Letter.) Cathet. Cardiovasc. Diagn. 7:341, 1981.
4. Page, H.L., Engel, H.J., Campbell, W.B., and Thomas, C.S.: Anomalous origin of the left circumflex coronary artery. Recognition, angiographic demonstration and clinical significance. Circulation 50:768, 1974.
5. Probst, P., Zangl, W., and Pachinger, O.: Relation of coronary arterial occlusion pressure during percutaneous transluminal coronary angioplasty to presence of collaterals. Am. J. Cardiol. 55:1264, 1985.

R

1. Radner, S.: An attempt at the Roentgenologic visualization of coronary blood vessels in man. Acta Radiol. 26:497, 1945.
2. Ricketts, H.J., and Abrams, H.L.: Percutaneous selective coronary cine arteriography. JAMA 181:620, 1962.
3. Richardson, J.V., Kouchoukos, N.T., Wright, J.O., III, and Karp, R.B.: Combined aortic valve replacement and myocardial revascularization: Results in 220 patients. Circulation 59:75, 1979.
4. Reynolds, G.: The electrocardiogram during angiocardiography. Br. Heart J. 15:74, 1953.
5. Rose, A.G.: Multiple coronary arterioventricular fistulae. Circulation 58:178, 1978.
6. Rare diseases of the coronary vasculature which can impair myocardial perfusion. *In* Marcus, M.L. (ed.): The Coronary Circulation in Health and Disease. McGraw-Hill, New York, 1983, p. 320.

S

1. Steckelberg, J.M., Vlietstra, R.E., Ludwig, J., and Mann, R.J.: Werner Forssman (1904–1979) and his unusual success story. Mayo Clin. Proc. 54:746, 1979.
2. Seldinger, S.I.: Catheter replacement of the needle in percutaneous arteriography. A new technique. Acta Radiol. 39:368, 1953.
3. Sones, F.M., Shirey, E.K., Proudfit, W.L., and Westcott, R.N.: Cine-coronary arteriography. Circulation 20:773, 1959.
4. Sones, F.M., Jr., and Shirey, E.K.: Cine coronary arteriography. Mod. Concepts Cardiovasc. Dis. 31:735, 1962.
5. Schoonmaker, F.W., and King, S.B., III: Coronary arteriography by the single catheter percutaneous femoral technique. Experience in 6,800 cases. Circulation 50:735, 1974.
6. Sos, T.A., Lee, T.G., Levin, D.C., and Baltaxe, H.A.: New lordotic projection for improved visualization of the left coronary artery and its branches. AJR 121:575, 1974.
7. Schlesinger, M.J.: Relation of anatomic pattern to pathologic conditions of the coronary arteries. Arch. Pathol. 30:403, 1940.
8. Sandhu, J.S., Uretsky, B.F., Zerbe, T.R., et al.: Coronary artery fistula in heart transplant patients: A potential complication of endomyocardial biopsy. (Abstract.) Circulation 78:II-253, 1988.
9. Schwarz, F., Flameng, W., Ensslen, R., et al.: Effect of coronary collaterals on left ventricular function at rest and during stress. Am. Heart J. 95:570, 1978.

T

1. Taliercio, C.P., Vlietstra, R.E., Fisher, L.D., and Burnett, J.C.: Risk for renal dysfunction with cardiac angiography. Ann. Intern. Med. 104:501, 1986.
2. Tubau, J.F., Chaitman, B.R., Bourassa, M.G., et al.: Importance of coronary collateral circulation in interpreting exercise test results. Am. J. Cardiol. 47:27, 1981.

V

1. Vlodaver, Z., Neufeld, H.N., and Edwards, J.E.: Pathology of coronary disease. Semin. Roengtenol. 7:376, 1972.
2. Vlodaver, Z., Frech, R., VanTassel, R.A., and Edwards, J.E.: Correlation of

the antemorten coronary arteriogram and the postmortem specimen. Circulation 47:162, 1973.

W

1. Williams, J.A., Littmann, D., Hall, J.H., et al.: Coronary arteriography. II. Clinical experiences with the loop-end catheter. N. Engl. J. Med. 262:328, 1960.
2. Weintraub, R.M., Voukydis, P.C., Aroesty, J.M., et al.: Treatment of preinfarction angina with intraaortic balloon counterpulsation and surgery. Am. J. Cardiol. 34:809, 1974.
3. White, C.W., Eckberg, D.L., Inasaka, T., and Abboud, F.M.: Effects of angiographic contrast media and sino-atrial nodal function. Cardiovasc. Res. 10:214, 1976.
4. Wolf, G.L., Kraft, L., and Kilzer, K.: Contrast agents lower ventricular fibrillation threshold. Radiology 129:215, 1978.
5. Weinrauch, L.A., Healy, R.W., Leland, O.S., Jr., et al.: Coronary angiography and acute renal failure in diabetic azotemic nephropathy. Ann. Intern. Med. 86:56, 1977.
6. Weidner, W., MacAlpin, R., Hanafee, W., and Kattus, A.: Percutaneous transaxillary selective coronary angiography. Radiology 85:652, 1965.
7. Wesselhoeft, H., Fawcett, J.S., and Johnson, A.L.: Anomalous origin of the left coronary artery from the pulmonary trunk. Its clinical spectrum, pathology, and pathophysiology, based on a review of 140 cases with seven further cases. Circulation 38:403, 1968.
8. Wilson, C.L., Dlabal, P.W., Holeyfield, R.W., et al.: Anomalous origin of left coronary artery from pulmonary artery. Case report and review of literature concerning teen-agers and adults. J. Thorac. Cardiovasc. Surg. 73:887, 1977.
9. Williams, D.O., Amsterdam, E.A., Miller, R.R., and Mason, D.T.: Functional significance of coronary collateral vessels in patients with acute myocardial infarction: Relation to pump performance, cardiogenic shock, and survival. Am. J. Cardiol. 37:345, 1976.
10. White, C.W., Wright, C.B., Doty, D.B., et al.: Does visual interpretation of the coronary arteriogram predict the physiologic importance of a coronary stenosis? N. Engl. J. Med. 310:819, 1984.
11. Webster, J.S., Moberg, C., and Rincan, G.: Natural history of severe proximal coronary artery disease as documented by coronary cineangiography. Am. J. Cardiol. 33:195, 1974.
12. Wilson, R.F., Holida, M.D., and White, C.W.: Quantitative angiographic morphology of coronary stenoses leading to myocardial infarction or unstable angina. Circulation 73:286, 1986.
13. Wyman, R.M., Safian, R.D., Portway, V., et al.: Current complications of diagnostic and therapeutic cardiac catheterization. J. Am. Coll. Cardiol. 12:1400, 1988.

Z

1. Zweiman, B., Mishkin, M.M., and Hildreth, E.A.: An approach to the performance of contrast studies in contrast material-reactive persons. Ann. Intern. Med. 83:159, 1975.
2. Zir, L.M., Dinsmore, R.E., Goss, C., and Harthorne, J.W.: Experience with preformed catheters for coronary angiography by the brachial approach. Cathet. Cardiovasc. Diagn. 1:303, 1975.
3. Zir, L.M., Miller, S.W., Dinsmore, R.E., et al.: Interobserver variability in coronary angiography. Circulation 53:627, 1976.

Chapter 13

Quantitative Coronary Angiography

JOHAN H.C. REIBER, Ph.D. ▪ PATRICK W. SERRUYS, M.D., Ph.D.
on behalf of the Thoraxcenter

PROBLEMS WITH INTERPRETATION OF THE CORONARY ANGIOGRAM 213
INTEROBSERVER AND INTRAOBSERVER VARIABILITY IN STENOSIS GEOMETRY BY VISUAL INTERPRETATION 213
REQUIRED NUMBER OF ANGIOGRAPHIC VIEWS 214
FURTHER LIMITATIONS IN ASSESSMENT OF GEOMETRIC LESION SEVERITY 214
PHYSIOLOGIC SIGNIFICANCE OF CORONARY OBSTRUCTIONS 215
SUMMARY 216

APPROACHES TO QUANTITATIVE CORONARY ANGIOGRAPHY 217
CALIPERS 218
BROWN-DODGE METHOD 218
IMAGE ACQUISITION AND DIGITIZATION OF 35-mm CINE FILM 219
ON-LINE DIGITAL CARDIAC SYSTEMS 220
COMPUTER HARDWARE AND SOFTWARE 221
CONTOUR DETECTION APPROACHES 222
Definition of Coronary Segment to Be Analyzed 222
Edge Definition 223
Pincushion Distortion and Correction 224
Calibration 224
CONTOUR ANALYSIS APPROACHES 225
Reference for Percent Diameter Stenosis Measurement 225
Roughness Measure of Arterial Segment 227
Derived Parameters of Coronary Arterial Segment 227
Interpretation of Results From Biplane Analyses 227
DENSITOMETRY 227
SUMMARY 230

QUALITY CONTROL IN QUANTITATIVE CORONARY ARTERIOGRAPHY 231
IMAGE ANALYSIS STEPS 231
SOURCES OF VARIATION AND APPROACHES TO STANDARDIZATION IN DATA ANALYSIS 231
SOURCES OF VARIATION AND APPROACHES TO STANDARDIZATION IN ANGIOGRAPHIC DATA ACQUISITION 232
On-Line Registration of X-Ray System Settings 232
Preangiographic Administration of Vasodilative Drugs 232
Use of Nonionic and Iso-osmolar Contrast Media 233
Administration of Contrast Medium by Electrocardiographically Triggered Injector ... 234
Selection of Catheter Material 234
Micrometric Measurement of Catheter Following Catheterization 234
SUMMARY 234

VALIDATION STUDIES 236
PROPOSED VALIDATION PROCEDURES 236
PARAMETERS DESCRIBING VALIDATION RESULTS 236
NONDENSITOMETRIC VALIDATION STUDIES OF ARTERIAL DIMENSIONS 236
Phantom Studies 236
In Vivo Validations 237
Variability in Repeated Analyses 237
DENSITOMETRIC VALIDATION STUDIES 237
Phantom Studies 237
In Vivo Validations 237
Variability in Repeated Analyses 238
Variability in Densitometric Results Assessed From Different Angiographic Views 238
VARIABILITY IN REPEATED CORONARY CINEANGIOGRAPHY AND COMPUTER ANALYSIS 238
Variability in Data Analysis 238
Overall Variability 238
Short-Term (5-Minute) Variability 239
Medium-Term (1-Hour) Variability 239
Long-Term (90-Day) Variability 240
IMPORTANCE OF FRAME SELECTION IN QUANTITATIVE CORONARY ANGIOGRAPHY 241
Results 241
SUMMARY 242

CORONARY FLOW RESERVE 243
BASIC PRINCIPLES FOR MEASUREMENT OF CORONARY BLOOD FLOW AND FLOW RESERVE 244
RADIOGRAPHIC TECHNIQUES 245
Angiographic Procedure and Induction of Maximal Hyperemic Response 246
Angiographic Image Processing and Coronary Flow Reserve Measurements 247
RELATIONSHIP BETWEEN CORONARY ARTERY DIMENSIONS AND CORONARY FLOW RESERVE 249
VARIABILITY IN CORONARY FLOW RESERVE MEASUREMENTS 250
Intraobserver Variability 250
Interobserver Variability 250
Short-Term (5-Minute) Variability 251
Medium-Term (1- to 3-Hour) Variability and Immediate Functional Result of Percutaneous Transluminal Coronary Angioplasty 251
Long-Term (3- to 5-Month) Variability and Long-Term Functional Result of Percutaneous Transluminal Coronary Angioplasty 251

CORONARY FLOW RESERVE AND PERCUTANEOUS TRANSLUMINAL CORONARY ANGIOPLASTY 255
COMPARISON OF INTRACORONARY DOPPLER TECHNIQUE WITH DIGITAL SUBTRACTION CINEANGIOGRAPHY IN MEASUREMENT OF CORONARY FLOW RESERVE IN THE SETTING OF CORONARY ANGIOPLASTY 255
ASSESSMENT OF CORONARY FLOW RESERVE BY MYOCARDIAL CONTRAST ECHOCARDIOGRAPHY 256
SUMMARY 258
APPLICATIONS OF QUANTITATIVE CORONARY ANGIOGRAPHY 259
RESTENOSIS 259
Angiographic Definitions 259
Incidence 260
Timing 262
Methodologic Considerations 263
Videodensitometric Analysis 263
Risk Factors 263
SUMMARY 263
EFFICACY OF ENDOLUMINAL PROSTHESES 263
Methods 264
Results 264
Discussion 266
Summary 267
PROGRESSION AND REGRESSION OF ATHEROSCLEROSIS 267
Angiographic Intervention Studies 267
Summary 270
CHAPTER SUMMARY 271

Despite the widespread and long-standing use of coronary angiography in clinical practice, the interpretation of angiograms has changed very little. Image quality continues to improve as a result of higher quality x-ray sources and image intensifiers, pulsed fluoroscopy, real-time image enhancement, and high-quality image digitization; however, most angiograms are still reviewed visually and therefore subjectively. In the almost exploding field of interventional catheterization procedures —including thrombolysis, balloon dilatation, and other rapidly evolving techniques for transluminal revascularization or recanalization—a more detailed and quantitative routine analysis of coronary arteriograms is urgently needed. Clearly, the visual interpretation of coronary obstructions as the basis for scientific studies is no longer acceptable. Spatial and temporal resolution of angiograms is relatively high, allowing the derivation of both anatomic and functional information of coronary obstructions. These quantitative data should be available not only off-line from cineangiographic film, but also on-line, during the patient's investigation, as they are urgently needed to facilitate the making of clinical decisions. The anatomic/geometric and functional/physiologic approaches are complementary; thus, using a combination of these approaches is far better than using either one alone. Furthermore, objective and reproducible analysis further enhances an understanding of pathophysiologic processes in coronary artery disease.

This chapter provides an overview of the field of quantitative coronary angiography. In the first section, we focus on the problems involved with the usual visual interpretation of coronary angiograms, which results in large interobserver and intraobserver variations. Investigators have shown that because of the complex spatial orientation of the coronary arterial system and the frequent occurrence of eccentric and asymmetric lesions, multiple angiographic views are required to describe qualitatively or quantitatively the morphology of the lesions. We also discuss why percent diameter stenosis is an inadequate approach to assess the severity of coronary obstructive disease, particularly in patients with multivessel coronary artery disease. Finally, we briefly describe the advantages and limitations of the available methods of assessing the functional significance of obstructions.

An extensive overview is given of the different techniques that are available or are being developed for the quantitative morphologic and densitometric computer-aided analysis of coronary obstructions. Both off-line and on-line approaches are discussed. The majority of the techniques have been developed for cineangiographic film analysis; however, in the same or a slightly modified format, they are also applicable to digitally acquired data. With rapid progress in improved hardware and software for digital systems, and the development of rapid, objective, and reproducible software application packages, the on-line approaches will play an increasingly dominant role in clinical decision-making and, possibly in the near future, in the assessment of the efficacy of interventional studies.

Evaluation of changes in arterial dimensions over time requires repeated performance and analysis of angiography. Various sources of error may interfere with the quality of the angiographic computer analysis, however. Approaches toward standardizing procedures for angiographic or cineangiographic acquisition and analysis are discussed. Variability in the measurement of absolute dimensions may increase dramatically unless such precautions are taken.

In addition, procedures are proposed for determining the accuracy, precision, and reproducibility of quantitative coronary angiographic methods. Extensive overviews of published data on nondensitometric and densitometric techniques are given. The results of our short-, medium-, and long-term validation studies on the overall variabilities in diameter measurements with repeated cineangiography and computer analysis are described as well. Variability in arterial dimensions due to the frame selection process is examined.

The concept of coronary flow reserve is introduced. Basically, two approaches have been developed to assess the coronary flow reserve of individual coronary arteries in the clinical setting: (1) the ratio of maximal to resting coronary blood flow, with the maximal flow produced by potent pharmacologic coronary vasodilation, and (2) coronary angiographic data. The basic principles of coronary flow measurement are presented.

Three techniques are now available for the first approach to assessing regional coronary flow reserve during cardiac catheterization: (1) the pulsed Doppler coronary artery catheter, which can measure intracoronary blood flow velocity, (2) radiographic assessment of myocardial perfusion using contrast medium, and (3) an indicator-dilution technique in which a platinum-tipped percutaneous transluminal coronary angioplasty (PTCA) guidewire is used with hydrogen as the indicator. In addition, positron emission tomography allows noninvasive assessment of flow reserve to specific vascular territories. At open heart surgery, coronary reserve can be measured in individual vessels with a suction Doppler probe.

Because of its great popularity, the radiographic technique is subsequently discussed in detail, followed by discussion of the relationships found between the resulting coronary flow reserve measurements and coronary anatomy. If this radiographic technique is to be used for the determination of the immediate or long-term functional results of pharmacologic therapy or revascularization procedures, data regarding the interobserver and intraobserver variations, and the short-, medium-, and long-term variabilities in the measurement of coronary flow reserve, must be available; results from our validation studies are therefore presented. Next, the application of coronary flow reserve measurements in the setting of PTCA is described, and comparative data on the results from use of this angiographic approach and Doppler catheterization are presented. Finally, the new developments in myocardial contrast echocardiography for the assessment of coronary flow reserve are discussed.

In the last section of this chapter, three typical areas of application are reviewed. The first application involves restenosis in the setting of PTCA. The definition of restenosis has been the subject of much debate; so far no consensus has been reached on how such restenosis studies should be performed, which has resulted in widely differing methodologic approaches that give diverse and conflicting data. The second area of application involves the efficacy of the endoluminal prosthesis (stent), which is described in terms of the early morphologic changes in stenosis geometry as assessed by quantitative coronary angiography in a group of 26 patients who had undergone PTCA. The stent has been proposed as an approach for preventing late restenosis after PTCA. The third area of application involves the progression and regression of atherosclerosis. A review of lipid-lowering intervention trials is provided, and the role of computer-supported analysis of atherosclerosis is described.

The conclusion to this chapter summarizes the basic approaches and results previously presented.

PROBLEMS WITH INTERPRETATION OF THE CORONARY ANGIOGRAM

The severity of a coronary obstruction can be expressed in terms of its geometric deviations from the normal size of the coronary vessel, as well as in terms of its functional or physiologic significance. In other words, the effect of the stenosis on the perfusion of the myocardial muscle at basal flow and at maximal flow levels can be used to express the severity of the obstruction. In clinical practice and in research studies, assessment of the morphology of the obstruction has been emphasized. Over the last few years, however, interest in the determination of the physiologic significance of obstructions has increased. This section begins with an overview of the problems in the visual interpretation of the morphology of the coronary system, which is followed by discussions of the required number of angiographic views and of further limitations in the geometric assessment of the lesion severity. Finally, the problems in estimating the physiologic significance of coronary obstructions are described.

INTEROBSERVER AND INTRAOBSERVER VARIABILITY IN STENOSIS GEOMETRY BY VISUAL INTERPRETATION

The use of 35-mm cine film for conventional visual evaluation of the geometric characteristics of coronary obstructions to assess their severity has been hampered by considerable interobserver and intraobserver variation.[C1, D1, D2, F1, M1, S1, S2, Z1, Z2] DeRouen and colleagues assessed interobserver variability by requesting 11 experienced cardiac angiographers to estimate from angiograms the percent diameter narrowing of the worst lesions in 10 different standard arterial segments, with 10 angiograms for each segment.[D2] Observed standard deviations for the total of 100 coronary segments ranged from zero percent to 51.32 percent; the largest deviation found involved the distal right coronary artery. The average standard deviation per vessel segment (taken over all 10 cases) ranged from 8.0 percent for the proximal right coronary artery to 28.5 percent for the diagonal branch. An overall average standard deviation of 18 percent was found for all 10 cases and 10 segments, which is a crude estimate of general variability. If two standard deviations are used to indicate the possible error in reading an obstruction, this value would indicate a possible error of 36 percent. Similar findings for the interobserver variability have been reported by Zir and associates.[Z1] These studies indicate that in addition to the problem of visually interpreting the severity of an obstruction, lack of uniformity in the designation of the location of lesions was an important cause of the large interobserver variations.

These variations can be reduced by means of a consensus opinion based on several observers reading the coronary angiograms at the same time.[Z2] Sanmarco and co-workers studied the reproducibility of a consensus panel in the interpretation of coronary cineangiograms and found an overall standard deviation of the differences in panel reading of 14 percent.[S1]

Shub and colleagues have demonstrated that the interobserver and intraobserver variabilities vary with the severity of the stenosis (Fig. 13–1).[S2] For stenoses of less than 20 percent or more than 80 percent of the diameter, the interobserver and intraobserver differences were relatively small (mean differences were less than 5 percent). For stenoses between 20 and 80 percent of the diameter, the differences were slightly greater (mean differences were 8 to 14 percent). The patterns of the interobserver and intraobserver variabilities were similar.

The interobserver variability in the interpretation of 870 coronary arteriograms by readers at two different clinics was determined as part of the Coronary Artery Surgery Study (CASS).[F1] Of the arteriograms for the seven segments studied, those of the left main coronary artery were the most difficult to read; arteriograms of the proximal right coronary artery were the easiest to read. Investigators in the study estimated that when one angiographer reports a stenosis of 50 percent or more in the left main coronary artery, a second angiographer reports no lesion, in 18.6 percent of cases. In 94.7 percent of the films, the number of vessels showing significant disease (stenoses greater than 70 percent of the diameter) was the same for both angiographers (72.1 percent) or differed by one vessel (22.6 percent). The reproducibility of interpretation of films of good or acceptable quality or of complete studies was better than the reproducibility of readings of arteriograms judged to be of poor quality or of incomplete studies.

Meier and associates assessed the interobserver and intraobserver variabilities in a PTCA study, using a calibrated magnifying glass for stenoses that were manually traced from a cine projector.[M1] The interobserver coefficients of variation in the determi-

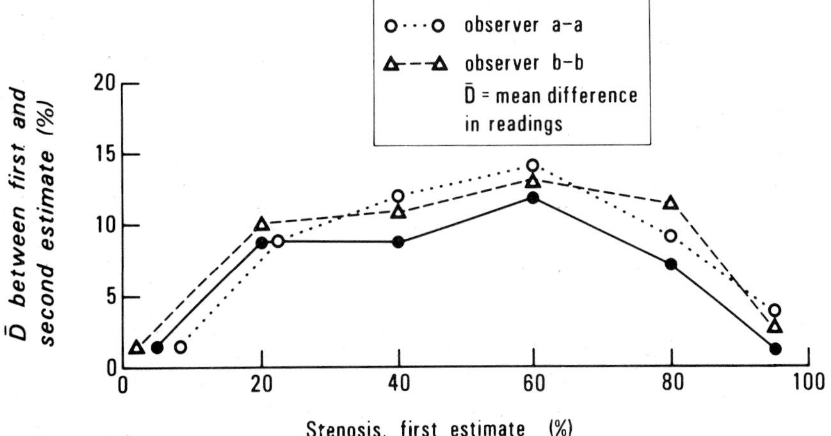

Figure 13–1. Reproducibility of angiographic interpretation. Twenty-five angiograms were randomly selected, read, and then reread 3 months later. Values for each stenosis were compared to assess interobserver (a-b) and intraobserver (a-a, b-b) variability. $\bar{D}$ represents the mean difference in readings between the first and second estimates. Lesions were grouped into the following ranges of percent diameter stenosis: 0 to 9, 10 to 29, 30 to 49, 50 to 69, 70 to 89, and 90 to 100 percent, as shown on the abscissa. (From Shub, C., et al.: The unpredictable progression of symptomatic coronary artery disease: A serial clinical-angiographic analysis. Mayo Clin. Proc. 56:155, 1981, with permission.)

nation of the percent diameter stenosis (which equal the standard deviations of differences between the measurements by the observers, divided by the mean value) were 7 percent for the projection showing the most severe stenosis and 6.4 percent for the mean of three projections. The intraobserver coefficient of variation was significantly reduced from 16.0 to 10.5 percent by using the mean of three projections. The investigators also made a visual selection of the projection that demonstrated the most severe stenosis and compared that with the projection measured to be the most severe. In only 7 of 30 (23 percent) of the angiograms was there complete agreement among the three readers regarding the projection that demonstrated the most severe coronary stenosis before angioplasty.

Cameron and colleagues demonstrated a 41 to 59 percent agreement on the severity of the lesion in the visual interpretation of left main coronary artery stenosis by three groups of experienced angiographers on a group consensus basis, with 80 percent agreement on whether the lesion was greater or less than 50 percent of the diameter.[C1] The severity of the lesion, its location, or the presence of calcium or ectasia did not affect the discrepancy rate, but arteriograms of segments that were unusually short, diffusely diseased, or obscured by overlapping vessels were especially difficult to interpret.

In summary, these studies demonstrate that interobserver and intraobserver variability severely limits the value of visual interpretation of coronary angiograms.

REQUIRED NUMBER OF ANGIOGRAPHIC VIEWS

Angiography of the major coronary arteries requires multiple projections (a minimum of two) for the following reasons: (1) Overlapping vessels can introduce substantial error unless multiple angulated views are obtained. (2) The luminal cross sections of coronary obstructions may be noncircular and eccentrically located, leading to overestimations and underestimations of their true severity.[F2, H1, L1, T1, V1, V2] (3) In each projection, only a limited number of coronary segments are approximately parallel to the input screen of the image intensifier; for the other segments, foreshortening occurs.

Histologic analyses of postmortem coronary arteries have shown that severity and incidence of lesions differ throughout the coronary artery system.[S3] Vlodaver and Edwards examined 200 consecutive sections of atheromatous coronary arteries histologically and found the following distribution of different shapes of lumen: central (30.5 percent), eccentric polymorphous (40.5 percent), and eccentric slit-like (29 percent).[V1] Investigators have argued, however, that the crescentic or slit-like lumen is a product of postmortem arterial fixation with sectioning in the unpressurized state.[A1, B1] Thomas and colleagues have shown that most stenotic lesions result in circular, elliptic, or D-shaped lumina if postmortem perfusion fixation of the coronary arteries occurs at physiologic pressures. Crescentic lumina in fully distended vessels were found to be associated only with acute mural thrombi projecting into the lumen or with massive intra-intimal thrombi and plaque fissuring.[T1] Freudenberg and Lichtlen found that 74 percent of all significantly stenosed vessels had eccentric lumina; the remaining 26 percent had central lumina.[F2] Ninety-five percent of all lumina in their study were approximately circular, elliptic, or D-shaped, while only 5 percent showed irregular star-shaped or crescentic lumina.

Alternatively, if the slit-like lumen is a true phenomenon in approximately one quarter (29 percent) of the atheromas studied, a severe obstruction might yield a luminal width that suggests no obstruction of the segment in certain angiographic views. Similarly, angiographic evaluation following angioplasty might be hampered by the eccentric nature of the mechanical disruption of the intima.[B2, E1, H2] On pure angiographic grounds, Ambrose and colleagues found that type II eccentric lesions (asymmetric lesions with a narrow neck or irregular borders, or both) are frequent in patients with unstable angina and probably represent ruptured atherosclerotic plaques or partially occlusive thrombi, or both.[A5] This type II eccentric lesion is also common in the progression of coronary artery disease.[A10] The concentric and type I eccentric lesions (asymmetric narrowing with smooth borders and a broad neck) were seen more frequently in patients with stable angina. In general, more complex stenoses are associated with future myocardial events.[C12, H14, L12] Falk demonstrated that the thrombotic process in patients with unstable angina is dynamic, and that recurrent mural thrombus formation in these patients alternates with intermittent thrombus fragmentation, which emphasizes the importance of quantitation of the lumen and plaque morphology.[F15]

The complex spatial orientation of the left coronary arterial system usually requires four or five projections, which should allow the filming of an obstruction in at least one projection en face. The right coronary arterial system has a much simpler configuration, for which two, preferably orthogonal, projections suffice. Recent work by Dodge and associates describing the intrathoracic spatial locations of all the coronary arterial segments may aid in selecting the best angiographic views to visualize the traditionally difficult parts of the coronary tree.[D16] Although densitometry should theoretically allow assessment of the severity of an obstruction from only one view, the results in practice have not yet been convincing for large-scale clinical use (see "Densitometry" in the section "Approaches to Quantitative Coronary Angiography").

FURTHER LIMITATIONS IN ASSESSMENT OF GEOMETRIC LESION SEVERITY

In addition to the problems mentioned earlier, other factors interfere with an accurate determination of the severity of coronary obstructions. Collateral flow to an obstructed segment may influence the estimation of distal vessel size.[L2] When the severity of an obstruction is expressed in terms of percent diameter reduction with respect to a so-called normal proximal or distal segment, diffuse atherosclerosis causes underestimation of the obstruction (Fig. 13–2). Studies have shown that coronary disease is often a diffuse process that involves the entire length of a coronary artery.[A1, I1, R1] Patients with multivessel coronary disease have substantial but variable diffuse coronary atherosclerosis, which may not be detectable without sophisticated quantitative

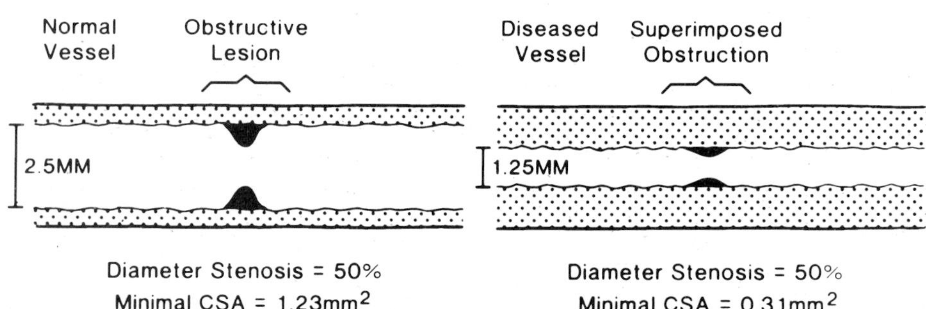

Figure 13–2. Both vessels would appear to contain 50 percent lesions at coronary angiography. The hemodynamic significance of the superimposed lesion on the right is greater than that of the lesion on the left. CSA—cross-sectional area. (From Harrison, D.G., et al.: The value of lesion cross-sectional area determined by quantitative coronary angiography in assessing the physiologic significance of proximal left anterior descending coronary arterial stenoses. Circulation 69:1111, 1984, with permission of the American Heart Association, Inc.)

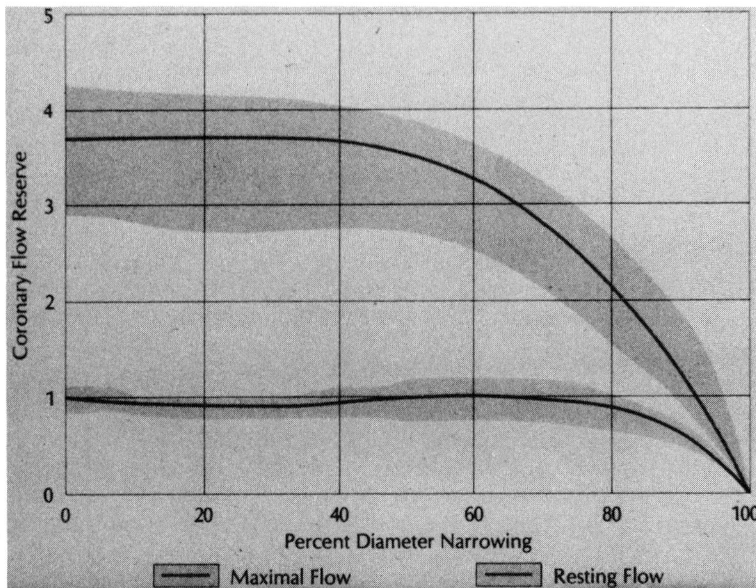

Figure 13–3. Coronary blood flow reserve in a stenotic artery under carefully controlled conditions is inversely proportional to the severity of stenosis. Resting coronary flow remains normal up to approximately 85 percent diameter narrowing, whereas maximal flow begins to fall at about 50 percent narrowing. With a stronger vasodilatory stimulus and a normal increase in flow of five times the resting levels, even 30 percent to 40 percent narrowing may be detectable. (From Kirkeeide, R.L., and Gould, K.L.: Cardiovascular imaging: Coronary artery stenosis. Hosp. Pract. 19:160, 1984. Reproduced with permission. Illustration by Albert Miller.)

coronary angiography.[A1, H3, M7] Therefore, percent stenosis measurement is an inadequate approach to assessing the severity of coronary obstructive disease in patients with multivessel coronary artery disease. Alternatively, diffuse disease undetectable by angiography is less common and less severe in patients with single-vessel disease.[W4]

More reasons exist, however, for the limited value of percent diameter measurements. First, cineangiography is now known to be incapable of reliably identifying the normal diameter of a coronary artery because of the general compensatory dilation associated with coronary artery disease.[G10] Second, because of the normal variation in diameter of diseased coronary arteries composed of stenotic and ectatic segments, the selected normal segment is subject to considerable individual variation; this problem is compounded when sequential analyses are performed on the same lesion. Third, between two analyses, the selected normal segment may undergo a significant change that is not recognized unless the segment is measured quantitatively.

Beatt and colleagues have shown in a quantitative PTCA study that the reference diameter may be involved in the dilation process, and that it therefore may be subject to the same restenotic process that takes place in initially stenotic segments (see "Restenosis" in the section "Applications of Quantitative Coronary Angiography").[B11] During angioplasty, the relatively normal coronary artery segments adjacent to the stenosis are inevitably involved in the angioplasty process, because the balloon is usually longer than the stenosis, and the balloon across the stenosis cannot always be positioned precisely. Percent diameter stenosis measurements tend to underestimate the change when a simultaneous reduction in the reference diameter occurs; thus, the percent diameter stenosis measurement fails to reflect the morphologic changes induced by balloon dilation. The use of the interpolated reference diameter minimizes these potential errors because it is not arbitrarily selected by the angiographer and is not based on an artery's behavior at one point alone, but it reflects the change in the segments adjacent to the stenosis, both proximally and distally.

Spontaneous or catheter-induced coronary spasm may exaggerate abnormalities by causing different reactions in vasomotility of normal and obstructed segments. Conversely, preferential dilatation of a nonobstructive segment with respect to the obstructed segment may lead to a misleading interpretation of the otherwise beneficial effect of the vasodilator, because the absolute dimension of the obstructive lumen is actually increased.

PHYSIOLOGIC SIGNIFICANCE OF CORONARY OBSTRUCTIONS

By means of coronary angiography, the morphology of the coronary arterial system can be visualized in great detail. A coronary obstruction potentially limits the coronary flow, however, and thus limits the perfusion of the distal bed. Therefore, highly accurate prediction of the flow reduction due to a coronary obstruction would be of great interest. Flow to a particular vascular bed is primarily a function of the resistance of the intramyocardial and epicardial vessels. Unless the stenosis in the epicardial vessel is severe, the flow through a vascular bed is controlled primarily by the bed resistance. As severity of the stenosis progresses, the resistance to flow as evidenced by the pressure drop across the stenosis becomes highly significant and can ultimately limit the flow to the peripheral bed, despite its maximal vasodilatation (Fig. 13–3).[S4]

In a narrowed segment, blood velocity (kinetic energy) increases, and pressure (static energy) decreases in accordance with the Bernoulli principle. The reduction in luminal size at a coronary obstruction results in a pressure drop or gradient over that obstruction, which is influenced by four factors: entrance effects, viscous friction, exit separation of vortex formation in the diverging portion of the stenosis, and inertia of the fluid (Fig. 13–4).[B3, G2, G3, K2, L3, L4, M2, M3, Y1–Y4] Abrupt changes in entrance and

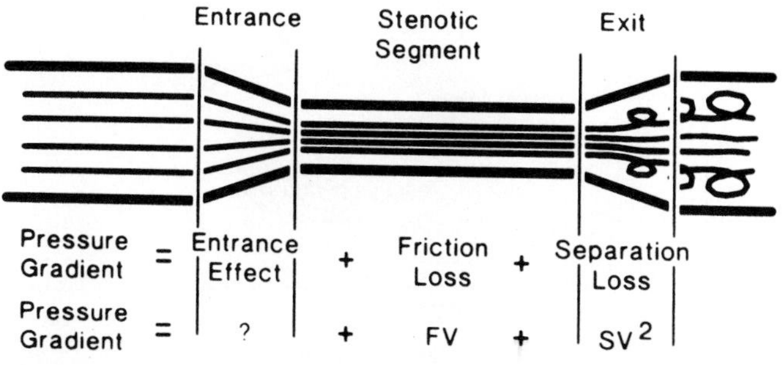

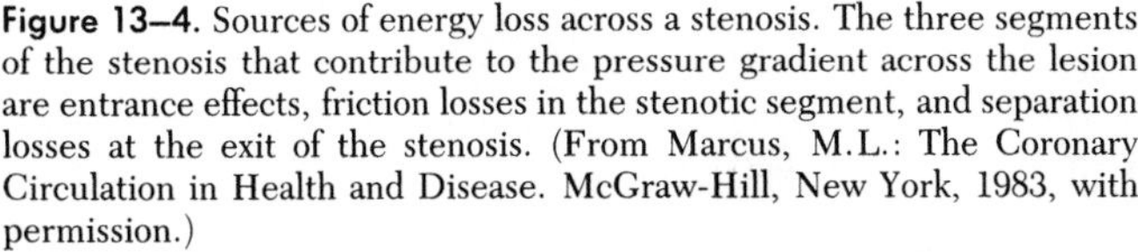
Figure 13–4. Sources of energy loss across a stenosis. The three segments of the stenosis that contribute to the pressure gradient across the lesion are entrance effects, friction losses in the stenotic segment, and separation losses at the exit of the stenosis. (From Marcus, M.L.: The Coronary Circulation in Health and Disease. McGraw-Hill, New York, 1983, with permission.)

exit angles are associated with substantial energy losses. These separation losses are usually greatest at the exit, where turbulence may occur; they are a function of the square of the blood flow velocity. Because myocardial oxygen delivery is proportional to coronary arterial blood flow, a severe stenosis in a major coronary artery can cause significant ischemia during periods of increased oxygen demand (e.g., exercise) by severely limiting flow, leading to either angina or myocardial infarction.

The functional significance of a lesion depends not only on the degree of coronary arterial narrowing, but also on its extent (Fig. 13–5),[F3–F5, S6] the degree of asymmetry of the lesion,[Y1, Y2] the effect of multiple occlusions in series,[F6, S6] the shapes of the entrance and exit from the narrowed segment,[C3] blood viscosity and density,[G3] residual vasomotor tone, collateral perfusion to the given myocardial region,[F7] coronary bed resistance, and blood flow velocity. Moreover, both active and passive increases in the severity of compliant coronary stenoses may occur.[B5, E2, M6, S7–S9] Active changes in coronary stenosis diameter may result from either localized vasomotion superimposed on an atherosclerotic plaque or generalized changes in coronary arterial diameter, which include those of the stenotic segment. Passive narrowing of a compliant coronary stenosis may occur in response to a fall in coronary pressure or to any intervention that dilates the coronary arterial bed and lowers distending pressure distal to and within the stenotic segment.

With the physiologic significance of coronary lesions depending on so many parameters, the fact that only poor correlations have been found with percent diameter stenosis measurements (or measurement of any other single stenosis dimension)—especially when interpreted visually—is not surprising.[M5, W2, W3] The percent diameter stenosis method ignores many important factors that contribute to the hydraulic effects of an obstruction.

Only under carefully controlled conditions, such as in animal experimental studies or in quantitative studies of stenosis severity in patients with single-vessel disease, have measurements of percent diameter stenosis, percent area stenosis, or the calculated pressure drop over the stenosis been found to be useful predictors of the physiologic significance of a lesion.[G2, G5–G8, Z3] In general, coronary flow reserve begins to decline when the diameter stenosis is greater than 50 percent, and it diminishes substantially when the diameter stenosis is greater than 75 percent. The reason for these measurements being useful in human studies is that diffuse disease undetectable by angiography is less common and less severe in patients with single-vessel disease.[W4] Clearly, however, the usefulness of visual interpretation of the severity of the stenosis is limited by interobserver and intraobserver variability, as discussed earlier. In patients with multivessel disease, visual[W3, M7] or quantitative[H3] estimates of percent diameter stenosis or percent area stenosis correlate poorly with the physiologic significance of coronary obstructive lesions, particularly when obstructions are of intermediate severity, which can be explained by the presence of diffuse coronary disease that is not detectable by angiography.

The physiologic significance is usually expressed in terms of coronary flow reserve, which is discussed in more detail in the section "Coronary Flow Reserve." Flow reserve can be measured in individual vessels with a suction Doppler probe at open heart surgery,[M4] with an intracoronary Doppler catheter at cardiac catheterization,[W1] with an indicator-dilution technique using hydrogen as the indicator and a platinum-tipped PTCA guidewire,[V9] and with digital angiographic techniques.[C2, V3, V4] The last approach has gained widespread interest and use and is discussed in more detail in the section "Coronary Flow Reserve." The great advantage of this technique is that it can be performed during routine cardiac catheterization without increasing the risk to the patient. The pressure drop over a stenosis calculated from the morphology has been found to be highly predictive of thallium-201 scintigraphic results in patients with single-vessel disease, with a sensitivity of 94 percent and a specificity of 90 percent.[Z3] Positron emission tomography allows the measurement of coronary flow reserve to specific vascular territories,[B4, G4, S5] and new approaches in cine computed tomography (or ultrafast computed tomography),[R2] contrast echocardiography,[A2] and magnetic resonance imaging[P1] are being actively investigated for their potential ability to measure coronary flow reserve.

SUMMARY

The data presented previously make clear that the visual interpretation of the severity of coronary obstructions, as the basis for scientific studies, is no longer acceptable. Quantitative coronary angiographic techniques, either off-line or on-line, have become available on a large scale; they allow the objective morphologic and physiologic assessment of the severity of obstructions (see the sections "Approaches to Quantitative Coronary Angiography" and "Coronary Flow Reserve"). Anatomic/geometric and functional/physiologic approaches are complementary; thus, using a combination of these approaches is far better than using either one alone.[G1, G8, G21]

Objective and reproducible techniques for the assessment of

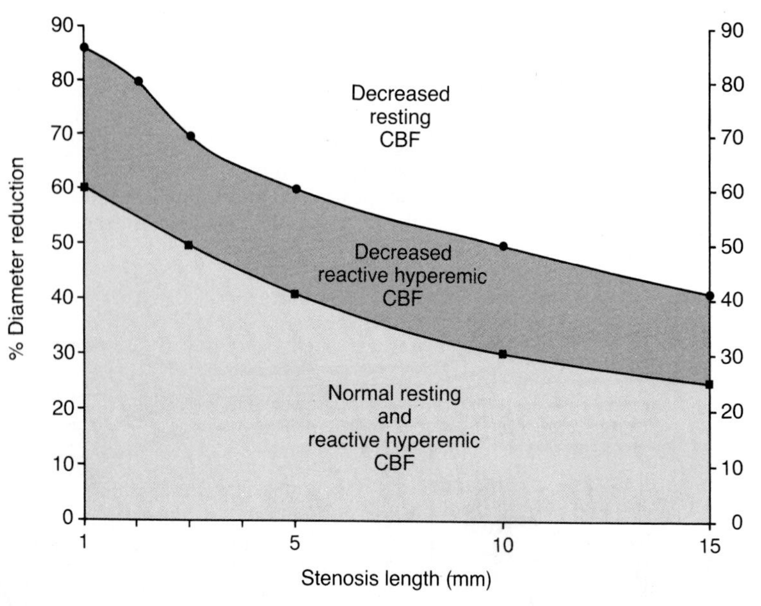

Figure 13–5. The effect of percent diameter reduction (vertical axis) and the length of diameter reduction (horizontal axis) on coronary blood flow. For example, an 85 percent stenosis greater than 1 mm long decreases resting and reactive hyperemic flows; a 50 percent stenosis greater than 5 mm long decreases reactive hyperemic flow, but not resting flow. If the length of a 50 percent stenosis is increased to 10 mm or greater, however, resting flow also decreases. A 20 percent stenosis 15 mm long or less does not decrease resting or hyperemic coronary blood flow. (Redrawn from Feldman R.L., et al.: The coronary hemodynamics of left main and branch coronary stenoses: The effects of reduction in stenosis diameter, stenosis length, and number of stenoses. J. Thorac. Cardiovasc. Surg. 77:377, 1979, with permission.)

coronary atherosclerosis have become indispensable for the evaluation of the efficacy of modern therapeutic procedures in the catheterization laboratory, the effects of vasoactive drugs on the size of coronary arterial segments, the effects of short- and long-term interventions on the regression or progression of coronary artery disease, and so forth. Such techniques provide absolute measurements of the minimal diameter and extent of the obstructions, as well as of mean diameters of nonobstructed coronary segments, which are assessed from multiple projections. Ultimately, densitometric analysis may provide the most relevant information on luminal obstruction area, regardless of the shape of the remaining cross section. Finally, developments should be directed toward the three-dimensional representation of coronary arterial segments.[B14, P12, P13, R4, R30, R31] The physiologic significance of the obstructions can be assessed either directly or indirectly.

The increased accuracy and precision in the assessment of coronary obstructions achieved with these newer techniques, as compared with the conventional visual interpretation, will greatly reduce the number of subjects needed in intervention studies to obtain desired confidence levels.

Approaches to Quantitative Coronary Angiography

At present, approximately a dozen groups worldwide are actively involved in the development of techniques for the objective and reproducible quantitative analysis of coronary angiograms. Such techniques should provide absolute measurements of the minimal and reference diameters, of extent and asymmetry of the obstructions, of percent diameter and percent area stenosis, of the area of the atherosclerotic plaque, and of the roughness of the entire coronary arterial segment or of subsegments, as well as data regarding the mean diameters of nonobstructed coronary segments, assessed from multiple angiographic views. By combining all stenosis measurements, the functional pressure-flow effects of the stenosis as well as stenotic flow reserve can be assessed.[G1] In situations in which the obstructions are extremely asymmetric, such as the period following PTCA, during which dissections frequently occur, and during and after thrombolytic therapy,[B6] the computation of relative and absolute cross-sectional narrowing by densitometry appears to be the ultimate goal.

The majority of the applications of quantitative coronary cineangiography require either the comparison of the arterial dimensions in a control group with those in a treated group, or the comparison of preinterventional data with postinterventional data, and possibly with the data from later angiograms at follow-up. The sample size of the number of patients that need to be investigated to demonstrate a certain effect is proportional to the variability of the measurement technique divided by the square of the number of years between the angiograms.[B7] Minimization of the variability of the angiographic data acquisition and computer analysis procedures is of great importance to the investigator who must consider the population size, duration, and cost-effectiveness of a study.

In general, the quantitative analysis of coronary obstructions is performed from 35-mm cine film. Great advantages of the off-line cine-film approach are that cine film has high spatial resolution and that regions of interest (e.g., the region encompassing an arterial segment) can be selected and digitized at a resolution optimally suitable for quantitative analysis through optical zooming. A disadvantage of the cine-film approach is the nonlinear density-log(exposure) transfer function. Because spatial resolution is the most important factor in obtaining high accuracy and precision in the geometric assessment of arterial dimensions, cine film is still the medium of choice for interventional studies, in which small morphologic changes need to be determined with as high a confidence level as possible.

Recent developments in digital cardiac imaging systems, however, have been directed toward obtaining such measurements on-line from videodigitized images during catheterization. A few centers have even completely replaced cine film with the digital approach.[T2] Because of the current limitations in spatial resolution of these on-line digitized images (512^2), this approach is of particular interest as a tool for diagnostic or therapeutic decision-making during catheterization. On the other hand, the digital systems are characterized by high-density resolution and a linear transfer function of the chain from the output of the image intensifier to the brightness levels in the digitized images, which makes them more suitable for densitometric analysis.

Extensive validation studies need to be performed to determine the accuracy and precision of these digital approaches as compared with the established off-line cine-film techniques with optical zooming. Higher resolutions (1024^2 digital images) may not necessarily result in improved accuracy and precision. With the use of modern small field-of-view (FOV) image intensifiers (4-inch and 5-inch FOV), the resolution of $512^2 \times 8$ bits or $512^2 \times 10$ bits images at 25 or 30 frames/sec may even be sufficient for on-line assessment of the efficacy of interventional studies, using the diameter and densitometric cross-sectional area measurements mentioned earlier.

An increasing number of publications are comparing the cine-film and the direct digital approaches. Bachmann and Gansser found an excellent correlation (r = 0.96) between the quantitatively assessed dimensions of angiographically normal coronary segments obtained from direct digital angiograms (Digitron II with 512^2 matrix) and those obtained from high-resolution digitized cineangiograms (Pie Data CAAS with 1330 × 1770 image resolution) (Fig. 13–6).[B8]

Vogel and associates have also compared 35-mm cine-film and digital radiographic images, with the latter digitized at 512 × 512 × 8 bit and at 1024 × 1024 × 8 bit resolution from a progressively scanned video system.[V5] For the quantitative analysis, optical and digital magnifications to an effective resolution of 2048 × 2048 pixels were used for the cine-film and the direct

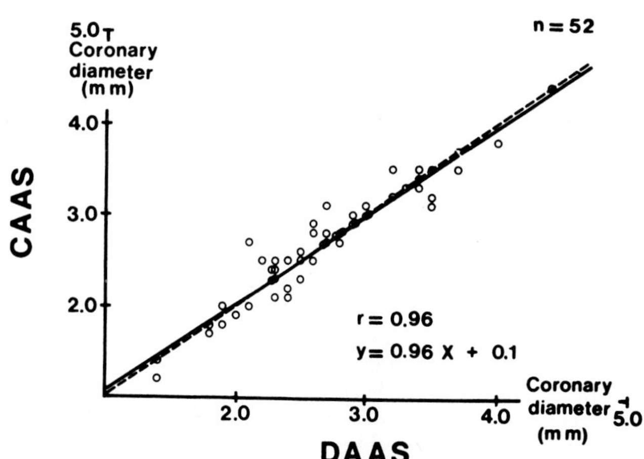

Figure 13–6. Comparison of the coronary diameters measured by quantitative digital angiography and coronary cineangiography. Quantitative studies were performed in 52 angiographically normal coronary segments from monoplane angiograms taken with 25 frames/sec simultaneously by digital angiographic and cineangiographic techniques. Analyses were carried out with computer-based systems that used fully automated coronary contour detection in direct digital angiograms (Siemens Digitron II) and in optically magnified and videodigitized cineangiographic frames (Pie Data CAAS). (From Bachman, K., and Gansser, R.: Digital angiography in coronary heart disease. *In* Heintzen, P.H., and Bürsch, J.H. (eds.): Progress in Digital Angiocardiography. Kluwer Academic, Dordrecht, 1988, p. 13, with permission.)

digital approaches. All images were analyzed with the same quantitation package, which is based on automated edge-detection techniques and densitometric analysis.[L5] The three imaging methods were concluded to be equivalently capable of measuring the diameter of arterial lumina. They all resulted in overestimation of lumina less than 1.0 mm in diameter. These experiments did not substantiate the hypothesized advantage of film's high spatial resolution compared with that of digital methods, or of an advantage of 1024^2 images over 512^2 images. The investigators found that the densitometric relative cross-sectional area analysis does not result in such problems of overestimation of small lumina. Digital techniques were concluded to be more precise than film in the application of densitometric methods for estimating the relative cross-sectional area of lumina in the diameter range tested.

Finally, Skelton and colleagues have compared the effects of digital image acquisition mode and subtraction techniques on 100 discrete lesions.[S31] Digital images were acquired using an ADAC 3100-C digital radiography system (resolution 512 × 512 × 8 bits). Subtracted digital images were also generated from unprocessed digital data using an electrocardiographic-phase–matched mask-mode subtraction. Selected cine frames were projected by a GE CAP35B projector equipped with the same videocamera as on the ADAC system, and the images were directly acquired by the digital imaging computer. Therefore, the optimal resolving power of the cine film was not used, because no optical zooming on the film was performed. Quantitation of the stenoses was performed with the automated edge-detection procedure on the ADAC system (including electronic bilinear interpolation by a factor of 4).[L5] The correlation coefficients for the minimal diameter (r = 0.90), percent diameter stenosis (r = 0.93), and densitometric percent area stenosis (r = 0.85) were found for the comparison of cine and unsubtracted digital methods; the relation between the cine and subtracted method was characterized by slightly lower correlation coefficients: r = 0.90, r = 0.91, and r = 0.80, respectively. The highest values were found for the subtracted versus the unsubtracted digital methods: r = 0.96, r = 0.94, and r = 0.89, respectively.

Although these initial publications indicate great promise for quantitative digital coronary angiography, extensive (in vivo) phantom as well as clinical studies need to be carried out to determine the definite advantages, disadvantages, and limitations of digital versus cine film methods. Until such information is obtained and these matters are resolved, one should be able to use 35-mm cine film simultaneously with digital acquisition without any limitations.

For the assessment of the arterial dimensions, the measurements are usually performed on the original nonsubtracted images. Difficulties in obtaining high-quality subtraction images include selection of background image in same phase of cardiac cycle and the occurrence of motion artifacts. No paper in the literature suggests any benefit from using such an approach for the accurate determination of coronary anatomy.

This section provides an overview of the different techniques now available for the quantitative morphologic and densitometric computer-aided analysis of coronary obstructions.[R3, R4] The majority of the techniques have been developed for cine-film analysis; however, in the same or a slightly modified format, these techniques are also applicable to the on-line digitally acquired data. This section begins with a brief overview of the different caliper techniques used in the early years of quantitative coronary angiography and of the first computer-aided technique, which was developed by Brown and colleagues.[B3] Next, the cine-film and direct digital acquisition techniques are discussed, as are the various computer hardware and software approaches of modern quantitation systems, the various contour detection and analysis techniques, and densitometry.

Most of the data presented in this chapter have been obtained by sending 12 widely known investigators a list containing 25 questions regarding different aspects of the previously mentioned topics: these data represent the state of their developments as of the end of 1987. All 12 principal investigators returned the questionnaire. They are, in alphabetical order:

Brown—University of Washington, Seattle, WA, USA
Collins—University of Iowa, Iowa City, IA, USA
Doriot—Hôpital Cantonal Université, Geneva, Switzerland
Kirkeeide—University of Texas, Houston, TX, USA
Marchand—Thomson CGR, Buc, France
Nichols—Columbia University, New York, NY, USA
Parker—University of Salt Lake City, Salt Lake City, UT, USA
Reiber—Erasmus University, Rotterdam, The Netherlands
Sanders—Stanford University, Palo Alto, CA, USA
Sandor—Harvard University, Boston, MA, USA
Selzer—Jet Propulsion Laboratory, Los Angeles, CA, USA
Vogel—University of Maryland, Baltimore, MD, USA

A summary of these results is presented in this section; further details can be found in reports by Reiber.[R5, R32] Where appropriate, information obtained from other investigators or other developments is included.

CALIPERS

One of the first systems for quantitative coronary angiography was developed by Gensini and colleagues. This system consisted of a projection head and a projection case containing a viewing screen and a cross-hair measuring system.[G9] The frame number and *x-y* coordinates were recorded on IBM punch cards for later analysis. These investigators claimed that the vessel diameter estimates were accurate to within ± 80 μm. MacAlpin and associates made direct estimates of coronary dimensions using caliper measurements and found a mean accuracy of ± 0.2 mm for the measurement of known objects,[M8] and Feldman and colleagues, using a comparable technique, reported a variability of ± 0.5 mm.[F8] Later, calipers were used on magnified projection images of the film, magnified approximately threefold, to assess severity of the stenoses.[K3, R6, S10] Also, an optical sixfold magnifying device applied to 105-mm spot film has been used.[F9]

Scoblionko and co-workers compared the effectiveness of a digital electronic caliper with visual estimates by four experienced angiographers and with measurements made according to the Brown-Dodge method of quantitative coronary angiography (see next section).[S10] They found that the variability, as defined by the standard deviation of multiple estimates of the stenosis minimum diameter and percent diameter reduction, averaged 0.09 mm and 3.1 percent for quantitative coronary angiography; 0.18 mm and 5.9 percent for the digital electronic caliper method; and 0.26 mm and 7.4 percent for the visual estimates. Compared with quantitative coronary angiography, the visual determination of percent diameter reduction resulted in underestimation of mild (−5 percent; $p < 0.02$) and overestimation of significant (+11 percent; $p < 0.002$) stenoses (Fig. 13–7). Visual estimates resulted in underestimation of the stenosis minimum diameter in significant lesions by 20 percent ($p < 0.04$). In contrast, the mean error for digital electronic caliper measurement of the stenosis minimum diameter and percent diameter reduction was not significantly different from zero. From these results, one may conclude that a digital caliper is superior to the visual interpretation of coronary stenoses, but inferior to the computer-assisted manual tracing procedure, with a variability of about twice that of manual tracing.

BROWN-DODGE METHOD

Brown and associates were the first to describe a computer-aided technique for the quantitative description of the geometry of coronary obstructions.[B3] In their approach, selected cine frames are projected by a Vanguard model M-35C cine projector onto a 52 × 67-cm screen with about a fivefold magnification. The borders of a selected coronary arterial segment are traced by hand from two projected perpendicular 35-mm cineangiographic views, and the *x-y* coordinates are digitized and stored into a PDP 11/45 computer. The computer program reduces the lesion

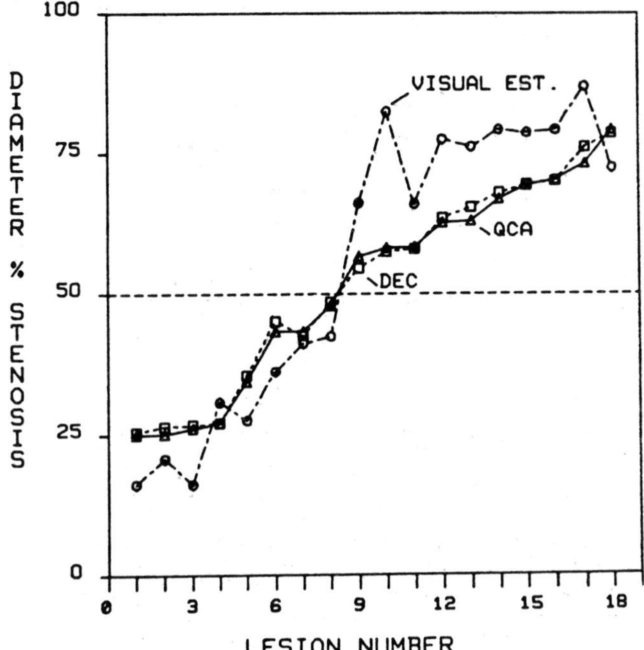

Figure 13–7. Measurements of percent diameter stenosis (%S) made by visual estimate, digital electronic caliper (DEC), and the computer-assisted methods (quantitative coronary angiography, QCA) for each of 18 lesions. The DEC measurements do not differ significantly from the QCA measurements, whereas the visual procedure tends to underestimate mild lesions and to overestimate significant lesions. (From Scoblionko, D.P., et al.: A new digital electronic caliper for measurement of coronary arterial stenosis: Comparison with visual estimates and computer-assisted measurements. Am. J. Cardiol. 53:689, 1984, with permission.)

image to true scale by compensating for pincushion distortion, out-of-plane magnification, and optical magnification, using the catheter and its location as a scaling device. The two views are matched and a spatial representation of the center line of the vessel is constructed mathematically; subsequently, orthogonal vessel diameters are computed at increments along this center line. If an elliptic lumen is assumed, the absolute and percentage reductions in diameter and in cross-sectional area of a stenosis are computed. In addition, more complex functions, such as integrated atheroma mass, Poiseuille and turbulent resistance values, and so forth are calculated. The performance of the system has been described in terms of absolute measurements being accurate to 0.1 mm, while the variability (standard deviation) averages ± 3 percent in estimates of percent stenosis and ± 0.1 mm in estimates of minimum lesion diameter.[B9, B17, K4, M9]

IMAGE ACQUISITION AND DIGITIZATION OF 35-mm CINE FILM

Two approaches to the digitization of selected cine frames have been taken: (1) optical magnification by means of a cine videoprojector with different lens systems and a videocamera, and (2) electronic magnification by means of a cine digitizer, either with a high-resolution linear or area array charge coupled device (CCD) camera or with a standard videocamera (either vidicon or CCD 512^2) (Table 13–1). The cine digitizers with optical magnification include a customized system (Collins), a self-modified Tagarno projector (Doriot), an Eyecom II from Spatial Data Systems (Table 13–1) (Kirkeeide), a videocamera attachment to a standard Vanguard model XR-35 35-mm projector (Nichols), a specially designed cine-to-video converter by Vanguard (Sanders,[S11] Vogel), a GE CAP35 cine projector modified by the addition of a 1000-line videocamera (Selzer[S12]), second-generation (CIVICO III) and third-generation (CIVICO IV) video-based cine-digitizing systems, developed at Erasmus University in Rotterdam, and finally, the commercially available Cine Video System SME-3300 from Sony.[R8]

In the CIVICO III, the cine film is mounted on a plateau with a film-guiding system that can be moved under computer control left/right and upward/downward; the selected portion of the image is then projected onto a high-resolution 1-inch pasecon videocamera (Fig. 13–8). The camera and the projection lens can each be moved independently by computer control, allowing the selection of the appropriate optical magnification (ranging from ×0.7 to ×4 in steps of $\sqrt{2}$). The light source consists of three light-emitting diodes (LEDs) with a narrow light spectrum; the emitted amount of light can be linearly adjusted. A user-controlled, motor-driven diaphragm and automated light-control system further provide optimal image quality in the selected region of interest.

At present, Reiber and colleagues are developing a third-generation cine digitizer, named CIVICO IV, which is based on the principles of CIVICO III, but is equipped with a state-of-the-art area-type CCD camera with matrix-size 512^2 pixels. Because of the rapid progress in the development of CCD cameras, which has resulted in light weight, high performance, and acceptable price, the mechanics of the cine digitizer can be simplified significantly, resulting in a system that performs the tasks much more quickly and at lower cost. The CIVICO IV will have three optical magnification factors: 0.7, 1, and 2.3.

Sanders is building a new CCD camera–based cine-film digitizer with a Siemens Cipro projector and a high-resolution area-type CCD camera (Videk Megaplus, 1300 × 1000 pixels) (Table 13–2).

The linear-array CCD-camera cine film digitizer developed by Reiber and colleagues is a standard cine projector (Tagarno 35 CX) with a field-installable modification package for high-resolution digitization of a selected cine frame.[R4, R9] This modification package consists of a film-guiding system, a specially developed optical chain, and a linear-array (1728-element) CCD camera; the array can be moved mechanically over a total of 2846 positions. The monochromatic light source consists of an array of four LEDs optimally suitable for densitometric analysis of the cine film with the present optical chain. Any area of 6.9 × 6.9 mm in a selected

Table 13–1. TWO APPROACHES FOR THE DIGITIZATION OF SELECTED CINE FRAMES

Approach	System	Investigator(s)
Optical magnification (cine videoprojector with different lens systems and video or CCD camera)	Customized system	Collins
	Modified Tagarno projector	Doriot
	Spatial Data Systems	Kirkeeide
	Vanguard	Nichols, Sanders, Vogel
	GE CAP35	Selzer
	CIVICO III and IV	Reiber
	Sony SME-3300 Cine Video System	
Electronic magnification	Modified Tagarno projector with linear-array (1728-element) CCD camera	Reiber
	Modified Siemens Cipro projector with 1300 × 1000-pixel area CCD camera	Sanders
	Tagarno projector with built-in standard videocamera	Reiber
	Standard slide projector with transparent screen with CCD-line sensor with 2000 × 3000 pixels	Sonoda

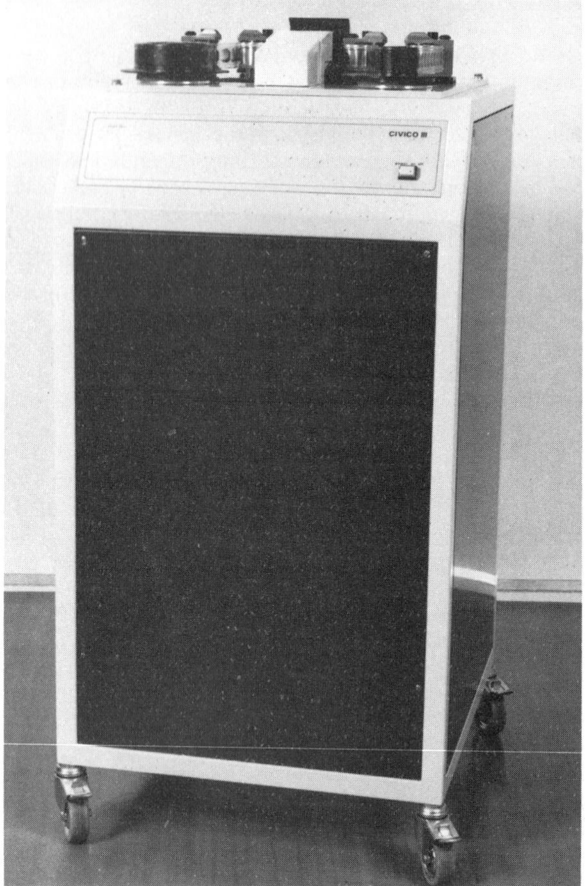

Figure 13–8. Second-generation video-based cineangiographic digitizing system, developed at Erasmus University Rotterdam, The Netherlands.

cine frame (size 18 × 24 mm) can be digitized by the CCD camera with a resolution of 512 × 512 pixels with 8 bits of gray levels. In other words, the entire cine frame of size 18 × 24 mm can be digitized at a resolution of 1329 × 1772 pixels. A homogeneity in the brightness distribution over the entire digitized image of better than 5 percent has been achieved.[K5]

The latest activities in this field by Reiber and colleagues are directed toward the development of a new, low-cost personal computer–based workstation CLAS (Coronary and Left Ventricular Analysis System) with a Tagarno projector with built-in standard videocamera for the quantitative analysis of coronary and left ventricular cineangiograms.[R7] Because no optical zooming is available, the images are digitized in CLAS with basically the same resolution (512 × 512) as with the direct on-line technique. Regions of interest encompassing the segment to be analyzed are interpolated linearly or cubically to obtain a sufficient number of pixels for the subsequent analysis with reasonable accuracy in the quantitative parameters. Validation studies are needed to demonstrate the accuracy and precision in the assessment of the

Table 13–2. TYPES OF CAMERAS USED IN CINE FILM DIGITIZING SYSTEMS

System	Camera	Investigator(s)
Standard video	Plumbicon (1-inch)	2 of 12 investigators
	Vidicon (1-inch)	6 of 12 investigators
	Pasecon (1-inch)	1 of 12 investigators
Nonstandard video	1000-line Vidicon camera	Selzer
CCD camera	1728-element linear array	Reiber
	512 × 512-pixel area–type CCD	Reiber
	1300 × 1000-pixel area–type CCD	Sanders
	2000-element linear array	Sonoda

obstruction parameters as compared with the optical magnification approaches.

Sony has recently produced the SME-3300 Cine Video System, featuring a CCD camera, maximally sixfold optical zooming, and vertical and horizontal positioning of the magnified region of interest, which make it an interesting system for quantitative coronary cineangiography.

Sonoda and associates have used a standard slide projector, transparent screen, and CCD line sensor with 2000 horizontal rows and 3000 vertical columns for their personal computer–based quantitation system.[S22]

In all but one of these videocamera-based systems, standard 1-inch videocameras have been used (see Table 13–2); in two systems, plumbicon tubes were installed; in six systems, a vidicon tube was installed; and in one system, a pasecon tube was installed. Selzer and associates have installed a 1000-line vidicon camera in their GE CAP35 projector.[S12] The CCD technology is progressing rapidly toward high-resolution area-type CCD cameras (512^2 and 1024^2 pixels).

Overall, the optical or electronic magnification factors that are available on these systems range from 0.7 to 7. In practice, however, twofold magnification is used most frequently. Selzer can use both optical (×1, ×1.6) and electronic (×2) zooming, resulting in a maximal magnification factor of 3.2.[S12] Brown and colleagues use a magnification factor of 5.5 with their analog projection system.[B3] In all of these cine digitizers, except for the ones developed at the Erasmus University in Rotterdam, the lens selection and camera positioning are performed manually.

ON-LINE DIGITAL CARDIAC SYSTEMS

The possibility of obtaining quantitative data about coronary morphology and functional significance immediately following an angiographic investigation is attractive to physicians who must make diagnoses and clinical decisions. This possibility is particularly appealing given the increasing application of recanalization techniques in the catheterization laboratory, such as PTCA,[B10, B17, L6, S13–S15] the use of thrombolytic agents,[B6, S15–S17] the introduction of the stent,[P4, S18, S23] the use of mechanical atherectomy devices,[R27, S52] and possibly in the near future, laser[I2, L7] and spark erosion techniques.[S19] Therefore, one may expect in the coming years a dramatic increase in the development and use of on-line digital cardiac systems, with more software packages of improved quality available for quantitative analysis. The improvement in image quality of the on-line digital systems through use of pulsed fluoroscopy and real-time image-enhancement techniques will also be beneficial and necessary for modern therapeutic procedures, such as stent implantation and subsequent follow-up angiographic studies.

Several questions on the questionnaire were related to the part of the digital systems involving image acquisition and digitization; the results are presented in Table 13–3. The items in this table have been updated according to the status as of 1989. The available software for quantitative analysis of the images is discussed later.

At present, only five groups (Doriot, Marchand, Parker, Reiber, and Vogel) are actively involved in the development of state-of-the-art quantitative software packages for on-line coronary angiography. Doriot and Parker use the Siemens Polytron 1000 VR and the Siemens Digitron III, respectively, Marchand uses the CGR system, Reiber uses the Philips DCI system, and Vogel uses the ADAC system (see Table 13–3, item 1). Vogel was the first one to develop and use high-quality software packages on an on-line digital system for the description of the morphologic and functional severity of coronary stenoses.[H4, L5, M10] The data from Reiber as presented in this chapter are all based on the off-line cine-film–based quantitation CAAS system. At present, new software packages for on-line quantification on the DCI system are being developed. Results of the DCI approach are not yet available, however.

The minimal requirement for image acquisition in quantitation of the coronary morphology is 512^2 matrices at a rate of 25 frames/sec (Europe) or 30 frames/sec (USA), with a density resolution of

Table 13–3. IMAGE ACQUISITION AND DIGITIZATION IN ON-LINE DIGITAL CARDIAC SYSTEMS

Questionnaire Item	Marchand	Doriot	Parker	Reiber	Vogel
1. Name of digital cardiac system	CGR	Siemens Polytron 1000 VR	Siemens Digitron III	Philips DCI	ADAC
2. Limitations in matrix acquisition					
Matrix size	512^2 1024^2	512 × 256 512^2 1024^2	512^2	512^2	256^2 512^2 1024^2
Maximum frame rate (pulse duration)	512^2:30 frames/sec (<10 msec) 1024^2:7.5 frames/sec	512 × 256:50 frames/sec (>10 msec) 512^2:25 frames/sec (>10 msec) 1024^2:6 frames/sec (>10 msec)	512^2:30 frames/sec (<8 msec)	512^2:50 frames/sec (3–8 msec), Europe 512^2:60 frames/sec (3–8 msec), USA	256^2:60 frames/sec (3–10 msec) 512^2:30 frames/sec (3–10 msec) 1024^2:4 frames/sec (3–10 msec)
Density resolution (bits)	8 or 10 bits	10 bits	10 bits	8 bits	8 bits
3. Features					
Type video camera	Primicon	Saticon	Saticon	Plumbicon	Vidicon
Size video tube	1 inch	1 inch	1 inch	2 inch	1 inch
Interlaced or noninterlaced scanning mode	Both interlaced and noninterlaced available	Noninterlaced	Noninterlaced	Noninterlaced	Noninterlaced
4. Is simultaneous 35-mm cine film acquisition with digital acquisition possible? If yes, what are the limitations?	Yes; no limitations	Yes	Yes; x-ray dose is reduced with simultaneous cine and digital acquisition as compared with digital acquisition only	Yes; film speed: 12.5, 25, and 50 frames/sec, Europe; 15, 30, and 60 frames/sec, USA; no limitations	Yes; no limitations

8 bits. In addition, pulsed x-ray radiation should be used to minimize motion blur in the images. From Table 13–3, item 2, it appears that all systems satisfy these minimal requirements with the Philips DCI in monoplane version even allowing 50 or 60 frames/sec. The ADAC system also provides 256^2 (at 60 frames/sec monoplane) and 1024^2 matrix sizes (at 4 frames/sec); the Siemens Polytron facilitates 512 × 256 (at 50 frames/sec) and 1024^2 matrices (at 6 frames/sec), and the CGR system the 1024^2 size matrix (at 7.5 frames/sec) in addition to the standard 512^2 matrices. The x-ray pulse width varies from short 3–8 msec values (Philips), < 8 msec (Siemens Digitron), 3–10 msec (ADAC), < 10 msec (CGR), to > 10 msec (Siemens Polytron), respectively; a short pulse width is necessary to minimize motion blur in the images.

The type and size of the videocameras used in the digital systems vary from a 1-inch vidicon tube on the ADAC system with noninterlaced readout, a 1-inch primicon with both standard interlaced and noninterlaced scanning on the CGR system, a 2-inch plumbicon with noninterlaced scanning on the Philips DCI, to a 1-inch saticon (noninterlaced readout) on the Siemens system (Table 13–3, item 3).[K10]

Item 4 in Table 13–3 shows that all current systems allow simultaneous cine-film and digital acquisition.

COMPUTER HARDWARE AND SOFTWARE

A great variety of host computers have been used in the development of the quantitative software (Table 13–4). The older systems are based on the DEC minicomputer systems (VAXs and PDPs), whereas the present trend is toward the more powerful personal computers (HP Vectra, IBM PC/AT compatible (80386), and Compaq 80386).

The video-converted frames or cine frames must be digitized and stored in an image processing system before any image processing functions can be applied. Again, the variety in complexity, and thus cost, is large (Table 13–5). Single-board image processing systems are now widely available for the personal computer–based systems (Data Translation, Imaging Technologies, Virtual Imaging, and so forth).

In the system developed by Brown (see the earlier section "Brown-Dodge Method"), selected cine frames are projected with a standard cine-film projector on a large writing tablet, which allows the manual tracing of the boundaries of the arterial segment of interest; the coordinates of these boundary points are sent to the host computer for subsequent analysis. As a result, Brown's system does not need an image processor. Kirkeeide

Table 13–4. HOST COMPUTERS USED IN QUANTITATIVE CORONARY ANGIOGRAPHIC APPLICATIONS

Computer	Investigator(s)
VAX-11/780	Kirkeeide
VAX-11/750	Brown, Doriot
MicroVax II	Collins, Sandor, Selzer
PDP 11/44	Reiber
PDP 11/73	Reiber, Vogel
HP 1000	Sanders
8086 μP	Parker
HP Vectra	Sanders
M68008/68010	Marchand, Nichols
20 MHz Compaq 80386 (CLAS)	Reiber
16 MHz 80386 IBM PC/AT-compatible (Quantim 2000I)	LeFree

Table 13–5. IMAGE PROCESSORS USED IN QUANTITATIVE CORONARY ANGIOGRAPHIC APPLICATIONS

Processing System	Investigator(s)
ADAC Array Processor	Vogel
Data Translation	Sanders
DeAnza Gould IP6400	Doriot, Sanders
DeAnza Gould IP8500	Collins
Imaging Technologies	Reiber, Sandor
MegaVision 1024 XM	Selzer
Pie Data VIP500	Reiber
Vicom VDP	Marchand
Virtual Imaging (Quantim 2000I)	LeFree
VTE	Reiber
None	Brown, Kirkeeide, Nichols

digitizes the selected frame and stores the data directly into the memory of the VAX computer for subsequent analysis. Nichols only displays the analog video image and uses a graphics overlay for the display of alphanumeric characters, contours, and lines on the screen. Parker uses a VAX-11/750 with the Digitron I as a display device.

With so many different host computer systems employed, the variety of operating systems is also large: VMS, RSX-11M(+), RTE, RT11, MS-DOS, Versados, and the Motorola VME/10 Development System (Table 13–6). Fortunately, a larger consensus is found regarding the high-level computer language in which the application software packages are written. The majority of the packages have been written in Fortran-(77), while Marchand uses Pascal and Assembly language, Brown uses Flex, and LeFree, Nichols, Reiber, and Sanders use the modern language C (see Table 13–6).

The last item on the questionnaire concerned the pixel size (μm) in the digitized image at the usual optical or electronic magnification and referred to the isocenter with the average focus-to-image intensifier distance. In other words, from this item, the pixel density (number of pixels per millimeter) in the image can be calculated. The pixel density is linearly related to the selected magnification and inversely linearly related to the image intensifier size. The original data from the investigators were difficult to compare because of the different magnifications and field-of-view sizes of the image intensifiers listed; however, after normalization of the given pixel sizes to an image intensifier size of 6 inches and a twofold optical magnification (for cine-film systems), the comparative data listed in Table 13–7 were obtained.

The pixel sizes in the majority of the cine-film–based systems are clearly in the range of 64 to 95 μm; in other words, the pixel density ranges from 15.6 to 10.5 pixels/mm. Doriot uses an exceptionally small pixel size (32 μm) or high pixel density (31.3 pixels/mm), while Nichols' system and the three digital systems (Parker, Reiber, Vogel) are characterized by large pixel sizes (111 to 156 μm) or low pixel density values (9.0 to 6.4 pixels/mm), as would be expected. Marchand did not specify the pixel size for the CGR digital system.

Of course, the higher the pixel density, the more pixels are available for contour detection. In general, however, one cannot state that a higher pixel density results in a more accurate edge-detection performance. As the pixel density increases, the quantum mottle (and for cine film, the film grain noise) increases as well. As a result, an optimal value in pixel size must be found. In our opinion, this optimal value is in the range of 64 to 80 μm/pixel or pixel density of 15.6 to 12.5 pixels/mm.

Table 13–6. OPERATING SYSTEMS AND COMPUTER LANGUAGES USED IN QUANTITATIVE CORONARY ANGIOGRAPHY

	Item Used	Investigator(s)
Operating system	Motorola VME/10 Development System	Nichols
	MS-DOS	LeFree, Reiber, Sanders
	RSX-11M(+)	Reiber
	RT11	Vogel
	RTE	Sanders
	Versados	Marchand
	VMS	Brown, Collins, Doriot, Kirkeeide, Parker, Sandor, Selzer
Computer language	C	LeFree, Nichols, Reiber, Sanders
	Flex	Brown
	Fortran	Collins, Doriot, Kirkeeide, Parker, Sandor, Selzer, Vogel
	Pascal	Marchand

Table 13–7. PIXEL SIZE IN DIGITIZED IMAGE NORMALIZED FOR A 6-INCH IMAGE INTENSIFIER AND TWOFOLD ELECTRONIC OR OPTICAL MAGNIFICATION

Investigator	Pixel Size (μm)
Collins	95
Doriot	32
Kirkeeide	77
Marchand	Unknown
Nichols	140
Parker (digital)*	118
Reiber	72
Reiber (digital)*	111
Sanders	93
Sandor	Magnification unknown
Selzer	64–80
Vogel (digital)*	156

*Digital refers to data obtained on digital imaging system; all other data apply to cine film–based system.

CONTOUR DETECTION APPROACHES

In general, the following steps can be distinguished for the computer-assisted definition of the boundaries of a selected coronary segment:

1. Definition of coronary segment to be analyzed
2. Edge definition

The different implementations of these steps are discussed in detail in the following sections.

Definition of Coronary Segment to Be Analyzed

In general, four approaches have been used:

1. User indicates approximate borders of vessel (Sanders).
2. User defines windows over stenotic and normal segments (Doriot and Nichols).
3. User indicates number of center points in arterial segment to be analyzed (Collins, Kirkeeide, Marchand, Reiber, Sandor, and Selzer).
4. Tracing of the center line is automated (Parker, Reiber, and Vogel).

By the first approach, Sanders' group manually traces the approximate borders of the vessel, and on the basis of these data, the boundary positions are detected more accurately by means of edge-detection techniques.[A4, E3]

Doriot[D3] and Nichols[N1, N2] and their colleagues place windows over the stenotic and normal segments, and the width of the arterial segment within these windows is computed with edge-detection techniques.

If the edge positions of an entire coronary segment must be computed, the best approach is detection of these points along scan lines that are perpendicular to the local center-line direction of the segment. The third approach, which is also user-interactive, requires that the operator defines a midline estimate for the arterial segment to be analyzed by indicating a few center points along the vessel by means of a sonic pen or writing tablet.[K6, L8, R4, S12, S20] This center line is then smoothed and defines the scan lines perpendicular to the local center line directions for the computation of the edge positions. Reiber and colleagues,[R4] and Selzer and associates,[S12] have advocated updating of this center line by a new one computed from the contour positions once these have been detected, and possibly corrected manually, and repetition of the contour detection procedure. By means of this iterative approach, the influence of the user definition of the center points on the detected contour positions can be minimized.

LeFree, Vogel, and associates have developed an automated procedure for the definition of the center line applied to digital cardiac images.[L5] A polar coordinate search algorithm is used to identify the center line of the artery, following operator assignment of the approximate center of the lesion and the diameter of a circle defining the region-of-interest, within which the center line is to be found. The arterial center line is determined by applying simple signal processing techniques to circular profiles of decreasing radii to locate the angular positions of the proximal and distal coronary segments at each radius.

In a recently developed automated center line tracing procedure, Reiber and associates require only the definition of the beginning and end points of the center line to be detected.[C5] The algorithm follows the points of maximal brightness levels in a low-resolution version (170^2 pixels) of the image. If the forward directed path cannot be completed, reverse tracing (from the end point to the beginning point) is initiated, and if the two tracers intersect, a definite center line is composed of the two connecting parts. If the two traces do not intersect, or if the center line partly follows another vessel, simple definition of a third point that must belong to the center line results in the requested center line in the majority of cases. Finally, the detected center line is projected back onto the original 512^2 image. A 200-point center line takes only 0.2 sec on the Compaq 386/20-based CLAS.

Barth and colleagues have developed a technique for the automated three-dimensional recognition of the coronary tree on subtracted digital (Siemens Digitron II) image pairs.[B13, B14] The tracing is started by marking the root of the tree with two points. The algorithm proceeds by looking for continuations in any direction, a method similar to that of a radar scanner. It requires manual interaction only for corrections in critical regions of the images, where vessels are superimposed in both views, or where the vessel dimensions are below detectability.

Edge Definition

To date, no consensus is found regarding the use of a first-derivative or a second-derivative, edge-detection approach or a combination of both approaches; nearly every research group has developed and used its own definitions. Basically, the following approaches can be distinguished:

1. Manual tracing (Brown).
2. First-derivative function (Kirkeeide, Sanders, and Selzer).
3. First-semiderivative function (Marchand).
4. Second-derivative function (Doriot).
5. First- and second-derivative functions (Collins, Reiber, Sandor, and Vogel).
6. Matched filter (Nichols and Parker).

On the other hand, investigators show a tendency toward using the minimal-cost contour detection approach for definition of the arterial contours.[R4]

The first approach, based on manual tracing of the arterial boundaries, is obvious and does not require computer-supported edge-detection techniques.[B3]

In the approach described by Kirkeeide and colleagues, the first-derivative function along a scan line is computed according to a least-squares convolution technique.[K6, W5] Two parameters of the edge-detection algorithm are important: the convolution kernel size and the edge threshold level in the first-derivative function. These investigators have shown that the errors in the diameter detection are hyperbolically related to the kernel size, for which correction can be obtained by simple empirical formulas.

Sanders and associates determine the positions with maximal first-derivative response along lines perpendicular to manually traced margins to improve upon these manually determined positions.[A4, E3]

Selzer and colleagues search for positions with maximal first-derivative response along scan lines that are perpendicular to the local direction of the center line defined earlier.[L8, S20] Marchand and colleagues use a first-semiderivative function.

These positions that are defined by the maximal values of the first-derivative functions correspond with the inflection points of the brightness profiles along the scan lines. Our experience has shown that such positions fit the arterial segments too tightly; if only the first-derivative response is used, certain correction factors should be employed so that the final contour positions are shifted toward the base of the brightness profiles.

Doriot and co-workers use the maximal values of the second-derivative functions to determine the edge positions.[D3] In our experience with this derivative approach, the contour points are too wide to fit the arterial segment.

To simplify and speed up the edge-enhancement and contour-definition procedures, Kooijman[K7] and Reiber and associates[R4] resampled the digital data along the scan lines, which resulted in a stretched version of the arterial segment (Fig. 13–9). In this resampled matrix, the center line has become a straight vertical line, whereas the scan lines are oriented horizontally. Edge enhancement can now easily be achieved by applying simple one-dimensional gradient functions along the horizontal lines. Second-derivative values can be obtained by applying the gradient function to the first-derivative matrix. Subsequently, a cost matrix is defined, in which the intensity value of a pixel is a measurement of the inverse value of the weighted sum of the first- and second-derivative values for that pixel (see Fig. 13–9*C*). Finally, the left and right contours are obtained by searching in a cost matrix from top to bottom for a minimal-cost path (satisfying some connectivity constraints) to the left and right of the center column, respectively (see Fig. 13–9*D*).[K7] The detected boundary positions can be superimposed in the stretched version of the segment (see Fig. 13–9*B*).

The great advantage of this minimum-cost contour-detection algorithm is the fact that the edge positions are not determined

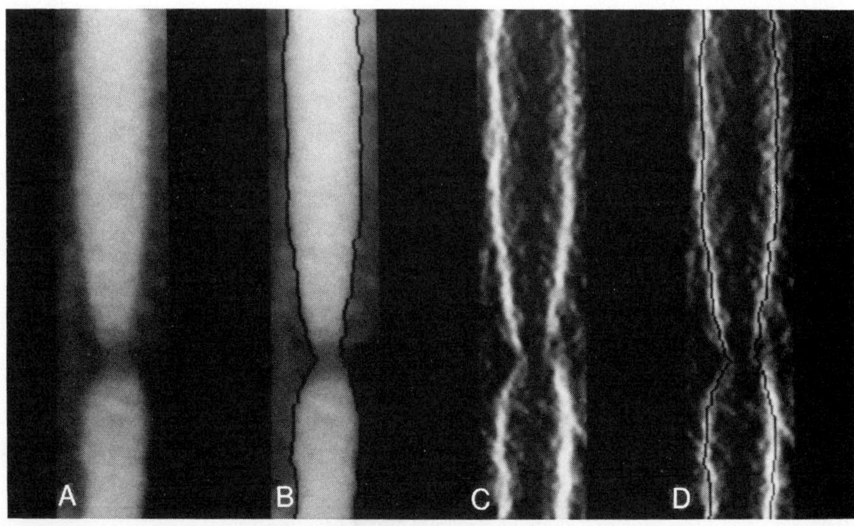

Figure 13–9. Minimal-cost contour-detection procedure. *A*, Transformed intensity matrix. *B*, Transformed intensity matrix with contours superimposed. *C*, Cost matrix. *D*, Cost matrix with contours superimposed.

per individual scan line; rather, information gathered from all of the other scan lines is considered. As a result, this approach is less sensitive than the local approach to intervening elements such as branches and overlying structures. As mentioned earlier, the contour-detection procedure is performed iteratively; following the first iteration of the contour-detection procedure, and possibly the manual correction of erroneous contour points, a new center line is computed as the midline of the detected points, and the contour-detection procedure is again repeated, resulting in the final arterial contours.

Collins and associates also search for minimum-cost paths in resampled matrices. Initially, they applied a Sobel operator over the entire image in two passes (horizontal and vertical) to determine the edge strength of individual pixels,[F10] but they later changed to a weighted sum of first- and second-derivative functions.

In the technique described by LeFree, Vogel, and associates, automatic edge detection is accomplished in two passes over the scan lines.[L5] During the first pass, the edge points are chosen between the locations defined by the extreme values of the first- (inflection point) and second- (base point) derivatives of the arterial profile, so that the brightness level of the edge points equals 75 percent of the difference between the brightness levels at these derivative extremes (i.e., weighted toward the first derivative extreme). Those initial edge points with a distance from neighboring edge points greater than an empirically determined distance are marked as not falling on the true arterial edge contour. During the second pass, the threshold values for the profiles corresponding to these spurious edge points are discarded and replaced by linear interpolation from the intensities at neighboring valid edge points. The final edge points thus use local gradient and intensity information.

Nichols and associates define the width of the arterial segment by the full-width-at-half-maximum (FWHM) value of the videodensitometric profile measured along a scan line.[N2]

Parker and colleagues apply a matched filter kernel to the density profiles that are defined perpendicular to the automatically detected center line of the vessel to obtain a likelihood matrix.[P2, P3] Dynamic programming techniques are then applied to the likelihood matrix to find the optimal paths and thus the optimal boundaries of the vessel.

Only Brown[B3] and Kirkeeide[K8] and their colleagues correct the arterial boundary positions for the line-spread function of the x-ray system.

Pincushion Distortion and Correction

It is well known that particularly the older types of image intensifiers introduce a geometric distortion, the so-called pincushion distortion. This distortion results in selective magnification of an object near the edges of the image as compared with its size in the center of the field. Correction for these differences is needed for absolute diameter measurements to be derived from coronary angiograms. The standard procedure for assessing the degree of distortion present is filming of a centimeter grid, which is positioned against the input screen of the image intensifier. This procedure needs to be performed only once for a given image intensifier tube at each of the available magnification modes.

A number of approaches to provide correction for pincushion distortion have been implemented. Theoretically, pincushion distortion is radially symmetric about the central x-ray beam, because of the rotational symmetry of the curved image intensifier's input screen and its internal fields.[L9] The first approach requires the assumption that the distortion is indeed radially symmetric about the center of the image intensifier, and that relative magnification can be determined from the distance of the pixel under consideration from the center of the image intensifier. An empirically determined analytic function of the radius is then used to provide correction for the distortion. This approach has been implemented by the groups of Brown[B3] and Kirkeeide.[W5]

The second method is also based on radial symmetry, but relative magnification factors for a single radial line are stored in the memory of the computer system. The relative magnification for each distance was obtained by averaging the four values measured in the four quadrants of the centimeter-grid image. Hence, no analytic function is employed; this approach has been taken by Sanders and colleagues.[A4, E3]

The third method, which we and Selzer use, involves no assumption about the geometric distribution of the distortion, but it requires storing of the relative magnifications of all the intersection points of the centimeter grid.[K7, L8, R4, S20] We developed a procedure that allows the fully automated detection of the wires and intersection points in the 1:1 projected cine frame. For a given point in the image that does not concur with one of the displayed intersection positions, the correction vector is determined by means of bilinear interpolation between the correction vectors of the four neighboring intersection points. Selzer also uses bilinear interpolation.

In their digital cardiac system, LeFree, Vogel, and associates have implemented a somewhat similar approach, except for the fact that they correct the entire image by piecewise linear warping, not only the contour positions of the catheter and arterial segment ("rubber sheet" transform).[L5] For these purposes, a 1-cm–spaced orthogonal array of bronze ball bearings is imaged at the image intensifier input screen. The "rubber sheet" transform is also optionally available from Selzer.

In institutes of five of the investigators (Collins, Doriot, Marchand, Nichols and Sandor), correction is not provided for the pincushion distortion in the detected contour positions.

Calibration

To compute absolute sizes of the arterial segment analyzed, a calibration factor needs to be determined. Basically, two different approaches have been used for the coronary arteries: (1) an analytic approach from geometric x-ray system parameters and (2) an approach based on the known diameter of the contrast catheter or the known size or distance of markers on the catheter. These techniques have been summarized in Table 13–8 and are described here in more detail.

Following the first approach, the size of an object in the plane through the center of rotation of the x-ray system (isocenter) and parallel to the image intensifier input screen can be determined from simple geometric principles from the height levels of the x-ray tube and image intensifier. For objects above or below the center of rotation, however, a slightly more complicated analysis must be carried out, which requires a second, preferably orthogonal view of the object. Wollschläger and associates have developed a method of calculating the exact radiologic magnification factors for each point in the fields of view of biplane multidirec-

Table 13–8. TWO APPROACHES FOR CALIBRATION TO CONVERT PIXEL MEASUREMENTS TO ABSOLUTE SIZES IN MILLIMETERS

	Technique	Investigator(s)
Analytic approach	Analytic calibration from geometric x-ray system settings in biplane images	Parker, Wollschläger
Catheter-based approach	Manual definition of boundaries of catheter segment	Brown
	Automated edge-definition of catheter segment	Collins, Doriot, Kirkeeide, Nichols, Reiber, Sandor, Selzer, Vogel
	Biplane assessment of distance of cardiomarker rings on catheter (1-cm spacing)	Kirkeeide
	Diameter metallic marker on catheter	Sanders

tional isocentric x-ray equipment.[W6, W7] By using this approach, they avoid two sources of error: contour detection of the catheter segment and the differential magnification of the scaling device and the arterial segment. Parker also determines the calibration factors from the geometric x-ray system settings in biplane images, and one of the options of Kirkeeide's method is also based on this approach.

If the catheter is used as a scaling device, either the contours of a short segment of the tip or shaft may be manually defined with a writing tablet, or contour detection techniques similar to those used for the coronary segments may be applied. The manual approach in biplane images is used by Brown and associates;[B3] Collins and Reiber allow both manual and automated definition of a catheter segment. Most authors apply the same kind of automated edge-detection technique to the catheter as used for a coronary segment (Collins, Doriot, Kirkeeide, Nichols, Reiber, Sandor, Selzer, and Vogel). In our routine practice, the catheter is magnified optically or electronically with a factor of $2\sqrt{2}$:1 or 2:1, respectively, and a priori information is included in the iterative edge-detection procedure, which is based on the fact that the selected part of the catheter is the projection of a cylindric structure (Fig. 13–10). In general, the size of the catheter as given by the manufacturer deviates from its actual size, especially in the case of disposable catheters. Therefore, for interventional studies, measuring the size of the catheter with a micrometer following the catheterization procedure may be advisable.[R10, R11]

Some time ago, several new types of catheters with cardiomarker rings were designed at the request of a number of investigators. Kirkeeide determines the distance between the cardiomarker rings (1 cm spacing) in biplane angiograms, and Sanders measures the diameter of a metallic marker on the catheter. In the latter case, the catheter manufacturer must assure that the outside shape of the rings is not convex or concave; the rings must be perfectly cylindric. Because of the high contrast of the marker in the x-ray images, the edges can be defined relatively reliably.

If the known size of the catheter in a single angiographic view is used for calibration, the computed calibration factor is applicable only to objects in the plane of the catheter that are parallel to the image intensifier input screen. The change in magnification for two objects located at different points along the x-ray beam axis is about 1.5 percent for each centimeter that separates the objects axially with the commonly used focus-image intensifier distances. For coronary segments lying in other planes, corrections of the calibration factor can be assessed from other views. Brown, Kirkeeide, Sanders, and Wollschläger provide the means on their systems to make correction for the differential magnification from biplane angiograms.

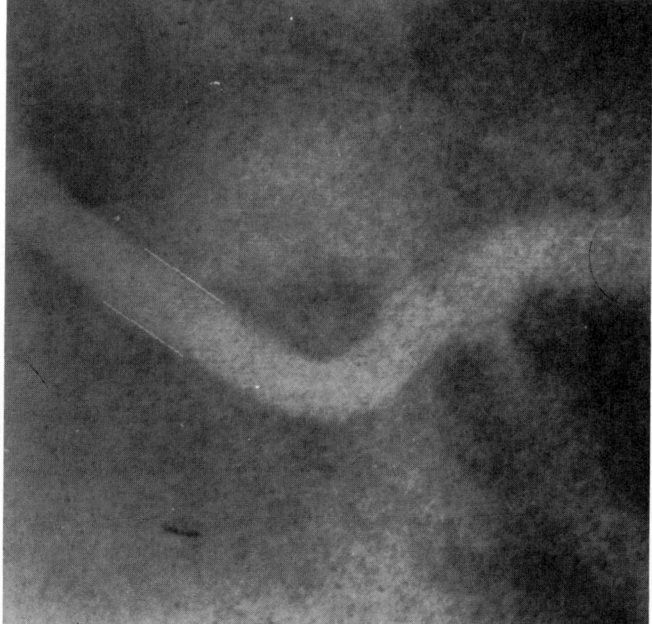

Figure 13–10. Detected contours along a user-defined portion of the contrast catheter.

The foregoing discussion makes clear that for the measurement of truly absolute sizes of coronary segments, two views, preferably but not necessarily orthogonal to each other, are required. If one is only interested in the changes in sizes of coronary segments as a result of short- or long-term interventions, however, excellent results can be achieved from single-plane views. In these situations, one must make sure that for the repeat angiogram the x-ray system is positioned in exactly the same geometric arrangement as during the first angiogram. Such assurance requires registration of the angles and height levels of the x-ray system, preferably on line with a microprocessor-based geometry readout system.[R10] Although the calibration factor used for a particular coronary arterial segment is then only an approximation of the true calibration factor, the same systematic error occurs for the first and repeat angiograms.

CONTOUR ANALYSIS APPROACHES

Following smoothing, pincushion correction, and calibration, a diameter function can be determined from the contours of the analyzed arterial segment by computing the distances between the left and right edges. From these data, several parameters may be calculated, such as minimal obstruction diameter, obstruction area, extent of the obstruction, percent diameter stenosis, percent area stenosis, symmetry of the stenosis, area of the atherosclerotic plaque, hemodynamic parameters of the obstruction, and mean diameter of a nonobstructive coronary segment. The minimal obstruction diameter is of particular importance, as it is present to the inverse fourth power in the formulas describing the pressure loss over a coronary obstruction. Moreover, to determine the effects of interventions on the severity of coronary obstructions, one should compute the changes in minimal obstruction diameter and not in percent diameter narrowing, as the reference position is also generally affected by the intervention.[B10, B11] The different approaches to measuring these and other parameters are described in the following sections.

Reference for Percent Diameter Stenosis Measurement

Although the absolute minimal obstruction diameter is one of the preferred parameters for describing the changes in the severity of an obstruction as a result of an intervention, percent diameter narrowing is a convenient parameter with which to work in individual cases.

The conventional method of determining the percent diameter stenosis of a coronary obstruction requires the user to indicate a reference position. A reference diameter is then usually computed as the average value of a number of diameter values in a symmetric region with a center at the user-defined reference position. This or a similar approach has been denoted the user-defined reference technique and has been adopted by Brown, Collins, Doriot, Kirkeeide, Nichols, Reiber, Sanders, Sandor, and Vogel.

Clearly, however, this computed percent diameter narrowing of an obstruction depends heavily on the selected reference position. In arteries with a focal obstructive lesion and a clearly normal proximal arterial segment, the choice of the reference region is straightforward and simple. In cases in which the proximal part of the arterial segment shows combinations of stenotic and ectatic areas, however, the choice may be difficult. This selection procedure is not always well standardized and, in practice, is difficult to reproduce reliably during sequential analysis.

To minimize these variations, alternative methods have been developed that do not depend on a user-defined reference region.[K7, L8, R4, S20] By these methods, estimates of the normal or pre-disease arterial size and luminal wall location are obtained on the basis of the computed center line and the 90th percentile of the diameter values (as done by Selzer's group)[L8, S12, S20] or on the basis of a first-degree polynomial, which is computed through the diameter values of the proximal and distal portions of the arterial segment followed by a translation to the 80th percentile level (reference diameter function) (as done by Reiber's group).[K7, R4] Tapering of the vessel to account for a decrease in arterial caliber associated with branches is accomplished in the latter approach. In this approach, the proximal and distal boundaries of the obstruction are determined from the diameter function on the basis of significant maxima in curvature using variable degrees of smoothing. If the user does not agree with either one or both of the proximal and distal obstruction boundaries, they can be corrected manually. The reference diameter is now taken as the value of the reference diameter function at the location of the minimal obstruction diameter. This approach is denoted as the interpolated or computer-defined reference technique. Gould and Kirkeeide also estimate the pre-disease dimensions at the obstruction.[G1]

The interpolated or computer-defined percent diameter stenosis is calculated by comparing the minimal diameter value at the obstruction with the corresponding value of the reference diameter. Figure 13–11 shows an example of our technique for an obstruction in the midportion of the left anterior descending (LAD) coronary artery in the right anterior oblique (RAO) projection. The actual contours as well as the estimated pre-disease reference contours of the arterial segment are superimposed in the image. The difference in area between the reference and the detected luminal contours is marked over the obstructive lesion; this area is a measure of the atherosclerotic plaque in this particular angiographic view. The upper function is the diameter function, and the straight line is the reference diameter function; the lower function is the densitometric area function (see the later section "Densitometry").

In addition, this interpolated or computer-defined reference diameter technique allows the assessment of the symmetry or asymmetry of the lesion in a given view with respect to a reconstructed center line.[A5, L12] Vessel midpoints for the proximal and distal "normal" portions are calculated by averaging the

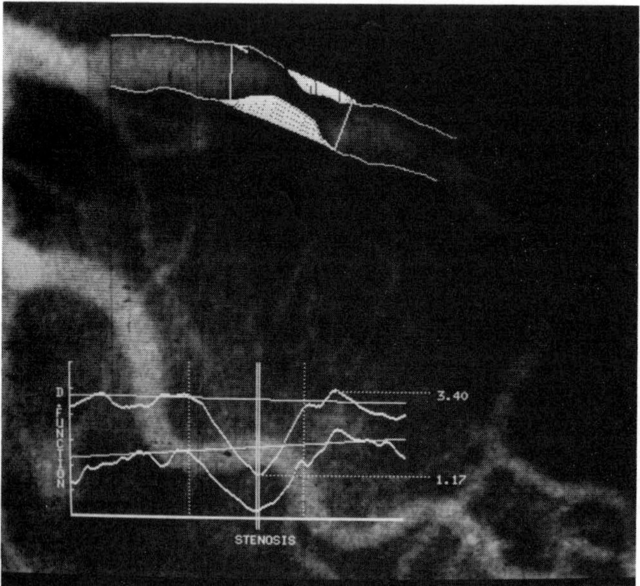

Figure 13–11. Example of the automatically detected luminal boundaries of a middle segment of the left anterior descending (LAD) artery and the estimated dimensions of the vessel at the site of the obstruction prior to disease (reference edges). The upper function is the diameter function, and the straight line through it is the reference diameter function; the lower function is that of the densitometric area. This example clearly shows that side branches close to the arterial segments to be analyzed cause artifacts, which can be recognized as dips, in the function of the densitometric area.

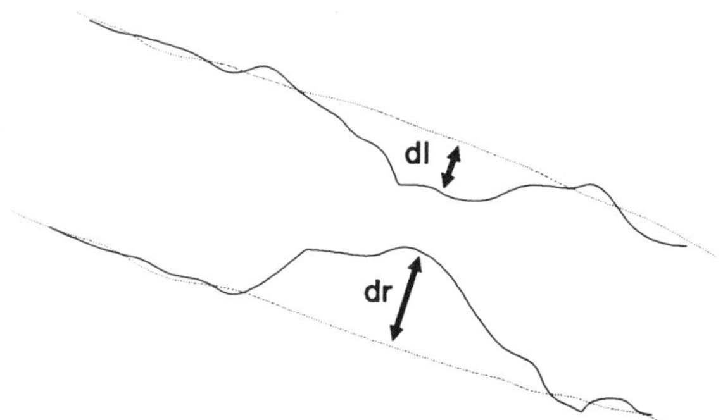

$$\text{SYMMETRY INDEX} = \frac{\min(dl,dr)}{\max(dl,dr)} = \frac{dl}{dr} \text{ in this example}$$

Figure 13–12. Diagrammatic example of an obstructed coronary artery illustrates the concept of the symmetry measure of an obstruction. The continuous lines represent the boundaries of the arterial segment; the outside broken lines represent the estimated original reference boundaries. At the site of the minimal diameter of the obstruction, the distances between the luminal and reference boundaries for the left-hand and right-hand sides are denoted dl and dr, respectively. The symmetry measure is defined by the minimum of dl and dr, divided by the maximum of dl and dr, which equals dl/dr for this particular example.

coordinates of the left and right contour points. For the obstructive region, the vessel midpoints are obtained by interpolation between the proximal and distal vessel midpoints with a second-degree polynomial. The symmetry measure is given as a value between 0 and 1, and defined as follows: The distance between the left-hand detected contour and the left-hand estimated contour at the obstruction is denoted dl, and similarly, the distance between the right-hand contours is denoted dr. Then, the symmetry measure is computed as the minimum of dl and dr, divided by the maximum of dl and dr. A symmetry measure of one denotes a concentric obstruction, and the number decreases with increasing asymmetry or eccentricity of the obstruction. Zero represents the most severe case of asymmetry or eccentricity. A typical example is presented in Figure 13–12. In addition to the fact that the interpolated technique provides data about the area of the atherosclerotic plaque and the lesion's symmetry in a given view, this approach has another practical advantage. When this technique is used, knowledge about the exact location of a reference, either proximal or distal to the stenosis, is not required for the analysis of repeated angiograms.

Vassanelli and co-workers have used the following definition of the eccentricity (EI) of a stenosis:

$$EI = B - 1/3A$$

where A is the radius of the "normal" vessel and B is the distance between the center of the "normal" vessel and the center line in the stenotic segment. EI is greater than zero in eccentric segments and less than zero in concentric ones.[V6] A stenosis is considered irregular if more than 25 percent of the nonadjacent segments are eccentric. Comparison with histologic data showed that 88 of 93 (94.6 percent) sections were correctly predicted as eccentric and 8 of 11 (72.7 percent) were correctly predicted as irregular.

From the available morphologic data of the obstruction, the Poiseuille and turbulent resistances at different flows, and thus the resulting transstenotic pressure gradients, can be computed on the basis of the well-known fluid-dynamic equations.[G1, R4, S21]

For the example given by Figure 13–11, the following quantitative measurements were obtained:

Extent obstruction	7.51 mm
Reference diameter	3.16 mm
Obstruction diameter	1.17 mm
Reference area (assuming circular cross sections)	7.86 mm^2
Obstruction area (densitometric)	0.84 mm^2
Area of atherosclerotic plaque	9.90 mm^2

Symmetry measure	0.53
Diameter stenosis	63.1%
Area stenosis (densitometric)	89.4%
Transstenotic pressure gradient at mean flow of 1 ml/sec	3.04 mmHg

The mean diameter of a nonobstructive coronary segment can easily be determined from the diameter data by requesting the user to indicate with the writing tablet, lightpen, or similar device the proximal and distal boundaries of the desired segment; the length of the segment in millimeters is usually also provided. For interventional studies, coronary branch points may be used to define the boundaries of the segment, because these determinations are fairly reproducible.

Roughness Measure of Arterial Segment

Information about the "roughness" of the arterial segment, and thus about diffuse coronary artery disease, may be obtained by dividing the coronary segment into an integer number of subsegments, each with a length of about 5 mm, and calculating for each subsegment the minimal, maximal, and mean diameters and the standard deviation of the diameter values.[R4] The ratio of the standard deviation value and the difference between minimal and maximal diameters can be used to determine whether a subsegment is focally or diffusely diseased, or normal. Clinical validation procedures need to be carried out, however, to determine the true value of this parameter. Figure 13–13 shows the four subsegments for the example of Figure 13–11; the derived subsegmental data are given in Table 13–9.

Sanders uses the variation of the vessel diameters as a measure of diffuse atherosclerosis, whereas Selzer and associates fit a least-squares straight line through the vessel width profile and use the residual variance as a measure of roughness. Crawford and colleagues have developed various edge-roughness measures for femoral arteries;[C4] the edge-roughness was defined by the root-mean-square difference between two sets of edge coordinates obtained by the use of filters of different lengths. The other investigators do not calculate a roughness index for diffuse atherosclerosis.

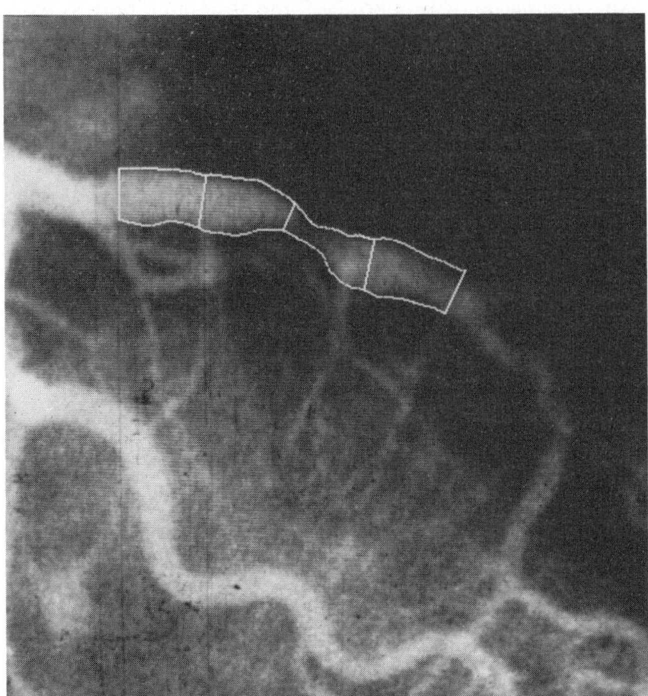

Figure 13–13. To obtain information about the "roughness" (irregularities) of the arterial segment, the segment is divided into an integer number of subsegments with lengths of approximately 5 mm. For each subsegment, the standard deviation with respect to the mean value is computed. The subsegmental data for this example are presented in Table 13–9.

Table 13–9. SUBSEGMENTAL DATA FOR THE EXAMPLE OF FIGURE 13–13

Segment	1	2	3	4
Length (mm)	5.51	5.51	5.51	5.51
Minimal diameter (mm)	2.92	1.74	1.17	2.68
Maximal diameter (mm)	3.29	3.27	3.03	3.40
Mean diameter (mm)	3.04	2.85	2.02	2.99
Standard deviation (mm)	0.12	0.48	0.69	0.24
Focal or diffuse disease	No	Yes	Yes	No

Segment 1 is the most proximal segment.

Derived Parameters of Coronary Arterial Segment

The investigators were requested to list all parameters that they compute and use to describe a coronary obstruction. From their information, the frequency of use was derived, as listed in Table 13–10. (For the individual data, see the report by Reiber.[R5])

Thus, almost all investigators use the "simple" parameters of obstruction diameter, reference diameter, percent diameter stenosis, obstruction area, and percent area stenosis, as assessed by different techniques. Less frequently used are the length of the obstruction, the area of the atherosclerotic plaque, the symmetry of the stenosis, and finally the transstenotic pressure gradient at a given flow.

Interpretation of Results From Biplane Analyses

In general, coronary obstructions are analyzed from at least two, preferably orthogonal, angiographic views, because of the eccentricity of lesions and because of the fact that the obstruction may be more visible in one view than in another as a result of foreshortening or overlap with other vessels or branches. According to the responses, six of the investigators (Brown, Kirkeeide, Sanders, Sandor, Selzer (optionally), and Vogel) compute elliptic cross sections from the biplane data, which requires that the two views be matched so that the positions of the stenosis in both views coincide.[B3] The points of minimum diameter in both views are generally assumed to correspond to the same site in the artery. Such an assumption can be a potential source of error, however. Collins, Reiber, and Sanders also use the data as separate items. On the other hand, Parker, Reiber, and Selzer average the results from the two views. Finally, Doriot and Nichols only perform single-plane analyses with densitometry.

DENSITOMETRY

Because the luminal cross section at a coronary obstruction is frequently irregular in shape, percent diameter reduction meas-

Table 13–10. FREQUENCY OF USE OF QUANTITATIVE PARAMETERS DESCRIBING THE SEVERITY OF CORONARY OBSTRUCTIONS

Derived Parameters for Coronary Arterial Segment	Frequency of Use (No. of Investigators of 12 Queried)
Obstruction diameter (mm)	9
Obstruction area (mm^2)	
Circular	
Elliptic	2
Densitometric	6
Reference diameter (mm)	10
Percent diameter stenosis	10
Percent area stenosis	
Circular	1
Elliptic	2
Densitometric	6
Length of obstruction (mm)	5
Symmetry of stenosis	2
Area of atherosclerotic plaque (mm^2)	5
Transstenotic pressure gradient (mmHg) at given flow	3

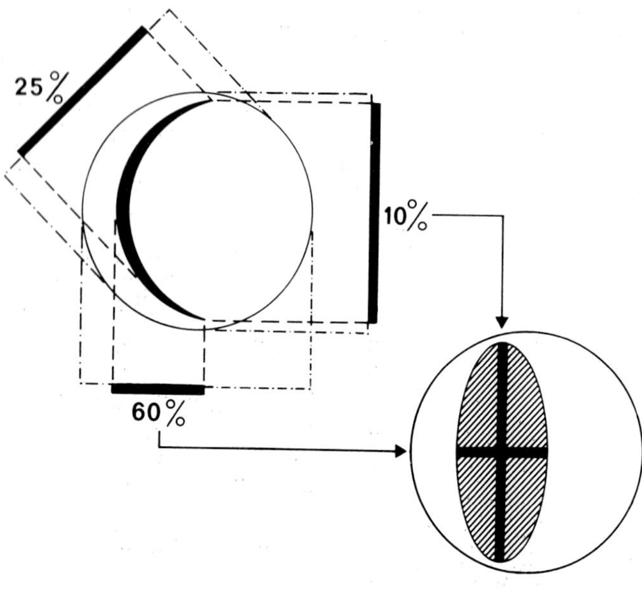

Figure 13–14. Potential errors in the evaluation of the severity of a crescent-like lesion from single and orthogonal views.

ured in a single angiographic view is of limited diagnostic value.[B6] The hemodynamic resistance of an obstruction is determined to a great extent by the minimal cross-sectional area. Computation of this cross-sectional area reduction from the percent diameter reduction measured in a single view requires the assumption of, for example, circular cross sections, an assumption that is hardly ever correct, particularly following PTCA, when dissections may be present.[S13, T3] The resulting error may be reduced by incorporating two orthogonal projections and computing elliptic cross sections. With the often occurring eccentric lesions, however, even this last approach may yield inaccurate results.

Figure 13–14 diagrammatically portrays the complex problems stemming from a slit-like stenosis having a crescent shape. In such cases, even three or more views do not "provide a faithful portrayal of their severity."[G12] A lateral view of the crescent would suggest a 10 percent reduction in lumen diameter; a left oblique view would yield a 25 percent narrowing and an anteroposterior view would imply a 60 percent stenosis. Even an elliptic model would fail to describe the severity of this lesion accurately.[B9]

The edge-detection techniques described previously are based, in general, on the measurement of changes in the brightness profiles along scan lines perpendicular to local center line segments. Therefore, if one could constitute the relationship between the path lengths of the x-rays through the artery and the absolute brightness values in the digitized image, one would obtain the information required to compute the cross-sectional areas from a single view (Fig. 13–15).[R4, S13] Clearly, a homogeneous mixing of the contrast agent with the blood must be assumed for the measurement to have any meaning. This approach is called the densitometric measurement technique. An additional advantage of the densitometric technique is that the stringent requirements regarding the accuracy of the edge detection can be diminished. If the detected boundaries are outside of the true edges, and if the background correction procedure (see later discussion) works well, then the true cross-sectional area can still be computed with the necessary accuracy. Eight investigators (Collins, Doriot, Marchand, Nichols, Parker, Reiber, Selzer, and Vogel) perform densitometric analyses of cross-sectional data from one angiographic view; Kirkeeide uses the density information only when orthogonal biplane views are available. A brief discussion of the common approaches and the differences between the various techniques follows.

A simplified block diagram of a complete x-ray-cineangiographic acquisition and analysis system is shown in Figure 13–16*A*. In a digital cardiac system, the videocamera at the output screen of the image intensifier (see Fig. 13–16*B*) is connected directly to the image processor via the analog-to-digital (A/D) converter. The image data are stored on a digital disk for later retrieval and analysis.

Constitution of the relationship between path length and brightness values requires detailed analysis of the complete imaging system. In a simplified approach, only the static properties of the system need to be considered. Analysis of the static transfer function of each link in the chain reveals that computation of the complete transfer function is difficult. A large number of parameters are involved, and many are spatially variant.[R4, R12] In practice, several simplifications are introduced to obtain usable techniques.

Eight of the nine investigators (Collins, Kirkeeide, Marchand, Nichols, Parker, Reiber, Selzer, and Vogel) assume that the x-ray absorption process, which constitutes the first part of the imaging chain from x-ray source to the image intensifier input screen, can be described by the Lambert-Beer law. Despite many potential sources of errors in the absorption process (nonmonochromatic x-ray spectrum, beam hardening, scattering, and so forth), Bürsch and Heintzen have demonstrated that by the use of appropriate filters and scatter grids the Lambert-Beer law can be applied to densitometric measurements in clinical studies with a sufficient degree of accuracy.[B12, H6]

On the other hand, Doriot and associates have indicated that the Lambert-Beer absorption law cannot account for the nonlinear relationship between the densitometric signal and logarithmic x-

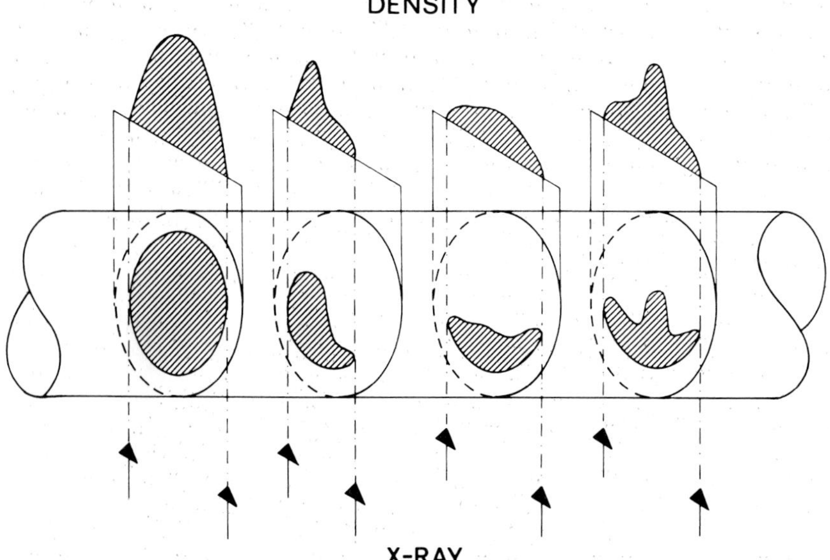

Figure 13–15. Schematic illustration of the relationship between the thickness of the irradiated object and the brightness level in the digitized angiographic image.

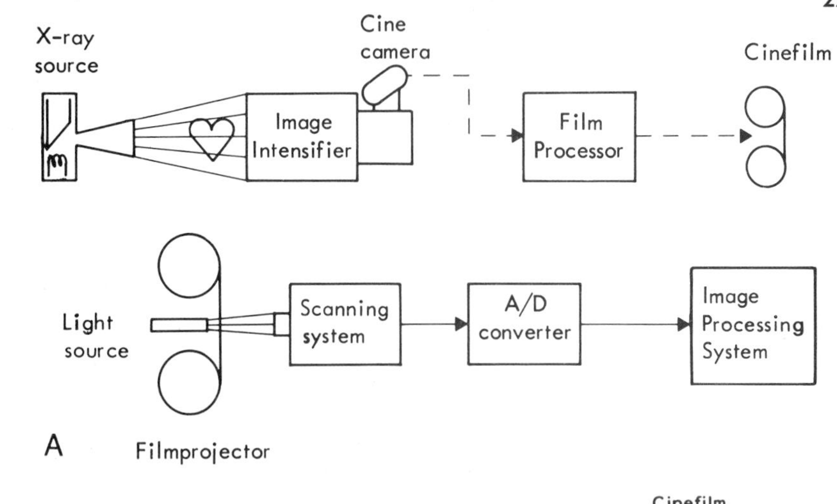

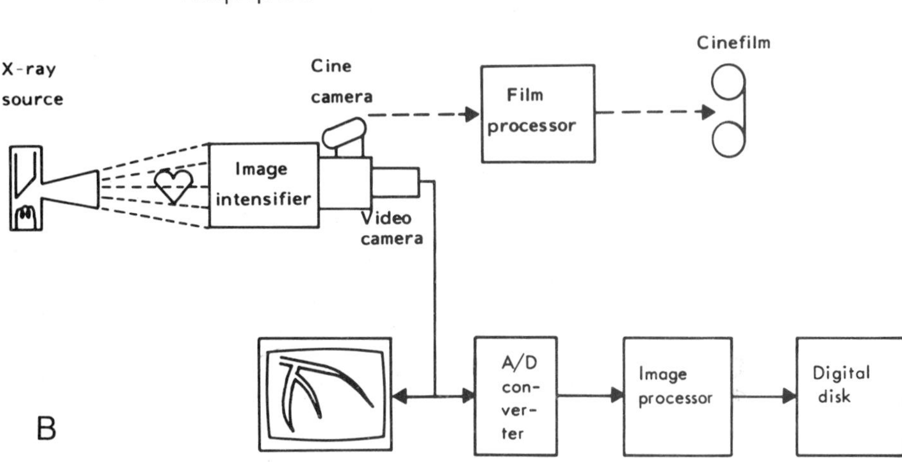

Figure 13–16. Block diagrams of an x-ray–cineangiographic acquisition and analysis system *(A)* and of an on-line digital cardiac system *(B)*.

ray transmission through the lumen of an opacified coronary artery.[D3–D5] Therefore, they have developed a physical model that considers the polychromatic and scattered radiation, and they have shown that this relationship can be approximated by a second-order polynomial. The coefficients of this polynomial depend primarily on the voltage applied to the x-ray tube and on the iodine concentration of the injected contrast medium. For a particular x-ray system, the coefficients of the polynomial can simply be obtained once by means of a linear wedge filled with contrast material. Doriot and associates have shown that the errors in the assessment of the densitometric percent area stenosis and obstruction area by the conventional densitometric technique (using the Lambert-Beer law and possibly compensating for the nonlinearity introduced by the cine film) depend on the actual size and shape of the intact and stenotic lumina, on their rotational orientation with respect to the incident x-rays, on the kV-level of the x-ray tube, and on the iodine concentration of the injected contrast medium.[D4]

In general, however, for the remaining subsystems of the cine film imaging chain, comprising the image intensifier, the cine film exposure and development process, and the film sampling process (which may be achieved via video and A/D conversion, with a CCD camera, or with another device), the simplified formulas that are used relate measured brightness levels to the irradiated object thicknesses and neglect the influence of spatially nonhomogeneous responses. By use of this approach, the response of film exposure—the density (D) versus log(exposure) (log [E]) curve—is linearized (linear transfer function). Kirkeeide, Reiber, Selzer, and their colleagues have implemented this approach.[G1, R13, W5] Nichols and associates[N1] assume a logarithmic transformation based on the photoelectric measurement technique of the light from the projector; they also use the characteristic curve of the cine film. Collins and co-workers determine the transfer function on the basis of a sensitometric strip.[J1]

We have also implemented a more complicated approach in an attempt to provide correction for the nonlinearities in the D versus log(E) plot and for the daily variations in the cine-film processing.[R4, R12] For this purpose, a special sensitometer has been developed that allows 21 full cine frames, covering the entire densitometric range of the film, to be exposed on each film cassette before the cassette is mounted on the image intensifier of the x-ray system.[R4, S13] The color temperature of the light source is the same as the one from the output screen of the image intensifier. The analysis procedure of a coronary cineangiogram therefore starts with the digitization of these 21 sensitometric frames, allowing the assessment of a nonlinear transfer function.

By means of this calibration procedure, many nonlinear, temporally and spatially variant effects in the film processing and the film-videocamera or film–CCD camera system are taken into account. This sensitometric approach has indeed been shown to improve the accuracy of measurement of cross-sectional area values as compared with the linear approach.[K5, R13]

In a digital cardiac system, the transfer function from the output of the image intensifier up to the digitized image can be approximated accurately by a linear function; this approach is taken by Doriot, Marchand, Parker, and Vogel.

The basic steps in the densitometric procedure to compute percent cross-sectional area reduction of a selected lesion can be summarized as follows (Fig. 13–17).[R4, R12] The contours of a selected arterial segment are detected as described earlier. On each scan line defined perpendicular to the center line, a profile of brightness values is measured. This profile is transformed into an absorption profile by means of the computed transfer functions (linear or nonlinear depending on the technique used). The background contribution is estimated by computing the linear regression line through the background points directly left and right of the detected contours. Recently, Nalcioglu and associates have compared three different background correction techniques

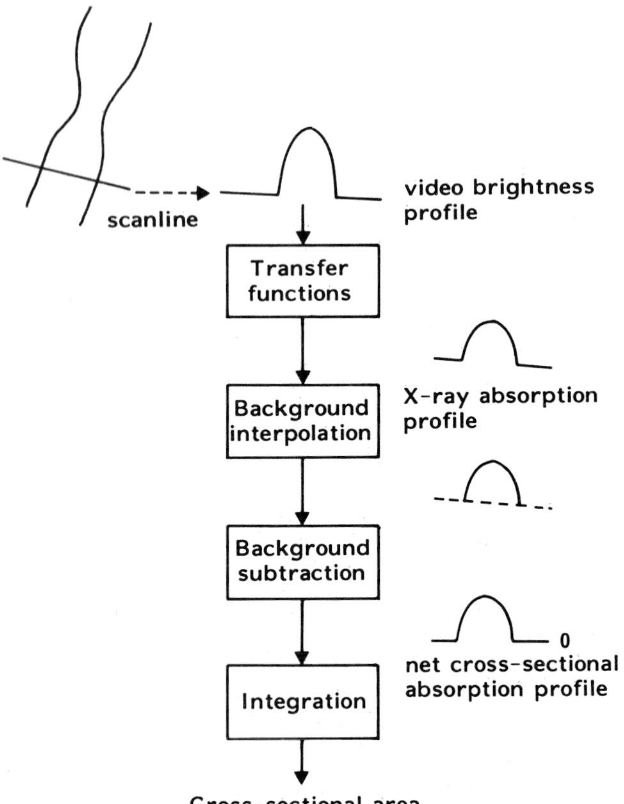

Figure 13–17. Schematic drawing for determining the cross-sectional area data from the densitometric data within the arterial segment.

(linear interpolation, a least-mean–squared error [LMSE] method, and a cubic spline interpolation [CSI] method) on phantom studies and concluded that all three algorithms allow a highly accurate determination of percent area stenosis.[N3, N11] If the background under the vessel varies rapidly, however, linear background subtraction may be inferior to the LMSE or CSI technique.

Subtraction of this background portion from the absorption profile within the arterial contours yields the net cross-sectional absorption profile. Integration of this function results in a measurement of the cross-sectional area at the particular scan line. By repeating this procedure for all the scan lines, the cross-sectional area function A(i) is obtained. Percent area reduction of an obstruction is determined by comparing the minimal area value at the obstruction with the mean value at a selected reference position. The interpolated approach mentioned earlier can also be applied to the estimation of the pre-disease area values. If one assumes that the cross section at the reference position is circular, absolute cross-sectional values for the arterial segments, (in square millimeters) and thus for the minimal cross section at the obstruction, can be obtained.[T3, W8]

The lower function in the example of Figure 13–11 is the densitometric area function for this segment. A densitometric cross-sectional area reduction of 89.4 percent was found, indicating that the obstruction is slightly more severe than one would estimate by assuming circular cross sections (86 percent area reduction).

The densitometric analysis of coronary arterial segments is difficult because of many potential problems. In addition to the possible sources of error mentioned previously, veiling glare and scatter, beam hardening, and the orientation of the vessel of interest to the x-ray beam should be mentioned.[P2, S24] In addition, side branches or branches lying close to the arterial segment to be analyzed cause significant errors in the background correction technique (see Fig. 13–11). Together with radiation scatter, veiling glare generates a low spatial–frequency component in the image-intensified video signal. This component nonuniformly biases the black level in videoangiography. In general, x-ray scatter and glare cause a suppression of contrast in the intensified image. A technique using a digital convolution algorithm has been proposed by Shaw and associates to approximate and provide correction for the scatter and glare.[S25]

Pfaff and colleagues have corrected for scatter and veiling glare by measuring the intensity beneath a 4-mm lead disk and subtracting it from each of the pixel intensities prior to logarithmic transformation.[P5] They concluded that errors in densitometric measurement of both absolute and relative iodine concentrations are substantial unless corrections are applied to the raw data.

Although various phantom studies of densitometric analysis of obstructions have been published,[N3, N4, N6, S26, T3] only three in vivo validation studies have been published to our knowledge (see the later section "Densitometric Validation Studies"). In a PTCA study using a digital angiographic system, Tobis and colleagues found no differences either prior to or following PTCA in the percent diameter stenosis values by the edge-detection or video-densitometric techniques (diameter stenosis derived from a reference diameter and a ratio of densitometric values at obstruction and reference).[T3] This finding contrasts sharply with the results from the PTCA study by Serruys and associates, which showed strong agreement between edge detection and densitometry prior to PTCA, but important discrepancies after PTCA, which were attributed to the asymmetric morphologic changes in luminal cross section occurring at PTCA.[S13] Nichols and associates concluded from pre- and post-PTCA data that the interobserver variability was significantly better for cine-videodensitometric ($r = 0.98$; SEE $= 6.4$ percent) than for caliper measurements ($r = 0.87$; SEE $= 13.1$ percent).[N4] In addition, videodensitometry provided comparable values for eccentric lesions filmed in right anterior oblique (RAO) and left anterior oblique (LAO) projections ($r = 0.99$, SEE $= 1.9$ percent).[N1]

A further demonstration of all the possible problems with densitometry can be given by the fact that only few investigators have been able to demonstrate that the densitometric results from different views of the same vessel agree closely, which is a requirement if densitometry is to work as well as one would hope (see the later section "Variability in Densitometric Results Assessed From Different Angiographic Views").

SUMMARY

In this section, an extensive overview of the major developments in off- and on-line quantitative coronary arteriography has been presented. Details provided in the text make clear that these developments are heterogeneous, but this heterogeneity should not be seen as only a negative point. So long as optimal results have not been achieved in certain areas, competition and new ideas are needed for development of better approaches.

Quantitative comparison of these systems at this time is very difficult, if not impossible. In other words, the question of how well all these systems work with routinely obtained coronary angiograms cannot be answered (see the later section "Validation Studies"). Data about the accuracy and precision of the edge-detection and analysis procedures, the success scores for images of different quality, the computation time, and so forth, are usually not provided in the publications; if they are provided, various parameters describing the validation results have been used, making comparisons difficult.[H5]

These computer-based systems also have definite interobserver and intraobserver variabilities, although these are usually not considered. The analysis procedures always contain several phases that result in observer variations, such as the definition of the center line of the coronary segment and the possibility of making manual corrections to the otherwise automatically detected contours.

In the coronary angiograms, the lumen of the artery is usually reasonably well visualized because of the administration of iodine-containing contrast medium, which means that one sees only the boundaries of the channel that is left open. One never can tell for sure whether or not a vessel is diffusely diseased, and thus whether the reference diameter that one is measuring represents the true original size of the vessel. Indications of the presence of diffuse disease may include a deviation in caliber of the vessel in relation to normal values (although normal values for all the coronary segments are not available) or the presence of irregularities in the contour as assessed by roughness measures of the segment (see the earlier section "Roughness Measure of Arterial Segment").[L13, M8, R6] Normal cross-sectional area of a specific vascular segment has also been found to be substantially influenced by the coronary branching pattern,[H15] left ventricular mass,[H16] and possibly other independent factors, such as gender, age, and ethnic origin. In patients with single-vessel disease with normal caliber coronary vessels and minimal irregularities, one may assume that diffuse disease plays a minor role. Under such circumstances, the use of the interpolated or computer-defined reference technique is acceptable; however, if any doubt exists regarding the presence of diffuse disease, this interpolated technique may also underestimate the original sizes of the vessel. To date, imaging of the intima of the coronary vessels by x-ray techniques has not been possible, nor is it likely to be possible in the future. Here exist excellent opportunities, however, for high-frequency echocardiographic approaches.[B18, J1]

Systems with facilities for densitometry usually also provide geometric data on the arterial dimensions (diameter values), because the densitometric data are derived from the brightness data within the arterial boundaries; these systems may be defined as hybrid systems. As discussed earlier, however, the accuracy of the edge-detection approaches in densitometric applications is less important provided that the boundaries are defined at or slightly outside of the true boundaries and that the background correction technique works well. The question then becomes whether in those systems that do have accurate contour detection facilities the densitometric data have made the geometric data completely obsolete. Gould and Kirkeeide automatically compare the cross-sectional area measurements by automated edge-detection techniques on biplane angiograms with the densitometric data.[G1] In addition, they have found that disagreements between the two methods may occur, especially for eccentric lesions in which the border recognition technique using the orthogonal biplane views is not as accurate as the densitometric technique,[K11, K12] or in cases in which other optically dense structures (catheters, other vessels, and so forth) are superimposed on the arterial segment of interest. In the latter circumstance, the diameter was best determined by the automated border recognition approach.

Given the present limitations in the accuracy and precision in densitometry, the use of only densitometric data may be helpful in selected studies in which a great number of conditions have been fulfilled, such as a coronary segment imaged en face with no intervening side branches, relatively homogeneous background, and so forth. In all other applications, especially in interventional studies, in which the pre- and post-intervention results must be compared from at least two angiographic views, the first choice at present must be the diameter data, and the second choice must be the densitometrically assessed cross-sectional area data. In other words, densitometric data may be used on a complementary basis, but should not replace the diameter data. Once the densitometric techniques have been improved so that the cross-sectional data can be measured under most clinical circumstances, with an accuracy and precision comparable to the current results of the best contour detection approaches, one may decide to rely only on the densitometric data.

The studies in which the on-line and off-line systems are compared will be of great interest. The question is whether one will be able to achieve the same accuracy and precision with on-line–acquired 512^2 images as with the off-line cine approaches. Appropriate interpolation schemes may prove to be extremely important in obtaining the required number of pixels with valuable information for automated edge-detection techniques.

Quality Control in Quantitative Coronary Arteriography

The previous section has presented an overview of the various computer-based techniques for the objective and reproducible assessment from coronary angiograms or cineangiograms of the quantitative parameters regarding the extent and severity of coronary artery disease. To evaluate changes in arterial dimensions over time, repeated angiographic or cineangiographic studies need to be performed and analyzed. The qualities of both the angiographic investigation and the subsequent computer analysis are hampered, however, by several sources of variation. If one is to obtain reliable and reproducible quantitative results from coronary angiograms or cineangiograms, these variations must be minimized as much as possible.

In this section, approaches toward standardized angiographic or cineangiographic acquisition and analysis procedures are presented.[R10, R14] Unless certain precautions are taken, the variabilities in absolute coronary dimensions may increase dramatically. On the other hand, if these precautions are followed, the variabilities in absolute dimensions from repeated cineangiography and analysis increase by a factor of only 1.5 to 2.2, as compared with those variabilities from repeated cine-film analysis alone. Although these data were established from validation studies on the cine film–based Cardiovascular Angiography Analysis System (CAAS), basically the same principles apply to all the other systems developed for quantitative coronary angiographic measurements (see previous section).[R4, R5, R15]

IMAGE ANALYSIS STEPS

In general, to analyze the dimensions of a coronary arterial segment quantitatively, the following steps need to be included in the application software packages (see the previous section, "Approaches to Quantitative Coronary Angiography"): (1) optical or electronic magnification of the region of interest encompassing the catheter or coronary segment by a high-quality cine digitizer or from the digitally acquired image; (2) computation of the calibration factor on the basis of the measured mean diameter in pixels (preferably from automatically detected boundaries) and the known size of the contrast catheter of metallic markers on the catheter, or on the basis of the distances between cardiomarker rings; (3) automated boundary detection of the arterial segment; (4) computation of the diameter function from the detected and pincushion-corrected contour positions; (5) computation of the cross-sectional area function if densitometry is available; and (6) determination of the severity of a coronary obstruction in terms of absolute and relative parameters.

SOURCES OF VARIATION AND APPROACHES TO STANDARDIZATION IN DATA ANALYSIS

In the procedures of cine-frame digitization and subsequent analysis, several sources of variation are apparent; these are listed in Table 13–11. The approaches that we have taken to minimize these variations are listed as well.[R10, R14] The noise sources (items 1 and 2, which are electronic noise and quantum noise, respectively) can be reduced by recursive digitization of the video-converted image, followed by spatial filtering. The recursive digitization is not applicable in a digital system, in which the x-ray–converted images are read out directly by a videocamera at

Table 13–11. SOURCES OF VARIATION AND APPROACHES TO STANDARDIZATION IN DATA ANALYSIS

Sources of Variation	Approaches to Standardization
1. Electronic noise contributions in cine-digitizing system	1. Recursive digitization of video image
2. Quantum noise in images	2. Spatial filtering of digital image data with a 5 × 5 median filter
3. Effects of resampling the data along scan lines through square grid of the digital image data	3. } Iterative edge-detection and correction procedures
4. Observer variations in definition of center positions within the catheter and the selected arterial segment	4. } Iterative edge-detection and correction procedures
5. Possible manual corrections to the detected contours	5. } Iterative edge-detection and correction procedures
6. Selection of reference positions	6. Computer-defined reference position (interpolated technique). For repeat studies, proper documentation of analysis data on Polaroid photographs or sheet film
7. Manual definition of starting and end points in nonobstructed arterial segments for measurement of overall mean diameter	7. Use of anatomic landmarks, such as bifurcations, as much as possible

the output screen of the image intensifier; however, these video-cameras are usually characterized by a high signal-to-noise ratio, so that the electronic noise contribution is minor. The variations in the contour-detection procedure (items 3 to 5) can be reduced by applying iterative edge-detection and correction procedures. The problem of the selection of the reference (normal) diameter of the arterial segment (item 6) can be alleviated by the use of the interpolated or computer-defined reference technique (see the earlier section "Reference for Percent Diameter Stenosis Measurement"), whereas anatomic landmarks should be used as much as possible for the manual definition of starting and end points of arterial segments (item 7).

These approaches have resulted in variabilities (standard deviations of the signed differences) in the repeated analysis of selected cine frames of more than 0.12 mm for the absolute measurements, and 3.94 percent for the percent diameter stenosis measurement by the computer-defined technique (see "Variability in Repeated Analyses" in the later section "Validation Studies.")[R4, R16]

SOURCES OF VARIATION AND APPROACHES TO STANDARDIZATION IN ANGIOGRAPHIC DATA ACQUISITION

The previous section discussed the sources of variation and the approaches to be taken in the data analysis procedure itself. The angiographic data acquisition procedure is also hampered by several sources of variation (Table 13–12). The approaches that we propose to minimize these variations in the data acquisition procedure are listed in the same order in Table 13–13; these are discussed in further detail in the following sections. We have shown that the variabilities in the coronary arterial measurements may increase dramatically if only a minimum or none of these precautions is taken.[R4, R16] (See "Long-Term [90-Day] Variability" in the later section "Validation Studies.")

On-Line Registration of X-Ray System Settings

A microprocessor system developed at the Thoraxcenter collects for each angiographic investigation a number of x-ray system

Table 13–12. SOURCES OF VARIATION IN ANGIOGRAPHIC DATA ACQUISITION

1. Differences between the angles and height levels of the x-ray gantry with respect to the patient at the time of repeated angiography and those used at the baseline study.
2. Differences in vasomotor tone of the coronary arteries.
3. Variations in the quality of mixing of the contrast agent with the blood.
4. Angiographic quality of catheter (image contrast).
5. Deviations in the size of the catheter as listed by the manufacturer from its actual size.

parameters, which are projected onto the patient film and printed on a line printer.[B15] Parameters describing the geometry of the x-ray gantry for a particular cine film run (rotation of U-arm and of object, as well as distances from isocenter to focus, film, and object) are projected onto the film immediately preceding the first angiographic image (Fig. 13–18*A*), while parameters describing the selected x-ray exposure factors (kV, mA, and pulse width), as well as film speed, focus, grid ratio, and the radiation dose, are projected onto the cine film immediately following the last angiographic image of this particular cine run (see Fig. 13–18*B*).

When repeat angiography is scheduled, the geometry of the x-ray system is set on the basis of the available data, so that approximately the same angiographic projection is obtained. This approach allows the accuracy and precision of the resettings to be controlled from the actual data projected onto the film and listed on the printout. In a clinical study with repositioning of the x-ray system, we found that the angular variability, defined by the standard deviation of the absolute differences of angular settings, was less than 4.2 degrees and that the variability in the various positions of image intensifier and x-ray source was less than 3.0 cm.[R10, R14] For each of the various x-ray system parameters, no significant differences were found between the average values of the initial and repeated settings. These results show that the x-ray system settings can be reproduced quite accurately in routine clinical practice if sufficient care is taken. If on-line registration of the x-ray system settings is not available, manual completion of appropriate forms for the x-ray system settings is a reasonable alternative.

Preangiographic Administration of Vasodilative Drugs

One of the most important variables in the quantitative assessment of coronary arterial dimensions is the vasomotor tone. If no precautions are taken, the vasomotor tone may differ even during consecutive coronary angiographic studies.

An optimal vasodilative drug for controlling the vasomotor tone of the epicardial vessel should produce a quick (within 30 seconds to 1 minute) and maximal response without influencing the hemodynamic state of the patient. Only nitrates and calcium antagonists satisfy these requirements. On isolated human coronary arteries, the calcium antagonists may be more vasoactive than nitrates, but they act more slowly.[G11] In the in vivo situation, however, the nitrates are more vasoactive than the calcium antagonists.[N5] Rafflenbeul and Lichtlen demonstrated that sublingually administered nitrate and nifedipine have cumulative ef-

Table 13–13. APPROACHES TO STANDARDIZATION IN ANGIOGRAPHIC DATA ACQUISITION

1. On-line registration of x-ray system settings, or manual completion of appropriate forms for x-ray system settings.
2. Administration of vasodilator immediately prior to angiographic investigation.
3. Use of nonionic and iso-osmolar contrast media. Administration of contrast medium by ECG-triggered injector.
4. Selection of acceptable catheter material (high angiographic image contrast and edge gradient).
5. Measurement of actual size catheter with micrometer following catheterization procedure.

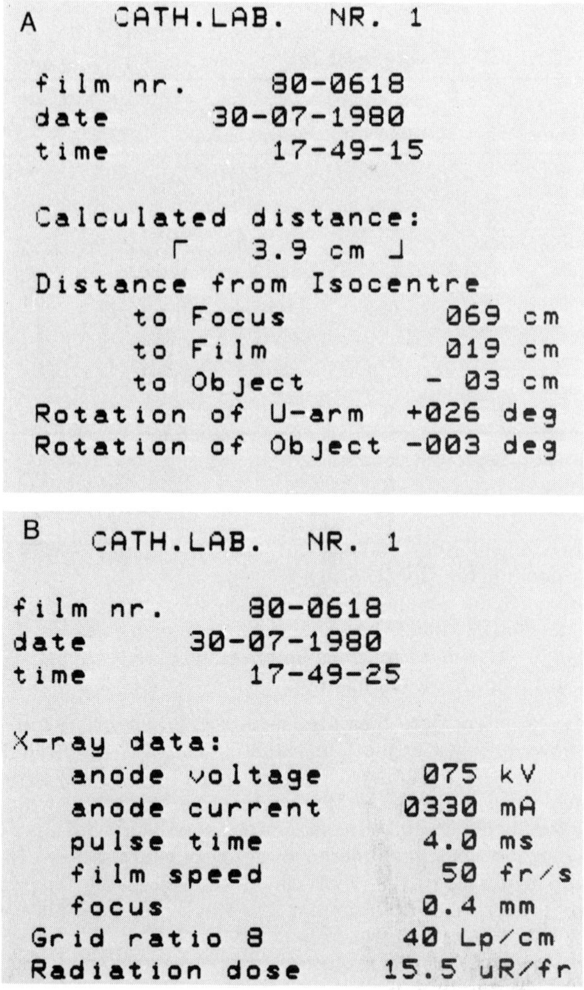

A CATH.LAB. NR. 1

film nr. 80-0618
date 30-07-1980
time 17-49-15

Calculated distance:
⌜ 3.9 cm ⌟
Distance from Isocentre
to Focus 069 cm
to Film 019 cm
to Object - 03 cm
Rotation of U-arm +026 deg
Rotation of Object -003 deg

B CATH.LAB. NR. 1

film nr. 80-0618
date 30-07-1980
time 17-49-25

X-ray data:
anode voltage 075 kV
anode current 0330 mA
pulse time 4.0 ms
film speed 50 fr/s
focus 0.4 mm
Grid ratio 8 40 Lp/cm
Radiation dose 15.5 uR/fr

Figure 13–18. Parameters describing the geometry of the x-ray gantry *(A)*, and those describing the selected x-ray exposure factors for a particular cineangiographic run *(B)* are projected onto the film for documentation purposes. (From Reiber J.H.C., et al.: Approaches towards standardization in acquisition and quantitation of arterial dimensions from cineangiograms. *In* Reiber, J.H.C., and Serruys, P.W. (eds.): State of the Art in Quantitative Coronary Angiography. Martinus Nijhoff, Dordrecht, 1986, p. 145, with permission.)

fects, which suggests that both agents should be used to obtain maximal vasodilation.[R17]

An alternative to the sublingual administration is the intracoronary injection of nitrate, calcium antagonist, or both.[S27] This route of administration has the advantage of allowing fast and complete action of the drug on the coronary vessel.[S28] In addition, possible negative inotropic effects of these drugs are less pronounced when the intracoronary route is followed. Figure 13–19 shows the effects of repeated intracoronary administrations of nifedipine on the mean diameters of normal and post-stenotic segments. Further vasodilation is observed after the second administration.

A dose of 3 mg isosorbide dinitrate (ISD) administered intracoronary has been shown to be well tolerated in clinical practice and is known to be 15 times stronger than the dose of nitroglycerin necessary to obtain maximal vasodilation.[F11] This dose of 3 mg ISD is equivalent to intracoronary administration of 0.3 mg of the nitrate nitroglycerin.[S29] A disadvantage of the nitroglycerin preparation is that it must be dissolved in an alcoholic solvent, because it is a lipophilic compound. Such alcoholic preparations may be deleterious to the myocardium and may induce hemolysis. In addition, some of the commercial preparations of nitroglycerin contain high levels of potassium, which could provoke spasm.[W9]

Isosorbide dinitrate is a hydrophilic preparation. Lablanche and associates have demonstrated that intracoronary and intrafemoral venous injections produce identical peripheral hemodynamic and coronary changes after the first minute following administration.[L10, L11] The effects were maximal between 2 and 4 minutes and continued after 10 minutes. The only difference was a more rapid decrease in systolic pressure after intrafemoral administration. With intracoronary injection, dilation preceded the occurrence of hemodynamic effects, which gives rise to an argument for using the intracoronary ISD (particularly in the treatment of spasm induced by ergonovine).

A potential advantage of choosing calcium antagonists over the nitrates is that small amounts of calcium antagonists injected by the intracoronary route produce coronary vasodilation without any systemic effect.[K13, S34] On the other hand, the calcium antagonists may produce transient negative inotropic, chronotropic, and dramatopic effects.

We may conclude that the vasomotor tone should be controlled in quantitative coronary angiographic studies. The only way to achieve such control is by attempting to reach the ceiling of vasodilation of the vessels by means of a vasodilatory drug that produces fast and complete vasodilation without any peripheral effects. Such results seem to be obtained most reliably by the intracoronary administration of nitrates or calcium antagonists. Investigators have not determined, however, which of these drugs is the single most potent vasodilator, and whether these drugs should be used in combination given their possibly synergistic actions.

Use of Nonionic and Iso-osmolar Contrast Media

Adverse effects of conventional contrast media are related to the single-valence cations such as sodium and meglumine, to an imbalance in the ratio of sodium ions to calcium ions, and to the high osmolality and hyperviscosity of the solutions.[B16, H7]

Much effort has been directed toward development of new water-soluble contrast media with iso- and low osmolality; these are either nonionic or contain physiologic concentrations of calcium ions.[F17] These agents cause less subjective discomfort, fewer hemodynamic and biochemical effects, and fewer blood pressure and rhythm disturbances in coronary angiography than conventional contrast media. Collective studies offer experimental and clinical evidence of the advantages of the low-osmolality agents in cardiac radiology.[C6, D12] Jost and associates have clearly demonstrated that the vasodilative changes in vessel dimensions due to the contrast medium administration are significantly smaller with use of a nonionic contrast medium than with use of an ionic contrast medium.[J3] Therefore, in quantitative coronary angiographic studies, nonionic contrast media with iso-osmolality

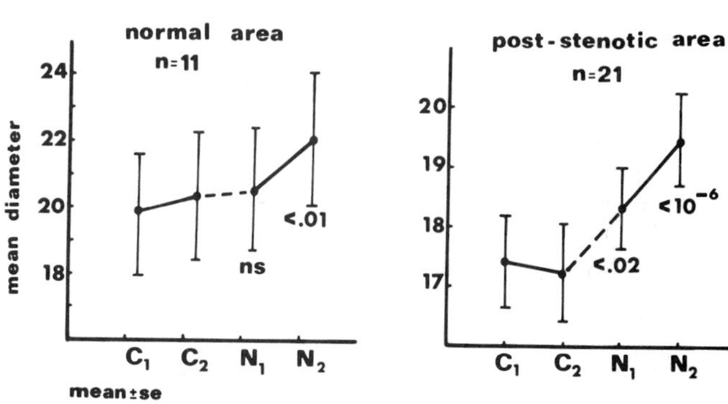

Figure 13–19. Effects of intracoronary administration of nifedipine on the mean diameter of 11 normal and 21 post-stenotic coronary segments during two control cineangiograms (C_1, C_2) and the two cineangiograms following nifedipine administration (N_1, N_2). The third angiogram (N_1) was obtained within 30 sec following nifedipine administration. The final angiogram (N_2) was recorded usually within 5 min from N_1. The mean diameter values along the ordinate of the figures are noncalibrated values expressed in pixels. (From Serruys, P.W., et al.: Unstable angina pectoris and coronary arterial vasomotion: Which role for nifedipine? *In* Rafflenbeul, W., et al. (eds.): Unstable Angina Pectoris. Georg Thieme Verlag, Stuttgart, 1981, p. 103, with permission.)

Table 13–14. SPECIFICATIONS OF FREQUENTLY USED CONTRAST MEDIA

	Generic Name	Percentage Solution	Trade Name	Iodine (mg/ml)	Osmolality (mosm/kg)	Viscosity	
						25°C	*37°C*
Ionic, high osmolality	Diatrizoate sodium 10% meglumine 66%	76	Renografin-76	370	1940	13.8	8.4
	Diatrizoate sodium 25% meglumine 50%	75	Hypaque-M, 75%	385	2108	12.69	7.99
Ionic, low osmolality	Ioxaglate sodium 19.6% meglumine 39.3%	58.9	Hexabrix	320	600	15.7	7.5
Nonionic, low osmolality	Iohexol	75.5	Omnipaque	350	862	18.50	11.15
	Iopamidol	76	Isovue 370	370	796	20.9	9.4

(From Fischer, H. W.: Catalog of intravascular contrast media. Radiology 159:561–563, 1986, with permission.)

should be applied; in addition, adequate injection intervals should be taken. The characteristics of some of the most frequently used contrast media are listed in Table 13–14.[F17, R4]

Administration of Contrast Medium by Electrocardiographically Triggered Injector

As part of their procedures to measure coronary flow, myocardial perfusion, and coronary flow reserve from coronary angiograms, Spiller and colleagues and Vogel and associates have been using ECG-synchronized, power contrast-medium injections to standardize the timing and flow rates of the contrast boluses.[S30, V7] When such injections are performed with a No. 8 or 9 Fr. catheter (for example, a guiding catheter for angioplasty), high flow rates can be achieved, resulting in angiograms of good quality. Modern injectors are relatively safe to use because upper limits for the flow rate and pressure can be set; pressure rise time is also adjustable. For quality-control purposes, registration of the pressure signal of the injector on paper is advisable. In our center, we have employed the power injector technique in a number of clinical research studies and for the assessment of coronary flow reserve. Our impression has been that the high flow rate contributes more to image quality than the timing of the contrast administration.

Selection of Catheter Material

Coronary contrast catheters have been used increasingly for purposes of calibration in the quantitative assessment of coronary arterial dimensions.[R5] We wished to determine the accuracy of such calibration measurements from coronary cineangiograms and the effects of catheter material, contrast filling of the catheter, and kilovolt setting of the x-ray source on image quality of the irradiated catheter and thus on the accuracy of the measurements. Therefore, we have analyzed four catheter materials, filmed under different conditions.[R11] The four catheters were fabricated from different materials:

Woven Dacron—Sones 7 French catheter (USCI Int., Inc., Billerica, MA, U.S.A.)

Polyvinylchloride—Judkins 7.3 French catheter (Cook Inc., Bloomington, IN, U.S.A.)

Polyurethane—Femoral-left coronary 8 French catheter (Cordis Corp., Miami, FL, U.S.A.)

Nylon—Alvaflo 7 French catheter (Mallinckrodt GmbH, Grossostheim, West Germany)

The catheters were measured with a micrometer. Figure 13–20 shows for each of the four catheter materials the brightness profile along a scan line across an analyzed catheter segment defined perpendicular to the center line direction, with the catheter filled with 100 percent contrast agent and with air. From these eight graphs, the differences in image contrast between the various materials can be appreciated, as well as the differences in the brightness distribution for a particular segment filled with 100 percent contrast agent or with air.

On the basis of our evaluation data, we concluded that the woven Dacron catheter is the one most suitable for quantitative coronary angiographic studies. Polyvinylchloride and polyurethane catheters produce similar levels of image quality, but lower than that achieved with the woven Dacron catheter. The nylon catheter should not be used for these types of studies.

Micrometric Measurement of Catheter Following Catheterization

In our experience, the size of the catheter as specified by the manufacturer often deviates from its actual size, especially in the case of disposable catheters. If the manufacturer cannot guarantee narrow ranges for the size of the catheter—for example, ± 0.05 Fr.—it should be measured with a micrometer following catheterization. This problem is even more significant for the tip of a catheter, which is often hand-made and thus poorly specified; we use the tip most often for the calibration. For a 5.5 Fr. tip of a Sones catheter, a deviation by 0.05 Fr. results in a 0.9 percent error in the computed calibration factor.

SUMMARY

The total variabilities in coronary arterial measurements with the CAAS have been assessed from repeated analyses on the

Table 13–15. MEAN AND STANDARD DEVIATION DIFFERENCES IN THE ABSOLUTE DIAMETER MEASUREMENTS AND INTERPOLATED PERCENT DIAMETER STENOSIS FOR REPEATED ANALYSIS

	Mean Difference			Standard Deviation Difference		
	Repeated Analysis	*Best-Controlled Study*	*Worst-Case Study*	*Repeated Analysis*	*Best-Controlled Study*	*Worst-Case Study*
Obstruction diameter (mm)	0.00	0.00	0.00	0.10	0.22	0.36
Interpolated reference diameter (mm)	−0.10	0.05	−0.13	0.10	0.15	0.66
Interpolated percent (%) diameter stenosis	−2.08	1.21	−1.92	3.94	7.23	6.52

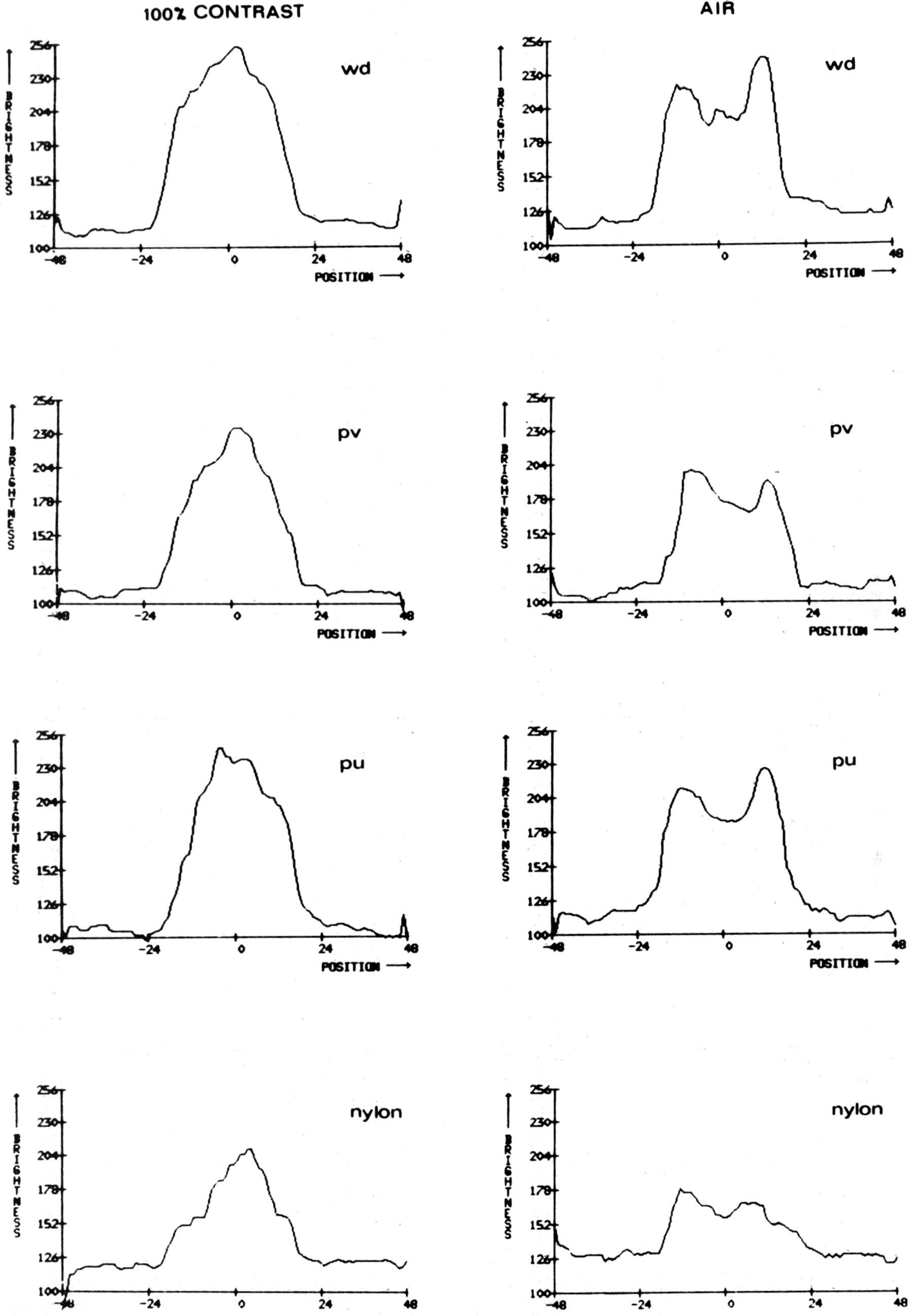

Figure 13–20. Examples of brightness distribution along scan lines that are perpendicular to the center-line directions for the four different catheters, which are filled with 100 percent contrast agent *(left column)* and with air *(right column)*. Graphs for the different materials are represented: woven Dacron (wd), polyvinylchloride (pv), polyurethane (pu), and nylon. In each graph, the pixel positions along the scan lines are plotted along the horizontal axis, and the brightness levels are plotted along the vertical axis. (From Reiber, J.H.C., et al.: Assessment of dimensions and image quality of coronary contrast catheters from cineangiograms. Cathet. Cardiovasc. Diagn. 11:521, 1985, with permission.)

same angiographic frames, from a best-controlled cineangiographic patient study in which most precautions mentioned previously were followed, as well as from a worst-case cineangiographic study, in which a minimum of precautions were taken (see the later section "Variability in Repeated Coronary Cineangiography and Computer Analysis").[R16] The results of these studies are summarized in Table 13–15.

The mean differences in absolute diameters were less than 0.13 mm in all studies. The variabilities (standard deviations of signed differences) in obstruction diameter for these three types of studies ranged from 0.10 mm for the repeated analysis only to 0.36 mm in the worst-case angiographic study. Likewise, the variability in the interpolated reference diameter was smallest for the repeated analysis and largest in the worst-case study (0.66 mm). The worst-case study clearly demonstrates that the variability in absolute dimensions increases if no special care is taken to reduce the potential sources of variation.

The variabilities in the interpolated percent diameter reduction were smallest for the repeated analysis study and were 84 percent and 65 percent higher for the best-controlled and worst-case angiographic studies, respectively. The mean differences were all less than 2.08 percent.

The data from Table 13–15 thus make clear that the variabilities in the obstruction diameters with repeated angiographic studies and analysis were 2.2 to 3.6 times greater than those from repeated analysis alone, and 1.5 to 6.6 times greater for the interpolated reference diameters. These increases are caused by the sources of variation in the data acquisition procedure described earlier. They make clear that the possible sources of variations in the data acquisition must be minimized as much as possible to obtain reliable and reproducible quantitative results from coronary cineangiograms. In addition, further attempts toward standardization of angiographic procedures are seriously needed to obtain further decreases in the remaining variabilities.

Validation Studies

Although different approaches to the morphologic and densitometric analysis of coronary obstructions have been reported in the literature (see the earlier section "Approaches to Quantitative Coronary Angiography"), quantitative comparison of these systems is difficult, if not impossible, at this time. The question of how well these systems work with routinely obtained coronary angiograms cannot yet be answered. The absence of data about the accuracy and precision of the edge-detection and analysis procedures; the success scores for different image qualities, computation times, and so forth; and the use of different parameters to describe the validation results make comparisons difficult.[H5] Recently, discussions among several groups active in this field have taken place in an attempt to define commonly accepted validation procedures for the quantitative coronary angiography analysis systems.

This section first proposes procedures for the determination of the accuracy, precision, and reproducibility of the edge-detection and densitometric techniques, and suggests ways in which these results should be presented. Next, an extensive overview of published data on the following topics is presented: (1) validation studies of arterial dimensions (nondensitometric) and (2) validation studies of the densitometric techniques. Thereafter, our results on the overall variabilities in diameter measurements with repeated cineangiographic studies and computer analysis (short-, medium-, and long-term variabilities) are described. Finally, we have investigated the critical nature of the frame selection in quantitative coronary angiography. A brief discussion on the topics mentioned concludes this section.

PROPOSED VALIDATION PROCEDURES

The following procedures should be carried out to validate a coronary quantitation system:

ASSESSMENT OF ACCURACY AND PRECISION OF EDGE-DETECTION AND DENSITOMETRIC TECHNIQUES

- Phantom studies of coronary obstructions with dimensions from 0.5 to 5.0 mm under different imaging conditions (e.g., various concentrations of the contrast agent, different kilovolt levels covering the routinely used range) and under static and dynamic flow conditions.
- In vivo animal studies with hollow plastic cylinders of various luminal shapes and sizes inserted in the coronary arteries.
- For densitometric studies, testing of the hypothesis that the results are independent of the angiographic views in which these studies were acquired.

REPRODUCIBILITY

- Repeated analysis of a set of clinical coronary angiograms obtained under various imaging conditions to assess interobserver and intraobserver variabilities, as well as short- and long-term variabilities in the angiographic data acquisition and image analysis.

PARAMETERS DESCRIBING VALIDATION RESULTS

A suggested procedure for describing the results of the validation studies involves expression of these results in terms of the mean differences (accuracy) and the standard deviations (precision) of the signed differences (measurement 1 minus measurement 2; not absolute differences) between the actual and measured values or between the values from repeated measurements.

In the following sections, the results of published data on such validation procedures are summarized. Details regarding the validation procedures performed by the various investigators listed in the earlier section "Approaches to Quantitative Coronary Angiography" can be found in the report by Reiber.[R5]

NONDENSITOMETRIC VALIDATION STUDIES OF ARTERIAL DIMENSIONS

Phantom Studies

As described in the previous section, "Proposed Validation Procedures," the first validation study to test a particular design and implementation of a quantitative coronary angiographic system should focus on the accuracy and precision of the actual edge-detection technique based on phantom studies of coronary obstructions. A brass model, or models made of any other material with a high x-ray absorption coefficient, should not be used, because these materials do not mimic the clinical situation; instead, perspex, Plexiglas, or Lucite models that can be filled with various concentrations of contrast medium are appropriate.

Only six investigators have presented results on the accuracy and precision of these techniques. The models used have been perspex models of various sizes, ranging from 0.3 to 5 mm (Collins, Kirkeeide, Nichols, Reiber, and Vogel), as well as brass arteries (Brown). The results on the accuracy of the different techniques are all good, ranging from 0.01 mm to 0.03 mm; however, owing to the different definitions used to describe the precision (absolute differences, signed differences, and standard error of the estimate), these data cannot simply be compared. These problems have also been recognized by Herrington and colleagues.[H5] In general, the studies mentioned previously were performed at different kilovolt levels, ranging from 50 to 110 kV, and at different concentrations of the contrast medium, varying from 50 to 100 percent. Simons and associates have performed the only dynamic phantom study: water was pumped through the phantom while contrast agent was administered through an injection port. They presented only densitometric results, however (see "Phantom Studies" in the later section "Densitometric Validation Studies").[S32] Therefore, the vast majority of the currently active groups did not validate their systems with a dynamic model.

In Vivo Validations

Three investigators (Brown, Nichols, and Vogel) have performed validations of their techniques on clinical material. Brown and Nichols used postmortem material and found correlation coefficients of 0.94 and 0.99, respectively; in Nichols's study, the standard error of the estimate for area stenosis was 0.71 mm^2.

Mancini, Vogel, and associates performed an in vivo study with dogs instrumented with precision-drilled, plastic cylinders to create intraluminal stenoses. The internal diameters of the cylinders ranged from 0.83 to 1.83 mm.[M10, M11] Performing on-line acquisition, they reported a standard error of the estimate of 0.09 mm ($r = 0.98$) for the minimal diameter of the "obstructions."

Finally, Kirkeeide and colleagues compared in vivo pressure drop and coronary flow reserve measurements with predicted values; unfortunately, no results are available.

Variability in Repeated Analyses

Limited data are available from seven investigators (Brown, Collins, Kirkeeide, Nichols, Reiber, Sanders, and Sandor) on the variability in repeated analyses of the same angiographic study. The mean differences (accuracy) ranged from 0.00 to 0.10 mm in the obstruction diameter, from 0.1 to 3 percent in the percent diameter stenosis, and from −0.2 to 4 percent in the percent area stenosis. The values for the standard deviation of the differences (precision) ranged from 0.06 to 0.18 mm in the obstruction diameters, from 2.5 to 6.2 percent in the percent diameter stenosis, and from 4.1 to 5.5 percent in the percent area stenosis. Again, one must be careful in comparing these numbers, because different definitions may have been used. (Our results are described in more detail in "Variability in Data Analysis" in the later section "Variability in Repeated Coronary Cineangiography and Computer Analysis.") Collins and associates compared their minimal luminal diameters obtained by automated edge-detection techniques with those obtained by the Brown-Dodge method (manual tracing on optically magnified images) and found a value for r of 0.88 and a standard error of the estimate of 0.32 mm.

DENSITOMETRIC VALIDATION STUDIES

Phantom Studies

Only Collins, Kirkeeide, Marchand, Parker, and Reiber responded on the questionnaire mentioned earlier, with some limited data, to questions regarding the accuracy and precision of the densitometric technique on the basis of phantom studies (i.e., data describing the size of the differences from truly known values). Parker used polyethylene tubing and Teflon rods for his experiments; the others used perspex models. The one parameter that three out of the five investigators measured was the accuracy of percent area stenosis, which ranged from 0.3 to 7 percent. The precision in percent area stenosis ranged from 1.76 to 5 percent, which is an acceptable result. Kirkeeide and Nichols also determined the precision in the measurement of the absolute area stenosis by densitometry and found values for standard error of the estimate of 0.24 and 0.32 mm^2, respectively. Nickoloff used the videodensitometric method for measuring the dimensions (diameter values) of small vessels based on the full-width-at-half-maximum (FWHM) values of the densitometric profiles.[N6] In Plexiglas cylinders, the diameters were measured to within 2 percent mean error. For clinical angiograms with nonconcentric lesions, however, this approach does not seem to have much practical use.

Two studies, however, addressed eccentric and concentric lesions. Selzer and associates have used a model with concentric holes (10 holes) and eccentric asymmetric holes placed inside and outside of an enbalmed chest; this validation study is in progress.

Simons and colleagues have performed both static and dynamic phantom studies over a wide range of iodine concentrations with digital subtraction videodensitometry.[S32] The dynamic phantom consisted of precision-drilled tubes within a set of interchangeable cylindric acrylic chambers; the lesions were concentric. Water was pumped at a known rate through the main chamber, from which it entered each of the coronary "vessels," and flow through each vessel could be regulated. Each of the 14 vessels, ranging from 1 to 3 mm in diameter with stenoses from 0.5 to 2.5 mm in diameter, was imaged after selective injection of contrast agent through an injection port. Eccentric stenoses were created in the static phantom study. Accuracy in the assessment of absolute cross-sectional area varied with iodine concentration and indicated a slight tendency to overestimate the area at high concentration and to underestimate the area at low concentration. Higher concentrations, on the other hand, improved the reproducibility, with standard deviations ranging from 2 to 7 percent of the measured value, compared with 7 to 27 percent at the lowest concentration. Accuracy and reproducibility of area measurements on either normal or stenotic segments were unchanged by rotation of the vessel by up to 25 degrees out of the plane of the image.

In Vivo Validations

To date, we know of only three in vivo densitometric validation studies published. Wiesel and co-workers described a study with closed-chest dogs in which 10 plastic cylinders with precisely machined circular and irregular lumina were inserted into the coronary arteries. Minimal cross-sectional area of the stenosis was determined by the edge-detection technique from two orthogonal views (ellipse method) and by densitometry from one view. The investigators concluded that the ellipse method is more accurate for circular stenoses, whereas the irregular stenoses were better quantitated by the videodensitometric method with an average absolute difference of 0.50 mm^2 and a standard error of the estimate of 0.47.[W8]

Johnson and colleagues have performed an in vivo validation study comparing the densitometric data with the results of intraoperative high-frequency epicardial echocardiography in a total of 36 arterial segments, which were uniformly filled with contrast and not markedly foreshortened.[J1] They found a correlation coefficient (r) of 0.86 between integrated optical density defined by videodensitometry and luminal area determined by high-frequency echocardiography. In addition, a good correlation ($r = 0.94$) was found between the integrated optical densities in the left anterior oblique and right anterior oblique views. (Note that the densitometric data are expressed in integrated optical densities, not in absolute square millimeters.)

Simons, Kruger, and associates tested a videodensitometric method in living dogs with coronary artery stenoses created surgically by placement of small Silastic cuffs.[K9, S32, S33] Their method is based on the assumption that the logarithmically subtracted attenuation value across a vessel filled with iodine and acquired on-line with a digital system is directly proportional to the product of the iodine concentration and the vessel thickness at any given point. Comparison of histologic data with the cross-sectional area at the site of the obstruction expressed in square millimeters (with calibration performed on the basis of the reference diameter and the reference area assumed to be circular) resulted in a slope of 0.948 with relatively wide 95 percent confidence limits ($r = 0.85$). The absolute cross-sectional areas of lesions as small as 1 mm^2 could be measured with an accuracy within 30 percent of the true absolute cross-sectional area in most cases. One should note that these results are based on approximately circular cross sections created surgically.

For the sake of completeness, the in vivo study with the dynamic spatial reconstructor (DSR) by Block and colleagues should also be mentioned.[B19] In this study, nine hollow plastic cylinders were positioned in the coronary arteries of mongrel dogs via percutaneous catheterization. Three of the plugs had irregular noncircular lumina. The percent area reduction caused by the hollow cylinders ranged from 53 to 92 percent and was underestimated by the DSR, on average, by 7 percent (r = 0.85; SEE = 5%).

Variability in Repeated Analyses

Only Collins, Nichols, and Vogel studied the variability in repeated analyses of densitometric studies. Collins found correlation coefficients in the cross-sectional area measurements of 0.88 for the interobserver variability on the same frames, and of 0.98 for the intraobserver variability on two consecutive frames. Nichols found interobserver and intraobserver variabilities in percent area stenosis of 5.3 percent (SEE) and 2.6 percent (SEE), with correlation coefficients of 0.96 and 0.99, respectively. The intraobserver variability in absolute area stenosis was found to be 0.26 mm^2 (SEE), with a correlation coefficient of 0.99. Vogel found a correlation coefficient of 0.999 in the repeated analysis of percent area stenosis.

Variability in Densitometric Results Assessed From Different Angiographic Views

Finally, we have examined the variability of densitometric measurements of the same obstructions assessed from different angiographic views. Earlier discussion in this chapter focused on the need for densitometric results to be independent of the angiographic view if the technique is to be considered to work well. Five investigators responded to questions on this topic—namely, Collins, Kirkeeide, Marchand, Nichols, and Vogel. Johnson, Collins, and associates found a correlation coefficient of 0.94 between the cross-sectional area data from right anterior oblique and left anterior oblique views; the relationship between the data could be described by the following equation:[J1, J2]

$$y = 1.04x + 0.002$$

Kirkeeide responded that the view selection is critical. In his experiences, the results are highly variable depending on whether other vessels become superimposed on the vessel of interest. This finding has been confirmed by other investigators. Marchand found an unlikely high accuracy and precision in percent area stenosis of 2 and 1 percent, respectively. In Nichols's study, the precision in the absolute area measurement was 0.11 mm^2 (SEE) with a correlation coefficient equal to 0.98, while Vogel found a precision in percent area stenosis of 13.3 percent. Finally, a correlation coefficient of 0.79 (SEE = 14.3) was obtained in the evaluation studies of Tobis and colleagues.[T3]

VARIABILITY IN REPEATED CORONARY CINEANGIOGRAPHY AND COMPUTER ANALYSIS

This section describes in more detail the results from our validation studies of the analysis procedure itself, and of both the angiographic acquisition and the computer analysis procedures.[R16]

Variability in Data Analysis

The variability of repeated analysis of cineangiograms was assessed from a total of 13 end-diastolic cine frames of 13 routinely performed coronary angiographic studies. These cine frames were analyzed twice by one technical analyst with a median time interval of 28 days. In each cine frame, one coronary obstruction was analyzed as well as several coronary segments showing no focal obstruction. As a result, a total of 13 coronary obstructions and 25 nonobstructed segments were analyzed twice. The mean difference and standard deviations of the repeated measurements,

Table 13–16. VARIABILITY IN MEASUREMENTS OF VARIOUS PARAMETERS OF CORONARY ARTERIAL SEGMENTS FROM REPEATED ANALYSIS OF 13 CINE FRAMES*

	Overall Mean Value	Mean Difference	*p* Value	Standard Deviation Difference
Calibration factor (mm/pixel)	0.096	0.0003	n.s.	0.002
User-defined reference (N = 13)				
Obstruction diameter (mm)	1.52	0.00	n.s.	0.10
Reference diameter (mm)	2.97	0.005	n.s.	0.12
Percent diameter stenosis (%)	48.40	0.23	n.s.	2.74
Extent (mm)	8.42	−0.38	n.s.	1.89
Interpolated reference (N = 13)				
Reference diameter (mm)	2.87	−0.10	<0.004	0.10
Percent diameter stenosis (%)	47.90	−2.08	n.s.	3.94
Nonobstructed segments (N = 25)				
Mean diameter (mm)	2.42	0.07	<0.005	0.11
Length segment (mm)	17.72	0.02	n.s.	0.97

*A total of 13 coronary obstructions and 25 nonobstructed coronary segments were analyzed twice.

n.s.—nonsignificant

(From Reiber, J. H. C., et al.: Quantitative Coronary and Left Ventricular Cineangiography: Methodology and Clinical Applications. Martinus Nijhoff, Boston, 1986, with permission.)

as well as the overall mean values of the parameters, are presented in Table 13–16. These data show that with the exception of the interpolated reference diameter measurement and the mean diameter of nonobstructed segments, no significant differences were found between the repeated measurements. The standard deviation of absolute measurements was less than 0.12 mm. The variabilities in the percent diameter stenosis measurements for the user-defined and interpolated procedures were 2.74 and 3.94 percent, respectively.

Overall Variability

Knowledge of overall variabilities of repeated coronary cineangiography and computer analysis is necessary to determine whether an observed change in the dimensions of a coronary arterial segment after an intervention is statistically significant. In this context, various situations must be distinguished. First, the effect of a selective injection of contrast medium on arterial dimensions must be studied under identical x-ray system settings (short-term variability). Second, one must determine the variability in arterial dimensions during one particular catheterization session that involves a relatively long time—for example, 1 hour—between contrast injections; during this period, other observations may be made (medium-term variability). Third, one must determine the worst-case changes in arterial dimensions between long-term observations—for example, over a period of several months (long-term variability).

Material to study the short-, medium-, and long-term variabilities in the acquisition and analysis of coronary cineangiograms was obtained from three interventional studies. The patient material is later described in more detail. For all studies, cine frames to be analyzed were selected at end-diastole when possible. In cases of overlap of a particular segment to be analyzed with other vessels, a different frame was selected near end-diastole. The user-determined beginning and end points of the major coronary segments were standardized according to definitions by the American Heart Association.[A8] The results from the various studies were analyzed for significant differences using Student's t-test for paired values (border of significance: $p = 0.01$).

Short-Term (5-Minute) Variability

The short-term variability was defined by the variability in measured arterial dimensions from repeated acquisition and analysis of coronary cineangiographic studies. These studies were performed 5 minutes apart with unchanged geometry of the x-ray system. Data were collected from 12 patients catheterized for suspected coronary artery disease. Two patients had normal coronary arteries, one patient had single-vessel disease, six patients had two obstructed vessels, and three patients had three obstructed vessels.

A total of 36 coronary segments were selected for quantitative angiographic analysis: eight were stenotic, and 28 were normal. The various parameters of the obstructions were measured for the eight stenotic segments, and the mean diameters of seven pre-stenotic and of four post-stenotic portions were determined, resulting in a total of 39 measurements for the mean diameters of nonobstructed portions of the coronary arterial system. Two baseline coronary angiograms (C_1 and C_2) were performed, 5 minutes apart. The second control angiogram (C_2) was carried out to study the effect of the contrast agent itself on the arteries. The patient's position was kept unchanged in relation to the x-ray equipment during both angiograms. All arteriograms were obtained via the Sones technique and were recorded on Kodak 35-mm cine film at the rate of 50 frames/sec. An ionic contrast medium, Urografin-76, was injected with a Medrad injector at a flow rate of 3 ml/sec. Peak systolic pressure remained constant during both control cineangiograms. Because the views were unchanged during the repeat angiographic studies, calibration was performed only for the first set of angiograms.

The data on the short-term (5-minute) variability as assessed from the two control cineangiograms (C_1 and C_2) are presented in Table 13–17. For the obstruction diameters, a small, nonsignificant increase of 0.05 mm (3.01 percent) was found between the repeat angiographic studies; the standard deviation of the differences was 0.34 mm. As a result of the contrast injection, four obstructions showed a decrease in the minimal obstruction diameter, and the four other obstructions showed an increase. The user-defined reference diameters, all taken at a point proximal to the obstructions, showed an average nonsignificant decrease of 0.1 mm with a standard deviation of 0.17 mm. On the average, the severity of the stenoses expressed in terms of user-defined percent diameter narrowing decreased by 2.46 percent with a standard deviation of 8.01 percent; in three of the cases, the percent diameter narrowing increased, and in the other five cases, it decreased. The variabilities in the reference diameter (0.21 mm) and percent diameter stenosis (8.30 percent) for the interpolated technique were slightly higher than for the user-defined technique; the mean differences in these parameters were also nonsignificant.

For the total of 39 nonobstructed segments, a small, nonsignificant decrease in mean diameter of 0.005 mm (0.18 percent) was found with a standard deviation of 0.16 mm; the average length of the segments was 11.37 mm. Seventeen segments showed an increase in the mean diameter, and the other 22 segments showed a decrease.

These data show that the short-term variability in the obstruction diameter (with a standard deviation of 0.34 mm) is about twice the variability of measurements at nonobstructed portions of the segments, for which the standard deviation of the reference diameter is 0.17 mm and that of the mean diameter is 0.16 mm. These last two variability measures are about 50 percent higher than the values obtained from repeated analysis of cine films alone (see Table 13–16).

Table 13–17. SHORT-TERM VARIABILITY IN MEASUREMENTS OF VARIOUS PARAMETERS OF CORONARY ARTERIAL SEGMENTS FOR TWO CONTROL CINEANGIOGRAMS (C_1 AND C_2)

	Overall Mean Value	Mean Difference	p Value	Standard Deviation Difference
User-defined reference (N = 8)				
Obstruction diameter (mm)	1.66	+0.05	n.s.	0.34
Reference diameter (mm)	3.33	−0.10	n.s.	0.17
Percent diameter stenosis (%)	46.50	−2.46	n.s.	8.01
Extent (mm)	6.60	+0.50	n.s.	1.31
Interpolated reference (N = 8)				
Reference diameter (mm)	3.17	+0.02	n.s.	0.21
Percent diameter stenosis (%)	44.90	−0.90	n.s.	8.30
Nonobstructed segments (N = 39)				
Mean diameter (mm)	2.82	−0.005	n.s.	0.16
Length segment (mm)	11.37	−0.33	n.s.	1.36

Difference values are computed as $C_2 - C_1$.
n.s.—nonsignificant
(From Reiber, J. H. C., et al.: Quantitative Coronary and Left Ventricular Cineangiography: Methodology and Clinical Applications. Martinus Nijhoff, Boston, 1986, with permission.)

Medium-Term (1-Hour) Variability

As part of a pharmacologic interventional study, we have assessed the 1-hour variability in the measurements of coronary arterial segments with repeated coronary angiography and analysis. Eleven patients were studied according to the following protocol. Initially, coronary angiography was performed in the control state (angio$_1$). The geometry of the x-ray gantry and the kilovolt and milliampere values of the x-ray generator were acquired on-line with each angiographic procedure.[B15] Immediately thereafter, the first metabolite of Molsidomine* (Sin1) was administered in the left main stem. Two minutes later, coronary angiography was performed in the same multiple views to study the immediate effect of the drug on the dimensions of the coronary arteries (angio$_2$).[S49] One hour later, these angiographic studies were repeated to assess the long-lasting effect of the drug (angio$_3$). A fourth angiographic procedure (angio$_4$) was carried out following a second intracoronary administration of the drug to assess whether further dilatation could be achieved by a second administration. Because other observations were performed during the 1-hour period, the x-ray system had to be repositioned

*Cassella, Frankfurt am Main, Germany.

in a projection corresponding as much as possible to the projection used during the first two angiographic studies. For such purposes, the angular settings of the x-ray gantry and the various height levels were readjusted according to the values recorded with the on-line registration system.

All arteriograms were obtained via the Judkins technique and were recorded on Kodak 35-mm cine film at a rate of 25 frames/sec. For this study, a nonionic contrast medium, Omnipaque,* was injected manually. By comparing the arterial dimensions from angio$_2$ and angio$_4$, we can assess the medium-term variability when standardization of the angiographic procedure is attempted (including "control" of the vasomotor tone). Each analyzed cine frame was separately calibrated on the basis of the displayed contrast catheter. Correction was made for pincushion distortion. A total of 16 coronary obstructions, as well as 90 nonobstructed segments, were analyzed.

The overall mean values and the variabilities in the x-ray gantry settings are presented in Table 13–18. The angular variability computed from the absolute differences of angular settings was less than 4.2 degrees. The variability in the various positions of image intensifier and x-ray source was less than 3.0 cm. No significant differences existed between the repeated x-ray system settings. These results show that the x-ray system settings can be reproduced quite accurately in routine clinical practice.

The mean differences in the measured parameters from angio$_2$ and angio$_4$ were all nonsignificant (Table 13–19). The overall mean values were computed from angio$_2$. The medium-term variabilities in the obstruction diameters are 35 percent lower than the short-term variabilities, and the variabilities in mean diameter and user-defined reference diameter increased by 50 percent and 65 percent, respectively. The medium-term variability in the interpolated reference diameter decreased by 29 percent from the short-term (5-minute) variability.

Long-Term (90-Day) Variability

Of 153 patients planned for percutaneous transluminal coronary angioplasty (PTCA), a subgroup of 26 PTCA candidates was selected. Candidates had had two good-quality cineangiograms performed in several standard views and were therefore suitable for paired analysis of the stenotic lesions.[W19] The first film was the diagnostic angiogram; the second measurements were obtained from the PTCA film, immediately prior to the actual PTCA procedure. At the time of the angiographic investigations, no attempt was made to standardize the inspiratory level, volume

*Nyegaard, Oslo, Norway.

Table 13–18. VARIABILITY IN X-RAY GANTRY SETTINGS WITH REPEATED CINEANGIOGRAPHIC STUDIES (N = 25 VIEWS)

	Overall Mean Value	Mean Difference	p Value	Standard Deviation Difference
Rotation U-arm (degrees)	31.2	0.3	n.s.	4.2
Rotation patient C-arm (degrees)	26.4	0.3	n.s.	2.2
Isocenter-image intensifier distance (IID) (cm)	22.6	1.1	n.s.	3.0
Focus-isocenter distance (FID) (cm)	72.8	−0.3	n.s.	0.8
Object-isocenter distance (OID) (cm)	5.3	0.2	n.s.	1.4

n.s.—nonsignificant

(From Reiber, J. H. C., et al.: Quantitative Coronary and Left Ventricular Cineangiography: Methodology and Clinical Applications. Martinus Nijhoff, Boston, 1986, with permission.)

Table 13–19. MEDIUM-TERM VARIABILITY IN MEASUREMENTS OF VARIOUS PARAMETERS OF CORONARY ARTERIAL SEGMENTS FROM REPEATED CORONARY ANGIOGRAPHIC STUDIES AND ANALYSIS

	Angio$_4$		Angio$_2$	
	Overall Mean	*Mean Difference*	*p Value*	*Standard Deviation Difference*
Calibration factor (N = 25; mm/pixel)	0.094	−0.001	n.s.	0.002
User-defined reference (N = 16)				
Obstruction diameter (mm)	2.13	0.00	n.s.	0.22
Reference diameter (mm)	3.57	0.06	n.s.	0.28
Percent diameter stenosis (%)	41.30	0.75	n.s.	8.09
Extent (mm)	6.28	−0.15	n.s.	2.03
Interpolated reference (N = 14)				
Reference diameter (mm)	3.32	0.05	n.s.	0.15
Percent diameter stenosis (%)	38.10	1.21	n.s.	7.23
Nonobstructed segments (N = 90)				
Mean diameter (mm)	3.05	0.07	n.s.	0.24
Length segment (mm)	14.03	−0.03	n.s.	1.02

The second and fourth angiograms (angio$_2$ and angio$_4$) were performed immediately after administration of a vasodilatory drug. Time between angio$_2$ and angio$_4$ was approximately 1 hour (see text).

n.s.—nonsignificant

(From Reiber, J. H. C., et al.: Quantitative Coronary and Left Ventricular Cineangiography: Methodology and Clinical Applications. Martinus Nijhoff, Boston, 1986, with permission.)

Table 13–20. LONG-TERM VARIABILITY IN MEASUREMENTS OF VARIOUS PARAMETERS OF CORONARY OBSTRUCTION

	Overall Mean	Mean Difference	p Value	Standard Deviation Difference
(N = 26)				
Obstruction diameter (mm)	1.25	0.00	n.s.	0.36
Extent (mm)	10.04	0.62	n.s.	4.34
Interpolated reference				
Reference diameter (mm)	3.72	−0.13	n.s.	0.66
Percent diameter stenosis (%)	66.19	−1.92	n.s.	6.52

n.s.—nonsignificant

(From Reiber, J. H. C., et al.: Quantitative Coronary and Left Ventricular Cineangiography: Methodology and Clinical Applications. Martinus Nijhoff, Boston, 1986, with permission.)

Table 13–21. MEAN DIFFERENCES AND STANDARD DEVIATIONS (MEAN ± SD) OF MEASUREMENTS IN FRAMES PRECEDING AND FOLLOWING FRAME 0 AND MEASUREMENTS OBTAINED IN FRAME 0*

	Preceding Optimal Frame			Following Optimal Frame			Preceding or Followed by
Measurement	−3	−2	−1	+1	+2	+3	±1c†
Obstruction diameter (mm)	−0.02 ± 0.24	0.02 ± 0.20	0.02 ± 0.22	0.006 ± 0.20	0.02 ± 0.19	0.009 ± 0.22	−0.05 ± 0.21
Reference diameter (mm)	0.03 ± 0.13	−0.007 ± 0.15	0.02 ± 0.09	0.02 ± 0.12	−0.03 ± 0.11	0.003 ± 0.13	−0.08 ± 0.18
Percent diameter stenosis (%)	1.07 ± 7.27	−0.71 ± 5.98	−0.20 ± 6.46	−0.07 ± 6.45	−1.14 ± 6.29	−0.12 ± 6.79	0.11 ± 7.11
Extent (mm)	−0.12 ± 0.58	0.06 ± 0.54	0.05 ± 0.40	0.13 ± 0.47	0.14 ± 0.50	0.20 ± 0.50	−0.10 ± 0.45
Area plaque (mm^2)	0.21 ± 2.17	0.09 ± 1.76	0.32 ± 1.77	0.34 ± 1.94	0.13 ± 1.53	0.43 ± 2.30	−0.70 ± 1.75

*All differences were not significant; border of significance at $p = 0.01$.
†Cardiac cycle.
(From Reiber, J. H. C., et al.: How critical is the frame selection in quantitative coronary angiographic studies? Eur. Heart J. 10:54, 1989, with permission.)

and rate of injection of the contrast agent, or the technical characteristics of the x-ray system. More important, the vasomotor tone in both conditions was unknown and neglected. These data therefore represent the worst case in terms of changes in arterial dimensions between long-term observations. The median delay between the diagnostic and the PTCA angiogram in these patients was 90 days (ranging from 1 to 250 days). The median percent diameter stenosis of the obstructions for this group as assessed from the diagnostic angiogram was 66.2 percent (ranging from 53 to 83 percent).

No significant differences were observed in the mean values of the obstruction and reference diameters, or in the mean values of percent diameter stenosis (Table 13–20). This finding suggests that no detectable progression or regression of atherosclerotic lesions had occurred over the period of 90 days. These paired data provide some insight into the total variability of the cineangiographic procedure and the computer analysis under worst-case circumstances, given that no special care had been taken to reduce the potential sources of variability (x-ray system settings, vasomotor tone, and so forth).

Under these uncontrolled conditions, the variations in absolute measurements were 0.36 mm for the obstruction diameter, 0.66 mm for the interpolated reference diameter, and 6.5 percent for the interpolated percent diameter stenosis.

IMPORTANCE OF FRAME SELECTION IN QUANTITATIVE CORONARY ANGIOGRAPHY

Usually, in quantitative coronary angiographic studies, an end-diastolic cine frame is selected for the quantitative analysis of a coronary obstruction. If the obstruction is not optimally visible in that particular frame, however—for example, because of overlap with another vessel—a neighboring frame in the sequence may be selected. Also, an aortic pressure signal or electrocardiographic marker on the cine film may not be available for the optimal selection of the end-diastolic frame; as a result, the visually selected cine frame may not be the true end-diastolic frame.

In addition, different cardiologists may select different (although usually neighboring) frames, even when the same selection criteria are followed. Another possibility is that the frames would be selected from different cardiac cycles, in relation to the moment of contrast injection. This uncertainty in the frame selection process raises the question of how the selection of a cine frame at another time in the cardiac cycle may affect the quantitative results. Uncertainty in the frame selection also occurs when corresponding frames in pre- and post-intervention angiographic studies, such as prior to and following administration of a vasoactive drug, must be selected. Motivated by these uncertainties, we planned a study to determine the variability in measurement of the obstructive arterial dimensions when different frames are proposed for the quantitative analysis in the end-diastolic phase of the cardiac cycle.[R18, R19]

Of a total of 38 consecutive patient films obtained at 25 frames/sec, with the frame 0 demonstrating the severity of a lesion optimally as judged by a senior cardiologist, selection consisted of the three preceding frames, the three following frames, and one frame exactly one cycle prior to or following frame 0. Frame 0 was always chosen in the end-diastolic phase of the cardiac cycle. In each film, one coronary arterial segment with a focal lesion was analyzed quantitatively in this total of eight frames with the Cardiovascular Angiography Analysis System (CAAS).

The calibration for this series of eight measurements per patient film was performed only once, because the geometry of the x-ray system with respect to the patient remained unchanged.

The variabilities in the measurements assessed from the frames other than frame 0 were defined by the standard deviations (s.d.) of the differences between these measurements and those from frame 0. Student's t-test for paired values was applied to determine the statistical significance of average differences between the measurements (border of significance: $p = 0.01$).

Results

We compared the minimal obstruction diameter, interpolated reference diameter, interpolated percent diameter stenosis, extent of the obstruction, and area of atherosclerotic plaque in a particular view. The results are presented in Table 13–21.

No consistent pattern could be found for a particular frame; none produced smaller values in terms of mean difference or standard deviation than any other frame. Also, reproducibility in analyzing a coronary obstruction one complete cardiac cycle earlier or later than the originally selected cine frame seemed to be as good as with a neighboring frame of frame 0.

Therefore, one may conclude that the selection of a cine frame for quantitative analysis in the end-diastolic phase of the cardiac cycle is not critical. One may argue that the quality of mixing of the contrast agent in the arterial segment is a major source of the observed variations; filling artifacts were potentially present in each of the selected frames.[R18] Therefore, we propose to define for each quantitative parameter a measure of variability arising

Table 13–22. VARIABILITY IN ASSESSMENT OF CORONARY OBSTRUCTION PARAMETERS DUE TO THE FRAME SELECTION PROCESS*

Obstruction diameter (mm)	0.24
Reference diameter (mm)	0.18
Percent diameter stenosis (%)	7.27
Extent obstruction (mm)	0.58
Plaque area (mm^2)	2.30

*The value presented for a particular parameter equals the maximal value of the seven standard deviations for that parameter from Table 13–21.
(From Reiber, J. H. C., et al.: How critical is the frame selection in quantitative coronary angiographic studies? Eur. Heart J. 10:54, 1989, with permission.)

Table 13–23. MINIMAL THRESHOLD VALUES FOR THE OCCURRENCE OF VASOMOTOR CHANGES AT THE INDIVIDUAL PATIENT LEVEL (95 PERCENT CONFIDENCE LEVEL)

Obstruction diameter (mm)	0.47
Reference diameter (mm)	0.35
Percent diameter stenosis (%)	14.25
Extent obstruction (mm)	1.14
Plaque area (mm^2)	4.51

(From Reiber, J. H. C., et al.: How critical is the frame selection in quantitative coronary angiographic studies? Eur. Heart J. 10:54, 1989, with permission.)

from the frame selection process, which is equal to the maximal value of the seven standard deviation values from Table 13–21 (Table 13–22).

For practical purposes, minimal threshold values for the changes in the obstruction parameters based on 95 percent confidence levels can be calculated at the individual patient level (Table 13–23), and at the group level, for the exclusion or inclusion of possible changes in coronary vasomotor tone.[R19]

SUMMARY

The data in this section clearly demonstrate that the validation data of most systems are still incomplete and that the individual results are described in different terms, so that comparison of the data is difficult if not impossible. A consensus must be found regarding which validation studies to perform, and particularly which parameters to use for description of the results. An ideal evaluation would require that certain phantoms and sets of films and digital data would be distributed to the investigators so that all validation studies could be performed on the same image data.

From the Tables 13–17, 13–19, and 13–20, the mean differences and standard deviations of the differences in the obstruction and interpolated reference diameters, as well as in the interpolated percent diameter stenosis, have been summarized in Table 13–24 for the short-, medium-, and long-term studies. One may conclude from all studies that the mean differences in absolute diameters are below 0.13 mm. The variabilities in the obstruction diameters for these three types of studies vary from 0.22 mm for the medium-term study to 0.36 mm for the least-controlled, long-term study. Likewise, the variabilities in the interpolated reference diameter are the smallest for the medium-term study (0.15 mm) and the largest for the long-term study (0.66 mm). The long-term study clearly demonstrates that the variabilities in absolute dimensions increase if no special care is taken to reduce their potential sources. Possible reasons the variabilities from the medium-term study are smaller than those from the short-term study are (1) controlled vasomotor tone and (2) the use of a nonionic versus ionic contrast medium.

Bentley and Henry, investigating the effect of Renografin-76 (1689 mosm/L) on animal arteries, demonstrated that the angiographic dye in concentrations not exceeding those during angiography has potent, dose-, and time-dependent vasomotor effects.[B16] In addition, in vivo experiments have shown that intracoronary injection of ionic, hyperosmolar, and hyperviscous contrast media produces direct myocardial depression, followed by a reflex effect, adrenergically mediated, which could potentially effect the vasomotor tone of the arteries.[H7] Bentley and associates have demonstrated that these deleterious effects can be prevented by the use of nonionic, iso-osmotic angiographic dye[B29] (such as Omnipaque), and that they may therefore account for the observed decrease in variability measures. This hypothesis has been confirmed by Jost and colleagues.[J3]

The variabilities in the interpolated percent diameter reduction are all of the same order of magnitude, ranging from 8.30 percent for the short-term study to 6.52 percent for the long-term study. Therefore, an upper limit of 8.30 percent for the variability in interpolated percent diameter stenosis from repeated angiography and analysis can be defined. The mean differences are less than 1.92 percent.

The data from Table 13–24 also make clear that the variabilities in the obstruction diameters with repeated angiography and analysis are 2.2 to 3.6 times greater than those from repeated analysis alone, and 1.5 to 6.6 times greater for the interpolated reference diameters. This finding is due to the various sources of variation in the data acquisition procedure described earlier. Alderman and colleagues found a threefold increase in variabilities in absolute sizes for a medium-term study compared with repeated analysis alone.[A4] We found an increase factor of 1.5 to 2.2. In the study by Alderman and colleagues, identical calibration factors, computed from the geometry of image intensifier and x-ray source, were used for the initial and repeat angiography. Thus, their actual variations in arterial size would be greater than those reported if the calibration factor was also assessed repeatedly from the catheter, as was done in our study.

Our data lead to the conclusion that the biologic variations are a source of major concern and that further attempts toward standardization of the angiographic procedure are seriously needed.

In summarizing the results of this study in terms of the sensitivity of the frame selection process in the quantitative measurements, one may conclude that the selection of a cine frame for quantitative analysis in the end-diastolic phase of the cardiac cycle is not critical. The measurements are not statistically significantly different if the selected frames in the same cineangiographic film sequence are out of phase by a maximum of three frames at a film speed of 25 frames/sec, or if a frame is selected exactly one cardiac cycle earlier or later. Most probably, the differences in the quality of the blood–contrast medium mixture are a major source of variation and are potentially present in each of the selected frames. Other possible error sources in the data acquisition procedure, such as changes in size and shape of the arterial segments and the pulsatile effect,[H8] probably contribute to the variation.

Therefore, the results from this study may reassure those involved in quantitative coronary angiographic studies. They show that when certain, not extremely demanding, precautions are followed, reliable quantitative data about coronary morphology can be obtained from cine film.

Table 13–24. SUMMARY OF THE MEAN AND STANDARD DEVIATIONS OF THE DIFFERENCES IN THE ABSOLUTE DIAMETER MEASUREMENTS AND IN INTERPOLATED PERCENT DIAMETER STENOSIS FOR THE SHORT-, MEDIUM-, AND LONG-TERM STUDIES

	Mean Difference			S.D. Difference		
	Short-Term Study	*Medium-Term Study*	*Long-Term Study*	*Short-Term Study*	*Medium-Term Study*	*Long-Term Study*
Obstruction diameter (mm)	0.05	0.00	0.00	0.34	0.22	0.36
Interpolated reference diameter (mm)	0.02	0.05	−0.13	0.21	0.15	0.66
Interpolated percent diameter stenosis (%)	−0.90	1.21	−1.92	8.30	7.23	6.52

(From Reiber, J. H. C., et al.: Quantitative Coronary and Left Ventricular Cineangiography: Methodology and Clinical Applications. Martinus Nijhoff, Boston, 1986, with permission.)

Coronary Flow Reserve

The concept of coronary flow reserve (CFR) as a functional measure of stenosis severity was initially proposed by Gould and colleagues.[G5, G6] Traditionally, CFR has been measured by the determination of coronary reactive hyperemia, which is defined as the increase in blood flow produced following temporary coronary occlusion. In the past, such determination was possible only by operative coronary exposure and therefore was not suitable for human application except during cardiac surgery. Today, the same principle can be applied by balloon occlusion during PTCA.[S42, Z11] In the meantime, however, other practical solutions for evaluating coronary reserve that do not require temporary vessel occlusion have been sought. Basically, two methodologic approaches have been developed to assess the CFR of individual coronary arteries in the clinical setting; as a result, the definition of CFR is method-dependent.

The first approach defines CFR as the ratio of maximal to resting coronary blood flow. Temporary occlusion of a coronary artery or potent pharmacologic coronary vasodilation produces maximal coronary hyperemia, which results in a hyperemic response. This response is characterized by a marked increase in flow that gradually subsides.[M4] Figure 13–21*A* is a schematic representation of this approach in a format proposed by Hoffman[H9] and Klocke.[K14] The actual flow measurements can be obtained following different techniques, which are described in more detail in the next section.

The second approach uses quantitative coronary angiography to determine the pressure-flow characteristics of coronary stenoses (see Fig. 13–4).[G13] Young and colleagues developed fluid dynamic equations that describe the relationship between the pressure distal to a stenosis and the flow.[Y1–Y3, Y5] When coronary flow increases, the coronary perfusion pressure distal to the stenosis decreases in a nonlinear fashion, according to the following equation:

$$P_c = P_{ao} - fQ - sQ^2$$

where P_c is the pressure distal to the stenosis, P_{ao} is the aortic pressure, f is the coefficient of viscous friction, s is the coefficient of exit separation, and Q is the flow. Viscous friction mainly depends on the absolute cross-sectional area of the artery at the site of the stenosis and on the length of the stenotic lesion. Exit separation mainly depends on the cross-sectional area at the site of obstruction and on the normal area distal to the stenosis.

Using the relationship between coronary perfusion pressure and coronary flow under conditions of maximal coronary vasodilation as described by Bache and Schwartz,[B21] and assuming a resting coronary blood velocity of 15 cm/sec, Kirkeeide and co-workers calculated a coronary flow reserve from the quantitative angiographic data.[G1, K8] This x-ray–predicted flow reserve is schematically shown in Figure 13–21*B*; more recently, Kirkeeide and co-workers have decided to use the term stenosis flow reserve (SFR) for this geometrically derived flow reserve parameter.[K26] The relationship between pressure and flow during maximal coronary vasodilation is represented by the dashed line. The dotted line represents the relationship between distal coronary pressure and coronary blood flow. The intersection of these curves is the SFR according to Kirkeeide and co-workers. The major advantage of this approach is that it integrates multiple angiographically defined anatomic characteristics of a coronary stenosis into a single parameter. The effect of a coronary stenosis on blood flow, however, is a response of an anatomic hemodynamic system of which the stenosis is only one component.[K8] Therefore, several important factors that may interfere with the CFR, such as the prevailing perfusion pressure, hypertrophy, collaterals, or previous myocardial infarction, are not taken into consideration.

Several important complexities of both approaches to assessing CFR should be considered; some of these are illustrated in Figure 13–21*C*.[H9, K14] At a constant level of myocardial metabolic demand, constancy of coronary flow is maintained over a wide range of coronary pressures. This phenomenon is called autoregulation. In this example, when maximal coronary vasodilation is induced by temporary occlusion of the artery or by pharmocologic means, coronary blood flow rises about threefold. Aside from the presence of the coronary stenosis, however, several other variables influence this ratio of resting and hyperemic coronary flow. These

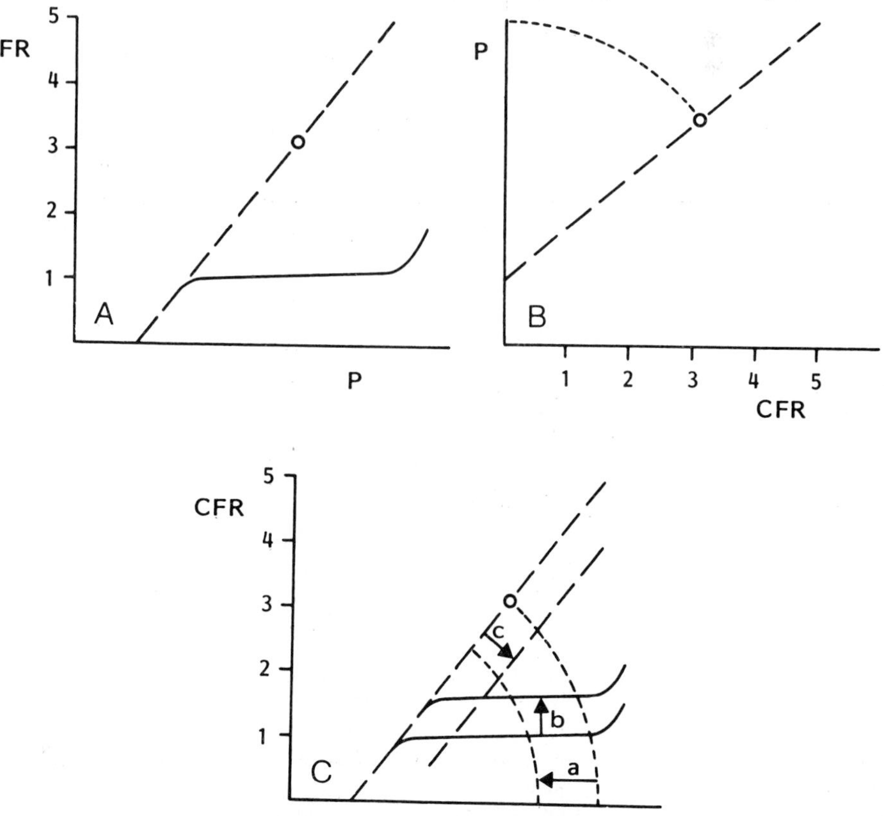

Figure 13–21. *A*, Schematic representation of the approach using the measurement of the ratio of maximal to resting coronary blood flow as a measure of coronary flow reserve (CFR) in a format used by Hoffman[H9] and Klocke.[K14] At a constant level of metabolic demand, coronary flow is maintained constant over a wide range of coronary perfusion pressure (P). This process is called autoregulation (*solid line*). The *open circle* represents a CFR of 3. *B*, The theory of the x-ray–predicted CFR as developed by Gould, Kirkeeide, and associates[G1,K8] is shown schematically. The *curved dashed line* represents the calculated distal coronary perfusion pressure as a function of coronary blood flow. The *straight dashed line* describes the relationship between coronary blood flow and perfusion pressure during maximal coronary vasodilation. The *open circle* represents a CFR of 3. *C*, Both approaches are combined to show the complexities of the concept of CFR. The *open circle* represents a CFR of 3, but small changes in perfusion pressure (a), an increase in resting blood flow (b), or an altered pressure-flow relationship during maximal vasodilation (c) can each result in a substantially lower CFR.

variables can be considered in terms of their effects on coronary pressure, resting coronary blood flow level, and the pressure-flow relationship during maximal coronary vasodilation.

Coronary blood flow during maximal vasodilation is linearly related to coronary perfusion pressure.[D6] Therefore, small changes in pressure result in significant changes in flow (a in Fig. 13–21*C*) even in a normal coronary artery. Likewise, small dynamic changes in stenosis geometry that result in changes in distal coronary perfusion pressure can change CFR substantially.[Z4] In the heart, increases in the metabolic rate are met by an increase in blood flow, rather than by an increase in metabolic substrate and oxygen extraction.[E4] An increase in resting flow (b in Fig. 13–21*C*) results in a decrease of the measured flow reserve. The pressure-flow relationship during maximal vasodilation varies substantially, owing to changes in hemodynamic variables. For instance, left ventricular hypertrophy shifts this relationship to the right (c in Fig. 13–21*C*). Several other variables are also important in this regard; these include heart rate, contractility, blood viscosity, and left ventricular end-diastolic pressure.[K14]

In the next section, the currently available techniques for measurement of coronary blood flow and flow reserve are discussed in more detail. Despite potential sources of uncertainty, the radiographic technique for the assessment of coronary flow in the manner proposed by Vogel and colleagues has advantages that have made it popular; this technique is described in detail in the later section "Radiographic Techniques." The relationships between coronary anatomy and flow reserve are discussed in the section "Relationship Between Coronary Artery Dimensions and Coronary Flow Reserve." The various variabilities of this angiographic approach are then presented in the section "Variability in Coronary Flow Reserve Measurements." The application of CFR measurements in the setting of PTCA is presented in that section and in the section "Coronary Flow Reserve and Percutaneous Transluminal Coronary Angioplasty." Comparative data of the angiographic approach and of the Doppler catheter are given in the subsequent section. Finally, recent developments in myocardial contrast echocardiography to determine CFR are described, and a summary concludes this discussion of CFR.

BASIC PRINCIPLES FOR MEASUREMENT OF CORONARY BLOOD FLOW AND FLOW RESERVE

Direct measurement by electromagnetic flowmeter and radionuclide particle distribution can be made only in experimental animals. With the exception of measurements made during open heart surgery, indirect approaches must be used to assess the severity of coronary obstructions in patients with coronary artery disease. At present, an ideal method for measuring coronary or myocardial blood flow in humans has not been found; each method has its own limitations.[M2, M15, W20] An ideal method would allow high spatial resolution, have a rapid frequency response (allowing it to detect phasic changes in flow), and be minimally invasive. To measure blood flow in *intact* animals and humans, the three classic principles (indicator-dilution, first-pass distribution, and inert-substance washout) have been adapted to the coronary circulation.[M2]

The indicator-dilution principle, introduced by Stewart in 1897 and developed by Hamilton in 1931, has been modified for the measurement of coronary blood flow during cardiac catheterization. Ganz and associates developed a thermodilution method for measuring coronary sinus flow.[G14] The basic principles of this technique are simple: A miscible fluid indicator (saline) with a known temperature lower than that of blood is infused into the coronary sinus or great cardiac vein. A thermistor mounted at a point at least 1.5 cm proximal to the infusion site records upstream the changes in the temperature of the fluid-blood mixture on the basis of which coronary blood flow can be calculated. Several conditions must be met, however, to obtain valid measurements. The infusion rate must be adequate, and sensitive thermistors and an insulated catheter system must be used. If multiple comparable measurements of flow must be acquired, a stable position of the catheter in the cardiac venous system is mandatory. Flow from the anterior left ventricular wall can be measured separately if the catheter is placed in the great cardiac vein.[G14, P6, S36] The main advantages of the technique are that it is simple, relatively inexpensive, and safe, and that it allows multiple measurements at short intervals with a frequency response sufficient to measure changes in flow occurring in 2 to 3 seconds.[G14] The major disadvantages of the technique are that a stable catheter position cannot always be obtained, and that small changes in catheter position induce large changes in measured flow and thus pose a difficulty in relating measured flow to a specific myocardial region.[B23] Therefore, the coronary sinus thermodilution technique is limited by crude spatial resolution and only modest temporal resolution.

Another application of this principle was recently developed by Vogel and colleagues.[V8–V10, V12] They measured absolute coronary blood flow with an angioplasty catheter or guidewire modified with microelectrodes on the basis of changes in electrical impedance that were induced by a 5 percent dextrose indicator bolus.

The principle of first-pass distribution was introduced by Sapirstein.[S37] When a diffusible indicator is infused into the arterial circulation, the concentration of the substance in an organ depends on the arterial concentration of the indicator, the organ extraction ratio of the indicator, and organ blood flow. Thallium-201 (^{201}Tl) scintigraphy is a widely used clinical application of this principle.[A6, G15, G16, J5] Relative coronary blood flow can be assessed following the same basic principles with tracers labeled with positron emitters such as rubidium-82 (^{82}Rb) or nitrogen-13 (^{13}N) ammonia.[B4, G4, K1, M2, S5, S38, W10] In particular, use of ^{82}Rb has increased, because it can be produced by a generator, which thus eliminates the need for an on-line cyclotron. This promising technique permits accurate and repeated measurement of transmural differences in myocardial perfusion in awake humans.[G20, M15, W11] The technique is expensive, however, and the resolution is limited to about 1 cm^2.[M2] In addition, both ^{82}Rb and ^{13}N ammonia have limitations: their extraction increases as the flow is augmented, and myocardial uptake depends on both metabolism and perfusion.

The method of inert-substance washout was developed by Kety and Schmidt for measuring cerebral blood flow.[K15] Two general categories of inert gas clearance techniques are in common use today for the measurement of myocardial blood flow: radioactive and nonradioactive tracers. The radioactive tracer currently used to measure myocardial perfusion in patients is xenon-133 (^{133}Xe). Nonradioactive tracers include nitrous oxide, helium, hydrogen, and argon.[E5] Major advantages of this technique are (1) that it can be used in humans to measure flow per gram of tissue in the left ventricle, and (2) that the technique is accurate over a wide range of flows. Several major disadvantages also exist, however, including poor spatial resolution, long measurement times, and the fact that the nonradioactive tracers are useful only under conditions in which coronary flow is known to be homogeneous. Because of this last limitation, regional localization of flow with nonradioactive gases is impossible.

The ^{133}Xe myocardial washout technique was introduced by Cannon and colleagues in 1977 and requires direct injection of the radioisotope into the coronary arteries;[C9, R22] as a result, it allows separation of flow through the right and left coronary circulations. In addition, flow values can be directly correlated to the anatomic findings obtained on coronary arteriography. Lesions with area obstructions greater than 75 percent[E6] and 80 percent[S44] have been found to cause reductions in coronary flow. A limitation of this technique is that maximum flow rates (greater than 200 ml/mg) cannot be determined accurately.

Grines and associates developed an application of this method for the measurement of absolute regional coronary blood flow.[G17] For this purpose, hydrogen-saturated saline is infused into a coronary artery. The hydrogen is detected during washout in the pulmonary artery by means of the voltage response of a platinum-tipped electrode, and volume flow is calculated according to the Kety-Schmidt method.[K15] This technique is potentially applicable during coronary angioplasty.[V9] The major disadvantages seem to be that subselective cannulation of the coronary arteries is necessary, and that greater than normal rates of volume flows are substantially underestimated.[G17]

Recently developed Doppler methods allow the assessment of coronary blood flow velocity or flow reserve, or both, for individual coronary arteries. The Doppler principle, described by Christian Johann Doppler in 1842, states that when sound waves are reflected from moving structures (such as moving red blood cells in the vascular tree), the frequencies of the reflected waves are shifted higher or lower;[D14] the frequency shifts are proportional to the velocities of the moving structures in relation to the transmitter. Ultrasonic flowmeters measure phasic and mean coronary blood flow velocity using this Doppler effect. To calculate an absolute velocity, one must know the precise angle between the crystal and the blood column. To convert measurements of flow velocity to volumetric flow, one must also know the cross-sectional area of the vessel and the velocity profile within the vessel. In most clinical situations, these considerations preclude the determination of absolute flow.

A piezoelectric crystal for the emission and detection of ultrasonic sound waves can be mounted in a suction cup and placed on epicardial coronary vessels during cardiac surgery.[M2, M4, W3, W12] Coronary flow reserve could be determined by transient (20-second) occlusion of the vessel, which would thus produce a reactive hyperemic response. A piezoelectric crystal can also be mounted on the tip of an angiography catheter,[W1] or on an angioplasty balloon catheter,[S39, S59, Z13] to assess coronary blood flow velocity and vasodilatory reserve during diagnostic or interventional catheterization (using an intracoronary Doppler catheter). The Iowa group claims that only side-mounted crystals produce consistently high-quality signals. The carefully validated studies with the Doppler catheter suggest that the maximal coronary blood flow of a normal coronary artery is four to six times the resting flow.[W1, W4, W13] Other advantages of the Doppler catheter are that it is an inexpensive device and that it is readily available from commercial sources. Currently, use of ultrasonic probes is the only available means of assessing phasic coronary blood flow velocity in the coronary arteries in awake humans.[Z13] As stated previously, the principal disadvantages of the technique are that absolute flow cannot be determined without knowledge of the angle between blood column and crystal and knowledge of the cross-sectional area of the coronary artery,[M2] and that the introduction of a Doppler catheter into a coronary artery entails risk.[W1] Also, diseased vessels with certain anatomic characteristics (e.g., extremely proximal obstructions or large branches prior to an obstruction) cannot be studied. Furthermore, only one vessel can be examined at a time, and the transmural distribution of perfusion cannot be assessed.

Other approaches, such as ultrafast computed tomography,[L15–L17, R2] contrast echocardiography,[A2] and magnetic resonance imaging,[P1] are being actively investigated for their potential ability to measure CFR. These three new approaches share one important characteristic, namely, that they can theoretically measure flow in different layers of the left ventricular wall. Many practical problems still need to be resolved, however. In a later section, a brief overview of myocardial contrast echocardiography as a means to determine coronary flow reserve is given (see "Assessment of Coronary Flow Reserve by Myocardial Contrast Echocardiography").

RADIOGRAPHIC TECHNIQUES

Selective coronary angiography is the standard means for obtaining anatomic information and is the physician's most important tool for making clinical decisions for patients with coronary artery disease. As a result, a radiologic technique that allows accurate measurements of CFR would be extremely welcome.

The injection of contrast medium into coronary arteries or bypass grafts induces an alteration of blood flow.[B26, B28, H13] The following phases can be distinguished: (1) Augmentation of the perfusion pressure in the vessel induced by the injection of contrast material causes an increase in the flow rate within the first second after injection. (2) The different hydromechanical properties (viscosity) of the contrast medium compared with those of blood cause a decrease in flow rate. (3) The pharmacologic effect of the contrast medium on the coronary vessels and the myocardium leads to a reactive hyperemia with an increase in flow. (4) The flow returns an average of 13 seconds after injection to the previous baseline level.[H10, S30] Therefore, measuring hyperemic responses in humans during cardiac catheterization requires a method for following rapid changes in coronary flow and for assessing its regional distribution.

Videodensitometry is a particularly promising approach to measuring flow velocities in human coronary arteries using differences in regional densities.[B27] At first, only mean flow velocities could be assessed by the measurement of the transit time of a bolus of contrast medium.[R23, R29, S45–S47] Further developments in this field have led to the determination of phasic flow pattern from electrocardiographically triggered contrast boluses,[F16] initially only in bypass grafts[H13, P11] and later in coronary arteries, also;[S30, S48] high film speeds of about 100 frames/sec are required.

The major limitations of these approaches are that they cannot be applied to branching or circuitous arterial segments, which are often present in the coronary arterial system of humans, and that multiple radiographic projections must be used if the arterial segment cannot be placed in a position parallel to the plane of the image intensifier. An indicator-dilution videodensitometric method was developed by Foerster and colleagues[F12] and recently validated by Nissen and associates.[N7] Subselective injection of contrast medium is necessary, however, and streaming or reflux of the contrast medium must be prevented.

The major drawback of all radiographic techniques is that contrast media cannot be used to measure coronary blood flow by the traditional methodologic approaches.[V4] An essential prerequisite of indicator-dilution (Stewart-Hamilton), inert-substance washout (Kety-Schmidt), or first-pass distribution (Sapirstein) techniques is that the indicator substance should not affect the flow being measured. Unfortunately, radiographic contrast media have substantial vascular effects,[B28] although nonionic and low-osmolality media may disturb blood flow less than ionic agents (see "Use of Nonionic and Iso-osmolar Contrast Media" in the previous main section of this chapter).[V4] Hodgson and associates studied the effects of a bolus injection of contrast medium on baseline and hyperemic coronary blood flow.[H10] They found that the ratio of baseline to hyperemic flow is approximately constant during the first 5 seconds after contrast injection. This effect is illustrated in Figure 13–22*A*.

Using electrocardiographically gated power injection of a contrast agent at a rate presumed to be sufficiently rapid to achieve its complete replacement of blood, Vogel and colleagues developed a mask-mode subtraction technique that allows determination of myocardial time-density curves before and during coronary vasodilation, before the vascular effects of the contrast medium disturb the ratio of resting to hyperemic coronary blood flow.[V3, V4] In these studies, the heart must be paced at a constant rate, just greater than the spontaneous heart rate. According to this radiographic technique, the "myocardial contrast appearance time" is measured. It is defined as the time from contrast injection to opacification of the myocardium. From these data and the peak opacification achieved in the myocardium, a contrast appearance time index is derived. Unlike the earlier transit-time approaches, this method of measuring the myocardial appearance time is used to calculate not total coronary blood flow, but rather coronary flow reserve, derived from flow changes measured in the basal state and following induction of coronary reactive hyperemia. This approach has been validated in the animal laboratory by Hodgson and associates[H4] and by Cusma and colleagues,[C2] and is illustrated in Figure 13–22*B*. If the injection rate is not adequate, an underestimation of flow ratio values results.[C2] Van der Werf and colleagues claim that the heart rate must be synchronized with the x-ray frequency ("apparent cardiac arrest") to obviate mismatching of the mask image and the subsequent contrast images.[W22] Under these conditions Pÿls and co-workers concluded that the mean transit time calculated by videodensitometry can be used to accurately assess changes in myocardial perfusion strictly according to the original principles of the indicator dilution technique.[P14]

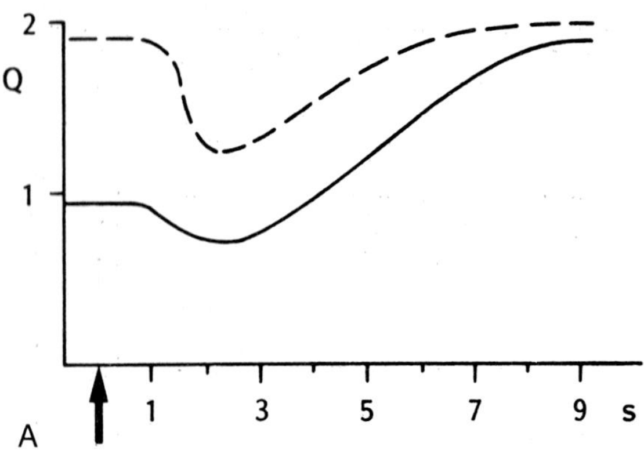

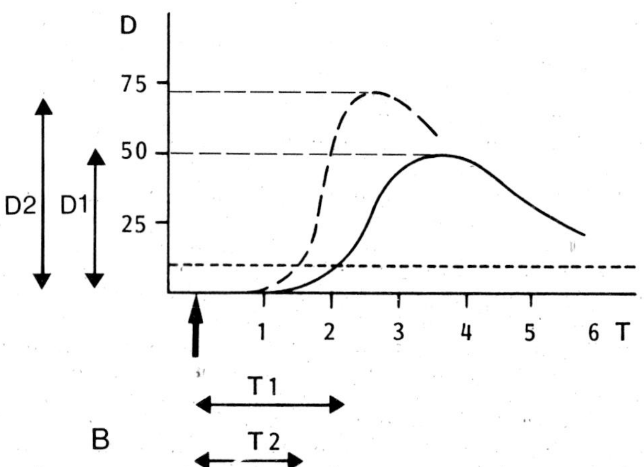

Figure 13–22. *A*, Sequence of events during seconds (s) following injection of radiographic contrast in a coronary artery during baseline (solid line) and already hyperemic (dashed line) coronary blood flow, as described by Hodgson and associates[H4] and by Cusma and colleagues.[C2] *Arrow* marks the timing of the contrast injections. Q—volume flow. *B*, In the myocardial region of interest, baseline (solid line) and hyperemic (dashed line) time-density curves can be generated with the use of digital subtraction of selected end-diastolic cineangiographic frames. After application of a fixed density threshold, a myocardial contrast appearance time *(T)* can be measured at baseline (T_1) and hyperemia (T_2). The maximal contrast density *(D)* is also measured at baseline (D_1) and hyperemia (D_2). Coronary flow reserve (CFR) can then be calculated according to the equation:

$$\text{CFR} = \frac{\text{Q (hyperemic)}}{\text{Q (baseline)}} = \frac{D_2}{T_2} \div \frac{D_1}{T_1}$$

The major advantage of the radiographic technique is that it can be performed during routine cardiac catheterization without increasing the risk to the patient.[B24, V4, Z5] Unfortunately, various definitions of the myocardial appearance time—including maximum density, time required to reach half of peak contrast, time of maximum change in contrast density,[V3] fixed threshold level at 5 percent of the density scale,[O1] mean-rise time,[B20] time of center of gravity[R20]—have been used, which impedes standardization of the technique.[B20] The relatively low temporal resolution can be improved by means of biharmonic Fourier fitting techniques[R20] or by linear interpolation of the contrast pass curves.[C2] In addition, Cusma and colleagues have proposed to generate and display a final parametric flow ratio image, defined by the ratio of the individual pixel values of the hyperemic and basal contrast medium appearance picture (CMAP) images.[C2] Although, at present, coronary flow reserve can only be assessed in a two-dimensional projection of the myocardium, developments toward three-dimensional reconstruction from biplane and multiplane angiographic views are in progress.[D7, D15, O2–O4]

An alternative approach to the assessment of coronary flow distribution and hyperemic flow reserve measurements is myocardial densitometry, which involves large regions of interest for summed density measurements of contrast agent in myocardial wall segments that are supplied by the branches of the main coronary artery.[B20] Calculation of coronary flow is based primarily on mass measurements of contrast medium. Enhancement of myocardial opacification, and the subsequent application of digital densitometry for one particular flow state, requires only simple mask-mode subtraction performed on a single image that is selected at the time of myocardial opacification prior to venous run-off. The image acquisition protocol requires a selective coronary injection with standardized flow rates that ensures retrograde contrast flow into the aorta. A practical advantage of this technique is that it is little affected by motion and superimposition artifacts.

Coronary flow reserve values assessed by the techniques just described, however, depend on several parameters, which should therefore be monitored during the acquisition procedure. For example, changes in preload and afterload that lead to different metabolic demands, as well as changes in the baseline perfusion pressure, may produce different values in a single patient.[S58]

To detect a limitation in coronary flow reserve due to an obstruction in a major epicardial coronary artery, one should obtain measurements when distal coronary resistance has been minimized; such minimization can be achieved by pharmacologic dilation of the arteriolar bed.[K2] A potent, short-acting vasodilator that induces a maximal hyperemic response is required. Wilson and White recently established the optimal dose of intracoronary papaverine needed to produce maximal coronary vasodilation; they found a maximal hyperemic response after administration of 8 mg in most coronary arteries and 12 mg in all coronary arteries.[W13] Zijlstra and associates found that an intracoronary dose of 10 mg of papaverine is ideally suited for investigation of CFR.[Z6] The maximal hyperemic response lasted from 24 to 37 seconds after the papaverine administration; moreover, no significant differences were found between two consecutive hyperemic responses ($r = 0.92$), which indicates excellent reproducibility. Because papaverine has a dilating effect on the major epicardial coronary arteries as well, maximal epicardial vasodilation should be obtained prior to the hyperemic investigation (e.g., by intracoronary administration of 3 mg of isorbide dinitrate).[G18, Z4] When this is not done, the CFR of a flow-limiting epicardial stenosis is overestimated by an average of 16 percent when papaverine is used to induce hyperemia. Although intracoronary adenosine is a potent and very short-acting vasodilator that could be used for studying CFR, it was found that side effects, including severe hypotension, and unpredictability of the dosage needed to produce maximal hyperemia limit its applicability.[Z7]

In our laboratory, we have implemented a technique for the quantitation of relative coronary blood flow from coronary *cine*-angiograms, based on the on-line approaches described by Vogel and associates;[H4, O1, R21, V3] this technique will be discussed in detail in the following section.

Angiographic Procedure and Induction of Maximal Hyperemic Response

The heart must be under atrial pacing at a constant rate just above the spontaneous heart rate. An electrocardiogram-triggered injection of contrast medium (Iopamidol at 37°C) into the coronary artery is done through a Medrad Mark IV infusion pump. This nonionic contrast agent has a viscosity of 9.4 cP at 37°C, an osmolality of 796 mosm/kg, and an iodium content of 370 mg/ml. For the left coronary artery, 7 to 10 ml is injected at a flow rate of 4 to 7 ml/sec; the coronary angiogram (film speed, 25 frames/sec) is obtained in a left anterior oblique projection. For the right coronary artery, 4 to 7 ml is injected at a flow rate of 3 to 5 ml/sec, and the angiogram is obtained in a left or right anterior oblique projection. The rate of injection of the contrast medium is judged to be adequate when backflow of contrast medium into the aorta occurs. The angiogram is repeated 30 seconds after a bolus injection of 12.5 mg of papaverine into the coronary artery.[W13]

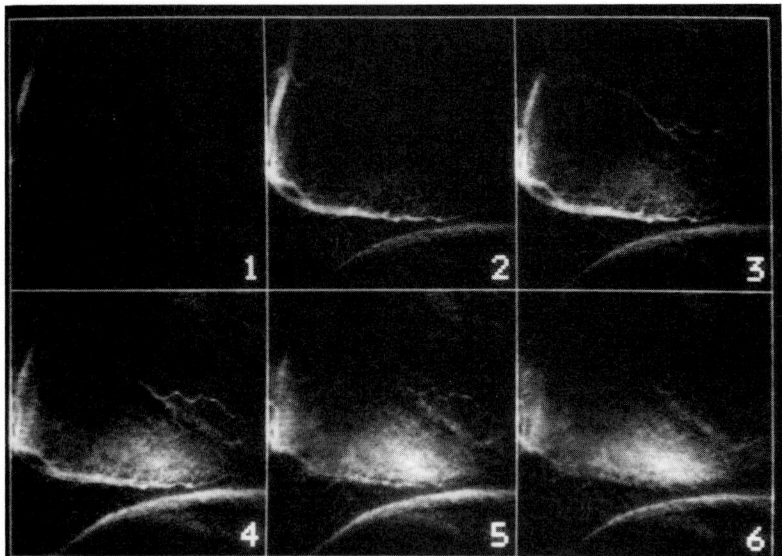

Figure 13–23. End-diastolic cineangiographic frames, digitized in 512 × 512 8-bit matrices from six consecutive heartbeats following contrast injection. Stationary background structures were eliminated by means of logarithmic mask-mode background subtraction, using the end-diastolic cineangiographic frame acquired prior to contrast administration as a mask.

Angiographic Image Processing and Coronary Flow Reserve Measurements

For the quantitation of relative coronary blood flow, 5 to 8 end-diastolic cineangiographic frames were selected from successive cardiac cycles (Fig. 13–23).[H4] Logarithmic nonmagnified mask-mode background subtraction was applied to the image subset to eliminate noncontrast medium densities (Fig. 13–24).[R21] The last end-diastolic frame prior to contrast administration was chosen as the mask. Each digitized image was also corrected for the dark current of the videocamera. From the sequence of background-subtracted images, a contrast arrival time image was determined based on a fixed density threshold. In this image, each pixel was labeled with the sequence number of the cardiac cycle in which the pixel intensity level exceeded the threshold for the first time, starting from the beginning of the ECG-triggered contrast injection. This contrast medium appearance in consecutive heart cycles is demonstrated in Figure 13–25. These arrival time numbers can be displayed color-coded: red was assigned to the pixels whose intensity surpassed the threshold during the first postinjection cycle, yellow for the second cycle, white for the third, green for the fourth, and so on. This intensity threshold was empirically derived by analyzing in 12 patients the relationship between the threshold and the baseline and hyperemic myocardial contrast medium appearance times, as well as the resulting coronary flow reserve.[Z8] The intensity level in more than 90 percent of the pixels exceeded threshold values of 4, 8, and 12 percent (Table 13–25). In 25 percent of patients, fewer than 90 percent of pixels reached the intensity level of 16 percent, making calculation of the contrast medium accumulation unreliable. With a threshold of 4 percent, and to a lesser extent with a threshold of 8 percent, background noise was not eliminated, resulting in very short contrast medium appearance times. Therefore, we used a threshold of 12 percent in all our patients.

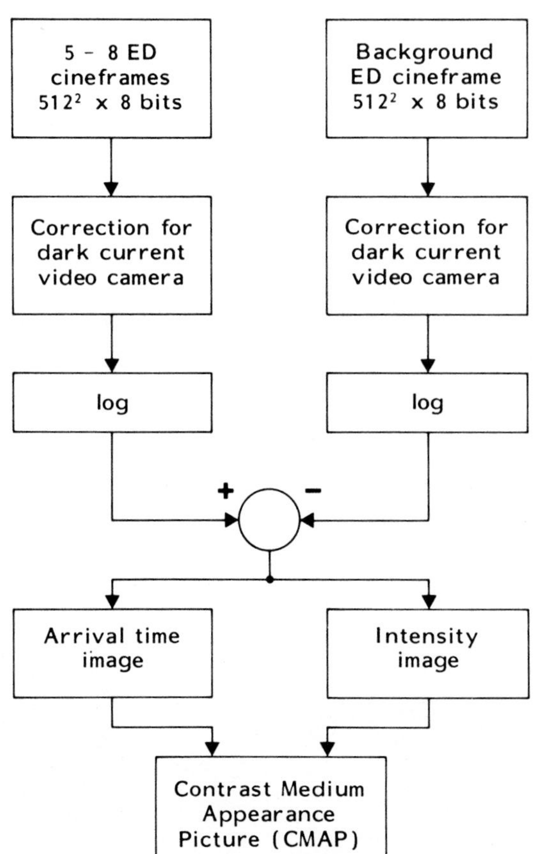

Figure 13–24. Flow diagram for the digitizing and processing of the end-diastolic (ED) cineangiographic frames for the assessment of the coronary flow reserve from 35-mm coronary cineangiograms.

For the calculation of relative regional blood flow within a user-defined myocardial region-of-interest (ROI), two parameters are required: the relative regional vascular volume and mean contrast appearance time. The relative regional vascular volume is calculated from a maximum intensity image, which is generated from the sequence of background subtracted cineangiograms. Each picture element (pixel) in this image represents the maximal intensity level found within the series of background-subtracted cine frames. As a result, the maximal intensity image contains information on the maximal contrast medium concentration within the displayed vessels as it occurred during the acquisition period. The maximal intensity image generated from the image series of Figure 13–23 is demonstrated in Figure 13–26. This maximal intensity image shows the distribution of contrast agent over the coronary tree. The intensity value in background-subtracted cineangiograms is proportional to the transradiated amount of contrast material within the vessels.[K5, R12] Therefore, the regional vascular volume (V) for a user-defined region-of-interest is proportional to the mean radiographic density within that ROI:

$$V = k \int_{ROI} D(p)\, dp = k'\overline{D},$$

where k and k′ are radiographic constants, D(p) the radiographic density per pixel, and $\overline{D}$ the mean radiographic density within the region-of-interest. In the second step, the information from these two images was combined into a dual parameter image, the contrast medium appearance picture (CMAP). In this picture,

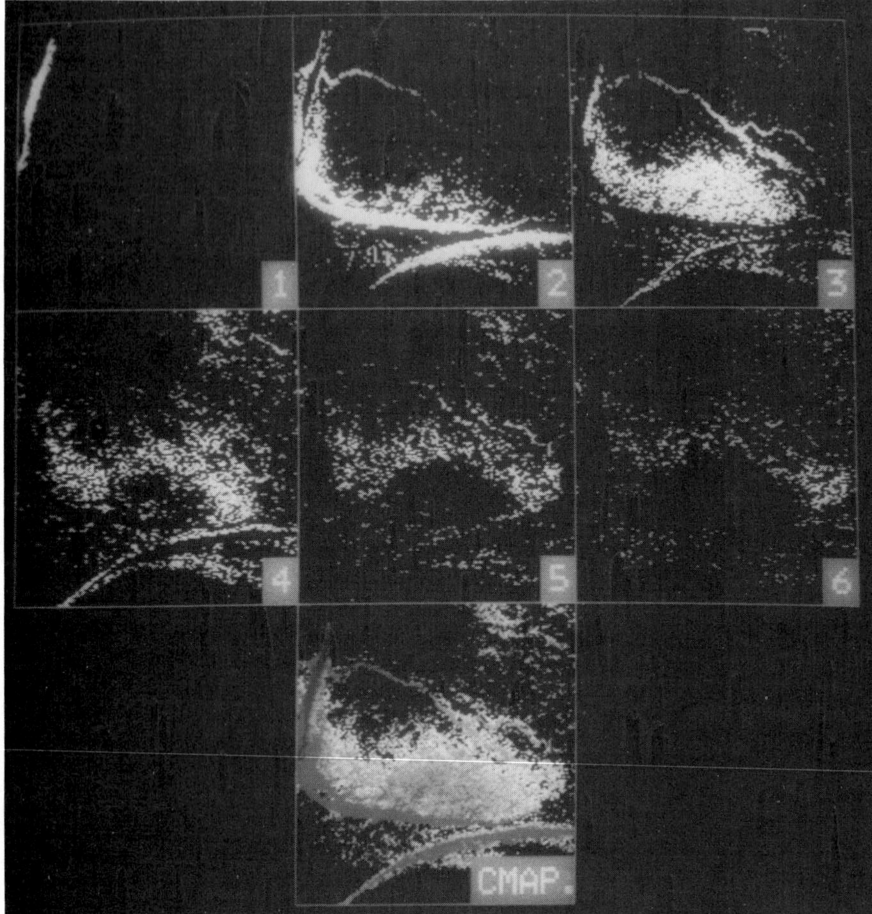

Figure 13–25. Contrast medium appearance in six consecutive cardiac cycles from the example of Figure 13–23. The first two cycles show the arterial phase, and the other cycles show the myocardial perfusion phase. The six individual cycles are finally combined into the last image, being the color-coded contrast medium appearance picture (CMAP) (shown here in black and white).

the appearance time was color coded, and the contrast medium accumulation was represented by the color intensity.

The coronary flow reserve was defined as the ratio of the regional flow computed from a hyperemic image divided by the regional flow of the corresponding baseline image. Regional flow values were quantitatively determined using the following video-densitometric principle:

$$Q = V/\bar{T}$$

where Q is the regional blood flow, V the regional vascular volume, and $\bar{T}$ the mean transit time.

As flow *ratios* are determined, only relative and not absolute regional flow values for baseline and hyperemic conditions are required. If the same regions of interest are used for baseline and hyperemic conditions, the coronary flow reserve can be determined from the regional blood flow values Q_h and Q_b at the hyperemic and baseline state, respectively:

$$CFR = \frac{Q_h}{Q_b} = \frac{V_h \cdot \bar{T}_b}{\bar{T}_h \cdot V_b} = \frac{\bar{D}_h \cdot \bar{T}_b}{\bar{T}_h \cdot \bar{D}_b}$$

where $\bar{D}$ is the mean contrast density and $\bar{T}$ the mean appearance time, at baseline (b) and hyperemia (h).

Table 13–25. INFLUENCE OF DENSITY THRESHOLD ON MYOCARDIAL CONTRAST MEDIUM APPEARANCE TIME AND CORONARY FLOW RESERVE (CFR)

	Percent						
DT	*4*		*8*		*12*		*16*
AT1	1.96		2.48		2.88		3.39
AT2	1.58		1.73		1.97		2.19
CFR	2.26	*	2.63	n.s.	2.66	*	2.82

DT—Density threshold in percentage of the brightness scale.
AT1—Baseline myocardial contrast medium appearance time.
AT2—Hyperemic myocardial contrast medium appearance time.
(AT1, AT2, and CFR are mean values calculated from 12 patients.)
*—$p < 0.01$; n.s.—not significant.
(From Zijlstra, F., et al.: Does the quantitative assessment of coronary artery dimensions predict the physiologic significance of a coronary stenosis? Circulation 75:1154, 1987, with permission of the American Heart Association, Inc.)

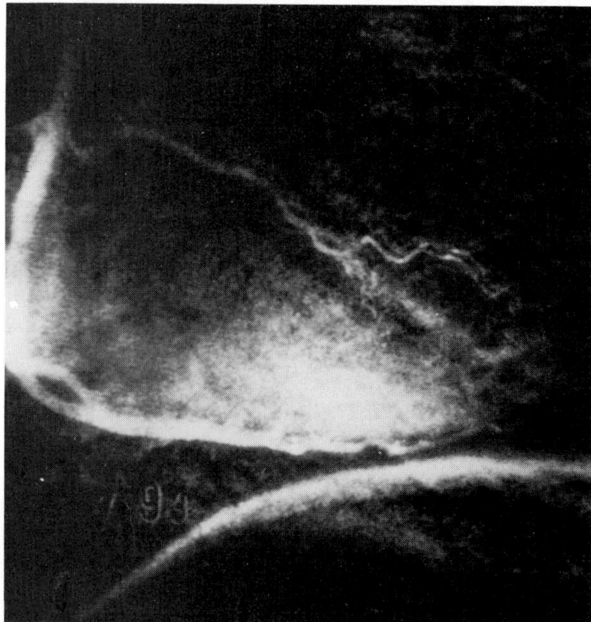

Figure 13–26. Maximal intensity image, generated from the image series of Figure 13–23. Intensity of each individual pixel in this image represents the maximal intensity for that particular pixel as it occurred over the entire image series.

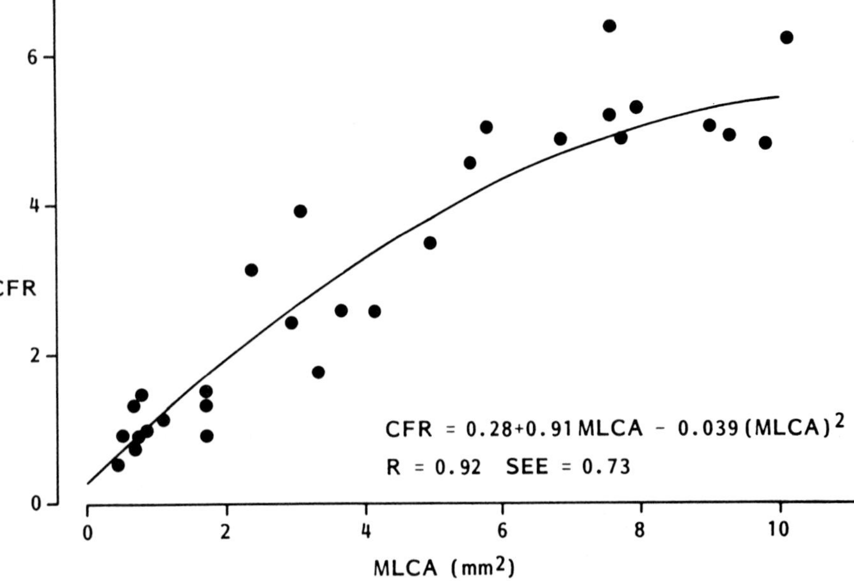

Figure 13–27. Relationship between coronary flow reserve (CFR) and minimal luminal cross-sectional area (MLCA). (From Zijlstra F., et al.: Does the quantitative assessment of coronary artery dimensions predict the physiologic significance of a coronary stenosis? Circulation 75:1154, 1987, with permission of the American Heart Association, Inc.)

Mean contrast medium appearance time and density were computed within user-defined regions-of-interest. These regions were chosen in such a way that the epicardial arteries visible on the angiogram, including diagonal and septal branches, the aortic root, the coronary sinus, and the great cardiac vein, were excluded from the analysis.

When coronary angiograms were repeated within 5 minutes, no significant differences were found in $\overline{T}$ and $\overline{D}$.[Z8] The mean difference between duplicate measurements of $\overline{T}$ was 7 percent, with a standard deviation of 8 percent. The mean difference between duplicate measurements of $\overline{D}$ was 6 percent, with a standard deviation of 5 percent.[Z8]

RELATIONSHIP BETWEEN CORONARY ARTERY DIMENSIONS AND CORONARY FLOW RESERVE

In the experimental animal, the physiologic significance of artificially produced arterial stenoses has been extensively studied.[G2, G5, K8, K16, S4] Gould and associates produced varying degrees of coronary narrowing and showed that stenoses with diameter narrowing in excess of 30 to 45 percent reduced coronary vasodilator response in a predictable fashion.[G5] In patients with single-vessel disease and with quantitative assessment of stenosis severity, percent diameter stenosis, percent area stenosis, or the calculated pressure drop over the stenosis has been found to be a useful predictor of the physiologic significance of a lesion.[Z3]

We have investigated 17 coronary arteries with a single discrete proximal stenosis and 12 normal coronary arteries, before and after intracoronary administration of papaverine.[Z8] In our patients, the interpolated reference cross-sectional area of the vessels with coronary artery disease was an average of 7.0 mm², and the cross-sectional areas of the 12 normal coronary arteries was an average of 7.6 mm², which indicates the isolated and focal character of the patients' coronary artery disease. Coronary flow reserve was curvilinearly related to minimal luminal cross-sectional area (r = 0.92, SEE = 0.73, Fig. 13–27) and to percent area stenosis (r = 0.92, SEE = 0.74, Fig. 13–28). Normal coronary arteries had a coronary flow reserve of 5.0 (s.d. = 0.8), which differed significantly from the coronary flow reserve of the coronary arteries with obstructive disease, in which values ranging from 0.5 to 3.9 were found (Table 13–26). Coronary arteries with a percent area stenosis of between 50 and 70 percent and a minimal luminal cross-sectional area of between 2 and 4.5 mm² (moderate coronary artery disease) differed significantly (p = 0.001) with respect to the coronary flow reserve from coronary arteries with

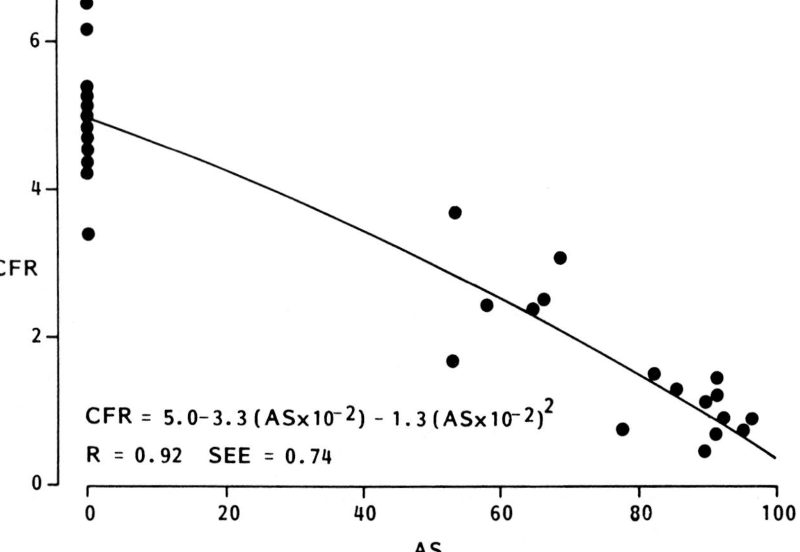

Figure 13–28. Relationship between coronary flow reserve (CFR) and percent area stenosis (AS). (From Zijlstra, F., et al.: Does the quantitative assessment of coronary artery dimensions predict the physiologic significance of a coronary stenosis? Circulation 75:1154, 1987, with permission of the American Heart Association, Inc.)

Table 13–26. RELATION BETWEEN QUANTITATIVELY ASSSESSED CORONARY ARTERY DIMENSIONS (CAD) AND CFR

	Normals (N = 12)		CAD: *Moderate* (*N = 6*)		CAD: *Severe* (*N = 11*)
MLCA (mm^2)	>4.5		2–4.5		<2
AS(%)	<50		50–70		>70
CFR (mean ± SD)	5.0 ± 0.8	*	2.6 ± 0.7	*	1.0 ± 0.3

CFR—coronary flow reserve; MLCA—minimal luminal cross-sectional area; AS—area stenosis, *—$p < 0.001$.

(From Zijlstra, F., et al.: Does the quantitative assessment of coronary artery dimensions predict the physiologic significance of a coronary stenosis? Circulation 75:1154, 1987, with permission of the American Heart Association, Inc.)

a percent area stenosis in excess of 70 percent and a minimal luminal cross-sectional area of less than 2 mm^2 (severe coronary artery disease).

In a previous study from our laboratory, the relation between the calculated pressure drop over a stenosis and the minimal lumen cross-sectional area (MLCA) was analyzed.[W14] A curvilinear relation was found, with a steep increase in pressure drop once the MLCA is less than 2 mm^2. The present study confirms the discriminant value of this criterion (see Table 13–26). These results are also in agreement with the data presented by Wilson and associates.[W4] In a more recent study, Zijlstra and colleagues found in a group of 38 patients with single-vessel disease that the calculated pressure drop over the stenosis is a better anatomic variable for assessing the functional significance of a stenosis, as assessed by digital cineangiography, than is percent diameter stenosis or obstruction area.[Z12] In addition, this pressure drop was highly predictive of thallium-201 scintigraphic results, with a sensitivity of 94 percent and a specificity of 90 percent. Thus, it may be concluded that, in single-vessel coronary artery disease, the consequent reduction in coronary flow reserve can be predicted with reasonable accuracy by quantitative assessment of coronary artery dimensions. However, in patients with multivessel disease, both visual[M7, W3] and quantitative[H3] estimates of percent diameter or area stenosis correlated poorly with the physiologic significance of a coronary obstructive lesion. This is particularly true for obstructions of intermediate severity, which can be explained by the presence of diffuse coronary artery disease that cannot be detected by angiography.[W3] In vessels with an expected normal cross-sectional area of between 7 and 10 mm^2, Harrison and associates found that a minimal luminal cross-sectional area below 3.5 mm^2 predicted a decreased coronary flow reserve. In vessels with an expected normal cross-sectional area of 7.0 mm^2 (s.d. = 1.7 mm^2), we observed that a minimal luminal cross-sectional area below 4.5 mm^2 was associated with a decreased coronary flow reserve.

As noted in the introduction to this section, Kirkeeide and associates calculated stenosis flow reserve values from the angiographic data.[W5] They showed in dogs the good correlation between such an angiographic approach and measured coronary flow reserve.[K8] In our patients, the calculated pressure-flow relationships were related to the reduction in coronary flow reserve (Table 13–27 and Fig. 13–29). A pressure drop over a stenosis at a flow of 3 ml/sec, resulting in a distal perfusion pressure below 40 mmHg, indicated the existence of a critical stenosis, defined as a vessel with a coronary flow reserve of 1 or less. With the use of this criterion, patients with severe CAD and a critical stenosis can be identified with a high sensitivity (83 percent) and specificity (82 percent) (Table 13–28). The rationale for use of this pressure value is based on previous observations that reactive coronary hyperemia is abolished when coronary artery perfusion pressure drops below this value.[D6]

VARIABILITY IN CORONARY FLOW RESERVE MEASUREMENTS

Although the radiographic assessment of myocardial perfusion is computer based, a crucial component of the analysis procedure is the user-dependent selection of the regions-of-interest (ROIs), resulting in inter- and intraobserver variations. Knowledge of the short-, medium-, and long-term variabilities in the measurement of coronary flow reserve, therefore, is an essential prerequisite if this radiographic technique is to be used for determination of the immediate or long-term functional results of pharmacologic therapy or revascularization procedures, such as PTCA. Zijlstra and associates have studied these variabilities from digitized coronary cineangiograms, as well as the immediate and long-term functional results of percutaneous transluminal coronary angioplasty.[Z9] The Student's t-test was used for the determination of statistically significant differences.

Intraobserver Variability

Intraobserver variability was assessed by measuring the coronary flow reserve in 11 different regions-of-interest in 6 patients twice, from the same cineangiograms by the same observer. In 5 patients, two ROIs in the myocardium supplied by the left coronary artery were analyzed, and in one patient one ROI was analyzed in the myocardium supplied by the right coronary artery. Care was taken to ensure that the ROIs in the duplicate determinations were identical. The results are presented in Figure 13–30*A*. No statistically significant differences were found between the first and second measurements; results from linear regression analysis were r = 0.99, SEE = 0.05.

Interobserver Variability

Interobserver variability was assessed by measuring the coronary flow reserve in 12 regions-of-interest in 7 patients from the same coronary cineangiograms by two observers. In 5 patients, two ROIs in the myocardium supplied by the left coronary artery were analyzed, and in 2 patients a ROI was analyzed in the myocardium supplied by the right coronary artery. The selected boundaries of the ROIs were unknown to the other observer. The results are presented in Fig. 13–30*B*. Again, no statistically significant differences were found between the two observers; linear regression analysis results were r = 0.91, SEE = 0.52.

Table 13–27. CALCULATED DISTAL CORONARY PERFUSION PRESSURE (mmHg) FOR THEORETIC CORONARY FLOWS OF 1 (P_1), 2 (P_2), AND 3 (P_3) ML/SEC OF VESSELS WITH CORONARY ARTERY DISEASE SUBDIVIDED ACCORDING TO CORONARY FLOW RESERVE

	No. of Patients	CFR: *Mean*	CFR: *Range*	AS (%)	MLCA (mm^2)	(mmHg): Ao	P_1	P_2	P_3
A	6	2.6	1.7–3.9	59	3.1	89	88	87	86
B	5	1.3	1.1–1.5	86	1.1	88	78	63	42
C	6	0.8	0.5–1.0	87	0.8	86	62	20	−41

CFR—coronary flow reserve; AS%—percent area stenosis; MLCA—minimal luminal cross-sectional area; Ao—mean aortic pressure.

A—CFR > 1.6; B—1.0 < CFR ≤ 1.6; C—CFR ≤ 1.0.

(From Zijlstra, F., et al.: Does the quantitative assessment of coronary artery dimensions predict the physiologic significance of a coronary stenosis. Circulation 75:1154, 1987, with permission of the American Heart Association, Inc.)

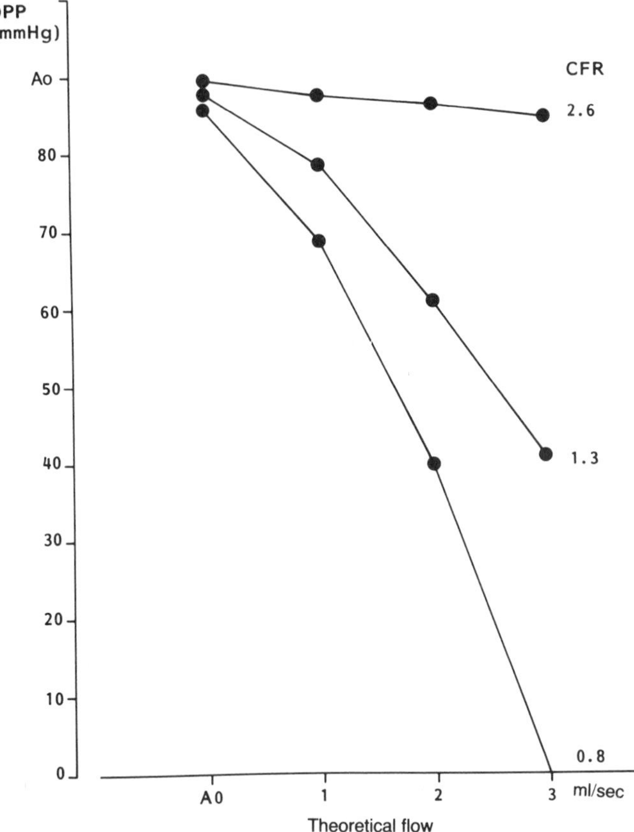

Figure 13–29. Calculated distal coronary arterial pressure–flow relationships for theoretic flows of 1, 2 and 3 ml/sec for vessels with coronary artery disease. Patients were divided into three groups according to the coronary flow reserve (CFR): Six patients had moderate coronary artery disease and CFR > 1.6, five patients had severe coronary artery disease and 1.0<CFR≤1.6, and six patients had severe coronary artery disease and CFR≤1.0. (DPP—distal coronary perfusion pressure; Ao—mean aortic pressure values for the three patient groups.)

Short-Term (5-Minute) Variability

The short-term variability was defined as the variation in measured coronary flow reserve values from two coronary cineangiograms taken 5 minutes apart, with identical position of the patient, x-ray source, and image intensifier. Coronary flow reserve was measured in 13 regions-of-interest in 7 patients. In 6 patients, two ROIs in the myocardium supplied by the left coronary artery were analyzed, and in one patient one ROI was analyzed in the myocardium supplied by the right coronary artery. Care was taken to ensure that the selected ROIs in the duplicate determinations were identical. The results are presented in Fig. 13–30*C*. No statistically significant differences were found between the two measurements; linear regression analysis results were r = 0.98, SEE = 0.26.

Table 13–28. IDENTIFICATION OF CORONARY ARTERIES WITH CRITICAL STENOSIS ON THE BASIS OF CALCULATED DISTAL CORONARY PERFUSION PRESSURE (DPP) AT A CORONARY FLOW OF 3 ML/SEC

DPP (*mmHg*)	CFR (*Mean ± SD*)		No. of Patients	
			CFR ≤ 1	*CFR > 1*
<40	0.96 ± 0.3	*p* = 0.01	5	2
>40	2.1 ± 0.9		1	9

Sensitivity = 5/6 × 100% = 83%
Specificity = 9/11 × 100% = 82%

(From Zijlstra, F., et al.: Does the quantitative assessment of coronary artery dimensions predict the physiologic significance of a coronary stenosis? Circulation 75:1154, 1987, with permission of the American Heart Association, Inc.)

Medium-Term (1- to 3-Hour) Variability and Immediate Functional Result of Percutaneous Transluminal Coronary Angioplasty

Coronary flow reserve was measured before and immediately after percutaneous transluminal coronary angioplasty (PTCA) in 25 patients. In 5 patients, the right coronary artery was dilated. In 20 patients undergoing PTCA of the left anterior descending coronary artery or the circumflex artery, coronary flow reserve was measured in both myocardial regions. To calculate the medium-term variability, regions-of-interest (N = 20) were chosen in the myocardium supplied by the nondilated coronary arteries. To assess the immediate alterations in coronary flow reserve caused by PTCA, regions-of-interest (N = 25) were chosen in the myocardium supplied by the dilated coronary arteries. During the PTCA procedure, various vasoactive drugs were administered (nitrates, calcium antagonists) as clinically indicated, probably resulting in changes in vasomotor tone. Care was taken to ensure that the cineangiographic projection and x-ray gantry settings, as well as the analyzed regions-of-interest, were identical before and after the PTCA. The results are presented in Figure 13–30*D*. No statistically significant differences were found between the measurements obtained before and after angioplasty; linear regression analysis results were r = 0.83, SEE = 0.52.

The diameter stenosis (mean ± SD) decreased from 65 ± 6 to 32 ± 10. The coronary flow reserve values (mean ± SD) of the dilated coronary arteries increased from 1.0 ± 0.3 to 2.3 ± 0.6, and the cross-sectional area at the site of obstruction (mean ± SD) increased from 0.9 ± 0.3 to 3.3 ± 0.7 mm^2. The data of the individual patients are shown in Figures 13–31 and 13–32. Eighteen of the 25 patients (72 percent) had an increase in coronary flow reserve greater than 2 standard deviations of the medium-term variability.

Long-Term (3- to 5-Month) Variability and Long-Term Functional Result of Percutaneous Transluminal Coronary Angioplasty

During follow-up coronary cineangiography 3 to 5 months (mean 4.2 months) later, coronary flow reserve was measured again in these 25 patients. To calculate the long-term variability, regions-of-interest (N = 20) were chosen in the myocardium supplied by the nondilated coronary arteries. To assess the long-term alterations in coronary flow reserve after percutaneous transluminal coronary angioplasty, ROIs (N = 25) were chosen in the myocardium supplied by the dilated coronary arteries. The follow-up investigation was always performed in a second cineangiographic room with different x-ray equipment. There was no standardized protocol for the administration of vasoactive medication before data acquisition; therefore, vasomotor tone in both conditions was unknown and ignored. Care was taken to ensure that identical regions-of-interest were analyzed. The results are presented in Figure 13–30*E*. No statistically significant differences were found between the measurements; linear regression analysis results were r = 0.72, SEE = 0.58.

Three to five months after percutaneous transluminal coronary angioplasty, the mean percentage diameter stenosis (mean ± SD) was 38 ± 18 percent. The coronary flow reserve (mean ± SD) of the dilated coronary arteries was 2.6 ± 1.0, and the cross-sectional area at the site of obstruction was 2.8 ± 1.4 mm^2. The alterations in these two parameters of the individual patients during the 3 to 5 months after percutaneous transluminal coronary angioplasty are shown in Figures 13–33 and 13–34. Nine of the 25 patients (36 percent) had restenosis defined as diameter stenosis greater than 50 percent during follow-up angiography. These 9 patients had an obstruction area (mean ± SD) of 1.3 ± 0.4 mm^2, and a coronary flow reserve of 1.5 ± 0.4. The patients without restenosis had an obstruction area of 3.6 ± 1.0 mm^2 and a coronary flow reserve of 3.3 ± 0.6. Seven of the 25 patients (28 percent) had an increase in coronary flow reserve greater than 2 standard deviations of the long-term variability, and 4 of the 25 patients (16 percent), all with restenosis, had a decrease

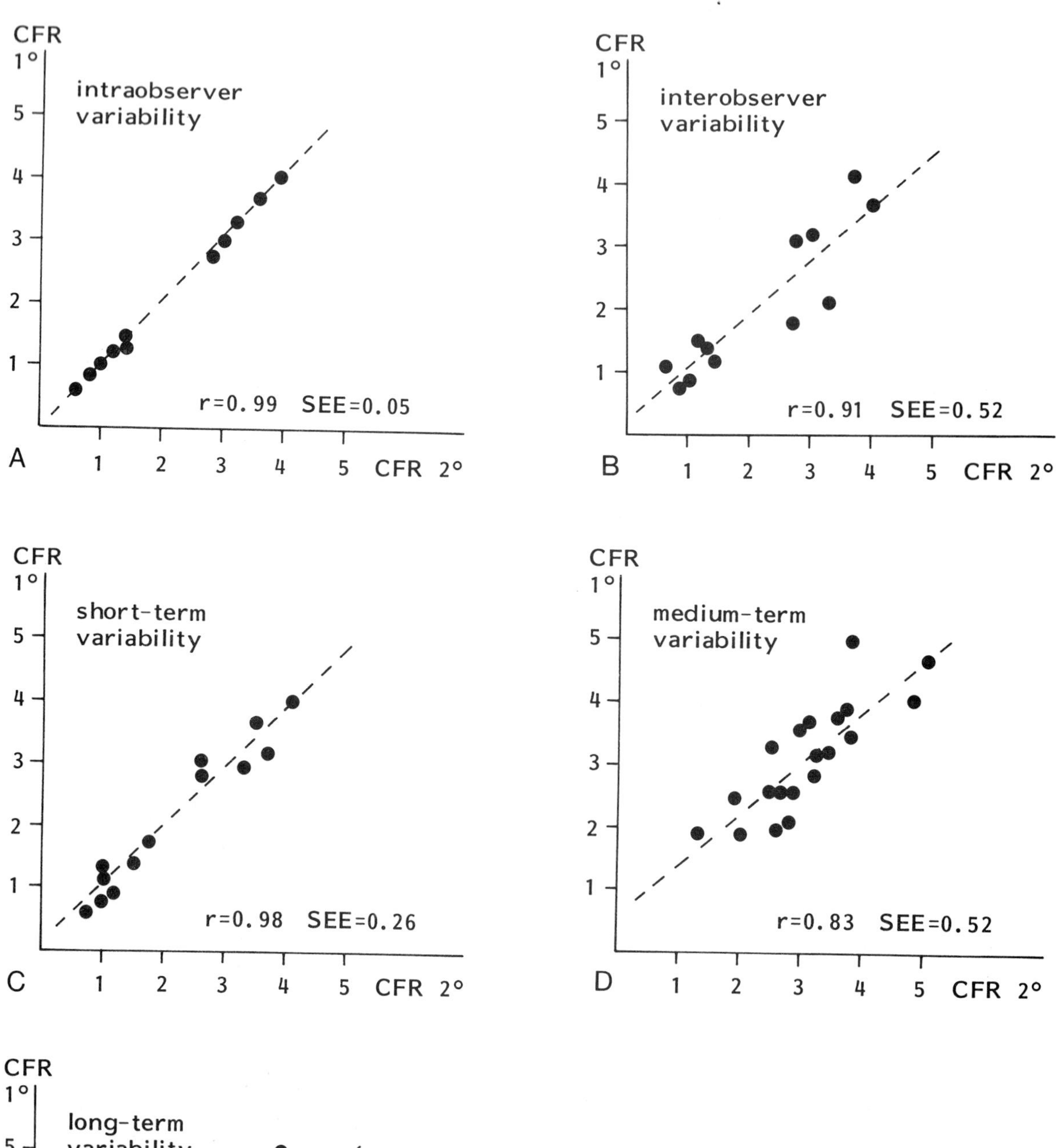

Figure 13–30. Scatter diagrams of the intraobserver variabilities *(A)*, interobserver variabilities *(B)*, short-term variabilities *(C)*, medium-term variabilities *(D)*, and long-term variabilities *(E)*. (r—correlation coefficient; SEE—standard error of the estimate.) (From Zijlstra F., et al.: Assessment of immediate and long-term functional results of percutaneous transluminal coronary angioplasty. Circulation 78:15, 1988, with permission of the American Heart Association, Inc.)

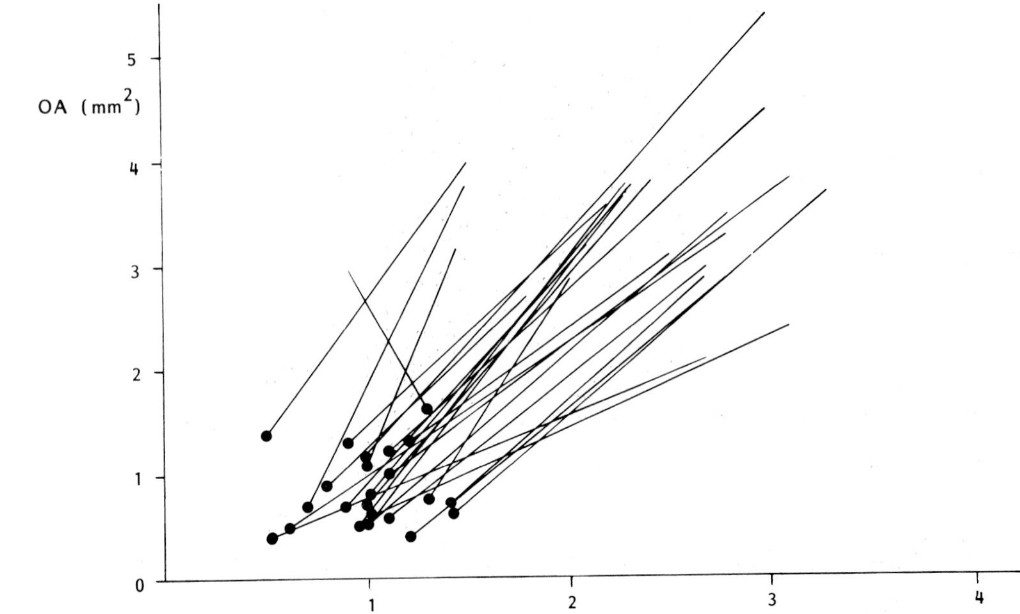

Figure 13–31. Cross-sectional area at the site of obstruction (OA) and coronary flow reserve (CFR) before and immediately after percutaneous transluminal coronary angioplasty. (From Zijlstra F., et al.: Assessment of immediate and long-term functional results of percutaneous transluminal coronary angioplasty. Circulation 78:15, 1988, with permission of the American Heart Association, Inc.)

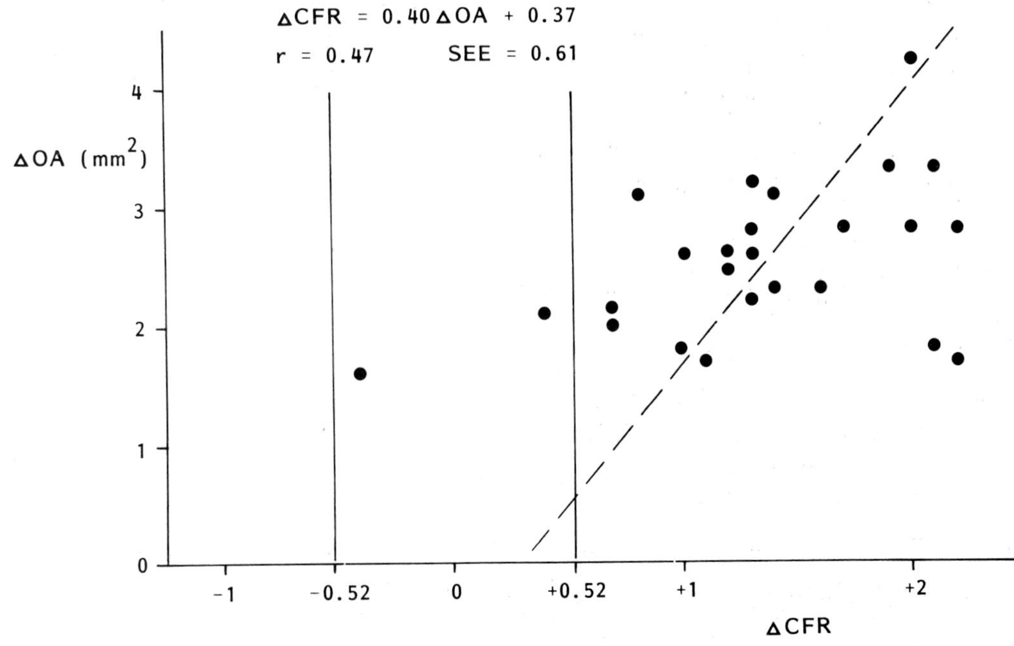

Figure 13–32. Relationship between change in obstruction-area (ΔOA) and change in coronary flow reserve (ΔCFR) as immediate result of percutaneous transluminal coronary angioplasty. The vertical lines mark 1 standard error of the estimate (SEE) of the medium-term variability. (r—correlation coefficient.) (From Zijlstra F., et al.: Assessment of immediate and long-term functional results of percutaneous transluminal coronary angioplasty. Circulation 78:15, 1988, with permission of the American Heart Association, Inc.)

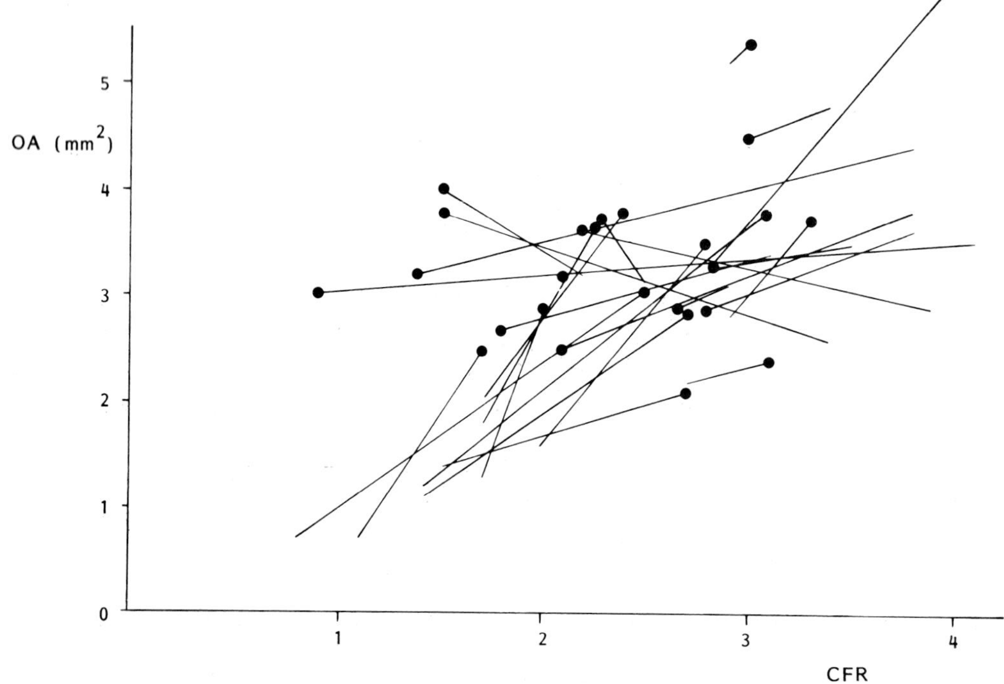

Figure 13–33. Cross-sectional area at the site of obstruction (OA) and coronary flow reserve (CFR) immediately after percutaneous transluminal coronary angioplasty and 3 to 5 months later. (From Zijlstra F., et al.: Assessment of immediate and long-term functional results of percutaneous transluminal coronary angioplasty. Circulation 78:15, 1988, with permission of the American Heart Association, Inc.)

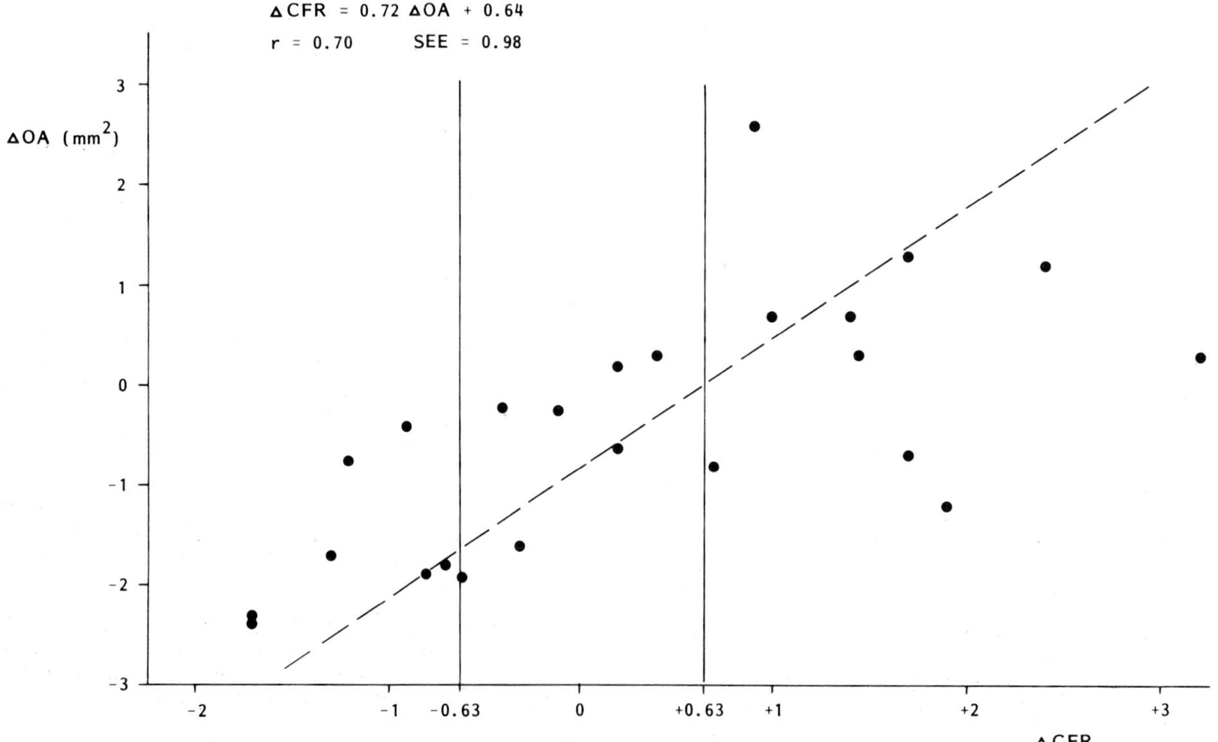

Figure 13–34. Relationship between change in obstruction area (ΔOA) and change in coronary flow reserve (ΔCFR) occurring from immediately following percutaneous transluminal coronary angioplasty to follow-up 3 to 5 months later. The vertical lines mark 1 standard error of the estimate (SEE) of the long-term variability. (r—correlation coefficient.) (From Zijlstra F., et al.: Assessment of immediate and long-term functional results of percutaneous transluminal coronary angioplasty. Circulation 78:15, 1988, with permission of the American Heart Association, Inc.)

of coronary flow reserve greater than 2 standard deviations of the long-term variability.

CORONARY FLOW RESERVE AND PERCUTANEOUS TRANSLUMINAL CORONARY ANGIOPLASTY

Although percutaneous transluminal coronary angioplasty (PTCA) has been shown to result in symptomatic, hemodynamic, and functional improvement,[K17, K18, S40] doubt has remained whether this procedure can restore coronary flow reserve of atherosclerotic coronary arteries to a normal level.[B24, H11, O5, W15] Therefore, we selected 15 patients who were free of angina and had a normal exercise thallium-201 scintigram 5 months after PTCA, and compared their radiographically measured coronary flow reserve with the flow reserve of 24 patients with angiographically normal coronary arteries.[Z10] In these 24 patients, flow reserve ranged from 3.4 to 6.5; the mean value was 5.0 (SD ± 0.8). The lower limit for a normal coronary flow reserve is therefore 3.4 (2 × SD below the mean coronary flow reserve). This is comparable to the normal values for flow reserve reported by other groups.[H11, W1] In the angioplasty patients, coronary flow reserve was measured in the myocardial region supplied by the dilated coronary artery before percutaneous transluminal coronary angioplasty, immediately after it, and 5 months later. Consecutive measurements were also obtained in 12 adjacent myocardial regions supplied by a nondilated coronary artery. The coronary flow reserve of these adjacent myocardial regions remained unchanged immediately after angioplasty and after 5 months' follow-up. Coronary flow reserve in the myocardial region supplied by the dilated coronary artery increased from 1.0 ± 0.3 to 2.5 ± 0.6 (mean ± SD) immediately after percutaneous transluminal coronary angioplasty ($p < 0.001$). In none of these patients was flow reserve restored to a normal level immediately after angioplasty. A substantial late improvement ($p < 0.01$) in coronary flow reserve occurred 5 months later. Coronary flow reserve in the myocardial region supplied by the dilated coronary artery 5 months after PTCA was of the same magnitude as the flow reserve in the myocardial region supplied by a nondilated coronary artery shown by angiography to be not diseased. In 11 (73 percent) of the 15 patients, coronary flow reserve of the dilated artery was restored to a normal level of ≥ 3.4, whereas in 4 (27 percent) of 15 patients, it was still abnormal (Figs. 13–35 and 13–36). Coronary flow reserve 5 months after PTCA was related to the change in minimal cross-sectional obstruction area occurring between immediate post-PTCA and follow-up (r = 0.61, SEE = 0.54).

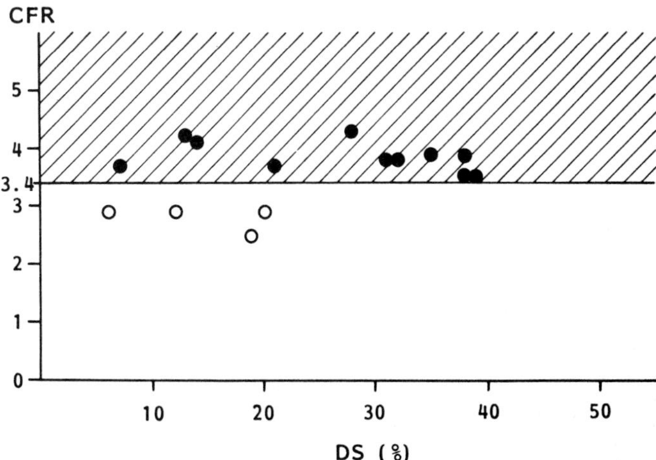

Figure 13–35. Coronary flow reserve (CFR) plotted against percent diameter stenosis (DS) 5 months after percutaneous transluminal coronary angioplasty. The lower limit of the normal value for CFR as measured with the digital subtraction cineangiographic technique is 3.4. (From Zijlstra, F., et al.: Normalization of coronary flow reserve by percutaneous transluminal coronary angioplasty. Am. J. Cardiol. 61:55, 1988, with permission.)

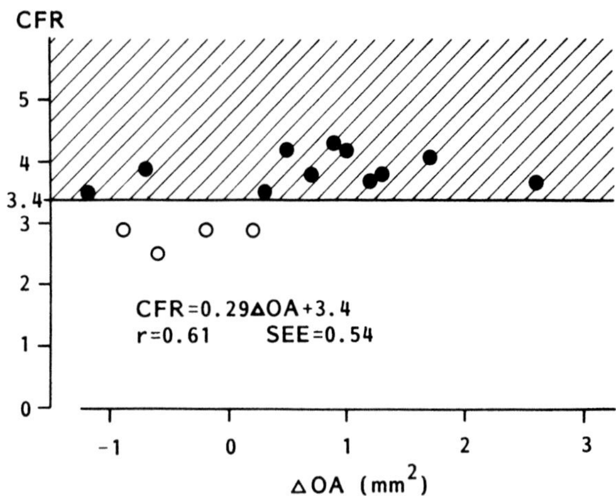

Figure 13–36. Relationship between coronary flow reserve (CFR) 5 months after percutaneous transluminal angioplasty and the change that occurred in minimal cross-sectional obstruction area (ΔOA) from immediately after percutaneous transluminal coronary angioplasty to 5 months later. The lower limit of the normal value for CFR as measured with the digital subtraction cineangiographic technique is 3.4. (r—correlation coefficient; SEE—standard error of the estimate.) (From Zijlstra F., et al.: Normalization of coronary flow reserve by percutaneous transluminal coronary angioplasty. Am. J. Cardiol. 61:55, 1988, with permission.)

Wilson and associates found slightly different results in a study with 31 patients with single-vessel disease in whom coronary flow reserve was measured with a 3 Fr. coronary Doppler catheter.[W21] Coronary flow reserve measured immediately after angioplasty returned to normal levels (> 3.5 peak/resting velocity ratio) in 14 of 31 patients and was improved, although not normal, in the remaining 17 patients. In the absence of restenosis, flow reserve eventually (7.5 months after PTCA) normalized in all patients. Wilson and colleagues concluded that measurements of coronary flow reserve immediately after angioplasty may not reflect the eventual success of the procedure in removing the physiologic obstruction to coronary blood flow.

Bates and associates reported that even though coronary flow reserve improved immediately and during the follow-up of patients who underwent PTCA, their values did not return to normal levels.[B24] Nevertheless, these values compared well with those found after bypass surgery and showed no sign of ischemia.

COMPARISON OF INTRACORONARY DOPPLER TECHNIQUE WITH DIGITAL SUBTRACTION CINEANGIOGRAPHY IN MEASUREMENT OF CORONARY FLOW RESERVE IN THE SETTING OF CORONARY ANGIOPLASTY

As noted earlier, the more widely employed methods to evaluate coronary flow reserve are the Doppler probe approach, and the just described radiographic technique.[B24, S41, V4, W1, Z8] Using a balloon catheter with a Doppler probe at the tip, Serruys and associates recently compared both techniques in the setting of percutaneous transluminal coronary angioplasty.[S39, S42, S59, Z11, Z13] Hyperemic response in these studies was obtained with the infusion of papaverine and a transitory transluminal occlusion.

Preangioplasty (N = 14) and postangioplasty (N = 19) measurements of coronary flow reserve were obtained by digital subtraction cineangiography in the myocardial region supplied by the dilated coronary artery, and with the Doppler probe in the proximal part of the dilated vessel. The reactive hyperemia following the final balloon inflation was recorded with the Doppler balloon catheter still positioned across the stenotic lesion. Intracoronary administrations of isosorbide dinitrate were repeated at regular intervals to ensure constant and maximal epicardial cor-

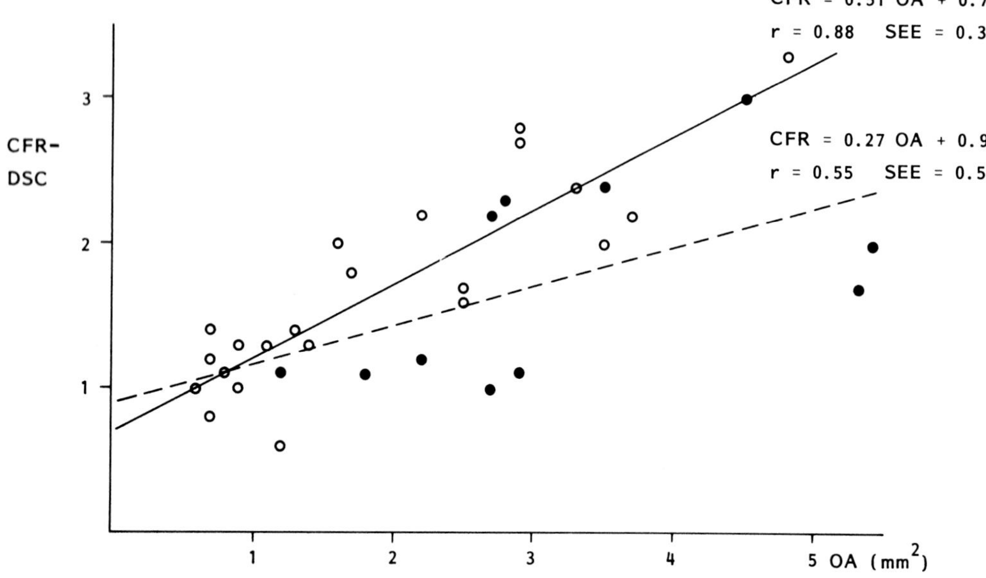

Figure 13–37. Relationship between coronary flow reserve measured with digital subtraction cineangiography (CRF-DSC) and cross-sectional area at the site of obstruction (OA). The open circles represent the patients with any of the following characteristics: left ventricular hypertrophy, hypertension, previous myocardial infarction, presence of collaterals, or dissection after percutaneous transluminal coronary angioplasty. The closed circles represent the patients without any of the foregoing characteristics. (From Serruys, P.W., et al.: A comparison of two methods to measure coronary flow reserve in the setting of coronary angioplasty: Intracoronary blood flow velocity measurements with a Doppler catheter and digital subtraction cineangiography. Eur. Heart J. 10:731, 1989, with permission.)

onary vasodilation during the entire procedure. Coronary stenosis geometry was quantified with the Cardiovascular Angiography Analysis System (CAAS).

When the epicardial stenosis was the only factor causing a reduction in coronary flow reserve, flow reserve measured with both digital subtraction cineangiography and with the Doppler probe correlated well with the cross-sectional area at the site of obstruction (r = 0.88, SEE = 0.36, and r = 0.77, SEE = 0.45, respectively) (Figs. 13–37 and 13–38). However, if other factors decreasing coronary flow reserve were present (intimal dissection, left ventricular hypertrophy, previous myocardial infarction, collaterals), measurements obtained with both techniques correlated poorly with the cross-sectional area (r = 0.55, SEE = 0.57, and r = 0.59, SEE = 0.50, respectively). Nevertheless, flow reserve measurements obtained with digital subtraction cineangiography correlated well with the measurements obtained with the Doppler probe in both groups of patients (r = 0.85, SEE = 0.38, and r = 0.87, SEE = 0.34) (Fig. 13–39), in spite of the fact that the two approaches have methodologically nothing in common and their respective regions-of-interest (myocardium for the radiographic technique and intracoronary lumen for the Doppler technique) are basically different. The relationships between the reactive hyperemia (RH), as assessed with the Doppler probe and recorded after the final balloon inflation with the angioplasty catheter still across the lesion, and the post-PTCA coronary flow reserve values measured with the angiographic technique (CFR − DSC = 0.27 + 0.95 RH, r = 0.85, SEE = 0.34) and with the Doppler catheter (CFR − DOP = 0.51 + 0.84 RH, r = 0.83, SEE = 0.32) are shown in Figures 13–40 and 13–41, respectively. As expected, the mean reactive hyperemia was somewhat lower than the coronary flow reserves measured with the angiographic technique or with the Doppler probe located proximal to the dilated stenosis. Reactive hyperemia was 1.9 ± 0.6; coronary flow reserve measured with the angiographic technique, 2.1 ± 0.6; and measured with the Doppler catheter, 2.1 ± 0.6. These data suggest that the hyperemia induced pharmacologically is similar to that obtained by ischemia following a transluminal occlusion.

ASSESSMENT OF CORONARY FLOW RESERVE BY MYOCARDIAL CONTRAST ECHOCARDIOGRAPHY

Recently, myocardial contrast echocardiography (MCE) has been used to study the perfusion bed of a coronary artery and the nutrient myocardial blood flow in experimental studies.[C14, K24, T5] Also, recent human studies have shown that the area of myocardial opacification and the rate of myocardial contrast

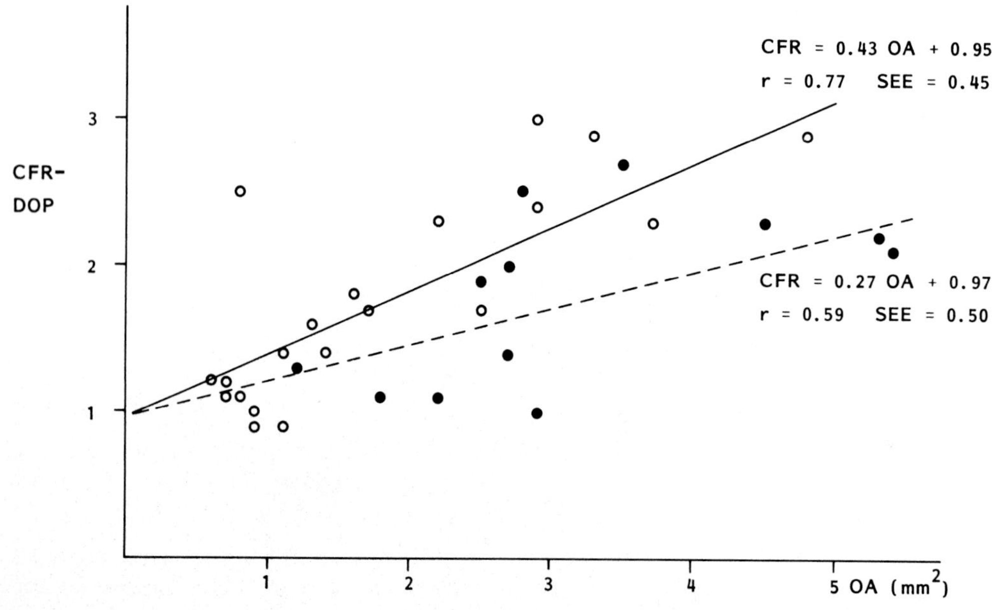

Figure 13–38. Relationship between coronary flow reserve measured with the Doppler probe (CFR-DOP) and cross-sectional area at the site of obstruction (OA). For explanation of open and closed circles, see legend for Figure 13–37. (From Serruys, P.W., et al.: A comparison of two methods to measure coronary flow reserve in the setting of coronary angioplasty: Intracoronary blood flow velocity measurements with a Doppler catheter and digital subtraction cineangiography. Eur. Heart J. 10:731, 1989, with permission.)

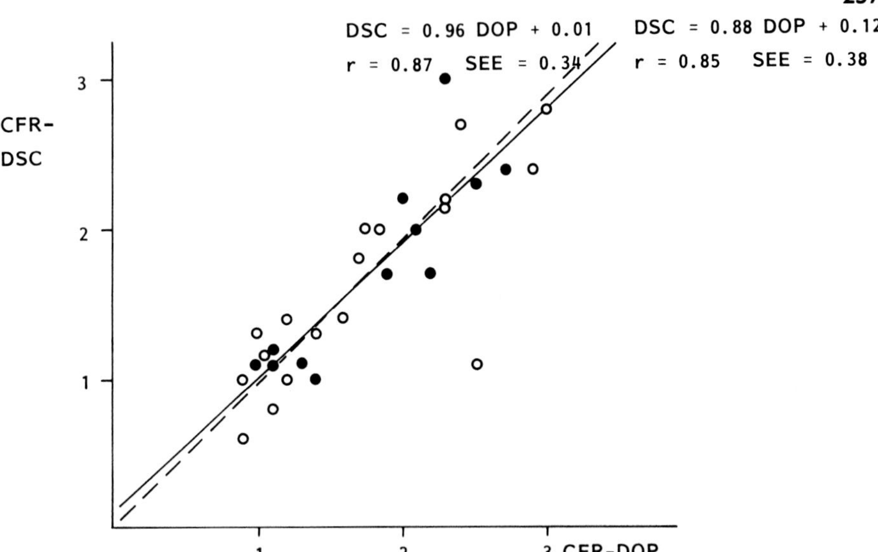

Figure 13–39. Relationship between coronary flow reserve measured with digital subtraction cineangiography (CFR-DSC) and coronary flow reserve measured with the Doppler probe (CFR-DOP). For explanation of open and closed circles, see legend for Figure 13–37. (From Serruys, P.W., et al.: A comparison of two methods to measure coronary flow reserve in the setting of coronary angioplasty: Intracoronary blood flow velocity measurements with a Doppler catheter and digital subtraction cineangiography. Eur. Heart J. 10:731, 1989, with permission.)

disappearance ("washout") correlate with the severity of coronary artery stenosis.[C15, L20, W26] Coronary blood flow reserve measurements have been performed in experimental studies and in humans, using different contrast agents.[K25, L21]

In the study of Cheirif and associates, sonicated meglumine was used as the echocontrast agent, which was given intracoronary.[C16, F19] Two-dimensional echocardiographic studies were performed before and after intracoronary administration of papaverine (8 mg for the right coronary artery and 10 mg for the left coronary artery). The resulting video images were digitized, and peak intensity values (following subtraction for baseline intensity) were determined. Cheirif and associates found that peak contrast intensity increased after the administration of papaverine in patients with normal coronary arteriograms, but this was not the case in patients with severe coronary artery disease. In addition, the method proved to be of value in determining the success of angioplasty. These findings were corroborated by our laboratory in patients not undergoing angioplasty.[S60]

Keller and colleagues determined coronary flow reserve in patients and in experimental animals with sonicated meglumine containing microbubbles of 4 to 10 μm ($500 \times 10^3 - 200 \times 10^3$/ml).[K25] In these studies, the areas under the echocardiographic time-intensity curves in regions perfused by the left anterior descending coronary artery and the circumflex artery were calculated and compared with absolute blood flows measured with radiolabeled microspheres. They found that the ratios of these areas under the curves from the two vascular beds (LAD and LCX) before and after papaverine correlated well with the ratios of blood flows between the two beds during the same stages ($r^2 = 0.73$ by linear regression and $r^2 = 0.85$ by an exponential function). The absolute values for the area under the curves did not correlate with the corresponding absolute coronary flows.

A recent study in patients and in experimental animals from our own laboratory confirmed the findings of Keller and associates concerning the absolute coronary flow correlations with data derived from echocardiographic time-intensity curves.[K25] Future developments in echocontrast agents that will pass the pulmonary circulation and produce no hyperemic effect are foreseen; with these agents it will be possible to assess the myocardial perfusion using an intravenous approach.[K25] These agents may expose a whole new area of studying coronary pathophysiology by myocardial contrast echocardiography.

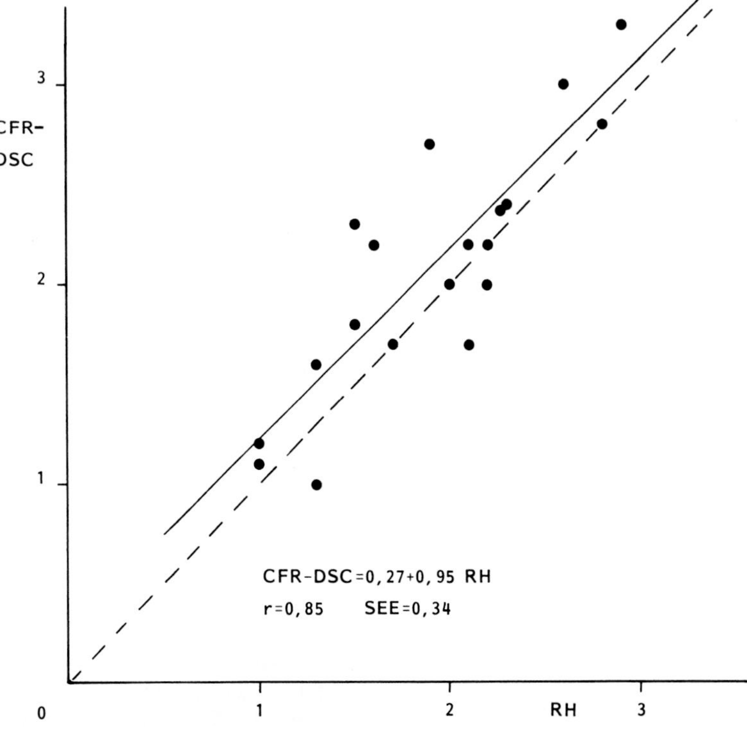

Figure 13–40. Relationship between coronary flow reserve measured with digital subtraction cineangiography (CFR-DSC) and the reactive hyperemia (RH) recorded with the Doppler probe across the dilated lesion after the final balloon inflation. (From Serruys, P.W., et al.: A comparison of two methods to measure coronary flow reserve in the setting of coronary angioplasty: Intracoronary blood flow velocity measurements with a Doppler catheter and digital subtraction cineangiography. Eur. Heart J. 10:731, 1989, with permission.)

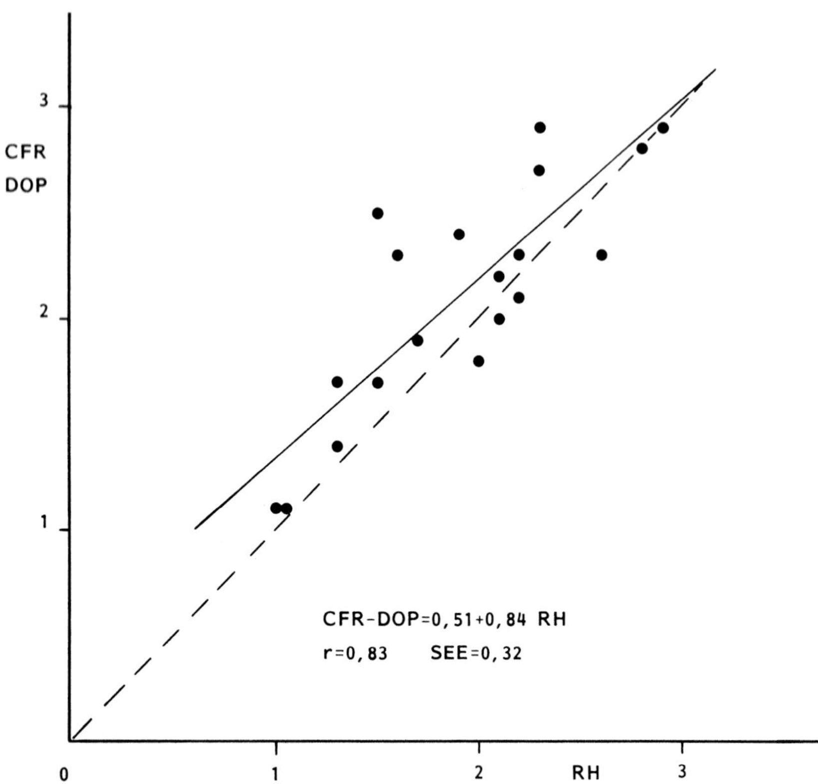

Figure 13–41. Relationship between coronary flow reserve measured with the Doppler technique (CFR-DOP) and the reactive hyperemia (RH) recorded with the Doppler probe across the dilated lesion after the final balloon inflation. (From Serruys, P.W., et al.: A comparison of two methods to measure coronary flow reserve in the setting of coronary angioplasty: Intracoronary blood flow velocity measurements with a Doppler catheter and digital subtraction cineangiography. Eur. Heart J. 10:731, 1989, with permission.)

SUMMARY

Three techniques are now available for the assessment of regional coronary flow reserve during cardiac catheterization. The first uses a pulsed Doppler coronary artery catheter that can measure intracoronary blood flow velocity.[W1] The second technique is based on the radiographic assessment of myocardial perfusion using contrast medium,[V4, Z8] and the third technique is an indicator-dilution technique with a standard angioplasty catheter or guidewire equipped with microelectrodes, using a 5 percent glucose solution (D5W) as the indicator.[V8–V10, V12] In addition, positron emission tomography allows a noninvasive assessment of flow reserve to specific vascular territories.

The intracoronary administration of contrast medium results in profound alterations in coronary blood flow, characterized by depression in the first seconds, followed by hyperemia.[B28, H10] The magnitude and timing of these changes depend primarily on the iodine concentration, injection rate, and amount of the contrast medium.[H10] The hyperemic to baseline coronary blood flow ratio nevertheless remains unchanged within the first 5 seconds after contrast medium injection when the infusion rate and the injected volume are constant.[C2, H10] The selection of the fixed-density threshold influences the measured myocardial contrast medium appearance time, and thus the resulting coronary flow reserve. However, when this threshold is chosen so that background noise is eliminated and more than 90 percent of pixels in the chosen region-of-interest reach the threshold, this influence is insignificant.[Z8]

Although we found a clear relationship among percent area stenosis (AS), absolute cross-sectional area (MLCA), and coronary flow reserve, individual coronary arteries with moderate disease may differ considerably in coronary flow reserve. Approaches that integrate all angiographic dimensions are conceptually attractive[K8] but are limited by the fact that coronary flow is estimated. We used theoretical flows of 1, 2, and 3 ml/sec to define the pressure-flow relationship, since resting coronary blood flow in a left anterior descending artery is 1.3 (range, 1.0 to 2.1) ml/sec.[S36]

Many other factors are potential causes of a decreased coronary flow reserve. Cardiac hypertrophy, previous myocardial infarction, anemia, polycythemia, valvular heart disease, and collateral circulation may influence coronary flow reserve; the patient population studied, therefore, always should be described carefully.[K2] Recently, Gould proposed to measure relative maximal flow as an index for the physiologic significance of an obstruction, defined as maximal flow of a stenotic artery divided (normalized) by the maximal flow of a nonstenotic artery; this index is independent of physiologic conditions and specifically reflects the physiologic stenosis severity.[G21, K21]

Applying the radiographic technique for the assessment of coronary flow reserve in our percutaneous transluminal coronary angioplasty (PTCA) study demonstrated that reserve was not restored to a normal level immediately after PTCA. There are several possible explanations for this limited restoration of coronary flow reserve. Since coronary flow reserve is a ratio of maximal and resting flow, an increase in resting flow results in a decrease of this ratio. Although several investigators using the thermodilution technique have reported comparable volume flows before and after PTCA,[R24, S36] recent work performed in our laboratory with intracoronary Doppler catheters suggests that resting coronary blood flow velocity increases during the PTCA procedure.[S39] Further studies are necessary to resolve this controversy. Metabolic, humoral, or myogenic factors may limit coronary flow reserve after PTCA. The metabolic derangements due to the PTCA seem quickly reversible, as shown by the fast decline of temporarily increased lactate, hypoxanthine, and K^+ concentrations.[S36, W17] The long-standing reduction in perfusion pressure distal to the stenotic lesion may induce alterations in the complex mechanism of coronary blood flow autoregulation,[B24] and a prolonged period of time might be needed before these abnormalities subside.[W18] Finally, the impaired coronary flow reserve could be directly related to the residual stenosis. The cross-sectional obstruction area measured immediately after percutaneous transluminal coronary angioplasty generally is about threefold increased as a result of the procedure but remains grossly abnormal.[J4, S13, Z10]

Multiple factors potentially contribute to the variability in the measurement of coronary flow reserve; these will be summarized briefly in the following paragraphs:[Z9]

First, *x-ray gantry settings and voltage and current of the x-ray generator must be identical* to permit a valid comparison of the myocardial contrast density measurements on both the baseline and hyperemic cineangiograms.

Cinefilm development must be very stable. This point, of course, is not present when using an on-line digital cardiac imaging system.

Many patient-related factors are important determiners of the measured coronary flow reserve. Changes in heart rate may influence the coronary flow reserve.[D8, F13] Furthermore, subtraction of the digitized selected end-diastolic frames is possible only when a strictly regular rhythm is present; therefore, atrial pacing is mandatory. Changes in blood pressure can influence coronary flow reserve in two ways.[H9] Firstly, myocardial oxygen consumption and therefore baseline coronary blood flow are to a large degree determined by the systemic arterial pressure. Since flow reserve is defined as the ratio of maximal to resting coronary blood flow, an increase in resting blood flow as a result of an increase in myocardial oxygen consumption results in a decrease of this ratio. Secondly, the coronary blood flow during maximal coronary vasodilation is linearly related to the coronary driving pressure.[D6] Angiograms that are used for the calculation of flow reserve during baseline and hyperemic conditions, or repeated radiographic coronary flow reserve measurements, should thus be obtained at the same blood pressure.

A prerequisite of this radiographic technique is the use of an electrocardiographically triggered pump to inject a fixed volume at a fixed contrast injection rate.[H10, V4] Although injection of a radiographic contrast agent induces profound alterations in coronary blood flow,[B28] the ratio of hyperemic coronary blood flow to baseline flow is unaffected by the contrast agent during the first 5 seconds after injection when injection rate and volume are identical in hyperemic and baseline conditions.[C2, H10] The injection rate and volume should be sufficient to ensure complete filling of the epicardial coronary arteries with contrast during pharmacologically induced hyperemia.[C2, H10, V4] The disturbance in coronary blood flow from the radiographic contrast agent lasts for less than 20 seconds, and sequential injections of contrast agent in doses as used in this investigation do not result in persisting changes in coronary blood flow.[B28, R24, S36]

The method of induction of a hyperemic response in the coronary circulation should be reproducible. Intracoronary papaverine induces a strong and short-lasting hyperemia that is reasonably reproducible in magnitude as well as in timing.[Z6] Wilson and White recently investigated the dose of intracoronary papaverine needed to produce maximal coronary vasodilation and reported a maximal hyperemic response after 8 mg in most coronary arteries and after 12 mg in all coronary arteries.[W13]

The analysis of the cineangiogram to permit calculation of coronary flow reserve from measured myocardial contrast appearance time and density involves the selection of end-diastolic cineangiographic frames and digitization and selection of a region-of-interest. The boundaries of the ROIs are drawn by the observer with a writing tablet that is interfaced with the computer. Although the entire analysis procedure can be performed with high reproducibility, the observer-dependent selection of the boundaries of the regions-of-interest introduces inter-observer variabilities. Consequently, rigid criteria should be applied to the selection of the boundaries of the regions-of-interest, preferably in an automated manner, not dependent on the user.

In conclusion, the development of a digital angiographic technique to measure regional coronary flow reserve and computer-based quantitative analysis of the coronary angiogram, including automated contour detection, has made the assessment of the relationship between a coronary artery stenosis and its physiologic consequences possible in human beings during cardiac catheterization. Although the reduction in coronary flow reserve as a result of coronary artery disease can be predicted with reasonable accuracy by quantitative angiography in selected patients with limited coronary artery disease, in the majority of patients the measurement of flow reserve by radiographic means or by intracoronary Doppler probe is a necessary addition to quantitative angiography to assess the functional capacity of coronary arteries and to assess the results of interventions, such as percutaneous transluminal coronary angioplasty.

Applications of Quantitative Coronary Angiography

RESTENOSIS

The acute results of medical treatments and interventions are, in general, relatively simple to assess; however, the long-term results are more difficult to determine and historically have frequently been unreliable, with the immediate results often differing greatly from those of the definitive studies. Innovators and exponents of new treatments may allow their enthusiasm to compromise their objectivity. It is therefore important that any new technique is assessed objectively using a methodology with known reproducibility and in which the technical limitations are known and understood. The past 2 to 3 years has seen an explosion of new devices and techniques designed to augment or replace conventional balloon angioplasty. With the progressive improvement in the immediate success rate and the decrease in complication rate of the procedure, it has become difficult to demonstrate the efficacy of new devices and interventions by showing an improvement in the immediate results; therefore, as with coronary artery bypass surgery in the past, the attention of investigators has rightly turned from the immediate results to the long-term outcome.

Restenosis following angioplasty, a recognized late complication since the introduction of the procedure in 1977, remains its main limitation. Studies addressing the problem of restenosis, consequently, have become important to the development of the procedure, but despite this there has been no consensus on how these studies should be performed. Widely differing methodologic approaches give diverse and conflicting results. Although the long-term clinical outcome will remain important in any assessment, the most objective means of assessing restenosis following angioplasty is by carefully controlled coronary angiography at the time of the procedure and at a defined follow-up time. In the past, visual estimation of the angiographic films has been used; fortunately, a consensus is now beginning to emerge that demands the use of a quantitative angiographic measuring system for assessing both the immediate and the long-term results of percutaneous transluminal coronary angioplasty. In addition, exercise-redistribution thallium-201 scintigraphy has been shown to be highly predictive of the occurrence of restenosis.[W24, W25]

Angiographic Definitions

The definition of choice of restenosis has been the subject of much debate; currently, no satisfactory definition takes into account both the functional and angiographic outcome of the patient after percutaneous transluminal coronary angioplasty.

The confusion and controversy that surround the subject of restenosis are essentially due to four factors. The first is that many angiographic definitions try to combine the angiographic outcome with a clinical outcome. This known discrepancy between these two parameters means that the objective will not be realized, particularly in multivessel disease.[V11] Secondly, a single "stenosis" measurement should not be confused with a measurement of "restenosis," which should represent the change in stenosis severity. Thirdly, definitions based on a cut-off value at follow-up, or related to the improvement in lesion diameter obtained at angioplasty, will preselect those lesions with a less satisfactory result postangioplasty. The definition of a $\geqslant$ 50 percent diameter stenosis at follow-up is used to illustrate this point in Figure 13–42. Fourthly, definitions based on percent diameter stenosis measurements may fail to identify lesions undergoing significant deterioration. These criteria are chosen to reflect the change in minimal luminal diameter in relation to the so-called "normal diameter" of the vessel in the immediate

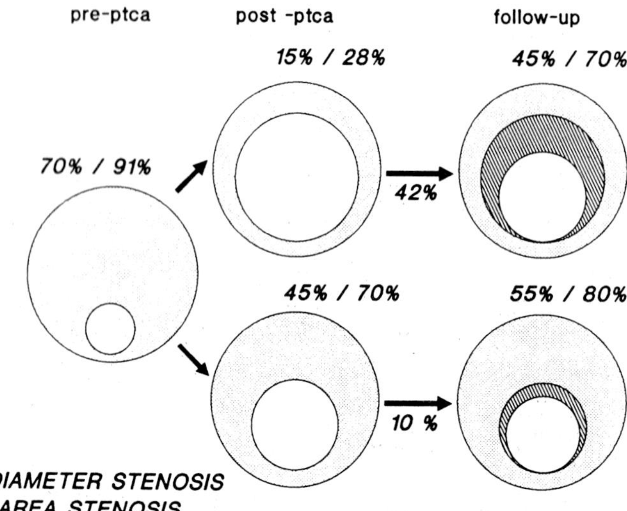

Figure 13–42. Two possible outcomes of an initially severe lesion following angioplasty are shown in terms of cross-sectional area. On the left, the lesion is shown prior to percutaneous transluminal coronary angioplasty (PTCA) with a 70 percent diameter stenosis (91 percent area stenosis). A good result, represented by the upper profile, leads to a 15 percent diameter stenosis (28 percent area stenosis). At follow-up, a 42 percent change in the area stenosis has occurred and is represented by the shaded area in the top circle on the right. Although a considerable increase in the plaque area is present, the follow-up diameter stenosis is only 45 percent; therefore, using the criterion of diameter stenosis greater than 50 percent at follow-up, one may designate this result as no restenosis. On the other hand, the lesion represented by the bottom circle, which is successfully dilated but to a lesser degree (45 percent diameter stenosis following PTCA), is designated as restenosis even if only a 10 percent deterioration occurs in the plaque area, which results in a diameter stenosis of 55 percent.

vicinity of the obstruction. It assumes that this normal diameter, or the reference diameter of the vessel, proximal or distal to the obstruction, does not change either as a result of angioplasty or during the immediate follow-up period when restenosis of the dilated lesion is a well-recognized phenomenon. Quantitative angiographic studies have shown this premise to be false, and these studies seriously question the use of percent diameter stenosis as the only index of restenosis.[B11] Figure 13–43 illustrates how the choice of reference diameter may influence the assessment of restenosis in what is a relatively simple segment to analyze. The "moving baseline" created by the fact that the reference diameter may decrease means that lesions that should be regarded as restenosis are not.

What is the rationale for the use of restenosis criteria in current use? Most are entirely arbitrary, some are based on doubtful logic, and some, although of some relevance for visual estimation of percent diameter stenosis, are unrealistic for the more accurate values obtained from quantitative angiography. The commonly used definitions of restenosis are:

- Loss of at least 50 percent of the initial gain achieved at percutaneous transluminal coronary angioplasty.
- Decrease of at least 30 percent in the lumen diameter, compared with the post-PTCA result.
- A return to within 10 percent of the preangioplasty diameter stenosis.
- An immediate post-PTCA diameter stenosis of less than 50 percent that increases to 50 percent or greater at follow-up.
- Same as the preceding, but for a diameter stenosis of 70 percent or greater at follow-up.
- Deterioration of 0.72 mm or greater in minimal luminal diameter from post-PTCA to follow-up.
- Deterioration of 0.5 mm or greater in minimal luminal diameter from post-PTCA to follow-up.

Let us consider again, for example, the commonly used definition of 50 percent or more diameter stenosis at follow-up. This is historically based on the physiologic concept of coronary flow reserve and is chosen because it represents the approximate value in animals with normal coronary arteries at which a blunting of the hyperemic response occurs.[G6] Although this value may be of some relevance in determining a significant stenosis in human atherosclerotic vessels, it tells us nothing of the way the lesion has behaved since the angioplasty procedure. It is clear from Figure 13–42 that no criterion defining the restenosis process, as such, can include the second example and not the first. Similar arguments concerning a bias in selection can be applied to the other commonly used definition of "a loss of greater than 50 percent of the gain."

Quantitative angiographic studies allowed the introduction of a new concept for the definition of restenosis based on the change in minimal luminal diameter.[S55] The change in this value from post-PTCA to follow-up can be expected to give a good quantitative measurement of the degree of restenosis. This restenosis criterion, or the cut-off point dividing the restenosis group from the nonrestenosis group, is then derived by determining the variability of measurement (1 SD of the difference in means) of the same lesion taken from separate catheterization sessions. Twice the variability (95 percent confidence intervals) reasonably differentiates those lesions that have undergone significant deterioration from those that have not. Reiber and associates found this value to be 0.72 mm, based on cineangiograms taken 90 days apart,[R16] whereas Nobuyoshi and colleagues, using a different measurement system and angiograms taken 7 to 10 days apart, found a value of 0.5 mm.[N10] It is important to realize that the variability will be greater for angiograms taken from repeat catheterizations as opposed to repeat angiograms from the same session,[R16] something that has not been appreciated by all investigators using this methodology.[S56]

Criteria on the absolute change in minimal luminal diameter are nevertheless limited, as they make no attempt to relate the extent of the restenosis process to the size of the vessel. What may be a significant increase in plaque area in a 1.5-mm-diameter vessel may be of no hemodynamic consequence in a larger vessel of 3.5 mm. Studies are needed to assess the variability of measurement in vessels of different diameter, creating "sliding scale" criteria that adjust for vessel size.

Incidence

The incidence of restenosis, therefore, depends greatly on the definition of restenosis used (Table 13–29); if based on changes in the percent diameter stenosis, the immediate post-PTCA result also will be an influencing factor. The choice of definition is responsible for the largest variation in the reported restenosis rates; similarly, as the method of analyzing an angiographic frame will influence the percent diameter stenosis measurement, it will influence the restenosis rate. Figure 13–44 shows the number of lesions fulfilling three different criteria of restenosis: although 43 of the lesions satisfying at least one criterion are included by all three, N = 39 (32 percent of N = 121) of those included in one of the criteria ("a loss of greater than half the gain") are not included in either of the other two. Despite this discrepancy, the incidence of restenosis is not too dissimilar, ranging from 21 to 34 percent. What should be clear is that a similar incidence of restenosis with different criteria may be defining different populations. This point has particular relevance when one determines the risk factors for restenosis: if restenosis cannot be determined reliably, then it is unlikely that the associated risk factors will be identified reliably.

The most sensitive index of restenosis is that of a loss of ≥ 50 percent of the gain, with reported incidences ranging from 16 to 52 percent. It follows that the definition of a loss of ≥ 20 percent of the gain generally will give higher restenosis rates. Conversely, a ≥ 50 percent diameter stenosis at follow-up will tend to give a lower incidence of restenosis, as lesions that deteriorate significantly but remain within the 0 to 50 percent range are not designated as restenosis. Of the two studies with larger numbers that document the change in minimal luminal diameter, only one uses this value to derive a restenosis value of 26 percent at 4 months.[S55]

The use of quantitative angiography has given valuable insight into the problem of defining an incidence of restenosis. Beatt

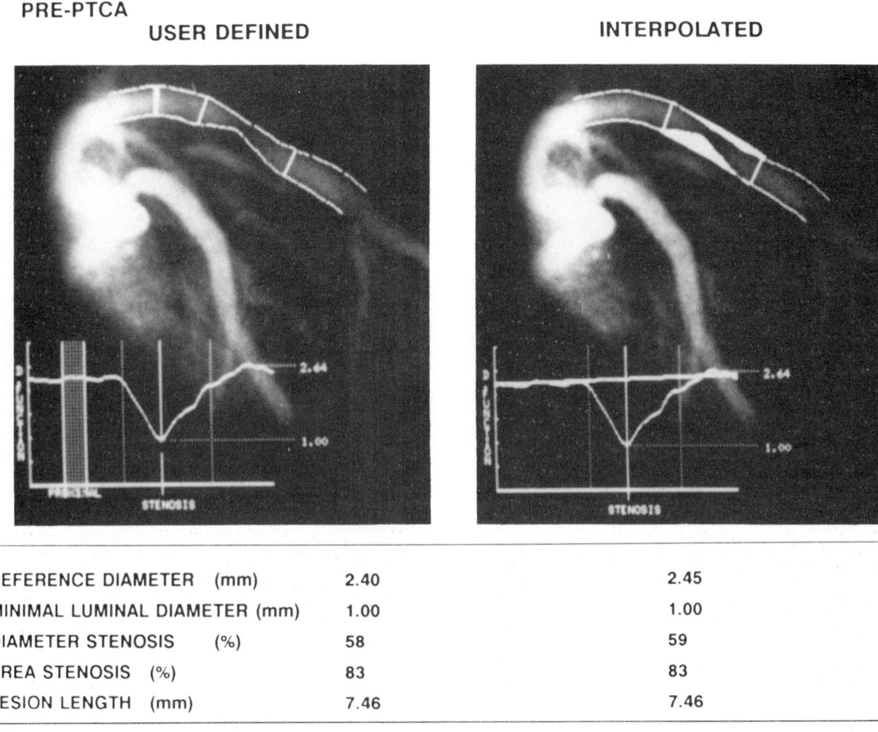

	USER DEFINED	INTERPOLATED
REFERENCE DIAMETER (mm)	2.40	2.45
MINIMAL LUMINAL DIAMETER (mm)	1.00	1.00
DIAMETER STENOSIS (%)	58	59
AREA STENOSIS (%)	83	83
LESION LENGTH (mm)	7.46	7.46

A

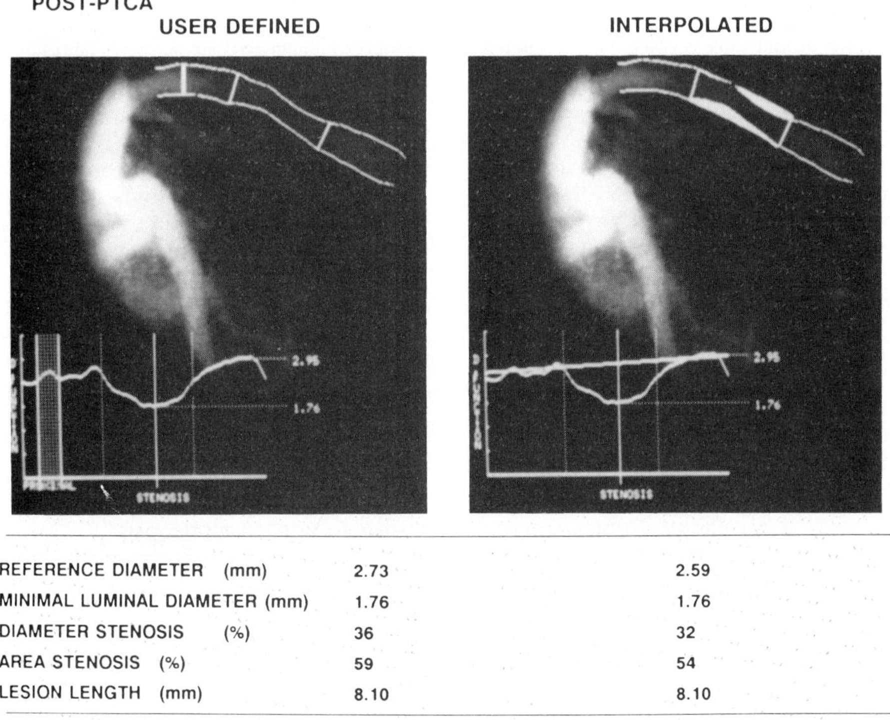

	USER DEFINED	INTERPOLATED
REFERENCE DIAMETER (mm)	2.73	2.59
MINIMAL LUMINAL DIAMETER (mm)	1.76	1.76
DIAMETER STENOSIS (%)	36	32
AREA STENOSIS (%)	59	54
LESION LENGTH (mm)	8.10	8.10

B

Figure 13–43. A series of single-frame angiograms shows a proximal left anterior descending stenosis prior to dilatation *(A)*, following dilatation *(B)*, and at follow-up *(C)*. Quantitative coronary analysis was performed with the Thoraxcenter CAAS system. The arterial boundaries detected by the system are shown on the angiogram, as are the diameter functions, derived from these contours. This example is chosen to illustrate the importance of the choice of the reference diameter, to emphasize the fact that the dilated but nonstenotic coronary artery may be involved in the restenosis process, and to demonstrate the value of the interpolated reference diameter for calculating the appropriate diameter stenosis.

A, Prior to percutaneous transluminal coronary angiography (Pre-PTCA), the lesion is relatively easy to analyze. The segments that are proximal and distal to the stenosis are of similar caliber, and the lesion is relatively discrete, so that the length of the lesion can be easily defined on the diameter function curve.

B, Following PTCA (Post-PTCA), the user-defined diameter stenosis decreases from 58 to 36 percent (area stenosis decreases from 83 to 59 percent), producing a satisfactory result. According to the interpolated technique, the percentages diameter and area stenoses decrease from 58 to 36 percent, and from 83 to 59 percent, respectively. Following PTCA, the interpolated technique indicates a slightly less severe obstruction compared with that indicated by the user-defined technique.

Illustration continued on following page

FOLLOW-UP

	USER DEFINED PROXIMAL	USER DEFINED DISTAL	INTERPOLATED

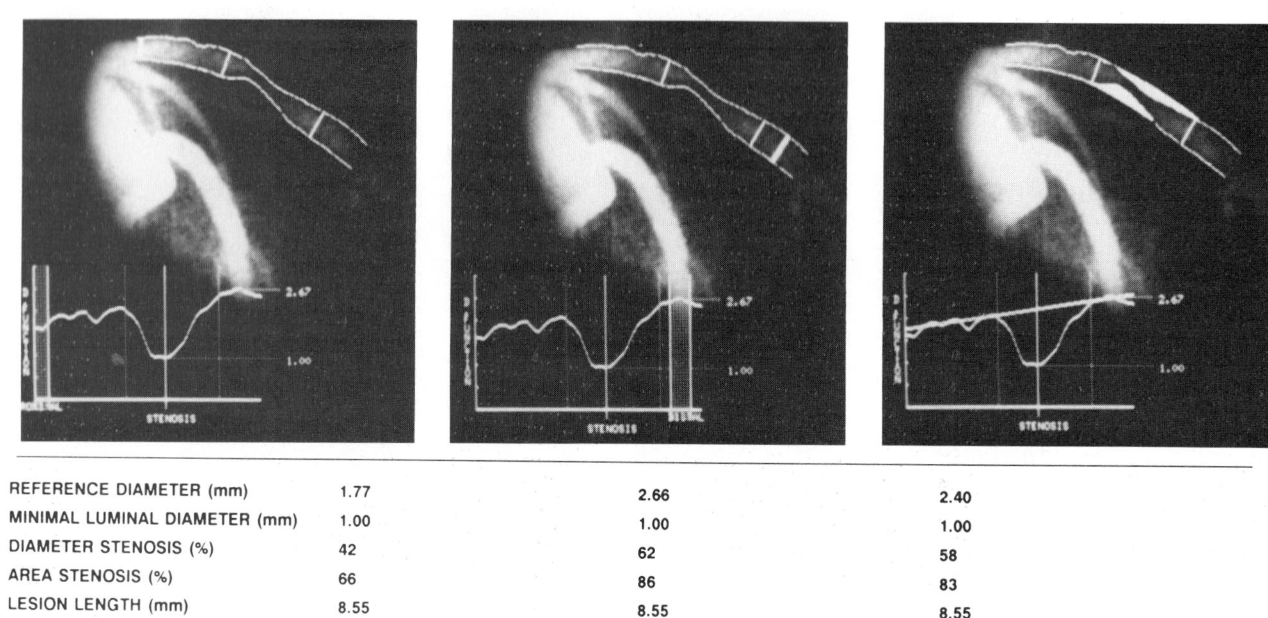

	USER DEFINED PROXIMAL	USER DEFINED DISTAL	INTERPOLATED
REFERENCE DIAMETER (mm)	1.77	2.66	2.40
MINIMAL LUMINAL DIAMETER (mm)	1.00	1.00	1.00
DIAMETER STENOSIS (%)	42	62	58
AREA STENOSIS (%)	66	86	83
LESION LENGTH (mm)	8.55	8.55	8.55

C

Figure 13–43. *Continued C*, At FOLLOW-UP, the result greatly depends on the method of analysis. Clearly the proximal artery has been involved in the restenosis process, and if this arterial portion is chosen as a reference diameter, a 42 percent diameter stenosis is found. The distal portion is of a larger caliber, and if this portion is chosen as a reference diameter, then the result is a 62 percent diameter stenosis. If the interpolated technique is used, a reference diameter similar to that of the post-PTCA value is obtained, and a 58 percent diameter stenosis is found. This finding accurately reflects the change occurring in the period between the PTCA and the follow-up. Even with this high-quality angiogram of a well-visualized segment with a discrete stenosis, however, considerable problems are encountered in attempts to obtain accurate and realistic results.

and associates have demonstrated that the restenosis process takes place to some extent in most of the lesions dilated; furthermore, it takes place in not only the stenotic portion, but also in the dilated but nonstenotic segments.[B11] This latter observation has been noted by others, but its implications have not been recognized by many investigators in the field. This observation in itself demands the use of a measurement system that will define the change in the minimal luminal diameter independent of the change in the "reference diameter."

Timing

It has been clear for some time that restenosis takes place within the first 6 months following dilatation.[H12, K22] Further progression after this time is unusual, with lesion improvement or deterioration occurring in a small number of lesions; this pattern is characteristic of coronary artery disease in general.[B36, K23] More detailed studies have shown that early "recoil" of the dilated artery occurs within 30 minutes of dilatation.[S57] This, together with some early remodeling, rather than the restenosis process, results in "restenosis" in 11 to 16 percent of lesions within the first 24 hours. It then appears that healing and remodeling may lead to improvement in an appreciable number of lesions, so that at 30 days the restenosis rate lies between 6 and 13 percent. Between 1 and 3 months, most lesions that will develop restenosis do so, with the restenosis rate reaching 25 to 37 percent. A small number may show further progression between 4 and 6 months. In reality, it seems likely that the

Table 13–29. STUDIES ADDRESSING THE INCIDENCE OF RESTENOSIS

Author (Ref.)	Year	No. of Patients	Follow-Up (%)	Interval PTCA–F.U. *(Months)*	Restenosis Criterion	Restenosis (%)
Corcos et al. (C13)	1985	92	100	8.2	DS ≥ 70%	18.5
Meyer et al. (M17)	1983	70	90	6	AS ≥ 85%	20
Leimgruber et al. (L14)	1986	1758	57	7	DS ≤ 50%	30.3
Thornton et al. (T4)	1984	248	72	6–9	NHLBI 4	31
Holmes et al. (H12)	1984	665	84	6.2	NHLBI 4	33.6
Levine et al. (L19)	1985	100	92	6	NHLBI 4	40
Galan et al. (G22)	1988	160	100	7 ± 7	DS ≥ 50%	47
Vandormael et al. (V11)	1987	129	62	7	≥20% reduction and ≥50% DS	33
STUDIES ADDRESSING THE TIMING AND INCIDENCE OF RESTENOSIS						
Serruys et al. (S55)	1988	400	85	1	≥0.72 mm	0.9
				2	≥0.72 mm	12.4
				3	≥0.72 mm	22.6
				4	≥0.72 mm	25.5
Nobuyoshi et al. (N10)	1988	185	81	24 hours	NHLBI 4	14.6
		229	100	1	NHLBI 4	12.7
		219	96	3	NHLBI 4	43.0
		149	65	6	NHLBI 4	49.4

DS—percent diameter stenosis; AS—percent area stenosis; NHLBI 4—loss of ≥50% of gain; F.U.—follow-up.

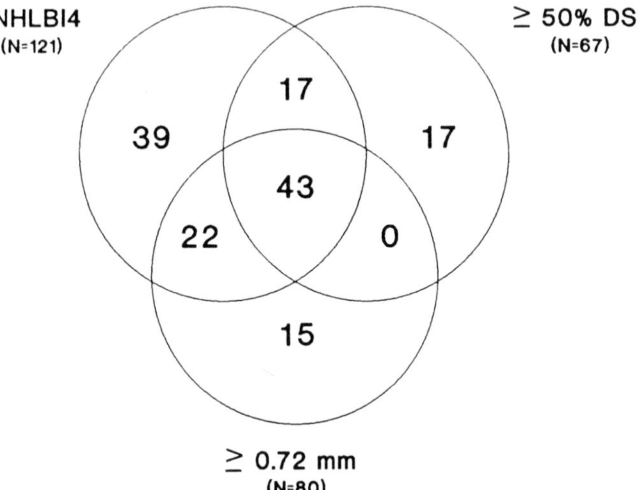

Figure 13–44. The numbers of lesions fulfilling three different restenosis criteria are illustrated. Lesions were taken from a population of 490 lesions followed up within 6 months of percutaneous transluminal coronary angioplasty. The total numbers of lesions that fulfill each criterion are shown in parentheses. Numbers of those lesions fulfilling only that particular criterion and none of the others are enclosed in the diagram by only one circle. The numbers of lesions satisfying two criteria are enclosed by two circles, and the number of lesions that fulfill all three criteria (N = 43) is shown overlapped by all three circles. One can see that lesions designated as restenotic depend greatly on the criteria for restenosis employed. Quantitative coronary angiography enables this type of comparison to be performed. DS = diameter stenosis; NHLBI4 = criterion 4 of the National Heart Lung and Blood Institute: loss of greater than 50 percent of the gain at angioplasty.

restenosis process begins early and is progressive over the first 3 to 4 months.[N10, S55] This early change has been shown in animals, in which there is evidence of smooth muscle cell proliferation as early as 7 to 14 days following dilatation. This same process has been identified in at least 7 postmortem hearts that were examined over a similar time period (17 to 150 days post-dilatation).[A11, E1, W23] However, with the presently known limitations of our measurement systems, we are not able to detect significant deterioration until after 30 days.

Methodologic Considerations

Clinical studies on restenosis are demanding of time and financial resources, as well as hard on the patient because of the need for repeat angiography, even if the patient is asymptomatic. It is important, therefore, particularly with studies that look at the impact of a new intervention on restenosis, that a suitable methodology be adopted—one capable of showing the effect of the intervention, if indeed one exists. Many of the studies published so far have failed to adopt an exacting methodology as a basis for their conclusions. In principle, three areas need to be addressed:

- *Population.* If the results are intended to apply to the PTCA population, the study population must reflect this. This means a high angiographic follow-up rate, with the time to restudy being predetermined at the time of percutaneous transluminal coronary angioplasty and not influenced by the recurrence of symptoms or the anatomy of the lesion post-PTCA. This will avoid a selection bias of symptomatic patients, or patients with borderline post-PTCA results.
- A well-validated *system of analysis* should be employed that has known accuracy and variability. The use of visual percent diameter stenosis measurements precludes meaningful results; edge tracing and visual techniques that produce physiologically impossible values are also unacceptable.
- The *measured parameters* must be chosen so as to reflect the restenosis process; the conventional assessment of percent diameter stenosis will not do this.

Videodensitometric Analysis

Videodensitometric analysis has not proved practical in large studies addressing the problem of restenosis. Although the technique is promising, the number of lesions that can be analyzed effectively by this technique is limited because of the present limitations (see "Densitometry" in the preceding section, "Approaches to Quantitative Coronary Angiography"). As a result, the use of a videodensitometric technique would mean that a large number of patients undergoing routine percutaneous transluminal coronary angioplasty would have to be excluded from restenosis studies. If further developments are successful, densitometry may become the method of choice for restenosis studies; the great advantage of this approach is that only one angiographic projection is necessary to obtain three-dimensional information about the vessel of interest.

Risk Factors

No studies using quantitative coronary angiography report on the risk factors in large numbers of patients. If restenosis cannot be reliably determined, it seems unlikely that the associated risk factors can be reliably identified. A small number of factors relating to the restenosis process have been identified and confirmed in more than one study. These include a proximal left anterior descending coronary artery stenosis, a totally occluded vessel pre-PTCA, and associated insulin-dependent diabetes. Risk factors that relate to the PTCA procedure, such as a residual stenosis of greater than 30 or 40 percent, should not be considered as risk factors for restenosis with our current knowledge. For most of the other risk factors described, it seems that as many studies do not identify a particular factor as studies that do. Quantitative angiography offers the possibility of objective measurement of lesion morphology, such as the length of the lesion and its eccentricity; when this more objective information is applied to large population studies, perhaps then it will be possible to identify lesion-related factors associated with restenosis.

SUMMARY

To date, quantitative coronary angiography has been used in a limited number of studies addressing the problem of restenosis. It has already provided valuable insight into the restenosis problem and has identified some of the sources of confusion surrounding this topic. It seems likely that with better measurement systems, particularly those that become available on-line in the catheterization laboratory, it will be easier to perform these studies; with more reliable data in smaller numbers of patients, the effect of various interventions to prevent restenosis will be assessed more accurately and efficiently.

EFFICACY OF ENDOLUMINAL PROSTHESES

Since the introduction of percutaneous transluminal coronary angioplasty (PTCA) in 1977,[G19] continuing improvements in the angioplasty technique have led to a high initial success rate and broad clinical application.[D9, F14] However, the rate of restenosis during the first 6 months after the procedure is still high (30 to 40 percent); thus, restenosis remains one of the main limitations of this therapeutic procedure.[B25, H12, L14, M12, M13]

Although other techniques—pharmacologic,[L14] mechanical,[R27, S52, S60] and thermal[A7, C7]—are currently under investigation, intravascular stenting of the dilated vessels has been proposed as an alternative approach for preventing late restenosis after percutaneous transluminal coronary angioplasty. Different prostheses have been developed and tested in animal experiments,[C8, D10, M14, P7–P9, R28, S18, S53, S54, W16] and recently intravascular stents have been implanted in patients.[P4, S18, S23] The endoprosthesis used in this open clinical trial consists of a self-expanding stainless steel mesh

(Medinvent), which exerts an active radial force on the vascular wall after deployment. However, no quantitative angiographic data indicate whether this ongoing outward force affects the immediate anatomic result of balloon angioplasty. On the other hand, since animal experiments have shown a neointimal proliferation totally encasing stent wires within a few weeks,[P8, P9, W16] it is crucial to demonstrate that the stenosis geometry of the human stented artery does not deteriorate at short-term follow-up.

We devised and carried out a study to assess early morphologic changes in stenosis geometry by quantitative coronary angiography after stenting of coronary arteries.[P10, S43]

Methods

PATIENTS. Twenty-six patients (twenty men, six women) were studied. They were treated and investigated in five European centers.* The endoprosthesis used in this study was provided by Medinvent SA, Lausanne, Switzerland, and inserted as previously described.[S18] The dilated and stented coronary artery was the left anterior descending artery in 19 cases, the left circumflex artery in 2 patients, the right coronary artery in 2 cases, and a coronary bypass vein graft in 3 cases. Informed consent was obtained from each patient before the intervention.

DESCRIPTION OF THE STENT.[P4, S18, S23, S43] The stent is woven from a surgical-grade stainless steel alloy formulated according to the specifications of the International Standards Organization. The prosthesis is geometrically stable, pliable, and self-expanding; it consists of 16 wire filaments, each 0.08 mm in diameter (Fig. 13–45). Its elastic and pliable properties are such that its diameter can be substantially reduced by moderate elongation. The prosthesis can be constrained on a small-diameter delivery catheter and, as the constraining membrane is progressively removed, the elastic device assumes its original (unconstrained) larger diameter. The constrained wire-mesh prosthesis is held at the distal end of the delivery catheter by a doubled-over membrane, the outer layer of which can be progressively withdrawn (Fig. 13–46). Two radiopaque metal markers on the delivery catheter facilitate identification of the end of the prosthesis at the time of its deployment. The outer diameter of the stent-catheter system mounted on this delivery device is 1.57 mm, using prostheses that expanded to a diameter of 6.5 mm.[P10]

In this study, unconstrained stent diameter ranged from 3.0 to 3.5 mm. The selection of stent sizes depended upon the size of the arterial segment, taking into consideration that the stent in its unconstrained form must have a diameter 0.5 mm larger than the stented vessel.

QUANTITATIVE ANALYSIS. The determination of coronary arterial dimensions from 35-mm cine film was performed with the computer-based Cardiovascular Angiography Analysis System.[R4, R16] The interpolated percent area stenosis and the minimal luminal cross-sectional area (mm^2) were averaged from at least two, preferably orthogonal, projections. The length of the lesion was determined from the diameter function on the basis of a curvature analysis (Fig. 13–47).

A change greater than the total long-term measurement variability of repeated coronary cineangiography and quantitative analysis (0.36 mm for obstruction diameter; i.e., 1 standard deviation of difference of duplicate measurements) was considered significant and indicative of restenosis. This change in absolute values corresponds to a change of 6.5 percent in percent diameter stenosis.

The theoretical transstenotic pressure drop was calculated from the stenosis geometry assessed by quantitative coronary angiography for theoretical coronary blood flows of 0, 5, 1, and 3 ml/sec.[R4]

STATISTICAL ANALYSIS. Comparison between measurements obtained after percutaneous transluminal coronary angioplasty and stenting was performed using the Student's t-test for paired observations.

Results

Twenty-six patients were studied, and a mean of 1.6 ± 0.5 angiographic projections per lesion were analyzed (see Fig. 13–

*Catheterization Laboratory and Laboratory for Clinical and Experimental Image Processing, Thoraxcenter, Rotterdam, The Netherlands: K. Beatt, M.R.C.P.; M. v.d. Brand, M.D.; P.J. de Feyter, M.D.; P.G. Hugenholtz, M.D.; Y. Juillière, M.D.; J.H.C. Reiber, Ph.D.; J.R.T.C. Roelandt, M.D.; and P.W. Serruys, M.D.

Department of Cardiology, Hôpital Cardiologique, Lille, France: M.E. Bertrand, M.D.; and J.M. Lablanche, M.D.

Department of Clinical Measurement, National Heart Institute, London, United Kingdom: A.F. Rickards, M.D.; and P. Urban, M.D.

Department of Clinical and Experimental Cardiology, CHRU Rangueil, Toulouse, France: J.P. Bounhoure, M.D.; A. Courtault, M.D.; F. Joffre, M.D.; J. Puel, M.D.; and H. Rousseau, M.D.

Division of Cardiology, Department of Medicine, CHUV, Lausanne, Switzerland: L. Kappenberger, M.D.; and U. Sigwart, M.D.

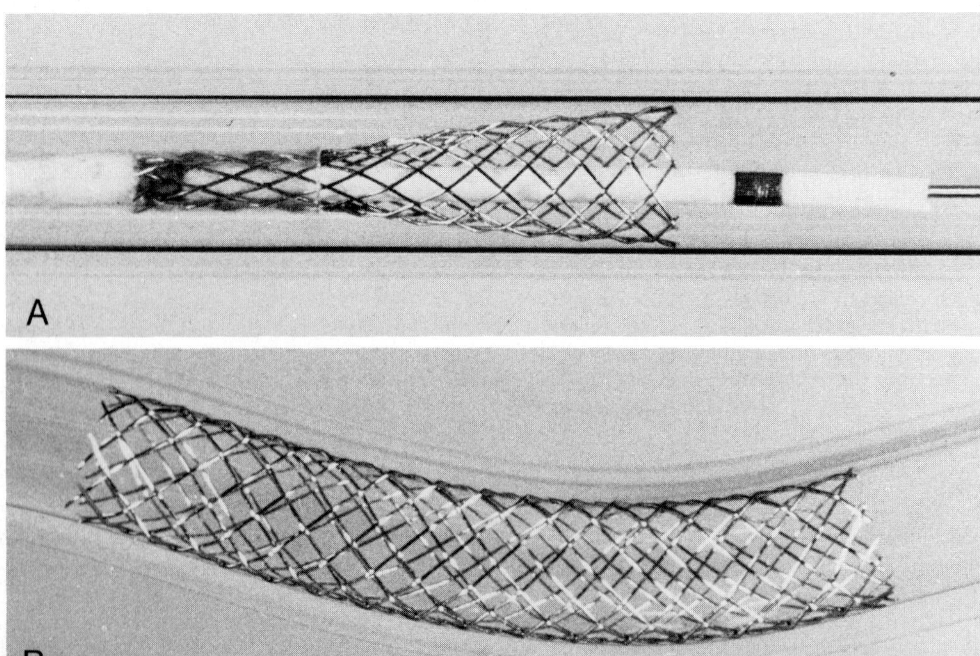

Figure 13–45. *A*, Simulated implantation in a plastic tube. A doubled-over membrane maintains the stent in a constrained elongated state. Retraction of this membrane allows the stent to be progressively released into the vascular lumen. As it is released, the stent gradually shortens and expands. *B*, Implantation within curvature of plastic tube demonstrates the stent's pliability. (From Serruys, P.W., et al.: Additional improvement of stenosis geometry in human coronary arteries by stenting after balloon dilatation. Am. J. Cardiol. 61:71G, 1988, with permission.)

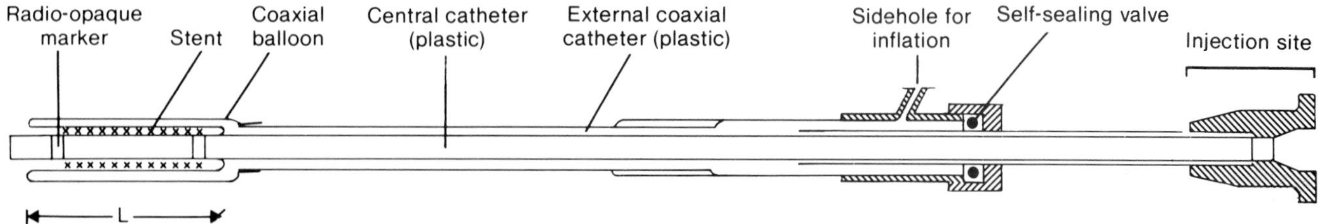

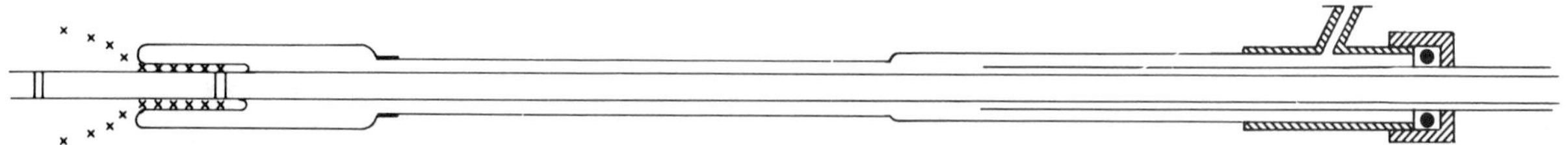

Figure 13–46. Longitudinal section of the stent delivery catheter showing the "constrained" stent surrounded by the coaxial balloon (top). After inflation of the balloon, the outer sheath of the coaxial system is retracted to allow the stent to expand within the arterial lumen (bottom). From Serruys, P.W., et al.: Additional improvement of stenosis geometry in human coronary arteries by stenting after balloon dilatation. Am. J. Cardiol. 61:71G, 1988, with permission.)

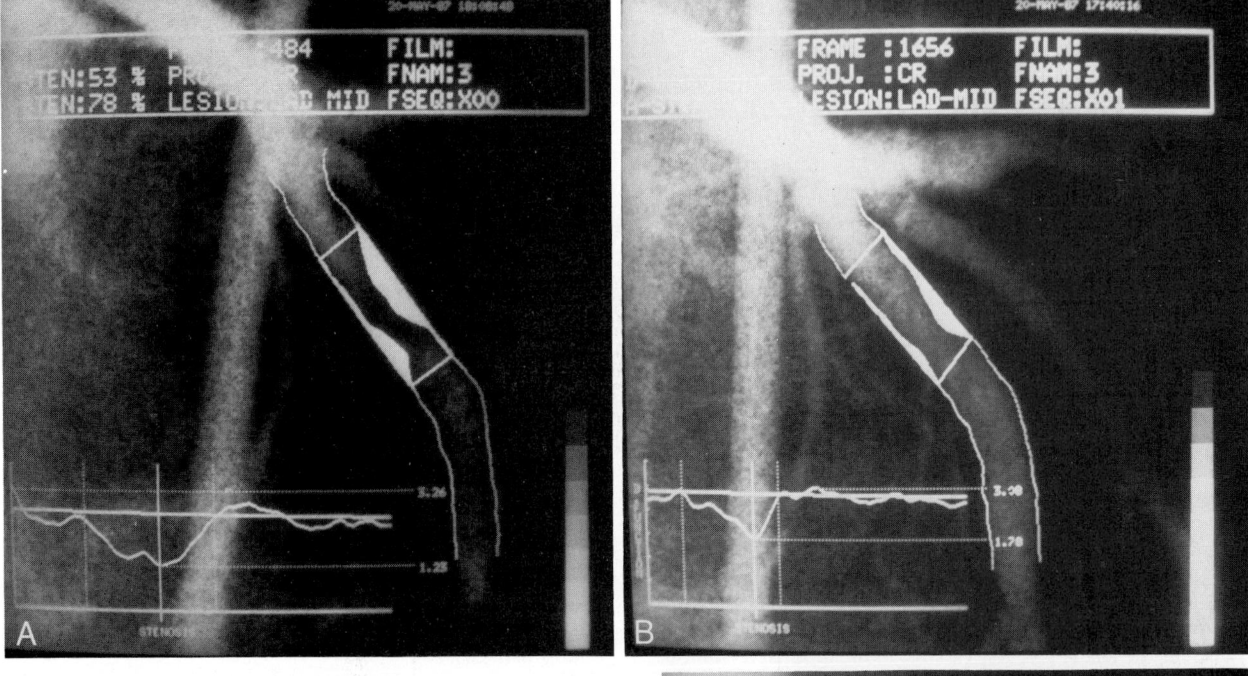

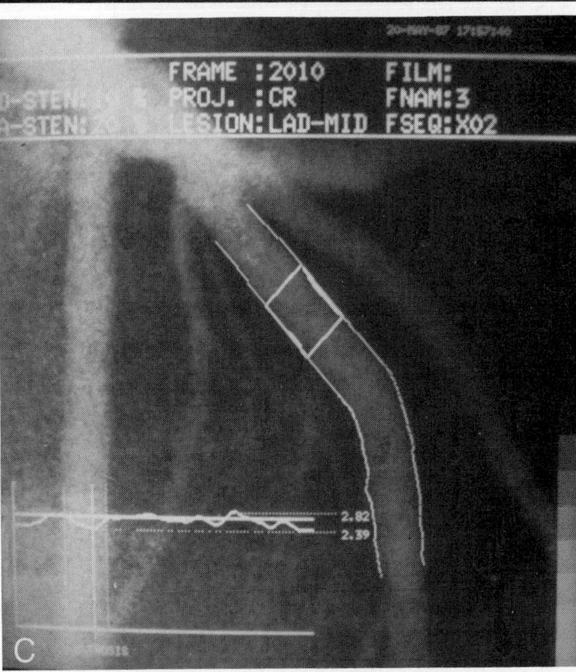

Figure 13–47. Angiograms of a left anterior descending coronary artery (cranial projection) before *(A)* and after *(B)* angioplasty, and immediately after stent implantation *(C)*, with superimposition of the automated contours of the coronary artery segment of interest. Also shown are the diameter functions of the detected contours of the coronary artery. The minimal luminal diameter (vertical line) and the interpolated reference diameter function (horizontal line) from which the reference diameter is derived are shown. (From Serruys, P.W., et al.: Additional improvement of stenosis geometry in human coronary arteries by stenting after balloon dilatation. Am. J. Cardiol. 61:71G, 1988, with permission.)

Table 13–30. MORPHOLOGIC RESULTS IMMEDIATELY AFTER STENTING

	Extent of Obstruction *(mm)*	Minimal Cross-Sectional Area *(mm₂)*	Percent Area Stenosis	Reference Area *(mm₂)*
Mean ± SD				
Pre-P	7.5 ± 0.5	1.2 ± 0.2	81 ± 2	7.3 ± 0.7
	**	*	*	n.s.
Post-P	6.9 ± 0.5	2.9 ± 0.2	55 ± 2	7.2 ± 0.7
	n.s.	*	*	n.s.
Post-S	7.3 ± 0.4	4.8 ± 0.5	36 ± 3	7.7 ± 0.7

$*p < 0.005$; $** p < 0.05$.
n.s.—not significant; P—percutaneous transluminal coronary angioplasty; S—stent; SD—standard deviation.

47). The morphologic and hemodynamic data (mean ± standard error of the mean) are presented in Tables 13–30 and 13–31, respectively.

Stent implantation following percutaneous transluminal coronary angioplasty resulted in an additional increase in minimal luminal cross-sectional area (Fig. 13–48) and obstruction diameter, and a decrease in percent area and percent diameter stenosis compared with the postangioplasty state. This morphologic improvement was associated with a decrease in both the turbulent and Poiseuille resistance, as well as in the theoretical transstenotic pressure drop for a theoretical flow of 1 ml/sec. The theoretical pressure gradient assumes a uniform reduction in the lumen over the entire length of the stenosis, which may not always apply to stenotic lesions, especially not to those with a more complex morphology. These data suggest that, immediately after PTCA, the endoprosthesis has an active dilating function in addition to its basic stenting (maintenance of dilated diameter) role.[S43]

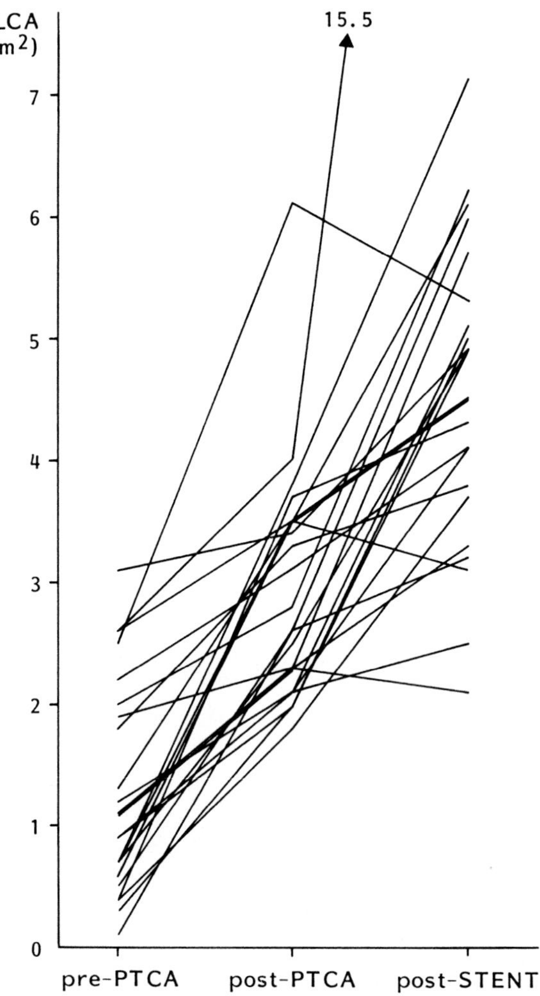

Figure 13–48. Minimal luminal cross-sectional area (MLCA) prior to percutaneous transluminal coronary angioplasty (pre-PTCA), after balloon dilatation (post-PTCA), and immediately after stent implantation (post-STENT). (From Serruys, P.W., et al.: Additional improvement of stenosis geometry in human coronary arteries by stenting after balloon dilatation. Am. J. Cardiol. 61:71G, 1988, with permission.)

Discussion

Although initial success rates for coronary angioplasty have improved, the problem of restenosis continues to compromise the overall results of the procedure.[D11] With restenosis rates ranging from 30 to 40 percent,[B25, H12, M12, R27] there is an evident need for new techniques to prevent restenosis.

A promising new approach to reduce the rate of restenosis and to help prevent abrupt reclosure is the implantation of an intravascular endoprosthesis. The principle of introducing intra-arterial grafts percutaneously was first described by Dotter in 1969.[D10] Over the last few years, variants of the original technique, using thermal-shaped memory alloys,[C8, D11, S54] expanding spring steel spirals,[S54] expanding stainless steel stents,[M16, W16] and expanding woven stainless steel meshes[P7–P9, S53] have been reported in animal experiments.

Recently, intravascular stents have been implanted in humans to prevent occlusion and restenosis after PTCA.[P4, S18, S23, S43] The endoprosthesis used in this first clinical series consisted of a new self-expandable stainless steel mesh.[S18] The present study has used quantitative coronary angiography to assess the early modifications in stenosis geometry after implantation of this new endoprosthesis.

The early assessment immediately after stent implantation showed an additional morphologic improvement over the results after balloon dilatation, demonstrating the intrinsic dilating force exerted by the stent. The questions arising with expandable vascular prostheses are (1) can a stable positioning be achieved only by expansile pressure against the vessel wall; and (2) what are the pressure thresholds to avoid serious injury, such as vessel

Table 13–31. HEMODYNAMIC RESULTS IMMEDIATELY AFTER STENTING

	Poiseuille Resistance *(dynes s cm⁻⁵)*	Turbulent Resistance *(dynes s cm⁻⁵)*	Pressure Gradient (mmHg) Flow (0.5 ml/sec)	Pressure Gradient (mmHg) Flow (1 ml/sec)	Pressure Gradient (mmHg) Flow (3 ml/sec)
Mean ± SD					
Pre-P	31.3 ± 21.2	20.1 ± 14.2	6.6 ± 1.7	16.3 ± 4.3	29.3 ± 7.1
			*	*	*
Post-P	0.7 ± 0.1	0.1 ± 0.0	3.0 ± 0.0	1.8 ± 0.1	3.2 ± 0.4
	*	*	*	*	*
Post-S	0.3 ± 0.0	0.0 ± 0.0	0.1 ± 0.0	0.3 ± 0.1	1.1 ± 0.2

$*p < 0.005$.
See abbreviations in Table 13–30.

wall pressure necrosis? Using an intravascular "double-helix" spiral prosthesis, Maass and associates showed that the preimplantation calculation of the fixation pressure can be estimated if the elasticity module of the material, the thickness of the metal wire, and the radii of the unconstrained as well as the partially expanded spiral prosthesis are known.[M16] Their experiments in dogs indicate that pressures up to 300 mmHg are well tolerated in the venous and arterial systems. In the former, however, this may represent an upper limit, whereas in the arterial system, a higher pressure probably can be sustained. Perforation, deep pressure marks, or cutting effects of the spiral coils were observed only in pressures exceeding 3000 mmHg. Sigwart and associates have indicated that this prosthesis has an elastic radial force that tends to dilate the artery when the vessel caliber is less than that of the unconstrained stent diameter.[S18] Dilatation continues until an equilibrium is achieved between the circumferential elastic resistance of the arterial wall and the dilating force of the prosthesis. Previously, Wright and Wallace and group showed that the expansile pressure depends on the recipient vessel diameter and on the intrinsic dilating force of the stent itself.[L18, W16] The present study confirms—in human beings—the dilating capacity of the stent.

All long-term experimental studies have shown that, in animals, neointimal proliferation produces a covering of the stent's luminal surface. The time taken for the endothelialization process to cover the stent surface depends on the thickness of the wire filaments (3 weeks for the prosthesis used in this study).[P7, P8, S18, W16] Neointimal thickening varies from 0.2 to 0.5 mm[P9, S18] and depends on the diameter of the prosthesis.[P8] However, most investigators have not found important angiographic reductions in vessel diameter after stent implantation,[C8, P8, S18, W16] except for Dotter in his initial study.[D10] In a previous study with conventional analysis of in vivo arteriograms, neointimal thickening was not described.[P9] In contradistinction, a recent study from our group demonstrated that a small, diffuse narrowing of the vessel's lumen is detectable by quantitative coronary angiography.[P10] In this latter study, neointimal proliferation was estimated to produce a 0.2-mm reduction in the vessel diameter, corresponding to an 11 ± 3 percent reduction in the percent diameter stenosis. These results are consistent with animal studies on neointimal thickening occurring after stent implantation.[P9, S18]

Summary

Percutaneous implantation of the self-expandable stainless steel endoprosthesis is a new technique to prevent restenosis after human coronary angioplasty. The dilating radial force of the stent is responsible for an additional improvement in the results of angioplasty. Intravascular stenting may be a promising complementary technique to coronary angioplasty to prevent abrupt closure and late restenosis after percutaneous transluminal coronary angioplasty.

PROGRESSION AND REGRESSION OF ATHEROSCLEROSIS

Jacques D. Barth, M.D., Ph.D.

This section reviews lipid-lowering intervention trials and the role of computed quantitative analysis of atherosclerosis.

The evolution and natural course of atherosclerosis can be studied by examining postmortem findings and by animal and human observational intervention studies. Although the natural course of atherosclerosis is a progressive one, there is also a process called regression, which reflects the reversal of the natural progressive mechanism. Total cholesterol and LDL cholesterol in particular are positively correlated to the progression of atherosclerosis; on the other hand, HDL cholesterol has an inverse correlation to coronary heart disease. Therefore, the latter has been identified as a possible antiatherosclerotic lipoprotein. Support for the notion of regression of atherosclerosis comes from the fact that reversal of the progressive mechanism has been observed in the aforementioned three approaches.

In this review we will restrict the concept of progression to the slow and steady progressive process of atherosclerosis within the arterial wall: the atheroma per se. This process leads to an increase in wall thickness, resulting in a decrease in the vessel luminal diameter. This process starts at an early age (second or even first decade of life) and ultimately gives rise to superimposed rapid phenomena like thrombosis, which may obstruct all blood flow through the artery.

A definition of regression of atherosclerosis should be reserved for any underlying mechanism that causes the natural progressive course to slow down or to reverse its course. Rapid reversal phenomena, such as breakage of the lining of the vessel wall or recanalization of the thrombus, may be thought of as mirror-image analogs of rapid phenomena of progression of atherosclerosis, as in thrombus formation. Thus a clear distinction should be made, both in progression and in regression, between slow and rapid phenomena.[A9]

In this review we will focus only on the cineangiographic lipid-lowering intervention studies; the role of the visual interpretation approach and the use of computer-supported quantitative analysis systems will be stressed. In addition, arguments confirming the occurrence of regression of atherosclerosis will be discussed, with particular reference to the likely relationship between cholesterol lowering and regression of atherosclerosis. Possible mechanisms will be presented and clinical implications stipulated.

Angiographic Intervention Studies

Invasive and noninvasive methods are available to assess the results of intervention studies in humans. Invasive methods rely on serial cineangiography, whereas noninvasive methods depend to a large extent on ultrasound techniques. Although angiography does not show the vessel wall itself, it nevertheless provides us with an indirect method by which one can investigate changes in luminal diameter over time. Various types of arteries have been studied: the coronaries, the carotid, and the femoral arteries. In the beginning, these intervention studies were evaluated solely by human visual interpretation. However, it became clear that the changes occurring in luminal diameter were very small, and that computer-supported quantitative methods would be necessary to obtain the required accuracy and precision in the measurements. All angiographic intervention studies reviewed here, with the exception of the study by Rafflenbeul, were aimed at lowering the serum cholesterol values (Table 13–32). However, only the studies by Blankenhorn and associates,[B30, B33] Duffield and associates,[D13] Arntzenius and associates,[A3] and Olsson and associates[O7] have been analyzed by computer-supported analysis systems with either automated contour detection of the arteries (Arntzenius, Blankenhorn) or by densitometric analysis of scan lines perpendicular to the axial line of the vessel, which allowed the assessment of an index of edge irregularity (Duffield) and of the amount of atherosclerosis (Olsson) (Table 13–33). All the other studies were interpreted either visually or by means of vernier calipers (Rafflenbeul and associates[R25] and Duffield and associates[D13]).

Öst and Stenson used sequential femoral angiograms in symptomatic patients and gave their patients the lipid-lowering drug nicotinic acid.[O6] Three of the 31 patients showed definite regression of disease.

The human coronary arterial system was studied for the first time by means of sequential angiography by Cohn and colleagues, who used nicotinic acid as the type of intervention in hyperlipemic patients.[C10] In the controlled study of 40 patients, which lasted for 1 year, no definite regression of atherosclerosis could be established.

Blankenhorn and group studied femoral arteries of hyperlipemic patients who were given clofibrate as the intervention medication; 14 of 25 patients showed definite regression.[B30]

Rafflenbeul and co-workers measured the coronary diameters with a vernier caliper in 25 patients with unstable angina pectoris, all of whom were given optimal medical treatment.[R25] Progression was seen in 11 patients; 9 patients demonstrated no changes; regression occurred in 5 of 25 patients.

Table 13–32. OVERVIEW OF HUMAN SEQUENTIAL ANGIOGRAPHIC INTERVENTION STUDIES IN ATHEROSCLEROTIC VASCULAR DISEASE

Author (*year*)	No. of Pts.	FH/N	Vessel	Interval (*yr*)	Intervention	Lipid Correlation	Definite Regression
Öst (1963)	31	?	FEM	0.9–5.6	Nic. acid	?	3
Cohn (1975)	40	FH	COR	1	Nic. acid	no	0
Blankenhorn (1978)	25	FH	FEM	1	Clofibrate	yes	14
Rafflenbeul (1979)	25	FH	COR	1	Antianginal	no	5
Kuo (1979)	25	FH	COR	3	Colestipol	yes	0
Nash (1982)	42	FH	COR	2	Colestipol	yes	0
Duffield (1983)	24	FH	FEM	1.6	Cholestyr. Nic. acid Clofibrate	yes	71/300 segments
Buchwald (1983)	22	FH	COR	3	PIB	yes	5
Nikkilä (1984)	28	FH	COR	7	Clofibrate Nic. acid	yes	9
Brensike (1984)	116	FH	COR	5	Cholestyr.	yes	18/59
Arntzenius (1985)	39	N	COR	2	Diet (PUFA)	yes	7
Olsson (1984)	63	FH	FEM	1	Nic. acid	yes	3/31
Blankenhorn (1987)	162	N	COR	2	Colestipol Nic. acid	yes	20/80

FH—Familiar hyperlipoproteinemia
N—Normal lipoprotein values
PUFA—Polyunsaturated fatty acids
FEM—Femoral artery
COR—Coronary
?—Unknown
Nic. acid—Nicotinic acid
Cholestyr.—Cholestyramine
PIB—Partial ileal bypass

Kuo and colleagues studied the lipid-lowering drug colestipol in hyperlipemic patients in a noncontrolled trial lasting 3 years.[K19] No definite regression could be detected. In a similar trial, almost identical results were presented by Nash and associates.[N8]

Duffield and group were the first to perform a controlled study on symptomatic peripheral disease with use of cholestyramine, nicotinic acid, and/or clofibrate as the intervention medication.[D13] They found definite signs of regression in 71 of 300 femoral segments.

Buchwald and associates used the partial ileal bypass (PIB) surgical technique as the lipid-lowering method. In this procedure about 2 meters of intestine were bypassed, which resulted in a profound reduction in serum cholesterol.[B31] Five of the 22 patients, who had proved to be resistant to conventional drug therapy, showed definite regression of atherosclerosis after this procedure.

Table 13–33. OVERVIEW OF TECHNIQUES USED IN INTERPRETATION OF SEQUENTIAL CINEANGIOGRAMS

Study	Measurement Technique	No. of Independent Visual Observers
Öst	visual	2
Cohn	visual	4
Blankenhorn	visual and computer*	2
Rafflenbeul	vernier calipers	—
Kuo	visual	3
Nash	visual	2
Duffield	vernier calipers and computer†	2
Buchwald	visual	2
Nikkilä	visual	2
Brensike	visual	3
Arntzenius	visual and computer*	2
Olsson	densitometric profile analysis‡	2
Blankenhorn	visual and computer§	2

*Automated contour detection method.
†Index of edge irregularity was measured based on integrated densitometric profiles defined perpendicular to axial line.
‡Assessment of atherosclerosis estimation based on computer-supported integrated densitometric profile analysis.
§Not yet published.

Nikkilä and colleagues, in a controlled study, obtained 9 cases of definite regression in a group of 28 hyperlipemic patients.[N9] The intervention lasted for 7 years and consisted of nicotinic acid and clofibrate.

Brensike and associates, in a 5-year controlled trial of hyperlipemic patients who were given cholestyramine, reported definite regression in 18 of 59 cases.[B32]

Arntzenius and associates used a low-fat diet enriched with polyunsaturated fatty acids as the intervention to lower serum cholesterol levels in a noncontrolled trial.[A3, B37, B38] The coronary cineangiograms were analyzed quantitatively with the CAAS in Rotterdam.[R4] A typical example of the quantitative analyses of the pre- and postintervention coronary angiograms is shown in Fig. 13–49. The large coronary arteries were divided into a total of nine coronary segments according to the recommendations by the American Heart Association.[A8] These nine coronary segments were analyzed in at least two angiographic views. For each analyzed coronary segment, the severity of an obstruction, if present, was computed in terms of relative and absolute measures; in addition, the mean diameters over the remaining normal proximal and distal parts were computed. From all quantitative diameter data two coronary scores were derived, a percentage coronary score and an absolute coronary score.

A patient was considered to have progressive disease if the absolute coronary score showed a decrease of 0.1 mm or more over the 2-year period (precoronary score minus postcoronary score). A change in the absolute coronary score of between -0.1 mm and $+0.2$ mm was considered no lesion growth; regression of the disease was defined by an increase in the absolute coronary score of 0.2 mm or more. The 2-year study demonstrated that in 7 (17 percent) of the 39 patients definite regression of coronary atherosclerosis had occurred. From this study several other interesting observations could be made:

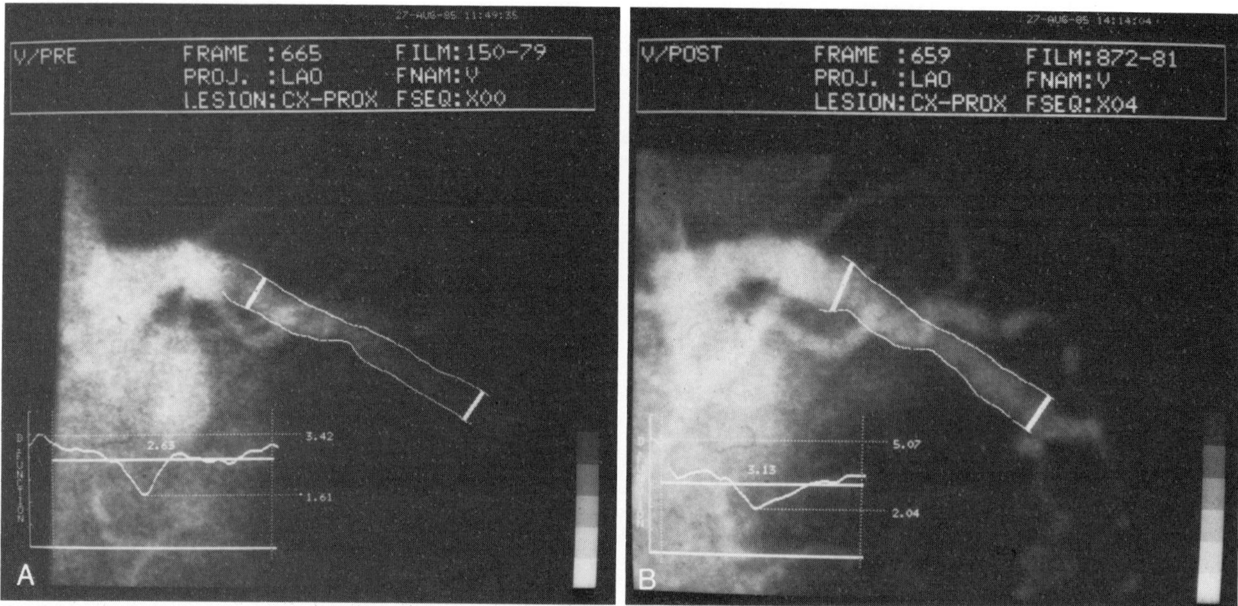

Figure 13–49. Example of quantitative results of one particular coronary segment (proximal part of right coronary artery) prior to *(A)* and following *(B)* intervention in angiographic study. Note that a decrease of approximately 0.1 mm in the minimal obstruction diameter was found at the end of the study (3.08 mm) as compared with the initial obstruction diameter (3.18 mm). Because the reference diameter showed a larger decrease than the obstruction diameter, the percent diameter stenosis also decreased, from 40 to 31 percent.

- A direct, linear, and positive correlation exists between the total cholesterol/HDL cholesterol ratio and the change over time in absolute coronary score (r = 0.50, $p<0.001$) (Fig. 13–50).[B37]
- All 5 deaths that had occurred 3.5 years following the termination of the intervention study were in the group of patients with progression of atherosclerosis ($p<0.05$) (see Fig. 13–50). No deaths occurred in the patients whose atherosclerosis was considered regressive.
- A direct and positive relationship was found between the computer-assessed positive change in absolute coronary scores and the persistence of the clinical feature of exertional angina pectoris (Table 13–34).

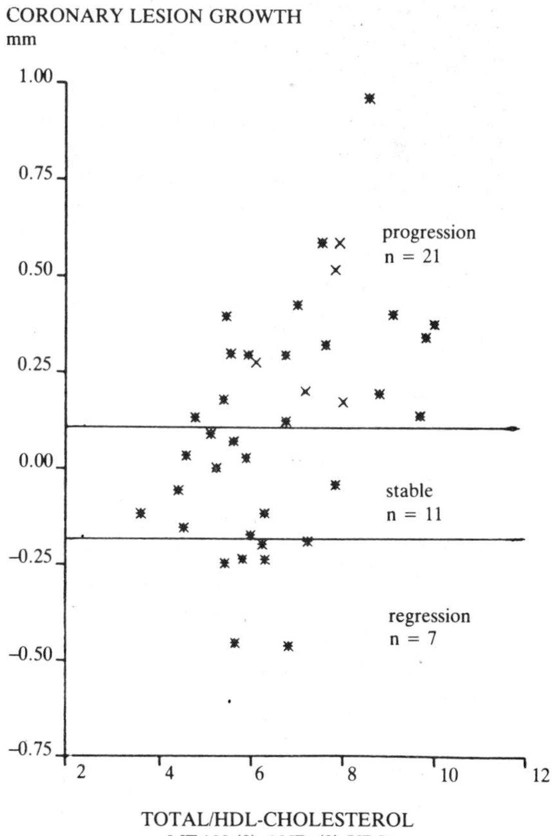

Figure 13–50. Computer assessment of change in absolute coronary score over 24-month intervention period in relationship to the lipid profile ratio of total cholesterol to HDL cholesterol (N = 39, r = 0.50, $p < 0.001$).

Values for the ratio of total cholesterol to HDL cholesterol were obtained by taking the average values of the baseline and the mean 2-year values for 39 patients. Progression of lesion growth (decrease in absolute coronary score by 0.1 mm or more) was associated with relatively high lipid ratios. Relatively low lipid ratios were more prone to appear in the stable situation (no lesion growth) with changes in absolute coronary score between +0.1 and −0.2 mm. Low lipid ratios occurred only in the regression of atherosclerotic patients (change in absolute coronary score greater than or equal to −0.2 mm). The deaths were assessed 3.5 years after termination of the trial.

- Coronary segment analysis showed that regression of atherosclerosis was more likely in left anterior descending coronary arteries than in right coronary or left circumflex arteries (Table 13–35). These trends appeared in a small group of segments; inference to a progression or regression preference after lipid-lowering therapy cannot yet be made. However, this finding may serve as an example of the possibilities that automated quantitative coronary analyses techniques may provide.

Olsson and associates also used a computerized quantitative method in the assessment of vessel lumen diameters.[O7] They found definite regression in 3 of the 31 hyperlipemic patients in a controlled study using nicotinic acid and fenofibrate for intervention.

The Cholesterol Lowering Atherosclerosis Study (CLAS) by Blankenhorn and co-workers also included sequential angiographic assessment of coronary, carotid, and femoral arteries.[B33] So far, no results have been published on the carotid or femoral artery, nor on the computerized quantitative analysis of the coronary arteries. The investigators, who used colestipol and nicotinic acid as the lipid-lowering intervention, saw definite signs of regression in 20 of the 80 patients after the 2-year study period. In this controlled study, both coronary arteries and venous aorta-coronary bypasses were analyzed.

Summary

A major concern when interpreting the results from all these intervention studies and trying to extrapolate them to the general public is that only the Leiden Intervention Trial and the Cholesterol Atherosclerosis Study included patients with normal blood lipid levels. In addition, the more accurate and reproducible quantitative analysis approaches with automated edge detection techniques were applied only in these two studies, with the results from the latter not yet published. The limitations of the visual interpretations of coronary cineangiograms have been discussed at length at the beginning of this chapter. Another confounding problem is the fact that dilation in the initial phase of atherosclerosis is a natural adaptive process, which is difficult to assess by visual analysis alone.

Glagov and group have pointed out that such initial dilation of coronary vessels during the natural progressive course of atherosclerosis may interfere with an accurate interpretation of its progression.[G10] In addition, the small changes in diameter over time and the superimposed oscillatory diameter changes during one complete heart cycle in one segment make visual interpretation alone inaccurate in lipid-lowering intervention trials.[S50]

A disadvantage of the computer approach is that usually only one frame per view is analyzed for a particular coronary segment; in the process of visual interpretation, the cardiologist incorporates mentally the data from the preceding and following frames.

Resorption of thrombotic lesions and recanalization of obstructed segments may further confound the interpretation of sequential angiograms. Interesting recent findings allow a better understanding of the phenomena of regression of atherosclerosis at the cellular level. In fact, two solubilizing systems may exist that can remove cholesterol crystals. Cholesterol, a crystalline solid at 37°C, has considerable solubility in phospholipid bilayers and cholesterol esters. After prolonged periods of low serum cholesterol, cholesterol esters disappear and crystalline cholesterol gradually dissolves, leading to true regression. As 60 percent of the total volume of the atherosclerotic plaque consists of lipids, and 95 percent of all lipids can regress, the potential removal of lipids may have a very considerable effect on the volume of the plaque.[S51] Cholesterol crystals dissolve gradually, and it may take up to 180 days to achieve complete resolution. During this period, a negative cholesterol flux must be maintained in the atherosclerotic plaque. It seems very likely that HDL cholesterol, which contains large amounts of phospholipids, may play a crucial role in lipid removal from the plaque, resulting in regression of atherosclerosis. Katz and colleagues have demonstrated that even in a severe atherosclerotic plaque the cholesterol turnover may be directed toward resolution.[K20]

It seems to us, therefore, that reversibility of atherosclerosis, from both the macroscopic and microscopic points of view, is attainable. On the basis of the data presented here, one may hypothesize that LDL cholesterol is primarily responsible for progression of atherosclerosis, whereas HDL cholesterol would be the main lipoprotein that may induce regression of atherosclerosis.[B34]

Furthermore, a problem to deal with is the fact that the original nomenclature for coronary vessels was aimed at facilitating surgical interventions and is unsuited for lipid-lowering intervention studies. A new method for assessing atherosclerotic lesion changes using sequential cineangiograms should be developed, as Conti has suggested.[C11]

A final point, assessment of changes in lesion size in atherosclerosis by repeated cineangiography remains a difficult problem. Since the development of new lesions has been shown to correlate significantly with serum cholesterol levels, we propose, as Blankenhorn has suggested, to focus on the evaluation of newly developed atherosclerotic lesions in future nonsurgical intervention studies.[B33, B35]

Table 13–34. RELATIONSHIP BETWEEN COMPUTER-ASSESSED CHANGES (2 YEARS) IN ABSOLUTE CORONARY SCORE AND THE INCIDENCE OF EXERTIONAL ANGINA PECTORIS IN THE LEIDEN INTERVENTION TRIAL[A3]

	Progression Group (N = 21)	Stable Group (N = 11)	Regression Group (N = 7)
Change in absolute coronary score (mm)	+0.35	−0.08	−0.29
Angina at termination of trial	N = 17	N = 5	N = 1 ($p < 0.001$)

Progression—decrease of 0.1 mm or more in absolute coronary score (mm) as defined by prestudy coronary score minus poststudy coronary score.

Stable—between a decrease of 0.1 and an increase of 0.2 mm in absolute coronary score.

Regression—increase of 0.2 mm or more in absolute coronary score.

Table 13–35. CORONARY SEGMENT ANALYSIS IN THE LEIDEN INTERVENTION TRIAL

Segments Studied	Number of Segments			
	Progression	*Stable*	*Regression*	*Total*
RCA Proximal	21	1	9	31
Mid	14	0	11	25
Distal	6	4	9	19
Total RCA lesions	41	5	29 (39%)	75
MAIN STEM	1	1	1 (33%)	3
LAD Proximal	15	0	9	24
Mid	8	0	11	19
Distal	5	0	2	7
Total LAD lesions	28	0	22 (44%)	50
LCX Proximal	9	2	6	17
Distal	11	5	2	18
Total LCX lesions	20	7	8 (23%)	35
Grand Total	90	13	60	163
Lesions with suspected recanalization				3
TOTAL LESIONS				166

For definitions of progression, stable, and regression, see text and Table 13–34.

RCA—right coronary artery; LAD—left anterior descending coronary artery; LCX—left circumflex coronary artery.

Chapter Summary

This chapter has presented an extensive overview of the major developments in off- and on-line quantitative coronary arteriography. It begins with the conclusion that sufficient evidence from the literature now indicates that the visual interpretation of the severity of coronary obstructions is no longer acceptable as the basis for scientific studies. Quantitative coronary angiographic techniques, either applied off-line or on-line, are now becoming available on a large scale, and they allow the objective morphologic and physiologic assessment of the severity of the obstructions. The anatomic/geometric and functional/physiologic approaches are complementary, so that a combination of these approaches is far better than using either one alone.

Because of the possible noncircular cross section of an obstruction, the problem of overlapping vessels, and the complex spatial orientation of the left coronary arterial system, usually four of five projections of this system are to be acquired, so that at the time of analysis the best two, preferably orthogonal, views can be selected. For the right coronary system with a much simpler configuration, two orthogonal angiographic views suffice. If it can be clearly demonstrated in the future that densitometry really provides reliable and reproducible data, a single view (optimally selected) will be all that is necessary; however, we have not achieved that point as yet. Work toward the goal of three-dimensional reconstruction and representation of coronary arterial segments should continue.

As mentioned earlier, the (user-defined) percent diameter reduction parameter is not a good parameter to describe the severity of a coronary obstruction. Several reasons can be formulated: (1) if diffuse coronary artery disease is present (most likely in patients with multivessel coronary artery disease), the reference diameter is underestimated, resulting in an underestimated percent diameter stenosis value; (2) the selection process of the normal diameter is subject to considerable individual variation, which could be minimized by the use of the interpolated percent diameter stenosis measurement; (3) in percutaneous transluminal coronary angioplasty, the reference diameter may be involved in the dilation process and therefore may be subject to the same restenosis process that takes place in initially stenotic segments; and (4) spontaneous or catheter-induced coronary spasm may exaggerate abnormalities by causing different reactions in vasomotility of normal and obstructed segments. Because of all these potential problems, the severity of a coronary obstruction should be described in absolute terms (minimal obstruction diameter, extent of the obstruction, asymmetry of the stenosis, area of the atherosclerotic plaque, and so on), all assessed from multiple angiographic views.

This section ends with a brief discussion of the possibilities and limitations of the measurement techniques for the assessment of the physiologic significance of coronary obstructions; details are presented in the section entitled "Coronary Flow Reserve." The functional significance of a lesion depends on many anatomic variables, as well as on blood viscosity and density, residual vasomotor tone, collateral perfusion, and so on; in addition, both active and passive increases in the severity of compliant coronary stenoses may occur. As a result, only under carefully controlled conditions, such as in animal experimental studies or in patients with single-vessel disease, has the quantitatively assessed percent diameter stenosis parameter, area stenosis, or the calculated pressure drop over the stenosis correlated reasonably well with coronary flow reserve measurements.

In the section titled "Approaches to Quantitative Coronary Angiography," an extensive overview is given of the different techniques that are now available for the quantitative assessment of morphologic and densitometric computer-aided analysis of coronary obstructions. The majority of the data presented were obtained from questionnaires sent to 12 widely known investigators. It was clear that most of the techniques have been developed for cine film analysis; however, these are in the same or a slightly modified format also applicable to the on-line digitally acquired data. Studies are under way to determine the differences in accuracy and precision between the digital and cine film approaches. To obtain optimal results in the digital approach, appropriate interpolation schemes may prove to be extremely important in obtaining the required number of pixels with valuable information for automated edge detection techniques; with cine film, the highest spatial resolution can be obtained with optical zooming approaches. At present, cine film is still the medium of choice for the assessment of changes in arterial dimensions in intervention studies, where very often small morphologic changes need to be determined with as high a confidence level as possible. The on-line direct digital approaches are particularly of interest as a tool for diagnostic and/or therapeutic decision-making during the catheterization procedure. However, with the use of modern small field-of-view image intensifiers (4- and 5-inch field-of-view) and these interpolation schemes, the present resolution of $512^2 \times 8$ or 10 bits may also be sufficient to perform such intervention studies using the diameter and densitometric cross-sectional area measures.

In this overview, the following topics were covered: calipers; Brown-Dodge method (the first computer-aided technique that became available); image acquisition and digitization of 35-mm cine film; on-line digital cardiac systems; computer hardware and software; contour detection approaches, including the definition of the coronary segment to be analyzed, edge definition, pincushion distortion and correction, and calibration; contour analysis approaches, including reference techniques for percent diameter stenosis measurement, roughness measures of an arterial segment, parameters derived from quantitatively analyzed segments and the combination of the results from biplane analyses; and finally densitometry. It has become clear from the overview that all these developments are rather heterogeneous and that the qualities of the various approaches are difficult to compare, because of the different evaluation studies performed and the fact that the results are often presented in different, noncomparable parameters.

In particular, the x-ray acquisition approach is hampered by many nonlinear effects, which makes a densitometric analysis of a coronary segment very difficult. The most important limitations are nonmonochromatic x-ray spectrum, beam hardening, scatter, veiling glare, for cine film the non-linear density-log(exposure) curve, overlapping vessels, and sidebranches (causing errors in the background-subtraction techniques). These difficulties can be demonstrated by the fact that so far only very few investigators have been able to show that the densitometric results from different views of the same vessel agree very closely, which must be a requirement if densitometry really works as well as one would hope. Therefore, we may conclude that with the present limitations in the accuracy and precision in densitometry, using only densitometric data to describe the severity of an obstruction may be useful in selected studies in which a great number of conditions have been fulfilled, such as coronary segment imaged en face, no intervening sidebranches, relatively homogeneous background, and so on. However, in all other applications, especially in intervention studies, where the results pre- and postintervention must be compared (from at least two angiographic views), the first choice at present must be the assessment of absolute diameter data, with the second choice being the densitometrically assessed cross-sectional area data. In other words, densitometric data may be used complementarily but should not replace the diameter data.

To evaluate changes in arterial dimensions over time, repeated (cine)angiography studies need to be performed and analyzed. It is shown in the section, "Quality Control in Quantitative Coronary Arteriography," that the angiographic investigation and the subsequent computer analysis procedure are hampered by various sources of variation. To obtain reliable and reproducible quantitative results from coronary (cine)angiograms, these variations should be minimized as much as possible. It is shown that without these precautions, the variabilities in absolute coronary dimensions may increase dramatically. On the other hand, if these precautions are followed, the variabilities in absolute dimensions from repeated cineangiographic acquisitions and analyses increase only by a factor of 1.5 to 2.2, compared with those from repeated cine film analysis alone. Topics that require the ultimate attention in this respect are (1) registration of x-ray system settings (particularly rotation and angulation); (2) administration of a vasodilative drug immediately prior to the angiographic investigation; (3) use of nonionic and iso-osmolar contrast media; (4) administration of contrast medium by ECG-triggered injector; and (5) selection of acceptable catheter material and measurement of the actual size of the catheter with a micrometer. From the viewpoint of the population size, duration, and cost-effectiveness of a study, it is of great importance to minimize this variability of the angiographic data acquisition and computer analysis procedures; therefore, further attempts toward standardization of the angiographic procedures should be taken to further decrease the remaining variabilities.

In the section on "Validation Studies," an extensive overview is given on published data on validation studies of arterial dimensions by the diameter and densitometric approaches discussed earlier. From this overview it may be concluded that it is very difficult if not impossible at this point to compare these techniques quantitatively. The absence of data on the accuracy and precision of the edge detection and analysis procedures, on the success scores under different image qualities, the computation times, and so on, as well as the use of different parameters to describe the validation results, makes comparisons very difficult. Therefore, validation procedures are proposed to validate a coronary quantification system. According to these proposals, phantom studies of coronary obstructions with dimensions of from 0.5 to 5.0 mm should be carried out under different imaging and under static and dynamic flow conditions, as well as in vivo animal studies with hollow plastic cylinders of various luminal shapes and sizes inserted in the coronary arteries, to assess the accuracy and precision of the edge detection techniques.

In addition, for densitometric studies, the hypothesis that the results are independent of the angiographic views in which these studies were acquired must be tested. To determine the reproducibility of a system, repeated analysis of a set of clinical coronary angiograms obtained under various imaging conditions must be performed to assess the inter- and intraobserver variabilities, as well as the short- and long-term variabilities in the angiographic data acquisition and image analysis. It is also proposed to describe the results from the validation studies in terms of the mean differences (accuracy) and the standard deviations (precision) of the signed differences between the true and measured values, or between the values from repeated measurements. Finally, it is shown in a cineangiographic study that the selection process of a cine frame for quantitative analysis in the end-diastolic phase of the cardiac cycle is not very critical. The variabilities in the measurements are not influenced statistically significantly if the selected frames in the same cineangiographic film sequence are out of phase by a maximum of three frames at a film speed of 25 frames/sec, or if a frame is selected exactly one cardiac cycle earlier or later.

In the section on "Coronary Flow Reserve," it is shown that three techniques are now available for the assessment of regional coronary flow reserve (CFR) during cardiac catheterization. The first uses a pulsed Doppler coronary artery catheter that can measure intracoronary blood flow velocity. The second technique is based on the radiographic assessment of myocardial perfusion using contrast medium, and the third technique is an indicator-dilution technique with a platinum-tipped PTCA guidewire, using hydrogen as the indicator; the last approach also allows the measurement of absolute coronary flow. In addition, positron emission tomography allows a noninvasive assessment of flow reserve to specific vascular territories. The implementation of the radiographic technique for cine film is described in more detail.

In patients with single-vessel coronary artery disease, good correlations have been found between the coronary flow reserve and the geometric descriptors of coronary obstructions (percent area stenosis, absolute cross-sectional area, and the calculated pressure drop). However, in patients with multivessel disease, the correlations are much lower, probably due to the presence of diffuse atherosclerosis.

In general, many potential causes exist for a decreased coronary flow reserve, one reason why the patient population studied should always be described carefully. The inter- and intraobserver variabilities, as well as the short-, medium-, and long-term variabilities in the assessment of coronary flow reserve as assessed in our laboratory are presented in detail. Again, it is shown that standardization of the angiographic acquisition technique is necessary to obtain the lowest variability values. The application of coronary flow reserve in the setting of percutaneous transluminal coronary angioplasty (PTCA) is also discussed. It is shown that the coronary flow reserve immediately after PTCA does not return to normal levels; however, in the absence of restenosis, coronary flow reserve eventually becomes normal. Comparison of the digital cineangiographic technique and the intracoronary blood flow velocity measurements with a Doppler catheter has shown high correlations. It is concluded that although the reduction in coronary flow reserve as a result of coronary artery disease can be predicted with reasonable accuracy by quantitative angiography (anatomic descriptors) in selected patients with limited coronary artery disease, in the majority of patients the measurement of flow reserve by radiographic means or by intracoronary Doppler probe is a necessary addition to quantitative angiography to assess the functional capacity of coronary arteries and to assess the results of interventions, such as percutaneous transluminal coronary angioplasty.

Recently, myocardial contrast echocardiography has been used to study the perfusion bed of a coronary artery and the nutrient myocardial blood flow. With intracoronary administration of the echocontrast agent, it seems that coronary flow reserve can be determined reasonably well. However, a true breakthrough will occur if such measurements can be obtained using an intravenous approach; this requires the development of new echocontrast agents that pass the pulmonary circulation and produce no hyperemic effects.

In the last section, three clinical applications of quantitative coronary angiography are described. The first topic relates to PTCA and the problem of restenosis. It is shown that at present there has been no consensus on how restenosis studies should be performed; in addition, currently no satisfactory definition takes into account both the functional and angiographic outcome of the patient after PTCA. As a result, diverse and conflicting data have been reported. It is concluded that three areas need to be addressed carefully in subsequent restenosis studies: (1) selection of the appropriate patient population; (2) employment of a well-validated system for quantitative analysis of the angiographic data; and (3) selection of the appropriate parameters to reflect the restenosis process (not percent diameter stenosis). It is expected that such studies will be easier to perform as on-line quantitation systems become more widely available in the catheterization laboratory.

The second study concerns the efficacy of endoluminal prostheses, which have been proposed as an alternative approach for preventing late restenosis after PTCA. In a group of 26 patients, the early morphologic changes in stenosis geometry after stenting were assessed by quantitative coronary angiography. It was demonstrated that the stent implantation following PTCA resulted in an additional increase in luminal cross-sectional area and obstruction diameter, and a decrease in percent area and percent diameter stenosis as compared with the postangioplasty state. These morphologic improvements were associated with decreases in both the turbulent and Poiseuille resistances, as well as in the theoretical transstenotic pressure drops at a flow of 1 ml/sec. These data suggest that immediately after PTCA, the endoprosthesis has an active dilating function in addition to its basic stenting (maintenance of dilated diameter) role.

Finally, in the last clinical application, a review of lipid-lowering intervention trials is presented, with particular emphasis on the role of computerized quantitative analysis of coronary atherosclerosis. From the data it follows that at present only two studies (with one yet unpublished) have been based on quantitative coronary angiography with the more sophisticated automated edge detection approaches. On the basis of the data available, it is concluded that reversibility of atherosclerosis, both from the macroscopic and microscopic points of view, seems attainable. In addition, one may hypothesize that LDL cholesterol is primarily responsible for progression of atherosclerosis, while HDL cholesterol would be the main lipoprotein that may induce regression of atherosclerosis. Finally, it is proposed to focus on the evaluation of newly developed atherosclerotic lesions in future nonsurgical intervention studies.

Acknowledgments

This work is based on the teamwork of many colleagues, both physicists and physicians, who have contributed over the last 20 years to the Thoraxcenter project "Quantitative Coronary Arteriography" and on an extensive literature search. The names of our colleagues can be found through the corresponding references of the Thoraxcenter papers that have been published over the years. However, a few colleagues should be acknowledged here, since they have contributed more specifically to this particular chapter.

These colleagues are Felix Zijlstra, M.D., who has done extensive work and written a Ph.D. thesis on coronary flow reserve assessed from coronary cineangiograms; Kevin Beatt, M.D., for his contribution of the section on restenosis; Folkert J. ten Cate, M.D., Ph.D., for the section on myocardial contrast echocardiography; and Imbraim Pinto, M.D., for his critical reading of the manuscript during his half-year stay at the Thoraxcenter. Jacques D. Barth, M.D., Ph.D., has contributed the section on the progression and regression of atherosclerosis. Finally, the authors wish to thank Mrs. B. Smit-van der Deure for her excellent secretarial assistance.

References

A

1. Arnett, E.N., Isner, J.M., Redwood, D.R., et al.: Coronary artery narrowing in coronary heart disease: Comparison of cineangiographic and necropsy findings. Ann. Intern. Med. 91:350, 1979.
2. Armstrong, W.F.: Assessment of myocardial perfusion with contrast enhanced echocardiography. Echocardiography 3:355, 1986.
3. Arntzenius, A.C., Kromhout, D., Barth, J.D., et al.: Diet, lipoproteins, and the progression of coronary atherosclerosis: The Leiden Intervention Trial. N. Engl. J. Med. 312:805, 1985.
4. Alderman, E.L., Berte, L.E., Harrison, D.C., and Sanders, W.: Quantitation of coronary artery dimensions using digital imaging processing. *In* Brody, W.R. (ed.): Digital Radiography. SPIE: Society of Photo-Optical Instrumentation Engineers 314, Bellingham, Wash., 1982, p. 273.
5. Ambrose, J.A., Winters, S.L., Stern, A., et al.: Angiographic morphology and the pathogenesis of unstable angina pectoris. J. Am. Coll. Cardiol. 5:609, 1985.
6. Albro, P.C., Gould, K.L., Westcott, R.J., et al.: Noninvasive assessment of coronary stenoses by myocardial imaging during pharmacologic coronary vasodilatation. III. Clinical trial. Am. J. Cardiol. 42:751, 1978.
7. Abela, G.S., Normann, S.J., Cohen, D.M., et al.: Laser recanalization of occluded atherosclerotic arteries in vivo and in vitro. Circulation 71:403, 1985.
8. Austen, W.G., Edwards, J.E., Frye, R.L., et al.: A reporting system on patients evaluated for coronary artery disease: Report of the Ad Hoc Committee for Grading of Coronary Artery Disease, Council on Cardiovascular Surgery, American Heart Association, 1975. Circulation 51:7, 1975.
9. Arntzenius, A.C.: Preventive aspects in angina pectoris. Eur. Heart J. 6(Suppl. F):41, 1985.
10. Ambrose, J.A., Hjemdahl-Monsen, C.E.: Arteriographic anatomy and mechanisms of myocardial ischemia in unstable angina. J. Am. Coll. Cardiol. 9:1397, 1987.
11. Austin, G.E., Ratliff, N.B., Hollman, J., et al.: Intimal proliferation of smooth muscle cells as an explanation for recurrent coronary artery stenosis after percutaneous transluminal coronary angioplasty. J. Am. Coll. Cardiol. 6:369, 1985.

B

1. Brown, B.G., Bolson, E., Frimer, M., and Dodge, H.T.: Computer-assisted measurements of coronary artery stenosis. (Letter.) Circulation 60:1196, 1979.
2. Block, P.C., Myler, R.K., Stertzer, S., and Fallon, J.T.: Morphology after transluminal angioplasty in human beings. N. Engl. J. Med. 305:382, 1981.
3. Brown, B.G., Bolson, E., Frimer, M., and Dodge, H.T.: Quantitative coronary arteriography: Estimation of dimensions, hemodynamic resistance, and atheroma mass of coronary artery lesions using the arteriogram and digital computation. Circulation 55:329, 1977.
4. Bergmann, S.R., Fox, K.A.A., Geltmann, E.M., and Sobel, B.E.: Positron emission tomography of the heart. Prog. Cardiovasc. Dis. 38:165, 1985.
5. Bove, A.A., Santamore, W.P., and Carey, R.A.: Reduced myocardial blood flow resulting from dynamic changes in coronary artery stenosis. Int. J. Cardiol. 4:301, 1983.
6. Brown, B.G., Gallery, C.A., Badger, R.S., et al.: Incomplete lysis of thrombus in the moderate underlying atherosclerotic lesion during intracoronary infusion of streptokinase for acute myocardial infarction: Quantitative angiographic observations. Circulation 73:653, 1986.
7. Blankenhorn, D.H., and Brooks, S.H.: Angiographic trials of lipid-lowering therapy. Arteriosclerosis 1:242, 1981.
8. Bachmann, K., and Gansser, R.: Digital angiography in coronary heart disease. *In* Heintzen, P.H., and Bürsch, J.H. (eds.): Progress in Digital Angiocardiography. Kluwer Academic, Dordrecht, 1988, p. 13.
9. Brown, B.G., Bolson, E.L., and Dodge, H.T.: Arteriographic assessment of coronary atherosclerosis: Review of current methods, their limitations and clinical applications. Arteriosclerosis 2:2, 1982.
10. Beatt, K.J., Luijten, H.E., Reiber, J.H.C., and Serruys, P.W.: Early regression and late progression in coronary artery lesions in the first 3 months following coronary angioplasty. *In* Reiber, J.H.C., and Serruys, P.W. (eds.): New Developments in Quantitative Coronary Arteriography. Martinus Nijhoff, Dordrecht, 1988, p. 167.
11. Beatt, K.J., Luijten, H.E., de Feyter, P.J., et al.: Change in diameter of coronary artery segments adjacent to stenosis after percutaneous transluminal coronary angioplasty: Failure of percent diameter stenosis measurement to reflect morphologic changes induced by balloon dilation. J. Am. Coll. Cardiol. 12:315, 1988.
12. Bürsch, J., Johs, R., and Heintzen, P.: Validity of Lambert-Beer's law in roentgendensitometry of contrast material (Urografin) using continuous radiation. *In* Heintzen, P.H. (ed.): Roentgen-, Cine- and Videodensitometry: Fundamentals and Applications for Blood Flow and Heart Volume Determinations. Georg Thieme Verlag, Stuttgart, 1971, p. 81.
13. Barth, K., Eicker, B., Koch, R., and Marhoff, P. Automated three-dimensional recognition of the coronary tree with clinical DSA image pairs. Comput. Cardiol. 187, 1988.
14. Barth, K., Koch, R., and Marhoff, P.: Fast automatic recognition and 3D reconstruction of the coronary tree from DSA-projection pairs. *In* Heintzen, P.H., and Bürsch, J.H. (eds.): Progress in Digital Angiocardiography. Kluwer Academic, Dordrecht, 1988, p. 193.
15. Boer, A. den: A microprocessor system for on-line registration of the x-ray system settings. Internal report. Thoraxcenter, Erasmus University, Rotterdam, 1982.
16. Bentley, K., and Henry, P.D.: Spasmogenic effect of angiographic dye on normal and atherosclerotic arteries. (Abstract.) Circulation 62(Suppl. III): III-218, 1980.
17. Brown, B.G., Bolson, E.L., and Dodge, H.T.: Percutaneous transluminal coronary angioplasty and subsequent restenosis: Quantitative and qualitative methodology for their assessment. Am. J. Cardiol. 60:34B, 1987.
18. Bom, N., Slager, C.J., van Egmond, F.C., et al.: Intra-arterial ultrasonic imaging for recanalization by spark erosion. Ultrasound Med. Biol. 14:257, 1988.
19. Block, M., Bove, A.A., and Ritman, E.L.: Coronary angiographic examination with the dynamic spatial reconstructor. Circulation 70:209, 1984.
20. Bürsch, J.H., and Heitzen, P.H.: Concepts for coronary flow and myocardial perfusion measurements. *In* Heintzen, P.H., and Bürsch, J.H. (eds.): Progress in Digital Angiocardiography. Kluwer Academic, Dordrecht, 1988, p. 201.
21. Bache, R.J., and Schwartz, J.S.: Effect of perfusion pressure distal to a coronary stenosis on transmural myocardial blood flow. Circulation 65:928, 1982.
22. Bookstein, J.J., and Higgins, C.B.: Comparative efficacy of coronary vasodilatory methods. Invest. Radiol. 12:121, 1977.
23. Bagger, J.P.: Coronary sinus blood flow determination by the thermodilution technique: Influence of catheter position and respiration. Cardiovasc. Res. 19:27, 1984.
24. Bates, E.R., Aueron, F.M., Legrand, V., et al.: Comparative long-term effects of coronary artery bypass graft surgery and percutaneous transluminal coronary angioplasty on regional coronary flow reserve. Circulation 72:833, 1985.
25. Bertrand, M.E., Marco, J., Cherrier, F., et al.: French percutaneous transluminal coronary angioplasty (PTCA) registry: Four years experience. (Abstract.) J. Am. Coll. Cardiol. 7:21A, 1986.
26. Bussmann, W.D., Rutishauser, W., Noseda, G., et al.: Influence of a new contrast medium (Metrizoate) on coronary blood flow. *In* Heintzen, P.H. (ed.): Roentgen-, Cine- and Videodensitometry: Fundamentals and Applications for Blood Flow and Heart Volume Determination. Georg Thieme Verlag, Stuttgart, 1971, p. 133.
27. Bürsch, J., Johs, R., Kirbach, H., et al.: Accuracy of videodensitometric flow measurement. *In* Heitzen, P.H. (ed.): Röntgen-, Cine- and Videodensitometry: Fundamentals and Applications for Blood Flow and Heart Volume Determination. Georg Thieme Verlag, Stuttgart, 1971, p. 119.
28. Bassan, M., Ganz, W., Marcus, H.S., and Swan, H.J.C.: The effect of intracoronary injection of contrast medium upon coronary blood flow. Circulation 51:442, 1975.
29. Bentley, K.I., Clark, M., and Henry, P.D.: Angiographic dye relaxes canine coronary artery by a nonosmotic mechanism. (Abstract.) Am. J. Cardiol. 47:407, 1981.

30. Blankenhorn, D.H., Brooks, S.H., Selzer, R.H., and Barndt, R., Jr.: The rate of atherosclerosis change during treatment of hyperlipoproteinemia. Circulation 57:355, 1978.
31. Buchwald, H., Moore, R.B., Rucker, R.D., Jr., et al.: Clinical angiographic regression of atherosclerosis after partial ileal bypass. Atherosclerosis 46:117, 1983.
32. Brensike, J.F., Levy, R.I., Kelsey, S.F., et al.: Effects of therapy with cholestyramine on progression of coronary arteriosclerosis: Results of the NHLBI Type II Coronary Intervention Study. Circulation 69:313, 1984.
33. Blankenhorn, D.H., Nessim, S.A., Johnson, R.L., et al.: Beneficial effects of combined colestipol-niacin therapy on coronary atherosclerosis and coronary venous bypass grafts. JAMA 257:3233, 1987.
34. Barth, J.D., Jansen, H., Kromhout, D., et al.: Progression and regression of human coronary atherosclerosis: The role of lipoproteins, lipases and thyroid hormones in coronary lesion growth. Atherosclerosis 68:51, 1987.
35. Blankenhorn, D.H., and the CLAS Study Group: In reply to letters to the editor: Colestipol-niacin therapy and coronary atherosclerosis. JAMA 258:2694, 1987.
36. Bruschke, A.V.G., Wijers, T.S., Kolsters, W., and Landmann, J.: The anatomic evolution of coronary artery disease demonstrated by coronary arteriography in 256 nonoperated patients. Circulation 63:527, 1981.
37. Barth, J.D.: Progression and regression of coronary atherosclerosis. Ph.D. dissertation. Erasmus University, Rotterdam, 1986.
38. Barth, J.D., Jansen, H., Kromhout, D., et al.: Progression and regression of human coronary atherosclerosis: The role of lipoproteins, lipases and thyroid hormones in coronary lesion growth. Atherosclerosis 68:51, 1987.

C

1. Cameron, A., Kemp, H.G., Fisher, L.D., et al.: Left main coronary artery stenosis: Angiographic determination. Circulation 68:484, 1983.
2. Cusma, J.T., Toggart, E.J., Folts, J.D., et al.: Digital subtraction angiographic imaging of coronary flow reserve. Circulation 75:461, 1987.
3. Clark, C.: The propagation of turbulence produced by a stenosis. J. Biomech. 13:591, 1980.
4. Crawford, D.W., Brooks, S.H., Selzer, R.H., et al.: Computer densitometry for angiographic assessment of arterial cholesterol content and gross pathology in human atherosclerosis. J. Lab. Clin. Med. 89:378, 1977.
5. Cuyck, P.J.H. van, Gerbrands, J.J., and Reiber, J.H.C.: Automated centerline tracing in coronary angiograms. *In* Gelsema, E.S., and Kanal, L.N. (eds.): Pattern Recognition and Artificial Intelligence. Elsevier Science, Amsterdam, 1988, p. 169.
6. Cumberland, D.C.: Low-osmolality contrast media in cardiac radiology. Invest. Radiol. 19:S301, 1984.
7. Choy, D.S.J., Stertzer, S., Rotterdam, H.Z., et al.: Transluminal laser catheter angioplasty. Am. J. Cardiol. 50:1206, 1982.
8. Cragg, A., Lund, G., Rysavy, J., et al.: Nonsurgical placement of arterial endoprostheses: A new technique using nitinol wire. Radiology 147:261, 1983.
9. Cannon, P.J., Weiss, M.B., and Sciacca, R.R.: Myocardial blood flow in coronary artery disease: Studies at rest and during stress with inert gas washout techniques. Prog. Cardiovasc. Dis. 20:95, 1977.
10. Cohn, K., Sakai, F.J., and Langston, M.F., Jr.: Effect of clofibrate on progression of coronary disease: A prospective angiographic study in man. Am. Heart J. 89:591, 1975.
11. Conti, C.R.: Discussion in diagnosis, prevention and the treatment of acute and chronic myocardial ischemia. Am. Coll. Cardiol. Highlights 3:1, 1987.
12. Conti, C.R., and Mehta, J.L.: Acute myocardial ischemia: Role of atherosclerosis, thrombosis, platelet activation, coronary vasospasm, and altered arachidonic acid metabolism. Circulation 75(Suppl. V):V84, 1987.
13. Corcos, T., David, P.R., Val, P.G., et al.: Failure of diltiazem to prevent restenosis after percutaneous transluminal coronary angioplasty. Am. Heart J. 109:926, 1985.
14. Cate, F.J. ten, Drury, J.K., Meerbaum, S., et al.: Myocardial contrast two-dimensional echocardiography: Experimental examination at different coronary flow levels. J. Am. Coll. Cardiol. 3:1219, 1984.
15. Cate, F.J. ten, Serruys, P.W., Huang, H., et al.: Is the rate of disappearance of echo contrast from the interventricular septum a measure of left anterior descending coronary artery stenosis? Eur. Heart J. 9:728, 1988.
16. Cheirif, J., Zoghbi, W.A., Raizner, A.E., et al.: Assessment of myocardial perfusion in humans by contrast echocardiography. I. Evaluation of regional coronary reserve by peak contrast intensity. J. Am. Coll. Cardiol. 11: 735, 1988.

D

1. Detre, K.M., Wright, E., Murphy, M.L., and Takaro T.: Observer agreement in evaluating coronary angiograms. Circulation 52:979, 1975.
2. DeRouen, T.A., Murray, J.A., and Owen, W.: Variability in the analysis of coronary arteriograms. Circulation 55:324, 1977.
3. Doriot, P.A., Pochon, Y., Rasoamanambelo, L., et al.: Densitometry of coronary arteries—an improved physical model. Comput. Cardiol. 91, 1985.
4. Doriot, P.A.: On the accuracy of densitometric measurements of coronary artery stenosis based on Lambert-Beer's absorption law. *In* Reiber, J.H.C., and Serruys, P.W. (eds.): New Developments in Quantitative Coronary Arteriography. Martinus Nijhoff, Dordrecht, 1988, p. 115.
5. Doriot, P.A., Pochon, Y., Welz, R., and Rutishauser, W.: Nonlinearity by densitometric measurements of coronary arteries. *In* Heintzen, P.H., and Bürsch, J.H. (eds.): Progress in Digital Angiocardiography. Kluwer Academic, Dordrecht, 1988, p. 173.
6. Dole, W.P., Montville, W.J., and Bishop, V.S.: Dependency of myocardial reactive hyperemia on coronary artery pressure in the dog. Am. J. Physiol. 240:H709, 1981.
7. Dumay, A.C.H., Minderhoud, H., Gerbrands, J.J., et al.: Three-dimensional reconstruction of myocardial contrast perfusion from biplane cineangiograms by means of linear programming techniques. Int. J. Cardiac Imag 3:141, 1988.
8. Domenech, R.J., and Goich, J.: Effect of heart rate on regional coronary blood flow. Cardiovasc. Res. 10:224, 1976.
9. Dorros, G., Cowley, M.J., Simpson, J., et al.: Percutaneous transluminal coronary angioplasty: Report of complications from the National Heart, Lung and Blood Institute PTCA Registry. Circulation 67:723, 1983.
10. Dotter, C.T.: Transluminally placed coilspring endarterial tube grafts: Long-term patency in canine popliteal artery. Invest. Radiol. 4:329, 1969.
11. Dotter, C.T., Buschmann, R.W., McKinney, M.K., and Rösch, J.: Transluminal expandable nitinol coil stent grafting: Preliminary report. Radiology 147:259, 1983.
12. Donadieu, A.M., Hartl, C., Cardinal, A., and Bonnemain, B.: Incidence of ventricular fibrillation during coronary arteriography in the rabbit: A comparative study of isotonic Ioxaglate and Iohexol. Invest. Radiol. 22:106, 1987.
13. Duffield, R.G.M., Lewis, B., Miller, N.E., et al.: Treatment of hyperlipidaemia retards progression of symptomatic femoral atherosclerosis. Lancet 2:639, 1983.
14. Doppler, C.J.: Über das farbige Licht der Doppelsterne und einiger anderen Gestirne des Himmels. Abhandlungen der Königl. Böhm. Gesellschaft der Wissenschaften zu Prag 2:467, 1842.
15. Dumay, A.C.M., Gerbrands, J.J., Zijlstra, F., et al.: Three-dimensional reconstruction of myocardial contrast perfusion from biplane cineangiograms. *In* Gelsema, E.S., and Kanal, L.N. (eds.): Pattern Recognition and Artificial Intelligence. Elsevier Science, Amsterdam, 1988, p. 155.
16. Dodge, J.T., Jr., Brown, B.G., Bolson, E.L., and Dodge, H.T.: Intrathoracic spatial location of specified coronary segments on the normal human heart: Applications in quantitative arteriography, assessment of regional risk and contraction, and anatomic display. Circulation 78:1167, 1988.

E

1. Essed, C.E., Brand, M. van den, and Becker, A.E.: Transluminal coronary angioplasty and early restenosis: Fibrocellular occlusion after wall laceration. Br. Heart J. 49:393, 1983.
2. Epstein, S.E., Cannon III, R.O., Watson, R.M., et al.: Dynamic coronary obstruction as a cause of angina pectoris: Implications regarding therapy. Am. J. Cardiol. 55:61B, 1985.
3. Ellis, S., Sanders, W., Goulet, C., et al.: Optimal detection of the progression of coronary artery disease: Comparison of methods suitable for risk factor intervention trials. Circulation 74:1235, 1986.
4. Eckenhoff, J.E., Hafkenschiel, J.H., Landmesser, C.M., and Harmel, M.: Cardiac oxygen metabolism and control of the coronary circulation. Am. J. Physiol. 149:634, 1947.
5. Eckenhoff, J.E., Hafkenschiel, J.H., Harmel, M.H., et al.: Measurement of coronary blood flow by the nitrous oxide method. Am. J. Physiol. 152:356, 1948.
6. Engel, H.J., Hundeshagen, H., and Lichtlen, P.: Auswirkungen von Koronarstenosen und ventrikulären Funktionsstörungen auf die regionale Myokarddurchblutung bei koronarer Herzkrankheit. Schweiz. Med. Wschr. 107:1920, 1977.

F

1. Fisher, L.D., Judkins, M.P., Lespérance, J., et al.: Reproducibility of coronary arteriographic reading in the Coronary Artery Surgery Study (CASS). Cathet. Cardiovasc. Diagn. 8:565, 1982.
2. Freudenberg, H., and Lichtlen, P.R.: The normal wall segment in coronary stenoses: A postmortem study. Z. Kardiol. 70:863, 1981.
3. Fiddian, R.V., Byar, D., and Edwards, E.A.: Factors affecting flow through a stenosed vessel. Arch. Surg. 88:83, 1964.
4. Feldman, R.L., Nichols, W.W., Pepine, C.J., and Conti, C.R.: Hemodynamic significance of the length of a coronary arterial narrowing. Am. J. Cardiol. 41:865, 1978.
5. Feldman, R.L., and Pepine, C.J.: Evaluation of coronary artery stenoses. Int. J. Cardiol. 4:185, 1983.
6. Feldman, R.L., Nichols, W.W., Pepine, C.J., and Conti, C.R.: Hemodynamic effect of long and multiple coronary arterial narrowings. Chest 74:280, 1978.
7. Feldman, R.L., and Pepine, C.J.: Determination of residual regional flow during acute coronary occlusion in conscious man. (Abstract.) J. Am. Coll. Cardiol. 1:684, 1983.
8. Feldman, R.L., Pepine, C.J., Curry, C., and Conty, C.R.: Case against routine use of glyceryl trinitrate before coronary angiography. Br. Heart J. 40:992, 1978.
9. Feldman, R.L., Pepine, C.J., Curry, R.C., and Conty, C.R.: Quantitative coronary arteriography using 105-mm photospot angiography and an optical magnifying device. Cathet. Cardiovasc. Diagn. 5:195, 1979.
10. Fleagle, S.R., Johnson, M.R., Skorton, D.J., et al.: Geometric validation of a robust method of automated edge detection in clinical coronary arteriography. Comput. Cardiol. 197, 1987.
11. Feldman, R.L., Marx, J.D., Pepine, C.J., and Conti, C.R.: Analysis of coronary responses to various doses of intracoronary nitroglycerin. Circulation 66:321, 1982.
12. Foerster, J.M., Link, D.P., Lantz, B.M.T., et al.: Measurement of coronary

reactive hyperemia during clinical angiography by video dilution technique. Acta Radiol. 22:209, 1981.

13. Forrester, J.S., Helfant, R.H., Pasternac, A., et al.: Atrial pacing in coronary heart disease: Effect on hemodynamics, metabolism and coronary circulation. Am. J. Cardiol. 27:237, 1971.
14. Faxon, D.P., Kelsey, S.F., Ryan, T.J., et al.: Determinants of successful percutaneous transluminal coronary angioplasty: Report from the National Heart, Lung and Blood Institute registry. Am. Heart J. 108:1019, 1984.
15. Falk, E.: Unstable angina with fatal outcome: Dynamic coronary thrombosis leading to infarction and/or sudden death. Autopsy evidence of recurrent mural thrombosis with peripheral embolization culminating in total vascular occlusion. Circulation 71:699, 1985.
16. Fermor, U., Huber, H., Neuhaus, K.L., et al.: Measurement of flow velocity in the model circulation by videodensitometry: Methodological investigations. Basic Res. Cardiol. 73:361, 1979.
17. Fischer, H.W.: Catalog of intravascular contrast media. Radiology 159:561, 1986.
18. Feldman, R.L., Nichols, W.W., Pepine, C.J., et al.: The coronary hemodynamics of left main and branch coronary stenoses: The effects of reduction in stenosis diameter, stenosis length, and number of stenoses. J. Thorac. Cardiovasc. Surg. 77:377, 1979.
19. Feinstein, S.B., Cate, F.J. ten, Zwehl, W., et al.: Two-dimensional contrast echocardiography. I. In vitro development and quantitative analysis of echo contrast agents. J. Am. Coll. Cardiol. 3:14, 1984.

G

1. Gould, K.L., and Kirkeeide, R.L.: Assessment of stenosis severity. *In* Reiber, J.H.C., and Serruys, P.W. (eds.): State of the Art in Quantitative Coronary Arteriography. Martinus Nijhoff, Dordrecht, 1986, p. 209.
2. Gould, K.L.: Pressure-flow characteristics of coronary stenoses in unsedated dogs at rest and during coronary vasodilation. Circ. Res. 43:245, 1978.
3. Gottwik, M.G., Siebes, M., Kirkeeide, R., and Schaper, W.: Hämodynamik von Koronarstenosen. Z. Kardiol. 73:47, 1984.
4. Gould, K.L., Schelbert, H.R., Phelps, M.E., et al.: Noninvasive assessment of coronary stenoses with myocardial perfusion imaging during pharmacologic coronary vasodilation. V. Detection of 47 percent diameter coronary stenosis with intravenous nitrogen-13 ammonia and emission-computed tomography in intact dogs. Am. J. Cardiol. 43:200, 1979.
5. Gould, K.L., Lipscomb, K., and Hamilton, G.W.: Physiologic basis for assessing critical coronary stenosis: Instantaneous flow response and regional distribution during coronary hyperemia as measures of coronary flow reserve. Am. J. Cardiol. 33:87, 1974.
6. Gould, K.L., and Lipscomb, K.: Effects of coronary stenoses on coronary flow reserve and resistance. Am. J. Cardiol. 34:48, 1974.
7. Gould, K.L., and Kelley, K.O.: Physiological significance of coronary flow velocity and changing stenosis geometry during coronary vasodilation in awake dogs. Circ. Res. 50:695, 1982.
8. Gould, K.L.: Quantification of coronary artery stenosis in vivo. Circ. Res. 47:341, 1985.
9. Gensini, G.G., Kelly, A.E., Da Costa, B.C.B., and Huntington, P.P.: Quantitative angiography: The measurement of coronary vasomobility in the intact animal and man. Chest 60:522, 1971.
10. Glagov, S., Weisenberg, E., Zarins, C.K., et al.: Compensatory enlargement of human atherosclerotic coronary arteries. N. Engl. J. Med. 316:1371, 1987.
11. Ginsburg, R.: The isolated human epicardial coronary artery. Am. J. Cardiol. 52:61A, 1983.
12. Gensini, G.G.: Coronary angiography. Futura, New York, 1975.
13. Gould, K.L., Kelley, K.O., and Bolson, E.L.: Experimental validation of quantitative coronary arteriography for determining pressure-flow characteristics of coronary stenosis. Circulation 66:930, 1982.
14. Ganz, W., Tamura, K., Marcus, H.S., et al.: Measurement of coronary sinus blood flow by continuous thermodilution in man. Circulation 44:181, 1971.
15. Gould, K.L.: Noninvasive assessment of coronary stenoses by myocardial perfusion imaging during pharmacologic coronary vasodilatation. I. Physiologic basis and experimental validation. Am. J. Cardiol. 41:267, 1978.
16. Gould, K.L., Westcott, R.J., Albro, P.C., and Hamilton, G.W.: Noninvasive assessment of coronary stenoses by myocardial perfusion imaging during pharmacologic coronary vasodilatation. II. Clinical methodology and feasibility. Am. J. Cardiol. 41:279, 1978.
17. Grines, C.L., Mancini, G.B.J., McGillem, M.J., et al.: Measurement of regional myocardial perfusion and mass by subselective hydrogen infusion and washout techniques: A validation study. Circulation 76:1373, 1987.
18. Gould, K.L., and Kelley, K.O.: Physiological significance of coronary flow velocity and changing stenosis geometry during coronary vasodilation in awake dogs. Circ. Res. 50:695, 1982.
19. Grüntzig, A.R., Senning, A., and Siegenthaler, W.E.: Nonoperative dilatation of coronary-artery stenosis. N. Engl. J. Med. 301:61, 1979.
20. Gould, K.L., Goldstein, R.A., Mullani, N.A., et al.: Noninvasive assessment of coronary stenoses by myocardial perfusion imaging during pharmacologic coronary vasodilation. VIII. Clinical feasibility of positron cardiac imaging without a cyclotron using generator-produced rubidium-82. J. Am. Coll. Cardiol. 7:775, 1986.
21. Gould, K.L.: Percent coronary stenosis: Battered gold standard, pernicious relic or clinical practicality? J. Am. Coll. Cardiol. 11:886, 1988.
22. Galan, K.M., Deligonul, U., Kern, M.J., et al.: Increased frequency of restenosis in patients continuing to smoke cigarettes after percutaneous transluminal coronary angioplasty. Am. J. Cardiol. 61:260, 1988.

H

1. Hort, W.: Anatomy and pathology of the human coronary circulation. *In* Schaper, W. (ed.): The Pathophysiology of Myocardial Perfusion. Elsevier, Biomedical Press, Amsterdam, 1979, p. 247.
2. Holmes, D.R., Vlietstra, R.E., Mock, M.B., et al.: Angiographic changes produced by percutaneous transluminal coronary angioplasty. Am. J. Cardiol. 51:676, 1983.
3. Harrison, D.G., White, C.W., Hiratzka, L.F., et al.: The value of lesion cross-sectional area determined by quantitative coronary angiography in assessing the physiologic significance of proximal left anterior descending coronary arterial stenoses. Circulation 69:1111, 1984.
4. Hodgson, J.M., LeGrand, V., Bates, E.R., et al.: Validation in dogs of a rapid digital angiographic technique to measure relative coronary blood flow during routine cardiac catheterization. Am. J. Cardiol. 55:188, 1985.
5. Herrington, D.M., Walford, G.A., and Pearson, T.A.: Issues of validation in quantitative coronary angiography. *In* Reiber, J.H.C., and Serruys, P.W. (eds.): New Developments in Quantitative Coronary Arteriography. Kluwer Academic, Dordrecht, 1988, p. 153.
6. Heintzen, P., and Moldenhauer, K.: The x-ray absorption by contrast material. *In* Heintzen, P.H. (ed.): Roentgen-, Cine- and Videodensitometry: Fundamentals and Applications for Blood Flow and Heart Volume Determinations. Georg Thieme Verlag, Stuttgart, 1971, p. 73.
7. Higgins, C.B., and Schmidt, W.: Direct and reflex myocardial effects of intracoronary administered contrast materials in the anesthetized and conscious dog: Comparison of standard and newer contrast materials. Invest. Radiol. 13:205, 1978.
8. Hori, M., Inoue, M., Shimazu, T., et al.: Clinical assessment of coronary arterial elastic properties by the image processing of coronary arteriograms. Comput. Cardiol.: 393, 1983.
9. Hoffman, J.I.E.: Maximal coronary flow and the concept of coronary vascular reserve. Circulation 70:153, 1984.
10. Hodgson, J.M.B., Mancini, G.B.J., LeGrand, V., and Vogel R.A.: Characterization of changes in coronary blood flow during the first six seconds after intracoronary contrast injection. Invest. Radiol. 20:246, 1985.
11. Hodgson, J.M., Riley, R.S., Most, A.S., and Williams, D.D.: Assessment of coronary flow reserve using digital angiography before and after successful percutaneous transluminal coronary angioplasty. Am. J. Cardiol. 60:61, 1987.
12. Holmes, D.R., Jr., Vliestra, R.E., Smith, H.C., et al.: Restenosis after percutaneous transluminal coronary angioplasty (PTCA): A report from the PTCA registry of the NHLBI. Am. J. Cardiol. 53:77C, 1984.
13. Hackbarth, W., Bircks, W., Pölitz, B., et al.: Vergleich videodensitometrischer und elektromagnetischer Flussmessungen in aortokoronaren Bypassgefässen. Fortschr. Röntgenstr. 132:554, 1980.
14. Horie, T., Sekiguchi, M., and Hirosawa, K.: Coronary thrombosis in pathogenesis of acute myocardial infarction: Histopathological study of coronary arteries in 108 necropsied cases using serial section. Br. Heart J. 40:153, 1978.
15. Hutchins, G.M., Miner, M.M., and Boitnott, J.K.: Vessel caliber and branch-angle of human coronary artery branch-points. Circ. Res. 38:572, 1976.
16. Hort, W., Lichti, H., Kalbfleisch, H., et al.: The size of human coronary arteries depending on the physiological and pathological growth of the heart, the age, the size of the supplying areas and the degree of coronary sclerosis: A postmortem study. Virchows Arch. (Pathol. Anat.) 397:37, 1982.

I

1. Isner, J.M., Wu, M., Virmani, R., et al.: Comparison of degrees of coronary arterial luminal narrowing determined by visual inspection of histologic sections under magnification among three independent observers and comparison to that obtained by video planimetry: An analysis of 559 five-millimeter segments of 61 coronary arteries from eleven patients. Lab. Invest. 5:566, 1980.
2. Isner, J.M., and Clarke, R.H.: Laser angioplasty: Unraveling the Gordian knot. J. Am. Coll. Cardiol. 7:705, 1986.

J

1. Johnson, M.R., McPherson, D.D., Fleagle, S.R., et al.: Videodensitometric analysis of human coronary stenoses: Validation in vivo using intraoperative high-frequency epicardial echocardiography. Circulation 77:328, 1988.
2. Johnson, M.R., McPherson, D.D., Hunt, M.M., et al.: Videodensitometry is independent of angiographic projection and lumen shape. (Abstract.) J. Am. Coll. Cardiol. 9:183A, 1987.
3. Jost, S., Rafflenbeul, W., Gerhardt, U., et al.: Influence of ionic and non-ionic radiographic contrast media on the vasomotor tone of epicardial coronary arteries. Eur. Heart J. 10(Suppl F):60, 1989.
4. Johnson, M.R., Brayden, G.P., Ericksen, E.E., et al.: Changes in cross-sectional area of the coronary lumen in the six months after angioplasty: A quantitative analysis of the variable response to percutaneous transluminal angioplasty. Circulation 73:467, 1986.
5. Jain, A., Mahmarian, J.J., Borges-Neto, S., et al.: Clinical significance of perfusion defects by thallium-201 single photon emission tomography following oral dipyridamole early after coronary angioplasty. J. Am. Coll. Cardiol. 11:970, 1988.

K

1. Kirkeeide, R.L., and Gould, K.L.: Cardiovascular imaging: Coronary artery stenosis. Hosp. Pract. 19:160, 1984.
2. Klocke, F.J.: Measurements of coronary blood flow and degree of stenosis: Current clinical implications and continuing uncertainties. J. Am. Coll. Cardiol. 1:31, 1983.
3. Kober, G., Spahn, G., Spitz, P., et al.: Weite der grossen Koronararterien im selektiven Arteriogramm bei Myocardhypertropie. Verh. Dtsch. Ges. Kreislaufforsch. 38:191, 1972.

4. Koh, D., Mitten, S., Stewart, D., et al.: Comparison between computerized quantitative coronary angiography and clinical interpretation. (Abstract.) Circulation 60(Suppl. II): II-160, 1979.
5. Kooijman, C.J., Kalberg, R., Slager, C.J., et al.: Densitometric analysis of coronary arteries. *In* Young, I.T., et al. (eds.): Signal Processing III: Theories and Applications. Elsevier, Amsterdam, 1986, p. 1405.
6. Kirkeeide, R.L., Fung, P., Smalling, R.W., and Gould, K.L.: Automated evaluation of vessel diameter from arteriograms. Comput. Cardiol. 215, 1982.
7. Kooijman, C.J., Reiber, J.H.C., Gerbrands, J.J., et al.: Computer-aided quantitation of the severity of coronary obstructions from single-view cine-angiograms. Proc. ISMIII '82. IEEE Computer Society Press, Silver Spring, MD 20910. IEEE Cat. No. 82 CH1804-4, 1982, p. 59.
8. Kirkeeide, R.L., Gould, K.L., and Parsel, L.: Assessment of coronary stenoses by myocardial perfusion imaging during pharmacologic coronary vasodilation. VII. Validation of coronary flow reserve as a single integrated functional measure of stenosis severity reflecting all its geometric dimensions. J. Am. Coll. Cardiol. 7:103, 1986.
9. Kruger, R.A.: Estimation of the diameter of and iodine concentration within blood vessels using digital radiography devices. Med. Phys. 8:652, 1981.
10. Kruger, R.A., and Riederer, S.J.: Basic Concepts of Digital Subtraction Angiography. G.K. Hall, Boston, 1984.
11. Kirkeeide, R.L., Smalling, R.W., and Gould, K.L.: Automated measurements of artery diameter from arteriograms. (Abstract.) Circulation 66:II-325, 1982.
12. Kirkeeide, R.L., Parsel, L., and Gould, K.L.: Prediction of coronary flow reserve of stenotic coronary arteries by quantitative arteriography. (Abstract.) Circulation 70:II-250, 1984.
13. Kaltenbach, M., Schultz, W., and Kober, G.: Effects of nifedipine after intravenous and intracoronary administration. Am. J. Cardiol. 44:832, 1979.
14. Klocke, F.J.: Measurements of coronary flow reserve: Defining pathophysiology versus making decisions about patient care. Circulation 76:1183, 1987.
15. Kety, S.S., and Schmidt, C.F.: The determination of cerebral blood flow in man by the use of nitrous oxide in low concentrations. Am. J. Physiol. 143:53, 1945.
16. Khouri, E.M., Gregg, D.E., and Lowensohn, H.S.: Flow in the major branches of the left coronary artery during experimental coronary insufficiency in the unanesthetized dog. Circ. Res. 23:99, 1968.
17. Kent, K.M., Bentivoglio, L.G., Block, P.C., et al.: Percutaneous transluminal coronary angioplasty: Report from the Registry of the National Heart, Lung and Blood Institute. Am. J. Cardiol. 49:2011, 1982.
18. Kent, K.M., Bonow, R.O., Rosing, D.R., et al.: Improved myocardial function during exercise after successful percutaneous transluminal angioplasty. N. Engl. J. Med. 306:441, 1982.
19. Kuo, P.T., Hayase, K., Kostis, J.B., and Moreyra, A.E.: Use of combined diet and colestipol in long-term (7–7½ years) treatment of patients with type II hyperlipoproteinemia. Circulation 59:199, 1979.
20. Katz, S.S., Small, D.M., Smith, F.R., et al.: Cholesterol turnover in lipid phases of human atherosclerotic plaque. J. Lipid Res. 23:733, 1982.
21. Kirkeeide, R.L., Buchi, M., Demer, L.L., and Gould, K.L.: Afterload effects on flow reserve of stenotic coronary arteries. (Abstract.) Circulation 76(Suppl. IV):IV-386, 1987.
22. Kaltenbach, M., Kober, G., Scherer, D., and Vallbracht, C.: Recurrence rate after successful coronary angioplasty. Eur. Heart J. 6:276, 1985.
23. Kramer, J.R., Matsuda, Y., Mulligan, J.C., et al.: Progression of coronary atherosclerosis. Circulation 63:519, 1981.
24. Kaul, S., Pandian, N.G., Okada, R.D., et al.: Contrast echocardiography in acute myocardial ischemia: I. In vivo determination of total left ventricular "area at risk." J. Am. Coll. Cardiol. 4:1272, 1984.
25. Keller, M.W., Glasheen, W., Smucker, M.L., et al.: Myocardial contrast echocardiography in humans. II. Assessment of coronary blood flow reserve. J. Am. Coll. Cardiol. 12:925, 1988.
26. Kirkeeide, R.L.: Coronary obstructions, morphology and physiologic significance. *In* Reiber, J.H.C., and Serruys P.W. (eds.): Quantitative Coronary Arteriography as of 1991. Kluwer Academic, Dordrecht, 1991 (in press).

L

1. Levin, D.C., Baltaxe, H.A., Lee, J.G., and Sos, T.A.: Potential sources of error in coronary arteriography. I. In performance of the study. AJR Rad. Ther. Nucl. Med. 124:378, 1975.
2. Levin, D.C., Baltaxe, H.A., and Sos, T.A.: Potential sources of error in coronary arteriography. II. In interpretation of the study. AJR Rad. Ther. Nucl. Med. 124:386, 1975.
3. Logan, S.E.: On the fluid mechanics of human coronary artery stenosis. IEEE Trans. Biomed. Eng. 22:327, 1975.
4. Lipscomb, K., and Hooten, S.: Effect of stenotic dimensions and blood flow on the hemodynamic significance of model coronary arterial stenoses. Am. J. Cardiol. 42:781, 1978.
5. LeFree, M.T., Simon, S.B., Lewis, R.J., et al.: Digital radiographic coronary artery quantification. Comput. Cardiol. 99, 1985.
6. Luyten, H.E., Beatt, K.J., de Feyter, P.J., et al.: Angioplasty for stable versus unstable angina pectoris: Are unstable patients more likely to get restenosis? A quantitative angiographic study in 339 consecutive patients. Int. J. Cardiac. Imag. 3:87, 1988.
7. Lee, G., Garcia, J.M., Chan, M.C., et al.: Clinically successful long-term laser coronary recanalization. Am. Heart J. 112:1323, 1986.
8. Ledbetter, D.C., Selzer, R.H., Gordon, R.M., et al.: Computer quantitation of coronary angiograms. *In* Miller, H.A., et al. (eds.): Noninvasive Cardiovascular Measurements. SPIE 167:17, 1978.
9. Lavayssière, B., Liénard, J., and Marchand, J.L.: RII geometrical distortion modelling and calibration. *In* Lemke, H.U., et al. (ed.): Computer Assisted Radiology. Springer-Verlag, Berlin, 1987, p. 225.
10. Lablanche, J.M., Delforge, M.R., Tilmant, P.Y., et al.: Effects hémodynamiques et coronaires du dinitrate d'isosorbide: Comparaison entre les voies d'injection intracoronaire et intraveineuse. Arch. Mal. Coeur. 75:303, 1982.
11. Lablanche, J.M., Delforge, M.R., Tilmant, P.Y., et al.: Action coronarodilatatrice de l'isosorbide dinitrate injectable. La Nouvelle Presse Médicale 11:2057, 1982.
12. Levin, D.C., Gardiner, G.A.: Complex and simple coronary artery stenoses: A new way to interpret coronary angiograms based on morphologic features of lesions. Radiology 164:675, 1987.
13. Lichtlen, P.R.: Koronar-Angiographie. Verlag, Dr. med. D. Straube, Erlangen, 1979.
14. Leimgruber, P.P., Roubin, G.S., Hollman, J., et al.: Restenosis after successful coronary angioplasty in patients with single-vessel disease. Circulation 73:710, 1986.
15. Lipton, M.J., and Boyd, D.P.: Contrast media in dynamic computed tomography of the heart and great vessels. *In* Felix, R.E., and Wegner, O.H.: Contrast Media in Computed Tomography. Elsevier, Amsterdam, 1981, p. 204.
16. Lipton, M.J., Higgins, C.B., Farmer, D.W., et al.: Real time cardiac CT scanning using a millisecond focused electron beam (cine/CT) scanner: Initial results in patients and animals. (Abstract.) J. Am. Coll. Cardiol. 3:539, 1984.
17. Lipton, M.J., Higgins, C.B., Farmer, D., and Boyd, D.P.: Cardiac imaging with a high-speed cine-CT scanner: Preliminary results. Radiology 152:579, 1984.
18. Lawrence, D.D., Charnsangavej, C., Wright, K.C., et al.: Percutaneous endovascular grafts: Experimental evaluation. Radiology 163:357, 1987.
19. Levine, S., Ewels, C.J., Rosing, D.R., and Kent, K.M.: Coronary angioplasty: Clinical and angiographic follow-up. Am. J. Cardiol. 55:673, 1985.
20. Lang, R.M., Feinstein, S.B., Feldman, T., et al.: Contrast echocardiography for evaluation of myocardial perfusion: Effects of coronary angioplasty. J. Am. Coll. Cardiol. 8:232, 1986.
21. Legrand, V., Mancini, G.B.J., Bates, E.R., et al.: Comparative study of coronary flow reserve, coronary anatomy and results of radionuclide exercise tests in patients with coronary artery disease. J. Am. Coll. Cardiol. 8:1022, 1986.

M

1. Meier, B., Gruentzig, A.R., Goebel, N., et al.: Assessment of stenoses in coronary angioplasty: Inter- and intraobserver variability. Int. J. Cardiol. 3:159, 1983.
2. Marcus, M.L.: The Coronary Circulation in Health and Disease. McGraw-Hill, New York, 1983.
3. Mates, R.E., Gupta, R.L., Bell, A.C., and Klocke, F.J.: Fluid dynamics of coronary artery stenosis. Circ. Res. 42:152, 1978.
4. Marcus, M., Wright, C., Doty, D., et al.: Measurements of coronary velocity and reactive hyperemia in the coronary circulation of humans. Circ. Res. 49:877, 1981.
5. Marcus, M.L., Skorton, D.J., Johnson, M.R., et al.: Visual estimates of percent diameter coronary stenosis: "A battered gold standard." J. Am. Coll. Cardiol. 11:882, 1988.
6. Maseri, A., Chierchia, S., Davies, G.J., and Fox, K.M.: Variable susceptibility to dynamic coronary obstruction: An elusive link between coronary atherosclerosis and angina pectoris. Am. J. Cardiol. 52:46A, 1983.
7. McPherson, D.D., Hiratzka, L.F., Lamberth, W.C., et al.: Delineation of the extent of coronary atherosclerosis by high-frequency epicardial echocardiography. N. Engl. J. Med. 316:304, 1987.
8. MacAlpin, R.N., Abbasi, A.S., Grollman, J.H., and Eber, L.: Human coronary artery size during life: A cinearteriographic study. Radiology 108:567, 1973.
9. McMahon, M.M., Brown, B.G., Cukingnan, R., et al.: Quantitative coronary angiography: Measurement of the "critical" stenosis in patients with unstable angina and single-vessel disease without collaterals. Circulation 60:106, 1979.
10. Mancini, G.B.J., Simon, S.B., McGillem, M.J., et al.: Automated quantitative coronary arteriography: Morphologic and physiologic validation in vivo of a rapid digital angiographic method. Circulation 75:452, 1987.
11. Mancini, G.B.J.: Morphologic and physiologic validation of quantitative coronary arteriography utilizing digital methods. *In* Reiber, J.H.C., and Serruys, P.W. (eds.): New Developments in Quantitative Coronary Arteriography. Martinus Nijhoff, Dordrecht, 1988, p. 125.
12. Mabin, T.A., Holmes, D.R., Jr., Smith, H.C., et al.: Follow-up clinical results in patients undergoing percutaneous transluminal coronary angioplasty. Circulation 71:754, 1985.
13. Mata, L.A., Bosch, X., David, P.R., et al.: Clinical and angiographic assessment 6 months after double vessel percutaneous coronary angioplasty. J. Am. Coll. Cardiol. 6:1239, 1985.
14. Maass, D., Zollikofer, C.L., Largiadèr, F., and Senning, A.: Radiological follow-up of transluminally inserted vascular endoprostheses: An experimental study using expanding spirals. Radiology 152:659, 1984.
15. Marcus, M.L., Wilson, R.F., and White, C.W.: Methods of measurement of myocardial blood flow in patients: A critical review. Circulation 76:245, 1987.
16. Maass, D., Kropf, L., Egloff, L., et al.: Transluminal implantation of intravascular "double-helix" spiral prostheses: Technical and biological considerations. Proc. Eur. Soc. Artif. Organs 9:252, 1982.
17. Meyer, J., Schmitz, H.J., Kiesslich, T., et al.: Percutaneous transluminal coronary angioplasty in patients with stable and unstable angina pectoris: Analysis of early and late results. Am. Heart J. 106:973, 1983.

N

1. Nichols, A.B., Gabrieli, C.F.O., Fenoglio, J.J., Jr., and Esser, P.D.: Quantification of relative coronary arterial stenosis by cinevideodensitometric analysis of coronary arteriograms. Circulation 69:512, 1984.
2. Nichols, A.B., Brown, C., Han, J., et al.: Effect of coronary stenotic lesions on regional myocardial blood flow at rest. Circulation 74:746, 1986.
3. Nalcioglu, O., Roeck, W.W., Reese, T., et al.: Interpolated background subtraction method for coronary stenosis quantification. SPIE Medical Imaging II, 914:690, 1988.
4. Nichols, A.B., Berke, A.D., Han, J., et al.: Cinevideodensitometric analysis of the effect of coronary angioplasty on coronary stenotic dimensions. Am. Heart J. 115:722, 1988.
5. Nellessen, U., Rafflenbeul, W., Daniel, W., et al.: Dilation of human epicardial coronary arteries after sublingual nifedipine and its relationship to blood levels. *In* Lichtlen, P.R. (ed.): 6th International Adalat Symposium. Excerpta-Medica, Amsterdam, 1986, p. 34.
6. Nickoloff, E.L., Han, J., Esser, P.D., and Nichols, A.B.: Evaluation of a cinevideodensitometric method for measuring vessel dimensions from digitized angiograms. Invest. Radiol. 22:875, 1987.
7. Nissen, S.E., Elion, J.L., Booth, D.C., et al.: Value and limitations of computer analysis of digital subtraction angiography in the assessment of coronary flow reserve. Circulation 73:562, 1986.
8. Nash, D.T., Gensini, G., and Esente, P.: Effect of lipid-lowering therapy on the progression of coronary atherosclerosis assessed by scheduled repetitive coronary arteriography. Int. J. Cardiol. 2:43, 1982.
9. Nikkilä, E.A., Viikinkoski, P., Valle, M., and Frick, M.H.: Prevention of progression of coronary atherosclerosis by treatment of hyperlipidaemia: A seven-year prospective angiographic study. Br. Med. J. 289:220, 1984.
10. Nobuyoshi, M., Kimura, T., Nosaka, H., et al.: Restenosis after successful percutaneous transluminal coronary angioplasty: Serial angiographic follow-up of 299 patients. J. Am. Coll. Cardiol. 12:616, 1988.
11. Nalcioglu, O., Roeck, W.W., Reese, T., et al.: Background subtraction algorithms for videodensitometric quantification of coronary stenosis. Machine Vision and Applications 1:155, 1988.

O

1. Ommeren, J. van, Zijlstra, F., Serruys, P.W., and Reiber, J.H.C.: A rapid angiographic technique to measure relative coronary blood flow. *In* Young, I.T., et al. (eds.): Signal Processing III: Theories and Applications. North-Holland, Amsterdam, 1986, p. 1375.
2. Onnasch, D.G.W., Lindenau, J., and Heintzen, P.H.: Reconstruction of the regional distribution of the myocardial perfusion from a few x-ray projections: First experimental results. *In* Lemke, H.U., et al. (eds.): Computer Assisted Radiology. Springer-Verlag, Berlin, 1985, p. 654.
3. Onnasch, D.G.W., Lindenau, J., Brossmann, J., et al.: Steps towards three-dimensional reconstruction of myocardial perfusion from multiple-view arteriography. Comput. Cardiol. 265, 1986.
4. Onnasch, D.G.W., Lindenau, J., Bürsch, J.H., and Heintzen, P.H.: Reconstruction of the spatial distribution of the myocardial perfusion from multiple-view arteriography. *In* Heintzen, P.H., and Bürsch J.H. (eds.): Progress in Digital Angiocardiography. Kluwer Academic, Dordrecht, 1988, p. 327.
5. O'Neill, W.W., Walton, J.A., Bates, E.R., et al.: Criteria for successful coronary angioplasty as assessed by alterations in coronary vasodilatory reserve. J. Am. Coll. Cardiol. 3:1382, 1984.
6. Öst, C.R., and Stenson, S.: Regression of peripheral atherosclerosis during therapy with high doses of nicotinic acid. Scand. J. Clin. Lab. Invest. (Suppl. 93):241, 1963.
7. Olsson, A.G., Erikson, U., Helmius, G., et al.: Regression of femoral atherosclerosis in humans: Methodological and clinical problems associated with studies on femoral atherosclerosis development as assessed by angiograms. *In* Malinow, M.R., and Blaton, V.H. (eds.): Regression of Atherosclerotic Lesions: Experimental Studies and Observations in Humans. Plenum Press, New York, 1984, p. 311.

P

1. Peshock, R.M., Malloy, C.R., Buja, L.M., et al.: Magnetic resonance imaging of acute myocardial infarction: Gadolinium diethylenetriamine pantaacetic acid as a marker of reperfusion. Circulation 74:1434, 1986.
2. Parker, D.L., Pope, D.L., Petersen, J.C., et al.: Quantitation in cardiac videodensitometry. Comput. Cardiol. 119, 1984.
3. Pope, D.L., Parker, D.L., Clayton, P.D., and Gustafson, D.E.: Left ventricular border recognition using a dynamic search algorithm. Radiology 155:513, 1985.
4. Puel, J., Joffre, F., Rousseau, H., et al.: Percutaneously implantable endocoronary prosthesis. *In* Reiber, J.H.C., and Serruys, P.W. (eds.): New Developments in Quantitative Coronary Arteriography. Kluwer Academic, Dordrecht, 1988, p. 271.
5. Pfaff, J.M., Whiting, J.S., Eigler, N.E., and Forrester, J.S.: Accurate densitometric quantification requires strict attention to the physical characteristics of x-ray imaging. *In* Reiber, J.H.C., and Serruys, P.W. (eds.): New Developments in Quantitative Coronary Arteriography. Martinus Nijhoff, Dordrecht, 1988, p. 22.
6. Pepine, C.J., Mehta, J., Webster, W.W., and Nichols, W.W.: In vivo validation of a thermodilution method to determine regional left ventricular blood flow in patients with coronary disease. Circulation 58:795, 1978.
7. Palmaz, J.C., Sibbitt, R.R., Reuter, S.R., et al.: Expandable intraluminal graft: A preliminary study. Radiology 156:73, 1985.
8. Palmaz, J.C., Sibbitt, R.R., Tio, F.O., et al.: Expandable intraluminal vascular graft: A feasibility study. Surgery 99:199, 1986.
9. Palmaz, J.C., Windeler, S.A., Garcia, F., et al.: Atherosclerotic rabbit aortas: Expandable intraluminal grafting. Radiology 160:723, 1986.
10. Puel, J., Juillière, Y., Bertrand, M.E., et al.: Early and late assessment of stenosis geometry after coronary arterial stenting. Am. J. Cardiol. 61:546, 1988.
11. Pannek, H., Neuhaus, K.L., Schmiel, F.K., and Spiller, P.: Röntgenvideodensitometrische Flussmessungen in aortokoronaren Bypass-Gefässen. Z. Kardiol. 67:787, 1978.
12. Parker, D.L., Pope, D.L., Van Bree, R.E., and Marshall, H.: Three-dimensional reconstruction and cross-section measurements of coronary arteries using ECG-correlated digital coronary arteriography. *In* Heintzen, P.H., and Bürsch, J.H. (eds.): Progress in Digital Angiocardiography. Kluwer Academic, Dordrecht, 1988, p. 181.
13. Parker, D.L., Wu, J., Pope, D.L., et al.: Three-dimensional reconstruction and flow measurements of coronary arteries using multi-view digital angiography. *In* Reiber, J.H.C., and Serruys, P.W. (eds.): New Developments in Quantitative Coronary Arteriography. Kluwer Academic, Dordrecht, 1988, p. 225.
14. Pÿls, N.H.J., Uÿen, G.J.H., Hoevelaken, A., et al.: Mean transit time for the assessment of myocardial perfusion by videodensitometry. Circulation 81:1331, 1990.

R

1. Roberts, W.C., and Buja, L.M.: The frequency and significance of coronary arterial thrombi and other observations in fatal acute myocardial infarction: A study of 107 necropsy patients. Am. J. Med. 52:425, 1972.
2. Rumberger, J.A., Feiring, A.J., Higgins, C.R., et al.: Use of ultrafast computed tomography to quantitate myocardial perfusion: A preliminary report. J. Am. Coll. Cardiol. 9:59, 1987.
3. Reiber, J.H.C., Kooijman, C.J., Slager, C.J., et al.: Computer-assisted analysis of the severity of obstructions from coronary cineangiograms: A methodological review. Automedica 5:219, 1984.
4. Reiber, J.H.C., Serruys, P.W., and Slager, C.J.: Quantitative Coronary and Left Ventricular Cineangiography: Methodology and Clinical Applications. Martinus Nijhoff, Boston, 1986.
5. Reiber, J.H.C.: Morphologic and densitometric quantitation of coronary stenoses: An overview of existing quantitation techniques. *In* Reiber, J.H.C., and Serruys, P.W. (eds.): New Developments in Quantitative Coronary Arteriography. Martinus Nijhoff, Dordrecht, 1988, p. 34.
6. Rafflenbeul, W., Heim, R., Dzuiba, M., et al.: Morphometric analysis of coronary arteries. *In* Lichtlen, P.R. (ed.): Coronary Angiography and Angina Pectoris. Georg Thieme, Stuttgart, 1976, p. 255.
7. Reiber, J.H.C., Mostert, M., Burken, G. van, and Dumay, A.: LVAS, a new PC-based left ventricular analysis system. Abstract book 54. Jahrestagung der Deutschen Gesellschaft für Herz- and Kreislauf-forschung, Mannheim, April 8–10, 1988, p. 150. (Abstract.) Steinkopff, Darmstadt Germany.
8. Reiber, J.H.C.: Morphologic and densitometric analysis of coronary arteries. *In* Heintzen, P. (ed.): Progress in Cardiovascular Angiography. Martinus Nijhoff, Dordrecht, 1987, p. 137.
9. Reiber, J.H.C., Kooijman, C.J., Slager, C.J., et al.: Taking a quantitative approach to cine-angiogram analysis. Diagn. Imag., April 1985, p. 87.
10. Reiber, J.H.C., Serruys, P.W., Kooijman, C.J., et al.: Approaches towards standardization in acquisition and quantitation of arterial dimensions from cineangiograms. *In* Reiber, J.H.C., and Serruys, P.W. (eds.): State of the Art in Quantitative Coronary Arteriography. Martinus Nijhoff, Dordrecht, 1986, p. 145.
11. Reiber, J.H.C., Kooijman, C.J., den Boer, A., and Serruys, P.W.: Assessment of dimensions and image quality of coronary contrast catheters from cineangiograms. Cathet. Cardiovasc. Diagn. 11:521, 1985.
12. Reiber, J.H.C., Slager, C.J., Schuurbiers, J.C.H., et al.: Transfer functions of the x-ray–cine-video chain applied to digital processing of coronary cineangiograms. *In* Heintzen, P.H., and Brennecke, R. (eds.): Digital Imaging in Cardiovascular Radiology. Georg Thieme Verlag, Stuttgart, 1983, p. 89.
13. Reiber, J.H.C., Kooijman, C.J., Slager, C.J., et al.: Improved densitometric assessment of percent area-stenosis from coronary cineangiograms. (Abstract.) Tenth World Congress of Cardiology, Washington, DC, 1986, p. 39.
14. Reiber, J.H.C., den Boer, A., and Serruys, P.W.: Quality control in performing quantitative coronary arteriography. Am. J. Cardiac Imag. 3:172, 1989.
15. Reiber, J.H.C.: An overview of morphologic and densitometric approaches for the quantitation of coronary stenoses. Automedica 10:171, 1989.
16. Reiber, J.H.C., Serruys, P.W., Kooijman, C.J., et al.: Assessment of short-, medium-, and long-term variations in arterial dimensions from computer-assisted quantitation of coronary cineangiograms. Circulation 71:280, 1985.
17. Rafflenbeul, W., and Lichtlen, P.R.: Release of residual vascular tone in coronary artery stenoses with nifedipine and glyceryl trinitrate. *In* Kaltenbach, M., and Neufeld, H.N. (eds.): Proceedings of the 5th International Adalat Symposium. New Therapy of Ischaemic Heart Disease and Hypertension. Excerpta-Medica, Amsterdam, 1983, p. 300.
18. Reiber, J.H.C., van Eldik-Helleman, P., Visser-Akkerman, N., et al.: Variabilities in measurement of coronary arterial dimensions resulting from variations in cineframe selection. Cathet. Cardiovasc. Diagn. 14:221, 1988.
19. Reiber, J.H.C., van Eldik-Helleman, P., Kooijman, C.J., et al.: How critical is frame selection in quantitative coronary angiographic studies? Eur. Heart J. 10(Suppl F):54, 1989.
20. Rutishauser, W., Ratib, O., Chappuis, F., et al.: Coronary blood flow and myocardial perfusion studied by digitized coronary angiograms. *In* Heintzen, P.H., and Bürsch, J.H. (eds.): Progress in Digital Angiocardiography. Kluwer Academic, Dordrecht, 1988, p. 221.

21. Reiber, J.H.C., Zijlstra, F., van Ommeren, J., and Serruys, P.W.: Relation between coronary flow reserve and severity of coronary obstruction, both assessed from coronary cineangiogram. *In* Heintzen, P.H., and Bürsch, J.H. (eds.): Progress in Digital Angiocardiography. Kluwer Academic, Dordrecht, 1988, p. 275.
22. Ross, R.S., Ueda, K., Lichtlen, P.R., and Rees, J.R.: Measurement of myocardial blood flow in animals and man by selective injection of radioactive inert gas into the coronary arteries. Circ. Res. 15:28, 1964.
23. Rutishauer, W., Noseda, G., Bussman, W.D., and Preter, B.: Blood flow measurement through single coronary arteries by röntgen densitometry. Part II. Right coronary artery flow in conscious man. AJR Rad. Ther. Nucl. Med. 109:21, 1970.
24. Rothman, M.T., Baims, D.S., Simpson, J.B., and Harrison, D.C.: Coronary hemodynamics during percutaneous transluminal coronary angioplasty. Am. J. Cardiol. 49:1615, 1982.
25. Rafflenbeul, W., Smith, L.R., Rogers, W.J., et al.: Quantitative coronary arteriography: Coronary anatomy of patients with unstable angina pectoris reexamined 1 year after optimal medical therapy. Am. J. Cardiol. 43:699, 1979.
26. Rutishauser, W.: Equipment for cinedensitometry for 35 mm film. *In* Heintzen, P.H. (ed.): Roentgen-, Cine- and Videodensitometry: Fundamentals and Applications for Blood Flow and Heart Volume Determinations. Georg Thieme Verlag, Stuttgart, 1971, p. 68.
27. Ritchie, J.L., Hansen, D.D., Vracko, R., and Auth, D.: In vivo rotational thrombectomy: Evaluation by angioscopy. (Abstract.) Circulation 74(Suppl II):II-457, 1986.
28. Roubin, G.S., Robinson, K.A., King III, S.B., et al.: Early and late results of intracoronary arterial stenting after coronary angioplasty in dogs. Circulation 76:891, 1987.
29. Rutishauser, W., Bussman, W.D., Noseda, G., et al.: Blood flow measurement through single coronary arteries by roentgen densitometry. Part I. A comparison of flow measured by a radiologic technique applicable in the intact organism and by electromagnetic flowmeter. AJR 109:12, 1970.
30. Reiber, J.H.C., Gerbrands, J.J., Booman, F., et al.: Objective characterization of coronary obstructions from monoplane cineangiograms and three-dimensional reconstruction of an arterial segment from two orthogonal views. *In* Schwartz, M.D. (ed.): Applications of Computers in Medicine. IEEE Cat No. TH 0095-0, 1982, p. 93.
31. Reiber, J.H.C., Gerbrands, J.J., Troost, G.J., et al.: 3-D reconstruction of coronary arterial segments from two projections. *In* Heintzen, P.H., and Brennecke, R. (eds.): Digital Imaging in Cardiovascular Radiology. Georg Thieme Verlag, Stuttgart, 1983, p. 151.
32. Reiber, J.H.C.: An overview of coronary quantitation techniques as of 1989. *In* Reiber, J.H.C., and Serruys, P.W. (eds.): Quantitative Coronary Arteriography as of 1989. Kluwer Academic, Dordrecht, 1990 (in press).

S

1. Sanmarco, M.E., Brooks, S.H., and Blankenhorn, D.H.: Reproducibility of a consensus panel in the interpretation of coronary angiograms. Am. Heart J. 96:430, 1978.
2. Shub, C., Vlietstra, R.E., Smith, H.C., et al.: The unpredictable progression of symptomatic coronary artery disease: A serial clinical-angiographic analysis. Mayo Clin. Proc. 56:155, 1981.
3. Schlesinger, M.J., and Zoll, P.M.: Incidence and localization of coronary artery occlusions. Arch. Pathol. 32:178, 1941.
4. Shipley, R.E., and Gregg, D.E.: The effect of external constriction of a blood vessel on blood flow. Am. J. Physiol. 141:289, 1944.
5. Schelbert, H.R., Wisenberg, G., Phelps, M.E., et al.: Noninvasive assessment of coronary stenoses by myocardial imaging during pharmacologic coronary vasodilation. VI. Detection of coronary artery disease in human beings with intravenous N-13 ammonia and positron computed tomography. Am. J. Cardiol. 49:1197, 1982.
6. Sabbah, H.N., and Stein, P.D: Hemodynamics of multiple versus single 50 percent coronary arterial stenoses. Am. J. Cardiol. 50:276, 1982.
7. Schwartz, J.S., Carlyle, P.F., and Cohn, J.N.: Effect of coronary arterial pressure on coronary stenosis resistance. Circulation 61:70, 1980.
8. Schwartz, J.S.: Fixed vs. nonfixed coronary stenosis: The response to a fall in coronary pressure in a canine model. Cathet. Cardiovasc. Diagn. 8:383, 1982.
9. Schwartz, J.S.: Compliant coronary stenoses. (Editorial note.) Int. J. Cardiol. 4:315, 1983.
10. Scoblionko, D.P., Brown, B.G., Mitten, S., et al.: A new digital electronic caliper for measurement of coronary arterial stenosis: Comparison with visual estimates and computer-assisted measurements. Am. J. Cardiol. 53:689, 1984.
11. Sanders, W.J., Alderman, E.L., and Harrison, D.C.: Coronary artery quantitation using digital image processing. Comput. Cardiol. 15, 1979.
12. Selzer, R.H., Shircore, A., Lee, P.L., et al.: A second look at quantitative coronary angiography: Some unexpected problems. *In* Reiber, J.H.C., and Serruys, P.W. (eds.): State of the Art in Quantitative Coronary Arteriography. Martinus Nijhoff, Dordrecht, 1986, p. 125.
13. Serruys, P.W., Reiber, J.H.C., Wijns, W., et al.: Assessment of percutaneous transluminal coronary angioplasty by quantitative coronary angiography: Diameter versus densitometric area measurements. Am. J. Cardiol. 54:482, 1984.
14. Serruys, P.W., Geuskens, R., de Feyter, P., et al.: Incidence of restenosis 30 and 60 days after successful PTCA: A quantitative coronary angiographic study in 200 consecutive patients. (Abstract.) Circulation 72(Supp. III):III-140, 1985.
15. Serruys, P.W., Wijns, W., van den Brand, M., et al.: Is transluminal coronary angioplasty mandatory after successful thrombolysis? A quantitative coronary angiographic study. Br. Heart J. 50:257, 1983.
16. Serruys, P.W., Arnold, A.E.R., Brower, R.W., et al.: Quantitative assessment of the effect of continued rt-PA infusion on the residual stenosis after initial recanalisation in acute myocardial infarction. (Abstract.) Circulation 74:II-368, 1986.
17. Serruys, P.W., Arnold, A.E.R., Brower, R.W., et al.: Effect of continued rt-PA administration on the residual stenosis after initially successful recanalization in acute myocardial infarction—a quantitative coronary angiography study of a randomized trial. Eur. Heart J. 8:1172, 1987.
18. Sigwart, U., Puel, J., Mirkovitch, V., et al.: Intravascular stents to prevent occlusion and restenosis after transluminal angioplasty. N. Engl. J. Med. 316:701, 1987.
19. Slager, C.J., Essed, C.A., Schuurbiers, J.C.H., et al.: Vaporization of atherosclerotic plaques by spark erosion. J. Am. Coll. Cardiol. 5:1382, 1985.
20. Selzer, R.H., Blankenhorn, D.H., Crawford, D.W., et al.: Computer analysis of cardiovascular imagery. Proceedings, Caltech./J.P.L. Conference on Image Processing Techniques, Data Sources, and Software for Commercial and Scientific Application. Pasadena, Cal., 1976, p. 1.
21. Siebes, M., D'Argenio, D.Z., and Selzer, R.H.: Computer assessment of hemodynamic severity of coronary artery stenosis from angiograms. Comput. Methods and Programs in Biomedicine 21:143, 1985.
22. Sonoda, Y., Mori, K., Yasue, H., and Horio, Y.: A simple quantitative analysis system for coronary cineangiograms using a personal computer. Jpn. Circ. J. 51:1157, 1987.
23. Sigwart, U., Golf, S., Kaufmann, U., and Kappenberger, L.: A coronary endoprosthesis to prevent restenosis and acute occlusion after percutaneous angioplasty: One and a half years of clinical experience. *In* Reiber, J.H.C., and Serruys, P.W. (eds.): New Developments in Quantitative Coronary Arteriography. Kluwer Academic, Dordrecht, 1988, p. 278.
24. Seibert, J.A., Nalcioglu, O., and Roeck, W.W.: Characterization of the veiling glare PSF in x-ray image intensified fluoroscopy. Med. Phys. 11:172, 1984.
25. Shaw, C.G., Ergun, D.I., Van Lysel, M.S., et al.: Quantitation techniques in digital subtraction videoangiography. *In* Brody, W.R. (ed): Digital Radiography. SPIE 314:121, 1982.
26. Simons, M.A., Bastian, B.V., Bray, B.E., and Dedrickson, D.R.: Comparison of observer and videodensitometric measurements of simulated coronary artery stenoses. Invest. Radiol. 22:562, 1987.
27. Serruys, P.W., Hooghoudt, T.E.H., Reiber, J.H.C., et al.: Influence of intracoronary nifedipine on left ventricular function, coronary vasomotility, and myocardial oxygen consumption. Br. Heart J. 49:427, 1983.
28. Serruys, P.W., Booman, F., Steward, R., et al.: Unstable angina pectoris and coronary arterial vasomotion: Which role for nifedipine? *In* Rafflenbeul, W., et al. (eds.): Unstable Angina Pectoris. Georg Thieme Verlag, Stuttgart, 1981, p. 103.
29. Strauer, B.E.: Isosorbide dinitrate: Its action on myocardial contractility in comparison with nitroglycerin. Int. J. Clin. Pharm. Ther. Toxicol. 8:30, 1973.
30. Spiller, P., Schmiel, F.K., Pölitz, B., et al.: Measurement of systolic and diastolic flow rates in coronary artery system by x-ray densitometry. Circulation 68:337, 1983.
31. Skelton, T.N., Kisslo, K.B., and Bashore, T.M.: Comparison of coronary stenosis quantitation results from on-line digital and digitized cine film images. Am. J. Cardiol. 62:381, 1988.
32. Simons, M.A., Kruger, R.A., and Power, R.L.: Cross-sectional area measurements by digital subtraction videodensitometry. Invest. Radiol. 21:637, 1986.
33. Simons, M.A., Muskett, A.D., Kruger, R.A., et al.: Quantitative digital subtraction coronary angiography using videodensitometry: An in vivo analysis. Invest. Radiol. 23:98, 1988.
34. Serruys, P.W., Brower, R.W., ten Katen, H.J., et al: Regional wall motion from radiopaque markers after intravenous and intracoronary injections of nifedipine. Circulation 63:584, 1981.
35. Spears, J.R., and Sandor, T.: Quantitation of coronary artery stenosis severity: Limitations of angiography and computerized information extraction. *In* Reiber, J.H.C., and Serruys, P.W. (eds.): State of the Art in Quantitative Coronary Arteriography. Martinus Nijhoff, Dordrecht, 1986, p. 103.
36. Serruys, P.W., Wijns, W., van den Brand, M., et al.: Left ventricular performance, regional blood flow, wall motion, and lactate metabolism during transluminal angioplasty. Circulation 70:25, 1984.
37. Sapirstein, L.A.: Regional blood flow by fractional distribution of indicators. Am. J. Physiol. 193:161, 1958.
38. Selwyn, A.P., Allan, R.M., L'Abatta, A., et al.: Relation between regional myocardial uptake of rubidium-82 and perfusion: Absolute reduction of cation uptake in ischemia. Am. J. Cardiol. 50:112, 1982.
39. Serruys, P.W., Juillière, Y., Zijlstra, F., et al.: Coronary blood flow velocity during percutaneous transluminal coronary angioplasty as a guide for assessment of the functional results. Am. J. Cardiol. 61:253, 1988.
40. Scholl, J.M., Chaitman, B.R., David, P.R., et al.: Exercise electrocardiography and myocardial scintigraphy in the serial evaluation of the results of percutaneous transluminal coronary angioplasty. Circulation 66:380, 1982.
41. Sibley, D.H., Millar, H.D., Hartley, C.J., and Whitlow, P.L.: Subselective measurement of coronary blood flow velocity using a steerable Doppler catheter. J. Am. Coll. Cardiol. 8:1332, 1986.
42. Serruys, P.W., Zijlstra, F., Reiber, J.H.C., et al.: A comparison of two methods to measure coronary flow reserve in the setting of coronary angioplasty: Intracoronary blood flow velocity measurements with a Doppler catheter and digital subtraction cineangiography. Eur. Heart J. 10:725, 1989.
43. Serruys, P.W., Juillière, Y., Bertrand, M.E., et al.: Additional improvement of stenosis geometry in human coronary arteries by stenting after balloon dilatation. Am. J. Cardiol. 61:71G, 1988.
44. Smith, S.C., Gorlin, R., Herman, M.V., et al.: Myocardial blood flow in man:

Effects of coronary collateral circulation and coronary artery bypass surgery. J. Clin. Invest. 51:2556, 1972.

45. Smith, H.C., Frye, R.L., Donald, D.E., et al.: Roentgen videodensitometric measure of coronary blood flow: Determination from simultaneous indicator-dilution curves at selected sites in the coronary circulation and in coronary artery–saphenous vein grafts. Mayo Clin. Proc. 46:800, 1971.
46. Simon, R., Amende, I., and Lichtlen, P.R.: Roentgen videodensitometry in the analysis of coronary angiograms. *In* Bruschke, G., et al. (eds.): Coronary Artery Disease Today: Diagnosis, Surgery and Prognosis. Excerpta-Medica, Amsterdam, 1982, p. 176.
47. Simon, R., Amende, I., Oelert, H., et al.: Blood velocity, flow and dimensions of aortacoronary venous bypass grafts in the postoperative state. Circulation 66(Supp. I):I34, 1982.
48. Sauer, G., Krause, H., Burmeister, A., et al.: Determination of coronary flow velocities in man by a computer-aided cine-videodensitometric system. Z. Kardiol. 72:207, 1983.
49. Schultz, W., Wendt, T., Scherer, D., and Kober, G.: Diameter changes of epicardial coronary arteries and coronary stenoses after intracoronary application of SIN 1, a Molsidomine metabolite. Z. Kardiol. 72:404, 1983.
50. Siebes, M., Selzer, R.H., and Blankenhorn, D.H.: Do coronary artery stenoses oscillate during a cardiac cycle? (Abstract.) J. Am. Coll. Cardiol. 11:48A, 1988.
51. Small, D.M.: Progression and regression of atherosclerotic lesions: Insights from lipid physical biochemistry. Arteriosclerosis 8:103, 1988.
52. Simpson, J.B., Zimmerman, J.J., Selmon, M.R., et al.: Transluminal atherectomy: Initial clinical results in 27 patients. (Abstract.) Circulation 74(Suppl II): II-203, 1986.
53. Schatz, R., Palmaz, J., Garcia, F., et al.: Balloon expandable intracoronary stents in dogs. (Abstract.) Circulation 74(Suppl II): II-458, 1986.
54. Sugita, Y., Shimomitsu, T., Oku, T., et al.: Nonsurgical implantation of a vascular ring prosthesis using thermal shape memory Ti/Ni alloy (Nitinol Wire). Trans. Am. Soc. Artif. Intern. Organs 32:30, 1986.
55. Serruys, P.W., Luijten, H.E., Beatt, K.J., et al.: Incidence of restenosis after successful coronary angioplasty: A time-related phenomenon. Circulation 77:361, 1988.
56. Schwartz, L., Bourassa, M.G., Lespérance, J., et al.: Aspirin and dipyridamole in the prevention of restenosis after percutaneous transluminal coronary angioplasty. N. Engl. J. Med. 318:1714, 1988.
57. Sanders, M.: Angiographic changes thirty minutes following percutaneous transluminal coronary angioplasty. Angiology 36:419, 1985.
58. Sibley, D., Bulle, T., Baxley, W., et al.: Acute changes in blood flow velocity with successful coronary angioplasty. (Abstract.) Circulation 74(Suppl. II):II-193, 1986.
59. Serruys, P.W., Zijlstra, F., Reiber, H.H.C., et al.: Assessment of coronary flow reserve during angioplasty using a Doppler tip balloon catheter: Comparison with digital subtraction cineangiography. J. Intervent. Cardiol. 1:19, 1988.
60. Simpson, J.B., Selmon, M.R., Robertson, G.C., et al.: Transluminal atherectomy for occlusive peripheral vascular disease. Am. J. Cardiol. 61:96G, 1988.

T

1. Thomas, A.C., Davies, M.J., Dilly, S., et al.: Potential errors in the estimation of coronary arterial stenosis from clinical arteriography with reference to the shape of the coronary arterial lumen. Br. Heart J. 55:129, 1986.
2. Tobis, J., Nalcioglu, O., Iseri, L., et al.: Detection and quantitation of coronary artery stenoses from digital subtraction angiograms compared with 35-millimeter film cineangiograms. Am. J. Cardiol. 54:489, 1984.
3. Tobis, J., Nalcioglu, O., Johnston, W.D., et al.: Videodensitometric determination of minimum coronary artery luminal diameter before and after angioplasty. Am. J. Cardiol. 59:38, 1987.
4. Thornton, M.A., Gruentzig, A.R., Hollman, J., et al.: Coumadin and aspirin in prevention of recurrence after transluminal coronary angioplasty: A randomized study. Circulation 69:721, 1984.
5. Tei, C., Kondo, S., Meerbaum, S., et al.: Correlation of myocardial echo contrast disappearance rate ("washout") and severity of experimental coronary stenosis. J. Am. Coll. Cardiol. 3:39, 1984.
6. Ten Cate, F.J., Serruys, P.W., Silverman, P.R., et al.: Current myocardial perfusion echo methodology precludes an accurate assessment of coronary vascular reserve. (Abstract.) JACC 13:116A, 1989.

V

1. Vlodaver, Z., and Edwards, J.E.: Pathology of coronary atherosclerosis. Prog. Cardiovasc. Dis. 14:256, 1971.
2. Vlodaver, Z., Neufeld, H.N., and Edwards, J.E.: Pathology of coronary disease. Semin. Roentgenol. 7:376, 1972.
3. Vogel, R., LeFree, M., Bates, E., et al.: Application of digital techniques to selective coronary arteriography: Use of myocardial contrast appearance time to measure coronary flow reserve. Am. Heart J. 107:153, 1984.
4. Vogel, R.A.: The radiographic assessment of coronary blood flow parameters. Circulation 72:460, 1985.
5. Vogel, R.A., LeFree, M.T., and Mancini, G.B.J.: Comparison of 35 mm cinefilm and digital radiographic image imaging for quantitative coronary arteriography. *In* Heintzen, P.H., and Bürsch, J.H. (eds.): Progress in Digital Angiocardiography. Kluwer Academic, Dordrecht, 1988, p. 159.
6. Vassanelli, C., Menegatti, G., Morando, G., et al.: The eccentricity and irregularity of coronary artery stenosis: Two additional computerized parameters of quantitative coronary angiography. Comput. Cardiol. 631, 1988.
7. Vogel, R.A., Bates, E.R., O'Neill, W.W., et al.: Coronary flow reserve measured during cardiac catheterization. Arch. Intern. Med. 144:1773, 1984.
8. Vogel, R.A., Grines, C.L., and Mancini, G.B.J.: Impedance measurement of coronary blood flow using a standard angioplasty catheter. (Abstract.) Circulation 76(Suppl. IV):402, 1987.
9. Vogel, R.A., Friedman, H.Z., Beauman, G.J., et al.: Measurement of absolute coronary blood flow using a standard angioplasty catheter. (Abstract.) J. Am. Coll. Cardiol. 9:69A, 1987.
10. Vogel, R.A., Martin, L.W., and Johnson, R.A.: Impedance measurement of absolute coronary blood flow using a standard angioplasty catheter. (Abstract.) Circulation 78(Suppl. II):II-104, 1988.
11. Vandormael, M.G., Deligonul, U., Kern, M.J., et al.: Multilesion coronary angioplasty: Clinical and angiographic follow-up. J. Am. Coll. Cardiol. 10:246, 1987.
12. Vogel, R.A., Martin, L.W.: Assessment of coronary blood flow and velocity in the catheterization laboratory. *In* Reiber, J.H.C., Serruys, P.W. (eds.): Quantitative Coronary Arteriography as of 1989. Kluwer Academic, Dordrecht, 1990 (in press).

W

1. Wilson, R.F., Laughlin, D.E., Ackell, P.H., et al.: Transluminal subselective measurement of coronary artery blood flow velocity and vasodilator reserve in man. Circulation 72:82, 1985.
2. Wright, C., White, C., Furda, J., et al.: Can the coronary arteriogram predict the functional significance of a coronary stenosis? (Abstract.) Circulation 62(Suppl. III):III-214, 1980.
3. White, C.W., Wright, C.B., Doty, D.B., et al.: Does visual interpretation of the coronary arteriogram predict the physiologic importance of a coronary stenosis? N. Engl. J. Med. 310:819, 1984.
4. Wilson, R.F., Marcus, M.L., and White, C.W.: Prediction of the physiologic significance of coronary arterial lesions by quantitative lesion geometry in patients with limited coronary artery disease. Circulation 75:723, 1987.
5. Wong, W.H., Kirkeeide, R.L., and Gould, K.L.: Computer applications in angiography. *In* Collins, S.M., and Skorton, D.J. (eds.): Cardiac Imaging and Image Processing. McGraw-Hill, New York, 1986, p. 206.
6. Wollschläger, H., Lee, P., Zeiher, A., et al.: Improvement of quantitative angiography by exact calculation of radiological magnification factors. Comput. Cardiol. 483, 1985.
7. Wollschläger, H.: Optimal biplane imaging of coronary segments with computed exact triple orthogonal projections. *In* Reiber, J.H.C., and Serruys, P.W. (eds.): New Developments in Quantitative Coronary Arteriography. Martinus Nijhoff, Dordrecht, 1988, p. 13.
8. Wiesel, J., Grunwald, A.M., Tobiasz, C., et al.: Quantitation of absolute area of a coronary arterial stenosis: Experimental validation with a preparation in vivo. Circulation 74:1099, 1986.
9. Webb, S.C., Canepa-Anson, R., Rickards, A.F., and Poole-Wilson, P.A.: High potassium concentration in a parenteral preparation of glyceryl trinitrate: Need for caution if given by intracoronary injection. Br. Heart J. 50:395, 1983.
10. Wilson, R., Shea, M., de Landsheere, C., et al.: Myocardial blood flow: Clinical application and recent advances. *In* Simoons, M.L., and Reiber, J.H.C. (eds.): Nuclear Imaging in Clinical Cardiology. Martinus Nijhoff, Boston, 1984, p. 39.
11. Walsh, W.F., Harper, P.V., Resnekov, L., and Fill, H.: Noninvasive evaluation of regional myocardial perfusion in 112 patients using a mobile scintillation camera and intravenous N-13 labeled ammonia. Circulation 54:266, 1976.
12. Wright, C.B., Doty, D.B., Eastham, C.L., and Marcus, M.L.: Measurements of coronary reactive hyperemia with a Doppler probe: Intraoperative guide to hemodynamically significant lesions. J. Thorax Cardiovasc. Surg. 80:888, 1980.
13. Wilson, R.F., and White, C.W.: Intracoronary papaverine: An ideal coronary vasodilator for studies of the coronary circulation in conscious humans. Circulation 73:444, 1986.
14. Wijns, W., Serruys, P.W., Reiber, J.H.C., et al.: Quantitative angiography of the left anterior descending coronary artery: Correlations with pressure gradient and results of exercise thallium scintigraphy. Circulation 71:273, 1985.
15. Wilson, R.F., Aylward, P.E., Talman, C.L., and White, C.W.: Does percutaneous transluminal coronary angioplasty restore coronary vasodilator reserve? (Abstract.) Circulation 72(Suppl. III):397, 1985.
16. Wright, K.C., Wallace, S., Charnsangavej, C., et al.: Percutaneous endovascular stents: An experimental evaluation. Radiology 156:69, 1985.
17. Webb, S.C., Rickards, A.F., and Poole-Wilson, P.A.: Coronary sinus potassium concentration recorded during coronary angioplasty. Br. Heart J. 50:146, 1983.
18. Wilson, R.F., Aylward, P.E., Leimbach, W.N., et al.: Coronary flow reserve late after PTCA—Do the early alterations persist? (Abstract.) J. Am. Coll. Cardiol. 7:212A, 1986.
19. Wijns, W., Serruys, P.W., van den Brand, M., et al.: Progression to complete coronary obstruction without myocardial infarction in patients who are candidates for percutaneous transluminal angioplasty: A 90-day angiographic follow-up. *In* Roskamm, H. (ed.): Prognosis of Coronary Heart Disease—Progression of Coronary Arteriosclerosis. Springer-Verlag, Berlin, 1983, p. 190.
20. White, C.W., Wilson, R.F., and Marcus, M.L.: Methods of measuring myocardial blood flow in humans. Progr. Cardiovasc. Dis. 31:79, 1988.
21. Wilson, R.F., Johnson, M.R., Marcus, M.L., et al.: The effect of coronary angioplasty on coronary flow reserve. Circulation 77:873, 1988.
22. van der Werf, T., Heethaar, R.M., Stegehuis, H., et al.: Comparison of time parameters derived from myocardial time-density curves in patients before and after percutaneous transluminal coronary angioplasty. *In* Heintzen, P.H.,

and Bürsch, J.H. (eds.): Progress in Digital Angiocardiography. Kluwer Academic, Dordrecht, 1988, p. 227.
23. Waller, B.F., McManus, B.M., Gorfinkel, H.J., et al.: Status of the major epicardial coronary arteries 80 to 150 days after percutaneous transluminal coronary angioplasty: Analysis of three necropsy patients. Am. J. Cardiol. 51:81, 1983.
24. Wijns, W., Serruys, P.W., Simoons, M.L., et al.: Predictive value of early maximal exercise test and thallium scintigraphy after successful percutaneous transluminal coronary angioplasty. Br. Heart J. 53:194, 1985.
25. Wijns, W., Serruys, P.W., Reiber, J.H.C., et al.: Early detection of restenosis after successful percutaneous transluminal coronary angioplasty by exercise-redistribution thallium scintigraphy. Am. J. Cardiol. 55:357, 1985.
26. Widimsky, P., Cornel, J.H., and Cate, F.J. ten: Evaluation of collateral blood flow by myocardial contrast enhanced echocardiography. Br. Heart J. 59:20, 1988.

Y

1. Young, D.F., and Tsai, F.Y.: Flow characteristics in models of arterial stenoses. I. Steady flow. J. Biomech. 6:395, 1973.
2. Young, D.F., and Tsai, F.Y.: Flow characteristics in models of arterial stenoses. II. Unsteady flow. J. Biomech. 6:547, 1973.
3. Young, D.F., Cholvin, N.R., and Roth, A.C.: Pressure drop across artificially induced stenoses in the femoral arteries of dogs. Circ. Res. 36:735, 1975.
4. Yongchareon, W., and Young, D.F.: Initiation of turbulence in models of arterial stenoses. J. Biomech. 12:185, 1979.
5. Young, D.F., Cholvin, N.R., Kirkeeide, R.L., and Roth, A.C.: Hemodynamics of arterial stenoses at elevated flow rates. Circ. Res. 41:99, 1977.

Z

1. Zir, L.M., Miller, S.W., Dinsmore, R.E., et al.: Interobserver variability in coronary angiography. Circulation 53:627, 1976.
2. Zir, L.M.: Observer variability in coronary angiography. (Editorial note.) Int. J. Cardiol. 3:171, 1983.
3. Zijlstra, F., Fioretti, P., Reiber, J.H.C., and Serruys, P.W.: Correlations between quantitative cineangiography, coronary flow reserve measured with digital subtraction cineangiography and exercise thallium perfusion scintigraphy. Int. J. Cardiac. Imag. 3:133, 1988.
4. Zijlstra, F., Reiber, J.H.C., and Serruys, P.W.: Does intracoronary papaverine dilate epicardial coronary arteries? Implications for the assessment of coronary flow reserve. Cathet. Cardiovasc. Diagn. 14:1, 1988.
5. Zijlstra, F., van Ommeren, J., Reiber, J.H.C., and Serruys, P.W.: Does the quantitative assessment of coronary artery dimensions predict the physiologic significance of a coronary stenosis? Circulation 75:1154, 1987.
6. Zijlstra, F., Serruys, P.W., and Hugenholtz, P.G.: Papaverine: The ideal coronary vasodilator for investigating coronary flow reserve? A study of timing, magnitude, reproducibility, and safety of the coronary hyperemic response after intracoronary papaverine. Cathet. Cardiovasc. Diagn. 12:298, 1986.
7. Zijlstra, F., Juillière, Y., Serruys, P.W., and Roelandt, J.R.T.C.: Value and limitations of intracoronary adenosine for the assessment of coronary flow reserve. Cathet. Cardiovasc. Diagn. 15:76, 1988.
8. Zijlstra, F., van Ommeren, J., Reiber, J.H.C., and Serruys, P.W.: Does quantitative assessment of coronary artery dimensions predict the physiologic significance of a coronary stenosis? Circulation 75:1154, 1987.
9. Zijlstra, F., den Boer, A., Reiber, J.H.C., et al.: Assessment of immediate and long-term functional results of percutaneous transluminal coronary angioplasty. Circulation 78:15, 1988.
10. Zijlstra, F., Reiber, J.H.C., Juillière, Y., and Serruys, P.W.: Normalization of coronary flow reserve by percutaneous transluminal coronary angioplasty. Am. J. Cardiol. 61:55, 1988.
11. Zijlstra, F.: Coronary flow reserve: A functional measure of stenosis severity. Ph.D. dissertation. Erasmus University, Rotterdam, 1988.
12. Zijlstra, F., Fioretti, P., Reiber, J.H.C., and Serruys, P.W.: Which cineangiographically assessed anatomic variable correlates best with functional measurements of stenosis severity? A comparison of quantitative analysis of the coronary cineangiogram with measured coronary flow reserve and exercise/redistribution thallium-201 scintigraphy. J. Am. Coll. Cardiol. 12:686, 1988.
13. Zijlstra, F., and Serruys, P.W.: Intracoronary blood flow velocity and transstenotic pressure drop in an awake human being during coronary vasodilation. J. Intervent. Cardiol. 1:43, 1988.

Part IV

Digital Angiography

Chapter 14

Physical Principles and Instrumentation in Digital Angiography

JAMES S. WHITING, Ph.D.

GENERAL PRINCIPLES OF DIGITAL IMAGING ... 281
Converting Images to Digital Form ... 282
Scanning ... 282
Sampling ... 282
Quantization ... 282
Bit Depth ... 282
Noise ... 282
Pixel Size ... 283
Digital Image Storage ... 283
DIGITAL ANGIOGRAPHY EQUIPMENT ... 283
Video for Digital Angiography ... 283
Linearity ... 283
Lag ... 284
Interlace ... 284
Progressive Scan ... 284
Digital Image Processor ... 284
Arithmetic Logic Unit ... 284
Intensity Transformation (Lookup) Table ... 284
Hardware Zoom ... 285
Host Computer ... 285
Array Processors ... 285
Real-Time Convolver ... 285
On-Line Image Storage ... 285
Solid-State Memory ... 285
Real-Time Digital Magnetic Disk ... 285
Archival Storage ... 286
Nine-Track Magnetic Tape ... 286
Analog Videotape ... 286
Cine Film ... 286
Digital Optical Disk ... 286
Helical Scan 8-mm Magnetic Tape ... 286
Developing Technologies ... 286
Image Workstations ... 286
ADVANTAGES OF DIGITAL ANGIOGRAPHY ... 287
Progressive Scan Fluoroscopy ... 287
Flicker-Free Cine ... 287
Image Manipulation and Immediate Display ... 287
Cine Loop Display ... 287
Quantification ... 287
DIGITAL SUBTRACTION ANGIOGRAPHY ... 287
Temporal Subtraction ... 288
Mask Mode Subtraction ... 288
Temporal Filters ... 288
Energy Subtraction ... 288
IMAGE ENHANCEMENT ... 288
Spatial Filtration ... 288
SPATIAL MEASUREMENTS ... 289
Accuracy and Calibration ... 290
Magnification ... 290
Pincushion Distortion ... 290
Edge Detection ... 290
DENSITOMETRY ... 290
Densitometric Correction Methods ... 291
Analog-to-Digital Conversion and Video Camera Response ... 291
Scatter and Veiling Glare ... 292
Beam Hardening ... 293
Density-Time Analysis ... 293

Although 35-mm cineangiography is the state of the art for diagnosis of coronary artery disease, film presents several limitations that are becoming more important as interventions make greater demands on x-ray imaging. The first of these limitations is that images are generally not available until 15 to 20 minutes following the procedure. As a result, the images cannot be used to guide therapy unless the procedure is interrupted for film processing. The adequacy of the images is not known until the end of the procedure, so more views than necessary are often obtained at a cost of contrast dose, radiation exposure, and time. Other problems related to the use of film are technical, including the limited dynamic range of x-ray film, densitometric nonlinearity, inconvenient quantitative analysis, and lack of control over display contrast.

GENERAL PRINCIPLES OF DIGITAL IMAGING

The basic concept of digital imaging is that an image is converted to numbers, the numbers are stored and possibly manipulated or analyzed by a computer, and then the numbers are converted back into a visual image for viewing. All current digital cardiac angiography systems use a video camera to provide an electronic video image from a conventional x-ray image intensifier. It is the analog signal from this video system that is viewed on the video monitor during conventional fluoroscopy. In digital imaging systems, the analog video signal is intercepted before it is displayed on the monitor. The signal is converted into a digital or numeric form and stored or manipulated by a computer before being reconverted to an analog video signal for display. Figure 14–1 is an overview of this process.

Converting Images to Digital Form

Converting an image into a finite set of numbers is called digitization. In all currently available digital angiography systems, digitization consists of three steps: scanning, sampling, and quantization.

Scanning

Scanning is accomplished by the video camera, which converts the continuous two-dimensional image into a number of horizontal scans, called rows or rasters. The details of this process are described in the section on video equipment below.

Sampling

The intensity along each raster scan is measured, or sampled, at evenly spaced points. Each of these measured values represents the brightness at one location in the image, known as a picture element, or pixel. Thus a digitized image consists of rows and columns of pixels, and the brightness of each pixel is represented by an intensity value.

Quantization

Finally, each pixel intensity is converted to an integer between 0 and $N_g - 1$, where N_g is the number of discrete gray levels the computer hardware can represent. This conversion of a continuous range of intensities to a set of discrete gray levels is called quantization.

Both the horizontal sampling and quantization are performed by the analog-to-digital (A/D) converter. Because a binary digital computer stores and manipulates these image data, it is efficient to choose the number of gray levels, N_g, and the number of rows and columns to be powers of 2. For reasons that have nothing to do with digital imaging, video standards[E1, E2] developed long ago call for 525 horizontal raster lines, so it turns out that all but 13 lines can be stored in a digital image with 512 (2^9) rows. In most digital angiography applications, the number of samples along each scan line (i.e., the number of columns) is chosen to be equal to the number of scan lines (rows), giving a square pixel matrix. Thus, the de facto standard digital image size for cardiac digital angiography is 512 rows by 512 columns.

Bit Depth

The number of gray levels, N_g, determines the precision with which the original image intensities are represented in the digital image. In turn, N_g is determined by the number of binary digits (bits) the A/D converter and the image memory use to represent the intensity: $N_g = 2^{(\#\ \text{bits})}$. The difference between a quantized gray level and the original intensity is called the quantization error and is at most one-half of the increment between gray levels. For a typical angiographic image the mean-square quantization error is equal to 1⁄12 the gray scale increment.[W1] This information is used in the design of a digital imaging system to choose the number of bits depending on the range and precision of intensities in the original image, that is, on its signal-to-noise ratio, as discussed below.

Noise

Image noise refers to random intensity variations added by the imaging processes, and it is a critically important measure of image quality because it fundamentally limits the detection of small, low-contrast features.[M1, W2] The primary types of noise in digital cardiac angiography are quantum noise, which is due to the statistical fluctuation of the finite number of x-ray photons in each pixel; electronic noise, which is added by the preamplifier of the video camera; and digitization noise, which is due to the discrete increment between gray levels in a digital image. In a properly designed and operated imaging system, the total image noise should be dominated by quantum noise; otherwise the x-ray dose to the patient could be reduced without sacrificing image quality. Low-noise video cameras are used in digital coronary angiography to keep electronic noise well below quantum noise. Quantization error can be made small compared to overall noise by choosing the increment between gray levels to be less than twice the quantum noise.[K1, S1]

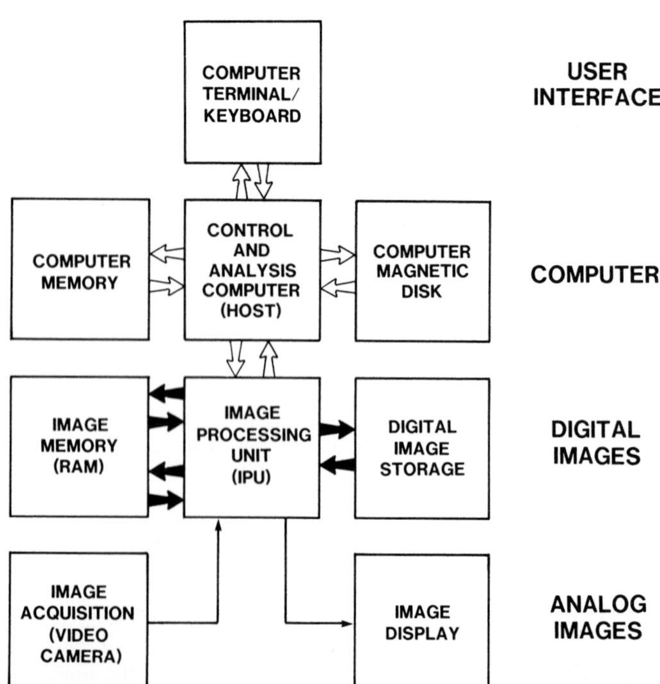

Figure 14–1. Overview of a digital image processing system for cardiac angiography. Open arrows represent computer control or data signals, filled arrows represent digital image data, and line arrows represent analog video signals.

The signal-to-noise ratio (SNR) is defined as the range of intensities to be digitized (the signal) divided by the root-mean-square deviation of intensity (the noise). The SNR is frequently expressed using the logarithmic decibel (dB) scale. An S/N ratio in decibels is calculated from the SNR as S/N (dB) = 20 $\log_{10}$(SNR), or SNR = $10^{(dB/20)}$. Thus, 60 dB corresponds to an SNR of 1000:1 and 48 dB to an SNR of 250:1. The number of gray levels, N_g, times the interval between gray levels must be sufficient to cover the range of intensities within the original image. Thus, the minimum number of gray levels needed is the dynamic range divided by the increment between gray levels. As an important example, cardiac angiography can be performed satisfactorily with an x-ray exposure of 30 microroentgens (μR) per image.[F1] This exposure produces an S/N of about 100:1, which, using our SNR/2 criterion, would require about 50 gray levels. However, this rule is complicated by the fact that the magnitude of the quantum noise is proportional to the square root of exposure. In a cardiac angiogram, the least intense area of the image typically receives 1/16 of the exposure and therefore the quantum noise is 1/4 of that corresponding to a 30-μR exposure, so the gray level increments must be made 1/4 as large. Thus, 200 gray levels are needed to digitize a 30-μR exposure image with a 16:1 intensity range, which requires a minimum of 8 bits (256 gray levels).

Pixel Size

The maximum resolving power of a digital imaging system is limited by the pixel size in accordance with the Nyquist sampling theorem, which states that a sinusoidally varying intensity can be accurately reproduced from sampled data only if the distance between samples is less than half the wavelength.[B1, P1] Actual pixel dimension is determined by the mapping of the pixel array onto the object being imaged and depends on radiographic magnification, image intensifier mode, the framing used in fitting the square or rectangular video image format to the circular image intensifier output phosphor, and matrix size (see Table 14–1). For example, a 512 × 512 digital image of an inscribed 15-cm (6-inch) diameter image intensifier (exact framing) has a pixel spacing of (15 cm)/512 = 0.29 mm, so the shortest wavelength that can be represented accurately is 0.58 mm and corresponds to a maximum spatial frequency of 1/(0.58 mm) = 1.7 cycles/mm. The size of the smallest feature that this system could resolve is about 0.6 mm. Modern intensifier tubes can image spatial frequencies greater than 3.5 cycles/mm. The number of pixels required for full resolution depends on the field of view, as shown at the left in Table 14–1.

Digital Image Storage

When an angiogram has been digitized, the data must be stored for later processing or display. There are four general classes of storage: (1) display buffer memory, which contains the image currently displayed on the video monitor; (2) high-speed image memory, from which images are transferred to the display buffer at rates of up to one image every 1/30 second ("real time" for standard video); (3) on-line mass storage, which may contain image series from examinations of several patients for direct access, but access is often slower than the real-time rate; and (4) archival storage, for long-term, off-line storage. The space required to store a digital image depends on the number of pixels and the bits per pixel. An image array of 512 rows by 512 columns has 512 × 512 = 262,144 pixels. When working with large powers of 2, it is convenient to define a slight modification of the standard scientific prefixes for powers of 10, making use of the fact that 2^{10} (= 1024) is close to 10^3 (= 1000), as shown in Table 14–2. Using this notation, a 512^2 digital image contains 256 kilopixels. If each pixel is quantized to 8 bits = 1 byte, the required storage space is 256 kilobytes (Kbytes).

Table 14–1. RELATIONSHIP BETWEEN IMAGE INTENSIFIER FIELD OF VIEW, MATRIX SIZE, AND SPATIAL RESOLUTION

Field of View (cm)	Image Intensifier Resolution (cycles/mm)	Required Matrix Size* (Nyquist)	512^2 Matrix *Resolution (cycles/mm)*	512^2 Matrix *Pixel Size (mm)*
23	3.5	1610^2	1.11	0.45
17	3.5	1190^2	1.51	0.33
15	3.5	1050^2	1.70	0.29
12	3.5	840^2	2.13	0.23

*Matrix size for equal analog and digital spatial resolution.

Table 14–2. DIGITAL AND BINARY PREFIXES

Prefix	Decimal Value		Binary Value	
Kilo (K)	10^3	1000	2^{10}	1024
Mega (M)	10^6	1000 K	2^{20}	1024 K = 1,048,576
Giga (G)	10^9	1000 M	2^{30}	1024 M = 1,073,741,824

DIGITAL ANGIOGRAPHY EQUIPMENT

Digital imaging equipment for cardiac angiography spans a wide range of function, flexibility, performance, and cost, yet there are elements in common from the simplest to the most complex equipment. In this section we describe the hardware building blocks of all digital imaging equipment, the parameters that specify each component's performance, and the combinations of these components used in the various types of digital angiographic devices.

Video for Digital Angiography

Linearity

Several of the important properties of a video camera are determined by the photoconducting target material used.[S2] Video camera tubes such as plumbicons (lead oxide), saticons, and chalnicons produce a linear response between light intensity and output signal. This eliminates a source of nonlinearity that would otherwise have to be corrected in quantitative applications. The response curve of video cameras consists of a power law relationship between input intensity and output signal: V = Iγ. Figure 14–2 shows typical response curves for cameras with γ values of 1.0 and 0.6, which correspond, respectively, to a linear lead oxide vidicon and a nonlinear antimony trisulfide vidicon commonly used for general fluoroscopy. A γ less than 1.0 produces increased contrast in darker areas of the image and decreased contrast in brighter areas. This is a good match with the video display monitor's γ of about 2.0, which means lower contrast in the dark areas and higher contrast in the bright areas. Thus, for

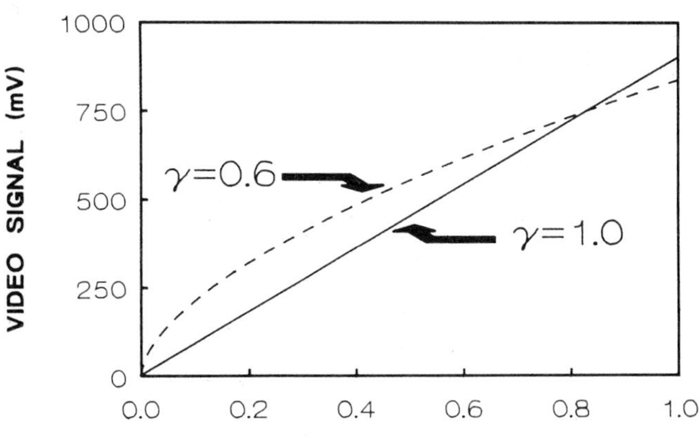

Figure 14–2. Relationship between video output signal and light intensity for a typical fluoroscopic vidicon (γ = 0.6) and a linear digital imaging vidicon (γ = 1.0).

direct fluoroscopy a γ of less than 1.0 produces a better displayed image. For digital imaging, a γ of 1.0 is needed for accurate subtraction and quantitation. Before the digital image is displayed its contrast can be manipulated to match the characteristics of the monitor.

Lag

Lead oxide and several other target materials used for digital angiography also have very low frame-to-frame image retention, or lag. Lag is produced when more than one scan is required to erase completely the image on the target. Cameras with relatively high lag are frequently used for general fluoroscopy because the lag reduces quantum noise by integrating several video frames. A camera with low lag is necessary for imaging of the coronary arteries, since lag produces multiple ghost images during pulsed cine exposures of rapidly moving objects.[S2]

Interlace

The way in which the camera target is electronically scanned also affects image quality. Conventional fluoroscopy cameras produce a complete image, called a frame, 30 times per second. Each 525-line frame is scanned by using a 2:1 interlace, which means that during the first 1/60 second the 262½ odd lines, called a field, are scanned, followed by the 262½-line even field. This is done to reduce the appearance of flicker, which is detectable when the intensity of a display oscillates at rates below about 45 Hz. Since the display screen is scanned twice during each 1/30 second frame time, once for each interlaced field, the overall intensity of the screen flickers at 60 Hz and the flicker is not perceived. There are two disadvantages of 2:1 interlace for coronary angiography. In order to obtain sharp images of the rapidly moving coronary arteries, the x-ray beam is operated in 5-msec (1/200 second) pulses. If the beam is pulsed only once for each video frame, the even field will be less intense than the odd field, since the odd field scan partially erases the even field. The result would be an objectionable amount of flicker and loss of verticle resolution. Therefore, the x-ray beam must be pulsed once for each video field, which results in a double exposure of the rapidly moving coronary arteries and increases the radiation dose to the patient. Thus, interlaced scanning is dose inefficient and reduces image resolution.

Progressive Scan

The preferred method for scanning the video camera for digital angiography is to scan all lines in sequence.[S3] This method, called progressive scan, reads all 525 lines of the image in order following each 5-msec x-ray pulse, so each frame consists of a single brief exposure. Progressive video camera scanning therefore produces images without artifacts due to motion of the coronary arteries and with a lower radiation dose. The image must still be displayed with 2:1 interlace to avoid the flicker problem, which requires a scan converter to reorder the scan lines. Alternatively, each frame can be displayed twice in progressive mode at 60 frames per second. The doubled display frame rate produces an image with even less flicker than an interlaced 30-Hz display, since all the lines are refreshed at 60 Hz.[S4] The disadvantage of this method is that the D/A converter, monitor, and videotape recorder must have double the bandwidth to preserve spatial resolution in the horizontal direction. This is one application of high-line video systems that is compatible with 512^2 digital acquisition.

Digital Image Processor

A representative block diagram of a digital angiographic system is shown in Figure 14–3. The block diagram shows the basic functional units of a digital image processor and their typical interconnection. Not all of the specific building blocks shown are used in all systems, and the actual configuration of the blocks in specific systems varies considerably. The capabilities of an image processing unit depend on its components and on how they are interconnected and controlled.

Arithmetic Logic Unit

The heart of an image processing unit is its arithmetic logic unit (ALU). This component performs operations such as addition, subtraction, and pixel-by-pixel intensity comparison of two images. The different operations that an ALU can perform make up its instruction set, which typically includes subtraction, addition, and logical "and," "or," "greater," and "lesser" operations. Some image processing units contain several ALUs working in parallel or in series so that more complex image processing algorithms can be implemented in one pass.

Intensity Transformation (Lookup) Table

Contrast enhancement is usually performed by an intensity transformation table (ITT). This device replaces the intensity of each pixel according to a predefined function of its original intensity. The host computer sets the entry values in the lookup table in response, for example, to setting of the display window and level controls by the user. The ITTs can also perform logarithmic or any other functional transformations of the image intensities for densitometry or subtraction.

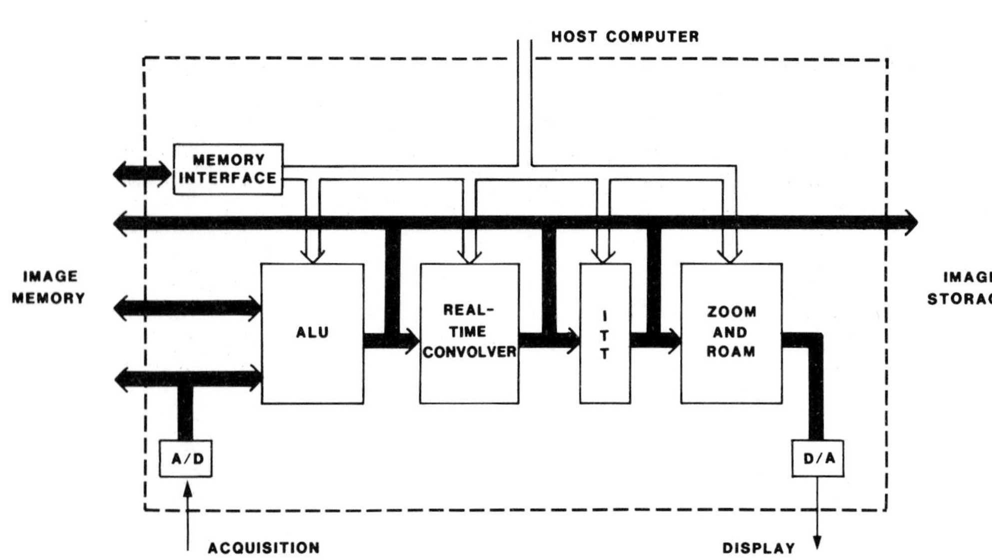

Figure 14–3. Schematic representation of the components of an image processing unit. Dark bus is for digital images; light bus is for digital computer control signals.

Hardware Zoom

An interpolated zoom device allows a portion of the digital image to be brought up to fill an entire frame. The zoom device fills in between the original pixels by using bilinear interpolation. To perform interpolated zoom in a single frame time requires special hardware. Noninterpolated, or pixel replication, zoom can usually be done in real time without special hardware, but the appearance of large pixels can be distracting.

Host Computer

The "host" computer is a general-purpose computer whose function is to control the activities of the system. The host interacts with the user and the x-ray imaging system, sends the appropriate instructions to the ALU, sets up the ITTs, and controls the flow of data between components of the system. In addition, the host computer is frequently used to perform image analyses that are unsuited for the ALU. Examples of tasks for which the ALU is not well suited are analysis of segmental wall motion and measurement of coronary artery stenosis. The speed of performance of these analytic algorithms depends on the speed of the general-purpose computer and on the way in which this computer accesses the image data. The image data may be transferred to the host computer one pixel, one row, one column, or one small rectangular region at a time. In some systems the programmer of the host computer can treat the entire image as though it were an array within its own memory. Although these factors do not always affect the clinical performance of a system, they may have a significant effect on the ease of programming new algorithms.

Array Processors

Some systems have a programmable array processor that the host computer uses to accelerate image analysis calculations. The performance of the array processor is slower than that of the ALU for image enhancement but much faster than that of the host computer for image analysis. Array processors are relatively expensive components and usually quite difficult to program directly.

Real-Time Convolver

Convolution is an important operation common to many image enhancement algorithms (see section on image enhancement). Generally, multiple passes through an ALU are required to perform convolution, which takes many frame times. Hardware is now available that can perform a convolution in a single frame time[D1] so that, for example, images can be edge-enhanced and displayed as they are being acquired. In some cases the type of enhancement (i.e., the convolution "kernel") may be adjustable by the user. These devices make possible real-time fluoroscopic edge enhancement, which many angiographers find helpful during angioplasty.

On-Line Image Storage

On-line image storage refers to storage of images so that they can be accessed without physically retrieving a storage medium and mounting it on a reading device. There are several types of on-line image storage devices, which differ in cost, capacity, and speed. Table 14–3 gives the capacity, speed, and cost per image of available on-line digital storage devices and archival storage media.

Solid-State Memory

The fastest and most expensive (per image) memory is solid-state (RAM) memory. RAM is volatile memory, which means that it is erased every time the computer's power is shut off. Digital angiography systems differ widely in amount of image RAM—from a single image (256 kilobytes) to 320 images (80 megabytes), enough for over 10 seconds of continuous recording at 30 frames per second of 512^2 by 8 bit images.

DISK BUFFER. In some systems the image RAM is used as a buffer for recording cine image sequences. Images are stored at real-time rates in the buffer and transferred to another storage medium such as magnetic disk at a different rate, which relaxes the requirement for rigid synchronization of the electromechanical disk drive with real-time digital-electronic image acquisition. If the buffer is large enough to hold an entire cine sequence, the magnetic disks can be much slower than real time, since the time between cine runs can be used to transfer the images. The extra time thus allowed for disk storage can also be used to perform image data compression, which can increase disk capacity by a factor of 2 to 4 times that for uncompressed data.

DISPLAY BUFFER. The display buffer consists of RAM connected directly to the digital-to-analog converter that drives the video monitor. Many systems are designed with space for more than one image in the display buffer, allowing an image to be displayed from one area of the buffer while a new image is being transferred to the other area. When the transfer is complete, the system can cause the area containing the new image to be displayed, so that the display instantaneously switches from one image to the next.

IMAGE MEMORY. Image memory, like the display buffer, consists of solid-state RAM memory, but is not connected directly to the D/A converter and so cannot be displayed directly. Image memory may be made large enough to hold one or more complete digital cineangiograms, which are loaded at rates determined by the speed of the on-line mass storage device, typically only a few images per second. Once loaded, the images can be transferred at a high rate to the display buffer for real-time display. In this way an image processing workstation can perform real-time display with slower conventional digital disk drives instead of more expensive real-time disk drives.

Real-Time Digital Magnetic Disk

On-line mass storage systems for cardiac digital angiography usually consist of special high-speed digital magnetic disk drives capable of recording images at 30 per second. This transfer rate can be achieved by modifying a conventional disk drive to enable data to be written to multiple heads in parallel.[V1] A system with such a disk does not need a separate large image memory, since images can be loaded directly from disk to the display buffer in

Table 14–3. DIGITAL IMAGE STORAGE MEDIA

Medium	Size	Image Capacity[1]	Images per Second	Cost (Dollars per Image)
Solid-state memory	48 Mbytes	192	30	130
Real-time disk	1 Gbyte	4,096	30	30
Conventional disk	1 Gbyte	4,096	6	6
Magnetic tape	2400 feet	80	0.5	0.2
Optical disk	2 Gbytes	8,192	0.5	0.02
Helical scan 8-mm tape	2 Gbytes	8,192	0.5	0.001
Analog Media				
Cine film	400 feet	6,400	30	0.01
Video analog tape[2]	30 minutes	54,000	30	0.0002

[1]Number of 512^2 8-bit images.
[2]Image quality significantly inferior to cine film.

real time. About 1800 images are acquired in a typical coronary angiogram and require 450 megabytes if they are digitized to 512^2 by 1 byte. Digital storage allows the image to be flexibly manipulated and processed, allows quantitative analysis to be performed, and allows random access to images for display. However, compared to analog image storage, as on film or videotape, digital image storage is currently more expensive, takes up more space, and is usually slower and less convenient to transport or transmit to a remote location. The main reason for these limitations is that a typical coronary angiogram contains a very large amount of data—about 1 minute of cine at 30 frames per second, or 1800 images. The storage required to record the angiogram at *full* resolution (see Table 14–1) is close to five times this amount! Thus, the storage device for even a single study of a patient at minimum acceptable resolution must have about 20 times the capacity of the hard disk drive of a typical personal computer. Digital storage devices differ greatly in speed, with solid-state memory the fastest and optical disk the slowest.

Archival Storage

Because of the large number of images created during cineangiography, long-term storage has been one of the major problems that have kept digital angiography from replacing film as the primary recording medium.

Nine-Track Magnetic Tape

Reels of magnetic tape, long the standard archival medium for digital data, have too little capacity and are too slow for routine practical archiving of complete digital cineangiograms. These tapes are 2400 feet long and can store 6250 bits per inch for a maximum capacity of 80 images ($512^2 \times 8$ bits). Since a typical coronary angiographic study contains about 1800 images, each patient would require 20 reels of standard magnetic tape and transferring the data would take several hours. One solution to this problem is to store only selected cine sequences (for example, a cardiac cycle, about 30 images) from each sequence (typically seven per patient), reducing the number of images to less than 240 and the number of reels to four. Another tactic is to store only a few selected images documenting the anatomy. In this case one reel of magnetic tape can archive perhaps 10 studies of patients. The disadvantage of this method is that accurate interpretation of coronary angiograms depends on dynamic information, which is discarded with the recording of single still frames.

Analog Videotape

Another approach to the archiving problem is to record the complete angiogram on videotape. This method has the advantages that all the dynamic data are preserved and the equipment for recording and playback is standard, widely available, and inexpensive. Although large-format videotape has sufficient bandwidth and signal-to-noise ratio to record 512^2 digital images with minimal degradation,[G1] the less expensive and more convenient videocassette recorders generally degrade both horizontal resolution and signal-to-noise ratio. However, this limitation can be minimized if the images are digitally enlarged and enhanced prior to recording. The disadvantage of this method is that the original digital image data are not stored, so the images have to be redigitized for enhancement or analysis, and redigitized data are not as accurate as the original data.

Cine Film

Most laboratories continue to use 35-mm cine film as the primary recording and archival medium because its spatial resolution is superior to that of digital imaging, the cost per archived frame is lower, and it is a universal format. In these laboratories digital imaging is used for instant storage and playback of images during the case and for quantitative analysis, but the images are routinely erased after the case to make room for the next study.

Digital Optical Disk

The digital optical disk, a larger relative of the audio compact disk, has adequate capacity (about 2 gigabytes) to store five patients' complete digital coronary angiograms on a single disk. The hardware for writing and reading these disks is not prohibitively expensive. "Jukebox" devices are available that can hold several hundred disks for automatic retrieval. Optical disk storage of 512^2 8-bit digital images is currently about twice as expensive as storage on cine film. Another disadvantage for cardiac imaging is that recording and playback speeds are slow, similar to those of magnetic tape.

Helical Scan 8-mm Magnetic Tape

This recently introduced technology provides large-capacity digital image storage at one-tenth the cost of cine film. The tape drives are comparable in cost to conventional nine-track tape drives and are already in wide use for backing up data on large disk drives. The physical size of the cassettes is much smaller than a roll of cine film. The drawbacks of helical scan 8-mm digital tape are the slow record/playback speed and lack of experience with its reliability for long-term archival.

Developing Technologies

Several recent technological advances are likely to find applications for archiving of digital angiograms. Magnetic tape cassette systems, which are being developed by several manufacturers, will have sufficient capacity for at least one complete study of a patient and will have record/playback rates close to 30 frames per second. The cost of the cassettes is likely to be much less than that of optical disks, but the tape drive itself will initially be more expensive than optical disk drives.

Another promising approach to increasing the speed and capacity of digital storage is the use of reversible or distortionless real-time data compression.

At present, a major disadvantage of all these digital recording media compared to cine film is the difficulty of interchanging images between laboratories because of the lack of accepted format and media standards.

Image Workstations

Digital angiograms are currently not as convenient to review as cine film angiograms because of the lack of inexpensive display devices analogous to cine film projectors. In some laboratories, review and analysis of digitally acquired coronary angiograms are done on the digital angiography system itself, but this creates a problem in busy laboratories because analysis, acquisition, and review cannot be done simultaneously. One solution to this problem is to record digital images on videotape, which can be reviewed on a second videotape recorder and monitor. By using a low-noise, high-bandwidth videotape recorder, these images can be reviewed without significant image degradation,[G1] particularly if some enhancement is performed prior to recording. The disadvantage of this approach is that the videotaped images cannot be manipulated or analyzed quantitatively.

The ideal way to review and process digital images is in digital format on an off-line digital image workstation with full analysis and display facilities. There are several ways to transport images from the acquisition system to a workstation. The workstation can be equipped to read any of the archival image storage media, such as nine-track tape, optical disk, or the emerging high-speed, high-capacity digital tapes. The workstation can also be networked with the acquisition system, with the advantage that storage media need not be physically transported and mounted on the workstation. However, current image network technology is limited to relatively slow transfer rates and would require about an hour for a complete coronary angiogram. One manufacturer currently offers a digital angiography system with a dual-ported real-time disk, which allows two systems to access the same disk. This allows the entire angiogram to be reviewed at the workstation as soon as the case is completed.

The development of high-speed, high-capacity digital archival media will enable rapid movement of digital images from the acquisition system to local or remote workstations for analysis and review. If the medical imaging community insists that the manufacturers adopt a standard format, digital images may someday be interchanged as conveniently as 35-mm cine film.

ADVANTAGES OF DIGITAL ANGIOGRAPHY

Digital angiography and film angiography employ identical imaging chains from the x-ray tube through to the image intensifier and therefore share the limitations of these systems in terms of resolution, contrast, and noise. The advantages of digital imaging during the angiographic procedure are the speed and ease with which the images can be replayed, the availability of image enhancement, random access to multiple reference frames from previous views, and increased contrast sensitivity with digital subtraction, with possible reduction of contrast material. The advantage of digital angiography for quantitation is that it is faster than quantitation from film because tracing and densitometry can be done directly from the digital data, without the delays involved in processing cine film and measuring the projected image. Finally, the display of digital images for review is more flexible than that of cine film.

Progressive Scan Fluoroscopy

In an analysis of progressive scan fluoroscopy, Seibert and associates found an improvement in fluoroscopic resolution (still frame) and a reduction of radiation dose for equal image quality of a factor of about four.[S3] This advantage can be achieved with a minimal digital imaging system consisting of a digital scan converter with the appropriate video camera, corresponding to the first system in Table 14–4.

Flicker-Free Cine

Removal of the 30-frame-per-second flicker during cine filming at 30 frames per second produces a much smoother and easier to interpret dynamic image. Flicker removal during live cine and videotape playback can be achieved with an inexpensive digital angiography system consisting of a digital frame store and scan converter, as described in column A of Table 14–4. In fact, progressive scan fluoroscopy with pulsed 30-Hz acquisition automatically provides for flicker removal in addition to the other advantages listed above. The same device provides stable full-frame static reference images, rather than the single-field still image usually obtained with a videotape recorder or analog videodisk. The still frame of a pulsed progressive video system with digital scan conversion thus has twice the vertical resolution of interlaced video. Digital still frames are more stable than videotape stills, which suffer from instabilities related to tape wear and stretching.

Table 14–4. TYPICAL CONFIGURATIONS OF CARDIAC DIGITAL ANGIOGRAPHY SYSTEMS

	System Configuration			
Features	*A*	*B*	*C*	*D*
A/D converter	Y	Y	Y	Y
Scan converter	Y	Y	Y	Y
RAM (512^2 images)	8	64	300	4—300
D/A converter	Y	Y	Y	Y
Real-time convolver	—	Y	Y	Y
Upscan to 1024 lines	—	Y	Y	Y
Lookup table	—	—	Y	Y
Disk (512^2 images)	—	—	—	3000
Programmable ALU	—	—	—	Y
Relative cost	1	2	3	6

Image Manipulation and Immediate Display

Digital images can be enhanced to sharpen edges and improve contrast, manipulations that have been found to improve detectability of simple patterns in radiographic noise[I1, L1] and may also improve detectability of atherosclerotic plaque morphology.[W3] Real-time image enhancement can be performed by the equipment described in column B in Table 14–4, which consists of A/D and D/A converters, a special-purpose real-time digital video convolver for performing the edge enhancement, and a lookup table for performing the contrast enhancement.

Cine Loop Display

Other advantages of digital coronary angiography are the ease with which previously acquired cine runs can be rapidly recalled for display and the way in which image sequences can be displayed smoothly as a loop or in a back-and-forth "yo-yo" format. With sufficient digital memory, all of the previous views acquired in a study can be available for random-access display as either still frames or cine loops much more quickly and smoothly than is possible with videotape recorders. It is also possible to select subsets of any image sequence to be stored or displayed separately. One use of this facility is to store a series of representative still frames throughout an angioplasty procedure to document the procedure and then to send these frames to a hardcopy printer for inclusion in the report on the patient or for producing slides. This type of functionality requires a digital imaging system with considerably more memory, as described in column C of Table 14–4. The memory requirement for a single angiographic cine run is about 45 megabytes (6 seconds × 30 frames per second × 0.25 megabytes per frame). Storage for one or two complete cine runs can be provided in digital RAM. If storage for more than one or two cine loops is desired, a real-time magnetic disk must be used to store the images. Such a system, described in column D of Table 14–4, has enough memory to allow completely random access to any image or image series throughout an entire study. This type of system is generally much more expensive than systems that use RAM for all real-time storage.

Quantification

Next to rapid and flexible display, quantification is digital angiography's strongest advantage over film. Analysis of left ventricular wall motion and quantitative coronary angiography are more easily and objectively performed with the aid of digital image processing. Many of the subjective steps, such as tracing edges, can be completely automated, increasing accuracy and reproducibility and decreasing analysis time.

The facility for quantitative analysis of angiographic data requires at a minimum that the system have frame store capability, and for most useful work it requires storage of at least a full cine run, allowing a frame to be chosen for analysis at peak opacification and at the optimum point in the cardiac cycle. Enough memory to store a cine run is, of course, the minimum requirement for analysis of density versus time data.

A second requirement for an analysis system is that the image data be available to a programmable computer, usually the host computer. As with image processing, many image analysis tasks can be accelerated by use of a pipeline processor or an array processor. Pipeline processors generally operate on the entire image and are faster than array processors, but array processors can usually be programmed to perform more kinds of operations.

DIGITAL SUBTRACTION ANGIOGRAPHY

Subtraction is a powerful technique for detecting subtle differences between two nearly identical images. In cardiology, images of the heart with and without contrast material are subtracted, which results in two major benefits. First, the range of intensities in the subtracted image is typically reduced by a factor of eight because the image consists only of the intensity changes due to the contrast material. This allows the subtracted image to be contrast enhanced without exceeding the dynamic range of the display monitor. Second, when stationary structures are subtracted from the image, features of the opacified cardiac anatomy become more conspicuous.[R1] Subtraction is therefore a method for removing a significant source of noise from angiographic images—patient structure noise due to overlying bone and soft tissue structures.

Subtraction does not reduce random noise, such as quantum mottle, since this noise changes from one frame to another. In fact, the quantum noise in a subtracted image is the square root of the sum of the squared quantum noise in the mask and that in the raw image.[K2]

Temporal Subtraction

Mask Mode Subtraction

In this method an image of the anatomy to be studied is acquired in the absence of contrast material. This mask image may be a single frame or the average of several frames either before the injection of contrast material or after its washout. The mask image is subtracted from each raw image in the cine series to obtain a new image series of the contrast material alone, which may then be enhanced. The advantage of mask mode subtraction is that a high-contrast image series can be produced with much less contrast material because patient structure noise is removed. A disadvantage is that motion of the patient between acquisition of the mask image and acquisition of the contrast images results in enhanced "misregistration" artifacts, which may obscure the angiogram more than the original, unenhanced image. As in all subtracted images, quantum noise is higher than in the raw images. This limitation can be minimized in subtraction studies where there is little motion, as in peripheral angiography, because a large number of frames can be averaged to obtain low-noise mask and raw images. In cardiac imaging, motion prevents averaging raw contrast frames. However, the mask image can be averaged because nonopacified thoracic structures move very little compared with the left ventricle and coronary arteries. In this way it is possible to produce a cardiac study with subtraction with about the same quantum noise as a study without subtraction.

Temporal Filters

Mask mode subtraction is a special example of the class of image processing algorithms known as time domain filtration. The intensity of each pixel, if plotted frame by frame, can be thought of as a digitally sampled time-varying signal, which may be processed with the highly developed tools of signal processing theory to enhance specific features of the signal, minimize noise and motion artifacts, or detect specific patterns in the signal. Mask mode subtraction corresponds to a very simple time domain filter in which, for each image in a series, the fixed value of the corresponding pixel in the mask image is subtracted.

Time interval difference (TID) imaging is very similar to mask mode subtraction. In TID imaging, the mask for each frame of a cine series is an image that was acquired a fixed number of frames earlier. The intensities in the TID image series therefore represent the change during the fixed time interval between images. This method has been applied to intravenous left ventriculography.[C2] TID is a simple form of high-pass filter, since parts of the signal that change slowly in time (low frequency) produce small TID intensities and rapidly changing signals (high frequency) produce large TID intensities. More sophisticated filters can be designed to overcome specific cardiac imaging problems. Kruger[K3] developed a recursive high-pass filter that minimizes the response to frequencies below about 0.2 Hz and thus reduces artifacts associated with respiration and table panning. Recursive filters are well suited for implementation in real time, since the output image is computed as a simple combination of a new input image and the last output image. Because slow, low-frequency changes are filtered out while rapid, high-frequency changes are displayed, a properly chosen time domain filter can produce enhanced coronary angiograms even with some respiration or panning.[H1, K4] Nevertheless, respiration, cardiac motion, and panning do produce some misregistration artifacts, which interfere with visibility.

Energy Subtraction

Unlike both mask mode and TID, energy subtraction does not depend on change in contrast over time to eliminate nonopacified structures. Instead, two nearly simultaneous images acquired with different x-ray energy spectra are subtracted. Because of the high effective atomic number of radiographic contrast material, the intensity of the image of opacified structures is much more sensitive to changes in x-ray spectrum than that of nonopacified structures. Therefore, energy subtraction enhances contrast material relative to soft tissue and bone. In fact, by using three different x-ray energies, images may be produced with soft tissue and bone eliminated.[K5] This process is analogous to taking black-and-white photographs of a scene with light sources of three different colors to record a full-color image. The major advantage of energy subtraction is that the images at different energies can be acquired in rapid succession, eliminating artifacts due to motion of the patient. This could be especially important in quantitative studies such as exercise left ventriculography or myocardial perfusion analysis, where time-density curves can be severely distorted by changes in normal tissue thickness due to respiration or other motion. Compared to mask-mode subtracted images, the signal-to-noise ratio of dual-energy subtracted images is two to three times less for equivalent radiation dose and x-ray tube heating.[M2] This problem makes this technique unpromising for coronary angiography, where detectability of small low-contrast features is important, but may not be such a limitation for large-area densitometric measurements used for ventriculographic and myocardial perfusion studies. At present, no x-ray equipment manufacturer supports energy subtraction as a clinical tool.

IMAGE ENHANCEMENT

When an image or series of images has been digitized and stored in the memory of a computer, a great variety of manipulations can be performed to enhance the image visually. Image manipulation may involve one or several images. An example of an operation on a single image is zooming a portion of the image to make it appear larger on the screen; an example of a multiple-image operation is digital subtraction angiography in which a new image is formed by subtracting two images. Image manipulations may also be divided into point operations, such as contrast enhancement or subtraction, which are performed on a pixel-by-pixel basis, and neighborhood operations, in which the intensity of a given pixel depends on the intensities of the pixels in its neighborhood.[C1] Examples of neighborhood operations are edge enhancement and smoothing or blurring. The time required to perform a manipulation depends on the complexity of the manipulation and the speed and design of the image processing computer. Some important image processing procedures are categorized in Table 14–5 according to the information used to calculate each pixel.

Spatial Filtration

Spatial filtration is a neighborhood operation in which the intensity of each pixel is replaced by some function of the intensities of other pixels, usually in its immediate neighborhood. In the most common types of spatial filtration, each pixel is

Table 14–5. CLASSIFICATION OF IMAGE PROCESSING PROCEDURES

Point Operations	Neighborhood Operations
Single Image	
Window, level	N × N smoothing
Histogram equalization	Edge enhancement
Logarithmic transform	Convolution
Pseudocolor	Median filter
Multiple Images	
Subtraction	
Mask mode	^
Time interval	|
Time domain filtration	<---+
Recursive	
Matched	
Functional images	

replaced with a weighted average of its original intensity and that of the pixels surrounding it. The effect of the filter on the image can be varied by selecting the size of the neighborhood to be averaged and the pattern of weights applied to each pixel within the neighborhood. The same pattern of weights, called a kernel, is applied equally to each pixel in the image, a process known as convolution.

Figure 14–4 shows examples of the effect of three simple kernels on a coronary angiogram and a resolution pattern. The first kernel specifies that each pixel shall be replaced by itself plus *zero* times the sum of its eight nearest neighbors. This is, of course, a trivial filter because it reproduces the original image.

The second kernel specifies that each pixel be replaced by an evenly weighted average of itself and its eight nearest neighbors. This filter has two noticeable effects on the images: it reduces random pixel-to-pixel fluctuations (noise), and it blurs image detail. Both effects are directly proportional to the size of the kernel. A 5 × 5 element, evenly weighted kernel will produce more smoothing and blurring than this 3 × 3 kernel. The processed images have the same overall intensity as the original images because the sum of the kernel elements is 1.0.

The third kernel specifies that each pixel be replaced by nine times the original pixel intensity *minus* the average of its eight nearest neighbors. If all nine pixels in the neighborhood have the same intensity, the central pixel value is unaffected. However, when the original pixel is just outside a region of increased intensity and several of its nearest neighbors have higher values, the original pixel is replaced by a lower value. Pixels just *inside* a region of increased intensity are replaced by higher values. Thus this is an edge enhancement filter. It noticeably enhances the contrast of the edges of the coronary arteries, the resolution pattern, and the quantum noise.

The action of spatial filters is often described in the language of time domain signal filtration. The second filter described above is a low-pass filter because it preserves the contrast of large areas (low spatial frequencies) while reducing the contrast of small details (high spatial frequencies), and it has an overall gain equal to the sum of the weights in the kernel. In fact, the highly developed theory of time domain signal filtration carries over in a straightforward way to two-dimensional spatial images. For example, we can easily design a high-pass filter to suppress large-area intensity differences while enhancing sudden (in the spatial sense!) intensity changes, such as those occurring at the edges of the coronary arteries.

SPATIAL MEASUREMENTS

Spatial dimensions are easily measured in digital images since each pixel has unique coordinates. By using a trackball, mouse, joystick, or lightpen as a pointer, features such as the ventricular wall may be outlined and ventricular volumes, stroke volume, and ejection fraction may be calculated automatically based on the desired algorithm. Outlining of the ventricle and tracing of

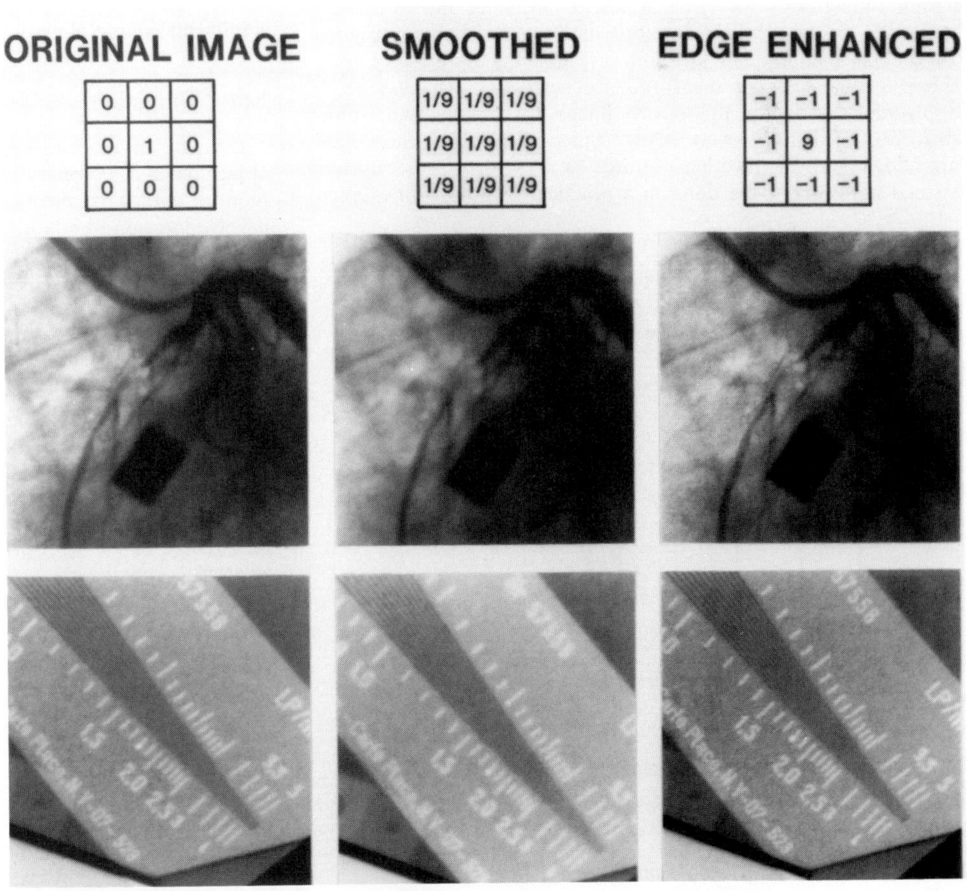

Figure 14–4. Image processing by convolution with a 3 × 3 pixel kernel. Each pixel of the processed image is the weighted sum of the original pixel and its eight nearest neighbors. The weights of the original pixel and its neighbors, specified by the kernels shown in the top row, determine the effect of the convolution, as shown in the processed angiogram (middle row) and resolution grid (bottom row). The kernel on the left does not change the image at all.

coronary artery stenoses can be automated by use of edge detection algorithms. This automation eliminates subjective variability and may improve absolute accuracy. In this section we discuss the fundamental basis for these methods.

Accuracy and Calibration

The pixels of a digital image form a highly accurate rectilinear array, so the x and y coordinates of a pixel are exact multiples of the pixel size. The distance between any two pixels is easily calculated using the theorem of Pythagorus. Although the smallest distance that can be measured is the pixel size, the actual limit of accuracy often is determined by unsharpness, noise, and distortions that occur in the radiographic imaging process before digitization[W4] rather than the pixel size itself.

Magnification

The pixel size is defined by the size of the object that maps exactly into one pixel of the image. This size depends on the radiographic magnification of the object, the electronic minification of the image by the image intensifier tube, the magnification of the image intensifier output by the video camera optics, and the way in which the video camera is scanned and the signal digitized. The overall effect of these magnifications can be calibrated by determining the number of pixels corresponding to an object of known size for a particular radiographic magnification and image intensifier mode. The error introduced by the finite pixel size can be minimized by using an object whose size corresponds to many pixels.

Pincushion Distortion

Pincushion distortion is an exaggeration of the distances measured from the center of the image as a result of the curvature of the input phosphor of the image intensifier. Distance measurements can be automatically corrected for pincushion distortion in a digital image by converting to polar coordinates and correcting the radial distances with calibration data such as shown in Figure 14–5. This technique is fast and easy to implement, since only the coordinates being measured are corrected. An alternative approach is to warp the entire image to remove pincushion distortion prior to measurement.[T1] Since all pixels in the image are affected, this correction requires an array processor or other special hardware to be done in a practical length of time, even on single frames. The pincushion distortion of most modern image intensifier tubes used for cardiac angiography is in the range of 1 or 2 percent,[C3] considerably less than the values of a decade ago,[B2] and for most routine measurements it is not a significant source of error.

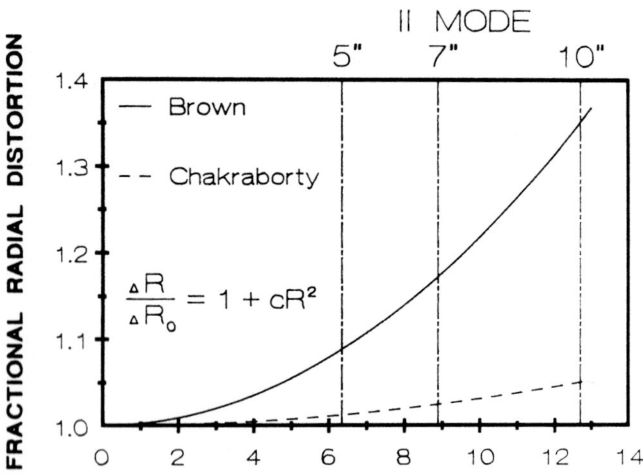

Figure 14–5. Pincushion distortion data as shown here can be used to correct measured dimensions. Modern image intensifiers (Chakraborty, 1986, *dashed line*)[C3] generally have less pincushion distortion than those of a decade ago (Brown, 1977, *solid line*).[B2]

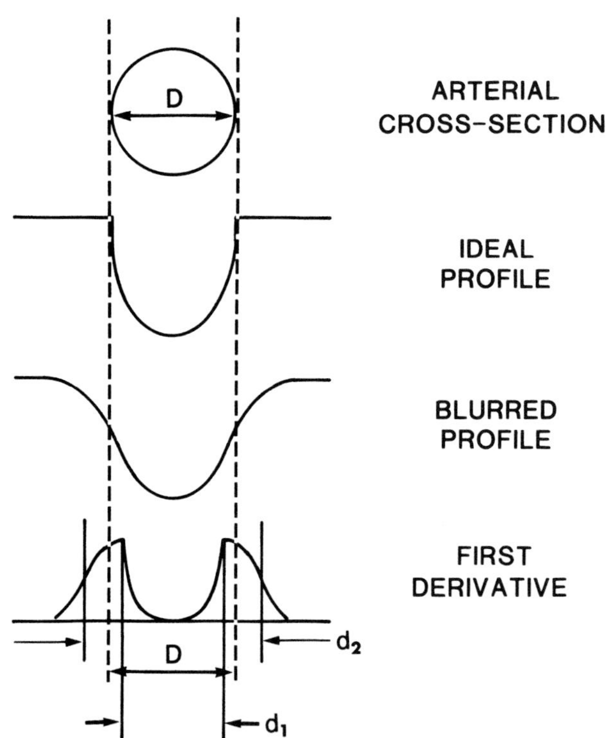

Figure 14–6. Schematic showing how image blur affects automatic vessel edge detection. Vessel diameter is underestimated by the maximum first-derivative edges (d_1) and overestimated by the maximum second-derivative edges (d_2). (From Whiting, J. S., Pfaff, J. M., and Eigler, N.: Effect of radiographic distortions on the accuracy of quantitative angiography. Am. J. Cardiac Imaging 2:244, 1988, with permission.)

Edge Detection

Because of the unsharpness of the borders of angiographic objects such as coronary arteries and the left ventricle, measurement accuracy is affected by subjective determination of the precise location of edges.

Digital edge detection methods are able to define these edges objectively. A variety of edge-selective criteria have been used to design edge detection algorithms.[F2, F3, R3] Some of these criteria are discussed in the chapter on quantitative coronary angiography. A common element in many of these methods is the first-derivative criterion. In this method the edge is identified by the maximum change in image intensity between adjacent pixels along a profile. A maximum second-derivative criterion has also been used. All edge detection methods depend on an assumed relationship between the shape of the edge intensity profile in the image and the true projected border of the object, as shown in Figure 14–6. The principal source of systematic error in relative coronary artery diameter is this dependence of profile shape on coronary artery cross-sectional shape and image system blur.[W5]

DENSITOMETRY

The concept of x-ray densitometry is to calculate the amount of contrast material along each ray through the patient from the x-ray intensity information recorded in the angiogram. Densitometry can be used to measure the thickness of any object containing a known concentration of contrast material or to measure the concentration of contrast material if the thickness is known.

Densitometry provides a way to measure vessel cross-sectional area and chamber volumes that is practically independent of imaging system unsharpness or motion blurring.[K6, P3] Fortunately, most applications of densitometry require only relative measurement of contrast material. Some measurements that would seem to require absolute densitometry, such as absolute cross-sectional areas of coronary arteries, can often be made relative to a calibration object. Relative densitometry is much easier because it does not require knowledge of the absolute concentration of contrast material and because some densitometric errors cancel out in the ratio of two measurements. However, several important errors are nonlinear, so some error will remain in relative measurements. Furthermore, most error sources are spatially and/or temporally variant, which leads to errors in relative densitometry when measurements are separated in time or space, even if the densitometry at each point is linear.

Densitometric Correction Methods

Figure 14–7 is a schematic representation of the factors that determine the intensity of a pixel in a digital angiogram. The primary intensity is determined by the output of the x-ray tube, the distance between the x-ray tube and the image intensifier, and the amount of attenuation of the primary beam by the patient. The relationship between the primary intensity and the amount of each kind of attenuating material in the patient is exponential. The coefficient of the exponent, known as the attenuation coefficient, depends on the atomic composition and density of the material and on the energy of the x-ray photons. Since the goal of densitometry is to determine the amount of contrast material in the beam, we must have a way of separating the attenuation due to normal tissues of the patient from that due to the contrast material. This may be done in one of two ways. The first method makes use of the change in pixel intensity between a preinjection "mask" image and the opacified image to isolate the attenuation due to the contrast material alone. The second method subtracts the average intensity of nearby non-opacified pixels from that of the artery.

Up to this point, we have been discussing the densitometric information in the x-ray beam prior to detection by the image intensifier. The imaging system itself further distorts and degrades the densitometric information. The detection of the input phosphor of the x-ray image intensifier is itself an absorption process similar to attenuation within the patient and is therefore affected by the x-ray energy spectrum. This effect may be lumped with beam hardening and is treated as a single artifact in the discussion of correction algorithms below. The image intensifier itself is a highly linear transducer, from absorbed x-ray energy at the input phosphor to visible light at the output phosphor. However, scattering of light within the image intensifier adds a nonuniform haze, known as veiling glare, which produces a densitometric error similar to that of radiation scatter. Finally, the image is recorded by the video camera and digitizer, which may produce another bias and/or nonlinear transformation.

Corrections for some of these errors can be accurately calibrated, whereas others are difficult to correct perfectly because they vary from patient to patient or even from pixel to pixel. Table 14–6 lists the corrections in the order in which they must be applied to the image data and their sources of error.

Table 14–6. DENSITOMETRIC TRANSFORMATIONS

Transformations	Corrections	Problems
1 A/D converter offset	Subtract offset	Miscalibration
2 Video tube response	Inverse	Miscalibration
3 Veiling glare (VG)	Subtract VG	VG not known
4 Scatter (S)	Subtract S	S not known
5 Lambert-Beers	Logarithm	Beam hardening
6 Beam hardening	Lookup table	Underdetermined

Analog-to-Digital Conversion and Video Camera Response

The final acquisition step is digitization of the video signal, and therefore any error in this step must be corrected first. A/D converters are highly linear devices that produce an output between 0 and $2^N - 1$, where N is the number of bits used to represent the signal in the computer, corresponding to a select-

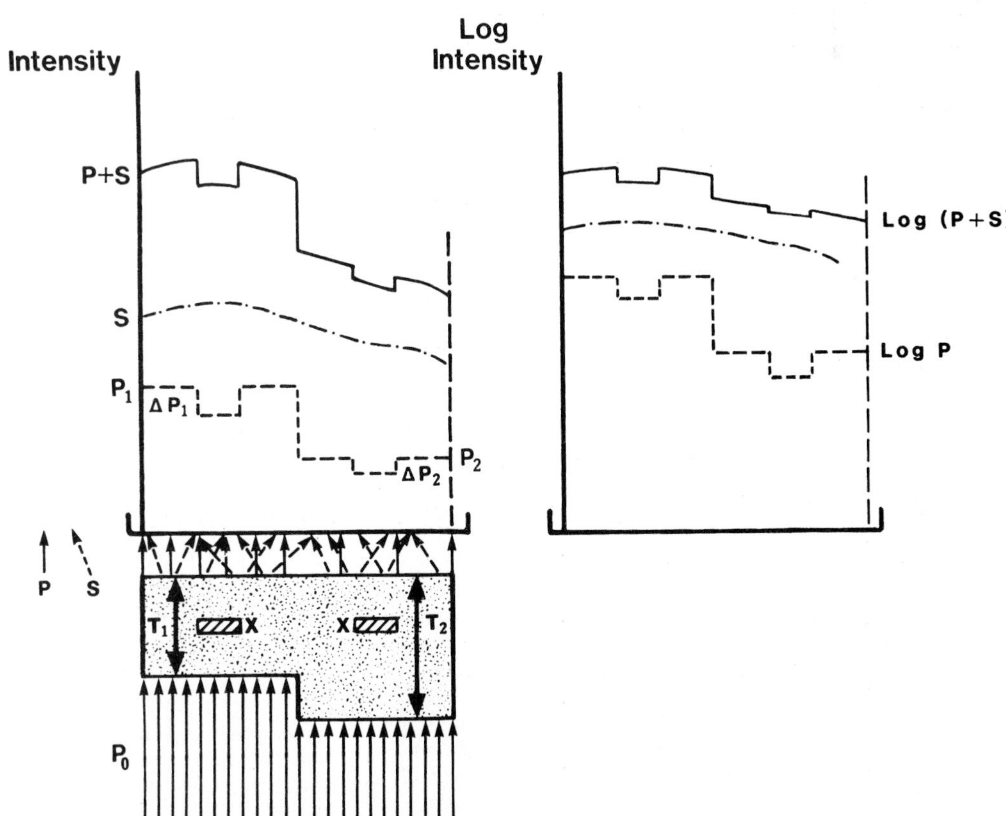

Figure 14–7. Illustration of fundamental factors affecting quantitative densitometry. X-rays that are transmitted without scattering through tissue thicknesses T_1 and T_2 produce primary intensities P_1 and P_2, respectively. Identical absorbers of thickness x produce changes in primary intensity, ΔP_1 and ΔP_2, which are directly proportional to P_1 and P_2 by the Lambert-Beers law. Thus, the change in the logarithm of the primary intensity is the same for both absorbers. Scattered radiation contributes a substantial intensity offset that results in differences between the log ΔP values corresponding to equal absorber thicknesses.

able input voltage range. Since both the level and gain of the video signal and the input range of the A/D converter are arbitrarily adjustable, it is important to remember that a digital pixel intensity of zero does not necessarily correspond to a primary x-ray intensity of zero. Failure to correct this offset produces densitometric nonlinearity similar to that produced by scatter and veiling glare.[M3, P3]

As discussed earlier, video cameras differ in their response to light. Even cameras with $\gamma = 1$ may deviate from linearity at very low or very high intensities. To avoid nonlinearity with these cameras, it is important to adjust the light intensity reaching the camera by using an aperture to make sure that the approximately 20:1 dynamic range of the image falls in the linear portion of the camera's dynamic range. If a camera with a nonlinear response is used, the image must be linearized with an intensity transformation function that is the inverse of the measured video camera response.

Scatter and Veiling Glare

Several important factors contribute to the intensity of a pixel by adding to the primary intensity. Scattered photons reaching the image intensifier add to the primary intensity. Thus, the intensity at any point on the image intensifier depends on the intensity of scatter originating from the rest of the x-ray beam. The scatter intensity depends on the cross-sectional area of the x-ray beam, the thickness of the patient, the imaging geometry, variations in thickness of the patient within the x-ray beam, and the beam energy. The scatter intensity is spatially variant across the image and typically is equal to or greater than the primary intensity. Failure to subtract scatter intensity will result in gross underestimation of absolute contrast material density and a nonlinear relationship between pixel intensity and relative contrast material density.

Scattering of light in the output phosphor,[R2] or veiling glare, also adds a significant spatially variant bias analogous to that of x-ray scatter. As with x-ray scatter, the contribution of veiling glare to an individual pixel depends on the intensity of the pixels in a large neighborhood around the pixel. The precise dependence on the surrounding intensities is different for veiling glare and x-ray scatter, so the determination of the magnitudes of these components requires two separate approaches. However, they affect densitometric accuracy in the same way and are often considered together as scatter and veiling glare (SVG). The contribution of scatter and veiling glare varies from point to point throughout an image. Both the intensity and spatial distribution of SVG depend on x-ray beam area, thickness and anatomy of the patient, distance between the patient and the image intensifier, type of antiscatter grid, and x-ray beam energy.

The contribution of SVG at a particular location in the image can be measured experimentally by using a small lead ball or disk to block the primary beam, leaving only the SVG component.[S6] The disadvantage of direct clinical application of this method is that it is valid only in the neighborhood of the lead disk, so several carefully placed lead disks may be needed to correct for scatter and veiling glare at the location of each region to be analyzed.

Shaw and associates[S7] and Seibert and associates[S8] have developed image processing methods to correct for the contribution of veiling glare at each pixel by assuming that the veiling glare can be characterized by a patient-independent point spread function (PSF). In Shaw's method the veiling glare was estimated by convolving this PSF with the image and multiplying the result by a constant weighting factor before subtracting it from the original image. Seibert derived an inverse filter that is calibrated to remove veiling glare when convolved with the original image.[S9]

Shaw and Plewes obtained direct measurements of scatter and veiling glare by moving one or several narrow lead bars across the field while imaging.[S10] The image series is passed through a "minimum pixels" algorithm, which constructs a single image in which each pixel has the value it had when the lead bar passed over it. This image is an approximate measurement of the SVG pattern throughout the image. This method has the disadvantages that the lead bars may obscure important transient detail as they scan across the image, changes in the scatter-glare field throughout due to cardiac motion during the scan may produce a rippling artifact, and the scatter-glare is underestimated because the long bar perturbs the field more than the small lead blockers described above.

Removal of x-ray scatter by convolution approaches has been studied by several investigators,[L2, M4, N1, S11] but the problem appears more difficult because the scatter point spread function itself depends on thickness of the patient, x-ray beam energy, and imaging geometry.[N1] Seibert and Boone[S11] modeled the scatter point spread function for a uniform-thickness homogeneous phantom as a modified Gaussian distribution. They studied the dependence of the scatter point spread function on phantom thickness and x-ray field size and concluded that practical clinical application of this method would require inverse convolution filters for specific imaging geometries, x-ray factors, and thicknesses.

Love and Kruger[L2] used a convolution filter with fixed parameters (as in Shaw's veiling glare method) and then used SVG measurements behind an array of 3-mm-diameter lead balls to adjust a constant weighting factor and bias. These "scaling parameters" were applied to the convolution-filtered image before it was subtracted from the original image. They found that good estimations of SVG in opacified regions could be obtained by convolution filtering the opacified image and using the scaling parameters derived from a nonopacified image. Thus, in clinical use the lead beam-stops could be removed from the field prior to the arrival of contrast material.

Malloi and Mistretta[M4] also developed a convolution SVG correction method with fixed filter parameters. However, prior to convolution they performed a gray scale transformation that converted the raw image intensities into approximate SVG intensities, based on measurements of SVG fraction versus gray level in a humanoid chest phantom in a 30-degree right anterior oblique projection. Variations of SVG fraction with thickness of the patient, field size, and beam energy were measured in the phantom, parameterized, and used to customize the gray level transformation to each patient. Minimum thickness of the patient was estimated from the x-ray factors and the distance from the

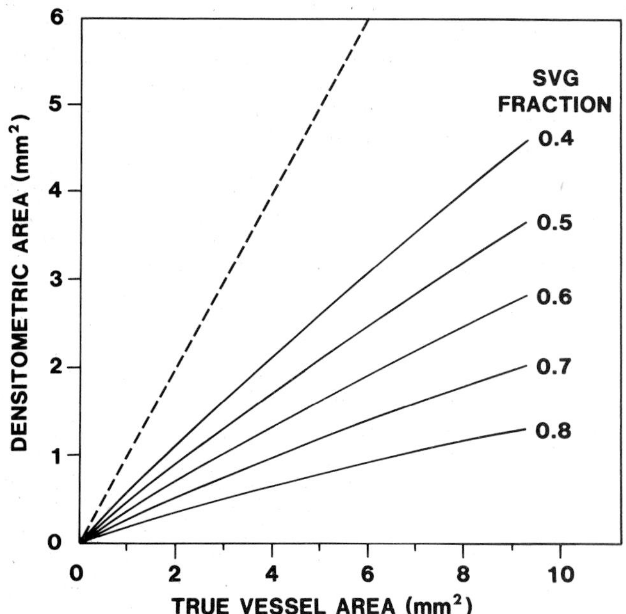

Figure 14–8. Densitometric versus true cross-sectional area for scatter and veiling glare (SVG) fractions typical of a clinical angiogram. Underestimation of area due to SVG increases with SVG fraction and with increasing vessel size (note the curvature of each plotted line).

focal spot to the image intensifier, and field size was measured in the image. The advantages of this method are that it does not use lead beam-stops for calibration and, since the calibration is based on the gray levels in the image, it can adjust to changes in SVG due to cardiac motion, respiration, or injection of contrast material.

The combined effects of scatter and veiling glare on absolute vessel cross-sectional area are illustrated in Figure 14–8. These errors also affect relative measurements when the scatter and veiling glare at the location of the stenosis is not the same as that at the reference vessel or catheter, as shown in Figure 14–9.

Beam Hardening

The beam produced by an x-ray tube contains a broad range of photon energies. This energy distribution depends on both the voltage applied to the tube and the amount of filtration of the beam before it reaches the patient. The problem is that the energy spectrum changes as the beam passes through the patient and contrast material, since the lower-energy photons are more readily attenuated than the higher-energy photons. Thus, the effective attenuation coefficient for a thick patient is lower than that for a thin patient. Likewise, the effective attenuation coefficient decreases with increasing amount of contrast material. This effect is known as beam hardening. If beam hardening is ignored and a fixed value for attenuation coefficient is used for each material, the result will be a nonlinear relationship between pixel intensity and the corresponding amount of contrast material. Beam hardening is influenced by several patient-dependent factors, so the correction cannot be determined exactly from a single x-ray projection.

Density-Time Analysis

Applications of density-time analysis currently in use or under development include measurements of coronary artery blood flow, left ventricular ejection fraction, mitral and aortic valve regurgitation, cardiac shunts, and myocardial perfusion.

Density-time analysis is subject to the densitometric errors discussed above. Nonlinear densitometry produces errors in most parameters derived from the density-time curves, including mean transit time, washout rate, full width at half-maximum, and area under the curve. An often overlooked source of error is that scatter and veiling glare is time dependent due to factors related to the patient, such as respiration, as well as to the reduced SVG that occurs because the injected contrast material attenuates the primary beam. Failure to correct for the latter effect results in nonlinear overestimation of the relative peak density, which leads to overestimation of rates of appearance and washout of as much as 20 percent.[P4]

Additional major sources of error in clinical application that are beyond the scope of this technical chapter include change in thickness of the patient with respiratory motion and problems related to the suitability of the contrast material as a blood flow tracer, such as its physiologic effect on cardiac function and the circulatory system, high viscosity and density, and incomplete mixing with blood.

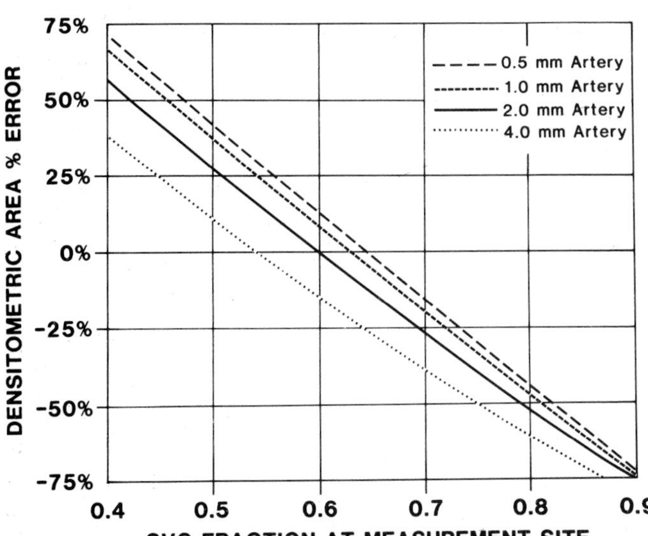

Figure 14–9. Error in densitometric cross-sectional area assuming calibration with a 2.0-mm-diameter catheter at an image location where the scatter and veiling glare (SVG) fraction is 0.6. The densitometric area of a 2.0-mm artery is overestimated by 58 percent at an SVG fraction of 0.4 and underestimated by 52 percent at an SVG fraction of 0.8. The relationship between percent error and SVG fraction is similar for all coronary luminal diameters and corresponds to a change in measured area of about 30 percent for each change of 0.1 in SVG fraction.

References

A

1. Arnold, B., Eisenberg, H., and Borger, D.: Digital video angiography system evaluation. Appl. Radiol. 10:81, 1981.

B

1. Brigham, E. O.: The Fast Fourier Transform. Prentice-Hall, Englewood Cliffs, New Jersey, 1974, p. 80.
2. Brown, G. B., Bolson, E., Frimer, M., and Dodge, H. T.: Quantitative coronary arteriography: Estimation of dimensions, hemodynamic resistance, and atheroma mass of coronary artery lesions using the arteriogram and digital computation. Circulation 55:329, 1977.

C

1. Castleman, K. R.: Digital Image Processing. Prentice-Hall, Englewood Cliffs, New Jersey, 1979.
2. Cox, G. G., Dwyer, S. J., III, and Templeton, A. W.: Computer networks for image management in radiology: An overview. CRC Crit. Rev. Diagn. Imaging 25:333, 1986.
3. Chakraborty, D. P.: Image intensifier distortion correction. Med. Phys. 14:249, 1987.

D

1. Dobbins, J. T., Van Lysel, M. S., Hasegawa, B. H., et al.: Spatial frequency filtering in digital subtraction angiography (DSA) by real-time digital convolution. SPIE J. 419:111, 1983.

E

1. EIA Standard RS-330: Electrical performance standards for closed circuit television camera 525/60 interlaced 2:1. Electronic Industries Association. Washington, D.C., 1966.
2. EIA Standard RS-170: Electrical performance standards—monochrome television studio facilities. Electronic Industries Association, Washington, D.C., 1957.

F

1. Friesinger, G. C., Adams, D. F., Bourassa, M.G., et al.: Optimal resources for examination of the heart and lungs: Cardiac catheterization and radiographic facilities. Circulation 68:893A, 1983.
2. Fleagle, S. R., Johnson, M. R., Skorton, D. J., et al.: Geometric validation of a robust method of automated edge detection in clinical coronary arteriography. Proc. IEEE Comput. Cardiol. October:197, 1986.
3. Fujita, H., Doi, K., and Fencil, L. E.: Image feature analysis and computer-aided diagnosis in digital radiography. 2. Computerized determination of vessel sizes in digital subtraction angiography. Med. Phys. 14:549, 1987.

G

1. Gray, J. E., Wondrow, M. A., Smith, H. C., and Holmes, D. R.: Technical considerations for cardiac laboratory high-definition video systems. Cathet. Cardiovasc. Diagn. 10:73, 1984.

H

1. Hardin, C. W., Kruger, R. A., Anderson, F. L., et al.: Real-time digital angiocardiography using a temporal high-pass filter. Radiology 151:517, 1984.
2. Holmes, D. R., Smith, H. C., Gray, J. E., and Wondrow, M. A.: Clinical evaluation and application of cardiac laboratory high-definition video systems. Cathet. Cardiovasc. Diagn. 10:63, 1984.

I

1. Ishida, M., Doi, K., Loo, L. N., et al.: Digital image processing: Effect on detectability of simulated low-contrast radiographic patterns. Radiology 150:569, 1984.

K

1. Kruger, R. A., Mistretta, C. A., and Riederer, S. J.: Physical and technical considerations of computerized fluoroscopy difference imaging. IEEE Trans. Nucl. Sci. NS-28:205, 1981.
2. Kruger, R. A., and Riederer, S. J.: Basic Concepts of Digital Subtraction Angiography, G. K. Hall Medical Publishers, Boston, 1984.
3. Kruger, R. A.: A method for time domain filtering using computerized fluoroscopy. Med. Phys. 8:466, 1981.
4. Kruger, R. A., Miller, F. J., Nelson, J. A., et al.: Digital subtraction angiography using a temporal bandpass filter: Associated patient motion properties. Radiology 145:315, 1982.
5. Kelcz, F., Mistretta, C. A., and Riederer, S. J.: Spectral considerations for absorption-edge fluoroscopy. Med. Phys. 4:26, 1977.
6. Kruger, R. A.: Estimation of the diameter of and iodine concentration within blood vessels using digital radiography devices. Med. Phys. 8:652, 1981.

L

1. Loo, L. N. D., Doi, K., and Metz, C. E.: Investigation of basic imaging properties in digital radiography. 4. Effect of unsharp masking on the detectability of simple patterns. Med. Phys. 12:209, 1985.
2. Love, A. L., and Kruger, R. A.: Scatter estimation for a digital radiographic system using convolution filtering. Med. Phys. 14:178, 1987.

M

1. Motz, J. W., and Danos, M.: Image information content and patient exposure. Med. Phys. 5:8, 1978.
2. Maher, K. P., O'Connor, M. K., and Malone, J. F.: Experimental examination of videodensitometry of large opacifications in digital subtraction angiography. Phys. Med. Biol. 32:1273, 1987.
3. Malloi, S. Y., and Mistretta, C. A.: Quantification techniques for dual-energy cardiac imaging. Med. Phys. 16:209, 1989.
4. Malloi, S. Y., and Mistretta, C. A.: Scatter-glare corrections in quantitative dual-energy fluoroscopy. Med. Phys. 15:289, 1988.

N

1. Naimuddin, S., Hasegawa, B., and Mistretta, C. A.: Scatter-glare correction using a convolution algorithm with variable weighting. Med. Phys. 14:330, 1987.

P

1. Pratt, W. K.: Digital Image Processing, Wiley-Interscience, New York, 1978.
2. Pfaff, J. M., Whiting, J. S., and Eigler, N. E.: Accurate densitometric quantification requires strict attention to the physical characteristics of x-ray imaging. *In:* Proceedings 2nd International Symposium on Coronary Arteriography. Rotterdam, June 1987.
3. Parker, D. L., Clayton, P. D., and Gustafson, D. E.: The effects of motion on quantitative vessel measurements. Med. Phys. 12:698, 1985.
4. Pfaff, J. M.: Quantitative coronary arteriography: Application of videodensitometric techniques for the evaluation of stenosis severity. Ph.D. Thesis, University of California, Los Angeles, University Microfilms International, 1988.

R

1. Revesz, G.: Conspicuity and uncertainty in the radiographic detection of lesions. Radiology 154:625, 1985.
2. Roehrig, H., Nudelman, S., and Fu, T.-Y.: Electro-optical devices for use in photoelectronic-digital radiology. *In:* Electronic Imaging in Medicine, AAPM Monograph No. 11. American Institute of Physics, New York, 1984.
3. Reiber, J. H. C., Kooijman, C. J., Slager, C. J., et al.: Computer assisted analysis of the severity of obstructions from coronary cineangiograms: A methodological review. Automedica 5:219, 1984.

S

1. Shroy, R. E.: Dependence of noise on array width and depth in digital radiography. Med. Phys. 15:64, 1988.
2. Sandrik, J. M.: The video camera for medical imaging. *In:* Electronic Imaging in Medicine, AAPM Monograph No. 11. American Institute of Physics, New York, 1984.
3. Seibert, J. A., Barr, D. H., Borger, D. J., et al.: Interlaced vs. progressive readout of television cameras for digital radiographic acquisitions. Med. Phys. 11:703, 1984.
4. Seibert, J. A.: Improved fluoroscopic and cine-radiographic display with pulsed exposures and progressive TV scanning. Radiology 159:277, 1986.
5. Suddarth, S. A., Johnson, G. A., Sherrier, R. H., and Ravin, C. E.: Performance of high-resolution monitors for digital chest imaging. Med. Phys. 14:253, 1987.
6. Seibert, J. A., Nalcioglu, O., and Roeck, W. W.: Deconvolution technique for the improvement of contrast of image intensifiers. SPIE J. 314:310, 1981.
7. Shaw, C. G., Ergun, D. L., Myerowitz, P. D., et al.: A technique of scatter and glare correction for videodensitometric studies in digital subtraction videoangiography. Rad. Phys. 142:209, 1982.
8. Seibert, J. A., Nalcioglu, O., and Roeck, W. W.: Characterization of the veiling glare PSF in x-ray image intensified fluoroscopy. Med. Phys. 11:172, 1984.
9. Seibert, J. A., Nalcioglu, O., and Roeck, W. W.: Removal of image intensifier veiling glare by mathematical deconvolution techniques. Med. Phys. 12:281, 1985.
10. Shaw, C. G., and Plewes, D. B.: Quantitative digital subtraction angiography: Two scanning techniques for correction of scattered radiation and veiling glare. Radiology 157:247, 1985.
11. Seibert, J. A., and Boone, J. M.: X-ray scatter removal by deconvolution. Med. Phys. 15:567, 1988.

T

1. Tehrani, S., LeFree, M. T., Sitomer, J., and Bourdillon, P. D. V.: High-speed digital radiologic pincushion distortion correction using an array processor. IEEE Proc. Comput. Cardiol. 615, 1986.

V

1. Van Lysel, M. S., Zarnstorff, W. C., Lancaster, J. C., et al.: Real-time digital video recording system, SPIE J. 314:389, 1981.

W

1. Widrow, B.: A study of rough amplitude quantization by means of Nyquist sampling theory. IEEE Trans. Circuit Theory CT-3:266, 1956.
2. Wagner, R. F.: Toward a unified view of radiological imaging systems. Part II: Noisy images. Med. Phys. 4:279, 1977.
3. Whiting, J. S., Eigler, N. L., Pfaff, J. M., et al.: Improved angiographic detection of coronary morphology in spatially filtered images. Circulation, 80(4):II-356, 1989.
4. Whiting, J. S., Pfaff, J. M., and Eigler, N. L.: Effect of radiographic distortions on the accuracy of quantitative angiography. Am. J. Cardiac Imaging 2:239, 1988.
5. Weber, D. M.: Absolute diameter measurements of coronary arteries based on the first zero crossing of the Fourier spectrum. Med. Phys. 16:188, 1989.

Z

1. Zulstra, F., Ommeren, J., Reiber, J. H. C., and Serruys, P. W.: Does the quantitative assessment of coronary artery dimensions predict the physiologic significance of a coronary stenosis? Circulation 75:1154, 1987.

Chapter 15

Ventricular Function Assessed with Digital Subtraction Angiography

▪ *JONATHAN M. TOBIS, M.D.* ▪ *ORHAN NALCIOGLU, Ph.D.*
▪ *WALTER L. HENRY, M.D.*

LEFT VENTRICULAR IMAGING WITH INTRAVENOUS ADMINISTRATION OF CONTRAST MEDIUM 295
LEFT VENTRICULAR IMAGING WITH VENTRICULAR ADMINISTRATION OF CONTRAST MEDIUM 297
ADVANTAGES AND DISADVANTAGES OF UTILIZING SUBTRACTION 297
VIDEODENSITOMETRY 300
Left Ventricular Ejection Fraction 300
ASSESSMENT OF RIGHT VENTRICULAR FUNCTION WITH DIGITAL SUBTRACTION ANGIOGRAPHY 302
ASSESSMENT OF LEFT VENTRICULAR FUNCTION WITH DIGITAL IMAGING DURING INTERVENTIONS 303
Ventricular Imaging During Bicycle Exercise 303
Atrial Pacing Studies 304
Correlation of Minimum Coronary Lumen Diameter with Left Ventricular Functional Impairment Assessed by Digital Angiography 306

Digital acquisition of cardiovascular images has intrigued angiographers ever since its inception.[H1] The benefit of converting radiographic images from a film-based method to a computerized format is that the digitized images can be manipulated with greater facility to enhance the contrast information within the image.[M1] In addition, conversion to a computerized imaging system increases the ability to perform quantitative analysis on cardiac structures.[K1] Nowhere is this more useful than in the assessment of left ventricular function and quantification of the severity of coronary artery stenosis.

Although the use of digital angiography was initially explored as a means for obtaining intravenous first-pass angiograms, this application is infrequently used because of the discomfort associated with a large intravenous injection of contrast material. Digital acquisition has proved to be most beneficial as an adjunct to invasive cardiac catheterization with intra-arterial injections.[T1] One reason for this change of emphasis is the computer's unique capacities to manipulate images and obtain functional information about blood flow, iodine contrast density, and ventricular performance. In the cardiac catheterization laboratory, digital angiography has been used to obtain left ventriculograms with a lower dose (12 ml) of iodinated contrast medium than is used during standard film-based angiography. This permits multiple left ventriculograms to be obtained, which in turn facilitates the performance of interventional studies such as atrial pacing to assess the functional significance of coronary artery stenosis. In addition, the digital format provides immediate access to enhance the ventricular or coronary images through computer processing techniques such as edge sharpening, contrast amplification, and fourfold image magnification.[M2] Computer software programs are also readily applied to facilitate the quantitation of coronary stenoses by either edge detection or videodensitometric analysis.[T2, T3]

The process of mask mode subtraction enhances low concentrations of contrast material, which enables first-pass right and left ventriculograms to be obtained with intravenous injections. Alternatively, left ventriculograms can be obtained with direct injections of smaller amounts of contrast material than would be required under conditions of film-based cineangiography.

This chapter summarizes the various methods that have been used to image the right and left ventricle with digital acquisition. The validation studies that were performed comparing standard film-based angiography with digital angiography are discussed, as well as different approaches that have been used to enhance the information obtained with digital acquisition with various types of mask acquisition, dual-energy subtraction, and videodensitometry. There is also a discussion of some of the methods in which digital subtraction angiography has been used to assess left ventricular function under conditions of stress to provide information about the physiologic significance of coronary artery obstructions.

LEFT VENTRICULAR IMAGING WITH INTRAVENOUS ADMINISTRATION OF CONTRAST MEDIUM

The prime motivating force behind the initial development of digital subtraction angiography was the desire to develop a means of visualizing the coronary arteries with intravenous administration of contrast material.[M3] Despite the concerted effort of many groups toward this end, it has not been possible to attain this goal because of the extreme dilution of contrast medium as it passes into the coronary arteries from an intravenous injection.[K2]

In order to understand and explore the capabilities of digital acquisition, the initial studies analyzed digitally processed left ventriculograms obtained with intravenous administration of contrast medium and compared them with images obtained by standard cine film–based methods during direct intraventricular injection of contrast medium.[T5] It was necessary to determine whether ventricular volumes and ejection fraction calculated from digitally acquired images correlated with the measurements obtained with standard film–based angiography. Comparison studies were initially performed with intravenous administration of iodine contrast medium as the left ventricle was imaged in a first-pass mode after the iodine bolus traveled through the right ventricular and pulmonary phases.[E1, G1, H2] Prior to these studies, digital acquisition of images of peripheral arteries with intravenous injection of contrast medium had been performed with framing rates of 2 to 8 per second. However, to follow the rapid motion during cardiac ventricular imaging, the digital images had to be acquired at 30 frames per second. The initial image processing computers available in 1981 did not have the capacity to store images in a digital format at this rapid framing rate. Therefore, initial comparison studies were performed by acquiring the images at 30 frames per second, subtracting a mask image in real time, and reconverting the digital information into an analog format for storage on videotape. Computer technology advanced rapidly, and by 1983 complete digital storage of 512 × 512 matrix images at 30 frames per second was accomplished. Digital storage made it easier for images to be recalled for postprocessing without degradation of the image by videotape noise.

Several different approaches were used for the intravenous administration of contrast medium, including peripheral locations such as the basilic vein, a centrally placed catheter in the vena cava, or the introduction of a catheter sheath into the femoral vein. During the first-pass angiograms, 30 to 40 ml of contrast medium was injected by hand over 2 to 3 seconds through a 6 Fr. introducing sheath. The angiograms were obtained with fluoroscopic exposure of 8 milliamperes (mA) and 70 to 90 kilovolts peak (kVp) with 4-mm aluminum filtration to diminish low-energy x-ray penetration. For the validation studies, standard 35-mm film–based cineangiograms were obtained in the 30-degree right anterior oblique projection with direct left ventricular injection of 40 ml of contrast medium. Left ventricular volumes were measured by the area-length technique from both the digital and film-based angiograms. Since the digital images were already in a computerized format, one of the inherent benefits of digital angiography was that quantitative analysis of left ventricular function could easily be accomplished with relatively simple software programs; the operator outlined the end-diastolic and end-systolic volumes of the left ventricle, and then the computer calculated left ventricular volumes and ejection fraction. In addition, wall motion analysis was easily performed by having the computer partition the left ventricular perimeter into multiple segments for the assessment of wall motion contractility.

Initial studies demonstrated good correlations in the measured volumes at end-diastole and end-systole and in the calculated ejection fractions.[N1, N2, V1] Of significance, there were no premature ventricular contractions during the left phase of the intravenous digital angiograms, whereas 18 percent of patients had ventricular tachycardia during the standard intraventricular injection of contrast medium with film-based angiograms and adequate wall motion analysis could not be performed during those studies.[T5] The quality of the initial first-pass digital left ventriculograms was not as good as that of the images from the direct intraventricular film-based studies because of the limitations of spatial resolution of the digital matrix compared to film acquisition, misregistration artifacts during the subtraction process, and the difficulty of adequate enhancement with very dilute boluses of contrast medium. However, the ability to measure volumes, calculate ejection fraction, and assess wall motion was adequate with the digital first-pass studies. In addition, for occasional patients with large apical aneurysms there was better visualization of the left ventricle in the digital study because there was improved mixing of the blood pool with the iodinated contrast medium following intravenous administration (Fig. 15–1). An acceptable correlation between the digital left ventriculograms and the film-based images persists even when the ejection fraction is below 30 percent. However, if the cardiac output is low or if tricuspid regurgitation is present, the bolus of contrast medium becomes too dilute and the image quality is degraded during the levo phase. It is perhaps more appropriate to compare these images with first-pass radionuclide images. From that perspective, first-pass digital angiograms have 10 times the spatial resolution of radionuclide images and therefore are very accurate for assessing ventricular wall motion at rest and during stressful interventions.

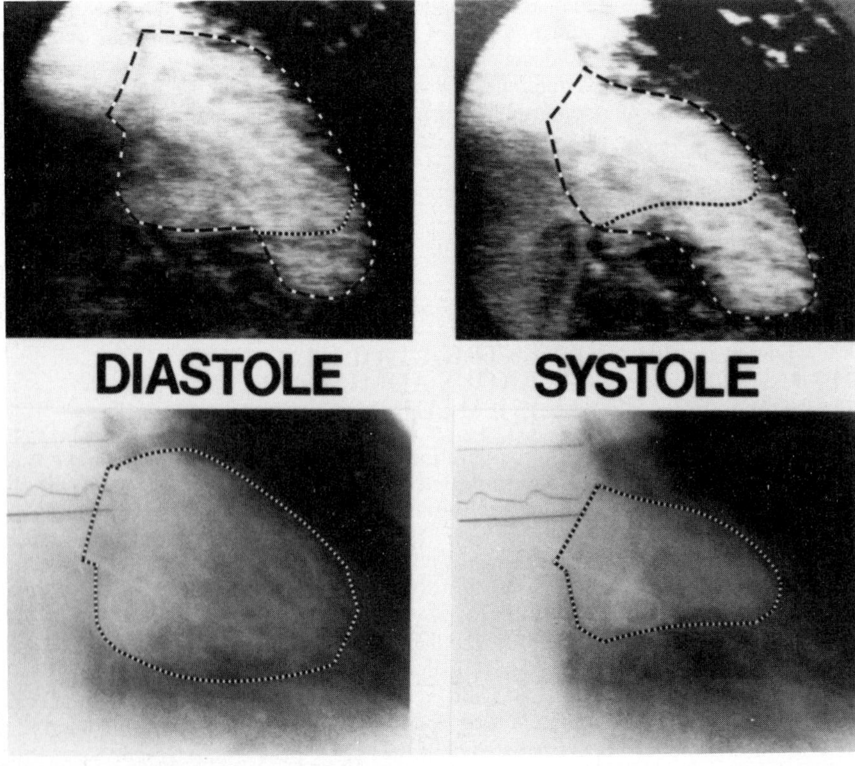

Figure 15–1. Intravenous digital angiograms *(upper panels)* and intraventricular cineangiograms *(lower panels)* from the same patient. Both studies were performed with 40 ml of contrast material. The intravenous technique provided better mixing of contrast material and allowed the apical aneurysm to be appreciated. The left ventricular boundaries that were seen on the standard intraventricular cineangiograms are superimposed on the digital angiograms and outlined with small dots; the boundaries appreciated on the digital angiograms are outlined by heavy dashed lines. (From Tobis, J. M., Nalcioglu, O., Johnston, W. D., et al.: Left ventricular imaging with digital subtraction angiography using intravenous contrast injection and fluoroscopic exposure levels. Am. Heart J. 104:25, 1982, with permission.)

Later developments in digital angiography permitted pulse mode cine acquisition with standard radiographic exposure, which improved the signal-to-noise ratio in the intravenous studies.

The use of first-pass digital angiography with intravenous administration of contrast medium to obtain left ventricular images had limited general applicability because of the less invasive nature of other imaging modalities such as echocardiography and radionuclide imaging. Moreover, the relatively large intravenous bolus of contrast medium caused discomfort for the patient and was associated with nausea and vomiting in approximately 5 percent of the cases. Also, an introducing catheter with a rather large lumen was required to inject the contrast medium within a short time to obtain a maximum bolus effect. Although the applications of digital angiography with intravenous administration are currently limited, these studies led to an understanding of the capabilities of digital acquisition and set the stage for the use of digital acquisition during invasive cardiac and coronary angiography.

LEFT VENTRICULAR IMAGING WITH VENTRICULAR ADMINISTRATION OF CONTRAST MEDIUM

The next area that was studied with digital angiography was the acquisition of left ventriculograms with low doses of contrast media administered directly into the left ventricle at the time of cardiac catheterization. Because of the enhancement of contrast by the mask mode subtraction process, digital left ventriculograms could be obtained with 10 to 15 ml of contrast medium, compared to the standard dose of 40 ml of undiluted contrast medium injected during standard film–based angiography (Fig. 15–2). In the early validation studies, several methods of administration of contrast medium were used.[S1] In order to obtain adequate mixing and filling of the left ventricle, our current practice is to dilute 15 ml of Hypaque-75 with 15 ml of water and to inject this amount at 10 ml/sec over 3 seconds. As with standard cineangiography, the rate of injection and amount of contrast medium injected to obtain the optimum digital left ventriculogram depend on the size of the ventricle under study.

The digital left ventriculograms were associated with less frequent episodes of ventricular tachycardia than the standard 40-ml injections (3 percent versus 20 percent).[T6] In addition, the lower doses used to obtain digital angiograms did not increase the mean left ventricular end-diastolic pressure, whereas the 40-ml injection increased the mean left ventricular end-diastolic pressure by an average of 6 mmHg ($p < 0.01$). Good correlations were found for the left ventricular volumes measured by the area-length technique at end-diastole and end-systole and the calculated ejection fractions obtained from the digital and film-based angiograms. The lower doses needed for digital left ventriculograms permit these studies to be performed with a lower total dose of iodine in diabetic patients and patients with renal or cardiac dysfunction. In addition, multiple left ventriculograms can be obtained without exceeding the recommended doses of iodinated contrast medium. This facilitates the assessment of left ventricular function during intervention studies such as atrial pacing during the cardiac catheterization study.[K3, M4, N3]

ADVANTAGES AND DISADVANTAGES OF UTILIZING SUBTRACTION

Although the technical aspects of mask mode subtraction are covered by Whiting in Chapter 14, a brief discussion of the various methods that have been studied for enhancement of digital left ventriculograms is appropriate here. The more common methods of acquiring digital images, along with their advantages, disadvantages, and clinical applications, are listed in Table 15–1. The major advantage of utilizing the subtraction process is that it enhances the visibility of iodinated contrast medium by deleting soft tissue and bone structures, which tend to impair visibility of cardiac structures within the region of interest. Subtraction imaging is a standard method for enhancing iodine contrast with radiographic cut films. A routine film-based angiogram is enhanced by superimposing the negative of a radiograph taken before administration of contrast medium over the negative of a radiograph obtained following the intra-arterial administration of contrast medium. This process is laborious and is useful only for selected cut films. The benefit of digital acquisition is that the images can be manipulated mathematically by the computer to perform the subtraction process. Once the images are in a digital matrix format, an image processing computer can compare the images and provide a subtracted image that accentuates differences between the initial and all subsequent images. Image processing computers operate at rates such that 8 million pieces of information are processed per second, which enables the computer to provide real-time subtraction of digital 512 × 512 matrix images at 30 frames per second.

The major disadvantage of using the mask mode subtraction technique is the presence of misregistration artifacts, which occur when there is motion of the underlying structures between the

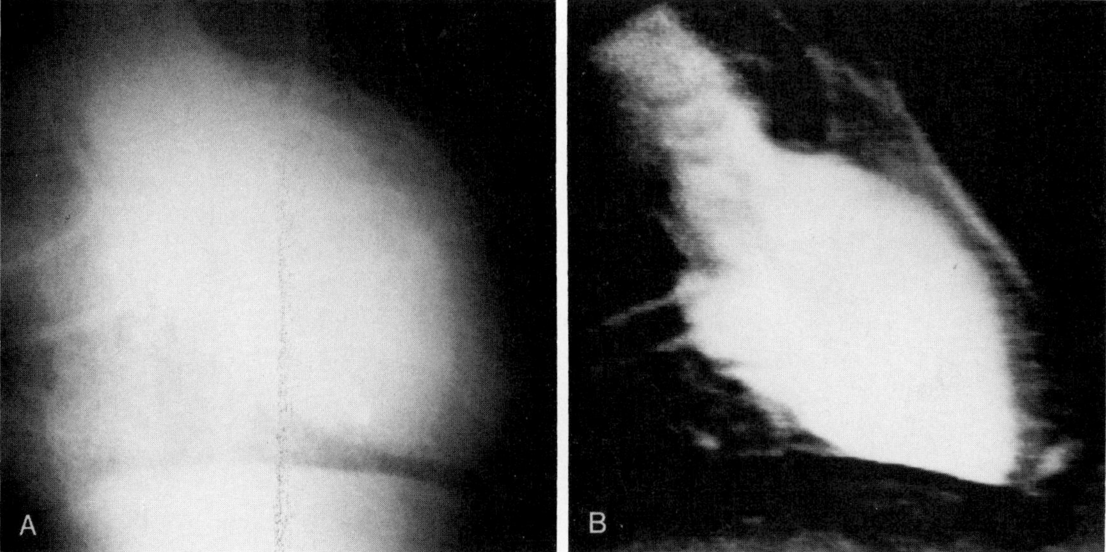

Figure 15–2. Digital left ventriculogram obtained with a low dose of contrast material. Both images were obtained with 12 ml of contrast medium injected directly into the left ventricle. *A*, Angiogram obtained with a standard cineangiographic film–based technique with 35-mm film. *B*, Image processed digitally and subtracted by the mask mode technique. Contrast enhancement is improved approximately fourfold with the digital subtraction method. (Reprinted by permission of the publisher from Rappaport, E. [ed.]: Cardiology Update 1984: Reviews for Physicians. Elsevier, New York, 1984, p. 206. Copyright 1984 by Elsevier Science Publishing Co., Inc.)

Table 15–1. DIGITAL ACQUISITION TECHNIQUES

Methods	Advantages	Useful Applications	Disadvantages
1. Unsubtracted digital acquisition	Digital matrix format	Quantitative analysis Coronary angiography Roadmap for PTCA	Contrast is not enhanced
2. Mask mode subtraction	Enhances contrast	Right and left ventriculograms First-pass studies Aortic root angiography Videodensitometry	Misregistration artifact
3. Summation mask subtraction	Diminishes minor misregistration due to cardiac motion	Same as mask mode subtraction	Large motion artifact
4. ECG-gated mask subtraction	Diminishes minor misregistration due to cardiac motion	Right and left ventriculograms	Need to digitize the ECG signal and initialize the digital image with ECG
5. Time interval difference	Diminishes motion artifact	Wall motion analysis	No significant clinical application over other methods
6. Dual-energy subtraction	No artifact due to motion Can pan image intensifier during acquisition	Coronary angiography First-pass left ventriculograms during bicycle exercise	Diminishes signal-to-noise ratio
7. Hybrid acquisition	Combines time and energy subtraction	Enhances contrast	No significant clinical application beyond other methods
8. Time-of-arrival mapping	Provides a relative measure of blood flow	Coronary artery studies of coronary flow reserve pre and post PTCA	Does not measure absolute blood flow; difficult to perform

PTCA—percutaneous transluminal coronary angioplasty.

time when the mask is obtained and the times when all subsequent images are recorded. The resulting subtracted images have light or dark streaks in the field of view and decreased visualization of the diluted iodine (Fig. 15–3). In addition, during digital coronary angiography, the misregistration streaks can be confused with arterial stenoses; thus the recognition of misregistration is important when using mask mode subtraction. One of the advantages of digital angiography over film-based radiography, in which the image cannot be altered after development, is that digital images can be restored from computer memory and manipulated after the angiogram is acquired.[K1] These postprocessing techniques can be used to improve image quality and reduce the problems caused by misregistration artifacts. For example, if a digitally subtracted left ventriculogram shows a significant misregistration streak in the subtracted image, a new mask taken from the series of images obtained prior to the injection of contrast medium can be recalled from computer memory and subtracted from the frames with iodine.[T6] A series of different

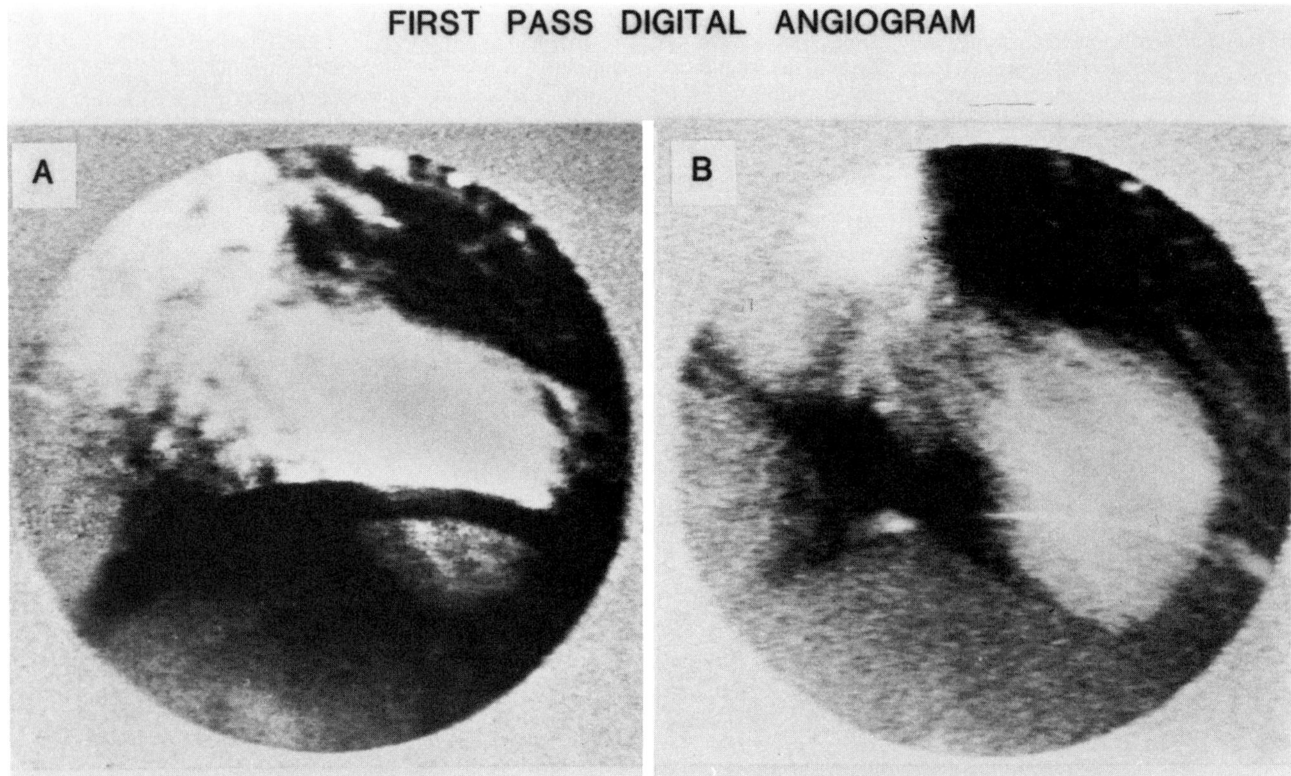

Figure 15–3. *A*, Misregistration artifact is present due to movement of the diaphragm between the time when the original mask image was taken and the times when subsequent images with contrast medium were obtained. *B*, The large black streak of misregistration artifact has been eliminated by choosing a new mask during the postprocessing period. The new mask is chosen from the series of images obtained prior to the levo phase, so the position of the diaphragm is more closely aligned. (From Tobis, J. M., Nalcioglu, O., and Henry, W. L.: Cardiovascular applications of digital subtraction angiography. Mod. Concepts Cardiovasc. Dis. 53:32, 1984, with permission from the American Heart Association, Inc.)

masks can be tried until one that has a minimum of misregistration is found. In addition, the mask can be moved by the computer relative to the second image during postprocessing of the digital angiogram to further reduce misregistration artifacts. Software algorithms have been written to permit movement of the mask horizontally or vertically by a fraction of a pixel or rotation of the mask around polar coordinates to decrease misregistration.

Another common method for obtaining subtracted mask mode left ventriculograms is to use a summation mask. During this process, 16 frames or ½ second of angiographic acquisition is obtained prior to the injection of contrast medium. The data from these 16 frames are averaged, and the average mask is then subtracted from all subsequent images. This method tends to decrease minor misregistration artifacts and provides an image that has less information from extraneous tissues.

An alternative approach has been to update the mask continuously in synchrony with the cardiac cycle.[B1] During this process, called dynamic mask subtraction, the electrocardiogram (ECG) signal is incorporated in the digital image and each image of the left ventricle that contains contrast medium is subtracted from a mask taken before injection of contrast medium that corresponds to the same part of the cardiac cycle.

A fourth method of subtracting images, called parametric imaging, utilizes all of the subtracted images with contrast medium. In this method, the end-diastolic subtracted image is recalled from computer memory and each subsequent image during the cardiac cycle is subtracted from the end-diastolic frame (Fig. 15–4). The difference image that is generated in this process represents the left ventricular shell or intracavitary space that has been displaced between end-diastole and end-systole. This geometric space corresponds to the stroke volume ejected with each heartbeat. In addition, parametric imaging highlights areas where wall motion abnormalities occur and clearly distinguishes between akinetic and dyskinetic segments. Although these figures are visually appealing, they have not often been used clinically because the quantitative information that they yield has not been any more useful than the information that can be obtained with standard quantitative analyses of wall motion function.

Because of the complexity of the mathematical functions that the image processing computers can perform, there is an alternative method of assessing left ventricular wall motion that involves the phase changes in the x-ray density in the z plane perpendicular to the two-dimensional projection image. Widmann and associates used a Fourier analysis of the x-ray density over the left ventricle versus time during intravenous digital ventriculography.[W1] The first-harmonic curve can be analyzed to quantitate the amplitude and phase angle of the x-ray absorption of iodinated contrast medium within the left ventricle. This analysis of the phase changes of the density of contrast medium within the two-dimensional digital image provides information about the synchronicity of wall motion in the z axis. With this method they were able to show that ischemic ventricular segments have a greater degree of asynchrony than ventricular segments perfused by normal coronary arteries.

Dual-energy subtraction is a more recent method that has been applied to enhance contrast and reduce motion artifacts.[M5] In this process, the images are acquired at two different energies. One image is obtained at a low energy (60 kVp) and a second image is obtained at a high energy (120 kVp). The low-energy image displays a greater variation in contrast because of the difference in x-ray attenuation at lower energies. This difference in x-ray attenuation at the two energy levels is utilized to decrease tissue densities when the images are subtracted from each other. In order to perform dual-energy subtraction, the x-ray tube voltage and the x-ray beam filtration are switched every 1/30 second. Because the pairs of high- and low-energy images are obtained every 1/30 second, there is minimal movement of cardiac structures between the image pairs, which negates the effect of misregistration due to motion artifact that so often plagues standard mask mode subtraction imaging. The reduction in motion artifact during dual-energy subtraction permits panning of the image intensifier over the thorax during the study. In addition, respiratory movement does not interfere with the image quality (Fig.

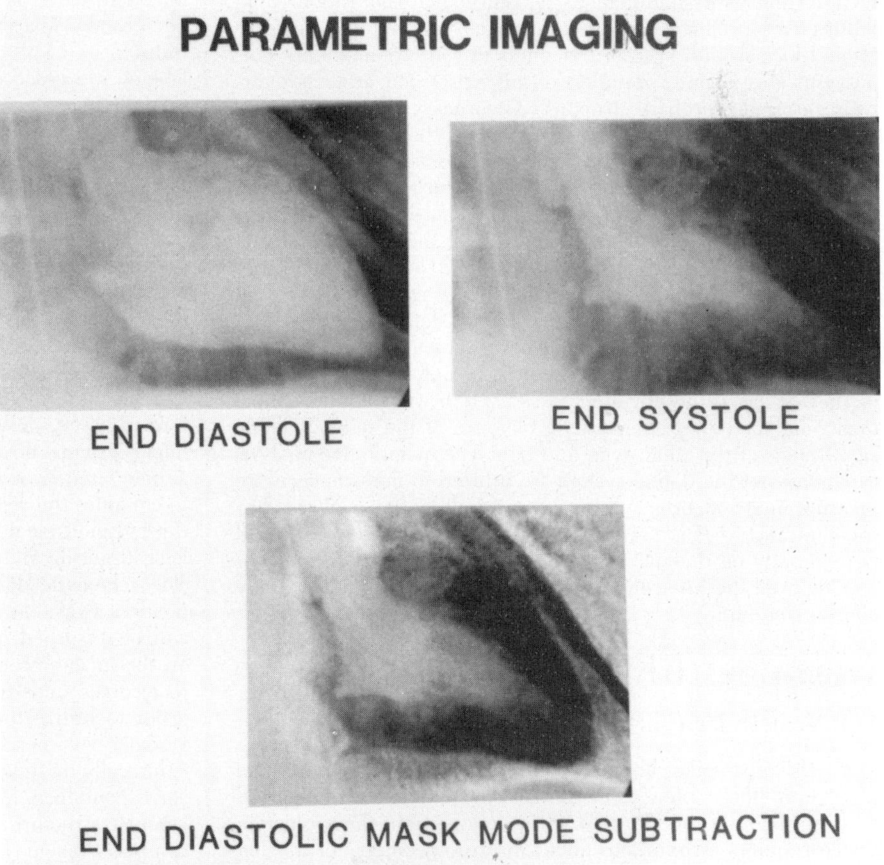

Figure 15–4. Composite figure demonstrating the method by which end-diastolic mask mode subtraction is performed to give both a qualitative and a functional image within the same picture. Instead of choosing a mask prior to the injection of contrast medium, one chooses an end-diastolic image when the left ventricle is maximally filled with contrast medium. This end-diastolic image is then used as the mask from which all subsequent images are subtracted. The images can be run through in a loop or the end-systolic image alone can be chosen and subtracted from the end-diastolic mask image to produce the image in the bottom panel. This image reveals the left ventricular outline at end-diastole in black and the end-systolic image in white, and the difference in wall motion between these two time periods is outlined as the black shell around the perimeter of the left ventricle. This geometric shell corresponds to the stroke volume that has been ejected. Thus, the same image provides a representation of end-diastole, end-systole, and stroke volume as well as a functional representation of any abnormalities in wall motion, which would be highlighted between the black and white contrast.

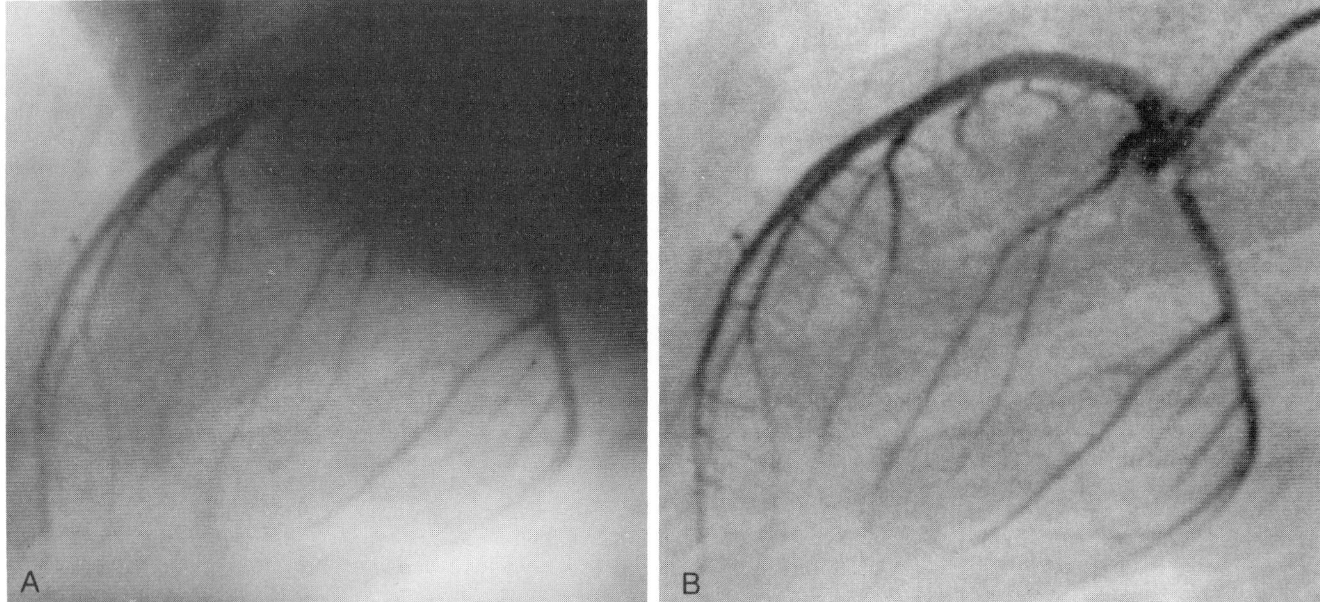

Figure 15–5. *A*, Unsubtracted coronary angiogram from a pig, showing interference in the iodine contrast caused by nonlinear distortion of soft tissue and bone densities. *B*, The same coronary angiogram processed with dual-energy subtraction. In this method, the soft-tissue densities and most of the bone densities are removed with enhancement of iodine contrast. There is no motion artifact, as there might be with a mask mode or time difference image.

15–5). Experimental studies have shown good image quality for thin subjects; whether the reduction in signal-to-noise ratio will interfere with image quality for thicker subjects remains to be tested.

With all of these digital acquisition capabilities, one might become overwhelmed by the choice of a technique for routine cardiology studies. Our current approach during routine cardiac catheterization is to obtain the left ventriculogram with a low dose of contrast medium with the image enhanced by summation mask mode subtraction. Our laboratory is equipped with a Philips DCI system with simultaneous biplane digital acquisition capabilities. We prefer to obtain coronary angiograms in an unsubtracted format with standard amounts of contrast medium. This prevents the misinterpretation of misregistration artifacts overlying the small coronary structures as coronary stenoses. During angioplasty procedures, selected frames of the coronary images are chosen from various views, and these "road maps" are displayed on the monitors next to the catheterization table within seconds of acquisition. The coronary road maps are extremely useful during angioplasty, and the digital format makes them easier to review and select than standard video images would be. In addition, the images can be digitally magnified fourfold in order to review a specific region in greater detail.

If there is a stenosis of uncertain severity, we prefer to perform a low-contrast digital subtraction atrial pacing study at the time of the cardiac catheterization to assess the wall motion abnormality induced by ischemia as a measure of the hemodynamic significance of the stenosis in question. The quantitative analysis capabilities of the digital system are utilized to perform accurate measurements of coronary stenosis and wall motion analysis after the clinical studies are acquired. The coronary images are stored permanently on digital tape. The DCI system splits the images coming from the intensifier, and they are recorded both digitally and on cine film.

VIDEODENSITOMETRY

Left Ventricular Ejection Fraction

A left ventricular angiogram represents a two-dimensional projection image of a three-dimensional object. Mathematical reconstruction of the left ventricular volume from the projection image requires assumptions about the true geometry of the left ventricular cavity. In area-length analysis, the shape of the left ventricular cavity is approximated by assuming that it is an ellipse in revolution. The stacked-coin method of calculating left ventricular volume does not assume that the left ventricle is an ellipse in revolution but estimates that the cross-sectional geometry is circular. By stacking the coins or cross-sectional segments of different radii, an approximation of the volume of the left ventricular cavity can be ascertained.

Densitometry is an alternative approach to left ventricular volume analysis that does not depend on the assumption that the left ventricle is a uniform geometric shape.[T7] This method has been used primarily during radionuclide angiography by counting the density of photons emitted from the volume of technetium-labeled red blood cells within a region of interest drawn around the left ventricle. A similar method can be used with radiographic images by counting the differential absorption of the x-ray photons as they pass through the iodine-filled left ventricular chamber.[B2] Because these images are usually displayed in a video format, the term that is used to describe this technique is videodensitometry. The benefit of videodensitometry over radionuclide imaging is that it combines the computational simplicity of radionuclide densitometry with the improved resolution capabilities of x-ray imaging devices so that the boundaries of the structures are clearly visible.[N4, N5]

Figure 15–6 demonstrates how the videodensitometric calculation is performed. When incident x-rays are transmitted through human tissue, they are attenuated in an exponential and not in a linear fashion, depending on the thickness of the tissue and the atomic number of the constituent elements in the tissue. In order to compute the relative absorption to derive the thickness of the three-dimensional object of interest, it is necessary to amplify logarithmically the x-ray signal that reaches the image intensifier. The schematic diagram in Figure 15–6 demonstrates that the incident x-rays, as they penetrate a step wedge filled with iodine, will be absorbed in an exponential fashion. This is represented on the image intensifier and television monitor as a video signal that corresponds to the exponentially absorbed x-ray signals. In order to utilize the density information for calculation of intravascular volumes, the incoming video signal is amplified logarithmically by the computer so that the output represents a linear correspondence between the depth of the iodine within the vascular structure and the resulting gray scale numbers on the computer image (Fig. 15–7).

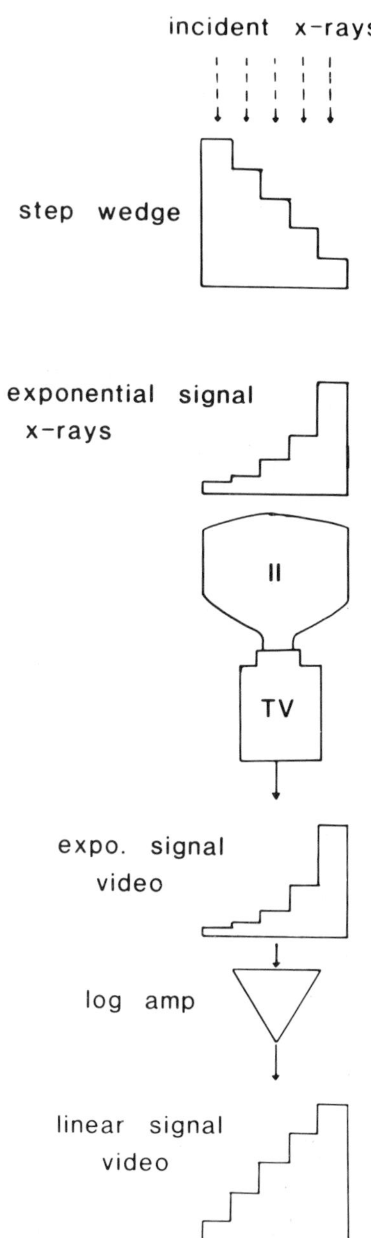

Figure 15–6. Incident x-rays that penetrate an object such as a step wedge are attenuated in an exponential fashion. The image intensifier (II) and television camera (TV) record the densities of the step wedge as an exponentially attenuated video signal. If this video signal is processed by a logarithmic amplifier (log amp), the exponential attenuation can be compensated for so that the contrast densities in the video signal output are linearly related to the depth of contrast material in the step wedge.

In order to obtain information on absolute left ventricular volume, the concentration of iodine in milligrams per milliliter of blood would have to be known to correlate the density levels with the chamber volume. However, since ejection fraction is a relative number, the densities in end-diastole and end-systole can be compared as a ratio without knowing the absolute concentration of the iodine within the chamber. Figure 15–8 demonstrates how the videodensitometric calculation is performed. An end-diastolic frame is chosen by the operator as the frame with the largest area of iodine in the left ventricle. The region of interest is outlined so that the border of the ventricle is included (approximately 1 cm beyond the visual border of the iodinated area). The aortic and mitral valve planes are used as the medial boundary. The digital images are played back from computer memory, and the end-systolic image is chosen. The area between the end-diastolic and end-systolic images is outlined and is used as the area from which to subtract background counts. This area was chosen for computing the average background density because it was thought that this area would correspond most closely to the densities due to x-ray attenuation by structures anterior or posterior to the left ventricular chamber and would include some of the tissue density due to the myocardium itself. The computer calculates the total density within the background region of interest and divides by the number of pixels within that region to derive the average background counts. This can be determined on a beat-to-beat basis to upgrade the calculation of background counts as the iodine bolus traverses the left ventricular phase.

The left ventriculograms are obtained with a first-pass bolus of iodinated contrast medium injected into the venous system, which provides for complete mixing and opacification of the left ventricular chamber without inducing any premature ventricular contractions. As the bolus of contrast medium passes through the left ventricular phase, the computer counts the densities and generates a curve of density versus time, analogous to the information that is generated during first-pass radionuclide studies. The maximal and minimal density values for each heartbeat are determined and correspond to the end-diastolic and end-systolic volumes. A separate density-time curve is also generated for the background area of interest so that beat-to-beat variations in the background can be accounted for. These density values are used to calculate an ejection fraction for each heartbeat using the formula

$$\mathrm{EF} = \frac{(\mathrm{ED} - [\mathrm{Bkg} \times \mathrm{ED\ area}]) - (\mathrm{ES} - [\mathrm{Bkg} \times \mathrm{ED\ area}])}{\mathrm{ED} - [\mathrm{Bkg} \times \mathrm{ED\ area}]}$$

where ED is the end-diastolic or maximal value, ES is the end-systolic or minimal value from the density-time curve, Bkg is the average value per pixel for the background region of interest, and ED area is the number of pixels in the end-diastolic region of interest. The total density values for the end-systolic or end-diastolic images are counted from the pixels within the original end-diastolic region of interest; therefore, the average background must be subtracted from the entire end-diastolic region (ED area). This formula is simplified to

$$\mathrm{EF} = \frac{\mathrm{ED} - \mathrm{ES}}{\mathrm{ED} - (\mathrm{Bkg} \times \mathrm{ED\ area})}$$

In order to validate the videodensitometric method for obtaining ejection fraction, the ejection fractions calculated from first-pass digital subtraction angiograms of 25 patients were compared to the ejection fractions calculated from direct ventricular cineangiograms by the area-length method. The correlation coefficient between the two techniques was 0.94, as demonstrated in Figure 15–9.[T8]

In addition to enhanced visibility of ventricular motion and ejection fraction analysis, digital angiography can be used to assess the diastolic function of the ventricles. As previously described, the digital subtraction angiogram can be used to generate a density-time curve as a bolus of iodine passes through the left ventricular cavity. The points along this curve represent relative volume in the ventricle. As previously determined with radionuclide imaging, the density-time pattern during the diastolic period provides a measure of ventricular filling that corresponds to the compliance of the ventricular chamber. In a similar manner, the densitometric filling curves generated with first-pass digital left ventriculography have correlated well with Doppler velocity patterns of flow across the mitral valve.[D3]

Most methods of measuring left ventricular volumes and ejection fraction are based on assumptions that may not be accurate under certain circumstances. For example, the area-length method, which assumes an ellipsoidal shape of the left ventricular cavity, may be a good approximation for normal ventricles; however, diseased hearts usually dilate and become more spherical. In addition, the two-dimensional projection images from cineangiograms tend to obscure volume-occupying structures in the left ventricular cavity, such as muscular trabeculations or papillary muscles and the mitral valve leaflets.

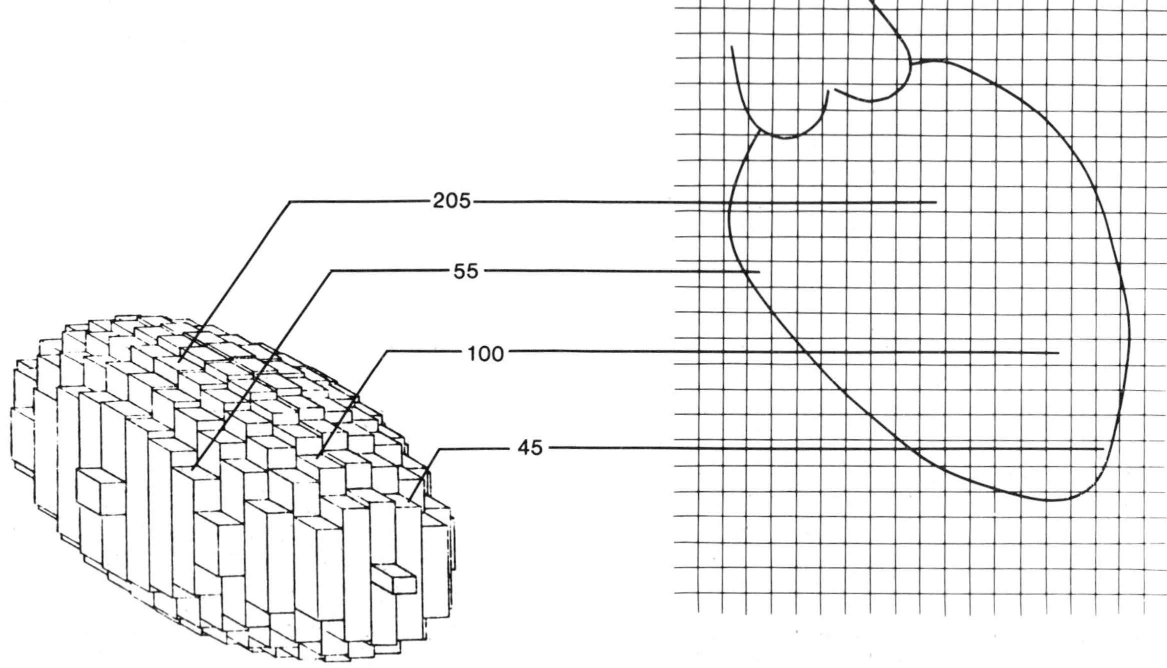

Figure 15–7. Relation between contrast depth and pixel density value. At the left is a three-dimensional model of a left ventriculogram that has been sectioned into boxes. The two-dimensional surfaces of these boxes correspond to the *x-y* coordinates of pixels on the digital angiographic image shown at the right. The density value of each pixel corresponds to the depth of the box represented in each pixel. By adding the density values on the digital image within the region of interest, a number is obtained that corresponds to the total volume of contrast medium within that region. (From Trenholm, B. G., Winter, D. A., Mymin, D., and Lansdown, E. L.: Computer determination of left ventricular volume using videodensitometry. Med. Biol. Eng. Comput. 10:163, 1972, with permission.)

Although videodensitometry is an alternative method of calculating left ventricular ejection fraction that does not depend on assumptions about ventricular geometry, other assumptions are used in the determination of densitometric volumes. The most sensitive term in determining the ejection fraction is the calculation of the average background density over the region of interest. In addition, it is necessary to have good-quality digital subtraction angiograms to be able to make the densitometric calculations. Therefore, it is important to exclude studies in which misregistration is caused by motion of the patient or when very low concentrations of iodine are present in the left ventricle. Other potential problems with the densitometric method are related to physical factors that could prevent x-ray attenuation by iodine from being proportional to the depth of iodine traversed by the x-ray beam. These physical factors include beam hardening, x-ray scatter, and veiling glare. Laboratory studies of these physical factors indicate that they may cause underestimation of ejection fraction by 5 to 15 percent.[N6, N7]

ASSESSMENT OF RIGHT VENTRICULAR FUNCTION WITH DIGITAL SUBTRACTION ANGIOGRAPHY

Digital subtraction angiography has proved to be beneficial in the assessment of right ventricular function. By using an intra-

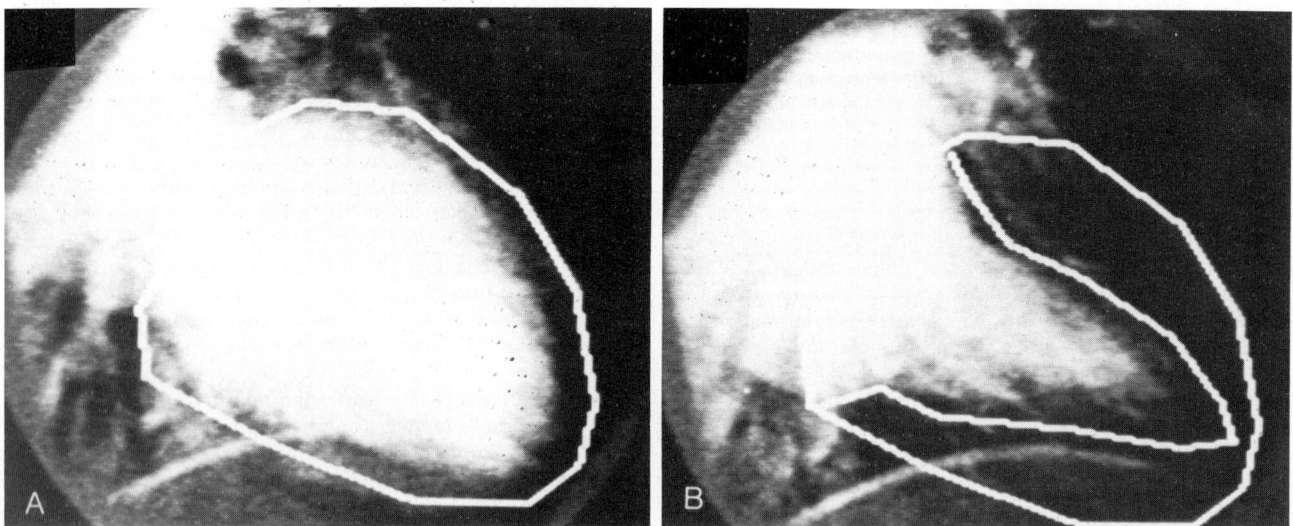

Figure 15–8. First-pass digital subtraction angiogram demonstrating the technique for obtaining the background area during the videodensitometric analysis. The end-diastolic frame (*A*) is outlined to include all the iodine within the left ventricle, and the boundary of the aorta and mitral valve plane is used as the medial border. The end-systolic frame (*B*) is then chosen and the area around the end-systolic border is outlined. The background region of interest is taken as the area between the end-diastolic and end-systolic regions of interest. (From Tobis, J., Nalcioglu, O., Seibert, J. A., et al.: Measurement of left ventricular ejection fraction by videodensitometric analysis of digital subtraction angiograms. Am. J. Cardiol. 52:873, 1983, with permission.)

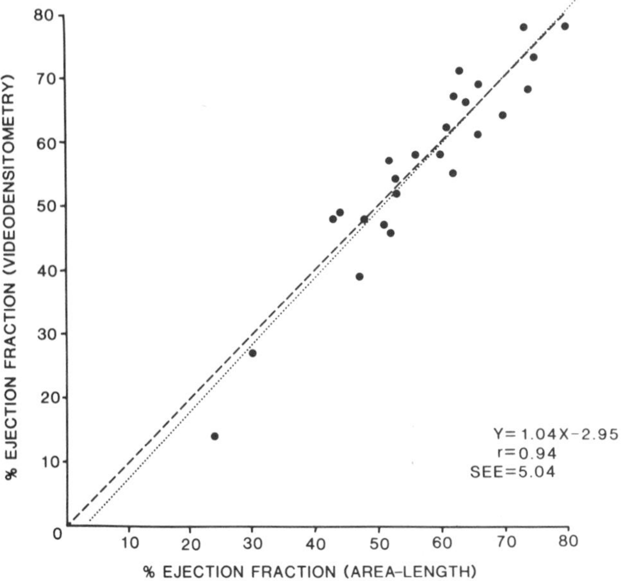

Figure 15–9. Correlation of ejection fraction determined by the area-length method with ejection fraction determined by videodensitometry (r = 0.94; SEE—standard error of the estimate). (From Tobis, J., Nalcioglu, O., Seibert, J. A., et al.: Measurement of left ventricular ejection fraction by videodensitometric analysis of digital subtraction angiograms. Am. J. Cardiol. 52:873, 1983, with permission.)

venous injection of contrast medium, the right ventricle can be imaged during a first-pass technique with excellent visibility and demarcation of the various anatomic structures. One of the difficulties in trying to measure right ventricular volumes by angiography is that the right ventricle does not conform to a simple geometric shape. In addition, the right ventricle has numerous trabeculae and interstices, which make it difficult to use a mathematic formula to derive its volume from a two-dimensional angiogram. The facility to perform a videodensitometric analysis with images that are acquired digitally offers unique advantages for assessing the right ventricular ejection fraction. Because the densitometric method can be used to derive the relative volume of any irregular object without using any assumptions about its three-dimensional geometry, this approach is well suited for the analysis of right ventricular volumes at end-diastole and end-systole.[N8]

Radionuclide imaging of the right ventricle has gained widespread support because the photon counting technique is based on densitometric principles. However, a major problem of radionuclide imaging is its limited spatial resolution. During intravenous first-pass digital studies, it was noted that the tricuspid valve annulus moved toward the apex and shortened the long axis of the right ventricle by about 20 percent. Densitometric methods such as radionuclide angiography, which use only one fixed region of interest to outline the right ventricle at end-diastole, neglect the apical displacement of the tricuspid valve annulus. The result of using one fixed region of interest is that some right atrial counts are included in the end-systolic volume calculation. The increased spatial resolution of digital angiograms permits excellent visualization of the tricuspid annulus and allows identification of the proper boundary of the right ventricle at end-diastole and end-systole (Fig. 15–10). In one study of 19 patients with first-pass digital right ventriculograms, the videodensitometric analysis with two separate regions of interest gave a closer correlation with the ejection fraction calculated by the area-length technique than did the method with only one region of interest, whereas the radionuclide data did not correlate very well with either the digital or the area-length method.[J1]

ASSESSMENT OF LEFT VENTRICULAR FUNCTION WITH DIGITAL IMAGING DURING INTERVENTIONS

The facility with which quantitative left ventricular analysis can be performed with digitally acquired images makes digital angiography an ideal means of assessing left ventricular function under conditions of stress as well as at rest. Two major approaches have been used to induce ischemia during digital angiographic imaging in patients with coronary artery disease. Quantitative analysis of left ventricular wall motion during the stress of bicycle exercise or atrial pacing has been used to assess the functional significance of a particular coronary artery obstruction.

Ventricular Imaging During Bicycle Exercise

In the first method, supine bicycle exercise has been used in an analogous manner to first-pass radionuclide exercise stress testing.[S2] Measurements of left ventricular volumes at end-diastole and end-systole and changes in the global ejection fraction

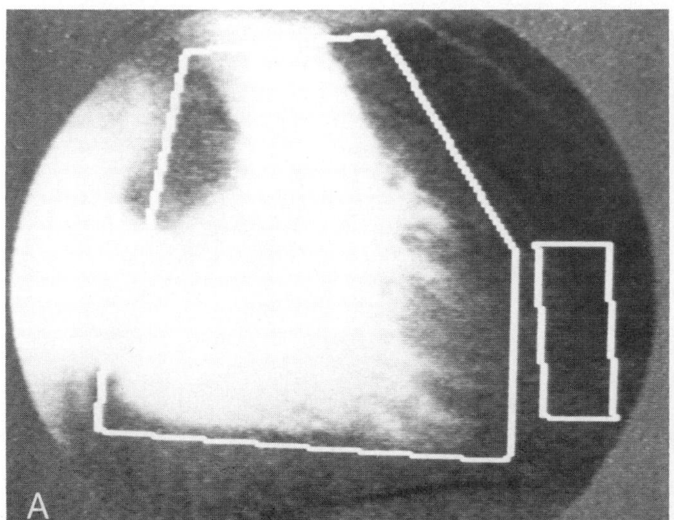

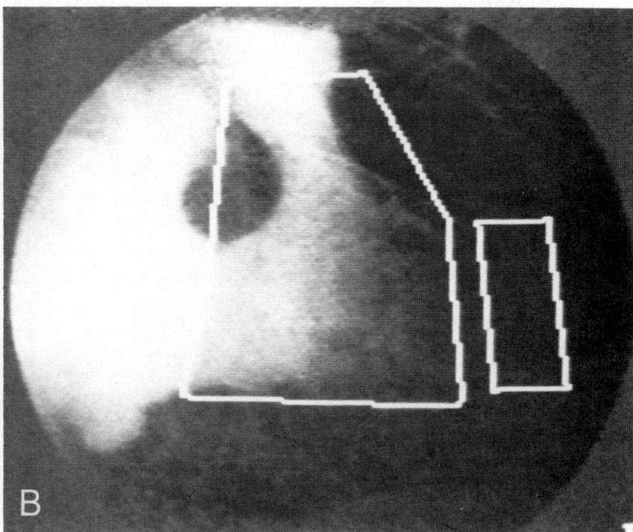

Figure 15–10. *A*, First-pass digital subtraction right ventriculogram with a region of interest generously outlining the boundary of the right ventricle. The plane of the tricuspid valve is demonstrated in this 30-degree right anterior oblique projection. *B*, The densitometric region of interest over the right ventricle during end-systole is outlined. The plane of the tricuspid valve has moved toward the right ventricular apex, but because the boundary definition is clear, the counts generated from the right atrium are separated for the densitometric calculation. The small rectangular box represents the region of interest used for determination of background densities.

or the development of segmental wall motion abnormalities from rest to peak exercise or after exercise are analyzed as a measure of exercise-induced ischemia. In one study of 19 patients who underwent coronary angiography for evaluation of chest pain, the assessment of the development of wall motion abnormalities and a fall in ejection fraction, as assessed by first-pass digital angiography, was more sensitive than the assessment of the development of chest pain or ST segment response on the ECG for identifying patients with coronary disease.[T9] Additional studies at the Cleveland Clinic and New York Hospital have demonstrated the validity of this method.[G2, Y1] However, supine bicycle exercise induces significant respiratory motion, which produces misregistration artifacts in the digital subtraction ventriculograms. Adequate first-pass digital ventriculograms could not be obtained for approximately 10 percent of patients because of problems with misregistration in the mask mode–subtracted angiograms. One way to overcome this problem of misregistration artifact during stress testing would be to use dual-energy subtraction instead of mask mode subtraction to obtain the left ventriculograms. Since the dual-energy images are obtained within 1/30 second of each other, misregistration artifacts due to respiratory motion are eliminated.

Atrial Pacing Studies

As an alternative approach to inducing ischemia in patients with coronary artery stenosis, atrial pacing can be performed in conjunction with digital subtraction angiography. Several methods have been explored for performing atrial pacing stress tests.[M6] We have found it most useful to obtain atrial pacing stress tests during cardiac catheterization. During these studies, the left ventriculogram is obtained with digital processing, which usually requires only 10 to 15 ml of contrast medium.[T10] After the baseline digital left ventriculogram and digital coronary angiograms have been obtained, the pigtail catheter is repositioned in the left ventricle and a pacing guidewire is placed in the right atrium. The atrium is stimulated at 2 mA starting at 10 to 20 beats per minute above the patient's resting heart rate. The pacemaker rate is increased by increments of 10 beats per minute every minute until the patient develops chest pain or until a maximum heart rate of 150 beats per minute is achieved. At the maximum heart rate, while the pacemaker is still stimulating the atrium, a second digital left ventriculogram is obtained. The pacemaker is then shut off.

During atrial pacing the left ventricular end-diastolic volume decreases in all patients, whether or not they have significant coronary artery disease. The distinction between patients with and patients without coronary artery disease occurs during the analysis of end-systolic volume. Patients with significant coronary artery disease are unable to contract the myocardial segment that becomes ischemic, and this alteration in systolic function is visualized as a segmental wall motion abnormality with inability to reduce the end-systolic volume appropriately (Figs. 15–11 and 15–12).

This method of assessing the hemodynamic significance of coronary artery disease is performed only in patients who have a stenosis of uncertain severity at the time of cardiac catheteriza-

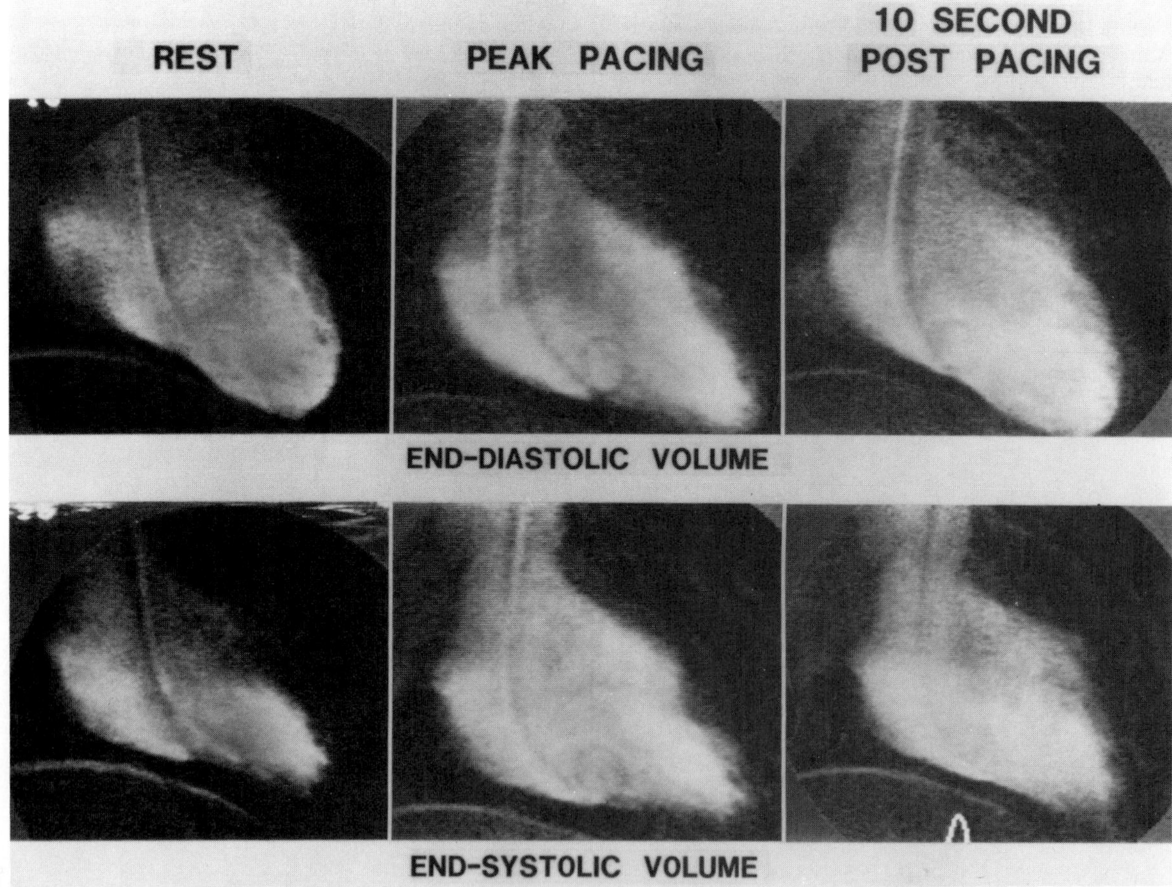

Figure 15–11. Composite figure showing isolated frames from the digital subtraction left ventriculograms obtained with 12 ml of contrast material during an atrial pacing study. Frames at end-diastole (*top row*) and end-systole (*bottom row*) are shown for the studies at rest, peak pacing, and 10 seconds after pacing was stopped. The baseline study revealed inferior wall hypokinesis with a global ejection fraction of 40 percent. At peak atrial pacing to a heart rate of 140, the patient had an abnormal ECG response but experienced no chest pain. However, the left ventricle demonstrates diffuse akinesis of the anterior, apical, and inferior walls with an ejection fraction of 16 percent. In the 10-second post-pacing study, there is still significant hypokinesis of the anterior and inferior walls and the ejection fraction is still depressed below rest at 34 percent but has improved compared to the value in the peak pacing study. (From Tobis, J., Iseri, L., Johnston, W. D., et al.: Determination of the optimal timing for performing digital ventriculography during atrial pacing stress tests in coronary heart disease. Am. J. Cardiol. 56:426, 1985, with permission.)

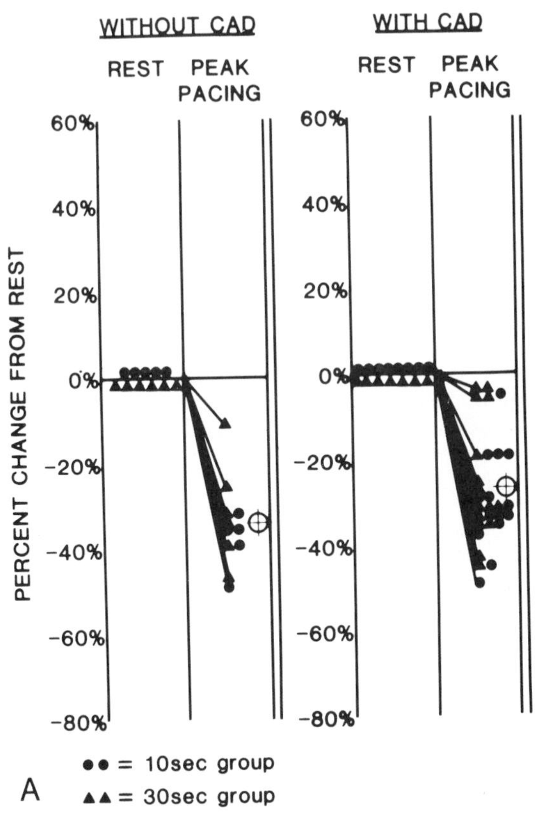

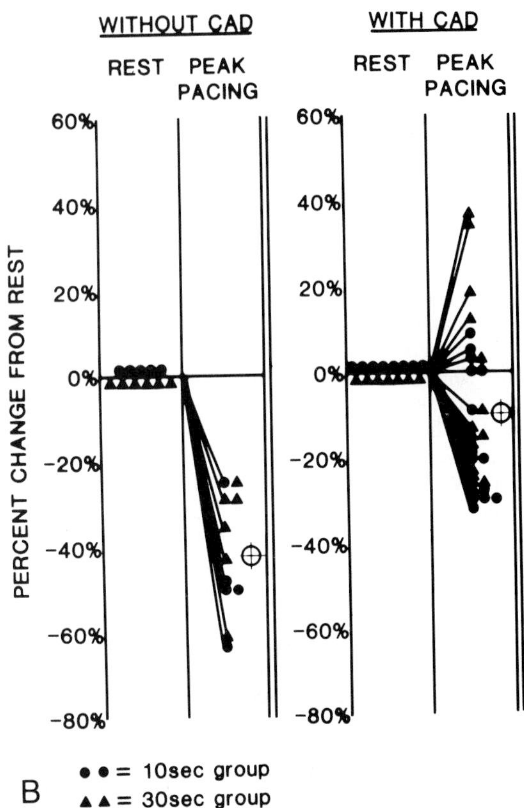

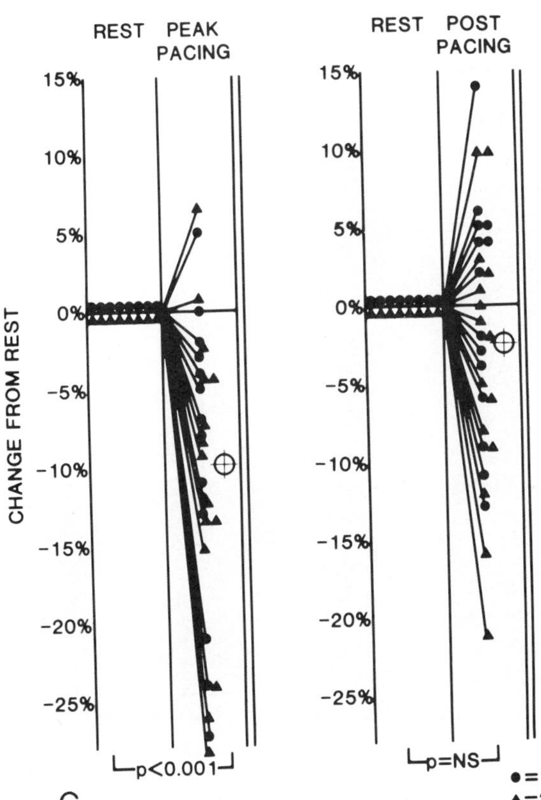

Figure 15–12. The optimal time for performing atrial pacing studies. The three graphs demonstrate the effect of atrial pacing on end-diastolic volume, end-systolic volume, and ejection fraction in patients with coronary artery disease (CAD) and patients with chest pain who did not have significant CAD on angiography. *A*, Percent change in end-diastolic volume from rest to the peak pacing rate for patients without and those with CAD. The circles represent patients who subsequently underwent left ventriculography 10 seconds after pacing, and triangles represent patients who subsequently underwent left ventriculography 30 seconds after pacing. There is no significant difference in the percent decrease in end-diastolic volumes between the patients with CAD and those without CAD. *B*, Percent change in end-systolic volume from rest to peak pacing. There is a significant difference ($p < 0.001$) in the decrease in end-systolic volume between patients without CAD and those with CAD. *C*, Data on ejection fraction (EF) response with patients with CAD. The EF response in the left ventriculogram was measured at the peak pacing rate compared to rest, as demonstrated at the left. At the right are the data for patients who had a third left ventriculogram performed at either 10 seconds or 30 seconds after atrial pacing was stopped. The mean decrease in EF was more pronounced during peak pacing, whereas the mean change in EF during the post-pacing study was not significantly different from the value at rest. This suggests that ischemia induced by atrial pacing is brief and studies should be performed at the peak heart rate.

tion. For patients with obvious critical obstructions, the decision to use angioplasty or bypass surgery is usually straightforward. However, for patients with obstructions in the range of 30 to 80 percent stenosis, at which there is often significant disagreement between observers about the severity of the anatomic narrowing,[D1, D2, D3] the atrial pacing stress test is frequently useful as a discriminating factor. If a large amount of myocardium is at jeopardy and shows a significant wall motion abnormality induced during atrial pacing, it may be preferable to perform revascularization with either angioplasty or bypass surgery. In 44 patients who had angiographic evidence of coronary artery obstructions with more than 50 percent diameter narrowing, the ejection fraction fell more than 2 percent in 38 (86 percent) of the patients.[T10, T11] The change in wall motion was more sensitive than the subjective sensation of chest pain or ECG abnormalities induced during atrial pacing. These findings are similar to those from radionuclide exercise stress tests. It is our current practice to perform an atrial pacing stress test with digital acquisition for patients whose obstruction, at the time of cardiac catheterization, is in the moderate range of 50 to 75 percent stenosis. If there is no drop in ejection fraction or no development of a significant localized wall motion abnormality, our recommendation is to continue with medical therapy and not use an interventional procedure.

Johnson and associates have used another approach in performing atrial pacing studies with first-pass intravenous injections of contrast medium.[J2] They pace the atrium first and then shut the pacemaker off just prior to the levo phase so that the left ventriculograms are obtained at the same heart rate before and after the atrial pacing stimulation. Although intravenous first-pass digital left ventriculograms can be obtained during bicycle exercise or with atrial pacing, these methods have not found wide clinical application because a large-bore intravenous puncture is still required. Moreover, 30 to 40 ml of contrast medium has to be injected rapidly, which causes nausea or emesis in approximately 5 percent of patients. Because of these difficulties, we prefer to perform atrial pacing stress tests with intraventricular injection of a low dose of contrast medium. In this setting, the test is used as an adjunct to the patient's cardiac catheterization and is clinically useful for determining the functional significance of a specific coronary artery stenosis.

Correlation of Minimum Coronary Lumen Diameter with Left Ventricular Functional Impairment Assessed by Digital Angiography

Quantitative analysis with digital processing of angiographic images has been beneficial in understanding the connection between the absolute cross-sectional area of a coronary artery stenosis and the resultant effect of impedance to blood flow on left ventricular function. The severity of coronary artery narrowing is assessed primarily by angiographic determination of the percent of diameter narrowing relative to a portion of the artery that is assumed to be normal. This determination may be misleading for several reasons. Of greatest importance, pathologic studies have demonstrated that atherosclerosis is a diffuse process, so that even when the angiogram demonstrates only a single stenosis, less than 25 percent of the length of the arteries will be free of disease and truly normal.[F1, W2] In addition, stenoses commonly occur at bifurcations, so it may be difficult to identify a normal proximal portion of the same arterial segment. White and associates reported that measurements of percent diameter narrowing correlate very poorly with a physiologic assessment of the severity of stenosis based on the hyperemic flow response

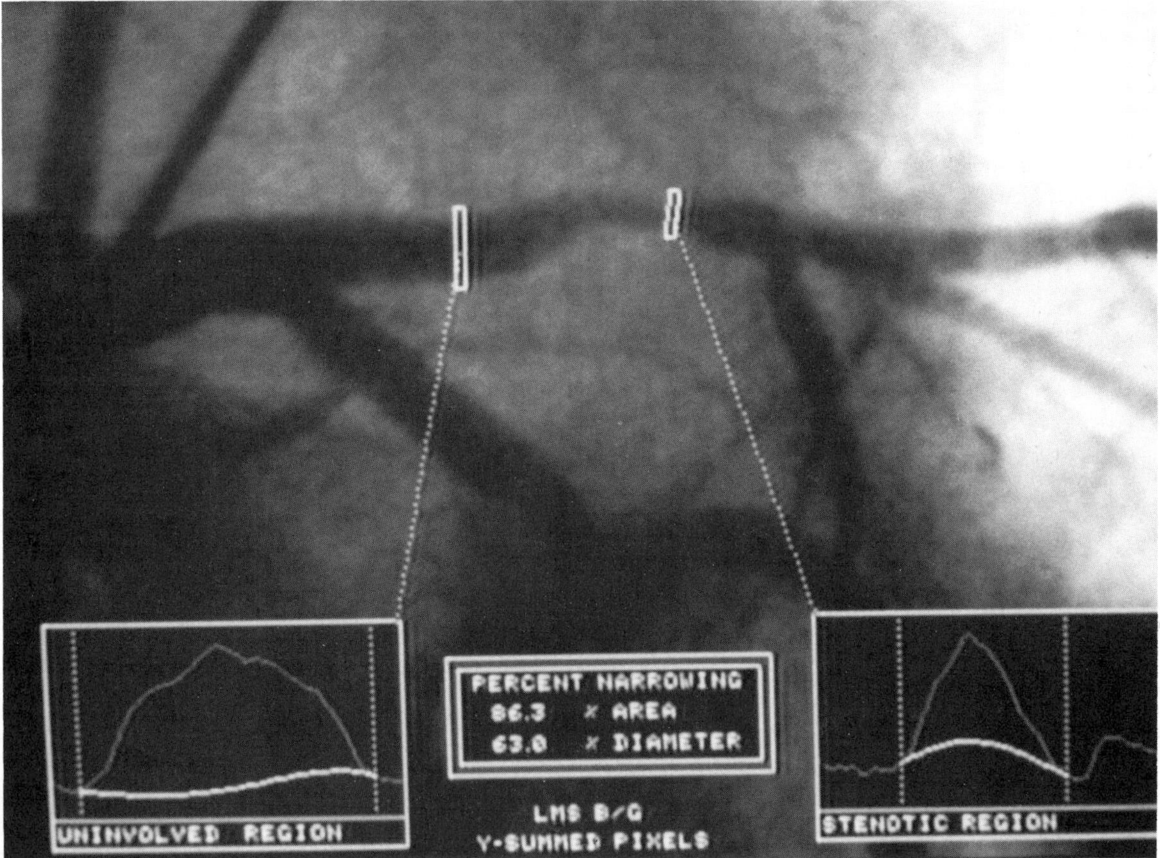

Figure 15–13. Minimum lumen diameter. This digital coronary angiogram of a left coronary artery demonstrates a moderate obstruction. Two regions of interest are defined at the obstruction and at a more proximal segment that is assumed normal. Because the image is already in a computerized format, the density of contrast medium within the lumen is calculated and plotted with the y axis representing relative density and the x axis corresponding to a 50-pixel-wide segment perpendicular to the long axis of the artery. The densitometric boundary of the artery is then chosen, and the percent area stenosis is calculated.

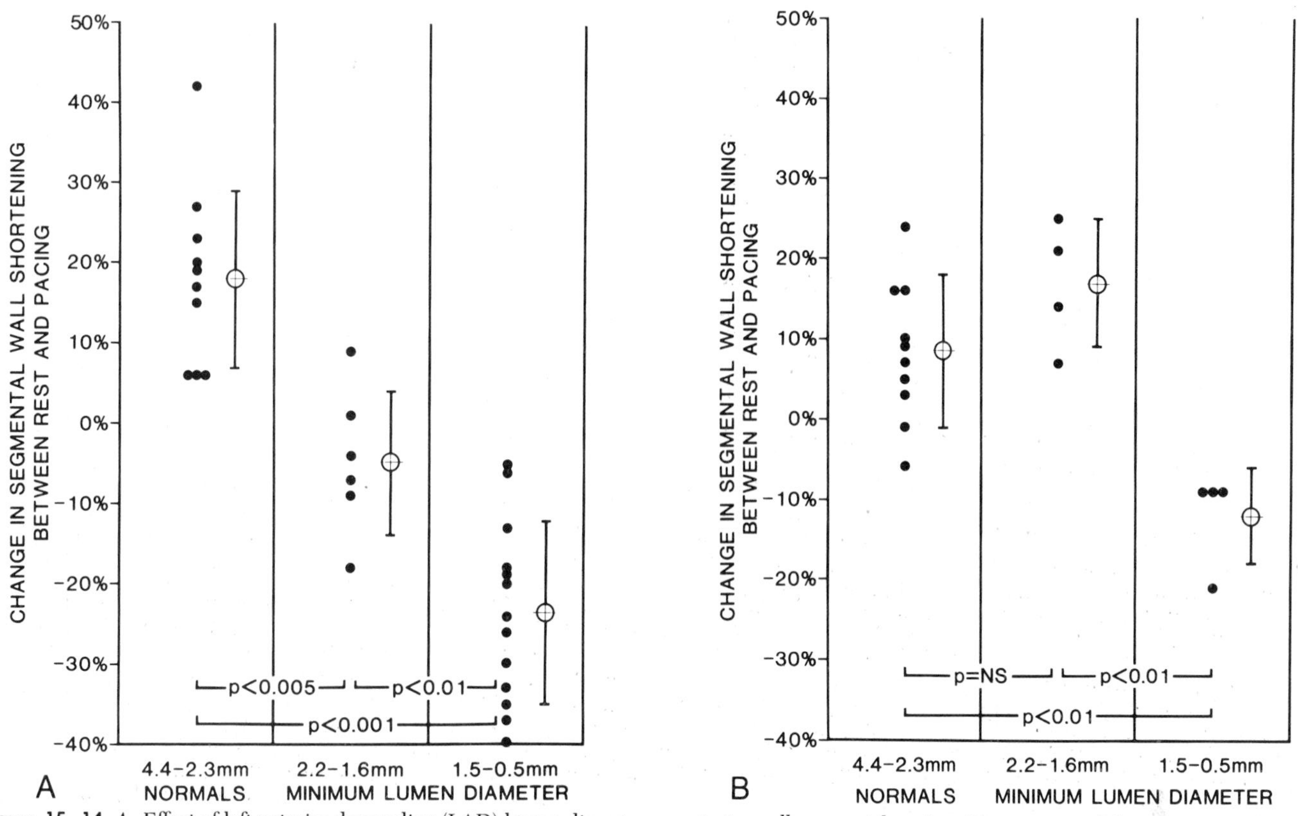

Figure 15–14. *A*, Effect of left anterior descending (LAD) lumen diameter on anterior wall segmental motion. The severity of the stenoses in the LAD artery demonstrated a progressively impaired response to atrial pacing as measured by the change in segmental anterior wall shortening. The group of patients with a minimal lumen diameter of 1.5 mm or less had a more severe functional response to stress induced by atrial pacing. *B*, Effect of right coronary artery (RCA) lumen diameter on diaphragmatic wall segmental motion. The RCA stenoses appeared to have a higher threshold than the LAD stenoses for demonstrating a functional impairment to atrial pacing by a reduction in segmental wall motion. Only stenoses of 1.5 mm or less had a significant response to atrial pacing.

following temporary coronary occlusion during open-heart surgery.[W3] Legrand and co-workers found a similar poor correlation between measurements of percent stenosis and coronary blood flow reserve as measured by digital flow maps following a hyperemic stimulus.[L1]

In trying to develop a better method for determining the functional significance of a stenosis, it is first necessary to be able to measure the stenosis accurately. One of the major advantages of digital acquisition of coronary angiograms is that the computerized format permits rapid quantitative determination of coronary stenosis. The operator can use computer graphics to outline the boundary of a coronary stenosis and quickly calculate the percent diameter narrowing. A second method of measuring stenotic segments uses a videodensitometric approach.[S4] In the densitometric method, the operator chooses a region of interest over a nonstenotic segment and a second region over the stenosis.[T3] Exact boundary detection is not necessary, since the computer subtracts background information and determines the relative density of contrast material between the two areas. Studies with phantom models suggest that the densitometric technique is independent of the eccentric or irregular geometries often found in atherosclerotic lesions. The densitometric analysis can be used with the edge detection method following calibration for magnification to derive the absolute minimum lumen diameter in terms of millimeters of a coronary stenosis (Fig. 15–13). This can be achieved densitometrically even if the boundary of the lesion is too small to be measured accurately with boundary detection methods.

Since digital coronary angiograms can readily provide measurements of stenosis in terms of percent narrowing or absolute cross-sectional area and minimum lumen diameter, the next step was to determine which measurement is more accurate for reporting stenoses. Measurements of percent stenosis and absolute minimum lumen diameter were analyzed to determine which was the better predictor of the functional significance of a specific narrowing, as reflected by the degree of dysfunction in left ventricular wall motion induced during the ischemic stress of atrial pacing. In a study of 27 patients with coronary artery disease, the effect of atrial pacing on segmental radial wall motion was analyzed and compared with the two methods of measurement of severity of stenosis.[T12] Percent diameter narrowing correlated with segmental wall motion with a coefficient of $r = -0.44$, but minimum lumen diameter correlated much more closely, with $r = 0.78$ ($p < 0.05$). The better correlation suggests that the absolute lumen diameter more accurately predicts the functional impairment induced by pacing because the absolute diameter is more directly related to the resistance of blood flow than is percent narrowing.

With regard to the amount of narrowing, the data from this study indicated that when a proximal epicardial coronary artery is narrowed to a diameter of less than 1.5 mm, a functional impairment induced by atrial pacing is more likely to occur in the myocardium supplied by the narrowed artery. If the artery was narrowed to less than 1.5 mm in diameter, there was a greater chance of having abnormal findings with both global ejection fraction and segmental wall motion. Thus, a minimum lumen diameter of less than 1.5 mm may be useful as a predictor of which patients will be symptomatic during stress (Fig. 15–14).

Digital angiographic acquisition has matured and is currently accepted as a useful adjunct in performing cardiac catheterization. The enhancement of contrast and the facility of performing quantitative analysis of both ventricular and coronary images provide additional means of optimizing these invasive diagnostic and therapeutic studies. As computer development improves, digital image processing will become faster and have better resolution and contrast definition. The immediate replay capabilities make digital angiography a welcome accessory in the interventional cardiology laboratory of today. The future for digital angiography is promising, as improvements in computers will be applied in the computerized catheterization laboratory of tomorrow.

References

B

1. Brennecke, R., Brown, T. K., and Bursch, J.: Digital processing of videoangiocardiographic image series using a minicomputer. Proceedings, Computers in Cardiology. IEEE Computer Society, Long Beach, California, 1976, p. 255.
2. Bursch, J. H., Heintzen, P. H., and Simon, R.: Videodensitometric studies by a new method of quantitating the amount of contrast medium. Eur. J. Cardiol. I:437, 1974.

D

1. Detre, K. M., Wright, E., Murphy, M. L., and Takaro, T.: Observer agreement in evaluating coronary angiograms. Circulation 52:979, 1975.
2. DeRouen, T. A., Murray, J. A., and Owen, W.: Variability in the analysis of coronary arteriograms. Circulation 55:324, 1977.
3. Dabestani, A., Johnston, W., Tobis, J. M., et al.: Relation between Doppler transmitral diastolic flow and left ventricular filling. J. Am. Coll. Cardiol. 3:612, 1984.

E

1. Engels, P. H. C., Ludwig, J. W., and Verhoeven, L. A. J.: Left ventricle evaluation by digital video subtraction angiography. Radiology 144:471, 1982.

F

1. Feldman, R. I., Nichols, W. W., Pepine, C. J., et al.: The coronary hemodynamics of left main branch coronary stenoses: The effects of reduction in stenosis diameter, stenosis length, and number of stenoses. J. Thorac. Cardiovasc. Surg. 77:377, 1979.

G

1. Goldberg, H. L., Borer, J. S., Moses, J. W., et al.: Digital subtraction intravenous left ventricular angiography: Comparison with conventional intraventricular angiography. J. Am. Coll. Cardiol. 1:858, 1983.
2. Goldberg, H. L., Moses, J. W., Borer, J. S., et al.: Exercise left ventriculography utilizing intravenous digital angiography. J. Am. Coll. Cardiol. 2:1092, 1983.

H

1. Heintzen, P. H., Brennecke, R., and Bursch, J. H.: Digital cardiovascular radiology. *In* Hohne, K. H. (ed.): Digital Image Processing in Medicine. Springer-Verlag, Berlin, 1981, p. 1.
2. Higgins, C. B., Norris, S. L., Gerber, K. H., et al.: Quantitation of left ventricular dimensions and function by digital video subtraction angiography. Radiology 144:461, 1982.

J

1. Johnston, W. D., Tobis, J. M., Seibert, J. A., et al.: A videodensitometric method for computing right ventricular ejection fraction from intravenous digital subtraction angiograms. (Abstract.) Circulation 66(Suppl. II):II-61, 1982.
2. Johnson, R. A., Wasserman, A. G., Leiboff, R. H., et al.: Intravenous digital left ventriculography at rest and with atrial pacing as a screening procedure for coronary artery disease. J. Am. Coll. Cardiol. 2:905, 1983.

K

1. Kruger, R. A., Mistretta, C. A., Houk, T. L., et al.: Computerized fluoroscopy techniques for intravenous study of cardiac chamber dynamics. Invest. Radiol. 14:279, 1979.
2. Kruger, R. A., Mistretta, C. A., Houk, T. L., et al.: Computer fluoroscopy in real time for noninvasive visualization of the cardiovascular system. Radiology 130:49, 1979.
3. Kronenberg, M. W., Price, R. R., Smith, C. W., et al.: Evaluation of left ventricular performance using digital subtraction angiography. Am. J. Cardiol. 51:837, 1983.

L

1. Legrand, V., Mancini, G. B. J., Bates, E. R., et al.: Comparative study of coronary flow reserve, coronary anatomy and results of radionuclide exercise tests in patients with coronary artery disease. J. Am. Coll. Cardiol. 8:1022, 1986.

M

1. Mistretta, C. A., and Crummy, A. B.: Diagnosis of cardiovascular disease by digital subtraction angiography. Science 214:761, 1981.
2. Mancini, G. B. J., and Higgins, C. B.: Digital subtraction angiography: A review of cardiac applications. Prog. Cardiovasc. Dis. 18:111, 1985.
3. Mistretta, C. A., Ort, M. G., Cameron, J. R., et al.: Multiple images subtraction technique for enhancing low contrast periodic objects. Invest. Radiol. 8:43, 1973.
4. Mancini, G. B. J., and Higgins, C. B.: Quantitative assessment of global and regional left ventricular function with low-contrast dose digital subtraction ventriculography. Chest 87:598, 1985.
5. Molloi, S., and Mistretta, C.: Quantification techniques for dual-energy cardiac imaging. Med. Phys. 16:209, 1989.
6. Mancini, G. B. J., Peterson, K. L., Gregoratos, G., et al.: Effects of atrial pacing in global and regional left ventricular function in coronary heart disease assessed by digital intravenous ventriculography. Am. J. Cardiol. 53:456, 1984.

N

1. Norris, S. L., Slutsky, R. A., Mancini, J., et al.: Comparison of digital intravenous ventriculography with direct left ventriculography for quantitation of left ventricular volumes and ejection fractions. Am. J. Cardiol. 51:1399, 1983.
2. Nissen, S. E., Booth, D., Waters, J., et al.: Evaluation of left ventricular contractile pattern by intravenous digital subtraction ventriculography: Comparison with cineangiography and assessment of interobserver variability. Am. J. Cardiol. 52:1293, 1983.
3. Nichols, A. B., Martin, E. C., Fles, T. P., et al.: Validation of the angiographic accuracy of digital left ventriculography. Am. J. Cardiol. 51:224, 1983.
4. Nalcioglu, O., Seibert, J. A., Roeck, W. W., et al.: Comparison of digital subtraction video densitometry and area length method in determination of left ventricular ejection fraction. SPIE J. 314:294, 1981.
5. Nissen, S. E., Waters, J., and Booth, D.: Determination of left ventricular ejection fraction by videodensitometry of intravenous digital subtraction angiograms: Experimental validation and initial clinical results. (Abstract.) J. Am. Coll. Cardiol. 1:617, 1983.
6. Nalcioglu, O., Seibert, J. A., and Roeck, W. W.: The requirements for and capabilities of x-ray video systems to provide quantitative information. SPIE J. 318:445, 1982.
7. Nalcioglu, O., Seibert, J. A., Boone, J. M., et al.: The effect of physical problems on the determination of ventricular ejection fraction by videodensiometry. *In* Heintzen, P. H., and Brennecke, R. (eds.): Digital Imaging in Cardiovascular Radiology. George Thieme Verlag, Stuttgart/New York, 1983, p. 104.
8. Nissen, S. E., Friedman, B., Waters, J., et al.: Right ventricular ejection fraction by videodensitometry of intravenous digital subtraction angiograms: Experimental validation and initial clinical results. (Abstract.) J. Am. Coll. Cardiol. 3:589, 1984.

S

1. Sasayama, S., Nonogi, H., Kawai, C., et al.: Automated method for left ventricular volume measurement by cineventriculography with minimal doses of contrast medium. Am. J. Cardiol. 48:746, 1981.
2. Spiller, P., Deetjen, W., Jehle, J., et al.: Quantitative evaluation of left ventricular function by digital subtraction and radionuclide angiocardiography at rest and during exercise. A comparison of both methods. (Abstract.) Circulation 68(Suppl. III):III-41, 1983.
3. Sanmarco, M. E., Brooks, S. H., and Blankenhorn, D. H.: Reproducibility of a consensus panel in the interpretation of coronary angiograms. Am. Heart J. 96:430, 1978.
4. Sandor, T., Als, A. V., and Paulin, S.: Cine-densitometric measurement of coronary arterial stenoses. Cathet. Cardiovasc. Diagn. 5:229, 1979.

T

1. Tobis, J. M., Nalcioglu, O., and Henry, W. L.: Digital angiography: The implementation of computer technology for cardiovascular imaging. Prog. Cardiovasc. Dis. 18:195, 1985.
2. Tobis, J., Nalcioglu, O., Iseri, L., et al.: Detection and quantitation of coronary artery stenoses from digital subtraction angiograms compared with 35mm film cine-angiograms. Am. J. Cardiol. 54:489, 1984.
3. Tobis, J., Nalcioglu, O., Johnston, W. D., et al.: Videodensitometric determination of minimum coronary artery luminal diameter before and after angioplasty. Am. J. Cardiol. 59:38, 1987.
4. Tobis, J., Johnston, W. D., Montelli, S., et al.: Digital coronary roadmapping as an aid for performing coronary angioplasty. Am. J. Cardiol. 56:237, 1985.
5. Tobis, J. M., Nalcioglu, O., Johnston, W. D., et al.: Left ventricular imaging with digital subtraction angiography using intravenous contrast injection and fluoroscopic exposure levels. Am. Heart J. 104:20, 1982.
6. Tobis, J., Nalcioglu, O., Johnston, W. D., et al.: Correlation of 10ml digital subtraction angiography compared with standard cineangiograms. Am. Heart J. 105:946, 1983.
7. Tobis, J., Nalcioglu, O., Seibert, J. A., et al.: Measurement of left ventricular ejection fraction by videodensitometric analysis of digital subtraction angiograms. Am. J. Cardiol. 52:871, 1983.

8. Tobis, J., Nalcioglu, O., Johnston, W. D., et al.: Exercise digital subtraction angiograms in patients with coronary artery disease. (Abstract.) Circulation 66(Suppl. II):II-229, 1982.
9. Tobis, J., Nalcioglu, O., Johnston, W. D., et al.: Digital angiography in assessment of ventricular function and wall motion during pacing in patients with coronary artery disease. Am. J. Cardiol. 51:668, 1983.
10. Tobis, J., Iseri, L., Johnston, W. D., et al.: Determination of the optimal timing for performing digital ventriculography during atrial pacing stress tests in coronary heart disease. Am. J. Cardiol. 56:426, 1985.
11. Tobis, J., Sato, D., Nalcioglu, O., et al.: Correlation of minimum lumen diameter with left ventricular functional impairment induced by atrial pacing. Am. J. Cardiol. 61:697, 1988.
12. Trenholm, B. G., Winter, D. A., Mymin, D., and Lansdown, E. L.: Computer determination of left ventricular volume using videodensitometry. Med. Biol. Eng. Comput. 10:163, 1972.

V

1. Vas, R., Diamond, G. A., Levisman, J. A., et al.: Computer enhanced digital angiography: Correlation of clinical assessment of left ventricular ejection fraction and regional wall motion. Am. Heart J. 104:732, 1982.

W

1. Widmann, T. F., Ashburn, W. L., Higgins, C. B. J., and Peterson, K. L.: Assessment of left ventricular wall motion by regional phase analysis of digital intravenous contrast fluoroangiography. Comput. Cardiol. IEEE:105–108, 1982.
2. Waller, B. F., and Roberts, W. C.: Amount of narrowing by atherosclerotic plaque in 44 nonbypassed and 52 bypassed major epicardial coronary arteries in 32 necropsy patients who died within 1 month of aortocoronary bypass grafting. Am. J. Cardiol. 46:956, 1980.
3. White, C. W., Creighton, B. W., Doty, D. B., et al.: Does visual interpretation of the coronary arteriogram predict the physiologic importance of a coronary stenosis? N. Engl. J. Med. 310:819, 1985.

Y

1. Yianakis, J., Simpfendorfer, C., Detrano, R., et al.: Stress digital subtraction angiography to assess presence of coronary artery disease in patients without myocardial infarction. (Abstract.) Circulation 68(Suppl. III):III-41, 1983.

Chapter 16

Applications of Digital Angiography to the Coronary Circulation

G.B. JOHN MANCINI, M.D.

INTRODUCTION AND HISTORICAL PERSPECTIVE 310
ANATOMIC ASSESSMENT OF THE CORONARY CIRCULATION 312
Coronary Arteries 312
Digital Fluoroscopy 312
Intravenous Angiography 312
Aortic Root Angiography 312
Direct Angiography 313
Bypass Grafts 324
Intravenous Angiography 324
Aortic Root Angiography 325
Direct Angiography 325
FUNCTIONAL ASSESSMENT OF THE CORONARY CIRCULATION 325
Methodology 325
Transit-Time Analysis 325
Indicator-Dilution Analysis 328
Contrast Washout Analysis 329
Impulse Response (Transfer Function) Analysis 331
Appearance Time and Density Analysis 334
General Comparative Summary 335
Achieving Maximal Hyperemia in the Clinical Setting 338
Physiologic Assessment of Coronary Artery Disease 339
Physiologic Assessment of Bypass Grafts 339
CONCLUSIONS 339

INTRODUCTION AND HISTORICAL PERSPECTIVE

Comprehensive evaluation of the coronary circulation ideally should include assessments of both anatomic and physiologic parameters. The exquisite temporal and spatial detail of film-based arteriography and the longitudinal images that it provides justify the technology's position as the best for evaluation of the anatomic aspects of coronary disease. However, it has long beeen recognized that subjective evaluation of coronary disease is marred by substantive intra- and interobserver variability[D2, 3, F4, G1, S4, Z2] and lack of correlation with postmortem findings.[G7, I3, V2] Although it is arguable whether or not these deficiencies have truly detracted from the value of film-based arteriography in helping clinicians tailor care for the majority of patients,[P1] there can be no question that such variability precludes the use of subjective evaluation of arteriograms in studies designed to evaluate new therapeutic methods or for documenting the effects of existing therapies. Moreover, since there is evidence demonstrating a lack of correlation between subjective arteriography and physiologic assessments of coronary disease, it is anticipated that more rigorous, reproducible, and quantitative analyses may be of substantive value in refining and documenting the delivery of cardiac care, particularly when mild or moderate stenoses are being evaluated.[L10, W2] At the very least, quantitative arteriography ensures that clinicians are using the same yardstick with which to evaluate angiograms and make therapeutic decisions.

Numerous early attempts at coronary quantification deserve review in order to put the digital approach discussed in this chapter into perspective. MacAlpin and associates[M1] and Feldman and colleagues[F1, 3] used hand-held calipers to make direct measurements of projected arteriographic coronary images and of a calibrating object to quantify cineangiograms. Feldman and colleagues further refined their technique by combining high quality 105-mm photospot arteriographic images with a magnifying vernier for quantification.[F2] Gensini and associates extended this film-based approach by using a viewing telescope that projects cross-hairs into the images.[G2] Rafflenbeul and associates used a vernier and image magnification for assessing coronary cineangiograms.[R1]

Brown and co-workers developed a method based on hand-tracings of film images magnified up to five times.[B14, 15] Orthogonal views are used to account for the irregular morphology of most lesions. These tracings are then subjected to computer-assisted coronary quantification that incorporates compensation for pincushion distortion and differential magnification and assumes an elliptic geometry of the lesions. The method of Brown and co-workers calculates the theoretic resistance to be expected at differing rates of coronary flow. This is of great importance as an initial attempt to try to span the gap between morphology and function. To overcome the use of subjective hand-tracing of arteriograms inherent in the Brown methodology, several more automated approaches have been developed.[L3, 7, M7, R6, S1, 15, 19] These methods automatically assess the abrupt gradients in optical density found at the edges of the vessels. These changes are analyzed to provide an automatically determined estimate of the location of the true edge. A further application of this concept is the use of the optical density information inherent in the luminal image as a representation of the volume of contrast within the arterial lumen and the volume of the arterial segment itself, since the densitometric profile is a function of luminal area, independent of its cross-sectional shape or its borders.[C2, H7, J1, K3, 6, N2, S2, 3] The latter is particularly attractive in the setting of angioplasty and thrombolysis, because lesions with intimal tears and clots are difficult to analyze solely by edge-based methods. The two approaches, however, are not mutually exclusive, and several investigators have combined the videodensity approach with the edge-detection approach for analysis of films.[C2]

Although all the film-based methods are extremely useful and accurate, they are not generally utilized in clinical practice because they are laborious and time-consuming. The initial delay in implementation is due to the need to develop the film. For the methods based on densitometry, meticulous calibration of the exposure and development process is needed to ensure that the gray scale corresponds linearly to known concentrations of contrast medium. Consequently, the only commonly employed quantitative approach in clinical practice is the use of hand-held calipers and rulers for the calculation of percent diameter stenosis. Although better than no quantitation at all, even this simple method can be cumbersome and variable, and it can be employed only after the films are developed, not during the course of catheterization when decisions regarding angioplasty, thrombolysis, or surgical intervention may be required.

The aforementioned method of Brown and associates was one of the first to relate morphologic measures to predictions of the actual functional impairment that a stenosis might produce. Such approaches have been further enhanced by other groups[K2] so that theoretic measures of coronary flow reserve, an index of the functional or physiologic significance of a stenosis, can be estimated more meticulously. Such calculations of coronary flow reserve take into account many morphologic features of a stenosis, such as length, entrance and exit angles, and absolute and relative cross-sectional areas (Fig. 16–1). Numerous circumstances, however, complicate the relation between morphologic measures of stenoses and the actual functional impairment that they produce. In the component analysis model proposed by Kirkeeide and colleagues, some of these factors are held constant (perfusion pressure, filling pressures, viscosity, and so on) and others are ignored (myocardial mass, collateral flow, and so on).[K2] These simplifications allow for lesion-to-lesion and patient-to-patient comparisons and replace the gradations from 0 to 100 percent diameter stenosis with a scale of 1 to 5 units of theoretic coronary flow reserve. However, since such predictions must necessarily be only approximations of the true functional importance of a lesion, other methods have been explored to assess coronary flow dynamics more directly from the angiogram.

Rutishauser and co-workers[R18, 19] and Smith and co-workers[S16, 17] were the first to investigate the use of cineangiograms for the measurement of coronary flow dynamics. By combining measures of length and diameter of proximal, noncircuitous arterial segments with videodensitometric measures of contrast media transit time, a calculation of epicardial blood flow was possible. Further, Spiller and co-workers more recently have used the same concept, together with high frame-rate cineangiography and timed power injection of contrast, to determine phasic coronary flow.[S20] Foerster and associates, instead of trying to measure absolute flow, proposed to measure relative coronary flow or coronary flow reserve with a less technically demanding approach employing radiographic arterial videodensitometry, independent of length and diameter measurements.[F5, 6] Robb and associates demonstrated the value of background subtraction for visualization of low concentrations of contrast material, especially in the coronary microcirculation.[R14]

These pioneering efforts provided the impetus and rationale for fuller computerization of x-ray cardiac imaging and automation of the intense image processing and computational requirements inherent in the comprehensive assessment of coronary artery and bypass graft morphology and function. With fuller integration of these processes in commercially available digital image processing units, the clinician, not just the investigator, has begun to gain greater and more routine access to complete anatomic and

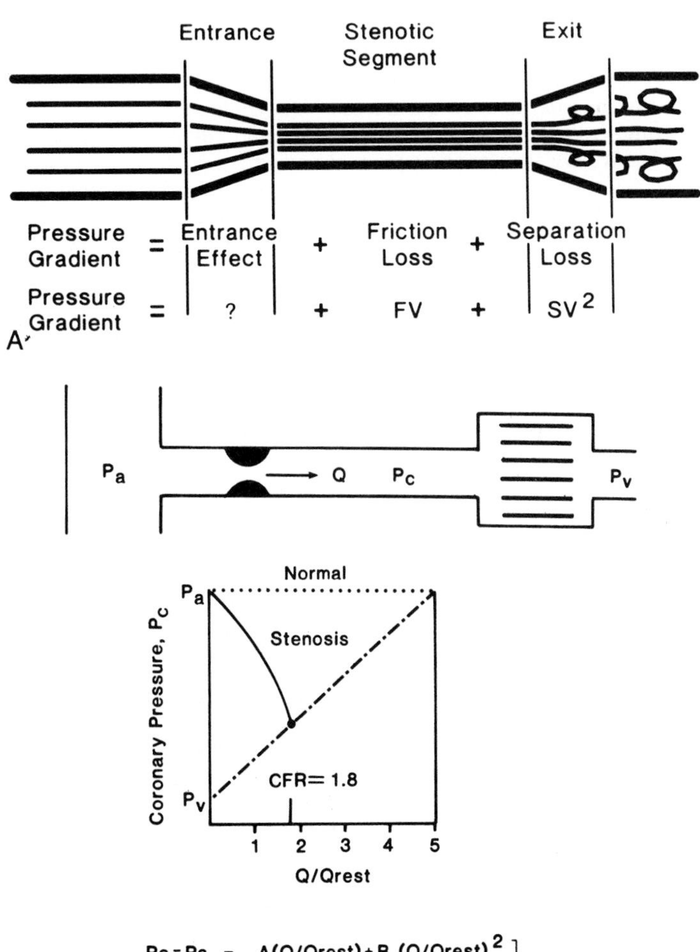

Figure 16–1. *A*, Sources of energy loss across a stenosis result from the entrance effects, friction losses in the stenotic segment, and separation losses at the exit of the stenosis. The pressure gradient generated by these factors can be predicted by mathematical equations. Entrance effects are ignored, and frictional losses (F) contribute directly as velocity (V) and exit effects due to separation losses (S) increase with the square of blood velocity. (From Marcus, M.L.: The Coronary Circulation in Health and Disease. McGraw-Hill, New York, 1988, p. 248, with permission.)
B, Under a given set of prevailing hemodynamic conditions, a theoretic calculation of coronary flow reserve (CFR) can be made. This value provides an integrated evaluation of all important geometric characteristics of a stenosis. The schematic of a stenotic coronary artery and distal bed is shown. Aortic pressure (P_a), coronary flow (Q), distal coronary perfusion pressure (P_c), and effective coronary back pressure (P_v) are represented. In the graph, P_c is plotted on the vertical axis, and coronary artery flow is plotted on the horizontal axis as a ratio to normal flow at rest (Q/Q_{rest}). The dash and dot line is used to plot the relationship between coronary perfusion pressure and coronary flow under conditions of maximal coronary vasodilatation in the presence of a stenosis. The solid line is used to plot the relationship between P_c and flow in the presence of a stenosis; this relationship is expressed by the equation at the bottom of the figure. (From Kirkeeide, R.L., et al.: Assessment of coronary stenoses by myocardial perfusion imaging during pharmacologic coronary vasodilation. VII. Validation of coronary flow reserve as a single integrated functional measure of stenosis severity reflecting all its geometric dimensions. J. Am. Coll. Cardiol. 7:103, 1986, with permission.)

functional analyses within the cardiac catheterization laboratory. This chapter summarizes the role of digital angiography in this process.

ANATOMIC ASSESSMENT OF THE CORONARY CIRCULATION

Coronary Arteries

Digital Fluoroscopy

An innovative application, not requiring catheterization or contrast injection, is the use of digital subtraction fluoroscopy for detecting coronary calcifications as a screening test for the presence of significant underlying coronary disease. Detrano and coworkers studied 191 subjects without history or electrocardiographic evidence of previous myocardial infarction, who were referred for coronary arteriography with both conventional and digital subtraction fluoroscopy.[D5] Subtraction was used to enhance the visibility of coronary calcium. Higher overall accuracy was achieved with the digital fluoroscopy technique than with regular fluoroscopy in predicting the presence of percent diameter stenoses greater than 50 percent, especially in younger patients.

Intravenous Angiography

Much of the initial clinical enthusiasm for the technology of digital angiography came from the prospect of imaging the coronary arteries by an intravenous contrast injection. The ability to provide sufficient anatomic detail in a familiar format that would be useful in following either progression or regression of disease or in determining the advisability of angioplasty or surgery by a relatively noninvasive means would have had tremendous impact on the clinical practice of cardiology. This very intriguing and important application of intravenous digital angiography has not yet been successfully achieved, for reasons recently elucidated by Mistretta and co-workers.[M10–12, P3, T7] The obstacles to successful achievement of this goal are formidable. Overlying iodinated pulmonary and cardiac structures obscure the contrast, which has undergone dilution by up to 20-fold, in the coronaries. There is a large dynamic range of x-ray transmission between lung fields and cardiac structures, leading to severe cross-scatter, image intensifier glare, increased television camera noise, and diminution in image contrast. Vessel motion and motion of noniodinated structures also detract from coronary visualization. Even high-pass temporal filtration techniques, dual energy subtraction, and hybrid subtraction have not provided practical solutions to these problems.[B13, R10–13, T7]

The largest clinical elucidation of the problems of intravenous digital angiography for coronary imaging is provided by Haggman and Detrano and co-workers from the Cleveland Clinic.[D4, H1] These investigators used a 30-degree right anterior oblique view and studied ideal thin candidates. Even so, they were not uniformly successful in obtaining diagnostic images. The technique provided information primarily involving proximal coronary artery disease segments and did not adequately detect distally located disease. The method appeared to be better in asssessing the right coronary artery than the left anterior descending artery even though the latter was seen in most patients as well. The circumflex artery was extremely difficult to image and only 84 percent of the studies demonstrated the left main trunk.

It is unlikely that intravenous digital coronary angiography using specialized processing of images generated by conventional x-rays will develop into a practical and widespread application, even for screening purposes. Synchrotron x-ray generation and energy subtraction techniques may rekindle this effort,[A1] but radiation doses are currently very high. Whether the use of cine-computed tomography or dynamic nuclear magnetic resonance imaging will provide images of sufficient anatomic detail and in a format usable by cardiologists and surgeons (i.e., longitudinal images of the coronaries and not just cross-sectional views) is also unknown, but much greater effort is being focused on these technologies for noninvasive coronary imaging than on digital angiography.

Aortic Root Angiography

Prior to the development of either selective angiography or digital angiography, several investigators examined the utility of aortic root angiography for visualization of the coronary arteries.[B7, N5, P2] Impressive film images were demonstrable provided several procedural details were observed. These details included the following: the Valsalva maneuver was necessary to slow aortic root outflow and washout of contrast; specially designed catheters with single or double coils perpendicular to the catheter shaft were needed to enhance delivery of contrast to the coronary ostia; and high flow rates of contrast were needed. Digital enhancement techniques were expected to alleviate some of these technical demands with respect to specialized catheters and volume of contrast. Clinical applications, however, generally have not demonstrated sufficiently detailed images, especially when these technical details are ignored.

Goldberg and colleagues were able to identify 18 of 20 stenoses with pulsed, high-energy fluoroscopic aortography; two lesions of 50 percent diameter stenosis were missed.[G3] Low-energy fluoroscopy identified only 15 of the lesions. Ross and colleagues used 5- to 20-ml of contrast injected into the aortic root to determine the ability to detect proximal coronary stenoses after digital enhancement.[R16] Additionally, they investigated whether delayed distal contrast arrival time and inappropriately poor opacification of a major artery could be used as ancillary evidence of significant coronary disease. Patients were studied using two views and time interval difference imaging. In 10 normal patients, one study was technically inadequate, and 7 of the remaining 9 (78 percent) were correctly classified as normal by analysis of the digital images. Of 13 patients with greater than 75 percent proximal stenosis, one study was technically inadequate, and 11 of 12 (92 percent) patients were felt to have at least one stenosis of this severity. Sensitivity for specific stenoses was 80 percent when all image criteria were considered. Discrimination of single from multivessel disease was much less accurate, demonstrating agreement between digital aortic root angiography and standard coronary angiography in only 8 of 13 patients (62 percent). The investigators concluded that improved catheter technology would be required to enhance delivery of contrast before such techniques would be useful in screening patients suspected of having coronary disease. Lassar and co-workers studied 41 patients by standard selective arteriography and by injecting 40 ml of half-strength ionic contrast at 20 ml per second via a supravalvular ring catheter.[L2] Density-gated mask-mode subtraction was utilized. They concluded that this procedure was a clinically adequate substitute for selective coronary arteriography in adequately visualizing all segments of native vessels, but optimization required using at least two views. Other centers have underscored the need for specialized aortic root catheters in increasing the yield of diagnostic images by this technique.[W4]

This particular technique has never been intended as a replacement for standard arteriography. However, since most of the studies have been performed in a traditional catheterization laboratory setting by cardiologists, it is obviously compelling to be less than satisfied with the diminished detail of aortic root angiography once arterial invasion has already occurred and to proceed, therefore, with selective direct angiography using much smaller doses of contrast. This accounts for much of the lack of enthusiasm for the potential role of this technique as an adjunctive screening test and the lack of large-scale comparative studies to assess this specific role. In this regard, comparison of this method to exercise testing with or without nuclear imaging, for example, would be more appropriate than comparisons of anatomic detail. It can be argued that high accuracy is not necessary for a screening technique applied in an outpatient setting or in noncardiac catheterization laboratories if the test results are going to be used only to gauge whether selective angiography by a cardiologist is going to be needed. There may be a definite role for this technique when the patient is already undergoing other vascular angiography, such as carotid or aortic angiography. A simple and rapid screening test performed by the radiologist may provide compelling evidence for the cardiologist that would justify subsequent coronary angiography. Such decisions are required frequently in a consultative practice and are often based on nonexercise stress test results, such as dypridamole thallium imaging. The demonstration of high-grade lesions with digital aortic root angiography might diminish the need for other noninvasive testing.

Direct Angiography

Digital angiography has a definite and important role in the morphologic quantitation of coronary stenoses and in facilitating interventional procedures. As outlined earlier, it is the only method that is rapid enough and simple enough to be acceptable in a clinical milieu. This section focuses on digitally based methods, since the film methods are described and discussed in detail elsewhere.

Roadmapping

The application that is most utilized and least technically demanding is that of "roadmapping" during percutaneous transluminal coronary angioplasty.[B10, T4, W6] In this application, a mask-mode subtracted image of the coronary artery is interlaced with the live fluoroscopic video image. The superimposition of the two allows greater confidence and ease in directing the guide wire and positioning the balloon.

Quantitative Arteriography

DEVELOPMENT OF METHODS. An exciting contribution of digital angiography is the ability to perform accurate, sophisticated, and rapid coronary quantification during the course of a procedure. The method developed at the University of Michigan is typical of digitally based methods and will be described in detail. The program determines the center line of an arterial segment within a region of interest by analyzing circular pixel density profiles of decreasing radii. Simple signal processing techniques are used to locate the angular positions of the proximal and distal portions of the arterial segment at each radius. Linear density profiles perpendicular to the arterial center line are extracted over the entire length of the arterial segment. Initial edge points are found by noting the density of points at the first and second derivatives of each perpendicular density profile and then determining the location of the points, which fall at a value of 75 percent of the difference between the densities at these derivative extrema (i.e., weighted toward the first derivative extrema) (Fig. 16–2). This method was found to give the best accuracy and precision of measurement of radiographic phantoms in the 0.5- to 5-mm diameter range.[L4] These initial gradient-determined edge points are then examined for spatial continuity, and outliers are discarded. The gray scale densities of initial edge points are then used to determine final edge points, using local thresholding. The set of accepted threshold densities for either edge (independently) is smoothed, and any threshold values discarded during the first pass are replaced by linear interpolation from neighboring valid edge points. Each perpendicular profile is reanalyzed, and the location of final edge points is determined using this locally adaptive threshold method. The geometric diameter at any point along the center line is the distance along each perpendicular profile between edge points on opposite sides of the artery. Calibration is achieved by measuring a magnification factor based on the known size of the angiographic catheter. Calibrations are obtained from nonsubtracted images. The catheter in subtracted images is not used for calibration because of the nearly routine occurrence of spatial misregistration. The computer program determines videodensitometric cross-sectional area at each point along the center line by integrating the densities across the perpendicular profile from edge to edge. Background corrections are made by subtracting a linearly interpolated background determined by the density values at the edge points. The final computer output consists of the arterial image with arterial edges and center line, plots of geometric diameter (calibrated with reference to the known diameter of the angiographic catheter), densitometric relative cross-sectional area, maximal percent diameter stenosis, and maximal area (densitometric) percent stenosis (Fig. 16–3). Approximately 1 minute is required to complete the analysis of each view of a single lesion.

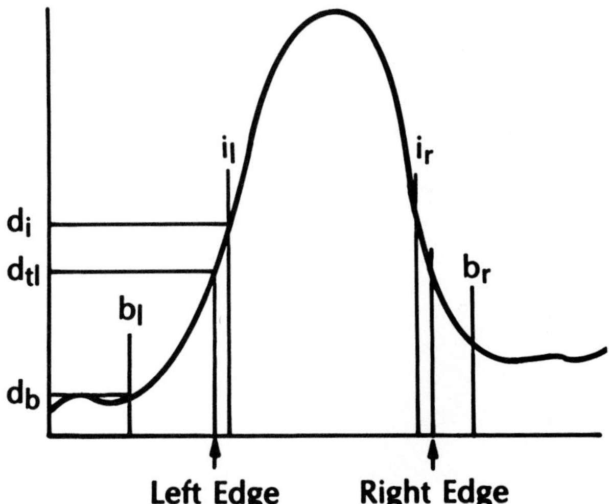

Figure 16–2. An idealized arterial cross-sectional densitometric image is illustrated with designation of the location of the first and second derivatives. In general, the first derivative location (d_i) provides an edge location that is too "tight," and the second derivative location (d_b) is often too "loose." Therefore, a weighted combination of these two locations (d_{tl}) is used to determine the initial approximation of the arterial edge. i, inflection; b, base; l, left; r, right.

Angiograms are acquired on a digital angiographic computer interfaced to a standard cineangiographic system. The radiographic input signal is kept constant (fixed kVp, mA, and pulse width x-ray exposure). A 12.5-cm field of view and a small focal spot size (0.6 mm, nominal) are used. Images are acquired at a minimum of 10 frames per second, and up to 30 frames per second in a 512 × 512 matrix with 256 gray levels. Images undergo logarithmic look-up transformation to account for Lambert-Beer exponential x-ray absorption. Care is taken to ensure that both the stenotic area and the angiographic catheter are within the central portion of the radiographic field in order to minimize any possible effects of pincushion distortion. Alternatively, a geometric image transformation that removes pincushion distortion can be used.[L3, T2]

The digital images can be processed and analyzed both with and without mask subtraction. The single mask frame and the image best demonstrating the stenosis are selected to minimize any misregistration artifacts in the region of the stenosis. R-wave gated cyclic mask-mode subtraction facilitates this process. Subtracted and nonsubtracted digital images undergo gray scale inversion to produce white-on-black pictures comparable with the gray scale of negative film images. All images are subjected to gray scale modifications to linearly expand their individual scene dynamic range and fill the full 8-bit dynamic range of the digital radiographic system. This preprocessing step is fully automated. All directly acquired digital images are then digitally magnified by a factor of 4. This was achieved by bilinear pixel interpolation using the system's array processor. Although this digital magnification does not improve the density of the spatial sampling of the electronic imaging methods, it does enhance precision. This magnification was experimentally determined to optimize the quantitative analyses. The analyzed effective pixel resolution is thus 2048 × 2048 for on-line digital images.

VALIDATION OF METHODS. Morphologic Considerations. The software was evaluated in phantoms and in vivo conditions for the measurement of minimal diameter stenosis. Phantom validation studies were performed using a precision-drilled Plexiglas plate with seven arterial models of "lesions" varying from

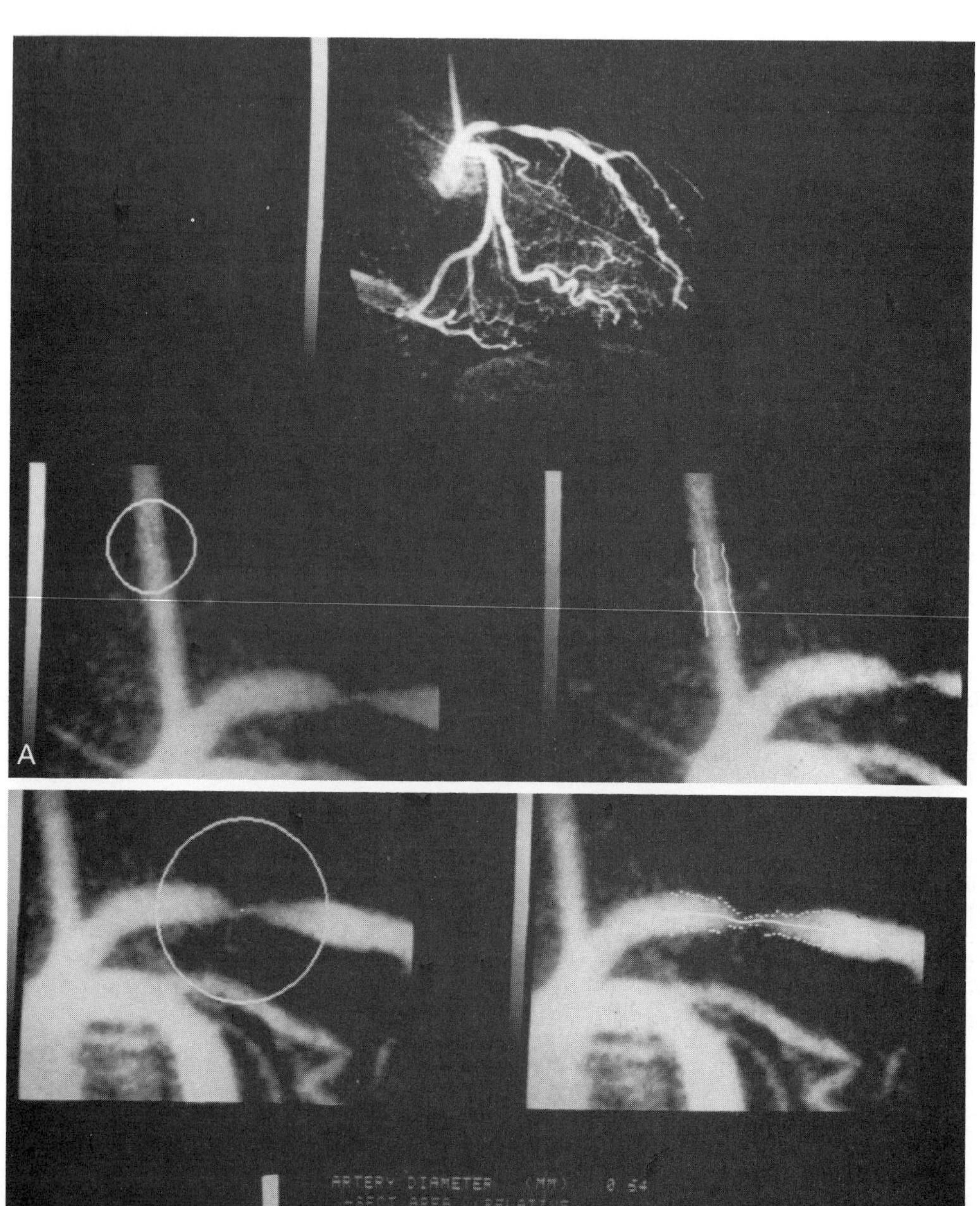

Figure 16–3. *A*, A clinical arteriogram illustrates the steps required for quantitative assessment. The initial frame, showing catheter and lesion in a central portion of the image, is magnified in the area of the catheter, and edge detection is performed to determine a calibration factor. *B*, The lesion to be quantitated is then magnified and automatic edge detection follows. The quantitative report at the bottom yields both geometric and videodensitometric results for single-plane analysis. Biplane analyses can also be performed.

0.5- to 3.0-mm diameter and proximal/distal lumina varying from 1.0- to 5.0-mm diameter.[L4–6] Using digital images of this phantom, highly accurate measurements were obtained. Slopes of the regressions were not different from 1.00. Correlation coefficients were not less than 0.998. Standard errors of the estimates (SEEs) were 0.135 mm for diameter measurements, 10.4 percent for percent diameter stenosis measurements, and 2.19 percent for percent area stenosis measurements (Fig. 16–4). The 10.4 percent standard error in percent diameter stenosis measurements was due to inclusion of "stenoses" with lumina of less than 1.0 mm that were overestimated, as anticipated, and this was at least partially due to the integration and averaging of diameter results over long lengths of the phantom.

The second phase of phantom validation involved a comparison of the accuracy of quantitation of the same phantom using both digital images (512 × 512 and 1024 × 1024) and analyses of digitized cineangiograms (effective pixel resolution of 1024 × 1024).[L5] The experiment demonstrated that the edge-detection algorithm could be applied to digitized film and still provide extremely accurate results in the measurement of absolute diameter (standard error of 0.189 mm, r = 0.992) and percent diameter stenosis (standard error of 13.4 percent, r = 0.776) (Fig. 16–5). Again, the latter results incorporate the effects of the anticipated overestimation of lumina that are less than 1.0 mm.

In vivo validation was in the form of a unique experiment.[M7] Animals were instrumented with intracoronary plastic "stenosis beads" with precision-drilled lumina ranging from 0.83 mm to 1.83 mm. This very small luminal range is uncommon in most other studies but is more consistent with the clinical range in which significant stenoses are likely to reside. Thus, the a priori characteristic of the sizes to be measured biased the study tremendously toward finding poor results. The second important feature is that the animals were imaged in a closed-chest preparation and the heart was beating—conditions that would also bias the experiment toward poor results (Fig. 16–6).

The study design also provided an opportunity to assess the effects of mask subtraction even in the absence of gross misregistration artifacts. Figure 16–7 shows the comparison of the measured minimal diameter as assessed by the automated technique and the known lumen diameters. A high correlation was

Table 16–1. REGRESSION RESULTS FOR ANALYSES OF DIFFERENT IMAGE MODALITIES IN DETERMINING MINIMAL DIAMETER

Image	r Value	Slope	y Intercept	SEE (mm)	p Value
Nonsubtracted	0.98	0.98	−0.02	0.09[a]	0.001
Subtracted	0.98	0.95	−0.01	0.09[a]	0.001
Film	0.87	0.97	−0.13	0.24	0.001

SEE—Standard error of the estimate in millimeters; [a]—$p < 0.03$ vs. SEE of film analysis.

From Mancini, G.B.J., et al.: Automated quantitative coronary arteriography: Morphologic and physiologic validation in vivo of a rapid digital angiographic method. Circulation 75:452, 1987, with permission of the American Heart Association, Inc.

obtained for both the subtracted and nonsubtracted on-line digital acquisitions. Automated analysis of film acquisitions showed a poorer overall correlation and almost a tripling of the standard error of the estimate. Table 16–1 summarizes the full regression results. Statistical analyses showed no significant differences among modalities with regard to slope, intercept, and r values. The standard error of the estimate was significantly greater with the use of film ($p < 0.03$ compared with subtracted and unsubtracted images).

Table 16–2 shows the results of inter- and intraobserver variability in measurement of the minimal stenosis diameter and geometric cross-sectional areas. All r values ranged from 0.90 to 0.97, with the best results occurring in nonsubtracted, on-line digital images (r = 0.97, SEE = 0.12 mm). No statistical differences were noted in r values, slopes, intercepts, or standard errors of the diameter measurements. However, in both the intra- and interobserver analyses, the standard errors of the estimate for cross-sectional area measurements were greater for the film analyses than for the nonsubtracted on-line digital image results (intraobserver variability: 0.56 mm^2 for film vs. 0.20 mm^2 for nonsubtracted images, $p < 0.02$; interobserver results: 0.50 mm^2 for film vs. 0.15 mm^2 for nonsubtracted images, $p < 0.005$). Although the standard error of the estimate for cross-sectional

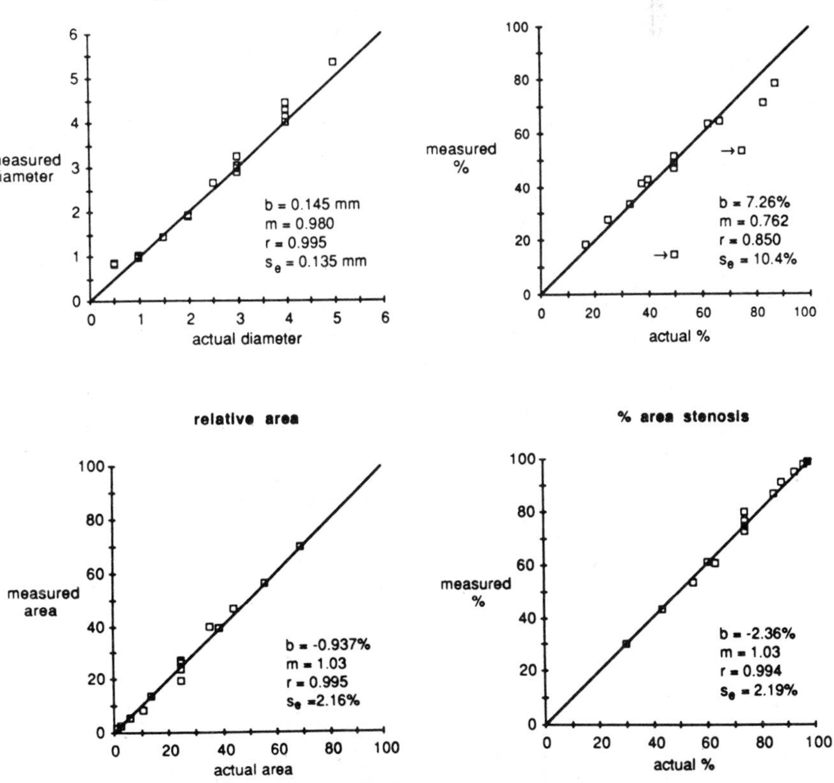

Figure 16–4. The results of linear regression analysis of measured versus actual geometric diameter, percent diameter stenosis, videodensitometric cross-sectional area, and percent area stenosis. The values shown are the y intercept (b), the slope (m), the coefficient of correlation (r), and the standard error of the estimate (s_e). (From LeFree, M.T., et al.: Digital radiographic coronary artery quantitation. *In* Proceedings of the IEEE Computer Society: Computers in Cardiology. IEEE Computer Society, Long Beach, CA, 1981, p. 99, with permission.)

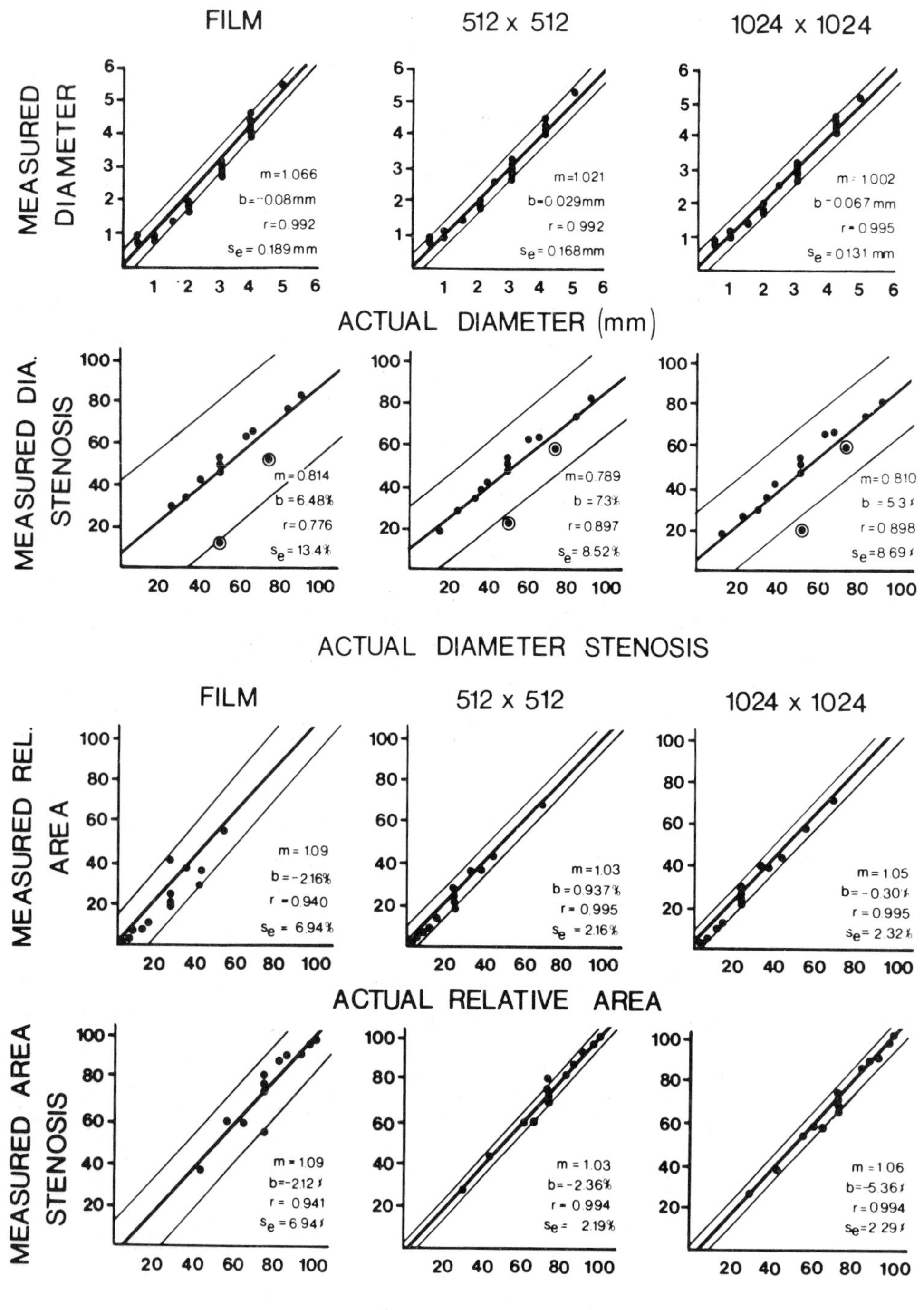

Figure 16–5. Geometric diameter and percent diameter stenosis, as well as densitometric relative cross-sectional area and percent area stenosis, linear regression results for cine film, 512 × 512 and 1024 × 1024 digital radiography. The regression lines are displayed along with 95 percent tolerance limits. Values shown are the y intercept (b), the regression slope (m), the coefficient of correlation (r), and the standard error of the estimate (s_e). (From LeFree, M.T., et al.: Quantitative coronary arteriography. *In* Mancini, G.B.J. (ed.): Clinical Applications of Cardiac Digital Angiography. Raven Press, New York, 1988, p. 219, with permission.)

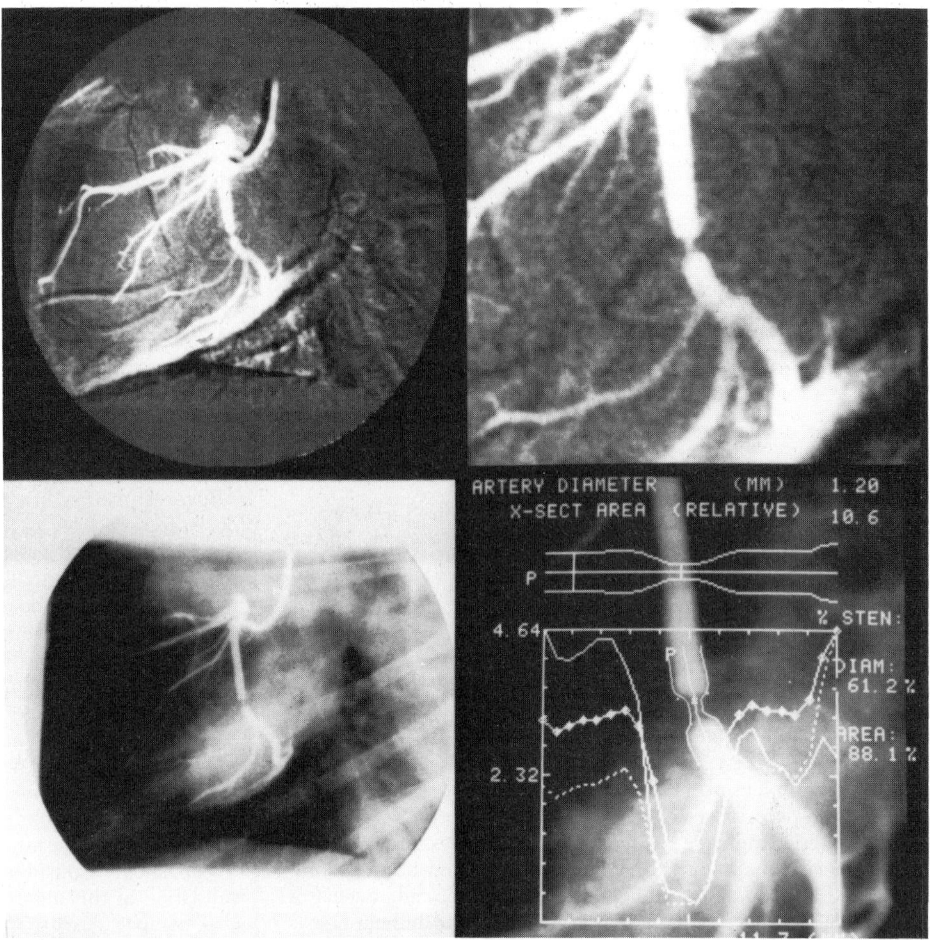

Figure 16–6. Images from a study in which a stenosing cylinder was placed in the circumflex artery of a dog. The *upper* and *lower panels* show the subtracted and nonsubtracted images, respectively. The *right-hand panels* show the magnified views. The *lower right-hand panel* shows the screen overlay with the quantitative variables, stylized arterial segment, and the plots of geometric diameter *(diamonds)*, densitometric relative cross-sectional area *(solid line)*, and the approximation of cross-sectional area as calculated from the geometric diameter data, with the assumption of the circular cross section *(dashed line)*. The automatically determined edge is shown on this image. (From Mancini, G.B.J., et al.: Automated quantitative coronary arteriography: Morphologic and physiologic validation in vivo of a rapid digital angiographic method. Circulation 75:452, 1987, with permission of the American Heart Association, Inc.)

area was smaller for the subtracted compared with film images, this difference was not statistically significant.

Another recent study shows that the results noted in the animal validation study appear also to be evident in analysis of clinical images by this technique.[M4] In consecutive, unselected patients, lesions were measured from images obtained in pairs after nitroglycerin dilatation, by film and on-line digital imaging. The latter were assessed in the subtracted and nonsubtracted modes. The on-line digital method was slightly superior to film with regard to reproducibility. Nonsubtracted images were superior to subtracted images. This study also demonstrated that power injection of contrast produced more reproducible images than hand injection.

Clinical validation was also undertaken in a population of patients undergoing angioplasty. Thirteen consecutive angiograms acquired in orthogonal views before and after angioplasty

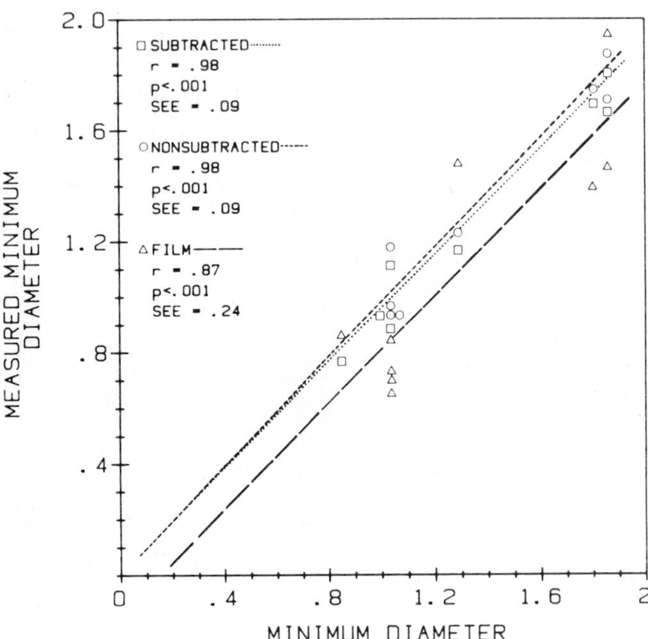

Figure 16–7. Regression analyses between known and measured stenosis diameters (in millimeters) from subtracted *(squares)*, nonsubtracted *(circles)*, and film *(diamonds)* images. Lines represent regression lines for each imaging technique. SEE—standard error of the estimate in millimeters. (From Mancini, G.B.J., et al.: Automated quantitative coronary arteriography: Morphologic and physiologic validation in vivo of a rapid digital angiographic method. Circulation 75:452, 1987, with permission of the American Heart Association, Inc.)

Table 16–2. RESULTS OF INTRA- AND INTEROBSERVER VARIABILITY ANALYSES

		Nonsubtracted (n = 8)	Subtracted (n = 8)	Film (n = 9)
Intraobserver	r	0.97	0.90	0.92
	SEE	0.12 mm	0.21 mm	0.23 mm
		0.20 mm^2	0.29 mm^2	0.56 mm^{2a}
	p	<0.0001	<0.003	<0.0005
Interobserver	r	0.97	0.90	0.92
	SEE	0.12 mm	0.19 mm	0.21 mm
		0.15 mm^2	0.25 mm^2	0.50 mm^{2b}
	p	<0.0001	<0.003	<0.0006

SEE—Standard error of the estimate. ^{a}—$p < 0.02$; ^{b}—$p < 0.005$ for film vs. nonsubtracted results.

(From Mancini, G.B.J., et al.: Automated quantitative coronary arteriography: Morphologic and physiologic validation in vivo of a rapid digital angiographic method. Circulation 75:452, 1987, with permission of the American Heart Association, Inc.)

were analyzed with the same algorithm (Fig. 16–8). Measures of absolute diameter stenosis were most reproducible from observer to observer, both before and after angioplasty. The overall observer variability was 0.19 mm, with a value of 0.16 mm before angioplasty and 0.23 mm after angioplasty. The interobserver variability for measurements of percent diameter stenosis was between 9.5 percent and 10.5 percent. The intraobserver variability for measuring percent diameter stenosis was 8.5 percent.[S5]

This specific method also has been validated in other laboratories and under different conditions. Skelton and associates assessed 39 coronary segments of excised dog and human hearts and compared the digital image quantitations with pathologic sections.[S14] This study used a coronary catheter as the calibration object. Correlations ranged between 0.85 and 0.91, and standard errors ranged from 0.23 to 0.27 mm (Fig. 16–9). Rosenberg and co-workers assessed the accuracy of the method in determining minimum diameter stenoses of excised, human coronary stenoses.[R15] The combined first and second derivative approach was found to be superior to algorithms using only the first derivative of the arterial density profile to determine edge points. Correlations of actual pathologic measurements and values calculated from digital images were excellent for both minimal and maximal stenotic diameters. This was an extremely rigorous test of the algorithm due to the complex asymmetric and eccentric nature of the stenoses studied and the limited views used to assess them.

The accuracy of the absolute measurements heavily depends on the reliability of the calibration system used. The angiographic catheter is generally used for this purpose, in preference to more elaborate methods that are more difficult to implement clinically. Inaccuracies of this approach have been shown to arise from several factors, including catheter material, manufacturing variabilities in lumen size, and the differential magnification that occurs when the stenosis and the catheter tip are at different distances from the x-ray source.[B14, R7, 8] Nevertheless, this remains the most convenient approach, and the results from our own study and others suggest that it yields values of sufficient accuracy. When an appropriate calibration is not available, only relative measures of stenosis severity are feasible.

Overestimation of diameters less than 1 mm has been previously reported for several automated techniques.[B14, L6, S3, 19] The diameters studied in our own investigation ranged from 0.71 to 1.83 mm, and the smallest diameter imaged successfully was 0.83 mm.[M7] The regression analyses did not suggest overestimation of sizes within this range. Figure 16–7 and Table 16–1 show regression slopes that were actually less than 1. It is postulated that this was due to measurement of only the minimal stenosis diameter, not average diameters over the entire length of the stenosis.[L4–6] Phenomena such as lack of sharpness due to motion, limited spatial resolution, oblique orientation of the vessel with respect to the x-ray beam, and geometric magnification would all lead to over-, not underestimation, thus providing the rationale for focusing on the minimal stenosis diameter.

Physiologic Considerations. One of the unique aspects in the validation of this algorithm is that the morphologic results were also compared with independent physiologic measures of the functional significance of stenoses.[M7]

Figures 16–10 and 16–11 show the relations between percent diameter stenosis and reactive hyperemia, and percent area (videodensitometric) stenosis and reactive hyperemia, respectively. All image modalities were highly correlated with the measured reactive hyperemia, and no significant differences were noted among the different methods. Moreover, no significant differences in the precision of correlation with reactive hyperemia was found between percent area and percent diameter measurements. All methods showed *r* values between 0.78 and 0.85.

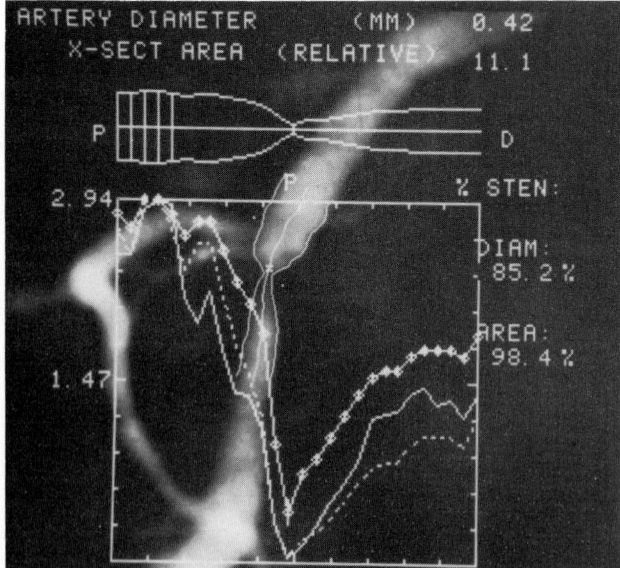

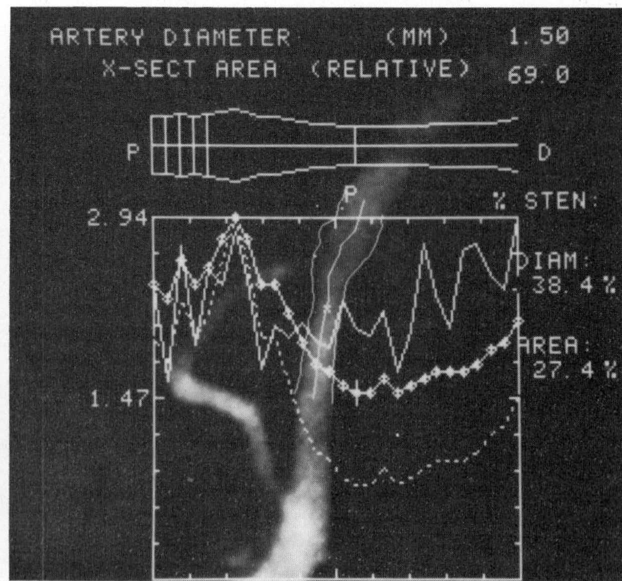

Figure 16–8. Automated digital analysis of coronary arterial stenosis before *(left)* and after *(right)* angioplasty. (From Bates, E.R., and Mancini, G.B.J.: Digital radiographic assessment of coronary angioplasty and bypass graft revascularization results. *In* Mancini, G.B.J. (ed.): Cardiac Applications of Digital Angiography. Raven Press, New York, 1988, p. 291, with permission.)

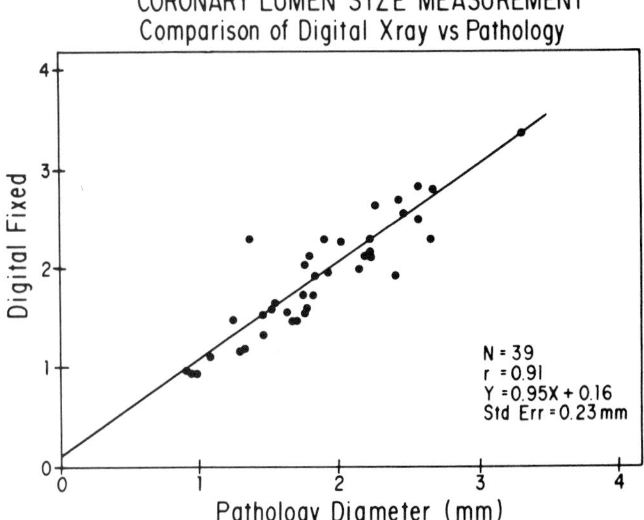

Figure 16–9. Comparison of diameter measurements from digital images of coronary segments after casting and fixation with diameter measurements from pathologic sections. The linear regression and correlation results are shown. (From Skelton, T.N., et al.: Accuracy of digital angiography for quantitation of normal coronary luminal segments in excised, perfused hearts. Am. J. Cardiol. 59:1261, 1987, with permission.)

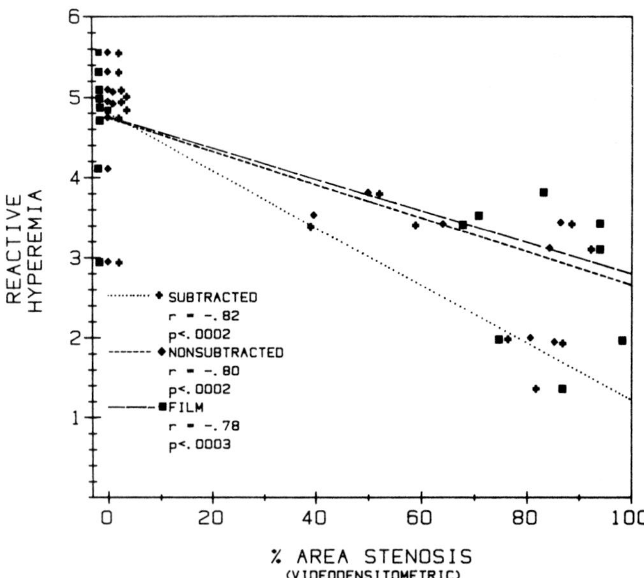

Figure 16–11. Relationship between reactive hyperemia and videodensitometrically determined percent area stenosis. No statistically significant differences in these regressions were found. (From Mancini, G.B.J., et al.: Automated quantitative coronary arteriography: Morphologic and physiologic validation in vivo of a rapid digital angiographic method. Circulation 75:452, 1987, with permission of the American Heart Association, Inc.)

Figures 16–12 and 16–13 show stenotic segment area, measured both geometrically and videodensitometrically, versus reactive hyperemia. As in the prior analyses, all image modalities yielded quantitative parameters that were highly correlated with reactive hyperemia (r = 0.77 to 0.83), and no statistical differences among modalities were noted.

Other investigators, using very accurate coronary quantification of cine images, have shown that quantitative parameters are useful in both reflecting and predicting coronary flow reserve.[H2] Thus, it was important to substantiate that the quantitative analysis of digital coronary angiograms bore some relation to the physiologic importance of the stenoses. As demonstrated in Figures 16–10 through 16–13, this was indeed the case. This establishes the potential usefulness of the automatic, digital program for studies designed to correlate morphologic parameters with physiologic aspects of coronary flow.

COMPARISONS OF DIGITAL AND CINE IMAGES FOR CORONARY QUANTIFICATION. Tobis and co-workers reported a study in which different observers independently identified and measured focal coronary narrowings in using digital subtraction angiograms and standard 35-mm cineangiograms.[T5] The digital angiograms used a 512 × 512 × 8-bit pixel matrix. Due to rapid evolution of digital hardware and software at that time, the study was undertaken in two parts. In Phase 1 of the study, 38 patients (35 with interpretable studies without misregistration artifacts) were studied with continuous fluoroscopic

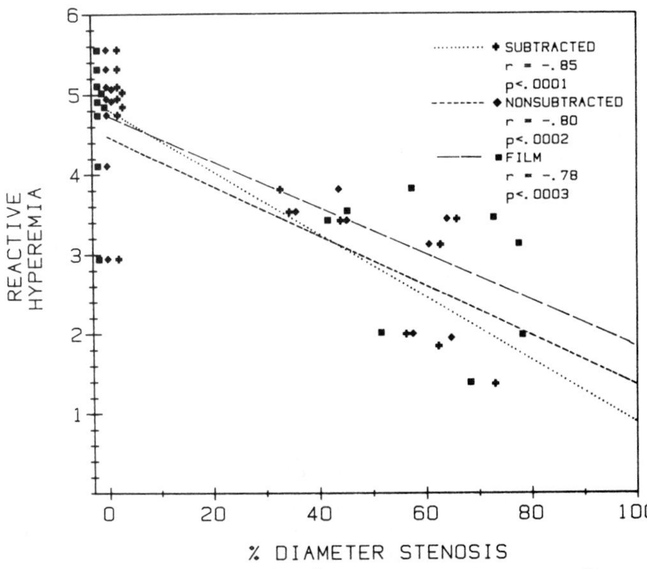

Figure 16–10. Regression analysis between quantitative percent diameter stenosis, determined from each image type, and reactive hyperemia. Regression lines are shown. No significant differences among these analyses were found. (From Mancini, G.B.J., et al.: Automated quantitative coronary arteriography: Morphologic and physiologic validation in vivo of a rapid digital angiographic method. Circulation 75:452, 1987, with permission of the American Heart Association, Inc.)

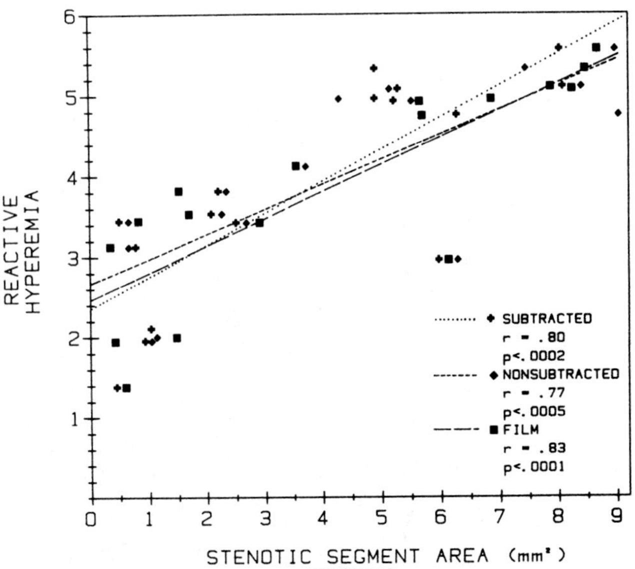

Figure 16–12. Relationship between reactive hyperemia and stenotic segment area. No statistically significant differences among results from different imaging methods were noted. (From Mancini, G.B.J., et al.: Automated quantitative coronary arteriography: Morphologic and physiologic validation in vivo of a rapid digital angiographic method. Circulation 75:452, 1987, with permission of the American Heart Association, Inc.)

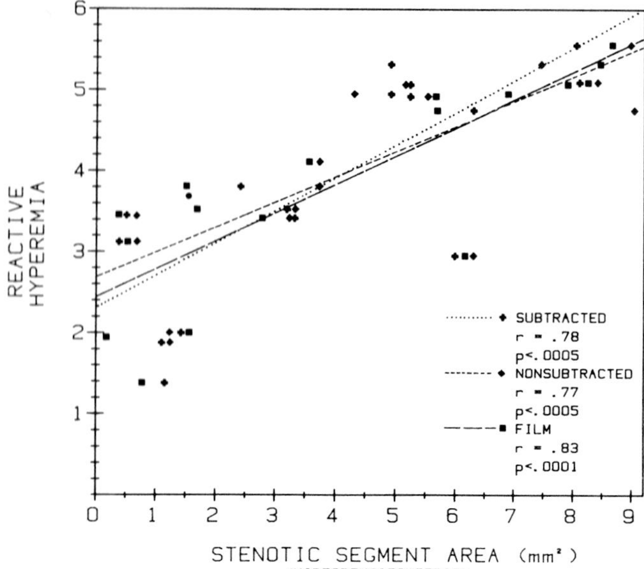

Figure 16–13. Relationship between reactive hyperemia and stenotic segment area determined from a combination of the videodensitometric data and catheter calibration. No statistical differences among the regressions were noted. (From Mancini, G.B.J., et al.: Automated quantitative coronary arteriography: Morphologic and physiologic validation in vivo of a rapid digital angiographic method. Circulation 75:452, 1987, with permission of the American Heart Association, Inc.)

exposures and an interlaced camera readout of 30 frames per second. Images were subjected to subtraction using a blurred mask and then converted back to videotape. Two observers analyzed both these images and the corresponding 35-mm cineangiograms with manually operated calipers. Results within 10 percent were considered equivalent; otherwise, results from the digital images were described as over- or underestimating the cineangiographic results that were used as the reference standard for this study. The results demonstrated that agreement in quantification within 10 percent occurred in 76 percent of cases. Underestimation by the digital technique occurred in 18 percent and overestimation in 6 percent of cases. Although these results were quite favorable, it was felt that the overall quality of film was better, because the image acquisition parameters and processing methods resulted in substantial noise in the video images.

In Phase 2 of this study, 19 patients were studied with more advanced techniques. Pulsed radiographic mode and a progressive scan camera were utilized. In addition, only a single-frame mask was used, and the observers were allowed to use an edge-enhancement algorithm and a 4× magnification algorithm. In this phase, four observers quantified the paired cineangiograms and digital angiograms, again using hand-held calipers. The results showed no significant difference in the mean percent diameter narrowing for all narrowings (53 ± 31 percent vs. 52 ± 31 percent, digital vs. film, respectively). No difference in variability of measurements between the two methods could be detected. In two patients, unsubtracted images were used because of excessive subtraction artifact. It was apparent that even when the digital images were suboptimally processed by older methodologies, including hand-held calipers, the digitally based quantifications compared favorably with the film-based results. This study suggested, however, that at least in some patients misregistration continued to be a problem and that fluoroscopic exposure levels and interlaced camera readout were not optimal for digital applications in coronary quantification.

Bray and co-workers analyzed 32 lesions in 15 patients using the technique of high-pass temporal filtration digital subtraction with a real-time recursive processor and videotape storage and display.[B12] An interlaced camera readout and radiographic exposure levels were utilized. A 480 × 792 × 8-bit image matrix and a framing rate of 30 Hz were used. Standard 35-mm cineangiograms were acquired simultaneously. Three observers using calipers analyzed the image sets, and the overall results demonstrated a correlation coefficient of 0.73 with a standard error of the estimate of 9.1 percent diameter stenosis. The average severity (49 percent for film images and 47 percent for digital images) and the variability of the measurements (average standard deviation for film of 6.6 percent and for digital of 7.7 percent) were indistinguishable. Twenty-eight percent of measurements were more than 10 percent different between methods, and 5 percent were more than 20 percent different. This variability was substantially reduced when multiple observations were averaged and then compared.

The recursive filtration technique utilized by Bray and coworkers has several attractive characteristics. It is relatively economical with dedicated hardware because of minimal image memory requirements; the temporal filtration is automatic, requiring no operator input to select frames for masks; results are seen in real-time without the need for postprocessing; and the subtraction method is more tolerant of patient motion. This latter characteristic is due to the continually updated "moving mask," which is a weighted average of the old mask image and the new input image in a recursive loop. This has the effect of suppressing stationary image structures while the more rapidly moving contrast bolus and cardiac structures are selectively enhanced. The effect of slow respiratory motion, a common cause of misregistration artifact, is partially suppressed. Unfortunately, this methodology is not widely available, and experience with it for coronary quantification is limited. It is anticipated that problems with absolute videodensity measurements may occur owing to temporal differences in background subtraction across the image field. Nevertheless, for routine quantification, this study was unable to demonstrate any striking loss of clinical information when digital imaging was compared with cineangiography. The study also confirms the merits of radiographic exposure levels, and the researchers suggest that progressive camera readout for such applications would improve results further.

Vas and group analyzed 36 coronary stenoses by three methods: visual interpretation of a single cineangiographic image, visual interpretation of a digital angiographic image (512 × 512 × 8-bit matrix, nonenhanced, nonfiltered, and nonmagnified), and quantification using a digital caliper system (2× magnification).[V1] The pixel size ranged from 0.22- to 0.46-mm/pixel in this study. Radiographic exposure levels were used, but the use of progressive or interlaced readout was not mentioned. No differences in the average percent diameter stenosis measurements were found (visual film analysis = 59.1 percent ± 22.7 percent, visual digital analysis = 60.8 ± 25.6 percent, caliper quantification = 55.5 ± 21.3 percent). Overall image quality was judged to be at least as good as the film, and no significant adverse effects on the perception and quantification of stenoses by angiographers were demonstrated. Overall, the digital calipers improved intraobserver and interobserver reproducibility and demonstrated that visual interpretation of both film and digital images overestimated the caliper results, especially in the 50 to 75 percent diameter stenosis range. The mean standard deviations of visual film analysis (12.6 percent) and digital analysis (10.7 percent) were equal but higher than for caliper analysis (3.8 percent). When the four angiographers used the caliper method, they agreed within a 10 percent diameter stenosis on all readings, whereas substantially poorer agreement occurred with visual interpretation irrespective of the type of image. Thus, using an improved electronic caliper method, nonsubtracted images, and radiographic exposure levels, digital images were comparable to film images in providing quantitative information. The value of even relatively crude quantitative methods in reducing intraobserver and interobserver variability was reconfirmed.

Goldberg and associates studied a total of 77 patients with mask-mode, 512 × 512 × 8-bit, 30 frame per second digital angiography using boosted fluoroscopy (i.e., the tube current was between fluoroscopic levels and full radiographic levels and ranged between 10 and 30 mA).[G3] Single views were compared with standard cineangiography in 27 patients (95 arteries). Two angiograms agreed with visual assessment within one grade of severity in 84 percent of cases, including comparisons of normal segments. Multiple-view digital angiograms were compared in 50 patients (144 arteries), and visual agreement within one grade occurred in 90 percent, including normal segments. It should be noted that the film images were acquired using the magnification mode, whereas digital images were acquired in a 9-inch mode so that the entire coronary tree could be seen without panning to avoid misregistration artifact during subtraction. Use of the 9-inch mode has the effect of yielding a larger pixel size in the digital images, but despite this bias against the digital images, the aforementioned comparisons were quite favorable. Moreover, the investigators reported that 95 percent of collateralized vessels noted on film images were also noted on the digital angiograms. The grade of the collateral vessels also agreed in 81 percent of instances with the cine assessment. As in the other studies, misregistration in several cases precluded analysis. Because only boosted fluorography was used, the investigators stated that mask subtraction was mandatory to provide sufficient contrast resolution. One can conclude from this study that, for practical purposes, the visual interpretation of coronary stenoses is quite comparable whether film or digital imaging is used.

Skelton and associates examined the effects of digital image acquisition mode and subtraction techniques on the quantification of coronary stenosis involving 100 discrete lesions in 45 patients.[S13] Each lesion was assessed from direct on-line digital, electrocardiogram-gated digital subtraction and digitized cine film images. Geometric measures of percent diameter stenosis and minimal lesion diameter showed correlations of between 0.90 and 0.98, with slopes of between 0.93 and 1.00 (Figs. 16–14 and 16–15). Thus, the measurements were not strongly affected by image acquisition mode nor by electrocardiogram-gated digital subtraction. These geometrically derived results were superior to similar comparisons using videodensitometric techniques.

Gurley and colleagues recently compared unprocessed digital angiograms and conventional cineangiograms for the diagnosis and quantification of coronary stenoses in both phantoms and clinical subjects.[G9] In contrast to the prior study, this group used unmagnified 512 × 512 digital images and caliper quantification of the stenoses. The effects of image subtraction were not assessed, and absolute minimal diameter measurements were not made. Additionally, the two images were acquired simultaneously, so that 85 percent of the image intensifier light intensity was used to expose film and only 15 percent of the light intensity was used to generate the digital image. Even under these conditions, phantom studies showed no differences in performance betweeen digital and film imaging. In analysis of patient images, the overall interobserver variability was also equivalent. However, the researchers noted that digital evaluation of percent stenosis in patients generally overestimated film results, and that this overestimation was progressively more severe with milder lesions, lesions in vessels of less than 2 mm, and branch stenoses. This study underscores the need for each laboratory to ascertain the equivalence of the two imaging techniques under the specific or likely conditions of use. For the most part, the lack of automated quantification, failure to use image magnification, and diminution in light source for the generation of digital images were strong biases against the digital imaging technique.

The reviewed studies suggest that analyses of digital and film-based coronary angiograms are essentially equivalent when several factors are taken into account. In our experience, subtracted images yield results of equivalent precision but with slightly higher inter- and intraobserver variability even when gross misregistration is not evident. This increase is believed to be due to increased image noise and the potential presence of subtraction artifacts; therefore, this laboratory does not recommend clinical use of subtraction techniques for coronary arteriography. Despite great advances in other aspects of digital imaging, misregistration artifact caused by patient motion remains one of the commonest causes of image degradation, and, therefore, the demonstrated accuracy of nonsubtracted quantitative digital angiography should enhance clinical implementation and acceptability. It is not yet clear whether the techniques outlined by Bray and co-workers[B12] will overcome this problem.

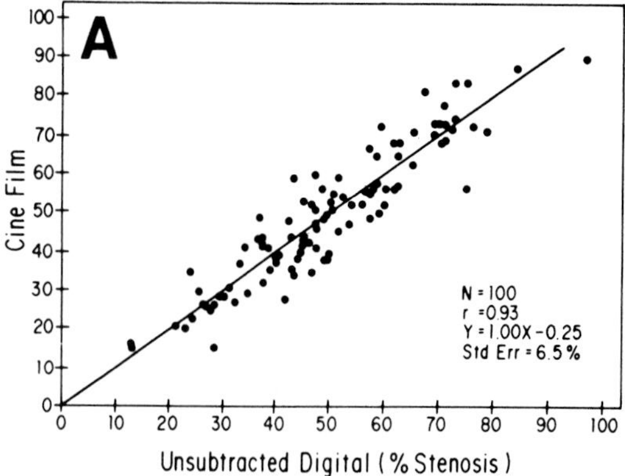

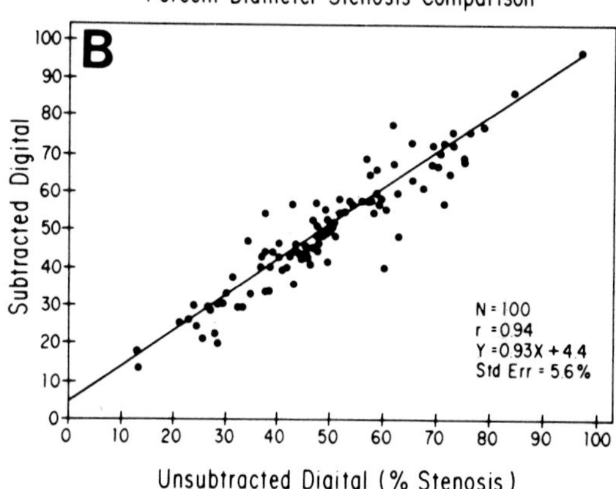

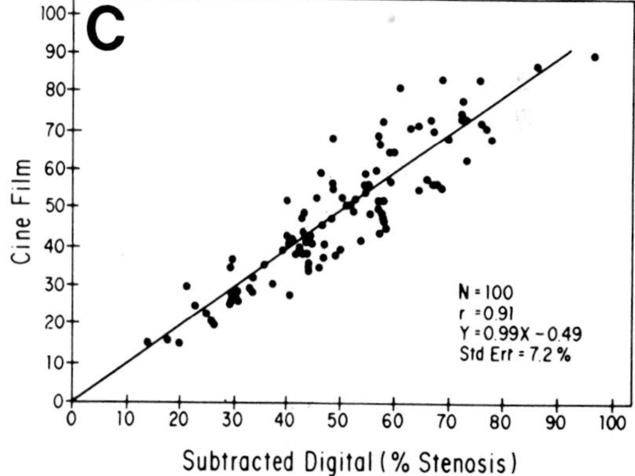

Figure 16–14. Regression analysis for percent diameter stenosis data. *A*, *B*, and *C* each represent a two-way comparison among the three image types. (From Skelton, T.N., et al.: Comparison of coronary stenosis quantitation results from on-line digital and digitized cine film images. Am. J. Cardiol. 62:381, 1988, with permission.)

Although film-based radiography has a very high theoretic resolution, numerous factors prevent attainment of this in clinical circumstances. The difference in attenuation coefficients between iodinated contrast medium and tissues is not great and may perturb edge detection in areas with significant variations in background density. The usual measurement of the resolving power of a system by using tungsten wires or lead strips does not truly reflect the much poorer object contrast in coronary angiograms. Moreover, the usable spatial resolution of film—considering the physical properties of cesium iodide image inten-

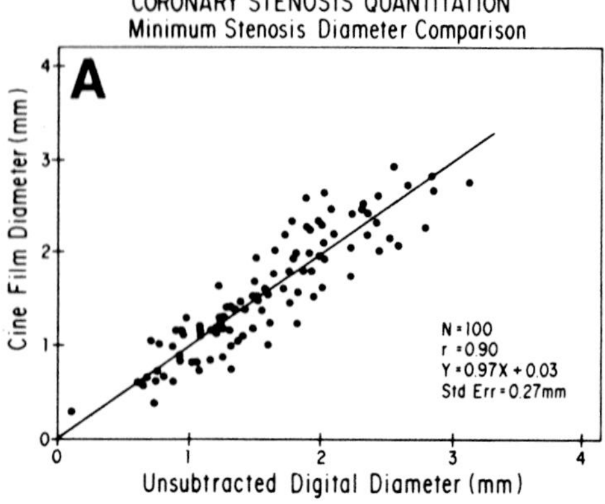

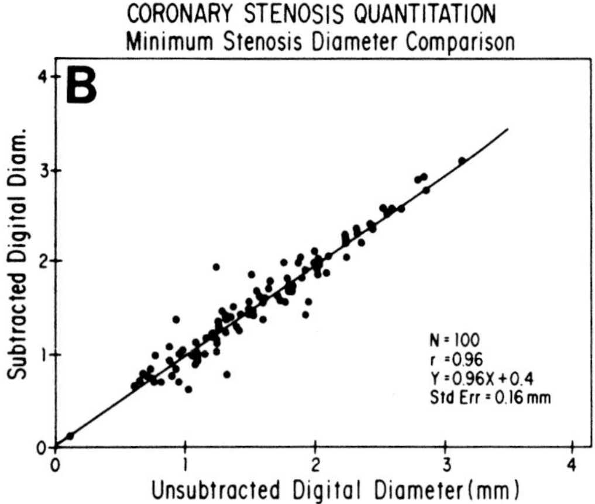

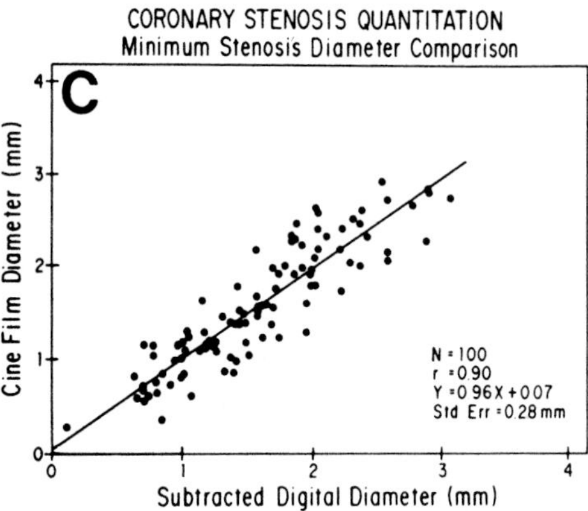

Figure 16–15. Regression analysis for minimal diameter stenosis data. *A*, *B*, and *C* each represent a two-way comparison among the three image types. (From Skelton, T.N., et al.: Comparison of coronary stenosis quantitation results from on-line digital and digitized cine film images. Am. J. Cardiol. 62:381, 1988, with permission.)

sifiers, the effects of the main objective lens in the image distributor, and the cine camera optics—is markedly deteriorated from the theoretic intrinsic resolution of cine film. The usable spatial resolution of film is approached by that of a high-quality video pickup tube.[M10] A second major factor is that the automated edge-detection scheme used in our investigation[M7] was optimized for the noise frequency of digital images. It should also be recognized that the reported investigations used different imaging systems, film types, and processing methods. Different processing systems and film types may alter the accuracy, compared with digital images. Thus, the small differences shown in some studies may not apply under all circumstances and in all laboratories, as evidenced by the work of Skelton and associates[S13] and Gurley and associates.[G9] Moreover, in spite of these differences, the relation between commonly measured parameters of coronary stenosis and reactive hyperemia have been shown to be equivalent among modalities, suggesting that no major clinical differences are present.[M7]

All the foregoing studies that compare the performance of quantitative arteriography from film to that from digital images utilized digital images with a matrix density of no greater than 512 × 512. Meticulous studies using a matrix density of 1024 × 1024 have failed to demonstrate any substantive improvement in quantitative accuracy when used in currently available x-ray systems.[G5, L5]

ACHIEVING OPTIMAL PERFORMANCE. Several recent publications and other chapters in this book contain reviews of the numerous factors affecting the accuracy and reproducibility of quantitative arteriography by film-based or digital-based methods.[B14, L7, M3, R8, 9, S7, 21] In general, sources of error in quantitative arteriography can be divided into those resulting from patient characteristics, from angiographic technique, from radiographic technique, and from the quantitative methodology itself.

Table 16–3 summarizes some of the more important patient characteristics that affect coronary quantification. To overcome variations in vasomotor tone, we currently use either sublingual tablets or a buccal spray of nitroglycerin before acquiring images to be quantified. Although this agent is not a maximal vasodilator, its use after several test injections or clinical image acquisitions with contrast material helps minimize effects of vasomotor tone. Cyclic variations in arterial size and contrast mixing, and the effects of cardiac and respiratory motion, can be ameliorated with ECG-gated acquisitions of images during diastasis and during held inspiration. When this is not possible, images during diastasis are visually selected. Other laboratories perform extensive frame-by-frame analyses and then average the results.[S7, 21] The most important patient characteristic that limits quantitative arteriography is the unique set of geometric relationships among vessel curvature, other vessels or branches, and the shape of the specific lesion of interest. Quantitative arteriography by geometric or videodensitometric methods requires more, not less, angiographic skill in selecting views that will optimize visualization of the stenosis. Attempts to aid this process of gantry positioning are under investigation in several laboratories[W10, S12] (Fig. 16–16).

Table 16–4 summarizes some of the important angiographic techniques that can affect quantitative arteriography. As already alluded to, the most important factor is the simple geometric one of optimally viewing the lesion in a view showing "triple orthogonality," so that gantry positions are orthogonal and the lesion is parallel to each image intensifier, thereby preventing foreshortening. Achieving truly orthogonal positions in patients is not easy. Moreover, in serial studies, it is absolutely necessary to reproduce the same view or sets of views to avoid large reproducibility errors.[R9] Displacement of blood by contrast is required, especially in large and/or high-flow conduits such as bypass grafts, to avoid spurious results owing to streaming.[S7] Power injection of contrast can achieve this, but this is often met with unfounded resistance in many laboratories.[K5] Nevertheless, it is the only method available that will give a precisely controlled bolus in a reproducible fashion. In lieu of this, rapid hand injection of a sufficient amount to cause some visible reflux is necessary before adequate coronary opacification can be guaranteed.

Table 16–3. SOURCES OF ERROR IN QUANTITATIVE ARTERIOGRAPHY: PATIENT CHARACTERISTICS

Patient size
Vessel motion (cardiac and respiratory)
Vasomotor tone
Cyclic variation in diameters
Geometric considerations (vessel curvature, stenosis irregularity, relation to other vessels/branches, including vasa vasorum)

Adapted from Mancini, G.B.J.: Quantitative coronary angiography: Development of methods, limitations, and clinical applications. Am. J. Cardiac Imag. 2:98, 1988.

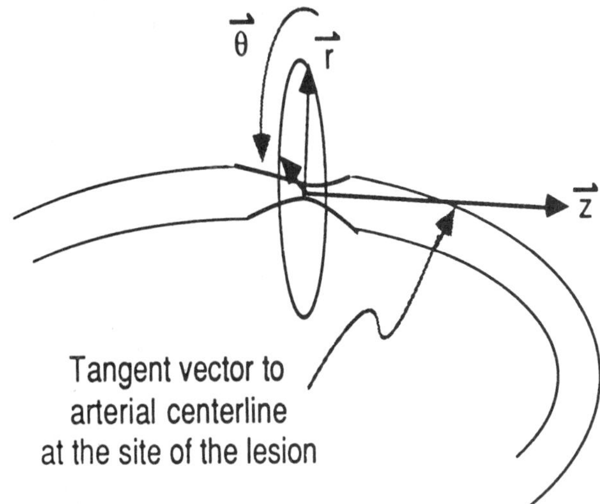

Figure 16–16. Cylindric coordinates about the arterial center line at the site of a hypothetic lesion. The tangent vector is perpendicular to the radial and angular vectors. "Triple orthogonality" allows accurate videodensitometry at the site of the lesion. Note, however, that other segments of the hypothetic artery may not conform to this requirement.

Reiber and colleagues have demonstrated that the catheter material itself and differences in stated versus actual lumen size may affect numerical results.[R7] We have shown that the overall size of the catheter is another critical factor. For example, based on our current observations, number five French catheters do not provide images that are sufficient for detailed studies of regression and/or progression of atherosclerosis, even though overall image quality is probably sufficient for most routine clinical purposes.[E3] Pincushion distortion can be largely avoided with most modern systems by obtaining images with the catheter tip centrally located and by panning only minimally, or if possible, not at all, during contrast injection so that the lesion of interest is also centrally located. This method has traditionally been considered to represent "poor technique," because most angiographers have been trained to include only the tip of the catheter at the upper edges of the image so that most, if not all, of the coronary tree fills the rest of the image, thereby minimizing the need to pan. However, absence of the catheter shaft or a sufficient portion of it is a very common deficiency of images considered for quantitative analysis. The differential magnification of the catheter shaft and the lesion of interest is a difficult problem to overcome, because all methods that incorporate external measurements and reimaging of grids or other objects are also prone to significant errors. Therefore, the catheter shaft remains the most convenient method of calibration.

Table 16–5 lists some of the radiographic aspects of image production that impact tremendously on image quality and image quantification.[L7] These are discussed more fully in other chapters related to film analyses. Table 16–6 demonstrates the numerous specific features of different methodologies that can affect coronary quantification dramatically.

Table 16–4. SOURCES OF ERROR IN QUANTITATIVE ARTERIOGRAPHY: ANGIOGRAPHIC TECHNIQUE

Geometric configuration and location of x-ray gantry with respect to patient and lesion of interest
Quality of mixing of contrast agents with blood
Quality and location of catheter image (susceptibility to pincushion distortion and differential magnification, effects on edge-detection)
Size of catheter (8 Fr. vs. 5 Fr.) and tolerance of specifications
Panning

Adapted from Mancini, G.B.J.: Quantitative coronary angiography: Development of methods, limitations, and clinical applications. Am. J. Cardiac Imag. 2:98, 1988.

Table 16–5. SOURCES OF ERROR IN QUANTITATIVE ARTERIOGRAPHY: RADIOGRAPHIC TECHNIQUE

X-ray generator (pulse width, dose, beam quality)
X-ray tube (focal spot size/shape, tube current, voltage, filtration, beam nonuniformity)
Image intensifier (magnification, resolution, gain factor, veiling glare, pincushion distortion)
Image distributor (objective lens focal length, blurring in main objective lens, aperture size, pincushion distortion)
Cine recording (cine camera lens focal length, blurring, film grain size, film speed, sensitometry, pincushion distortion)
Electronic recording (progressive/interlaced television tube, image matrix size, video noise)

Adapted from Mancini, G.B.J.: Quantitative coronary angiography: Development of methods, limitations, and clinical applications. Am. J. Cardiac Imag. 2:98, 1988.

Our own experience to date can be summarized as follows: (1) We have not been able to show a definite advantage of film-based imaging over digital imaging using a 512 × 512 matrix size when fully automated quantification is performed. (2) A definite advantage of 1024 × 1024 digital image matrix size has not been shown. (3) Subtracted images in clinical subjects are severely vulnerable to misregistration artifacts and cannot be recommended for quantitative analyses. (4) Film images must be averaged to reduce sufficiently image noise inherent in video digitization. (5) Because nearly all sources of error (lack of sharpness due to motion, limited spatial resolution, oblique orientation of the vessel with respect to the x-ray beam, geometric magnification) serve to cause overestimates in actual luminal dimensions, and because truly orthogonal views are difficult to achieve clinically, a strong case can be made for assessing minimal luminal diameters in a view showing the lesion to its best advantage. (6) When serial studies are anticipated, the view must be reproduced as closely as possible.

Of the six factors, the most important aspects over which the clinician can exercise significant control are

- use of radiographic exposure levels and progressive scan readout,
- use of full contrast doses, preferably injected with a power injector,
- framing rates of not less than 10 Hz,
- avoidance of subtraction-dependent image processing,
- alignment of catheter and stenosis as close to the central portion of the image field as possible to reduce effects of pincushion distortion,
- utilization of fully automated and quantitative programs that analyze digital images magnified up to fourfold with a 512 × 512 image matrix,
- and use of minimum diameter measurements in preference to average diameters over extended lengths.

Table 16–6. SOURCES OF ERROR IN QUANTITATIVE ARTERIOGRAPHY: QUANTITATIVE METHODOLOGY

Film vs. digital
Image processing (subtracted, nonsubtracted)
Video frame averaging
Matrix size and magnification
Filtering
Fully automated vs. computer-assisted analyses (observer variation)
Edge-detection algorithm (first or second derivative, combined algorithms, smoothing, interpolation)
Definition of normal (observer vs. interpolated)
Calibration technique
Quantitative output (average diameters, minimum diameters, orthogonal data, minimum areas, length, integrated indexes [theoretic flow reserve], videodensitometry)

Adapted from Mancini, G.B.J.: Quantitative coronary angiography: Development of methods, limitations, and clinical applications. Am. J. Cardiac Imag. 2:98, 1988.

VIDEODENSITOMETRY USING DIGITAL ANGIOGRAPHY. Validation of Methods. The previous discussion focused predominantly on the geometric quantification of coronary stenoses. Videodensitometry is an important and attractive method theoretically unaffected by the commonly irregular luminal morphology of coronary lesions. Therefore, videodensitometry may provide a rotationally invariant measure of relative cross-sectional area or absolute area of an irregular lumen. Chapters 12, 13, and 14 deal with the complex corrections required to begin to use this methodology, and applications using cineangiography are provided. Digital angiography is particularly suited to this application because the complex image preprocessing required to linearize the relation between contrast depth and x-ray transmission can be easily implemented. Such applications, however, are few, and they serve to highlight several practical, residual limitations of current techniques.

Wiesel and co-workers evaluated a combined geometric and videodensitometric approach for measuring stenoses created in dogs.[W5] They used edge detection applied to the normal segment and videodensitometry applied to the stenosis to determine the absolute luminal cross-sectional area by the following relationship: stenotic area = An = (1 − S/100), when An is the area of a normal segment determined geometrically and S is the relative severity of the stenosis based on the density profiles over the normal and stenotic segments. Relatively few stenoses were imaged, and the minority were truly irregular. A moderately good correlation could be shown between known lesion area and the combined edge detection/videodensity approach (r = 0.76, standard error = 0.71 mm^2, absolute area deviation = 0.65 mm^2).

Tobis and co-workers studied 19 patients before and after percutaneous transluminal coronary angioplasty (PTCA).[T5] They compared geometric and videodensitometric stenosis measurements obtained from digital angiograms. Although intimal tears and dissections are expected to make edge-detection methods inaccurate after angioplasty, in fact the mean stenotic measurements by either technique both before and after angioplasty were not significantly different. Interobserver variability was similar in each method. Since videodensitometry, in theory, should provide a rotationally invariant assessment of percent stenosis, they also compared results from orthogonal views of single lesions. Although the densitometry showed a good correlation of results, the performance of the edge-detection methodology was no worse. There was, therefore, no apparent added value of densitometry in this clinical application.

Klein and co-workers provided a pathoanatomic validation of videodensitometric analyses in 15 stenotic segments of excised human coronary arteries imaged by digital techniques.[K4] These investigators showed good results with videodensitometry when percentage area narrowing results were compared with analyses of pathologic sections (r = 0.93). This performance was somewhat better than a similar comparison using purely geometric methods. Measures of absolute area narrowing were not undertaken.

Sanz and associates analyzed 13 consecutively, acquired biplane digital subtraction angiograms before and after percutaneous transluminal coronary angioplasty (PTCA) to determine intra- and interobserver variability of absolute lesion diameter, relative videodensitometric cross-sectional area, automated percent diameter stenosis, and visual percent diameter stenosis.[S5] Both before and after angioplasty, measures of absolute diameter showed less interobserver variability than densitometry or percent automated diameter stenosis measurements. It is important to note that in these routinely acquired clinical images, the relative videodensitometric cross-sectional area correlated poorly with images from the orthogonal view.

Skelton and co-workers undertook a large clinical study of 100 discrete lesions in 45 patients.[S13] Comparisons were made among direct on-line digital, electrocardiogram-gated digital subtraction and digitized cine film images. Videodensitometric percent area stenosis data showed correlation coefficients among the different modalities of between 0.80 and 0.89. These correlations were less and the apparent variability was greater than for similar comparisons of geometric measurements. No standard was available to evaluate the significance of these results, but the investigators point out that many more factors contribute to nonlinearity of cineangiograms than on-line digital images. Other experience suggests that the inferior relation between film-derived and on-line digital-derived videodensitometric measurements is a result of larger errors in the film-derived data.[L3–5]

Katritsis and associates studied 73 lesions in 63 patients who had undergone coronary angioplasty.[K1] Digital subtraction coronary angiograms were analyzed with an automated border-detecting computer program capable of simultaneous geometric and densitometric cross-sectional area estimation. They showed good agreement between geometric and densitometric area percent stenoses calculated by the program on the pre-PTCA digital angiograms. After PTCA, however, important discrepancies between the two methods existed. Densitometric evaluation demonstrated a significantly greater mean coefficient of variation between different views after PTCA but not before. This degree of variation was much larger than noted for geometric evaluations on the same views. The results are similar to those demonstrated by Sanz and group, except for the finding that the deficiencies in densitometry from different views were limited only to the post-PTCA analyses.[S5] In general, although the distortion of the vessel lumen after angioplasty is assumed to render geometric methods potentially inaccurate, the altered geometry after angioplasty cannot fully explain the results of Katritsis and co-workers, since a high degree of variability was not noted for geometric measurements either before or after angioplasty. The investigators postulated that distortion of the vessel as a result of angioplasty may have interfered with the mixing of contrast medium and blood, hence invalidating any assumptions about uniform dye distribution and thereby also invalidating densitometry measurements. Further studies will be required to elucidate more fully these practical problems.

Limitations of Videodensitometry. The foregoing studies were performed either in in vivo models, in vitro models of actual human coronary arteries, or patients undergoing routine catheterization. They represent extremely rigorous tests of the current applicability of densitometry in clinical practice. The results, although in general promising, are quite different from the excellent results noted almost routinely in phantom studies or in studies using highly selected images demonstrating optimal background conditions, meticulous density calibrations to ensure linearity, and absence of foreshortening of either normal or stenotic segments.[K6, L5, 6, S9–11] In biplane images, one must be confident that the long axis of the lesion and normal segments are parallel to the image intensifier planes and perpendicular to the x-ray beams. This "triple orthogonality" can be achieved in new-generation catheterization laboratories,[W10] and the process can be automated substantially in digital catheterization laboratories[S12] (see Fig. 16–6).

Some of the numerous impediments to videodensitometry are summarized in Table 16–7. At this point, it is felt that the role of videodensitometry should be in rapid calculation of relative cross-sectional areas in a single view, and if repeated studies are anticipated, then the same view must be utilized to avoid large errors owing to potential differences in foreshortening, background, veiling glare, and scatter. The latter problems are spatially variable within isolated frames and temporally variable as contrast moves in and out of the field and as brightness automatically changes in response to different backgrounds caused by panning. Accordingly, substantially increased efforts will be required before robust methods are devised that will allow for successful and rapid clinical application of videodensitometric techniques even with on-line digital images.

Bypass Grafts

Intravenous Angiography

The problems of using intravenous angiography for delineating coronary arteries outlined previously also apply to the imaging of

Table 16–7. SOURCES OF ERROR IN QUANTITATIVE ARTERIOGRAPHY: VIDEODENSITOMETRY

Foreshortening increases contrast thickness
Determination of edge gradients may affect integration of densities of relevance
Inhomogeneities of contrast mixing
Inhomogeneities of background thickness
Nonlinear relation between optical density and contrast medium thickness (spectral beam hardening, image intensifier gamma, vignetting, veiling glare)
Nature of the nonlinear relation spatially variable in a single image
Nonlinear relation also both temporally and spatially variable

Adapted from Mancini, G.B.J.: Quantitative coronary angiography: Development of methods, limitations, and clinical applications. Am. J. Cardiac Imag. 2:98, 1988.

coronary bypass grafts. However, grafts are larger, farther away from the left ventricular cavity, and subject to less motion, so the problems encountered in imaging them are somewhat less severe. Even so, difficulties continue to arise, especially since the grafts are in close proximity to the aortic contrast pool.

In general, clinical studies have focused on the detection of graft patency because the fine detail of graft stenoses and anastomoses cannot be assessed using this technique. In a comparison of graft patency using intravenous and selective angiography, Myerowitz and colleagues found that 11 of 15 truly patent grafts could be visualized by the digital technique (sensitivity of 73 percent) and that all of 11 truly occluded grafts were correctly identified digitally (100 percent specificity).[M13–15] Drury and associates identified 9 of 13 patent grafts (sensitivity of 69 percent) with a specificity of 100 percent.[D6] Guthaner and associates identified only 13 of 32 patent grafts.[G10] Thus, although the technique appears to be highly specific, low sensitivity relative to cine-CT has generally tempered the enthusiasm for this approach. More recently, however, Lupon-Roses and colleagues studied 101 venous grafts and 7 internal mammary grafts and were able to positively identify 95 of 97 patent grafts and all 11 occluded grafts (98 percent sensitivity and 100 percent specificity).[L15] These excellent results were attributed to the routine use of two views, a priori knowledge of the location of each graft, and the use of radiographic x-ray exposures instead of lower fluoroscopic exposure levels. Similarly, Guiraudon and co-workers demonstrated 100 percent specificity and 98 sensitivity in the detection of internal mammary grafts in 42 patients.[G8] These results are, in part, attributed to the fact that internal mammary grafts are farther from the heart and great vessels, and their position varies less from patient to patient. In addition, these investigators achieved good-to-excellent imaging without significant misregistration in nearly 90 percent of cases.

Aortic Root Angiography

In keeping with the trend toward intra-arterial contrast administration, aortic root digital angiography has been shown to be highly accurate for detecting saphenous vein bypass grafts. Two groups have reported 100 percent specificity and sensitivity for detecting patent grafts using this technique, although graft detail cannot be analyzed.[D6, G4] Guthaner and groups reported a sensitivity of 98 percent (101 of 103 patent grafts).[G10] Steffenino and colleagues demonstrated an overall sensitivity of 83 percent and a specificity of 100 percent, but performance varied considerably depending on the site and type of graft.[S22] Greatest success was achieved with venous grafts to the left anterior descending artery. The worst performance was in assessing internal mammary grafts to this artery. Additional views were helpful in delineating the status of venous grafts to the right or circumflex arteries. Improved evaluation of internal mammary grafts was obtained by Kuttler and colleagues, who successfully and safely used ipsilateral brachial artery injections of contrast postoperatively to assess early patency.[K8] In this application, details of anastomotic adequacy and perfusion were evident.

Anecdotal reports of digital detection of patent grafts that were not found by selective angiography suggest that such methods may even be superior to standard catheterization methods if graft patency alone is to be assessed. But even this procedure does not routinely provide sufficient detail to allow accurate assessment of stenoses, anastomoses, and adequacy of distal run-off (Fig. 16–17). Moreover, because this procedure entails the same risk and preparation as selective catheterization, this laboratory uses the method only as a quick screening test at the time of regular catheterization, especially in individuals who do not have implanted graft markers. The use of this procedure early in the course of the catheterization helps expedite the examination. In many instances, the amount of contrast used for the aortogram is offset by the time and contrast saved in trying to find unmarked grafts with selective catheters. The concept of aortographic digital "roadmapping" also could expedite the procedure.

Direct Angiography

The specific use of digital angiography for assessing graft anatomy by direct contrast injection is not different from that for assessing the native coronary circulation, and this topic was discussed earlier. The major additional information that digital angiography has to offer with direct contrast injection is the assessment of graft function and flow. These latter aspects are discussed later.

FUNCTIONAL ASSESSMENT OF THE CORONARY CIRCULATION

Methodology

Transit-Time Analysis

The concept of using transit-time analysis to measure coronary velocity and flow is summarized in Figure 16–18. The passage of contrast past two arterial regions of interest at a known distance apart can be used to calculate velocity of a contrast bolus. Measurement of the mean cross-sectional area of the arterial segment allows conversion of the velocity measurement to a flow measurement. The transit time can be measured from the peaks of the contrast density profile within each region of interest or other portions of the curve (e.g., the point at which half the maximal contrast density is achieved, see later).

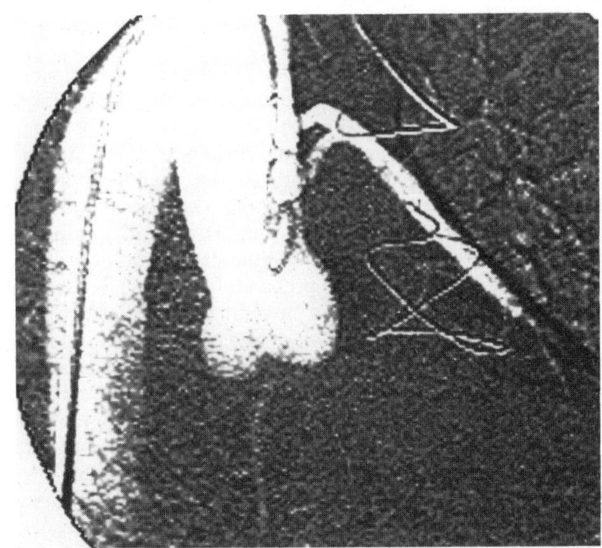

Figure 16–17. A direct, digital aortogram obtained with 20 ml of a 50 percent solution of contrast material. This patient had aortocoronary bypass grafts to the left anterior descending and first diagonal branches of the left coronary artery. Note that although the proximal segments are clearly visible, no definite anatomic information about the anastomoses or distal vessels is available from this image. In addition, the main bodies of the grafts are overlapped in this projection. Despite these limitations, selective catheterization of grafts can be expedited by first screening for graft patency by this technique. (From Mancini, G.B.J., and Higgins, C.B.: Digital subtraction angiography: A review of cardiac applications. Prog. Cardiovasc. Dis. 18:111, 1985, with permission.)

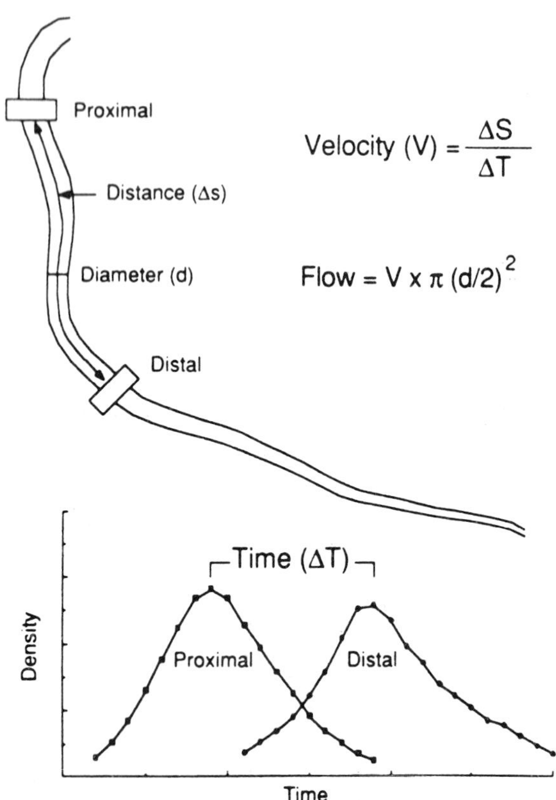

Figure 16–18. Schematic illustration of the scientific basis for calculation of coronary flow from the transit time. The time (ΔT) for passage of a contrast bolus from a proximal to a distal coronary region of interest is measured. The velocity (V) and flow can be calculated from the distance (ΔS) between the regions of interest and the diameter of the coronary segment. (From Nissen, S.E., et al.: Methods for calculation of coronary flow reserve by computer processing of digital angiograms. *In* Heintzen, P.H., and Bürsch, J.H. (eds.): Progress in Digital Angiocardiography. Kluwer Academic, Dordrecht, 1988, p. 237, with permission.)

The insightful and progressive work of Rutishauser provides all workers in the field of digital angiography with probably the largest body of concentrated effort toward extraction of dynamic, quantitative data from angiographic images.[R17–19] His dedication to this work is a testament both to the wealth of untapped information inherent in cineangiographic images and to the difficulty in extracting it accurately and consistently. Rutishauser and colleagues validated a transit-time–based method of measuring coronary flow in a canine preparation and also demonstrated its application to measurement of right coronary artery flow in patients.[R18, 19] The densograms measured at two regions of interest in the arterial image were calibrated by filming a contrast wedge prior to image acquisitions, so that contrast depth and density could be linearized. The calculation of blood flow required geometric measurement of the distance between the two regions of interest and the volume of the coronary segment.

Smith and associates[S16] used essentially the same technique as Rutishauser and also demonstrated applications in humans.[S17] These investigators emphasized the need for background subtraction to correct contrast densograms.

More than a decade after the aforementioned investigations, the transit-time approach continues to be one of the commonest fundamental applications in digital imaging for measuring blood flow. Kruger and colleagues described a method of temporal filtration of 30 frame per second fluoroscopic video sequences to establish a parametric image demonstrating the time to maximal opacification of arterial segments after contrast injection. Geometric length measurements were required to calculate flow velocity.[K7]

Spiller and associates expanded upon the combined transit-time and geometric measurement technique in two distinct ways.[S20] First, multiple contrast injections were used to enable calculations of *phasic* coronary flow, and second, the leading edge of the contrast bolus (appearance time) was tracked instead of the peak of the contrast densograms (mean transit time). These investigators used the leading edge of the contrast bolus to avoid the errors inherent in calculations of mean transit time in a pulsatile system and the alterations in densogram shape (and therefore mean transit-time calculations) caused by layering and incomplete washout of contrast. The appearance time was defined as the time at which the contrast density was half the peak value in the regions of interest studied. The method showed a strong linear correlation with saphenous vein bypass blood flow measured by electromagnetic probe at the time of surgery (Fig. 16–19). A systematic overestimation of approximately 20 percent was noted. This technique was developed with high-frame rate angiography (50 frames per second) and the calculations of phasic flow required repeated contrast injection at different phases of the cardiac cycle (Fig. 16–20).

Swanson and co-workers measured the linear distance that the contrast material waveform moved in each of 60 video fields per second[S24] and combined this with a densitometrically based volume calculation[K6] to establish phasic flow measurements. That is, instead of using two fixed regions of interest to calculate mean transit time, these investigators examined the changes in the distribution of contrast material along the arterial segment on a frame-by-frame basis. Excellent results for measures of phasic femoral flow in dogs were reported. A subsequent investigation[S23] employed this technique to quantify absolute phasic and mean flow in coronary artery bypass grafts (Fig. 16–21). Correlations for mean and peak flows were high (r = 0.91 and 0.88, respec-

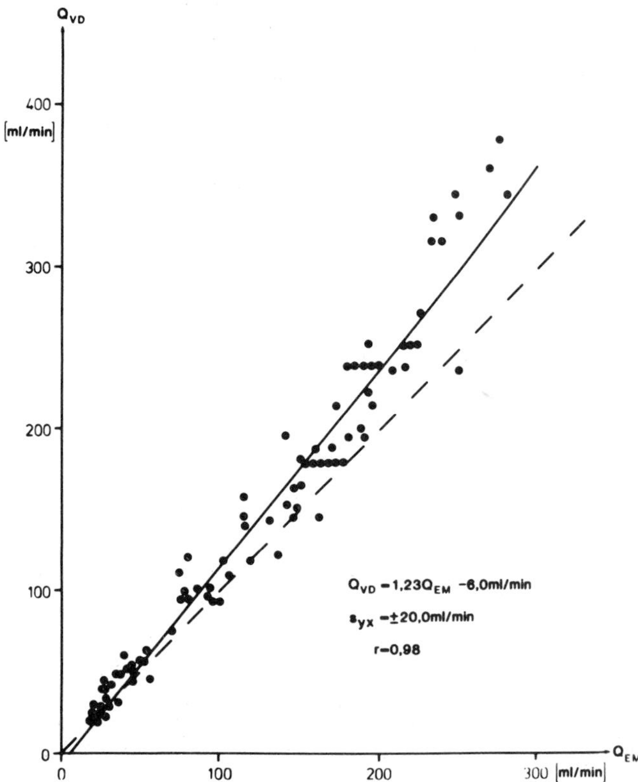

Figure 16–19. Relationship between videodensitometrically determined flow (ordinate) and the electromagnetically determined flow (abscissa) in 16 aortocoronary bypass grafts (80 single measurements). The electromagnetically measured flow is overestimated by about 20 percent on the basis of the videodensitometrically measured flow. The *solid line* represents regression; the *dashed line* represents the line of identity. (From Spiller, P., et al.: Measurement of systolic and diastolic flow rates in the coronary artery system by x-ray densitometry. Circulation 68:337, 1983, with permission of the American Heart Association, Inc.)

Figure 16–20. Pattern of flow in a left anterior descending coronary artery before *(solid line)* and after *(dashed line)* a bifurcation. *Top*, flow velocity (V, cm/sec); *bottom*, flow rate (Q, ml/min). The patient's electrocardiogram is depicted as a reference signal. The flow velocities measured in the distal branch of the vessel are similar to those measured in the proximal branch. The flow rates are considerably lower in the distal vessel segment. (From Spiller, P., et al.: Measurement of systolic and diastolic flow rates in the coronary artery system by x-ray densitometry. Circulation 68:337, 1983, with permission of the American Heart Association, Inc.)

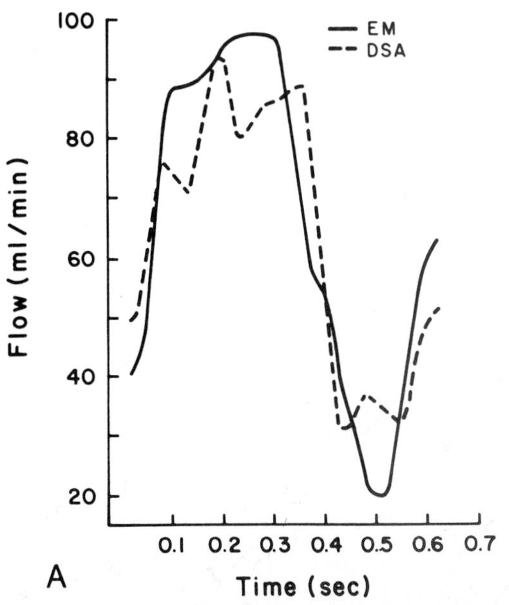

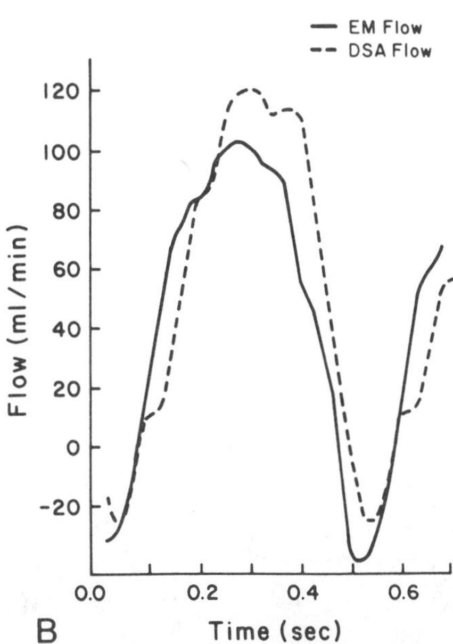

Figure 16–21. Direct comparison of blood-flow waveforms measured simultaneously with digital subtraction angiography (DSA) and electromagnetic (EM) methods under baseline flow conditions *(A)* and under high-flow conditions *(B)*. (From Swanson, D.K., et al.: Quantitation of absolute flow in coronary artery bypass grafts using digital subtraction angiography. J. Surg. Res. 44:326, 1988, with permission.)

tively). In contrast to the method of Spiller, this technique requires only a single contrast injection to measure phasic flow.

Shaw and Plewes published a novel pulsed-contrast injection method for measuring the velocity of blood flow.[55] Contrast material is injected with a specially modified injector at a pulsing frequency as high as 15 Hz, so that two or more boluses can be imaged simultaneously. Contrast injections are gated to an electrocardiographic signal. The velocity of flow is determined by measuring the spacing between the boluses and multiplying this distance by the pulsing frequency (Fig. 16–22). In this application, the actual time measurement, therefore, is not obtained from the contrast densogram, as it is in the usual transit-time applications. Instead, it is obtained from the known injection frequency. The multiple contrast densograms are analyzed solely to determine the distance traveled by each bolus. In vivo coronary applications have not yet been performed with this method.

These techniques are most suitable for assessments in relatively straight, long and nonbranching arterial segments or bypass grafts imaged parallel to the image intensifier, so that foreshortening will not affect arterial volume calculations and so that velocity changes at branch points will not alter transit-time measurements. Alternatively, biplane images and geometric corrections for foreshortening can be employed. The methods require a high frame-rate image acquisition to ensure adequate temporal resolution. The proposal of Shaw and Plewes requires both high-frame rate angiography and high pulsatile rates of contrast injection. Because the contrast bolus must be compact, all the methods are best applied with power injection of contrast material. More important, the transit-time techniques assume constant flow even though flow is phasic. Consequently, mean transit times must be measured over at least one cardiac cycle, or precise gating of the contrast injection during a specified phase of the cardiac cycle is required. Arrhythmias or contrast-induced heart rate changes also will invalidate the transit-time calculations, so atrial pacing should be used with these techniques.

Indicator-Dilution Analysis

This method utilizes the theory embodied in the standard Stewart and Hamilton equations, which predict that the area under an indicator density versus time curve will be directly proportional to the quantity of indicator injected and inversely proportional to flow (Fig. 16–23). For angiographic applications, the indicator is contrast material itself, and the density is measured in an arterial region of interest. This method can be used to measure both absolute and relative flow. If cardiac output is known, then absolute flow can be calculated if indicator dilution curves are obtained from both a reference injection into the aorta and a separate injection of the same amount into the artery of interest. The technique requires precise knowledge of the amount of contrast injected and full mixing of the indicator with blood. Alternatively, the measurement of absolute flow from single injections into an artery can be performed if complex corrections are made. These are needed for the effects of radiographic scatter, veiling glare, and beam hardening in order to optimize and linearize the effective mass absorption coefficient, the conversion factor of the image intensifier, the transfer function of the television system, the intensity of incident radiation, and the gains of the densitometry detectors. However, if the same quantity of contrast can be administered under both basal and

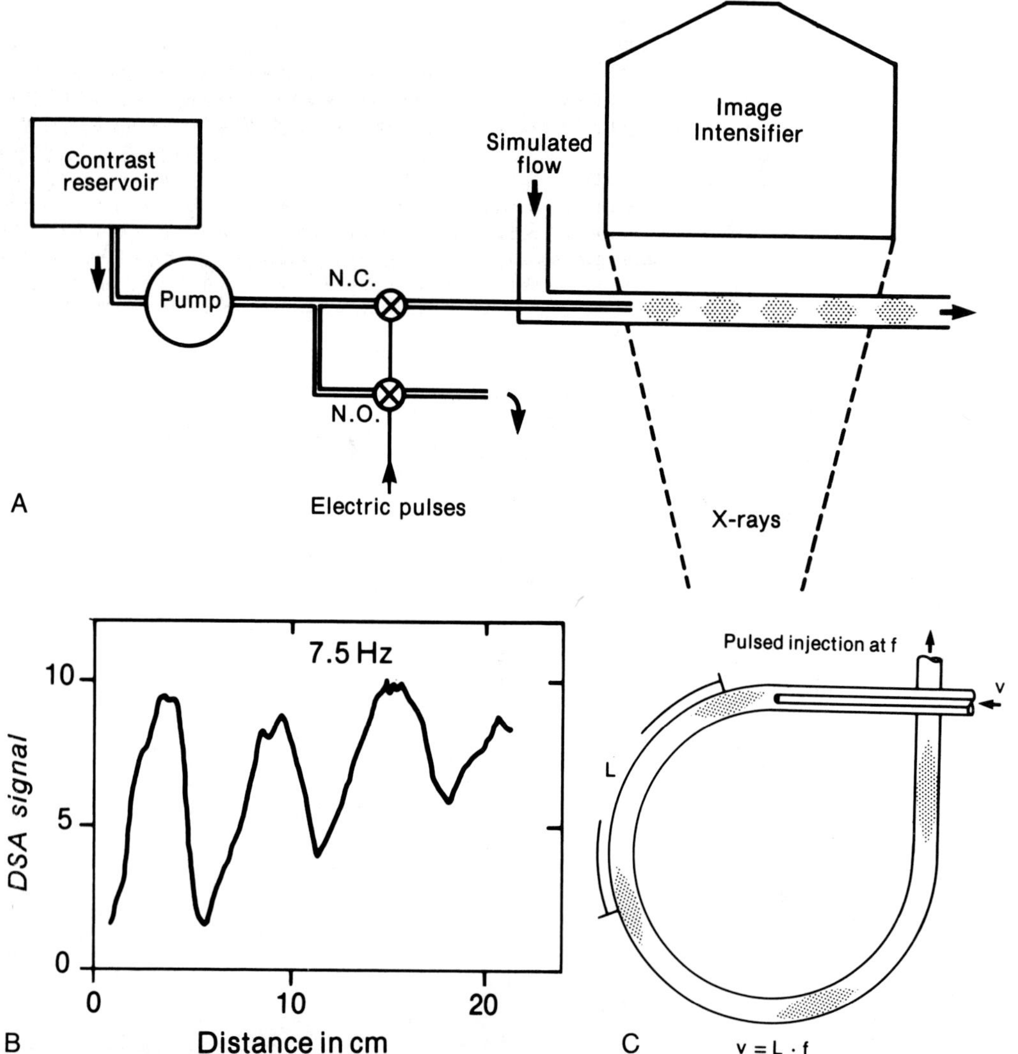

Figure 16–22. *A*, Prototype injector and experimental setup used in the pulsed-injection studies. N.C.—normally closed valve; N.O.—normally open valve. *B*, Contrast material profile for boluses generated by injections pulsed at 7.5 Hz. *C*, Velocity measurement (v) with the pulsed-injection method is determined by measuring the spacing (L) between two adjacent boluses and multiplying by the pulsing frequency (f). (From Shaw, C.G., and Plewes, D.B.: Pulsed-injection method for blood flow velocity measurement in intra-arterial digital subtraction angiography. Radiology 160:556, 1986, with permission.)

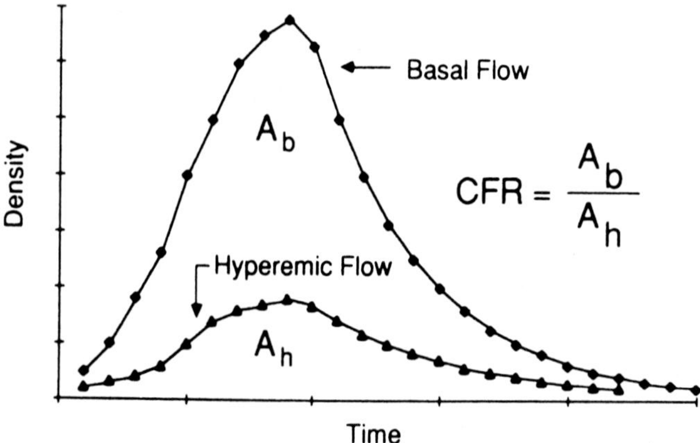

Figure 16–23. Calculation of coronary flow reserve from indicator-dilution curves. Coronary flow reserve is equal to the ratio of the area under a time-density curve for a coronary region of interest obtained under basal conditions (A_b) divided by the area of the curve of an identical region of interest obtained under hyperemic flow conditions (A_h). CRF—coronary flow reserve. (From Nissen, S.E., et al.: Methods for calculation of coronary flow reserve by computer processing of digital angiograms. *In* Heintzen, P.H., and Bürsch, J.H. (eds.): Progress in Digital Angiocardiography. Kluwer Academic, Dordrecht, 1988, p. 237, with permission.)

hyperemic conditions, and if the radiographic technique is relatively constant so that any effects are effectively canceled out, then a much less technically demanding measure of relative flow is possible.

A series of investigations from the University of California, Davis, extensively investigated the indicator-dilution technique for measures of blood flow.[F5, 6, L1, 13] In the early applications, the method was used to measure the flow into any artery that is selectively injected as a fraction of proximal reference flow, usually the cardiac output. This required two contrast injections. One injection was made into the aortic root as the reference injection for representation of the cardiac output, and the second was made into the specific artery of interest, such as the renal artery. Videodilution curves from the artery of interest were analyzed after each injection. The ratio of the two curves gave an estimate of the proportion of cardiac output perfusing the specific artery. If the absolute value of the cardiac output is known by another method, then a calculation of absolute flow can be made. The method was then extended to measure flow sequentially in the same artery, with results expressed as a fraction of the baseline measurement. This provided a measure of reactive hyperemia.

Foerster and colleagues applied this method in animals and human beings.[F5, 6] Lois and associates also demonstrated its validity in a phantom model and found it to be suitable for measuring either absolute or relative coronary flow.[L14] Optimal results were achieved primarily when measuring relative coronary flow. Nissen and associates have re-evaluated the method more recently, using digital angiography in a canine model.[N3, 4] They demonstrated a correlation of 0.86 between electromagnetic measures of coronary flow reserve and ratios obtained from the integration of the time-density curves (Fig. 16–24).

The most important technical prerequisite of this technique is that the administered contrast dose must be known precisely, and it should be constant between injections. This mandates *subselective* cannulation of the coronary artery for the delivery of the contrast and avoidance of reflux. Complete mixing must also occur, so the sampling site must be sufficiently distal to the site of contrast injection. This method is also best applied with power injection of contrast and utilization of atrial pacing. The temporal resolution required for this application is not as great as with the transit-time methods described earlier. For example, Nissen and colleagues have used analysis of a single end-diastolic frame per cardiac cycle to produce the time versus density curves (Fig. 16–25).[N3]

Contrast Washout Analysis

The aforementioned methods focus regions of interest over the arteries, whereas contrast washout methods analyze the disappearance of contrast from the myocardial bed. Digital subtraction enhances the evaluation of this technique, because visualization of the myocardial blush phase is augmented. These analyses are predicated upon utilization of an inert indicator and measurement of its monoexponential washout, as embodied in the Kety-Schmidt relations (Fig. 16–26).

Ikeda and associates studied 53 patients with variable degrees of coronary stenosis isolated to the left anterior descending artery.[I1, 2] One third of the patients had prior myocardial infarction. These investigators manually injected 2 to 3 ml of contrast material into the left main coronary artery and recorded an image run for 20 seconds at 30 frames per second. Mask node subtraction was utilized to provide background correction and enhancement of the myocardial phase of contrast. Eight 45-degree sectors emanating from the center of gravity of the diastolic left ventricular silhouette were analyzed to produce sectorial time-density curves, and the sectors corresponding to the left anterior descending perfusion bed were analyzed (Fig. 16–27). The disappearance half-life (T½) was calculated after fitting the descending slope of the densograms to a monoexponential function. The T½ was given by: T½ = ln 2/k, where ln is the natural logarithm and k is the exponential disappearance rate. Whenever the curves exhibited two components during the disappearance phase, T½ was calculated from the initial fast portion of the curve. In a subset of patients, a strong inverse correlation was noted between the T½ value and great cardiac vein flow (Fig. 16–28*A*). The washout T½ was notably shortened by the presence of collateral vessels and lengthened by the presence of infarction, despite a comparable degree of stenosis of the left anterior descending coronary artery. A curvilinear relation was noted between the T½ and caliper-determined coronary stenosis (excluding patients with collaterals) such that prolonged half-times were associated, in general, with stenoses of greater than 75 percent (see Fig. 16–28*B*). The number of instances in which the descending limb appeared to have two components was not provided, although this is generally recognized as a common problem. Moreover, since the T½ was calculated 3 to 10 seconds after injection of contrast, it can be anticipated that the measures were obtained during some degree of hyperemia.[F8, 9] This has two potential

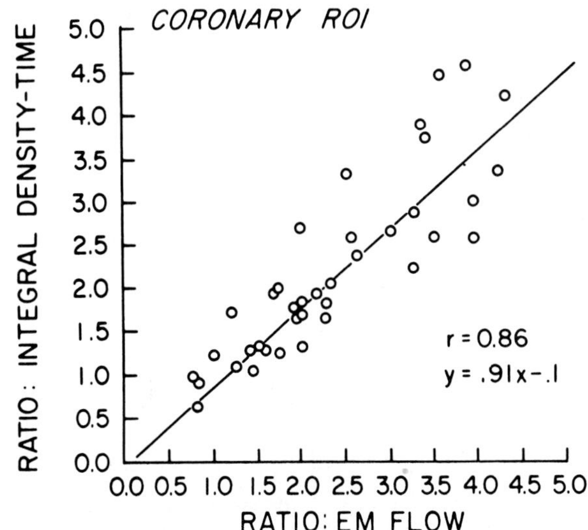

Figure 16–24. Results of linear regression analysis comparing coronary reserve measured by the electromagnetic (EM) flow probe to that obtained by the integral of the coronary density-time curve. A close correlation was observed, with a slope of the regression line near unity. (From Nissen, S.E., et al.: Value and limitations of computer analysis of digital subtraction angiography in the assessment of coronary flow reserve. Circulation 73:562, 1986, with permission of the American Heart Association, Inc.)

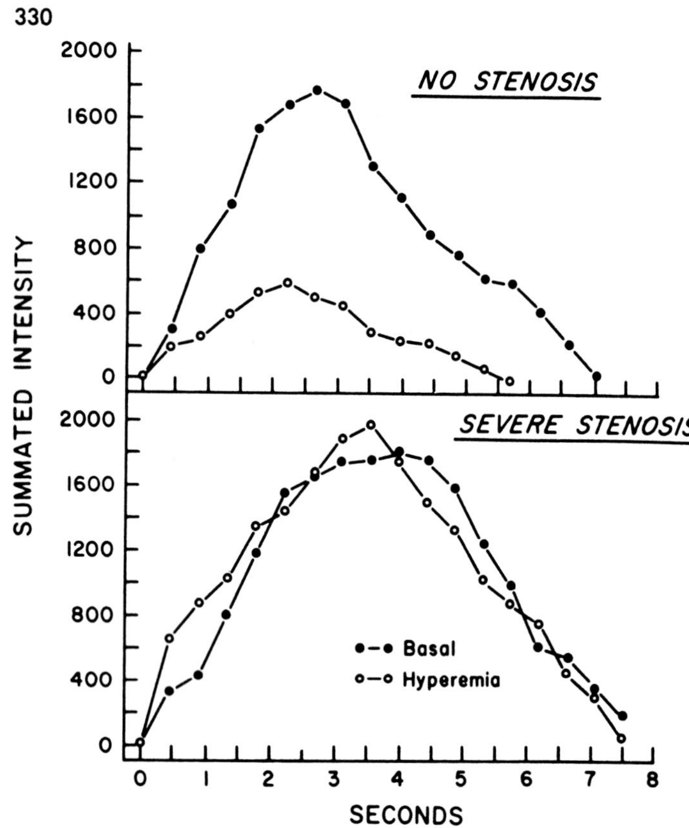

Figure 16–25. Representative density-time curves for a proximal circumflex coronary region of interest. The *top panel* illustrates the curves obtained in the absence of coronary stenosis, showing a marked decrease in the area under the curve for the hyperemic image *(open circles)* and for the basal image *(closed circles)*. The *(bottom panel)* shows similar curves obtained under basal and hyperemic conditions in the presence of a severe coronary stenosis. (From Nissen, S.E., et al.: Value and limitations of computer analysis of digital subtraction angiography in the assessment of coronary flow reserve. Circulation 73:562, 1986, with permission of the American Heart Association, Inc.)

effects on the results. First, it may account for the outstanding separation of patients based on coronary stenosis, collateral status, and presence of wall motion abnormalities. Such separation based on coronary flow that is truly basal would not be anticipated until very severe stenoses are present. Second, and more problematic, the T½ measurements were very likely made during a time when flow was not in a steady state.[B9]

Takeda and associates employed a similar technique in 10 control subjects and 8 patients with anterior myocardial infarction.[T1] Atrial pacing was used to avoid heart rate variability. In contrast to the aforementioned study, the washout time constants were calculated on a pixel by pixel basis and displayed as a parametric image. Washout time constant images were nearly homogeneous in the normal cases except at the basal region, where heterogeneity was felt to be due to superimposed contrast material in the coronary sinus, right ventricle, and pulmonary arteries. In patients with myocardial infarction, regional heterogeneity was demonstrated with prolonged washout times localized to the zones of contraction abnormality. It is interesting that the discrete areas with abnormal washout agreed more closely with discrete areas of wall thickening abnormalities than with the much broader areas of abnormal wall motion.[M9]

Investigators at the University of California, Los Angeles, have provided an extensive evaluation of the role of washout analysis for measures of coronary flow and flow reserve. Whiting and colleagues studied a dog model and developed algorithms for

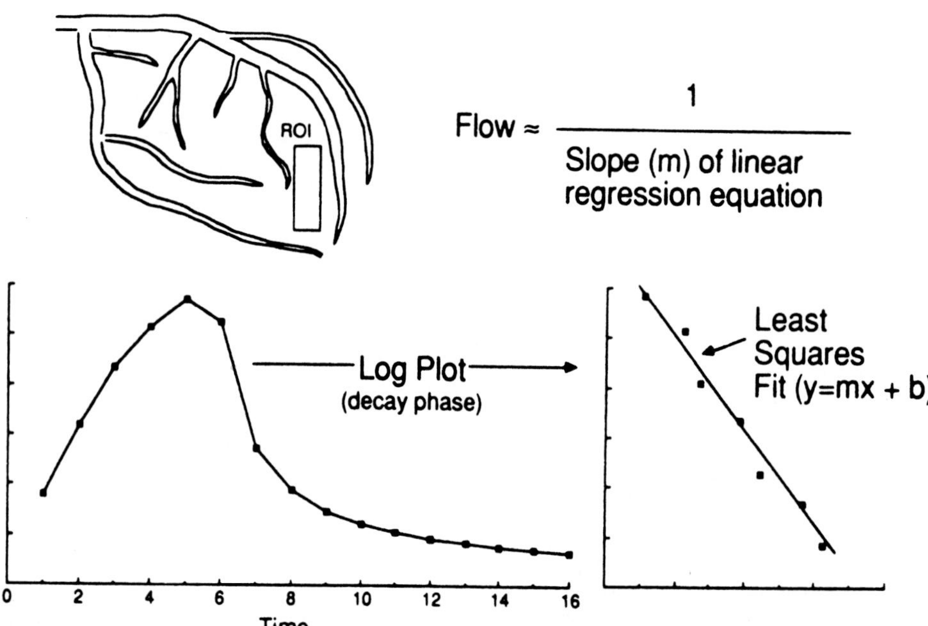

Figure 16–26. Measurement of coronary flow from the washout phase of myocardial contrast. The decay phase is assumed to be monoexponential and is plotted on a logarithmic scale. A linear regression least squares fit is determined for the decay phase. Flow is proportional to the inverse of the slope m of the regression equation. (From Nissen, S.E., et al.: Methods for calculation of coronary flow reserve by computer processing of digital angiograms. *In* Heintzen, P.H., and Bürsch, J.H. (eds.): Progress in Digital Angiocardiography. Kluwer Academic, Dordrecht, 1988, p. 237, with permission.)

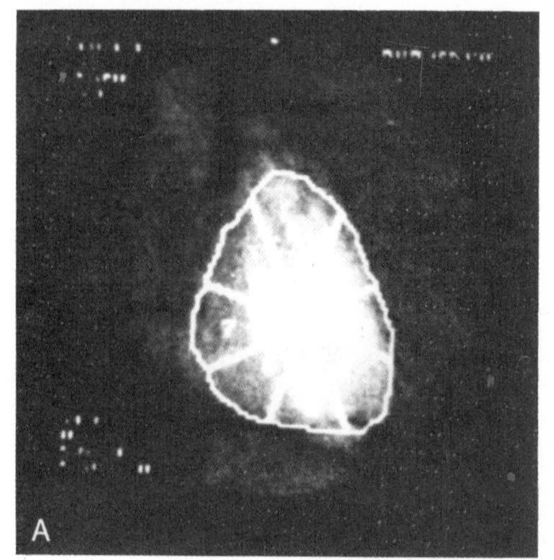

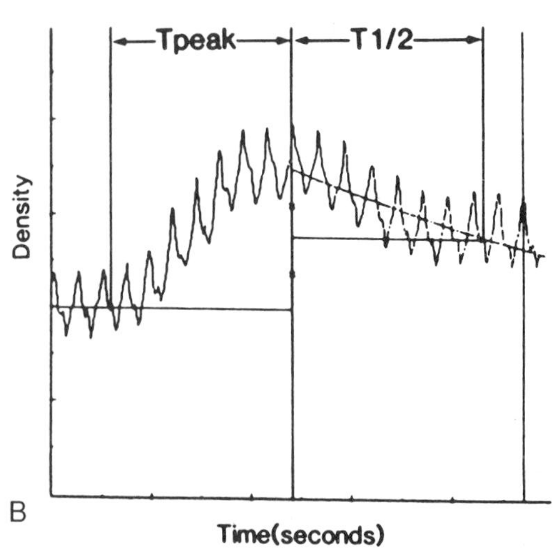

Figure 16–27. Computerized time-density analysis of digital subtraction coronary arteriograms. After computer-aided epicardial outlining and automatic subdivision into eight sectors *(A)*, a sectorial time-density curve *(B)* was constructed in four sectors of the myocardium perfused by the left anterior descending coronary artery. The descending slope of the time-density curve was fitted to a monoexponential function with a standard least-squares method and the contrast disappearance half-life (T½) was calculated. (From Ikeda, H., et al.: Quantitative evaluation of regional myocardial blood flow by videodensitometric analysis of digital subtraction coronary arteriography in humans. J. Am. Coll. Cardiol. 8:809, 1986, with permission.)

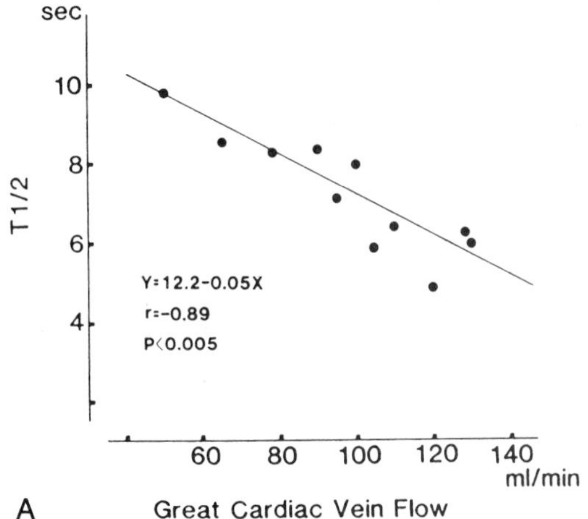

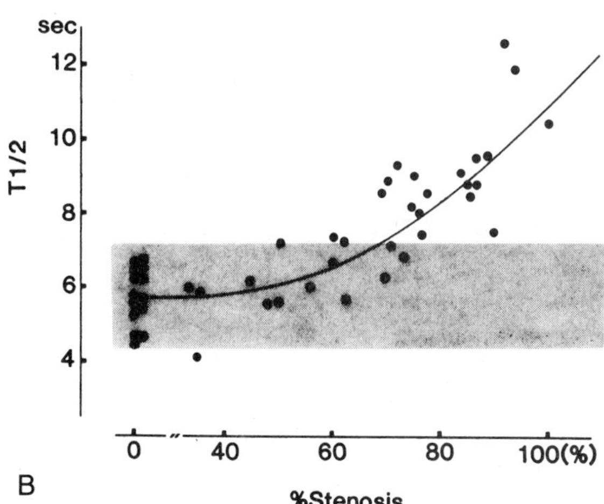

Figure 16–28. *A*, Relationship between the mean contrast disappearance half-life (T½) and great cardiac vein flow. The mean T½ exhibited a high correlation with great cardiac vein flow: r = −0.89. *B*, Relationship between the mean T½ and percent stenosis of the left anterior descending coronary artery when patients with coronary collateral vessels were excluded. A normal range of mean T½ *(shaded area)* was defined as that inside the ±2 standard deviation band around the mean from the control subjects. An abnormally high T½ occurred when stenosis of the left anterior descending coronary artery was 75 percent or greater. (From Ikeda, H., et al.: Quantitative evaluation of regional myocardial blood flow by videodensitometric analysis of digital subtraction coronary arteriography in humans. J. Am. Coll. Cardiol. 8:809, 1986, with permission.)

generating time-intensity curves from several regions of interest.[W3] These were placed over the proximal coronary artery to time contrast bolus onset accurately and obviate ECG-gated power injection, and over the myocardium to calculate time from injection to peak concentration and exponential washout rates. A region over a small lead blocker was analyzed to partially correct for scatter and veiling glare before logarithmic transformation of intensity data, thereby allowing assessment of absolute flow (Fig. 16–29). Analyses were made on images acquired at 30 frames per second before and after hand injection of contrast material, and densograms were constructed from 10 sample per second data. Some of the time-concentration curves displayed a secondary maximum 5 to 10 seconds after peak opacification, coincident with the arrival of contrast in overlying pulmonary vessels. Therefore, the densogram analysis was limited to the arrival and initial washout portions of the curve. Analysis was considered possible only if three strict criteria were met: (1) the postinjection concentration had to remain above the preinjection baseline, (2) the curve had to exhibit a single smooth peak, and (3) the correlation coefficient of the logarithmic fit of the washout portion had to be greater than $r = 0.995$. Sixty-seven percent of all curves obtained were suitable for analysis. Respiratory motion or low myocardial iodine contrast detection were the commonest causes for exclusion. A linear correlation was found between absolute coronary arterial blood flow and both the washout rate ($r = 0.85$) and the inverse of the time to peak myocardial concentration ($r = 0.85$) (Fig. 16–30). Analyses during hyperemia significantly improved the ability of both indexes to distinguish between normal and ischemic regions, and the effect was most marked in the washout rate analysis. The investigators argue that the measurement of the time to peak concentration should be less affected by delayed contrast-induced hyperemia than the washout rate calculation that is obtained slightly later in time. The comparable relation of both indexes to absolute coronary flow suggested, therefore, that delayed contrast effects did not importantly affect the washout portion of the densograms in this study.

Impulse Response (Transfer Function) Analysis

Eigler and associates[E1, 2] extended the work of Whiting and colleagues by introducing the concept of transfer function analysis and linear systems theory.[B1, 2, 3, N1] The approach is intended to address several unsolved problems, including lack of a validated physiologic model of contrast flow, systematic errors in densitometry, dependence on contrast agent injection technique, and the transient or variable effects of contrast material, or other hyperemic stimuli, on flow. In the linear systems theory, the transfer function predicts the output of the system (obtained from a myocardial region of interest) to any input signal (obtained from a region of interest near the injection catheter tip) if the param-

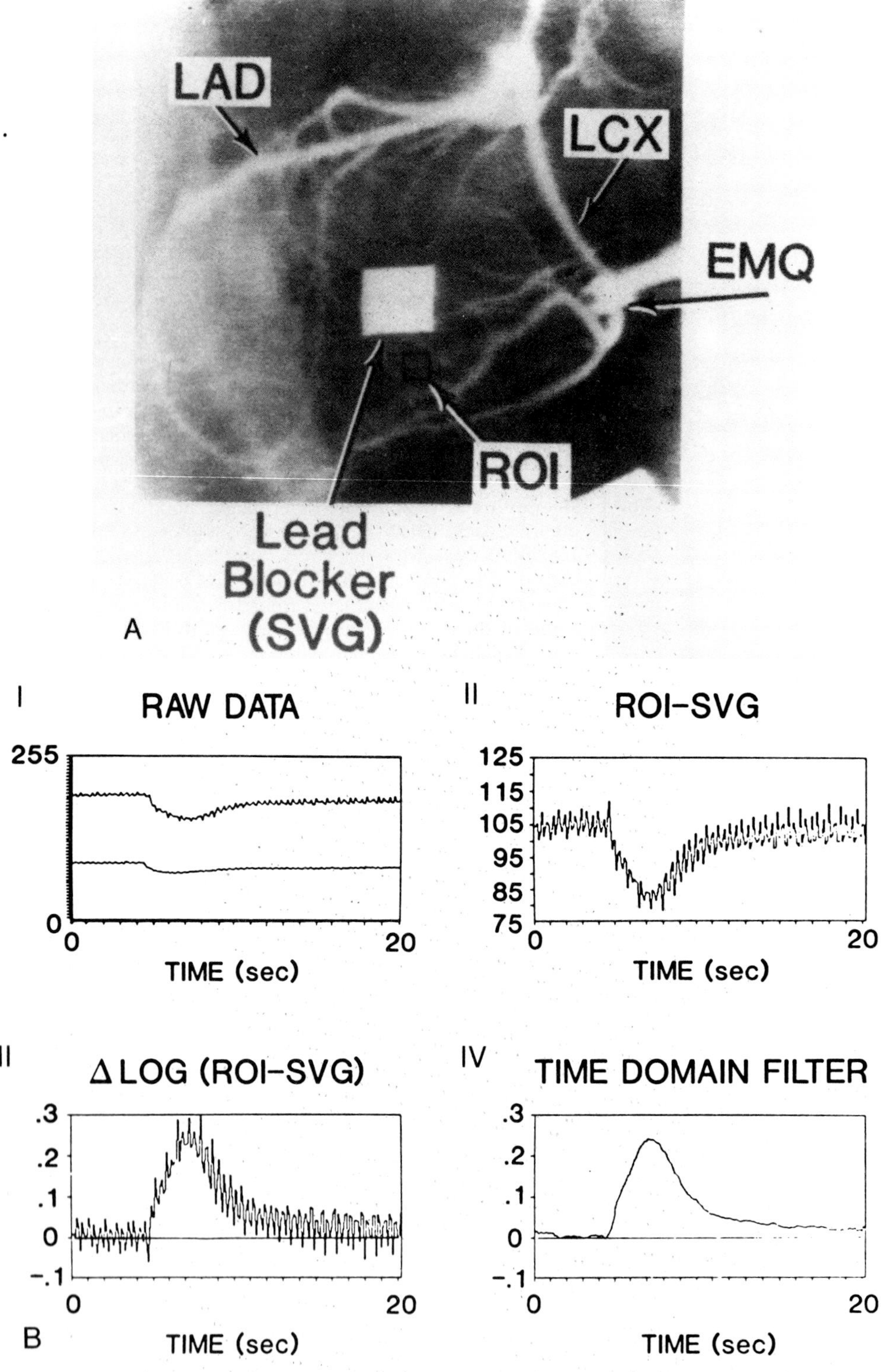

Figure 16–29. *A*, Digital angiogram illustrating the experimental configuration. Contrast material was injected into the left main coronary artery. The electromagnetic flowmeter probe (EMQ) was placed around the left circumflex coronary artery (LCX), and the snare occluder (not visualized) was placed just distal to the probe. The lateral projection was used to minimize overlap of the LCX and left anterior descending (LAD) perfusion beds. A 10 × 10 pixel region of interest (ROI) was placed over the myocardium served by the LCX. Scatter and veiling glare (SVG) were determined by measuring the intensity over a lead blocker placed adjacent to the myocardial region of interest. *B*, Processing steps used to obtain accurate time-concentration curves include I, raw data over myocardium (region of interest, ROI) and lead blocker (scatter and veiling glare, SVG); II, subtraction of SVG; III, logarithmic subtraction of data from pre-injection intensity; IV, moving average (two cardiac cycles) applied to each point in III to filter high-frequency intensity variations. (From Whiting, J.S., et al.: Digital angiographic measurements of radiographic contrast material kinetics for estimation of myocardial perfusion. Circulation 73:789, 1986, with permission of the American Heart Association, Inc.)

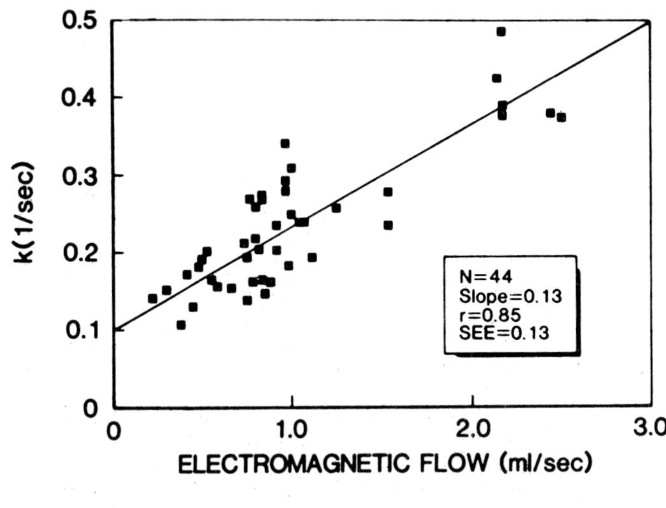

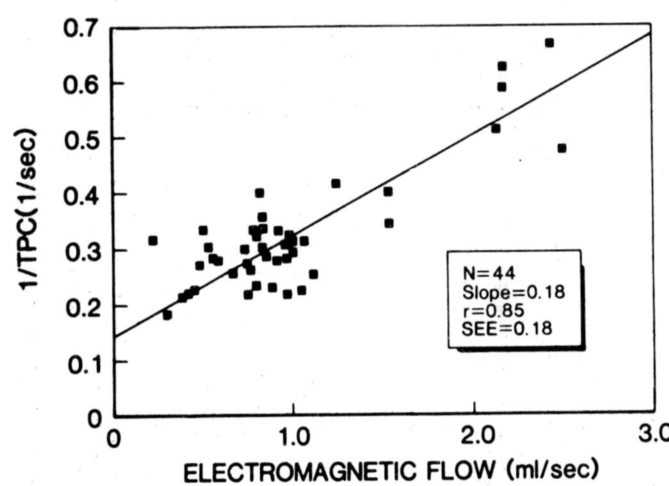

Figure 16–30. Perfusion indexes versus coronary arterial blood flow measured by electromagnetic flowmeter for 31 studies in six dogs. Flow was varied from 0.2 to 2.4 ml/sec by snare occluder and dipyridamole. Washout rate *(upper panel)* varied from approximately 0.1 to 0.4/sec, and the inverse of time to peak concentration (TPC; *lower curve*) varied from 0.2 to 0.6/sec. The differences in slope and correlation coefficient between the two indexes were not significant. (From Whiting, J.S., et al.: Digital angiographic measurement of radiographic contrast material kinetics for estimation of myocardial perfusion. Circulation 73:789, 1986, with permission of the American Heart Association, Inc.)

eters describing the system have two essential characteristics. First, they must remain constant (principle of stationarity) and, second, the output function in response to a combination of simultaneous inputs must equal the sum of the outputs in response to each input applied separately (principle of superposition). Unlike the washout method, this method uses the entire washin and washout curve obtained from both the input (proximal arterial) and output (myocardial) regions of interest (Fig. 16–31). By investigating both phantom and animal models, they were able to demonstrate that this approach is insensitive to differences in hyperemic stimuli and contrast injection technique. Thus, differences in the effects of hyperemic stimuli on vascular volume do not affect the analysis, in contrast to techniques listed in the next section. In addition, gated power injection of contrast becomes unnecessary. They demonstrated that the mean transit time of the coronary system (the mean system transit time) obtained by this calculation is inversely proportional to actual flow per contrast distribution volume, normalized for myocardial mass (Fig. 16–32). In these experiments, the time to peak concentration and the washout time were found to be inferior to the system transit time as indexes of flow. Thus, this method utilizes the entire washin and washout curve, but an overall system transit time, not washout time, is calculated. The relation between the mean system transit-time calculation and myocardial flow, however, was bimodal (see Fig. 16–32), in that the analysis yielded higher flow per distribution volume in perfusion zones supplied by nonstenotic arteries than in zones supplied by stenotic arteries, even though actual flow per gram of myocardium was similar. This was interpreted to reflect the normal, autoregulatory vascular vasodilation that is expected to occur in the

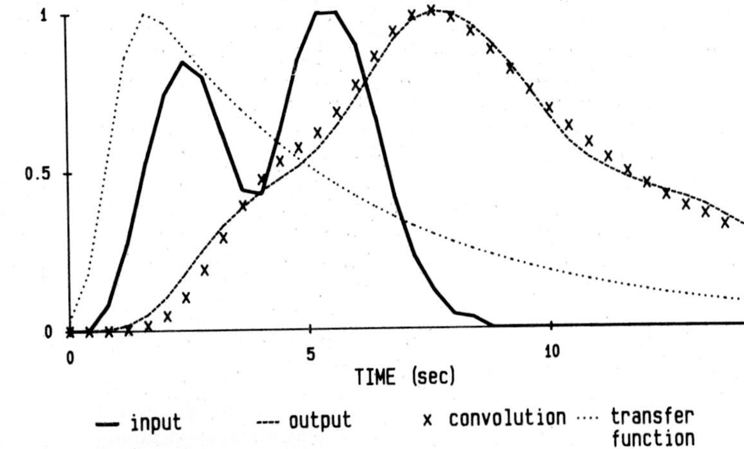

Figure 16–31. Derivation of the system transfer function by iterative convolution. The input time-density function over the left main coronary artery has a complex double-peaked bolus shape, owing to deliberate, double-hand injection of contrast agent. Such injection is also reflected in the output function acquired over the left circumflex artery–supplied microcirculation. A lagged-normal density model was iteratively convolved with the input curve, and its parameters were serially adjusted until the result of the convolution converged on the observed output function. The final model is the system transfer function. (From Eigler, N.L., et al.: Digital angiographic transfer function analysis of regional myocardial perfusion. Measurement system and coronary contrast transit linearity. *In* Heintzen, P.H., and Bürsch, J.H. (eds.): Progress in Digital Angiocardiography. Kluwer Academic, Dordrecht, 1988, p. 265, with permission.)

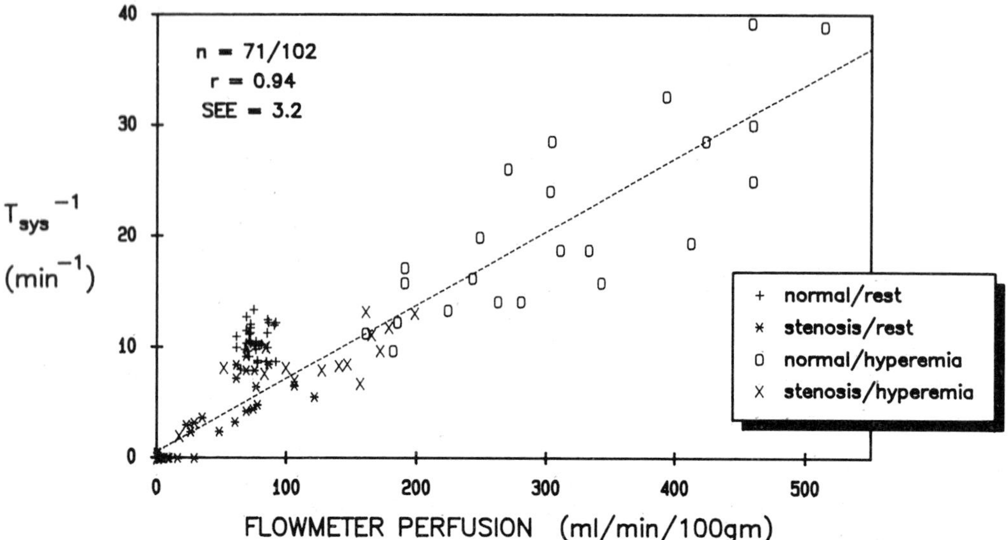

Figure 16–32. Animal study comparing angiographic mean system transit time (T_{sys}^{-1}) with flowmeter perfusion for all injections during four flow states. A bimodal relationship is evident with normal/rest values of T_{sys}^{-1} greater than stenosis/rest values for the same flow. The regression line has been plotted for all states except normal/rest state. (From Eigler, N.L., et al.: Digital angiographic transfer function analysis of regional myocardial perfusion: Measurement system and coronary contrast transit linearity. *In* Heintzen, P.H., and Bürsch, J.H. (eds.): Progress in Digital Angiocardiography. Kluwer Academic, Dordrecht, 1988, p. 265, with permission.)

presence of a coronary stenosis. They hypothesized that the observed flow-dependent changes in distribution volume were a consequence of the normal mechanism that regulates coronary flow.

As the myocardial microcirculation vasodilates to decrease vascular resistance and thus maintain flow in the presence of stenosis, or to augment flow following a hyperemic stimulus, vascular capacitance simultaneously increases, as reflected by an increased distribution volume of the contrast material. This sensitivity of the mean transit time to autoregulatory vasodilatation represents a new finding that may help differentiate normal and stenotic arteries at rest without requiring a prior hyperemic stimulus.

Appearance Time and Density Analysis

This approach was developed empirically at the University of Michigan in two distinct stages. In the first phase of development, the concept that appearance of contrast in the myocardium was inversely proportional to flow was explored. This method is an outgrowth of the transit-time method, but it had the advantage of not requiring potentially inaccurate geometric calculations of arterial segments, was geared toward measurement of relative, not absolute, flow, did not require high temporal resolution or precise dosages of contrast, and did not require subselective injection of contrast. Additionally, the early phase of contrast washin was analyzed to avoid the potential problems inherent in washout analyses that may coincide with the time when flow has been substantially perturbed by contrast material. The results with this early approach showed a good correlation with measures of coronary sinus and great cardiac vein flow in patients in whom variations in flow were induced with atrial pacing.[V3, 4] Some degree of underestimation of flow ratios was noted in this early application, although the method was useful as a gauge of stenosis severity. Similarly, Rutishauser's group demonstrated that a variation of the appearance-time technique based on pixel by pixel calculation of the time to maximal opacification or the time to mean ascending time[B16] was effective in stratifying normal and ischemic myocardium.[D1, R3, 4]

Animal validation studies, however, demonstrated a substantial underestimation of flow reserve values by the appearance-time method when flow was altered by papaverine or contrast material instead of atrial pacing[H3] (Fig. 16–33). Hodgson and colleagues highlighted the potential importance of the density information in helping rectify this problem[H3] (Fig. 16–34). In the absence of incorporation of the density information, appearance time can be considered to be inversely proportional to flow only if the contrast concentration remains constant and if the volume of dispersion remains constant. That is, Q1 = RVV/t1, Q2 = RVV/t2, so that Q1/Q2 = t2/t1, where Q = flow, RVV = regional vascular volume, and t = transit time (appearance time in this application).

Whereas this was apparently adequate with the relatively weak stimulus provided by atrial pacing,[V3, 4] in the presence of papaverine and/or contrast material, the effects on regional vascular volume were much more significant. Indeed, subjective analysis of the images revealed a distinctly brighter, more intense image after contrast- or papaverine-induced hyperemia induction than after atrial pacing, and this suggested that the volume of distribution was not constant in the face of the profound, pharmacologically induced hyperemia.

Recruitment of capillaries,[T3] capillary dilatation,[B11, R5] fluid shifts into the vascular compartment,[F10, L10] dilation of epicardial arteries,[G6] and increases in the total myocardial vascular volume[C1, 3, H8, W1, 11] have all been observed during pharmacologically induced hyperemia. Accordingly, an estimate of RVV for both the baseline and hyperemic images was obtained as follows: RVV = (k/c) $\int$ D, where k is a radiographic constant, c = contrast medium con-

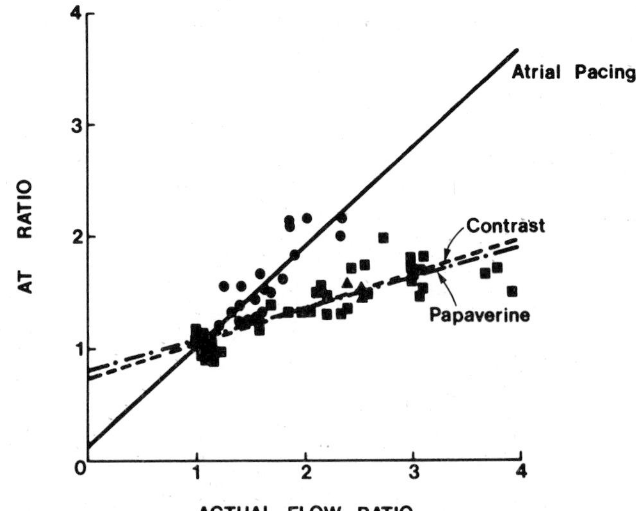

Figure 16–33. Comparison of appearance time (AT) ratios calculated for differing methods of inducing hyperemia. Actual flow ratios were calculated from coronary sinus flow measurements for atrial pacing and from electromagnetic flow measurements for both contrast- and papaverine-induced hyperemia. Note the marked underestimation of actual flow ratios for both methods of pharmacologically induced hypermia. The *circles* represent atrial pacing hyperemia; the *squares* represent contrast-induced hyperemia; the *triangles* represent papaverine-induced hyperemia. (From Hodgson, J.M., et al.: Validation in dogs of a rapid digital angiographic technique to measure relative coronary blood flow during routine cardiac catheterization. Am. J. Cardiol. 55:188, 1985, with permission.)

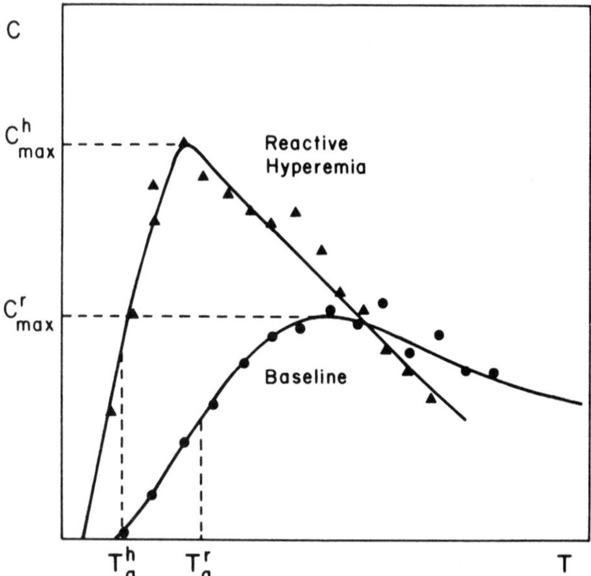

Figure 16–34. Contrast pass curve measured in a myocardial region of interest using videodensitometry for normal resting flow (r) and for flow during reactive hyperemia (h). The abscissa represents time (T), and the ordinate represents contrast density (C). (From Cusma, J.T., Toggart, E.J., Folts, J.D., et al.: Digital subtraction angiographic imaging of coronary flow reserve. Circulation 75:461, 1987, with permission of the American Heart Association, Inc.)

centration, and D = radiographic density. The radiographic constant (k) is a function of the attenuation coefficient of the iodine medium, the transfer function of the image intensifier and plumbicon, the radiographic parameters used, and the analog-to-digital conversion function. If sufficient contrast is injected under both basal and hyperemic conditions, then c can be considered to be 100 percent under both conditions, and it cancels out. Similarly, if radiographic technique is maintained constant and if the same region of the image is analyzed in the basal and hyperemic states, then k also cancels out. Accordingly, an estimate of RVV is given by the accumulated radiographic density within a region. Thus, the relation between two flows can be given by $Q1/Q2 = \{D1/t1\}/\{D2/t2\}$. To compensate for uncertainties in timing due to the limited temporal resolution of the images (1 per cycle), ECG-gated contrast injections were used and appearance times were assigned as 0.5, 1.5, 2.5, and so on, for each consecutive cardiac cycle after contrast injection. Whenever heart rate stability could not be maintained by atrial pacing, then cycle length appearance times were converted to absolute seconds. Using these empiric approaches, Hodgson and co-workers demonstrated a marked improvement over the previous method based solely on appearance times. A strong linear correlation with simultaneously measured electromagnetic flow was demonstrated in the animal model (Fig. 16–35). Figure 16–36 is an example from a patient with normal coronary reserve.

Figure 16–36. See Color Plate 1.

Cusma, Mistretta, and co-workers investigated a refinement of the Hodgson technique in an animal model that included single vessel coronary stenoses.[C4] Several differences are noteworthy. The image acquisition was at a higher frame rate (15/sec), giving greater flexibility in selecting frames for analysis and in temporal precision. The analyzed frames usually consisted of 8 to 10 end-diastolic images. Each pixel of the image was analyzed to create two separate data sets that encoded the time of peak opacification and the peak intensity (Fig. 16–37). The time of arrival of contrast was determined on a pixel by pixel basis with a linear interpolation algorithm to estimate the time at which contrast density reached half its maximal value (Fig. 16–38). The peak opacification data set was divided by the time of arrival data set to obtain a composite parametric "flow" image, being inversely proportional to flow and directly proportional to peak opacification. This process was repeated for a hyperemic image. The two resultant parametric images encoded the ratio of contrast density to arrival time, analogous to the method of Hodgson. The basal image encoded a pixel by pixel index of resting "flow," and the hyperemic image encoded the index of maximal flow. A final parametric image was produced by dividing the results from the basal analysis into the hyperemic analysis, thereby creating a single parametric image that encoded a "flow reserve" estimate for each pixel (Fig. 16–39). Excellent image registration was mandatory to create this final image. These investigators developed an explicit mathematical model emphasizing the importance of adequate contrast administration to ensure that the contrast concentration was virtually 100 percent during both basal and hyperemic conditions. That is, a sufficient bolus was required to prevent mixing between blood and contrast. Under such conditions, excellent correlations with measured flow reserves were demonstrated (Fig. 16–40). Because mixing is more likely to occur during hyperemic flow, the result of insufficient contrast administration is an underestimation of the flow ratio at high values (Figs. 16–40 and 16–41). Using this mathematical model, the investigators were also able to demonstrate the relative constancy of the effects of the radiographic parameters discussed earlier and the small effects of uncorrected scatter and veiling glare when measuring relative flow parameters.

General Comparative Summary

As is evident from the foregoing discussion, the interest in the application of digital angiography to the measurement of coronary dynamics is intense and has led to a great variety of approaches. No consensus currently exists as to which method is most reliable or most applicable in a clinical setting. Each method presents counterbalancing advantages and disadvantages. These can be summarized as follows: all methods designed to measure actual flow or flow per distribution volume must correct meticulously

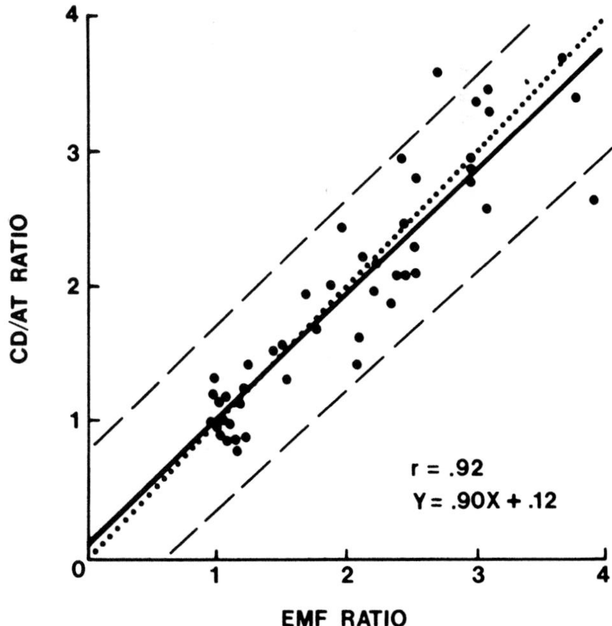

Figure 16–35. Correlation of coronary flow reserve ratios measured by electromagnetic flow (EMF) probe, and ratios calculated digitally using both contrast density and appearance time (CD/AT) (in seconds) information. Confidence limits (95 percent) are represented by the dashed lines. Digital CD/AT ratios correlated well with EMF ratios and were more accurate than appearance time ratios alone. (From Hodgson, J.Mc.B., Legrand, V., Bates, E.R., et al.: Validation in dogs of a rapid digital angiographic technique to measure relative coronary blood flow during routine cardiac catheterization. Am. J. Cardiol. 55:188, 1985, with permission.)

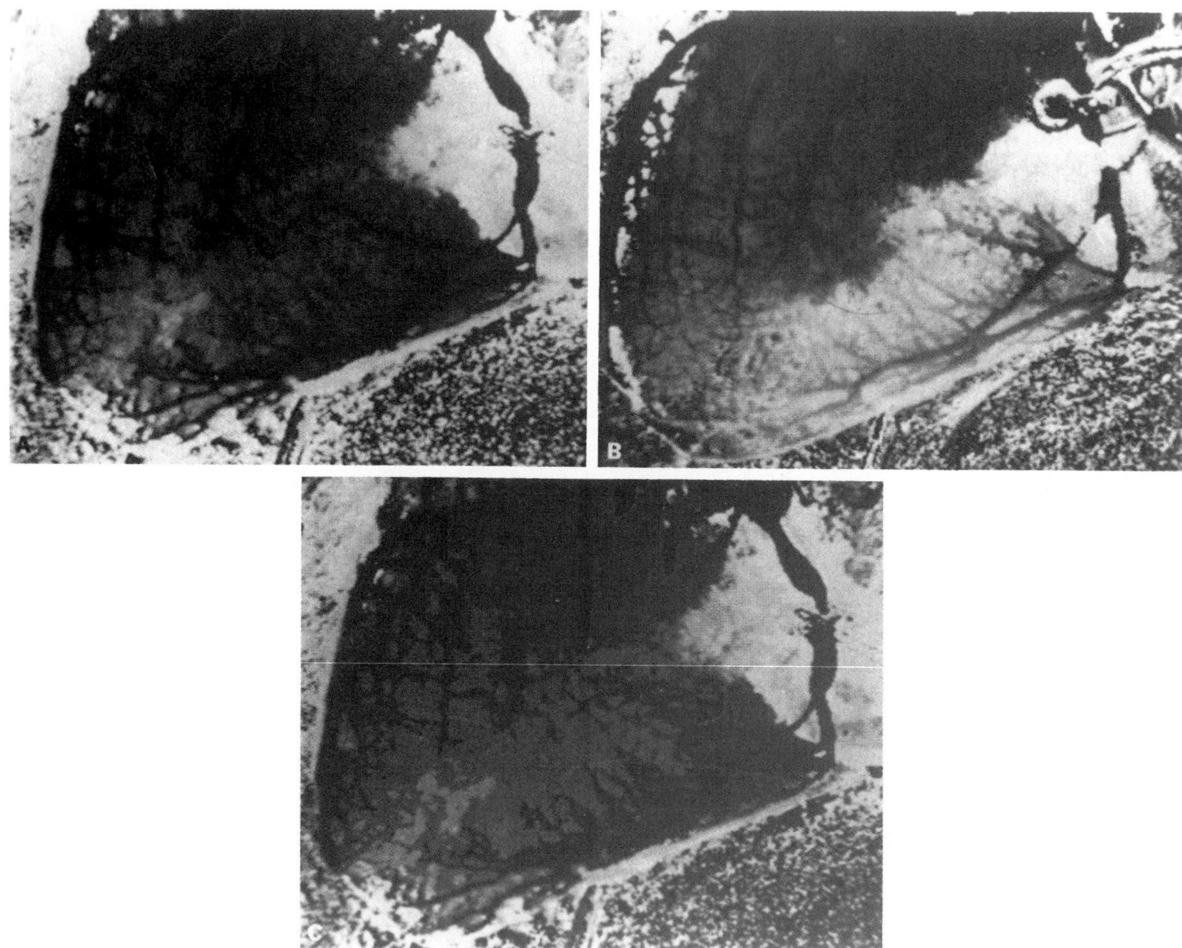

Figure 16–37. Interpolated time of arrival images produced during hyperemia. *A*, Time of arrival image for a normal canine heart. *B*, Time of arrival image for the same heart with a severe stenosis produced on the circumflex artery. *C*, Time of arrival image produced without temporal interpolation, i.e., using one sample per cardiac cycle. (From Cusma, J.T., Toggart, E.J., Folts, J.D., et al.: Digital subtraction angiographic imaging of coronary flow reserve. Circulation 75:461, 1987, with permission of the American Heart Association, Inc.)

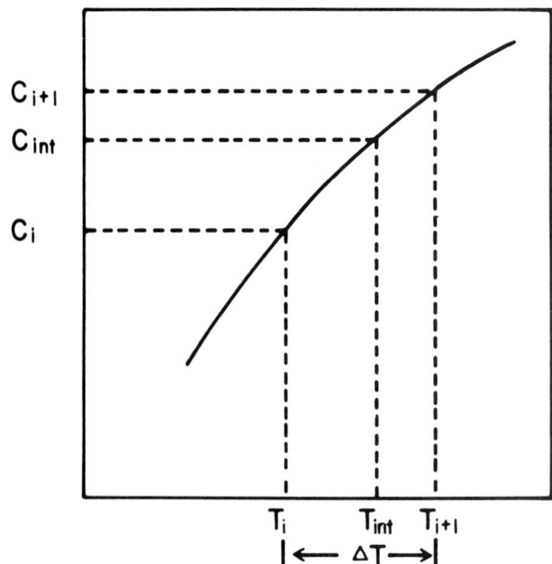

Figure 16–38. Interpolation algorithm used to calculate contrast values during the cardiac cycle. Values measured once every heart cycle are used to determine the contrast values for intermediate points in the cycle. (From Cusma, J.T., Toggart, E.J., Folts, J.D., et al.: Digital subtraction angiographic imaging of coronary flow reserve. Circulation 75:461, 1987, with permission of the American Heart Association, Inc.)

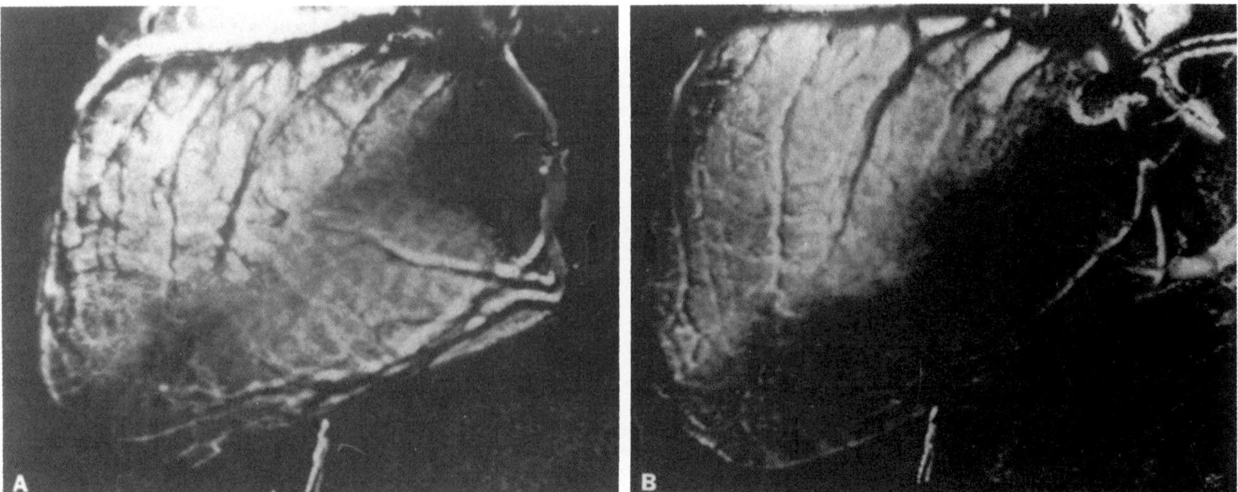

Figure 16–39. Parametric flow ratio images. *A*, Flow ratio image for a normal dog heart. *B*, Image for the same heart with a severe stenosis placed on the circumflex branch, which reduced the coronary reserve in that vessel to unity. (From Cusma, J.T., Toggart, E.J., Folts, J.D., et al.: Digital subtraction angiographic imaging of coronary flow reserve. Circulation 75:461, 1987, with permission of the American Heart Association, Inc.)

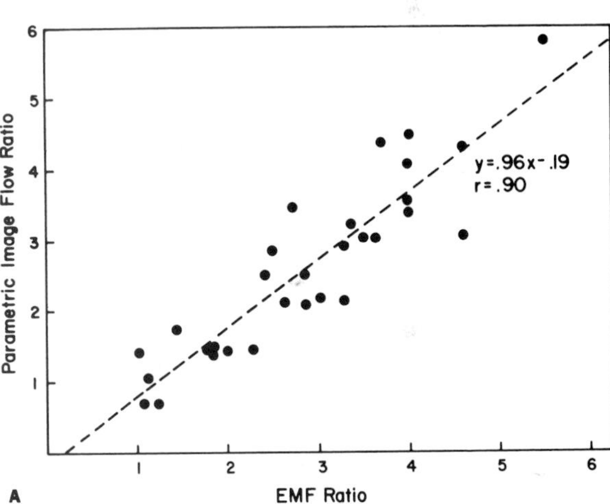

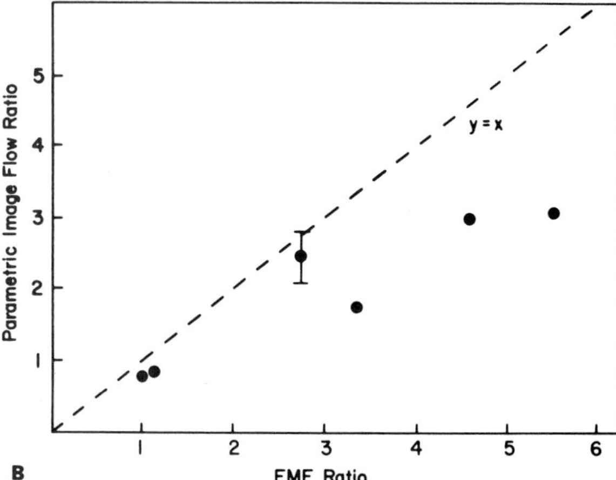

Figure 16–40. Results of flow ratio calculations using parametric images plotted against ratios calculated from electromagnetic flow probe (EMF) measurements. *A*, Results obtained with a contrast injection rate chosen to avoid dilution of contrast. *B*, Results obtained with an injection rate of 3 ml/sec. (From Cusma, J.T., Toggart, E.J., Folts, J.D., et al.: Digital subtraction angiographic imaging of coronary flow reserve. Circulation 75:461, 1987, with permission of the American Heart Association, Inc.)

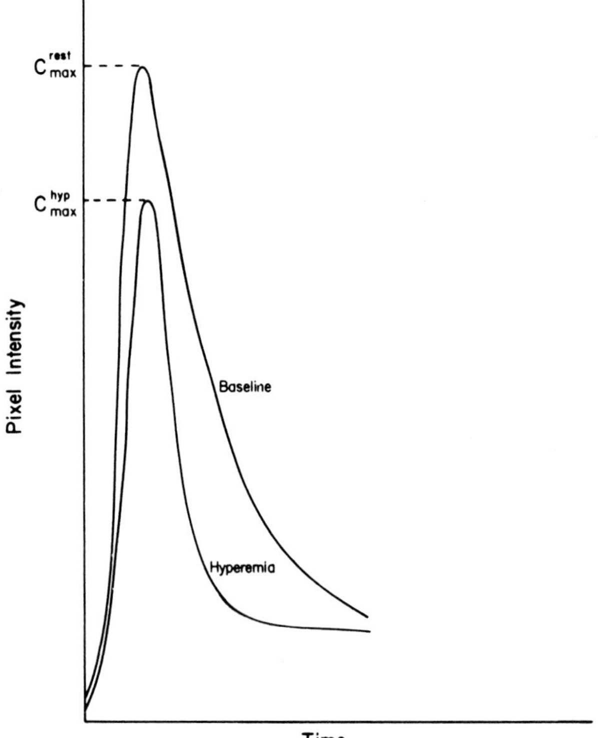

Figure 16–41. Contrast pass curve measured in the circumflex artery after injection at a rate of 3 ml/sec during baseline flow and during hyperemia. (From Cusma, J.T., Toggart, E.J., Folts, J.D., et al.: Digital subtraction angiographic imaging of coronary flow reserve. Circulation 75:461, 1987, with permission of the American Heart Association, Inc.)

for the nonlinear relation between x-ray attenuation and iodine depth. All methods that do not employ atrial pacing and gated-ECG power injection must compensate by utilizing high-frame rate image acquisitions and/or complex mathematical corrections. Methods based solely on transit time or appearance time are prone to errors caused by potential changes in vessel cross-sectional area or changes in regional vascular volume that are produced by coronary vasodilators. These methods, in addition, must either be constrained to measures of mean transit time because of the phasic nature of coronary flow, or they must be applied after repeated boluses of contrast at different phases of the cardiac cycle. These methods are even further compromised when coupled with geometric vessel volume measurements to calculate flow because of inaccuracies in quantifying the volume of arterial segments that may be tortuous or foreshortened. Methods based solely on the washout portion of contrast densograms must use high frame rate acquisitions and must invoke mathematical corrections to avoid errors caused by perturbations of the tail of the curves that can be caused by superimposition of contrast-laden structures, recirculation, and the delayed effects of contrast material itself on flow. Strict indicator-dilution methods mandate subselective injection of precise volumes of contrast. Only additional research will determine which trade-offs are appropriate for achieving an acceptable degree of accuracy in the clinical application of this important digital technique.

Achieving Maximal Hyperemia in the Clinical Setting

Aside from the technical issues noted, the accurate assessment of coronary flow reserve is also dependent upon achievement of maximal coronary hyperemia so that mild-to-moderate impairments in flow reserve can be differentiated from normal. In practice, the choice of agents is currently limited to essentially three: hyperosmolar contrast media, intravenous dipyridamole, and intracoronary papaverine. Although contrast material itself has been used to achieve hyperemia, it has long been recognized that the hyperemia is not maximum, and, moreover, the hyperemia is very short lived. Since timing of the digital image acquisition is crucial, this latter factor also detracts from the use of hyperosmolar contrast media for induction of hyperemia.

Foult and Nitenberg assessed intravenous dipyridamole (0.56 mg/kg) and intracoronary doses of ioxaglate (8 ml) and showed a very close correlation of coronary flow and resistance reserve values by each method.[F7] However, a better separation between normals and patients was achieved after dipyridamole infusion. Although intravenous dipyridamole does achieve maximal or near-maximal hyperemia when used in doses of between 0.56 and 0.84 mg/kg, several disadvantages are associated with its use. First, its long-lasting effects make repeated assessment of the hyperemic response of a coronary vascular bed or assessment of different coronary vascular beds during the same procedure impractical. Second, the long-lasting endoepicardial redistribution of coronary blood flow in conjunction with an increase in myocardial oxygen consumption may induce ischemia, requiring termination by the intravenous administration of aminophylline.

Intracoronary papaverine in doses of between 8 and 12 mg is currently the agent of choice for the assessment of coronary flow reserve by selective angiographic methods. Bookstein and Higgins have shown in dogs that the coronary hyperemic response after a bolus injection of papaverine into a coronary artery is of the same magnitude as after a 15-sec occlusion of the coronary artery.[B8] Hodgson and Williams compared induction of hyperemia in humans administered papaverine and hyperosmolar contrast media and showed a twofold greater hyperemic response after papaverine.[H6] Wilson and White assessed doses of 4, 8, 12, and 16 mg of intracoronary papaverine and demonstrated a maximal hyperemic response after 8 mg in most left coronary arteries and after 12 mg in all left coronary arteries.[W7] In the right coronary artery, the equivalent doses were 6 and 8 mg, respectively. The onset of maximal vasodilation after papaverine injection was around 16 seconds. It peaked and was maintained for 49 seconds on average, and the effects had nearly dissipated completely by approximately 128 seconds (Fig. 16–42). Zijlstra and colleagues demonstrated excellent reproducibility of the coronary hyperemic response after intracoronary papaverine.[Z1] The maximal hyperemic response occurred between 24 and 37 seconds after injection, and effects completely dissipated within 5 minutes, thus allowing repeated assessments of coronary flow reserve.

Intracoronary injection of papaverine appears to be a safe procedure when it is used in doses of 12 mg or less. Practitioners should be aware of transient ST-T changes, Q-T prolongation, and the appearance of U waves. Anecdotal cases of ventricular tachycardia and fibrillation, as well as elucidation of enhancement of stimulated ventricular arrhythmias, have been reported.[L12, M2] These effects on myocardial repolarization may not be due to subendocardial ischemia or "coronary steal," since they have been seen in normal individuals. In over 300 cases, Wilson and White demonstrated only two instances of serious ventricular dysrhythmias, and one occurred in a patient with normal coronary arteries.[W9]

Some contrast material may interact with papaverine to form a potentially toxic precipitate.[P4] This has not been noted with nonionic contrast materials.[M6] It is recommended that doses should not exceed 12 mg for the left coronary system and 8 mg for the right coronary system. Additionally, the drug should not be flushed into the coronary artery with solutions other than normal saline or other physiologic solutions unless drug incompatibilities have been deliberately examined and excluded.[P4, M6]

Directly administered vasodilators, such as papaverine, and systemically administered agents, such as dipyridamole, may affect established or potential collateral flow differently. These potential differences have not been elucidated. Since the presence of collateral flow, either at rest or during hyperemia, substantially affects the measurement of myocardial vascular reserve by digital techniques and catheter techniques, fuller investigation of the consequences of these potential differences on the accuracy of parametric digital imaging is needed. Currently, for techniques using selective angiographic digital angiography, papaverine is the agent of choice.

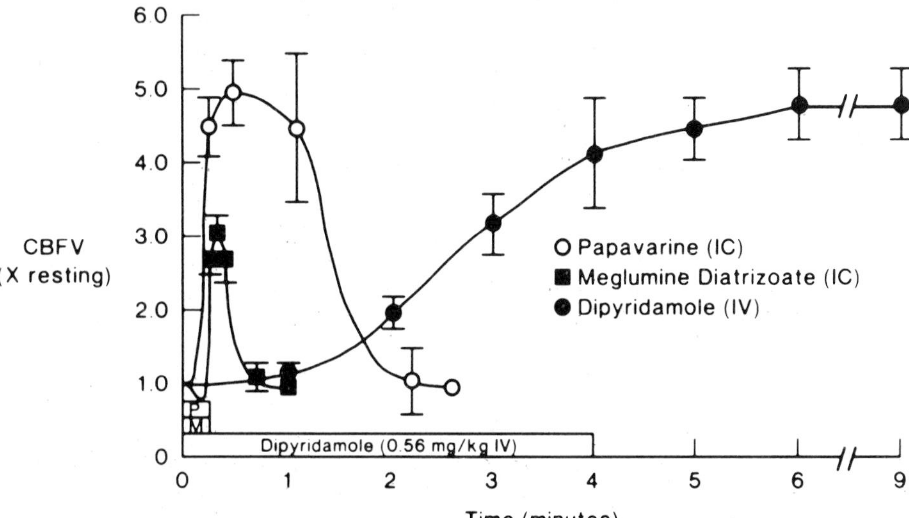

Figure 16–42. Schematic display of the average change in coronary blood flow velocity (CBFV) after administration of each coronary vasodilator. (From Wilson, R.F., and White, C.W.: Intracoronary papaverine: An ideal coronary vasodilator for studies of the coronary circulation in conscious humans. Circulation 73:444, 1986, with permission of the American Heart Association, Inc.)

Physiologic Assessment of Coronary Artery Disease

As outlined earlier, several of the various methods of measuring coronary flow or flow reserve have been applied in clinical settings. The bulk of digital applications has been with the method described by Vogel and colleagues[V3, 4] and its refinement proposed by Hodgson and associates[H3, L8] and others.[D1, R3, 4] The methods have also been applied in humans through postprocessing of cineangiograms (see Chapter 13).

Legrand and co-workers undertook a comparative study of flow reserve, quantitative percent stenosis, and exercise test measurements in patients with coronary disease.[L10] Two broad groups were investigated—those with and those without prior infarction and/or collateralized zones. In patients without prior infarction or collateral vessels, a rough correlation between percent stenosis measurement and flow reserve values was found. There was strong concordance among exercise-induced regional wall motion abnormalities or thallium defects, percent diameter stenosis greater than 50 percent in the artery serving that region, and flow reserve values of less than 2 measured by contrast-induced hyperemia and digital angiography. Strongest concordance was noted with very severe (>75 percent) and very mild (<25 percent) stenoses. The clinical and diagnostic value of the flow reserve and exercise test results was greatest in determining the functional significance of the intermediate-grade lesions, especially when single-vessel disease was present. In the presence of multivessel disease, the exercise test results tended to reflect congruity only with the vascular bed showing the most severely depressed flow reserve and/or percent stenosis (Figs. 16–43 through 16–45).

In the setting of prior infarction or collateral flow or both, there was a significant relation between abnormal exercise test results and stenoses greater than 50 percent. Coronary flow reserve measurements, however, tended to be extremely low and, therefore, correlated less well with percent diameter stenosis. Moreover, the exercise-induced regional abnormalities were associated with lower flow reserve values (<1.3) than in the group without infarction or collaterals (see Figs. 16–43 through 16–45).

These studies underscore the value of coronary flow reserve measurememts in assessing the true significance of moderate stenoses and the caution required when evaluating the meaning of isolated flow reserve measurements in the presence of prior infarction or collateralization.

Legrand and co-workers also studied patients with atypical chest pain and normal coronary arteries and demonstrated that those individuals with exercise-induced radionuclide abnormalities also tended to have abnormal vasodilator reserve (Fig. 16–46).[L9] These radionuclide abnormalities, sometimes considered to represent false-positive results, were actually true-positive results revealing underlying functional abnormalities of flow not attributable to epicardial stenoses.

Hodgson and co-workers determined flow reserve before and after angioplasty in 20 patients with single vessel disease.[H4] Using papaverine as the hyperemic stimulus, they demonstrated a doubling of the flow reserve value after the procedure that was of a similar magnitude in adjacent nonstenotic and nondilated arteries. The flow reserve in these arteries, however, was decidedly less than that measured by the same technique in totally normal individuals, thereby suggesting the presence of unrecognized coronary disease in angiographically normal coronary arteries.

Physiologic Assessment of Bypass Grafts

Bates and co-workers used digital angiography to assess the adequacy of bypass grafts soon and late after surgery.[B4–6] Immediate and sustained improvements were measured that were equivalent to results achieved by angioplasty, but flow reserve measurements were still depressed relative to normal values (Fig. 16–47). This latter finding remains controversial.[W8] It possibly reflects residual, diffuse atherosclerosis, alterations of adrenergic tone, arteriolar intimal thickening and fibrosis, or chronic microembolization of platelet aggregates. Others have argued that methodologic limitations may have precluded measurements of high flow reserves due to the use of contrast material as the vasodilator.[W8]

Hodgson and colleagues compared the flow reserve of sequential internal mammary bypass grafts to that of sequential and single saphenous vein grafts.[H5] All results were comparable, but overall the values achieved were less than expected in totally normal patients, a finding similar to that of Bates and colleagues.

CONCLUSIONS

The ultimate role of cardiac digital angiography will rest upon the demonstration that quantitative arteriography and functional imaging provide diagnostically important information that may also be of prognostic benefit, and that this information can be obtained, stored, and communicated in an efficient and cost-effective manner. Although scientific information about the former continues to accrue at a rapid rate, the latter, more practical issues have prevented broader and faster acceptance of the technique in clinical practice. The rapid availability of images and the ability to quantify them quickly have not provided sufficient motivation to allow full acceptance of the existing technology. Accordingly, continued vigorous scientific and engineering efforts over the next decade will be necessary to determine the ultimate role of digital angiography in assessing both the morphologic and functional aspects of the coronary circulation.

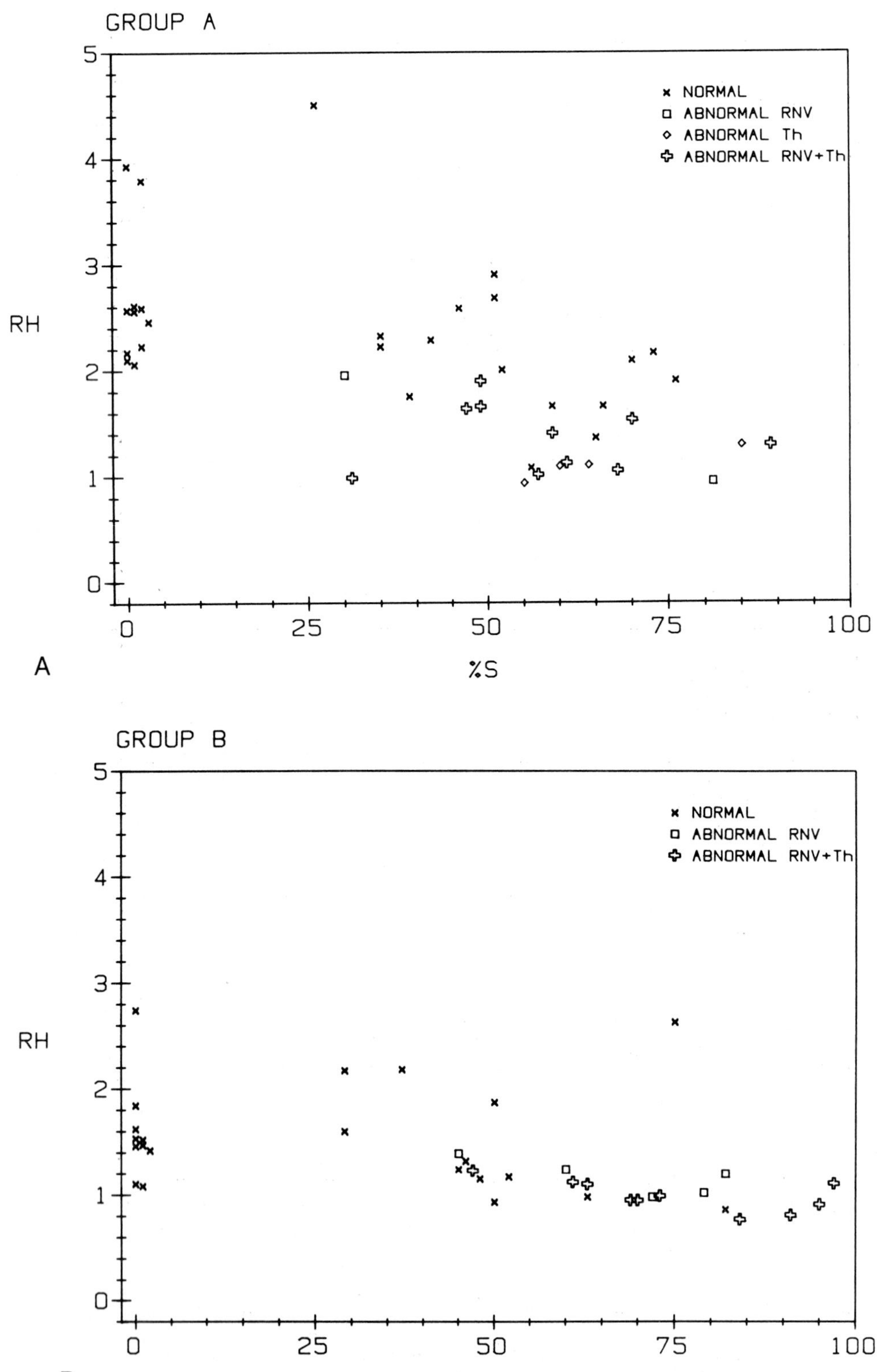

Figure 16–43. Relation between quantitative percent diameter stenosis (%S) and reactive hyperemia (RH) in Group A (without collaterals) and Group B (with collaterals). x—normal exercise test results, □—abnormal radionuclide ventriculography result (RNV), ◇—abnormal thallium (Th) result, ✜ —both tests were abnormal. (Adapted from Legrand, V., Mancini, G.B.J., Bates, E.R., et al.: Comparative study of coronary flow reserve, coronary anatomy and results of radionuclide exercise tests in patients with coronary artery disease. J. Am. Coll. Cardiol. 8:1022, 1986. Reprinted with permission of the American College of Cardiology.)

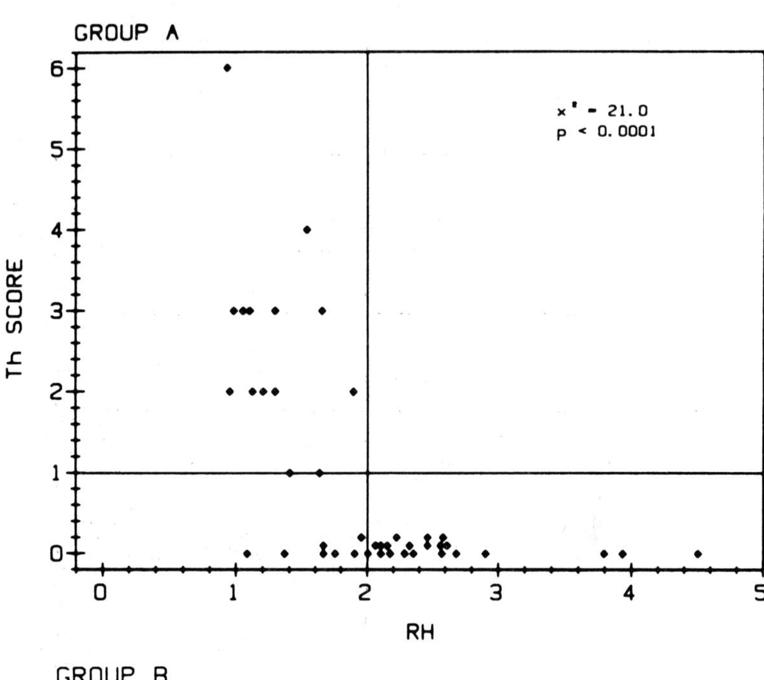

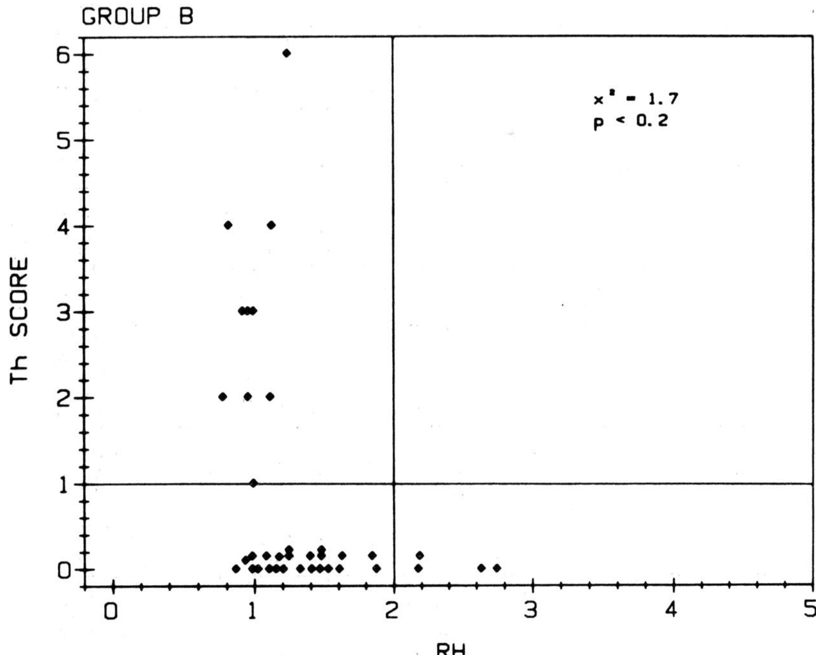

Figure 16–44. Relation between exercise thallium-201 tests and reactive hyperemia (RH). Th score—the difference in regional thallium scores between exercise and redistribution images, with a score of 1 or greater signifying a positive test. (From Legrand, V., Mancini, G.B.J., Bates, E.R., et al.: Comparative study of coronary flow reserve, coronary anatomy and results of radionuclide exercise tests in patients with coronary artery disease. J. Am. Coll. Cardiol. 8:1022, 1986. Reprinted with permission of the American College of Cardiology.)

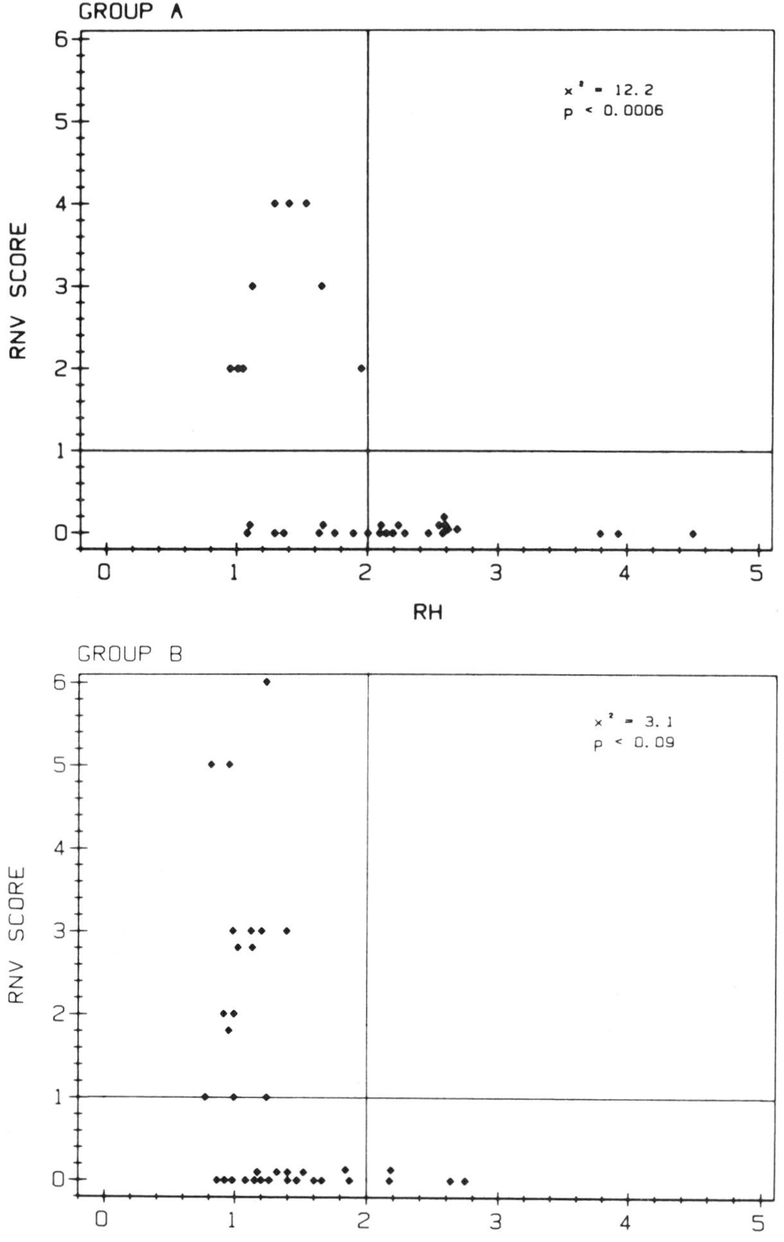

Figure 16–45. Relation between reactive hyperemia and exercise radionuclide ventriculography, demonstrated as in Figure 16–44. (From Legrand, V., Mancini, G.B.J., Bates, E.R., et al.: Comparative study of coronary flow reserve, coronary anatomy and results of radionuclide exercise tests in patients with coronary artery disease. J. Am. Coll. Cardiol. 8:1022, 1986. Reprinted with permission of the American College of Cardiology.)

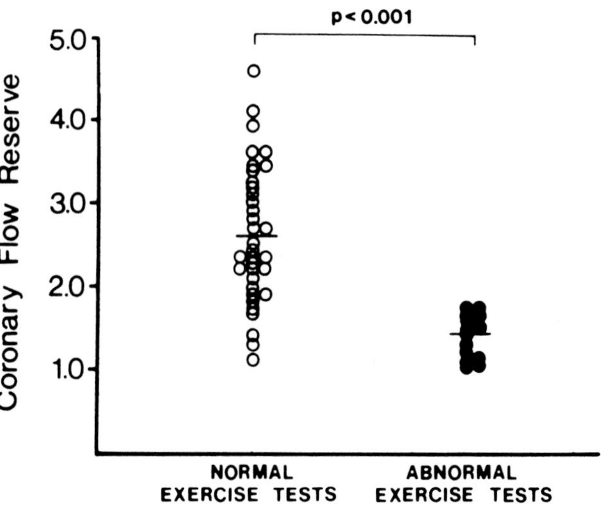

Figure 16–46. Coronary flow reserve for arterial distributions without *(open circles)* and with *(closed circles)* radionuclide abnormalities (exercise thallium-201 scintigraphy or radionuclide ventriculography, or both). (From Legrand, V., Hodgson, J.McB., Bates, E.R., et al.: Abnormal coronary flow reserve and abnormal radionuclide exercise tests in patients with normal coronary angiograms. J. Am. Coll. Cardiol. 6:1245, 1985. Reprinted with permission of the American College of Cardiology.)

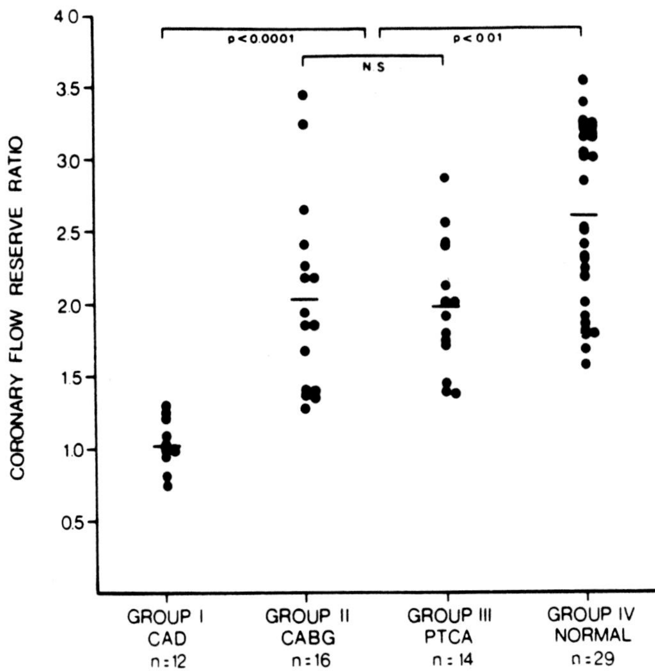

Figure 16–47. Long-term coronary flow reserve values for different patient groups. CAD—coronary artery disease; CABG—coronary artery bypass grafts, PTCA—percutaneous transluminal coronary angioplasty. (From Bates, E.R., and Mancini, G.B.J.: Digital radiographic assessment of coronary angioplasty and bypass graft revascularization results. *In* Mancini, G.B.J. (ed.): Cardiac Applications of Digital Angiography. Raven Press, New York, 1988, p. 291, with permission.)

APPLICATIONS OF DIGITAL ANGIOGRAPHY TO THE CORONARY CIRCULATION

References

A

1. Akisada, M., Hyodo, K., Ando, M., et al.: Synchrotron radiation at the photon factory for non-invasive coronary angiography: Experimental studies. J. Cardiol. 16:527, 1986.

B

1. Bassingthwaighte, J.B.: Plasma indicator dispersion in arteries of the human leg. Circ. Res. 19:332, 1966.
2. Bassingthwaighte, J.B., Ackerman, F.S., and Wood, E.H.: Applications of the lagged normal density curve as a model for arterial dilution curves. Circ. Res. 18:398, 1966.
3. Bassingthwaighte, J.B., Warner, H.R., and Wood E.H.: A mathematical description of the dispersion in blood traversing an artery. Physiologist 4:8, 1961.
4. Bates, E.R., Aueron, F.M., LeGrand, V., et al.: Comparative long-term effects of coronary artery bypass graft surgery and percutaneous transluminal coronary angioplasty on regional coronary flow reserve. Circulation 72:833, 1985.
5. Bates, E.R., and Mancini, G.B.J.: Digital radiographic assessment of coronary angioplasty and bypass graft revascularization results. *In* Mancini, G.B.J. (ed.): Cardiac Applications of Digital Angiography. Raven Press, New York, 1988, p. 291.
6. Bates, E.R., Vogel, R.A., LeFree, M.T., et al.: The chronic coronary flow reserve provided by saphenous vein bypass grafts as determined by digital coronary radiography. Am. Heart J. 108:462, 1984.
7. Bellman, S., Frank, H.A., Lambert, P.B., et al.: Coronary arteriography. I. Differential opacification of the aortic stream by catheters of special design. N. Engl. J. Med. 262:325, 1960.
8. Bookstein, J.J., and Higgins, C.B.: Comparative efficacy of coronary vasodilatory methods. Invest. Radiol. 12:121, 1977.
9. Booth, D.C., Nissen, S.E., and DeMaria, A.N.: The promise of digital cardiac angiography. J. Am. Coll. Cardiol. 8:817, 1986.
10. Boxt, L.M., Meryerovitz, M.F., Taus, R.H., et al.: Use of digital video coronary arteriography in the performance of percutaneous transluminal coronary angioplasty. Cardiovasc. Intervent. Radiol. 10:55, 1987.
11. Branemark, P.L., Jacobsson, B., and Sorensen, S.E.: Microvascular effects of topically applied contrast media. Acta. Radiol. (Diagn.) (Stockh.) 8:547, 1969.
12. Bray, B.E., Anderson, F.L., Hardin, C.W., et al.: Digital subtraction coronary angiography using high-pass temporal filtration: A comparison with cineangiography. Cathet. Cardiovasc. Diagn. 11:17, 1985.
13. Brody, W.R.: Hybrid subtraction for improved arteriography. Radiology 141:828, 1981.
14. Brown, B.G., Bolson, E.L., and Dodge, H.T.: Quantitative computer techniques for analyzing coronary arteriograms. Prog. Cardiovasc. Dis. 28:403, 1986.
15. Brown, B.G., Bolson, E., Frimer, J., and Dodge, H.T.: Quantitative coronary arteriography: Estimation of dimensions, hemodynamic resistance, and atheroma mass of coronary artery lesions using the arteriogram and digital computation. Circulation 55:329, 1977.
16. Bursch, J.H., and Heintzen, P.H.: Parametric imaging. Radiol. Clin. North Am. 23:321, 1985.

C

1. Corsini, G., Puri, P.B., Duran, P.V., and Bing, M.J.: Effect of nicotine on capillary flow and terminal vascular capacity of the heart in normal dogs and in animals with restricted coronary circulation. J. Pharmacol. Exp. Ther. 163:353, 1968.
2. Crawford, D.W., Brooks, S.H., Barndt, R., and Blankenhorn, D.H.: Measurement of atherosclerotic luminal irregularity and obstruction by radiographic densitometry. Invest. Radiol. 12:307, 1977.
3. Crystal, G.J., Downey, H.F., and Bashour, F.A.: Small vessel and total coronary blood volume during intracoronary adenosine. Am. J. Physiol. 241:H194, 1981.
4. Cusma, J.T., Toggart, E.J., Folts, J.D., et al.: Digital subtraction angiographic imaging of coronary flow reserve. Circulation 75:461, 1987.

D

1. DeBruyne, B., Dorsaz, P.A., Doriot, P.A., et al.: Assessment of regional coronary flow reserve by digital angiography in patients with coronary artery disease. Int. J. Cardiac. Imag. 3:47, 1988.
2. DeRouen, T.A., Murray, J.A., and Owen, W.: Variability in the analysis of coronary arteriograms. Circulation 55:324, 1977.
3. Detre, K.M., Wright, P.H., Murphy, M.L., et al.: Observer agreeement in evaluating coronary angiograms. Circulation 52:979, 1975.
4. Detrano, R., Haggman, D.L., Simpfendorfer, C., et al.: Digital fluoroscopy and intravenous cardiac angiography for the detection of coronary artery disease in selected subjects. Cleve. Clin. J. Med. 55:129, 1988.
5. Detrano, R., Markovic, D., Simpfendorfer, C., et al.: Digital subtraction fluoroscopy: A new method of detecting coronary calcifications with improved sensitivity for the prediction of coronary disease. Circulation 71:725, 1985.
6. Drury, J.K., Gray, R., Diamond, G.A., et al.: Computer-enhanced digital angiography visualizes coronary bypass grafts without need for selective injection. (Abstract.) Circulation (Suppl.) 66:229, 1982.

E

1. Eigler, N.L., Pfaff, J.M., Whiting, J.S., et al.: Digital angiographic transfer function analysis of regional myocardial perfusion: Measurement system and coronary contrast transit linearity. *In* Heintzen, P.H., and Bursch, J.H., (eds.): Progress in Digital Angiocardiography. Kluwer Academic Publishers, Dordrecht, 1988, p. 265.
2. Eigler, N.L., Pfaff, J.M., Zeiher, A., et al.: Digital angiographic impulse response analysis of regional myocardial perfusion: Linearity, reproducibility, accuracy, and comparison with conventional indicator dilution curve parameters in phantom and canine models. Circ. Res. 64:853, 1989.
3. Ellis, S.G., DeBoe, S.F., Sanz, M.L., and Mancini, G.B.J.: Accuracy and reproducibility of 5 Fr. catheter systems for outpatient use compared with 8 Fr. systems. (Abstract.) Circulation 76:369, 1987.

F

1. Feldman, R.L., Pepine, C.J., Curry, R.C., and Conti, C.R.: Case against routine use of glyceryl trinitrate before coronary arteriography. Br. Heart J. 40:992, 1978.
2. Feldman, R.L., Pepine, C.J., Curry, R.C., and Conti, C.R.: Quantitative coronary arteriography using 105mm photospot angiography and an optical magnifying device. Cathet. Cardiovasc. Diagn. 5:195, 1979.
3. Feldman, R.L., Pepine, C.J., Curry, R.C., and Conti, C.R.: Coronary arterial responses to graded doses of nitroglycerin. Am. J. Cardiol. 43:91, 1979.
4. Fisher, L.K., Judkins, M.P., Lesperance, J., et al.: Reproducibility of coronary arteriographic reading in the coronary artery surgery study (CASS). Cathet. Cardiovasc. Diagn. 8:565, 1982.
5. Foerster, J., Lantz, B.M.T., Holcroft, J.W., et al.: Angiographic measurement of coronary blood flow by video dilution technique. Acta Radiol. (Diagn.) (Stockh.) 22:121, 1981.
6. Foerster, J., Link, D.P., Lantz, B.M.T., et al.: Measurement of coronary reactive hyperemia during clinical angiography by video dilution technique. Acta Radiol. (Diagn.) (Stockh.) 22:209, 1981.
7. Foult, J.M., and Nitenberg, A.: Dipyridamole versus intracoronary injection of contrast medium for the evaluation of coronary reserve in man: A comparative study. Cathet. Cardiovasc. Diagn. 12:304, 1986.
8. Friedman, H.Z., DeBoe, S.F., McGillem, M., and Mancini, G.B.J.: The immediate effects of iohexol on coronary blood flow and myocardial function. Circulation 74:1416, 1986.
9. Friedman, H.Z., DeBoe, S.F., McGillem, M.J., and Mancini, G.B.J.: Immediate effects of graded ionic and nonionic contrast injections on coronary blood flow and myocardial function: Implications for digital coronary angiography. Invest. Radiol. 22:722, 1987.
10. Friesinger, G.C., Schaffer, J., Crilley J.M., et al.: Hemodynamic consequences of the injection of radiopaque material. Circulation 31:730, 1965.

G

1. Galbraith, J.E., Murphy, M.L., and DeSoyza, N.: Coronary angiogram interpretation: Interobserver variability. JAMA 240:2053, 1978.
2. Gensini, G.G., Kelly, A.E., DaCosta, B.C.B., and Huntington, P.P.: Quantitative angiography; The measurement of coronary vasomobility in the intact animal and man. Chest 60:522, 1971.
3. Goldberg, H.L., Moses, J.W., Fisher, J., et al.: Diagnostic accuracy of coronary angiography utilizing computer-based digital subtraction methods: Comparison to conventional cineangiography. Chest 90:793, 1986.
4. Goldberg, H.L., Moses, J.W., Borer, J.S., et al.: The role of digital subtraction angiography in coronary and bypass graft arteriography. (Abstract.) Circulation 66 (Suppl. II):II–229, 1982.
5. Gomes, A.S., Papin, P.J., Mankovich, N.J., and Lois, J.F.: Digital subtraction angiography: A comparison of 512^2 and 1024^2 imaging. AJR 146:853, 1986.
6. Gould, K.L., and Kelley, K.O.: Physiologic significance of coronary flow velocity and changing stenosis geometry during coronary vasodilation in awake dogs. Circ. Res. 50:695, 1982.
7. Grondin, C.M., Dydra, I., Pasternac, A., et al.: Discrepancies between cineangiographic and post-mortem findings in patients with coronary artery disease and recent myocardial revascularization. Circulation 49:703, 1974.
8. Guiraudon, G.M., Rankin, R.N., Kostuk, W.J., et al.: Visualization of internal mammary artery bypass graft by digital intravenous angiography. Experience with 42 consecutive patients. (Abstract.) J. Am. Coll. Cardiol. 7:152A, 1986.
9. Gurley, J.C., Nissen, S.E., Booth, D.C., et al.: Comparison of simultaneously performed digital- and film-based angiography in assessment of coronary artery disease. Circulation 78:1411, 1988.
10. Guthaner, D.F., Wexler, L., and Bradley, B.: Digital subtraction angiography of coronary grafts: Optimization of technique. AJR 145:1185, 1985.

H

1. Haggman, D., Detrano, R., and Simpfendorfer, C.: The value of coronary artery visualization during routine intravenous digital subtraction ventriculography. Cathet. Cardiovasc. Diagn. 12:5, 1986.
2. Harrison, D.G., White, C.W., Hiratzka, L.F., et al.: The value of lesion cross-sectional area determined by quantitative coronary angiography in assessing the physiologic significance of proximal left anterior descending coronary arterial stenoses. Circulation 69:1111, 1984.
3. Hodgson, J.McB., Legrand, V., Bates, E.R., et al.: Validation in dogs of a rapid digital angiographic technique to measure relative coronary blood flow during routine cardiac catheterization. Am. J. Cardiol. 55:188, 1985.
4. Hodgson, J.McB., Riley, R.S., Most, A.S., and Williams, D.O.: Assessment of coronary flow reserve using digital angiography before and after successful percutaneous transluminal coronary angioplasty. Am. J. Cardiol. 60:61, 1987.

5. Hodgson, J.McB., Singh, A.K., Drew, T.M., et al.: Coronary flow reserve provided by sequential internal mammary artery grafts. J. Am. Coll. Cardiol. 7:32, 1986.
6. Hodgson, J.McB., and Williams, D.O.: Superiority of intracoronary papaverine to radiographic contrast for measuring coronary flow reserve in patients with ischemic heart disease. Circulation 72:III-453, 1985.
7. Hoornstra, K., Hanselman, J.M.H., Holland, W.P.J., et al.: Videodensitometry for measuring blood vessel diameter. Acta Radiol. Diagn. 21:155, 1980.
8. Howe, B.B., and Winbury, M.M.: Effect of pentrinitrol, nitroglycerin and propranolol on small vessel blood content of the canine myocardium. J. Pharmacol. Exp. Ther. 187:465, 1973.

I

1. Ikeda, H., Koga, Y., Utsu, F., and Toshima, H.: Quantitative evaluation of regional myocardial blood flow by videodensitometric analysis of digital subtraction coronary arteriography in humans. J. Am. Coll. Cardiol. 8:809, 1986.
2. Ikeda, H., Shibao, K., Okabe, K., et al.: Functional myocardial perfusion imaging by digital subtraction coronary arteriography: Comparison of contrast decay rates in normal and ischemic myocardium. Heart Vessels 2:45, 1986.
3. Isner, J.M., Kishel, J., Kent, K.M., et al.: Accuracy of angiographic determination of left main coronary arterial narrowing. Circulation 63:1056, 1981.

J

1. Johnson, M.R., Brayden, G.P., Ericksen, E.E., et al.: Changes in cross-sectional area of the coronary lumen in the six months after angioplasty: A quantitative analysis of the variable response to percutaneous transluminal angioplasty. Circulation 73:467, 1986.

K

1. Katritsis, D., Lythall, D.A., Anderson, M.H., et al.: Assessment of coronary angioplasty by an automated digital angiographic method. Am. Heart J. 116:1181, 1988.
2. Kirkeeide, R.L., Gould, K.L., and Parsel, L.: Assessment of coronary stenoses by myocardial perfusion imaging during pharmacologic coronary vasodilation. VII. Validation of coronary flow reserve as a single integrated functional measure of stenosis severity reflecting all its geometric dimensions. J. Am. Coll. Cardiol. 7:103, 1986.
3. Kishan, Y., Yerushalmi, S., Deutsh, V., and Neufeld, H.N.: Measurement of coronary arterial lumen by densitometric analysis of angiograms. Angiology 30:304, 1979.
4. Klein, L.W., Agarwal, J.B., Rosenberg, M.C., et al.: Assessment of coronary artery stenoses by digital subtraction angiography: A pathoanatomic validation. Am. Heart J. 113:1011, 1987.
5. Koppes, G.M.: Complication rate of power coronary angiography injection. Angiology 31:130, 1980.
6. Kruger, R.A.: Estimation of the diameter of and iodine concentration within blood vessels using digital radiography devices. Med. Phys. 8:652, 1981.
7. Kruger, R.A., Bateman, W., Lin, P.Y., et al.: Blood flow determination using recursive processing: A digital radiographic method. Radiology 149:293, 1983.
8. Kuttler, H., Hauestern, K.H., Kameda, T., et al.: Significance of early angiographic follow-up after internal thoracic artery anastomosis in coronary surgery. Thorac. Cardiovasc. Surg. 36:96, 1988.

L

1. Lantz, B.M.T., Foerster, J.M., Link, D.P., and Holcroft, J.W.: Determination of relative blood flow in single arteries: New video dilution technique. AJR 134:1161, 1980.
2. Lassar, T., Roden, R., Grenier, R., et al.: Nonselective coronary artery and bypass graft angiography utilizing density-gated aortic root digital subtraction angiography. (Abstract.) Clin. Res. 34:318A, 1986.
3. LeFree, M.T., Mulvancy, J.A., and Vogel, R.A.: Image corrections for digital radiographic geometric and videodensitometric distortions. (Abstract.) Radiology 157:36, 1985.
4. LeFree, M.T., Simon, S.B., Lewis, R.J., et al.: Digital radiographic coronary artery quantitation. *In* Proceedings of the IEEE Computer Society, Computers in Cardiology. IEEE Computer Society, Long Beach, Cal. 1987, pp. 99-102.
5. LeFree, M.T., Simon, S.B., Mancini, G.B.J., et al.: A comparison of 35 mm cine film and digital radiographic image recording: Implications for quantitative arteriography. Invest. Radiol. 23:176, 1988.
6. LeFree, M.T., Simon, S.B., Mancini, G.B.J., and Vogel, R.A.: Digital radiographic assessment of coronary arterial geometric diameter and videodensitometric cross-sectional area. Proc. SPIE 626:334, 1986.
7. LeFree, M.T., Simon, S.B., Sanz, M.L., et al.: Quantitative coronary arteriography. *In* Mancini, G.B.J. (ed.): Clinical Applications of Cardiac Digital Angiography. Raven Press, New York, 1988, pp. 219–237.
8. Legrand, V., Aueron, F.M., Bates, E.R., et al.: Value of exercise radionuclide ventriculography and thallium-201 scintigraphy in evaluating successful coronary angioplasty: Comparison with coronary flow reserve, translesional gradient and percent diameter stenosis. Eur. Heart J. 8:329, 1987.
9. Legrand, V., Hodgson, J.Mc.B., Bates, E.R., et al.: Abnormal coronary flow reserve and abnormal radionuclide exercise tests in patients with normal coronary angiograms. J. Am. Coll. Cardiol. 6:1245, 1985.
10. Legrand, V., Mancini, G.B.J., Bates, E.R., et al.: Comparative study of coronary flow reserve, coronary anatomy and results of radionuclide exercise tests in patients with coronary artery disease. J. Am. Coll. Cardiol. 8:1022, 1986.
11. Lehan, P.H., Harman, M.A., and Oldewurtel, H.A.: Myocardial water shifts induced by coronary arteriography. (Abstract.) J. Clin. Invest. 42:950, 1963.
12. Lindner, E., and Katz, L.N.: Papaverine hydrochloride and ventricular fibrillation. Am. J. Physiol. 133:155, 1941.
13. Link, D.P., Foerster, J.M., Lantz, B.M.T., and Holcroft, J.W.: Assessment of peripheral blood flow in man by video dilution technique: A preliminary report. Invest. Radiol. 16:298, 1981.
14. Lois, J.F., Mankovich, N.J., and Gomes, A.S.: Blood flow determinations utilizing digital densitometry. Acta Radiol. 28:635, 1987.
15. Lupon-Roses, J., Montana, J., Domingo, E., et al.: Venous digital angioradiography: An accurate and useful technique for assessing coronary bypass graft patency. Eur. Heart J. 7:979, 1986.

M

1. MacAlpin, R.N., Abbasi, A.S., Grothman, J.H., and Eber, L.: Human coronary artery size during life. Radiology 108:567, 1973.
2. Mahomed, Y., Moorthy, S.S., Brown, J.W., and King R.D.: ECG changes with papaverine injection into coronary artery bypass grafts. Anesthesiology 61:350, 1984.
3. Mancini, G.B.J.: Quantitative coronary arteriography: Development of methods, limitations and clinical applications. Am. J. Cardiac Imag. 2:98, 1988.
4. Mancini, G.B.J., DeBoe, S.F., McGillem, M.J., and Ellis, S.G.: Comparative clinical assessment of quantitative coronary arteriography using digital and film-based methods. J. Am. Coll. Cardiol. 11:63A, 1988.
5. Mancini, G.B.J., and Higgins, C.B.: Digital subtraction angiography: A review of cardiac applications. Prog. Cardiovasc. Dis. 18:111, 1985.
6. Mancini, G.B.J., and McGillem, M.J.: Papaverine as a coronary vasodilator. AJR 147:1095, 1986.
7. Mancini, G.B.J., Simon, S.B., McGillem, M.J., et al.: Automated quantitative coronary arteriography: Morphologic and physiologic validation in vivo of a rapid digital angiographic method. Circulation 75:452, 1987.
8. Marcus, M.L.: The coronary circulation in health and disease. McGraw-Hill, New York, 1988, p. 248.
9. McGillem, M.J., Mancini, G.B.J., DeBoe, S.F., and Buda, A.J.: Modification of the centerline method for assessment of echocardiographic wall thickening and motion: A comparison with areas of risk. J. Am. Coll. Cardiol. 11:861, 1988.
10. Mistretta, C.A.: X-ray image intensifiers. *In* Haus, A.G. (ed.): The Physics of Medical Imaging: Recording System Measurements and Techniques. American Institute of Physics, New York, 1979, p. 182.
11. Mistretta, C.A., and Crummy, A.B.: Basic concepts of digital angiography. Prog. Cardiovasc. Dis. 28:245, 1986.
12. Mistretta, C.A., Peppler, W.W., Van Lysel, M., et al.: Recent advances in digital angiography. Ann. Radiol. (Paris) 26:537, 1983.
13. Myerowitz, P.D.: Digital subtraction angiography: Present and future uses in cardiovascular diagnosis. Clin. Cardiol. 5:623, 1982.
14. Myerowitz, P.D., Turnipseed, W.D., Shaw, C.-G., et al.: Computerized fluoroscopy: New technique for the non-invasive evaluation of the aorta, coronary artery bypass grafts, and left ventricular function. J. Thorac. Cardiovasc. Surg. 83:65, 1982.
15. Myerowitz, P.D., Turnipseed, W.D., Swanson, D.K., et al.: Digital subtraction angiography as a method for screening for coronary artery disease during peripheral vascular angiography. Surgery 92:1042, 1982.

N

1. Nicholes, K.R.K., Warner, H.R., and Wood, E.H.: A study of dispersion of an indicator in the circulation. Ann. N.Y. Acad. Sci. 115:721, 1964.
2. Nichols, A.B., Gabrich, C.F.O., Fenoglio, J.J., and Esser, P.D.: Quantification of relative coronary arterial stenosis by cinevideodensitometric analysis of coronary arteriograms. Circulation 69:512, 1984.
3. Nissen, S.E., Elion, J.L., Booth, D.C., et al.: Value and limitations of computer analysis of digital subtraction angiography in the assessment of coronary flow reserve. Circulation 73:562, 1986.
4. Nissen, S.E., Elion, J.L., and DeMaria, A.N.: Methods for calculation of coronary flow reserve by computer processing of digital angiograms. *In* Progress in Digital Angiocardiography. Heintzen, P.H. and Bürsch, J.H. (eds.): Kluwer Academic Publishers, Dordrecht, 1988, p. 237.
5. Nordenstrom, B.: Contrast examination of the cardiovascular system during increased intrabronchial pressure. Acta Radiol. (Stockh) (Suppl.) No. 200, 1960.

P

1. Paulin, S.: Assessing the severity of coronary lesions with angiography. N. Engl. J. Med. 316:1405, 1987.
2. Paulin, S.: Nonselective coronary arteriography. Semin. Roentgenol. 7:369, 1972.
3. Peppler, W.W., Van Lysel, M.S., Dobbins, J.T., et al.: Progress report on the University of Wisconsin Digital Video Image Processor (DVIP 11). *In* Heintzen, P.H., and Brennecke, R. (eds.): Digital Imaging in Cardiovascular Radiology. George Thieme Verlag, Stuttgart/New York, 1983, pp. 56–66.
4. Pilla, T.J., Beshany, S.E., and Shields, J.B.: Incompatibility of Hexabrix and papaverine. AJR 146:1300, 1986.

R

1. Rafflenbeul, W., Heim, R., Dzeuiba, M., et al.: Morphometric analysis of coronary arteries. *In* Lichtlen, P. (ed.): Coronary Angiography and Angina Pectoris; Symposium of the European Society of Cardiology. Georg Thieme Verlag, Stuttgart, 1976, pp. 255–265.

2. Rafflenbeul, W., Smith, L.R., Rogers, W.J., et al.: Quantitative coronary arteriography: Coronary anatomy of patients with unstable angina pectoris reexamined 1 year after optimal medical therapy. Am. J. Cardiol. 43:699, 1979.
3. Ratib, O., Chappuis, F., and Rutishauser, W.: Digital angiographic technique for the quantitative assessment of myocardial perfusion. Am. Radiol. 28:193, 197, 1985.
4. Ratib, O., and Rutishauser, W.: Parametric imaging in cardiovascular digital angiography. *In* Mancini, G.B.J. (ed.): Cardiac Application of Digital Angiography. Raven Press, New York, 1988, p. 239.
5. Read, R.C., Johnson, J.A., Vick, J.A., and Meyer, M.W.: Vascular efffects of hyperionic solutions. Circ. Res. 8:538, 1960.
6. Reiber, J.H.C., Booman, F., Tan, H.S., et al.: A cardiac image analysis system: Objective quantitative processing of angiograms. IEEE Comput. Cardiol. pp. 239–242, 1978.
7. Reiber, J.H.C., Kooijman, C.J., den Boer, A., and Semuys, P.W.: Assessment of dimensions and image quality of coronary contrast catheters from cineangiograms. Cathet. Cardiovasc. Diagn. 11:521, 1985.
8. Reiber, J.H.C., Kooijman, C.J., Slager, C.J., et al.: Computer assisted analysis of the severity of obstructions from coronary cineangiograms: A methodological review. Automedica 5:219, 1984.
9. Reiber, J.H.C., Serruys, P.W., Kooijman, C.J., et al.: Approaches toward standardization in acquisition and quantitation of arterial dimensions from cineangiograms. *In* Reiber, J.H.C., and Serruys, P.W. (eds.): State of the Art in Quantitative Coronary Arteriography. Martinus Nijhoff Publishers, Boston, 1986, p. 145.
10. Riederer, S.J., Brody, W.R., Enzmann, D.R., et al.: Work in progress: The application of temporal filtering techniques to hybrid subtraction in digital subtraction angiography. Radiology 147:859, 1983.
11. Riederer, S.J., Enzmann, D.R., Hall, A.L., et al.: The application of matched filtering to x-ray exposure reduction in digital subtraction angiography: Clinical results. Radiology 146:349, 1983.
12. Riederer, S.J., Hall, A.L., Maier, J.K., et al.: The technical characteristics of matched filtering in digital subtraction angiography. Med. Phys. 10:209, 1983.
13. Riederer, S.J., and Krager, R.A.: Intravenous digital subtraction: A summary of recent developments. Radiology 147:633, 1983.
14. Robb, R.A., Wood, E.H., Ritman, E.L., et al.: Three-dimensional reconstruction and display of the working canine heart and lungs by multiplanar x-ray scanning video densitometry. IEEE Comput. Cardiol. pp. 151–163, 1974.
15. Rosenberg, M.C., Klein, L.W., Agarwal, J.B., et al.: Quantification of absolute luminal diameter by computer-analyzed digital angiography: An assessment in human coronary arteries. Circulation 77:484, 1988.
16. Ross, A.M., Johnson, R.A., Katz, R.J., et al.: Diagnosis of coronary disease by aortic digital subtraction angiography. Circulation 63:III–43, 1983.
17. Rutishauser, W., Bussman, W.D., Noseda, G., et al.: Blood flow measurement through single coronary arteries by roentgen densitometry. Part I. A comparison of flow measured by radiologic techniques applicable in the intact organism and by electromagnetic flowmeter. AJR 109:12, 1970.
18. Rutishauser, W., Noseda, G., and Bussman, W.D.: Blood flow measurements through single coronary arteries by roentgen densitometry. Part II. Right coronary artery flow in conscious man. AJR 109:21, 1970.
19. Rutishauser, W.: Kreislanganalyse mettels Montgendensitometrie. Verlag Hans Huber, Bern/Stuttgart, 1969.

S

1. Sanders, W.J., Alderman, E.L., and Harrison, D.C.: Coronary artery quantitation using digital image processing techniques. IEEE Comput. Cardiol. pp. 15–20, 1979.
2. Sandor, T., Als, A.V., and Paulin, S.: Cinedensitometric measurement of coronary arterial stenosis. Cathet. Cardiovasc. Diagn. 5:229, 1979.
3. Sandor, T., Sridharb, R., and Paulin, S.: Remote densitometric analysis of stenotic lesions. Int. J. Bio. Med. Comp. 10:15, 1979.
4. Sanmarco, M.E., Brooks, S.H., and Blankenhorn, D.H.: Reproducibility of a consensus panel in the interpretation of coronary angiograms. Am. Heart J. 96:430, 1978.
5. Sanz, M.L., Mancini, G.B.J., LeFree, M.T., et al.: Variability of quantitative digital subtraction coronary angiography before and after percutaneous transluminal coronary angioplasty. Am. J. Cardiol. 60:55, 1987.
6. Schwartz, J.N., Kong, Y., Hackel, D.B., and Bartel, A.G.: Comparison of angiographic and post-mortem findings in patients with coronary artery disease. Am. J. Cardiol. 36:174, 1975.
7. Selzer, R.H., Shircore, A., Lee, P.L., et al.: A second look at quantitative coronary angiography: Some unexpected problems. *In* Reiber, J.H.C., and Serruys, P.W. (eds.): State of the Art in Quantitative Coronary Arteriography. Martinus Nijhoff, Dordrecht, 1986, pp. 125–144.
8. Shaw, C.G., and Plewes, D.B.: Pulsed-injection method for blood flow velocity measurement in intra-arterial digital subtraction angiography. Radiology 160:556, 1986.
9. Simons, M.A., Bastion, B.V., Bray, B.E., and Dedrickson, D.R.: Comparison of observer and videodensitometric measurements of simulated coronary artery stenoses. Invest. Radiol. 22:562, 1987.
10. Simons, M.A., and Kruger, R.A.: Vessel diameter measurement using digital subtraction radiography. Invest. Radiol. 20:510, 1985.
11. Simons, M.A., Kruger, R.A., and Power, R.L.: Cross-sectional area measurements by digital subtraction videodensitometry. Invest. Radiol. 21:637, 1986.
12. Sitomer, J., Anselmo, E.G., Feldt, D.A., et al.: On line mathematical model of bi-plane x-ray gantry. IEEE Comput. Cardiol. 659, 1986.
13. Skelton, T.N., Kisslo, K.B., and Bashore, T.M.: Comparison of coronary stenosis quantitation results from on-line digital and digitized cine film images. Am. J. Cardiol. 62:381, 1988.
14. Skelton, T.N., Kisslo, K.B., Mikat, E.M., and Bashore, T.M.: Accuracy of digital angiography for quantitation of normal coronary luminal segments in excised, perfused hearts. Am. J. Cardiol. 59:1261, 1987.
15. Smith, D.N., Colfer, H., Brymer, J.F., et al.: A semiautomatic computer technique for processing coronary angiograms. IEE Comput. Cardiol. pp. 325–328, 1981.
16. Smith, H.C., Frye, R.I., Donald, D.E., et al.: Roentgen videodensitometric measurement of coronary blood flow. Determination from simultaneous indicator-dilution curves to selected sites in the coronary circulation and in coronary artery saphenous vein grafts. Mayo Clin. Proc. 46:800, 1971.
17. Smith, H.C., Sturm, R.E., and Wood, E.H.: Videodensitometric system for measurement of vessel blood flow, particularly in the coronary arteries, in man. Am. J. Cardiol. 32:144, 1973.
18. Spears, J.R.: Rotating step-wedge technique for extraction of luminal cross-sectional area information from single plane coronary cineangiograms. Acta Radiol. Diagn. 22:217, 1985.
19. Spears, J.R., Sandor, T., Als, A.V., et al.: Computerized image analysis for quantitative measurement of vessel diameter from cineangiograms. Circulation 68:453, 1983.
20. Spiller, P., Schmeil, F.K., Politz, B., et al.: Measurement of systolic and diastolic flow rates in the coronary artery system by x-ray densitometry. Circulation 68:337, 1983.
21. Spears, J.R., and Sandor, T.: Quantitation of coronary artery stenosis severity: Limitations of angiography and computerized information extraction. *In* Reiber, J.H.C., and Serruys, P.W. (eds.): State of the Art in Quantitative Coronary Arteriography. Martinus Nijhoff, Dordrecht, 1986, pp. 103–124.
22. Steffenino, G., Meier, B., Bopp, P., et al.: Non-selective intra-arterial digital subtraction angiography for the assessment of coronary artery bypass grafts. Int. J. Cardiac Imag. 1:209, 1985.
23. Swanson, D.K., Kress, D.C., Pasaoglu, I., et al.: Quantitation of absolute flow in coronary artery bypass grafts using digital subtraction angiography. J. Surg. Res. 44:326, 1988.
24. Swanson, O.K., Myerowitz, P.D., Hegge, J.D., and Watson, K.M.: Arterial blood-flow waveform measurement in intact animals: New digital radiographic technique. Radiology 161:323, 1986.

T

1. Takeda, T., Matsuda, M., Akatsuka, T., et al.: Clinical validity of wash-out time constant images obtained by digital subtraction angiography. J. Cardiol. 16:841, 1986.
2. Tehrani, S., LeFree, M.T., Sitomer, J., and Bourdillon, P.D.V.: High-speed digital radiographic pincushion distortion correction using an array-processor. *In* Proceedings of the IEEE Computer Society. Computers in Cardiology. IEEE Computer Society, Long Beach, Cal. 1986.
3. Tillmans, H., Steinhausen, M., Dart, A., et al.: New aspects of myocardial capillary recruitment during hypoxia and reactive hyperemia. (Abstract.) Circulation 66(Suppl.)II:11–43, 1982.
4. Tobis, J., Johnston, W.D., Montelli, S., et al.: Digital coronary roadmapping as an aid for performing coronary angioplasty. Am. J. Cardiol. 56:237, 1985.
5. Tobis, J., Nalcioglu, O., Iseri, L., et al.: Detection and quantitation of coronary artery stenoses from digital subtraction angiograms compared with 35 millimeter film cineangiograms. Am. J. Cardiol. 54:489, 1984.
6. Taggart, E.J., and Mistretto, C.A.: Digital coronary angiography: Approaches using intravenous and direct methods. *In* Mancini, G.B.J. (ed.): Clinical Applications of Cardiac Digital Angiography. Raven Press, New York, 1988, pp. 253–279.
7. Tobis, J., Nalcioglu, O., Johnston, W.D., et al.: Videodensitometric determination of minimum coronary artery luminal diameter before and after angioplasty. Am. J. Cardiol. 59:38, 1987.

V

1. Vas, R., Eigler, N., Miyazono, C., et al.: Digital quantification eliminates intraobserver and interobserver variability in the evaluation of coronary artery stenosis. Am. J. Cardiol. 56:718, 1985.
2. Vlodaver, Z., Frech, R., Van Tassel, R.A., et al.: Correlation of the antemortem coronary arteriogram and the postmortem specimen. Circulation 47:162, 1973.
3. Vogel, R., LeFree, M., Bates, E., et al.: Application of digital techniques to selective coronary arteriography: Use of myocardial contrast appearance time to measure coronary flow reserve. Am. Heart J. 107:153, 1984.
4. Vogel, R.A., Bates, E.R., O'Neill, W.W., et al.: Coronary flow reserve measured during cardiac catheterization. Arch. Intern. Med. 144:1773, 1984.

W

1. Weiss, H.R., Winbury, M.M.: Nitroglycerin and chromonar on small-vessel blood content of the ventricular walls. Am. J. Physiol. 228:838, 1974.
2. White, C.W., Wright, C.B., Doty, D.B., et al.: Does visual interpretation of the coronary arteriogram predict the physiologic importance of a coronary stenosis? N. Engl. J. Med. 310:819, 1984.
3. Whiting, J.S., Drury, J.K., Pfaff, J.M., et al.: Digital angiographic measurement of radiographic contrast material kinetics for estimation of myocardial perfusion. Circulation 73:789, 1986.
4. Wholey, M.H.: Cardiovascular applications of digital subtraction angiography. Radiol. Clin. North Am. 23:627, 1985.
5. Wiesel, J., Grunwald, A.M., Tobiasz, C., et al.: Quantitation of absolute area of a coronary arterial stenosis: Experimental validation with a preparation in vivo. Circulation 74:1099, 1986.

6. Williams, D.O., and Thomas, E.S.: Use of digital angiography for percutaneous transluminal coronary angioplasty. Am. J. Cardiac Imag. 2:233, 1988.
7. Wilson, R.F., and White, C.W.: Intracoronary papaverine: An ideal coronary vasodilator for studies of the coronary circulation in conscious humans. Circulation 73:444, 1986.
8. Wilson, R.F., and White, C.W.: Does coronary artery bypass surgery restore normal maximal coronary flow reserve? The effect of diffuse atherosclerosis and focal obstructive lesions. Circulation 76:563, 1987.
9. Wilson, R.F., and White, C.W.: Serious ventricular dysrhythmias after intracoronary papaverine. Am. J. Cardiol. 62:1301, 1988.
10. Wollschlager, H., Zeiher, A.M., Bonzel, T., et al.: Optimal biplane imaging of coronary segments with computed exact triple orthogonal projections. Proceedings of the Second International Symposium on Coronary Arteriography, June 1987. Martinus Nijhoff, Dordrecht, 1987, p. 19.
11. Wueten, B., Busa, D.D., Deiet, H., and Schaper, W.: Dilatory capacity of the coronary circulation and its correlation to the arterial vasculature in the canine left ventricle. Basic Res. Cardiol. 72:636, 1977.

Z

1. Zijlstra, F., Serruys, P.W., and Hugenholtz, P.G.: Papaverine: The ideal coronary vasodilator for investigating coronary flow reserve? A study of timing, magnitude, reproducibility and safety of the coronary hyperemic response after intracoronary papaverine. Cathet. Cardiovasc. Diagn. 12:298, 1986.
2. Zir, L.M., Miller, S.W., Dinsmore, R.E., et al.: Interobserver variability in coronary angiography. Circulation 52:627, 1976.

Part V

Echocardiography

Chapter 17

Echocardiography: Physics and Instrumentation

EDWARD A. GEISER, M.D.

HISTORICAL PERSPECTIVE 348
WAVES AND PERIODIC MOTION 349
PIEZOELECTRICITY AND THE GENERATION OF ULTRASOUND 350
ULTRASOUND TRANSMISSION 351
Measurement of Sound Amplitude 351
Mechanical Wave Transmission in an Imperfect Medium 351
Reflection and Refraction 351
Scatter 352
INSTRUMENTATION 353
Pulse Transmission, Beam Insertion 353
Other Determinants of Axial Resolution 354
Beam Patterns and Determinants of Lateral Resolution 354
Electronic Focusing: The Annular Array 355
Transmission 355
Dynamic Focusing During Reception 356
DISPLAY FROM SINGLE-BEAM SYSTEMS 356
MECHANISMS FOR FORMING REAL-TIME B-MODE IMAGES 356
Electronic Beam Steering: Linear Array 356
Electronic Beam Steering: Phased Array 357
Electronic Beam Steering: The Orthogonal Phased Array/Three-Dimensional Beam Formation 359
RECEPTION, AMPLIFICATION, AND IMAGE FORMATION 359
DIGITAL SCAN CONVERSION 360
PRE- AND POSTPROCESSING 363
FREEZE-FRAME AND CONTINUOUS LOOP DISPLAY 363
CONCLUSION 363

Ultrasonic imaging of the heart has become one of the mainstays of diagnosis, treatment evaluation, and research in cardiology. Part of the reason for this acceptance is the safety, portability, and versatility of the technique. Undoubtedly, although all of these can be listed as factors in the growth and development of new applications of ultrasound, the true reason for its tremendous success is the fact that the information it provides is helpful in understanding the mechanisms and evaluating the status and causes of cardiovascular disease in patients. The important consideration is having knowledge of a patient's cardiac anatomy in terms of chamber size, chamber function, valvular structure and motion, and pericardial structure and knowledge of blood flow patterns and velocities.

The versatility of echocardiography continues to grow as advances in material science, biomechanics, and computers affect instrumentation. Transesophageal echocardiography is already improving diagnostic accuracy in special cases and improving the early diagnosis of ischemia. Intravascular ultrasound imaging is now readily available. The utility of all of these devices and features is discussed elsewhere.

Although there are great promise and great utility in all of these applications, there are also limitations. Through a better understanding of the physical principles and instrumentation utilized in ultrasound, those who use it for care of patients will come to a better understanding of both the strengths and weaknesses of the technique.

HISTORICAL PERSPECTIVE

From the scientific point of view, understanding of the transmission of sound waves has paralleled that of light waves. For this reason, many of the same names are associated with elucidation of the physical principles of both light and ultrasound transmission. Such names as Doppler, Rayleigh, Fresnel, Fraunhofer, and Huygens are frequently encountered. Their particular contributions to our understanding will be described later in the chapter, but it is appropriate here to recall that over a century of dedicated hypothesis generation and experimentation took place before Langevin was able to develop sonar in the early part of the 20th century. In its early form, sonar was used mainly to map the ocean floor or to detect submerged objects. By the 1940's other methods for producing sound waves had been explored. Furthermore, measurements of sound velocities in various media, including human tissues, had been carried out by Ludwig.[L1] At about the same time, pulsed-echo techniques were developed.[F1] In 1954 Edler and Hertz[E1] described the application of ultrasound for dynamic cardiac imaging. The information obtained was displayed by the use of A-mode and B-mode methods; B-mode displays were developed by Wild and Reid in the early 1950's.[W1] Continuous-wave Doppler ultrasound was subsequently applied to the cardiovascular system in the late 1950's by Nimura and co-workers in Japan.[Y1] Further improvements in piezoelectric materials, computer materials, and electronic design made two-dimensional real-time B-mode imaging practical by the late 1960's. Some of the two-dimensional images were produced with wobbling or rotating mechanical head scanners. The phased-array radar technology was adapted to produce two-dimensional B-mode scans by Somer.[S1] This technology was specifically applied to imaging of the heart in the mid-1970's by Kisslo and associates.[K1]

In spite of the technological developments, ultrasound images remained noisy because of poor penetration of sound through the lung. Intravascular approaches were discussed in the early 1960's, and catheter-mounted transducers were developed and tested into the late 1970's. Also, in the early 1970's Frazin and associates[F2] used the esophagus as a window to the heart. The 1980's have been dominated by advances in computer technology and speed that have allowed the development of color flow imaging and improved image processing and scan conversion.

Other imaging techniques have developed concurrently with echocardiography over the past 30 years. The use of x-rays has progressed to computed tomography and fast computed tomography. Magnetic resonance imaging has been developed, and now "flash" magnetic resonance imaging can also provide near-real-time information. Many new isotope sources have been developed, and the techniques for tomographic reconstruction using these labeled sources have become more sophisticated. In all of these techniques, electromagnetic energy is used to form the images. In the case of computed tomography and magnetic resonance, images with extremely high resolution are obtained. Echocardiography is unique among the imaging techniques in that it utilizes a mechanical wave, that is, an energy that must be transmitted in a medium and that cannnot traverse a vacuum. Although sound waves can produce extremely high energy concentrations, as in the case of lithotripsy, the sound waves used to create images are high-frequency, low-energy waves.

Echocardiography also differs from the other imaging modalities in that the energy that produces the image is reflected. Sound traveling into the body is reflected from structures and returns along the same path before being received at the transducer. With x-ray techniques the energy penetrates completely, and with magnetic resonance and nuclear methods the energy source is within the tissue being imaged. Furthermore, because ultrasound is a mechanical wave, its propagation within tissue is slow; with other imaging techniques, transmission occurs at the speed of light. Therefore, while x-ray, magnetic resonance, and nuclear images are usually formed by using some type of back-projection technique, ultrasound images are based on line-of-sight and time-of-flight information. In addition, mechanical waves are much more susceptible to attenuation than light waves. Therefore, image quality differs greatly with ultrasound, and attenuation correction, which depends on the distance traversed, becomes extremely important.

All of these not-so-subtle features of ultrasound have provided unique challenges in the development of the imaging technique. Yet it is because of these challenges that echocardiography has its unique features of safety, portability, and versatility. In the remainder of this chapter, the causes, magnitude, and some of the solutions to these basic problems are discussed.

WAVES AND PERIODIC MOTION

A wave is a cyclic disturbance that is nature's way of moving energy from one place to another. In the case of mechanical waves, the energy must be passed through matter or a medium and not through a vacuum. Waves are cyclic in nature. This means that each particle in the medium is displaced as the energy disturbance passes through. Subsequently, the displaced particle experiences a restoring force that is dependent on the properties of the medium and proportional to the displacement. This restoring force tends to return each particle to its predisturbance position. In an ideal situation in which there are no frictional forces, each particle is again at its original position after the wave has passed, so there has been no net movement of particles nor permanent changes in the medium. Such a cyclic disturbance of particles is sinusoidal in nature and in its simplest form can be expressed as

$$A = A_0 \sin kt \qquad (1)$$

where A is the amplitude of the displacement at any point in time, t; A_0 is the original amplitude of the wave; and k is a constant that depends on both the frequency of the disturbance and the properties of the medium through which the disturbance travels.

Mechanical waves can be of two types: transverse and longitudinal. With transverse waves the particle's displacement is perpendicular to the direction of propagation of the wave. Waves of this type are usually on the surface of the medium. An example is a wave on the ocean; displacement of the water particles is up and down while the wave travels slowly along the surface. Figure 17–1*A* shows such a transverse displacement of particles around a zero resting position. The vertical or perpendicular restoring forces are represented by the vertical springs. The transverse energy is stored in the vertical springs but is passed along by the horizontal springs that tether the particles together. Figure 17–1*B* shows an example of a longitudinal wave through the same

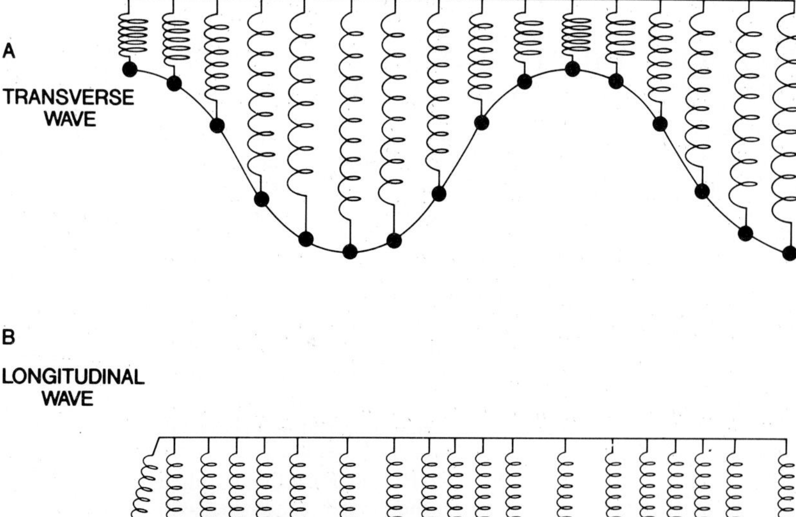

Figure 17–1. Diagrammatic representation of the two types of mechanical wave motion. *A*, A transverse wave moving from left to right. Particle motion is perpendicular to the direction of propagation of the wave. *B*, A longitudinal wave analogous to that of sound. Particle motion oscillates in a direction parallel to the propagation of energy in the wave. The time to complete one cycle is referred to as the period, T. The length of one complete cycle is referred to as the wavelength, λ.

particles. In this case, the energy propagation is parallel to the direction of motion of the particles. The restoring force on the particles is now supplied by the tethering springs as the particles move back and forth in an oscillatory pattern.

Waves, whether transverse or longitudinal, are described by several parameters, including the frequency, f; the period, T; the wavelength, λ; the amplitude, A; and the propagation velocity, v. The wavelength is defined as the distance between any two particles simultaneously experiencing the same displacement amplitude. The wavelength is usually expressed in meters, but in applications of ultrasound the wavelength is often given in millimeters. The period is expressed in seconds and is defined as the time that it takes for a particle to undergo one complete cycle of oscillation. The number of complete cycles of oscillation that occur in 1 second is called the frequency and expressed in hertz (Hz); 1 Hz is defined as one cycle per second. The propagation velocity can be either measured or calculated from the relationship

$$v = \lambda f \qquad (2)$$

The human ear can hear mechanical waves in its environment that are between the limits of 20 Hz and 20 kilohertz (kHz). Frequencies below 20 Hz are called subsonic; those greater than 20 kHz are out of the range of audible sound and are referred to as ultrasound. Diagnostic ultrasound frequencies are the range of 1 to 12 megahertz (MHz).

The velocity of sound in various materials depends on the properties of the materials. This difference in velocity is related to the forces between molecules in the materials, since these intermolecular forces are the basic restoring forces that return the disturbed particles toward their equilibrium position. The velocity in a material can be expressed as

$$v = K/\rho \qquad (3)$$

where ρ is the density of the material and K is the elastic modulus. This relationship implies that as the density of the material increases, so does the velocity. In general, this proves to be true; the velocity of sound in the air is approximately 330 m/sec and in soft tissue is approximately 1540 m/sec.[W2] Although this relationship seems simple, in practice it is somewhat more complex. Consider that the density of most materials changes with temperature; for example, ice has a lower density than water. Therefore, the velocity of sound in the medium is also dependent on the temperature of the medium. For this reason normal saline at 40°C is used to test ultrasound equipment, since at 40°C the propagation velocity is 1540 m/sec.

PIEZOELECTRICITY AND THE GENERATION OF ULTRASOUND

The longitudinal wave depicted in Figure 17–1*B* was initiated by pulling on the particle at the left-hand side. The displacement could have been initiated by compression, or pushing on the particle with a piston. This mechanism would be analogous to the introduction of ultrasound into the body by using a piezoelectric crystal. Piezoelectricity refers to the generation of a small electrical current in certain materials when pressure is placed on them. One of the first substances in which this phenomenon was recognized was quartz. When pressure is applied to thin wafers of ground quartz crystal, a current is generated. One of the first uses of quartz crystals was in the microphone, where the voice waves supplied the pressure on the quartz crystal and the small current generated from the crystal was then amplified.

The inverse is also true in piezoelectric materials; that is, when a very high voltage is placed across the crystal, the crystal will expand. The reason for this is that piezoelectric materials consist of microscopic, asymmetric, molecular structures that are highly polarized. When a piezoelectric material is subjected to a high electric potential, the molecules' long axes become oriented toward the surfaces of the wafer and the thickness of the wafer increases. This concept is shown diagrammatically in Figure 17–2. When the electrical charge is removed, the particles return to their resting position and the thickness of the wafer decreases. Thinning of the wafer when the charge is removed does not stop abruptly but "rings down" in the manner of a damped oscillation. The frequency of this oscillation depends on multiple factors, but the most important are the nature of the material itself and the thickness of the wafer. Other ceramic materials with the property of piezoelectricity, such as lead-zirconate-titanate (PZT) and barium titanate, have now replaced the quartz crystal in ultrasound applications.

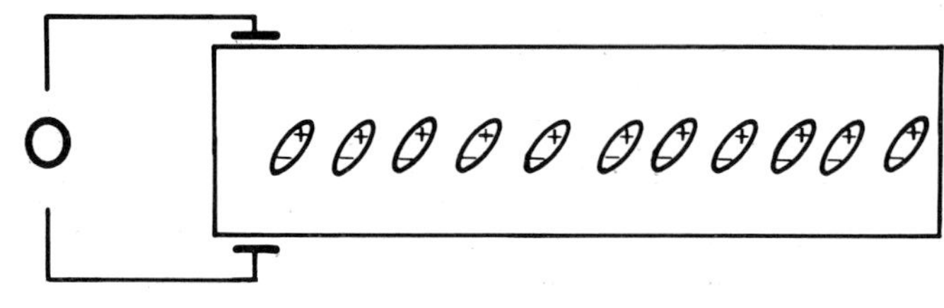

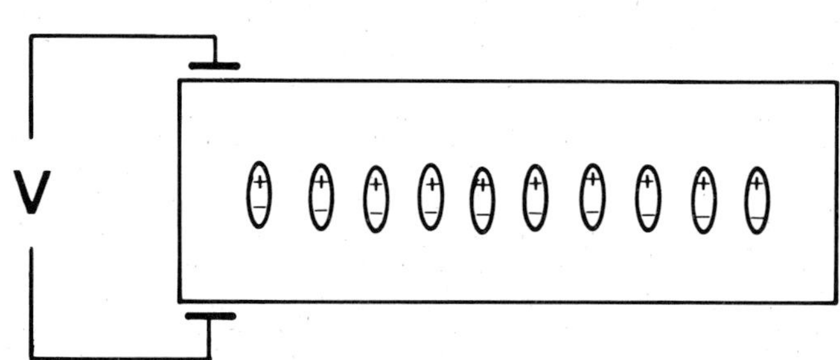

Figure 17–2. Diagrammatic representation of a piezoelectric crystal. In the resting state, with no voltage applied, the crystal and particles may be aligned but the particles are not parallel to faces of the crystal. When a voltage, V, is applied to the surfaces of the crystal, the polarized particles align in the electrical field, more perpendicular to the faces of the crystal, and cause it to expand.

Since the frequency of oscillation of the crystal is fixed by the material and the thickness, the wavelength of the sound traveling through a medium must vary directly with the propagation velocity of the medium in order to maintain the relationship of $v = \lambda f$. Table 17–1 shows the wavelengths of a distribution of frequencies commonly utilized in diagnostic ultrasound; in the table a propagation velocity of 1540 meters per second is assumed. These wavelengths in part determine the axial resolution of the ultrasound system. Many other factors come into play, however. Therefore, before considering the basic elements of transducer design, it is important to consider in more detail the factors that influence movements of these mechanical waves through the many complex media found in the human thorax.

Table 17–1. WAVELENGTHS AT VARIOUS ULTRASOUND FREQUENCIES*

Frequency (MHz)	Wavelength (mm)
1.6	0.962
2.5	0.616
3.5	0.440
5.0	0.308
7.5	0.205
10.0	0.154
12.0	0.128

*In tissue with 1540 m/sec propagation velocity.

ULTRASOUND TRANSMISSION

Measurement of Sound Amplitude

Prior to considering transmission characteristics and the problems in ultrasound image formation, it is important to understand how ultrasound amplitude (or intensity) is measured. The basic unit of measurement is the decibel (dB). The decibel is not an absolute amplitude measurement. Rather it is a unit that expresses the ratio between sound intensities (or amplitudes) at two different points. Because the difference in ultrasound energy varies over many orders of magnitude, the decibel scale is logarithmic rather than linear. The decibel is defined as

$$\text{decibel (dB)} = 10 \log_{10}(I_2/I_1) \tag{4}$$

where I_1 and I_2 are the sound intensities to be compared. Since intensity is proportional to the square of the amplitude, A, the decibel can also be expressed in terms of the ratio of amplitudes

$$\text{dB} = 20 \log_{10}(A_2/A_1) \tag{5}$$

Whether attenuation or amplification has occurred is indicated by the sign. For instance, if the measured amplitude of sound is one-half of the transmitted amplitude, then

$$\text{dB} = 20 \log_{10}(0.5)$$

or, since log 0.5 = −0.3,

$$\text{dB} = -6$$

Similarly, if the amplitude of a sound wave is increased by a factor of 2 by an amplifier, this is expressed as

$$\text{dB} = 20 \log_{10}(2)$$

Since $\log_{10}$ of 2 is 0.3, a doubling of the amplitude is expressed as a 6-dB gain. Table 17–2 shows the corresponding decibel values and amplitude ratios for both attenuation and amplification over a range that is commonly encountered in ultrasound images. As an example, the range of returning amplitudes encountered in a B-mode scan is approximately 100 dB. This means that the largest returning amplitude is 100,000 times greater than the smallest reflected amplitude.

Mechanical Wave Transmission in an Imperfect Medium

The equation of a periodic sinusoidal wave has been given above. The point was also made that in the absence of frictional forces within the medium, the amplitude of the wave would remain the same regardless of the distance of propagation. Body tissues, however, are not perfect media. Muscle, lung, fat, cardiac muscle, and blood all have internal friction and viscous forces between their molecules. Therefore, part of the energy of the propagating mechanical wave is lost. The overall loss of wave amplitude is referred to as attenuation. The major factors contributing to the loss of amplitude are (1) scattering by very small targets, which disperse the wave in many directions; (2) mode conversion, which is represented principally by conversion of the wave fronts into shear waves in large specular targets such as bone; and (3) absorption, which refers to the conversion of wave energy into heat, primarily due to frictional forces.

Table 17–2. INTENSITY RATIOS AND CORRESPONDING DECIBEL VALUES FOR ATTENUATION AND AMPLIFICATION

Attenuation		Amplification	
dB	*Ratio*	*dB*	*Ratio*
0	1.000	0	1.000
−1	0.794	+1	1.259
−2	0.631	+2	1.585
−3	0.501	+3	1.995
−6	0.251	+6	3.981
−20	0.01	+20	100.000
−25	0.003	+25	316.000
−30	0.001	+30	1000.000
−50	10^{-5}	+50	10^{5}
−100	10^{-10}	+100	10^{10}
−120	10^{-12}	+120	10^{12}

Table 17–3. ATTENUATION COEFFICIENTS (α) AND CHARACTERISTIC IMPEDANCES (Z) OF SELECTED TISSUES

Tissue	$\alpha(\text{cm}^{-1})$*	Z
Water	0.0003	1.52
Blood	0.02	1.62
Heart	0.25–0.38	1.65–1.74
Liver	0.07–0.13	1.64–1.68
Lung		0.26
Fat	0.04–0.09	1.35
Bone		7.80

*At 1 MHz

The overall attenuation of ultrasound by a specific medium is characterized by the attenuation coefficient. The sound amplitude A along any path of propagation in the medium may be expressed as

$$A(x) = A_0 e^{-\alpha x} \tag{6}$$

where A_0 is again the initial displacement amplitude, α is the attenuation coefficient, and x is the distance traversed in the medium. Since absorption is due to frictional and viscous forces in the medium, it seems reasonable that the faster particles move in the medium, the more resistance they will encounter. Therefore, one expects that as the frequency is increased, more viscous and inertial opposition to motion will be present and the attenuation will be greater. This, indeed, is true, so the attenuation is dependent on both the frequency of the transmitted wave and the properties of the medium. Thus, the values for attenuation are often given in units of decibels per centimeter per megahertz (dB/cm/MHz). Table 17–3 gives the attenuation coefficients for tissues of interest in echocardiography.

The foregoing discussion has been oriented toward the amplitude of displacement of the particles in the medium or tissue. Much of the literature on the safety of ultrasound refers to the intensity. Intensity is the concentration of energy in a mechanical wave front, that is, the power divided by the wave's cross-sectional area. Therefore, the units of intensity are watts per centimeter squared. Because of attenuation, the intensity varies and is again dependent on the medium, the frequency of oscillation, and the distance traversed. With diagnostic ultrasound equipment, these intensities are quite low and within defined safety limits.[C1, A1]

Reflection and Refraction

Thus far, only propagation of ultrasound in a single homogeneous medium has been considered. In imaging, however, ultrasound must encounter and, in part, traverse the boundaries between multiple types of tissues. Although the shapes of the interfaces between tissues in the body may be quite complex, the laws that determine reflection and refraction at any point on the surface are similar to those that govern the reflection and refraction of light passing through prisms or lenses. It is well known that ultrasound images are formed by a process of reflection of a portion of the energy at an interface while the rest of the energy propagates into the next tissue. The amount of ultrasound that is reflected and the amount that continues depend on the difference in characteristic impedance, Z, between the two types of tissue. This type of interaction, reflection or refraction, occurs only at interfaces that are referred to as specular (from the Latin word for mirror). A specular reflector (of light or sound waves) is an approximately planar surface that is greater in size than the wavelength of the incident energy and that has irregularities much smaller than the wavelength of the incident energy. For instance, light is not reflected from paper because the irregularities in the surface of paper are much larger than the wavelength of light. Light is reflected from a mirror because the irregularities in the surface of the glass and between the silver molecules are much smaller than the wavelength of light. Similarly, since the wavelength of microwaves is measured in meters, a parabolic television dish that appears to be made out of wire screen is actually a perfect parabolic mirror because the irregularities of the screen are much smaller than the wavelength of broadcast television.

When the specular surface conditions of size and smoothness are met, the intensity, I, of the reflected wave is given by

$$I_r = I_i\left(\frac{Z_2 - Z_1}{Z_2 + Z_1}\right)^2 \quad (7)$$

where r refers to the reflected wave, i refers to the incident wave, and 1 and 2 refer to the tissues on either side of the interface. The quantity

$$\left(\frac{Z_2 - Z_1}{Z_2 + Z_1}\right)^2 \quad (8)$$

is the reflection coefficient. Some characteristic impedances for biologic tissues are given in Table 17–3. Insertion of the appropriate values from this table into equation (7) shows that only 0.06 percent of the incident beam is reflected at a blood-muscle interface; but approximately 54 percent of the beam is reflected at the interface between pericardium and lung.

Like light waves, sound waves are reflected from a specular interface at an angle that is equal to the angle of incidence, as shown diagrammatically in Figure 17–3. The sound energy that continues on does not necessarily continue in the same direction, and a change in direction is referred to as refraction. The relationship between the angle of incidence, θ_i, and the angle of refraction, θ_t, is dependent on the propagation velocity in the two tissues

$$\sin \theta_i/\sin \theta_t = v_1 / v_2 \quad (9)$$

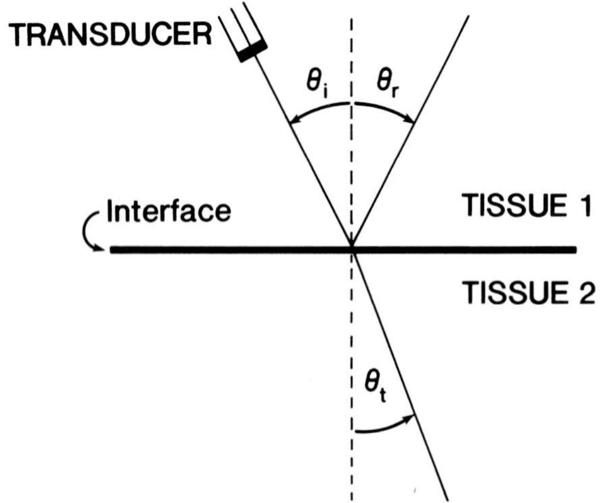

Figure 17–3. Reflection and refraction at a specular (mirrorlike) acoustic interface. The ultrasound coming from the transducer encounters the interface at an angle of incidence, θ_i, and is reflected at the same angle, θ_r, with respect to the surface normal. Sound transmitted through the interface does not necessarily continue in a straight line but may be bent at an angle, θ_t, depending on the acoustic impedance of the two tissues.

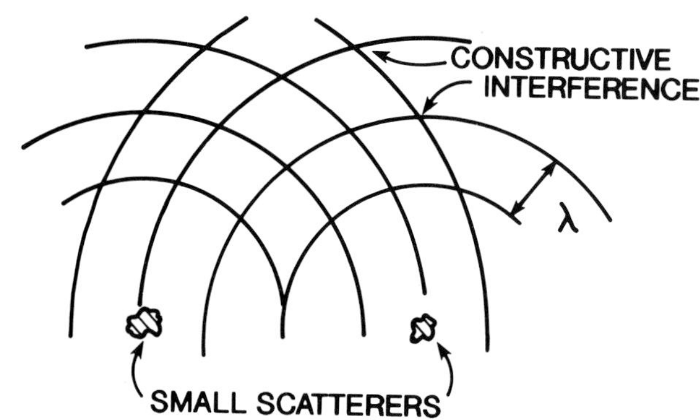

Figure 17–4. Diagrammatic representation of acoustic scatter. The two small scatterers serve as point sources of the reflected ultrasound and give rise to a standing wave interference pattern with nodes of constructive interference.

where v_1 and v_2 refer to the velocity of sound in tissue 1 and tissue 2, respectively.

As mentioned early in this chapter, ultrasound image formation is along lines of sight. Therefore, only sound that is incident on a specular target that is perpendicular to the line of sight will be imaged. In actuality, since the face of the transducer is large (approximately 1 cm^2), ultrasound that undergoes only a small angular change during reflection and refraction can still contribute to image formation. An example of image degradation due to excessive reflection is frequently noted in the lateral left ventricular wall on the parasternal short-axis view. In this region, not only is there increased attenuation due to lung tissue but also the epicardial and pericardial surfaces are oriented so that much of the beam energy is reflected out of the line of sight.

Scatter

Obviously, reflection from specular targets accounts for only a portion of the interaction of the ultrasound beam with tissue in the body. Most of the time, the beam is interacting with various tissues during its propagation. Each of these tissues consists of cellular structures that are much smaller than the wavelength of incident ultrasound. The interaction of ultrasound with these much smaller targets is very different. Huygens' principle states that all points on a wave front can be considered as point sources for the production of spherical secondary wavelets. Indeed, energy incident on a small spherical particle of radius r is scattered in all directions such that the intensity, I, of the scattered wave is inversely proportional to the fourth power of the wavelength and directly proportional to the sixth power of the radius, that is,

$$I \propto (2\pi/\theta)^4 r^6 \quad (10)$$

Figure 17–4 shows two small scatterers at a small distance apart. After the wave energy reaches the two particles, each particle serves as a secondary source, generating spherical wave fronts that radiate in all directions. As these spherical wave fronts propagate from the two particles, they eventually overlap. At points where the maximum amplitudes of oscillation occur together—that is, the oscillations are in phase—the wave amplitudes sum together. At points where the overlapping waves are out of phase by 180 degrees, cancellation occurs. This phenomenon of interaction is known as constructive and destructive interference. A familiar example of interference is seen in the high school physics experiment in which two point sources generate waves at the same frequency in a water tank; the positions of points of constructive and destructive interaction between the waves do not change and the result is called a standing wave pattern. In the case of an ultrasound image, literally thousands of point scatterers contribute but the resultant standing wave pattern follows the same principle. The standing wave interference pattern is detected by the ultrasound transducer and displayed in the image. This portion of the image is referred to as acoustic speckle, or noise, and is the major contributor to the "noisy" appearance of ultrasound images.

As can be seen from equation (10), the coarseness of the speckle is related to the wavelength and thus the frequency of the transducer. It is also related to the radius, r, of the scatterers and thus to the microscopic structure of the tissue causing the scatter. It is this relationship between the pattern of backscatter energy and the microscopic properties of the scattering particles that forms the basis for research on ultrasonic characterization of tissues.

INSTRUMENTATION

Pulse Transmission, Beam Insertion

In the section on historical perspective, reference was made to the development of pulsed-echo techniques. The importance of this development for modern ultrasound imaging cannot be overestimated. In order to understand this point, it is helpful to approach the problem of transducer design from an engineering perspective in which the objective is to optimize both energy introduction into the body and the resolution capabilities of the system.

Piezoelectric materials act as a piston to inject or insert ultrasound into the body. In applications of ultrasound, the current is applied to the crystal in what is called "shock excitation." The shock is normally on the order of several hundred volts, and its duration is roughly 1 microsecond (μsec). Following a short burst, the crystal resonates or "rings down." This ring-down time may be of the order of 10 μsec. If the speed of sound in the medium is 1540 m/sec, the 10-μsec ring-down would produce a pulse 15.4 mm in length. The effect of pulse length on axial resolution is shown diagrammatically in Figure 17–5*A*. In the figure the two targets have been placed in the line of sight of the generated pulse at 10 and 10.5 cm from the surface of the crystal. Figure 17–5*B* shows the returning pulse at some time after encountering both targets. Because of the long pulse length, the echoes from the two targets are superimposed and the system would not be able to resolve the two targets in the image. In fact, the axial resolution is defined as the minimum reflector separation along the sound path required to produce separate reflections. The primary determinants of axial resolution are the frequency of the transducer (the wavelength), the bandwidth (the range of frequencies contained in the pulse), and the pulse length. Although all of these factors contribute, a safe general approximation of the axial resolution is that it is equal to one-half of the spatial pulse length.

To shorten the pulse length, the ring-down time must be shortened, which is accomplished by applying a sound-absorbing backing to the piezoelectric crystal. This process is referred to as damping. With this technique, most ultrasound systems can cut the ring-down time to approximately 1 μsec. Thus, using a common frequency such as 3 MHz as an example, only three waves of sound are injected into the body. Figures 17–5*C* and 17–5*D* show diagrammatically this short burst following transmission and the two separate wave packets returning. These two packets can be resolved into two separate targets by the system.

Damping, however, is not without its limitations. Although damping decreases the pulse length, it also increases the bandwidth. Furthermore, more than 90 percent of the acoustic energy of the output of the piezoelectric material may be lost in the damping material and not transmitted into the body. Thus, optimal damping requires a trade-off between transmitted energy, increased resolution due to shortened pulse length, and decreased resolution due to increased bandwidth. One of the descriptors of transducer design is the quality factor, which is expressed as

$$Q = f/BW$$

where f is the operating frequency of the transducer and BW is the bandwidth.

Another problem in injecting sound into the body is the acoustic mismatch between the piezoelectric material and the skin. For the piezoelectric ceramic, a typical acoustic impedance, Z, is approximately 30 rales. An average acoustic impedance for the skin and body tissues is close to 1.6 rales. Insertion of these values into equation (7) shows that more than 80 percent of the energy at the surface of the transducer will be reflected back into the transducer and will not enter the body. One way to overcome this mismatch is to place another layer of material with an intermediate impedance value between the piezoelectric crystal and the skin. This concept of impedance matching is common in many types of electronic equipment.

How thick should the impedance-matching layer be? This seemingly small question turns out to be very important. With the impedance-matching layer in place, there are both an interface between the piezoelectric material and the matching layer and an interface between the matching layer and the skin. Sound is thus trapped and reflected back and forth within the matching layer, a phenomenon referred to as reverberation. If the matching layer thickness was random, this reverberation would result in a loss of energy and an increase in pulse length. Consider, however, that when a wave is reflected from a high-impedance medium to a medium of lower impedance, there is a 180-degree phase shift in the reflected portion of the wave. If the matching layer is made one-quarter wavelength thick, the reflected wave will undergo another shift of one-quarter wavelength as a result of round-trip propagation within the matching layer. Thus, when the reflected portion of the wave returns to its point of origin on the surface of the piezoelectric material, it will be exactly in phase with the motion of the surface at that point in time. The use of one-quarter wavelength impedance-matching layers has

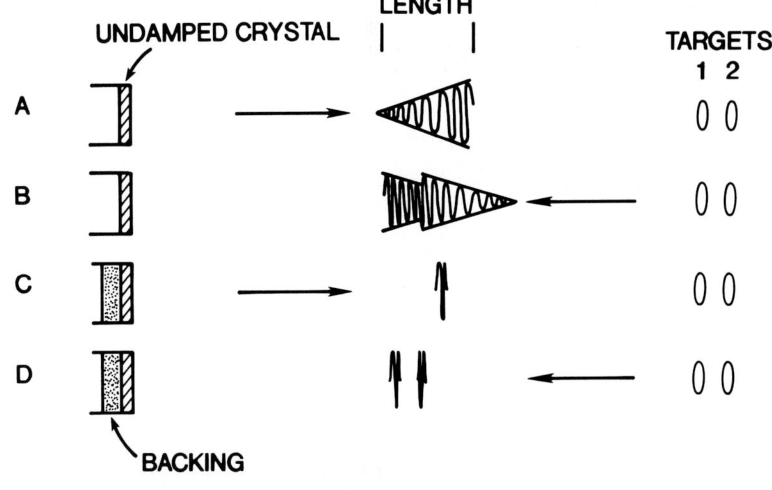

Figure 17–5. Effect of pulse length on axial resolution. *A*, The undamped crystal gives rise to a burst of ultrasound whose pulse length is greater than 15 mm. Targets 1 and 2 are separated by 5 mm. *B*, The reflected pulses, after encountering targets 1 and 2, are indistinguishable. *C*, Since the reflected pulse from target 2 has merged with that from target 1, a sound-absorbing backing has been applied to the transmitting crystal. Ring-down is markedly shortened so that spatial pulse length is now approximately 1 mm. *D*, Pulses reflected from targets 1 and 2 remain separate and easily distinguishable.

been an important step in the improvement of image quality. More complete descriptions of the theory behind impedance matching are given by Wells[W3] and Kinsler and Frey.[K2]

Impedance-matching layers do not result in 100 percent insertion of the ultrasound energy into the body. Even in the presence of multiple matching layers, some portion of the wave is still reflected; and since there is a finite bandwidth, the one-quarter wavelength matching is not perfect. Impedance-matching layers are now commonplace in all types of ultrasound systems. The principles are the same whether they are applied to single crystals, linear arrays, or phased arrays.

Other Determinants of Axial Resolution

The transmitted ultrasound pulse injected into the body has a center frequency and a bandwidth. The foregoing discussion of the physics of transmission brought attention to the fact that higher frequencies are attenuated to a higher degree as they pass through tissues. Therefore, as the ultrasound pulse propagates through tissue, there is an apparent decrease in the center frequency of the pulse. This frequency downshift is more pronounced in pulses reflected from deeper structures, since it also depends on the distance of propagation. Therefore, the axial resolution is, in part, also dependent on the ability of the transducer to respond to a wider range of frequencies than its designed natural center frequency. In other words, a wider bandwidth can provide better axial resolution of deeper structures.

Beam Patterns and Determinants of Lateral Resolution

Lateral resolution is defined as the minimum reflector separation perpendicular to the direction of propagation that will produce separate representations in the image. Since the lateral resolution is defined perpendicular to each line of sight, the lateral resolution can be thought of as sweeping across the image in an arc and is, therefore, frequently referred to as azimuthal resolution. Factors that determine the lateral resolution are the frequency of the transducer, focusing, aperture (width) of the transducer, bandwidth, and finally side lobe and grating lobe levels (these are defined later). Of these, the dominant factor is the focusing or beam width at any particular depth.

In the single-crystal, circular-face transducer as used for M-mode echocardiography, the beam pattern is fairly simple. The pattern consists of a near zone, called the Fresnel zone, in which the beam remains columnar, and a far zone, called the Fraunhofer zone, in which the beam starts to diverge. The length of the Fresnel zone, F_1, is defined by

$$F_1 = D^2/4\lambda \tag{11}$$

where D is the transducer diameter. In the Fraunhofer zone, the beam diverges at an angle defined by

$$\sin \Theta = 1.22\lambda/D \tag{12}$$

where θ is the divergence angle. These equations show the dependence on both frequency (and therefore wavelength) and the size of the transducer face.

Figure 17–6 shows the near- and far-field dependence on both frequency and diameter. In Figure 17–6*A* the piezoelectric crystal face is assumed to have a diameter of 10 mm and a frequency of 2.25 MHz. Thus, the near zone is 36.5 mm in length and the far-field divergence is approximately 5 degrees. Figure 17–6*B* shows that with a decrease in diameter to 7 mm, a transducer of the same frequency will have half the near-field depth and a wider divergence angle of approximately 7 degrees. The effect of increasing frequency to 5 MHz is to increase the near-field length

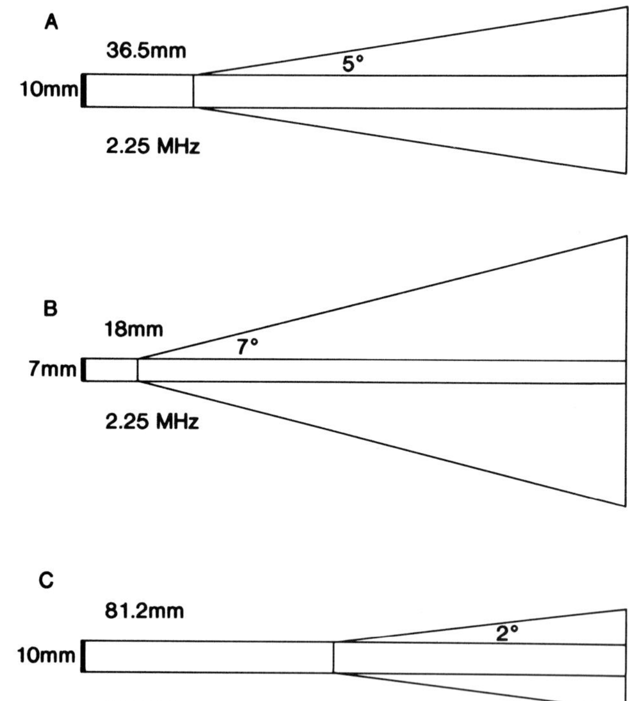

Figure 17–6. Effect of crystal diameter and crystal frequency on beam pattern. *A*, A 10-mm-diameter crystal with a frequency of 2.25 MHz. The near field (Fresnel zone) is 36.5 mm in length, while the far field (Fraunhofer zone) diverges at approximately 5 degrees. *B*, The crystal diameter has been decreased to 7 mm with the frequency kept constant. The near-field length is reduced by 50 percent and the far-field divergence angle is increased. *C*, The crystal diameter is 10 mm but the crystal frequency is increased to 5 MHz. The near field is now increased in length to 81 mm and the far-field divergence has decreased to only 2 degrees.

to 81.2 mm and decrease the far-field divergence to only 2 degrees, as shown in Figure 17–6*C*. The effects of both aperture and transducer frequency on lateral resolution for targets at varying depths are apparent.

In the foregoing discussion it was assumed that the transducer is unfocused. One method of focusing, and thus improving the lateral resolution, is to make the surface of the piezoelectric material concave, as shown in Figure 17–7*A*. The concavity forces the radiation at all points on the surface of the transducer to converge toward a point—the focal point. The beam width at that point may be quite narrow. The technique of accomplishing focusing by modifying the surface of the crystal is referred to as internal focusing.

A second method of focusing is to leave the surface of the

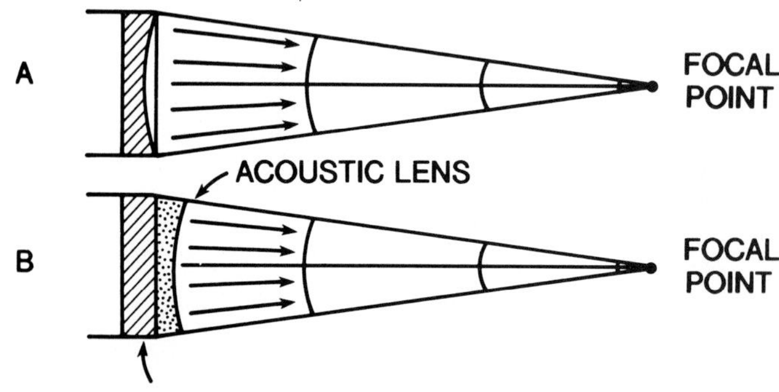

Figure 17–7. Focusing of the single-crystal transducer. *A*, Focusing is achieved by grinding the surface of the crystal itself. This method of forcing convergence of the transmitted sound pulse toward a focal point is referred to as internal focusing. *B*, The acoustic pulse is focused by an added epoxy lens. This method is referred to as external focusing.

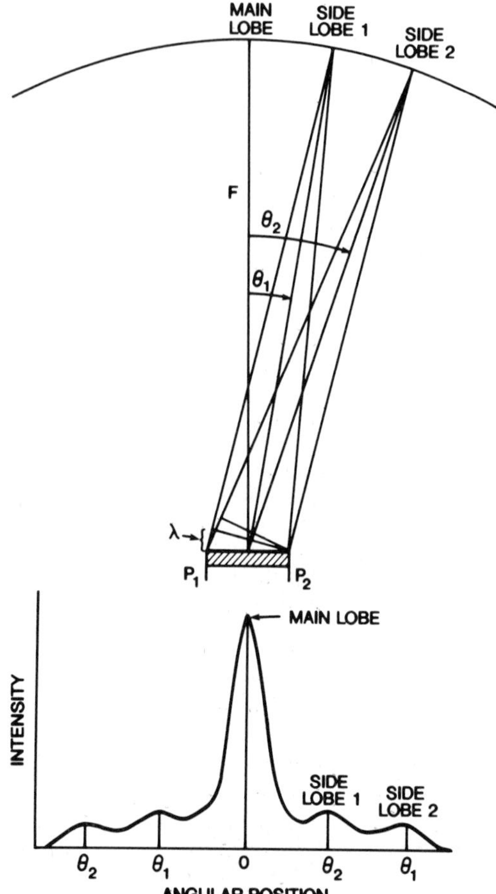

Figure 17–8. *Top*, Diagram showing the positions at which side lobes will form. Side lobes occur at points at which the distances traversed by the ultrasound pulse from each edge of the crystal face differ by exactly one wavelength. Note that the distance from the left edge of the crystal at point P_1 to the position of side lobe 1 is exactly one wavelength longer than the distance from point P_2 at the extreme right edge of the crystal to the position of the side lobe 1. *Bottom*, The beam intensity plot formed by sweeping along an arc at the focal length, F.

piezoelectric material flat but apply an acoustic lens to the front surface of the crystal. The acoustic lens can be made of a material with refraction properties appropriate to force beam convergence. These lenses are analogous to optical lenses made for focusing light. This method of focusing is referred to as external focusing and is shown in Figure 17–7*B*. Again, the beam is much narrower at the focal point of the transducer.

No matter which method of focusing is utilized, the beam width at the focal point and the depth of the focal point can be controlled, which is an advantage in the near field and in the focal zone. The disadvantage of focusing is that the far-field divergence occurs more rapidly than with an unfocused transducer. Thus, lateral resolution in the far field is sacrificed.

Lateral resolution is also diminished by the presence of secondary lobes, which in the case of single-crystal transducers are frequently referred to as side lobes. Side lobes exist because not all the acoustic energy is propagated in the direction perpendicular to the face of the transducer, that is, parallel to the central axis of the beam. Figure 17–8 shows an unfocused single-crystal transducer. From Huygens' principle we know that any point on the surface of the crystal can be considered as a point source for the transmitted ultrasound. Therefore, at any point at which the path lengths from the opposite ends of the transducer differ by exactly one wavelength, there will be a node of constructive interference or a secondary lobe. From Figure 17–8 it can be appreciated that the angle between the side lobes and the central axis of the beam is given by

$$\sin \Theta = m\lambda/D \tag{13}$$

where θ is the angle at which the side lobe occurs, m is an integer (1, 2, 3, . . .), and D is the diameter of the transducer.

Transducers are frequently evaluated by using a beam intensity plot as shown in Figure 17–8. In order to form this plot, which characterizes the beam quality of the transducer, the transducer is placed in a bath that contains a liquid with a conduction velocity of approximately 1540 m/sec, similar to that of tissue. A device known as a hydrophone probe, which measures sound intensity, is swept in an arc at a constant distance near the focal length, F, from the surface of the transducer. A specific method of testing single-element transducers has been standardized by the American Institute of Ultrasound in Medicine (AIUM).[A2] The resulting beam intensity plot shows the normal beam width, which is defined as the width of the main lobe at the point where the intensity has fallen to one-half of the maximum intensity, or at the point where the main lobe has fallen off by 3 dB in intensity. The beam intensity plot also shows the characteristics of the side lobes, which should be more than 50 dB below the main lobe.

Electronic Focusing: The Annular Array

Transmission

Thus far, only single-crystal transducers have been considered. One final method of focusing a single-beam, circular-faced transducer is based on Huygens' principle. The focusing is accomplished by placing multiple circular crystal elements in the face of the transducer and firing them at slightly different times. This arrangement is referred to as an annular array.

Such a transducer face consists of a small circular element and multiple concentric elements placed around it, as shown in Figure 17–9*A*. Figure 17–9*B* shows a cross section of the set of circular crystal elements. If all three of the elements are fired simultaneously, the characteristics of the resulting beam are the same as those for an unfocused circular transducer. If the outer circular crystal is fired slightly ahead of the intermediate crystal and the central crystal is fired last, the summation of the wave fronts results in focusing of the beam at some distance, F, from the face of the transducer. Thus focusing has been accomplished by purely electronic means, as opposed to the external and internal methods described above. Although this may seem somewhat unimportant at first glance, the results are far-reaching. For instance, a laboratory that performs both pediatric and adult echocardiography may require 3.25-MHz transducers with both 4-cm and 8-cm focal lengths. With a single annular-array transducer, both needs could be met simply by changing the time delay between the outer and inner elements. Focal lengths of 4

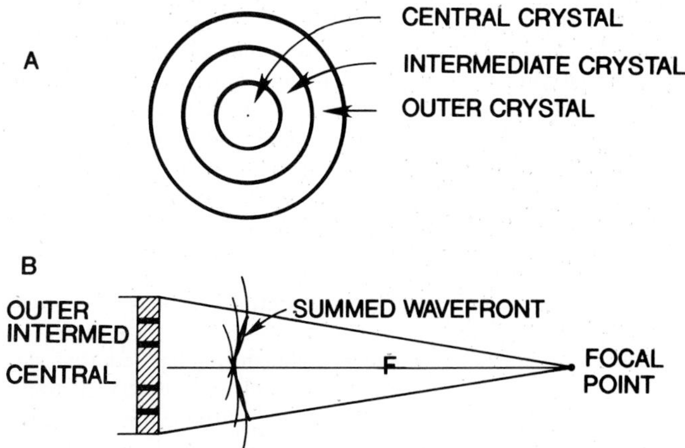

Figure 17–9. Focusing in the annular-array transducer. *A*, Face of a simple annular-array transducer consisting of three independent crystals. *B*, Cross section of the crystal face. The outer crystal has been fired first, followed by the intermediate and central crystals, so that the wave fronts sum to form a single focused wave front. Note that in this case the focusing is electronic, rather than mechanical as in the internal and external focusing methods depicted in Figure 17–7.

cm and 8 cm are used here as examples, but it is clear that the focal point of the transmitted beam can be set to any depth simply by changing the timing of the shocks to the circular array elements. All of the foregoing discussion regarding backing of the elements to damp ring-down and impedance matching applies to the surface of the individual annular-array elements. Therefore, when a focal point for the transmitted wave is chosen, a single pulse of sound of approximately 1 μsec is injected into the body toward a single focal point.

Dynamic Focusing During Reception

Up to this point, pulse generation, impedance matching, and focusing have been discussed. These processes are involved in insertion of the ultrasound beam into the body, which takes only 1 to 2 μsec. After generation of the pulse, the transducer's function is inverted and it operates essentially as a microphone to listen for the returning pulses. As mentioned before, any reflecting target along the path of the beam serves as a point source of radiation of sound back toward the transducer. In a single-crystal transducer the external or internal focusing lens is still attached to the front of the transducer. If a reflector is close to the transducer, the reflected wave fronts will be quite curved. In this case of excessive curvature, sound will arrive at the center of the transducer crystal slightly before it arrives at the edges. On the other hand, the reflected wave front from a very distant target will have a large radius of curvature and thus will be nearly planar when it arrives back at the crystal. This radius of curvature will be larger than that accommodated by the focusing lens; therefore, the reflected wave front will arrive at the edges of the transducer slightly before it arrives at the center. Thus, reflected waves from both very near and very far targets will be slightly "smeared" in time, and only reflected waves from targets in the focal zone of the transducer will arrive so that the whole wave front reaches the crystal face in phase and causes maximum vibration of the crystal.

In the annular-array transducer, the returning sound activates the center, intermediate, and outer circular crystals. The small voltage outputs from the compression of all three of these crystals must be added to produce a single output analogous to that of the single-crystal transducer. In fact, if the outputs of the three crystals were simply added together, the results would be the same as for a single unfocused crystal. On the other hand, the signals from the individual crystals can be delayed before they are added, just as the shock exitation voltages were delayed in order to produce focusing. In the case of a reflector close to the transducer, where the wave front is quite curved, the sound arriving at the central crystal can be delayed slightly before being added to the sound arriving at the intermediate crystal, which in turn can be delayed slightly before being added to the sound arriving at the outer crystal. These delays before summation ensure that the voltages produced by the wave front reflected from a nearby object are placed in phase and thus sum to form a maximum estimate of the amplitude of the reflected wave front. The wave front reflected from a very distant target will have a large radius of curvature, and no time delays will be necessary to ensure the highest possible sum since the wave front will be nearly planar. This process of changing the focal point along the scan line during reception to ensure optimal response is referred to as dynamic focusing.

The ability to change the focal point, during both transmission and reception, is a marked advantage of multiple-crystal transducers. These concepts are expanded further in subsequent sections.

DISPLAY FROM SINGLE-BEAM SYSTEMS

From the preceding discussions, it can be seen that echocardiography systems are phase-sensitive ultrasound systems designed to measure the distance from the transducer face to structures within and surrounding the heart. This distance measurement is accomplished by measuring the time between pulse generation and reception of a reflected signal and assuming a velocity of sound propagation through tissue.

The time-of-flight information or distance can be displayed in several ways. In one method the depth is displayed on one axis and the relative amplitude of the returning sound on the other axis. This type of display is frequently placed at the side of the two-dimensional image and is referred to as an A-mode or amplitude-mode display. A second method is to display a peak in amplitude as a spot whose brightness is proportional to the amplitude of ultrasound returning from that depth. This type of display is referred to as the B-mode or brightness mode. If the B-mode display is routed through a fiber optic cable onto photographic paper while the paper is moved along at a constant speed, an M-mode or motion-mode display is obtained. The A-, B-, and M-mode displays are all designed to provide a graphic representation of the positions of the reflecting sites along single beam paths. Recall that the pulse generated along a single line requires only 1 μsec. The transducer is switched into a receive or listening mode for 999 μsec. This means that a single line of sight, such as an M-mode line, can be obtained in 1/1000 of a second. This speed results in the very high temporal resolution of the M-mode tracing, which allows accurate measurement of very short time intervals, such as the time for opening of the mitral valve. In most cardiac applications, the display of anatomic structure and spatial relationships is more important than the extremely high temporal resolution. When multiple B-mode lines are displayed on the screen at the time when a two-dimensional image is formed, the methods by which these lines are generated and displayed are varied, as discussed in the next section.

MECHANISMS FOR FORMING REAL-TIME B-MODE IMAGES

Three basic methods are used to form images from multiple B-mode scan lines. The first and simplest method is to move a single-crystal transducer back and forth through an arc of interest. The second is to rotate several crystals and allow each to form a portion of the image as they rotate through the arc of interest. The third is to form and move the beam electronically using multiple-phased crystals. In both the wobbling transducer and the rotating-head transducer, the same principles that were applied to single-crystal beam formation and single-crystal reception continue to apply. Specifically, the limitations imposed by a fixed focal length are present. In more recent wobbling-head mechanical scanners, the annular-array transducer has replaced the single-crystal transducer previously utilized. Thus, variable-transmit focusing and dynamic focusing during reception can be implemented while the two-dimensional image itself is formed by mechanical means. Although this type of transducer overcomes some of the disadvantages inherent in single-crystal transducers of fixed focal length, the problems of impedance matching through the medium in which oscillation or rotation occurs (usually mineral oil) and maintenance of the moving parts within the plastic housing that provides the contact with the skin continue to be obstacles to acceptance. It is not surprising that the competing technology of electronic beam steering in stationary-array transducers has developed.

Electronic Beam Steering: Linear Array

Besides the annular-array transducer described above, two other types of array technology are commonplace. These are the linear array and the phased array. The linear array is used mostly in obstetrics and abdominal ultrasound, and phased-array systems are most common in cardiac applications. The linear-array transducer has a rectangular face of width W and height H. Within the face of the transducer are multiple small rectangular crystals that are placed parallel to each other and parallel to the height dimension of the transducer as pictured in Figure 17–10A. The linear-array image is formed along multiple scan lines that are perpendicular to the face of the transducer. If the number of transducer elements activated is chosen so that the total active surface is approximately a square of dimensions H × H, then the same near- and far-field equations apply as if the beam were formed by a single circular crystal. Again, the beam travels in a line of sight perpendicular to the face of the transducer. Since the linear-array image is formed by multiple parallel B-mode lines that are perpendicular to the face of the transducer, the first B-mode line in Figure 17–10 would be formed by firing elements 1, 2, 3, and 4. The next line would be formed by firing elements 2, 3, 4, and 5. Thus, each of the B-mode lines that make up the image would be formed by sequential activation of the individual elements down the face of the array.

The individual beams formed for each line in this situation would be unfocused. At this point it becomes necessary to introduce the third dimension, or resolution, which becomes a factor in forming two-dimensional echocardiographic images. Axial resolution and lateral resolution have already been discussed. The third dimension is the cross-plane resolution or beam thickness, which is the thickness of the beam perpendicular to the plane of the image. In other words, the plane of the scan is not thin like a sheet of paper but may be 2 mm to more than 1 cm thick. The image is then formed from the average reflection of all structures contained within this thickness. It follows that the larger the cross-plane thickness, the more blurred the image will be. In comparable tomographic techniques, such as magnetic resonance imaging and computed tomography, this effect is also seen and is referred to as volume averaging. In general, the narrower the cross-plane beam thickness, the sharper the image will be. Since mechanical sector scans are formed by using either a single crystal or rotating circular crystals with cylindrical beam shapes, the elevation resolution is generally the same at any depth as the lateral resolution.

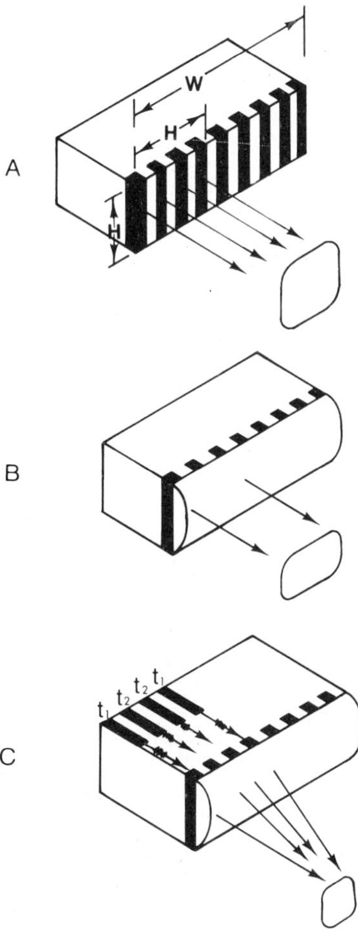

Figure 17–10. Diagrammatic representation of beam formation and focusing along each B-mode line generated by a linear-array transducer. A, The four parallel crystal elements are fired simultaneously to form the beam. In this case the beam is unfocused and the cross-sectional beam shape is depicted as approximately square. *B*, Adding an acoustic external focusing lens in the elevation dimension results in a rectangular beam cross section. For this illustration, it has been assumed that the propagation velocity of sound through the lens is less than the propagation velocity through tissue, so a convex lens is appropriate. *C*, Crystals 1 and 4 have been fired slightly earlier than crystals 2 and 3 in order to obtain focusing in the lateral (azimuthal) direction. Thus, focusing in the elevation dimension is accomplished by means of fixed external focusing, while focusing in the lateral dimension is accomplished electronically. (From Geiser, E. A., and Oliver, L. O.: Echocardiography physics and instrumentation. *In* Collins, S. M., and Skorton, D. J. [eds.]: Cardiac Imaging and Image Processing. McGraw-Hill, New York, 1986, with permission.)

Notice that neither of the fixed methods of focusing, external or internal, nor the variable technique of focusing described for the annular array can solve the problems of focusing in the linear-array transducer. Therefore, a combination of the techniques must be used. In the elevation dimension, the thickness of the beam must be focused by one of the fixed methods. In Figure 17–10*B* an external focusing lens has been applied to the surface of the array. Note the narrowing of the cross-plane dimension and the more rectangular shape of the beam. The lateral or azimuthal focusing cannot be accomplished in the same manner. Therefore, in a manner similar to that described for the annular array, elements 1 and 4 can be fired earlier than 2 and 3, forcing convergence toward a point, as shown in Figure 17–10*C*. Again, the time interval between the firing of the lateral elements and the firing of the central elements can be changed, so the azimuthal focal point is variable.

The linear-array transducer accomplishes focused two-dimensional image generation by rapidly producing parallel B-mode scan lines with no moving parts. Side lobes still exist, but their positions become more complex. In the elevation dimension, side lobe positions are determined by the frequency of the transducer elements and by the height, H, of the transducer. In the lateral dimension, however, side lobe positions are determined by the number of elements fired to form an individual beam, since this determines the width of the active transducer face for each beam.

In addition to the side lobes, a new problem develops in transducers with multiple crystal arrays. One of these problems is a secondary lobe that degrades the resolution of the images and is usually more serious than the side lobe. This secondary lobe is usually referred to as a grating lobe. Figure 17–11 shows the cause of these grating lobes in the format used in Figure 17–8 to show the development of side lobes. Each of the crystal elements in the face of the transducer is again considered a point source for sound, and the beam is formed by the summation of these wave fronts, again according to Huygens' principle. However, at some angle θ to the side of the main beam, the first wave front emitted from element 1, having traveled a longer distance, will arrive exactly in phase with the second wave front emitted from element 4. At this point there will be constructive interference and the appearance of a grating lobe. The position of the grating lobes is given by the equation

$$\sin \Theta = m\lambda/S$$

where θ is now the angle at which the grating lobe will appear, m is again an integer, and S is the center-to-center spacing between the individual transducer crystal elements.

Since grating lobes may have a serious effect on quality, careful matching of transducer frequency to element spacing is a critical point in transducer design. Other critical points include electrical isolation, sealing of the transducer, and aspects of element isolation to suppress resonance modes.[A3, L2]

Electronic Beam Steering: Phased Array

In the linear-array transducer the B-mode lines were formed parallel to each other and by firing a limited number of the transducer array elements. In the phased-array transducer, the individual 110 to 130 B-mode lines are formed as if from the same point source and through an arc of usually 90 degrees.

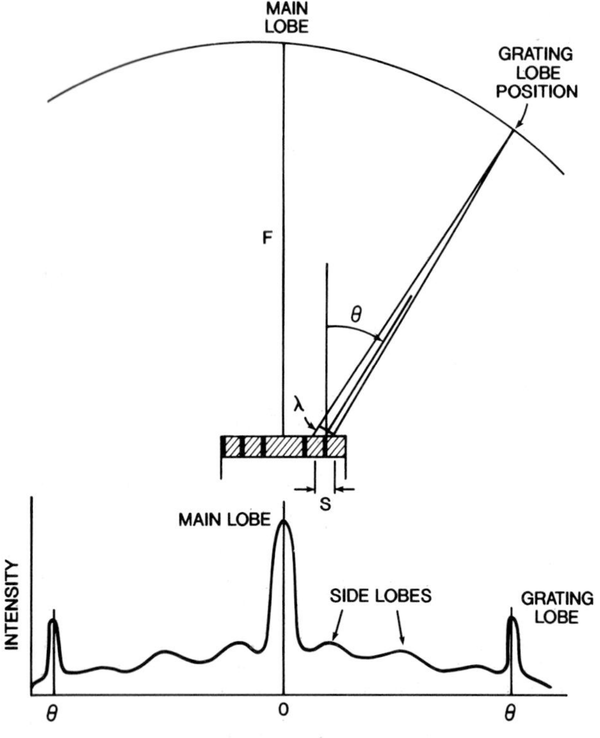

Figure 17–11. *Top,* Diagram showing the position of grating lobes in array transducers. The position of grating lobes is determined by the spacing between the centers of independent crystal elements in the transducer. At any point where the path length between the two crystal elements differs by one wavelength, a grating lobe is formed. The grating lobe is formed at an angle θ that depends on the wavelength (λ) of the crystals and the spacing (S) between the crystal elements. *Bottom,* The beam intensity plot formed at the focal length, F.

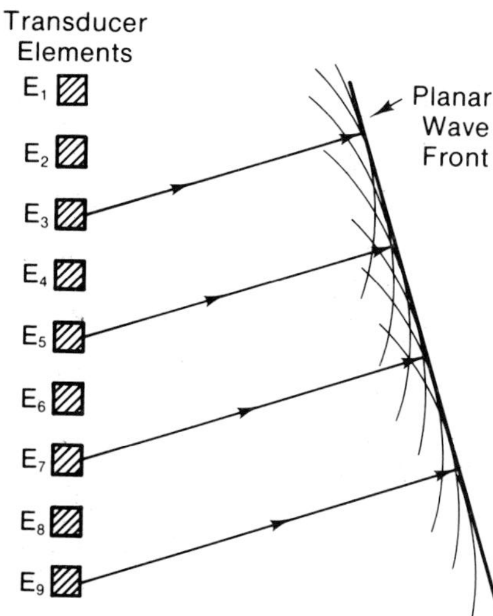

Figure 17–12. Diagrammatic representation of the formation of a planar wave front moving away from a transducer array at an angle. In this situation, transducer element E_9 would have been fired first and each successive crystal element fired at a slightly delayed time after its predecessor. The individual wave fronts have summed according to Huygens' principle into a single planar wave front. The formation of this single wave front moving away from the transducer face at an angle is an example of electronic beam steering. (From Geiser, E. A., and Oliver, L. O.: Echocardiography physics and instrumentation. *In* Collins, S. M., and Skorton, D. J. [eds.]: Cardiac Imaging and Image Processing. McGraw-Hill, New York, 1986, with permission.)

Since each line is considered to have as its origin the center of the transducer face, each line is formed by firing all the elements (usually 32 to 64) in the array. Figure 17–12 depicts a simple nine-element transducer array. If element 9 is fired first and each lower-numbered element is fired at a slightly later time, the wave fronts sum to a single planar wave front moving at an angle to the face of the transducer that is determined by the delay in time between firing the individual successive elements. This planar wave front would form an unfocused beam at that angle with characteristics similar to those of a beam from a single crystal aimed in the same direction. By compounding the time delay patterns, this beam can be focused in the lateral direction as were the linear-array and annular-array beams. This is shown diagrammatically in Figure 17–13. As for the linear-array transducer, the elevation or cross-plane focusing must be accomplished by use of a fixed external or internal acoustic lens. Therefore, the depth of field focus is again variable in the lateral or azimuthal direction but fixed in the cross-plane direction and the two focal points may not coincide, as seen in Figure 17–14. Dynamic focusing during listening can also be accomplished, as explained for the annular array. Side lobes and grating lobes continue to be present and are generally found at the locations predicted by the foregoing equations.

Because it has no moving parts and both the transmit and receive focal points can easily be adjusted, the phased-array transducer has become the transducer most widely utilized for cardiology. The compact size of the crystal arrays not only accommodates transmission between the ribs but also allows adaption to other windows. Rotating-head technology has been utilized for transesophageal imaging,[F3] but phased-array transesophageal transducers are most commonly used.

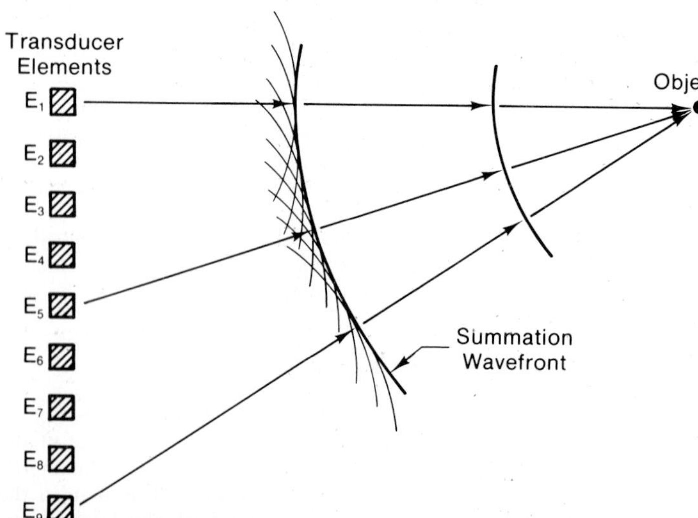

Figure 17–13. Diagrammatic representation of the formation of a curved wave front. Here the time delay between elements is not constant. The delay is set so that the summation of the individual waves forms a circular or parabolic wave front that will converge at the focal point in addition to moving away from the transducer at an angle. This is an example of simultaneous electronic beam steering and electronic focusing. (From Geiser, E. A., and Oliver, L. O.: Echocardiography physics and instrumentation. *In* Collins, S. M., and Skorton, D. J. [eds.]: Cardiac Imaging and Image Processing. McGraw-Hill, New York, 1986, with permission.)

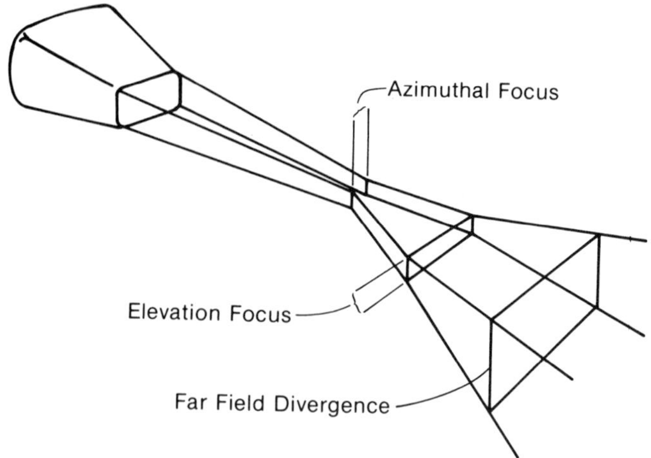

Figure 17–14. Focusing of the main lobe in a phased-array transducer. The elevation focus is accomplished with an acoustic lens. The focus in the azimuthal direction is determined in the manner of electronic focusing shown in Figure 17–13. Note that the azimuthal focal point and the elevation focal point are not necessarily the same. (From Geiser, E. A., and Oliver, L. O.: Echocardiography physics and instrumentation. *In* Collins, S. M., and Skorton, D. J. [eds.]: Cardiac Imaging and Image Processing. McGraw-Hill, New York, 1986, with permission.)

Electronic Beam Steering: The Orthogonal Phased Array/Three-Dimensional Beam Formation

In the past several years, development has proceeded on transducers that contain crystal arrays in two different directions. This new type of transducer facilitates display of two-dimensional orthogonal B-mode images, which is referred to as O-mode scanning. The design of one such crystal face and the resulting orthogonal planes are shown in Figure 17–15*A*. This work was first reported and has continued to develop under the direction of von Ramm and associates.[52] In the original form of this transducer, the cross-plane resolution was dependent primarily on fixed techniques. Simultaneous short- and long-axis images could be obtained at the same point in time. Although these two simultaneous views are helpful in assessing the cardiac geometry, the methodology remained merely a modification or union of two phased-array transducers.

More recently, the investigators have succeeded in building a transducer that provides true three-dimensional volumetric imaging. Within a transducer face of approximately 15 × 15 mm, multiple square crystal elements are positioned so that the scan lines can be directed through two-dimensional phasing in any direction within a pyramidal volume, as shown diagrammatically in Figure 17–15*B*. This transducer appears to represent the final step in accomplishing variable-transmit focusing and dynamic focusing during reception along any desired line of sight.

One interesting feature is that the received signals can be gated so that only reflecting structures at a predetermined depth from the transducer face are displayed. Thus, it is possible to display a plane that is parallel to the surface of the transducer. Furthermore, the thickness of this plane is now dependent on the axial resolution. Display of a plane parallel to the transducer face is referred to as C-scan imaging, and since the cross-plane resolution is approximately the axial resolution, the scan thickness is on the order of 1 to 2 mm. Obviously, display of an entire three-dimensional volumetric image is not a trivial task, and image quality is still limited with these first-generation three-dimensional transducers. However, continued research in this area will undoubtedly influence the importance of echocardiography as an imaging tool in the future.

RECEPTION, AMPLIFICATION, AND IMAGE FORMATION

The process of converting the returning ultrasound into a visible image in television format is no less complicated than the process of beam formation. Figure 17–16 is a generalized flow diagram of the processes involved. The process of dynamic focusing during reception, which has been described above, is carried out in the first five blocks of the flow diagram. The actual delay that forms the dynamically focused line occurs in block 4. Prior to this, there are three other steps.

In the first step, the reflected ultrasound returning to the face of the transducer crosses the impedance-matching layer and causes oscillation of each piezoelectric crystal. The oscillation of the crystal (which has now been placed in listening mode) produces an electric voltage. These oscillations are slightly downshifted in frequency because of the frequency dependence of attenuation, but they are still quite close to the nominal frequency of the transducer. These high-frequency signals coming from each transducer element (referred to as single-crystal receiver in Figure 17–16) are extremely weak and must be linearly amplified before any further processing is performed.

Recall that attenuation is expressed as dB/cm/MHz. Therefore, sound reflected from deeper structures is much weaker than that received from a shallower depth. Frequently, this difference is great enough that the amplitude of sound returning from the deeper portions of the image is 1/10 to 1/100 of the amplitude of that returning from the near field. Thus, more amplification must be performed on signals returning to the transducer at a later time. This process of applying increased gain to signals returning

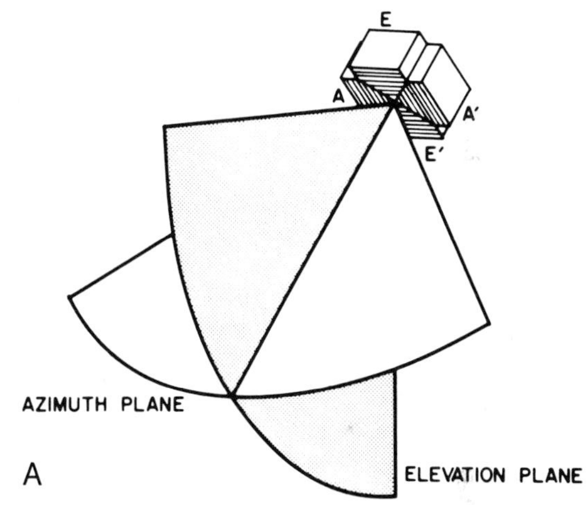

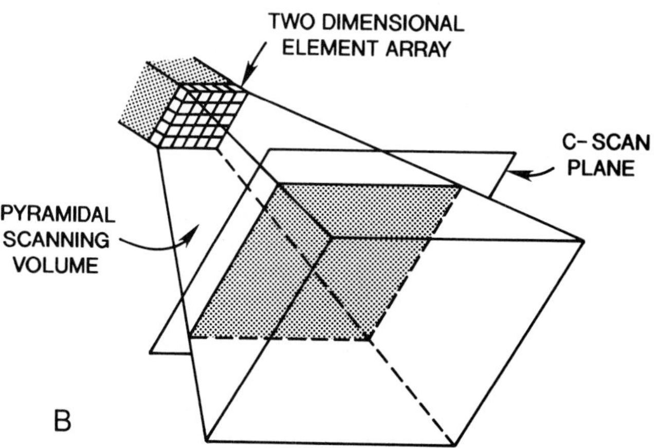

Figure 17–15. *A*, The "bow-tie" arrangement of transducer elements for simultaneous two-dimensional echocardiographic scanning in orthogonal planes. (Reprinted with permission from the American College of Cardiology [Journal of the American College of Cardiology, Vol. 7, No. 6, June 1986, p. 1280].) *B*, A two-dimensional crystal array transducer in which the transducer face consists of a 5×5 crystal array. Such a transducer is capable of three-dimensional pyramidal volumetric scanning. With this type of scanning it is possible to reconstruct an image that represents the echoes returning at a chosen distance from the transducer. This type of imaging in which the plane is parallel to the face of the transducer is referred to as C-scan imaging.

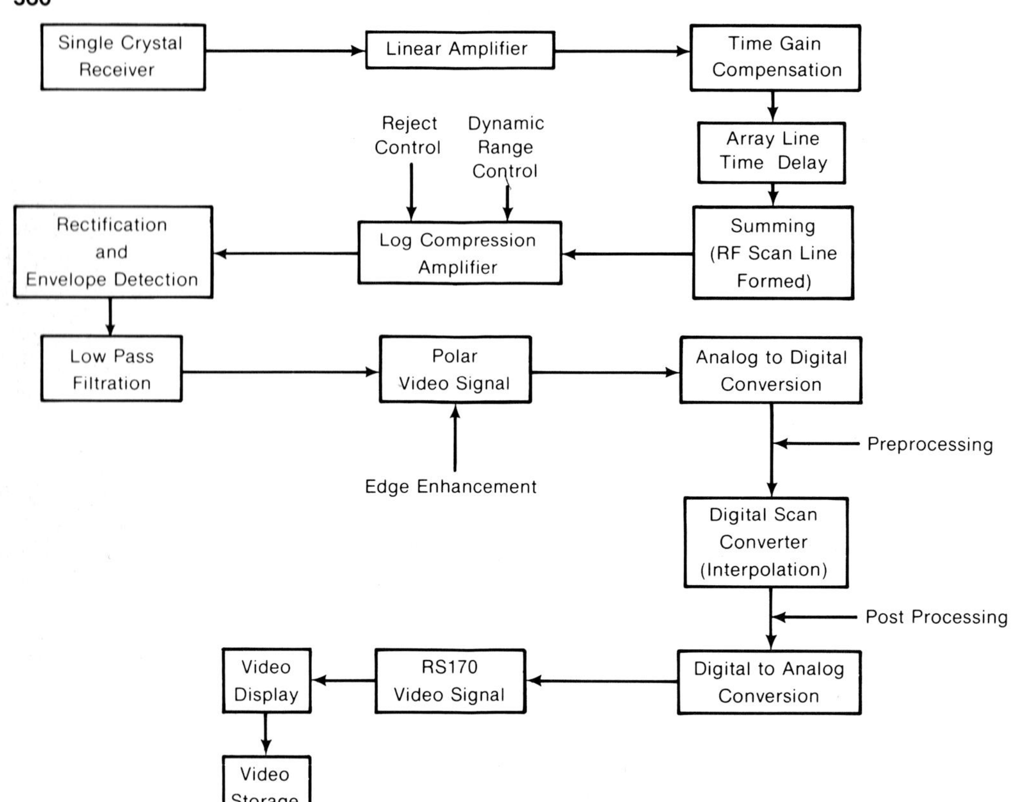

Figure 17–16. Block flow diagram of the steps involved in reception of the reflected ultrasound and formation of a two-dimensional cardiographic image. (From Geiser, E. A., and Oliver, L. O.: Echocardiography physics and instrumentation. *In* Collins, S. M., and Skorton, D. J. [eds.]: Cardiac Imaging and Image Processing. McGraw-Hill, New York, 1986, with permission.)

at a later time is referred to as time gain compensation (TGC). In single-crystal transducers, TGC is accomplished with a ramp that allows separate gain factors to be set for the near and far fields. This principle is also utilized in rotating-head or oscillating two-dimensional ultrasound systems. In the phased-array system, TGC is usually accomplished by setting slide potentiometers on the control panel, which allows individual selection of amplification factors at varying depths during the performance of the study. Figure 17–16 shows TGC being applied to the output of each crystal element. Whether the TGC is applied to scan line formation or after the dynamic-focusing time delay and summation depends on the manufacturer.

After linear amplification and TGC, the outputs of the individual crystal elements in the transducer are appropriately phased to accomplish dynamic focusing and summed to form a single scan line. This scan line still contains the very high-frequency information. Thus, the scan line formed at this point is called the radio frequency (RF) scan line.

The information contained in the RF scan line is still too complex to be displayed. The difference between the lowest-amplitude and highest-amplitude signals along the scan line may be as much as 80 to 100 dB, whereas video display devices and the human eye have the ability to display and perceive 25 to 30 dB of information. Therefore, the 80 to 100 dB must be compressed into 25 to 30 dB of dynamic range for the display device. Many of the low-amplitude signals in the scan line may represent background noise; and it would be inappropriate to use part of the display capabilities unnecessarily for this portion of the signal. Therefore, the lower-level background is thresholded or rejected from the RF scan line and the remaining dynamic range is compressed into the capabilities of the display device. This compression can be done linearly or logarithmically. In most situations, linear amplification would result in failure to display most of the very low-level signals. Hence, logarithmic amplification, which favors enhancement of the lower-level signals in the RF data, is preferred.

Following amplification, the polar scan line RF data still contain radio frequency sinusoidal waves with both positive and negative values. Since only the positive values can be displayed, the next step in signal processing consists of rectification of the RF scan line to remove or invert all values below zero. When rectification has been accomplished, individual echocardiographic specular targets consist of groups of high-frequency spikes. In order to display these sets of spikes as single targets, envelope detection is performed on the RF signal. In this process the best curve outlining each set of high-frequency spikes—that is, the envelope—is chosen. In some of the newer scanners, more complex mathematical methods are used for full-wave envelope detection and rectification is not needed as a first step. Whichever method is used, these processes consolidate multiple spikes into single outlines that represent the targets. The targets are displayed as single bright spots on the scan line instead of series of tiny bright spots.

Following envelope detection, the signal undergoes a final low-pass filtration that removes much of the remaining high-frequency signal. The resulting envelope-detected and filtered signal is referred to as the video signal or the polar scan line data.

When all of the individual polar lines have been obtained, the data necessary to form one two-dimensional echo image have been obtained. In the polar image data, each scan line has been obtained at a different angle and the data along each line are a radial distance, R, from the theoretical center point of the transducer. Figure 17–17 shows a polar video image. In this format the data are not particularly useful and appear distorted. Only when the data have been redisplayed at the appropriate angles and depths will appropriate target positions be placed in their correct anatomic locations.

DIGITAL SCAN CONVERSION

As mentioned, the polar scan line data cannot be presented in standard video format. In early two-dimensional ultrasound machines, these data were presented on an oscilloscope that had independent steering of the beam in the x and y directions so that the lines could be displayed at the angles at which they had been obtained. However, display of this type of image cannot be placed on videotape, since it is not a standard horizontal and vertical video signal (RS170). The only way to store the scan was to photograph the screen or to place a television camera in front

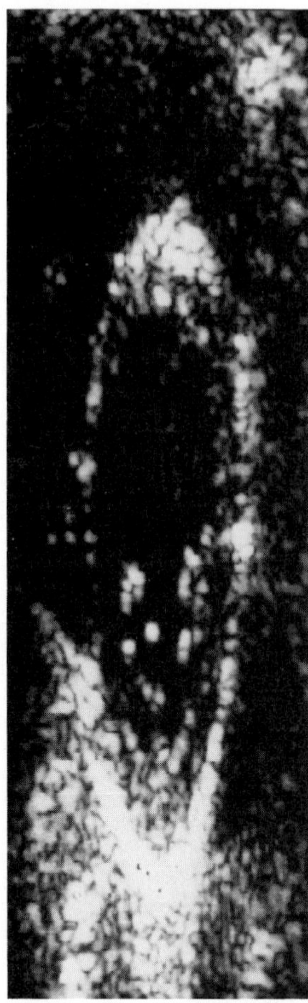

Figure 17–17. Display of polar video data without scan conversion. Values along the ordinate represent axial distance from the face of the transducer. Values along the abscissa represent the angle along which the individual B-mode lines were obtained.

of the screen and record it on videotape. Furthermore, the overlap of the scan lines in the near field made this portion of the picture extremely bright, while there were wide gaps in the far field. This display was not visually optimal.

To circumvent these problems, digital scan conversion was developed. Scan conversion refers to conversion from analog polar scan line data to analog standard video by means of a digital computerized process. In this process each analog polar video line first goes through analog-to-digital conversion. In most modern equipment the voltage amplitude of the polar video signal is converted to a numeric (digital) value at 512 equally spaced points along each scan line. Each of these digital values is then mapped into the nearest Cartesian (x, y) location in a rectangular image that has 512 × 512 points. Since a picture is to be produced, each of these points is referred to as a picture element or pixel. In the near field close to the apex of the scan, the polar lines overlap. Thus, much of the information from the polar data must be deleted or averaged to fit the digitized data into the limited number of Cartesian matrix positions. Conversely, in the far field the polar scan lines are quite separated in the Cartesian space, so there is only enough data to fill one-half to one-third of the available matrix positions. Figure 17–18 shows this 1:1 mapping of the polar scan line points to the appropriate x, y pixel locations that correspond to their positions in the sector scan. The figure can be thought of as the digital equivalent of the older analog x, y, z oscilloscope displays. In Figure 17–18 the polar scan line data presented in Figure 17–17 have, in part, been mapped into a 256 × 200 Cartesian array. This lower resolution was chosen so that the individual pixel elements in mapping would be more easily illustrated. Notice that the process of mapping the polar data to the discrete locations

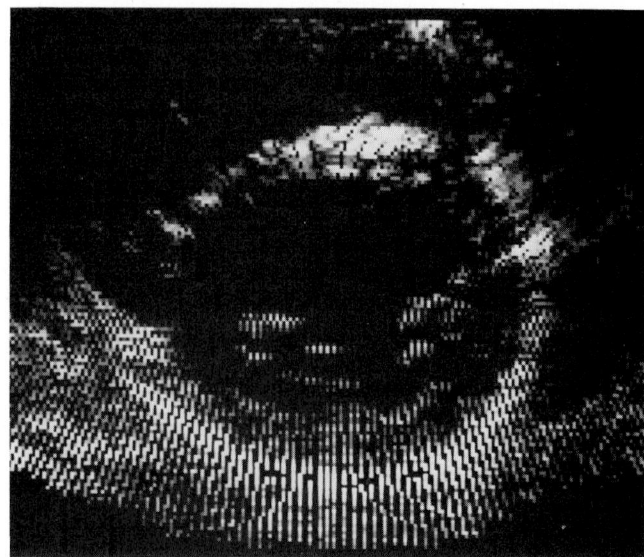

Figure 17–18. Simple digital scan conversion without interpolation. Here the brightness values from Figure 17–17 have been placed in the nearest appropriate x, y location in Cartesian space. Note the symmetric curved pattern of unfilled pixels around the central axis of the scan. This is referred to as a moiré pattern.

in the Cartesian array produces a regular pattern of unfilled matrix elements between and through scan lines. These curved lines sweeping upward and outward are referred to as a moiré pattern.

Clinicians find both the unfilled regions between scan lines and the moiré pattern distracting in evaluating clinical studies. Therefore, various schemes have been developed to fill in or interpolate the existing data in order to smooth the image.

The simplest way to fill in blank matrix elements is to perform a linear interpolation in the horizontal or x direction. If only one pixel value was to be filled, as in the case of matrix element M_{AB} in Figure 17–19, the digital gray level value assigned to matrix element M_{AB} would be

$$M_{AB} = (M_A + M_B)/2$$

If two matrix elements were to be interpolated, the values assigned to pixels M_{AB2} and M_{AB3} would be given by

$$M_{AB2} = M_B + (M_B - M_A)/3$$
$$M_{AB3} = M_B + 2(M_B - M_A)/3$$

In this linear interpolation, it is assumed that the actual spacing between the known gray levels along scan lines is equal in the x direction and the nearest gray levels in the y direction are not considered. For this reason simple linear interpolation in the horizontal direction produces a somewhat coarse quality in the image. Because this coarseness is also objectionable to most observers, simple interpolation has been replaced by a more complex form of interpolation referred to, in general, as R, θ scan conversion.[1,3] In the more complex interpolation scheme, the gray level assignment for a matrix element is derived by interpolation of the digital gray level values of the four nearest positions in the digital polar scan line data. In addition, the contribution of each of the four is dependent on its relative distance to the new pixel in both radial and azimuthal directions. In Figure 17–19, the value of matrix element M_{AB} would now be filled by interpolating new gray level values along scan line A and scan line B in the radial directions. The two new points corresponding to the radial length to the center of M_{AB} are labeled G_{AI} and G_{BI} and their values are given by

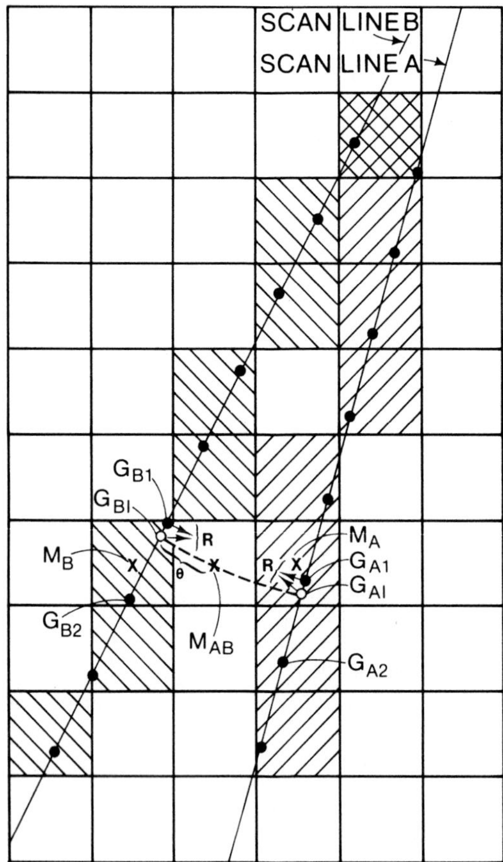

Figure 17–19. Schematic representation of the mapping of polar scan line data into Cartesian coordinates by the digital scan converter. The digitized gray levels or brightnesses at equally spaced positions along polar scan lines are represented by the letter G. The gray level assigned to a position in the scan converter Cartesian matrix is designated by the letter M. Position M_{AB} is an unfilled position in the matrix and must be interpolated. Two methods for determining the gray level of position M_{AB} are described in the text. (From Geiser, E. A., and Oliver, L. O.: Echocardiography physics and instrumentation. *In* Collins, S. M., and Skorton, D. J. [eds.]: Cardiac Imaging and Image Processing. McGraw-Hill, New York, 1986, with permission.)

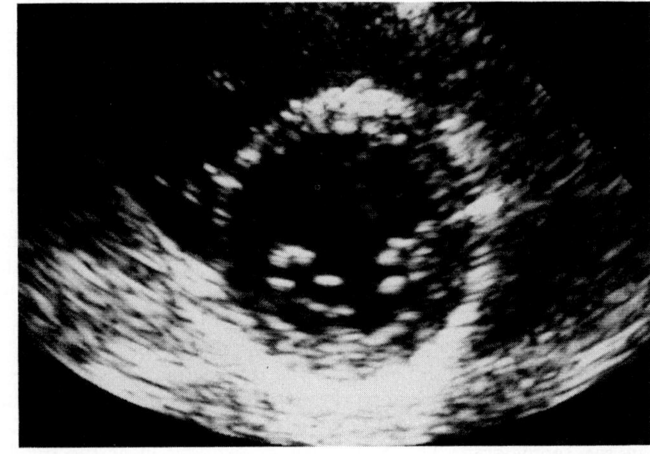

Figure 17–20. Final two-dimensional echocardiographic image formed from the data in Figure 17–17. Scan conversion has been accomplished in a larger matrix scan converter than was used for Figure 17–18, and all the matrix elements have been filled by an R, θ scan conversion similar to that described in the text.

$$G_{AI} = \frac{1 - R}{\Delta R} G_{AI} + \frac{R}{\Delta R} G_{A2}$$

$$G_{BI} = \frac{1 - R}{\Delta R} G_{B2} + \frac{R}{\Delta R} G_{B2}$$

The value of M_{AB} is then calculated as

$$M_{AB} = \frac{1 - \Theta}{\Delta\Theta} G_{BI} + \frac{\Theta}{\Delta\Theta} G_{AI}$$

which shows that the relative contribution of G_{AI} and G_{BI} is again proportional to the distance to these respective points. This method of filling the matrix and forming a final image in which the gray level of each picture element is proportional to the relative position of that pixel in relation to the original digitized amplitudes from the polar video signal produces a very smooth image, as shown in Figure 17–20.

From the preceding discussion it should be clear that the actual image content in terms of real data is identical in the analog polar oscilloscope presentation, the digital interpolated image, and the R, θ scan converted image. The image quality, however, varies greatly. Thus, image quality may to a large extent be cosmetic and a matter of preference, since the image content is the same.

PRE- AND POSTPROCESSING

The advent of the digital scan converter has made possible almost limitless variation in the display of the image to satisfy user preference. The foregoing discussion showed that the polar video signal arriving at the scan converter is a logarithmically compressed, envelope-detected, and low-pass-filtered varying voltage in which the amplitude at any point is proportional to the amplitude (actually phase) of the returning ultrasound waves. Logarithmic compression was done partly to reduce the range of amplitudes in the polar video signal. Even after this compression, however, patient-to-patient variation makes it desirable to manipulate the amplitudes and thereby enhance some low-level signals or decrease very high-level signals that may saturate the display. This further manipulation of gray scale can be accomplished at one of two points. The first point is at analog-to-digital conversion, when the polar scan line data are placed into image memory. Manipulation of gray levels at this point means that the modified gray levels will be utilized in the R, θ interpolation scheme and will thus modify the image. The second point is at digital-to-analog conversion, when the digital scan converter matrix is read horizontally along each sequential line and converted into horizontal video signals. Modification at this point produces slightly different control such that all pixels having the same value after interpolation can be either suppressed or enhanced. Modifying the image during polar analog-to-digital conversion as the image is acquired is referred to as preprocessing, and modifying the image during digital-to-analog formation of the standard video signal is referred to as postprocessing. The point at which each of these is applied is shown in Figure 17–16.

Both preprocessing and postprocessing are generally done with a computerized lookup table. For example, during preprocessing, if the polar video signal had an amplitude variation between 0 and 5 volts (V) and digital scan conversion was taking place at an 8-bit gray scale resolution (256 levels of gray), a voltage of 0 would be assigned a digital gray level of 0 and a voltage of 5 would be assigned a digital gray level of 255.

A target of intermediate amplitude in the polar video signal might have a voltage of 2.5 V. In a linear system this would be assigned a digital gray level in the scan converter of 127. If one wished to enhance these intermediate-level targets, a value greater than 127 could be assigned to an incoming analog voltage of 2.5. This analog-to-digital conversion is handled through a lookup table. In the system, the computer that is managing the analog-to-digital conversion looks at an incoming voltage of 2.5 V and looks at the table to see what digital value is to be assigned to that voltage. Most manufacturers supply four to six of these lookup tables, which are referred to as preprocessing curves.

Postprocessing is analogous, but in this case the digital value prompts assignment of a voltage. An interesting application of postprocessing is inversion of the image. In this situation, a value of 255 can be assigned a voltage of 0 and a value of 0 can be assigned a voltage of 5. Thus, the image is converted from white on black to black on white.

FREEZE-FRAME AND CONTINUOUS LOOP DISPLAY

One of the disadvantages of analog or early digital scan conversion equipment was that an image could not be saved on the screen and analyzed. The incorporation of analog-to-digital conversion and scan converter technology has substantially increased the ability to study and make measurements within the two-dimensional ultrasound equipment. In the preceding section, the polar video signal was considered to be digitized and the digital gray levels were mapped into the appropriate x, y location in the Cartesian coordinate image in the scan converter. If, instead of going directly into the scan converter, the digital gray levels at every point along each scan line are kept in random-access memory (RAM), then at any point the digital polar data can be fed into the scan converter and displayed in video format for the operator. Thus, it is possible to store images while continuing the examination and to restore previous images for comparison at a different point in time.

The concept of storing images in RAM for later recall can be expanded by increasing the available RAM storage capabilities of the ultrasound machine. It is possible to store 16, 32, or even 128 polar images in digital format. Any sequence or portion of a sequence of these stored images can then be read in real time into the scan converter and displayed. This capability is commonly referred to as continuous loop memory.

Finally, a polar digital image stored in RAM can be read into one-half or even one-quarter of the rectangular scan converter memory. Such manipulation allows side-by-side or four-quadrant simultaneous comparison of images.

When an image is in the rectangular scan converter and interpolated, various structures can be marked by using a cursor. Since the depth of the scan is known from other machine settings, both the number of pixels per centimeter and the number of pixels per square centimeter can be calculated. Thus, measurements of distance and area can be made with relative ease from the screen.

Since any output from the scan converter is in standard video format, whatever is seen on the screen can be recorded on videotape, which is the usual mode of storage for two-dimensional echocardiography. Many contemporary systems allow review of videotapes through the system. During this process of review, any video frame obtained from tape can be passed through a video analog-to-digital converter and passed to a section of memory that is similar to the scan converter. Postprocessing curves can then be applied, so even after a videotape is made some changes in gray scale can be accomplished to enhance visual appreciation of structures. This digitization process also allows measurements to be made from the videotape images.

CONCLUSION

The basic principles of ultrasound and the methods that allow formation of diagnostic images have been reviewed. In brief, contemporary ultrasound machines are quite sophisticated and powerful computers that are designed specifically to provide real-time visualization of structure and motion in the heart. Although the specifics of implementation may differ somewhat between manufacturers, the individual components and methods remain fairly constant. It is hoped that, through a better understanding of these principles, the reader will develop a better understanding of the strengths and weaknesses of the technique.

References

A

1. American Institute of Ultrasound in Medicine: Safety considerations for diagnostic ultrasound. J. Ultrasound Med. 3(Suppl.):S1, 1984.
2. American Institute of Ultrasound in Medicine: Standard methods for testing single-element pulsed-echo ultrasonic transducers. J. Ultrasound Med. 1(Suppl.):S1, 1982.
3. Aero-Tech Reports: Linear arrays: Theory of operation and performance. KB-AEROTECH 2(1), 1981.

C

1. Carson, P.L., Fischella, P.R., and Oughton, T.V.: Ultrasonic power and intensities produced by diagnostic ultrasound equipment. Ultrasound Med. Biol. 3:341, 1978.

E

1. Edler, I., and Hertz, C.H.: Use of ultrasonic reflectoscope for continuous recording of movement of heart walls. K. Fysiogr. Sallsk. Lund Forh. 24:40, 1954.

F

1. Firestone, F.A.: The supersonic reflectoscope for interior inspection. Met. Prog. 48:505, 1945.
2. Frazin, L., Talano, J.V., Stephanides, L., et al.: Esophageal echocardiography. Circulation 54:102, 1976.
3. Fearnot, N.E., Babbs, C.F., Bourland, J.D., and Geddes, L.A.: Dynamic intraesophageal imaging of the heart with ultrasound. Ultrasonic imaging 2:78, 1980.

K

1. Kisslo, J., von Ramm, O.T., and Thurstone, F.L.: Cardiac imaging using a phased array ultrasound system. II. Clinical technique and application. Circulation 53:262, 1976.
2. Kinsler, L.E., and Frey, A.R.: Fundamentals of Acoustics, 2nd ed. Wiley, New York, 1962.

L

1. Ludwig, G.D.: The velocity of sound through tissues and the acoustic impedances of tissues. J. Acoust. Soc. Am. 22:862, 1950.
2. Larson, J.D., III: An acoustic transducer array for medical imaging: Part I. Hewlett-Packard J. 34:17, 1983.
3. Leavitt, S.C., Hunt, B.F., and Larsen, H.G.: A scan conversion algorithm for displaying ultrasound images. Hewlett-Packard J. 34:32, 1983.

S

1. Somer, J.C.: Electronic sector scanning for ultrasonic diagnosis. Ultrasonics 6:153, 1968.
2. Snyder, J.E., Kisslo, J., and von Ramm, O.T.: Real-time orthogonal mode scanning of the heart. I. System design. J. Am. Coll. Cardiol. 7:1279, 1986.

W

1. Wild, J.J., and Reid, J.M.: Further pilot echographic studies on the histologic structure of tumors of the living intact human breast. Am. J. Pathol. 28:839, 1952.
2. Wells, P.N.T.: Wave fundamentals. *In* Biomedical Ultrasonics. Academic Press, New York, 1977, pp. 1–25.
3. Wells, P.N.T.: Biomedical Ultrasonics. Academic Press, New York, 1977, p. 20.

Y

1. Yoshiba, T., Mori, M., Nimura, Y., et al.: Study on examining the heart with ultrasonics. III. Kinds of Doppler beats. IV. Clinical applications. Jpn. Circ. J. 20:228, 1956.

Chapter 18

Principles and Physics of Doppler

■ *SCOTT R. CANNON, Ph.D.* ■ *KENT L. RICHARDS, M.D.*

THE DOPPLER EFFECT 365
Waves and Propagation 365
Frequency Shifts 365
The Cosine Factor 366
CARDIOVASCULAR DOPPLER PHYSICS 367
Reflection 367
Point and Blood Backscatter 367
Doppler Frequency Ambiguity 367
PHYSICS OF BLOOD FLOW 367
Viscosity and Flow Profiles 367
Turbulence 368
BASIC DOPPLER INSTRUMENTATION 368
Doppler Transducers 368
Continuous-Wave Doppler 369
Pulsed Doppler 369
Color Flow Doppler 371
DOPPLER PROCESSING AND DISPLAY 371
Time-Based Processing 371
Spectral Analysis 371

Significant developments in the application of noninvasive Doppler ultrasound techniques in cardiovascular medicine have taken place over the last 20 years. Doppler instrumentation is now capable of providing easily obtainable hemodynamic data based on blood flow velocities, which has proved extremely useful in the clinical assessment and management of cardiovascular disease. Doppler methods have been introduced for the recognition of cardiac shunts and congenital or acquired abnormal morphology. Quantitative assessment methods for valvular stenosis and regurgitation, shunts, and cardiac output have been proposed. The recent development of real-time color flow imaging with two-dimensional ultrasound imaging has further enhanced the utility of Doppler technology.

As with any technology, it is important that physicians and technicians understand the basic concepts, the capabilities, and, perhaps most important, the limitations inherent in this tool. The purpose of this chapter is to present these three attributes of cardiovascular Doppler. This discussion begins with a simple explanation of wave propagation and the Doppler effect. Then practical considerations related to the application of the Doppler effect in cardiovascular hemodynamics are mentioned. The basic physics of blood flow is introduced for an appreciation of the phenomena that Doppler methods attempt to measure. The common modes of Doppler instrumentation are discussed, and methods of signal processing and display of basic Doppler information are presented. The basic similarities, differences, strengths, and limitations of continuous-wave, pulsed, and color flow Doppler instrumentation are discussed.

THE DOPPLER EFFECT

Waves and Propagation

Sound waves propagating through a uniform medium can be represented by a simple natural analogy. Consider a pebble dropped into the middle of a still pond. One can imagine ripples moving away from the disturbance at a constant rate and in concentric circles.

We commonly characterize wave propagation using the terms *wavelength, frequency, propagation velocity, magnitude, phase,* and *attenuation.* Wavelength is the distance between successive peaks. Frequency is the rate at which successive peaks travel past any fixed point. Propagation speed is the rate at which any one peak moves across the pond. Magnitude is a measure of the height of the peaks.

If we were able to view the pond from the side, this series of peaks and valleys (or the wave) would take the shape of the trigonometric sine function. As the wave travels out from the disturbance, magnitudes become progressively smaller because of energy loss. The water is attenuating the wave. Wave propagation speed is a constant for a particular medium and frequency. Fluids with different viscosities and densities exhibit different propagation velocities and attenuation in response to the same disturbance.

If three small bubbles are floating on the pond surface and arranged in a line along the direction of wave propagation, the bubbles will oscillate up and down as they follow the peaks and valleys of the waves passing underneath. Each bubble, however, oscillates slightly out of synchronization with its neighbors; the bubble closest to the disturbance leads the middle bubble and the middle bubble leads the last. The position of one bubble relative to another or to a particular wave position is a measurement of phase.

Mathematically, frequency (f) and wavelength (λ) are related to propagation speed (c) by the following:

$$c = f\lambda \quad (1)$$

As ultrasound propagates through the body, tissues vibrate similarly to the bubbles of the pond.

Frequency Shifts

An interesting phenomenon now occurs if a disturbance generating waves also happens to be moving. Imagine a continuously sounding horn on a moving car (Fig. 18–1). Sound waves leaving the horn and traveling forward along the direction of the car are moving at a constant speed through the air. After the generation of one wave peak, the car moves forward slightly prior to the generation of the next peak. Consequently, the two peaks are closer together and arrive at an observer ahead of the car at a higher rate. In other words, the original frequency of the horn is shifted higher and the observer hears a slightly higher note.

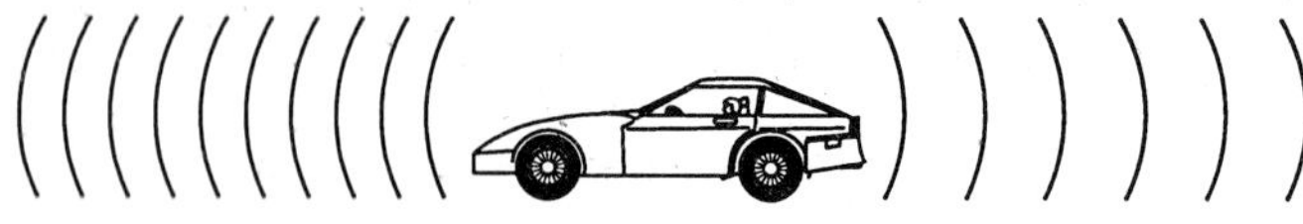

Figure 18–1. Sound waves originating from the horn of a moving car are Doppler-shifted because of the motion of the car relative to the listener.

On the other hand, a second observer listening to the car from behind would find the opposite to be true. The car has now added distance between wave peaks. Although the sound is traveling at the same speed to the front and rear of the car, sound peaks arrive at the second observer at a lower rate and the frequency is shifted slightly lower. This is commonly known as the Doppler effect. One can also easily imagine that this motion is relative; the same Doppler effect is present when the sound source is stationary and the listener is moving.

Consider now what would happen if the moving car reflected sound from a stationary horn some distance in front of the car. Suppose the stationary horn emits f_1. Observers in the car would note a Doppler shift because of the motion of the car relative to the stationary source. The moving observers hear f_2. The car now reflects this Doppler-shifted sound (f_2), causing a *second* equal Doppler shift. An observer at the stationary horn now hears f_3 or a Doppler-shifted f_2 coming from the car. The original sound is reflected back with a double shift: $f_1 < f_2 < f_3$.

This relationship can be more formally expressed as in Figure 18–2. When both source and receiver are stationary, a frequency f produces a wavelength λ. When the source moves toward the receiver, λ is reduced by dλ or the distance traveled during one wave cycle or period. If v_s is the velocity of the source toward the receiver and f_s is the frequency at the source, the source will move $1/f_s$ between two peaks;

$$d\lambda = v_s * (1/f_s) \quad (2)$$

The wavelength detected by the receiver is then

$$\lambda_r = \lambda_s - d\lambda = (c/f_s) - (v_s/f_s) \quad (3)$$

where the subscript r refers to the receiver. The frequency of this wavelength can then be written as

$$(c/f_r) = (c/f_s) - (v_s/f_s) \quad (4)$$

so now

$$f_r = (f_s)c/(c - v_s) \quad (5)$$

If we divide equation (5) by c we find

$$f_r = (f_s)1/(1 - v_s/c) \quad (6)$$

The last part of this equation can be approximated with a series:

$$1/(1 - x) = 1 + x + x^2/2 + \ldots \quad (7)$$

Since v/c is normally very small if we are well below the sound barrier, we will use only the first term of this series:

$$f_r = f_s + (f_s)(v_s/c) \quad (8)$$

The Doppler shift, f_d, is then given by the relationship

$$f_d = f_r - f_s = (f_s)v_s/c \quad (9)$$

If the source is now stationary and the receiver is a moving reflector, the receiver hears a Doppler-shifted frequency f_r, which is then reflected back to an observer at the original source for a second Doppler shift. If the frequency heard by the observer is f'_r,

$$f'_r = f_r + (f_r)\,v_s/c$$
$$=(f_s + (f_s)v_r/c) + (f_s + v_r/c)(v_s/c) \quad (10)$$

Now, $|v_r| = |v_s|$ and $(v/c)^2$ is very small, so equation (10) can be written as

$$f'_r = f_s + (f_s)2v/c \quad (11)$$

and the Doppler shift becomes

$$f_d = (f_s)2v/c \quad (12)$$

If the source frequency and c are constant, the Doppler shift is then directly proportional to the velocity of the reflector. Solving equation (12) for v allows us to predict the velocity for a given shift.

The Cosine Factor

In the foregoing discussion it is assumed that the observer and source are directly in front of or behind the moving reflector. If the observer is off to one side of the road, a Doppler effect may still be noticed, since the v represents the *relative velocity* of the moving reflector with respect to the observer and source. This relative velocity can be calculated by using the cosine of the angle α between the line from observer to reflector and the reflector's direction of motion (Fig. 18–3).

$$f_d = (f_s)2v\cos(\alpha)/c \quad (13)$$

If the reflector is moving perpendicular to the observer, $\cos(90°) = 0$ and no Doppler shift is noticed. However, it should be noted (particularly for cardiovascular applications) that for angles

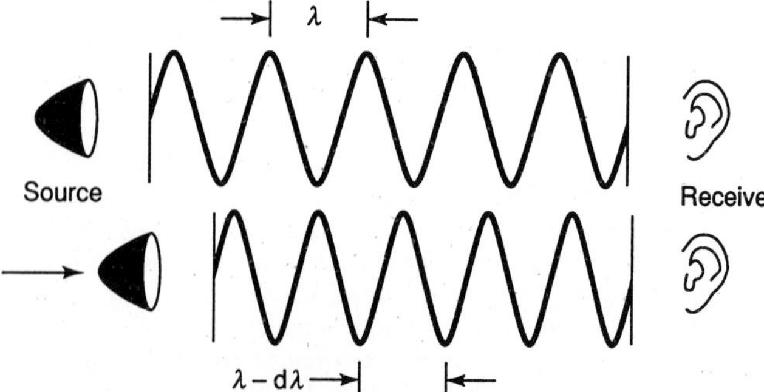

Figure 18–2. The wavelength of sound originating from a moving source is reduced by dλ, representing the distance traveled during one wave period.

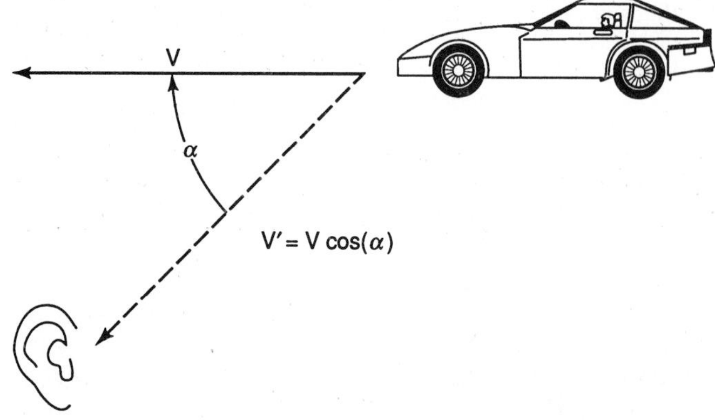

Figure 18–3. Doppler shift is calculated from relative velocity, which is the velocity of the moving source corrected by the cosine of the angle between the direction of motion and the observer.

less than approximately 25 degrees, the cosine is 0.9 or greater and the cosine effect is small. For angles greater than 25 degrees, very small changes (or errors in measurement) in angle can produce significant changes (or errors) in Doppler shift calculations.

In summary: Doppler frequency shifts are directly proportional to the velocity of a moving reflector. Assuming that the propagation velocity and transmission frequency are known and constant, the velocity of the moving reflector can be calculated. If the observer is at an angle to the direction of motion, correction must be made by using the cosine of the angle.

CARDIOVASCULAR DOPPLER PHYSICS

Cardiovascular ultrasound frequencies are typically in the range of 1.5 to 7 megahertz (MHz, or 1 million cycles or periods per second). Above 7 MHz, ultrasound attenuation is generally too great to allow sufficient penetration for noninvasive cardiac use, although intracardiac applications may range to 20 MHz. Below 1.5 MHz, Doppler frequency shifts are normally small and transducers become bulky. In relatively homogeneous soft tissue, the propagation velocity of ultrasound is similar to that in water, approximately 1580 m/sec.[H1]

Reflection

Ultrasound waves travel through tissue in a straight line until they encounter tissue interfaces—the borders between tissues with different densities and/or wave propagation speeds. At these interfaces, a portion of the sound energy is reflected. In general, a term known as the acoustic impedance, Z, defines the mechanical propagation property of a medium:

$$Z = \rho c \tag{14}$$

where ρ represents density and c again represents propagation speed. The greater the difference in impedances between two tissues at a boundary, the greater the reflection of ultrasound. Bone and air or lung boundaries represent large impedance differences with tissue and thus tend to block transmission of ultrasound energy. In addition, air is a strong attenuator at ultrasound frequencies. For these reasons, Doppler ultrasound examinations are done through soft-tissue paths with a gel interface between the transducer and the skin.

Point and Blood Backscatter

Although some studies have attempted to examine ventricular wall and valve leaflet motion with Doppler ultrasound, its primary clinical use is in the characterization of blood flow. Human blood consists primarily of erythrocytes, leukocytes, and platelets, in addition to plasma. At a hematocrit value of 45 percent, the erythrocyte concentration is approximately 5×10^6 per mm^3. The erythrocytes are probably the major source of reflection, since leukocytes (although much larger) are relatively sparse, at approximately 8×10^3 per mm^3. Platelets, at approximately 4×10^5 per mm^3, are almost as dense as red cells but are significantly smaller.[G1]

Erythrocytes have a concave disklike shape, but this shape plays no part in the reflecting characteristics of blood. The red cell is so small with respect to ultrasound wavelengths that it effectively serves as a point reflector. That is, each cell reflects ultrasound as if the cell were a very small sphere.[S1, W1] The primary source of reflected or backscattered ultrasound energy is the impedance difference between erythrocytes and plasma. In vivo differences in hematocrit value and aggregations of red cells known as rouleaux do not significantly affect ultrasound reflections. It should be noted, however, that in studies in vitro even minor clotting can significantly affect ultrasound characteristics and backscatter.[A1]

Doppler Frequency Ambiguity

The accuracy of the Doppler shift from a moving blood pool is limited by several important factors. First, in the Doppler equation (equation (13)) it is assumed that the reflector is infinitely large and the source sound wave is infinitely wide.[K1, W1] In moving blood, Doppler shifts are due to randomly distributed point sources. Practical observations demonstrate that ultrasound reflected from blood moving at constant velocity exhibits random fluctuations and that these fluctuations are independent of the cosine of the angle of incidence (the angle between the ultrasound and blood velocity vectors).[S2] These random fluctuations are occasionally referred to as "granular echo."

As might be imagined, blood moving through a finite volume contains a distribution of cell velocities rather than a fixed single velocity for all cells. In addition, cells in cardiac applications are frequently accelerating or changing velocity during the volume transit time.

Another simple explanation of at least a component of granular echo concerns fluctuations in cell density. Since blood cells are randomly distributed, each small volume of an arbitrary size will contain cell densities that fluctuate about the mean density.[M1] Smaller volumes will have larger fluctuations. This phenomenon is supported by statistical diffraction theory studies.[A2, F1, F2, S3] Even small variations in density are significant; the power of reflected ultrasound is a function of the square of the mean cell density. As previously mentioned, the random orientation of the disk-shaped erythrocytes has no effect on backscatter.

In summary: The speed of ultrasound in soft tissue is relatively constant. Bone and air block significant transmission. Moving red cells are primary reflectors of Doppler-shifted ultrasound. The relatively small size of red cells causes them to appear as point reflectors. Granular echo and random cell distributions cause distortion in Doppler shifts and limit the accuracy of Doppler in cardiovascular applications. Other significant limitations on the accuracy of determinations of blood flow velocity with Doppler are discussed in later sections concerning the physics of blood flow, transducers, instrumentation, and display processing.

PHYSICS OF BLOOD FLOW

Blood is a mixture of solid cells and liquid plasma. The treatment of flow patterns in such a fluid is quite complex. For arteries with a radius of at least 1 mm, it has been shown that blood behaves similarly to a uniform fluid with a linear viscosity. Such a fluid is called *Newtonian.* The following arguments are based on such an assumption.

Viscosity and Flow Profiles

Two small neighboring volumes of blood flowing at differing velocities generate frictional forces between them that oppose the flow. Higher viscosities and velocities produce correspondingly higher frictional forces. These frictional forces tend to smooth fluid motion along regular lines. Studies have shown that in a long column these frictional forces between adjacent flow elements and between the fluid and the column wall produce a symmetric profile (Fig. 18–4).[C1] As shown by the arrows of Figure 18–4 representing velocities, flow elements travel in parallel lines along the column. Flow at the center is at a higher velocity than flow near the edges. In general, the distribution of this profile is parabolic in shape. Such a flow profile is termed "laminar." Flow profiles in cardiac chambers and across valves are quite complex, with eddies, swirls, and varied flows in drastically different directions. Normal morphology, however, still produces fairly laminar flow because there are few distinctly defined flow boundaries. Transitions from one flow region to another are smooth.

In vitro experiments and mathematical models have shown that acceleration and converging geometry tend to flatten a parabolic flow profile (Fig. 18–5).[C1] A bend or change in direction tends to skew a parabolic profile first to the inner wall and then

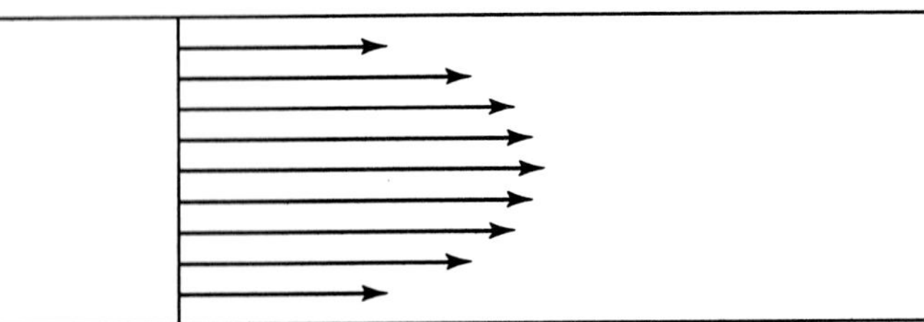

Figure 18–4. Blood flowing in a straight vessel produces a symmetric parabolic profile of velocities.

to the outer wall of the bend. Diverging geometry tends to peak the profile beyond the parabolic shape. If the divergence is extreme, eddies may form along the wall.

Turbulence

As velocity increases in a column of fluid, a point may be reached where the laminar nature of flow changes drastically and the flow becomes turbulent. Turbulent flow is characterized by flow velocities with two terms: a slowly varying term representing the forward motion of fluid along the column and a rapidly varying term representing random eddies and fluctuations in direction and speed for any particular small volume. The rapid component produces Doppler reflections that are relatively independent of the cosine of the angle between ultrasound direction and net forward flow.[A3] There is no simple flow rate at which turbulence can be expected for a given viscosity. Rather, a tendency for turbulence increases as flow rate increases. Flow is said to become less stable. At low flow rates, small disturbances tend to smooth out quickly or decay as flow progresses. At higher flow rates, small disturbances may produce rapid degradation into turbulent flow, which may persist far into the flow column. Without disturbances, however, flow may persist in a laminar condition at even higher rates. In addition, a certain hysteresis condition exists because flow at rates significantly lower than the rate at which turbulence began may be required to return to laminar flow.

The Reynolds number, Re, is frequently used to express the stability of flow:

$$Re = \rho dv/\mu \tag{15}$$

where ρ is density, d is column diameter, v is velocity, and μ is viscosity. Turbulent flow usually develops with a disturbance at Reynolds numbers greater than 2000. Without a disturbance, Reynolds numbers as great at 20,000 can be produced in laminar flow conditions.[C2]

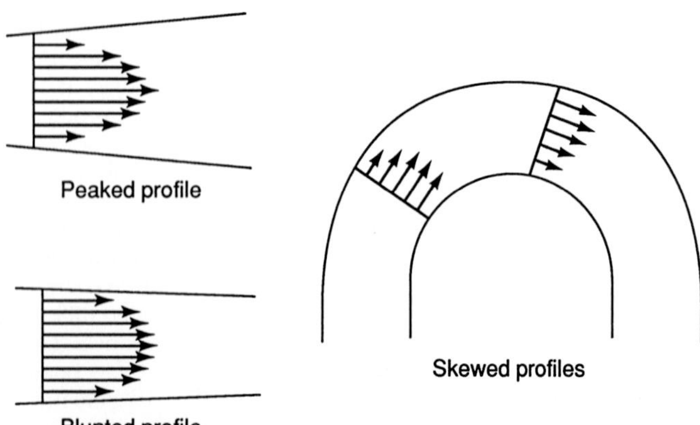

Figure 18–5. Diverging vessel walls produce a more peaked velocity profile, whereas converging walls produce a blunted profile. A bend tends to skew the profile, first toward the inner wall and then toward the outer wall.

Although the definition of true turbulent flow is statistical in nature, the general term "disturbed" flow can be used in cardiovascular applications to indicate areas containing nonparallel flow lines or areas of random fluctuations in direction and speed including small swirls and eddies.[M2] This definition may include flow that is not truly turbulent according to mathematical definitions, but it is significant in Doppler applications because it represents all flow that contains a broad distribution of velocity components.[A4, F1]

In flow across a stenotic aortic valve a complex set of spatial conditions may occur, with a high-velocity laminar jet bordered by a region of disturbed flow extending to the sides and front of the jet and with random, laminar, low-velocity flow beyond and at the aortic walls.[C1, C2] In general, ultrasound reflections from regions of disturbed flow contain a broad spectrum of both positive and negative Doppler shifts with little tendency toward a common mean.

In summary: Geometry, viscosity, and acceleration may combine to produce a distribution of velocities in any given volume of blood producing Doppler ultrasound reflections. The determination of blood flow velocity from Doppler is then somewhat more complex than might originally be imagined. Doppler reflections will, however, represent a similar distribution of shifts approximately corresponding to the velocity profile of the blood volume producing the reflection. Doppler shifts tend to be narrow-banded and cluster around a central mean frequency in laminar flow. In conditions of disturbed flow, a broad band of both positive and negative shifts is seen and determinations of net forward velocity or peak velocity are difficult.

BASIC DOPPLER INSTRUMENTATION

This section discusses the basics of ultrasound generation and reception as well as the specific modalities of continuous-wave, pulsed, and color flow instrumentation.

Doppler Transducers

Ultrasound is generated with a piezoelectric crystal. Such a crystal has the property that it vibrates at a resonance frequency if excited by an electrical signal of similar frequency. Conversely, if vibrated externally at nearly the resonance frequency, the crystal produces a corresponding electrical signal of the same frequency. A typical 2-MHz Doppler transducer is cylindrical in shape with a 15-mm (approximately 20 wavelengths) diameter. The front face vibrates much like a piston. Since ultrasound can be refracted similarly to light, a lens is placed at the crystal front to direct and focus the sound into a beam.

The focal point of the beam is defined as the position at which the beam is narrowest (Fig. 18–6). This point is a function of the lens, the transducer frequency, and the crystal diameter, all of which are fixed for a particular transducer. Proximal and distal to this focal point, the beam is considerably wider. The edges of the beam are not sharp, however, and diffraction effects tend to produce a fairly diffuse boundary. Ultrasound energy is not uniform across the beam. In addition, side lobes of ultrasound are typically generated at low angles away from the main beam and can produce noticeable reflections from areas not of interest. In general, then, the cross-sectional area of the beam varies with

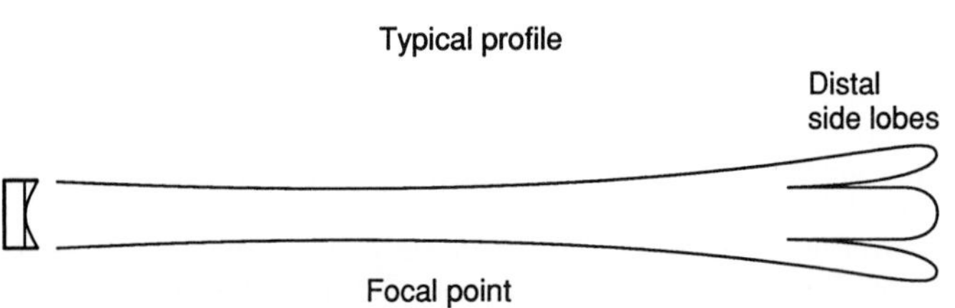

Figure 18–6. A typical beam profile showing beam narrowing at the focal point and distal side lobes. Beam edges are fairly diffuse, and ultrasound energy is not uniform across the beam profile.

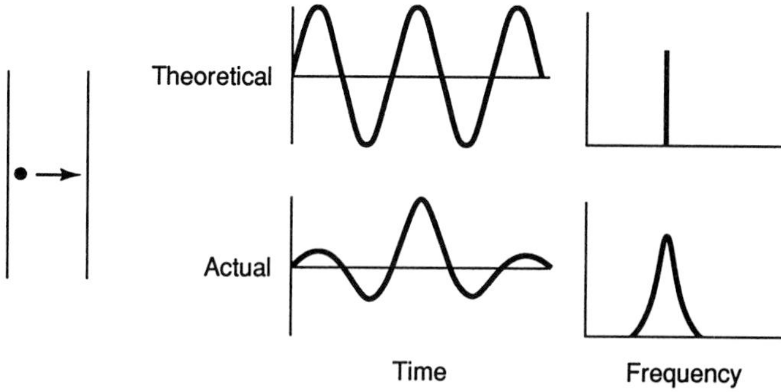

Figure 18–7. Theoretical and actual Doppler shifts for a point of reflector moving across a beam, plotted in both time and frequency. Diffuse beam borders and changes in ultrasound energy across the beam profile produce transit-time spectral broadening.

both depth and transducer focus and may not be a simple circle at depths where side lobes are significant.[A3, K1]

A single red cell moving through an ultrasound beam will represent two velocity components: a velocity with respect to the beam that produces the primary Doppler shift and a velocity normal to the beam. The velocity normal to the beam, or *transit velocity*, is responsible for amplitude fluctuations in ultrasound reflections as the red cell moves across the beam and for subsequent changes in ultrasound energy. Therefore, if a moving red cell is to produce no Doppler shift, it should have no velocity components toward the transducer center. This is possible only if the red cell moves along an arc of a circle around the transducer. If the red cell is moving in a straight line perpendicular or normal to the finite-width beam, it will have velocity components toward the transducer (except at the beam center). In other words, as the red cell crosses the beam in a straight line, its *apparent* velocity toward the transducer center is continually changing.[F3, N1]

In addition, ultrasound power is not evenly distributed across the beam cross section but tapers off at the edges to produce a "fuzzy" beam. The amplitude or strength of Doppler reflections from the single red cell varies with changes in beam power as the cell moves across the beam. The combination of transit velocity and fuzzy beam effects produces distortion artifacts by smoothing the true Doppler shift across neighboring frequencies. This effect is commonly known as "spectral broadening." Mathematically, if the amplitude of the Doppler-shifted ultrasound is being modulated, Fourier analysis dictates that the resulting wave must contain more than one frequency (Fig. 18–7).[A5]

Since a density of red cells is moving through the ultrasound beam, each cell reflects and Doppler-shifts the sound energy. Because of the distribution of velocities of red cells in any flow field (as previously discussed), ultrasound reflections contain a distribution of Doppler shift frequencies. Frequency is, of course, proportional to red cell velocity. If we assume that all cells reflect equally, the *power* or strength of a particular Doppler shift is proportional to the number of red cells moving at the respective velocity.[A1]

Continuous-Wave Doppler

In continuous-wave Doppler instruments, two crystals are utilized in the transducer: one for continuous transmission and one for continuous reception. Both crystals are mounted side by side and focused for beam overlap at some distance from the transducer. For all practical purposes, it is blood moving through the intersection of the two beams that produces significant ultrasound reflections. Doppler shifts are directly proportional to blood velocity components and crystal frequencies according to equation (13). Although Doppler reflections from blood nearer the transducer are stronger than returns from more distant locations along the beam, there are no practical methods for accurately determining the range of a particular Doppler-shifted reflection. In other words, it is not possible to determine the position of blood with a particular velocity.[A3, A4]

Pulsed Doppler

By transmitting a single pulse of ultrasound and timing the Doppler-shifted returns, one can determine the beam distance at which the reflection occurred.[B1, F4] Typically, a single transducer crystal is utilized. A time delay between transmission and reception (known as sample volume range or depth) is chosen by the operator. A reception time (specifying the sample volume length) is also chosen or fixed by the instrument. A single burst of ultrasound is transmitted by the crystal. After the selected delay (representing the sample volume depth), the crystal is monitored by the instrument for the chosen reception time (representing the sample volume length). Typically, bursts are extremely short, consisting of only three to six full wavelengths. As previously mentioned, the sample volume cross-sectional area varies with depth. Power is not evenly distributed across the sample volume area but tapers off toward the sides.[A3, K1]

This process is then repeated at a rate know as the *pulse repetition frequency*. Doppler returns are thus selectively chosen from a small "sample" volume cylinder along the beam (Fig. 18–8). For example, at a propagation speed of 1580 m/sec, a selected sample volume depth of 10 cm, and a sample volume length of 1 cm, reception would occur between 127 and 139 μsec after transmission. Waves reflected from the front of the sample volume would travel 20 cm, and waves reflected from the rear would travel 22 cm. If an additional 1 μsec is allowed for transmission of the burst, the maximum pulse repetition frequency would then be approximately one cycle every 140 μsec, or about 7 kHz. In practice, the sample volume tends to be shaped like a teardrop with fuzzy or diffuse borders, and pulsed Doppler exhibits the same transit-time broadening artifacts as continuous-wave Doppler.

Two additional problems occur as a trade-off with this technology. First, pulsing the transmitted ultrasound represents additional amplitude modulation.[A3] In other words, the continuous-wave ultrasound is being shaped by another wave to form the bursts. This implies that frequencies in addition to the primary frequency are being transmitted. These additional frequencies are, of course, also Doppler-shifted by moving blood. The result is that returns are now somewhat more ambiguous and less specific to the actual blood velocity profile.

Mathematically, if the pulse is square (with an abrupt beginning and end), the primary frequency has effectively been multiplied by a square wave. It can be shown by Fourier analysis that this square contains an extremely broad range of frequencies that can produce significant spectral broadening.[E1] Most instruments attempt to produce a burst with rise and fall times more nearly of a cosine shape, which helps to reduce this spectral broadening.

The second problem is more significant. If the pulse repetition frequency is less than one-half of a Doppler shift frequency, a

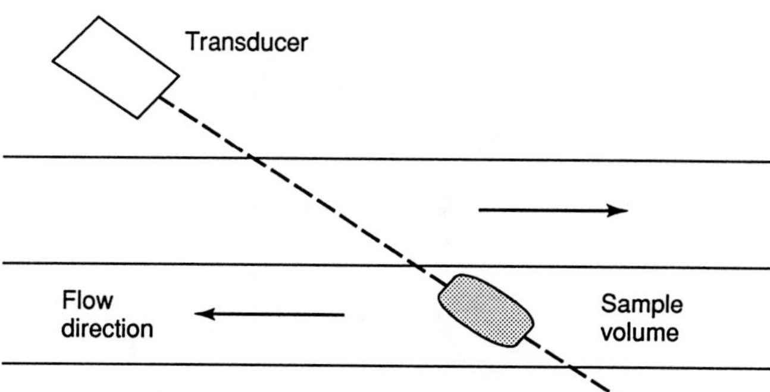

Figure 18–8. By range-gating the reception of ultrasound backscatter, returns can be chosen from a selected depth or sample volume. Returns from flow more proximal (or distal) to the transducer are excluded.

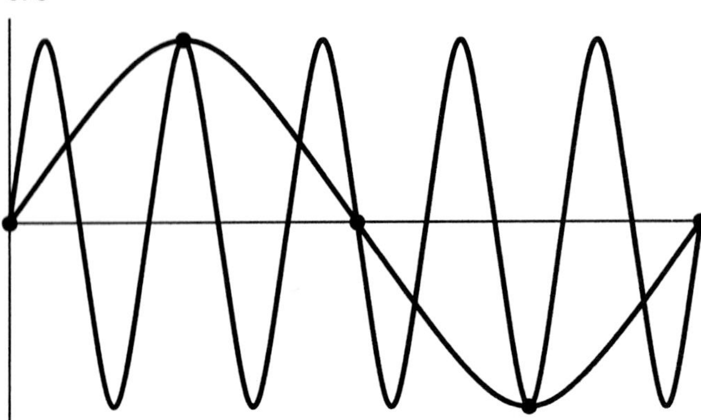

Figure 18–9. For a set of evenly spaced samples of a particular frequency, an infinite number of frequencies will fit the same samples. This plot demonstrates two frequencies of the same magnitude for the same five sample points.

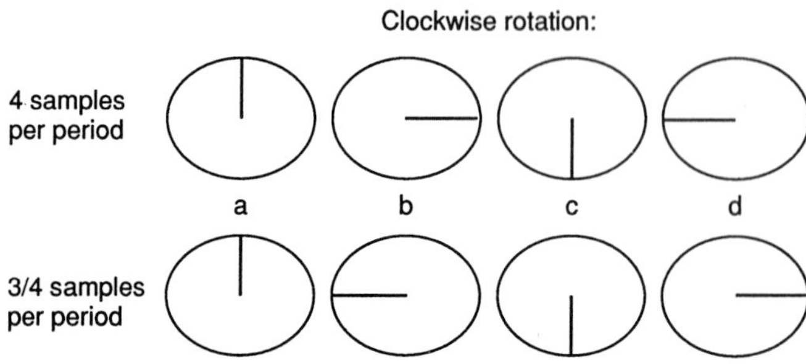

Figure 18–11. A strobe light is used to sample the position of a disk rotating in a clockwise direction. At four samples per period, the disk appears to be correctly moving in a clockwise or forward direction. At three-fourths sample per period, the disk rotates three-fourths of a revolution between strobes and now appears to be rotating in a negative direction.

phenomenon known as aliasing causes the true Doppler shift to appear as a different frequency. This is known as the Nyquist theorem.[E1] Each short reflected burst of ultrasound can be thought of as a single sample of the distribution of Doppler shifts returning from the sample volume. The problem is analogous to one that might arise in attempting to plot the graph of a function with evenly spaced dots. If the dots are close together, we are reasonably confident of the shape of the function. If the dots are far apart, however, ambiguity occurs.

Consider the hypothetical case of a single frequency being sampled or measured at evenly spaced intervals. We know the function has the shape of a sine wave. For any series of samples of the single frequency, an infinite number of other frequencies will exactly fit the same series of points! Figure 18–9 shows two such frequencies. If we make the basic assumption that the correct answer is always the lowest frequency that will fit our series of sample points, we must then sample at least twice per period or cycle. Suppose we are attempting to determine the frequency of the unknown sine wave of Figure 18–10. At three samples per period, the correct frequency is the lowest frequency that will fit the sample points. At 1.5 samples per period, however, a lower frequency will fit and our assumption forces us to choose this lower frequency as the correct answer. The true frequency is then assumed to be a lower value and our answer is *aliased.*

Aliasing can make positive Doppler shifts (representing flow towards the transducer) appear to be negative (flow away from the transducer). Consider a simple experiment involving a strobe light and a spinning disk with a single spoke (Fig. 18–11). The strobe represents our sampling bursts and the rotating disk represents a single frequency. At four samples per period, the disk is correctly assumed to be rotating forward. At three-fourths sample per period, the disk rotates too far between samples for correct visualization and now appears to be rotating backward. In general, the graphic relationship between sampling rate or pulse repetition frequency and aliasing found in Figure 18–12 applies.

According to equation (13), Doppler shifts are directly proportional to the transducer frequency. Lower transducer frequencies produce correspondingly lower Doppler shifts for the same blood flow velocity. For this reason, lower-frequency transducers allow better determination of high blood velocities wihout problems of aliasing. The trade-off is now in frequency or velocity resolution. Separate Doppler shifts may no longer be detectable for two closely spaced blood flow velocities.[B2, C3]

Pulsed transmission and range-gated reception are intended to allow Doppler shift frequencies from a single specific sample volume to be accepted. In practice, however, returns from multiple sample volumes at evenly spaced intervals are present. Consider the case of a sample volume at a depth of 5 cm. Only a portion of the ultrasound energy is Doppler-shifted and reflected back from the designated sample volume to the transducer. The remainder continues on along the beam. When the returns from the designated sample volume arrive back at the transducer, the unreflected waves are at a depth of 10 cm. If they are now reflected back by a moving blood pool at this depth, they will arrive at the designated sample volume at the same time as the second burst. At this point, they combine. When the second burst arrives back at the transducer, it now contains Doppler shifts from depths of 5 and 10 cm—a second sample volume. This is known as range ambiguity, since the operator cannot be certain from which volume a return was reflected.[B1]

Fortunately, returns from secondary sample volumes, having propagated twice the distance, are attenuated to levels lower than returns from the designated sample volume. Artifacts from secondary sample volumes can be a problem, however, if the secondary blood pool is a significantly stronger reflector. Secondary sample volumes not within moving blood pools produce no artifacts.

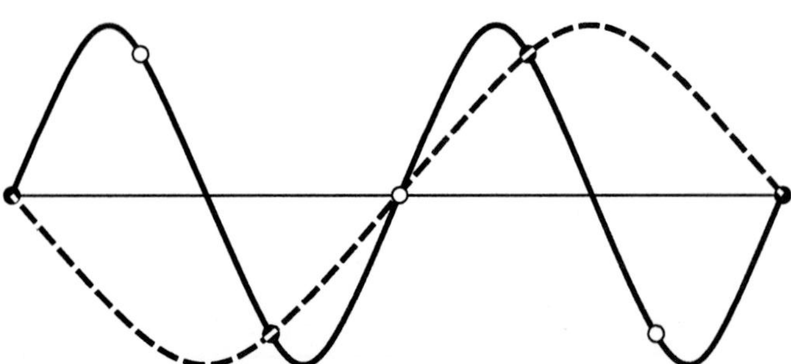

Figure 18–10. Circles represent samples of unknown frequency *(solid line).* When samples are taken at a rate of three per period *(all circles),* the correct frequency is the lowest to fit the sample points. At 1.5 samples per period *(filled circles),* a lower frequency *(dashed line)* fits the points and the choice is aliased.

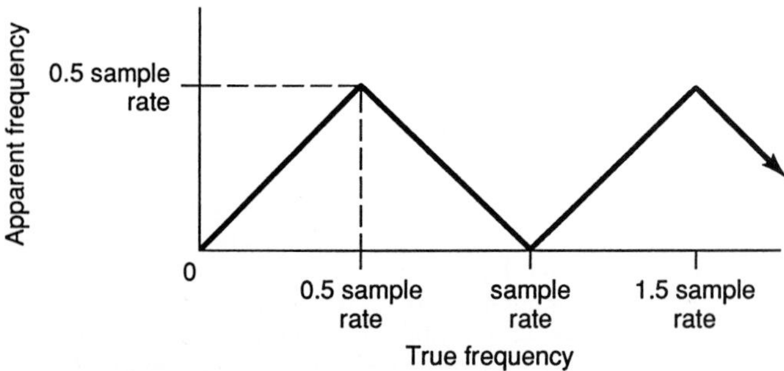

Figure 18–12. Graphic relationship between true and apparent frequency as a result of sampling rate. Note that the apparent or calculated frequency is never more than one-half the sampling rate.

Some instruments allow an operator to select a pulse repetition frequency twice (or occasionally three or four times) as high as normal.[C4, C5, R1] In this case, a second burst is transmitted prior to the return of the Doppler-shifted first burst. At twice-normal pulse repetition frequency, the second burst is sent as the first arrives at the designated sample volume. If the designated sample volume is again at 5 cm, secondary sample volumes now occur at 2.5 cm, 7.5 cm, 10 cm, and farther. The operator now needs to be particularly careful to prevent the proximal sample volume at 2.5 cm from residing in a moving blood pool, since these returns would be significantly stronger than returns from the sample volume of interest.

Color Flow Doppler

An extension of the basic pulsed Doppler instrument permits mapping of Doppler information with two-dimensional ultrasound imaging.[A3, H1] In such a system, Doppler shifts are collected from an entire sector plane rather than a single small sample volume. The technique is referred to (somewhat erroneously) as "real-time two-dimensional Doppler." Instead of a desired two-dimensional field being scanned by the operator using basic pulsed Doppler techniques, an entire field is scanned and presented in a two-dimensional format.

In this technique, multiple gates allow a string of sample volumes along the ultrasound beam during reception of the reflected burst. After returns from the farthest sample volume reach the transducer, the beam direction is mechanically or electronically changed to allow sampling along another path. After a particular sector of a few to perhaps 128 different angles has been scanned, the original beam path is again sampled to repeat the process. Each sector may contain a matrix of several thousand sample volume sites. In mechanical systems, the transducer is rotated through the desired sector angle. In electronic or phased-array systems, the beam is directed by receiving with multiple crystals. By choosing the appropriate relative phases of returns to separate crystals from a single burst, the origin (the sample volume) of the reflections can be specified.

There are two approaches to treating individual sample volumes within a sector. Multigate systems treat each sample volume similarly to basic pulsed Doppler instruments and produce a complete (although somewhat coarse) distribution of blood velocities.[S4] Other systems utilize a radar technique known as "moving-target indication" to produce a single magnitude for the dominant or mean frequency and perhaps a single measure of the spread or variation of frequencies within each volume.[A3] Both systems typically display Doppler information with color coding on a gray scale two-dimensional image.

As well as the limitations of basic Doppler technology mentioned previously, three additional concerns should be understood when using this technology. First, the aliasing problem of basic pulsed Doppler is compounded. The number of sample volumes that must be scanned severely limits the rate at which each individual volume is sampled. Aliasing may be significant even within normal cardiovascular flow rate limits. Second, regardless of the display resolution for individual flow elements, the basic limitations of Doppler (problems of beam geometry, fuzzy sample volume size, acceleration, random density, transit time smoothing, etc.) combine to produce significant overlap of adjacent sample volume cells in a two-dimensional display. Third, a slight phase lag may exist between Doppler signals from opposite sides of the two-dimensional sector due to the time required to sweep or steer the beam for one full scan. This artifact is normally not a significant concern. However, if full sector width is selected for a significant depth during a rapid heart rate, this artifact could affect results. Consider a 128-angle sector at a depth of 10 cm. Assuming that there is no instrument overhead time, a single scan would require approximately 140 μsec and a full sector approximately 18 msec. At a heart rate of 120, this time may represent as much as 12 percent of systole.

Regardless of limitations, these instruments appear to be a significant aid as scanning and screening tools for subsequent basic Doppler examinations.

DOPPLER PROCESSING AND DISPLAY

Doppler shift frequencies are typically in the audio range and are commonly played over instrument speakers or headphones. Trained operators can easily distinguish between low and high velocities and between laminar and turbulent flow. Graphic displays provide additional aids to quantitative measurements.

Time-Based Processing

Some early instruments calculated the rates of zero crossings of Doppler-shifted signals. These rates were then plotted in a histogram format to produce an approximation to the frequency distribution of the original signal. Such a calculation is called a "time interval histogram." Although simple to implement, this technique tends to treat low-magnitude frequencies on an equal basis with strong or large-magnitude frequencies. As might be expected, such an approach is quite sensitive to noise. Modest estimates of the mean Doppler shift and the width of the distribution may be obtained from the time interval histogram, but it is of questionable value in calculating maximum frequency shifts and in comparing separate distributions.[B2, L1]

Spectral Analysis

To obtain a more complete representation of the distribution of Doppler shifts in a signal, spectral analysis techniques are more commonly employed.[R2, R3] A digital or discrete Fourier transform (DFT)[E1] algorithm or analog Chirp-Z[B3] circuitry is usually implemented within the processing and display component of the Doppler instrument. The DFT calculations are frequently referred to as *fast Fourier transform*. More correctly, the fast Fourier transform is simply an efficient algorithm for the calculation of a DFT. Several important characteristics and limitations of spectral analysis must be understood to intepret Doppler displays correctly.

The DFT transforms a Doppler signal to the frequency domain. This means simply that a graph of the function now represents the relative magnitude of each frequency component. (In the original time domain, the function graph represents the magnitudes of the Doppler signal at each point in time.) The DFT cannot, however, distinguish when a particular frequency component occurred within the signal or whether the corresponding reflector was accelerating.[C3, C6] Accordingly, each Doppler signal is typically divided into a series of segments representing small slices of time. A DFT is then calculated for each time slice. Displaying sequential DFTs allows an operator to visualize the temporal nature of flow.

Continuous-wave Doppler signals must be digitized or sampled to produce a series of discrete values for the DFT. Once again, sampling must be done at a rate greater than twice the highest frequency in the signal to prevent aliasing. Pulsed Doppler signals by nature have already been sampled at the pulse repetition frequency. Continuous-wave systems can arbitrarily increase the sampling rate for spectral analysis to prevent aliasing, whereas pulsed systems are limited by the pulse repetition frequency. However, if an inappropriate sampling rate or display range is chosen by the operator, aliasing will occur in a continuous-wave display just as in pulsed systems.

The period of time represented by each time slice of signal is now the reciprocal of spectral resolution or the ability to distinguish between two closely spaced Doppler shifts. For example, if DFTs are calculated every 10 msec, spectral resolution is 1/0.01 or 100 Hz. For a 2-MHz crystal, this corresponds to a velocity difference of approximately 4 cm/sec. Therefore, a trade-off exists between frequency resolution and temporal resolution. Longer time slices produce better frequency resolution, but there is greater ambiguity about when a particular frequency component occurred. Some systems attempt to bypass this problem by overlapping DFT time slices.[E1] The effect of this approach is somewhat cosmetic, as it simply smooths or reduces the unique

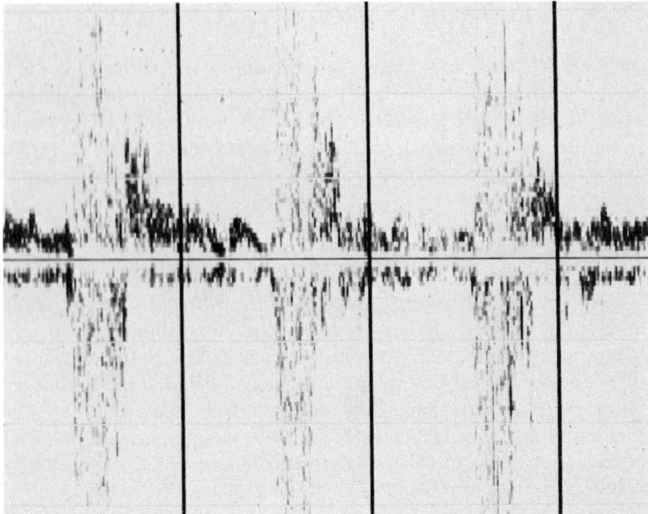

Figure 18–13. A pulsed Doppler display with forward flow shown above the centerline and reverse flow below the centerline. Each vertical step or bar represents one DFT of Doppler returns to show the temporal nature of flow. DFT magnitudes are shown in shades of gray.

information available in each DFT. Changing the sampling rate in continuous-wave systems has no effect on frequency resolution.

Pulsed and continuous-wave systems commonly display each DFT (or the analog equivalent, Chirp-Z) as a vertical bar with each point represented by a shade of gray—dark indicating large magnitudes and light indicating small magnitudes (Fig. 18–13). Forward flow is generally above and reverse flow below a centerline. Successive DFT bars are then scrolled across a dynamic display to show the temporal nature of flow velocity changes. Typically, each bar point (commonly called a pixel in a video image) can be represented by 16 or 32 shades of gray or color. Although more amplitude resolution is technically possible, the typical human eye cannot resolve more than 32 shade differences. Some systems allow a single DFT function (representing a single time slice) to be displayed as a simple graph to allow greater amplitude resolutions for special circumstances.

Most systems allow the operator to adjust the zero line of this display. The net effect of the adjustment is to wrap the display around to move reverse frequencies to forward and vice versa. If the operator is confident that no reverse flow is present, for example, some aliasing effects can be eliminated simply by shifting the display to move reverse frequencies to their assumed appropriate positions. It should be emphasized that this is simply a cosmetic change; no real changes are occurring in Doppler signal generation or the calculation of the DFT. If true reverse frequency shifts are also present, they are moved along with everything else.

It should be emphasized again that the DFT display does not represent the true velocity distribution within the sample volume.[A3, A5, H1] The representation is at best approximate. In addition to the distorting effects inherent in Doppler measurements, the DFT calculation adds additional uncertainty of its own. One such uncertainty results from the fact that in the DFT each time slice is assumed to be exactly periodic. That is, each time slice function begins and ends at exactly the same value. Any deviation from this assumption tends to introduce both ripple and smoothing distortion, which can be quite apparent.

A technique known as "windowing" can be applied to reduce some of this distortion, or the computational expense can be ignored with the simple assumption that this distortion is no worse than that already present from other Doppler artifacts. The reader is referred to another text for a more complete discussion of windowing algorithms.[E1] Mathematically, this distortion from nonperiodic time slices is the same as the effect of allowing abrupt or square pulses in pulsed Doppler systems, as previously mentioned. Additional ambiguity in the DFT representation can also be caused by truncation errors in sampling and mathematics in the algorithm implementation. In general, it should be noted that a significant portion of any spectral broadening noted in a DFT display is an artifact of the combined limitations of the system itself.

Color flow Doppler system displays are more limited. Each pixel in a two-dimensional sector display must now represent an entire velocity distribution function. Typically, color is chosen to differentiate between forward and reverse flow. Red usually represents forward flow and blue reverse flow. Shade is then used to represent the magnitude of one parameter of the velocity distribution such as mean or peak frequency (or some combination of these). Occasionally, a mode velocity can be displayed. Mode velocity is the velocity corresponding to the Doppler shift with the greatest power, or the velocity common to the most red cells within the sample volume. A separate "orthogonal" color (such as green) is usually chosen to represent a second parameter such as degree of variation in the velocity distribution. The final color display for each pixel is then the sum of these two orthogonal colors. High velocities toward the transducer would appear as areas of bright red, low velocities away from the transducer as areas of dark blue. Areas of turbulence may appear as a scatter of many colors and shade referred to as a "mosaic" pattern. The pulse repetition frequency and scan rates as well as processing requirements may combine to reduce the display update time to fewer than five frames per second in some situations.

In summary: Doppler transducers produce beams with diffuse borders and may have side lobes. Transit-time effects produce ambiguity in Doppler shifts from sampling volumes. Continuous-wave Doppler is able to detect large shifts but allows no range determinations. Pulsed systems provide range information but suffer from aliasing when shifts exceed half the pulse repetition frequency. The pulse repetition frequency that is possible is determined by the maximum depth of the desired sample volume. Additional ambiguity caused by pulse shaping can be present. Secondary sample volumes can interfere with signals from a depth of interest, particularly in systems with high pulse repetition frequencies.

Real-time color flow systems allow simultaneous visualization of a two-dimensional sector blood flow and aid in mapping complex flow patterns over large areas. Typically, only the peak or mean velocity from each sample volume is displayed. These systems suffer from serious aliasing effects, which are frequently present even in normal flow conditions. Display sector update times may be quite slow with respect to the cardiac cycle. Regardless of the resolution of the display, significant overlap occurs between adjacent sample volumes, which adds ambiguity to velocity determinations at specific points.

References

A

1. Angelsen, B.A.: A theoretical study of the scattering of ultrasound from blood. IEEE Trans. Biomed. Eng. BME-27:61, 1980.
2. Atkinson, P., and Berry, M.V.: Random noise in ultrasonic echoes diffracted by blood. J. Phys. A 7:1293, 1974.
3. Atkinson, P., and Woodcock, J.P.: Doppler Ultrasound and Its Use in Clinical Measurement. Academic Press, London, 1982.
4. Angelsen, B.A., and Brubakk, A.O.: Transcutaneous measurement of blood flow velocity in the human aorta. Cardiovasc. Res. 10:368, 1976.
5. Atkinson, P., and Follett, D.H.: Problems of signal extraction in ultrasonic Doppler systems. *In* Woodcock, F. (ed.): Clinical Blood Flow Measurement. Sector Publications, London, 1976.

B

1. Baker, D.W., Gubenstein, G.A., and Lorch G.S.: Pulsed Doppler echocardiography: Principles and applications. Am. J. Med. 63:69, 1977.
2. Burckhardt, C.B.: Comparison between spectrum and time-interval histogram of ultrasound Doppler signals. Ultrasound Med. Biol. 7:79, 1981.
3. Brodersen, R.W., Hewes, C.R., and Buss, D.D.: A 500-stage CCD transversal filter for spectral analysis. IEEE Trans. Electron Devices ED-23:143, 1976.

C

1. Clark, C., and Schultz, D.L.: Velocity distribution in aortic flow. Cardiovasc. Res. 7:601, 1973.
2. Caro, C.G., Pedley, T.J., Schroter, R.C., and Seed, W.A.: The Mechanics of the Circulation. Oxford University Press, Oxford, 1978.

3. Cannon, S.R., Richards, K.L., and Rollwitz, W.: Digital Fourier techniques in the diagnosis and quantitation of aortic stenosis with pulsed Doppler echocardiography. J. Clin. Ultrasound 10:101, 1982.
4. Cannon, S.R., and Richards, K.L.: Quantification of mean aortic gradients by high pulse repetition frequency Doppler. J. Cardiol. Ultrasound 3:488, 1984.
5. Cannon, S.R., Richards, K.L., and Morgann, R.: Comparison of continuous wave and high pulse repetition frequency Doppler for quantifying aortic stenosis. Circulation 68:228, 1983.
6. Cannon, S.R., Richards, K.L., and Morgann, R.: Comparison of Doppler peak frequency and turbulence parameters in the quantitation of aortic stenosis in a pulsatile flow model. Circulation 71:129, 1985.

E

1. Elliot, D.F.: Handbook of Digital Signal Processing. Academic Press, San Diego, 1987.

F

1. Flax, S.W., Webster, J.G., and Updike, S.J.: Statistical evaluation of the Doppler ultrasonic blood flowmeter. Biomed. Sci. Instrum. 7:201, 1973.
2. Furgason, E.S., Newhouse, V.L., Bilgutay, N.M., and Cooper, G.R.: Applications of random signal correlation techniques to ultrasonic flow detection. Ultrasonics 13:11, 1975.
3. Flax, S.W., Webster, J.G., and Updike, S.J.: Noise and functional limitations of the Doppler blood flowmeter. *In* Reneman, S.W. (ed.): Cardiovascular Applications of Ultrasound. North-Holland, Amsterdam, 1974.
4. Follett, D.H.: Electronic Instrumentation in Ultrasound Diagnosis. Faraday House, London, 1977.

G

1. Guyton, A.C.: Textbook of Medical Physiology. W.B. Saunders, Philadelphia, 1971.

H

1. Hatle, L., and Angelsen, B.: Doppler Ultrasound in Cardiology. Lea & Febiger, Philadelphia, 1982.

K

1. Kinsler, L.E., and Frey, A.R.: Fundamentals of Acoustics, 2nd ed. Wiley, New York, 1962.

L

1. Lunt, M.J.: Accuracy and limitations of the ultrasonic Doppler blood velocimeter and zero crossing detector. Ultrasound Med. Biol. 2:1, 1975.

M

1. Marion, J.B.: Classical Dynamics of Particles and Systems. Academic Press, New York, 1970.
2. McDonald, D.A.: Blood Flow in Arteries. Edward Arnold, London, 1974.

N

1. Newhouse, V.L., Bendick, P.J., and Varner, L.W.: Analysis of transit time effects on Doppler flow measurement. IEEE Trans. Biomed. Eng. BME-23:381, 1976.

R

1. Richards, K.L., Cannon, S.R., and Crawford, M.H.: Noninvasive quantification of mitral valve area using high pulse repetition frequency Doppler. J. Am. Coll. Cardiol. 3:493, 1984.
2. Richards, K.L., Cannon, S.R., Crawford, M. H., and Sorensen, S.G.: Noninvasive diagnosis of aortic and mitral valve disease with pulsed Doppler spectral analysis. Am. J. Cardiol. 51:1122, 1983.
3. Richards, K.L., and Cannon, S.R.: Comparison of continuous wave and pulsed Doppler in diagnosis of mitral and aortic stenosis in adults. *In* Spencer, M.P. (ed.): Cardiac Doppler Diagnosis. Martinus Nijhoff, Boston, 1983.

S

1. Shung, K.K., Sigelmann, R.A., and Reid, J.M.: Scattering of ultrasound by blood. IEEE Trans. Biomed. Eng. BME-23:460, 1976.
2. Skidmore, R., and Woodcock, J.P.: Physiological interpretation of Doppler shift waveforms. Ultrasound Med. Biol. 6:7, 1980.
3. Snedecor, G.W., and Cochran, W.G.: Statistical Methods. Iowa State University Press, Ames, 1967.
4. Stevenson, J.G.: Multigate Doppler visualization of intracardiac flow disturbances in congenital heart disease. *In* Spencer, M.P. (ed.): Cardiac Doppler Diagnosis. Martinus Nijhoff, Boston, 1983.

W

1. Wells, P.N.T.: Wave fundamentals. *In* Wells, P.N.T. (ed.): Biomedical Ultrasonics. Academic Press, New York, 1977.

Chapter 19

Echocardiographic Assessment of Ventricular Function

■ *THOMAS L. FORCE, M.D.* ■ *EDWARD D. FOLLAND, M.D.*
■ *NICOLE AEBISCHER, M.D.* ■ *SATISH SHARMA, M.D.*
■ *ALFRED F. PARISI, M.D.*

GLOBAL LEFT VENTRICULAR FUNCTION 374
Background Considerations 374
Models for Estimation of Volume 375
Echocardiographic Measurements of Left Ventricular Volume 375
Left Ventricular Ejection Fraction 377
End-Systolic Pressure-Volume Relationship 379
Left Ventricular Mass 380
REGIONAL LEFT VENTRICULAR FUNCTION 381
Relation of Systolic Dysfunction to Ischemia and Infarction 382
Analysis Algorithms 382
Preliminary Considerations 382
Endocardial Motion 383
Reference Systems 383
Types of Measurements 386
Numbers of Measurements 387
Sampling Frequency in the Cardiac Cycle 387
Reference-Independent Systems 387
Quantification of Infarct Size with Endocardial Motion 388
Single Plane 388
Integrative Approaches to the Whole Ventricle 388
Analysis of Apical Endocardial Motion 388
Systolic Wall Thickening Analysis 390
Summary 391
RIGHT VENTRICULAR FUNCTION 391
Echocardiographic Examination 392
M-Mode Echocardiography 392
Two-Dimensional Echocardiography 392
Right Ventricular Dimensions 392
Global Right Ventricular Function: Volumes and Ejection Fraction 393
Regional Right Ventricular Function 396

GLOBAL LEFT VENTRICULAR FUNCTION

Echocardiography is well suited to assessment of left ventricular function because it can accurately resolve endocardial and epicardial targets throughout the cardiac cycle in multiple well-defined anatomic planes. The current state of two-dimensional echocardiography enables formation of left ventricular images that are useful for quantitative analytic purposes in about three-quarters of adults and nearly all children. From these images it is possible to derive clinically useful indices of left ventricular function, including volumes, ejection fraction, pressure-volume relationship, and myocardial mass.

Although recent interest has properly focused primarily on two-dimensional echocardiography, M-mode display remains a useful tool and should be included as a complementary part of the echocardiographic examination. Chamber dimensions are easily measured from M-mode images; normal values for these dimensions have become familiar to cardiologists and internists alike. The hard-copy display usually generated from M-mode studies also facilitates side-by-side comparison of serial examinations. Such comparisons for two-dimensional studies require video storage and playback systems that are presently unavailable in most laboratories.

Background Considerations

Virtually all indices of left ventricular pump performance have been derived from measurements of volume and pressure. Traditionally, this has required cardiac catheterization and contrast left ventricular angiography. The indices derived from volume measurements have proved to be of greatest clinical value.[K1] End-diastolic volume is useful for evaluating and following the course of patients with left ventricular volume overloading lesions or myocardial disease. In both of these conditions, effective stroke volume delivered to the systemic circulation may be initially reduced. In the case of left ventricular volume overload, the total stroke volume actually delivered to the circulation is reduced by the regurgitant volume; in myocardial disease the total stroke volume is diminished by impaired myocardial contractility. As a compensatory mechanism, the left ventricle dilates to maintain effective stroke volume and hence cardiac output. In general, end-diastolic volume increases in direct proportion to the severity of the underlying lesion and the magnitude of preload.

End-systolic volume is determined by end-diastolic volume, myocardial contractility, and afterload. Thus it is often ambiguous as an isolated measurement. When both end-diastolic and end-systolic volumes (EDV and ESV) are measured, however, left ventricular stroke volume (SV) can be estimated:

$$SV_{cc} = EDV_{cc} - ESV_{cc} \tag{1}$$

In the absence of valvular regurgitation, cardiac output (CO) can be estimated as the product of stroke volume and heart rate (HR):

$$CO_{cc/min} = HR_{beats/min} \times SV_{cc/min} \tag{2}$$

When end-diastolic and end-systolic volumes are known, ejection fraction (EF) can be calculated as the ratio of stroke volume to end-diastolic volume:

$$EF = \frac{SV}{EDV} \tag{3}$$

Ejection fraction is a widely used index of left ventricular function and is generally considered to be the best single predictor of prognosis in both coronary and valvular heart disease, whether treated medically[M1, N1] or surgically.[C1, H1]

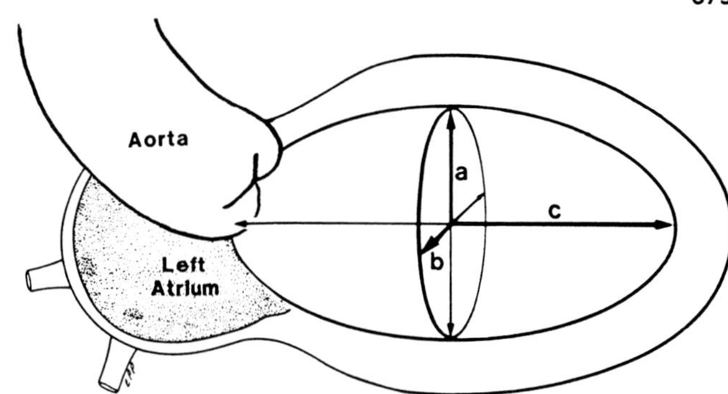

Figure 19–1. The ellipsoid model for left ventricular volume. This model is commonly used to estimate left ventricular volume from angiographic and/or echocardiographic images. The minor hemiaxes (a and b) and the major hemiaxis (c) are indicated by heavy arrows. The minor hemiaxes can be either directly measured from appropriate views or derived from the respective area and largest length of the appropriate views. (From Folland, E.D., and Parisi, A.F.: Ventricular volume and function. *In* Talano, J.V., Gardin, J.M. (eds.): Textbook of Two-Dimensional Echocardiography. Grune & Stratton, New York, 1983, p. 165, with permission.)

Models for Estimation of Volume

Angiographic estimates of left ventricular volume are usually based on the assumption that the left ventricle approximates the geometry of an ellipsoid—that is, a three-dimensional figure created by rotating an ellipse on its long axis (Fig. 19–1). The volume of such a figure can be calculated if the lengths of its three hemiaxes, a, b, and c, are known:

$$\text{Volume} = \tfrac{4}{3}\,\pi a \times b \times c \tag{4}$$

In the earliest application of this model, the hemiaxes were measured directly from angiographic anteroposterior and lateral projections of the left ventricle. Dodge and associates,[D1] in comparing the angiographic volume with the true volume of barium-filled left ventricles from fresh autopsy hearts, found that accuracy was enhanced if the minor axes were derived arithmetically from idealized ellipses of the same area and length as the two respective angiographic projections. The area of an ellipse is the product of π and its two hemiaxes. Thus, if c is the major hemiaxis, a the minor hemiaxis in the anteroposterior plane, b the minor hemiaxis in the lateral plane, and A_{AP} and A_{lat} the respective measured angiographic areas, the minor hemiaxes can be expressed as follows:

$$a = \frac{A_{AP}}{\pi c} \tag{5}$$

$$b = \frac{A_{lat}}{\pi c} \tag{6}$$

Then, by substitution in equation (4), volume is derived from the respective areas of the two projections and their common major hemiaxis:

$$\text{Volume} = \frac{4\pi}{3} \times \frac{A_{AP}}{\pi c} \times \frac{A_{lat}}{\pi c} \times c \tag{7}$$

which simplifies to

$$\text{Volume} = \frac{4A_{AP}A_{lat}}{3\pi c} \tag{8}$$

This formula is commonly referred to as a biplane area-length volume model. In applications where angiography is performed only in a single plane, the formula is simplified by assuming that both minor hemiaxes (a and b) are equal. Thus, volume can be derived from the length and area of the single ventricular silhouette:

$$\text{Volume} = \frac{4A^2}{3\pi c} \tag{9}$$

This formula is commonly referred to as the single-plane area-length volume model.

An alternative model for measuring left ventricular volume employs the concept of Simpson's rule, whereby the volume of a solid may be estimated by subdividing it along one axis into a series of slices, each with a finite thickness and measureable area. The volume of each slice is the product of its area and thickness. The volume of the complete solid is the sum of the volumes of all its slices. The greater the number of slices, the greater is the accuracy of the volume estimation. According to Simpson's rule, the left ventricle can be envisioned as a series of slices from the base to the apex, analogous to a stack of coins with uniform thickness but variable area (Fig. 19–2). In estimating the volume of Dodge's barium-filled hearts,[D1] this method proved to be slightly less accurate than the area-length method. Although Simpson's rule is theoretically attractive, its use is cumbersome without computer assistance and it has not gained wide acceptance among clinical angiographers.

Echocardiographic Measurements of Left Ventricular Volume

Image formation is fundamentally different in angiography and ultrasound. Angiographic images are silhouettes or shadows, whereas ultrasound images are tomographic slices. Nevertheless, there is ample evidence that left ventricular dimensions measured with the two techniques correlate well, provided that the ultrasound section is properly oriented.

Figure 19–3 shows a plot of 100 corresponding linear measurements from right anterior oblique angiograms and two-dimensional echocardiograms performed in our laboratory.[M2] The echocardiographic long axis (in the apical four-chamber view) was measured from the midpoint of the mitral valve to the apex. The short axis (in a parasternal short-axis view at mitral valve level) was measured at the tips of the mitral valve leaflets perpendicular to the long axis. Echocardiographic and angiographic measurements were made at end-diastole and end-systole for a total of four measurements in each patient. The plot shows excellent agreement ($r = 0.92$, standard error of the estimate [SEE] = 0.97 cm); however, as evident from the relationship to the line of identity, the echocardiographic measurements consistently tended to underestimate the angiographic measurements, which

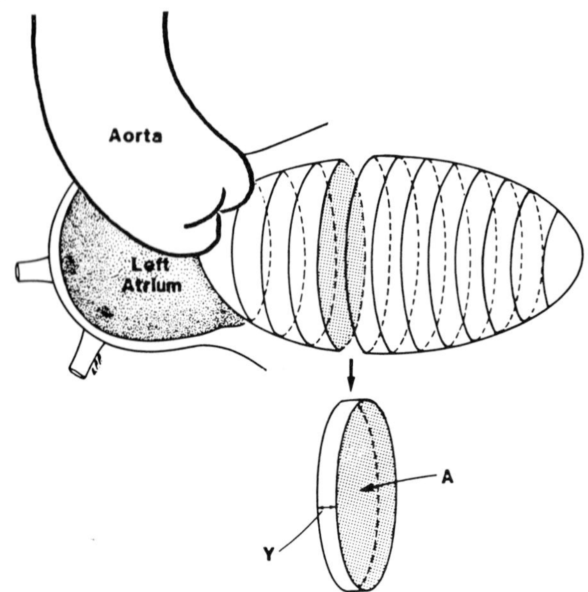

Figure 19–2. Simpson's rule model for left ventricular volume with the left ventricle sliced perpendicular to the long axis. The total left ventricular volume is the sum of volumes of individual slices, each with known thickness (Y) and area (A). (From Folland, E.D., and Parisi, A.F.: Ventricular volume and function. *In* Talano, J.V., Gardin, J.M. (eds.): Textbook of Two-Dimensional Echocardiography. Grune & Stratton, New York, 1983, p. 165, with permission.)

is not surprising in view of the differences in projection in the respective techniques. An x-ray silhouette represents the largest area of the ventricle perpendicular to the x-ray beam. The analogous ultrasound slice is very likely to be smaller unless it is perfectly oriented through the central axis to the true anatomic apex of the ventricle. In fact, it is usually impossible to locate the transducer precisely at the anatomic cardiac apex. When Barrett and associates performed simultaneous x-ray contrast and two-dimensional echocardiographic imaging of a series of patients, they attributed uniform underestimation of x-ray contrast volumes by echocardiography to the finding that the apical ultrasound window was 33 degrees cephalad to the true cardiac apex.[B1] In addition, angiographic images are ordinarily traced at the outermost boundary of contrast, which tends to include trabeculae within the cavity profile. Echocardiographic images are traced along the innermost edge of endocardial echoes, which would tend to exclude trabeculae from the cavity. Despite these differences, the correlation in measurement between the two techniques is good enough so that formulas for angiographic volume should apply equally well to echocardiographic volume determination, provided that systematic differences are corrected by regression formulas.

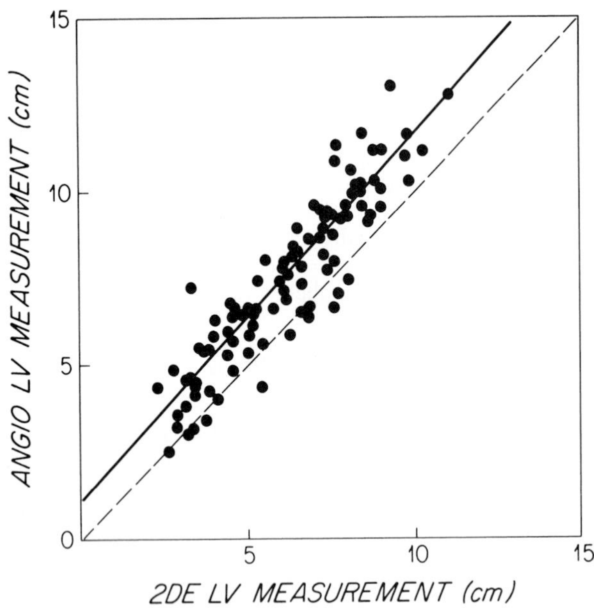

Figure 19–3. Correlation of 100 analogous measurements of left ventricular dimensions made from angiograms (ANGIO) and echocardiograms (2DE) in 25 patients. The short axis from parasternal view at mitral valve level and long axis from apical four-chamber view were measured at end-diastole and end-systole and compared to analogous measurements from the right anterior oblique left ventricle (LV) angiogram, as shown by the solid regression line (r = 0.92, SEE = 0.97). The dashed line of identity is shown for reference. (Reprinted with permission of the publisher from Moynihan, P.F., Parisi, A.F., Folland E.D., et al.: A system for quantitative evaluation of left ventricular function with two-dimensional ultrasonography. Medical Instrumentation 14:113, 1980. Copyright 1980 by the Association for the Advancement of Medical Instrumentation, Arlington, Virginia.)

The earliest attempt to estimate left ventricular volumes from echocardiography utilized left ventricular short-axis dimensions from M-mode echocardiograms. This method employed the single-plane area-length volume formula, which required several assumptions: (1) that the left ventricular dimension in the standard position at the level of the chordae tendineae coincides with the minor axis of the left ventricle, (2) that both minor axes are equal in length, and (3) that the long axis is twice the length of the minor axis. This approach is commonly referred to as the "cube method" for left ventricular volume determination.[P1] If D represents the short-axis dimension (at end-diastole or end-systole), then volume is estimated as follows:

$$\text{Volume} = \frac{4\pi}{3} \times \frac{D}{2} \times \frac{D}{2} \times D \qquad (10)$$

which simplifies to

$$\text{Volume} = D^3 \qquad (11)$$

Modifications of this formula have been proposed in order to compensate for systematic deviations from the foregoing assumptions in unusually large and unusually small ventricles.[F1, T1] Although formulas based on the cube assumption produce fair correlations with angiographic volume (r = 0.64 to 0.74),[F1, P1, T1] they suffer from the inherent inaccuracy of making multiple geometric assumptions in an attempt to derive three-dimensional data from a single measurement. Furthermore, an important degree of correlation is expected only in the absence of asynergy.

Two-dimensional echocardiography offers a considerable advantage over the M-mode technique because it enables direct measurement of left ventricular contours and dimensions in the planes of all three hemiaxes. It also allows application of other volume formulas, such as Simpson's rule. It has been well demonstrated that correlations between angiographic and echocardiographic volumes are improved if two-dimensional rather than M-mode methods are used.[C3, F2, P2, S1] Both Simpson's rule[F2, G1, M3, N2, P2, S2, W1] and single-plane and biplane area-length methods[C3, F2, G2, O1, P2, S1] have yielded such results. Furthermore, correlations between two-dimensional echocardiographic and angiographic volumes have been equally good (r = 0.80 to 0.90) regardless of the presence of left ventricular asynergy.[G1, O1]

Simpson's rule can be used with tomographic slicing of the ventricle perpendicular to the long axis (see Fig. 19–2) or parallel to the long axis. When the left ventricle is sliced with short-axis images perpendicular to the long axis, there are insufficient recognizable landmarks to allow full application of Simpson's rule.[F2, G1, N2, P2, W1] Consequently, when this method is applied with only two or three slices, it is usually referred to as "modified" Simpson's rule. In our laboratory, we have found that tomograms recorded at the mitral leaflet tips and papillary muscle bodies are sufficiently reproducible for this application.[F2, P2] Studies in which slices are taken parallel to the long axis have allowed a more classic application of Simpson's rule.[E1, S2] Schiller and associates[S2] successfully applied this approach to patients who underwent biplane angiography and had technically adequate two-dimensional echocardiograms in the apical two-chamber and parasternal short-axis views. The ventricle was sliced at 20 levels along the vertical axis common to both views, and the total volume was calculated from the sum of these 20 slices. Using this method for both the echocardiographic and angiographic images, they obtained correlations of $r = 0.90$ for end-systolic volume and $r = 0.80$ for end-diastolic volume. As usual, the echocardiographic volumes tended to underestimate the angiographic volumes.

The ellipsoid model has been tested with both direct measurements of the minor axis[M3, W1] and derived estimates of the minor axis from the previously discussed area-length formula.[C3, F2, K2, S1, W1] Comparison of Simpson's rule and ellipsoid formulations has generally indicated comparable accuracy in estimating left ventricular volumes,[F2, M3, P2, S1] with one study slightly favoring the ellipsoid approach[S1] and others slightly favoring Simpson's rule.[F2, P2, W1]

Our experience favors Simpson's rule.[F2, P2] We estimated left ventricular volume by two-dimensional echocardiography in a series of 50 patients undergoing single-plane angiography. Apical four-chamber and parasternal short-axis views at both mitral valve and papillary muscle levels were employed, as illustrated in Figure 19–4. Volume was estimated with the five formulas illustrated in Figure 19–5. The best correlation with angiography was obtained with the modified Simpson's rule formula ($r = 0.84$, SEE = 43 ml; Fig. 19–6).

In general, correlation with angiographic volume is improved by using the area-length method rather than direct minor-axis measurement and by using biplane rather than single-plane imaging.[F2, P2, W1] In theory, the accuracy of volume estimation increases with the number of image planes sampled. Computer-generated three-dimensional reconstructions of left ventricular geometry can be derived from multiplane two-dimensional images. Most approaches to three-dimensional reconstruction have employed four or more radial image planes along the apical long axis of the left ventricle[F3, N3] or reconstruction systems that combine parasternal and apical views.[G19, M14] Others have employed integration of numerous images obtained from a single transducer position as the transducer is progressively tilted through a sweep of the left ventricle.[B10] Figure 19–7 depicts an example of such a reconstruction. The advantage of such reconstructions currently is not great enough to justify the time and expense required for their application in clinical practice.

A summary of angiographic-echocardiographic correlations for various two-dimensional methods is presented in Table 19–1. Although the correlations are good, some of the estimating errors are rather large. Appropriate judgment should be exercised, therefore, in applying these echocardiographic estimates of left ventricular volume to individual patients.

Measurement of left ventricular volume has been simplified by inclusion of quantitative software programs in most commercially available two-dimensional echocardiography systems. Images must still be traced by hand, which is often tedious and time consuming. Technically good images and painstaking care are required to achieve the results presented in this chapter. Consequently, many laboratories, including our own, perform full quantitation only in selected cases and routinely report M-mode dimensions as indicators of volume. Laboratories may develop their own normal values for these dimensions or rely on comprehensive normal values developed by others,[P13] keeping in mind that normal ranges vary with sex and body surface area.[D2]

Left Ventricular Ejection Fraction

The reliability of the echocardiographic estimate of ejection fraction depends on the accuracy of the method used to measure end-diastolic and end-systolic volumes. M-mode echocardiography is a particularly weak method because of the adverse influence of left ventricular asynergy on its accuracy. Fair correlations with angiographic ejection fraction have been obtained for patients with symmetric contraction patterns ($r = 0.64$ to 0.74), but poor correlations have been found for ischemic heart disease patients with segmental contraction abnormalities.[F1, P1, T1] Ejection fractions derived from two-dimensional echocardiography correlate well with those derived from angiography ($r = 0.73$ to 0.93; see Table 19–1). Furthermore, two-dimensional echocardiographic estimates are relatively accurate even in the presence of asynergy when either Simpson's rule or the area-length method is used. In our series of 50 patients, a modified Simpson's rule algorithm (see Fig. 19–5, top) provided good results ($r = 0.80$, SEE = 0.90) despite the fact that 25 patients had documented asynergy.[P2] In 35 of our patients whose ejection fractions were

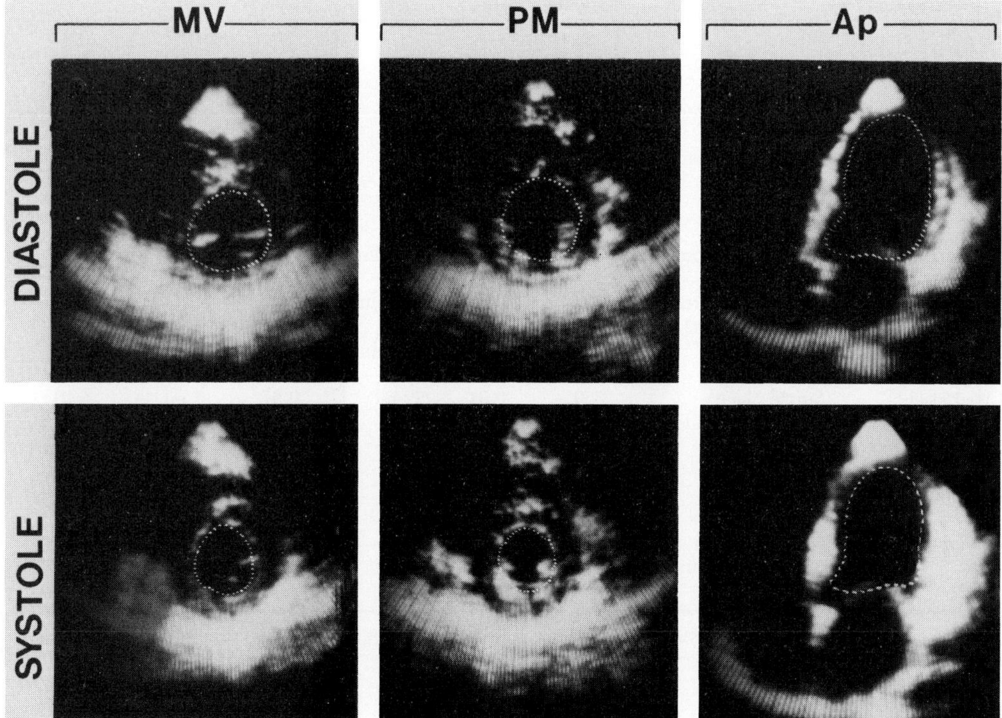

Figure 19–4. Examples of echocardiographic images from a normal heart at end-diastole and end-systole from the parasternal short-axis view at the mitral valve (MV) and papillary muscle (PM) levels and the apical four-chamber view (Ap). The endocardial outlines have been traced as described in the text for volume analysis.[F2, P2] Because of echo dropout, tracing of these outlines required fast- and slow-motion playback of frames immediately preceding and succeeding the still end-diastolic and end-systolic frames shown here. (From Folland, E.D., Parisi, A.F., Moynihan, P.F., et al.: Assessment of left ventricular ejection fraction and volumes by real-time, two-dimensional echocardiography. A comparison of cineangiographic and radionuclide techniques. Circulation 60:760, 1979, with permission of the American Heart Association, Inc.)

Algorithm	Formulation
Simpson's Rule	$V=(A_m)\frac{L}{3}+\left(\frac{A_m+A_p}{2}\right)\frac{L}{3}+\frac{1}{3}(A_p)\frac{L}{3}$
Ellipsoid–Biplane	$V=\frac{\pi}{6}L\left(\frac{4A_m}{\pi D}\right)\left(\frac{4A_l}{\pi L}\right)$
Ellipsoid–Single Plane	$V=\frac{8(A_l)^2}{3\pi L}$
Hemisphere–Cylinder	$V=(A_m)\frac{L}{2}+\frac{2}{3}(A_m)\frac{L}{2}$
Modified Ellipsoid	$V=\left(\frac{7.0}{2.4+D}\right)D^3$

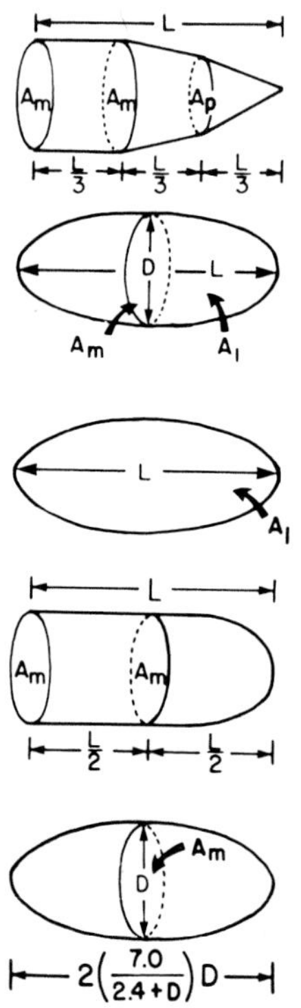

Figure 19–5. Geometric models used to derive left ventricular volumes from two-dimensional echocardiographic data. A denotes area measurements, L the long-axis length from the apical view, and D the septal-lateral diameter from the high cross section of the ventricle. Subscripts m, p, and l refer to the mitral valve, papillary muscle, and long-axis sections, respectively. The modified Simpson's rule model (top) agreed most closely with angiographic volume and ejection fraction. (From Parisi, A.F., Moynihan, P.F., Folland, E.D., et al.: Approaches to determination of left ventricular volume and ejection fraction by real-time two-dimensional echocardiography. Clin. Cardiol. 2:259, 1979. © Appleton & Lange. Used by permission.)

Table 19–1. COMPARISON BETWEEN ECHOCARDIOGRAPHIC AND ANGIOGRAPHIC VOLUMES AND EJECTION FRACTIONS

Investigators	Method	No. of Patients	EDV		ESV		EF		Comments
			r	*SEE*	*r*	*SEE*	*r*	*SEE*	
Teichholz et al.[T2]	B scan	25	—	—	—	—	0.87	—	14 of 25 had asynergy
Folland et al.[F2]	Modified Simpson's rule	35	0.76	43 ml	0.86	32 ml	0.78	0.10	10 of 35 had asynergy
Parisi et al.[P2]	Modified Simpson's rule	50	0.82	39 ml	0.90	29 ml	0.80	0.09	25 of 50 had asynergy
Carr et al.[C3]	Biplane area-length	22	0.93	—	—	—	0.93	—	23 of 24 volumes clustered: EDV *r* fell to 0.46 if 1 patient excluded; 6 of 22 had asynergy
Schiller et al.[S2]	Modified Simpson's rule	30	0.80	15 ml/m²	0.90	8.5 ml/m²	0.87	0.08	16 of 30 had asynergy
Ohuchi et al.[O1]	Single plane area-length	38	0.84 (for all volumes)				0.88	—	Patients with and without asynergy
		18	0.86 (for all volumes)				0.88	—	Only patients with asynergy
Erbel et al.[E1]	Single plane Simpson's rule	50	0.94	22 ml	0.97	15 ml	0.91	0.06	Same model and view (RAO equivalent) used for both echo and angiographic volumes
Kan et al.[K2]	Single plane area-length	30	0.84	—	0.85	—	0.91	—	RAO equivalent view
Quinones et al.[Q1]	Mulitple linear measurements in three planes	35	—	—	—	—	0.91	0.07	See Figure 19–8

EDV—end-diastolic volume; ESV—end-systolic volume; EF—ejection fraction; *r*—correlation coefficient; SEE—standard error of the estimate; RAO—right anterior oblique.

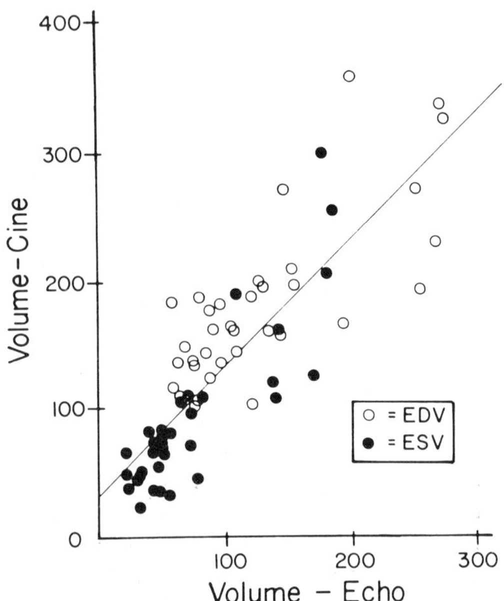

Figure 19–6. Relationship of end-diastolic volumes (EDV) and end-systolic volumes (ESV) as measured by cineangiography (Cine) and two-dimensional echocardiography (Echo) using the modified Simpson's rule approach shown in Figure 19–5 (r = 0.84, SEE = 43 ml). (From Folland, E.D., Parisi, A.F., Moynihan, P.F., et al.: Assessment of left ventricular ejection fraction and volumes by real-time, two-dimensional echocardiography. A comparison of cineangiographic and radionuclide techniques. Circulation 60:765, 1979. By permission of the American Heart Association, Inc.)

also measured by radionuclide angiocardiography, the standard error of the estimate (0.10) approached that of the radionuclide technique (0.07) when each method was compared to cineangiography.[F2]

Quinones and associates[Q1] have developed a simplified method of measuring left ventricular ejection fraction from two-dimensional images without the need for planimetry and/or computer processing. The apical four-chamber, apical two-chamber, and parasternal long-axis views are used, and multiple diameters are measured by calipers in each of these views at end-diastole and end-systole. Diameters (D) are measured at the following locations: two in the parasternal long-axis view—at the tips of the mitral valve and halfway to the most distal point of the left ventricle; and three each in the two apical views—1 cm below the tips of the mitral valve, halfway from the mitral valve to the apex, and a more distal dimension at the same distance from the second dimension that the second is from the first. All of these dimensions are averaged in diastole and in systole and the fractional shortening is calculated (% ΔD). Finally, an arbitrary contraction factor (% ΔL) is assigned to the apex according to its visual grading (normal apical contraction, +15%; hypokinetic, +5%; akinetic, 0%; mild dyskinesis, −5%; and severe dyskinesis, −10%). When these values are substituted into the formula

$$EF = (\%\ \Delta D^2) + [(1 - \%\ D^2)(\%\ \Delta L)]$$

an estimate of ejection fraction results that agrees well with the ejection fractions determined by both gated radionuclide and cineangiographic techniques for the same patients (Fig. 19–8). By averaging fractional shortening at multiple locations, regional contraction defects are taken into account and the shortcomings of the unidimensional M-mode fractional shortening measurement are avoided. Good correlations are shown in Figure 19–8 in spite of the fact that 42 of 55 patients had coronary artery disease.

In the clinical setting, visual estimation of left ventricular ejection fraction has become a common practice. Figure 19–9 displays the correlation between ejection fractions visually estimated from echocardiography and measured radionuclide angiography in 48 patients studied in our laboratory. The visual estimates were the averages of two independent observers who were blinded to the radionuclide results and were asked to estimate the left ventricular ejection fraction to the nearest 5 percent. The correlation between the ejection fractions determined by the two methods is surprisingly good, especially for patients with impaired ejection fraction. The standard error of the estimate (0.11) in this comparison is similar to the estimating error quoted earlier when quantitative echocardiographic and cineangiographic ejection fractions were compared (0.10). In spite of this, many prefer not to report a discrete number for ejection fraction unless a quantitative or semiquantitative method has been employed, because a numeric report conveys the impression of quantitative even when explicitly denoted as an estimate. A visually graded report may simply state that left ventricular ejection fraction is normal or mildly, moderately, or severely impaired.

End-Systolic Pressure-Volume Relationship

The left ventricular pressure-volume relationship has received increasing interest as an index of left ventricular performance that takes into account loading conditions and therefore is thought to be more indicative of intrinsic muscle function than is ejection fraction. This is particularly true in conditions in which augmented afterload may depress ejection fraction (aortic stenosis) or diminished afterload may enhance ejection fraction (mitral regurgitation). In either case, interpretation of ejection fraction

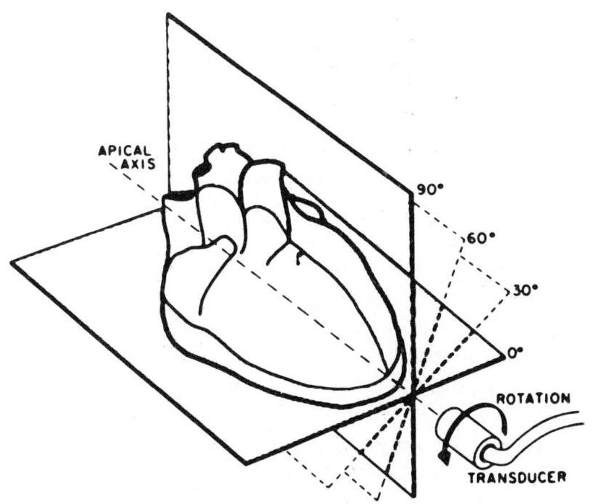

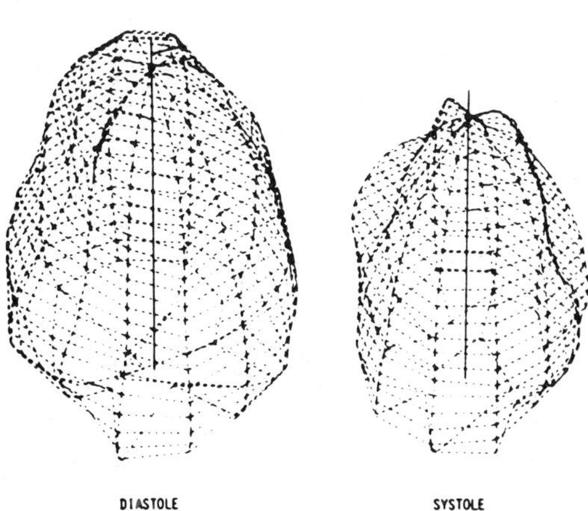

Figure 19–7. Three-dimensional reconstruction, apical axis rotation method. The transducer rotation and different planes intersecting the heart are shown on the left. Three-dimensional end-diastolic and end-systolic computer reconstructions of the left ventricle are shown on the right. These images represent a viewing angle of 45 degrees from the apical axis. (Reprinted with permission from Nanda, N.C., and Maurer, G.: Three dimensional reconstruction of echocardiographic images using the rotation method. Ultrasound Med. Biol. 8:659, 1982. Copyright 1982, Pergamon Press, Inc.)

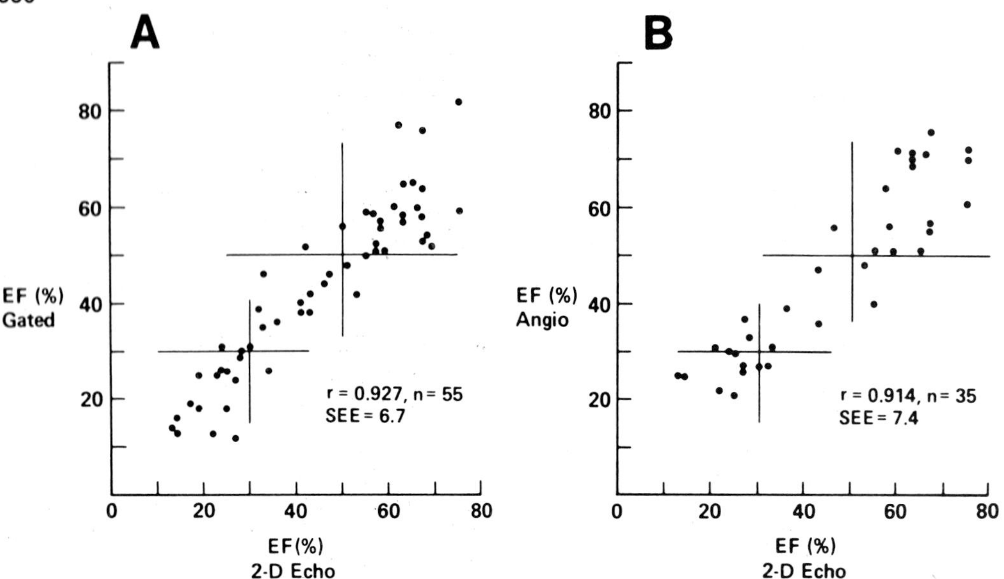

Figure 19–8. Results of a simplified method for measuring left ventricular ejection from two-dimensional images. This method utilized linear measurements alone, avoiding the need for planimetry (see text). Correlation of ejection fraction (EF) by two-dimensional echocardiography (2-D Echo) with (A) gated cardiac blood pool imaging (gated) and (B) single-plane cineangiography (Angio). Two-dimensional echo versus gated, $y = 0.90x + 3.0$; versus angio, $y = 0.95x + 7.1$. Cross bars are shown at ejection fractions of 50 and 30 percent. (From Quinones, M.A., Waggoner, A.D., Reduto, L.A., et al.: A new, simplified and accurate method for determining ejection fraction from two-dimensional echocardiography. Circulation 64:749, 1981, with permission of the American Heart Association, Inc.).

in isolation from loading conditions may lead to an incorrect impression of the true state of left ventricular myocardial contractility.

This measurement of left ventricular function entails plotting end-systolic meridional wall stress against end-systolic volume (or short-axis dimension in M-mode applications) at various loading states. The slope of this plot is nearly linear and indicates the intrinsic contractile state: the steeper the slope, the greater the contractility.[G3] Different loading states required for the plot are generated by administration of vasodilators or pure systemic pressors.

In its original form, this analysis was performed in the cardiac catheterization laboratory by obtaining end-systolic volumes and pressures from simultaneous left ventricular contrast cineangiography and pressure recording by high-fidelity catheter tip manometry.[G3] The noninvasive approach to systolic pressure-volume relations substitutes arm cuff systolic pressure for left ventricular end-systolic pressure. The validity of this substitution is a subject of controversy, with some investigators finding that systolic cuff pressures do not alter the stress-volume slope[R1] and others advising against such a substitution.[B2] In any case, assessment of left ventricular function by measurement of the stress-volume relationship is time consuming and tedious and has not yet found much application in general clinical practice.

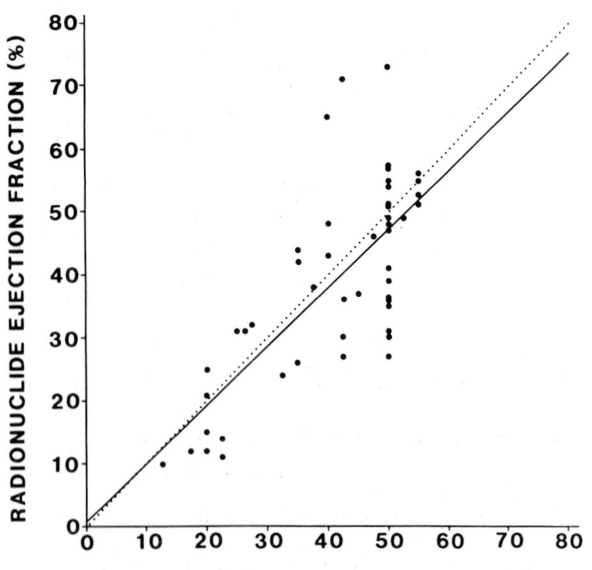

Figure 19–9. Comparison of left ventricular ejection fraction estimated visually from two-dimensional echocardiography and ejection fraction measured by radionuclide angiography. Each estimate was the average of two independent observers who were blinded to the radionuclide results. $n = 48$, $r = 0.73$, SEE $= 10.8$. The solid line is the linear regression ($y = 0.94x + 0.61$), and the dotted line is the line of identity.

Left Ventricular Mass

Left ventricular mass is estimated most simply from the M-mode dimensions of interventricular septum and left ventricular posterior wall. A more quantitative approach to estimating mass from M-mode data employs these dimensions in a modification of the cube volume formula:

$$\text{Mass} = 1.05 \text{ g/cc } [(D + IVS + PW)^3 - D^3] \text{ g}$$

In this formula D is the left ventricular internal dimension, IVS the thickness of interventricular septum, and PW the thickness of the posterior wall; all these dimensions are measured at the level of chordae tendineae at end-diastole in units of centimeters. Basically, in this formula the difference between total left ventricular volume (including walls) and left ventricular chamber volume is multiplied by the specific gravity of heart muscle (1.05 g/cc).

This simple technique has been validated anatomically by correlation of premortem echocardiographic measurements with postmortem left ventricular mass in 34 patients. The best agreement ($r = 0.96$) was obtained by using a modified convention (Penn convention) for measuring left ventricular dimensions that *excluded* the thickness of endocardial echoes from wall thickness and included these echoes in the left ventricular internal dimension (D) (Fig. 19–10).[D3] Corrected left ventricular mass calculated from measurements in which the Penn convention was used is as follows:

$$\text{Mass} = 1.04 \text{ g/cm } [(D + IVS + PW)^3 - D^3] - 14 \text{ g}$$

Other investigators have had equally good results with standard convention (leading edge) measurements in this formula.[W2] This technique has been shown to be a more accurate indicator of left ventricular hypertrophy than electrocardiography.[R2, W2] Devereux has defined left ventricular hypertrophy by this method as a mass index over 134 g/M^2 in men and 110 g/M^2 in women.[D4] Woythaler and associates have developed a practical nomogram (Fig. 19–11) for determining the presence of left ventricular hypertrophy from standard M-mode measurements.[W2] This nomogram was developed from a comparison of premortem echocardiographic data

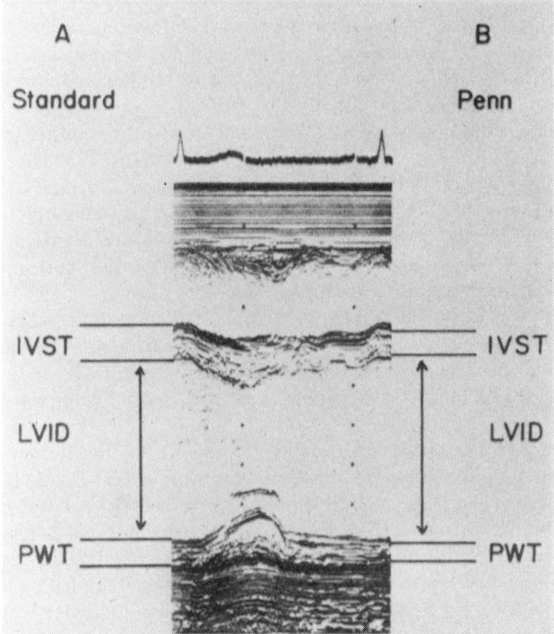

Figure 19–10. Methods for echocardiographic measurement of interventricular septal thickness (IVST), left ventricular internal dimension (LVID), and posterior wall thickness (PWT). *A*, Standard measurement convention includes the thickness of the right and left septal endocardial echoes in IVST and includes posterior wall endocardial echoes in PWT. *B*, The Penn convention excludes right and left septal endocardial echo thickness from IVST and excludes posterior wall endocardial echo thickness from PWT—these structures are thus included in LVID by this method. (From Devereux, R.B., and Reichek, N.: Echocardiographic determination of left ventricular mass in man. Anatomic validation of the method. Circulation 55:613, 1977, with permission of the American Heart Association, Inc.)

with postmortem left ventricular mass in 50 patients of both sexes.

The M-mode approach is theoretically limited by its unidimensional nature, which assumes that the walls measured are representative of the general thickness of the left ventricular wall. Consequently, this technique should be applied cautiously to hearts with regional left ventricular dysfunction or distorted geometry.

The limitations of M-mode data can be largely overcome by use of two-dimensional echocardiographic approaches to measurement of left ventricular mass.[B3, H2, R3] Typical approaches entail calculating the total left ventricular volume (including the walls), subtracting the left ventricular cavity volume, and multiplying the difference by the specific gravity of muscle. Any of the two-dimensional volume formulations described earlier (see Fig. 19–5, Table 19–1) may be employed. Formulas that have been validated include the concentric truncated ellipsoid,[B3, S3] Simpson's rule,[H2] and area-length.[H2] Helak and Reichek demonstrated that the Simpson's rule and area-length formulations are equally accurate with in vitro validation.[H2] Because of its simplicity, the area-length formulation seems preferable for clinical application:

$$V = 5/6 A_{pap} L$$

where A_{pap} is the area of the parasternal short-axis image at the level of papillary muscle determined by planimetry and L is the maximum length from mitral valve to apex measured from an apical view. Reichek and associates obtained better agreement between premortem echocardigraphic measurements and postmortem left ventricular mass with this two-dimensional formulation (area-length) than with their own M-mode formulation described earlier.[R3]

Both M-mode and two-dimensional echocardiography have been shown to be superior to electrocardiography in detecting left ventricular hypertrophy[R2, W2] and have accuracy similar to that of contrast angiography.[D4, R3] Because of the ease of application of ultrasound, it has an extremely important role in the determination of left ventricular mass for evaluation of therapy of patients with hypertension.

REGIONAL LEFT VENTRICULAR FUNCTION

Abnormalities of regional systolic function are important consequences of coronary artery disease. These abnormalities may

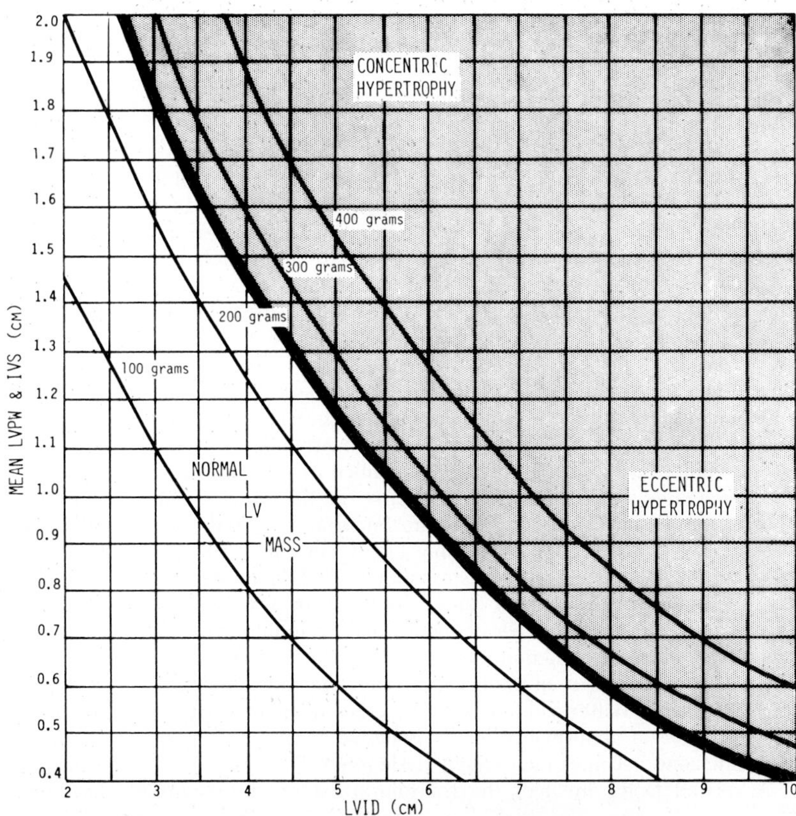

Figure 19–11. Nomogram for the clinical determination of left ventricular (LV) mass from M-mode echocardiographic measurements. After end-diastolic M-mode measurements are made, the mean of interventricular septal (IVS) and left ventricular posterior wall (LVPW) thickness is found on the vertical axis and followed to where it intersects the left ventricular internal chamber diameter (LVID) on the horizontal axis. Left ventricular mass is estimated from the relation of this point to the four plotted left ventricular mass meridians. All points above the 254-g mass meridian (*gray zone*) reflect an abnormally heavy left ventricle. Coordinates that lie in the upper left of the gray zone reflect concentric left ventricular hypertrophy with thickened left ventricular walls and no corresponding chamber dilation. Toward the middle and lower right of the gray zone lie regions where the chamber dilation is in proportion with the wall thickening in the situation of eccentric left ventricular hypertrophy. (From Woythaler, J.N., Singer, S.H., Kwan, O.H., et al.: Accuracy of echocardiography versus electrocardiography in detecting left ventricular hypertrophy: Comparison with post mortem mass measurements. J. Am. Coll. Cardiol. 2:310, 1983, with permission.)

be acutely precipitated by ischemia but will be temporally limited if the ischemia resolves without concomitant myocardial necrosis. If necrosis ensues, a permanent regional contraction abnormality will result. The extent and severity of the latter abnormalities strongly predict subsequent clinical outcomes.[G4, H3, N4]

By virtue of its noninvasive nature and in particular its ease of application, portability, repeatability, and safety, two-dimensional echocardiography is, in theory, an ideal technique for assessing systolic function during and after acute myocardial infarction or thrombolytic therapy. Multiple studies have confirmed that qualitative analysis of two-dimensional echocardiograms can be used reliably to identify regional contraction abnormalities.[G4, H3, K3, N4, N5] When applied in a semiquantitative manner by experienced observers, the technique provides important short-term prognostic information on patients with acute myocardial infarction.[G4, H3, H4, I3, N4] For patients who survive the hospital phase of acute myocardial infarction, predischarge semiquantitative two-dimensional echocardiography predicts 1- to 2-year outcomes as well.[B4, N6, V1]

Division of the left ventricle into standardized segments,[E2] use of standard nomenclature for degree of asynergy,[H5] and other conventions promote a unified approach and allow interstudy comparisons to be made. Furthermore, the reproducibility of qualitative review of echocardiograms used to identify regional wall motion abnormalities[H4, N4, N5] generally compares favorably with that of qualitative angiography.[C5, Z1] Nevertheless, qualitative and semiquantitative wall motion analyses are inferior to quantitative methods because of poorer reproducibility even when trained observers are used.[C5, Z1] In nonquantitative methods, a ventricular region is identified as abnormal primarily by visually comparing its systolic function to that of the remainder of the ventricle rather than to a normally contracting ventricle or to segmental data averaged from a group of normal ventricles. The process of visually classifying subtle motion abnormalities is particularly difficult.[G5, P3] When interventions are made (e.g., to alter infarct size) and/or serial studies are done to identify subtle changes in regional systolic function, accurate quantitative methods are necessary. The various quantitative analytic algorithms for examining regional left ventricular systolic function, and the theoretical and practical advantages and limitations of each, are explained here in further detail.

Relation of Systolic Dysfunction to Ischemia and Infarction

Historically, the accuracy of most techniques used to examine regional systolic function has been evaluated by how closely they reflect the pathologic extent of ischemia or infarction. Several factors disrupt the linear relationship between size of the ischemic region and extent of regional systolic dysfunction, irrespective of the method used to examine the latter.[F4] Most of these factors cause the extent of systolic dysfunction to exceed the extent of ischemia.

The first of these factors is tethering, that is, systolic dysfunction of nonischemic myocardium adjacent to ischemic or infarcted myocardium.[K4, W3] On the basis of a spherical mathematical model of the ventricle, tethering has been explained as resulting from local increases in afterload.[B5] Irrespective of the mechanism, recent studies have indicated that the importance of tethering has been overstated by studies using two-dimensional echocardiography.[F5] When tethering was examined using sonomicrometry, the extent of dysfunction caused by tethering was minimal (less than 8 mm or 30 degrees of endocardial circumference) and the degree of this dysfunction was modest.[C6, C7, G6, G17, H6] However, the extent and severity of tethering can be expected to increase with increases in afterload and with increases in the severity of the wall motion abnormality of the ischemic zone (i.e., as the ischemic zone becomes increasingly dyskinetic).[G18, W10]

A related factor involves the transmural extent of ischemia compared to the transmural extent of dysfunction. Gallagher and associates have shown that systolic wall thickening deteriorates significantly when blood flow to the subendocardium only is impaired.[G7] A number of factors appear to account for this. First, the epicardial one-third of the wall contributes minimally to overall wall thickening (approximately 17 percent).[M4, S4] Therefore, even if the epicardium continued to function normally during periods of subendocardial ischemia, overall wall thickening would be significantly reduced. Second, there is some evidence that epicardial function is "tethered" to endocardial and midwall function, at least in the anterior wall of the heart.[G8, G9, W4] Thus, not only does circumferential extent of dysfunction exceed circumferential extent of ischemia, but also transmural extent of dysfunction exceeds transmural extent of ischemia.

A third factor is the temporal relationship between resolution of ischemia and return of systolic function. The return of systolic function consistently lags behind the resolution of ischemia, often by prolonged periods (myocardial "stunning").[H7, K5, T3] The time to complete return of systolic function is inversely related to but significantly greater than the duration of ischemia. A transient 15-minute occlusion may produce changes in systolic function that persist for up to 6 hours[H7] or more.[T3] These data have obvious implications for examining return of function following reperfusion.[B6, E3, H8, T4, W5]

Analysis Algorithms

Preliminary Considerations

The ideal system for analyzing regional ventricular function should be reproducible (i.e., intraobserver and interobserver, intersubject, and day-to-day variability should all be low) and accurate compared to some standard. Unfortunately, even the choice of an ideal standard is problematic. Pathologic data are suboptimal because of the factors (discussed above) that disrupt the linear relationship between infarct size and extent of dysfunction and cause the latter to exceed the former. Therefore the accuracy of two-dimensional echocardiography (or any method that examines systolic function) should not be determined solely by comparison to pathology.

One is left with in vivo methods of wall motion analysis that are in reality only historic standards (i.e., the "standard" technique predated two-dimensional echocardiography). Contrast ventriculography, one of the historic standards, also has problems with defining ideal analysis systems.[C8, C9, F4, G10, I1, K9, S5, U1] In addition, contrast ventriculography is very difficult to equate one-to-one with two-dimensional echocardiography. Two-dimensional echocardiography images a tomographic cross section of the ventricle, whereas contrast ventriculography produces a silhouette of the ventricle. Thus, volume of the ventricle predicted by two-dimensional echocardiography is consistently less than that predicted by contrast ventriculography, even with model hearts.[E4] Considerations such as these have led different investigators to choose widely differing reference standards—electrocardiography,[H10] quantitative contrast ventriculography,[F6, L1, P6] qualitative two-dimensional echocardiographic wall motion analysis,[G11, S6] or some combination of these standards. These limitations should be kept in mind as various analytic algorithms for measuring regional function are considered. Observer variability is easy to define, but values for quantitative two-dimensional echocardiography rarely have been compared directly to values for other quantitative methods. However, with occasional exceptions,[Z2] most investigators have reported values for intraobserver and interobserver variability that compare favorably to values for quantitative contrast ventriculography.[C5, L1, S5, Z3] In general, 5 to 10 percent interobserver variability for regional fractional area change is an acceptable value.

The definition of the range of normal regional ventricular function (intersubject variability) from which to define abnormal regional function poses more difficult problems. The first problem is the wide range of normal or the large variability (defined here as standard deviation divided by the mean) reported for populations of normal subjects. Normal segmental cavity area shrinkage has been reported to vary from 0 percent (i.e., akinesis) to 100 percent and segmental wall thickening to vary from 0 percent to 150 percent.[P4] Such extreme variability makes differentiation of normal and abnormal difficult in individual patients. If correct, these data suggest that quantitative wall motion analysis may be of little value as a marker of ischemia in an individual and would be of value only for comparing groups of subjects.[Z2] Even in studies in which variability was not found to be so extreme,[F6, M5, N7] the lower limit of normal for cavity area shrinkage and systolic thickening, as defined by the mean minus two standard deviations, is near 0 percent for some regions. In reality, akinesis and failure of myocardium to thicken are rarely observed qualitatively in the hearts of normal humans or healthy animals.

It is this disagreement between mathematically derived quantitative ranges of normal for two-dimensional echocardiography and what one observes qualitatively that raises important concerns about the quantitative analysis algorithms currently used. Further problems arise in technical execution of these algorithms (e.g., tracing of endocardial borders). Because of this extreme variability of regional performance, a conservative lower limit of normal is often chosen (arbitrarily) to be 0 percent thickening[N7, P4, P5] and some minimal amount of endocardial motion (e.g., 0 to 10 percent radial shortening or cavity area shrinkage).[P5] However, there is no consensus about this arbitrary cutoff and other values (10 to 20 percent shortening) have been used.[G5, K6, M6] Sensitivity and specificity for detecting regional abnormalities thus will change significantly as different cutoffs for the normal range are chosen.

Several physiologic factors also compound the difficulties with quantitative analysis. First, there is considerable heterogeneity of endocardial motion and thickening from level to level within the same ventricle. Left ventricular systolic thickening and endocardial motion increase from base to apex.[F13, H9, L2, M5, N7] Intersegmental variation within the same level has also been shown with numerous techniques.[H9, K7, K8, P4] Finally, temporal asynergy of contraction may contribute significantly to regional variability, especially in ventricles with regional wall motion abnormalities.[M7, P4] Variability may be decreased by disregarding temporal asynergy and analyzing the maximum contraction of each segment, irrespective of when it occurred in the cardiac cycle. The problems related to temporal asynergy can be solved by analyzing multiple frames within the cardiac cycle, but this approach creates new difficulties (see below).

Endocardial Motion

Analysis of endocardial motion antedated systolic thickening analysis for several reasons. First, endocardial targets were better imaged than epicardial targets by using stop-frame tracing. Second, endocardial motion analysis is similar to the approach that had been used to evaluate regional motion with contrast ventriculography. Despite the fact that endocardial motion analyses with contrast ventriculography have been performed for a number of years, the true course of endocardial motion in the 30 degree right anterior oblique plane has been elucidated only recently using endocardial markers implanted in experimental animals (Fig. 19–12).[S7] This motion is a complex combination of inward transverse motion of the anterior and inferior wall and descent of the base toward the apex. It is clear from this study that none of the analysis algorithms currently in use track motion of individual endocardial points. Rather, they are simply a representation of endocardial motion. With this caveat in mind, we proceed to a discussion of these analysis systems.

As in contrast ventriculography, there are numerous choices in deciding on an analysis algorithm[C9]—choices involving reference systems relating diastole to systole, the type of measurement to make, the number of such measurements to be made per ventricular section, and the frequency of such measurements.

Reference Systems

Analysis of wall motion must account for the intrinsic centripetal motion ("contractile" motion) of the walls as well as for the extrinsic or translational and rotational motion of the entire heart (Fig. 19–13). Systems with a fixed or external frame of reference ignore the heart's translational and rotational motion. Systems with a floating or internal frame of reference attempt to control

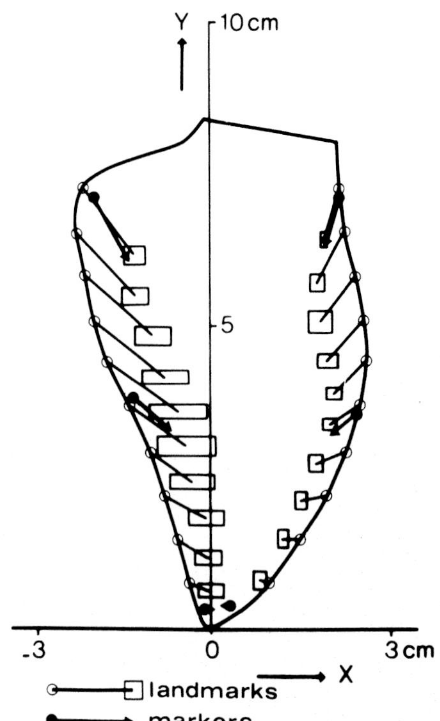

Figure 19–12. Mean end-diastolic contour and mean systolic pathways of implanted metal endocardial markers (*filled circles with arrows*) and of endocardial landmarks (*open circles*) in the right anterior oblique view in eight pigs. Boxes represent standard deviations of endocardial landmark motion. (From Slager, C.J., Hooghoudt, T.E.H., Serruys, P.W., et al.: Quantitative assessment of regional left ventricular motion using endocardial landmarks. J. Am. Coll. Cardiol. 7:317, 1986. Reprinted with permission from the American College of Cardiology.)

for or correct for translation and rotation so that only intrinsic motion is analyzed (Fig. 19–14). In general, as translational and rotational motion increases, fixed reference systems become less reliable and floating systems more reliable.[C9] Hence, the need to choose one system in preference to another depends on the degree of translational and rotational motion occurring in a specific clinical or experimental setting.[C9]

Fluoroscopic studies of myocardial markers implanted in the left ventricular midwall in the 30 degree right anterior oblique (RAO) plane in humans indicate that there is very little rotational motion of the ventricular long axis in either the 30 degree RAO plane (roughly approximating the echocardiographic apical two-chamber view) (Fig. 19–13*C*) or the 60-degree left anterior oblique plane (approximately the apical four-chamber view) (Fig. 19–13*D*)[I1, I2] and for practical purposes it can be ignored. Similarly, with two-dimensional echocardiography, the amount of rotational and translational motion of the ventricle (as measured by the amount of change in the position of the long axis in the apical four-chambers and two-chamber planes) in normal subjects and in preoperative coronary bypass patients is insignificant.[F7, F8] In theory, since translation and rotation are minimal in these patients, one would expect a fixed reference system to outperform a floating system, especially since the process of "floating" introduces unavoidable variability of its own.[I2, S5, S6, U1] In practice, this has not always been the case for the apical views, and in some cases floating systems correcting for translation have performed better than fixed analysis. It is difficult to reconcile the theoretical advantage of fixed systems with the reported superiority of floating systems. The reason for this may be that the range of normal is smaller with floating systems in apical views. Even in normal individuals in whom translational motion is minimal, there is variability from individual to individual. Consequently, with a fixed external frame of reference, systems in the apical views have greater ranges of normal.[F8, G11, S6] Thus smaller intersubject variability of floating systems in the apical views probably accounts for their superior performance.[G11, S6]

For patients following cardiac surgery in whom there is marked

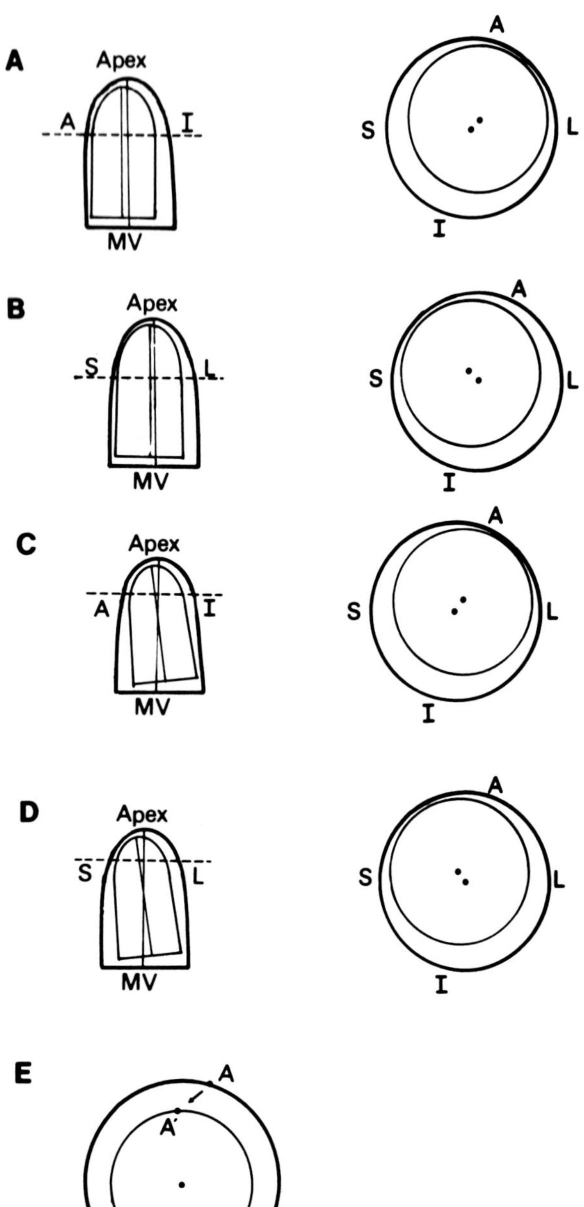

Figure 19–13. Schematic drawings of possible systolic translational and rotational motions of the ventricle as described by movement of the ventricular long axis (*solid line*) in the apical four-chamber (A4C) *or* apical two-chamber (A2C) views (left) and parasternal short-axis (SAX) view (right). The ventricular level of the short-axis section is identified by a dashed line on the A2C or A4C images. *A*, Anterior translation of the long axis of the ventricle seen in the A2C and SAX views. *B*, Medial translation of the long axis seen in the A4C (left) and SAX views. *C*, Rotation of the long axis in the A2C plane as seen in A2C and SAX views. *D*, Rotation of the long axis in the A4C plane as seen in the A4C and SAX views. *E*, Rotation of the ventricle about the long axis seen in the SAX view. S—septum; A—anterior wall; L—lateral wall; I—inferior wall; MV—mitral valve. (From Force, T.L., and Parisi, A.F.: Quantitative methods for analyzing regional systolic function with two-dimensional echocardiography. *In* Kerber, R. E. (ed.): Echocardiography in Coronary Artery Disease. Futura Publishing Company, Inc., Mount Kisco, NY, 1988, p. 193, with permission.)

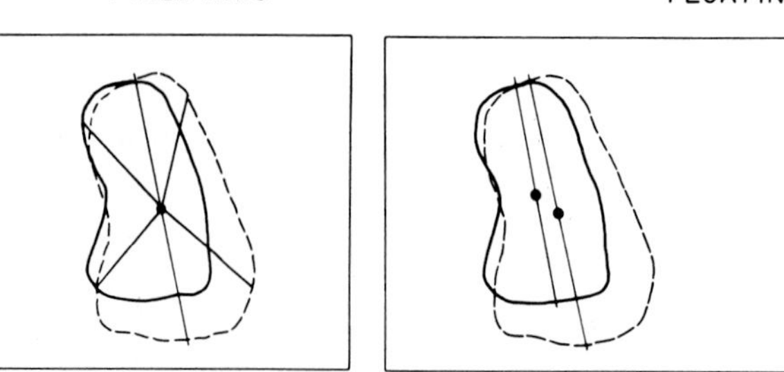

Figure 19–14. Schematic of the fixed- and floating-axis systems used to analyze regional wall motion in the apical four-chamber view. For the fixed-axis system, radii are generated from the midpoint of the diastolic long axis. For the floating-axis system, the long axes of both diastolic and systolic images are defined, the midpoint is identified, the long axes are then superimposed, and radii are again generated from the midpoint. (From Force, T., Bloomfield, P., O'Boyle, J.E., et al.: Quantitative two-dimensional echocardiographic analysis of motion and thickening of the interventricular septum after cardiac surgery. Circulation 68:1013, 1983. By permission of the American Heart Association, Inc.)

anteromedial translational motion of the ventricle, a floating reference system is clearly superior. The floating system has proved to be significantly better than a fixed system for differentiating patients with perioperative infarction from those without and for localizing the area of infarction (Fig. 19–15).[F7–F9] Thus, in the apical views, superiority of fixed versus floating-axis systems largely depends on the degree of translational motion of the ventricle in a particular clinical setting. Although the process of floating introduces a potential source of error, the smaller range of normal may allow more accurate identification of abnormal regions, especially where translational motion is great.

The choice of an analysis system is more difficult for the *parasternal short-axis view*, in which analysis systems must rely on a "centroid" as the internal reference to correct for translation. The centroid or center of mass (area) is a point in space that is defined by the endocardial or epicardial contour. Although a number of techniques exist for generating a centroid, all floating systems suffer from similar limitations. Figure 19–16 illustrates the problem. With normal, symmetric, and equal contractions and some anterior translation of the ventricle, the fixed reference system will lead to the conclusion that there is anterior hypokinesis. The floating endocardial center-of-mass system corrects for this and normalizes wall motion. Figure 19–16*B* is a schematic of a ventricle with an anterior wall motion abnormality and no translation. Here the fixed analysis system correctly localized the wall motion abnormality. The floating endocardial center-of-mass system falsely normalizes anterior wall motion because the centroid moves toward the abnormally contracting segment.

Not surprisingly, these theoretical concerns have been borne out repeatedly in experimental animal and human studies. Although fixed and floating systems may not differ in their abilities to detect the presence of a regional abnormality or to separate patients with an abnormality from those without, the floating system localizes the abnormality and quantifies it far less accurately than the fixed system.[F6, M5, S6] Floating systems may incorrectly localize wall motion abnormalities more than 50 percent of the time.[S6] These negative features of floating-axis analyses in the parasternal short-axis view more than outweigh the smaller range of normal compared to that obtained with fixed analyses. However, an epicardial floating center-of-mass system may be a compromise that reduces the range of normal (albeit not to the extent that endocardial center systems do[F13]) but does not falsely enhance motion of abnormal regions as much.[S8, Z3] With this system, the centroid still moves toward the wall motion abnormality but less so than with an endocardial center-of-mass analysis (Fig. 19–17). With increasing degrees of dyskinesis, even the epicardial center of mass will increasingly falsely improve apparent wall motion, although not to normal. Thus, identification of regional dysfunction will remain good but quantitation of the degree of asynergy will be suspect.

In summary, the choice of a fixed or floating reference system and, if floating, the choice of what type of centroid are the most problematic decisions in quantitative two-dimensional echocardiography. Use of a fixed external frame of reference system is limited by a wider range of normal that is probably responsible for the suboptimal sensitivity for the apical four-chamber[G11, S6] and apical two-chamber[G11] views. In these views with more consistent internal landmarks to construct the long axis of the left ventricle, a floating analysis system may be superior. In the parasternal short-axis views, however, where a centroid must be used, endocardial center-of-mass floating-axis analysis leads to false normalization of regional wall motion abnormalities and poor localization. Use of an epicardial center-of-mass system will lead to less movement of the centroid and less false normalization of wall motion. However, it produces inherent alterations that will not reflect true wall motion.

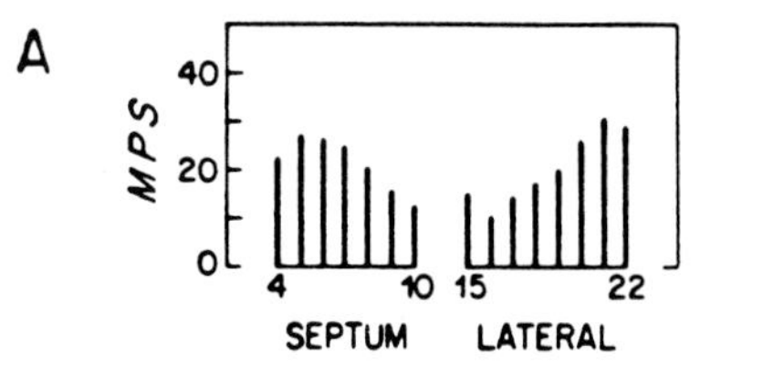

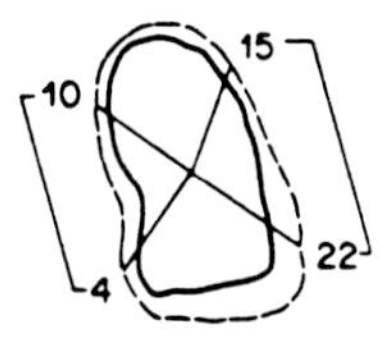

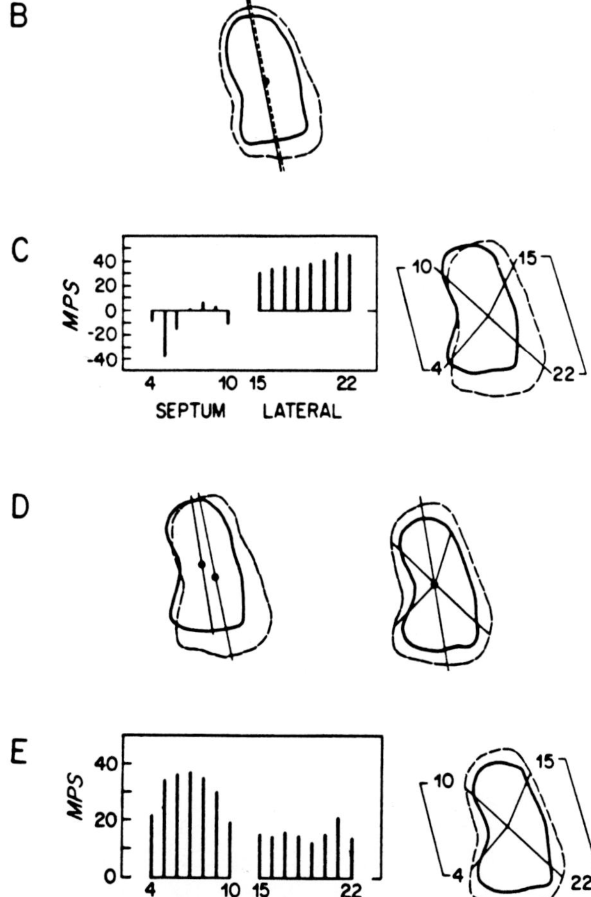

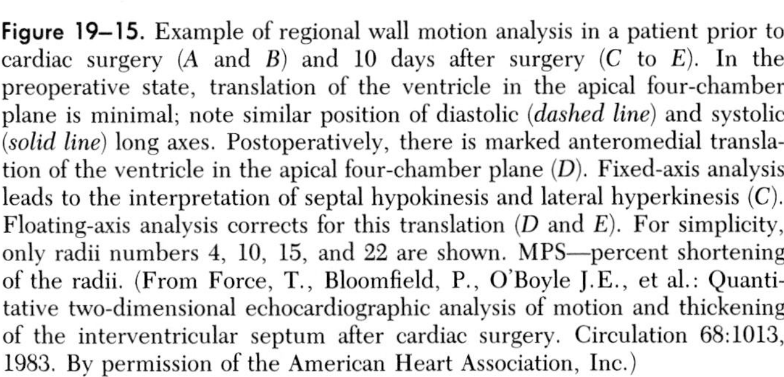

Figure 19–15. Example of regional wall motion analysis in a patient prior to cardiac surgery (*A* and *B*) and 10 days after surgery (*C* to *E*). In the preoperative state, translation of the ventricle in the apical four-chamber plane is minimal; note similar position of diastolic (*dashed line*) and systolic (*solid line*) long axes. Postoperatively, there is marked anteromedial translation of the ventricle in the apical four-chamber plane (*D*). Fixed-axis analysis leads to the interpretation of septal hypokinesis and lateral hyperkinesis (*C*). Floating-axis analysis corrects for this translation (*D* and *E*). For simplicity, only radii numbers 4, 10, 15, and 22 are shown. MPS—percent shortening of the radii. (From Force, T., Bloomfield, P., O'Boyle J.E., et al.: Quantitative two-dimensional echocardiographic analysis of motion and thickening of the interventricular septum after cardiac surgery. Circulation 68:1013, 1983. By permission of the American Heart Association, Inc.)

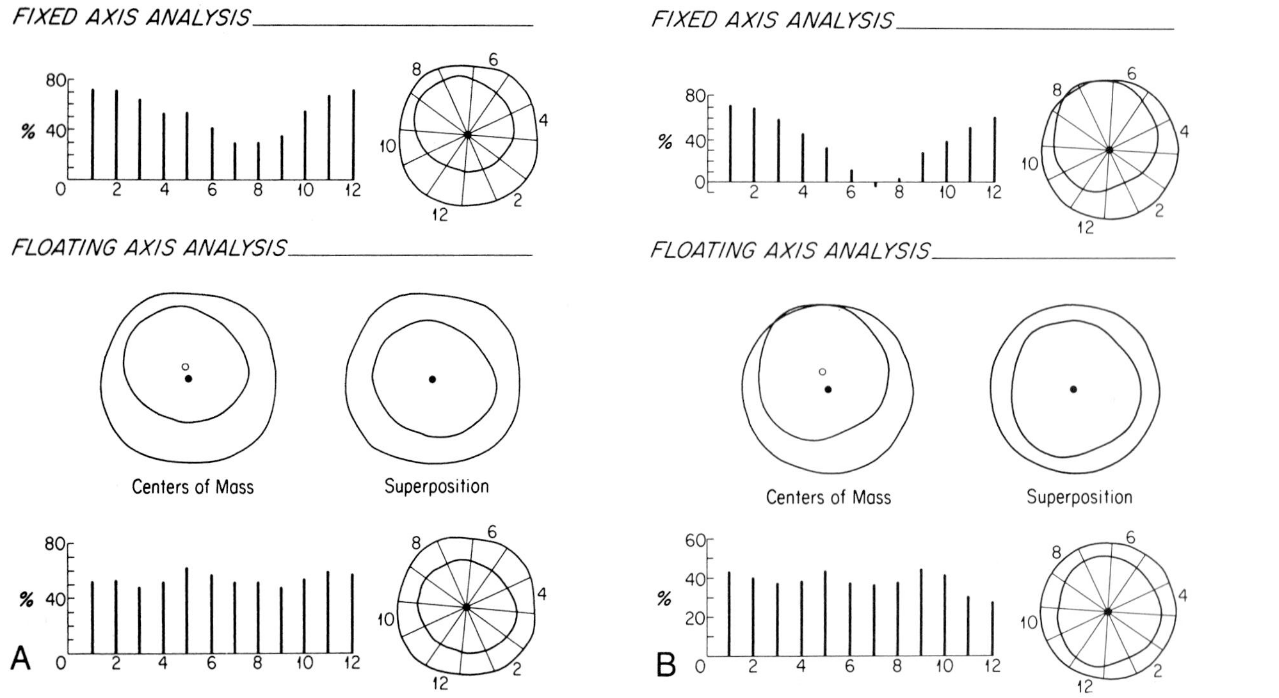

Figure 19–16. *A*, Fixed- and floating-axis wall motion analyses (area shrinkage) of a normally contracting ventricle with anterior translation of the ventricle. Fixed-axis analysis leads to the conclusion that anterior hypokinesis is present. Floating-axis analysis superimposes the diastolic (*filled circle*) and systolic (*open circle*) centroids and normalizes wall motion. *B*, Fixed- and floating-axis analyses of a ventricle with an anterior wall motion abnormality and no translation of the ventricle. Fixed-axis analysis correctly localizes the abnormality. Because the centroid moves toward the wall motion abnormally in systole, superimposition of the diastolic and systolic centroids falsely normalizes anterior endocardial motion. (From Force, T.L., and Parisi, A.F.: Quantitative methods for analyzing regional systolic function with two-dimensional echocardiography. *In* Kerber, R. E. (ed.): Echocardiography in Coronary Artery Disease. Futura Publishing Company, Inc., Mount Kisco, NY, 1988, p. 193, with permission.)

A related though less problematic issue is correction for systolic rotation of the ventricle about the long axis (see Fig. 19–13*E*). Normally, the ventricle "twists" slightly with ejection (i.e., more apical segments rotate relative to the base).[S19] If the degree of systolic rotation is sufficient, analogous portions of the ventricle will not be examined in diastole as compared to systole. The usual approach to this problem is to correct for such rotation by realigning the diastolic and systolic contours based on the position of some internal landmarks (usually the papillary muscles). In general, the basal two-thirds of the heart rotates minimally (only 3 to 4 degrees).[F5, M8] This suggests that correction for rotation about the long axis of the heart is unnecessary for short-axis views of the basal two-thirds of the heart unless precise alignment of papillary muscle contours is desired (i.e., if motion of the papillary muscles is being analyzed). This issue has not been examined adequately at the cardiac apex. It is our impression that rotation here may be a more significant factor, as it may be with inotropic stimulation.[S19] If this is so, it will pose a significant problem to quantitative analysis of short-axis apical images, since there are no internal landmarks with which to realign the diastolic and systolic contours.

Types of Measurements

The next choice to be made is between types of measurements—change in length of a chord or a radius emanating from a center point or change in a cavity area. Intuitively, area-based methods should be superior, since they sample a region more completely than a single linear measurement and thus would be less susceptible to errors due to minor geometric aberrations.[P6] In general, area methods are more reproducible, more accurate, and have smaller ranges of normal than length-based methods.[G10, G11, P6] However, as the number of areas into which the ventricle

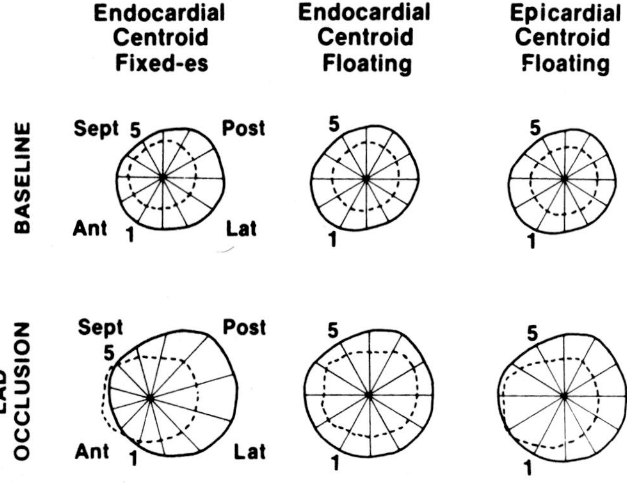

Figure 19–17. Reference systems used to determine radial shortening along 12 equidistant radii. Only one of the four fixed reference systems (endocardial centroid fixed at end-systole [es]) and the two floating reference systems are shown. The endocardial contours at end-diastole and end-systole are from before and after experimental coronary occlusion. Radius 1 is at the level of the anterolateral papillary muscle during end-diastole and end-systole. In this figure, the endocardial contours are already rotated so that the respective radii are superimposed. In the case of floating references, the contours are furthermore translated to superimpose the respective end-diastolic and end-systolic centroids. During baseline, using either floating centroid system, radial shortening adequately reflects regional function, whereas the fixed reference delineates hypokinesia in the anteroseptal (Ant-Sept) area secondary to cardiac translation. During left anterior descending (LAD) coronary occlusion, radial shortening in the involved region shows evidence of dyskinesia with the fixed reference, no abnormality with the floating endocardial centroid, and akinesia/hypokinesia with the floating epicardial centroid. Lat—lateral; Sept—septum; Ant—anterior; Post—posterior. (From Zoghbi, W.A., Charlat, M.L., Bolli, R., et al.: Quantitative assessment of left ventricular wall motion by two-dimensional echocardiography: Validation during reversible ischemia in the conscious dog. J. Am. Coll. Cardiol. 11:851, 1988. Reprinted with permission from the American College of Cardiology.)

is subdivided increases, and the size of each such area decreases, the area methods increasingly resemble length methods and any superiorities of the former are lost.

An alternative to these coordinate systems is the "coordinateless" centerline method developed for contrast ventriculography but applicable to two-dimensional echocardigraphy as well.[B7, M12] In this system, radii are not generated from a predefined center point. Instead, a line is generated midway between the end-diastolic and end-systolic contours and then multiple chords are constructed perpendicular to this line (Fig. 19–18). Wall motion is assessed as the length of these chords. This system avoids the problem, albeit of minor practical importance,[11] of where to place the center point for generation of radii. It also prevents tangential intersection of radii with endocardium that may give a false impression of the extent of motion in a region. More importantly, motion is absolute and can be more reliably compared from region to region than when referenced to an end-diastolic radius or area and expressed as a percent change. However, this system does not solve the major problem of quantitative two-dimensional echocardiography: whether to correct for translation and rotation and how to accomplish this.

Numbers of Measurements

There are few data regarding the optimum number of measurements in assessing regional ventricular function (i.e., the number of subdivisions of the left ventricle). Infarctions with small circumferential extent may be difficult to detect even if they are transmural.[Q2, P5] Theoretically, systems with more subdivisions would be more likely to detect small regional wall motion abnormalities. In practice, it is not clear that more subdivisions increase detection of small infarctions significantly,[P6] even when the ventricle is subdivided into 72 segments (at 5 degree intervals).[S6] Balanced against any possible increase in sensitivity is the fact that reproducibility and variability deteriorate with greater subdivision of the left ventricle; that is, the signal-to-noise ratio increases.[M5] Hence, as the number of subdivisions decreases, so does the number of false-positive wall motion abnormalities.

Sampling Frequency in the Cardiac Cycle

Early attempts to quantify regional wall motion with radionuclide ventriculography or two-dimensional echocardiography examined only end-diastole and end-systole. This approach does not account for temporal heterogeneity of contraction. Dyskinesis is maximal in early systole in the vast majority of patients with previous infarction.[G12, J1, L3, S9, S10, W6] In one study only 1 percent of regions were maximally dyskinetic at end-systole.[W6] Thus, important regional wall motion abnormalities can clearly be missed by sampling only end-diastole and end-systole.

Weyman and associates have extensively evaluated a system that samples endocardial motion every 16.7 msec and integrates the entire temporal course of systolic radial motion (Fig. 19–19). At present, this approach requires the operator to digitize manually multiple frames throughout the cardiac cycle and is thus extremely tedious and time consuming. Reproducibility with this approach is surprisingly good if echocardiograms are of sufficiently high quality.[K6, Z2] However, a significantly greater amount of "noise" is inherent in such analyses. Such noise can be from irregularities of the endocardial surface, from the video image, and from errors in the digitization process (whether automated or manual). Fourier analysis is a logical approach to reducing the intraframe (spatial) and interframe (temporal) noise.[T5] Unfiltered analyses show a large number of regional endocardial direction reversals for each systolic contraction sequence that are largely due to errors in tracing (Fig. 19–20). Smoothing via Fourier transformation reduces the number of these endocardial direction reversals and produces an image that more closely resembles what the echocardiographer sees qualitatively (i.e., smooth, symmetric, centripetal contraction) (see Fig. 19–20). At present, such analyses are far too cumbersome and require very high-quality images for applications other than research. As automated edge detection systems become increasingly accurate, clinical applications should be possible.

Reference-Independent Systems

Because all of the approaches to wall motion analysis discussed above must deal with the issue of whether (and how) to correct for translation of the ventricle and what type of coordinate system to use, attempts have been made to develop systems that are truly independent of reference points. One such approach to identifying ischemic or infarcted segments is to analyze regional radius of curvature rather than wall motion.[M13] Curvature clearly changes when a region becomes ischemic or is infarcted.[F12] However, it is far too soon to determine whether analysis of

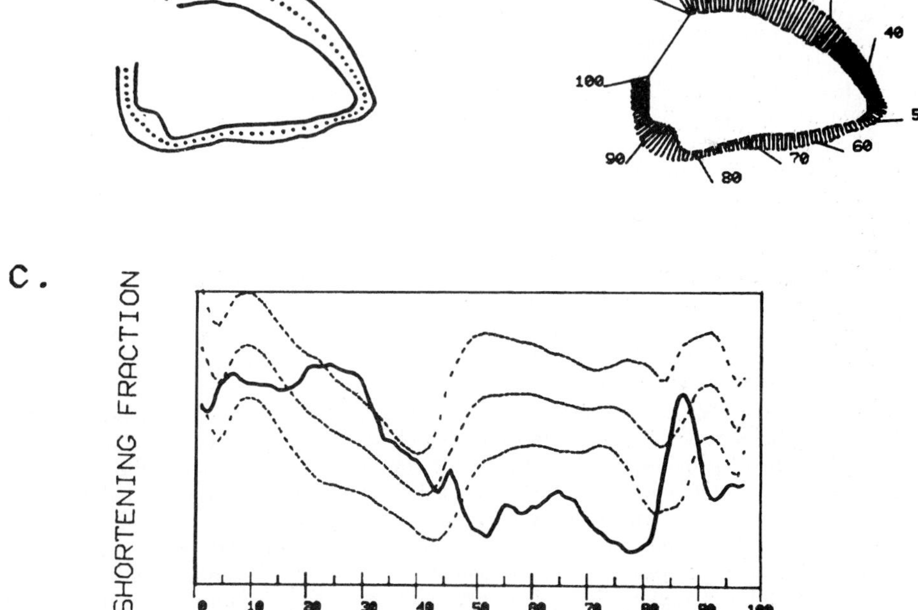

Figure 19–18. Centerline method of Bolson and associates. *A*, End-diastolic and end-systolic contours with dotted centerline. *B*, Chords constructed perpendicular to the centerline. *C*, Wall motion in a patient (*heavy solid line*) with inferior hypokinesis and anterior hyperkinesis plotted compared to the normal range. (From Sheehan, F.H., Stewart, A.K., Dodge, H.T., et al.:[S5] Variability in the measurement of regional left ventricular wall motion from contrast angiograms. Circulation 68:550, 1983. By permission of the American Heart Association, Inc.)

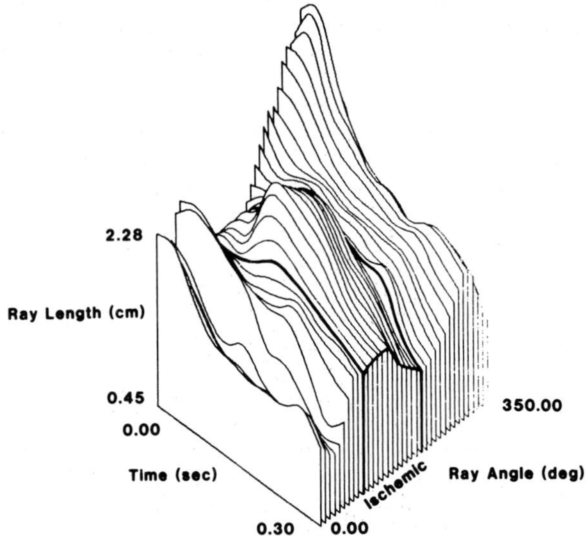

Figure 19–19. Plot of radial wall motion (expressed as ray length) from end-diastole (left) to end-systole (right) for 36 radii around the circumference of the ventricle. There is mid-systolic dyskinesis (ray lengthening) within the ischemic zone (demarcated by *dark solid lines*). (From Weyman, A.E., Franklin, T.D., Hogan, R.D., et al.:[W5] Importance of temporal heterogeneity in assessing the contraction abnormalities associated with acute myocardial ischemia. Circulation 70:102, 1984. By permission of the American Heart Association, Inc.)

curvature will allow differentiation of normal from abnormal segments and accurate quantification of abnormal region size.

Quantification of Infarct Size with Endocardial Motion

Single Plane

To this point we have been concerned only with using echocardiographic imaging to determine whether or not a regional abnormality is present. While there are some limitations in comparing extent of regional wall motion abnormalities to observations of pathologic material, pathology at least offers an easily quantifiable and unequivocal standard. Numerous investigators have examined the accuracy of two-dimensional echocardiographic wall motion analyses for determining infarct size. In general, semiquantitative approaches (Fig. 19–21)[H12, M9, W5, W7] (i.e., the echocardiographer qualitatively estimates the percent circumference that is dysfunctional) reasonably predict pathologic infarct size[H12, M9, W5, W7] even in humans.[W7] Accuracy is, of course, critically dependent on the echocardiographer's experience, and all the problems of qualitative analysis will be apparent. Nevertheless, such approaches, as noted above, have been used successfully to classify patients according to risk after myocardial infarction.

In general, although purely quantitative systems can identify normal and abnormal regional contraction reliably,[H4, L4] they are less successful in quantifying the extent of a contraction abnormality as related to another standard. Several studies using quantitative analyses have consistently found the same problem: the size of the ischemic region is overestimated, and there is a large amount of "scatter"—the standard error of the estimate is often 15 to 20 percent of the circumference of the left ventricle. One must realize that overestimation of ischemic region size is not necessarily a limitation, since the functional sequelae of myocardial infarction (i.e., the severity of left ventricular dysfunction) are excellent predictors of prognosis and are not necessarily inferior to measures of ischemic region size.[K12] The two should be viewed as complementary. However, although some of the overestimation occurs because extent of dysfunction truly exceeds pathologic extent of infarction, at least some of the overestimation is certainly due to limitations of analysis algorithms (Fig. 19–22). Furthermore, the inaccuracy implicit in the largely reported standard errors of the estimate is certainly a limitation.

It is not clear whether systems that examine for temporal heterogeneity of contraction by sampling multiple times in the cardiac cycle will improve infarct size determinations. Initial reports have been encouraging.[G5, K6] However, since the major advantage of the technique is that it increases the ability to detect abnormalities along individual radii by sampling all of systole, it would seem that overestimation of infarct size might be a greater problem than with standard end-diastolic/end-systolic approaches.

Integrative Approaches to the Whole Ventricle

The problems of single-plane analyses are multiplied when attempting to combine uniplanar images to reconstruct the entire ventricle. The most common approach is to use a Simpson's rule algorithm for summating data from individual short-axis planes. However, in order to derive a percent of the left ventricle that is infarcted, either one must know the "height" of the two-dimensional echocardiographic section (or more accurately the distance between sections) in order to calculate percent of myocardial mass infarcted (which is rarely possible clinically) or one must make assumptions concerning the height of the section or the relative proportion of mass represented by each section (also impossible clinically). Even in the experimental setting, such approaches have produced suboptimal correlations.[N7]

A novel approach to this problem is the endocardial surface mapping technique.[G14, G15] With this technique, the endocardial surface area of the ventricle is determined by using a computer algorithm with measured input from three short-axis views (circumference at each level) and two apical views (length of the long axis in the apical four-chamber and two-chamber views). The extent of dysfunction is determined qualitatively in each view, and then extent of dysfunction is calculated by the algorithm as a percent of the total left ventricular surface area for the whole ventricle. Finally, for ease of viewing, the surface area of the ventricle is displayed as a planar map similar to a Mercator projection of the globe (Fig. 19–23).

In the hands of trained operators, this approach accurately determines total endocardial surface area and extent of infarction in experimental animals and in autopsied human hearts.[G14, G15, W11] This technique has some important advantages over other approaches to combining data from multiple views to express global left ventricular dysfunction. First, it is free of major assumptions concerning the geometry of the ventricle (i.e., the ventricle does not have to be modeled as a geometric figure, the resemblance to which may be minimal, especially in the distorted ventricle). Second, regional aneurysmal dilations are handled easily when this system is used.[W11] Although the initial reports used qualitative analysis of abnormal wall motion and no allowance was made for the severity of the wall motion abnormality, the algorithm can also easily be adapted to quantification.

Analysis of Apical Endocardial Motion

Apical regional wall motion abnormalities are extremely common with disease of the left anterior descending coronary artery. Unfortunately, the apex of the left ventricle is the most difficult area to evaluate, irrespective of the technique used. With contrast ventriculography, magnitude of motion is low and variability is high at the apex.[S5] Therefore reliability of motion measurement is worse there than in any other ventricular region and motion must be nearly dyskinetic to be abnormal.[S5]

Two-dimensional echocardiography has additional problems vis-à-vis the cardiac apex. In the short-axis, lack of internal landmarks below the papillary muscles makes it difficult to define a reproducible section. In the apical views the true apex of the left ventricle is often truncated, since the operator-defined echocardiographic apex is often not identical to the anatomic apex. Since truncating the apex may falsely enhance wall motion, one would expect limited sensitivity to be a problem.[Z2] Similar to the findings of contrast ventriculography,[S5] apical endocardial motion in the four-chamber view is minimal, making differentiation of

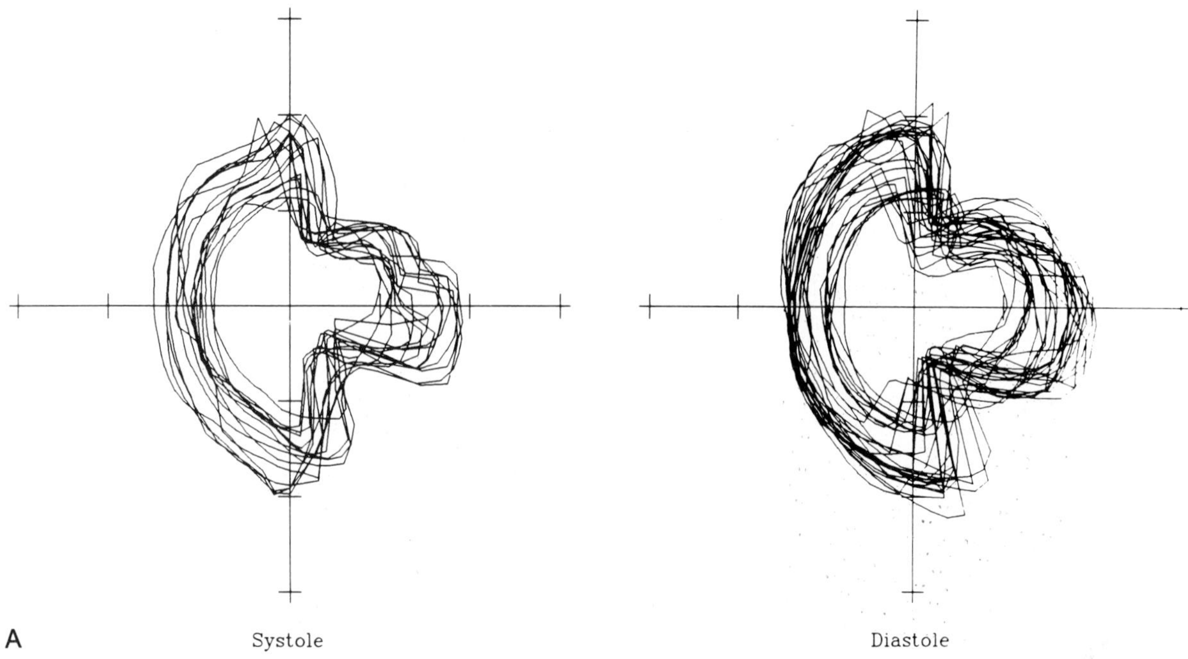

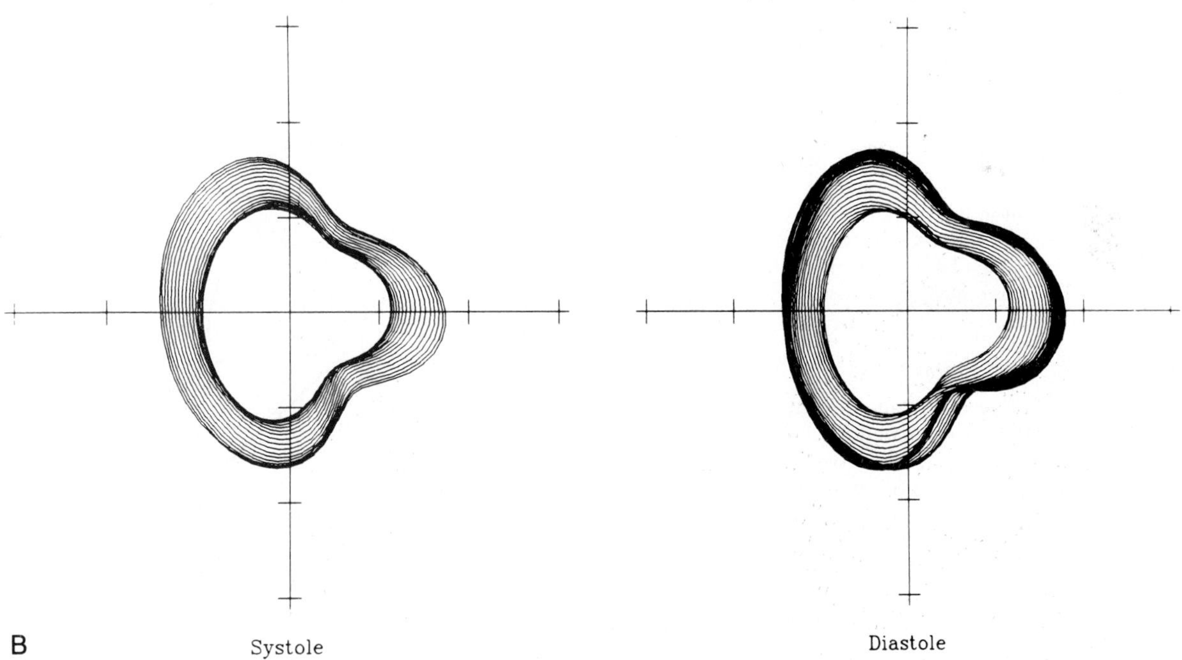

Figure 19–20. *A*, Polar display of raw echocardiographic data. Hand-traced endocardial borders from a single cardiac cycle at the midpapillary level in the dog are shown. Successive video fields (16.7-msec intervals) are drawn concentrically for systole (left) and diastole (right). Tick marks on horizontal and vertical axes are at centimeter intervals. The papillary muscles are identifiable at 2:00 and 4:00 in the tracings, but a considerable amount of random variation in endocardial positioning is evident. *B*, Filtered reconstruction of echocardiographic data. Shown is the smoothed reconstruction of the data in *A* with cutoff frequencies $T_c = 7$ and $O_c = 9$. Systolic borders are on the left and diastolic borders on the right. (From Thomas, J.D., Hagege, A.A., Choong, C.Y., et al.: Improved accuracy of echocardiographic endocardial borders by spatiotemporal filtered Fourier reconstruction: Description of the method and optimization of filter cutoffs. Circulation 77:415, 1988. By permission of the American Heart Association, Inc.)

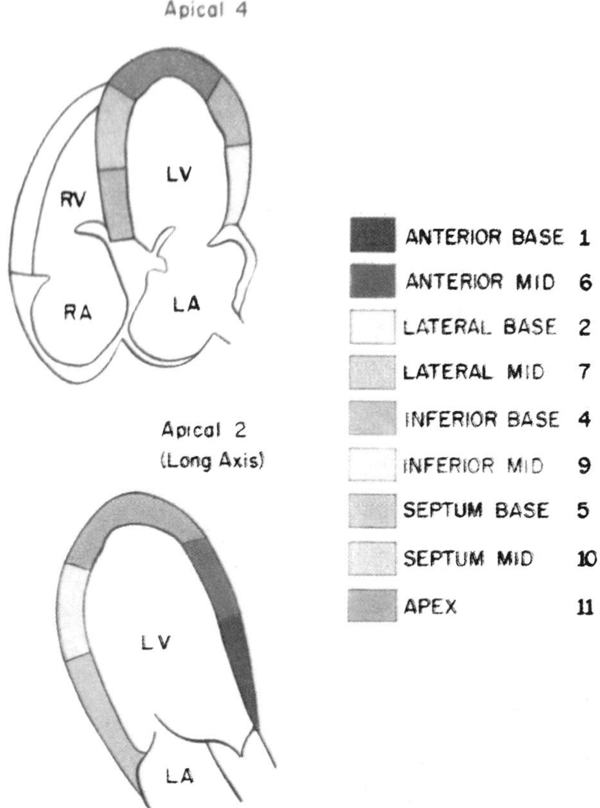

Figure 19–21. Schematic diagram showing the method used to identify visually myocardial segments from the apical four- and two-chamber echocardiographic views. RA—right atrium; LA—left atrium; LV—left ventricle; RV—right ventricle. (From Gibson, R.S., Bishop, H.L., Stamm, R.B., et al.: Value of early two-dimensional echocardiography in patients with acute myocardial infarction. Am. J. Cardiol. 49:1110, 1982, with permission.)

abnormal and normal difficult.[F8] Part of the reason for this may be difficulty in identifying endocardium.[G13, M10, S11] Endocardial dropout is most prominent apico-laterally due to overlying lung. For this reason, one can expect false-positive wall motion abnormalities of the apex or apico-lateral region if the criterion of hypokinesis is used.[S6] Therefore we consider isolated apical hypokinesis as normal.[F9]

Systolic Wall Thickening Analysis

Quantitative analysis of systolic wall thickening is the major alternative to analyzing the extent of endocardial motion. Thickening analysis has some important theoretical and practical advantages over motion analysis. Quantification of systolic thickening is relatively uninfluenced by translation of the ventricle, and correction for this with some sort of floating-axis system is unnecessary.[F10, L4, L5, W8] Furthermore, thickening analyses are thought to be more independent of the particular center of mass chosen for the analysis. Endocardial motion may have passive components,[L4] whereas systolic thickening does not. In addition, the analysis of systolic thickening has sounder experimental support: systolic wall thickening (determined with sonomicrometry) correlates closely with subendocardial shortening, subendocardial blood flow, and transmural blood flow.[G6, G7, S12] In addition, it accurately separates infarcted and noninfarcted tissue.[H13, S12] Finally, there is excellent qualitative agreement between systolic wall thickening determined by two-dimensional echocardiography and that determined by sonomicrometry.[P7, P8] Several studies have confirmed very good correlations between extent of abnormal systolic thickening and infarct size.[N7, O2, P9]

In direct comparisons, however, systolic thickening analyses have not consistently outperformed endocardial motion analyses. Specifically, the sensitivity for detecting presence or absence of infarction is not significantly different[H10, O2, P5] and the sensitivity of both is limited when infarction is small.[O2, P5] Furthermore, systolic thickening analyses are no more accurate at quantifying extent of infarction.[O2] However, although both thickening and endocardial motion clearly separate infarcted from distant normal myocardium, systolic thickening is superior to wall motion analysis at distinguishing infarct zones from adjacent noninfarcted ones.[L4, O2] Consequently, endocardial wall motion analyses systematically overpredict the circumferential extent of infarction more than thickening analyses.

Systolic thickening analysis has some additional problems. It is often difficult to identify the epicardial targets sufficiently to trace them, even in experimental animals. This problem may produce large interobserver variabilty.[F10] When the normal change from end-diastolic to end-systolic wall thickness can be only 1 to 2 mm, small errors in identifying epicardium can become important sources of variability. Definition of the range of normal systolic thickening has all the same problems as endocardial motion analyses. Intersubject, intersegment, and interlevel variability are just as high with systolic thickening, and temporal asynergy is also present.[P4]

In addition, systolic thickness analyses may be subject to the "threshold phenomenon."[L4] As the percentage of the transmural extent of ischemia or myocardial infarction exceeds some figure, systolic thickening deteriorates no further.[E6, G7, G9, L4, S13, W4] Clarification is still needed on the transmural extent of infarction at which the threshold is reached. This does prevent precise sizing of transmural extent of infarction (although not necessarily circumferential extent of infarction). This phenomenon should not be viewed as a limitation of systolic thickening analyses but rather as another factor disrupting the linear relationship between extent of infarction and extent of dysfunction.

Finally, there are some problems with systolic thickening analysis algorithms. First, systolic thickening is often measured along radii generated from a center of mass. It is assumed that

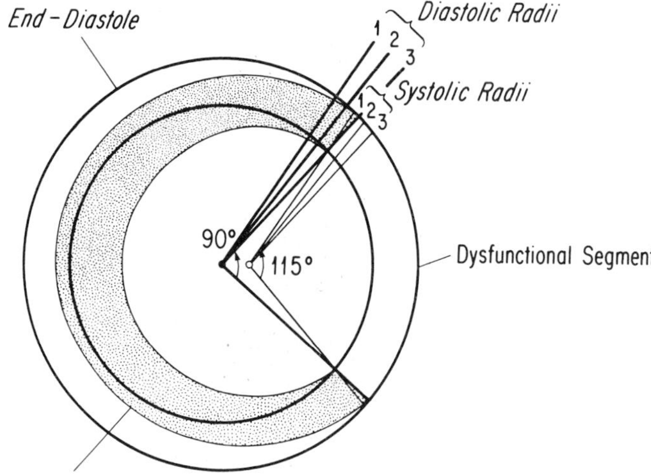

Figure 19–22. Schematic of short-axis echocardiographic systolic wall motion or thickening analysis. Radii are generated from the centers of mass for the diastolic and systolic contours. Equivalent radii are determined by their position on the radial coordinate plot (i.e., diastolic radius 1 is matched with systolic radius 1) rather than by any myocardial landmark. In the example, the dysfunctional segment subtends an angle of 90 degrees or 25 percent of the diastolic circumference versus 115 degrees or 32 percent of the systolic circumference. Since diastolic radii 1, 2, and 3 intersect abnormally contracting myocardium, the extent of dysfunction would be 32 percent rather than the 25 percent predicted from the diastolic image. Systolic expansion of the dysfunctional segment or hypercontractility of the normal segment would lead to further overestimation of dysfunctional region size compared to pathology. (From Force, T., Kemper, A.J., Perkins, L., et al.: Overestimation of infarct size by quantitative two-dimensional echocardiography—the role of tethering and of analytic procedures. Circulation 73:1360, 1986, with permission of the American Heart Association, Inc.)

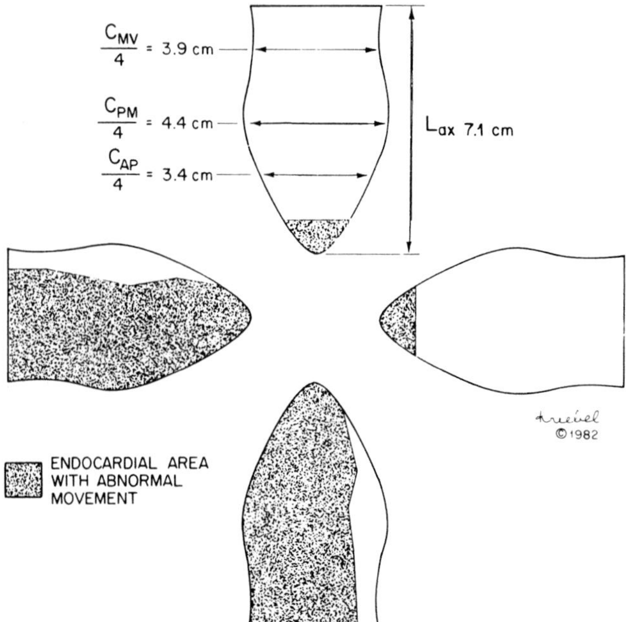

Figure 19–23. Planar map for an animal with a myocardial infarction from occlusion of a left circumflex coronary artery. C_{MV}, C_{PM}, C_{AP}—short-axis circumference at the mitral valve level, papillary muscle level, and apex, respectively. Endocardial area with abnormal wall motion was 43.2 cm^2 and total endocardial area was 101.9 cm^2. (From Guyer, D. E., Foale, R. A., Gillam, L. D., et al.: An echocardiographic technique for quantifying and displaying the extent of regional ventricular dyssynergy. J. Am. Coll. Cardiol. 8:830, 1986. Reprinted with permission from the American College of Cardiology.)

these radii will intersect the wall nearly perpendicular to tangents to endocardium and epicardium, which may not be the case when contraction is asymmetric (Fig. 19–24). Although this will introduce only small absolute errors in end-systolic thickness, it may be an important source of error when examining percent thickening. An adaptation of the centerline method of analysis (see Fig. 19–18)[G9, G16, L4, M12] might be superior, since even with asymmetric contraction, the minimum thickness of the wall in both diastole and systole will be measured and the problem of tangential intersection of radii will be avoided.

Of potentially greater importance is that, like short-axis wall motion analyses (see Fig. 19–22), all systems reported to date use an analysis based on the percent of circumference of the left ventricle that is dysfunctional in systole. Thus overestimation of extent of dysfunction (compared to pathologic extent of infarction) is inherent in these systems. Systolic expansion of the dysfunctional segment would lead to larger estimates of dysfunctional region size, since the abnormal segment would then occupy an even larger percent of the systolic left ventricular circumference. The importance of tethering has been exaggerated by these flaws in analysis systems,[A1, F5] since two-dimensional echocardiographic estimates of amount of myocardium "tethered" significantly exceed estimates from sonomicrometry.[G6, H6]

Summary

Two-dimensional echocardiographic wall motion or systolic thickening analyses compare favorably in terms of reproducibility and accuracy with the established technique of contrast ventriculography. Choice of type of analysis (motion versus thickening) and choice of analysis system (fixed versus floating) are to some extent arbitrary, but some general conclusions can be drawn. In order to identify the presence or absence of a contraction abnormality, either motion or thickening analysis is adequate. When quantitation of ischemic region or infarct size is required and two-dimensional echocardiograms are of sufficiently high quality, systolic thickening analysis is superior to motion analysis primarily because there is less overlap of adjacent normally perfused regions and infarct regions. Consequently, there is less overestimation of ischemic region size with thickening analyses. For wall motion in the parasternal short-axis view, where motion is measured relative to a centroid, fixed-axis analysis systems or possibly epicardial center-of-mass floating-axis systems are superior to endocardial center-of-mass floating systems. In the apical views, where motion is analyzed relative to the long axis of the ventricle, floating-axis analyses may be superior because they reduce variability in normal individuals. Certain clinical situations (such as the postoperative cardiac surgery state) dictate the use of a floating system. Area change methods are probably better than radial change methods in all views. Although there may be no unanimity of opinion about the optimum analysis algorithm, we think these viewpoints represent a consensus of the investigators working in this area. One point on which there is a clear consensus is that analysis algorithms free from the limitations of currently available ones must continue to be developed.

Quantitative analysis of two-dimensional echocardiograms is a reproducible and accurate noninvasive technique for identifying and quantifying abnormalities of systolic function. It has clearly been validated by comparisons to other accepted techniques. From this point on, the use of qualitative and semiquantitative analyses for research purposes should continue to decline, particularly for analyzing serial studies. When used properly, quantitative two-dimensional echocardiography has great potential for expanding our understanding of fundamental pathophysiologic processes in the experimental laboratory, intensive care unit, and operating room.

RIGHT VENTRICULAR FUNCTION

Until a few short years ago there was a paucity of information on right ventricular function in the literature. Several factors explain this lack of attention to the right heart as compared to the left.

First, the left ventricle has been considered the "main" chamber of the heart, since it is responsible for producing systemic

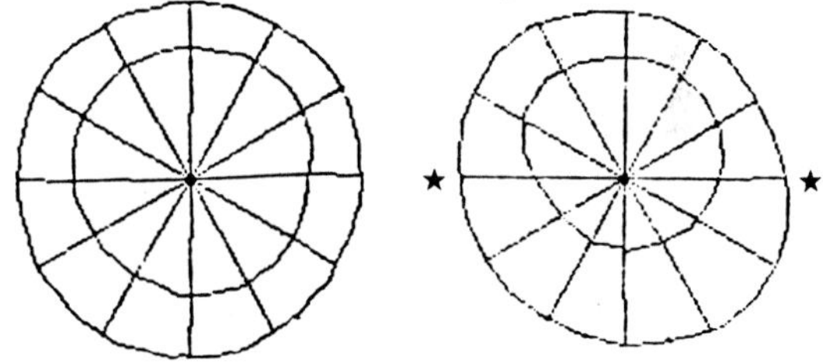

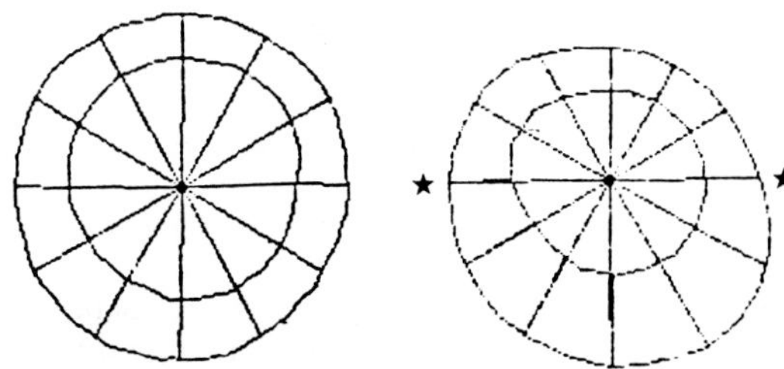

Figure 19–24. Analysis of systolic thickening along radii generated from the end-diastolic and end-systolic epicardial (top) and endocardial (bottom) centers of mass. In diastole (left), the radii intersect the walls approximately perpendicular to the tangents. In systole, with asymmetric contraction (right), this is not the case with the epicardial center of mass system (note starred radii). (From Guyer, D.E., Foale, R.A., Gillam, L.D., et al.: An echocardiographic technique for quantifying and displaying the extent of regional left ventricular dyssynergy. J. Am. Coll. Cardiol. 8:830, 1986. Reprinted with permission of the American College of Cardiology.)

cardiac output. The right ventricle, on the other hand, was regarded as a "passive conduit," not playing an important role in normal cardiac output. This notion was based on early canine experiments demonstrating lack of hemodynamic compromise despite severe damage to the right ventricular wall by cauterization.[K10, S14] More recent clinical studies of right ventricular function in various disease states, especially right ventricular infarction, have demonstrated that severe hemodynamic compromise can occur without significant left ventricular involvement. These data have laid the passive-conduit theory to rest.[C10]

Second, in comparison to the left ventricle, the right ventricle has a more complicated geometric shape that has defied full characterization by simple mathematical models. Consequently, quantitative evaluation of right ventricular function has been fraught with difficulty. As a result, despite the availability of several different geometric methods for evaluating left ventricular function, a historic standard or "gold standard" for quantifying right ventricular function has not emerged. The development and widespread availability of two-dimensional echocardiography has provided a new opportunity to image the right ventricular chamber noninvasively and hence a new opportunity for further study of its structure and function.

Echocardiographic Examination

The echocardiographic examination of the normal right ventricle has some limitations related to accessibility. A major portion of the normal right ventricle is obscured by the sternum, which interferes with the transmission of ultrasound. An enlarged or dilated right ventricle is easier to image. This enlargement typically occurs in conditions that cause right ventricular volume overload, such as tricuspid regurgitation, atrial septal defect, and Ebstein's anomaly.[M11] In addition, depending on the patient's position, there can be an important variation in the location of the right ventricle within the chest cavity in relationship to the chest wall.[F11] This can lead to a significant variation in the measured dimension along a single axis, depending on the angle of the ultrasonic beam to the chamber.

M-Mode Echocardiography

M-mode echocardiography has been commonly used to estimate the internal right ventricular dimension. However, owing to the difficulty in obtaining clear images of the right ventricular endocardium anteriorly, accurate measurement of the true anteroposterior dimension of the right ventricle is quite difficult. Since the initial study by Popp and associates,[P10] it has been commonly estimated that the anterior wall of the right ventricle begins approximately 5 mm from the chest wall. However, the American Society of Echocardiography recommends that the dimensions of the right ventricle should be reported only if the endocardium of the anterior right ventricular wall and the right side of the septum are clearly visualized.[S15] A second problem is that the right ventricular dimension is larger when the patient is in left lateral decubitus than in a supine position. To standardize the dimensions, it is recommended that only the supine measurements be reported.

In summary, although M-mode echocardiography is not highly accurate for the measurement of right ventricular dimension in all patients, it can usually separate patients with a clearly dilated from those with a normal right ventricle.

Two-Dimensional Echocardiography

Two-dimensional echocardiography, with its ability to image a single chamber in multiple planes, offers a considerable advantage over M-mode echocardiography in qualitative and quantitative assessment of right ventricular size, shape, and function.

Right Ventricular Dimensions

Qualitatively, with two-dimensional echocardiography the size of the right ventricle is usually assessed by visual comparison with the left ventricle. Normally, the transverse dimension of the right ventricle in the parasternal short-axis and apical four-chamber views is smaller than that of the left ventricle. Figure 19–25 shows the parasternal short-axis and apical four-chamber views of a normal heart. Note the crescent-like shape of the right ventricle in the short-axis view. Figure 19–26 shows the short-axis and four-chamber views of the heart in a patient with volume overload of the right ventricle. Note that the transverse right ventricular dimension appears equal to or larger than the left ventricular dimension. In addition, the left ventricle has lost its normal round shape in the parasternal short-axis view due to a change in the septal curvature at end-diastole.

Bommer and associates[B8] were the first to attempt to determine right ventricular size by two-dimensional echocardiography. Initially, right ventricular area and short- and long-axis dimensions obtained from human right ventricular casts were compared to the actual right ventricle cast volume. The maximum short-axis dimension and the area yielded better correlation, with coefficients of correlation of 0.93 and 0.95, respectively, compared to 0.70 and 0.82 for the mid-short-axis and long-axis dimensions. In

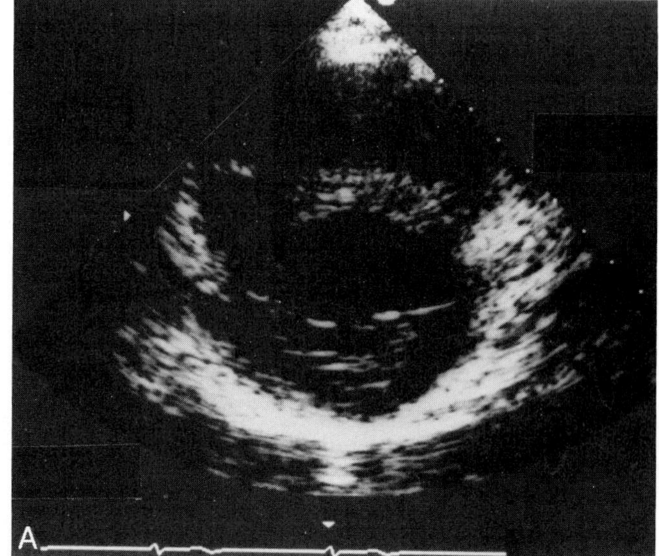

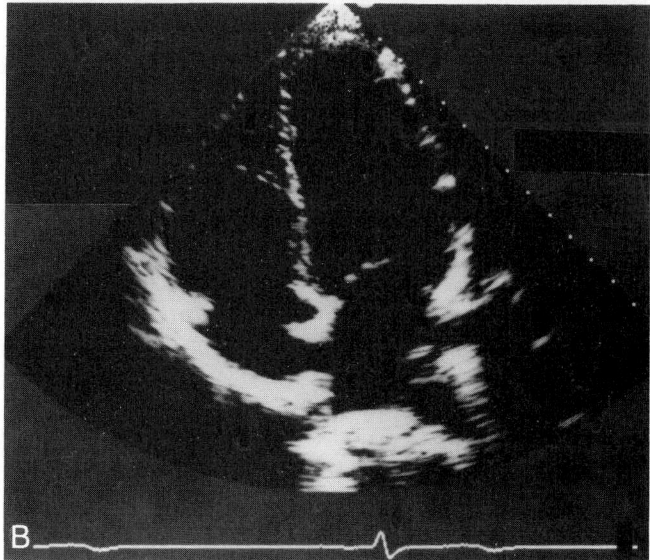

Figure 19–25. Normal heart. *A*, Parasternal short-axis view illustrating the cross-sectional crescentic shape of the right ventricle. *B*, Apical four-chamber view demonstrating the tapering configuration of the right ventricle.

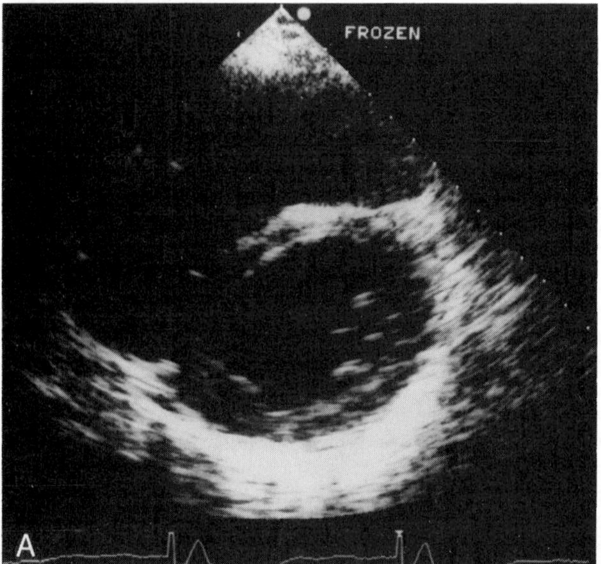

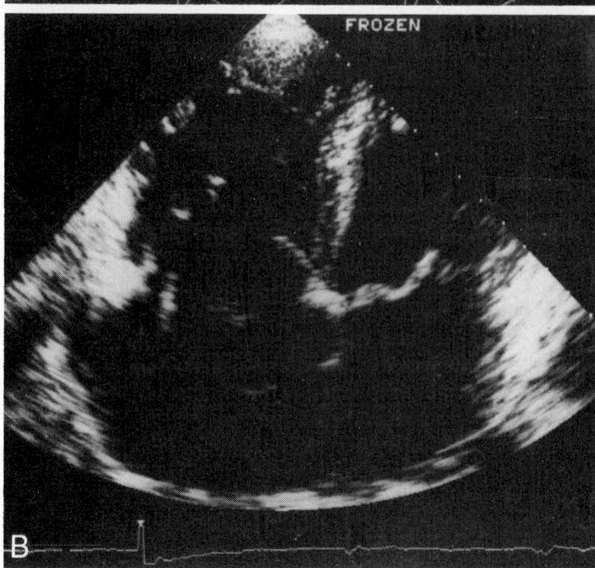

Figure 19–26. Volume-overloaded right ventricle. *A*, The parasternal short-axis view shows the increase in the width of the right ventricle as well as the change in septal curvature. *B*, Apical four-chamber view with enlarged right ventricle and right atrium.

the second part of the study, the echocardiographic dimensions and area of the right ventricle of 25 patients with right ventricle volume overload were compared to those of 25 patients with normal right ventricles. The echocardiographic measurements were obtained from the apical four-chamber view. In the patients evaluated, the right ventricle short-axis dimensions and the area better separated normal from overloaded right ventricle than did the long-axis or the standard M-mode study.

Global Right Ventricular Function: Volumes and Ejection Fraction

One approach to the complex geometric shape of the right ventricle is to consider it as comprising two chambers: a body extending from the tricuspid annulus to the apex and an outflow tract, which is situated anteriorly and medially. The body of the right ventricle in short-axis section is shaped like a crescent and its outflow tract is cylindrical. Because of this peculiar configuration, several different approaches have been used to quantify right ventricular function, including geometric models,[A2, K11, L6, N8, P11, S16–S18, T6, W8] tricuspid valve systolic excursion index,[K11] and even contrast echocardiography.[W9]

Saito and associates[S16] were the first to use geometrical assumptions to measure right ventricular volume by two-dimensional echocardiography. Two proposed methods used two subcostal views in a population of children with congenital heart disease (Fig. 19–27). In the first model, based on the assumption that the cross section of the right ventricle was circular or elliptic, the authors used a modified Simpson's rule method to get right ventricular volume, the volume of each slice being equal to (π/4)ABH. In the second model, the right ventricle was considered as an ellipsoid. To obtain this volume, the authors used a modified area-length method. The correlations between end-diastolic volumes obtained by echocardiography and by angiography were good (r = 0.86 for the area-length method; r = .085 for the Simpson's rule method); nevertheless, because of the difficulty in tracing the right ventricular cavity, they thought that further work should be done before application to individual clinical cases.

Ninomiya and associates[N8] used a Simpson's rule method to calculate right ventricular volume in 24 children after Mustard repair. They showed that the echocardiographic ejection fraction correlated well with the angiographic ejection fraction (r = 0.98) but that the volumes did not. The ratio of angiographic volume to echocardiographic volume varied from 1.08 to 3.33 for both end-diastole and end-systole, with systematic underestimation by echocardiography of more than 40 percent. The discrepancy in the volumes may be explained in part by the exclusion of the right ventricular outflow tract from the echocardiographic measurement. Watanabe and associates,[W8] applying the Simpson's rule method on two perpendicular apical views, found a coefficient of correlation of 0.94 for end-diastolic volumes and 0.84 for the end-systolic volumes when echocardiographic right ventricular volumes were compared to angiographic right ventricular body volumes. However, the echocardiographic volumes were still smaller, averaging 68 percent of the angiographic volumes in the group of patients with normal right ventricular volume and 61 percent in the groups with right ventricular volume and right ventricular pressure overload. They attributed these differences to the difficulty in tracing the right ventricular chamber and suggested that maximal right ventricular dimensions are not fully represented by the tomographic nature of the ultrasonic examination.

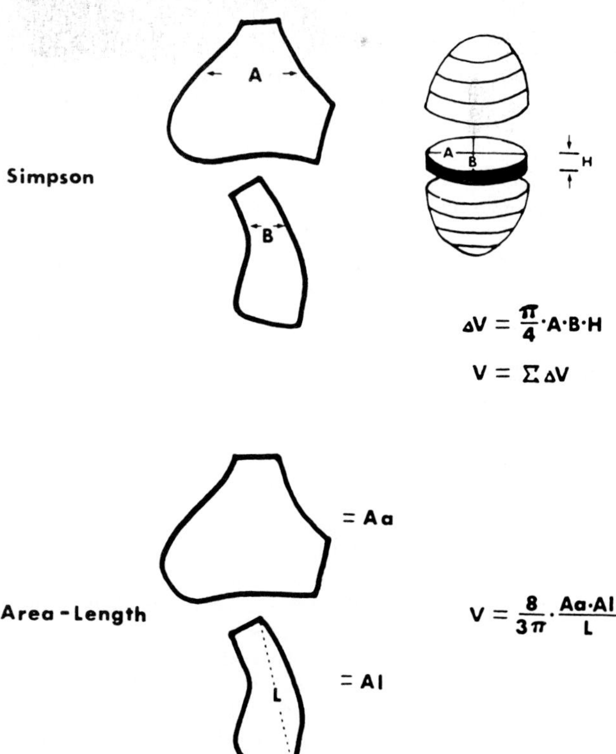

Figure 19–27. Diagram of mathematical models—Simpson's rule and area-length methods—for the calculation of right ventricular volume. (From Saito, A., Veda, K., and Nakano, H.: Right ventricular volume determination by two-dimensional echocardiography. J. Cardiogr. 11:1159, 1987, with permission.)

Starling and associates[S17] proposed a simple pyramidal model of the right ventricle in which the triangular base was obtained from an inflow view and the height from an outflow view, both obtained from the subcostal approach. As they compared the echocardiogaphic volumes with background-corrected end-diastolic and end-systolic counts from radionuclide angiography, no conclusion can be drawn about the ability of their model to estimate right ventricular volume. However, good correlations were reported between the echocardiographic end-diastolic and end-systolic volumes and ejection fraction and the corresponding radionuclide measures (Table 19–2). This approach was good enough to detect significant variations in right ventricular size after administration of isosorbide dinitrate in a selected population of patients with chronic obstructive pulmonary disease.

Another approach that takes into consideration the two separate components of the right ventricle was proposed by Silverman and Hudson.[S18] They found that the end-diastolic and end-systolic volumes obtained with a single-plane area-length method from the apical four-chamber view and the short-axis view underestimated the angiographic volumes. However, echocardiographically derived values for end-diastolic and end-systolic volumes and ejection fractions obtained from both single views correlated well with the angiographic values. Considering that the two views they chose passed through different portions of the right ventricle, namely the inlet portion for the apical view and the outlet portion for the short-axis view, they assumed that a summation of the two volumes would be more appropriate. Indeed, looking at their data, the echocardiographic end-diastolic volumes derived from the apical view and the short-axis view taken separately averaged 34.8 and 41 percent of the angiographic volumes. After addition of the volumes obtained from the two single planes, the echocardiographic volumes averaged 76.5 percent of the angiographic volumes. Although the concept of adding two complementary volumes to obtain a total right ventricular volume was novel and interesting, their results showed that once again the echocardiographic determination underestimated the volume obtained by angiography.

Hiraishi and associates[H14] compared echocardiographic right ventricular dimensions and areas for children with congenital heart disease with similar angiographic data (right ventricular body). They showed that the echocardiographic longest length and area obtained from the apical four-chamber view underestimated the same dimensions obtained from either the anteroposterior or lateral angiogram, with one exception. Therefore, they introduced corrected echocardiographic dimensions for the angiographic views in the area-length formula to obtain total right ventricular volume. The correlations between right ventricular volumes and ejection fractions obtained by echocardiography and angiography were good (see Table 19–2); unfortunately, right ventricular volumes were not reported. In their earlier angiographic study, the same authors introduced an important concept.[H14] They found that the ratio of the right ventricular body volume to the total right ventricular volume measured angiographically averaged 0.75 at end-diastole and end-systole in patients with normal ventricles, with right ventricular volume overload, with right ventricular pressure overload, with volume-overloaded right and left ventricles, and with only left ventricular volume overload. The only exception was the group of patients with tetralogy of Fallot, for whom this ratio was 0.81. These findings suggested that the increased right ventricular volume seen in diverse pathologic conditions is proportionately distributed between the right ventricular body and its outflow tract. Therefore, it does not appear critical to include the right ventricular outflow tract in the echocardiographic analysis in order to obtain accurate total right ventricular volume, since this volume can easily be derived from the right ventricular body volume.

Validation of the echocardiographic right ventricular volume determination has been complicated by lack of consensus on a reference standard or "gold standard." Most of the studies assessing right ventricular function have reported the ejection fraction. Ejection fraction can be more easily compared with angiographic studies as well as with radionuclide techniques including first-pass and gated equilibrium scintigraphy. The latter techniques have the inherent advantage of being independent of a fixed geometric assumption, since they depend solely on radionuclide counts in a defined area of interest. However, the use of radioisotopes and the high price of these tests make serial studies impractical.

Panidis and associates[P11] compared echocardiographic right ventricular ejection fractions calculated from biplane area lengths and Simpson's rule methods on paired orthogonal views in 39 patients with coronary artery disease and those derived from radionuclide studies. Ejection fractions obtained by two-dimensional echocardiography correlated well with those derived from radionuclide angiograms; echocardiography adequately separated patients with impaired right ventricular systolic function from those with normal right ventricular function. In this study, patients with acute or old inferior myocardial infarction had lower right ventricular ejection fractions than did patients with anterior myocardial infarction and patients with right coronary artery obstruction without right ventricular infarction. Trowitzsch and associates[T6] employed two subcostal views in a population of infants with a systemic right ventricle. Besides volumes derived by the Simpson's rule method, the authors reported the fractional area change in each of the two views as well as a mean total area change. The echocardiographic ejection fraction and the total area change correlated better with the angiographic ejection fraction (r = 0.83 and 0.78, respectively) than did volumes (r = 0.65 for end-diastolic volume and 0.56 for end-systolic volume).

Other interesting approaches have been proposed to overcome the difficulties inherent in right ventricular assessment by echocardiography. To avoid mathematical modeling based on geometric assumptions, Kaul and associates[K11] proposed a simple index, the tricuspid annular plane systolic excursion (TAPSE) measured from the apical four-chamber view to assess right ventricular function. The TAPSE index showed a better correlation with right ventricular radionuclide ejection fraction (r = 0.92) than did other simple measures taken from the same view, such as right ventricular end-diastolic area (r = −0.76) or percent systolic change in area (r = 0.81). Interestingly, in the patients studied, this single and simple index allowed semi-quantitative estimation of the right ventricular function.

To improve the outline of the right ventricular cavity, Wann and associates[W9] applied digital processing of contrast echocardiograms to right ventricular area and volume determination. They found a wide range of correlation coefficients (0.59 to 0.84), depending on geometric assumptions used to process four-chamber views, when compared to radionuclide ejection fraction (see Table 19–2).

Levine and associates,[L6] using measurements of postmortem casts of human right ventricles, found that the area-length formula that takes into account two-thirds of the right ventricular area in one view times the long axis obtained from the other view was the area-length formula that gave the best correlation when compared to the actual cast volumes. This formula was then applied to the echocardiographic apical four-chamber and subcostal right ventricular outflow tract images of hollow latex molds made from casts. The correlation between the actual cast volumes and the echocardiographic volumes involving the area derived from either view with the corresponding orthogonal length was similarly high (r = 0.95). The high correlation is probably related to the fact that this area-length formula described several tapering geometric volumes (Fig. 19–28). This approach describing tapered configuration of the right ventricle in one direction is new; however, as pointed out by the authors, the ideal model should have a crescentic shape with a double tapering configuration to describe the right ventricular body and its outflow tract.

Recently, Aebischer and Czegledy[A2] developed a model based on the crescentic shape of the cross section of the right ventricle tapering toward the apex (Fig. 19–29). The intersection of two circles whose curvature depicts, respectively, the right ventric-

Table 19–2. QUANTITATIVE ECHOCARDIOGRAPHIC STUDIES OF THE RIGHT VENTRICLE

Authors	Population*	Echo View†	Geometric‡	Reference Study	Coefficient of Correlation§
Saito 1981[S16]	31 children CHD	subcost front LAT	AL ellipsoid $V = \frac{8}{3\pi} \frac{A_1A_2}{L}$ Simpson $\Delta V = \frac{\pi}{3} A \cdot B \cdot H$	Angiogram	EDV $r = 0.86$ $y = 1.32x - 7.39$ EDV $r = 0.85$ $y = 0.91x + 7.35$
Ninomiya 1981[N8]	24 children CHD	PSA Ap_4	Simpson $\Delta V = \frac{\pi}{3} x \cdot y \cdot h$	Angiogram	EF $r = 0.98$ $y = 0.97x + 0.02$
Watanabe 1982[W8]	33 patients N RVVO RVPO	Ap_4 Ap_2RV	Simpson $\Delta V = \frac{\pi}{3} A \cdot B \cdot H$	Angiogram Body volume	EDV $r = 0.94$ $y = 0.56x + 10.1$ ESV $r = 0.84$ $y = 0.55x + 8.0$
Starling 1982[S17]	19 patients COPD	subcost inflow outflow	AL pyramid $V = A\frac{H}{3}$	Radionuclide ED, ES counts EF	EDV $r = 0.76$ $y = 1.54x + 21$ ESV $r = 0.82$ $y = 1.71x + 10$ EF $r = 0.83$ $y = 0.74x + 12$
Silverman 1983[S18]	20 children CHD	Ap_4	AL single volume $V = 0.849A/L$ Addition of $V(Ap_4)$ and $V(PSA)$	Angiogram	EDV $r = 0.81$ $y = 0.62x + 7.0$ ESV $r = 0.85$ $y = 0.82x + 1.4$ EF $r = 0.82$ $y = 0.66x + 17.8$
Hiraishi 1982[H14]	22 children CHD	Ap_4	AL formula echo length and area corrected pr angiographic values (two biplanes = I, II 1 uniflow = III)	Angiogram	I EDV $r = 0.92$ $y = 0.96x - 1.14$ ESV $r = 0.84$ $y = 0.94x - 0.27$ EF $r = 0.78$ $y = 1.03x - 0.01$ II $r = 0.91$ $y = 0.97x - 0.32$ $r = 0.83$ $y = 1.02x - 0.74$ $r = 0.74$ $y = 0.90 + 0.07$ III $r = 0.93$ $y = 0.93x + 1.46$ $r = 0.88$ $y = 0.94x + 0.33$ $r = 0.77$ $y = 0.87x + 0.33$
Panidis 1983[P11]	39 patients CHD	Ap_4 Ap_2RV subcost 4 Ap_4/Ap_2RV = I Ap_4/subcost II	A · L (I, II) $V = \frac{8A_1A_2}{3\pi L}$ Simpson (I, II) $V = \frac{\pi}{3} A \cdot B \cdot H$	Radionuclide	I EF $r = 0.76$ $y = 0.71x + 8.2$ EF $r = 0.78$ $y = 0.78x + 4.1$ II $r = 0.76$ $y = 0.69x + 11.4$ $r = 0.74$ $y = 0.66x + 6.2$
Trowitzsch 1984[T6]	19 children CHD	subcost LA SA	Simpson $V = \frac{L}{20} * \frac{\pi}{4} * \sum_{i=1} a_ib_i$	Angiogram	EDV $r = 0.65$ ESV $r = 0.56$ EF $r = 0.83$ $y = 0.94x + 4.43$
Kaul 1984[K11]	30 patients CAD, N	Ap_4	TAPSE	Radionuclide EF	TAPSE $r = 0.92$ $y = 0.31x + 0.30$ EDA $r = -0.76$ $y = -0.2x + 18.8$ % area change $r = 0.81$ $y = 0.98x + 4.8$
Wann 1984[W9]	13 patients CAD COPD ICM	Ap_4 PSA	% area change Ap_4 % area change SA Ellipsoid Ap $V = 4/3\pi\, a \cdot b \cdot c$ Pyramid Ap $V = A\frac{H}{3}$ Simpson $V = \frac{h(\text{base} \cdot \text{height})}{2}$	Radionuclide	$r = 0.79$ $y = 0.6x + 11.5$ $r = 0.59$ $y = 0.58x + 3$ $r = 0.84$ $y = 0.82x + 6.4$ $r = 0.79$ $y = 0.69x + 11$ $r = 0.62$ $y = 0.72x + 10$
Levine 1984[L6]	12 human casts	Ap_4 subcost	AL $V = ⅔\, A(Ap_4) \cdot L(\text{subcost})$ $V = ⅔\, A(\text{subcost}) \cdot L(Ap_4)$	Cast volume	$r = 0.95$ $y = 1.1x - 3.9$ $r = 0.95$ $y = 1.02x - 2.1$
Aebischer 1988[A2]	14 dog casts	PSA Ap_4	basal vol. = AL apical vol. = integration	Cast volume	$r = 0.96$ $y = 0.81x - 1.31$

*CHD—congenital heart disease; N—normal; RVVO—right ventricular volume overload; RVPO—right ventricular pressure overload; COPD—chronic obstructive pulmonary disease; ICM—idiopathic cardiomyopathy; CAD—coronary artery disease.

†subcost—subcostal; front—frontal; LAT—lateral; PSA—parasternal short axis; Ap_4—apical form-chamber view; Ap_2RV—apical two-chamber view, right ventricle; LA—long axis; SA—short axis.

‡AL—area-length method; TAPSE—tricuspid annular plane systolic excursion; Ap—approximation; V—volume.

§EDV—end-diastolic volume; ESV—end-systolic volume; EF—ejection fraction; EDA—end-diastolic area.

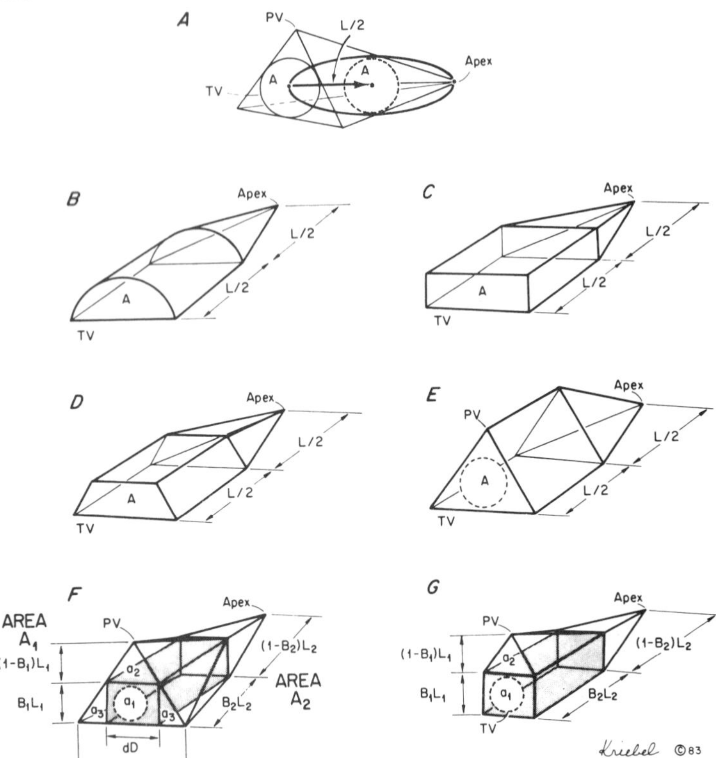

Figure 19–28. Geometric models with volumes of 2A · L/3. *A*, Prolate ellipsoid. *B*, Half cylindrical, half conical structure. *C–E*, Tapering structures with rectangular *(C)*, trapezoidal *(D)*, and triangular *(E)* bases. *F*, Flexible right ventricular model. *G*, Similar model without flanking structures that taper. (From Levine, R.A., Gibson, T.C., Aretz, T., et al.: Echocardiographic measurement of right ventricular volume. Circulation 69:497, 1983, with permission of the American Heart Association, Inc.)

ular free wall and the interventricular septum was used to describe the crescentic area. A conventional short-axis view at the mitral valve level and an apical four-chamber view were used to evaluate fixed canine hearts. The echocardiographic volumes were compared with cast volumes of the same hearts (Fig. 19–30). The coefficient of correlation was excellent ($r = 0.96$), with an echocardiographic volume/cast volume ratio averaging 0.76. The difference between the echocardiographic volumes and cast volumes was explained by the exclusion of the right ventricular outflow tract from the echocardiographic model. This new approach suggests that accurate volume determination is approachable when the complex geometry of the right ventricle is taken into consideration.

Since the original studies of Saito and associates, the echocardiographic approach to measurement of right ventricular volume has evolved toward more realistic spatial representation of the right ventricular cavity. The results of the last two studies,[A2, L6] in which the authors compared right ventricular volumes with actual cast volumes of the right ventricle for more accuracy, are promising in this sense.

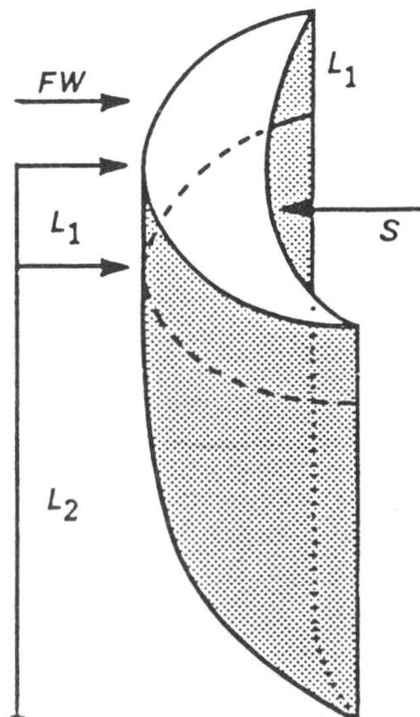

Figure 19–29. Schematic representation of the right ventricle using a crescentic mode. L_1—length of the basal portion; L_2—length of the apical portion; FW—right ventricular free wall; S—septum. The basal crescentic area is displayed in white. The dashed line separates a basal volume where the mid-width of the crescent is constant from the apical volume where the crescentic width decreases progressively toward the apex. (From Aebischer, N.M., and Czegledy, F.: Determination of right ventricular volume by two-dimensional echocardiography with a crescentic model. J. Am. Soc. Echo. 2:110, 1989, with permission.)

Regional Right Ventricular Function

In coronary artery disease with right ventricular myocardial infarction, two-dimensional echocardiography can be used to confirm right ventricular involvement. The three most common echocardiographic findings associated with right ventricular infarction are right ventricular dilation, regional wall motion abnormality, and paradoxic septal motion. Of these three conditions, regional wall motion abnormality is probably the most useful. Although right ventricular enlargement has been reported commonly in the setting of acute right ventricular infarction,[D5, J2, P12, S20] Arditti and associates[A3] did not find significant differences in the two-dimensional right ventricular end-diastolic dimension in patients with inferoposterior myocardial infarction and right ventricular dysfunction compared to patients with inferoposterior myocardial infarction without right ventricular dysfunction and patients with normal hearts. However, the two-dimensional echocardiographic right ventricular end-systolic dimensions and the percent fractional shortening in the long and short axes of the right ventricle taken from the apical four-chamber view were significantly different in the group of patients with right ventricular dysfunction compared to the other two groups. The percent fractional shortening of the long-axis, maximal, and mid-short-axis dimensions, were (mean ± standard deviation) 31.25 ± 9.60, 33.12 ± 7.80, and 30.68 ± 9.10 percent, respectively, in the normal group; 13.10 ± 8.20, 5.75 ± 13.80, and 5.80 ± 20.30 percent, respectively, in the group of patients with right ventricular dysfunction; and 20.42 ± 7.06, 35.30 ± 11.58, and 38.95 ± 16.70 percent, respectively, in patients with inferoposterior myocardial infarction but without right ventricular dysfunction.

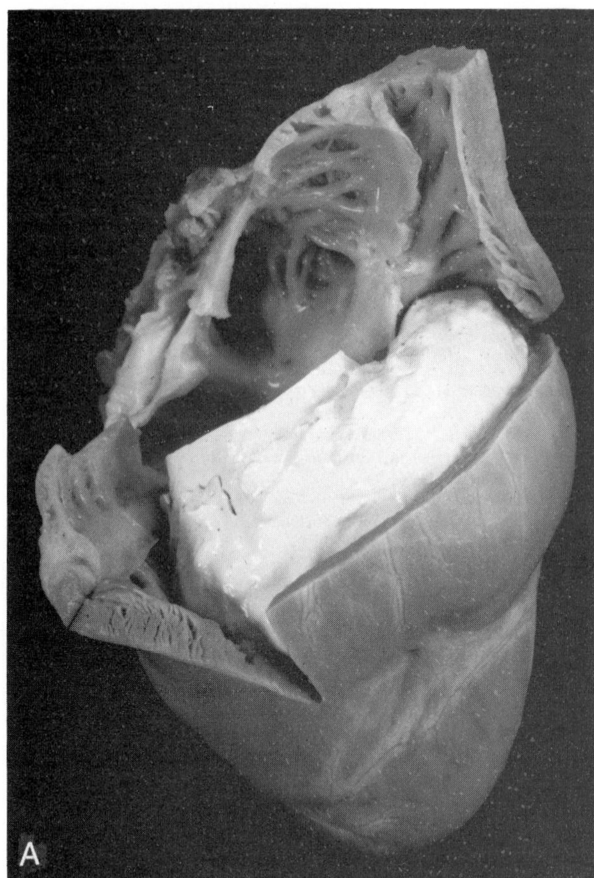

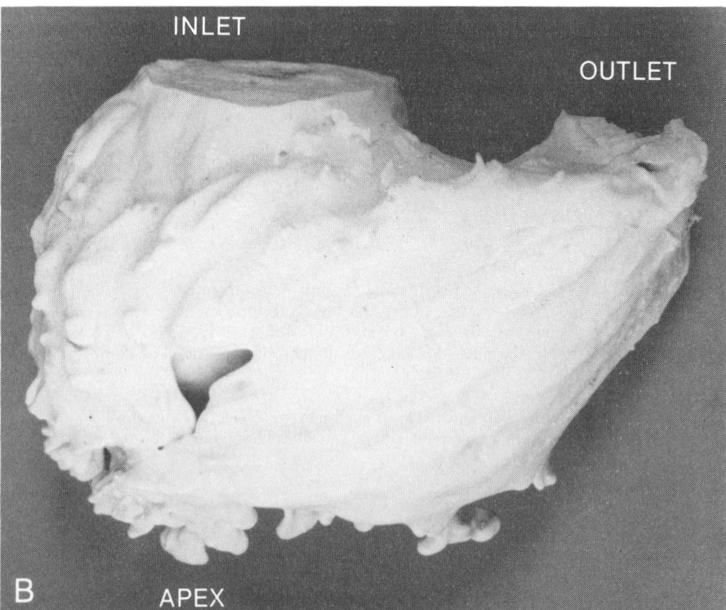

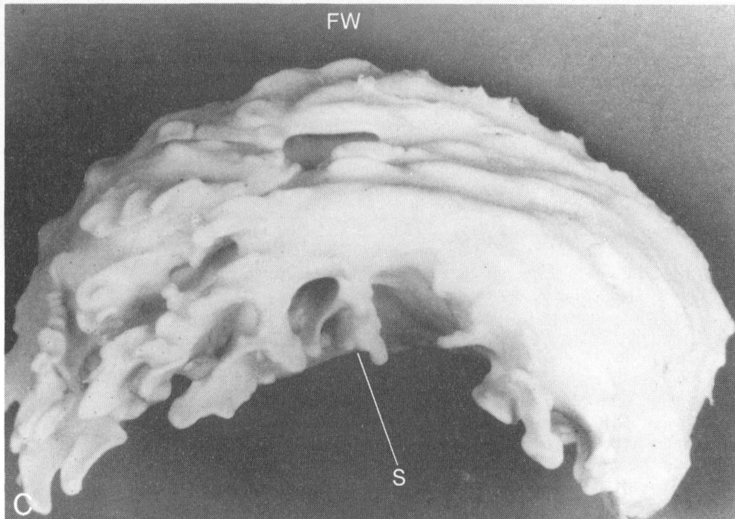

Figure 19–30. *A*, Right ventricle cast in the right ventricular cavity. *B*, The anterior view of the right ventricle cast illustrates the separate inflow and outflow regions of the right ventricle. *C*, The apical view shows the crescentic aspect of the right ventricle delineated anteriorly by the right ventricular free wall (FW) and posteriorly by the interventricular septum (S).

Only recently, right ventricular infarction per se has been reported as a cause of paradoxic septal motion. In a closed-chest canine experiment, Sharkey and associates[S21] showed that isolated infarction of the right ventricular free wall produced by right coronary artery embolization was associated with right ventricular dilatation, right ventricular free wall dyskinesis, and paradoxic septal motion with preserved systolic thickening. The paradoxic septal motion coincided with reversal of the transseptal end-diastolic pressure gradient due to an isolated increase in right ventricular end-diastolic pressure. To avoid paradoxic septal motion related to the opening of the pericardium, the authors chose a closed-chest canine model. Significant tricuspid regurgitation with right ventricular volume overload was ruled out as a cause of the paradoxic septal motion.

Regional wall motion abnormality has been commonly reported in the setting of right ventricular infarction[A3, B9, C11, D5, J2, L7, P12] and compared to clinical findings, electrocardiograms, hemodynamic data, or radionuclide studies. In a study of 50 patients with acute inferior myocardial infarction in which equilibrium gated blood pool study was used as a standard, Bellamy and associates[B9] found that 20 of 50 patients had regional wall motion abnormality by two-dimensional echocardiography compared to 22 by gated blood pool study. The sensitivity and specificity for the detection of right ventricular infarction were 82 and 93 percent for two-dimensional echocardiography compared to 50 and 71 percent for ST elevation in V_{4R}, 77 and 85 percent for elevation of venous pressure, and 59 and 89 percent for a positive Kussmaul's sign.

In the study by Arditti and associates,[A3] two-dimensional echocardiography and multigated acquisition radionuclide study revealed right ventricular dysfunction in 60 of 104 patients with acute inferoposterior myocardial infarction. Right ventricular dysfunction was diagnosed by two-dimensional echocardiography in the presence of regional wall motion abnormality and by multigated acquisition radionuclide study by a right ventricular ejection fraction lower than 2 standard deviations from the normal value. Eight patients presented with regional wall motion abnormality by two-dimensional echocardiography and normal ejection fraction by the radionuclide study, and five patients without regional wall motion abnormality showed a low right ventricular ejection fraction. Compared to the radionuclide study, two-dimensional echocardiography had a sensitivity of 92 percent and a specificity of 79 percent in the detection of right ventricular dysfunction. However, in this study a depressed ejection fraction but not regional wall motion abnormality was included in the diagnosis of right ventricular dysfunction by the radionuclide method. As the authors pointed out, the eight false-positive diagnoses of right ventricular dysfunction by two-dimensional echocardiography may, in fact, represent a higher sensitivity of this test.

In summary, two-dimensional echocardiography can provide valuable information about right ventricular global and regional function in a variety of clinical settings such as coronary artery disease, congenital heart disease, valvular heart disease with secondary pulmonary hypertension, and chronic obstructive lung disease. In the near future, new developments in echocardiography such as three-dimensional reconstruction may provide the needed "gold standard" for right ventricular volume determination.

References

A

1. Armstrong, W.F., Conley, M.J., Dillon, J.C., and Feigenbaum, H.: Systolic expansion of infarcted myocardium explains the overestimation of infarct size by wall motion analysis. (Abstract.) J. Am. Coll. Cardiol. 3:513, 1984.
2. Aebischer, N.M., and Czegledy, F.: Determination of right ventricular volume by two dimensional echocardiography with a crescentic model. J. Am. Soc. Echo. 2:110, 1989.
3. Arditti, A., Lewin R.F., Hellman, C., et al.: Right ventricular dysfunction in acute inferoposterior myocardial infarction. An echocardiographic and isotopic study. Chest 87:307, 1985.

B

1. Barrett, M.J., Jacobs, L., Gomberg, J., et al.: Simultaneous contrast imaging of the left ventricle by two-dimensional echocardiography and standard ventriculography. Clin. Cardiol. 5:208, 1982.
2. Borow, K.M., Neumann, A., and Wynne, J.: Sensitivity of end-systolic pressure-dimension and pressure-volume relations to the inotropic state in humans. Circulation 65:988, 1982.
3. Byrd, B.F., Wahr, D., Wang, Y.S., et al.: Left ventricular mass and volume/mass ratio determined by two-dimensional echocardiography in normal adults. J. Am. Coll. Cardiol. 6:1021, 1985.
4. Bhatnagar, S.K., Moussa, M.A.A., and Al-Yusut, A.: The role of prehospital discharge two-dimensional echocardiography in determining the prognosis of survivors of first myocardial infarction. Am. Heart J. 109:472, 1985.
5. Bogen, D.K., Rabinowitz, S.A., Needleman, A., et al: An analysis of the mechanical disadvantage of myocardial infarction in the canine left ventricle. Circ. Res. 47:728, 1980.
6. Blumenthal, D.S., Becker, L.C., Bulkley, B.H., et al.: Impaired function of salvaged myocardium: Two-dimensional echocardiographic quantification of regional wall thickening in the open-chest dog. Circulation 67:225, 1983.
7. Bolson, E.L., Kliman, S., Sheehan, F., et al.: Left ventricular segmental wall motion—a new method using local direction information. IEEE Comput. Cardiol. 1980, p 245.
8. Bommer, W., Weinert, L., Neumann, A., et al.: Determination of right atrial and right ventricular size by two-dimensional echocardiography. Circulation 60:91, 1979.
9. Bellamy, G.R., Rasmussen, H.H., Nasser, F.N., et al.: Value of two-dimensional echocardiography, electrocardiography, and clinical signs in detecting right ventricular infarction. Am. Heart J. 112:304, 1986.
10. Buckey, J.C., Beattie, J.M., Nixon, J.V., et al.: Right and left ventricular volumes in vitro by a new nongeometric method. Am. J. Cardiac Imag. 1:277, 1987.

C

1. Cohn, P.F., Gorlin, R., Cohn, L.H., and Collins, J.J.: Left ventricular ejection fraction as a prognostic guide in surgical treatment of coronary and valvular heart disease. Am. J. Cardiol. 34:136, 1974.
2. Chapman, C.B., Baker, O., Reynolds, J., and Bonte, F.J.: Use of biplane cinefluorography for measurement of ventricular volume. Circulation 18:1105, 1958.
3. Carr, K.W., Engler, R.L., Forsythe, J.R., et al.: Measurement of left ventricular ejection fraction by mechanical cross-sectional echocardiography. Circulation 59:1196, 1979.
4. Chaudry, K.R., Ogawa, S., Pauletto, F.J., et al.: Biplane measurements of left ventricular volumes using wide-angle, cross-sectional echocardiography. (Abstract.) Am. J. Cardiol. 41:391, 1978.
5. Chaitman, B.R., DeMots, H., Brislow, J.D., et al.: Objective and subjective analysis of left ventricular angiograms. Circulation 52:420, 1975.
6. Cox, D., and Vatner, S.F.: Disparity between regional myocardial function and blood flow at the ischemic border. Circ. Suppl. II 66:II-1, 1982.
7. Cox, D.A., and Vatner, S.F.: Myocardial function in areas of heterogeneous perfusion after coronary artery occulsion in conscious dogs. Circulation 66:1154, 1982.
8. Chaitman, B.R., Bristow, J.D., and Rahimtoola, S.H.: Left ventricular wall motion assessed by using fixed external reference systems. Circulation 48:1043, 1973.
9. Clayton, P.D., Jeppson, G.M., and Klausner, S.C.: Should a fixed external reference system be used to analyze left ventricular wall motion? Circulation 65:1518, 1982.
10. Cohn, J.N., Guiha, N.H., Broder, M.I., and Limas, C.J.: Right ventricular infarction. Clinical and hemodynamic features. Am. J. Cardiol. 33:209, 1974.
11. Cecchi, F., Zuppiroli, A., Favilli, S., et al.: Echocardiographic features of right ventricular infarction. Clin. Cardiol. 7:405, 1984.

D

1. Dodge, H.T., Sandler, H., Ballew, D.W., and Lord, J.D., Jr.: Use of biplane angiocardiography for the measurement of left ventricular volume in man. Am. Heart J. 60:762, 1960.
2. Devereux, R.B., Lutas, E.M., Casale, P.N., et al.: Standardization of M-mode echocardiographic left ventricular anatomic measurements. J. Coll. Cardiol. 4:1222, 1984.
3. Devereux, R.B., and Reichek, N.: Echocardiographic determination of left ventricular mass in man. Anatomic validation of the method. Circulation 55:613, 1977.
4. Devereux, R.B.: Detection of left ventricular hypertrophy by M-mode echocardiography. Anatomic validation, standardization, and comparison to other methods. Hypertension 9:II, 1987.
5. D'Arcy, B., and Nanda, N.C.: Two-dimensional echocardiographic features of right ventricular infarction. Circulation 65:167, 1982.

E

1. Erbel, R., Schweizer, P., Meyer, J., et al.: Left ventricular volume and ejection fraction determination by cross-sectional echocardiography in patients with coronary artery disease: A prospective study. Clin. Cardiol. 3:377, 1980.
2. Edwards, W.D., Tajik, A.J., and Seward, J.B.: Standardized nomenclature and anatomic basis for regional tomographic analysis of the heart. Mayo Clin. Proc. 56:479, 1981.
3. Ellis, S.G., Henschke, C.I., Sandor, T., et al.: Time course of functional and biochemical recovery of myocardium salvaged by reperfusion. J. Am. Coll. Cardiol. 1:1047, 1983.
4. Erbel, R., Krebs, W., Henn, G., et al.: Comparison of single-plane and biplane volume determination by two-dimensional echocardiography. I. Asymmetric model hearts. Eur. Heart J. 3:469, 1982.
5. Erbel, R., Schweizer, P., Lambertz, H., et al.: Echoventriculography—a simultaneous analysis of two-dimensional echocardiography and cinveventriculography. Circulation 67:205, 1983.
6. Ellis, S.G., Henschke, C.I., Sandor, T., et al.: Relation between the transmural extent of acute myocardial infarction and associated myocardial contractility two weeks after infarction. Am. J. Cardiol. 55:1412, 1985.
7. Eaton, L.W., Weiss, J.L., Bulkley, B.H., et al.: Regional cardiac dilation after acute myocardial infarction. Recognition by two-dimensional echocardiography. N. Engl. J. Med. 300:57, 1979.

F

1. Fortuin, N.J., Hood, W.P., Jr., Sherman, M.E., and Craige, E.: Determination of left ventricular volumes by ultrasound. Circulation 44:575, 1971.
2. Folland, E.D., Parisi, A.F., Moynihan, P.F., et al.: Assessment of left ventricular ejection fraction and volumes by real-time, two dimensional echocardiography. A comparison of cineangiographic and radionuclide techniques. Circulation 60:760, 1979.
3. Fazzalari, N.L., Davidson, J.A., Mazumdar, J., et al.: Three dimensional reconstruction of the left ventricle from four anatomically defined apical two-dimensional echocardiographic views. Acta Cardiol. 34:409, 1984.
4. Falsetti, H.L., Marcus, M.L., Kerber, R.E., and Skorton, D.J.: Quantification of myocardial ischemia and infarction by left ventricular imaging. (Editorial.) Circulation 63:747, 1981.
5. Force, T., Kemper, A.J., Perkins, L., et al.: Overestimation of infarct size by quantitative two-dimensional echocardiography—the role of tethering and of analytic procedures. Circulation 73:1360, 1986.
6. Fujii, J., Sawada, H., Aizawa, T., et al.: Computer analysis of cross sectional echocardiogram for quantitative evaluation of left ventricular asynergy in myocardial infarction. Br. Heart J. 51:139, 1984.
7. Force, T., Bloomfield, P., O'Boyle, J.E., et al.: Quantitative two-dimensional echocardiographic analysis of motion and thickening of the interventricular septum after cardiac surgery. Circulation 68:1013, 1983.
8. Force, T., Bloomfield, P., O'Boyle, J.E., et al.: Quantitative two-dimensional echocardiographic analysis of regional wall motion in patients with perioperative myocardial infarction. Circulation 70:233, 1984.
9. Force, T., Kemper, A.J., Bloomfield, P., et al.: Non-Q wave perioperative myocardial infarction: Assessment of the incidence and severity of regional dysfunction with quantitative two-dimensional echocardiography. Circulation 72:781, 1985.
10. Fedele, F., Penco, M., and Dagianti, A.: Quantification of left ventricular regional wall thickening in two-dimensional echocardiography: Analysis of a new semiautomated method. J. Cardiovasc. Ultrasongr. 4:201, 1985.
11. Feigenbaum, H.: Echocardiography. Lea & Febiger, Philadelphia, 1986.
12. Force, T., Kemper, A., Leavitt, M., and Parisi, A.F.: Acute reduction in functional infarct expansion with late reperfusion. Assessment with quantitative two-dimensional echocardiography. J. Am. Coll. Cardiol. 11:192, 1988.
13. Feiring, A.J., Rumberger, J.A., Reiter, S.J., et al.: Sectional and segmental variability of left ventricular function—experimental and clinical studies using ultrafast computed tomography. J. Am. Coll. Cardiol. 12:2, 415, 1988.

G

1. Gueret, P., Meerbaum, S., Wyatt, H.L., et al.: Two-dimensional echocardiographic quantitation of left ventricular volumes and ejection fraction. Importance of accounting for dyssynergy in short axis reconstruction mode. Circulation 62:1308, 1980.
2. Gehrke, J., Leeman, S., Raphael, M., and Pridie, R.B.: Non-invasive left ventricular volume determination by two-dimensional echocardiography. Br. Heart J. 37:911, 1975.
3. Grossman, W., Braunwald, E., Mann, T., et al.: Contractile state of the left ventricle in man as evaluated from end-systolic pressure-volume relations. Circulation 56:845, 1977.
4. Gibson, R.S., Bishop, H.L., Stamm, R.B., et al.: Value of early two-dimensional echocardiography in patients with acute myocardial infarction. Am. J. Cardiol. 49:1110, 1982.

5. Gillam, L.D., Hogan, R.D., Foale, R.A., et al.: A comparison of quantitative echocardiographic methods for delineating infarct-induced abnormal wall motion. Circulation 70:113, 1984.
6. Gallagher, K.P., Gerren, R.A., Stirling, M.C., et al.: The distribution of functional impairment across the lateral border of acutely ischemic myocardium. Circ. Res. 58:570, 1986.
7. Gallagher, K.P., Kumada, T., Koziol, J.A., et al.: Significance of regional wall thickening abnormalities relative to transmural myocardial perfusion in anesthetized dogs. Circulation 62:1266, 1980.
8. Gallagher, K.P., Stirling, M.C., and Choy, M.: Dissociation between epicardial and transmural function during acute myocardial ischemia. Circulation 71:1279, 1985.
9. Gallagher, K.P., Osakada, G., Hess, O.M., et al.: Subepicardial segmental function during coronary stenosis and the role of myocardial fiber orientation. Circ. Res. 50:352, 1982.
10. Gelberg, H.J., Brundage, B.H., Glantz, S., and Parmley, W.W.: Quantitative left ventricular wall motion analysis: A comparison of area, chord and radial methods. Circulation 59:991, 1979.
11. Grube, E., Hanisch, H., Neumann, G., and Simon, H.: Quantitative evaluation of LV-wall motion by two-dimensional echocardiography (2-DE). (Abstract.) J. Am. Coll. Cardiol. 1:581, 1983.
12. Gibson, D.G., Doran, J.H., Traill, T.A., and Brown, D.J.: Abnormal left ventricular wall movement during early systole in patients with angina pectoris. Br. Heart J. 40:758, 1978.
13. Geiser, E.A., Skorton, D.J., and Conetta, D.A.: Quantification of left ventricular function by two-dimensional echocardiography: Consideration of factors restricting image quality. Am. Heart J. 103:905, 1982.
14. Guyer, D.E., Gibson, T.C., Gillam, L.D., et al.: A new echocardiographic model for quantifying three-dimensional endocardial surface area. J. Am. Coll. Cardiol. 8:819, 1986.
15. Guyer, D.E., Foale, R.A., Gillam, L.D., et al.: An echocardiographic technique for quantifying and displaying the extent of regional left ventricular dyssynergy. J. Am. Coll. Cardiol. 8:830, 1986.
16. Garrison, J.B., Weiss, J.L., Maughan, W.L., et al.: Quantitative regional wall motion and thickening in two-dimensional echocardiography with a computer-aided contouring system. *In* Ostrow, H., and Ripley, K. (eds): Proceedings of Computers in Cardiology. IEEE, Long Beach, Calif. 1977.
17. Gallagher, K.P., Gerren, R.A., Ning, X-H., et al.: The functional border zone in conscious dogs. Lab. Invest. 76:4, 1987.
18. Gallagher, K.P., McClanahan, T.B., Lynch, M.J., et al.: Occlusion of the left anterior descending artery produces a larger functional border zone than circumflex occlusion. (Abstract). Circ. Suppl. IV 76:IV-373, 1987.
19. Geiser, E.A., Ariet, M., Conetta, D.A., et al.: Dynamic three-dimensional reconstruction of the human left ventricle in vivo: Technique and initial observation in patients. Am. Heart J. 103:1056, 1982.

H

1. Hammermeister, K.E., and Kennedy, J.W.: Predictors of surgical mortality in patients undergoing direct myocardial revascularization. Circ. Suppl. II 49,50:112, 1974.
2. Helak, J.W., and Reichek, N.: Quantitation of human left ventricle mass and volume by two-dimensional echocardiography: In vitro anatomic validation. Circulation 63:1398, 1981.
3. Heger, J.J., Weyman, A.E., Wann, L.S., et al.: Cross-sectional echocardiography in acute myocardial infarction: Detection and localization of regional ventricular asynergy. Circulation 60:531, 1979.
4. Horowitz, R.S., Morganroth, J., Parrotto, G., et al.: Immediate diagnosis of acute myocardial infarction by two-dimensional echocardiography. Circulation 65:323, 1982.
5. Herman, M.V., and Gorlin, R.: Implications of left ventricular asynergy. Am. J. Cardiol. 23:538, 1969.
6. Homans, D.C., Asinger, R., Elsperger, J., et al.: Regional function and perfusion at the lateral border of ischemic myocardium. Circulation 71:1038, 1985.
7. Heyndrickx, G.R., Millard, R.W., McRitchie, R.J., et al.: Regional myocardial function and electrophysiologic alterations after brief coronary artery occlusion in conscious dogs. J. Clin. Invest. 56:978, 1975.
8. Hammerman, H., O'Boyle, J.E., Cohen, C., et al.: Dissociation between two-dimensional echocardiographic left ventricle wall motion and myocardial salvage in early experimental acute myocardial infarction in dogs. Am. J. Cardiol. 54:875, 1964.
9. Haendchen, R.V., Wyatt, H.L., Maurer, G., et al.: Quantitation of regional cardiac function by two-dimensional echocardiography. I. Patterns of contraction in the normal left ventricle. Circulation 67:1234, 1983.
10. Henschke, C.I., Risser, T.A., Sandor, T., et al.: Quantitative computer assisted analysis of left ventricular wall thickening and motion by 2-dimensional echocardiography in acute myocardial infarction. Am. J. Cardiol. 52:960, 1983.
11. Herman, M.V., Heinle, R.A., Klein, M.D., and Gorlin, R.: Localized disorders in myocardial contraction, asynergy and its role in congestive heart failure. N. Engl. J. Med. 277:222, 1967.
12. Heng, M.K., Lang, T.W., Takashi, T., et al.: Quantification of myocardial ischemic damage by two-dimensional echocardiography. (Abstract.) Circ. Suppl. III 56:III-125, 1977.
13. Heikkila, J., Tabakin, B.S., and Hugenholtz, P.G.: Quantification of function in normal and infarcted regions of the left ventricle. Cardiovas. Res. 6:516, 1972.
14. Hiraishi, S., DiSessa, T.G., Jarmakani, J.M., et al.: Two-dimensional echocardiographic assessment of right ventricular volume in children with congenital heart disease. Am. J. Cardiol. 50:1368, 1982.

I

1. Ingels, N.B., Jr., Daughters, G.T., II, Stinson, E.B., and Alderman, E.L.: Evaluation of methods for quantitating left ventricular wall motion in man using myocardial markers as a standard. Circulation 61:966, 1980.
2. Ingels, N.B., Daughters, G.T., II, Stinson, E.B., and Alderman, E.L.: Measurement of mid-wall myocardial dynamics in intact man by radiography of surgically implanted markers. Circulation 52:859, 1975.
3. Isaacsohn, J.L., Earle, M.G., Kemper, A.J., and Parisi, A.F.: Postmyocardial infarction pain and infarct extension in the coronary care unit: Role of two-dimensional echocardiography. J. Am. Coll. Cardiol. 11:246, 1988.

J

1. Johnson, L.L., Ellis, K., Schmidt, O., et al.: Volume ejected in early systole, a sensitive index of left ventricular performance in coronary artery disease. Circulation 52:378, 1975.
2. Jugdutt, B.I., Sussex, B.A., Sivaram, C.A., and Rossall, R.E.: Right ventricular infarction: Two-dimensional echocardiographic evaluation. Am. Heart J. 107:505, 1984.

K

1. Kreulen, T.M., Bove, A.A., McDonough, M.T., et al.: The evaluation of left ventricular function in man. A comparison of methods. Circulation 51:677, 1975.
2. Kan, G., Visser, C.A., Lie, K.I., and Durrer, D.: Left ventricular volumes and ejection fraction by single plane two-dimensional apex echocardiography. Eur. Heart J. 2:337, 1981.
3. Kisslo, J.A., Robertson, D., Gilbert, B.W., et al.: A comparison of real-time, two-dimensional echocardiography and cineangiography in detecting left ventricular asynergy. Circulation 55:134, 1977.
4. Kerber, R.E., Marcus, M.L., Ehrhardt, J., et al.: Correlation between echocardiographically demonstrated segmental dyskinesis and regional myocardial perfusion. Circulation 52:1097, 1975.
5. Kloner, R.A., DeBoer, L.W.V., Darsee, J.R., et al.: Recovery of cardiac function and adenosine triphosphate requiring 7 days of reperfusion following 15 minutes of ischemia. Clin. Res. 29:562A, 1981.
6. Kaul, S., Pandian, N.G., Gillam, L.D., et al.: Contrast echocardiography in acute myocardial ischemia. III. An in vivo comparison of the extent of abnormal wall motion with the area at risk for necrosis. J. Am. Coll. Cardiol. 7:383, 1986.
7. Kong, Y., Morris, J.J., Jr., and McIntosh, H.D.: Assessment of regional myocardial performance from biplane cineangiograms. Am. J. Cardiol. 27:529, 1971.
8. Klausner, S.C., Blair, T.J., Bulawa, W.F., et al.: Quantitative analysis of segmental wall motion throughout systole and diastole in the normal human left ventricle. Circulation 65:580, 1982.
9. Karsch, K.R., Lamm, U., Blanke, H., and Rentrop, K.D.: Comparison of nineteen quantitative models for assessment of localized left ventricular wall motion abnormalities. Clin. Cardiol. 3:123, 1980.
10. Kagan, A.: Dynamic responses of the right ventricle following extensive damage by cauterization. Circulation 5:816, 1952.
11. Kaul, S., Tei., C., Hopkins, J.M., and Shah, P.M.: Assessment of right ventricular function using two-dimensional echocardiography. Am. Heart J. 107:526, 1984.
12. Kaul, S., Glasheen, W., Ruddy, T.D., et al.: The importance of defining left ventricular area at risk in vivo during acute myocardial infarction: an experimental evaluation with myocardial contrast two-dimensional echocardiography. Circulation 75:1249, 1987.

L

1. Loperfido, F., Mongiardo, R., Pennestri, F., et al.: Variability of normal regional wall motion and recognition of dyssynergy by angiography and two-dimensional echocardiography in myocardial infarction. J. Cardiovasc. Ultrasongr. 4:175, 1985.
2. LeWinter, M.M., Kent, R.S., Kroener, J.M., et al.: Regional differences in myocardial performance in the left ventricle of the dog. Circ. Res. 37:191, 1975.
3. Leighton, R.F., Pollack, M.E.M., and Welch, T.G.: Abnormal left ventricle wall motion at mid-ejection in patients with coronary heart disease. Circulation 52:238, 1975.
4. Lieberman, A.N., Weiss, J.L., Jugdutt, B.J., et al.: Two-dimensional echocardiography and infarct size: Relationship of regional wall motion and thickening to the extent of myocardial infarction in the dog. Circulation 63:739, 1981.
5. Lima, J.A.C., Becker, L.C., Melin, J.A., et al.: Impaired thickening of nonischemic myocardium during acute regional ischemia in the dog. Circulation 71:1048, 1985.
6. Levine, R.A., Gibson, T.C., Aretz, T., et al.: Echocardiographic measurement of right ventricular volume. Circulation 69:497, 1983.
7. Lopez-Sendon, J., Garcia-Fernandez, M.A., Coma-Canella, I., et al.: Segmental right ventricle function after acute myocardial infarction: Two-dimensional echocardiographic study in 63 patients. Am. J. Cardiol. 51:390, 1983.

M

1. Murray, J.A., Chinn, N., and Peterson, D.R.: Influence of left ventricular function on early prognosis in atherosclerotic heart disease. (Abstract.) Am. J. Cardiol. 33:159, 1974.
2. Moynihan, P.F., Parisi, A.F., Folland, E.D., et al.: A system for quantitative

evaluation of left ventricular function with two-dimensional ultrasonography. Med. Instrum. 14:111, 1980.
3. Mercier, J.C., DiSessa, T.G., Jarmarani, J.M., et al.: Two-dimensional echocardiographic assessment of left ventricular volume and ejection fraction in children. Circulation 65:962, 1982.
4. Myers, J.H., Stirling, M.C., Choy, M., et al.: Direct measurement of inner and outer wall thickening dynamics with epicardial echocardiography. Circulation 74:164, 1986.
5. Moynihan, P.F., Parisi, A.F., and Feldman, C.L.: Quantitative detection of regional left ventricular contraction abnormalities by two-dimensional echocardiography. I. Analysis of methods. Circulation 63:752, 1981.
6. Mann, D.L., Foale, R.A., Ascah, K.J., et al.: Persistence of abnormal wall motion in the canine ventricle after subacute infarction: Implications for reperfusion therapy. (Abstract.) J. Am. Coll. Cardiol. 5:425, 1985.
7. Marier, D.L., and Gibson, D.G.: Limitations of two frame method for displaying regional left ventricular wall motion in man. Br. Heart J. 44:555, 1980.
8. Mirro, M.J., Rogers, E.W., Weyman, A.E., and Feigenbaum, H: Angular displacement of the papillary muscles during the cardiac cycle. Circulation 60:327, 1979.
9. Meltzer, R.S., Woythaler, J.N., Buda, A.J., et al.: Non-invasive quantification of experimental canine myocardial infarct size using two-dimensional echocardiography. Eur. J. Cardiol. 11:215, 1980.
10. Meister, S.G., Casey, P.R., Jacobs, L., and Barrett, M.J.: 2D echo definition of endocardium. Circ. Suppl III 62:III-132, 1980.
11. Matsumoto, M., and Matsuo, H.: Echocardiography for the evaluation of the tricuspid valve, right ventricle, and atrium. Prog. Cardiovasc. Dis. 21:1, 1978.
12. McGillem, M.J., Mancini, G.B.J., DeBoe, S.F., and Buda, A.J.: Modification of the centerline method for assessment of echocardiographic wall thickening and motion: A comparison with areas of risk. J. Am. Coll. Cardiol. II:4, 861, 1988.
13. Mancini, G.B.J., DeBoe, S.F., Lefree, M.T., et al.: Quantitative regional curvature: A comparison of shape vs wall motion analysis. (Abstract.) Circ. Suppl. II:II-498, 1986.
14. Matsumoto, M., Inoue, M., Tamura, S., et al.: Three-dimensional echocardiography for spatial visualization and volume calculation of cardiac structures. J. Clin. Ultrasound 9:157, 1981.

N

1. Nelson, G.R., Cohn, P.F., and Gorlin, R.: Prognosis in medically treated coronary artery disease. Influence of ejection fraction compared to other parameters. Circulation 52:408, 1975.
2. Nixon, J.V., and Saffer, S.I.: Three-dimensional echoventriculography. (Abstract.) Circulation 57, 58:II-57, 1978.
3. Nanda, N.C., and Maurer, G.: Three-dimensional reconstruction of echocardiographic images using the rotation method. Ultrasound Med. Biol. 8:655, 1982.
4. Nixon, J.V., Brown, C.N., and Smitherman, T.C.: Identification of transient and persistent segmental wall motion abnormalities in patients with unstable angina by two-dimensional echocardiography. Circulation 65:1497, 1982.
5. Nixon, J.V., Narahara, K.A., and Smitherman, T.C.: Estimation of myocardial involvement in patients with acute myocardial infarction by two-dimensional echocardiography. Circulation 62:1248, 1980.
6. Nishimura, R.A., Reeder, G.S., Miller, F.A., Jr., et al.: Prognostic value of predischarge 2-dimensional echocardiogram after acute myocardial infarction. Am. J. Cardiol. 53:429, 1984.
7. Nieminen, M., Parisi, A.F., O'Boyle, J.E., et al.: Serial evaluation of myocardial thickening and thinning in acute experimental infarction: Identification and quantification using two-dimensional echocardiography. Circulation 66:174, 1982.
8. Ninomiya, K., Duncan, W.J., Cook, D.H., et al.: Right ventricular ejection fraction and volumes after Mustard repair: Correlation of two dimensional echocardiograms and cineangiograms. Am. J. Cardiol. 48:317, 1981.

O

1. Ohuchi, Y., Kuwako, K., Umeda, T., et al.: Real-time, phased-array, cross-sectional echocardiographic evaluation of left ventricular asynergy and quantitation of left ventricular function. A comparison with left ventricular cineangiography. Jpn. Heart J. 21:1, 1980.
2. O'Boyle, J.E., Parisi, A.F., Nieminen, M., et al.: Quantitative detection of regional left ventricular contraction abnormalities by two-dimensional echocardiography. Comparison of myocardial thickening and thinning and endocardial motion in a canine model. Am. J. Cardiol. 51:1732, 1983.

P

1. Pombo, J.F., Troy, B.L., Russell, R.O., Jr.: Left ventricular volumes and ejection fraction by echocardiography. Circulation 43:480, 1971.
2. Parisi, A.F., Moynihan, P.F., Folland, E.D., et al.: Approaches to determination of left ventricular volumes and ejection fraction by real-time two-dimensional echocardiography. Clin. Cardiol. 2:257, 1979.
3. Parisi, A.F.: Two-dimensional echocardiographic examination for quantitative detection of regional wall motion abnormalities. *In* Giuliani, E.R. (ed.): Two-Dimensional Real-time Ultrasonic Imaging of the Heart. Martinus Nijhoff, Boston, 1985, p. 221.
4. Pandian, N.G., Skorton, D.J., Collins, S.M., et al: Heterogeneity of left ventricular segmental wall thickening and excursion in 2-dimensional echocardiograms of normal human subjects. Am. J. Cardiol. 51:1667, 1983.
5. Pandian, N.G., Skorton, D.J., Collins, S.M., et al.: Myocardial infarct size threshold for two-dimensional echocardiographic detections: Sensitivity of systolic wall thickening and endocardial motion abnormalities in small versus large infarcts. Am. J. Cardiol. 55:551, 1985.
6. Parisi, A.F., Moynihan, P.F., Folland, E.D., and Feldman, C.L.: Quantitative detection of regional left ventricular contraction abnormalities by two-dimensional echocardiography. II. Accuracy in coronary artery disease. Circulation 63:761, 1981.
7. Pandian, N.G., and Kerber, R.E.: Two-dimensional echocardiography in experimental coronary stenosis. I. Sensitivity and specificity in detecting transient myocardial dyskinesis: Comparison with sonomicrometers. Circulation 66:597, 1982.
8. Pandian, N.G., Kieso, R.A., and Kerber, R.E.: Two-dimensional echocardiography in experimental coronary stenosis. II. Relationship between systolic wall thinning and regional myocardial perfusion in severe coronary stenosis. Circulation 66:603, 1982.
9. Pandian, N.G., Koyanagi, S., Skorton, D.J., et al.: Relations between 2-dimensional echocardiographic wall thickening abnormalities, myocardial infarct size and coronary risk area in normal and hypertrophied myocardium in dogs. Am. J. Cardiol. 52:1318, 1983.
10. Popp, R.L., Wolfe, S.B., Hirata, T., and Feigenbaum, H.: Estimation of right and left ventricular size by ultrasound. A study of the echoes from the interventricular septum. Am. J. Cardiol. 24:523, 1969.
11. Panidis, I.P., Ren, J.F., Kotler, M.N., et al.: Two-dimensional echocardiographic estimation of right ventricular ejection fraction in patients with coronary artery disease. J. Am. Coll. Cardiol. 2:911, 1983.
12. Panidis, I.P., Kotler, M.N., Mintz, G.S., et al.: Right ventricular function in coronary artery disease as assessed by two-dimensional echocardiography. Am. Heart J. 107:1187, 1984.
13. Pearlman, J.D., Triulzi, M.O., King, M.E., et al.: Limits of normal left ventricular dimensions in growth and development: Analysis of dimensions and variance in the two-dimensional echocardiograms of 268 normal healthy subjects. J. Am. Coll. Cardiol. 12:1432, 1988.

Q

1. Quinones, M.A., Waggoner, A.D., Reduto, L.A., et al.: A new, simplified and accurate method for determining ejection fraction with two-dimensional echocardiography. Circulation 64:744, 1981.

R

1. Reichek, N., Wilson, J., St. John Sutton, M., et al.: Noninvasive determination of left ventricular end-systolic stress: Validation of the method and initial application. Circulation 65:99, 1982.
2. Reichek, N., and Devereux, R.B.: Left ventricular hypertrophy: Relationship of anatomic, echocardiographic and electrocardiographic findings. Circulation 63:1391, 1981.
3. Reichek, N., Helak, J., Plappert, T., et al.: Anatomic validation of left ventricular mass estimates from clinical two-dimensional echocardiography: Initial results. Circulation 67:348, 1983.

S

1. Silverman, N.H., Ports, T.A., Snider, A.R., et al.: Determination of left ventricular volume in children: Echocardiographic and angiographic comparisons. Circulation 62:548, 1980.
2. Schiller, N.B., Acquatella, H., Ports, T.A., et al.: Left ventricular volume from paired biplane two-dimensional echocardiography. Circulation 60:547, 1979.
3. Schiller, N.B., Skioldebrand, C.G., Schiller, E.J., et al.: Canine left ventricular mass estimation by two-dimensional echocardiography. Circulation 68:210, 1983.
4. Sabbah, H.N., Marzilli, M., Stein, P.D.: The relative role of subendocardium and subepicardium in left ventricular mechanics. Am. J. Physiol. 240:4920, 1981.
5. Sheehan, F.H., Stewart, A.K., Dodge, H.T., et al.: Variability in the measurement of regional left ventricular wall motion from contrast angiograms. Circulation 68:550, 1983.
6. Schnittger, I., Fitzgerald, P.J., Gordon, E.P., et al.: Computerized quantitative analysis of left ventricular wall motion by two-dimensional echocardiography. Circulation 70:242, 1984.
7. Slager, C.J., Hooghoudt, T.E.H., Serruys, P.W., et al.: Quantitative assessment of regional left ventricular motion using endocardial landmarks. J. Am. Coll. Cardiol. 7:317, 1986.
8. Sakamaki, T., Lang, D., Wong, O.Y., et al.: Comparative validation of two-dimensional echocardiographic segmental wall motion analysis methods. (Abstract.) J. Am. Coll. Cardiol. 1:581, 1983.
9. Sniderman, A., Marpole, D., and Fallen, E.: Regional contraction patterns in the normal and ischemic left ventricle in man. Am. J. Cardiol. 31:484, 1973.
10. Slutsky, R., Karliner, J.S., Battler, A., et al.: Comparison of early systolic and holosystolic ejection phase indexes by contrast ventriculography in patients with coronary artery disease. Circulation 61:1083, 1980.
11. Skorton, D.J., McNary, C.A., Child, J.S., et al.: Digital image processing of two-dimensional echocardiograms: Identification of endocardium. Am. J. Cardiol. 48:479, 1981.
12. Sasayama, S., Franklin, D., Ross, J., Jr., et al.: Dynamic changes in left ventricular wall thickness and their use in analyzing cardiac function in the conscious dog. A study based on modified ultrasonic technique. Am. J. Cardiol. 38:870, 1976.

13. Savage, R.M., Guth, B., White, F.C., et al.: Correlation of regional myocardial blood flow and function with myocardial infarct size during acute myocardial ischemia in the conscious pig. Circulation 64:699, 1981.
14. Starr, I., Jeffers, W.A., and Meade, R.H., Jr.: The absence of conspicuous increments of venous pressure after severe damage to the right ventricle of the dog., with a discussion of the relationship between clinical congestive heart failure and heart disease. Am. Heart J. 26:291, 1943.
15. Sahn, D.J., DeMaria, A., Kisslo, J., and Weyman, A.: Recommendations regarding quantitation in M-mode echocardiography: Results of a survey of echocardiographic measurements. Circulation 58:1072, 1978.
16. Saito, A., Ueda, K., and Nakano, H.: Right ventricular volume determination by two-dimensional echocardiography. J. Cardiogr. 11:1159, 1981.
17. Starling, M.R., Crawford, M.H., Sorensen, S.G., and O'Rourke, R.A.: A new two-dimensional echocardiographic technique for evaluating right ventricular size and performance in patients with obstructive lung disease. Circulation 66:612, 1982.
18. Silverman, N.H., and Hudson, S.: Evaluation of right ventricular volume and ejection in children by two-dimensional echocardiography. Pediatr. Cardiol. 4:197, 1983.
19. Shapiro, E.P., Buchalter, M.B., Rogers, W.J., et al.: LV twist is greater with inotropic stimulation and less with regional ischemia. (Abstract.) Circ. Suppl. II:II-466, 1988.
20. Sharpe, D.N., Botvinick, E.H., Shamos, D.M., et al.: The noninvasive diagnosis of right ventricular infarction. Circulation 57:483, 1978.
21. Sharkey, S.W., Shelley, W., Carlyle, P.F., et al.: M-mode and two-dimensional echocardiographic analysis of the septum in experimental right ventricular infarction: Correlation with hemodynamic alterations. Am. Heart J. 110:1210, 1985.

T

1. Teichholz, L.E., Kreulen, T., Herman, M.V, and Gorlin, R.: Problems in echocardiographic volume determinations: Echocardiographic-angiographic correlations in the presence or absence of asynergy. Am. J. Cardiol. 37:7, 1976.
2. Teichholz, L.E., Cohen, M.V., Sonnenblick, E.H., and Gorlin, R.: Study of left ventricular geometry and function by B-scan ultrasonography in patients with and without asynergy. N. Engl. J. Med. 291:1220, 1974.
3. Theroux, P., Ross, J., Jr., Franklin, D., et al.: Regional myocardial function in the conscious dog during acute coronary occlusion and responses to morphine, propranolol, nitroglycerin, and lidocaine. Circulation 53:302, 1976.
4. Taylor, A.L., Kieso, R.A., Melton, J., et al.: Echocardiographically detected dyskinesis, myocardial infarct size, and coronary risk region relationships in reperfused canine myocardium. Circulation 71:1292, 1985.
5. Thomas, J.D., Hagege, A.A., Choong, C.Y., et al.: Improved accuracy of echocardiographic endocardial borders by spatiotemporal filtered Fourier reconstruction: Description of the method and optimization of filter cutoffs. Circulation 77:415, 1988.
6. Trowitzsch, E., Colan, S.D., and Sanders, S.P.: Two-dimensional echocardiographic estimation of right ventricular area change and ejection fraction in infants with systemic right ventricle (transposition of the great arteries or hypoplastic left heart syndrome). Am. J. Cardiol. 55:1153, 1985.

U

1. Urie, P.M., Jensen, R.L., Clayton, P.D., et al.: Comparison of methods for quantifying segmental wall motion. (Abstract.) Circ. Suppl. III 56:III-238, 1977.

V

1. Van Reet, R.E., Quinones, M.A., Poliner, L.R., et al.: Comparison of two-dimensional echocardiography with gated radionuclide ventriculography in the evaluation of global and regional left ventricular function in acute myocardial infarction. J. Am. Coll. Cardiol. 3:243, 1984.
2. Vatner, S.F.: Correlation between acute reductions in myocardial blood flow and function in conscious dogs. Circ. Res. 47:201, 1980.

W

1. Wyatt, H.L., Heng, M.K., Meerbaum, S., et al.: Cross-sectional echocardiography. II. Analysis of mathematical models for quantifying volume of the formalin-fixed left ventricle. Circulation 61:1119, 1980.
2. Woythaler, J.N., Singer, S.L., Kwan, O.L., et al.: Accuracy of echocardigraphy versus electrocardiography in detecting left ventricular hypertrophy: Comparison with post-mortem mass measurements. J. Am. Coll. Cardiol. 2:305, 1983.
3. Wyatt, H.L., Forrester, J.S., daLuz, P.L., et al.: Functional abnormalities in nonoccluded regions of myocardium after experimental coronary occlusion. Am. J. Cardiol. 37:366, 1976.
3. Weintraub, W.S., Hattori, S., Agarwal, J.B., et al.: The relationship between myocardial blood flow and contraction by myocardial layer in the canine left ventricle during ischemia. Circ. Res. 48:430, 1981.
4. Wyatt, H.L., Meerbaum, S., Heng, M.K., et al.: Experimental evaluation of the extent of myocardial dyssynergy and infarct size by two-dimensional echocardiography. Circulation 63:607, 1981.
5. Weyman, A.E., Franklin, T.D., Hogan, R.D., et al.: Importance of temporal heterogeneity in assessing the contraction abnormalities associated with acute myocardial ischemia. Circulation 70:102, 1984.
6. Weyman, A.E., Franklin, T.D., Egenes, K.M., and Green, D.: Correlation between extent of abnormal regional wall motion and myocardial infarct size in chronically infarcted dogs. Circ. Suppl. III 56:III-72, 1977.
7. Weiss, J.L., Bulkley, B.H., Hutchins, G.M., and Mason, S.J.: Two-dimensional echocardiographic recognition of myocardial injury in man: Comparison with postmortem studies. Circulation 63:401, 1981.
8. Watanabe, T., Katsume, H., Matsukubo, H., et al.: Estimation of right ventricular volume with two dimensional echocardiography. Am. J. Cardiol. 49:1946, 1982.
9. Wann, L.S., Stickels, K.R., Bamrah, V.S., and Gross, C.M.: Digital processing of contrast echocardiograms: A new technique for measuring right ventricular ejection fraction. Am. J. Cardiol. 53:1164, 1984.
10. Weiss, R.M., and Marcus, M.L.: The extent of regional systolic dysfunction during acute ischemia is load-dependent. (Abstract.) Circ. Suppl. II 78:II-484, 1988.
11. Wilkins, G.T., Southern, J.F., Choong, C.Y., et al.: Correlation between echocardiographic endocardial surface mapping of abnormal wall motion and pathologic infarct size in autopsied hearts. Circulation 77:978, 1988.

Z

1. Zir, L.M., Miller, S.W., Dinsmore, R.E., et al.: Interobserver variability in coronary angiography. Circulation 53:627, 1976.
2. Zanolla, L., Marino, P., Golia, G., et al.: Intraobserver reproducibility of quantitative two-dimensional echocardiography. Analysis of left ventricular area-time curve and of regional wall motion with two-frame and frame-by-frame methods. J. Cardiovasc. Ultrasonogr. 4:211, 1980.
3. Zoghbi, W.A., Charlat, M.L., Bolli, R., et al.: Quantitative assessment of left ventricular wall motion by two-dimensional echocardiography: Validation during reversible ischemia in the conscious dog. J. Am. Coll. Cardiol. II:185, 1988.

Chapter 20

Evaluation of Cardiac Function by Doppler Echocardiographic Techniques

ALAN S. PEARLMAN, M.D.

RELATIVE ROLE OF ULTRASONIC DOPPLER AND IMAGING TECHNIQUES 402
ASSESSMENT OF LEFT VENTRICULAR EJECTION 403
Measures of Interest 403
Clinical Applications 403
Measurement of Ventricular Systolic Function at Rest 403
Measurement of Ventricular Systolic Function After Interventions 407
Doppler Indices of Systolic Performance—Caveats 407
ASSESSMENT OF LEFT VENTRICULAR FILLING ... 408
Measures of Interest 408
Clinical Applications 409
Assessment of Diastolic Left Ventricular Function 409
Detection of Altered Diastolic Function Induced by Ischemia 410
Doppler Indices of Diastolic Performance—Caveats 410
Influence of Sampling Site 410
Influence of Age 410
Influence of Respiratory Cycle 410
Influence of Heart Rate 410
Influence of Left Atrial Pressure 412
Influence of Atrioventricular Sequence 412
ASSESSMENT OF RIGHT VENTRICULAR EJECTION 413
Measures of Interest 413
Associated Hemodynamics 414
Clinical Applications 414
ASSESSMENT OF RIGHT VENTRICULAR FILLING 415
Measures of Interest 415
Clinical Applications 415
SUMMARY 415

Since its inception, Doppler echocardiography has been used to evaluate cardiac function. Nearly 30 years ago, Franklin and associates[F1] described how the ultrasonic Doppler shift could be used to measure blood flow as a means to determine cardiac performance. In the late 1960's and early 1970's, Light and his colleagues[C1, L1–L3, S1] used suprasternal Doppler echocardiography to measure the velocity of ascending aortic blood flow in order to quantitate left ventricular systolic performance. In the past 10 years, a large number of investigators have applied both pulsed-wave and continuous-wave Doppler techniques to assess ventricular ejection and filling. This chapter reviews the Doppler echocardiographic methods that can be used, the clinical questions that can be studied, and the technical cautions that must be kept in mind by the investigator who wants to evaluate ventricular performance noninvasively.

RELATIVE ROLE OF ULTRASONIC DOPPLER AND IMAGING TECHNIQUES

As described in Chapter 19, echocardiographic imaging also can be used to evaluate ventricular performance. It therefore seems appropriate to comment on the comparative utility of these related but different ultrasonic techniques. Both techniques are properly referred to as "echocardiography." However, echocardiographic imaging assesses cardiac performance by using tomographic images of ventricular structure that result from ultrasound *reflected* at myocardium-blood interfaces, whereas Doppler echocardiography uses frequency shifts in the ultrasound *backscattered* from moving blood cells to assess blood flow within the cardiac chambers and great vessels. In essence, ultrasonic imaging uses the change in ventricular chamber size during systole (or diastole) to evaluate the volume and time course of ventricular emptying (or filling), whereas ultrasonic Doppler measures the velocity, timing, and volume of blood flow leaving (or entering) the ventricle directly.

Imaging techniques provide valuable data about both global and regional ventricular performance, although global measures generally are less accurate when regional abnormalities are present. Doppler techniques for measuring blood flow cannot quantitate regional ventricular function, but they do provide a simple and practical means of measuring global performance that is relatively insensitive to regional nonuniformity. This chapter focuses exclusively on Doppler techniques, but it is important to remember that echocardiographic imaging and Doppler are largely complementary rather than competing techniques; they are best used in conjunction, with the results of one technique interpreted in the context of the findings from the other technique.

Doppler methods can be used to evaluate both left and right ventricular function. The majority of clinical applications described to date have focused on left ventricular behavior. Hence, this chapter emphasizes the Doppler techniques and applications used to assess left ventricular function. Similar methods also can be used to evaluate right ventricular performance.

ASSESSMENT OF LEFT VENTRICULAR EJECTION

A major use of early Doppler techniques was in evaluating ventricular systolic function.[C1, C2, H1, L1–L3, S1] Although many important applications in judging valvular and shunt lesions have since evolved,[C3, H2, H3, O1, P1, S2, V1, W1] assessment of systolic performance remains an area of major clinical as well as research interest.

Measures of Interest

Various Doppler measures can be helpful in evaluating ventricular function during the ejection phase (Table 20–1). In general, all are based on determination of the velocity of blood flow out of the ventricle during systole. This can be done either by using range-gated, pulsed-wave Doppler to examine selectively in the left ventricular outflow tract or ascending aorta, or by using continuous-wave Doppler to examine flow through the aortic valve. The technical details of the echocardiographic measurement of blood flow velocities and the differences between pulsed-wave and continuous-wave Doppler are discussed in detail in Chapter 18.

Representative pulsed-wave and continuous-wave Doppler recordings for a normal subject are illustrated in Figure 20–1. In the graphic output, flow velocity (on the ordinate) is plotted against time (on the abscissa), with signal intensity shown in gray scale. From such tracings, a variety of measurements can be made directly: velocities, time intervals, and velocity-time integrals. Doppler measures also can be combined with anatomic dimensions (determined by echocardiographic imaging) to compute flow volumes and flow rates.

In Figure 20–2, maximum systolic ejection velocity is indicated. The instantaneous velocity at any desired point during the ejection phase also can be measured. The duration of ejection can be determined, as can fractional durations. Finally, the systolic velocity-time integral (VTI) can be determined by planimetry, as can fractional integrals. Note that since velocity is a derivative measure expressing distance per unit time, the integral of velocity (as a function of time) represents distance. Accordingly, the systolic velocity-time integral is equivalent to the distance downstream through which a representative red blood cell is propelled during systole. Use of the term "stroke distance" instead of velocity-time integral is thus intuitively sensible.

Table 20–1. DOPPLER MEASURES OF SYSTOLIC VENTRICULAR FUNCTION

Ejection velocity
Peak
Mean
Ejection duration
Acceleration
Maximum
Average
Acceleration time
Deceleration time
Systolic velocity-time integral ("stroke distance")
Stroke volume
Cardiac output
Ventricular dP/dt

Physiologists have long recognized that volumetric flow rate can be computed by multiplying the average flow velocity (in cm/sec) by the area filled by flow (in cm^2), the product of these two terms being expressed in units of ml/sec. The average flow velocity can be determined by dividing the velocity-time integral by the duration of flow. Alternatively, the product of systolic velocity-time integral (in cm/beat) and flow cross-sectional area (in cm^2) yields the volume of flow ejected per beat (in ml/beat), which is the stroke volume. Thus, as illustrated in Figure 20–3, Doppler measures can be combined with anatomic area determinations to calculate volumetric flow. It is important to remember that area and velocity integral measures should be made at the same anatomic site. Thus, if pulsed-wave Doppler is used to record systolic ejection velocity in the left ventricular outflow tract, flow area should be measured at that same site.[G1, G2, I1, L4, O2] If continuous-wave Doppler is used, the site of area measurement should take into account that in this situation peak instantaneous velocities will be recorded from the narrowest area of the ejection flow stream[B1, C4, H4, N1] as long as flow direction and the ultrasound beam are nearly coaxial. In either case, flow area typically is computed from the measured diameter of the outflow tract or aorta by assuming that the area filled by flow is circular in cross section and that the measured diameter is equivalent to the average systolic diameter. The centerline systolic velocity profile is recorded and assumed to represent the spatial average velocity of a laminar plug of flow. Experimental observations[O2] suggest that these assumptions generally are reasonable.

For patients with mitral regurgitation, theoretical considerations and observations in patients[B2, C5, H5] suggest that the rate of rise of left ventricular systolic pressure (dP/dt) can be estimated noninvasively from the rate of increase in mitral regurgitant jet velocity during systole (Fig. 20–4). Since left atrial pressure changes relatively little during early ventricular systole, the rate of change of mitral regurgitant velocity (which is proportional to the square root of the left ventricular–left atrial pressure difference) is determined primarily by the rate of change of simultaneous left ventricular pressure. Hence, if one measures the time interval Δt (in seconds) during which mitral regurgitant velocity increases from 1 to 3 m/sec (corresponding to a change in pressure difference from 4 to 36 mmHg), the *average* rate of change of pressure is $32/\Delta t$, expressed in m/sec/sec. Preliminary studies[B2, C5] support the validity of this approach.

Clinical Applications

Measurement of Ventricular Systolic Function at Rest

A number of the measures just described can be used to this end. Stroke volumes and cardiac outputs are perhaps the most intuitively logical measures of systolic ventricular emptying (Fig. 20–5). A number of experimental[C2, M1, S3, V1, V2] and clinical[C4, G1, G2, H4, I1, L4, L5, N1, S2, V2] studies have demonstrated convincingly that Doppler measures of stroke volume and cardiac output agree well with measures obtained by invasive (Fick or indicator dilution) techniques.

Several points are noteworthy. First, Doppler stroke volumes can be determined with either pulsed-wave[G2, L4, L5, S3, V1] or continuous-wave[C2, C4, H4, N1] techniques and at a number of measurement sites, including the ascending aorta, left ventricular outflow tract, descending aorta, main pulmonary artery, and mitral orifice.[F2, G1, G2, H4, H6, L1, L4, L5, S2, S4, V1, V2] Second, notwithstanding the high correlations generally reported in the studies cited, some individual data points do show significant disagreement between the methods tested. It should be recognized that stroke volume and cardiac output are dynamic variables that can change from moment to moment and that the majority of studies comparing Doppler to invasive measures of volume flow were *not* done

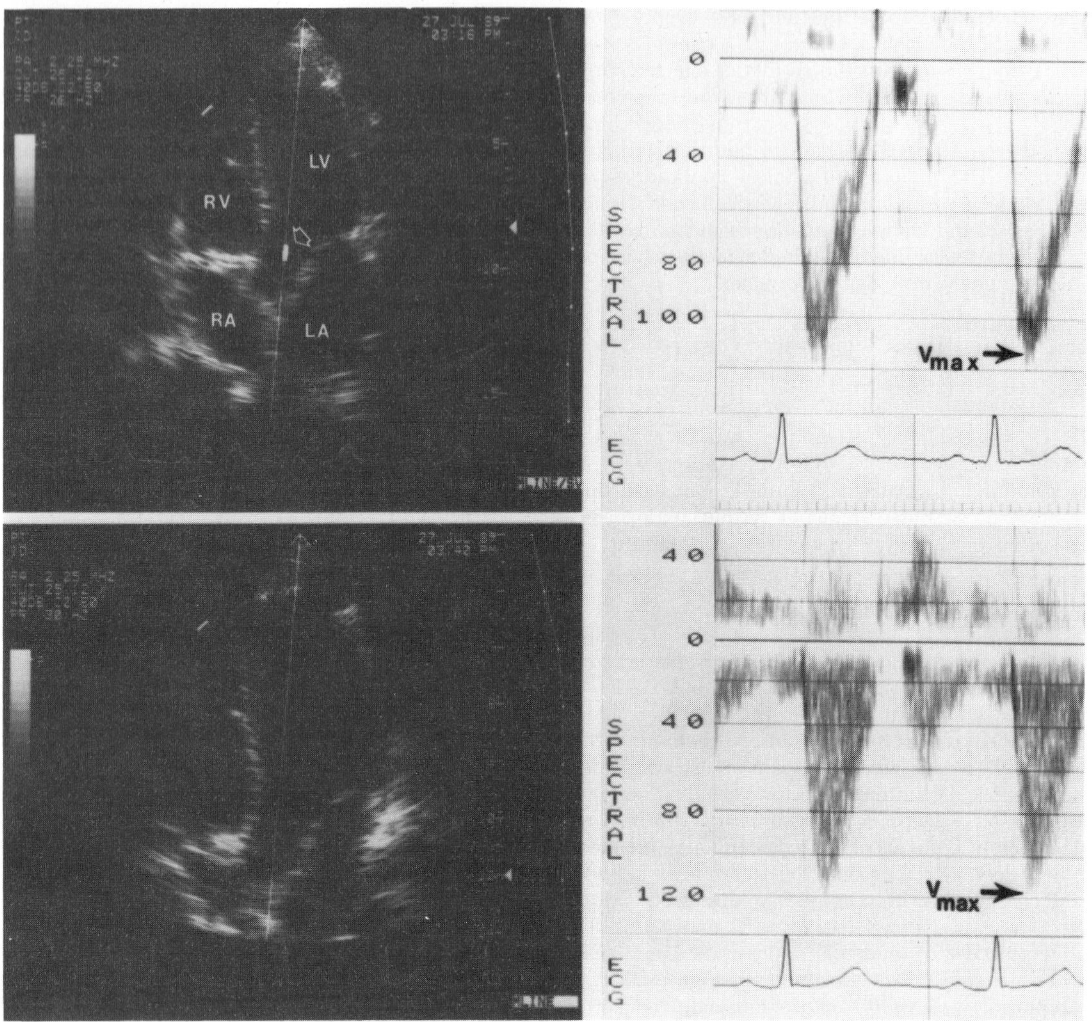

Figure 20–1. Left ventricular ejection flow in a normal 30-year-old woman. *Top panels*, Pulsed-wave Doppler. *Left*, Systolic freeze-frame, apical four-chamber plane. The Doppler sample volume *(open arrow)* is positioned along the Doppler interrogation cursor in the high left ventricular outflow tract, just proximal to the aortic leaflets. Doppler velocities are recorded from blood cells moving through this region. LA—left atrium; LV—left ventricle; RA—right atrium; RV—right ventricle. *Right*, Graphic output of Doppler velocity (y axis) as a function of time (x axis), with simultaneous electrocardiogram (ECG) recorded for timing. Velocities are calibrated in cm/sec, small time markers are 0.04 second apart. The narrow band of velocities at each instant in systole denotes organized ejection flow through the region of sampling. Maximum ventricular ejection velocity (V_{max}) is indicated. *Bottom panels*, Continuous-wave Doppler. *Left*, Systolic freeze-frame, apical four-chamber plane. The Doppler cursor is oriented parallel to the direction of ventricular outflow. Doppler velocities are recorded all along this line of interrogation, with the highest instantaneous velocities coming from the region of the aortic valve and proximal ascending aorta. *Right*, Graphic output, same format as above. The broad band of velocities at each instant in systole denotes recording of simultaneous Doppler shifts from blood cells at multiple depths along the cursor line. Maximum ejection velocity (V_{max}) is indicated and typically is slightly higher than that measured proximal to the aortic valve.

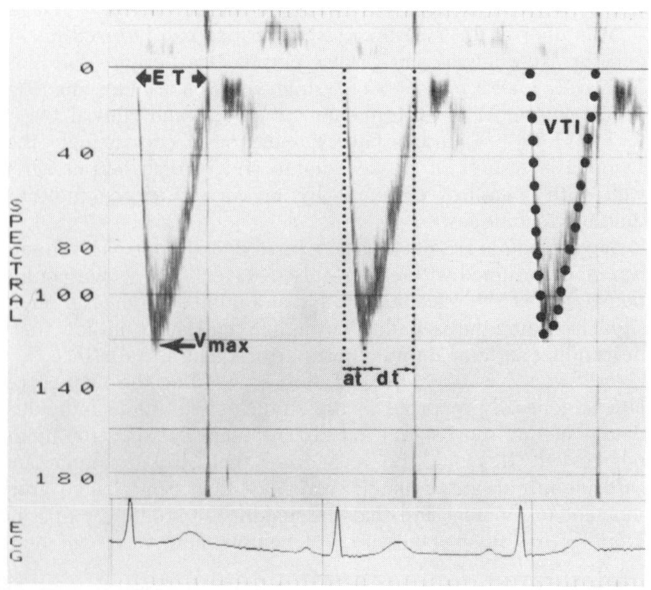

Figure 20–2. Ejection velocities in a normal subject, recorded from the left ventricular outflow tract (apical examining window) with pulsed-wave Doppler. Maximum ejection velocity (V_{max}) is 120 cm/sec (first complex), and instantaneous velocities also can be determined throughout systole (third complex). The duration of ejection (ET—ejection time) is 0.33 second. The time from onset to peak ejection (at—acceleration time) and from peak to end-ejection (dt—deceleration time) also can be measured. The area enclosed by the velocity curve (VTI—velocity-time integral) can be determined by planimetry and represents the "stroke distance."

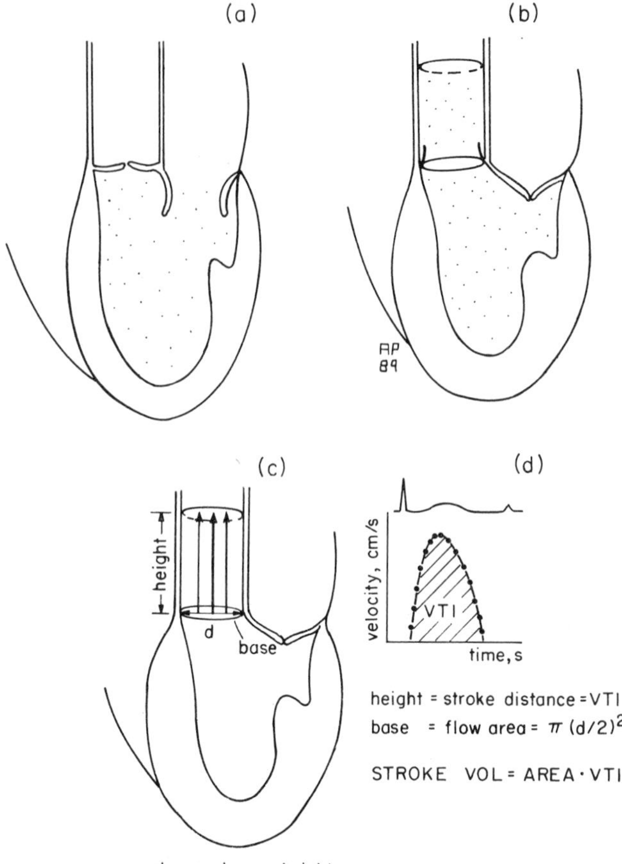

Figure 20–3. Diagram illustrating determination of systolic left ventricular stroke volume with Doppler echocardiographic data. *a*, Frontal view showing the left ventricle in diastole; for purposes of illustration, blood in the ventricular cavity is stippled. *b*, In late systole, the ventricle has emptied into the ascending aorta, filling a cylindrical segment of this vessel with stippled blood. *c*, The volume of the cylindrical segment of aorta filled during systole can be measured as the product of its base times height. The area of the base can be calculated from the diameter (d) as $\pi(d/2)^2$. *d*, The height of the cylinder is equivalent to the distance downstream through which an average blood cell is propelled during systole (the "stroke distance"). This distance is equivalent to the velocity-time integral (VTI) measured with a planimeter as the area enclosed by the ejection velocity curve. The product of flow area and stroke distance yields stroke volume.

simultaneously. Moreover, the available standards of reference are not ideal, since cardiac outputs determined by thermodilution, Fick, and angiographic techniques can be substantially different for individual patients.[C6, G3, H7, R1] Even when a single "reference standard" technique is used for the same patient, duplicate measures show imperfect agreement; for example, repeat determinations of cardiac output by thermodilution often differ from each other[G3] as much as determinations by Doppler and thermodilution methods differ. These considerations suggest that although Doppler stroke volumes and cardiac outputs do have technical limitations, they may in practical terms be generally as accurate as other available methods for measuring volumetric flow.

Measures of ejection velocity, systolic time intervals, and velocity-time integrals also reflect resting systolic left ventricular function. More than 25 years ago, Rushmer suggested that since the ventricles acted as impulse generators, "initial ventricular impulse" could be used as an indicator of systolic ventricular performance.[R2] Ultrasonic Doppler methods were not then available, but Rushmer and associates used electromagnetic flowmeters to show that measures of systolic ejection velocity and acceleration increased with treadmill exercise and decreased with ischemia-induced systolic dysfunction.[R3] These studies also showed that measures of the velocity and timing of blood ejection into the systemic and pulmonary circulations reflected selective changes in left and right ventricular systolic function, respectively.

Gardin and associates[G4] extended these observations by using pulsed-wave Doppler echocardiography to study normal subjects and patients with dilated cardiomyopathy (some ischemic, some idiopathic). These investigators found that peak Doppler left ventricular ejection velocity, measured in the ascending aorta, was significantly lower in patients with cardiomyopathy than in normal individuals, as were measures of average acceleration and ejection time (Fig. 20–6). It is noteworthy that although Gardin and associates found no overlap in peak velocities between individuals with normal and those with depressed left ventricular function, the patients they studied had impairment of systolic left ventricular function that was obvious clinically as well as by two-dimensional echocardiography (Gardin, J. M., personal communication). Clinical experience shows that although ejection velocities generally are depressed in patients with systolic ventricular dysfunction, there may be overlap between patients with impaired global function and subjects with normal ventricles (unpublished observations). In other words, normal ventricular systolic performance indices at rest do not preclude significant heart disease, a caveat that long has been recognized by advocates of stress testing.[B3, G5]

A number of authors have suggested that measures of systolic acceleration of blood flow in the ascending aorta correlate well with traditional indices of global systolic performance.[B4, C7, N2, S5–S7, W2] Several experimental[B4, N2] and clinical[S5] studies have concluded that maximum acceleration may be better than peak ejection velocity for measuring systolic ventricular function. Moreover, since maximum acceleration is relatively unaffected

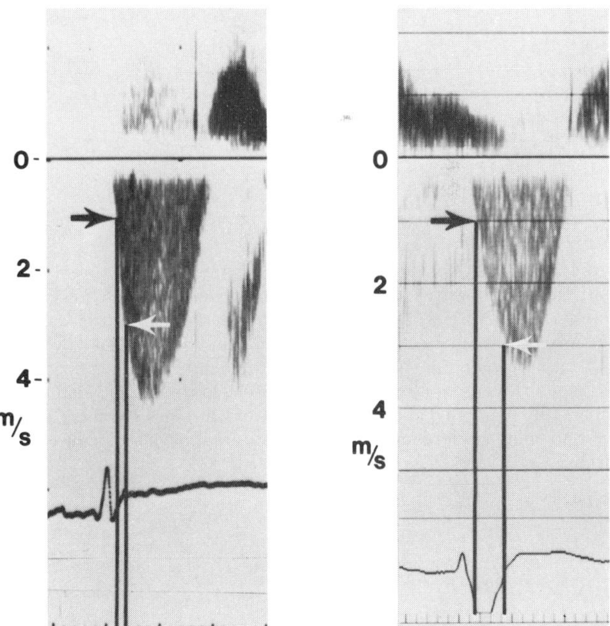

Figure 20–4. Mitral regurgitation, continuous-wave Doppler, recorded from the cardiac apex. *Left*, Recording from a 56-year-old man with moderate mitral regurgitation and normal left ventricular systolic function. Regurgitant velocity increases from 1 m/sec *(black arrow)* to 3 m/sec *(white arrow)* in 0.015 second, corresponding to an average dP/dt of 2133 mmHg/sec. See text for details. *Right*, Recording from a 49-year-old man with an aortic prosthesis, moderate mitral regurgitation, and markedly decreased global left ventricular systolic function (ejection fraction 15 to 20 percent). In this case, regurgitant velocity increases from 1 m/sec *(black arrow)* to 3 m/sec *(white arrow)* in 0.055 second, corresponding to a depressed average dP/dt of 582 mmHg/sec.

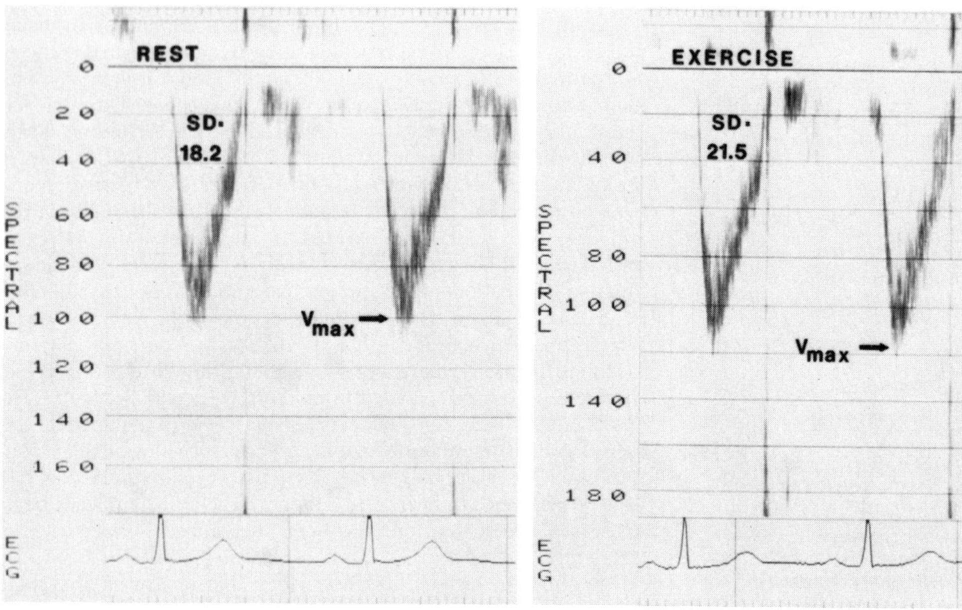

Figure 20–5. Left ventricular ejection velocities in a normal 30-year-old woman, recorded from the left ventricular outflow tract (apical examining window) with pulsed-wave Doppler. *Left*, At rest, maximum velocity (V_{max}) is 100 cm/sec, stroke distance (SD) is 18.2 cm, and calculated stroke volume is 76 ml per beat. Heart rate is 63 beats per minute and thus cardiac output is 4.8 liters/min. *Right*, After mild exercise, maximum velocity has increased to 120 cm/sec and stroke distance to 21.5 cm. Calculated stroke volume has increased to 89 ml, heart rate to 74 beats per minute, and cardiac output to 6.6 liters/min.

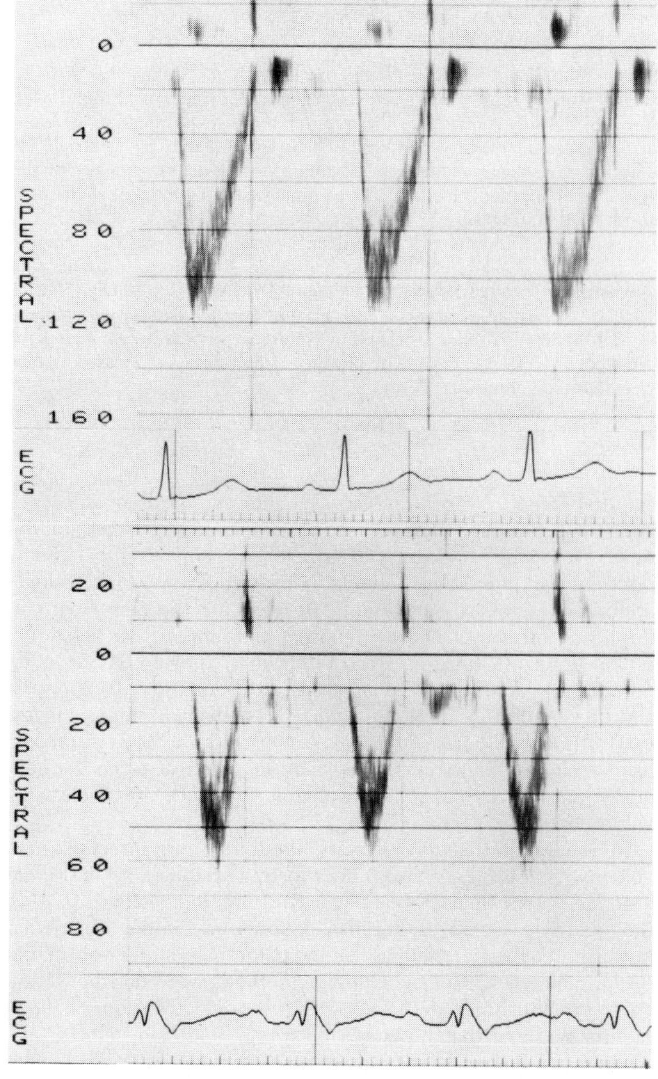

Figure 20–6. Left ventricular ejection velocities, recorded from the left ventricular outflow tract (apical examining window) with pulsed-wave Doppler. *Top*, Normal 30-year-old woman with normal ventricular systolic function. Maximum ejection velocity is 115 cm/sec and stroke distance is 18.2 cm. *Bottom*, 46-year-old man with dilated cardiomyopathy and severe global ventricular systolic dysfunction. Maximum ejection velocity is markedly depressed at 60 cm/sec and stroke distance is 8.0 cm; ejection duration and acceleration measures also are obviously reduced from normal.

by changes in preload but is sensitive to altered inotropic state,[B4, N2] this measure may be particularly attractive as a marker of ventricular contractile performance. Maximum acceleration is, however, influenced by alterations in afterload.[B5]

Measurement of Ventricular Systolic Function After Interventions

The preceding considerations suggest that the use of Doppler echocardiographic methods to measure ventricular function during (or immediately after) interventions would be of paramount interest. A number of investigators have used Doppler techniques to demonstrate exercise-induced increases in stroke volume and cardiac output[C8, D1, G6, 12, L6, M2, M3, R4, S8] that agree well with those measured by traditional invasive procedures, which suggests that Doppler methods can be used not only to define basal systolic ventricular function but also to document changes in function as a result of intervention. Other workers have demonstrated that significant increases in peak ejection velocity and acceleration accompany supine bicycle ergometer exercise[D1, G6, L6, M2, M3, R4] and upright bicycle or treadmill exercise[B6, H8, M4, M5, S8] when patients with normal ventricular function are studied, whereas patients with ventricular systolic dysfunction generally show a blunted response or an actual decline in ejection phase measures. Accordingly, exercise Doppler measures have been touted as a means of detecting ischemic heart disease[B6, D2, M4, M5] and as a useful adjunct to conventional exercise testing.

A related application involves the use of Doppler methods to study changes in systolic performance after therapies designed to improve depressed ventricular function (Fig. 20–7). Elkayam and associates[E1] studied patients with heart failure and reported increases in peak ejection velocity and stroke distance after treatment with vasodilator agents. These workers also noted that the degree of improvement in the Doppler measures correlated well with the magnitude of change in invasive indicators of systolic ventricular performance. Sabbah and associates[S9] also studied patients with congestive heart failure and reported that depressed measures of maximum acceleration increased toward normal during treatment in patients whose failure improved but not in the subgroup whose failure persisted. Labovitz and associates[L7] evaluated left ventricular function in patients undergoing percutaneous transluminal coronary angioplasty. These investigators noted a fall in Doppler systolic ejection velocities during balloon inflation, with a return toward normal after reperfusion, as evidence for reversible depression of systolic ventricular function due to transient ischemia. Harrison and associates[H8] used Doppler techniques to study the hemodynamic effects of cardioactive drugs. They noted increases during exercise in both peak ejection velocity and maximum acceleration measured by continuous-wave Doppler. These increases were blunted significantly by propranolol therapy (with more blunting of acceleration than of peak velocity), indicating the negative inotropic effect of this drug. In contrast, acute administration of verapamil did not alter exercise-induced increases in ejection velocity or acceleration. These studies show the role of Doppler measures as a practical means of assessing the effect of interventions on global systolic left ventricular performance.

Doppler Indices of Systolic Performance—Caveats

It is appealing to use Doppler measures to assess global ventricular systolic function, in part because these measures are physiologically meaningful and in part because they are atraumatic, noninvasive, and widely available. Notwithstanding their practical utility, however, Doppler echocardiographic measures have several noteworthy limitations that should not be ignored.

Accurate Doppler velocity measures depend on examining flowing blood with an ultrasound beam that is oriented nearly parallel to the direction of blood flow; angular errors in ultrasonic orientation will lead to underestimates of velocity, acceleration, and velocity-time integrals. In addition, Doppler shifts measured in one area of a cardiac chamber or great vessel are representative of the average behavior of blood flow at that site and time during the cardiac cycle only when the flow is laminar and blunt in its spatial profile. Potential physiologic variations in the actual behavior of blood flow are perhaps even more important. The volume and time course of ventricular ejection, which vary with changes in ventricular systolic performance, also change with heart rate and ventricular loading conditions. Alterations in heart rate may occur without obvious changes in clinical status, and so may changes in ventricular preload and afterload. Accordingly, Doppler measures of velocity and stroke distance can change even though ventricular contractile function remains fundamentally unaltered. Maximum acceleration may provide a more sensitive indicator of systolic contractile performance that is less influenced by loading conditions,[B4, N2] but acceleration is also affected by changes in afterload.[B5] Thus, interpretation of Doppler measures for a patient with suspected ventricular malfunction must take into consideration the hemodynamic as well as the clinical context in which these measures were obtained.

The multiple Doppler measures of systolic performance that can be obtained raise a question: which measure is "best"? This question has not been answered by comparative studies of different diagnostic protocols in the same patients, and we cannot assume that what is most appropriate for one clinical application

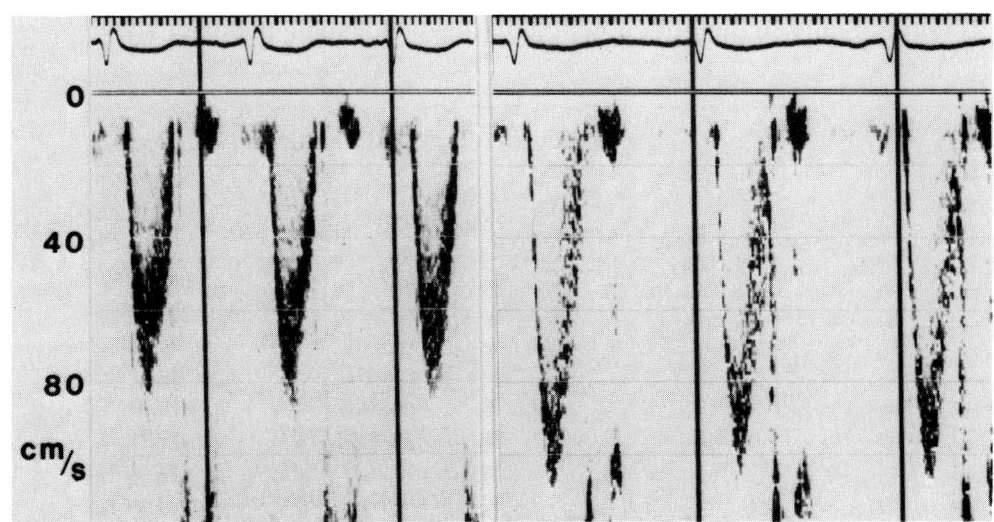

Figure 20–7. Left ventricular ejection velocities from a 31-year-old man with an infiltrative cardiomyopathy due to hemochromatosis, recorded from the left ventricular outflow tract (apical examining window) with pulsed-wave Doppler. *Left,* Before treatment, depressed measures of systolic function parallel clinical symptoms and signs of left ventricular failure; maximum ejection velocity is 80 cm/sec, stroke distance is 10.9 cm, stroke volume is 54 ml, and cardiac output is 4.3 liters/min. *Right,* After treatment, clinical improvement in ventricular systolic function is accompanied by increases in maximum ejection velocity to 105 cm/sec, stroke distance to 15.7 cm, and stroke volume to 77 ml. Although heart rate has slowed, cardiac output has increased to 5.1 liters/min.

will necessarily be useful for another. Depending on the application, different characteristics may be desirable: for detecting systolic dysfunction as an early marker of ischemic disease, a measure with high sensitivity would be most helpful; for demonstrating improved function resulting from treatment of heart failure with a vasodilator agent, a measure with narrow confidence limits would be best suited. With our current state of knowledge it is not possible to identify an individual Doppler echocardiographic measure, or set of such measures, that is ideal for any particular application, let alone for all potential applications. Further research will be needed to help define the relative clinical utility of different Doppler measures of ventricular systolic function.

ASSESSMENT OF LEFT VENTRICULAR FILLING

Cardiologists recognize increasingly that abnormalities of diastolic ventricular function are clinically relevant[D3, H9, L8, N3]; indeed, in some clinical disorders they antedate alterations in systolic function.[D4, D5, S10] The advent of quantitative noninvasive radionuclide[B7, B8] and M-mode echocardiographic[G7, H10] methods for defining diastolic ventricular function has made it practical to analyze the prevalence and significance of abnormal ventricular filling in various disease states. A number of investigators have emphasized the use of Doppler echocardiography to evaluate the volumetric rate and time course of ventricular filling[A1, B9, F3, F4, G8, G9, K1, K2, M6, M7, N2, P2–P4, R5, S11, T1, T2, W2] and thereby to assess ventricular diastolic performance.

Measures of Interest

Familiar categories of Doppler variables are used to assess diastolic ventricular performance (Table 20–2): velocities, time intervals, velocity-time integrals, and volumetric flow rates. Again, both pulsed-wave and continuous-wave Doppler techniques can be used to record ventricular inflow velocities during diastole.

Normally, the left ventricle fills rapidly during early diastole, as a result of a small initial diastolic pressure gradient between the left atrium and ventricle coupled with ventricular relaxation and elastic recoil. As the atrium empties and the ventricle fills, the atrioventricular pressure gradient abates and reverses, causing a period of diastasis (with little or no filling) during mid-diastole. In normal sinus rhythm, atrial contraction results in a small late-diastolic atrioventricular pressure difference and increase in filling.

Table 20–2. DOPPLER MEASURES OF DIASTOLIC VENTRICULAR FUNCTION

Filling velocities
Peak early diastolic velocity (E)
Peak atrial contraction velocity (A)
E/A ratio
Diastolic intervals
Isovolumic relaxation period
Rapid filling period
Slow filling period (diastasis)
Atrial contraction period
Fractional intervals (first-third, half-filling, etc.)
Early diastolic deceleration
Deceleration slope
Deceleration time
Diastolic velocity-time integral ("stroke distance")
Peak rapid filling rate
Stroke volume
Cardiac output

Figure 20–8 illustrates the early rapid filling, diastasis, and atrial contraction phases that characterize the normal pattern of ventricular filling. From such curves of diastolic Doppler flow velocity as a function of time, one can measure a number of variables. Instantaneous velocities can be determined throughout diastole; maximum velocities typically are measured during the early (E) rapid filling phase and during the atrial (A) contribution to ventricular filling. The rate of decay of early diastolic peak velocity can be expressed as the slope of this curve or as the deceleration time. The duration of diastole and of its component phases can be determined, as can integrals of diastolic velocity during all or part of the filling period (i.e., from onset to peak of rapid filling). Filling volumes can be calculated by combining velocity-time integral measures (diastolic "stroke distance") with flow cross-sectional areas.

In the case of ventricular filling, dynamic changes in the area filled by flow during diastole must be borne in mind. It appears that the mitral leaflet tips open as far as they need to as the flow volume changes during the different phases of diastole. Thus, an accurate measure of transmitral volume flow during diastole at the tip of the mitral leaflets requires that the *average* diastolic mitral orifice area be determined. This could be done by measuring the instantaneous mitral orifice area with a planimeter on a frame-by-frame basis during diastole, a process that is at best tedious. In reality, this approach sometimes is rendered impractical by difficulties in imaging the actual leaflet tips throughout diastole. Alternatively, one can measure the maximum mitral orifice area during diastole and then compute the mean orifice area.

Fisher and associates[F2] reasoned that the mean diastolic orifice area could be calculated by multiplying the maximum area measured with a planimeter by the ratio of mean to maximum leaflet separation during diastole and determined the latter ratio from M-mode echocardiographic tracings. Mean orifice area determined in this manner, when multiplied by the diastolic velocity-time integral recorded (using pulsed-wave Doppler) at the level of the leaflet tips, yielded a measure of stroke volume that agreed well with thermodilution measures in a series of animal experiments.[F2, V1] More recently, de Zuttere and associates[D6] have proposed an elliptical correction for determining mean mitral orifice area at the level of the leaflet tips, since the orifice diameter changes primarily in the anteroposterior dimension and little in the mediolateral dimension. Hoit and associates[H6] also have devised a method that couples Doppler velocities with M-mode echocardiographic measures of mitral leaflet separation and timing to calculate transmitral stroke volume.

An alternative approach evolves from the fact that normal mitral leaflets are pliable and offer little resistance to left ventricular filling; the leaflets open as needed to accommodate volumetric flow. Accordingly, the limiting flow orifice actually is found at the level of the mitral annulus. In this circumstance, annular diameters can be used to determine the flow orifice area and thus the diastolic filling volume. Although echocardiographic studies[O3] suggest that the normal mitral annulus diameter changes during diastole, it does appear that the mid-diastolic annular area approximates the average diastolic orifice with sufficient accuracy for clinical use.[L4] Whether the annulus is circular[F2, L4] or elliptical[D6, P3] in shape is debated. The circular model requires measurement of a single diameter, whereas the elliptical model requires both anteroposterior and medial-lateral diameters, to determine orifice area.

Mean mitral annular area, multiplied by the diastolic velocity-time integral recorded at the level of the annulus (Fig. 20–9), yields transmitral diastolic stroke volume. In the absence of aortic and mitral insufficiency, this volume should be identical to the stroke volume ejected across the left ventricular outflow tract and aortic valve during systole.[L4] Moreover, if the mitral annular cross-sectional area varies relatively little during diastole, the product of annular area (in cm^2) and instantaneous transmitral

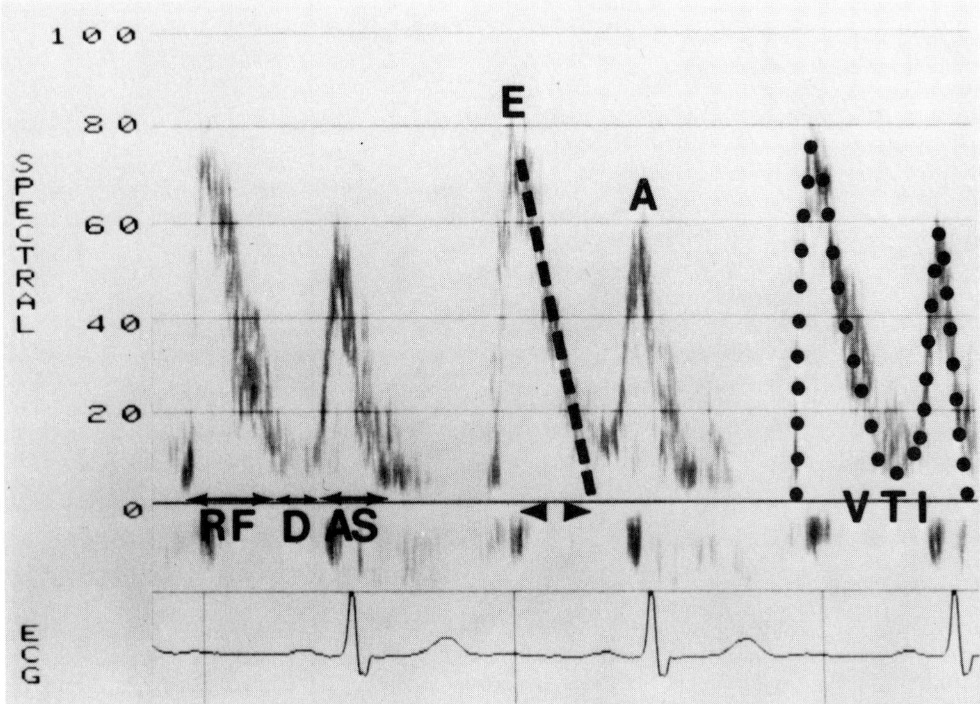

Figure 20–8. Left ventricular filling velocities from a normal middle-aged man, recorded at the level of the mitral leaflet tips (apical examining window) with pulsed-wave Doppler. In the first diastolic complex, the periods of rapid filling (RF), diastasis (D), and atrial systole (AS) are labeled. In the second complex, early diastolic (E) and atrial systolic (A) maximum velocities are indicated. The dashed line denotes the slope of decay of peak early diastolic velocity, and the arrowheads mark the deceleration time (from peak E velocity to the point at which the linear decay slope crosses the zero-velocity baseline). The third complex shows how planimetry of the diastolic velocity curve as a function of time yields the velocity-time integral (VTI), which indicates diastolic "stroke distance." Rapid filling and atrial systolic integrals also can be determined.

velocity (in cm/sec) yields a measure of instantaneous diastolic flow rate.[R5] Accordingly, peak rapid filling rate, maximum atrial filling rate, or the fraction of filling due to atrial contraction can be determined.

Finally, Doppler records can be used to measure the period of isovolumic relaxation,[A1, S12] an important marker of early ventricular diastolic behavior. Since isovolumic relaxation begins at aortic valve closure and ends at mitral valve opening, the onset of this period can be noted from the cessation of ejection flow recorded by Doppler echocardiography and the end of isovolumic relaxation is marked by the onset of diastolic transmitral flow.

Clinical Applications

Assessment of Diastolic Left Ventricular Function

Doppler measurements of left ventricular filling have been shown to agree well with measurements by other techniques used to assess left ventricular diastolic function. Rokey and associates[R5] used frame-by-frame analysis of angiographic left ventricular volumes during diastole to derive filling curves and compared these curves to diastolic transmitral flow velocity curves recorded by pulsed-wave Doppler. For patients with various disorders, these two approaches yielded quite similar results. Moreover, peak rapid filling rates computed from mitral annular Doppler velocities and echocardiographic diameters showed good agreement ($r = 0.87$) with angiographic peak filling rates. Spirito and associates[S12] and Friedman and associates[F4] demonstrated that Doppler measures of the peak rapid filling rate and of the time course and relative early and atrial contributions to ventricular filling correlated well with radionuclide angiographic measures for normal subjects and patients with different cardiac disorders. Using Doppler and M-mode echocardiographic techniques, Pearson and associates[P3] found similar abnormalities of ventricular filling in patients with ventricular hypertrophy. The practicality of using Doppler ventricular filling curves to assess diastolic left ventricular function has made this approach increasingly popular.

In the past 3 years, abnormal diastolic Doppler indices have been used to show evidence for abnormal diastolic left ventricular function in patients with a number of different cardiac disorders (Fig. 20–10). Maron and associates[M7] reported shortening of the isovolumic relaxation time, blunting of the Doppler rapid filling (E) wave, flattening of the velocity decay slope, and decreases in the Doppler E/A ratio in patients with hypertrophic cardiomyopathy. Other authors also have reported decreased early filling velocities and increased atrial contributions to ventricular filling

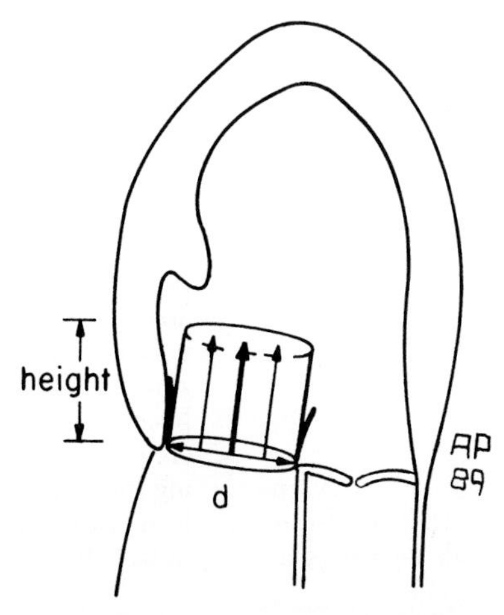

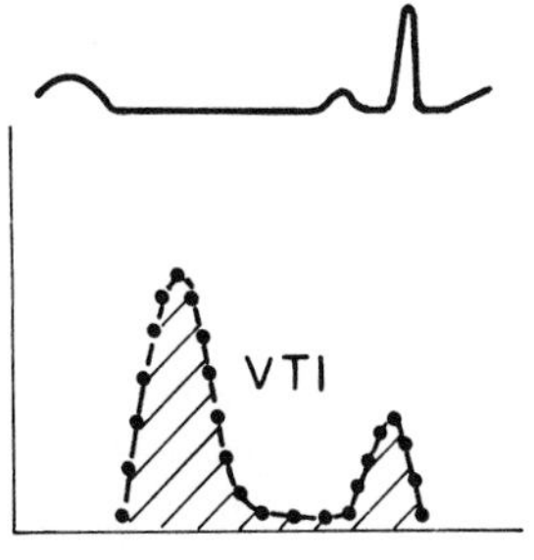

height = stroke distance = VTI

base = flow area = $\pi (d/2)^2$

STROKE VOL = AREA · VTI

Figure 20–9. Diagram illustrating calculation of diastolic stroke volume from mitral annular area and velocity measures. *Left,* Diagram of left ventricular diastolic filling as seen from an apical examining window. Diastolic blood flow across the mitral annulus fills a segment of the left ventricle whose volume is equivalent to that of a cylinder; the base and height of the cylinder can be used to measure filling volume. Mitral cross-sectional flow area is determined from annulus diameter (d). *Right,* Diastolic stroke distance is determined by planimetry of the diastolic velocity-time integral (VTI). Stroke volume is the product of annulus area times stroke distance and (in the absence of both mitral and aortic incompetence) is identical to the stroke volume ejected through the ventricular outflow tract during systole. Note that annulus area times peak rapid filling velocity yields peak rapid filling rate; see text for details.

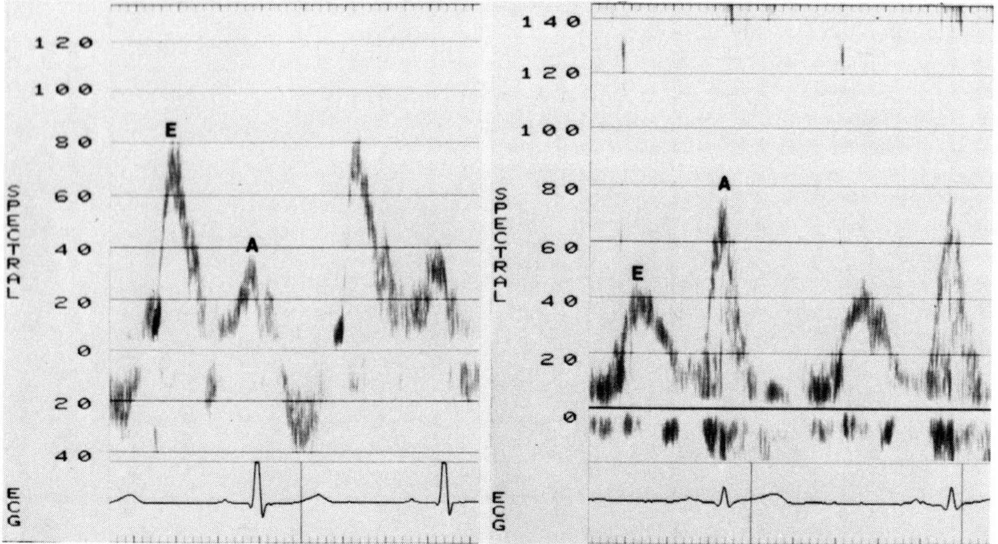

Figure 20–10. Left ventricular filling velocities, recorded at the level of the mitral leaflet tips (apical examining window) with pulsed-wave Doppler. *Left*, Velocity curve from a normal 25-year-old woman; the early diastolic velocity is 80 cm/sec, the E/A ratio exceeds 1, and the deceleration time is approximately 150 msec. *Right*, Velocity curve from a 53-year-old man with coronary artery disease causing an anteroapical left ventricular aneurysm and also abnormal diastolic ventricular filling; the early diastolic velocity is depressed, peak atrial velocity is augmented, the E/A ratio is less than 1, and deceleration time is prolonged at 260 msec.

in hypertrophic cardiomyopathy.[B9, K2, P3, T2] These Doppler findings have suggested that slowed ventricular relaxation and increased chamber stiffness result from left ventricular hypertrophy. Studies of hypertensive patients[F4, G9, K2, P3, P4, S13, S14] have documented similar Doppler abnormalities, which presumably indicate similar defects in diastolic chamber function, again resulting from ventricular hypertrophy. Abnormal Doppler filling measures have also been noted in patients with ischemic heart disease[F3] and diabetes,[Z1] indicating that these patients too have abnormalities of diastolic function. For patients with aortic stenosis, Otto and associates[O2] documented a decrease in the mid-diastolic velocity decay slope and increase in the A velocity, particularly in patients with increased wall thickness. The findings of these and other studies suggest that many cardiac disorders cause defects in diastolic left ventricular filling; these abnormalities probably contribute to symptoms and signs of congestive heart failure and may be particularly important in patients with normal systolic function.

Detection of Altered Diastolic Function Induced by Ischemia

The ability of Doppler transmitral flow velocities to reflect left ventricular filling on a beat-by-beat basis makes this approach ideal for studying the alterations in diastolic left ventricular function that result from acute myocardial ischemia. Labovitz,[L7,] Nishimura,[N5] Wind,[W3] and their associates all used Doppler transmitral velocity recordings to study patients with coronary artery disease during percutaneous transluminal coronary angioplasty. Balloon inflation was accompanied by decreases in peak Doppler E velocity, the velocity decay slope, and the E/A ratio, which returned toward baseline values with deflation of the angioplasty balloon. The alterations in diastolic measures were considered to indicate abnormal ventricular relaxation and slowed diastolic filling induced (albeit reversibly) by transient myocardial ischemia.

Doppler Indices of Diastolic Performance—Caveats

Doppler measures of ventricular filling velocities, rates, and volumes provide a physiologic assessment that otherwise is not readily available. However, recent work by a number of investigators shows several notable limitations and suggests that Doppler measures of diastolic function should be used cautiously.

Influence of Sampling Site

The pattern of transmitral velocities during diastole varies significantly with the site of sampling (Fig. 20–11). Pulsed-wave Doppler studies show that mitral E and A peak velocities are higher at the tips of the open leaflets than at the annulus level.[G10] Of course, continuous-wave Doppler records the highest instantaneous velocities throughout the cardiac cycle, so the peak E and A velocities measured by this technique might occur at different levels of the ventricular inflow tract. It seems sensible to employ pulsed-wave Doppler to record the ventricular filling pattern and use anatomic landmarks to establish the site of sampling; this approach would facilitate meaningful serial comparisons and would be requisite for volumetric flow measures. Unfortunately, some studies of diastolic function have used Doppler recordings at the annulus level,[F3, F4, M7, P3, R5] whereas others have recorded at the leaflet tips.[P4, T2] There is no consensus as to what recording site is "correct."

Influence of Age

The transmitral diastolic velocity pattern also appears to vary with the age of the subjects being studied.[B10, K2, M6, P3, S14] In young normal individuals the early rapid filling peak is large and dominates the atrial filling peak (Fig. 20–12), so the E/A velocity and integral ratios exceed unity. When older clinically normal subjects are studied, however, the E/A velocity and integral ratios decrease, and in normal individuals in their late sixties and older, E/A ratios typically are less than one. Since what is "normal" for an elderly subject may be "abnormal" for a young subject, Doppler diastolic indices must be interpreted in light of the age of the patient.

Influence of Respiratory Cycle

During inspiration, venous return to the right heart is augmented and left ventricular filling and stroke volume are reduced. Hence, inspiratory decreases in early diastolic peak mitral flow velocities and intervals have been reported.[D7] Although the magnitude of these changes usually is small, it appears sensible to standardize the phase of the respiratory cycle at which ventricular filling velocities are measured.

Influence of Heart Rate

Diastolic Doppler velocities are to some extent affected by changes in heart rate.[H11, P5] At relatively slow heart rates, a distinct period of diastasis is noted in mid-diastole. During this time, the atrioventricular gradient is minimal and transmitral velocities are very low. The late diastolic A velocity increase starts from a near-zero baseline. As heart rate increases, the period of diastasis becomes shorter and eventually ends, so the late-diastolic increase in velocity due to atrial contraction begins on the descending limb of the rapid filling wave (Fig. 20–13). At extremely rapid heart rates, the E and A components of the Doppler curve may, in fact, be superimposed. Thus, all other influences being equal,

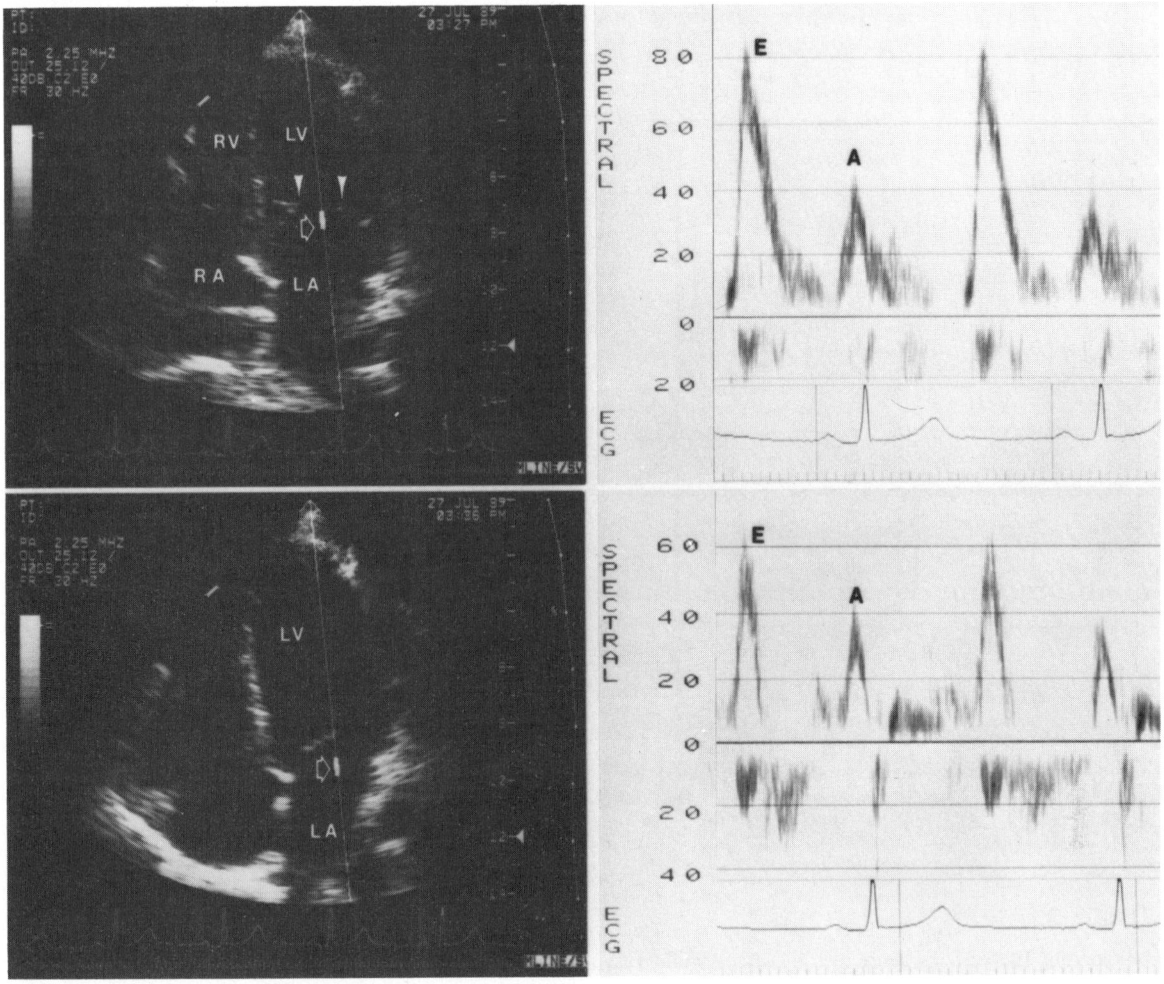

Figure 20–11. Left ventricular filling in a normal 30-year-old woman, recorded with pulsed-wave Doppler. *Top panels,* Leaflet tips level. *Left,* Diastolic freeze-frame, apical four-chamber plane. The tips of the open mitral leaflets are indicated by solid arrowheads. The Doppler sample volume *(open arrow)* is positioned at the level of the mitral leaflet tips. Abbreviations as in Figure 20–1. *Right,* Graphic output demonstrating normal early (E) and atrial systolic (A) maximum velocities. *Bottom panels,* Annular level. *Left,* Diastolic freeze-frame, apical four-chamber plane. The Doppler sample volume *(open arrow)* now is positioned just to the ventricular side of the mitral annulus. *Right,* Graphic output shows (compared to the leaflet tip level) a lower peak E velocity, a lower E/A ratio, and a shortened deceleration time. While the values are still normal, they do demonstrate the importance of selecting a standardized sampling site for comparing data from patient to patient or from study to study in the same individual.

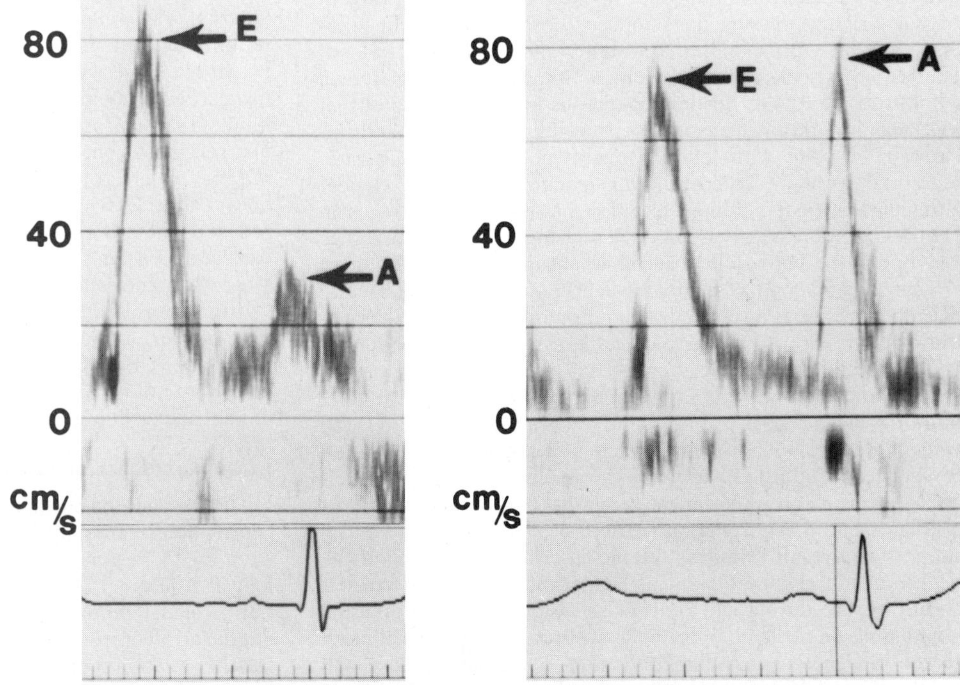

Figure 20–12. Left ventricular filling velocities, recorded at the level of the mitral leaflet tips (apical examining window) with pulsed-wave Doppler. *Left,* Velocity curve from a 25-year-old woman with normal left ventricular systolic and diastolic function, demonstrating dominance of the rapid filling peak, a small atrial systolic velocity, and an E/A ratio well in excess of 1. *Right,* Velocity curve from a 69-year-old man with normal ventricular function, demonstrating a prominent atrial component and an E/A ratio less than 1. This pattern is *not* abnormal for patients in their mid-sixties or older.

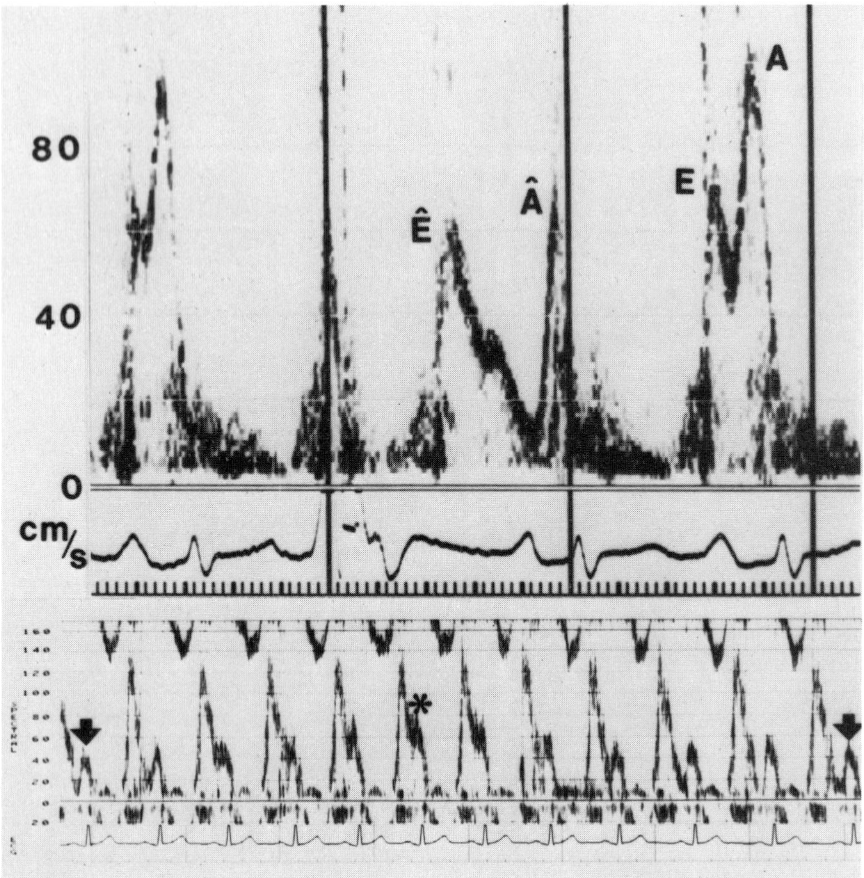

Figure 20–13. Left ventricular filling velocities, recorded at the level of the mitral leaflet tips (apical examining window) with pulsed-wave Doppler. *Top*, Velocity curve from a 79-year-old man with aortic stenosis (valve area, 0.6 cm^2; mean transvalvular gradient, 70 mmHg). The first and fourth diastolic periods show a dominant atrial velocity of 100 cm/sec, a depressed E/A ratio, and a deceleration time of 220 msec. The second diastolic period is interrupted by a ventricular premature contraction, following which the third diastolic period shows compensatory prolongation, with an Ê velocity that decays to zero, an Â velocity of 68 cm/sec, and an Ê/Â ratio that is normal for age. *Bottom*, Velocity curve from a 42-year-old man with mitral prolapse and moderate mitral regurgitation. The condensed record shows sinus arrhythmia probably related to the respiratory cycle. At longer R-R intervals (approximately 800 msec, first and last complexes), there is diastasis prior to atrial contraction, and peak A velocity is 50 cm/sec *(dark arrows)*. At shorter R-R intervals (630 msec, middle of record), there is no diastasis; atrial contraction augments the residual mid-diastolic velocity so that peak A velocity is 80 cm/sec *(asterisk)*. Since E velocity remains relatively constant throughout, E/A ratios vary inversely with heart rate although ventricular diastolic properties presumably do not change.

Doppler A velocities increase as heart rate increases while E/A ratios decrease (Fig. 20–13, bottom).

Influence of Left Atrial Pressure

Transmitral flow velocities reflect atrioventricular driving pressure. The relation between the left atrial–left ventricular pressure difference and transmitral flow velocity probably does not correspond exactly to the simplified Bernoulli equation ($\Delta P = 4v^2$) because the effects of flow acceleration, inertial forces, and viscous friction are not negligible in relation to the small pressure differences present. Nonetheless, the net instantaneous atrioventricular driving pressure does appear to exert a significant influence on the corresponding transmitral flow velocity. Indeed, Ishida and associates[I3] used volume infusion and angiotensin administration to alter loading conditions in dogs and found that the maximum atrioventricular pressure difference correlated linearly ($r = 0.90$) with left ventricular peak rapid filling rate, measured with implanted electromagnetic flowmeters. Hence, although ventricular filling velocities may vary with changes in ventricular properties, simultaneous changes in atrial pressure can modify the net result to an important degree.

This phenomenon is evident when abnormal left ventricular diastolic function is associated with mitral regurgitation. Consider the patient with hypertrophic cardiomyopathy and abnormal ventricular filling as a consequence. Pulsed Doppler echocardiographic and radionuclide angiographic studies have shown that blunting of the peak rapid filling wave, prolongation of the velocity decay slope, and augmentation of the atrial contribution to ventricular filling can be expected in this situation.[B9, K2, M7, P3, S12, T2] However, it is important to recall that many of these patients also have mitral regurgitation because of deformity of submitral support as a result of mitral systolic anterior motion. When the degree of mitral regurgitation is significant, the increase in left atrial pressure during late ventricular systole may be substantial (depending on atrial compliance as well as regurgitant volume). In the presence of mitral regurgitation, left atrial pressure will be elevated at the point of atrioventricular pressure crossover at the beginning of diastole. Even if the decline of ventricular pressure is slow as a result of delayed relaxation, the net effect often is an increase in the maximum net atrioventricular pressure difference, so the peak rapid filling rate is maintained or even increased[T2] in these patients (Fig. 20–14).

Conversely, as demonstrated by Choong and associates in patients[C9] as well as experimental animals,[C10] ventricular rapid filling velocities may decrease as a result of lowered atrial pressure when preload is decreased by nitroglycerin therapy. In this circumstance, a lowered E velocity and a depressed E/A ratio might erroneously be taken as evidence that diastolic ventricular function was abnormal. The complexity of the relation between rapid filling rate and ventricular relaxation has been emphasized by Morgan and associates,[M8] who studied the effects of transient myocardial ischemia on ventricular relaxation and ventricular filling. Transient myocardial ischemia did lead to slowed ventricular relaxation, but it also caused an increase in left atrial pressure at pressure crossover. Hence, although the ventricular pressure decay slope was prolonged, the peak rapid filling rate was *not* reduced but was slightly enhanced by Doppler measures. Stoddard and associates[S15] and Levine and Thomas[L9] also have emphasized that coexisting alterations in preload may mask slowed ventricular relaxation, so that early diastolic ventricular *filling* may appear to be normal even when ventricular *function* is abnormal. These findings emphasize the need to consider the important influence of left atrial pressure in interpreting measures of ventricular filling (Fig. 20–15).

Influence of Atrioventricular Sequence

The preceding considerations indicate that the timing of atrial contraction relative to the preceding rapid filling period will also alter the A velocity and E/A ratio.[F5, H9, P5] In the presence of a long P-R interval, A velocity will be augmented if atrial contraction occurs before diastasis begins. In second-degree or third-degree atrioventricular block, both E and A velocities will depend on the relation between atrial and ventricular contraction. If atrial activation and contraction occur during ventricular systole,

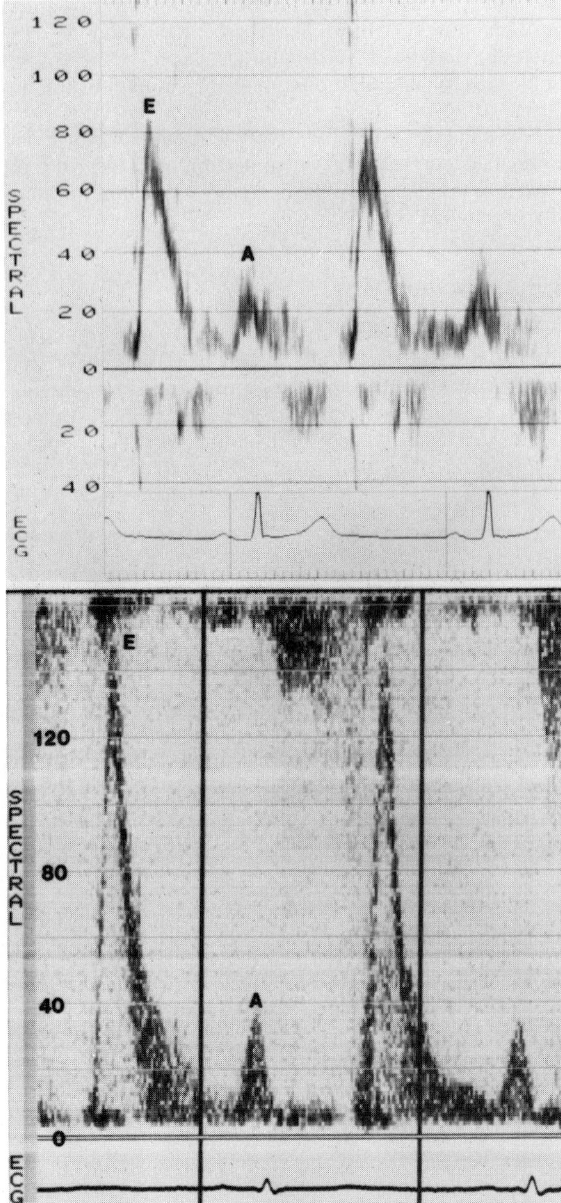

Figure 20–14. Left ventricular filling velocities, recorded at the level of the mitral leaflet tips (apical examining window) with pulsed-wave Doppler. *Top*, Velocity curve from a normal 25-year-old woman. The E velocity is dominant, deceleration time is 200 msec, and the E/A ratio is normal. *Bottom*, Velocity curve from a 56-year-old man with moderate mitral regurgitation and diffuse left ventricular systolic dysfunction (coronary artery disease and aortic stenosis requiring aortic valve replacement). Peak E velocity is increased at 150 cm/sec, E/A ratio is higher than normal, and deceleration time is short at 110 msec, even though diastolic ventricular function probably is abnormal.

the atrioventricular gradient at mitral valve opening will increase and so will the peak E velocity during the ensuing rapid filling period. If atrial contraction occurs before rapid filling has ended, the A velocity will be augmented (see Fig. 20–13). If the timing of atrial contraction is delayed into very late diastole, just preceding ventricular contraction, the A velocity might be decreased by virtue of the concomitant rise in end-diastolic ventricular pressure.

Clearly, the multiple factors that influence diastolic ventricular filling require careful consideration in interpreting the significance of transmitral Doppler velocities. An abnormal filling curve probably denotes abnormal diastolic performance. However, in an individual patient, a normal-appearing filling curve should not be considered as solid evidence that diastolic ventricular function is normal.

ASSESSMENT OF RIGHT VENTRICULAR EJECTION

The Doppler techniques used to evaluate left ventricular systolic function can be adapted to assess global right ventricular performance during systole.

Measures of Interest

Both pulsed-wave and continuous-wave Doppler can be used to record ejection velocities in the right ventricular outflow tract

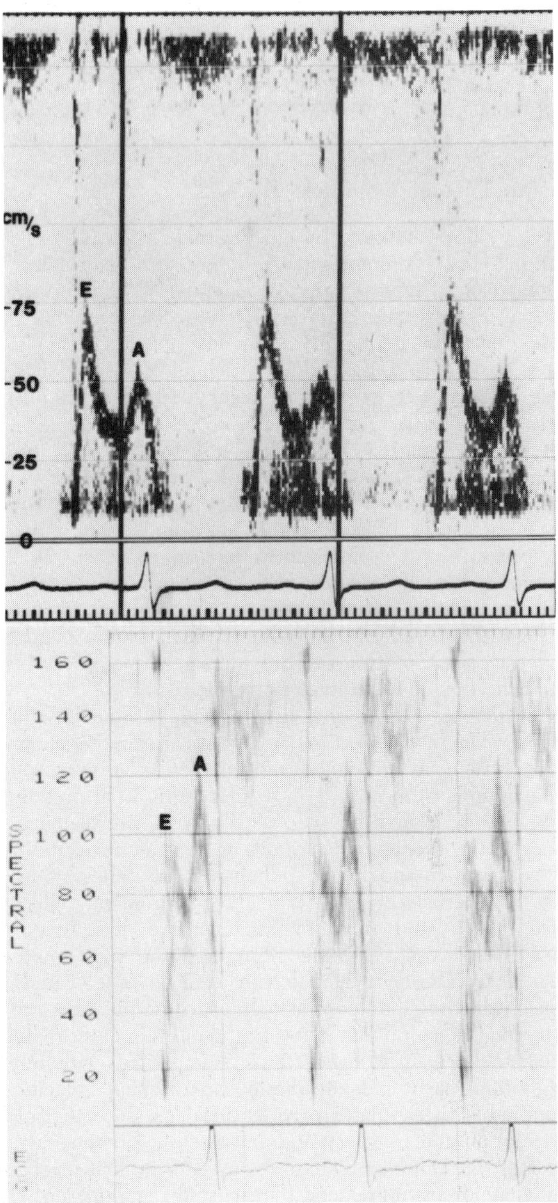

Figure 20–15. Left ventricular filling velocities in a 59-year-old man with aortic stenosis (valve area, 1.0 cm^2; mean transvalvular gradient, 70 mmHg), mild mitral stenosis, and moderate mitral regurgitation leading to concentric ventricular hypertrophy, ventricular enlargement, and pulmonary hypertension (systolic peak pressure, 45 mmHg). Systolic ventricular function is normal. Velocity curves recorded at the level of the mitral valve tips (apical examining window) with pulsed-wave Doppler. *Top*, Preoperative record showing a normal filling pattern. *Bottom*, Postoperative record after replacement of both aortic and mitral valves, regression of ventricular hypertrophy, normalization of ventricular size and pulmonary pressure, and preservation of systolic ventricular function. Despite these favorable hemodynamic changes, the velocity curve shows an augmented A velocity and "reversal" of the E/A ratio. It is likely that diastolic ventricular function was abnormal, preoperatively as well as postoperatively, but that the simultaneous influence of mitral regurgitation caused "pseudo-normalization" of the preoperative curve that was unmasked after insertion of a competent mitral prosthesis.

and main pulmonary artery. Measures of systolic flow velocity, acceleration, and deceleration, as well as systolic time intervals and velocity-time integrals, provide useful insight into global ventricular function. By combining measures of anatomic diameter and velocity-time integral recorded in the proximal pulmonary artery, right ventricular stroke volume can be determined noninvasively.[G1, S2, V2] A similar approach can be applied to diameter and velocity-time integral measures proximal to the pulmonic valve,[M9] high in the right ventricular outflow tract. Several groups of investigators compared echo-Doppler measures of right and left ventricular stroke volume in children and adults with intracardiac shunts and found these measures to provide pulmonary/systemic flow ratios that compared favorably with those determined by invasive procedures.[B11, D8, K3, S2, V2]

Associated Hemodynamics

Acceleration of flow by the ejecting right ventricle provides a useful marker of pulmonary artery pressure. Normally, peak ejection velocity typically occurs in mid-systole (approximately 120 msec or more after the onset of ejection), and the systolic velocity curve has a smoothly "rounded" appearance. With pulmonary hypertension, the right ventricle develops pressure more quickly, so peak ejection velocity occurs earlier in systole and an early systolic "spike" appears in the velocity curve.[D9] When pulmonary acceleration time (from onset to peak velocity) is 60 msec or shorter, substantial pulmonary hypertension can be inferred. Several investigators have reported inverse relations between measures of acceleration time and mean pulmonary artery pressure,[D9, I4, K4] although there is no consensus about the ideal site for velocity recording, the need to normalize for heart rate or pre-ejection period, or the merits of expressing pressure on a logarithmic rather than a linear scale. Many investigators consider acceleration times to provide a semiquantitative assessment of the range of pulmonary artery pressure.

Other Doppler techniques can provide further insight into pulmonary hemodynamics. When tricuspid regurgitation is present, peak tricuspid regurgitant velocity can be used to compute the maximum systolic right ventricular–right atrial pressure difference.[B12, C11, Y1] When coupled with an estimate of mean right atrial pressure, this approach yields an accurate measure of peak right ventricular (and hence pulmonary arterial) systolic pressure.[C11, Y1] Alternatively, the time interval from pulmonic valve closure to tricuspid valve opening can be determined from Doppler velocity curves; this represents the right ventricular isovolumic relaxation time. In the absence of elevated atrial pressure, this time lengthens as pulmonary systolic pressure rises and it can be combined with heart rate to determine peak pulmonary systolic pressure.[H12] Finally, in patients with pulmonic regurgitation, early and end-diastolic regurgitant velocities can be coupled with estimates of right atrial pressure to yield (respectively) pulmonary mean and end-diastolic pressures.[M10]

Most of the Doppler techniques used to evaluate right-sided hemodynamics are influenced by tricuspid regurgitation. Determination of the peak right ventricular–right atrial pressure difference requires the presence of enough tricuspid regurgitation for its maximum velocity to be recorded accurately. When substantial tricuspid regurgitation is present, mean right atrial pressure is elevated. This affects the calculation of right-sided pressures regardless of whether tricuspid regurgitant velocity, right ventricular isovolumic relaxation time, or pulmonic regurgitant velocity data are used. Thus, the severity of tricuspid regurgitation must be considered in using Doppler methods to assess right-sided hemodynamics. Pulsed-wave and color flow Doppler techniques can be used to determine the spatial distribution of regurgitant signals within the right atrium[M11, S16]; localized signals imply mild regurgitation, and widespread signals indicate severe regurgitation. Assessment of the systolic flow velocity pattern in the hepatic vein[P6, S17] also may be helpful. Normally, the middle hepatic vein empties into the right atrium during ventricular systole. This systolic pattern is blunted by moderate tricuspid regurgitation, and severe regurgitation causes frank reversal of systolic flow (implying a large regurgitant volume) in the hepatic veins (Fig. 20–16).

Although all of these Doppler approaches for studying tricuspid and pulmonary flow do have shortcomings, they do permit noninvasive assessment of right heart hemodynamics in the large majority of patients.[C12]

Clinical Applications

Doppler measures of global right ventricular function have been reported infrequently but should in theory prove valuable in a number of situations. For example, measurement of right ventricular ejection fraction from two-dimensional echocardiographic images can be accomplished,[L10] but this approach is

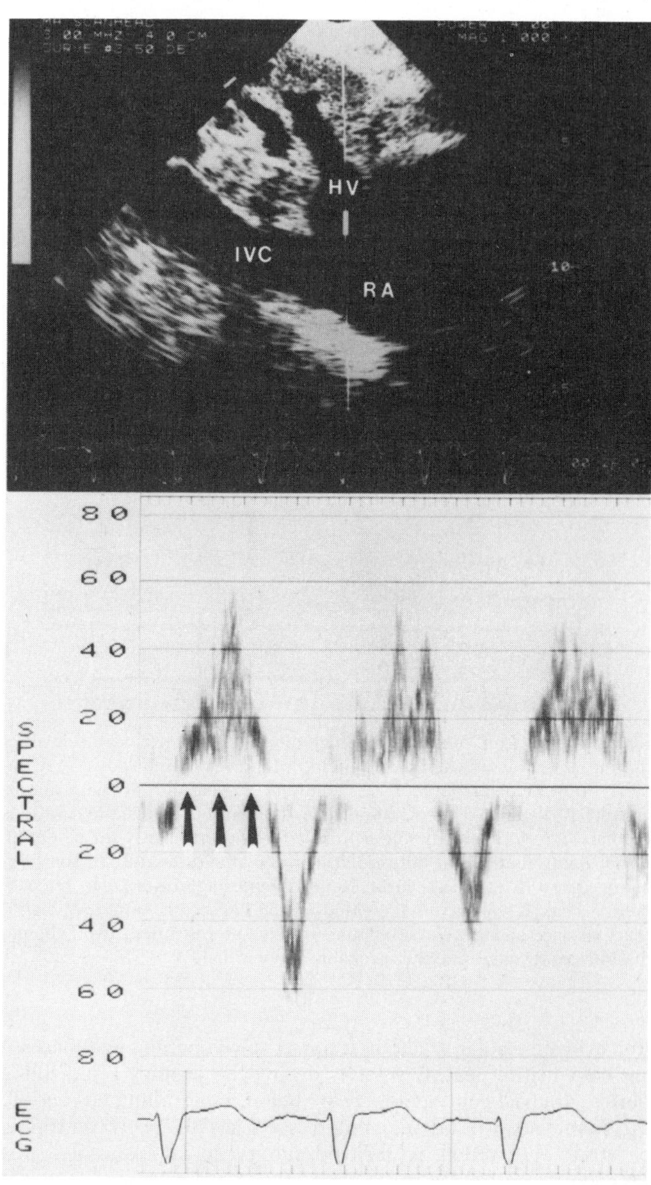

Figure 20–16. Right atrial filling velocities from a 71-year-old man with pulmonary hypertension and right ventricular failure. *Top*, Velocity curve recorded (subcostal examining window) from the middle hepatic vein (HV), near its junction with the right atrium (RA), by pulsed-wave Doppler. IVC—inferior vena cava. *Bottom*, Velocity record shows reversed systolic flow *(arrows)* upward into the hepatic vein, followed by diastolic flow out of the hepatic veins and through the right atrium into the right ventricle. Systolic reversal of flow into the systemic veins denotes significant tricuspid regurgitation.

rendered difficult by the shape of the right ventricle, which does not lend itself to simple geometric formulas for volume computation. It might be possible to use Doppler measures to define global right ventricular systolic performance and use this approach to detect and study the functional consequences of right ventricular infarction or to assess right ventricular decompensation in patients with pulmonary hypertension. Measures of relative right and left ventricular stroke volumes have proved useful in the assessment of shunt size in children and adults with atrial septal defect,[B11, S2, V2] and similar approaches can be used for other shunt lesions.[B11, S4] Doppler measures of pulmonary artery pressure are valuable in judging the significance of mitral valve disease and the suitability of patients with severe heart failure as potential cardiac transplant recipients, among other potential clinical applications.

ASSESSMENT OF RIGHT VENTRICULAR FILLING

Doppler measures of ventricular filling have been used largely in connection with left ventricular disorders because of their relatively high prevalence in adults with heart disease, but similar approaches permit assessment of right ventricular diastolic function.

Measures of Interest

Doppler velocities, time intervals, and velocity-time integrals can be measured from recordings made at the level of the tricuspid valve leaflets and annulus with either pulsed-wave or continuous-wave techniques and either apical or precordial examining windows. When coupled with tricuspid annular diameter, tricuspid flow velocities can be used to compute peak filling rate as well as stroke volume. These measures have been discussed above in relation to left ventricular filling.

Clinical Applications

Abnormal Doppler right ventricular filling patterns have been reported in right ventricular infarction,[F3, 15] and abnormal patterns presumably would occur if right ventricular distensibility were reduced by hypertrophy or infiltrative processes. The influence of confounding variables such as age, heart rate, atrioventricular sequence, and right atrial pressure has not yet been investigated. However, it seems reasonable to expect that these variables will influence right as well as left ventricular filling, as described earlier.

SUMMARY

Doppler recordings of flow velocity during ventricular ejection and filling provide an attractive means of quantitating ventricular function during both systole and diastole. The technique is completely noninvasive, atraumatic, and well suited to serial studies. The necessary equipment is widely available and relatively inexpensive compared to the equipment used for other cardiac imaging modalities. Acceptance by patients is excellent. Doppler blood flow velocities provide a direct means of measuring the time course, rate, and volume of ventricular emptying and filling. Cardiac function can be evaluated by Doppler echocardiographic techniques in outpatients as well as inpatients, at basal state, and during interventions. Thus, this approach is well suited for use in studying a wide variety of cardiac disorders.

However, although the concept of "evaluating cardiac function" sounds deceptively simple, ventricular systole and diastole are quite complex. Thus, it probably is naive to expect to use relatively simple Doppler measures to define ventricular function without considering the hemodynamic context in which these measures are obtained. Systolic performance varies not only with the state of the ventricle but also with loading conditions (especially afterload), which may change significantly from moment to moment. Other clinical and hemodynamic variables, such as age and heart rate, also exert an influence on some systolic performance indices. Diastolic measures likewise vary with age, heart rate, atrioventricular sequence, and loading conditions (especially preload). Using Doppler data to assess cardiac function requires several assumptions: that blood flow is relatively laminar and blunt in profile, that the cross-sectional area filled by flow is relatively constant, and that the direction of blood flow is stable during the cardiac cycle as well as relatively coaxial with the examining ultrasound beam. Although reasonable, these assumptions are not always *strictly* true. Also, Doppler measures of global function cannot demonstrate regional abnormalities. Finally, it is difficult to judge the "true" accuracy of Doppler measures, since the available reference standard methods have their own technical limitations.

Although much remains to be learned about the various factors that influence systolic and diastolic cardiac function and how these factors alter ventricular ejection and filling velocities, Doppler techniques hold great promise for evaluating patients with cardiac disease. Functional abnormalities are prevalent in a great number of disorders and cause clinical symptoms and signs. A practical way to detect, quantitate, and follow these abnormalities during treatment would have considerable clinical benefit. It seems reasonable to expect Doppler echocardiographic techniques to fill that role.

References

A

1. Appleton, C. P., Hatle, L. K., and Popp, R. L.: Relation of transmitral flow velocity patterns to left ventricular diastolic function: New insights from a combined hemodynamic and Doppler echocardiographic study. J. Am. Coll. Cardiol. 12:426, 1988.

B

1. Bouchard, A., Blumlein, S., Schiller, N. B., et al.: Measurement of left ventricular stroke volume using continuous wave Doppler echocardiography of the ascending aorta and M-mode echocardiography of the aortic valve. J. Am. Coll. Cardiol. 9:75, 1987.
2. Bargiggia, G. S., Bertucci, C., Recusani, F., et al.: A new method for calculation of left ventricular dP/dt by continuous wave Doppler-echocardiography: Validation studies at cardiac catheterization. Circulation 80:1287, 1989.
3. Bruce, R. A., Blackmon, J. R., Jones, J. W., and Strait, G.: Exercise testing in adult normal subjects and cardiac patients. Paediatrics 32:742, 1963.
4. Bennett, E. D., Barclay, S. A., Davis, A. L., et al.: Ascending aorta blood velocity and acceleration using Doppler ultrasound in the assessment of left ventricular function. Cardiovasc. Res. 18:632, 1984.
5. Berk, M. R., Evans, J., Knapp, C., et al.: Influence of alterations in loading produced by lower body negative pressure on aortic blood flow acceleration. J. Am. Coll. Cardiol. 15:1069, 1990.
6. Bryg, R. J., Labovitz, A. J., Mehdirad, A. A., et al.: Effect of coronary artery disease on Doppler-derived parameters of aortic flow during upright exercise. Am. J. Cardiol. 58:14, 1986.
7. Bonow, R. O., Bacharach, S. L., Green, M. V., et al.: Impaired left ventricular diastolic filling in patients with coronary artery disease: Assessment with radionuclide angiography. Circulation 64:315, 1981.
8. Bonow, R. O., Vitale, D. F., Maron, B. J., et al.: Regional left ventricular asynchrony and impaired global left ventricular filling in hypertrophic cardiomyopathy: Effect of verapamil. J. Am. Coll. Cardiol. 9:1108, 1987.
9. Bryg, R. J., Pearson, A. C., Williams, G. A., and Labovitz, A. J.: Left ventricular systolic and diastolic flow abnormalities determined by Doppler echocardiography in obstructive hypertrophic cardiomyopathy. Am. J. Cardiol. 59:925, 1987.
10. Bryg, R. J., Williams, G. A., and Labovitz, A. J.: Effect of aging on left ventricular diastolic filling in normal subjects. Am. J. Cardiol. 59:971, 1987.
11. Barron, J. V., Sahn, D. J., Valdes-Cruz, L. M., et al.: Clinical utility of two-dimensional Doppler echocardiographic techniques for estimating pulmonary to systemic blood flow ratios in children with left to right shunting atrial septal defect, ventricular septal defect or patent ductus arteriosus. J. Am. Coll. Cardiol. 3:169, 1984.
12. Berger, M., Haimowitz, A., Van Tosh, A., et al.: Quantitative assessment of pulmonary hypertension in patients with tricuspid regurgitation using continuous wave Doppler ultrasound. J. Am. Coll. Cardiol. 6:359, 1985.

C

1. Cross, G., and Light, L. H.: Non-invasive intra-thoracic blood velocity measurement in the assessment of cardiovascular function. Biomed. Eng. 9:464, 1974.
2. Colocousis, J. S., Huntsman, L. L., and Curreri, P. W.: Estimation of stroke volume changes by ultrasonic Doppler. Circulation 56:914, 1977.
3. Callahan, M. J., Tajik, A. J., Su-Fan, Q., and Bove, A. A.: Validation of

instantaneous pressure gradients measured by continuous-wave Doppler in experimentally induced aortic stenosis. Am. J. Cardiol. 56:989, 1985.
4. Chandraratna, P. A., Nanna, M., McKay, C., et al.: Determination of cardiac output by transcutaneous continuous-wave ultrasonic Doppler computer. Am. J. Cardiol. 53:234, 1984.
5. Cordoba, M., Pai, R. G., Bansal, R. C., and Shah, P. M.: Comparisons of Doppler derived rate of left ventricular pressure rise with traditional echocardiographic parameters of left ventricular function. (Abstract.) Circulation 78(Suppl. II):II-549, 1988.
6. Croft, C. H., Lipscomb, K., Mathis, K., et al.: Limitations of qualitative angiographic grading in aortic or mitral regurgitation. Am. J. Cardiol. 53:1593, 1984.
7. Chandraratna, P. A. N., Silveira, B., and Aronow, W. S.: Assessment of left ventricular function by determination of maximum acceleration of blood flow in the aorta using continuous Doppler ultrasound. Am. J. Cardiol. 45:398, 1980.
8. Christie, J., Sheldahl, L. M., Tristani, F. E., et al.: Determination of stroke volume and cardiac output during exercise: Comparison of two-dimensional and Doppler echocardiography, Fick oximetry, and thermodilution. Circulation 76:539, 1987.
9. Choong, C. Y., Herrmann, H. C., Weyman, A. E., and Fifer, M. A.: Preload dependence of Doppler-derived indexes of left ventricular diastolic function in humans. J. Am. Coll. Cardiol. 10:800, 1987.
10. Choong, C. Y., Abascal, V. M., Thomas, J. D., et al.: Combined influence of ventricular loading and relaxation on the transmitral flow velocity profile in dogs measured by Doppler echocardiography. Circulation 78:672, 1988.
11. Currie, P. J., Seward, J. B., Chan, K.-L., et al.: Continuous wave Doppler determination of right ventricular pressure: A simultaneous Doppler-catheterization study in 127 patients. J. Am. Coll. Cardiol. 5:750, 1985.
12. Chan, K.-L., Currie, P. J., Seward, J. B., et al.: Comparison of three Doppler ultrasound methods in the prediction of pulmonary artery pressure. J. Am. Coll. Cardiol. 9:549, 1987.

D

1. Daley, P. J., Sagar, K. B., and Wann, L. S.: Supine versus upright exercise: Doppler echocardiographic measurement of ascending aortic flow velocity. Br. Heart J. 54:562, 1985.
2. Daley, P. J., Sagar, K. B., Collier, B. D., et al.: Detection of exercise induced changes in left ventricular performance by Doppler echocardiography. Br. Heart J. 58:447, 1987.
3. DeMaria, A. N., and Wisenbaugh, T.: Identification and treatment of diastolic dysfunction: Role of transmitral Doppler recordings. J. Am. Coll. Cardiol. 9:1106, 1987.
4. Dodek, A., Kassenbaum, D. G., and Bristow, J. D.: Pulmonary edema in coronary artery disease without cardiomegaly. N. Engl. J. Med. 25:1347, 1972.
5. Dougherty, A. M., Naccarelli, G. V., Gray, E. L., et al.: Congestive heart failure with normal systolic function. Am. J. Cardiol. 54:778, 1984.
6. de Zuttere, D., Touche, T., Saumon, G., et al.: Doppler echocardiographic measurement of mitral flow volume: Validation of a new method in adult patients. J. Am. Coll. Cardiol. 11:343, 1988.
7. Dabestani, A., Takenaka, K., Allen, B., et al.: Effects of spontaneous respiration on diastolic left ventricular filling assessed by pulsed Doppler echocardiography. Am. J. Cardiol. 61:1356, 1988.
8. Dittmann, H., Jacksch, R., Voelker, W., et al.: Accuracy of Doppler echocardiography in quantification of left to right shunts in adult patients with atrial septal defect. J. Am. Coll. Cardiol. 11:338, 1988.
9. Dabestani, A., Mahan, G., Gardin, J. M., et al.: Evaluation of pulmonary artery pressure and resistance by pulsed Doppler echocardiography. Am. J. Cardiol. 59:662, 1987.

E

1. Elkayam, U., Gardin, J. M., Berkley, R., et al.: The use of Doppler flow velocity measurement to assess hemodynamic response to vasodilators in patients with heart failure. Circulation 67:377, 1983.

F

1. Franklin, D. L., Schlegel, W., and Rushmer, R. F.: Blood flow measured by Doppler frequency shift of backscattered ultrasound. Science 134:564, 1961.
2. Fisher, D. C., Sahn, D. J., Friedman, M. J., et al.: The mitral valve orifice method for noninvasive two-dimensional echo Doppler determinations of cardiac output. Circulation 67:872, 1983.
3. Fujii, J., Yazaki, Y., Sawada, H., et al.: Noninvasive assessment of left and right ventricular filling in myocardial infarction with a two-dimensional Doppler echocardiographic method. J. Am. Coll. Cardiol. 5:1155, 1985.
4. Friedman, B. J., Drinkovic, N., Miles, H., et al.: Assessment of left ventricular diastolic function: Comparison of Doppler echocardiography and gated blood pool scintigraphy. J. Am. Coll. Cardiol. 8:1348, 1986.
5. Freedman, R. A., Yock, P. G., Echt, D. S., and Popp, R. L.: Effect of variation in PQ interval on patterns of atrioventricular valve motion and flow in patients with normal ventricular function. J. Am. Coll. Cardiol. 7:595, 1986.

G

1. Goldberg, S. J., Sahn, D. J., Allen, H. D., et al.: Evaluation of pulmonary and systemic blood flow by 2-dimensional Doppler echocardiography using fast Fourier transform spectral analysis. Am. J. Cardiol. 50:1394, 1982.
2. Gardin, J. M., Tobis, J. M., Dabestani, A., et al.: Superiority of two-dimensional measurement of aortic vessel diameter in Doppler echocardiographic estimates of left ventricular stroke volume. J. Am. Coll. Cardiol. 6:66, 1985.
3. Ganz, W., Donoso, R., Marcus, H. S., et al.: A new technique for measurement of cardiac output by thermodilution in man. Am. J. Cardiol. 27:392, 1971.
4. Gardin, J. M., Iseri, L. E., Elkayam, U., et al.: Evaluation of dilated cardiomyopathy by pulsed Doppler echocardiography. Am. Heart J. 106:1057, 1983.
5. Goldschlager, N., Selzer, A., and Cohn, K.: Treadmill stress tests as indicators of presence and severity of coronary artery disease. Ann. Intern. Med. 85:277, 1976.
6. Gardin, J. M., Kozlowski, J., Dabestani, A., et al.: Studies of Doppler aortic flow velocity during supine bicycle exercise. Am. J. Cardiol. 57:327, 1986.
7. Gibson, D. G., Prewitt, T. A., and Brown, D. J.: Analysis of left ventricular wall movement during isovolumic relaxation and its relation to coronary artery disease. Br. Heart J. 38:1010, 1976.
8. Gidding, S. S., Snider, A. R., Rocchini, A. P., et al.: Left ventricular diastolic filling in children with hypertrophic cardiomyopathy: Assessment with pulsed Doppler echocardiography. J. Am. Coll. Cardiol. 8:310, 1986.
9. Gardin, J. M., Drayer, J. I. M., Weber, M., et al.: Doppler echocardiographic assessment of left ventricular systolic and diastolic function in mild hypertension. (Abstract.) Hypertension 9 (Suppl. II):II-90, 1987.
10. Gardin, J. M., Dabestani, A., Takenaka, K., et al.: Effect of imaging view and sample volume location on evaluation of mitral flow velocity by pulsed Doppler echocardiography. Am. J. Cardiol. 57:1335, 1986.

H

1. Huntsman, L. L., Gams, E., Johnson, C. C., and Fairbanks, E.: Transcutaneous determination of aortic blood flow velocities in man. Am. Heart J. 89:605, 1975.
2. Hatle, L., Angelsen, B., and Tromsdal, A.: Noninvasive assessment of atrioventricular pressure half-time by Doppler ultrasound. Circulation 60:1096, 1979.
3. Hatle, L., Angelsen, B., and Tromsdal, A.: Non-invasive assessment of aortic stenosis by Doppler ultrasound. Br. Heart J. 43:284, 1980.
4. Huntsman, L. L., Stewart, D. K., Barnes, S. R., et al.: Noninvasive Doppler determination of cardiac output in man. Clinical validation. Circulation 67:593, 1983.
5. Hatle, L., and Angelsen, B.: Doppler Ultrasound in Cardiology—Physical Principles and Clinical Applications. 2nd ed. Lea & Febiger, Philadelphia, 1985, p. 188.
6. Hoit, B. D., Rashwan, M., Watt, C., et al.: Calculating cardiac output from transmitral volume flow using Doppler and M-mode echocardiography. Am. J. Cardiol. 62:131, 1988.
7. Hodges, M., Downs, J. B., and Mitchell, L. A.: Thermodilution and Fick cardiac index determinations following cardiac surgery. Crit. Care Med. 3:182, 1975.
8. Harrison, M. R., Smith, M.D., Nissen, S. E., et al.: Use of exercise Doppler echocardiography to evaluate cardiac drugs: Effects of propranolol and verapamil on aortic blood flow velocity and acceleration. J. Am. Coll. Cardiol. 11:1002, 1988.
9. Hammermeister, K. E., and Warbasse, J. R.: The rate of change of left ventricular volume in man. II. Diastolic events in health and disease. Circulation 49:739, 1974.
10. Hanrath, P., Mathey, D. G., Siegert, R., and Bleifeld, W.: Left ventricular relaxation and filling pattern in different forms of left ventricular hypertrophy. An echocardiographic study. Am. J. Cardiol. 45:15, 1980.
11. Herzog, C. A., Elsperger, K. J., Manoles, M., et al.: Effect of atrial pacing on left ventricular diastolic filling measured by pulsed Doppler echocardiography. (Abstract.) J. Am. Coll. Cardiol. 9 (Suppl. A):197A, 1987.
12. Hatle, L., Angelsen, B. A. J., and Tromsdal, A.: Non-invasive estimation of pulmonary artery systolic pressure with Doppler ultrasound. Br. Heart J. 45:157, 1981.

I

1. Ihlen, H., Amlie, J. P., Dale, J., et al.: Determination of cardiac output by Doppler echocardiography. Br. Heart J. 51:54, 1984.
2. Ihlen, H., Endresen, K., Golf, S., and Nitter-Hauge, S.: Cardiac stroke volume during exercise measured by Doppler echocardiography: Comparison with the thermodilution technique and evaluation of reproducibility. Br. Heart J. 58:455, 1987.
3. Ishida, Y., Meisner, J. S., Tsujioka, K., et al.: Left ventricular filling dynamics: Influence of left ventricular relaxation and left atrial pressure. Circulation 74:187, 1986.
4. Isobe, M., Yazaki, Y., Takaku, F., et al.: Prediction of pulmonary arterial pressure in adults by pulsed Doppler echocardiography. Am. J. Cardiol. 57:316, 1986.
5. Isobe, M., Yazaki, Y., Takaku, F., et al.: Right ventricular filling detected by pulsed Doppler echocardiography during the convalescent stage of inferior wall acute myocardial infarction. Am. J. Cardiol. 59:1245, 1987.

K

1. Kitabatake, A., Inoue, M., Asao, M., et al.: Transmitral blood flow reflecting diastolic behavior of the left ventricle in health and disease: A study by pulsed Doppler technique. Jpn. Circ. J. 46:92, 1982.
2. Kuo, L. C., Quinones, M. A., Rokey, R., et al.: Quantification of atrial contribution to left ventricular filling by pulsed Doppler echocardiography and the effect of age in normal and diseased hearts. Am. J. Cardiol. 59:1174, 1987.
3. Kitabatake, A., Inoue, M., Asao, M., et al.: Noninvasive evaluation of the ratio of pulmonary to systemic flow in atrial septal defect by duplex Doppler echocardiography. Circulation 69:73, 1984.
4. Kitabatake, A., Inoue, M., Asao, M., et al.: Noninvasive evaluation of pulmonary hypertension by a pulsed Doppler technique. Circulation 68:302, 1983.

L

1. Light, L. H.: Non-injurious ultrasonic technique for observing flow in the human aorta. Nature (London) 224:119, 1969.
2. Light, L. H., and Cross, G.: Cardiovascular data by transcutaneous aortovelography. *In* Roberts, C. (ed.): Blood Flow Measurement. Sector Publishing, London, 1972, p. 60.
3. Light, L. H.: Transcutaneous aortovelography—a new window on the circulation. Br. Heart J. 38:433, 1976.
4. Lewis, J. F., Kuo, L. C., Nelson, J. G., et al.: Pulsed Doppler echocardiographic determination of stroke volume and cardiac output: Clinical validation of two new methods using the apical window. Circulation 70:425, 1984.
5. Labovitz, A. J., Buckingham, T. A., Habermehl, K., et al.: The effect of sampling site on the two-dimensional echo Doppler determination of cardiac output. Am. Heart J. 109:327, 1985.
6. Loeppky, J. A., Greene, E. R., Hoekenga, E. D., et al.: Beat-by-beat stroke volume assessment by pulsed Doppler in upright and supine exercise. J. Appl. Physiol. 50:1173, 1981.
7. Labovitz, A. J., Lewen, M. K., Kern, M., et al.: Evaluation of left ventricular systolic and diastolic dysfunction during transient myocardial ischemia produced by angioplasty. J. Am. Coll. Cardiol. 10:748, 1987.
8. Labovitz, A. J., and Pearson, A. C.: Evaluation of left ventricular diastolic function: Clinical relevance and recent Doppler echocardiographic insights. Am. Heart J. 114:836, 1987.
9. Levine, R. A., and Thomas, J. D.: Insights into the physiologic significance of the mitral inflow velocity pattern. J. Am. Coll. Cardiol. 14:1718, 1989.
10. Levine, R. A., Gibson, T. C., Aretz, T., et al.: Echocardiographic measurement of right ventricular volume. Circulation 69:497, 1984.

M

1. Magnin, P. A., Stewart, J. A., Myers, S., et al.: Combined Doppler and phased array echocardiographic estimation of cardiac output. Circulation 63:388, 1981.
2. Marx, G. R., Hicks, R. W., Allen, H. D., and Kinzer, S. M.: Measurement of cardiac output and exercise factor by pulsed Doppler echocardiography during supine bicycle ergometry in normal young adolescent boys. J. Am. Coll. Cardiol. 10:430, 1987.
3. Maeda, M., Yokota, M., Iwase, M., et al.: Accuracy of cardiac output measured by continuous wave Doppler echocardiography during dynamic exercise testing in the supine position in patients with coronary artery disease. J. Am. Coll. Cardiol. 13:76, 1989.
4. Mehta, N., Bennett, D., Mannering, D., et al.: Usefulness of noninvasive Doppler measurement of ascending aortic blood velocity and acceleration in detecting impairment of the left ventricular functional response to exercise three weeks after acute myocardial infarction. Am. J. Cardiol. 58:879, 1986.
5. Mehdirad, A. A., Williams, G. A., Labovitz, A. J., et al.: Evaluation of left ventricular function during upright exercise: Correlation of exercise Doppler with postexercise two-dimensional echocardiographic results. Circulation 75:413, 1987.
6. Miyatake, K., Okamoto, M., Kinoshita, N., et al.: Augmentation of atrial contribution to left ventricular inflow with aging as assessed by intracardiac Doppler flowmetry. Am. J. Cardiol. 53:586, 1984.
7. Maron, B. J., Spirito, P., Green, K. J., et al.: Noninvasive assessment of left ventricular diastolic function by pulsed Doppler echocardiography in patients with hypertrophic cardiomyopathy. J. Am. Coll. Cardiol. 10:733, 1987.
8. Morgan, D. E., Pearlman, A. S., Otto, C. M., et al.: Enhanced Doppler peak rapid filling rate despite delayed ventricular relaxation post-ischemia: Influence of atrial pressure (Abstract.) Circulation 78(Suppl. II):II-114, 1988.
9. Meijboom, E. J., Valdes-Cruz, L. M., Horowitz, S., et al.: A two-dimensional Doppler echocardiographic method for calculation of pulmonary and systemic blood flow in a canine model with a variable-sized left-to-right extracardiac shunt. Circulation 68:437, 1983.
10. Masuyama, T., Kodama, K., Kitabatake, A., et al.: Continuous-wave Doppler echocardiographic detection of pulmonary regurgitation and its application to noninvasive estimation of pulmonary artery pressure. Circulation 74:484, 1986.
11. Miyatake, K., Okamoto, M., Kinoshita, N., et al.: Evaluation of tricuspid regurgitation by pulsed Doppler and two-dimensional echocardiography. Circulation 66:777, 1982.

N

1. Nishimura, R. A., Callahan, M. J., Schaff, H. V., et al.: Noninvasive measurement of cardiac output by continuous-wave Doppler echocardiography: Initial experience and review of the literature. Mayo Clin. Proc. 59:484, 1984.
2. Noble, M. I. M., Trenchard, D., and Guz, A.: Left ventricular ejection in conscious dogs—measurement and significance of the maximum acceleration of blood from the left ventricle. Circ. Res. 19:139, 1966.
3. Nishimura, R. A., Housmans, P. R., Hatle, L. K., and Tajik, A. J.: Assessment of diastolic function of the heart: Background and current applications of Doppler echocardiography. Part I. Physiologic and pathophysiologic features. Mayo Clin. Proc. 64:71, 1989.
4. Nishimura, R. A., Abel, M. D., Hatle, L. K., and Tajik, A. J.: Assessment of diastolic function of the heart: Background and current applications of Doppler echocardiography. II. Clinical studies. Mayo Clin. Proc. 64:181, 1989.
5. Nishimura, R. A., Holmes, D. R., Jr., Reeder, G. S., et al.: Doppler echocardiographic observations during percutaneous aortic balloon valvuloplasty. J. Am. Coll. Cardiol. 11:1219, 1988.

O

1. Otto, C. M., Pearlman, A. S., Comess, K. A., et al.: Determination of the stenotic aortic valve area in adults using Doppler echocardiography. J. Am. Coll. Cardiol. 7:509, 1986.
2. Otto, C. M., Pearlman, A. S., and Amsler, L. C.: Doppler echocardiographic evaluation of left ventricular diastolic filling in isolated valvular aortic stenosis. Am. J. Cardiol. 63:313, 1989.
3. Ormiston, J. A., Shah, P. M., Tei, C., and Wong, M.: Size and motion of the mitral valve annulus in man. I. A two-dimensional echocardiographic method and findings in normal subjects. Circulation 64:113, 1981.

P

1. Pearlman, A. S., and Otto, C. M.: Quantification of valvular regurgitation. Echocardiography 4:271, 1987.
2. Pearson, A. C., Schiff, M., Mrosek, D., et al.: Left ventricular diastolic function in weight lifters. Am. J. Cardiol. 58:1254, 1986.
3. Pearson, A. C., Labovitz, A. J., Mrosek, D., et al.: Assessment of diastolic function in normal and hypertrophied hearts: Comparison of Doppler echocardiography and M-mode echocardiography. Am. Heart J. 113:1417, 1987.
4. Phillips, R. A., Coplan, N. L., Krakoff, L. R., et al.: Doppler echocardiographic analysis of left ventricular filling in treated hypertensive patients. J. Am. Coll. Cardiol. 9:317, 1987.
5. Parker, T. G., Cameron, D., Serra, J., et al.: The effect of heart rate and A-V interval on Doppler ultrasound indices of left ventricular diastolic function (Abstract.) Circulation 76(Suppl. IV):IV-124, 1987.
6. Pennestri, F., Loperfido, F., Salvatori, M. P., et al.: Assessment of tricuspid regurgitation by pulsed Doppler ultrasonography of the hepatic veins. Am. J. Cardiol. 54:363, 1984.

R

1. Reddy, P. S., Curtis, E. I., Bell, B., et al.: Determinants of variation between Fick and indicator dilution estimates of cardiac output during diagnostic catheterization. Fick vs. dye cardiac outputs. J. Lab. Clin. Med. 87:568, 1976.
2. Rushmer, R. F.: Initial ventricular impulse—a potential key to cardiac evaluation. Circulation 39:268, 1964.
3. Rushmer, R. F., Watson, N., Harding, D., and Baker, D.: Effects of acute coronary occlusion on performance of right and left ventricles in intact unanesthetized dogs. Am. Heart J. 66:522, 1963.
4. Rose, J. S., Nanna, M., Rahimtoola, S. H., et al.: Accuracy of determination of changes in cardiac output by transcutaneous continuous-wave Doppler computer. Am. J. Cardiol. 54:1099, 1984.
5. Rokey, R., Kuo, L. C., Zoghbi, W. A., et al.: Determination of parameters of left ventricular diastolic filling by pulsed Doppler echocardiography: Comparison with cineangiography. Circulation 71:543, 1985.

S

1. Sequeira, R. F., Light, L. H., Cross, G., and Raftery, E. B.: Transcutaneous aortovelography—a quantitative evaluation. Br. Heart J. 38:443, 1976.
2. Sanders, S. P., Yeager, S., and Williams, R. G.: Measurement of systemic and pulmonary blood flow and QP/QS ratio using Doppler and two-dimensional echocardiography. Am. J. Cardiol. 51:952, 1983.
3. Steingart, R. M., Meller, J., Barovick, J., et al.: Doppler echocardiographic measurement of beat-to-beat changes in stroke volume in dogs. Circulation 62:542, 1980.
4. Sahn, D. J.: Determination of cardiac output by echocardiographic Doppler methods: Relative accuracy of various sites for measurement. J. Am. Coll. Cardiol. 6:663, 1985.
5. Sabbah, H. N., Khaja, F., Brymer, J. F., et al.: Noninvasive evaluation of left ventricular performance based on peak aortic blood acceleration measured with a continuous-wave Doppler velocity meter. Circulation 74:323, 1986.
6. Sabbah, H. N., Przbylski, J., Albert, D. E., and Stein, P. D.: Peak aortic blood acceleration reflects the extent of left ventricular ischemic mass at risk. Am. Heart J. 113:885, 1987.
7. Stein, P. D., Sabbah, H. N., Albert, D. E., and Snyder, J. E.: Continuous wave Doppler for the noninvasive evaluation of aortic blood velocity and rate of change of velocity: Evaluation in dogs. Med. Instrum. 21:177, 1987.
8. Shaw, J. G., Johnson, E. C., Voyles, W. F., and Greene, E. R.: Noninvasive Doppler determination of cardiac output during submaximal and peak exercise. J. Appl. Physiol. 59:722, 1985.
9. Sabbah, H. N., Gheorghiade, M., Smith, S. T., et al.: Serial evaluation of left ventricular function in congestive heart failure by measurement of peak aortic blood acceleration. Am. J. Cardiol. 61:367, 1988.

10. Soufer, R., Wohlgelernter, D., Vita, N. A., et al.: Intact systolic left ventricular function in clinical congestive heart failure. Am. J. Cardiol. 55:1032, 1985.
11. Spirito, P., Maron, B. J., Chiarella, F., et al.: Diastolic abnormalities in patients with hypertrophic cardiomyopathy: Relation to magnitude of left ventricular hypertrophy. Circulation 72:310, 1985.
12. Spirito, P., Maron, B. J., and Bonow, R. O.: Noninvasive assessment of left ventricular diastolic function: Comparative analysis of Doppler echocardiographic and radionuclide techniques. J. Am. Coll. Cardiol. 7:518, 1986.
13. Snider, A. R., Gidding, S. S., Rochini, A. P., et al.: Doppler evaluation of left ventricular diastolic filling in children with systemic hypertension. Am. J. Cardiol. 56:921, 1985.
14. Sartori, M. P., Quinones, M. A., and Kuo, L. C.: Relation of Doppler-derived left ventricular filling parameters to age and radius/thickness ratio in normal and pathologic states. Am. J. Cardiol. 59:1179, 1987
15. Stoddard, M. F., Pearson, A. C., Kern, M. J., et al.: Influence of alteration in preload on the pattern of left ventricular diastolic filling as assessed by Doppler echocardiography in humans. Circulation 79:1226, 1989.
16. Suzuki, Y., Kambara, H., Kadota, K., et al.: Detection and evaluation of tricuspid regurgitation using a real-time, two-dimensional, color-coded, Doppler flow imaging system: Comparison with contrast two-dimensional echocardiography and right ventriculography. Am. J. Cardiol. 57:811, 1986.
17. Sakai, K., Nakamura, K., Satomi, G., et al.: Evaluation of tricuspid regurgitation by blood flow pattern in the hepatic vein using pulsed Doppler technique. Am. Heart J. 108:516, 1984.

T

1. Takenaka, K., Dabestani, A., Gardin, J. M., et al.: Pulsed Doppler echocardiographic study of left ventricular filling in dilated cardiomyopathy. Am. J. Cardiol. 58:143, 1986.
2. Takenaka, K., Dabestani, A., Gardin, J. M., et al.: Left ventricular filling in hypertrophic cardiomyopathy: A pulsed Doppler echocardiographic study. J. Am. Coll. Cardiol. 7:1263,1986.

V

1. Valdes-Cruz, L. M., Horowitz, S., Mesel, E., et al.: A pulsed Doppler echocardiographic method for calculation of pulmonary and systemic flow: Accuracy in a canine model with ventricular septal defect. Circulation 68:597, 1983.
2. Valdes-Cruz, L. M., Horowitz, S., Mesel, E., et al.: A pulsed Doppler echocardiographic method for calculating pulmonary and systemic blood flow in atrial level shunts: Validation studies in animals and initial human experience. Circulation 69:80, 1984.

W

1. Wilkins, G. T., Gillam, L. D., Kritzer, G. L., et al.: Validation of continuous-wave Doppler echocardiographic measurements of mitral and tricuspid prosthetic valve gradients: A simultaneous Doppler-catheter study. Circulation 74:786, 1986.
2. Wallmeyer, K., Wann, L. S., Sagar, K. B., et al.: The influence of preload and heart rate on Doppler echocardiographic indexes of left ventricular performance: Comparison with invasive indexes in an experimental preparation. Circulation 74:181, 1986.
3. Wind, B. E., Snider, R., Buda, A. J., et al.: Pulsed Doppler assessment of left ventricular diastolic filling before and immediately after coronary angioplasty. Am. J. Cardiol. 59:1041, 1987.

Y

1. Yock, P. G., and Popp, R. L.: Noninvasive estimation of right ventricular systolic pressure by Doppler ultrasound in patients with tricuspid regurgitation. Circulation 70:657, 1984.

Z

1. Zarich, S. W., Arbuckle, B. E., Cohen, L. R., et al.: Diastolic abnormalities in young asymptomatic diabetic patients assessed by pulsed Doppler echocardiography. J. Am. Coll. Cardiol. 12:114, 1988.

Chapter 21

Echocardiographic Evaluation of Valvular Heart Disease

■ *LYLE J. OLSON, M.D.* ■ *A. JAMIL TAJIK, M.D.*

NATIVE VALVULAR HEART DISEASE 419
Historical Perspective 419
Aortic Stenosis 419
Doppler Echocardiography in Aortic Stenosis 421
Role of Echocardiography in Clinical Decision Making in Aortic Stenosis 425
Aortic Regurgitation 425
Doppler Echocardiography in Aortic Regurgitation 427
Role of Echocardiography in Clinical Decision Making in Aortic Regurgitation 430
Mitral Stenosis 430
Doppler Echocardiography in Mitral Stenosis 431
Role of Echocardiography in Clinical Decision Making in Mitral Stenosis 433
Mitral Regurgitation 433
Doppler Echocardiography in Mitral Regurgitation 435
Role of Echocardiography in Clinical Decision Making in Mitral Regurgitation 436
Tricuspid Stenosis 436
Doppler Echocardiography in the Evaluation of Tricuspid Stenosis 436
Role of Echocardiography in Clinical Decision Making in Tricuspid Stenosis 436
Tricuspid Regurgitation 437
Doppler Echocardiography in the Evaluation of Tricuspid Regurgitation 438
Doppler Echocardiographic Estimation of Right Ventricular Systolic Pressure 438
Role of Echocardiography in the Evaluation of Tricuspid Regurgitation 440
Pulmonary Stenosis and Regurgitation 440
Doppler Echocardiography in the Evaluation of Pulmonary Valve Disease 440
Role of Echocardiography in the Evaluation of Pulmonary Valve Disease 440
ASSESSMENT OF VALVE FUNCTION AFTER INTERVENTION 440
Prosthetic Stenosis and Regurgitation 440
Doppler Echocardiography in the Evaluation of Prosthetic Valves 441
Valvuloplasty 441
SUMMARY 443

NATIVE VALVULAR HEART DISEASE

Historical Perspective

The modern era of evaluation and management of valvular heart disease began with the development of cardiac catheterization and surgical intervention more than 3 decades ago. Cardiac catheterization has remained the standard for the detection and assessment of the severity of valvular stenosis and regurgitation. However, the primary role of cardiac catheterization has been challenged over the past 5 years by combined two-dimensional (2D) and Doppler echocardiography.

Since the first descriptions of M-mode echocardiography for the evaluation of mitral stenosis more than 30 years ago, echocardiography has evolved from a technique limited to analysis of valve motion to a comprehensive tomographic and hemodynamic method that uses 2D and Doppler echocardiography. Moreover, the emergence of Doppler echocardiography has dramatically altered the approach to patient management. The detection and the assessment of cause and hemodynamic severity of stenotic and regurgitant valvular disease now can be reliably performed noninvasively. Therefore, early diagnosis and accurate characterization of the natural history of valvular heart disease in symptomatic and asymptomatic patients can be accomplished by serial examination without the risk or cost of cardiac catheterization.

In this chapter, we describe the utility and the complementary roles of M-mode, 2D, and spectral and color flow Doppler echocardiography for the evaluation of valvular disease in adult patients, including prosthetic valve dysfunction and valvular disease treated by valvuloplasty. The use of transesophageal echocardiography is also cited in selected clinical settings, and the role of echocardiography in clinical decision making for patients with valvular heart disease is reviewed.

Aortic Stenosis

The anatomic hallmark of aortic valvular stenosis is reduced orifice dimension, which may be associated with valve calcification and commissural fusion.[C1, D1, D2, E1, E2, P1, R1, R2, S1] The morphologic appearance of the aortic valve depends on the cause of aortic stenosis. In the past, most cases of fibrocalcific aortic stenosis were considered to be rheumatic in origin, [C1, D2] but it is now recognized that other causes account for most cases. The three most common causes of aortic stenosis are degenerative (senile) calcification, calcification of a congenital bicuspid aortic valve, and postinflammatory disease.[D1, P1, P2, S1] These three causes account for 95 percent of the patients undergoing operation for pure aortic stenosis at our institution.[P2, S1] The single most common cause is senile aortic stenosis, accounting for almost half the cases.[H1] The increase in relative frequency of senile aortic stenosis has been attributed to the decline in rheumatic fever observed in Western nations.[A1, D3]

Senile aortic stenosis is characterized morphologically by a trileaflet aortic valve free of commissural fusion, with calcified nodular excrescences within the valve pockets that restrict motion. The congenitally bicuspid aortic valve is identified by two leaflets of unequal size, the larger of which is conjoined and often contains a fibrous ridge (raphe) at the site of congenital fusion. Calcification of the raphe, annulus, and valve pockets produces a narrowed orifice shaped like an ellipse. Postinflammatory aortic stenosis is characterized by commissural fusion and by cuspid fibrosis and calcification.[P2, S1] Stenosis becomes more severe with fusion of more commissures and progressive calcification.

Two-dimensional echocardiography reliably demonstrates valve thickening and calcification and may identify reduced leaflet excursion in systole, thereby qualitatively differentiating valvular stenosis from left ventricular outflow obstruction due to subvalvular or supravalvular disease.[C2, D4, G1, W1–W3] This assessment is best performed from the parasternal long-axis view.[B1, T1] Typically, severe calcification of the aortic valve leaflets on echocardiographic examination is associated with significant stenosis. However, the severity of calcification is not a reliable predictor of the hemodynamic severity of stenosis, and calcification may be absent, especially in young patients with obstruction due to congenital or rheumatic disease. Systolic doming of the valve leaflets is frequently observed in association with significant stenosis when calcification is not prominent.[D4, W2] Echocardiographic evaluation from the parasternal short-axis view enables characterization of valve leaflet morphology with high sensitivity, including identification of a congenitally bicuspid aortic valve[B2, N1] and commissural fusion associated with rheumatic disease (Fig. 21–1). However, dense calcification may make identification of cusp number, and hence morphology, difficult. Assessment of morphology is important for patients considered candidates for balloon valvuloplasty, as results of valvuloplasty may be best in elderly patients with senile degenerative disease in which there is no commissural fusion or in patients with rheumatic disease without dense calcification.[K1]

Other anatomic abnormalities frequently associated with aortic valvular stenosis demonstrated by 2D echocardiography are left ventricular hypertrophy, poststenotic dilatation of the aorta, other associated valvular heart disease, and subaortic muscular hypertrophy, which may contribute to left ventricular outflow obstruction. The risk of aortic dissection is increased in patients with congenitally bicuspid aortic valves, whether or not stenosis is present.[L1] Hence, patients with a congenitally bicuspid aortic valve should have serial echocardiographic evaluation, including

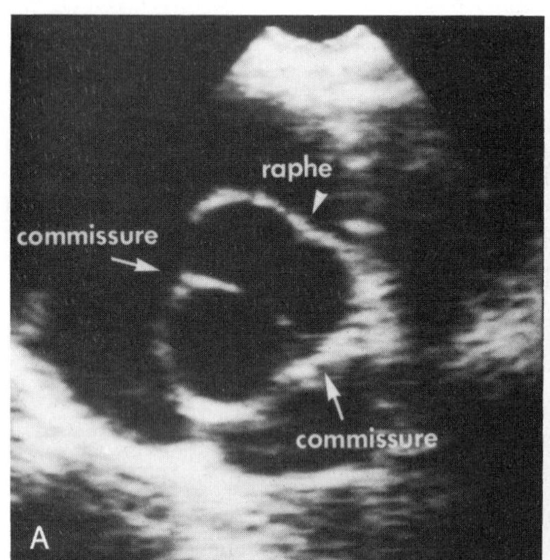

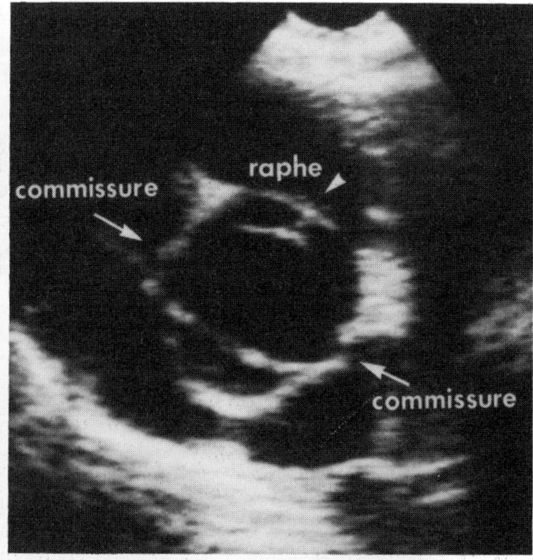

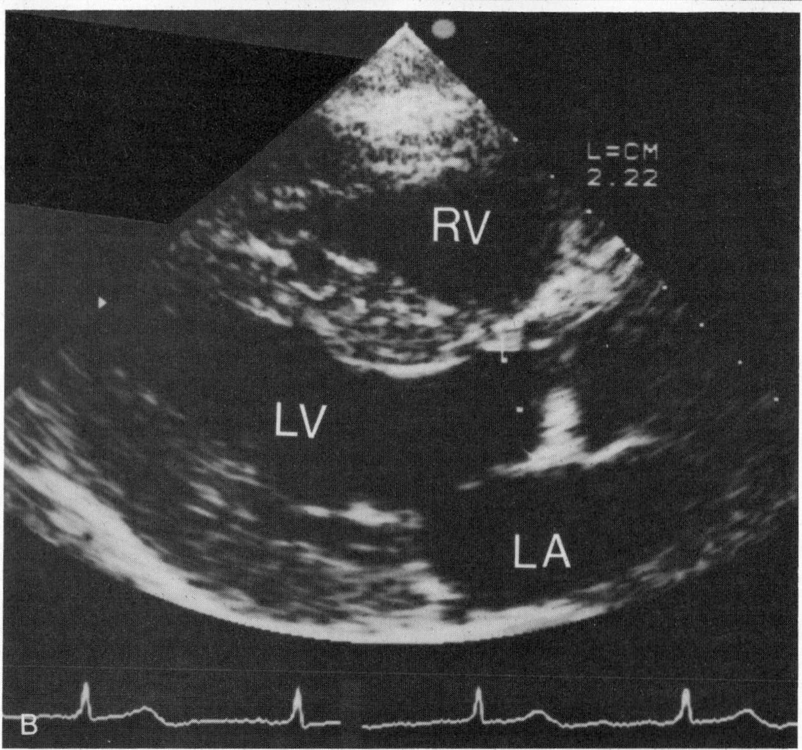

Figure 21–1. *A*, Parasternal short-axis view of the bicuspid aortic valve in diastole (*left*) and systole (*right*). Commissures are abnormally located at 4 o'clock and nearly 10 o'clock, with a raphe at 1 o'clock (*arrowhead*). Note the oval appearance of the valve orifice during systole. Study of valve opening and closing on real-time 2D echocardiographic examination enables distinction of the bicuspid from the tricuspid valve. (From Brandenburg, R. O., Jr., et al.: Accuracy of 2-dimensional echocardiographic diagnosis of congenitally bicuspid aortic valve: Echocardiographic-anatomic correlation in 115 patients. Am. J. Cardiol. 51:1469, 1983. By permission of Cahners Publishing Company.) *B*, Parasternal long-axis view in systole from a patient with aortic valvular stenosis. The noncoronary cusp appears thickened and calcified. LA—left atrium; LV—left ventricle; RV—right ventricle.

careful evaluation of the aorta.[S2] M-mode echocardiography is used to quantify the dimensions of the aortic root, ventricular wall thickness, and left ventricular cavity dimension in diastole and systole, enabling quantification of left ventricular function.

The hemodynamic severity of valvular aortic stenosis may be estimated with confidence by combined 2D and M-mode echocardiography in some patients.[D4, G1, W1] In patients with densely calcific aortic stenosis, severely decreased leaflet motion, and left ventricular hypertrophy, 2D echocardiography reliably predicts severe obstruction. Similarly, in patients with minimal aortic valve calcification, normal valve motion, and no left ventricular hypertrophy, 2D echocardiography reliably predicts that aortic stenosis is absent or trivial. However, many patients are not in either of these categories. In these patients, 2D echocardiography is unreliable for prediction of the transvalvular gradient or semiquantitative assessment of the severity of stenosis.[D4, G1, S3, W1] Definitive assessment of the hemodynamic severity of aortic stenosis requires estimation of the transvalvular pressure gradient and aortic valve area by Doppler echocardiography.

Doppler Echocardiography in Aortic Stenosis

The aim of the Doppler echocardiographic evaluation of the patient with aortic valve stenosis is measurement of both the transvalvular pressure gradient and the aortic valvular orifice area. This may be accomplished in more than 97 percent of patients.[O1] Pressure gradient estimation in aortic stenosis by Doppler echocardiography requires measurement of the velocity of blood flow distal to the stenotic valve. This is accomplished by directing the continuous-wave ultrasound beam so that it is within the flow jet and parallel to the velocity vector of transvalvular blood flow. Most often, this is accomplished from an apical transducer position, but occasionally the best site is either right parasternal or axillary.[N2]

Transvalvular aortic velocity is increased in the presence of aortic stenosis. The measurement of transvalvular aortic velocity by continuous-wave Doppler echocardiography enables estimation of *maximal instantaneous* and mean transvalvular pressure gradients by application of the *modified Bernoulli equation*.[C3, C4, H1, H2, S4] The modified Bernoulli equation is expressed as $P = 4V^2$, in which P represents the pressure gradient and V is the velocity of transvalvular blood flow measured by continuous-wave Doppler echocardiography. The pressure gradient is estimated by substituting the measured velocity for V in the modified Bernoulli equation. In addition to providing quantification of the transvalvular gradient, the characteristic Doppler echocardiographic profile aids in the discrimination of valvular or supravalvular stenosis from subvalvular obstruction.[S5, Y1] However, the anatomic cause of stenosis is optimally characterized by 2D echocardiography.

Proper interpretation of data obtained by the Doppler echocardiographic method requires appreciation that the maximal instantaneous gradient represents an *instantaneous* pressure difference between the left ventricle and the aorta, whereas the commonly used peak-to-peak gradient obtained by pull-back of a single catheter at catheterization reflects the difference between peak left ventricular systolic and ascending aortic pressures, which are *nonsynchronous* events[C3] (Fig. 21–2). The Doppler-determined *maximal* instantaneous gradient always exceeds the peak-to-peak gradient obtained at cardiac catheterization. The peak-to-peak gradient is an arbitrary convention, is not physiologic, and is not directly comparable to the Doppler-derived *maximal instantaneous* gradient. The clinical utility of the catheterization-measured peak-to-peak gradient may be attributed to the fortuitous correlation between peak-to-peak and mean gradients.

The validation of the Doppler method for gradient measurement has been proved in *simultaneous* Doppler echocardiographic and dual cardiac catheterization studies of aortic valve gradients in animals[C5, S6] and humans.[C3] They have demonstrated extremely high correlation between maximal instantaneous gradients measured by Doppler echocardiography and those measured by dual catheters in the left ventricle and aorta. The correlation of mean gradient measurements by catheterization and Doppler echocardiography in simultaneous studies has also been extremely high[C3] (Fig. 21–3). The hemodynamic severity of aortic valve stenosis by measurement of catheter pressure gradient is typically expressed as a peak-to-peak or mean gradient. Hence, the most useful expression for the severity of aortic stenosis by Doppler echocardiography is provided by the mean gradient, because it is directly comparable to the mean gradient estimated by catheterization.

Pressure gradient determination by either Doppler echocardiography or cardiac catheterization provides only partial assessment of the severity of aortic stenosis because of the flow-dependence of gradient determinations.[C6] Simultaneous Doppler echocardiographic and dual catheter studies in patients have shown that pressure gradient data alone correctly classify the hemodynamic severity of aortic stenosis in less than 50 percent of patients compared with estimates of aortic valve area.[O1] Hence, it is prudent to determine valve area in all patients with aortic stenosis.

The preferred method for the Doppler echocardiographic determination of aortic valve area is provided by the continuity equation. Although aortic valve area may be determined by the Gorlin formula from data obtained by Doppler echocardiography,[T2] the advantages of the continuity equation are that it is completely noninvasive and requires only two Doppler velocity measurements. The method is based on the physiologic principle that laminar flow through a conduit is equal to the *mean* velocity multiplied by the cross-sectional orifice dimension. At constant flow, the ratio of cross-sectional areas at two different sites is inversely proportional to the ratio of the respective mean velocities at those sites. This relationship is expressed by the equation:

$$A_1 \times V_1 = A_2 \times V_2$$

in which A_1 is the cross-sectional area of the left ventricular outflow tract, A_2 is the cross-sectional area of the stenotic valve, V_2 is the *mean* velocity of blood flow distal to the obstruction, and V_1 is the *mean* velocity proximal to the obstruction. If the mean velocity at the stenotic valve and the flow are known, the stenotic area can be derived as flow divided by the mean velocity of the stenotic jet. Rearrangement of the continuity equation yields the aortic valve area:

$$A_2 = A_1 \times (V_1/V_2)$$

Because the systolic ejection time is the same and the time-velocity curves have a similar course for the left ventricular outflow tract and aortic valve flow, the *peak* aortic velocity and *peak* left ventricular outflow tract velocity may be substituted for the mean velocities in the continuity equation.[O1] In practice, A_1 is determined by 2D echocardiography, and peak V_1 and peak V_2 are measured by pulsed and continuous-wave Doppler echocardiography, respectively (Fig. 21–4). When the aortic outflow jet is eccentric, color flow imaging may improve the accuracy of the continuous-wave method for measurement of the aortic velocity by guiding the placement of the continuous-wave ultrasound beam.[F1]

Using this method, investigators have consistently demonstrated the accuracy of Doppler echocardiography for the estimation of aortic valve area in adults with aortic stenosis, when compared with measurement of aortic valve area by cardiac catheterization using the Gorlin formula[O1–O3, S7, Z1] (Fig. 21–5). For patients in whom it is not possible to estimate the left ventricular outflow tract diameter by 2D echocardiography (and, hence, impossible to estimate valve area), a highly sensitive index for the detection of severe aortic stenosis is provided by the ratio of V_1 to V_2. Severe aortic stenosis has been demonstrated to be present in 92 percent of patients in whom V_1/V_2 is less than 0.25.[O1] This index is independent of cardiac output and therefore may be used for serial evaluation.

Invasive and Doppler echocardiographic estimates of aortic valve area may yield discordant data. Pitfalls that may contribute to potential discrepancies are associated with either method. Invasive estimates of aortic valve area require measurement of

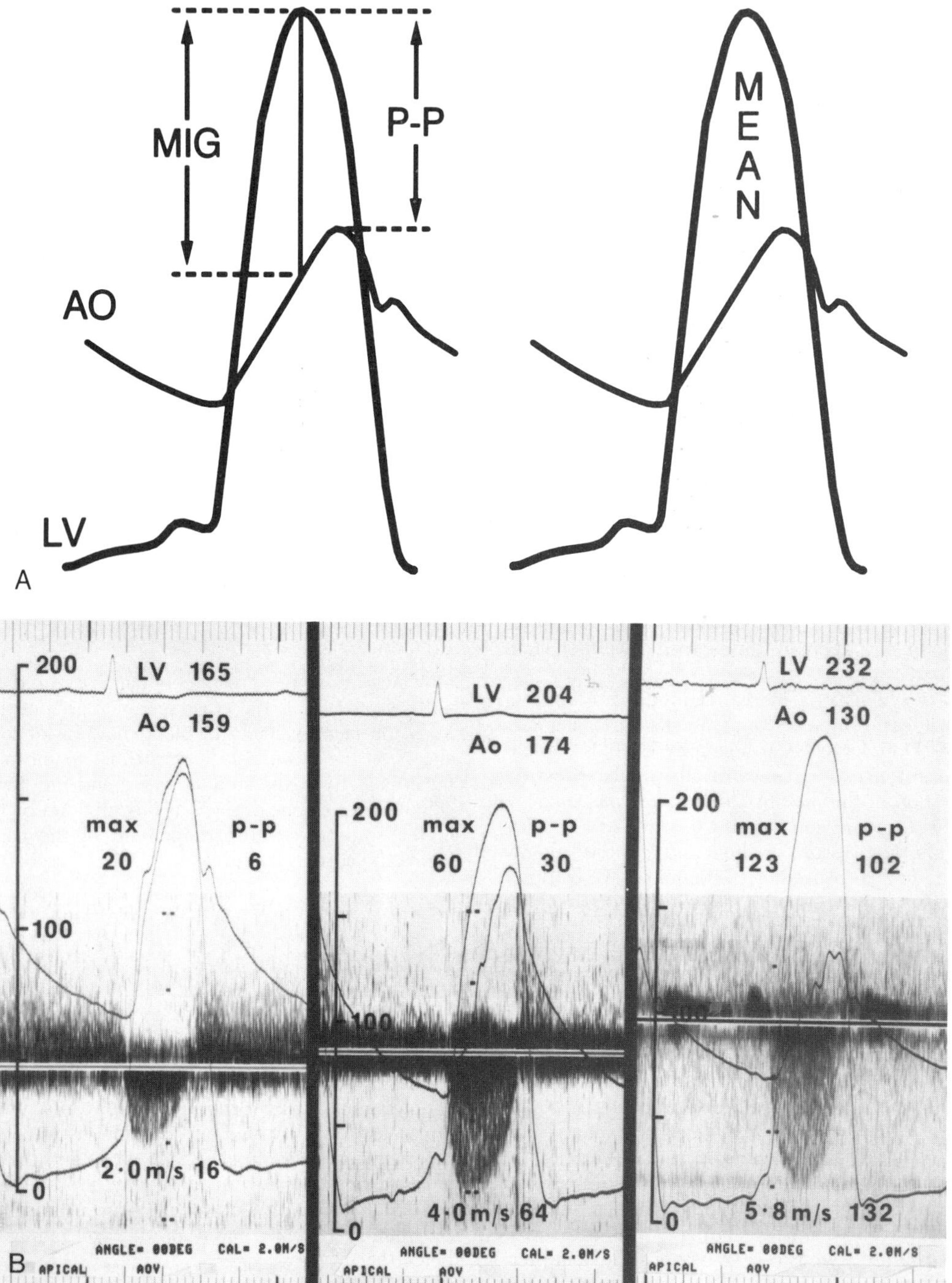

Figure 21–2. *A*, Schematic representation of peak-to-peak aortic transvalvular gradients (P-P) and maximum instantaneous gradient (MIG), measured simultaneously, and mean gradient. *Left*, Catheter-determined peak left ventricular systolic pressure and peak aortic systolic pressure are nonsynchronous events; maximum instantaneous pressure gradient determined by continuous-wave Doppler echocardiography reflects simultaneous events. Hence, peak-to-peak and maximum instantaneous measurements do not measure the same gradient, and the maximum instantaneous gradient always will be greater than the peak-to-peak gradient. *Right*, Mean gradient is obtained by planimetry of the area between pressure curves. *B*, Composite of simultaneous Doppler-catheter pressure measurements in three patients with mild, moderate, and severe elevations of transvalvular aortic gradients due to aortic stenosis. Pressure gradients were measured by dual catheters in the left ventricle and ascending aorta. The maximal (max) catheter gradient is greater than the peak-to-peak (p-p) catheter gradient at each level of stenosis. The maximal Doppler-derived gradients accurately measure the simultaneously recorded maximal catheter gradient but overestimate the peak-to-peak catheter gradient. The Doppler calibrations are in 2-m/sec increments. Ao—ascending aorta; LV—left ventricle. (From Currie, P. J., et al.: Continuous-wave Doppler echocardiographic assessment of severity of calcific aortic stenosis: A simultaneous Doppler-catheter correlative study in 100 adult patients. Circulation 71:1162, 1985, with permission of the American Heart Association, Inc.)

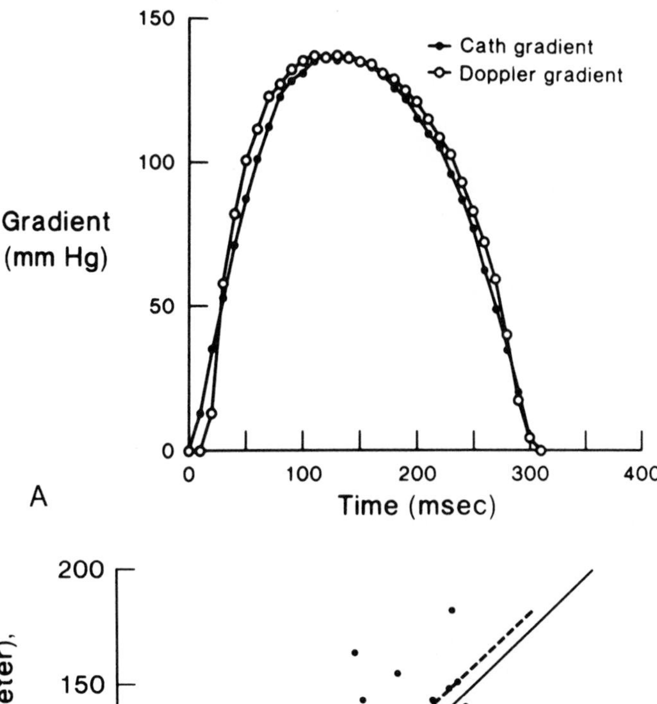

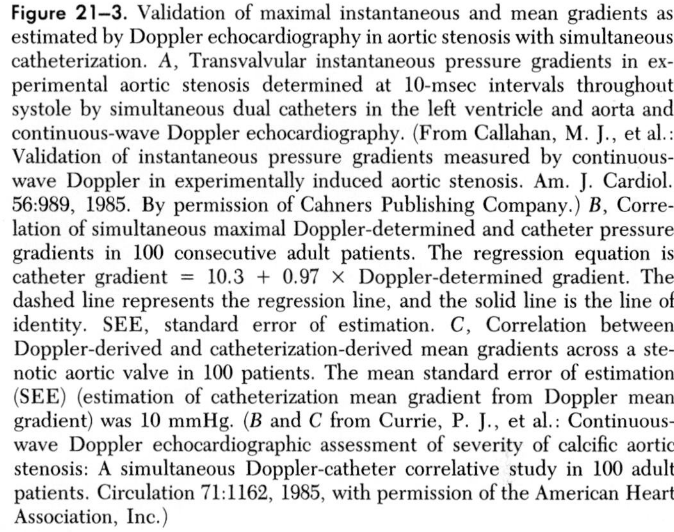

Figure 21–3. Validation of maximal instantaneous and mean gradients as estimated by Doppler echocardiography in aortic stenosis with simultaneous catheterization. *A*, Transvalvular instantaneous pressure gradients in experimental aortic stenosis determined at 10-msec intervals throughout systole by simultaneous dual catheters in the left ventricle and aorta and continuous-wave Doppler echocardiography. (From Callahan, M. J., et al.: Validation of instantaneous pressure gradients measured by continuous-wave Doppler in experimentally induced aortic stenosis. Am. J. Cardiol. 56:989, 1985. By permission of Cahners Publishing Company.) *B*, Correlation of simultaneous maximal Doppler-determined and catheter pressure gradients in 100 consecutive adult patients. The regression equation is catheter gradient = 10.3 + 0.97 × Doppler-determined gradient. The dashed line represents the regression line, and the solid line is the line of identity. SEE, standard error of estimation. *C*, Correlation between Doppler-derived and catheterization-derived mean gradients across a stenotic aortic valve in 100 patients. The mean standard error of estimation (SEE) (estimation of catheterization mean gradient from Doppler mean gradient) was 10 mmHg. (*B* and *C* from Currie, P. J., et al.: Continuous-wave Doppler echocardiographic assessment of severity of calcific aortic stenosis: A simultaneous Doppler-catheter correlative study in 100 adult patients. Circulation 71:1162, 1985, with permission of the American Heart Association, Inc.)

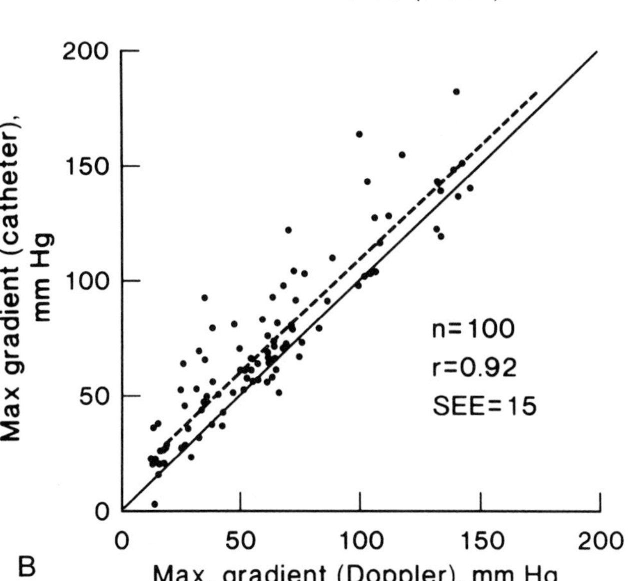

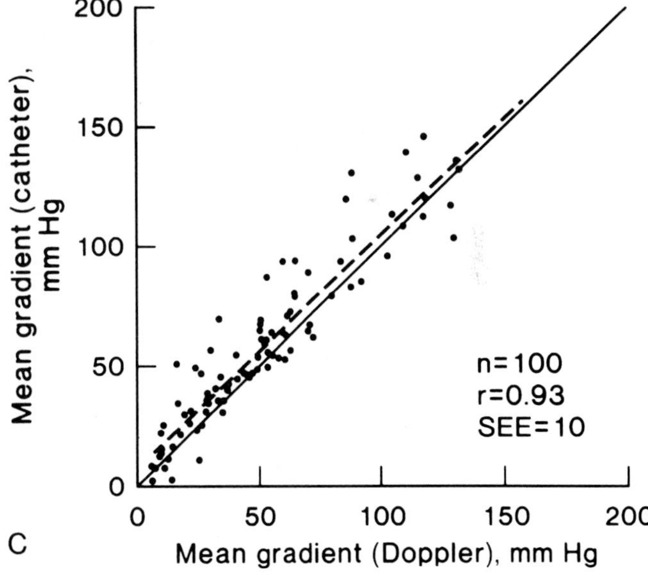

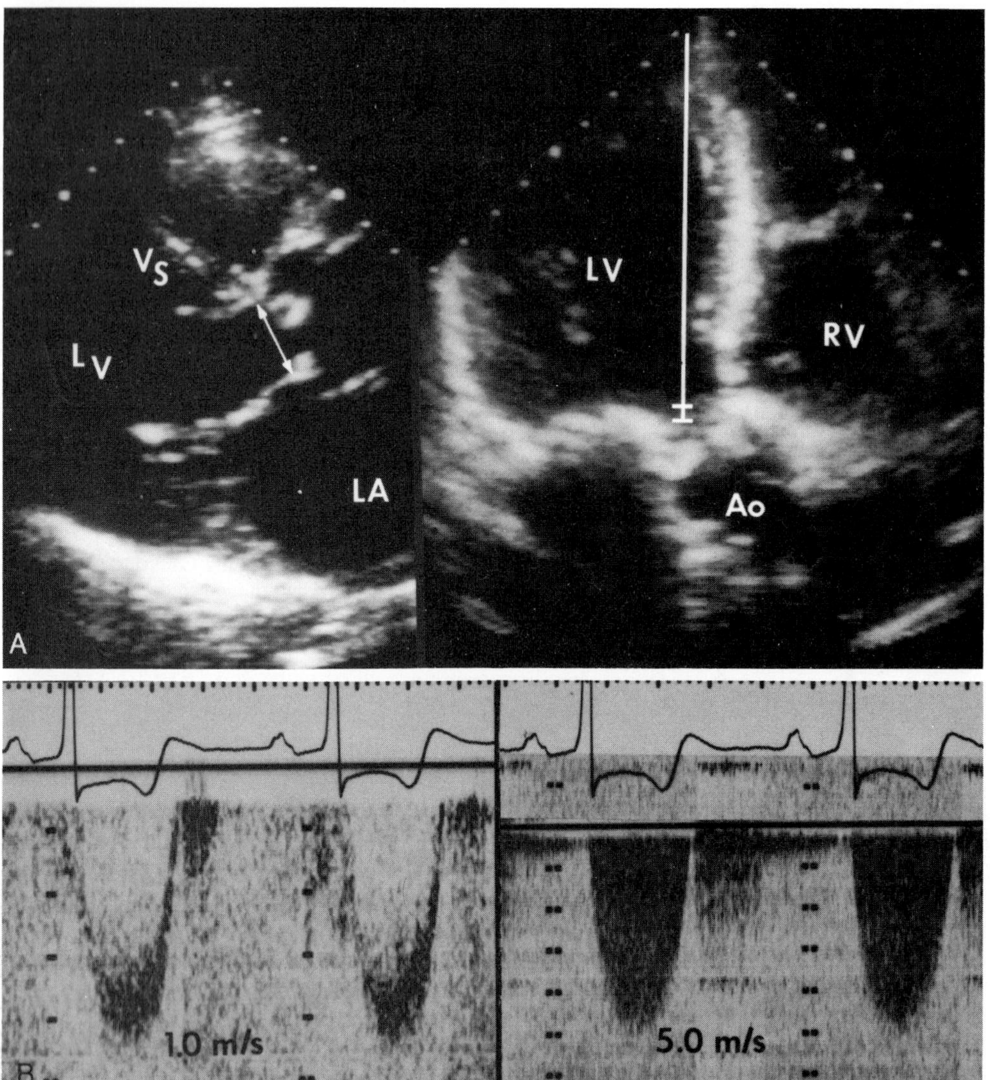

Figure 21–4. Determination of the aortic valve area by use of the continuity equation. *A*, *Left*, Parasternal long-axis view of a heart in systole. Diameter (d) of the left ventricular outflow tract is measured (*double-headed arrow*). The cross-sectional area of the left ventricular outflow tract, A_1, of the continuity equation is then calculated by the formula $\pi(d/2)^2$. *Right*, Left ventricular outflow velocity (V_1 of the continuity equation) is measured by pulsed-wave Doppler echocardiography with the sample volume in the subvalvular area from an apical position. Ao—aorta; LA—left atrium; LV—left ventricle; RV—right ventricle; VS—ventricular septum. *B*, Velocity profiles of the left ventricular outflow tract (*left*) and aorta (*right*) measured by Doppler echocardiography in a patient with aortic stenosis. (From Olson, L. J., et al.: Aortic valve stenosis: Etiology, pathophysiology, evaluation, and management. Curr. Probl. Cardiol. 12:455, 1987. By permission of Mayo Foundation.)

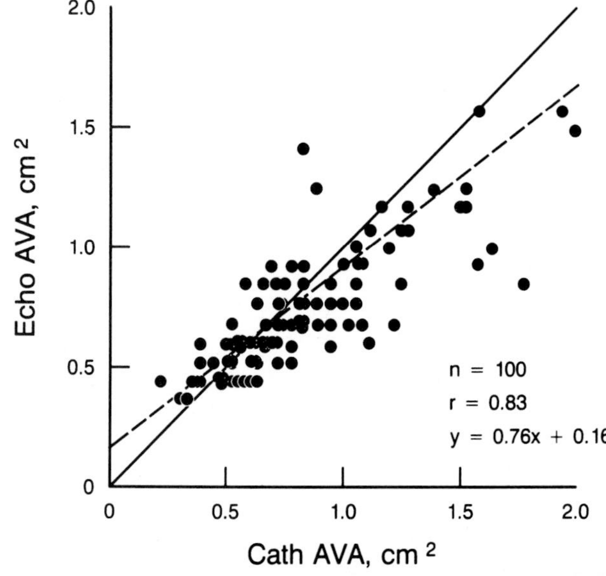

Figure 21–5. Correlation between catheterization-derived aortic valve area (Cath AVA) and Doppler echocardiography–derived aortic valve area (Echo AVA) in 100 patients. Mean standard error of estimation was 0.19 cm². (From Oh, J. K., et al.: Prediction of the severity of aortic stenosis by Doppler aortic valve area determination: Prospective Doppler-catheterization correlation in 100 patients. J. Am. Coll. Cardiol. 11:1227, 1988. By permission of the American College of Cardiology.)

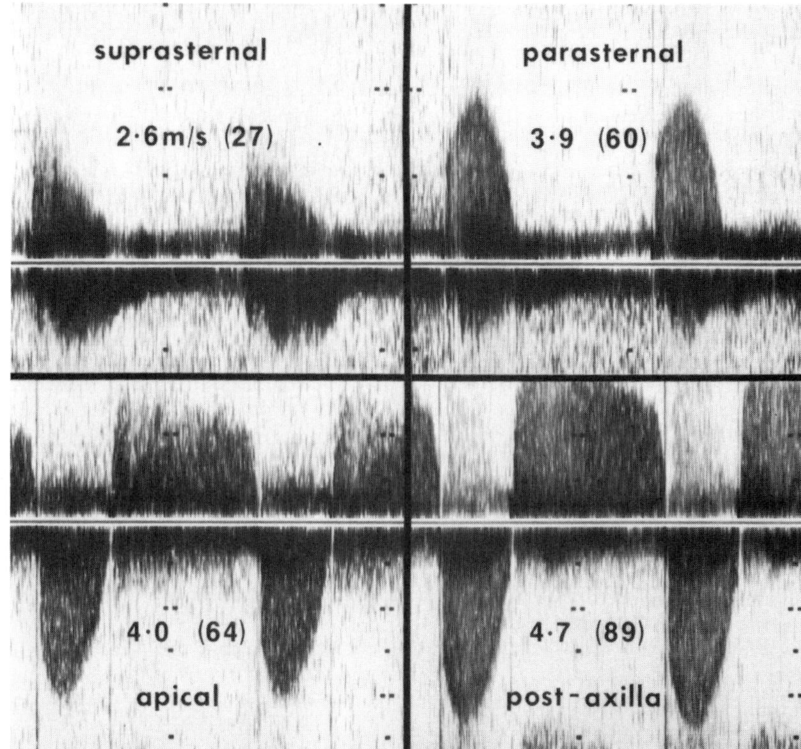

Figure 21–6. Underestimation of aortic valve gradient by Doppler echocardiography, illustrated with Doppler signals from one patient with aortic stenosis. Maximal velocity varies with the position of the transducer. The examiner must systematically search for the anatomic window that yields the highest maximal instantaneous velocity. Velocity is given in meters per second (m/s); Doppler-determined instantaneous gradients (mmHg) are shown in parentheses. (From Olson, L. J., et al.: Aortic valve stenosis: Etiology, pathophysiology, evaluation, and management. Curr. Probl. Cardiol. 12:455, 1987. By permission of Mayo Foundation.)

cardiac output by either Fick or indicator dilution technique, each of which is subject to considerable error.[S8, T3, V1, V2] Furthermore, cardiac output may vary substantially during a single invasive procedure, with alterations in sympathetic tone and loading conditions confounding the estimate of valve area because of beat-to-beat variation in cardiac output and gradient, which are not simultaneously measured. Finally, the hydraulic constants of the Gorlin formula[G2] are not truly constant, particularly in low-flow states, in which error in estimates of aortic valve area may exceed 50 percent,[C7, S9] and the presence of associated more-than-mild aortic regurgitation may cause overestimation of the severity of aortic stenosis.[C6]

Advantages of the continuity equation and Doppler echocardiography for estimation of aortic valve area are that the continuity equation does not require measurement of cardiac output and that aortic valve area estimates are not affected by aortic regurgitation. However, there are also practical and theoretic limitations to the Doppler echocardiographic method. The measurement of aortic valve gradient depends on the Doppler beam being parallel to blood flow. Thus, a small, nonimaging transducer with multiple angulations from various positions is required to obtain peak aortic velocity (Fig. 21–6). Small errors in the measurement of left ventricular outflow tract diameter cause relatively large errors in estimation of aortic valve area, because the diameter is squared in the continuity equation. Other potential problems are related to assumptions made in the application of the modified Bernoulli equation. Energy loss across the stenosis, pressure recovery distal to the stenosis, acceleration of blood flow, and the velocity of blood flow proximal to the stenosis are factors that are neglected when the modified Bernoulli equation is applied. These factors may cause overestimation of the gradient in mild stenosis and underestimation of the gradient in severe stenosis.[R3] Nevertheless, the performance of the Doppler echocardiographic examination by experienced, well-trained echocardiographers yields reliable hemodynamic data.

Role of Echocardiography in Clinical Decision Making in Aortic Stenosis

In patients in whom 2D and Doppler echocardiography has established the cause and hemodynamic severity of aortic valvular stenosis, cardiac catheterization for determination of the transvalvular gradient and valve orifice area adds little information to aid in clinical decision making. We believe that use of Doppler echocardiography makes cardiac catheterization unnecessary for evaluation of aortic stenosis in those patients. Furthermore, serial assessment by combined 2D and Doppler echocardiography poses no risk to the patient. Echocardiographic evaluation may assist the surgeon by identification of subaortic hypertrophy requiring myectomy and by assessment of aortic root dimension, which may limit the size of prosthesis used for valve replacement. Preoperative catheterization is indicated only for evaluation of coronary disease or for resolution of discordant clinical and Doppler echocardiographic data.

Aortic Regurgitation

Aortic regurgitation is classified as either acquired or congenital and is due to disease of the valve or of the aortic root or combination thereof.[E3, E4, R4] Regurgitation is subclassified as acute or chronic, each form with characteristic 2D, M-mode, and Doppler echocardiographic findings. Two-dimensional echocardiography identifies the anatomic abnormality underlying regurgitation and hence forms the basis of diagnostic classification.

Rheumatic disease of the aortic valve produces leaflet thickening, fibrosis, and retraction and often causes combined regurgitation and stenosis.[O4, S10] Leaflet calcification is prominent if stenosis is present.[S10] Characteristic echocardiographic features include leaflet thickening and calcification, reduced leaflet excursion, and leaflet doming when stenosis is present, best demonstrated in the parasternal long-axis view. Incomplete diastolic leaflet coaptation may be demonstrated in the parasternal short-axis view, especially when aided by color flow imaging.

Infectious endocarditis may cause aortic valve regurgitation owing to vegetations that prevent proper leaflet coaptation or damage to the leaflets that produces perforation or dehiscence. Combined 2D and color flow imaging is used to characterize anatomic abnormalities from the parasternal long-axis and short-axis views. Valvular vegetations less than 3 mm in diameter frequently are not identified by transthoracic 2D echocardiography, especially if there is thickening of the valve leaflets. Transesophageal echocardiography aids in the detection of vegetations because of high image resolution, and, in combination with color flow imaging, it is useful for localization of the regurgitant jet to the valvular orifice or perivalvular region.[E5, S11] Transesophageal echocardiography may also demonstrate perivalvular abscess. Less common causes of acquired aortic valvular regurgitation identified by 2D echocardiography are spontaneous dehiscence of an aortic valve leaflet,[S12] diastolic leaflet prolapse,[C8] and ankylosing spondylitis, which is recognized by aortic root dilatation and characteristic nodules in the vicinity of the aortic-mitral junction with associated leaflet fibrosis and retraction.[B3, S13, T4]

Enlargement of the aortic root is frequently associated with aortic regurgitation, regardless of cause. Aortic root dilatation may be primary and cause regurgitation, or it may be acquired as a consequence of increased total flow. In chronic aortic regurgitation, idiopathic dilatation of the aortic root is the leading indication for surgical replacement of the aortic valve at the Mayo Clinic.[O4] The anatomy of the root and ascending aorta, best evaluated from the parasternal long-axis and short-axis views, should be studied systematically in all patients undergoing 2D echocardiography.[D5] Careful inspection of the root, ascending aorta, arch, and descending thoracic aorta should be performed in all patients with aortic regurgitation.

Acquired aortic root dilatation causing regurgitation may be due to idiopathic dilatation of the annulus and root, with subsequent inadequate aortic valve leaflet coaptation in diastole,[D6, E6] disruption of the aortic valve apparatus due to aortic dissection,[R5] or rupture of a sinus of Valsalva aneurysm.[C8] Two-dimensional echocardiography suggests aortic dissection in the presence of aortic dilatation and an associated intraluminal linear echo, which represents the intimal flap separating the true from the false lumen (Fig. 21–7). Typically, the flap moves in unison with the remnant of the aortic wall, and color flow imaging demonstrates flow in the false lumen.[K2] Retrograde dissection may disrupt the aortic valve apparatus to produce flail aortic leaflets easily identified by 2D echocardiography. Dilatation of an aortic sinus associated with a sinus of Valsalva aneurysm may cause prolapse of an aortic leaflet and associated aortic regurgitation, identified echocardiographically by the characteristic appearance of the dilated sinus and diastolic leaflet prolapse.[E7]

Congenital disease of the aortic valve or root may produce aortic regurgitation in the young or middle-aged adult. The prevalence of the congenital bicuspid aortic valve is 1 to 2 percent, and it frequently becomes stenotic, regurgitant, or involved by endocarditis.[E6, O4, R6, S10] Its characteristic appearance is identified with high sensitivity from the parasternal short-axis view. Similarly, the rare quadricuspid aortic valve may be identified from the parasternal short-axis view and is also frequently associated with aortic regurgitation.[D7] Other congenital disorders associated with aneurysms or dilatation of the aortic root and secondary aortic regurgitation are Marfan's syndrome,[P3] Ehlers-Danlos syndrome,[L2] and coarctation of the aorta.[S14] In the adult with Marfan's syndrome, the aortic root may be massively dilated, and the wall

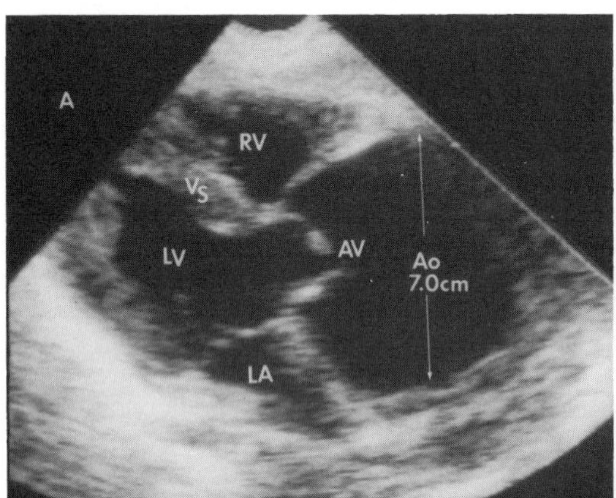

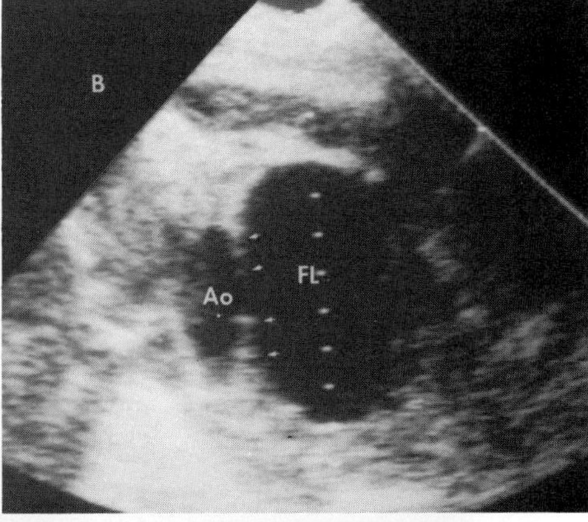

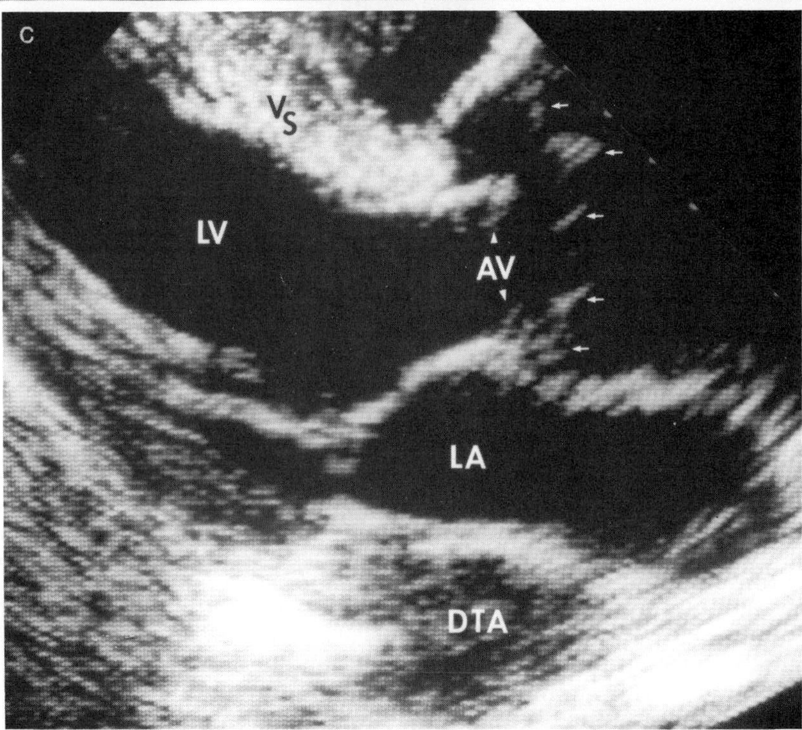

Figure 21–7. Type I aortic dissection. *A*, Long-axis view demonstrating markedly dilated aortic root (7.0 cm). *B*, Short-axis view shows intimal flap (*arrowheads*) separating false lumen (FL) from true lumen (Ao). *C*, Systolic frame from another patient. Parasternal long-axis view shows intimal flap (*arrows*) immediately above the aortic valve (AV) in a markedly dilated aortic root. DTA—descending thoracic aorta; LA—left atrium; LV—left ventricle; RV—right ventricle; VS—ventricular septum. (From Khandheria, B. K., et al.: Aortic dissection: Review of value and limitations of two-dimensional echocardiography in a six year experience. J. Am. Soc. Echo. 2:17, 1989. By permission of the American Society of Echocardiography.)

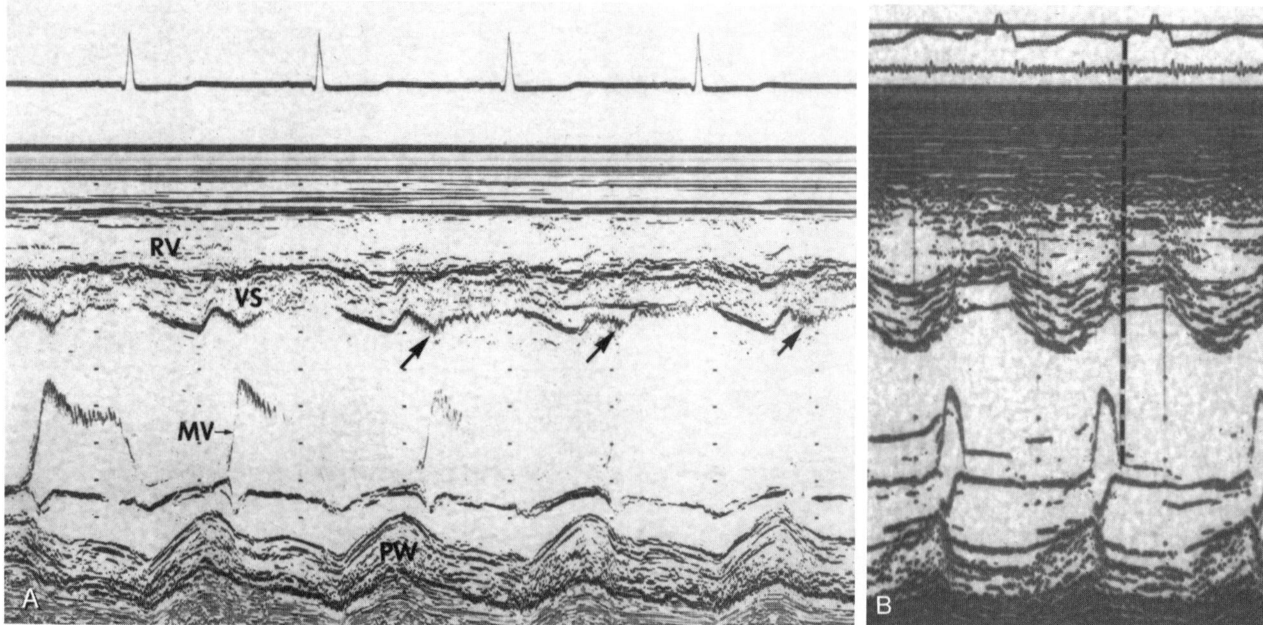

Figure 21–8. M-mode echocardiographic features of chronic (*A*) and acute (*B*) aortic regurgitation. *A*, Indirect features of aortic regurgitation include diastolic flutter of the mitral valve (MV) and ventricular septum (VS) (*arrows*) and an enlarged left ventricle. PW, posterior wall; RV, right ventricle. *B*, Mitral valve closure before the onset of the QRS complex (*interrupted vertical line*) indicates premature closure of mitral valve, characteristic of acute, severe aortic regurgitation. (*B* from Shub, C.: The role of echocardiography in clinical practice. *In* Spittell, J. A., Jr. (ed.): *Clinical Medicine.* Vol. 6. Harper & Row, Philadelphia, 1982, pp. 1–44. By permission of the publisher.)

appears thin. Dilatation also involves the annulus, sinuses of Valsalva, and aorta. The aortic leaflets are enlarged and yet are often unable to occlude the aortic valve orifice. The dilated root also frequently causes compression of the left atrium, which appears small from the parasternal long-axis view. Mitral valve prolapse is also frequently seen in patients with Marfan's syndrome.[P4]

In chronic aortic regurgitation, characteristic 2D and M-mode echocardiographic findings are left ventricular volume overload[M1, M2] and diastolic fluttering of the anterior leaflet of the mitral valve and interventricular septum.[C9, D8, J1] In acute severe aortic regurgitation, premature closure of the mitral valve may be observed on M-mode echocardiography; left ventricular cavity size is typically normal, and function is normal or hyperdynamic[B4, M3] (Fig. 21–8). Combined 2D and M-mode echocardiography has proved useful for the serial evaluation of the patient with known aortic regurgitation, for monitoring of left ventricular size and function, and for decision making about the timing of surgical intervention.[C10, D9, F2, G3, H3, H4, K3, N3] Although useful for the serial assessment of left ventricular size and systolic function in the patient with known chronic aortic regurgitation, combined M-mode and 2D echocardiography has not proved consistently reliable in either the detection or the assessment of the severity of aortic regurgitation, because the findings are nonspecific and indirectly related to the hemodynamic abnormality. For the direct detection and assessment of severity of aortic regurgitation, Doppler echocardiography is necessary.

Doppler Echocardiography in Aortic Regurgitation

In aortic regurgitation, diastolic reverse flow occurs in the left ventricular outflow tract, with a primary velocity vector opposite to normal systolic outflow. Typically, it is holodiastolic and of high velocity, corresponding to the large diastolic pressure gradient between the aorta and the left ventricle. For the *detection* of aortic regurgitation, pulsed-wave Doppler echocardiography has been shown to be more than 95 percent sensitive and 96 percent specific compared with aortography.[C11, G4, W4] Continuous-wave and color flow Doppler are similarly sensitive.[M4, O5, S11] The absence of diastolic regurgitation demonstrated by Doppler echocardiography has been reported to be 99 to 100 percent specific for the absence of aortic regurgitation compared with aortography.[G4] Therefore, a discrepancy between Doppler echocardiographic findings and auscultatory evidence of aortic regurgitation by physical diagnosis should be attributed to the limitations of auscultation.

Assessment of the severity of aortic regurgitation may be accomplished by *semiquantitative* Doppler echocardiographic methods, including pulsed-wave mapping, demonstration of aortic flow reversal, and color flow imaging. Pulsed-wave mapping of the severity of aortic regurgitation is performed by 2D echocardiography–guided placement of the sample volume in the left ventricular outflow tract and left ventricular cavity, searching for a high-velocity diastolic jet. Sampling is performed in multiple orthogonal imaging planes, thereby mapping the three-dimensional spatial extent of regurgitation. The severity of regurgitation has been defined as the depth at which the signal is found in the left ventricle.[C11] Although reasonable correlation between pulsed-wave Doppler and aortography for semiquantitative estimate of the severity of regurgitation was observed in initial studies,[C11] subsequent investigation demonstrated that estimates of the severity of regurgitation by pulsed-wave mapping may overlap considerably with grading by aortography. Estimates of the severity of aortic regurgitation based on pulsed-wave signal depth alone often underestimate the three-dimensional distribution of regurgitant flow and, hence, the severity of the hemodynamic abnormality.[P5, S15] Our practice is to sample in the left ventricular outflow tract, using the pulsed-wave method for *detection* of aortic regurgitation, but to estimate severity by alternative Doppler echocardiographic methods.

Detection of thoracic aortic flow reversal by pulsed-wave Doppler echocardiography has been proposed as a semiquantitative method for the assessment of the severity of aortic regurgitation (Fig. 21–9). Quinones and associates showed that if the area of the reverse thoracic aortic flow profile was greater than 30 percent of that of the forward flow profile, pulsed-wave Doppler echocardiography reliably differentiated mild from moderate aortic regurgitation in patients with aortic regurgitation proved by aortography.[Q1] In a separate study, the detection of reverse flow in the abdominal aorta was observed to correlate well with severe aortic regurgitation demonstrated at aortography, although the number of patients in the study was small.[T5] Flow reversal in the descending aorta may also be demonstrated

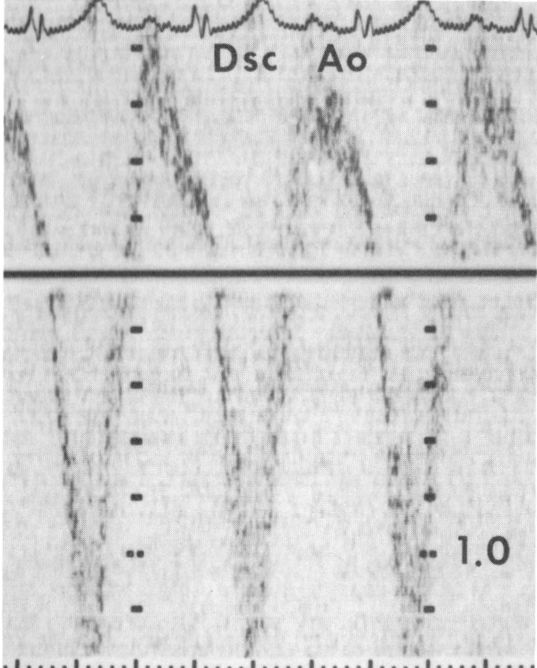

Figure 21–9. Velocity profiles of blood flow in descending aorta (Dsc Ao) in a patient with severe aortic regurgitation. A flow profile above the baseline occurs in diastole and represents regurgitant flow, which in this patient is holodiastolic. The flow profile below the baseline is systolic and represents forward flow.

by color flow imaging from the suprasternal notch. The region of brightest color or any region of aliasing may be used to guide the placement of the pulsed-wave Doppler sample volume for recording of flow velocities (Fig. 21–10). The abdominal aorta or iliac and femoral arteries may be examined in similar fashion if the suprasternal window is inadequate. Color M-mode aids in the timing of the regurgitant signal and demonstrates that it is pandiastolic.

Figure 21–10. See Color Plate 1.

Semiquantitative estimate of the severity of aortic regurgitation by color flow imaging is based on the spatial extent of detected regurgitation (Fig. 21–11). Orthogonal imaging planes are used to characterize the severity of regurgitation in both parasternal long- and short-axis views. Regurgitant flow appears as a jet of mosaic turbulent signals extending from the left ventricular outflow tract into the ventricular cavity during diastole. In clinical practice, measures of the color jet used to estimate severity have included maximal width, area, and length. However, experimental studies comparing known regurgitant *volumes* with maximal width, area, and length have demonstrated poor correlation. The discrepancies observed in the experimental setting have been attributed to the dependence of the spatial extent of the regurgitant jet on velocity rather than on volume.[S15] However, the proximal minimal width of the color jet in the parasternal long-axis view or the area in the left ventricular outflow tract has been demonstrated to correlate well with quantitative measures of regurgitant volume; this correlation has been attributed to the relationship of the proximal width of the color jet to the regurgitant orifice area. Although the minimal proximal width and area of the regurgitant color jet are not direct measures of the volume of regurgitation, correlation with semiquantitative estimates of severity by aortography has also been excellent.

Figure 21–11. See Color Plate 2.

Perry and associates, using a ratio of the minimal proximal regurgitant jet width divided by left ventricular outflow width in the parasternal long-axis view, described four grades of aortic regurgitation by color flow imaging: grade I corresponded to a ratio of less than 0.25; grade II, from 0.25 to 0.46; grade III, from 0.47 to 0.64; and grade IV, 0.65 or greater. Using this method, these investigators correctly classified the severity of aortic regurgitation in more than 90 percent of patients, using aortography as the standard.[P5]

Potential limitations of color flow imaging include variation of the spatial extent of the color jet with transducer frequency, gain setting, and pulse repetition frequency and physiologic factors not directly related to the severity of regurgitation that may affect the dimension of the regurgitant jet, including the driving pressure of the aorta, compliance of the left ventricle, the duration of diastole, and left ventricular end-diastolic pressure.[P5, W5] Furthermore, color flow Doppler echocardiography is highly operator-dependent. Small alterations in transducer angulation may substantially influence the dimensions of the regurgitant jet. The dimension of the regurgitant jet must be maximized to avoid underestimation of the severity of the hemodynamic abnormality. Despite these limitations, the semiquantitative estimate of the severity of aortic regurgitation by color flow imaging is widely accepted and used because of its excellent correlation with semiquantitative estimates by aortography. However, it is prudent to use color flow imaging in conjunction with other echocardiographic variables for assessment of the severity of the hemodynamic abnormality.

Quantitative methods for the assessment of the severity of aortic regurgitation include analysis of the continuous-wave Doppler profile of regurgitation and measurement of regurgitant fraction and regurgitant volume. Doppler echocardiographic methods for the evaluation of regurgitant orifice area have also been described.[S16, Y2]

Continuous-wave Doppler is used to measure the velocity of regurgitant blood flow throughout diastole. According to the principles of Bernoulli hydrodynamics, the pressure gradient across a restricting orifice is proportional to the square of the velocity gradient. Hence, the deceleration slope of the aortic regurgitant signal detected by continuous-wave Doppler is a measure of the rate of pressure decay between aorta and left ventricle, which reflects the severity of regurgitation in the absence of left ventricular dysfunction or rapid peripheral runoff. In mild aortic regurgitation, aortic diastolic pressure declines slowly, left ventricular pressure rises slowly, and a large pressure gradient persists at end-diastole. Accordingly, the Doppler profile of aortic regurgitant velocity also decays slowly. In contrast, in severe aortic regurgitation, there is a rapid decrease in the pressure gradient between the aorta and left ventricle, corresponding to a rapid collapse of aortic diastolic pressure and a simultaneous rapid rise in left ventricular diastolic pressure, manifested by a rapid fall in aortic regurgitant velocity by Doppler echocardiography (Fig. 21–12).

The rate of pressure decline has been demonstrated to be directly related to the severity of regurgitation by measurement of the deceleration slope[G5, L3, S16] or derivation of the pressure half-time[T6] from the continuous-wave Doppler signal. Generally, a diastolic velocity decay slope of greater than 3 m/sec^2 is indicative of severe aortic regurgitation. The pressure half-time method was originally described with use of invasive techniques[L4]; the use of Doppler echocardiography to derive the pressure half-time has been clinically validated by simultaneous Doppler echocardiography and catheterization studies.[N4] Pressure half-time measurements correlate well with the severity of aortic regurgitation as assessed by semiquantitative invasive methods (Fig. 21–13). A pressure half-time of less than 350 msec is usually indicative of

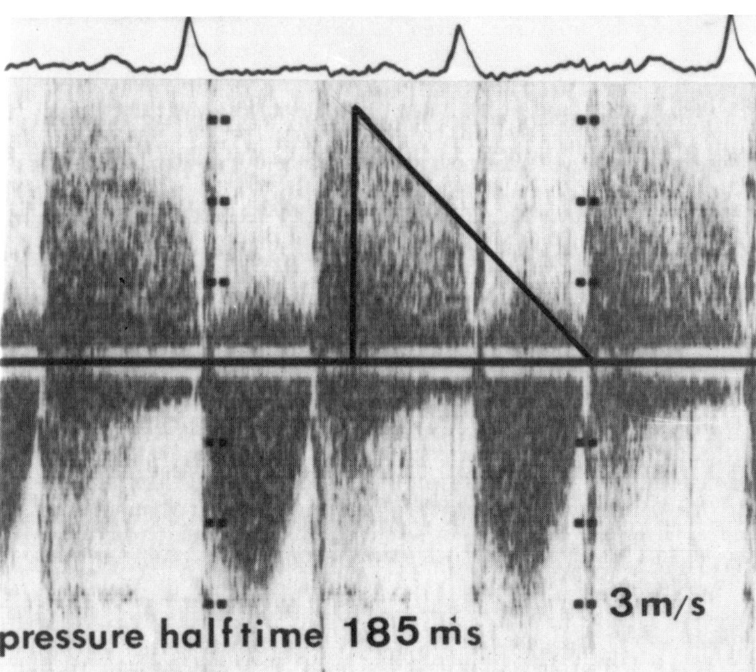

Figure 21–12. Severe aortic regurgitation demonstrated by continuous-wave echocardiography. Signals are obtained from the apical window such that regurgitant flow is directed toward the transducer and is displayed above baseline. The slope of deceleration is indicated by the solid line. The deceleration rate exceeds 3 m/sec², and pressure half-time is less than 300 msec; each value is consistent with severe aortic regurgitation.

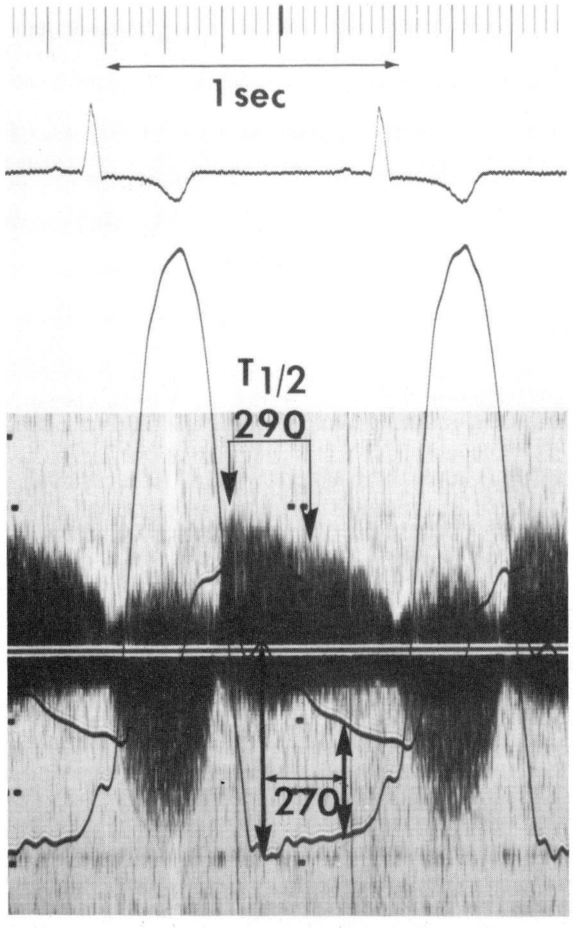

Figure 21–13. Simultaneous dual-catheter and Doppler tracings from a patient with aortic regurgitation, illustrating the correlation between diastolic half-times measured by Doppler (290 msec) and catheterization (270 msec). (From Nishimura, R. A., and Tajik, A. J.: Determination of left-sided pressure gradients by utilizing Doppler aortic and mitral regurgitant signals: Validation by simultaneous dual catheter and Doppler studies. J. Am. Coll. Cardiol. 11:317, 1988. By permission of the American College of Cardiology.)

severe regurgitation.[T6] The method appears to be independent of heart rate, pulse pressure, left ventricular ejection fraction, and the incident angle between the Doppler beam and the regurgitant jet.[T6]

Potential limitations of the analysis of the continuous-wave profile of regurgitation include acquisition of an analyzable signal, which may not be possible in approximately 10 percent of patients, and increased left ventricular end-diastolic pressure, which may cause overestimation of the severity of aortic regurgitation because of more rapid equalization of the aortic–left ventricular diastolic pressure difference.

Quantitative assessment of the severity of aortic regurgitation is also possible by the use of combined 2D and Doppler echocardiography for the measurement of either regurgitant fraction or regurgitant volume. Estimation of regurgitant fraction or regurgitant volume requires estimates of total stroke volume and forward stroke volume. The difference between the two measurements represents regurgitant stroke volume, and regurgitant fraction is given by the regurgitant stroke volume divided by the total stroke volume. The total stroke volume is obtained by 2D echocardiographic measurement of the left ventricular outflow tract area multiplied by the time-velocity integral of left ventricular outflow measured by pulsed-wave Doppler; forward stroke volume is similarly measured by evaluation of a second, nondiseased valve. In practice, forward stroke volume is estimated by 2D echocardiographic measurement of the right ventricular outflow area multiplied by the time-velocity integral of right ventricular outflow measured by pulsed-wave Doppler echocardiography. Limitations of the echocardiographic determination of regurgitant fraction or regurgitant volume include cardiac cycle–dependent variation in annular cross-sectional area, coexistent disease affecting other valves, and intracardiac or extracardiac shunts.[R7] Regurgitant orifice area may be derived by applying the continuity equation to reverse diastolic flow signals associated with aortic regurgitation at the supravalvular and subvalvular levels. Preliminary reports in patients suggest that this method will provide another useful measure for the quantitative assessment of the severity of aortic regurgitation.[Y2]

Although echocardiographic methods for the estimation of regurgitant fraction and regurgitant volume have correlated well with invasive techniques, the quantitative methods are not used routinely in clinical practice. This may be attributed to the technical limitations and measurement error associated with the use of invasive methods for the quantitative assessment of aortic regurgitation, including catheter position, volume and rate of injection of contrast medium, left ventricular size, the volume of forward flow, ventricular ectopic activity, and the effects of variation in peripheral arterial pressure.[A2, C12, F3, S17] Quantitative assessment of the severity of regurgitation by invasive methods really provides only semiquantitative categories of regurgitant severity (mild, moderate, severe) rather than true volumetric assessment. Hence, the chief limitation of the clinical implementation of noninvasive estimates of regurgitant fraction or regurgitant volume has been the lack of a reliable method to establish a precedent for their use in routine clinical decision making.

Role of Echocardiography in Clinical Decision Making in Aortic Regurgitation

Doppler echocardiographic information is used in conjunction with M-mode and 2D echocardiographic data for the detection and assessment of the cause and severity of aortic regurgitation. Serial combined M-mode and 2D echocardiography provides quantitative assessment of aortic root and left ventricular cavity dimensions and systolic function necessary for decisions on the timing of surgery.[C10, D9, G3, H4, K3, N3]

Doppler echocardiography enables semiquantitative or quantitative assessment of the severity of aortic regurgitation. The availability of several methods makes assessment of the hemodynamic severity of aortic regurgitation possible in virtually all patients. The estimate of the severity of regurgitation may be presumed to be accurate if different methods provide concordant results. Similar to the evaluation of patients with aortic valvular stenosis, cardiac catheterization for determination of severity of aortic regurgitation adds little to influence clinical decision making. Transesophageal echocardiography or aortography is indicated for complete preoperative evaluation of patients in whom resection or repair of the aortic root is contemplated. Preoperative catheterization is indicated in patients in whom there may be underlying coronary artery disease and coronary angiography in patients in whom echocardiographic data are not optimal.

Mitral Stenosis

Mitral stenosis is characterized by a reduced mitral orifice dimension with associated impairment of left ventricular filling. Rheumatic disease remains the most common cause despite the declining incidence of rheumatic fever in Western nations.[O6, R8, R9] Rare causes of valvular obstruction include congenital mitral stenosis and the parachute mitral valve. Other unusual causes of obstruction to left ventricular filling not affecting the mitral valve and easily recognized by 2D echocardiography include tumors, thrombi, dense mitral annulus calcification, cor triatriatum, and supravalvular rings.[H5, O7, W6]

The echocardiographic features of rheumatic mitral stenosis are best appreciated from the parasternal long-axis and short-axis views and include thickened and deformed leaflets with fusion of the commissures and subvalvular apparatus. Frequently, there is associated calcification of the valvular and subvalvular apparatus.[P6, R8, R9, Z2] Characteristic motion abnormalities are reduced leaflet excursion in diastole with doming and the so-called hockey-stick deformity of the anterior leaflet due to tethering by the subvalvular apparatus (Fig. 21–14). The posterior leaflet is frequently immobile or severely restricted in its motion.

Congenital mitral stenosis is characterized by thickened and fibrotic mitral valve leaflets with fused or absent commissures and fibrotic and shortened chordae and papillary muscles.[R10] In contrast to acquired rheumatic mitral stenosis, calcification of the mitral apparatus is not typically seen. Motion abnormalities of the leaflets of the mitral valve are similar to those observed in patients with rheumatic disease.[W6] A second form of congenital mitral stenosis is the parachute mitral valve, in which there is a single, large papillary muscle with normal chordae and valve leaflets. The convergence of the chordae to insert on a single papillary muscle may produce obstruction at the subvalvular level.[R10, S18, S19]

Associated morphologic abnormalities frequently observed by 2D echocardiography in the patient with chronic obstruction to left ventricular filling are left atrial and right ventricular enlargement. Coexistent left atrial thrombus is not an uncommon finding in the patient with long-standing mitral stenosis, especially in the presence of chronic atrial fibrillation. However, thrombus in the left atrial appendage frequently cannot be demonstrated by transthoracic 2D echocardiography. Transesophageal echocardiography should be performed in patients in whom left atrial thrombus is suspected, especially if transseptal catheterization is anticipated.

Assessment of the hemodynamic severity of mitral valvular stenosis by 2D echocardiography is performed by direct measurement of the mitral orifice area from the parasternal short-axis view (Fig. 21–14). The accuracy of the 2D echocardiographic method for the assessment of mitral valve area has been validated by comparison with data obtained at surgery,[G6, H6] at pathologic examination,[W7] and at cardiac catheterization.[G6, M5, W7] The smallest orifice is detected by slow, methodical scanning superiorly to inferiorly, and a reproducible estimate of mitral valve area is possible in 85 to 90 percent of patients. In the remainder of patients, assessment of mitral valve area is either not possible or unreliable because of suboptimal images, dense calcification, prior commissurotomy,[S20] or predominant subvalvular obstruction. Whenever possible, estimations of mitral valve area by 2D and Doppler echocardiographic methods should be correlated.

Two-dimensional echocardiography has been used for the iden-

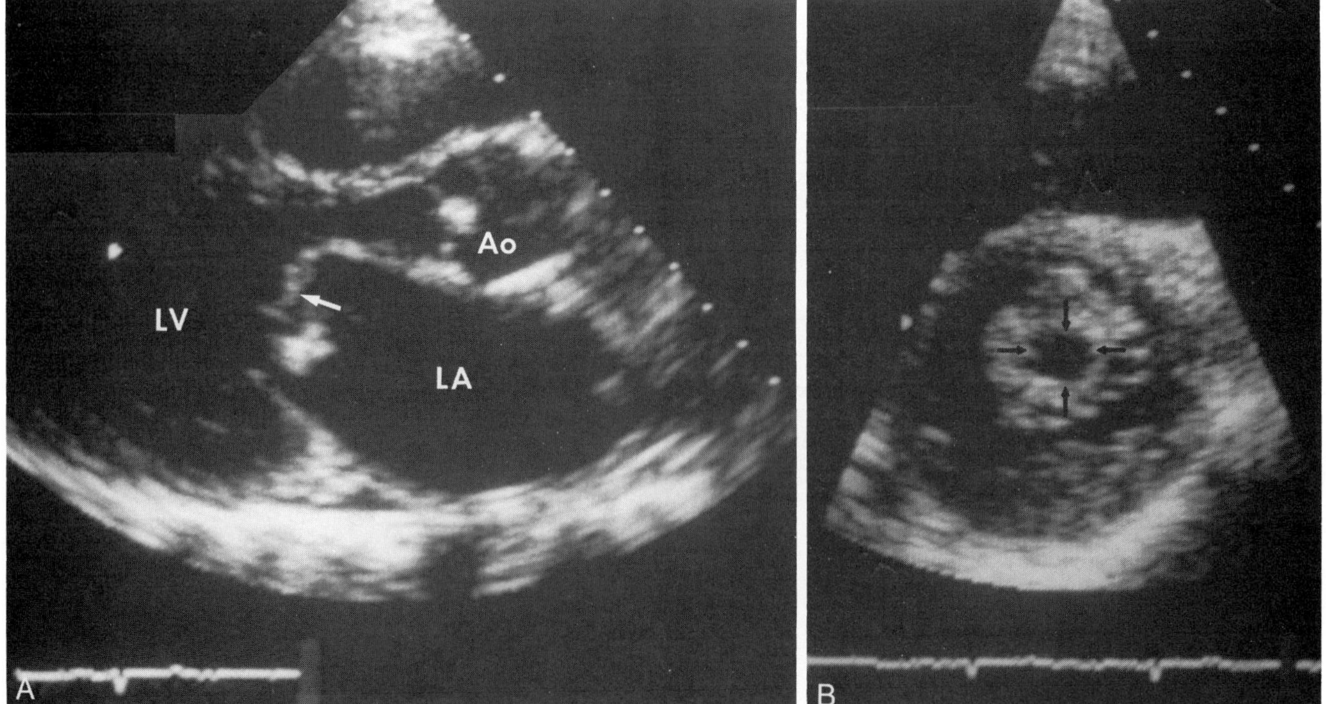

Figure 21–14. *A*, Two-dimensional echocardiographic evaluation of rheumatic mitral stenosis. A parasternal long-axis view demonstrates the typical appearance of a stenotic mitral valve. The anterior leaflet of the mitral valve (*arrow*) has a doming configuration (also referred to as a "hockey-stick" appearance) in diastole. Full excursion of the valve leaflet is prevented by the tethering effect of the subvalvular apparatus. The posterior leaflet is immobile. The left atrium (LA) is enlarged. Ao—aorta; LV—left ventricle. *B*, Parasternal short-axis view of a stenotic mitral valve. Restriction of the opening of anterior and posterior leaflets causes a reduced mitral orifice area (*arrows*). There is minimal calcification of valve leaflets. The mitral orifice area may be measured directly by planimetry from a freeze-frame image on modern equipment.

tification of patients who may benefit from mitral balloon valvuloplasty. A scoring system based on 2D echocardiographic criteria has been proposed to characterize the suitability of the valve for valvuloplasty.[W8] The system scores (grades 1 through 4) each of four 2D echocardiographic characteristics: valve mobility, valve thickness, valve calcification, and subvalvular thickening. Patients with a score of 8 or less have a greater than 90 percent chance of a satisfactory result. The most important factors in predicting the initial success and long-term outcome of valvuloplasty are the severity of calcification and subvalvular fibrosis.[W8] Evidence of left atrial thrombus is a contraindication to the procedure. Because 2D echocardiography usually does not visualize the left atrial appendage, transesophageal echocardiography should be performed to exclude thrombus.

Doppler Echocardiography in Mitral Stenosis

Analysis of the mitral valve inflow velocity profile by Doppler echocardiography provides direct hemodynamic assessment of the severity of obstruction to mitral inflow. The optimal Doppler flow profile is obtained from an apical window and in the absence of valvular disease demonstrates low-velocity diastolic flow toward the transducer, with a peak velocity of less than 1.3 m/sec.

Impediment to mitral inflow causes an increase in left atrial pressure, thereby increasing the driving pressure from left atrium to ventricle, and also slows emptying of the left atrium. Continuous-wave Doppler echocardiography is used to assess mitral inflow because velocity aliasing occurs with pulsed-wave Doppler in moderate-to-severe stenosis. Continuous-wave Doppler demonstrates an increased diastolic flow velocity and a reduced rate of velocity decay corresponding directly to the severity of the pressure gradient throughout diastole.[H7–H9, K4] Color flow imaging is helpful in optimizing the parallel placement of the continuous-wave cursor by identification of the direction of the jet, which may be eccentric.[K5]

The left atrial–left ventricular diastolic pressure gradient is obtained from the mitral inflow velocity profile by application of the *modified Bernoulli equation*. The *instantaneous* pressure gradient between the left atrium and the left ventricle can be estimated at any point in diastole. As has been the convention by invasive techniques, hemodynamic severity is assessed by estimation of the transvalvular left atrial–left ventricular peak, mean, and end-diastolic gradients. If the gradient is mild to moderate at rest, our practice is to exercise the patient while supine and repeat the Doppler examination immediately after exercise. Because the gradient is flow-dependent, it is always necessary to estimate mitral valve area.

Mitral valve area may be estimated by two different Doppler echocardiographic methods: estimation of the pressure half-time or measurement of valve area by the continuity equation. The pressure half-time method, originally described by invasive methods,[L5] has been adapted for the estimation of mitral valve area by Doppler echocardiography. The rate of decline of the diastolic pressure gradient may be described by the pressure half-time, which is the time required for the initial diastolic gradient to decline by 50 percent. Estimation of mitral valve area is based on the observation that as the degree of stenosis becomes more severe, the diastolic gradient is maintained for a longer period and the pressure half-time is prolonged. On continuous-wave Doppler echocardiographic examination, this effect is manifested as a reduced rate of decline and prolongation of the diastolic flow-velocity profile.

According to the principles of Bernoulli hydrodynamics, the relationship between pressure drop and velocity is quadratic. Hence, the pressure half-time is obtained from the Doppler velocity profile by dividing peak velocity by the square root of 2 and then measuring the time from peak velocity to the time of peak velocity divided by the square root of 2. The pressure half-time is directly related to mitral valve area; the more prolonged the half-time, the more severe the reduction in orifice area. Hatle and associates[H10] derived an empiric constant that relates pressure half-time to mitral valve area (MVA):

$$\text{MVA} = 220/\text{pressure half-time}$$

In normal individuals, pressure half-time is less than 60 msec, whereas it is 100 to 400 msec in patients with mitral stenosis

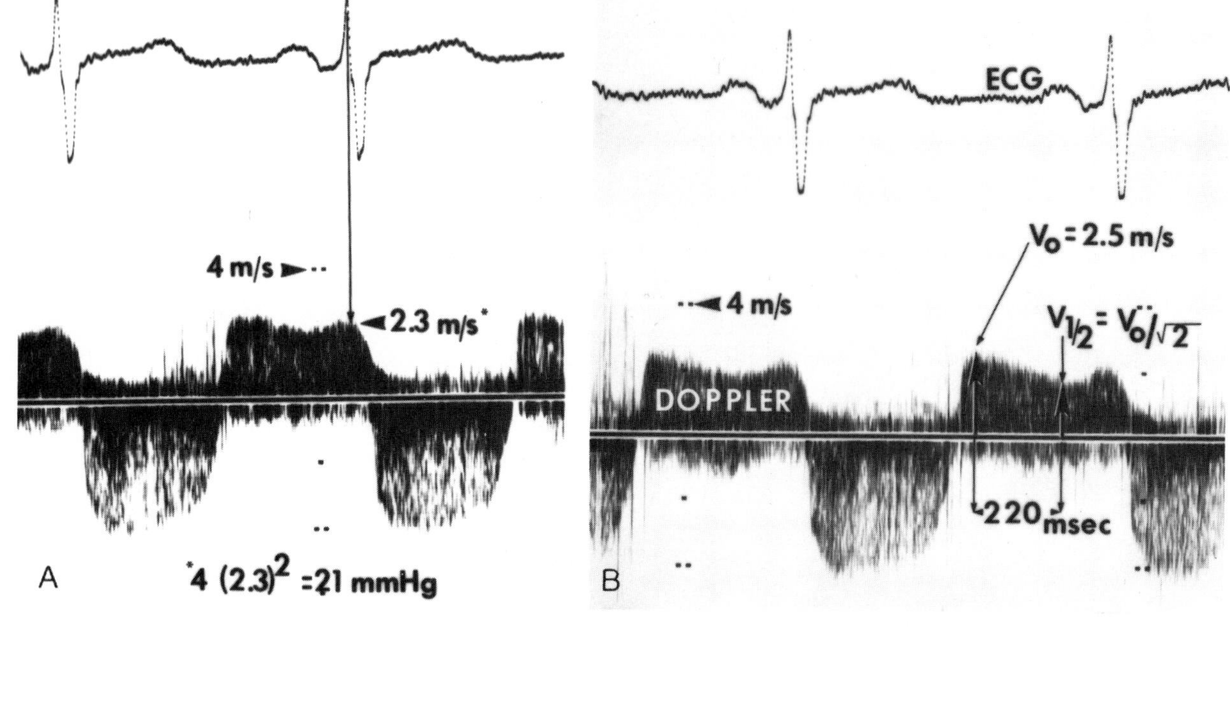

$$\text{MVA (cm}^2) = \frac{220}{\text{pressure halftime (msec.)}} = \frac{220}{220} = 1.0 \text{ cm}^2$$

C

Figure 21–15. Continuous-wave Doppler echocardiography for the hemodynamic evaluation of mitral stenosis. *A*, Estimation of the end-diastolic gradient by continuous-wave Doppler evaluation. End-diastolic velocity measured at the peak of the electrocardiographic R wave equals 2.3 m/sec, yielding an end-diastolic pressure gradient between the left atrium and the left ventricle of 21 mmHg. *B*, Initial peak velocity (V_0) is 2.5 m/sec. Peak velocity divided by the square root of 2 equals approximately 1.8 m/sec. The time elapsed between the initial peak velocity of 2.5 m/sec and the half-time velocity of 1.8 m/sec equals approximately 220 msec. *C*, Calculation of the mitral valve area: The diastolic half-time (220 msec) is divided into an empirically derived constant of 220, yielding an estimated valve area of 1 cm². (From Callahan, M. J., et al.: Continuous-wave Doppler assessment of mitral stenosis: Case example and technique. Echocardiography 1:102, 1984. By permission of Futura Publishing Company.)

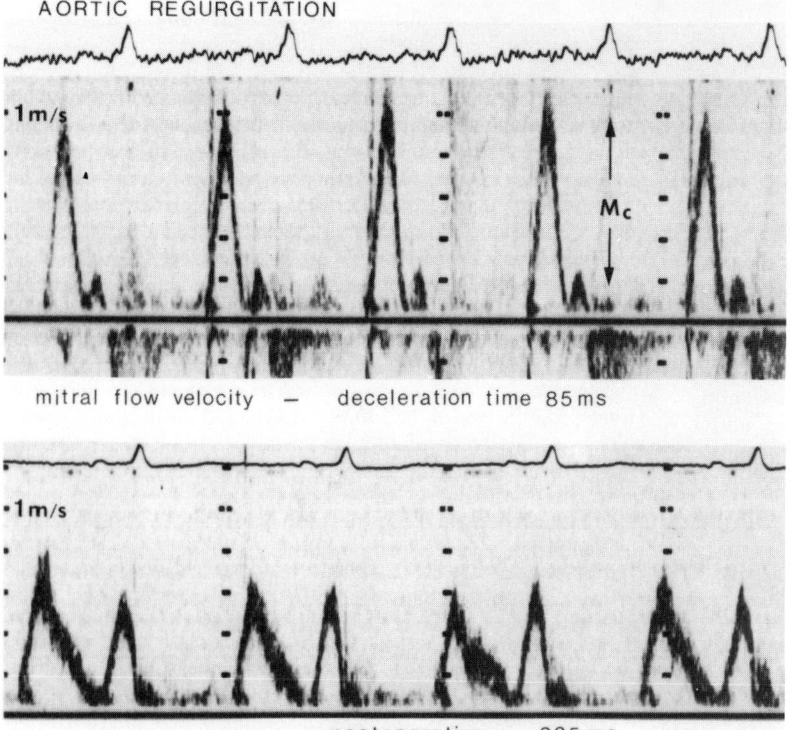

Figure 21–16. Effect of severe aortic regurgitation on the profile of mitral flow velocity obtained by Doppler echocardiography. *Top*, Mitral flow velocity profile in a patient with a normal mitral valve and severe aortic regurgitation. The peak velocity of early mitral inflow is increased, and deceleration time is markedly shortened. Abbreviation of the inflow signal would lead to a shortened half-time estimate and, hence, overestimation of the mitral valve area. *Bottom*, Same patient after aortic valve replacement. Mitral valve inflow has become normal.

(Fig. 21–15). Mitral valve area determined by the pressure half-time method has been demonstrated to correlate extremely well with mitral valve area determination at cardiac catheterization by the Gorlin formula in patients without other associated valvular disease or coronary artery disease.[H10, H11] The pressure half-time method is also independent of heart rate and mitral regurgitation.[B5]

Although estimation of mitral valve area by the Doppler half-time method is widely used, it cannot be applied to all patients with mitral stenosis. In patients with a prolonged P-R interval, increased velocity from atrial contraction in early diastole makes it impossible to separate the mitral inflow E and A waves and, hence, to measure pressure half-time. Similar problems are encountered in patients with sinus tachycardia, atrial flutter, and atrial tachycardia.[H10] In patients with atrial fibrillation, pressure half-time should be estimated from an average of at least five inflow signals. Use of the Doppler pressure half-time method is also precluded after recent mitral valvuloplasty[R11] and if moderate or severe aortic regurgitation is present.[M6, N5] In these two situations, estimates of mitral valve area by the half-time method may differ significantly from estimates based on the Gorlin formula. Significant aortic regurgitation is associated with a rapidly rising left ventricular diastolic pressure, which may decrease the transmitral pressure gradient, thereby abbreviating the pressure half-time and causing overestimation of valve area (Fig. 21–16). The discrepancy between valve area estimated immediately after valvuloplasty by pressure half-time and the Gorlin formula is not entirely explained. Furthermore, it has been demonstrated in experimental models and in patients with mitral stenosis that the pressure half-time depends on chamber stiffness and the peak pressure difference as well as orifice area. Accordingly, in patients with mitral stenosis and coexistent coronary artery disease or aortic valvular stenosis with increased left ventricular stiffness, the pressure half-time method may also overestimate mitral valve area.[K6]

The limitations of the pressure half-time method for estimation of mitral valve area may be overcome by use of the continuity equation. The continuity equation may be applied to mitral stenosis to yield valve area estimates that correlate extremely well with Gorlin formula estimates despite coexistent moderate or severe aortic regurgitation.[N5] The method assumes that flow volume through the mitral annulus in one cardiac cycle is equal to left ventricular stroke volume. Hence, mitral valve area can be determined as the stroke volume (SV) divided by the time-velocity integral of mitral flow (TVIm): MVA = SV/TVIm. Because stroke volume is the product of the cross-sectional area of the aortic or pulmonary annulus and the time-velocity integral of aortic (TVIa) or pulmonary (TVIp) flow velocity, MVA = aortic (or pulmonary) annular cross-sectional area × TVIa (or TVIp)/TVIm. In the presence of significant mitral regurgitation, this method underestimates mitral valve area.

In addition to measurement of transvalvular gradients and mitral valve area, complete Doppler echocardiographic evaluation of mitral stenosis requires assessment of right ventricular pressures. Assessment of the pulmonary artery systolic pressure is performed by measurement of the peak tricuspid regurgitant jet velocity by continuous-wave echocardiography and application of the modified Bernoulli equation, which yields the pressure gradient between the right ventricle and the right atrium. The estimated right atrial pressure is added to the measured right ventricular–right atrial gradient to yield right ventricular systolic pressure, which is equivalent to pulmonary artery systolic pressure in the absence of obstruction to right ventricular outflow. Determination of pulmonary artery systolic pressure by this method is possible in approximately 90 percent of patients (see subsequent section on tricuspid regurgitation for details). Assessment of right ventricular pressures should be performed in the resting and postexercise states in patients with mitral stenosis to completely assess the hemodynamic severity of the lesion.

Role of Echocardiography in Clinical Decision Making in Mitral Stenosis

Combined 2D and Doppler echocardiography is the preferred method for the detection and assessment of severity of mitral stenosis, because of proven efficacy and safety. Two-dimensional echocardiography is used for the detection, morphologic characterization, and initial assessment of the hemodynamic severity of obstruction to left ventricular filling. Doppler echocardiographic methods for estimate of mitral valve area are superior to invasive methods in the presence of mitral or aortic regurgitation. Mitral valve area can be determined by the continuity equation if the pressure half-time method cannot be applied. Serial study enables assessment of the progression of disease. Invasive studies are unnecessary except in the rare patient in whom 2D and Doppler data are unsatisfactory. Cardiac catheterization (coronary angiography) is indicated only in patients who have suspected coronary artery disease.

Mitral Regurgitation

Proper coaptation of the mitral valve leaflets depends on the normal function of the leaflets, papillary muscles, chordae tendineae, and subjacent ventricular myocardium. Dysfunction of any of these components of the mitral valve apparatus may produce mitral regurgitation.[P7, R12] Hence, mitral regurgitation has many causes.

Structural abnormalities of the valve apparatus are readily identified by 2D echocardiography. The most frequent cause of isolated mitral regurgitation is leaflet prolapse.[O6, P8] The prevalence of mitral prolapse, the variability of clinical findings, and the skill required to detect midsystolic clicks or a late systolic murmur have made M-mode and 2D echocardiography extremely important for the detection of mitral prolapse.[P8] The 2D echocardiographic diagnosis is based on the demonstration of a systolic arching (billowing) motion of one or both of the valve leaflets above the mitral annulus into the left atrium (Fig. 21–17). However, clinical echocardiographic investigation has demonstrated that M-mode and 2D echocardiography can overdiagnose prolapse. The diagnosis should be limited to patients in whom there is late systolic prolapse by M-mode or 2D echocardiographic evidence of prolapse from the parasternal long-axis view. Two-dimensional echocardiographic evaluation for prolapse from apical views alone is associated with false-positive diagnosis.[L6] Prolapse of the valve leaflets is also frequently associated with exaggerated motion of the posterior aspect of the mitral annulus[G7, M7] and increased thickness and redundancy of the leaflets.[M8, N6]

A great spectrum of anatomic abnormalities is associated with mitral valve prolapse demonstrated by M-mode and 2D echocardiography.[D10, M8, N6, P9] Routine assessment of severity is based on the magnitude of leaflet prolapse and degree of leaflet thickness.[M8, N6] Other patient groups may be identified in whom there is annular and leaflet enlargement.[P10] Quantitative assessment of prolapse, leaflet thickness, and leaflet and annular size by combined 2D and M-mode echocardiography has demonstrated that the severity of prolapse is related to subsequent morbid events, including endocarditis, thromboembolism, sudden death, and the need for surgical valve repair or replacement.[D11, M8, M9, N6, P10, W9] Men and patients older than 45 years appear to be at greatest risk for severe mitral regurgitation.[D12]

Chordal rupture is a frequent complication of mitral valve prolapse and may be associated with acute, severe decompensation or chronic progressive regurgitation.[G8, G9, H12, O8, O9, R13] Ruptured chordae tendineae are the most common cause of acute, severe mitral regurgitation and may also be associated with infectious endocarditis, rheumatic disease, myocardial infarction, or trauma or may occur in isolation. A ruptured chord is recognized echocardiographically as a highly mobile linear density that may appear to move primarily with the leaflet or subvalvular structures, depending on the site of rupture.[M10] It should be sought carefully in all patients with mitral regurgitation associated with exaggerated prolapse or flail segments of the mitral valve. Transesophageal echocardiography will establish the diagnosis when transthoracic echocardiographic findings are indeterminate. Other echocardiographic abnormalities associated with chordal rupture depend on the underlying disease, duration, and hemodynamic severity of mitral regurgitation.

A flail mitral valve leaflet is associated with acute, severe

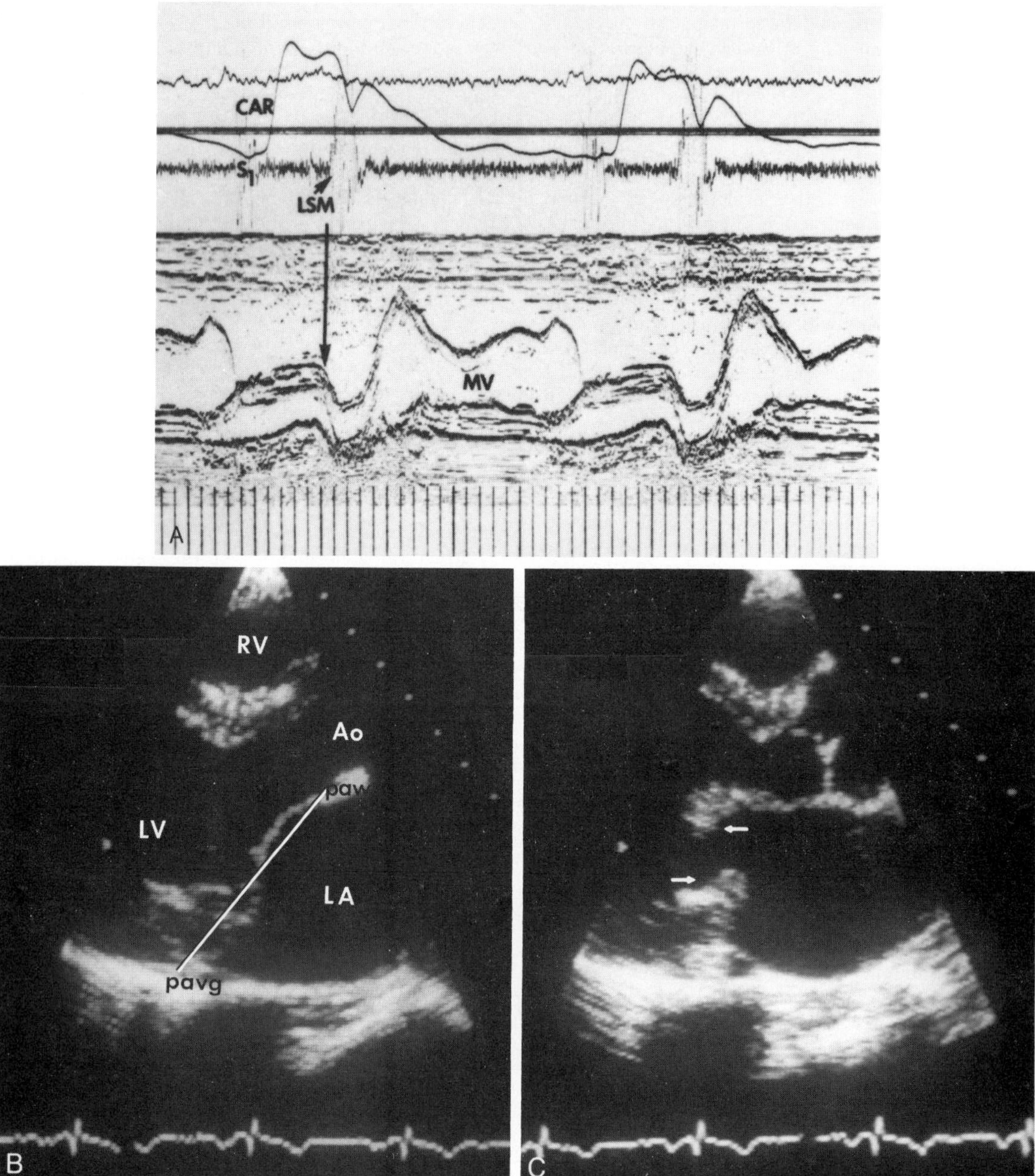

Figure 21–17. Mitral valve prolapse. *A*, M-mode echocardiogram demonstrates posterior motion of mitral valve leaflets in late systole. (From Shub, C.: The role of echocardiography in clinical practice. *In* Spittell, J. A. (ed.): Clinical Medicine. Vol. 6. Harper & Row, Philadelphia, 1982, p. 18. By permission of the publisher.) *B*, Two-dimensional echocardiogram from the parasternal long-axis view demonstrates prolapse of the posterior mitral valve leaflet into the left atrium (LA) during systole. Prolapse is defined as detection of motion of one or both leaflets superior to an imaginary line between the posterior atrioventricular groove (pavg) and the posterior aortic wall (paw). Ao—aorta; LV—left ventricle; RV—right ventricle. *C*, Two-dimensional echocardiogram from the parasternal long-axis view in diastole demonstrates redundant anterior and posterior leaflets characteristic of mitral valve prolapse (*arrows*).

regurgitation due to disruption of either the chordae tendineae or the papillary muscles. The motion of the flail leaflet is best demonstrated from either the parasternal long-axis or the apical four-chamber view.[E8] The motion is exaggerated and not easily missed, because the valve whips between the left ventricular cavity and the left atrium. The portion of the subvalvular apparatus that is affected is usually recognized on transthoracic 2D echocardiographic examination.[E8, N7] Transesophageal echocardiography is useful in selected cases in which the diagnosis is uncertain.

Papillary muscle dysfunction of any cause may produce mitral regurgitation. Abnormalities of the papillary muscles associated with regurgitation and identified by 2D echocardiography include fibrosis, calcification, dysfunction of the subjacent myocardium, and papillary muscle rupture.[E9, G10, N7] Dysfunction of the papillary muscle produces mitral regurgitation because of consequent improper systolic leaflet coaptation.

Infectious endocarditis produces mitral regurgitation by prevention of proper function of the mitral valve apparatus because of damage to the leaflets or subvalvular structures (Fig. 21–18). Complications of infectious endocarditis detected by 2D echocardiography include large vegetations preventing leaflet coaptation, leaflet prolapse, chordal rupture, leaflet perforation, and flail leaflets.[O6] The demonstration of vegetations less than 3 mm in diameter is generally not possible.[M11] Furthermore, because bacterial endocarditis frequently involves previously diseased valves, it is often impossible to distinguish between valvular vegetations and leaflet thickening, calcification, or myxomatous degeneration. Transesophageal echocardiography is useful for identification of small vegetations and characterization of valvular

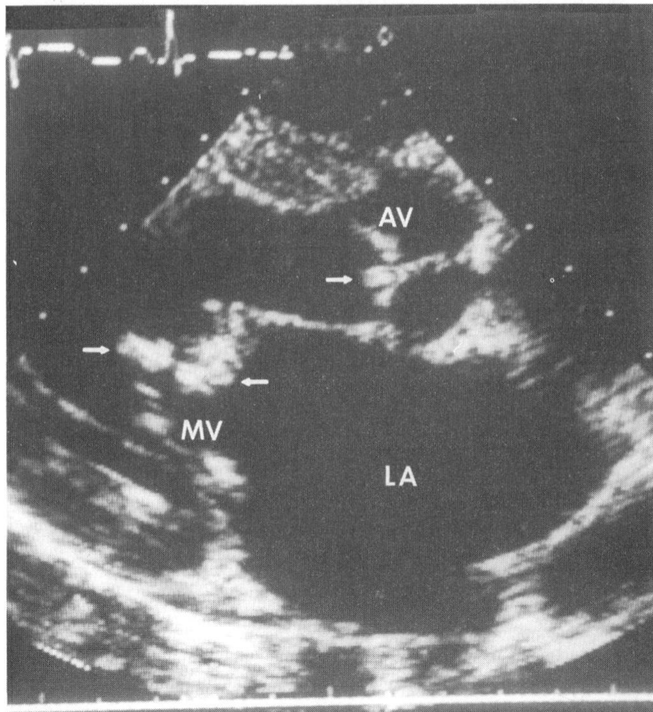

Figure 21–18. Parasternal long-axis views in diastole of mitral and aortic valvular vegetations (*arrows*) from a patient with bacterial endocarditis. AV—aortic valve; LA—left atrium; MV—mitral valve.

abnormalities, including leaflet perforation, perivalvular abscess, and damage to the subvalvular apparatus.[D13]

Mitral annular calcification is a degenerative disorder, is a frequent echocardiographic finding in elderly patients, and is often associated with mitral regurgitation. It is recognized echocardiographically by the presence of dense echoes in the region of the annulus. It may be mild or severe and is typically most severe at the posterior aspect of the annulus.[N8] Less commonly, it is associated with mitral stenosis.[H5]

Rheumatic mitral regurgitation is recognized echocardiographically from the parasternal long- and short-axis views by the presence of thickened, deformed leaflets and subvalvular apparatus with or without associated calcification. Frequently, mitral stenosis and aortic valve disease are associated. In the absence of mitral stenosis, there is little leaflet calcification and no commissural fusion.[B6, D14]

A congenital anomaly of the mitral valve that may be responsible for mitral regurgitation in the adult is a cleft of the anterior leaflet, which may be partial or complete.[D15] Accessory chordae from the anterior leaflet attach to the crest of the ventricular septum, effectively preventing coaptation and causing regurgitation. The cleft is best appreciated from the parasternal short-axis view in diastole, is frequently associated with an ostium primum atrial septal defect, and only occasionally occurs as an isolated anomaly.

In the evaluation of the patient with suspected or proved mitral regurgitation, combined 2D and M-mode echocardiography is used to evaluate left atrial and left ventricular size and function and to detect associated valvular heart disease. Serial studies are useful for the longitudinal follow-up of patients with known chronic mitral regurgitation for evaluation of the timing of surgical intervention.[M12, Z3, Z4] However, neither M-mode nor 2D echocardiography is useful for the detection or estimation of severity of mitral regurgitation, because the findings are nonspecific and indirectly related to the severity of the hemodynamic abnormality.

Doppler Echocardiography in Mitral Regurgitation

Detection of mitral regurgitation by pulsed-wave Doppler echocardiography is performed by placement of the sample volume within the left atrium immediately superior to the mitral valve leaflets. Normally, no systolic signal is detected other than the clicks of the mitral valve. The presence of mitral regurgitation is confirmed by the detection of a systolic signal of high velocity. Mitral regurgitation is detected with very high sensitivity by pulsed-wave[A3, B7, V3] and color flow Doppler echocardiography.[M13, M14] Physiologic mitral regurgitation is detected in more than 40 percent of normal patients by Doppler echocardiography.[Y3] This does *not* represent "false-positive" evidence of mitral regurgitation. Instead, it represents subclinical regurgitation, detected by an extremely sensitive technique. Our practice is to describe this as physiologic or trivial regurgitation.

A *semiquantitative* estimate of the severity of mitral regurgitation is performed by pulsed-wave and color flow Doppler echocardiography. Pulsed-wave mapping of regurgitant flow within the territory of the left atrium is performed in a manner similar to that described for aortic regurgitation. Mild mitral regurgitation has been characterized as systolic flow detected immediately posterior and superior to the mitral valve leaflets only.[A3, V3] More severe regurgitation is associated with larger areas of turbulent systolic flow detected within the left atrium.[A4] Complete mapping by pulsed-wave echocardiography requires examination from multiple tomographic orientations to accurately characterize the three-dimensional spatial extent of regurgitation. The regurgitant jet may be narrow or broad and is frequently eccentric. However, when compared with semiquantitative assessment by ventriculography, pulsed-wave mapping frequently overestimates or underestimates the severity of regurgitation.[A4] As in the evaluation of aortic regurgitation, pulsed-wave mapping is laborious and time-consuming and has been supplanted by color flow imaging.

Color flow imaging is accurate for the semiquantitative assessment of the severity of mitral regurgitation. The regurgitant flow signals characteristically have a mosaic appearance because of turbulence and aliasing associated with high-velocity flow due to the large systolic pressure gradient between the left ventricle and atrium (Fig. 21–19). Helmcke and colleagues demonstrated high correlation between color flow imaging and semiquantitative grading by angiography, correctly classifying grade I, II, or III mitral regurgitation in 77 of 82 patients.[H13] In their study, the spatial extent of the regurgitant jet was analyzed in three different tomographic planes, and the severity was expressed as the maximum jet area indexed by left atrial area. A ratio of less than 0.2 corresponded to angiographic grade I (mild), a ratio of between 0.2 and 0.4 represented grade II (moderate), and a ratio greater than 0.4 corresponded to grade III (severe) regurgitation. In the same study, evaluation of the severity of mitral regurgitation by color flow imaging correlated well with invasive estimates of regurgitant fraction. Other investigators have demonstrated acceptable reproducibility and interobserver variability in the quantification of Doppler color flow jet area and correlation with the angiographic grade of mitral regurgitation.[S21, S22]

Figure 21–19. See Color Plate 2.

Continuous-wave Doppler enables measurement of the peak mitral regurgitant velocity, which typically is 4 to 5 m/sec. The instantaneous pressure difference between the left ventricle and the left atrium can be measured at any point in systole by application of the *modified Bernoulli equation* and correlates extremely well with instantaneous pressure gradients measured by simultaneous dual catheterization of the left atrium and left ventricle.[N4] However, the maximum instantaneous pressure gradient is *not* a measure of the severity of mitral regurgitation. The gradient is determined chiefly by the left ventricular systolic (driving) pressure and reflects the left ventricular–left atrial gradient in systole, which may have little relation to the severity of regurgitation. However, it has been suggested that the severity of mitral regurgitation may be semiquantitatively estimated by visual inspection of the intensity of the continuous-wave Doppler profile of regurgitation relative to the mitral diastolic inflow signal. When regurgitation is mild, the Doppler signal appears faint, and when regurgitation is severe, the signal appears intense. However, other semiquantitative and quantitative methods are superior for the assessment of the severity of mitral regurgitation.

Quantitative evaluation of the severity of mitral regurgitation requires estimation of regurgitant volume or regurgitant fraction. Combined pulsed-Doppler and 2D echocardiography has been used to calculate regurgitant fraction and volume from the difference between mitral and aortic stroke volume, and the results correlate well with angiographic and scintigraphic estimates.[B8] Aortic stroke volume is derived as the product of the aortic time-velocity integral and aortic annular cross-sectional area. Similarly, mitral stroke volume is derived as the product of the mitral time-velocity integral and mitral cross-sectional annulus area. The diameter of the mitral annulus is measured from the apical four-chamber view at maximal diastolic leaflet excursion, from the medial inner edge to the lateral inner edge of the annulus just below the insertion of the leaflets. Cross-sectional areas for each valve are calculated using $\pi \cdot r^2$, assuming circular valve orifices, with r equivalent to one half the measured diameter. Regurgitant flow is the difference between mitral and aortic flow, and regurgitant fraction is regurgitant flow divided by mitral inflow.

The major limitation of echocardiographic methods for the estimation of regurgitant fraction or volume is the exclusion of patients with other left-sided valvular heart disease. The most important potential sources of error include measurement of aortic and mitral orifice area, which may lead to estimates of regurgitant fraction as high as 20 percent for normal valves.[L7] However, this is similar to the error inherent in measurement of regurgitant fraction by invasive methods.[L8] The chief problem with the use of any invasive or noninvasive quantitative method for the assessment of the severity of regurgitation is that no criteria have been defined for the evaluation of disease progression, reproducibility of the techniques, or usefulness in assisting decision making about the timing of valve surgery.

Role of Echocardiography in Clinical Decision Making in Mitral Regurgitation

Combined 2D and M-mode echocardiography provides anatomic and quantitative information that enables classification of the cause of mitral regurgitation and assessment of cardiac chamber dimension and left ventricular function necessary for longitudinal follow-up in the patient with chronic mitral regurgitation. Doppler echocardiography enables detection and assessment of the hemodynamic severity of regurgitation. Complete Doppler echocardiographic assessment should include estimation of pulmonary artery pressure for the assessment of possible pulmonary hypertension (see section on tricuspid regurgitation). Cardiac catheterization is reserved for patients in whom suboptimal data are obtained, clinical and echocardiographic data are discordant, or there is suspected coronary artery disease.

Tricuspid Stenosis

The tricuspid valve is larger and more complex than the mitral valve. It consists of three leaflets, an annular ring, and subvalvular components, including chordae tendineae, papillary muscles, and subjacent right ventricular myocardium. It is differentiated from the mitral valve by its trileaflet structure, multiple separate papillary muscles, and annular insertion inferior to the mitral annulus.[S23] As in mitral stenosis, tricuspid stenosis is characterized by reduced orifice dimension, which impairs right ventricular filling. Obstruction to right ventricular inflow may be due to congenital or acquired disease and may be primarily valvular, subvalvular, or supravalvular in location.[S24]

Rheumatic heart disease is the most common cause of tricuspid stenosis.[H14, S24] Stenosis is produced by leaflet fibrosis, commissural fusion, and fibrosis and thickening of the chordae; calcification is unusual.[C13, H14, S24] There are virtually always associated tricuspid regurgitation and rheumatic mitral disease. Echocardiographic evaluation of the tricuspid valve is best performed from the right ventricular inflow view, in long- and short-axis positions. Rheumatic stenosis is recognized by demonstration of thickened and deformed leaflets, abnormal leaflet motion, and reduced orifice dimension. Unlike rheumatic mitral disease, tricuspid stenosis is uncommonly accompanied by calcification. As in other stenotic valvular lesions, abnormal leaflet motion is characterized by doming at maximal excursion.[D16]

Less frequent causes of acquired tricuspid valvular stenosis are carcinoid, methysergide toxicity, endomyocardial fibrosis, and endomyocardial fibroelastoma.[H14, H15, W10] Each of these disorders is characterized pathologically by deposition of fibrous material on the tricuspid leaflet, producing combined stenosis and regurgitation. Two-dimensional echocardiography demonstrates a thickened valve and shortened supporting structures and diastolic doming of the leaflets. In severe cases, the tricuspid valve is immobile, fixed in a semiopen position[C14] (Fig. 21–20). These disorders may not always be easily distinguishable from rheumatic disease by echocardiography. However, associated findings suggest specific diagnoses. In rheumatic disease, there will virtually always be associated mitral valve disease, whereas in carcinoid and methysergide toxicity, combined pulmonary stenosis and regurgitation are frequent and left-sided valvular disease is extremely unusual. Similarly, endomyocardial fibrosis and fibroelastosis are frequently associated with obliteration of the right ventricular apex, easily demonstrated by 2D echocardiography.

The hemodynamic severity of tricuspid stenosis cannot be assessed directly by combined 2D and M-mode echocardiography. Short-axis recording of the tricuspid orifice is seldom possible. Hence, estimation of the orifice area cannot be performed routinely as in mitral stenosis. Enlargement of the right atrium, inferior vena cava, and hepatic veins is frequently seen but is an indirect marker of right atrial hypertension. Therefore, an estimate of the severity of tricuspid stenosis requires Doppler echocardiography.

Doppler Echocardiography in the Evaluation of Tricuspid Stenosis

The tricuspid inflow Doppler signals are best demonstrated in the right ventricular inflow view or the apical four-chamber view. The normal tricuspid valve flow profile is qualitatively similar to that of mitral inflow but of lesser magnitude.

Tricuspid stenosis causes an increased gradient from the right atrium to the right ventricle throughout diastole. Pressure gradients by continuous-wave Doppler echocardiography may be reliably estimated. Doppler echocardiography demonstrates increased velocity and slowed decay of the inflow signal, as in mitral stenosis[D17, H16, V4] (Fig. 21–21). However, the velocities observed are usually not as high as those in mitral stenosis. The ease of the Doppler method contrasts with the difficulty of verifying the pressure gradient at cardiac catheterization, especially in the presence of atrial fibrillation, because of effects of respiration, unless right atrial and right ventricular pressures are recorded simultaneously by the dual-catheter technique. The pressure half-time method is used to estimate tricuspid valve area, as in mitral stenosis, with use of the empiric formula of Hatle and associates,[H10] described for mitral stenosis. Noninvasive estimates of severity correlate well with invasive estimates.[D17]

Role of Echocardiography in Clinical Decision Making in Tricuspid Stenosis

Two-dimensional echocardiography demonstrates the anatomic location and cause of obstruction to right ventricular filling. Evaluation of associated valvular pathologic conditions and chamber size and function is helpful in determining the cause of disease and provides indirect assessment of hemodynamic sever-

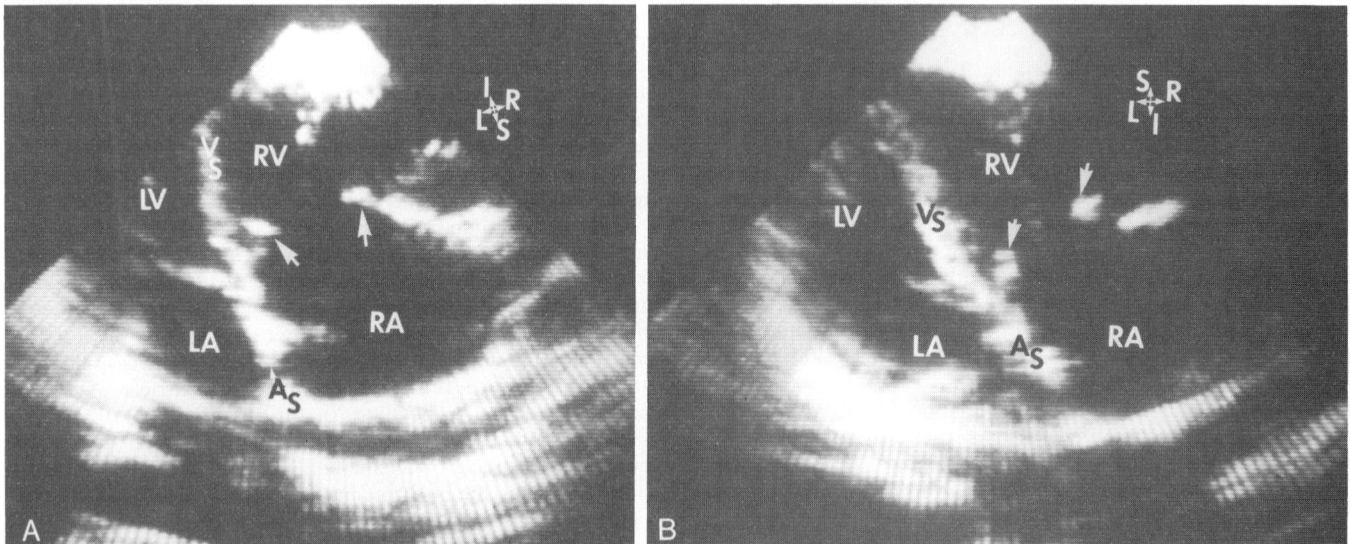

Figure 21–20. Carcinoid syndrome. Four-chamber view demonstrates enlarged right ventricle (RV) and right atrium (RA). *A*, Diastolic frame; *B*, systolic frame. Anterior and septal leaflets of the tricuspid valve are thickened and retracted as well as fixed in a semiopen position. AS—atrial septum; I—inferior; L—left; LA—left atrium; LV—left ventricle; R—right; S—superior; VS—ventricular septum. (From Callahan, J. A., et al.: Echocardiographic features of carcinoid heart disease. Am. J. Cardiol. 50:762, 1982. By permission of Cahners Publishing Company.)

ity. Doppler echocardiography confirms the presence and severity of stenosis.

Tricuspid Regurgitation

Tricuspid valve regurgitation may be due to either intrinsic valvular disease or tricuspid annular dilatation.[E10, W11, W12] Functional tricuspid regurgitation is caused by right ventricular hypertension of any cause, with associated dilatation of the right ventricle and the tricuspid annulus.

Valvular abnormalities producing tricuspid regurgitation are associated with many diseases, in part because of the anatomic and functional complexity of the valve apparatus. Proper closure of the tricuspid valve requires coordinated function of the leaflets, chordae, papillary muscles, and subjacent ventricular myocardium. Functional or anatomic abnormality of any component of the tricuspid valve apparatus may produce tricuspid regurgitation. Two-dimensional echocardiography identifies the morphologic abnormality causing tricuspid regurgitation and also associated anatomic abnormalities of the right side of the heart.

Valvular disease diagnosed by 2D echocardiography includes leaflet prolapse, endocarditis, carcinoid, and Ebstein's anomaly. Prolapse of the tricuspid valve, like mitral prolapse, is recognized by systolic buckling of one or more leaflets beyond the plane of the tricuspid annulus into the right atrium, best appreciated in either the parasternal long-axis view of the right ventricular inflow tract or the apical four-chamber view. Isolated tricuspid valve prolapse is unusual and occurs most commonly in association with mitral valve prolapse.[O10]

Infectious endocarditis of the tricuspid valve is relatively uncommon. As in endocarditis of the left side of the heart, the diagnosis is primarily clinical. Echocardiographic findings characteristic of tricuspid endocarditis include large vegetations with a so-called shaggy appearance. In the presence of severe leaflet

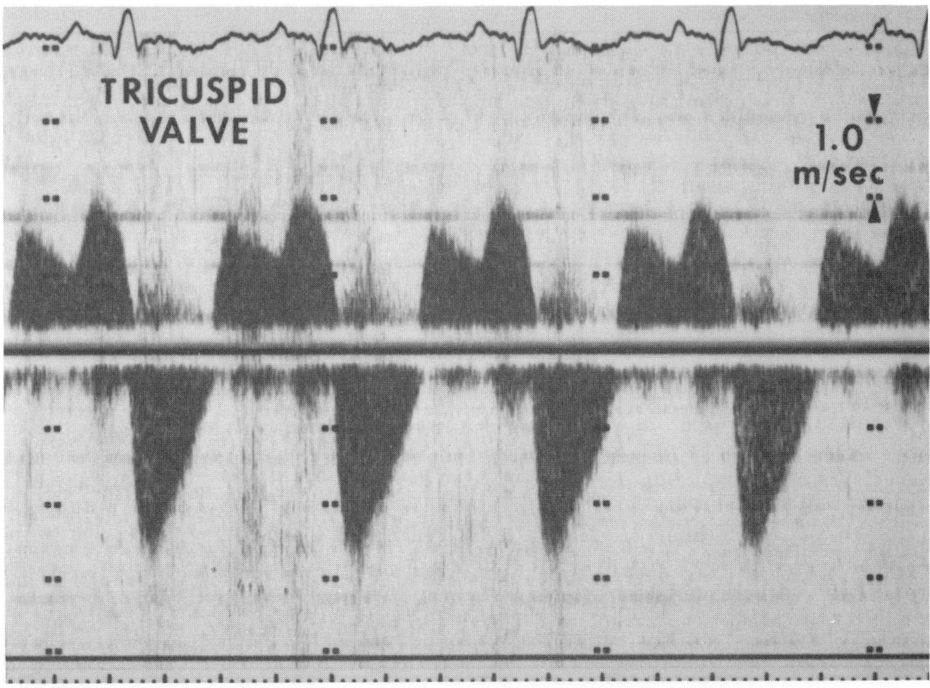

Figure 21–21. Combined tricuspid stenosis and regurgitation in a patient with a carcinoid evaluated by continuous-wave Doppler. Examination was performed from an apical window; hence, signals above the baseline correspond to diastolic antegrade tricuspid flow and systolic signals below the baseline indicate tricuspid regurgitation (2.7 m/sec). Peak and mean diastolic gradients measured 16 and 9 mmHg, respectively. The estimated right ventricular systolic pressure was 42 mmHg.

and subvalvular damage, there may be flail motion of the valvular apparatus.[B9, M15] If chronic disease occurs, there will be associated right atrial and ventricular enlargement.

Echocardiographic characteristics of carcinoid heart disease include thickening and retraction of the leaflets due to leaflet and subvalvular involvement. The valve leaflets may become fixed in a semiopen position, producing combined tricuspid stenosis and regurgitation.[O11, S25] There is frequently associated pulmonary valve involvement. Other unusual causes of tricuspid regurgitation are nonpenetrating chest trauma with disruption of the tricuspid chordal apparatus[B10, K7, W13] and sinus of Valsalva aneurysms.[G11]

Ebstein's anomaly is a congenital abnormality of the tricuspid valve and right side of the heart characterized by apical displacement of deformed tricuspid leaflets.[L9, Z5] The characteristic echocardiographic findings have been extensively reviewed[S26] and are described elsewhere in this text.

The presence of tricuspid regurgitation is suggested on combined M-mode and 2D echocardiography by valvular anatomic abnormalities and associated dilatation of the right heart chambers and central veins. Volume overload of the right side of the heart also shifts the interventricular septum toward the left side, producing paradoxic systolic septal motion.[W14] The severity of tricuspid regurgitation is best evaluated by combined 2D and Doppler echocardiography. In severe tricuspid regurgitation, 2D echocardiography invariably demonstrates right ventricular and right atrial enlargement as well as dilatation of the inferior vena cava and hepatic veins. Doppler echocardiography enables direct detection and assessment of the severity of the flow abnormality.

Doppler Echocardiography in the Evaluation of Tricuspid Regurgitation

Pulsed-wave, continuous-wave, and color flow imaging are all extremely sensitive for the detection of tricuspid regurgitation.[M16, P11, S27, W15] However, tricuspid regurgitation is detected in at least 60 to 70 percent of normal individuals and is attributed to normal physiologic, but subclinical, tricuspid regurgitation.[K8] These regurgitant jets are localized and narrow, corresponding to a relatively low volume of regurgitant flow, and are easily differentiated from pathologic regurgitation.

Validation of the accuracy of Doppler echocardiography for the assessment of severity of tricuspid regurgitation has not been possible because there is no reliable reference standard. Ventriculography requires placement of a catheter across the tricuspid orifice, which induces regurgitation. A practical semiquantitative approach uses pulsed-wave Doppler and color flow imaging in combination with anatomic assessment by 2D echocardiography for assessment of the severity of regurgitation, whereas continuous-wave Doppler echocardiography is used to estimate right ventricular systolic pressure. If the right heart chambers are of normal dimension, the likelihood of significant tricuspid regurgitation is low. Conversely, patients with moderate-to-severe tricuspid regurgitation typically have enlarged right heart chambers with large-volume tricuspid regurgitation, manifested by pulsed-wave Doppler and color flow imaging as a broad systolic right atrial signal.

Tricuspid regurgitation by color flow imaging has an appearance similar to that of mitral regurgitation (Fig. 21–22). Flow signal originates from the valve annulus and extends into the right atrium. From the apical four-chamber view and the right ventricular inflow view, the regurgitant jet is directed away from the transducer and appears in shades of blue. When tricuspid regurgitation is severe, the right atrium and ventricle essentially function as a single chamber. In this situation, there is a low pressure gradient from the right ventricle to the right atrium and the color flow image will not demonstrate aliasing and mosaic colors characteristic of turbulent flow. However, the severity of regurgitation is recognized because the low-velocity regurgitant signals fill most of the right atrium.

Figure 21–22. See Color Plate 2.

Assessment of hepatic vein flow by pulsed-wave Doppler and color flow imaging is a useful adjunct for the characterization of the severity of regurgitation. Normally, hepatic blood flow is antegrade and toward the right side of the heart, producing a signal below the baseline when examined from the subcostal view[A5] (Fig. 21–23). In the presence of severe tricuspid regurgitation, right ventricular systole may produce retrograde flow through the tricuspid orifice into the right atrium, inferior vena cava, and hepatic veins. The detection of systolic flow reversal in the hepatic veins by pulsed-wave Doppler or color flow imaging is indicative of severe tricuspid regurgitation.[P11, W16] Conversely, the absence of flow reversal in the hepatic veins does not necessarily imply that tricuspid regurgitation is not severe, especially in the presence of an enlarged and compliant right atrium.

Doppler Echocardiographic Estimation of Right Ventricular Systolic Pressure

Continuous-wave Doppler echocardiographic characterization of tricuspid regurgitation facilitates diagnosis and clinical decision making in patients with a wide spectrum of cardiac disease by

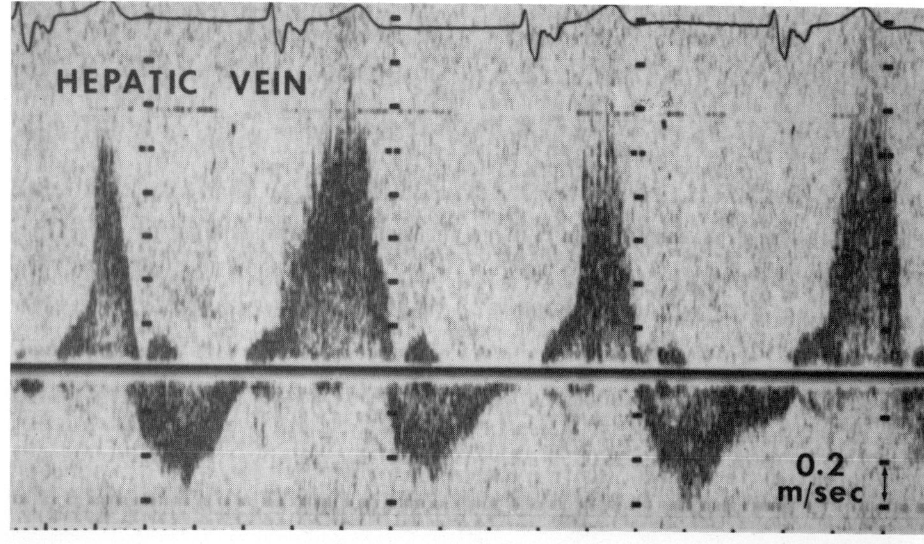

Figure 21–23. Pulsed-wave Doppler evaluation of hepatic vein flow in a patient with tricuspid regurgitation. The examination was performed from a subcostal window, short-axis view. Marked systolic flow reversal (flow signals above baseline) is seen, indicative of severe tricuspid regurgitation.

enabling noninvasive quantitative estimation of right ventricular systolic pressure and pulmonary artery pressure.

The velocity of the tricuspid regurgitant jet is related to the systolic right ventricular–right atrial pressure gradient by the principles of Bernoulli hydrodynamics. Hence, estimation of the systolic maximal instantaneous right ventricular–right atrial pressure gradient is performed by application of the modified Bernoulli equation to velocity data obtained by continuous-wave Doppler. Currie and colleagues demonstrated high correlation between Doppler echocardiographic estimates and simultaneous dual-catheter measurements of the right ventricular–right atrial pressure gradient in 111 patients with a wide spectrum of cardiac disease, severity of tricuspid regurgitation, and right heart pressures (Fig. 21–24).[C15] On the basis of their investigation, simple regression equations were devised that enable accurate assessment of right ventricular systolic pressure; in patients with normal right heart pressures, right ventricular systolic pressure is obtained by the addition of 14 to the right ventricular–right atrial pressure gradient. In patients with moderately or severely elevated right heart pressure, the best estimate of right ventricular

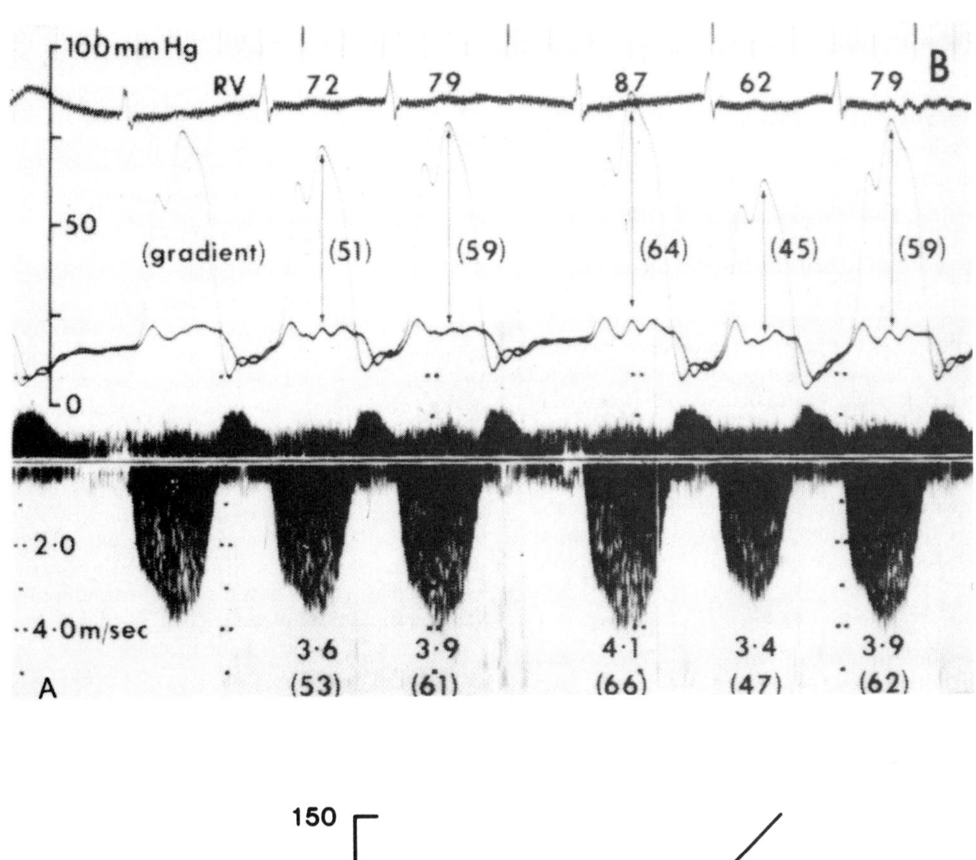

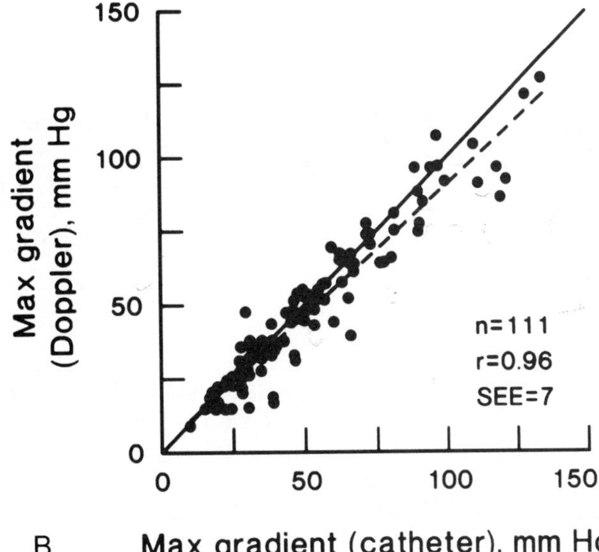

Figure 21–24. Assessment of right ventricular–right atrial systolic pressure gradients by continuous-wave Doppler echocardiography. *A*, Simultaneous Doppler and right ventricular and right atrial tracings. The patient was in atrial fibrillation; the fourth beat was chosen for analysis. The right ventricular (RV) systolic pressure was 87 mmHg, and the maximal catheter right ventricular–right atrial gradient was 64 mmHg. The maximal Doppler velocity was 4.1 m/sec, and the maximal Doppler gradient was 66 mmHg. Note the excellent beat-to-beat correlation between the Doppler and the catheter maximal gradients. *B*, Correlation of simultaneous Doppler and right ventricular–right atrial maximal (Max) systolic pressure gradient in 111 patients with tricuspid regurgitation. The dashed line is the regression line, and the solid line is the line of identity. The regression equation is Doppler gradient = 2.2 + 0.88 × catheter gradient. SEE—standard error of estimation. (From Currie, P. J., et al.: Continuous-wave Doppler determination of right ventricular pressure: A simultaneous Doppler-catheterization study in 127 patients. J. Am. Coll. Cardiol. 6:750, 1985. By permission of the American College of Cardiology.)

systolic pressure is obtained by the addition of 20 to the right ventricular–right atrial gradient. Other investigators have demonstrated analyzable tricuspid regurgitation signals by continuous-wave Doppler echocardiography in up to 90 percent of patients with congestive heart failure, and a high proportion of normals as well.[S28, Y4] Therefore, measurement of peak tricuspid regurgitant jet velocity should be attempted routinely in patients undergoing echocardiographic examination.

As in the evaluation of mitral regurgitation by continuous-wave Doppler echocardiography, the magnitude of regurgitant velocity is not a measure of the severity of tricuspid regurgitation. Instead, the velocity is determined primarily by right ventricular–right atrial pressure gradient.

Role of Echocardiography in the Evaluation of Tricuspid Regurgitation

Combined 2D and color flow imaging provides anatomic and hemodynamic information that enables diagnostic classification and assessment of the severity of tricuspid regurgitation. Echocardiography is the diagnostic method of choice for the evaluation of the patient with tricuspid regurgitation. Invasive methods requiring catheterization induce regurgitation, because the catheter must be placed across the tricuspid orifice to perform ventriculography. In the absence of obstruction to right ventricular outflow, estimated peak right ventricular systolic pressure is equivalent to pulmonary artery pressure. Noninvasive assessment of pulmonary artery pressure is useful for the assessment of patients with a wide spectrum of disease, including mitral stenosis, mitral regurgitation, and malfunctioning mitral or aortic prostheses. The ability to perform serial noninvasive assessment of right heart pressures at rest and at exercise is extremely useful in these patient groups.

Pulmonary Stenosis and Regurgitation

Acquired pulmonary valve disease is extremely uncommon in adult patients. Most often, pulmonary valve stenosis or significant pulmonary valve regurgitation is associated with congenital heart disease recognized in childhood. However, an increasing adult population with treated congenital heart disease may come under the care of the adult cardiologist.

Congenital pulmonary valve stenosis may occur in isolation or in association with other congenital cardiac abnormalities.[A6, D18, G12] Acquired disease of the pulmonary valve in adult patients is usually associated with combined stenosis and regurgitation due to rheumatic heart disease or carcinoid.[A6, D18, G12] Rheumatic disease should be suspected in the patient in whom there are typical left-sided valvular abnormalities suggestive of previous rheumatic fever. Carcinoid heart disease is most often isolated to the right side of the heart. Pulmonary valvular regurgitation is most often functional and acquired because of underlying pulmonary hypertension of any cause. Endocarditis of the pulmonary valve is relatively rare but may produce isolated regurgitation.[C16, N9]

Echocardiographic assessment of the pulmonary valve is performed from the parasternal long- and short-axis and subcostal long-axis views. Pulmonary valve stenosis is suspected on the basis of 2D echocardiography if systolic doming of the valve leaflets is observed.[W17, W18] Doppler echocardiography increases the sensitivity of the detection of pulmonary valve stenosis and provides accurate hemodynamic assessment.[L10]

Pulmonary valve regurgitation is suspected on 2D echocardiographic examination if valvular vegetations are demonstrated or if there is rapid oscillatory motion of the free edges of the valve during diastole.[B11, K9] In patients with carcinoid heart disease, the pulmonary valve may be relatively fixed in a semiopen position, the leaflets appear retracted, and the pulmonary annulus may be narrowed, producing outflow obstruction. There is usually associated involvement of the tricuspid valve.[B11, C16, K9] Another abnormality demonstrated by 2D echocardiography may be right ventricular enlargement, depending on the duration and severity of regurgitation.

Doppler Echocardiography in the Evaluation of Pulmonary Valve Disease

Pulmonary valve stenosis causes alteration in blood flow qualitatively similar to that seen in other valvular stenoses. Blood flow accelerates proximal to the valve and flows through the stenotic orifice in a laminar jet. The peak velocity of flow in the jet measured by continuous-wave Doppler echocardiography allows estimation of the transvalvular gradient by application of the modified Bernoulli equation.[H17] Gradient estimations of discrete nonvalvular right ventricular outflow obstruction by continuous-wave Doppler echocardiography have been clinically validated by simultaneous invasive examination in several studies.[F4, R14] Color flow imaging aids in the assessment of the transvalvular gradient by guiding the placement of the ultrasonic beam to a position parallel to flow. Estimation of pulmonary valve area is possible by the continuity equation, but at present there are no established criteria for estimate of severity of stenosis on the basis of valve area.

Pulmonary valve regurgitation may be detected in most normal patients by Doppler echocardiography, corresponding to subclinical, physiologic regurgitation as also seen in normal mitral and tricuspid valves.[K10, M17] In the normal population, pulmonary regurgitation is detected by pulsed-wave echocardiography only in the region immediately below the valve, whereas in those with significant pulmonary valve regurgitation, color flow imaging demonstrates a wide regurgitant jet extending deep into the right ventricle, with associated right ventricular enlargement. The appearance of pulmonary regurgitation by color flow imaging is qualitatively similar to aortic regurgitation (Fig. 21–25). It is best demonstrated from the parasternal short-axis view and appears as a pandiastolic jet of red signals extending from the pulmonary valve into the right ventricular outflow tract and cavity. The dimensions of the color jet increase with increasing severity of pulmonary regurgitation.

Role of Echocardiography in the Evaluation of Pulmonary Valve Disease

Combined 2D and Doppler echocardiography is reliable for the identification of the cause of pulmonary valve disease and for assessment of hemodynamic severity. Abnormalities of valvular structure and cardiac chamber dimensions are helpful in diagnostic classification. Doppler echocardiography provides definitive assessment of hemodynamic severity.

Figure 21–25. See Color Plate 2.

ASSESSMENT OF VALVE FUNCTION AFTER INTERVENTION

Prosthetic Stenosis and Regurgitation

Prosthetic valves have either bioprosthetic or mechanical components. Bioprosthetic valves are more easily evaluated, because the valve leaflets are composed of tissue and have echocardiographic characteristics somewhat similar to those of native valves. However, the struts and ring to which the leaflets are attached are metallic, so that they cause ultrasonic reverberations and sidelobes that may obscure anatomic abnormalities. Mechanical valves are composed entirely of inert, highly reflective materials that tend to saturate the recording system and make evaluation more difficult than that for bioprosthetic valves. Acoustic shadowing from bioprostheses and mechanical valves may limit the usefulness of transthoracic 2D echocardiography for the detection of leaflet vegetations, ring abscess, valve-associated thrombus, and left atrial thrombus.[S29]

In the assessment of tissue valves by 2D echocardiography, the bioprosthetic portion of the valve normally moves in concert with the highly echo-reflective struts and sewing ring. Bioprosthetic valves are normally subject to degeneration over a span of 8 to 10 years, and this is clinically manifested as stenosis or regurgitation or both.[C17, S30] Bioprosthetic valve degeneration appears echocardiographically as increased leaflet thickness and calcification.[F5] Other abnormalities of the leaflets identified by echocardiography include focal masses, perforations, prolapse, and fluttering due to endocarditis and thrombosis.[A7, E11, G13, K11, S30] For mitral prostheses, leaflet motion detected within the body of the left atrium indicates disruption of the leaflet from the valve apparatus, which may be due to endocarditis or degeneration.[E11, G13, K11] Abnormalities of the sewing ring are also demonstrated by 2D echocardiography and include excessive rocking due to dehiscence of the sewing ring from the annulus.[E11]

Two-dimensional echocardiographic evaluation of mechanical prostheses is more difficult. Although the valves have a characteristic appearance and are easily recognized by 2D echocardiography, the individual components of the valve apparatus are difficult to distinguish because of the highly echo-reflective materials used in their construction. Furthermore, because of acoustic "masking," structures beyond the valve relative to the incident ultrasound beam are poorly visualized, especially in the mitral position.[N10, W19] Despite these difficulties, gross evaluation of valve motion, detection of large masses associated with the valve, and detection of perivalvular abnormalities are routinely possible.[E11, S30]

Doppler Echocardiography in the Evaluation of Prosthetic Valves

Normal Doppler echocardiographic findings for prosthetic valves have been described and reviewed.[N11, R15, R16] It has been suggested that the complex and multiple orifices of prosthetic valves may invalidate the assumptions of the modified Bernoulli equation for the evaluation of prosthetic stenosis; in vitro work has indicated that correlation between Doppler-derived and manometric pressure gradients varies with the size and type of prosthesis.[Y5] Another in vitro investigation has demonstrated the validity of the Doppler echocardiographic method for the evaluation of irregular, tunnel-like obstructions.[T7] Furthermore, the use of the modified Bernoulli equation and Doppler echocardiography has been validated by comparison with catheterization for the evaluation of stenosis of a variety of bioprosthetic and mechanical valves.[B12, W20]

Close correlation between Doppler-derived and simultaneous catheter-measured gradients in patients with mitral and tricuspid prostheses has been described in small numbers of patients.[B12, H18, H19, W20] Nonsimultaneous studies in patients with aortic prostheses have yielded conflicting results.[R17, S31, W19] However, simultaneous echocardiographic and dual-catheter study of 42 prosthetic valves, including 20 in the aortic position, has demonstrated extremely high correlation between catheter- and Doppler-derived maximal instantaneous and mean gradients, regardless of prosthetic position or type[B12] (Fig. 21–26). Furthermore, in this same study, Doppler echocardiography correlated better with estimation of transmitral prosthetic gradients when direct left atrial measurement was used instead of pulmonary capillary wedge pressure, a result suggesting that overestimation of transmitral gradients may occur when pulmonary capillary wedge pressure is used.[B12, S32] As in native valve disease, the transvalvular pressure gradient alone may be insufficient to characterize the severity of prosthetic dysfunction because of the flow-dependence of the measured gradients. Hence, an estimate of prosthetic valve area is indicated. However, in studies of a limited number of patients with mitral prostheses, correlation between Doppler- and catheter-derived valve areas has been poor.[W20] It has been suggested that this may represent a limitation of the Gorlin formula in the assessment of prosthetic valve area.[W20]

Aortic prosthetic regurgitation is detected with high sensitivity, and severity is accurately assessed by Doppler echocardiography.[A8, P12] In contrast, acoustic "masking" by the inert materials used in construction of bioprostheses and mechanical valves severely limits the usefulness of transthoracic Doppler echocardiography for the assessment of prosthetic mitral regurgitation.[C18, N10, S29] However, transesophageal echocardiography provides an unimpeded ultrasonic window to the left atrium, allowing easy characterization of left atrial anatomy and mitral regurgitation. Furthermore, sensitivity for detection of mitral regurgitation is markedly enhanced compared with conventional transthoracic imaging.[N10, S33] In suspected endocarditis, vegetations and perivalvular disease are also identified with much greater sensitivity.[E5, N10]

Valvuloplasty

Experience with surgical valvuloplasty preceded the development and use of prosthetic valves.[M12] Although surgical valvuloplasty was performed at only a few centers after the development of prosthetic valves, there has been renewed interest in the technique in the past 10 years. Surgical repair, rather than replacement, of the mitral valve is frequently feasible and offers many advantages. Done by experienced surgeons, the procedure is associated with increased survival and improved left ventricular function as well as a lower frequency of valve-related complications.[B13, C19, G14, P13] Operative repair of the aortic valve has been performed by mechanical[K12] and ultrasonic[F6] decalcification of stenotic valves, with consistent relief of stenosis. Tricuspid annuloplasty is routinely performed at many centers and is generally favored over valve replacement whenever possible. Data obtained by intraoperative transesophageal echocardiographic assessment guide the surgeon in making the repair, are directly comparable with data obtained postoperatively, and are useful for follow-up.[G15] The intraoperative assessment of valvuloplasty by echocardiography is described elsewhere in this text.

Combined 2D and Doppler echocardiography has also been used for patient selection and the assessment of the morphologic and hemodynamic alterations associated with percutaneous aortic, mitral, and pulmonary balloon valvuloplasty.[B14, M18, R18] Echocardiographic criteria for identification of patients who are optimal candidates for mitral valvuloplasty are described earlier in this chapter. Two-dimensional echocardiography has demonstrated that the mechanism of successful mitral balloon valvuloplasty is due to splitting of fusion along one or both leaflets' commissures. This is associated with an increase in the transverse diameter and an increased opening of the angle between the commissures.[B15, R11] In patients with calcification of the mitral leaflets or commissures, incomplete splitting of commissures and less increase in the angle of opening are observed, with less associated improvement in mitral valve area.

The pressure half-time method immediately after valvuloplasty has been demonstrated to correlate poorly with Gorlin formula estimates of mitral valve area by invasive techniques.[C20] However, the half-time method may be applied with confidence from 24 to 48 hours after valvuloplasty.[C20] Doppler echocardiography is also useful for estimation of valve gradient immediately after intervention and for the detection of mitral regurgitation.[A9]

Combined 2D and Doppler echocardiography is ideal for long-term follow-up of patients with valvuloplasty, because the techniques are noninvasive and provide accurate morphologic and hemodynamic assessment, including estimates of valve area. The discrepancy between estimates of mitral valve area by catheterization and the Doppler half-time method immediately after valvuloplasty is not observed at 6 months.[A10] Restenosis occurs in some patients, and patients at risk are identified by the same 2D echocardiographic scoring system described for the identification of optimal candidates for valvuloplasty.[B14, P14]

Echocardiographic evaluation of aortic valvular morphology has not been used for the selection of patients for aortic balloon valvuloplasty. The morphologic abnormalities of the stenotic aortic valve are not as heterogeneous as those in mitral stenosis,

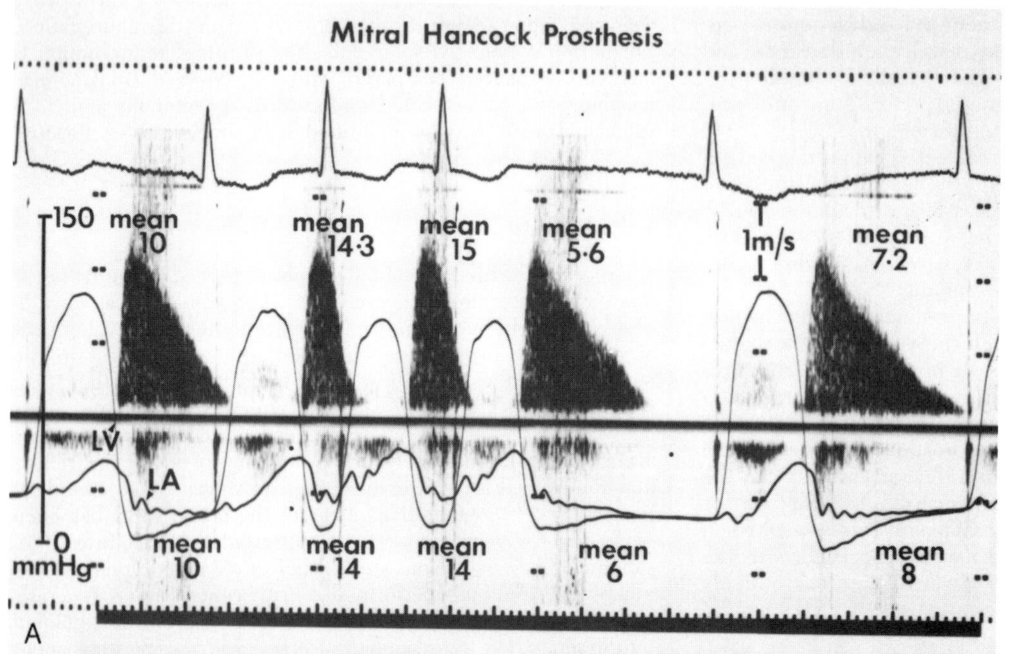

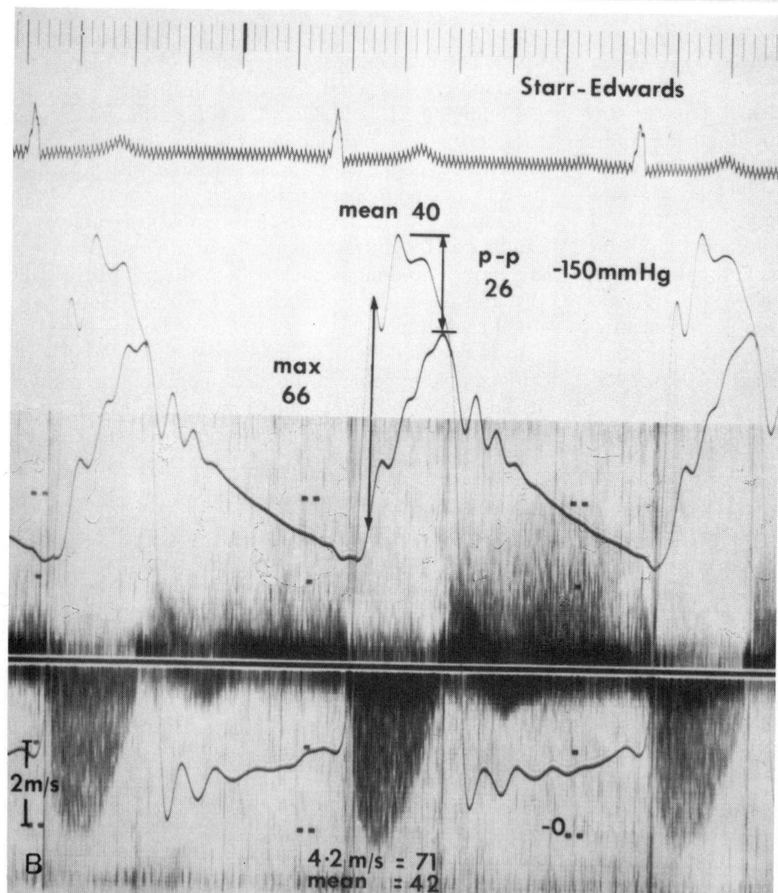

Figure 21–26. *A*, Simultaneous Doppler and catheter pressure estimates in a patient with a stenotic mitral Hancock prosthesis. The pressure gradient was measured by the dual-catheter technique, with catheters in the left ventricle (LV) and the left atrium (LA). Note the excellent beat-to-beat correlation in estimated mean gradients by Doppler echocardiography and cardiac catheterization. *B*, Simultaneous Doppler and catheter pressure estimates in a patient with a stenotic Starr-Edwards aortic prosthesis. The pressure gradient was measured by the dual-catheter technique, with catheters in the left ventricle and the aorta. Note that maximum (max) instantaneous and mean gradients exceed peak-to-peak (p-p) gradient. There is excellent correlation between Doppler and catheter-determined mean gradients.

and hence an anatomic scoring system would not be expected to stratify patients. Some experience has suggested that the stenotic valve due to degenerative disease may be more successfully dilated than the calcified, congenitally bicuspid or rheumatic aortic valve.[K1] However, if calcification is dense, this distinction cannot always be made by 2D echocardiography.

The early postintervention hemodynamic effects of aortic balloon valvuloplasty have been described by Doppler echocardiography. Nishimura and associates reported a significant reduction in the aortic mean gradient and valve area within 24 to 48 hours after the procedure, but restenosis was frequently observed in patients seen at 6-month follow-up.[N12] These investigators cautioned against hemodynamic assessment immediately after intervention because of transient left ventricular dysfunction due to the procedure, with associated alterations in cardiac output, gradient, and valve area. However, Doppler-derived aortic valve area more than 24 to 48 hours after balloon valvuloplasty correlates well with valve area determined by invasive methods.[C21, N12] Trivial-to-mild aortic regurgitation is frequently observed by Doppler echocardiography after intervention, but significant regurgitation has been described infrequently.[N12, S34]

Morphologic alterations of the aortic valve associated with aortic balloon valvuloplasty have been characterized in intraoperative[M19, R19, S35] and postmortem[I1, M19, S35] studies. The mechanism of successful aortic valvuloplasty has been attributed to fracture of calcific deposits of the aortic valve leaflets, with associated increased leaflet mobility.[I1, K1, M19, S35] Small postmortem studies suggest that fracture of fused commissures associated with rheumatic or senile stenosis does not occur.[K1] These observations have not been corroborated by 2D echocardiography, probably because most patients who undergo the procedure have senile aortic stenosis and because the detection of fracture of calcium deposits is not possible.

SUMMARY

Echocardiography has become the preferred diagnostic modality for the evaluation of patients with valvular heart disease. Although there are limitations to the techniques, interpretive errors may be avoided by a thorough understanding of the methods. Careful attention to detail on the part of the operator performing the study ensures data of high quality for analysis. Combined 2D and Doppler echocardiography with color flow imaging provides comprehensive, accurate, and noninvasive assessment of the cause and hemodynamic severity of valvular heart disease. Doppler echocardiographic methods have been proved to be extremely accurate for the assessment of valvular stenosis, yielding data that are directly comparable to those obtained by cardiac catheterization. For the evaluation of valvular regurgitation, Doppler echocardiography provides a semiquantitative estimate of hemodynamic severity that compares favorably with semiquantitative invasive estimation by angiography. It is now possible to perform accurate serial evaluation of the hemodynamic progression of valvular heart disease without the cost or risk of cardiac catheterization.

References

A

1. Annegers, J. F., Pillman, N. L., Weidman, W. H., and Kurland, L. T.: Rheumatic fever in Rochester, Minnesota, 1935–1978. Mayo Clin. Proc. 57:753, 1982.
2. Arvidsson, H., and Karnell, J.: Quantitative assessment of mitral and aortic insufficiency by angiocardiography. Acta Radiol. 2:105, 1964.
3. Abbasi, A. S., Allen, M. W., DeCristofaro, D., and Ungar, I.: Detection and estimation of the degree of mitral regurgitation by range-gated pulsed Doppler echocardiography. Circulation 61:143, 1980.
4. Ascah, K. J., Stewart, W. J., Jiang, L., et al.: A Doppler–two-dimensional echocardiographic method for quantitation of mitral regurgitation. Circulation 72:377, 1985.
5. Appleton, C. P., Hatle, L. K., and Popp, R. L.: Superior vena cava and hepatic vein Doppler echocardiography in healthy adults. J. Am. Coll. Cardiol. 10:1032, 1987.
6. Altrichter, P. M., Olson, L. J., Edwards, W. D., et al.: Surgical pathology of the pulmonary valve: A study of 116 cases spanning 15 years. Mayo Clin. Proc. 64:1352, 1989.
7. Alam, M., Lakier, J. B., Pickard, S. D., and Goldstein, S.: Echocardiographic evaluation of porcine bioprosthetic valves: Experience with 309 normal and 59 dysfunctioning valves. Am. J. Cardiol. 52:309, 1983.
8. Alam, M., Rosman, H. S., Lakier, J. B., et al.: Doppler and echocardiographic features of normal and dysfunctioning bioprosthetic valves. J. Am. Coll. Cardiol. 10:851, 1987.
9. Abascal, V. M., Wilkins, G. T., Choong, C. Y., et al.: Mitral regurgitation after percutaneous balloon mitral valvuloplasty in adults: Evaluation by pulsed Doppler echocardiography. J. Am. Coll. Cardiol. 11:257, 1988.
10. Abascal, V. M., Wilkins, G. T., Choong, C. Y., et al.: Echocardiographic evaluation of mitral valve structure and function in patients followed for at least 6 months after percutaneous balloon mitral valvuloplasty. J. Am. Coll. Cardiol. 12:606, 1988.

B

1. Bansal, R. C., Tajik, A. J., Seward, J. B., and Offord, K. P.: Feasibility of detailed two-dimensional echocardiographic examination in adults: Prospective study of 200 patients. Mayo Clin. Proc. 55:291, 1980.
2. Brandenburg, R. O., Jr., Tajik, A. J., Edwards, W. D., et al.: Accuracy of 2-dimensional echocardiographic diagnosis of congenitally bicuspid aortic valve: Echocardiographic-anatomic correlation in 115 patients. Am. J. Cardiol. 51:1469, 1983.
3. Bulkley, B. H., and Roberts, W. C.: Ankylosing spondylitis and aortic regurgitation: Description of the characteristic cardiovascular lesion from study of eight necropsy patients. Circulation 48:1014, 1973.
4. Botvinick, E. H., Schiller, N. B., Wickramasekaran, R., et al.: Echocardiographic demonstration of early mitral valve closure in severe aortic insufficiency: Its clinical implications. Circulation 51:836, 1975.
5. Bryg, R. J., Williams, G. A., Labovitz, A. J., et al.: Effect of atrial fibrillation and mitral regurgitation on calculated mitral valve area in mitral stenosis. Am. J. Cardiol. 57:634, 1986.
6. Byram, M. T., and Roberts, W. C.: Frequency and extent of calcific deposits in purely regurgitant mitral valves: Analysis of 108 operatively excised valves. Am. J. Cardiol. 52:1059, 1983.
7. Blanchard, D., Diebold, B., Peronneau, P., et al.: Non-invasive diagnosis of mitral regurgitation by Doppler echocardiography. Br. Heart J. 45:589, 1981.
8. Blumlein, S., Bouchard, A., Schiller, N. B., et al.: Quantitation of mitral regurgitation by Doppler echocardiography. Circulation 74:306, 1986.
9. Banks, T., Fletcher, R., and Ali, N.: Infective endocarditis in drug heroin addicts. Am. J. Med. 55:444, 1973.
10. Berkery, W., Hare, C., Warner, R. A., et al.: Nonpenetrating traumatic rupture of the tricuspid valve: Formation of ventricular septal aneurysm and subsequent septal necrosis: Recognition by two-dimensional Doppler echocardiography. Chest 91:778, 1987.
11. Berger, M., Delfin, L. A., Jelveh, M., and Goldberg, E.: Two-dimensional echocardiographic findings in right-sided infective endocarditis. Circulation 61:855, 1980.
12. Burstow, D. J., Nishimura, R. A., Bailey, K. R., et al.: Continuous-wave Doppler echocardiographic measurement of prosthetic valve gradients: A simultaneous Doppler-catheter correlative study. Circulation 80:504, 1989.
13. Bochek, L. I.: Correction of mitral valve disease without mitral valve replacement. Am. Heart J. 104:865, 1982.
14. Block, P. C.: Who is suitable for percutaneous balloon mitral valvotomy? (editorial). Int. J. Cardiol. 20:9, 1988.
15. Block, P. C., Palacios, I. F., Jacobs, M. L., and Fallon, J. T.: Mechanisms of percutaneous mitral valvotomy. Am. J. Cardiol. 59:178, 1987.

C

1. Clawson, B. J.: Rheumatic heart disease: An analysis of 796 cases. Am. Heart J. 20:454, 1940.
2. Chang, S., Clements, S., and Chang, J.: Aortic stenosis: Echocardiographic cusp separation and surgical description of aortic valve in 22 patients. Am. J. Cardiol. 39:499, 1977.
3. Currie, P. J., Seward, J. B., Reeder, G. S., et al.: Continuous-wave Doppler echocardiographic assessment of severity of calcific aortic stenosis: A simultaneous Doppler-catheter correlative study in 100 adult patients. Circulation 71:1162, 1985.
4. Currie, P. J., Hagler, D. J., Seward, J. B., et al.: Instantaneous pressure gradient: A simultaneous Doppler and dual catheter correlative study. J. Am. Coll. Cardiol. 7:800, 1986.
5. Callahan, M. J., Tajik, A. J., Su-Fan, Q., and Bove, A. A.: Validation of instantaneous pressure gradients measured by continuous-wave Doppler in experimentally induced aortic stenosis. Am. J. Cardiol. 56:989, 1985.
6. Carabello, B., and Grossman, W.: Calculation of stenotic valve orifice area. *In* Grossman, W. (ed.): Cardiac Catheterization and Angiography. Lea & Febiger, Philadelphia, 1986, pp. 143–154.
7. Cannon, S. R., Richards, K. L., and Crawford, M.: Hydraulic estimation of stenotic orifice area: A correction of the Gorlin formula. Circulation 71:1170, 1985.
8. Carter, J. B., Sethi, S., Lee, G. B., and Edwards, J. E.: Prolapse of semilunar cusps as causes of aortic insufficiency. Circulation 43:922, 1971.
9. Cope, G. D., Kisslo, J. A., Johnson, M. L., and Myers, S.: Diastolic vibration of the interventricular septum in aortic insufficiency. Circulation 51:589, 1975.
10. Cunha, C. L. P., Giuliani, E. R., Fuster, V., et al.: Preoperative M-mode echocardiography as a predictor of surgical results in chronic aortic insufficiency. J. Thorac. Cardiovasc. Surg. 79:256, 1980.
11. Ciobanu, M., Abbasi, A. S., Allen, M., et al.: Pulsed Doppler echocardiography

in the diagnosis and estimation of severity of aortic insufficiency. Am. J. Cardiol. 49:339, 1982.
12. Croft, C. H., Lipscomb, K., Mathis, K., et al.: Limitations of qualitative angiographic grading in aortic or mitral regurgitation. Am. J. Cardiol. 53:1593, 1984.
13. Chopra, P., and Tandon, H. D.: Pathology of chronic rheumatic heart disease with particular reference to tricuspid valve involvement. Acta Cardiol. 32:423, 1977.
14. Callahan, J. A., Wroblewski, E. M., Reeder, G. S., et al.: Echocardiographic features of carcinoid heart disease. Am. J. Cardiol. 50:762, 1982.
15. Currie, P. J., Seward, J. B., Chan, K.-L., et al.: Continuous wave Doppler determination of right ventricular pressure: A simultaneous Doppler-catheterization study in 127 patients. J. Am. Coll. Cardiol. 6:750, 1985.
16. Cremieux, A.-C., Witchitz, S., Malergue, M.-C., et al.: Clinical and echocardiographic observations in pulmonary valve endocarditis. Am. J. Cardiol. 56:610, 1985.
17. Cohn, L. H., Mudge, G. H., Pratter, F., and Collins, J. J., Jr.: Five to eight-year follow-up of patients undergoing porcine heart-valve replacement. N. Engl. J. Med. 304:258, 1981.
18. Come, P. C.: Pitfalls in the diagnosis of periprosthetic valvular regurgitation by pulsed Doppler echocardiography. J. Am. Coll. Cardiol. 9:1176, 1987.
19. Carpentier, A.: Cardiac valve surgery—the "French correction." J. Thorac. Cardiovasc. Surg. 86:323, 1983.
20. Chen, C., Wang, Y., Guo, B., and Lin, Y.: Reliability of the Doppler pressure half-time method for assessing effects of percutaneous mitral balloon valvuloplasty. J. Am. Coll. Cardiol. 13:1309, 1989.
21. Come, P. C., Riley, M. F., McKay, R. G., and Safian, R. D.: Echocardiographic assessment of aortic valve area in elderly patients with aortic stenosis and of changes in valve area after percutaneous balloon valvuloplasty. J. Am. Coll. Cardiol. 10:115, 1987.

D

1. Davies, M. J.: Pathology of Cardiac Valves. Butterworths, London, 1980, pp. 18–35.
2. Dry, T. J., and Willius, F. A.: Calcareous disease of the aortic valve: A study of two hundred twenty-eight cases. Am. Heart J. 17:138, 1939.
3. DiSciasco, G., and Taranta, A.: Rheumatic fever in children. Am. Heart J. 99:635, 1980.
4. DeMaria, A. N., Bommer, W., Joye, J., et al.: Value and limitations of cross-sectional echocardiography of the aortic valve in the diagnosis and quantification of valvular aortic stenosis. Circulation 62:304, 1980.
5. DeMaria, A. N., Bommer, W., Neumann, A., et al.: Identification and localization of aneurysms of the ascending aorta by cross-sectional echocardiography. Circulation 59:755, 1979.
6. Davies, M. J.: Pathology of Cardiac Valves. Butterworths, London, 1980, pp. 37–61.
7. Davia, J. E., Fenoglio, J. J., DeCastro, C. M., et al.: Quadricuspid semilunar valves. Chest 72:186, 1977.
8. D'Cruz, I., Cohen, H. C., Prabhu, R., et al.: Flutter of left ventricular structures in patients with aortic regurgitation, with special reference to patients with associated mitral stenosis. Am. Heart J. 92:684, 1976.
9. Daniel, W. G., Hood, W. P., Jr., Siart, A., et al.: Chronic aortic regurgitation: Reassessment of the prognostic value of preoperative left ventricular end-systolic dimension and fractional shortening. Circulation 71:669, 1985.
10. Devereux, R. B., Kramer-Fox, R. B., Shear, M. K., et al.: Diagnosis and classification of severity of mitral valve prolapse: Methodologic, biologic, and prognostic considerations. Am. Heart J. 113:1265, 1987.
11. Düren, D. R., Becker, A. E., and Dunning, A. J.: Long-term follow-up of idiopathic mitral valve prolapse in 300 patients: A prospective study. J. Am. Coll. Cardiol. 11:42, 1988.
12. Devereux, R. B., Hawkins, I., Kramer-Fox, R., et al.: Complications of mitral valve prolapse: Disproportionate occurrence in men and older patients. Am. J. Med. 81:751, 1986.
13. Daniel, W. G., Schröder, E., Mügge, A., and Lichtlen, P. R.: Transesophageal echocardiography in infective endocarditis. Am. J. Cardiac Imag. 2:78, 1988.
14. Davies, M. J.: Pathology of Cardiac Valves. Butterworths, London, 1980, pp. 73–99, 105–114.
15. Di Segni, E., and Edwards, J. E.: Cleft anterior leaflet of the mitral valve with intact septa: A study of 20 cases. Am. J. Cardiol. 51:919, 1983.
16. Daniels, S. J., Mintz, G. S., and Kotler, M. N.: Rheumatic tricuspid valve disease: Two-dimensional echocardiographic, hemodynamic, and angiographic correlations. Am. J. Cardiol. 51:492, 1983.
17. Denning, K., Henneke, K.-H., and Rudolph, W.: Assessment of tricuspid stenosis by Doppler-echocardiography. (Abstract.) J. Am. Coll. Cardiol. (Suppl. A):237A, 1987.
18. Davies, M. J.: Pathology of Cardiac Valves. Butterworths, London, 1980, pp. 8–18, 24–35, 131–137.

E

1. Edwards, J. E.: Calcific aortic stenosis: Pathologic features. Proc. Staff Meet. Mayo Clin. 36:444, 1961.
2. Edwards, J. E.: Pathology of left ventricular outflow tract obstruction. Circulation 31:586, 1965.
3. Edwards, J. E.: Pathologic aspects of cardiac valvular insufficiencies. Arch. Surg. 77:634, 1958.
4. Edwards, J. E.: Pathology of acquired valvular disease of the heart. Semin. Roentgenol. 14:96, 1979.
5. Erbel, R., Rohmann, S., Drexler, M., et al.: Improved diagnostic value of echocardiography in patients with infective endocarditis by transoesophageal approach. A prospective study. Eur. Heart J. 9:43, 1988.
6. Edwards, J. E.: Pathology of aortic incompetence. *In* Silver, M. D. (ed.): Cardiovascular Pathology. Vol. 1. Churchill-Livingstone, New York, 1983, pp. 619–631.
7. el Haitem, N., Chaara, A., Mesbahi, R., and Benomar, M.: Rupture traumatique du sinus de Valsalva antéro-droit dans le ventricule droit, associée à une insuffisance aortique. Arch. Mal. Coeur 81:793, 1988.
8. Erbel, R., Schweizer, P., Bardos, P., and Meyer, J.: Two-dimensional echocardiographic diagnosis of papillary muscle rupture. Chest 79:595, 1981.
9. Edwards, J. E.: Pathology of mitral incompetence. *In* Silver, M. D. (ed.): Cardiovascular Pathology. Vol. 1. Churchill-Livingstone, New York, 1983, pp. 575–598.
10. Edwards, J. E.: The spectrum and clinical significance of tricuspid regurgitation. Pract. Cardiol. 6:86, 1980.
11. Effron, M. K., and Popp, R. L.: Two-dimensional echocardiographic assessment of bioprosthetic valve dysfunction and infective endocarditis. J. Am. Coll. Cardiol. 2:597, 1983.

F

1. Fan, P.-H., Kapur, K. K., and Nanda, N. C.: Color-guided Doppler echocardiographic assessment of aortic valve stenosis. J. Am. Coll. Cardiol. 12:441, 1988.
2. Fioretti, P., Roelandt, J., Bos, R. J., et al.: Echocardiography in chronic aortic insufficiency: Is valve replacement too late when left ventricular end-systolic dimension reaches 55 mm? Circulation 67:216, 1983.
3. Fifer, M. A., and Grossman, W.: Measurement of ventricular volumes, ejection fraction, mass, and wall stress. *In* Grossman, W. (ed.): Cardiac Catheterization and Angiography. Lea & Febiger, Philadelphia, 1986, pp. 282–300.
4. Fyfe, D. A., Currie, P. J., Seward, J. B., et al.: Continuous-wave Doppler determination of the pressure gradient across pulmonary artery bands: Hemodynamic correlation in 20 patients. Mayo Clin. Proc. 59:744, 1984.
5. Forman, M. B., Phelan, B. K., Robertson, R. M., and Virmani, R.: Correlation of two-dimensional echocardiography and pathologic findings in porcine valve dysfunction. J. Am. Coll. Cardiol. 5:224, 1985.
6. Freeman, W. K., Schaff, H. V., and Orszulak, T. A.: Ultrasonic aortic valve decalcification: Serial Doppler echocardiographic follow-up. Circulation 78 (Suppl. II):II-379, 1988.

G

1. Godley, R. W., Green, D., Dillon, J. C., et al.: Reliability of two-dimensional echocardiography in assessing the severity of valvular aortic stenosis. Chest 79:657, 1981.
2. Gorlin, R., and Gorlin, S. G.: Hydraulic formula for calculation of the area of the stenotic mitral valve, other cardiac valves, and central circulatory shunts. I. Am. Heart J. 41:1, 1951.
3. Gaasch, W. H., Carroll, J. D., Levine, H. J., and Criscitiello, M. G.: Chronic aortic regurgitation: Prognostic value of left ventricular end-systolic dimension and end-diastolic radius/thickness ratio. J. Am. Coll. Cardiol. 1:775, 1983.
4. Grayburn, P. A., Smith, M. D., Handshoe, R., et al.: Detection of aortic insufficiency by standard echocardiography, pulsed Doppler echocardiography, and auscultation: A comparison of accuracies. Ann. Intern. Med. 104:599, 1986.
5. Grayburn, P. A., Handshoe, R., Smith, M. D., et al.: Quantitative assessment of the hemodynamic consequences of aortic regurgitation by means of continuous wave Doppler recordings. J. Am. Coll. Cardiol. 10:135, 1987.
6. Glover, M. U., Warren, S. E., Vieweg, W. V. R., et al.: M-mode and two-dimensional echocardiographic correlation with findings at catheterization and surgery in patients with mitral stenosis. Am. Heart J. 105:98, 1983.
7. Gilbert, B. W., Schatz, R. A., VonRamm, O. T., et al.: Mitral valve prolapse: Two-dimensional echocardiographic and angiographic correlation. Circulation 54:716, 1976.
8. Goodman, D., Kimbiris, D., and Linhart, J. W.: Chordae tendineae rupture complicating the systolic click-late systolic murmur syndrome. Am. J. Cardiol. 33:681, 1974.
9. Grenadier, E., Alpan, G., Keidar, S., and Palant, A.: The prevalence of ruptured chordae tendineae in the mitral valve prolapse syndrome. Am. Heart J. 105:603, 1983.
10. Godley, R. W., Wann, L. S., Rogers, E. W., et al.: Incomplete mitral leaflet closure in patients with papillary muscle dysfunction. Circulation 63:565, 1981.
11. Gibbs, K. L., Reardon, M. J., Strickman, N. E., et al.: Hemodynamic compromise (tricuspid stenosis and insufficiency) caused by an unruptured aneurysm of the sinus of Valsalva. J. Am. Coll. Cardiol. 7:1177, 1986.
12. Gikonyo, B. M., Lucas, R. V., and Edwards, J. E.: Anatomic features of congenital pulmonary valvular stenosis. Pediatr. Cardiol. 8:109, 1987.
13. Grenadier, E., Sahn, D. J., Roche, A. H. G., et al.: Detection of deterioration or infection of homograft and porcine xenograft bioprosthetic valves in mitral and aortic positions by two-dimensional echocardiographic examination. J. Am. Coll. Cardiol. 2:452, 1983.
14. Galloway, A. C., Colvin, S. B., Baumann, F. G., et al.: Current concepts of mitral valve reconstruction for mitral insufficiency. Circulation 78:1087, 1988.
15. Galloway, A. C., Colvin, S. B., Baumann, F. G., et al.: Long-term results of mitral valve reconstruction with Carpentier techniques in 148 patients with mitral insufficiency. Circulation 78 (Suppl. I):I-97, 1988.

H

1. Hegranaes, L., and Hatle, L.: Aortic stenosis in adults: Non-invasive estimation of pressure differences by continuous wave Doppler echocardiography. Br. Heart J. 54:396, 1985.
2. Hatle, L., Angelsen, B. A., and Tromsdal, A.: Non-invasive assessment of aortic stenosis by Doppler ultrasound. Br. Heart J. 43:284, 1980.
3. Henry, W. L., Bonow, R. O., Borer, J. S., et al.: Observations on the optimum time for operative intervention for aortic regurgitation: I. Evaluation of the results of aortic valve replacement in symptomatic patients. Circulation 61:471, 1980.
4. Henry, W. L., Bonow, R. O., Rosing, D. R., and Epstein, S. E.: Observations on the optimum time for operative intervention for aortic regurgitation: II. Serial echocardiographic evaluation of asymptomatic patients. Circulation 61:484, 1980.
5. Hammer, W. J., Roberts, W. C., and DeLeon, A. C., Jr.: "Mitral stenosis" secondary to combined "massive" mitral annular calcific deposits and small, hypertrophied left ventricles: Hemodynamic documentation in four patients. Am. J. Med. 64:371, 1978.
6. Henry, W. L., Griffith, J. M., Michaelis, L. L., et al.: Measurement of mitral orifice area in patients with mitral valve disease by real-time, two-dimensional echocardiography. Circulation 51:827, 1975.
7. Holen, J., Aaslid, R., Landmark, K., and Simonsen, S.: Determination of pressure gradient in mitral stenosis with a non-invasive ultrasound Doppler technique. Acta Med. Scand. 199:455, 1976.
8. Hatle, L., Brubakk, A., Tromsdal, A., and Angelsen, B.: Noninvasive assessment of pressure drop in mitral stenosis by Doppler ultrasound. Br. Heart J. 40:131, 1978.
9. Holen, J., and Simonsen, S.: Determination of pressure gradient in mitral stenosis with Doppler echocardiography. Br. Heart J. 41:529, 1979.
10. Hatle, L., Angelsen, B., and Tromsdal, A.: Noninvasive assessment of atrioventricular pressure half-time by Doppler ultrasound. Circulation 60:1096, 1979.
11. Holen, J., Aaslid, R., Landmark, K., et al.: Determination of effective orifice area in mitral stenosis from non-invasive ultrasound Doppler data and mitral flow rate. Acta Med. Scand. 201:83, 1977.
12. Hickey, A. J., Wilcken, D. E. L., Wright, J. S., and Warren, B. A.: Primary (spontaneous) chordal rupture: Relation to myxomatous valve disease and mitral valve prolapse. J. Am. Coll. Cardiol. 5:1341, 1985.
13. Helmcke, F., Nanda, N. C., Hsuing, M. C., et al.: Color Doppler assessment of mitral regurgitation with orthogonal planes. Circulation 75:175, 1987.
14. Hauck, A. J., Freeman, D. P., Ackermann, D. M., et al.: Surgical pathology of the tricuspid valve: A study of 363 cases spanning 25 years. Mayo Clin. Proc. 63:851, 1988.
15. Harley, J. B., McIntosh, C. L., Kirklin, J. J. W., et al.: Atrioventricular valve replacement in the idiopathic hypereosinophilic syndrome. Am. J. Med. 73:77, 1982.
16. Hatle, L. K., and Angelsen, B. A.: Doppler Ultrasound in Cardiology: Physical Principles and Clinical Applications, 2nd ed. Lea & Febiger, Philadelphia, 1985, pp. 151–153.
17. Hatle, L. K., and Angelsen, B. A.: Doppler Ultrasound in Cardiology: Physical Principles and Clinical Applications, 2nd ed. Lea & Febiger, Philadelphia, 1985, p. 109.
18. Holen, J., Simonsen, S., and Frøysaker, T.: An ultrasound Doppler technique for the noninvasive determination of the pressure gradient in the Björk-Shiley mitral valve. Circulation 59:436, 1979.
19. Holen, J., Simonsen, S., and Frøysaker, T.: Determination of pressure gradient in the Hancock mitral valve from noninvasive ultrasound Dopper data. Scand. J. Clin. Lab. Invest. 41:177, 1981.

I

1. Isner, J. M., Samuels, D. A., Slovenkai, G. A., et al.: Mechanism of aortic balloon valvuloplasty: Fracture of valvular calcific deposits. Ann. Intern. Med. 108:377, 1988.

J

1. Johnson, A. D., and Gosink, B. B.: Oscillation of left ventricular structures in aortic regurgitation. J. Clin. Ultrasound 5:21, 1977.

K

1. Kennedy, K. D., Hauck, A. J., Edwards, W. D., et al.: Mechanism of reduction of aortic valvular stenosis by percutaneous transluminal balloon valvuloplasty: Report of five cases and review of literature. Mayo Clin. Proc. 63:769, 1988.
2. Khandheria, B. K., Tajik, A. J., Taylor, C. L., et al.: Aortic dissection: Review of value and limitations of two-dimensional echocardiography in a six year experience. J. Am. Soc. Echo. 2:17, 1989.
3. Kumpuris, A. G., Quinones, M. A., Waggoner, A. D., et al.: Importance of preoperative hypertrophy, wall stress and end-systolic dimension as echocardiographic predictors of normalization of left ventricular dilatation after valve replacement in chronic aortic insufficiency. Am. J. Cardiol. 49:1091, 1982.
4. Knutsen, K. M., Bae, E. A., Sivertssen, E., and Grendahl, H.: Doppler ultrasound in mitral stenosis: Assessment of pressure gradient and atrioventricular pressure half-time. Acta Med. Scand. 211:433, 1982.
5. Khandheria, B. K., Tajik, A. J., Reeder, G. S., et al.: Doppler color flow imaging: A new technique for visualization and characterization of the blood flow jet in mitral stenosis. Mayo Clin. Proc. 61:623, 1986.
6. Karp, K., Teien, D., Bjerle, P., and Eriksson, P.: Reassessment of valve area determinations in mitral stenosis by the pressure half-time method: Impact of left ventricular stiffness and peak diastolic pressure difference. J. Am. Coll. Cardiol. 13:594, 1989.
7. Katz, N. M., and Pallas, R. S.: Traumatic rupture of the tricuspid valve: Repair by chordal replacements and annuloplasty. J. Thorac. Cardiovasc. Surg. 91:P310, 1986.
8. Klein, A. L., Burstow, D. J., Taliercio, C. P., et al.: Age-related prevalence of valvular regurgitation in normal subjects. (Abstract.) Circulation 78 (Suppl. II):II-133, 1988.
9. Kramer, N. E., Gill, S. S., Patel, R., and Towne, W. D.: Pulmonary valve vegetations detected with echocardiography. Am. J. Cardiol. 39:1064, 1977.
10. Kostucki, W., Vandenbossche, J.-L., Friart, A., and Englert, M.: Pulsed Doppler regurgitant flow patterns of normal valves. Am. J. Cardiol. 58:309, 1986.
11. Kotler, M. N., Mintz, G. S., Panidis, I., et al.: Noninvasive evaluation of normal and abnormal prosthetic valve function. J. Am. Coll. Cardiol. 2:151, 1983.
12. King, R. M., Pluth, J. R., Giuliani, E. R., and Piehler, J. M.: Mechanical decalcification of the aortic valve. Ann. Thorac. Surg. 42:269, 1986.

L

1. Larson, E. W., and Edwards, W. D.: Risk factors for aortic dissection: A necropsy study of 161 cases. Am. J. Cardiol. 53:849, 1984.
2. Leier, C. V., Call, T. D., Fulkerson, P. K., and Wooley, C. F.: The spectrum of cardiac defects in the Ehlers-Danlos syndrome, types I and III. Ann. Intern. Med. 92:171, 1980.
3. Labovitz, A. J., Ferrara, R. P., Kern, M. J., et al.: Quantitative evaluation of aortic insufficiency by continuous wave Doppler echocardiography. J. Am. Coll. Cardiol. 8:1341, 1986.
4. Libanoff, A. J.: A hemodynamic measure of aortic regurgitation: Half-time of the rate of fall in aortic pressure during diastole. Cardiology 58:162, 1973.
5. Libanoff, A. J., and Rodbard, S.: Atrioventricular pressure half-time: Measure of mitral valve orifice area. Circulation 38:144, 1968.
6. Levine, R. A., Stathogiannis, E., Newell, J. B., et al.: Reconsideration of echocardiographic standards for mitral valve prolapse: Lack of association between leaflet displacement isolated to the apical four chamber view and independent echocardiographic evidence of abnormality. J. Am. Coll. Cardiol. 11:1010, 1988.
7. Lewis, J. F., Kuo, L. C., Nelson, J. G., et al.: Pulsed Doppler echocardiographic determination of stroke volume and cardiac output: Clinical validation of two new methods using the apical window. Circulation 70:425, 1984.
8. Lopez, J. F., Hanson, S., Orchard, R. C., and Tan, L.: Quantification of mitral valvular incompetence. Cathet. Cardiovasc. Diagn. 11:139, 1985.
9. Lev, M., Liberthson, R. R., Joseph, R. H., et al.: The pathologic anatomy of Ebstein's disease. Arch. Pathol. 90:334, 1970.
10. Lima, C. O., Sahn, D. J., Valdes-Cruz, L. M., et al.: Noninvasive prediction of transvalvular pressure gradient in patients with pulmonary stenosis by quantitative two-dimensional echocardiographic Doppler studies. Circulation 67:866, 1983.

M

1. McDonald, I. G.: Echocardiographic assessment of left ventricular function in aortic valve disease. Circulation 53:860, 1976.
2. McDonald, I. G., and Jelinek, V. M.: Serial M-mode echocardiography in severe chronic aortic regurgitation. Circulation 62:1291, 1980.
3. Morganroth, J., Perloff, J. K., and Zeldis, S. M.: Acute severe aortic regurgitation: Pathophysiology, clinical recognition, and management. Ann. Intern. Med. 87:223, 1977.
4. Masuyama, T., Kodama, K., Kitabatake, A., et al.: Noninvasive evaluation of aortic regurgitation by continuous-wave Doppler echocardiography. Circulation 73:460, 1986.
5. Martin, R. P., Rakowski, H., Kleiman, J. H., et al.: Reliability and reproducibility of two-dimensional echocardiographic measurement of the stenotic mitral valve orifice area. Am. J. Cardiol. 43:560, 1979.
6. Moro, E., Nicolosi, G. L., Zanuttini, D., et al.: Influence of aortic regurgitation on the assessment of the pressure half-time and derived mitral valve area in patients with mitral stenosis. Eur. Heart J. 9:1010, 1988.
7. Mintz, G. S., Kotler, M. N., Segal, B. L., and Parry, W. R.: Two-dimensional echocardiographic evaluation of patients with mitral insufficiency. Am. J. Cardiol. 44:670, 1979.
8. Marks, A. R., Choong, C. Y., Sanfilippo, A. J., et al.: Identification of high-risk and low-risk subgroups of patients with mitral-valve prolapse. N. Engl. J. Med. 320:1031, 1989.
9. MacMahon, S. W., Roberts, J. K., Kramer-Fox, R., et al.: Mitral valve prolapse and infective endocarditis. Am. Heart J. 113:1291, 1987.
10. Mintz, G. S., Kotler, M. N., Segal, B. L., and Parry, W. R.: Two-dimensional echocardiographic recognition of ruptured chordae tendineae. Circulation 57:244, 1978.
11. Martin, R. P., Meltzer, R. S., Chia, B. L., et al.: Clinical utility of two-dimensional echocardiography in infective endocarditis. Am. J. Cardiol. 46:379, 1980.
12. McGoon, D. C.: Repair of mitral insufficiency due to ruptured chordae tendineae. J. Thorac. Cardiovasc. Surg. 39:357, 1960.
13. Miyatake, K., Izumi, S., Okamoto, M., et al.: Semiquantitative grading of severity of mitral regurgitation by real-time two-dimensional Doppler flow imaging technique. J. Am. Coll. Cardiol. 7:82, 1986.
14. Miyatake, K., Okamoto, M., Kinoshita, N., et al.: Clinical applications of a new type of real-time two-dimensional Doppler flow imaging system. Am. J. Cardiol. 54:857, 1984.
15. McKinsey, D. S., Ratts, T. E., and Bisno, A. L.: Underlying cardiac lesions in

adults with infective endocarditis: The changing spectrum. Am. J. Med. 82:681, 1987.
16. Miyatake, K., Okamoto, M., Kinoshita, N., et al.: Evaluation of tricuspid regurgitation by pulsed Doppler and two-dimensional echocardiography. Circulation 66:777, 1982.
17. Miyatake, K., Okamoto, M., Kinoshita, N., et al.: Pulmonary regurgitation studied with the ultrasonic pulsed Doppler technique. Circulation 65:969, 1982.
18. Marantz, P. M., Huhta, J. C., Mullins, C. E., et al.: Results of balloon valvuloplasty in typical and dysplastic pulmonary valve stenosis: Doppler echocardiographic follow-up. J. Am. Coll. Cardiol. 12:476, 1988.
19. McKay, R. G., Safian, R. D., Lock, J. E., et al.: Balloon dilatation of calcific aortic stenosis in elderly patients: Postmortem, intraoperative, and percutaneous valvuloplasty studies. Circulation 74:119, 1986.

N

1. Nanda, N. C., and Gramiak, R.: Evaluation of bicuspid valves by two-dimensional echocardiography. (Abstract.) Am. J. Cardiol. 41:372, 1978.
2. Nishimura, R. A., Miller, F. A., Jr., Callahan, M. J., et al.: Doppler echocardiography: Theory, instrumentation, technique, and application. Mayo Clin. Proc. 60:321, 1985.
3. Nishimura, R. A., McGoon, M. D., Schaff, H. V., and Giuliani, E. R.: Chronic aortic regurgitation: Indications for operation—1988. Mayo Clin. Proc. 63:270, 1988.
4. Nishimura, R. A., and Tajik, A. J.: Determination of left-sided pressure gradients by utilizing Doppler aortic and mitral regurgitant signals: Validation by simultaneous dual catheter and Doppler studies. J. Am. Coll. Cardiol. 11:317, 1988.
5. Nakatani, S., Masuyama, T., Kodama, K., et al.: Value and limitations of Doppler echocardiography in the quantification of stenotic mitral valve area: Comparison of the pressure half-time and the continuity equation methods. Circulation 77:78, 1988.
6. Nishimura, R. A., McGoon, M. D., Shub, C., et al.: Echocardiographically documented mitral-valve prolapse: Long-term follow-up of 237 patients. N. Engl. J. Med. 313:1305, 1985.
7. Nishimura, R. A., Schaff, H. V., Shub, C., et al.: Papillary muscle rupture complicating acute myocardial infarction: Analysis of 17 patients. Am. J. Cardiol. 51:373, 1983.
8. Nestico, P. F., Depace, N. L., Morganroth, J., et al.: Mitral annular calcification: Clinical, pathophysiology, and echocardiographic review. Am. Heart J. 107:989, 1984.
9. Naidoo, D. P., Seedat, M. A., and Vythilingum, S.: Isolated endocarditis of the pulmonary valve with fragmentation haemolysis. Br. Heart J. 60:527, 1988.
10. Nellessen, U., Schnittger, I., Appleton, C. P., et al.: Transesophageal two-dimensional echocardiography and color Doppler flow velocity mapping in the evaluation of cardiac valve prostheses. Circulation 78:848, 1988.
11. Nellessen, U., Masuyama, T., Appleton, C. P., et al.: Mitral prosthesis malfunction: Comparative Doppler echocardiographic studies of mitral prostheses before and after replacement. Circulation 79:330, 1989.
12. Nishimura, R. A., Holmes, D. R., Jr., Reeder, G. S., et al.: Doppler evaluation of results of percutaneous aortic balloon valvuloplasty in calcific aortic stenosis. Circulation 78:791, 1988.

O

1. Oh, J. K., Taliercio, C. P., Holmes, D. R., Jr., et al.: Prediction of the severity of aortic stenosis by Doppler aortic valve area determination: Prospective Doppler-catheterization correlation in 100 patients. J. Am. Coll. Cardiol. 11:1227, 1988.
2. Otto, C. M., Pearlman, A. S., Comess, K. A., et al.: Determination of the stenotic aortic valve area in adults using Doppler echocardiography. J. Am. Coll. Cardiol. 7:509, 1986.
3. Otto, C. M., Pearlman, A. S., and Gardner, C. L.: Hemodynamic progression of aortic stenosis in adults assessed by Doppler echocardiography. J. Am. Coll. Cardiol. 13:545, 1989.
4. Olson, L. J., Subramanian, R., and Edwards, W. D.: Surgical pathology of pure aortic insufficiency: A study of 225 cases. Mayo Clin. Proc. 59:835, 1984.
5. Omoto, R., Yokote, Y., Takamoto, S., et al.: The development of real-time two-dimensional Doppler echocardiography and its clinical significance in acquired valvular diseases: With special reference to the evaluation of valvular regurgitation. Jpn. Heart J. 25:325, 1984.
6. Olson, L. J., Subramanian, R., Ackermann, D. M., et al.: Surgical pathology of the mitral valve: A study of 712 cases spanning 21 years. Mayo Clin. Proc. 62:22, 1987.
7. Osterberger, L. E., Goldstein, S., Khaja, F., and Lakier, J. B.: Functional mitral stenosis in patients with massive annular calcification. Circulation 64:472, 1981.
8. Osmundson, P. J., Callahan, J. A., and Edwards, J. E.: Ruptured mitral chordae tendineae. Circulation 23:42, 1961.
9. Oliveira, D. B. G., Dawkins, K. D., Kay, P. H., and Paneth, M.: Chordal rupture: I: Aetiology and natural history. Br. Heart J. 50:312, 1983.
10. Ogawa, S., Hayashi, J., Sasaki, H., et al.: Evaluation of combined valvular prolapse syndrome by two-dimensional echocardiography. Circulation 65:174, 1982.
11. Okada, R., Ewy, G. A., and Copeland, J. G.: Echocardiography and surgery in tricuspid and pulmonary valve stenosis due to carcinoid syndrome. Cardiovasc. Med. 4:871, 1979.

P

1. Pomerance, A.: Pathogenesis of aortic stenosis and its relation to age. Br. Heart J. 34:569, 1972.
2. Passik, C. S., Ackermann, D. M., Pluth, J. R., and Edwards, W. D.: Temporal changes in the causes of aortic stenosis: A surgical pathologic study of 646 cases. Mayo Clin. Proc. 62:119, 1987.
3. Pyeritz, R. E., and McKusick, V. A.: The Marfan syndrome: Diagnosis and management. N. Engl. J. Med. 300:772, 1979.
4. Pyeritz, R. E., and Wappel, M. A.: Mitral valve dysfunction in the Marfan syndrome: Clinical and echocardiographic study of prevalence and natural history. Am. J. Med. 74:797, 1983.
5. Perry, G. J., Helmcke, F., Nanda, N. C., et al.: Evaluation of aortic insufficiency by Doppler color flow mapping. J. Am. Coll. Cardiol. 9:952, 1987.
6. Pomerance, A.: Chronic rheumatic and other inflammatory valve disease. *In* Pomerance, A., and Davies, M. J. (eds.): The Pathology of the Heart. Blackwell Scientific Publications, London, 1975, pp. 307–326.
7. Perloff, J. K., and Roberts, W. C.: The mitral apparatus: Functional anatomy of mitral regurgitation. Circulation 46:227, 1972.
8. Procacci, P. M., Savran, S. V., Schreiter, S. L., and Bryson, A. L.: Prevalence of clinical mitral-valve prolapse in 1169 young women. N. Engl. J. Med. 294:1086, 1976.
9. Pini, R., Greppi, B., Kramer-Fox, R., et al.: Mitral valve dimensions and motion and familial transmission of mitral valve prolapse with and without mitral leaflet billowing. J. Am. Coll. Cardiol. 12:1423, 1988.
10. Pini, R., Devereux, R. B., Greppi, B., et al.: Comparison of mitral valve dimensions and motion in mitral valve prolapse with severe mitral regurgitation to uncomplicated mitral valve prolapse and to mitral regurgitation without mitral valve prolapse. Am. J. Cardiol. 62:257, 1988.
11. Pennestrí, F., Loperfido, F., Salvatori, M. P., et al.: Assessment of tricuspid regurgitation by pulsed Doppler ultrasonography of the hepatic veins. Am. J. Cardiol. 54:363, 1984.
12. Panidis, I. P., Ross, J., and Mintz, G. S.: Normal and abnormal prosthetic valve function as assessed by Doppler echocardiography. J. Am. Coll. Cardiol. 8:317, 1986.
13. Perier, P., Deloche, A., Chauvaud, S., et al.: Comparative evaluation of mitral valve repair and replacement with Starr, Björk, and porcine valve prostheses. Circulation 70 (Suppl. I):I-87, 1984.
14. Palacios, I. F., Block, P. C., Wilkins, G. T., and Weyman, A. E.: Follow-up of patients undergoing percutaneous mitral balloon valvotomy: Analysis of factors determining restenosis. Circulation 79:573, 1989.

Q

1. Quinones, M. A., Young, J. B., Waggoner, A. D., et al.: Assessment of pulsed Doppler echocardiography in detection and quantification of aortic and mitral regurgitation. Br. Heart J. 44:612, 1980.

R

1. Roberts, W. C.: The structure of the aortic valve in clinically isolated aortic stenosis: An autopsy study of 162 patients over 15 years of age. Circulation 42:91, 1970.
2. Roberts, W. C.: The congenitally bicuspid aortic valve: A study of 85 autopsy cases. Am. J. Cardiol. 26:72, 1970.
3. Rijsterborgh, H., and Roelandt, J.: Doppler assessment of aortic stenosis: Bernoulli revisited. Ultrasound Med. Biol. 13:241, 1987.
4. Roberts, W. C.: Left ventricular outflow tract obstruction and aortic regurgitation. Monogr. Pathol. 15:110, 1974.
5. Roberts, W. C.: Aortic dissection: Anatomy, consequences, and causes. Am. Heart J. 101:195, 1981.
6. Roberts, W. C., Morrow, A. G., McIntosh, C. L., et al.: Congenitally bicuspid aortic valve causing severe, pure aortic regurgitation without superimposed infective endocarditis: Analysis of 13 patients requiring aortic valve replacement. Am. J. Cardiol. 47:206, 1981.
7. Rokey, R., Sterling, L. L., Zoghbi, W. A., et al.: Determination of regurgitant fraction in isolated mitral or aortic regurgitation by pulsed Doppler two-dimensional echocardiography. J. Am. Coll. Cardiol. 7:1273, 1986.
8. Roberts, W. C.: Morphologic features of the normal and abnormal mitral valve. Am. J. Cardiol. 51:1005, 1983.
9. Rusted, I. E., Scheifley, C. H., and Edwards, J. E.: Studies of the mitral valve: II. Certain anatomic features of the mitral valve and associated structures in mitral stenosis. Circulation 14:398, 1956.
10. Ruckman, R. N., and Van Praagh, R.: Anatomic types of congenital mitral stenosis: Report of 49 autopsy cases with consideration of diagnosis and surgical implications. Am. J. Cardiol. 42:592, 1978.
11. Reid, C. L., McKay, C. R., Chandraratna, P. A. N., et al.: Mechanisms of increase in mitral valve area and influence of anatomic features in double-balloon, catheter balloon valvuloplasty in adults with rheumatic mitral stenosis: A Doppler and two-dimensional echocardiographic study. Circulation 76:628, 1987.
12. Roberts, W. C., and Perloff, J. K.: Mitral valvular disease: A clinicopathologic survey of the conditions causing the mitral valve to function abnormally. Ann. Intern. Med. 77:939, 1972.
13. Roberts, W. C., Braunwald, E., and Morrow, A. G.: Acute severe mitral regurgitation secondary to ruptured chordae tendineae: Clinical, hemodynamic, and pathologic considerations. Circulation 33:58, 1966.
14. Reeder, G. S., Currie, P. J., Fyfe, D. A., et al.: Extracardiac conduit obstruction: Initial experience in the use of Doppler echocardiography for noninvasive estimation of pressure gradient. J. Am. Coll. Cardiol. 4:1006, 1984.

15. Ryan, T., Armstrong, W. F., Dillon, J. C., and Feigenbaum, H.: Doppler echocardiographic evaluation of patients with porcine mitral valves. Am. Heart J. 111:237, 1987.
16. Reisner, S. A., and Meltzer, R. S.: Normal values of prosthetic valve Doppler echocardiographic parameters: A review. J. Am. Soc. Echo. 1:203, 1988.
17. Rothbart, R. M., Smucker, M. L., and Gibson, R. S.: Overestimation by Doppler echocardiography of pressure gradients across Starr-Edwards prosthetic valves in the aortic position. Am. J. Cardiol. 61:475, 1988.
18. Rediker, D. E., Block, P. C., Abascal, V. M., and Palacios, I. F.: Mitral balloon valvuloplasty for mitral restenosis after surgical commissurotomy. J. Am. Coll. Cardiol. 11:252, 1988.
19. Robicsek, F., and Harbold, N. B., Jr.: Limited value of balloon dilatation in calcified aortic stenosis in adults: Direct observations during open heart surgery. Am. J. Cardiol. 60:857, 1987.

S

1. Subramanian, R., Olson, L. J., and Edwards, W. D.: Surgical pathology of pure aortic stenosis: A study of 374 cases. Mayo Clin. Proc. 59:683, 1984.
2. Seward, J. B., and Tajik, A. J.: Noninvasive visualization of the entire thoracic aorta: A new application of wide-angle two-dimensional sector echocardiographic technique. (Abstract.) Am. J. Cardiol. 43:387, 1979.
3. Schwartz, A., Vignola, P. A., Walker, H. J., et al.: Echocardiographic estimation of aortic-valve gradient in aortic stenosis. Ann. Intern. Med. 89:329, 1978.
4. Stamm, R. B., and Martin, R. P.: Quantification of pressure gradients across stenotic valves by Doppler ultrasound. J. Am. Coll. Cardiol. 2:707, 1983.
5. Sasson, Z., Yock, P. G., Hatle, L. K., et al.: Doppler echocardiographic determination of the pressure gradient in hypertrophic cardiomyopathy. J. Am. Coll. Cardiol. 11:752, 1988.
6. Smith, M. D., Dawson, P. L., Elion, J. L., et al.: Correlation of continuous wave Doppler velocities with cardiac catheterization gradients: An experimental model of aortic stenosis. J. Am. Coll. Cardiol. 6:1306, 1985.
7. Skjaerpe, T., Hegrenaes, L., and Hatle, L.: Noninvasive estimation of valve area in patients with aortic stenosis by Doppler ultrasound and two-dimensional echocardiography. Circulation 72:810, 1985.
8. Selzer, A., and Sudrann, R. B.: Reliability of the determination of cardiac output in man by means of the Fick principle. Circ. Res. 6:485, 1958.
9. Segal, J., Lerner, D. J., Miller, D. C., et al.: When should Doppler-determined valve area be better than the Gorlin formula? Variation in hydraulic constants in low flow states. J. Am. Coll. Cardiol. 9:1294, 1987.
10. Subramanian, R., Olson, L. J., and Edwards, W. D.: Surgical pathology of combined aortic stenosis and insufficiency: A study of 213 cases. Mayo Clin. Proc. 60:247, 1985.
11. Stewart, W. J., Agler, D. A., Koch, J. M., and Currie, P. J.: Color flow mapping diagnosis and localization of paravalvular aortic regurgitation. (Abstract.) Circulation 76 (Suppl. IV):IV-448, 1987.
12. Silverman, K. J., and Hutchins, G. M.: Spontaneous dehiscence of an aortic commissure complicating idiopathic aortic root dilatation. Am. Heart J. 97:367, 1979.
13. Stewart, S. R., Robbins, D. L., and Castles, J. J.: Acute fulminant aortic and mitral insufficiency in ankylosing spondylitis. N. Engl. J. Med. 299:1448, 1978.
14. Sahn, D. J., Allen, H. D., McDonald, G., and Goldberg, S. J.: Real-time cross-sectional echocardiographic diagnosis of coarctation of the aorta: A prospective study of echocardiographic-angiographic correlations. Circulation 56:762, 1977.
15. Switzer, D. F., Yoganathan, A. P., Nanda, N. C., et al.: Calibration of color Doppler flow mapping during extreme hemodynamic conditions in vitro: A foundation for a reliable quantitative grading system for aortic incompetence. Circulation 75:837, 1987.
16. Slørdahl, S. A., Solbakken, J. E., Angelsen, B. J., et al.: Estimation of aortic regurgitant orifice size and volume by measurements available noninvasively: In vivo validation in pigs. (Abstract.) Circulation 78 (Suppl. II):II-133, 1988.
17. Sandler, H., Dodge, H. T., Hay, R. E., and Rackley, C. E.: Quantitation of valvular insufficiency in man by angiocardiography. Am. Heart J. 65:501, 1963.
18. Snider, A. R., Roge, C. L., Schiller, N. B., and Silverman, N. H.: Congenital left ventricular inflow obstruction evaluated by two-dimensional echocardiography. Circulation 61:848, 1980.
19. Shone, J. D., Sellers, R. D., Anderson, R. C., et al.: The developmental complex of "parachute mitral valve," supravalvular ring of left atrium, subaortic stenosis, and coarctation of aorta. Am. J. Cardiol. 11:714, 1963.
20. Smith, M. D., Handshoe, R., Handshoe, S., et al.: Comparative accuracy of two-dimensional echocardiography and Doppler pressure half-time methods in assessing severity of mitral stenosis in patients with and without prior commissurotomy. Circulation 73:100, 1986.
21. Spain, M. G., Smith, M. D., Grayburn, P. A., et al.: Quantitative assessment of mitral regurgitation by Doppler color flow imaging: Angiographic and hemodynamic correlations. J. Am. Coll. Cardiol. 13:585, 1989.
22. Smith, M. D., Grayburn, P. A., Spain, M. G., et al.: Observer variability in the quantitation of Doppler color flow jet areas for mitral and aortic regurgitation. J. Am. Coll. Cardiol. 11:579, 1988.
23. Silver, M. D., Lam, J. H. C., Ranganathan, N., and Wigle, E. D.: Morphology of the human tricuspid valve. Circulation 43:333, 1971.
24. Silver, M. D.: Obstruction to blood flow related to tricuspid, pulmonary, and mitral valves. *In* Silver, M. D. (ed.): Cardiovascular Pathology. Vol. 1. Churchill-Livingstone, New York, 1983, pp. 551–574.
25. Strickman, N. E., Rossi, P. A., Massumkhani, G. A., and Hall, R. J.: Carcinoid heart disease: A clinical, pathologic, and therapeutic update. Curr. Probl. Cardiol. 6:1, 1982.
26. Shiina, A., Seward, J. B., Tajik, A. J., et al.: Two-dimensional echocardiographic-surgical correlation in Ebstein's anomaly: Preoperative determination of patients requiring tricuspid valve plication vs. replacement. Circulation 68:534, 1983.
27. Skjaerpe, T., and Hatle, L.: Diagnosis and assessment of tricuspid regurgitation by Doppler ultrasound. *In* Rijsterbough, H. (ed.): Echocardiography. Martinus Nijhoff, The Hague, 1981, pp. 299–304.
28. Skjaerpe, T., and Hatle, L.: Noninvasive estimation of pulmonary artery pressure by Doppler ultrasound in tricuspid regurgitation. *In* Spencer, M. P. (ed.): Cardiac Doppler Diagnosis, Vol 1. Martinus Nijhoff, Boston, 1984, pp. 247–254.
29. Sprecher, D. L., Adamick, R., Adams, D., and Kisslo, J.: In vitro color flow, pulsed and continuous wave Doppler ultrasound masking of flow by prosthetic valves. J. Am. Coll. Cardiol. 9:1306, 1987.
30. Schoen, F. J., Collins, J. J., Jr., and Cohn, L. H.: Long-term failure rate and morphologic correlations in porcine bioprosthetic heart valves. Am. J. Cardiol. 51:957, 1983.
31. Sagar, K. B., Wann, L. S., Paulsen, W. H. J., and Romhilt, D. W.: Doppler echocardiographic evaluation of Hancock and Björk-Shiley prosthetic valves. J. Am. Coll. Cardiol. 7:681, 1986.
32. Schoenfeld, M. H., Palacios, I. F., Hutter, A. M., Jr., et al.: Underestimation of prosthetic mitral valve areas: Role of transseptal catheterization in avoiding unnecessary repeat mitral valve surgery. J. Am. Coll. Cardiol. 5:1387, 1985.
33. Seward, J. B., Khandheria, B. K., Oh, J. K., et al.: Transesophageal echocardiography: Technique, anatomic correlations, implementation, and clinical applications. Mayo Clin. Proc. 63:649, 1988.
34. Safian, R. D., Warren, S. E., Berman, A. D., et al.: Improvement in symptoms and left ventricular performance after balloon aortic valvuloplasty in patients with aortic stenosis and depressed left ventricular ejection fraction. Circulation 78:1181, 1988.
35. Safian, R. D., Mandell, V. S., Thurer, R. E., et al.: Postmortem and intraoperative balloon valvuloplasty of calcific aortic stenosis in elderly patients: Mechanisms of successful dilation. J. Am. Coll. Cardiol. 9:655, 1987.

T

1. Tajik, A. J., Seward, J. B., Hagler, D. J., et al.: Two-dimensional real-time ultrasonic imaging of the heart and great vessels: Technique, image orientation, structure identification, and validation. Mayo Clin. Proc. 53:271, 1978.
2. Teirstein, P., Yeager, M., Yock, P. G., and Popp, R. L.: Doppler echocardiographic measurement of aortic valve area in aortic stenosis: A noninvasive application of the Gorlin formula. J. Am. Coll. Cardiol. 8:1059, 1986.
3. Thomasson, B.: Cardiac output in normal subjects under standard conditions: The repeatability of measurements by the Fick method. Scand. J. Clin. Lab. Invest. 9:365, 1957.
4. Tucker, C. R., Fowles, R. E., Calin, A., and Popp, R. L.: Aortitis in ankylosing spondylitis: Early detection of aortic root abnormalities with two-dimensional echocardiography. Am. J. Cardiol. 49:680, 1982.
5. Takenaka, K., Dabestani, A., Gardin, J. M., et al.: A simple Doppler echocardiographic method for estimating severity of aortic regurgitation. Am. J. Cardiol. 57:1340, 1986.
6. Teague, S. M., Heinsimer, J. A., Anderson, J. L., et al.: Quantification of aortic regurgitation utilizing continuous wave Doppler ultrasound. J. Am. Coll. Cardiol. 8:592, 1986.
7. Teirstein, P. S., Yock, P. G., and Popp, R. L.: The accuracy of Doppler ultrasound measurement of pressure gradients across irregular, dual, and tunnellike obstructions to blood flow. Circulation 72:577, 1985.

V

1. Visscher, M. B., and Johnson, J. A.: The Fick principle: Analysis of potential errors in its conventional application. J. Appl. Physiol. 5:635, 1953.
2. Van Grondelle, A., Ditchey, R. V., Groves, B. M., et al.: Thermodilution method overestimates low cardiac output in humans. Am. J. Physiol. 245:H690, 1983.
3. Veyrat, C., Ameur, A., Bas, S., et al.: Pulsed Doppler echocardiographic indices for assessing mitral regurgitation. Br. Heart J. 51:130, 1984.
4. Veyrat, C., Kalmanson, D., Farjon, M., et al.: Non-invasive diagnosis and assessment of tricuspid regurgitation and stenosis using one and two dimensional echo-pulsed Doppler. Br. Heart J. 47:596, 1982.

W

1. Weyman, A. E., Feigenbaum, H., Dillon, J. C., and Chang, S.: Cross-sectional echocardiography in assessing the severity of valvular aortic stenosis. Circulation 52:828, 1975.
2. Weyman, A. E., Feigenbaum, H., Hurwitz, R. A., et al.: Localization of left ventricular outflow obstruction by cross-sectional echocardiography. Am. J. Med. 60:33, 1976.
3. Wong, M., Tei, C., Sadler, N., et al.: Echocardiographic observations of calcium in operatively excised stenotic aortic valves. Am. J. Cardiol. 59:324, 1987.
4. Wautrecht, J. C., Vandenbossche, J. L., and Englert, M.: Sensitivity and specificity of pulsed Doppler echocardiography in detection of aortic and mitral regurgitation. Eur. Heart J. 5:404, 1984.
5. Welch, G. H., Jr., Braunwald, E., and Sarnoff, S. J.: Hemodynamic effects of quantitatively varied experimental aortic regurgitation. Circ. Res. 5:546, 1957.
6. Weyman, A. E.: Cross-Sectional Echocardiography. Lea & Febiger, Philadelphia, 1982, pp. 150–157.

7. Wann, L. S., Weyman, A. E., Feigenbaum, H., et al.: Determination of mitral valve area by cross-sectional echocardiography. Ann. Intern. Med. 88:337, 1978.
8. Wilkins, G. T., Weyman, A. E., Abascal, V. M., et al.: Percutaneous balloon dilatation of the mitral valve: An analysis of echocardiographic variables related to outcome and the mechanism of dilatation. Br. Heart J. 60:299, 1988.
9. Wilcken, D. E. L., and Hickey, A. J.: Lifetime risk for patients with mitral valve prolapse of developing severe valve regurgitation requiring surgery. Circulation 78:10, 1988.
10. Weyman, A. E., Rankin, R., and King, H.: Loeffler's endocarditis presenting as mitral and tricuspid stenosis. Am. J. Cardiol. 40:438, 1977.
11. Waller, B. F., Moriarty, A. T., Eble, J. N., et al.: Etiology of pure tricuspid regurgitation based on annular circumference and leaflet area: Analysis of 45 necropsy patients with clinical and morphologic evidence of pure tricuspid regurgitation. J. Am. Coll. Cardiol. 7:1063, 1986.
12. Waller, B. F.: Etiology of pure tricuspid regurgitation. Cardiovasc. Clin. 17:53, 1987.
13. Watanabe, T., Katsume, H., Matsukubo, H., et al.: Ruptured chordae tendineae of the tricuspid valve due to nonpenetrating trauma: Echocardiographic findings. Chest 80:751, 1981.
14. Weyman, A. E., Wann, S., Feigenbaum, H., and Dillon, J. C.: Mechanism of abnormal septal motion in patients with right ventricular volume overload: A cross-sectional echocardiographic study. Circulation 54:179, 1976.
15. Waggoner, A. D., Quinones, M. A., Young, J. B., et al.: Pulsed Doppler echocardiographic detection of right-sided valve regurgitation: Experimental results and clinical significance. Am. J. Cardiol. 47:279, 1981.
16. Wranne, B., and Marklund, T.: Evaluation of tricuspid regurgitation. A comparison between pulsed Doppler, jugular vein and liver pulse recordings, contrast echocardiography and angiography. *In* Spencer, M. P. (ed.): Cardiac Doppler Diagnosis, Vol. 1. Martinus Nijhoff, Boston, 1984, pp. 255–262.
17. Weyman, A. E., Dillon, J. C., Feigenbaum, H., and Chang, S.: Echocardiographic differentiation of infundibular from valvular pulmonary stenosis. Am. J. Cardiol. 36:21, 1975.
18. Weyman, A. E., Hurwitz, R. A., Girod, D. A., et al.: Cross-sectional echocardiographic visualization of the stenotic pulmonary valve. Circulation 56:769, 1977.
19. Williams, G. A., and Labovitz, A. J.: Doppler hemodynamic evaluation of prosthetic (Starr-Edwards and Björk-Shiley) and bioprosthetic (Hancock and Carpentier-Edwards) cardiac valves. Am. J. Cardiol. 56:325, 1985.
20. Wilkins, G. T., Gillam, L. D., Kritzer, G. L., et al.: Validation of continuous-wave Doppler echocardiographic measurements of mitral and tricuspid prosthetic valve gradients: A simultaneous Doppler-catheter study. Circulation 74:786, 1986.

Y

1. Yock, P. G., Hatle, L., and Popp, R. L.: Patterns and timing of Doppler-detected intracavitary and aortic flow in hypertrophic cardiomyopathy. J. Am. Coll. Cardiol. 8:1047, 1986.
2. Yeung, A. C., Plappert, T., and St. John Sutton, M. G.: Calculation of aortic regurgitation orifice area by Doppler echocardiography: A new application of the continuity equation. (Abstract.) Circulation 78 (Suppl. II):II-39, 1988.
3. Yoshida, K., Yoshikawa, J., Shakudo, M., et al.: Color Doppler evaluation of valvular regurgitation in normal subjects. Circulation 78:840, 1988.
4. Yock, P. G., and Popp, R. L.: Noninvasive estimation of right ventricular systolic pressure by Doppler ultrasound in patients with tricuspid regurgitation. Circulation 70:657, 1984.
5. Yoganathan, A. P., Jones, M., Sahn, D. J., et al.: Bernoulli gradient calculations for mechanical prosthetic aortic valves: In vitro Doppler studies. (Abstract.) Circulation 74 (Suppl. II):II-391, 1986.

Z

1. Zoghbi, W. A., Farmer, K. L., Soto, J. G., et al.: Accurate noninvasive quantification of stenotic valve area by Doppler echocardiography. Circulation 73:452, 1986.
2. Zanolla, L., Marino, P., Nicolosi, G. L., et al.: Two-dimensional echocardiographic evaluation of mitral valve calcification: Sensitivity and specificity. Chest 82:154, 1982.
3. Zile, M. R., Gaasch, W. H., Carroll, J. D., and Levine, H. J.: Chronic mitral regurgitation: Predictive value of preoperative echocardiographic indexes of left ventricular function and wall stress. J. Am. Coll. Cardiol. 3:235, 1984.
4. Zile, M. R., Gaasch, W. H., and Levine, H. J.: Left ventricular stress-dimension-shortening relations before and after correction of chronic aortic and mitral regurgitation. Am. J. Cardiol. 56:99, 1985.
5. Zuberbuhler, J. R., Allwork, S. P., and Anderson, R. H.: The spectrum of Ebstein's anomaly of the tricuspid valve. J. Thorac. Cardiovasc. Surg. 77:202, 1979.

Chapter 22

Echocardiography in Cardiomyopathies

■ *PRAVIN M. SHAH, M.D.* ■ *RAMESH C. BANSAL, M.D.*

Definitions and Classification 449
ECHOCARDIOGRAPHY IN HYPERTROPHIC CARDIOMYOPATHY 449
Role in Diagnosis 449
Summary 453
ECHOCARDIOGRAPHY IN DILATED CARDIOMYOPATHY 453
Role in Diagnosis 453
Role in Differential Diagnosis 456
Role in Prognosis 456
Summary and Conclusions 456
ECHOCARDIOGRAPHY IN RESTRICTIVE CARDIOMYOPATHY 457
Role in Diagnosis 457
ECHOCARDIOGRAPHY IN OBLITERATIVE CARDIOMYOPATHY 458
SUMMARY 459

Definitions and Classification

Echocardiography combined with Doppler techniques provide important information on the disorders classified under the title of cardiomyopathies. A report of the WHO/ISFC Task Force defines cardiomyopathy as a disorder of the heart muscle of unknown etiology.[R1] A commonly used classification is based on pathophysiologic differences and common clinical presentations. This classification, popularized by Goodwin,[G1] attempts to categorize cases of cardiomyopathy under one of four types: hypertrophic, dilated, restrictive-infiltrative, or obliterative.

Although this classification serves a useful purpose, considerable overlap exists between types. The following descriptions of typical features are based on commonly encountered differences:

- *Hypertrophic cardiomyopathy* is characterized by hypertrophy of unknown cause, not accompanied by cavitary dilation, and generally associated with hyperdynamic or normal systolic function and some evidence of diastolic filling abnormalities indicative of reduced compliance.[B1, C1] Hypertrophy involves both ventricles, although the left ventricle is commonly predominantly affected. The hypertrophy may be concentric, with uniform distribution, or asymmetric. The hyperdynamic left ventricle may be associated with the development of intraventricular gradients[B1, C1, M1] and of cavity obliteration.[C2] Predominant involvement of the right ventricle may be associated with features of infundibular pulmonary stenosis.
- *Dilated cardiomyopathy* is characterized by cavitary dilation without increase in wall thickness. Both ventricles are commonly affected, although the left ventricle may be more severely diseased. The systolic pump function is depressed, and in advanced cases, all four cardiac chambers are dilated, with atrioventricular valvular insufficiency. The abnormalities in diastolic function are secondary to systolic dysfunction and resulting elevations in end systolic and end diastolic volumes and pressures. The increase in muscle mass is characterized pathologically as eccentric hypertrophy resulting from cavitary dilation with little or no increase in wall thickness.
- *Restrictive-infiltrative cardiomyopathy* is characterized by increased wall thickness, commonly as a result of infiltration, reduced ventricular cavity sizes, and dilation of atria. The systolic function, although preserved in the early course of the disease, is subsequently reduced. There is a marked and early diastolic impairment of function. Insufficiency of the atrioventricular valves is common.
- *Obliterative cardiomyopathy* is characterized by reduction in ventricular cavity size secondary to endocardial fibrosis and thrombus formation. A stereotypical disorder is termed *endomyocardial fibrosis*, which may involve either one or both ventricles and is commonly associated with atrioventricular valve insufficiency.

It is important to re-emphasize that although typical aspects of each category of cardiomyopathy are sufficiently different, an overlap of some features is frequently observed. For instance, an early case of infiltrative-restrictive cardiomyopathy may mimic hypertrophic cardiomyopathy, including the presence of intraventricular gradients. Similarly, rare instances of advanced hypertrophic cardiomyopathies with depressed ventricular function and cavity dilation simulating dilated cardiomyopathy have been described. Some infiltrative processes may have combined features of dilated and restrictive forms.

Echocardiography is ideally suited to define with considerable accuracy the anatomic pathology as well as functional abnormalities. Cross-sectional imaging with real-time two-dimensional echocardiography permits assessment of cavity size, wall thickness, and corresponding volume and mass, as well as determination of ejection fraction. The use of Doppler methods allows assessment of stroke volume, the presence and severity of regurgitation, and intraventricular pressure gradients, as well as characterization of diastolic inflow abnormalities associated with diastolic dysfunction. Echocardiography is also useful to determine the presence and severity of associated valvular or congenital heart disease.

ECHOCARDIOGRAPHY IN HYPERTROPHIC CARDIOMYOPATHY

Role in Diagnosis

HYPERTROPHY. A most constant feature is the presence of hypertrophy, which may be concentric, i.e., uniform in distribution, or asymmetric with varied distribution. The asymmetric type may involve different distributions. Commonly, the interventricular septum is markedly thickened. This may involve the upper, mid, or apical third of the septum, singly or in combinations. Less commonly, the free wall may be predominantly involved, especially the anterior and the lateral walls and much less commonly the inferior wall. Predominantly apical asymmetric hypertrophy has also been described, which in whites is associated with some involvement of the basal aspect of the left ventricle, while in Japanese people, the basal portion of the ventricle is spared and structurally normal (Fig. 22–1).[S1] The two types appear to have differing prognoses; the Japanese variety is associated with an exceptionally benign long-term prognosis. In most cases of hypertrophic cardiomyopathy, the posterobasal wall adjacent to the posterior aspect of the mitral annulus remains thin. The exact reason for this is unknown. Although the presence of hypertrophy is evident from multiple cross-sections by echocardiography, the estimation of muscle mass can be made only with accuracy in patients with concentric hypertrophy. The current approaches to derivations of muscle mass are not suitable in the presence of asymmetric hypertrophy.

The wall thickness may be measured with calipers from the video monitor; however, M-mode echo permits a more accurate measurement. In either event, it is important to avoid cross-sections from oblique planes, since these may overestimate the measurements. The typical asymmetric septal hypertrophy (ASH) is defined as a septal thickness 1.5 or more times the free wall from M-mode echo. This measurement is generally unnecessary, since more accurate information can be gleaned from multiple cross-sections by two-dimensional echocardiography.

CAVITARY SIZE. The left ventricular cavity dimension may be assessed from appropriate M-mode echo derived from the 2-D by placing a cursor through the center of the cavity at the level of the chordae tendineae, utilizing parasternal short or long axis cross-sections. Direct measurements from the video monitor can also be made from the appropriate cross-sections with use of calipers. A quantitative assessment of volume can be made from appropriate apical views using the modified Simpson's rule. The left ventricular dimension and volumes are nearly always normal or small. The left atrial size may be increased or normal. The right ventricle and atrium are similarly normal in size.

Even when the left ventricular end diastolic cavitary dimensions are normal, the end systolic dimensions are markedly reduced, with near obliteration of the midventricular cavity owing to hyperdynamic systolic function.

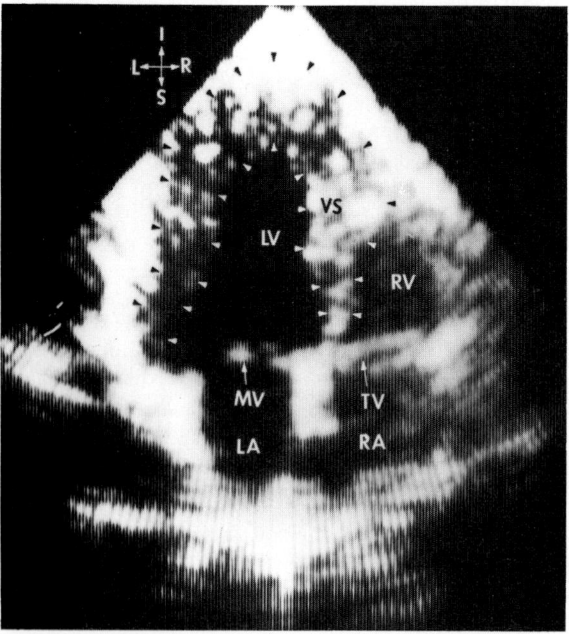

Figure 22–1. Apical four-chamber view in a patient with apical asymmetric hypertrophy designated by *arrowheads* surrounding the left ventricular (LV) walls. The walls are greatly hypertrophied nearer the apex compared with the base. RV—right ventricle, MV—mitral valve, TV—tricuspid valve, LA—left atrium, RA—right atrium, VS—ventricular septum.

LEFT VENTRICULAR SYSTOLIC FUNCTION (EJECTION FRACTION). The left ventricular ejection fraction can be assessed readily by visual analysis or quantified by the modified Simpson's approach, using two nearly orthogonal apical views. The ejection fraction is nearly always increased and may reach values up to 90 per cent, with resultant cavity obliteration. The pattern of ejection is such that a large fraction of stroke volume is generally discharged within the first half of the ejection period.

LEFT VENTRICULAR DIASTOLIC FUNCTION. Although left ventricular diastolic function has been evaluated from digitized M-mode echo analysis, its accuracy in an asymmetric ventricle with a heterogeneous relaxation pattern remains in question. The overall diastolic properties may be reflected from the mitral inflow pattern. Typically, the inflow pattern shows a reduced early diastolic filling with a decrease in E amplitude and slowed deceleration rate. The A wave is augmented, and the ratio of E/A is abnormally reduced.[M2] This pattern is observed characteristically in the presence of severe hypertrophy unaccompanied by significant elevations in the mean left atrial pressure, mitral regurgitation, or loss of atrial contractile function. When significant mitral regurgitation is present, or the left atrial pressure is elevated, the E wave is augmented and the E/A ratio may normalize. If the atrial contractile function is reduced—generally observed late in the course—the A wave may become markedly reduced in size. Thus, no diastolic mitral inflow pattern can be considered truly characteristic. Several hemodynamic factors influence it and should be considered.

INTRAVENTRICULAR PRESSURE GRADIENTS. Left ventricular intracavitary pressure gradients may be observed at one of three different sites. The commonest is a left ventricular outflow obstruction occurring a few centimeters below the aortic valve. A second site of obstruction is at the midventricular level. A third form of pressure gradient is associated with cavity obliteration. Combined pulsed and continuous wave Doppler with duplex scanning can be used to locate the site and timing of obstruction. The two-dimensional echocardiographic features also provide substantial clues about the site of obstruction.

Left Ventricular Outflow Obstruction or Muscular Subaortic Stenosis

Echo Assessment. The characteristic outflow obstruction develops as a result of systolic anterior motion (SAM), commonly involving the anterior mitral leaflet and rarely the posterior mitral leaflet (Fig. 22–2). The apposition of mitral leaflet against the septum results in a pressure drop across the outflow tract. The severity of obstruction is related to the duration and extent of mitral leaflet/septal contact.

The initial description of SAM was made using M-mode echocardiogram.[S2] Currently, this is best evaluated by two-dimensional echocardiography; a cursor-derived M-mode may be used to confirm the presence of SAM in doubtful cases.[S3] Although parasternal views may indicate the presence of SAM, the apical views are best suited to study the presence and timing of SAM when anteriorly directed to include the aortic root. The distal portion of the elongated anterior leaflet remains in the left ventricle during early systolic valve closure. Shortly after the onset of ejection, this distal portion angulates anteromedially toward the interventricular septum. At the end of ejection, the leaflet returns to its original position just prior to the mitral valve opening in early diastole. In some instances, an elongated posterior leaflet participates in or forms a sole basis of SAM. It must be emphasized that an association between SAM and left ventricular outflow obstruction exists when a portion of the mitral leaflet is involved in the formation of SAM. The so-called chordal SAM, which refers to anterior displacement of redundant chordae in a rapidly emptying ventricle, does not correlate well with the presence of an intraventricular pressure gradient.

Doppler Assessment. A site of localized obstruction is associated with increased velocity of flow, which indicates a pressure drop across the stenosis. An increase in velocity of systolic outflow can be examined by Doppler techniques. The pulsed Doppler allows accurate localization of increased velocity by moving a sample volume gradually from the apex of the left ventricle to the aortic root, utilizing the anteriorly directed apical imaging planes inclu-

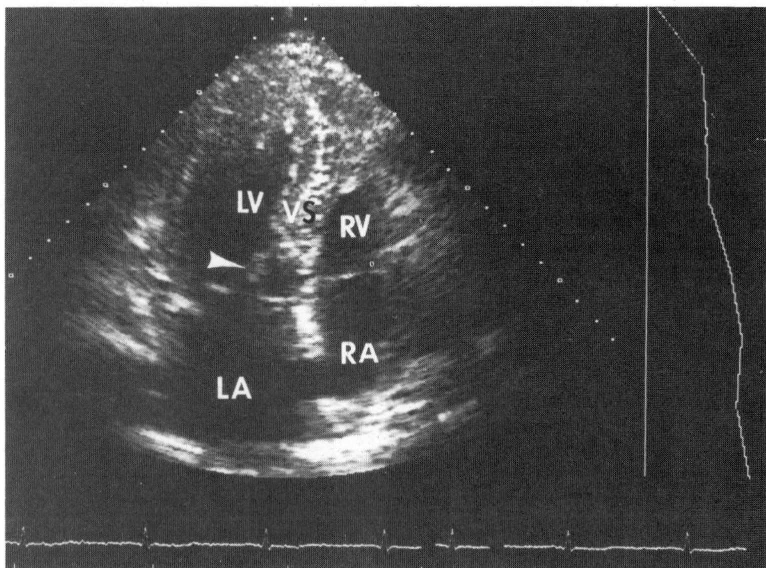

Figure 22–2. Apical four-chamber cross-section showing systolic anterior motion (SAM) of the mitral valve *(arrowhead)*. SAM comes in contact with the interventricular septum (VS) in this freeze frame at midsystole. LV—left ventricle, RV—right ventricle, LA—left atrium, RA—right atrium.

sive of the aortic root. A sudden increase in velocity and evidence of disturbed flow can be established at the site of SAM-septal contact. This also may be well appreciated by color flow imaging, which in real time shows an augmentation of outflow velocity as seen by color reversal, followed by disturbed or turbulent flow as seen by a mosaic pattern of flow (Fig. 22–3). The latter

Figure 22–3. See Color Plate 3.

immediately follows the SAM-septal contact. This characteristic appearance in real-time color flow imaging leaves little room for doubt as to the localization of obstruction and gradient development in the left ventricular outflow tract. The continuous wave Doppler provides an accurate assessment of peak outflow velocity, which reflects the magnitude of pressure drop. The continuous wave Doppler profile of left ventricular outflow obstruction is highly characteristic (Fig. 22–4). The initial outflow velocity is mildly increased to between 1.5 and 2.0 m/sec, which then increases to a peak in midsystole. This is sustained until the end of ejection, when the flow rapidly decelerates. The earlier in the systolic ejection period the peak of outflow velocity is achieved, the earlier is the development of outflow pressure gradient. It appears that both the magnitude and duration of the pressure gradient are likely to have important pathophysiologic significance in hypertrophic obstructive cardiomyopathy (Fig. 22–5). The magnitude of the pressure gradient can be determined by using a simplified Bernoulli equation, in which pressure drop $= 4 \times$ velocity^2. The Doppler-derived pressure gradients correlate well with those measured directly.

Midventricular Obstruction

Echo Assessment. A diagnosis of midventricular obstruction may be considered when an apical cavity is separated from the

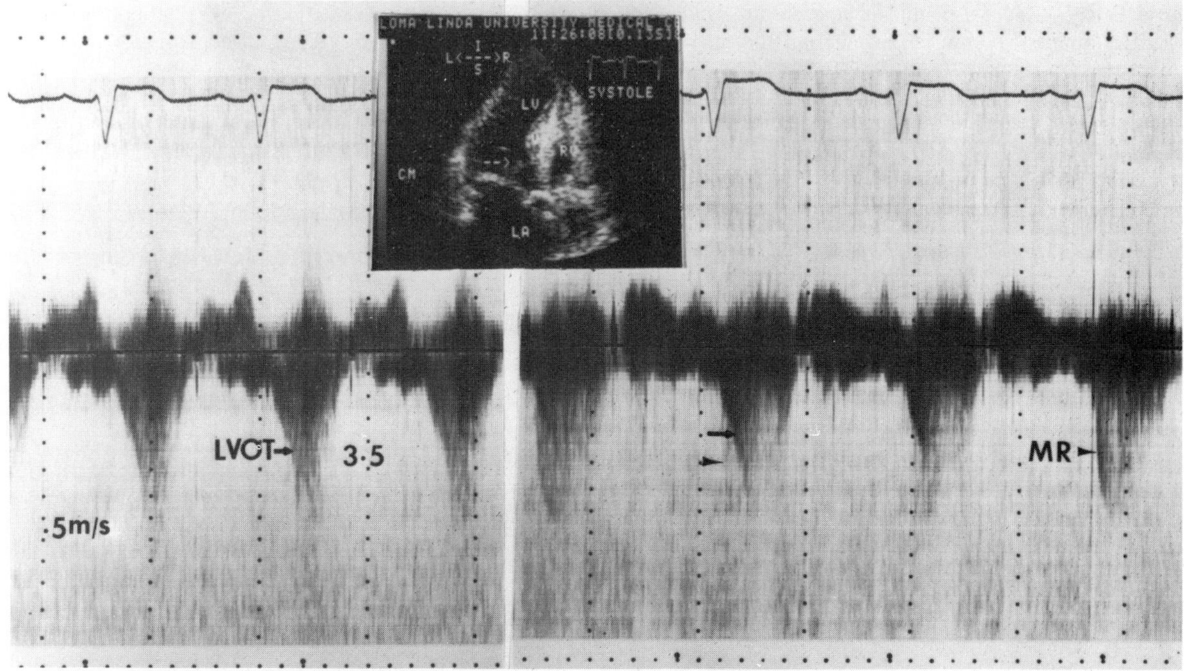

Figure 22–4. A composite showing an apical long-axis cross-section *(upper center)* and continuous-wave Doppler recordings of left ventricular outflow tract (LVOT) in the *lower left panel* and mitral regurgitation (MR) flow in the *lower right panel*. The typical mid to late systolic peaking jet is seen in LVOT at a peak velocity of 3.5 m/sec, which, using a simplified Bernoulli equation, corresponds to a pressure gradient of 50 mmHg. The MR jet shown by *arrowheads* starts in early systole but contains the LVOT jet shown by the arrow in the *lower right panel*. The SAM is shown by the *arrow* in the two-dimensional echocardiographic cross-section. The calibration marks are 0.5 m/sec apart.

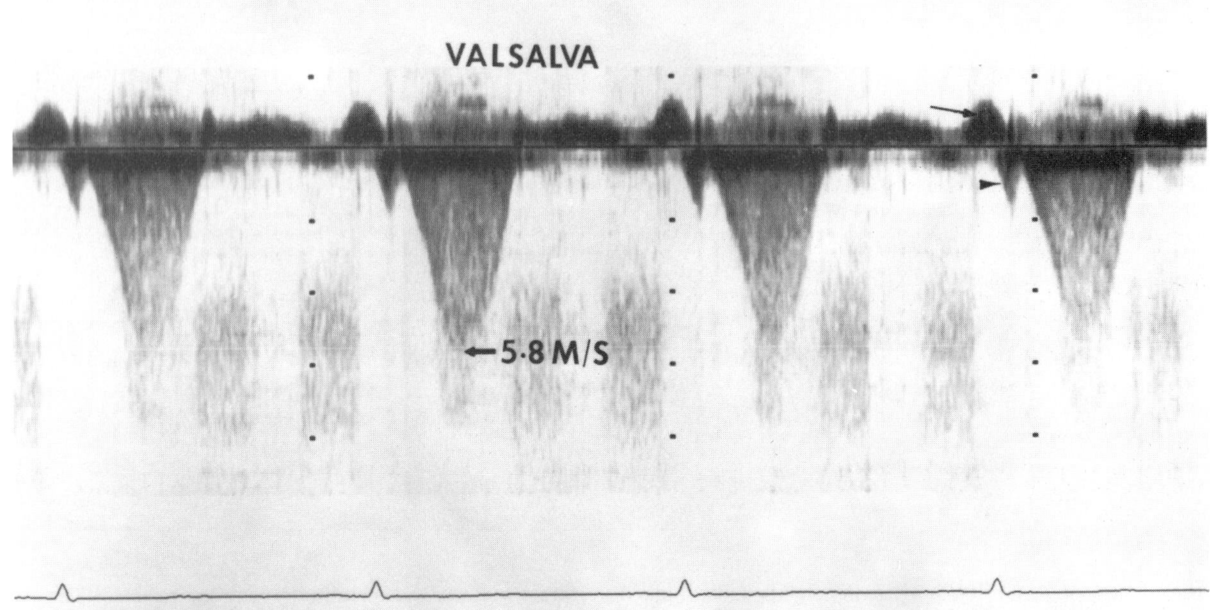

Figure 22–5. The LVOT jet velocity increased from a resting value of 3.5 to a peak of 5.8 m/sec during a Valsalva maneuver, suggesting a peak gradient of 134 mmHg. The calibration marks denote 2 m/sec.

basal (inflow-outflow) portion of the left ventricle by apposition of midventricular walls (generally at the level of papillary muscles) during ventricular ejection. The pressure in the apical cavity is higher. The apical walls are often thinner than the rest of the ventricle (Fig. 22–6). The echocardiographic assessment requires demonstration of midsystolic cavity obliteration at the papillary muscle level (visualized in parasternal short-axis or apical cross-sections) and the presence of an apical cavity (best demonstrated in carefully obtained apical views with recognition of endocardial outline) (Fig. 22–7).

Doppler Assessment. As with the outflow tract obstruction, the midventricular obstruction is associated with an increase in velocity at the site of obstruction (see Fig. 22–5). Thus, mapping with pulsed Doppler reveals a sudden increase in systolic flow velocity as the sample volume is moved from the apex slowly toward the base at the level of the papillary muscles. The color flow imaging in real time shows an increase in velocity (color reversal) and disturbed flow (mosaic appearance) just downstream to the site of obstruction at the papillary muscle level. The continuous wave Doppler permits assessment of an increased velocity, generally occurring in mid or late systole. The peak velocity reflects a pressure drop across the obstruction, and its magnitude can be derived by using the simplified Bernoulli equation. It appears that the hemodynamic significance of this obstruction is related to the timing as well as the magnitude of the pressure drop.

Cavity Obliteration

Echo Assessment. The hyperdynamic left ventricle with rapid emptying results in cavity obliteration, which may be associated with intraventricular pressure gradients. Multiple cross-sectional imaging planes permit visualization of cavity obliteration associated with an ejection fraction in excess of 90 percent.

Doppler Assessment. The pulsed Doppler recording of intraventricular systolic flow patterns shows a higher than normal peak velocity (between 1 and 2 m/sec) progressively increasing toward the aortic root, but without a sudden transition. The color

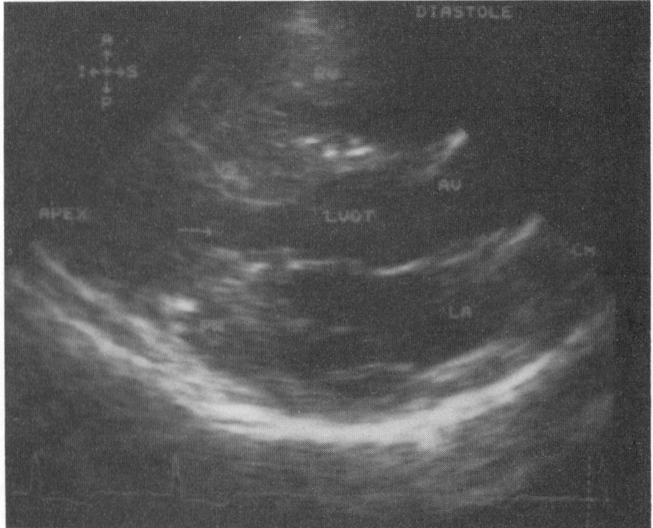

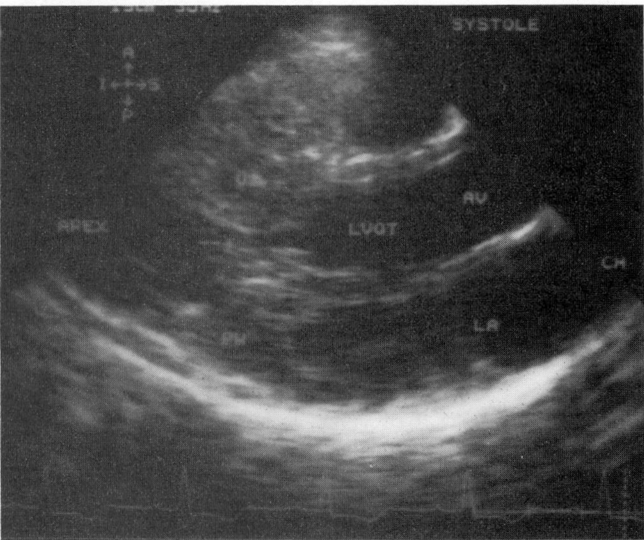

Figure 22–6. Parasternal long-axis cross-sections show freeze frames at end diastole *(left)* and midsystole *(right)*. Note the midsystolic obstruction at the papillary muscle level *(arrow)*. The apical cavity is separated from the left ventricular outflow tract (LVOT).

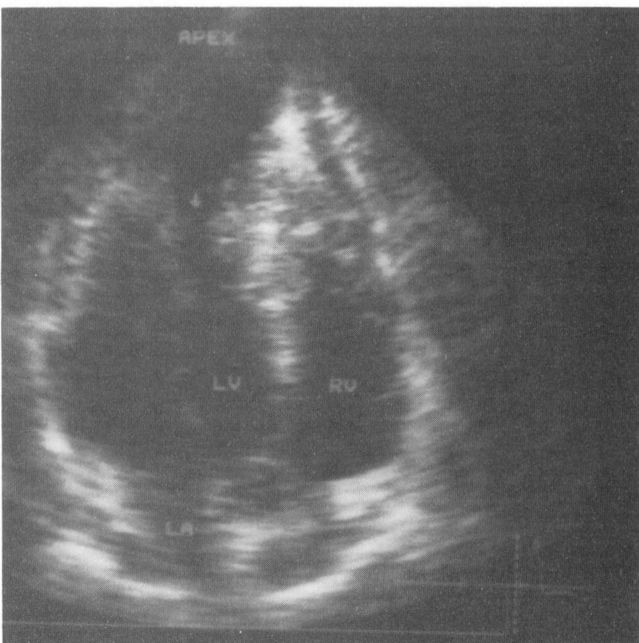

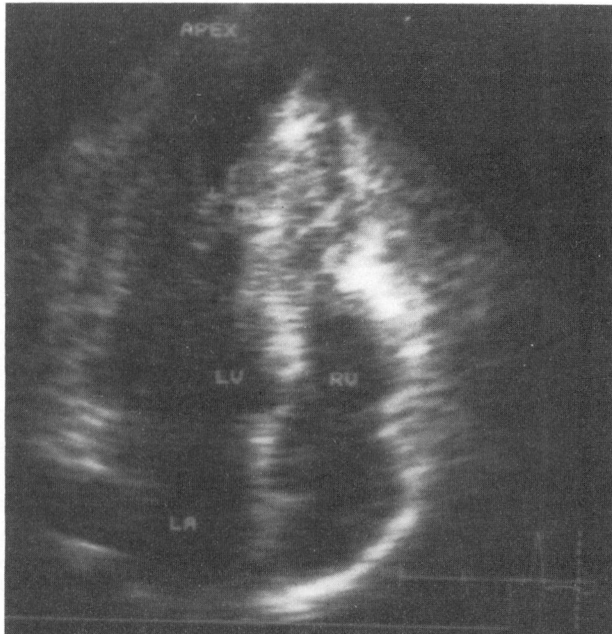

Figure 22–7. Apical four-chamber cross-sections showing midventricular obstruction in the freeze frames at end diastole *(left panel)* and midsystole *(right panel)*. The apex is composed of a thin-walled akinetic cavity separated from the LV by midventricular obstruction *(arrow)*, as seen in the right panel.

flow imaging shows color reversal within the left ventricular cavity without evidence of localized turbulence. The continuous wave Doppler often shows a characteristic sharp peak in late systole during the last few milliseconds of ejection. The systolic intraventricular pressure gradients develop in late systole, corresponding with a short-lived late increase in velocity. This transient late systolic pressure gradient results from cavity obliteration rather than obstruction to flow.

Mixed Patterns of Gradients

Any combination of the aforementioned patterns of intraventricular pressure gradient may coexist in some patients. Thus, midventricular and outflow tract obstruction may be present in the same patient. Similarly, a patient with outflow obstruction may also show features of cavity obliteration. The echocardiographic and Doppler assessment, therefore, should be carried out to consider a possibility of more than one type of intraventricular gradients.

Mitral Regurgitation. A nearly constant accompaniment of left ventricular outflow obstruction is the presence of mitral regurgitation, which is mild or moderate in severity. The underlying mechanism appears to be related to distortion of the mitral valve apparatus resulting from systolic anterior motion of the valve leaflet. The pulsed Doppler technique confirms the presence and timing of mitral regurgitation. The continuous wave Doppler recording of regurgitant flow provides a peak velocity from which left ventricular systolic pressure may be estimated, using the simplified Bernoulli equation. The regurgitation signal is pansystolic; however, the mid and late systolic portion of the jet signal is more intense, indicating a larger volume of regurgitant flow. The presence, timing, and severity of regurgitation generally are related to the presence, timing, and extent of systolic anterior motion. In some patients with hypertrophic cardiomyopathy, the mitral regurgitation is independent of outflow obstruction, and alternate mechanisms are involved. Occasionally, nonobstructive cases may also have an insufficient mitral valve. The pulsed and color Doppler approaches assess severity.

Associated and Complicating Features. Hypertrophic cardiomyopathy may be associated with coexistent valvular heart disease or complicated by infective endocarditis. Echocardiography plays an important role in diagnosis of these conditions, which may not be apparent on clinical evaluation of patients.

Summary

Echocardiography, combined with conventional and color Doppler methods, permits accurate, noninvasive diagnosis of disease, including its hemodynamic profile and consequences. In the majority of cases, it is not necessary to undertake additional tests, invasive or noninvasive, for diagnostic assessment. In patients undergoing surgical treatment or with refractory anginal syndromes, selective coronary arteriography may be needed for comprehensive evaluation.

ECHOCARDIOGRAPHY IN DILATED CARDIOMYOPATHY

Role in Diagnosis

M-mode and cross-sectional echocardiography are well suited to detect the presence and severity of dilation of all four chambers of the heart and to provide quantitative assessment of left ventricular function.[84] Doppler ultrasound techniques provide additional information on the competence of the atrioventricular valves and some insights into systolic and diastolic function of the left ventricle (Fig. 22–8).

VENTRICULAR SIZE. Although dilation of both ventricles is a common feature, occasionally predominant or isolated enlargement of one ventricle may be observed. The left ventricular dilation often dominates. The left ventricular internal dimension at end diastole may in severe cases exceed 8 cm (normal, $\leq$ 5.6 cm). Two-dimensional echocardiography is used to assess end diastolic volume with the modified Simpson's rule. The appropriate diastolic frames in the apical four- and two-chamber views are used to trace endocardiac outlines, and the long axis of the left ventricle is obtained by a line that joins the mitral anulus to the left ventricular apex. The end diastolic volumes are computed readily with the modified Simpson's rule approach. The left ventricular end diastolic volumes may exceed 200 ml in patients with advanced stages of cardiomyopathy. The ventricular volumes may also be estimated from M-mode measurement of end diastolic dimension at the chordal level. Two common approaches use either the cube method (with an assumed ellipsoid geometry) or

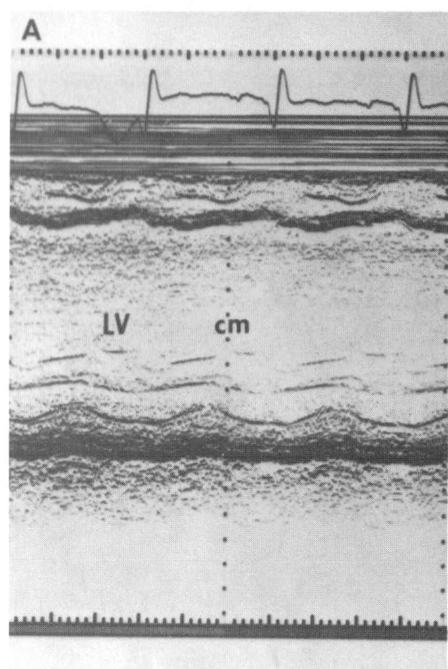

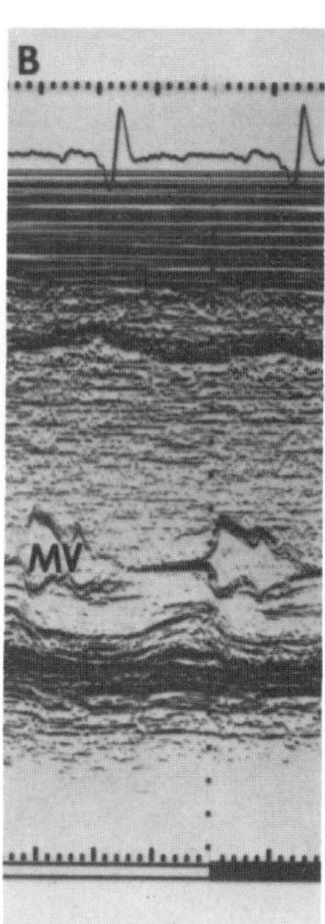

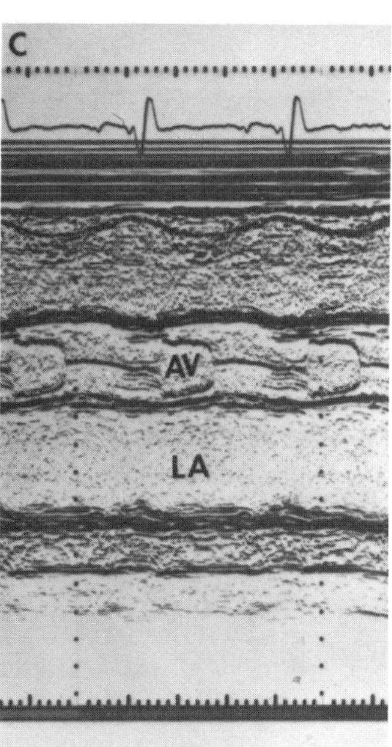

Figure 22–8. A composite of typical M-mode echocardiograms of the left ventricle (LV) in *A*, the mitral valve (MV) in *B*, and the aortic valve (AV) and left atrium (LA) in *C* in a patient with dilated cardiomyopathy. Note the markedly dilated left ventricle with thin walls and reduced systolic function, the incomplete mitral valve opening with increased E point to septal separation, and the short-lived and incompletely open aortic valve with dilation of LA.

the Teichholz method. The latter tends to be more accurate for dilated ventricles that are more spherical in shape.

In a subgroup of patients (between 5 and 10 percent), the left ventricular dilation may be minimal or absent.[T1, K1] These patients are best designated as having minimally dilated congestive cardiomyopathy.

The right ventricular dilation is more difficult to quantify because of its unusual geometry. M-mode measurement of the right ventricular dimension is a less reliable indicator of ventricular dilation, except for advanced cases. Measurements of cross-sectional areas in apical four-chamber views are also less dependable. A qualitative assessment of right ventricular dilation is often made by comparison with the left ventricle.

ATRIAL SIZE. The left atrial size can be readily determined from M-mode measurement behind the aortic root at the level of the aortic valve. Although generally reliable, it may be subject to errors depending on the direction of the ultrasound beam. Thus an obliquely directed beam with a lower transducer position may overestimate this dimension, and a medially directed beam may foreshorten the left atrial size along the interatrial septum. The left atrial volume may be determined with apical four- and two-chamber views. This is generally unnecessary in routine clinical use. Left atrial enlargement is commonly present in symptomatic patients with advanced stages of the disease and is absent in early and less severe cases.

The right atrial size is even more difficult to quantify. It is generally evaluated with apical and subcostal four-chamber views. The right parasternal approach to image the interatrial septum has also been used for this assessment.

LEFT VENTRICULAR FUNCTION. Left ventricular ejection fraction is readily determined by measuring end diastolic and end systolic volumes. Although global hypokinesia as a feature of dilated or congestive cardiomyopathy has been used to differentiate it from left ventricular dysfunction caused by ischemic heart disease, this is by no means a constant sign. Echocardiographically derived ejection fraction correlates well with contrast angiography or radionuclide angiography. The methods that use two-dimensional echocardiography provide accurate results even when segmental or focal asynergy exists. Alternatively, M-mode echocardiography may be used to estimate end diastolic and end systolic volumes. The ejection fraction as estimated assumes absence of asynergy. The current techniques of two-dimensional echocardiography make it possible to obtain volumes and ejection fractions in well over 80 percent of adult patients and nearly all patients in the pediatric age group (Fig. 22–9).

Figure 22–9. See Color Plate 3.

A simple parameter of left ventricular ejection consists of mitral E-point–septal separation (EPSS). In the presence of a normal ejection fraction (>55 percent), this distance does not exceed 6 mm. The increase in EPSS correlates with a decreasing ejection fraction. This end point cannot be used in the presence of mitral stenosis or aortic regurgitation, in which the anterior mitral leaflet may be mechanically prevented from full opening; however, it works equally well for asynergic and uniformly contracting ventricles. An EPSS of 1 cm or greater is distinctly abnormal and is uniformly associated with a depressed ejection fraction. When the EPSS exceeds 2 cm, it generally signifies an ejection fraction of less than 30 percent. Another M-mode echocardiographic clue of left ventricular dysfunction consists of a prominent B notch on the mitral valve, which is indicative of increased end diastolic pressure. This sign in the presence of a normal PR interval carries a high specificity for elevated left ventricular end diastolic pressure.

INTRACAVITARY THROMBUS. Formation of intracavitary thrombus is a common complication in patients with congestive or dilated cardiomyopathy. It is generally seen in the left ventricular apex, although it may occasionally be noted in the right ventricular apex (Fig. 22–10). Stasis resulting from reduced flow velocity appears to be a condition for formation of thrombus. Two-dimensional echocardiography is demonstrated to be highly diagnostic in the detection of intracavitary left ventricular thrombus, with sensitivity and specificity in excess of 90 percent. The size and shape of left ventricular thrombi may be varied; they may appear as layered and organized thrombus or be spherical or irregularly shaped and pedunculated. The overlying left ventricular wall is severely hypokinetic or akinetic. Special care in technique is required to prevent errors in diagnosis. The apical views are generally most useful in diagnosis. Care should be taken to differentiate rib cage reverberations from apical thrombus.

Thrombus may also be present in the left atrial appendage in patients in atrial fibrillation. This is generally not detectable by two-dimensional echocardiography unless the thrombus extends into the wall of the left atrium. Transesophageal echocardiography appears to be well suited for detection of left atrial thrombus.

MITRAL AND TRICUSPID VALVE FUNCTION. Ventric-

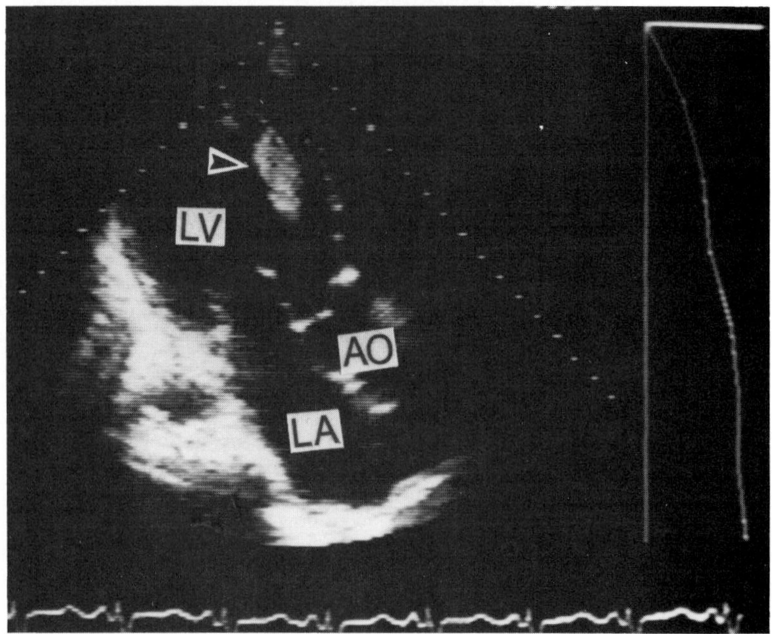

Figure 22–10. Apical thrombus *(arrowhead)* is seen in the left ventricle (LV) of a patient with minimally dilated cardiomyopathy with depressed systolic function in this apical long-axis cross-section. LA—left atrium, AO—aorta.

ular dilation, a most common occurrence in congestive cardiomyopathy, is frequently associated with incompetence of the atrioventricular valves. Thus mitral and/or tricuspid regurgitation is commonly present in the patients. Although valvular regurgitation is generally mild or moderate, it may be severe in some patients.

Mitral Regurgitation. The precise mechanism of mitral regurgitation in congestive cardiomyopathy has been controversial and a subject of several studies.[B2, B3] Two-dimensional echocardiography is suitable for quantitative evaluation of various components of the mitral valve apparatus. Doppler methods are well suited to detect and quantify the severity of mitral regurgitation.

The mitral anulus may be dilated in congestive cardiomyopathy, and its dilation appears to be related to the presence of mitral regurgitation. Although annular dilation accompanies left ventricular dilation, there does not appear to be a direct and proportional relationship between the two. Because the presence of mitral regurgitation was a more important correlate of annular dilation than left ventricular size, the two may be causally related. The annular size may be readily assessed with two-dimensional echocardiography. The apical views are generally more suitable. The normal systolic reduction in mitral annular size is reduced in congestive cardiomyopathy and shows a rough correlation with the degree of depression in ejection fraction.

The mitral leaflet opening excursion, especially of the anterior leaflet, is reduced. This reduction in diastolic opening of the mitral valve can be correlated with reduced stroke volume. The apical views reveal abnormality in leaflet coaptation, so that the point of the tip coaptation is transposed deeper into the left ventricle. In severe cases, a failure of the tips to coapt may be observed. This tented or inverted V appearance of the closed mitral valve in the apical views is a result of ventricular dilation and displacement of the papillary muscles. The resulting distortion of geometry of the papillary-chordal-valve apparatus combined with annular dilation best explains the occurrence of mitral regurgitation, which develops when a critical surface area of the valve tissue, required to produce an effective seal, is no longer available.

The advent of Doppler techniques provides objective evidence of the presence and severity of mitral regurgitation. The pulsed Doppler method allows the placement of sample volume on the left atrial side of the closed mitral valve to scan parts of the left atrium for systolic regurgitant jet. Use of multiple apical cross-sections permits mapping of the jet in the left atrium to reconstruct its direction, size, and shape. Pulsed Doppler mapping of the left atrium may also be carried out in the parasternal views. Color flow imaging with the multigated pulsed Doppler system allows ready visualization of the jet size. Both these methods have proved useful in the semiquantitative assessment of the severity of regurgitation. The continuous wave Doppler technique registers a regurgitant velocity profile that is generally pansystolic. The peak velocity in excess of 4 m/sec is attained in early systole, which reflects the left ventricular to left atrial pressure gradient, and its shape in systole follows the systolic pressure gradient profile. Because the left ventricular pressure is substantially higher than the left atrial pressure throughout ventricular systole, the velocity profile reaches a plateau in early systole, and this is retained until the end of ventricular ejection and early relaxation. The velocity profile reflects the pressure gradient profile between the left ventricle and left atrium throughout systole. When the left atrial V wave is markedly elevated, as in acute or acutely worsening mitral regurgitation, the velocity profile reaches a peak in early systole and decelerates in late systole, reflecting an altered pressure gradient profile. The early acceleration of the regurgitant velocity profile has been used to assess left ventricular rate of pressure rise, which in the presence of dilated cardiomyopathy is invariably reduced (i.e., <1200 mmHg/sec).

Tricuspid Regurgitation. Although tricuspid regurgitation is commonly associated with right ventricular dilation, its pathogenetic mechanisms have been less rigorously studied. It has been demonstrated that tricuspid annular size, measured by two-dimensional echocardiographic analysis of multiple tricuspid inflow views, is significantly enlarged in patients with functional tricuspid regurgitation. This could serve as a major mechanism of tricuspid regurgitation in congestive cardiomyopathy.

The Doppler methods are useful in the detection and quantification of regurgitation and estimation of right ventricular systolic pressure. The pulsed Doppler technique reveals a systolic jet directed toward the right atrium, with sample volume placed behind the tricuspid valve. As with mitral regurgitation, the severity of tricuspid regurgitation may be evaluated from the size and area of the regurgitant velocity map in the right atrium. Mapping of the inferior vena cava and hepatic vein is useful to confirm more severe forms of tricuspid regurgitation, which shows a systolic flow disturbance moving away from the right atrium. These findings, obtained by careful mapping with the pulsed Doppler technique, are more readily evaluated by multigated color flow imaging systems. The continuous wave Doppler method shows a complete profile that is used to estimate right ventricular systolic pressure. The peak velocity is a measure of peak right ventricular–right atrial pressure drop. The right atrial pressure may be estimated by examination of jugular venous pressure, or it may be assumed to be 10 mmHg in the absence of clinical right heart failure. The simplified Bernoulli equation states that peak pressure gradient = 4 × peak velocity^2. Thus peak RV–RA pressure = 4 × tricuspid regurgitation velocity^2. Hence, peak RV systolic pressure = 4 × tricuspid regurgitation velocity^2 + RA pressure. The right ventricular systolic pressure so determined correlates with that measured by cardiac catheterization. This approach provides important and accurate determination of the presence and severity of pulmonary hypertension in patients with congestive cardiomyopathy.

DOPPLER EVALUATION OF SYSTOLIC AND DIASTOLIC LEFT VENTRICULAR FUNCTION

Systolic Function. The flow velocity profile of the left ventricular outflow or aortic root has been used to evaluate systolic left ventricular function in congestive cardiomyopathy. The peak acceleration of the aortic flow pulse shows prolongation with decreasing pump function. The duration of flow velocity profile and its magnitude are decreased, which reflects a reduction in stroke volume.

Doppler measurements of cardiac output have been validated in a number of studies. A commonly used approach in adults consists of recording flow velocity in the ascending aorta and measuring aortic dimension by echocardiography. Because flow equals velocity integral times the area of the vessel (aorta), the stroke volume times the heart rate gives cardiac output. Some of the modifications of this method include obtaining the velocity profile across the aortic valve and planimetered aortic valve area from the M-mode recording of the open aortic valve, or obtaining flow velocity across the left ventricular outflow tract and measuring its diameter just below the aortic root from the parasternal long axis view. All these approaches have yielded reliable estimates of cardiac output. Although cardiac output measurement has limited usefulness in the diagnosis of congestive cardiomyopathy, it may serve to evaluate short-term effects of drug intervention.

Diastolic Function. The mitral diastolic inflow velocity provides one indirect measure of the rate of left ventricular filling, which reflects its diastolic function. In patients with congestive cardiomyopathy and elevated left atrial pressures, the E wave generally dominates. There is little useful diagnosic information in this measurement.

Role in Differential Diagnosis

Congestive cardiomyopathy may need to be differentiated from heart failure caused by coronary artery disease or hypertensive heart disease. Echocardiography may provide some diagnostic clues, although these are by no means specific. Segmental asynergy typically favors underlying coronary artery disease with infarction or severe ischemia. However, pronounced focal asynergy has been reported in patients with congestive cardiomyopathy and angiographically normal coronary arteries. Similarly, patients with multivessel coronary artery disease and advanced heart failure may show diffuse global asynergy. Involvement of both left and right ventricles with four-chamber dilation is a feature of congestive cardiomyopathy. However, right heart dilation may be seen as a result of prior right ventricular free wall infarction or of pulmonary hypertension in advanced cases of left ventricular failure caused by coronary artery disease. A hyperdynamic right ventricle associated with a dilated and asynergic left ventricle in a patient with heart failure strongly favors coronary artery disease as a likely cause. Hypertensive heart disease is associated with marked concentric hypertrophy with early involvement of the left ventricle. A differentiation in advanced cases is often difficult and may be purely academic. Similarly, viral myocarditis and toxic cardiomyopathies (e.g., cytotoxic agents, cobalt, alcohol, radiation damage) cannot be distinguished from echocardiographic appearances.

Role in Prognosis

It has been reported in patients with dilated cardiomyopathy that global estimates of left ventricular systolic function, that is, ejection fraction or left ventricular minor axis fractional shortening, are independent predictors of survival, although the overall size as estimated by end diastolic dimension is not.[U1] Furthermore, Benjamin and associates reported in an autopsy study that lower heart weights and thinner left ventricular free walls were associated with poorer survival.[B4] These observations imply that compensatory hypertrophy, which results in reduced diastolic wall stress, may provide a favorable compensatory adaptation in these patients.

Echocardiography has the potential to provide assessment of left ventricular function, size, and wall thickness and thus may yield independent predictors of survival among patients with congestive cardiomyopathy. This question was addressed in a recently completed Veterans Administration multicenter cooperative study (VHEFT study), which evaluated the prognostic value of echocardiography in patients with chronic congestive heart failure.[S5] All patients' conditions were stabilized with digitalis and diuretics. An M-mode echocardiogram was obtained before random assignment to one of three treatment regimens consisting of placebo, isosorbide dinitrate and hydralazine, or prazosin. The cause of heart failure was considered idiopathic or congestive cardiomyopathy in approximately 55 percent and coronary artery disease in 45 percent of patients. Various echocardiographic dimensions of left ventricular size and function were measured.

Univariate analysis of the predictive value of survival in 390 patients demonstrated the highest predictive significance ($p < 0.001$) for the ratio of left ventricular end systolic dimension over wall thickness (interventricular septum plus posterior wall). This was followed by EPSS ($p < 0.0001$) and left ventricular internal dimension at end systole ($p < 0.0001$). The other echocardiographic parameters of significant predictive value included dimension-to-wall thickness ratio at end diastole ($p < 0.0003$); fractional shortening ($p < 0.0005$); and left ventricular end-diastolic dimension ($p < 0.003$). A multivariate analysis of the prognostic significance of these echo parameters demonstrated the most powerful predictive measurement to be the left ventricular dimension-over-thickness ratio at end systole ($p < 0.0001$), followed by EPSS ($p < 0.013$). The remaining measurements did not have significant additional predictive power.

The left ventricular ejection fraction is a global estimate of systolic function, and dimension-to-thickness ratio is an estimate of myocardial wall stress. The greater the reduction in ejection fraction and the higher the wall stress, the worse the prognosis. In this study, when a left ventricular ejection fraction of 28 or more percent was associated with an internal dimension-to-thickness ratio of 4.0 or less in diastole and 2.5 or less in systole, a lower annual mortality of 9.3 percent and 9.9 percent per year, respectively, was observed. In contrast, the left ventricular internal dimension-over-thickness ratio at end diastole of over 4 with an ejection fraction of less than 28 percent was associated with an annual mortality of nearly 25 percent per year. The additive value of ejection fraction and left ventricular dimension-to-thickness ratio in projecting subsequent mortality was clearly demonstrated. The actuarial survival statistics showed a continued effect on mortality over a follow-up period in excess of 3 years from entry into the study, when these measurements were made. The echocardiographic parameters proved useful in the assessment of prognosis and may be used in prospective therapeutic trials. It remains to be seen whether improvement in these parameters can be achieved by long-term treatment and, further, whether such improvement indicates increased survival.

Summary and Conclusions

Echocardiographic methods are diagnostically useful in congestive cardiomyopathy for assessment of (1) chamber dimensions

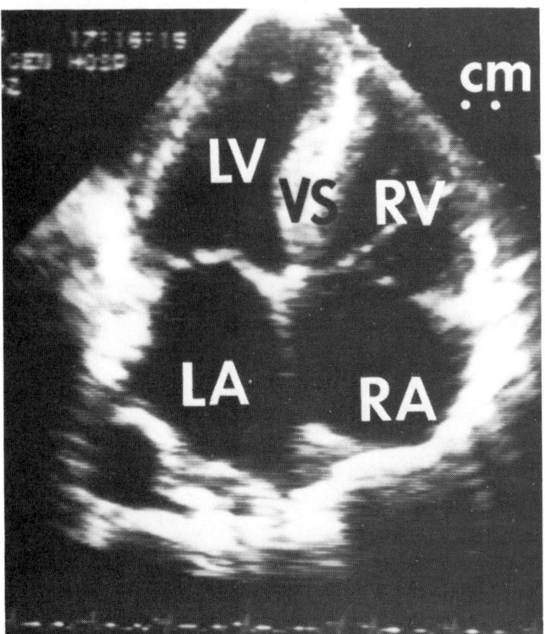

Figure 22–11. Apical four-chamber cross-section in a patient with biopsy-proved amyloid heart disease. Small ventricular and enlarged atrial cavities with increased brightness of the ventricular septum (VS) are quite typical.

and ventricular volumes; (2) global left ventricular ejection fraction and segmental wall motion abnormalities; (3) wall thickness measurements and estimation of mass; (4) the presence of intracavitary thrombus; (5) anatomic and functional abnormalities of atrioventricular valves, such as thickening, anular dilation, and leaflet coaptation; (6) Doppler estimates of cardiac output; (7) Doppler detection and quantification of mitral regurgitation; and (8) Doppler quantification of pulmonary hypertension. In addition, echocardiographic methods have been shown to provide predictors of survival. Among the more powerful prognostic indicators of survival are the ratio of left ventricular internal dimension-to-wall thickness and left ventricular ejection fraction.

Echocardiographic methods should be used routinely to provide important diagnostic and prognostic information in patients suspected of having congestive or dilated cardiomyopathy. Furthermore, these methods may be used to characterize subsets of patients with varying severity and prognosis in future randomized therapeutic trials.

ECHOCARDIOGRAPHY IN RESTRICTIVE CARDIOMYOPATHY

Role in Diagnosis

VENTRICULAR WALL THICKNESS AND CAVITY DIMENSIONS. The infiltrative disorders, such as amyloid heart disease, are typically associated with increased wall thickness. This gives a gross appearance of concentric hypertrophy, although at microscopic level no true hypertrophy is observed. The increase in wall thickness is uniform and generally involves the right ventricular free wall as well. A characteristic sparkling or ground glass appearance of the left ventricular wall is commonly seen.[S6] This appearance is highly suggestive, although not diagnostic, of the presence of an infiltrative disorder, such as amyloid heart disease (Fig. 22–11). It may also be seen in hypertrophic cardiomyopathy or secondary left ventricular hypertrophy. The left ventricular cavity dimension is typically small.

ATRIAL SIZE. Commonly, both the left and the right atria are dilated.[C3] The atrial dilation is largely due to reduced compliance with elevations in filling pressures, although atrioventricular valve incompetence may also contribute. The presence of small ventricular cavity dimensions and enlarged atria involving both left- and right-sided chambers is highly characteristic and should raise a diagnostic suspicion of restrictive cardiomyopathy (Fig. 22–12).

VENTRICULAR SYSTOLIC FUNCTION. Both left and right ventricular pump functions are depressed as a result of myocardial infiltration with amyloid deposits. The extent of functional impairment is related to the severity and chronicity of the illness. In early cases, left ventricular ejection fraction may be preserved, but this is rarely seen in clinically symptomatic cases. The depression in ejection fraction is progressive.

VENTRICULAR DIASTOLIC FUNCTION. The ventricular walls are stiff and less compliant and have a reduced rate of relaxation. This diastolic function may be assessed by digitized M-mode echo or more conveniently by Doppler examination.[A1, K2, N1, N2] Pulsed Doppler recording of mitral valve inflow shows characteristic changes and provides an insight into diastolic

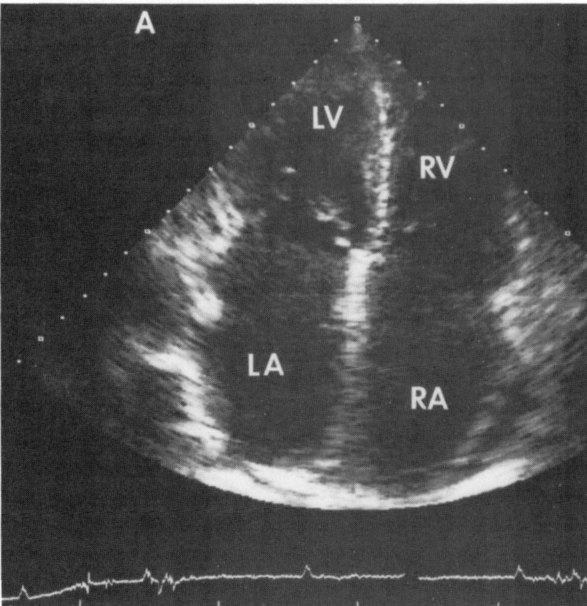

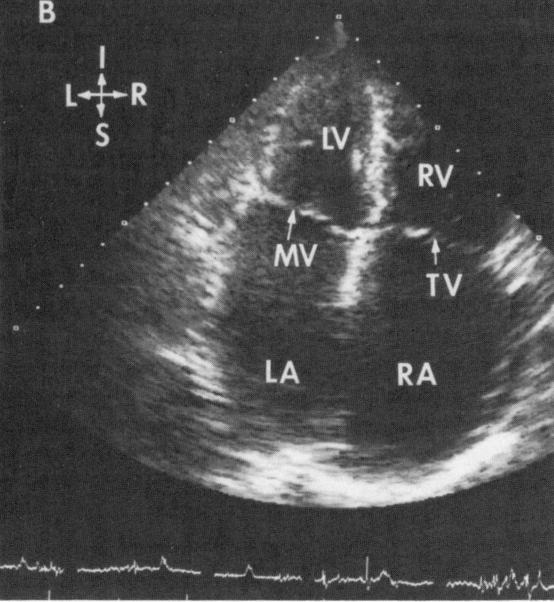

Figure 22–12. Apical four-chamber cross-sections in diastole *(A)* and in systole *(B)* in a patient with restrictive cardiomyopathy. Note the marked biatrial enlargement and the normal size of the LV.

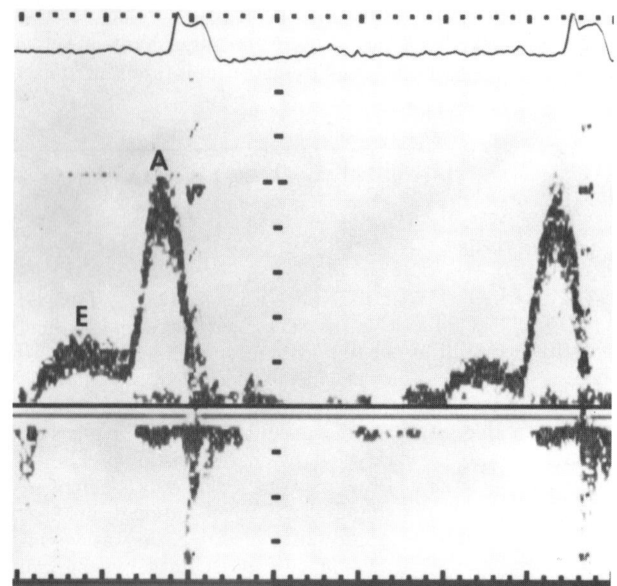

Figure 22–13. Pulsed-wave Doppler tracing of a mitral inflow signal in a patient with restriction to early filling and a markedly augmented atrial filling wave (A). This appearance may be seen in hypertrophied LV or with early restrictive cardiomyopathy. E, early filling wave.

function. In early cases with relaxation abnormality, the early diastolic E wave is reduced in amplitude and its deceleration time prolonged. The A wave velocity is augmented with strong atrial contraction (Fig. 22–13). In later stages, the left atrial mean pressure increases, resulting in progressive augmentation of the E wave. Thus, E/A ratio is reduced abnormally in the early phase of predominant diastolic abnormality. This ratio increases gradually with elevations of filling pressures to become normal and subsequently increases to values in excess of 1.5 or 2.0. At a late stage in the disease, diastolic filling demonstrates a tall sharp E wave with short deceleration time and a small A wave (Fig. 22–14). The latter may result from chronic atrial dilation or amyloid infiltration of the atrial wall.

In the presence of atrial fibrillation, the E wave is typically tall with rapid deceleration. This is generally indicative of elevations in atrial pressures but may also result from atrioventricular valve incompetence.

A-V VALVE INCOMPETENCE. Mitral and tricuspid valve incompetences of mild or moderate severity are commonly seen. The underlying mechanisms are not clear, although marked atrial dilation may result in anular dilatation and valve dysfunction. The severity of mitral and tricuspid regurgitation can be evaluated by pulsed Doppler mapping or color flow imaging.

PERICARDIAL EFFUSION. Small or moderate-sized effusions are commonly seen. When present, no additional hemodynamic impairment is noted.

ADDITIONAL CONSIDERATIONS. Besides amyloid heart disease, other infiltrative and storage disorders likely to involve the myocardium include sarcoidosis, hemochromatosis, glycogen storage disorders, Fabry's disease, and scleroderma. Hemochromatosis may result in a predominant picture of restrictive or congestive cardiomyopathy but often has mixed features of both. Similarly, sarcoidosis and scleroderma may result in a cor pulmonale type of presentation secondary to extensive pulmonary involvement, although a restrictive form of cardiomyopathy may be noted. Glycogen storage disease may simulate hypertrophic cardiomyopathy or may have predominant features of restrictive physiology.

ECHOCARDIOGRAPHY IN OBLITERATIVE CARDIOMYOPATHY

The characteristic echocardiographic features of endomyocardial fibrosis (EMF) have been described from regions of the world where this disorder is commonly seen. It is extremely rare in Western Europe and the United States.

1. Right ventricular endomyocardial fibrosis is characterized by obliteration of the apical cavity with endocardial thickening and thrombus formation. The outflow tract is generally hyperactive. The tricuspid valve leaflets are thickened and often incompetent.

2. Left ventricular endomyocardial fibrosis is also associated with endocardial thickening and intracavitary thrombus formation. The mitral valve is often involved in thickening with associated mitral regurgitation. The disease process may involve one or both ventricles and is generally progressive in nature.

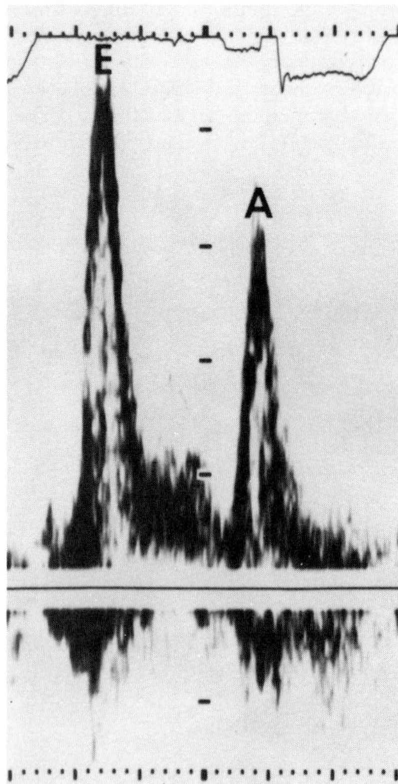

Figure 22–14. Pulsed-wave Doppler tracing of mitral inflow in a patient with a more advanced stage of restriction than in Figure 22–13, showing a peaked early filling wave (E) and rapid deceleration to baseline. This pattern is generally seen in restrictive cardiomyopathy, with marked elevations of mean left atrial pressures in later stages of the disease.

SUMMARY

Echocardiography, including current Doppler techniques, is extremely useful in diagnostic and functional evaluation of patients with different forms of cardiomyopathies. In patients with hypertrophic cardiomyopathy, the extent and severity of hypertrophy, the presence and location of intraventricular pressure gradients, the presence and severity of mitral regurgitation, and diastolic and systolic function may be evaluated. In those with dilated cardiomyopathy, the degree of chamber dilation, systolic dysfunction, and mitral and tricuspid regurgitation may be determined. In restrictive cardiomyopathies, the extent of systolic and of diastolic dysfunction can be assessed. Thus, echocardiography is ideally suited for imaging patients with the suspected diagnosis of cardiomyopathy.

References

A

1. Appleton, C.P., Hatle, L.K., and Popp, R.L.: Demonstration of restrictive ventricular physiology by Doppler echocardiography. J. Am. Coll. Cardiol. 11:757, 1988.

B

1. Braunwald, E., Lambert, C.T., Rockoff, S.D., et al.: Idiopathic hypertrophic subaortic stenosis: I. A description of the disease based on an analysis of 64 patients. Circulation 30 (Suppl. 4):3, 1964.
2. Boltwood, C.M., Tei, C., Wong, M., et al.: Quantitative echocardiography of the mitral complex in dilated cardiomyopathy: The mechanism of functional mitral regurgitation. Circulation 68:498, 1983.
3. Ballester, M., Jajoo, J., Rees, S., et al.: The mechanism of mitral regurgitation in dilated left ventricle. Clin. Cardiol. 6:333, 1983.
4. Benjamin, I.J., Schuster, E.H., and Bulkley, B.H.: Cardiac hypertrophy in idiopathic dilated congestive cardiomyopathy: A clinicopathologic study. Circulation 64:442, 1981.

C

1. Cohen, J., Effat, H., Goodwin, J.F., et al.: Hypertrophic obstructive cardiomyopathy. Br. Heart J. 26:16, 1964.
2. Criley, J.M., Lewis, K.B., White, R.I., Jr., and Ross, R.S.: Pressure gradients without obstruction: A new concept of "hypertrophic subaortic stenosis." Circulation 32:881, 1965.
3. Child, J.S., Levisman, J.A., Abbasi, A.S., and MacAlpin, R.N.: Echocardiographic manifestations of infiltrative cardiomyopathy. A report of seven cases due to amyloid. Chest 70:726, 1976.

G

1. Goodwin, J.F.: Prospects and predictions for the cardiomyopathies. Circulation 50:210, 1974.

K

1. Keren, A., Billigham, M.E., Weintraub, D., et al.: Mildly dilated congestive cardiomyopathy. Circulation 72:302, 1985.
2. Klein, A.L., Hatle, L.K., Burstow, D.J., et al.: Doppler characterization of left ventricular diastolic function in cardiac amyloidosis. J. Am. Coll. Cardiol. 13:1017, 1989.

M

1. Maron, B.J., Gottdiener, J.S., Arce, J., et al.: Dynamic subaortic obstruction in hypertrophic cardiomyopathy: Analysis by pulsed Doppler echocardiography. J. Am. Coll. Cardiol. 6:1, 1985.
2. Maron, B., Arce, J., Bonow, R., et al.: Non-invasive assessment of left ventricular relaxation and filling by pulsed echocardiography in hypertrophic cardiomyopathy (Abstract). Circulation 70:18, 1984.

N

1. Nishimura, R.A., Housmans, P.R., Hatle, L.K., and Tajik, A.J.: Assessment of diastolic function of the heart: Background and current applications of Doppler echocardiography. Part I: Physiologic and pathophysiologic features. Mayo Clin. Proc. 64:71, 1989.
2. Nishimura, R.A., Abel, M.D., Hatle, L.K., and Tajik, A.J.: Assessment of diastolic function of the heart: Background and current applications of Doppler echocardiography. Part II: Clinical studies. Mayo Clin Proc 64:181, 1989.

R

1. Report of the WHO/ISFC Task Force on the definition and classification of cardiomyopathies. Br. Heart J. 44:672, 1980.

S

1. Sakamoto, T., Tei, C., Murama, M., et al.: Giant negative T-wave inversion as a manifestation of asymmetric apical hypertrophy (AAH) of the left ventricle. Echocardiographic and ultrasonocardiotomographic study. Jpn. Heart J. 17:611, 1976.
2. Shah, P.M., Gramiak, R., and Kramer, D.H.: Ultrasound localization of left ventricular outflow obstruction in hypertrophic obstructive cardiomyopathy. Circulation 40:3, 1969.
3. Shah, P.M., Taylor, R.D., and Wong, M.: Abnormal mitral valve coaptation in hypertrophic obstructive cardiomyopathy: Proposed role in systolic anterior motion of the mitral valve. Am. J. Cardiol. 48:258, 1981.
4. Shah, P.M.: Echocardiography in congestive or dilated cardiomyopathy. J. Am. Soc. Echo. 1:20, 1988.
5. Shah, P.M., Archibald, D., Lopez, B., and Cohn, J.N.: Prognostic value of echocardiographic parameters in chronic congestive heart failure. The VHEFT study (Abstract). J. Am. Coll. Cardiol. 9:202, 1987.
6. Smith, T.J., Kyle, R.A., and Lie, J.T.: Clinical significance of histopathologic pattern of cardiac amyloidosis. Mayo Clin. Proc. 59:547, 1984.

T

1. Tei, C., Boltwood, C.M., and Shah, P.M.: Minimally dilated cardiomyopathy: A distinct subset of severe systolic dysfunction (Abstract). Circulation 68 (Suppl. 3):III–336, 1983.

U

1. Unverferth, D.V., Margorien, R.D., Moeschberger, M.L., et al.: Factors influencing the one-year mortality of dilated cardiomyopathy. Am. J. Cardiol. 54:147, 1984.

Chapter 23

Echocardiography in Pericardial Diseases

- *GARY M. BROCKINGTON, M.D.* ▪ *STEVEN L. SCHWARTZ, M.D.*
- *NATESA G. PANDIAN, M.D.*

ECHOCARDIOGRAPHIC APPEARANCE OF THE NORMAL PERICARDIUM 460
PERICARDIAL EFFUSION 460
Detection of Pericardial Effusion 460
Localization of Pericardial Fluid 460
Quantitation of the Amount of Pericardial Fluid 463
Assessment of the Contents of Pericardial Effusion 463
Cardiac Motion Abnormalities in Pericardial Effusion 464
Conditions That May Mimic Pericardial Effusion 464
CARDIAC TAMPONADE 464
Pathophysiology 464
Echocardiographic Signs of Tamponade 464
Echocardiography During Pericardiocentesis 470
CONSTRICTIVE PERICARDITIS 470
ECHOCARDIOGRAPHIC FINDINGS IN CERTAIN SPECIFIC DISORDERS 475
Acute and Chronic Pericarditis 475
Neoplastic Pericardial Disease 475
Traumatic Pericardial Disease 476
Pericardial Cysts 476
Absence of Pericardium 476
CONCLUSION 476

Pericardial involvement in disease processes is manifested in a multitude of ways ranging from innocuous, trivial, pericardial effusion to life-threatening cardiac tamponade. Echocardiography has proved to be highly valuable in evaluating pericardial disorders. This technique aids in the detection, localization, and quantitation of pericardial effusion; diagnosis of cardiac tamponade; identification of the presence of pericardial thickening; diagnosis of constrictive pericarditis; evaluation of pericardial neoplasms; and detection of congenital abnormalities of the pericardium such as absence of the pericardium and pericardial cysts. All the different modalities of cardiac ultrasound, including two-dimensional echocardiography, M-mode echocardiography, pulsed-wave and continuous-wave Doppler, and color flow imaging, are used in the comprehensive evaluation of patients with pericardial diseases. The echocardiographic instrumentation and technical aspects related to the use of these various modalities have been described in earlier chapters. In this chapter we review the utility and limitations of echocardiography in the evaluation of pericardial diseases.

ECHOCARDIOGRAPHIC APPEARANCE OF THE NORMAL PERICARDIUM

The appearance of the pericardium in M-mode and two-dimensional echocardiography is that of a bright, dense layer of echoes inseparable from the epicardial echo. This echo layer covers the entire surface of the heart except for the posterior aspect of the left atrium and is composed of signals from the epicardium, or visceral pericardium, and the parietal pericardium. Signals generated by this layer are generally the brightest signals originating from the heart. Figure 23–1 illustrates that even when the ultrasound gain is low and the signals from other cardiac structures are not apparent, the pericardial echo is often persistent. Although the morphologic thickness of the pericardium is 1 mm or less, the pericardial echo is generally greater than 2 mm thick. The dimension of this echo may be discrepant in different views because of the variation between axial and lateral resolution inherent in two-dimensional echocardiography. Motion of the pericardial echo is congruent with that of the posterior wall throughout the cardiac cycle. This normal appearance of the epi-pericardial echo is altered in the presence of pericardial disorders such as pericardial effusion and constrictive pericarditis.

PERICARDIAL EFFUSION

Detection of Pericardial Effusion

A number of disease states may be associated with the development of a pericardial effusion. Echocardiography is the most sensitive technique for detection of fluid in the pericardial space.[F1] Pericardial fluid is seen on two-dimensional echocardiographic images and M-mode recordings as a relatively echo-free space between the epicardium and pericardium (Figs. 23–2 to 23–5).[F1, F2, M1] If the fluid contains clots or fibrinous material, then granular, strand-like, or masses of echo signals can be visualized on the two-dimensional echocardiogram (Fig. 23–6).[M2] Although M-mode echocardiography is useful in the detection of an effusion, two-dimensional echocardiography is the method of choice for assessing a pericardial effusion, since it presents a two-dimensional spatial display of the pericardial fluid. If the effusion is trivial, the separation between the epicardial and pericardial echoes and the consequent echo-free space are apparent only during systole. In the presence of a small effusion, a small echo-free space is seen both during diastole and systole. The size of the echo-free space varies with the amount of fluid present, as demonstrated in Figure 23–4, which shows images recorded from patients with small, moderate, and large pericardial effusions.

Localization of Pericardial Fluid

Most pericardial effusions are circumferential, as seen in Figure 23–4. The majority of small effusions are seen only posteriorly

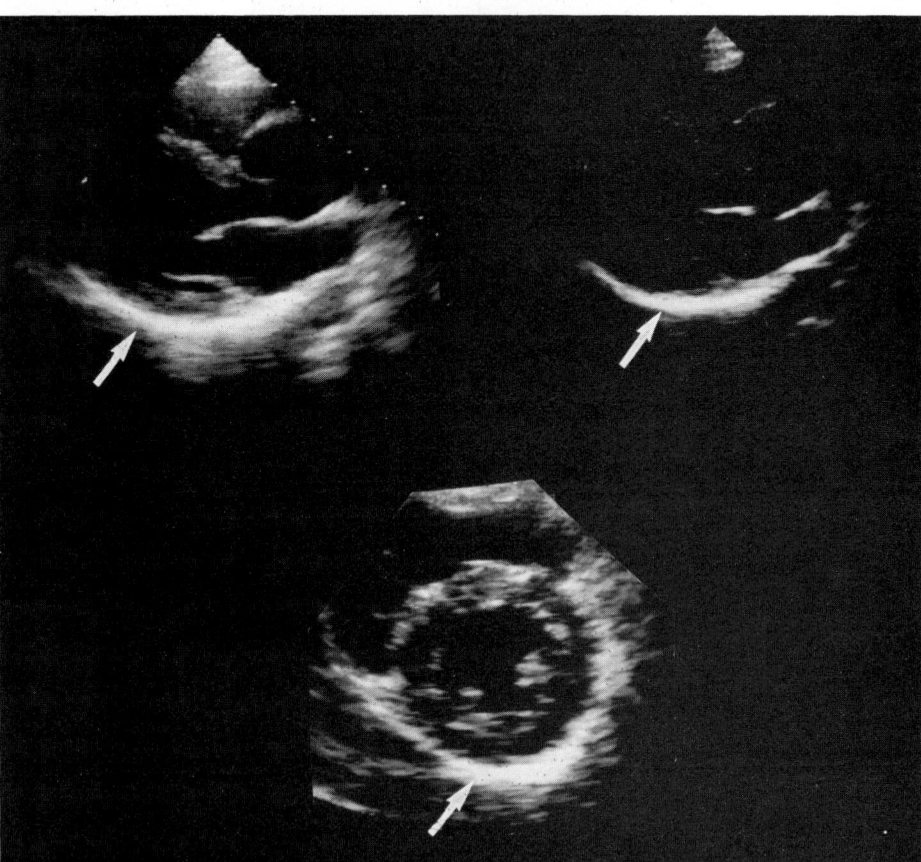

Figure 23–1. Two-dimensional echocardiographic images from a normal subject: parasternal long-axis image (above) and parasternal short-axis image (below). Normal pericardium is seen as a bright linear echo (*arrow*) surrounding the cardiac chambers. The pericardial echo is the brightest structure in a normal heart and is seen even when the ultrasound gain is turned low (above right).

because this region is most dependent during the routine echocardiographic study performed with the patient in the supine position. Moderate-sized and large effusions result in echo-free spaces both anteriorly and posteriorly in the parasternal long-axis view and circumferentially in the parasternal short-axis and apical views (see Figs. 23–3 and 23–4). Because of the lack of pericardial reflection over the left atrium, pericardial fluid is generally not seen behind this chamber if the effusion is small. Large effusions, however, can stretch and bulge the pericardium to such a degree that an echo-free space can be seen posterior to the left atrium as well. Fluid confined to the anterior region is uncommon; posteriorly loculated effusions are more frequently encountered. Posterior loculation is particularly common in patients after cardiac surgery.[P1] In these patients, the right ventricular epicardium and pericardium are often adherent to the inner surface of the chest wall and thus pericardial fluid collection does not develop in this region. These findings are illustrated in Figure 23–7, from a patient who had recently undergone bypass surgery.

To recognize the presence of fluid and delineate its distribution, it is of prime importance to attempt to visualize the heart from as many planes as possible when a pericardial effusion is suspected. It is also imperative that the person performing the echocardiographic examination become familiar with the variety of gain settings and attenuation factors in the ultrasound equipment. Proper use of these controls can eliminate the chance of missing an effusion. Very high ultrasound gain setting can cause blooming echo signals that may obliterate the echo-free space caused by a small effusion. It is recommended that the initial

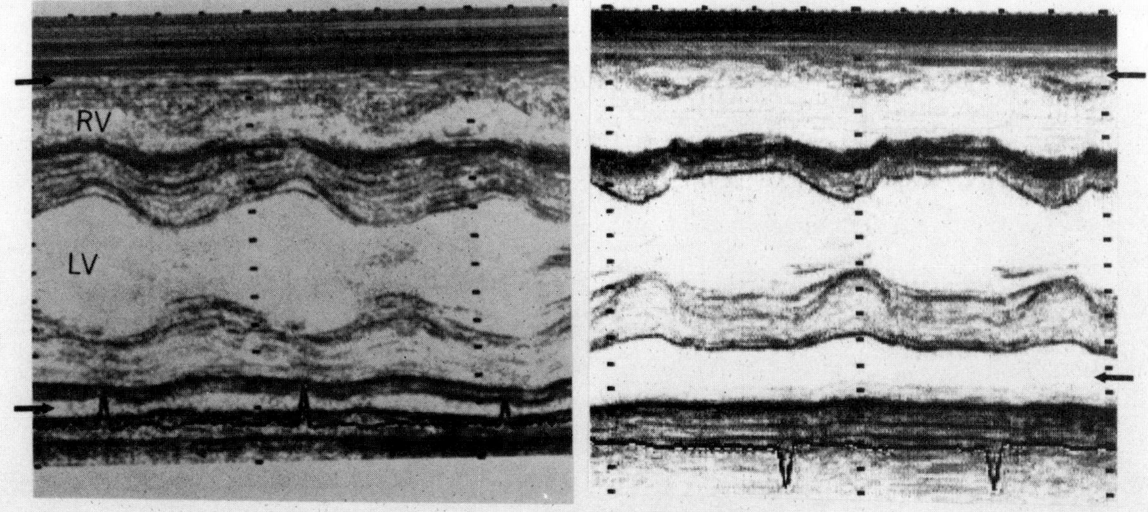

Figure 23–2. M-mode echocardiographic tracing from two patients with pericardial effusion. In the recording at the left, a small echo-free space is seen between the epicardium and pericardium both anteriorly and posteriorly (*arrows*). In the recording on the right, from a patient with a moderate-sized effusion, a larger anterior and posterior space is noted (*arrows*). LV—left ventricle; RV—right ventricle.

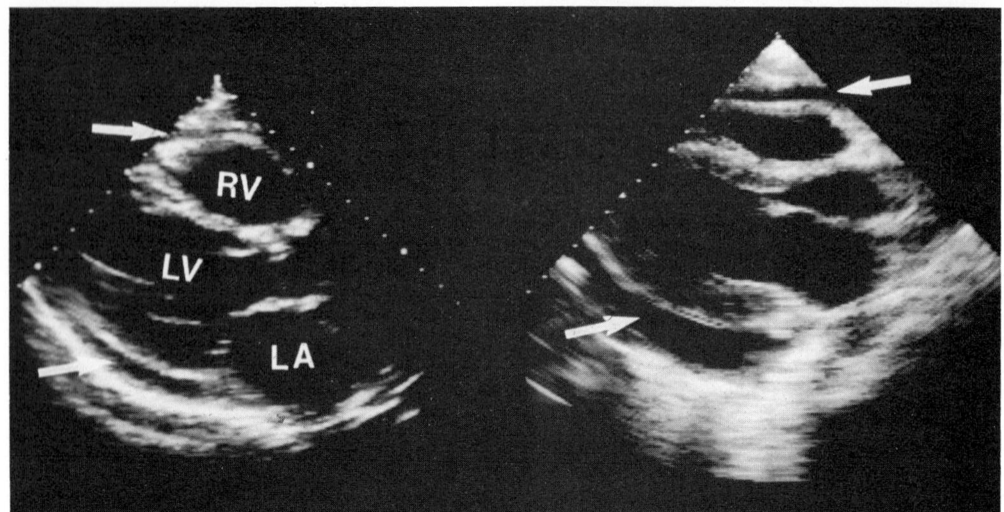

Figure 23–3. Parasternal long-axis images from two patients with pericardial effusions. A small echo-free space surrounding both the right and left ventricles is seen (*arrows*), indicating the presence of a pericardial effusion. A larger effusion is noted in the image on the right. RV—right ventricle; LV—left ventricle; LA—left atrium.

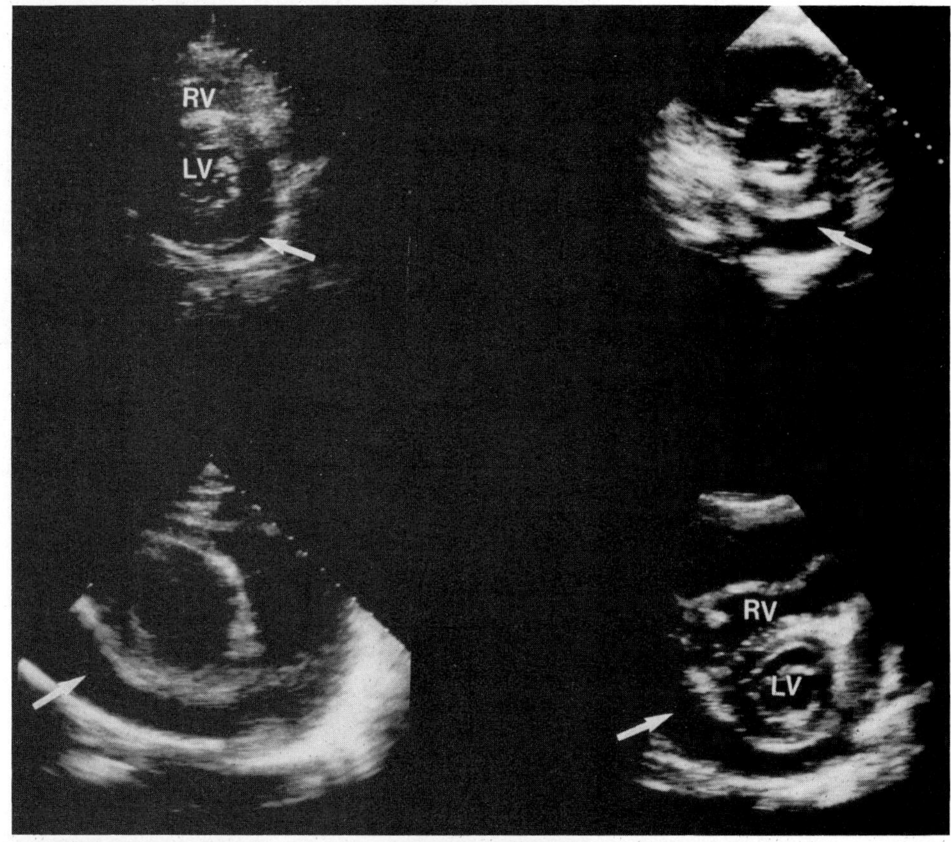

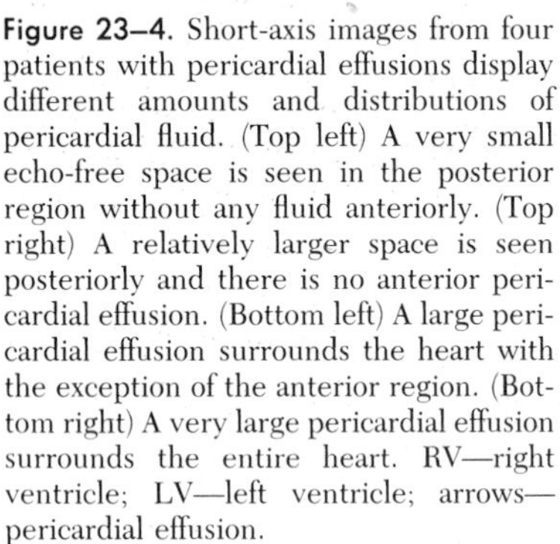

Figure 23–4. Short-axis images from four patients with pericardial effusions display different amounts and distributions of pericardial fluid. (Top left) A very small echo-free space is seen in the posterior region without any fluid anteriorly. (Top right) A relatively larger space is seen posteriorly and there is no anterior pericardial effusion. (Bottom left) A large pericardial effusion surrounds the heart with the exception of the anterior region. (Bottom right) A very large pericardial effusion surrounds the entire heart. RV—right ventricle; LV—left ventricle; arrows—pericardial effusion.

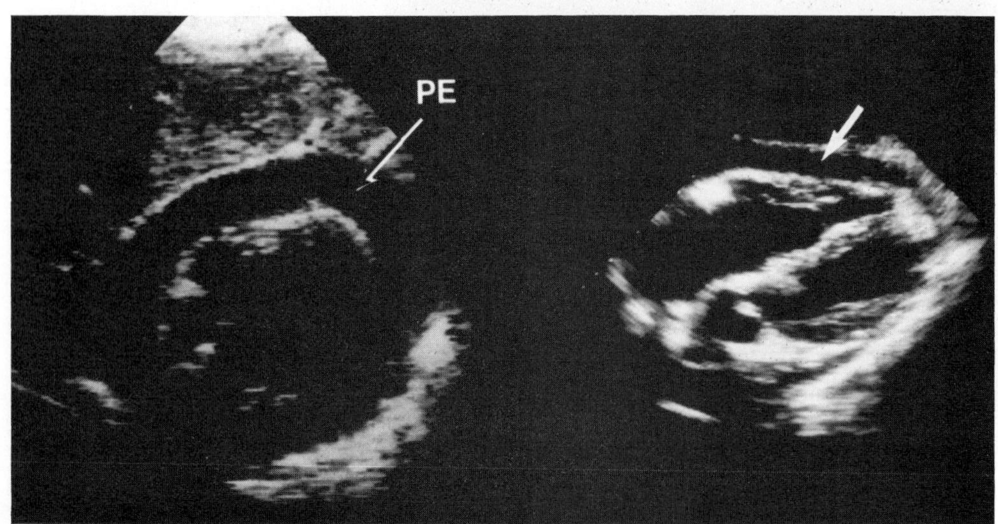

Figure 23–5. Subcostal images from two patients with pericardial effusions. The effusion seen in the left image is circumferential and is very large. The effusion seen in the right image is of moderate size (*arrow*). PE—pericardial effusion.

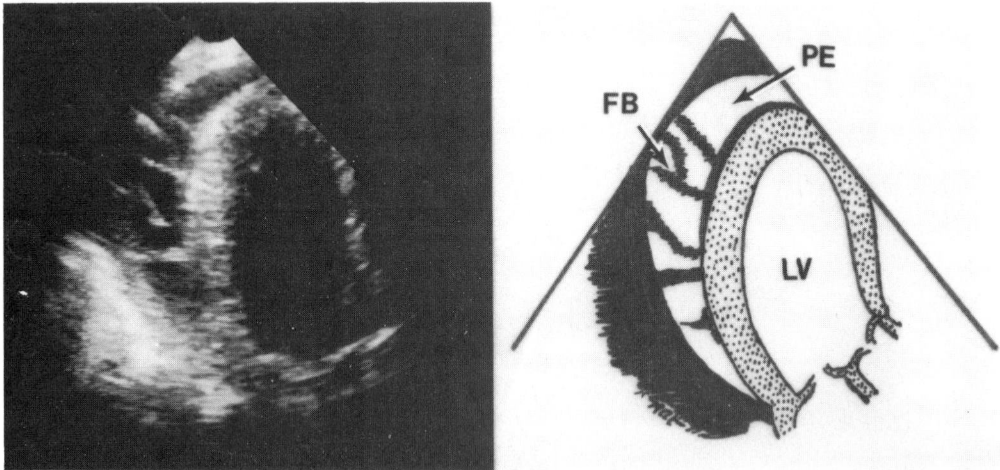

Figure 23–6. Apical long-axis image from a patient with an organized pericardial effusion. A moderate-sized pericardial effusion is seen posteriorly and around the cardiac apex. Within the effusion, multiple linear bandlike echoes indicate the presence of fibrinous bands within the pericardal cavity. PE—pericardial effusion; FB—fibrinous bands; LV—left ventricle.

gain be set low so that only the posterior pericardium is visualized. This setting should then be raised to allow slow visualization of the posterior epicardium and other structures. By using this technique, small posterior effusions can be more precisely defined. Typically, there is a paucity of pericardial motion relative to the epicardium in the presence of a pericardial effusion, and this can be more easily observed using the technique mentioned above. Fibrin structures and clots within the pericardial cavity may be missed if the gain is too low or if the gray scale, or compression, is not optimal. Hence it is important to utilize varying ultrasound gain and gray scale levels when a pericardial effusion is examined.

Quantitation of the Amount of Pericardial Fluid

The sensitivity of echocardiography is such that as little as 20 ml of pericardial fluid can be detected if proper ultrasound techniques are used. Since even healthy individuals occasionally may have up to 50 ml of pericardial fluid, echocardiographic visualization of a very small amount of pericardial fluid in an otherwise healthy individual should not be cause for concern.[B1, H1] Accurate quantitation of pericardial fluid is not possible by echocardiography, or any noninvasive technique, but echocardiography allows discrimination between small, moderate, and large quantities of fluid.[H1] The images in Figures 23–4 and 23–8 are examples of how two-dimensional echocardiography can be used to semiquantify the volume of an effusion. In general, if a circumferential effusion is seen clearly, it indicates the presence of an effusion usually exceeding 300 ml. If the average width of the space circumferentially exceeds 1 cm, the effusion is likely to be larger than 500 ml; and if the average width is close to 2 cm, the fluid collection is likely to be more than 700 ml.[H1]

Assessment of the Contents of Pericardial Effusion

It is not possible to assess the character of the fluid by echocardiography. Serous effusions, hemopericardium, and chylopericardium all appear as similar clear spaces. If hematomas are present within the effusion, solid masses of granular echoes may be seen interspersed with zones of clear space. A honeycomb appearance, caused by fibrous strands, is often observed in a purulent pericardial effusion. Fibrous strands are frequently present even in nonpurulent effusions.[M2] Figure 23–6 illustrates these strands, which appear as small linear bands that in real time may exhibit mobility. In an effusion undergoing organization, granular and layer-like echo signals may be seen in a space that was previously clear. In neoplastic diseases, solid masses of echoes caused by metastatic deposits may occasionally be visualized within the pericardial cavity.[C1] Frequently, the masses are

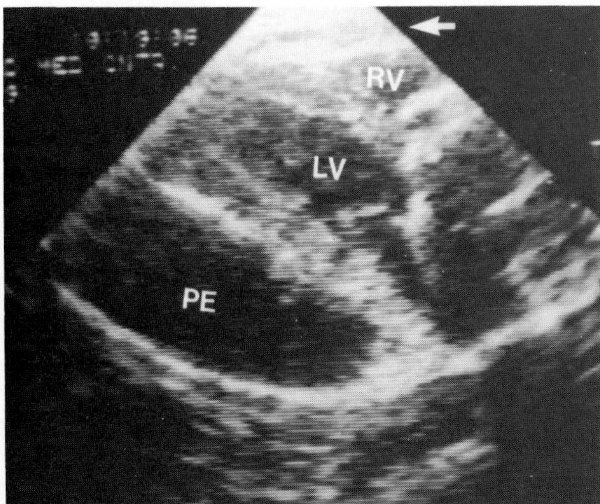

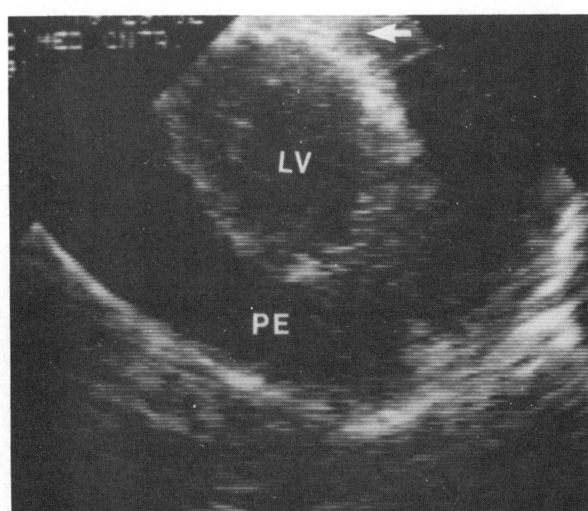

Figure 23–7. Parasternal long-axis (left) and parasternal short-axis (right) images from a patient with a postoperative pericardial effusion. A large echo-free space is seen posteriorly and laterally in this patient, but no fluid is seen anteriorly. The anterior right ventricular wall *(arrow)* adheres to the chest wall, which is usually the case in postoperative pericardial effusions. RV—right ventricle; LV—left ventricle; PE—pericardial effusion.

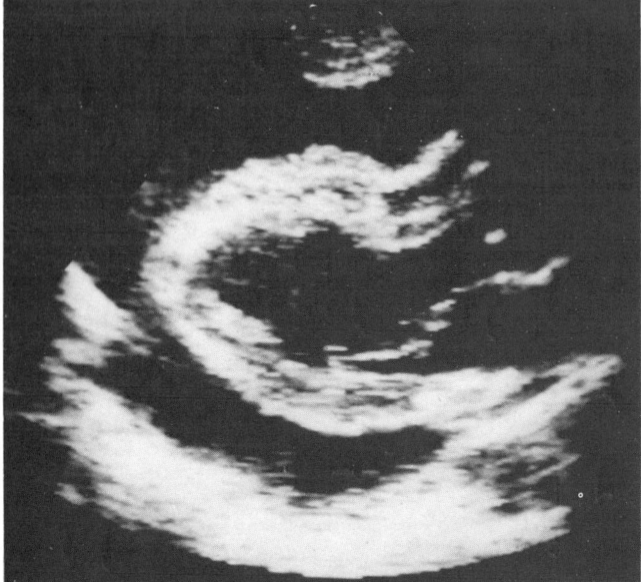

Figure 23–8. Parasternal long-axis image from a patient with a large pericardial effusion and tamponade. A large echo-free space is seen surrounding both ventricles. The right ventricle appears very small and compressed. The anterior right ventricular wall is indented, indicating the presence of right ventricular diastolic collapse.

seen to be adherent to the epicardial surface, as shown in Figure 23–9.

Cardiac Motion Abnormalities in Pericardial Effusion

Cardiac motion abnormalities are often seen with large effusions.[F3, G2, L1, M1] Prominent excursions of the anterior right ventricular wall and posterior left ventricular free wall have been described. The entire heart moves back and forth within the pericardial space.[F3, G1, K1, M2, U1] Figure 23–10 is an M-mode tracing for a patient with a large effusion that illustrates this to-and-fro motion. This motion is thought to be the basis for the electrocardiographic voltage variability observed in patients with large effusions, known as electrical alternans.[G1] The cause of such cardiac motion abnormalities may be multifactorial and may include loss of the tethering effect of the pericardium as well as interactions between heart rate, rhythm, and pericardial pressures.

Abnormal motions of the cardiac valves have also been described with effusive states. These motions include systolic anterior motion of the mitral valve, pseudoprolapse of the atrioventricular valves, and abnormal excursion of the semilunar valves.[D1, L2, N1] These valvular phenomena are thought to be the result of abnormal "swaying" of the heart within the effusion. They are primarily M-mode echocardiographic findings and are partly artifactual because of the fixed transducer reference. These findings are generally not seen on two-dimensional echocardiograms.

Conditions That May Mimic Pericardial Effusion

Certain conditions and pitfalls in echocardiographic examination techniques may result in apparent echo-free spaces that may mimic the presence of a pericardial effusion.[C2, L3, M3, R1, R2] A prominent epicardial fat pad may sometimes be mistaken for pericardial fluid. Layers of fat, although more common on the anterior surface of the heart, can be present surrounding both ventricles. Space caused by a fat pad is generally devoid of echo signals but often contains granular echoes, whereas a pericardial effusion causes a clear echo-free space.[R2] An organized effusion, however, can exhibit echo signals within the pericardial space and may appear similar to an epicardial fat pad. Close observation of the motion of the pericardial echo layer, appropriate adjustment of the gain, and examination from various views are often helpful in differentiating a pericardial effusion from an epicardial fat pad. Similar maneuvers would help in the discrimination of an effusion from certain tumors that may encircle the heart.[L4] A dilated coronary sinus may mimic a posterior pericardial effusion in an off-axis view recorded from short-axis or apical orientations.

Left pleural effusions may occasionally be difficult to discern from pericardial fluid collections. Several points of differentiation are noteworthy. Fluid isolated behind the left ventricle, without extension to the area behind the left atrium, is usually of pericardial origin. The echo-free space caused by a pericardial effusion is often aligned with the anterior and lateral aspect of the descending aorta, whereas the clear space due to pleural effusion is aligned with the posterior and lateral aspects of the descending aorta (Fig. 23–11).[L3] Other conditions that may be confused with pericardial effusions include pericardial cysts, mediastinal tumors, pericardial masses, pneumopericardium, and diaphragmatic hernias.[C2, L4, N2] Most of the difficulties in differentiating these entities can be eliminated by optimizing the technical and practical aspects (gain attenuation, avoidance of "off-axis" views, etc.) of ultrasound imaging.

CARDIAC TAMPONADE

Pathophysiology

The output of both ventricles depends on adequate diastolic filling. Normally, intrapericardial pressure is zero or slightly negative. Since the intraventricular diastolic pressures are higher, there is a positive transmural pressure gradient across the myo-

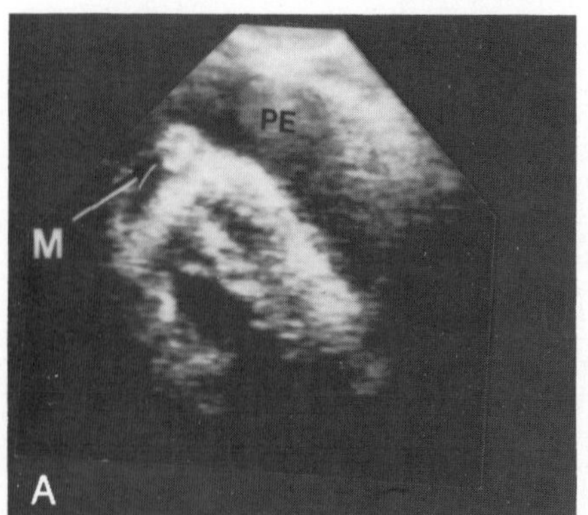

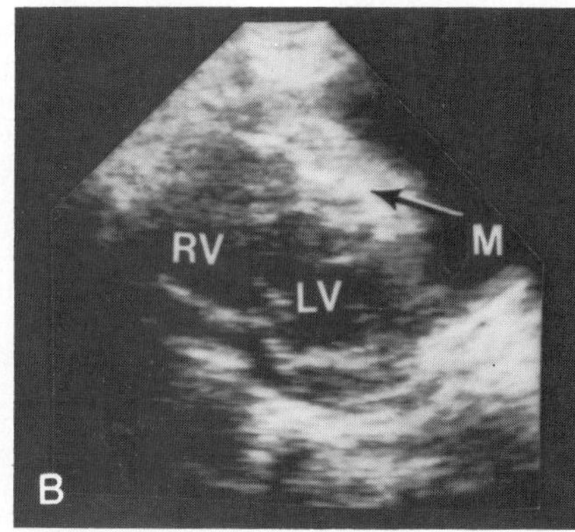

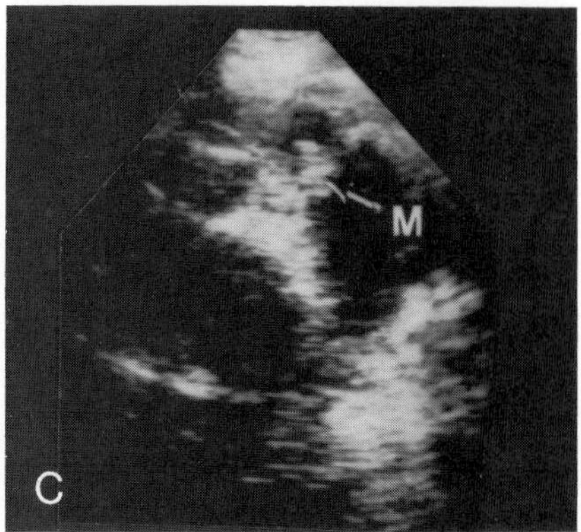

Figure 23–9. Two-dimensional echocardiographic images from a patient with neoplastic pericardial disease, showing a pericardial effusion and tumor deposits at the left ventricular apex (*A*), in the anterior intraventricular root area (*B*), and near the right ventricular outflow tract area (*C*). RV—right ventricle; LV—left ventricle; PE—pericardial effusion; M—mass.

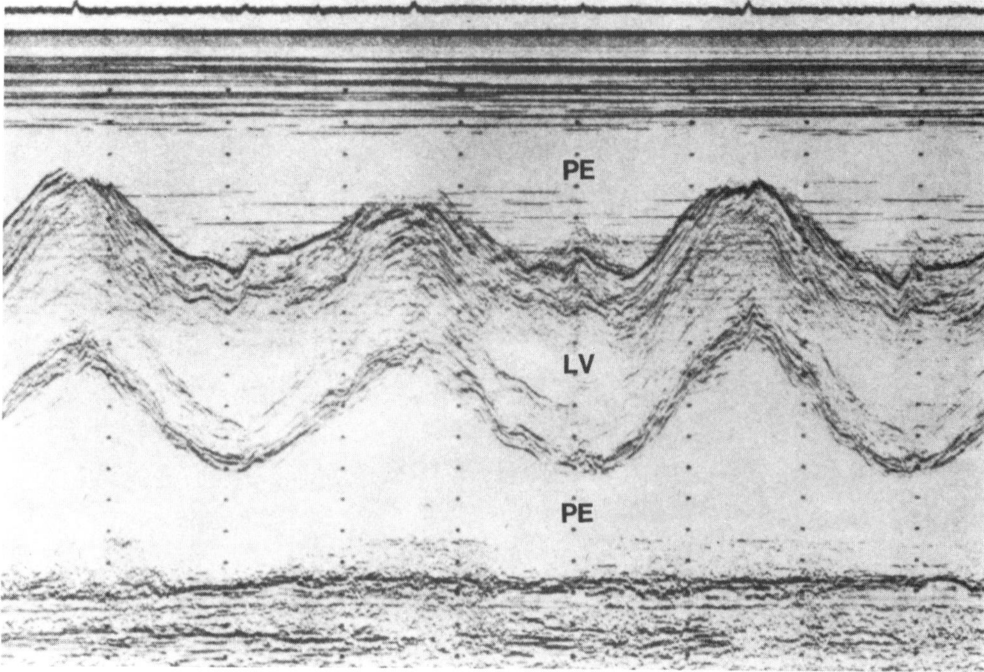

Figure 23–10. An M-mode echocardiographic tracing from a patient with a large pericardial effusion, demonstrating a swinging motion of the heart. The cardiac chambers are small with compression of the right ventricle. The whole heart moves anteriorly with every other beat. LV—left ventricle; PE—pericardial effusion.

cardium during diastole that aids ventricular filling. As pericardial fluid accumulates, both the intrapericardial pressure and intracardiac pressure increase but the difference between them narrows, reducing the distending force for ventricular filling. Although the pericardial effusion surrounds both ventricles, the hemodynamic effects of tamponade are considered to be primarily the result of right heart compression. With a decreasing transmural gradient, ventricular filling and therefore stroke volume and cardiac output fall. Up to a point, various circulatory mechanisms can compensate, contributing to the familiar clinical signs of tamponade such as elevated jugular venous pressure, narrow pulse pressure, pulsus paradoxus, and poorly perfused extremities. When the intrapericardial pressure becomes almost equal to the filling pressures, compensatory mechanisms reach their limit and marked hemodynamic deterioration can occur.[G2, S1–S6] Pulsus paradoxus, an important clinical sign of tamponade, is observed because inspiration increases the filling gradient across the right heart but not the left heart. The augmented right ventricular filling occurs at the expense of reduced filling and stroke output of the left ventricle. These pathophysiologic alterations in tamponade are also responsible for the many echocardiographic findings.[L1, P1–P4, R3, S4–S7]

Echocardiographic Signs of Tamponade

Several M-mode echocardiographic studies described a number of findings as indicators of cardiac tamponade. These findings include reciprocal respiratory variation in ventricular dimensions (exaggerated inspiratory expansion of the right ventricle and compression of the left ventricle), diminution of mitral valve E-F slope, systolic notching of the right ventricular epicardium, and compression of the right ventricle.[K2, M4, S1, S2, S6] Right ventricular compression is a late sign of tamponade, noted only in advanced cases. The reciprocal changes in ventricular dimensions with inspiration noted above are seen only in a minority of patients with tamponade. An example of these changes is seen in Figure 23–12. Overall, the M-mode echocardiographic signs are relatively insensitive and occur predominantly in advanced stages of tamponade. These signs are also nonspecific and can occur in association with other conditions.

Two-dimensional echocardiography has a greater application in assessing cardiac tamponade. Besides demonstrating the presence and distribution of pericardial fluid, two-dimensional echocardiography provides two useful signs in tamponade. These signs are right ventricular diastolic collapse and right atrial collapse, which

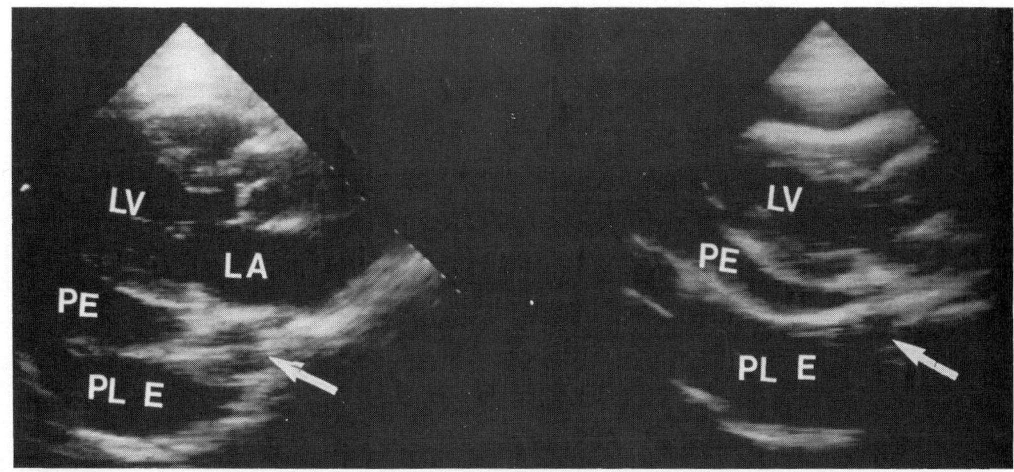

Figure 23–11. Parasternal long-axis images from two patients demonstrating the presence of both pericardial and pleural effusions. The pericardial effusion is seen posterior to the left ventricle aligned with the anterior aspect of the descending thoracic aorta (*arrow*); the pleural effusion extends beyond the posterior aspect of the left ventricle and is aligned with the posterior aspect of the descending thoracic aorta. L—left ventricle; LA—left atrium; PE—pericardial effusion; PLE—pleural effusion.

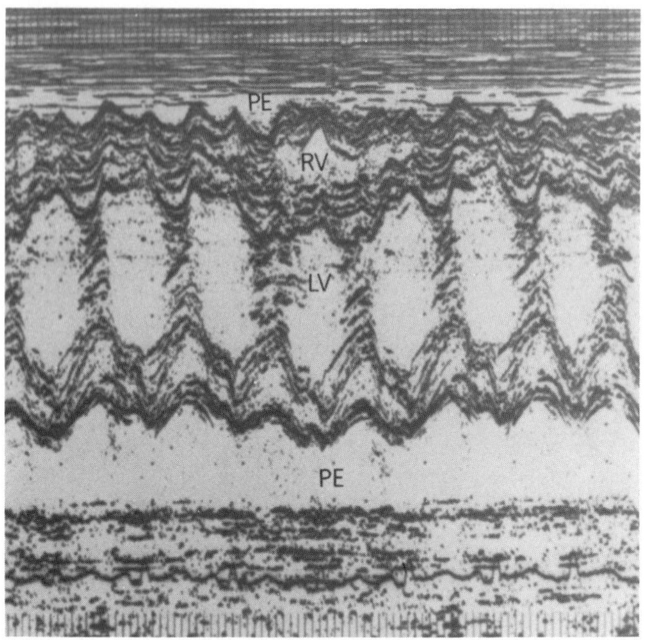

Figure 23–12. An M-mode echocardiographic recording from a patient with cardiac tamponade. A large pericardial effusion is seen anteriorly and posteriorly. There is cyclic variation in the dimensions of the right ventricle and the left ventricle related to respiration. The right ventricle is markedly compressed during expiration but increases in size during inspiration, whereas the left ventricular dimension decreases during inspiration. RV—right ventricle; LV—left ventricle; PE—pericardial effusion.

are illustrated in Figures 23–8, 23–13, and 23–14.[G3, K2, R3, S1, S6] In normal individuals and in patients with pericardial effusion without tamponade, the free walls of the cardiac chambers maintain a rounded contour. During tamponade, the normal convex shape of the cardiac chambers becomes distorted. A transient invagination of the right ventricular free wall occurs in tamponade; this finding is known as right ventricular diastolic collapse (Figs. 23–8 and 23–14.[M4, R3, S1] Right atrial collapse, a transient invagination of the right atrial free wall, is also noted during tamponade (Figs. 23–13 and 23–14).[G3, R3] Chamber collapse occurs when intracavitary pressures are lowest: early diastole for the right ventricle and late diastole or early systole for the right atrium. It has been proposed that when the pericardial pressure approaches intracavitary pressure, the transmural gradient may reverse transiently during diastole, leading to indentation of the myocardium. In the presence of right atrial and right ventricular collapse, the cardiac walls are acting as visual transducers of the transmural pressure gradient. Since this gradient is the basis for cardiac tamponade, it is not surprising that collapse of the right atrium or right ventricle is more reliable than the previously described clinical and M-mode signs for the diagnosis of tamponade. In general, right atrial collapse is highly sensitive (100 percent) but relatively less specific for the diagnosis of tamponade.[R3] The specificity is improved when the duration of right atrial collapse occupies a longer portion of the cardiac cycle. Right ventricular diastolic collapse is a more specific sign of tamponade than right atrial collapse and is also highly sensitive.[R3, S1, S6] Diastolic collapse of the right ventricle has been found to develop when tamponade causes a decline of 20 percent in cardiac output. Right atrial and right ventricular collapse may precede the development of pulsus paradoxus; both occur prior to the reduction of mean arterial pressure.[R3] Presence of both of these signs almost always indicates that the effusion is hemodynamically significant. These signs are present even in the setting of low-pressure tamponade, since the transient relative changes in the pressure gradients between the pericardial cavity and the chambers persist despite low absolute pressures.[L5] If tamponade is caused by a large or posteriorly localized effusion, the left atrial free wall also may manifest an inward motion; this is referred to as left atrial collapse. An example of right atrial, right ventricular, and left atrial collapse in the presence of a large pericardial effusion and tamponade is shown in Figure 23–14.

In patients who have had cardiac surgery, the right ventricular and right atrial walls are often adherent to the inner chest wall, in which case collapse of these chambers may not be evident despite tamponade. Pericardial fluid in these patients is usually posterior. If such an effusion causes regional tamponade, even the thick-walled left ventricle can be deformed and collapse during diastole.[P1] This sign, left ventricular diastolic collapse, is useful in the diagnosis of postoperative tamponade caused by a loculated pericardial effusion (Figs. 23–15 and 23–16). Localized compression of a single cardiac chamber by hematoma may also

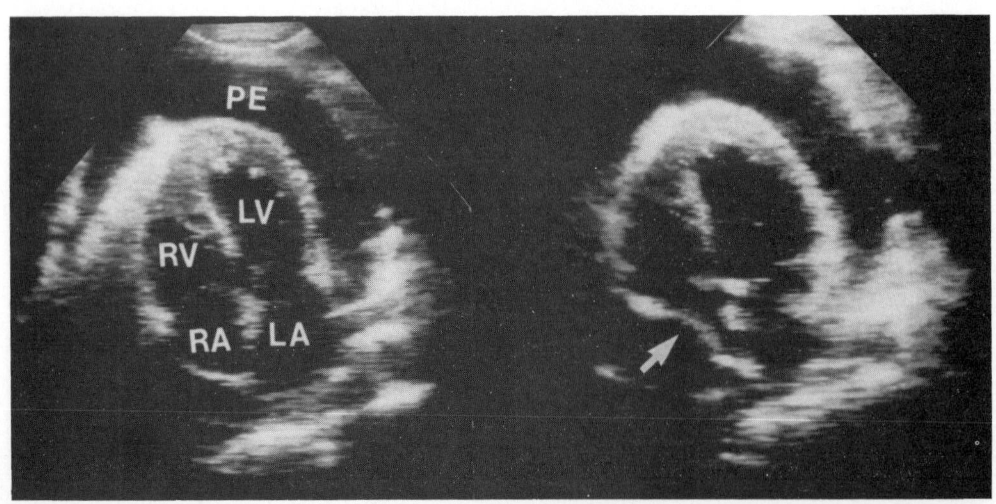

Figure 23–13. Apical four-chamber images from a patient with cardiac tamponade. A large pericardial effusion is noted surrounding almost the entire heart. The right atrial wall has a rounded contour during mid-diastole (left) but exhibits indentation during late diastole. The arrow points to right atrial collapse. RV—right ventricle; LV—left ventricle; RA—right atrium; LA—left atrium; PE—pericardial effusion.

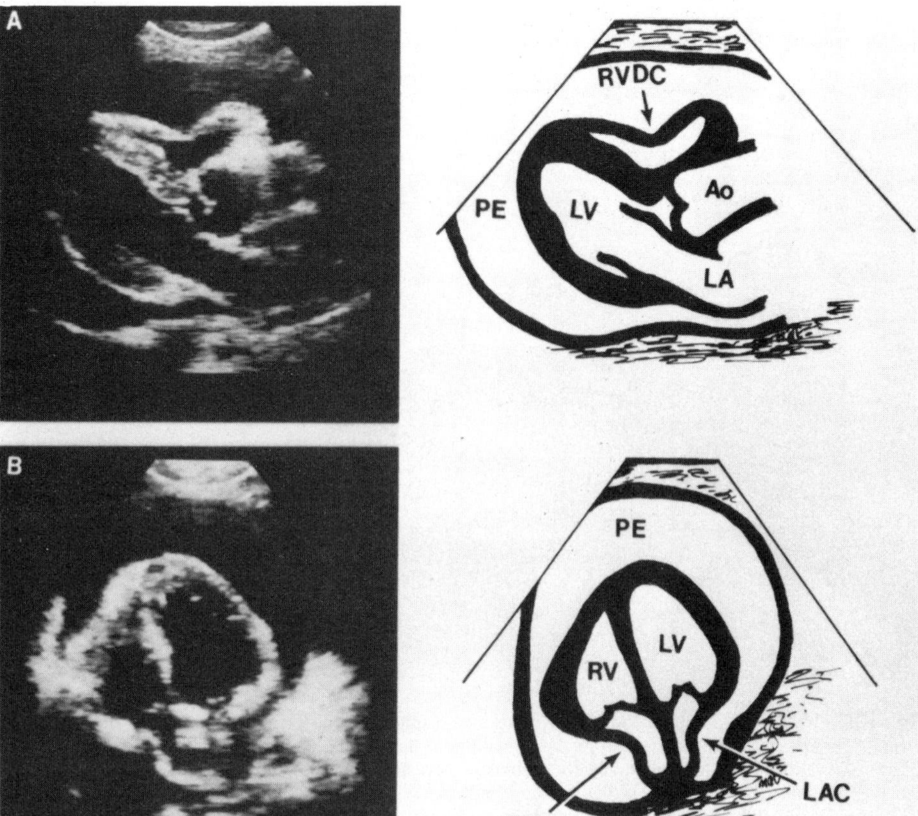

Figure 23–14. Parasternal long-axis (*A*) and apical four-chamber (*B*) images from a patient with cardiac tamponade, demonstrating the presence of right ventricular diastolic collapse and right atrial collapse. In this patient even the left atrium is seen to collapse because of tamponade. LV—left ventricle; LA—left atrium; Ao—aorta; PE—pericardial effusion; RVDC—right ventricular diastolic collapse; RAC—right atrial collapse; LAC—left atrial collapse.

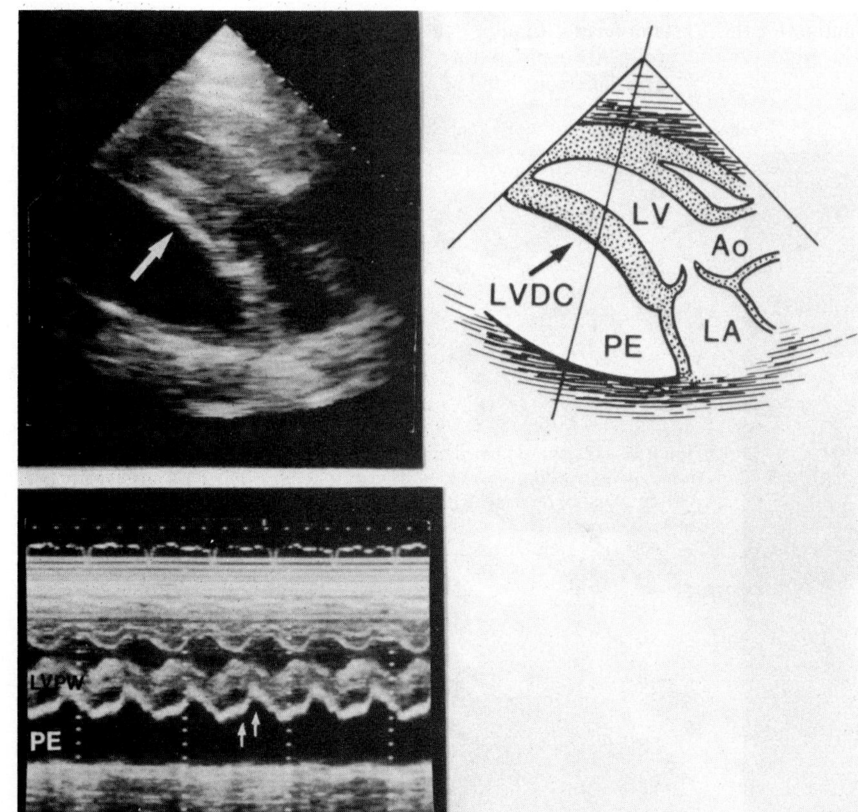

Figure 23–15. Low parasternal long-axis image from a patient with postoperative pericardial effusion and cardiac tamponade demonstrates a large posterior effusion and the presence of left ventricular diastolic collapse. Anteriorly, the right ventricular wall is adherent to the chest wall. The left ventricular posterior wall exhibits an invagination during early ventricular diastole (*large arrow*). Left ventricular diastolic collapse is seen in the M-mode echocardiographic recording as well (*second small arrow*). The first arrow points to the end of ventricular systole. LV—left ventricle; LA—left atrium; Ao—aorta; LVPW—left ventricular posterior wall; LVDC—left ventricular diastolic collapse; PE—pericardial effusion.

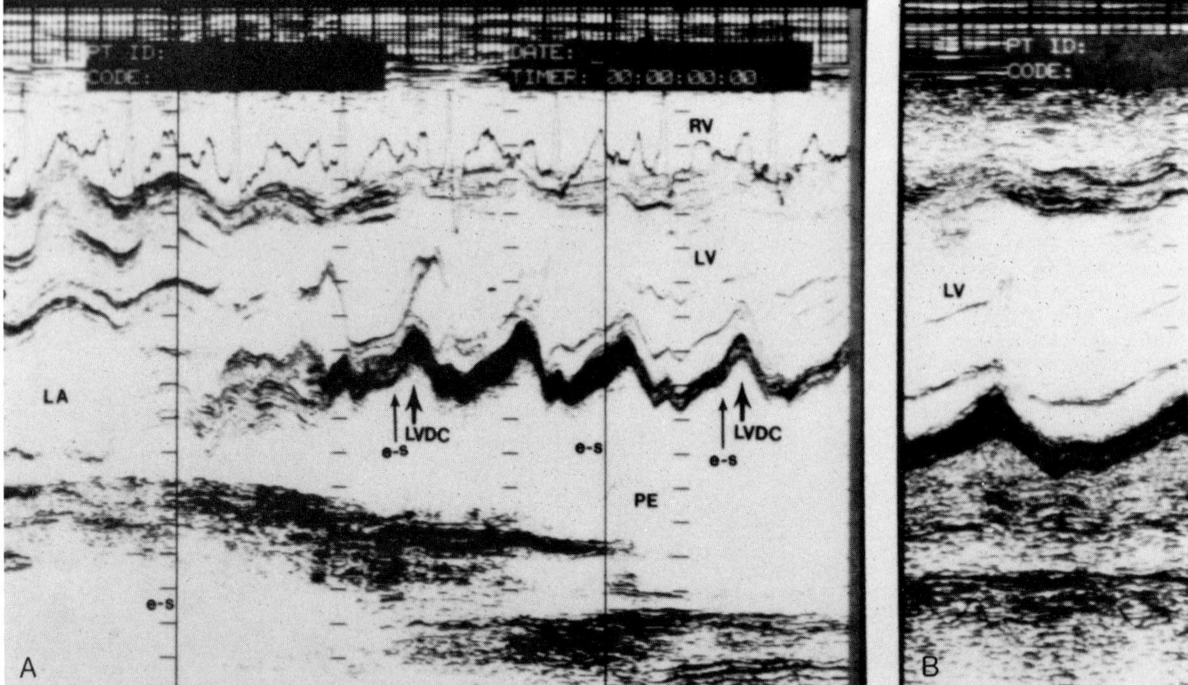

Figure 23–16. M-mode echocardiographic recordings from a patient with a postoperative pericardial effusion and cardiac tamponade, before (left) and after (right) pericardiocentesis. During tamponade, the left ventricular posterior wall exhibits a marked inward motion during the early portion of diastole because of the hemodynamically significant pericardial effusion. Following pericardiocentesis, a small amount of residual fluid is seen but the left ventricular diastolic motion has become normal without any diastolic collapse. RV—right ventricle; LV—left ventricle; LA—left atrium; PE—pericardial effusion; LVDC—left ventricular diastolic collapse; e-s—end systole.

produce a syndrome suggestive of tamponade without the presence of right ventricular diastolic collapse, as demonstrated in Figure 23–17. Right ventricular diastolic collapse may also be absent despite tamponade when the right ventricular wall is thickened and stiff or when pulmonary hypertension is present. Since the right atrial wall is generally more compliant than the right ventricular wall, right atrial collapse might occur without right ventricular collapse, which may be the explanation for the higher sensitivity of right atrial collapse compared to right ventricular diastolic collapse.

Visualization of the inferior vena cava is of diagnostic value when tamponade is suspected. Normally, the diameter of this vessel decreases with inspiration. Inferior vena caval plethora, defined as dilation or engorgement of the inferior vena cava associated with an inspiratory reduction in diameter of less than 50 percent, may often be demonstrated.[H2] Inferior vena caval plethora is thought to be a sensitive sign for the presence of tamponade, though it may occur with constrictive pericarditis as well. Absence of this finding in a patient who is not being artificially ventilated makes the diagnosis of tamponade less likely.

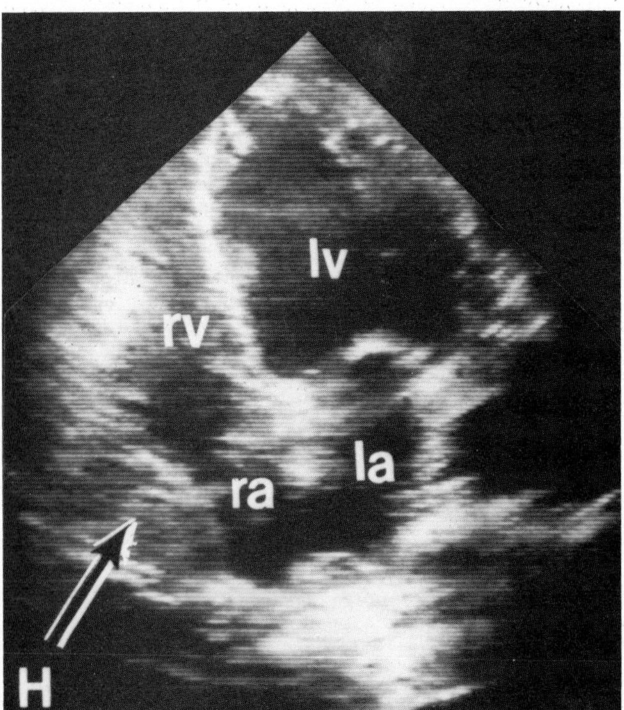

Figure 23–17. Apical four-chamber two-dimensional echocardiographic image from a patient who presented with features suggestive of cardiac tamponade. A large mass (*arrow*), which proved to be a hematoma, is seen compressing the right atrium. There is no pericardial effusion. rv—right ventricle; lv—left ventricle; ra—right atrium; la—left atrium; H—hematoma.

Respiration profoundly influences cardiac hemodynamics and intracardiac flow dynamics. Normally, inspiration causes a minimal increase in systemic venous, tricuspid valvular, and pulmonary valvular blood flow velocities and a corresponding decrease in pulmonary venous, mitral valvular, and aortic blood flow velocities.[D1, K3, L6] This inspiratory change is usually less than 20 percent. Minimal inspiratory change in blood flow velocities is noted in patients with pericardial effusions as well.[A1] In the setting of cardiac tamponade, however, there is a pronounced increase in the magnitude of inspiratory change in blood flow velocity. With inspiration, right-sided flow velocities are increased by more than 40 percent, while left-sided flow velocities are decreased by more than 40 percent. Figures 23–18 through 23–20 demonstrate this finding, which is known as flow velocity paradoxus.[L6, P2] These variations in flow velocity can be recorded by both pulsed-wave and continuous-wave Doppler. Another measurement that can be derived from spectral Doppler tracings is the isovolumic relaxation time, which is prolonged during inspiration in patients with tamponade. This feature is primarily a result of an inspiratory decrease in the pressure gradient between pulmonary capillary wedge pressure and left ventricular diastolic pressure.[A1] Color Doppler flow mapping can also demonstrate the changes in blood flow velocity caused by cardiac tamponade. Right-sided filling is greatest during inspiration. The tricuspid flow jet by color Doppler appears correspondingly larger during inspiration than during expiration. Conversely, the mitral flow jet is smaller during inspiration.[P4] Thus, the various Doppler modalities are very useful in showing instantly the flow variations associated with respiration during tamponade. However, an exaggerated inspiratory change in blood flow velocities may be noted in patients with obstructive lung disease or even in normal individuals if respiration is highly labored.

A comprehensive cardiac ultrasound examination involving all modalities is necessary to make the diagnosis of tamponade with maximal confidence. By its ability to detect early tamponade, echocardiography is an extremely valuable tool in assessing the hemodynamic significance of a pericardial effusion. However, some patients with a pericardial effusion and wall motion abnormalities consistent with cardiac tamponade appear otherwise stable. Thus, when early tamponade is suspected on the basis of echocardiography, the decision to perform pericardiocentesis rests on additional considerations. These patients warrant very careful observation. Further experience will help identify other causes of falsely positive or falsely negative right atrial collapse and right ventricular diastolic collapse in patients with pericardial effusions.

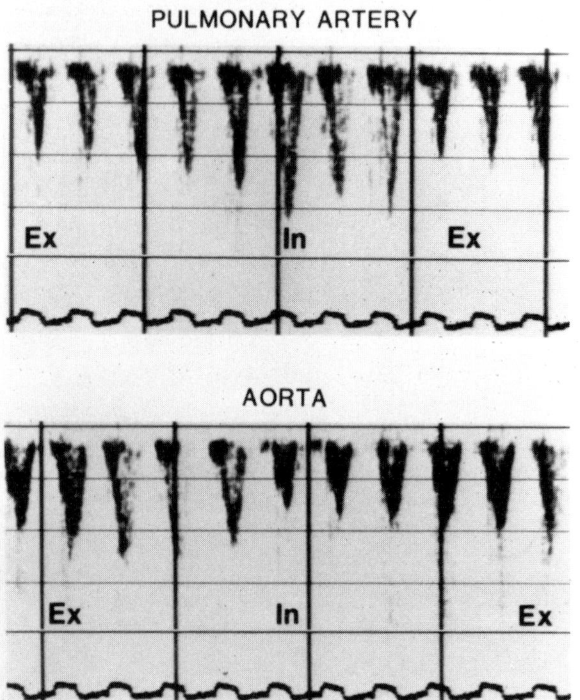

Figure 23–18. Pulmonary artery and aortic blood flow velocity recordings in cardiac tamponade. There is a marked increase in the pulmonary flow velocity during inspiration. Simultaneously, there is a marked decrease in aortic flow velocity. In—inspiration; Ex—expiration.

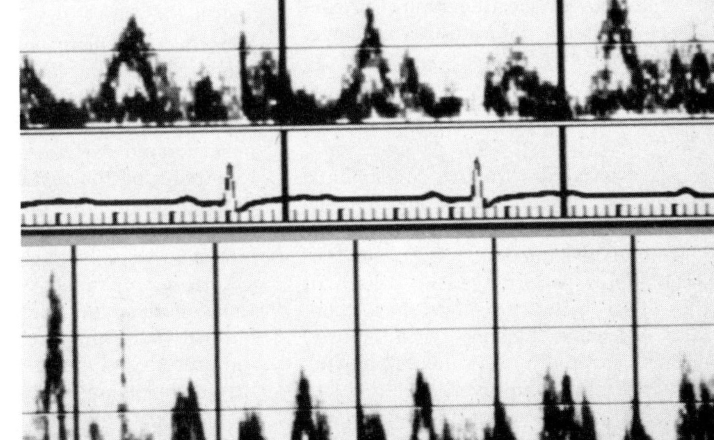

Figure 23–19. Tricuspid flow velocity recordings from a patient with cardiac tamponade, recorded at a fast paper speed on top and at a slower paper speed on the bottom. Both tracings exhibit a marked variation in tricuspid flow velocity. There is a decrease in flow velocity during expiration but an increase in flow velocity during inspiration. TV—tricuspid valve.

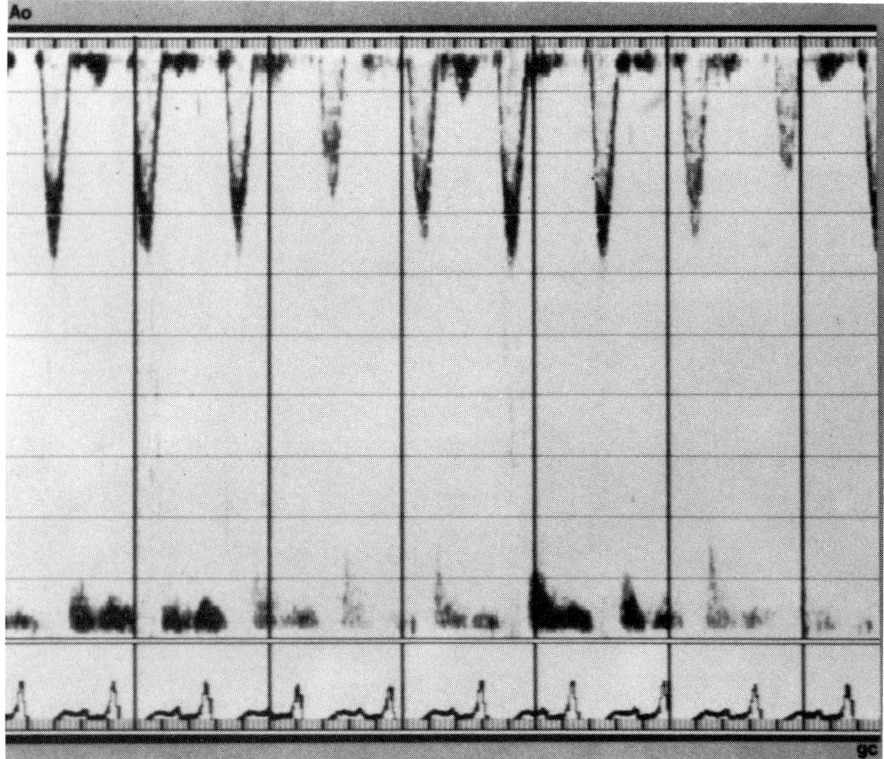

Figure 23–20. Blood flow velocity recording from the aorta of a patient with cardiac tamponade, demonstrating exaggerated cyclic variation in the flow velocity during respiration. Ao—aorta.

Echocardiography During Pericardiocentesis

Once the diagnosis of tamponade has been made, echocardiography may be instrumental in aiding with therapeutic modalities to relieve hemodynamic compromise.[K4, P1, P5] Pericardiocentesis is the preferred procedure for relieving hemodynamic compromise, since previous studies have indicated that temporizing measures (i.e., fluid loading) may not be effective.[K5] When pericardiocentesis is contemplated, it is important to obtain a two-dimensional echocardiographic image of the planned path of the aspiration needle to confirm the presence of fluid in that orientation. Two-dimensional echocardiography is also frequently used as an aid during pericardiocentesis. Under echocardiographic guidance, proper needle and catheter position in the pericardial cavity can be confirmed with confidence, as shown in Figure 23–21.[C3, C4, S8] It is particularly useful during drainage of loculated effusions.[P5] Figure 23–22 shows images before and after pericardiocentesis and illustrates how echocardiography can confirm resolution of chamber compression, indicate the efficacy of drainage, and delineate residual fluid.

CONSTRICTIVE PERICARDITIS

Constrictive pericarditis is associated with two fundamental abnormalities, one anatomic and the other physiologic. The fundamental anatomic feature is a thickened pericardium; the physiologic abnormality is filling dysfunction.[A2, H3, I1, M5, S3, S4, S9] Several M-mode echocardiographic patterns can be consistent with pericardial thickening. They include a single thick echodense line, a double line of echoes moving synchronously, multiple parallel moving lines, and multiple parallel nonmoving lines (Fig. 23–23).[E1, H4, S10] None of these, however, has proved to be reliably diagnostic of thickened pericardium or constrictive pericarditis. The sensitivity and specificity of M-mode features have not been verified in any systematic prospective studies.

Two-dimensional echocardiography may show a bright, thick pericardial echo in patients with thickened pericardium (Figs. 23–24 and 23–25).[P6] In patients with advanced calcific constrictive pericarditis, the pericardium may appear like a shell encompassing the heart, similar to that seen in Figure 23–24. A strong suggestion of constrictive pericarditis can be inferred from this finding. Accurate assessment of pericardial thickness, however, is not possible by M-mode or two-dimensional echocardiographic techniques. Instrument settings such as gain and gray scale profoundly influence the echocardiographic appearance of this structure and make it difficult to assess the presence of a thickened pericardium. In general, two-dimensional echocardiography tends to overestimate the thickness of the pericardial layer. Computed tomography probably is a better approach to quantify pericardial thickness.[I1]

Although limited in assessing pericardial thickness, echocardiographic techniques are useful in defining the filling impairment associated with constrictive pericarditis. The physiologic abnormality in constriction is characterized by impediment to filling during middle and late periods of diastole, when ventricular diastolic expansion is suddenly restricted by the thick, noncompliant pericardium. Consequently, most of the filling occurs early in diastole.[H5, I1] Computer digitization of diastolic left ventricular wall motion may be helpful in demonstrating the degree of abnormality in ventricular expansion. Various qualitative M-mode echocardiographic findings have been reported to be consistent with constrictive physiology. Figure 23–23 shows an example of one of these signs. The left ventricular posterior wall, after normal rapid early-diastolic outward motion, demonstrates flattening during the rest of diastole.[E1, H4, I1] Other M-mode echocardiographic findings reported in constrictive pericarditis include a rapid E-F slope in the mitral valve echogram, paradoxic septal motion, diastolic notching of the interventricular septum, and premature opening of the pulmonic valve.[C5, E2, H3, H6, I1, T1] Mitral valve motion and paradoxic septal motion are nonspecific and insensitive. Premature opening of the pulmonic valve indicates the presence of elevated right ventricular diastolic pressure, but this feature is not specific for constrictive pericarditis and can be found in patients with restrictive cardiomyopathy as well.[T1] The finding of an early and/or late diastolic notch in the interventricular septum, shown in Figure 23–26, is relatively more frequently observed in constrictive pericarditis.[C5, E2, I1] The sensitivity and specificity of this M-mode echocardiographic sign, however, are not known.

Two-dimensional echocardiography in patients with constriction usually demonstrates a normal-sized heart with preserved left and right ventricular systolic function. As pointed out earlier,

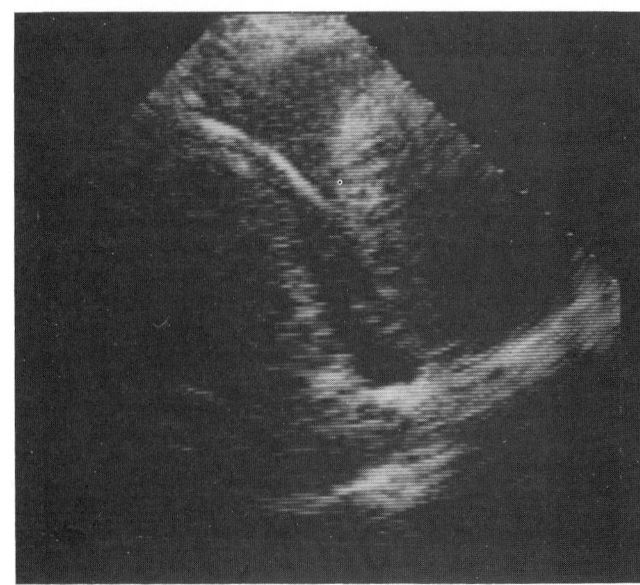

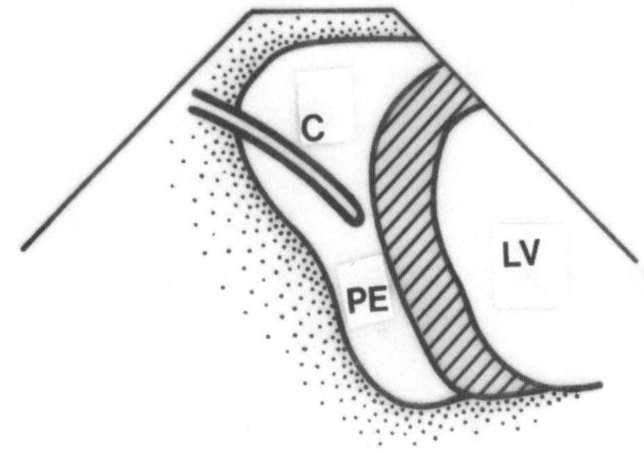

Figure 23–21. Two-dimensional echocardiographic images obtained during pericardiocentesis. A large effusion is seen surrounding the left ventricle. A catheter that has been introduced into the pericardial cavity is seen as a bright linear echo. LV—left ventricle; PE—pericardial effusion; C—catheter.

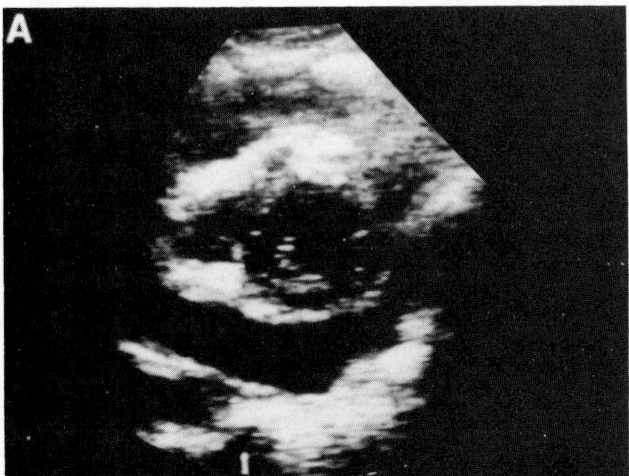

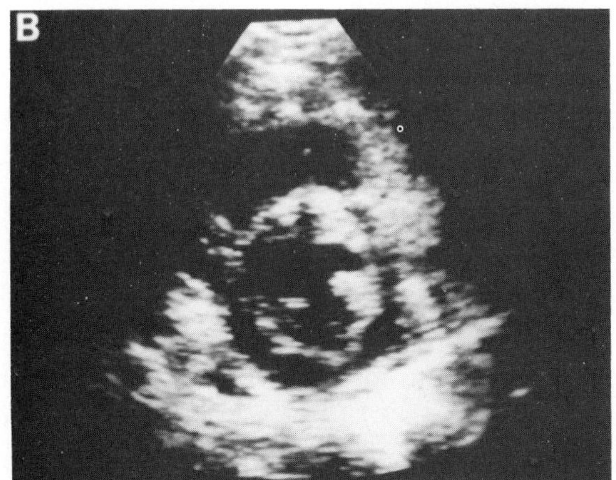

Figure 23–22. Parasternal short-axis images from a patient with cardiac tamponade before (*A*) and after (*B*) pericardiocentesis. A large pericardial effusion is seen prior to pericardiocentesis. The image obtained following the procedure demonstrates absence of fluid in the pericardial cavity.

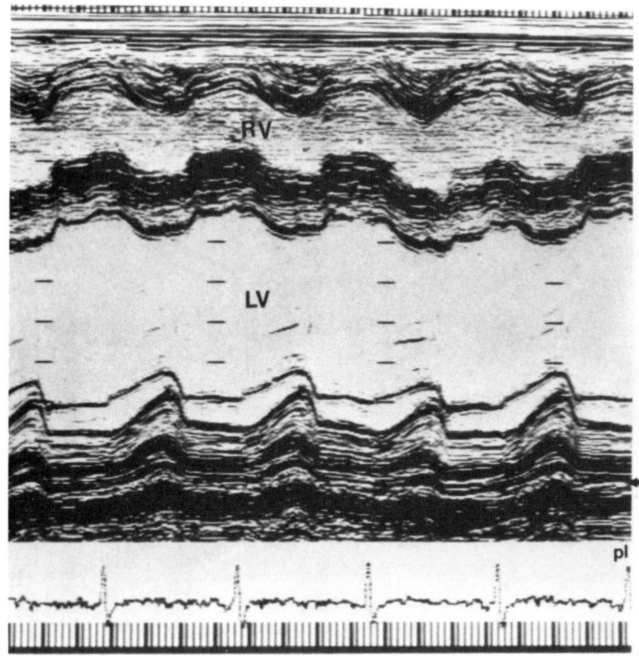

Figure 23–23. M-mode echocardiographic recording from a patient with constrictive pericarditis. The pericardial echo (*arrow*) is seen as multiple dense layers moving in concert. The left ventricular posterior wall demonstrates a rapid relaxation at early diastole but appears flattened during the rest of diastole. RV—right ventricle; LV—left ventricle.

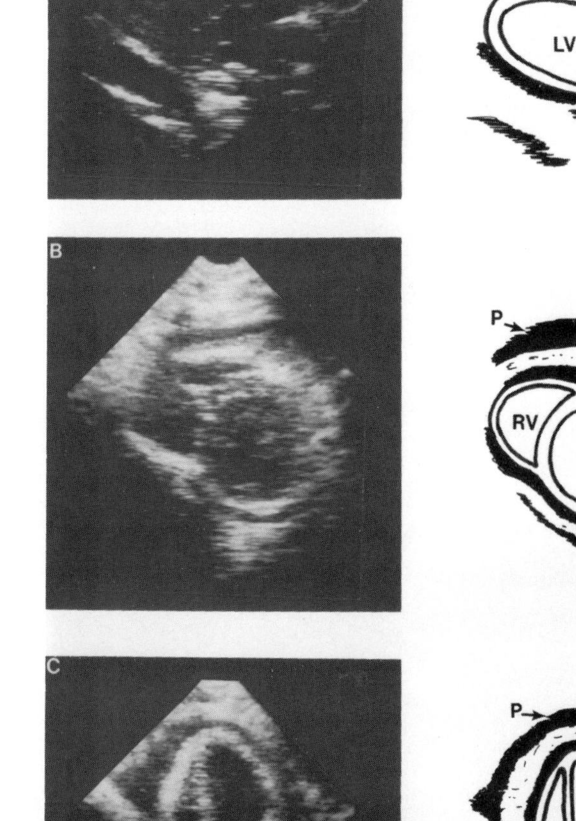

Figure 23–24. Two-dimensional echocardiographic images from a patient with constrictive pericarditis. *A*, Parasternal long-axis view; *B*, parasternal short-axis view; *C*, apical four-chamber view. The pericardial echo appears thickened and bright. There is a shell-like appearance around the heart. Computed tomography demonstrated markedly thickened pericardium and no pericardial effusion. RV—right ventricle; LV—left ventricle; P—pericardium.

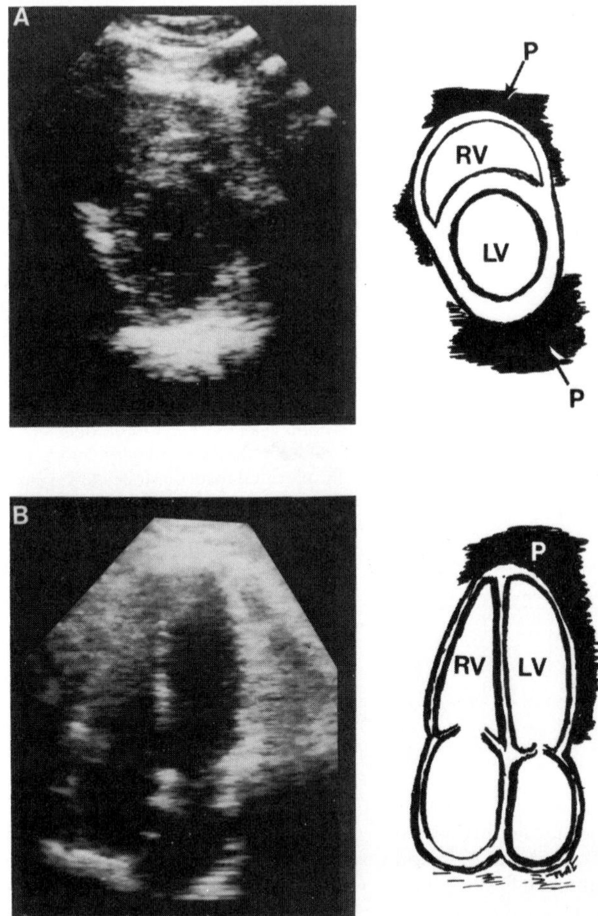

Figure 23–25. Parasternal short-axis *(A)* and apical four-chamber *(B)* two-dimensional echocardiographic images from a patient with constrictive pericarditis. In both images, the pericardium appears bright and thickened. Computed tomography in this patient demonstrated a markedly thickened pericardium. RV—right ventricle; LV—left ventricle; P—pericardium.

the pericardial echo generally appears bright and thick. A repeated finding in patients with constriction is a brisk, early diastolic bouncing motion of the interventricular septum, evident particularly during inspiration.[H2, P6] This finding has been reported to have 93 percent specificity and 62 percent sensitivity. Plethora of the inferior vena cava, described earlier, is another two-dimensional echocardiographic sign noted in constrictive pericarditis.[H2]

Filling dysfunction associated with constrictive pericarditis can be assessed by two-dimensional echocardiography. With frame-by-frame measurement of the cavity area during the cardiac cycle, a filling curve can be constructed. Such analysis may reveal that most of the diastolic filling occurs during the first third or half of diastole. Although this approach demonstrates the characteristic filling pattern of constrictive pericarditis, the method is tedious and may be impossible to perform when the endocardial borders of the left ventricle are indistinct.[P6]

Both the filling dysfunction of constrictive pericarditis and the abnormal respiratory influence on filling are reflected in the pattern of intracardiac and venous flows. Doppler echocardiography allows evaluation of such abnormalities, as illustrated in Figure 23–27. Examination of the mitral flow velocity in constrictive pericarditis shows a markedly increased early diastolic filling velocity (E velocity) with a rapid deceleration and a decreased late diastolic filling velocity following atrial contraction (A velocity), resulting in an increased E/A ratio.[A2, A3, H5, K3] This finding, however, is not specific for constriction and may be noted with restrictive cardiomyopathy and with severe mitral regurgitation. Such analysis of mitral flow may be difficult in patients who are tachycardic and is not possible in the presence of atrial fibrillation. Nevertheless, in a patient known to have a thickened pericardium who has sinus rhythm and does not have severe mitral regurgitation, observation of an increased E/A ratio and a rapid deceleration slope of the early filling wave strongly suggests constrictive physiology.

The filling dysfunction in constrictive pericarditis is associated with elevated ventricular diastolic pressures. Certain Doppler findings can indicate the presence of elevated ventricular diastolic pressure. If right ventricular diastolic pressure exceeds right atrial pressure, diastolic tricuspid regurgitation can occur. Right

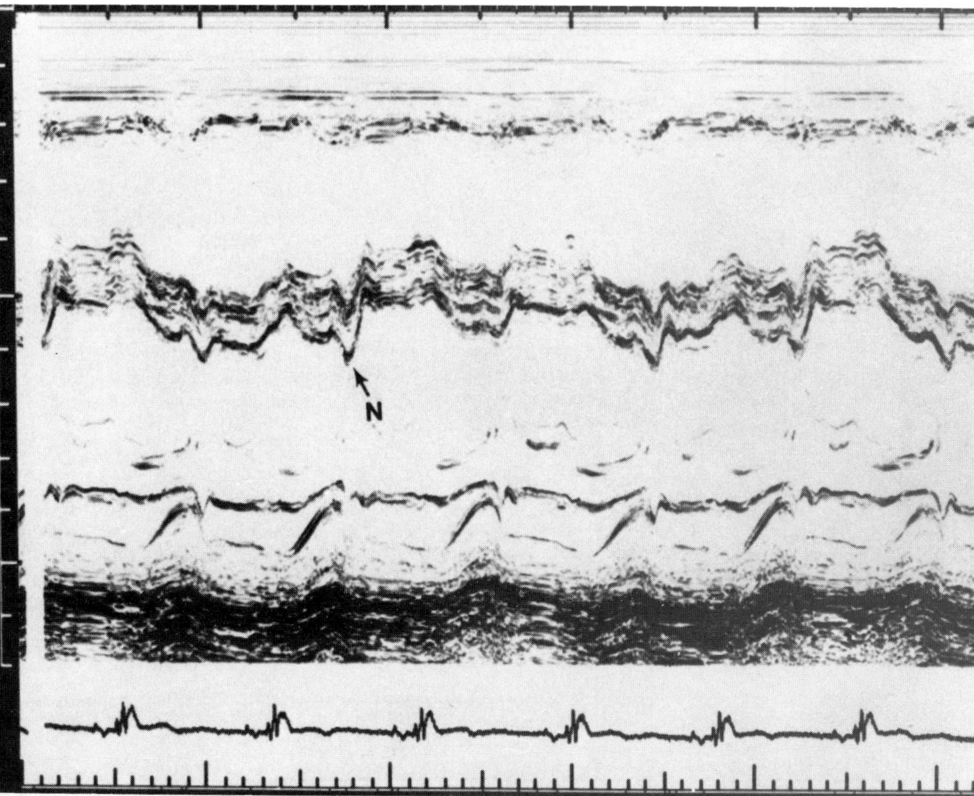

Figure 23–26. M-mode echocardiographic tracing in a patient with constrictive pericarditis. An early diastolic notch (*N*) is evident on the interventricular septum.

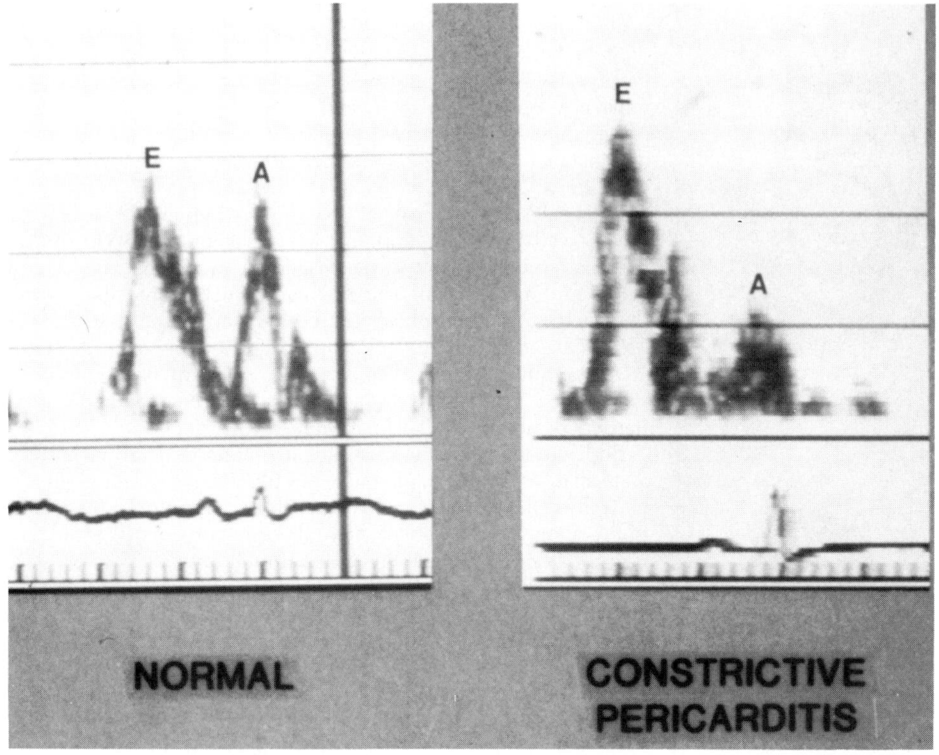

Figure 23–27. Pulsed Doppler recording of mitral flow velocity from a normal subject and from a patient with constrictive pericarditis. Compared to the normal pattern, the patient with constrictive pericarditis exhibits a markedly increased early diastolic velocity (E), a rapid deceleration of the early diastolic velocity, and a markedly elevated late diastolic flow velocity (A).

ventricular diastolic pressure may also transiently exceed pulmonary artery pressure. This reversal of the usual pressure gradient leads to premature opening of the pulmonary valve with resulting diastolic antegrade flow into the pulmonary artery (Fig. 23–28).[K3] Diastolic mitral regurgitation may also be found in some patients. These findings, however, are encountered in patients with restrictive cardiomyopathy as well.[K6]

Another feature noted in patients with constrictive pericarditis is an exaggerated respiratory variation in the velocity of right-sided and left-sided flows, with more than 25 percent difference between inspiratory and expiratory values.[P2] During inspiration, there is an increase in right-sided flow velocities and a corresponding decrease in left-sided flow velocities. The mitral valve tracings shown in Figure 23–29 demonstrate these changes.

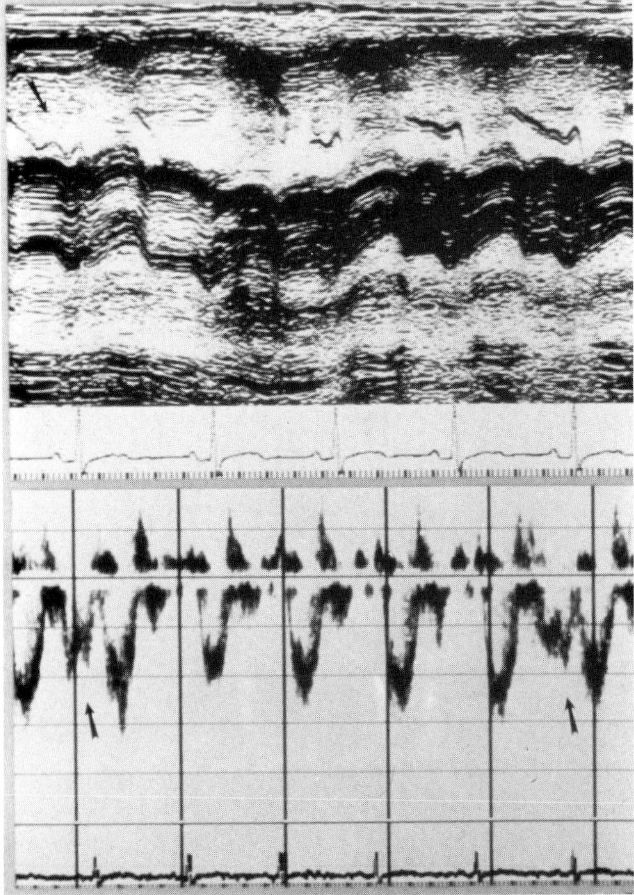

Figure 23–28. M-mode recording of the pulmonary valve and pulsed Doppler recording of pulmonary artery blood flow velocity. The pulmonary valve shows premature opening, and the pulmonary blood flow velocity recording shows intermittent diastolic antegrade flow into the pulmonary artery (*arrows*). This diastolic flow pattern occurred during inspiration.

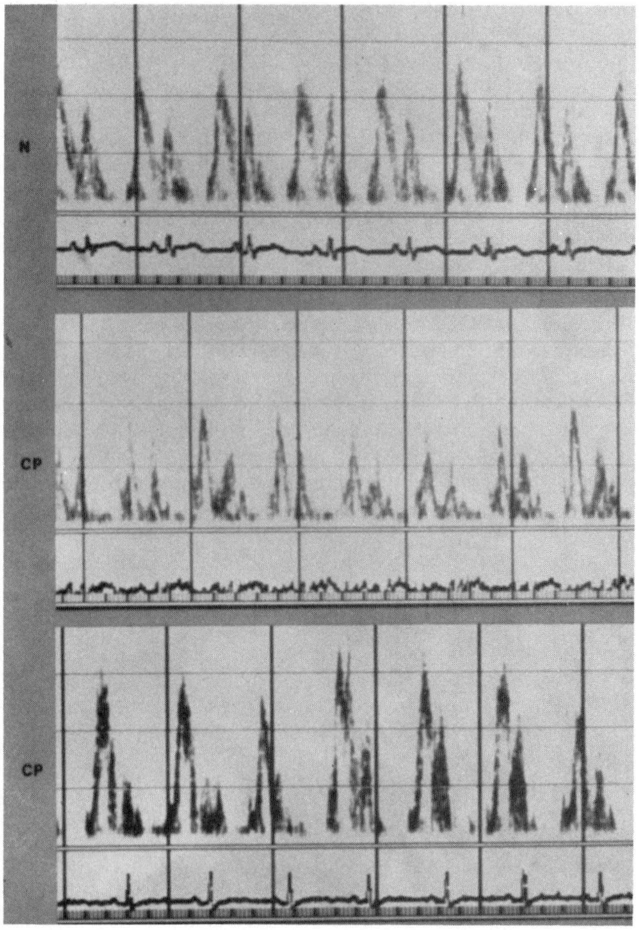

N

CP

CP

Figure 23–29. Mitral flow velocity recordings from a normal subject (N) and from two patients with constrictive pericarditis (CP). In contrast to the minimal respiratory variation in mitral flow velocity seen in the normal patient, a markedly exaggerated variation in the mitral flow velocity is noted in the patients with constrictive pericarditis.

Respiratory variation is seen in the left ventricular isovolumic relaxation time as well; this parameter decreases during expiration and increases during inspiration.[H5] These respiratory changes in flow dynamics are also useful in differentiating constrictive pericarditis from restrictive cardiomyopathy. In contrast to patients with constrictive pericarditis, patients with restrictive cardiomyopathy do not exhibit the exaggerated respiratory changes in flow velocities and isovolumic relaxation time.[H5] Analysis of superior vena caval and hepatic vein flow velocity recordings is also useful in differentiating constriction from restriction. In patients with constriction, the systolic component of the systemic venous flow velocity is increased, corresponding to the deep *x* descent on pressure tracings. Alternatively, the diastolic antegrade component, which corresponds to the *y* descent, is prominent in restrictive cardiomyopathy.[A3]

In effusive-constrictive pericarditis, echocardiography demonstrates the presence of a clear or organized pericardial effusion. There are usually echocardiographic features consistent with cardiac tamponade or constriction. In contrast to tamponade, in which the flow abnormalities registered by Doppler typically resolve after pericardiocentesis, there is persistent evidence of elevated diastolic pressures in patients with effusive-constrictive pericarditis.

ECHOCARDIOGRAPHIC FINDINGS IN CERTAIN SPECIFIC DISORDERS

Acute and Chronic Pericarditis

Acute pericarditis is diagnosed clinically on the basis of the symptom of respirophasic pain, the presence of a pericardial friction rub, and characteristic electrocardiographic features. The causes of acute pericarditis are legion and include viral illness, bacterial and mycobacterial infection, myocardial infarction, systemic disease, drugs, and radiation.[A4, B2–B4, C6, H6, J1, K7, K8, R4, R5, T2, Y1] Pericardial effusion may be noted in patients with acute pericarditis, but its absence does not exclude the diagnosis. When present, the effusion is usually small, but occasionally a large amount of fluid accumulates and cardiac tamponade may result. The size of the effusion and the presence of tamponade can be evaluated by echocardiography based on the features previously described. However, the etiology of the effusion cannot be determined echocardiographically. Not infrequently, the inflammatory process may progress and lead to the development of constrictive pericarditis.[C6, C7] Close echocardiographic follow-up may be warranted in these patients.

Neoplastic Pericardial Disease

Pericardial involvement in malignant disease can occur via contiguous spread or metastatic implants. Carcinoma of the breast and lung, leukemia, lymphoma, and melanoma have the highest incidence of cardiac involvement. Primary malignant tumors of the heart, including angiosarcoma, mesothelioma, fibrosarcoma, and rhabdomyomas, may involve the pericardium. The pericardium is the predominant site of neoplasm in 85 percent of patients with cardiac malignancies.[E3] Pericardial effusion with or without tamponade is the major manifestation of neoplastic pericardial disease. In addition, solid tumor masses occupying the pericardial cavity have been visualized with two-dimensional echocardiography, as shown in Figure 23–10.[C1] Besides revealing the presence of pericardial effusion and offering guidance during pericardiocentesis, repeat post-pericardiocentesis studies are useful because the fluid frequently reaccumulates. Cardiac constriction secondary to encasement of the heart by a tumor may occur, and this can also be identified.[L4] Thus, echocardiography provides diagnostic information regarding pericardial neoplasms and can be instrumental in facilitating their treatment.

Traumatic Pericardial Disease

Several previously described disorders of the pericardium (cardiac tamponade, constrictive pericarditis, etc.) have been associated with trauma.[P7] Since the echocardiographic findings in these disorders were mentioned earlier, attention here is given only to traumatic entities that were not previously discussed. Penetrating wounds of the chest or inadvertent surgical disruption of the thoracic duct can result in a chylous effusion that is echocardiographically indistinct from other effusions.[E3] However, if fat globules or fibrinous debris is present in the effusion, echo densities may be observed within the echo-free space. As always, analysis of the fluid is necessary to confirm the diagnosis. Pneumopericardium can be seen secondary to penetrating wounds of the chest, esophageal rupture, gastric rupture, or infections involving gas-producing organisms and may result in cardiac tamponade.[B5] Echocardiography may demonstrate an "air gap" in the pericardium, although on a plain chest film air can usually be seen between the heart and the pericardium.[R6]

Pericardial Cysts

Pericardial cysts are uncommon, round or oval-shaped dilations of the pericardium containing varying amounts of pericardial fluid. The congenital type is most often located at the right cardiophrenic angle but can be seen in almost any position.[F4] Acquired cysts can be caused by neoplastic infiltration of the pericardium, trauma, or infection. The pericardial cyst may resemble a ventricular aneurysm, cardiac mass, mediastinal tumor, or hiatal hernia on a plain chest film. Confirmation of a fluid-filled outpouching of pericardium seen echocardiographically allows the diagnosis of a cyst to be made.[N2] Calcium deposits in the cyst wall may also be noted.[P8] Occasionally, such cysts may rupture and therefore not be present on follow-up studies.[K9]

Absence of Pericardium

Complete absence of the pericardium is a rare congenital anomaly. Most of these patients are asymptomatic despite the loss of the stabilizing effect of the pericardium.[S11] Without the pericardium, there is no ability to contain expansion of the ventricles during cardiac filling. Congenital absence of the left pericardium, while rare, does occur more frequently than absence of the entire pericardium. In individuals with complete absence of the pericardium, echocardiographic imaging reveals apparent enlargement of the right ventricle and paradoxic septal motion, mimicking right ventricular volume overload. These findings are also noted in patients who have undergone surgical removal of the pericardium.[P9] Rare cases of strangulation and/or herniation of portions of the heart have been reported in patients with partial absence of the pericardium.[C8, M6] Protrusion of the left atrial appendage through the pericardial defect may lead to expansion or aneurysm formation of the left atrium, which can be visualized on the two-dimensional echocardiogram. The low specificity of many of these echocardiographic features makes it difficult to diagnose absence of the pericardium with confidence. Computerized tomography can more accurately identify this anomaly.

CONCLUSION

Echocardiography has become the technique of choice for the assessment of most disorders involving the pericardium. A comprehensive examination with multiple echocardiographic modalities is necessary for proper delineation of the morphologic and physiologic abnormalities associated with pericardial diseases. In addition to its diagnostic capability, echocardiography contributes by guiding and monitoring therapeutic interventions.

References

A

1. Appleton, C.P., Hatle, L.K., and Popp, R.L.: Cardiac tamponade and pericardial effusion: Respiratory variation in transvalvular flow velocities studied by Doppler echocardiography J. Am. Coll. Cardiol. 11: 1020, 1988.
2. Agatson, A.S., Rao, A., Price, R.J., and Kenney, E.L.: Diagnosis of constrictive pericarditis by pulsed Doppler echocardiography. Am. J. Cardiol. 54:929, 1984.
3. Appleton, C.P., Hatle, L.K., and Popp, R.L.: Central venous flow velocity patterns can differentiate constrictive pericarditis from restrictive cardiomyopathy. (Abstract.) J. Am. Coll. Cardiol. 9 (Suppl. A):119A, 1987.
4. Applefield, M.M., Cole, J.F., Pollack, S.H., et al.: The late appearance of chronic pericardial disease in patients treated by radiotherapy for Hodgkin's disease. Ann. Intern. Med. 94:338, 1981.

B

1. Braunwald, E. (ed.): Heart Disease. A Textbook of Cardiovascular Medicine. 3rd ed. W.B. Saunders, Philadelphia, 1988, p. 83.
2. Baldwin, J.J., and Edwards, J.E.: Uremic pericarditis as a cause of cardiac tamponade. Circulation 53:896, 1976.
3. Berger, H.W., and Seckler, S.G.: Pleural and pericardial effusions in rheumatoid disease. Ann. Intern. Med. 64:1291, 1966.
4. Botti, R.E., Driscol, T.E., Pearson, O.H., and Smith, J.C.: Radiation myocardial fibrosis simulating constrictive pericarditis. Cancer 22:1254, 1968.
5. Bedotto, J.B., McBride, W., Abraham, M., and Taylor, A.I.: Echocardiographic diagnosis of pneumopericardium and hydropneumopericardium. J. Am. Soc. Echo. 1:359, 1988.

C

1. Chandraratna, P.A., and Aronow, W.S.: Detection of pericardial metastasis by cross-sectional echocardiography. Circulation 63:54, 1981.
2. Cummings, R.G., Wesley, R.L.R., Adams, D.H., and Lowe, J.E.: Pneumopericardium resulting in cardiac tamponade. Ann. Thorac. Surg. 37:511, 1984.
3. Callahan, J.A., Seward, J.B., and Tajik, A.J.: Pericardiocentesis assisted by two-dimensional echocardiography. J. Thorac. Cardiovasc. Surg. 85:877, 1983.
4. Callahan, J.A., Seward, J.B., and Tajik, A.J.: Cardiac tamponade pericardiocentesis directed by two dimensional echocardiography. Mayo Clin. Proc. 60:344, 1985.
5. Candell-Riera, J., DelCastillo, A.G., Dermanger-Miralda, G., and Soler-Soler, J.: Echocardiographic features of the interventricular septum in chronic constrictive pericarditis. Circulation 57:1154, 1978.
6. Cameron, J., Osterle, S.N., Baldwon, J.C., and Hancock, E.W.: The etiologic spectrum of constrictive pericarditis. Am. Heart J. 113:354, 1987.
7. Cohen, M.V., and Greenberg, M.A.: Constrictive pericarditis: Early and late complication of cardiac surgery. Am. J. Cardiol. 43:657, 1979.
8. Cassosla, L., and Katz, J.A.: Management of cardiac herniation after intrapericardial pneumonectomy. Anesthesiology 60:362, 1984.

D

1. D'Cruz, I.A., Cohen, H.C., Prabbu, R., and Glick, G.: Diagnosis of cardiac tamponade by echocardiography: changes in mitral valve motion and ventricular dimensions with special reference to paradoxical pulse. Circulation 52:460, 1975.
2. Dabestani, A., Takenak, K., Allen, B., et al.: Effects of spontaneous respiration on diastolic left ventricular filling assessed by pulsed Doppler echocardiography. Am. J. Cardiol. 61:1356, 1988.
3. D'Cruz, I.A., Cohen, H.C., Prabbu, R., and Glick, G.: Potential pitfalls in quantification of pericardial effusion by echocardiography. Br. Heart J. 39:529, 1977.

E

1. Engel, P.J., Fowler, N.O., Tei, C., et al.: M-mode echocardiography in constrictive pericarditis. J. Am. Coll. Cardiol. 6:471, 1985.
2. Elkayam, U., Kotler, M.N., Segal, B., and Parry, W.: Echocardiographic findings in constrictive pericarditis: A case report. J. Med. Sci. 12:1308, 1976.
3. Eagle, K.A., Haber, E., DeSanctis, R.W., and Austen, G.W. (eds.): The Practice of Cardiology. 2nd ed. Little Brown, Boston, 1989, p. 977.

F

1. Feigenbaum, H. (ed.): Echocardiography. 4th ed. Lea & Febiger, Philadelphia, 1986, p. 548.
2. Feigenbaum, H., Waldhauser, J.A., and Hyde, L.P.: Ultrasonic diagnosis of pericardial effusion. JAMA 191:107, 1965.
3. Feigenbaum, H., Zacky, A., and Grabborn, L.: Cardiac motion in patients with pericardial effusion: A study using ultrasound cardiography. Circulation 34:611, 1966.
4. Feign, D.S.Z., Ferrogli, J.J., McCallister, H.A., and Madewell, J.E.: Pericardial cyst: A radiologic pathologic correlation and review. Radiology 15:125, 1977.

G

1. Gabor, G.E., Winsberg, F., and Bloom, H.S.: Electrical and mechanical alternation in pericardial effusion. Chest 59:341, 1971.
2. Gaffney, F.A., Keller, A.M., Perchock, R.M., et al.: Pathophysiologic mechanisms of cardiac tamponade and pulsus alternans shown by echocardiography. Am. J. Cardiol. 53:1662, 1984.
3. Gillam, L.D., Guyer, D.E., Gibson, T.E., et al.: Hydrostatic compression of the right atrium: A new echocardiographic sign of cardiac tamponade. Circulation 68:294, 1983.

H

1. Horowitz, M.S., Schully, C.S., Stinson, E.B., et al.: Sensitivity and specificity of echocardiographic diagnosis of pericardial effusion. Circulation 50:239, 1974.
2. Himelman, R.B., Lee, E., and Schiller, N.B.: Septal bounce, vena cava plethora and pericardial adhesion: Informative two-dimensional echocardiographic signs in the diagnosis of pericardial constriction. J. Am. Soc. Echo. 1:333, 1988.
3. Hancock, W.E.: On the elastic and rigid forms of constrictive pericarditis. Am. Heart J. 100:917, 1980.
4. Horowitz, M.S., Rossen, R., and Harrison, D.C.: Echocardiographic diagnosis of pericardial disease. Am. Heart J. 97:420, 1979.
5. Hatle, L.K., Appleton, C.P., and Popp, R.L.: Constrictive pericarditis and restrictive cardiomyopathy, differentiation by Doppler recording of atrioventricular flow velocities. (Abstract.) J. Am. Coll. Cardiol. 9 (Suppl. A):119A, 1987.
6. Hochberg, M.S., Merrill, W.H., Bruber, M., et al.: Delayed cardiac tamponade associated with prophylactic anticoagulation in patients undergoing coronary bypass grafting: Early diagnosis with two-dimensional echocardiography. J. Thorac. Cardiovasc. Surg. 75:777, 1978.

I

1. Isner, J.M., Pandian, N.G., McInerney, K.P., et al.: The pericardial tourniquet: Evaluation of the anatomic and physiologic features of constrictive pericarditis by combined use of computed tomography and cardiac ultrasound. Echocardiography 2:197, 1985.

J

1. John, T.J., Hough, A., and Sergent, J.S.: Pericardial disease in rheumatoid arthritis. Am. J. Med. 66:383, 1979.

K

1. Kraeger, S.K., Zucker, R.P., Ozindzro, B.S., and Forker, A.D.: Swinging heart syndrome with predominant anterior pericardial effusion. J. Clin. Ultrasound 4:113, 1976.
2. Kronzon, I., Cohen, M.L., and Winer, H.E.: Diastolic atrial compression: A sensitive echocardiographic sign of cardiac tamponade. J. Am. Coll. Cardiol. 2:770, 1983.
3. King, W.S., Pandian, N.G., and Gardin, J.M.: Doppler echocardiographic findings in pericardial tamponade and constriction. Echocardiography 5:361, 1988.
4. Kopecky, S.L., Callahan, J.A., Tajik, A.J., and Seward, J.B.: Percutaneous pericardial catheter drainage: Report of 42 consecutive cases. Am. J. Cardiol. 50:633, 1986.
5. Kerber, R.E., Gascho, J.A., Litchfield, R., et al.: Hemodynamic effects of volume expansion and nitroprusside compared with pericardiocentesis in patients with acute cardiac tamponade. N. Engl. J. Med. 307:929, 1982.
6. Klein, A.L., Hatle, L.K., Bursytow, D.J., et al.: Doppler characterization of left ventricular function in cardiac amyloidosis. J. Am. Coll. Cardiol. 13:1017, 1989.
7. Kottiner, M.P., Ritkaranta, D.P., Heikineuf, L.O., et al.: Esophagia-pericardial fistula. A case report and review of the literature. Thorac. Cardiovasc. Surg. 33:341, 1985.
8. Krikorian, J.G., and Hancock, E.W.: Pericardiocentesis. Am. J. Med. 65:808, 1978.
9. King, J.F., Corby, I., Pugh, D., and Reed, W.: Rupture of pericardial cyst. Chest 60:611, 1971.

L

1. Leimbruger, P.P., Klopfenstein, S., Wann, L.S., and Brooks, H.L.: The hemodynamic derangement associated with right ventricular collapse in cardiac tamponade: An experimental echocardiographic study. Circulation 689:612, 1983.
2. Levisman, J.A., and Abbas, A.A.: Abnormal motion of the mitral valve with pericardial effusion: Pseudoprolapse of the mitral valve. Am. Heart J. 91:18, 1976.
3. Lewandowski, B.J., Jaffer, N.M., and Winsberg, F.: Relationship between the pericardial and pleural spaces in cross sectional imaging. J. Clin. Ultrasound 9:272, 1981.
4. Lin, T.K., Stech, J.M., Echert, W.G., et al.: Pericardial angiosarcoma simulating pericardial effusion by echocardiography. Chest 73:881, 1978.
5. Labib, S., Udelson, J., and Pandian, N.G.: Echocardiography in low pressure cardiac tamponade. Am. J. Cardiol. 63:1156, 1989.
6. Leeman, D.E., Levine, M.J., and Come, P.C.: Doppler echocardiography in cardiac tamponade: Exaggerated respiratory variation in transvalvular flow velocity integrals. J. Am. Coll. Cardiol. 11:572, 1988.

M

1. Matuso, H., Matsumoto, M., Hamarrha, Y., et al.: Rotational excursion of the heart in massive pericardial effusion studied by phased-array echocardiography. Br. Heart J. 41:513, 1979.
2. Martin, R.P., Bowden, R., Filly, K., and Popp, R.L.: Intrapericardial abnormalities in patients with pericardial effusion: Findings by two-dimensional echocardiography. Circulation 61:568, 1980.
3. Millman, A., Meller, J., Motro, M., et al.: Pericardial tumor or fibrosis mimicking pericardial effusion by echocardiography. Ann. Intern. Med. 86:434, 1977.
4. Martins, J.B., and Kerber, R.E.: Can cardiac tamponade be diagnosed by echocardiography?; experimental studies. Circulation 60:733, 1979.
5. Marsa, R., Mehta, S., Willis, W., and Baily, L.: Constrictive pericarditis after myocardial revascularization: Report of 3 cases. Am. J. Cardiol. 44:177, 1979.
6. Minocha, G.K., Falicon, R.E., and Nyensohn, E.: Partial right sided congenital pericardial defect with herniation of the right atrium and right ventricle. Chest 76:484, 1979.

N

1. Nanda, N.C., Gramiak, R., and Gross, C.M.: Echocardiography of cardiac valves in pericardial effusion. Circulation 54:50, 1976.
2. Nasser, W.K.: Congenital disease of the pericardium. Cardiovasc. Clin. 7:271, 1976.

P

1. Pandian, N.G., Rosenfield, K., and Mohanty, P.K.: Left ventricular diastolic collapse—an echocardiographic sign of cardiac tamponade caused by loculated pericardial effusion in post operative patients. Circulation. (Suppl. IV) 76:IV–192, 1987.
2. Pandian, N.G., Rifkin, R.D., and Wang, S.S.: Flow velocity paradoxus—a Doppler echocardiographic sign of cardiac tamponade: Exaggerated respiratory variation in pulmonary and aortic blood flow velocities. (Abstract.) Circulation (Suppl. II) 70:II–381, 1984.
3. Pandian, N.G., Wang, S.S., McInerney, K., et al.: Doppler echocardiography in cardiac tamponade abnormalities in tricuspid and mitral flow response to respiration in experimental and clinical tamponade. (Abstract.) J. Am. Coll. Cardiol. 5:485, 1985.
4. Pandian, N.G., Wang, S.S., Moten, M., et al.: Color Doppler study of tricuspid and mitral flow changes in cardiac tamponade. (Abstract.) Circulation (Suppl. IV) 76: IV–525, 1987.
5. Pandian, N.G., Brockway, B., Simonetti, J., et al.: Pericardiocentesis under two-dimensional echocardiographic guidance in loculated pericardial effussion. Ann. Thorac. Surg. 45:99, 1988.
6. Pandian, N.G., Skorton, D.J., Kiesco, R.A., and Kerber, R.E.: Diagnosis of constrictive pericarditis by two-dimensional echocardiography; studies in a new experimental model and in patients. J. Am. Coll. Cardiol. 4:1164, 1984.
7. Pandian, N.G., Weintraub, A., Kusay, B.S., et al.: Emergency echocardiography. Echocardiography 6:1, 1989.
8. Pugatch, R.D., Braner, J.H., Robbins, A.H., and Failing, L.J.: CT diagnosis of pericardial cysts. AJR 131:515, 1978.
9. Payvandi, N.M., and Kerber, R.E.: Echocardiography in congenital and acquired absence of the pericardium. Circulation 53:86, 1976.

R

1. Ratshin, R.A., Smith, M.K., and Hood, W.P., Jr.: Possible false positive diagnosis of pericardial effusion by echocardiography in the presence of large left atrium. Chest 65:112, 1974.
2. Rifkin, R.D., Isner, J.M., Carter, B.L., and Bankoff, M.S.: Combined posteroanterior subepicardial fat simulating the echocardiographic diagnosis of pericardial effusion. J. Am. Coll. Cardiol. 3:1333, 1984.
3. Rifkin, R.D., Pandian, N.G., Funai, J.T., et al.: Sensitivity of right atrial collapse and right ventricular diastolic collapse in the diagnosis of graded cardiac tamponade. Am. J. Noninvas. Cardiol. 1:73, 1987.
4. Roberts, W.C., and Spray, T.L.: Pericardial heart disease: A study of its causes, consequences, and morphologic features. Cardiovasc. Clin. 7:67, 1976.
5. Rooney, J.J., Crocco, J.A., and Lynon, H.A.: Tuberculous pericarditis. Ann. Intern. Med. 64:1291, 1966.
6. Reid, C.L., Chandraratna, A.W., Kawanishi, D., et al.: Echocardiographic detection of pneumomediastinum and pneumopericardium: The air gap sign J. Am. Coll. Cardiol. 1:916, 1983.

S

1. Schiller, N.B., and Botvinich, E.H.: Right ventricular compression as a sign of cardiac tamponade: An analysis of echocardiographic ventricular dimensions and their clinical implications. Circulation 56:774, 1977.
2. Settle, H.P., Adolph, R.J., Fowler, N.O., et al.: Echocardiographic study of cardiac tamponade. Circulation 56:951, 1977.
3. Shabetai, R.: The pathophysiology of cardiac tamponade and constriction. Cardiovasc. Clin. 7:67, 1976.

4. Shabetai, R., Fowler, N.O., and Guntheroth, W.G.: The hemodynamics of cardiac tamponade and constrictive pericarditis. Am. J. Cardiol. 26:480, 1970.
5. Shiina, S., Yagirymat, T., Kondo, K., et al.: Echocardiographic evaluation of inpending cardiac tamponade. J. Cardiogr. 9:555, 1979.
6. Singh, S., Wann, S., Schuchard, G.H., et al.: Right ventricular and right atrial collapse in patients with cardiac tamponade—a combined echocardiographic and hemodynamic study. Circulation 68:294, 1983.
7. Schiavone, W.A., Calafiore, P.A., and Salcedo, E.E.: Transesophageal Doppler echocardiographic demonstration of pulmonary venous flow velocity in restrictive cardiomyopathy and constrictive pericarditis. Am. J. Cardiol. 63:1286, 1989.
8. Santos, G.H., and Rrater, R.W.M.: The subxyphoid approach in the treatment of pericardial effusion. Ann. Thorac. Surg. 23:467, 1977.
9. Siegel, R.J., Shak, P.K., and Fishbein, M.C.: Idiopathic restrictive cardiomyopathy. Circulation 70:163, 1984.
10. Siqueira-Fihlo, A.G., Cunha, C.L.P., Tajik, A.J., et al.: M-mode and two-dimensional echocardiographic features in cardiac amyloidosis. Circulation 63:188, 1981.
11. Southworth, H., and Stevenson, C.S.: Congenital defects of the pericardium. Arch. Intern. Med. 61:223, 1938.

T

1. Tanaka, C., Nishimoto, M., Takeudi, K., et al.: Presystolic pulmonary valve opening in constrictive pericarditis. Jpn. Heart J. 20:419, 1979.
2. Thadani, U., Ivenson, J.M.I., and Wright, V.: Cardiac tamponade, constrictive pericarditis and pericardial resection in rheumatoid arthritis. Medicine 54:261, 1975.

U

1. Usher, B.W., and Popp, R.L.: Electrical alternans, mechanisms in pericardial effusion. Am. Heart J. 83:459, 1972.

Y

1. Yurchak, P.M., Levine, S.A., and Gorlin, R.: Constrictive pericarditis complicating disseminated lupus erythematosus. Circulation 31:113, 1965.

Chapter 24

Two-Dimensional and Doppler Echocardiography in the Evaluation of Congenital Heart Disease

▪ *A. REBECCA SNIDER, M.D.* ▪ *A. RESAI BENGUR, M.D.*

CONGENITAL HEART DISEASE WITH ACYANOSIS AND INCREASED PULMONARY BLOOD FLOW 479
Ventricular Septal Defects 479
Atrial Septal Defects 483
Patent Ductus Arteriosus 483
Atrioventricular Septal Defects 486
Doppler Quantitation of Left-to-Right Shunts 487
CONGENITAL HEART DISEASE WITH VENTRICULAR OUTFLOW OBSTRUCTION 489
Left Ventricular Outflow Obstruction 489
Right Ventricular Outflow Obstruction 492
CONGENITAL HEART DISEASE WITH CYANOSIS AND DECREASED PULMONARY VASCULARITY 492
Defects With a Right-to-Left Shunt at Ventricular Level 492
Defects With a Right-to-Left Shunt at Atrial Level 495
CONGENITAL HEART DISEASE WITH CYANOSIS AND INCREASED PULMONARY VASCULARITY 496
Increased Pulmonary Arterial Markings 496
Increased Pulmonary Venous Markings 499
ECHOCARDIOGRAPHIC APPROACH TO COMPLEX CONGENITAL HEART DISEASE 499
SUMMARY 502

In recent years, the noninvasive technique of echocardiography has had a major influence on the diagnostic and therapeutic management of children with congenital heart disease. M-mode echocardiography provided a method for the assessment of wall thickness, chamber size, and valve motion. The development of two-dimensional echocardiography provided a technique for spatial anatomic display of cardiac structures and, thus, led to more exact definition of cardiac anatomy, even in the most complex congenital cardiac defects. Recent advances in equipment and image processing have allowed improved visualization of cardiac structures even in small preterm infants. The recent addition of Doppler ultrasonography to the two-dimensional echocardiographic examination has provided a technique for the quantitative assessment of valve gradients, cardiac output, and shunt size. Because of these rapid advances in technology, two-dimensional echocardiography and Doppler echocardiography have allowed cardiac catheterization for diagnostic purposes to be eliminated in many instances and, in other cases, to be postponed until the infant or child is better able to withstand this invasive procedure.

In this chapter, we review the echocardiographic findings in the more common congenital cardiac defects and discuss briefly the echocardiographic approach to the segmental diagnosis of complex congenital cardiac abnormalities.

CONGENITAL HEART DISEASE WITH ACYANOSIS AND INCREASED PULMONARY BLOOD FLOW

Ventricular Septal Defects

Children with a large ventricular septal defect and normal pulmonary vascular resistance have evidence of left ventricular volume overload (enlarged left atrium and left ventricle) on the two-dimensional echocardiogram. Because of the increase in left ventricular diastolic filling, left ventricular stroke volume is increased and septal and posterior wall motion is exaggerated. On the two-dimensional echocardiogram, ventricular septal defects can be imaged directly as areas of echocardiographic dropout in the ventricular septum.[C1] These defects can occur in any of the four portions of the ventricular septum that have different embryologic derivations but usually occur along the fusion lines between the different portions of the septum.[S9] The different portions of the ventricular septum are (1) the membranous septum, which is subaortic and beneath the septal leaflet of the tricuspid valve; (2) the muscular or trabeculated septum, which includes the inferior two-thirds of the septum; (3) the outlet or infundibular septum, which is subaortic and subpulmonic; and (4) the inlet or sinus septum, which is the superior and posterior one-third of the septum between the atrioventricular valves (Figs. 24–1 and 24–2). With two-dimensional echocardiography, defects are classified as being entirely within a portion of the ventricular septum (i.e., muscular defects) or as being on a fusion line between two or more portions of the ventricular septum (i.e., perimembranous outlet defects, perimembranous inlet defects).

Two-dimensional echocardiography has been reported to be 100 percent sensitive in the detection of outlet and inlet ventricular septal defects. In infants less than 1 year of age, the sensitivity for detecting membranous ventricular septal defects has ranged from 74 to 87 percent.[B5, C1, C3] Muscular ventricular septal defects are the most difficult to detect with two-dimensional echocardiography, and sensitivity has been reported to be as low as 30 percent in some prospective studies. Several factors make direct visualization of muscular ventricular septal defects very difficult. First, these defects can occur anywhere in the wide area of the

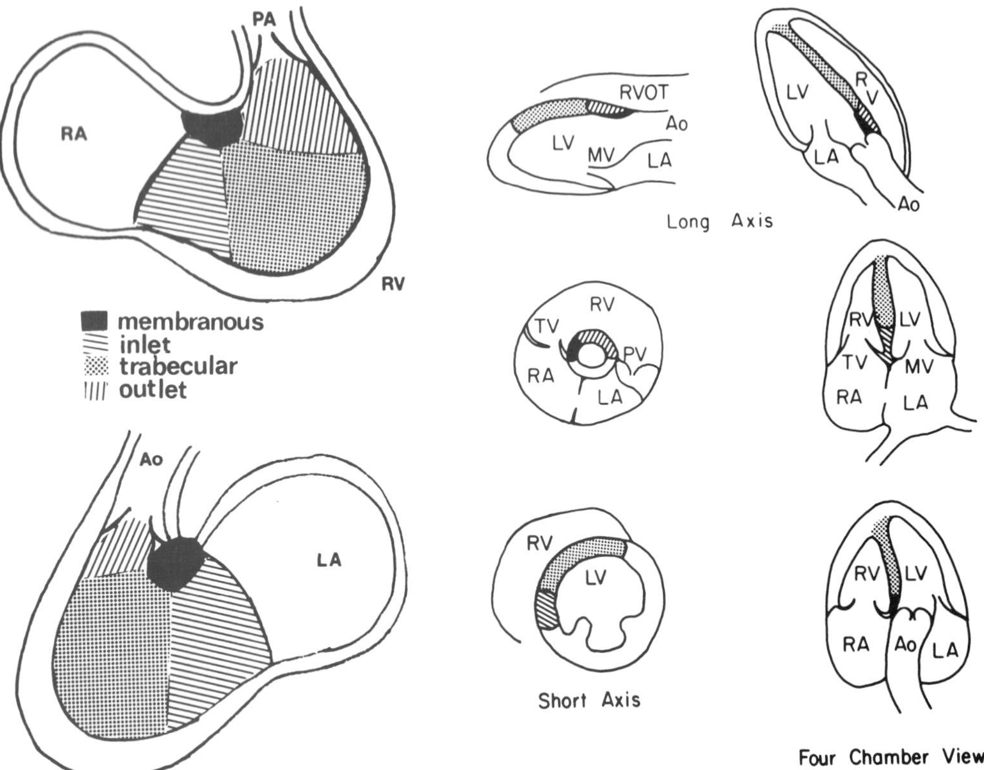

Figure 24–1. (Left) Diagrammatic representation of the parts of the ventricular septum as viewed from the right ventricle (above) and left ventricle (below). (Right) Diagrammatic representation of the parts of the ventricular septum as viewed in the long-axis, short-axis, and four-chamber views. Abbreviations: Ao—aorta; LA—left atrium; LV—left ventricle; MV—mitral valve; PA—pulmonary artery; PV—pulmonary valve; RA—right atrium; RV—right ventricle; RVOT—right ventricular outflow tract; TV—tricuspid valve. (From Silvermann, N. H., and Snider, A. R.: Two-Dimensional Echocardiography in Congenital Heart Disease. Appleton-Century-Crofts, Norwalk, Conn., 1982, p. 71, with permission.)

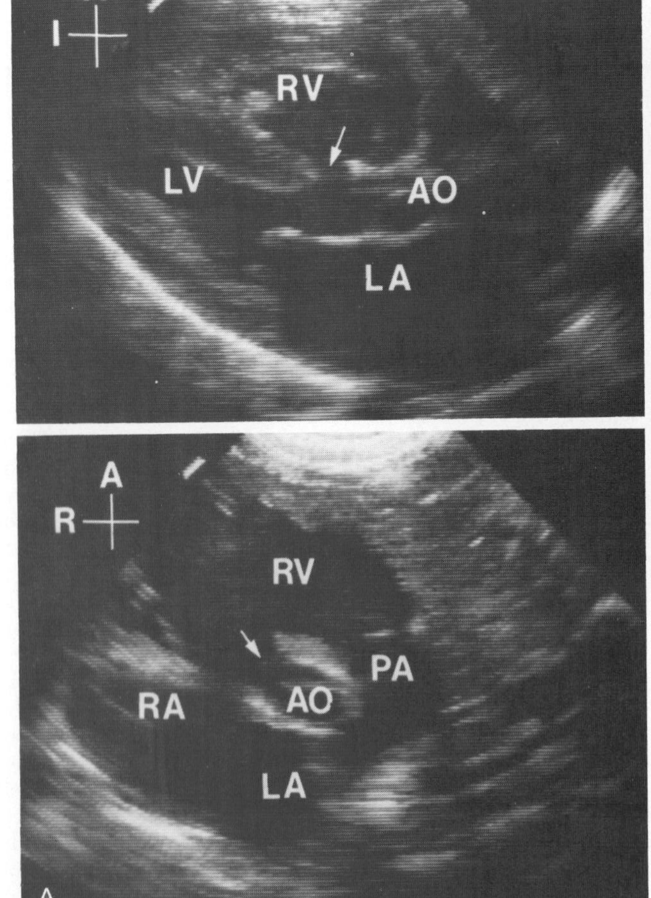

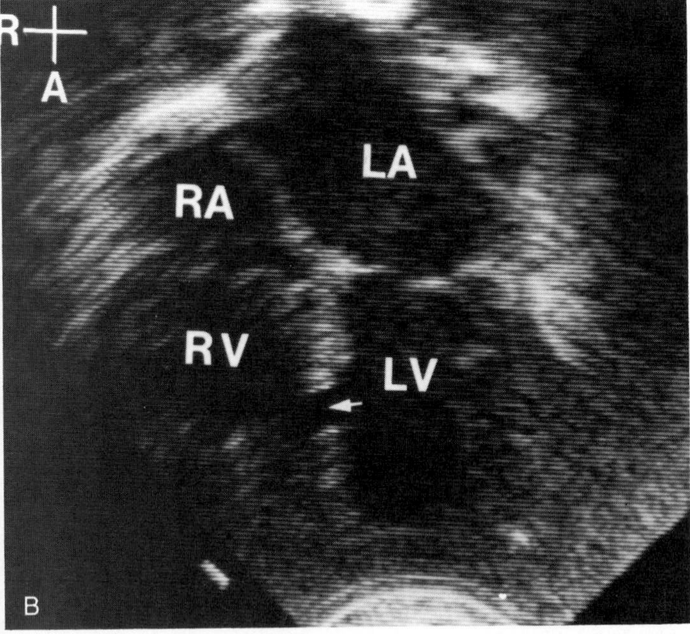

Figure 24–2. *A*, Parasternal long-axis (top) and short-axis (bottom) views of a child with a large membranous ventricular septal defect (*arrow*). The defect is located just beneath the aortic valve and adjacent to the tricuspid valve septal leaflet. Abbreviations: A—anterior; AO—aorta; I—inferior; LA—left atrium; LV—left ventricle; PA—pulmonary artery; R—right; RA—right atrium; RV—right ventricle. *B*, Apical four-chamber view of a patient with a large muscular ventricular septal defect (*arrow*). The defect is located in the inferior two-thirds of the ventricular septum. Abbreviations: A—apex; LA—left atrium; LV—left ventricle; R—right; RA—right atrium; RV—right ventricle.

septum that is the muscular septum. Second, these defects are often serpiginous, so the right septal surface of the defect may not be visualized simultaneously with the left septal surface of the defect. Third, these defects may change size and be virtually obliterated in systole. Finally, these defects may be hidden on the right septal surface by septoparietal muscle bundles within the right ventricle.

With the introduction of pulsed, continuous-wave, and color flow Doppler techniques, the sensitivity for detection of ventricular septal defects has improved considerably. In children with a ventricular septal defect and left ventricular pressure higher than right ventricular pressure, a systolic jet can be recorded in the right ventricle on the Doppler examination (Fig. 24–3).[H3, H5, M1, S18] Usually, the jet extends throughout systole and has a very high peak velocity because left ventricular systolic pressure is much higher than right ventricular systolic pressure; however, with very large defects and systemic right ventricular pressure, systolic velocities may be low (less than 2.5 m/sec) or not recorded at all.[M6] In patients with a very large left-to-right ventricular shunt, Doppler examination of the main pulmonary artery shows an increased velocity (due to increased flow) and spectral broadening (due to the persistence of disturbed flow downstream from the defect).

Doppler color flow mapping has had a major application in the rapid detection of septal defects (Fig. 24–4). With this technique, blood flow can be seen crossing defects that are too small to be visualized directly on the two-dimensional echocardiogram. In a recent study, the abilities of color Doppler and angiography to detect multiple muscular ventricular septal defects were compared. The color Doppler technique correctly identified 72 percent of all patients proved by angiography to have multiple muscular defects. No false-positive diagnoses were made with the color Doppler technique.[L4]

Figure 24–4. See Color Plate 4.

In patients with a ventricular septal defect and no right or left ventricular outflow obstruction, the pressure difference between the left and right ventricles can be calculated from the peak velocity of the systolic jet.[H3] For this calculation, a simplified Bernoulli equation is used:

$$\text{Pressure gradient} = 4 \times (\text{peak velocity})^2$$

If the arm blood pressure is obtained at the time of the Doppler examination, the right ventricular systolic pressure can be calculated as

$$\text{RV systolic pressure} = \text{systolic arm blood pressure} - 4\times(\text{peak velocity})^2$$

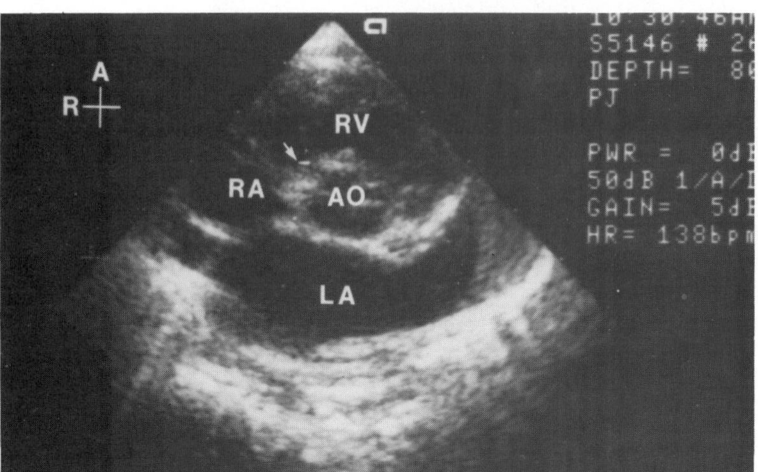

Figure 24–3. Simultaneous two-dimensional image and continuous-wave Doppler recording from a child with a membranous ventricular septal defect. The parasternal short-axis view (top) shows the position of the continuous-wave beam (*arrow*) at the time of the Doppler recording. The Doppler tracing (bottom) shows a high-velocity jet in systole directed toward the transducer and above the baseline. The peak velocity of the jet is 3.2 m/sec, which predicts a pressure gradient of 40 mmHg across the septal defect. Abbreviations: A—anterior; Ao—aorta; LA—left atrium; R—right; RA—right atrium; RV—right ventricle.

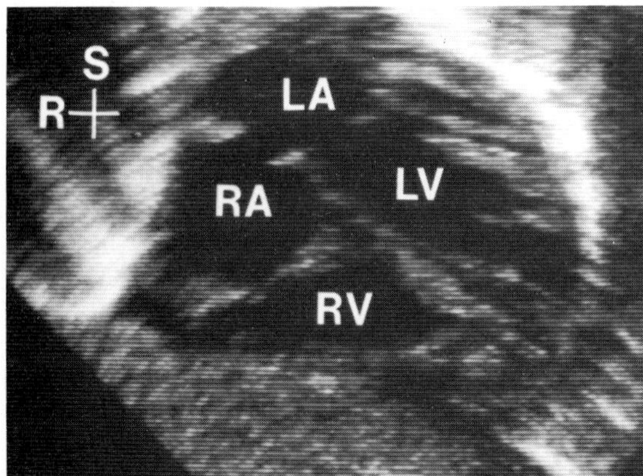

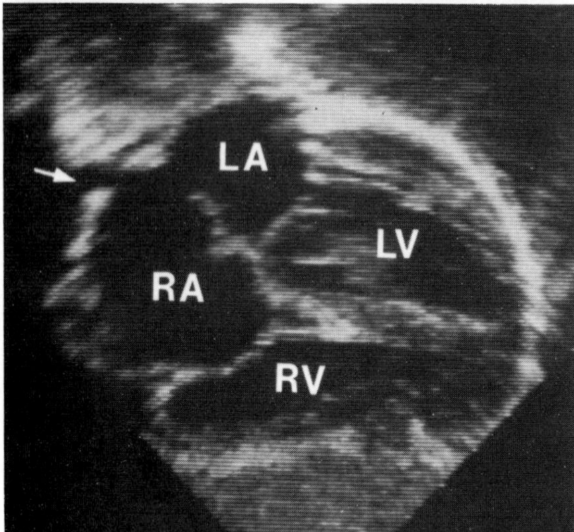

Figure 24–5. (Top) Subcostal four-chamber view of a patient with a secundum atrial septal defect. The secundum atrial septal defect appears as an area of echocardiographic dropout in the middle portion of the atrial septum. (Bottom) Subcostal four-chamber view of a child with a sinus venosus atrial septal defect and anomalous drainage of the right upper pulmonary vein (*arrow*). The sinus venosus atrial septal defect is seen as an area of echocardiographic dropout in the superior portion of the atrial septum. The right upper pulmonary vein drains just to the right of the atrial septal defect. Abbreviations: LA—left atrium; LV—left ventricle; R—right; RA—right atrium; RV—right ventricle; S—superior.

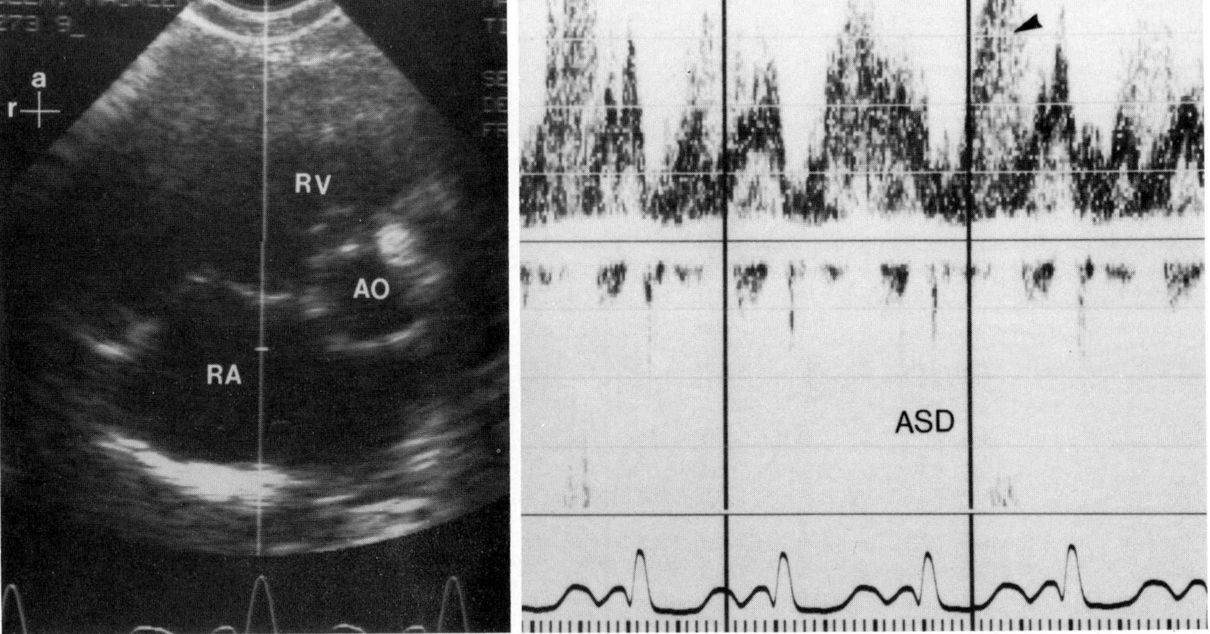

Figure 24–6. Pulsed Doppler recording from the parasternal short-axis view of a small child with an atrial septal defect. The freeze-frame image (left) shows the position of the sample volume in the right atrium at the time of the Doppler recording. The Doppler tracing (right) shows disturbed flow above the baseline (toward the transducer) beginning in mid-systole and extending into early diastole. This flow reaches its peak velocity in late systole (*arrow*). A second short period of left-to-right shunting appears as disturbed flow above the baseline at the time of atrial contraction. Abbreviations: a—anterior; AO—aorta; r—right; RV—right ventricle; RA—right atrium; ASD—atrial septal defect. (Reprinted from Snider, A. R.: Doppler echocardiography in congenital heart disease. *In* Berger, M. [ed.]: Doppler Echocardiography in Heart Disease. Marcel Dekker, Inc., New York, 1987, p. 271, by courtesy of Marcel Dekker, Inc.)

Using this equation, good correlations have been found between Doppler and cardiac catheterization measurements of right ventricular systolic pressure.[M6, S10] If an adequate recording of the peak velocity of the jet through the ventricular septal defect cannot be obtained, the right ventricular systolic pressure can be estimated from the peak velocity of the tricuspid insufficiency jet using the following equation:

$$\text{RV systolic pressure} = 4 \times (\text{peak velocity})^2 + \text{right atrial pressure}$$

Most children (and especially those with right ventricular hypertension) have, at least, a small tricuspid insufficiency jet that can be used to estimate right ventricular systolic pressure. Right atrial pressure can be estimated from the amount of jugular venous distention, can be assumed to be normal (8 to 10 mmHg), or can be measured if a central venous line is in place.

Atrial Septal Defects

Children with a large atrial septal defect show evidence of right ventricular volume overload (right atrial and right ventricular dilatation, paradoxic septal motion) on the two-dimensional echocardiogram. Atrial septal defects can be visualized directly as an area of echocardiographic dropout in the atrial septum (Fig. 24–5). These defects can occur in the midportion of the atrial septum (ostium secundum defect), in the lower third of the atrial septum adjacent to the atrioventricular valves (ostium primum defect), or in the superior portion of the atrial septum near the superior vena cava (sinus venosus defect). The low parasternal and subcostal four-chamber views are the best views for direct visualization of septal defects because the atrial septum is perpendicular to the plane of sound in these views.[B6]

On Doppler examination of the right atrium (from either a subcostal or a right parasternal position), the left-to-right shunt across an atrial septal defect causes disturbed flow above the baseline (toward the transducer) in midsystole extending into early diastole (Fig. 24–6). Maximal velocity generally occurs in late systole. A second short period of left-to-right shunt appears as disturbed flow above the baseline during atrial contraction. In addition, all simple atrial septal defects have a short period of right-to-left shunting, which produces disturbed flow signals directed away from the transducer (below the baseline) in early systole. Variations in the pressure differences between the left and right atria throughout the cardiac cycle account for these variations in the direction of shunt flow.[A1, G4, H3, K1, L2, M4]

Usually, the peak velocity of the left-to-right shunt in late systole is between 1 and 1.5 m/sec, indicating a peak pressure gradient between the atria of about 5 mmHg. With a restrictive atrial communication and a large pressure difference between the atria (i.e., stretched open patent foramen ovale), a high-velocity jet can be recorded across the atrial septum.

In patients with an atrial septal defect, the increased volume of flow through the right heart chambers causes an increase in flow velocity across the tricuspid and pulmonary valves.[H3, M4] Often, flow velocities across the mitral and aortic valves are decreased. Close correlations have been found between the ratios of right-sided and left-sided flow velocities (i.e, pulmonary artery/aorta and tricuspid/mitral) and the pulmonary-to-systemic flow ratio measured at cardiac catheterization.[H3]

Doppler color flow mapping techniques can be used to detect shunting across an atrial septal defect (Fig. 24–7). This technique is particularly useful for confirming the presence of an atrial septal defect in patients for whom direct imaging of the atrial septum is technically inadequate and in distinguishing a true atrial septal defect from artifactual echocardiographic dropout in the thin region of the fossa ovalis.

Figure 24–7. See Color Plate 4.

Patent Ductus Arteriosus

Patent ductus arteriosus, a communication between the main pulmonary artery and the descending aorta, is a common cardiac abnormality that can occur as an isolated defect or in association with various congenital cardiac defects. The medical and surgical management of infants with a patent ductus arteriosus requires knowledge of the direction and magnitude of the ductal shunts.[G3, S1] In most instances, two-dimensional echocardiography can accurately define the presence and morphologic characteristics of the patent ductus arteriosus; however, the hemodynamic characteristics of the patent ductus arteriosus cannot usually be defined with two-dimensional echocardiography alone. Doppler echocardiography provides a method for diagnosing the direction and magnitude of ductal shunts, for assessing the relative pulmonary and systemic vascular resistances, and for estimating pulmonary artery systolic, mean, and diastolic pressures.

As pulmonary vascular resistance decreases after birth, the left-to-right shunt through the patent ductus arteriosus increases, leading to increased pulmonary blood flow, increased pulmonary venous return, and, consequently, left atrial and left ventricular volume overload. On the two-dimensional echocardiogram of children with a large patent ductus arteriosus, the left atrium is considerably larger than the right atrium or the aortic root and the atrial septum bulges toward the right due to left atrial dilatation. The left ventricle is dilated and hypercontractile, and the descending aorta pulsations are increased.[G3, S8]

The patent ductus arteriosus can be imaged directly from left parasternal, high left parasternal, and suprasternal locations.[S1] In the parasternal short-axis view, the patent ductus arteriosus is seen connecting the main pulmonary artery and the descending aorta (Fig. 24–8). In this view, visualization of the patent ductus arteriosus can often be optimized by rotating the transducer slightly clockwise toward a long-axis plane. This maneuver allows one to visualize more of the descending aorta and, usually, the entire length of the patent ductus arteriosus. The patent ductus arteriosus is imaged in the direction of the lateral resolution of the equipment in this view; thus, even with the use of a high-frequency transducer such as a 7.5-MHz probe, a ductus lumen of 1 mm or less will not be visualized directly by two-dimensional echocardiography.

In most cases of isolated patent ductus arteriosus, the ductus cannot be imaged in the suprasternal long-axis view without tilting the plane of sound toward the left pulmonary artery. In this projection, the patent ductus arteriosus is seen between the origin of the left pulmonary artery and the descending aorta (see Fig. 24–8). In patients without a patent ductus arteriosus, one must be careful not to mistakenly diagnose the area where the left pulmonary artery crosses over the descending aorta as a patent ductus arteriosus.

Figure 24–8 contains a high left parasternal view of a patent ductus arteriosus. This view is obtained by sliding the transducer down from the suprasternal notch toward the left parasternal position. The plane of sound is oriented in the same direction as a suprasternal long-axis view.

Doppler interrogation of the main pulmonary artery was the first technique used to confirm the presence of a left-to-right shunt through the patent ductus arteriosus. Several different flow patterns can be seen on the Doppler examination of the main pulmonary artery. If the Doppler sample volume is positioned distally in the main pulmonary artery near the origin of the left pulmonary artery, continuous disturbed flow directed toward the transducer (above the baseline) can be seen.[G2, S20] These signals represent the shunt flow throughout systole and diastole. If the sample volume is placed in the main pulmonary artery adjacent to the pulmonary valve, the systolic portion of the left-to-right shunt may be directed away from the sample volume. Instead, signals arising from the forward flow through the pulmonary valve are seen below the baseline. Signals from the diastolic portion of the left-to-right shunt are seen above the baseline when the pulmonary valve closes. With the sample volume positioned in the midportion of the main pulmonary artery, it is even possible to record diastolic flow signals below the baseline. Presumably,

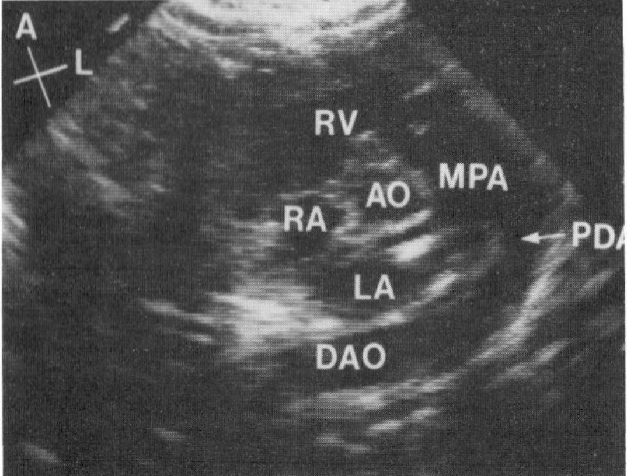

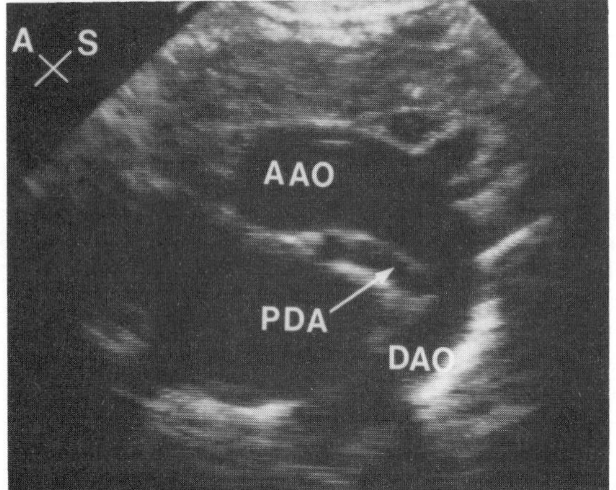

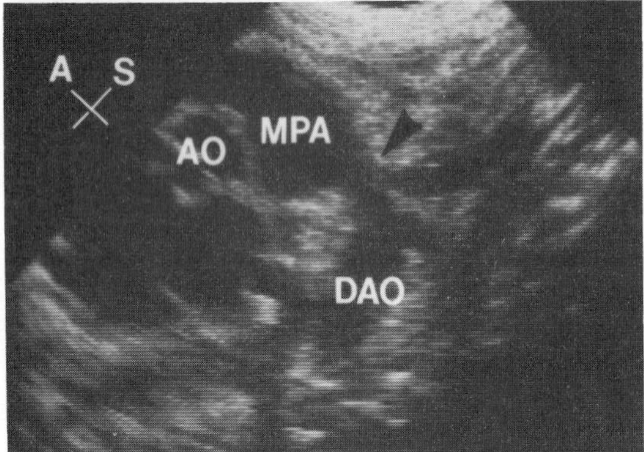

Figure 24–8. (Top) Parasternal short-axis view of an infant with a large patent ductus arteriosus (PDA). In this view, the PDA is seen connecting the main pulmonary artery (MPA) and the descending aorta (DAO). The bright echoes in the left atrium (LA) arise from an umbilical venous catheter that was inadvertently placed across the foramen ovale into the LA. (Middle) Suprasternal long-axis view of a child with pulmonary atresia and a PDA. Note the long tortuous appearance of the PDA and the lack of aortic isthmus narrowing, which is commonly seen in children with severe right ventricular outflow tract obstruction. (Bottom) High left parasternal view (also known as the ductus view) of a child with a large PDA (*arrow*). The PDA is seen communicating between the MPA and DAO. This view is obtained by placing the transducer in a parasternal short-axis position and sliding the transducer up toward the suprasternal notch. Abbreviations: A—anterior; AAO—ascending aorta; AO—aorta; L—left; LA—left atrium; RA—right atrium; RV—right ventricle; S—superior.

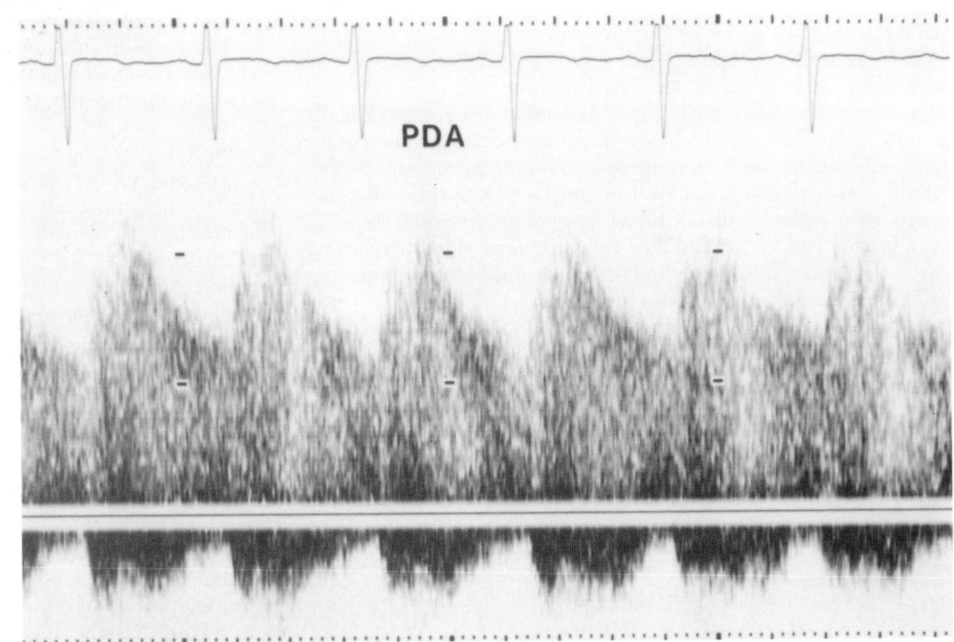

Figure 24–9. Continuous-wave Doppler examination of a patent ductus arteriosus (PDA). The Doppler transducer is placed in the second left intercostal space and aimed toward the pulmonary artery. High-velocity continuous disturbed flow is seen above the baseline, indicating flow through a restricted PDA toward the transducer. The peak velocity of the flow in systole is greater than 4 m/sec, indicating a pressure difference of greater than 64 mmHg between the aorta and pulmonary artery in systole. This pattern of continuous disturbed flow directed toward the transducer is typical of a PDA with a pure left-to-right shunt.

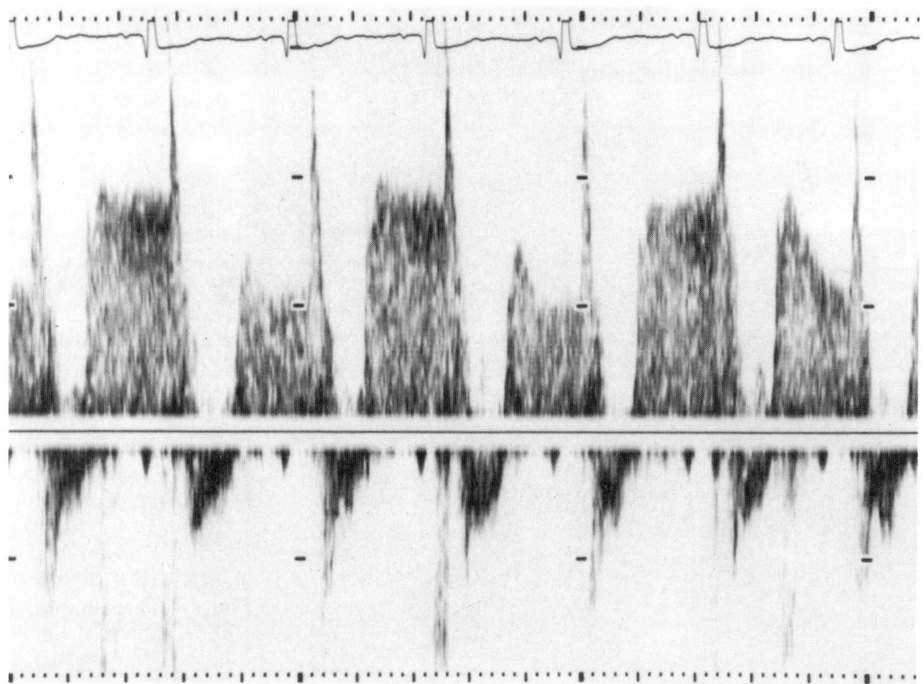

Figure 24–10. Continuous-wave Doppler examination of an infant with a patent ductus arteriosus, severe pulmonary artery hypertension, and bidirectional ductal shunting. The left-to-right shunt occurs as a positive deflection (above the baseline) beginning in late systole and extending into late diastole. Note that the peak velocity of the left-to-right shunt is approximately 1 m/sec, indicating no pressure difference between the aorta and pulmonary artery at this time in the cardiac cycle. The right-to-left shunt is seen as a negative deflection below the baseline in systole.

these signals arise as the jet flow from the patent ductus arteriosus strikes the closed pulmonary valve in diastole and swirls back on itself, giving rise to Doppler signals directed away from the transducer.[D1]

Following the initial descriptions of the Doppler findings in the main pulmonary artery in patients with a patent ductus arteriosus, several investigators reported the results of direct interrogation of the ductus arteriosus with pulsed and continuous-wave Doppler.[H7, M7]

Direct Doppler interrogation of the ductus arteriosus has many advantages over Doppler interrogation of the pulmonary artery. First, a small patent ductus arteriosus shunt can be missed by sampling only in the pulmonary artery. Second, direct ductus examination has the advantage of being able to differentiate a patent ductus arteriosus from other defects that cause disturbed diastolic flow in the pulmonary artery (e.g., aortopulmonary window, anomalous origin of a coronary artery from the pulmonary artery, or bronchial collateral vessels). Third, Doppler sampling in the main pulmonary artery does not permit detection of a right-to-left ductus shunt.

Several different flow patterns can be observed when the patent ductus arteriosus is sampled directly with pulsed or continuous-wave Doppler.[C4] Patients with an isolated left-to-right patent ductus arteriosus shunt and no other cardiac abnormalities have continuous positive flow with a peak velocity in late systole (Fig. 24–9). Peak systolic pressure gradients across the patent ductus arteriosus can be calculated by substituting the peak velocity in late systole in the simplified Bernoulli equation. If one measures the blood pressure at the time of the Doppler examination, the pulmonary artery systolic pressure can be

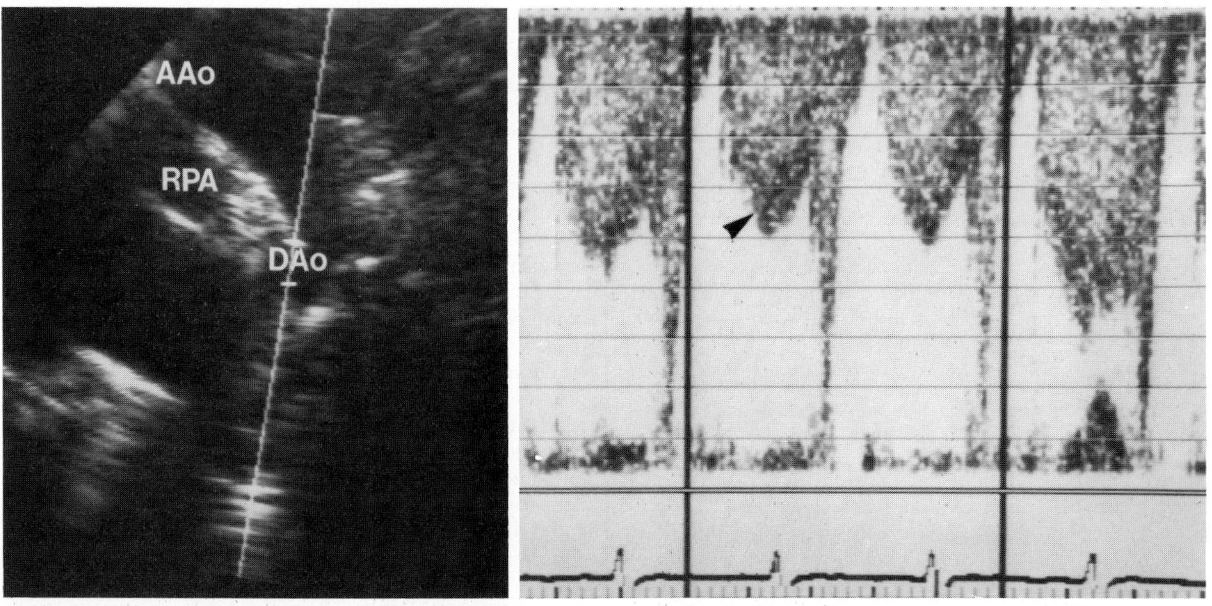

Figure 24–11. Doppler spectral recording from the suprasternal notch view of an infant with a patent ductus arteriosus, markedly elevated pulmonary vascular resistance, and a pure right-to-left ductal shunt. The freeze-frame image on the left shows the position of the sample volume at the descending aortic (DAo) end of the patent ductus arteriosus at the time of the Doppler recording. The Doppler spectral tracing on the right shows evidence of forward flow in systole down the descending aorta. In diastole, there are Doppler flow signals below the baseline (*arrow*), indicating a right-to-left shunt from the ductus arteriosus to the DAo. Abbreviations: AAo—ascending aorta; RPA—right pulmonary artery. (Reprinted from Snider, A. R.: Doppler echocardiography in congenital heart disease. *In* Berger, M. [ed]: Doppler Echocardiography in Heart Disease. Marcel Dekker, Inc., New York, 1987, p. 294, by courtesy of Marcel Dekker, Inc.)

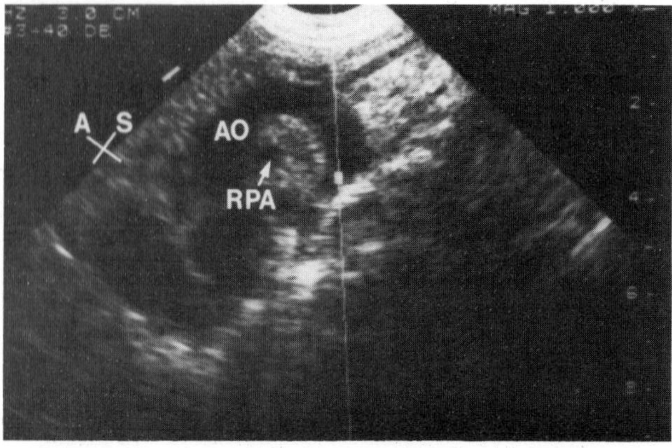

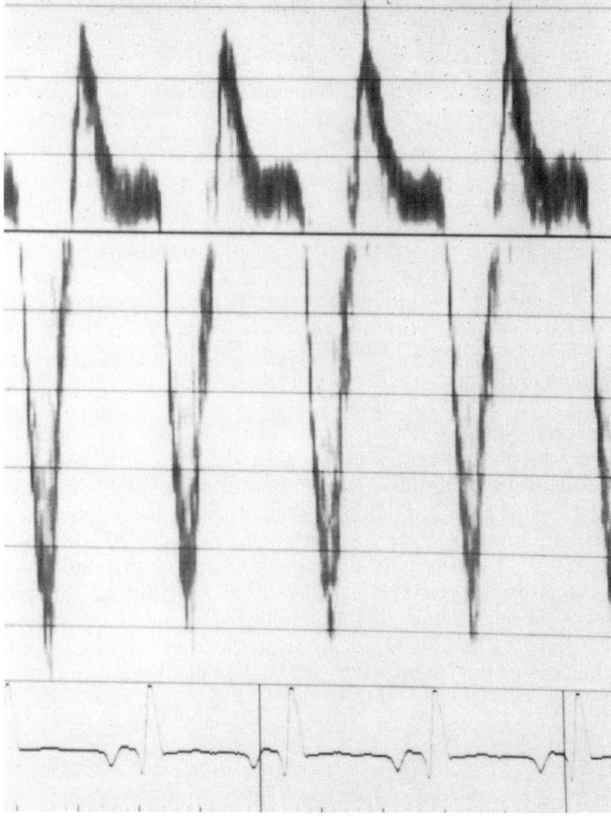

Figure 24–12. Pulsed Doppler recording from the suprasternal long-axis view of an infant with a large patent ductus arteriosus. The freeze-frame image at the top shows the position of the sample volume in the descending aorta (AO) at the time of the Doppler recording. The Doppler spectral tracing (bottom) shows normal forward flow down the aorta (away from the transducer and below the baseline) in systole. In diastole, there are flow signals above the baseline, indicating retrograde flow up the descending aorta toward the transducer. These retrograde diastolic flow signals are caused by a steal of blood in diastole from the aorta to the pulmonary artery. Abbreviations: A—anterior; RPA—right pulmonary artery; S—superior.

calculated as the systolic blood pressure minus the Doppler peak gradient.

Patients with an isolated right-to-left patent ductus arteriosus shunt (as may occur in infants with aortic arch interruption and severe pulmonary hypertension) have continuous negative flow away from the transducer with a peak velocity in early systole.

Bidirectional ductal shunting is detectable in infants with patent ductus arteriosus and very severe pulmonary artery hypertension (Fig. 24–10). In these cases, the right-to-left shunt occurs as a negative deflection in systole and the left-to-right shunt occurs as a positive deflection beginning in late systole and extending into late diastole.[S19] Patients with no oxygen saturation differences above and below the patent ductus arteriosus have a right-to-left shunt that peaks in early systole, whereas patients with a difference in oxygen saturation of 5 to 30 percent above and below the patent ductus arteriosus have a right-to-left shunt that peaks in middle-to-late systole. When diagnosing a right-to-left ductal shunt (especially when using continuous-wave Doppler), care must be taken not to confuse normal systolic flow in the adjacent left pulmonary artery with a right-to-left patent ductus arteriosus shunt.

In patients with bidirectional patent ductus arteriosus shunt and high pulmonary vascular resistance (Fig. 24–11), the right-to-left shunt begins in diastole, abbreviates the left-to-right diastolic shunt, and extends into early systole as a high-velocity reverse flow. The left-to-right shunt (if present) is present in late systole to early diastole.

Pulsed and continuous-wave Doppler interrogation of the descending aorta is also useful for assessing the magnitude of the left-to-right patent ductus arteriosus shunt. With a large patent ductus arteriosus and low pulmonary artery diastolic pressures, blood flows from the aorta into the pulmonary artery in diastole. Evidence of a diastolic runoff or "steal" of blood from the aorta can be seen on the Doppler examination of the aorta.[A2, F1, M3, P3, S6] If the Doppler sample volume is positioned in the descending aorta below the ductus arteriosus, forward flow signals are seen in systole below the baseline. In diastole, flow signals are seen above the baseline, indicating flow up the descending aorta toward the ductus arteriosus and main pulmonary artery (Fig. 24–12). Good correlation has been found between clinical estimates of the shunt size and the ratio of the retrograde flow area to the forward flow area.[S6]

Color flow Doppler has improved the ease and quickness with which one can visualize the patent ductus arteriosus. With color flow Doppler, flow can be detected in a patent ductus arteriosus that is too small to be imaged clearly on the two-dimensional echocardiogram (Fig. 24–13). With the color Doppler display of the patent ductus arteriosus jet, one can obtain better alignment of the pulsed or continuous-wave Doppler beam with the jet flow and thus improve the estimation of pulmonary artery pressures. One limitation of two-dimensional color flow mapping is that it lacks the temporal resolution to identify clearly the exact timing of bidirectional patent ductus arteriosus shunts.

Figure 24–13. See Color Plate 4.

Atrioventricular Septal Defects

Atrioventricular septal defects occur because of failure of partitioning of the embryonic atrioventricular canal. This results in a confluent defect that involves the ostium primum, atrioventricular canal, and interventricular foramen. Atrioventricular septal defects have a common atrioventricular valve that contains superior (anterior) and inferior (posterior) bridging leaflets as well as left lateral, right lateral, and right accessory leaflets.[G6] The common atrioventricular valve can have an undivided common orifice or can be divided into right-sided and left-sided orifices by a tongue of tissue connecting the superior and inferior bridging leaflets. The common atrioventricular valve can be displaced downward into the ventricle and anchored to the crest of the muscular septum, thus allowing left-to-right shunting to occur only above the valve at atrial level (so-called partial form), or can float freely in the septal defect, allowing shunting to occur above and below the valve at atrial and ventricular levels (so-called complete form). In addition, intermediate forms of atrioventricular septal defects (incomplete forms) can occur, depending on the position and attachments of the valve leaflets.[B3]

Two-dimensional echocardiography has been particularly useful for definition of the morphology and attachments of the atrioventricular valve leaflets, determination of the level of the left-to-right shunt, and estimation of the sizes of the right and left ventricles (Figs. 24–14 through 24–16).[H1] Some two-dimensional echocardiographic findings common to all variants of atrioventric-

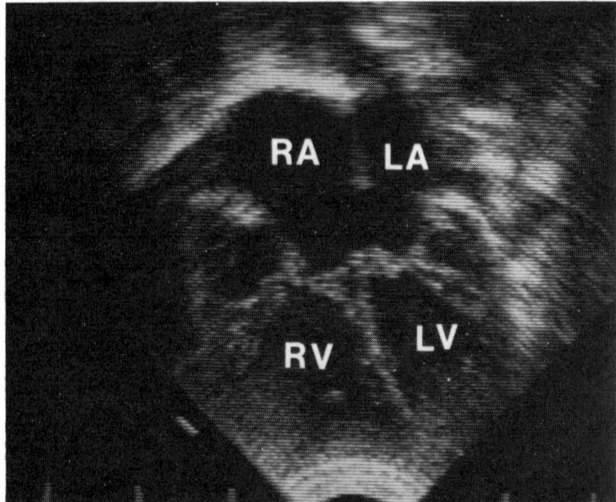

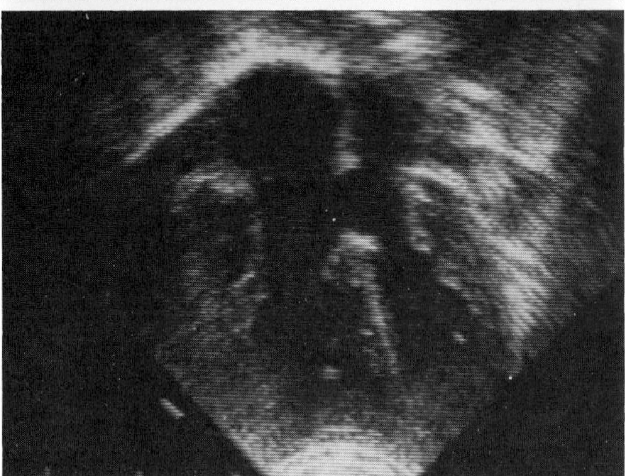

Figure 24–14. Apical four-chamber views in systole (above) and diastole (below) of a patient with a primum atrial septal defect. The primum atrial septal defect is seen as an area of echocardiographic dropout in the lower portion of the atrial septum adjacent to the atrioventricular valve. In this case, the common atrioventricular valve is tethered to the crest of the ventricular septum so that no shunting can occur at ventricular level. Note that there are not separate atrioventricular valve fibrous rings at separate levels; rather there is a single atrioventricular valve ring with the leaflets positioned lower in the heart than usual. Abbreviations: LA—left atrium; LV—left ventricle; RA—right atrium; RV—right ventricle.

ular septal defect include (1) deficiency of the inlet portion of the ventricular septum, (2) displacement of the atrioventricular valve inferiorly, (3) lack of two separate fibrous valve rings at different distances from the cardiac apex, and (4) attachment of the left half of the common atrioventricular valve to the ventricular septum, with resulting orientation of the valve into the left ventricular outflow tract.

Pulsed and color flow Doppler techniques have been especially useful for defining the complex patterns of intracardiac shunting and valve regurgitation that occur in patients with atrioventricular septal defects. Deformities of the common atrioventricular valve are such that insufficiency jets can be directed anywhere in the left or right atrium. Color flow mapping has provided a technique for rapid visualization of these eccentric jets.

Doppler Quantitation of Left-to-Right Shunts

Both systemic and pulmonary blood flows can be calculated from the two-dimensional and Doppler echocardiograms in patients with a left-to-right shunt by using these equations for volumetric flow:[G5, S21, V1, V2]

$$SV = \frac{V \times CSA \times RR}{1000 \text{ ml/L}}$$

where SV is stroke volume (ml/beat), V is mean velocity (cm/sec), CSA is vessel cross-sectional area $(cm)^2$, and RR is the R-to-R interval (seconds per beat). Since the cardiac output equals the stroke volume times the heart rate and heart rate equals 60/R-R interval,

$$\text{Volumetric flow (L/min)} = \frac{V \times CSA \times 60 \text{ sec/min}}{1000 \text{ ml/L}}$$

Commonly, the pulmonary artery mean velocity and diameter are used to calculate pulmonary blood flow and the ascending aorta mean velocity and diameter are used to calculate systemic blood flow; however, other sites can be used, depending on the location of the left-to-right shunt. The magnitude of the left-to-right shunt can be calculated directly as pulmonary blood flow minus systemic blood flow or can be assessed indirectly by calculating the ratio of the pulmonary and systemic blood flows or the Qp/Qs.

The calculation of volumetric flow requires measurement of the mean velocity and the vessel cross-sectional area. In measuring the mean velocity, one fundamental assumption is that flow is laminar and organized and that the velocity profile is uniform across the vessel or valve inlet. Under these circumstances, a single sampling of the flow velocity in the center of the vessel is recorded. Care is taken to align the Doppler beam parallel with flow in the vessel so that the maximal velocities are recorded and no correction for intercept angle need be made. The mean velocity is then calculated as the integrated area under the Doppler curve or the velocity time integral divided by the flow period of the traced beats. A computer program is used to integrate the Doppler velocity curve by tracing the densest area of the Doppler curve or the modal velocity over several consecutive cardiac cycles.

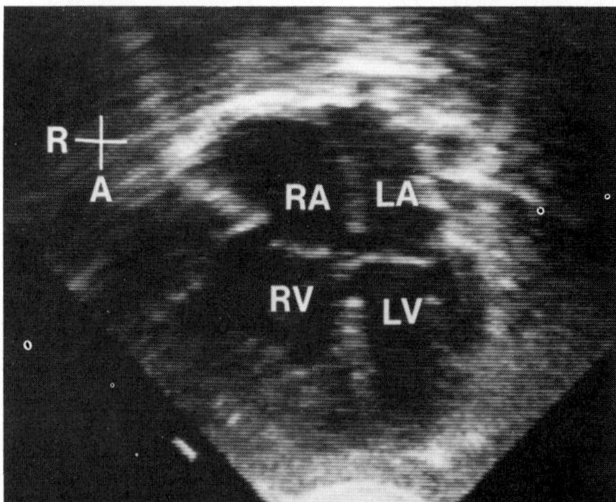

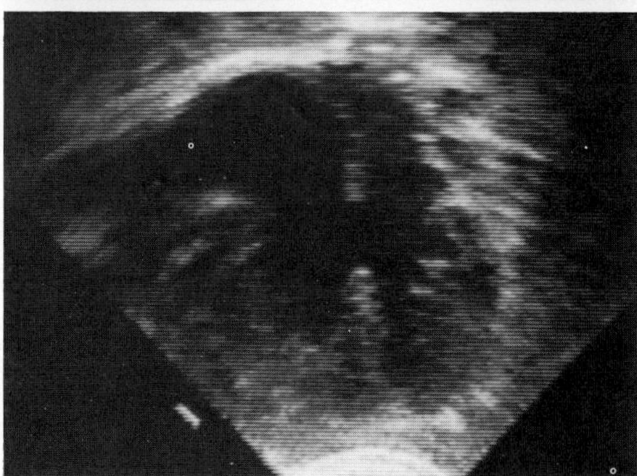

Figure 24–15. Apical four-chamber views in systole (above) and diastole (below) of a child with the so-called complete form of an atrioventricular septal defect. When the common atrioventricular valve is closed in systole, shunting can occur at atrial and ventricular levels. When the atrioventricular valve is open in diastole, a large central confluent defect is seen in the atrioventricular septum. Note the deficiency of the ventricular septum in this view. Abbreviations: A—apex; LA—left atrium; LV—left ventricle; R—right; RA—right atrium; RV—right ventricle.

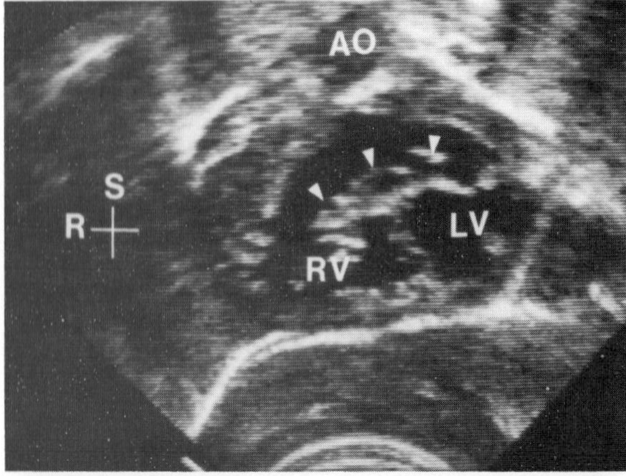

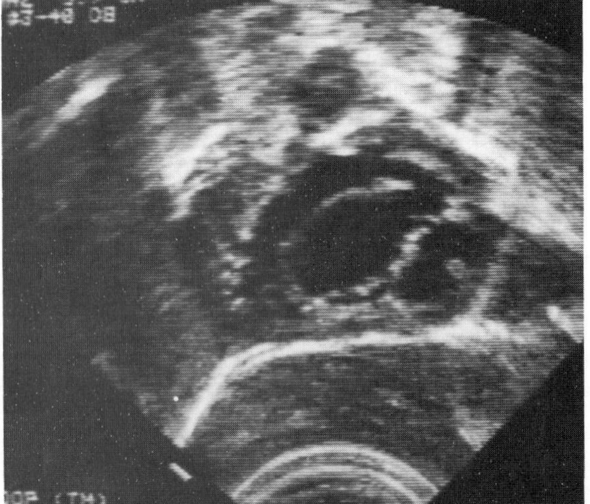

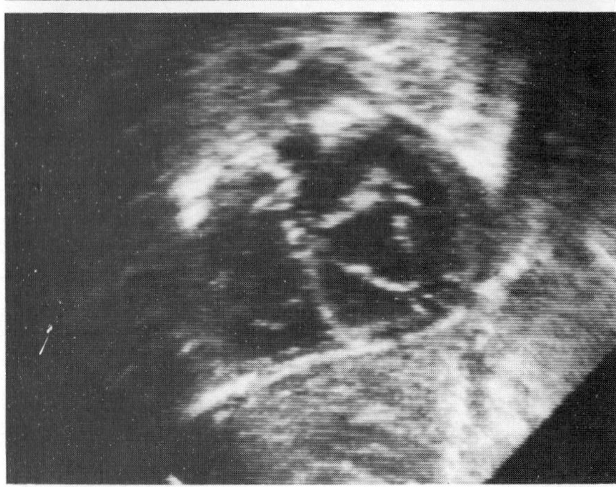

Figure 24–16. Subcostal sagittal views at the level of the common atrioventricular valve in two patients with atrioventricular septal defect. The top frame shows the atrioventricular valve (*arrows*) of one patient in the closed position in systole. The middle frame shows the atrioventricular valve of the same patient in the open position in diastole. Note that the common atrioventricular valve bridges from the right ventricle (RV) to the left ventricle (LV). In this patient, the common atrioventricular valve has a common orifice. The bottom frame is a subcostal sagittal view of a different patient with an atrioventricular septal defect. In this patient, the common atrioventricular valve is divided by a bridging tongue of tissue into two separate valve orifices. These frames show how the two-dimensional echocardiogram can be used to determine the morphology of the common atrioventricular valve in patients with atrioventricular septal defect. Abbreviations: AO—aorta; R—right; S—superior. (From Snider, A. R.: Two-dimensional and Doppler echocardiographic evaluation of heart disease in the neonate and fetus. Clin. Perinatol. 15:534, 1988, with permission.)

If one does not have a computer program for integrating the area under the Doppler curve, this area can be calculated manually. If a straight line is drawn from the peak velocity to the baseline, the Doppler spectral tracing can be divided into two right-angle triangles. The area of a right-angle triangle is one-half the base times the height, both of which can be measured directly from the Doppler tracings. The areas of the forward and reverse triangles are then added to obtain the total area under the Doppler spectral tracing.

For systemic blood flow, aortic velocity can be recorded from many windows including suprasternal, apical, and subcostal approaches. In most cases, the apical view is preferable because it is easily obtainable in most patients and because one can position the sample volume parallel with flow across the aortic annulus and close to the valve leaflets. In the suprasternal view, it is often not possible to sample aortic flow just at the valve leaflets at an acceptable angle and often flow has to be sampled in the ascending aorta several centimeters above the valve. If aortic mean velocity is measured in the ascending aorta, the vessel cross-sectional area should be measured at the same location. It is difficult to measure the aortic diameter accurately at this location because of difficulties in imaging the anterior aortic wall from the suprasternal notch and because the aortic diameter is measured in the direction of the lateral resolution of the equipment. The pulmonary artery mean velocity is calculated in a similar manner from the pulmonary artery Doppler tracing. Usually, acceptable pulmonary artery Doppler tracings can be obtained from the parasternal short-axis view or the subcostal view of the right ventricular outflow tract. Frequently, with a large shunt or a shunt whose location is close to the pulmonary artery (i.e., ventricular septal defect), the Doppler tracing shows spectral broadening or signs of disturbed flow. In these instances, one cannot assume a uniform velocity profile in the main pulmonary artery and another site should be chosen to calculate pulmonary blood flow (i.e., mitral valve for ventricular septal defect). Also, the main pulmonary artery Doppler tracing cannot be used to calculate pulmonary blood flow if there is any pulmonary stenosis accompanying the shunt because, in this instance as well, the velocity profile is not uniform across the vessel lumen.

The vessel cross-sectional area is usually calculated by measuring the vessel diameter from the two-dimensional echocardiogram and assuming that the vessel is circular so that cross-sectional area equals $\pi(d^2)/4$. There are many different techniques for measuring vessel diameters. It is recommended that the aorta and pulmonary artery be measured from inner edge to inner edge in early systole at the level of the valve annulus. The inner-edge measurements should be used because they provide the closest approximation of the actual flow diameter. It is known that systolic expansion accounts for a 5 to 10 percent change in aortic cross-sectional area and a 2 to 18 percent change in pulmonary artery cross-sectional area throughout systole. The increase in cross-sectional area occurs early in systole and is simultaneous with the upstroke of the pressure curve, so most of the flow in the aorta or pulmonary artery occurs when the vessel is at or near its peak systolic dimension. The vessel diameter is measured at the valve annulus because the annulus is the smallest area or the flow-limiting point in the vessel where maximal flow velocity should theoretically occur.[S21]

For the aorta, the parasternal long-axis view provides a diameter that is measured in the direction of the axial resolution of the equipment. For the pulmonary artery flow diameter, the parasternal long-axis view of the right ventricle can be used. In this view, it is easier to visualize the origin of the pulmonary valve leaflets and the left lateral wall of the main pulmonary artery away from the lung. Accurate measurement of the pulmonary artery diameter is much more difficult than accurate measurement of the aortic diameter. First, it is usually not possible to image the pulmonary artery in a view that will allow one to measure the diameter in the direction of the axial resolution. Second, it may be difficult to visualize the left lateral border of the main pulmonary artery because of the adjacent lung tissue. Placing the patient in a steep left lateral decubitus position will optimize visualization of the left border of the pulmonary artery. Third, Stewart and associates have shown that with increasing volumetric flow, pulmonary artery diameter increases to a far greater extent than aortic diameter.[S21] With increasing volume flow from 0.5 to 1 L/min, aortic mean velocity increased linearly and aortic diameter increased very slightly. No further changes were observed with increasing flow rates from 2 to 5 L/min. With increasing pulmonary blood flow, there was a consistent increase in pulmonary artery diameter throughout the entire range of flows. Pulmonary artery mean velocity increased as well, but the percent increase in pulmonary artery mean velocity was less than the percent increase in aortic mean velocity for the same change in volumetric flow. Thus, there is far greater variability in pulmonary artery diameter at different volume flows than there is in aortic diameter. Pulmonary artery diameter, then, can never be assumed to be constant in a particular patient when assessing serial changes in pulmonary blood flow.

In patients with a ventricular septal defect, systemic blood flow can be calculated at the aortic and tricuspid valve sites and pulmonary blood flow can be calculated at the pulmonary and mitral valve sites. With an atrial septal defect, mitral and aortic valve flow reflects systemic output and tricuspid and pulmonary valve flow reflects pulmonary blood flow. In the case of a patent ductus arteriosus, the left-to-right shunt is downstream from the pulmonary valve; therefore, the pulmonary and tricuspid valve sites reflect systemic blood flow and the mitral and aortic valve sites reflect pulmonary blood flow.

In general, in patients with left-to-right shunts, Doppler-derived values for pulmonary and systemic blood flows and Qp/Qs have correlated well with the same values determined at cardiac catheterization by the Fick technique.[B1, S4] For systemic blood flow, correlation coefficients in several clinical studies have ranged from 0.78 to 0.91 and standard errors of the estimate have ranged from 0.60 to 0.81 L/min. For pulmonary blood flow, correlation coefficients have ranged from 0.72 to 0.88 and standard errors from 1.11 to 2.4 L/m. For Qp/Qs, correlation coefficients have been 0.85 with standard errors of around 0.48. There are several possible explanations for the errors or discrepancies noted between Doppler calculations of shunt magnitude and values measured at cardiac catheterization. First, errors can occur in the measurement of the mean velocity from the Doppler spectral tracing. Gardin and associates have shown that in general there is good reproducibility in measurement of the mean velocity.[G1] For the aortic mean velocity, intraobserver variability in their study was 3.2±2.9 percent, interobserver variability was 5.4±3.4 percent, and the day-to-day variability was 3.8±3.1 percent. Potential sources of error in measuring the Doppler mean velocity include errors in determining the intercept angle and the lack of a uniform velocity profile across the vessel lumen. Determination of vessel cross-sectional area is the largest source of error in the Doppler technique. Errors can occur in determination of vessel cross-sectional area because the instrument's gain settings may be too high or too low to optimize visualization of the vessel walls; the vessel cross-sectional area changes throughout the cardiac cycle (especially the main pulmonary artery) and these changes depend on factors such as pressure, flow, and elasticity in the vessel; and it may be necessary to measure the vessel in the direction of the lateral resolution of the equipment.

Errors in the calculation of flow can occur because of the presence of additional defects. For example, an additional undetected shunt such as a patent ductus arteriosus located downstream from the pulmonary artery sampling site will lead to underestimation of the total pulmonary flow and Qp/Qs ratio. Semilunar valve regurgitation results in overestimation of flow due to failure to measure the regurgitant volume. Finally, discrepancies can occur between the Doppler and catheterization measurements of flow because of errors in the use of the Fick technique as the gold standard. Variability in the measurement of blood flow by the Fick technique occurs because this technique requires the patient to be in a steady state for several minutes, which does not often occur, and because the Fick technique is influenced by the patient's ventilatory rate, room temperature, barometric pressure, and the patient's respiratory exchange ratio.

CONGENITAL HEART DISEASE WITH VENTRICULAR OUTFLOW OBSTRUCTION

Ventricular outflow obstruction causing symptoms in childhood is usually hemodynamically severe, and children with these defects are often critically ill. Two-dimensional echocardiography and Doppler echocardiography provide a noninvasive technique for rapid diagnosis of the anatomic type of obstruction and its severity. In many cases, the noninvasive techniques have eliminated the need for diagnostic cardiac catheterization prior to surgical therapy. This approach has been especially useful in the care of sick infants with severe left ventricular obstruction, in whom dye injections at the time of cardiac catheterization may be poorly tolerated because of low systemic output and poor renal perfusion.[H8, K2]

Left Ventricular Outflow Obstruction

Left ventricular outflow obstruction can occur beneath the aortic valve (subvalvular), at the level of the aortic valve (valvular), or above the aortic valve (supravalvular aortic stenosis, coarctation and interruption of the aorta). In the most severe form, the entire left side of the heart can be underdeveloped, a condition known as hypoplastic left heart syndrome. On the two-dimensional echocardiogram, all of these defects can cause left ventricular hypertrophy and decreased left ventricular shortening fraction (caused by increased afterload). Often, left atrial and pulmonary venous distention develops as left ventricular compliance decreases.

Aortic valve stenosis can occur with a normal valve annulus size and fused commissures or with a small valve annulus and dysplastic leaflets (Fig. 24–17).[W3] The aortic valve can be tricuspid, bicuspid, or unicuspid, and the left ventricle can be dilated and poorly contractile, small and somewhat underdeveloped, or concentrically hypertrophied. Often, bright echoes arising from areas of endocardial fibroelastosis can be seen in the bases of the papillary muscles or throughout the endocardium. Doppler echo-

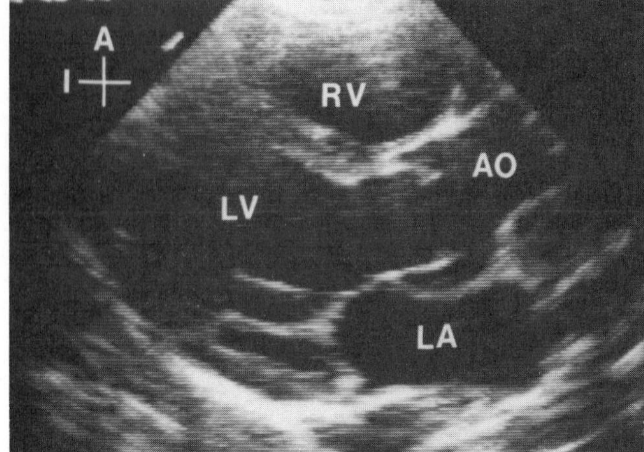

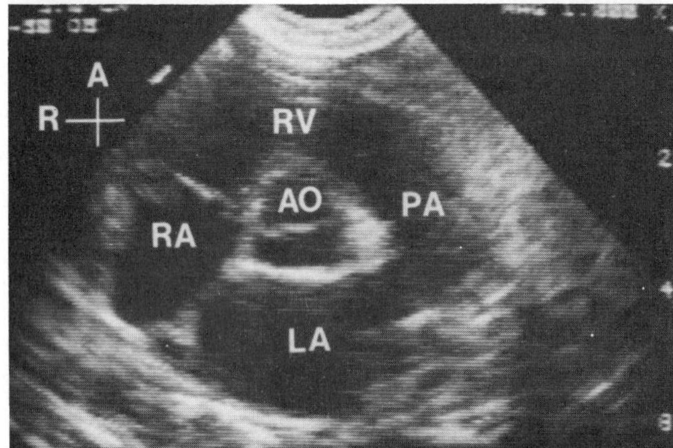

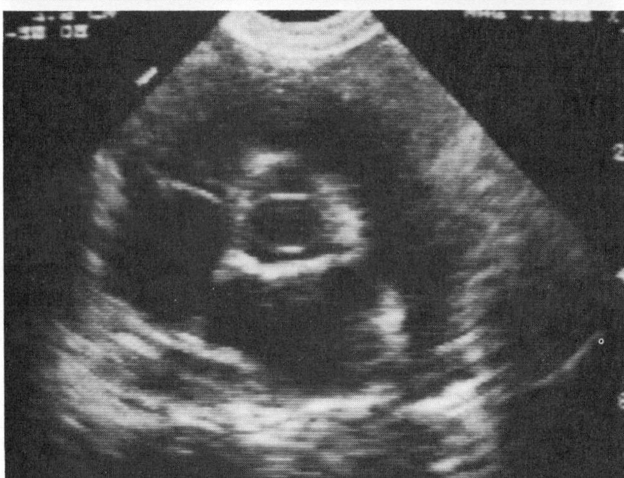

Figure 24–17. (Top) Parasternal long-axis view of a child with aortic valve stenosis. In this view, the aortic valve is thickened and domed in systole. (Middle and bottom) Parasternal short-axis views of the same patient. In this view, the aortic valve is bicuspid, forms a single closure line in the closed position, and is "fish-mouthed" in shape in the open position. Abbreviations: A—anterior; AO—aorta; I—inferior; LA—left atrium; LV—left ventricle; PA—pulmonary artery; R—right; RA—right atrium; RV—right ventricle.

cardiography is especially useful for estimating the peak systolic pressure gradient across the aortic valve (Fig. 24–18). For this calculation, Doppler recordings of the systolic jet through the aortic valve are obtained from apical, right parasternal, and suprasternal notch transducer positions. The highest value of the peak velocity is used in the simplified Bernoulli equation ($4V^2$) to predict the peak instantaneous pressure gradient across the aortic valve. The Doppler peak gradient is always larger than the peak-to-peak pressure gradient measured at catheterization. The difference between the two is greatest in mild aortic stenosis and is less marked in severe aortic stenosis. Nevertheless, excellent correlations have been found between Doppler peak gradients and peak-to-peak pressure gradients measured at cardiac cathe-

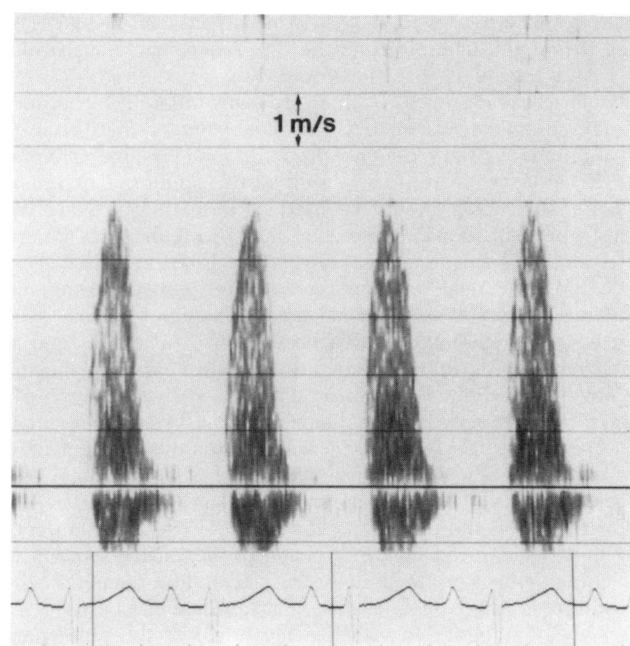

Figure 24–18. Continuous-wave Doppler examination from the suprasternal notch of a newborn infant with severe aortic valve stenosis. A high-velocity jet that peaks in late systole is present. The peak velocity of the jet is 5 m/sec, which indicates a pressure gradient of 100 mmHg across the valve.

terization.[B4, H4, S16, S17, Y1] One should keep in mind that in the presence of myocardial dysfunction and low cardiac output, the peak gradient may not reflect the severity of the aortic stenosis.

Subvalvular aortic stenosis can occur as a discrete membrane (Fig. 24–19) or as a long area of muscular thickening (tunnel type). Subaortic stenosis can be an isolated defect but most often occurs in association with other cardiac defects (i.e., along with multiple left heart obstructive lesions or along with ventricular septal defect and double-chambered right ventricle). As with valvular aortic stenosis, the severity of discrete membranous subaortic stenosis can be estimated from the simplified Bernoulli equation. The highest value for the peak velocity of the subaortic stenosis jet is usually recorded from an apical transducer position. An accurate estimate of the pressure drop across a long tunnel type of subaortic stenosis cannot be obtained with the simplified

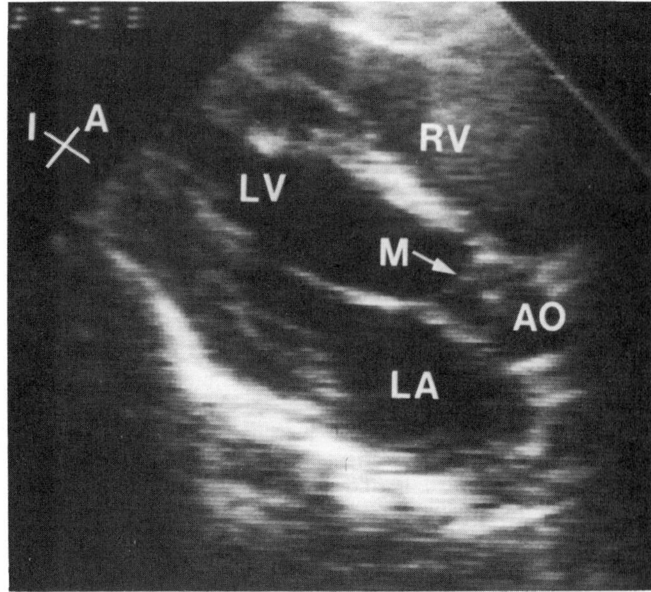

Figure 24–19. Parasternal long-axis view of a child with a discrete subaortic membrane (M). The membrane is seen just beneath the aortic valve. Abbreviations: A—anterior; AO—aorta; I—inferior; LA—left atrium; LV—left ventricle; RV—right ventricle.

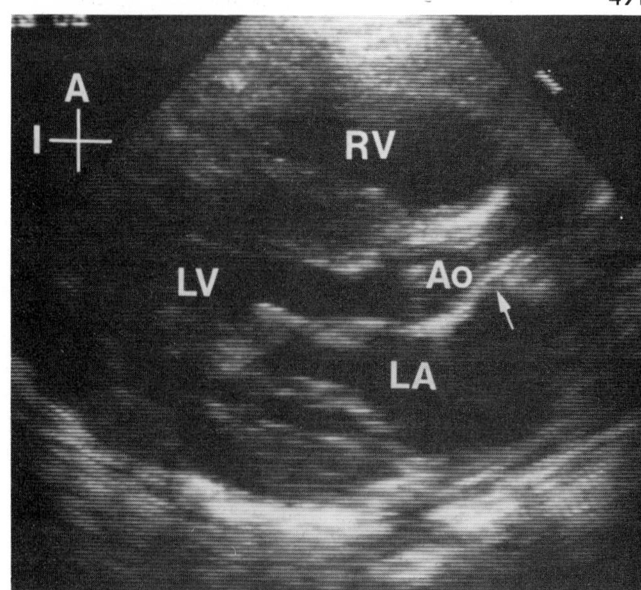

Figure 24–20. Parasternal long-axis view of a child with severe supravalvular aortic stenosis. In this view, an area of severe narrowing can be seen above the aortic valve (*arrow*). Note the marked concentric hypertrophy of the left ventricle (LV). Abbreviations: A—anterior; Ao—aorta; I—inferior; LA—left atrium; RV—right ventricle.

Bernoulli equation because this equation neglects the pressure drop caused by viscous friction along the flow path.

Supravalvular aortic stenosis occurs in three anatomic forms: (1) a discrete membrane above the aortic sinuses of Valsalva, (2) an hourglass constriction in the ascending aorta, and (3) a long tubular hypoplasia of the ascending aorta.[G6] Usually, the exact location and extent of the obstruction can be visualized on the two-dimensional echocardiogram from parasternal and suprasternal views (Fig. 24–20). Since the simplified Bernoulli equation does not apply to a pressure drop across a long tubular narrowing, it can be successfully used to predict the pressure gradient only when the supravalvular obstruction is a discrete membrane.

Supravalvular aortic stenosis is often associated with bilateral, severe peripheral pulmonary artery stenosis. Thus, when using a continuous-wave Doppler transducer without image orientation to estimate the severity of supravalvular aortic stenosis, care must be taken not to mistake a high-velocity jet from a peripheral pulmonary artery for the jet flow in the ascending aorta.

The suprasternal notch views have been especially useful for the diagnosis of coarctation and interruption of the aorta.[M5, N1, S3, S14, W1, W2] In the suprasternal long-axis view, coarctation of the aorta can be visualized as a narrowing in the descending aorta just beyond the left subclavian artery caused by a prominent posterior endothelial shelf (Fig. 24–21). Poststenotic dilatation of the descending aorta is seen just distal to the narrowed area. Unless there is a large right-to-left shunt through a patent ductus arteriosus, descending aorta pulsations are decreased. Interruption of the aorta is seen as an area of discontinuity between the ascending aorta and descending aorta in the suprasternal long-axis view. If the plane of sound is tilted slightly leftward of the standard suprasternal long-axis view, the main pulmonary artery can be seen connecting to the descending aorta via the patent ductus arteriosus. In the newborn infant, the suprasternal views can be obtained by placing the transducer directly over the manubrium sternum, which is not heavily ossified at this age. With this transducer position, there is no need to hyperextend the neck—a maneuver that can be risky in an intubated infant.

In coarctation of the aorta, a high-velocity jet usually can be recorded in the descending aorta when the transducer is positioned in the suprasternal notch. Figure 24–22 is a continuous-wave Doppler tracing from the suprasternal notch of a patient with severe coarctation. The lower-velocity signals from the descending aorta proximal to the obstruction are seen superimposed on the higher-velocity signals from the jet flow distal to the obstruction. In this patient, the peak velocity of 4 m/sec predicts a 64-mmHg gradient across the coarctation. If the peak velocity proximal to the coarctation is greater than 1 m/sec, the expanded Bernoulli equation (pressure gradient $= 4V_2^2 - 4V_1^2$) should be used in order to obtain an accurate estimate of the pressure gradient across the coarctation. Since a high percentage of patients with aortic coarctation have a bicuspid aortic valve and aortic valve stenosis, the peak velocity proximal to the

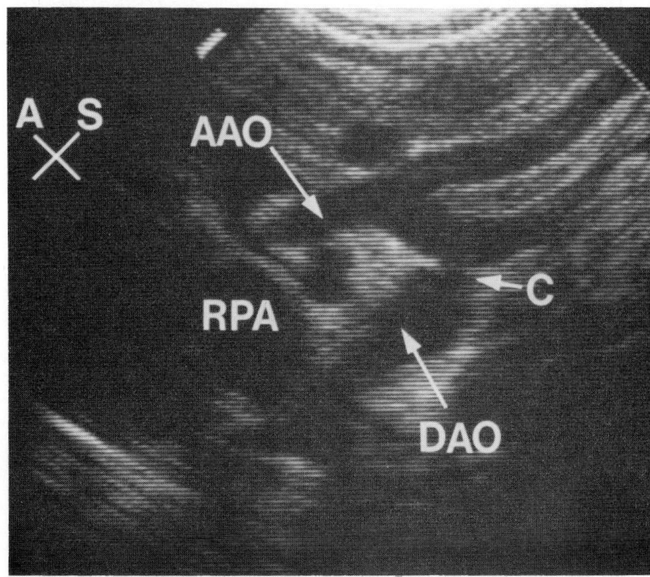

Figure 24–21. Suprasternal long-axis view of an infant with a severe coarctation of the aorta. The coarctation (C) is seen as a discrete narrowing just beyond the takeoff of the left subclavian artery. Distal to the coarctation, there is poststenotic dilatation of the descending aorta (DAO). Abbreviations: A—anterior; AAO—ascending aorta; RPA—right pulmonary artery; S—superior.

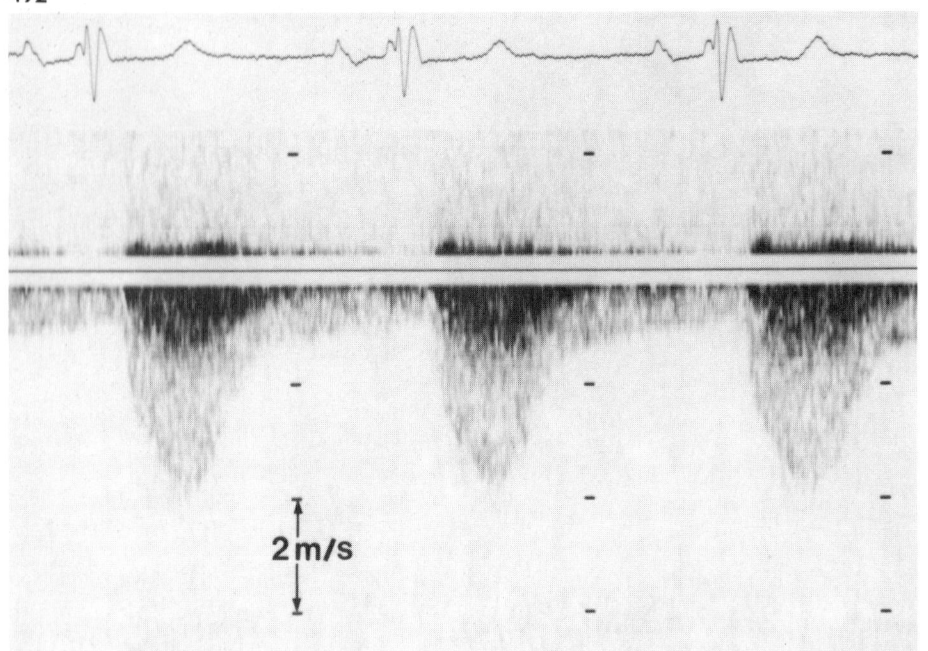

Figure 24–22. Continuous-wave Doppler examination from the suprasternal notch of an adolescent female with a severe coarctation of the aorta. There is a high-velocity jet in systole with a peak velocity of nearly 4 m/sec. This predicts a pressure gradient of 64 mmHg down the descending aorta. Forward flow continues throughout diastole in this patient, indicating a very severe coarctation of the aorta with a pressure gradient across the coarctation that persists throughout diastole. Note the darker low-velocity signals in systole superimposed on the signals from the jet flow. These low-velocity signals indicate normal flow in the descending aorta proximal to the coarctation.

coarctation is likely to be increased and should be measured (with pulsed Doppler).

With a mild coarctation, the high-velocity jet extends throughout systole only. With increasing severity of the obstruction, the jet extends throughout diastole as well. This finding occurs because, with severe obstruction, the pressure above the coarctation remains elevated throughout diastole.[H3]

The most severe form of left ventricular outflow obstruction is hypoplastic left heart syndrome. This defect has many anatomic variations but, in the most common form, both the aortic and mitral valves are atretic and the left ventricle is a small, slitlike cavity with no obvious contractions in real time (Fig. 24–23). The ascending aorta is extremely small and a coarctation is usually present.[B2, L1]

Right Ventricular Outflow Obstruction

Right ventricular outflow obstruction can occur beneath the pulmonary valve (subvalvular), at the level of the pulmonary valve (valvular), or above the pulmonary valve (supravalvular pulmonary stenosis and peripheral or branch pulmonary stenosis). On the two-dimensional echocardiogram, severe right ventricular outflow obstruction results in right ventricular hypertrophy, right atrial dilatation (due to decreased right ventricular compliance), and decreased right ventricular fractional shortening (due to increased afterload).

In children with valvular pulmonary stenosis, the two-dimensional echocardiogram shows thickened valve leaflets with restricted lateral mobility (doming).[W4] The pulmonary valve annulus varies in size from small to normal (Fig. 24–24), and there is poststenotic dilatation of the main pulmonary artery. Doppler echocardiography can be used to record the peak velocity of the pulmonary stenosis jet and, thus, estimate the peak instantaneous gradient across the pulmonary valve. The parasternal and subcostal views provide the best positions for recording the peak velocity of the jet.[J1, L3, S16]

Subvalvular pulmonary stenosis is most commonly found in association with a ventricular septal defect in the setting of tetralogy of Fallot, which is discussed in a later section of this chapter. The most common form of isolated subvalvular pulmonary stenosis is double-chambered right ventricle, a defect in which an anomalous muscle bundle traverses the right ventricular cavity and causes obstruction to forward flow out the right ventricle. The anomalous muscle bundle can be located high in the infundibulum of the right ventricle (so-called napkin ring type) or low in the body of the right ventricle (Fig. 24–25). Double-chambered right ventricle is often associated with discrete membranous subaortic stenosis.

Because of the fetal circulatory patterns, the pulmonary artery branches are considerably smaller in diameter than the main pulmonary artery at birth.[S12] This normal discrepancy in size between the main and branch pulmonary arteries should not be mistaken for pathologic peripheral pulmonary stenosis. When there is uniform hypoplasia of both pulmonary artery branches, the diagnosis depends on an accurate measurement of the branch pulmonary artery diameter from the two-dimensional echocardiogram and a comparison of this measurement with normal values for the branch pulmonary artery diameter at various body surface areas. Localized areas of branch stenosis are more easily diagnosed by two-dimensional echocardiography because they appear as a discrete area of narrowing in the pulmonary artery branch followed distally by poststenotic dilatation.

CONGENITAL HEART DISEASE WITH CYANOSIS AND DECREASED PULMONARY VASCULARITY

Infants who present with cyanosis and decreased pulmonary vascularity on chest x-ray have some form of right ventricular outflow obstruction associated with a right-to-left shunt at the atrial or ventricular level. Two-dimensional echocardiography is especially useful for defining the anatomic type of outflow obstruction and the level of intracardiac shunt.

Defects With a Right-to-Left Shunt at Ventricular Level

Decreased pulmonary blood flow and a right-to-left ventricular shunt are characteristic features of several different anatomic types of cyanotic congenital heart disease. One group of defects, the conotruncal defects, is characterized by the following anatomic features: (1) anterior discontinuity between the septum and the anterior aortic root, (2) an outlet ventricular septal defect, (3) underdevelopment of the entire right ventricular outflow tract (subvalvular, valvular, and branch pulmonary stenosis), and (4) severe right ventricular hypertrophy. Defects that belong to this category include tetralogy of Fallot, pulmonary atresia with a ventricular septal defect, and double-outlet right ventricle with normally related great arteries and severe pulmonary stenosis. These defects have in common several two-dimensional echocardiographic features including (1) a dilated, dextroposed aorta that

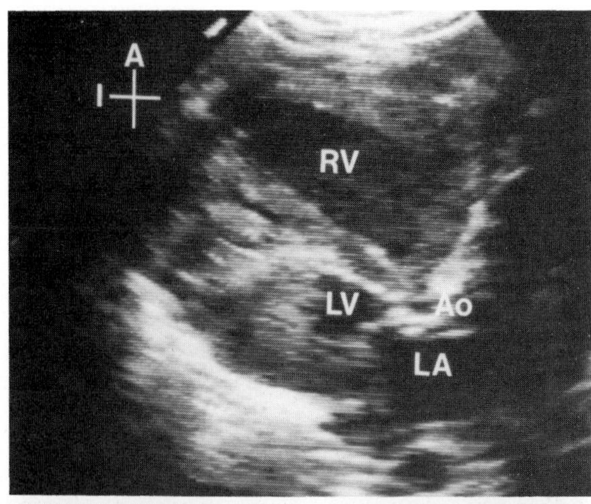

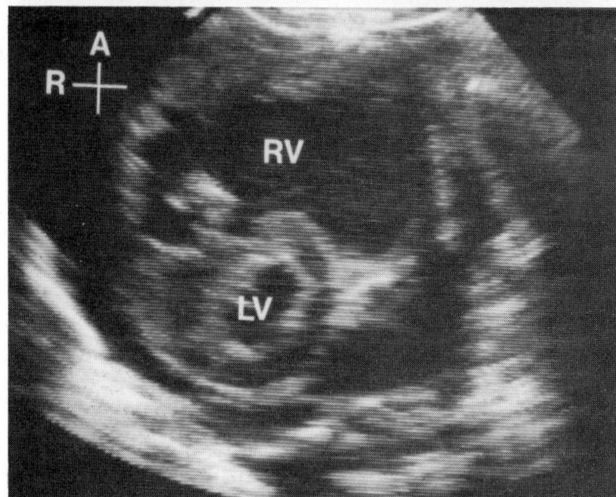

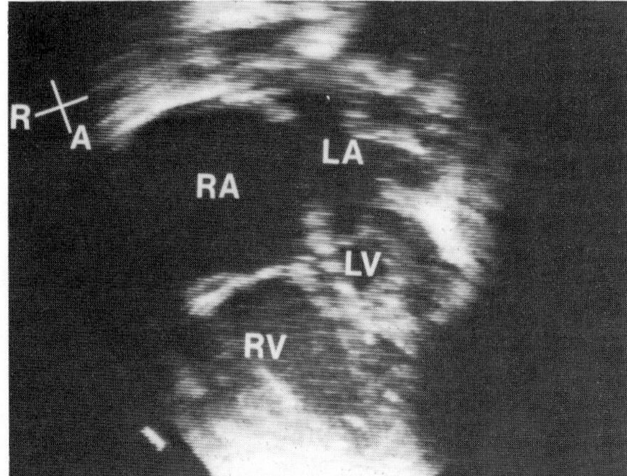

Figure 24–23. Parasternal long-axis (top), short-axis (middle), and four-chamber (bottom) views of a newborn infant with a hypoplastic left heart syndrome. The ascending aorta (Ao) is diminutive and the left ventricle (LV) is a small muscle-bound chamber. Abbreviations: A—anterior; I—inferior; LA—left atrium; R—right; RA—right atrium; RV—right ventricle.

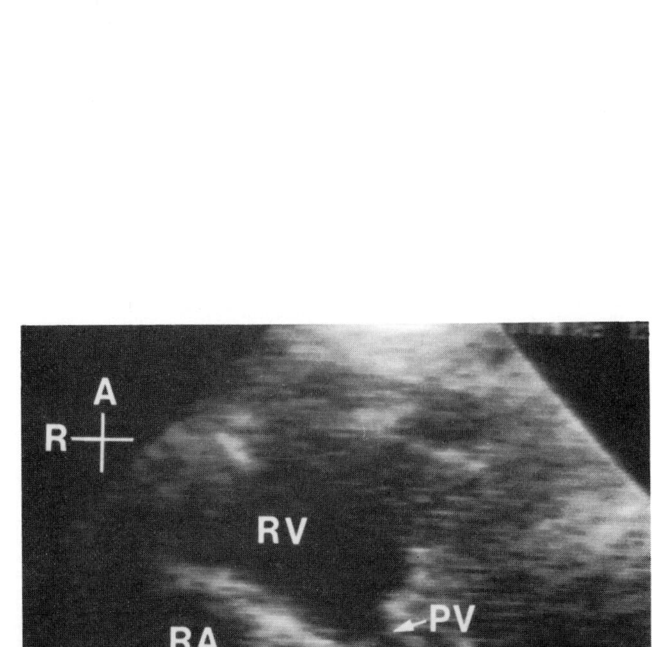

Figure 24–24. Parasternal short-axis view of a child with stenosis of the pulmonary valve (PV). There is narrowing of the PV annulus and poststenotic dilatation of the main pulmonary artery (MPA). Abbreviations: A—anterior; AO—aorta; R—right; RA—right atrium; RV—right ventricle.

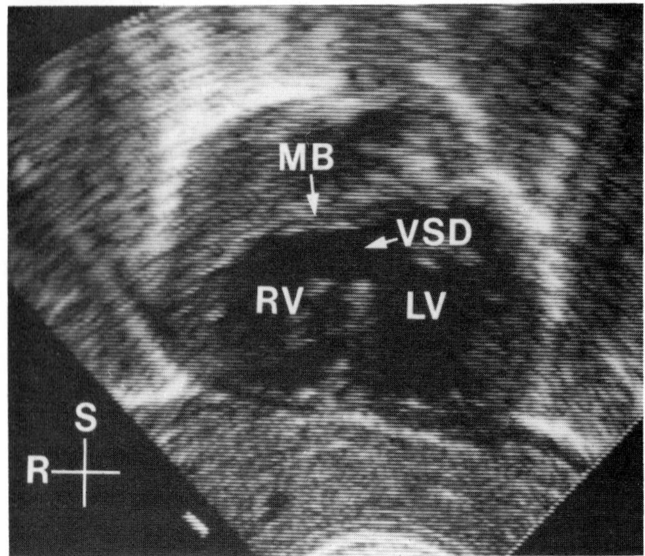

Figure 24–25. Subcostal sagittal view of a child with a large ventricular septal defect (VSD) and an anomalous muscle bundle (MB) obstructing the right ventricle (RV). Abbreviations: LV—left ventricle; R—right; S—superior.

overrides the ventricular septum (Fig. 24–26); (2) a large outlet ventricular septal defect; (3) a narrowed infundibulum, pulmonary valve annulus, main pulmonary artery, and branches; and (4) severe hypertrophy of the right ventricular anterior wall and septum.[H2] These defects each have several distinguishing echocardiographic features. In tetralogy of Fallot and pulmonary atresia with a ventricular septal defect, the posterior aortic root and anterior mitral valve leaflet are in fibrous continuity and the aorta is primarily committed to the left ventricle. In the parasternal short-axis view in tetralogy of Fallot, the pulmonary valve is small but patent (see Fig. 24–26) and antegrade flow is shown by Doppler examination of the main pulmonary artery. In the parasternal short-axis view in pulmonary atresia with a ventricular septal defect, no pulmonary valve leaflet motion can be detected and Doppler examination of the main pulmonary artery shows no evidence of antegrade blood flow. Usually, an imperforate membrane occupies the position where the pulmonary valve would normally be found; however, occasionally the right ventricular outflow tract ends blindly and there is no evidence of a main pulmonary artery segment. Pulmonary blood flow is supplied by way of a patent ductus arteriosus or bronchial collateral vessels. In both of these defects, the two-dimensional echocardiogram is particularly useful for assessing the exact anatomy and measurements of the pulmonary artery branches and for determining whether the branches are confluent. In addition, in tetralogy of Fallot the two-dimensional echocardiogram is useful for detecting

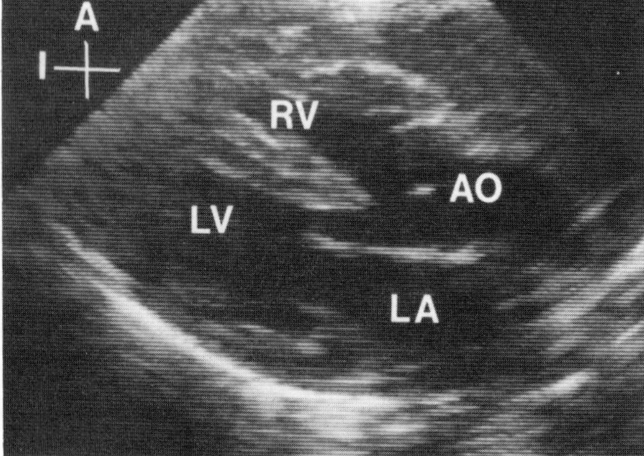

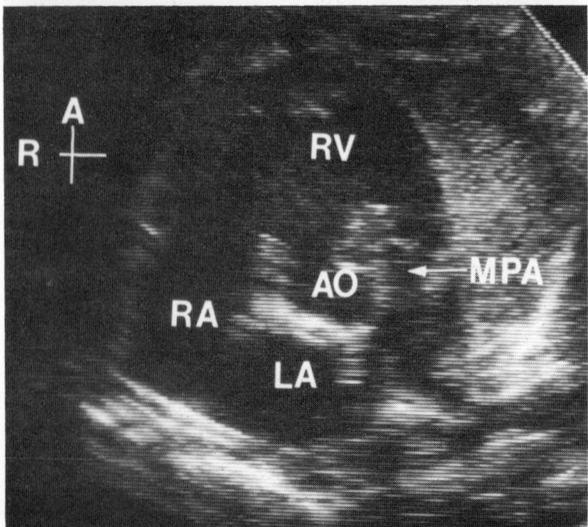

Figure 24–26. Parasternal long-axis (top) and short-axis (bottom) views of an infant with tetralogy of Fallot. Note the lack of anterior continuity between the septum and the anterior aortic (AO) root. This represents aortic override. In the short-axis view, a large ventricular septal defect is seen extending from the membranous to the outlet septum. The right ventricular outflow tract, main pulmonary artery (MPA), and pulmonary artery branches are small. The pulmonary valve is clearly seen. Abbreviations: A—anterior; I—inferior; LA—left atrium; LV—left ventricle; R—right; RA—right atrium; RV—right ventricle.

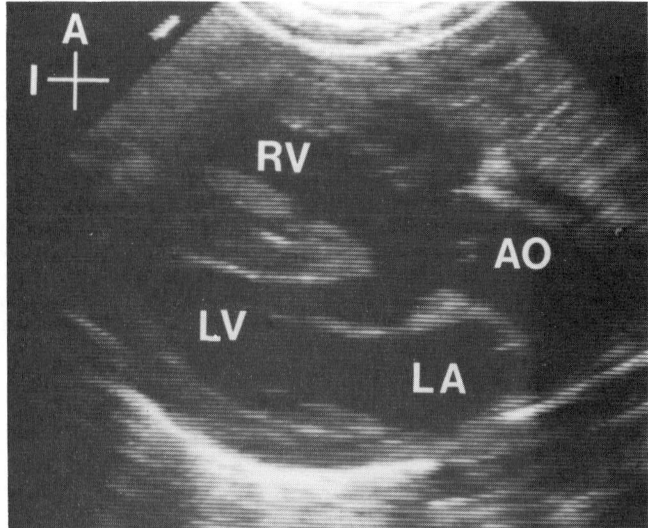

Figure 24–27. Parasternal long-axis view of an infant with double-outlet right ventricle. There is anterior discontinuity between the septum and the anterior aortic (AO) root. In addition, there is posterior discontinuity between the anterior leaflet of the mitral valve and the aortic valve. The fibrous area between these two structures represents persistent subaortic conus. Abbreviations: A—anterior; I—inferior; LA—left atrium; LV—left ventricle; RV—right ventricle.

associated lesions (i.e., additional muscular ventricular septal defects or anomalous origin of the left anterior descending coronary artery from the right coronary artery) prior to complete repair. In double-outlet right ventricle and normally related great arteries, the aorta arises predominantly from the right ventricle and there is, in addition, lack of continuity between the aortic valve and the anterior mitral valve leaflet because of persistent conus tissue beneath the aortic valve (Fig. 24–27). In the parasternal short-axis view, the great arteries are seen in cross section as double circles side by side. Both semilunar valves are anterior to the level of the ventricles and are at the same height above the ventricles (Fig. 24–28).

Tricuspid atresia with normally related great arteries, small ventricular septal defect, and pulmonary stenosis is another example of a cyanotic defect with a right-to-left ventricular shunt. In the apical and subcostal four-chamber views, the atretic tricuspid valve, small right ventricular chamber, ventricular septal defect, and large right atrium can be visualized (Fig. 24–29). The two-dimensional echocardiogram is useful for assessment of the adequacy of the atrial septal defect and for detection of commonly associated abnormalities (i.e., left juxtaposition of the right atrial appendage, right aortic arch, persistent left superior vena cava to the coronary sinus).

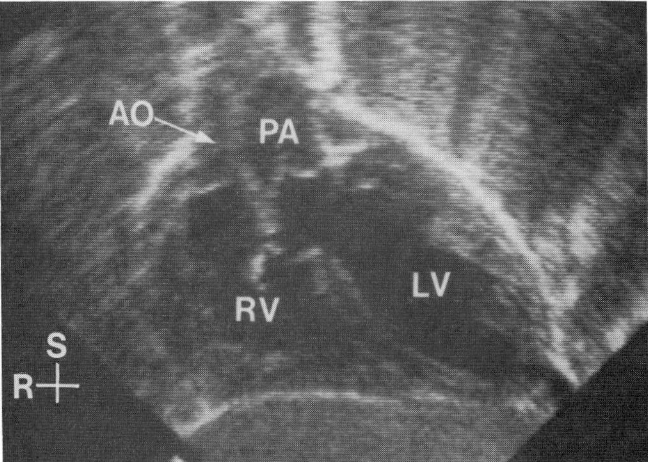

Figure 24–28. Subcostal view in a coronal body plane of a child with double-outlet right ventricle and d-transposition of the great arteries. The aorta (AO) is entirely committed to the right ventricle (RV). The pulmonary artery (PA) overrides the ventricular septum, and there is a large subpulmonary ventricular septal defect. Note that the aortic and pulmonic valves are at the same heights above the ventricles. This is because of the persistence of bilateral conus beneath the semilunar valves. Abbreviations: LV—left ventricle; R—right; S—superior.

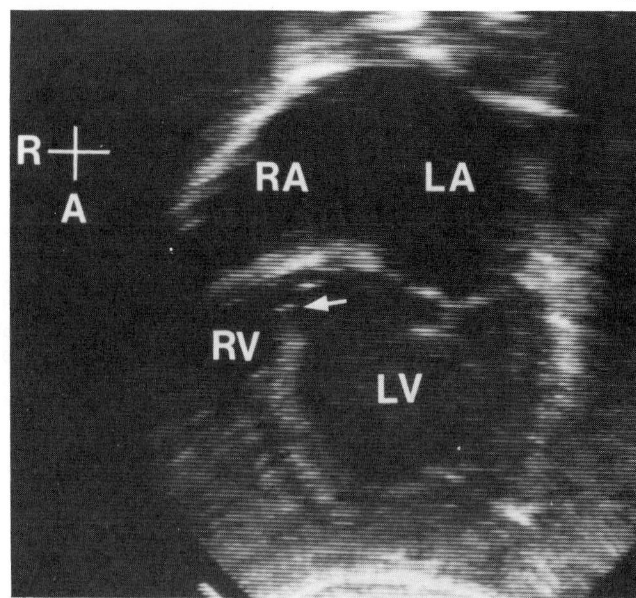

Figure 24–29. Apical four-chamber view of a child with tricuspid atresia, normally related great vessels, and severe pulmonary stenosis. An imperforate thick membrane is seen in the area that would normally be occupied by a tricuspid valve. The right ventricle (RV) is extremely small, and there is a moderate-sized inlet ventricular septal defect (*arrow*). Abbreviations: A—apex; LA—left atrium; LV—left ventricle; R—right; RA—right atrium.

Defects With a Right-to-Left Shunt at Atrial Level

Several cyanotic congenital heart defects are characterized by having severe right ventricular outflow obstruction, an intact ventricular septum, and a right-to-left atrial shunt. Included in this category of defects are Ebstein malformation of the tricuspid valve, critical pulmonary stenosis, and pulmonary atresia with an intact ventricular septum.

In Ebstein malformation, the tricuspid valve apparatus is displaced downward away from the annulus fibrosis. The tricuspid valve septal leaflet can be seen in the apical four-chamber view arising from the ventricular septum near the cardiac apex and away from the annulus (Fig. 24–30).[P4] The anterior leaflet of the tricuspid valve, which usually arises normally from the fibrous annulus, is large and sail-like and spirals downward and outward toward the right ventricular outflow tract. The large redundant anterior leaflet can obstruct forward flow out the right ventricle and, thus, cause pulmonary stenosis. In the most severe cases, there may be true anatomic pulmonary atresia. In infants with a widely patent ductus arteriosus and severe tricuspid insufficiency, the main pulmonary artery systolic pressure can exceed right ventricular systolic pressure, causing a functional pulmonary atresia. In these patients, no pulmonary valve leaflet motion can be detected on the two-dimensional echocardiogram and no antegrade flow across the pulmonary valve can be detected on the Doppler examination. Under these circumstances, it can be very difficult to distinguish true anatomic pulmonary atresia from functional pulmonary atresia by echocardiographic examination.

Additional valuable information that can be obtained from the two-dimensional and Doppler echocardiographic examination in patients with Ebstein malformation includes (1) the size of the atrialized portion of the right ventricle, (2) the size of the functioning portion of the right ventricle, (3) the size of the atrial septal defect, (4) the presence and severity of tricuspid insufficiency, and (5) the presence of a patent ductus arteriosus.

Pulmonary atresia with an intact ventricular septum (hypoplas-

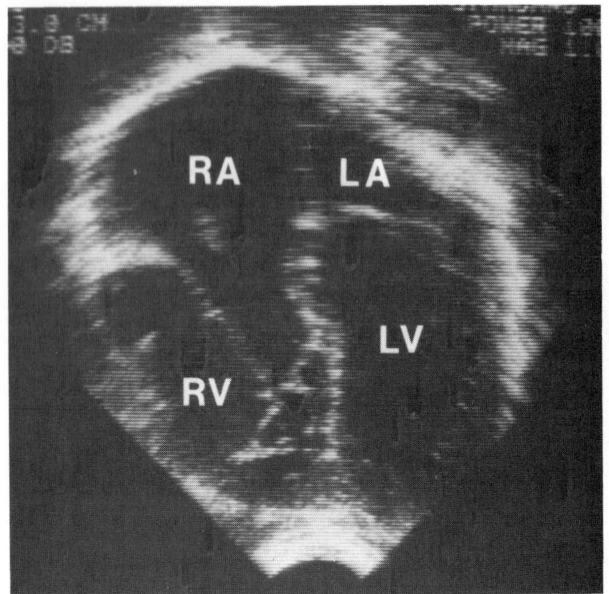

Figure 24–30. Apical four-chamber view of a child with Ebstein deformity of the tricuspid valve. The anterior leaflet of the tricuspid valve arises normally from the fibrous annulus; however, the septal leaflet of the tricuspid valve is displaced inferiorly in the right ventricle (RV) and arises from the lower portion of the ventricular septum. This displacement results in atrialization of a large portion of the RV and loss of total functioning RV mass. Abbreviations: LA—left atrium; LV—left ventricle; RA—right atrium.

tic right heart syndrome) is another defect with right ventricular obstruction and right-to-left atrial shunting. On the two-dimensional echocardiogram in these infants (Fig. 24–31), the right ventricle is severely hypertrophic and has bright endocardial echoes (fibroelastosis). The right ventricular cavity varies in size from diminutive to nearly normal and, frequently, large sinusoids are seen connecting the cavity of the right ventricle to the coronary arteries. Usually, the tricuspid valve is thickened and immobile and has an annulus size that is smaller than normal. The right atrium is enlarged and the amount of tricuspid insufficiency (if present) varies considerably. There is also a great deal of variability in the size of the right ventricular infundibulum, main pulmonary artery, and pulmonary artery branches.

CONGENITAL HEART DISEASE WITH CYANOSIS AND INCREASED PULMONARY VASCULARITY

Increased Pulmonary Arterial Markings

Children with cyanosis and increased pulmonary arterial markings on chest x-ray have mixing of venous and arterial blood,

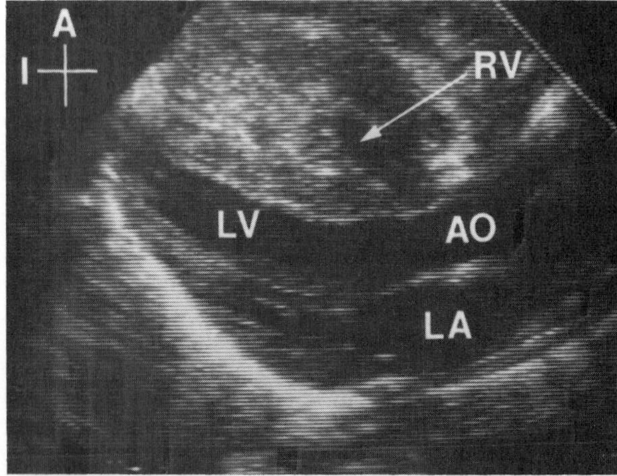

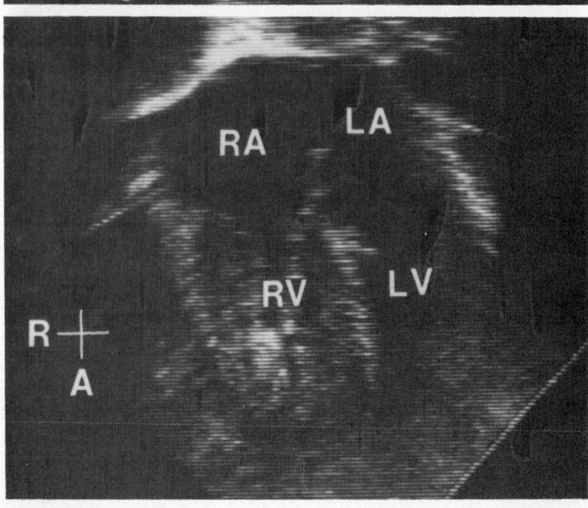

Figure 24–31. Parasternal long-axis (top) and apical four-chamber (bottom) views of an infant with pulmonary atresia and an intact ventricular septum. Note that the right ventricle (RV) is very hypertrophic and has a diminutive cavity. Abbreviations: A—anterior; AO—aorta; I—inferior; LA—left atrium; LV—left ventricle; R—right; RA—right atrium. (From Snider, A. R.: Two-dimensional and Doppler echocardiographic evaluation of heart disease in the neonate and fetus. Clin. Perinatol. 15:547, 1988, with permission.)

increased pulmonary blood flow, and no significant pulmonary stenosis. Some of the more common congenital heart defects that fall into this category are d-transposition of the great arteries, truncus arteriosus, single ventricle, and single atrium.

In simple or d-transposition of the great arteries, there are concordant atrioventricular connections (right atrium connected to the morphologic right ventricle) and discordant ventriculoarterial connections (aorta arising from the morphologic right ventricle). The morphology of the cardiac chambers is readily determined on the two-dimensional echocardiogram. The techniques for determining cardiac chamber morphology are discussed in detail in a later section. Multiple echocardiographic views are necessary for a complete diagnosis of d-transposition; however, the subcostal views are especially useful for demonstrating the abnormal ventriculoarterial connections. In these views, the aorta is identified as the vessel that arches and the pulmonary artery is identified as the vessel that bifurcates (Fig. 24–32).[B7] D-transposition of the great arteries is caused by lack of rotation of the embryonic conotruncus; therefore, the great arteries exit the heart in a parallel fashion rather than being coiled around one another. This abnormal parallel arrangement of the great arteries can be seen in the parasternal long-axis and short-axis views. In the short-axis view, the great vessels are seen as double circles in cross section with the aorta anterior and rightward of the pulmonary artery.[H6]

In severely cyanotic and acidotic newborn infants, the diagnosis of d-transposition can be made rapidly and safely with two-dimensional echocardiography. The arterial switch procedure has gained widespread acceptance as the preferred surgical repair of transposition in the first month of life. Part of the success of this operation is based on a clear identification of coronary artery anatomy. Initial reports suggest that coronary artery anatomy can be correctly diagnosed by two-dimensional echocardiography in most infants with simple transposition of the great arteries.[P1]

In persistent truncus arteriosus, a large artery exits the heart from both ventricles and gives rise to the aortic arch, coronary arteries, and pulmonary arteries. On the two-dimensional echocardiogram, the truncus arteriosus overrides the ventricular septum and there is discontinuity between the anterior truncal wall and the ventricular septum (Fig. 24–33).[H2] Usually, the truncal valve is in fibrous continuity with the anterior mitral valve leaflet. A large outlet ventricular septal defect is usually present. The right ventricle is hypertrophic and the pulmonary valve is absent. The parasternal short-axis views and the suprasternal views are useful for identifying the connections of the pulmonary arteries to the truncus arteriosus. In truncus arteriosus Type I, the pulmonary artery branches arise via a short main pulmonary segment from the left lateral aspect of the ascending aorta (Fig. 24–34). In truncus arteriosus Type II, the two pulmonary artery branches arise from the posterior wall of the ascending aorta via

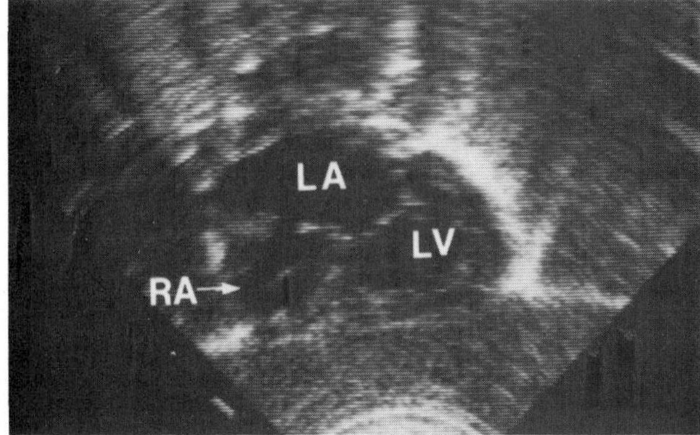

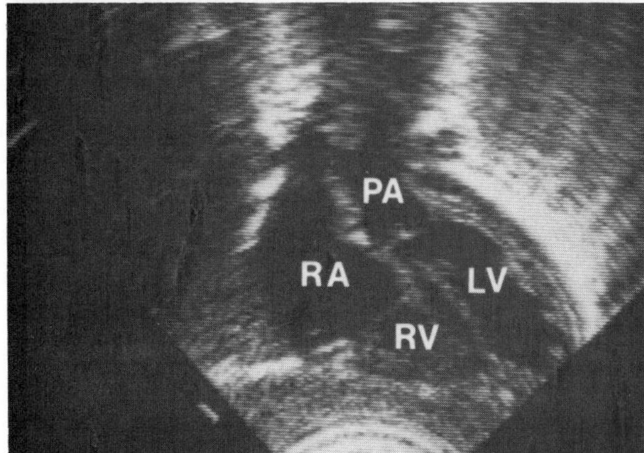

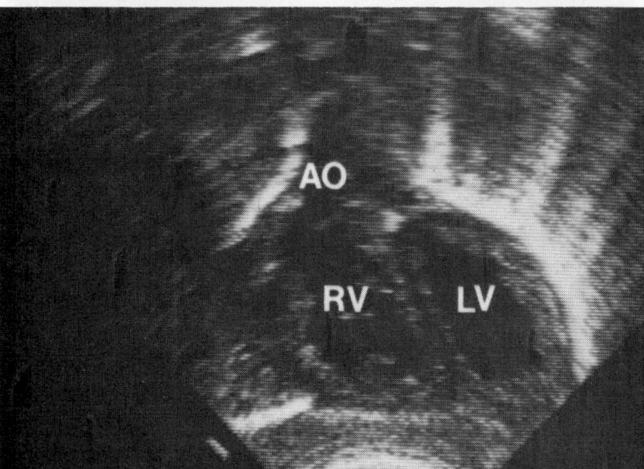

Figure 24–32. Subcostal views in coronal body planes of a newborn infant with d-transposition of the great arteries. From top to bottom, these frames represent a progressive tilt of the plane of sound from a posterior to a very anterior position. The top frame is a coronal view taken with the plane of sound oriented posteriorly through the inlet of the heart. The eustachian valve can be imaged in the morphologic right atrium (RA), and the pulmonary veins can be seen draining to the morphologic left atrium (LA). The echocardiographic dropout in the atrial septum represents a secundum atrial septal defect. The middle frame represents a slight anterior tilt of the plane of sound so that the entire left ventricular (LV) outflow tract can be imaged. The pulmonary artery (PA) and its bifurcation into two pulmonary artery branches can be seen arising from the LV. Imaging of a vessel that bifurcates arising from the LV is echocardiographic proof of discordant ventriculoarterial connection or transposition of the great arteries. The bottom frame represents the most anterior coronal plane. In this plane, a vessel that does not bifurcate and is, therefore, the aorta (AO) is seen arising from the right ventricle (RV).

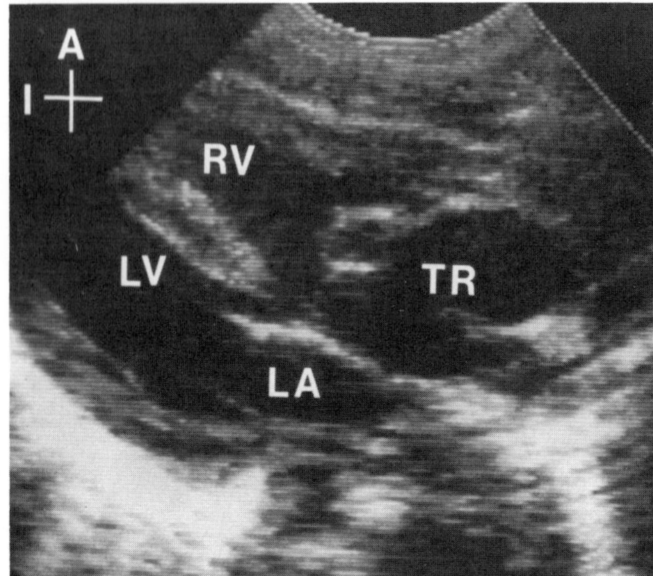

Figure 24–33. Parasternal long-axis view of an infant with truncus arteriosus. The discontinuity between the septum and the anterior wall of the truncus arteriosus (TR) represents a large outlet ventricular septal defect. The truncal vessel overrides the ventricular septum so that both the right ventricle (RV) and the left ventricle (LV) eject into the truncus arteriosus. Abbreviations: A—anterior; I—inferior; LA—left atrium.

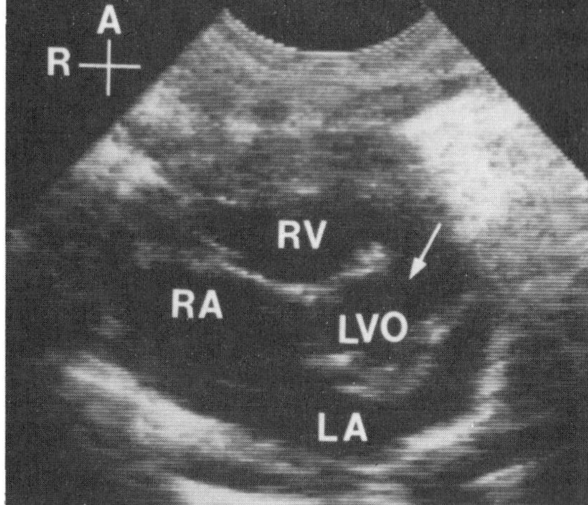

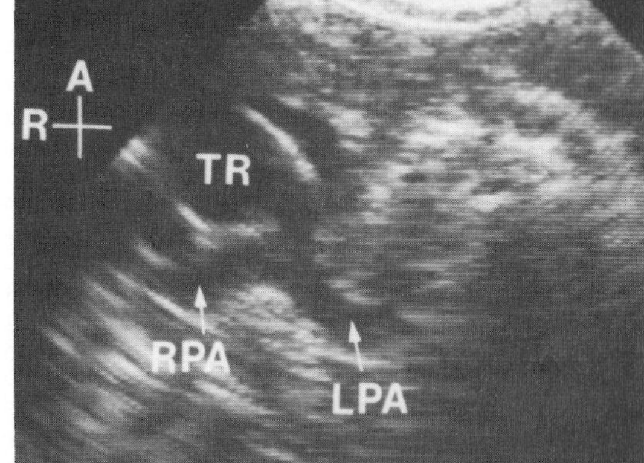

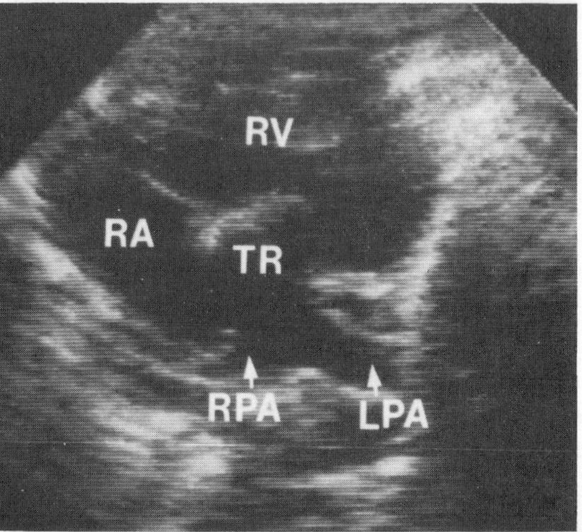

Figure 24–34. Parasternal short-axis views of several infants with truncus arteriosus. The top frame shows a short-axis view at the base of the heart and demonstrates a large ventricular septal defect (*arrow*) in the outlet portion of the ventricular septum. The position of the defect in this patient is very typical of that found in truncus arteriosus. The middle frame shows a cross section through the truncal vessel (TR) of an infant with truncus arteriosus Type I. In this form of truncus arteriosus, there is a short main pulmonary artery segment that arises from the left lateral aspect of the TR and gives rise to both right and left pulmonary artery branches (RPA and LPA). The bottom frame is a short-axis view through the truncal vessel of an infant with Type II truncus arteriosus. In Type II truncus arteriosus, both great arteries arise from the posterior aspect of the truncal vessel by way of side-by-side but separate orifices. Abbreviations: A—anterior; LA—left atrium; LVO—left ventricular outflow tract; R—right; RA—right atrium; RV—right ventricle.

separate (but side-by-side) orifices. In truncus arteriosus Type III, the pulmonary artery branches arise from the truncal vessel via two widely separated orifices.

In children with truncus arteriosus, the two-dimensional echocardiogram is especially useful for detecting associated abnormalities, including (1) the presence of a right aortic arch, present in about one-third of patients with truncus arteriosus; (2) the number of truncal valve cusps (quadricuspid truncal valves are common); (3) the presence of a patent ductus arteriosus; and (4) the presence of additional muscular ventricular septal defects. The Doppler examination is particularly helpful for determining (1) whether the truncal valve is stenotic and, if so, the degree of stenosis; (2) whether the truncal valve is insufficient and, if so, the severity of insufficiency; and (3) whether the pulmonary artery branches are stenotic at their origins.

Increased Pulmonary Venous Markings

Cyanotic infants with increased pulmonary venous markings on chest x-ray have intracardiac right-to-left shunting and obstruction to pulmonary venous return. The most common defect in this category is total anomalous pulmonary venous return, a condition in which the pulmonary veins join to form a confluence that drains back to the right atrium rather than the left atrium. Clinically, this defect can be difficult to differentiate from persistent pulmonary artery hypertension or pulmonary disease of the newborn, and prior to the use of echocardiography, cardiac catheterization was often required for a definitive diagnosis. With two-dimensional and Doppler echocardiography, total anomalous pulmonary venous return usually can be diagnosed rapidly and with certainty. Thus, potentially risky cardiac catheterizations can be avoided in unstable newborn infants with lung disease or primary pulmonary hypertension.

Total anomalous pulmonary venous return can be diagnosed on the two-dimensional echocardiogram by identifying the pulmonary venous confluence that is situated posterior and separated from the left atrium (Fig. 24–35).[S9] Usually, the final site of drainage of the pulmonary venous confluence into the right atrium can be visualized.[S2] In total anomalous pulmonary venous return to the coronary sinus (intracardiac type), the pulmonary venous confluence can be seen connecting to a very dilated coronary sinus in the parasternal long-axis and short-axis views.[S13] In total anomalous pulmonary venous return to the superior vena cava by way of a left vertical vein and innominate vein (supracardiac type), the entire anomalous connection can be seen in the suprasternal short-axis view (Fig. 24–36).[S14]

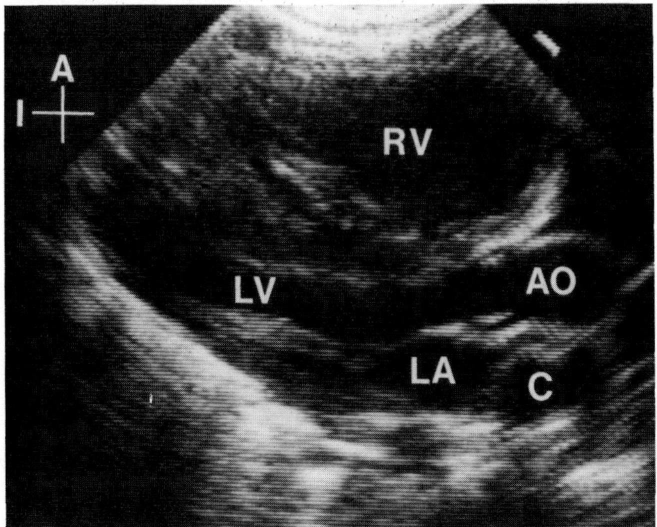

Figure 24–35. Parasternal long-axis view of an infant with total anomalous pulmonary venous connection. The pulmonary veins come together to form a confluence (C) that is located behind and separate from the left atrium (LA). Abbreviations: A—anterior; AO—aorta; I—inferior; LV—left ventricle; RV—right ventricle.

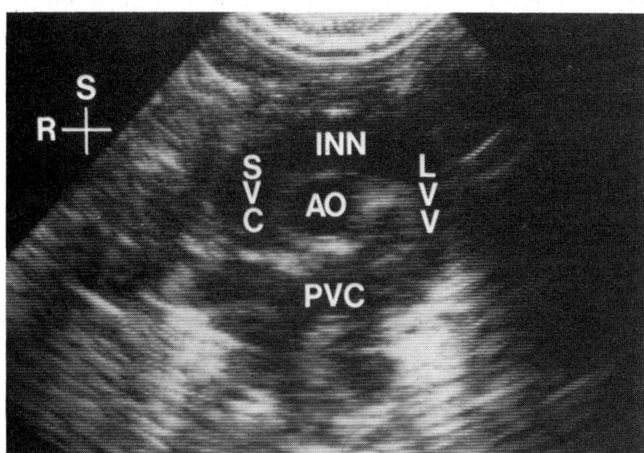

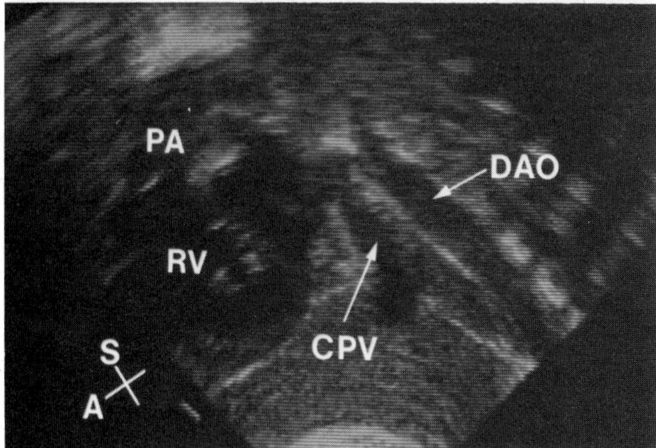

Figure 24–36. (Top) Suprasternal short-axis view of an infant with total anomalous pulmonary venous return to the right superior vena cava (SVC) by way of a left vertical vein (LVV) and innominate vein (INN). In this view, the pulmonary venous confluence (PVC) can be seen draining to the LVV and eventually to the SVC. This anomalous pulmonary venous connection surrounding the aorta (AO) creates the appearance of a snowman-shaped heart on the chest x-ray. (Bottom) Subcostal sagittal view of an infant with infradiaphragmatic total anomalous pulmonary venous connection. In this view, the pulmonary veins drain together to form a common pulmonary vein (CPV) that then drains anterior to the descending aorta (DAO), through the diaphragm, and into the abdomen. Once in the abdomen, the CPV immediately turned anteriorly and drained into the left hepatic vein. Abbreviations: A—anterior; PA—pulmonary artery; R—right; RV—right ventricle; S—superior.

In infradiaphragmatic total anomalous pulmonary venous return (infracardiac type), the common pulmonary vein can be visualized in the subcostal views as it leaves the pulmonary venous confluence, passes anterior to the aorta through the diaphragm, and drains into a systemic vein in the adomen—usually the hepatic portal venous system (see Fig. 24–36).[S15] In children with total anomalous pulmonary venous return, Doppler interrogation of the left vertical vein or common pulmonary vein shows venous flow directed away from the heart. Thus, the Doppler examination is useful for confirming that the unusual venous structure seen on the two-dimensional echocardiogram is the common pulmonary vein and not some other anomalous systemic vein (in which flow would be directed toward the heart).[S11]

ECHOCARDIOGRAPHIC APPROACH TO COMPLEX CONGENITAL HEART DISEASE

Two-dimensional echocardiography has had a major impact on our ability to diagnose complex congenital heart defects. With this technique, one can image detailed structural anatomy even more precisely than with cardiac catheterization in the majority of patients. The echocardiographic approach to the diagnosis of complex congenital heart disease is a very logical and systematic approach that requires a basic knowledge of how cardiac chambers are identified on the two-dimensional echocardiogram.

The echocardiographic approach to the diagnosis of complex congenital disease involves a segmental analysis of the heart. In this type of analysis, one can think of the heart as being much like a house. To describe a house completely, one must describe where the rooms or chambers are on each floor. For the cardiac house, then, one must describe where each atrium is located on the ground floor, where the ventricles are located on the second story, and where each great artery is positioned at the top of the house. In addition, one must describe where the staircases are that connect the floors. In other words, one must describe the atrioventricular connections and the ventriculoarterial connections. If one does not describe the atria correctly, the entire house comes tumbling down.

Thus, the approach to the echocardiographic diagnosis of the patient with complex congenital heart disease is begun by determining the atrial situs. In atrial situs solitus, the morphologic right atrium is on the right and the morphologic left atrium is on the left. In situs inversus, the morphologic left atrium is on the right and the morphologic right atrium is on the left. In situs ambiguus, the atria do not differentiate into right and left atria. Instead, both atria can have features of a morphologic right atrium, a condition called asplenia, or both atria can have features of a morphologic left atrium, a condition called polysplenia. The echocardiographic findings used to identify the morphology of the atria are reviewed later in this section.

The next step in diagnosing complex congenital heart disease is determination of the bulboventricular loop. The bulboventricular loop describes the locations of the ventricles. In a d-loop (dextro loop) the morphologic right ventricle is on the right and the morphologic left ventricle is on the left. In an l-loop (levo loop), the morphologic right ventricle is on the left and the morphologic left ventricle is on the right. These definitions of d-loop and l-loop apply regardless of what the atrial situs is.

The final step in the diagnosis of complex congenital heart disease is a description of the great artery connections. In normal or concordant connections, the pulmonary artery arises from the right ventricle and the aorta arises from the left ventricle. In transposition, the aorta arises from the morphologic right ventricle and the pulmonary artery arises from the morphologic left ventricle. Transposition is a discordant ventriculoarterial connection. Other types of great artery connections include double-outlet right ventricle, double-outlet left ventricle, and single outlet from the heart. Three common forms of single outlet from the heart include truncus arteriosus, aortic atresia, and pulmonary atresia.

Concordant or normal connections between the atria and ventricles (right atrium to right ventricle, left atrium to left ventricle) occur when there is situs solitus with a d-loop or situs inversus with an l-loop. Discordant or abnormal connections between the atria and ventricles (right atrium to left ventricle, left atrium to right ventricle) occur when there is situs solitus with an l-loop or situs inversus with a d-loop. Before reviewing how cardiac chambers are identified on the two-dimensional echocardiogram, we should review the rule of 50 percent. The rule of 50 percent states that a chamber is a ventricle if it receives 50 percent or more of an inlet. A chamber need not have an outlet to be a ventricle. For example, the left ventricle in double-outlet right ventricle is a ventricle because it receives the mitral valve even though it does not have an outlet. Second, if 50 percent or more of a great artery arises above a chamber, it is defined as being connected to that chamber. Rudimentary chambers are chambers that receive less than 50 percent of an inlet and, therefore, do not qualify to be ventricles (Figs. 24–37 and 24–38). There are two types of rudimentary chambers. An outlet chamber is a chamber that has less than 50 percent of an inlet but 50 percent or more of an outlet or great artery. A trabeculated pouch is a chamber that has less than 50 percent of an inlet and less than 50 percent of an outlet.[H9]

In order to diagnose complex congenital heart disease, one must know how cardiac chambers are identified on the two-dimensional echocardiogram. The cardiac chambers are largely defined by the anatomic landmarks on their septal surfaces. The right atrium has a septal surface that receives the tendinous insertion of the eustachian valve and has the limbus of the fossa ovalis. The eustachian valve crosses the floor of the right atrium from the orifice of the inferior vena cava and inserts into the septum primum (the lower portion of the atrial septum adjacent to the atrioventricular valves). This tendinous insertion is along the lower border of the fossa ovalis and is called the inferior limbic band (Fig. 24–39). In real time, the eustachian valve moves rapidly back and forth in the right atrium and can be visualized in virtually all infants and in many older children and adults.

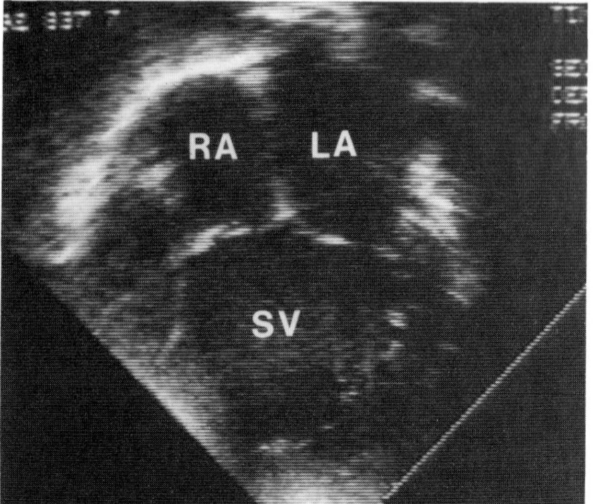

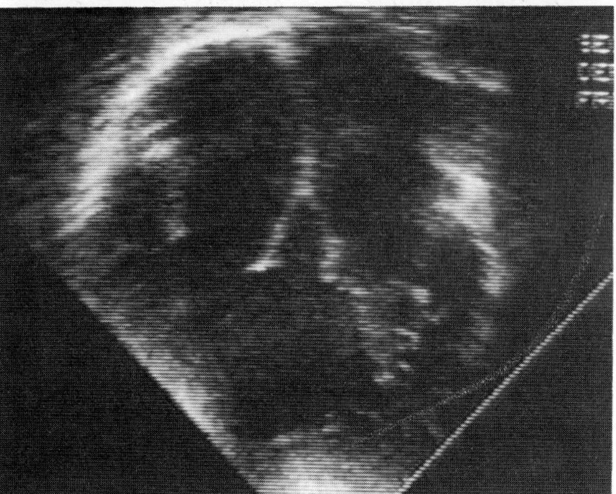

Figure 24–37. Apical four-chamber views in systole (above) and diastole (below) of a child with a single ventricle (SV) of the left ventricular type, l-transposition of the great arteries, and an outlet chamber situated at the left basal aspect of the heart giving rise to the aorta. In the apical four-chamber views, both atrioventricular valves can be seen emptying into a large posterior single ventricle. Abbreviations: LA—left atrium; RA—right atrium.

The left atrial septal surface has the flap valve of the fossa ovalis. This is the septum primum tissue that covers the foramen ovale and seals it closed after birth. The flap valve can be seen on the two-dimensional echocardiogram protruding into the left atrium in the fetus when the foramen ovale is open; however, the flap valve cannot ordinarily be identified after birth on the two-dimensional echocardiogram. Therefore, other methods must be used to identify the left atrium.

The right ventricle is the chamber whose septal surface has prominent muscle bundles crossing from the septum to the parietal free wall (Fig. 24–40). The largest of these septoparietal muscle bundles is the moderator band. In addition, the septal surface of the right ventricle receives chordal insertions from the tricuspid valve septal leaflet (Fig. 24–41).

The left ventricle is the chamber whose septal surface is smooth. There are no septoparietal free wall muscle bundles,

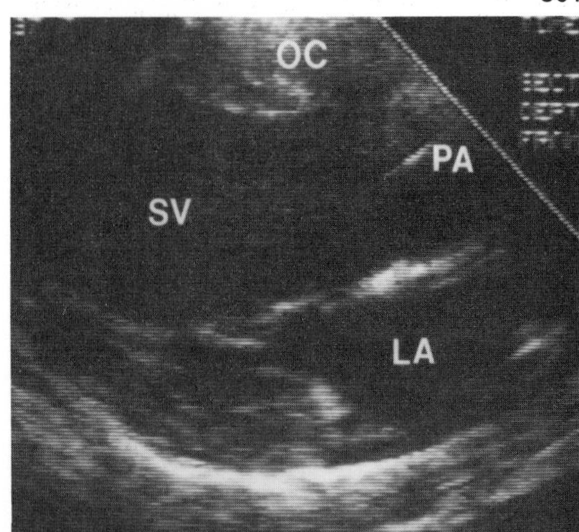

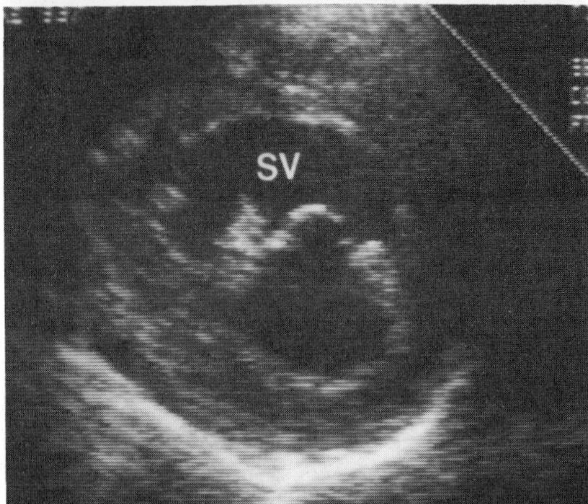

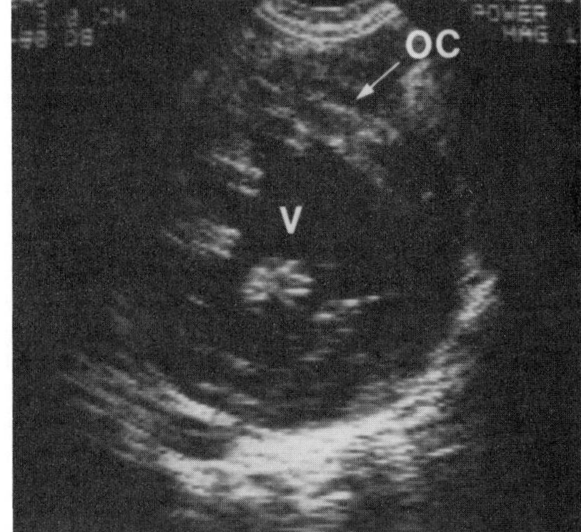

Figure 24–38. Parasternal long-axis (top) and short-axis (middle and bottom) views of the same patient as in Figure 24–37. In the parasternal long-axis view, the single ventricle (SV) can be seen communicating with the outlet chamber (OC) by way of the bulboventricular foramen. The pulmonary artery (PA) is seen arising from the posterior single ventricle. Other views showed the aorta arising from the OC. The middle frame shows that both atrioventricular valves empty into the SV. The bottom frame shows that the OC is located at the leftward and basal aspect of the heart. With these views, it is obvious that the OC does not receive any portion of an inlet and, therefore, does not qualify to be a ventricle. Abbreviation: LA—left atrium.

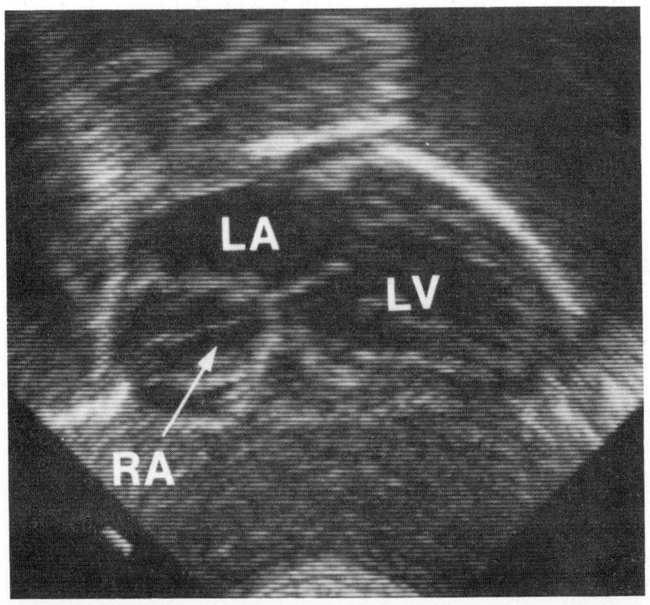

Figure 24–39. Subcostal four-chamber view through the inlet of the heart in a normal patient. The eustachian valve can be seen crossing the floor of the right atrium (RA) from its origin at the orifice of the inferior vena cava to its insertion in the lowermost portion of the atrial septum. The eustachian valve is an anatomic marker of a morphologic right atrium. Abbreviations: LA—left atrium; LV—left ventricle.

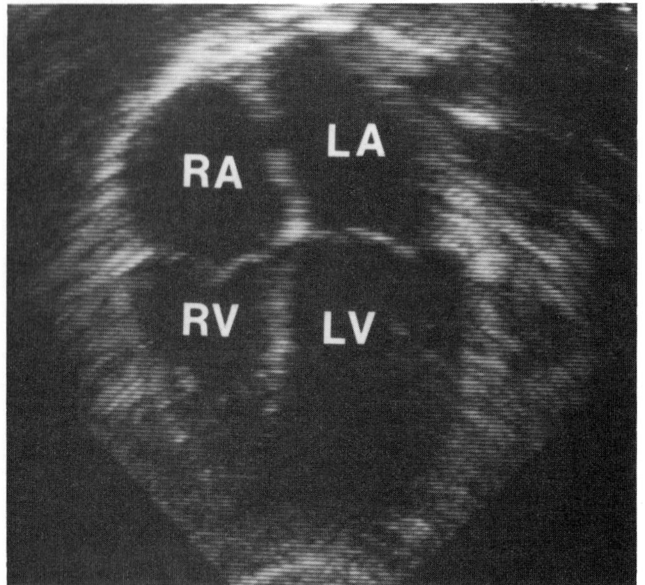

Figure 24–40. Apical four-chamber view of a normal patient. The ventricle on the patient's right has an atrioventricular valve that is closer to the cardiac apex and has heavy trabeculations crossing from the septum to the parietal free wall. These anatomic features indicate that the right-sided ventricle is a morphologic right ventricle (RV). The ventricle on the patient's left has a smooth septal surface and no muscle bundles coursing from the septum to the parietal free wall. In addition, its atrioventricular valve is farther from the cardiac apex. These features are landmarks of a morphologic left ventricle (LV). Abbreviations: LA—left atrium; RA—right atrium.

and the mitral valve normally has no chordal insertions into the septum.

Another anatomic feature that is useful in identifying the cardiac chambers is that the atrioventricular valve always belongs to the appropriate ventricle. Thus, the tricuspid valve is always found in the morphologic right ventricle and the mitral valve is always found in the morphologic left ventricle. The tricuspid valve is closer to the cardiac apex (see Fig. 24–40), has three leaflets, and has chordal insertions into the ventricular septum (see Fig. 24–41). The mitral valve is farther from the cardiac apex, is a fish-mouth bicuspid valve, and has chordal insertions only into two papillary muscles in the left ventricle.

Systemic and pulmonary venous return can be helpful in identifying the atria. The pulmonary veins usually drain to the left atrium; however, this is not a constant feature of the left atrium, as the pulmonary veins can drain anomalously. If three or more pulmonary veins are visualized draining by separate orifices to a chamber and there is no evidence of a pulmonary venous confluence, then that chamber is most likely a morphologic left atrium. The inferior vena cava usually drains to the morphologic right atrium. This relationship is constant in the majority of cases except in patients with situs ambiguus. The superior vena cava usually drains to the right atrium; however, this relationship is not constant as the superior vena cava can drain to either or both atria (Figs. 24–42 through 24–44).

The morphology of the atrial appendages can be helpful in identifying the atria. The right atrial appendage is short and stout (resembling "Snoopy's" nose), and the left atrial appendage is long and fingerlike (resembling "Snoopy's" ear) (Fig. 24–45).

In addition, the situs of the abdomen may be helpful in determining the atrial situs. In atrial situs solitus, the inferior vena cava is to the right of the spine, the descending aorta is to the left of the spine, the stomach bubble is on the left, and the liver is on the right. In atrial situs inversus, the inferior vena cava is usually to the left of the spine and the descending aorta is usually to the right of the spine. The stomach bubble is on the right and the liver is on the left (Fig. 24–46). In situs ambiguus, there are several types of anomalies of systemic venous drainage that are often present.[S5, S7] For example, in asplenia, the inferior vena cava and aorta may be on the same side of the spine (Fig. 24–47). Also, in situs ambiguus, it is common to find an interrupted inferior vena cava. In this case, the hepatic veins usually drain to the right side of the common atrium and inferior vena cava drainage is usually by way of an azygous or hemiazygous vein (Fig. 24–48).

Figures 24–49 through 24–51 show examples of how the echocardiogram can be used to define cardiac chamber morphology and thus diagnose complex congenital defects.[C2, M2, P2]

SUMMARY

Two-dimensional echocardiography and Doppler echocardiography are important noninvasive techniques for the diagnosis and subsequent management of children with congenital heart dis-

Text continued on page 508

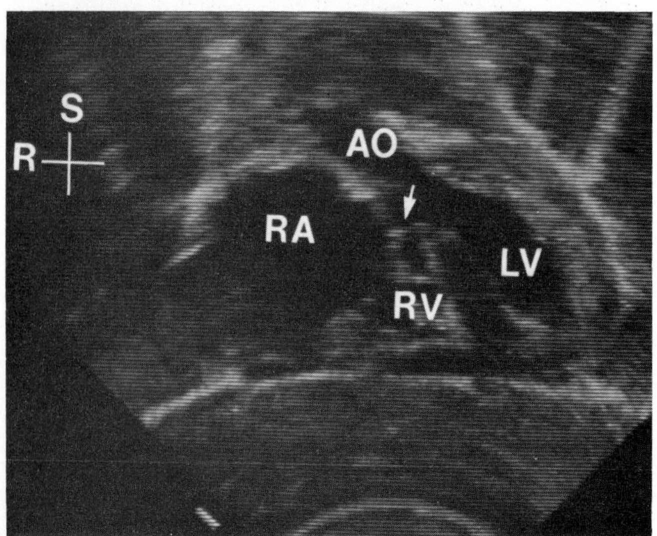

Figure 24–41. Subcostal coronal view through the left ventricular (LV) outflow tract of a child with a large membranous ventricular septal defect (*arrow*). Note that the tricuspid valve has chordal insertions into the right ventricular side of the ventricular septum at the lower border of the ventricular septal defect. This anatomic feature identifies the morphologic right ventricle (RV). Abbreviations: AO—aorta; R—right; RA—right atrium; S—superior.

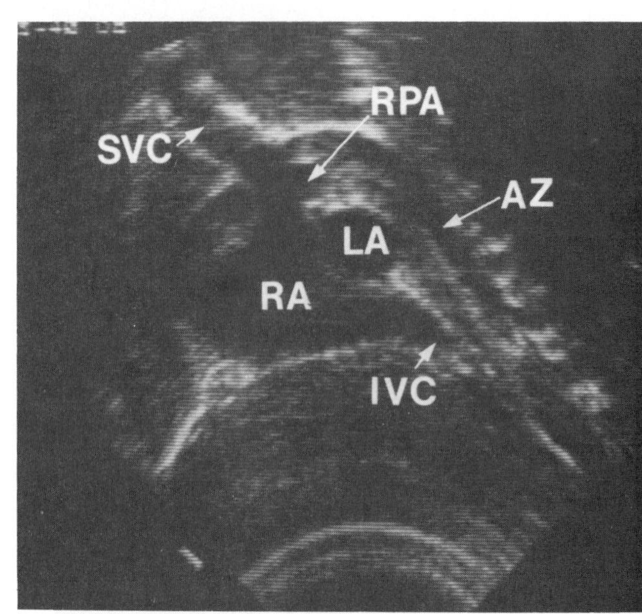

Figure 24–42. Subcostal sagittal view of a normal patient showing the normal pattern of systemic venous return. This plane was obtained by positioning the plane of sound in a sagittal body plane and orienting the transducer toward the patient's right atrium (RA). The superior vena cava (SVC) and inferior vena cava (IVC) can be seen draining to the RA. Posteriorly, the azygous vein (AZ) can be seen entering the SVC posterior and superior to the right pulmonary artery (RPA). Abbreviation: LA—left atrium.

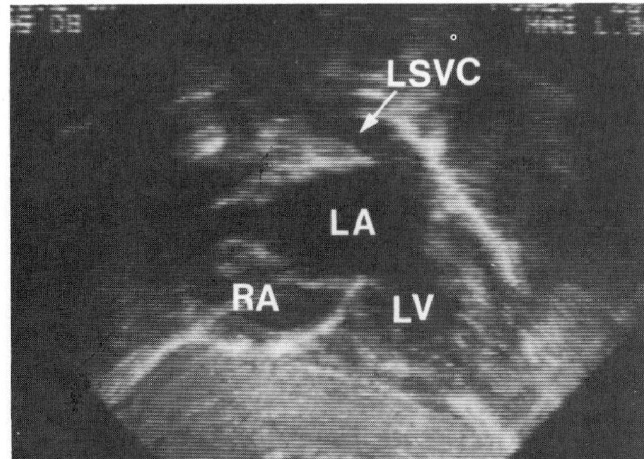

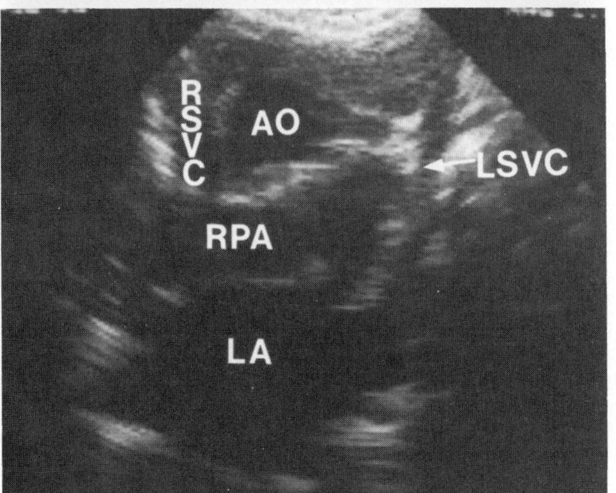

Figure 24–43. Subcostal four-chamber (top) and suprasternal short-axis (bottom) views of a patient with a persistent left superior vena cava (LSVC) draining directly to the left atrium (LA). In these views, the persistent LSVC-to-LA communication can be seen. In addition, this patient had a right superior vena cava (RSVC). Abbreviations: AO—aorta; LV—left ventricle; RA—right atrium; RPA—right pulmonary artery.

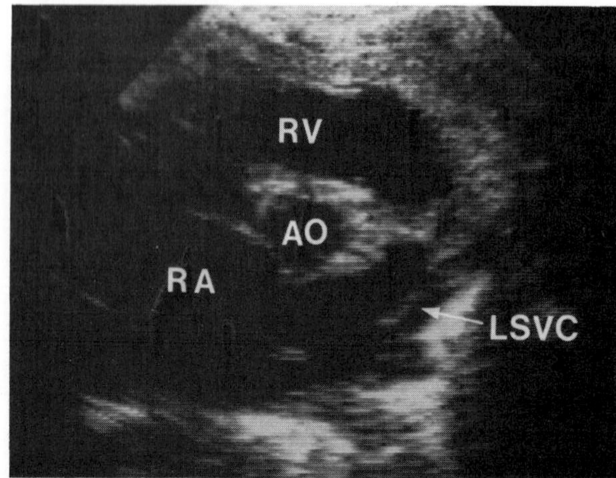

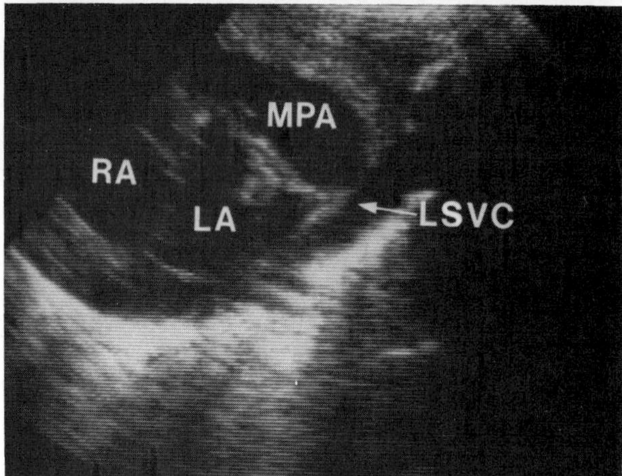

Figure 24–44. Parasternal short-axis (top) and suprasternal long-axis (bottom) views of a patient with a persistent left superior vena cava (LSVC) draining to the coronary sinus. In these views, the anomalous connection between the persistent LSVC, coronary sinus, and right atrium (RA) can be visualized. Abbreviations: AO—aorta; LA—left atrium; MPA—main pulmonary artery; RV—right ventricle.

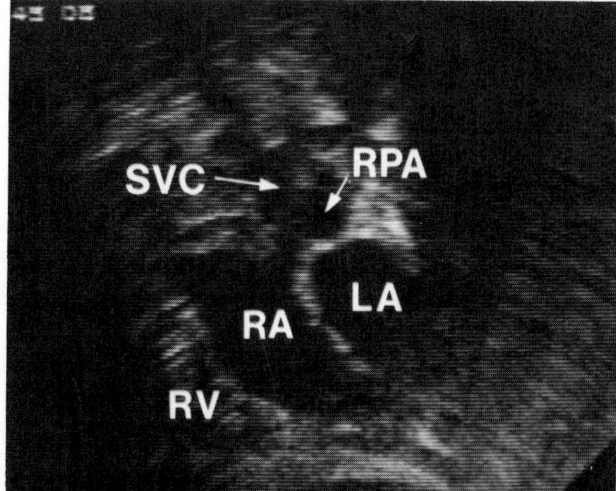

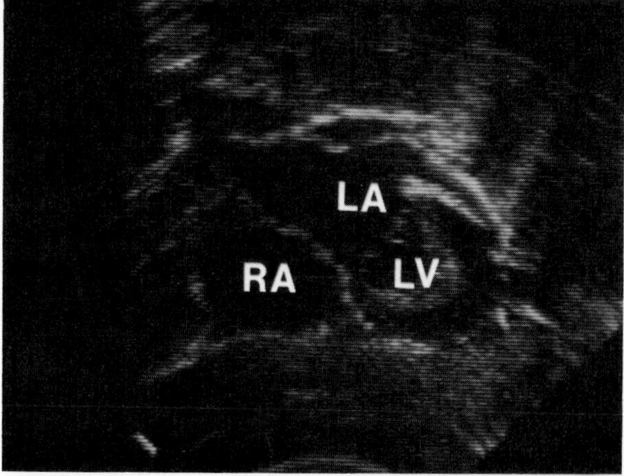

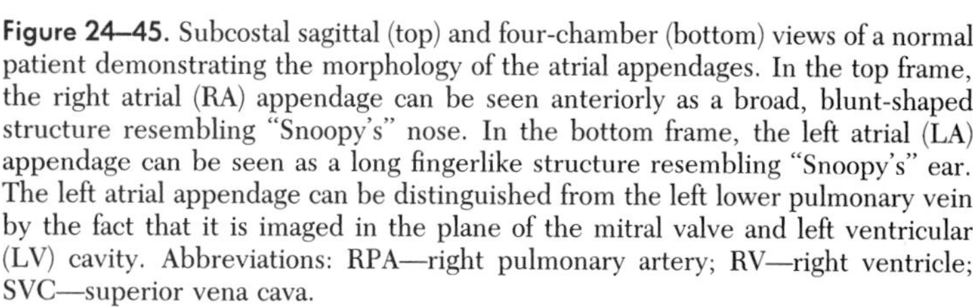

Figure 24–45. Subcostal sagittal (top) and four-chamber (bottom) views of a normal patient demonstrating the morphology of the atrial appendages. In the top frame, the right atrial (RA) appendage can be seen anteriorly as a broad, blunt-shaped structure resembling "Snoopy's" nose. In the bottom frame, the left atrial (LA) appendage can be seen as a long fingerlike structure resembling "Snoopy's" ear. The left atrial appendage can be distinguished from the left lower pulmonary vein by the fact that it is imaged in the plane of the mitral valve and left ventricular (LV) cavity. Abbreviations: RPA—right pulmonary artery; RV—right ventricle; SVC—superior vena cava.

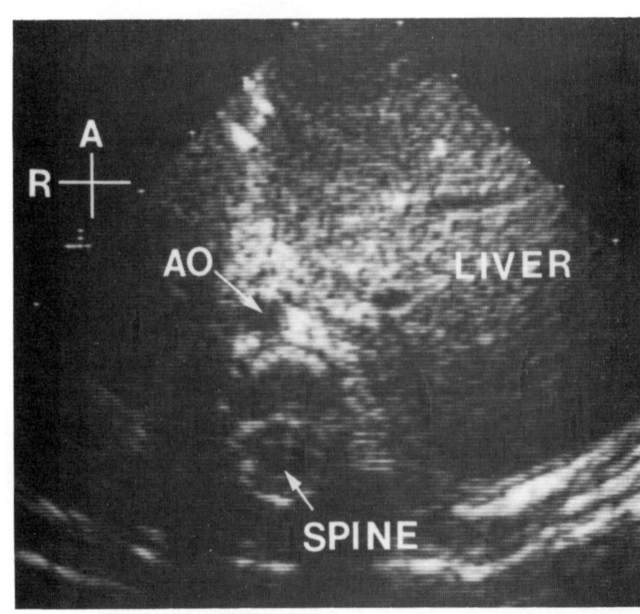

Figure 24–46. Subcostal short-axis view of the abdomen of a patient with situs inversus of the atria. In this patient, findings of situs inversus of the abdomen are a clue that there is probably situs inversus of the atria. Note that the liver is on the patient's left, as is the inferior vena cava. The aorta (AO) is to the right of the spine. Abbreviations: A—anterior; R—right.

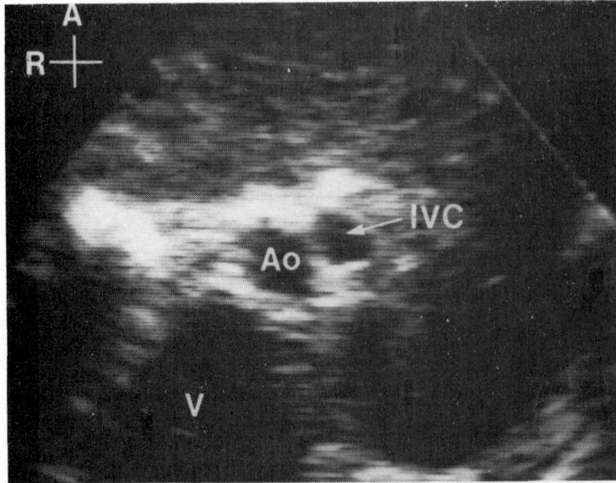

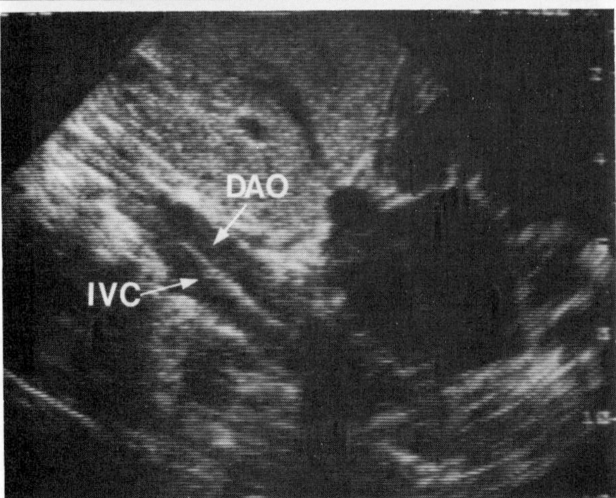

Figure 24–47. Subcostal short-axis (top) and long-axis (bottom) views of two patients with situs ambiguus (asplenia). In these two patients, the inferior vena cava (IVC) was on the same side of the vertebral body (V) as the descending aorta (DAO). The IVC is anterior and to the left of the DAO. This arrangement of the vessels in the abdomen is frequently seen in patients with situs ambiguus. Abbreviations: A—anterior; R—right; Ao—aorta.

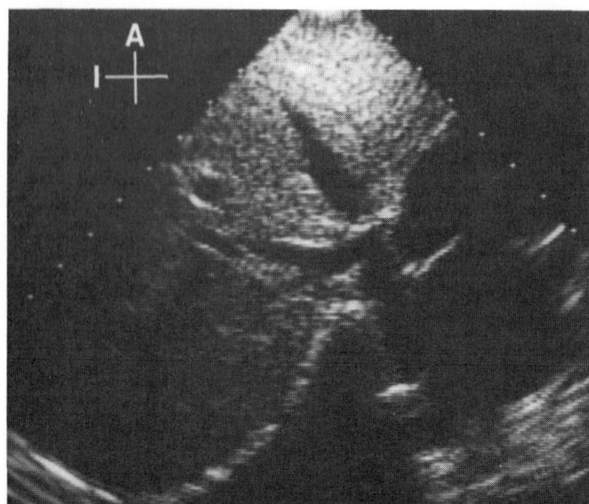

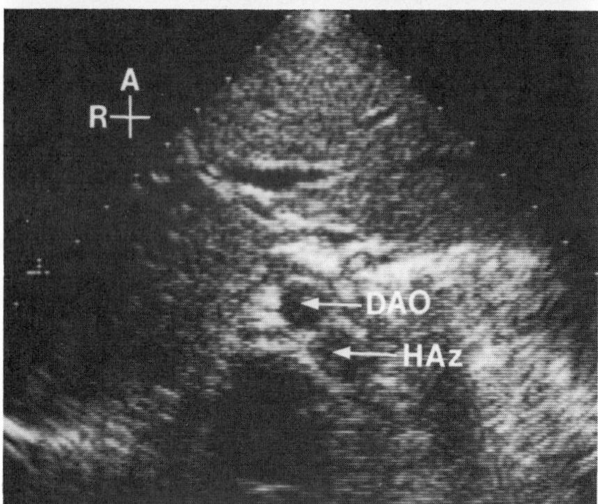

Figure 24–48. Subcostal long-axis (top) and short-axis (bottom) views of the abdomen in a patient with situs ambiguus (polysplenia). The subcostal long-axis view in this patient showed the hepatic veins draining directly to the right side of a common atrium. The inferior vena cava was interrupted in this patient. The bottom frame shows that inferior vena caval drainage was by way of a hemiazygous (HAz) vein that drained to the left side of the common atrium. The hemiazygous vein is situated to the left and posterior of the descending aorta (DAO). This posterior position differentiates it from the inferior vena cava. Abbreviations: A—anterior; I—inferior; R—right.

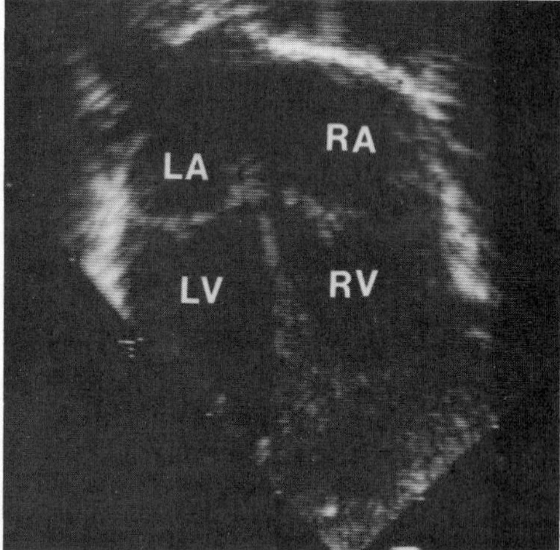

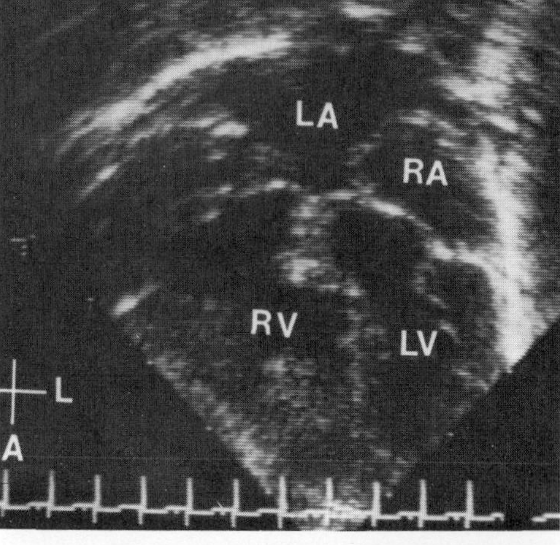

Figure 24–49. (Top) Apical four-chamber view of a patient with situs inversus of the atria, l-loop, and normally connected great arteries. In this patient, the pulmonary veins are seen draining to the right-sided atrium, suggesting that this atrium is a morphologic left atrium (LA). The ventricle on the patient's left has an atrioventricular valve closer to the cardiac apex and has a prominent moderator band. These findings suggest that the left-sided ventricle is a morphologic right ventricle (RV). Thus, the patient has atrial situs inversus with an l-loop. (Bottom) Apical four-chamber view of a patient with atrial situs inversus, d-loop, and d-transposition of the great arteries. In this patient, the pulmonary veins are seen draining to the right-sided atrium, indicating that it is a morphologic LA. The ventricle on the patient's right side has prominent muscle bundles coursing from the septum to the parietal free wall and has an atrioventricular valve with chordal insertions into the ventricular septum. These findings suggest that the ventricle on the patient's right side is a morphologic RV and that there is a d-bulboventricular loop. Thus, the patient has atrial situs inversus with a d-loop (discordant atrioventricular connections). Note the large inlet ventricular septal defect in this patient. Abbreviations: A—apex; L—left; RA—right atrium; LV—left ventricle.

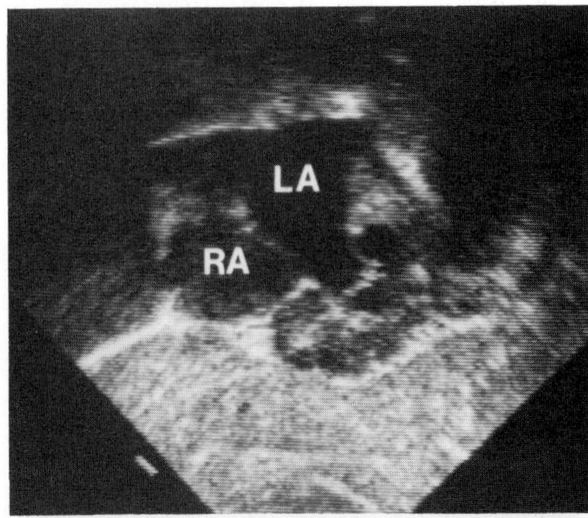

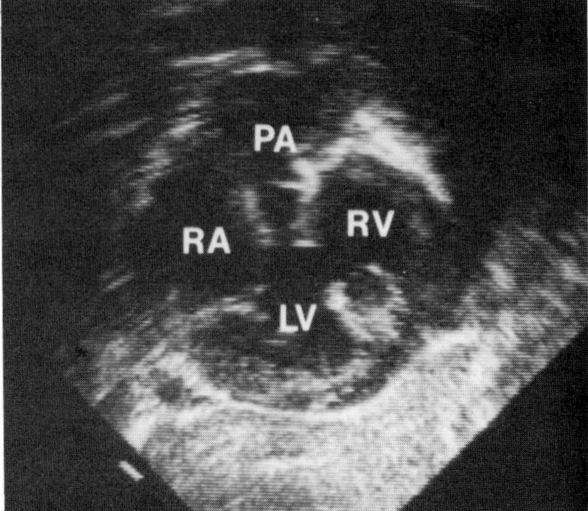

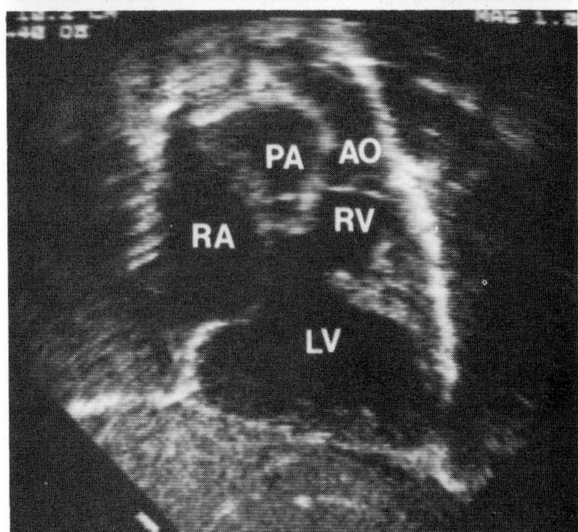

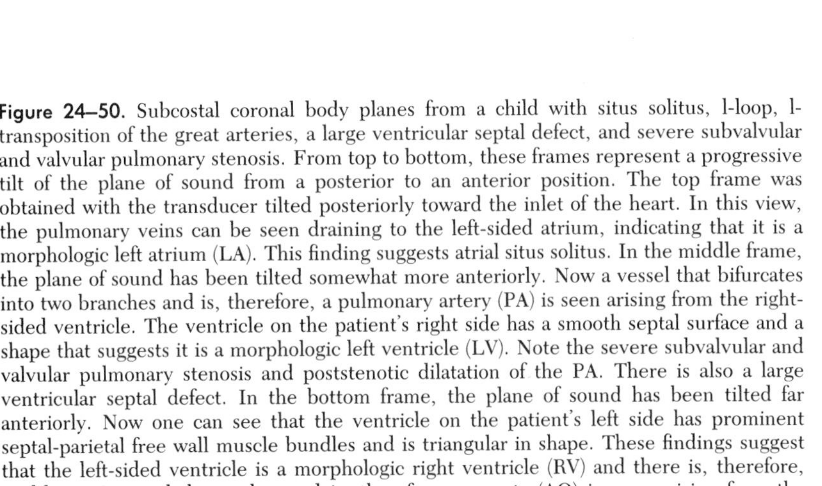
Figure 24–50. Subcostal coronal body planes from a child with situs solitus, l-loop, l-transposition of the great arteries, a large ventricular septal defect, and severe subvalvular and valvular pulmonary stenosis. From top to bottom, these frames represent a progressive tilt of the plane of sound from a posterior to an anterior position. The top frame was obtained with the transducer tilted posteriorly toward the inlet of the heart. In this view, the pulmonary veins can be seen draining to the left-sided atrium, indicating that it is a morphologic left atrium (LA). This finding suggests atrial situs solitus. In the middle frame, the plane of sound has been tilted somewhat more anteriorly. Now a vessel that bifurcates into two branches and is, therefore, a pulmonary artery (PA) is seen arising from the right-sided ventricle. The ventricle on the patient's right side has a smooth septal surface and a shape that suggests it is a morphologic left ventricle (LV). Note the severe subvalvular and valvular pulmonary stenosis and poststenotic dilatation of the PA. There is also a large ventricular septal defect. In the bottom frame, the plane of sound has been tilted far anteriorly. Now one can see that the ventricle on the patient's left side has prominent septal-parietal free wall muscle bundles and is triangular in shape. These findings suggest that the left-sided ventricle is a morphologic right ventricle (RV) and there is, therefore, an l-loop. A vessel that arches and is, therefore, an aorta (AO) is seen arising from the morphologic RV. This finding indicates transposition of the great arteries. In summary, this patient has atrial situs solitus, l-loop (discordant atrioventricular connections), and l-transposition of the great arteries (discordant ventriculoarterial connections). Abbreviation: RA—right atrium.

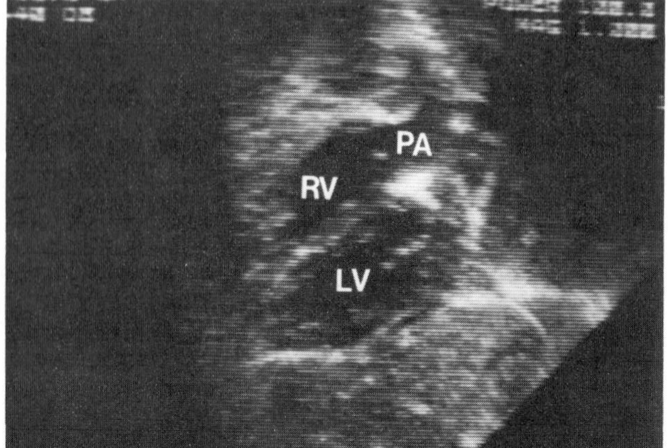

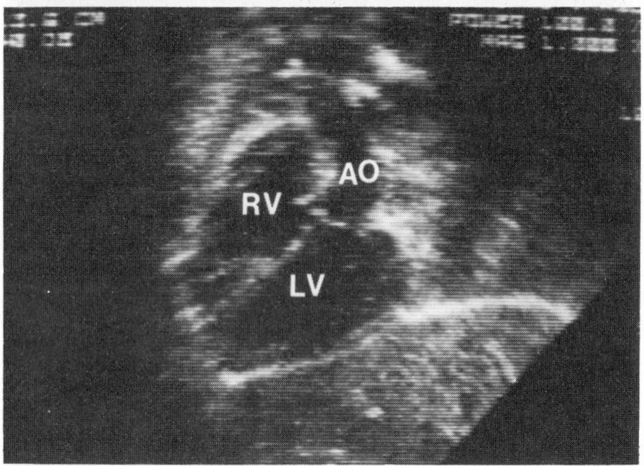

Figure 24–51. Subcostal coronal views of a patient with dextrocardia. In these views, the cardiac apex is seen pointing toward the patient's right. The top frame shows that the right-sided ventricle has a prominent moderator band and is, therefore, a morphologic right ventricle (RV). It gives rise to a vessel that bifurcates and is, therefore, a pulmonary artery (PA). The bottom frame shows that the left-sided ventricle has a smooth septal surface and is a morphologic left ventricle (LV). This ventricle gives rise to a vessel that arches and is, therefore, the aorta (AO). Other echocardiographic views in this patient demonstrated atrial situs solitus. In summary, the patient has atrial situs solitus, a d-loop, and normally related great vessels. This patient had normal atrioventricular connections and normal ventriculoarterial connections with isolated dextroversion of the cardiac apex.

ease. The spatial anatomic display of cardiac structures provided by two-dimensional echocardiography has led to a more exact definition of cardiac anatomy, even in the most complex congenital cardiac defects. The addition of Doppler echocardiography has provided a noninvasive method for quantitation of the size of intracardiac shunts and the severity of ventricular outflow obstructions. These rapid developments in ultrasound technology have allowed cardiac catheterization for diagnostic purposes to be eliminated in most instances and, in other cases, to be postponed until the infant or child is better able to tolerate this invasive procedure.

References

A

1. Alexander, J. A., Reinbert, J. C., Sealy, W. C., et al.: Shunt dynamics in experimental atrial septal defects. J. Appl. Physiol. 39:281, 1975.
2. Alverson, D. C., Eldridge, M., Aldrich, M., et al.: Effect of patent ductus arteriosus on lower extremity blood flow velocity patterns in preterm infants. Am. J. Perinatol. 1:216, 1984.

B

1. Barron, J. V., Sahn, D. J., Valdes-Cruz, L. M., et al.: Clinical utility of two-dimensional Doppler echocardiographic techniques for estimating pulmonary to systemic blood flow ratios in children with left to right shunting atrial septal defect, ventricular septal defect, or patent ductus arteriosus. J. Am. Coll. Cardiol. 3:169, 1984.
2. Bash, S. E., Huhta, J. C., Vick, G. S., III, et al.: Hypoplastic left heart syndrome: Is echocardiography accurate enough to guide surgical palliation? J. Am. Coll. Cardiol. 7:610, 1986.
3. Becker, A. E., and Anderson, R. H.: Atrioventricular septal defects: What's in a name? J. Thorac. Cardiovasc. Surg. 83:461, 1982.
4. Berger, M., Berdoff, R. L., Gallerstein, P. E., et al.: Evaluation of aortic stenosis by continuous wave Doppler ultrasound. J. Am. Coll. Cardiol. 3:150, 1984.
5. Bierman, F. Z., Fellows, K., and Williams, R. G.: Prospective identification of ventricular septal defects in infancy using subxiphoid two-dimensional echocardiography. Circulation 62:807, 1980.
6. Bierman, F. Z., and Williams, R. G.: Subxiphoid two-dimensional imaging of the interatrial septum in infants and neonates with congenital heart disease. Circulation 60:80, 1979.
7. Bierman, F. Z., and Williams, R. G.: Prospective diagnosis of d-transposition of the great arteries in neonates by subxiphoid two-dimensional echocardiography. Circulation 60:1496, 1979.

C

1. Canale, J. M., Sahn, D. J., Allen, H. D., et al.: Factors affecting real-time cross-sectional echocardiographic imaging of perimembranous ventricular septal defects. Circulation 63:689, 1981.
2. Carminati, M., Valsecchi, O., Borghi, A., et al.: Cross-sectional echocardiographic study of criss-cross hearts and superoinferior ventricles. Am. J. Cardiol. 59:114, 1987.
3. Cheatham, J. P., Latson, L. A., and Gutgesell, H. P.: Ventricular septal defect in infancy: Detection with two-dimensional echocardiography. Am. J. Cardiol. 47:85, 1981.
4. Cloez, J. L., Isaaz, K., and Pernot, C.: Pulsed Doppler flow characteristics of ductus arteriosus in infants with associated congenital anomalies of the heart or great arteries. Am. J. Cardiol. 57:845, 1986.

D

1. Daniels, O., Hopman, J. C. W., Stelinga, G. B. A., et al.: Doppler flow characteristics in the main pulmonary artery and LA/Ao ratio before and after ductal closure in healthy newborns. Pediatr. Cardiol. 3:99, 1982.

F

1. Feldtman, R. W., Andrassy, R. J., Alexander, J. A., et al.: Doppler ultrasonic flow detection as an adjunct in the diagnosis of patent ductus arteriosus in premature infants. J. Thorac. Cardiovasc. Surg. 72:288, 1976.

G

1. Gardin, J. M., Tobis, J. M., Dabestani, A., et al.: Superiority of two-dimensional measurement of aortic vessel diameter in Doppler echocardiographic estimates of left ventricular stroke volume. J. Am. Coll. Cardiol. 6:66, 1985.
2. Gentile, R., Stevenson, G., Dooley, T., et al.: Pulsed Doppler echocardiographic determination of time of ductal closure in normal newborn infants. J. Pediatr. 98:443, 1981.
3. Goldberg, S. J., Allen, H. D., and Sahn, D. J.: Echocardiographic detection and management of patent ductus arteriosus and neonates with respiratory distress syndrome: A two-and-one-half year prospective study. J. Clin. Ultrasound 5:161, 1977.
4. Goldberg, S. J., Areias, J. C., Spitaels, S. E. C., et al.: Use of time interval histographic output from echo-Doppler to detect left-to-right atrial shunts. Circulation 58:147, 1978.

5. Goldberg, S. J., Sahn, D. J., Allen, H. D., et al.: Evaluation of pulmonary and systemic blood flow by 2-dimensional Doppler echocardiography using fast Fourier transform spectral analysis. Am. J. Cardiol. 50:1394, 1982.
6. Goor, D. A., and Lillihei, C. W.: Congenital Malformations of the Heart. Grune & Stratton, New York, 1975.

H

1. Hagler, D. J., Tajik, A. J., Seward, J. B., et al.: Real-time wide-angle sector echocardiography: Atrioventricular canal defects. Circulation 59:140, 1979.
2. Hagler, D. J., Tajik, A. J., Seward, J. B., et al.: Wide-angle two-dimensional echocardiographic profiles of conotruncal abnormalities. Mayo Clin. Proc. 55:73, 1980.
3. Hatle, L., and Angelsen, B.: Doppler Ultrasound in Cardiology. Lea & Febiger, Philadephia, 1985.
4. Hatle, L., Angelsen, B. A., and Tromsdal, A.: Non-invasive assessment of aortic stenosis by Doppler ultrasound. Br. Heart J. 43:284, 1980.
5. Hatle, L., and Rokseth, R.: Noninvasive diagnosis and assessment of ventricular septal defect by Doppler ultrasound. Acta Med. Scand. Suppl. 645:47, 1981.
6. Henry, W. L., Maron, B. J., Griffith, J. M., et al.: Differential diagnosis of anomalies of the great arteries by real-time two-dimensional echocardiography. Circulation 51:283, 1975.
7. Hiraishi, S., Horiguchi, Y., Misawa, H., et al.: Noninvasive Doppler echocardiographic evaluation of shunt flow dynamics of the ductus arteriosus. Circulation 75:114, 1987.
8. Huhta, J. C., Glasow, P., Murphy, D. J., et al.: Surgery without catheterization for congenital heart defects: Management of 100 patients. J. Am. Coll. Cardiol. 9:823, 1987.
9. Huhta, J. C., Seward, J. B., Tajik, A. J., et al.: Two-dimensional echocardiographic spectrum of univentricular atrioventricular connection. J. Am. Coll. Cardiol. 5:149, 1985.

J

1. Johnson, G. L., Kwan, O. L., Handshoe, S., et al.: Accuracy of combined two-dimensional echocardiography and continuous wave Doppler recordings in the estimation of pressure gradient in right ventricular outlet obstruction. J. Am. Coll. Cardiol. 3:1013, 1984.

K

1. Kalmanson, D., Veyrat, C., Derai, C., et al.: Non-invasive technique for diagnosing atrial septal defect and assessing shunt volume using directional Doppler ultrasound. Br. Heart J. 34:981, 1972.
2. Krabill, K. A., Ring, S., Foker, J. E., et al.: Echocardiographic versus cardiac catheterization diagnosis of infants with congenital heart disease requiring cardiac surgery. Am. J. Cardiol. 60:351, 1987.

L

1. Lange, L. W., Sahn, D. J., Allen, H. D., et al.: The utility of cross-sectional echocardiography in the evaluation of hypoplastic left ventricle syndrome—echocardiographic/angiographic/anatomic correlations. Pediatr. Cardiol. 1:287, 1980.
2. Levin, A. R., Spach, M. S., Boineau, J. P., et al.: Atrial pressure-flow dynamics in atrial septal defects (secundum type). Circulation 37:476, 1968.
3. Lima, C. O., Sahn, D. J., Valdes-Cruz, L. M., et al.: Noninvasive prediction of transvalvular pressure gradients in patients with pulmonary stenosis by quantitative two-dimensional echocardiographic Doppler studies. Circulation 67:866, 1983.
4. Ludomirsky, A., Huhta, J. C., Vick, G. W., III, et al.: Color Doppler detection of multiple ventricular septal defects. Circulation 74:1317, 1986.

M

1. Magherini, A., Azzolina, G., Wiechmann, V., et al.: Pulsed Doppler echocardiography for diagnosis of ventricular septal defects. Br. Heart J. 43:143, 1980.
2. Marino, B., Sanders, S. P., Pasquini, L., et al.: Two-dimensional echocardiographic anatomy in criss-cross heart. Am. J. Cardiol. 58:325, 1986.
3. Martin, C. G., Snider, A. R., Katz, S. M., et al.: Abnormal cerebral blood flow patterns in preterm infants with a large patent ductus arteriosus. J. Pediatr. 101:587, 1982.
4. Minagoe, S., Tei, C., Kisanuki, A., et al.: Noninvasive pulsed Doppler echocardiographic detection of the direction of shunt flow in patients with atrial septal defect: Usefulness of the right parasternal approach. Circulation 71:745, 1985.
5. Morrow, W. R., Huhta, J. C., Murphy, D. J., et al.: Quantitative morphology of the aortic arch in neonatal coarctation. J. Am. Coll. Cardiol. 8:616, 1986.
6. Murphy, D. J., Jr., Ludomirsky, A., and Huhta, J. C.: Continuous-wave Doppler in children with ventricular septal defect: Noninvasive estimation of interventricular pressure gradient. Am. J. Cardiol. 57:428, 1986.
7. Musewe, N. N., Smallhorn, J. F., Benson, L. N., et al.: Validation of Doppler-derived pulmonary arterial pressure in patients with ductus arteriosus under different hemodynamic states. Circulation 76:1081, 1987.

N

1. Nihoyannopoulos, P., Karas, S., Sapsford, R. N., et al.: Accuracy of two-dimensional echocardiography in the diagnosis of aortic arch obstruction. J. Am. Coll. Cardiol. 10:1072, 1987.

P

1. Pasquini, L., Sanders, S. P., Parness, I. A., et al.: Diagnosis of coronary artery anatomy by two-dimensional echocardiography in patients with transposition of the great arteries. Circulation 75:557, 1987.
2. Pasquini, L., Sanders, S. P., Parness, I., et al.: Echocardiographic and anatomic findings in atrioventricular discordance with ventriculoarterial concordance. Am. J. Cardiol. 62:1256, 1988.
3. Perlman, J., Hill, A., and Volpe, J.: The effect of patent ductus arteriosus on flow velocity in the anterior cerebral arteries: Ductal steal in the premature newborn infant. J. Pediatr. 99:767, 1981.
4. Ports, T. A., Silverman, N. H., and Schiller, N. B.: Two-dimensional echocardiographic assessment of Ebstein's anomaly. Circulation 58:336, 1978.

S

1. Sahn, D. J., and Allen, H. D.: Real-time cross-sectional echocardiographic imaging and measurement of the patent ductus arteriosus in infants and children. Circulation 58:343, 1978.
2. Sahn, D. J., Allen, H. D., Lange, L. W., et al.: Cross-sectional echocardiographic diagnosis of the sites of total anomalous pulmonary venous drainage. Circulation 60:1317, 1979.
3. Sahn, D. J., Allen, H. D., McDonald, G., et al.: Real-time cross-sectional echocardiographic diagnosis of coarctation of the aorta. A prospective study of echocardiographic-angiographic correlations. Circulation 56:762, 1977.
4. Sanders, S. P., Yeager, S., and Williams, R. G.: Measurement of systemic and pulmonary blood flow and Qp/Qs ratio using Doppler and two-dimensional echocardiography. Am. J. Cardiol. 51:952, 1983.
5. Sapire, D. W., Ho, S. Y., Anderson, R. H., et al.: Diagnosis and significance of atrial isomerism. Am. J. Cardiol. 58:342, 1986.
6. Serwer, G. A., Armstrong, B. E., and Anderson, P. A. W.: Noninvasive detection of retrograde descending aortic flow in infants using continuous wave Doppler ultrasonography. J. Pediatr. 97:394, 1980.
7. Sharma, S., Devine, W., Anderson, R. H., et al.: Identification and analysis of left atrial isomerism. Am. J. Cardiol. 60:1157, 1987.
8. Silverman, N. H., Lewis, A. B., Heymann, M. A., et al.: Echocardiographic assessment of ductus arteriosus shunt in premature infants. Circulation 50:821, 1974.
9. Silverman, N. H., and Snider, A. R.: Two-dimensional Echocardiography in Congenital Heart Disease. Appleton-Century-Crofts, Norwalk, Conn., 1982, p. 142.
10. Skjaerpe, T., Hegrenaes, L., and Hatle, L.: Noninvasive estimation of right ventricular pressure by Doppler ultrasound in VSD. (Abstract.) *In* Fifth Symposium on Echocardiology, Rotterdam, 1983. Ultrasonar Bull. 1983, p. 92.
11. Smallhorn, J. F., and Freedom, R. M.: Pulsed Doppler echocardiography in the preoperative evaluation of total anomalous pulmonary venous connection. J. Am. Coll. Cardiol. 8:1413, 1986.
12. Snider, A. R., Enderlein, M. E., Teitel, D. F., et al.: Two-dimensional echocardiographic determination of aortic and pulmonary artery sizes from infancy to adulthood in normal subjects. Am. J. Cardiol. 53:218, 1984.
13. Snider, A. R., Ports, T. A., and Silverman, N. H.: Venous anomalies of the coronary sinus: Detection by M-mode, two-dimensional and contrast echocardiography. Circulation 60:721, 1980.
14. Snider, A. R., and Silverman, N. H.: Suprasternal notch echocardiography: A two-dimensional technique for evaluating congenital heart disease. Circulation 63:165, 1981.
15. Snider, A. R., Silverman, N. H., Turley, K., et al.: Evaluation of infradiaphragmatic total anomalous pulmonary venous connection with two-dimensional echocardiography. Circulation 66:1129, 1982.
16. Snider, A. R., Stevenson, J. G., French, G. W., et al.: Comparison of high pulse repetition frequency and continuous-wave Doppler for velocity measurement and gradient prediction in children with valvular and congenital heart disease. J. Am. Coll. Cardiol. 7:873, 1986.
17. Stamm, R. B., and Martin, R. P.: Quantification of pressure gradients across stenotic valves by Doppler ultrasound. J. Am. Coll. Cardiol. 2:707, 1983.
18. Stevenson, J. G., Kawabori, I., Dooley, T., et al.: Diagnosis of ventricular septal defect by pulsed Doppler echocardiography: Sensitivity, specificity, and limitations. Circulation 58:322, 1978.
19. Stevenson, J. G., Kawabori, I., and Guntheroth, W. G.: Noninvasive detection of pulmonary hypertension in patent ductus arteriosus by pulsed Doppler echocardiography. Circulation 60:355, 1979.
20. Stevenson, J. G., Kawabori, I., and Guntheroth, W. G.: Pulsed Doppler echocardiographic diagnosis of patent ductus arteriosus: Sensitivity, specificity, limitations, and technical features. Cathet. Cardiovasc. Diagn. 6:255, 1980.
21. Stewart, W. I., Jiang, L., Mich, R., et al.: Variable effects of changes in flow rate through the aortic pulmonary, and mitral valves on valve area and flow velocity: Impact on quantitative Doppler flow calculations. J. Am. Coll. Cardiol. 6:653, 1985.

V

1. Valdes-Cruz, L. M., Horowitz, S., Mesel, E., et al.: A pulsed Doppler echocardiographic method for calculating pulmonary and systemic blood flow in atrial level shunt: Validation studies in animals and initial human experience. Circulation 69:80, 1984.
2. Valdes-Cruz, L. M., Horowitz, S., Mesel, E., et al.: A pulsed Doppler echocardiographic method for calculation of pulmonary and systemic flow: Accuracy in a canine model with ventricular septal defect. Circulation 68:597, 1983.

W

1. Weyman, A. E., Caldwell, R. L., Hurwitz, R. A., et al.: Cross-sectional echocardiographic characterization of aortic obstruction. 1. Supravalvar aortic stenosis and aortic hypoplasia. Circulation 57:491, 1978.
2. Weyman, A. E., Caldwell, R. L., Hurwitz, R. A., et al.: Cross-sectional echocardiographic detection of aortic obstruction. 2. Coarctation of the aorta. Circulation 57:498, 1978.
3. Weyman, A. E., Feigenbaum, H., Hurwitz, R. A., et al.: Cross-sectional echocardiographic assessment of the severity of aortic stenosis in children. Circulation 55:773, 1977.
4. Weyman, A. E., Feigenbaum, H., Hurwitz, R. A., et al.: Cross-sectional echocardiographic visualization of the stenotic pulmonary valve. Circulation 56:769, 1977.

Y

1. Young, D. B., Quinones, M. A., Waggoner, A. D., et al.: Diagnosis and quantification of aortic stenosis with pulsed Doppler echocardiography. Am. J. Cardiol. 45:987, 1980.

Chapter 25

Cardiac and Extracardiac Masses: Echocardiographic Evaluation

INGELA SCHNITTGER, M.D.

NORMAL VARIANTS 511
TUMORS 512
Primary Cardiac Tumors 512
Primary Benign Cardiac Tumors 512
Primary Malignant Cardiac Tumors 517
Metastatic Tumors 519
Extracardiac Masses Adjacent to the Heart 520
THROMBI 520
Intracardiac Thrombi 520
MISCELLANEOUS MASSES AND ARTIFACTS 528

Echocardiography, particularly two-dimensional echocardiography,[F1, F2] is the preferred method for detection of cardiac masses.[P1, F3] It is a pain-free, frequently available, and an inexpensive way to image the heart. Serial studies easily can be obtained.

Size, shape, mobility, point of attachment, and location of tumor can also often be provided by echocardiography.[B1, S1, R1] Although one cannot make a tissue diagnosis by ultrasound, the appearance of a cardiac mass is often suggestive of a particular process so that further diagnostic tests can be avoided. Frequently, patients can be recommended for surgery without being submitted to invasive angiography. The recent addition of transesophageal echocardiography to our diagnostic tools in the noninvasive laboratory has further enhanced the detection of intracardiac masses.[M1]

Extracardiac masses can be visualized by echocardiography if adjacent to the heart, but the extension of such masses often requires the additional use of magnetic resonance imaging, computed tomography, angiography, and so forth.

In this chapter the following cardiac/extracardiac masses are discussed: normal variants, primary cardiac tumors (benign and malignant), metastatic tumors, extracardiac masses adjacent to the heart, intracardiac thrombi, and miscellaneous masses and artifacts. Infective endocarditis is discussed elsewhere.

NORMAL VARIANTS

Several normal structures in the heart can mimic a cardiac mass. To avoid an incorrect interpretation of these normal variants, the echocardiographer must be familiar with the location, size, shape, and motion of these normal structures. It is important to separate these normal structures from abnormal masses, especially when a patient is referred to the noninvasive laboratory for exclusion of a cardiac mass.

The right ventricular *moderator band* is a muscular structure that traverses the right ventricular cavity. This structure originates from the trabecula septomarginalis and runs an oblique course anteriorly through the right ventricular chamber toward the base of the anterior papillary muscle. The moderator band is usually best seen in the apical four-chamber view (Fig. 25–1). In a study by Keren and associates[K1] the moderator band was seen in 26 of 33 patients (79 percent) with cardiomyopathy whose hearts were subsequently examined at transplantation for pathologic correlation. The moderator band may mimic right ventricular thrombi, mural masses, or hypertrophy of the interventricular septum.[K2]

The *eustachian valve* of the right atrium is commonly seen in adults and is a remnant of the embryonic right sinus venosus valve. This structure appears as a linear density at the junction of the inferior vena cava and the right atrial posterior wall.[L1, P2] The eustachian valve is often best seen in the mid-precordial parasternal long-axis view with the transducer tilted medially to image the right heart (Fig. 25–2) or in the apical four-chamber view. If it is large enough, it may obstruct venous inflow and it may mimic a tumor. The eustachian valve is often prominently seen when the right atrium is dilated.

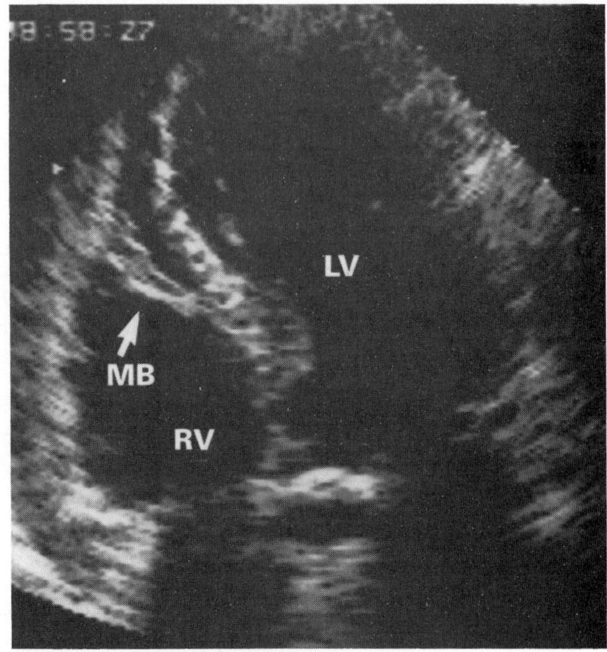

Figure 25–1. An apical four-chamber view demonstrating a moderator band (MB) traversing the right ventricular cavity. Abbreviations: LV—left ventricle; RV—right ventricle.

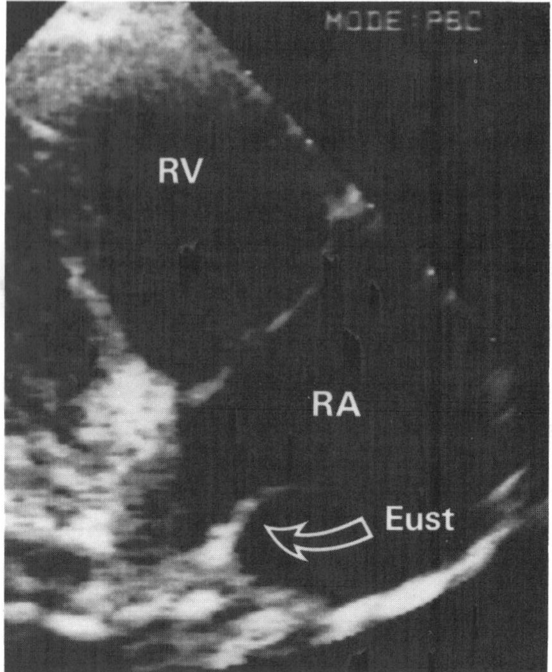

Figure 25–2. A parasternal long-axis view. The transducer is angled medially to visualize clearly the right ventricle (RV) and right atrium (RA). A prominent eustacian valve (Eust) is seen in the right atrium.

Chiari's network is found in the right atrium in 2 to 3 percent of normal hearts.[C1] This is a fine filamentous network of no clinical importance other than its mimicking a right atrial clot, ruptured chordae tendineae of the tricuspid valve, tricuspid valve vegetation, or a tumor.[C2, P2, W1] This structure is a highly mobile echo that usually arises from the orifice of the inferior vena cava. It is separated from the tricuspid valve and interatrial septum. The Chiari's network is best imaged in the apical four-chamber view (Fig. 25–3) or in a subcostal long-axis scan plane.

Numerous other miscellaneous masses and artifacts can mimic intracardiac tumors or clots. They are discussed at the end of the chapter.

TUMORS

Primary Cardiac Tumors

Primary tumors of the heart and pericardium are very rare. The incidence is less than 0.08 percent of all tumors in autopsy series.[B2] Approximately 75 percent of cardiac tumors and cysts are benign and 25 percent are malignant.[M2] The most common benign and malignant tumors are listed in decreasing frequency[M2] in Table 25–1.

Primary *myocardial* tumors are more common than primary *pericardial* tumors, but pericardial tumors are more frequently malignant. *In adults* the most common cardiac tumor is the myxoma, and it accounts for approximately one-third of the benign tumors of the heart and pericardium.[M2] In *children* (patients less than 15 years old), the most common cardiac tumor is the rhabdomyoma and it accounts for approximately 40 percent of the benign tumors of the heart and pericardium in this group.[M2] In *infants* (patients less than 1 year old), the most commonly found tumor is again the rhabdomyoma (58 percent of all benign tumors) and the second most common tumor is the teratoma.[F4, M2, S2] One study reports on the use of *fetal* echocardiography in the diagnosis of intrapericardial teratoma.[D1]

Table 25–1. MOST COMMON PRIMARY CARDIAC TUMORS

Benign Tumors	Malignant Tumors
Myxoma	Angiosarcoma
Lipoma	Rhabdomyosarcoma
Papillary fibroelastoma	Mesothelioma
Rhabdomyoma	Fibrosarcoma
Fibroma	Malignant lymphoma
Hemangioma	Extraskeletal osteosarcoma
Teratoma	Neurogenic sarcoma
Mesothelioma of the atrioventricular node	Malignant teratoma
Granular cell tumor	Thymoma
Neurofibroma	Leiomyosarcoma
Lymphangioma	Liposarcoma

Of the malignant tumors, 33 percent are angiosarcoma, 20 percent rhabdomyosarcoma, 15 percent mesothelioma, and 10 percent fibrosarcoma.[M2] These tumors occur mostly in adults. Malignant tumors of the heart and pericardium are very rare in children.

The myxoma is the most frequent primary tumor of the heart. It arises from the endocardium as a polypoid mass that is generally pedunculated but occasionally broad-based. Myxomas are either papillary or smooth. The cells are derived from mesenchymal cells of the subendocardial layer and primitive mesenchyme. Myxomas are most commonly located in the atria, preferably the left atrium (75 percent). Myxoma also occurs in the right atrium (18 percent), right ventricle (4 percent), and left ventricle (3 percent).[M2] There are even reports of myxomas found in the inferior vena cava,[D2] and occasionally they are biatrial[F5, G1, N1, S3, T1] or multifocal.[A1]

The most common tumor in children is the rhabdomyoma. This tumor is derived from cardiac muscle and probably originates from embryonic cardiac myoblasts.[M2] The rhabdomyoma is nearly always multiple. In approximately 30 percent of patients, this tumor is associated with tuberous sclerosis.[M2] Rhabdomyomas are a rare occurrence in adults. The tumor usually is intramural with a portion of the tumor extending into the cavity.

Primary Benign Cardiac Tumors

Left Atrium

The most common primary tumor of the left atrium is the myxoma. M-mode echocardiography was used in 1959 for the first diagnosis of myxoma by ultrasound.[E1] Since then, two-dimensional echocardiography has proved to be a sensitive and often specific method for diagnosis of these tumors and indeed echocardiography has become the diagnostic method of choice.[F6, G2, K3, M3, P3–P5, S4, W2] Often, the patients can be recommended for surgery without further evaluation with invasive techniques.

The left atrial myxoma is usually pedunculated (90 percent) and attached via a stalk to the interatrial septum at the fossa ovalis. The stalk allows the tumor to move freely about in the atrium and prolapse through the mitral valve into the left ventricle in diastole (Fig. 25–4). Clinically, this tumor often presents as an obstruction to the left ventricular inflow tract, mimicking mitral stenosis.[G3, P6] A prominent symptom may be dyspnea accompanied by a diastolic murmur on physical examination. However, constitutional symptoms such as fever, malaise, and peripheral emboli frequently accompany the tumor. Occasionally these tumors give the patient no significant cardiac symptoms[G4] or no murmur.[N2] Although M-mode echocardiography demonstrates an absolutely classic pattern in the case of myxoma,[B3] two-dimensional echocardiography provides a more complete evaluation of the precise shape, motion, and location of the tumor.[L2] The atrial myxoma is not attached to the mitral valve. As the mitral valve opens in early diastole, the tumor mass will always follow behind the leaflet by a few frames. The atrial myxoma can be visualized in most of the standard echocardiographic views. Figure 25–4 shows a myxoma in the parasternal long axis view, and Figure 25–5 shows a myxoma in the apical four-chamber view. The movement of these tumors in systole and diastole may be dramatic and is best appreciated in real time. These tumors may be smooth surfaced (Figs. 25–4 and 25–6) or villose (Figs. 25–7 and 25–8). The patient whose echocardiogram is shown in Figure 25–7 had two peripheral emboli prior to the diagnosis of cardiac myxoma.

In the past, before echocardiography was widely used and competently interpreted, patients were referred to our echocardiography laboratory with suspected mitral stenosis. Occasionally such a patient turned out to have a myxoma. Although obviously

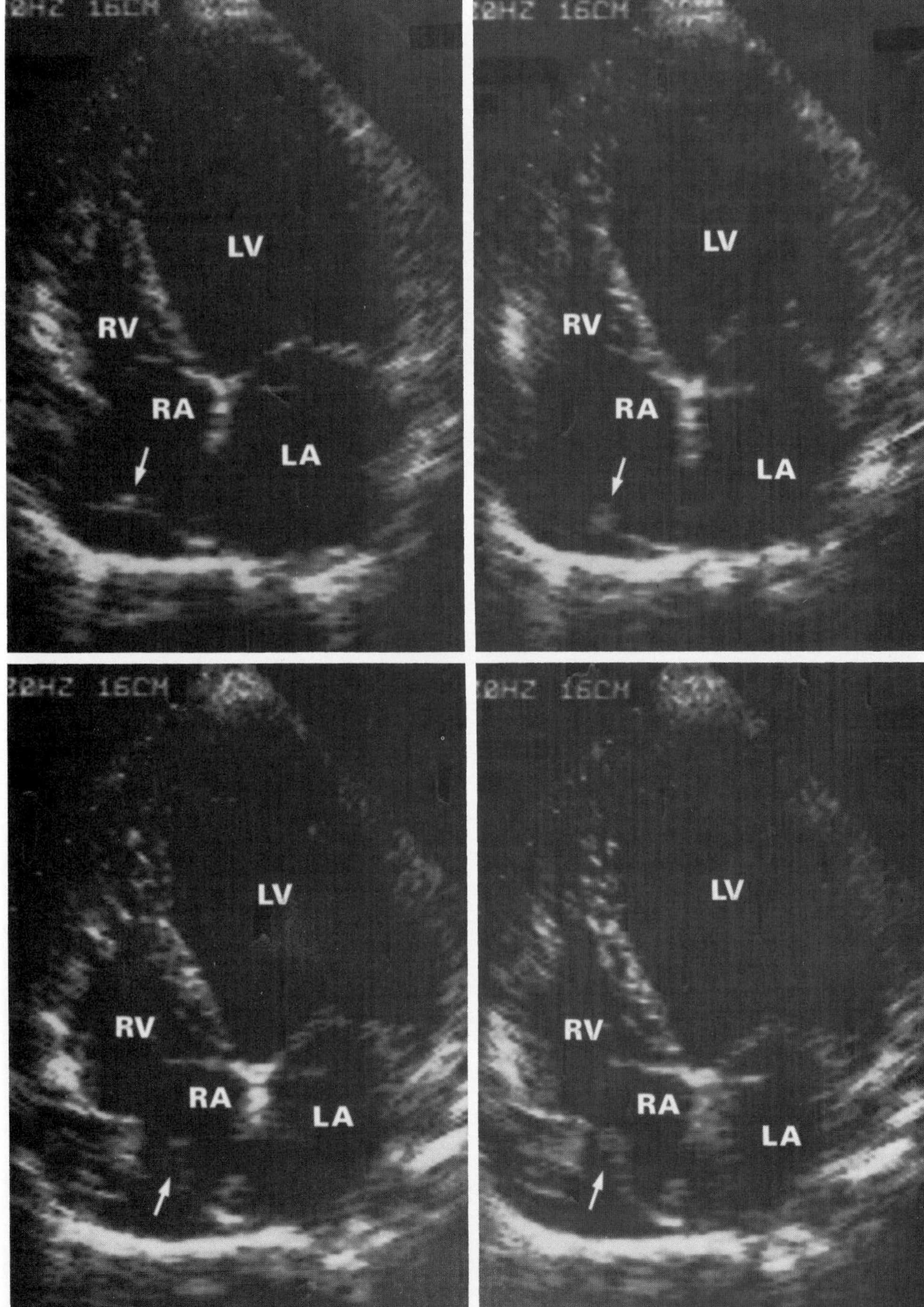

Figure 25–3. Four panels of an apical four-chamber view demonstrating a fine filamentous network, Chiari's network, in the right atrium, marked by the arrows. The four frames demonstrate the different positions of this highly mobile network throughout the cardiac cycle. Abbreviations: LV—left ventricle; RV—right ventricle; LA—left atrium; RA—right atrium.

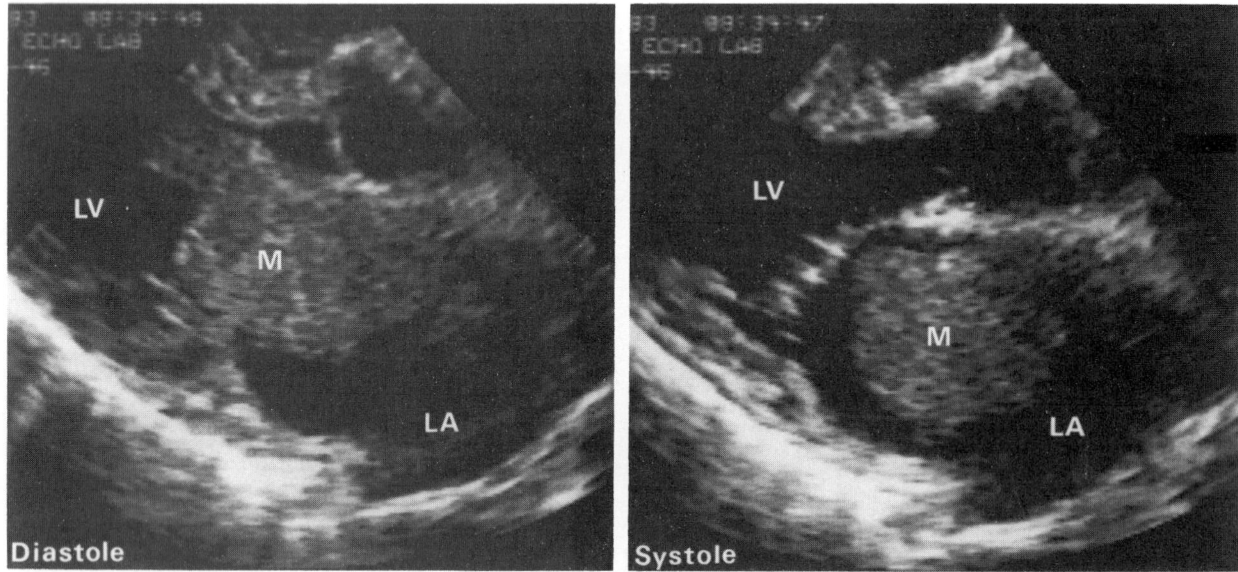

Figure 25–4. A parasternal long-axis view of a patient with a large myxoma (M) anchored in the left atrium (LA) and prolapsing through the mitral valve into the left ventricle (LV) in diastole.

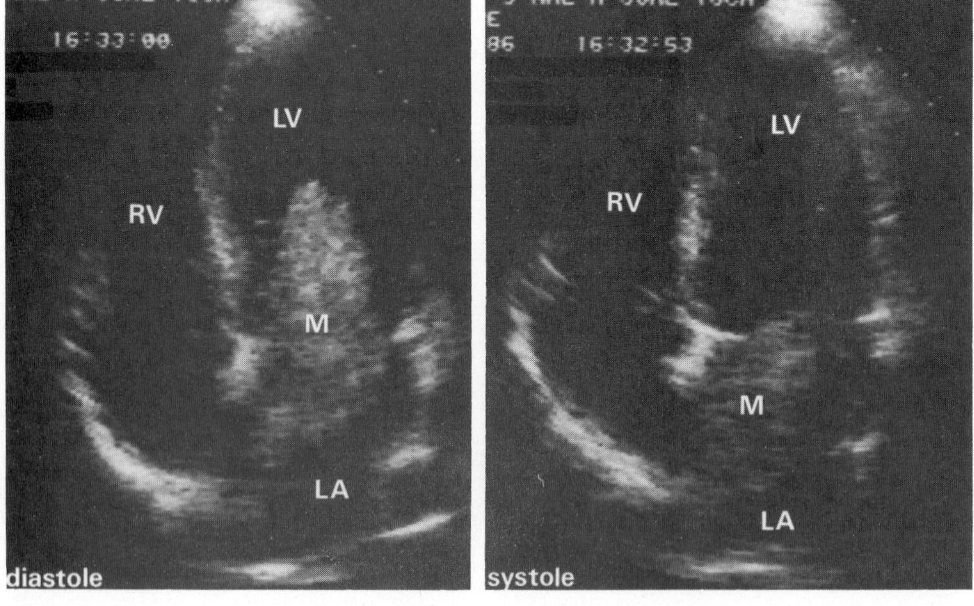

Figure 25–5. An apical four-chamber view of a patient with a large myxoma (M) prolapsing into the left ventricle (LV) during diastole and contained within the left atrium (LA) during systole. Abbreviation: RV—right ventricle.

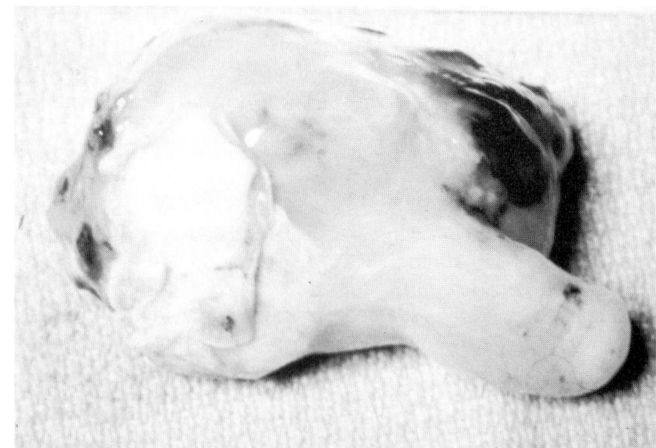

Figure 25–6. The myxoma excised from the patient in Figure 25–4 in the operating room. Note the prominent stalk and the smooth surface of the myxoma.

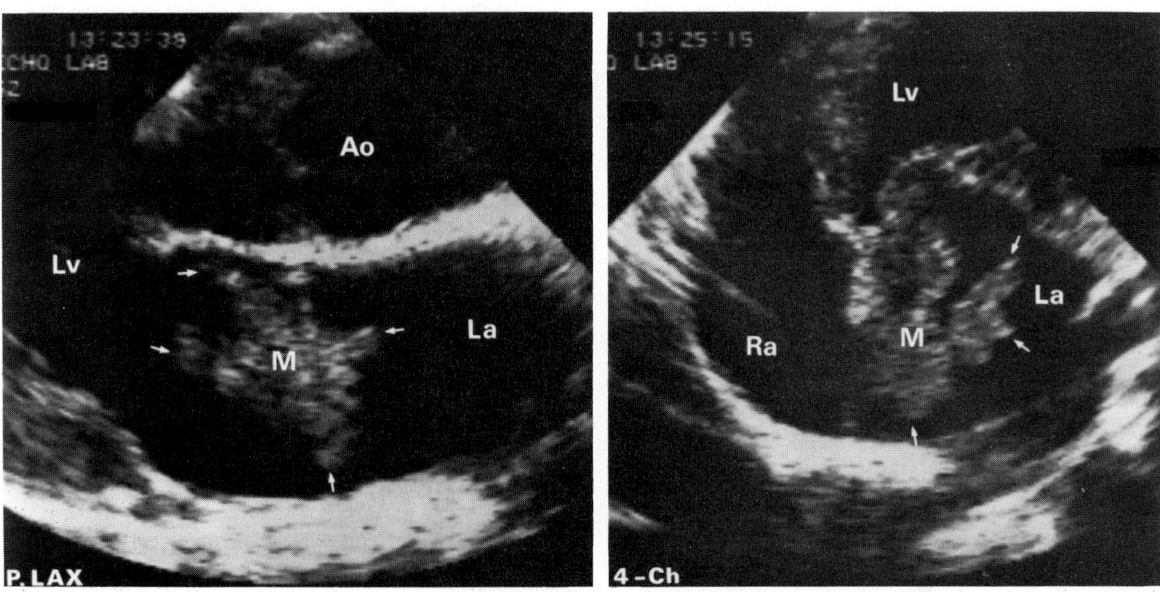

Figure 25–7. A parasternal long-axis view (P.LAX) in the left panel and an apical four-chamber view (4-Ch) in the right panel. This patient has a villose myxoma (M) and had two embolic episodes prior to diagnosis of the myxoma. Abbreviations: La—left atrium; Lv—left ventricle; Ao—aorta; Ra—right atrium.

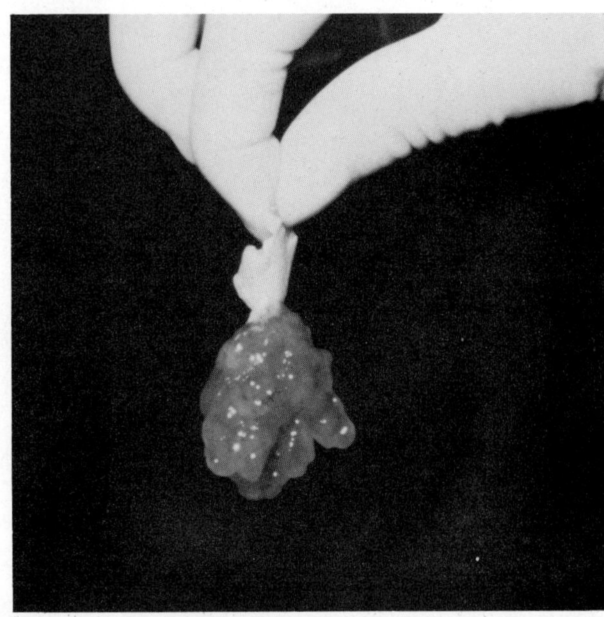

Figure 25–8. The surgeon demonstrating the myxoma after excision from the patient whose echocardiogram is shown in Figure 25–7.

rare, we have seen one case of coexisting atrial myxoma and rheumatic mitral stenosis.

The left atrial myxoma can occasionally be located in other parts of the atrium: free wall, posterior wall, and lateral wall. In those cases it is more difficult to differentiate the myxoma from other tumors or a clot. This is especially true when the myxoma is sessile (as it is in 10 percent of the cases) and does not prolapse into the left ventricle in diastole.[L3]

Echocardiography is ideally suited for serial follow-up.[R2] Recurrence of atrial myxoma has been reported but is very rare.[Z1] It may be difficult to prove whether such "recurrence" represents a second occurrence of the tumor or inadequate removal of the tumor at surgery. Intraoperative echocardiography may be of use in evaluation of the operative site at the time of surgery. Left atrial myxomas also occasionally become infected[Q1] and may mimic a vegetation. Myxomas arising from the mitral valve also have been diagnosed by ultrasound.[B4, G5]

Another benign tumor of the heart and preferably the cardiac valves is the papillary fibroelastoma. This tumor is derived from endocardium and consists of the normal components of such tissue: fibrous tissue, elastic fibers, and smooth muscle cells. The fibroelastoma is usually a small, well-rounded mass that appears attached to the atrioventricular or semilunal valves. If the tumor is attached to the mitral (or tricuspid) valve leaflets, it is usually an incidental finding on an echocardiogram.[A2, S5] The tumor is often clinically silent but can occasionally embolize.[F7, T2] Figure 25–9 illustrates an echocardiogram from a patient with a fibroelastoma attached to the tricuspid valve.

Hemangiomas of the left atrium are rare but benign tumors that potentially can mimic a cardiac myxoma.[W3]

Left atrial thrombi attached to a wall or freely floating clots may also mimic a cardiac myxoma. Thrombi usually occur in the presence of mitral valve disease, mitral valve replacement, or atrial fibrillation/flutter. (See discussion below.) Extrinsic processes such as esophageal cancer and hiatal hernias may mimic a left atrial tumor.[N3]

Transesophageal echocardiography probably will emerge as the technique of choice for diagnosing intracardiac tumors, particularly tumors of the atria.[T3]

Left Ventricle

The most common primary left ventricular tumors are fibromas and rhabdomyomas.[M2] These tumors are more common in the pediatric age group than in adults. The rhabdomyoma is the most common tumor in the child[B5, M2, P7] and usually presents as multiple intracavitary nodules, sometimes protruding into the cavity.[F8] It can also be intramural.[B6, F9, P7] In children rhabdomyomas are often associated with tuberous sclerosis.[B7, D3, G6, G7, S6]

The fibroma is the most common benign tumor of the left ventricle in adults.[M2] It is usually intramural and appears as a localized area of "irregular hypertrophy" of the septum, apex, or free wall.[T4] The involved wall segment is often hypocontractile with an inhomogeneous echocardiographic texture. Frequently these tumors are visualized in the apical views or subcostal long-axis scan plane. The echocardiographic features of a fibroma in a 17-year-old girl are illustrated in Figure 25–10. This patient presented with symptoms of dyspnea and fatigue. She underwent open-heart surgery for direct cardiac biopsy and confirmation of diagnosis; otherwise no treatment was given. If the patient deteriorates, she will be considered for cardiac transplantation. Other than dyspnea and fatigue, these patients may have arrhythmias and electrocardiographic changes.

Left ventricular fibroma localized to the apex may be particularly difficult to differentiate from left ventricular hypertrophy of the apex or a thrombus. Keren and associates[K4] noted that underlying wall motion abnormalities were present in patients with fibroma and thrombus but not in patients with apical hypertrophy. Apical hypertrophy usually demonstrates normal myocardial texture, whereas thrombi and fibroma frequently exhibit an abnormal ultrasonic appearance. Other masses and artifacts that may be mistaken for ventricular tumors include papillary muscles, anomalous bands, false tendons, or off-axis scan planes. The latter are discussed below. Myxomas of the left ventricle are rare, but several case reports exist in the literature.[C3, M4, M5] They occur in the left ventricle in 3 percent of all cases of myxoma.[M2] Left ventricular lipomas have also been observed by echocardiography.[B8]

Right Atrium

Echocardiography, and more specifically two-dimensional echocardiography, has substantially increased the antemortem diagnosis of right atrial masses.[G8, H1] The most common right atrial tumor is the myxoma, which occurs in the right atrium in approximately 18 percent of all cases of myxoma.[M2] The right atrial myxoma is usually larger than the left atrial myxoma by the time of discovery, since the patients usually become symptomatic much later. These tumors, as in the case of the left atrium, usually originate from the interatrial septum but they have also been found at other sites in the right atrium. We recently

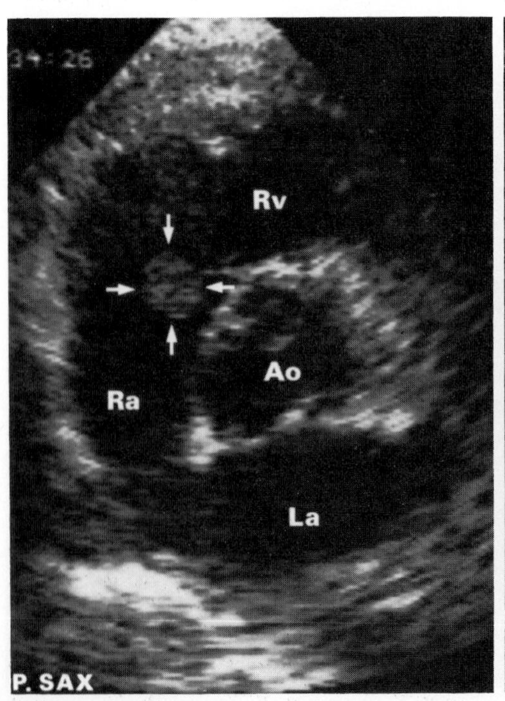

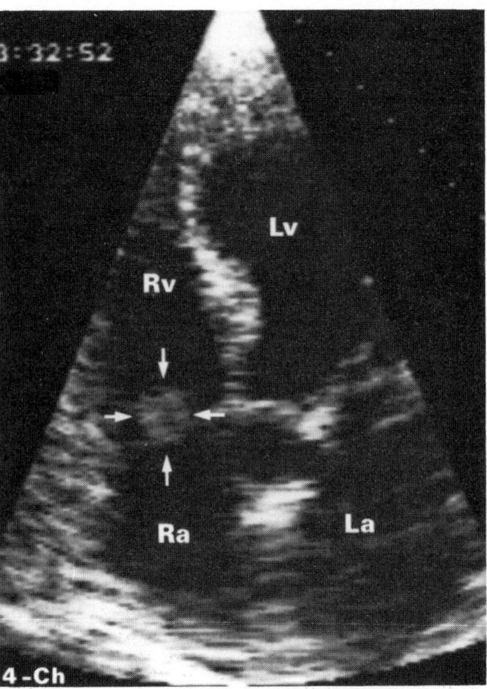

Figure 25–9. Parasternal short-axis view (P.SAX) in left panel and apical four-chamber (4-Ch) view in panel right showing a patient with a tricuspid valve papillary fibroelastoma (*arrows*). Abbreviations: Rv—right ventricle; Lv—left ventricle; Ao—aorta; La—left atrium; Ra—right atrium.

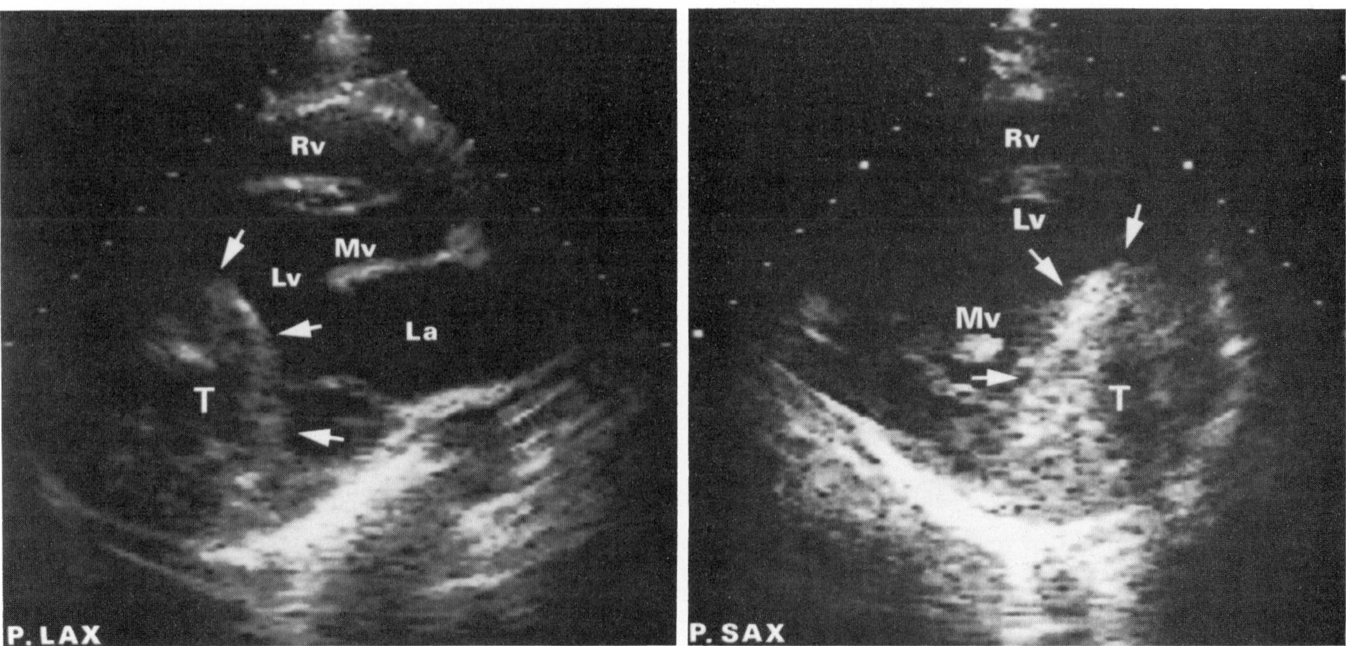

Figure 25–10. Parasternal long-axis (P.LAX) and parasternal short-axis (P.SAX) views of a patient with a large left ventricular (Lv) tumor (T) occupying most of the anterolateral and posterior wall of the left ventricle. Open biopsy showed fibroma. Abbreviations: Mv—mitral valve; Rv—right ventricle; La—left atrium.

diagnosed a right atrial tumor by transthoracic echocardiography (Fig. 25–11) but could not clearly delineate the attachment of this mass in the right atrium. A transesophageal echocardiogram (Fig. 25–12) clearly demonstrated that the tumor was attached to the right atrial lateral wall and free from the interatrial septum. The tumor was surgically removed and histologically proved to be a myxoma.

Since right atrial myxomas are less frequently seen than left atrial myxomas, a major echocardiographic problem is that of differentiating myxoma from a number of other masses.[P2] Neoplasms that extend from below the diaphragm to the heart, such as hepatoma,[C4] nephroma, renal cell carcinoma,[G9] and leiomyoma,[M6] may mimic a right atrial myxoma. Infradiaphragmatic tumors extending to the heart will fill up the inferior vena cava and may therefore potentially be separated from primary cardiac neoplasms. However, there has been one report of a myxoma arising from the inferior vena cava.[D2] Right atrial clots, Chiari's network, eustachian valve, catheters, and so forth may also confuse the echocardiographer.

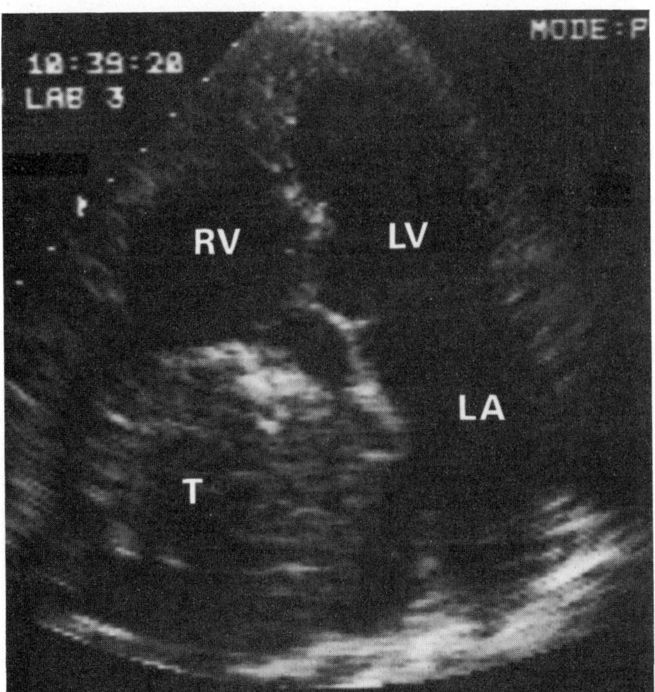

Figure 25–11. Apical four-chamber view with a large tumor (T) located in the right atrium, which is markedly enlarged. No clear attachment of this tumor to the wall is identified. Abbreviations: LA—left atrium; RV—right ventricle; LV—left ventricle.

Large vegetations on the tricuspid valve may simulate a right atrial mass.[C5] As always in echocardiography, it is important to obtain multiple views of every area of interest to reduce the possibility of diagnostic errors. Tricuspid valve papillary fibroelastoma (see Fig. 25–9) has also been reported[F10] and may be confused with a myxoma.

The best echocardiographic scan planes for viewing the right atrium are the parasternal short-axis, apical four-chamber, and subcostal positions. Transesophageal echocardiography offers an advantage when poor resolution from transthoracic imaging precludes optimal visualization of the atrium.

Right Ventricle

Primary benign tumors of the right ventricle identified by echocardiography include myxoma,[V1, C6, C7] fibroma,[M7] rhabdomyoma,[F8, R3, S7] and eosinophilic myocardial infiltration.[P8] Occasionally these tumors can prolapse into the outflow tract and mimic pulmonary stenosis. Intramural tumors may appear as localized areas of hypertrophy, as in the case of the left ventricle. Figure 25–13 shows an example of a right ventricular rhabdomyoma in a 25-year-old man with tuberous sclerosis. Rhabdomyoma of the right ventricle may also obstruct the tricuspid valve and result in early death in the pediatric age group. Indwelling catheters and pacemaker lines may mimic right ventricular tumors.[C8] Ultrasound color image processing may aid in the diagnosis of ventricular rhabdomyoma.[A3]

Primary Malignant Cardiac Tumors

Malignant primary tumors of the heart are less frequent than benign tumors and account for only 25 percent of primary tumors of the heart.[M2] Primary malignant tumors of the heart are more frequently found in the right than the left side of the heart.

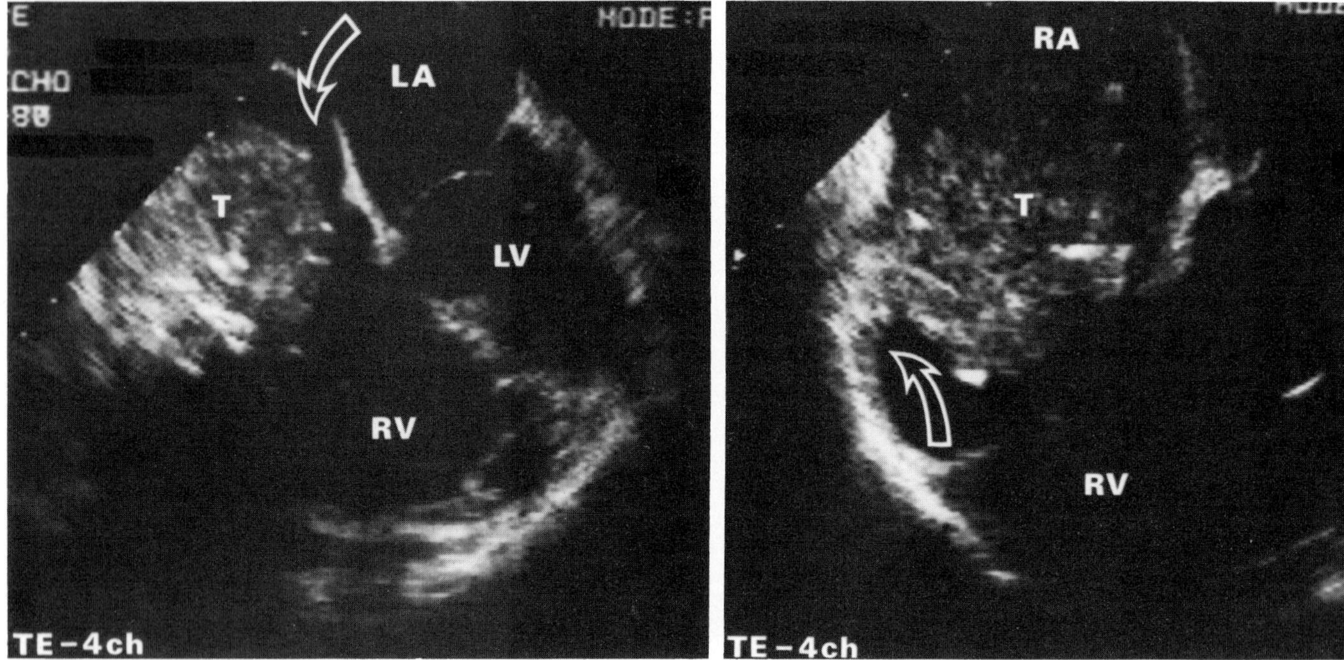

Figure 25–12. A transesophageal four-chamber view (TE–4ch) showing all four chambers in the left panel and focused on the right heart in the right panel. This echocardiogram was obtained from the same patient as Figure 25–11. The transesophageal echocardiogram demonstrates that this tumor was not attached to the interatrial septum (*arrow*, left panel) but instead was attached to the right atrial free wall (*arrow*, right panel). Abbreviations: LA—left atrium; RA—right atrium; LV—left ventricle; RV—right ventricle; T—tumor.

Angiosarcomas, fibrosarcomas, and rhabdomyosarcomas are the most common malignant tumors of the heart, and the mesothelioma[A4] is the most common malignant tumor of the pericardium. Echocardiographically, the sarcomas[F11, F12, W4, W5] are visualized as intramural masses and it may be difficult to distinguish them from their benign counterpart.[M8] Direct biopsy is usually necessary. Often these tumors can be seen penetrating the pericardium and extrapericardial structures.[C9, L4] Conversely, extracardiac processes may invade the heart from the outside and a metastatic process can then mimic a primary cardiac neoplasm. When the pericardium is involved, a pericardial effusion is often present on the echocardiogram.

Figure 25–14 demonstrates a small angiosarcoma of the right atrium. Figure 25–15 illustrates a larger diffuse mass, also an angiosarcoma, in a patient who presented with symptoms and signs of acute pericarditis. Figure 25–16 shows an angiosarcoma

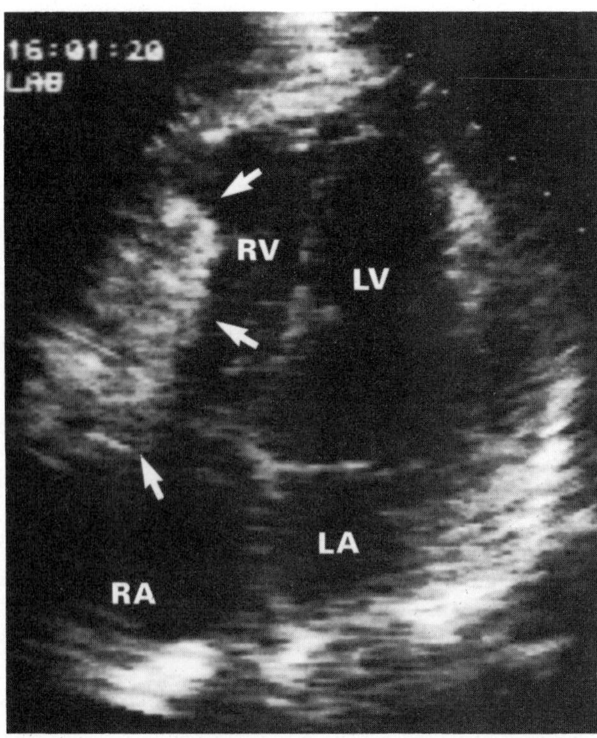

Figure 25–13. An apical four-chamber view of a patient with an intramural and intracavitary rhabdomyoma. The patient also had tuberous sclerosis. Abbreviations: RV—right ventricle; LV—left ventricle; RA—right atrium; LA—left atrium.

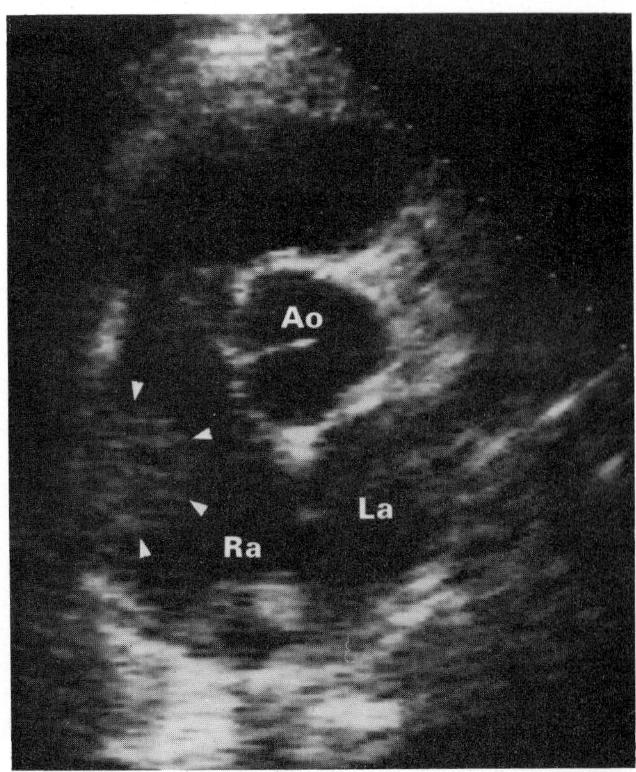

Figure 25–14. A parasternal short-axis view of a patient with a 2 × 2 cm right atrial angiosarcoma attached to the right atrial free wall. Abbreviations: Ra—right atrium; La—left atrium; Ao—aorta.

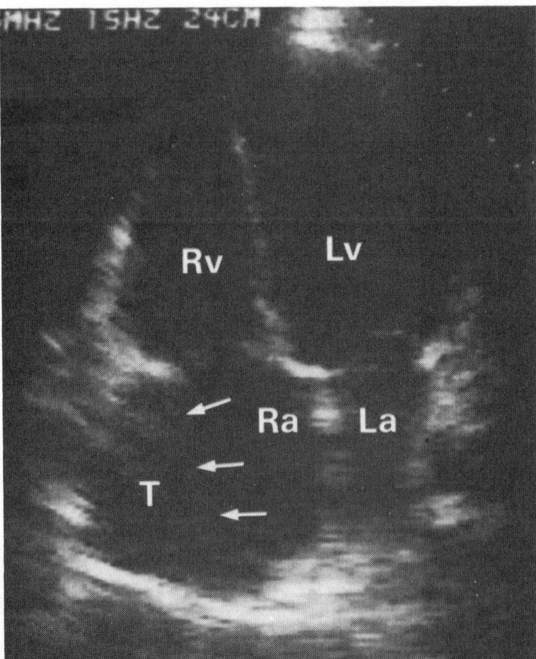

Figure 25–15. An apical four-chamber view of a patient with a large right atrial angiosarcoma infiltrating the enlarged right atrium (Ra). The tumor (T) had the appearance of a cloud of echoes in the posterolateral aspect of the right atrium (Ra). Abbreviations: La—left atrium; Rv—right ventricle; T—tumor.

of the right atrium and right ventricle. Depending on the size and location of the tumor in the heart, different symptomatology may occur.[I1, L5, M9, W5] Other malignant tumors of the heart that have been noted by echocardiography include malignant lymphoma and extraskeletal osteosarcoma.[R4] Figure 25–17 shows a case of malignant fibrous histiocytoma in the ascending pulmonary artery.

Table 25–2. MOST COMMON MALIGNANCIES THAT METASTASIZE TO THE HEART

Carcinoma of lung
Carcinoma of breast
Leukemia/lymphoma
Malignant melanoma
Renal cell carcinoma

Metastatic Tumors

Metastatic tumors to the heart and pericardium are the most frequently encountered cardiac tumors. The incidence of secondary tumors of the heart and pericardium is 20 to 40 times greater than that of primary cardiac tumors.[M2] At necropsy, cardiac metastases are found in 1 to 5 percent of all cases of cancer. Cardiac metastases have been reported from nearly every known malignancy except for the central nervous system. There are numerous reports in the literature of cardiac metastases diagnosed by echocardiography.[A5, C10, C11, D4, G10, H2, J1, K5–K7, L6, M10, N4, P9, S8, S9, T5, W6, Z2] The most common malignancies to metastasize to the heart are shown in Table 25–2. Pericardial metastases[K8] are much more common than myocardial metastases.[M2] Clinical symptoms and signs of cardiac involvement of neoplasm include pericarditis, pericardial effusion, tamponade, electrocardiographic changes, arrhythmias, and heart failure. Pericardial effusion is the most common echocardiographic finding in metastatic cardiac disease. Figure 25–18 represents a patient with pericardial effusion and metastatic adenocarcinoma of the colon. Echocardiographic visualization of visceral and parietal pericardial mestatases has been reported by several investigators. They may look like irregularly shaped "cauliflowers" of the pericardium, as seen in Figure 25–18. These masses may be difficult to diagnose as tumors, and one should be cautious because they may represent blood clots or fibrous strands. Direct cytologic examination of the pericardial fluid is essential for diagnosis of malignancy spread to the pericardial space. Figure 25–19 shows a case of poorly differentiated adenocarcinoma metastasizing to the right and left ventricles and to the pericardium. This patient presented with constrictive pericarditis. Figure 25–20 shows a case of adenocarcinoma

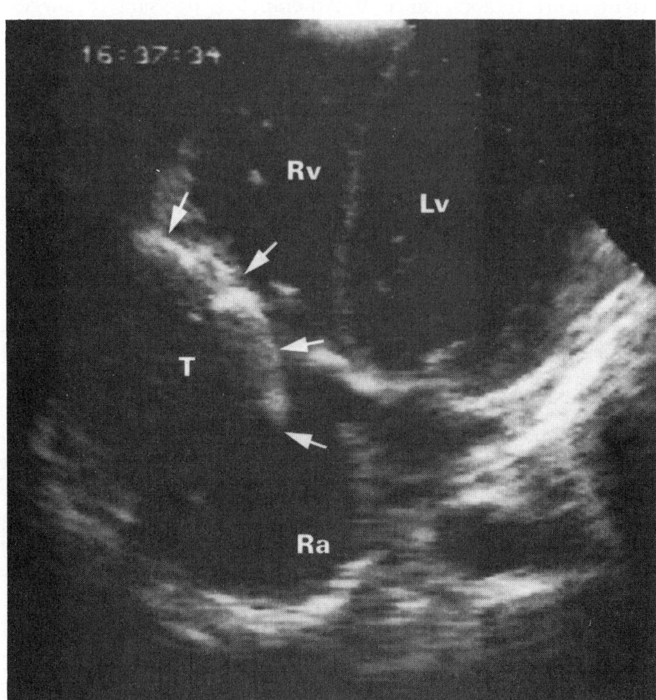

Figure 25–16. An apical four-chamber view of a patient with a large angiosarcoma infiltrating the right atrium (Ra) and right ventricle (Rv). Abbreviations: Lv—left ventricle; T—tumor.

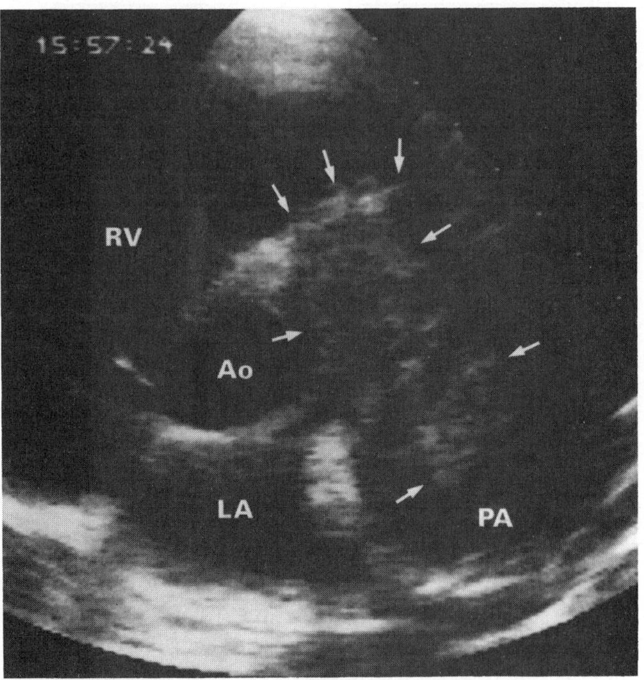

Figure 25–17. Parasternal short-axis view at the level of the aorta (Ao) and pulmonary artery (PA) from a patient with a malignant fibrous histiocytoma of the pulmonary artery. The pulmonary artery is markedly dilated. The tumor cloud is shown within the arrows. Abbreviations: LA—left atrium; RV—right ventricle.

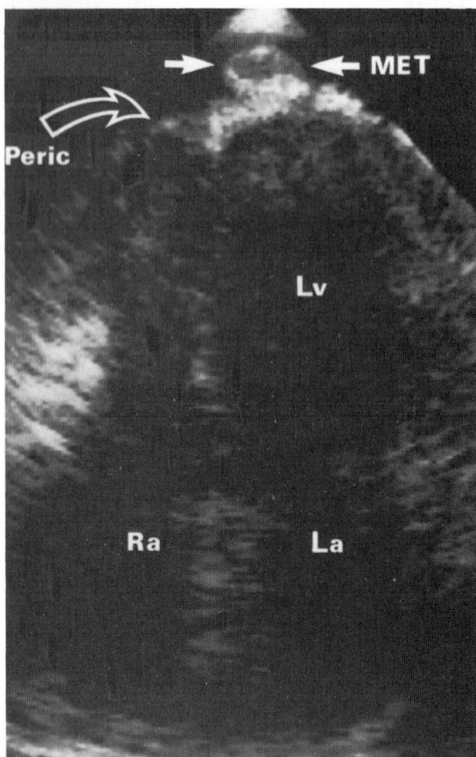

Figure 25–18. An apical four-chamber view of a patient with adenocarcinoma of the colon metastasizing to the pericardium with characteristic "cauliflower" tumors attached to the pericardium. Abbreviations: MET—metastases; Peric—pericardium; Lv—left ventricle; La—left atrium; Ra—right atrium.

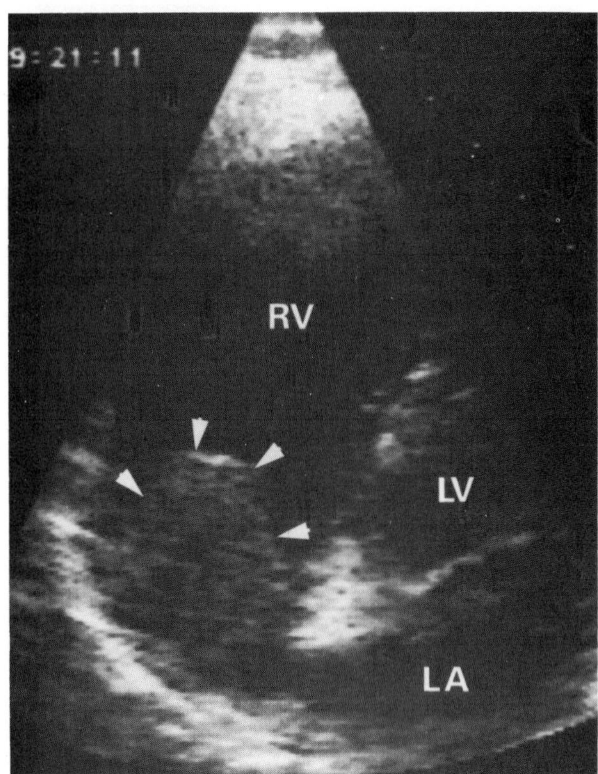

Figure 25–20. A slightly off-axis four-chamber view of a patient with adenocarcinoma of the rectum metastasizing to the right atrium. The tumor is shown within the arrows. Abbreviations: RV—right ventricle; LV—left ventricle; LA—left atrium.

of the rectum metastasizing to the right atrium. Figure 25–21 shows a case of a 25-year-old man with embryonal carcinoma metastasizing to the right ventricle.

Direct invasion of the right heart from infradiaphragmatic tumors has been reported to occur in cases of hepatoma, leiomyoma, and nephroma. These tumors, although of benign histology, can pose serious problems for the patient because of their local spread to the heart. Figure 25–22 shows a case of nephroma invading the right atrium that may be mistaken for a myxoma. This tumor was prolapsing into the right ventricle during diastole but was contained within the right atrium during systole. Careful evaluation of the inferior vena cava, as was done in this case, demonstrated a tumor present in this vessel. Ultrasonic scanning below the diaphragm should always be performed in cases of right heart tumors, since the therapeutic decision or surgical approach may be different if the tumor is known to be infradiaphragmatic.

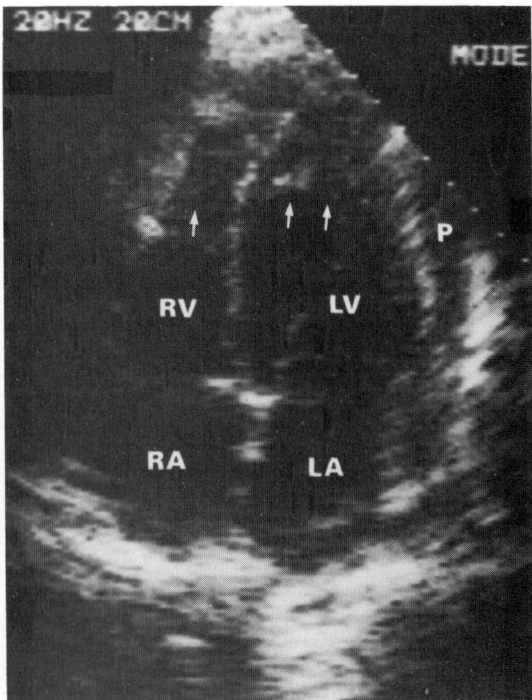

Figure 25–19. An apical four-chamber view of a patient with a tumor infiltrating the right ventricular (RV) and left ventricular (LV) apexes as well as the pericardium (P). The tumor was a poorly differentiated adenocarcinoma causing constrictive pericarditis. Abbreviations: RA—right atrium; LA—left atrium.

Extracardiac Masses Adjacent to the Heart

Mediastinal tumors and intrathoracic neoplasms have been detected by echocardiography.[C12, D5, Y1] These tumors may compress one or several chambers of the heart, with or without direct involvement of the heart.[G11, P10, S10] Depending on the location of such tumor, the patient may present with superior vena cava syndrome,[C13] pericarditis, tamponade,[C13] constriction,[S11] or obstruction to venous filling. Hodgkin's disease with involvement of the mediastinal lymph nodes may result in an extra large distance between the chest wall and the heart, as seen in Figure 25–23. A large cystic mass in the mediastinum was noted in several echocardiographic views in another patient with Hodgkin's disease and necrosis of the lymph tissue (Fig. 25–24). Figure 25–25 illustrates a lymphoma compressing the left atrium and left ventricle in a young man.

Magnetic resonance imaging and computed tomographic scanning can offer additional information in the evaluation of extracardiac masses.

THROMBI

Intracardiac Thrombi

Intracardiac thrombi are detected in all four cardiac chambers, including attachments to the valves, and occur when there is

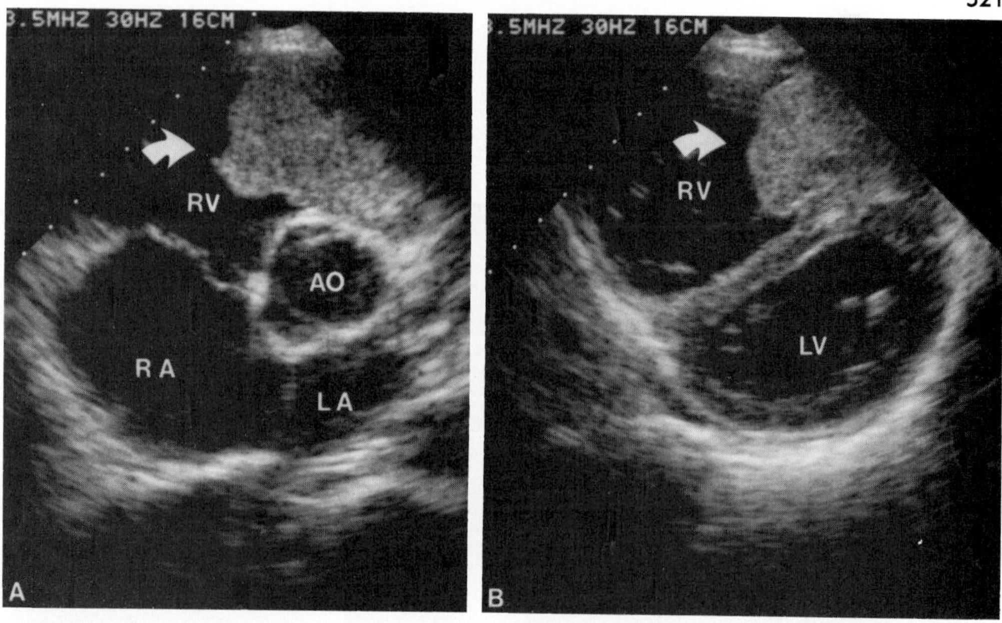

Figure 25–21. *A*, Parasternal short-axis view at the level of the aorta (AO) demonstrating a large tumor (*arrow*) in a patient with embryonal carcinoma metastasizing to the right ventricle (RV). *B*, The same tumor at the level of the left ventricular (LV) chordae tendineae. Abbreviations: LA—left atrium; RA—right atrium.

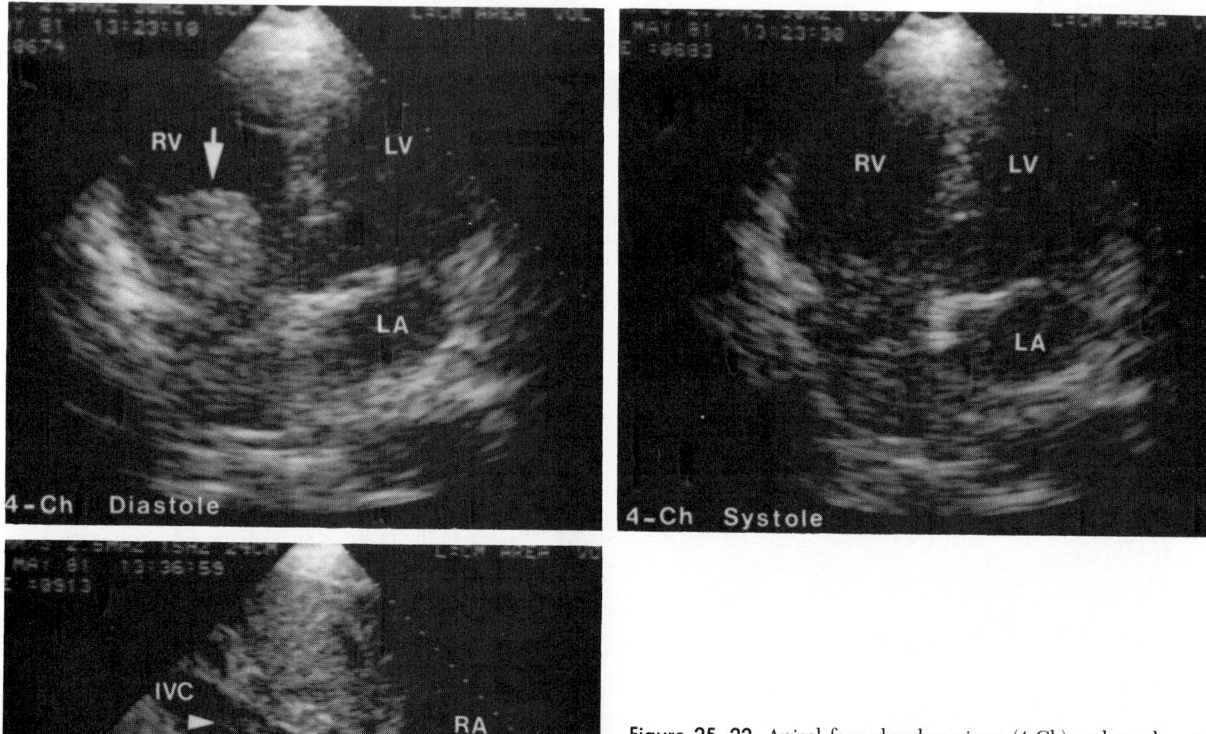

Figure 25–22. Apical four-chamber views (4-Ch) and a subcostal view (SubC) from a patient with hypernephroma invading the right heart. The upper left panel shows the tumor prolapsing through the tricuspid valve during diastole and contained within the right atrium (RA) during systole. The lower panel represents a subcostal view showing the tumor (*arrows*) in the inferior vena cava (IVC) and extending into the right atrium. Abbreviations: RV—right ventricle; LV—left ventricle; LA—left atrium.

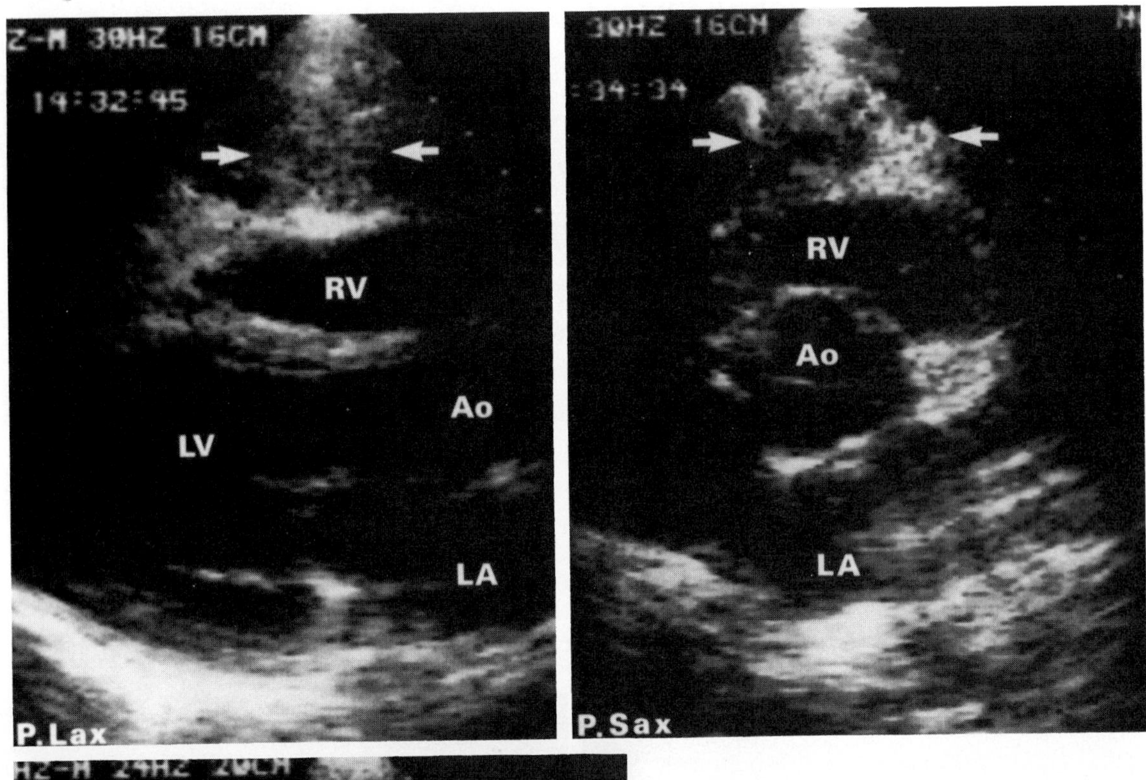

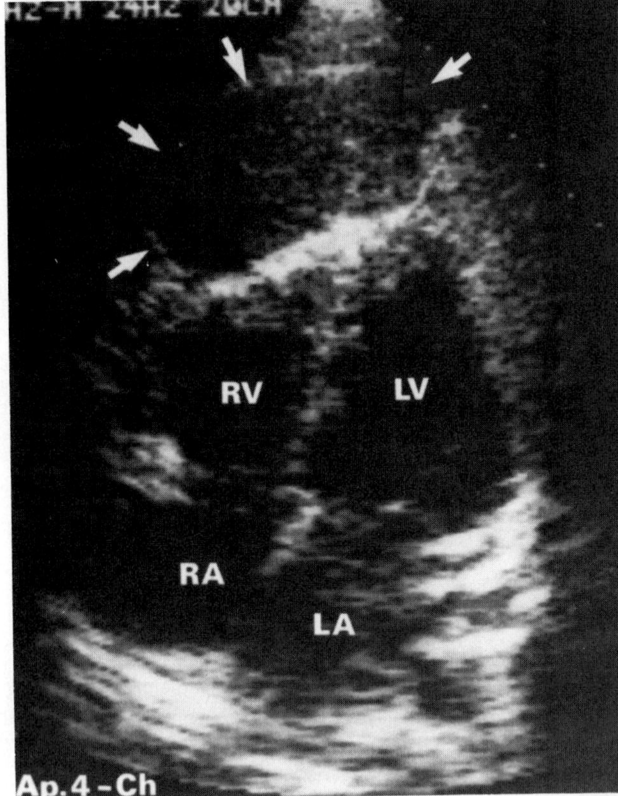

Figure 25–23. Three panels from a patient with mediastinal Hodgkin's disease. The upper left panel is a parasternal long-axis view (P.Lax) with the tumor anterior to the right ventricle (RV) and the upper right panel is the parasternal short-axis view (P.Sax). The lower panel shows an apical four-chamber view (Ap.4-Ch) demonstrating a large tumor mass anterior and apical to the heart. Abbreviations: RA—right atrium; LA—left atrium; LV—left ventricle; Ao—aorta.

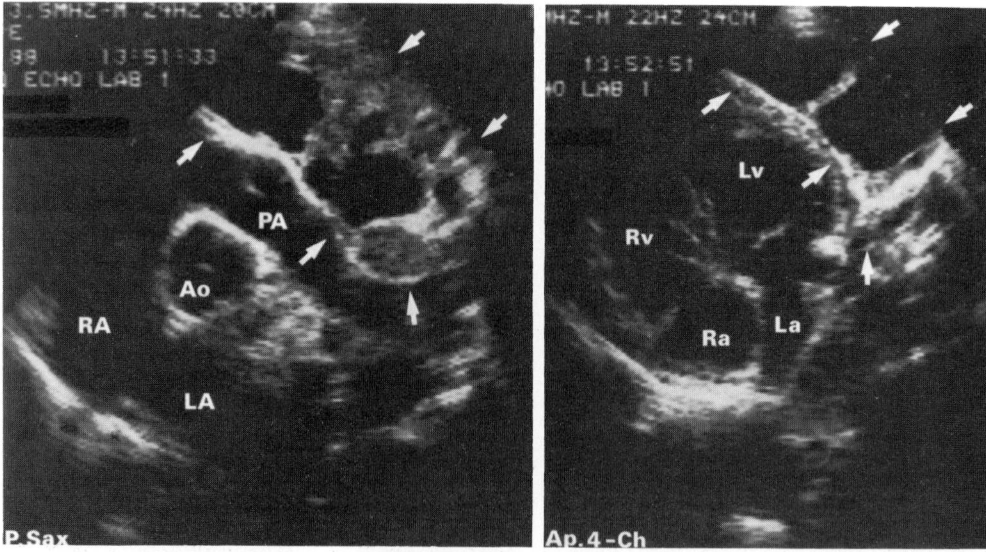

Figure 25–24. A parasternal short-axis view (P.Sax) in the left panel and an apical four-chamber view (Ap.4-Ch) in the right panel, demonstrating a large cystic mass anterior and lateral to the heart. This patient had biopsy-proven Hodgkin's disease. Abbreviations: RA and Ra—right atrium; Rv—right ventricle; LA and La—left atrium; Lv—left ventricle; Ao—aorta; PA—pulmonary artery.

stagnation of blood flow within the chamber or endocardial injury. Thrombi appear as intracardiac masses that usually differ from the surrounding myocardium in acoustic density and texture. Based on location, motion, texture, and underlying cardiac abnormalities, these clots usually can be distinguished from other cardiac masses and tumors. Intracardiac thrombi attached to the cardiac valves are discussed elsewhere. Intracavitary thrombi are discussed below for each chamber.

Left Ventricle

Echocardiographic detection of left ventricular thrombi has been described in several reports.[A6, D6, F13, G12, K9, L7, S12–S14, V2, V3] Two-dimensional echocardiography is the method of choice in diagnosing left ventricular thrombi and is superior to left ventricular angiography.[T6] Recently, color Doppler echocardiography has been shown to aid in the diagnosis of left ventricular thrombus.[M11] Left ventricular thrombi typically occur where there is an underlying wall motion abnormality, due to either acute ischemia,[S15] infarct,[F14, J2, K10] or aneurysm,[R5] as well as in idiopathic cardiomyopathy.[G13] In rare instances, left ventricular thrombi can form where the underlying wall segment moves normally but there are abnormal clotting parameters. This is unusual, however, and one should probably be hesitant to make the diagnosis of left ventricular thrombus in the absence of wall motion abnormalities. Left ventricular thrombi are most commonly seen in the left ventricular apex. In acute anterior myocardial infarctions they form in as many as 22 to 46 percent [A7, F14] of all cases, compared to 0 to 5 percent[A7, W7] in acute inferior myocardial infarctions. Although a large number of these clots do resolve spontaneously, we frequently see mural thrombi in chronic infarcts and in left ventricular aneurysms.

The left ventricular thrombus may be flat (Figs. 25–26, 25–27) or protruding (Figs. 25–28, 25–29), mobile (Fig. 25–30) or immobile (see Fig. 25–26), very dense (see Fig. 25–27) or echolucent (Fig. 25–31), and with or without an echo-dense margin (Fig. 25–32). There may be a single thrombus or multiple thrombi (see Fig. 25–28). If the thrombus is flat or layered, it can be difficult to detect. However, if the wall thickness in an area of suspicion is greater than normal, there is high likelihood that a thrombus is present since the underlying wall segment is usually thinner than normal. The mural flat thrombi are usually immobile or occasionally may have a loose flap. The protruding thrombi are often highly mobile and exhibit a characteristic undulating motion.

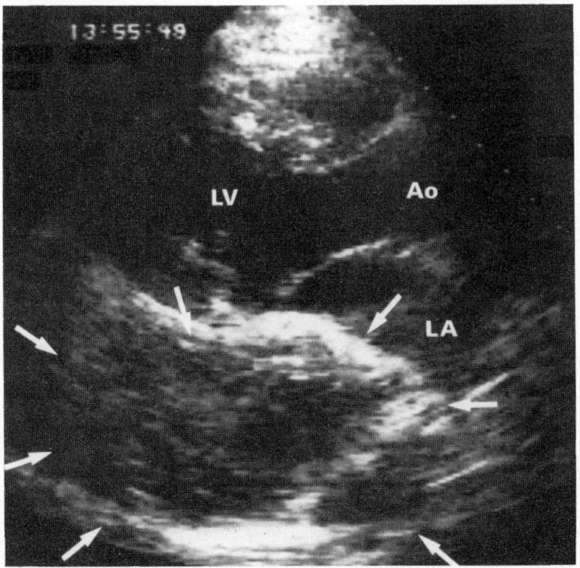

Figure 25–25. A parasternal long-axis view of a patient with a large retrocardiac mass. Biopsy proved this to be a "small round cell" tumor, probably lymphoma. Abbreviations: LA—left atrium; LV—left ventricle; Ao—aorta.

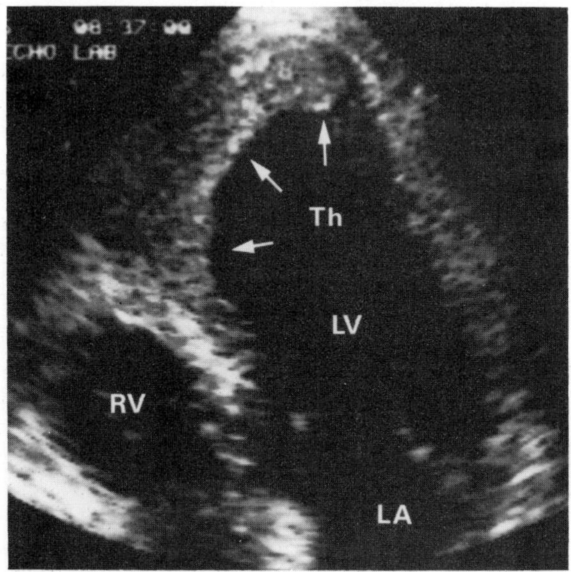

Figure 25–26. Apical four-chamber view demonstrating a large apical aneurysm in a patient status post myocardial infarction with a large layered thrombus (Th) in the left ventricular (LV) apex. Abbreviations: LA—left atrium; RV—right ventricle.

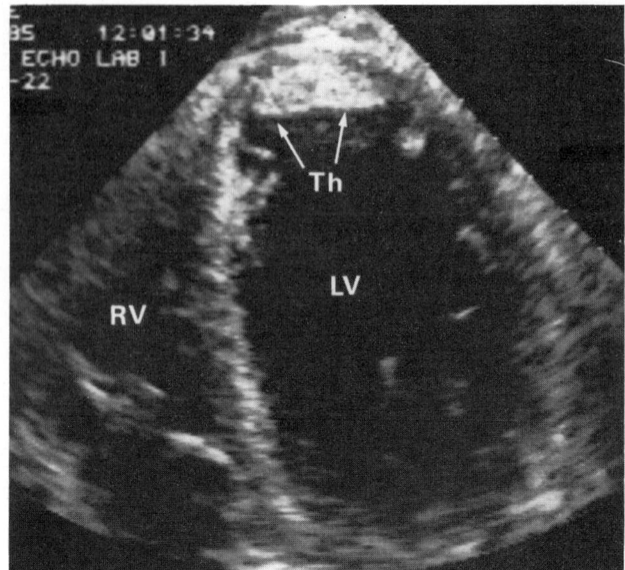

Figure 25–27. An apical four-chamber view of a patient with an apical infarct and a layered mural thrombus in the apex. Abbreviations: Th—thrombus; LV—left ventricle; RV—right ventricle.

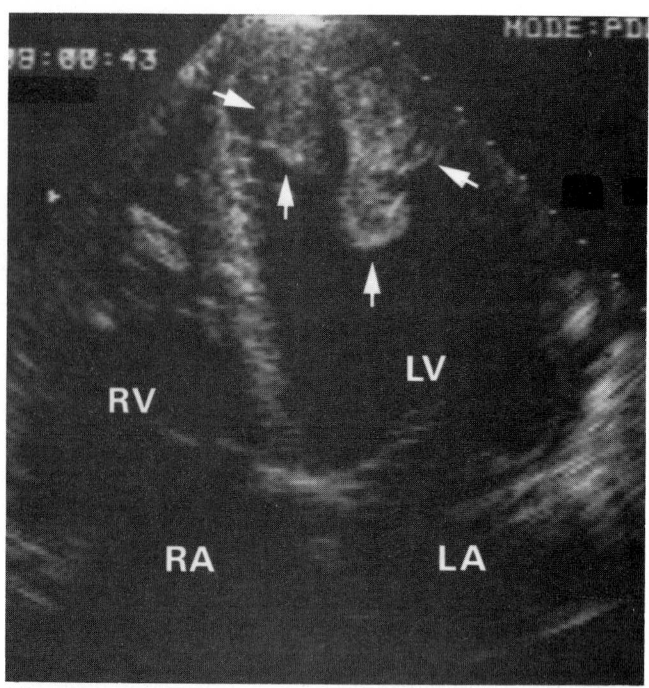

Figure 25–29. An apical four-chamber view of a patient with congestive cardiomyopathy and a large horseshoe-shaped thrombus in the left ventricle (LV). Abbreviations: RV—right ventricle; RA—right atrium; LA—left atrium.

If in doubt about the diagnosis, it is helpful to obtain several different echocardiographic views and often unconventional two-dimensional echocardiographic views with the transducer tilted slightly inferiorly to image the cardiac apex clearly (see Fig. 25–31). Mural thrombi, especially in the left ventricular apex, must be differentiated from trabeculae, anomalous bands, and papillary muscles.[A8] The apical thrombi are typically seen in the apical four-chamber and two-chamber views. They often "disappear" into the near-focus artifact. A short-focus transducer or a shallow focal point may reduce the noise level. Also, the near-focus artifact moves independently of the heart, "cutting across" both left and right ventricular apices. Ultrasonic tissue characterization of the reflected amplitudes from left ventricular apical masses has been reported as a means of differentiating a thrombus from a tumor or artifact[G14]; however, clinically this has not yet become a useful tool.

Several investigators have shown that there is an increased risk of embolization in patients with left ventricular thrombi compared with patients who have no demonstrable thrombus.[S16] The tendency to embolize is greatest for protruding and mobile thrombi.[M12, H3, N5] However, Domenecci and associates[D7] showed that left ventricular thrombi change shape over time.

Left ventricular thrombi do regress spontaneously,[S17] but warfarin seems to hasten their disappearance.[T7] Figure 25–33 represents a patient with dilated congestive cardiomyopathy who was admitted to the hospital with an acute stroke. An echocardiogram (August 1988) showed a large, protruding, mobile thrombus in the left ventricular apex. The patient was started on anticoagulation therapy, and a subsequent echocardiogram (September 1988) showed disappearance of the thrombus without another diagnosed embolic episode in the interim. Whether anticoagulation can prevent thrombus formation is more doubtful.[A9, N6] The risk of peripheral emboli in acute myocardial infarction is definite[V4] but low,[V5] and in chronic myocardial infarction/

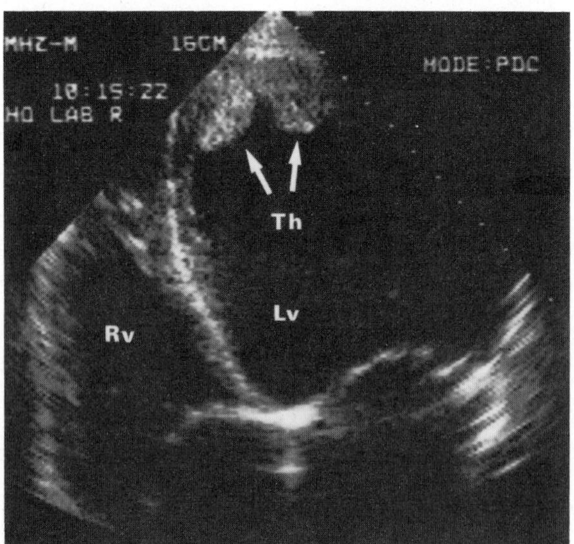

Figure 25–28. Apical four-chamber view of a patient with a dilated congestive cardiomyopathy and two large thrombi in the left ventricular (Lv) apex. Abbreviations: Th—thrombi; Rv—right ventricle.

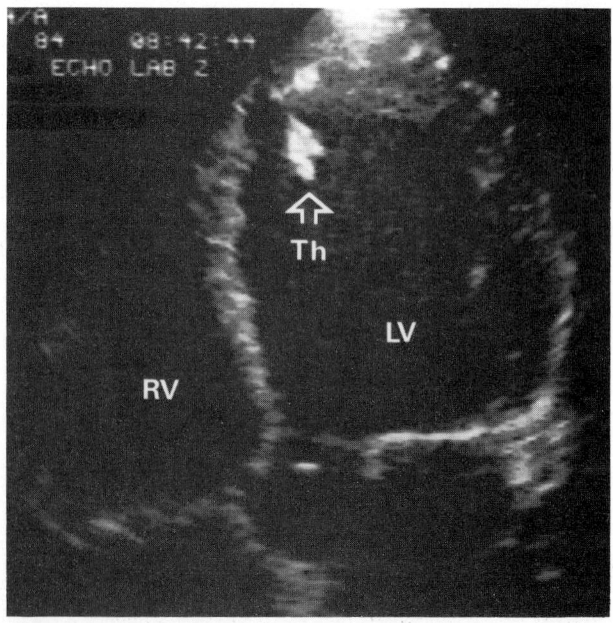

Figure 25–30. An apical four-chamber view of a patient with congestive cardiomyopathy demonstrating a highly mobile thrombus in the left ventricular (LV) apex. Abbreviations: RV—right ventricle; Th—thrombus.

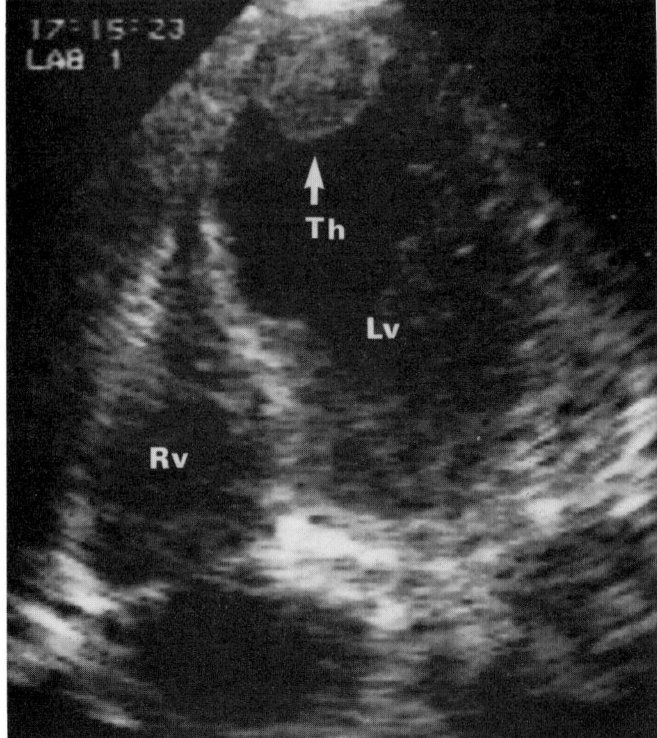

Figure 25–31. An apical four-chamber view of a patient with an anterior myocardial infarction demonstrating a mobile echo-lucent clot in the apex. Note how an unconventional scan plane optimized visualization of the thrombus with the transducer tilted more inferiorly than for a standard apical four-chamber view. Abbreviations: Th—thrombus; Lv—left ventricle; Rv—right ventricle.

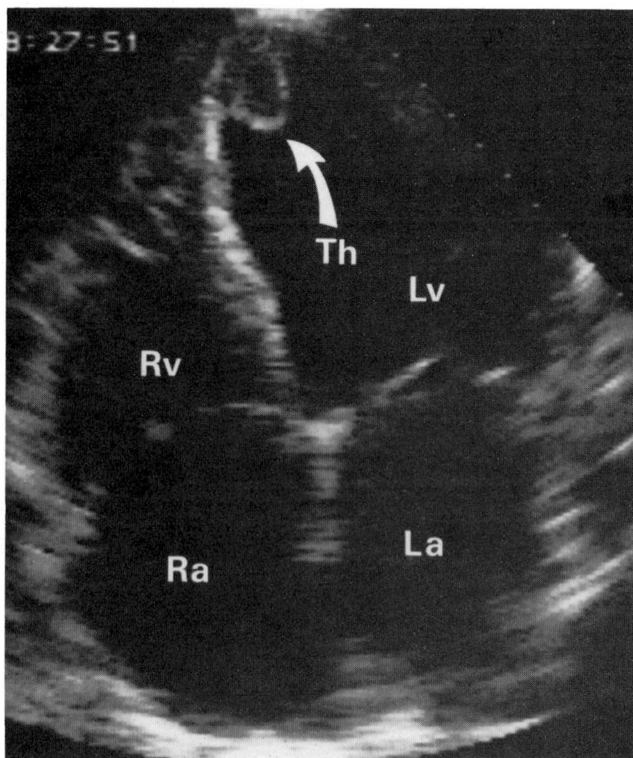

Figure 25–32. An apical four-chamber view of a patient with dilated cardiomyopathy. A large mobile thrombus (Th) was found in the left ventricular (Lv) apex. Note the center lucency with the prominent edge. Abbreviations: Ra—right atrium; La—left atrium; Rv—right ventricle.

aneurysm[R5] the risk is even lower. However, one study has demonstrated that hematologically active thrombi can be observed up to a year after their appearance.[B9] Since there is a bleeding risk of 5 percent with warfarin, it is not clear that everyone with a mural thrombus should be so treated.[M13, S18] Patients with highly mobile and protruding thrombi, however, should definitely be considered for anticoagulation therapy. Most investigators agree that patients with congestive cardiomyopathy and left ventricular thrombi should be treated with warfarin because of very low output and tendency for slow flow. There are several reports of surgical removal of left ventricular thrombi.[L8, N7] This approach, however, carries a high risk and should be considered investigational. Left ventricular thrombi may become infected, although this is exceedingly rare.[S19]

"Swirling" of blood flow (Fig. 25–34) is typically seen when there is very low cardiac output and stagnation of blood flow.

Left Atrium

Thrombi or clots in the left atrium occur mainly in three settings: in mitral valve disease, usually rheumatic heart disease; status post mitral valve replacement[C14]; and in atrial fibrillation/flutter.[C15] The left atrium usually is enlarged. An atrial clot in a patient with rheumatic heart disease is demonstrated in Figure 25–35. This clot was located just behind the valve. Commonly

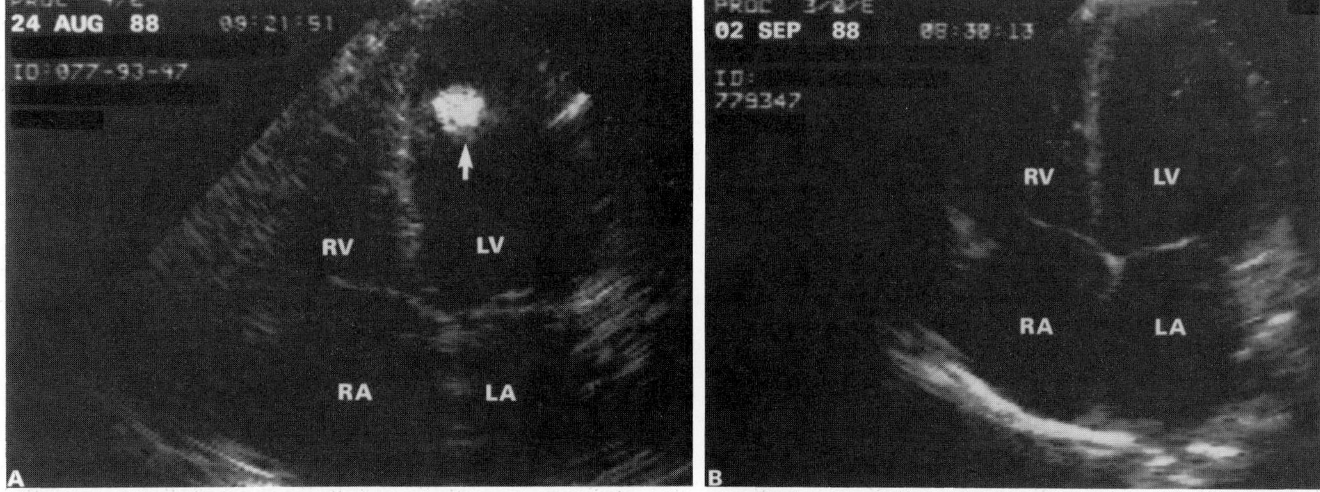

Figure 25–33. An apical four-chamber view of a patient with congestive cardiomyopathy and history of multiple strokes. On August 24, 1988, the patient was admitted to the hospital with a stroke. Echocardiogram demonstrated a large dense mass in the left ventricular (LV) apex. On September 2, 1988, this thrombus was gone after warfarin (Coumadin) treatment was started. The patient suffered no further stroke between the first and second echocardiograms. Abbreviations: RA—right atrium; RV—right ventricle; LA—left atrium.

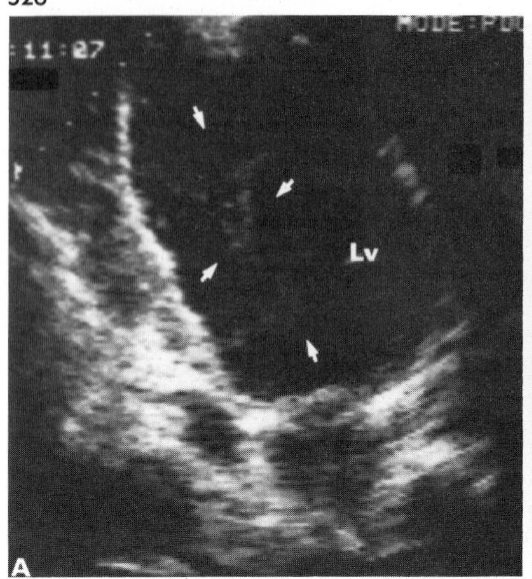

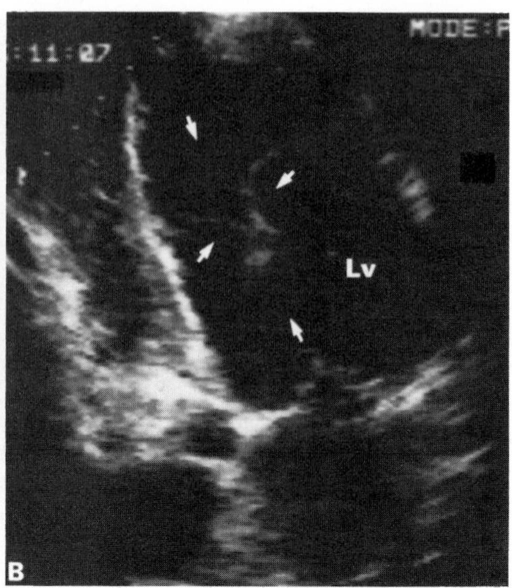

Figure 25–34. An apical two-chamber view of a patient with congestive cardiomyopathy and "swirling" secondary to slow blood flow in the left ventricle (Lv). Two consecutive frames (*A* and *B*) demonstrate the rapid change in the "swirling" pattern.

these clots are located on the posterior wall of the left atrium, as illustrated in a patient with an artificial mitral valve in Figure 25–36. Left atrial thrombi may also be located at the orifice to the left atrial appendage (Fig. 25–37). The patient whose echocardiogram is shown in Figure 25–37 had a history of intermittent atrial fibrillation and a transischemic attack. The echocardiogram demonstrated a 1½ × 1½ cm clot in the left atrium. This clot was highly mobile. The day after the echocardiogram was obtained, the patient suffered an acute embolism to the right leg. Clots secondary to arrhythmia alone without enlargement of the chamber usually are located in the left atrial appendage.

The sensitivity and specificity of standard two-dimensional echocardiography in detecting left atrial thrombi are not nearly as good as for left ventricular thrombi. The left atrium is farther from the transducer, and the left atrial appendage is difficult to image.[R6] The best way to view the left atrial appendage is probably with the short-axis parasternal view. However, the advent of transesophageal echocardiography has greatly improved the possibility of visualization of the left atrial appendage.[A10, T8] Figure 25–38 represents a patient with intermittent atrial fibrillation, a history of multiple cerebral emboli, and a small serpentine clot in the appendage detected only by transesophageal echocardiography. Other investigators have reported freely floating left atrial thrombi,[B10, C16, F15, G15, G16, J3] which can mimic left atrial myxoma. Stagnation of blood flow in the atrium will cause "swirl,"[D8, E2] as is the case in the left ventricle. Figure 25–39 demonstrates a transesophageal echocardiogram from a patient with atrial flutter and a prominent swirling pattern in the left atrium and through the mitral valve.

Figure 25–35. A parasternal long-axis view of a patient with rheumatic mitral valve disease and a mobile clot in the left atrium (La). Abbreviations: MV—mitral valve; Ao—aorta; Rv—right ventricle.

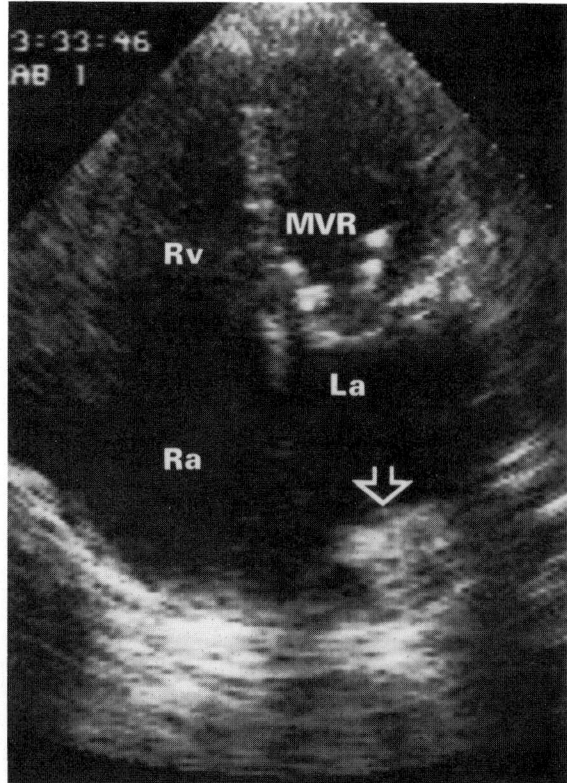

Figure 25–36. An apical four-chamber view of a patient status post mitral valve replacement with an enlarged left atrium (La) and a large mass in the posterior aspect of the left atrium (*arrow*), presumed to be thrombus. The patient had a history of two recent transischemic attacks. Abbreviations: Ra—right atrium; MVR—mitral valve replacement; Rv—right ventricle.

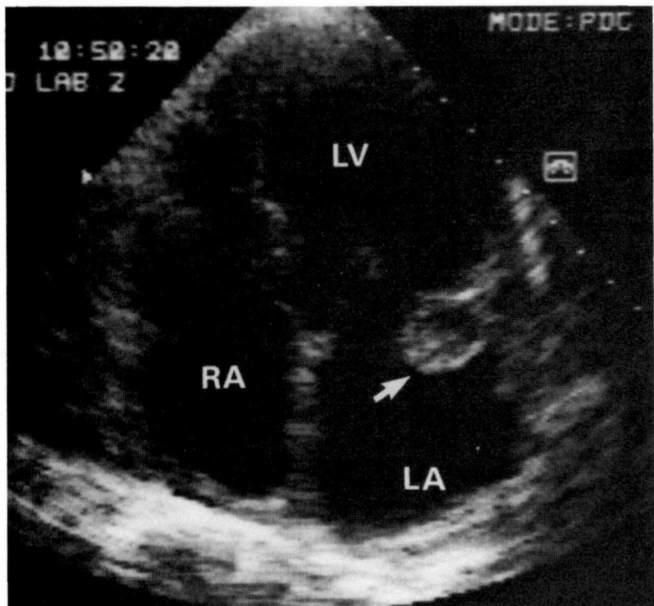

Figure 25–37. An apical four-chamber view of a patient with atrial fibrillation and a mobile clot at the junction of the left atrium (LA) and the left atrial appendage. This clot embolized to the patient's leg a few hours after this study. Abbreviations: RA—right atrium; LV—left ventricle.

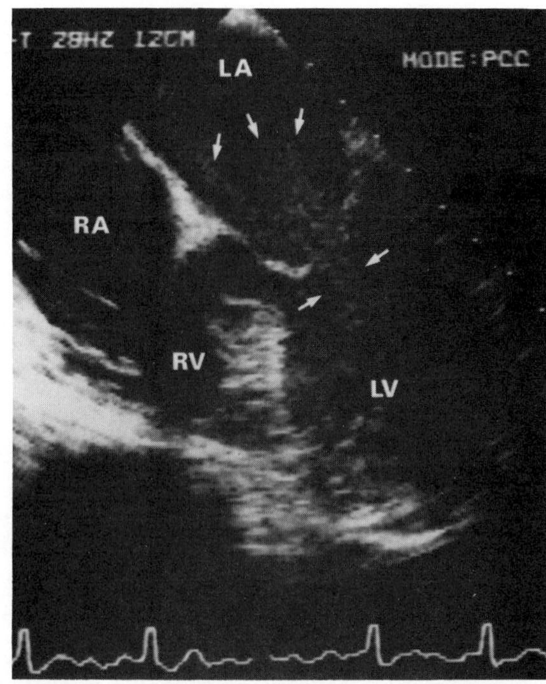

Figure 25–39. A transesophageal echocardiogram of a patient with atrial flutter and a prominent "swirling" pattern in the left atrium (LA) and through the mitral valve. Abbreviations: RA—right atrium; RV—right ventricle; LV—left ventricle.

Right Ventricle

Right ventricular thrombi are rare and infrequently encountered in echocardiography. They occur typically in the setting of acute right ventricular infarct,[S20] low output as in cor pulmonale[J4] or cardiomyopathy, trapping of peripheral emboli, chest trauma,[K11] and endomyocardial fibrosis.[W8] Right ventricular thrombi in the setting of an acute infarct and in cor pulmonale are usually of the same type as in the left ventricle. Trapped peripheral emboli may be highly mobile or serpentine-like. Figure 25–40 shows a right ventricular apical thrombus in a patient with a history of vasculitis, pulmonary hypertension, cor pulmonale, and pulmonary emboli. In the setting of pulmonary emboli, the heart should be routinely examined for right heart clots, since the presence of a clot, especially if it is mobile, is an ominous sign associated with a poor prognosis. The right ventricular clot should be differentiated from right ventricular trabeculae and the right ventricular moderator band.

Right Atrium

Right atrial clots occur as an in situ development in rheumatic heart disease, status post tricuspid valve replacement, and arrhythmias.[B11] There are also reports of right atrial thrombus

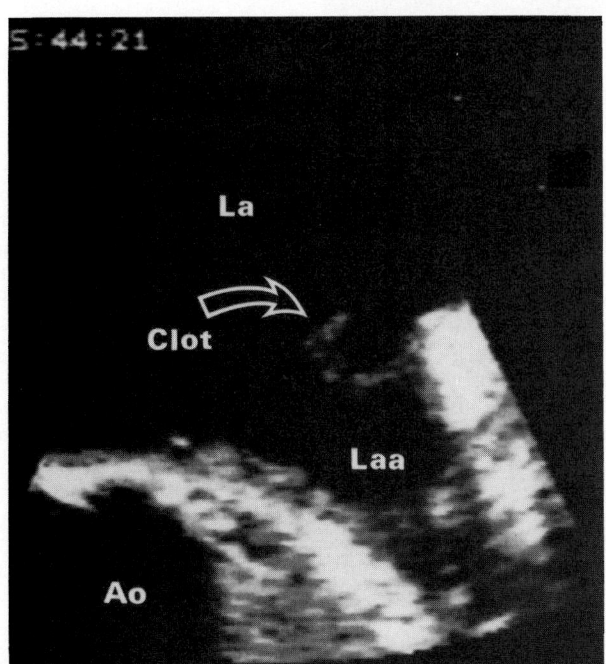

Figure 25–38. A transesophageal echocardiogram focusing on the left atrium (La) and left atrial appendage (Laa) of a patient with a history of intermittent atrial fibrillation and a recent stroke. In the left atrial appendage a small serpentine clot was found which had been missed on the transthoracic echocardiogram. Abbreviation: Ao—aorta.

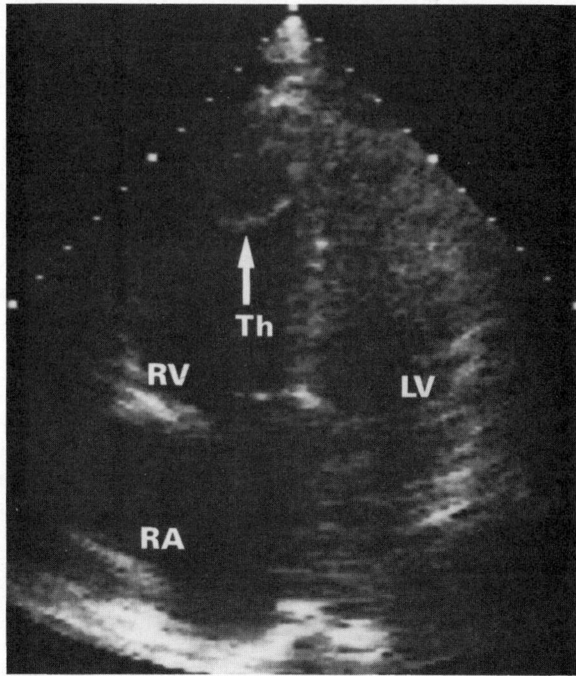

Figure 25–40. An apical four-chamber view of a patient with recent pulmonary emboli and collagen vascular disease. A large thrombus (Th) was found in the right ventricular (RV) apex. Abbreviations: RA—right atrium; LV—left ventricle.

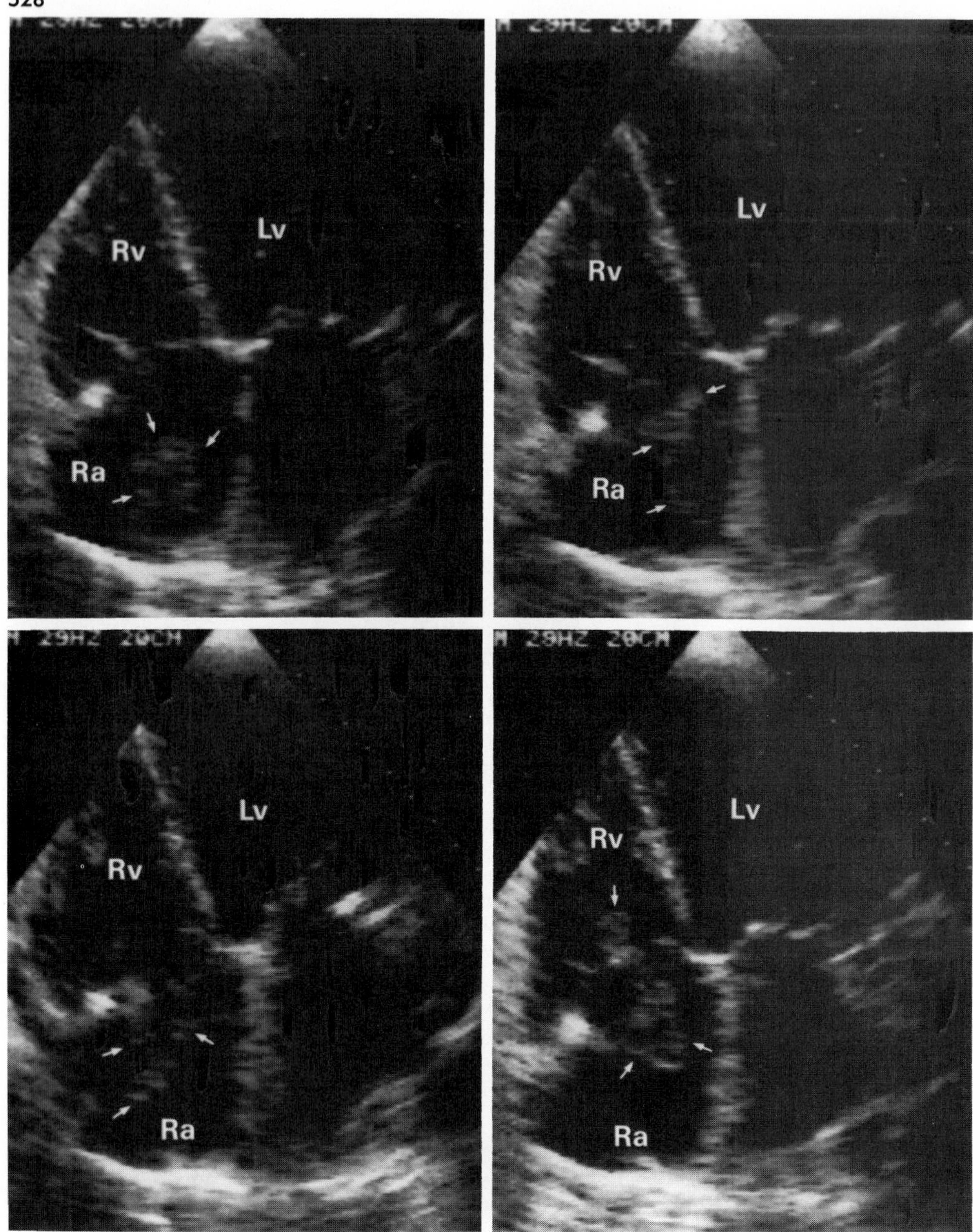

Figure 25–41. An apical four-chamber view with four frames throughout the cardiac cycle demonstrating the highly mobile free-floating clot in the right atrium (Ra) prolapsing through the tricuspid valve in diastole. Abbreviations: Rv—right ventricle; Lv—left ventricle.

formation after transvenous catheter ablation[K12] and after cardiac surgery.[A11] As in the right ventricle, these clots may be trapped from peripheral circulation[S21] or may be developed on the intravenous lines[S22, U1] or catheters.[M14] Figure 25–41 shows a right atrial clot in a patient with multiple pulmonary emboli who expired shortly after this echo was obtained. Autopsy showed a thrombus in the left iliac vein, which was thought to be the source. Figure 25–42 shows a right atrial clot, again highly mobile, in a patient with an acute pulmonary embolus. Thrombi found in the right atrium in association with acute pulmonary embolism are often serpentine-like and highly mobile. They have a propensity to form emboli[S23] and probably should be treated aggressively.[T9] Right atrial clots typically can mimic Chiari's network or a eustachian valve.

MISCELLANEOUS MASSES AND ARTIFACTS

Several other masses and artifacts can mimic neoplasms and thrombi in the heart. A carefully obtained history and physical examination of the patient can often give a clue to the diagnosis. Normal variants have been discussed at the introduction. Table 25–3 lists the structures that are discussed below.

LIPOMATOUS HYPERTROPHY. Lipomatous hypertrophy of the interatrial septum is characterized by abnormal accumulations of adipose tissue that form a recognizable mass. The mass of adipose tissue in the atrial septum is in continuity with the epicardial fat and probably represents atypical hyperplasia rather than a true tumor. These hyperplasias are usually "dumbbell" in shape, sparing the fossa ovalis.[S24] The echocardiographic appearance is quite specific,[F16] and ultrasound can be used for prospective follow-up of patients with this known entity. These hyperplasias are best seen in the subcostal view (Fig. 25–43) but may

Table 25–3. MASSES AND ARTIFACTS THAT MIMIC CARDIAC NEOPLASMS AND THROMBI

Lipomatous hypertrophy
Aneurysm of the interatrial septum
Trabeculae and anomalous bands
Foreign bodies
Hiatal hernia
Extracardiac structures
Giant valve vegetations
Surgical suture lines
Cardiac hypertrophy
Calcified cardiac structures

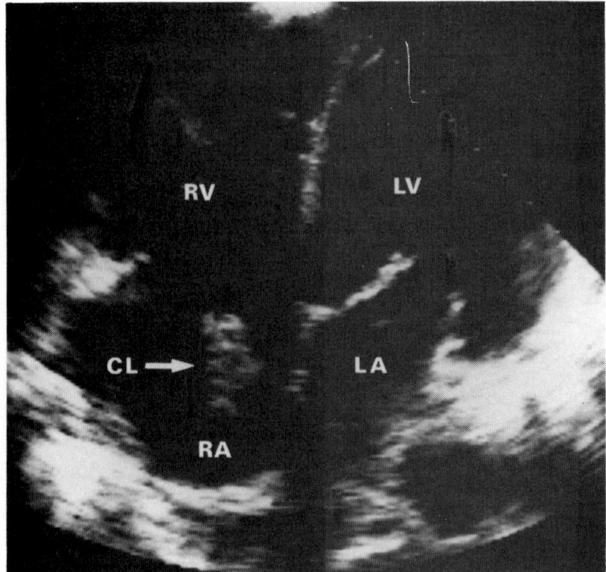

Figure 25–42. An apical four-chamber view of a patient with severe biventricular failure and multiple pulmonary emboli. A large mobile nonattached clot was found in the right atrium (RA). Abbreviations: RV—right ventricle; LV—left ventricle; LA—left atrium; CL—clot.

also be seen in the four-chamber view. They should be differentiated from "dropout" of the middle section of the interatrial septum. Transesophageal echocardiography may be helpful. These hyperplasias should also be differentiated from other tumors or masses. The clue to lipomatous hypertrophy is intractable congestive heart failure or persistent rhythm disturbances without other definable causes. Magnetic resonance scanning may show tissue as fat.

ANEURYSM OF THE INTERATRIAL SEPTUM. Interatrial septal aneurysms are thinned areas of the fossa ovalis resulting in redundant wall tissue. The interatrial septal aneurysm is usually highly mobile and may have the appearance of a serpentine-like clot (Fig. 25–44).

FALSE TENDONS, VENTRICULAR TRABECULAE, AND ANOMALOUS BANDS. False tendons,[G17, P11] ventricular trabeculae, and anomalous bands[K1, K2] occur within the left and right ventricular cavities and may mimic thrombus margins or tumors (Fig. 25–45). In one report[K2] correlating echocardiographic and pathologic data for 35 patients, right ventricular trabeculae were found in 28 percent and left ventricular trabeculae in 43 percent

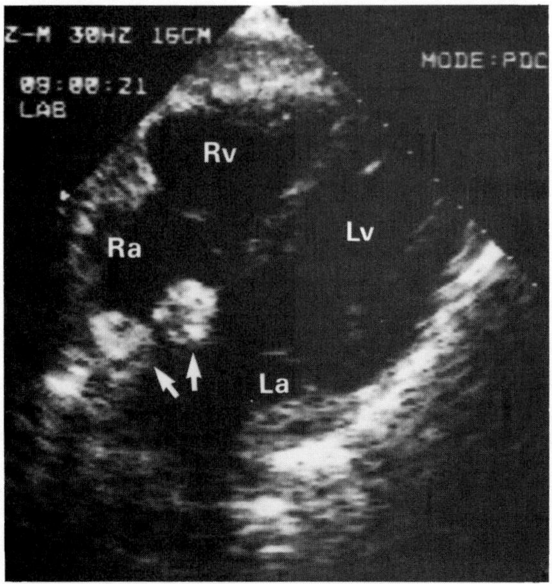

Figure 25–43. An apical four-chamber view of a patient with lipomatous hypertrophy with the characteristic "dumbbell"-shaped interatrial septum (*arrows*). Abbreviations: La—left atrium; Lv—left ventricle; Ra—right atrium; Rv—right ventricle.

of the cases. Aberrant bands were found in the right ventricle in 10 percent and in the left ventricle in 37 percent.

FOREIGN BODIES. Foreign bodies in the heart, such as catheters (Fig. 25–46), pacemaker lines (Fig. 25–47), and prosthetic valves, often give rise to prominent, bright, echo-dense reverberations. Indwelling catheters usually can be differentiated easily from tumors or clots because of excessive mobility.

HIATAL HERNIA. Large hiatal hernias of the esophagus can mimic intracavitary left atrial masses.[N3] The large mass seen in Figure 25–48 was initially thought to be a left atrial myxoma. However, careful examination, including an apical four-chamber view, showed this mass over an area of both right and left atria, which made an extrinsic mass more likely than an intrinsic mass. This patient had a very large esophageal hiatal hernia. Differentiation between a hiatal hernia and a left atrial mass may be achieved by having the patient drink water, which will appear as targets in the mass if it is a hiatal hernia.

EXTRACARDIAC STRUCTURES INDENTING THE HEART. Extracardiac structures can mimic an intracardiac mass. A prominent pectus excavatum, as shown in Figure 25–49, gave the appearance of a right atrial and right ventricular intracardiac tumor. Occasionally we have seen collapsed vertebrae altering the position and shape of the heart.

GIANT VALVE VEGETATIONS. A giant valve vegetation may mimic a myxoma[H4, Z3] or clot, especially if it is attached to the atrial aspect of the atrioventricular valve. The echocardiogram shown in Figure 25–50 was obtained from a patient with fungal endocarditis. Staphylococcal and fungal valvular infections are typically large and fluffy. Clinical correlation is very important, and positive results of blood culture make the diagnosis of endocarditis more likely than the diagnosis of other mass or tumor.

SURGICAL SUTURE LINES. In cardiac transplantation, the suture line between the donor and recipient atria can be very prominent and may mimic an atrial mass or clot.[G18] This is important to note, since cardiac transplant patients treated with cyclosporine have an increased risk of developing lymphoma. Figure 25–51 illustrates such a prominent suture line. Transesophageal echocardiography was helpful for improved resolution and to define this structure (Fig. 25–52).

CARDIAC HYPERTROPHY. Left ventricular[K4] and right ventricular hypertrophy,[J5] especially apical, can mimic tumors and clots. An important differential diagnosis includes left ventricular fibroma. Figure 25–53 represents a case of left ventricular apical hypertrophy of the "spade-shaped" type associated with giant negative precordial T waves in the electrocardiogram. Underlying wall motion abnormalities usually are not present in apical hypertrophy but are frequently found when tumors or thrombi are present.

CALCIFIED CARDIAC STRUCTURES. Calcified papillary muscles and mitral valve annulus can appear as prominent bright calcified masses (Fig. 25–54).[B12]

Finally, there have been reports of cardiac echinococcosis[O1] and hydatid cysts[A12, D9] diagnosed by two-dimensional echocardiography and mimicking cardiac tumors. Giant Lambl's excrescences also have been noted by several investigators.[C17, C18]

Detection of cardiac masses has substantially improved since echocardiography was introduced 35 years ago. Prior to the ultrasound era, angiography could provide an antemortem diagnosis of a cardiac tumor or mass in a limited number of patients.

Echocardiography has gained universal acceptance among physicians and patients alike. It is a frequently available, easily tolerated, safe, and relatively inexpensive technique. Although ultrasound cannot provide a histologic diagnosis of a certain disease process, an experienced echocardiographer can often make a presumptive diagnosis of a cardiac mass based on motion, location, texture, and other characteristics.

The addition of transesophageal echocardiography has further enhanced the ultrasound technique. With the esophageal approach, clearer images can be recorded from patients that are difficult to examine for a variety of reasons and improved images also can be obtained from areas of the heart not usually well seen by standard echocardiography.

Text continued on page 534

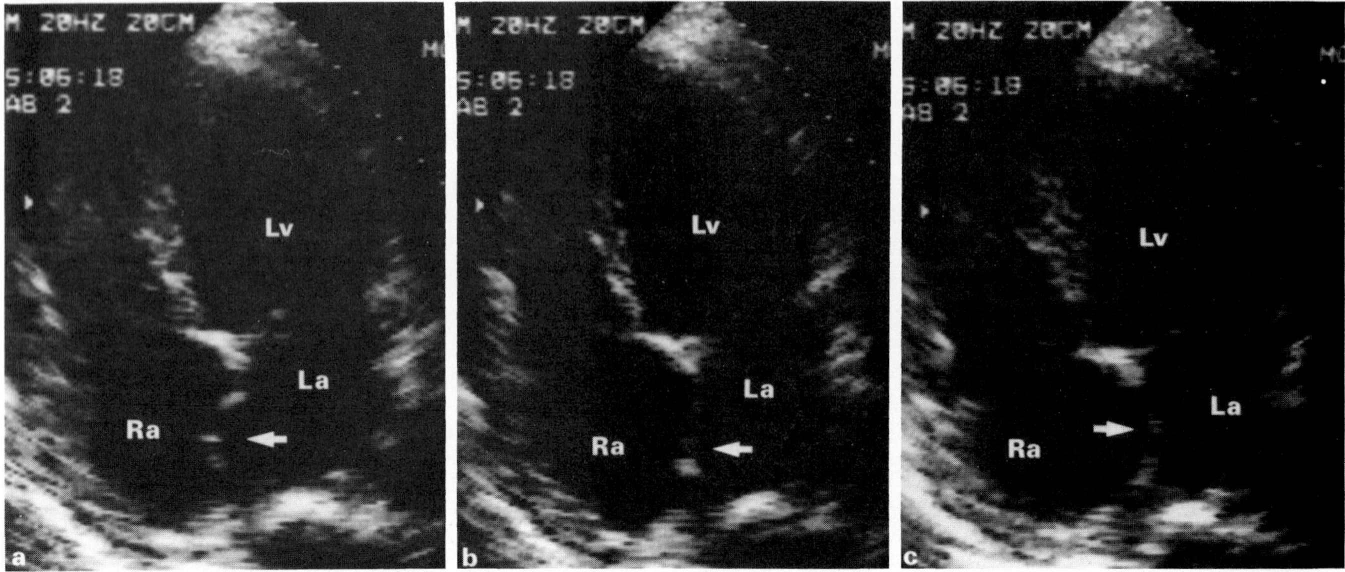

Figure 25–44. Three frames (*a, b, c*) from an apical four-chamber view of a patient with an aneurysmal dilatation of the interatrial septal wall. The highly mobile septum may mimic an atrial clot. Abbreviations: Lv—left ventricle; La—left atrium; Ra—right atrium.

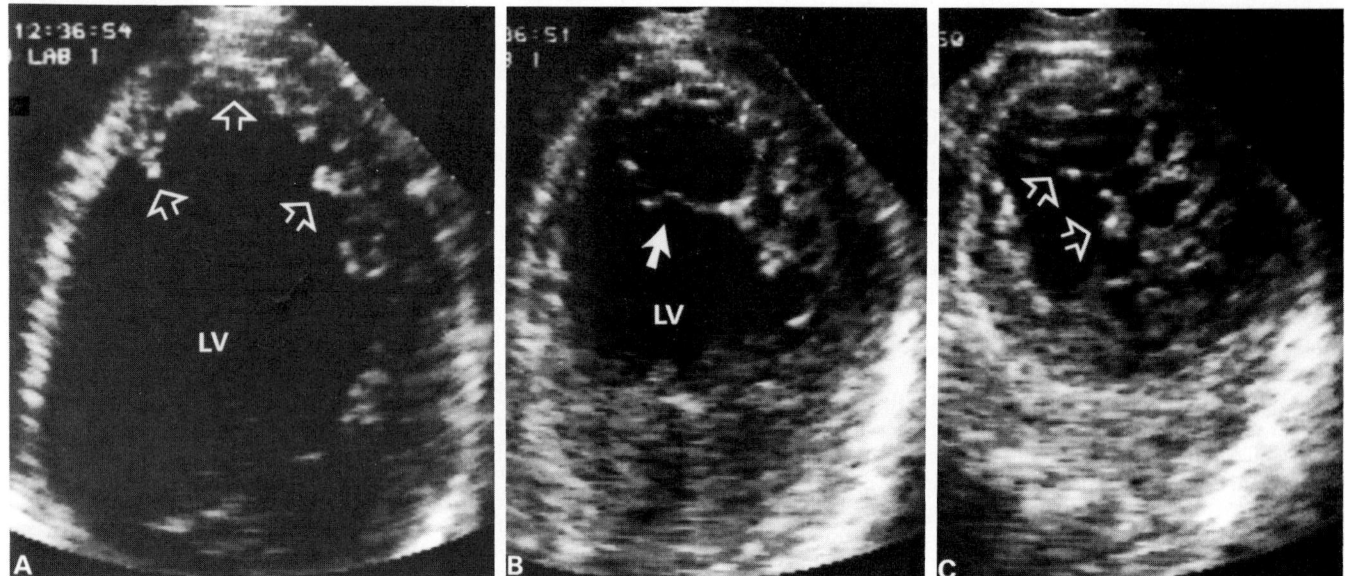

Figure 25–45. Three frames (*A, B, C*) from the left ventricular apex in an apical four-chamber view of a patient with dilated cardiomyopathy. *A*, Marked trabeculations are seen in the left ventricular (LV) apex (*arrows*). *B*, As the transducer is tilted more inferiorly, an anomalous band (*solid arrow*) is seen. A more marked trabecular network (*arrows*) is seen in panel *C* as the transducer was angled further inferiorly. Abbreviation: LV—left ventricle.

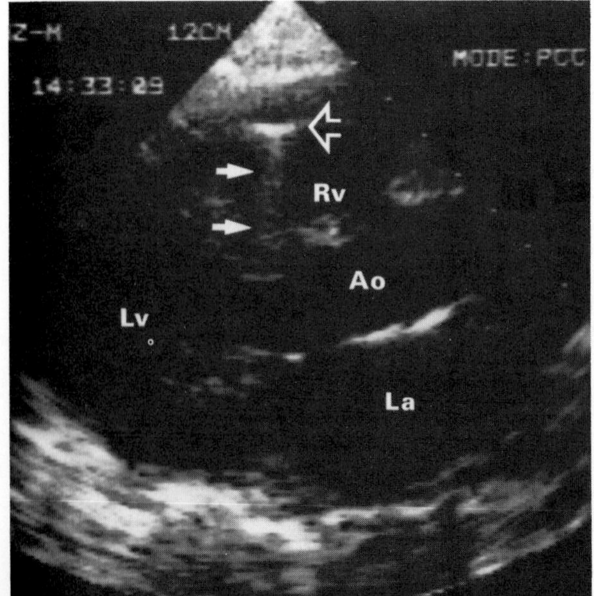

Figure 25–46. Parasternal long-axis view of a patient with a Swan-Ganz catheter placed in the right ventricle (Rv). This catheter appears as a highly mobile mass (*open arrow*) in the anterior right ventricle reverberating into the body of the right ventricle (*filled arrows*). Abbreviations: La—left atrium; Lv—left ventricle; Ao—aorta.

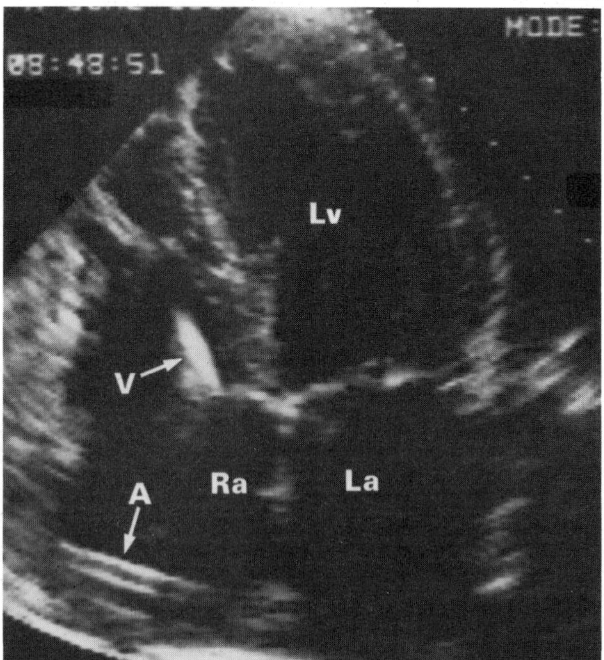

Figure 25–47. An apical four-chamber view of a patient with a dual-chamber pacemaker with the atrial pacemaker wire (A) resting in the right atrium (Ra) casting multiple artifactual echoes. The ventricular pacemaker wire (V) can be seen passing through the tricuspid valve. Abbreviations: Lv—left ventricle; La—left atrium.

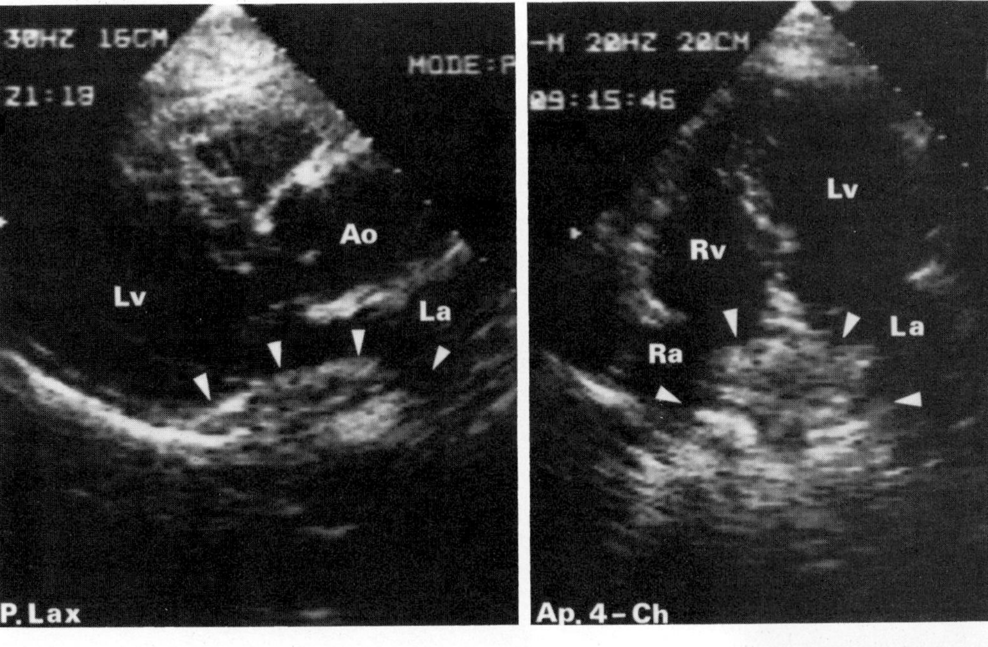

Figure 25–48. A parasternal long-axis view (P. Lax) in the left panel and an apical four-chamber view (Ap.4-Ch) in the right panel demonstrating a large hiatal hernia compressing the left atrium (La) and left ventricle (Lv) as well as the right atrium (Ra). Note that in the four-chamber view this mass seems to occupy part of both atria. Abbreviations: Rv—right ventricle; Ao—aorta.

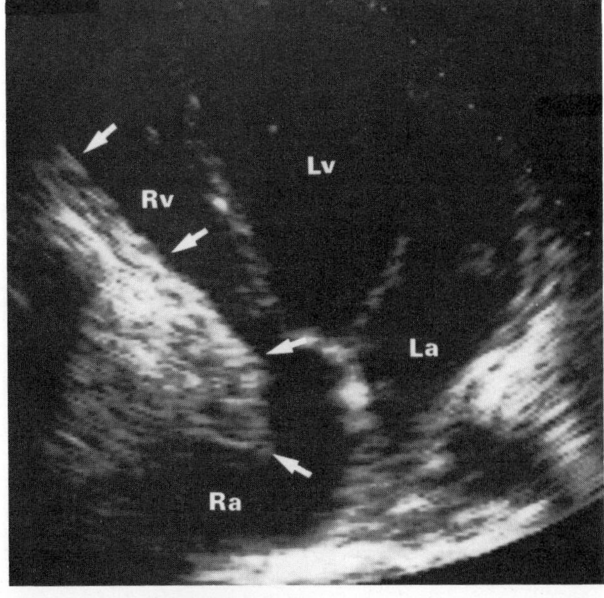

Figure 25–49. An apical four-chamber view demonstrating a very prominent pectus excavatum indenting the right atrium (Ra) and right ventricle (Rv). Abbreviations: Lv—left ventricle; La—left atrium.

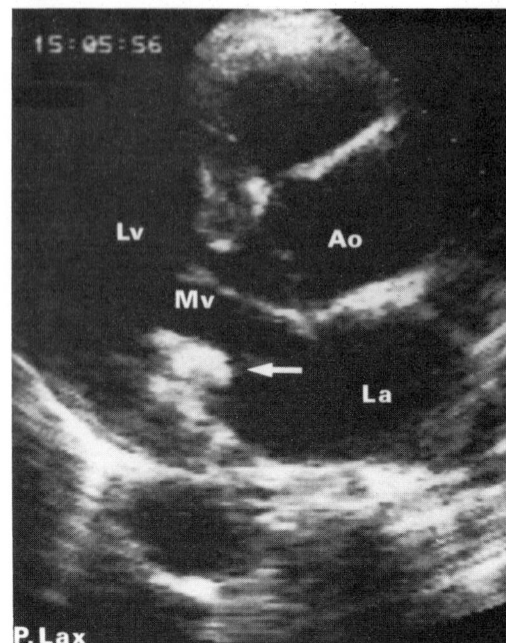

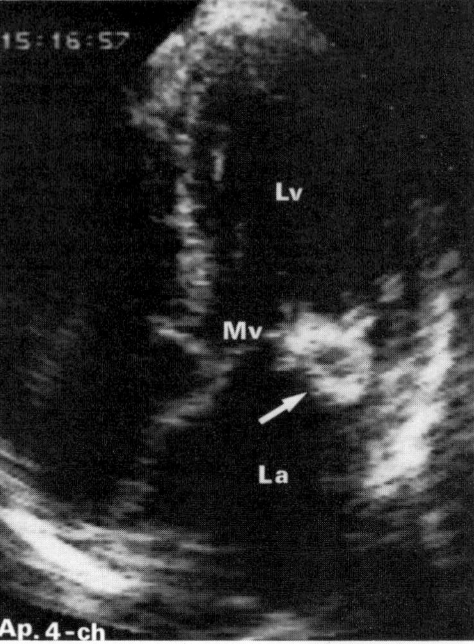

Figure 25–50. A parasternal long-axis view (P.Lax) in the left panel view and an apical four-chamber view (Ap.4-ch) in the right panel demonstrating a large mass attached to the posterior mitral valve leaflet in this patient with fungal endocarditis. This giant valve endocarditis may mimic myxoma or calcified clot. Abbreviations: Mv—mitral valve; Lv—left ventricle; La—left atrium; Ao—aorta.

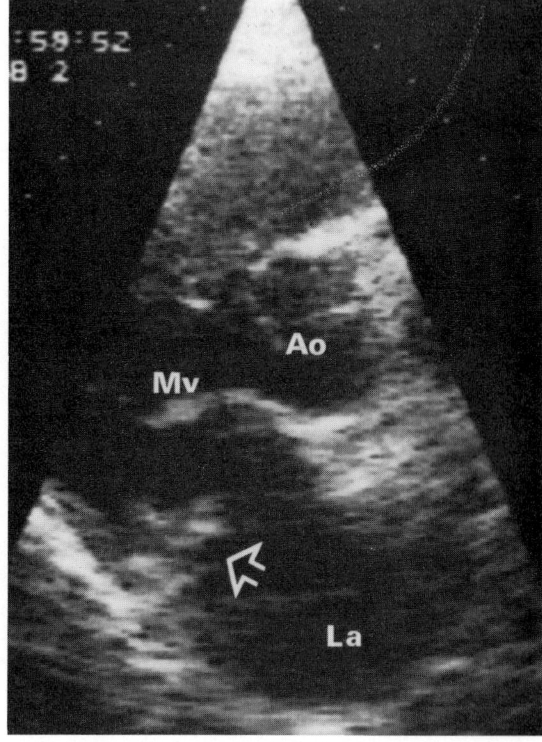

Figure 25–51. A parasternal long-axis view of a patient status post cardiac transplantation. A mass is detected in the left atrium (La). In subsequent transesophageal studies (see Fig. 25–52) this was proved to be a suture line between the donor and recipient atria. Abbreviations: La—left atrium; Mv—mitral valve; Ao—aorta.

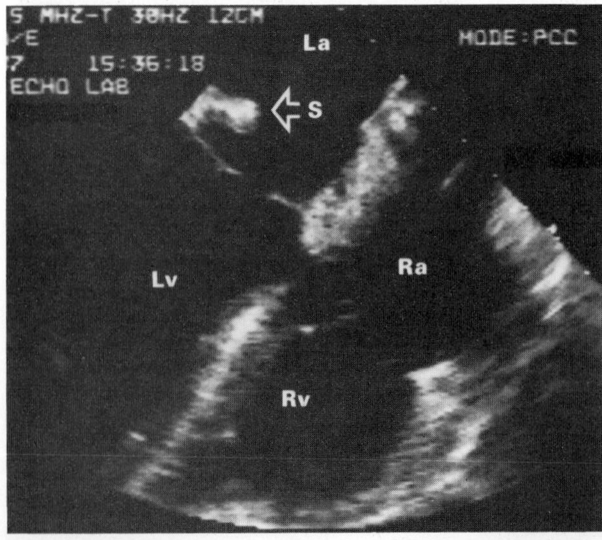

Figure 25–52. A transesophageal four-chamber view of the patient in Figure 25–51 demonstrating a suture line (S) in the left atrium. This suture line was traversing the left atrium (La) from the free wall to the interatrial septum. Abbreviations: Ra—right atrium; Rv—right ventricle; Lv—left ventricle.

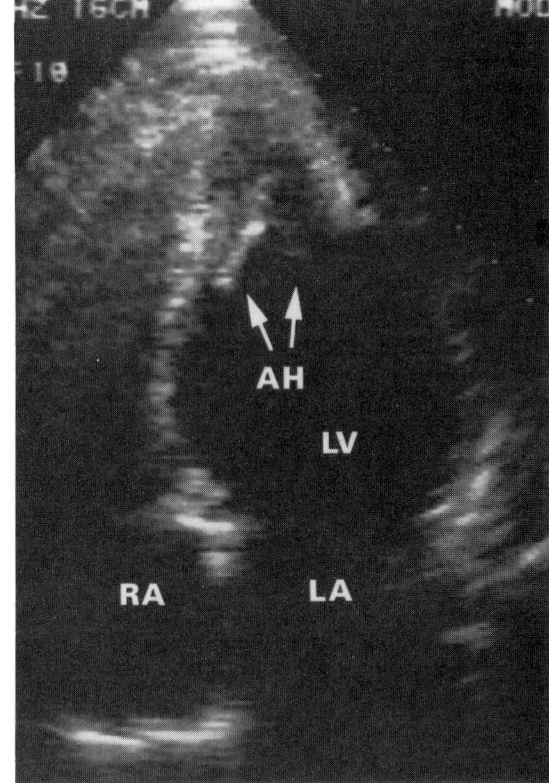

Figure 25–53. An apical four-chamber view of a patient with a localized left ventricular (LV) apical hypertrophy (AH) and giant negative T waves on the electrocardiogram. This spade-shaped left ventricle may give a clue to this variant of hypertrophic obstructive cardiomyopathy, although it can mimic left ventricular fibroma. Abbreviations: LA—left atrium; RA—right atrium.

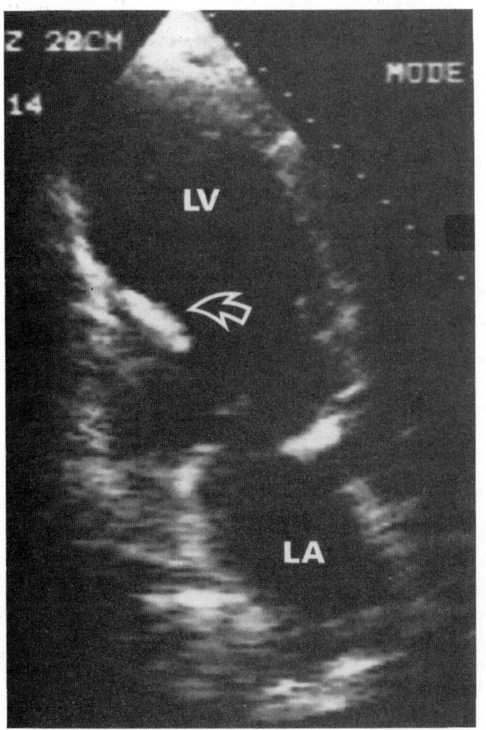

Figure 25–54. An apical two-chamber view of a patient with a markedly calcified posteromedial papillary muscle (*arrow*). This structure may mimic a left ventricular (LV) tumor. Abbreviation: LA—left atrium.

CARDIAC AND EXTRACARDIAC MASSES: ECHOCARDIOGRAPHIC EVALUATION

References

A

1. Abramowitz, R., Majdan, J. F., Plzak, L. F., and Berger, B. C.: Two-dimensional echocardiographic diagnosis of separate myxomas of both the left atrium and left ventricle. Am. J. Cardiol. 53:379, 1984.
2. Almargo, U. A., Perry, L. S., Choi, H., and Pintar, K.: Papillary fibroelastoma of the heart. Report of six cases. Arch. Pathol. Lab. Med. 106:318, 1982.
3. Allan, L. D., Joseph, M. C., and Tynan, M.: Clinical value of echocardiographic colour image processing in two cases of primary cardiac tumour. Br. Heart J. 49:154, 1983.
4. Agatston, A. S., Robinson, M. J., Trigo, L., et al.: Echo-cardiographic findings in primary pericardial mesothelioma. Am. Heart J. 111:986,1986.
5. Armstrong, W. F., Buck, J. D., Hoffman, R., and Waller, B. F.: Cardiac involvement by lymphoma: Detection and follow-up by two-dimensional echocardiography. Am. Heart J. 112:627,1986.
6. Arvan, S.: Mural thrombi in coronary artery disease. Recent advances in pathogenesis, diagnosis and approaches to treatment. Arch. Intern. Med. 144:113, 1984.
7. Asinger, R. W., Mikell, F. L., Elsperger, J., and Hodges, M.: Incidence of left-ventricular thrombosis after acute transmural myocardial infarction. Serial evaluation by two-dimensional echo-cardiography. N. Engl. J. Med. 305:297, 1981.
8. Asinger, R. W., Mikell, F. L., Sharma, B., and Hodges, M.: Observations on detecting left ventricular thrombus with two dimensional echocardiography: Emphasis on avoidance of false positive diagnoses. Am. J. Cardiol. 47:145, 1981.
9. Arvan, S., and Boscha, K.: Prophylactic anticoagulation for left ventricular thrombi after acute myocardial infarction: A prospective randomized trial. Am. Heart J. 113:688, 1987.
10. Aschenberg, W., Schluter, M., Kremer, P., et al.: Transesophageal two-dimensional echocardiography for the detection of left atrial appendage thrombus. J. Am. Coll. Cardiol. 7:163, 1986.
11. Amsel, B. J., Dion, R., and Gillebert, T. C.: Right heart thromboembolism after cardiac surgery. Eur. Heart J. 7:86, 1986.
12. Antonelli, G., Chiddo, A., Bortone, A., et al.: Hydatid cyst of the interventricular septum causing obstruction of the right ventricular outflow tract: Cross-sectional echocardiographic, angiographic and pathological findings. Eur. Heart J. 7:1083, 1986.

B

1. Bhandari, A. K., Nanda, N. C., and Hicks, D. G.: Two-dimensional echocardiography of intracardiac masses: Echo pattern-histopathology correlation. Ultrasound Med. Biol. 8:673,1982.
2. Bogren, H. G., DeMaria, A. N., and Mason, D. T.: Imaging procedures in the detection of cardiac tumors with emphasis on echocardiography: A review. Cardiovasc. Intervent. Radiol. 3:107, 1980.
3. Bass, N. M., and Sharratt, G. P.: Left atrial myxoma diagnosed by echocardiography with observations on tumor movement. Br. Heart J. 35:1332, 1973.
4. Barold, S. S., Hicks, G. L., Nanda, N. C., et al.: Mitral valve myxoma diagnosed by two-dimensional echocardiography. Am. J. Cardiol. 59:182, 1987.
5. Bini, R. M., Westaby, S., Bargeron, L. M., et al.: Investigation and management of primary cardiac tumors in infants and children. J. Am. Coll. Cardiol. 2:351, 1983.
6. Biancariello, T. M., Meyer, R. A., Gaum, W. E., et al.: Primary benign intramural ventricular tumors in children: Pre and postoperative electrocardiographic, echocardiographic and angiographic evaluation. Am. Heart J. 103:852, 1982.
7. Bass, J. L., Breningstall, G. N., and Swaiman, K. F.: Echocardiographic incidence of cardiac rhabdomyoma in tuberous sclerosis. Am. J. Cardiol. 55:1379, 1985.
8. Bradford, J. H., Nomeir, A. M., and Watts, L. E.: Left ventricular lipoma: Echocardiographic and angiographic features. South. Med. J. 73:663, 1980.
9. Bellotti, P., Claudiani, F., Chiarella, F., et al.: Activity of left ventricular thrombi of different ages. Assessment with indium-oxine platelet imaging and cross-sectional echocardiography. Eur. Heart J. 8:855, 1987.
10. Balbarini, A., Pugliese, P., and Mariani, M.: Echocardiographic and surgical findings of a ball-like thrombus floating freely in the left atrium. J. Cardiovasc. Surg. 28:135, 1987.
11. Boulay, F., Danchin, N., Neimann, J. L., et al.: Echocardiographic features of right atrial thrombi. J. Clin. Ultrasound 14:601, 1986.
12. Berger, I., Levine, O. R., and Antillon, J.: Echocardiographic diagnosis of pseudotumor of the left ventricle: A calcified posterior papillary muscle. J. Med. Soc. N.J. 76:758, 1979.

C

1. Chiari, H.: Ueber Netzbildungen im rechten vorhofe des herzens. Beitr. Pathol. Anat. 22:1, 1897.
2. Clopz, J. L., Neimann, J. L., Chivoret, G., et al.: Echocardiographic rediscovery of an anatomical structure: The Chiari network. A propos of 16 cases. Arch. Mal. Coeur 76:1284, 1983.
3. Camesas, A. M., Lichtstein, E., Kramer, J., et al.: Complementary use of two-dimensional echocardiography and magnetic resonance imaging in the diagnosis of ventricular myxoma. Am. Heart J. 114:440, 1987.
4. Chua, S. O., Chiang, C. W., Lee, Y. S., et al.: Moving right atrial mass associated with hepatoma. Two cases detected by echocardiography. Chest 89:149, 1986.
5. Come, P. C., Kurland, G. S., and Vine, H. S.: Two-dimensional echocardiography in differentiating right atrial and tricuspid valve mass lesions. Am. J. Cardiol. 44:1207,1979.
6. Chia, B. L., Lim, C. H., Sheares, J. H., and Choo, M. H.: Echocardiographic findings in right ventricular myxoma. Am. J. Cardiol. 58:663, 1986.
7. Chandravatua, P. A. N., San Pedro, S., Elkin, S. R. C., et al.: Echocardiographic, angiocardiographic and surgical correlations in right ventricular myxoma simulating valvular pulmonic stenosis. Circulation 55:619, 1977.
8. Charuzi, Y., Kraus, R., and Swan, H. J. C.: Echocardiographic interpretation in the presence of Swan-Ganz intracardiac catheters. Am. J. Cardiol. 40:989, 1977.
9. Caralis, D. G., Kennedy, H. L., Bailey, I., and Bulkley, B. H.: Primary right cardiac tumor. Detection by echocardiographic and radioisotopic studies. Chest 77:100,1980.
10. Cohen, D. E., Mora, C., and Keefe, D. L.: Echocardiographic findings of metastatic chondrosarcoma involving the left atrium. Am. Heart J. 111:993, 1986.
11. Corris, P. A., Kertes, P. J., Jennings, K., et al.: Detection of occult cardiac invasion by two dimensional echocardiography in patients with bronchial carcinoma. Thorax 41:138, 1986.
12. Chandraratna, P. A. N., Littman, B. B., Serafini, A., et al.: Echocardiographic evaluation of extracardiac masses. Br. Heart J. 40:741, 1978.
13. Canedo, M. I., Otkeu, L., and Stefadouros, M. A.: Echocardiographic features of cardiac compression by a thymoma simulating cardiac tamponade and obstruction of the superior vena cava. Br. Heart J. 39:1038, 1977.
14. Chambers, J., Whaley, A., and Campbell, S.: Doppler echocardiography in massive left atrial thrombus before and after successful thrombolysis. Int. J. Cardiol. 18:427, 1988.
15. Chesebro, J. H., Ezekowitz, M., Badimon, L., and Fuster, V.: Intracardiac thrombi and systemic thromboembolism: Detection, incidence and treatment. Annu. Rev. Med. 36:579, 1985.
16. Chen, C. C., Hsiung, M., and Chiang, B. N.: Variable diastolic rumbling murmur caused by floating left atrial thrombus. Br. Heart J. 50:190, 1983.
17. Cogswell, T. L., Komorowski, R. A., Galbraith, T. A., and Singh, S.: Giant Lambl's excresences of the left ventricular outflow tract in rheumatic heart disease. Echocardiography 4:424, 1987.
18. Cha, S. D., Incarvito, J., Fernandez, J., et al.: Giant Lambl's excrescences of papillary muscle and aortic valve: Echocardiographic, angiographic, and pathologic findings. Clin. Cardiol. 4:51, 1981.

D

1. DeGeeter, B., Kretz, J. G., Nisand, I., et al.: Intrapericardial teratoma in a newborn infant: Use of fetal echocardiography. Ann. Thorac. Surg. 35:664, 1983.
2. Devig, P. M., Clark, T. A., and Aaron, B. L.: Cardiac myxoma arising from the inferior vena cava. Chest 78:784, 1980.
3. Diamant, S., Sharoz, J., Holtzman, M., et al.: Echocardiographic diagnosis of cardiac tumors in symptomatic tuberous sclerosis patients. Clin. Pediatr. 22:297, 1983.
4. D'Cruz, I. A., and Roth, R. B.: Left atrial extension of pulmonary adenocarcinoma mimicking left atrial myxoma. Echocardiography 4:59, 1987.
5. D'Cruz, I. A., and Chiemmongkoltip, P.: Echocardiographic diagnosis of an unusual anterior mediastinal mass. Clin. Cardiol. 5:464, 1982.
6. DeMaria, A. N., Bommer, W., Neumann, A., et al.: Left ventricular thrombi identified by cross-sectional echocardiography Ann. Intern. Med. 90:14, 1979.
7. Domenicucci, S., Bellotti, P., Chiarella, F., et al.: Spontaneous morphologic changes in left ventricular thrombi: A prospective two-dimensional echocardiographic study. Circulation 75:737, 1987.
8. Daniel, W. G., Nellessen, U., Schroder, E., et al.: Left atrial spontaneous echo contrast in mitral valve disease: An indicator for an increased thromboembolic risk. J. Am. Coll. Cardiol. 6:1204, 1988.
9. DeMartini, M., Nador, F., Binda, A., et al.: Myocardial hydatid cyst ruptured into the pericardium: Cross-sectional echocardiographic study and surgical treatment. Eur. Heart J. 9:819, 1988.

E

1. Effert, S., and Domanig, E.: The diagnosis of intraatrial tumor and thrombus by the ultrasonic echo method. German Med. Mth 4:1, 1959.
2. Erbel, R., Stern, H., Ehrenthal, W., et al.: Detection of spontaneous echocardiographic contrast within the left atrium by transesophageal echocardiography: Spontaneous echocardiographic contrast. Clin. Cardiol. 9:245, 1986.

F

1. Fyke, F. E.,III, Seward, J. B., Edwards, W. D., et al.: Primary cardiac tumors: Experience with 30 consecutive patients since the introduction of two-dimensional echocardiography. J. Am. Coll. Cardiol. 5:1465, 1985.
2. Feigenbaum, H. (ed.): Echocardiography. 4th ed. Lea & Febiger, Philadelphia, 1986, p. 579.
3. Felner, J. M., and Knopf, W. D.: Echocardiographic recognition of intracardiac and extracardiac masses. Echocardiography 2:3, 1985.
4. Farooki, Z. Q., Arciniegas, E., Hakimi, M., et al.: Real-time echocardiographic features of intrapericardial teratoma. J. Clin. Ultrasound 10:125, 1982.
5. Fittever, J. D., Spicer, M. J., and Nelson, W. P.: Echocardiographic demonstration of bilateral atrial myxomas. Chest 70:282, 1976.

6. Finegan, R. E., and Harrison, D. C.: Diagnosis of left atrial myxoma by echocardiography. N. Engl. J. Med. 282:1022, 1970.
7. Fowles, R. E., Miller, D. C., Egbert, B. M., et al.: Systemic embolization from a mitral valve papillary endocardial fibroma detected by two-dimensional echocardiography. Am. Heart J. 102:128, 1981.
8. Fischer, D. R., Beerman, L. B., Park, S.C., et al.: Diagnosis of intracardiac rhabdomyoma by two-dimensional echocardiography. Am. J. Cardiol. 53:978, 1984.
9. Farooki, Z. Q., Adelman, S., and Garen, E. W.: Echocardiographic differentiation of cystic and solid tumors of the heart. Am. J. Cardiol. 39:107, 1977.
10. Frumin, H., O'Donnell, L., Kerin, N. Z., et al.: Two-dimensional echocardiographic detection and diagnostic features of tricuspid papillary fibroelastoma. J. Am. Coll. Cardiol. 2:1016, 1983.
11. Fitzmorris, S. J., Seward, J. B., Sheedy, P. F., II, and Schaff, H. V.: Clinical presentation and diagnosis of angiosarcoma of the right atrium: Noninvasive recognition of a rare cardiac tumor. Echocardiography 2:105, 1985.
12. Fye, W. B., and Molina, J. E.: Right atrial angiosarcoma: Echocardiographic diagnosis and surgical correlation. Johns Hopkins Med. J. 147:111, 1980.
13. Foster, C. J., Sekiya, T., Love, H. G., et al.: Identification of intracardiac thrombus: Comparison of computed tomography and cross-sectional echocardiography. Br. J. Radiol. 60:327, 1987.
14. Friedman, M. J., Carlson, K., Marcus, F. I., and Woolfenden, J. M.: Clinical correlations in patients with acute myocardial infarction and left ventricular thrombus detected by two-dimensional echocardiography. Am. J. Med. 72:894, 1982.
15. Fraser, A. G., Angelini, G. D., Ikram, S., and Butchart, E. G.: Left atrial ball thrombus: Echocardiographic features and clinical implications. Eur. Heart J. 9:672, 1988.
16. Fyke, F. E., III, Tajik, A. J., Edwards, W. D., and Seward, J. B.: Diagnosis of lipomatous hypertrophy of the atrial septum by two-dimensional echocardiography. J. Am. Coll. Cardiol. 1:1352, 1983.

G

1. Gustavson, A. G., Edler, I. G., and Dahlback, O. K.: Bilateral atrial myxomas diagnosed by echocardiography. Acta Med. Scand. 201:391, 1977.
2. Gustavson, A., Edler, I., Dahlback, O., et al.: Left atrial myxoma diagnosed by ultrasound cardiography. Angiology 24:554, 1973.
3. Goli, V. D., Thadani, U., Thomas, S. R., et al.: Doppler echocardiographic profiles in obstructive right and left atrial myxomas. J. Am. Coll. Cardiol. 9:701, 1987.
4. Galton, B. B.: Left atrial myxoma without significant cardiac manifestations. J. Med. Soc. N. J. 76:754, 1979.
5. Gosse, P., Herpin, D., Roudaut, R., et al.: Myxoma of the mitral valve diagnosed by echocardiography. Am. Heart J. 111:803, 1986.
6. Gibbs, J. L.: The heart and tuberous sclerosis. An echocardiographic and electrocardiographic study. Br. Heart J. 54:596, 1985.
7. Gresser, C. D., Shime, J., Rakowski, H., et al.: Fetal cardiac tumor: A prenatal echocardiographic marker for tuberous sclerosis. Am. J. Obstet. Gynecol. 156:689, 1987.
8. Gladden, J. R., Dreiling, R. J., Gollub, S. B., et al.: Two-dimensional echocardiographic features of multiple right atrial myxomas. Am. J. Cardiol. 52:1364, 1983.
9. Goldman, A., Parmeswaran, R., Kotler, M. N., et al.: Renal cell carcinoma and right atrial tumor diagnosed by echocardiography. Am. Heart J. 110:183, 1985.
10. Green, C., Alam, M., Rosman, H. S., and Lakier, J. B.: Echocardiographic features of metastatic pericardial and myocardial malignancy. Henry Ford Hosp. Med. J. 34:288, 1986.
11. Gottdiener, J. S., and Maron, B. J.: Posterior cardiac displacement by anterior mediastinal tumor. Chest 77:784, 1980.
12. Gur, H., Keren, G., Averbuch, M., and Levo, Y.: Severe congestive lupus cardiomyopathy complicated by an intracavitary thrombus: A clinical and echocardiographic followup. J. Rheumatol. 15:1278, 1988.
13. Gottdiener, J. S., Gay, J. A., Van Voorhees, L., et al.: Frequency and embolic potential of left ventricular thrombi in dilated cardiomyopathy: Assessment by two-dimensional echocardiography. Am. J. Cardiol. 52:1281, 1983.
14. Green, S. E., Joynt, L. F., Fitzgerald, P. J., et al.: In vivo ultrasonic tissue characterization of human intracardiac masses. Am. J. Cardiol. 51:231, 1983.
15. Gillmer, D., and Campanella, C.: Echocardiographic diagnosis of left atrial ball-valve thrombus. A case report. S. Afr. Med. J. 65:662, 1984.
16. Gottdiener, J. S., Temeck, B. K., Patterson, R. H., and Fletcher, R.D.: Transient ("hole-in-one") occlusion of the mitral valve orifice by a free-floating left atrial ball thrombus: Identification by two-dimensional echocardiography. Am. J. Cardiol. 53:1730, 1984.
17. Geggel, R. L., Fulton, D. R., and Chernoff, H. L.: Left ventricular false tendons: Unusual cause of diastolic murmur in a child. Echocardiography 4:69, 1987.
18. Guthaner, D. F., Schnittger, I., Wright, A., and Wexler, L.: Diagnostic challenges following cardiac transplantation. Radiol. Clin. North Am. 25:367,1987.

H

1. Harbold, N. B., Jr., and Gan, G. T.: Echocardiographic diagnosis of right atrial myxoma. Mayo Clin. Proc. 48:284, 1973.
2. Henuzet, C., Franken, P., Polis, O., and Fievez, M.: Cardiac metastasis of rectal adenocarcinoma diagnosed by two-dimensional echocardiography. Am. Heart J. 104:637, 1982.
3. Haugland, M. J., Asinger, R. W., Mikell, F. L., et al.: Embolic potential of left ventricular thrombi detected by two-dimensional echocardiography. Circulation 70:588, 1984.
4. Heydarian, M., Werthammer, J. W., and Kelly, P. J.: Echocardiographic diagnosis of *Candida* mass of the right atrium in a premature infant. Am. Heart J. 113:402, 1987.

I

1. Isner, J. M., Falcone, M. W., Virmani, R., and Roberts, W.C.: Cardiac sarcoma causing "ASH" and simulating coronary heart disease. Am. J. Med. 66:1025, 1979.

J

1. Johnson, M. H., and Soulen, R. L.: Echocardiography of cardiac metastases. AJR 141:677, 1983.
2. Johannessen, K. A.: Peripheral emboli from left ventricular thrombi of different echocardiographic appearance in acute myocardial infarction. Arch. Intern. Med. 147:641, 1987.
3. Jansyn, E. M., Pandian, N. G., Isner, J. M., et al.: Free-floating left atrial thrombus producing intermittent exacerbation of mitral valvular stenosis. Echocardiography 3:47, 1986.
4. Johnson, D. E., Vacek, J., Gollub, S. B., et al.: Comparison of gated cardiac magnetic resonance imaging and two-dimensional echocardiography for the evaluation of right ventricular thrombi: A case report with autopsy correlation. Cathet. Cardiovasc. Diagn. 14:266, 1988.
5. Jaramillo, L. S. A., Vargas-Barroń, J., Gonzalez, A. S., et al.: Hipertrofia ventricular derecha que simula un tumor intracavitario diagnostico ecocardiografico. Arch. Inst. Cardiol. Mex. 57:395, 1987.

K

1. Keren, A., Billingham, M. E., and Popp, R. L.: Echocardiographic recognition of paraseptal structures. J. Am. Coll. Cardiol. 6:913, 1985.
2. Keren, A., Billingham, M. E., and Popp, R. L.: Echocardiographic recognition and implications of ventricular hypertrophic trabeculations and aberrant bands. Circulation 70:836, 1984.
3. Kronzon, I., Rosenzweig, B., and Dack, S.: Diagnosis of a large left atrial myxoma: The role of two-dimensional echocardiography. J. Clin. Ultrasound 10:39, 1982.
4. Keren, A., Takamoto, T., Harrison, D. C., and Popp, R. L.: Left ventricular apical masses: Noninvasive differentiation of rare from common ones. Am. J. Cardiol. 56:697, 1985.
5. Koiwaya, Y., Kawachi, Y., Orita, Y., et al.: Echocardiographic detection of metastatic cardiac mural tumor. J. Clin. Ultrasound 8:443, 1980.
6. Kutalek, S. P., Panidis, I. P., Kotler, M. N., et al.: Metastatic tumors of the heart detected by two-dimensional echocardiography. Am. Heart J. 109:343, 1985.
7. Kubac, G., Doris, I., Ondro, M., and Davey, P. W.: Malignant granular cell myoblastoma with metastatic cardiac involvement: Case report and echocardiogram. Am. Heart J. 100:227, 1980.
8. Kurkjian, K., Naber, S. P., McInerney, K. P., et al.: Echocardiographic evaluation of metastatic pericardial disease. Echocardiography 3:273, 1986.
9. Küpper, A. J. F., Verheugt, F. W. A., Jaarsma, W., et al.: Detection of ventricular thrombosis in acute myocardial infarction: Value of indium–111 platelet scintigraphy in relation to two-dimensional echocardiography and clinical course. Eur. J. Nucl. Med. 12:337,1986.
10. Keating, E. C., Gross, S. A ., Schlamowitz, R. A., et al.: Mural thrombi in myocardial infarctions. Am. J. Med. 74:989, 1983.
11. Kessler, K. M., Mallon, S. M., Bolooki, H., and Myerburg, R. J.: Pedunculated right ventricular thrombus due to repeated blunt chest trauma. Am. Heart J. 102:1064, 1981.
12. Kunze, K. P., Schluter, M., Costard, A., et al.: Right atrial thrombus formation after transvenous catheter ablation of the atrioventricular node. J. Am. Coll. Cardiol. 6:1428, 1985

L

1. Leon, M., Pechacek, L. W., Solana, L. G., et al.: Identification of a prominent eustachian valve by means of contrast two dimensional echocardiography. Texas Heart Inst. 10:219, 1983.
2. Liu, H. Y., Pauidis, I., Soffer, J., et al.: Echocardiographic diagnosis of intracardiac myxomas: Present status. Chest 84:62, 1983.
3. Lee, Y. C., and Magran, M. Y.: Nonprolapsing left atrial tumor: The M-mode echocardiographic diagnosis. Chest 78:332, 1980.
4. Lin, T. U., Stech, J. M., Ecbert, W. G., et al.: Pericardial angiosarcoma simulating pericardial effusion by echocardiography. Chest 73:881, 1978.
5. Lutas, E. M., and Stelzer, P.: Echocardiographic demonstration of right atrial rupture in a patient with right-sided cardiac tumor. Chest 83:921, 1983.
6. Lestuzzi, C., Biasi, S., Nicolosi, G. L., et al.: Secondary neoplastic infiltration of the myocardium diagnosed by two-dimensional echocardiography in seven cases with anatomic confirmation. J. Am. Coll. Cardiol. 9:439, 1987.
7. Lloret, R. L., Cortada, X., Bradford, J., et al.: Classification of left ventricular thrombi by their history of systemic embolization using pattern recognition of two-dimensional echocardiograms. Am. Heart J. 110:761, 1985.
8. Lew, A. S., Federman, J., Harper, R. W., et al.: Operative removal of mobile pedunculated left ventricular thrombus detected by 2-dimensional echocardiography. Am. J. Cardiol. 52:1148, 1983.

M

1. Mitchell, M. M., Sutherland, G. R., Gussenhoven, E. J., et al.: Transesophageal echocardiography. J. Am. Soc. Echo. 1:362, 1988.
2. McAllister, H. A., Jr., and Fenoglio, J. J., Jr.: Tumors of the cardiovascular

system. *In* Atlas of Tumor Pathology, Fascicle 15, Second Series. Armed Forces Institute of Pathology, 1978.

3. Millman, A. E., Federici, E. E., and Miskovits, C.: Left atrial myxoma: Two-dimensional echocardiographic, angiographic, and pathological correlations. J. Med. Soc. N.J. 76:749, 1979
4. Meller, J., Teichholz, L. E., Pichard, A. D., et al.: Left ventricular myxoma. Echocardiographic diagnosis and review of the literature. Am. J. Med. 63:816, 1977.
5. Mazer, M. S., and Harrigan, P. R.: Left ventricular myxoma: M-mode and two-dimensional echocardiographic features. Am. Heart J. 104:875, 1982.
6. Maurer, G., and Nanda, N. C.: Two-dimensional echocardiographic identification of intracardiac leiomyomatosis. Am. Heart J. 103:915, 1982.
7. Maria-Garcia, J., Fitch, C. W., and Shenefelt, R. E.: Primary right ventricular tumor (fibroma) simulating cyanotic heart disease in a newborn. J. Am. Coll. Cardiol. 3:868, 1984.
8. Mich, R. J., Gillam, L. D., and Weyman, A. E.: Osteogenic sarcomas mimicking left atrial myxomas: Clinical and two-dimensional echocardiographic features. J. Am. Coll. Cardiol. 6:1422, 1985.
9. Malcolm, A. D., Shiu, M. F., and Jenkins, B. S.: Sarcoma obstructing right ventricular cavity: Clinical, echocardiographic, haemodynamic and angiographic features. Postgrad. Med. J. 55:203, 1979.
10. Molajo, A. O., McWilliam, L., Ward, C., and Rahman, A.: Cardiac lymphoma: An unusual case of myocardial perforation—clinical, echocardiographic, haemodynamic and pathological features. Eur. Heart J. 8:549, 1987.
11. Maze, S. S., Kotler, M. N., and Parry, W. R.: The contribution of color Doppler flow imaging to the assessment of a left ventricular thrombus. Am. Heart J. 115:479, 1988.
12. Meltzer, R. S., Visser, C. A., Kan, G., and Roelandt, J.: Two-dimensional echocardiographic appearance of left ventricular thrombi with systemic emboli after myocardial infarction. Am. J. Cardiol. 53:1511, 1984.
13. Meltzer, R. S., Visser, C. A., and Fuster, V.: Intracardiac thrombi and systemic embolization. Ann. Intern. Med. 104:689, 1986.
14. Marsh, D., Wilkerson, S. A., Cook, L. N., and Pietsch, J. B.: Right atrial thrombus formation screening using two-dimensional echocardiograms in neonates with central venous catheters. Pediatrics 81:284, 1988.

N

1. Nicholson, K. G., Prior, A. L., Norman, A. G., et al.: Bilateral atrial myxomas diagnosed preoperatively and successfully removed. Br. Med. J. 2:440, 1977.
2. Nihoyannopoulos, P., Venkatesan, P., David, J., et al.: Left atrial myxoma: New perspectives in the diagnosis of murmur free cases. Br. Heart J. 56:554, 1986.
3. Nishimura, R. A., Tajik, A. J., Schattenberg, T. T., and Seward, J.B.: Diaphragmatic hernia mimicking an atrial mass: A two-dimensional echocardiographic pitfall. J. Am. Coll. Cardiol. 5:992, 1985.
4. Norell, M. S., Sarvasvaran, R., and Sutton, G. C.: Solitary tumor metastasis: A rare cause of right ventricular outflow tract obstruction and sudden death. Eur. Heart J. 5:684, 1984.
5. Narvaez, R., Strauss, C., Kotler, M. N., et al.: Embolization of a large left ventricular thrombus during two-dimensional and color flow Doppler examination in idiopathic dilated cardiomyopathy. Am J Cardiol 60:402, 1987.
6. Nordrehaug, J. E., Johannessen, K. A., and von der Lippe, G.: Usefulness of high-dose anticoagulants in preventing left ventricular thrombus in acute myocardial infarction. Am. J. Cardiol. 55:1491, 1985.
7. Nili, M., Deviri, E., Jortner, R., et al.: Surgical removal of a mobile, pedunculated left ventricular thrombus: Report of 4 cases. Ann. Thorac. Surg. 46:396, 1988.

O

1. Oliver, J. M., Sotillo, J. F., Dominguez, F. J., et al.: Two-dimensional echocardiographic features of echinococcosis of the heart and great blood vessels. Clinical and surgical implications. Circulation 78:327, 1988.

P

1. Pietro, D.: Echocardiographic detection of intracardiac masses. Echocardiography 1:165, 1984.
2. Panidis, I. P., Kotler, M. N., Mintz, G. S., and Ross, J.: Clinical and echocardiographic features of right atrial masses. Am. Heart J. 107:745, 1984.
3. Pandian, N. G., Isner, J. M., McInerney, K. P., et al.: Left atrial myxoma—implications of site, size, mobility and tissue structure. Echocardiography 2:113, 1985.
4. Popp, R. L., and Harrison, D. C.: Ultrasound in the diagnosis of atrial tumor. Ann. Intern. Med. 71:785, 1969.
5. Perry, L. S., King, J. F., Zett, H., et al.: Two-dimensional echocardiography in the diagnosis of left atrial myxoma. Br. Heart J. 45:667, 1981.
6. Panidis, I. P., Mintz, G. S., and McAllister, M.: Hemodynamic consequences of left atrial myxomas as assessed by Doppler ultrasound. Am. Heart J. 111:927,1986.
7. Ports, T. A., Cogan, J., Schiller, N. B., et al.: Echocardiography of left ventricular masses. Circulation 58:528, 1978.
8. Presti, C., Ryan, T., and Armstrong, W. F.: Two-dimensional and Doppler echocardiographic findings in hypereosinophilic syndrome. Am. Heart J. 114:172, 1987.
9. Patel, A. K., Moorthy, A. V., Yap, V. U., and Thomsen, J. H.: Cardiac metastasis from transitional cell carcinoma: A subtle echocardiographic entity. J. Clin. Ultrasound 8:49:1980.
10. Percy, R. F., Conetta, D. A., and Miller, A. B.: Esophageal compression of the heart presenting as an extracardiac mass on echocardiography. Chest 85:826, 1984.
11. Pierard, L. A., Henrard, L., and Noel, J. -F.: Detection of left ventricular false tendons by two-dimensional echocardiography. Acta Cardiol. 60:229. 1985.

Q

1. Quinn, T. J., Codini, M. A., and Harris, A. A.: Infected cardiac myxoma. Am. J. Cardiol. 53:381, 1984.

R

1. Roudaut, R., Gosse, P., Aquizerate, E., and Dallocchio, M.: The diagnosis of intraatrial masses with two-dimensional echocardiography: Experience with 64 patients. Echocardiography 4:431, 1987.
2. Roudaut, R., Gosse, P., and Dallocchio, M.: Rapid growth of a left atrial myxoma shown by echocardiography. Br. Heart J. 58:413, 1987.
3. Riggs, T. W., Ilbawi, M., DeLeon, S., and Paul, M. H.: Echocardiographic diagnosis of right ventricular rhabdomyoma in two infants. Pediatr. Cardiol. 3:31, 1982.
4. Reynard, J. S., Jr., Gregoratos, G., Gordon, M. J., and Bloor, C. M.: Primary osteosarcoma of the heart. Am. Heart J. 109:598, 1985.
5. Reeder, G. S., Lengyel, M., Tajik, A. J., et al.: Mural thrombus in left ventricular aneurysm. Incidence, role of angiography, and relation between anticoagulation and embolization. Mayo Clin. Proc. 56:77, 1981.
6. Rousso, I., Deviri, E., Lerner, M. A., et al.: CT diagnosis of left atrial thrombus undiagnosed by echocardiography. Comput. Radiol. 8:293, 1984.

S

1. Sheiban, I., Casarotto, D., Trevi, G., et al.: Two-dimensional echocardiography in the diagnosis of intracardiac masses: A prospective study with anatomic validation. Cardiovasc. Intervent. Radiol. 10:157, 1987.
2. Seguin, J. R., Coulon, P. L., Perez, M., et al.: Echocardiographic diagnosis of an intrapericardial teratoma in infancy. Am. Heart J. 113:1239, 1987.
3. Schäfer, R. O., Heine, H., Bohm, J., et al.: Bilateral atrial myxomas. Surgical correction after echocardiographic diagnosis. Eur. Heart J. 8:1032, 1987.
4. Salcedo, E. E., Adams, K. V., Lever, H. M., et al.: Echocardiographic findings in 25 patients with left atrial myxoma. J. Am. Coll. Cardiol. 1:1162, 1983.
5. Shub, C., Tajik, A. J., Seward, J. B., et al.: Cardiac papillary fibroelastomas. Two-dimensional echocardiographic recognition. Mayo Clin. Proc. 56:629, 1981.
6. Shiraishi, H., Yanagisawa, M., Kuramatsu, T., et al.: Cardiac tumor in a neonate with tuberous sclerosis: Echocardiographic demonstration and magnetic resonance imaging. Eur. J. Pediatr. 148:50, 1988.
7. Schmaltz, A. A., and Apitz, J.: Primary rhabdomyosarcoma of the heart. Pediatr. Cardiol. 2:73, 1982.
8. Sonotani, N., Takatsu, T., and Sawada, K.: Conventional and two-dimensional real-time echocardiographic diagnosis of osteosarcoma. A case report. Jpn. Heart J. 21:281, 1980.
9. Schmekel, B., Landelius, J., Aberg, T., and Enghoff, E.: Extensive surgery for left atrial leiomyosarcoma diagnosed by echocardiography. Scand. J. Thorac. Cardiovasc. Surg. 21:277, 1987.
10. Shah, A., and Schwartz, H.: Echocardiographic features of cardiac compression by mediastinal pancreatic pseudocyst. Chest 77:440, 1980.
11. Schloss, M., Kronzon, I., Gelber, P. M., et al.: Cystic thymoma simulating constrictive pericarditis. The role of echocardiography in the differential diagnosis. J. Thorac. Cardiovasc. Surg. 70:143, 1975.
12. Stratton, J. R., Lighty, G. W., Jr., Pearlman, A. S., and Ritchie, J. L.: Detection of left ventricular thrombus by two-dimensional echocardiography: Sensitivity, specificity, and causes of uncertainty. Circulation 66:156, 1982.
13. Seabold, J. E., Schroder, E., Conrad, G. R., et al.: Indium–111 platelet scintigraphy and two-dimensional echocardiography for detection of left ventricular thrombus: Influence of clot size and age. J. Am. Coll. Cardiol. 9:1057, 1987.
14. Stratton, J. R., Lighty, G. W., Jr., Pearlman, A. S., and Ritchie, J. L.: Detection of left ventricular thrombus by two-dimensional echocardiography: Sensitivity, specificity, and causes of uncertainty. Circulation 66:156, 1982
15. Stratton, J. R., Speck, S. M., Caldwell, J. H., et al.: Late effects of intracoronary streptokinase on regional wall motion, ventricular aneurysm and left ventricular thrombus in myocardial infarction: Results from the Western Washington Randomized Trial. J. Am. Coll. Cardiol. 5:1023, 1985.
16. Stratton, J. R., and Resnick, A. D.: Increased embolic risk in patients with left ventricular thrombi. Circulation 75:1004, 1987.
17. Spirito, P., Bellotti, P., Chiarella, F., et al.: Prognostic significance and natural history of left ventricular thrombi in patients with acute anterior myocardial infarction: A two-dimensional echocardiographic study. Circulation 72:774, 1985.
18. Stratton, J. R., Nemanich, J. W., Johannessen, K. A., and Resnick, A.D.: Fate of left ventricular thrombi in patients with remote myocardial infarction or idiopathic cardiomyopathy. Circulation 78:1388, 1988.
19. Schofield, P. M., Rahman, A. N., Ellis, M. E., et al.: Infection of cardiac mural thrombus associated with left ventricular aneurysm. Eur. Heart J. 7:1077, 1986.
20. Stowers, S. A., Leiboff, R. H., Wasserman, A. G., et al.: Right ventricular thrombus formation in association with acute myocardial infarction: Diagnosis by 2-dimensional echocardiography. Am. J. Cardiol. 52:912, 1983.

21. Singh, A., Fein, S., Daudiss, K., et al.: Passage of mobile right heart thrombus to the left cardiac chambers: Echocardiographic detection and surgical removal. J. Clin. Ultrasound 16:592, 1988.
22. Schuster, A. H., Zugibe, F., Jr., Nanda, N. C., and Murphy, G. W.: Two-dimensional echocardiographic identification of pacing catheter–induced thrombosis. PACE 5:124, 1982.
23. Spirito, P., Bellotti, P., Chiarella, F., et al.: Right atrial thrombus detected by two-dimensional echocardiography after acute pulmonary embolism. Am. J. Cardiol. 54:467, 1984.
24. Simons, M., Cabin, H. S., and Jaffe, C. C.: Lipomatous hypertrophy of the atrial septum: Diagnosis by combined echocardiography and computerized tomography. Am. J. Cardiol. 54:465, 1984.

T

1. Tway, K. P., Shah, A. A., and Rahimtoola, S. H.: Multiple biatrial myxomas demonstrated by two-dimensional echocardiography. Am. J. Med. 71:896, 1981.
2. Topol, E. J., Biern, R. O., and Reitz, B. A.: Cardiac papillary fibroelastoma and stroke. Echocardiographic diagnosis and guide to excision. Am. J. Med. 80:129, 1986.
3. Thier, W., Schluter, M., Krebber, H. J., et al.: Cysts in left atrial myxomas identified by transesophageal cross-sectional echocardiography. Am. J. Cardiol. 51:1793, 1983.
4. Takahashi, K., Imamura, Y., Ochi, T., et al.: Echocardiographic demonstration of an asymptomatic patient with left ventricular fibroma. Am. J. Cardiol. 53:981, 1984.
5. Tominaga, K., Shinkai, T., Eguchi, K., et al.: The value of two-dimensional echocardiography in detecting malignant tumors in the heart. Cancer 58:1641, 1986.
6. Takamoto, T., Kim, D., Murie, P., et al.: Comparative recognition of left ventricular thrombi by echocardiography and cineangiography. Br. Heart J. 53:36, 1985.
7. Tramarin, R., Pozzoli, M., Febo, O., et al.: Two-dimensional echocardiographic assessment of anticoagulant therapy in left ventricular thrombosis early after acute myocardial infarction. Eur. Heart J. 7:482, 1986.
8. Taams, M. A., Gussenhoven, E. J., and Lanceé, C. T.: Left atrial vascularised thrombus diagnosed by transoesophageal cross sectional echocardiography. Br. Heart J. 58:669, 1987.
9. Torbicki, A., Pasierski, T., Uchman, B., and Miskiewicz, Z.: Right atrial mobile thrombi: Two-dimensional echocardiographic diagnosis and clinical outcome. Cor Vasa 29:293, 1987.

U

1. Ugolini, V., Norcross, J. F., Schreiber, J. T., et al.: Intracardiac thrombus causing peritoneovenous shunt failure: Detection by two-dimensional echocardiography. J. Am. Coll. Cardiol. 7:1174, 1986.

V

1. Valdivieso, E. Z. M., Barker, A. M. H., Cerna, J. L. G., et al.: Mixoma del ventriculo derecho. Informe de un caso operado. Arch. Inst. Cardiol. Mex. 57:141, 1987.
2. Visser, C. A., Kan, G., David, G. K., et al.: Two dimensional echocardiography in the diagnosis of left ventricular thrombus. A prospective study of 67 patients with anatomic validation. Chest 83:228, 1983.
3. Visser, C., and Roelandt, J.: Left ventricular thrombus. Echocardiography 2:245, 1985.
4. Visser, C. A., Kan, G., Meltzer, R. S., et al.: Embolic potential of left ventricular thrombus after myocardial infarction: A two-dimensional echocardiographic study of 119 patients. J. Am. Coll. Cardiol. 5: 1276, 1985.
5. Visser, C. A., Kan, G., Meltzer, R. S., et al.: Long-term follow-up of left ventricular thrombus after acute myocardial infarction. A two-dimensional echocardiographic study in 96 patients. Chest 86:532, 1984.

W

1. Werner, J. A., Cheitlin, M. D., Gross, B. W., et al.: Echocardiographic appearance of the Chiari network: Differentiation from right-heart pathology. Circulation 63:1104, 1981.
2. Wolfe, S. B., Popp, R. L., and Feigenbaum, H.: Diagnosis of atrial tumors by ultrasound. Circulation 39:615, 1969.
3. Weir, I., Mills, P., and Lewis, T.: A case of left atrial haemangioma: Echocardiographic, surgical, and morphological features. Br. Heart J. 58:665, 1987
4. Wright, E. C., Wellons, H. A., and Martin, R. P.: Primary pulmonary artery sarcoma diagnosed non-invasively by two-dimensional echocardiography. Circulation 67:459, 1983.
5. Winer, H. E., Kronzon, I., Fox, A., et al.: Primary cardiac chondromyxosarcoma—clinical and echocardiographic manifestations. A case report. J. Thorac. Cardiovasc. Surg. 74:567, 1977.
6. Weg, I. L., Mehra, S., Azueta, V., and Rosner, F.: Cardiac metastasis from adenocarcinoma of the lung. Echocardiographic-pathologic correlation. Am. J. Med. 80:108, 1986.
7. Weinreich, D. J., Burke, J. F., and Pauletto, F. J.: Left ventricular mural thrombi complicating acute myocardial infarction. Long-term follow-up with serial echocardiography. Ann. Intern. Med. 100:789, 1984.
8. Wiseman, M. N., Giles, M. S., and Camm, A. J.: Unusual echocardiographic appearance of intracardiac thrombi in a patient with endomyocardial fibrosis. Br. Heart J. 56:179, 1986.

Y

1. Yoshikawa, J., Sabah, I., Yanagihara, K., et al.: Cross-sectional echocardiographic diagnosis of large left atrial tumor and extracardiac tumor compressing the left atrium. Am. J. Cardiol. 42:853, 1978.

Z

1. Zackia, A. H., Weber, D. J., Ramsey, C., and Wong, B.: Recurrence of left atrial myxoma. J. Cardiovasc. Surg. 25:467, 1974.
2. Zuppiroli, A., Cecchi, F., Ciaccheri, M., et al.: Two-dimensional echocardiographic findings in a case of massive cardiac involvement by malignant lymphoma. Acta Cardiol. 60:485, 1985.
3. Zee-Cheng, C. S., Gibbs, H. R., Johnson, K. P., and Smith, J. C.: Giant vegetation due to *Staphylococcus aureus* endocarditis simulating left atrial myxoma. Am. Heart J. 111:414, 1986.

Chapter 26

Ultrasonic Characterization of Cardiovascular Tissue

■ *DAVID J. SKORTON, M.D.* ■ *JAMES G. MILLER, Ph.D.*
■ *SAMUEL WICKLINE, M.D.* ■ *BENICO BARZILAI, M.D.*
■ *STEVE M. COLLINS, Ph.D.* ■ *JULIO E. PEREZ, M.D.*

BASIC CONCEPTS OF ULTRASONIC TISSUE CHARACTERIZATION 539
Definition of Acoustic Terms 539
Approaches to Tissue Characterization and Measurement Techniques 540
Methods Based on Radio-Frequency Data Analysis (Including Integrated Backscatter Imaging) 540
Methods That Display Acoustically Abnormal Tissue 541
Methods That Quantitate Echocardiographic Gray Level (Image) Data 542
BIOLOGIC DETERMINANTS OF MYOCARDIAL ACOUSTIC PROPERTIES 543
Collagen 543
Scatterer Geometry 544
Fiber Orientation 544
Blood Flow/Water Content 544
Other Determinants 545
Dynamic Aspects of Scattering 545
SPECIFIC DISEASE PROCESSES STUDIED BY ULTRASONIC TISSUE CHARACTERIZATION ... 545
Ischemic Heart Disease 545
Acute Ischemia/Infarction 545
Reperfused Myocardium 546
Subacute and Chronic Infarction 548
Cardiomyopathy 549
Dilated Cardiomyopathy 549
Infiltrative/Restrictive Cardiomyopathy 551
Hypertrophic Cardiomyopathy 551
Experimental Cardiomyopathy 551
Intracardiac Masses 553
Intracardiac Thrombus 553
Myxoma 553
Vegetations 553
Myocardial Contusion 553
Atherosclerosis 553
CONCLUSIONS 554

One of the important but unmet goals of cardiac diagnosis is the direct, noninvasive identification of tissue composition of cardiac structures. Certainly, abundant indirect information can be used to identify abnormal regions of the myocardium. For example, alterations in left ventricular contraction appearing in the setting of chest discomfort and electrocardiographic abnormalities suggest acute myocardial ischemia. Unfortunately, regional wall motion abnormalities are somewhat nonspecific and may appear in acute ischemia,[F1] infarction, scar, and even nonischemic cardiomyopathy.[W1] Similarly, alterations in cardiac enzymes in the same setting establish the presence of myocardial necrosis but do not differentiate between relatively diffuse subendocardial damage and localized transmural infarction. Thus, identifying the precise site, extent, and chronicity of ischemic myocardial injury is one of many possible situations in which current diagnostic techniques leave an important gap in the identification and characterization of regional myocardial abnormalities. At present, only endomyocardial biopsy, with its inherent limitations, permits the clinician to identify myocardial composition in a direct fashion.

Toward the goal of direct, yet noninvasive, myocardial tissue characterization, there has been increasing interest in the use of quantitative analysis of transmitted or reflected diagnostic ultrasound.[L1, M1, S1] In particular, much information from experimental animal studies and a growing clinical investigative literature suggest that ultrasound interacts differently with abnormal and normal tissue. Thus, there has been interest in the use of ultrasound to identify acute and chronic abnormalities of myocardial composition and physiologic state—a field of investigation termed ultrasonic tissue characterization.[L1] Ultrasonic cardiac tissue characterization may be defined as the *identification and characterization of abnormalities in the physical or physiologic state of myocardium based on analyzing interactions between ultrasound and tissue.* The rationale for this field of study is that sufficient information is available in the ultrasound signal passing through or returning from myocardial tissue to identify the tissue as normal or abnormal and to indicate the nature of the abnormality.

Is the field of ultrasonic tissue characterization a new one? In fact, observations suggesting that ultrasound analyses might be capable of identifying abnormal soft tissue date back to the 1950's.[W2] In the early 1970's, studies of experimental myocardial ischemia suggested that some acoustic properties were altered within minutes after acute coronary occlusion.[N1] Why, then, has ultrasound tissue characterization not yet risen to the clinical horizon? Among many other problems, to be discussed subsequently, there has until recently been relatively little *clinical* research using ultrasound tissue characterization techniques. However, recent progress by several groups suggests the potential for clinical application in the near future. That there is a need for noninvasive tissue characterization is clear when one considers the examples cited above or other clinical scenarios in which a precise knowledge of tissue state would greatly influence clinical management decisions. This need for information on tissue composition and physiologic state is particularly relevant in the present era of interventions to minimize acute ischemic injury. The ultimate success or failure of interventions designed to limit infarct size will be judged by their effect on the amount of infarcted tissue resulting from a given decrement in myocardial perfusion to a particular perfusion field. Unless precise identification of the presence and extent of abnormalities such as infarction is available, judgments as to the efficacy of interventional procedures will continue to be based on useful but relatively imprecise measures such as global and regional left ventricular contractile function, angiographic coronary arterial anatomy, and survival of patients.

In this chapter we first describe some basic physical and physiologic concepts relevant to ultrasound tissue characterization, including instrumentation-related considerations and common approaches used in prior investigations. Biologic determinants of normal and abnormal myocardial acoustic properties are also discussed. The majority of the chapter is devoted to the results of ultrasonic tissue characterization studies of specific disease processes including ischemic heart disease, cardiomyopathy, intracardiac masses, and vessel wall atherosclerosis. Finally, we attempt to place the present status of ultrasonic tissue characterization in a clinical perspective with our projections for the future of this promising diagnostic technique.

BASIC CONCEPTS OF ULTRASONIC TISSUE CHARACTERIZATION

Definition of Acoustic Terms

In this section, we define several concepts in acoustics as they apply to ultrasonic interrogation of tissue. Many of these concepts have been used to develop quantitative parameters that convey information about the physical state of the tissue that is characteristic of its normal or abnormal condition.

Ultrasound travels within myocardium with a *propagation speed* that is determined by its density and compressibility. Other tissues that are much less compressible than myocardium, such as bone, exhibit much higher ultrasound propagation speeds.[K1] Even among soft tissues, there are small differences in the velocity of ultrasound. For example, ultrasound velocity values increase progressively as waves travel through fat, water, liver, and muscle. All values of propagation speed for soft tissue are, however, close to the conventionally accepted value of approximately 1540 m/sec. Even though this property may potentially lend itself to tissue differentiation, commercially available echocardiographic scanners assume a fixed propagation speed and therefore negate any role for acoustic velocity variations in characterizing tissue. Thus far, there has been very little work on differentiation of myocardial physical state based on differences in propagation speed.

The *ultrasonic wavelength* is the length of one cycle of the ultrasonic wave. The wavelength is given by the ratio of the propagation speed to the ultrasonic frequency employed. The frequency is conveyed as a nominal or center frequency, as all transducers have some useful bandwidth or range extending from below to above this center frequency. Although, theoretically, decreasing the wavelength will improve resolution, this effect is limited by the fact that higher transmitted frequencies will achieve *less penetration* through the chest wall into the myocardial region of interest. The diminished penetration of ultrasound with increasing frequency is due to higher *attenuation* as a function of frequency. Attenuation reduces the intensity and amplitude of the waves as the sound travels into the tissue of interest (i.e., it is depth related). The losses from attenuation can be due to *reflection, scattering,* or *absorption* (conversion into heat). We shall return to these concepts.

The product of propagation speed times the density of tissue yields the *acoustic impedance.* This is somewhat characteristic for a given tissue, although physiologic and dynamic interactions within the tissue may in theory modify the impedance and thus it should not be considered as a constant factor. One of the cardinal features of ultrasound that makes it powerful as a diagnostic tool is its property of being *reflected* when the waves reach a boundary between tissues (or areas within the same tissue) with different acoustic impedance values (e.g., different density and/or propagation speed values; an *acoustic impedance mismatch*). When the incident wavelength is smaller than the dimension of the boundary, the reflection occurring is termed *specular.* In echocardiography, for example, specular reflection occurs at the interface between endocardium and blood and defines the borders or edges of cardiac muscle with respect to the cavities.

On the other hand, when the boundary (between the different tissues or components of a given tissue) is smaller than the wavelength of the incident wave, the type of reflection that takes place is called *scattering.* As opposed to specular reflections, scattering is a multidirectional phenomenon, in particular for heterogeneous media or in suspensions with particles such as the blood stream. Among the multidirectional waves that result from scattering, those that are redirected back to the transmitting transducer are defined as being *backscattered.* Both the extent of backscatter and the degree of attenuation of a given tissue can be expressed in quantitative terms and are useful parameters for tissue characterization, in particular of myocardium. Both attenuation and backscatter are frequency dependent, although not necessarily in a linear fashion. Backscatter can be expressed as a function of frequency over the useful bandwidth of frequencies for a particular transducer. By averaging data over a range of frequencies, the variability in backscatter measurement related to *phase cancellation effects* is minimized.[M1] The phenomenon of phase cancellation compromises measurements performed with transducers that contain piezoelectric elements (the only type used in clinical echocardiographic systems). The effects are caused by distortions of the ultrasonic wave front resulting from inhomogeneities in the tissue and lead to degradation of the signal as it is received at the transducer. Furthermore, reflected waves interfere with each other (i.e., *constructive* or *destructive* interference), also contributing to phase cancellation effects.[S2]

To put into perspective the ultrasonic backscatter measurements of myocardium, we shall define three additional related parameters[M2, O1]: *backscatter transfer function, backscatter coefficient,* and *integrated backscatter.* The detailed measurement techniques for these parameters are described in the next section. Briefly, the transducer is excited with an electrical voltage and the power spectrum received from tissue is referenced to the power spectrum obtained from measured reflection from a reference reflector such as a steel plate (a perfect reflector) to obtain the *backscatter transfer function.* In this context, power spectrum refers to the plot of the ultrasonic energy returned from the tissue or reflector, with power as ordinate and frequency as abscissa. *Integrated backscatter* is defined as the frequency average of the backscatter transfer function (over the bandwidth of the transducer).

Although backscatter transfer function and integrated backscatter are useful relative measurements of the scattering efficiency of a selected volume of tissue, they are influenced by the aperture and focusing properties of the transducer utilized and by the attenuation of tissue. The *backscatter coefficient* can be obtained by multiplying the backscatter transfer function by factors that compensate for attenuation and the inverse solid angle subtended by the scattering volume.[M2] The backscatter coefficient is an absolute measurement of the scattering properties of the volume of tissue.

Estimates of backscatter of tissue can be compromised by both phase cancellation effects at piezoelectric receivers and interference effects in the ultrasonic field. These effects combine to produce a phenomenon known as *speckle* in two-dimensional ultrasonic imaging.[A1, B1] Speckle is also described in laser imaging and is defined as the pattern of gray shades in the image resulting from interference among the scattered waves.[S2] It occurs whenever sound scatters from a surface whose irregularities are approximately equal to the wavelength of the sound. The interference pattern generated by the complex interaction between the ultrasonic beam and the individual scatterers or targets in tissue causes an uneven amplitude of noise, which gives a grainy or granular appearance to the image scan. This grainy pattern is superimposed on the tissue structural information. As the grainy pattern degrades the resolution of an image, it is considered to be noise, and for imaging purposes several attempts have been made to reduce speckle in the image. Two of these approaches are spatial averaging (making multiple discrete measurements within a region of tissue to provide a more reliable estimate of the average scattering properties of that region) and expressing the measurements in terms of integrated backscatter (frequency averaging).[M2]

Approaches to Tissue Characterization and Measurement Techniques

Methods Based on Radio-Frequency Data Analysis (Including Integrated Backscatter Imaging)

Progress in quantitative myocardial tissue characterization to date has been possible because of significant advances in electrical engineering and physics applied to improving and modifying ultrasonic measurement and imaging systems. This technical evolution has been coupled with the interest of noninvasive cardiologists in providing echocardiography with quantitative power to distinguish normal from abnormal myocardium on the basis of intrinsic acoustic properties rather than myocardial dimensions or motion. Different groups of investigators have approached the problem of ultrasonic myocardial characterization with different instrumentation techniques and analysis systems. The strong dependence of standard echocardiographic data on specific instrumentation and operator system adjustments adds considerable subjectivity and thus variability to information extracted from these scans.

One important direction of research has relied on the analysis of unprocessed radio-frequency signals returning from myocardium. This approach has been used to quantify the degree of ultrasonic attenuation in *transmission* studies (in which excised tissue is studied in vitro with a transmitting transducer at one side of the tissue and a receiver at the other). Radio-frequency data analysis has also been used to quantify the extent of ultrasonic backscatter in *reflection* studies (i.e., using the same transducer as transmitter and receiver) as in conventional echocardiography (Fig. 26–1). Attenuation is quantified by measuring the signal loss due to transmission through a given thickness of tissue (in vitro) normalized to the signal loss due to transmission through the same thickness of saline. By a substitution technique, the *attenuation coefficient* as a function of frequency is obtained (Fig. 26–2). The resulting slope (least-square fit) is expressed in decibels per centimeter thickness of tissue, per megahertz of useful frequency (dB/cm/MHz).

Although attenuation is an important quantitative descriptor of tissue architecture, it is difficult to adapt to the heart in vivo. Thus, measurements of backscatter have been developed by detecting the signals reflected from a selected segment of myocardium. An electronic gate (typically 3 μsec in duration) and the beamwidth define the volume of tissue of interest for measurements, avoiding specular reflections from endocardial and epicardial surfaces.[O1] The *backscatter transfer function* (see above) is obtained from the reflection from a standard perfect-reflector surface (steel plate). As mentioned, *integrated backscatter* is the frequency average of the transfer function over the useful bandwidth of the transducer (Fig. 26–3) and is a measure of the total energy in the signal returned from the myocardium. These quantitative approaches offer the advantage of reducing the variability in measurements (i.e., due to phase cancellation effects) and minimizing the effects of operator-dependent alteration of system controls that influence information derived from conventional echocardiographic data. Furthermore, integrated backscatter measurements have the potential to lend themselves to serial evaluation of the same segment of tissue. In addition, integrated backscatter can be estimated in the time domain, as well as in the more time-consuming approach of frequency-domain analysis with Fourier transforms alluded to above. The estimate can be done by simply squaring and summing the time-domain signal. The result is normalized to the total energy obtained from the signal reflected from a steel plate to obtain an approximate value of integrated backscatter.[P1]

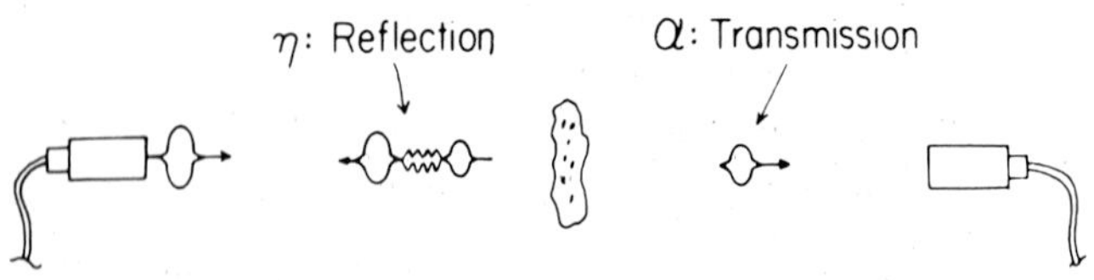

Figure 26–1. Attenuation (α) is measured in transmission with separate transmitting and receiver transducers. Backscatter (η) is measured in reflection with the same transducer serving as both transmitter and receiver.

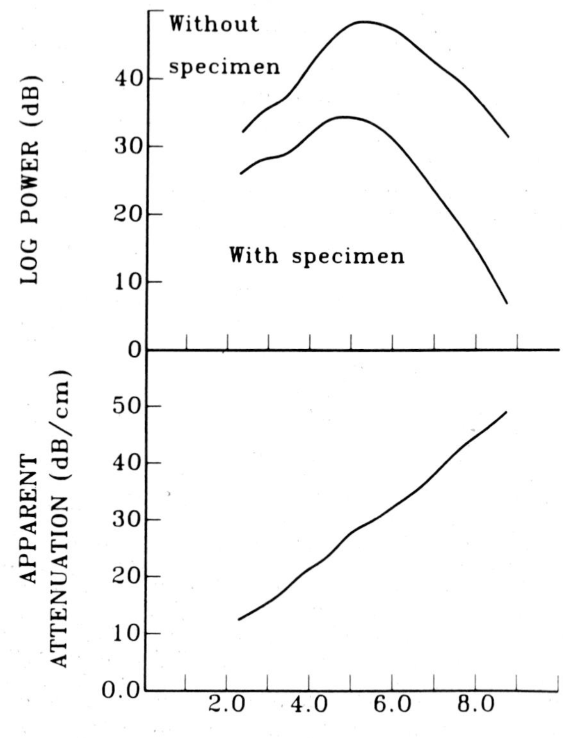

Figure 26–2. Plot of the ultrasonic energy transmitted with no specimen in the system and that obtained with a specimen present *(top)*. The attenuation versus frequency plot *(bottom)* is determined by subtracting the two curves shown at the top and correcting for the thickness of the specimen. (From Miller, J.G., Yuhas, D.E., Mimbs, J.W., et al.: Ultrasonic tissue characterization: Correlation between biochemical and ultrasonic indices of myocardial injury. Proc. IEEE Ultrasonics Symp. Vol. 76, CH1120–5SU:33, 1976, © 1976 IEEE.)

Real-Time Backscatter Imaging

To translate these quantitative measurements of acoustic properties of tissue into a clinically acceptable measurement or image format, a transitional step was taken to construct an M-mode–based system capable of measuring integrated backscatter in real time.[T1] The next generation of this system was based on the adaptation of a commercial two-dimensional imaging device that uses conventional phased-array transducers and computes in real time the integrated backscatter along each individual line of sight in the sector.[B2, T2, V1, V2] In the current implementation, once the summed intermediate-frequency signal has been formed from the output of the phased-array transducer, it can be sent to either the conventional video processing path or the integrated backscatter processor (Fig. 26–4). The processor incorporates digital hardware that produces a continuous signal that is proportional to the logarithm of integrated backscatter along each acoustic line in the image. The dynamic range of the integrated backscatter

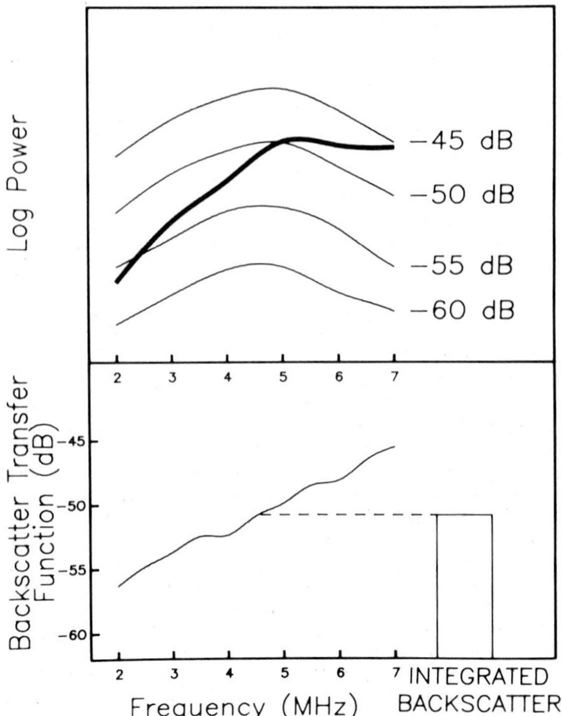

Figure 26–3. Backscatter transfer function and integrated backscatter obtained by interpolating the received power spectrum (bold curve in *top panel*) backscattered from myocardium with respect to the reference spectra from a stainless steel plate measured at 5-dB intervals. (From Miller, J.G., Perez, J.E., Mottley, J.G., et al.: Myocardial tissue characterization: An approach based on quantitative backscatter and attenuation. Proc. IEEE Ultrasonics Symp. 83CH1947–1:782, 1983, © 1983 IEEE.)

processor is more than 40 dB. The full dynamic range of the integrated backscatter data is mapped in 0.5-dB increments into the approximately 30-dB dynamic range available in the displayed video images. The output of the processor follows the remaining signal path through the scan converter as in the conventional image. Thus, the resulting image is created on the basis of integrated backscatter, and image resolution is reasonably well preserved (Fig. 26–5). The image is a quantitative, parametric image in which each picture element represents the value of relative integrated backscatter at a particular point in the field, with data obtained in real time. The magnitude of the cyclic variation of integrated backscatter of a specific myocardial site is defined quantitatively in decibels as the logarithm of the ratio of backscattered energy in diastole to that in systole (see below for definition of the cyclic variation of myocardial backscatter). Over the range of transmit power employed in the system, the magnitude of cyclic variation of integrated backscatter is essentially independent of transmit power.

In this system the data can be analyzed with a separate computer that records up to 2 megabytes of data in real time, yielding storage of 44 frames of backscatter images (1.5 seconds of real-time data). Off-line analysis of the backscatter images acquired in real time is done by an interactive program in which regions of interest are constructed, avoiding the specular reflections of endocardium and epicardium. Subsequently, the data are analyzed by frame-by-frame tracking of the stored image information. The spatially averaged integrated backscatter from each site expressed in decibels is generated and displayed along with the electrocardiogram. Recently, M-mode–derived integrated backscatter data from selected segments have been obtained in real time from the integrated backscatter two-dimensional image.[M3] The data can be analyzed directly while displayed on the screen for documentation of the cyclic variation of backscatter within seconds of data acquisition.

The current implementation of the system permits computation of the physiologic cardiac cycle–dependent variation in myocardial integrated backscatter (see below). Additional refinements in the future may permit quantitative comparison of absolute (or time-averaged) backscatter from patient to patient and among populations of patients with dissimilar myocardial pathology.

Methods That Display Acoustically Abnormal Tissue

Marked alterations in tissue structure are known to produce alterations in the echocardiographic appearance of conventional images. Thus, increased brightness of a portion of the image may be interpreted as increases in ultrasonic amplitude that may be related to specific pathologic alterations of tissue. For example, calcified or fibrotic valvular tissue reflects ultrasound strongly, producing an increase in regional image brightness. However, echo strength or amplitude depends not only on the absolute scattering strength of the tissue but also on tissue absorption and instrumentation settings.

In addition to changes in overall echo amplitudes in the image (*gray level*), there are many recognizable changes in the spatial distribution or *texture* of these gray levels. Qualitative, subjective descriptions of texture have employed terms such as coarse or fine, uniform or nonuniform, and high-amplitude or low-amplitude echoes.[B3] Obviously, these descriptions are strongly influenced by the experience and training of the operator and by equipment settings. Yet this display-based approach has been used successfully by many investigators to describe the peculiar

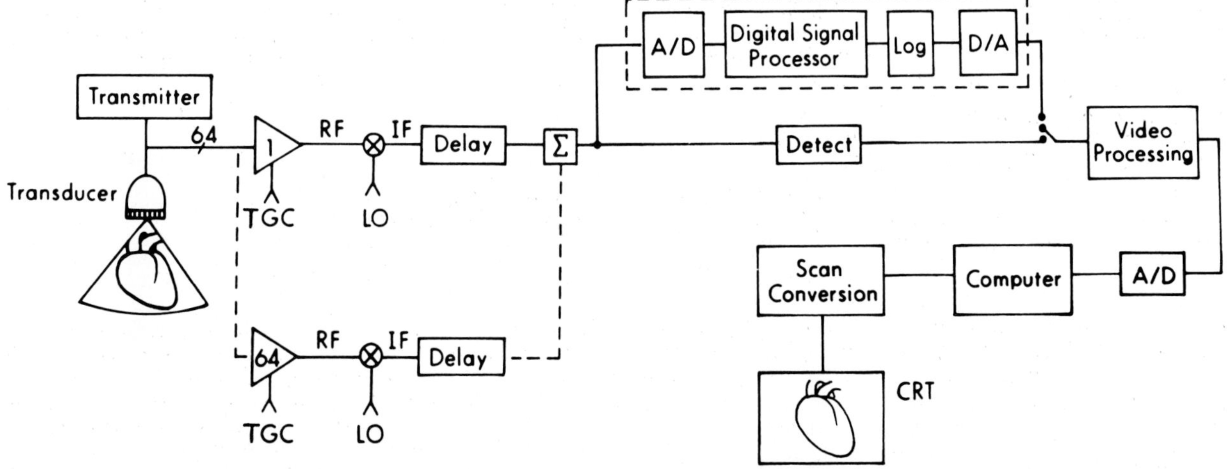

Figure 26–4. Diagram showing the modified signal processing path for the two-dimensional integrated backscatter imaging system. As in conventional imaging, the usual time-gain compensation (TGC) is employed for attenuation. IF—intermediate-frequency signal; A/D—analog-to-digital conversion; D/A—digital-to-analog conversion; LO—low-pass filter; CRT—cathode ray tube. (From Vered, Z., Barzilai, B., Gessler, C.J., et al.: Ultrasonic integrated backscatter tissue characterization of remote myocardial infarction in human subjects. J. Am. Coll. Cardiol. 13:84, 1989. Reprinted with permission of the American College of Cardiology.)

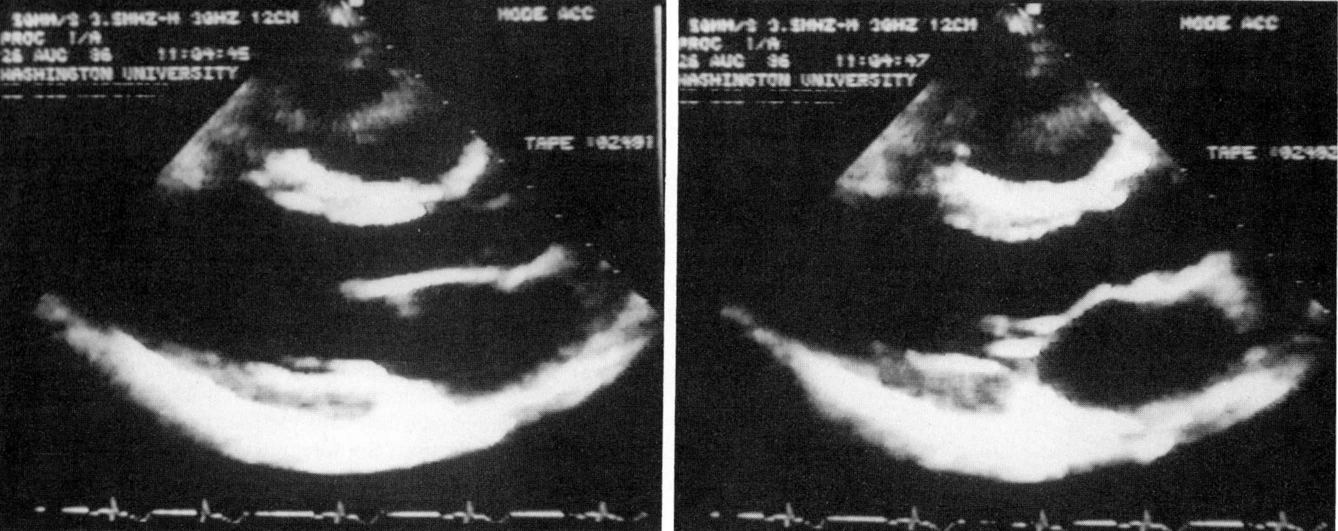

Figure 26–5. Diastolic *(left)* and systolic *(right)* still frames obtained with real-time integrated backscatter imaging in normal subject. Diastolic-to-systolic decrease in myocardial integrated backscatter can be appreciated in the posterobasal and septal-basal segments. (From Perez, J.E., Miller, J.G., Barzilai, B., et al.: Progress in quantitative ultrasonic characterization of myocardium: From the laboratory to the bedside. J. Am. Soc. Echo. 1:294, 1988, with permission.)

appearance of the ventricular septum in patients with hypertrophic cardiomyopathy[M4] and the myocardium of patients with amyloid heart disease,[B3] as well as the increased echogenicity of the ventricular septum (M-mode) in patients with remote myocardial infarction.[R1]

Color encoding of conventional echocardiographic images with or without additional brightness modulation, as an alternative to gray scale displays, has been employed by Logan-Sinclair, Davies, and associates to describe increased amplitude in segments of remote myocardial infarction[L2] or eosinophilic myocardial disease.[D1] These investigators, like Tanaka and associates,[T3] have defined the pericardial reflection on two-dimensional views as exhibiting maximal intensity (or 100 percent). This pericardial reference has then been used to describe in percentage values the relative signal strength of normal versus abnormal regions. Since the human visual system is better able to distinguish among colors than among subtle changes in gray scale, this methodology has been employed by other investigators as well. Parisi and associates[P2] described the evolution of scar maturation in dogs followed serially with color-encoded images after experimental myocardial infarction. Serial measurements were required, as opposed to a single set of observations of any one dog, to establish conclusively abnormal scar content.

The principal difficulty in these descriptive techniques is the subjective nature of the interpretation, which can be greatly altered by manipulation of the equipment settings. Other instrumentation-related considerations pertinent to this problem (and certainly to all other current approaches) involve changes in the time-gain compensation settings that may alter the acoustic signal, the use of nonlinear signal compression schemes, and reject and damping settings. Subjective setting of these controls in the system may mask or mimic pathologic processes. Melton and Skorton[M5] have proposed the use of "rational" (as opposed to conventional) time-gain compensation to better compensate for the attenuation suffered by round-trip travel of the signals into the tissue segment of interest. Conventional time-gain compensation may overcompensate, undercompensate, or both, leading to false differences in brightness (related to ultrasonic amplitude) that do not arise from true alterations in tissue structure.[M5] In rational gain compensation, previously measured values for attenuation of blood and myocardium are assigned to define attenuation of a region along each line of sight in the image. This approach may improve detection of small scars in myocardium due to remote infarction[M5] and has been implemented in the real-time integrated backscatter imaging[V1] system to enable comparison of cyclic variation of myocardial integrated backscatter at different depths in the field (e.g., ventricular septum versus posterior wall values).

Methods That Quantitate Echocardiographic Gray Level (Image) Data

As opposed to the use of data derived from radio-frequency signals (as used in the calculation of integrated backscatter) or visual inspection of images, a third approach has attempted to utilize quantitative analysis of video or image data. The motivations for this approach include (1) the smaller data storage and processing requirements for video (as opposed to radio-frequency) data and (2) the previously described abnormalities that may be seen by simple visual inspection of standard images, which suggests that information relevant to tissue ultrasonic properties may be extracted from images. The general approach consists of computer analysis of regional echo amplitude including the spatial distribution *(texture)* of amplitudes in a quantitative, statistical fashion.[A2] Assessment of regional echo amplitude first took the form of evaluating so-called first-order gray level attributes, such as average gray level (similar to image brightness), variance, skewness, and kurtosis of gray levels.[S3] Quantitative analysis of

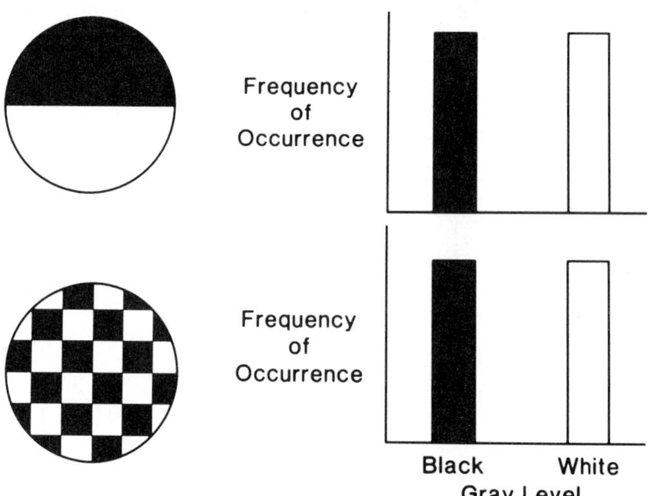

Figure 26–6. Concept of two-dimensional gray level texture. Two stylized digital regions of interest are shown *(left)*. Because each region is half black and half white, the regions will display the same average gray level and identical gray level histograms *(right)*. The obvious differences in the spatial distribution of black and white in the two regions, termed gray level texture, are not appreciated by simple inspection of average gray level or gray level histograms. (From Collins, S.M., and Skorton, D.J.: Cardiac Imaging and Image Processing. McGraw-Hill, New York, 1986, p. 199, with permission.)

first-order gray level data has proved useful for identification of infarction,[S3] reperfusion,[H1] and other abnormalities.

In contrast to the first-order gray level measurements, several groups have utilized quantitative analysis of *spatial* echo amplitudes in so-called texture analysis. Texture can be assessed by a number of measures involving calculation of features of the two-dimensional spatial pattern of regional image gray levels (Fig. 26–6). One useful category of gray level texture measures includes the run-length measures. A gray level run is defined as the number of pixels in a given direction that have the same or similar gray levels.[G1] A run-length matrix representing the number of runs of varying lengths and gray levels can be calculated. From the run-length matrix, one can compute statistics such as short-run emphasis, long-run emphasis, gray level nonuniformity, run-length nonuniformity, and run percentage.[G1] These measures give information concerning the heterogeneity of the gray levels and the relative size of the individual echo reflections and thus characterize the image texture. Other categories of quantitative texture measures, such as gray level difference measures, have also proved useful in echocardiographic image analysis.[W3]

These quantitative texture measures have been used to demonstrate tissue changes due to myocardial contusion in closed-chest dogs[S4] and cardiomyopathic changes in humans.[C1] The methods can be applied in vivo to images from standard echocardiographic systems. The main disadvantage lies in their dependence on instrumentation settings and probable lack of reproducibility among different laboratories.

BIOLOGIC DETERMINANTS OF MYOCARDIAL ACOUSTIC PROPERTIES

Rational use of ultrasonic tissue characterization methods for clinical diagnosis requires an understanding of the biologic determinants of tissue acoustic properties. A substantial body of research has identified diverse structural components of myocardium that influence its acoustic properties under physiologic and pathologic conditions.[M2, P3] Ultrasonic tissue characterization for clinical application is directed primarily at delineation of the scattering properties of myocardial tissue. Properties of ultrasonic attenuation are not measured directly in present clinical applications but require thorough definition for accurate characterization of intrinsic scattering properties of myocardium.

As mentioned earlier, when sound waves travel through a material such as heart tissue, they are reflected or scattered where local regions of different acoustic impedance are encountered. Thus, tissue elements responsible for scattering (i.e., scatterers) represent local regions of acoustic impedance mismatch.[W4] The intensity of scattering depends on a number of factors, including (1) the size, shape, and concentration of scatterers; (2) the difference in intrinsic acoustic impedance of the scatterers relative to the medium in which they reside; and (3) the spatial distribution of individual scatterers (e.g., random versus highly ordered). Myocardial elements responsible for scattering are much smaller than the wavelengths of ultrasound used for clinical imaging (wavelengths are 300 and 600 μm for 5-MHz and 2.5-MHz ultrasound, respectively). Various microstructural elements have been proposed as scatterers, including blood vessels, intact myocytes, and sarcomeres.

Collagen

Early work in the field of quantitative ultrasonic tissue characterization identified collagen as a primary determinant of both scattering and attenuation of myocardial tissue. Miller and associates described the dependence of ultrasonic attenuation and scattering on myocardial collagen content and structure after experimental myocardial infarction. Attenuation measurements were made in excised canine hearts 2, 4, and 6 weeks after coronary occlusion. Collagen content in regions of infarction was determined by assay of hydroxyproline. The attenuation coefficient increased and paralleled the hydroxyproline content in the infarct zone at each time interval.[M6] Mimbs and associates also studied the relationship between collagen content and ultrasonic attenuation and backscatter in dogs after myocardial infarctions of approximate age 5, 10, and 15 weeks. Backscatter, attenuation, and hydroxyproline content increased significantly at each time interval in the infarct regions (Fig. 26–7).[O2]

Further studies of isolated rabbit hearts excised 5 to 7 weeks after coronary artery occlusion and perfused with collagenase solutions were performed to determine the dependence of scattering and attenuation on the structural integrity of collagen in scar tissue after infarction.[M6] Perfusion of infarct regions with collagenase for 30 minutes reduced ultrasonic backscatter measured at 2.25 MHz from −39.2 ± 1.2 to −45.1 ± 1.2 dB, representing a fourfold decrease in the intensity of scattering from the collagenase-perfused infarct zones. The concentration of hydroxyproline measured in the infarct regions remained unchanged after collagenase treatment. Therefore, these investigators postulated that fragmented but measurable collagen peptide products persist in the infarct region despite the structural dissolution of collagen. Thus, intact collagen with its complex

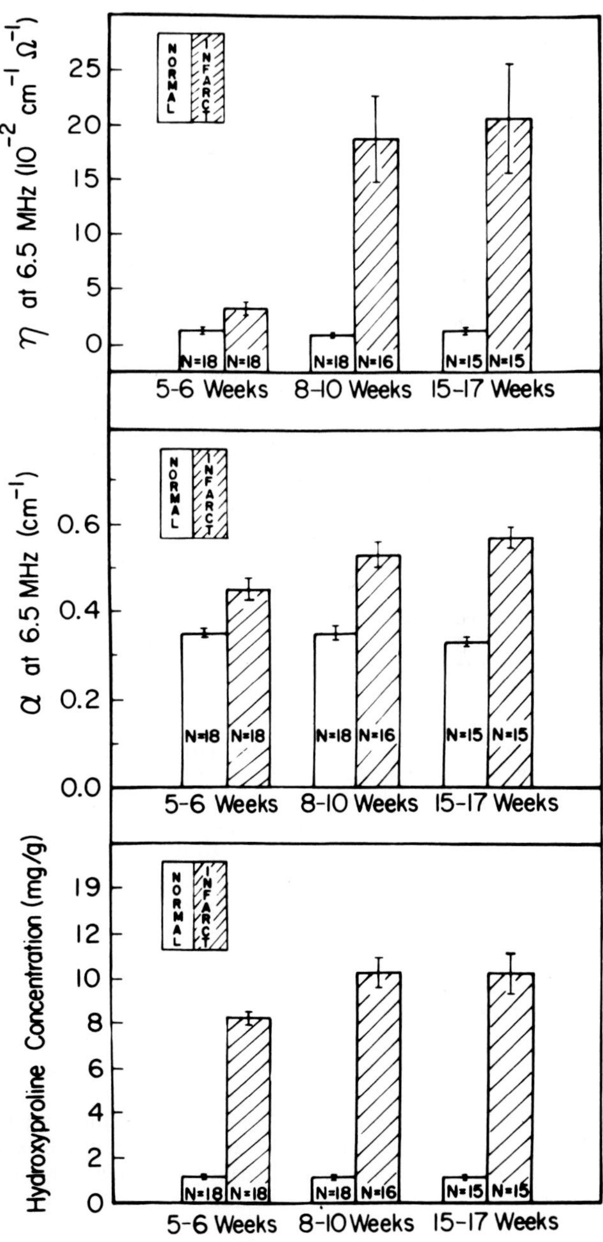

Figure 26–7. Comparison of the backscatter coefficient at 6.5 MHz (η, *top*), the attenuation coefficient at 6.5 MHz (α, *middle*), and the hydroxyproline concentration *(bottom)* in normal dog myocardium to values obtained from zones of infarction at three intervals after coronary artery occlusion. (From O'Donnell, M., Mimbs, J.W., and Miller, J.G.: The relationship between collagen and ultrasonic backscatter in myocardial tissue. J. Acoust. Soc. Am. 69:580, 1981, with permission.)

structural organization in regions of infarct scar tissue appears to represent an important contributor to scattering. In contrast, *attenuation* remained unchanged after perfusion with collagenase. Thus, the complex structural organization of collagen may not represent as significant a determinant for ultrasonic attenuation as it does for scattering.

Other investigators also have made observations supporting the idea that collagen is an important determinant of ultrasonic backscatter. Hoyt and associates studied autopsied human hearts with fibrotic changes associated with remote infarction and demonstrated a linear relationship between integrated backscatter measured at 2.25 MHz and hydroxyproline content.[H2] These investigators also showed that the magnitude of backscatter is greater in excised normal right ventricular segments than in normal left ventricular segments and that this difference corresponds to a higher collagen content in the right ventricle than in the left ventricle.[H3] Numerous other investigators have confirmed that the magnitude of backscatter is elevated in regions of myocardial infarction in both experimental animals and patients[C2, H4, L2, P2, S5, S6] and is presumably related to increased collagen content.

Scatterer Geometry

The geometric attributes of myocardial scatterers have been investigated by a number of groups. On the basis of measurements of the frequency dependence of scattering for normal myocardium, Shung and Reid[S7] and O'Donnell and associates[O2] postulated that myocardial scatterers are comparable in size to cardiac myocytes. The relationship between the intensity of scattering and the frequency (f) of insonification can be described by a power law in which backscatter increases approximately as f^3 for normal myocardium.[M2, O3] Theoretically, scatterers that are much smaller than a wavelength of sound are characterized by f^4 (so-called Rayleigh scattering), and scatterers much larger than a wavelength of sound by f^0 (specular scattering). The reduction of frequency dependence from approximately f^3 to f^2 after myocardial infarction may indicate that the dominant myocardial scatterers are larger for infarcted than for normal myocardium and demonstrates the sensitivity of measurements of the frequency dependence of backscatter to pathologic replacement of normal myocytes by scar tissue after infarction.

More detailed definition of the acoustic properties of biologic tissue has been attempted by the use of acoustic microscopy.[K2] Linker and associates insonified thin histologic sections of autopsied normal and cardiomyopathic human myocardium with 200-MHz continuous-wave ultrasound to produce high-resolution two-dimensional images of heart tissue.[L3] These images reveal spatial variations of acoustic properties that are on the order of the size of cardiac myocytes for normal human myocardium. Furthermore, the dimensions of acoustic inhomogeneities increased significantly in cardiomyopathic hearts. Fei and Shung also reported that scattering intensity depends directly on cell size for a variety of tissues.[F2] Thus, myocardial elements approximately the size of intact myocytes may be responsible in part for ultrasonic scattering under physiologic conditions. Elegant electron micrographs by Caulfield and Borg have shown that cardiac myocytes are invested externally by a complex collagen matrix that provides structural support.[C3] This microstructural arrangement (Fig. 26–8) of cells embedded in a collagen matrix may provide a sufficient local acoustic impedance mismatch to account for the scattering from normal myocardium.[W4]

Fiber Orientation

Myocardial acoustic properties also are influenced by the orientation of ventricular muscle fibers. Streeter and Hanna have demonstrated that transmural ventricular muscle fiber bands spiral from endocardium to epicardium such that the predominant orientation of endocardial fiber bands is nearly perpendicular to the orientation of epicardial fibers.[S8] The middle portion of the ventricular wall comprises mainly circumferentially oriented fiber bands. Mottley and Miller have demonstrated that the magnitude of both ultrasonic attenuation and backscatter in excised heart tissue depends critically on the angle of insonification.[M7] Attenuation is maximal when sound waves propagate parallel to or along the major fiber orientation and minimal in a direction perpendicular to the fiber orientation. Ultrasonic backscatter is maximal in a direction perpendicular to the fibers and minimal in a direction parallel to or along the fiber axis. Madaras and associates have shown that integrated backscatter from canine myocardium measured in open-chest dogs is angle dependent but that the cardiac cycle–dependent variation of backscatter persists regardless of the angle of insonification.[M8] However, the amplitude of cyclic variation is significantly enhanced for insonification at an angle of 60 degrees as compared with perpendicular to myocardial fibers. Also, the backscatter remains minimal at end-systole regardless of the angle of insonification.

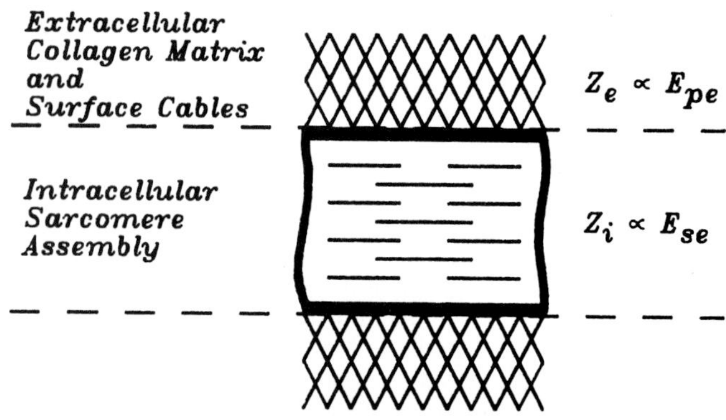

Figure 26–8. Proposed anatomic structure of myocardial scatterers. Myocardial scatterers are theorized to be approximately the size of myocytes. The Z_e (extracellular acoustic impedance) is proportional to the appropriate E_{pe} (extracellular parallel elastic modulus) and is identified with the extracellular collagen matrix and surface cables. The Z_i (intracellular acoustic impedance) is proportional to the appropriate E_{se} (series elastic element stiffness) and is identified with the intracellular sarcomere assembly and associated intracellular elastic fibers. If Z_e differs from Z_i at baseline, the juxtaposition of extracellular and intracellular elastic domain forms a scattering interface composed of elastic elements with different baseline acoustic impedances. (From Wickline, S.A., Thomas, L.J., III, Miller, J.G., et al.: A relationship between ultrasonic integrated backscatter and myocardial contractile function. J. Clin. Invest. 76:2151, 1985, by copyright permission of the American Society for Clinical Investigation.)

Blood Flow/Water Content

Although nutritive blood flow per se may not be necessary for the production of cardiac cycle–dependent variation of backscatter (see below), tissue water content and hematocrit both influence myocardial scattering and attenuation. Mimbs and associates perfused normal isolated rabbit hearts with either Krebs-Henseleit buffer or whole blood and observed that integrated backscatter increased by 200 percent after a 30-second washout with Krebs-Henseleit solution and returned to normal after perfusion with whole blood.[M9] Perfusion with Krebs-Henseleit solutions of differing osmotic strengths for 30 minutes to promote the formation of tissue edema resulted in increased tissue wet weight accompanied by increased integrated backscatter that paralleled the extent of tissue edema. The accumulation of tissue edema early in the course of acute infarction results in decreased attenuation, in contrast to the increased attenuation observed in established infarct scars. Thus, both tissue water content and microvascular hematocrit may influence acoustic properties of myocardium. The presence or absence of blood flow itself may have a small impact on the absolute level of integrated backscatter. Wickline and associates reported a 4-dB decrease of cyclic variation of integrated backscatter immediately following restoration of blood flow after 1 hour of coronary artery occlusion in dogs, associated with a lack of recovery of wall thickening after reperfusion.[W5]

Other Determinants

Myocardial acoustic properties may be influenced profoundly by disease entities that alter normal histologic architecture. A classic example is cardiac amyloidosis, which has been described in terms of textural alterations consisting of bright and speckled patterns manifest on conventional two-dimensional echocardiograms.[B3] Other pathologic entities that entail infiltration or reorganization of myocardial tissue manifest by distinctive textural changes include idiopathic hypertrophic subaortic stenosis, hemochromatosis, and eosinophilic endomyocardial disease.[S9]

Dynamic Aspects of Scattering

So far, our discussion has focused on determinants of backscatter in excised tissue or in vivo, averaged throughout the heart cycle. Additional evidence that supports a dynamic contribution of myocytes to the scattering process was reported by Madaras and associates.[M10] These investigators observed that backscatter intensity varies throughout the cardiac cycle, with maximal levels of scattering at end-diastole and minimal levels at end-systole (Fig. 26–9). The presence of cardiac cycle–dependent variation of backscatter intensity (or other measures of echo amplitude) has been confirmed by many other investigators in both experimental animals and human subjects.[A3, C4, F3, H5, O4, S10] The average magnitude of cyclic variation of backscatter is approximately 5 dB. Cyclic variation of backscatter decreases substantially as a consequence of ischemic injury and may recover after reperfusion of injured but viable myocardial tissue in both experimental animals and human subjects.[F4, G2, H5, S10, W5, W6] Wickline and associates have demonstrated that the magnitude and rate of change of physiologic cyclic variation of backscatter are related to intrinsic myocardial contractile performance.[W7] These investigators also have shown that the magnitude and rate of change of cyclic variation are greater in subendocardial than in subepicardial regions of the myocardium. These results have been confirmed by Sagar and associates[S10] and are consistent with the expectation of enhanced contractile performance in the subendocardium as compared with the subepicardium.[S11, W4] Isolated preparations of superfused canine myocardial papillary and frog skeletal gastrocnemius muscle also demonstrate a dependence of scattering intensity on muscle contractile state, independent of perfusion with blood.[G3, W8]

These observations indicate that acoustic properties of myocardium can vary according to contractile performance. Several hypotheses have been advanced to explain the cyclic alteration of myocardial acoustic properties and include cyclic alterations of myocardial elastic characteristics[W4] and alterations of myocardial scatterer geometry.[W8] However, no simple explanation yet appears sufficient to account for the entire gamut of experimental observations.

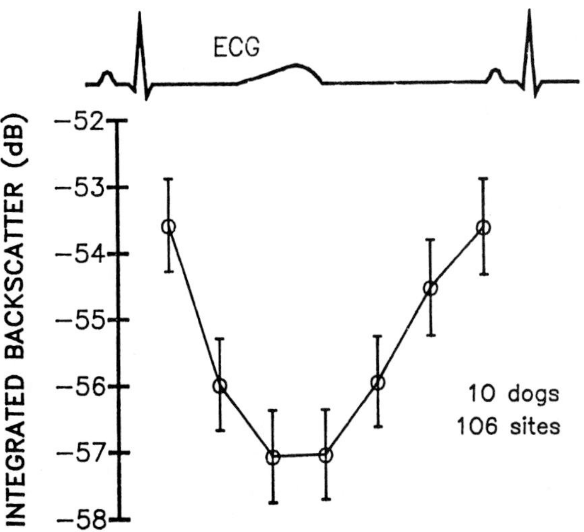

Figure 26–9. Cyclic variation of integrated backscatter in normal canine myocardium. (From Miller, J.G., Perez, J.E., Mottley, J.G., et al.: Myocardial tissue characterization: An approach based on quantitative backscatter and attenuation. Proc. IEEE Ultrasonics Symp. 83CH1947–1:782, 1983, © 1983 IEEE.)

SPECIFIC DISEASE PROCESSES STUDIED BY ULTRASONIC TISSUE CHARACTERIZATION

Ischemic Heart Disease

At present, with effective methods for restoration of coronary blood flow at the time of acute myocardial infarction, it is increasingly important to assess the extent of myocardium at risk, the intensity and severity of segmental ischemia, the ultimate size of irreversible damage, and the amount of residual functional myocardium. Conventional parameters such as serial electrocardiograms and enzymatic evaluation, although accurate, may suffer from shortcomings when evaluating the severity and precise location of ischemia or infarction. In addition, conventional imaging such as x-ray ventriculography, two-dimensional echocardiography, and radionuclide ventriculography cannot differentiate viable but stunned myocardium from irreversibly damaged tissue on the basis of motion or thickening, as segmental function is impaired in both entities. Therefore, ultrasonic tissue characterization has been employed to ascertain whether the diagnosis of segmental myocardial viability after ischemia or infarction can be improved.

Acute Ischemia/Infarction

Among the qualitative observations from conventional echocardiograms, Fraker and associates[F5] detected early increases in regional echo amplitude as soon as 15 minutes after coronary occlusion. The approximate size of the region exhibiting increased echo amplitude correlated with infarct size in experimental animals as determined by histochemical techniques. Werner and associates [W9] identified a subset of patients with acute myocardial infarction who exhibited a decrease in regional echo amplitude. These patients had a higher risk of severe complications including free wall rupture and death. Other investigators have attempted to improve the visual perception of differences in regional echo amplitude by using color encoding of the amplitude information. Thus, Parisi and associates [P2] reported increases in echo amplitude during the evolution of myocardial infarction in experimental animals.

In a series of studies utilizing quantitative analysis of radiofrequency signals, various aspects of the acoustic characteristics of ischemia in experimental animals have been delineated. Lele and Namery[L4, N1] reported decreases in acoustic impedance soon after coronary artery occlusion in dogs. In other early radiofrequency experiments, attenuation through excised myocardial specimens was measured in transmission studies. Mimbs and associates identified significant decreases in attenuation through ischemic tissue as soon as 15 minutes after coronary artery occlusion in the dog.[M11] Decreased attenuation was noted up to 24 hours after coronary artery occlusion and was thereafter replaced by an increase in attenuation. This study suggested that ischemic myocardial injury could be detected as early as 15 minutes after coronary occlusion, much sooner than light microscopic evidence of ischemic damage could be expected, and that the early decrease followed by a later increase in attenuation suggested that the stage of an acute injury could be estimated by using ultrasound methods (Fig. 26–10).

With the use of reflected ultrasound, as opposed to attenuation measurements, Mimbs and associates showed that integrated backscatter increased as soon as 1 hour after acute coronary artery occlusion in dogs.[M9] Schnittger and associates[S12] utilized a fundamentally different calculation technique and identified an increase in the ratio of mean regional echo amplitude to the standard deviation of echo amplitudes (the mean-to-standard-deviation ratio) within 30 minutes after coronary occlusion in dogs (Fig. 26–11).

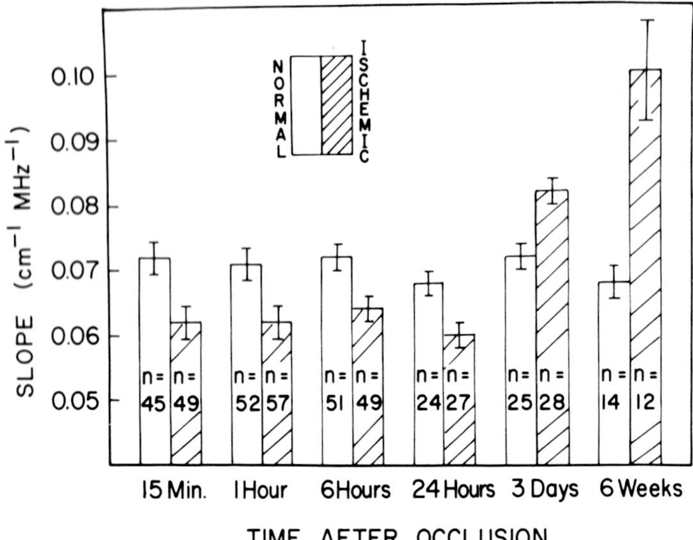

Figure 26–10. A quantitative index of ultrasonic attenuation is plotted for zones of ischemic injury and normal zones from the same hearts in groups of canine hearts studied in vitro at specified intervals after coronary occlusion. (From Mimbs, J.W., O'Donnell, M., Miller, J.G., and Sobel, B.E.: Changes in ultrasonic attenuation indicative of early myocardial ischemic injury. Am. J. Physiol. 236:H340, 1979, with permission.)

Most of these results were based on the total amount of ultrasonic energy returning to the transducer, averaged throughout the cardiac cycle. The *cyclic variation of ultrasound backscatter* with cardiac contraction has been employed as a variable to assess ischemic damage. Studies by Barzilai and associates[B4] and confirmed by Fitzgerald[F3] and Sagar[S10] and their associates demonstrated that the normal cyclic variation of backscatter (decreasing with contraction) is blunted by ischemia (Fig. 26–12). This finding is now generally accepted to be an indication of the acute ischemic process. The physiologic basis of normal cardiac cycle–dependent backscatter variation has not been completely elucidated, but it may be related to cardiac contractile performance,[W7] the elasticity of myocardial tissue,[W4] and/or contraction-dependent variations in myocardial scatterer geometry.

Promising results have also been obtained in acute infarction by studying echocardiographic image gray level characteristics. McPherson and associates[M12] have used quantitative texture analysis to identify acute ischemia 2 hours after coronary occlusion in closed-chest dogs (Fig. 26–13). Chandrasekaran and associates confirmed these findings.[C5]

Reperfused Myocardium

The ability to identify successfully reperfused tissue (i.e., segments that remain viable despite temporary contractile abnormalities) and the ability to identify potentially viable myocardium to decide whether to attempt reperfusion are extremely important clinical issues in cardiovascular medicine at present. Recent echocardiographic tissue characterization data suggest that acoustic analysis techniques may aid in these determinations. To this end, Rasmussen and associates demonstrated in an experimental canine preparation that alterations in ultrasound backscatter that occur following 20 minutes of coronary artery occlusion were reversed following 30 minutes of reperfusion.[R2] In a study evaluating regional echo amplitude (gray level) data, Haendchen and associates evaluated the effect of 3 hours of coronary occlusion followed by 1 hour of reperfusion.[H1] Viable myocardium demonstrated characteristic differences in mean echo amplitudes and skewness of gray level distributions compared to regions that were infarcted (Fig. 26–14). Glueck and associates[G2] have shown that the cardiac cycle–dependent variation in backscatter that is blunted by ischemia returns toward normal values after reperfusion. These findings were confirmed by Sagar and associates.[S10] Furthermore, Wickline and associates have demonstrated that the extent of alterations in the cyclic variation of backscatter resulting from ischemia (Fig. 26–15) and the magnitude of subsequent recovery after reperfusion are not merely related to the level of segmental wall thickening.[W5] Similarly, Milunski and associates demonstrated in dogs[M13] and patients [M14] that cyclic variation of backscatter may recover after

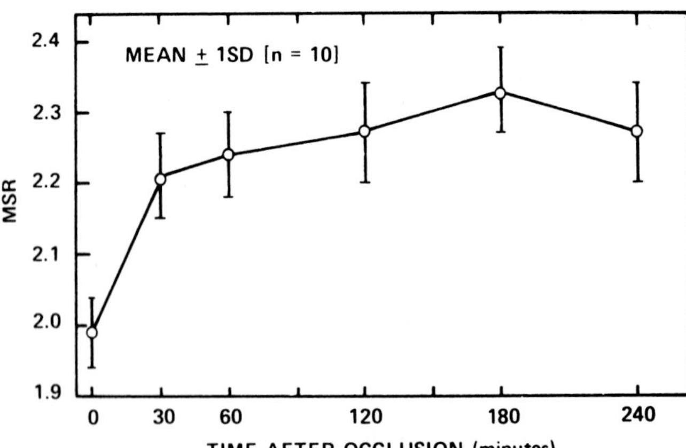

Figure 26–11. Alteration in ultrasound backscatter after acute coronary occlusion. The graph shows a plot of the ratio of mean echo amplitude to standard deviation of echo amplitude (MSR) against time after coronary occlusion. Within 30 minutes after coronary occlusion, the MSR increased and remained elevated throughout the remainder of the experiment. (From Schnittger, I.A., Vieli, A., Heiserman, J.E., et al.: Ultrasonic tissue characterization: Detection of acute myocardial ischemia in dogs. Circulation 72:193, 1985, with permission of the American Heart Association, Inc.)

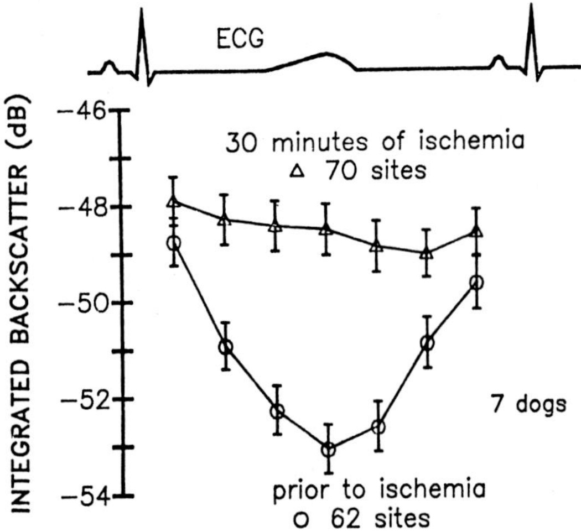

Figure 26–12. Blunting of the cyclic variation of backscatter and elevation of the time-averaged integrated backscatter after 30 minutes of myocardial ischemia in dogs. (From Miller, J.G., Perez, J.E., Mottley, J.G., et al.: Myocardial tissue characterization: An approach based on quantitative backscatter and attenuation. Proc. IEEE Ultrasonics Symp. 83CH1947–1:782, 1983, © 1983 IEEE.)

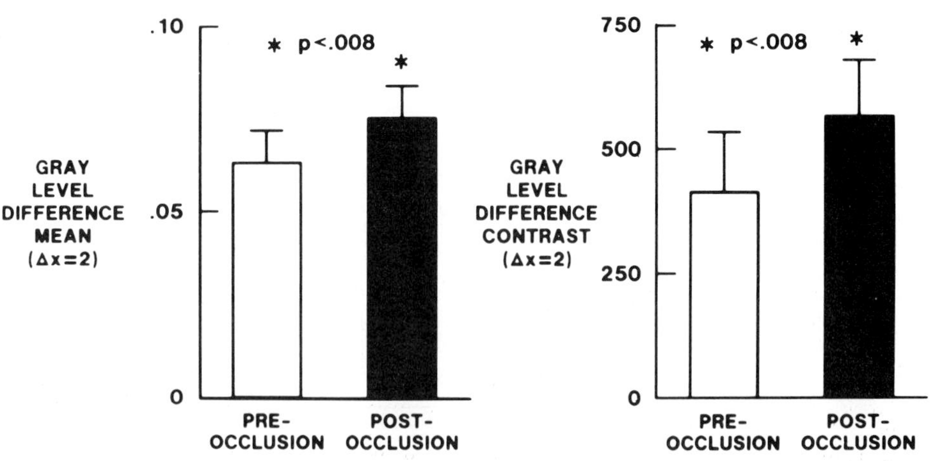

Figure 26–13. Efficacy of quantitative texture analysis in identifying acute ischemia. The data shown are for two quantitative texture parameters (gray level difference mean and contrast, both measured at a horizontal spacing [Δx] of two pixels) measured before and after occlusion through the chest wall in nine dogs. Both texture parameters show significant alteration 2 hours after coronary occlusion. (From McPherson, D.D., Aylward, P.E., Knosp, B.M., et al.: Ultrasound characterization of acute myocardial ischemia by quantitative texture analysis. Ultrason. Imag. 8:227, 1986, with permission.)

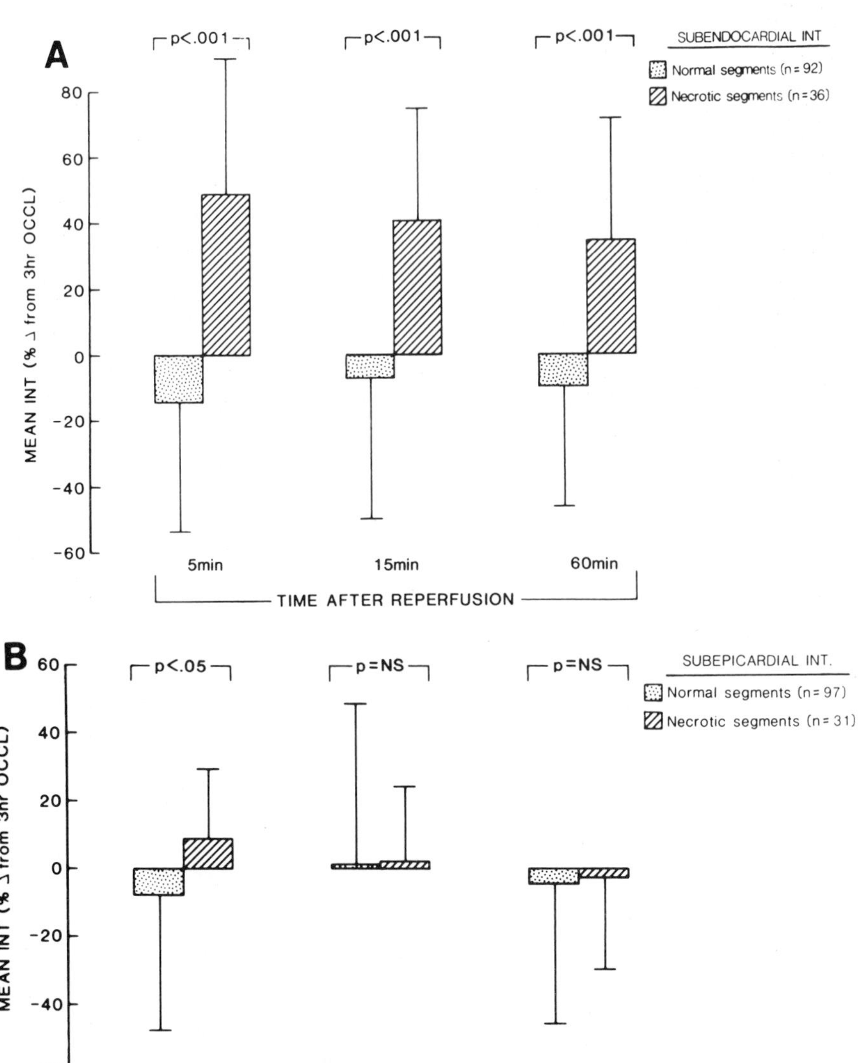

Figure 26–14. Alterations in mean echo intensities after coronary occlusion and reperfusion in dogs. *A* and *B* show data for subendocardial and subepicardial regions, respectively. The percent change in mean intensity in the subendocardial regions from 3 hours of coronary occlusion to 5, 15, and 60 minutes of reperfusion were significantly greater in necrotic tissue than in segments eventually shown to be salvaged. Results were somewhat similar only at 5 minutes of reperfusion in subepicardial regions. (From Haendchen, R.V., Ong, K., Fishbein, M.C., et al.: Early differentiation of infarcted and noninfarcted reperfused myocardium in dogs by quantitative analysis of regional myocardial echo amplitudes. Circ. Res. 57:718, 1985, with permission of the American Heart Association, Inc.)

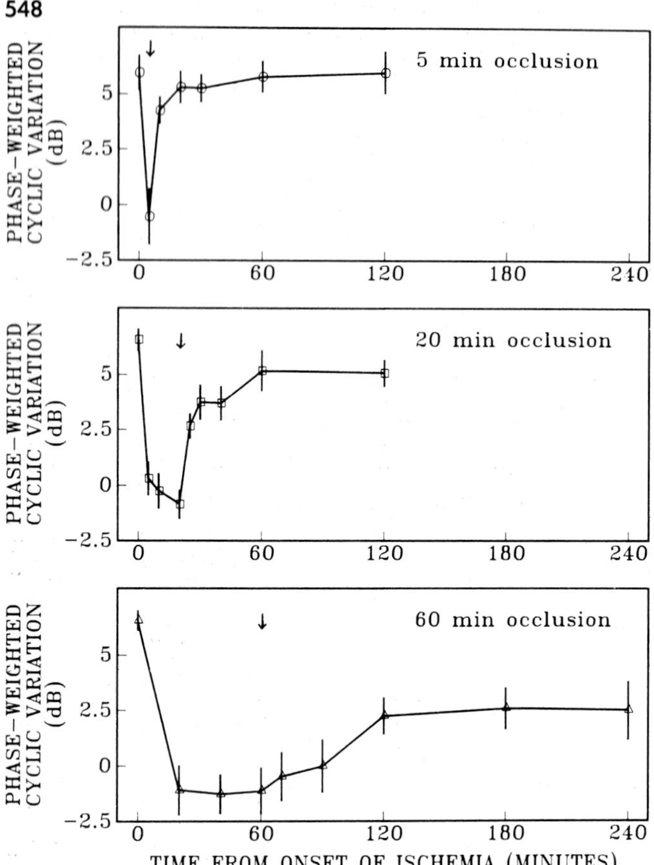

Figure 26–15. Changes in the phase-weighted amplitude of cyclic variation after coronary occlusion followed by reperfusion. The top, middle, and bottom panels represent responses of the phase-weighted amplitude for 5-, 20-, and 60-minute occlusions, respectively. The onset of reperfusion is denoted by an arrow. Each data point represents an average value for five dogs. Error bars represent standard error of the mean. (From Wickline, S.A., Thomas, L.J., III, Miller, J.G., et al.: Sensitive detection of the effects of reperfusion on myocardium by ultrasonic tissue characterization with integrated backscatter. Circulation 74:389, 1986, with permission of the American Heart Association, Inc.)

reperfusion at a time when wall motion and thickening abnormalities persist. Thus, preliminary observations suggest that reperfused, viable, but "stunned" myocardium may be differentiated from necrotic tissue by ultrasound tissue characterization methods.

One inherent difficulty in the use of cyclic backscatter variation measurements to identify acute infarction is the nonspecific nature of blunted cyclic variation. Decreases in cyclic variation of backscatter may occur in acute or chronic infarction. Recently, Wear and associates[W10] have shown that analysis based on the frequency dependence of integrated backscatter can differentiate recently ischemic tissue from remotely infarcted myocardium in the same animal (Fig. 26–16), which suggests that future refinements in the assessment of parameters derived from radiofrequency data may be more specific for this differentiation.

Subacute and Chronic Infarction

Myocardial infarction that has been present for a few days (but not sufficiently long to result in significant deposition of collagen) also results in characteristic acoustic changes. For example, Mimbs and associates noted that attenuation through infarcted myocardium was greater than that in normal tissue, beginning approximately 3 days after coronary occlusion.[M11] In contrast, measurements earlier (15 minutes to at least 24 hours) after occlusion demonstrated decreased attenuation compared to normal. Therefore, very early changes in acoustic properties may be related to changes in myocardial perfusion, alterations in the formed elements of blood within the tissue region, and edema, whereas alterations in acoustic properties two or more days after coronary occlusion may be due to early cellular infiltration and other features of the necrotic process. The analysis performed by Parisi and associates[P2] demonstrated progressive increases in echo image amplitude as displayed by a color-encoding technique during evolving infarction. Logan-Sinclair and associates[L2] and Shaw and associates[S5] also used color encoding to detect regions of fibrosis in patients with remote myocardial infarction. Skorton and associates demonstrated in a closed-chest dog preparation of 48-hour-old myocardial infarction that the distribution of regional echo amplitudes differentiated infarcted from normal tissue.[S3] Regions of myocardial infarction showed a decrease in the kurtosis (peakedness) of the echo amplitude distribution as compared to normal myocardium (Fig. 26–17).

Utilizing in vitro measurements of attenuation through excised myocardial specimens, O'Donnell and associates demonstrated marked increases in attenuation of the ultrasound signal that correlated well with increased collagen content at 2, 4, or 6 weeks after an acute myocardial infarction in dogs.[O3] Studies of ultrasonic attenuation in excised tissue specimens by Mimbs and associates had earlier established that the amount of change in attenuation in remote infarction correlated with the extent of injury assessed by creatine kinase levels.[M15] Furthermore, integrated backscatter showed a substantial increase in remote experimental myocardial infarction.[O2] Hoyt and associates studied specimens of fibrotic human myocardium and demonstrated a correlation between collagen content (assessed by hydroxyproline concentration) and integrated ultrasound backscatter (Fig. 26–18).[H2] Barzilai and associates[B2] have demonstrated the applicability of integrated backscatter imaging for the precise localization of chronic experimental myocardial infarction correlated with gross pathology. Scarred myocardium lacked cyclic variation of integrated backscatter and exhibited higher values of relative backscatter. More recently, Vered and associates,[V2] using the same instrumentation, have extended these observations to humans with chronic myocardial infarction (Figs. 26–19 and 26–20). Identification of scarred tissue was based on diminished cyclic variation of integrated backscatter and a prolonged time period from the R wave of the electrocardiogram to the nadir of the segmental integrated backscatter waveform.

In summary, these studies of chronic infarction suggest that the deposition of collagen as scar was responsible in part for the acoustic alterations manifested as increased attenuation and backscatter of abnormal tissue.

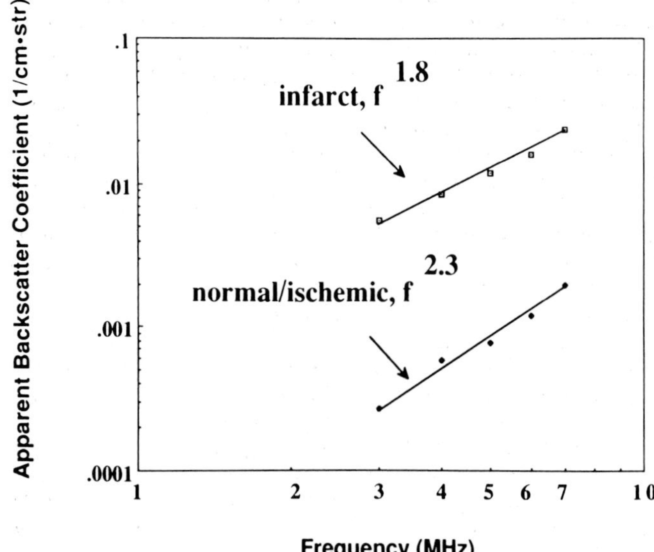

Figure 26–16. Backscatter coefficients for infarct and normal/ischemic myocardium. The backscatter coefficient for infarct is larger in magnitude and rises less rapidly with frequency (not compensated for attenuation). (From Wear, K.A., Milunski, M.R., Wickline, S.A., et al.: Differentiation between acutely ischemic myocardium and zones of completed infarction on the basis of frequency dependent backscatter. J. Acoust. Soc. Am. 85:2634, 1989, with permission.)

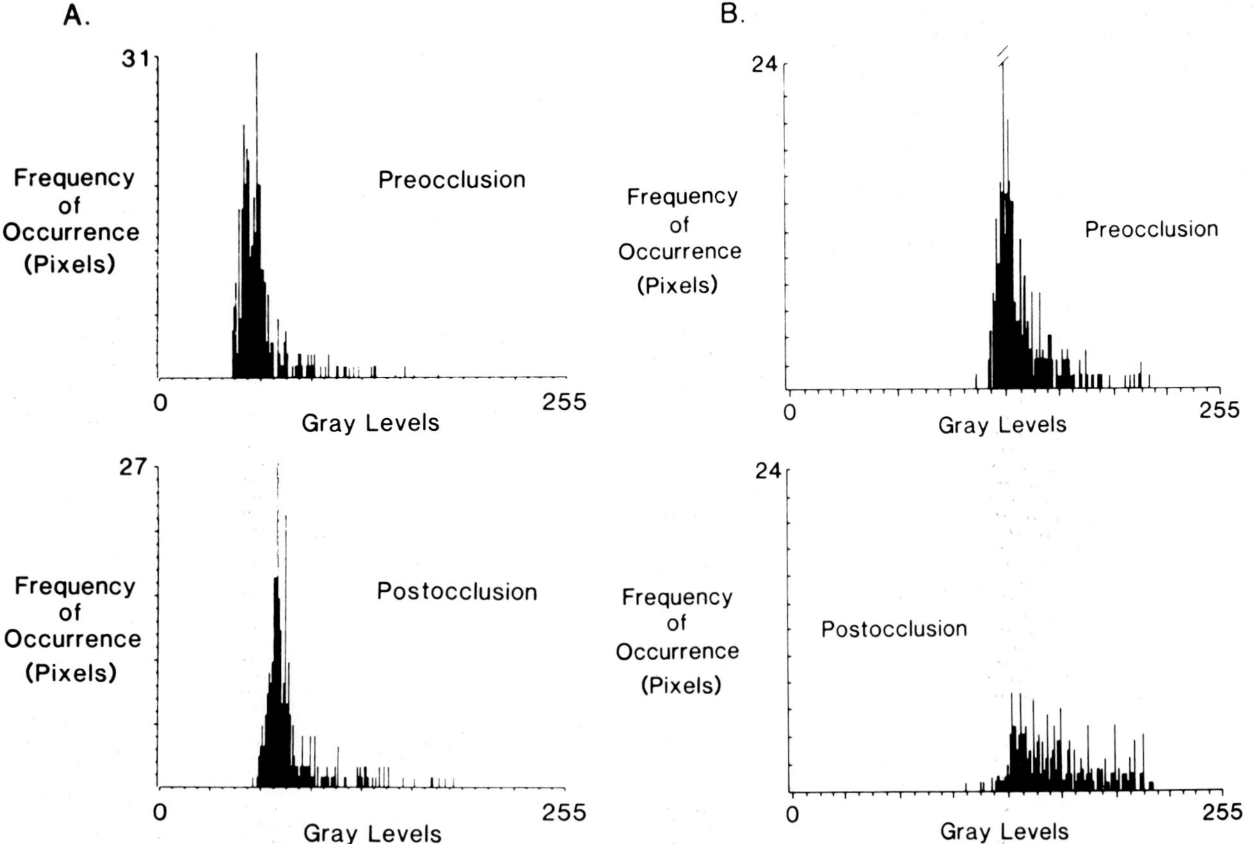

Figure 26–17. Gray level histograms (echo amplitude distributions) from infarcted and control myocardial regions before and 2 days after coronary occlusion in data acquired through the chest wall in dogs. *A*, Preocclusion and postocclusion gray level histograms from a control region; the shape of the histogram does not change between the two studies. *B*, Histograms from an infarcted region; the gray level distribution changes with a relatively higher frequency of higher gray levels postocclusion. (From Skorton, D.J., Melton, H.E., Jr., Pandian, N.G., et al.: Detection of acute myocardial infarction in closed-chest dogs by analysis of regional two-dimensional echocardiographic gray-level distributions. Circ. Res. 52:36, 1983, with permission of the American Heart Association, Inc.)

Cardiomyopathy

The majority of investigative observations using ultrasonic tissue characterization techniques have been made in ischemic heart disease; however, cardiomyopathies are also amenable to assessment with acoustic analyses. *Why might cardiomyopathies be amenable to ultrasonic tissue characterization?* Abnormalities in myocardial function and/or composition occur across the spectrum of cardiomyopathies. For example, dilated cardiomyopathies are commonly manifest as disorders of systolic function. Thus, contraction-dependent variation in myocardial backscatter might be expected to be abnormal in the dilated, myopathic heart. Similarly, calcification and fibrosis in the wall of the dilated myopathic heart may increase backscatter and alter other acoustic properties. Deposition of other abnormal substances (including amyloid and iron) may alter ultrasound backscatter and echocardiographic image texture, as may abnormal myofibrillar architecture, as in hypertrophic cardiomyopathy. Thus, some of the functional and structural abnormalities common to cardiomyopathies have been shown experimentally to alter the interaction between ultrasound and biologic tissue.

Are the techniques of ultrasonic tissue characterization necessary for the noninvasive diagnosis of cardiomyopathy? Certainly, conventional echocardiographic analysis usually permits identification of the major dilated, hypertrophic, and restrictive cardiomyopathies. However, some of the morphologic findings considered pathognomonic of particular cardiomyopathies may in fact be somewhat nonspecific. For example, hypertensive left ventricular hypertrophy may be difficult to discriminate from concentric, nonobstructive hypertrophic cardiomyopathy, particularly in the elderly.[T4] Similarly, amyloid heart disease may simulate hypertrophic cardiomyopathy.[S13] Other diagnostic ambiguities may blur the distinctions among the various cardiomyopathies. Thus, there appears to be a role for further noninvasive characterization of cardiomyopathies, whether by ultrasound or other diagnostic methods.

Dilated Cardiomyopathy

The gross anatomic and echocardiographic appearance of the dilated cardiomyopathy is that of a thin-walled, poorly contractile heart with increased ventricular mass and with the process commonly involving both ventricles. Histologic evaluation of the myocardium in dilated cardiomyopathy reveals irregular hyper-

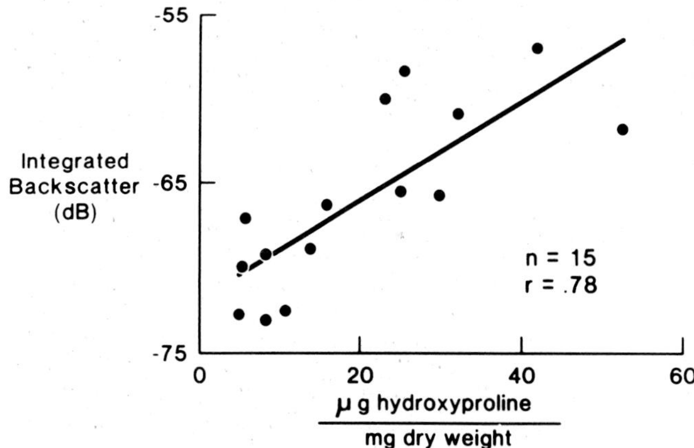

Figure 26–18. Relationship between ultrasound integrated backscatter and collagen content in fibrotic myocardium. The data show a linear relationship between backscatter and hydroxyproline concentration in fibrotic human myocardium evaluated in vitro. (From Hoyt, R.H., Collins, S.M., Skorton, D.J., et al.: Assessment of fibrosis in infarcted human hearts by analysis of ultrasonic backscatter. Circulation 71:740, 1985, with permission of the American Heart Association, Inc.)

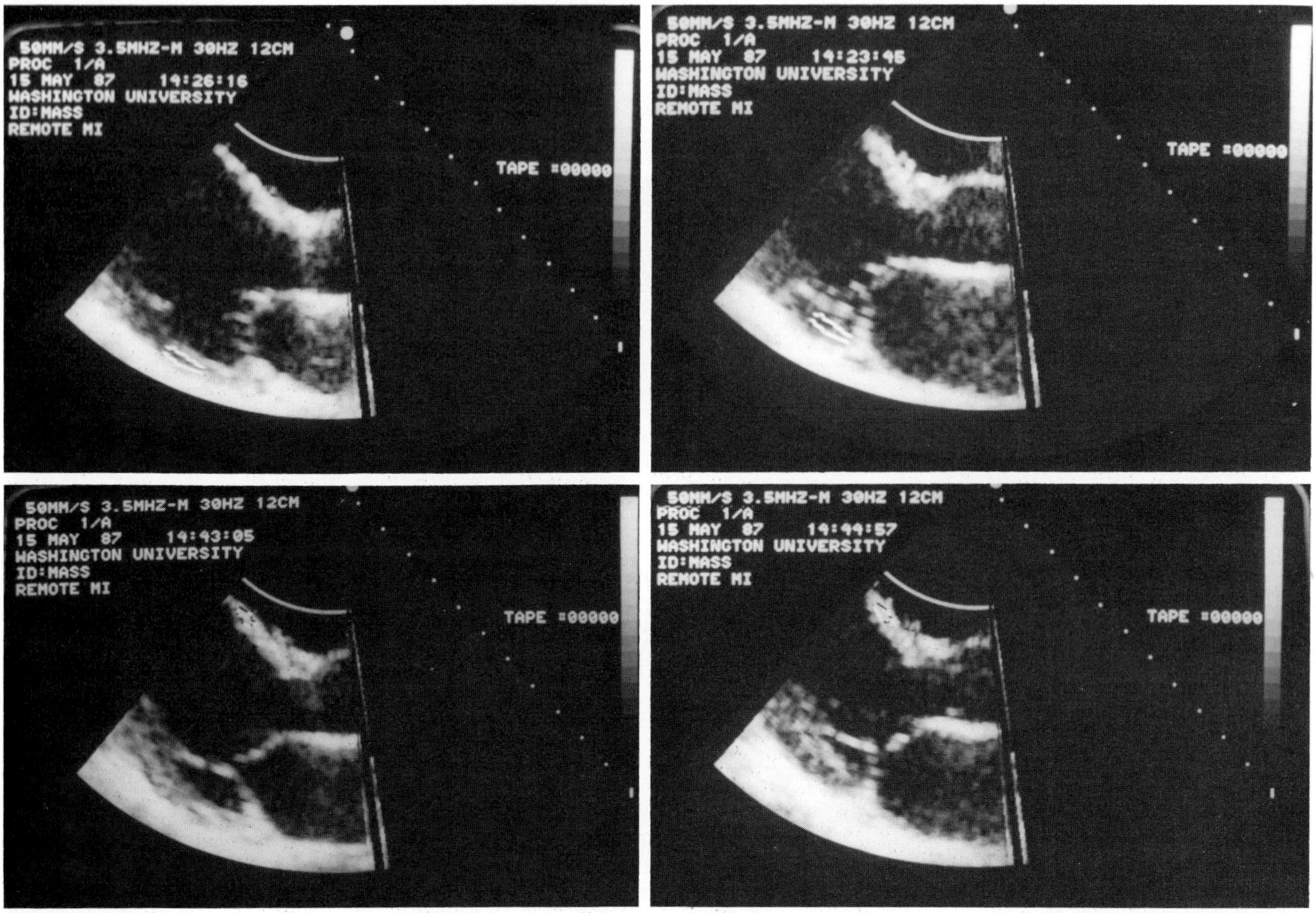

Figure 26–19. Real-time two-dimensional integrated backscatter images from a patient with septal infarction. End-diastolic frame *(top left)* shows the site of analysis for integrated backscatter in a normal posterior wall region. End-systolic frame *(top right)* demonstrates the relative decrease in integrated backscatter (as indicated by decreased image brightness) characteristic of cyclic variation in normal myocardium. End-diastolic frame *(bottom left)* shows the site of analysis in an infarct segment within the septum. This region appears brighter than the normal zone shown in the top left panel. End-systolic frame *(bottom right)* exhibits very little change in brightness (that is, cyclic variation of backscatter) in this infarct site. (From Vered, Z., Barzilai, B., Gessler, C.J., et al.: Ultrasonic integrated backscatter tissue characterization of remote myocardial infarction in human subjects. J. Am. Coll. Cardiol. 13:84, 1989. Reprinted with permission of the American College of Cardiology.)

trophy and degeneration of myocardial fibers as well as varying degrees of myocardial fibrosis.[W11] In the late stages of idiopathic congestive cardiomyopathy, myofibrils are converted to granular, amorphous degenerated fibers.

Based on previous acoustic observations in animals and in patients with chronic myocardial infarction, one might expect the acoustic properties of dilated cardiomyopathies to include increased time-averaged ultrasound backscatter and a decrease in the cyclic variation of backscatter. Although, to our knowledge, absolute time-averaged backscatter has not been measured in dilated cardiomyopathies, Vered and associates[V1] have recently noted that patients with dilated cardiomyopathy do exhibit a significant decrease in cyclic backscatter variation (Fig. 26–21).

Other observations in dilated cardiomyopathy also support a role for ultrasound tissue characterization. Utilizing color encoding of echocardiographic data to enhance the perception of regional differences in backscatter, Davies and associates[D1] noted increased echo brightness in patients with endomyocardial involvement due to hypereosinophilic cardiomyopathy. Angermann and associates[A3] utilized quantitative texture analysis to differentiate dilated cardiomyopathies from normal myocardium in patients.

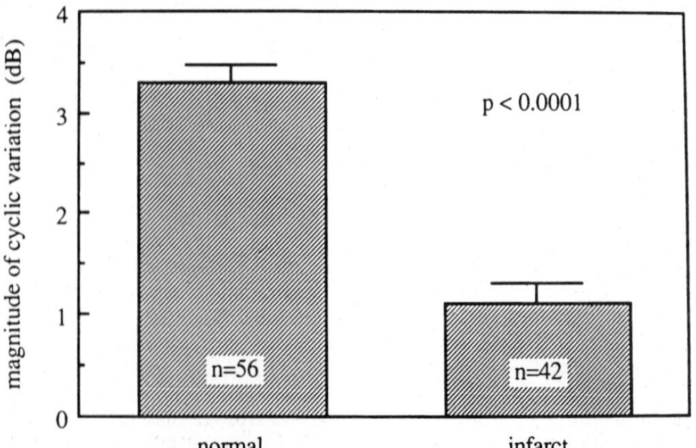

Figure 26–20. Magnitude of cyclic variation of integrated backscatter in normal versus remotely infarcted myocardium in clinical real-time backscatter imaging studies. Previously infarcted myocardium exhibited significantly less cardiac cycle–dependent variation in backscatter than did normal myocardium. (From Vered, Z., Barzilai, B., Gessler, C.J., et al.: Ultrasonic integrated backscatter tissue characterization of remote myocardial infarction in human subjects. J. Am. Coll. Cardiol. 13:84, 1989. Reprinted with permission of the American College of Cardiology.)

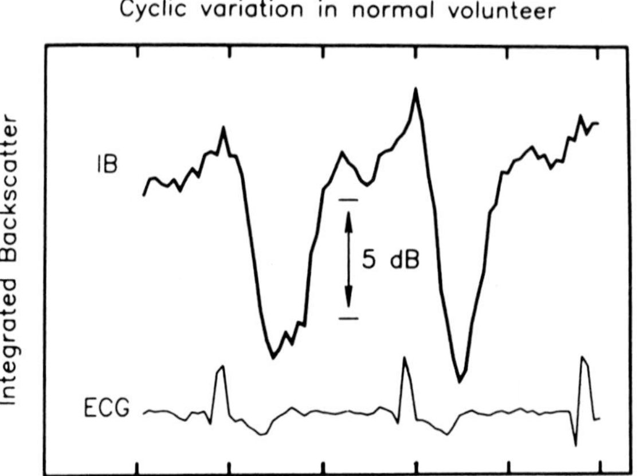

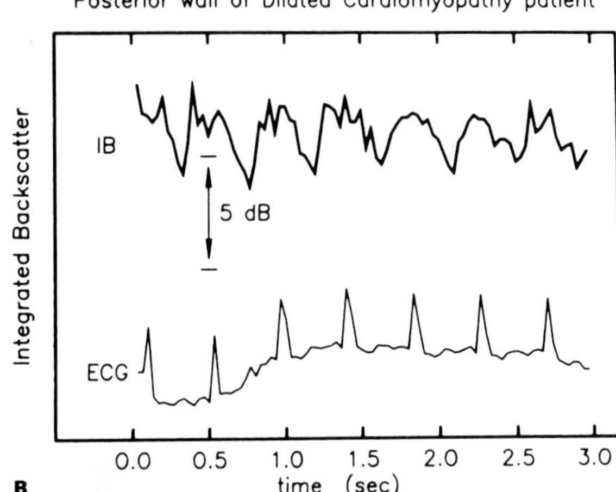

Figure 26–21. Cyclic variation of integrated backscatter in the myocardium of a normal volunteer *(A)* and in the posterior wall of a patient with dilated cardiomyopathy *(B)*. The patient with dilated cardiomyopathy exhibits significantly less cyclic variation of backscatter than does the normal volunteer. (From Vered, Z., Barzilai, B., Mohr, G.A., et al.: Quantitative ultrasonic tissue characterization with real-time integrated backscatter imaging in normal human subjects and in patients with dilated cardiomyopathy. Circulation 76:1067, 1987, with permission of the American Heart Association, Inc.)

In summary, the data on dilated cardiomyopathies indicate that regional echo intensity appears to be increased (although absolute measurements of backscatter have not been accomplished), cyclic variation in backscatter is blunted, and quantitative texture parameters are altered.

Infiltrative/Restrictive Cardiomyopathy

The best-studied infiltrative/restrictive cardiomyopathy is cardiac amyloidosis. Amyloid infiltration of the heart produces increased thickness of chamber walls and valves, which exhibit a waxy, homogeneous appearance on gross examination. On histologic examination, amyloid deposits are found either primarily in the blood vessel walls or diffusely in the myocardial interstitium.[R3] Advanced amyloidosis produces nuclear degeneration and myofibrillar necrosis with atrophy of myofibrils and deposition of lipid or pigment as well as variable myocardial fibrosis.[R3]

The gross echocardiographic morphology of amyloid heart disease is that of concentric left ventricular hypertrophy with a small chamber and abnormal diastolic and, eventually, systolic function.[S14] In addition to these findings, qualitative and quantitative abnormalities of myocardial acoustic properties have been demonstrated.

Qualitative echocardiographic abnormalities in cardiac amyloidosis supplied some of the early motivation for ultrasound myocardial tissue characterization. That is, the common clinical observation of abnormal tissue appearance in echocardiograms of patients with amyloidosis suggested that sufficient information was available in the ultrasound signal to differentiate these patients from normal persons. For example, Siqueira-Filho and associates[S14] noted an unusual "granular sparkling" appearance of the myocardium in 90 percent of their amyloid cases. Chiaramida and associates[C6] reported bright regional myocardial texture in a patient with amyloidosis. In a systematic study of qualitative abnormalities in echocardiographic image texture, Bhandari and Nanda[B3] assessed the histologic and clinical correlates of abnormal texture as displayed on standard two-dimensional echocardiograms. Of seven patients with amyloidosis in their study, three demonstrated "highly refractile echoes" (Fig. 26–22).

Quantitation of acoustic abnormalities in amyloidosis has been limited. Recently, Chandrasekaran and associates evaluated the quantitative characteristics of echocardiographic image texture in patients with amyloid heart disease, hypertrophic cardiomyopathy, and hypertensive left ventricular hypertrophy and in normal persons.[C1] These investigators found that quantitative image texture analysis differentiated amyloidosis from hypertrophic cardiomyopathy and from normal myocardium (Fig. 26–23). Pinamonti and associates[P4] also used quantitative texture measures to differentiate amyloid-infiltrated myocardium from normal tissue in patients.

In summary, qualitative observations and preliminary quantitative analyses support a role for ultrasonic tissue characterization techniques in the diagnosis of infiltrative myopathy. This capability would be especially valuable in cases in which amyloid cardiomyopathy may mimic hypertrophic cardiomyopathy.

Hypertrophic Cardiomyopathy

Hypertrophic cardiomyopathy is characterized by a variable distribution of myofibrillar disarray within the left ventricle. "Classic" hypertrophic cardiomyopathy primarily involves the base of the ventricle septum. However, the idea that abnormal myofibrillar architecture may occur in other regions is supported by more recent observations, including cases in which it is found only in the left ventricular apex and others with fibrillar disarray found diffusely throughout the left ventricular myocardium.[W11] Histologically, muscle fiber hypertrophy, focal fiber degeneration, a "whorled" arrangement of myocardial fibers, and variable areas of fibrosis are observed.

Qualitative echocardiographic observations in hypertrophic cardiomyopathy include ventricular hypertrophy, a normal to small left ventricular cavity, and usually preserved or augmented systolic function. Early in the echocardiographic evaluation of hypertrophic myopathy, abnormalities in qualitative tissue appearance were noted. Martin and associates reported an unusual "ground-glass" texture in the ventricular septum of some patients with hypertrophic cardiomyopathy.[M4] In the study mentioned above, Bhandari and Nanda[B3] noted that the majority of cases of hypertrophic cardiomyopathy in their review exhibited bright echoes (which was, unfortunately, a somewhat nonspecific finding).

In the quantitative texture analytic study mentioned above, Chandrasekaran and associates[C1] were able to differentiate hypertrophic cardiomyopathy from amyloidosis and from normal myocardium based on quantitative features of echocardiographic image texture (see Fig. 26–23).

In summary, a small number of studies suggest that the altered architecture and fibrosis of hypertrophic cardiomyopathy may produce diagnostic abnormalities in cardiac acoustic properties.

Experimental Cardiomyopathy

Two sets of observations in animal models of cardiomyopathy also support a place for ultrasound tissue characterization in these disorders. Mimbs and associates[M16] administered doxorubicin to rabbits to produce an anthracycline-induced cardiomyopathy. Increases in ultrasound integrated backscatter were found in cardiomyopathic and fibrotic tissue in this model. Perez and associates[P5] reported the acoustic accompaniments of the spontaneous cardiomyopathy that occurs in the Syrian hamster; the investigators noted increased regional ultrasound backscatter and

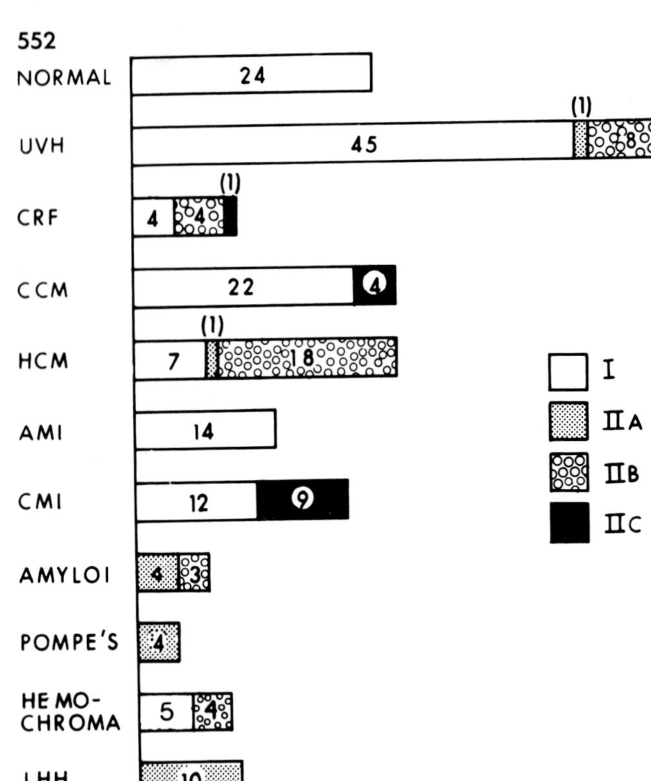

Figure 26–22. Qualitative texture analysis based on clinical echocardiographic data. The graph shows types of myocardial texture observed in various categories of diseases. Myocardial texture is classified as normal (I—a fine, speckled homogeneous appearance) or abnormal (IIA and IIB—multiple small and discrete highly refractile echoes superimposed on finely speckled echoes; IIC—long, linear or broad patches of bright myocardium). Note that in several disorders the majority of patients exhibited qualitative abnormalities of myocardial texture. UVH—uncomplicated ventricular hypertrophy; CRF—chronic renal failure; CCM—congestive cardiomyopathy; HCM—hypertrophic cardiomyopathy; AMI—acute myocardial infarction; CMI—chronic myocardial infarction; AMYLOI—amyloidosis; LHH—left heart hypoplastic syndrome. (From Bhandari, A.K., and Nanda, N.C.: Myocardial texture characterization by two-dimensional echocardiography. Am. J. Cardiol. 51:817, 1983, with permission.)

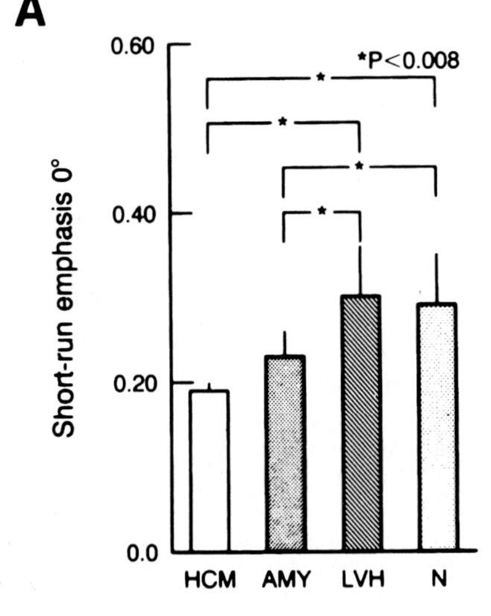

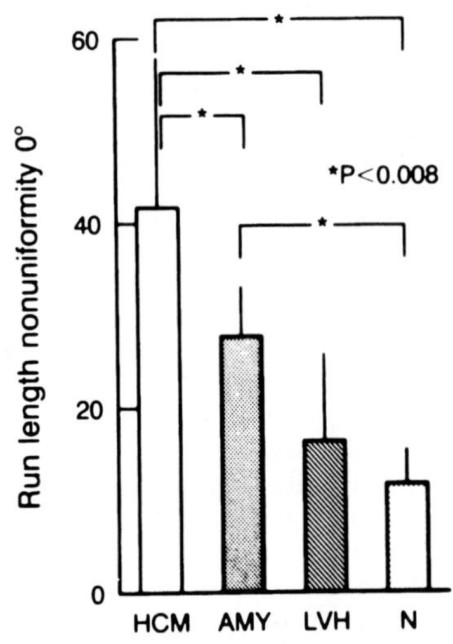

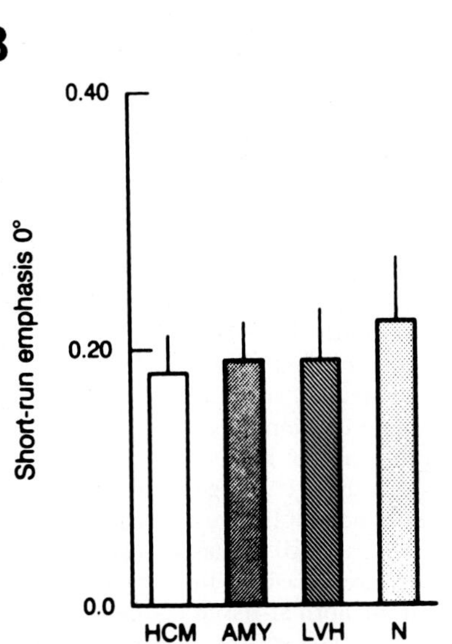

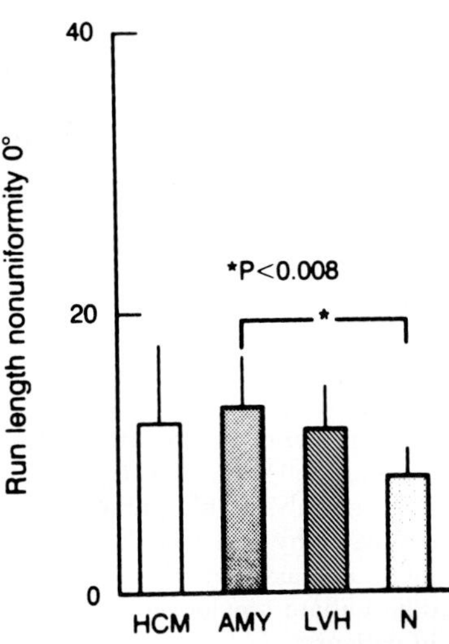

Figure 26–23. Differentiation of cardiomyopathies from normal myocardium in clinical echocardiograms based on quantitative texture analysis. The graphs show selected gray level run length data obtained from end-diastolic long-axis clinical echocardiographic views of the ventricular septum *(A)* and posterior left ventricular wall *(B)* in patients with hypertrophic cardiomyopathy (HCM), amyloidosis (AMY), and left ventricular hypertrophy (LVH) and in normal persons (N). Quantitative parameters were able to differentiate both cardiomyopathies from normal and from each other. (From Chandrasekaran, K., Aylward, P.E., Fleagle, S.R., et al.: Feasibility of identifying amyloid and hypertrophic cardiomyopathy with the use of computerized quantitative texture analysis of clinical echocardiographic data. J. Am. Coll. Cardiol. 13:832, 1989. Reprinted with permission of the American College of Cardiology.)

increased heterogeneity of backscatter within regions of calcification and fibrosis.

In summary, ultrasound tissue characterization techniques show promise for identifying each of the major categories of clinical cardiomyopathies. Clinical data are preliminary, however, and standardization techniques have not yet been achieved.

Intracardiac Masses

Echocardiography is widely used to identify the presence and some characteristics of intracardiac masses. Conventional two-dimensional echocardiography is generally accepted to be one of the most sensitive techniques for the identification of left atrial myxomas[F6] and ventricular thrombi.[V3] Nonetheless, definitive identification of an intracardiac mass may sometimes be difficult because of confounding echocardiographic reverberations or other sources of noise. Further, layered, nonprotruding ventricular thrombi or false tendons may sometimes be difficult to distinguish from a thickened myocardium, particularly when walls are imaged through an oblique plane. For these reasons, there has been interest in ultrasound characterization of intracardiac masses. Most of the work in this area has focused on intracardiac thrombi or cardiac myxomas.

Intracardiac Thrombus

The acoustic properties of blood change substantially with the process of thrombus formation. Shung and associates[S15] found that by 24 hours after clot formation, ultrasound backscatter from human blood increased by almost 19 dB when evaluated with a 7.5-MHz transducer. Bhandari and associates[B5] noted an unusual, speckled echocardiographic texture in thrombi (which was somewhat nonspecific and similar to that found in tumors). In a more quantitative approach to assessment of the acoustic properties of ventricular thrombus, Green and associates[G4] utilized stochastic analysis of radio-frequency ultrasound data to differentiate thrombus from artifact and intracardiac tumor. McPherson and associates[M17] evaluated the first-order gray level statistics of experimental ventricular thrombi in acutely infarcted dogs. These investigators showed that mean gray level, standard deviation, and skewness of regional gray levels all distinguished thrombus from intracavitary blood and that mean gray level and standard deviation distinguished thrombus from adjacent myocardium in views in which the regions of interest could be placed at similar depths of field (thus yielding data at approximately the same point along the time-gain compensation profile). Recent preliminary work with a real-time backscatter imaging system suggests that ventricular thrombi exhibit no significant cyclic variation of backscatter and have increased localized integrated backscatter compared to surrounding blood and adjacent myocardium.[V4] In addition to the identification of a cardiac mass as a thrombus, ultrasound tissue characterization techniques may offer insight into the embolic potential of a thrombus. Lloret and associates[L5] showed that selected quantitative texture features of human intraventricular thrombi were of value in classifying thrombi as potentially embolic.

Myxoma

Only very preliminary data have been gathered on the acoustic properties of atrial myxomas. Green and associates,[G4] using the stochastic analysis method mentioned above, were able to differentiate tumor from thrombus within the heart; the tumor was, however, not differentiated from artifact in that study.

Vegetations

Recently, Tak and associates[T5] evaluated the echo amplitude characteristics of active versus healed valvular vegetations due to infective endocarditis. Active (acute, culture-positive) vegetations exhibited relatively low echo amplitude, and the echo amplitude increased during healing. Presumably, these changes in echo amplitude were due to collagen deposition as vegetations healed.

Myocardial Contusion

Acute myocardial contusion causes a variety of pathologic sequelae including intramyocardial hematomas and hemopericardium. Using an experimental model of myocardial contusion, Skorton and associates showed that the quantitative features of echocardiographic image texture differentiated contused from normal myocardium.[S4]

Atherosclerosis

There has been growing interest in characterization of the acoustic properties of the vascular wall in order to identify and define the composition of atherosclerotic plaque noninvasively. Wolverson and associates utilized a high-resolution scanner to image aortic and iliac vessels in vitro.[W12] Fibrous, fibrofatty, and calcified lesions could be qualitatively differentiated by their characteristic ultrasonic image. Picano and associates[P6] quantitatively assessed normal and atherosclerotic specimens of excised abdominal aorta. They demonstrated increased integrated backscatter index in fibrofatty and calcified regions.

Barzilai and associates[B6] have shown that quantitative measurements of integrated backscatter differentiated calcified and fibrous regions from fibrofatty regions of human aorta (Fig. 26–24). McPherson and associates[M18] utilized high-frequency epicardial echocardiography intraoperatively to assess the acoustic characteristics of coronary arteries of patients at the time of cardiac surgery. They demonstrated significant differences in the average gray level between atherosclerotic and normal coronary arterial wall. Early experience with intravascular ultrasound methods (i.e., catheter-mounted transducers) has also shown differences between qualitative and quantitative acoustic features of normal and atherosclerotic tissue.[G5, L6] Thus, quantitative estimates of the energy reflected by the arterial wall give some insight into the composition of normal and atherosclerotic plaque in aorta, iliac, and coronary arteries.

Other investigators have utilized the angle dependence of scattering to characterize arterial tissue. Shung and associates[S16] described a technique in which an oblique beam angle is used to limit the effect of the initial specular echo. Picano and associates measured the angle dependence of ultrasonic backscatter in arterial tissues.[P7] A very directive pattern with a strongly angle-dependent backscatter was typical of calcified and fibrous plaques. Fatty samples were characterized by a nondirective pattern that was not significantly dependent on the angle of incidence of the ultrasonic beam.

These observations suggest that definition of the composition of atherosclerotic plaque may be feasible with quantitative ultrasonic techniques. These methods are potentially applicable for the identification of peripheral vascular atherosclerosis and coronary atherosclerosis when used intraoperatively or with the use of intravascular ultrasonic catheters in the future.

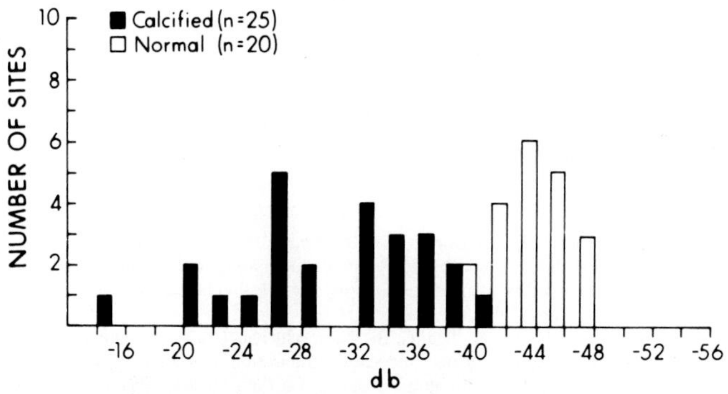

Figure 26–24. Distribution of echo amplitudes in normal and calcified aortic tissue. Calcified tissue exhibited significantly higher integrated backscatter values than normal aortic tissue. (From Barzilai, B., Saffitz, J.E., Miller, J.G., and Sobel, B.E.: Quantitative ultrasonic characterization of the nature of atherosclerotic plaques in human aorta. Circ. Res. 60:459, 1987, with permission of the American Heart Association, Inc.)

CONCLUSIONS

Abundant experimental evidence supports the idea that ultrasound interacts differently with normal and abnormal cardiovascular tissue. Ultrasonic tissue characterization techniques have been shown by a variety of methods and different investigative groups to be accurate in identifying acute myocardial ischemia, reperfusion, infarction, and scar deposition. Cardiomyopathies, intracardiac masses, and atherosclerotic plaque also may be characterized by using ultrasonic analysis methods. Although these techniques are still considered investigational, very promising recent clinical results support their potential in the clinical setting. Certainly, much further work remains to be accomplished before widespread clinical application can be strongly endorsed. In particular, the various stages of acute myocardial infarction cannot currently be differentiated solely on the basis of time-averaged backscatter or cyclic backscatter variation. Adding information on the frequency dependence of backscatter may help to make this clinically critical distinction.[W10] Techniques based on analysis of echocardiographic image (gray level) data are quite dependent on instrumentation variables such as user adjustments of the imaging system. These instrumentation-related sources of variability will need to be minimized by standardization of the data acquisition method or by correction for variations in instrument settings. Improvements in methods of gain compensation for attenuation will also be an important step toward more routine utilization of ultrasonic tissue characterization.

Despite these remaining problems, the long history of successful experimental observations with ultrasonic tissue characterization techniques and recent clinical observations support further development of this diagnostic approach to myocardial and vascular structural characteristics.

References

A

1. Abbot, J. G., and Thurstone, F. L.: Acoustic speckle: Theory and experimental analysis. Ultrason. Imag. 1:303, 1979.
2. Aylward, P. E., McPherson, D. D., Kerber, R. E., et al.: Ultrasound tissue characterization in ischemic heart disease. Echocardiography 3:385, 1986.
3. Angermann, C. E., Hart, F. J., Stempfle, U., et al.: Frame-by-frame quantitation of myocardial backscatter: Analysis of standard 2D echo images and radiofrequency signals. (Abstract.) Circulation 74:II–270, 1987.

B

1. Burckhardt, C. B.: Speckle in ultrasound B-mode scans. IEEE Trans. Sonics Ultrasonics SU–25:1, 1978.
2. Barzilai, B., Thomas, L. J., III, Glueck, R. M., et al.: Detection of remote myocardial infarction with quantitative real-time ultrasonic tissue characterization. J. Am. Soc. Echo. 1:179, 1988.
3. Bhandari, A. K., and Nanda, N. C.: Myocardial texture characterization by two-dimensional echocardiography. Am. J. Cardiol. 51:817, 1983.
4. Barzilai, B., Madaras, E. I., Sobel, B. E., et al.: Effects of myocardial contraction on ultrasonic backscatter before and after ischemia. Am. J. Physiol. 247:H478, 1984.
5. Bhandari, A. K., Nanda, N. C., and Hicks, D. G.: Two-dimensional echocardiography of intracardiac masses: Echo pattern–histopathology correlation. Ultrasound Med. Biol. 8:673, 1982.
6. Barzilai, B., Saffitz, J. E., Miller, J. G., and Sobel, B. E.: Quantitative ultrasonic characterization of the nature of atherosclerotic plaques in human aorta. Circ. Res. 60:459, 1987.

C

1. Chandrasekaran, K., Aylward, P. E., Fleagle, S. R., et al.: Feasibility of identifying amyloid and hypertrophic cardiomyopathy with the use of computerized quantitative texture analysis of clinical echocardiographic data. J. Am. Coll. Cardiol. 13:832, 1989.
2. Chandraratna, P. A. N., Ulene, R., Nimalasuriya, C., et al.: Differentiation between acute and healed myocardial infarction by signal averaging and color-encoding echocardiography. Am. J. Cardiol. 56:381, 1984.
3. Caulfield, J. B., and Borg, T. K.: The collagen network of the heart. Lab. Invest. 40:364, 1979.
4. Collins, S. M., Skorton, D. J., Prasad, N. V., et al.: Quantitative echocardiographic image texture: Normal contraction-related variability. IEEE Trans. Med. Imag. 4:185, 1985.
5. Chandrasekaran, K., Chu, A., Greenleaf, J. F., et al.: 2D echo quantitative texture analysis of acutely ischemic myocardium. (Abstract.) Circulation 74:II–271, 1986.
6. Chiaramida, S. A., Goldman, M. A., Zema, M. J., et al.: Real-time cross-sectional echocardiographic diagnosis of infiltrative cardiomyopathy due to amyloid. J. Clin. Ultrasound 8:58, 1980.

D

1. Davies, J., Gibson, D. G., Foale, R., et al.: Echocardiographic features of eosinophilic endomyocardial disease. Br. Heart J. 48:434, 1982.

F

1. Falsetti, H.L., Marcus, M.L., Kerber, R. E., and Skorton, D. J.: Quantification of myocardial ischemia and infarction by left ventricular imaging. (Editorial.) Circulation 63:747, 1981.
2. Fei, D. Y., and Shung, K. K.: Ultrasonic backscatter from mammalian tissues. J. Acoust. Soc. Am. 78:871, 1985.
3. Fitzgerald, P. J., McDaniel, M. M., Rolett, E. L., et al.: Two-dimensional ultrasonic variation in myocardium throughout the cardiac cycle. Ultrason. Imag. 8:241, 1986.
4. Fitzgerald, P. J., McDaniel, M. D., Rolett, E. L., et al.: Two-dimensional ultrasonic tissue characterization: Backscatter power, endocardial wall motion and their phase relationship for normal, ischemic and infarcted myocardium. Circulation 76:850, 1987.
5. Fraker, T. D., Jr., Nelson, A. D., Arthur, J. A., and Wilkerson, R. D.: Altered acoustic reflectance on two-dimensional echocardiography as an early predictor of myocardial infarct size. Am. J. Cardiol. 53:1699, 1984.
6. Fyke, F. E., Seward, J. B., Edwards, W. D., et al.: Primary cardiac tumors: Experience with 30 consecutive patients since the introduction of two-dimensional echocardiography. J. Am. Coll. Cardiol. 5:1465, 1985.

G

1. Galloway, M. M.: Texture analysis using gray level run lengths. Comput. Graph. Image Process. 4:172, 1975.
2. Glueck, R. M., Mottley, J. G., Miller, J. G., et al.: Effect of coronary artery occlusion and reperfusion on cardiac cycle–dependent variation of myocardial ultrasonic backscatter. Circ. Res. 56:683, 1985.
3. Glueck, R. M., Mottley, J. G., Sobel, B. E., et al.: Changes in ultrasonic attenuation and backscatter of muscle with state of contraction. Ultrasound Med. Biol. 11:605, 1985.
4. Green, S. E., Joynt, L. F., Fitzgerald, P. J., et al.: In vivo ultrasonic tissue characterization of human intracardiac masses. Am. J. Cardiol. 51:231, 1983.
5. Gussenhoven, E. J., Essed, C. E., Lancee, C. T., et al.: Arterial wall characteristics determined by intravascular ultrasound imaging: An in vitro study. (Abstract.) J. Am. Coll. Cardiol. 14:947, 1989.

H

1. Haendchen, R. V., Ong, K., Fishbein, M. C., et al.: Early differentiation of infarcted and noninfarcted reperfused myocardium in dogs by quantitative analysis of regional myocardial echo amplitudes. Circ. Res. 57:718, 1985.
2. Hoyt, R. H., Collins, S. M., Skorton, D. J., et al.: Assessment of fibrosis in infarcted human hearts by analysis of ultrasonic backscatter. Circulation 71:740, 1985.
3. Hoyt, R. H., Skorton, D. J., Collins, S. M., and Melton, H. E.: Ultrasonic backscatter and collagen in normal ventricular myocardium. Circulation 69:775, 1984.
4. Hikichi, H., and Tanaka, M.: Ultrasono-cardiotomographic evaluation of histologic changes in myocardial infarction. Jpn. Heart J. 22:287, 1981.
5. Hajduczki, I., Jaffe, M., Areeda, J., et al.: Ultrasonic backscatter and 2D echocardiographic wall motion analysis during PTCA. (Abstract.) Circulation 778:II–442, 1988.

K

1. Kremkau, F. W.: Ultrasound. *In* Kremkau, F.W. (ed.): Diagnostic Ultrasound: Physical Principles and Exercises. Grune & Stratton, New York, 1980, p. 5.
2. Kolosov, O. V., Levin, V. M., Mayev, R. G., and Senjushkina, T. A.: The use of acoustic microscopy for biological tissue characterization. Ultrasound Med. Biol. 13:477, 1987.

L

1. Linzer, M. (ed.): Ultrasonic tissue characterization. II. National Bureau of Standards Special Publication 525. U.S. Government Printing Office, Washington, D.C., 1979.
2. Logan-Sinclair, R. B., Wong, C. M., and Gibson, D. G.: Clinical applications of amplitude processing of echocardiographic images. Br. Heart J. 45:621, 1981.
3. Linker, D. T., Angelsen, B. A. J., and Popp, R. L.: Acoustic microscopy of normal and myopathic human myocardium: Implications for ultrasonic tissue characterization. (Abstract.) J. Am. Coll. Cardiol. 9:211A, 1987.
4. Lele, P. P., and Namery, J.: A computer-based ultrasonic system for the detection and mapping of myocardial infarcts. Proc. San Diego Biomed. Symp. 13:121, 1974.
5. Lloret, R. L., Cortada, X., Bradford, J., et al.: Classification of left ventricular thrombi by their history of systemic embolization using pattern recognition of two-dimensional echocardiograms. Am. Heart J. 110:761, 1985.

6. Linker, D. R., Yock, P. G., Thapliyal, H. V., et al.: In vitro analysis of backscattered amplitude from normal and diseased arteries using a new intraluminal ultrasonic catheter. (Abstract.) J. Am. Coll. Cardiol. 11:4A, 1988.

M

1. Miller, J. G., Perez, J. E., and Sobel, B. E.: Ultrasonic characterization of myocardium. Prog. Cardiovasc. Dis. 28:85, 1985.
2. Miller, J. G., Perez, J. E., Mottley, J. G., et al.: Myocardial tissue characterization: An approach based on quantitative backscatter and attenuation. Proc. IEEE Ultrason. Symp. 83CH1947–1:782, 1983.
3. Milunski, M., Canter, C. E., Wickline, S. A., et al.: Cardiac cycle–dependent variation of integrated backscatter is not distorted by abnormal myocardial wall motion in human subjects with paradoxical septal motion. Ultrasound Med. Biol. 15:311, 1989.
4. Martin, R. D., Rakowski, H., French, J., and Popp, R. L.: Idiopathic hypertrophic subaortic stenosis viewed by wide-angle phased-array echocardiography. Circulation 59:1206, 1979.
5. Melton, H. E., and Skorton, D. J.: Rational gain compensation for attenuation in cardiac ultrasonography. Ultrason. Imag. 5:214, 1983.
6. Mimbs, J. W., O'Donnell, M., Bauwens, D., et al.: The dependence of ultrasonic attenuation and backscatter on collagen content in dog and rabbit hearts. Circ. Res. 47:49, 1980.
7. Mottley, J. G., and Miller, J. G.: Anisotropy of the ultrasonic backscatter of myocardial tissue. I. Theory and measurements in vitro. J. Acoust. Soc. Am. 83:755, 1988.
8. Madaras, E. I., Perez, J. E., Sobel, B. E., et al.: Anisotropy of the ultrasonic backscatter of myocardial tissue. II. Measurements in vivo. J. Acoust. Soc. Am. 83:762, 1988.
9. Mimbs, J. W., Bauwens, D., Cohen, R. D., et al.: Effects of myocardial ischemia on quantitative ultrasonic backscatter and identification of responsible determinants. Circ. Res. 49:89, 1981.
10. Madaras, E. I., Barzilai, B., Perez, J. E., et al.: Changes in myocardial backscatter throughout the cardiac cycle. Ultrason. Imag. 5:229, 1983.
11. Mimbs, J. W., O'Donnell, M., Miller, J. G., and Sobel, B. E.: Changes in ultrasonic attenuation indicative of early myocardial ischemic injury. Am. J. Physiol. 236:H340, 1979.
12. McPherson, D. D., Aylward, P. E., Knosp, B. M., et al.: Ultrasound characterization of acute myocardial ischemia by quantitative texture analysis. Ultrason. Imag. 8:227, 1986.
13. Milunski, M. R., Mohr, G. A., Wear, K. A., et al.: Early identification with ultrasonic integrated backscatter of viable but stunned myocardium in dogs. J. Am. Coll. Cardiol. 14:462, 1989.
14. Milunski, M. R., Mohr, G. A., Perez, J. E., et al.: Ultrasonic tissue characterization with integrated backscatter: Acute myocardial ischemia, reperfusion, and stunned myocardium in patients. Circulation 80:491, 1989.
15. Mimbs, J. W., Yuhas, D. E., Miller, J. G., et al.: Detection of myocardial infarction in vitro based on altered attenuation of ultrasound. Circ. Res. 41:192, 1977.
16. Mimbs, J. W., O'Donnell, M., Miller, J. G., and Sobel, B. E.: Detection of cardiomyopathic changes induced by doxorubicin based on quantitative analysis of ultrasonic backscatter. Am. J. Cardiol. 47:1056, 1981.
17. McPherson, D. D., Knosp, B. M., Kieso, R. A., et al.: Ultrasound characterization of acoustic properties of acute intracardiac thrombi: Studies in a new experimental model. J. Am. Soc. Echo. 1:264, 1988.
18. McPherson, D. D., Sirna, S. J., Haugen, J. A., et al.: Acoustic properties of normal and atherosclerotic human coronary arteries: In vitro and in vivo observations. (Abstract.) Circulation 76:IV–43, 1987.

N

1. Namery, J., and Lele, P. P.: Ultrasonic detection of myocardial infarction in dog. Proc. IEEE Ultrason. Symp. 72CH0708–8 SU:491, 1972.

O

1. O'Donnell, M., Bauwens, D., Mimbs, J. W., and Miller, J.G.: Broadband integrated backscatter: An approach to spatially localized tissue characterization in vivo. Proc. IEEE Ultrason. Symp. 79CH1482–9:175, 1979.
2. O'Donnell, M., Mimbs, J. W., and Miller, J. G.: The relationship between collagen and ultrasonic backscatter in myocardial tissue. J. Acoust. Soc. Am. 69:580, 1981.
3. O'Donnell, M., Mimbs, J. W., and Miller, J. G.: The relationship between collagen and ultrasonic attenuation in myocardial tissue. J. Acoust. Soc. Am. 65:512, 1979.
4. Olshansky, B., Collins, S. M., Skorton, D. J., and Prasad, N. V.: Variation of left ventricular myocardial gray level in two-dimensional echocardiograms as a result of cardiac contraction. Circulation 70:972, 1984.

P

1. Perez, J. E., Madaras, E. I., Sobel, B. E., and Miller, J.G.: Quantitative myocardial characterization with ultrasound. Automedica 5:201, 1984.
2. Parisi, A. F., Nieminen, M., O'Boyle, J. E., et al.: Enhanced detection of the evolution of tissue changes after acute myocardial infarction using color-coded two-dimensional echocardiography. Circulation 66:764, 1982.
3. Perez, J. E., Miller, J. G., Barzilai, B., et al.: Progress in quantitative ultrasonic characterization of myocardium: From the laboratory to the bedside. J. Am. Soc. Echo. 1:294, 1988.
4. Pinamonti, B., Picano, E., Ferdeghina, E. M., et al.: Quantitative texture analysis in two-dimensional echocardiography: Application to the diagnosis of myocardial amyloidosis. J. Am. Coll. Cardiol. 14:666, 1989.
5. Perez, J. E., Barzilai, B., Madaras, E. I., et al.: Applicability of ultrasonic tissue characterization for longitudinal assessment and differentiation of calcification and fibrosis in cardiomyopathy. J. Am. Coll. Cardiol. 4:88, 1984.
6. Picano, E., Landini, L., Distante, A., et al.: Different degrees of atherosclerosis detected by backscattered ultrasound: An in vitro study on fixed human aortic walls. J. Clin. Ultrasound 11:375, 1983.
7. Picano, E., Landini, L., Distante, A., et al.: Angle dependence of ultrasonic backscatter in arterial tissues: A study in vitro. Circulation 72:572, 1985.

R

1. Rasmussen, S., Corya, B. C., Feigenbaum, H., and Knoebel, S.B.: Detection of myocardial scar tissue by M-mode echocardiography. Circulation 57:230, 1978.
2. Rasmussen, S., Lovelace, E., Knoebel, S. B., et al.: Echocardiographic detection of ischemic and infarcted myocardium. J. Am. Coll. Cardiol. 3:733, 1984.
3. Rubinow, A.: Amyloidosis. *In* Stein, J. H. (ed.): Internal Medicine. 2nd ed. Little, Brown, Boston, 1987, p. 1354.

S

1. Skorton, D. J., and Collins, S. M.: Characterization of myocardial structure with ultrasound. *In* Greenleaf, J. (ed.): Tissue Characterization with Ultrasound. Vol. II. Results and Applications. CRC Press, Boca Raton, Fla., 1986, p. 123.
2. Shawker, T. H., Garra, B. S., and Insana, M. F.: Ultrasonic tissue characterization: Fundamental concepts and clinical applications. *In* Sanders, R. C., and Hill, M. C. (eds.): Ultrasound Annual 1985. Raven Press, New York, 1985, p. 93.
3. Skorton, D. J., Melton, H. E., Jr., Pandian, N. G., et al.: Detection of acute myocardial infarction in closed-chest dogs by analysis of regional two-dimensional echocardiographic gray-level distributions. Circ. Res. 52:36, 1983.
4. Skorton, D. J., Collins, S. M., Nichols, J., et al.: Quantitative texture analysis in two-dimensional echocardiography: Application to the diagnosis of experimental myocardial contusion. Circulation 68:217, 1983.
5. Shaw, T. R. D., Logan-Sinclair, R. B., Surin, C., et al.: Relation between regional echo intensity and myocardial connective tissue in chronic left ventricular disease. Br. Heart J. 51:46, 1984.
6. Shimazu, T., Nishioka, H., Fujiwara, M., et al.: Quantitative integrated backscatter characterization in canine myocardium. J. Cardiogr. 16:799, 1986.
7. Shung, K. K., and Reid, J. M.: Ultrasonic scattering from tissue. Proc. IEEE Ultrason. Symp. CH12364-ISU:230, 1977.
8. Streeter, D. D., Jr., and Hanna, W. T.: Engineering mechanics for successive states in canine left ventricular myocardium. II. Fiber angle and sarcomere length. Circ. Res. 33:656, 1973.
9. Skorton, D. J., and Collins, S. M.: Clinical potential of ultrasound tissue characterization in cardiomyopathies. J. Am. Soc. Echo. 1:69, 1988.
10. Sagar, K. B., Rhyne, T. L., Wartlier, D. C., et al.: Intramyocardial variability in integrated backscatter: Effects of coronary occlusion and reperfusion. Circulation 75:436, 1987.
11. Sabbah, H. N., Marzilli, M., and Stein, P. D.: The relative role of subendocardium and subepicardium in left ventricular mechanics. Am. J. Physiol. 240:H920, 1981.
12. Schnittger, I. A., Vieli, A., Heiserman, J. E., et al.: Ultrasonic tissue characterization: Detection of acute myocardial ischemia in dogs. Circulation 72:193, 1985.
13. Sedlis, S. P., Saffitz, J. E., Schwob, V. S., and Jaffe, A. S.: Cardiac amyloidosis simulating hypertrophic cardiomyopathy. Am. J. Cardiol. 53:969, 1984.
14. Siqueira-Filho, A. G., Cunha, C. L. P., Tajik, A. J., et al.: M-Mode and two-dimensional echocardiographic features in cardiac amyloidosis. Circulation 63:188, 1981.
15. Shung, K. K., Fei, D. Y., Yuan, Y. W., and Reeves, W. C.: Ultrasonic characterization of blood during coagulation. J. Clin. Ultrasound 12:147, 1984.
16. Shung, K. K., Hughes, D., Yujani, Y. W., and Thiele, B. L.: C-mode imaging of arterial atherosclerotic lesion surfaces using oblique incidence. (Abstract.) Ultrason. Imag. 9:47, 1987.

T

1. Thomas, L. J., III, Wickline, S. A., Perez, J. E., et al.: A real-time integrated backscatter measurement system for quantitative cardiac tissue characterization. IEEE Trans. Ultrason. Ferroelectric Freq. Control UFFC–33:27, 1986.
2. Thomas, L. J., III, Barzilai, B., Perez, J. E., et al.: Quantitative real-time imaging of myocardium based on ultrasonic integrated backscatter. IEEE Trans. Ultrason. Ferroelectric Freq. Control 36:466, 1989.
3. Tanaka, M., Teresawa, Y., and Hikichi, H.: Qualitative evaluation of the heart tissue by ultrasound. J. Cardiogr. 7:515, 1977.
4. Topol, E. G., Traill, T. A., and Fortuin, N. J.: Hypertensive hypertrophic cardiomyopathy of the elderly. N. Engl. J. Med. 312:277, 1985.
5. Tak, T., Rahimtoola, S. H., Kumar, A., et al.: Value of digital image processing of two-dimensional echocardiograms in differentiating active from chronic vegetations of infective endocarditis. Circulation 78:116, 1988.

V

1. Vered, Z., Barzilai, B., Mohr, G. A., et al.: Quantitative ultrasonic tissue characterization with real-time integrated backscatter imaging in normal human subjects and in patients with dilated cardiomyopathy. Circulation 76:1067, 1987.
2. Vered, Z., Barzilai, B., Gessler, C. J., et al.: Ultrasonic integrated backscatter tissue characterization of remote myocardial infarction in human subjects. J. Am. Coll. Cardiol. 13:84, 1989.
3. Visser, C. A., Kan, G., David, G. K., et al.: Two-dimensional echocardiography in the diagnosis of left ventricular thrombus: A prospective study of 67 patients with anatomic validation. Chest 83:228, 1983.
4. Vandenberg, B. F., Kieso, R. A., Fox-Eastham, K., et al.: Characterization of acute experimental left ventricular thrombi with quantitative backscatter imaging. Circulation 81:1017, 1990.

W

1. Wallis, D. E., O'Connell, J. B., Henkin, R. E., et al.: Segmental wall motion abnormalities in dilated cardiomyopathy: A common finding and good prognostic sign. J. Am. Coll. Cardiol. 4:674, 1984.
2. Wild, J. J., Crafford, H. D., and Reid, J. M.: Visualization of the excised human heart by means of reflected ultrasound or echography. Am. Heart J. 54:903, 1957.
3. Weszka, J. S., Dyer, C. R., and Rosenfeld, A.: A comparative study of texture measures for terrain classification. IEEE Trans. Syst. Man Cybern. SMC-6:269, 1976.
4. Wickline, S. A., Thomas, L. J., III, Miller, J. G., et al.: A relationship between ultrasonic integrated backscatter and myocardial contractile function. J. Clin. Invest. 76:2151, 1985.
5. Wickline, S. A., Thomas, L. J., III, Miller, J. G., et al.: Sensitive detection of the effects of reperfusion on myocardium by ultrasonic tissue characterization with integrated backscatter. Circulation 74:389, 1986.
6. Wickline, S. A., Mohr, G. A., Shoup, T. A., et al.: Delineation of improved contractile performance after thrombolysis in acute myocardial infarction with real-time two-dimensional ultrasonic integrated backscatter. (Abstract.) J. Am. Coll. Cardiol. 11:99A, 1988.
7. Wickline, S. A., Thomas, L. J., III, Miller, J. G., et al.: The dependence of myocardial ultrasonic integrated backscatter on contractile performance. Circulation 72:183, 1985.
8. Wear, K. A., Shoup, T. A., and Popp, R. L.: Ultrasonic characterization of canine myocardial contraction. IEEE Trans. Ultrason. Ferrelectric Freq. Control 33:347, 1986.
9. Werner, J. A., Speck, S. M., Greene, H. L., et al.: Discrete intramural sonolucency: A new echocardiographic finding in acute myocardial infarction. (Abstract.) Am. J. Cardiol. 47:404, 1981.
10. Wear, K. A., Milunski, M. R., Wickline, S. A., et al.: Differentiation between acutely ischemic myocardium and zones of completed infarction on the basis of frequency dependent backscatter. J. Acoust. Soc. Am. 85:2634, 1989.
11. Wynne, J., and Braunwald, E.: The cardiomyopathies and myocarditides. *In* Braunwald, E. (ed.): Heart Disease: A Textbook of Cardiovascular Medicine, Vol. 2, 3rd ed. W. B. Saunders, Philadelphia, 1988, p. 1410.
12. Wolverson, M. K., Bashiti, H. M., and Peterson, G. J.: Ultrasonic tissue characterization of atheromatous plaques using a high resolution real-time scanner. Ultrasound Med. Biol. 9:599, 1983.

Chapter 27

Contrast Echocardiography

▪ *STEVEN B. FEINSTEIN, M.D.* ▪ *PAOLO VOCI, M.D.*
▪ *LAWRENCE J. SEGIL, M.D.* ▪ *PAUL V. HARPER, M.D.*

CONTRAST AGENT DEVELOPMENT 558
Manually Produced Contrast Agents (Hand-Agitated) 558
Sonicated Contrast Agents 558
Hand-Agitation and Sonication Techniques Compared 559
Safety and Efficacy Studies 559
QUANTIFICATION 560
The Contrast Agent 560
Ultrasound Equipment 560
Mathematical Model for Perfusion Imaging 561
EXPERIMENTAL AND CLINICAL PERFUSION STUDIES 565
Assessment of Area at Risk 565
Assessment of Perfusion of Cardioplegic Solutions 565
Detection of Myocardial Ischemia 567
Studies of the Coronary Collateral Circulation .. 568
Advantages and Disadvantages of Contrast Echocardiography for Studies of Myocardial Perfusion 568
OTHER CARDIAC APPLICATIONS OF CONTRAST ECHOCARDIOGRAPHY 568
Measurement of Cardiac Output 568
Right Heart Studies 568
Intracardiac Shunts 568
Left Heart Studies 569
SUMMARY 572

Current contrast echocardiography research focuses on the development of a relatively simple, safe and economic method of noninvasively imaging and quantifying regional myocardial perfusion and blood volume distribution in patients. This chapter discusses recent developments in contrast echocardiography and associated issues requiring continued research. Theoretic, experimental, and clinical work is described. In particular, this chapter focuses on (1) the development of an intravenously injectable contrast agent, (2) recent design improvements in ultrasound hardware to enable mathematical analysis of perfusion data, based on linearization of the ultrasound signal, and eventual quantification of regional perfusion, and (3) newly derived and validated mathematical models calculating blood flow based upon classic dye dilution theory. In addition, this chapter describes current and future clinical applications of contrast echocardiography, as well as early clinical applications that were primarily limited to the study of gross cardiac structures and abnormalities.

Perfusion imaging studies at present are being performed on an experimental basis in patients in the setting of cardiac catheterization, angioplasty, and cardiac operations. The combined use of contrast echocardiography and angioplasty or surgical therapy provides anatomic and functional perfusion parameters for the evaluation of coronary artery disease. In addition, intravenously injectable contrast agents are being developed and tested clinically; if successful, they will permit the use of contrast echocardiography for perfusion assessment in outpatients for screening and follow-up purposes, because of the noninvasive nature of the procedure and the portability and safety of the ultrasound equipment. Transthoracic and transesophageal contrast echocardiographic techniques also are being developed. If these contrast echocardiographic techniques and agents withstand rigorous safety and efficacy studies, this imaging modality may become a useful tool in the management of patients with ischemic heart disease, either in combination with interventional therapy or potentially as a screening technique.

Contrast echocardiographic perfusion imaging would be particularly important to the clinical management of patients with ischemic heart disease because the majority of cardiovascular diseases are characterized by the alteration of blood flow and volume. Coronary angiography, an accepted standard for evaluating coronary artery disease, provides a planar image of the lumen of epicardial arteries but does not reliably predict the physiologic impact of coronary stenoses[W1] or the extent of myocardium at risk for coronary occlusion.[F1] Moreover, coronary blood flow is affected not only by the anatomic configuration of the coronary arteries, but also by other variables such as the status of the microcirculation, the viability of the underlying myocardium, and regional wall stress. In addition, the interpretation of coronary angiograms usually lacks standardization and may present significant inter- and intra-observer variability. Although computed angiography may overcome some of these limitations, it will not satisfy the need for quantitative regional blood flow data.

Although newly developing techniques, such as magnetic resonance imaging, positron emission tomography, and fast computed tomography, are capable of measuring regional myocardial perfusion to some extent, as yet they are not routinely available, and their use, at least in the immediate future, will be restricted by the relatively high cost and complexity of the required equipment.

Echocardiography is based upon the relatively simple principles of ultrasound, as employed by the military service for "sonar" tracking and subsequently in the medical context by Edler, who used ultrasound to detect the mitral valve in 1953.[E1] Sound waves are reflected from adjacent structures of different densities. Ultrasound "noise" depends upon this acoustic mismatch, as well as the characteristics of the ultrasound beam and the absolute number of reflecting interfaces.

However, conventional ultrasound, without the use of contrast agents, does not detect blood flow or blood volume, because blood is relatively homogeneous with respect to tissue and appears essentially "silent" to ultrasound because of this lack of acoustically mismatched interfaces. Accordingly, ultrasound was not capable of tracking blood flow, or evaluating certain cardiac structures, until the discovery by Gramiak and Shah in 1968 of the first contrast tracking agent which, when injected, provided the necessary acoustic mismatch with blood and reflected the ultrasound signals.[G1] Over the years,[M1, O1, Z1] various contrast agents have been studied, most recently air-filled microbubbles produced by "sonicating" a variety of solutions.[F2] These microbubbles reflect a bright ultrasound signal owing to the differing densities between the air and the blood. In addition, their flow patterns through the microvasculature are equivalent to those of red blood cells.[C1, F3] Based on this physiologic behavior, the microbubbles may be considered surrogate red blood cells as they distribute throughout the tissue, and they may be suitable for regional microcirculation studies in a variety of organs. The intravascular path taken by the microbubbles is reflected by the ultrasound energy emitted from the external ultrasound transducer. The regional variability of tissue perfusion, as assessed by examination of reflected ultrasound energy, may chart previously unresolved perfusion issues. These contrast echocardiographic techniques, if successfully developed, will enable clinicians to sample regional perfusion patterns at a rapid rate (30 frames per second) with high spatial resolution (1 to 2 millimeters) and in a noninvasive, serial manner.

CONTRAST AGENT DEVELOPMENT

Approximately 15 years after Edler's first description of transthoracic imaging of cardiac structures, Gramiak and Shah found that, during cardiac catheterization, an aortic root injection of indocyanine green dye produced an echocardiographic contrast effect based upon agitation of the solution; microcavitation at the catheter tip caused ultrasound "noise" at the interfaces of the fluid and air.[G1] Subsequently, contrast echocardiographic techniques were used with intracardiac or intravenous injections for a variety of purposes, including the identification of cardiac structures[F4] or shunts,[S1] the detection of valvular regurgitation,[K1] the evaluation of complex congenital diseases,[V1] and the assessment of cardiac output and flow.[D1]

Traditionally, contrast echocardiography focused on the identification of cavity blood flow patterns. Contrast agents consisted of hand-agitated solutions of normal saline, dextrose, or indocyanine green. Ziskin and associates[Z1] in 1972 identified a variety of solutions that could be used as ultrasound agents. Over the years, the uses of ultrasound contrast agents have expanded, as described in a recent review by Ophir and Parker.[O1]

The early hand-agitated contrast agents contained bubbles that were too large and unstable for pulmonary capillary passage; nevertheless, they could be used to detect right heart chambers or valvular abnormalities.[S1] If the microbubbles were visualized in left heart chambers following an intravenous bolus, it was presumed that a right-to-left intracardiac shunt existed (atrial septal defect, sinus venosus defect, ventricular septal defect, patent foramen ovale, and so on). The degree of left heart opacification and the duration of contrast effect suggested the degree of shunting. However, it was not possible to quantify the degree of valvular regurgitation or shunts owing to the variability in the ultrasound contrast effects. In addition, left heart cavity flow patterns, anatomy, and valvular competence could not be identified following intravenous injections because of failure of the contrast agent to pass the pulmonary vasculature.

With the development of Doppler techniques (pulsed, continuous, and color Doppler), the use of contrast echocardiography to detect intracardiac shunts and valvular competence has been greatly reduced. However, contrast ultrasound techniques may be combined with Doppler procedures. In principle, the Doppler techniques are based upon the reflection of ultrasound energy from the flowing red blood cells. If microbubbles are mixed with blood following an intravascular injection, it has been shown by Beard and Byrd that the Doppler signal is enhanced.[B1] The Doppler signal indicates flow patterns and/or velocity of the red blood cells. The contrast effect and enhancement of the Doppler signal induced by the presence of microbubbles may serve as a flow indicator, so that quantification of shunts or regurgitant blood volumes may be possible using combined techniques.

Although it is too early to predict whether the use of contrast material and Doppler techniques will be synergistic for the detection and quantification of blood volumes, regurgitant lesions, or shunts, the potential is exciting and further development is needed.

Manually Produced Contrast Agents (Hand-Agitated)

Early echocardiographic contrast agents were prepared by hand-agitating a variety of solutions, including saline, indocyanine green, hydrogen peroxide, intralipid, 5 percent dextrose, and even blood.[Z1, O1, M1] Virtually any liquid that can be forcibly agitated contains bubbles and, therefore, could potentially serve as an echo reflector.

The methods of preparing hand-agitated contrast agents were relatively simple. Accordingly, contrast echocardiography developed rapidly and became a familiar imaging tool in nearly all echocardiographic laboratories. One such technique employed plastic disposable syringes joined by a three-way stopcock and filled with a 3:2 mixture of 0.9 percent saline and diatrizoate sodium and meglumine (Renografin–76) and 0.1 to 0.2 ml of air.[T1] The contents were flushed from one syringe to another. The turbulence and hydraulic cavitation generated by this process resulted in a tremendous mixture of air and liquid that ultimately led to bubble formation.

Contrast echocardiographic techniques using hand-agitated microbubble solutions were found to produce relatively few side effects. In a retrospective study of 51,180 patients, transient complaints such as respiratory or neurologic symptoms (including two cases of transient hemiparesis) were reported in only 32 patients (0.062 percent).[B2] Generally, most of the side effects were considered trivial and nonspecific. In addition, pathologic animal studies found no histologic changes 24 hours after multiple injections of hand-agitated microbubbles into the myocardium, kidney, and brain of dogs.[G2]

However, the use of hand-agitated microbubbles has two significant limitations: (1) their relatively short and variable half-lives, and (2) their relatively large diameters, which generally appear to preclude transpulmonary passage. In 1979, Reale and associates showed that in order to accomplish transpulmonary passage of hand-agitated microbubbles it was necessary to inject the contrast agent forcefully through a Swan-Ganz catheter placed in a branch of a pulmonary artery.[R1, R2] That same year, Bommer and colleagues also described successful transpulmonary passage of protein-stabilized microbubbles that reached the left ventricular cavity following intravenous injection.[B3, B4] Subsequently, DeMaria and associates showed that it was possible to use an intracoronary injection of relatively large bubbles (30 microns in diameter) to obtain ultrasonic enhancement of the left ventricular myocardium.[D2] This report was the first to describe the use of contrast echocardiography to represent myocardial perfusion.

Sonicated Contrast Agents

More recently, smaller and more stable microbubbles have been produced using a sonicator instead of hand-agitation techniques.[F2] Sonicated microbubbles have been shown to be capable of crossing the pulmonary capillary bed following intravenous injection[F5, K2, T2] and accordingly have expanded the potential uses of contrast echocardiography to include perfusion assessment, both outside as well as within the context of catheterization or surgery. Nevertheless, although sonication can be reproducibly performed in experimental laboratories,[F6] it remains an operator-dependent technique. Although sonication has significant advantages over hand agitation, certain limitations remain.

The sonication process uses an electromechanical "sonicator," a machine otherwise used in laboratories for a variety of nonclinical purposes. The sonicator produces ultrasonic cavitation in liquids[W2] and was applied to echocardiography by Feinstein.[F2] Specifically, ultrasound energy is applied to a liquid solution using a modified lead zirconate-titanate electrostrictive (piezoelectric) crystal. This triggers ultrasound compression and rarefaction waves. Microimpurities present in the solution serve as "motes," or foci, for the initial production of energy-dependent cavitation bubbles, which subsequently collapse and generate a myriad of nonenergy-dependent by-product microbubbles (Fig. 27–1).

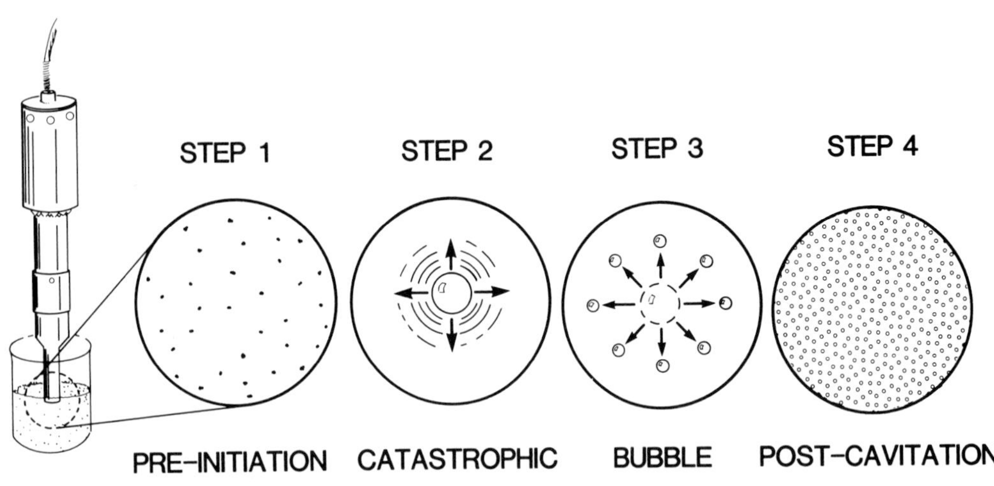

Figure 27–1. The steps involved in ultrasonic microcavitation are shown schematically. The solution filled with impurities, microparticles, air cavities, and so on, serves as the focus for the development of microcavities when energy is applied. The second step, or catastrophic phase, follows the application of energy. Resonant bubbles are induced from compression and rarefaction created by the sonicator. Following the collapse of the energy-dependent resonant bubble, a myriad of smaller, non-energy-dependent bubbles remain in solution, resulting in the post-cavitation phase. (From Powsner, S., Wood, J., Prieto, P., et al.: High speed interface for myocardial sonicated echo contrast studies. SPIE 845:384, 1987, with permission.)

To begin sonication, a 10-ml plastic syringe is filled with 8 ml of a solution (which will serve as the carrier solution). After removal of the plunger, the tip of the sterilized sonicator horn is immersed approximately 1 to 2 cm below the surface of the liquid, and power is turned on. After 10 seconds, the syringe is briefly lowered to permit the tip of the horn to touch the surface, producing surface agitation. After an additional 20 seconds, the energy is turned off. Care should be taken to avoid excessive contact between the horn tip and the surface; otherwise, large bubbles (foam) will be generated, and the solution will appear opaque and white (or "milky"). However, if the solution has been correctly sonicated, it will appear gray and translucent and will be ready for injection.[F6]

The ultimate size and stability of the sonicated by-product microbubbles depend upon the physical and chemical properties of the carrier solutions.[B3, B4, F2] In the past, a variety of surfactants have been used to stabilize microbubbles for transpulmonary passage.[B3, B4] In particular, proteins such as albumin and gelatin have produced stable microbubbles. Albumin used as a surfactant for sonicated 70 percent dextrose was subsequently sonicated, resulting in the production of microbubbles. Unlike sonicated microbubbles of radiopaque compounds, sonicated albumin microbubbles are isotonic to serum and therefore would not result in reactive hyperemia following intracoronary injections. In addition, the albumin molecule is biodegradable and biocompatible. Commercial efforts are underway to produce a reliable contrast agent. If successful, standardized sonicated agents would lessen problems associated with the preparation of the agent, which include operator-dependence, sterility, and preparation time. However, no contrast agent has yet completed regulatory scrutiny and become commercially available.

Hand-Agitation and Sonication Techniques Compared

Although hand-agitated microbubbles have been considered safe and useful for the limited purposes just described, sonicated microbubbles present certain advantages and permit expanded uses for contrast echocardiography. They are smaller and more uniform in size,[F2] and thus capable of unimpeded flow through the pulmonary microcirculation. Peripheral venous injections of sonicated contrast agents[F5, K2, T2] and other agents[B5, R1, R2] have produced left ventricular opacification.

In addition, unlike hand-agitated microbubbles that may become "trapped" in the pulmonary capillaries, sonicated microbubbles flow through the vasculature at physiologic transit times.

Doppler measurements of intracavitary flow velocity have been made in patients before and after injection of ultrasound agents, and these measurements have shown the similarity between the flow patterns of red blood cells and microbubbles.[L1] In addition, studies of the cat mesentery showed that most of the hand-agitated bubbles become trapped in the capillaries and thus temporarily interrupted blood flow; however, sonicated microbubbles uniformly crossed the microcirculation with the red blood cells, at the same velocity.[F3] Cheirif and associates used a frame-by-frame cinemicroscopic analysis of a microvascular preparation of rabbit chremaster muscle and confirmed that the intracapillary velocity of the microbubbles is similar to that of red blood cells.[C1] Because of their physiologic transit times, sonicated microbubbles serve as vascular ultrasound "tracers," and, therefore, the principles of dye dilution theory may be applied for purposes of quantification of regional perfusion.

Safety and Efficacy Studies

The safety and efficacy of sonicated microbubble contrast agents are undergoing clinical and animal testing, with apparent success.[F7, L2, M2, R3, S2] Recently, three medical centers have reported upon their initial clinical safety and efficacy studies using intravenous injections of Albunex (Molecular Biosystems, Inc., San Diego, CA), a commercially prepared contrast agent consisting of sonicated albumin.[F7] These centers (University of Chicago, Baylor College of Medicine, and Thoraxcenter in Rotterdam) reported minor, nonspecific problems, such as discomfort and irritation at the injection site and transient taste alteration. Researchers also have found that intravenous injections of Albunex in humans, with doses of up to 0.12 ml/kg, did not cause significant cardiovascular, neurologic, or serum chemistry alterations,[F7] and that the intracoronary injection of 2 to 3 ml of an independently prepared sonicated albumin solution in patients with severe coronary artery disease did not produce any symptom, arrhythmia, or hemodynamic changes.[S2] The multicenter Albunex studies evaluated left ventricular opacification following intravenous injections in 71 patients. Sixty-three percent (151/240 injections) produced at least moderate cavity opacification; 1+, trace; 2+ moderate, and 3+, full opacification. However, at present, detecting an enhancement of the left ventricular myocardium following intravenous contrast injections is less common using current commercially available video image processing. Nevertheless, recent advances in ultrasound equipment design may overcome this limitation. Considerable testing remains to be done.

In general, sonicated microbubbles do not appear to alter myocardial performance. Any negative inotropic effect is believed to be directly related to microbubble dimensions. Gillam and colleagues used coronary artery injections of hand-agitated bubbles in dogs and found transient but consistent regional hypokineses, ST-T changes, a slight decrease in left ventricular DP/DT, and an increase in end-diastolic pressure.[G2] Depressant effects on the myocardium were subsequently estimated by

Shapiro and colleagues to be proportional to the microbubble diameter.[S2] The microbubbles used in these studies were larger (12 ± 3 microns, and 20 ± 6 microns) in diameter than sonicated microbubbles, which are similar in size to red blood cells. In addition, Lang and associates compared the effects of Renografin on the myocardium with and without sonicated bubbles of 4.5 ± 2.8 microns in diameter.[L2] The study concluded that any negative inotropic effect on the sonicated microbubbles was secondary only to the radiopaque carrier and not to the presence of microbubbles in the solution. More recent studies found that intracoronary injections of a noncommercially prepared sonicated albumin solution did not appear to alter coronary blood flow or result in reactive hyperemia.[K3]

QUANTIFICATION

Before rigorous approaches to quantification of perfusion may be developed, researchers must address these issues: (1) the characteristics of the contrast agent, and their effects on the ultrasound signal; (2) the design of the ultrasound equipment, and in particular the ability of the equipment to receive and reliably display the range of ultrasound information; and (3) the validation of the mathematical model for perfusion analysis.

The Contrast Agent

The size, variability, and concentration of the microbubble greatly influence ultrasound response. The larger the microbubble, the more pronounced the ultrasound backscatter, since the reflected backscatter varies directly with the sixth power of the radius of the microbubble.[P1] Similarly, when microbubbles vary widely in size, there will be considerable variation in the ultrasound signal. The greater the variability of the microbubble sizes, the more difficult it will be to calibrate the ultrasound signal.

One difficulty currently encountered with the use of contrast echocardiography for intravenous perfusion assessment is that the smaller microbubbles are required for unimpeded passage through the pulmonary microcirculation. The ultrasound equipment currently available has not been sufficiently tested for use with sonicated microbubbles, and as such may not present the full range of ultrasound information generated by smaller microbubbles within the myocardial tissue. However, technology is being developed to increase the sensitivity and reliability of the ultrasound equipment to the point at which perfusion analyses have been performed successfully in experimental settings. These efforts will be discussed more fully.

With regard to calibration of the microbubble's ultrasound signal, it should be noted that a linear response to ultrasound is a sine qua non for perfusion analysis using a mathematical model. The direct calibration of a system must take into consideration the acoustic response of reflected ultrasound from the microbubbles found in various tissues and cavities, and the electronic calibration response of the reflected signal (ultrasound system response). These two important components may be individually characterized and analyzed, or their combined effects may be treated as a "black box" approach. However, ultimately a direct and linear ultrasound response from the microbubbles must be determined. Linearity has been maintained to concentrations of 10^4 per ml, as demonstrated by Heidenreich and associates in vitro.[H1] The range of concentrations they tested appears to be reasonable estimates of doses required in the experimental and clinical setting. It is important to recognize that the microbubbles or air-filled microspheres used for perfusion studies have a rather uniform diameter and a small range of sizes, because the reflected signal will vary directly with the radius of the microbubble.

Therefore, before quantification can be reproducibly performed, the concentration and microbubble size must be standardized. When the microbubble concentration is significantly increased, acoustic shadowing or attenuation phenomena appear to dominate, and thus linearity is lost. This noteworthy effect causes a substantial alteration in the calculation of flow and must be carefully considered in analytical perfusion studies. It appears that in the selection of an ideal contrast agent, rigorous analysis of in vitro and in vivo persistence are of critical importance to determining whether the contrast effect is constant over time in a variety of physiologic and pathologic conditions.

Ultrasound Equipment

The design of current commercial ultrasound equipment has focused on identification of cardiac anatomic structures (e.g., endocardial borders, valve leaflets, edge detection, and so on). The returning ultrasound signal undergoes a logarithmic compression and distortion that permits optimal visualization of the cardiac anatomy but significantly alters the linear display of the "gray tones" of tissue. In order for ultrasound equipment to be capable of quantitative perfusion assessment, equipment design modifications will likely be necessary to allow access to an expanded dynamic range of linear, digital signal[P2]—perhaps similar to the requirements used for ultrasound tissue characterization.[B6, H2, M3, R4, R5] The increasing availability of inexpensive electronic components now makes it feasible to acquire and process a larger dynamic range of ultrasound reflected energy, and the development of a transpulmonary contrast agent makes these design modifications potentially clinically useful.

However, as discussed by Zwehl and co-workers, significant problems remain before a true quantitative approach to perfusion imaging can be achieved.[Z2] It is important to note that the effects of acoustic shadowing (with and without contrast agents) will materially affect the reflected signal. All the technical limitations involved in ultrasound imaging techniques in general must be addressed in the specific context of ultrasound perfusion imaging. Lateral resolution ("dropout"), depth compensation, motion artifacts, operator variability, and basic ultrasound processing variabilities will require substantial testing before a reliable perfusion index can be developed.

The complex interaction of the ultrasound energy within a tissue matrix is the subject of intense scientific investigation.[B6, H2, R5] Reports by Miller and colleagues[M3] have noted the cyclic nature of reflected ultrasound energy from the myocardial tissue. Figure 27–2 shows schematically the ultrasound energy originating from a transducer and subsequently penetrating a tissue prior to being variably reflected back to the transducer. It also demonstrates the interaction of ultrasound energy within the cardiac tissue, and the variability of reflectance at different points along the cardiac cycle. Figure 27–3 illustrates the radiofrequency (amplitude) energy returning from a cross-sectional slice of myocardial tissue perfused with microbubbles during diastole and subsequently during systole. The amplitude of reflected energy is plotted on the ordinate axis and time (or cardiac cycle) on the abscissa. While several possible explanations may be advanced regarding the cyclic nature of the reflected energy, it may be useful to ascribe the changes in reflectance simply to cardiac tissue orientation and tissue blood volume. During systole, the total myocardial fiber orientation and tissue blood volume are likely to be significantly different from those during diastole, and this has been shown to alter the reflected energy obtained from the cardiac tissue.

In contrast echocardiography, when microbubbles or air-filled microspheres are injected into the vasculature, significant alterations in the acoustic properties of the vascular bed occur (Fig. 27–3). Figure 27–4 illustrates the marked increase in ultrasound reflected energy following the intracoronary introduction of 1.5 ml of sonicated Renografin–76 into the left coronary arteries of a patient undergoing cardiac catheterization. The cyclic variation present within normally contracting myocardial tissue is disrupted, and the total amount of energy reflected from the microsphere-filled tissue is significantly increased. The magnitude of the increase in reflected ultrasound signal depends upon rate of injection, microbubble size, and concentration within the myocardial tissue.

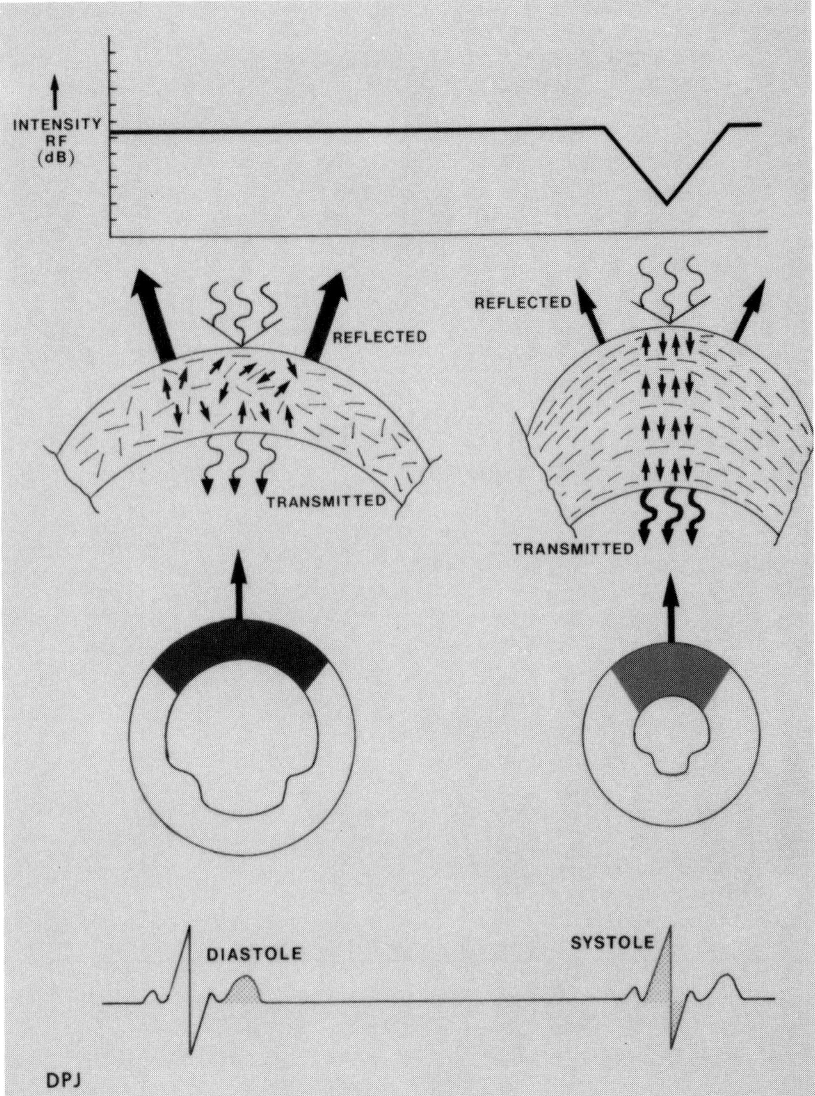

Figure 27–2. At the bottom, a single cardiac cycle (two electrocardiographic complexes) is displayed. Above the ECG tracings are two corresponding cross-sectional images of the left ventricle (as seen by two-dimensional echocardiography). A cutaway enlargement of the anterior wall of the left ventricle is depicted above the short axis left ventricular views. The magnitude of the reflected ultrasound energy is indicated by the arrows emanating from the anterior surface of the myocardium. A graph at the top illustrates the change in reflected energy or intensity (radiofrequency signal) during systole or diastole. Note that in diastole, the left ventricle has the largest diameter, and the reflected ultrasound signals register higher intensity than those of systole.

Mathematical Model for Perfusion Imaging

Quantification of myocardial perfusion with contrast echocardiography requires a new implementation of conventional indicator-dilution theory. The need for a new approach arises from the technical advances in modern imaging equipment. The foundation for the current development is contained in the work of Meier and Zierler[M4] and Zierler.[Z3] The original formulations were based on the ability to measure quantities of indicator at the vascular inlet and outlet from a tissue of interest. The new model differs from the original in two basic ways. First, an intravascular indicator is observed as it transits tissue, not at an *outlet* from tissue. Second, external tomographic imaging devices, such as modern ultrasound, can measure a signal proportional to indicator concentration in tissue or blood, but not an absolute quantity of indicator. Therefore, the original premises and mathematics have been extended to include the opportunities for perfusion measurement made available by contrast echocardiography.

An external tomographic imaging device creates a two-dimensional representation of a three-dimensional slice of an organ. For example, an ultrasound beam is typically between 0.5 and 1 cm in width. This essential third dimension is compressed into two dimensions at the transducer lens. Therefore, any image produced by the transducer has an implicit depth and represents a volume rather than an area. If an indicator produces a response in the imaging system that is proportional to the quantity of indicator (i.e., a change in pixel intensity) in a region of interest, the imaging system is then capable of measuring an indicator concentration in that region (concentration = quantity/volume) (Fig. 27–5). The capability of measuring an indicator concentration in a constant volume of tissue or blood suggests the possibility of calculating regional perfusion in any organ that permits the simultaneous imaging of both an afferent blood supply and tissue region of interest.

Current research makes several assumptions: (1) the indicator behaves as a blood component of physiologic interest in its flow patterns; (2) the indicator must remain entirely within the vascular space and not be trapped at any level of the vascular system; (3) the indicator produces a response in the imaging system that is linear or capable of being made linear with indicator concentration in tissue and blood; (4) the indicator does not perturb the physiologic parameters being measured; and (5) the measured parameters are either constant during the measurement process, or the observations can be gated so that the parameters are constant in the images used for calculations. In addition, other potential problems, such as a variation in system response to indicator concentration depending on image geometry or depth, are important in implementation of the measurement theory but have no impact on the theory itself. It is of special note that the new model is quite general and in theory can be applied to any type of indicator bolus or infusion.

Actual blood flow is calculated from the mean transit time theorem.[M4] The theorem states that the blood flow (ml/sec) through a tissue region is given by the ratio of the volume of distribution of an indicator in a tissue region to the mean transit time of the indicator through the region:

$$F = \frac{V_d}{\bar{t}_s}$$

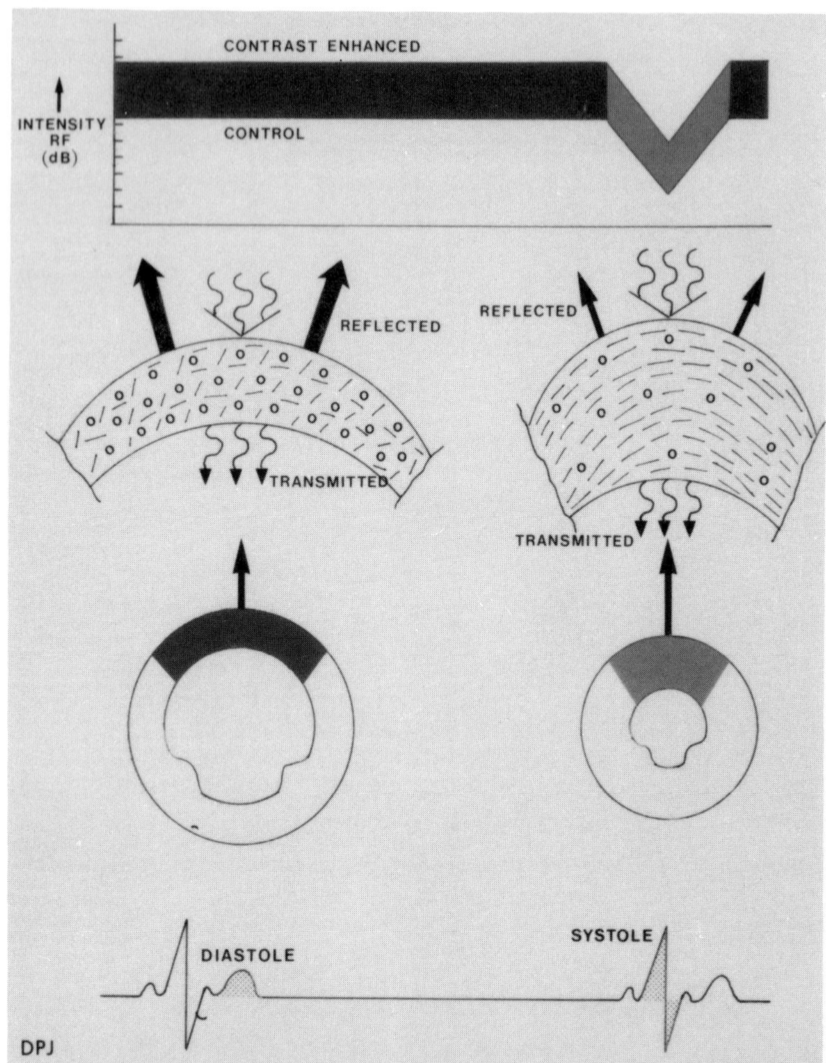

Figure 27–3. On the same framework as in Figure 27–2, it can be seen that the introduction of microbubbles into the myocardial vasculature results in an increase in reflected ultrasound signal intensity. The increase in the reflected signal corresponds to microbubble size, concentration, and fiber orientation (cardiac cycle).

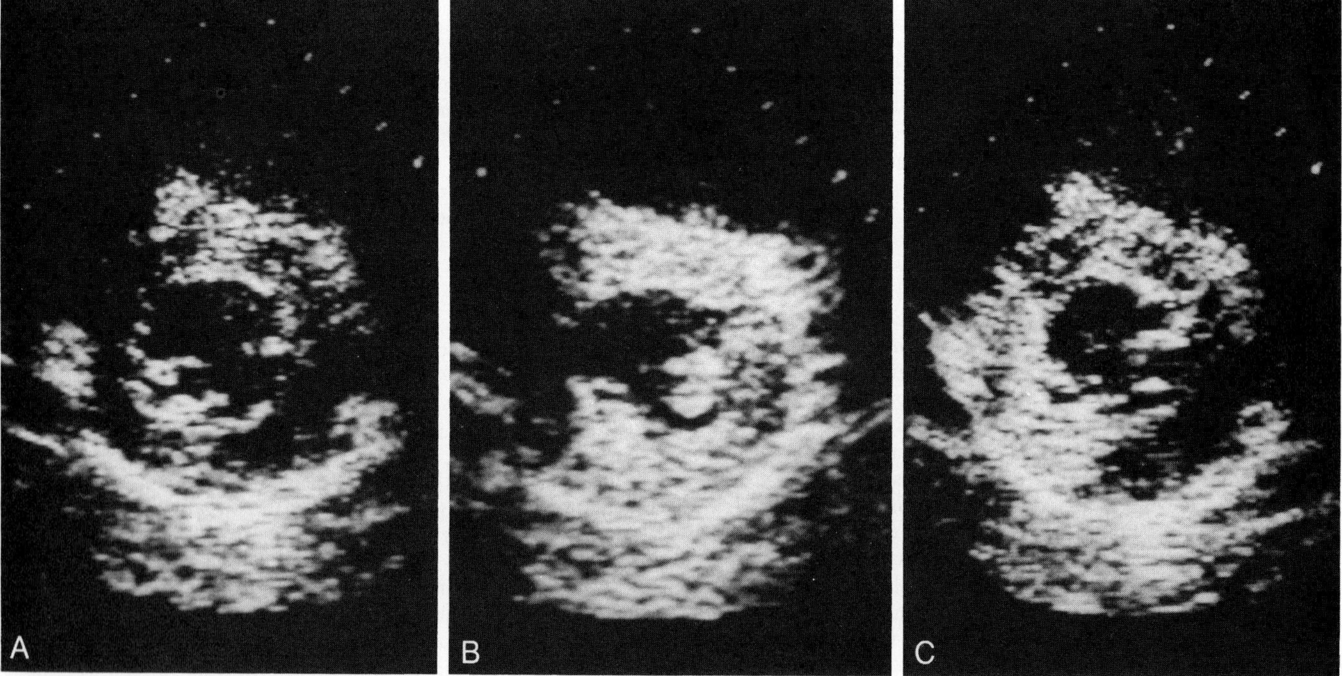

Figure 27–4. Clinical myocardial perfusion studies in a patient without significant angiographically demonstrated atherosclerosis. *A*, A two-dimensional, cross-sectional echocardiographic study of the patient during coronary angiography. Beginning at the top of the image and continuing clockwise, the anterior, lateral, posterior, and interventricular septal regions can be identified. This echocardiographic view was obtained at the papillary muscle level. *B*, Following a direct intracoronary injection of 1.5 ml of sonicated Renografin–76, the anterior, lateral, and posterior lateral myocardial regions demonstrate marked contrast enhancement. *C*, The inferior and inferoseptal regions (posterior-medial papillary muscle level) demonstrate marked contrast enhancement following right coronary injection of 1.5 ml of sonicated Renografin–76.

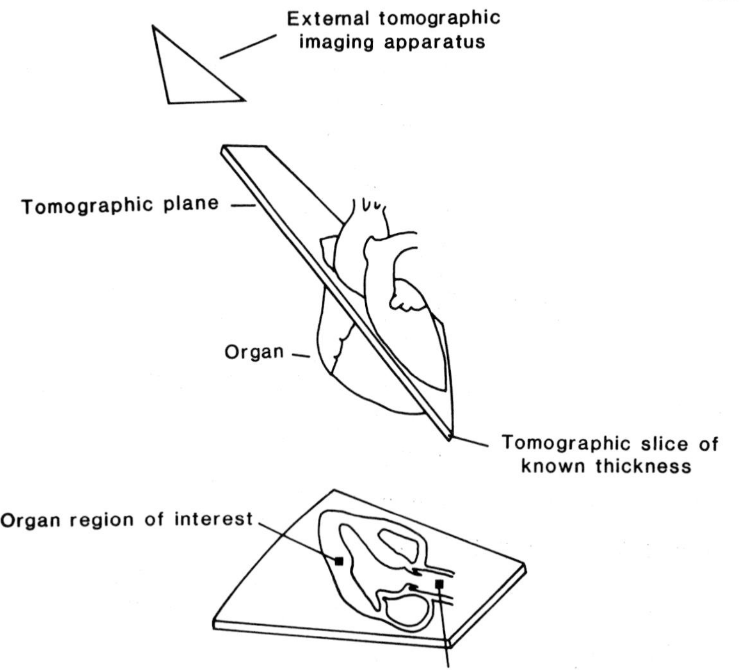

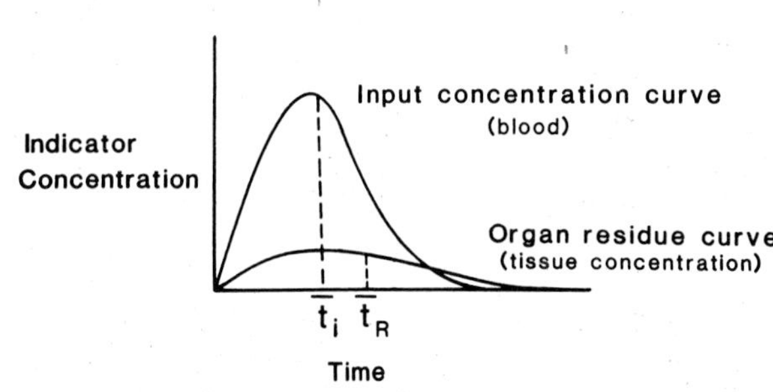

Figure 27–5. The model for calculation of tissue perfusion with an external tomographic imaging device. This device produces tomographic images of the organ and afferent vessel supplying blood to the organ. The tomographic plane has a known finite thickness, which is compressed into the two dimensions of the image. Regions of interest in the organ tissue and the afferent vessel can be identified and analyzed to produce intensity/time curves, which provide information on indicator concentration versus time in the regions of interest. The plots of indicator concentration versus time can be analyzed to produce the necessary parameters for the calculation of tissue perfusion (see text). The figure shows hypothetic regions of interest with appropriate curves of indicator concentration. In the afferent blood vessel, the input curve will have a higher peak concentration, a greater area, and a shorter mean transit time, t_i, than the tissue indicator concentration, or residue, curve.

Therefore, the implementation of the new model is an exercise in deriving the contrast volume of distribution and mean transit time from the sequential images. In the case of contrast echocardiography, the microbubbles reside entirely within the vascular space and are evenly distributed through the plasma volume, so the volume of distribution of the indicator is the blood volume of the region of interest. The mean transit time of the microbubbles through the tissue is the average time that a microbubble requires to pass through that vascular volume. If a microbubble injection does not enter the tissue instantaneously, the finite time required for all the indicator to enter the tissue must be taken into account in deriving the mean transit time from the recorded images. Thus, simultaneous imaging of the indicator bolus in an arterial vessel supplying the tissue region is essential.

Implicit in any implementation of the mean transit time theorem is the importance of the indicator volume of distribution, or the tissue blood volume for contrast echocardiography. As the tissue blood volume changes, an average indicator particle will take more or less time to traverse the tissue at the same blood flow. Conversely, if the blood volume is unchanged, a change in blood flow will cause an indicator particle to require more or less time to traverse the tissue. Any attempt to calculate blood flow from indicator transit times or image pixel intensity must take into account the interdependence of transit time and blood volume. A model that neglects blood volume may produce a correlation with blood flow, but the model will break down to the extent that blood flow and volume can vary independently.

However, accurately obtained contrast echocardiographic images potentially can contain enough information to derive the tissue blood volume and indicator mean transit time and then explicitly calculate blood flow. To accomplish the measurement, it is necessary to observe the indicator in an afferent vessel, and the complete transit of the indicator through the tissue. The amount of indicator entering the tissue region at any time is given by the indicator concentration (which will vary with time), $C_i(t)$, multiplied by the blood flow, F, into the tissue (quantity/time = (quantity/volume)(volume/time) and is the input function of indicator into the tissue:

$$i(t) = C_i(t) \cdot F$$

If an infinitesimally brief input of a known quantity of indicator into the tissue could be accomplished and the number of particles exiting the tissue at all times is measured, the mean transit time simply would be the average time it took for all particles to traverse the tissue. The total number of particles that had exited the tissue also could be counted. The number of particles remaining in the tissue at any time t would be the difference between the number that instantaneously entered the tissue and the number that had exited. The last quantity is what is actually visualized by the ultrasound system in contrast echocardiography: the indicator actually in the tissue at any time t. In indicator dilution theory, the first function, the frequency distribution of indicator transit times, is denoted by h(t) and known as the unit impulse response if the input has a unit area. The quantity of indicator remaining in the tissue after an instantaneous unit input is known as the residue function of the tissue R(t). The family of unit impulse response functions is shown in Figure 27–6.

In reality, a unit impulse injection of indicator is not possible. In the general case for any type of input function, the amount of indicator remaining in the tissue at time t is given by the convolution of the input with the residue function R(t). In other words, the actual concentration of indicator $C_R(t)$, seen by an

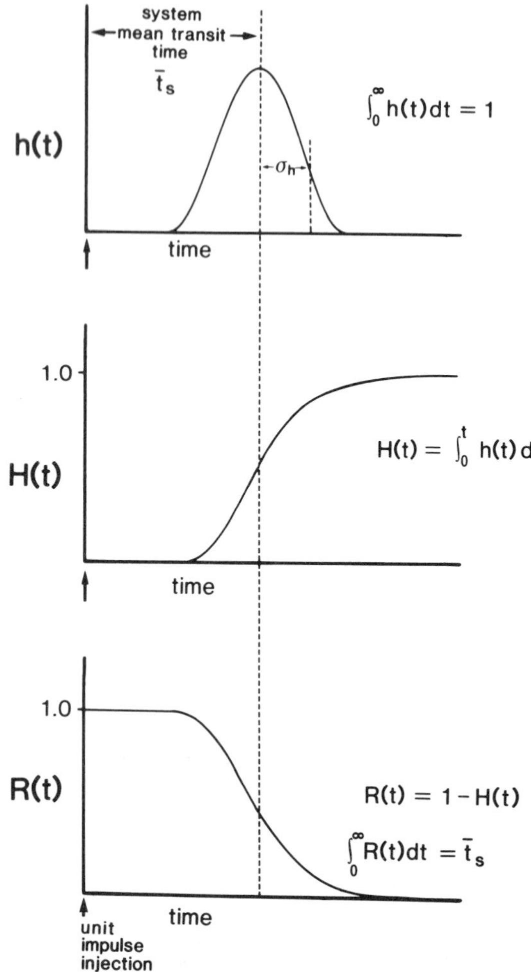

Figure 27–6. The family of unit impulse response functions. These curves represent the theoretic functions obtained after a unit impulse injection of an indicator into a tissue. A unit impulse injection is infinitesimal in duration and unit area and is not achievable in practice. h(t) is the frequency function of tissue transit times. It represents the number of indicator particles that would be seen exiting a tissue region of interest as a function of time after injection of a unit impulse of indicator into the tissue. Since it is a probability, h(t) has an area of 1. The mean transit time of indicator through the tissue is represented as $\bar{t}_s$ and is the average time for the indicator to exit the tissue. The standard deviation of indicator transit times from the mean σ_h can be measured from the curve. H(t) is calculated as the definite integral of h(t) from time 0, indicator injection, to any time t after injection. H(t) is the amount of indicator that has exited from the tissue at time t and must equal one, or all the indicator after enough time has passed. R(t), the residue function, is calculated as 1 − H(t). Since H(t) is the amount of indicator that has exited a tissue at time t, R(t) gives the amount of indicator remaining in the tissue at any time t following a unit impulse injection of indicator at time t = 0. The external tomographic imaging device detects indicator remaining in the tissue, which is a function of R(t). The integral of R(t) is equal to the mean transit time of the tissue, $\bar{t}_s$.

external tomographic imaging system at any time t varies from that theoretically seen after a unit impulse injection in a way that is determined by the shape of the actual input and the theoretic residue function:

$$C_R(t) = F \cdot C_i(t) * R(t)$$

The input concentration curve $C_i(t)$ and the tissue transit curve $C_R(t)$ are what an ultrasound machine actually can record after a contrast injection. An example calculated from an arbitrarily chosen $C_i(t)$ and R(t) produces the tissue transit curve $C_R(t)$ shown in Figure 27–7. If R(t) could be solved by deconvolution, determination of the mean transit is equal to the integral of R(t) over time. However, deconvolution is in practice too noise-producing a procedure to be clinically useful, so an alternative method of solving for the mean transit time must be found. The tissue blood volume must also be calculated in order to apply the mean transit time theorem.

If the convolution is integrated, and the volume of distribution V_d is substituted from the mean transit time theorem as flow multiplied by the mean transit time, the result is:

$$V_d = \frac{\int_0^\infty C_R(t)\,dt}{\int_0^\infty C_i(t)\,dt}$$

Both integrals are obtained directly from the observed input and tissue concentration curves, so the tissue blood volume can be explicitly calculated.

A formula for calculating the mean transit time ($\bar{t}_s$) through the tissue can be found by substituting into the formula which defines a mean transit time:

$$\bar{t}_R = \frac{\int_0^\infty t \cdot C_R(t)\,dt}{\int_0^\infty C_R(t)\,dt}$$

If the appropriate substitutions from the original convolution for $C_R(t)$ and its integral are made and the result expanded and simplified, the general result can be derived:

$$\bar{t}_s = \frac{2\,(\bar{t}_R - \bar{t}_i)}{1 + \frac{\sigma_h 2}{\bar{t}_s^{\,2}}}$$

The formula provides a relationship between the tissue mean transit time ($\bar{t}_s$), which would be observed after a theoretic unit impulse injection, and the actual input and tissue mean transit times, $\bar{t}_R$ and $\bar{t}_i$, which will be observed after realistic input boluses, and thus permits calculation of $\bar{t}_s$. With $\bar{t}_s$ and V_d calculated from observable data, the calculation of tissue blood flow is done by simply substituting these derived values into the mean transit time theorem.

The expression in the denominator represents the ratio of the variance of the impulse response function to its mean value and may frequently be small compared with 1. The expression then simplifies to:

$$\bar{t}_s = 2 \cdot [\bar{t}_R - \bar{t}_i]$$

Of important note, in all the foregoing development all measurements are made from the first appearance of indicator in the artery or tissue region of interest, not from the time of indicator injection as in the classic theory. A consequence of this difference is that the transfer function R(t) of the tissue has the general shape shown in Figures 27–6 and 27–7, instead of an arbitrary function such as a lagged normal distribution.

The general shape of R(t) leads to several useful results. At the time of first appearance of indicator in the tissue region of interest, (t = 0), no indicator will have yet exited, and R(t) must equal 1. It will continue to do so until indicator begins to exit the region, the shortest transit time. Since R(t) is constant prior to this shortest transit time, the basic convolution equation simplifies to:

$$F_v = \frac{C_R(t)}{\int_0^t C_i(t)dt} \quad t < \text{shortest transit time}$$

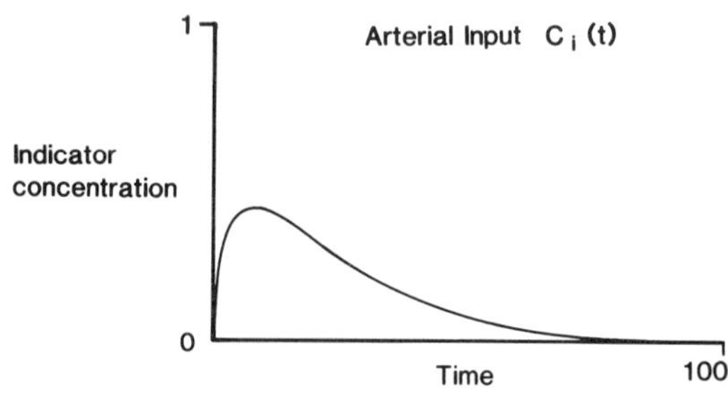

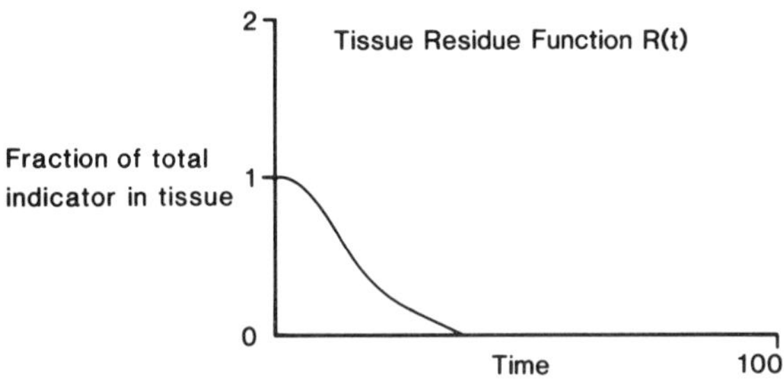

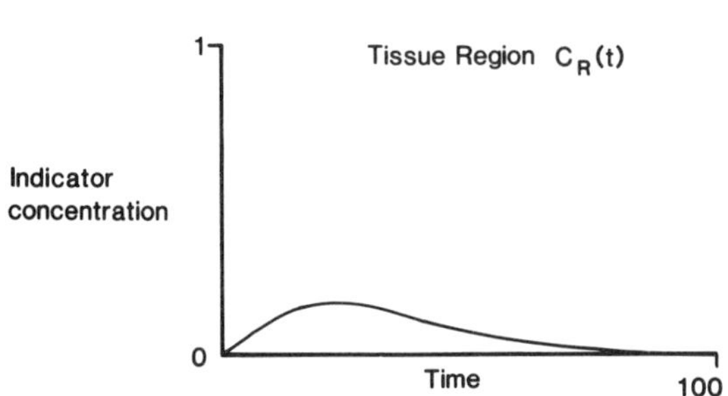

Figure 27–7. Theoretical input and tissue concentration curves. The concentration of indicator versus time in a tissue is calculated from the convolution of the input curve with the residue function of the tissue region (see text). The figure shows a plausible input function into a tissue, generated from an arbitrary mathematical function. The input function, $C_i(t)$, is obtained by observing the concentration of indicator over time in the arterial vessel supplying the tissue region. The tissue residue function R(t) represents the amount of indicator that would remain in the tissue after a unit impulse indicator at time 0, at any time t (see text and Figure 27–6). The residue function shown in the figure is also an arbitrary mathematical function. The bottom panel of the figure shows the tissue concentration curve that is actually calculated from the convolution of the arbitrary arterial input and tissue residue curves shown in the top two panels.

This equation allows a simple method for calculation of flow directly from the observed tissue concentration curves. In practice, it gives a contrast flow value until the shortest transit time is exceeded, at which point the calculated value begins to decrease. Worth noting also is that the peak height of an indicator tissue transit curve is useful for calculation of flow only if no indicator has exited the tissue before all the bolus has entered the tissue, an assumption that is frequently not met in experimental studies and results in misapplication of equations of this general form.

If the arterial input into an organ cannot be observed, it is still possible to obtain some measure of relative blood flow and volume in different regions of the same organ. Assuming that the afferent arterial concentration curves are equal in each region, the relative blood volumes are given by:

$$\frac{V_{d1}}{V_{d2}} = \frac{\int_0^\infty C_{R1}(t)\,dt}{\int_0^\infty C_{R2}(t)\,dt}$$

If measurements are made prior to shortest transit time through the tissue, the flow ratio in two regions is

$$\frac{F_{V1}}{F_{V2}} = \frac{C_{R1}(t)}{C_{R2}(t)} \quad t < \text{shortest transit time}$$

or, for a short bolus relative to the tissue transit time, an approximate expression for the flow ratio between two regions is given by:

$$\frac{F_{V1}}{F_{V2}} = \frac{V_{d1}}{V_{d2}} \cdot \frac{\bar{t}_{R2}}{\bar{t}_{R1}}$$

In summary, the classic indicator dilution theory has been extended in a rigorous mathematical fashion to enable perfusion measurements to be performed using modern imaging technology. The formulation is general, not dependent on any particular imaging system or site of indicator injection. The mathematical results lead to specific predictions for measurement calculations and ought to be readily confirmed experimentally, unlike earlier empiric formulations for perfusion calculations.

EXPERIMENTAL AND CLINICAL PERFUSION STUDIES

Assessment of Area at Risk

De Maria and colleagues performed the initial contrast echocardiographic perfusion studies, using intracoronary injections of microbubble solutions to evaluate regional myocardial perfusion.[D2] Subsequent reports by Armstrong and co-workers,[A1] Tei and co-workers,[T1] and Kaul and associates[K4] demonstrated the feasibility of using a variety of contrast techniques to identify perfusion. Regional perfusion patterns have been validated, using autoradiography or vascular dye, and have yielded significant correlations between ultrasound and postmortem autoradiographic findings on corresponding slices of the left ventricle.[K4] These early reports generated a rebirth of interest in contrast echocardiographic research for myocardial perfusion identification. A variety of reports were published describing the use of contrast echocardiography for assessing tissue viability and the degree of left ventricle at risk for coronary occlusion (Fig. 27–8). Feinstein and colleagues used contrast echocardiography to delineate regional variability in myocardial perfusion in patients found to have normal coronary anatomy during coronary angiography.[F1] The study concluded that regional perfusion patterns could be approximated but not necessarily or accurately predicted from the epicardial coronary artery anatomy alone (Fig. 27–9). In addition, perfusion patterns as identified by contrast echocardiography have been correlated with fixed perfusion deficits demonstrated at the time of coronary angiography and later by thallium–201 perfusion studies[B7] (Fig. 27–10).

These observations suggest the lack of a physiologic component to the anatomic descriptors previously used to evaluate tissue viability. With further development, contrast echocardiography could supply this dynamic physiologic component.

Assessment of Perfusion of Cardioplegic Solutions

The relatively high degree of myocardial infarction during cardiac surgery suggests a need for a reliable, quantitative method of assessing perfusion during coronary bypass grafting or other coronary surgical procedures. As early as 1984, Goldman, Mindich, and colleagues proposed the use of contrast echocardiography for guiding selective cardioplegia delivery beyond severe coronary stenosis, in order to protect poorly perfused ventricular areas.[G3] Recent studies have shown transesophageal echocardiography to be highly useful for monitoring patients undergoing cardiac surgery. Smith and co-workers recently published an abstract describing the use of transesophageal echocardiography to detect regional perfusion during bypass surgery, using left

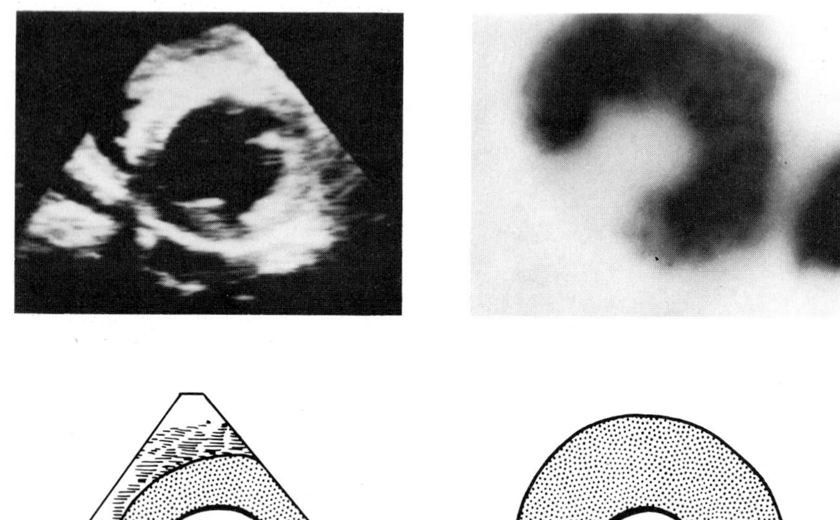

Figure 27–8. Estimation of coronary perfusion bed, or "area at risk." *A*, An area at risk in an experimental animal preparation following an intracoronary injection of a manually agitated ultrasound contrast solution. *B*, The corresponding technetium autoradiograph revealed a similar deficit in flow as measured by radiolabeled microspheres in the same animal. (From Kaul, S., Pandian, N.G., Okada, R.D., et al.: Contrast echocardiography in acute myocardial ischemia: I. In vivo determination of total left ventricular "area at risk." J. Am. Coll. Cardiol. 4:1272, 1984. Reprinted with permission of the American College of Cardiology.)

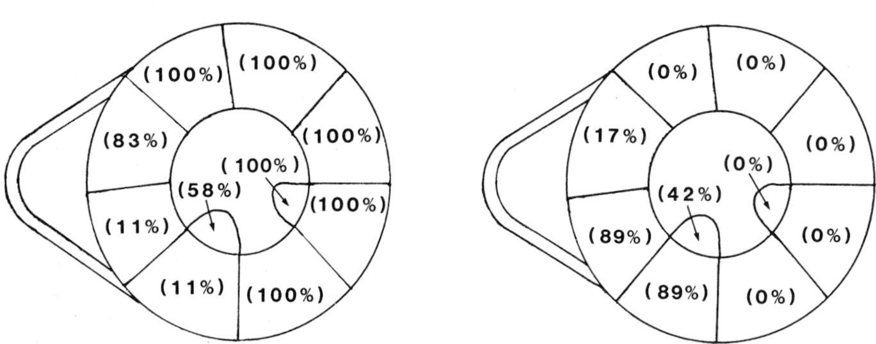

Figure 27–9. Regional myocardial perfusion in 12 normal patients following intracoronary ultrasound contrast injections of sonicated Renografin-76. The percentage of regional myocardial opacification following an intracoronary injection is identified. As an example, the inferior septal region was considered perfused owing to contrast enhancement after a right coronary injection in 89 percent of the patients with a dominant right coronary artery. In 11 percent of the patients with evidence of a right dominant coronary artery, the inferior septal region was perfused by the left coronary system following contrast injections into the left main artery. Of particular note, in all 12 patients the anterior septum and anterior anterolateral and posterolateral walls were perfused from the left coronary artery system. In addition, the anterolateral papillary muscle was uniformly perfused from the left coronary injection, whereas the posteromedial papillary muscle was perfused approximately equally (58 percent from the left coronary system, 42 percent from the right coronary artery). (From Feinstein, S.B., Lang, R.M., Dick, C.D., et al.: Contrast echocardiography during coronary arteriography in humans: Perfusion and anatomic studies. J. Am. Coll. Cardiol. 11:59, 1988. Reprinted with permission of the American College of Cardiology.)

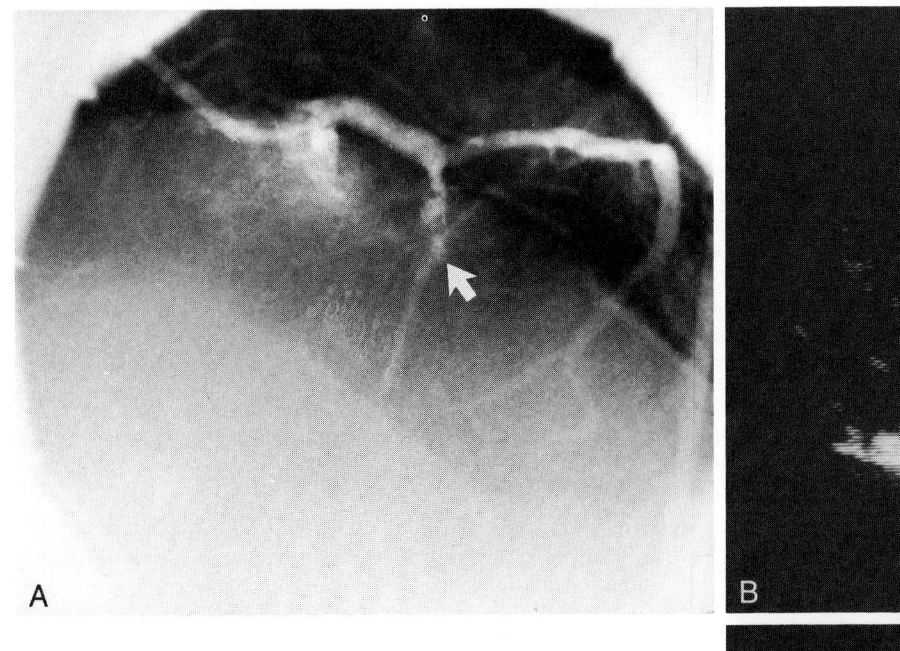

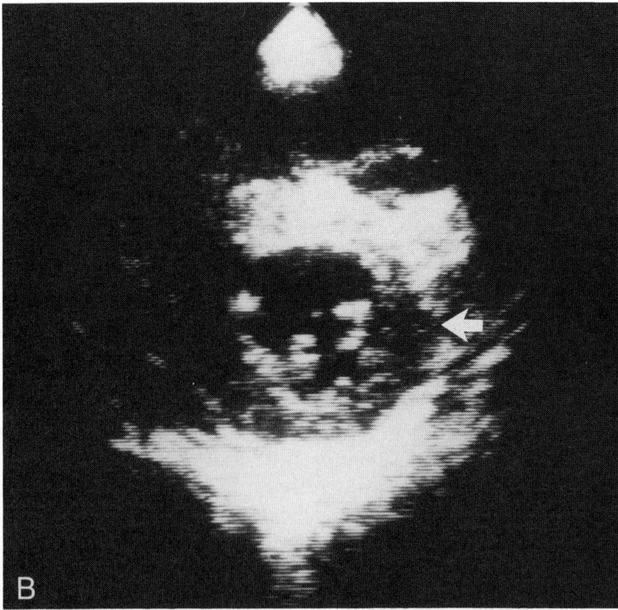

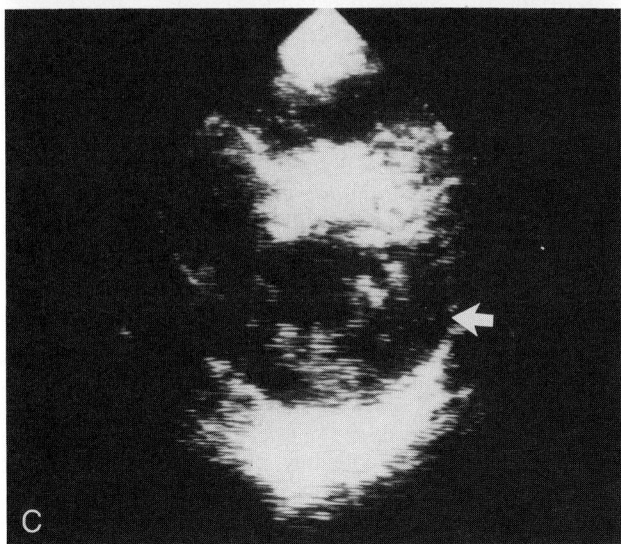

Figure 27–10: Angiographic correlate of contrast echocardiographic perfusion patterns. *A*, A coronary angiogram illustrating complete blockage of a mid-left anterior descending coronary artery (arrow). This angiogram was obtained from a young patient thought to have suffered an embolic myocardial infarction. *B* and *C*, Cross-sectional echocardiographic images taken following an intracoronary injection of 1.5 ml of sonicated Renografin–76. In *B*, the arrow is pointing to an absence of contrast effect in the posterior lateral regions. *C* similarly illustrates a perfusion defect in the posterolateral region in the same patient. The cross-sectional echocardiographic view of *C* was taken at the mid-papillary muscle level, whereas the images obtained in *B* were photographed at the mitral valve level. These perfusion deficits illustrate the area subtended from the occlusion of the mid-left anterior descending artery.

atrial injections of sonicated Renografin–76.[S4] They found that regions with less ultrasound contrast before surgery overlapped with areas of wall motion abnormalities. Following the bypass surgery, the distribution of pixel intensity was uniformly enhanced, thus qualitatively suggesting that contrast echocardiography may be used to evaluate the success of revascularization procedures.

These clinical observations have been supported in animal (canine) experiments.[S5] Although much progress is being made in the intraoperative use of contrast echocardiography, considerable work remains in order to establish a firm scientific basis for intraoperative contrast echocardiographic perfusion assessment.

Detection of Myocardial Ischemia

In an effort to define the presence or absence of myocardial ischemia, a variety of qualitative analyses have been performed, based upon observed time/intensity curves derived from digitized contrast-enhanced ultrasound images. However, none of these empiric approaches has used calibrated direct ultrasound acquisition systems, and, accordingly, only relative perfusion parameters have been identified. In addition, in many of these studies rigorous validation techniques have not been applied. Nonetheless, these studies, while of limited scope, have yielded some encouraging results. Berwing and colleagues described a prolonged myocardial contrast washout curve after right ventricular pacing and intracoronary contrast injections in patients having significant coronary artery stenosis without wall motion abnormalities.[B8] However, no independent measure of coronary reserve was uniformly applied, and the degree of coronary stenosis that may be correlated with the loss of contrast effect within the myocardium remains to be established. In addition, Rovai and associates attempted to use contrast echocardiography to quantify ischemia and showed that the slope of washout curves and mean transit time (i.e., half-life of intensity appearance) correlated well with different flows.[R5] Further, the investigators affirmed the possibility of differentiating the spatial (subendocardial versus subepicardial) and temporal distribution of coronary blood flow through the entire cardiac cycle[R8] in the canine model. Lim and colleagues suggested similar findings in patients using contrast echocardiography.[L4]

In addition, Ten Cate and colleagues found that digital echocardiographic parameters (i.e., area under the curve, duration of the curve, half-life of intensity disappearance) were prolonged in patients who had coronary stenoses greater than 50 percent as determined by quantitative coronary angiogram.[T3] Indirect assessments of vascular reserve were performed by Cheirif and associates, using contrast echocardiography during angiography in patients undergoing coronary angioplasty.[C2] Ultrasound contrast material was injected into the coronary arteries prior to and after artery dilatation. Papaverine was used to test vascular reserve in early experimental condition. The peak intensity of the contrast effect, determined by off-line videointensity measurements, served as the end point for assessing increased vascular reserve. From measurements made in patients before and after percutaneous balloon angioplasty, Cheirif and associates concluded: (1) The presence of a statistically significant increase in background signal was 80 percent sensitive and 92 percent specific in separating patients with normal coronary arteries from patients with angiographically demonstrated coronary artery disease; (2) the peak reflected ultrasound intensity significantly improved in those patients with proven coronary artery disease, following successful coronary angioplasty procedures.[C2]

Although these initial clinical studies support the potential use of contrast echocardiography in assessing myocardial perfusion, rigorously controlled clinical studies, using independent measures of regional perfusion, will be required prior to full clinical applicability.

Contrast echocardiography also has been utilized to evaluate the efficacy of invasive therapy.[S3] Researchers at the University of Chicago first used contrast echocardiography during percutaneous transluminal coronary angioplasty to evaluate the efficacy of therapy.[L3] Of seven patients with single-vessel disease, five patients whose treatment had been deemed effective (based on angiographic improvement of the stenosis) showed an increased contrast effect in regions that had been underperfused prior to angioplasty. Reisner and associates described similar findings using peak contrast intensity as a quantitative perfusion marker.[R6] The changes in coronary gradient were found to correlate well with the changes in peak pixel intensity ($r = 0.82$). However, these reports, while intriguing, are based on small numbers of patients, and controlled studies using larger patient bases would be required to establish the role that contrast echocardiography could play in evaluating interventional therapies.

Studies of the Coronary Collateral Circulation

To date, studies of the coronary collateral circulation have not been the focus of interest in investigators working with contrast echocardiography. However, in one study, Widimsky and coworkers demonstrated during angioplasty that contrast echocardiography may be used to identify collateral vessels not seen by conventional coronary angiography.[W3] In addition, Grill and coworkers described, in an abstract, changes in collateral flow prior to and after coronary angioplasty using contrast echocardiographic techniques.[G4] Kemper and associates studied changes in collateral blood flow patterns after occlusion of the canine circumflex coronary artery, using serial intra-aortic injections of hand-agitated microbubbles.[K5] After 1 minute of occlusion, no contrast was visible in the area of the perfusion defect, but after 20 minutes a small amount of contrast effect appeared (primarily in the subepicardial aspect of the "recipient" region). After 2 hours, full opacification occurred in the area of coronary occlusion (with a brief delay after injection).

Although these initial reports concerning the use of contrast echocardiography to study the coronary collateral circulation are of some interest, much more work needs to be done in this area before the value of this technique for studying the coronary collateral circulation can be established.

Advantages and Disadvantages of Contrast Echocardiography for Studies of Myocardial Perfusion

Contrast echocardiographic studies of myocardial perfusion could be extremely helpful if they could be done with an intravenous injection of bubbles and if the studies could be validated under a variety of conditions utilizing rigorous standards. Under these circumstances, contrast echocardiography would be extremely useful in the clinical care of patients with heart disease.

At present, however, formidable problems remain, including

- difficulties with echocardiographic instrumentation, which presently does not reveal a signal that is linear with respect to bubble concentration;
- difficulties with three-dimensional reconstruction of the entire left ventricle;
- lateral dropout;
- validation of estimating blood volume within the myocardium with echocardiographic contrast;
- lack of rigorously controlled validation studies;
- problems with the ultrasonic contrast media that have been used in the great majorities of studies published thus far;
- many unresolved problems concerning the appropriate algorithm to measure myocardial perfusion with echocardiographic contrast.

OTHER CARDIAC APPLICATIONS OF CONTRAST ECHOCARDIOGRAPHY

Measurement of Cardiac Output

In the past, contrast echocardiography has been used to evaluate static as well as dynamic volumes with principles of indicator-dilution theory. DeMaria and co-workers, using 30-micron plastic balloons, established a linear correlation between concentration and backscatter and subsequently found a direct correlation between videodensitometric and thermodilution measurements at various cardiac outputs in an animal model (Fig. 27–11).[D1] In addition, Rovai and co-workers[R7] correlated left ventricular contrast echo washout curves with ejection fraction (determined by angiography) in animals.

In the future, the use of transpulmonary contrast injections for determination of left ventricular ejection indices (i.e., cardiac output, stroke volumes, and so on) will require the establishment of a direct, linear relationship between microbubble concentration and reflected ultrasound energy. If these calibration steps can be performed and utilized successfully, cardiac ultrasound imaging will be useful in providing significant additional information regarding global left ventricular function.

Right Heart Studies

Contrast echocardiographic techniques continue to be used in the management of patients with difficult or confusing cardiac anatomy.[S1, V1] The earliest described uses of contrast ultrasound were designed to identify cardiac chambers. Even today, with the development of Doppler techniques, contrast ultrasound techniques compare favorably in economy and clinical utility. Furthermore, the simultaneous use of contrast echocardiography and Doppler enhances information relating to identification of the right heart structures. Figure 27–12 provides an example.

Intracardiac Shunts

Recent thorough reviews by Van Hare and Silverman[V1] and Sahn and Valdez-Cruz[S1] have discussed the utility of contrast echocardiographic techniques for diagnosing congenital cardiac abnormalities. Van Hare and Silverman described their experience in studying over 14,000 pediatric patients with two-dimensional echocardiographic examinations from 1976 to 1988.[V1] Approximately 6 percent of these studies involved contrast echocardiography, one third of which were performed following cardiac surgery. The majority of the cardiac abnormalities detected consisted of ventricular septal defects, transposition of the great vessels, and atrial septal defects. A vast array of other congenital abnormalities was noted, including double outlet right ventricle, total anomalous pulmonary venous connection, pulmonary atresia and critical pulmonary stenosis, single ventricle and tricuspid atresia, and so on. A variety of other congenital cardiac anatomy abnormalities were also identified.

In the adult cardiology practice, the primary use of contrast echocardiography has been to identify atrial or ventricular septal defects. The use of contrast echocardiography to identify an intra-atrial shunt was recently reported by Lechat and colleagues.[L5]

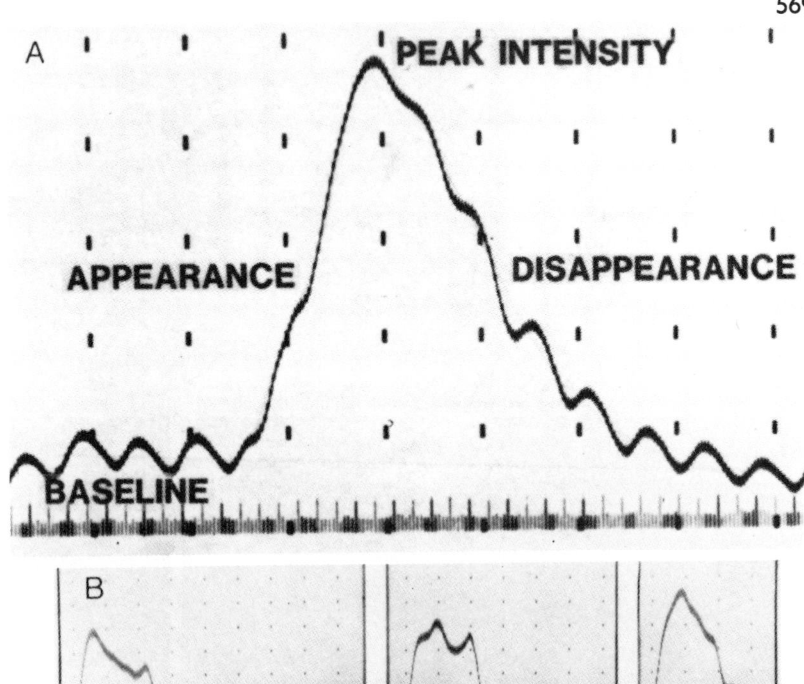

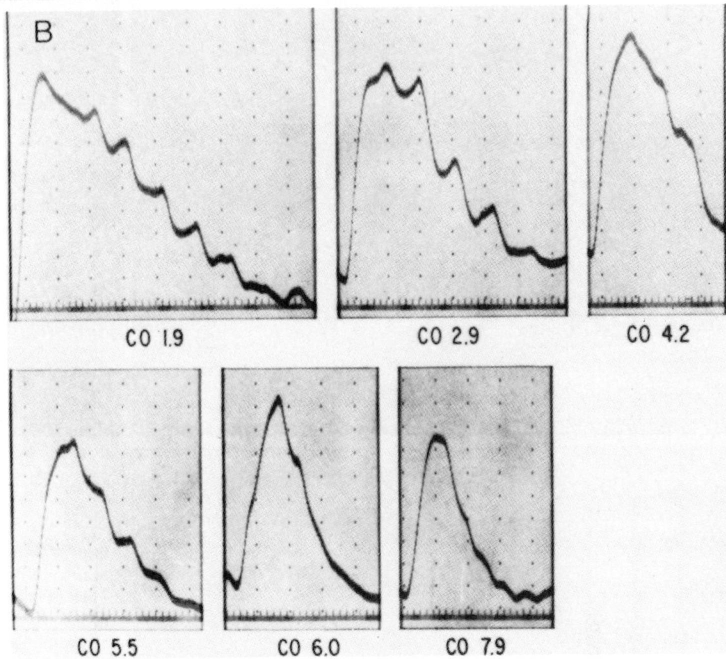

Figure 27–11. Kinetics of left ventricular contrast indicator curves correlated with the cardiac output as determined with thermodilution techniques. *A*, Contrast material was directly injected into the left ventricular cavity of an animal and revealed a brisk appearance, a peak effect, and, ultimately, a decay. *B* illustrates the effect of varying cardiac output (measured by thermodilution techniques) correlated with the video-intensity signal obtained following direct left ventricular ultrasound contrast injections. Note the decrease in area under the time intensity graph as the cardiac output increases. (From DeMaria, A. N., Bommer, W., Kwan, O. L., et al.: In vivo correlation of thermodilution cardiac output and video-densitometric indicator-dilution curves obtained from contrast 2-dimensional echocardiograms. J. Am. Coll. Cardiol. 3:999, 1984. Reprinted with permission of the American College of Cardiology.)

They suggested that contrast echocardiographic techniques could detect the presence of a patent foramen ovale, with the possibility that paradoxic emboli emanating from a patent foramen ovale may lead to a cerebrovascular accident. They noted a disproportionate prevalence of right-to-left atrial shunts proved by contrast echocardiography in a significant portion of patients who had suffered an ischemic stroke as compared with a normal (nonstroke) population. Further, in the subgroup of patients in whom a source of the emboli could not be identified, 54 percent of the 26 patients demonstrated a patent foramen ovale at rest or during provocation maneuvers (Valsalva test). The reports by Van Hare[V1] and Lechat[L5] continue to emphasize the clinical utility of performing contrast echocardiography.

Left Heart Studies

Ultimately, the ability to assess left heart function and structures following an intravenous injection of an ultrasound contrast material could improve markedly the ability to diagnose cardiac disease with noninvasive imaging techniques. Ironically, the first reported use of contrast echocardiography was to identify left heart structures. In 1968, Gramiak and Shah used manually agitated microbubbles to identify the LV cavity and aortic root of patients undergoing cardiac catheterization.[G1] Due to the relatively large and unstable nature of these microbubbles, it was necessary to inject the contrast material directly into the aorta or left ventricle in order to visualize the left heart structures by echocardiography.

Important clinical information can be obtained from the use of left-side contrast echo injections. Qualitative assessments of mitral valve regurgitation, aortic root delineation, or LV cavity identification can be performed at coronary angiography or cardiac operation.

Figure 27–13 illustrates the application of contrast echocardiographic techniques during coronary angiography in a patient with a dilated congestive cardiomyopathy. The volume of radiopaque dye required to opacify the left ventricular cavity fully posed a risk to the patient because of the potentially deleterious effects of the dye load on renal function. In this case, 0.5 ml of sonicated Renografin–76 dye (microbubble diameter, 10 ± 4 microns[F1]) was injected through a catheter inserted into the left ventricular cavity. Simultaneous two-dimensional echocardiographic imaging during the injection revealed the endocardial surface of the heart and thus permitted an assessment of left ventricular systolic function. In addition, it was possible to note that the degree of mitral regurgitation was minimal, as evidenced by the small fan of contrast material in the left atrium during systolic function.

With the development of stabilized ultrasound contrast agents, the ability to identify the left heart structures via an intravenous injection of a contrast agent may obviate the need in certain situations to perform invasive studies. As an example of the use

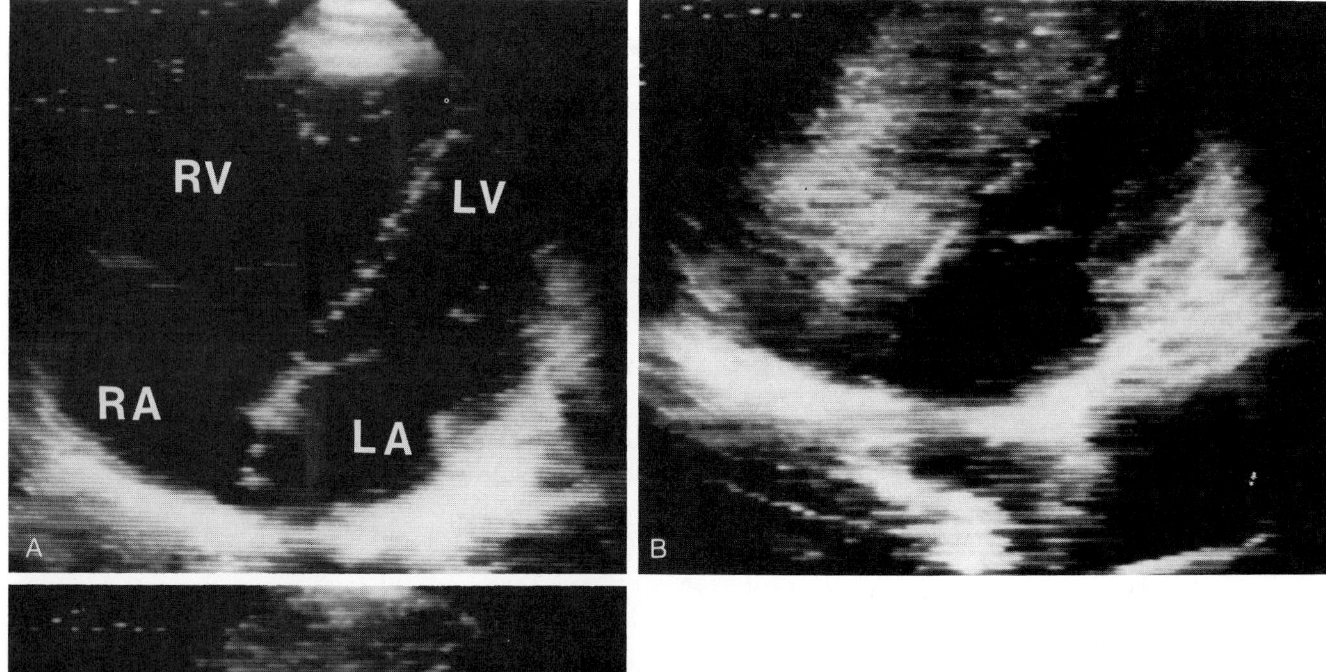

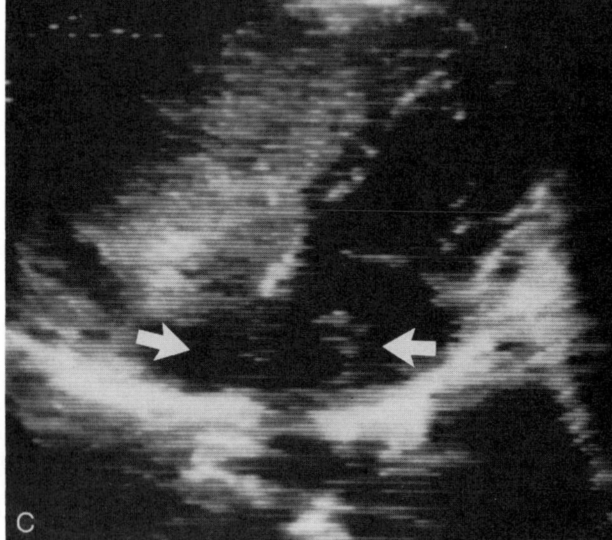

Figure 27–12. Contrast echocardiography in the evaluation of right heart abnormality. *A*, A two-dimensional echocardiographic apical four-chamber view of a 31-year-old patient with symptoms of palpitations and mild shortness of breath with ex exertion; right-sided chambers appear moderately enlarged. Doppler studies revealed no abnormalities. *B*, Following a peripheral intravenous injection of 3.0 ml of a sterile sonicated solution (dextrose 50 percent [mean microbubble size, 12 ± 6 microns][F2]), the right heart chambers appear opacified. *C*, Several cardiac cycles following the initial opacification of the right heart chambers, a wisp of contrast material was identified in the posterior aspect of the left atrium (arrow denotes contrast material in the left atrium). In addition, note the "negative" contrast in the right atrium (arrow in right atrium). The presence of a "negative contrast effect" suggested to-and-fro shunting at the atrial level. A sinus venosus atrial septal defect was diagnosed at cardiac catheterization and subsequently confirmed at cardiac operation.

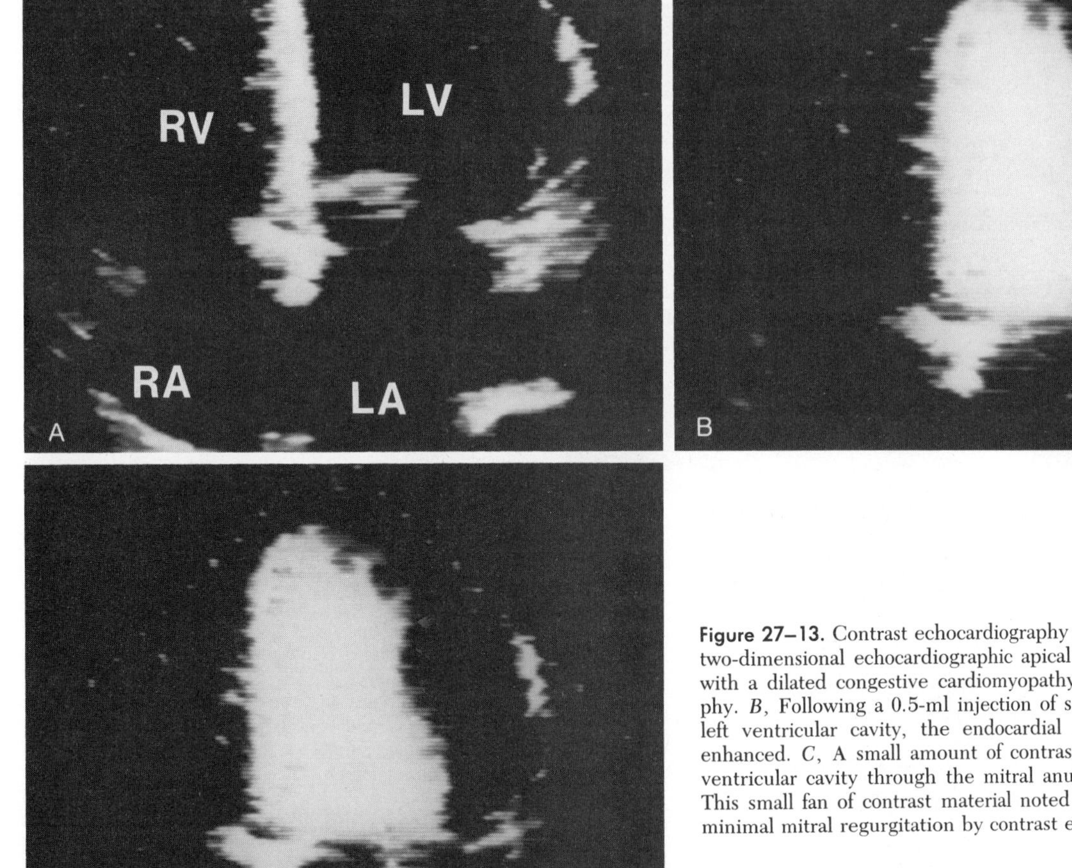

Figure 27–13. Contrast echocardiography in dilated cardiomyopathy. *A*, A two-dimensional echocardiographic apical four-chamber view of a patient with a dilated congestive cardiomyopathy undergoing coronary angiography. *B*, Following a 0.5-ml injection of sonicated Renografin-76 into the left ventricular cavity, the endocardial surface of the left ventricle is enhanced. *C*, A small amount of contrast material extends from the left ventricular cavity through the mitral anulus into the left atrium (arrow). This small fan of contrast material noted in the left atrium demonstrates minimal mitral regurgitation by contrast echocardiography.

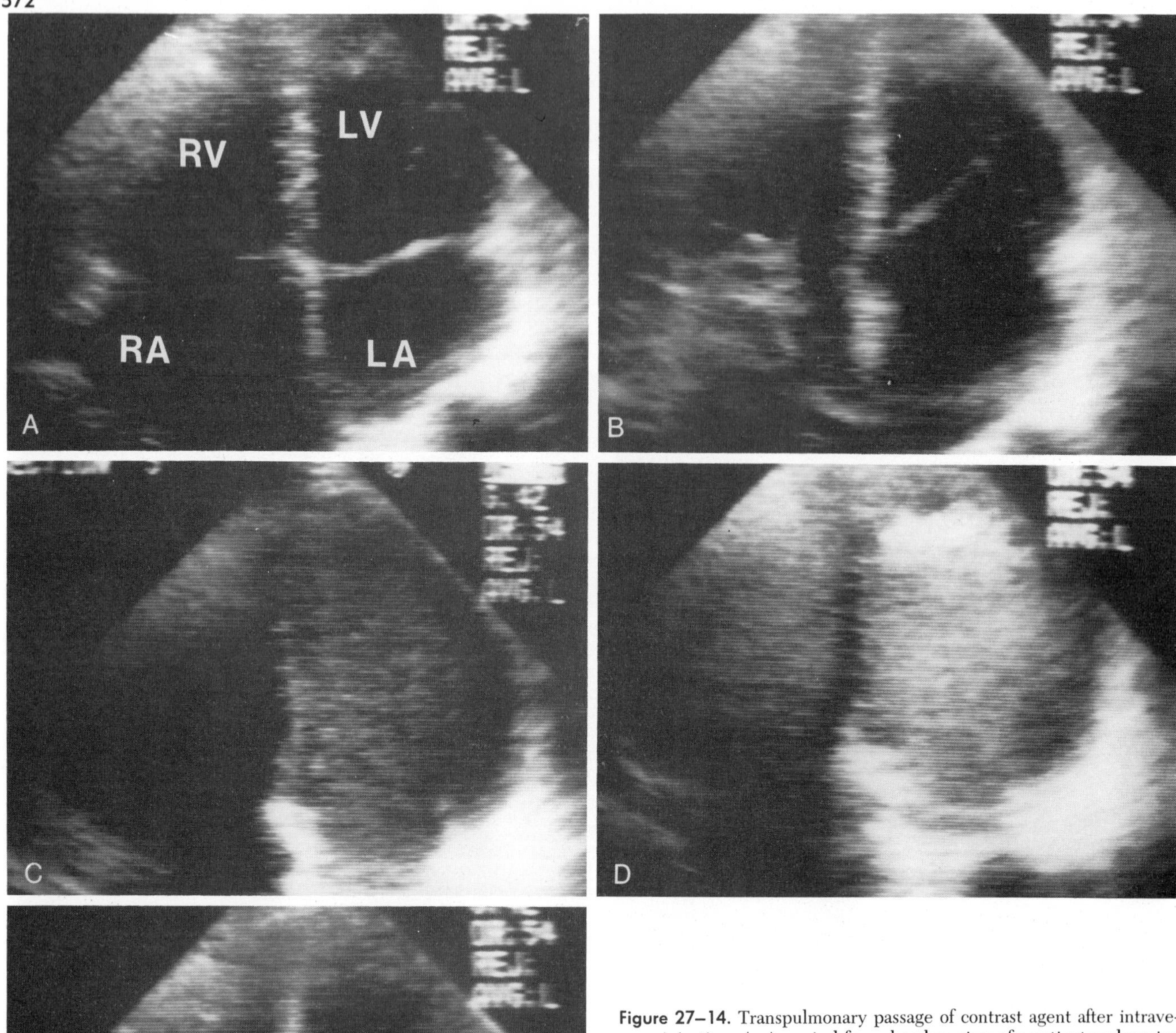

Figure 27–14. Transpulmonary passage of contrast agent after intravenous injection. *A*, An apical four-chamber view of a patient undergoing an echocardiographic examination. *B*, The first appearance of contrast is seen in the right atrium following the intravenous injection of a commercially prepared ultrasound contrast agent capable of transpulmonary passage. *C* illustrates complete right heart attenuation due to contrast overload, with minimal appearance of the contrast agent in the left ventricle. *D*, Several cardiac cycles later, the contrast material had substantially cleared the right ventricular cavity and is predominantly seen in the left ventricular cavity. *E* shows the clearance of contrast material from both the right and left ventricular cavities.

of an intravenous contrast agent, Figure 27–14 demonstrates the use of a commercially prepared echo contrast agent (Albunex, Molecular Biosystems, Inc., San Diego, CA) that successfully crosses the lung vasculature in patients.[F7] Following a peripheral intravenous injection of the ultrasound contrast agent, dense opacification and attenuation of the right heart structures could be noted. Within six to seven cardiac cycles after noting the contrast effect in the right ventricle, contrast material is identified in the left heart. After several heart beats, the entire left and right ventricular cavities are filled with the ultrasound contrast material. Following the clearance of contrast material from the right ventricle, the delay in clearing the left ventricular cavity opacification is evidenced in Figure 27–14*D*. Figure 27–14*E* illustrates complete clearance of the contrast material from the right and left ventricular cavities.

SUMMARY

Numerous potential uses of contrast echocardiography may significantly improve the clinical management of cardiac, and even noncardiac, patients. The primary potential uses include better definition of cardiac structure and function and measurement of regional myocardial perfusion. Perhaps the most ambitious goal of current contrast echocardiography research is the development of an intravenous technique for perfusion screening and follow-up evaluation that could be employed outside the operating room and catheterization laboratory. Contrast echocardiography appears to be a safe, reliable, and convenient technique.[F7] Ongoing work in these areas is promising and should be encouraged.

Acknowledgment

We are grateful to and thank Ms. Fran Murphy for her expert assistance in preparing this chapter.

References

A

1. Armstrong, W. F., Mueller, T. M., Kinney, E. L., et al.: Assessment of myocardial perfusion abnormalities with contrast enhancement two-dimensional echocardiography. (Abstract.) Circulation 4 (Suppl. II):566, 1988.

B

1. Beard, J. T., and Byrd, B. R.: Saline contrast enhancement of trivial Doppler tricuspid regurgitation signals for estimating pulmonary artery pressure. Am. J. Cardiol. 62:486, 1988.
2. Bommer, W. J., Shah, P. M., Allen, H., et al.: The safety of contrast echocardiography: Report of Committee on Contrast Echocardiography of the American Society of Echocardiography. J. Am. Coll. Cardiol. 3:6, 1984.
3. Bommer, W. J., Mason, D. T., and DeMaria, A. N.: Studies in contrast echocardiography. Development of new agents with superior reproducibility and transmission through lungs. (Abstract.) Circulation 60 (Suppl. II):II–17, 1979.
4. Bommer, W. J., Tickner, E. G., Rasor, J., et al.: Development of a new echocardiographic contrast agent capable of pulmonary transmission and left heart opacification following peripheral venous injection. (Abstract.) Circulation 62 (Suppl. III):III–34, 1980.
5. Berwing, K., and Schlepper, M.: Echocardiographic imaging of the left ventricle by peripheral intravenous injection of echo contrast agent. Am. Heart J. 115:399, 1988.
6. Buda, A. J., Delp, E. J., Meyer, C. R., et al.: Automatic computer processing of digital 2-dimensional echocardiograms. Am. J. Cardiol. 52:384, 1983.
7. Bach, D. S., Feinstein, S. B., Williams, K. A., and Carroll, J. D.: Comparative imaging modalities in patients with coronary artery disease: Coronary angiography, thallium–201 and contrast echocardiography. Dynamic Cardiovasc. Imaging 2:15, 1989.
8. Berwing, K, Schlepper, M., Kremer, P., and Bahavar, H.: Assessment of myocardial perfusion abnormalities in patients with coronary heart disease by intracoronary injection of new echo contrast agent. (Abstract.) Circulation 74 (Suppl. II):475, 1986.

C

1. Cheirif, J., Yamamoto, H., Zoghbi, W. A., et al.: Demonstration of physiologic transit time of sonicated meglumine diatrizoate in a microvascular preparation. J. Cardiovasc. Ultrasound 6:245, 1987.
2. Cheirif, J., Zoghbi, W. A., Raizner, A. E., et al.: Assessment of myocardial perfusion in humans by contrast echocardiography. I. Evaluation of regional coronary reserve by peak intensity. J. Am. Coll. Cardiol. 11:735, 1988.

D

1. DeMaria, A. N., Bommer, W., Kwan, O. L., et al.: In vivo correlation of thermodilution cardiac output and video-densitometric indicator-dilution curves obtained from contrast 2-dimensional echocardiograms. J. Am. Coll. Cardiol. 3:999, 1984.
2. DeMaria, A. N., Bommer, W. J., Riggs, K., et al.: Echocardiographic visualization of myocardial perfusion by left heart and intracoronary injection of echo contrast agent. (Abstract.) Circulation 62 (Suppl. III):III–143, 1980.

E

1. Edler, I., Gustafson, A., Karlefors, T., and Christensson, B: Ultrasound cardiography. Acta Med. Scand. (Suppl.) 370:68, 1961.

F

1. Feinstein, S. B., Lang, R. M., Dick, C. D., et al.: Contrast echocardiography during coronary arteriography in humans: Perfusion and anatomic studies. J. Am. Coll. Cardiol. 11:59, 1988.
2. Feinstein, S. B., Ten Cate, F., Zwehl, W., et al.: Two-dimensional contrast echocardiography. I. In vitro development and quantitative analysis of echo contrast agents. J. Am. Coll. Cardiol. 3:14, 1984.
3. Feinstein, S. B., Shah, P. M., Bing, R. J., et al.: Microbubble dynamics visualized in the intact capillary circulation. J. Am. Coll. Cardiol. 4:595, 1984.
4. Feigenbaum, H., Stone, J. M., Lee, D. A., et al.: Identification of ultrasound echoes from the left ventricle by the use of indocyanine green. Circulation 41:615, 1970.
5. Feinstein, S. B., Keller, M. W., Dick, C. D., et al.: Successful transpulmonary contrast echocardiography in monkeys. (Abstract.) J. Am. Coll. Cardiol. 9:111A, 1987.
6. Feinstein, S. B., Keller, M. W., Kerber, R. E., et al.: Sonicated echocardiographic contrast agents: Reproducibility studies. J. Am. Soc. Echo. 2:125, 1989.
7. Feinstein, S. B., Heidenrich, P. A., Dick, C. D., et al.: Albunex: a new intravascular ultrasound contrast agent; Preliminary safety and efficacy results. (Abstract.) Circulation 4 (Suppl. II):565, 1988.

G

1. Gramiak, R., and Shah, P. M.: Echocardiography of the aortic root. Invest. Radiol. 3:356, 1968.
2. Gillam, L. D., Kaul, S., Fallan, J., et al.: Functional and pathologic effect of multiple echocardiographic contrast injections on the myocardium, brain and kidney. J. Am. Coll. Cardiol. 6:687, 1985.
3. Goldman, M. E., Mindich, B. P., Teichholz, L. E., et al.: Intraoperative cardioplegia contrast echocardiography for assessing perfusion during open heart surgery. J. Am. Coll. Cardiol. 4:1029, 1984.
4. Grill, H. P., Brinker, J. A., Cadden, J., et al.: Contrast echocardiography demonstration of coronary collateral flow in humans. (Abstract.) Circulation 4 (Suppl. II):463, 1988.

H

1. Heidenreich, P. A., Harper, P. V., Chen, T. W., et al.: Contrast echo measurement of myocardial perfusion: Standardization. (Abstract.) Circulation 4 (Suppl. II):566, 1988.
2. Hoyt, R. H., Collins, S. M., Skorton, D. J., et al.: Assessment of fibrosis in infarcted human hearts by analysis of ultrasonic backscatter. Circulation 71:740, 1985.

K

1. Kerber, R. E., Kioschos, J. M., and Lauer, R. M.: Use of an ultrasonic contrast method in the diagnosis of valvular regurgitation and intracardiac shunts. Am. J. Cardiol. 34:722, 1974.
2. Keller, M. W., Feinstein, S. B., and Watson, D. D.: Successful left ventricular opacification following peripheral venous injection of sonicated contrast agent: An experimental evaluation. Am. Heart J. 114:570, 1987.
3. Keller, M. W., Glasheen, W. P., Teja K., et al.: Myocardial contrast echocardiography without significant hemodynamic effects or reactive hyperemia: A major advantage in the imaging of myocardial perfusion. J. Am. Coll. Cardiol. 12:1039, 1988.
4. Kaul, S., Pandian, N. G., Okada, R. D., et al.: Contrast echocardiography in acute myocardial ischemia: I. In vivo determination of total left ventricular "area at risk." J. Am. Coll. Cardiol. 4:1272, 1984.
5. Kemper, A. J.: Animal studies: Part II. *In* Feinstein SB (ed.): Workshop on contrast echocardiography. Echocardiography 5:8, 1988.

L

1. Levine, R. A., Teicholz, L. E., Goldman, M. E., et al.: Microbubbles have intracardiac velocities similar to those of red blood cells. J. Am. Coll. Cardiol. 3:28, 1984.
2. Lang, R. M., Borow, K. M., Neumann, A., and Feinstein, S. B.: Echocardiographic contrast agents: Effects of microbubbles and carrier solutions on left ventricular contractility. J. Am. Coll. Cardiol. 9:910, 1987.
3. Lang, R. M., Feinstein, S. B., Feldman, T., et al.: Contrast echocardiography for evaluation of myocardial perfusion: Effects of coronary angioplasty. J. Am. Coll. Cardiol. 8:232, 1986.
4. Lim, Y.-J., Nanto, S., Masuyama, T., et al.: Visualization of subendocardial myocardial ischemia with myocardial contrast echocardiography in humans. Circulation 79:233, 1989.
5. Lechat, P., Mas, J. L., Lascault, G., et al.: Prevalence of patent foramen ovale in patients with stroke. N. Engl. J. Med. 318:1148, 1988.

M

1. Meltzer, R. S., Tickner, E. G., Sahines, T., and Popp, R. L.: The source of ultrasound contrast effect. J. Clin. Ultrasound 18:121, 1980.
2. Moore, C. A., Smucker, M. L., and Kaul, S.: Myocardial contrast echocardiography in humans: I. Safety in comparison with routine coronary arteriography. J. Am. Coll. Cardiol. 8:1066, 1986.
3. Miller, J. G., Perez, J. E., and Sobel, B. E.: Ultrasonic characterization of myocardium. Prog. Cardiovasc. Dis. 28:85, 1985.
4. Meier, P., and Zierler, K. L.: On the theory of the indicator-dilution method for measurement of blood flow and volume. J. Appl. Physiol. 6:731, 1954.

O

1. Ophir, J., and Parker, K. J.: Contrast agents in diagnostic ultrasound. Ultrasound Med. Biol. 15:319, 1989.

P

1. Powsner, S. M., Feinstein, S. B., and Samie, J.: Quantitative radiofrequency analysis of sonicated echo contrast agents. (Abstract.) J. Am. Coll. Cardiol. 5:474, 1985.
2. Powsner, S., Wood, J., Prieto, P., et al.: High speed interface for myocardial sonicated echo contrast studies. SPIE 845:384, 1987.
3. Preuss, K. C., Gross, G. J., Brooks, H. L., and Warltier, D. C.: Time course of recovery in "stunned" myocardium following variable periods of ischemia in conscious and anesthetized dogs. Am. Heart J. 114:696, 1987.

R

1. Reale, A.: Visualizzazione ecocontrastografica delle sezioni sinistre del cuore mediante iniezione di anidride carbonica in arteria polmonare. Policlin. Prat. 67:585, 1979.
2. Reale, A., Pizzuto, F., Gioffre, P. A., et al.: Contrast echocardiography: Transmission of echoes to the left heart across the pulmonary vascular bed. Eur. Heart J. 1:101, 1980.
3. Reisner, S. A., Ong, L. S., Shapiro, J. R., et al.: Efficacy and safety of myocardial perfusion imaging using intracoronary sonicated albumin in humans. (Abstract.) Circulation 4 (Suppl. II):565, 1988.
4. Rasmussen, S., Lovelace, D. E., Knoebel, S. B., et al.: Echocardiographic detection of ischemic and infarcted myocardium. J. Am. Coll. Cardiol. 3:733, 1984.
5. Rovai, D., Lombardi, M., De Pieri, G., et al.: Accurate flow quantitation by radiofrequency analysis of contrast echo. (Abstract.) Circulation 4 (Suppl. II):566, 1988.
6. Reisner, S. A., Ong, L. S., Lichtenberg, G. S., et al.: Quantitative assessment of the immediate results of coronary angioplasty by myocardial contrast echocardiography. J. Am. Coll. Cardiol. 13:852, 1989.
7. Rovai, D., Nissen, S. E., Elion, J., et al.: Contrast echo washout curves from the left ventricle: Application of basic principles of indicator-dilution theory and calculation of ejection fraction. J. Am. Coll. Cardiol. 10:125, 1987.
8. Rovai, D., Lombardi, M., Nissen, S. E., et al.: Spatial and temporal heterogeneity of coronary blood flow by myocardial contrast echocardiography. (Abstract.) J. Am. Coll. Cardiol. 9:112A, 1987.

S

1. Sahn, D. J., and Valdez-Cruz, L. M.: Ultrasound contrast studies for the detection of cardiac shunts. J. Am. Coll. Cardiol. 3:978, 1984.
2. Shapiro, J. R., Xie, F., and Meltzer, R. S.: Myocardial contrast two-dimensional echocardiography: Dose-myocardial effect relations of intracoronary microbubbles. J. Am. Coll. Cardiol. 3:765, 1988.
3. Smalling, R. W.: Can the immediate efficacy of coronary angioplasty be adequately addressed? J. Am. Coll. Cardiol. 10:261, 1987.
4. Smith, J., Feinstein, S. B., Kapelanski, D. P., et al.: Transesophageal echocardiographic determination of myocardial perfusion during cardiac surgery. (Abstract.) Circulation 74 (Suppl. II):475, 1986.
5. Spotnitz, W. D., Keller, M. W., Watson, D. D., et al.: Success of internal mammary bypass grafting can be assessed intraoperatively using myocardial contrast echocardiography. J. Am. Coll. Cardiol. 12:196, 1985.

T

1. Tei, C., Sakamaki, T., Shah, P. M., et al.: Myocardial contrast echocardiography: A reproducible technique of myocardial opacification for identifying regional perfusion deficits. Circulation 67:585, 1983.
2. Ten Cate, F. J., Feinstein, S. B., Zwehl, W., et al.: Two-dimensional contrast echocardiography. II. Transpulmonary studies. J. Am. Coll. Cardiol. 3:21, 1984.
3. Ten Cate, F. J., Cornell, J. H., Surruys, P. W., et al.: Quantitative myocardial perfusion imaging using contrast two-dimensional echocardiography. (Abstract.) J. Am. Coll. Cardiol. 9:112A, 1987.

V

1. Van Hare, G. F., and Silverman, N. H.: Contrast two-dimensional echocardiography in congenital heart disease: Techniques, indications and clinical utility. J. Am. Coll. Cardiol. 13:673, 1989.

W

1. White, C. W., Wright, C. B., Doty, D. B., et al.: Does visual interpretation of the coronary arteriogram predict the physiologic importance of a coronary stenosis? N. Engl. J. Med. 310:819, 1984.
2. Willard, G. E.: Ultrasonically induced cavitation in water: A step-by-step process. J. Acoust. Soc. Am. 25:669, 1953.
3. Widimsky, P., Cornel, J. H., and Ten Cate, F. J.: Evaluation of collateral blood flow by myocardial contrast-enhanced echocardiography. Br. Heart J. 59:20, 1988.

Z

1. Ziskin, M. C., Bonakdapour, A., Weinstein, D. P., and Lynch, P. R.: Contrast agents for diagnostic ultrasound. Invest. Radiol. 7:500, 1972.
2. Zwehl, W., Areeda, J., Schwartz, G., et al.: Physical factors influencing quantitation of two-dimensional contrast echo-amplitudes. J. Am. Coll. Cardiol. 4:157, 1984.
3. Zierler, K. L.: Equations for measuring blood flow by external measurement of radioisotopes. Circulation Res. 14:309, 1965.

Chapter 28

Stress Echocardiography

▪ *CHARLES F. PRESTI, M.D.* ▪ *MICHAEL H. CRAWFORD, M.D.*

ECHOCARDIOGRAPHIC TECHNIQUES 575
M-Mode Echocardiography 575
Two-Dimensional Echocardiography 575
Doppler Echocardiography 577
Analysis of Exercise Echocardiographic Studies 580
CLINICAL APPLICATIONS OF EXERCISE ECHOCARDIOGRAPHY 580
Application to Ischemic Heart Disease 580
Diagnosis of Ischemic Heart Disease 582
Use of Left Ventricular Ejection Fraction in the Diagnosis of Coronary Artery Disease 584
Comparison With Exercise Electrocardiography 585
Comparison With Radionuclide Techniques 585
Exercise Doppler Echocardiography in the Assessment of Ischemic Heart Disease 586
Risk Stratification Post Myocardial Infarction 588
NON-EXERCISE STRESS ECHOCARDIOGRAPHY 589
Techniques That Increase Myocardial Oxygen Demand 589
Techniques That Alter Coronary Blood Flow 589
Dipyridamole 589

Exercise electrocardiography has proved to be a valuable technique in the evaluation of patients with known or suspected cardiac disease. Several different techniques have been used in conjunction with exercise electrocardiographic testing either to enhance its diagnostic accuracy or to objectively assess left ventricular function during exercise. These techniques include radionuclide angiography, thallium-201 scintigraphy, M-mode and two-dimensional echocardiography, and, more recently, Doppler echocardiography. Echocardiography offers several unique advantages when applied to the exercising patient. It is totally noninvasive, requires no radiation exposure, permits the analysis of left ventricular function on a beat-by-beat basis, and can be applied to several different exercise protocols. In addition, as in any echocardiographic study, the information obtained from an exercise echocardiogram is related not only to regional and global left ventricular function but also to valvular structure and function, chamber size and wall thickness, and pericardial abnormalities. Finally, advances in both imaging and computer technologies have significantly improved the ability to obtain acceptable echocardiographic images both at rest and during exercise and rapidly assess segmental and global left ventricular function. These features combine to make exercise echocardiography a useful modality for the investigation of left ventricular function in a research setting as well as in the clinical arena. This chapter discusses the use of a variety of stress echocardiographic techniques from a technical standpoint and as a practical approach to the assessment of cardiac disease.

ECHOCARDIOGRAPHIC TECHNIQUES

M-Mode Echocardiography

M-mode echocardiography was the ultrasound technique initially used to study the left ventricular response to exercise. Using an early form of this technique, Kraunz and Kennedy in 1970 and Smithen and associates in 1972 demonstrated a significant increase in posterior wall velocity and amplitude of excursion in normal subjects following isotonic exercise.[K1, S2] Fogelman and associates, using a similar technique, demonstrated a significant decrease in maximal diastolic velocity of the posterior left ventricular endocardium during exercise-induced ischemia in patients with angina pectoris.[F1] M-mode echocardiography was subsequently used by Stefadouros and associates in 1974 to investigate the effect of isometric exercise on left ventricular performance in normal subjects.[S2] In 1978, Stein and associates used M-mode echocardiography to evaluate changes in left ventricular dimensions and performance during and immediately following low-level supine bicycle exercise in 10 normal subjects.[S3] Following these initial reports, several investigators utilized M-mode echocardiography to study the left ventricular response to various types of exercise in normal subjects, in patients with ischemic heart disease, and in patients with valvular and myopathic heart disease.[A1, B1, B2, C1, E1, L1, M1, P1, S4–S6, W1]

Although these early investigations demonstrated the ability of M-mode echocardiography to assess left ventricular performance during exercise, certain limitations have precluded its widespread clinical use. Technical difficulties due to exaggerated chest wall motion during exercise frequently result in inability to obtain high-quality M-mode echocardiograms suitable for measurement. Although Sugishita and Koseki reported an 83 percent success rate in obtaining M-mode echocardiograms during submaximal supine bicycle exercise in a population of normal subjects and patients with cardiac disease,[S4] others have reported a substantially lower imaging success rate.[C1, M1] In addition, since small changes in angulation of the M-mode beam can lead to relatively larger changes in dimensional measurements, consistency of transducer position and axis becomes important in the performance of exercise M-mode echocardiography. However, the major limitation of this technique is that M-mode echocardiography provides only an "ice-pick" view of the heart. Hence, it is likely that many patients with ischemic heart disease will develop exercise-induced regional wall motion abnormalities that will not be detected with M-mode echocardiography. Similarly, in patients with regional myocardial dysfunction or dilated left ventricles, the narrow view of M-mode echocardiography does not provide a reliable estimate of left ventricular function. For these reasons, M-mode echocardiography is not routinely used to provide information about the global or regional left ventricular response to exercise.

Two-Dimensional Echocardiography

The development of two-dimensional echocardiography provided a technique that overcame many of the problems associated with M-mode echocardiography. Since two-dimensional echocardiography allows for imaging of the heart in multiple tomographic planes, in theory all myocardial segments can be evaluated. In addition, measurements made by two-dimensional echocardiography are less dependent than those made by M-mode echocardiography on the relationship between the axis of the ultrasound beam and the position of the heart in the chest. Therefore, left ventricular function can be more accurately quantified with two-dimensional echocardiography. As noted above, this is especially important in patients with regional wall motion abnormalities or dilated left ventricles. Finally, two-dimensional echocardiography allows a much higher imaging success rate during and immediately following exercise than M-mode echocardiography. All of these factors have combined to make two-dimensional echocardiography the dominant echocardiographic technique used to evaluate left ventricular function during exercise.

Two-dimensional echocardiography has been used as an imaging technique in combination with a variety of exercise techniques. In 1979, Wann and associates used a 30-degree mechanical sector scanner to demonstrate the feasibility of performing two-dimensional echocardiography during supine bicycle exercise.[W2] Technically adequate echocardiographic studies were obtained in 71 percent of a population of patients with ischemic heart disease studied at rest and during exercise and in 80 percent of patients who had adequate resting echocardiograms. These authors commented that the major technical limitation of obtaining echocardiographic studies during exercise appeared to be hyperventilation rather than chest wall motion. The interposition of the lung between the heart and chest wall made recording of the parasternal views especially difficult during exercise (success rate of 55 percent in patients with adequate examinations); however, the apical window remained readily accessible during exercise (success rate of 95 percent).[W2] Zwehl and associates in 1981 used two-dimensional echocardiography to quantitate left ventricular function in normal subjects during bicycle exercise in a 30-degree left lateral decubitus position.[Z1] These investigators demonstrated that during exercise there was a significant reduction in end-systolic volume without a significant change in end-diastolic volume, which resulted in an increase in left ventricular ejection fraction. Subsequent studies by Morganroth and associates and Visser and associates demonstrated that two-dimensional echocardiography during supine bicycle exercise could be useful in the diagnosis of coronary artery disease.[M2, V1] The overall imaging success rates for these studies with supine bicycle exercise ranged from 71 to 80 percent.[M2, V1, W2, Z1] Performing exercise in the left lateral decubitus position did not appear to enhance the imaging success rate significantly.[V1, Z1]

Upright bicycle exercise has also been used in conjunction with two-dimensional echocardiographic imaging (Fig. 28–1). Studies by Crawford and associates demonstrated that two-dimensional echocardiographic imaging from the apical window was practical for the assessment of wall motion and quantitation of left ventricular function during upright bicycle exercise in a group of patients with coronary artery disease.[C2, C3] They obtained adequate images for quantitating left ventricular performance in two apical views in 72 percent of patients.[C2] Other investigators have subsequently utilized this technique to evaluate left ventricular function in both normal subjects and patients with ischemic heart disease.[G1, C2, P2] Using the subcostal approach, Ginzton and associates had a 95 percent success rate in obtaining adequate images of normal subjects during upright bicycle exercise, and they found that all subjects who had adequate two-dimensional echocardiograms at rest had adequate exercise studies.[G1] Finally, Simard and associates used a device to hold the echocardiographic transducer in the apical plane during semi-upright bicycle exercise and reported an imaging success rate of 95 percent in a group of normal volunteers.[S7]

Two-dimensional echocardiography has also been used as an adjunct to treadmill exercise testing. Maurer and Nanda in 1981 described the use of two-dimensional echocardiography before and immediately following graded exercise treadmill testing in 48 patients being evaluated for suspected coronary artery disease.[M3] They used a technique in which the patient was imaged in the left lateral decubitus position before and after exercise and reported a success rate for obtaining diagnostic images of 85 percent of patients. Subsequently, Limacher and associates, using a similar technique, had an imaging success rate of 100 percent in a group of patients with suspected coronary artery disease.[L2] Robertson and associates performed two-dimensional echocardiography with the patient in the sitting position before and immediately after treadmill exercise testing and reported a 92 percent imaging success rate.[R1] These authors noted that the success rate and quality of post-exercise echocardiograms would probably have been improved if imaging had been done with the patient in the supine or left lateral decubitus position. In all of these studies the apical window usually provided the best images after exercise. Using the fixed transducer device originally described by Simard and associates,[S7] Heng and associates had an 87 percent imaging success rate during treadmill exercise testing.[H1] More recently, several studies have confirmed the clinical utility of echocardiographic imaging immediately following treadmill exercise.[A2, A3, R2]

The type of exercise employed is usually determined by the preference of the exercise laboratory. Patients appear to be more accustomed to treadmill-type exercise and hence are more often able to do it for a relatively longer period of time than bicycle

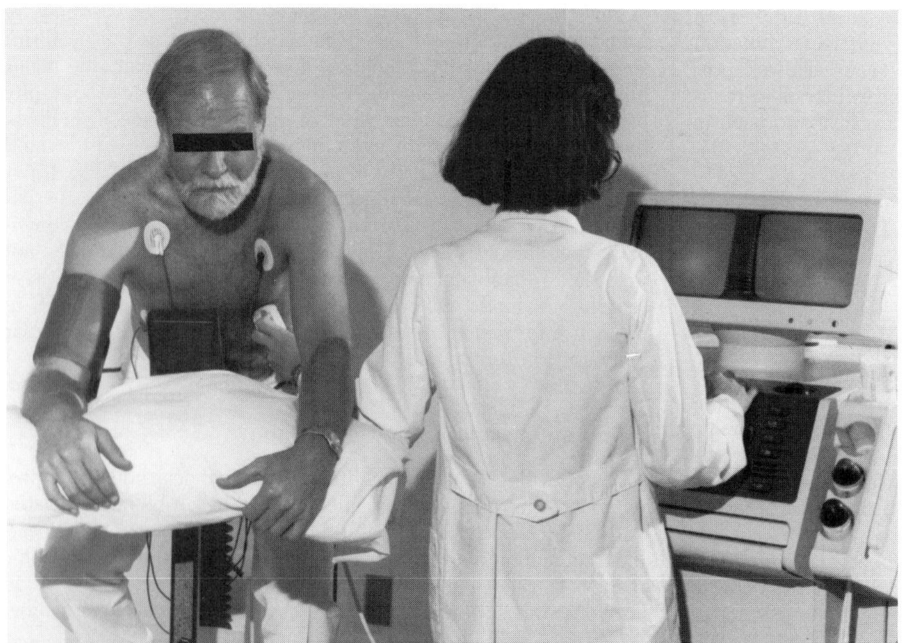

Figure 28–1. Positions of operator, subject, and equipment during performance of an upright exercise echocardiographic examination.

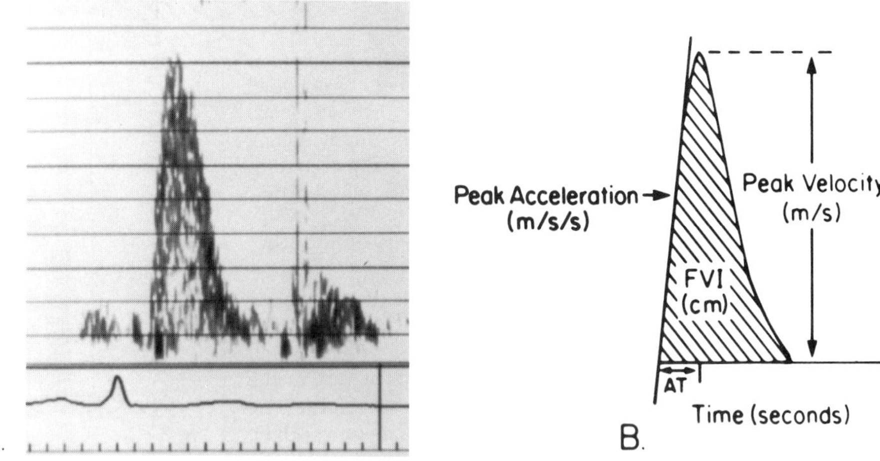

Figure 28–2. *A*, Spectral display of a normal aortic flow velocity recording. *B*, Schematic of the flow velocity signal demonstrating the variables measured. AT—acceleration time; FVI—flow velocity integral.

exercise. However, similar maximal double products are achieved with both types of exercise. The ability to perform continuous echocardiographic imaging during bicycle exercise as opposed to treadmill exercise appears to play a small role in the diagnostic accuracy for significant coronary artery disease, as discussed later. The type of exercise does, however, influence the transducer locations used to image the heart during and following exercise. Supine bicycle exercise allows imaging in all available planes, although the apical window is generally superior to the parasternal window for imaging during exercise.[W2] The apical and subcostal windows provide biplane assessment of left ventricular function and are the most commonly used transducer locations during upright bicycle exercise. The use of immediate post-treadmill exercise echocardiography generally allows imaging in all planes and may provide improved imaging success and quality compared with imaging during exercise. Also, since the parasternal views have more axial resolution than the apical views, they provide better definition of endocardial thickening[F2] and may result in improved diagnostic accuracy, especially in the detection of subtle regional wall motion abnormalities.[P2]

Despite significant advances in ultrasound equipment and imaging quality, exercise two-dimensional echocardiography is unable to image successfully 100 percent of patients, and this is its major limitation. However, with further refinements in technique and equipment and the introduction of digital computer analysis systems, as discussed later in this chapter, it is anticipated that it will be possible to evaluate the vast majority of patients referred for the assessment of left ventricular function at rest and during exercise with two-dimensional echocardiography.

Doppler Echocardiography

Doppler echocardiography is a noninvasive technique for the evaluation of intracardiac blood flow patterns. Studies using Doppler echocardiographic analysis of blood flow in the ascending aorta have demonstrated that peak aortic acceleration and, to a lesser extent, peak aortic blood flow velocity are accurate indicators of global left ventricular systolic function and are independent of changes in preload or heart rate (Fig. 28–2).[S8, W3] By using the product of the aortic systolic velocity integral from Doppler echocardiography and the proximal ascending aorta area from two-dimensional echocardiographic imaging it is possible to measure left ventricular stroke volume and cardiac output.[C4, H2]

Doppler aortic flow profiles of the exercising patient are obtained relatively easily. The small non-imaging continuous-wave Doppler ultrasound transducer available with most ultrasound equipment conveniently fits into the suprasternal notch and allows continuous monitoring of aortic flow velocity during both supine and upright exercise testing (Fig. 28–3). Because the Doppler ultrasound beam traverses the mediastinum to reach the ascending aorta, many of the problems that limit the application of imaging echocardiography to exercise, such as hyperventilation and chest wall motion, are avoided. By using both the graphic display and the audio signal it is possible to localize the peak

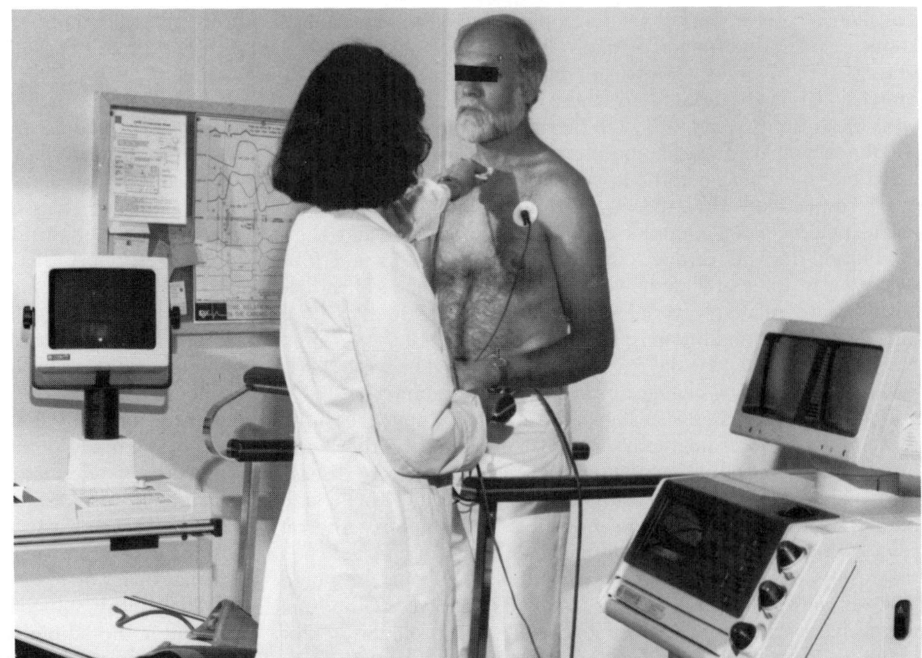

Figure 28–3. Positions of operator, subject, and equipment during performance of an exercise aortic flow Doppler examination during treadmill exercise. Note that the continuous-wave Doppler ultrasound transducer is placed in the suprasternal notch.

aortic velocity envelope with the non-imaging continuous-wave transducer. Despite the problems that may be encountered, such as optimizing flow signals in elderly patients with tortuous aortas, studies of the use of aortic flow Doppler echocardiography during exercise have achieved success rates of 81 to 100 percent in populations of both normal subjects and patients with cardiac disease.

Loeppky and associates applied this technique to measure changes in stroke volume during exercise.[L3] Using a pulsed Doppler instrument, they measured the aortic flow velocity integral at rest and during steady-state low-level supine and upright bicycle exercise in eight healthy volunteers. Derived left ventricular stroke volume was significantly higher at rest in the supine than in the upright position; however, during exercise there was a significant increase in stroke volume only in the upright position. Peak aortic velocity increased approximately 24 percent during exercise in both the supine and upright positions. Daley and associates confirmed and extended these findings in ten normal subjects during maximal supine and upright bicycle exercise.[D1] Although left ventricular stroke volume as determined from aortic flow Doppler echocardiography during rest was significantly lower in the upright than in the supine position, during peak exercise stroke volume did not differ significantly between the two positions (Fig. 28–4*A*). Similarly, peak aortic flow velocity was also lower at rest in the upright than in the supine position but rose significantly during exercise in both positions and did not differ significantly between positions at peak exercise (Fig. 28–4*B*). Mean acceleration of flow in the ascending aorta did not differ significantly between the supine and upright positions either at rest or at peak exercise, which provided further evidence that this parameter is relatively independent of preload (see Fig. 28–4*B*). Subsequent studies of normal volunteers have demonstrated similar changes in aortic flow parameters in the supine and upright positions (Fig. 28–5).[G3, M4, R3, S9] These studies confirm that aortic flow measurements made with the Doppler technique reflect the positional changes in left ventricular stroke volume that were previously observed with invasive techniques, two-dimensional echocardiography, and radionuclide angiography.[P3, W4]

Although stroke volume measured by Doppler echocardiography correlates well with stroke volume measured by invasive methods at rest, the correlation during exercise is more variable. Christie and associates made simultaneous estimates of cardiac output with aortic flow Doppler echocardiography, two-dimensional echocardiographic imaging, thermodilution, and Fick oximetry in 10 healthy volunteers during upright bicycle exercise.[C5] The linear correlation between Doppler-derived stroke volume and invasively determined stroke volume (Fick and thermodilution) was 0.67, and for stroke volume estimated from two-dimensional echocardiography there was a correlation of 0.72 with Fick oximetry and 0.81 with thermodilution. The correlation of Doppler-derived cardiac output with that measured by Fick oximetry and thermodilution was somewhat better—0.78 and 0.81, respectively (Fig. 28–6). Within individual subjects the correlation between Doppler-derived cardiac output and thermodilution-derived cardiac output ranged from 0.75 and 0.96 with a mean value of 0.86; however, Doppler estimates of cardiac output were relatively variable, ranging from 6.1 to 12.8 liter/min for a thermodilution output estimate of 10.0 liter/min. Nevertheless, changes in invasive flow estimates were fairly reliably predicted by changes in Doppler flow parameters.

Ihlen and associates also compared stroke volume measured by Doppler echocardiography with that measured by thermodilution in a group of patients with severe coronary artery disease during low-level supine and upright bicycle exercise.[I1] They found no systematic differences between the two techniques either at rest or during exercise, despite considerable variation between the results obtained with the two methods. It should be noted that, although they are widely accepted, invasive methods of measuring cardiac output are not without their problems.[S10] For example, in the study by Christie and associates adequate Doppler tracings could be obtained at all levels of exercise, whereas in subjects with large cardiac outputs thermodilution measurements could not be made at higher work loads.[C5] Nevertheless, the results of these studies suggest that Doppler echocardiography may be more useful for predicting changes in flow over exercise than for making quantitative flow predictions in individual subjects.

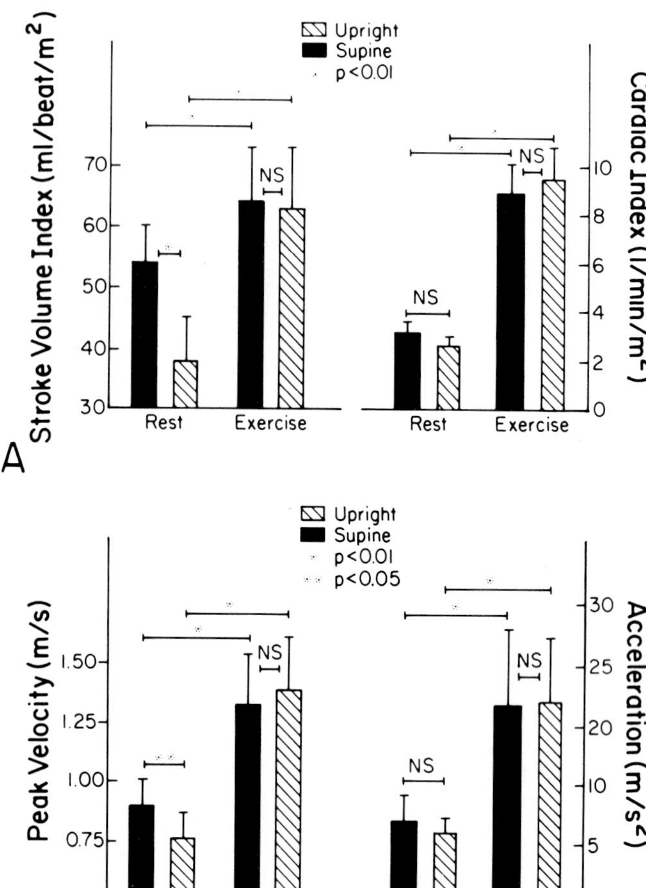

Figure 28–4. *A*, Changes in Doppler-derived mean stroke volume index and cardiac index in normal subjects during supine and upright bicycle exercise. *B*, Changes in mean peak flow velocity and mean acceleration of flow in the ascending aorta during exercise. (From Daley, P. J., Sagar, K. B., and Wann, L. S.: Doppler echocardiographic measurement of flow velocity in the ascending aorta during supine and upright exercise. Br. Heart J. 54:565, 1985, with permission.)

The Doppler estimate of stroke volume involves measurement of the proximal ascending aortic area. Many of the studies that have used aortic flow Doppler to measure changes in left ventricular stroke volume have measured aortic diameter only at rest. Thus, it is assumed that no significant changes occur in aortic diameter during exercise. Several studies have provided data to support this assumption. Ihlen and associates demonstrated no significant change in aortic diameter when cardiac output was increased severalfold by dobutamine infusion.[I2] Studies by Christie and associates[C5] and Rassi and associates[R3] also found no changes in aortic diameter measured by two-dimensional echocardiography during exercise in normal subjects. Since measurement of aortic diameter during high levels of exercise is not feasible in many subjects, it appears that the use of resting aortic diameter is adequate for estimating changes in stroke volume during exercise.

Harrison and associates have demonstrated the usefulness of exercise Doppler echocardiography for evaluating the effects of cardiac drugs on myocardial function.[H3] They studied the response of 20 healthy subjects during exercise treadmill testing before and after the administration of propranolol and verapamil. Propranolol, but not verapamil, resulted in significant alterations of

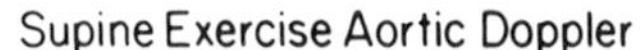

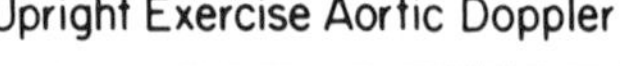

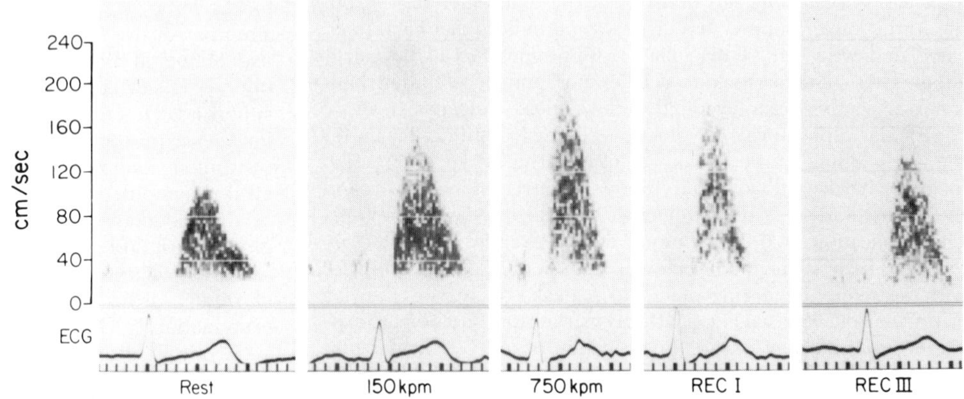

Figure 28–5. Aortic Doppler velocity recordings obtained at rest and during supine and upright bicycle exercise in normal subjects. kpm—kilopond-meters; REC—recovery stage. (From Rassi, A., Crawford, M. H., Richards, K. L., and Miller, J. F.: Differing mechanisms of exercise flow augmentation at the mitral and aortic valves. Circulation 77:550, 1988, by permission of the American Heart Association, Inc.)

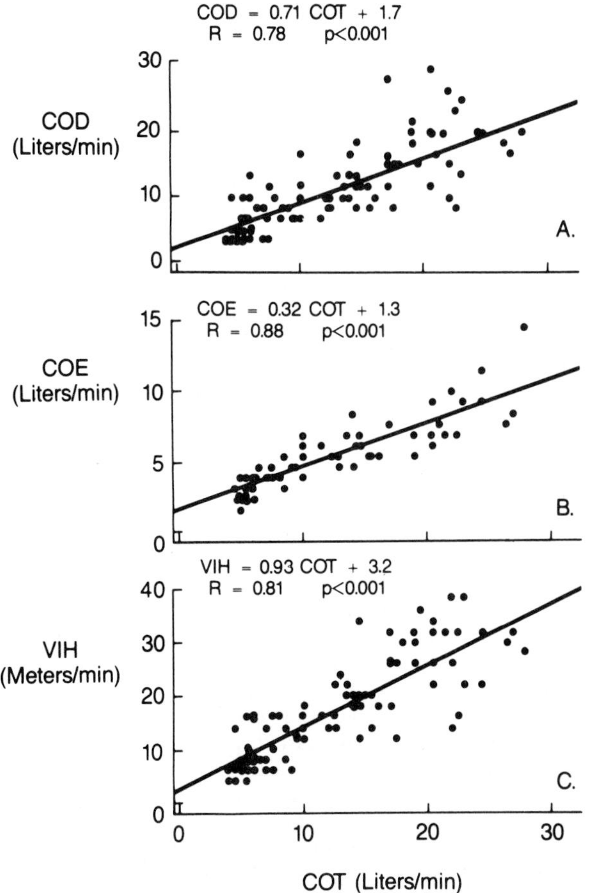

Figure 28–6. Regression plots comparing Doppler-derived cardiac output estimates (COD), cross-sectional echocardiographic cardiac output estimates (COE), and the product of velocity integral and heart rate (VIH) with thermodilution cardiac output estimates (COT) in normal subjects during upright exercise. (From Christie, J.G., Shildahl, L. M., Tristani, F. E., et al: Determination of stroke volume and cardiac output during exercise: Comparison of two-dimensional and Doppler echocardiography, Fick oximetry, and thermodilution. Circulation 76:543, 1987, by permission of the American Heart Association, Inc.)

aortic flow parameters both at rest and during exercise, with a significant depression of peak aortic velocity and acceleration and a significant increase in exercise flow velocity integral. The results of this study imply that Doppler echocardiography can be used to assess changes in left ventricular hemodynamics in response to cardiac medication both at rest and during exercise. In addition, studies involving the analysis of patients with cardiac disease states need to consider the effects of cardiac drugs on aortic Doppler flow parameters.

Doppler echocardiography of aortic flow has also been used during exercise to investigate patients with various types of cardiac disease, particularly ischemic heart disease. This use of Doppler echocardiography is discussed later.

Just as Doppler analysis of aortic valve flow has provided information regarding left ventricular systolic function, mitral valve inflow Doppler parameters have been used to derive information regarding left ventricular diastolic function.[L4] From the mitral valve Doppler tracings, several indices that have been correlated with left ventricular diastolic function can be calculated. These indices include acceleration and deceleration half-times of early diastolic rapid inflow, peak velocity at rapid ventricular filling (peak E velocity), flow velocity integral under the early filling curve, peak velocity during atrial contraction (peak A velocity), flow velocity under the atrial filling curve, and the ratios of E to A peak velocities and flow velocity integrals. The application of this technique during exercise is limited by the rapid increase in and high levels of heart rates during exercise, with subsequent merging of E and A peaks. However, the use of transmitral flow velocity patterns during the immediate post-exercise period may permit investigation of left ventricular diastolic behavior in patients with various types of cardiac disease.[I3, M5]

Rassi and associates used Doppler echocardiography combined with imaging echocardiography to investigate the mechanisms of exercise flow augmentation at the mitral and aortic valves.[R3] As in previous studies investigating stroke volume changes during exercise with aortic flow Doppler, these investigators demonstrated an increase in aortic stroke volume during exercise that was accomplished by an increase in systolic velocity time integral and no significant change in aortic cross-sectional area. In contrast, the increase in flow measured at the mitral valve was due predominantly to an increase in mean diastolic mitral valve area (approximately 30 percent from rest to exercise) with no significant increase in diastolic velocity time integral. This study emphasizes the dynamic properties of the mitral valve, in contrast to the aortic valve, and shows that mitral valve cross-sectional area must be known to assess changes in cardiac output from diastolic velocities.

The use of Doppler echocardiography to assess changes in left ventricular function involves both assumptions and limitations. First, it is assumed that the ultrasound beam is parallel to flow at rest and remains parallel throughout exercise. Second, the accuracy of measured flow periods at high exercise levels may be less because of deterioration of signal quality. Finally, it is unlikely that Doppler flow parameters reflect only left ventricular contractility; as with ejection fraction, they probably reflect a combination of contractility, afterload, and, to a lesser extent, preload. Nevertheless, aortic Doppler flow can be obtained in almost all patients during exercise and is a relatively simple means of assessing global left ventricular systolic function. The use of Doppler mitral flow parameters also may provide a unique tool for assessing the diastolic properties of the left ventricular response to exercise.

The most recently developed echocardiographic technique, color flow Doppler imaging, allows noninvasive analysis of the direction, spatial distribution, and relative velocity of intracardiac blood flow. Application of this technique with exercise has to date been somewhat limited. However, Zachariah and associates described the presence of exercise-induced mitral regurgitation detected by color flow Doppler imaging during supine bicycle exercise as an additional diagnostic criterion in the evaluation of patients with known or suspected ischemic heart disease.[Z2]

Analysis of Exercise Echocardiographic Studies

Just as exercise echocardiography can be performed in a variety of ways, interpretation of exercise echocardiographic studies can be accomplished by several different methods. Evaluation of the exercise echocardiogram can be done off-line with videotape in much the same way that routine two-dimensional echocardiograms are interpreted. This method requires that each view be recorded for a sufficient period of time to allow adequate analysis. In addition, one must contend with respiratory artifact, which may be substantial at high levels of exercise.

Where available, the use of digital acquisition techniques to obtain a single high-quality cardiac cycle and display it in a continuous loop format is advantageous. This technique allows elimination of the respiratory artifact and permits side-by-side display of rest and exercise echocardiograms, which may improve the ability to detect subtle regional wall motion abnormalities. This technique also allows the interpreter to view a cardiac cycle for as long as desired and to display several different views simultaneously. A continuous loop recording is obtained with the use of digital frame-grabbing equipment.[F3] Generally, the sequence is started at the R wave of the electrocardiogram, and subsequent frames are digitized at a given time interval to allow for the acquisition of all of systole and a little of diastole. The continuous loop recording can be acquired with either on-line or off-line computer equipment. Off-line acquisition requires review of the videotape after completion of the exercise echocardiographic test and selection of a specific cardiac cycle or cycles for analysis.[A2] The on-line acquisition technique allows digitization of single cardiac cycles during the exercise echocardiographic examination.[P2] These cycles are stored in memory and can then be reviewed after the exercise test is finished. With both the on-line and off-line acquisition techniques, the videotape is always available for backup analysis, if needed. Use of the continuous loop technique in the evaluation of regional wall motion abnormalities is discussed in more detail below.

CLINICAL APPLICATIONS OF EXERCISE ECHOCARDIOGRAPHY

Application to Ischemic Heart Disease

The application of echocardiographic imaging as an adjunct to stress testing for diagnosing coronary artery disease is based on the premise that exercise-induced myocardial ischemia results in segmental wall motion abnormalities that are detectable with echocardiography. The concept of ischemia-induced regional myocardial dysfunction is well supported by numerous clinical and experimental studies dating back to the classic study in which Tennant and Wiggers demonstrated the appearance of paradoxic ventricular wall motion immediately following coronary artery occlusion.[T1] The use of two-dimensional echocardiographic imaging to detect regional wall motion abnormalities is well supported by numerous studies of echocardiographic imaging in the setting of acute myocardial infarction.[H5, H6, V2, W5] Because of the multiple tomographic imaging planes available with two-dimensional echocardiography, it is possible to assess the regional function of all myocardial segments.

Several wall motion schemes have been constructed for use with two-dimensional echocardiography for the evaluation of regional left ventricular function (Fig. 28–7).[K2, P4, S11, S12] The basis for these regional wall motion scoring systems is that specific myocardial segments are, in general, supplied by specific coronary arteries (Fig. 28–8). This regional myocardial perfusion pattern underscores the advantages of being able to assess the left ventricle in multiple tomographic planes with two-dimensional echocardiography. For example, the left ventricular apex, an area commonly affected by ischemic heart disease, is not routinely visualized from the parasternal window but can be examined from the apical window. Conversely, the proximal anterior interventricular septum, an area usually perfused by the proximal left anterior descending coronary artery, is best evaluated from the parasternal long-axis view. The true inferior wall, usually supplied by the right coronary artery, is best visualized

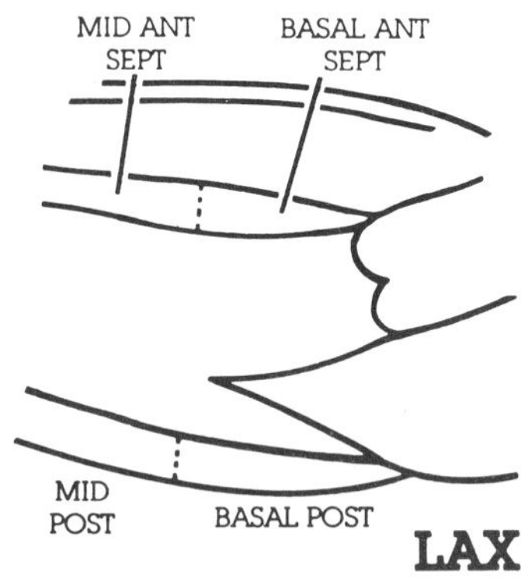

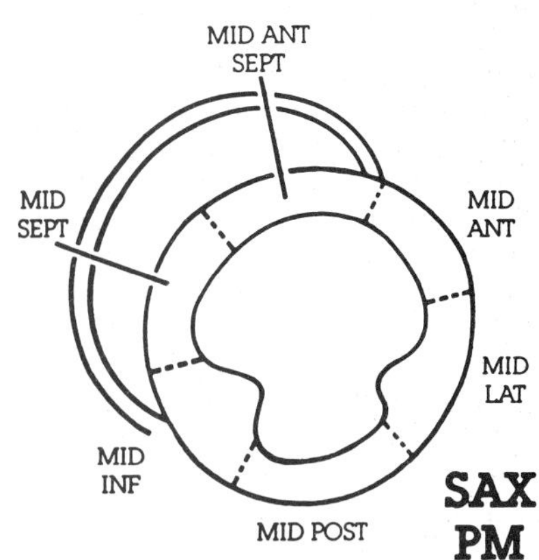

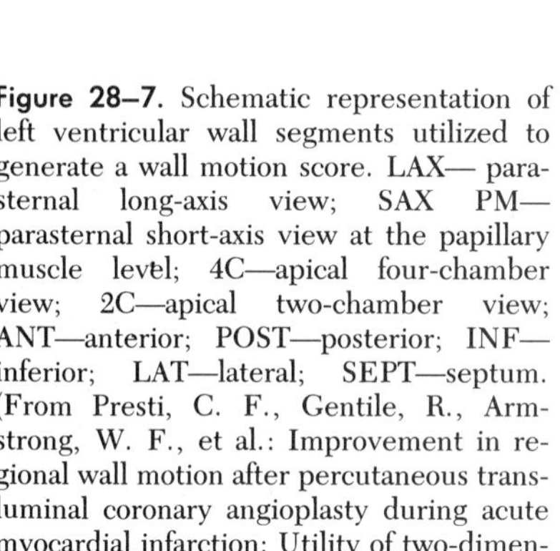

Figure 28–7. Schematic representation of left ventricular wall segments utilized to generate a wall motion score. LAX— parasternal long-axis view; SAX PM— parasternal short-axis view at the papillary muscle level; 4C—apical four-chamber view; 2C—apical two-chamber view; ANT—anterior; POST—posterior; INF—inferior; LAT—lateral; SEPT—septum. (From Presti, C. F., Gentile, R., Armstrong, W. F., et al.: Improvement in regional wall motion after percutaneous transluminal coronary angioplasty during acute myocardial infarction: Utility of two-dimensional echocardiography. Am. Heart J. 115:1150, 1988, with permission.)

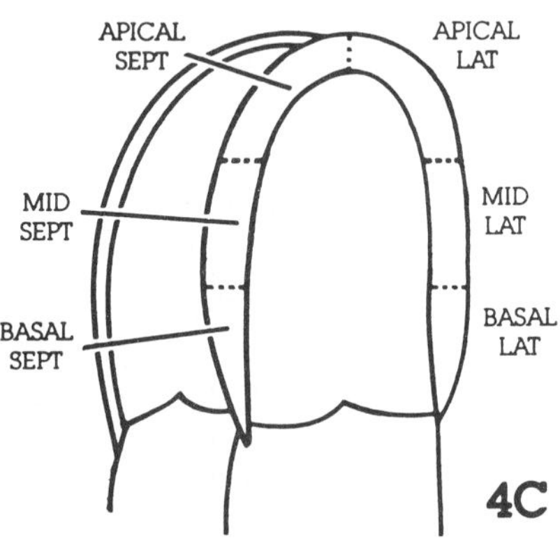

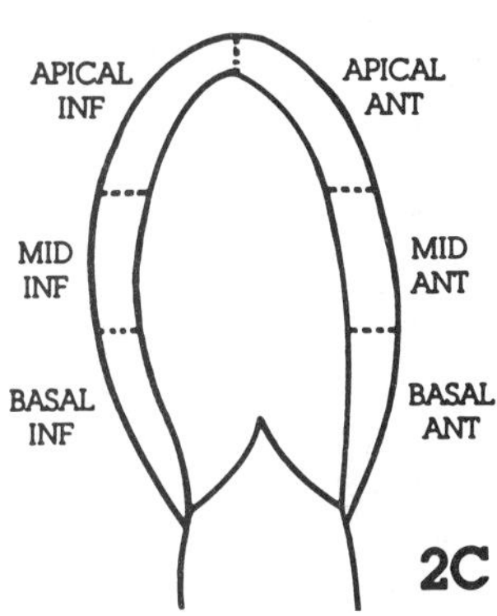

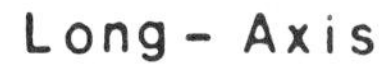

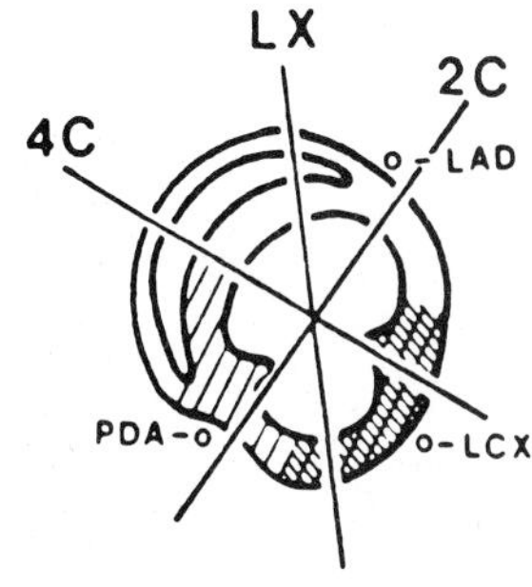

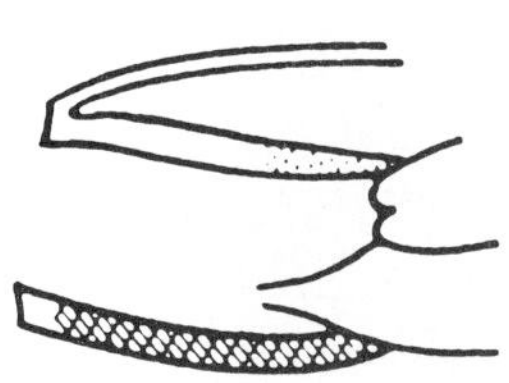

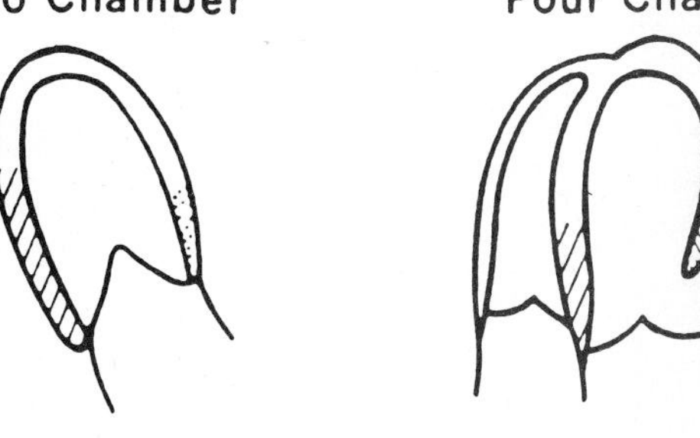

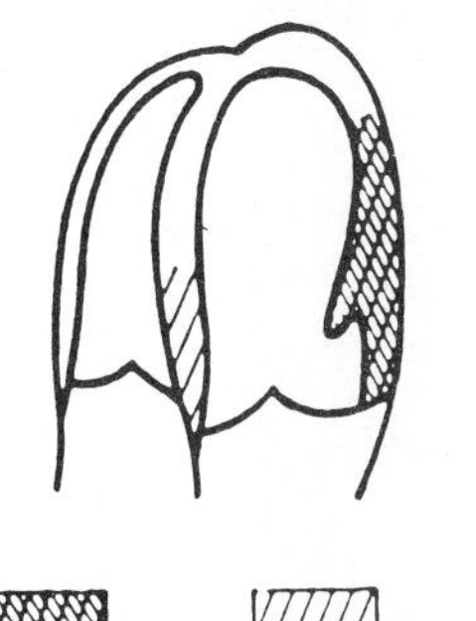

Figure 28–8. Diagram illustrating the relationship between two-dimensional echocardiographic views and coronary artery perfusion. 4C—four-chamber; LX—long-axis; 2C—two-chamber; LAD—left anterior descending artery; PROX—proximal; LCX—left circumflex artery; RCA—right coronary artery; PDA—posterior descending artery. (From Feigenbaum, H.: Echocardiography, 4th ed. Lea & Febiger, Philadelphia, 1986, p. 467, with permission.)

from the parasternal short-axis and apical two-chamber views. Hence, by using multiple imaging planes it is possible to evaluate regional left ventricular function more completely.

As discussed earlier, the use of the continuous loop technique aids in the analysis of stress echocardiograms. With this technique it is possible to display rest and exercise echocardiographic views in a side-by-side format. This format allows a direct comparison of individual myocardial segments pre-exercise and post-exercise and may aid in the delineation of subtle regional wall motion abnormalities. Regional wall motion can then be analyzed by using a qualitative, semiquantitative, or quantitative approach. The qualitative approach involves visual grading of the motion of individual myocardial segments, classifying them as normal, hypokinetic, akinetic, or dyskinetic. This approach has the advantage of speed of interpretation and has proved to be reliable in the assessment of patients with ischemic heart disease. By using a regional wall motion scoring system, it is possible to generate a semiquantitative analysis of left ventricular function. In this format, which has been used in the evaluation of patients in the setting of acute myocardial infarction[K2, P4, S11, S12] as well as in the analysis of patients with ischemic heart disease undergoing exercise echocardiography,[C2, G1, L2] each myocardial segment is given a numerical score according to its regional wall motion. A wall motion score (or score index) can then be calculated and used to provide a semiquantitative estimate of the extent of abnormal wall motion.

Further quantitative analysis of regional wall motion can be obtained by the determination of changes in endocardial excursion from end-diastole to end-diastole.[M6] With this technique it is possible to divide the left ventricle into multiple radial segments and calculate the percent area change for each segment. More sophisticated analytical techniques evaluate the entire systolic contraction sequence instead of only end-diastole and end-systole.[G4] These techniques involve consideration of the temporal heterogeneity of ischemia-induced wall motion abnormalities and evaluation of wall motion at the time of maximal dyskinesis. With newer automated edge-detection equipment, these quantitative methods may become more widely applicable to the analysis of exercise echocardiograms.

Using quantitative analysis of segmental wall motion, Ginzton and associates demonstrated variability in left ventricular segmental wall motion during maximal upright bicycle exercise in normal subjects.[G2] These investigators demonstrated wide ranges at peak exercise in segmental area reduction of the same segment between different normal subjects and between segments in the same subject. Because of this significant variability, it was concluded that segmental hypokinesis during exercise may be a normal event. Segmental akinesis or dyskinesis, however, never occurred at peak exercise. Thus, it appears that although regional hypokinesis during exercise may occasionally be a normal finding, akinetic or dyskinetic wall motion is a distinctly abnormal event (Fig. 28–9).

Diagnosis of Ischemic Heart Disease

Imaging echocardiography during or immediately following exercise testing has been used in the diagnosis of coronary artery disease. As discussed previously, although early studies with the M-mode technique demonstrated the ability of echocardiography to assess exercise-induced wall motion abnormalities,[F1, M1, S6] the limited view and technical problems associated with this technique have made it less useful than two-dimensional echocardiography for this purpose. Several studies have investigated the utility of exercise two-dimensional echocardiography in the diagnosis of coronary artery disease. Three criteria have been used to diagnose coronary artery disease with two-dimensional echo-

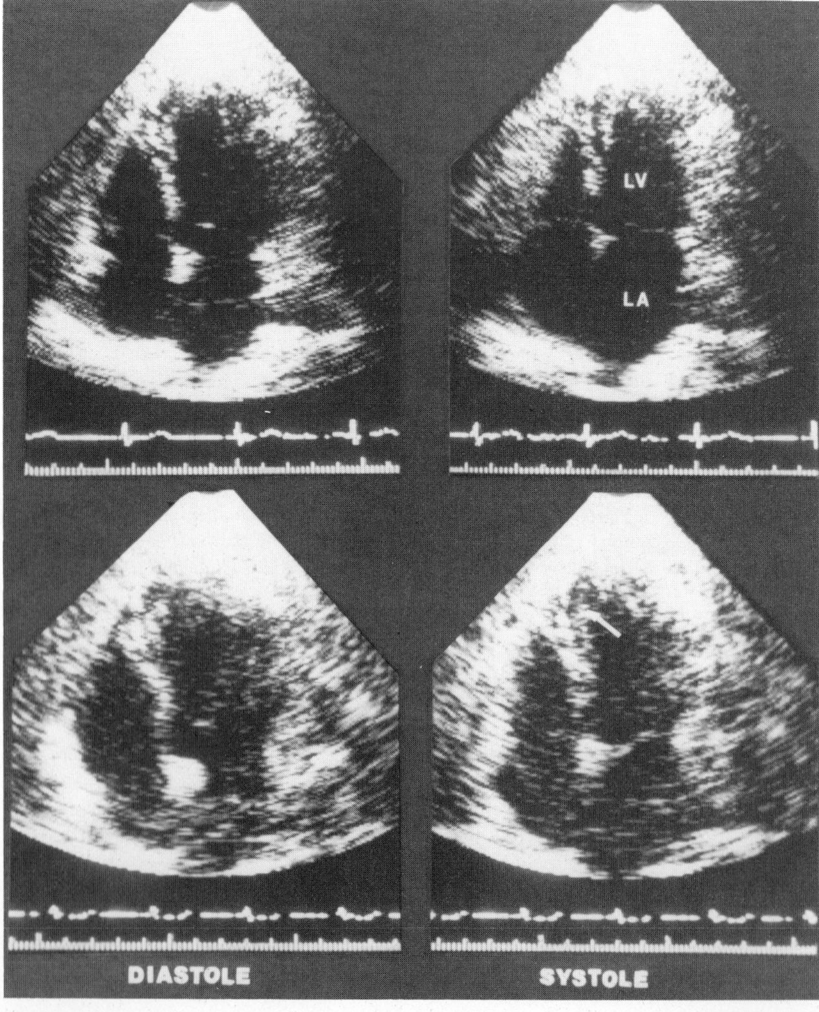

Figure 28–9. Apical four-chamber views demonstrating an exercise-induced wall motion abnormality. Resting images are displayed on top, and images at peak bicycle exercise are displayed on bottom. Wall motion is normal at rest but the apical septum becomes akinetic during exercise (*arrow*). LA—left atrium; LV—left ventricle.

Table 28–1. STUDIES USING ASSESSMENT OF REGIONAL WALL MOTION IN DIAGNOSIS OF CORONARY ARTERY DISEASE

							Coronary Angiography			Exercise Echocardiography†							
										SVD		*MDV*		*All CAD*			
										Sens. (%)		Spec. (%)		Sens. (%)		Spec. (%)	
Study	(Year)	N	Exercise Type	Analysis Technique*	Success Rate (%)	Percent Stenosis	*Normal*	*SVD*	*MVD*	all WMA	new WMA	all WMA	new WMA	all WMA	new WMA	all WMA	new WMA
Wann	(1979)	28	Supine bicycle	1	71	50	5	2	13	50	50	92	69	87	67	60	100
Morganroth	(1981)	55	Supine bicycle	1	78	50	11	7	25	71	57	64	60	66	59	91	91
Mitamura	(1981)	45	Handgrip	2	100	50	7	12	26	50	42	77	88	74	62	86	100
Maurer	(1981)	48	Post-TME‡	1	85	50	13	6	17	50§	50§	9§	94§	83§	83§	69§	90§
Limacher	(1983)	73	Post-TME	1	100	50	17	11	45	64	27	98	71	91	63	88	88
Robertson	(1983)	30	Post-TME	1	92	75	4	8	13	100	63	100	92	100	81	75	75
Visser	(1983)	52	Supine bicycle	1	75	50	13	11	15	73	73	80	73	77	73	92	92
Ginzton	(1984)	41	Upright bicycle	1	95	ND	16	23¶		—	—	—	—	100	57	100	100
Armstrong	(1986)	95	Post-TME	3	100	50	15	35	45	NS	NS	NS	NS	88	NS	87	NS
Armstrong	(1987)	123	Post-TME	3	NA	50	22	42	59	81	NS	93	NS	88	NS	86	NS
Ryan	(1988)**	64	Post-TME	3	NA	50	24	25	15	—	76	—	80	—	78	—	100
Voelker	(1988)	56	Supine bicycle	1	86	50	6	12	22	NS	NS	NS	NS	41	NS	96	NS

*1—Analysis performed using video playback (real time, slow motion, stop-frame formats); 2—analysis performed from single cardiac cycle using end-diastolic and end-systolic endocardial contours; 3—analysis performed using digital acquisition and side-by-side comparison of rest/exercise single cardiac cycles.

†SVD—single vessel disease; MVD—multivessel disease; CAD—coronary artery disease; Sens.—sensitivity; Spec.—specificity; WMA—wall motion abnormality; ND—not done; NS—not stated; NA—not applicable (nonconsecutive series of patients).

‡TME—treadmill exercise.

§Includes right ventricular wall motion abnormalities.

¶All patients post myocardial infarction.

**All subjects had normal resting wall motion.

cardiography: (1) the presence of a resting wall motion abnormality, (2) exercise-induced wall motion abnormality, and (3) an abnormal ejection fraction response to exercise.

Table 28–1 reviews the studies that have utilized the assessment of regional wall motion in making the diagnosis of coronary artery disease. As shown in this table, the imaging success rate, exercise protocol, severity of coronary artery disease, and use of resting wall motion abnormalities as a diagnostic criterion are all factors that influence the results of these studies. Mitamura and associates studied 45 patients with suspected coronary artery disease with two-dimensional echocardiography during submaximal handgrip exercise.[M7] They found that although the development of an exercise-induced wall motion abnormality predicted the presence of significant coronary artery disease with a specificity of 100 percent, only 65 percent of patients with coronary artery disease and normal resting wall motion demonstrated such a response. This low sensitivity is at least partially attributable to the relative insensitivity of handgrip exercise compared with isotonic exercise for the diagnosis of coronary artery disease.[H7, L5]

In studies using various forms of isotonic exercise, sensitivities of exercise two-dimensional echocardiography ranged from 41 to 100 percent in the diagnosis of coronary artery disease with specificities ranging from 60 to 100 percent. Use of a resting wall motion abnormality as a diagnostic criterion for coronary artery disease results in increased sensitivity compared with the use of only exercise-induced wall motion abnormalities or the worsening of a resting wall motion abnormality with exercise (see Table 28–1). Patients with resting wall motion abnormalities have a higher pre-test likelihood of ischemic heart disease than patients with normal resting wall motion. Conversely, use of the presence of a resting wall motion abnormality as a diagnostic criterion results in a somewhat lower specificity for the diagnosis of coronary artery disease (see Table 28–1), as occasional patients with nonischemic cardiomyopathy have regional wall motion abnormalities at rest.[M8, W6] Ryan and associates attempted to define the sensitivity and specificity of exercise echocardiography in a group of patients with suspected coronary artery disease who had normal resting wall motion.[R2] The presence of an exercise-induced wall motion abnormality in this population predicted the presence of coronary artery disease with a sensitivity of 78 percent and specificity of 100 percent. Thus, the detection of a new exercise-induced wall motion abnormality by two-dimensional echocardiography appears to be highly specific for the diagnosis of coronary artery disease with a sensitivity in the range 70 to 80 percent.

The sensitivity of exercise echocardiography is also influenced by the severity of underlying coronary artery disease. In general, exercise echocardiography is more sensitive for the detection of patients with multivessel coronary artery disease than of patients with single-vessel disease (see Table 28–1). This finding is similar for all exercise techniques used to diagnose coronary artery disease[C6, O1] and is presumably due to the increased number of potentially ischemic areas in patients with multivessel disease. Armstrong and associates investigated the diagnostic utility of exercise echocardiography in relation to the severity of angiographic coronary artery disease and found that the overall sensitivity of exercise echocardiography was 93 percent in patients with multivessel disease and 81 percent in patients with single-vessel disease.[A3] The sensitivity was higher in patients who had a prior myocardial infarction, most of whom had resting wall motion abnormalities on two-dimensional echocardiography. In patients who had single-vessel disease without prior myocardial infarction the sensitivity of exercise echocardiography was only 72 percent, compared to 86 percent in patients with multivessel disease and no prior infarction. This suggests that patients with single-vessel disease have a smaller amount of potentially ischemic myocardium. An interesting result of this study was that although exercise echocardiography was highly accurate in detecting patients with multivessel disease, its ability to identify these patients specifically as having multivessel disease was limited. Only 54 percent of this subset of patients was diagnosed by exercise echocardiography as having multivessel disease, the majority of the remainder being classified as having single-vessel disease. Similar results have been noted with thallium-201 imaging[R4] and are probably related to the development of ischemia during exercise in only one myocardial region among several potentially ischemic areas in patients with multivessel disease. The development of ischemia in a single area may lead to chest pain or electrocardiographic changes that result in termination of exercise prior to the development of ischemia in other myocardial regions. Thus, although exercise echocardiography appears to be highly sensitive for the detection of patients with multivessel coronary artery disease, it is somewhat limited at identifying these patients specifically as having multivessel disease.

As discussed earlier, one approach to exercise echocardiography is to perform imaging prior to and immediately following exercise testing. The advantages of this approach are that all imaging planes can be used and that respiratory and motion artifacts are reduced compared with those at peak exercise. However, a potential disadvantage of imaging immediately after exercise is that transient exercise-induced wall motion abnormalities may resolve quickly in the recovery period and hence be missed. Several exercise echocardiographic studies have demonstrated that patients with ischemic heart disease have exercise-induced wall motion abnormalities that persist for 1 to 5 minutes during recovery[M3, W2] and that patients with multivessel coronary artery disease may have abnormalities that persist even longer.[R1] Presti and associates studied patients with two-dimensional echocardiography during peak upright bicycle exercise and immediately following exercise and concluded that in the majority of patients post-exercise imaging and imaging at peak exercise provided equivalent information with regard to regional wall motion analysis, particularly if all imaging planes were used post-exercise.[P2] However, whereas the overall sensitivity for the detection of patients with significant coronary artery disease was 100 percent for peak exercise imaging, it was only 70 percent when imaging was performed during the post-exercise period (Fig. 28–10). Similar results have been obtained with radionuclide angiography[D3] and two-dimensional echocardiographic imaging during transesophageal atrial pacing.[14] Applegate and associates, in a study of patients recovering from acute myocardial infarction, found that the wall motion response on recovery from treadmill exercise was predictive of the wall motion response at peak bicycle exercise in 81 percent of patients and that 13 percent of patients had wall motion abnormalities detected during bicycle exercise but not during recovery from treadmill exercise.[A4] These studies suggest that imaging during the immediate recovery period is capable of detecting the majority of exercise-induced wall motion abnormalities but that a significant minority of patients with coronary artery disease will not be detected with this approach.

Finally, it is important to emphasize that the use of regional wall motion analysis with exercise echocardiography in the diagnosis of coronary artery disease requires the end effect of myocardial ischemia, namely abnormal wall motion. Exercise echocardiography does not provide direct information concerning myocardial perfusion or metabolism. In addition, the calculation of sensitivity and specificity of exercise echocardiography based on coronary arteriography alone has significant shortcomings, as coronary arteriography, which describes anatomy, provides somewhat different information from exercise echocardiography, which assesses left ventricular function and depends on the induction of myocardial ischemia. The use of coronary arteriography as a gold standard, especially when visual interpretation of percent luminal stenosis is used, suffers from several potential limitations, including intraobserver and interobserver variability, underdiagnosis of diffuse coronary artery disease, and lack of consideration of other factors that may be involved in the precipitation or amelioration of myocardial ischemia (such as alterations in vasomotor tone, anemia, coronary collateral circulation, and antianginal medications).[M9] However, these problems are not unique to exercise echocardiography but also apply to other noninvasive methods used in the diagnosis of coronary artery disease, including exercise electrocardiography and radionuclide techniques. A combination of quantitative coronary angiography and physiologic studies measuring coronary flow reserve (such as intracoronary Doppler ultrasound or positron emission tomography) provides a more exact measure of the functional significance of a coronary arterial stenosis and would serve as a superior reference standard with which to determine the accuracy of exercise echocardiography for the detection of coronary artery disease. Although much work remains to be done in this area, studies to date suggest that echocardiographic imaging during or immediately following exercise may prove to be a useful technique for the diagnosis of ischemic heart disease.

Use of Left Ventricular Ejection Fraction in the Diagnosis of Coronary Artery Disease

Studies utilizing radionuclide angiography have demonstrated that a fall in left ventricular ejection fraction during exercise and

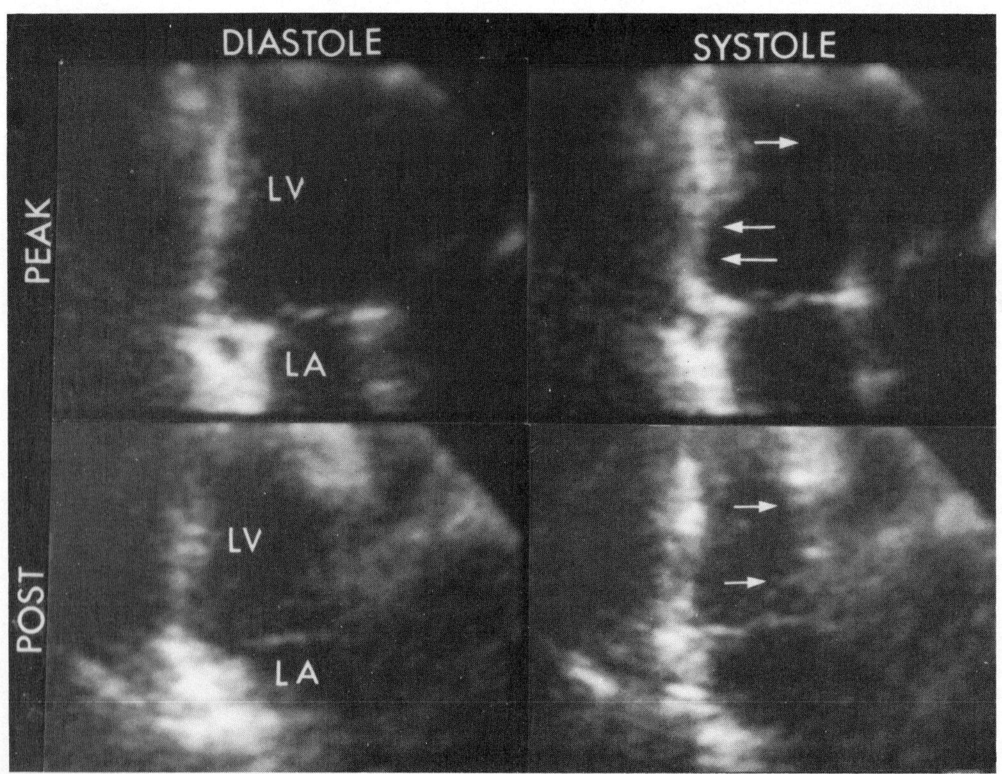

Figure 28–10. Apical two-chamber views from a patient with an exercise-induced wall motion abnormality confined to peak exercise. Images obtained at peak exercise are on top, and images taken immediately post-exercise are on bottom. At peak exercise (*top right*) there is akinesis of the proximal inferior wall (*arrows*) that was resolved by the time of imaging after exercise (*bottom right*). LA—left atrium; LV—left ventricle. (From Presti, C. F., Armstrong, W. F., and Feigenbaum, H.: Comparison of echocardiography at peak exercise and after bicycle exercise in evaluation of patients with known or suspected coronary artery disease. J. Am. Soc. Echo. 1:121, 1988, with permission.)

a failure to increase ejection fraction with exercise are predictive of ischemic heart disease, although the criteria for an abnormal ejection fraction response to exercise vary from laboratory to laboratory.[B4, P5] Two-dimensional echocardiography can also be used to calculate left ventricular volumes and ejection fraction. Studies comparing two-dimensional echocardiography with radionuclide angiography and left ventricular cineangiography have shown that two-dimensional echocardiography underestimates left ventricular volumes as compared with these alternative techniques but that the ejection fractions correlate well.[S13, S14] The application of two-dimensional echocardiographic imaging to exercise testing allows quantitative assessment of global left ventricular function on a beat-by-beat basis.

Limacher and associates, using a technique for calculating ejection fraction from a series of minor-axis dimensions and an assessment of apical contraction,[Q1] evaluated the left ventricular ejection fraction response to exercise.[L2] By using two-dimensional echocardiographic imaging before and immediately after treadmill testing, these investigators noted an increase in ejection fraction from 66 ± 9 percent at rest to 73 ± 8 percent after exercise in patients without angiographic coronary artery disease. As a group, patients with coronary artery disease had a fall in ejection fraction, from 56 ± 13 percent at rest to 53 ± 16 percent after exercise (Fig. 28–11A). However, the overall sensitivity of the ejection fraction response for the detection of coronary artery disease in this study was only 70 percent. The overall fall in post-exercise ejection fraction for the entire group of patients with coronary artery disease was due primarily to the substantial decrease in ejection fraction in patients with three-vessel disease (from 55 ± 14 percent to 47 ± 13 percent) (Fig. 28–11B). Seven of the 11 patients with single-vessel disease had a rise in post-exercise ejection fraction. These data are consistent with the greater magnitude of exercise-induced ischemia in patients with multivessel disease and are substantiated by a worse regional wall motion score in this group of patients.[L2] These results illustrated how the ejection fraction response to exercise, an indicator of global left ventricular function, may be less sensitive indicator of coronary artery disease than is analysis of regional wall motion.

Crawford and associates compared ejection fraction measured by two-dimensional echocardiography with that obtained by gated equilibrium radionuclide angiography in a group of patients with coronary artery disease.[C3] These investigators noted a discordance between the two techniques, with the percent change in ejection fraction during exercise determined by two-dimensional echocardiography being significantly greater than that determined by radionuclide angiography (—25 percent versus − 13 percent) (Fig. 28–12A). This discrepancy appeared to be explained by the different time course of data collection for the ejection fraction determination by the two techniques. Radionuclide angiography involves averaging counts over many cardiac cycles, whereas two-dimensional echocardiography allows analysis of ejection fraction on a beat-by-beat basis. Analysis of ejection fraction values during the last minute of exercise showed that they were significantly greater than the values obtained at peak exercise (Fig. 28–12B). Thus, two-dimensional echocardiography may be more accurate than radionuclide angiography in measuring ejection fraction at peak exercise.

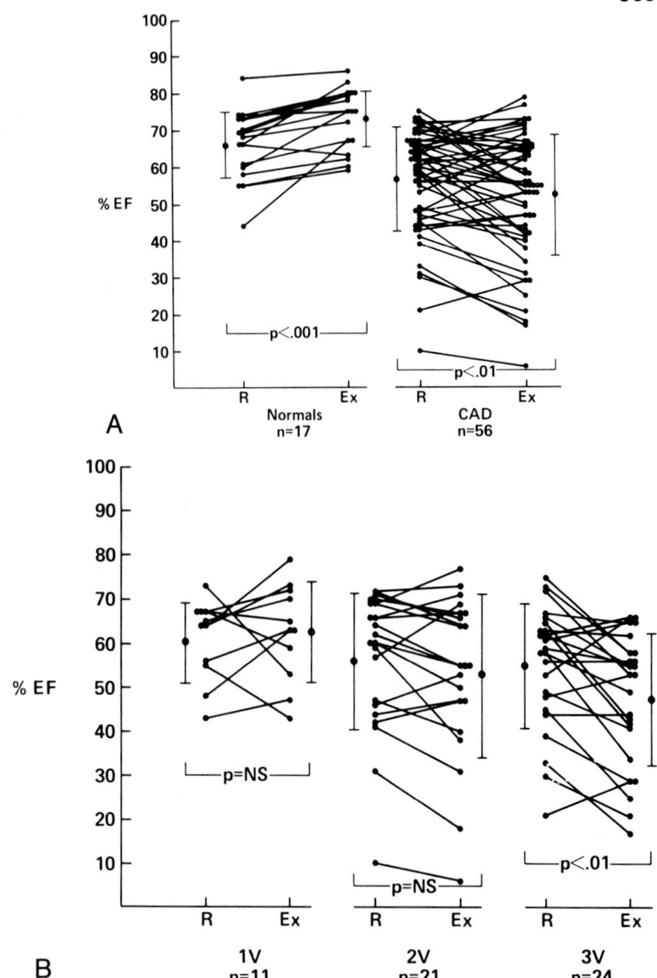

Figure 28–11. *A*, Resting (R) and post-exercise (Ex) ejection fraction (% EF) in normal subjects and patients with coronary artery disease (CAD). Ejection fraction increased significantly with exercise in normal subjects but fell in patients with CAD. *B*, Ejection fraction response in patients with CAD, grouped by the number of vessels involved. Note the significant decrease in ejection fraction in patients with three-vessel (3V) disease compared to those with one- and two-vessel (1V and 2V) involvement. (From Limacher, M. C., Quinones, M. A., Poliner, L. R., et al.: Detection of coronary artery disease with exercise two-dimensional echocardiography. Circulation 67: 1214, 1215, 1983, by permission of the American Heart Association, Inc.)

Comparison With Exercise Electrocardiography

Segmental left ventricular dysfunction has been shown to precede electrocardiographic changes following the induction of myocardial ischemia.[V1, W7] Sugishita and associates, using M-mode echocardiography, demonstrated that segmental wall motion abnormalities precede ST-T changes by an average of 60 seconds during exercise in patients with coronary artery disease.[S6] In addition, the presence of abnormal resting electrocardiograms due to prior infarctions, left ventricular hypertrophy, conduction disturbances, drug effects, or electrolyte disturbances reduces the specificity of exercise electrocardiographic changes in a significant proportion of patients evaluated for myocardial ischemia. Although factors such as conduction abnormalities or large prior infarctions also may make its interpretation difficult, exercise echocardiography has the potential of being both more sensitive and more specific than electrocardiographic testing for the detection of coronary artery disease.

Armstrong and associates investigated the complementary value of exercise echocardiography with routine treadmill testing in a group of patients referred for the evaluation of chest pain.[A2] In 14 of 18 patients (78 percent) who had a nondiagnostic electrocardiographic treadmill response, exercise echocardiography was able to diagnose correctly or exclude significant coronary artery disease. Thus, patients with abnormal baseline electrocardiograms who are likely to have a nondiagnostic exercise electrocardiographic response appear to be particularly likely to benefit from the addition of echocardiographic imaging for diagnosing coronary artery disease.

Comparison With Radionuclide Techniques

Exercise echocardiography has been compared with planar thallium–201 scintigraphy in a small number of studies.[M3, V1, W2] In general, there has been excellent concordance between reversible thallium-201 defects and exercise-induced wall motion abnormalities detected by two-dimensional echocardiography. As noted by Maurer and Nanda, the ability of two-dimensional echocardiography to detect right ventricular wall motion abnor-

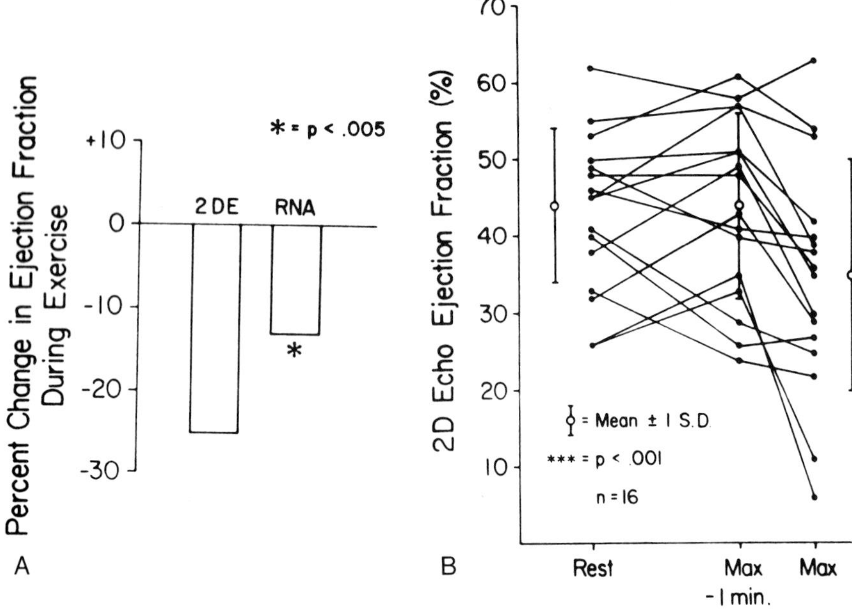

Figure 28–12. *A*, Percent change in ejection fraction during exercise as measured with two-dimensional echocardiography (2DE) and radionuclide angiography (RNA) in patients with coronary artery disease. *B*, Ejection fraction measured by two-dimensional echocardiography (2D Echo) at rest, at 1 minute before maximal exercise (Max − 1 min), and at maximal exercise (Max). SD—standard deviation. (Reprinted by permission from Crawford, M. H., et al: Comparative value of two-dimensional echocardiography and radionuclide angiography for quantitating changes in left ventricular performance during exercise limited by angina pectoris. Am. J. Cardiol. 53:42, 1984).

malities may be an added advantage.[M3] Although the two imaging techniques are based on different end points (thallium-201 scintigraphy assesses abnormalities of myocardial flow, and two-dimensional echocardiography relies on abnormal wall motion), the good correlation between them helps substantiate the ischemic basis of exercise-induced wall motion abnormalities as detected by two-dimensional echocardiography.

Radionuclide angiography, like two-dimensional echocardiography, can also be used to assess regional wall motion and left ventricular ejection fraction. Studies comparing the two techniques for the detection of patients with significant coronary artery disease have demonstrated similar sensitivities and specificities.[C3, G1, L2, V1] Advantages of two-dimensional echocardiography are that it allows imaging in multiple views throughout exercise and it allows the evaluation of both global and regional left ventricular function on a beat-by-beat basis. As noted above, this may be important in detecting changes in left ventricular ejection fraction or abnormal wall motion at peak exercise.[C3, P2] On the other hand, radionuclide angiography provides images for nearly 100 percent of patients, whereas a small percentage of subjects cannot be adequately imaged with two-dimensional echocardiography.

Exercise Doppler Echocardiography in the Assessment of Ischemic Heart Disease

As discussed previously, the velocity and acceleration of blood flow in the ascending aorta have been shown to be reliable indicators of global left ventricular performance at rest and during exercise in normal subjects. Bryg and associates compared the exercise response as assessed by Doppler echocardiography of a group of normal subjects with that of a group of patients with coronary artery disease studied during treadmill exercise.[B3] Normal subjects had a significant increase in peak aortic flow velocity during and immediately following exercise, whereas the peak velocity in the group of patients with coronary artery disease increased much less during exercise (Fig. 28–13). However, within the group of patients with coronary artery disease, various responses were noted. Patients with single-vessel disease had a larger increase in peak ejection velocity than patients with multivessel disease (Fig. 28–14). The majority of patients with the least rise in peak ejection velocity from rest to exercise had multivessel disease and abnormal left ventricular function at rest.

Harrison and associates confirmed and extended these findings in their investigation of aortic flow parameters during exercise in

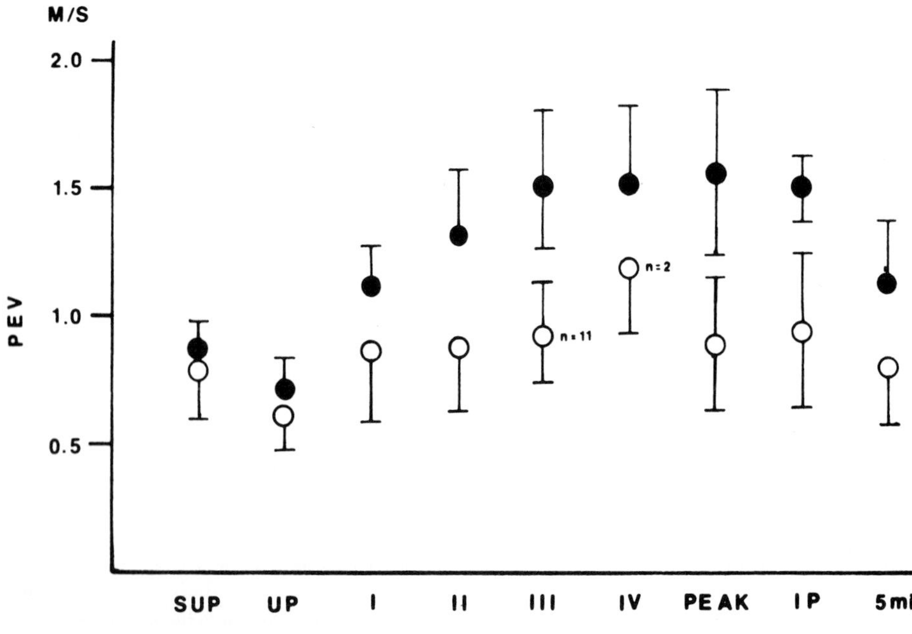

Figure 28–13. Peak ejection velocity (PEV) response (mean ± standard deviation) in normal subjects (filled circles) and patients with coronary artery disease (open circles) at rest in the supine (SUP) and upright (UP) positions, at each stage of exercise, at peak exercise, immediately post-exercise (IP) in the upright position, and 5 minutes after exercise in the supine position. The rise in peak ejection velocity during exercise in the patients with coronary artery disease is significantly less than in the control subjects. (From Bryg, R. J., Labovitz, A. J., Mehdirad, A. A., et al: Effect of coronary artery disease on Doppler-derived parameters of aortic flow during upright exercise. Am. J. Cardiol. 58:14, 1986, with permission.)

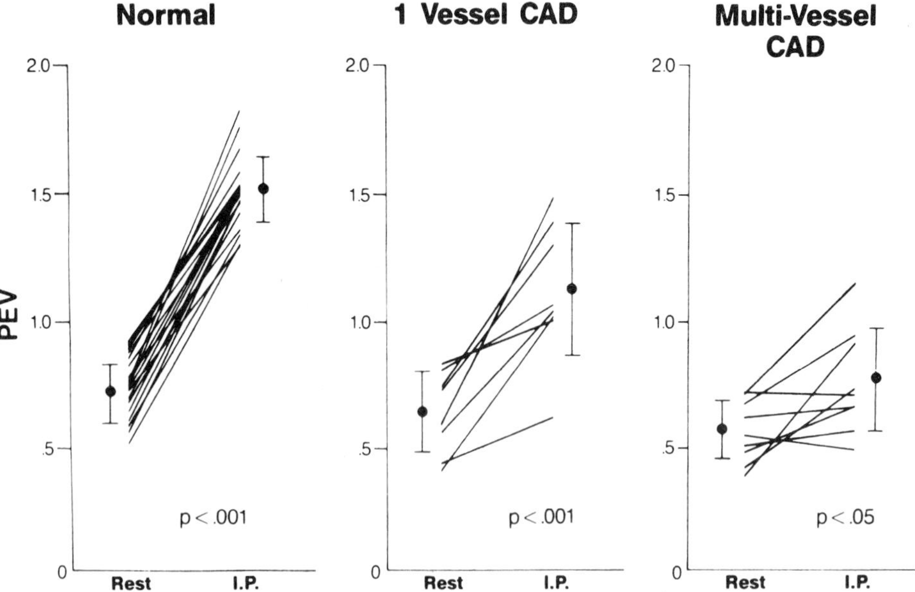

Figure 28–14. Change in peak ejection velocity (PEV) from rest to immediate post-exercise (IP) in normal subjects, patients with one-vessel coronary artery disease (CAD), and patients with two- and three-vessel CAD. (From Bryg, R. J., Labovitz, A. J., Mehdirad, A. A., et al.: Effect of coronary artery disease on Doppler-derived parameters of aortic flow during upright exercise. Am. J. Cardiol. 58:14, 1986, with permission.)

normal subjects and patients with or without myocardial ischemia based on thallium-201 perfusion scintigraphy.[H4] These investigators demonstrated that, as a group, patients with coronary artery disease and abnormal thallium scans had a reduced peak ejection velocity and aortic acceleration in response to exercise as compared with healthy volunteers. However, they found qualitatively similar responses in peak aortic flow velocity and maximal acceleration in patients with normal and ischemic responses based on thallium scintigraphy (Fig. 28–15). As a group, the patients with abnormal thallium perfusion scans had lower peak acceleration than the patients with normal scans, and when corrected for exercise capacity, this difference was most pronounced in patients with multivessel disease.

These two studies indicate that the use of aortic flow assessment by Doppler echocardiography as an aid to the diagnosis of ischemic heart disease is compromised by the same factors that limit the use of exercise ejection fraction. Although they are different, left ventricular ejection fraction and aortic flow velocity are both measures of global left ventricular systolic function. Several studies have demonstrated that Doppler-determined changes in peak aortic flow velocity and acceleration during exercise tend to mirror changes in ejection fraction.[D2, M10, T2]

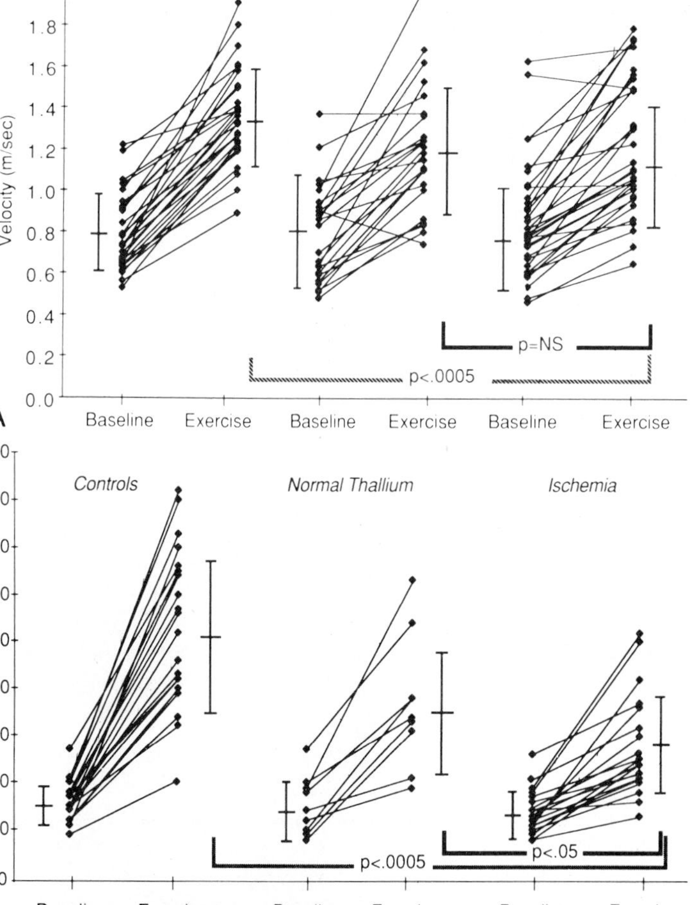

Figure 28–15. Values for maximal aortic blood velocity (*A*) and peak acceleration of aortic blood flow (*B*) at baseline and immediately after exercise for control subjects, patients with normal thallium-201 scans, and patients with ischemia by thallium-201 imaging. The p values refer to the difference between groups for the mean change in Doppler variables. NS—no statistical significance. (Reprinted with permission from The American College of Cardiology [J. Am. Coll. Cardiol. 10:811, 1987].)

Therefore, the response in a particular patient is related to both resting left ventricular function and the severity of exercise-induced left ventricular dysfunction. Thus, this technique appears most likely to be helpful in identifying the presence of advanced coronary artery disease.

Risk Stratification Post Myocardial Infarction

The prognosis of patients who survive the acute phase of acute myocardial infarction has been extensively investigated in an attempt to identify high-risk subsets. Risk stratification prior to hospital discharge improves the identification of patients with an increased likelihood of future cardiac events. Recognition of such a high-risk subgroup may permit appropriate therapeutic interventions to be undertaken. Although the presence of resting left ventricular dysfunction, post-infarction angina, and significant ventricular arrhythmias are all predictors of an adverse outcome post myocardial infarction, many patients with "uncomplicated" infarctions are still at an increased risk for subsequent cardiac events. In these intermediate-risk and low-risk subgroups, evidence for residual myocardial ischemia is the most important predictor of outcome. Therefore, exercise stress testing soon after recovery from an acute myocardial infarction has become useful for detecting inducible ischemia, and the safety of low-level exercise testing after acute myocardial infarction has been established. However, studies of the predictive value of electrocardiographic changes alone for subsequent mortality have yielded conflicting results. The addition of thallium-201 scintigraphy or radionuclide angiography to the exercise test appears to enhance the ability to detect high-risk patients.[B5]

Exercise echocardiography has also been used to evaluate patients with post myocardial infarction (Fig. 28–16).[A4, J1, M10, R5] In studies utilizing two-dimensional echocardiography in combination with exercise testing, the development of a new wall motion abnormality remote from the area of infarction or a significant deterioration of a resting wall motion abnormality predicted the development of a future cardiac event with a sensitivity of 63 to 80 percent and specificity of 78 to 95 percent (Table 28–2). Similarly, exercise echocardiography was able to detect multivessel coronary artery disease with a sensitivity of 77 to 82 percent and specificity of 88 to 95 percent.[J1, R5] In addition, most of the false-negative results for patients with multivessel disease were for patients who did not suffer a subsequent cardiac event[R5] or who had obstructions of only branch vessels of major coronary arteries.[J1] Changes in left ventricular ejection fraction during exercise were less predictive of subsequent events than was regional wall motion. Thus, it appears that the use of two-dimensional echocardiography during low-level exercise testing following an uncomplicated myocardial infarction is capable of defining the subgroup of patients at risk for subsequent cardiac events. One potential limitation of this method is for patients with single-vessel disease and myocardial infarction who still have viable myocardium within the infarct zone. This subgroup of patients may be particularly difficult to diagnose, since a resting wall motion abnormality is already present and worsening of motion with exercise may or may not be present with ischemia.

Mehta and associates evaluated the application of exercise-induced changes in aortic Doppler flow parameters in the evaluation of patients following myocardial infarction.[M11] Peak aortic flow velocity, maximal acceleration, and systolic velocity integral were significantly lower at peak exercise in a group of patients who had a positive electrocardiographic stress test. Maximal acceleration and peak velocity of flow at peak exercise were 65 percent predictive of three-vessel disease, and when they were combined with the time to onset of ST segment depression the predictive value increased to 80 percent. Thus, exercise Doppler may also prove to be useful in the evaluation of patients following myocardial infarction for the detection of advanced coronary artery disease.

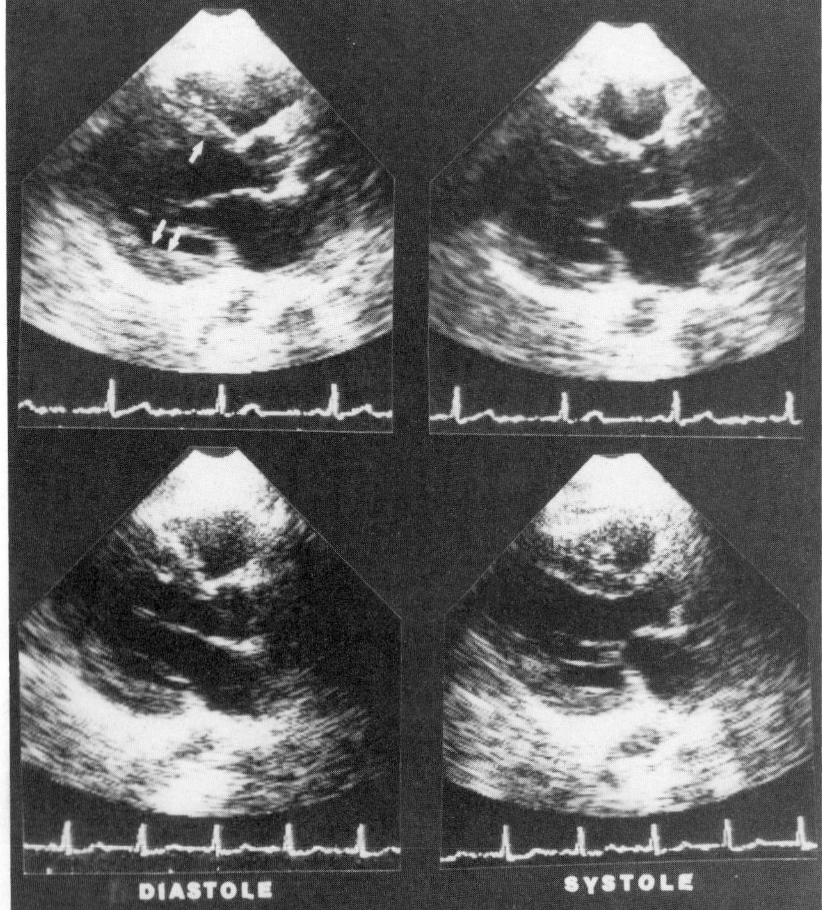

Figure 28–16. Exercise echocardiographic study from a patient with recent inferior-posterior myocardial infarction. Parasternal long-axis views at rest (*top*) and immediately post-exercise (*bottom*). Inferior-posterior akinesis is present at rest and after exercise (*double arrows*), while the interventricular septum moves normally at rest and becomes hyperdynamic after exercise (*single arrow*). Short-axis and apical views confirmed normal hyperdynamic anterior wall and apical motion following exercise. At cardiac catheterization this patient had an isolated occlusion of the left circumflex coronary artery.

Table 28–2. EXERCISE ECHOCARDIOGRAPHY FOR THE EVALUATION OF PATIENTS WITH POST MYOCARDIAL INFARCTION

					Exercise Echocardiography†			
					MVD‡		*Cardiac Events*§	
Study	(Year)	Technique	Success (%)	Follow-up (range, mean)	Sens.	Spec.	Sens.	Spec.
Jaarsma	(1986)	2DE* post-TME*	88	8–16 wk (12)	77	95	75	78
Applegate	(1987)	2DE upright bike post-TME	74	3–24 mo (11)	—	—	63	80
Ryan	(1987)	2DE post-TME	—	6–10 mo (7.2)	82	88	80	95
Mehta	(1986)	aortic Doppler TME	91	—	77¶	53¶	—	—

*2DE—two-dimensional echocardiography; TME—treadmill exercise.
†Development of a new wall motion abnormality with exercise or worsening of existing wall motion abnormality.
‡MVD—multivessel disease; Sens.—sensitivity; Spec.—specificity.
§Recurrent angina; reinfarction; need for coronary artery bypass grafting; cardiac death.
¶Based on peak aortic velocity at peak exercise.

NON-EXERCISE STRESS ECHOCARDIOGRAPHY

Other forms of stress echocardiography are used most often for patients who cannot exercise because of physical limitations. The major purpose of non-exercise stress echocardiography is the same as that of exercise echocardiography: to diagnose the presence of ischemic heart disease or evaluate specific questions concerning cardiac function in those with known heart disease. Most non-exercise stress interventions involve increasing myocardial oxygen demand by altering heart rate and blood pressure. A few approaches are designed to alter coronary blood flow. The latter techniques are better suited to imaging modalities that take advantage of differences in coronary blood flow, such as thallium-201 scintigraphy. Methods that increase myocardial oxygen demand mimic exercise and are best suited for the echocardiographic evaluation of wall motion.

Techniques That Increase Myocardial Oxygen Demand

A popular form of non-exercise stress testing that has been used frequently in the cardiac catheterization laboratory is atrial pacing.[A5] In the non-invasive laboratory, pacing can be accomplished by use of a transesophageal catheter or transcutaneous electrodes.[G5] Although the latter is the least invasive approach to atrial pacing, transcutaneous methods cause considerable chest wall muscle activation, which can interfere with obtaining high-quality echocardiograms. A study of esophageal pacing in 19 patients with known coronary artery disease found that one patient had an inadequate echocardiogram, two could not be paced, and one had excessive discomfort with pacing. In the 15 patients studied, 13 developed wall motion abnormalities, giving a sensitivity in this select group of 87 percent. Only nine patients developed chest pain, and three had ST-T wave changes on the electrocardiogram.[C7] A larger study showed similar results; sensitivity 80 percent in those with normal resting wall motion and specificity 88 percent.[15] The same authors compared esophageal pacing to post-supine bicycle exercise echocardiography and found similar results in a select group of subjects undergoing coronary angiography.[14] Thus, echocardiography during esophageal pacing is an alternative to exercise echocardiography in those who cannot exercise. Overall, the sensitivity is less than that reported for exercise echocardiography, probably because an increase in heart rate alone does not raise myocardial oxygen demand sufficiently to cause ischemia in some patients with significant coronary artery disease. Also, approximately 5 percent of patients with good echocardiograms cannot be studied because of failure to pace or esophageal pain.

A more popular approach for increasing myocardial oxygen demand in the echocardiographic laboratory has been the intravenous infusion of catecholamines.[M12] Isoproterenol has been employed with some success but, like pacing, it has a high specificity and lower sensitivity, since the major effect of isoproterenol is to increase heart rate without significant changes in blood pressure. Thus, as with pacing, myocardial oxygen demand is not increased as much as it is with exercise. More recently, dobutamine has been employed because of experimental studies suggesting that dobutamine increases myocardial oxygen demand more than dopamine and often results in demonstrable abnormalities of wall motion in situations where there is critical narrowing of coronary arteries.[M13]

Techniques That Alter Coronary Blood Flow

The cold pressor response has been applied to the evaluation of patients with suspected ischemic heart disease. The technique involves placing the patient's hand in an ice-water bath for as long as the patient can tolerate it, which is usually between 1 and 4 minutes. This stimulus results in considerable α-adrenergic discharge, which increases arterial pressure, and in the normal coronary circulation the increase in myocardial oxygen demand is met with an appropriate degree of coronary dilatation. In severely obstructed coronary vessels the α-adrenergic tone can sometimes override the metabolic vasodilatation, and the cold pressor test can result in a decrease in perfusion of the severely obstructed vascular bed secondary to α-adrenergic constriction. Gondi and Nanda applied this test to 20 patients with normal resting left ventricular wall motion on two-dimensional echocardiography.[G6] They noted that the product of heart rate and blood pressure increased by 49 percent, but this was mainly due to an increase in blood pressure with only mild changes in heart rate. None of their patients developed angina or electrocardiographic changes. Using the detection of wall motion abnormalities by two-dimensional echocardiography as a criterion for ischemic heart disease compared with the results of cardiac catheterization, they found a sensitivity of 69 percent and a specificity of 86 percent. Thus, like pacing and catecholamine infusion, the cold pressor test seems to be most useful if it is positive. A negative test has less discriminatory value.

Dipyridamole

The most popular technique for altering coronary blood flow has been intravenous administration of dipyridamole. This drug is a potent vasodilator that acts mainly on normal coronary arteries and diverts blood flow away from areas subtended by arteries with significant coronary stenoses. The drug may also cause significant systemic vasodilatation and lead to a reduction in blood pressure. The usual dose employed is 0.56 mg/kg over 4 minutes, but larger doses over longer periods of time have been used. The drug also can be administered orally at a dose of 200 or 400 mg, but the onset of action and maximal effect of the drug are delayed for 60 to 90 minutes.[T3] Thus, the intravenous approach is more efficient. At this writing, intravenous dipyridamole is not available in the United States.

Dipyridamole also has certain adverse effects that vary with the dose administered. Headaches are the most common adverse effect, followed by flushing and nausea. The incidence of severe hypotension and severe angina pectoris is low, largely because the antidote aminophylline is administered immediately if chest pain or falling blood pressure is noted. The major use of dipyridamole echocardiography is in the detection of ischemic heart disease. Two-dimensional echocardiography is done during the 4- to 10-minute infusion of the drug and for up to 20 minutes after the drug has been administered. The criterion for the diagnosis of ischemic heart disease is the development of wall motion abnormalities.

A group at the Institute of Clinical Physiology in Pisa, Italy, have the largest reported experience with intravenous dipyridamole echocardiography and report sensitivities for the detection of arteriographically proven coronary disease of 56 to 74 percent, depending on the dosage used.[P6, P7] The higher sensitivities were found with doses between 0.56 and 0.84 mg/kg. Also, patients with more severe coronary artery disease were identified more frequently than those with one-vessel disease (Table 28–3). In addition, the group did not exclude patients with prior myocardial infarction in whom the diagnosis of coronary artery disease is almost certain. In their hands, the specificity has consistently been 100 percent, with no false-positives either in young normal individuals or in age-matched normals with angiographically proven normal coronary arteries.

Other investigators have reported lower sensitivities for the detection of myocardial ischemia. Margonato and associates studied 21 patients with severe angina pectoris, positive Bruce exercise tolerance tests, and angiographically proven multivessel coronary artery disease by using 0.6 mg/kg of intravenous dipyridamole and multiview two-dimensional echocardiography.[M14] They detected new wall motion abnormalities in only 11 patients, for a sensitivity of 52 percent. However, they noted that the area of the transient wall motion abnormality identified the culprit vessel, which was helpful in the management of patients whose results were positive. They concluded that the test was most useful if the patient's exercise capacity was restricted.

The Pisa group compared dipyridamole to exercise echocardiography in 55 patients with chest pain syndromes who subsequently underwent coronary arteriography to determine the presence or absence of coronary artery disease.[P8] In this study they used 0.56 mg/kg of dipyridamole unless the study was negative, in which case they used 0.84 mg/kg on another day. Supine bicycle exercise was employed. Sensitivity in this study for dipyridamole was 72 percent and for exercise echocardiography was 76 percent. Specificity was again 100 percent with dipyridamole and 87 percent with exercise echocardiography. The success rate of dipyridamole echocardiography was 100 percent, whereas they could use exercise echocardiography in only 73 percent of patients. The group concluded that the two

Table 28–3. DETECTION OF CORONARY ARTERY DISEASE WITH INTRAVENOUS DIPYRIDAMOLE ECHOCARDIOGRAPHY

	Vessel Disease (+Echo/Total Number)			
Dipyridamole	*0*	*1*	2	3
Low dose*	0/25	11/30 (37%)	10/31 (71%)	7/7 (100%)
High dose†	0/31	12/24 (50%)	29/36 (81%)	12/12 (100%)

*Data from Picano, E., Distante, A., Masini, M., et al.: Dipyridamole-echocardiography test in effort angina pectoris. Am. J. Cardiol. 56:452, 1985.

†Data from Picano, E., Lattanzi, F., Masini, M., et al.: High dose dipyridamole echocardiography test in effort angina pectoris. J. Am. Coll. Cardiol. 8:848, 1986.

test results were similar but that dipyridamole had a greater success rate with this type of patient. Their exercise echocardiography results are less than those reported by other investigators as discussed above.

It is well known that dipyridamole has a profound effect on the distribution of coronary blood flow, but in animal models of ischemia it does not reliably produce segmental wall motion abnormalities.[F4] One reason for this may be that the drug can induce differences in regional blood flow that are detectable by perfusion imaging techniques but do not result in sufficient myocardial ischemia to alter the mechanical function of the heart. Thus, intravenous dipyridamole stress has been very popularly employed with thallium-201 imaging, especially in patients who cannot exercise. Several studies suggest that use of intravenous dipyridamole with thallium-201 imaging is of value for detecting significant coronary artery disease. The data of Okada and associates confirm earlier experience with animals, in which transient thallium-201 defects could be found in those with normal rest and exercise radionuclide angiographic results. Okada and associates reported an overall sensitivity of dipyridamole thallium of 94 percent and a specificity of 84 percent.[O2] Thus, dipyridamole thallium imaging appears to have greater sensitivity for the detection of coronary artery disease than dipyridamole echocardiography.

Dipyridamole echocardiography has also been applied in specific situations for evaluating patients with known ischemic heart disease. Picano and associates evaluated 19 patients with known left anterior descending coronary artery disease.[P9] Nine of these patients had a positive dipyridamole echocardiography test at a dose of 0.56 mg/kg. These patients had reduced great cardiac vein coronary blood flow as determined by thermodilution following dipyridamole, and the investigators concluded that dipyridamole echocardiography can predict reductions in coronary artery reserve despite similar anatomic one-vessel coronary artery disease. Also, Masini and associates evaluated the utility of dipyridamole echocardiography compared with upright bicycle electrocardiographic testing in 83 women with chest pain syndromes.[M15] The sensitivity of dipyridamole echocardiography for angiographically significant coronary artery disease was 79 percent and that of exercise electrocardiography was 72 percent. However, the specificity of the dipyridamole echocardiography test was 93 percent, versus 52 percent for exercise electrocardiography. They concluded that dipyridamole echocardiography was superior to the exercise electrocardiographic test in women, who are known to have less good results on exercise electrocardiographic testing. Thus, in specific situations, dipyridamole echocardiography may be a useful adjunct to the diagnostic armamentarium. The combination of high-dose dipyridamole and exercise echocardiographic testing may result in improved sensitivity over either technique alone in the diagnosis of ischemic heart disease.[P10]

The available data suggest that the diagnosis of coronary artery disease in patients who cannot exercise is best accomplished by use of intravenous dipyridamole combined with thallium-201 imaging. If this test is not available or gives equivocal results, either dobutamine echocardiography or dipyridamole echocardiography may be of value. However, at the present time in the United States, only dobutamine is available for intravenous administration. Dipyridamole can be given orally, but this is less convenient. There may be specific clinical situations in which non-exercise stress approaches are of particular value, but there are few data to support this concept at present. Also, there is currently interest in using non-exercise stress echocardiography for risk stratification in patients who have had myocardial infarction, coronary artery bypass, or chronic coronary artery disease, especially those who cannot exercise adequately. However, available data suggest that patients who cannot exercise adequately have a poor prognosis no matter what the reason for their lack of ability to exercise. Whether non-exercise stress echocardiography can further stratify these patients into high- and low-risk groups and whether there is any appropriate therapeutic intervention for the potential high-risk groups so identified remain to be proved. Finally, there is interest in non-exercise stress techniques for the determination of myocardial viability. Whether any of the techniques mentioned above will prove to be useful for this purpose remains to be determined.

References

A

1. Amon, K. W., and Crawford, M. H.: Upright exercise echocardiography. J. Clin. Ultrasound 7:373, 1979.
2. Armstrong, W. F., O'Donnell, J., Dillon, J. C., et al.: Complementary value of two-dimensional exercise echocardiography to routine treadmill exercise testing. Ann. Intern. Med. 105:829, 1986.
3. Armstrong, W. F., O'Donnell, J., Ryan, T., and Feigenbaum, H.: Effect of prior myocardial infarction and extent and location of coronary disease on accuracy of exercise echocardiography. J. Am. Coll. Cardiol. 10:531, 1987.
4. Applegate, R. J., Dell'Italia, L. J., and Crawford, M. H.: Usefulness of two-dimensional echocardiography during low-level exercise testing early after uncomplicated acute myocardial infarction. Am. J. Cardiol. 60:10, 1987.
5. Aroesty, J. M., McKay, R. G., Heller, G. V., et al.: Simultaneous assessment of left ventricular systolic and diastolic dysfunction during pacing-induced ischemia. Circulation 71:889, 1985.

B

1. Berberich, S. N., and Zager, J. R. S.: Hybrid exercise echocardiography. Angiology 32:1, 1981.
2. Berberich, S. N., Zager, J. R. S., Plotnick, G. D., and Fisher, M. L.: A practical approach to exercise echocardiography: Immediate postexercise echocardiography. J. Am. Coll. Cardiol. 3:284, 1984.
3. Bryg, R. J., Labovitz, A. J., Mehdirad, A. A., et al.: Effect of coronary artery disease on Doppler-derived parameters of aortic flow during upright exercise. Am. J. Cardiol. 58:14, 1986.
4. Borer, J. S., Kent, K. M., Bacharach, S. L., et al.: Sensitivity, specificity and predictive accuracy of radionuclide cineangiography during exercise in patients with coronary artery disease. Circulation 60:572, 1979.
5. Beller, G. A., and Gibson, R. S.: Risk stratification after myocardial infarction. Mod. Concepts Cardiovasc. Dis. 55:5, 1986.

C

1. Crawford, M. H., White, D. H., and Amon, K. W.: Echocardiographic evaluation of left ventricular size and performance during handgrip and supine and upright bicycle exercise. Circulation 79:1188, 1979.
2. Crawford, M. H., Amon, K. W., and Vance, W. S.: Exercise 2-dimensional echocardiography: Quantitation of left ventricular performance in patients with severe angina pectoris. Am. J. Cardiol. 51:1, 1983.
3. Crawford, M. H., Petru, M. A., Amon, K. W., et al.: Comparative value of 2-dimensional echocardiography and radionuclide angiography for quantitating changes in left ventricular performance during exercise limited by angina pectoris. Am. J. Cardiol. 53:42, 1984.
4. Colocousis, J. S., Huntsman, L. L., and Curreri, P. W.: Estimation of stroke volume changes by ultrasonic Doppler. Circulation 56:914, 1977.
5. Christie, J. G., Sheldahl, L. M., Tristani, F. E., et al.: Determination of stroke volume and cardiac output during exercise: Comparison of two-dimensional and Doppler echocardiography, Fick oximetry, and thermodilution. Circulation 76:539, 1987.
6. Chaitman, B. R., Bourassa, M. G., Wagniart, P., et al.: Improved efficiency of treadmill exercise testing using a multiple lead ECG system and basic hemodynamic exercise response. Circulation 57:71, 1978.
7. Chapman, P. D., Doyle, T. P., Troup, P. J., et al.: Stress echocardiography with transesophageal atrial pacing: Preliminary report of a new method for detection of ischemic wall motion abnormalities. Circulation 70:445, 1984.

D

1. Daley, P. J., Sagar, K. B., and Wann, L. S.: Doppler echocardiographic measurement of flow velocity in the ascending aorta during supine and upright exercise. Br. Heart J. 54:562, 1985.
2. Daley, P. J., Sagar, K. B., Collier, B. D., et al.: Detection of exercise induced changes in left ventricular performance by Doppler echocardiography. Br. Heart J. 58:447, 1987.
3. Dymond, D. S., Foster, C., Grenier, R. P., et al.: Peak exercise and immediate postexercise imaging for the detection of left ventricular functional abnormalities in coronary artery disease. Am. J. Cardiol. 53:1532, 1984.

E

1. Ehsani, A. A., Heath, G. W., Hagberg, J. M., and Schechtman, K.: Noninvasive assessment of changes in left ventricular function induced by graded isometric exercise in healthy subjects. Chest 80:51, 1981.

F

1. Fogelman, A. M., Abbasi, A. S., Pearce, M. L., and Kattus, A. A.: Echocardiographic study of the abnormal motion of the posterior left ventricular wall during angina pectoris. Circulation 46:905, 1972.
2. Feigenbaum, H.: Echocardiography, 3rd ed. Lea & Febiger, Philadelphia, 1981, p. 3.
3. Feigenbaum, H.: Exercise echocardiography. J. Am. Soc. Echo. 1:161, 1988.
4. Fung, A. F., Gallagher, K. P., and Buda, A. J.: The physiologic basis of dobutamine as compared with dipyridamole stress interventions in the assessment of critical coronary stenosis. Circulation 76:943, 1987.

G

1. Ginzton, L. E., Conant, R., Brizendine, M., et al.: Exercise subcostal two-dimensional echocardiography: A new method of segmental wall motion analysis. Am. J. Cardiol. 53:805, 1984.
2. Ginzton, L. E., Conant, R., Brizendine, M., et al.: Quantitative analysis of segmental wall motion during maximal upright dynamic exercise: Variability in normal adults. Circulation 73:268, 1986.
3. Gardin, J. M., Kozlowski, J., Dabestani, A., et al.: Studies of Doppler aortic flow velocity during supine bicycle exercise. Am. J. Cardiol. 57:327, 1986.
4. Gillam, L. D., Hogan, R. D., Foale, R. A., et al.: A comparison of quantitative echocardiographic methods for delineating infarct-induced abnormal wall motion. Circulation 70:113, 1984.
5. Gallagher, J. J., Smith, W. M., Kerr, C. R., et al.: Esophageal pacing: A diagnostic and therapeutic tool. Circulation 65:336, 1982.
6. Gondi, B., and Nanda, N. C.: Cold pressor test during two-dimensional echocardiography: Usefulness in detection of patients with coronary disease. Am. Heart J. 107:278, 1984.

H

1. Heng, M. K., Simard, M., Lake, R., and Udhoji, V. H.: Exercise two-dimensional echocardiography for diagnosis of coronary artery disease. Am. J. Cardiol. 54:502, 1984.
2. Huntsman, L. L., Stewart, D. K., Barnes, S. R., et al.: Noninvasive Doppler determination of cardiac output in man. Circulation 67:593, 1983.
3. Harrison, M. R., Smith, M. D., Nissen, S. E., et al.: Use of exercise Doppler echocardiography to evaluate cardiac drugs: Effects of propranolol and verapamil on aortic blood flow velocity and acceleration. J. Am. Coll. Cardiol. 11:1002, 1988.
4. Harrison, M. R., Smith, M. D., Friedman, B. J., and DeMaria, A. N.: Uses and limitations of exercise Doppler echocardiography in the diagnosis of ischemic heart disease. J. Am. Coll. Cardiol. 10:809, 1987.
5. Heger, J. J., Weyman, A. E., Wann, L. S., et al.: Cross-sectional echocardiography in acute myocardial infarction: Detection and localization of regional left ventricular asynergy. Circulation 60:531, 1979.
6. Horowitz, R. S., Morganroth, J., Parrotto, C., et al.: Immediate diagnosis of acute myocardial infarction by two-dimensional echocardiography. Circulation 65:323, 1982.
7. Haissly, J.-C., Messin, R., Degre, S., et al.: Comparative response to isometric (static) and dynamic exercise tests in coronary disease. Am. J. Cardiol. 33:791, 1974.

I

1. Ihlen, H., Endresen, K., Golf, S., and Nitter-Hauge, S.: Cardiac stroke volume during exercise measured by Doppler echocardiography: Comparison with the thermodilution technique and evaluation of reproducibility. Br. Heart J. 58:455, 1987.
2. Ihlen, H., Amlie, J. P., Dale, J., et al.: Determination of cardiac output by Doppler echocardiography. Br. Heart J. 51:54, 1984.
3. Iwase, M., Sotobata, I., Takagi, S., et al.: Effects of diltiazem on left ventricular diastolic behavior in patients with hypertrophic cardiomyopathy: Evaluation with exercise pulsed Doppler echocardiography. J. Am. Coll. Cardiol. 9:1099, 1987.
4. Iliceto, S., D'Ambrosio, G., Sorino, M., et al.: Comparison of postexercise and transesophageal atrial pacing two-dimensional echocardiography for detection of coronary artery disease. Am. J. Cardiol. 57:547, 1986.
5. Iliceto, S., Sorino, M., D'Ambrosio, G., et al.: Detection of coronary artery disease by two-dimensional echocardiography and transesophageal atrial pacing. J. Am. Coll. Cardiol. 5:1188, 1985.

J

1. Jaarsma, W., Visser, C. A., Kupper, A. J. F., et al.: Usefulness of two-dimensional exercise echocardiography shortly after myocardial infarction. Am. J. Cardiol. 57:86, 1986.

K

1. Kraunz, R. F., and Kennedy, J. W.: Ultrasonic determination of left ventricular wall motion in normal man. Am. Heart J. 79:36, 1970.
2. Kan, G., Visser, C. A., Koolen, J. J., and Dunning, A. J.: Short and long term predictive value of admission wall motion score in acute myocardial infarction. A cross sectional echocardiographic study of 345 patients. Br. Heart J. 56:422, 1986.

L

1. Laird, W. P., Fixler, D. E., and Huffines, F. D.: Cardiovascular response to isometric exercise in normal adolescents. Circulation 59:651, 1979.
2. Limacher, M. C., Quinones, M. A., Poliner, L. R., et al.: Detection of coronary artery disease with exercise two-dimensional echocardiography. Circulation 67:1211, 1983.
3. Loeppky, J. A., Greene, E. R., Hoekenga, D. E., et al.: Beat-by-beat stroke volume assessment by pulsed Doppler in upright and supine exercise. J. Appl. Physiol. 50:1173, 1981.

4. Labovitz, A. J., and Pearson, A. C.: Evaluation of left ventricular diastolic function: Clinical relevance and recent Doppler echocardiographic insights. Am. Heart J. 114:836, 1987.
5. Lowe, D. K., Rothbaum, D. A., McHenry, P. L., et al.: Myocardial blood flow response to isometric (handgrip) and treadmill exercise in coronary artery disease. Circulation 51:126, 1975.

M

1. Mason, S. J., Weiss, J. L., Weisfeldt, M. L., et al.: Exercise echocardiography: Detection of wall motion abnormalities during ischemia. Circulation 59:50, 1979.
2. Morganroth, J., Chen, C. C., David, D., et al.: Exercise cross-sectional echocardiographic diagnosis of coronary artery disease. Am. J. Cardiol. 47:20, 1981.
3. Maurer, G., and Nanda, N. C.: Two dimensional echocardiographic evaluation of exercise-induced left and right ventricular asynergy: Correlation with thallium scanning. Am. J. Cardiol. 48:720, 1981.
4. Marx, G. R., Hicks, R. W., and Allen, H. D.: Measurement of cardiac output and exercise factor by pulsed Doppler echocardiography during supine bicycle ergometry in normal young adolescent boys. J. Am. Coll. Cardiol. 10:430, 1987.
5. Mitchell, G. D., Brunken, R. C., Schwaiger, M., et al.: Assessment of mitral flow velocity with exercise by an index of stress-induced left ventricular ischemia in coronary artery disease. Am. J. Cardiol. 61:536, 1988.
6. Moynihan, P. F., Parisi, A. F., and Feldman, C. L.: Quantitative detection of regional left ventricular contraction abnormalities by two-dimensional echocardiography. Circulation 63:752, 1981.
7. Mitamura, H., Ogawa, S., Hori, S., et al.: Two dimensional echocardiographic analysis of wall motion abnormalities during handgrip exercise in patients with coronary artery disease. Am. J. Cardiol. 48:711, 1981.
8. Medina, R., Panidis, I. P., Morganroth, J., et al.: The value of echocardiographic regional wall motion abnormalities in detecting coronary artery disease in patients with or without a dilated left ventricle. Am. Heart J. 109:799, 1985.
9. Marcus, M. L., White, C. W., and Kirchner, P. T.: Isn't it time to reevaluate the sensitivity of noninvasive approaches for the diagnosis of coronary artery disease? J. Am. Coll. Cardiol. 8:1033, 1986.
10. Mehdirad, A. A., Williams, G. A., Labovitz, A. J., et al.: Evaluation of left ventricular function during upright exercise: Correlation of exercise Doppler with postexercise two-dimensional echocardiographic results. Circulation 75:413, 1987.
11. Mehta, N., Bennett, D., Mannering, D., et al.: Usefulness of noninvasive Doppler measurement of ascending aortic blood velocity and acceleration in detecting impairment of the left ventricular functional response to exercise three weeks after acute myocardial infarction. Am. J. Cardiol. 58:879, 1986.
12. Mancini, G. B. J., Friedman, H. Z., Hramiec, J. E., and Deboe, S. F.: Relation between graded, subcritical impairments of coronary flow reserve and regional myocardial dysfunction induced by isoproterenol infusion in dogs. Am. Heart J. 113:906, 1987.
13. McGillem, M. J., DeBoe, S. F., Friedman, H. Z., and Mancini, G. B. J.: The effects of dopamine and dobutamine on regional function in the presence of rigid coronary stenoses and subcritical impairments of reactive hyperemia. Am. Heart J. 115:970, 1988.
14. Margonato, A., Chierchia, S., Cianflone, D., et al.: Limitations of dipyridamole-echocardiography in effort angina pectoris. Am. J. Cardiol. 59:225, 1987.
15. Masini, M., Picano, E., Lattanzi, F., et al.: High dose dipyridamole-echocardiography test in women: Correlation with exercise-electrocardiography test and coronary arteriography. J. Am. Coll. Cardiol. 12:682, 1988.

O

1. Osbakken, M. D., Okada, R. D., Boucher, C. A., et al.: Comparison of exercise perfusion and ventricular function imaging: An analysis of factors affecting the diagnostic accuracy of each technique. J. Am. Coll. Cardiol. 3:272, 1984.
2. Okada, R. D., Bendersky, R., Strauss, W., et al.: Comparison of intravenous dipyridamole thallium cardiac imaging with exercise radionuclide angiography. Am. Heart J. 114:524, 1987.

P

1. Paulsen, W. J., Boughner, D. R., Friesen, A., and Persaud, J. A.: Ventricular response to isometric and isotonic exercise: Echocardiographic assessment. Br. Heart J. 42:521, 1979.
2. Presti, C. F., Armstrong, W. F., and Feigenbaum, H.: Comparison of echocardiography at peak exercise and after bicycle exercise in evaluation of patients with known or suspected coronary artery disease. J. Am. Soc. Echo. 1:119, 1988.
3. Poliner, L. R., Dehmer, G. J., Lewis, S. E., et al.: Left ventricular performance in normal subjects: A comparison of the responses to exercise in the upright and supine positions. Circulation 62:528, 1980.
4. Presti, C. F., Gentile, R., Armstrong, W. F., et al.: Improvement in regional wall motion after percutaneous transluminal coronary angioplasty during acute myocardial function: Utility of two-dimensional echocardiography. Am. Heart J. 115:1149, 1988.
5. Port, S., Cobb, F. R., Coleman, R. E., and Jones, R. H.: Effect of age on the response of the left ventricular ejection fraction to exercise. N. Engl. J. Med. 303:1133, 1980.
6. Picano, E., Distante, A., Masini, M., et al.: Dipyridamole-echocardiography test in effort angina pectoris. Am. J. Cardiol. 56:452, 1985.
7. Picano, E., Lattanzi, F., Masini, M., et al.: High dose dipyridamole echocardiography test in effort angina pectoris. J. Am. Coll. Cardiol. 8:848, 1986.
8. Picano, E., Lattanzi, F., Masini, M., et al.: Comparison of the high-dose dipyridamole-echocardiography test and exercise two-dimensional echocardiography for diagnosis of coronary artery disease. Am. J. Cardiol. 59:539, 1987.
9. Picano, E., Simonetti, I., Masini, M., et al.: Transient myocardial dysfunction during pharmacologic vasodilation as an index of reduced coronary reserve: A coronary hemodynamic and echocardiographic study. J. Am. Coll. Cardiol. 8:84, 1986.
10. Picano, E., Lattanzi, F., Masini, M., et al.: Usefulness of the dipyridamole-exercise echocardiography test for diagnosis of coronary artery disease. Am. J. Cardiol. 62:67, 1988.

Q

1. Quinones, M. A., Waggoner, A. D., Reduto, L. A., et al.: A new, simplified and accurate method for determining ejection fraction with two-dimensional echocardiography. Circulation 64:744, 1981.

R

1. Robertson, W. S., Feigenbaum, H., Armstrong, W. F., et al.: Exercise echocardiography: A clinically practical addition in the evaluation of coronary artery disease. J. Am. Coll. Cardiol. 2:1085, 1983.
2. Ryan, T., Vasey, C. G., Presti, C. F., et al.: Exercise echocardiography: Detection of coronary artery disease in patients with normal left ventricular wall motion at rest. J. Am. Coll. Cardiol. 11:993, 1988.
3. Rassi, A., Crawford, M. H., Richards, K. L., and Miller, J. F.: Differing mechanisms of exercise flow augmentation at the mitral and aortic valves. Circulation 77:543, 1988.
4. Rigo, P., Bailey, I. K., Griffith, L. S. C., et al.: Value and limitations of segmental analysis of stress thallium myocardial imaging for localization of coronary artery disease. Circulation 61:973, 1980.
5. Ryan, T., Armstrong, W. F., O'Donnell, J. A., and Feigenbaum, H.: Risk stratification after acute myocardial infarction by means of exercise two-dimensional echocardiography. Am. Heart J. 114:1305, 1987.

S

1. Smithen, C. S., Wharton, C. F. P., and Sowton, E.: Independent effects of heart rate and exercise on left ventricular wall movement measured by reflected ultrasound. Am. J. Cardiol. 30:43, 1972.
2. Stefadouros, M. A., Grossman, W., Shahawy, M. E., et al.: Noninvasive study of effect of isometric exercise on left ventricular performance in normal man. Br. Heart J. 36:988, 1974.
3. Stein, R. A., Michielli, D., Fox, E. L., and Krasnow, N.: Continuous ventricular dimensions in man during supine exercise and recovery. Am. J. Cardiol. 41:655, 1978.
4. Sugishita, Y., and Koseki, S.: Dynamic exercise echocardiography. Circulation 60:743, 1979.
5. Stein, R. A., Michielli, D., Diamond, J., et al.: The cardiac response to exercise training: Echocardiographic analysis at rest and during exercise. Am. J. Cardiol. 46:219, 1980.
6. Sugishita, Y., Koseki, S., Matsuda, M., et al.: Dissociation between regional myocardial dysfunction and ECG changes during myocardial ischemia induced by exercise in patients with angina pectoris. Am. Heart J. 106:1, 1983.
7. Simard, M., Heng, M. K., Udhoji, V. N., and Weber, L.: Exercise two-dimensional echocardiography: A technique for improving ultrasound images during exercise stress. Clin. Cardiol. 6:318, 1983.
8. Sabbah, H. N., Khaja, F., Brymer, J. F., et al.: Noninvasive evaluation of left ventricular performance based on peak aortic blood acceleration measured by a continuous-wave Doppler velocity meter. Circulation 74:323, 1986.
9. Shaw, J. G., Johnson, E. C., Voyles, W. F., and Greene, E. R.: Noninvasive Doppler determination of cardiac output during submaximal and peak exercise. J. Appl. Physiol. 59:722, 1985.
10. Schuster, A. H., and Nanda, N. C.: Doppler echocardiographic measurement of cardiac output: Comparison with a non-golden standard. Am. J. Cardiol. 53:257, 1984.
11. Stamm, R. B., Gibson, R. S., Bishop, H. L., et al.: Echocardiographic detection of infarct-localized asynergy and remote asynergy during acute myocardial infarction: Correlation with the extent of angiographic coronary disease. Circulation 67:233, 1983.
12. Shiina, A., Tajik, A. J., Smith, H. C., et al.: Prognostic significance of regional wall motion abnormality in patients with prior myocardial infarction: A prospective correlative study of two-dimensional echocardiography and angiography. Mayo Clin. Proc. 61:254, 1986.
13. Schiller, N. B., Acquatella, H., Ports, T. A., et al.: Left ventricular volume from paired biplane two-dimensional echocardiography. Circulation 60:547, 1979.
14. Starling, M. K., Crawford, M. H., Sorensen, S. G., et al.: Comparative accuracy of apical biplane cross-sectional echocardiography and gated equilibrium radionuclide angiography for estimating left ventricular size and performance. Circulation 63:1075, 1981.

T

1. Tennant, R., and Wiggers, C. J.: The effect of coronary occlusion on myocardial contraction. Am. J. Physiol. 112:351, 1935.
2. Teague, S. M., Corn, C., Sharma, M., et al.: A comparison of Doppler and radionuclide ejection dynamics during ischemic exercise. Am. J. Card. Imag. 1:145, 1987.
3. Taillefer, R., Lette, J., Phaneuf, D. C., et al.: Thallium-201 myocardial imaging during pharmacologic coronary vasodilation: Comparison of oral and intravenous administration of dipyridamole. J. Am. Coll. Cardiol. 8:76, 1986.

U

1. Upton, M. T., Rerych, S. K., Newman, G. E., et al.: Detecting abnormalities in left ventricular function during exercise before angina and ST-segment depression. Circulation 62:341, 1980.

V

1. Visser, C. A., van der Wieken, R. L., Kan, G., et al.: Comparison of two-dimensional echocardiography with radionuclide angiography during dynamic exercise for the detection of coronary artery disease. Am. Heart J. 106:528, 1983.
2. Visser, C. A., Lie, K. I., Kan, G., et al.: Detection and quantification of acute, isolated myocardial infarction by two dimensional echocardiography. Am. J. Cardiol. 47:1020, 1981.
3. Voelker, W., Jacksch, R., Dittmann, H., and Karsch, K. R.: Diagnostic accuracy of 2-D echocardiography for detection of exercise-induced wall motion abnormalities in patients with coronary artery disease: Comparison to biplane cineventriculography. Clin. Cardiol. 11:547, 1988.

W

1. Weiss, J. L., Weisfeldt, M. L., Mason, S. J., et al.: Evidence of Frank-Starling effect in man during severe semisupine exercise. Circulation 59:655, 1979.
2. Wann, L. S., Faris, J. V., Childress, R. H., et al.: Exercise cross-sectional echocardiography in ischemic heart disease. Circulation 60:1300, 1979.
3. Wallmeyer, K., Wann, L. S., Sagar, K. B., et al.: The influence of preload and heart rate on Doppler echocardiographic indexes of left ventricular performance: Comparison with invasive indexes in an experimental preparation. Circulation 74:181, 1986.
4. Wang, Y., Marshall, R. J., and Shepherd, J. T.: The effect of changes in posture and of graded exercise on stroke volume in man. J. Clin. Invest. 39:1051, 1960.
5. Weiss, J. L., Bulkley, B. H., Hutchins, G. M., and Mason, S. J.: Two-dimensional echocardiographic recognition of myocardial injury in man: Comparison with postmortem studies. Circulation 63:401, 1981.
6. Wallis, D. E., O'Connell, J. B., Henkin, R. E., et al.: Segmental wall motion abnormalities in dilated cardiomyopathy: A common finding and good prognostic sign. J. Am. Coll. Cardiol. 4:674, 1984.
7. Waters, D. D., Luz, P. D., Wyatt, H. L., et al.: Early changes in regional and global left ventricular function induced by graded reductions in regional coronary perfusion. Am. J. Cardiol. 39:537, 1977.

Z

1. Zwehl, W., Gueret, P., Meerbaum, S., et al.: Quantitative two dimensional echocardiography during bicycle exercise in normal subjects. Am. J. Cardiol. 47:866, 1981.
2. Zachariah, Z. P., Hsiung, M. C., Nanda, N. C., et al.: Color Doppler assessment of mitral regurgitation induced by supine exercise in patients with coronary artery disease. Am. J. Cardiol. 59:1266, 1987.

Chapter 29

Echocardiography in Coronary Artery Disease: Myocardial Ischemia and Infarction

RICHARD E. KERBER, M.D.

REGIONAL CONTRACTION ABNORMALITIES—DETECTION AND QUANTIFICATION 594
PROGNOSIS AFTER MYOCARDIAL INFARCTION 598
COMPLICATIONS OF MYOCARDIAL INFARCTION 599
OTHER APPLICATIONS OF ECHOCARDIOGRAPHY IN CORONARY ARTERY DISEASE 602
CONCLUSION 603

Coronary atherosclerosis, the most common cause of cardiac disease in adults, characteristically manifests by interrupting or reducing myocardial perfusion, causing ischemia or infarction. Echocardiography can be used in a variety of ways to detect ischemic heart disease:[K1] it can demonstrate regional contraction abnormalities, manifest as changes in wall motion or thickening. It can display the complications of myocardial infarction, such as ventricular thrombi, ventricular aneurysms, and ventricular septal or papillary muscle rupture. These are the uses of echocardiography that are emphasized in this chapter. Many other applications of echocardiography related to coronary artery disease—exercise ventricular function, intraoperative coronary arterial imaging, myocardial perfusion by contrast techniques and tissue characterization methods to detect myocardial fibrosis—are discussed in detail elsewhere in this book. They are reviewed here briefly for the sake of comprehensiveness.

REGIONAL CONTRACTION ABNORMALITIES—DETECTION AND QUANTIFICATION

Reductions in myocardial perfusion result in abnormalities of contraction, typically on a local or regional basis. Such reductions may be acute or chronic and yield hypokinesis (reduced systolic contraction), akinesis (absence of systolic contraction), or dyskinesis (systolic thinning or bulging) (Fig. 29–1). Such abnormalities are easy to detect by echocardiography and have been well studied experimentally and clinically for almost 20 years.[K2]

The presence of regional contraction abnormalities at rest strongly suggests the diagnosis of coronary disease. Not only can echocardiography demonstrate the presence of infarction, but also it may be used to quantify the extent of infarction. Several experimental and clinical studies[P1, T1, W1] have shown a very good correlation between the extent of wall motion abnormalities, as demonstrated by echocardiography, and the size or mass of an infarction (Fig. 29–2). All these studies have shown that the extent of regional dyskinesis overestimates the infarct size. This is probably due to the phenomenon of "adjacent nonischemic dyskinesis"—that is, the observation that noninfarcted areas immediately adjacent to regions of ischemia or infarction develop contraction abnormalities—perhaps because of tethering effects.

Does the absence of regional contraction abnormalities exclude infarction? Lieberman and associates showed, in experimental studies, that a "threshold" phenomenon exists: absence of dyskinesis did not exclude infarction involving less than 20 percent of the left ventricular wall[L1] (Fig. 29–3). Furthermore, when dyskinesis is present the extent of transmurality cannot be calculated simply from the extent of thinning.

The Lieberman study implies that echocardiography may be insensitive to the presence of small infarcts, but this was an open-chest study. Do the conclusions apply to transthoracic echocardiographic imaging? In our laboratory we studied a closed-chest canine model of varying infarct size (Fig. 29–4) and showed that echocardiography was highly sensitive for the detection of large infarcts but often could not demonstrate dyskinesis in small, nontransmural infarctions.[P2] This is consonant with the Lieberman study.

The methods of analysis used to evaluate regional contraction in echocardiographic recordings are many and are of considerable importance in determining the accuracy of the technique.[B1, C1, F1] Regional contraction indices are illustrated in Figure 29–5. Most are load dependent and cannot distinguish between true regional contraction abnormalities and other causes of distorted motion, such as electrical conduction abnormalities, volume overload, and previous thoracotomy and cardiac surgery. Additional factors to be considered include the manner in which the reference center is defined (usually end diastolic), whether the center of the comparison frame (usually end systolic) is aligned on the reference frame (i.e., fixed vs. "floating" analysis) (Figs. 29–6 and 29–7), and what corrections are made for translational and rotational motion and for respiratory changes. Different situations require different corrections.

Regional wall *thickening* analysis has been used by some investigators; this measurement reflects segmental performance independent of a reference axis and is relatively unaffected by rotational or translational cardiac motion.[B1] The presence of normal wall thickening can clarify endocardial motion alterations caused by noncoronary factors (e.g., bundle branch block). Such measurements, however, are still load dependent.

Supported in part by NHLBI grants #HL32295 and HL14388.

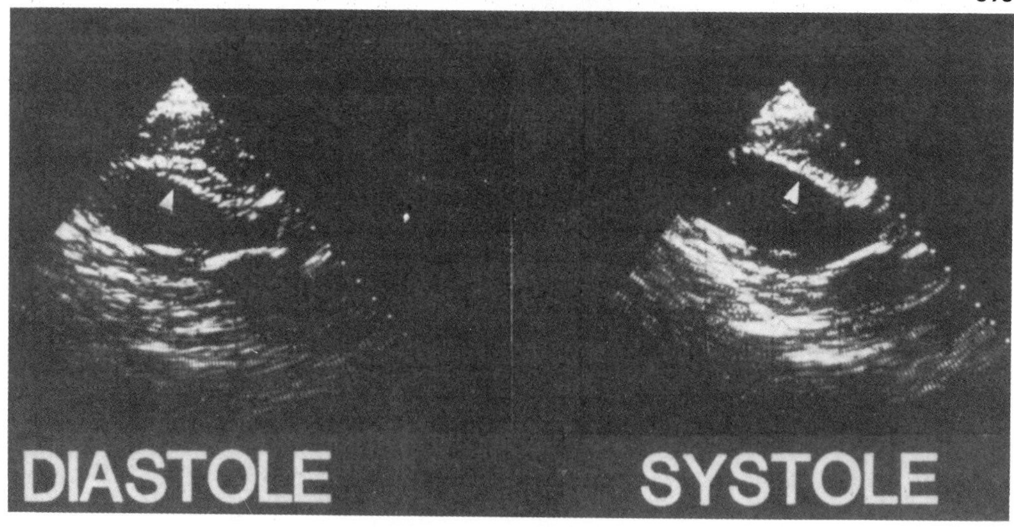

Figure 29–1. Two-dimensional echocardiogram, parasternal long-axis view. This view of a patient with an acute anteroseptal infarction shows systolic thinning and anterior bulging of the interventricular septum *(arrowhead)*. (From Pandian, N. P., et al.: Ischemic heart disease. *In* Talano, J. V., and Gardin, J. M. (eds.): Textbook of Two-Dimensional Echocardiography. Grune & Stratton, New York, 1983, with permission.)

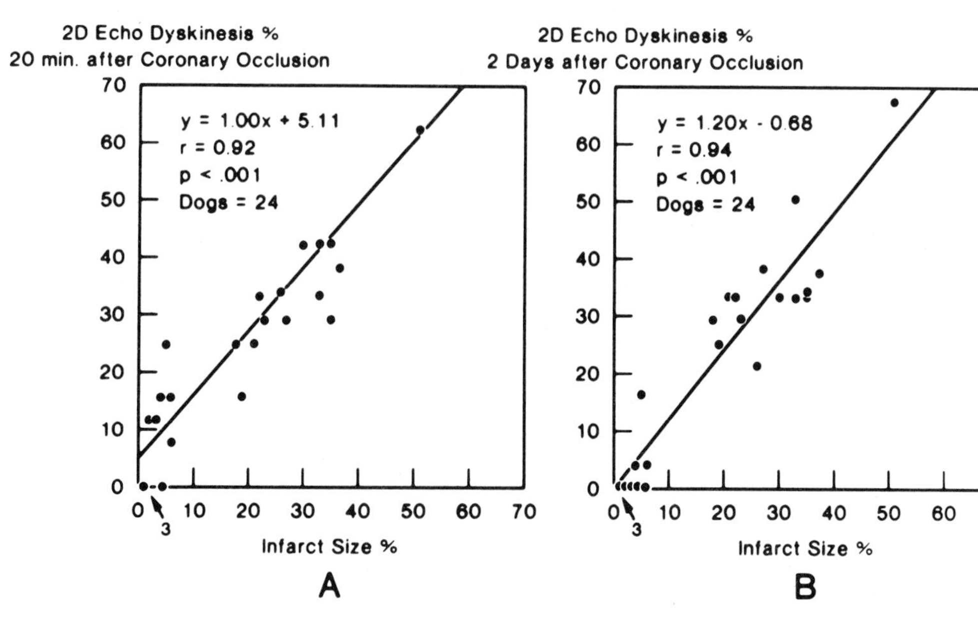

Figure 29–2. Relation between infarct size and the extent of dyskinesia by two-dimensional echocardiography at 20 minutes (*A*) and 2 days (*B*) after coronary occlusion. The percent dyskinesia was highly correlated with infarct size at both 20 minutes and 2 days, but echo-measured dyskinesia overestimated the size of infarction. (From Pandian, N. G., et al.: Relationships between two-dimensional echocardiographic wall thickening abnormalities, infarct size, and coronary risk area in normal and hypertrophied myocardium in dogs. Am. J. Cardiol. 52:1318, 1983, with permission.)

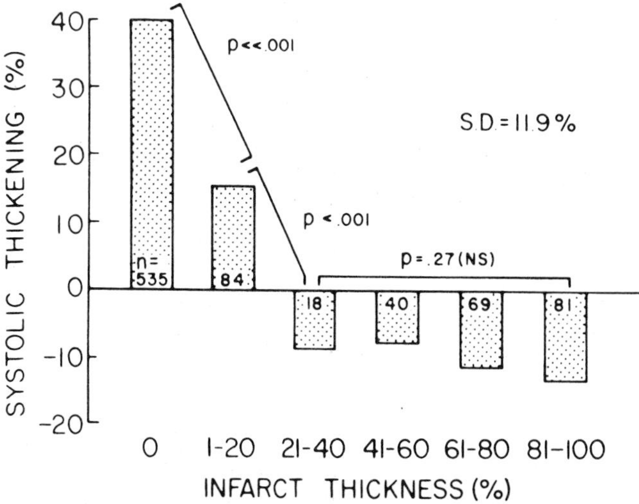

Figure 29–3. Relationship of percent wall thickening and transmural extent of necrosis. Systolic thinning did not appear until the extent of necrosis exceeded 20 percent of the wall thickness. (From Leberman, A. N., et al.: Two-dimensional echocardiography and infarct size: Relationship of regional wall motion and thickening to the extent of myocardial infarct in the dog. Circulation 63:739, 1981, with permission of the American Heart Association, Inc.)

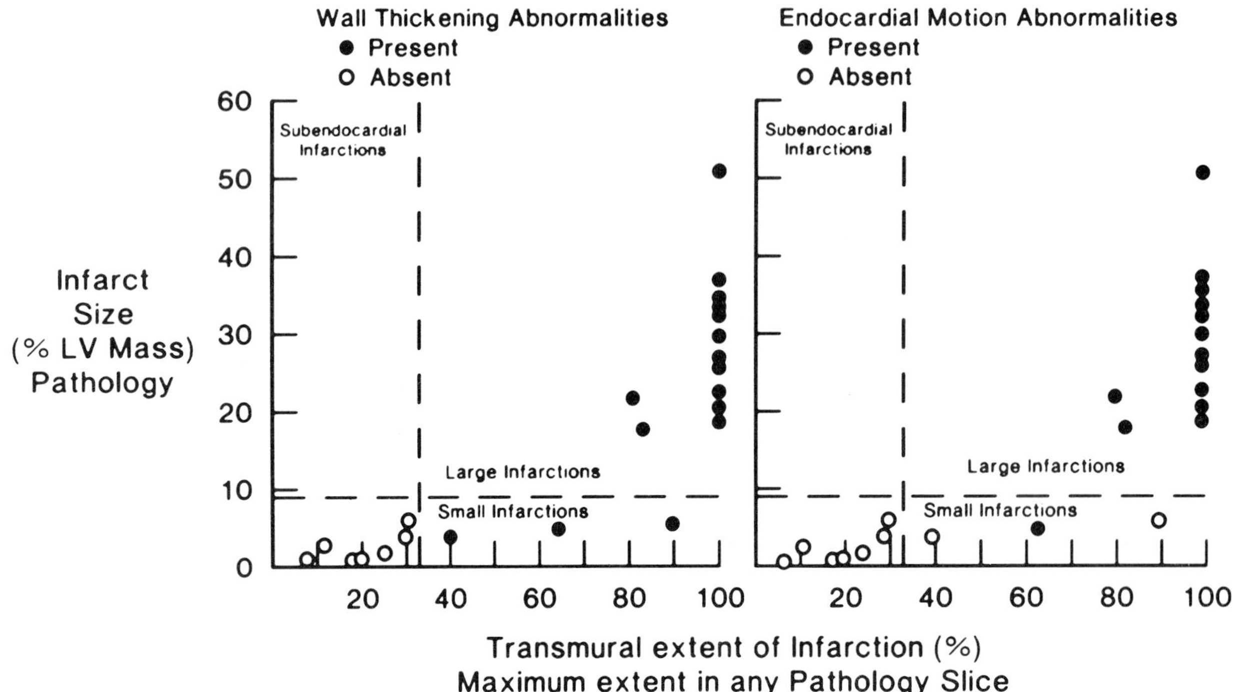

Figure 29–4. Relation between infarct size (% LV mass), maximal transmural extent of infarct, and two-dimensional echocardiographic abnormalities. Wall thickening and endocardial motion remained normal in slices with only small subendocardial infarcts but were invariably abnormal in larger infarcts that extended into the subepicardium. (From Pandian, N. G., et al.: Myocardial infarct size threshold for two-dimensional echocardiographic detection. Sensitivity of systolic wall thickening and endocardial motion abnormalities in small vs. large infarctions. Am. J. Cardiol. 55:551, 1985, with permission.)

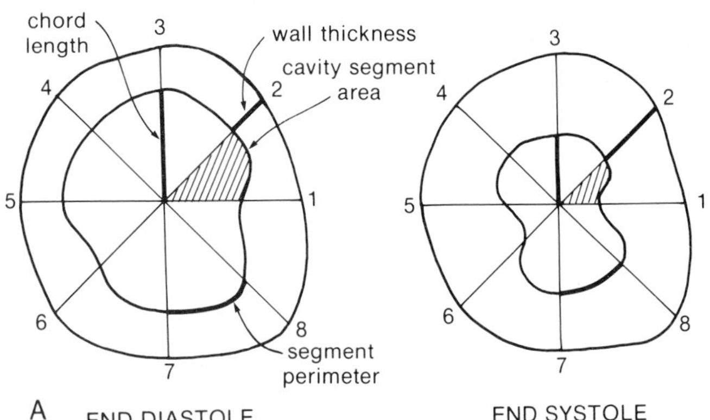

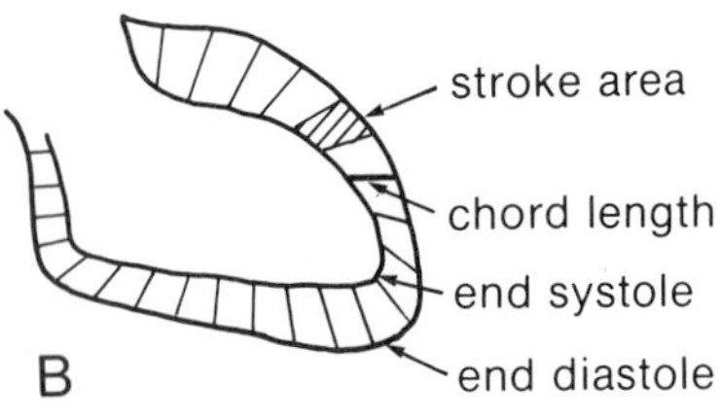

Figure 29–5. Indexes of regional left ventricular performance. *A*, Short-axis representation of LV at end diastole and end systole, showing deviation in chord length, wall thickness, cavity segment area, and segment perimeter. *B*, Right anterior oblique representation of endocardial borders at end diastole and end systole, showing change of chord length and stroke area. (From Collins, S. M., et al.: Quantitative analysis of left ventricular function by imaging methods. *In* Miller, D. D., (ed.): Clinical Cardiac Imaging. McGraw-Hill, New York, 1988, pp. 233–259, with permission.)

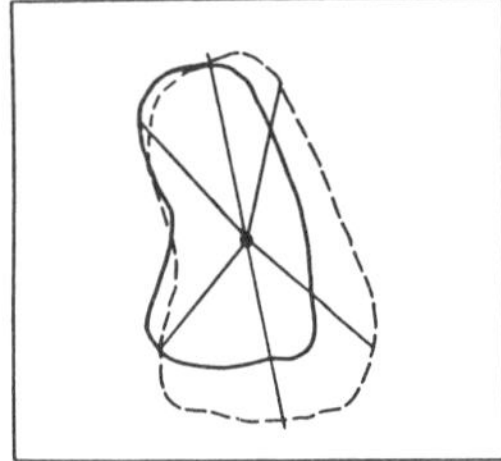

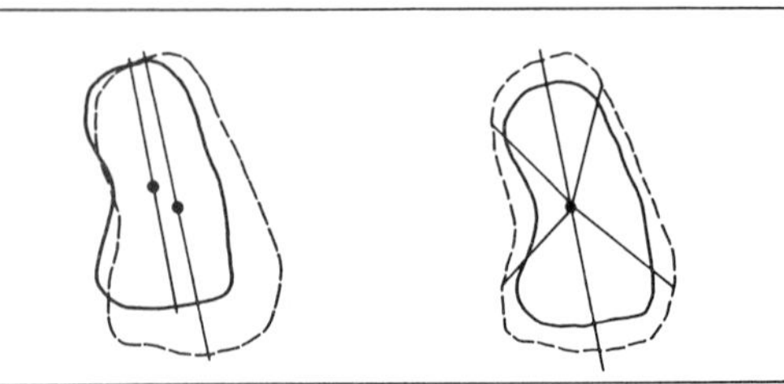

Figure 29–6. Representation of long-axis imaging of the left ventricle, showing the difference between fixed-axis and floating-axis approaches to regional wall motion analysis. In floating axis, end systolic and end diastolic long axes are defined, midpoint is identified, and long axes then superimposed. (From Force, T., et al.: Quantitative two-dimensional echocardiographic analysis of regional wall motion in patients with perioperative myocardial infarction. Circulation 70:233, 1984, with permission of the American Heart Association, Inc.)

The use of end diastolic and end systolic points to quantify regional motion is convenient, but it is an oversimplification; much of the dyskinesis of ischemia/infarction occurs in midsystole and is overlooked by focusing on only two points in the cardiac cycle. This point has been emphasized by Gillam and associates[G1] and Weyman and associates.[W2] Integrating two-dimensional images to develop three-dimensional quantification of infarct size has been explored by Guyer and associates[G2] and Wilkins and associates.[W3] These approaches have yielded good correspondence between echo and autopsy estimates of infarct volume.

Table 29–1 from Borow summarizes the advantages and limitations of various indices of left ventricular contraction.[B1]

The phenomenon of infarct expansion has been emphasized.[H1] This occurs when a transmural infarct dilates and expands so that a greater proportion of the ventricular circumference is occupied by the infarct, even though the mass of the infarct does not increase—as distinct from extension of an existing infarct (i.e., new necrosis). Such infarct expansion may result in aneurysm formation and cardiac rupture. Since the end diastolic shape of the ventricle is altered by the process of infarct expansion, this complicates the use of analytic algorithms that employ echocardiographic dyskinesis to determine infarct size.

An additional complicating factor in the use of contraction abnormalities to quantify infarct size is the phenomenon of myocardial stunning—the postischemic dyskinesis of non-necrotic myocardium. In an experimental reperfusion model, we showed that the good correlation between dyskinesis and infarct size in

Table 29–1. CAUSES OF REGIONAL LEFT VENTRICULAR ENDOCARDIAL WALL MOTION ABNORMALITIES

Intrinsic	Extrinsic
Active myocardial ischemia	Inappropriate reference system rotation, correction, and so on
Prior myocardial infarction with tissue fibrosis	Abnormalities in regional afterload (wall stress)
Intraventricular conduction abnormality due to bundle branch block, premature ventricular contraction, or ventricular pacing	Adjacent nonischemic dyskinesis (tethering)
	RV-LV interaction (e.g., RV volume overload, pericardial restraint)

From Borow, K. M.: Clinical assessment of contractility in the ischemic left ventricle. Mod. Concepts Cardiovasc. Dis. 57:35, 1988, with permission of the American Heart Association, Inc.

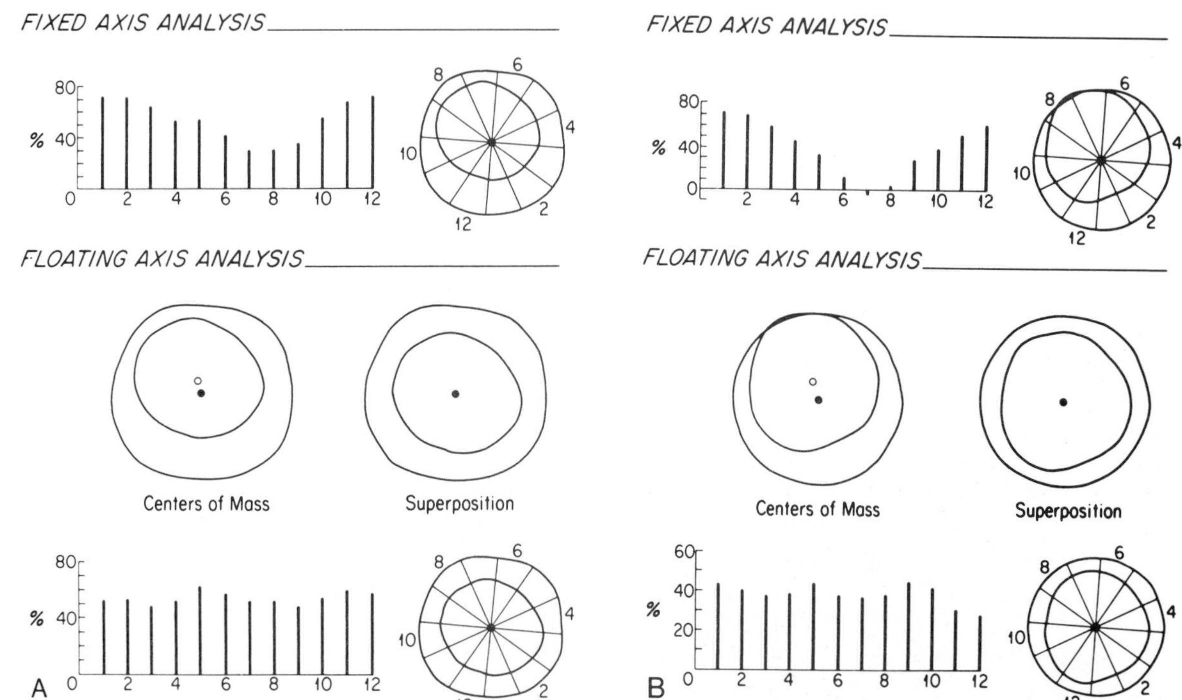

Figure 29–7. *A*, Fixed and floating axis wall motion analyses (area shrinkage) of a normal contracting ventricle, with anterior translation of the ventricle. Fixed axis analysis leads to the conclusion that anterior hypokinesis is present. Floating axis analysis superimposes the diastolic (*closed circle*) and systolic (*open circle*) centroids and normalizes wall motion. *B*, Fixed and floating axis analyses of a ventricle with an anterior wall-motion abnormality and no translation of the ventricle. Fixed axis analysis correctly localizes the abnormality. Because the centroid moves toward the wall motion abnormality in systole, superimposition of the diastolic and systolic centroids falsely normalizes anterior endocardial motion. (From Force, T. L., and Parisi, A. F.: Quantitative methods for analyzing regional systolic function with two-dimensional echocardiography. In Kerber, R. E. (ed.): Echocardiography in Coronary Artery Disease. Futura Publishing Company, Mt. Kisco, N.Y., 1988. pp. 193–219.)

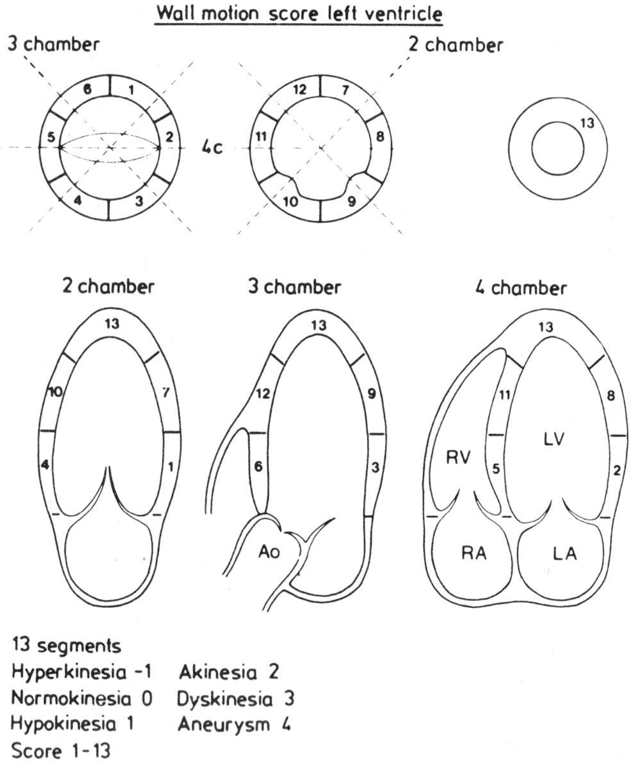

Wall motion score left ventricle

3 chamber 2 chamber 4c

2 chamber 3 chamber 4 chamber

13 segments
Hyperkinesia -1 Akinesia 2
Normokinesia 0 Dyskinesia 3
Hypokinesia 1 Aneurysm 4
Score 1-13

Figure 29–8. Diagram of the three apical long-axis views *(lower panel)* used for calculation of a wall motion score index. In each of the three views, the left ventricle was divided into five segments; the apex was considered to be common to all three apical views. If the apical views were not adequate for analysis, the same segments could be evaluated from short-axis cross-sections *(upper panel)*. Ao—aorta; LA—left atrium; LV—left ventricle; RA—right atrium; RV—right ventricle. (From Kan, G., et al.: Short- and long-term predictive value of admission wall motion score in acute myocardial infarction: A cross-sectional echo study of 345 patients. Br. Heart J. 56:422, 1986, with permission.)

the setting of permanent coronary occlusion was lost once reperfusion was undertaken; the residual dyskinesis substantially overestimated the myocardium subsequently shown to be necrotic.[T1] Presumably, the discordance between postreperfusion dyskinesis and infarct size disappears as the "stunned" myocardium gradually recovers its function, but we found that dyskinesis still overestimated infarct size 10 days after the occlusion-reperfusion sequence.

The phenomenon of stunning complicates the use of echocardiography to monitor the effect of *any* potentially therapeutic intervention, not only reperfusion. Because of this, indices of benefit apart from regional contraction have been explored. These include end diastolic wall thickness and brightness, both of which increase markedly upon reperfusion in canine experiments.[H2] This may be in part due to reperfusion-induced damage, and thus an ideal intervention might restore preocclusion end diastolic wall thickness and regional contraction but *avoid* edema and increased thickness and brightness. The clinical applicability of these experimental observations remains to be determined.

PROGNOSIS AFTER MYOCARDIAL INFARCTION

Prognosis after myocardial infarction is determined by the extent of global dysfunction and residual functioning myocardium.[V1] Several investigators have utilized echocardiographic techniques to derive prognostic information in postinfarct patients. The most common approach has been the development of a wall motion score index. Typically, the ventricle is divided into 9 to 14 segments, each of which is assigned a score based on severity of dysfunction (usually endocardial motion abnormalities). A typical scoring system, developed by Kan and associates, is illustrated in Figure 29–8.[K3] In most systems, the higher the

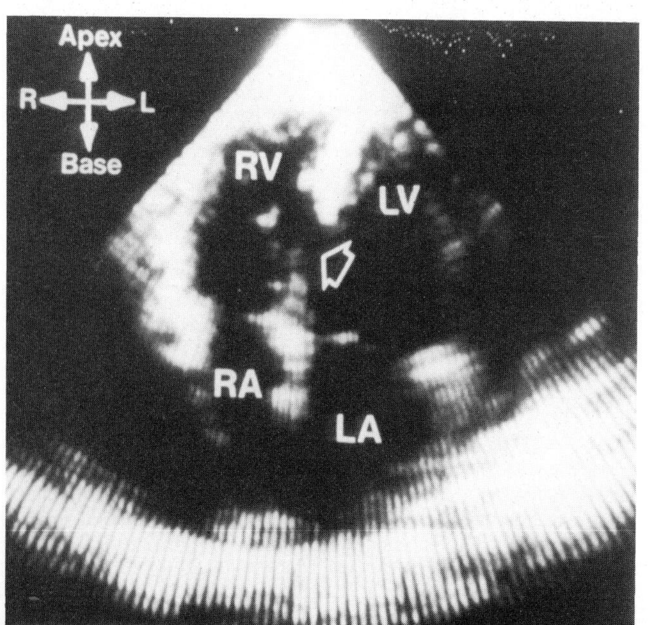

Figure 29–9. Apical four-chamber view in a patient with acute ventricular septal rupture secondary to myocardial infarction. The arrow shows the break in continuity between the junction of the proximal one third and distal two thirds of the septum. The right side of the septum actually was flail and moved in a chaotic manner. LA—left atrium; LV—left ventricle; RA—right atrium; RV—right ventricle. (From Mintz, G. S., et al.: Two-dimensional echocardiographic identification of surgically correctable complications of acute myocardial infarction. Circulation 64:91, 1981, with permission of the American Heart Association, Inc.)

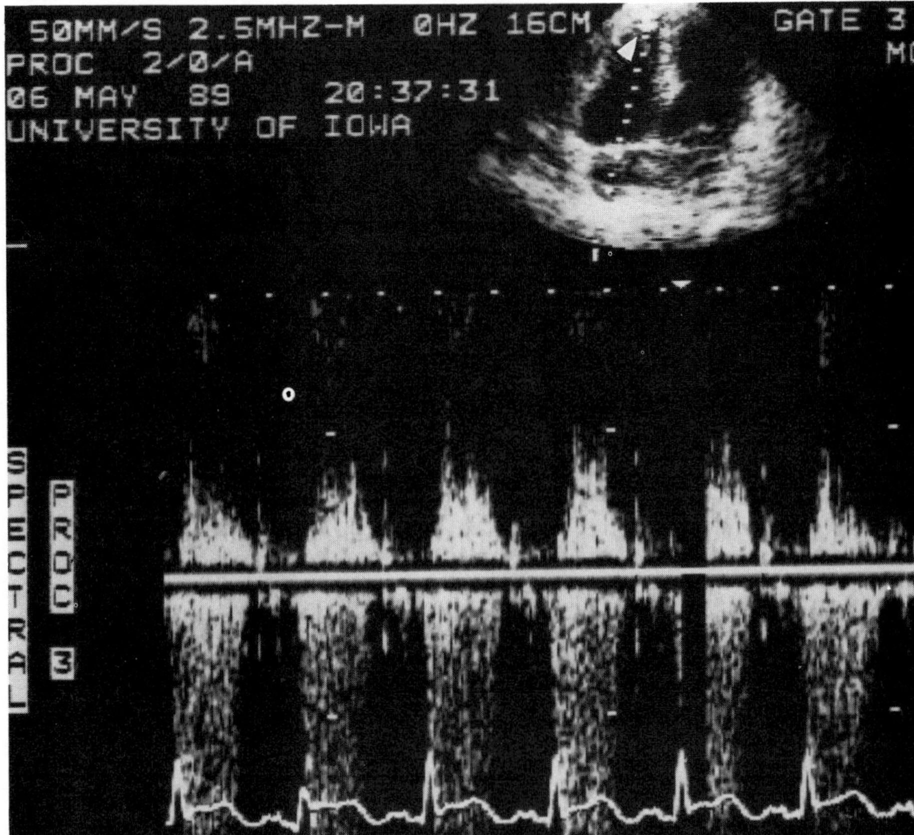

Figure 29–10. An example of a pulsed-wave Doppler recording in a patient with a postinfarction ventricular septal defect. *Upper panel,* The sample gate *(arrow)* is in the right ventricle adjacent to the septum. *Lower panel,* There is an abnormal flow pattern in systole away from the transducer at the sampling point in the right ventricle, indicating left ventricular to right ventricular flow across a septal defect.

numerical score, the more severe or extensive the dysfunction. High scores identify patients at risk for malignant ventricular arrhythmias, pump failure, and death during hospitalization for their acute infarction and during their posthospitalization course. Visser and associates found a 1-year 80 percent mortality in patients who developed a ventricular aneurysm (demonstrated by echocardiography) within 5 days of acute infarction.[V2] A similar outcome was found using radionuclide techniques.[M1]

COMPLICATIONS OF MYOCARDIAL INFARCTION

Echocardiography can be used to detect and demonstrate numerous complications of myocardial infarction. These include ventricular septal defect, papillary muscle rupture with acute mitral regurgitation, infarct expansion (already discussed), ventricular aneurysm, and pseudoaneurysm and left ventricular thrombi.

Ventricular septal rupture typically occurs in a setting of single vessel coronary disease, initial infarction, and absence of septal collateral vessels.[K4] The rupture typically occurs in the center of a septal aneurysm (Fig. 29–9), but the actual defect may not always be visualized. Doppler echocardiography is invaluable in demonstrating the high velocity jet across the defect, either by using single-dimension pulsed-wave Doppler (Fig. 29–10) or by two-dimensional "color Doppler" techniques (Fig. 29–11). The left-to-right shunt volumes and interventricular pressure gradients can be measured and calculated.[B2]

Figure 29–11. See Color Plate 5.

Papillary muscle rupture often presents in a fashion that mimics that of ventricular septal rupture: acute infarction, a new systolic murmur, pulmonary edema, and/or shock. Echocardiography can establish the correct diagnosis, showing an abnormal papillary muscle appearance, often with a mobile mass attached to the mitral leaflet/chordae apparatus (Fig. 29–12). The leaflets may be flail. Doppler and color Doppler techniques show the mitral regurgitation well (Fig. 29–13); if there is rapid equilibration of left ventricular and atrial pressures, the instantaneous Doppler

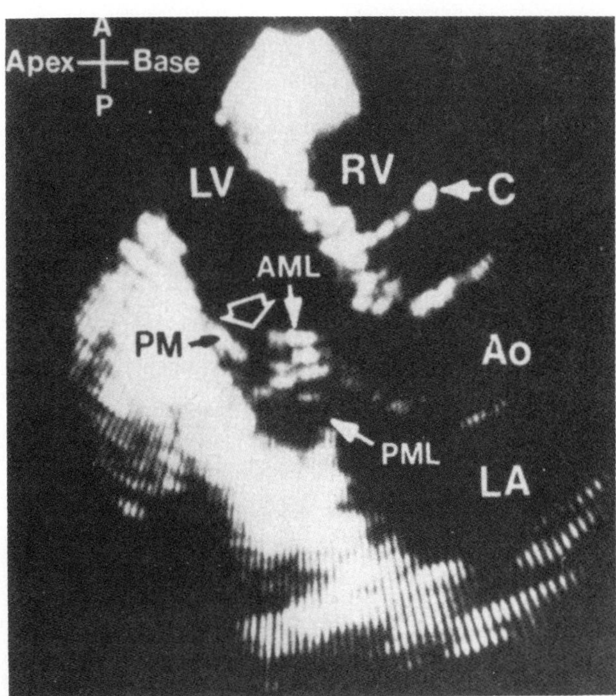

Figure 29–12. Parasternal long axis view. The head of a ruptured papillary muscle (PM) is attached to the anterior mitral leaflet (AML). LV—left ventricle; RV—right ventricle; C—catheter; PML—posterior mitral leaflet; Ao—aorta; LA—left atrium. (From Mintz, G. S., et al.: Two-dimensional echocardiographic identification of surgically correctable complications of acute myocardial infarction. Circulation 64:91, 1981, with permission of the American Heart Association, Inc.)

velocity decreases very rapidly from early to late systole (Fig. 29–14). Papillary muscle *dysfunction* functionally yields mitral regurgitation even when there is no anatomic rupture of the papillary muscle (Fig. 29–13).

Figure 29–13. See Color Plate 5.

Left ventricular aneurysms are generally defined as well-demarcated bulging segments, present in diastole as well as systole but expanding even more in systole (Fig. 29–15). These occur in up to one third of acute infarction patients,[W4] most often at the ventricular apex. Consequently, they are best demonstrated by apical views; often oblique, nonstandard tomographic planes are required. In this respect, echocardiography has an advantage, since multiple planes are available to the operator, as opposed to radiographic techniques that utilize standardized, fixed tomographic slices. Nonstandard planes can be obtained by angiographic or computed tomographic techniques, but often additional angiographic dye injections are required. On the other hand, the number of echocardiographic planes available is often limited by the size and location of the ultrasound "window"—i.e., the transducer placement in the intercostal spaces.

The term *aneurysm* is sometimes applied to an extensively dyskinetic apex that expands in systole but does not show a diagnostic diastolic contour abnormality; functionally, these behave like a true aneurysm.

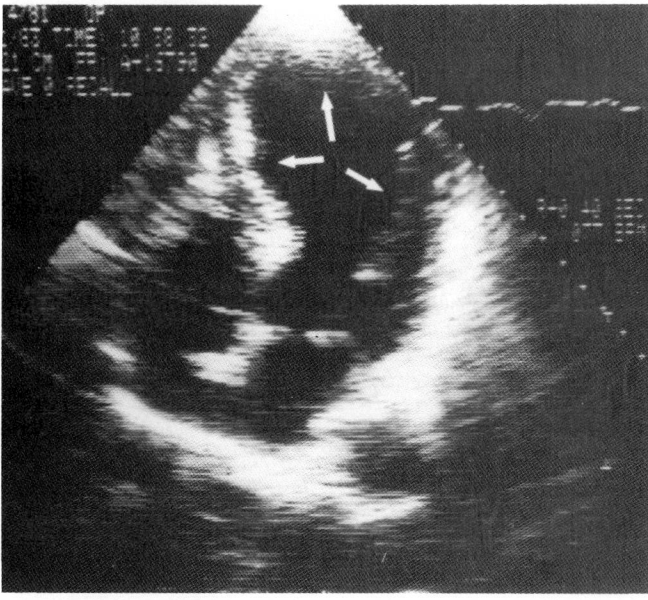

Figure 29–15. Apical four-chamber view. An apical left ventricular aneurysm is demonstrated by the arrows. (From McPherson, D. D., et al.: Two-dimensional echocardiography in coronary artery disease: Present status and new directions. *In* Kotler, M.N., and Steiner, R.M. (eds.): Cardiac Imaging: New Technologies and Clinical Applications. F.A. Davis, Philadelphia, 1986; with permission.)

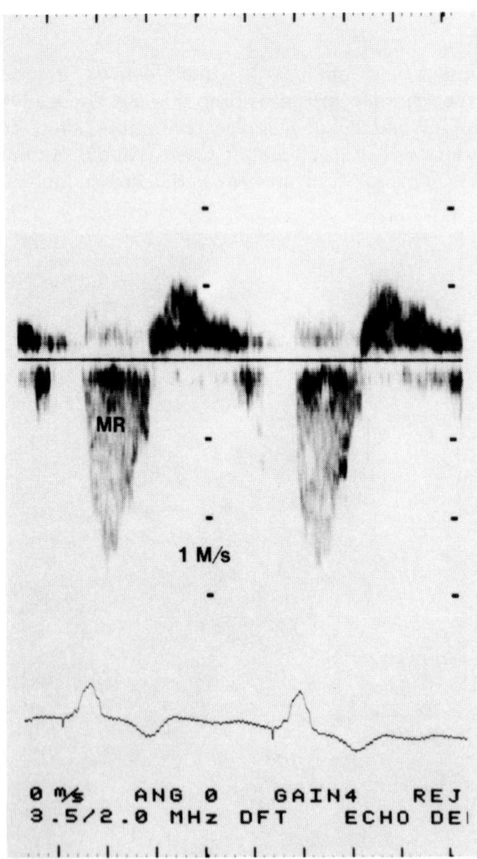

Figure 29–14. Continuous wave Doppler in a patient with acute mitral regurgitation. The maximal velocity peaks early in systole and then decreases abruptly. This occurs presumably on the basis of a large "V" wave with rapid reduction of the pressure difference between the LA and the LV in mid-to-late systole. (From Kotler, M. N., et al.: Acute consequences and chronic complications of acute myocardial infarction. *In* Kerber, R. E. (ed.): Echocardiography in Coronary Artery Disease. Futura Publishing Company, Mt. Kisco, NY, 1988, p. 17, with permission.)

It may be important to distinguish between thin- and thick-walled aneurysms; a recent preliminary CT report suggests that the former are more amenable to surgical resection.[G3] Whether this is correct, and whether echocardiography allows accurate measurement of the wall thickness of apical aneurysms, must be determined by further clinical experience.

Left ventricular pseudoaneurysms occur when an infarcted segment of myocardium ruptures but the hemopericardium is contained by adherent parietal pericardium; thus, in contrast to a true aneurysm, there is no myocardial tissue in the wall surrounding and containing the aneurysm. Most investigators have emphasized that by echocardiography the entrance or "neck" of the pseudoaneurysm is narrow in relation to the size of the pseudoaneurysm itself; this is in contrast to the wide opening into a true aneurysm (Fig. 29–16).

Other unique characteristics of pseudoaneurysms by two-dimensional echocardiography include a sharp discontinuity of the endocardial image at the site of the pseudoaneurysm's communication with the left ventricular chamber, as compared with true aneurysms in which there is not usually such a sharp discontinuity but rather a more gradual dilation at the communicating site. A saccular or globular contour of the pseudoaneurysm is often present, as is thrombotic material in the pseudoaneurysm. Catherwood and associates, using these criteria, found that two-dimensional echocardiography correctly diagnosed four of five pseudoaneurysms originally diagnosed by ventriculography, and 22 true left ventricular aneurysms.[C2] Surgical and pathologic confirmation was obtained in 2 of the 5 pseudoaneurysms and 12 of the 22 true aneurysms. Similar findings have been noted by Weyman and associates[W4] and Gatewood and Nanda.[G4] Pseudoaneurysms are much less common than true aneurysms, and differentiation between an atypically appearing true aneurysm and a pseudoaneurysm may be difficult.

Left ventricular thrombi are a common complication of myocardial infarction. Thrombi typically occur in association with anterior infarction, usually in a dyskinetic left ventricular apex. In such patients, the incidence of thrombi is 30 percent.[V3] Thrombi appear as echo-dense masses adjacent to but distinct from the underlying endocardium. Most investigators require visualization in at least two distinct planes to establish the diagnosis. Since the acoustic characteristics of thrombi and myocardium differ, ultrasonic tissue characterization techniques may

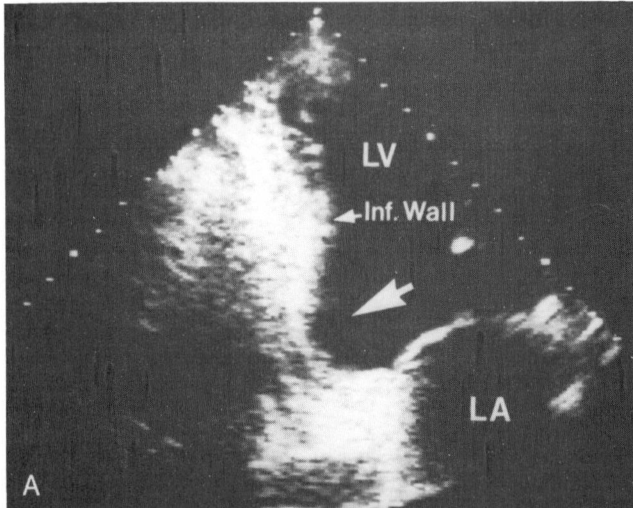

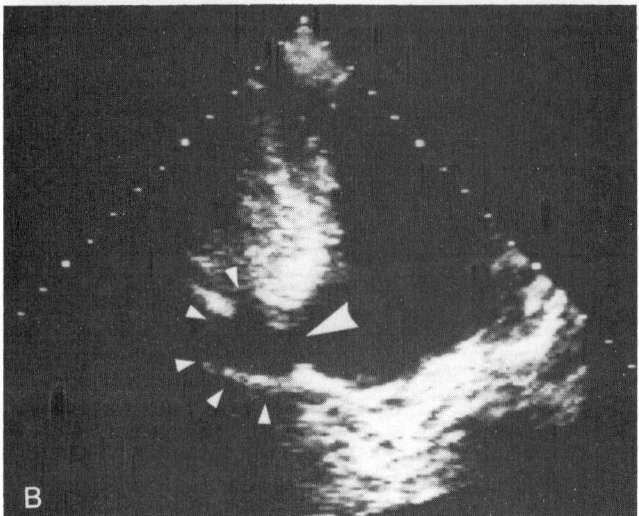

Figure 29–16. *A*, An apical two-chamber view in a patient with a large inferior wall infarction (*large arrow*). *B*, An off-axis view reveals a narrow communicating orifice (*large arrow*). The pseudoaneurysm is outlined by the *smaller arrows*. (From Kotler, M. N., et al.: Acute consequences and chronic complications of acute myocardial infarction. *In* Kerber, R. E. (ed.): Echocardiography in Coronary Artery Disease. Futura Publishing Company, Mt. Kisco, NY, 1988, p. 17, with permission.)

afford another method of diagnosing thrombi.[A1, M2, V4] Echocardiography has been found to be highly sensitive (77 to 95 percent) and specific (86 to 93 percent) in the detection of experimental and clinical left ventricular thrombi.[E1, S1, S2, V3] Thrombi rarely occur in inferior infarctions. They occur in 4 to 5 days following anterior infarction; more rapid development is associated with larger infarcts and higher mortality.[A2, K5, S3]

The appearance of thrombi varies. They may be flat and layered, in part assuming the contour of the underlying infarcted myocardium, or they may protrude into the left ventricular cavity. The centers of established thrombi may liquefy, yielding a sonolucent appearance. Examples of these varying configurations are shown in Figures. 29–17, 29–18, and 29–19. Thrombi may be mobile (especially those that protrude into the ventricular cavity) or immobile. These varying morphologies have prognostic significance with regard to the risk of embolization. Thrombi that protrude into the left ventricular cavity, which are mobile and which have sonolucent centers, have a substantially higher rate of embolization than do flat, layered, immobile thrombi.[E1, H3, S4, V4] For example, Visser and associates reported 119 patients with left ventricular thrombi complicating acute myocardial infarction; 26 of these patients experienced embolic events.[V4] A protruding thrombus was encountered in 23 (88 percent) of the 26 patients with embolism, but only 17 (18 percent) of 93 without emboli. Free mobility of the thrombus was seen in 15 (58 percent)

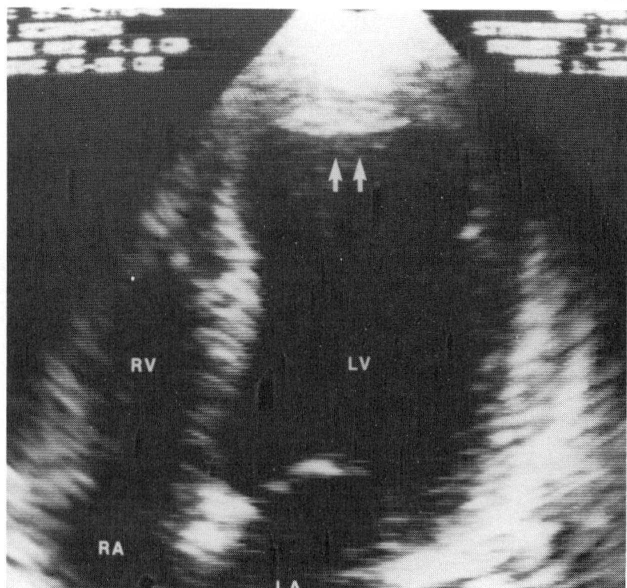

Figure 29–17. Apical four-chamber view illustrating a flat, layered ventricular thrombus located in the apex *(arrows)*. LA—left atrium; LV—left ventricle; RA—right atrium; RV—right ventricle. (From Vandenberg, B. F., et al.: Noninvasive imaging of left ventricular thrombi: Two-dimensional echocardiography and indium–111 platelet scintigraphy. Am. J. Cardiac Imag. 1:289, 1987, with permission.)

of the 26 embolism patients, compared with 3 (3 percent) of 93 nonembolism patients. In all patients with a freely mobile thrombus, the thrombus was also protruding. Similar results have been reported by other investigators.

If thrombi with a high embolic potential are detected, should the patient receive anticoagulant therapy? Prospective but nonrandomized studies have suggested a beneficial effect; anticoagulated patients had a much lower rate of embolic events.[K6, W5] However, Visser and associates found that of 12 patients with embolism complicating thrombus in acute infarction, 7 were already receiving oral anticoagulant therapy.[V4] Large scale prospective randomized studies of anticoagulation in echo-detected

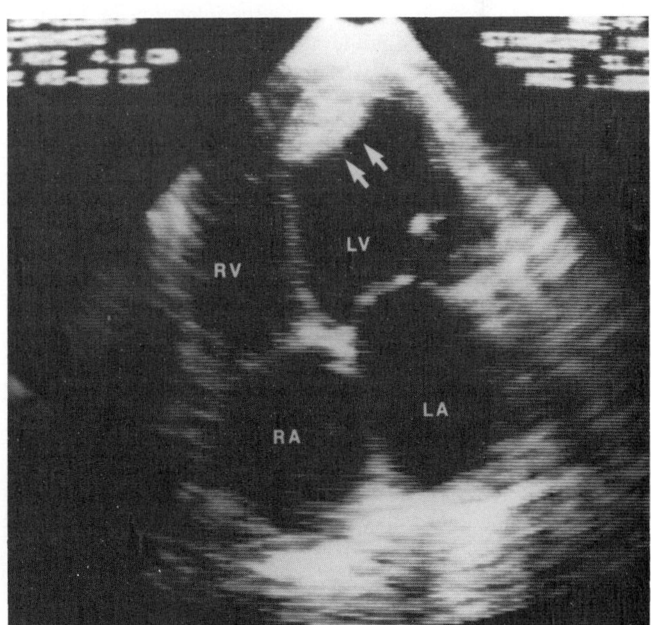

Figure 29–18. Four-chamber apical view illustrating an apical thrombus protruding into the left ventricular cavity *(arrows)*. LV—left ventricle; LA—left atrium; RV—right ventricle; RA—right atrium. (From Vandenberg, B.F., et al.: Noninvasive imaging of left ventricular thrombi: Two-dimensional echocardiography and indium–111 platelet scintigraphy. Am. J. Cardiac Imag. 1:289, 1987, with permission.)

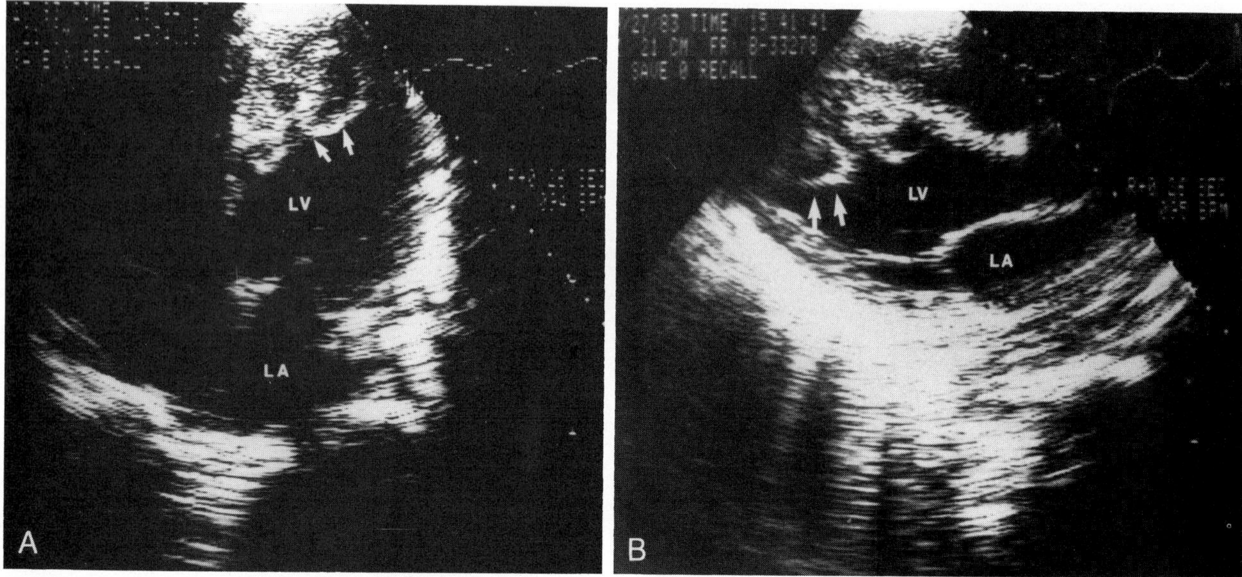

Figure 29–19. An apical left ventricular thrombus with areas of sonolucency *(arrows)*. *A*, Four-chamber apical view. *B*, Parasternal long-axis view. LV—left ventricle; LA—left atrium. (From Vandenberg, B. F., et al.: Noninvasive imaging of left ventricular thrombi: Two-dimensional echocardiography and indium–111 platelet scintigraphy. Am. J. Cardiac Imag. 1:289, 1987, with permission.)

high-risk thrombi are needed; at present, however, there seems enough clinical evidence to recommend systemic anticoagulation (if there are no contraindications) for patients with acute infarction and mobile or protruding or sonolucent left ventricular thrombi. To search for these thrombi, Vandenberg and associates recommend an initial echocardiogram during the first week of admission after acute infarction; if the initial study ,shows no thrombus but apical dyskinesis is noted, the echocardiogram should be repeated prior to discharge.[V5, V6]

Does anticoagulation of acute infarct patients prevent the formation of mural thrombi? Turpie and associates performed a randomized trial of low-dose versus high-dose subcutaneous heparin in 221 patients with acute anterior infarction.[T2] The detection of left ventricular thrombus by echocardiography rather than the occurrence of systemic embolism was used as the primary outcome. Ventricular thrombi were observed by two-dimensional echocardiography on the tenth day after infarction in 10 of 95 patients (11 percent) in the high-dose heparin (12,500 units q 12 hours) group, versus 28 of 88 patients (32 percent) in the low-dose (5000 units q 12 hours) group, $p = 0.0004$. There was no difference in the frequency of hemorrhagic complications. Thus, high-dose subcutaneous heparin appears to be an appropriate therapy for anterior infarction patients.

Does anticoagulation affect *existing* thrombi? Kupper and associates found that in patients with established thrombi, 93 percent showed resolution or change in thrombus size and shape on treatment with oral anticoagulants.[K5]

What is the effect of coronary artery thrombolytic therapy on the incidence of ventricular thrombus formation? Two prospective studies have provided different answers to this question: Eigler and associates showed a reduction in the rate of left ventricular mural thrombus formation after systemic thrombolysis.[E2] More recently, however, Held and associates showed no difference in mural thrombus incidence in patients receiving systemic tissue plasminogen activator versus streptokinase versus no thrombolytic agent.[H4] Patients with anterior infarctions in this series had a thrombus incidence of 33 percent, similar to the rate found in most other studies.

OTHER APPLICATIONS OF ECHOCARDIOGRAPHY IN CORONARY ARTERY DISEASE

ULTRASONIC CONTRAST TECHNIQUES. Microbubbles contained in an injected solution are strong ultrasonic reflectors that can be easily detected using commercially available ultrasonic equipment. Such microbubbles can be easily created by the intravascular injection of hand-agitated saline solutions, indocyanine green dye, sodium diatrizoate, dextrose, sorbitol, gelatin-encapsulated spheres, albumin microspheres, and other agents. Extensive animal experimentation and initial human experience with these agents have shown that intra-aortic and intracoronary injections can be used to demonstrate risk area and infarct size, and it may be possible to determine myocardial perfusion. This technique is discussed in detail in Chapter 27.

EXERCISE ECHOCARDIOGRAPHY. Coronary arterial stenosis may have minimal effects at rest but be profoundly flow-limiting during exercise. Exploiting this, electrocardiographic changes during exercise have long been sought as a marker of ischemic heart disease. Similarly, echocardiographically demonstrated exercise-induced dyskinesis is a marker for myocardial ischemia. This use of echocardiography is examined extensively in Chapter 28.

DIPYRIDAMOLE ECHOCARDIOGRAPHY. Pharmacologic methods to unmask myocardial ischemia in patients without resting wall motion abnormalities have been explored. The Pisa group has extensively evaluated the use of dipyridamole for this purpose.[P3] Dipyridamole causes a reduction in subendocardial blood flow in the presence of coronary stenosis, with ST depression on electrocardiogram, and a fall in left ventricular dp/dt. If the echocardiogram is monitored continuously, new asynergy can be detected.

INTRAOPERATIVE ESOPHAGEAL ECHOCARDIOGRAPHY. Echocardiography can be used to detect myocardial ischemia and infarction during cardiac surgery, via the transesophageal approach. Generally the probe is inserted after the patient is anesthetized and manipulated to an appropriate esophageal position. Short-axis and four-chamber views can be obtained and monitored. Changes in ventricular size and regional contractility can be recognized and appropriate adjustments made to correct hypovolemia and improve coronary perfusion. Transient segmental wall abnormalities have been associated with transient ischemia: persistent abnormalities with infarction. An extensive discussion of this approach is found in Chapter 30.

CORONARY ARTERIAL IMAGING BY ULTRASOUND. The coronary arteries and bypass graft–native vessel anastomoses can be imaged during cardiac surgery using 12 MHz epicardial transducers, placed on the exposed coronary arteries. This is discussed in Chapter 31.

A new application of ultrasound uses very high frequency (20 to 40 MHz) miniaturized probes inserted into arteries and veins, to image from an intraluminal position. Preliminary animal and

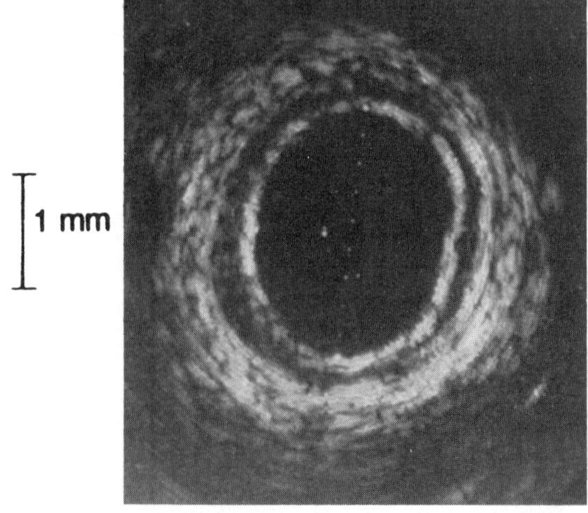

Figure 29–20. Intravascular ultrasonic image of an excised bovine coronary artery, obtained with a 20-MHz transducer. Note the hypoechoic media, typical of a muscular artery. (Courtesy of Dr. Charles McKay.)

human studies have shown excellent demonstration of the normal and diseased arterial wall and atheromatous plaques.[B3]

Measurements of lumen diameter and arterial wall thickness by this technique have been validated by histologic and angiographic techniques.[M5] The composition of the arterial wall alters the appearance of the image; elastic arteries (aorta, pulmonary artery, carotids, iliacs) show an echogenic media, whereas in muscular arteries (coronaries, femorals) the media is hypoechoic (Fig. 29–20).[G5] Potential applications of this approach include assessment of cross-sectional lumen area, the effect of interventions such as angioplasty or atherectomy, and, if combined with Doppler techniques, assessment of the functional severity of anatomic lesions by measurements of flow reserve.[Y1] Possible limitations, including the effect of off-center catheter position within the lumen on the quality and accuracy of the image, remain to be determined.[M6]

ULTRASONIC TISSUE CHARACTERIZATION. As the ultrasonic pulse traverses tissue, the signal is attenuated by absorption and scattering. The degree of attenuation, absorption and backscattering that occurs is specific for the tissue or medium traversed and is determined by physical properties of the tissue itself. Changes in the tissue, such as those induced by ischemia or infarction, may result in characteristic alterations of these properties. The relationship of ultrasound–tissue interaction to tissue structure is known as ultrasound tissue characterization and is discussed in Chapter 26.

CONCLUSION

Echocardiography can be used to detect and characterize myocardial ischemia and infarction. It can be used in settings of acute infarction and chronic coronary disease, with or without angina. Because echocardiography is noninvasive, without side effects, and portable, it is uniquely suitable for use in multiple settings—emergency department, coronary care unit, ward, clinic, and operating room. It is accurate and well validated and in most circumstances should be the initial imaging technique used to evaluate the coronary patient.

References

A

1. Asinger, R. W., Mikell, F. L., Sharma, B., and Hodges, M.: Observations on detecting left ventricular thrombus with two-dimensional echocardiography. Emphasis on avoidance of false-positive diagnoses. Am. J. Cardiol. 47:145, 1981.
2. Asinger, R. W., Mikell, F. L., Elsperger, J., and Hodges, M.: Incidence of left ventricular thrombus after acute transmural myocardial infarction. N. Engl. J. Med. 305:297, 1981.

B

1. Borow, K. M.: Clinical assessment of contractility in the ischemic left ventricle. Mod. Concepts Cardiovasc. Dis. 57:35, 1988.
2. Barron, J. V., Sahn, D. J., Valdes-Cruz, L. M., et al.: Clinical utility of two-dimensional Doppler echocardiographic techniques for estimating pulmonary to systemic blood flow ratios in children with left-to-right shunting, atrial septal defect, ventricular septal defect or patent ductus arteriosus. J. Am. Coll. Cardiol. 3:169, 1984.
3. Bom, N., and Roelandt, J. R. T. C.: Intravascular ultrasound: Techniques, developments, clinical perspectives (Symposium). Int. J. Cardiac Imag. 4:79, 1989.

C

1. Collins, S. M., Kerber, R. E., and Skorton, D. J.: Quantitative analysis of left ventricular function by imaging methods. *In* Miller, D. D. (ed.): Clinical Cardiac Imaging. McGraw-Hill, New York, 1988, pp. 233–259.
2. Catherwood, E., Mintz, G. S., Kotler, M. N., et al.: Two-dimensional echocardiographic recognition of left ventricular pseudoaneurysm. Circulation 62:294, 1980.

E

1. Ezekowitz, M. D., Wilson, D. A., Smith, E. O., et al.: Comparison of Indium-111 platelet scintigraphy and two-dimensional echocardiography in the diagnosis of left ventricular thrombi. New. Engl. J. Med. 306:1509–1513, 1983.
2. Eigler, N., Maurer G., Shah, P. E.: Effect of early systemic thrombolytic therapy on left ventricular mural thrombus formation in acute myocardial infarction. Am. J. Cardiol. 54:261–263, 1984.

F

1. Force, T. L., and Parisi A. F.: Quantitative methods for analyzing regional systolic function with two-dimensional echocardiography, *In* Kerber, R. E. (ed.): Echocardiography in Coronary Artery Disease. Futura Publishing, Mt. Kisco, N.Y., 1988, pp. 193–219.
2. Force, T., Bloomfield P., O'Boyle, J. E., Khuri S. F., Josa, M., Parisi, A. F.: Quantitative two-dimensional echocardiographic analysis of regional wall motion in patients with perioperative myocardial infarction. Circulation 70:233–241, 1984.

G

1. Gillam, L. D., Hogan, R. D., Foale, A., et al.: A comparison of quantitative echocardiographic methods for delineating infarct-induced abnormal wall motion. Circulation 70:113–122, 1984.
2. Guyer, D. E., Foale, R. A., Gillam, L. D., et al.: An echocardiographic technique for quantifying and displaying the extent of regional left ventricular dysynergy. J. Am. Coll. Cardiol. 8:830–835, 1986.
3. Grenadier, E., Weiss, R., Lemmer, H. H., et al.: Surgically resectable left ventricular aneurysm: specific characteristics by ultrafast computerized tomography (Abst). J. Am. Coll. Cardiol. 13:47A, 1989.
4. Gatewood, R. P., and Nanda, N.: Differentiation of left ventricular pseudoaneurysm from true aneurysm with two-dimensional echocardiography. Am. J. Cardiol. 46:869, 1980.
5. Gussenoven, W. J., Essed, C. E., Frietman, P., et al.: Intravascular echocardiographic assessment of vessel wall characteristics: A correlation with histology. Int. J. Cardiac Imag. 4:105, 1989.

H

1. Hutchins, G. M., and Bulkley, B. H.: Infarct expansion versus extension. Two different complications of acute myocardial infarction. Am. J. Cardiol. 41:1127, 1978.
2. Haendchen, R. V., Corday, E., Torres, M., et al.: Increased regional end-diastolic wall thickness early after reperfusion. A sign of irreversibly damaged myocardium. J. Am. Coll. Cardiol. 3:1444, 1984.
3. Haugland, J. M., Asinger, R. W., Mikell, F. L., et al.: Embolic potential of left ventricular thrombi detected by two-dimensional echocardiography. Circulation 70:588, 1981.
4. Held, A. C., Gore, J. M., Parasakos, J., et al.: Impact of thrombolytic therapy on left ventricular mural thrombi in acute myocardial infarction. Am. J. Cardiol. 62:310, 1988.

K

1. Kerber, R. E. (ed.): Echocardiography in Coronary Artery Disease. Futura Publishing Company, Mt. Kisco, N.Y., 1988.
2. Kerber, R. E., and Abboud, F. M.: Echocardiographic detection of regional myocardial infarction. An experimental study. Circulation 47:997, 1973.
3. Kan, G., Visser, C. A., Koolen, J., et al.: Short- and long-term predictive value of admission wall motion score in acute myocardial infarction: A cross-sectional echo study of 345 patients. Br. Heart J. 56:422, 1986.
4. Kotler, M. N., Goldman, A. P., and Parry, W. R.: Acute consequences and chronic complications of acute myocardial infarction. *In* Kerber, R. E. (ed.): Echocardiography in Coronary Artery Disease. Futura Publishing Company, Mt. Kisco, N.Y., 1988, pp. 17–51.
5. Kupper, A. J. F., Verheught, F. W. A., Peels, C. H., et al.: Left ventricular thrombus incidence and behavior studied by serial two-dimensional echocardiography in acute anterior myocardial infarction: Left ventricular wall motion,

systemic embolism and oral anticoagulation. J. Am. Coll. Cardiol. 13:1514, 1989.
6. Keating, E. C., Gross, S. A., Schlamowitz, R. A., et al.: Mural thrombi in myocardial infarction. Am. J. Med. 74:989, 1983.

L

1. Lieberman, A. N., Weiss, J. L., Jugdutt, B. I., et al.: Two-dimensional echocardiography and infarct size: Relationship of regional wall motion and thickening to the extent of myocardial infarct in the dog. Circulation 63:739, 1981.

M

1. Meiztish, J. L., Berger, H. J., Plankey, M., et al.: Functional left ventricular aneurysm formation after acute anterior transmural myocardial infarction. N. Engl. J. Med. 311:1001, 1984.
2. McPherson, D. D., Knosp, B. M., Kieso, R., et al.: Ultrasound characterization of acoustic properties of acute intracardiac thrombi: Studies in a new experimental model. J. Am. Soc. Echocardiog. 1:264, 1988.
3. Mintz, G. S., Victor, M. F., Kotler, M. N., et al.: Two-dimensional echocardiographic identification of surgically correctable complications of acute myocardial infarction. Circulation 64:91, 1981.
4. McPherson, D. D., Taylor, A. L., Collins, S. M., et al.: Two-dimensional echocardiography in coronary artery disease: Present status and new directions. *In* Kotler, M. N., and Steiner, R. M. (eds.): Cardiac Imaging: New Technologies and Clinical Applications. F. A. Davis. Philadelphia, 1986.
5. McKay, C., Waller, B., Gessert, J., et al.: Quantitative analysis of coronary artery morphology using intracoronary high frequency ultrasound: Validation by histology and quantitative coronary angiography. (Abstract.) J. Am. Coll. Cardiol. 13:228A, 1989.
6. McKay, C. R., Griffith, J., Kerber, R. E., Marcus, M. L.: Factors influencing intraluminal ultrasound image quality and arterial wall morphology. Circulation 80:II-581, 1989.

P

1. Pandian, N. G., Koyanagi, S., Skorton, D. J., et al.: Relationships between two-dimensional echocardiographic wall thickening abnormalities, infarct size, and coronary risk area in normal and hypertrophied myocardium in dogs. Am. J. Cardiol. 52:1318, 1983.
2. Pandian, N. G., Skorton, D. J., Collins, S. M., et al.: Myocardial infarct size threshold for two-dimensional echocardiographic detection. Sensitivity of systolic wall thickening and endocardial motion abnormalities in small vs. large infarctions. Am. J. Cardiol. 55:551, 1985.
3. Picano, E., Distante, F., Masini, M., et al.: Dipyridamole-echocardiography test in effort angina pectoris. Am. J. Cardiol. 56:452, 1985.
4. Pandian, N. G., Skorton, D. J., and Kerber, R. E.: Ischemic heart disease. *In* Talano, J. V., and Gardin, J. M. (eds.): Textbook of Two-Dimensional Echocardiography. Grune & Stratton, New York, 1983.

S

1. Stratton, J. R., Lighty, G. W., Pearlman, A. S., and Ritchie, J. L.: Detection of left ventricular thrombus by two-dimensional echocardiography: Sensitivity, specificity, and causes of uncertainty. Circulation 66:156, 1982.
2. Seabold, J. E., Schroder, E., Conrad, G. R., et al.: Indium–111 platelet scintigraphy and two-dimensional echocardiography for detection of left ventricular thrombus: Influence of clot size and age. J. Am. Coll. Cardiol. 9:1057, 1987.
3. Spirito, P., Bellotti, P., Chiarella, F., et al.: Prognostic significance and natural history of left ventricular thrombi in patients with acute anterior myocardial infarction—a two-dimensional echocardiographic study. Circulation 72:774, 1985.
4. Stratton, J. R., and Resnich, A. D.: Increased embolic risk in patients with left ventricular thrombi. Circulation 75:1004, 1987.

T

1. Taylor, A. L., Kieso, R., Melton, J., et al.: Echocardiographically detected dyskinesis, myocardial infarct size, and coronary risk region relationships in reperfused canine myocardium. Circulation 71:1292, 1985.
2. Turpie, A. G. G., Robinson, J. G., Doyle, D. J., et al.: Comparison of high-dose with low-dose subcutaneous heparin to prevent left ventricular mural thrombosis in patients with acute transmural anterior myocardial infarction. N. Engl. J. Med. 320:352, 1989.

V

1. Vandenberg, B. F., and Kerber, R. E.: Regional wall-motion abnormalities and coronary artery disease: Prognostic implications. *In* Kerber, R. E. (ed.): Echocardiography in Coronary Artery Disease. Futura Publishing Company, Mt. Kisco, N.Y., 1983.
2. Visser, C. A., Kan, G., Meltzer, R. S., et al.: Incidence, timing and prognostic value of left ventricular aneurysm formation after myocardial infarction: A prospective, serial echocardiographic study of 158 patients. Am. J. Cardiol. 57:729, 1986.
3. Visser, C. A., Kan, G., David, G. K., et al.: Two-dimensional echocardiography in the diagnosis of left ventricular thrombus: A prospective study of 67 patients with anatomic validation. Chest 83:228, 1983.
4. Visser, C. A., Kan, G., Meltzer, R. S., et al.: Embolic potential of left ventricular thrombus after myocardial infarction: A two-dimensional echocardiographic study of 119 patients. J. Am. Coll. Cardiol. 5:1276, 1985.
5. Vandenberg, B. F., Seabold, J. E., Schroder, E., and Kerber, R. E.: Noninvasive imaging of left ventricular thrombi: Two-dimensional echocardiography and indium–111 platelet scintigraphy. Am. J. Cardiac. Imag. 1:289, 1987.
6. Vandenberg, B. F., and Kerber, R. E.: Left ventricular thrombi in acute and chronic coronary artery disease: The role of two-dimensional echocardiography. *In* Kerber, R. E. (ed.): Echocardiography in Coronary Artery Disease. Futura Publishing Company, Mt. Kisco, N.Y., 1988.

W

1. Weiss, J. L., Buckley, B. H., Hutchins, G. M., and Mason, S. J.: Two-dimensional echocardiographic recognition of myocardial injury in man. Comparison with post-mortem studies. Circulation 63:401, 1981.
2. Weyman, A. E., Franklin, T. D., Jr., Hogan, R. D., et al.: Importance of temporal heterogeneity in assessing the contraction abnormalities associated with acute myocardial ischemia. Circulation 70:102, 1984.
3. Wilkins, G. T., Southern, J. F., Choong, C. Y., et al.: Correlation between echocardiographic endocardial surface mapping of abnormal wall motion and pathologic infarct size in autopsied hearts. Circulation 77:978, 1988.
4. Weyman, A. E., Peskoe, S. N., Williams, E. S., et al.: Detection of left ventricular aneurysms by cross-sectional echocardiography. Circulation 54:936, 1976.
5. Weinrich, D. J., Burke, J. F., and Ferrel, J. P.: Left ventricular mural thrombi complicating acute myocardial infarction. Ann. Intern. Med. 100:789, 1984.

Y

1. Yock, P. G., Linker, D. T., White, N. W., et al.: Clinical applications of intravascular ultrasound imaging in atherectomy. Int. J. Cardiac Imag. 4:117, 1989.

Chapter 30

Transesophageal Echocardiography in Clinical Cardiology

▪ EDMOND LEE, M.D. ▪ NELSON B. SCHILLER, M.D.

Historical Development 605
Current Transesophageal Echocardiographic Probe Technology 606
Performance 606
Anatomic Imaging Views 607
Indications for Ambulatory Transesophageal Echocardiography 609
Transesophageal Echocardiography Training 612
Safety 613
Future Developments 614
Conclusion 616

Transesophageal echocardiography (TEE) is a new and rapidly expanding technique that allows ultrasonic imaging of the cardiac structures and great vessels via the esophagus.[G1, M1, S1–S3] Although advances in two-dimensional echocardiography, pulsed and continuous wave Doppler, and color flow imaging have revolutionized noninvasive assessment of cardiac disorders,[F1, H1, M2] in many patients these modalities may be limited by several factors: acoustic attenuation from structures in the thorax (lungs, subcutaneous tissues, and ribs) and heart (prosthetic valve construction materials and calcification of native valves). It is common for prosthetic strut and sewing ring artifacts to shadow and compromise almost completely the interrogation of most cardiac structures lying beyond the ultrasound beam.[C1, S4] Image resolution may be further limited by the use of low-frequency transducers necessary to achieve far-field penetration in adults. In addition, in evaluating thoracic aortic diseases, the ascending and descending aorta is difficult to visualize from the precordium. Transesophageal echocardiography represents an ideal method of circumventing many of these limitations. Commercially available probes, capable of two-dimensional imaging, real time Doppler color flow imaging, and pulsed Doppler interrogation have been incorporated into small (9 mm), flexible, gastroscope-like devices that allow easy and safe esophageal introduction into both awake and anesthetized patients. From this retrothoracic vantage point, in close juxtaposition to the heart, high-resolution images of the ventricles, atria, valvular structures, and thoracic aorta can be obtained that are otherwise unobtainable from precordial imaging. This review will focus on this new technique of performing transesophageal echo, its historical development, current clinically useful indications for ambulatory transesophageal echocardiography, and potential future developments.

Historical Development
(Table 30–1)

In 1975, Frazin and co-workers developed the first transesophageal echocardiographic imaging probes, consisting of a 3.5-mHz, 9-mm, lozenge-shaped M-mode crystal attached to a 3-mm coaxial cable.[F2] Although their probe design enabled acquisition of M-mode images only at the aortic root and mitral valve level and failed to image the left ventricle consistently, these investigators demonstrated the incremental utility of this technique in patients with chronic obstructive lung disease and are to be credited with the conceptual leap of having recognized the esophagus as a new acoustic window to the heart.

In 1977, Hisanaga and associates developed the first transesophageal echocardiographic probes capable of real-time two-dimensional imaging.[H2–H4] Their probe consisted of a high-speed rotating mechanical scan head immersed in an oil-filled bag. Although high-quality 180- to 260-degree sector images could be obtained, this probe was not adopted because of its rigid shaft design, the need for injection-inflation of the oil bag offset to obtain optimal mucosal contact, and patient discomfort from vibration of the scan head.

In 1980 and 1981, Hanrath and colleagues[H5] and Souquet and associates[S5] developed the first two-dimensional transesophageal probes by incorporating a 32-element phased-array imaging crystal into the tip of a modified adult gastroscope-like device. The improved flexibility of this device enabled reliable acquisition of a number of standard imaging views.[S6] Hanrath, at Eppendorf School of Medicine (Hamburg, FRG), and our colleagues at the University of California, San Francisco, performed the seminal research that demonstrated that these probes could serve as a means for the continuous on-line intraoperative monitoring of left ventricular function and ischemia.[B1, K1, R1, S7, S8] In 1982, Hanrath and colleagues extended this work by demonstrating that transesophageal echocardiography could be performed in ambulatory outpatients in a manner similar to that of upper gastric endoscopy.[S9] Despite a modest popularity of this technique in Europe and Japan during the early 1980s, explosive proliferation of this technique in the United States did not occur until the development of smaller and higher-resolution (64-element, 5-mHz)

Table 30–1. HISTORICAL DEVELOPMENT OF TRANSESOPHAGEAL ECHOCARDIOGRAPHY

Year	Development
1975	M-mode TEE (Frazin et al.)
1977	2-D mechanical sector TEE probe (Hisanaga et al.)
1980	2-D phased-array TEE probe (Hanrath and Souguet)
1982	Pulsed Doppler TEE (Schlüter et al.)
1986	Color flow imaging TEE (de Bruijn et al.)
1989	Biplane TEE (Omoto and Kyo)
1989	Pediatric TEE probes (Omoto and Kyo)

TEE—Transesophageal echocardiography.

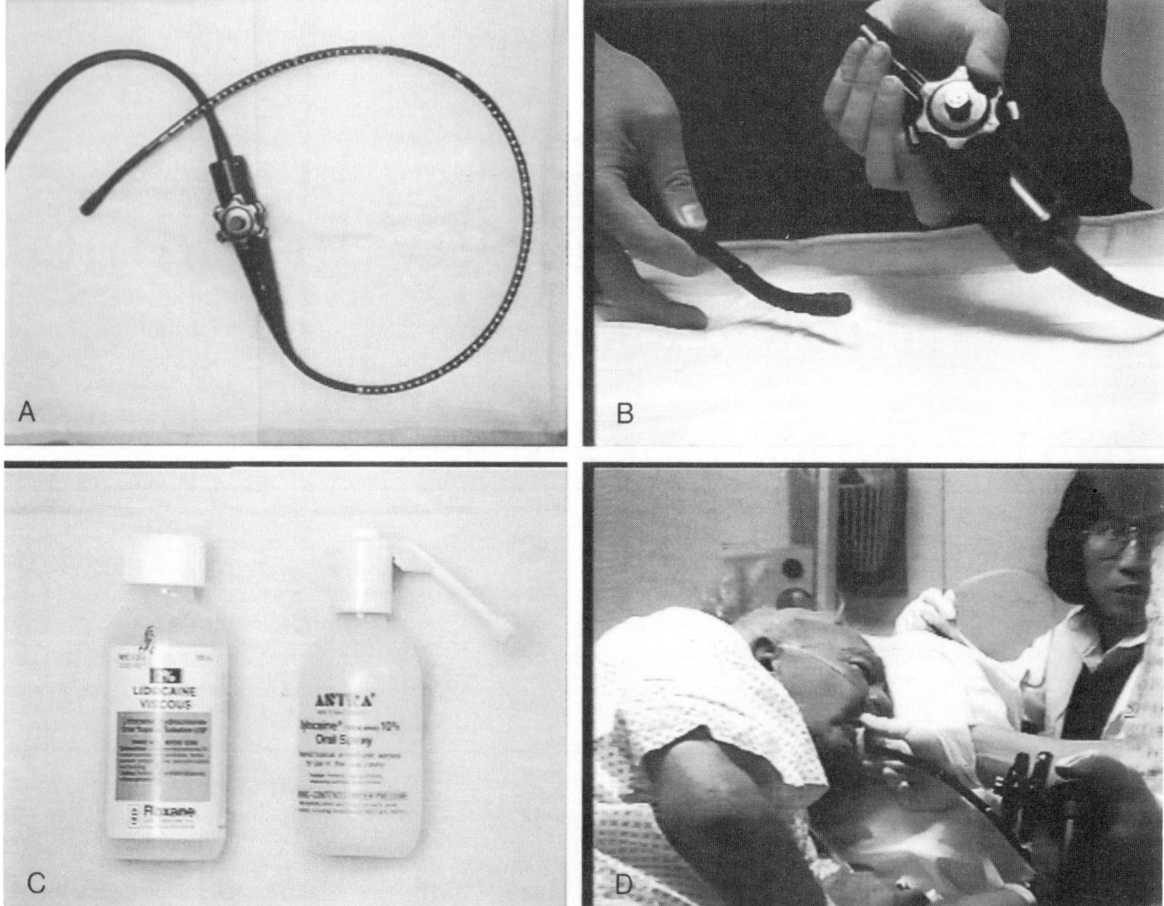

Figure 30–1. Technique of performing transesophageal echocardiography (TEE). *A*, A commercially available 64-element phased-array TEE probe/gastroscope-like device. *B*, Basal control knobs allow anterior/posterior and right/left tip flexion. *C*, Viscous lidocaine (2 percent diluted 5:1) and 10 percent lidocaine spray are used for topical anesthesia. *D*, Probe is introduced with the patient in the left lateral decubitus position.

probes that incorporated pulsed Doppler[S10] and color flow imaging modalities.[D1, O1] Now over 500 major institutions worldwide are performing transesophageal echocardiography as a routine clinical procedure. A plethora of forthcoming data and publications and a large backlog of orders for probes demonstrate how enthusiasm for this technique has proliferated.

Current Transesophageal Echocardiographic Probe Technology

Most commercially available transesophageal echocardiographic probes utilize 3.5- to 5.6-mHz, 32- to 64-element phased-array imaging crystals incorporated into moderate-sized (9-mm shaft; 100-cm length) adult gastroscope-like devices (Fig. 30–1) interfaced with echocardiographic machines to provide two-dimensional sector, M-mode, pulsed Doppler and color flow imaging. Basal control knobs enable anterior and posterior (90 to 120 degrees) as well as right and left lateral (60 to 120 degrees) tip flexion (Fig. 30–1). These maneuvers, along with manipulating the probe by gentle advancement and withdrawal and rotating it axially along its shaft, enable image optimization.

Most probes incorporate thermistors to monitor probe temperatures and automatically shut down when temperatures exceed 42° C to safeguard against esophageal mucosal thermal injury that may occur from malfunctioning ultrasound crystals converting electrical energy into heat. This feature may be important in intraoperative patients in whom prolonged probe use may result in overheating, but the need for this safety precaution is unproved in the outpatient setting. In fact, in febrile patients automatic shutdown may prove a problem, preventing completion of the examination. Other safety features in some probes have included suction and fiberoptic ports, which enable direct visualization during probe insertion and manipulation. The necessity of such modifications is also unproved, and they require larger and stiffer probe shaft designs; it is likely that such modifications soon will be abandoned.

Performance

In the outpatient laboratory, transesophageal echocardiographic probes can be introduced in awake cooperative patients in a manner similar to performing gastric endoscopy (Table 30–2). It is the procedure in our laboratory to obtain informed consent in all patients. Fasting is required for at least 4 to 6 hours to minimize the risk of aspiration. Local anesthesia (Fig. 30–1) of the hypopharynx is achieved by having the patient gargle and swallow 50 ml of 0.4 percent viscous lidocaine (2 percent lidocaine diluted 5:1 with water) in divided aliquots. The throat

Table 30–2. TRANSESOPHAGEAL ECHOCARDIOGRAPHY PROCEDURE

Standard Procedure
Informed consent
Fasting for 4–6 hours
Topical anesthesia (lidocaine)
BP, HR, ECG monitoring
Procedure performed in left lateral decubitus position
Other Options
Intravenous sedation (midazolam)
Anticholinergic drying agents (glycopyrrolate)
Antibiotic prophylaxis (prosthetic valves)
Nasal oxygen
Transcutaneous pulse oximetry monitoring
Patient guidance of probe insertion (difficult esophageal intubation)

BP—blood pressure; HR—heart rate; ECG—electrocardiographic.

is then sprayed with aerosolized 10 percent lidocaine, and, when adequate gag suppression is achieved, the patient is turned into the left lateral decubitus position and the probe introduced by a combination of gentle operator advancement and patient swallowing (Fig. 30–1). Suctioning of oral secretions is performed as needed, and the patient's vital signs, such as cardiac rhythm and blood pressure, are monitored by blood pressure cuff and a single-lead ECG displayed on the echocardiographic monitor. Most ambulatory studies can be completed in 15 minutes, with a success rate of performing the procedure in over 97 percent of patients with high patient tolerance.

In many laboratories, sedation with intravenous midazolam or diazepam is useful in anxious and young patients and may be associated with greater patient acceptance of the procedure due to a postsedative amnestic effect. The routine use of intravenous sedation must be performed with caution, for although judicious use of intravenous sedation is generally safe, adverse morbidity and mortality, including respiratory arrest and death from anoxic brain injury, have been reported with use of short-acting diazepam-like agents.[R2] Despite these admonishments, one clinical situation in which sedation is routinely recommended is in patients undergoing evaluation for aortic dissection. Here, use of intravenous sedation is particularly useful in allaying anxiety and blunting modest but possibly detrimental rises in heart rate and blood pressure during probe introduction.[G2]

There are a variety of other variations in the technique of performing transesophageal echocardiography in the outpatient setting. If optimal esophageal mucosal and probe contact and images cannot be easily obtained, it is often useful to turn patients into supine (after adequate suctioning of oral secretions), right decubitus, or even sitting upright positions to better optimize images. If repeated difficulty is encountered in passing the esophageal probe past the upper esophageal junction, a useful maneuver in nonsedated patients is to have patients actually guide the probe insertion themselves. Some laboratories routinely use intravenous anticholinergic drying agents, such as glycopyrrolate (2 mg) to decrease salivary secretions.[S1] If routinely employed, these agents should be used with caution in elderly patients with glaucoma or urinary retention. Antibiotic prophylaxis for endocarditis should also be given routinely to patients with prosthetic valves and other high risk lesions such as mitral regurgitation and complex congenital heart diseases. It is our practice to administer antibiotic prophylaxis in accordance with the guidelines of the American Heart Association[S11] and the current practice of the gastroendoscopists at our institution. Patients with prosthetic valves who are being evaluated for endocarditis are not given antibiotics, to avoid interference with analysis of blood culture data.

Anatomic Imaging Views

Standard transesophageal echocardiographic views (Fig 30–2) that can be obtained include (1) short-axis images of the aortic valve, (2) a long-axis equivalent view that includes the left atrium, mitral valve, and left ventricle, (3) a four-chamber equivalent view that provides excellent visualization of the left and right atria, interatrial septum, mitral and tricuspid valves, and the left and right ventricles, and (4) left ventricular short-axis images at the mitral valve, midpapillary muscle, and apex levels.[S6] Additional structures that can be imaged in over 90 percent of patients include (1) the left atrial appendage, (2) the superior vena cava, (3) the right and left upper pulmonary veins, (4) the coronary sinus, (5) the ascending, transverse, and descending thoracic aorta, and (6) the proximal coronary vasculature.[S6]

After the esophageal probe is introduced past the upper oral pharyngeal–esophageal junction, images can be obtained first at a level 30 cm from the teeth (measured by centimeter markings on the probe). Here, the probe is situated behind the left atrium, and highly resolved short-axis images of the aortic valve (Fig. 30–2) can be obtained. By advancing the probe 1 to 2 cm, images

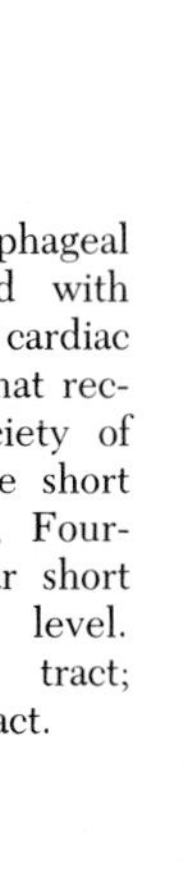

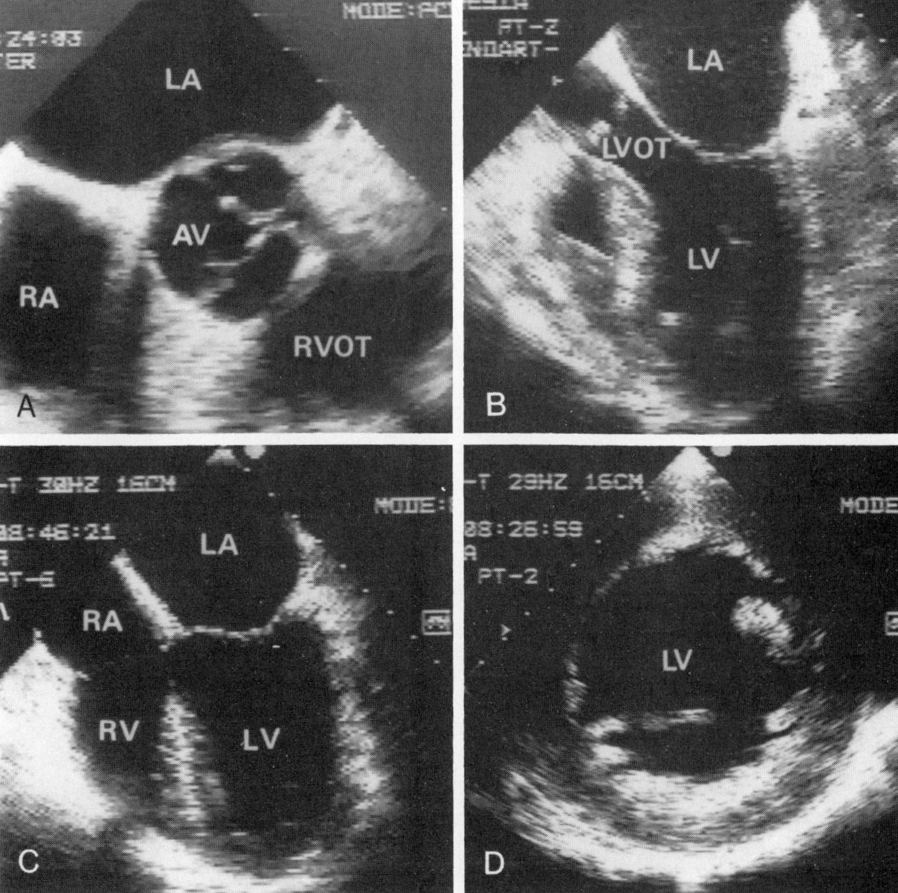

Figure 30–2. Standard transesophageal echocardiographic views displayed with atria in the near field and left-sided cardiac structures to the right (display format recommended by the American Society of Echocardiography). *A*, Aortic valve short axis. *B*, Long axis equivalent. *C*, Four-chamber view. *D*, Left ventricular short axis at the midpapillary muscle level. LVOT—left ventricular outflow tract; RVOT—right ventricular outflow tract.

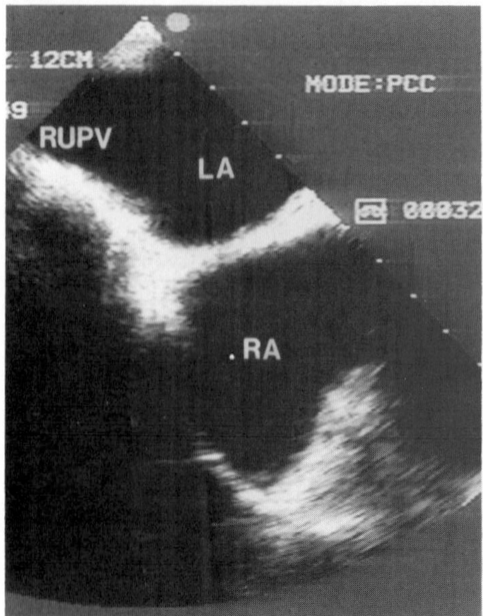

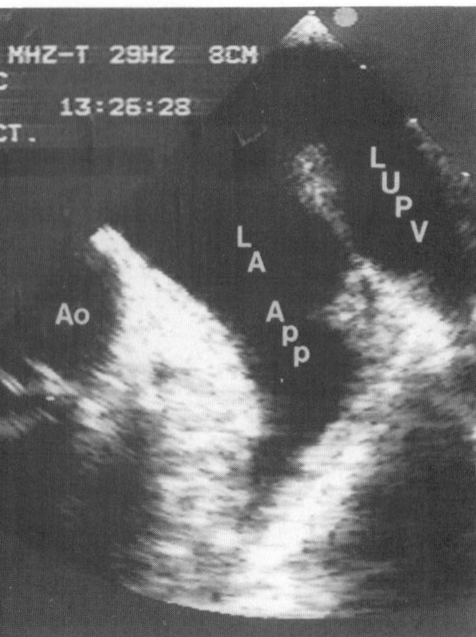

Figure 30–3. Transesophageal echocardiographic views showing right (RUPV) and left (LUPV) upper pulmonary veins and left atrial appendage (LA app). Ao—aortic root; RA—right atrium.

of the left ventricular outflow tract can be obtained in a long-axis view (Fig. 30–2) that includes the left atrium, mitral valve, and left ventricle. With further probe advancement of 1 to 2 cm and retroflexion of the tip, a four-chamber equivalent view (Fig. 30–2) can be obtained. By advancing the probe into the lower esophagus and past the gastroesophageal junction, anteroflexion of the probe tip allows imaging through the gastric fundus and diaphragm (transgastric echocardiography), producing a family of tomographic left ventricular short-axis planes at the level of the mitral valve, midpapillary muscle level (Fig. 30–2), and apex. These views are particularly useful for intraoperative monitoring of the left ventricular function.

Imaging of the thoracic aorta is best begun at the short-axis level of the aortic valve with the probe turned anteriorly. Slow withdrawal of the probe enables visualization of 5 to 10 cm of the ascending aorta in short axis until the level of the bronchus intermedius is reached, where further visualization is often obscured by an air-cartilage interface. By returning to the level of the aortic valve and rotating the probe counterclockwise 90 to 150 degrees posteriorly, the midthoracic descending aorta is imaged. With gentle advancement and withdrawal of the probe in the esophagus, serial short-axis images of the entire thoracic aorta can be recorded. The major part of the transverse aorta can be imaged in long axis in continuity with the ascending aorta. However, in awake patients, obtaining images at the transverse aortic level is sometimes frustrated by probe tip stimulation of cough and gag reflexes. Thus this portion of the procedure is best performed just prior to the completion of the study, at the time of probe withdrawal.

The left atrial appendage can be best seen starting at the level of the aortic valve in short axis. Counterclockwise probe rotation will give excellent visualization of the typical "dog ear" or triangular appearance of the atrial appendage (Fig. 30–3). Continuation of counterclockwise rotation exposes the adjacent left upper pulmonary vein (Fig. 30–3). The right upper pulmonary vein can be visualized by starting at the aortic valve level and rotating clockwise (Fig. 30–3). The right and left lower pulmonary veins are more difficult to visualize consistently. The proximal trunks of the left and right coronary arterial systems are best seen at slightly different tomographic planes just above the level of the aortic valve (Fig. 30–4); the superior vena cava can also be seen at this level (Fig. 30–4). The inferior vena cava and coronary sinus can be best seen at the level of the lower esophagus just prior to crossing the gastroesophageal junction (Fig. 30–5).

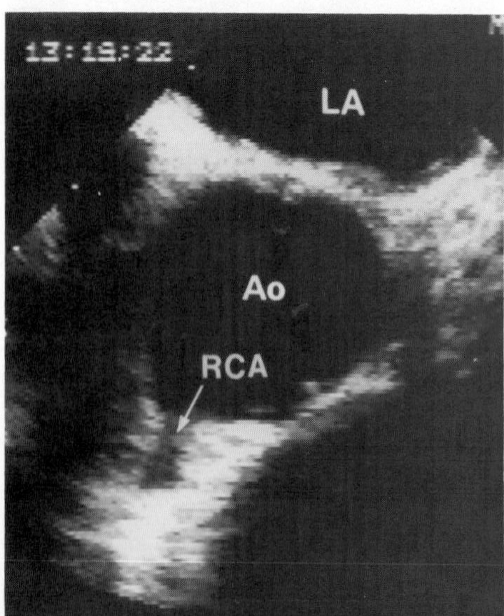

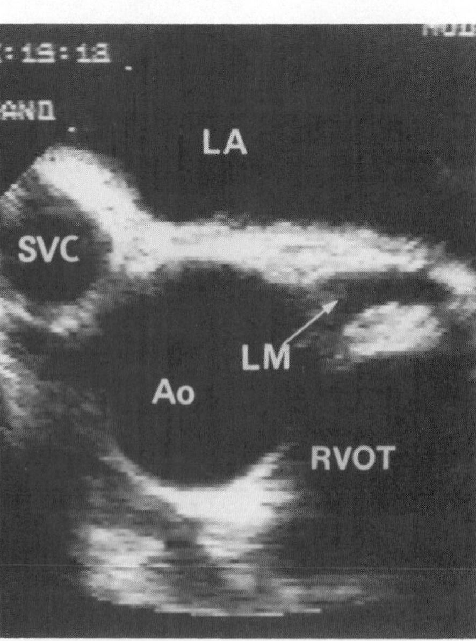

Figure 30–4. Transesophageal echocardiographic demonstration of the right coronary artery (RCA), left main coronary artery (LM), and superior vena cava (SVC). Ao—aortic root; RVOT—right ventricular outflow tract.

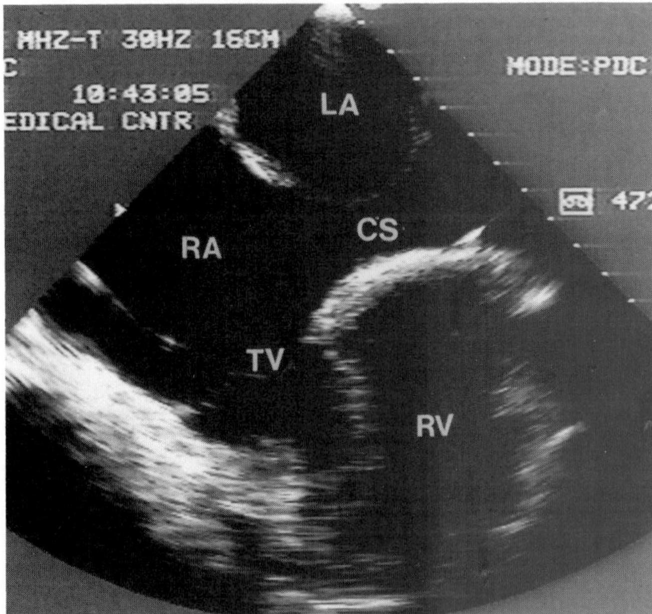

Figure 30–5. Transesophageal echocardiographic view of a prominent coronary sinus (CS) in a patient with a persistent left superior vena cava. LA—left atrium; RA—right atrium; RV—right ventricle; TV—tricuspid valve.

Indications for Ambulatory Transesophageal Echocardiography

Although transesophageal echocardiography is a relatively new technique, its indications in clinical cardiology are rapidly expanding (Table 30–3).

Table 30–3. INDICATIONS FOR AMBULATORY/ICU TRANSESOPHAGEAL ECHOCARDIOGRAPHY

Aortic dissection/aneurysms
Native valve endocarditis
Flail mitral/tricuspid valves
Mitral/aortic prosthetic dysfunction
Detection and quantification of regurgitation
Central vs. paravalvular regurgitation
Endocarditis (abscesses, vegetations)
Systemic thromboemboli (LA thrombi, spontaneous contrast)
Intracardiac masses (tumors)
Congenital heart disease (ASDs, VSDs, subaortic membranes)
Other
Postinfarction complications (VSD, papillary muscle rupture)
Pericardial disease (tamponade, tumors)
LV function

ASD—atrial septal defect; ICU—intensive care unit; LA—left atrium; VSD—ventricular septal defect; LV—left ventricle.

AORTIC DISSECTION. Most likely transesophageal echocardiography will become one of the standards for assessing acute and chronic aortic dissection. Not only can aortic regurgitation, pericardial effusion, and aneurysmal aortic dilatation be detected, but intimal dissection flaps can be visualized with high spatial and temporal resolution[B2, E1–E5] (Fig. 30–6), and color flow imaging can clearly demonstrate blood flow across entry and re-entry tears[H6, T1] (Fig. 30–7). Preliminary data from a European cooperative study[E3, E4] demonstrate that this method is equivalent, if not superior, to angiography and cine computed tomography in the evaluation of acute dissection. In a study of 164 consecutive patients with aortic dissection, the sensitivity and specificity of transesophageal echocardiography were 99 percent and 98 percent, respectively. For computed tomography, the sensitivity measured 83 percent and the specificity, 100 percent. Aortography demonstrated a sensitivity and specificity of 88 percent and

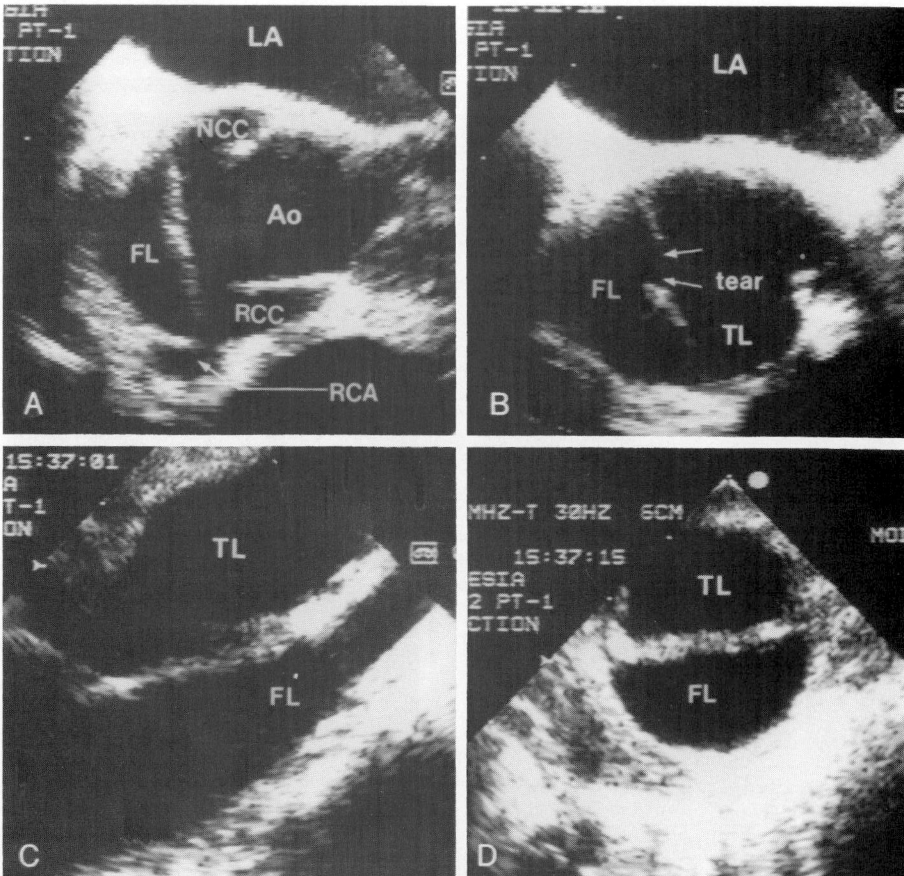

Figure 30–6. Transesophageal echocardiographic evaluation of an ascending aortic dissection. *A*, At the aortic valve level, the false lumen (FL) can be seen adjacent to the right coronary ostium (RCA). *B*, A large intimal flap entry tear (tear) connecting the true lumen (TL) and false lumen can be seen in the ascending aorta. The dissection can be demonstrated to extend distally involving the entire transverse (*C*) and descending (*D*) aorta. Ao—aorta; NCC—noncoronary cusp; RCC—right coronary cusp.

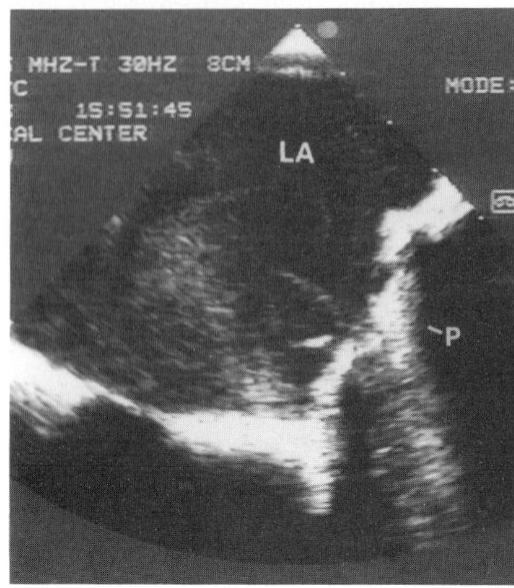

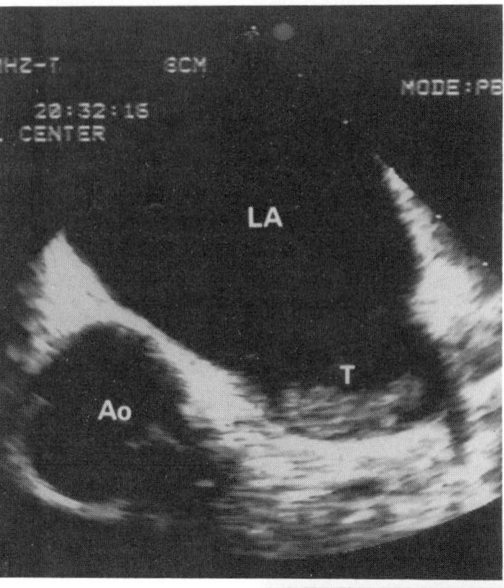

Figure 30–8. Transesophageal echocardiographic demonstration of left atrial spontaneous contrast (*left*) in a patient with a normal functioning mitral prosthesis (P). A left atrial appendage thrombus (T) is illustrated in a patient with a recent peripheral thromboembolic event (*right.*) Ao—aortic root.

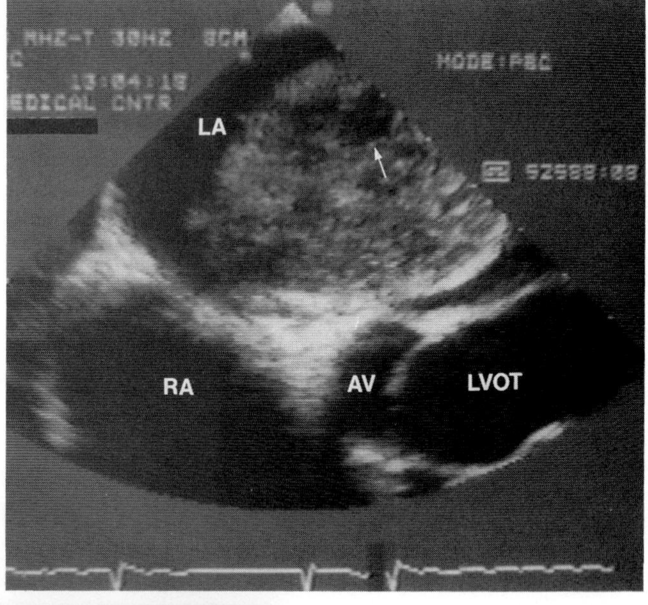

Figure 30–9. Transesophageal echocardiographic view illustrating characteristic cystic (*arrow*) acoustic findings that may be seen in benign myxomas. LVOT—left ventricular outflow tract; LA—left atrium; RA—right atrium; AV—aortic valve.

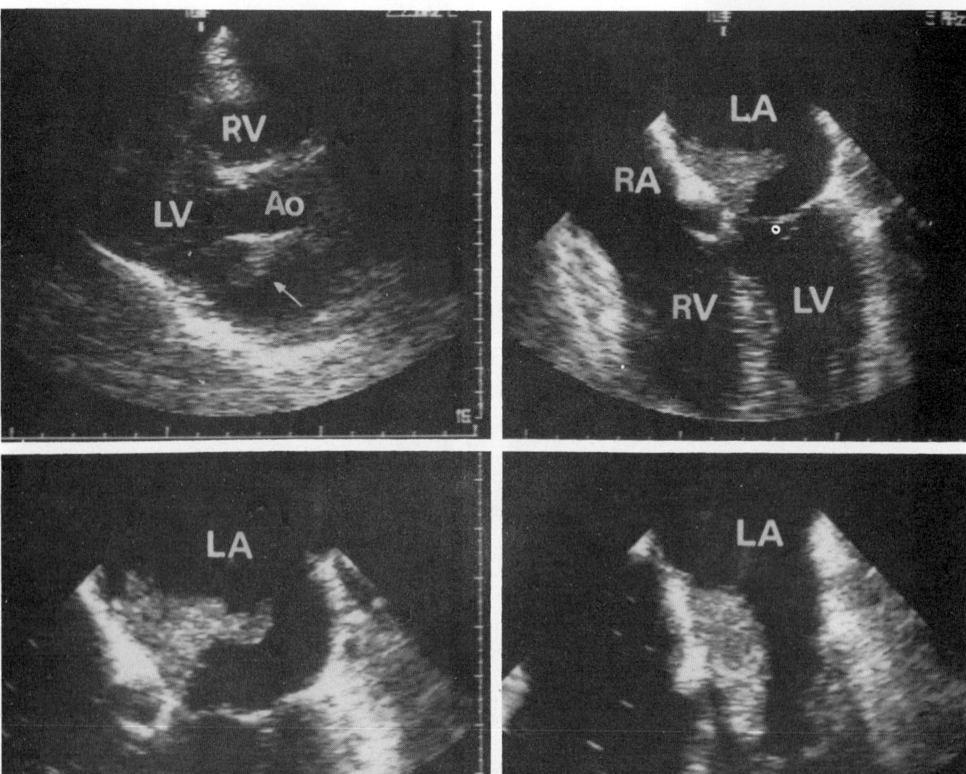

Figure 30–10. A left atrial myxoma in a young patient with recurrent cerebrovascular accidents. Precordial imaging (*upper left*) showed a nonspecific mass in the left atrium (*arrow*). Transesophageal echocardiographic imaging (*remaining views*) clearly demonstrated a highly mobile mass arising from the interatrial septum and provided important preoperative information to the surgeon. Ao—aortic root; LA—left atrium; RA—right atrium; LV—left ventricle.

94 percent, respectively. Furthermore, in these critically ill patients, transesophageal echocardiography could be performed more rapidly, while at the same time avoiding risks associated with the administration of radiopaque contrast material and transporting patients from heavily monitored critical care units to radiology suites. The portability of transesophageal echocardiography allows its performance anywhere in the hospital, and it requires fewer hospital personnel to operate. Preliminary data from the European cooperative study also suggest that the time saved by using it as the primary imaging modality decreases mortality by 5 to 10 percent per hour.

Figure 30–7. See Color Plate 5.

INTRA-ATRIAL THROMBI. Transesophageal echocardiography is a powerful technique for evaluating intra-atrial thrombi.[A1, N1] Despite the common finding of intra-atrial thrombi at operation or necropsy in patients with rheumatic valvular disease or atrial fibrillation, precordial imaging is rarely able to demonstrate thrombi successfully. In patients with a high clinical suspicion of a cardiac source for peripheral emboli, transesophageal echocardiography may demonstrate (1) thrombi in the left atrium or left atrial appendage[D2, D3, Z1] (Fig. 30–8, right) or (2) the unique appearance of spontaneous left atrial contrast (due to sluggish blood flow), a sign of embolic potential[D4] (Fig. 30–8, left). A particularly valuable use is in patients with recently recognized atrial fibrillation present for an indeterminate time, who are being considered for elective cardioversion to sinus rhythm. If left atrial or appendage thrombi or marked spontaneous contrast is identified by transesophageal echocardiography patients should undergo a 2- to 3-week course of anticoagulation prior to attempted cardioversion.

TUMOR MASSES. In the evaluation of cardiac tumor masses, transesophageal echocardiography can provide important information, not available by precordial imaging, about acoustic characteristics of tumors, their mobility and morphology, and precise sites of attachment[G3, H7, T2] (Figs. 30–9 and 30–10).

PROSTHETIC VALVES. Transesophageal echocardiography is a valuable technique for evaluating patients with mitral and aortic prosthetic valve dysfunction; this task is currently the most common reason for performing it. Clinical and in vitro studies have demonstrated that shadowing by mechanical prosthetic valves may mask Doppler and color flow interrogation from precordial imaging approaches.[C1, S4] By imaging from a retrocardiac approach, it can circumvent much of this masking during evaluation of patients with aortic and mitral prosthetic valve dysfunction.[C2, C3, K2, L1]

In patients with mitral prostheses, not only can previously unrecognized mitral prosthetic regurgitation be detected and semiquantified, but, in addition, a clear distinction between central and paravalvular leaks can be made (Figs. 30–11 and 30–12). Transesophageal echocardiography may be particularly valuable in the subgroup of patients with both mitral and aortic prostheses, because in this situation interrogation of the left atrium and mitral prosthetic function is blocked in both apical and parasternal approaches.

A note of caution in evaluating mitral prostheses: it has been observed that almost all normally functioning mechanical valves (with the exception of Starr-Edwards ball and cage valves) exhibit mild leaks where the valve leaflets seat with the sewing ring[K3, T3]

Figure 30–11. See Color Plate 6.

Figure 30–12. See Color Plate 6.

Figure 30–13. See Color Plate 6.

(Fig. 30–13). Recognition of this normal finding is important to avoid misinterpreting this retrograde flow as signifying the presence of pathology. In addition to its superiority in evaluating mitral prosthetic regurgitation, esophageal echocardiography is also effective in delineating vegetations or thrombi on the atrial side of a prosthesis.

In the aortic prosthetic position, transesophageal echocardiography is useful in evaluation of complications of endocarditis, such as posterior ring abscesses (Fig. 30–14), flail porcine cusps (Fig. 30–15), sewing ring dehiscence, and detection of paravalvular reguritant leaks (Fig. 30–16). However, in the aortic position, the success of imaging is somewhat less than in the mitral position, because the only available tomographic planes are short-axis planes that require interrogation through the sewing ring. In this setting, the internal architecture of the prosthesis and its anterior attachment site may be masked by shadowing from the posterior side of the prosthesis.

Figure 30–14. See Color Plate 7.

Figure 30–15. See Color Plate 7.

Figure 30–16. See Color Plate 7.

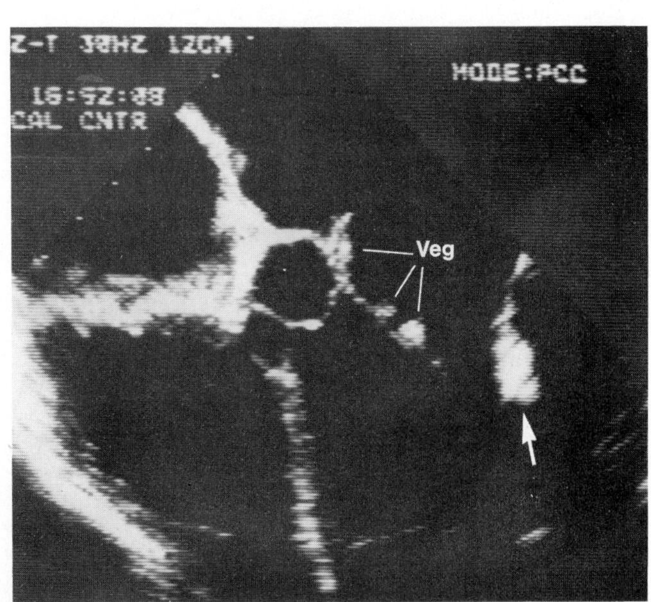

Figure 30–17. Transesophageal echocardiographic 4-chamber view in a patient with infectious endocarditis. Multiple small vegetations are seen studding the anterior mitral leaflet (Veg). Only the large vegetation on the posterior leaflet (*arrow*) was seen by precordial imaging.

NATIVE VALVE ENDOCARDITIS. In patients with clinical evidence of endocarditis, precordial imaging may fail to demonstrate the presence of vegetations. Transesophageal echocardiography may be useful in recognizing vegetations smaller than those that can be detected by precordial imaging. In addition, multiple vegetations may be demonstrated (Fig. 30–17), and complications such as annular abscesses (Fig. 30–18), valve perforations or aneurysms, intracardiac fistulas (Fig. 30–19), or the presence of mycotic aneurysms may be detected.[D5, D6, E6, G1]

Figure 30–18. See Color Plate 8.

Figure 30–19. See Color Plate 8.

FLAIL LEAFLETS. Transesophageal echocardiography has been demonstrated to be a useful technique in detecting mitral and tricuspid valve chordal ruptures or flail leaflets not seen by precordial surface imaging[S12] (Fig. 30–20). Preoperative recognition in patients with ruptured mitral chordae is becoming increasingly important.[A2, B3, C4, O2, O3] Currently, myxomatous disease is the most common cause of hemodynamically significant regurgitation in patients referred for mitral valve surgical corrective procedures.[W1] With growing enthusiasm for mitral repair procedures and increasing evidence of a morbidity and mortality comparable to or even lower than that of valve replacement,[B4, G4, G5, O4, S13] transesophageal echocardiography represents an important advancement in the preoperative evaluation of candidates for valve surgery.

CONGENITAL HEART DISEASE. Transesophageal echocardiography may provide an important adjunct in evaluation of young adults with congenital heart disease.[D7, H8, I1, R3, Z2] In atrial septal defects, the diameter of the defects can be directly visualized and shunt flow confirmed by color flow and saline contrast imaging (Fig. 30–21). Transesophageal echocardiography is particularly useful in differentiating sinus venosus from secundum or primum defects.[O5]

Figure 30–21. See Color Plate 9.

In patients with ventricular defects, the morphology of the defect can be directly visualized with high resolution; the use of color flow Doppler or saline contrast can be used to delineate the extent and timing of both right-to-left and left-to-right shunting (Fig. 30–22).

INTENSIVE CARE UNIT PATIENTS. In these patients, transesophageal echocardiography has been useful for the evaluation of catastrophic postinfarction complications, such as ventricular septal defects and mitral regurgitation caused by extensive wall damage or papillary muscle rupture.[K4] Other potential uses in the intensive care unit include evaluation of right ventricular function in patients with precordial chest trauma, tamponade in postcardiothoracic surgical patients, and global left and right ventricular function in patients with limited acoustic windows.[B5, C5, K3]

PERCUTANEOUS VALVULOPLASTY. As a research tool, transesophageal echocardiography has been used as a technique for evaluating patients prior to and during percutaneous aortic and mitral balloon valvuloplasty.[C6, H9, V1] In candidates for mitral balloon valvuloplasty, precatheterization transesophageal echocardiography may detect unsuspected left atrial thrombi; such findings will alter management, in that surgical commissurotomy should be recommended in lieu of balloon dilatation. During actual mitral valvuloplasty procedures, it has been demonstrated to be helpful in guiding transseptal puncture, assessing the extent of postdilatation mitral regurgitation, and detecting such complications as myocardial perforation and pericardial tamponade. During balloon aortic valvuloplasty, it has been useful in observing the time course of recovery of myocardial depression after balloon inflation and deflation.[E7] Monitoring has resulted in altering procedures: the duration of balloon inflations is shorter, and the time allowed between inflations is prolonged to allow adequate recovery of depression of myocardial contractility. As with mitral valvuloplasty, the extent of iatrogenically induced regurgitation can be detected, as well as catastrophic complications.

Transesophageal Echocardiography Training

Standard training requirements for competency in performing transesophageal echocardiography remain to be established. Obviously the operators should be competent and adept at performing and interpreting routine precordial two-dimensional, Doppler, and color flow imaging. In our experience, performing a minimum of 25 to 50 procedures is desirable before an individual becomes comfortable in his or her ability to do this procedure independently. A parallel recommendation is that of the American

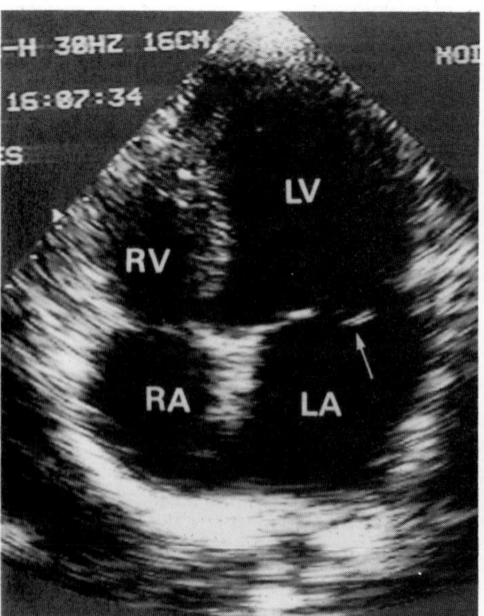

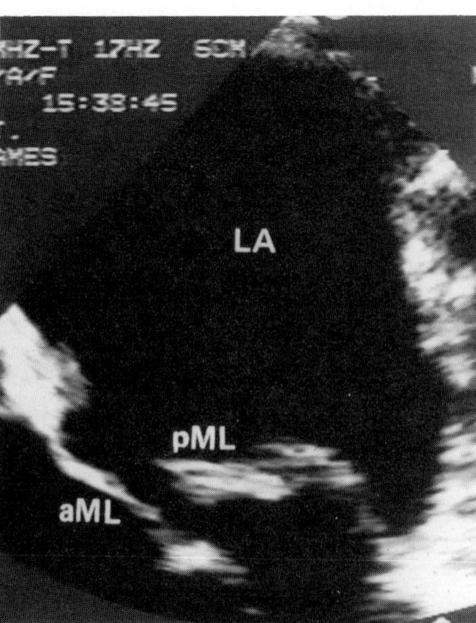

Figure 30–20. Transesophageal echocardiographic demonstration of a flail posterior mitral leaflet (*right*) that was misinterpreted as mitral valve prolapse (*arrow*) by precordial imaging (*left*.) aML—anterior mitral leaflet; pML—posterior mitral leaflet; LA—left atrium; RA—right atrium; LV—left ventricle; RV—right ventricle.

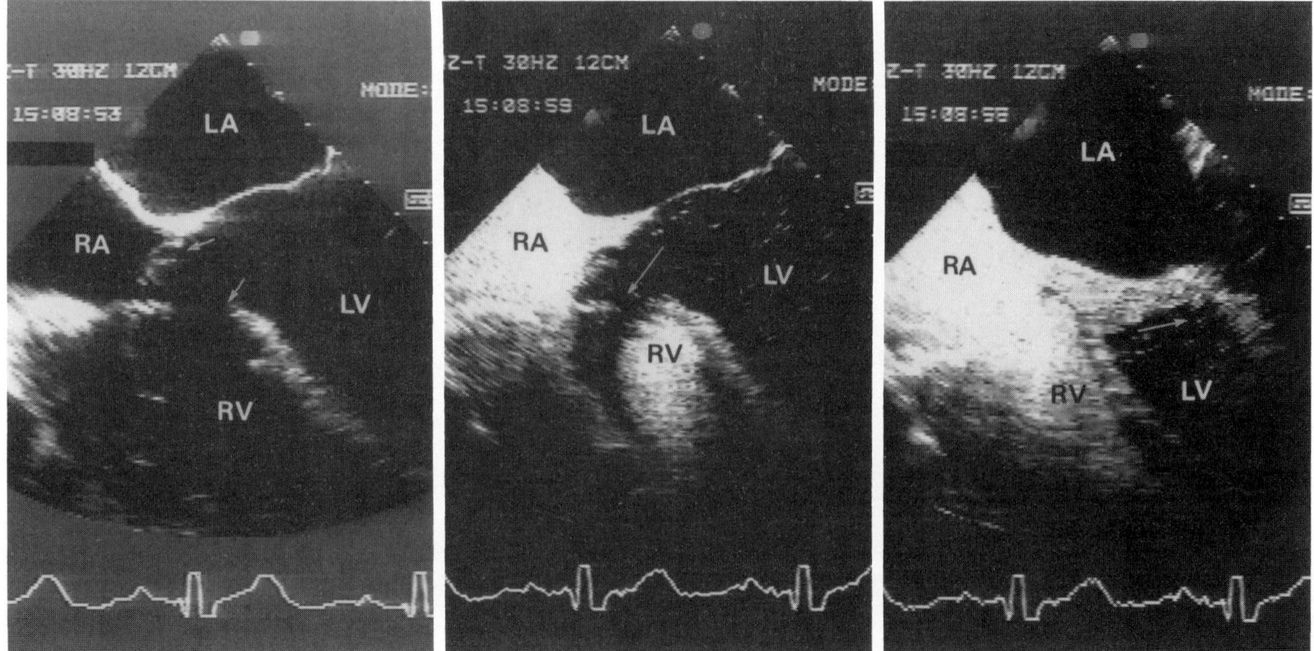

Figure 30–22. Direct visualization of a perimembranous ventricular septal defect by transesophageal echocardiography (*left*). Saline contrast demonstrated a large "negative contrast effect" of left-to-right shunting (*middle*) and moderate "positive contrast effect" of right-to-left shunting (*right.*)

Society of Gastroenterology, requiring a minimum of 50 upper endoscopy procedures to achieve competency in diagnostic gastroesophageal endoscopy.[H10]

Learning this technique from a trained cardiologist is the most efficient means of gaining competence. Alternatively, experience with probe manipulation and an understanding of anatomic image orientation and pathology can be gained by working intraoperatively with an anesthesiologist. Working with a gastroenterologist is additionally useful to help learn esophageal probe intubation in ambulatory patients.

Safety

COMPLICATIONS. The safety of this technique is well established. Worldwide, over 20,000 transesophageal echocardiographic procedures have been performed without report of serious complications. To date, the only complications reported have been transient recurrent laryngeal nerve paralysis in two neurosurgical patients undergoing intraoperative transesophageal echocardiography in the sitting–cervical neck flexion position.[C7] It is now believed that it should be avoided in intubated patients in this position. Although no known major catastrophic complications in alert, conscious patients have been reported, the potential for perforation of the esophagus exists. The American Society of Gastroenterology estimated the risk of esophageal perforation in upper gastric endoscopy to be approximately 1 in 3000.[S14] The rate of perforation may be significantly lower in transesophageal echocardiography than in gastric endoscopy, for the highest complication rates during endoscopy are seen in those with active esophageal disease or undergoing biopsy. Performing transesophageal echocardiography in these subgroups is generally avoided. Other minor complications that may occur with low (1 to 2 percent) frequency include atrial and ventricular arrhythmias, vasovagal reactions, transient bronchospasm, hypoxemia, and minor bleeding.

CONTRAINDICATIONS. Important relative contraindications are listed in Table 30–4. If a transesophageal echocardiogram is deemed necessary in a patient with known prior esophageal pathology, prior delineation of precise pathology by fiberoptic endoscopy or barium swallow may be useful.

OTHER CONCERNS. Excessive force should never be used with probe insertion and manipulation. In a conscious ambulatory patient, the procedure should be discontinued if a particular maneuver results in significant pain or discomfort. The probe should not be withdrawn or advanced with forced flexion or extension of the probe tip. In addition, great care must be taken that the probe is never moved with the basal control knobs in the locked position.

Ambulatory esophageal echocardiographic procedures are optimally performed with appropriate ancillary personnel and equipment. In addition to the physician operator, a nurse is important to assist with patient positioning, monitoring of vital signs, and suctioning of oral secretions and to provide moral support and comfort for the patient. A third person, such as an echo technician, is useful to assist in video recording and optimization of imaging parameters and gain settings. Routine placement of an intravenous line or heparin lock is recommended if sedation is used and to safeguard against the possibility of occasional vasovagal responses seen during esophageal intubation. In addition, resuscitation equipment, such as a defibrillator, crash cart (including a laryngoscope, venting bag, and resuscitation drugs), and oxygen should be available. Intermittent monitoring of heart rate, blood pressure, and respiratory status is also mandatory in sedated patients. Transcutaneous pulse oximetry and automated blood pressure cuffs are useful adjuncts in monitoring.

Prior to each use, probe inspection for mechanical and operational defects is mandatory. After a procedure is completed, careful probe cleaning is necessary to avoid transmission of

Table 30–4. RELATIVE CONTRAINDICATIONS FOR TRANSESOPHAGEAL ECHOCARDIOGRAPHY

Active upper gastrointestinal bleeding
Known esophageal pathology
Strictures, webs, rings
Varices
Diverticula
Fistulas
Esophagitis
Carcinoma
Prior esophageal-gastric surgery
Esophagectomy
Fundal-plication procedures
Gastric stapling procedures (transgastric imaging contraindicated)
Prior mediastinal irradiation
Penetrating or blunt thoracic esophageal trauma
Uncooperative patient

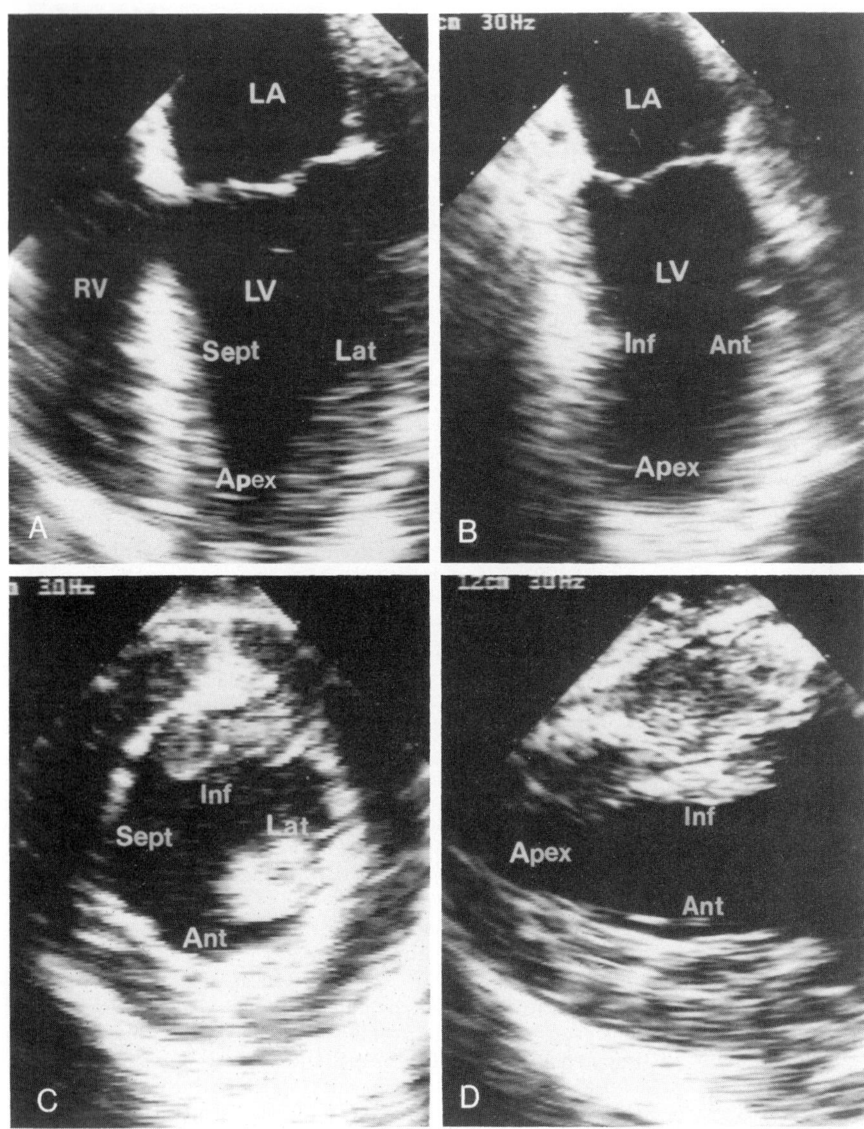

Figure 30–23. Biplane transesophageal echocardiographic imaging of the left ventricle. Near-simultaneous apical 4-chamber (*A*) and 2-chamber (*B*) views enable imaging of the septal (Sept), lateral (Lat), inferior (Inf), anterior (Ant), and apical (Apex) walls. These wall segments also can be imaged in high resolution in near-simultaneous short-axis (*C*) and long-axis (*D*) views. LA—left atrium; LV—left ventricle; RV—right ventricle.

infectious agents. Immersion of the distal half of the probe shaft (the basal control knobs should not be immersed) for 15 to 20 minutes in an aldehyde-based solution (Cidex, Wavicide) is recommended for disinfection. For intraoperative patients, a disposable rubber sheath for the probe may be used to protect against transmission of infectious disease. However, such sheaths are not recommended in ambulatory patients, for the bulky size of existing sheaths prohibit their use.

Future Developments

Transesophageal echocardiography is clearly continuing to evolve as a powerful new and exciting diagnostic technique.

Table 30–5. FUTURE DEVELOPMENTS IN TRANSESOPHAGEAL ECHOCARDIOGRAPHY

Continuous wave Doppler
Biplane imaging probes
Smaller/pediatric probes
Proximal coronary artery assessment
Myocardial contrast imaging
Higher/multiple frequency transducers
Tissue characterization
Three-dimensional reconstruction

Further advances in probe development (Table 30–5) will result in the inclusion of continuous wave Doppler imaging, permitting hemodynamic measurements such as transvalvular pressure gradients. The development of smaller probes for pediatric and adult use will extend the use of the technique to groups that cannot currently be studied. The most exciting advancement, soon to be available, is the development of orthogonal biplane imaging crystals.[96] This will enable acquisition of new acoustic views that include (1) near-simultaneous two- and four-chamber views (Fig. 30–23), (2) long-axis imaging of the left ventricular apex (Fig. 30–23), (3) imaging of the ascending, transverse, and descending aorta in both long- and short-axis views, and (4) long-axis imaging of both the aortic root and the right ventricular outflow tract (Figs. 30–24 and 30–25). Such views will be important in allowing improved evaluation of (1) regional wall motion abnormalities, (2) flail mitral leaflets, (3) paravalvular mitral and aortic prosthetic regurgitation, (4) left ventricular masses and thrombi, (5) thoracic aortic dissection flaps and entry tears (Fig. 30–26), and (6) congenital heart disease including atrial septal defects and conditions associated with right ventricular outflow tract obstruction.

Figure 30–26. See Color Plate 9.

Figure 30–27. See Color Plate 10.

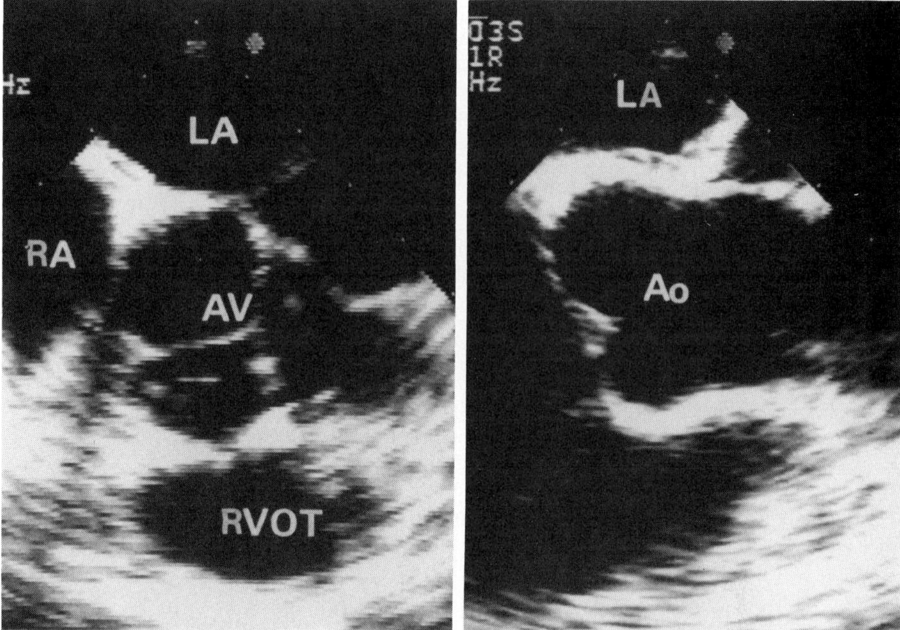

Figure 30–24. Biplane transesophageal echocardiographic imaging of the aortic valve and root. Aortic valve (AV) in short axis (*left*.) Aortic root (Ao) in long axis (*right*.) RVOT—right ventricular outflow tract; LA—left atrium; RA—right atrium.

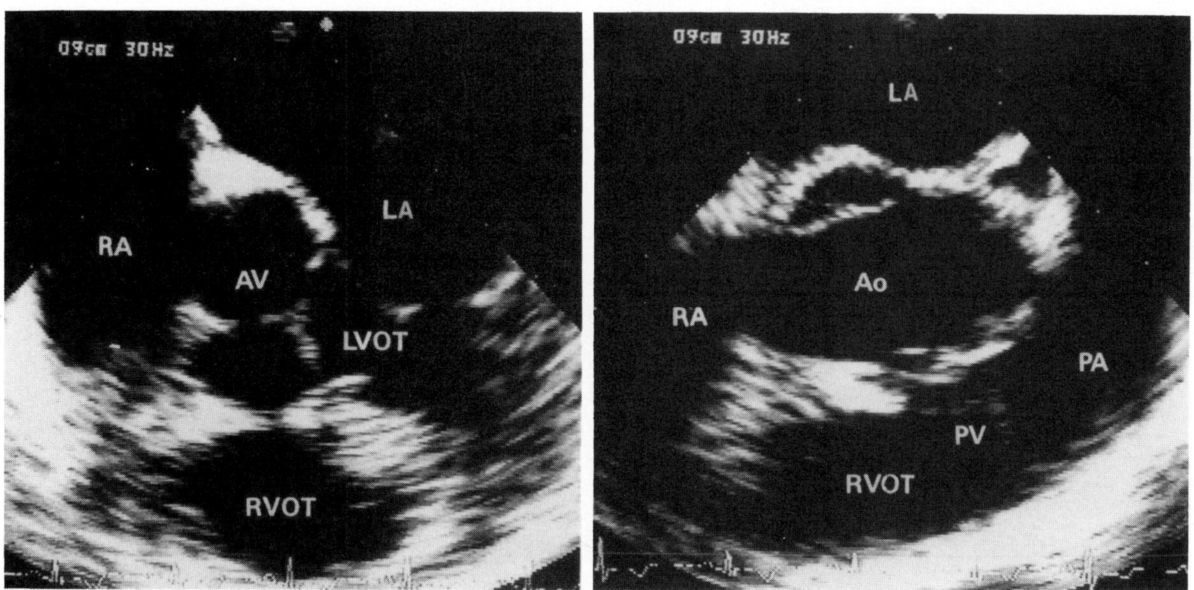

Figure 30–25. Biplane transesophageal echocardiographic imaging of the right ventricular outflow tract (RVOT) in short axis (*left*) and long axis (*right*.) Ao—aortic root; AV—aortic valve; LVOT—left ventricular outflow tract; PA—main pulmonary artery; PV—pulmonic valve; LA—left atrium, RA—right atrium.

The potential ability to image right and left coronary trunks leads to the intriguing possibility that this technique may eventually evolve into a method of detecting proximal coronary artery stenoses. The development of higher-frequency probes, detection of calcific plaques, or phasic analysis of pulsed and color Doppler coronary flow patterns[Y1, Z3] may be valuable in this endeavor (Fig. 30–27). In the intraoperative arena, transesophageal echocardiography is being investigated in conjunction with intracoronary or aortic root injection of sonicated Renografin or albumin contrast agents to assess the success of regional myocardial reperfusion post coronary artery bypass grafting.[S15] This technique may find wide application in the intraoperative evaluation of the extent of coronary revascularization. Other potential future advances include development of higher or multiple frequency enabling greater resolution, application of this technique to the field of ultrasonic tissue characterization, and possible three-dimensional image reconstruction.[W2]

Conclusion

Transesophageal echocardiography is a relatively new imaging technique that is rapidly evolving into a major tool for general cardiac imaging in a variety of venues. This technique can be easily learned and safely performed. Future advances in probe technology will continue to expand its possibilities.

References

A

1. Aschenberg, W., Schlüter, M., Kremer, P., et al.: Transesophageal two-dimensional echocardiography for detection of left atrial appendage thrombus. J. Am. Coll. Cardiol. 7:163, 1986.
2. Adebo, O. A., and Ross, J. K.: Surgical treatment of ruptured mitral valve chordae: A comparison between valve replacement and valve repair. Thorac. Cardiovasc. Surg. 32:139, 1984.

B

1. Beaupre, P. N., Kremer, P., Cahalan, M., et al.: Intraoperative detection of changes in left ventricular segmental wall motion by transesophageal two-dimensional echocardiography. Am. Heart J. 107:1021, 1984.
2. Börner, N., Erbel, R., Braun, V., et al.: Diagnosis of aortic dissection by transesophageal echocardiography. Am. J. Cardiol. 54:1157, 1984.
3. Bashour, T. T., Andraei, G. E., Hanna, E. S., et al.: Reparative operations for mitral valve incompetence: An emerging treatment of choice. Am. Heart J. 113:1199, 1987.
4. Bonchek, L. I., Olinger, G. N., Siegel, R., et al.: Left ventricular performance after reconstruction for mitral regurgitation. J. Thorac. Cardiovasc. Surg. 88:122, 1984.
5. Beppu, S., Nakatani, S., Tanaka, N., et al.: Transesophageal echocardiographic diagnosis of localized pericardial coagula: A special cause of cardiac tamponade. (Abstract.) Circulation 78(Suppl. II)4:299, 1988.

C

1. Come, P. C.: Pitfalls in the diagnosis of periprosthetic valvular regurgitation by pulsed Doppler echocardiography. J. Am. Coll. Cardiol. 9:1176, 1987.
2. Currie, P. J., Calafiore, R., Stewart, W. J., et al.: Transesophageal echo in mitral prosthetic dysfunction: Echo-surgical correlation. (Abstract.) J. Am. Coll. Cardiol. 13:69A, 1989.
3. Currie, P. J., Schiavone, W. A., Stewart, W. J., et al.: Evaluation of mitral prosthetic dysfunction with transesophageal color flow Doppler in ambulatory patients. (Abstract.) Circulation 76(Suppl. IV):39, 1987.
4. Carpentier, A., Chauvaud, S., Fabiani, J. N., et al.: Reconstructive surgery of mitral valve incompetence: Ten year appraisal. J. Thorac. Cardiovasc. Surg. 79:338, 1980.
5. Chan, K. L.: Transesophageal echocardiography in the management of intubated cardiac patients. (Abstract.) Circulation 78(Suppl. II):299, 1988.
6. Cormier, B., Vahanian, A., Michel, P.-L., et al.: The contribution of transesophageal echocardiography in the ultrasound assessment of percutaneous mitral valvuloplasty. (Abstract.) J. Am. Coll. Cardiol. 13:51A, 1989.
7. Cucchiara, R. F., Nugent, M., Seward, J. B., and Messick, J. M.: Air embolism in upright neurosurgical patients: Detection and localization by two-dimensional transesophageal echocardiography. Anesthesiology 60:353, 1984.

D

1. De Bruijn, N. P., Clements, F. M., and Kisslo, J. A.: Intraoperative transesophageal color flow mapping: Initial experience. Anesth. Analg. 66:386, 1987.
2. Daniel, W. G., Engberding, R., Erbel, R., et al.: Transesophageal echocardiography in unexplained arterial embolism—a European multicenter study. (Abstract.) International Symposium on Transesophageal Echocardiography, Mainz, 1988, p. 25.
3. Daniel, W. G., Nikutta, P., Schröder, E., and Nellessen, U.: Transesophageal echocardiography detection of left atrial appendage thrombi in patients with unexplained arterial embolism. (Abstract.) Circulation 74(Suppl. II):391, 1986.
4. Daniel, W. G., Nellessen, U., Schröder, E., et al.: Left atrial spontaneous contrast in mitral valve disease: An indicator for an increased thromboembolic risk. J. Am. Coll. Cardiol. 11:1204, 1988.
5. Daniel, W. G., Schröder, E., Mügge, A., and Lichtlen, P. R.: Transesophageal echocardiography in infective endocarditis. Am. J. Card. Imag. 2:78, 1988.
6. Daniel, W. G., Schröder, E., Nonnast-Daniel, B., and Lichtlen, P. R.: Conventional and transesophageal echocardiography in the diagnosis of infective endocarditis. Eur. Heart J. 8(Suppl. J):287, 1987.
7. Dreysse, S., Dougherty, F. C., Loos, D., et al.: Transesophageal color flow mapping in patients with atrial septal defects. (Abstract.) International Symposium on Transesophageal Echocardiography, Mainz, 1988, p. 11.

E

1. Engberding, R., Bender, F., Grosse-Heitmeyer, W., et al.: Identification of dissection or aneurysm of the descending thoracic aorta by conventional and transesophageal two-dimensional echocardiography. Am. J. Cardiol. 59:717, 1987.
2. Erbel, R., Börner, N., Steller, D., et al.: Detection of aortic dissection by transesophageal echocardiography. Br. Heart J. 58:45, 1987.
3. Erbel, R., Rennollet, H., Engberding, R., et al.: Detection of aortic detection by transesophageal echocardiography. A multicenter cooperative study. (Abstract.) Circulation 78(Suppl. II):4, 1988.
4. Erbel, R., Rennollet, H., Engberding, R., et al.: A cooperative trial: Complementary role of echocardiography in the diagnosis of aortic dissection including transesophageal echocardiography. (Abstract.) International Symposium on Transesophageal Echocardiography, Mainz, 1988, p. 17.
5. Erbel, R., Mohr-Kahaly, S., Rennollet, H., et al.: Diagnosis of aortic dissection: Value of transesophageal echocardiography. Thorac. Cardiovasc. Surg. 35(Special Issue 2):126, 1987.
6. Erbel, R., Rohmann, S., Drexler, M., et al.: Improved diagnostic value of echocardiography in patients with infective endocarditis by transesophageal approach. A prospective study. Eur. Heart J. 9:43, 1988.
7. Erbel, R.: Personal communication, 1988.

F

1. Feigenbaum, H.: Echocardiography. 4th ed. Lea & Febiger, Philadelphia, 1986.
2. Frazin, L., Talano, J. V., Stephanides, L., et al.: Esophageal echocardiography. Circulation 54:102, 1975.

G

1. Gussenhoven, E. J., Taams, M. A., Roelandt, J., et al.: Transesophageal two-dimensional echocardiography: Its role in solving clinical problems. J. Am. Coll. Cardiol. 8:975, 1986.
2. Geibel, A., Kasper, W., Behroz, A., et al.: Risk of transesophageal echocardiography in awake patients with cardiac diseases. Am. J. Cardiol. 62:337, 1988.
3. Grossegger, C., Globits, S., Mlczoch, J., and Gloga, D.: Intracardiac masses: Detection and characterization by transesophageal versus other methods. (Abstract.) International Symposium on Tranesophageal Echocardiography, Mainz, 1988, p. 27.
4. Galloway, A. C., Colvin, S. B., Baumann, G., et al.: Long-term results of mitral valve reconstruction with Carpentier techniques in 148 patients with mitral insufficiency. Circulation 78(Suppl. II):97, 1988.
5. Goldman, M. E., Mora, F., Guarino, T., et al.: Mitral valvuloplasty is superior to valve replacement for preservation of left ventricular function: An intraoperative two-dimensional echocardiographic study. J. Am. Coll. Cardiol. 10:568, 1987.

H

1. Hatle, H., and Angelsen, B.: Doppler Ultrasound in Cardiology: Physical Principles and Clinical Applications. 2nd ed. Lea & Febiger, Philadelphia, 1985.
2. Hisanaga, K., Hisanaga, A., Nagata, K., and Yoshida, S.: A new transesophageal real-time two-dimensional echocardiographic system using a flexible tube and its clinical application. Proc. Jpn. Soc. Ultrason. Med. 32:43, 1977.
3. Hisanaga, K., Hisanaga, A., Nagata, K., and Ichie, Y.: Transesophageal cross-sectional echocardiography. Am. Heart J. 100:605, 1980.
4. Hisanaga, H., Hisanaga, A., Hibi, N., et al.: High speed rotating scanner for transesophageal cross-sectional echocardiography. Am. J. Cardiol. 46:837, 1980.
5. Hanrath, P., Kremer, P., Langenstein, B. A., et al.: Transösophageale Echokardiographie: Ein neues Verfahren zur dynamischen Ventrikelfunktionsanalyse. Dtsch. Med. Wochenschr. 106:533, 1981.
6. Hashimoto, S., Kumada, T., Osakada, G., et al.: Detection of the entry by color Doppler in dissecting aortic aneurysm: Clinical significance of the transesophageal color Doppler. (Abstract.) Circulation, 76(Suppl. IV):37, 1987.
7. Hofmann, T., Behroz, A., Köster, W., and Kasper, W.: Detection of intracardiac masses by two-dimensional transesophageal echocardiography. (Abstract.) Circulation 76(Suppl. IV):37, 1987.

8. Hanrath, P., Schlüter, M., Langenstein, B. A., et al.: Detection of ostium secundum atrial septal defects by transesophageal cross-sectional echocardiography. Br. Heart J. 49:350, 1983.
9. Henrichs, K. J., and Klinik, M.: TEE monitoring of aortic valvuloplasty. (Abstract.) International Symposium on Transesophageal Echocardiography, Mainz, 1988, p. 29.
10. Health and Public Policy Committee, American College of Physicians: Clinical competence in diagnostic esophagogastroduodenoscopy. Ann. Intern. Med. 107:937, 1987.

I

1. Isaji, F.: Diagnosis of atrial septal defect (secundum type) with transesophageal echocardiography: Special references to size and type of ASD. Nippon Kyobu Geka Gakkai Zasshi 32:37, 1984.

K

1. Kremer, P., Schwartz, L., Cahalan, M. K., et al.: Intraoperative monitoring of left ventricular performance by transesophageal M-mode and 2-D echocardiography. (Abstract.) Am. J. Cardiol. 49:956, 1982.
2. Khanderia, B., Seward, J., Oh, J., et al.: Mitral prosthesis malfunction: Utility of transesophageal echocardiography. (Abstract.) J. Am. Coll. Cardiol. 13:69A, 1989.
3. Kyo, S., Takamoto, S., Matsumura, M., et al.: Immediate and early postoperative evaluation of results of cardiac surgery by transesophageal two-dimensional Doppler echocardiography. Circulation 76(Suppl. V):13, 1987.
4. Koenig, K., Kasper, W., Hofmann, M., et al.: Transesophageal echocardiography for diagnosis of rupture of the ventricular septum or left ventricular papillary muscle during acute myocardial infarction. Am. J. Cardiol. 59:362, 1987.

L

1. Lee, E., Kee, L., and Schiller, N. B.: Transesophageal echocardiography and color flow imaging assessment of prosthetic and native valve dysfunction. (Abstract.) Circulation (Suppl. II)78:607, 1988.

M

1. Mitchell, M. M., Sutherland, G. R., Gussenhoven, E. J., et al.: Transesophageal echocardiography. J. Am. Soc. Echo. 1:362, 1988.
2. Miyatake, K., Okamoto, M., Kinnoshita, N., et al.: Clinical applications of a new real-time two-dimensional Doppler flow imaging system. Am. J. Cardiol. 9:952, 1987.

N

1. Nellessen, U., Daniel, W. G., Matheis, G., et al.: Impending paradoxical embolism from atrial thrombus: Correct diagnosis by transesophageal echocardiography and prevention by surgery. J. Am. Coll. Cardiol. 5:1002, 1985.

O

1. Oh, J. K., Khandheria, B. K., Seward, J. B., et al.: Transesophageal color flow imaging. Echocardiography 5:407, 1988.
2. Oliveria, D. B. G., Kawkins, K. D., Kay, P. H., and Paneth, M.: Chordal rupture: Comparison between repair and valve replacement. Br. Heart J. 50:318, 1983.
3. Olson, L. J., Subramanian, R., Ackerman, D. M., et al.: Surgical valve repair. J. Thorac. Cardiovasc. Surg. 89:491, 1985.
4. Orszulak, T. A., Schaff, H. V., Danielson, G. K., et al.: Mitral regurgitation due to ruptured chordae tendineae: Early and late results of pathology of the mitral valve: A study of 712 cases spanning 21 years. Mayo Clin. Proc. 62:22, 1987.
5. Oh, J. K., Seward, J. B., Khandheria, B. K., et al.: Visualization of sinus venosus defect by transesophageal echocardiography. J. Am. Soc. Echo. 1:275, 1988.
6. Omoto, R., Kyo, S., Matsumura, M., et al.: Biplane color transesophageal Doppler echocardiography (color TEE): Its advantages and limitations. Int. J. Cardiac Imag. 4:57, 1989.

R

1. Roizen, M. F., Beaupre, P. N., Alpert, R. A., et al.: Monitoring with two-dimensional transesophageal echocardiography: Comparison of myocardial function in patients undergoing supraceliac, suprarenal-infraceliac, or infrarenal aortic occlusion. J. Vasc. Surg. 1:300, 1984.
2. Roche Laboratories Nutley, NJ: Important new information on the administration of Versed (midazolam hydrochloride) injection for conscious sedation. (Letter.) Nov, 1987.
3. Reifart, N., Strohm, W. D.,: Detection of atrial septum defects by transesophageal two-dimensional echocardiography with a mechanical scanner. In Hanrath, P., Bleifeld, W., and Souquet, J. (eds.): Cardiovascular Diagnosis by Ultrasound: Transesophageal, Computerized, Contrast, Doppler Echocardiography. Martinus Nijhoff Publishers, The Hague, 1982, p. 247.

S

1. Seward, J. B., Khandheria, B. K., Oh, J. K., et al.: Transesophageal echocardiography: Technique, anatomic correlations, implementation and clinical applications. Mayo Clin. Proc. 63:649, 1988.
2. Schiller, N. B., Cahalan, M. K., and Lee, E.: Intraoperative assessment of left ventricular function and wall motion by transesophageal echocardiography. Echocardiography 6:79, 1989.
3. Shively, B. K., and Schiller, N. B.: Intraoperative transesophageal echocardiography in left ventricular function analysis in the detection of myocardial ischemia and infarction. Am. J. Cardiac Imag. 1:160, 1987.
4. Sprecher, D. L., Adamick, R., Adams, D., and Kisslo, J.: In vitro color flow and continuous wave Doppler ultrasound masking of flow by prosthetic valves. J. Am. Coll. Cardiol. 9:1306, 1987.
5. Souquet, J., Hanrath, P., Zitelli, L., et al.: Transesophageal phased array for imaging the heart. IEEE Trans. Biomed. Eng. 29:707, 1982.
6. Schlüter, M., Hinrichs, A., Their, W., et al.: Transesophageal two-dimensional echocardiography: Comparison of ultrasonic and anatomic sections. Am. J. Cardiol. 53:1173, 1984.
7. Smith, S. S., Cahalan, M. K., Benefiel, D. J., et al.: Intraoperative detection of myocardial ischemia in high risk patients: Electrocardiography versus two-dimensional transesophageal echocardiography. Circulation 72:1015, 1985.
8. Schlüter, M., Langenstein, B. A., Polster, J., et al.: Ventricular function analysis in the detection of myocardial ischemia and infarction. Am. J. Cardiac Imag. 1:160, 1987.
9. Schlüter, M., Langenstein, B. A., Polster, J., et al.: Transesophageal cross-sectional echocardiography with a phased array transducer system: Technique and initial clinical results. Br. Heart J. 48:67, 1982.
10. Schlüter, M., Langenstein, B. A., Hanrath, P., et al.: Assessment of transesophageal pulsed Doppler echocardiography in the detection of mitral regurgitation. Circulation 66:784, 1982.
11. Shulman, S. T., Amren, D. P., Bisno, A. L., et al.: Prevention of bacterial endocarditis: A statement for health professionals by the Committee on Rheumatic Fever and Infective Endocarditis of the Council on Cardiovascular Disease in the Young. Circulation 70:1123A, 1984.
12. Schlüter, M., Kremer, P., and Hanrath, P.: Transesophageal 2-D echocardiography feature of flail mitral leaflet due to ruptured chordae tendineae. Am. J. Cardiol. 108:609, 1984.
13. Spencer, F. C., Colvin, S. B., Culliford, A. T., and Isom, O. W.: Experiences with the Carpentier techniques of mitral valve reconstruction in 103 patients (1980–1985). J. Thorac. Cardiovasc. Surg. 90:341, 1985.
14. Silvis, S. E., Nebel, O., Rogers, G., et al.: Endoscopic complications: Results of the 1974 American Society of Gastroenterology Survey. JAMA 135:928, 1976.
15. Smith, J., Feinstein, S. B., Kapelanski, D. P., et al.: Transesophageal echocardiography determination of myocardial perfusion during surgery. (Abstract.) Circulation 74(Suppl. II):475, 1986.

T

1. Takamoto, S., and Omoto, R.,: Visualization of thoracic dissecting aortic aneurysm by transesophageal Doppler color flow mapping. Herz 12:187, 1987.
2. Their, W., Schlüter, M., Krebber, H., et al.: Cysts in left atrial myxomas identified by transesophageal cross-sectional echocardiography. Am. J. Cardiol. 51:1793, 1983.
3. Taams, M. A., Gussenhoven, E. J., Cahalan, M. K., et al.: Transesophageal Doppler color flow imaging in the detection of native and Björk-Shiley mitral valve regurgitation. J. Am. Coll. Cardiol. 13:95, 1989.

V

1. Visser, C., Jaarsma, W., Ernst, S., et al.: Transesophageal color Doppler echocardiography during mitral valvuloplasty. (Abstract.) International Symposium on Transesophageal Echocardiography, Mainz, 1988, p. 30.

W

1. Waller, B. F., Morrow, A. G., Maron, B. J., et al.: Etiology of clinically isolated, severe, chronic, pure mitral regurgitation: Analysis of 97 patients over 30 years of age having mitral valve replacement. Am. Heart J. 104:276, 1982.
2. Wollschläger, H., Zeiher, A. M., Klein, H.-P., et al.: Transesophageal echocardiography computed tomography: A new method for dynamic 3-D imaging of the heart. (Abstract.) J. Am. Coll. Cardiol. 13:68A, 1989.

Y

1. Yamagishi, M., Miyatake, K., Beppu, S., et al.: Assessment of coronary blood flow by transesophageal two-dimensional pulsed Doppler echocardiography. Am. J. Cardiol. 62:641, 1988.

Z

1. Zenker, G., Erbel, R., Krämer, G., et al.: Transesophageal two-dimensional echocardiography in young patients with cerebral ischemic events. Stroke 19:345, 1988.
2. Zatz, R., Wittlich, N., Erbel, R., and Meyer, J.: Value of transesophageal echocardiography in ventricular septal defects. (Abstract.) International Symposium on Transesophageal Echocardiography, Mainz, 1988, p. 22.
3. Zwicky, P., Daniel, W. G., Mügge A., and Lichtlen, P. R.: Imaging of coronaries by color-coded transesophageal Doppler echocardiography. Am. J. Cardiol. 62:639, 1988.

Chapter 31

Intraoperative Echocardiography

■ *WILLIAM J. STEWART, M.D.* ■ *RICHARD E. KERBER, M.D.*

Unique Applicability of Echocardiography to Intraoperative Use 618
Technology of Two-Dimensional and Color Doppler Echocardiography 618
Imaging Planes for Epicardial Echocardiography 618
Transducer Preparation for Epicardial Imaging 620
Transesophageal Echocardiography in the Operating Room 620
Transesophageal Image Planes 621
Intraoperative Echocardiography in Patients Undergoing Valvular Surgery 622
Coronary Arterial Imaging by Ultrasound 625
Determination of Left Ventricular Function and Myocardial Perfusion 630
Intraoperative Echocardiography in Congenital Heart Disease 630
Conclusion 631

Unique Applicability of Echocardiography to Intraoperative Use

The use of cardiac ultrasound to image the heart and great vessels during cardiac surgery is a logical extension of its increasing role outside the echocardiographic laboratory. In comparison with other types of cardiovascular imaging, intraoperative echocardiography has a most dramatic potential to affect the outcome of the patient. Studies performed immediately prior to cardiopulmonary bypass help formulate the surgical plans on the basis of accurate anatomic and physiologic information and provide a baseline for comparison after intervention. The findings of post-cardiopulmonary bypass echocardiography may mandate immediate changes in surgical therapy in a small percentage of cases, which may prevent the need for subsequent reoperation.[C1, G1, G2, M1, S1–S5] This chapter focuses on the ability of intraoperative echocardiography to assist with decision making in patients undergoing surgery for valve repair and valve replacement and coronary, myocardial, and congenital abnormalities.

Echocardiography is uniquely applicable during cardiac surgery because it provides anatomic and physiologic data about intracardiac dynamics that are not obtainable with other techniques, such as inspection or palpation of the external surface of the heart, intraluminal pressure waveform analysis, or other hemodynamic measurements.[F1, F2, K1, K2, N1, P1, P2] The technique may have an advantage over other imaging modalities potentially applicable intraoperatively, because the small ultrasound transducer can be applied easily directly to the epicardial surface or introduced via the transesophageal approach. To be useful, intraoperative imaging must be performed without major disruptions of the operative process. Although it is bulky, the echocardiographic equipment can be positioned outside the sterile field, adjacent to the head of the table. It should be placed where the surgeon and anesthesiologist can readily see the images.

The echo information should be integrated with the technology and clinical expertise from numerous disciplines. In addition, intraoperative echocardiography should be applied with a good understanding of the individual patient, the operative process, the ultrasound technology, and the pertinent clinical questions at hand. The rapid expansion of technology in ultrasound promises to make the area of intraoperative echocardiography a most interesting one for the future.

Technology of Two-Dimensional and Color Doppler Echocardiography

Ultrasound technology currently involves numerous types of image processing. We can image the structure of the heart with M-mode and two-dimensional echocardiography (in the amplitude domain) and flow within the heart with Doppler echocardiography (in the frequency domain).[K3, O1, S6] Principles of cardiac ultrasound derived from standard precordial imaging are equally applicable during cardiac surgery.[H1] One must be careful to address the right question with the appropriate ultrasound tool: Two-dimensional imaging should be utilized to determine the thickness and motion of walls, valves, or vascular structures. M-mode echocardiography (standard or color) is useful for timing events. Continuous wave Doppler ultrasound should be used to measure maximal velocity to estimate gradients, which requires parallel or nearly parallel alignment between the ultrasound beam and the direction of high-velocity flow. Pulsed Doppler and color flow imaging are useful for spatial mapping of intracardiac shunts and valvular regurgitation. Structural imaging of coronary anatomy requires high-frequency imaging and specially adapted transducers. For intraoperative echocardiography of valvular, myocardial, and congenital abnormalities we use standard equipment and transducer frequencies of 2.0 to 5.0 MHz. For epicardial imaging of coronary arteries, we use higher transducer frequencies, such as 12 MHz.

Instrument controls, such as gain, transducer frequency, pulse repetition frequency, image angle, and pulses per line and depth, must be appropriately chosen and used optimally.[B1, S7–S10] Attention must be given to the potential for ultrasound artifacts and other limitations, such as sampling rate and aliasing. When surveying three-dimensional flow disturbances or cardiac structures with a two-dimensional tomographic technique, the importance of utilizing multiple image planes cannot be overemphasized.[H2]

Imaging Planes for Epicardial Echocardiography

For individuals accustomed only to standard transthoracic echocardiography, the prospect of cardiac imaging during an operation implies an ideal setting with a limitless number of available image planes and freedom from the problems of poor

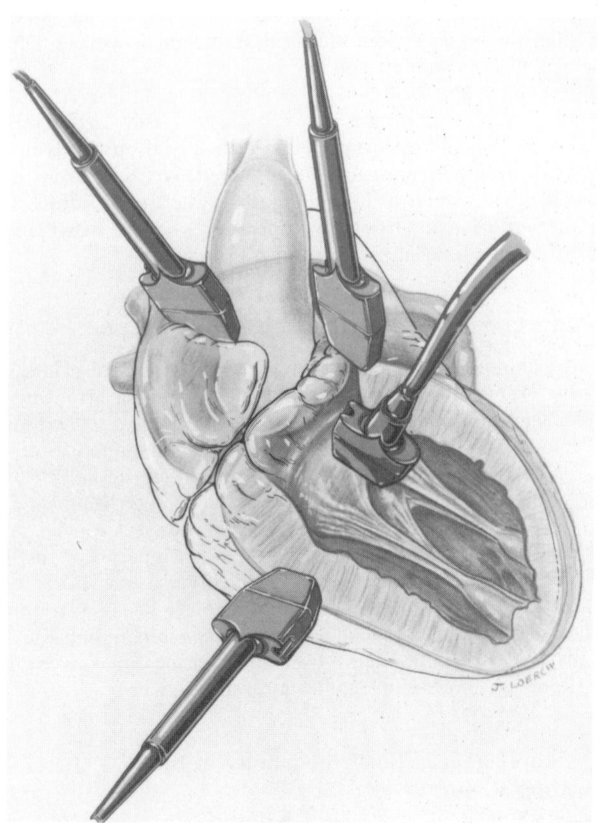

Figure 31–1. Artist's drawing of the four locations for transducer placement during epicardial intraoperative echocardiography.

ultrasound transmission through bone and lung. Unfortunately, a new set of difficulties unique to intraoperative echocardiography emerges. In particular, during epicardial imaging, the heart is a moving target, which may result in intermittent transducer contact. Inordinate transducer pressure can induce arrhythmias and disturb hemodynamics. Therefore, we have developed a set of usable epicardial imaging planes that comprise a complete intraoperative examination of the heart.[51] Some of the available transducer windows are quite different from those used for transthoracic imaging. For example, some new windows are available that cannot be obtained from transthoracic imaging windows. With the size of transducers presently available, the apical window is unavailable; this makes it impossible to orient a continuous wave beam parallel to the mitral inflow. In addition, because of its large size, the epicardial imaging transducer does not have good access to the posterior surface of the heart for imaging the circumflex and posterior descending coronary arteries without substantial perturbation of hemodynamics.

The transducer positions we have found useful for general cardiac imaging during a midsternal thoracotomy are described next (Fig. 31–1). These positions must be adapted or individualized in order to address specific questions or adapt to differences in an individual patient's anatomy.

THE PARASTERNAL EQUIVALENT TRANSDUCER POSITION (Fig. 31–2). This is the easiest and most obvious window. It is obtained by placing the transducer against the most anterior portion of the heart, the right ventricular outflow tract. Firm contact with the heart without causing significant hemodynamic disruption is quite feasible. The image planes available are similar to those obtainable from the left parasternal window during transthoracic imaging. However, the operator has more latitude to slide the transducer to various positions on the heart in order to concentrate on specific cardiac structures, rather than to simply make changes in angulation from a fixed transducer position as is done in transthoracic imaging. The transducer may be angled medially to evaluate the right ventricular inflow tract and tricuspid valve.

Figure 31–2. See Color Plate 10.

From the same parasternal equivalent transducer position, short-axis views may be obtained by rotation of the transducer 90 degrees clockwise. We generally pan in the short-axis orientation from the cardiac apex up through the base of the heart in order to completely interrogate each level. Short-axis views give a better appreciation of the medial versus lateral spatial orientation of valvular or flow abnormalities, which are particularly useful in guiding surgical technique.

THE AORTA–PULMONARY SULCUS TRANSDUCER POSITION (Fig. 31–3). This is obtained by placing the longer side

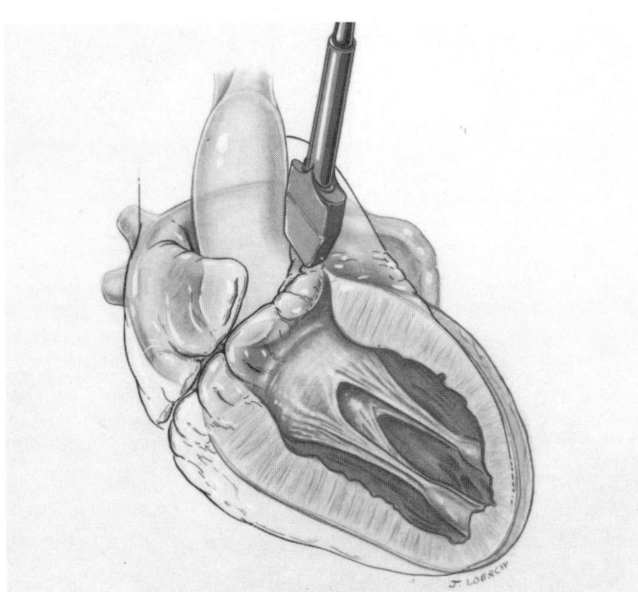

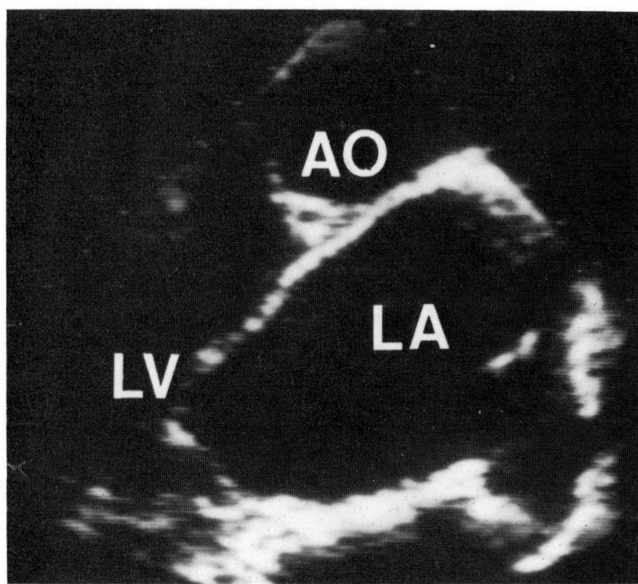

Figure 31–3. Artist's drawing (left) and two-dimensional echo image (right) of the aorta–pulmonary sulcus imaging plane used during intraoperative echocardiography. AO—aorta, LA—left atrium, LV—left ventricle. (From Stewart, W. J., et al.: Intraoperative epicardial echocardiography: Technique, imaging planes, and use in valve repair for mitral regurgitation. Dynam. Cardiovasc. Imag. 1:179, 1987, with permission.)

of the transducer against the left side of the ascending aorta in the sulcus between the aorta and the pulmonary artery. As the transducer is oriented inferiorly and medially, the left ventricular outflow tract, left atrium, mitral valve, and aortic valve are well delineated. The image resembles the parasternal equivalent long-axis image, but the aorta is angled more sharply to the top of the screen.

THE SUBCOSTAL EQUIVALENT TRANSDUCER POSITION (Fig. 31–4). This is obtained by placing the transducer against the right ventricular free wall at the inferior portion of the incision of the midsternal thoracotomy. The subcostal equivalent four-chamber view is useful for evaluation of all four chambers, the mitral valve, the tricuspid valve, the pulmonary artery, the systemic veins, and intracardiac shunts. One may angulate medially (to the right) to image the vena cavae, the atrial septum, and the left and right atria. Lateral angulation permits imaging of the right ventricle, the pulmonic valve, the pulmonary artery, and the left ventricular apex. Angling superiorly brings out a five-chamber view, including the aortic valve. Short-axis views obtained from the subcostal equivalent transducer position may be obtained by panning the image plane superiorly and inferiorly to provide another systematic overview from apex to base of the heart.

Figure 31–4. See Color Plate 10.

THE AORTA–SUPERIOR VENA CAVA TRANSDUCER POSITION (Fig. 31–5). This is the most difficult and the most important image plane that differs from standard precordial imaging. It is obtained by placing the long side of the transducer against the right side of the ascending aorta and pointing inferiorly and to the left. The ascending aorta is utilized as a "stand-off" device to put intracardiac structures, such as the aortic and mitral valves, at approximately the focal zone of the transducer (4 to 7 cm). This is the best view to evaluate outflow tract velocity for estimation of gradients because the continuous wave Doppler beam can be aligned parallel to flow. The entire left atrium, including the superior dome of the left atrium, is well visualized from this view. Although one can turn the transducer superiorly to image the aortic arch and descending aorta, these structures are better delineated with transesophageal echocardiography. Imaging the ascending aorta itself is difficult because it is in the near field; better images may be obtained by using an artificial stand-off device, such as a rubber glove filled with saline. This puts the aorta farther from the transducer, so the structures of interest are at the focal zone of the transducer.

Transducer Preparation for Epicardial Imaging

Two techniques have been employed for epicardial echocardiography. Our preference is to use nonsterile standard transducers by inserting them into two sterile sleeves. We use a second inner sleeve for added insurance against inadvertent puncture of the plastic that could cause contamination of the sterile field.[S11] Our techniques for transducer preparation have been published in video form.[S1] Alternatively, ultrasound transducers can be sterilized by "cold gas sterilization" using ethylene oxide at 100 degrees. However, damage to transducers is more likely with such sterilization. Furthermore, 48 hours of shelf time is required to allow gases to escape. The sterile sleeve technique also has the advantage of immediacy; transducers used for conventional transthoracic echo can be readily interchanged.

Transesophageal Echocardiography in the Operating Room

The transesophageal transducer uses a set of crystals mounted on the tip of a flexible endoscope. After induction of anesthesia and endotracheal intubation, we suction the stomach and remove the nasogastric tube. The transesophageal transducer is easier to introduce before placement of the anesthetic curtain and sterile drapes. Baseline transesophageal (or epicardial) images prior to cardiopulmonary bypass are useful as a reference even if major diagnostic decisions will not occur until the postpump study. Transesophageal echocardiography provides another window to the heart and great vessels that is complementary to epicardial

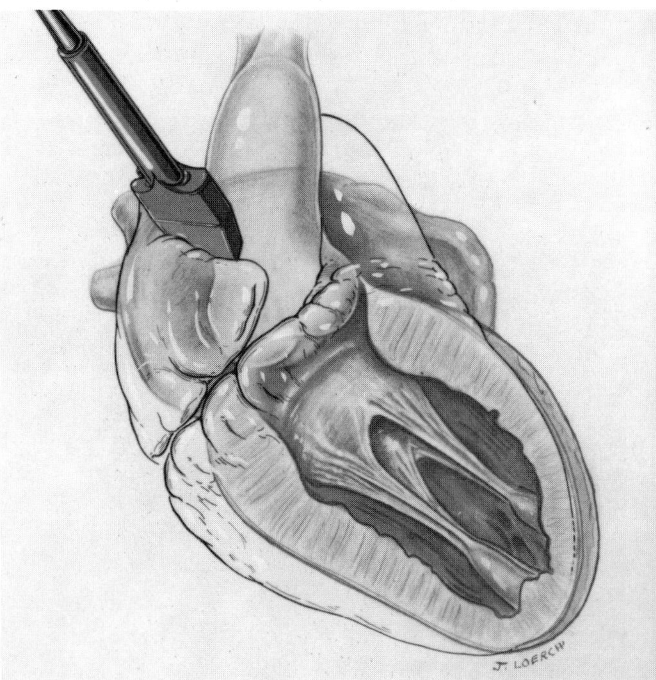

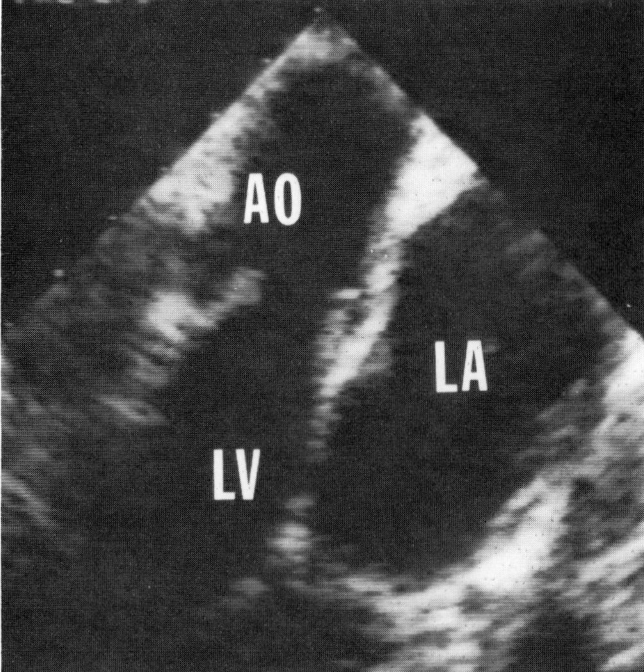

Figure 31–5. Artist's drawing (left) and two-dimensional echo image (right) of the aorta–superior vena cava image plane used during intraoperative echocardiography. AO—aorta, LA—left atrium, LV—left ventricle. (From Stewart, W. J., et al.: Intraoperative epicardial echocardiography: Technique, imaging planes, and use in valve repair for mitral regurgitation. Dynam. Cardiovasc. Imag. 1:179, 1987, with permission.)

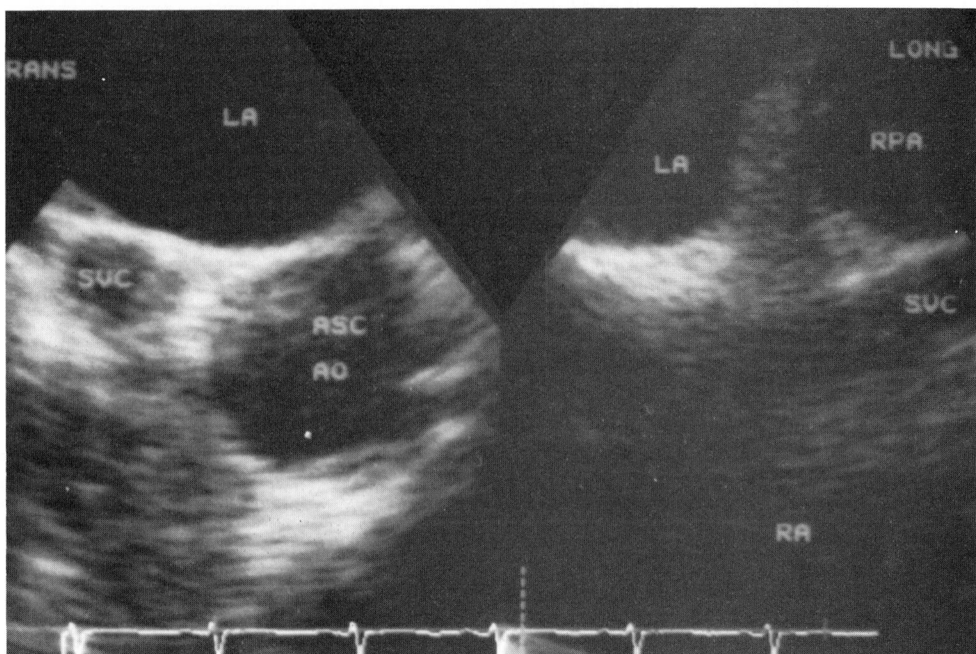

Figure 31–6. Biplane transesophageal echo images in the standard transverse (TRANS) plane (left) and the new longitudinal (LONG) plane (right), oriented to visualize the superior vena cava (SVC) to exclude thrombus. ASC AO—ascending aorta, RA—right atrium, RPA—right pulmonary artery, LA—left atrium.

imaging for intraoperative diagnosis and monitoring. Our expe- of color flow mapping from the transesophageal window. However, our operative routine has increasingly utilized transesophageal echocardiography as the method of choice for routine, intraoperative imaging. Some types of abnormalities are most amenable to transesophageal echocardiographic diagnosis. Transesophageal echocardiography images cardiac structures in the posterior part of the heart better than any other imaging technique because they are in the near field of the instrument. Transesophageal echocardiography has several advantages over epicardial imaging. Because the transducer does not enter the sterile field, it interferes less with the surgeon's activities. Transesophageal echocardiography may be performed simultaneously with surgical activities. However, simultaneous electrocautery or major surgical manipulation of the heart results in image degradation or distortion. If echocardiography is to be used in the operating room as a diagnostic procedure to answer the appropriate questions, it is important not to subjugate the quality of diagnostic imaging. The operating room lights should be dimmed and activities such as electrocautery suspended during the echocardiographic imaging.

Transesophageal Image Planes

The standard transesophageal planes[D1] emanate from the endoscope in a transverse orientation, with the image oriented perpendicular to the axis of the endoscope, as viewed from above. The standard image planes are related to each other like a stack of coins. Variations in each plane may be obtained by slight rotations of the endoscope and minor flexion of its tip. Anterior flexion may be necessary for certain planes important for intraoperative diagnosis, such as short-axis views at the mitral valve and aortic valve levels. By pushing the endoscope farther in or pulling it farther out of the esophagus, the heart can be scanned from the most inferior portion of the left ventricle (45- to 50-cm depth) to the top of the aortic arch (20- to 25-cm depth).

Recently, biplane transesophageal technology has been developed. A longitudinal image plane is oriented parallel to the long axis of the endoscope. These image planes are related to each other like the positions of a door on a hinge. Switching back and forth from the transverse to the longitudinal plane (Figs. 31–6 and 31–7) may be particularly useful for understanding the three-dimensional topography of structure or flow.

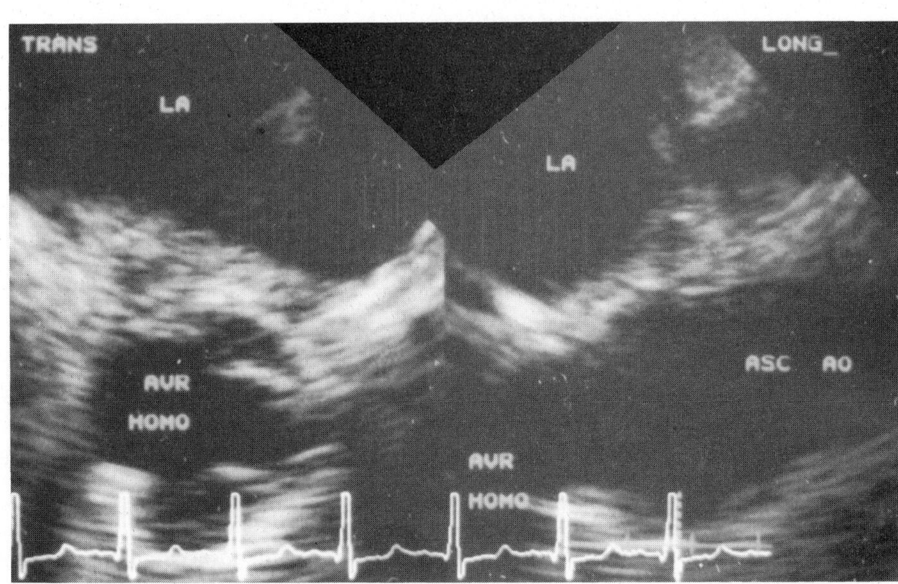

Figure 31–7. Biplane transesophageal images in transverse (TRANS) (left) and longitudinal (LONG) (right) image planes immediately after implantation of an aortic homograft (AVR HOMO). ASC AO—ascending aorta, LA—left atrium. Note the increased thickness of the aortic annulus, typical of normal homografts representing adjacent tissues of donor and recipient.

Intraoperative Echocardiography in Patients Undergoing Valvular Surgery

Surgery for valvular disease has been the primary arena in which the clinical utility of intraoperative echocardiography has been demonstrated.[C1, C2, E1, G1–G6, J1, M1–M4, S1, S4, S5, S11–S13, T1, V1] Many patients undergoing valvular surgery, particularly patients undergoing valve repair, can benefit from a judicious use of intraoperative echocardiography, prior to or after cardiopulmonary bypass or both.

Prior to cardiopulmonary bypass, intraoperative echocardiography is useful to further refine the valvular dysfunction in order to give the surgeon a more dynamic appraisal of the valve, the ventricles, the prosthesis, the shunt, or the coronary artery in question. In most circumstances, we do not advocate using the prepump intraoperative echo to decide on whether valvular surgery should be done. We advocate obtaining complete cardiac catheterization and angiographic studies and preoperative two-dimensional and Doppler echocardiographic studies in the echocardiography laboratory prior to surgery. In many cases, however, the information gained on the precardiopulmonary bypass intraoperative echocardiographic examination surpasses the preoperative data in understanding the mechanism of an abnormality. In rare cases, we have taken an emergency patient to the operating room, where the intraoperative echocardiogram has been the primary diagnostic abnormality to determine what type of surgery is performed. In borderline cases, when the preoperative clinical angiographic and echocardiographic data are equivocal and the patient requires a thoracotomy on account of another cardiac problem, we have utilized the prepump intraoperative echocardiographic studies to make a final decision on whether another valve should be repaired, replaced, or left alone.

The postpump intraoperative echocardiographic examination serves primarily to detect persistent dysfunction not adequately corrected by surgery. Additionally, the postpump study uncovers unexpected complications of surgery. Intraoperative echocardiography also is useful when weaning patients from cardiopulmonary bypass becomes difficult. For example, we have used postpump echocardiography to detect unsuspected posterior hematoma, new myocardial infarction, and iatrogenic atrial septal defect. In addition, the usefulness of documenting the absence of significant problems prior to chest closure should not be underestimated.

It is important not to distract the surgeon, the anesthesiologist, and other people from their hemodynamic observations and judgments at key times. In particular, if imaging is required in the minute immediately following cessation of cardiopulmonary bypass, it may be best to use a third individual, possibly a cardiologist/echocardiographer, who can concentrate on the imaging information. Just as distractions to the pilot and co-pilot during the take-off and landing of an airplane should be avoided, so the surgeon and anesthesiologist must be attentive to the patient at the times crucial to intraoperative imaging.

VALVE REPAIR FOR MITRAL REGURGITATION. The primary factor fueling the recent increase in popularity of intraoperative echocardiography has been the simultaneous development of Doppler color flow imaging technology and improved surgical techniques allowing nonprosthetic repair for mitral regurgitation. The techniques of Carpentier and colleagues,[C3–C5] Duran and colleagues,[D2, D3] Kay and colleagues,[K4, K5] and Cosgrove and colleagues[C6, C7] have advanced the field of valve conservation surgery substantially. Valve repair is increasingly the surgical procedure of choice in patients with mitral regurgitation. Valve repair has lower perioperative mortality, fewer perioperative complications, a lower thromboembolic risk, an improved effect on left ventricular function,[A1, B2, G5] and probably an improvement in durability and long-term survival compared with the results of mitral valve replacement.[B2, R1, S14]

However, valve repair is more technically demanding than valve replacement. In order to repair the mitral valve, the surgeon must understand the components of normal valvular function and address the specifics of each patient's particular dysfunction.

Table 31–1. UTILITY OF COLOR FLOW JET DIRECTION IN DETERMINING THE MECHANISM OF MITRAL REGURGITATION

Jet Direction	Mechanism	Most Common Etiology
Anterior	PL flail	Myx or SBE
	PL prolapse	Myx
Posterior	AL flail	Myx or SBE
	AL prolapse	Myx
	AL override with PL restriction	Rheumatic
Central	Annular dilation	Cardiomyopathy or ischemia
	Balanced restriction	Rheumatic
Commissural	Pap muscle elongation	Ischemia
	Pap muscle disruption	Ischemia
	Pap muscle fibrosis	Rheumatic
Eccentric origin	Leaflet perforation	SBE

PL—posterior leaflet; AL—anterior leaflet; Pap—papillary; SBE—endocarditis; Myx—myxomatous degeneration.

Preoperative echocardiography is the most useful tool available to determine the dynamic pathology of the valve and the dynamics of the regurgitant jet. The improved image resolution afforded by the intraoperative approach may add to the surgeon's understanding of the techniques required for valve repair. We have found a good correlation between the findings of preoperative echocardiography and the direct inspection of the valve by the surgeon.[S15] The "tool box" required for repair of various valves for mitral regurgitation varies from quite simple to quite complex maneuvers.[C3, C4, C6, C7] Accurate data obtained in the echocardiographic laboratory can be used to determine the feasibility of repair and to select a surgeon who has experience with the specific surgical maneuvers required to repair that patient's valve.

Determination of the direction of the mitral regurgitant jet with color flow mapping is useful in learning which leaflet suffers from inadequate chordal support (Table 31–1).[S16] The majority of patients who have ruptured or elongated chordae to the anterior leaflet show a posterior jet direction by color flow mapping. The majority of patients who have similar posterior leaflet abnormalities show an anterior jet direction by color flow mapping (Fig. 31–8). A second cause of posterior jet direction is the common pattern of anterior leaflet overriding seen in rheumatic mitral regurgitation, in which the posterior leaflet is more severely restricted than the anterior leaflet.

Figure 31–8. See Color Plate 11.

Another pattern of jet direction is observable when the mitral regurgitant jet emanates from the medial or lateral commissure. Izumi and associates reported jet direction recorded with color flow mapping in patients with ischemic mitral regurgitation.[I1] When the posteromedial papillary muscle was infarcted, the jet emanated from the medial commissure and angled laterally across the mid-left atrium. When the anterolateral papillary muscle was infarcted (a less common occurrence), the jet emanated from the lateral commissure and traversed across the mid-left atrium in a medial direction.

When restricted leaflet motion, affecting both leaflets equally, is the primary abnormality causing mitral regurgitation, a central jet direction is usually seen. This occurs most commonly in patients with rheumatic heart disease in whom the chordae to both mitral leaflets become contracted. Like a door that is too small for the door frame, the leaflets become too small, compared with a normal-sized annulus. A similar common phenomenon resulting from multiple etiologies is isolated mitral annular dilatation, which also causes a central jet direction. Although the leaflets are normal in size, like an oversized door frame, the annulus is too large for the leaflets.

The last type of jet seen in mitral regurgitation is the eccentric jet origin. In leaflet perforation, the jet origin is displaced away from the leaflet coaptation site.

The prepump intraoperative echocardiogram in our institutions has been a primary motivating influence in improved communication between echocardiographers and cardiac surgeons. The availability of images with improved anatomic detail in the operating room has led to an improved understanding and trust on the part of our surgical team in echocardiographic diagnosis. In addition, familiarity with the operating theater has motivated the echocardiographers to obtain a direct correlation of their results with the operative inspection of the valve.

THE POSTPUMP INTRAOPERATIVE ECHO IN VALVE REPAIR FOR MITRAL REGURGITATION. Echocardiography after repair for mitral regurgitation is an extremely useful addition to the surgical process. In the majority of cases, when the results of the postpump echocardiogram show a satisfactory result (Figs. 31–2 and 31–9), the surgical team is reassured that subsequent hemodynamic changes are not due to failure of the surgical repair itself. Unfortunately, in approximately 8 percent of our patients, the echocardiograph has revealed persistent regurgitation (see Fig. 31–4) or other data that lead to a change in operative plans.[M2, S3] Certainly, the entire clinical picture of that patient must be taken into account. Our policy is to return patients to cardiopulmonary bypass when they have persistent mitral regurgitation that is moderate in severity (2 plus on a 4 plus scale) or greater on the postpump echocardiograph.

Figure 31–9. See Color Plate 11.

Intraoperative echocardiography is a reliable way to predict which patients will have a satisfactory clinical outcome and which will fare poorly. Early in our experience, two patients' postpump intraoperative echocardiogram showed significant mitral regurgitation after repair. Because the left atrial pressure and cardiac index were borderline normal, we chose to close the chest and not operate further. Both patients required reoperation within 5 days, because of failure to wean from mechanical ventilation and persistent pulmonary edema.[S3]

In a subset of patients undergoing valvuloplasty with the Carpentier technique using a stiff annular ring, the phenomenon of dynamic left ventricular outflow tract obstruction with systolic anterior motion has been observed[K6, K7, S17] (Fig. 31–10). We have noted this intraoperatively in approximately 3 to 4 percent of patients undergoing this procedure.[S3, S17] Continuous wave Doppler echocardiography performed from the aorta–superior vena cava transducer position is useful in estimating the severity of obstruction.[S18] In some patients with mild obstruction, the outflow tract gradient and concomitant mitral regurgitation can be reduced by volume loading and discontinuing all catecholamine administration. In others, the amount of mitral regurgitation, the severity of obstruction, and the difficulty in weaning from cardiopulmonary bypass may require a second pump run for correction of the difficulty. Successful correction has entailed removal of the annular ring in some patients and replacement of the mitral valve with a prosthesis in others.[S1, S3, S17]

When mitral regurgitation is found on the postpump study after an initial attempt at valve repair, the detailed evaluations of valvular motion and jet direction are even more important in understanding the mechanism of regurgitation. In these settings, the surgeon has already done his or her best attempt at repair of the problem and needs guidance in determining whether the same dynamic pathology persists or whether a new mechanism of dysfunction has occurred as a consequence of the surgical maneuvers.

INTRAOPERATIVE ECHOCARDIOGRAPHIC EVALUATION IN AORTIC VALVE REPAIR. Although less advanced than mitral repairs, techniques of repairing abnormal aortic valves have been reported.[F3] The aortic valve is more difficult than the mitral valve to repair because of less valvular tissue and material with which to work. Accordingly, the frequency of failed repair discovered on the postpump intraoperative echocardiograph is higher in aortic repair than in mitral repair. Nevertheless, the potential advantages of avoiding implantation of prosthetic material may still be considerable.

In patients undergoing valve repair for aortic stenosis, we find it very useful before and after cardiopulmonary bypass to document the gradient with continuous wave Doppler, recorded from the aorta–superior vena cava transducer position (Fig. 31–11). The improvement in maximal instantaneous gradient in our series of patients undergoing valve repair for aortic stenosis was substantial, from an average of 56 mmHg to an average of 21 mmHg. However, in approximately 12 percent of cases, the postpump intraoperative echocardiograph showed moderate (2 plus or more) aortic regurgitation, necessitating further surgery for aortic valve replacement during the same thoracotomy.[S13]

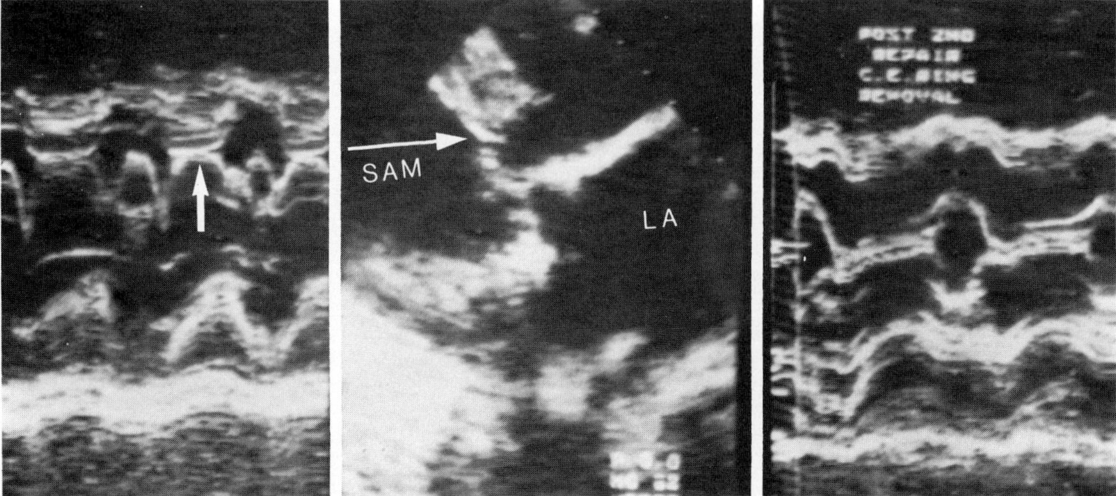

Figure 31–10. Sequential intraoperative M-mode echocardiograph studies in failed valve repair for mitral regurgitation caused by dynamic outflow tract obstruction. *Left*, After repair showing mitral systolic anterior motion *(vertical arrow)*. *Middle*, Parasternal long axis two-dimensional echocardiograph showing systolic anterior motion of the mitral valve *(arrow)*. *Right*, After removal of Carpentier-Edwards ring during a second pump run, the systolic anterior motion resolved completely. (From Cosgrove, D. M., and Stewart, W. J.: Mitral valvuloplasty. Curr. Prob. Cardiol. 14:355, 1989, with permission.)

Figure 31–11. See Color Plate 11.

Figure 31–12. See Color Plate 12.

In our series of patients undergoing valve repair for aortic regurgitation (Fig. 31–12), 10 to 15 percent also required a second pump run due to persistent (2 plus or more) aortic regurgitation on the postpump intraoperative echocardiogram.[S13] Again, the two-dimensional echocardiograph (Fig. 31–13) and color flow mapping examinations help define the mechanism of aortic regurgitation and show exactly what surgical tools are available to remedy the problem. The transesophageal echocardiograph also affords a new diagnostic tool that is particularly helpful for patients whose aortic insufficiency is due to aneurysm or dissection[G7] (Fig. 31–14).

Figure 31–14. See Color Plate 12.

The aortic valve homograft is an increasingly attractive alternative to aortic valve replacement, particularly in individuals who are young or have endocarditis. The operation is technically more demanding and reimplantation of the coronary arteries is often required. A major difficulty in successfully implanting an aortic homograft is in achieving adequate support of the implanted annulus and commissures (see Fig. 31–7). When distortion of the aortic valve occurs during implantation, the resultant aortic regurgitation may be substantial. Intraoperative echocardiography after implantation of a homograft may provide useful reassurance of its competency.

INTRAOPERATIVE ECHOCARDIOGRAPHY DURING OPEN MITRAL COMMISSUROTOMY FOR MITRAL STENOSIS. Echocardiography has been used to predict the feasibility of balloon valvuloplasty, based on a grading system of the amount of subvalvular disease, leaflet immobility, leaflet calcification, and leaflet thickening.[W1] Similarly, the prepump echocardiograph in patients with mitral stenosis shows the extent of debridement that will be required in addition to simple commissurotomy. Although uncommon, we have seen some patients in whom the severity of mitral regurgitation has increased after mitral commissurotomy. In some cases, placement of an annular ring during a second pump run may provide adequate mitral competence.[S1]

INTRAOPERATIVE ECHOCARDIOGRAPHY DURING SURGERY FOR HYPERTROPHIC CARDIOMYOPATHY. For patients with persistent symptoms despite maximal medical therapy and significant dynamic outflow tract obstruction, myectomy is an effective way to reduce symptoms and improve prognosis. Baseline studies in the operating room prior to cardiopulmonary bypass are essential, with estimation of gradient based on the maximal velocity from continuous wave Doppler (Fig. 31–15). On the postpump studies, the amount of mitral regurgitation, the outflow tract gradient, and the absence of induced ventricular septal defect are important parameters for echocardiographic study.[S18, S19] On these studies, we routinely administer isoproterenol infusions to bring out latent obstruction. A postpump gradient of over 50 mmHg (either at rest or with provocation) warrants a second pump run for further myectomy.

PROSTHETIC VALVE REPLACEMENT. Transesophageal echocardiography is an important tool in preoperative workup of prosthetic dysfunction. However, most patients who have simple, first-time prosthetic valve replacement do not benefit substantially from intraoperative echocardiography. Epicardial or transesophageal studies of normally functioning prosthetic valves commonly show a small regurgitant jet (Fig. 31–16), caused by "physiologic" regurgitation, representing the blood required to close the poppet. In occasional patients, we have detected perivalvular leaks early after surgery that have been repaired on a second cardiopulmonary bypass run. In patients whose indication for surgery was a periprosthetic leak (Fig. 31–17), the echocardiograph can pinpoint the location of the perivalvular regurgitation.[C8, S20, S21] Postpump echocardiography after suture closure of the leak is useful in verifying its resolution or pointing out the need for further surgery.

Figure 31–16. See Color Plate 12.

Figure 31–17. See Color Plate 12.

VALVE REPAIR FOR TRICUSPID REGURGITATION. For patients undergoing surgery for tricuspid regurgitation, valve repair is a common choice.[C5] Preoperative echocardiography is useful in documenting the type of tricuspid valvular disease, the

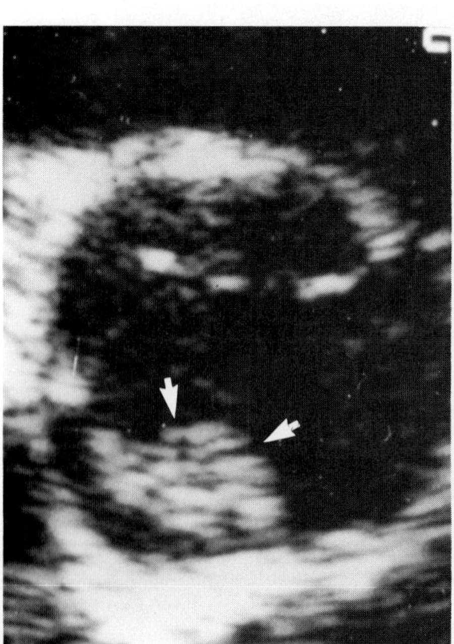

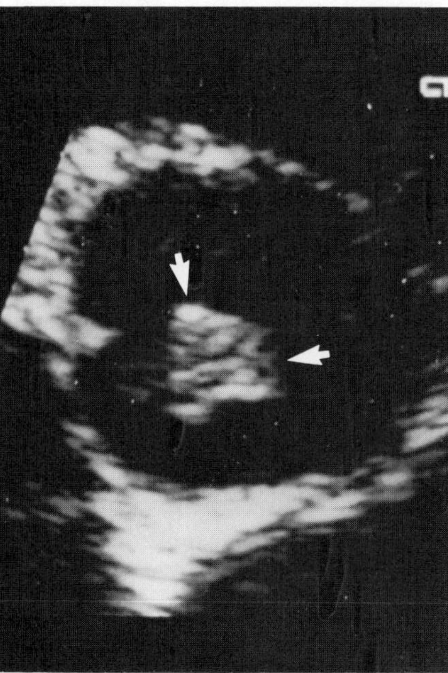

Figure 31–13. Short-axis views of the aortic valve in systole (left), and diastole (right, at slightly less magnification) showing a mobile 1.5-cm vegetation (arrowheads) attached to the noncoronary cusp.

DOPPLER ESTIMATED GRADIENT = 96 mmHg

VELOCITY SPECTRUM

4.9m/sec

PRESSURES

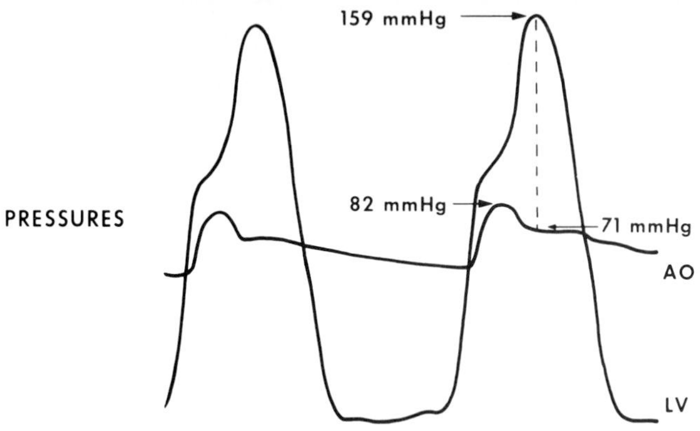

INSTANTANEOUS GRADIENT = 88 mmHg

Figure 31–15. Intraoperative Doppler determination of outflow tract gradient in hypertrophic cardiomyopathy, showing simultaneous spectral tracing of the high-velocity jet (top) and the left ventricular (LV) and aortic (AO) pressures. (From Stewart, W. J. et al.: Intraoperative Doppler echocardiography in hypertrophic cardiomyopathy: Correlations with the obstructive gradient. J. Am. Coll. Cardiol. 10(2):327–335, 1987. Reprinted with permission of the American College of Cardiology.)

presence of leaflet thickening, and the degree to which leaflet support is abnormal. Intraoperative echocardiography can document the amount of regurgitation prior to cardiopulmonary bypass, and the resolution of the regurgitation afterward[G3, S2] (Fig. 31–18). The amount of tricuspid regurgitation is even more dependent than mitral regurgitation on the loading conditions present at the time of study. For this reason, not all patients who reveal tricuspid regurgitation on Doppler or color flow mapping should have tricuspid surgery. In patients undergoing operation for left-sided valvular or myocardial problems, "functional" tricuspid regurgitation is common, in which the amount of regurgitation improves merely with correction of the left-sided cardiac abnormality. Tricuspid surgery is indicated in patients who have right-sided heart failure and structural tricuspid leaflet or annular abnormalities that cause severe tricuspid insufficiency. After tricuspid repair, when the postpump intraoperative echocardiogram shows substantial tricuspid regurgitation, consideration should be made for a second cardiopulmonary bypass run with tricuspid valve replacement or further repair. This alternative is far better than discovering postoperatively that the patient's left-sided valvular problem is improved but the tricuspid regurgitation warrants another operation at a future date.

Figure 31–18. See Color Plate 13.

Coronary Arterial Imaging by Ultrasound

Intraoperative coronary angiography can be used for coronary visualization, but it requires fixed radiographic installations in the operating room, which are uncommon and expensive. In patients with coronary artery disease, intraoperative echocardiography may be useful to determine physiology, such as coronary flow reserve (using Doppler techniques), to assess myocardial perfusion (using contrast echo), and to image the coronary arteries directly. Imaging coronary arteries and coronary bypass grafts intraoperatively is an area that may be fruitful for practical intraoperative decisions, to evaluate immediately the results of intraoperative revascularization procedures. Such imaging has also been utilized to study the physiology of atherosclerosis.

Because the coronary arterial walls and lumen are so small, higher frequency probes are required for direct imaging that can resolve small arterial structures. The 12-MHz instrument has a resolution of 0.1 to 0.2 mm at imaging depths of 1 to 2 cm.[M5, M6, S22] The transducer is hand-held by the surgeon and placed on the exposed left anterior descending or right coronary arteries on the anterior surface of the heart. Filling the pericardial well with saline creates a stand-off between the imaging site and the probe; compression of vein grafts is thereby avoided and images improved. Unfortunately, imaging of the lateral and posterior arteries is more difficult due to the size of the present device.

Intraoperative images from the beating heart are made just prior to the institution of cardiopulmonary bypass. This is necessary in order to image the arteries at physiologic distending pressure. Imaging during cardiopulmonary bypass yields views of collapsed arteries that are difficult to interpret. The images are recorded on videotape; a simultaneous audio recording allows the surgeon to describe the location of the image by reference to external landmarks (distance from the coronary arterial origin, distance from lateral margins) and by branch points.

After the completion of cardiopulmonary bypass, imaging can again be done of native arteries and of bypass grafts. The bypass graft–native vessel anastomosis and the bypass graft–aorta anastomosis can also be visualized.

Examples of normal and diseased native coronary arteries are shown in Figure 31–19. Images in either longitudinal or transverse planes are obtainable. In general, we have chosen to image native arteries in the transverse plane in order to more easily quantify the degree of atherosclerosis. The normal coronary arteries appear as a sonolucent lumen surrounded by bright arterial walls; the latter are in turn surrounded by loose adventitial tissue. Atherosclerotic lesions protrude into the coronary lumen to varying degrees, resulting in residual lumina that are round, oval, or complex in shape and variably located within the original lumen. Calcified atheromatous plaques result in shadowing, that is, loss of images of more distal structures because of the highly reflective calcification.

Quantitative measurements can be made of arterial wall thickness, lumen diameters, and lumen area from transverse arterial images. The accuracy of these images has been verified in both animals and humans.[M7] In animal studies, echocardiographic lumen diameters correlate well with diameters estimated by sonomicrometry. Measurements of lumen areas and wall thickness obtained by echocardiography correlate well with similar measurements from pressure-distended histologic preparations. Intraoperative echocardiography images from normal and diseased coronary arteries obtained from fresh human postmortem coronary arterial specimens were compared with histologic preparations from the same specimens, with excellent correlations.

HIGH-FREQUENCY EPICARDIAL ECHOCARDIOGRAPHY FOR EVALUATION OF GRAFT–NATIVE VESSEL CORONARY ANASTOMOSES. Epicardial echocardiography has been useful for evaluating graft–native vessel bypass anastomoses. The probe is placed on the anastomotic site, using either longitudinal or transverse image orientation. Good correlations were demonstrated in a canine model between graft–native vessel anastomosis diameter measurements by the high-frequency echo-

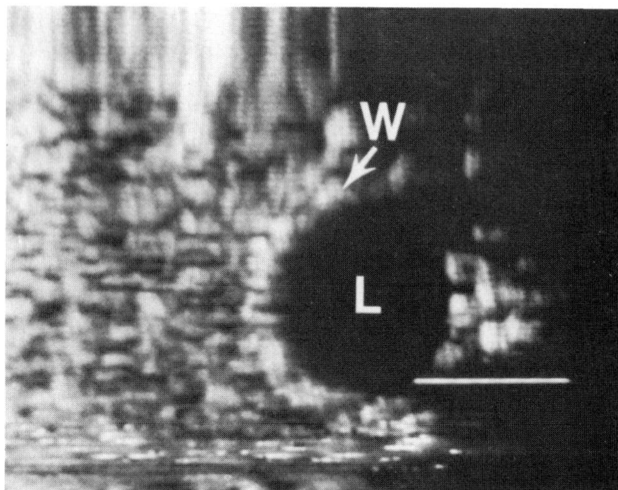

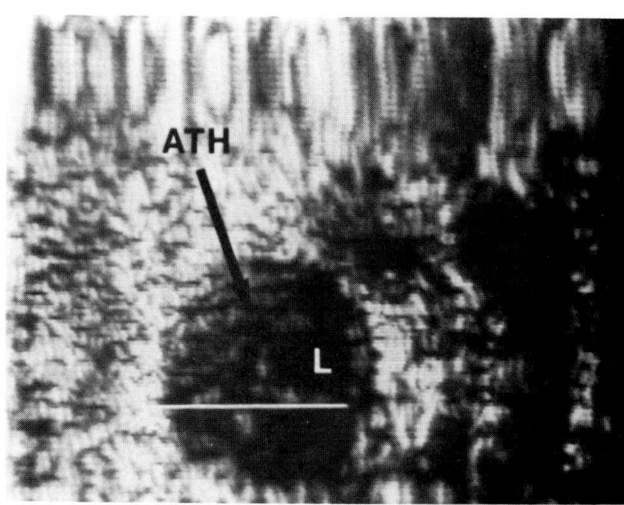

Figure 31–19. Examples of high-frequency epicardial echocardiographic coronary arterial images recorded intraoperatively. A transverse section of a normal coronary artery is shown on the left, and a diseased coronary artery is shown on the right. The arterial lumen is much reduced because of atherosclerosis, and the residual lumen is eccentrically placed. W—wall, L—lumen, ATH—atheroma. Calibration bar—3 mm. (From McPherson, D. D., and Kerber, R. E.: High frequency epicardial echocardiography for the intraoperative demonstration and evaluation of coronary atherosclerosis. Echocardiography 3:371, 1986, with permission.)

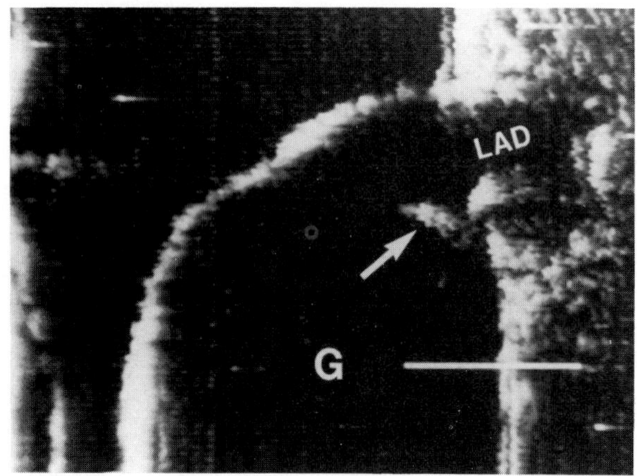

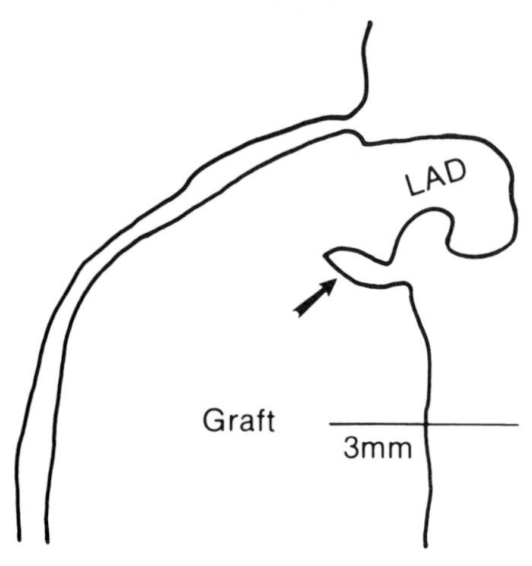

Figure 31–20. Experimental vein graft coronary artery anastomosis: High-frequency epicardial echocardiographic study of a deliberate technical error. A large vein graft (G) was sutured end-to-side to a small coronary artery (LAD) with a venous valve flap *(arrow)* deliberately incorporated into the anastomosis and partially obstructing it. (From Hiratzka, L. F., et al.: Intraoperative evaluation of coronary artery bypass graft anastomoses using high frequency epicardial echocardiography: Experimental validation and initial patient studies. Circulation 73:1199, 1986, with permission of the American Heart Association, Inc.)

cardiography technique and by histologic preparations taken from the same area (r = 0.92).[M5] In addition, deliberately created technical deficiencies or errors could be demonstrated. Such deliberate mistakes included incorporation of venous valves into the anastomotic opening (Fig. 31–20) and also excessively deep suturing resulting in "tenting" of the posterior arterial wall into the anastomotic opening.

Examples of the intraoperative images are shown in Figures 31–21 and 31–22. Figure 31–21 shows a good end-to-side anastomosis. An example of a less satisfactory anastomosis is shown in Figure 31–22, which demonstrates an atherosclerotic plaque in the native coronary artery opposite the graft anastomosis and a relatively small side-to-side anastomosis. The criteria for a satisfactory result are that the size of anastomosis of the graft to the native vessel should be larger than the native vessel diameter at the point of bypass. This seems better accomplished by end-to-side anastomosis[H3] (Fig. 31–23) than by side-to-side anastomosis.

The proximal anastomosis (Fig. 31–24) between the vein and aorta also can be imaged.[H4] Occasional instances of unsatisfactory anastomosis between grafts and native vessels have been encountered. Figure 31–25 shows almost total occlusion of an anastomosis between an internal mammary artery and a native coronary artery.[H4] On the basis of this echocardiogram, this stenotic anastomosis was immediately revised.

At present, internal mammary arteries are preferred to native vein bypass grafting because of greater durability.[L1] However, these arteries are smaller than saphenous veins. We compared anastomosis from internal mammary arteries to native coronary vessels versus similar saphenous vein–native coronary anastomosis to be certain that the smaller size of the internal mammary artery did not result in an anastomosis too small, which might be prone to subsequent occlusion. We found that although internal mammary arteries are indeed smaller than saphenous vein grafts upon high-frequency epicardial echocardiographic imaging, the size of the distal anastomoses is the same. This supports the use of internal mammary arteries for bypass procedures.[S23]

High-frequency echocardiography can also be used to demonstrate the position and location of arteries deeply embedded in epicardial fat, thereby avoiding prolonged dissection that would otherwise be necessary to locate such arteries.[H5] This is particularly applicable on reoperations.

PATHOLOGIC AND PHYSIOLOGIC CORRELATIONS WITH HIGH-FREQUENCY EPICARDIAL ECHOCARDIOGRAPHY. In addition to practical surgical applications of the high-frequency echocardiographic technique, other scientific information has been obtained that furthers our understanding of the atherosclerotic process. Comparisons with angiography have shown that the angiogram frequently underestimates the degree of coronary atherosclerosis. Particularly when atherosclerosis is diffuse rather than discrete, its severity is often not appreciated from the angiographic images. An example of this is shown in Figure 31–26, in which a diffuse encircling atheroma is well visualized by high-frequency echocardiography but less apparent by angiographic examination.[M5]

Coronary atherosclerotic lesions vary markedly in size and shape.[W2] The high-frequency echocardiographic technique can also obtain detailed information in vivo regarding the shape of atherosclerotic lumina, which can be oval, circular, or complex. Circular lumina have been defined as those with a major-to-minor lumen diameter ratio of 1.5:1 or less, whereas oval lumina have a diameter ratio greater than 1.5:1. In one study of 31 lesions, circular lumina were found in 15, oval lumina in 13, and complex lumina in 3. Even in these atherosclerotic arteries, a portion of the arterial wall was within the range of normal wall thickness (< 0.7 mm) in 16 of the 31 lesions; such preserved segments of arterial wall may retain vasoreactivity and/or contribute to coronary spasm.[M8]

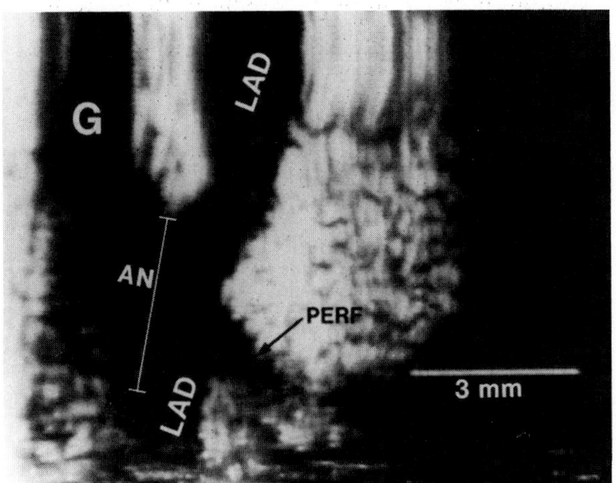

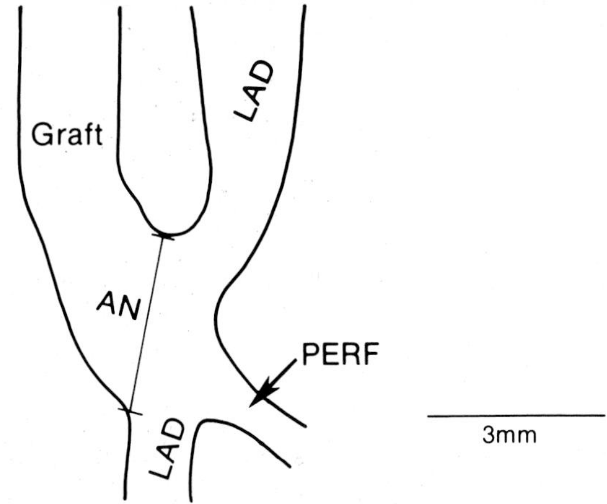

Figure 31–21. Intraoperative recording of an end-to-side anastomosis (AN) of a vein graft (G) to a native left anterior descending coronary artery (LAD). There is mild narrowing of the proximal portion of the LAD at the anastomosis, but the luminal diameters of the anastomosis and native artery are not compromised. Also note a septal perforator (PERF) opposite the anastomosis. (From Hiratzka, L. F., et al.: Intraoperative evaluation of coronary artery bypass graft anastomoses using high frequency epicardial echocardiography: Experimental validation and initial patient studies. Circulation 73:1199, 1986, with permission of the American Heart Association, Inc.)

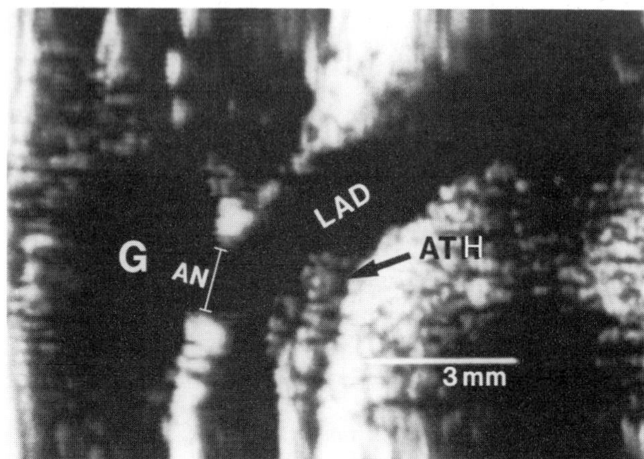

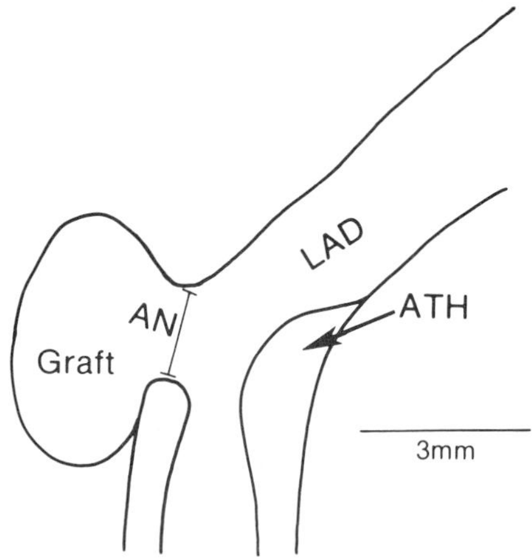

Figure 31–22. Intraoperative recording of a side-to-side vein graft (G) to a left anterior descending coronary artery (LAD) anastomosis (AN). Note the atherosclerotic plaque (ATH) opposite the anastomotic site. Also note that the luminal diameter of this side-to-side anastomosis is relatively small in comparison with the LAD diameter. Compare with the end-to-side anastomosis of Fig. 31–21. (From Hiratzka, L. F., et al.: Intraoperative evaluation of coronary artery bypass graft anastomoses using high frequency epicardial echocardiography: Experimental validation and initial patient studies. Circulation 73:1199, 1986, with permission of the American Heart Association, Inc.)

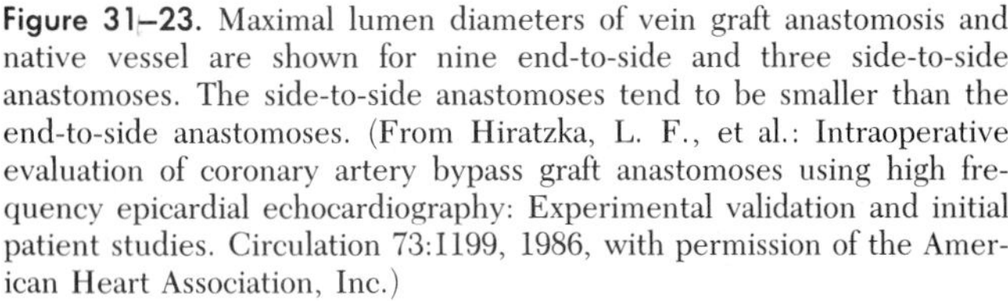
Figure 31–23. Maximal lumen diameters of vein graft anastomosis and native vessel are shown for nine end-to-side and three side-to-side anastomoses. The side-to-side anastomoses tend to be smaller than the end-to-side anastomoses. (From Hiratzka, L. F., et al.: Intraoperative evaluation of coronary artery bypass graft anastomoses using high frequency epicardial echocardiography: Experimental validation and initial patient studies. Circulation 73:1199, 1986, with permission of the American Heart Association, Inc.)

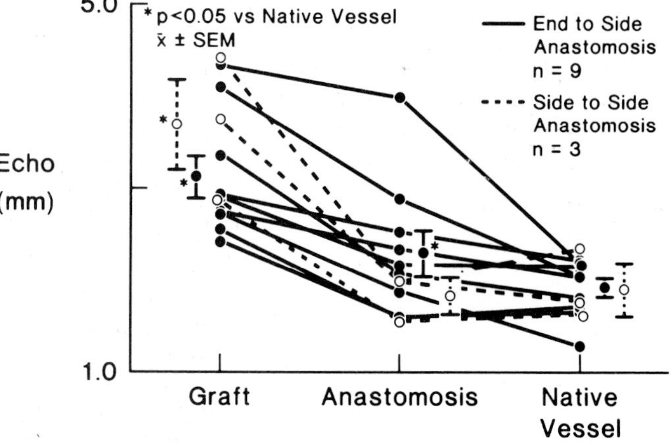

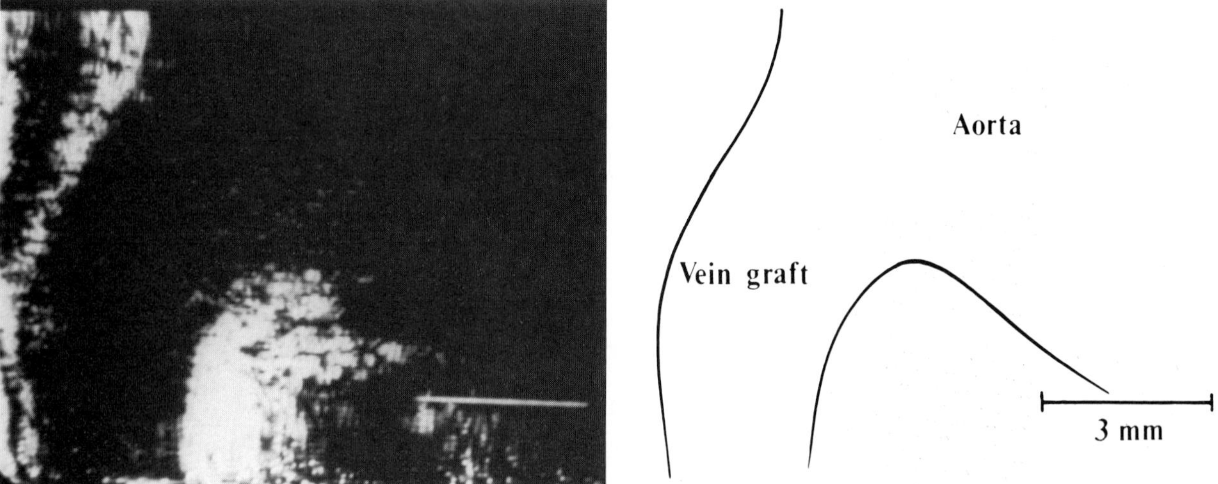

Figure 31–24. Intraoperative recording of an anastomosis between an aorta and a saphenous vein. (From Hiratzka, L. F., et al.: The role of intraoperative high frequency epicardial echocardiography during coronary revascularization. Circulation 76(Suppl. II):V–33, 1987, with permission of the American Heart Association, Inc.)

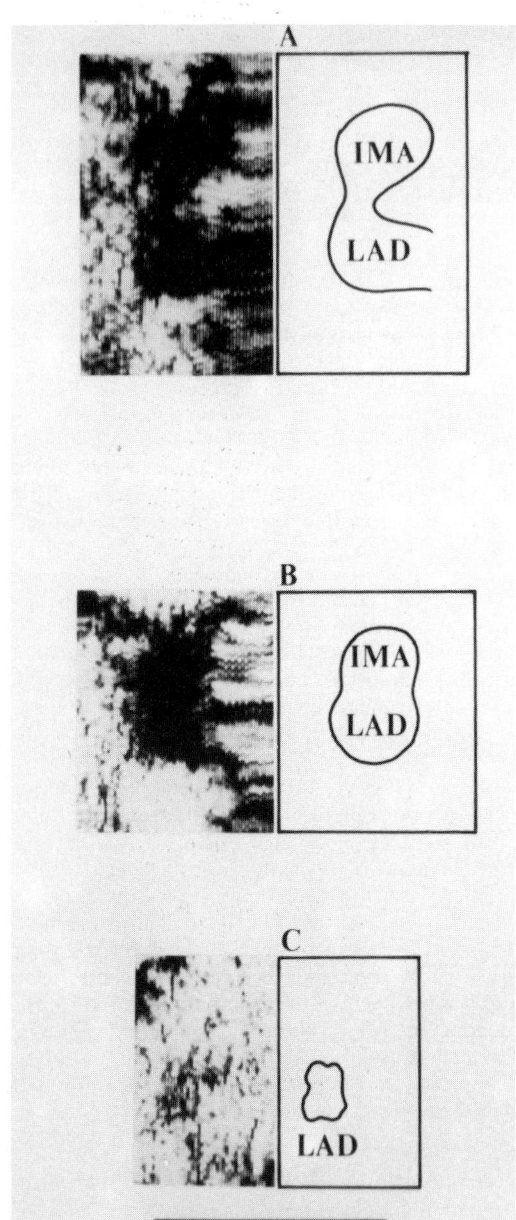

Figure 31–25. Intraoperative recording of an unsatisfactory anastomosis between an internal mammary artery and a native coronary artery. *A*, *B*, and *C* show progressively more severe stenosis of the anastomoses in different imaging planes. This technically inadequate anastomosis was immediately revised after this recording was obtained. IMA—Internal mammary artery, LAD – left anterior descending coronary artery. (From Hiratzka, L. F., et al.: The role of intraoperative high frequency epicardial echocardiography during coronary revascularization. Circulation 76(Suppl. II):V–33, 1987, with permission of the American Heart Association, Inc.)

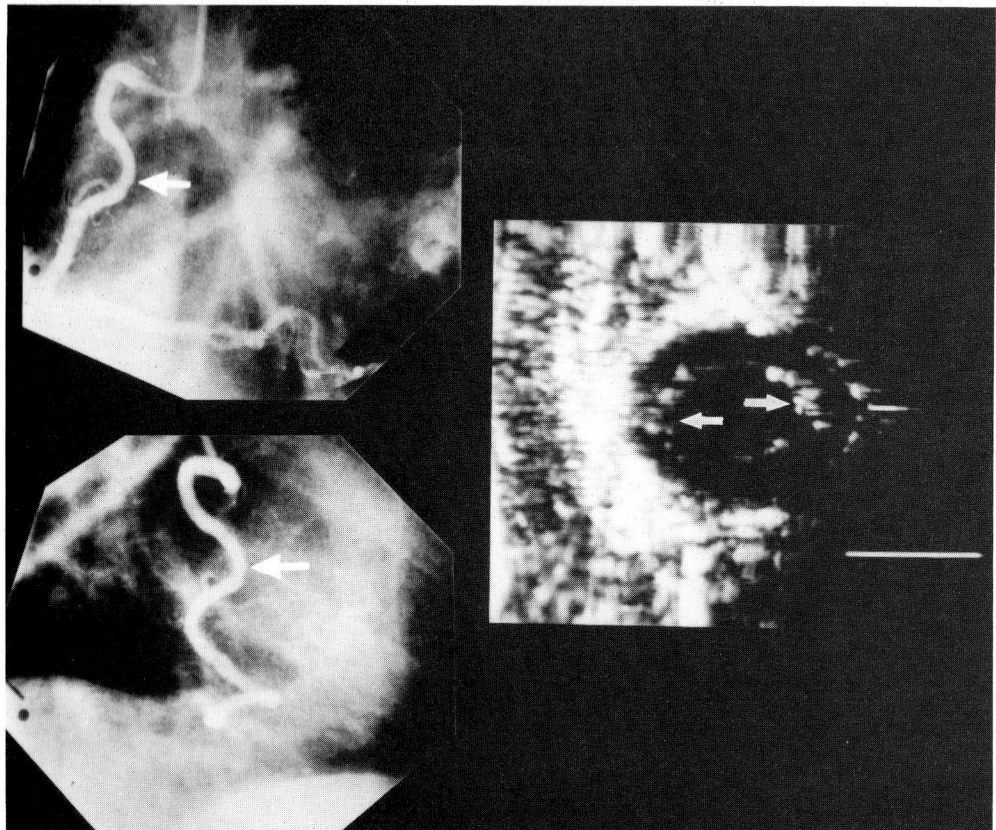

Figure 31–26. Echocardiographic image of a right coronary artery *(right panel)* with corresponding cine angiograms in the left anterior oblique *(upper left)* and right anterior oblique *(lower left)* projections. The arrows on the cine angiograms indicate the point at which the echocardiographic image was recorded. Although only minimal irregularity is demonstrated by cine angiography, the high-frequency echocardiographic recording shows that an encircling atheromatous lesion is present *(white arrows)*. (From McPherson, D. D., et al.: Delineation of the extent of coronary atherosclerosis by high frequency epicardial echocardiography. N. Engl. J. Med. 316:304, 1987, with permission.)

During the development of coronary atherosclerosis, the coronary artery size and shape may change, a process we have referred to as arterial remodeling. This process may minimize the obstructive effect of developing atherosclerotic plaques by preserving lumen size. The process has been previously demonstrated by pathologic studies in coronary arteries of atherosclerotic primates[A2] and humans.[G8] Using the high-frequency echocardiographic technique, we have demonstrated remodeling in the coronary arteries of patients coming to surgery.[M9] This remodeling process occurs earlier than the development of angiographically visible collaterals.[M10]

We have also correlated coronary lumen size assessed by the high-frequency echocardiographic technique with the degree of reactive hyperemia following a brief period (20 seconds) of coronary occlusion deliberately induced intraoperatively by the surgeon. Significant differences occur between the reactive hyperemia of echocardiographically normal coronary vessels compared with arteries that have high-frequency echo-demonstrated coronary atherosclerosis. Thus, there is a good correspondence between echo-demonstrated anatomic abnormalities and Doppler functional assessment of coronary flow reserve.[M11]

Ultrasonic catheters that can image arteries from within the arterial lumen are currently being developed.[M12, P3, Y1] Such probes can image at 20 to 40 MHz and may provide images of unparalleled detail. It is quite likely that intraoperative intra-arterial coronary imaging using such devices will be of major assistance in assessing coronary artery pathology, both before and during coronary revascularization procedures. At present, high-frequency epicardial echocardiographic visualization of coronary arteries is a useful technique for assisting the surgeon intraoperatively and for enhancing our understanding of the pathologic anatomy of coronary atherosclerosis.

Determination of Left Ventricular Function and Myocardial Perfusion

Intraoperative echocardiography also can be useful in determining left ventricular function during cardiac and noncardiac surgery.[P4, S24–S26, T2] The left ventricle can be imaged using the transesophageal or epicardial approach, in order to determine improvement in dysfunctional segments,[T2] the effects of anesthetic agents, or the development of new wall motion abnormalities induced by ischemia or acute changes in loading conditions.[S25] The echocardiogram provides a direct estimate of preload from the end-diastolic ventricular size, which appears to be more reliable than pulmonary capillary wedge pressure in determining requirements for volume expansion.

Contrast echocardiography to evaluate myocardial perfusion may be useful during coronary bypass operations.[G9, K8, L2, M13, S27, S28] Demonstration of the perfusion territory of a coronary vessel, its "area of risk," by means of contrast echocardiography has been useful in documenting the success of coronary grafting.[S28] Identifying areas with the lowest perfusion in ischemic heart disease may lend itself to appraisal with contrast-enhanced echocardiography in order to avoid perioperative infarction. Spontaneous intraluminal microbubbles are quite common after cardiopulmonary bypass, despite efficient venting and effective surgical technique.[R2]

Intraoperative Echocardiography in Congenital Heart Disease

Intraoperative echocardiography has an important role in surgery for a variety of congenital cardiac problems.[H6] The prepump intraoperative echocardiogram is an important avenue for exchange of communication between cardiologist and surgeon, particularly in patients with complex congenital heart disease. The preoperative data can often be refined because of improved acoustic access and the absence of volitional movement. Some specific questions can be addressed that are not answerable with the preoperative data. For example, a key question we have answered is the size of great vessels to which the surgeon wants to construct a shunt (Fig. 31–27).

Figure 31–27. See Color Plate 13.

The postpump intraoperative assessment with echocardiography may detect new or residual abnormalities. After placement of a baffle or patch, it may be useful to look for residual shunting before closure of the chest (Fig. 31–28). It may also be useful to monitor gradients before and after adjustments in a pulmonary artery band. More complex repairs have more potential for shortcomings that can be determined by the echocardiogram and corrected, saving the patient a second thoracotomy.

Figure 31–28. See Color Plate 13.

Conclusion

Intraoperative echocardiography is an extremely useful tool. We consider it a mandatory portion of the surgery in patients undergoing valve repair. The prepump study is the best way to define the dynamic abnormalities of anatomy and physiology that are present. Two-dimensional echocardiography and color flow mapping provide the "road map" for valve repair, in the same way that the coronary arteriogram provides the road map for coronary bypass surgery. Postpump intraoperative studies may demonstrate important abnormalities that can be corrected during a second run of cardiopulmonary bypass. Intraoperative echocardiography remains an exciting and rapidly developing field of great importance to the process of cardiac surgery.

Acknowledgments

We thank Paula LaManna, Jo Rolph, and Peggy Cornell for their help in preparation of this manuscript.

References

A

1. Angell, W. W., Oury, J. H., and Shah, P.: A comparison of replacement and reconstruction in patients with mitral regurgitation. J. Thorac. Cardiovasc. Surg. 93:665, 1987.
2. Armstrong, M. L., Heistad, D. D., Marcus, M. L., et al.: Structural and hemodynamic responses of peripheral arteries of macaque monkeys to atherogenic diet. Arteriosclerosis 5:336, 1985.

B

1. Bolger, A. F., Eigler, N. L., Pfaff, J. M., and Maurer, G.: Quantitative color flow imaging: In vitro assessment of new and conventional parameters of flow. Echocardiography 5:417, 1988.
2. Bonchek, L. I., Olinger, G. N., Siegel, R., et al.: Left ventricular performance after mitral reconstruction for mitral regurgitation. J. Thorac. Cardiovasc. Surg. 88:122, 1984.

C

1. Currie, P. J., Stewart, J. W., Salcedo, E. E., et al.: Comparison of intraoperative transesophageal and epicardial color flow Doppler in mitral valve repair. (Abstract.) J. Am. Coll. Cardiol. 11:2A, 1988.
2. Czer, L. S., Maurer, G., Bolger, A. F., et al.: Intraoperative evaluation of mitral regurgitation by Doppler color flow mapping. Circulation 76:III–108, 1987.
3. Carpentier, A.: Cardiac valve surgery—The "French correction." J. Thorac. Cardiovasc. Surg. 86:323, 1983.
4. Carpentier, A., Chauvaud, S., Fabianai, J. N., et al.: Reconstructive surgery of the mitral valve incompetence: Ten-year appraisal. J. Thorac. Cardiovasc. Surg. 79:338, 1980.
5. Carpentier, A., Deloche, A., Dauptain, J., et al.: A new reconstructive operation for correction of mitral and tricuspid insufficiency. J. Thorac. Cardiovasc. Surg. 61:1, 1971.
6. Cosgrove, D. M., Chavez, A. M., Gill, C. C., et al.: Mitral valvuloplasty at The Cleveland Clinic Foundation. Cleveland Clin. J. Med. 55:37, 1988.
7. Cosgrove, D. M., Chavez, A. M., Lytle, B. W., et al.: Results of mitral valve reconstruction. Circulation 74(Suppl. I):I–82, 1986.
8. Currie, P. J., Schiavone, W. A., Stewart, W. J., et al.: Evaluation of mitral prosthetic dysfunction with transesophageal color flow Doppler in ambulatory patients. (Abstract.) Circulation 76:IV–39, 1987.

D

1. DeBruijn, N. P., and Clements, F. M.: Transesophageal Echocardiography. Martinus Nijhoff Publishing, The Hague, Netherlands, 1987.
2. Duran, C. G., Pomar, J. L., Revuelta, J. M., et al.: Conservative operation for mitral insufficiency: Critical analysis supported by postoperative hemodynamic studies of 72 patients. J. Thorac. Cardiovasc. Surg. 79:326, 1980.
3. Duran, C. G., and Ubago, J. L.: Clinical and hemodynamic performance of a totally flexible prosthetic ring for atrioventricular valve reconstruction. Ann. Thorac. Surg. 22:458, 1976.

E

1. Eguaras, M. G., Pasalodos, J., Gonzalez, V., et al.: Intraoperative contrast two-dimensional echocardiography: Evaluation of the presence and severity of aortic and mitral regurgitation during cardiac operations. J. Thorac. Cardiovasc. Surg. 89:573, 1985.

F

1. Fairly, K. F.: Influence of atrial size and elasticity of the left atrial pressure tracing. Br. Heart J. 23:512, 1961.
2. Fuchs, R. M., Heuser, R. R., Yin, F. C. P., and Brinker, J. A.: Limitations of pulmonary wedge V-waves in diagnosing mitral regurgitation. Am. J. Cardiol. 49:849, 1982.
3. Freeman, W. K., Schaff, H. V., and Orszulak, T. A.: Ultrasonic aortic valve decalcification serial Doppler echocardiographic follow-up. Circulation 78:II–379, 1988.

G

1. Goldman, M. E., Mindich, B. P., and Nanda, N. C.: Intraoperative echocardiography: Who monitors the flood once the flood gates are opened? J. Am. Coll. Cardiol. 11:1362, 1988.
2. Goldman, M. E., Mindich, B. P., Teichholz, L. E., et al.: Intraoperative contrast echocardiography to evaluate mitral valve operations. J. Am. Coll. Cardiol. 4:1035, 1984.
3. Goldman, M. E., Fuster, V., Guarino, T., and Mindich, B. P.: Intraoperative echocardiography for the evaluation of valvular regurgitation experience in 263 patients. Circulation 74:I–143, 1986.
4. Goldman, M. E., and Mindich, B. P.: Intraoperative two-dimensional echocardiography: New application of an old technique. J. Am. Coll. Cardiol. 7:374, 1986.
5. Goldman, M. E., Mora, F., Guarino, T., et al.: Mitral valvuloplasty is superior to valve replacement for preservation of left ventricular function: An intraoperative two-dimensional echocardiographic study. J. Am. Coll. Cardiol. 10:568, 1987.
6. Gussenhoven, E. J., Van Herwerden, L. A., Roelandt, J., et al.: Intraoperative two-dimensional echocardiography in congenital heart disease. J. Am. Coll. Cardiol. 9:565, 1987.
7. Goldman, M. E., Guarino, T., and Mindich, B. P.: Localization of aortic dissection intimal flap by intraoperative two-dimensional echocardiography. J. Am. Coll. Cardiol. 6:1155, 1985.
8. Glacov, S., Weisenberg, E., Zarins, C. K., et al.: Compensatory enlargement of human atherosclerotic coronary arteries. N. Engl. J. Med. 316:1371, 1987.
9. Goldman, M. E., and Mindich, B. P.: Intraoperative cardioplegic contrast echocardiography for assessing myocardial perfusion during open heart surgery. J. Am. Coll. Cardiol. 4:1029, 1984.

H

1. Hatle, L., and Angelson, B.: Doppler Ultrasound in Cardiology; Physical Principles and Clinical Applications. Lea and Febiger, Philadelphia, 1985.
2. Helmcke, F., Nanda, N. C., and Hsiung, M. C.: Color Doppler assessment of mitral regurgitation with orthogonal planes. Circulation 75:175, 1987.
3. Hiratzka, L. F., McPherson, D. D., Lamberth, W. C., et al.: Intraoperative evaluation of coronary artery bypass graft anastomoses using high frequency epicardial echocardiography: Experimental validation and initial patient studies. Circulation 73:1199, 1986.
4. Hiratzka, L. F., McPherson, D. D., Brandt, B., et al.: The role of intraoperative high frequency epicardial echocardiography during coronary revascularization. Circulation 76(Suppl. II):V–33, 1987.
5. Hiratzka, L. F., McPherson, D. D., Brandt, B., et al.: Intraoperative high frequency epicardial echocardiography in coronary revascularization: Locating deeply embedded coronary arteries. Ann. Thorac. Surg. 442:S9, 1986.
6. Hagler, D. J., Tajik, A. J., Seward, J. B., et al.: Intraoperative two-dimensional Doppler echocardiography: A preliminary study for congenital heart disease. J. Thorac. Cardiovasc. Surg. 95:516, 1988.

I

1. Izumi, S., Miyatake, K., Beppu, S., et al.: Mechanism of mitral regurgitation in patients with myocardial infarction: A study using real time two-dimensional Doppler flow imaging and echocardiography. Circulation 76:777, 1987.

J

1. Johnson, M. L., Holmes, J. H., Spangler, R. D., and Paton, B. C.: Usefulness of echocardiography in patients undergoing mitral valve surgery. J. Thorac. Cardiovasc. Surg. 64:922, 1972.

K

1. Kent, E. M., Ford, W. B., Fisher, D. L., and Childs, T. B.: Estimation of the severity of mitral regurgitation, correlation of direct left atrial pressure

recording with observations made during surgical palpation of valve area. Ann. Surg. 141:47, 1955.
2. King, H., Csicsko, J., and Leshnower, A.: Intraoperative assessment of the mitral valve following reconstructive procedures. Ann. Thorac. Surg. 29:81, 1980.
3. Kisslo, J.: Color Doppler Echocardiography. Lea and Febiger, Philadelphia, 1987.
4. Kay, E. B., Nogueira, C., Head, L. R., et al.: Surgical treatment of mitral insufficiency. J. Thorac. Cardiovasc. Surg. 36:677, 1958.
5. Kay, G. L., Kay, J. H., Zubiate, P., et al.: Mitral valve repair for mitral regurgitation secondary to coronary artery disease. Circulation 74(Suppl. I):I–88, 1986.
6. Kreindel, M. S., Schiavone, W. A., Lever, H. M., and Cosgrove, D.: Systolic anterior motion of the mitral valve after Carpentier ring valvuloplasty for mitral valve prolapse. Am. J. Cardiol. 57:408, 1986.
7. Kronzon, I., Cohen, M. L., Winer, H. E., and Calvin, S. B.: Left ventricular outflow obstruction: Complication of mitral valvuloplasty. J. Am. Coll. Cardiol. 4:825, 1984.
8. Keller, M. W., Kaul, S., Spotuitz, W. D., and Duling, B. R.: Perfusion with cardioplegia solution changes microbubble rheology: Implications for intraoperative myocardial contrast echocardiography. (Abstract.) Circulation 80:II–371, 1989.

L

1. Loop, F. D., Lytle, B. W., Cosgrove, D. M., et al.: Influence of the internal mammary artery graft on 10 year survival and other cardiac events. N. Engl. J. Med. 314:1, 1986.
2. Lim, Y. J., Nanto, S., Masuyama, T., et al.: Visualization of subendocardial myocardial ischemia with myocardial contrast echocardiography in humans. Circulation 79:233, 1989.

M

1. Mindich, B. P., Goldman, M. E., Fuster, V., et al.: Improved intraoperative evaluation of mitral valve operations utilizing two-dimensional contrast echocardiography. J. Thorac. Cardiovasc. Surg. 90:112, 1985.
2. Marwick, T., Currie, P. J., and Stewart, W. S.: Echo evaluation of immediate and late failed mitral valve repair. (Abstract.) J. Am. Coll. Cardiol. 13:114A, 1989.
3. Mary, D. A. S., Catchpole, L. A., and Ionescu, M. I.: Intraoperative echocardiographic studies of the mitral valve; Assessment of commissurotomy and repair. JCU 4:349, 1976.
4. Maurer, G., Czer, L. S. C., Chaux, A., et al.: Intraoperative Doppler color flow mapping for assessment of valve repair for mitral regurgitation. Am. J. Cardiol. 60:333, 1987.
5. McPherson, D. D., Hiratzka, L. F., Lamberth, W. C., et al.: Delineation of the extent of coronary atherosclerosis by high frequency epicardial echocardiography. N. Engl. J. Med. 316:304, 1987.
6. McPherson, D. D., and Kerber, R. E.: High frequency epicardial echocardiography for the intraoperative demonstration and evaluation of coronary atherosclerosis. Echocardiography 3:371, 1986.
7. McPherson, D. D., Armstrong, M., Rose, E., et al.: High frequency epicardial echocardiography for coronary arterial evaluation: In vitro and in vivo validation of arterial lumen and wall thickness measurements. J. Am. Coll. Cardiol. 8:600, 1986.
8. McPherson, D. D., Collins, S. M., Hunt, M., et al.: Ultrasonic intraoperative evaluation of coronary lesions. (Abstract.) J. Am. Coll. Cardiol. 7:1A, 1986.
9. McPherson, D. D., Hunt, M., Hiratzka, L. F., et al.: Coronary atherosclerosis causes remodeling of arterial geometry. Demonstration by high frequency epicardial echocardiographic studies. (Abstract.) Circulation 74:II–468, 1986.
10. McPherson, D. D., Hiratzka, L. F., Meng, R., et al.: Coronary arterial remodeling precedes collateral formation and obstructive coronary atherosclerosis: High frequency intraoperative epicardial echocardiographic studies. (Abstract.) Circulation 76:IV–42, 1987.
11. McPherson, D. D., Hiratzka, L. F., Brandt, B., et al.: Relationship of echo-demonstrated atherosclerosis to reactive hyperemia. (Abstract.) Circulation 74:II–85, 1986.
12. McKay, C., Waller, B., Gessert, J., et al.: Quantitative analysis of coronary artery morphology using intracoronary high frequency ultrasound: Validation by histology and quantitative coronary arteriography. (Abstract.) J. Am. Coll. Cardiol. 13:228A, 1989.
13. Matthew, T. L., Keller, M. W., Kaul, S., and Spotuitz, W. D.: Assessment of myocardial perfusion during coronary artery bypass operations in humans using myocardial contrast echocardiography. Surg. Forum 40:248, 1989.

N

1. Nair, K. K., and Yates, A. K.: Direct evaluation of mitral valve function during surgery following conservation procedures. J. Thorac. Cardiovasc. Surg. 73:684, 1977.

O

1. Omoto, R.: Color Atlas of Real-Time Two-Dimensional Doppler Echocardiography. Shindan-to-Chiryo Company, Ltd., Tokyo, 1984.

P

1. Pagliero, K. M., and Yates, A. K.: Preoperative assessment of mitral valve function. J. Thorac. Cardiovasc. Surg. 63:458, 1972.
2. Pomar, J. L., Cucchiara, G., Gallo, I., and Duran, C. M. G.: Intraoperative assessment of mitral valve function. Ann. Thorac. Surg. 25:354, 1978.
3. Pandian, N., Kreis, A., Desnoyers, M., et al.: In vivo ultrasound angioscopy in humans and animals: Intraluminal imaging of blood vessels using a new catheter-based high resolution ultrasound probe. (Abstract.) Circulation 78:II–22, 1988.
4. Panidis, I. P., and Morganroth, J.: The use of echocardiography in the operating room. *In* Pohost, G. M., Higgins, C. B., Morganroth, J., et al. (eds.): New Concepts of Cardiac Imaging 1986. Year Book Medical Publishers, Chicago, 1986, p. 91.

R

1. Rankin, J. S., Feneley, M. P., Hicky, M. S. J., et al.: A clinical comparison of mitral valve repair versus valve replacement in ischemic mitral regurgitation. J. Thorac. Cardiovasc. Surg. 95:165, 1988.
2. Rodigas, P. C., Meyer, R. J., Haasler, G. B., et al.: Intraoperative 2-dimensional echocardiography: Ejection of microbubbles from the left ventricle after cardiac surgery. Am. J. Cardiol. 50:1130, 1982.

S

1. Stewart, W. J., Currie, P. J., Agler, D. A., and Cosgrove, D. M.: Intraoperative epicardial echocardiography: Technique, imaging planes, and use in valve repair for mitral regurgitation. Dynam. Cardiovasc. Imag. 1:179, 1987.
2. Stewart, W. J., Currie, P. J., Lytle, B. W., et al.: The role of intraoperative echocardiography during cardiac valvular surgery. (Abstract.) J. Am. Coll. Cardiol. 11:217A, 1988.
3. Stewart, W. J., Currie, P. J., Salcedo, E. E., et al.: Intraoperative Doppler color flow mapping for decision making in valve repair for mitral regurgitation: Technique and results in 100 patients. Circulation 81:556, 1990.
4. Stewart, W. J., Gill, C. C., Currie, P. J., et al.: Intraoperative Doppler color flow mapping in valve conservation surgery. (Abstract.) Circulation 74:II–145, 1986.
5. Stewart, W. J., Salcedo, E. E., Schiavone, W. A., et al.: Intraoperative assessment of mitral regurgitation using Doppler color flow mapping. (Abstract.) Tenth World Congress of Cardiology, Washington, D.C., 1986, p. 247.
6. Stewart, W. J., Levine, R. A., Main, J., and King, M. E.: Initial experience with color-coded Doppler flow mapping. Echocardiography 2:511, 1985.
7. Sahn, D. J.: Instrumentation and physical factors related to visualization of stenotic and regurgitant jets by Doppler color flow mapping. J. Am. Coll. Cardiol. 12:1254, 1988.
8. Sahn, D. J., Chungk, J., Tamurat, R., et al.: Factors affecting jet visualization by color flow mapping Doppler echo: In vitro studies. (Abstract.) Circulation 74:II–271, 1986.
9. Stewart, W. J., Schiavone, W. A., and From, J. A.: In vitro studies of Doppler color flow mappings: Dependence of spatial distribution on instrument settings. (Abstract.) Circulation 72:III–98, 1985.
10. Switzer, D. F., Yoganathan, A. P., and Nanda, N. C.: Calibration of color Doppler flow mapping during extreme hemodynamic conditions in vitro: A foundation for a reliable quantitative grading system for aortic incompetence. Circulation 75:837, 1987.
11. Stewart, W. J., Currie, P. J., Agler, D. A., et al.: Intraoperative echocardiography does not increase the incidence of postoperative sternal wound infections. (Abstract.) Echocardiography 4:458, 1987.
12. Spotnitz, H. M., Malm, J. R., King, D. L., et al.: Outflow tract obstruction in tetralogy of Fallot: Intraoperative analysis by echocardiography. N.Y. State J. Med. 78:1100, 1978.
13. Stewart, W. J., Currie, P. H., Salcedo, E. E., et al.: Intraoperative echocardiography in aortic valve repair. Circulation 78:II–435, 1988.
14. Sand, M. E., Naftel, D. C., Blackstone, E. H., et al.: A comparison of repair and replacement for mitral valve incompetence. J. Thorac. Cardiovasc. Surg. 94:208, 1987.
15. Stewart, W. S., Chavez, A. M., Currie, P. J., et al.: Echo determination of mitral pathology and feasibility of repair for mitral regurgitation. (Abstract.) Circulation 76:III–434, 1987.
16. Stewart, W. J., Currie, P. J., Salcedo, E. E., et al.: Jet direction by color flow mapping accurately depicts the mechanism of mitral regurgitation. (Abstract.) Circulation 78:II–434, 1988.
17. Schiavone, W. A., Cosgrove, D. M., Lever, H. M., et al.: Long-term follow-up of patients with left ventricular outflow tract obstruction following Carpentier ring mitral valvuloplasty. Circulation 78:I–60, 1988.
18. Stewart, W. J., Schiavone, W. A., Salcedo, E. E., et al.: Intraoperative Doppler echocardiography in hypertrophic cardiomyopathy: Correlations with the obstructive gradient. J. Am. Coll. Cardiol. 10:327, 1987.
19. Syracuse, D. C., Gaudiani, V. A., Kastl, D. G., et al.: Intraoperative, intracardiac echocardiography during left ventriculomyotomy and myectomy for hypertrophic subaortic stenosis. Circulation 58(Suppl. I):I–24, 1978.
20. Stewart, W. J., Agler, D. A., Koch, J. M., and Currie, P. J.: Color flow mapping diagnosis and localization of paravalvular aortic regurgitation. (Abstract.) Circulation 76:IV–448, 1987.
21. Stewart, W. J., Currie, P. J., Agler, D. A., et al.: Peri-prosthetic mitral and aortic regurgitation: Utility of pre- and intraoperative Doppler color flow mapping. (Abstract.) J. Am. Coll. Cardiol. 11:20A, 1988.

22. Sahn, D. J., Barrett-Boyes, B. G., Graham, K., et al.: Ultrasonic imaging of the coronary arteries in open chest humans: Evaluation of atherosclerotic lesions during cardiac surgery. Circulation 66:1034, 1982.
23. Sirna, S. J., McPherson, D. D., Meng, R., et al.: Intraoperative high frequency echo comparison of internal mammary artery vs. saphenous vein to native coronary anastomosis. (Abstract.) Circulation 78(Suppl. II):II–419, 1988.
24. Sahn, D. J.: Intraoperative applications of two-dimensional and contrast two-dimensional echocardiography for evaluation of congenital, acquired, and coronary heart disease in open-chested humans during cardiac surgery. *In* Rijstergorgh, H. (ed.): Echocardiology. Martinus Nijhoff Publishers, The Hague, Netherlands, 1981, p. 9.
25. Smith, J. S., Cahalan, M. K., Benefiel, D. J., et al.: Intraoperative detection of myocardial ischemia in high-risk patients: Electrocardiography versus two-dimensional transesophageal echocardiography. Circulation 72:1015, 1985.
26. Spotnitz, H. M.: Two-dimensional ultrasound and cardiac operations. J. Thorac. Cardiovasc. Surg. 83:43, 1982.
27. Sahn, D. J.: Cardiovascular diagnosis by ultrasound: Transesophageal, computerized, contrast, Doppler echocardiography. *In* Hanrath, P., Bleifeld, W., and Souquet, J. (eds.): Developments in Cardiovascular Medicine. Martinus Nijhoff Publishers, The Hague, Netherlands, 1982, p. 294.
28. Spotnitz, W. D., Keller, M. W., Watson, D. D., et al.: Success of internal mammary bypass grafting can be assessed intraoperatively using myocardial contrast echocardiography. J. Am. Coll. Cardiol. 12:196, 1988.

T

1. Takamoto, S., Kyo, S., Adachi, H., et al.: Intraoperative color flow mapping by real-time two-dimensional Doppler echocardiography for evaluation of valvular and congenital heart disease and vascular disease. J. Thorac. Cardiovasc. Surg. 90:802, 1985.
2. Topol, E. J., Weiss, J. L., Guzman, P. A., et al.: Immediate improvement of dysfunctional myocardial segments after coronary revascularization: Detection by intraoperative transesophageal echocardiography. J. Am. Coll. Cardiol. 4:1123, 1984.

V

1. Van Herwerden, L. A., Gussenhoven, W. J., Roelandt, J., et al.: Intraoperative epicardial two-dimensional echocardiography. Eur. Heart J. 7:386, 1986.

W

1. Wilkens, G. T., Weymman, A. E., Abascal, V. M., et al.: Percutaneous mitral valvuloplasty related to outcome and the mechanism of dilatation. Br. Heart J. (in press).
2. Waller, B. F.: The eccentric coronary atherosclerotic plaque. Morphologic observations and clinical relevance. Clin. Cardiol. 12:14, 1989.

Y

1. Yock, P., Linker, D., Saether, O., et al.: Intravascular two-dimensional catheter ultrasound: Initial clinical studies. (Abstract.) Circulation 78:II–21, 1988.

Part VI

Ultrafast Computed Tomography

Chapter 32

Principles and Instrumentation for Dynamic X-Ray Computed Tomography

R. A. ROBB, Ph.D. ▪ *R. L. MORIN, Ph.D.*

HISTORY 634
BASIC PRINCIPLES 635
Fundamental Radiation Physics 635
Reconstruction from Projections 637
Image Quality 639
ENGINEERING SYNTHESIS 641
The Gantry 641
The Couch 641
The X-Ray Tube 641
The Detector 641
The Computer 643
The Display 643
DYNAMIC THREE-DIMENSIONAL COMPUTED TOMOGRAPHY 643
Needs 643
Gated Computed Tomography of the Heart 644
Stop-Action Computed Tomography of Moving Organs 645
The Fast Computed Tomography Scanner 645
Radiation Dosimetry 647
Slice Thickness and Contiguity 648
Spatial Resolution 648
Low-Contrast Resolution 648
Uniformity 649
Noise 649
Hounsfield Unit Linearity 649
Half-Value Layer 650
The Mayo Dynamic Spatial Reconstructor 650
The Scanner 652
Analysis and Display 656
Basic Imaging Performance 656
Applications 657
Image Display and Analysis 659
CONCLUSION 665

The discovery[G1] of x-rays in 1895 opened a new era in the practice of medicine: visualization into the body without painful and often life-threatening surgery. The discovery was almost immediately recognized and accepted for its potential as a new medical diagnostic technique. During the past 95 years, there have been numerous improvements in the methodology. These advances have been spurred by the development of more sophisticated and powerful instruments and techniques that have broadened and refined the utilization of x-rays for medical imaging.

X-ray imaging is essentially noninvasive. Modest risks are incurred due to the ionizing effect of the x-ray,[S1] but these risks are usually acceptable because of the diagnostic advantages provided by direct visualization of intracorporeal structures when such examination is indicated by illness and associated symptoms.

However, conventional x-ray imaging techniques have several important limitations: (1) much detail is lost in the radiographic process because of superposition of three-dimensional structural information on a two-dimensional detector, (2) small characteristic differences (1–2 percent) in x-ray attenuation by various body tissues are not detectable in recordings on x-ray film or fluoroscopic screens, and (3) a large percentage of the radiation detected is scattered from the patient, which reduces the true signal-to-noise ratio of the recorded information. The development of x-ray computed tomography (CT) in the 1970's had a revolutionary impact on diagnostic imaging with x-rays because it eliminated or greatly minimized these problems and provided a capability for noninvasive examination of internal structures of the body with an accuracy and specificity previously unavailable.

HISTORY

The mathematical basis for computed tomography is known as image reconstruction. In 1917 an Austrian mathematician, J. Radon, derived an analytic formulation applicable to the problem of reconstructing an object from its projections.[R1] Radon's formulation is the basis for the now most commonly used image reconstruction technique—the convolution method, sometimes known as filtered back projection.

In the 1950's, mathematical image reconstruction techniques were independently developed and applied in a variety of scientific investigations. These applications included solar radio astronomy[B1, C1] and electron microscopy,[C2, D1] although significant efforts in the latter field were not published until nearly a decade later. Bracewell[B1] first discussed a Fourier transform method for image reconstruction of solar microwave emissions, and the method was later described mathematically by Crowther and associates[C2] for reconstruction in electron microscopy.

The applicability of mathematical image reconstruction techniques in radiographic medical imaging was first studied in the late 1950's and early 1960's independently by Oldendorf and Cormack. Oldendorf published[O1] the first attempt at a medical application of image reconstruction and suggested that the technique could be used to image transverse sections of the head. Cormack was interested in determining the distribution of attenuation coefficients in tissues of the body in order to improve radiation treatment planning. His early studies[C3, C4] led to a mathematically accurate method for quantitative reconstruction of images from x-ray projections (radiographs), for which he received the Nobel Prize in 1979.[D2]

In the 1960's, Kuhl and Edwards developed the first practical, clinically applied gamma emission (not x-ray transmission) CT scanner,[K1] which detected the transaxial distribution of radionuclides in the brain. They recognized the limitations associated with conventional tomography and introduced transverse section scanning to avoid these problems. This technique is a form of the basic reconstruction method known as summation, or *simple back projection*, but it is limited by the blurring of sharp features inherent in the method.

In 1967, Bracewell and Riddle[B2] proposed the mathematical basis for a direct approximation of Radon's integral formula, which came to be known as the *convolution method*. This approach was also discovered by Ramachandran and Lakshminarayanan,[R2] who derived a numerically implementable formulation. The convolution method, modified and refined in one way or another by several investigators, was to become the method of choice for implementation with most x-ray CT scanners developed in the latter half of the 1970's.

Also in the late 1960's, British scientist Godfrey Hounsfield was independently developing ideas that mathematical techniques could be used to reconstruct the internal structure of the body from a number of different x-ray measurements. He showed that a quantitative tomographic technique could produce up to 100 times more accurate measurements of the absolute value of x-ray attenuation coefficients within the body than conventional radiographic methods.[H1] These efforts eventually resulted in construction of the first clinical x-ray CT scanner, the EMI brain scanner, which was installed at Atkinson Morleys Hospital, Wimbledon, England, in 1971. The results obtained with the EMI brain scanner were presented in 1972, followed by the now-classic publications in 1973[A1, H2] that heralded the revolutionary era of diagnostic x-ray computed tomography. Hounsfield accomplished the remarkable synthesis of (1) recognizing the diagnostic need, (2) developing a numerically implementable mathematical solution to the image reconstruction problem, and (3) organizing electromechanical and x-ray technology in a precisely engineered instrument that resulted in a successful clinical machine. The award to Hounsfield in 1979 of the Nobel Prize,[D2, H1] which was shared with Cormack, recognized perhaps the greatest advance in diagnostic imaging in over 75 years and provided significant scientific credibility to the field of computed medical imaging.

With the successful introduction of the EMI brain scanner in the clinical arena, an explosive development and marketing of CT scanners by a variety of manufacturers followed. Notable was Robert Ledley's development,[L1] in the academic environment of Georgetown University, of the first CT scanner for the body as well as the head, called the ACTA scanner. This development opened the door to a variety of designs of computed tomographic scanners directed at improving scan speed and accuracy while maintaining the comfort and safety of the patient.

By 1976, more than 20 companies were producing one or more models of x-ray CT scanners for commercial purposes. By 1980, this number had decreased significantly, as smaller companies realized they could not compete with major radiographic equipment manufacturers. The decade of the 1980's saw CT scanners installed in more than 1000 medical institutions throughout the world and a prodigious accumulation of published data,[D3] and experience related to a wide variety of clinical applications of these and newer-generation computed tomography systems in biomedical research is just beginning to be realized.

BASIC PRINCIPLES

Fundamental Radiation Physics

A beam of x-rays passing through the body is differentially absorbed and scattered by structures in the beam path. The amount of absorption depends on the physical density and atomic composition of these structures and on the energy of the x-ray beam. For equivalent x-ray energy, a more dense structure will attenuate the beam more than a less dense structure. This pattern of differential absorption by tissues within the body is carried in the transmitted x-ray beam and recorded by the x-ray detector, usually film.

Even though two spatially separated x-ray beams of equal energy may be recorded by the detector as having nearly equal total attenuation, they may have passed through entirely different materials. This is because attenuation is dependent on path length through an object as well as on the object's physical density and atomic composition. In such cases, it is impossible to "see" or determine from the detector (film) the different materials through which the beam passed. The attenuations at different points along the beam path accumulate and are superimposed on the same points on the detector, as illustrated in the left panel of Figure 32–1, with the result that only in regions where high density differences exist between adjacent structures can details be clearly discerned in the film, as in the case of the ribs (bone) against the lungs (air).

Conventional longitudinal (axial) tomography, which was developed in the 1930's,[E1, K2] attempts to overcome the superposition problem, as illustrated in the center panel of Figure 32–1. However, the problem of superposition is not eliminated. Small density differences are difficult to detect or estimate in conventional tomograms, owing to superposition and scattering, even under favorable conditions of small field size and low x-ray energy.[E1]

In computed (transaxial) tomography, scatter is minimized by collimating the beam and superposition is eliminated by scanning around a transaxial plane, as shown in the right panel of Figure 32–1. The x-ray transmitted through the plane or slice is measured with detectors, which can record intensity differences less than 0.1 percent, and the individual attenuation coefficients of structures in the beam path can be determined to within 0.5 percent accuracy from a mathematically analyzed set of these measurements.

Techniques for calculating the cross-sectional distribution of attenuation coefficients are based, in part, on a well-known law of radiation physics (Lambert-Beer's law[B3]), which states that when a monoenergetic x-ray beam (i.e., a beam with a single x-ray wavelength) passes through an object of varying density, the beam is attenuated according to the exponential relationship

$$I_t = I_0 e^{-\int \mu \, dl} \qquad (1)$$

where I_0 is the incident intensity, I_t is the transmitted intensity, dl is the differential length of the path of the beam through the object, and μ is the different absorption coefficient (often called the linear attenuation coefficient) in computed tomography in the object along the beam path. The μ values are determined by the physical density and atomic composition of the object and are dependent on the energy (voltage or wavelength) of the x-ray beam.[M1]

In computed tomography, I_0 and I_t are measured from many different angles of view by x-ray detectors, and dl is mathematically defined to be arbitrarily small in order to assume uniform-

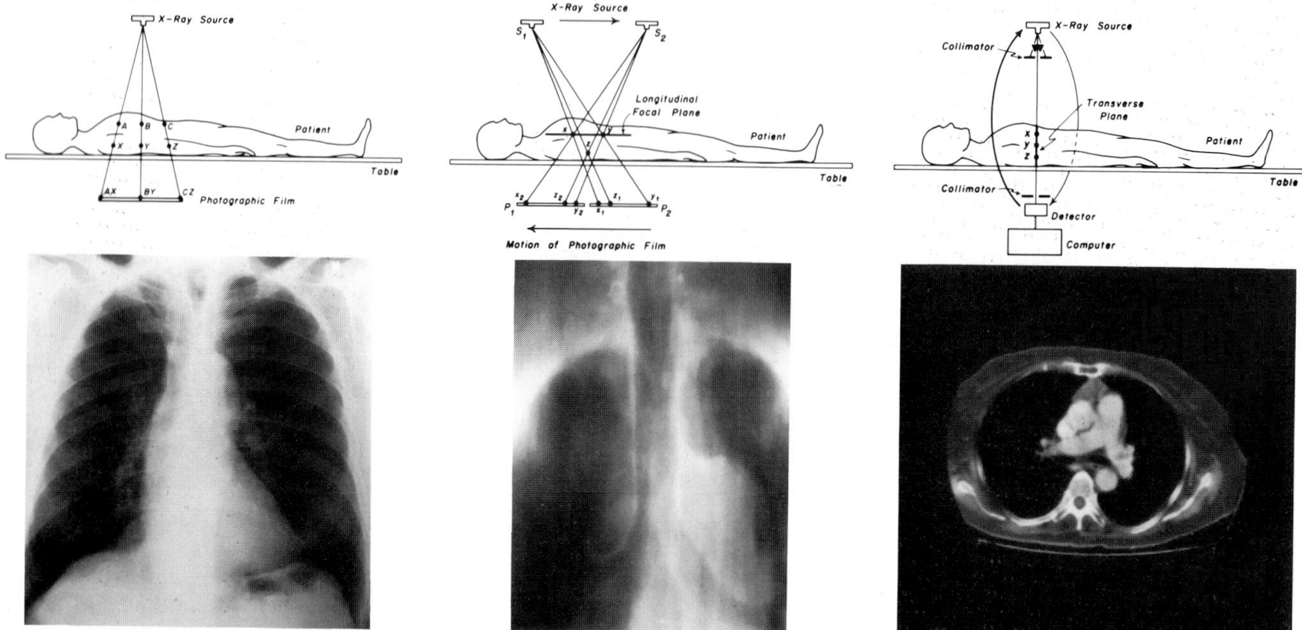

Figure 32–1. *Left,* Conventional x-radiographic technique. All points in the path of any ray (e.g., A and X) are projected onto the same point on the film (e.g., AX), resulting in superposition of structures on the photographic images. This is demonstrated in the conventional chest x-ray, where ribs, heart, and spine are superimposed on one another, rendering detailed visualization of these separate structures difficult. *Center,* Conventional tomographic technique. X-ray source and detector (film) are moved in opposite directions at appropriate relative speeds such that only points in a longitudinal plane (e.g., X) are projected onto the same points (e.g., $X_1 = X_2$) on the photographic film, resulting in a sharper focus on the film of structures within the plane than of structures not within the plane (e.g., point Z). The tracheal tomogram shown illustrates the sharpened features of the trachea, which lie within the focal plan, but structures from outside this plane, which degrade image quality, are also superimposed on the film. *Right,* Computed tomography technique. X-ray source and detector are collimated to define a beam that passes only through a transverse plane or "slice" of the body and are rotated about the body so that x-ray absorption patterns are recorded from many different directions about the transverse plane. These recordings are used by the computer to determine accurately the correct distribution of attenuation values at all points within the plane. The computed tomographic transverse image of the thorax shows sternum, heart, spine, and ribs in correct position, permitting visualization of anatomic detail without superposition of these structures. (From Robb, R. A.: X-ray computed tomography: An engineering synthesis of multiscientific principles. CRC Critical Reviews in Biomedical Engineering 7[4]:265–334, 1982, with permission.)

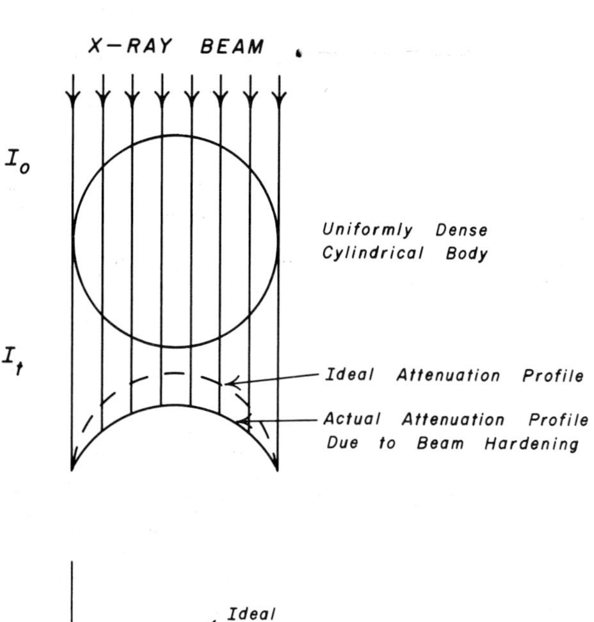

Figure 32–2. Effect of x-ray beam hardening on relationship between measured x-ray attenuation profiles and body thickness. As x-ray beam passes through a uniformly dense but variably shaped body, longer paths through the body result in greater attenuation of the lower energies present in the incident polyenergetic beam, I_0, than for shorter paths. Thus, the transmitted beam, I_t, has higher average energy for longer pathways than for shorter pathways, resulting in an attenuation profile that is nonlinear with respect to body thickness. (From Robb, R. A.: X-ray computed tomography: An engineering synthesis of multiscientific principles. CRC Critical Reviews in Biomedical Engineering 7[4]:265–334, 1982, with permission.)

density segments throughout an object. These measurements give multiple equations in the same unknowns, the individual attenuation coefficients μ, which are solved by various mathematical approaches called image reconstruction. This description is idealized, since in the practical situation monoenergetic x-ray sources of sufficient intensity to irradiate the body are not available and tissues within the body, particularly bone, may alter beam direction, resulting in the detection of scattered as well as directly transmitted x-rays. However, the latter problem is significantly reduced in computed tomography by appropriate collimation of the x-ray beam at the source and at the detector. Problems due to x-ray spectral changes during irradiation of an object with a polyenergetic x-ray source (often called "beam hardening")[B4, Z1] are minimized by mathematical corrections[J1, M2] to the measured projection data before image reconstruction.

The problem of beam hardening is illustrated in Figure 32–2. Ideally, the beam attenuation is directly proportional to the thickness of the body traversed by the beam. However, the x-ray beam is polyenergetic (i.e., has a distribution of energies), and lower-energy x-rays are preferentially absorbed as the beam passes through the object; the continuing x-rays are more penetrating because of their increased average energy, which causes the object to appear less dense than if a monoenergetic beam equivalent to the average incident energy of the polyenergetic beam was used. Relative to the average energy of the incident beam, the average energy of the transmitted beam is increased more for longer pathways through the body than for shorter pathways, and thus the relationship to body thickness departs from linearity.

This problem has been well described in x-ray computed tomography,[B4, M1, Z1] and several approaches have been proposed and implemented to correct it.[H6, J1, M2, R6] The initial approach used in the first CT scanner[H2] was to place a water bag around the head to serve as a "compensating" filter.[M1] The water bag made all beam path lengths similar, so that beam hardening was made linear. The same linear correction can be obtained by mathematical processing[H6, M2] of the measured transmission data within the computer, eliminating the need for and inconvenience of the water bag. However, more sophisticated mathematical approaches[J1, R6] are needed for adequate correction of the decidedly nonlinear beam hardening caused by dense material within the body, such as compact bones, x-ray contrast agents, or prosthetic implants.

Generally, these more exact methods for correction of beam hardening involve the use of an iterative approach to approximate the distribution and amount of dense material (e.g., bone) in the scan region, followed by correction of the absorption measurements relative to the known (assumed or measured) x-ray energy spectrum before making the final reconstruction. Therefore, these procedures increase the computational time required for image reconstruction, but this is generally an acceptable trade-off for obtaining improved image quality.

Several investigators have performed tissue attenuation studies both in vitro and in vivo and with both monoenergetic photons generated by isotope sources and polyenergetic x-ray beams in computed tomography systems.[F1, M3, N1, P1, P2, R4] Current x-ray CT methods that include beam-hardening corrections provide excellent accuracy in measurement of tissue attenuation coefficients compared with other radiographic techniques (10 to 100 times better).[H1] A typical standard deviation in measurement of absorption coefficients of tissue is about ½ percent relative to water, which is an accuracy of ±¼ percent.

Reconstruction from Projections

Figure 32–3 illustrates the concept of generating projections of a slice of an object by scanning an x-ray beam and detector across and about the object. Several different schemes and geometries for scanning have been used and have various advantages for speed and calibration, as discussed in the next section. Two of these are known as parallel-beam geometry and fan beam geometry. For simplicity, the parallel scanning geometry scheme, as illustrated in Figure 32–3, will be used to describe the basic

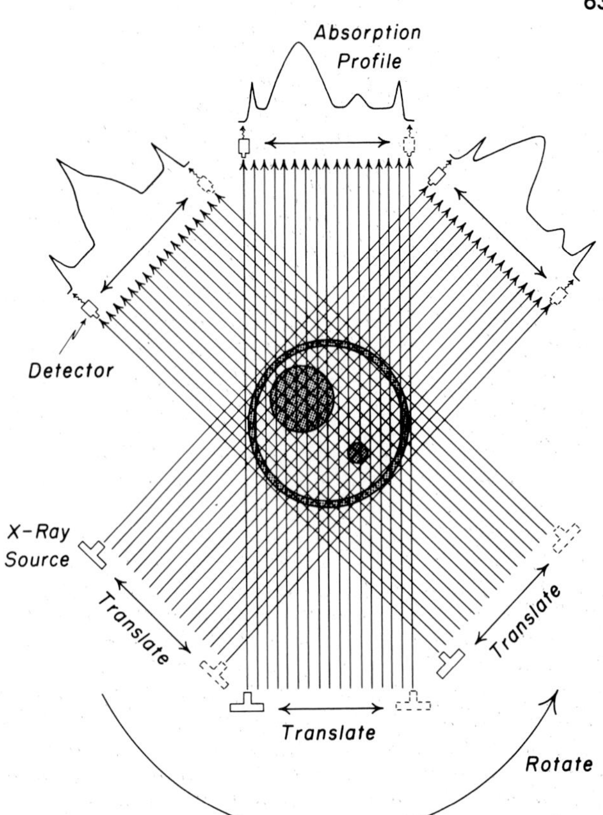

Figure 32–3. Procedure for generation of multidimensional x-ray attenuation profiles. X-ray source and detector are translated across the body as the transmitted x-ray is measured at successive points. These measurements, when divided by (or logarithmically subtracted from) the amount of x-ray measured incident on the body, can be expressed as profiles of absorption versus position. The amplitude at each point on the absorption profile is proportional to the total absorption along the corresponding ray path through the object. These absorption profiles are recorded for many directions of x-ray passing through the body by incrementally rotating the x-ray source and detector in tandem about the body. (From Robb, R. A.: X-ray computed tomography: An engineering synthesis of multiscientific principles. CRC Critical Reviews in Biomedical Engineering 7[4]:265–334, 1982, with permission.)

mathematical approach to reconstruction. Fan beam geometry can be reduced to parallel-beam geometry,[D4] or appropriate geometric calculations can be used to do fan beam reconstructions directly.[H7, R7]

Figure 32–4 illustrates the basic geometric concept used in image reconstruction. All conventional image reconstruction algorithms require that, during computed tomographic scanning, the x-ray source and detector lie in the same plane as the slice to be reconstructed. X-ray transmission measurements, called projection data, are made at many different discrete positions of the x-ray source and detector relative to the body. The set of projection data collected at each angular setting of the x-ray source and detector is often called a profile or view (the terms *projection, profile,* and *view* are used interchangeably). The discrete projection samples are often called line integral values or ray sums (the terms *profile sample, line integral value,* and *ray sum* are used interchangeably). The image reconstruction algorithm implemented on a computer specifies a finite planar region in the space irradiated that contains all structures of interest to be reconstructed; attenuation of the beam outside this region is assumed to be zero. This planar region is usually bounded by a square or a circle and is partitioned into a matrix (grid) of small, nonoverlapping regions (usually square) called pixels (for picture elements), each of which is assumed to have a uniform x-ray attenuation coefficient (or x-ray density). The number and size of pixels are based on the spatial resolution desired in the picture and on the spatial resolution that is

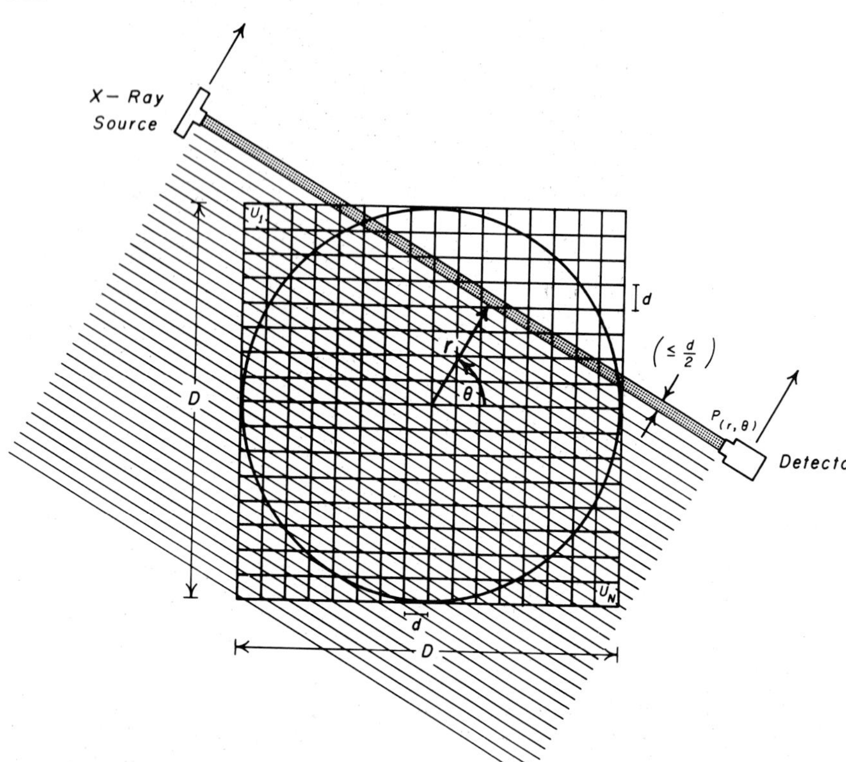

Figure 32–4. Geometry of image reconstruction space. Region of diameter D to be reconstructed is subdivided into a grid of N small squares (d × d) called pixels (picture elements), and x-ray attenuation in any given pixel (U_1) is assumed to be uniform. Width and spacing of the measured x-ray beam should be small (≤d/2) relative to size of pixels. Each absorption value, or projection sample, P(r, θ) is a function of the distance r of each corresponding ray from the center of the grid and of the angle θ that each ray makes relative to the *x*, *y* axis of the grid. (From Robb, R. A.: X-ray computed tomography: An engineering synthesis of multiscientific principles. CRC Critical Reviews in Biomedical Engineering 7[4]:265–334, 1982, with permission.)

practically achievable.[G2, H3] Since the detected x-ray beam has finite width, the pixels are really small volume elements (voxels) and the reconstruction plane is really a slice or slab.

The task of the reconstruction algorithm is to determine geometrically the paths of the x-ray beams passing through the voxels of the reconstruction matrix and to relate the measurements mathematically to total attenuation (ray sums) for many such intersecting paths obtained from different views in such a way as to solve for the fractional attenuation by each voxel. The result is a map of the attenuation coefficient within the object that can be displayed as an image by assigning brightness values proportional to the attenuation values determined at individual points throughout the matrix.

$$P(r,\theta) = \int_{-\infty}^{\infty} U(x,y)dl \qquad (2)$$

where the path of integration is along a beam line and $P(r,\theta)$ is the measured value of the corresponding transmitted x-ray. The set of $P(r,\theta)$, projection data, are expressed in polar coordinates relative to the reconstruction plane. $U(x,y)$ is a function of position within the reconstruction plane whose magnitude evaluated at any point (x,y) is the linear attenuation coefficient at that point, and dl is the differential path length along a ray. This equation forms the basis for all approaches to image reconstruction and may be called the general projection formula. The problem is to invert equation (2) to solve for $U(x,y)$. It is generally not practical to solve the projection equations by direct matrix inversion. In typical applications, the number of unknowns may be on the order of 10^4 to 10^5 and the number of measurements on the order of 10^5 to 10^6.

Radon proved[R1] the existence of a valid inversion formula for equation (2), assuming ideal conditions of continuity and compact support of the function, U, and infinite, noiseless projections, P. One approach to evaluating Radon's transform by using Fourier integrals[S2] results in the inversion formula

$$U(x,y) = \frac{1}{4\pi^2}\int_0^{\pi}\int_{-\infty}^{\infty} P(w,\theta)e^{iwr}|w|dw \qquad (3)$$

where $P(w,\theta)$ is the Fourier transform of the projection data. A wide variety of mathematical approaches[C5, G3, G4, R2, S3, V1] to the reconstruction problem have been developed. Most approaches can be classified[G4] in one or more of the following four categories: (1) summation methods (e.g., simple back projection), (2) series expansion methods (e.g., iterative estimate-correct), (3) transform methods (e.g., Fourier transform), and (4) direct analytic methods (e.g., convolution or filtered back projection).

The method most used for image reconstruction from projections is called the convolution, or filtered back projection, method. It has fundamental components in categories 1, 3, and 4 but is considered primarily a direct analytic solution in closed form to the integral equations derived from the basic projection formula. As the name suggests, it is related to the simple back-projection method but with a significant important difference: it corrects the blurring produced when the projections are simply overlapped[G4] by appropriate prefiltering (convolution with a "deblurring" function) of the projection data before the back-projection (summation) process. The approach has proved to be both accurate and computationally efficient and is a direct solution to the inverse integral equations derived from the projection formula. According to this method, the two basic procedures, which are readily implemented on a computer, are (1) to filter (the convolution step) the projection data with a function selected to negate the blurring effect of the summation process and (2) to sum (the back-projection step) the filtered projections. The convolution step may be expressed by

$$P^*(r,\theta) = \int_{-\infty}^{\infty} P(r',\theta)h(r - r')dr' \qquad (4)$$

where P^* denotes convolved projection and $h(r)$ is the deblurring function, or convolution kernel. The second step is to integrate (back-project) the filtered projections over all projection angles (zero to 180 degrees):

$$U(x,y) = \int_0^{\pi} P^*(x \cos \theta = y \sin \theta,\theta)d\theta \qquad (5)$$

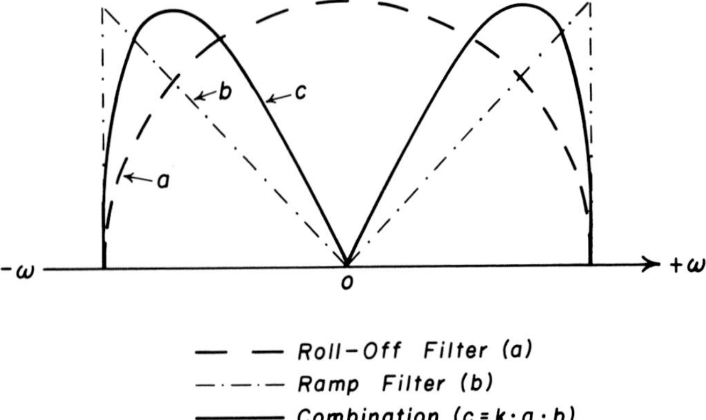

Figure 32–5. Frequency-space plots of three idealized filters for image reconstruction. Roll-off filter (curve a) produces a gradual cutoff of high-frequency components but is not suitable for image reconstruction because it is not a ramp function. However, a pure ramp filter (curve b) has a sharp cutoff, which can result in "overshoot" artifacts at regions of high spatial frequency (e.g., sharp edges) in the reconstruction. A combination of the two filters (curve c, which is the normalized product of curves a and b) can produce the desired effect of smoothly attenuating high-frequency data (i.e., noise) and avoiding overshoot artifacts. (From Robb, R. A.: X-ray computed tomography: An engineering synthesis of multiscientific principles. CRC Critical Reviews in Biomedical Engineering 7[4]:265–334, 1982, with permission.)

Under appropriate conditions,[S3] equations (4) and (5) may be numerically implemented by replacing the integrals with sums; the convolution sum is performed over the number of projection samples in each view, and the back-projection sum is performed over the number of views available. The resultant discrete equations constitute the filtered back-projection algorithm and are computationally efficient; they are amenable to very rapid parallel processing, since projections can be filtered and back-projected independently of each other.

The number of multiplications and additions involved is approximately $4M(m^2 + N)$, where M is the number of views, m is the number of ray sums, and N is the number of pixels to be reconstructed.[S3] The projected data may be interpolated to increase the number of ray sums required for back projection. The accuracy of the method is excellent if sufficient samples are available and an appropriate filter function is used.[S3]

To ensure convergence of equation (4), the filter function is generally defined to be a ramp for frequencies up to a specified limit and zero beyond that limit. However, to avoid artifacts due to the sharp cutoff and to save the extra computation time required to smooth the final image, a modified filter, which is the product of a ramp and roll-off filter, is commonly used. Idealized ramp, roll-off, and combination filters are depicted in Figure 32–5.

Figure 32–6 shows two examples of commonly used convolution filter functions.[R2, S2] The purpose of the negative side lobes in each filter is to compensate for the positive side lobes or spokes of the l/r point spread distribution introduced by back projection. If the filter is carefully chosen, these negative and positive side lobes cancel each other out when the filtered projections are summed, resulting in an unblurred image of the original object. This result, in effect, is a deconvolution of the point spread function and the blurred picture obtained by simple back projection and is, under appropriate sampling conditions, equivalent to convolution of the inverse point spread function with the simple back-projected image.[B8]

Image Quality

The quality of a computed tomographic image is affected by many factors. These include but are not limited to (1) initial beam characteristics, (2) total dose (energy levels and number of views used), (3) transmissivity of subject, (4) thickness of section scanned, (5) x-ray beam scatter, (6) efficiency of conversion of detector readings to numbers of the computer, (7) pixel size in the reconstruction, (8) reconstruction algorithm used, and (9) display resolution. Many articles[B5, B6, C6, G2, H4, J2, V2] have been published on these parameters and their effect on resolution and accuracy in x-ray computed tomography. One formula that expresses image quality in x-ray computed tomographic images based on several of these parameters is the following:

$$\sigma^2(\mu) \simeq kT/(td^3R)$$

where the variance $\sigma^2(\mu)$, due to noise in the reconstructed value of the linear attenuation coefficient at any given point in the body, is directly proportional to the transmissivity T of the subject (transmissivity is a general term that represents the inverse of attenuation and incorporates the composition and distribution of tissues in the beam path) and inversely proportional to the slice thickness t, the cube of the attenuation element size d, and the x-ray dose R; k is the factor used to convert from incident (skin) dose R to the absorbed dose at a given point.

Since the transmissivity of the subject cannot generally be changed and for any scan setting the slice thickness would be fixed, two separate, important relationships can be extracted from the equation that can be selectively modified to attempt to improve image quality:

$$\sigma \simeq R^{-1/2}, \qquad \sigma \simeq d^{-3/2}$$

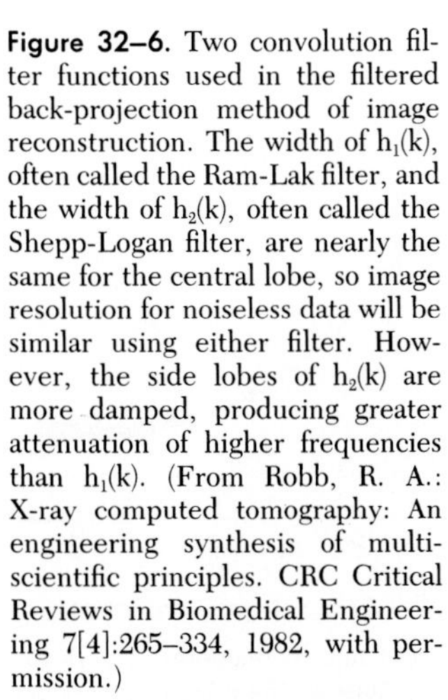

Figure 32–6. Two convolution filter functions used in the filtered back-projection method of image reconstruction. The width of $h_1(k)$, often called the Ram-Lak filter, and the width of $h_2(k)$, often called the Shepp-Logan filter, are nearly the same for the central lobe, so image resolution for noiseless data will be similar using either filter. However, the side lobes of $h_2(k)$ are more damped, producing greater attenuation of higher frequencies than $h_1(k)$. (From Robb, R. A.: X-ray computed tomography: An engineering synthesis of multiscientific principles. CRC Critical Reviews in Biomedical Engineering 7[4]:265–334, 1982, with permission.)

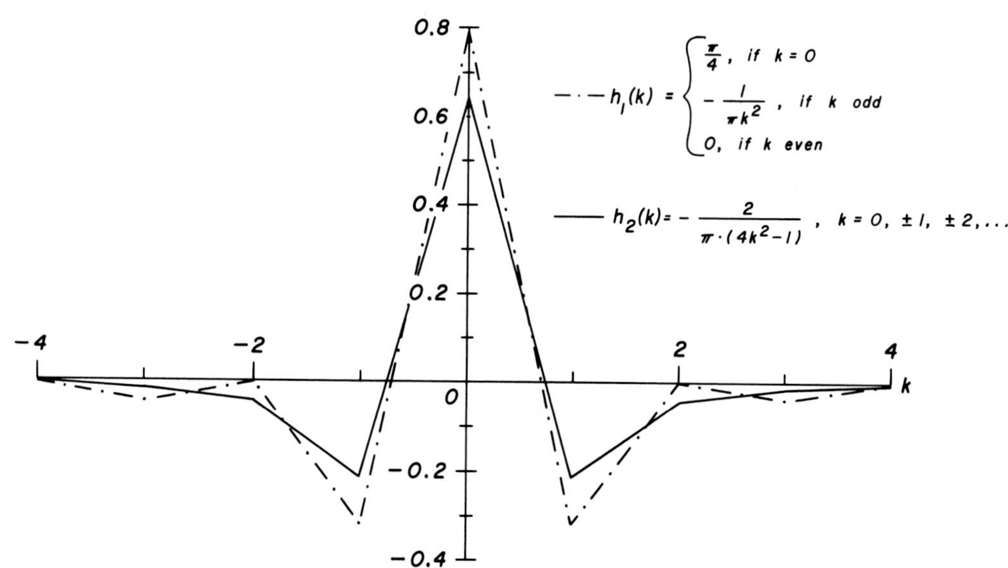

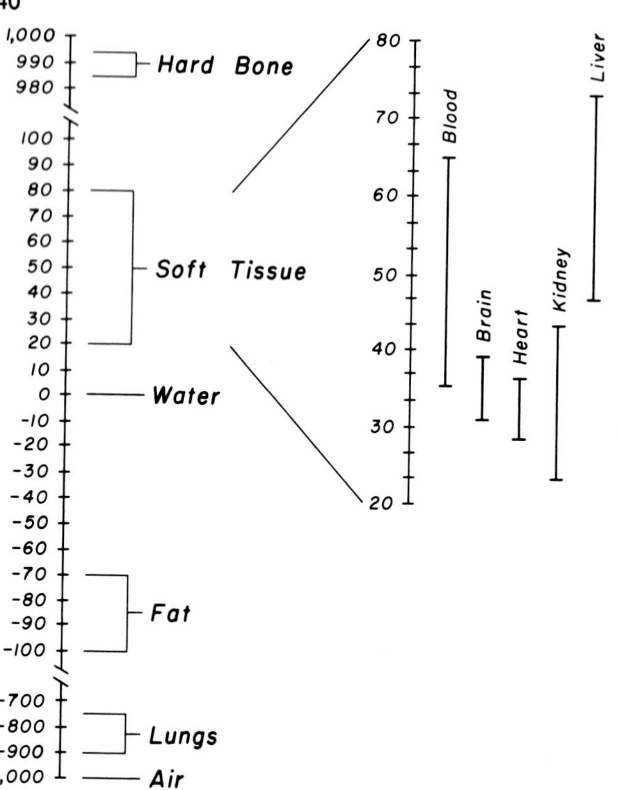

Figure 32–7. Typical computed tomography number scale and values for various body tissues. Values are based on measurements with an effective x-ray energy of 72 keV. The range of values for a given tissue reflects both measurement errors and actual attenuation differences among samples. Data include both in vitro measurements made with monoenergetic sources and in vivo measurements made with actual computed tomography scanners. (From Robb, R. A.: X-ray computed tomography: An engineering synthesis of multiscientific principles. CRC Critical Reviews in Biomedical Engineering 7[4]:265–334, 1982, with permission.)

Thus, image noise (standard deviation σ) is inversely proportional to both the square root of the dose used and the $3/2$ power of the element size used.

The practical question regarding dose efficiency in computed tomography is, how much radiation is actually captured and converted to signal for use in the image reconstruction? The overall dose efficiency of computed tomography systems is the product of capture efficiency (how much radiation is detected) and conversion efficiency (how much of the captured radiation is converted to signal). An overall dose efficiency of 70 percent or better would be considered excellent in current systems, but the typical value is around 50 percent or lower.[S4] Higher doses must be delivered by low-efficiency systems to produce image quality comparable to that provided by higher-efficiency systems. Typical radiation dose levels in current computed tomography systems may range from 2 to 10 rads per slice scanned.

As mentioned earlier, in tissue attenuation studies with monoenergetic photons and polyenergetic x-ray beams, the typical standard deviation in measurement of absorption coefficients of tissue was about $1/2$ percent relative to water, or an accuracy of $\pm 1/4$ percent. Figure 32–7 shows a typical scale of numbers used to represent the computed values of attenuation coefficients of human body tissues and organs and illustrates the precision with which they can be obtained by current x-ray CT scanners.

It has been shown[C2, H3] that if d is the linear dimension (side) of a resolution element (pixel), D is the linear dimension (diameter) of the region to be reconstructed (refer to Fig. 32–4), and M is the number of projection views recorded around 180 degrees, with each view sampled (ray sums) at intervals of $d/2$ or smaller, the *theoretically* achievable spatial resolution is given by

$$d = \pi D/2M$$

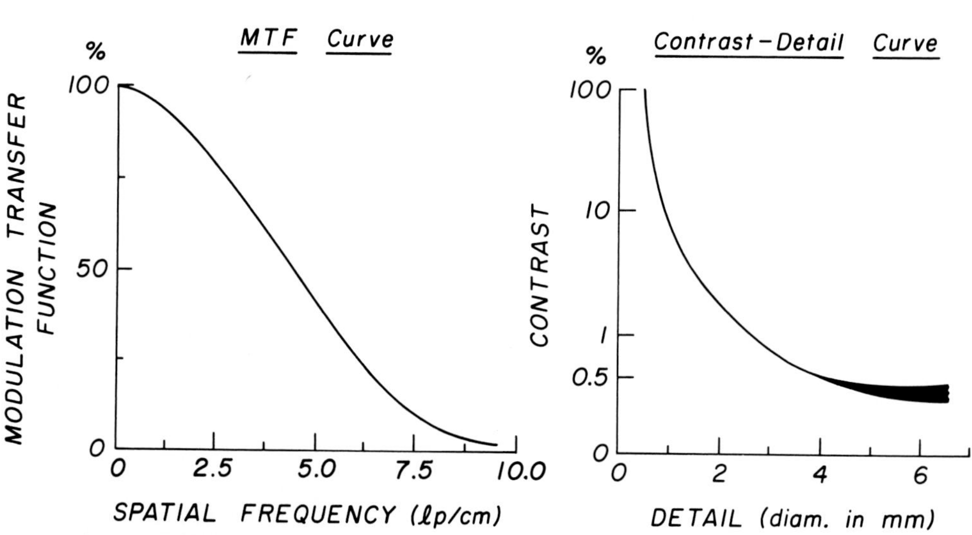

Figure 32–8. Typical modulation transfer function (MTF) and contrast-detail curves for x-ray computed tomography systems. The MTF curve is one way of expressing the *spatial resolution* of a computed tomography system. It is a measure of the ability to discriminate objects of varying density a small distance apart against a uniform background. Spatial resolution of up to 10 line pairs/cm (1-mm resolution) can be obtained in some systems. The contrast-detail curve is a way of expressing the *contrast resolution* of a computed tomography system; it is a measure of the ability to image structures of a given size and contrast that can be detected by an observer. Current computed tomography scanners can detect (i.e., produce for visualization in the reconstructed image) structures of 0.5 mm diameter at very high contrast relative to background (approaching 100 percent) and structures 3 to 4 mm in diameter at very low contrast relative to background (about 0.5 percent). The detectability of objects below 0.5 percent contrast is limited by noise in the image, as depicted by the broadened lower end of the contrast-detail curve. (From Robb, R. A.: X-ray computed tomography: An engineering synthesis of multiscientific principles. CRC Critical Reviews in Biomedical Engineering 7[4]:265–334, 1982, with permission.)

However, the actual resolution achievable in a reconstruction is highly dependent on the asymmetry of the object being reconstructed, the frequency and distribution of projection data samples, the noise in the sampled projection data, and the reconstruction algorithm used.

Spatial resolution in x-ray computed tomographic images is influenced by at least five intrinsic factors: (1) x-ray focal spot size, (2) detector element aperture, (3) sample spacing, (4) form of the convolution filter, and (5) size of the reconstructed pixels. The modulation transfer function of the overall imaging system ultimately determines the spatial resolution of a scanner. Curves of the form shown at the left in Figure 32–8 are typical for current-generation systems and are readily measured by using phantoms designed to test high- and low-contrast spatial resolution.[G5, M4] High-contrast resolution nominally implies object-to-background contrast of 10 percent or above, and spatial resolution between 0.5 and 1.0 mm is attainable at these contrast levels in current systems. Low-contrast resolution is nominally taken as 0.1 to 3.0 percent, and typical spatial resolution at such contrast ranges between 2 and 4 mm, with detectability lost because of noise at a contrast level of about 0.2 to 0.5 percent. A convenient way to represent detectability is the contrast-detail curve,[C7] as illustrated at the right in Figure 32–8, which is a graph of background-to-object contrast as a function of object size. Accuracy of high-contrast detail is limited primarily by the modulation transfer function of the system, whereas low-contrast sensitivity is limited primarily by dose. To improve low-contrast sensitivity in computed tomography, higher doses must be used.

Image quality in computed tomography is significantly influenced by factors other than intrinsic spatial and contrast resolution of the imaging process. These factors give rise to artifacts[K3, S5] that are either scanner related or subject related. Scanner-related artifacts can result from malfunction, misalignment, and/or poor calibration of system components and from the geometry and physics of the system. Physical adjustments are required to correct component-induced artifacts, and some mathematical corrections can be used to minimize geometry- and physics-related artifacts. Subject-related artifacts can result from motion of the patient, either biologic or voluntary, or from a dense object in the patient (e.g., bone, contrast material, or a prosthesis). Body and/or organ motion is perhaps the most critical source of artifacts and degradation of image quality in x-ray computed tomography applications.

ENGINEERING SYNTHESIS

X-ray computed tomography is thought of primarily as the precisely engineered machines that embody the requisite physics and mathematical principles to provide routine, noninvasive, clinical diagnostic transaxial images of the body. Many papers and proceedings of workshops[B9, K4, W1, W2] provide detailed information regarding the evolution and current status of engineering accomplishments in x-ray computed tomography.

The systems may include a variety of components, but generally six modular subsystems are basic to an x-ray CT scanner:

1. The rotating gantry, which supports the x-ray source and detectors
2. The subject table or "couch"
3. The x-ray source and collimation assembly (with associated power supply and cooling system)
4. The detector/collimation system (including electronic amplifiers)
5. The computer system (including the analog-to-digital converter)
6. The display and analysis console

The Gantry

The gantry has been constructed in a variety of configurations to achieve optimal performance. It is subject to strict mechanical tolerances (e.g., wobble less than 0.1 mm) during scanning to ensure precise alignment of the x-ray source and detectors relative to the body section being imaged. In their relatively short history, commercial x-ray CT scanners have evolved through five distinct geometries. The first four geometries are illustrated in Figure 32–9. (The fifth geometry is the subject of the next section on dynamic systems.) These changes have been motivated primarily by the desire for high-resolution images and the need for faster scanning to reduce blurring and eliminate streak artifacts due to biologic motion[A2] and have resulted in improved detection efficiency, calibration techniques, and image quality.[H4]

The Couch

The couch is designed to present the subject to the scanner. Generally, in body scanners, the couch is motorized to move the patient into the gantry. Special devices are often added to facilitate subject positioning, such as a laser beam that illuminates a line on the surface of the body indicating the section of anatomy to be scanned. Angulation of the couch (typically ±20 degrees) and/or tilting of the gantry (typically ±30 degrees) provides the capability for scanning sections oblique to the long axis of the body. The couch is made of radio-translucent material so that it does not significantly interfere with the transmission of the x-ray beam through the body. In many scanners, the couch can be continuously moved through the gantry during rapidly repeated rectilinear scans to provide a high-resolution digital radiograph of the part of the body passed through the gantry. This image, sometimes called a "scout view," provides anatomic information to facilitate selection of the range and spacing of scan slice levels desired in a scan sequence and also facilitates accurate positioning of the patient.

The X-Ray Tube

Typical x-ray tubes in first-generation and second-generation CT scanners are oil-cooled, fixed-anode, continuous x-ray sources. Air-cooled, rotating-anode (pulsed) x-ray sources are most commonly used in third-generation and fourth-generation scanners. The x-ray tubes operate between 100 and 160 kVp. The photon spectrum is polyenergetic with an average energy of approximately 50 keV before entry into the subject.[M1] Pulsed x-ray sources have a typical duty cycle of about 20 percent, with pulses of 2 to 3 msec at a current of 600 to 650 mA. Focal spot sizes are typically 0.6 to 1.2 mm in diameter, with target angles of 15 to 30 degrees.[W1] The focal spot size has a direct bearing on the limiting resolution of a computed tomography system. Aluminum filters of approximately 2.5 mm thickness are typically used to meet federal standards for filtration of x-ray beams in the range 70 to 150 kVp. X-ray beam collimation on the source side of the patient restricts exposure of the patient to the area scanned by eliminating off-focus radiation (e.g., limiting the conical beam to a fan beam). The entry beam is also shaped to compensate for size and dynamic range of the detector. One commonly used compensating filter is the "bowtie" filter, so called because of its characteristic shape, as shown in Figure 32–10.

The Detector

The detector used in x-ray computed tomography is perhaps the single most important element in the system. To a major extent, the detector aperture size determines spatial resolution and detector efficiency determines contrast resolution.

Aperture sizes of the detectors on scanners range from 0.5 to 2.0 mm. This size, along with the x-ray source focal spot size (0.6 to 1.2 mm), defines the beam width used for image reconstruction and generally dictates the maximum absolute spatial resolution attainable. In fourth-generation systems, spatial resolution is determined by the frequency of position samples of the continuously rotating x-ray source. In such systems, the spatial resolution is a function of the width of the fan beam at the center of the scan region and the number of samples recorded across the

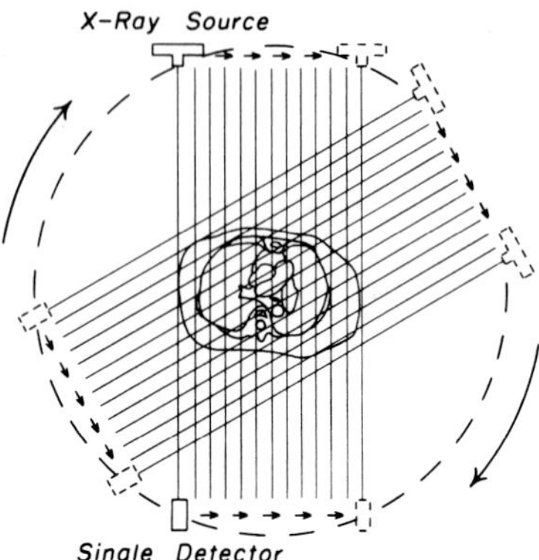

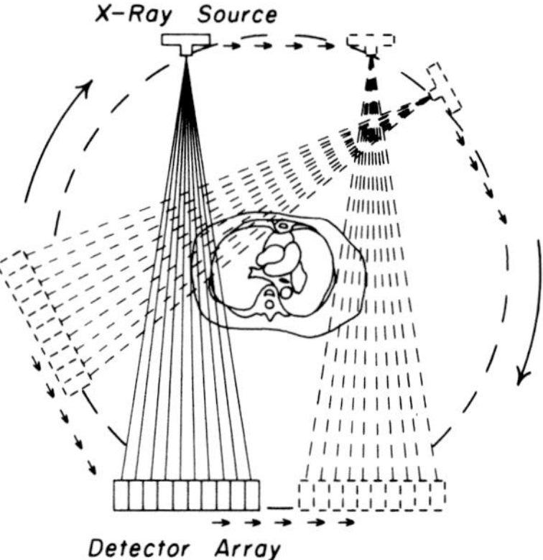

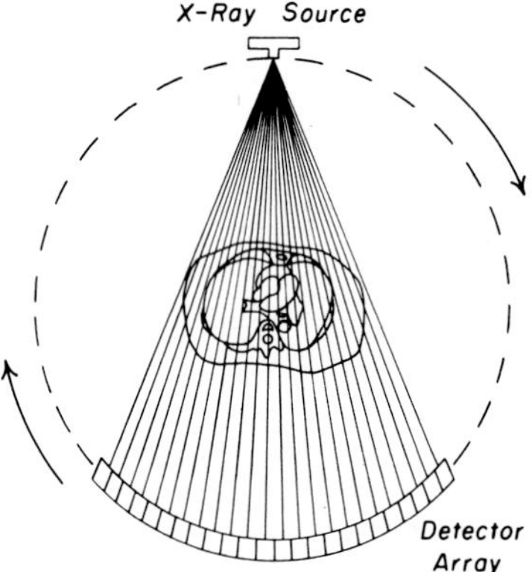

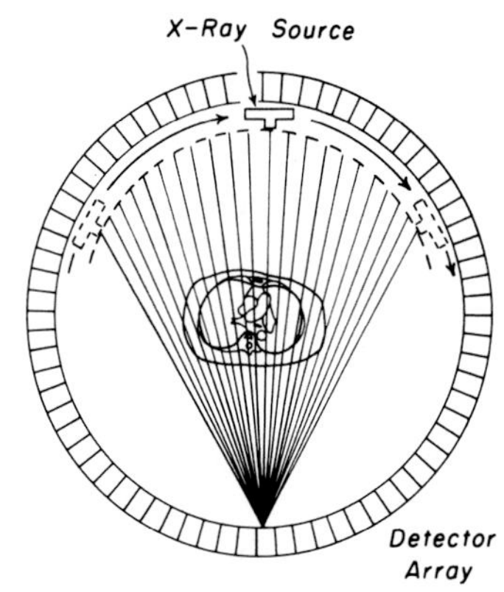

Figure 32–9. Diagram of evolution of computed tomography scanner geometries. First-generation scanners used a pencil beam defined by a well-collimated x-ray source and a single detector. The source and detector are first translated in tandem in a rectilinear pattern, with successive beam measurements parallel to each other. Then the source and detector are rotated through a small angle and the rectilinear scan repeated. This translate-rotate procedure continues for 180 degrees. Second-generation scanners use a small linear array of detectors instead of a single detector to speed up data acquisition with fan beam geometry, but still a translation and rotation of source and detectors are required. Third-generation systems use a larger array of detectors (usually circular) so that the entire body is subtended by the x-ray fan beams, and only rotation of the source and detector array is required to obtain the readings for image reconstruction. Fourth-generation systems use a fixed circular array of many detectors and a rotating x-ray source inside (or outside) the detector ring. In this geometry, each detector position defines the apex of the fan beam as x-rays are recorded from the various source positions. The geometry considerations for image reconstruction are the same, however, as for third-generation systems, where the source position defines the apex of the fan beam. (From Robb, R. A.: X-ray computed tomography: An engineering synthesis of multiscientific principles. CRC Critical Reviews in Biomedical Engineering 7[4]:265–334, 1982, with permission.)

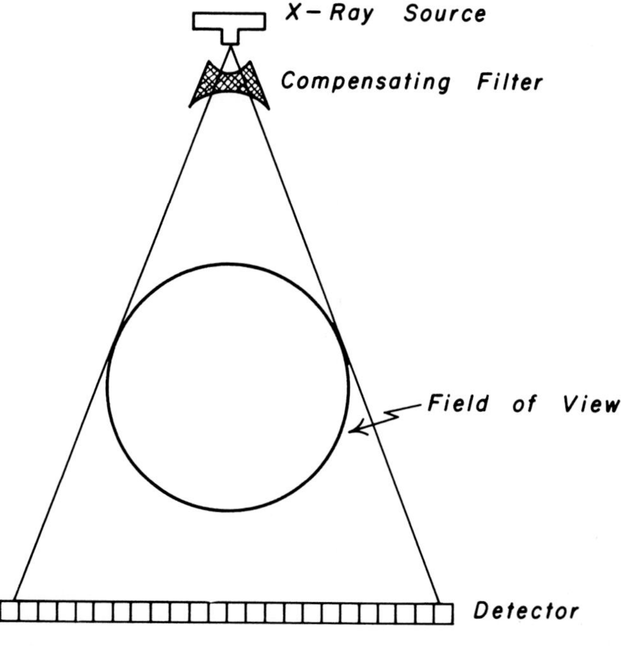

Figure 32–10. Compensating filter for fan beam x-ray computed tomographic scanning. X-ray attenuating material (usually aluminum) is shaped (somewhat like a bow tie) to absorb proportionally more of the x-rays as a function of distance from the center of the field of view. This shaping is done primarily to reduce the dynamic range (i.e., the range of accurate linear response) required of the detectors. The assumption is made that the subject to be scanned is approximately round, so that less x-ray would be attenuated toward the periphery of the field of view. The compensating filter attempts to equalize the attenuation across the entire field. (From Robb, R. A.: X-ray computed tomography: An engineering synthesis of multiscientific principles. CRC Critical Reviews in Biomedical Engineering 7[4]:265–334, 1982, with permission.)

fan. Ray spacing can be as small as 0.1 mm, but this does not necessarily mean that 0.1-mm spatial resolution is produced in the system. Other factors, such as the modulation transfer function of the overall imaging system, the accuracy of analog-to-digital conversion, and the reconstruction algorithm used, also influence spatial resolution.

X-ray beam collimation is performed on the detector side of the subject as well as on the source side. The purpose of detector collimation is to reject scattered radiation; careful design and alignment of the collimator are critically important to overall image quality. Collimators also help determine the aperture size of the detector. Pixel sizes in the reconstruction matrix may be two, three, or four times smaller than the detector aperture size to ensure true aperture resolution and/or to produce a more aesthetically pleasing effect in the reconstructed image.[H4]

The electronic signal from the detector, after appropriate amplification, is converted to digital form by an analog-to-digital converter. To be able to reconstruct to 0.5 percent density resolution, the conversion process must accurately convert detector readings representing differences in tissue absorption of at least 1 part in 200 as well as accurately convert much higher detector signals when no absorption takes place (i.e., the incident signal). Current scanner systems employ up to 22-bit (4×10^6 parts) analog-to-digital conversion to capture accurately the dynamic range of the detector signal[W1] and thus provide up to 0.5 percent contrast resolution in the reconstructed image.

The Computer

The computer is the key to computed tomographic image reconstruction. Images with a total number of pixels ranging from 65,536 (256×256) to 262,144 (512×512) may be reconstructed from 500,000 to over 1,000,000 measurements. It is within the capability of current minicomputers, aided by special-purpose, high-speed arithmetic hardware (often called array processors), to perform such reconstructions in a few seconds. Some systems perform the reconstruction in parallel with the scan and have the reconstruction completed within fractions of a second after the scan is finished. For the convolution method of reconstruction, fewer than $4M(m^2 + N)$ multiplications and additions are required,[S3] where M is the number of views, m is the number of samples per view, and N is the number of pixels to be reconstructed. ($M \bullet m \bullet N$ multiplications and additions are required for the generalized inversion solution.) For $M = 180$, $m = 256$, and $N = 65{,}536$, the number of multiplications and additions would be over 94 million. Assuming that the speed of the central processing unit in a minicomputer is 1 second for additions and 4 seconds for multiplications, almost 8 minutes would be required to do a 256×256 reconstruction with system software alone. However, the special-purpose hardware array processors can perform floating-point (real number) arithmetic operations at rates of 15 million operations per second or more and can perform multiplications and additions simultaneously (i.e., in parallel). For the problem stated, a 256×256 reconstruction with such a device could be performed in about 6 seconds, instead of 8 minutes!

The computer software on most current x-ray CT computer systems permits the flexibility of selection of several different reconstruction parameters, generally including matrix size (typically 256×256 or 512×512), pixel size (typically a factor of 4 variability), and algorithm used (this generally means use of different filter functions and/or corrections for such problems as beam hardening). In addition to reconstruction and display of the images, the computer system handles the scanning tasks as well, including tracking positions of source and detectors, monitoring voltage (kV) and current (mA), converting detector signals to numbers, and correcting for variations in detector response. Multiple central processing units may be used to facilitate simultaneous parallel control of scanning, reconstruction, and display.

The Display

The display console of a modern x-ray computed tomography system provides a wide variety of operator-interactive image manipulation and diagnostic capabilities. Images can be displayed with up to 512 gray levels (or color) on 512×512 or 1024×1024 screens with alpha-numeric and/or graphic information displayed on the same screen, either adjacent to or superimposed on the image, as desired. Simple keystrokes invoke complex image processing and analysis functions via advanced software programs. Rapidly positioned cursors provide identification of specific points in the image or outlining of desired regions. For these selected regions, one can obtain plots of mean density values, histograms, standard deviations, magnified images, distance measurements, enhancement of selected "windows" or CT numbers, and so forth. Sagittal and coronal sections can be computed and displayed from a series of transaxial slices stored in the computer memory. Through programming, the computer provides the flexibility for readily expanding the scope and detail of procedures for displaying and analyzing the data. The image data are stored on large magnetic disks (approximately 300 million values) for rapid retrieval, manipulation, display, and analysis. The data are also recorded on magnetic computer tape for archival storage. Permanent hard-copy records of the images can be recorded on x-ray film in a variety of sizes, numbers, and formats by use of special devices attached to the display console.

DYNAMIC THREE-DIMENSIONAL COMPUTED TOMOGRAPHY

Needs

The function and performance of the heart, lungs, and circulation are intrinsically related to their motion in three dimensions. Direct and simultaneous measurement of the instant-to-instant changes in size, shape, and perfusion of the heart and lungs over their entire anatomic extent is required for accurate and comprehensive assessment of their normal physiologic or pathophysiologic status.[W3] Such measurements would provide capabilities for detailed synergistic analyses of regional, global, and integrated function within the cardiopulmonary system. In addition to providing elucidation of a myriad of investigative physiologic questions, these capabilities would facilitate clinically applicable estimations of cardiac reserve and increase the ability to detect and treat congenital or acquired cardiovascular disabilities. Similarly, quantitative synchronous measurements of regional lung tissue mechanics and perfusion, chest wall displacement, and diaphragm dynamics would facilitate accurate studies and diagnosis of respiratory function and disease.

However, no satisfactory noninvasive method has been available for direct quantitative measurement of the fundamental determinants of cardiovascular and respiratory function, namely the full temporal and spatial distribution of heart muscle and lung dynamics and simultaneously the spatial distribution and magnitude in all regions of the heart and lungs of blood flow, on which myocardial and pulmonary dynamics depend.

In general terms, two major problems of x-ray computed tomographic scanners for full-volume imaging of moving organs are limitation of spatial resolution due to the partial volume effect[H10] and temporal resolution due to motion blurring.[11] Increased density resolution can be achieved by increasing imaged slice thickness; increased slice thickness tends to increase the signal-to-noise ratio of the tomographic image (because more x-ray photons per picture element [voxel] are available). However, increased slice thickness results in blurring of edges due to the partial volume effect. As shown in Figure 32–11, these opposing relationships would be expected to result in a slice thickness that is optimal. The importance of the partial volume effect depends on slice thickness relative to the anatomic detail of interest and the angle of the surface (to be detected) relative to the plane of the imaged slice. In addition to the slice thickness, the spatial intervals between contiguous slices are important, especially for evaluating three-dimensional shape.

Analogous to the effect of slice thickness on spatial resolution is the effect of scan duration on temporal resolution. In general, the longer the scan, the greater the number of x-ray photons detected and the greater the image signal-to-noise ratio. On the

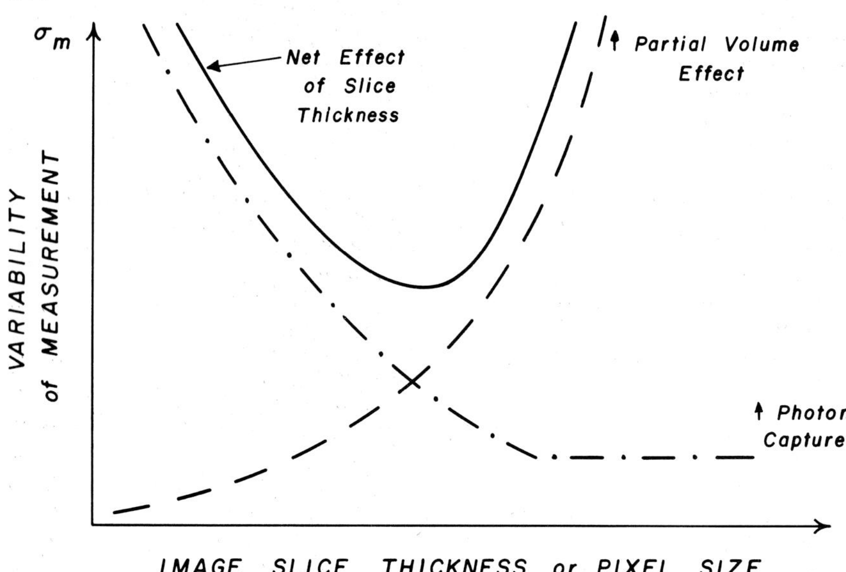

Figure 32–11. Schematic representation of the role of image slice thickness in spatial resolution. When the number of x-ray photons detected per pixel is increased by increasing slice thickness, the photon noise in the image decreases approximately as the square root of the increased slice thickness (shown by the dashed and dotted line). When the slice thickness is increased, the partial volume effect increases (shown by the dashed line); the rate of rise of this line depends somewhat on the detailed geometry of the object relative to the slice thickness. The sum of these two opposing effects results in the relationship depicted by the solid line. Spatial resolution is expressed as the uncertainty of the spatial location of a detected edge in the image. (From Kim, K. H., Hoffman, E. A., and Ritman, E. L.: Needs and requirements for accurate measurement of dynamic 3-D geometry of the in situ heart. *In* Sideman, S., and Beyar, R., [eds.]: Simulation and Control of the Cardiac System, Vol. 1, Chap. 4. CRC Critical Press, Boca Raton, Fla., 1987, pp. 41–50, with permission.)

other hand, the longer the scan, the greater the motion that can occur, hence the loss of spatial resolution due to motion blurring. As shown in Figure 32–12, these two factors would be expected to oppose each other, resulting in an optimal scan duration that depends on the speed of motion of the anatomic structure scanned and the number of photons needed to provide the desired signal-to-noise ratio. In addition to scan duration, the timing of the scan relative to the phase of the cardiac cycle and the time interval between sequential scans are important for accurate analysis of the moving heart.

Gated Computed Tomography of the Heart

Several reports have described the potential use of x-ray computed tomography for dynamic studies of the heart, lungs, and circulation.[B10, G6, G7, H8, H9, L2, R8, R9, S6, T1, Y1] However, most approaches using conventional computed tomography systems are inadequate for true dynamic structural/functional studies of moving organs, either because they ignore the motion and suffer the inevitable deleterious effects on image resolution or because they use gating techniques[B10, H8, S6] in an attempt to reduce motion artifacts, but these too are subject to significant image degradation.

As an illustration, Figure 32–13 is a schematic diagram of two strategies for computed tomography of the heart by scan gating. In retrospective gating, appropriate angles of view are assembled for reconstruction after the scan on the basis of the electrocardiogram recorded during the scan. In prospective gating, the scan is performed at preselected cardiac intervals, using on-line electrocardiographic detection. In both methods, to collect enough angles of view to achieve reasonable resolution in the reconstructed transaxial image, several cardiac cycles must be recorded during several rotations of the scanner.

The advantage of retrospective gating is that different sets of projection data can be assembled following the continuous recording procedure to reconstruct the same cross section of the heart during different cycle segments. The advantage of prospective gating is the smaller dose to the patient required to obtain any single cardiac segment, since the x-ray exposure is required only during the portion of successive cardiac cycles selected for reconstruction prior to the scan. However, even though these cardiac gating techniques may provide "better" images of regions of the body contiguous to the heart and therefore are subject to displacement by its motion, both techniques suffer a serious disadvantage for imaging of the heart itself. Electrocardiographic gated scanning requires that there be physiologic stationarity—that is, exact reproducibility of the position of the thorax and the intrathoracic position, shape, dimensions, and density distribution within the heart—during the several heartbeats required for the scan and that the rate, amplitude, and position of the heart be independent of respiratory effects. These conditions are gen-

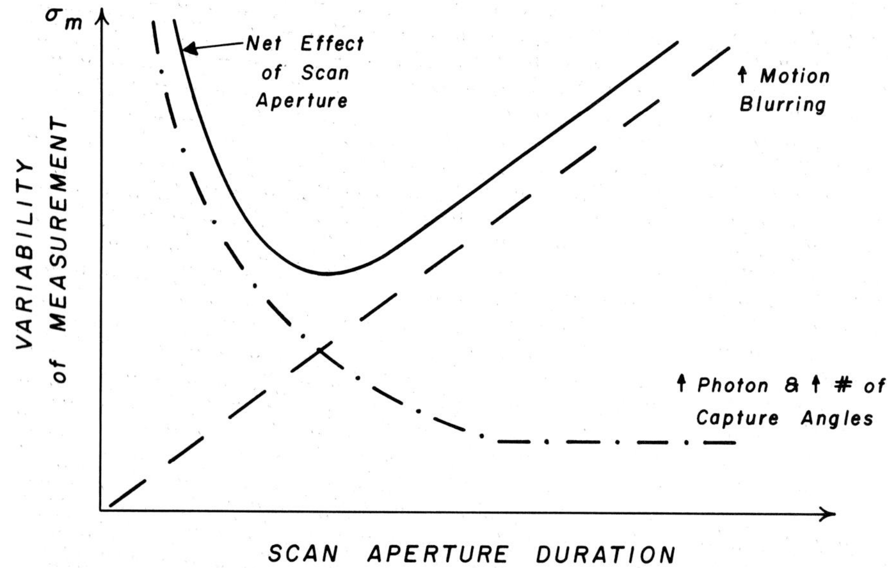

Figure 32–12. Schematic representation of the role of scan aperture duration in spatial resolution when the number of x-ray photons detected per pixel is increased by increasing the duration of the scan. The photon noise in the image decreases approximately as the square root of the increased scan duration (shown by the dashed and dotted line). When the scan duration is increased, motion "blurring" results in loss of spatial resolution of the structure's edge, as shown by the dashed line. The rate of rise of this line depends on the rate of movement of the structure of interest relative to the scan duration. The sum of these two opposing effects results in the relationship depicted by the solid line. Spatial resolution is expressed as the uncertainty of the spatial location of a detected edge in the image. (From Kim, K. H., Hoffman, E. A., and Ritman, E. L.: Needs and requirements for accurate measurement of dynamic 3-D geometry of the in situ heart. *In* Sideman, S., and Beyar, R., [eds.]: Simulation and Control of the Cardiac System, Vol. 1, Chap. 4. CRC Press, Boca Raton, Fla., 1987, pp. 41–50, with permission.)

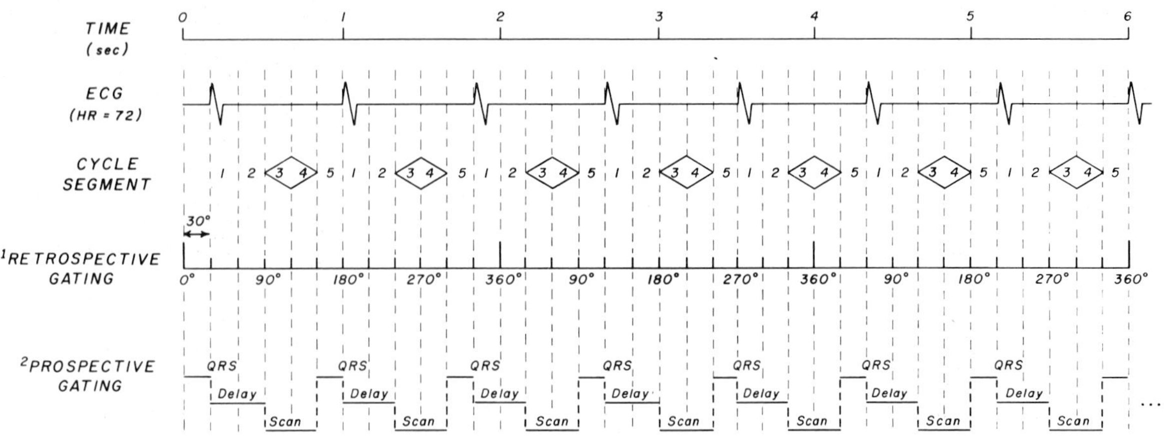

1. *Cardiac Cycle Segments Reconstructed from Post-Scan Selection of Different Projections Recorded during Same Segment of Successive Heart Beats*

2. *Cardiac Cycle Segment Reconstructed by Pre-Scan Selection of the Projection Recording Interval in Successive Heart Beats, Relative to the QRS Complex*

Figure 32–13. Examples of two gating techniques for computed tomographic imaging of the heart. The electrocardiogram is recorded simultaneously with the scan. By using the QRS complex of the electrocardiographic signal, successive cardiac cycles can be partitioned into several separate segments for reconstruction, as shown in the graph. In retrospective gating, the angles of view recorded during the same segment of successive cardiac cycles are assembled after the scan from enough cardiac cycles to provide all (or sufficient) angles of view required for the reconstruction. In prospective gating, the QRS complex of the electrocardiogram is detected during the scan, a predetermined delay is enacted, and the scan is performed only during the segment of the cardiac cycle that is preselected. Assuming a complete 360-degree scan in 2 seconds and a heart rate of 72 beats per minute, seven total heartbeats and three rotations of the scanner are required by both methods to collect all angles of view for reconstruction of segments 3 and 4 combined. (From Robb, R. A., Ritman, E. L., Harris, L. D., and Wood, E. H.: Dynamic three-dimensional x-ray computed tomography of the heart, lungs and circulation. IEEE Trans. Nucl. Sci. 26:1646, 1979, with permission.)

erally not true for extended periods of time, even in the presence of cardiac pacing. The fact that these conditions are not true presents a paradox for gated scanning of the heart, since to improve resolution in the images, more views must be collected, which means that more heartbeats must be used, which in turn degrades resolution because of lack of physiologic stationarity.

Gated scanning, even if each profile scan at each angle of view is virtually instantaneous, cannot be used for angiographic imaging of vascular anatomy or circulatory function. The transient dynamic distribution pattern and concentration of the contrast medium during and following its injection vary continuously and nonreproducibly. Moreover, the pharmacologic effect of the contrast medium alters the hemodynamic and cardiodynamic status considerably, so that beat-to-beat constancy of the heartbeat cannot be achieved during or for a considerable period after the injection of contrast materials.

Stop-Action Computed Tomography of Moving Organs

The capability for measurement of cardiac, pulmonary, and circulatory dynamics is now available and is based on the development of three-dimensional, x-ray computed tomography systems with high temporal resolution. These systems offer the potential for measurement in the intact thorax of the instant-to-instant regional changes in shape and dimensions of the heart and lungs and of the spatial distribution of myocardial and pulmonary blood flow, which are the fundamental determinants of cardiac and pulmonary function and reserve. In addition, dynamic spatial computed tomography of the heart facilitates accurate diagnostic assessment of the localization, extent, and nature of cardiovascular abnormalities and pathology such as coronary artery disease, myocardial ischemia, and myocardial infarction.

Two different approaches to true high-temporal-resolution three-dimensional imaging of the heart have been developed into what might be termed fifth-generation x-ray computed tomography systems. These systems are known as the Imatron, a commercially available fast scanner originally developed at the University of California, San Francisco, and the Dynamic Spatial Reconstructor, a biomedical research system developed at the Mayo Clinic.

The Fast Computed Tomography Scanner

In this section, the fundamental principles and operating parameters of a fast computed tomography scanner first described by Boyd and associates[B7, H5] will be discussed. This fifth-generation scanner is unique in several aspects, the most important of which is that it has no x-ray tube but has an electron beam that scans four stationary rings, allowing the acquisition of relative x-ray attenuation information in as little as 50 msec. This design is fundamentally different from that of other conventional CT scanners, including those which are capable of subsecond scanning. As might be suspected, the ability to acquire information so rapidly involves trade-offs with regard to the performance of this system compared with conventional CT scanners. The fundamental principles of data acquisition, image reconstruction, and data processing as well as the operational performance of this system with respect to other CT scanners will be described.

In conventional computed tomography, the necessity to rotate the gantry back to its original position following data acquisition and other mechanical and electrical considerations limit the scan acquisition time to about 2 seconds and the interscan delay time to about 3 seconds. Fast computed tomography may be performed with an x-ray tube by eliminating the cabling of high voltage to the x-ray tube ("Slip-ring" technology), thus allowing the gantry to rotate continuously and allowing acquisition times as short as 0.6 second with interscan delay.

The acquisition geometry for the fast scanner that uses a scanning electron beam with stationary targets, termed the fifth-generation scanner, is shown diagrammatically in Figure 32–14. In this design, a conventional x-ray tube does not exist; rather, an electron beam is scanned over stationary tungsten targets to produce a moving fan beam of x-rays as the electrons are stopped in the tungsten target (this process is the same as that found in conventional x-ray tubes and the x-ray radiation produced is

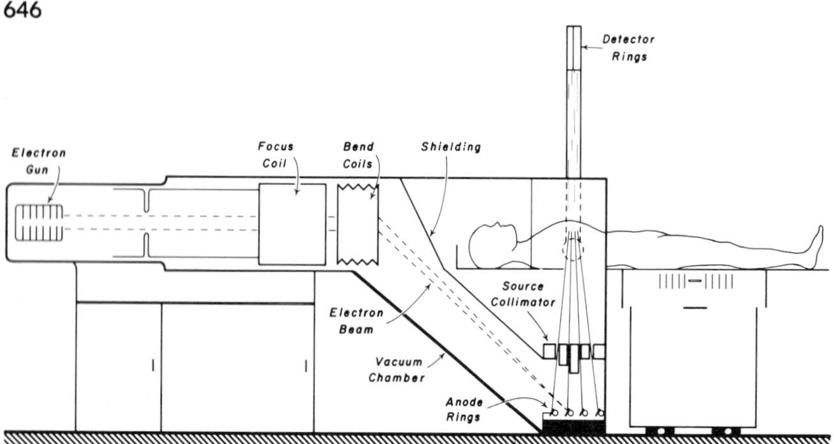

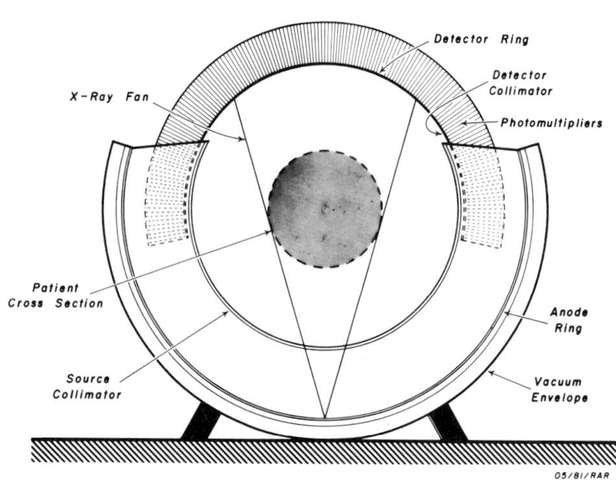

Figure 32–14. Acquisition technique for fifth-generation fast x-ray computed tomography systems. (From Robb, R. A.: X-ray computed tomography: An engineering synthesis of multiscientific principles. CRC Critical Reviews in Biomedical Engineering 7[4]:265–334, 1982, with permission.)

called bremsstrahlung).[C8] These targets encompass an angle of 180 degrees about the patient, and the total area of acquisition is 210 degrees about the patient (180 degrees plus the fan angle of 30 degrees). Above the patient, a ring of detectors extends 180 degrees about the patient. This detector ring comprises two separate banks of solid-state detectors, which allow two image slices to be reconstructed from x-ray production on one of the target rings. Hence, eight image slices are obtained after the four targets are scanned in succession by the electron beam in this multiple-slice mode. An individual target can be scanned in as short a time as 50 msec with a 5-msec interscan delay time. To improve resolution, a special set of collimators (devices to limit the x-ray beam width) can be placed mechanically about the patient. In this single-slice mode, scans as short as 100 msec can be obtained. In either case, it is possible to average multiple data sets to produce acquisition times that range from 50 to 1400 msec in increments of 50 or 100 msec, depending on the mode used (single slice or multiple slice). Since only one detector ring is actually coplanar with the detectors, special care and techniques must be used to account for this geometry during reconstruction.[B7] Also, since data are not acquired completely about the patient (as in conventional computed tomography), special techniques must be utilized to reconstruct the image following data acquisition.[P7] These two facets of cone beam geometry and limited angle reconstruction also differentiate this type of fast computed tomography from conventional techniques.

The precise selection of acquisition mode (multiple slice without collimator versus single slice with collimator), slice width, and scan time can have a marked effect on image quality, as demonstrated with the test object shown in Figure 32–15. To

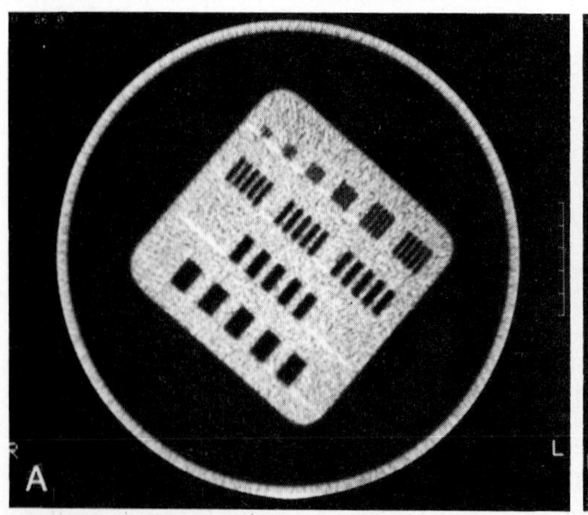

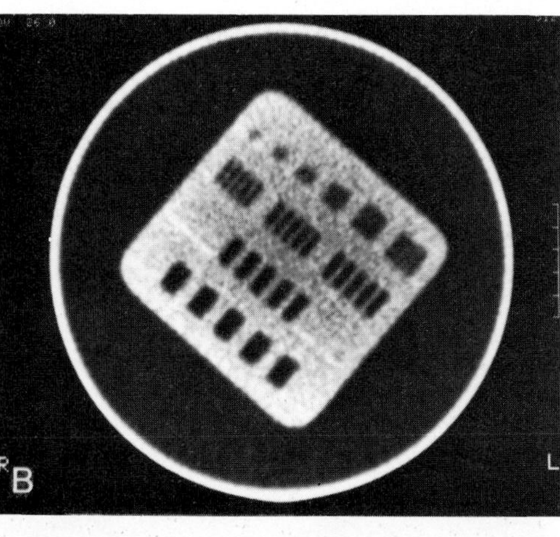

Figure 32–15. Resolution test objects for fast computed tomography in the single-slice, *A*, and multiple-slice, *B*, modes.

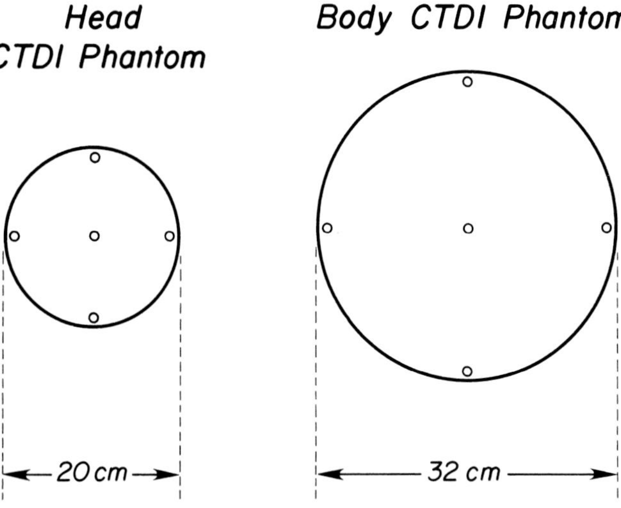

Figure 32–16. Diagram of phantom positions for computed tomography dose index (CTDI) measurements.

better appreciate the interrelationship among these variables, we shall next examine the performance measurements and characteristics of this system compared to conventional systems. We shall describe the traditional physics performance tests commonly used in computed tomography and compare the results obtained with scanning electron beam fast CT and conventional CT systems. The tests to be described include the following:

1. Radiation dosimetry
2. Slice thickness and contiguity
3. Spatial resolution
4. Low-contrast resolution
5. Uniformity
6. Noise
7. Hounsfield unit linearity
8. Half-value layer
9. Accuracy of scanned projection radiograph
10. Accuracy of quantitative measurements.

The purpose of these measurements is to discover and define the performance of the computed tomography system with respect to optimum image quality and most efficient use of radiation dose.

Radiation Dosimetry

The radiation dose of computed tomography systems is commonly measured by using the computed tomography dose index (CTDI). This method was first presented by Shope and associates[S10] and is performed with a special ionization chamber[S11] that is capable of accurately measuring the radiation exposure for x-ray beams of variable beam width. This measurement is performed in a Plexiglas phantom (to simulate the scatter of radiation within a patient) at various positions within the scan circle as diagrammed in Figure 32–16. Two sizes of phantoms are used to simulate doses encountered in examination of the head or small body parts and examinations of the chest, abdomen, and pelvis. In general, the computed tomography dose index is designed to measure the total integral dose the patient would receive from a series of contiguous slices. This value is not identical to a single-slice exposure because the dose profile does not decrease abruptly to zero at the edges of the slice but rather follows a more Gaussian distribution,[M5, S10] as shown in Figure 32–17. The measured exposure value is divided by the slice width, which makes the measurement much more robust because it is independent of slice width. This independence becomes important for scanning electron beam fast computed tomography because the slice width, particularly in the multiple-slice mode, is dependent on table height and other factors owing to the cone beam geometry and the limited sweep of the fan beam. For this reason, it often is important to measure the radiation slice width accurately by wrapping radiographic film around the CTDI phantom to produce images of the radiation beam as shown in Figure 32–18. It is important to distinguish this radiation slice thickness from the image slice thickness, which we shall discuss later; it is possible for the image slice thickness to be significantly smaller than the radiation slice thickness. This procedure is commonly not necessary in conventional computed tomography because of the coplanar geometry and rotation of the fan beam completely about the patient. Comparative dosimetry for head and body scanning for conventional and fast computed tomography is given in Table 32–1. Note that the dose distribution for the scanning electron beam fast technique is very different from that for the conventional technique. This difference is due to the fact that the fan beam does not rotate completely about the patient in scanning electron beam fast computed tomography. As a result, the radiation exposure of anterior structures for a supine patient is

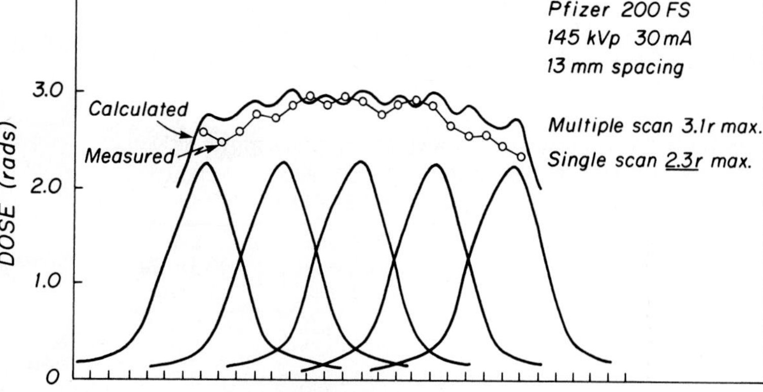

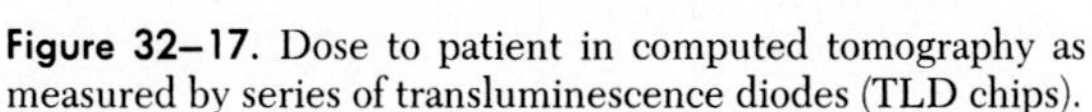
Figure 32–17. Dose to patient in computed tomography as measured by series of transluminescence diodes (TLD chips).

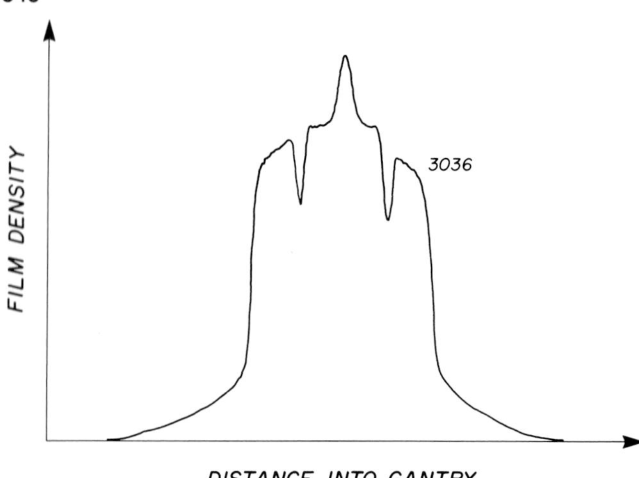

Figure 32–18. Radiation slice profiles for fifth-generation scanning electron beam fast computed tomography.

Table 32–2. SLICE THICKNESS AND CONTIGUITY FOR CONVENTIONAL (PICKER 1200) AND FAST (PICKER FASTRAC) COMPUTED TOMOGRAPHY

Slice Location	Desired (8 mm)	Conventional (5 mm)	Fast, Single Slice (6 mm)	Fast, Multiple Slice (8 mm)
1	8	5	6	7
1–2	0	0	0	1
2	8	5	6	5
2–3	0	0	0	6
3	8	5	6	6
3–4	0	0	0	1
4	8	5	6	7
4–5	0	0	0	1
5	8	5	6	8
5–6	0	0	0	1
6	8	5	6	7
6–7	0	0	0	10
7	8	5	6	7
7–8	0	0	0	1
8	8	5	6	2

approximately 83 percent less with stationary-target fast computed tomography.

Slice Thickness and Contiguity

The purpose of this test is to measure the slice thickness and the adjacency (contiguity) of successive slices. This measurement is compared with the selected slice thickness and table movement if applicable. The reference test phantom[G12] consists of a cylinder with a spiral staircase of Plexiglas disks. Each disk is 2 mm thick and has one section (vane) milled every 12 degrees. These disks are then stacked on one another to produce a spiral staircase effect. This assembly is encased in a Plexiglas cylinder that is filled with water. Hence, the slice thickness measurement is performed by counting the number of vanes and multiplying by 2 to obtain the slice thickness in millimeters. The adjacency of successive slices is measured by determining the number of missing vanes between successive slices. This phantom is somewhat different from the traditional "ramp" phantom that is used with conventional computed tomography. It is used in fast computed tomography because of its accuracy and ease of use in examining slice thickness and contiguity in the multiple-slice mode. The relative performance of the conventional and fast techniques is given in Table 32–2. Representative images are shown in Figure 32–19. The slice thickness and contiguity in the multiple-slice mode can vary substantially, which is an important observation with regard to the clinical utility of images obtained with this acquisition geometry. It is important to determine this exact relationship on a specific machine, particularly if the detection of small anatomic detail is an important diagnostic criterion.

Spatial Resolution

The purpose of this test is to determine how a system is able to resolve small, dense objects, or how close together small objects can be before a system can no longer determine the presence of two or more objects. The test phantom utilized in this procedure is the General Electric 8800 resolution pattern. This phantom, shown diagrammatically in Figure 32–20, consists of a Plexiglas block in which lines of variable width and interspacing have been milled. The groups span a range of resolution from 0.63 to 10.0 line pairs (lp)/cm. The performance of both conventional and fast computed tomography is summarized in Table 32–3. Representative images are shown in Figures 32–21 and 32–22. Since by definition the objects to be used for testing are of high contrast (in this case, relatively dense), the overall signal difference measured is great and therefore does not appreciably depend on scan time for fast computed tomography, as shown in Table 32–4 and Figure 32–23.

Low-Contrast Resolution

The purpose of this test is to determine the ability of a system to record faithfully the presence of an object that does not differ from its surrounding to a great degree. The test object used (RMI Corp., Madison, Wisconsin) consists of a cylinder that differs from its surroundings by 6 Hounsfield units. Holes ranging

Table 32–1. COMPARATIVE RADIATION DOSIMETRY FOR CONVENTIONAL (PICKER 1200) AND FAST (PICKER FASTRAC) COMPUTED TOMOGRAPHY SYSTEMS

Scanner	Mode	Entrance Exposure (R/sec)	Midline Exposure (R/sec)	Exit Exposure (R/sec)
Conventional	Body	1.9	0.8	1.9
Conventional	Head	1.9	1.8	1.9
Fast	Body	10.0	2.5	1.7
Fast	Head	10.0	6.0	4.1

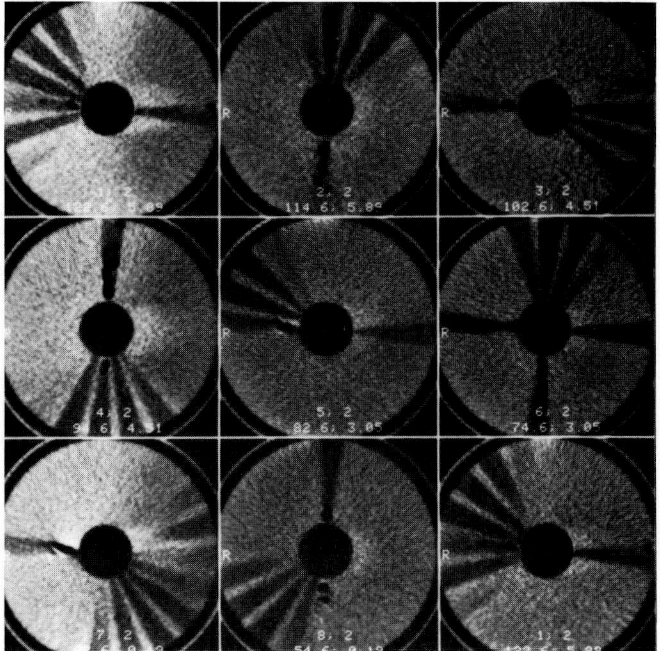

Figure 32–19. Slice thickness and contiguity for multiple-slice fast computed tomography (Picker FASTRAC).

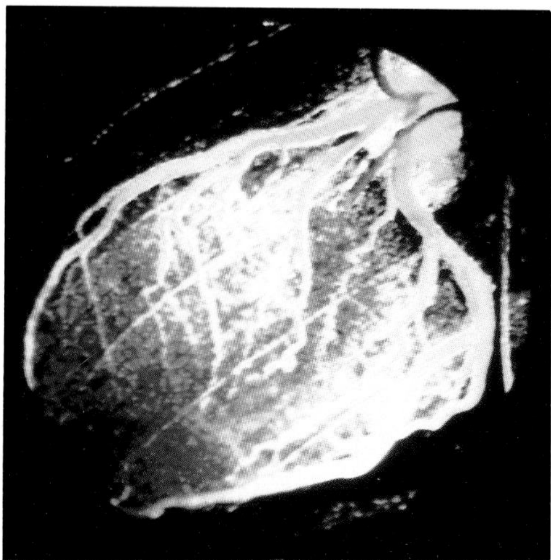

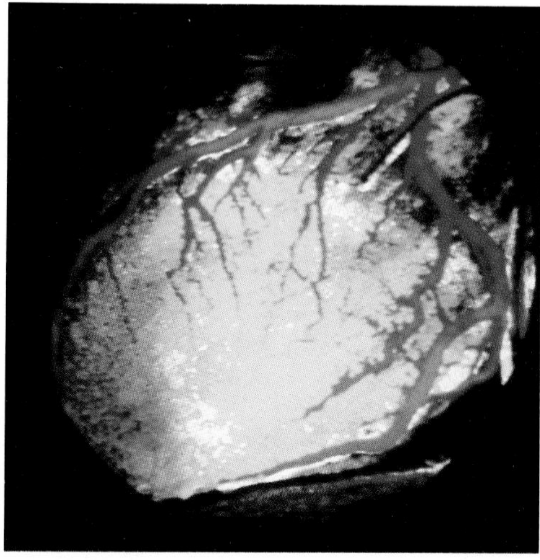

Figure 16–36.
A set of contrast myocardial appearance pictures taken in the basal state *(left)* and after papaverine-induced hyperemia *(right)*. Color coding depicts the transit of contrast per cycle (cycle 1 = red, cycle 2 = yellow, and so on). Density information is encoded in the intensity of each pixel. Analyses from regions of interest in both coronary beds showed normal flow reserve in this patient.

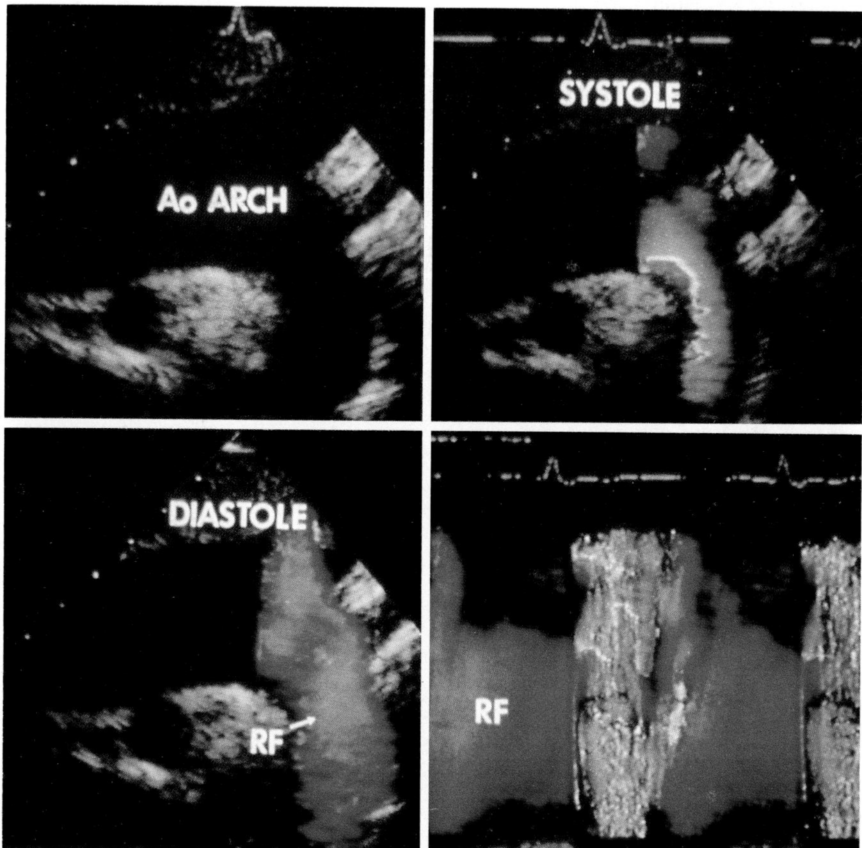

Figure 21–10.
Flow reversal in the descending aorta in a patient with severe aortic regurgitation demonstrated from the suprasternal window. *Top left,* Two-dimensional image of the aortic arch and descending aorta. *Top right,* Systolic frame demonstrates anterograde flow, which appears blue, in descending aorta. *Bottom left,* Diastolic frame demonstrates retrograde flow, which appears red, in descending aorta. *Bottom right,* Color M-mode demonstrates holodiastolic regurgitant flow. Ao arch—aortic arch; RF—regurgitant flow.

Plate 2

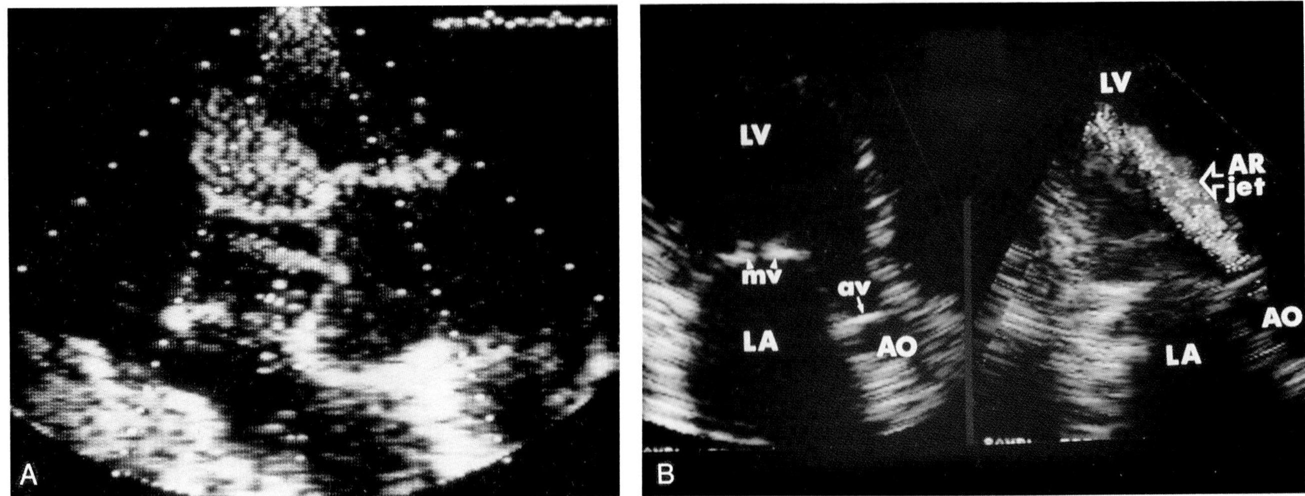

Figure 21–11.
Assessment of severity of aortic regurgitation by color-flow imaging. *A*, Parasternal long-axis view. The proximal minimal width of the regurgitant jet is less than 20 per cent of the width of the left ventricular outflow tract, indicative of mild aortic regurgitation. *B*, Apical long-axis views, with and without color flow. A long, broad jet of aortic regurgitation is seen in a patient with moderate aortic regurgitation. AO—aorta; AR—aortic regurgitation; av—aortic valve; LA—left atrium; LV—left ventricle; mv—mitral valve.

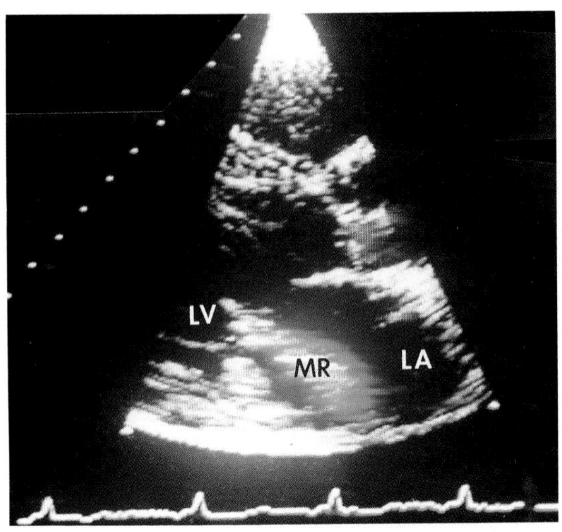

Figure 21–19.
Moderate mitral regurgitation from a parasternal long-axis view. High-velocity, turbulent flow (mosaic pattern) is characteristic because of the large systolic pressure gradient between the left ventricle and left atrium. LA—left atrium; LV—left ventricle; MR—mitral regurgitation.

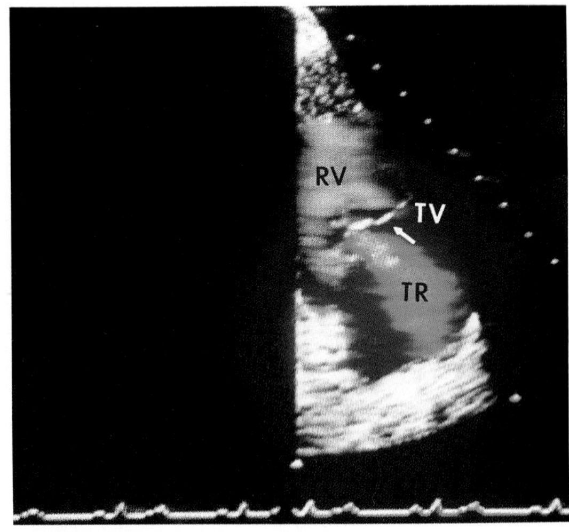

Figure 21–22.
Moderate tricuspid regurgitation. Color-flow imaging from an apical four-chamber view demonstrates systolic regurgitant flow through the tricuspid orifice into the right atrium. RV—right ventricle; TR—tricuspid regurgitation; TV—tricuspid valve.

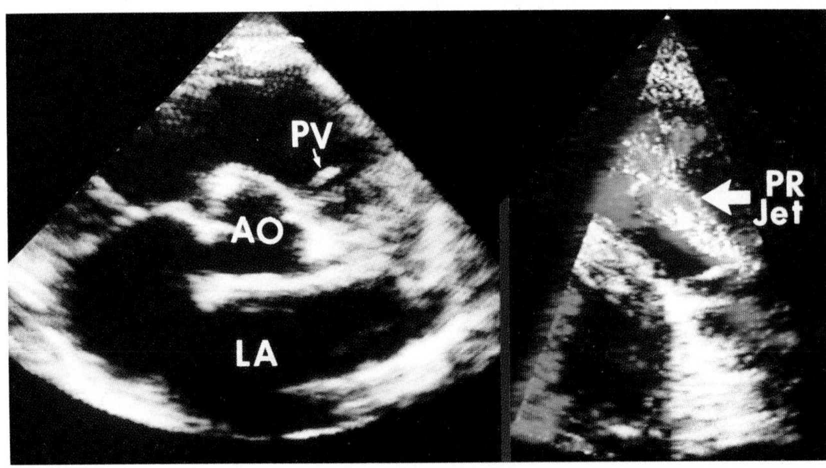

Figure 21–25.
Pulmonary regurgitation (PR) by color-flow imaging. A parasternal short-axis view demonstrates a diastolic red encoded jet in the right ventricular outflow tract representing a mild-to-moderate degree of pulmonary regurgitation. Ao—aorta; LA—left atrium; PV—pulmonary valve.

Plate 3

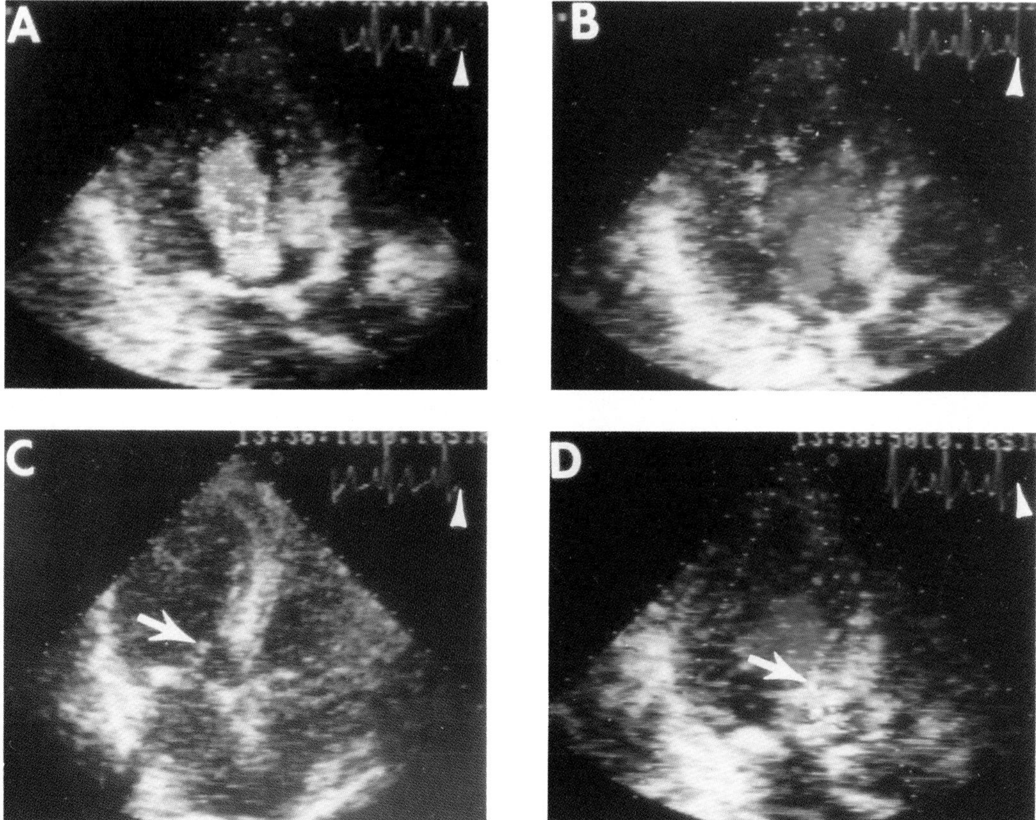

Figure 22–3.
A color flow imaging sequence using an apical long-axis cross-sectional view in a patient with hypertrophic cardiomyopathy. *A* is in early diastole with mitral inflow (red color) coming into the left ventricle. *B* is taken at end diastole when eddy formation results in flow pointed toward outflow tract (blue color). *C* and *D* are both in midsystole; the image in *C* is without color flow and shows SAM as pointed by *arrow*. As the color is turned on, *D* at the same phase of this cardiac cycle shows turbulence (mosaic coloration) at the site of the SAM–septal contact *(arrow)*.

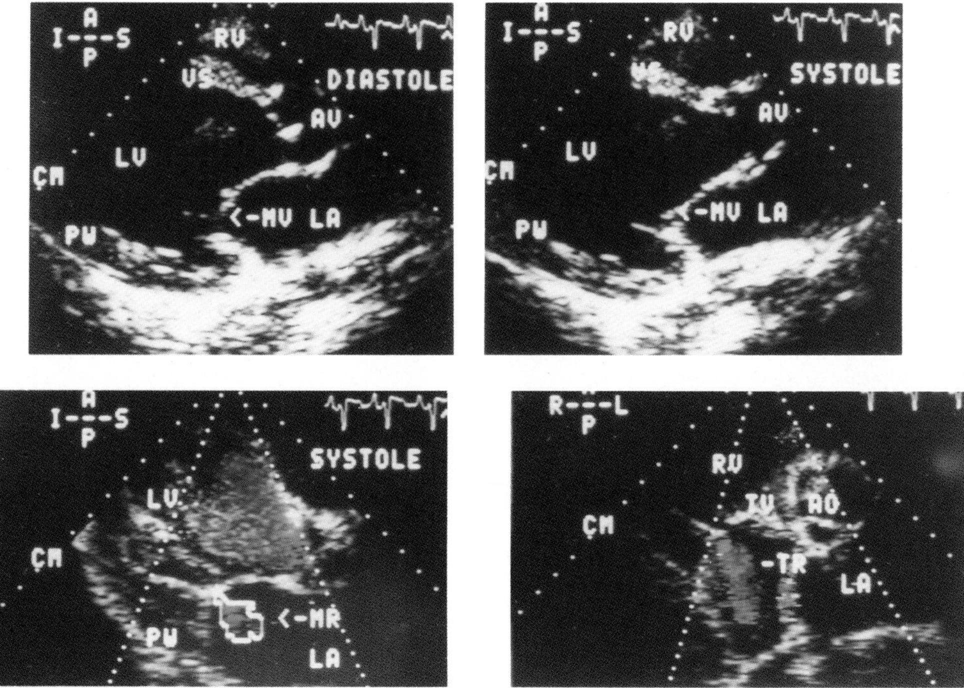

Figure 22–9.
A composite showing parasternal long-axis views in the *upper panels* and color flow images of mitral regurgitation and tricuspid regurgitation in the *lower panels* in a patient with dilated cardiomyopathy. Poor systolic excursion with displacement of mitral valve coaptation in the left ventricle is seen in the *upper right panel*. The central jet of mitral regurgitation (blue color) is seen in the parasternal long-axis view *(lower left)*, and the jet of tricuspid regurgitation (blue color) is seen in the parasternal short-axis view *(lower right)*.

Plate 4

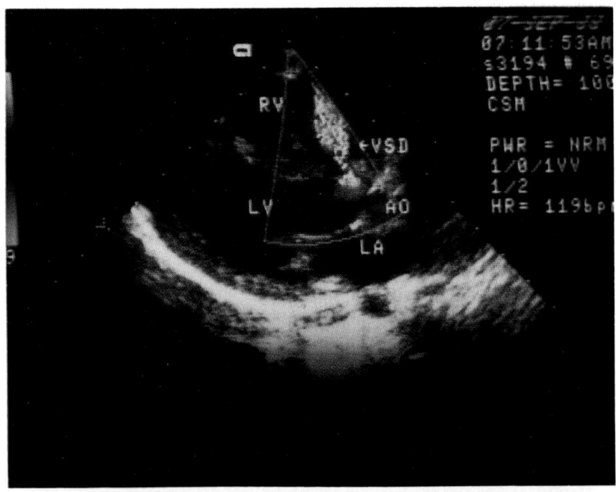

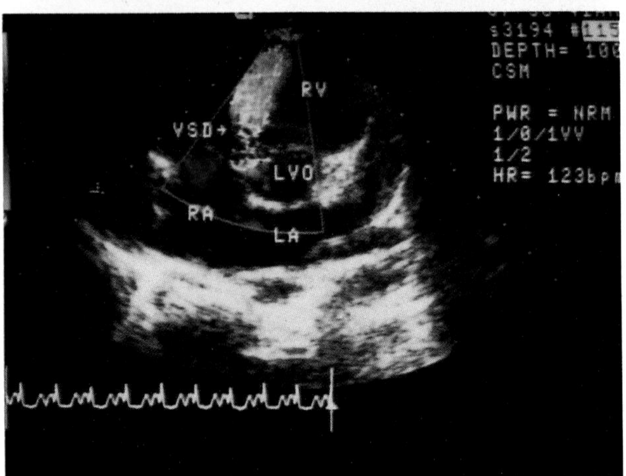

Figure 24–4.
Color flow Doppler examination of a patient with a small membranous ventricular septal defect (VSD). The jet flow through the VSD is seen in the parasternal long-axis *(top)* and short-axis *(bottom)* views. The mosaic appearance of the jet is caused by the presence of high-velocity disturbed flow. Abbreviations: AO—aorta; LA—left atrium; LV—left ventricle; LVO—left ventricular outflow tract; RA—right atrium; RV—right ventricle.

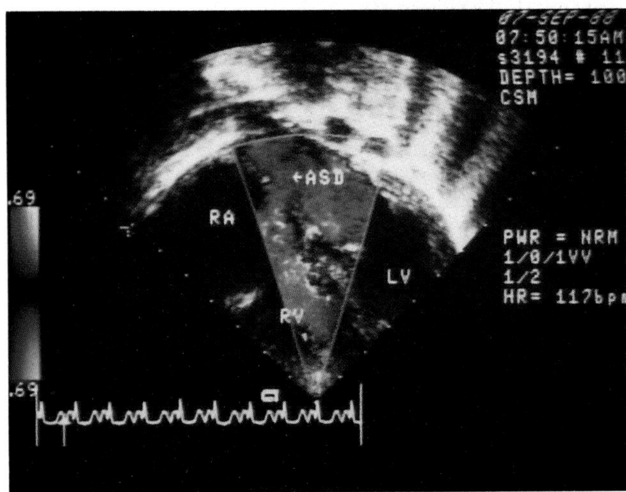

Figure 24–7.
Doppler color flow examination of a child with a large secundum atrial septal defect (ASD). In the four-chamber view, the jet flow through the ASD is seen. The red color of the jet indicates low-velocity flow directed toward the transducer. The yellow areas within the jet indicate variance or disturbed flow. Abbreviations: LV—left ventricle; RA—right atrium; RV—right ventricle.

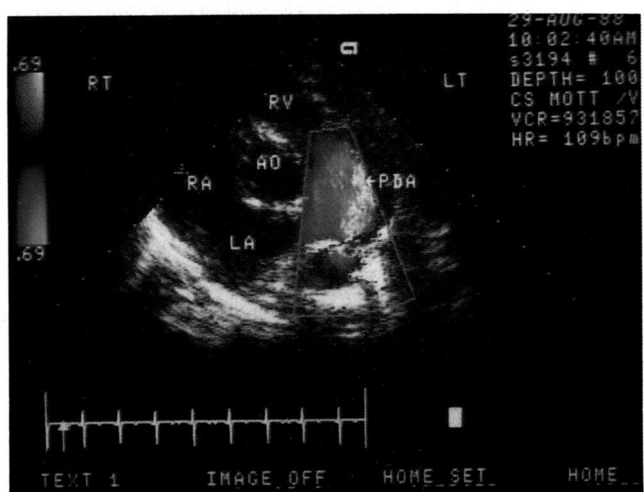

Figure 24–13.
Doppler color flow examination in the parasternal short-axis view of a child with a patent ductus arteriosus (PDA). The jet flow through the PDA appears as a mosaic of colors, which indicates disturbed high-velocity flow toward the transducer. Abbreviations: AO—aorta; LA—left atrium; LT—left; RA—right atrium; RT—right; RV—right ventricle.

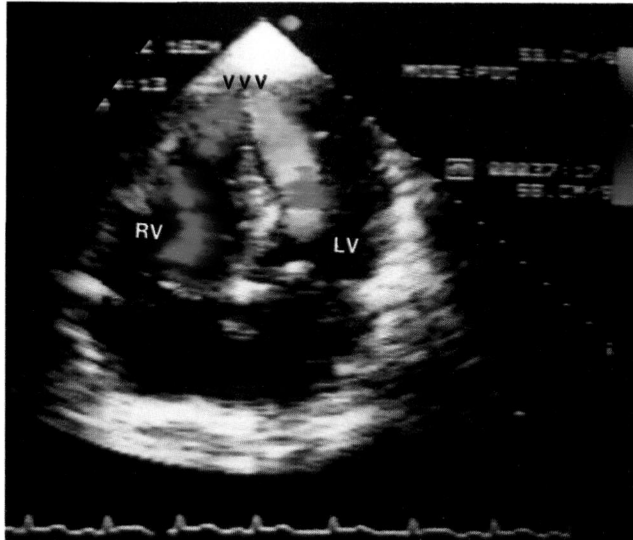

Figure 29–11.
Color Doppler demonstration of ventricular septal defect secondary to myocardial infarction. Abnormal left ventricle to right ventricular flow across the defect is depicted by *arrowheads*. The orange color indicates blood flow toward the transducer; blue indicates flow away from the transducer. LV—left ventricle. RV—right ventricle.

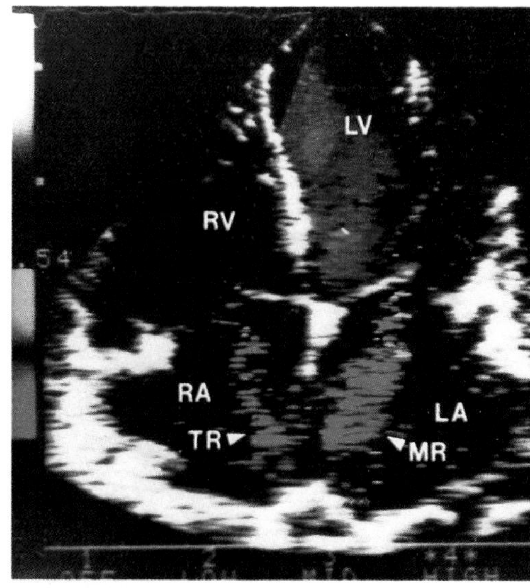

Figure 29–13.
Color Doppler echocardiogram obtained from the apical four-chamber view. An eccentric turquoise mitral regurgitant jet (MR) and a tricuspid regurgitant jet (TR) are evident in this patient with ischemic myocardiopathy and papillary muscle dysfunction. LA—left atrium; LV—left ventricle; RA—right atrium; RV—right ventricle. (From Kotler, M. N., Goldman, A. P., and Parry, W. R.: Acute consequences and chronic complications of acute myocardial infarction. *In* Kerber, R. E. (ed.): Echocardiography in Coronary Artery Disease. Futura Publishing Company, Mt. Kisco, NY, 1988, p. 17, with permission.)

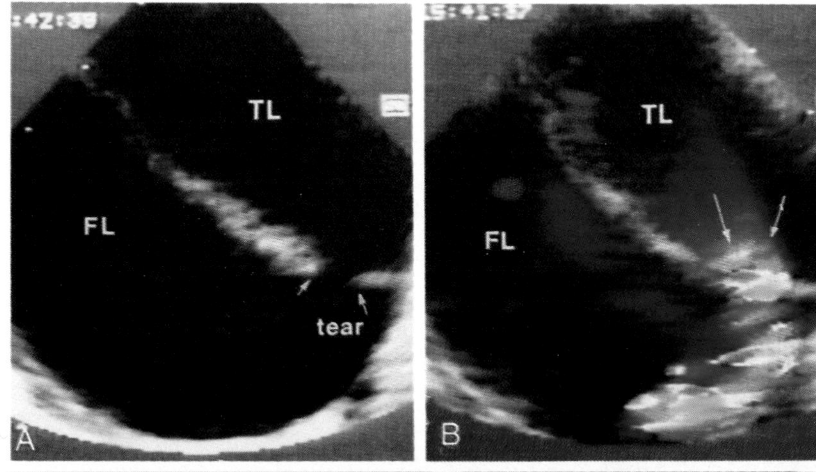

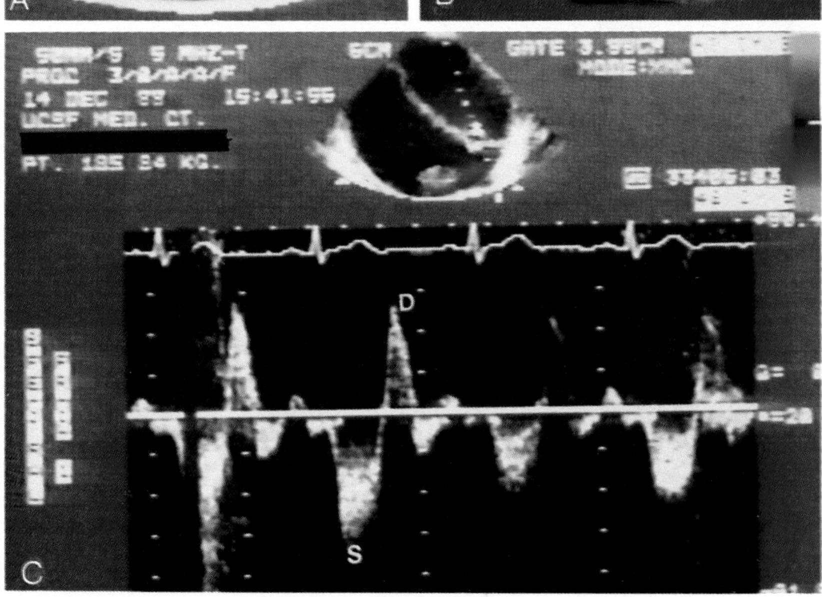

Figure 30—7.
Transesophageal echocardiographic evaluation of a descending aortic dissection. *A*, Two-dimensional imaging demonstrates a 0.5-cm intimal tear. *B*, Blood flow through this intimal flap is illustrated by color Doppler imaging. *C*, Pulsed Doppler interrogation demonstrates that flow is predominantly systolic (S) from the true lumen (TL) to the false lumen (FL); there is a component of diastolic (D) reverse flow from the false lumen to the true lumen.

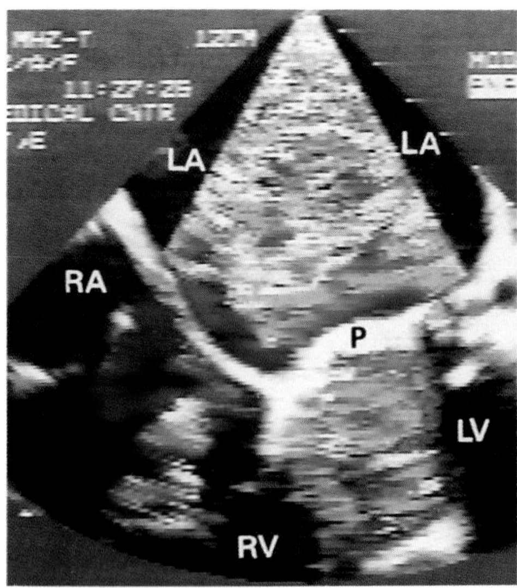

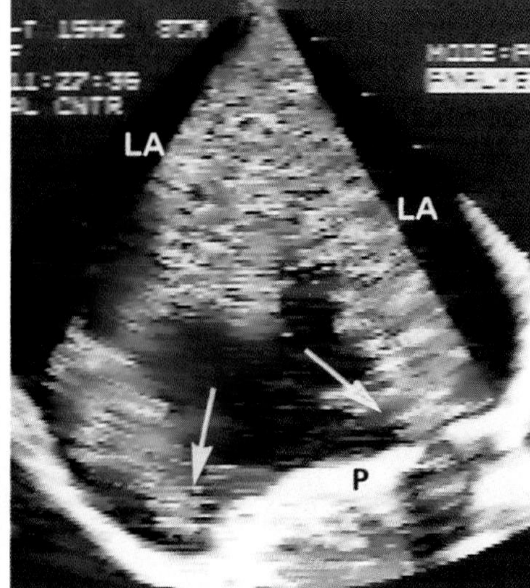

Figure 30–11.
Transesophageal echocardiographic demonstration of severe paravalvular mitral prosthetic regurgitation. Two separate, distinct paravalvular regurgitant jets can be seen *(arrows)*. P — mitral valve prosthesis. LA—left atrium; RA—right atrium; LV—left ventricle, RV—right ventricle.

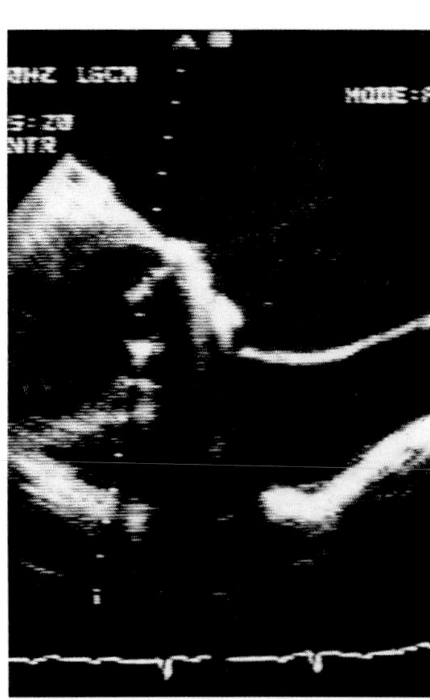

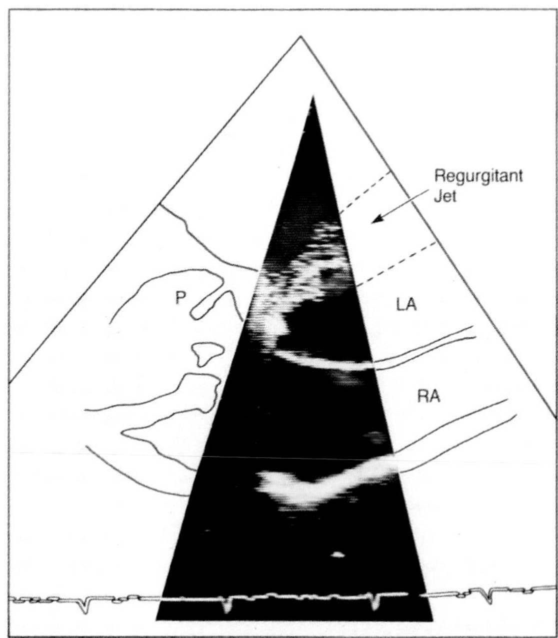

Figure 30–12.
Central mitral prosthetic regurgitation. Transesophageal echocardiographic view of a patient with a Starr-Edwards mitral prosthesis and a "giant" left atrium (10 cm) compressing the right atrium *(left)*. Schematic and photo composite *(right)* demonstrates a moderate central regurgitant jet not detected by TTE (dual aortic and mitral prostheses block *both* parasternal and apical interrogation). LA—left atrium; P—mitral valve prosthesis; RA—right atrium.

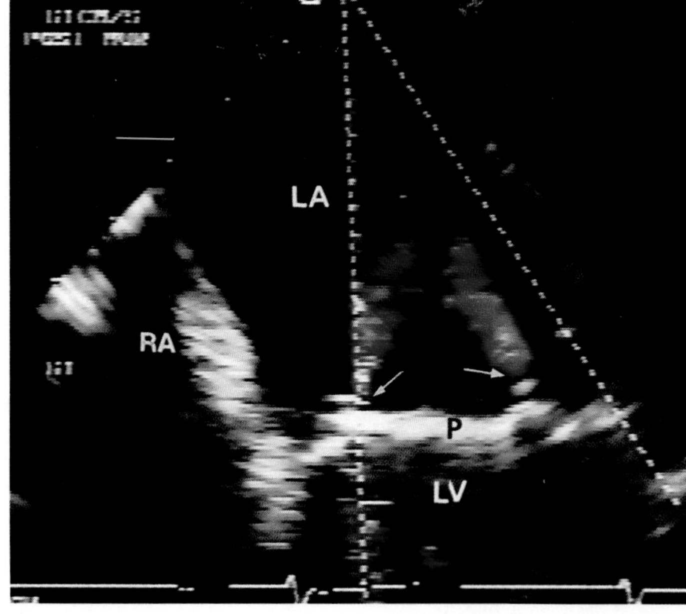

Figure 30–13.
Transesophageal echocardiographic image of normal "physiologic" regurgitation *(arrows)* in a St. Jude mitral prosthesis. P—prosthesis; LA—left atrium; RA—right atrium; LV—left ventricle.

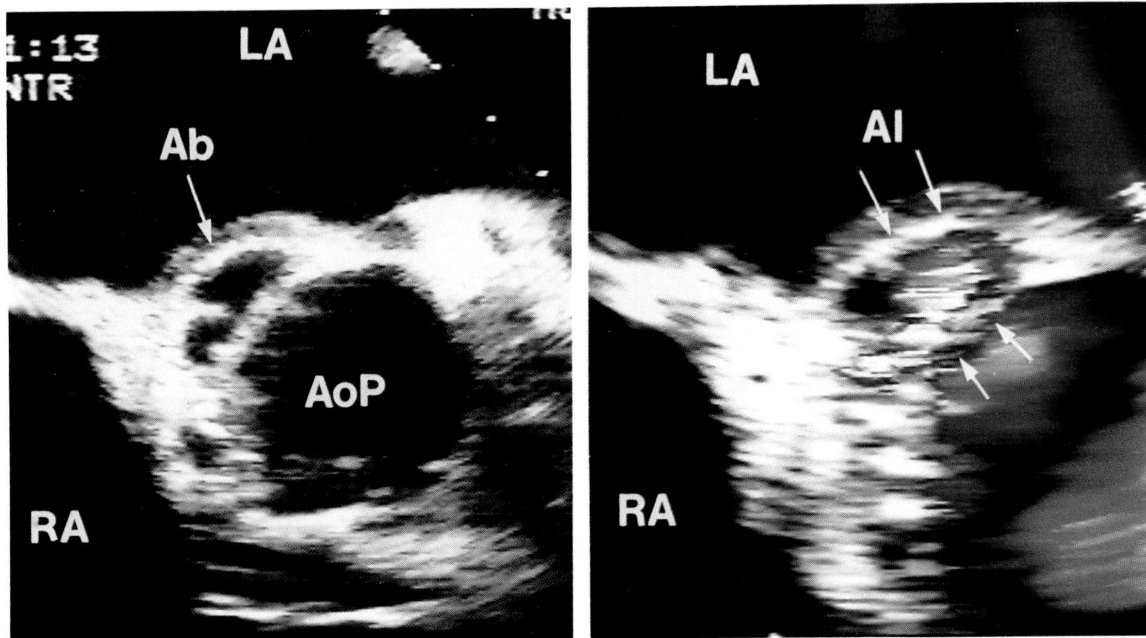

Figure 30–14.
Transesophageal echocardiographic views of a posterior aortic prosthetic (AoP) sewing ring abscess (Ab) in the region of the fibrous trigone (region of His bundle crossing) in a patient with prosthetic endocarditis and a new second-degree heart block. Color flow images demonstrate paravalvular aortic regurgitation (AI) *(arrows)* through the ring abscess.

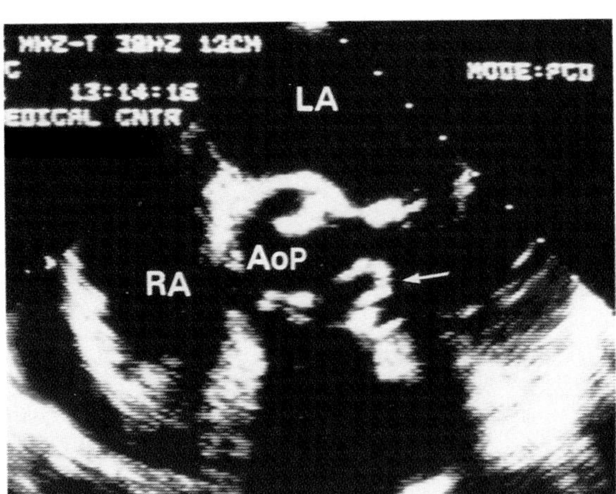

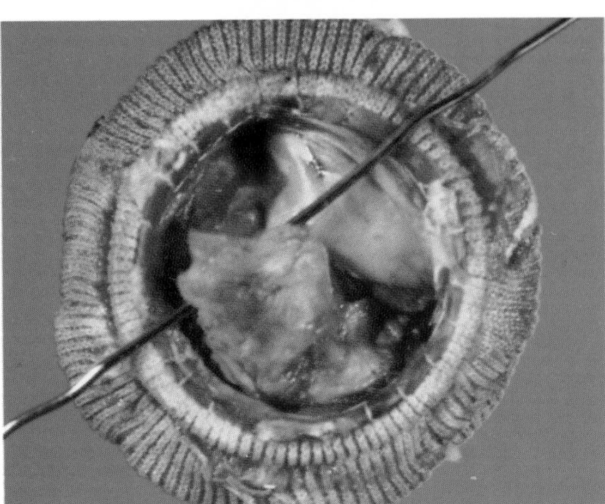

Figure 30–15.
In this patient with severe aortic regurgitation due to prosthetic valve endocarditis, transesophageal echocardiography demonstrated a flail porcine cusp *(arrow)* prolapsing into the left ventricular outflow tract. The torn cusp was confirmed at surgery. Pathologic specimen at *bottom*. AoP—aortic prosthesis; LA—left atrium; RA—right atrium.

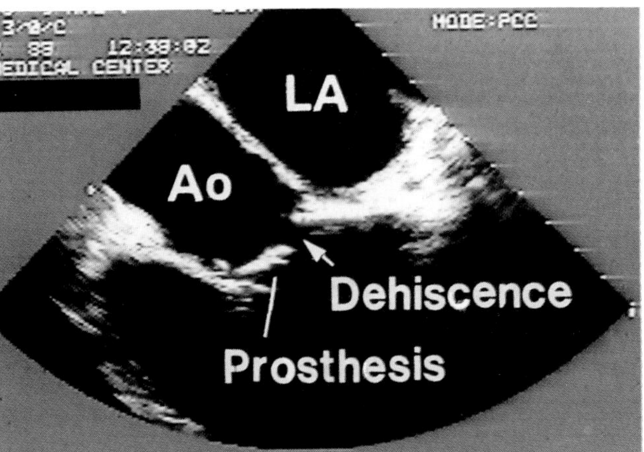

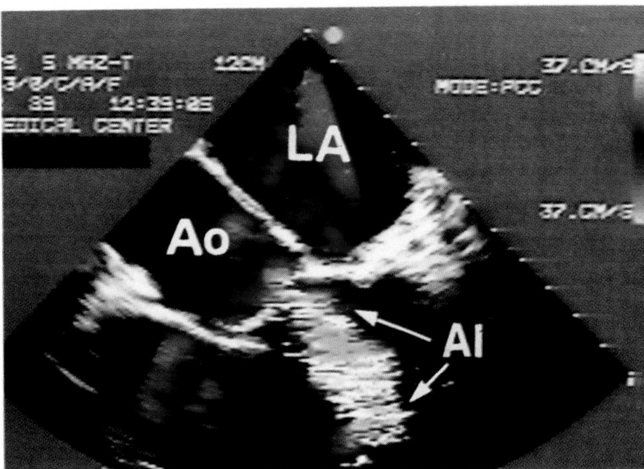

Figure 30–16.
Modified transesophageal echocardiographic long-axis view of the aortic root (Ao) demonstrating paravalvular aortic prosthetic regurgitation *(bottom)* due to sewing ring dehiscence *(top)*. AI—aortic insufficiency; LA—left atrium.

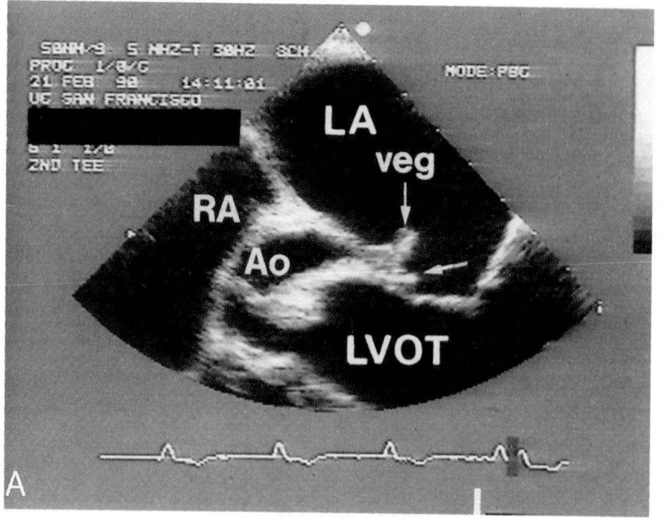

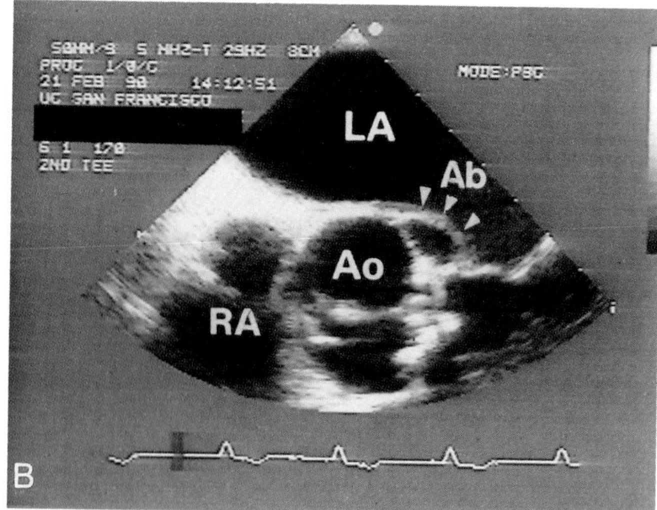

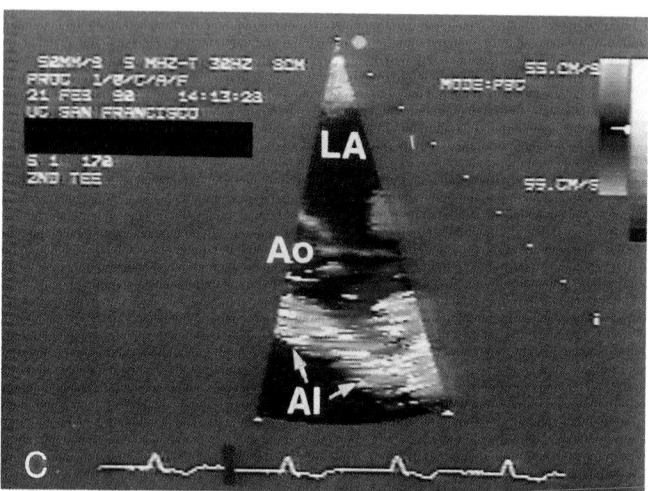

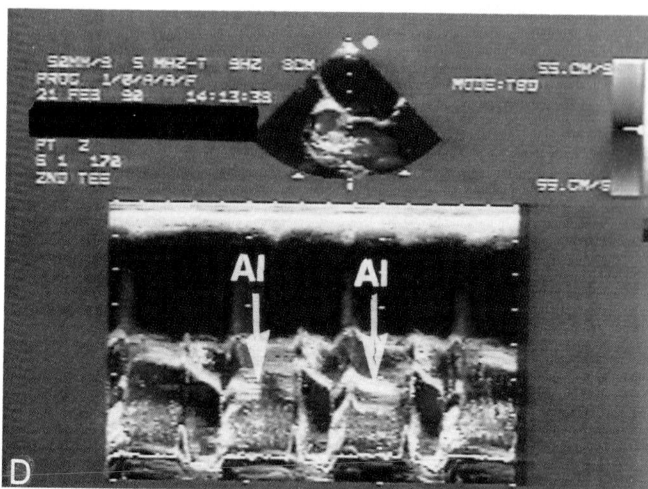

Figure 30–18.
Transesophageal echocardiographic views in a patient with aortic valve endocarditis. *A*, There is marked thickening of the aortic leaflets, with a vegetation (veg) involving the aortic annulus and base of the anterior mitral leaflet. An annular ring abscess (Ab) can also be seen in this region *(B)*, as well as aortic insufficiency *(C* and *D)*. AI—aortic insufficiency; Ao—aortic root; LVOT—left ventricular outflow tract; LA—left atrium; RA—right atrium.

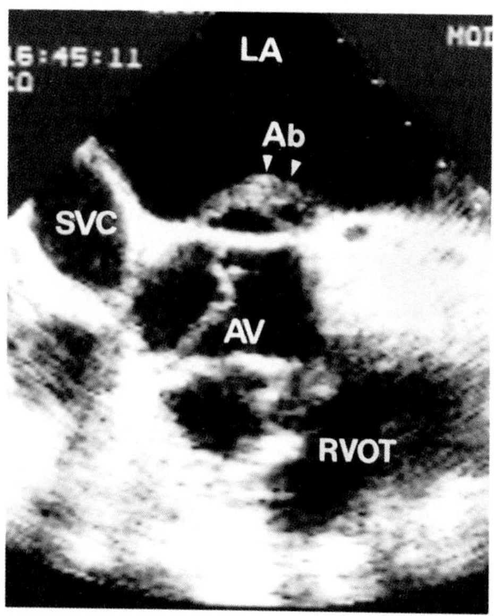

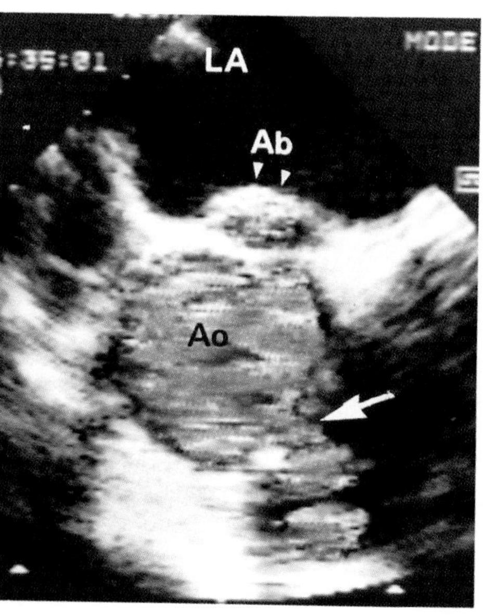

Figure 30–19.
Complications of endocarditis. Transesophageal echocardiographic visualization of an aortic root (Ao) to right ventricular outflow tract fistula (large arrow) and an abscess (Ab) involving the left coronary sinus. SVC—superior vena cava; RVOT—right ventricular outflow tract; LA—left atrium; AV—aortic valve.

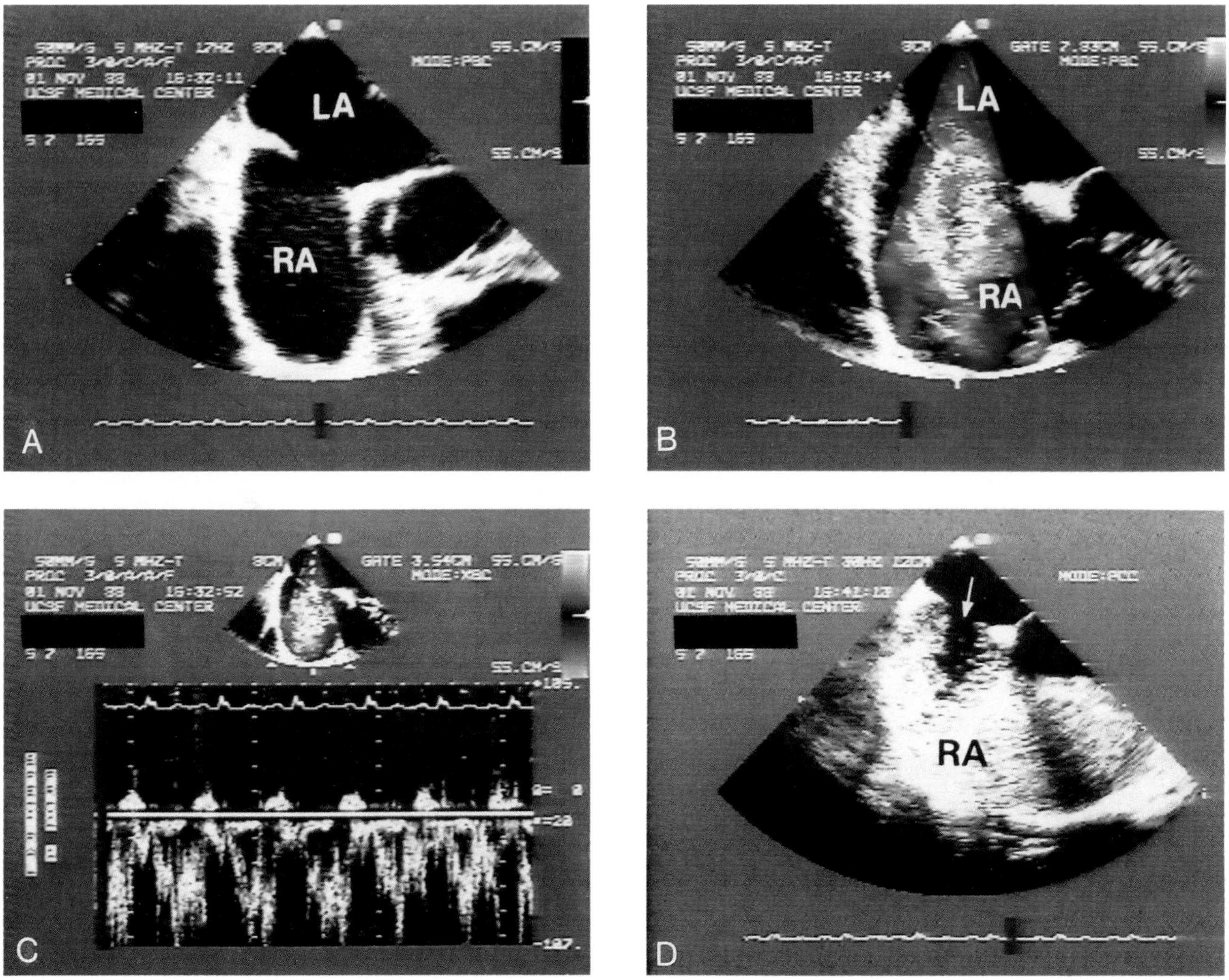

Plate 9

Figure 30–21.
A, Direct visualization of a large secundum atrial septal defect by two-dimensional transesophageal echocardiographic imaging. *B*, Predominant left-to-right shunting can be seen by color flow and pulsed Doppler interrogation *(C)*. *D*, Saline contrast administration demonstrated a "negative contrast effect" *(arrow)* of left-to-right shunting. LA—left atrium; RA—right atrium.

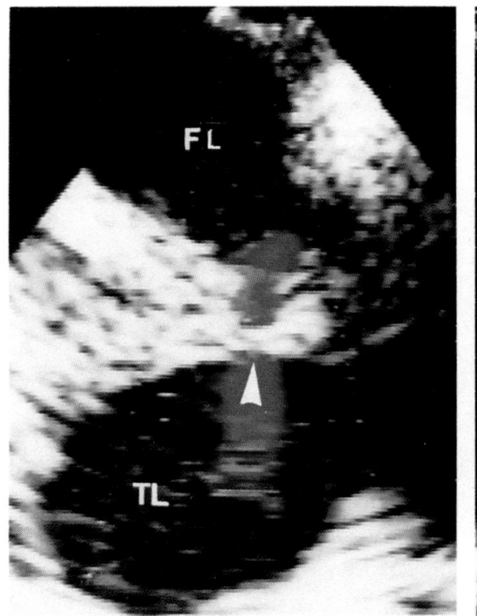

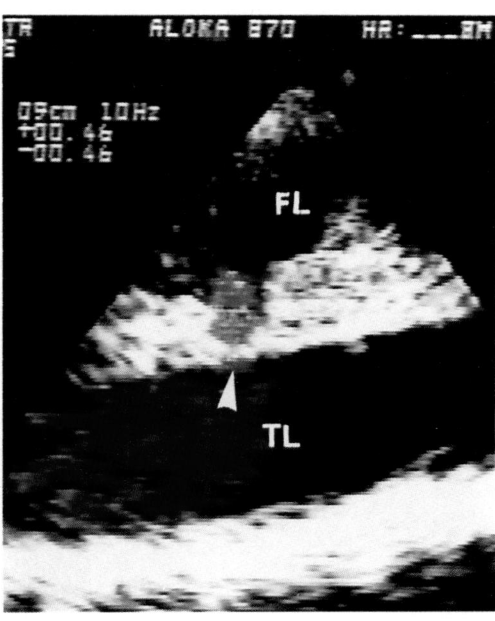

Figure 30–26.
Biplane transesophageal echocardiographic imaging of a descending aortic dissection. True (TL) and false lumina (FL), intimal flaps, and blood flow from true to false lumen *(arrowhead)* can be visualized in both short axis *(left)* and long axis *(right)*.

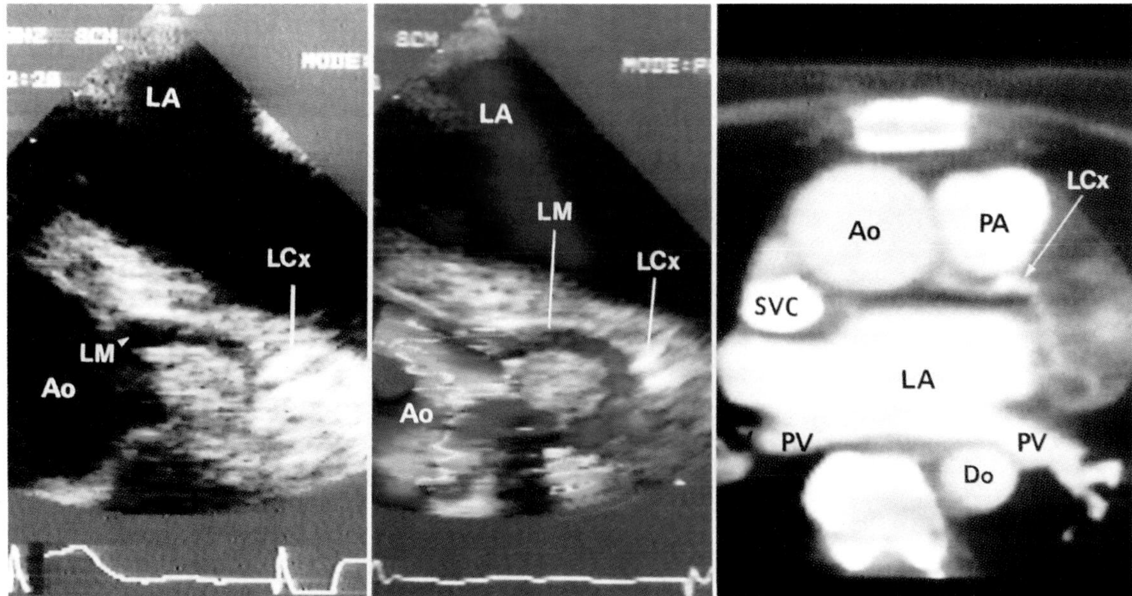

Figure 30–27.
Transesophageal echocardiographic imaging of the left coronary vasculature *(left)*. Color Doppler detection of blood flow in the left main (LM) can be seen, as well as a calcific plaque at the take-off of the left circumflex (LCx) *(middle)*. A cine computed tomography scan of the thorax *(right)* in the same patient confirmed a calcific plaque at the take-off of the left circumflex *(arrow)*. Ao—ascending aorta; Do—descending aorta; PA—pulmonary artery; PV—pulmonary vein; SVC—superior vena cava; LA—left atrium.

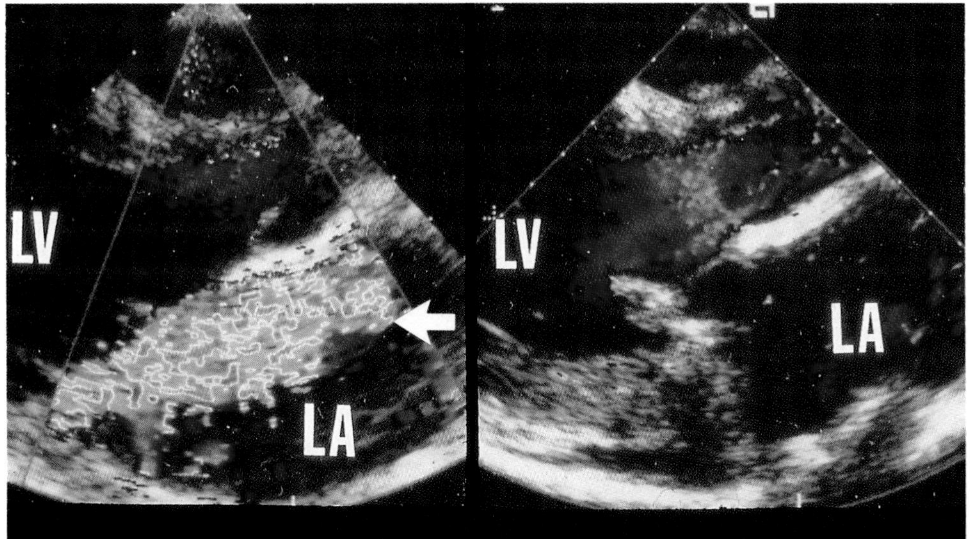

Figure 31–2.
Intraoperative epicardial echocardiography in mitral valve repair, parasternal long axis equivalent views in systole. *Left side:* Prepump echo showing moderately severe mitral regurgitation directed anteriorly in the left atrium (LA). *Right side:* Post-pump echo after valve repair showing no mitral regurgitation. LV—left ventricle.

Figure 31–4.
Subcostal equivalent epicardial echo showing failed mitral valve repair. *Left*, 4+ mitral regurgitation *(arrow)* prerepair. *Right*, 4+ mitral regurgitation *(arrow)* after repair. LA—left atrium, LV—left ventricle.

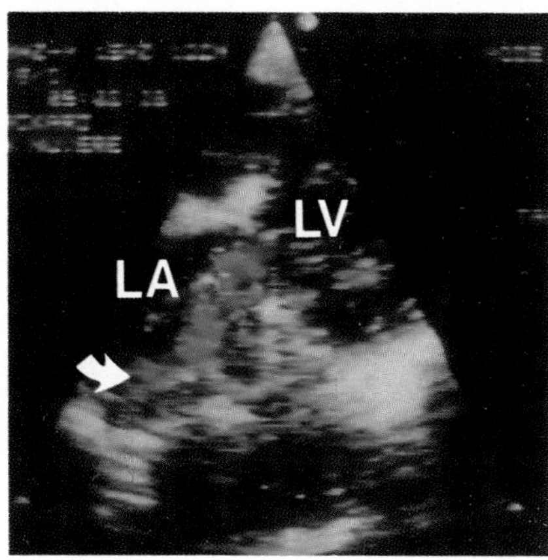

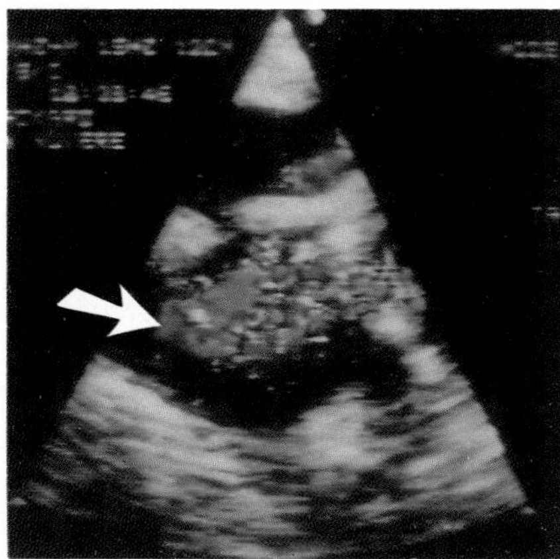

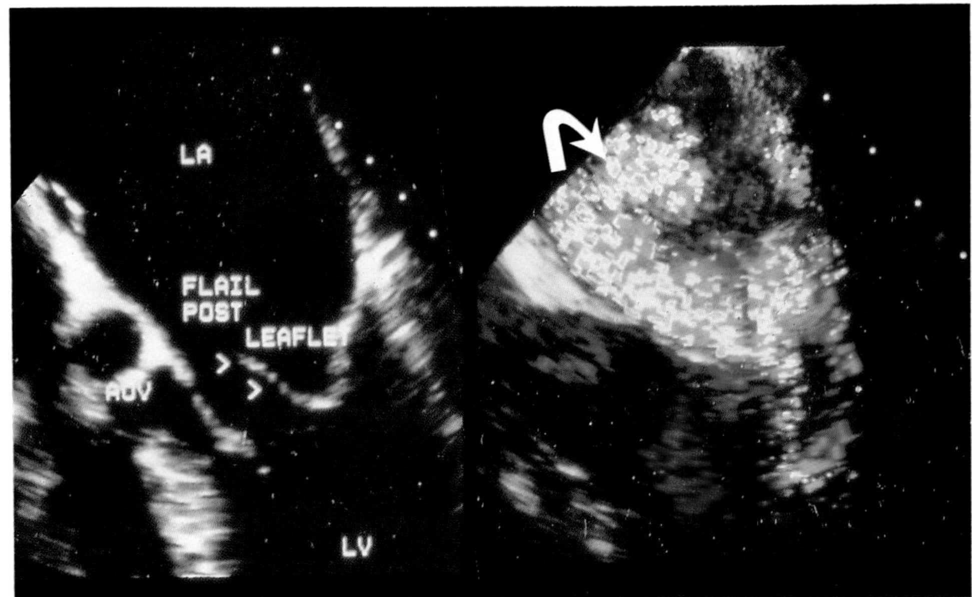

Figure 31–8.
Transesophageal echocardiogram of a patient prior to mitral valve repair. The two-dimensional echocardiogram *(left)* shows a flail posterior (post) leaflet *(arrowheads)*. On the right, the mitral regurgitant jet *(arrow)* is deflected anteriorly and medially by the posterior leaflet flail. AOV—aortic valve, LA—left atrium, LV—left ventricle.

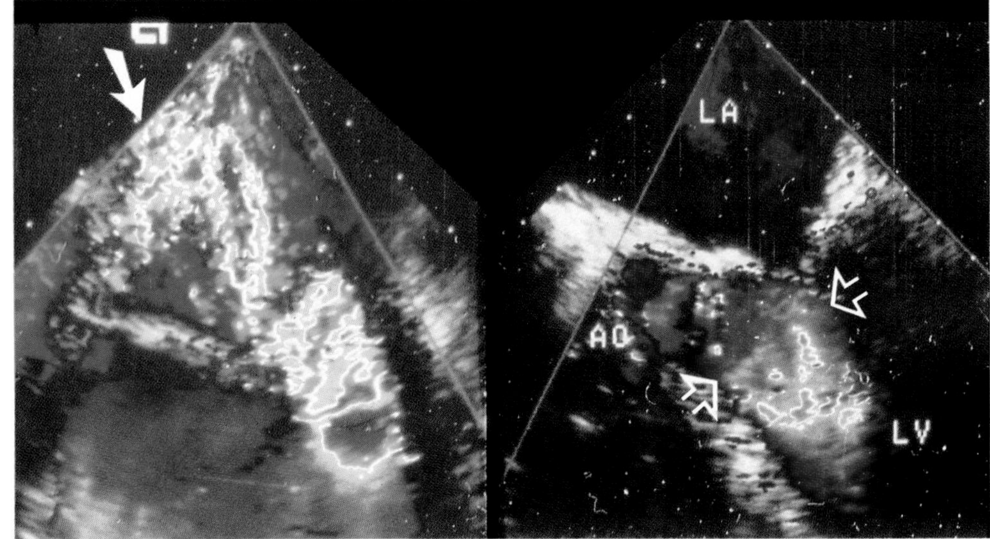

Figure 31–9.
Intraoperative transesophageal echo five-chamber view in mitral valve repair. *Left,* Severe mitral regurgitation *(arrow)* prior to repair. *Right,* After valve repair (slightly less magnification), no mitral regurgitation. The homogeneous orange color *(arrowheads)* is normal flow in the left ventricular outflow tract. AO—aorta, LA—left atrium, LV—left ventricle.

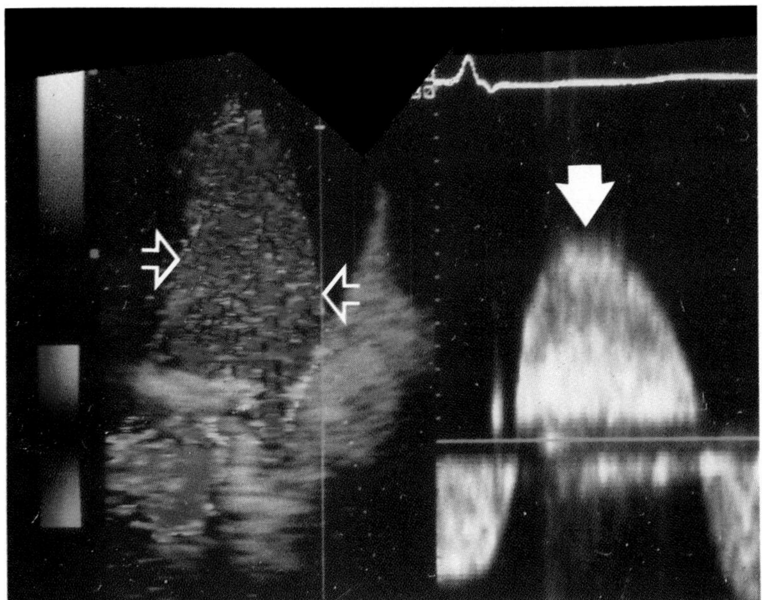

Figure 31–11.
Intraoperative image from the aorta–superior vena cava position, prepump measurement of aortic stenosis gradient. *Left,* Color flow image of postjet high-velocity jet *(arrows)*. *Right,* Continuous-wave Doppler recording indicating severe aortic stenosis with a 4.5 m/sec maximum velocity *(arrow)*. Calibration marks are 0.5 m/sec each.

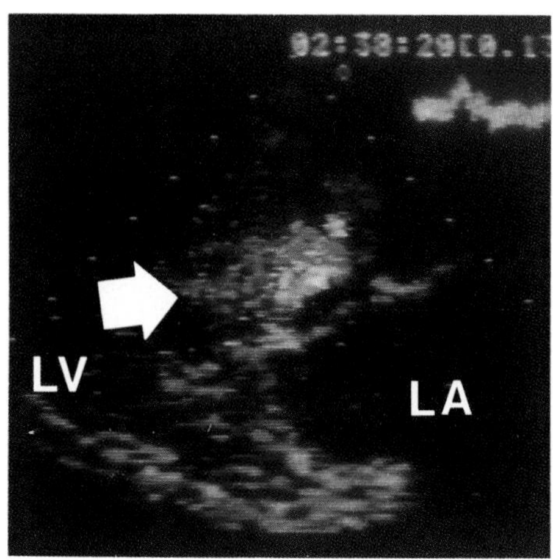

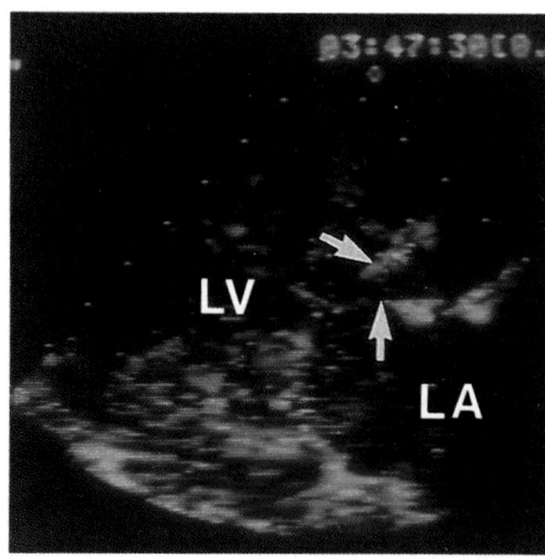

Figure 31–12.
Intraoperative echo in valve repair for aortic regurgitation, showing 3+ aortic regurgitation *(arrow)* before repair *(left)*, and 1+ aortic regurgitation *(small arrows) (right)* after repair.

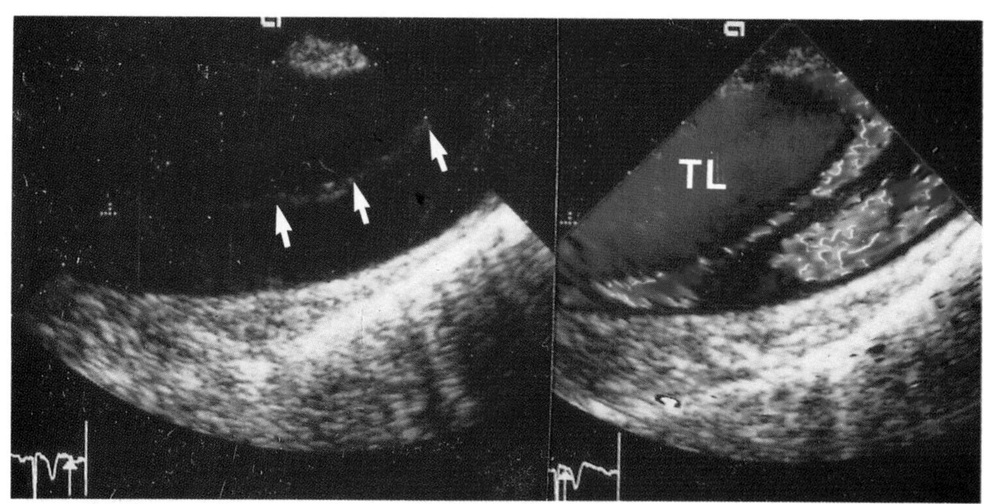

Figure 31–14.
Transesophageal echocardiogram of the ascending aorta in a type I dissection due to Marfan's syndrome. *Left,* Two-dimensional echo showing intimal flap *(arrows)*. *Right,* Color flow image showing differential flow between the true lumen (TL) in red and false lumen (multicolor).

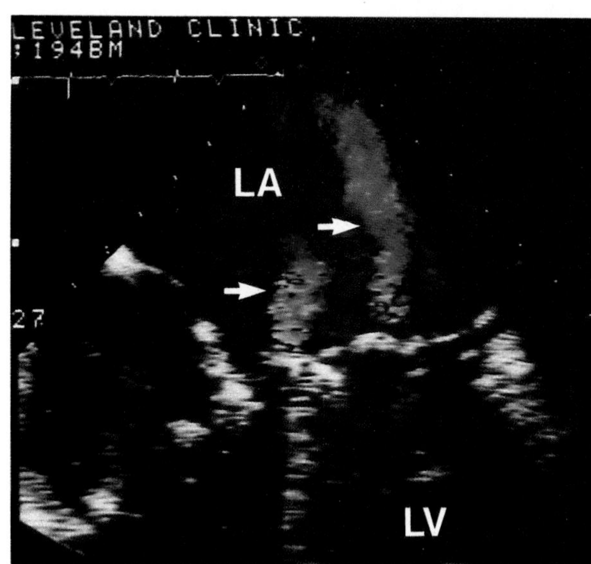

Figure 31–16.
Transesophageal echo after implantation of a normally functioning St. Jude mitral prosthesis, showing two small jets *(arrowheads)*. This amount of regurgitation of the mechanical valve is physiologic, and the jets are characterized by short duration and homogeneous orange color, indicating relative little regurgitation. LA—left atrium, LV—left ventricle.

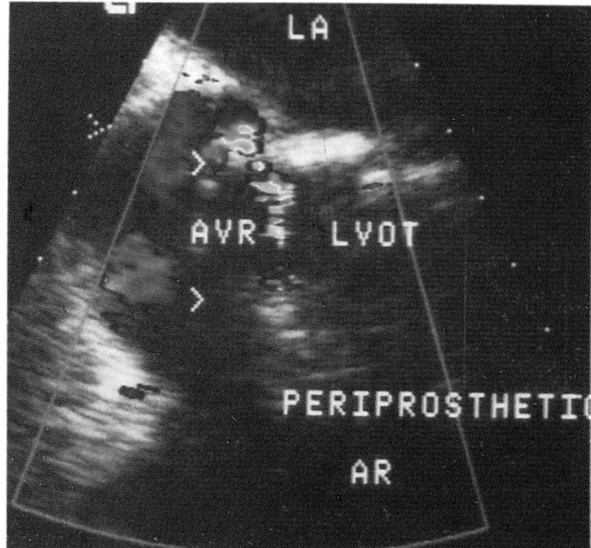

Figure 31–17.
Transesophageal echo five chamber view, with zoom magnification, of an aortic prosthesis (AVR), with *arrowheads* showing the locations of the prosthetic annulus and a periprosthetic aortic regurgitant (AR) jet (shown in mosaic turquoise) posterior to the valve. LA—left atrium, LVOT—left ventricular outflow tract.

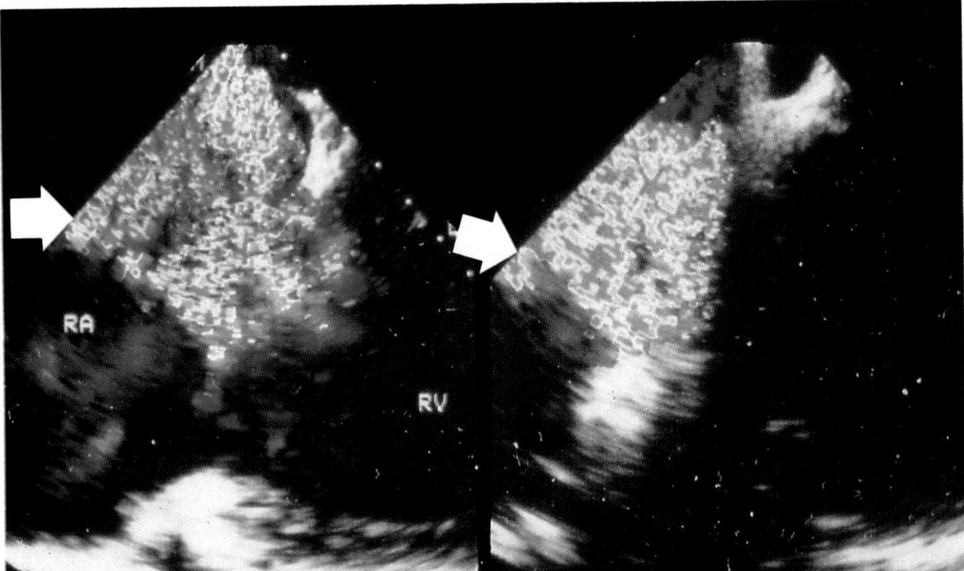

Figure 31–18.
Transesophageal echocardiogram in severe tricuspid insufficiency *(arrow)* on the prepump study *(left)*. The post-pump study using the same image plane *(right)* shows persistent severe tricuspid insufficiency *(arrow)* after attempted valve repair. The patient was subsequently placed back on the pump for placement of a tricuspid prosthesis. RA—right atrium, RV—right ventricle.

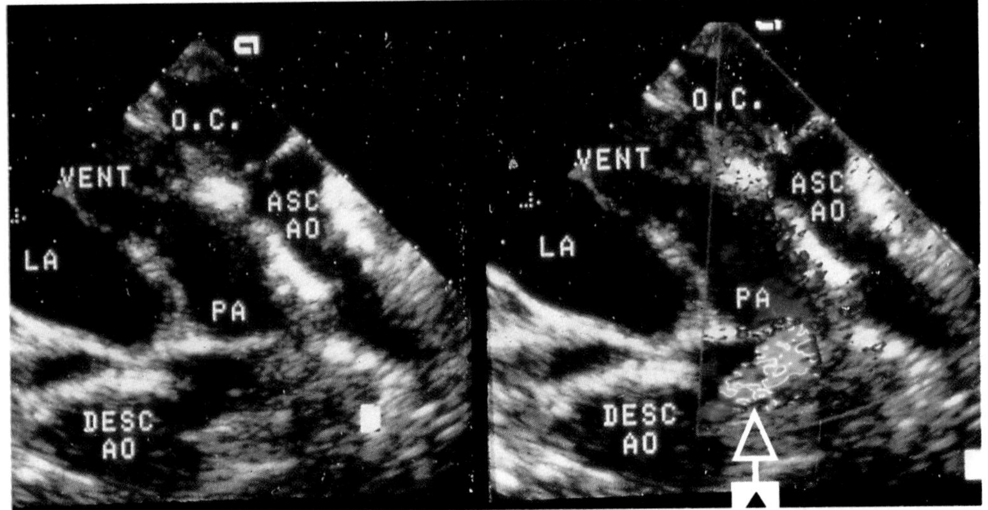

Figure 31–27.
Prepump intraoperative epicardial two-dimensional echocardiogram *(left)* and color flow image *(right)* in a patient with transposition of the great vessels, interrupted aortic arch, single ventricle with outflow chamber (O.C.), and a surgical shunt between the main pulmonary artery and the descending aorta *(arrow)*. ASC AO—ascending aorta, DESC AO—descending aorta, LA—left atrium, PA—pulmonary artery, VENT—double inlet left ventricle.

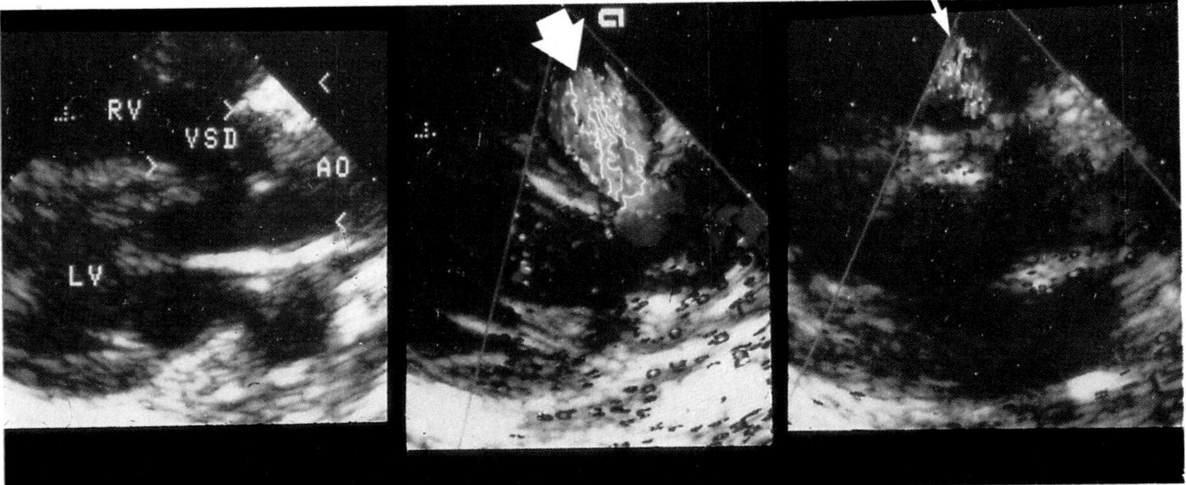

Figure 31–28.
Intraoperative echocardiographic studies on a patient with tetralogy of Fallot. *Left*, two-dimensional echocardiogram prior to repair, showing a large aorta (AO) overriding a ventricular septal defect (VSD). The middle view shows the prepump color flow image displaying the ventricular septal defect flow *(large arrow)*. The right view shows the color flow image after repair with a patch closure of the defect, and a small residual VSD jet *(small arrow)*. LV—left ventricle, RV—right ventricle.

Plate 14

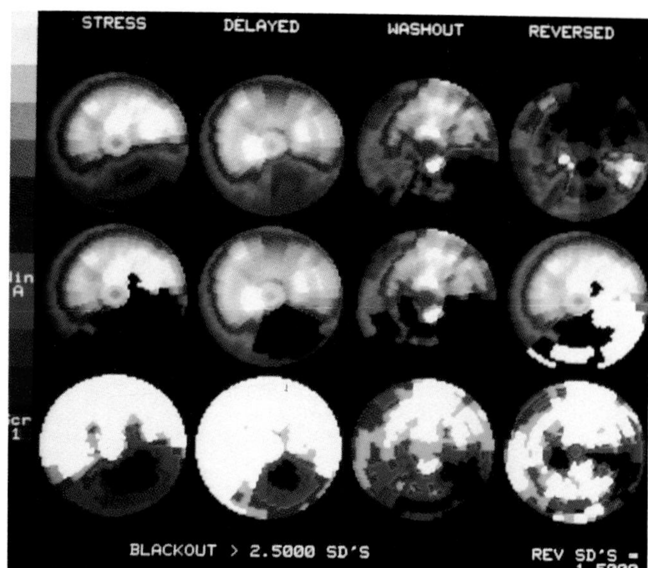

Figure 55–19.
Bull's eye polar representation of myocardial perfusion. Complete set of 12 bull's eye polar maps for a patient with an inferolateral, reversible perfusion defect. The top four polar maps are the raw bull's eyes before comparison with normal limits. The four polar maps (blacked out and whited out bull's eyes) in the middle row represent the raw data after a single threshold cutoff criteria for abnormality (2.5 standard deviations from the mean for the stress, delayed, and washout; 1.5 for reversibility). Note blacked out region in the inferolateral wall of the stress bull's eye corresponding to the perfusion defect. Although the defect appears to remain fixed in the delayed bull's eye, the large whited out region in the reversibility map corresponds to significant reversibility. The four polar maps in the bottom row are the standard deviation bull's eyes in which the deviation of each pixel from the mean normal response is color-coded from white (least) to black (most).

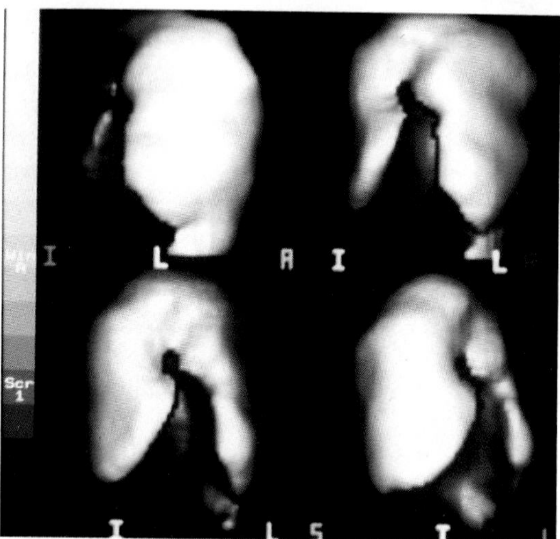

Figure 55–22.
Surface rendering of three-dimensional thallium-201 (^{201}Tl) perfusion distribution of a patient with left circumflex coronary artery disease. Each panel demonstrates a slightly different rotation (apex pointing up) of a hypoperfused inferolateral myocardial wall. Perfusion defect is demonstrated by the missing region between the inferior (I) and lateral (L) walls. A—anterior wall; S—septal wall. (Results courtesy of David Nowak, General Electric Co.)

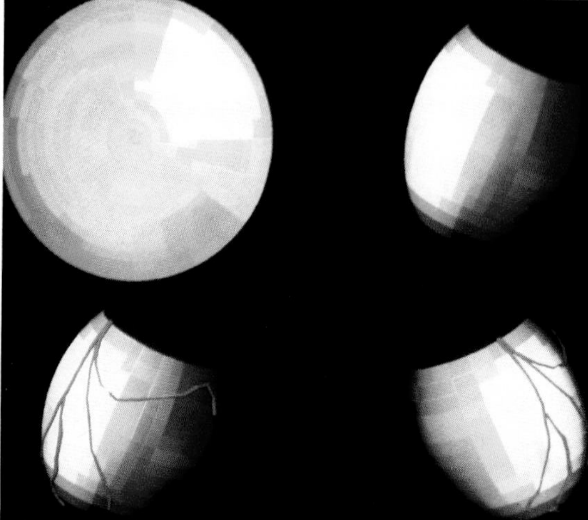

Figure 55–23.
Three-dimensional heart models of a patient exhibiting hypoperfusion of the inferior and inferolateral myocardial walls. *Top left panel* illustrates the patient's bull's eye polar map, in which the perfusion defect is represented by shades of blue. *Top right panel* represents the corresponding three-dimensional ellipsoidal model of the myocardium. *Bottom panels* show two different orientations of a unified model for which the patient's own left coronary arteries have been registered onto the ellipsoidal perfusion model. On the *bottom left panel*, note the high grade lesion at the midcourse of the left circumflex coronary artery. (Results generated by C. David Cooke and John Peifer.)

Figure 55–31.
Phase-analysis of a normal Tc-99m multiple-gated equilibrium study. *Top right panel* is a filtered end-diastolic frame. *Top left panel* is the stroke count or amplitude image. *Bottom right panel* is the phase image. Left-ventricular edges are superimposed in all three images. Bottom left panel illustrates a phase histogram in which the color-coded phase *(x-axis)* is plotted versus the number of pixels in the phase image with that phase. Note bimodal peaks corresponding to synchronous contractions of ventricles (blue-green) and atria (red-white). (Figure courtesy of John Almasi, General Electric Co.)

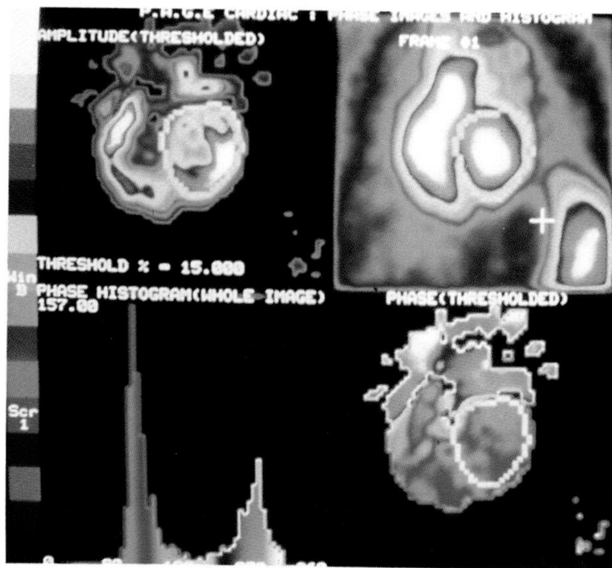

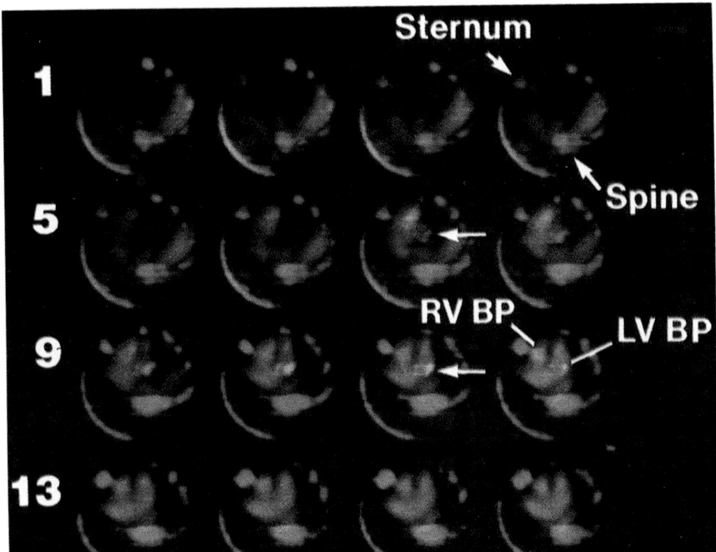

Figure 59–12.
Color-coded overlay of PPi (in orange) on the ungated blood pool (in blue). Images are of transaxial sections through the volume of the thorax, including the heart. Sections 1 to 16 begin caudal to the heart and progress cephalad through the thorax. Sections are in standard computed tomographic format, i.e., head in face up, except that the sections have been rotated counterclockwise so that the ventricular apex is at 12 o'clock. Note the sternum at 10 o'clock and the spine at 4 o'clock. An intense area of 99m-Tc-PPi uptake (⟶) along the posterior segment of the left ventricle can be seen in images up to 12. (From Corbett, J. R., et al.: 99m-Tc-pyrophosphate imaging in patients with acute myocardial infarction: comparison of planar imaging with single-photon tomography with and without blood pool overlay. Circulation 69:1120, 1984, with permission.)

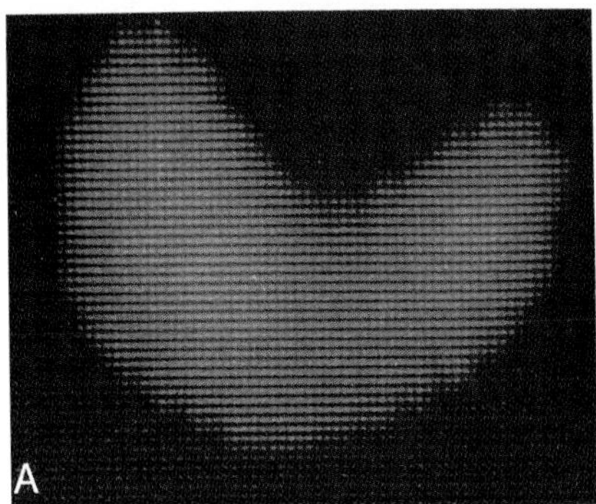

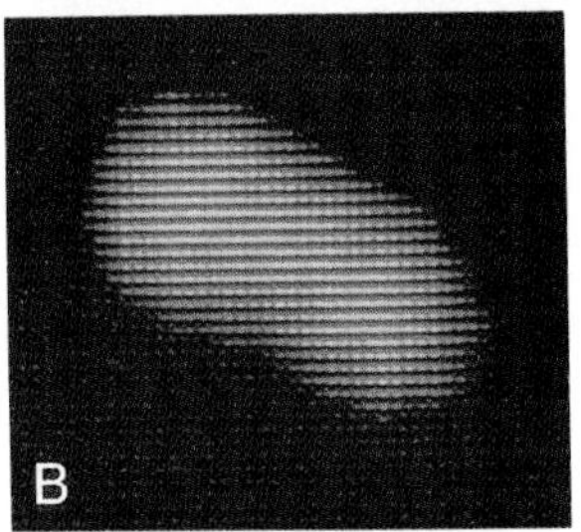

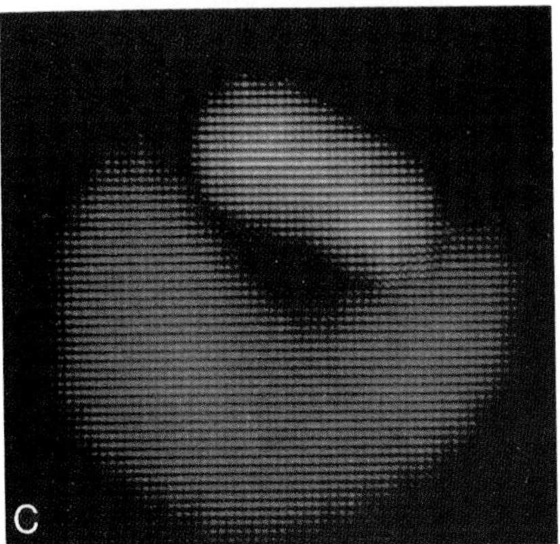

Figure 59–18.
A representative set of transverse sections from a dog with a left anterior descending artery occlusion. *A*, Thallium-201, *B*, Tc-99m-PPi, and *C*, thallium/technetium pyrophosphate (overlay) images. (From Wolfe, C. L., et al.: Measurement of myocardial infarction fraction using single photon emission computed tomography. J. Am. Coll. Cardiol. 6:145, 1985, with permission.)

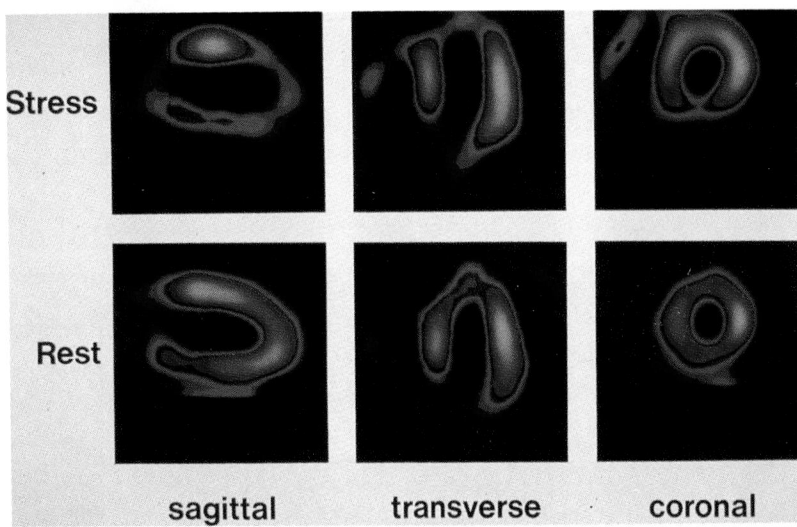

Figure 61–8.
Tc-sestamibi SPECT images of the patient with 95 percent right coronary artery stenosis, performed using the same-day rest-stress protocol. Note the reversible defects in the inferior and apical wall of the left ventricle. (Courtesy of Raymond Taillefer, M.D., Hotel Dieu, Montreal, Canada.)

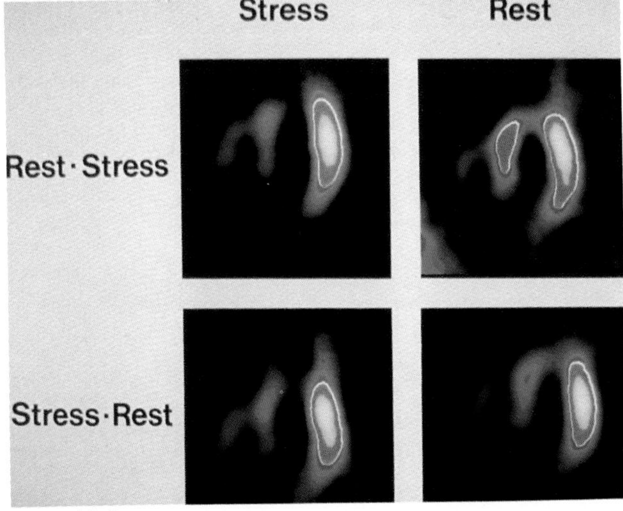

Figure 61–9.
Comparison of same day Tc-sestamibi protocols, using the rest-stress *(top)* and stress-rest *(bottom)* injection sequences in a patient with prior apical myocardial infarction and ischemia in the intraventricular septum. The reversible defect in the septum is clearly detected by the rest-stress sequence and is not readily perceived on the stress-rest sequence. (Courtesy of Raymond Taillefer, M.D., Hotel Dieu, Montreal, Canada.)

Plate 16

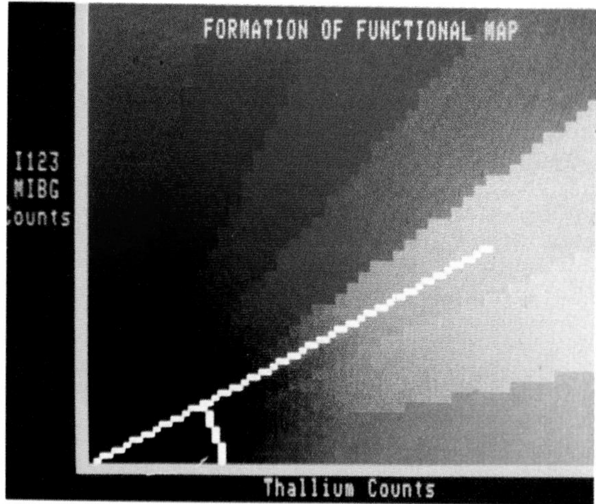

Figure 64–2.
This figure illustrates the method for generating the MIBG/Tl functional maps. Thallium counts are plotted on the horizontal axis, and MIBG counts on the vertical axis. For areas that show an equivalent amount of MIBG and thallium, an angle of 45 degrees is defined and is color-coded red. Areas where thallium counts exceed MIBG counts are coded green, indicating MIBG deficiency, or denervation. When MIBG counts exceed ^{201}Tl, the color is blue, indicating a greater degree of innervation. In this manner, a color relates to the proportion of MIBG versus thallium on a pixel-by-pixel basis. An additional feature of this method is the representation of relative intensity or brightness. As the color scale approaches the origin, there is a reduction in intensity. In this manner, areas of scar would be identifiable in the functional maps as low-intensity regions. (From Dae, M. W., O'Connell, J. W., Botvinick, E. H., et al.: Scintigraphic assessment of regional cardiac adrenergic innervation. Circulation 79:634–644, 1989, with permission.)

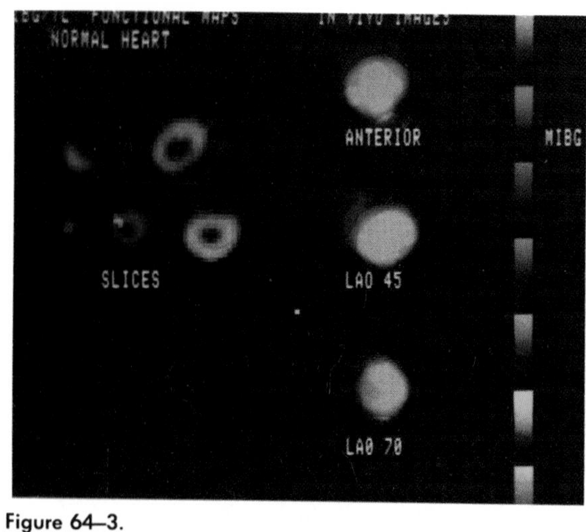

Figure 64–3.
This is an example of functional maps from a normal heart. On the right are in vivo planar images, and on the left are myocardial slices. The major left ventricular mass appears red, indicating a similar and parallel distribution of MIBG and thallium (normal innervation). The right ventricle shows increased MIBG to thallium, consistent with increased innervation, relative to the left ventricle. (From Dae, M. W., O'Connell, J. W., Botvinick, E. H., et al.: Scintigraphic assessment of regional cardiac adrenergic innervation. Circulation 79:634–644, 1989, with permission.)

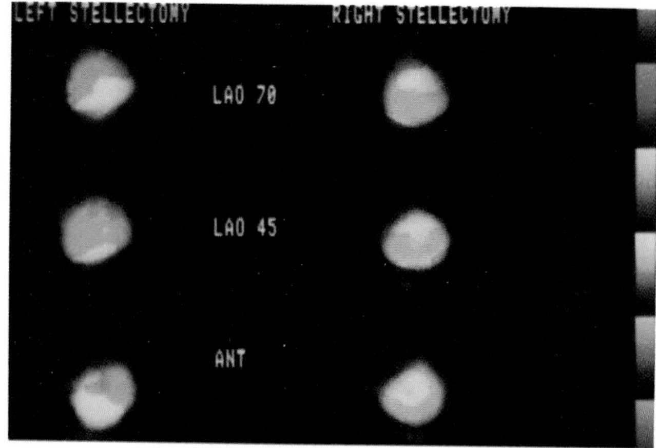

Figure 64–5.
Shown are functional maps from in vivo planar images in a dog with left stellectomy *(on the left)* and right stellectomy *(on the right)*. The area coded green is consistent with relative denervation of the posterior left ventricle in the left-stellectomized heart, and relative denervation of the anterior left ventricle in the right stellectomized heart. (From Dae, M. W., O'Connell, J. W., Botvinick, E. H., et al.: Scintigraphic assessment of regional cardiac adrenergic innervation. Circulation 79:634–644, 1989, with permission.)

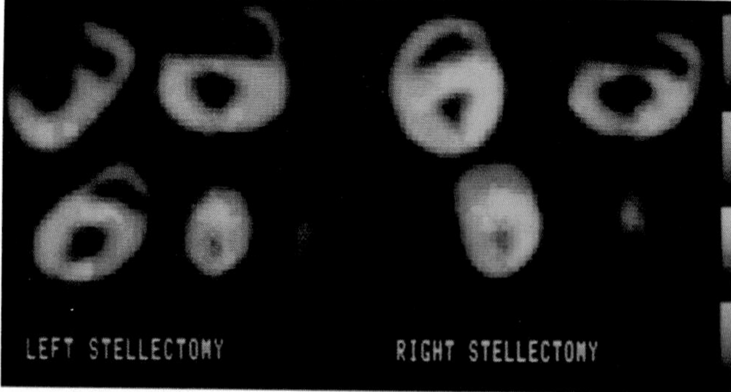

Figure 64–6.
The myocardial slices from the hearts illustrated in Figure 64–5 are shown here; these also show denervation of the posterior left ventricle in left stellectomy, and anterior left ventricle in right stellectomy. Both studies show involvement of the septum as well. (From Dae, M. W., O'Connell, J. W., Botvinick, E. H., et al.: Scintigraphic assessment of regional cardiac adrenergic innervation. Circulation 79:634–644, 1989, with permission.)

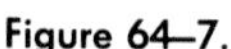

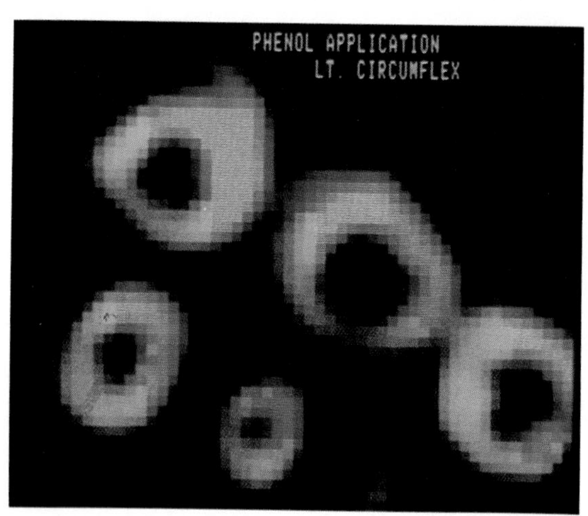

Figure 64–7.
Functional maps of myocardial slices from a dog with regional denervation (yellow-to-green color), produced by epicardial application of phenol. (From Dae, M. W., O'Connell, J. W., Botvinick, E. H., et al.: Scintigraphic assessment of regional cardiac adrenergic innervation. Circulation 79:634–644, 1989, with permission.)

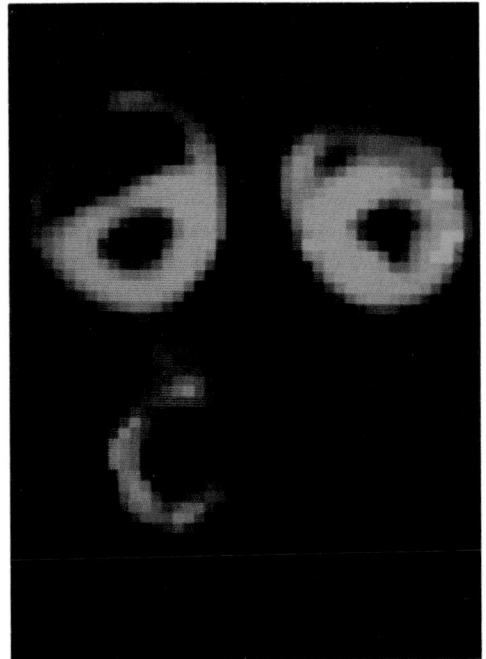

Figure 64–8.
Shown are functional maps of myocardial slices from a dog with myocardial infarction. Note the area of absent activity in the slice proximal to the apex. This represents a region of transmural scar. Adjacent and distal to this region of scar is an area of denervated myocardium, represented by the yellow-to-green color. (From Dae, M. W., O'Connell, J. W., Botvinick, E. H., et al.: Scintigraphic assessment of regional cardiac adrenergic innervation. Circulation 79:634–644, 1989, with permission.)

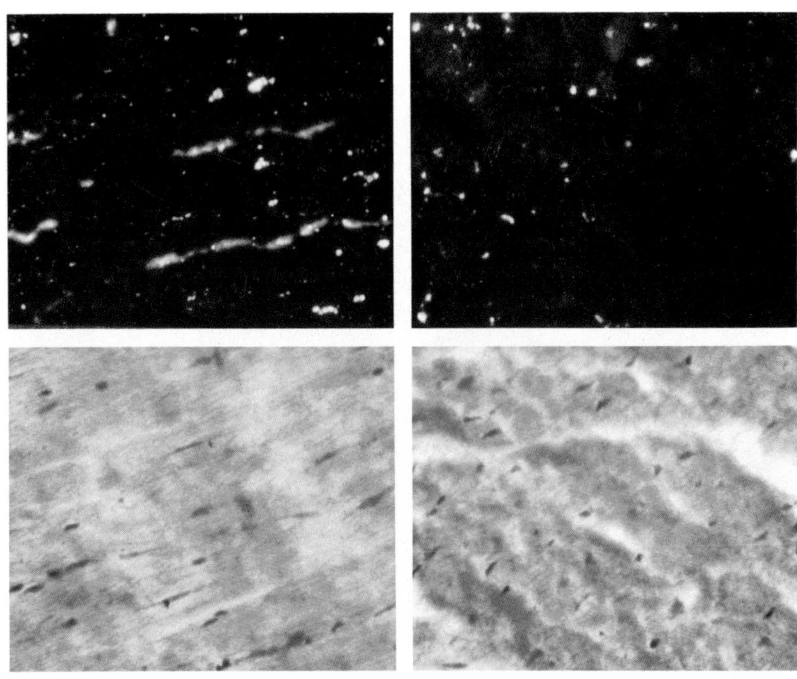

Figure 64–9.
Histofluorescence miscroscopy. Shown are histofluorescence micrographs *(above)* and corresponding H & E micrographs *(below)*, from a normal basal region *(left)*, and a region of denervated myocardium *(right)*. Note the blue-green fluorescence of the sympathetic nerves from the normal region, and their absence from the denervated region. Muscle histology is normal in both areas.

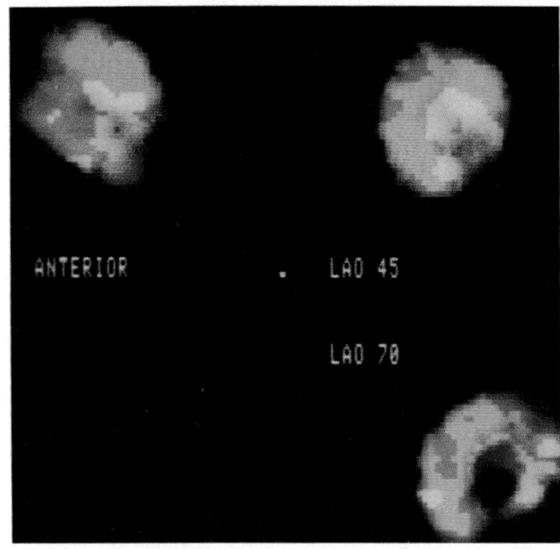

Figure 64–10.
Shown are planar functional maps from a patient who was imaged two years after an apical lateral infarction. Note in the LAO 70 projection the region of scar defined by the absence of intensity, and the surrounding area of denervation illustrated by the yellow-to-green color.

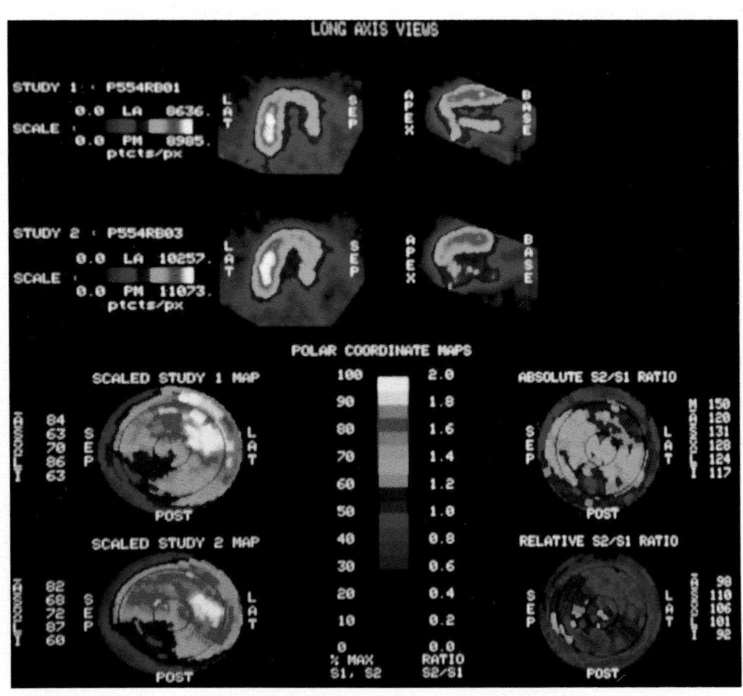

Figure 66–6.
Positron emission tomographic perfusion images in horizontal and vertical long-axis views, before (study 1) and after (study 2) dipyridamole stress *(top)*. Bull's eye format *(below)* is used to depict the perfusion at rest and stress *(left)*, and the absolute and relative ratios of stress to rest perfusion *(right)*. A severe inferior defect is present at rest that worsens slightly with stress. (From Gould, K. L.: Identifying and measuring severity of coronary artery stenosis: Quantitative coronary angiography and positron emission tomography. Circulation 78:242, 1988, with permission. Courtesy of KL Gould, University of Texas Medical School, Houston, Texas.)

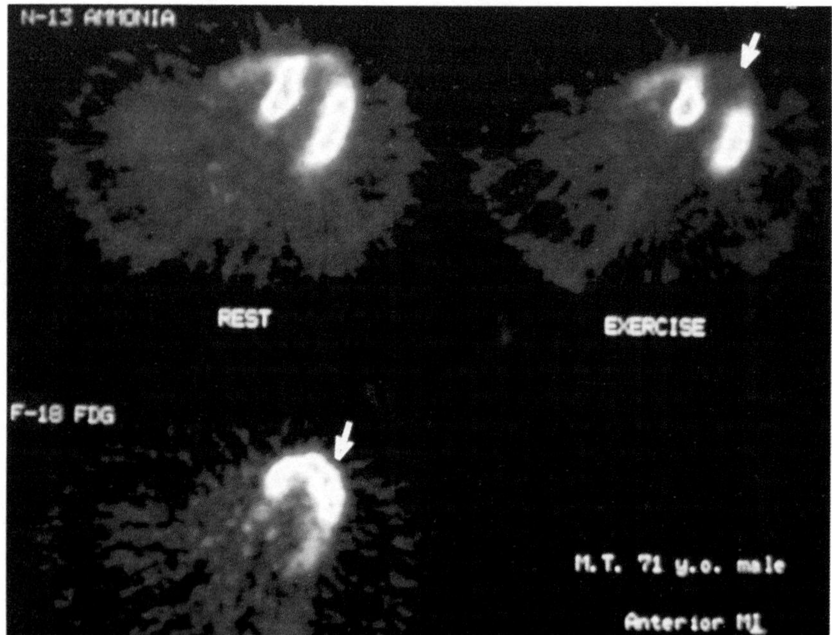

Figure 67–13.
Representative rest and stress ammonia perfusion images and rest ^{18}F 2-fluoro 2-deoxyglucose metabolic images in a patient 8 weeks after anterior myocardial infarction. The resting perfusion images demonstrate a decrease in relative myocardial perfusion in the anterior region of the ventricle. With exercise, the perfusion defect extends peripherally and is more pronounced. On metabolic imaging with ^{18}F 2-fluoro 2-deoxyglucose on a different day augmented uptake of the glucose analog is identified in the anteroseptal and anterolateral regions of the ventricle, corresponding to the territory encompassed by the stress-induced perfusion defect. (Reproduced by permission from Yonekura et al: Detection of metabolic alterations in ischemic myocardium by F-18 deoxyglucose uptake with positron emission tomography. Am. J. Cardiac Imaging 2:122–132, 1988.)

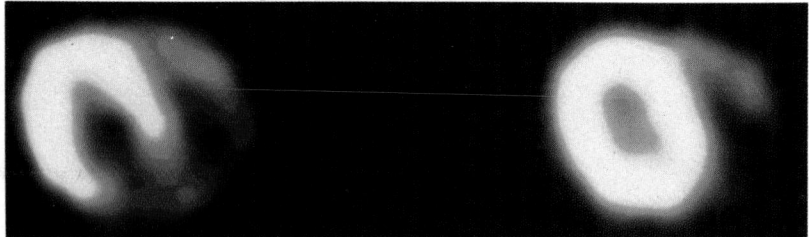

Figure 69–1.
PET transverse sections at two anatomic levels from the same subject after intravenous injection of ^{11}C-MQNB, an antagonist of the muscarinic acetylcholine receptor. The PET scans were obtained 12 minutes after injection of ^{11}C-MQNB (14 mCi, 625 Ci/mmole). The lateral left ventricular wall is to the left, apex uppermost. A high activity is seen in the lateral wall, septum *(left and right panels)* and inferior wall *(right panel)*. Activity in the right ventricle is lower than that in the left ventricle. Lungs and blood are not visualized.

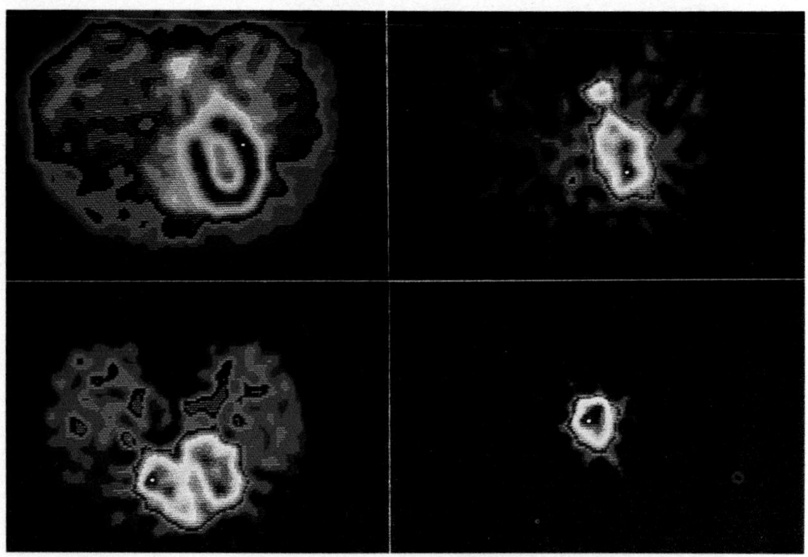

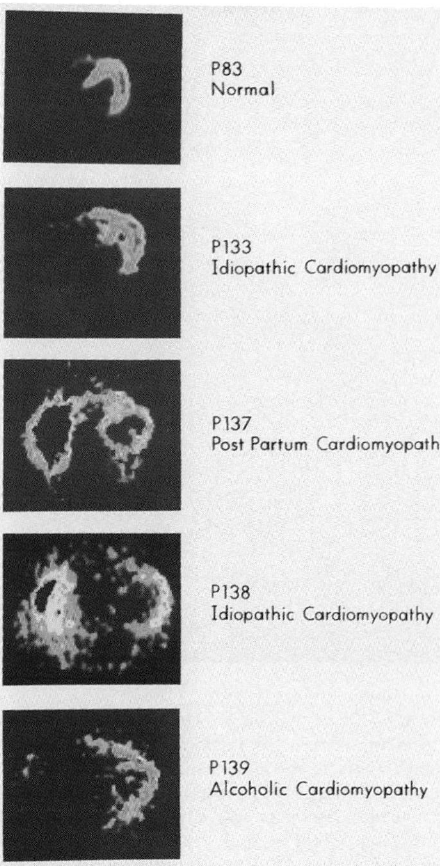

Figure 68–2.
Positron emission tomographic images obtained after the intravenous administration of ^{11}C-palmitate at the midventricular level of a normal subject and patients with dilated cardiomyopathy from the causes indicated. The top of each image represents the anterior; the right of each image represents the patient's left. Areas in red represent areas of greatest accumulation of tracer, areas in blue the least. The posterior discontinuity is due to the mitral valve apparatus and atria, which are below the spatial resolution of the instrument. Accumulation of radioactivity in the normal subject was homogeneous, with smooth transition between regions with intense to regions of only modest accumulation of tracer. Patients with cardiomyopathy demonstrate marked spatial heterogeneity in the accumulation of ^{11}C-palmitate. The regions of accumulation on the left of each image represent activity in the dome of the liver. (From Geltman, E. M., Smith, J. L., Beecher, D., et al.: Altered regional myocardial metabolism in congestive cardiomyopathy detected by positron tomography. Am. J. Med. 74:773–785, 1983, with permission.)

Figure 69–6.
Tomograms of ^{11}C-CGP 12177 studies from a normal subject. Images were obtained at the same anatomic level 1 second *(upper left panel)*, 3 seconds *(upper right panel)*, 5 seconds *(lower left panel)* and 10 minutes *(lower right panel)* after intravenous injection of ^{11}C-CGP 12177 (11 mCi, 407 MBq). The first image shows the ^{11}C-CGP blood activity in the right heart chamber; the second image displays activity in both chambers. The activity is then concentrated in the left chamber and the aorta *(lower left panel)*. The *lower right panel* shows the uptake of the beta-blocking agent in the septum and lateral wall of the left ventricle. Good contrast between myocardium, blood, and lung is present.

Location	Line Pairs/cm	Resolution in mm
A	9.80	.51
B	7.81	.64
C	6.17	.81
D	4.90	1.02
E	3.85	1.30
F	3.07	1.63
G	2.43	2.06
H	1.93	2.59
I	1.54	3.25
J	1.05	4.76
K	.63	7.94

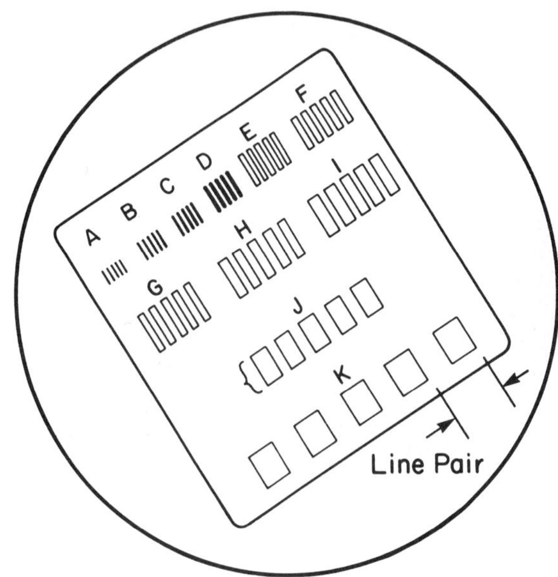

Figure 32–20. Diagram of General Electric 8800 resolution test object.

from 3.5 to 5.0 mm in diameter have been drilled in this block, and the diameter of the smallest holes that are visualized is the measurement variable. The phantom is shown diagrammatically in Figure 32–24. Comparative results for a conventional and fast computed tomography are given in Table 32–5 and Figure 32–25. Representative images are shown in Figures 32–26 to 32–28. As demonstrated, this measurement is very dependent on available photon flux and therefore is strongly related to the scan time in the case of fast computed tomography in particular. The superior resolution possible with longer scan times must be weighed against an increase in radiation dose and an increase in blurring due to motion, which may be particularly acute in the case of conventional computed tomography.

Uniformity

This test is done to determine whether a system faithfully produces a uniform image of a uniform test object. The test phantom is a Plexiglas cylinder 32 cm or 20 cm in diameter. A large cylinder filled with water may also be used for the test object. The test measurement is performed by determining the mean Hounsfield unit for a region of interest located in the center and a similar region at the periphery or in the area of greatest nonuniformity. The measurement variable is the difference in Hounsfield units between the center and the edge. Comparative performance for conventional and fast systems is given in Table 32–6. Representative images are shown in Figures 32–29 to 32–31. The relative performance of fast computed tomography is quite close to that of conventional computed tomography in the single-slice mode. In the multiple-slice mode, there is a substantial difference between the two techniques, again owing largely to the difference in the distribution of scattered radiation and the manner in which this software correction is performed.

Noise

The test object used in this measurement is the same as that described for the uniformity measurement. The variable used as a noise measurement is the standard deviation of a region of interest located in the center. Hence, noise values are characterized in Hounsfield units. The relative performance of conventional and fast systems is shown in Table 32–7.

Hounsfield Unit Linearity

The intensity of pixel values for computed tomography has a specific meaning. Each pixel in an image is represented by a specified number of Hounsfield units (HU). The Hounsfield unit is defined as

$$HU = \frac{u_{H_2O} - u}{u_{H_2O}} \times 1000$$

With this relative scale, the intensity values are linearly related to the attenuation coefficient of water (u_{H_2O}). Water by definition has a Hounsfield unit of zero, air (or other substances with virtually no attenuation) has a Hounsfield unit of -1000, and dense bone has a large positive Hounsfield unit. The purpose of this measurement is to determine that objects of known attenuation coefficients are faithfully rendered with the proper Hounsfield unit and that the relationship among various objects is linear. The test object is the General Electric 8800 test phantom

Table 32–3. RESOLUTION FOR CONVENTIONAL (PICKER 1200) AND FAST (PICKER FASTRAC) COMPUTED TOMOGRAPHY

System	Resolution with Clinical Technique
Conventional	6.3 lp/cm
Fast (Single Slice)	5.0 lp/cm
Fast (Multiple Slice)	3.1 lp/cm

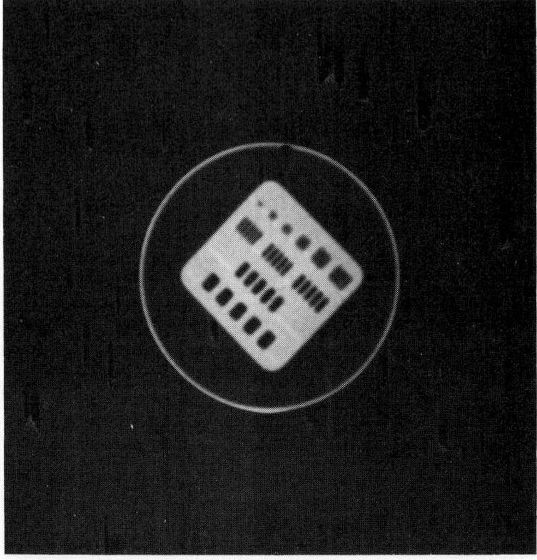

Figure 32–21. Resolution for fast computed tomography (Picker FASTRAC) with multiple-slice acquisition.

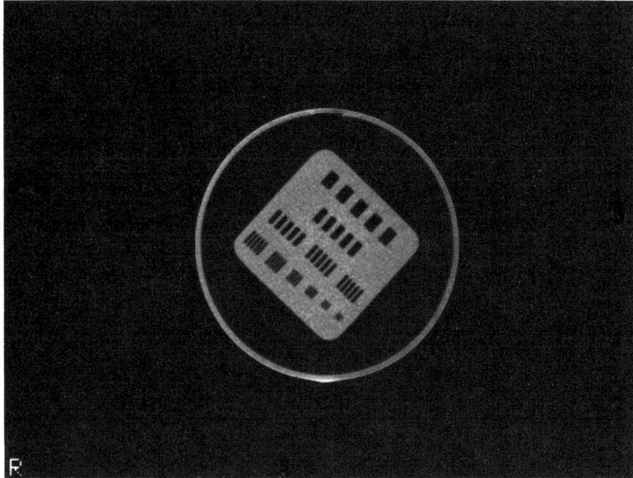

Figure 32–22. Resolution for fast computed tomography (Picker FASTRAC) with single-slice acquisition.

and consists of three cylinders of Teflon, Plexiglas, and polyethylene. Measurements are made in regions of interest over each object and over an area of water within the phantom, providing a range of Hounsfield units from 0 to 920. Comparative performance for conventional and fast computed tomography is given in Table 32–8 and Figure 32–32. Note that although the absolute scaling may not be correct, the relationship among various materials may still be accurate. This situation simply means that the calibration for water has not been determined correctly.

Half-Value Layer

The purpose of this measurement is to determine the energy quality of the bremsstrahlung beam. X-ray beams produced by the deceleration of electrons in a target material actually produce a spectrum of x-ray energy, as shown in Figure 32–33. Hence, there is no single x-ray energy that enters the patient but rather a distribution of these energies. Beams with higher average energies are called "harder" and have a higher half-value layer, whereas beams of lower average energy are called "softer" and have a lower half-value layer. This beam quality can be important in parameters such as uniformity, beam-hardening artifacts, and radiation dose. This test is performed by placing successive thicknesses of aluminum in the x-ray beam and measuring their relative transmissions.[C8] For a number of technical reasons, this is a difficult measurement to perform with common radiation detectors in the case of fast computed tomography. Therefore, a different measurement technique involving the scanner system radiation detectors is utilized in fast computed tomography.[C13] This technique involves inspecting the sinogram and determining the relative x-ray transmission through the central ray, which encounters aluminum, and a peripheral ray that encounters only air. The half-value layer for the fast system was 10.2-mm aluminum, compared to approximately 7 mm for a typical conventional system.

Table 32–4. RESOLUTION AS A FUNCTION OF TIME FOR CONVENTIONAL (PICKER 1200) AND FAST (PICKER FASTRAC) COMPUTED TOMOGRAPHY

Scan Time (seconds)	Conventional CT (lp/cm)	Fast, Single Slice—6 mm (lp/cm)	Fast, Multiple Slice (lp/cm)
0.05	—	—	1.9
0.10	—	3.9	—
0.20	—	3.9	2.4
0.40	—	5.0	2.4
0.65	—	—	3.1
0.80	—	5.0	—
1.0	—	5.0	—
1.4	—	5.0	—
3.3	6.3	—	—

Table 32–5. LOW-CONTRAST RESOLUTION FOR CONVENTIONAL (PICKER 1200) AND FAST (PICKER FASTRAC) COMPUTED TOMOGRAPHY

Scan Time (seconds)	Conventional (mm)	Fast, Single Slice—3 mm (mm)	Fast, Single Slice—10 mm (mm)
0.05	—	—	>20
0.1	—	20	—
0.2	—	20	—
0.4	—	20	—
0.8	—	20	—
1.0	—	5	—
1.4	—	3	—
3.3	3	—	—

As demonstrated by the previous performance measurements, the typical armamentarium of physics test objects and analysis indicates that the overall performance of fast computed tomography is somewhat below that of conventional computed tomography. However, it is the improved temporal resolution that is of fundamental importance in assessing the relative performance of the fast technique. This is most graphically demonstrated by clinical images that demonstrate the marked superiority of fifth-generation fast computed tomography in thoracic and abdominal imaging. At present, the materials and methodologies for assessing the performance of computed tomography systems are undergoing a reassessment. It appears that static test objects will be of less value in the future and that acquisition and analysis techniques must include regular and predictable motion of the test object. It is apparent that there are substantial benefits of less than 1 second. Further development and availability of fast CT scanning systems may well alter the manner and nature of medical imaging by x-ray computed tomography.

The Mayo Dynamic Spatial Reconstructor

Dynamic volume computed tomography with the Dynamic Spatial Reconstructor (DSR) has been under development since 1975 in the Biodynamics Research Unit at the Mayo Clinic.[K5, R10–R13] Figure 32–34 is a diagram of the multiple-source, multiple-detector scanning concept on which the DSR system is based. The design is different from that of other x-ray computed tomog-

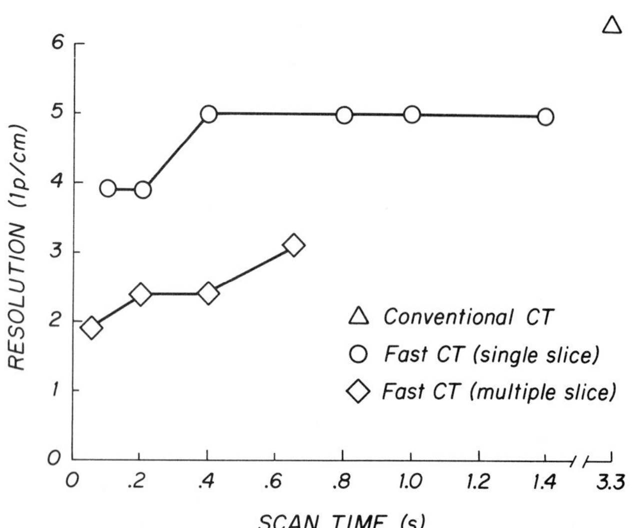

Figure 32–23. Resolution as a function of time for fast computed tomography (Picker FASTRAC) with multiple-slice and single-slice acquisition.

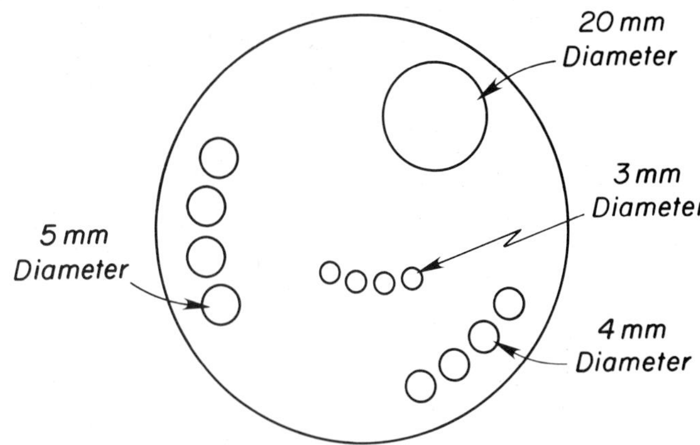

Figure 32–24. Diagram of RMI low-contrast-resolution test phantom.

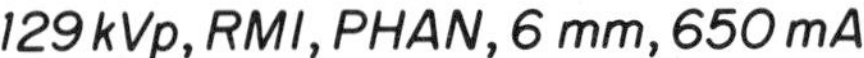

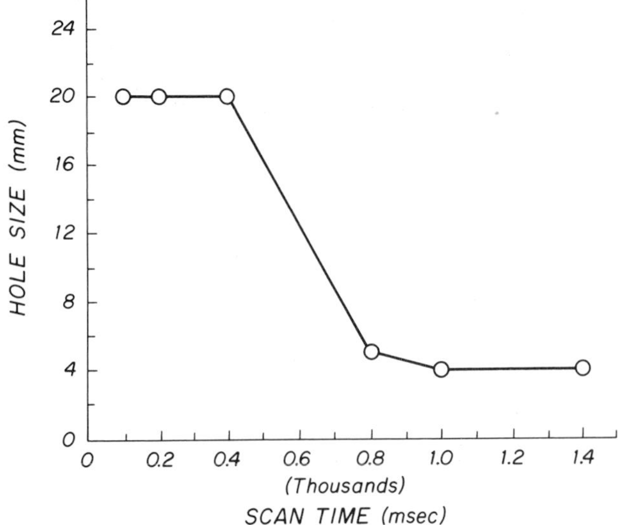

Figure 32–25. Contrast resolution as a function of time for conventional (Picker 1200) and fast (Picker FASTRAC) computed tomography.

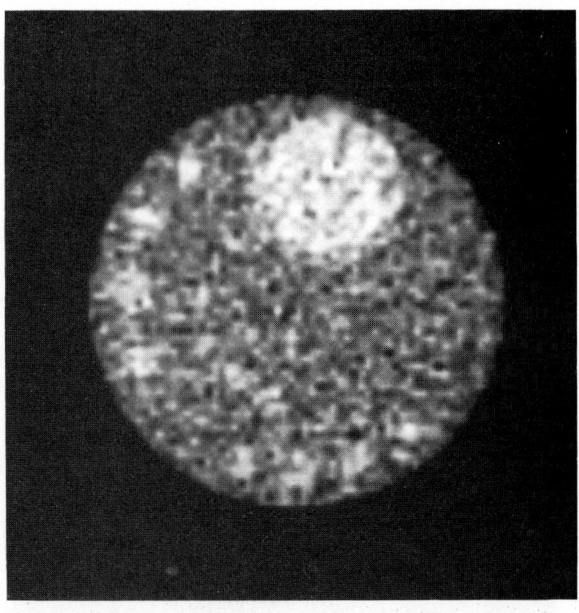

Figure 32–26. Low contrast resolution for conventional computed tomography (Picker 1200).

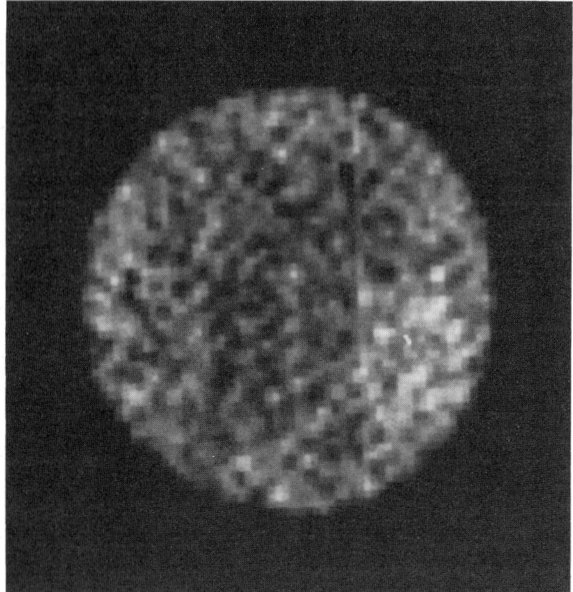

Figure 32–27. Low contrast resolution for fast computed tomography (Picker FASTRAC) with multiple-slice acquisition.

raphy systems in two major respects: (1) many angles of view are rapidly (nearly simultaneously) obtained from an "electronic scan" by multiple x-ray tubes placed around a 160-degree arc of a circular gantry that mechanically rotates about the patient, and (2) a fluorescent screen and multiple video imaging systems record two-dimensional projection images for each x-ray source, providing the data for reconstruction of dynamic three-dimensional volumes of the body.

Even though the DSR is based on the physics and mathematical principles of x-ray computed tomography, it is designed to achieve *dynamic volume scanning*, in contrast to the static cross-sectional scanning performed by conventional x-ray CT scanners. The DSR can simultaneously scan up to 240 adjacent 1-mm-thick cross sections at rates up to 60 per second. Desired trade-offs between temporal, spatial, and density resolution can be achieved by retrospective selection and processing of appropriate subsets of the total data recorded during a scan sequence. This capability permits detailed evaluation of the important relationships between temporal, spatial, and contrast resolution in computed tomography of the body, allowing imaging of nonmoving structures with high spatial or density resolution, or imaging of moving organs such as the heart, lungs, and circulation with high temporal resolution. Figure 32–35 is a depiction of the DSR system.

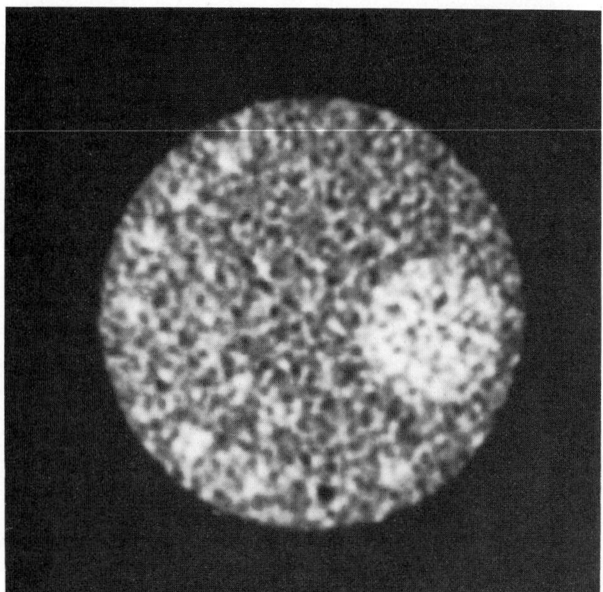

Figure 32–28. Low contrast resolution for fast computed tomography (Picker FASTRAC) with single-slice acquisition.

Table 32–6. UNIFORMITY FOR CONVENTIONAL (PICKER 1200) AND FAST (PICKER FASTRAC) COMPUTED TOMOGRAPHY

Scan Time (seconds)	Conventional (HU)	Fast, Single Slice—6 mm (HU)	Fast, Multiple Slice (HU)
0.05	—	—	19
0.1	—	19	—
0.4	—	18	—
0.8	—	17	—
1.0	—	18	—
1.4	—	17	—
3.3	3	—	—

The Scanner

The DSR scanner provides the capabilities for collecting two-dimensional projection data at high temporal resolution to generate dynamic images of selected volumes of the body. As illustrated in Figure 32–36, 14 x-ray tubes and 14 television cameras (of the 28 for which it is designed) are attached to the scanner. The x-ray tubes are arranged 12 degrees apart along a semicircular array with television cameras positioned opposite each x-ray source. As each x-ray tube is pulsed for 350 msec, a 30 cm × 30 cm image is generated on a portion of the curved fluorescent screen. The corresponding image isocon television camera is gated on for 762 msec to read out the fluoroscopic image. The subject or animal scanned is positioned inside the machine at the center of rotation as indicated in the schematic in Figure 32–36. The 14 television images of the fluoroscopic images, generated in one scan by the 14 x-ray pulses over an 11-msec period, are recorded on seven videodisk channels at a repetition rate of 60 scans per second. Each television image consists of 240 horizontal lines, but since only seven recording channels are currently available, sets of two views are recorded on each channel by combining every other line in each view into one video field. Therefore, up to 120 horizontal scan lines of each of the 14 video fields can be used to reconstruct the image of a corresponding anatomic cross section.

The DSR simultaneously scans a cylindrical volume 22 cm in axial height and 22 to 38 cm in transaxial diameter. Using the 14 x-ray source system, the 22-cm-diameter volume can be scanned in 0.011 second for a 14-view reconstruction, 0.127 second for a 112-view reconstruction, or 2.244 seconds for a 240-view recon-

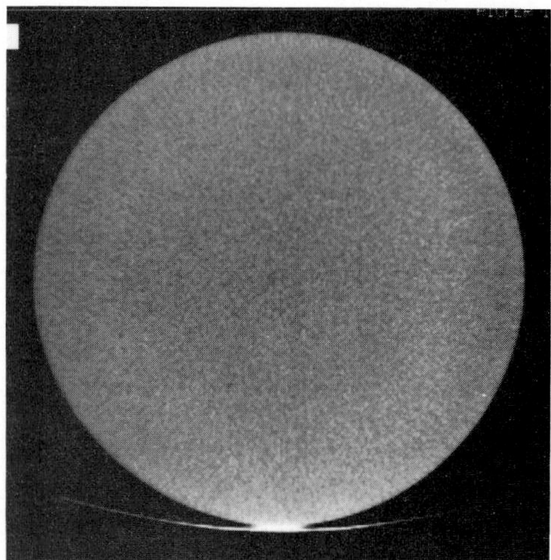

Figure 32–29. Uniformity for conventional computed tomography (Picker 1200).

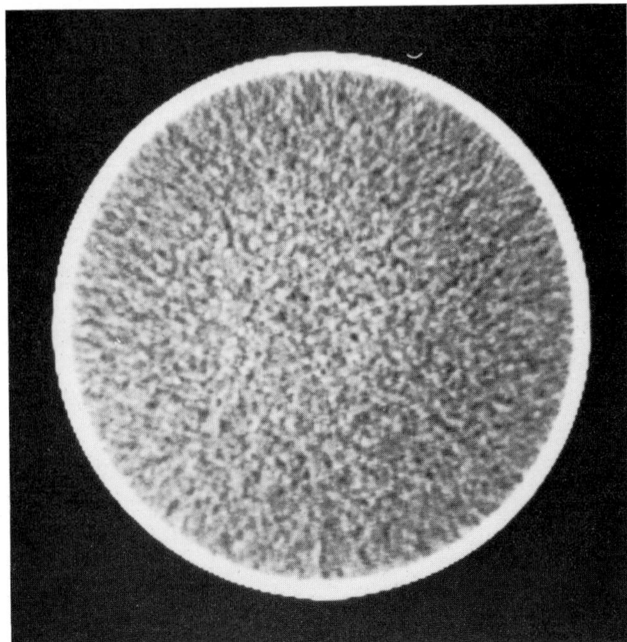

Figure 32–30. Uniformity for fast computed tomography with multiple-slice acquisition (Picker FASTRAC).

struction from a complete 360-degree range of views. The 38-cm-diameter volume is scanned in 0.06 second for a 16-view reconstruction or 0.57 second for a 135-view reconstruction. (In this mode, three adjacent cameras are simultaneously exposed and subsequently combined to provide a "wide-angle" view, so that only four total angles of view are recorded every 1/60 second.)

The volume can be scanned repetitively at selected rates, ranging between the highest rate of 60 scans per second to 1 scan in 2.2 seconds. If desired, the sequential scans can be retrospectively selected to overlap in time. The repetitive scans can continue for up to 20 total seconds—the recording capacity of the videodisks.

An Alderson Rando phantom was used to evaluate DSR x-ray exposure.[K6] At 100 kVp and 1000 mA for each x-ray pulse, the radiation entrance exposure for the 14 x-ray tube system was 0.9 R/sec in the thoracic region of interest. The thyroid region was exposed to less than 300 mR/sec, the eye to 7 mR/sec, and the gonads to less than 1 mR/sec. Consequently, for a scan of 4 to 5

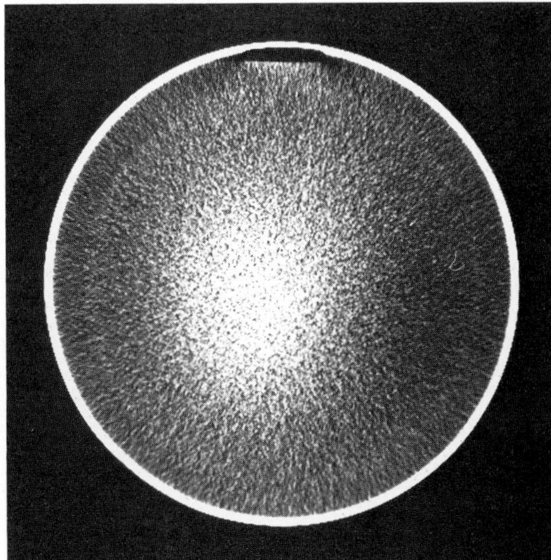

Figure 32–31. Uniformity for fast computed tomography with single-slice acquisition (Picker FASTRAC).

Table 32–7. NOISE FOR CONVENTIONAL (PICKER 1200) AND FAST (PICKER FASTRAC) COMPUTED TOMOGRAPHY

Scan Time (seconds)	Conventional (HU)	Fast, Single Slice—6 mm (HU)	Fast, Multiple Slice (HU)
0.05	—	—	15
0.1	—	29	—
0.8	—	14	—
1.4	—	12	—
3.3	12	—	—

seconds encompassing several heart cycles, which are required to evaluate cardiac function during the passage of contrast agent through the myocardium and through the lung, a total exposure of 4 to 5 R might be required. For similar scan times, this is about the level of radiation exposure used in conventional computed tomography to produce a single cross section. (The DSR can produce 300 volumes of 120 cross sections each in 5 seconds!) In conventional clinical cardiac angiography, patients are exposed to 5 to 10 times this level of radiation and may receive up to 100 R if cine imaging is used.

A special-purpose reconstruction program has been developed to integrate and execute efficiently all required steps in producing DSR volume images for analysis. This program allows the user to select interactively and retrospectively (after the scan) the time increments and spatial extent of recorded projection data to be processed. Options are available to combine recorded time points (to obtain more views per reconstruction) and/or adjacent lines in each view (for thicker cross sections) to obtain the temporal, spatial, or contrast resolution desired in the reconstructed volume image. This very useful capability for retrospective recombining of the reconstructed volume images is possible because the projection data acquisition and image reconstruction processes are linearly dependent.[R14] The program provides a special feature for "zoom" or "target" reconstructions to obtain high-spatial-resolution images of selected regions of interest within the scan volume. If specified, the program will also calculate the volume image(s) in cubic dimensions by appropriately interpolating between sections (generally the spacing between adjacent sections [0.9 mm] is greater than the pixel size within sections). This feature capitalizes on the intrinsic capability of the DSR to scan many adjacent thin cross sections of the body and facilitates efficient and accurate computation of arbitrarily oriented sections (oblique) without loss of spatial resolution.

A cone beam of x-rays is used in the DSR to produce the two-dimensional x-ray video projection images used for reconstruction of the three-dimensional volumes. True cone beam image reconstruction algorithms are being investigated.[A3] However, since the relatively large x-ray source-to-object distance (145 cm) of the DSR results in a small subtended angle (3 degrees) in forming the two-dimensional projection image, the video lines above and below the centerline of the image represent x-ray projections of near-parallel sets of fan beams. Therefore, fan beam reconstruction algorithms have been successfully applied to data digitized from video lines spanning the entire axial extent (22 cm) of the video projection image and have obtained satisfactory reconstructions, particularly over the extent of the heart.[R14] The same fan

Table 32–8. HOUNSFIELD LINEARITY FOR CONVENTIONAL (PICKER 1200) AND FAST (PICKER FASTRAC) COMPUTED TOMOGRAPHY

Material	HU	Conventional (HU)	Fast, Single Slice—6 mm (HU)	Fast, Multiple Slice (HU)
Polyethylene	−97	−102	−83	−85
Water	0	2	1	−5
Lucite	124	124	126	116
Teflon	908	930	876	816

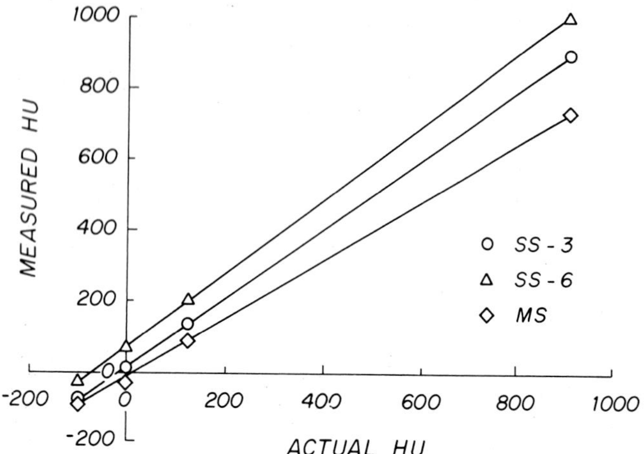

Figure 32–32. Hounsfield linearity for conventional (Picker 1200) and fast (Picker FASTRAC) computed tomography. HU—Hounsfield unit.

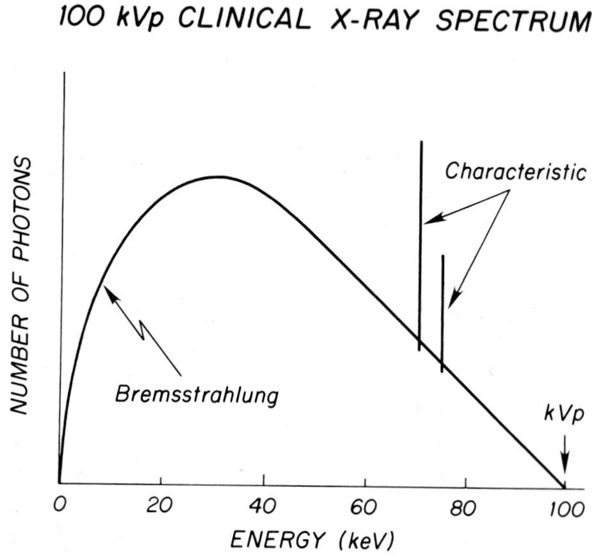

100 kVp CLINICAL X-RAY SPECTRUM

NUMBER OF PHOTONS

Characteristic

Bremsstrahlung

kVp

0 20 40 60 80 100

ENERGY (keV)

Figure 32–33. Diagrammatic representation of a bremsstrahlung x-ray spectrum.

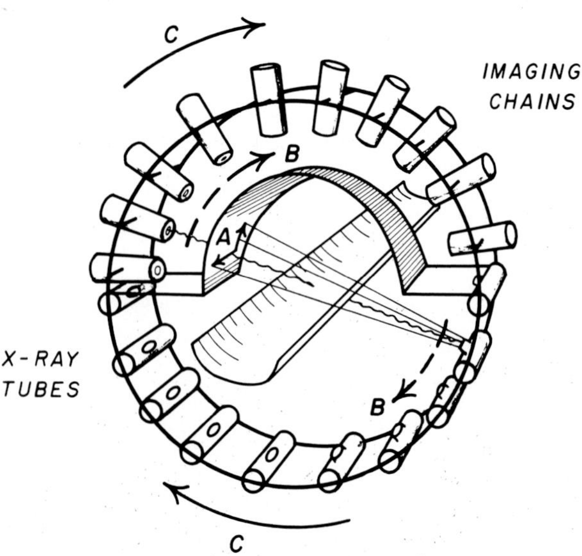

Figure 32–34. Scanning geometry concept for high-temporal-resolution volume computed tomography scanning system. Two-dimensional detector simultaneously records projection data (A) for reconstruction of multiple cross sections. Multiple x-ray sources perform high-speed electronic scan (B) for stop-action high-repetition-rate reconstructions, and mechanical rotation of the entire system (C) provides more data for reconstructions with high spatial and density resolution. (From Ritman, E. L.: Quantitative transaxial imaging of the heart. Eur. J. Cardiol. 5:203, 1977, with permission.)

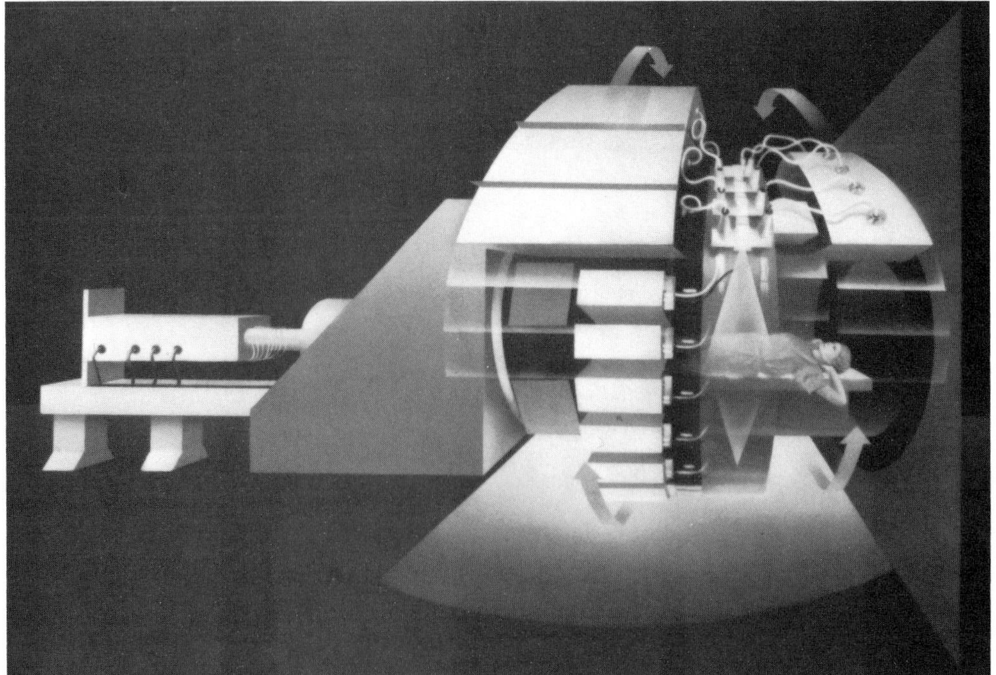

Figure 32–35. Artistic depiction of Dynamic Spatial Reconstructor (DSR), a four-dimensional image scanner at the Mayo Clinic. (From the Raytheon Magazine, Fall 1983, p. 28, with permission.)

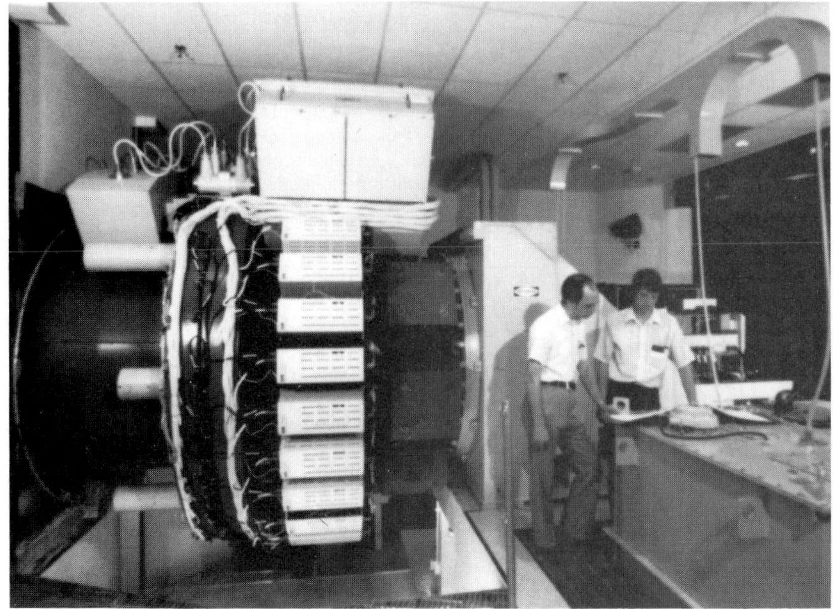

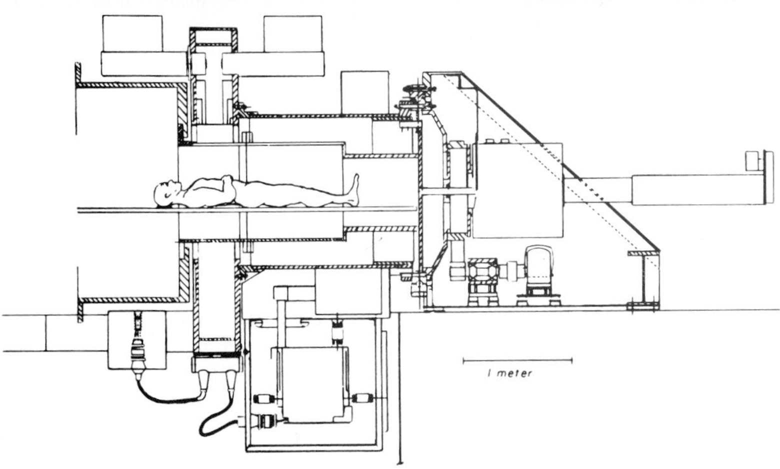

Figure 32–36. *Upper panel*, Dynamic Spatial Reconstructor scanner assembly. The entire structure to the left of the men is cantilevered from the triangular base. Multiple-image isocon television cameras and corresponding x-ray sources are arranged along a vertical plane. Rotation of the cantilevered section increases the number of angles of view per scan in proportion to the programmed duration of the scan. *Lower panel*, Midline longitudinal section of the scanner shows relationship of human subject lying on table and the surrounding gantry. (From Behrenbeck, T., Sinak, L. J., Robb, R. A., et al.: Some imaging characteristics of the Dynamic Spatial Reconstructor x-ray scanner system. *In* Reba, R. C., Goodenough, D. J., and Davidson, H. F., [eds.]: Diagnostic Imaging in Medicine. NATO ASI Series, Series E: Applied Sciences, Naples, Italy, No. 61, 1981, with permission.)

beam reconstruction algorithms have been modified to produce improved images from limited projection data sets, including limited number of views, limited range of views, and limited field of view.[R14]

Analysis and Display

The quantitative analysis of four-dimensional DSR image data (three spatial plus one temporal dimension) requires the development of new multidimensional display methods, primarily because (1) the tremendous amount of image data generated by the DSR must be edited and analyzed quantitatively in order to extract useful information and (2) the structures and processes studied are most often four-dimensional by nature. Multidimensional display facilitates quantitative analysis of these data by providing direct visualization of three-dimensional shapes and spatial relationships among imaged structures. This direct visual feedback in turn facilitates (1) detection of the presence or absence of imaged features, (2) cognition (understanding) of three-dimensional shapes, (3) identification of the optimal orientation of oblique cross-sectional images, and (4) measurement of organ shape and dimensions. A special software package for multidimensional image display and analysis, ANALYZE, will be described in a subsequent section.

Basic Imaging Performance

The DSR is made up of several separate components, including x-ray tubes, television cameras, and electronic amplifiers, which can be independently controlled and have unique effects on image characteristics. Therefore, there is some variation of image characteristics from scan to scan due to the independent setting and calibration of each component. However, variability of these characteristics during one or more scans of several seconds with the same component settings is negligible.

The noise in the cross-sectional images is stochastic and can therefore be reduced by summing the signals generated by a number of adjacent video scan lines, that is, increasing image slice thickness. This, however, accentuates the problem of partial volume effects, which reduce image quality and accuracy due to blurring of structure edges. The solution to this paradox is to compute a number of appropriately oriented, thin oblique sections from the stack of thin transaxial sections and then sum the thin oblique sections (to enhance the signal-to-noise ratio in the resultant image) over an extent that does not result in a serious partial volume effect. The partial volume effect becomes more and more severe as the slice thickness approaches the size of complex-shaped structures.[S7] This deleterious effect has to be weighed against the advantage of improved signal-to-noise ratio that results from increasing image slice thickness. Appropriate consideration of these opposing factors can result in images for which maximum quality is obtained through minimized noise and tolerable partial volume effects. The optimal trade-off between these factors is dependent on the structure of interest, the scanning conditions, and the amount of contrast present, and capabilities for retrospective determination of this optimal trade-off for any scan are very valuable.

As illustrated in Figure 32–37, if such a procedure is followed, the image quality of transaxial slices of varying thickness *computed* through a phantom scanned in an axial or oblique direction is quite comparable to that of slices obtained from a transaxial scan of the phantom. For this phantom, the limiting high-contrast spatial resolution is approximately 1.25 mm. Images such as those shown in Figure 32–37 were used to compute a modulation transfer function for the DSR, as illustrated in Figure 32–38. The limiting high-contrast spatial resolution of the DSR approaches 1 mm in both transaxial and axial directions under "near-ideal" scanning conditions. The air-to-Plexiglas x-ray attenuation difference is approximately equivalent to that of 30 mg of iodine per milliliter of blood. Such concentrations are readily achieved in

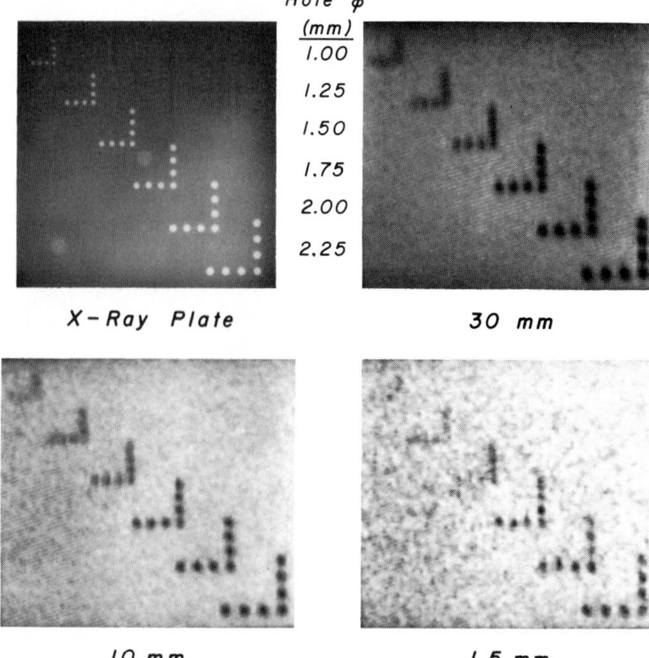

Figure 32–37. Plexiglas cube with air-filled holes was scanned with the holes oriented parallel to the scan plane. That is, the structures to be imaged, the holes, were not perpendicular to the scan plane, as would be done in conventional single-slice computed tomography. However, since the entire cube was scanned by the Dynamic Spatial Reconstructor, multiple adjacent slices were reconstructed (from 120 views around 360 degrees) and represented in the computer as a three-dimensional array of attenuation coefficients, from which slices through the cube at any orientation relative to the scan plane could be computed. This figure shows variable-thickness images of the cube computed from multislice images (i.e., three-dimensional images) obtained from the Dynamic Spatial Reconstructor so that the selected plane of the images is perpendicular to the holes, or resolution elements. After computation of these appropriately oriented images of thin slices in the "transaxial" plane, images of adjacent slices were added to provide improved signal-to-noise ratio. The reconstructed images are displayed with pixel size of 0.8 mm. (From Behrenbeck, T., Sinak, L. J., Robb, R. A., et al.: Some imaging characteristics of the Dynamic Spatial Reconstructor x-ray scanner system. *In* Reba, R. C., Goodenough, D. J., and Davidson, H. F. [eds.]: Diagnostic Imaging in Medicine. NATO ASI Series, Series E: Applied Sciences, Naples, Italy, No. 61, 1981, with permission.)

vivo by bolus injections of iodinated x-ray contrast agent into blood vessels upstream of the anatomic site of the scan.

When the image data recorded under *practical* conditions are appropriately manipulated so that the signal-to-noise ratio is maximized and the partial volume effect is minimized, the characteristic imaging capabilities of the DSR[B11] may be summarized as follows:

1. Maximum spatial resolution of high-contrast, stationary structures is 8 lines per centimeter in transaxial (transverse) and axial (cephalocaudal) directions.
2. For the 14 x-ray tube configuration, the spatial resolution of a high-contrast structure moving at 80 mm/sec is 4 line pairs per centimeter in the transverse and cephalocaudal directions.
3. For a 112-view scan (i.e., 0.127 second in duration) of a 10-cm-diameter water-equivalent test phantom, the density resolution (defined as the smallest resolvable difference between the reconstructed linear attenuation coefficients of a structure of a given size and its uniformly dense surroundings) is 100 percent of the roentgen opacity of water in a 1-mm^3 volume (i.e., average data from 100 voxels). Density resolution of 3 percent in 1 mm^3 can be achieved in images produced from 2.24-second scans of 240 views around 360 degrees.
4. The small increments of volume in a balloon during successive 0.06-second scans produced by injection of 100 ml of contrast

Figure 32–38. Spatial resolution in line pairs per millimeter expressed as a function of image contrast (modulation transfer function, or MTF) determined from reconstructed Dynamic Spatial Reconstructor images of high-contrast phantom (see Fig. 32–37). Image noise was also measured as a percentage of peak-to-peak differences between regional reconstructed values for water and air. The limiting resolution (intersection of MTF and noise curves) is approximately 0.8 lp/mm. (From Behrenbeck, T., Sinak, L. J., Robb, R. A., et al.: Some imaging characteristics of the Dynamic Spatial Reconstructor x-ray scanner system. *In* Reba, R. C., Goodenough, D. J., and Davidson, H. F. [eds.]: Diagnostic Imaging in Medicine. NATO ASI Series, Series E: Applied Sciences, Naples, Italy, No. 61, 1981, with permission.)

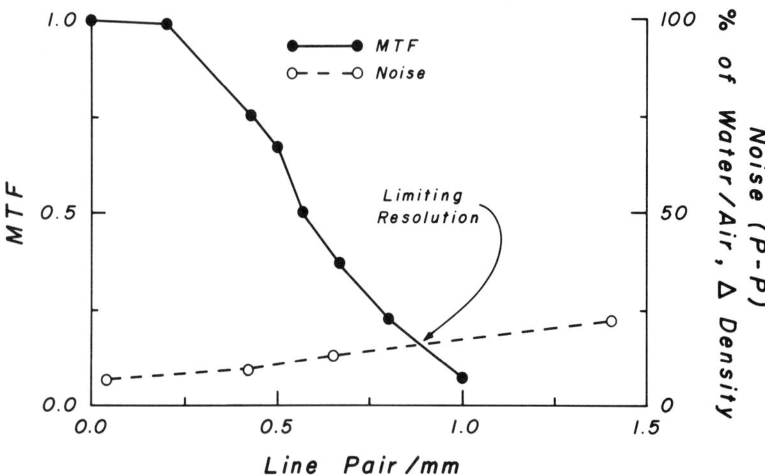

agent into the balloon at the rate of 150 ml/sec were estimated correctly from reconstructed images of the balloon to within 3 percent of the known values.

5. Lung volume (air plus parenchyma) and total heart muscle mass estimated from images of intact anesthetized experimental animals were correct to within 3 and 5 percent of postmortem measurements, respectively.

6. Estimates of blood flow in carotid arteries of anesthetized dogs from dynamic DSR images were correct to within 10 percent of electromagnetic flowmeter measurements. Similarly, the relative cardiac output of anesthetized dogs calculated from dynamic images was correct to within 10 percent of the outputs determined with conventional techniques for estimation of cardiac output, such as dye dilution curves.[W3]

7. Stenoses (constrictions or blockages) as small as 0.6 mm (diameter) by 1.5 mm (length) placed in 3.2-mm-diameter plastic tubing sutured to the heart of an anesthetized dog were calculated correctly from images of the intact thorax.

These imaging performance capabilities may be decreased somewhat as the size of the subject being scanned is increased, primarily because of the limited sensitivity and dynamic range of the fluoroscopic video detector system.[K5, R13] Therefore, the DSR in its present form (the detection system is modular and can be upgraded) may be more useful for children and slender adults than for large adults.

Applications

The DSR has unique capabilities for cognitive visualization and accurate measurement of shapes and dimensions of the thoracic contents, such as cardiac chambers, pleural surfaces, airways (down to three levels of branching), diaphragm, kidneys, and pulmonary and systemic blood vessels. Such measurements obtained throughout a cardiac and respiratory cycle, in conjunction with simultaneous recording[S8] of physiologic parameters such as blood pressures, pleural pressure, and electrocardiogram, hold promise for yielding new insights into the function of the heart and lungs and their interaction. Preliminary experience with the DSR has shown that adequate delineation of these structures can be achieved from images reconstructed with as few as 56 views. With the present 14-imaging-chain system, 56 views are obtained for every successive 1⁄15 second of scanning time. These 56-view reconstructions are obtained by adding together four successive 14-view reconstructions. Alternatively, each 14-view reconstruction can be obtained during a specific physiologic event, such as a specific point in the cardiac cycle (as determined from the electrocardiogram), before summing. The latter method is similar to "gated" imaging.

Images obtained from the DSR involve no assumptions about size and shape of organs. True three-dimensional structure of the heart and cardiac chambers can be detected by imaging radiopaque contrast agent, injected peripherally, as it passes through the various chambers and vascular structures. Figure 32–39 illustrates such a capability. A 12-kg dog was anesthetized with pentobarbital, placed supine in the DSR, and scanned during injection of radiopaque contrast agent (Renovist, 1.2 ml/kg) into the inferior vena cava. In the upper panel, an 8-mm-thick sagittal section selected from the reconstructed volume image is shown; the right atrium, right ventricle, and inferior vena cava are clearly

Sagittal Section

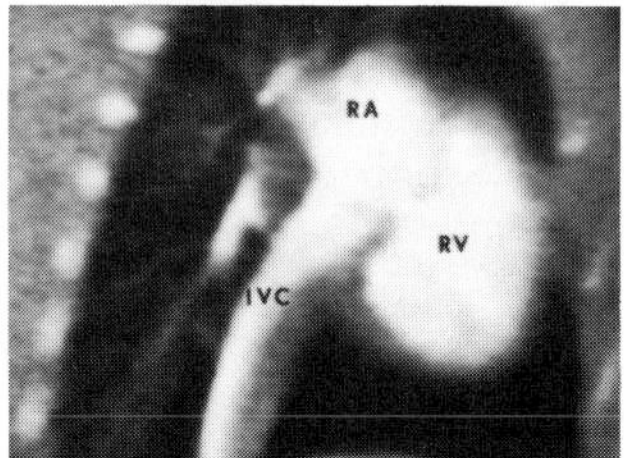

8 mm THICK

Shaded Surface Display

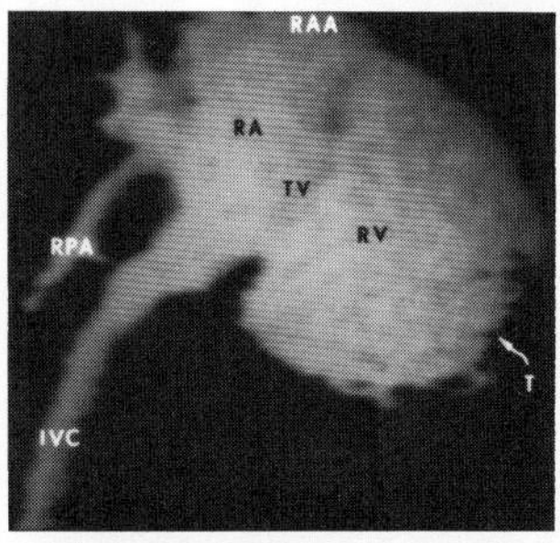

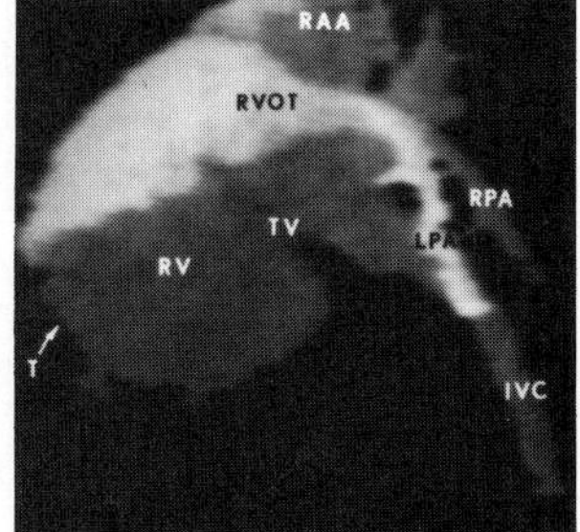

RIGHT LATERAL ASPECT   LEFT LATERAL ASPECT

Figure 32–39. Visualization of right heart chambers and major vessels. The top panel shows an 8-mm-thick sagittal section reconstructed from a 240-view Dynamic Spatial Reconstructor (DSR) scan, viewed from the right side of the 12-kg, supine, anesthetized dog following contrast injection (Renovist, 1.2 ml/kg) into the inferior vena cava (IVC). Because of the slow heart rate (produced by vagal stimulation), dye settled into the dorsal portion of the inferior vena cava. Also visible are the right atrium and right ventricle (RA and RV). Right and left lateral aspects of a shaded-surface display of the right heart chambers and associated vessels of the same dog are displayed in the lower panels. Structures of interest are the right atrium and right ventricle (RA and RV); tricuspid valve region (TV); right atrial appendage (RAA); right ventricular outflow tract (RVOT); right and left pulmonary arteries (RPA and LPA); inferior vena cava (IVC); and negative cast of trabeculae (T). (From Robb, R. A., Hoffman, E. A., Sinak, L. J., et al.: High-speed three-dimensional x-ray computed tomography: The Dynamic Spatial Reconstructor. Proc. IEEE 71:308, (March) 1983, with permission.)

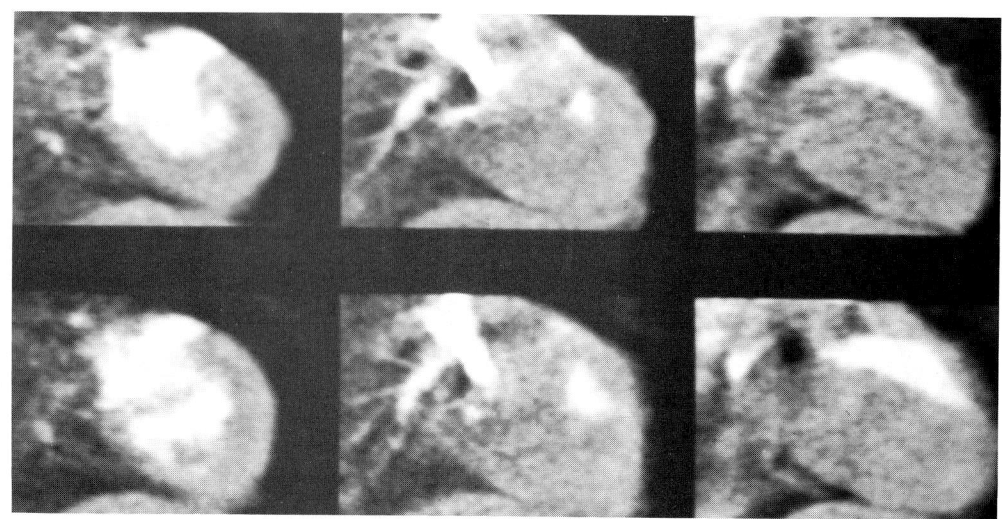

Figure 32–40. Dynamic images of sagittal sections of dog's heart obtained from synchronous volume scans (15 per second) performed by the Dynamic Spatial Reconstructor throughout one complete cardiac cycle during injection of x-ray contrast material into the superior vena cava. *Top row*, Three different 1-mm-thick sagittal sections, 8 mm apart, all in the right half of the heart. These sections were obtained at an instant in the cardiac cycle near end-systole (minimum volume of chambers). *Bottom row*, The same three sagittal sections obtained at an instant near end-diastole (maximum volume of chambers) of the same heartbeat. Left-hand images show right atrium and a small part of the right ventricle filled with contrast material; center images show superior vena cava and pulmonary artery with small branching vessels; right-hand images show more of right ventricular chamber and demonstrate the marked difference in chamber area between systole (*top*) and diastole (*bottom*). (From Robb, R. A.: X-ray computed tomography: An engineering synthesis of multiscientific principles. CRC Critical Reviews in Biomedical Engineering 7[4]:265–334, 1982, with permission.)

visible. By using a computer-aided three-dimensional surface detection and shaded-surface display algorithm,[A5] the three-dimensional surface of the contrast agent detected within the right heart chambers can be displayed, as shown in the lower panels of Figure 32–39. Note the detail of the right atrium and right ventricle, the trabeculae at the ventricular surface, the tricuspid valve region, the left and right branches of the pulmonary arteries, the inferior vena cava, the right atrial appendage, and the right ventricular outflow tract.

Figure 32–40 illustrates the capability of the DSR for rapid three-dimensional imaging of the heart and circulation for study of the dynamic distributions of blood flow to, within, and from

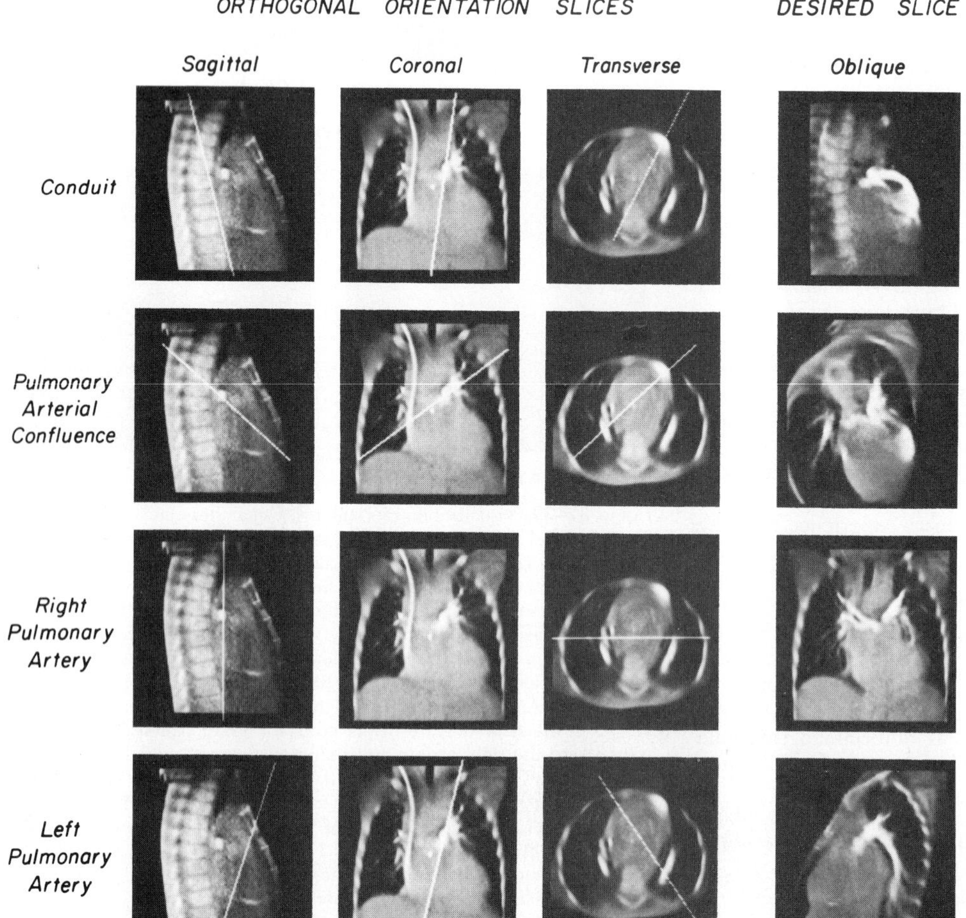

Figure 32–41. The midsagittal, midcoronal, and midtransverse sections in the left three sets of images are selected to provide the observer with orientation information. The bright lines in these images indicate the intersection of the oblique cross section displayed in the rightmost panel. Orientation of oblique sections is along axis of selected pulmonary arteries (1.5-mm-thick sections; 0.3-second scan aperture, patient 1). (From Spyra, W. J. T., Bove, A. A., and Ritman, E. L.: Some technical considerations in tomographic coronary arteriography. Int. J. Cardiac Imag. 2:223, 1987, with permission.)

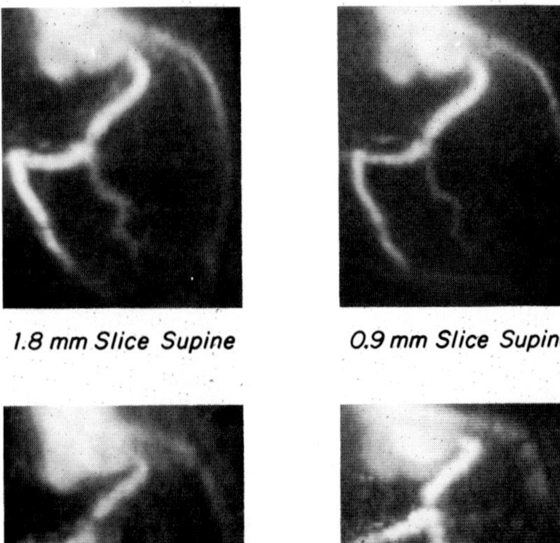

Figure 32–42. Computer-generated projection dissolution display of coronary arteries of a dog during an aortic root injection of a bolus of iohexol contrast medium. In this instance, the left anterior descending coronary artery is particularly blurred compared with the left circumflex coronary artery. This blurring was somewhat diminished when the Dynamic Spatial Reconstructor (DSR) was programmed to scan with 0.9-mm-thick slices (*right upper panel*) versus 1.8-mm-thick slices (*left upper panel*). The lower two panels show no significant difference in blurring of the left anterior descending coronary artery when the dog is scanned in the prone or 30-degree head-up supine orientation. (From Liu, Y.-H., Hoffman, E. A., Hagler, D. J., et al.: Accuracy of pulmonary vascular dimensions estimated with the Dynamic Spatial Reconstructor. Am. J. Physiol. Imag. 1:201, 1986, with permission.)

the heart with circulatory contrast agents. The entire heart was dynamically imaged with successive 0.067-second volume scans for one complete heartbeat (about 0.7 second) during infusion of contrast material into the superior vena cava.

Figure 32–41 shows images of midline sagittal, coronal, and transverse sections from one point in time during the injection of contrast material in a patient scanned with the DSR. The volume image may also be used to create planar images at oblique angles to the transverse scanning plane. The rightmost panels of Figure 32–41 show such oblique sections passing through the main course of the pulmonary arteries. This figure also demonstrates how the operator-interactive sectioning program works for retrospective selection of a sectioning plane through a structure of interest. The leftmost three panels are midsagittal, midcoronal, and midtransverse orientation sections. The bright line intersecting these orientation images indicates the location of the oblique section shown at the right in the figure.

Figure 32–42 is an example of a projection dissolution display of the left main, left anterior descending, and left circumflex coronary arteries of a dog scanned in the DSR during an aortic root injection. Note the blurring of the left anterior descending coronary artery compared with the left circumflex coronary artery. The contrast of this blurring is reduced when 0.9-mm-thick slices are scanned (rather than 1.8-mm-thick slices) and when the dog is scanned in the 30-degree head-up (supine) position. The prone image is not different from the supine image. These images suggest that viscosity and specific gravity of the contrast medium are not major causes of this blurring.

Regional renal perfusion may be observed and measured by following changes in the regional concentration of roentgen contrast agent over time or by following the variation in roentgen density caused by the passage of a bolus of contrast material. Figure 32–43 shows a 0.5-cm-thick coronal section of a kidney during the time course of an injection of contrast agent into the renal artery.

Image Display and Analysis

The ability to extract objective and quantitatively accurate information from three-dimensional images produced by dynamic computed tomography (and other medical image scanners) has not kept pace with the ability to produce the images themselves. What are required are capabilities to display, manipulate, and measure efficiently the intrinsic and relevant information contained in the multidimensional image data (i.e., the true morphologic, pathologic, biologic, physiologic, and/or metabolic meaning of the numbers) produced by these new three-dimensional imaging modalities.

Display techniques for conveying three-dimensional information include integrated projections of the volume onto the display screen, sometimes with prior dissolution of structures from the volume,[H11] stereo displays generated from projection images,[H12, H13]

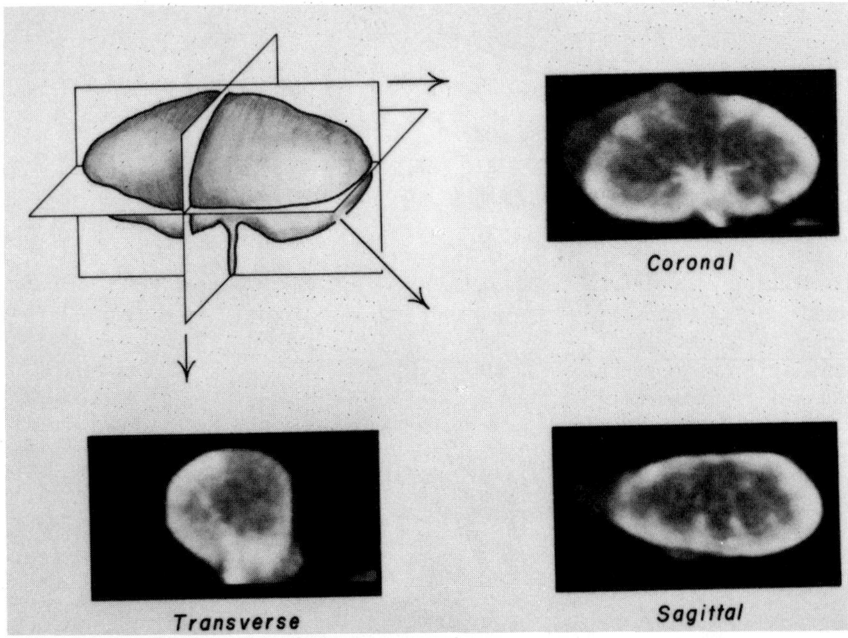

Figure 32–43. Three orthogonal 5-mm-thick sections of sodium-replete dog kidney determined from Dynamic Spatial Reconstructor (DSR) volume scan following injection of contrast material into the renal artery. These images were determined at a point following the injection where much of the renal cortex remains perfused but the medullary bed is clearing. (From Robb, R. A.: X-ray computed tomography: Advanced systems and applications in biomedical research and diagnosis. *In* Robb, R. A. [ed.]: Three-Dimensional Biomedical Imaging, Vol. I, Chap. 5. CRC Press, Boca Raton, Fla., 1985, pp. 107–166, with permission.)

and shaded-surface display.[H14–H16] One of the most popular techniques for presenting three-dimensional structures involves depth shading of object surfaces. An important precursor to shaded-surface display is the extraction of a three-dimensional surface description from a raw three-dimensional volume image. This segmentation step is often required not only for display but also for measurement. However, the segmentation step is an area that is in need of improved algorithms,[H16, P3] particularly for the extraction of soft tissue structures and for images such as those produced by magnetic resonance imaging and ultrasound. Shaded-surface display algorithms for medical applications have been based on conventional polygonal models,[F2] a cuberille model for the surface,[H17] a contour model for the surface,[F2, H17, H18] and an octree model of the three-dimensional object.[H17]

Another three-dimensional display technique, often called ray casting or volume rendering,[T2] has been implemented in several applications.[F3, H14] This technique has the advantage of using the entire three-dimensional data set ("volume image") in the process. The challenge heretofore has been to exploit this powerful technique in an interactive implementation.

Integrated systems (workstations) for the analysis of two-, three-, and four-dimensional images are beginning to appear in the commercial and research markets. As yet, there is no system that is satisfactory for both biomedical research and clinical diagnostic applications, possibly because the focuses of the two areas have been different. The medical imaging systems and hence the commercial image analysis workstations have been targeted at the practice of radiology, where it may be sufficient simply to visualize structures within the body. This philosophy has led to the development of so-called PACS (picture archiving and communications systems).[G8, H19, M7] Such systems aim to duplicate the capabilities of a film-based radiology department but without the use of film.[B12, G9, N2, P4, R15] This limited focus has diluted general enthusiasm for such systems, particularly in view of the high cost required to achieve the desired performance. Some systems are now available that are aimed at medical specialties other than radiology. For example, several companies sell workstations or services designed for surgery planning.[A4, F2, R16] Various image analysis workstations have been developed for a range of research applications, and these systems vary widely in their goals and capabilities. Some of the systems have been designed to handle volume images from a variety of sources and so could find application in a variety of medical circumstances.[G10, L3, O2, S9]

Various multidimensional image analysis software modules have been integrated into a comprehensive, highly interactive, intuitive software system called ANALYZE.[R5, R17] This software is written in "C," is well documented, and will run on most standard workstation systems supported by UNIX. The ANALYZE system consists of a hierarchical set of processes, each process representing a particular analysis task, as indicated in Figure 32–44. The modules share image memory segments and communicate with each other to pass related image information. The integration of these subprocesses allows for multiple analyses in which the output of one process may be in the input to another.

Figure 32–45 shows a display of 12 sections from a Dynamic Spatial Reconstructor chest scan displayed with the sections module in ANALYZE. Each row of sections is a different slice orientation. The sections can be selected orthogonal to any major axis and displayed with arbitrary increments between sections. The image(s) can be processed before display by using any of several transforms, including windowing, thresholding, smoothing, inverting, contouring, and rotating, none of which alters the original data set. This module is used to review, select, and nondestructively process image data prior to further analysis. Figure 32–46 shows a different way to display orthogonal sections—as a cubic volume with interactive dissection at any depth in the transverse, coronal, and/or sagittal directions.

An important part of multidimensional image analysis is selection of the optimal viewing orientation for the image data. One process in ANALYZE, called *oblique*, provides an interactive method for entirely arbitrary viewpoint selection by providing the user with pictorial feedback cues to indicate the current orientation of the volume image data.

Figure 32–47 depicts a typical screen in the *oblique* process using a full Dynamic Spatial Reconstructor volume scan of the chest for display. The upper three images are orthogonal central sections of the three-dimensional image volume (sagittal, coronal, and transverse), with the intersection of the current selected oblique image indicated by the line drawn on each reference image. A diagram indicating the current position of the oblique plane within the volume image is shown at the lower right. The current thin oblique image is displayed in the center of the screen, with a "thickened" image consisting of 10 parallel oblique

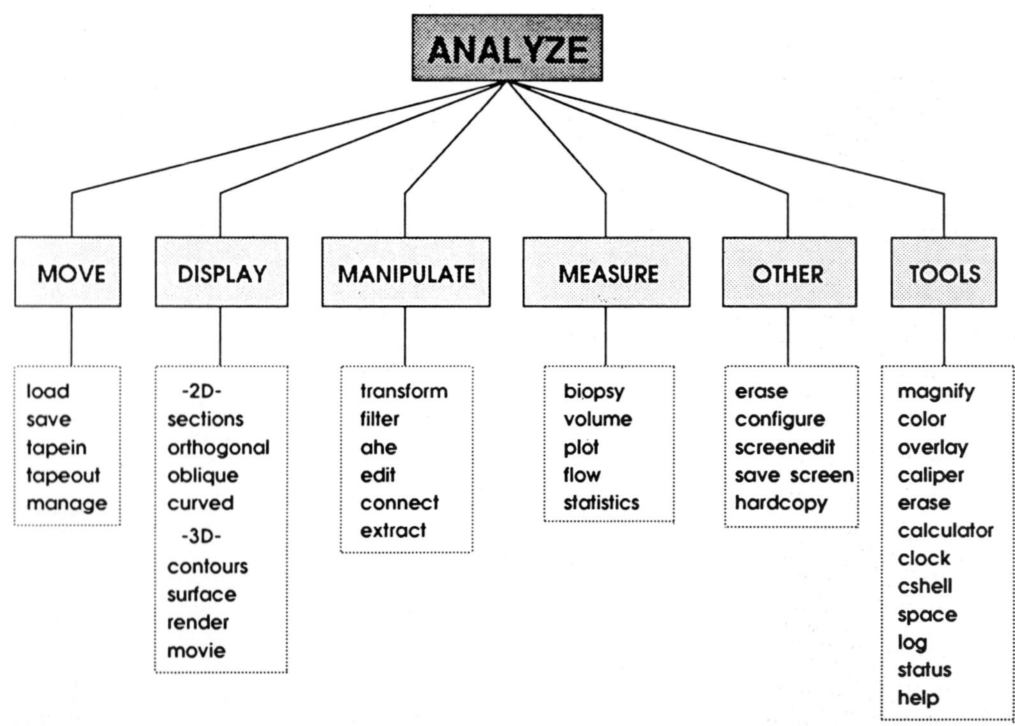

Figure 32–44. Diagram of ANALYZE software system. (From Robb, R. A., and Barillot, C.: Interactive 3-D image display and analysis. *In* Casasent, D. P., and Tescher, A. G. [eds.]: SPIE, Hybrid Image and Signal Process. 939:173, 1988, with permission.)

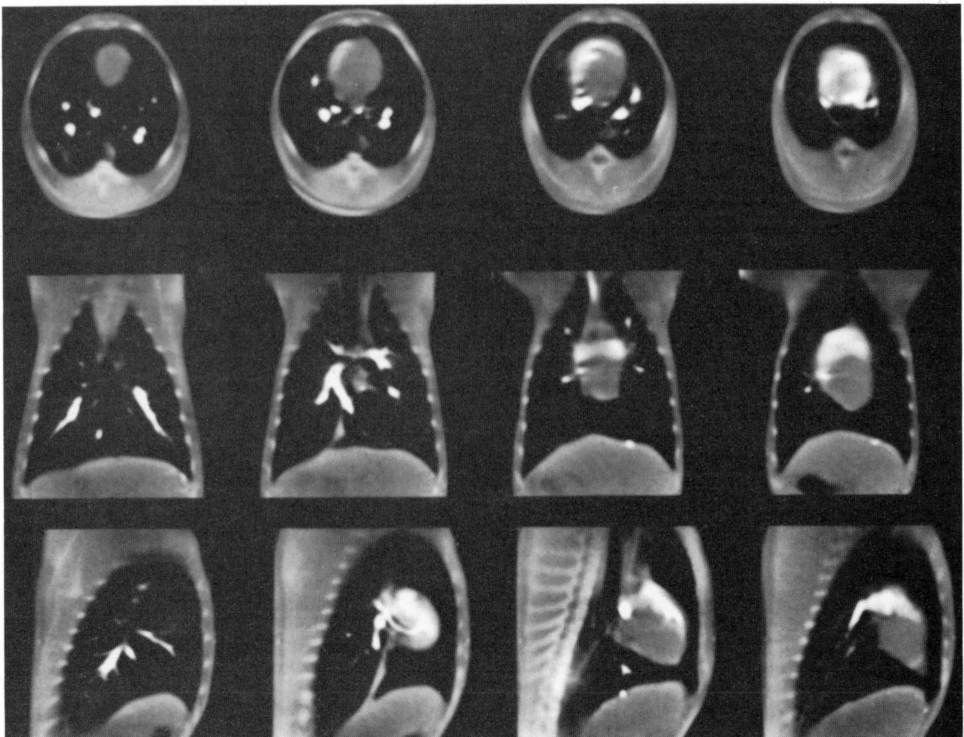

Figure 32–45. Montage produced by the *sections* module illustrating a set of intensity-windowed transverse, coronal, and sagittal slices through the chest from a Dynamic Spatial Reconstructor volume scan. (From Robb, R. A., and Barillot, C.: Interactive display and analysis of 3-D medical images. IEEE Trans. Med. Imag. MI-8:217–226, 1989, with permission.)

sections summed together at the left. Any sequence of parallel oblique sections can be selectively added together to produce thicker sections, or a stack of adjacent sections parallel to the current oblique section can be generated. This new oriented three-dimensional image can be stored in the data base for subsequent analysis.

Figure 32–48 shows the display of an ANALYZE process called *curved sections* in which a curved line can be drawn on one of the standard orthogonal planes (transverse, coronal, or sagittal) and sections perpendicular to this line interactively computed and displayed adjacent one to another to yield an image of any curvilinear section through the volume.

The MANIPULATE processes allow the user to modify the image data in memory by using a set of interactive editing and/or transform tools. Addition, subtraction, multiplication, and division can be performed in linear combinations on sets of volume image data. Interpolation, scaling, and partitioning of the image data can be performed. Special techniques for image warping and image mapping are available. Other processes include normalization of image data sets with control images, correction for a nonlinear distribution of image densities, selected enhancement of objects in the image data, and correlation of image data produced by different imaging modalities. The editing tools include interactive global and regional windowing, intensity thresholding, erasing, painting, and cut-and-paste operations. The transforms include a wide variety of standard and customized image processing functions for contrast enhancement, edge detection, and segmentation. A powerful feature in this set of tools is "image algebra," through which the user can generate complex formulas with different images as operands. Combinations of arithmetic and logical operations can be performed.

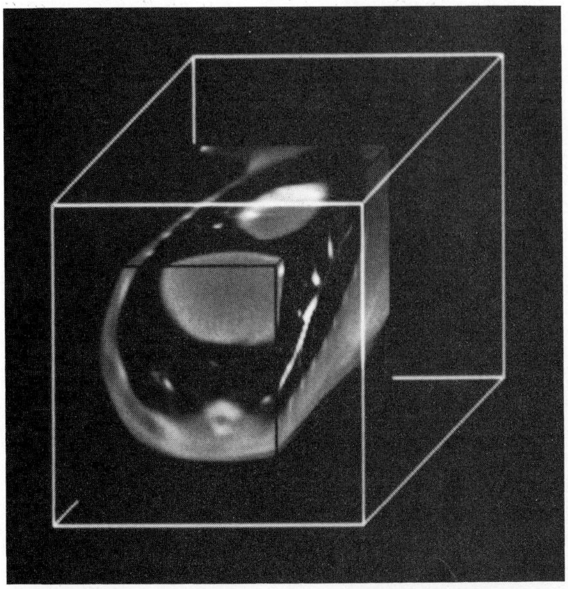

Figure 32–46. Interactive dissection of cubic volume along the perpendicular planes using *ortho* module. (From Robb, R. A., and Barillot, C.: Interactive display and analysis of 3-D medical images. IEEE Trans. Med. Imag. MI-8:217–226, 1989, with permission.)

When the data have been selected and manipulated to the point where region-of-interest measurements or specific parametric information about the image data is desired, the MEASURE processes can be used. One such process is called *biopsy*. This module displays a set of serial two-dimensional sections on which measurements can be made. These serial sections can be interactively selected from any portion of the multidimensional image data set by using a variable increment factor to scan through the sections. Repeated measurements through the multidimensional image data set can be performed by specifying a range of image slices to process. The screen shown in Figure 32–49 is an example of the use of the *biopsy* module on a DSR chest scan. Three basic types of regions of interest or "numerical samples" can be specified in *biopsy* to provide image data measurements: point samples, line samples, and area samples. A sampling threshold may be set to specify a range of information to include in the sampling functions.

The information generated from a point sample consists of the multidimensional coordinate of the point (three- or four-dimensional) and the image pixel value (e.g., density) at that point. Line profiles can be generated and displayed along any arbitrarily oriented line, which is selected by interactively specifying its end points in an image. Sampling areas can be specified as regular shapes, such as rectangles and ellipses, or by tracing a free-form area on the image. Multiple sampling areas can be specified on

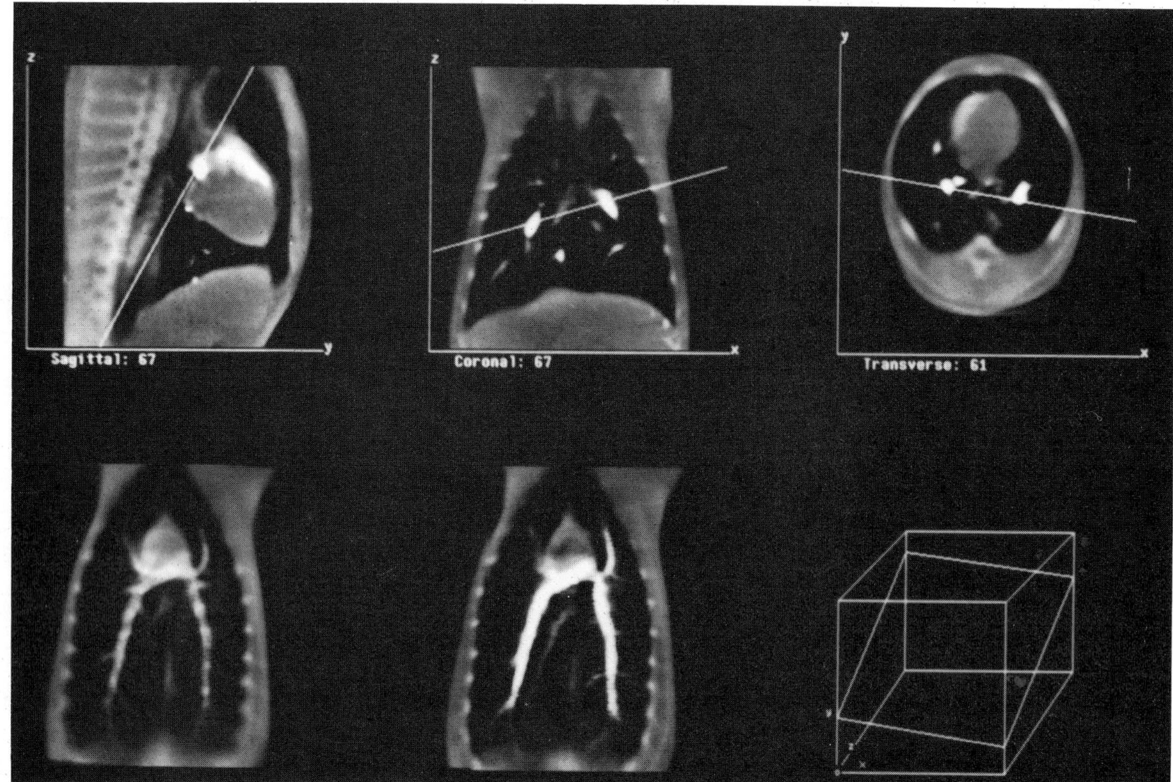

Figure 32–47. A typical screen in the *oblique* module during selection of arbitrary slices through a three-dimensional chest image. Bottom center image is oblique slice computed through volume at orientation indicated by lines on orthogonal reference images (*top row*). Image at lower left is "thickened" oblique slice. (From Robb, R. A., and Barillot, C.: Interactive display and analysis of 3-D medical images. IEEE Trans. Med. Imag. MI-8:217–226, 1989, with permission.)

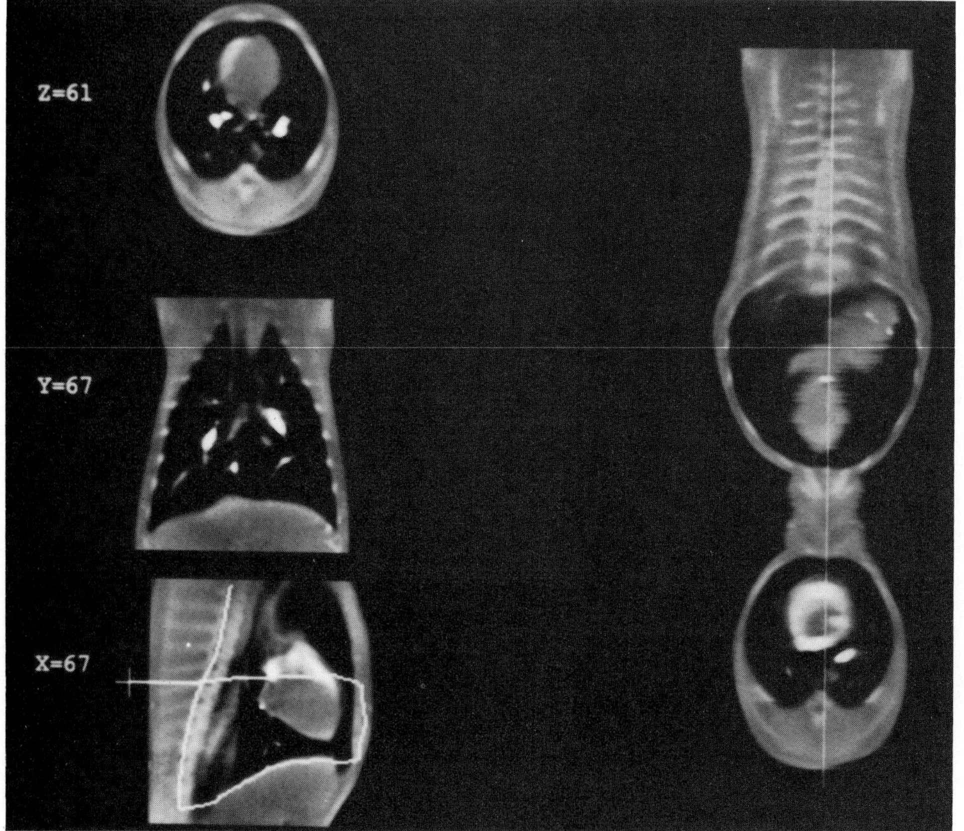

Figure 32–48. Example of interactive curved sectioning wherein a trace along an arbitrary curved path on a lateral chest section *(bottom left)* shows the spinal canal, diaphragmatic surface, and mid-thoracic cross sections *(right top to bottom)*. (From Robb, R. A., and Barillot, C.: Interactive display and analysis of 3-D medical images. IEEE Trans. Med. Imag. MI-8:217–226, 1989, with permission.)

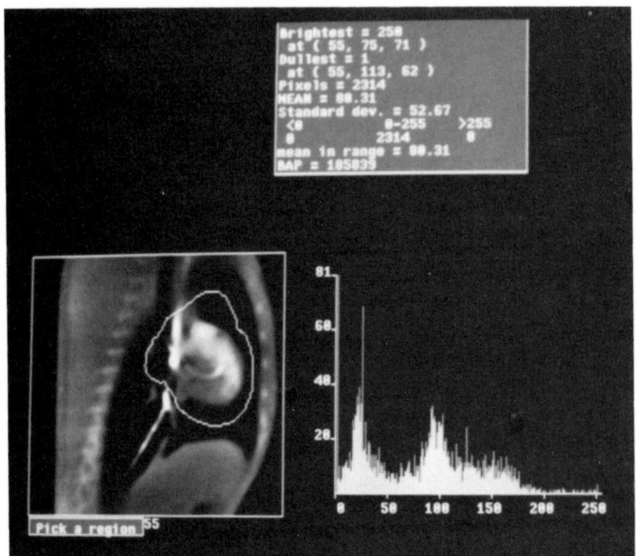

Figure 32–49. Example of the statistics and histogram computed by the biopsy module for a selected region of interest in a Dynamic Spatial Reconstructor image of the chest. (From Robb, R. A., and Barillot, C.: Interactive display and analysis of 3-D medical images. IEEE Trans. Med. Imag. MI-8:217–226, 1989, with permission.)

a single image. Information provided by area sampling includes the area; maximum and minimum values within the area; area coordinates; sum, standard deviation, and mean of image pixel values; brightness-area product; and number of image data elements above and below a selected threshold. A histogram of the data within the specified area sampled is plotted on the display screen. Areas can be automatically sampled through a set of serial sections to provide a volumetric sampling function. Individually traced area samples can be summed to provide an arbitrarily shaped volumetric sample through the multidimensional image data. Traces may be saved and recalled for future reference or use.

Arguably the most important problem and challenge in three-dimensional biomedical imaging is the efficient extraction of accurate and relevant quantitative information from the images. The problem is both conceptual and practical in scope; that is, extrapolations of two-dimensional approaches to three dimensions are not necessarily straightforward or theoretically valid, and even if they are, their implementation in an efficient, useful way is not readily achieved. The ANALYZE approach to three-dimensional object definition and tissue characterization is heuristic but based on fundamentally sound principles, which in some cases have been proved meritorious in two-dimensional image processing and for which generalizations to higher dimensionality are possible. These methods include manual outlining, multiresolution techniques,[P5, P6] relaxation,[G11] mathematical modeling,[K7] and fractals.[M6]

The objective of segmentation for isolation of anatomic structures is often to produce shaded-surface displays of the structure(s). Display of the surface of three-dimensional objects is often useful for conveying shape and relative dimensions and for verifying that a particular object has been properly identified. Hard tissue surfaces may often be successfully segmented by interactive thresholding alone, without the need for outlining. Figure 32–50 shows the interactive thresholding of several adjacent DSR slices through a chest to segment the heart. Figure 32–51 shows a montage of shaded-surface displays of the segmented heart from several angles of view.

One of the most versatile and powerful image display and manipulation tools in ANALYZE is the *volume-rendering* module. Our implementation of this technique[R17] has several unique features and advantages compared with shaded-surface display and other volume-rendering methods. We therefore will describe this module in some detail.

Volume-rendering display techniques are able to display surfaces with shading *and* other parts of the volume simultaneously. An important advantage is that of displaying data *directly* from the gray scale volume. The data that will appear on the screen are selected during the projection of the voxels (sometimes called ray casting). A function of different attributes of the voxels, such as their density or gradient values and/or spatial coordinates, can be invoked during the projection process to produce "on-the-fly" segmented surfaces, cutting planes anywhere in the volume, and/or selected degrees of transparency or opacity within the volume. Volume set operations (union, intersection, difference of volume) can also be invoked during the projection process.

Figure 32–52 shows a sequence of volume-rendered images of a dog chest obtained from a DSR scan. The soft tissue image (top left) shows the skin surface, including the distinctive nipples. The top center image reveals the skeletal framework, and the top right image shows the dye-filled heart and pulmonary vessels. Each image required only 2 seconds for computation. The bottom row of images shows a coronal dissection plane, a transparency image, and a brightest-voxel projection of the same volume, respectively.

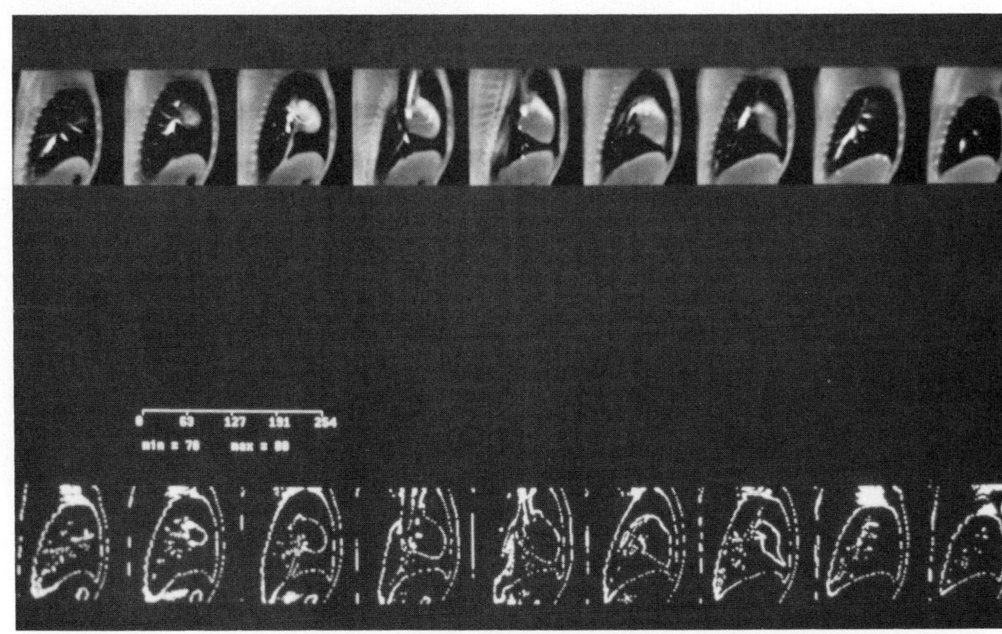

Figure 32–50. Multiple slices through volume scan of chest, showing original data (*top*) and simultaneously thresholded data (*bottom*) with EDIT module used to segment bone from soft tissue. (From Robb, R. A.: Multidimensional biomedical image display and analysis in the Biotechnology Computer Resource at the Mayo Clinic. Machine Vision Appl. 1:75, 1988, with permission.)

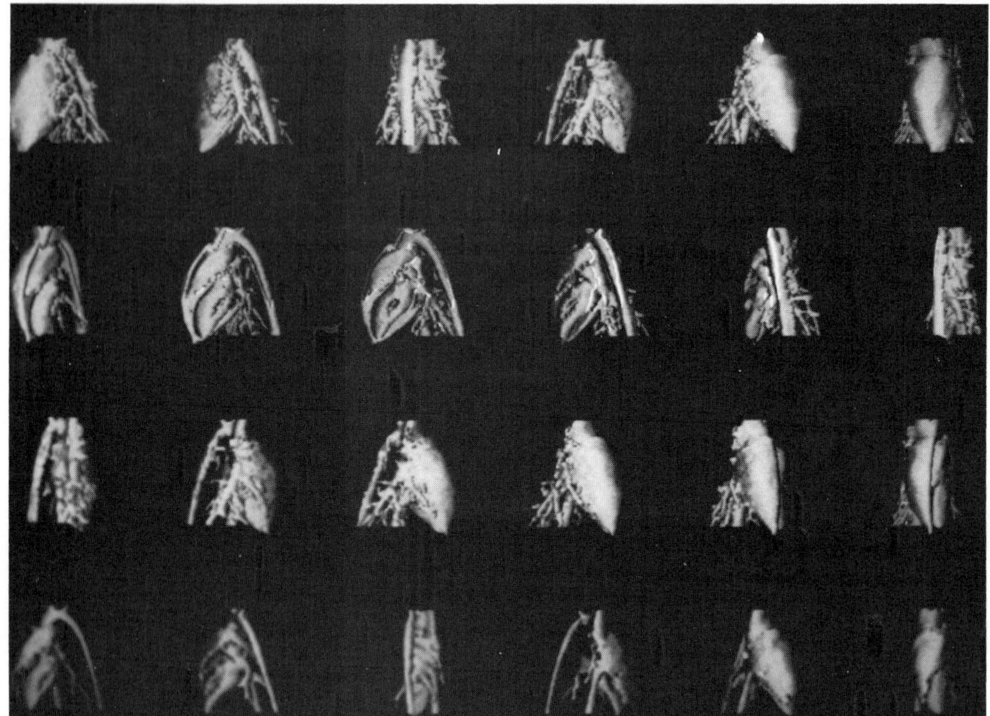

Figure 32–51. Shaded-surface displays of heart and chambers segmented from Dynamic Spatial Reconstructor volume scan of chest. Top row shows different views of epicardial surface and great vessels, second and third rows show heart bisected to reveal inner surfaces of left and right ventricular chambers and the myocardium, and bottom row is a display of chambers alone. (From Robb, R. A.: Multidimensional biomedical image display and analysis in the Biotechnology Computer Resource at the Mayo Clinic. Machine Vision Appl. 1:75, 1988, with permission.)

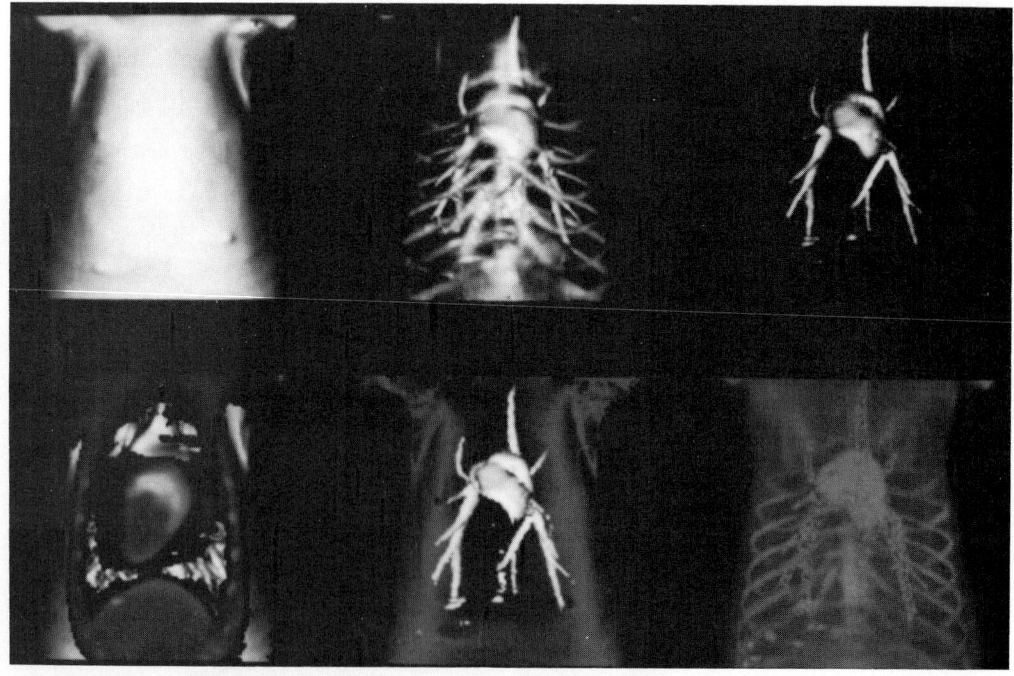

Figure 32–52. Volume-rendered images of dog chest with increasing threshold on gradient shading parameters to reveal successively skin (*top left*), rib cage (*top center*), and dye-filled heart and pulmonary vessels (*top right*). Images on the bottom row show a cut plane, transparency, and brightest voxel projection from left to right, respectively. (From Robb, R. A., and Barillot, C.: Interactive display and analysis of 3-D medical images. IEEE Trans. Med. Imag. MI-8: 217–226, 1989, with permission.)

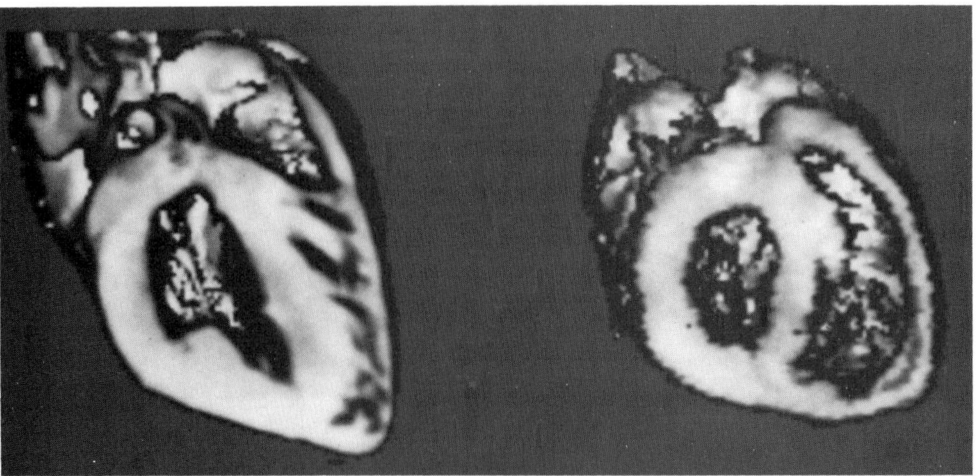

Figure 32–53. Volume-rendered images of heart showing cut planes from long-axis view (*left*) and short-axis view (*right*), revealing ventricular cavities and myocardial walls. (From Robb, R. A., and Barillot, C.: Interactive 3-D image display and analysis. *In* Casasent, D. P., and Tescher, A. G. [eds.]: Proc. SPIE, Hybrid Image and Signal Process. 939:173, 1988, with permission.)

Figure 32–53 shows a volume-rendered display of the heart with cut planes from a long-axis view (left) and a short-axis view (right), revealing the myocardial walls and ventricular chambers. These images have a realistic resemblance to actual gross pathology specimens.

Figure 32–54 shows volume-rendered images of another heart, with successive dissolution (top row) to reveal the branching network of the dye-filled coronary arteries. Successive dissection planes (bottom row) reveal the thick muscles of the left ventricular chamber walls and the chamber itself. These images depict the capability of interactive volume rendering to explore three-dimensional images as a surgeon or pathologist would an actual organ.

CONCLUSION

The trend in development of x-ray computed tomography systems has been toward faster and faster scanners, with concomitant improvement in image quality. However, conventional computed tomography systems do not scan rapidly enough to eliminate motion blurring in images of moving organs such as the heart and circulation and still produce only one or two two-dimensional slices in each scan. The results obtained with the Imatron and Dynamic Spatial Reconstructor scanners suggest the advent of two new powerful dimensions in x-ray computed tomography—high temporal resolution and synchronous volume scanning. That is, true stop-action, full three-dimensional imaging at a high repetition rate is possible with CT scanners. Such imaging capabilities, coupled with powerful computer workstations and comprehensive display and analysis software, promise to make possible new basic investigative and clinical studies of the structure-function relationships of moving organ systems like the heart and lungs and of the circulation in any organ of the body. This state-of-the-art computed tomography technology holds promise of exciting new clinical and research capabilities, such as quantitative analysis of regional blood flow and perfusion, simultaneous measurement of physiologic function and anatomic structure, and differential diagnosis of disease based on determination of tissue composition and dynamics in any organ of region of the body, with a sensitivity and specificity not possible before.

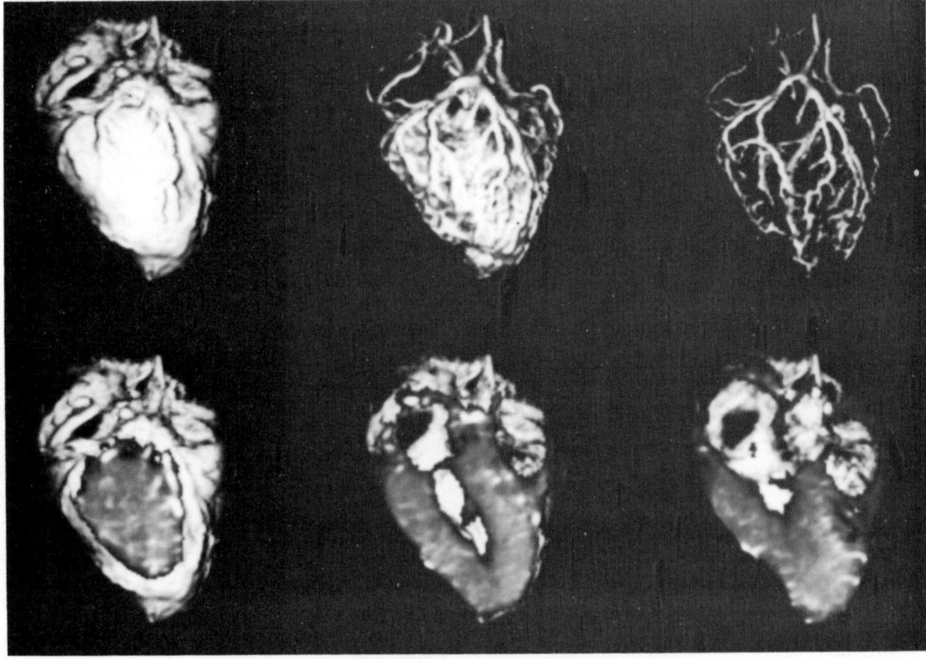

Figure 32–54. Volume-rendered images of heart with successive dissolution to reveal coronary artery network (*top row*) and with dissection planes to examine the left ventricular myocardial wall and chamber (*bottom row*). (From Robb, R. A., and Barillot, C.: Interactive display and analysis of 3-D medical images. IEEE Trans. Med. Imag. MI-8:217–226, 1989, with permission.)

References

A

1. Ambrose, J.: Computerized transverse axial scanning (tomography). II. Clinical application. Br. J. Radiol. 46:1034, 1973.
2. Alfidi, R. J., MacIntyre, W. J., and Haager, J. R.: The effects of biological motion on CT resolution. Am. J. Roentgenol. 127:11, 1976.
3. Altschuler, M. D., Censor, Y., Eggermont, P. P. B., et al.: Demonstration of a software package for the reconstruction of the dynamically changing structure of the human heart from cone beam x-ray projections. J. Med. Syst. 4:289, 1980.
4. Austin, J. D., and Pizer, S. M.: A multiprocessor adaptive histogram equalization machine. Proc. Xth IPMI Int. Conf., 375, 1987.
5. Artzy, E., Frieder, G., and Herman, G. T.: The theory, design, implementation and evaluation of a three-dimensional algorithm. Comput. Graph. Image Process. 15:1, 1981.

B

1. Bracewell, R. N.: Strip integration in radioastronomy. Aust. J. Phys. 9:198, 1956.
2. Bracewell, R. N., and Riddle, A. C.: Inversion of fan-beam scans in radioastronomy. Astrophys. J. 150:427, 1967.
3. Bursch, J., Johs, R., and Heintzen, P. H.: Validity of Lambert-Beer's law in roentgen-densitometry of contrast material using continuous radiation. *In* Heintzen, P. H. (ed.): Roentgen-, Cine, and Videodensitometry. Georg Thieme Verlag, Stuttgart, 1971, p. 81.
4. Brooks, R. A., and DiChiro, G.: Beam hardening in x-ray computed tomography. Phys. Med. Biol. 21:390, 1976.
5. Barrett, H. H., Bowen, T., Hershel, R. S., et al.: Noise and dose considerations. *In* Image Processing for 2-D and 3-D Reconstruction from Projections, WB2.1–WB2.4. IEEE Computer Society Press, Stanford, Calif., August 1975.
6. Brooks, R. A., and DiChiro, G.: Statistical limitations in x-ray reconstruction tomography. Med. Phys. 3:237, 1976.
7. Boyd, D. P., Gould, R. G., Quinn, J. R., et al.: A proposed dynamic cardiac 3-D densitometer for early detection and evaluation of heart disease. IEEE Trans. Nucl. Sci. NS-26:2724, 1979.
8. Budinger, T. F., and Gullberg, G. T.: Three-dimensional reconstruction in nuclear medicine imaging. IEEE Trans. Nucl. Sci. 21:2, 1974.
9. Boyd, D. P., Korbin, M. T., and Moss, A.: Engineering status of computerized tomographic scanning. Opt. Eng. 16:37, 1977.
10. Beringer, W. H., Redington, R. W., Doherty, D., et al.: Gated cardiac scanning: Canine studies. J. Comput. Assist. Tomogr. 3:155, 1979.
11. Behrenbeck, T., Kinsey, J. H., Harris, L. D., et al.: Three-dimensional spatial, density and temporal resolution of the DSR. J. Comput. Assist. Tomogr. 6:1138, 1982.
12. Birkner, D. A.: Design considerations for a user oriented PACS. Proc. ISMII '84, 89, 1984.

C

1. Christiansen, W. N., and Warburten, J. A.: The distribution of radio brightness over the solar disk at a wavelength of 21 centimeters. III. The quiet sun—two-dimensional observations. Aust. J. Phys. 8:474, 1955.
2. Crowther, R. A., deRosier, D. J., and Klug, A.: The reconstruction of three-dimensional structure from projections and its application to electron microscopy. Proc. R. Soc. London Ser. A 317:319, 1970.
3. Cormack, A. M.: Representation of a function by its line integrals, with some radiological applications. J. Appl. Phys. 34:2722, 1963.
4. Cormack, A. M.: Early two-dimensional reconstruction (CT scanning) and recent topics stemming from it. Nobel Lecture, December 8, 1979. J. Comput. Assist. Tomogr. 4:658, 1980.
5. Cho, Z. H., Ahn, I., Bohm, C., and Huth, G.: Computerized image reconstruction methods with multiple photon/x-ray transmission scanning. Phys. Med. Biol. 19:511, 1974.
6. Chesler, D. A., Rieder, S. J., and Pelc, N. J.: Noise due to photon counting statistics in computed x-ray tomography. J. Comput. Assist. Tomogr. 1:64, 1977.
7. Cohen, G., and DiBianca, F. A.: The use of contrast-detail-dose evaluation of image quality in a computed tomography scanning. J. Comput. Assist. Tomogr. 3:189, 1979.
8. Curry, T. S., Dowdey, J. E., and Murry, R. C.: Christensen's Introduction to the Physics of Diagnostic Radiology. Lea & Febiger, Philadelphia, 1984.

D

1. DeRosier, D. J., and Klug, A.: Reconstruction of three-dimensional images from electron micrographs. Nature (London) 217:130, 1968.
2. DiChiro, G., and Brooks, R. A.: The 1979 Nobel Prize in Physiology and Medicine. J. Comput. Assist. Tomogr. 4:241, 1980.
3. Dwyer, S. J., III, Brenner, D. J., Takasugi, S., and Goldberg, H.: Annotated Bibliography of Computed Tomography. Special Publication Series UMC-HCTC/E-001, University of Missouri, Columbia, Mo., 1979.
4. Drieke, P., and Boyd, D.: Convolution reconstruction of fan beam projections. Comput. Graph. Image Process. 5:459, 1976.

E

1. Edholm, P.: The tomogram—its formation and content. Acta Radiol. Suppl. 193:1, 1960.

F

1. Fullerton, G. D.: Fundamentals of CT tissue characterization. *In* Medical Physics of CT and Ultrasound Tissue Imaging and Characterization, AAPM. Med. Phys. Monogr. 6:125, 1980.
2. Fellingham, L. L., Vogel, J. H., Lau, C., and Dev, P.: Interactive graphics and 3-D modeling for surgical planning and prosthesis and implant design. Proc. NCGA '86 3:132, 1986.
3. Farrell, E. J., Watson, T. J., Zappulla, R. A., and Spigelman, M.: Imaging tools for interpreting two- and three-dimensional medical data. Proc. NCGA '87 3:60, 1987.

G

1. Glasser, O.: Wilhelm Conrad Rontgen and the Early History of the Roentgen Rays. Charles C Thomas, Springfield, Ill., 1934.
2. Glover, G. H., and Eisner, R. L.: Theoretical resolution of computed tomography systems. J. Comput. Assist. Tomogr. 3:85, 1979.
3. Gilbert, P. F. C.: Iterative methods for the reconstruction of three-dimensional objects from projections. J. Theor. Biol. 36:105, 1972.
4. Gordon, R., and Herman, G. T.: Three-dimensional reconstruction from projections: A review of algorithms. Int. Rev. Cytol. 38:111, 1974.
5. Goodenough, D. J., Weaver, K. G., and Davis, D. O.: Development of a phantom for evaluation and assurance of image quality in CT scanning. Opt. Eng. 16:52, 1977.
6. Guthaner, D. F., Wexler, L., and Harell, G.: Computed tomography demonstration of cardiac structures. Am. J. Roentgenol. 133:75, 1979.
7. Gur, D., Drayer, B. P., Borovetz, H. S., et al.: Dynamic computed tomography of the lung: Regional ventilation measurements. J. Comput. Assist. Tomogr. 3:749, 1979.
8. Gray, M. J., and Rutherford, H.: Functional specifications of a useful digital multimodality image workstation. Proc. ISMII '84, 8, 1984.
9. Grewer, R., Monnich, K. J., Schmidt, J., et al.: Design of interactive workstations for the interpretation of medical images in pictorial information systems. Proc. Int. Symp. CAR '85, 679, 1985.
10. Goldwasser, S. M., Reynolds, R. A., Bapty, T., et al.: Physician's workstation with real-time performance. IEEE NC&A 4:43, 1985.
11. Grossberg, S., and Mingolla, E.: Neural dynamics of perceptual groupings: Textures, boundaries, and emergent segmentation. Percent. Psychophys. 38:141, 1985.
12. Gray, J. E., and Felmlee, J. P.: Section thickness and contiguity phantom for MR imaging. Radiology 164:193, 1987.
13. Gould, R. G.: Personal communication, 1987.

H

1. Hounsfield, G. N.: Computed medical imaging. Nobel Lecture, December 8, 1979. J. Comput. Assist. Tomogr. 4:665, 1980.
2. Hounsfield, G. N.: Computerized transverse axial scanning (tomography). I. Description of system. Br. J. Radiol. 46:1016, 1973.
3. Huesman, R. H.: The effects of a finite number of projection angles and finite lateral sampling of projections on the propagation of statistical errors in transverse section reconstruction. Phys. Med. Biol. 22:511, 1977.
4. Hounsfield, G. N.: Picture quality of computed tomography. Am. J. Roentgenol. 127:3, 1976.
5. Hounsfield, G. N.: Method and apparatus for measuring x- or gamma-radiation absorption or transmission at plural angles and analyzing the data. U.S. Patent No. 3778614, 1973.
6. Herman, G. T., and Simmons, R.: Illustrations of a beam hardening correction method in computerized tomography. Appl. Opt. Instrum. Med. III, SPIE 173:264, 1979.
7. Herman, G. T., Lakshminarayanan, A. V., and Naparstek, A.: Convolution reconstruction techniques for divergent beams. Comput. Biol. Med. 6:259, 1976.
8. Harell, G. S., Guthaner, D. F., Breiman, R. S., et al.: Stop-action cardiac computed tomography. Radiology 123:515, 1977.
9. Heinz, E. R., Dubois, P. J., Drayer, B. P., and Hill, R.: A preliminary investigation of the role of dynamic computed tomography in renovascular hypertension. J. Comput. Assist. Tomogr. 4:63, 1980.
10. Hoffman, E. A., and Ritman, E. L.: Shape and dimensions of cardiac chamber via computed tomography: Role of imaged slice thickness and orientation. Radiology 739:155, 1985.
11. Harris, L. D., Robb, R. A., Yuen, T. S., and Ritman, E. L.: Non-invasive numerical dissection and display of anatomic structure using computerized x-ray tomography. Proc. SPIE 152:10, 1978.
12. Harris, L. D., Robb, R. A., Yuen, T. S., and Ritman, E. L.: Stereo display of computed tomographic data. *In* Emlet, H. A., Jr. (ed.): Challenges and Prospects for Advanced Medical Systems. Symposia Specialists, Minneapolis, MN, 1978, p. 127.
13. Hodges, L. F., and McAllister, D. F.: Stereo and alternating-pair techniques for display of computer-generated images. IEEE Comput. Graph. Appl. 5:38, 1985.
14. Hohne, K. H., Riemer, M., Tiede, U., and Bomans, M.: Volume rendering of 3D-tomographic imagery. Proc. Xth IPMI Int. Conf. 403, 1987.
15. Herman, G. T.: Computer produced stereoscopic display in radiology. Proc. NCGA '86, 3:71, 1986.

16. Heffernan, P. B., and Robb, R. A.: Display and analysis of 4-D medical images. Proc. Int. Symp. CAR '85, 583, 1985.
17. Herman, G. T., and Liu, H. K.: Display of three-dimensional information in computed tomography. J. Comput. Assist. Tomogr. 1:155, 1977.
18. Heffernan, P. B., and Robb, R. A.: A new method for shaded surfaced display of biological and medical images. IEEE Trans. Med. Imag. MI-4:26, 1985.
19. Huang, H. K., Mankovich, N. J., Taira, R., et al.: Picture archiving and communication systems for Radiology. *In* Lemke, H. U., Rhodes, M. L., Jaffee, C. C., and Felix, R. (eds.) Proc. Int. Symp. CAR '87, 487, 1987.

I

1. Iwasaki, T., Sinak, L. J., Hoffman, E. A., et al.: Mass of left ventricular myocardium estimated with the Dynamic Spatial Reconstructor. Am. J. Physiol. H138:15, 1984.

J

1. Joseph, P. M., and Spital, R. A.: A method for correcting bone induced artifacts in computed tomography scanners. J. Comput. Assist. Tomogr. 2:100, 1978.
2. Johnson, S. A.: Total body exposure, pixel size, and signal-to-noise ratio considerations for three-dimensional x-ray attenuation reconstructions. *In* Ter-Pogossian, M. M., Phelps, M. E., Brownell, G. L., Cox, J. R., Jr., Davis, D. O., and Evens, R. G. (eds.): Reconstruction Tomography in Diagnostic Radiology and Nuclear Medicine. University Park Press, Baltimore, 1977, p. 199.

K

1. Kuhl, D. E., and Edwards, R. Q.: Rapid brain scanner with self contained computer and CRT display for both rectilinear and transverse section viewing. J. Nucl. Med. 9:332, 1968.
2. Kieffer, J.: The laminagraph and its variations: Applications and implications of the planigraphic principle. AJR 39:497, 1938.
3. Kowalski, D. G., and Wagner, W.: Artifacts in CT pictures. Medicamundi 22:13, 1977.
4. Kinlaks, J. R.: Computer tomographic equipment survey. Appl. Radiol. 4:81, 1976.
5. Kinsey, J. H., Robb, R. A., Ritman, E. L., and Wood, E. H.: The DSR—a high temporal resolution volumetric roentgenographic CT scanner. Herz 5:177, 1980.
6. Kinsey, J. H., and Orvis, A. L.: High repetition rate volumetric x-ray CT scanning. IEEE Trans. Nucl. Sci. 28:1732, 1981.
7. Kohonen, T.: Self-Organization and Associative-Memory, Springer-Verlag, Berlin, 1984, p. 255.

L

1. Ledley, R. S., DiChiro, G., Leussenhop, A. J., and Twigg, H. L.: Computerized transaxial x-ray tomography of the human body. Science 186:207, 1974.
2. Lipton, M. J., Brundage, B. H., Doherty, P. W., et al.: Contrast medium-enhanced computed tomography for evaluating ischemic heart disease. J. Comput. Assist. Tomogr. 4:571, 1980.
3. Lenz, R.: Processing and presentation of 3-D images. Proc. ISMII '84, 298, 1984.

M

1. McCullough, E. C., Baker, H. L., Houser, O. W., and Reese, D. F.: An evaluation of the quantitative and radiation features of a scanning x-ray transverse axial tomography: The EMI scanner. Radiology 111:709, 1974.
2. McDavid, W. D., Waggener, R. G., Payne, W. H., and Dennis, M. J.: Correction for spectral artifacts in cross-sectional reconstructions from x-rays. Med. Phys. 4:54, 1977.
3. Mategsano, V. C., Petasnick, J., Clark, J., et al.: Attenuation values in computed tomography of the abdomen. Radiology 125:135, 1977.
4. McCullough, E. C.: Specifying and evaluating the performance of computed tomography (CT) scanners. J. Comput. Assist. Tomogr. 7:291, 1980.
5. McCullough, E. C., and Payne, J. T.: Patient dosage in computed tomography. Radiology 129:457, 1978.
6. Mandelbrot, B. B.: Fractals: Form, Chance, and Dimension. Freeman, San Francisco, 1977, p. 365.
7. Maguire, G. Q., Jr., Noz, M. E., Bakker, A., et al.: Introduction of PACS for those interested in image processing. Proc. Xth IPMI Int. Conf. 403, 1987.

N

1. New, P. E. J., and Aronow, S.: Attenuation measurements of whole blood and blood fractions in computed tomography. Radiology 121:635, 1976.
2. News: AT&T ventures into radiology market with DIM system. Diag. Imag. 7:45, 1985.

O

1. Oldendorf, W. H.: Isolated flying spot detection of radio-density discontinuities displaying the internal structural pattern of a complex object. IRE Trans. Bio-Med. Electron. BME8:68, 1961.
2. Oswald, H.: A medical workstation for three-dimensional display of computed tomogram images. Proc. Int. Symp. CAR '85, 565, 1985.

P

1. Phelps, M. E., Hoffmann, G. J., and Ter-Pogossian, M. M.: Attenuation coefficients of various body tissues, fluids, and lesions at photon energies of 18 to 136 KeV. Radiology 117:573, 1975.
2. Pullan, B. R., Fawcett, R. H., and Isherwood, I.: Tissue characterization by an analysis of the distribution of attenuation values in computed tomography scans. J. Comput. Assist. Tomogr. 2:49, 1978.
3. Pizer, S. M., Oliver, W. R., and Bloomberg, S. H.: Hierarchical shape description via a multiresolution symmetric axis transform. Technical Report, Department of Computer Science, University of North Carolina, 1986.
4. Peters, J. H., Roos, P., van Kijky, M. C. A., and Viergever, M. A.: Loss-less image compression methods applicable to PACS. Proc. Xth IPMI Int. Conf., 335, 1987.
5. Pizer, S. M., Gauch, J. M., and Lifshitz, L. M.: Interactive 2D and 3D object definition in medical images based on multiresolution image descriptions. University of North Carolina Technical Report, 88-005, 1988.
6. Peleg, S., Naor, J., Hartley, R., and Avnir, D.: Multiple resolution texture analysis and classification. IEEE Pattern Anal. Machine Intell. 6:518, 1984.
7. Parker, D. L.: Optimal short scan convolution reconstruction for fanbeam CT. Med. Phys. 9:254, 1982.

R

1. Radon, J.: Uber die Bestimmung von Funktionen durch ihre integralwerte langs gewisser Manningfaltigkeiten. Berichte Saechsische Akad. Wiss. Leipzig Math. Phys. K 69:262, 1917.
2. Ramachandaran, G. N., and Lakshminarayanan, A. V.: Three-dimensional reconstruction from radiographs and electron micrographs: Application of convolutions instead of Fourier transforms. Proc. Natl. Acad. Sci. USA 68:2236, 1971.
3. Ring, B. A.: An overview: Computed axial tomography. Appl. Radiol. 8(5):110, 1979.
4. Rao, P. S., and Gregg, E. C.: Attenuation of mono-energetic gamma rays in tissues. AJR 123:631, 1975.
5. Robb, R. A.: A workstation for interactive display and analysis of multidimensional biomedical images. *In* Lemke, H. U., Rhodes, M. L., Jaffee, C. C., and Felix, R. (eds.): Proc. Int. Symp. CAR '87, 642, 1987.
6. Ruegsegger, P., Hangartner, Th., Keller, H. U., and Hinderling, Th.: Standardization of computed tomographic images by means of a material-selective beam hardening correction. J. Comput. Assist. Tomogr. 2:184, 1978.
7. Robb, R. A., Greenleaf, J. F., Ritman, E. L., et al.: Three-dimensional visualization of the intact thorax and contents: A technique for cross-sectional reconstruction for multiplanar x-ray views. Comp. Biomed. Res. 7:395, 1974.
8. Robb, R. A., and Ritman, E. L.: High-speed synchronous volume computer tomography of the heart. Radiology 133:655, 1979.
9. Ritman, E. L., Robb, R. A., Johnson, S. A., et al.: Quantitative imaging of the structure and function of the heart, lungs, and circulation. Mayo Clin. Proc. 53:3, 1978.
10. Robb, R. A., Ritman, E. L., Gilbert, B. K., et al.: The DSR: A high-speed three-dimensional x-ray computed tomography system for dynamic spatial reconstruction of the heart and circulation. IEEE Trans. Nucl. Sci. NS-26:2713, 1979.
11. Ritman, E. L., Kinsey, J. H., Robb, R. A., et al.: Three-dimensional imaging of heart, lungs, and circulation. Science 210:273, 1980.
12. Robb, R. A., and Gilbert, B. K.: Description and evaluation of a system for high-speed three-dimensional computed tomography of the body: The Dynamic Spatial Reconstructor. NCC-80 Natl. Comput. Conf. Am. Fed. Inform. Process. Soc. 49:427, 1980.
13. Ritman, E. L., Kinsey, J. H., Robb, R. A., et al.: Physics and technical considerations in the design of the DSR: A high temporal resolution volume scanner. AJR 134:369, 1980.
14. Robb, R. A., Lent, A. H., Gilbert, B. K., and Chu, A.: The Dynamics Spatial Reconstructor: A computed tomography system for high-speed simultaneous scanning of multiple cross sections of the heart. J. Med. Syst. 4:253, 1980.
15. Risser, T.: Processing and presentation of 3-D images. Proc. ISMII '84, 61, 1984.
16. Rhodes, M. L., Glenn, W. V., Rothman, S. L. G., et al.: CT image processing using commercial digital networks. Proc. 1984 Int. Joint Alpine Symp. 37, 1984.
17. Robb, R. A., and Barillot, C.: Interactive 3-D image display and analysis. Proc. SPIE, Hybrid Image and Signal Processing 939:173, 1988.

S

1. Symposium on Biological Effects, Imaging Techniques, and Dosimetry of Ionizing Radiations. Department of Health and Human Sciences, 80-8126 (July), Federal Drug Administration, Washington, D.C., 1980.
2. Shepp, L. A., and Logan, E. C.: The Fourier reconstruction of a head section. IEEE Trans. Nucl. Sci. 21:21, 1974.
3. Shepp, L. A., and Kruskal, J. B.: Computerized tomography: The new medical x-ray technology. Am. Math. Mon. 85:420, 1978.
4. Skalnik, R.: CT radiation dose. Appl. Radiol. 8:69, 1979.
5. Shepp, L. A., and Stein, J. A.: Simulated reconstruction artifacts in computerized x-ray tomography. *In* Ter-Pogossian, M. M., Phelps, M. E., Brownell, G. L., Cox, J. R., Jr., Davis, D. O., and Evens, R. G. (eds.): Reconstruction Tomography in Diagnostic Radiology and Nuclear Medicine. University Park Press, Baltimore, 1977, p. 33.
6. Sagal, S. S., Weiss, E. S., Gillard, R. G., et al.: Gated computed tomography of the human heart. Invest. Radiol. 12:554, 1977.
7. Scanlan, J. G., Gustafson, D. E., Chevalier, P. A., et al.: Evaluation of ischemic heart disease with a prototype volume imaging computed tomographic (CT) scanner: Preliminary experiments. Am. J. Cardiol. 46:1263, 1980.
8. Sturm, R. E., Ritman, E. L., Hansen, R. J., and Wood, E. H.: Recording of multichannel analog data and video images on the same video tape or disc. J. Appl. Physiol. 36:761, 1974.
9. Scharnweber, H., and Tonnie, K. D.: Three-dimensional reconstruction and display of complex anatomical objects. Proc. 1984 Int. Joint Alpine Symp. 7, 1984.
10. Shope, T. B., Gagne, R. M., and Johnson, R. C.: A method for describing the

doses delivered by transmission x-ray computed tomography. Med. Phys. 8:488, 1981.

11. Suzuki, A., and Suzuki, M. N.: Use of a pencil-shaped ionization chamber for measurement of exposure resulting from a computed tomography scan. Med. Phys. 5:536, 1978.

T

1. Taber, P., Chang, L. W. M., and Campion, G. M.: Left brachycephalic vein simulating aortic dissection on computed tomography. Radiology 133:562, 1979.
2. Talton, D. A., Goldwasser, S. M., Reynolds, R. A., and Walsh, E. S.: Volume rendering algorithms for the presentation of 3-D medical data. Proc. NCGA '87, 3:119, 1987.

V

1. Vainshtein, B. K.: Finding the structure of objects from projections. Kristallografiya 15:894, 1970.
2. Vasseur, J. P.: Quality of image and irradiation in reconstruction tomography. *In* Ter-Pogossian, M. M., Phelps, M. E., Brownell, G. L., Cox, J. R., Jr., Davis, D. O., and Evens, R. G. (eds.): Reconstruction Tomography in Diagnostic Radiology and Nuclear Medicine. University Park Press, Baltimore, 1977, p. 67.

W

1. Waggener, R., and McDavid, W.: Transmission computed tomographic system components. *In* Medical Physics of CT and Ultrasound Tissue Imaging Characteristics, AAPM. Med. Phys. Monogr. 6:94, 1980.
2. Workshop on Physics and Engineering in Computerized Tomography. IEEE Trans. Nucl. Sci. NS-26(April):1979.
3. Wood, E. H., Ritman, E. L., Sturm, R. E., et al.: The problem of determination of the roentgen density, dimensions and shape of homogeneous objects from biplane roentgenographic data with particular reference to angiocardiography. Proc. San Diego Biomed. Symp. 2:3, 1972.

Y

1. Young, S. W., Noon, M. A., Nassi, M., and Castellino, R. A.: Dynamic computed tomography body scanning. J. Comput. Assist. Tomogr. 4:168, 1980.

Z

1. Zatz, L. M., and Alvarez, R. G.: An inaccuracy in computed tomography: The energy dependence of CT values. Radiology 124:91, 1977.

Chapter 33

Evaluation of Cardiac Structure and Function with Ultrafast Computed Tomography

■ *MELVIN L. MARCUS, M.D.* ■ *ROBERT M. WEISS, M.D.*

ADVANTAGES AND DISADVANTAGES OF STUDIES OF CARDIAC STRUCTURE AND FUNCTION WITH ULTRAFAST COMPUTED TOMOGRAPHY 669
Advantages 669
Disadvantages 670
LEFT VENTRICLE 671
Left Ventricular Volume 671
Left Ventricular Mass 672
Regional Left Ventricular Function 672
Assessment of Diastolic Left Ventricular Function 675
Three-Dimensional Reconstruction of Left Ventricular Geometry 676
RIGHT VENTRICLE 676
Right Ventricular Volume 676
Right Ventricular Mass 677
RIGHT AND LEFT ATRIAL VOLUMES 678
MEASUREMENTS OF CARDIAC OUTPUT 678
SHUNT CALCULATIONS 678
EVALUATION OF CARDIAC VALVES 678
INTERVENTIONAL STUDIES OF LEFT VENTRICULAR FUNCTION 679
CORONARY ANATOMY 680
CONCLUSIONS 680

Conventional computed tomographic (CT) images of the heart are not useful in assessing cardiac structure and function because image acquisition takes 1 to 3 seconds. Because the normal heart contracts at the rate of one cycle or greater per second, conventional CT images of the heart invariably result in blurred pictures of the cardiac chambers. Images of the cardiac chambers require rapid scan acquisition. This can be achieved in several ways, described in Chapter 32. Rapid computed tomographic images of the heart may be obtained radiographically using one of two devices: The Imatron C-100 computed tomography scanner and the Dynamic Spatial Reconstructor.[11] The latter device is not commercially available at this time. Thus this chapter describes the results of studies of cardiac structure and function with the C-100 Imatron scanner. The central focus of this discussion is the accuracy of quantitative data achievable with this device.

ADVANTAGES AND DISADVANTAGES OF STUDIES OF CARDIAC STRUCTURE AND FUNCTION WITH ULTRAFAST COMPUTED TOMOGRAPHY

Advantages

Of the several potential applications of ultrafast computed tomography to the evaluation of patients with heart disease, the one that has been most extensively validated concerns the evaluation of cardiac structure and function. For this purpose, ultrafast computed tomography has many advantages. Because the technique produces tomographic images that are nearly parallel to one another, calculations of chamber volumes are not hampered by assumptions concerning the presumed shape of the cardiac chamber in question. In the standard cardiac mode, resolution in the imaging plane (1.5 mm) and slice thickness (8 mm) are sufficient to achieve very accurate estimates of size and function of cardiac structures, such as the ventricular and atrial cavities that are much larger than the resolving power of this technique. Smaller cardiac structures—coronary vessels, valve leaflets, free wall of the right ventricle, atrial walls, and pericardium—cannot be measured precisely in the standard cardiac mode. These smaller structures can be defined if the high resolution mode of the Imatron scanner is employed. In this mode, resolution is 0.7 mm in the image plane, and effective slice thickness is 3 mm. In the standard mode, multiple contiguous slices can be obtained, whereas in the high-resolution mode only one tomographic slice can be obtained unless the scanning table is moved.

The temporal resolution of ultrafast computed tomography (17 frames per second) is sufficient to obtain reasonably precise end-diastolic and end-systolic images and to calculate left ventricular ejection and filling rates in humans under control conditions.[B1] Although increases in ejection and filling rates of the left ventricle during stress can be measured with ultrafast computed tomography, studies by Bacharach and associates suggest that during stress, filling and ejection rates of the left ventricle in humans are too rapid to be accurately measured with a technique that has a temporal resolution of only 17 frames per second.[B2] In addition, phase imaging, although possible with ultrafast computed tomography,[A1, C1] has obvious limitations because scan acquisition rate is restricted to 17 frames per second.

Another advantage of ultrafast CT that contributes to the accuracy of measurements of cardiac structure and function is that the images of any given tomographic slice are obtained in one cardiac cycle. Hence, unlike conventional radionuclide imaging, positron emission tomography, and cardiac magnetic resonance imaging, images from multiple cycles are not superimposed to produce a single composite image. Thus, errors derived from patient motion and respiratory excursion are minimized. Prototype advanced nuclear magnetic resonance imaging devices that can obtain cardiac pictures in a single cardiac cycle are under development.[K1]

Disadvantages

Ultrafast computed tomography has several inherent limitations that are in part responsible for the deficiencies this method has in assessing cardiac structure and function. The most important of these is that there is no accepted method to account fully for some of the complex motions of the heart during systole. When the heart contracts, five specific types of motion occur: inward motion of the endocardium; rotation; torsion or wringing; translocation; and an "accordion-like" base-to-apex shortening motion. With ultrafast computed tomography, the element of the motion that is primarily assessed is by far the dominant one—inward motion of the endocardium. By utilizing internal and external reference points, such as the right ventricular–left ventricular junction, valve planes, and skeletal structures, image-processing algorithms can compensate in a limited manner for rotation and translocation but have not compensated for torsion or the accordion-like apex-to-base motion that is prominent in the left ventricle. Compensations are imprecise and involve theoretical assumptions and approximations that are difficult to standardize. Fortunately, the elements of cardiac motion that are not precisely measured with ultrafast computed tomography or other tomographic methods in the aggregate constitute a minor component of overall cardiac motion in the normal heart.[S1] As expected, failure to assess these components of cardiac motion accurately is most apparent when small changes in the dimensions of small cardiac structures are measured or when these normally minor movements are exaggerated by pericardial effusion or absence of the pericardium. These factors are probably only significant when *regional* function is assessed, since assessment of global function requires only that the entire heart be interrogated throughout the cardiac cycle.

A second limitation of ultrafast computed tomography that has bearing on the accuracy of assessing cardiac structure and function is the 8-mm-thick tomographic images obtained in sequential pairs and the gaps (4-mm) between image pairs. Because the heart of an adult human often extends over 12 cm and occasionally up to 16 cm, images of the entire heart can involve data from eight cardiac cycles. In addition, as much as 2.8 cm (4 mm × 7) of the cardiac mass lies within the interslice gaps and is thus never imaged. Finally, because of the current limitations in system memory, only 8 to 12 tomographic slices can be obtained per imaging sequence, and hence, two separate contrast injections usually separated by 5 to 10 minutes are required. Thus, one must assume that conditions during these two separate contrast injections were identical. This latter problem may be overcome by adding additional memory to the computer system so that the entire cardiac structure can be imaged during one contrast injection. Any imaging sequence that requires information from multiple cardiac cycles can be affected by gross patient movement or respiratory motion. In addition, alterations in cardiac rhythm, changes in the physiologic function of the heart, or errors in patient positioning between contrast injections also can contribute to inaccuracy of this technique. In practice, respiratory motion is minimized by instructing the patient to hold the breath at end-inspiration during the scanning sequence. Also, studies in patients with irregular cardiac rhythms (atrial fibrillation, frequent atrial premature contractions, or ventricular premature contractions) may contain inaccuracies. This latter problem is common to all imaging techniques.

A third limitation of ultrafast computed tomography that can influence the precision of measurement of cardiac structure and function is that the imaging planes are fixed in space. Hence, in contrast to nuclear magnetic resonance imaging, the image orientation must be achieved by patient positioning in the scanner prior to image acquisition. This is frequently a problem because the long axis of the left ventricle differs variably from the long axis of the body. In addition, the long axis of the left ventricle shifts slightly during the cardiac cycle. Tomographic images that are perpendicular to the long axis of the left ventricle are necessary for quantitative evaluation of the size and structure of the cardiac chambers. Despite these problems, with the use of short-axis views skilled operators can obtain tomographic images that are approximately perpendicular to the long axis of the left ventricle in the great majority of patients studied.

A fourth limitation of ultrafast computed tomography that contributes error to the evaluation of cardiac structure and function is the necessity of injecting contrast medium to visualize most cardiac structures adequately. If conventional contrast media are injected, cardiac function changes sufficiently during image acquisition to contribute significantly to errors in the calculation of cardiac volumes[R1] (Fig. 33–1). This is a lesser problem if nonionic contrast media are employed. Also, the contrast injection must be timed so that the proper sequence of opacification of the cardiac chambers is achieved, depending upon the imaging protocol being employed. To obtain quantitative measurements of cardiac chamber volumes, the right and left cardiac chambers need to be well opacified during image acquisition. In practice, measurement of the patient's circulation time, either with earlobe densitometry following injection of green dye or with arm-to-tongue circulation time with magnesium sulfate, is utilized to assist operators in proper timing of scan acquisition. This approach works reasonably well in most patients but can lead to poor

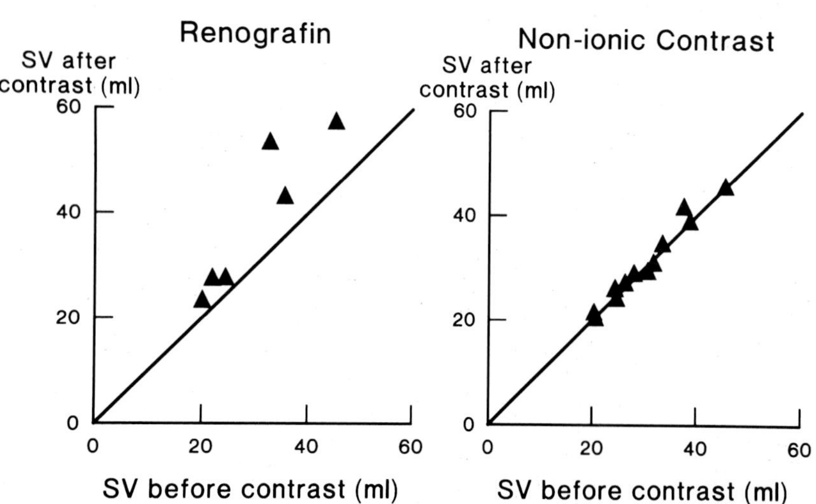

Figure 33–1. Comparison of thermodilution stroke volumes obtained immediately before and after intravenous infusion of iodinated contrast medium. The *left panel* shows a significant increase in stroke volume following infusion of ionic contrast. The *right panel* shows that when non-ionic contrast medium is used there is negligible perturbation of stroke volume. These data were obtained in closed-chest anesthetized dogs. (From Reiter, S. J., et al.: Precision of measurements of right and left ventricular volume by cine computed tomography. Circulation 74:890, 1986, with permission of the American Heart Association, Inc.)

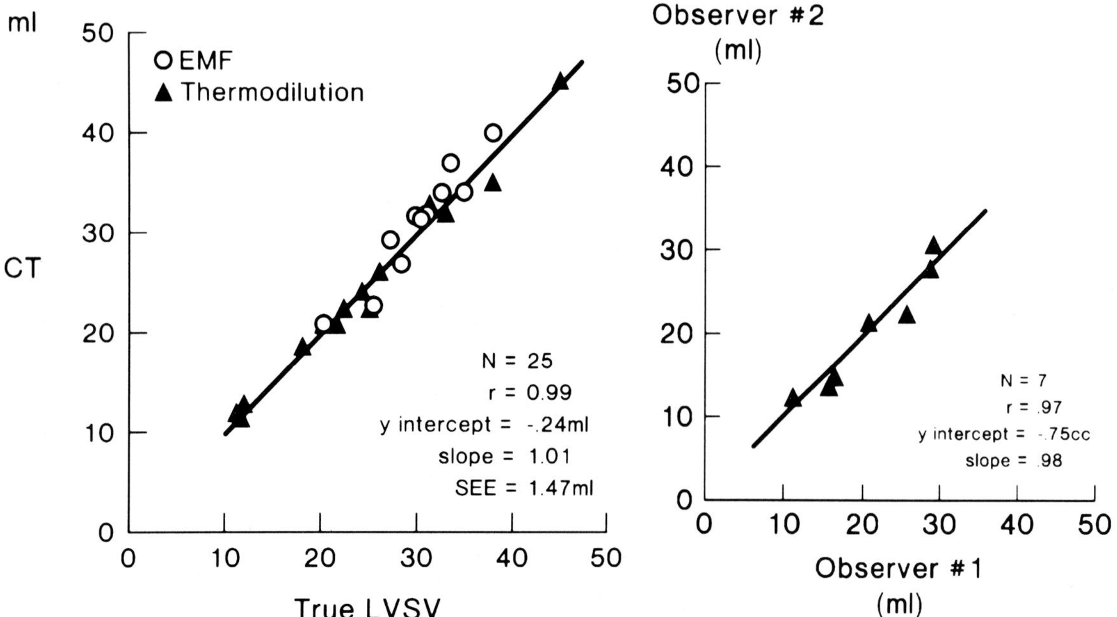

Figure 33–2. *Left panel*—Comparison of global left ventricular stroke volume measured by ultrafast CT with thermodilution or chronically implanted aortic electromagnetic flowmeter as the reference standard. *Right panel*—Interobserver variability of left ventricular stroke volume measurements with ultrafast CT. These studies were performed in closed-chest anesthetized dogs. (From Reiter, S. J., et al.: Precision of measurements of right and left ventricular volume by cine computed tomography. Circulation 74:890, 1986, with permission of the American Heart Association, Inc.)

images if circulation time changes (e.g., rest versus dobutamine infusion) between the measurement of circulation time and scan acquisition or if the circulation time is very long and has a poorly defined end point. The latter is a problem in patients with severe congestive heart failure. If chamber opacification is suboptimal, border recognition will be difficult and quantification of structures will suffer. Nevertheless, with careful attention to technique, adequate images can be obtained in over 95 percent of patients, which compares favorably with other imaging modalities. Finally, an occasional patient has an adverse reaction to injection of contrast medium. Studies in patients with renal dysfunction (creatinine level greater than 1.5 mg percent) or diabetes can be associated with serious deterioration in renal function.[H1]

Despite the problems that limit the precision with which cardiac structure and function can be defined with ultrafast computed tomography (complex cardiac motion, sequential image acquisition, non–three-dimensional format, and contrast medium injection), remarkably accurate measurements of the heart can be obtained with this technology.

In the following sections of this chapter, the application of ultrafast computed tomography to making specific measurements in various cardiac structures is defined.

LEFT VENTRICLE

Left Ventricular Volume

Three approaches have been employed to determine the accuracy with which left ventricular chamber volume could be measured with ultrafast computed tomography. First, postmortem left ventricles from various-sized animals were filled with a radiopaque casting medium. Computed tomographic images of the casts were obtained and volume estimates based on Simpson's rule for reconstruction of outlined tomographic images were compared with the volume of the left ventricular cast measured by water displacement. These studies demonstrated that the volume of a nonmoving left ventricular chamber could be accurately estimated from analysis of ultrafast computed tomographic images. Second, left ventricular stroke volumes (left ventricular end-diastolic volume minus end-systolic volume) measured from the analysis of computed tomographic images obtained in closed-chest dogs were compared with nearly simultaneous measurements of stroke volume, either with a chronically implanted electromagnetic flowprobe on the ascending aorta or with thermodilution.[R1] Left ventricular stroke volume measurements with ultrafast computed tomography correlated very well with directly measured left ventricular stroke volume (Fig. 33–2). Measurements of left ventricular stroke volume were accurate both in normally contracting left ventricles and in left ventricles with major regional wall motion abnormalities secondary to coronary occlusion.[R2] Furthermore, the left ventricular stroke volume measurements with ultrafast computed tomography were very reproducible (Fig. 33–2). Third, to validate measurements of left ventricular chamber volumes against a standard that could be readily employed in patients, left ventricular ejection fraction measurements with computed tomography were compared with left ventricular ejection fraction measurements with equilibrium radionuclide angiography (Fig. 33–3). Although the measure-

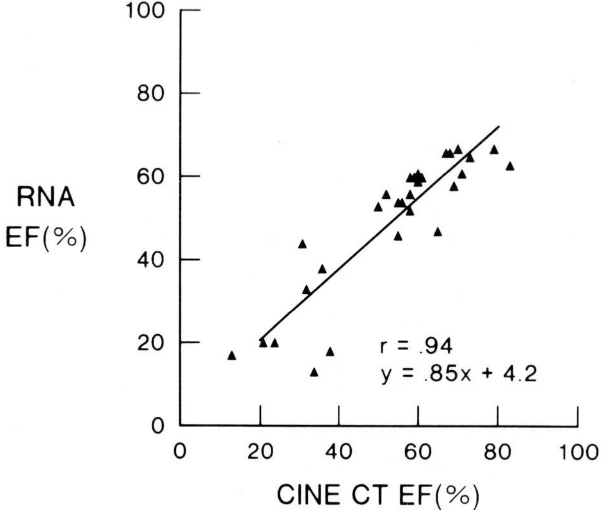

Figure 33–3. Comparison of measurements of left ventricular ejection fraction (EF) with radionuclide angiography (RNA) and with ultrafast CT (Cine CT). These measurements were made several days apart. Nevertheless, there is a very good correlation between the two methods.

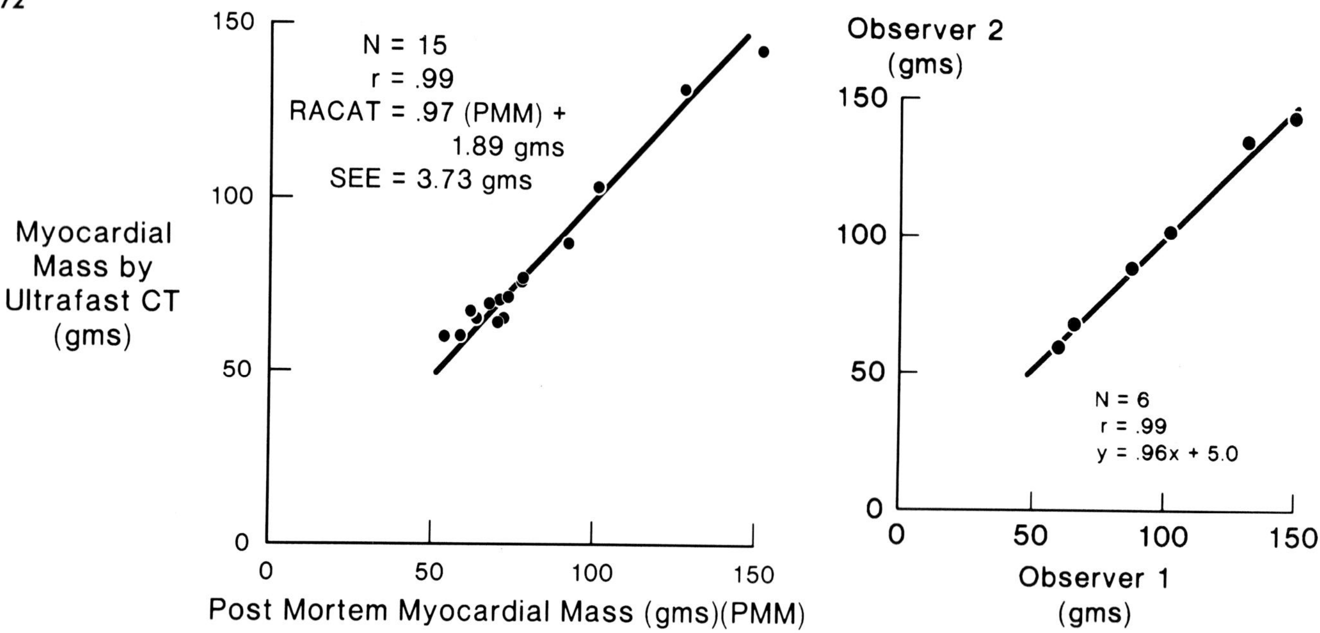

Figure 33–4. *Left panel*—Correlation between ultrafast CT measurements of left ventricular mass and actual postmortem mass. *Right panel*—Interobserver variability of left ventricular mass measurements with ultrafast CT. This study was done in closed-chest anesthetized dogs. (From Feiring, A. J., et al.: Determination of left ventricular mass in dogs with rapid-acquisition cardiac computed tomographic scanning. Circulation 72:1355, 1985, with permission of the American Heart Association, Inc.)

ments with these two techniques were obtained several days apart, there was a close relationship between left ventricular ejection fraction measured by these two approaches. Taken together, these three approaches to validating the precision of computed tomographic measurements of left ventricular chamber volume indicate that the CT data are remarkably precise and probably within 5 percent of the true value.

Left Ventricular Mass

Left ventricular mass measurements with ultrafast computed tomography have been compared with postmortem weights of the left ventricle.[F1] These experiments, performed in closed-chest anesthetized dogs, indicate that left ventricular mass can be precisely measured with ultrafast computed tomography (Fig. 33–4). The measurements of left ventricular mass are highly reproducible. Furthermore, repeated measurements of left ventricular mass, performed on successive days, have demonstrated excellent reproducibility.[R3]

Normal values for left ventricular volume and mass measured with ultrafast computed tomography have been reported (Table 33–1). Unfortunately, these data were obtained in a small group

Table 33–1. NORMAL VALUES FOR CARDIAC CHAMBER SIZE AND FUNCTION WITH ULTRAFAST COMPUTED TOMOGRAPHY

	LV	RV	LA	RA
EDV (ml)	141 ± 17	167 ± 24	27 ± 5	43 ± 16
ESV (ml)	41 ± 10	72 ± 18	60 ± 10	86 ± 21
SV (ml)	10 ± 12	95 ± 14	34 ± 9	43 ± 14
EF (%)	70 ± 5	57 ± 6		
Mass g/m^2	80 ± 10	27 ± 4		

LV—Left ventricle
RV—Right ventricle
LA—Left atrium, including appendage
RA—Right atrium, including appendage
EDV—Volume at the end of ventricular diastole
ESV—Volume at the end of ventricular systole
SV—Stroke volume
EF—Ejection fraction = (end-diastolic volume–end systolic volume)/end-diastolic volume
Values are expressed as mean ± SD.

of young, healthy male volunteers. Normal values in a broader population are needed.

These studies strongly support the opinion that ultrafast computed tomography can provide reproducible and precise measurements (±5 percent) of global left ventricular chamber volumes and mass.

Regional Left Ventricular Function

The parameters of regional left ventricular function that have been evaluated thus far, utilizing ultrafast computed tomography, are sectional performance (contraction of individual tomographic "slices"), segmental cavity performance (regional endocardial excursion within a single tomographic slice), wall-thickening, and phase sequence of contraction. The results obtained with each of these indices of regional left ventricular function are reviewed.

SECTIONAL PERFORMANCE. When ultrafast computed tomographic images of the left ventricle are obtained in the "short axis" (approximately perpendicular to the long axis of the left ventricle), typically 7 to 11 tomograms are needed to encompass the entire left ventricle in an adult patient. When the performances of these serial tomographic sections are compared, they provide information about "sectional performance" of the left ventricle. Studies of sectional function in anesthetized closed-chest dogs and in normal young male volunteers indicate a substantial heterogeneity of sectional performance from apex to base of the normal left ventricle.[F2] Tomographic sections at the base of the left ventricle have lower ejection fractions and those at the apex have higher ejection fractions than the ejection fraction of the entire left ventricle (Fig. 33–5). The sectional heterogeneity of function proceeds in an orderly manner that can be described by a third-order polynomial equation.

These observations have several implications. First, estimates of total left ventricular ejection fraction based on calculation of ejection fraction from one tomographic slice obtained with any technique (ultrafast CT, two-dimensional echocardiography, or nuclear magnetic resonance imaging) are unlikely to produce a precise assessment of global left ventricular ejection fraction. Such errors will be greatest when single-slice ejection fractions are employed in ventricles with major shape or regional wall motion abnormalities. Second, contributions of the various sections to total stroke volume are quite heterogeneous. The cardiac volume ejected from the basal sections of the left ventricle is

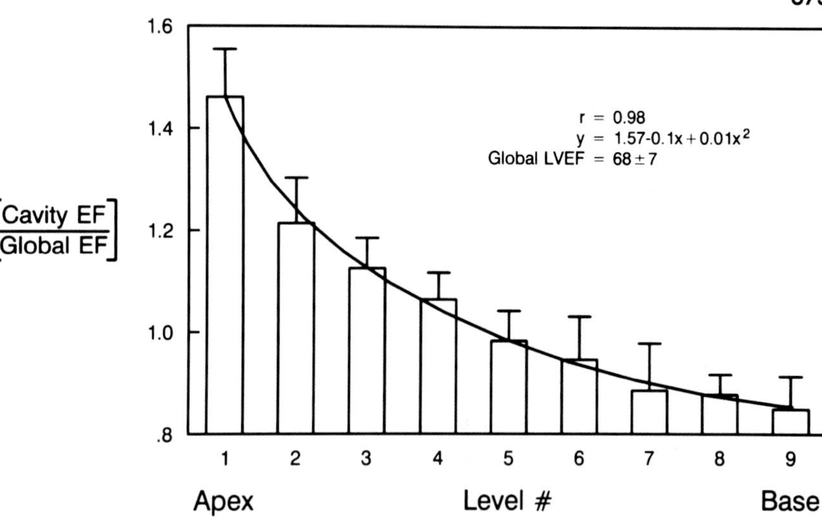

Figure 33–5. Sectional tomographic ejection fraction (cavity EF) normalized for global left ventricular ejection fraction (y axis) by ventricular region (x axis). Level 1 represents the cardiac apex; level 8 represents the base. There is an orderly decrement in sectional ejection fraction progressing from apex-to-base. Data are pooled from 11 normal human subjects. (From Feiring, A. J., et al.: Sectional and segmental variability of left ventricular function: Experimental and clinical studies using ultrafast computed tomography. J. Am. Coll. Cardiol. 12:415, 1988, with permission of the American Heart Association, Inc.)

responsible for most of the stroke volume ejected. This probably explains why many patients with myocardial infarctions that involve the apical half of the left ventricle maintain nearly normal stroke volume and cardiac output. Third, when calculations of sophisticated indices of left ventricular performance are made (left ventricular wall stress, volume/mass ratio), the site in the ventricle where the measurements of wall thickness and chamber dimensions are obtained will profoundly influence the calculated value. Hence, calculations based on data from a single section should not be assumed to represent the entire left ventricle, and comparison between ventricles or of the same ventricle measured at different times must be made only if the sections from which the data are obtained are carefully matched. These critical points are frequently ignored by investigators in this field, although in a few studies complex analyses based on complete three-dimensional reconstructions from tomographic x-ray data have been accomplished.[A2, C2] Finally, the extent of apex-to-base heterogeneity of ventricular function is not fixed. When afterload is substantially increased,[W1] apex-to-base heterogeneity of contraction diminishes (Fig. 33–6). Thus, the left ventricle adapts to an increased load by more uniform contraction.

SEGMENTAL ENDOCARDIAL MOTION. The performance of arbitrarily defined segments of a particular tomographic slice is usually assessed by dividing the tomogram into a predetermined number of radial "pie-slice" segments (Fig. 33–7), by extending equally spaced radial lines from a geometrically defined centroid. The placement of this centroid is critical. Most investigators employ either an epicardial or an endocardial centroid, which may be fixed throughout the cardiac cycle regardless of cavity movement (fixed centroid) or repositioned throughout the cycle in each tomographic image (floating centroid). Floating centroids or endocardial centroids may alter apparent segmental wall motion abnormalities. In addition, some investigators realign images, using internal reference points (right ventricular–left ventricular junction or papillary muscles) to compensate for rotational movement.

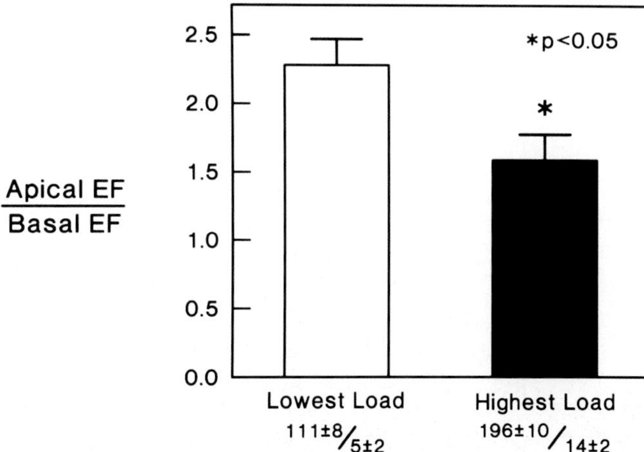

Figure 33–6. The regional heterogeneity of sectional ejection fraction as a function of left ventricular loading conditions. Ratio of ejection fraction in the apical section (apical EF) to that at the base (basal EF), an index of heterogeneity, is lower when left ventricular pressure is increased. These studies were conducted in closed-chest anesthetized dogs. Loading conditions were altered using an inferior vena cava balloon and aortic snare. The numbers below each column represent left ventricular pressure in mmHg (mean ± S.E.).

When segmental function is measured in this general manner, a great deal of heterogeneity is observed.[F2] The heterogeneity is less if an endocardial as opposed to an epicardial centroid is utilized (Fig. 33–7). Elimination of segments containing the papillary muscle, a scheme often employed by echocardiographers, does not alter significantly the extent of segmental heterogeneity observed on ultrafast computed tomographic images.

The marked heterogeneity of segmental contraction that characterizes normal left ventricular performance is not fixed. If afterload is significantly increased, the heterogeneity of segmental contraction decreases.[W1] Furthermore, if the inotropic state of the left ventricle is enhanced by dobutamine infusion, there is a marked decrease in the heterogeneity of segmental ventricular contraction.[S2]

The segmental heterogeneity of contraction observed in normal ventricles confounds any approach to identification of ischemic myocardium that is based on regional wall motion abnormalities. This problem is further amplified if changes in loading conditions on the ventricular chamber occur, because such hemodynamic alterations greatly alter segmental ventricular function.

SEGMENTAL WALL THICKENING. When left ventricular wall thickening is measured between end-diastole and end-systole from ultrafast computed tomographic images,[L1, F3] investigators have assessed either the change in the area of a given segment of the left ventricular wall or a linear dimension, such as the distance along an arbitrarily defined radial line or the shortest distance between the epicardial and endocardial surface at a given point on the circumference of the tomographic slice. With any of these approaches to measuring left ventricular wall thickening, if small ventricular segments from ultrafast computed tomographic images are employed, results suggest that left ventricular wall thickening in normal ventricles is extremely heterogeneous[F3] (Fig. 33–8). This apparent heterogeneity is related to a variety of factors. The normal left ventricular wall thickness of adult humans is between 8 and 11 mm. The pixel size on a typical cardiac computed tomographic image is 1 to 2 mm^2. Hence, if the left ventricular border definition is in error by one pixel, this results in a 9 to 12 percent error in the estimation of wall thickening. In addition, the left ventricle can rotate slightly during the cardiac

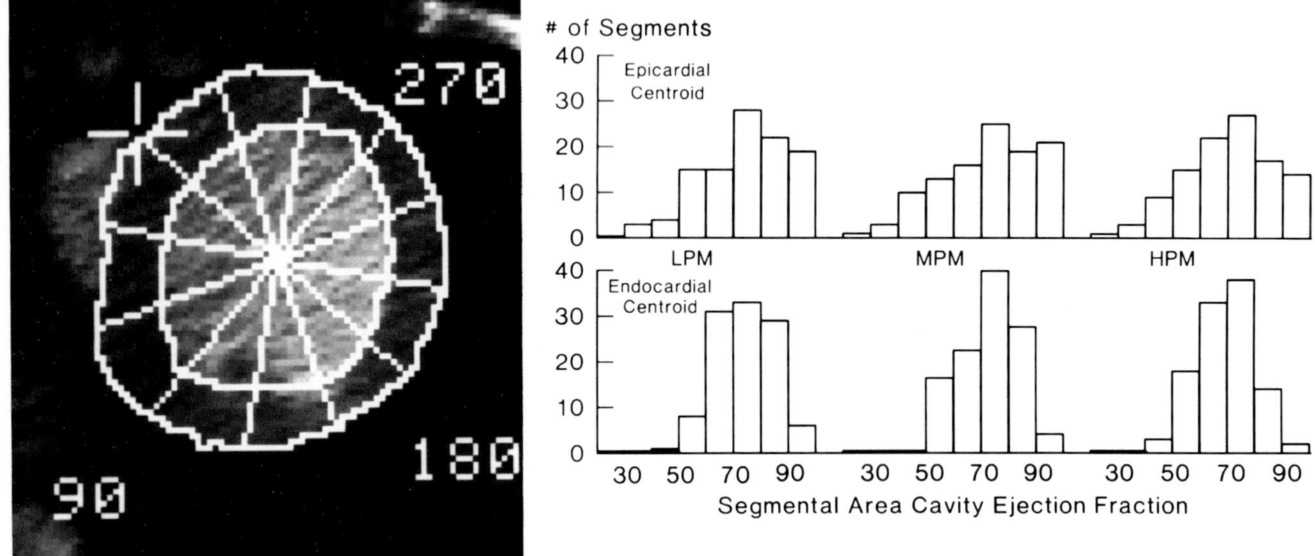

Figure 33–7. Assessment of regional left ventricular function within a tomographic slice. The *left panel* shows division of the left ventricular wall into 12 segments, each representing 30° of the total circumference. The *right panel* shows the frequency distribution of segmental ejection fractions obtained in 11 normal human subjects using this approach. Different results are obtained when an epicardial center of mass (centroid) is used to assign individual segments than when an endocardial centroid is used. Results are pooled for all 11 subjects. LPM—low papillary muscle; MPM—mid-papillary muscle; HPHM—high papillary muscle. (From Feiring, A. J., et al.: Sectional and segmental variability of left ventricular function: Experimental and clinical studies using ultrafast computed tomography. J. Am. Coll. Cardiol. 12:415, 1988. Reprinted with permission of the American College of Cardiology.)

cycle, and this artifactually alters the apparent ventricular wall thickening by changing the obliquity of the tomographic image. Also, papillary muscles and apex-to-base motion through the imaging plane of the short-axis tomographic slices makes it nearly impossible to assess wall thickness in exactly the same segment of the left ventricle both at end-diastole and end-systole. When all these potential sources of artifact are added to the inherent heterogeneity of left ventricular function, the final result is an extremely broad range of segmental left ventricular wall thickening.

Measurements of left ventricular wall thickening in larger circumferential segments of the left ventricle are less heterogeneous and can be useful in defining the location of left ventricular aneurysms[G1] or in diagnosing such conditions as idiopathic hypertrophic subaortic stenosis.

Although measurements of left ventricular wall thickening could be of great diagnostic value, at present these measurements with ultrafast computed tomography have limited utility. The problems that affect ultrafast computed tomography measurements of wall thickness in small ventricular segments throughout the cardiac cycle are common to all tomographic imaging techniques.

LEFT VENTRICULAR CONTRACTION PHASE ANALYSIS. By carefully examining the sequence of contraction of individual left ventricular segments, characteristic contraction sequences can be defined. These sequences can be utilized to predict the presence and location of bypass tracts in patients with Wolff-Parkinson-White syndrome[A1] and those with conduction disturbances.[C1] Although this application of ultrafast computed tomography is interesting, it has not been determined how well it compares with phase imaging with other modalities, such as digital subtraction angiography and conventional nuclear imaging, which inherently have greater temporal resolution than ultrafast computed tomography.

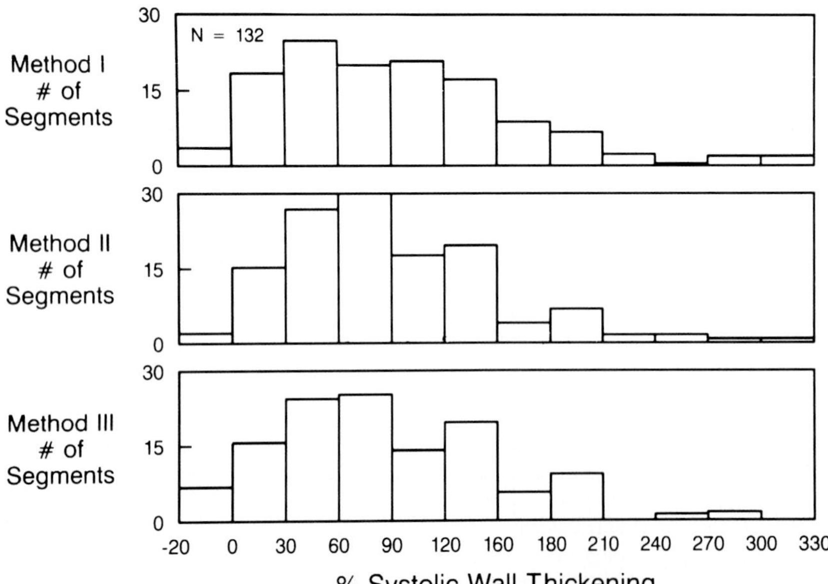

Figure 33–8. Heterogeneity of segmental left ventricular systolic function when percent change in wall thickness is measured. Figure shows frequency distribution of percent ΔT in mid-ventricular levels using three different methods (see text). Data are pooled from normal human subjects. (Data from Feiring, A. J., et al.: Regional ventricular function with cine CT. J. Am. Coll. Cardiol. 7:44A, 1986.)

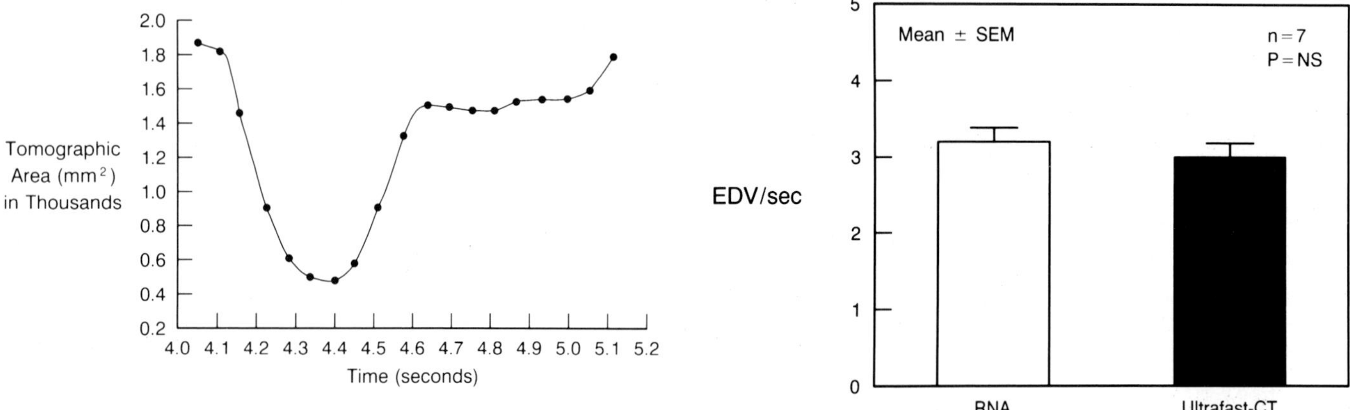

Figure 33–9. *Left panel*—Plot of cavity area versus time for a single tomographic slice in a normal volunteer. *Right panel*—Global left ventricular peak filling rate, normalized for end-diastolic volume (EDV/sec), using radionuclide angiography (RNA) and ultrafast CT. These studies were sequentially performed in 7 normal human subjects. There is no significant difference between the values obtained with these two methods. (From Rumberger, J. A., et al.: Patterns of regional diastolic function in the normal human left ventricle: An ultrafast CT study. J. Am. Coll. Cardiol. 14:119, 1989. Reprinted with permission of the American College of Cardiology.)

Assessment of Diastolic Left Ventricular Function

By measuring volume in either individual tomographic slices of the left ventricle or the entire left ventricle (by summation of individual slice volumes), the pattern of left ventricular ejection and filling can be reasonably well defined from computed tomographic imaging data[R4] (Fig. 33–9). Under unstressed conditions, global ventricular filling rates are slow enough to be accurately measured with ultrafast computed tomography at imaging rates of 17 frames per second. Peak left ventricular filling is usually defined by fitting a polynomial equation to the points that define the early diastolic phase of the left ventricle. A similar approach to defining peak filling rate is utilized with radionuclide techniques.[B3]

When peak filling rate normalized for left ventricular volume was measured in normal young male volunteers with both the radionuclide angiogram approach and ultrafast computed tomography, similar values for normalized peak filling rates were obtained (Fig. 33–9). Furthermore, as expected, normalized peak filling rate measured with ultrafast computed tomography increased significantly during stimulation with intravenous infusion of dobutamine.[W2]

Measurement of left ventricular diastolic filling with ultrafast computed tomography has several advantages versus that obtained with the radionuclide method. With ultrafast computed tomography, filling rates of individual tomographic sections of the left ventricle can be assessed. Such measurements indicate that when peak filling rate is normalized for the end-diastolic volume of the tomographic slice being analyzed, the normalized peak filling rate is greater in apical segments of the left ventricle compared with basal segments (Fig. 33–10). A number of other factors have been identified that appear to influence peak filling rate in various sections of the left ventricle. These factors include heart rate, systolic function, and ventricular loading conditions.[W2]

With ultrafast computed tomography, absolute as opposed to relative diastolic filling rates can be calculated. This cannot ordinarily be accomplished with radionuclide angiography. Measurement of absolute peak filling rates may be of importance because peak filling rate normalized for end-diastolic volume is unlikely to be normal if the left ventricle is dilated, even if the absolute rate of diastolic filling is well within the acceptable range.[R5] It should be recognized that ultrafast computed tomographic studies of diastolic filling performed thus far have been limited mainly to measurements of early diastolic changes in volume of the left ventricle. A more complete evaluation of diastolic function would include measurements of all three phases of diastole (early filling, diastasis, and atrial contraction), as well as simultaneous measurements of both pressure and volume.

Studies of diastolic filling with ultrafast computed tomography will be facilitated when technical improvements in the imaging

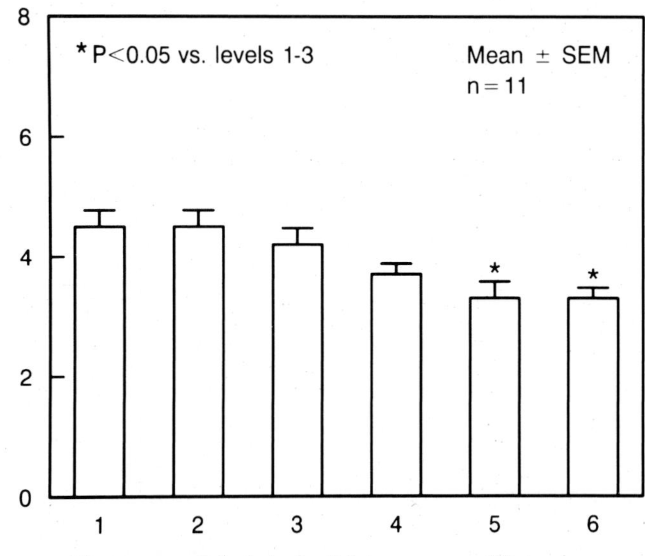

Figure 33–10. Sectional peak filling rate, normalized for end-diastolic volume (EDV/sec), as a function of cardiac region. Diastolic function, using this parameter, is significantly greater at the cardiac apex than at the base. Data are pooled from studies in 11 normal human subjects. (From Rumberger, J. A., et al.: Patterns of regional diastolic function in the normal human ventricle: An ultrafast CT study. J. Am. Coll. Cardiol. 14:119, 1989. Reprinted with permission of the American College of Cardiology.)

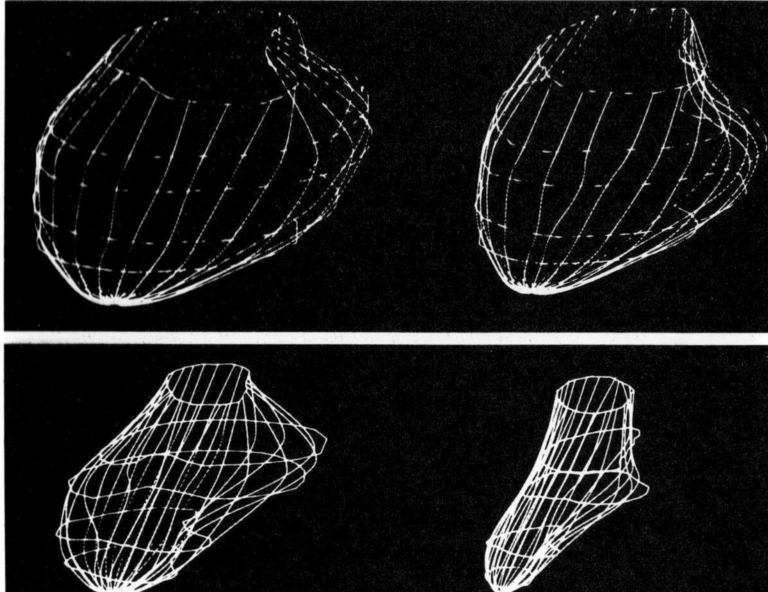

Figure 33–11. Three-dimensional depiction of left ventricular epicardium (*top*) and endocardium (*bottom*) in diastole (*left*) and systole (*right*) based on images obtained with ultrafast CT. (From Collins, S. J., et al.: Three-dimensional reconstruction of the contracting canine heart using cine computed tomography. Proceedings of the IEEE Computers in Cardiology, 1985, p. 67, © 1985 IEEE.)

system (expanded immediate memory; fully automated left ventricular border recognition) are implemented. When these changes become a reality, it may be possible to obtain routine assessment of left ventricular diastolic filling rates with ultrafast computed tomography.

Three-Dimensional Reconstruction of Left Ventricular Geometry

The ultrafast computed tomographic images of the left ventricle can be utilized to generate three-dimensional reconstruction of the left ventricular chamber (Fig. 33–11).[A2, C2] These reconstructions are visually impressive and permit easy appreciation of abnormalities in regional shape and function. However, investigators have not yet demonstrated that these reconstructions provide important information that cannot be gleaned from examination of the original tomographic images, although some sophisticated measurements of wall stress have utilized information from x-ray computed tomographic images. This area of investigation is at an early stage. It is possible that three-dimensional reconstructions of the left ventricular chamber will be useful in both clinical and research applications that involve an analysis of structure and function of the left ventricular chamber.

RIGHT VENTRICLE

Right Ventricular Volume

Validation studies have been performed to assess the accuracy with which right ventricular volume can be measured with ultrafast computed tomography. These validation studies were similar to those performed for the left ventricle. Radiopaque casts of the right ventricle were imaged in the CT scanner, and

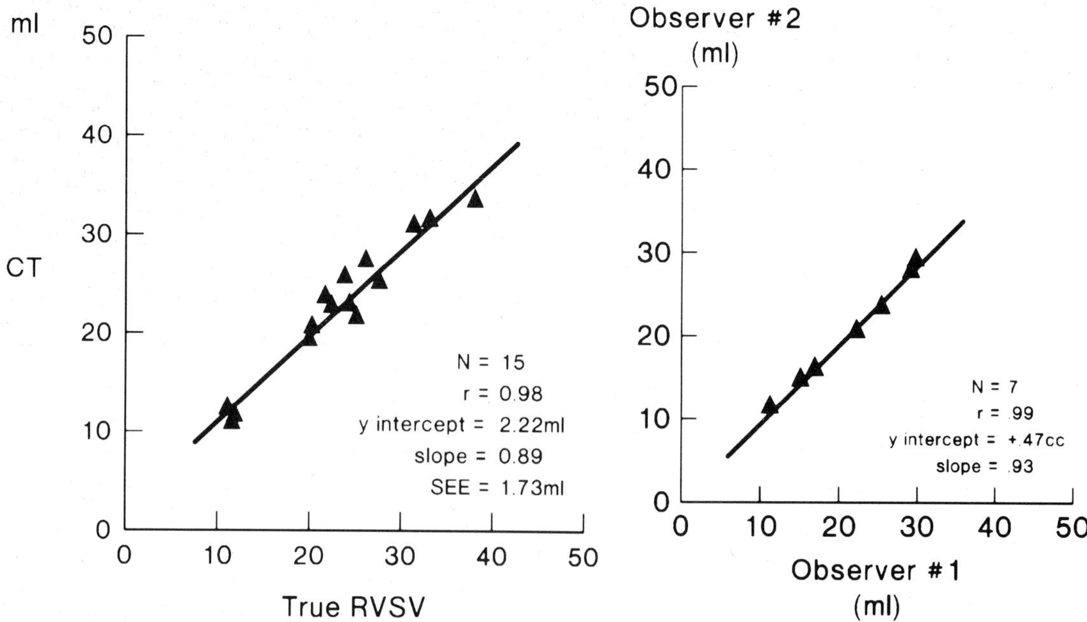

Figure 33–12. *Left panel*—Right ventricular stroke volume measured with ultrafast CT compared with simultaneous measurement by thermodilution (true RVSV). There is a very close correlation between the two methods. *Right panel*—Interobserver variability in measurement of right ventricular stroke volume with ultrafast CT. These studies were conducted in closed-chest anesthetized dogs. (From Reiter, S. J., et al.: Precision of measurements of right and left ventricular volume by cine computed tomography. Circulation 74:890, 1986, with permission of the American Heart Association, Inc.)

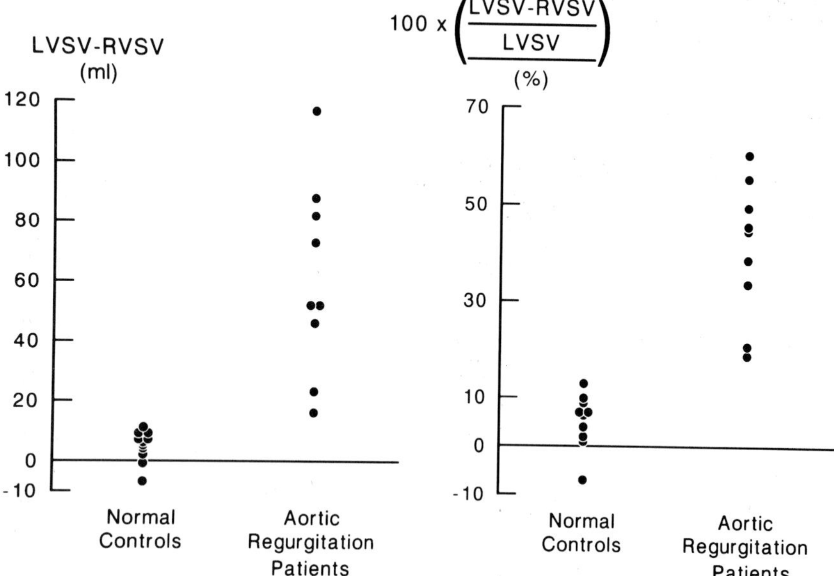

Figure 33–13. Difference between stroke volumes of the left and right ventricles as measured by ultrafast CT in normal human subjects and in patients with aortic regurgitation. The *left panel* shows the absolute difference in stroke volumes measured in ml; the *right panel* shows percent difference. Normal human subjects had little or no difference in stroke volumes, whereas patients with aortic regurgitation showed substantially greater left ventricular stroke volume than right ventricular stroke volume. (Data from Stark, C. A.: Dobutamine stress CT. Circulation 74:II-242, 1986.)

calculated right ventricular volume was compared with cast volume measured by water displacement. An excellent relationship between these estimates of static right ventricular volume was observed. To measure the ability of ultrafast computed tomography to define accurately dynamic changes in right ventricular volume, right ventricular stroke volume measurements based on the analysis of CT images (right ventricular end-diastolic volume minus end-systolic volume) were compared with direct and nearly simultaneous measurements of right ventricular stroke volume, obtained with thermodilution.[R1] Ultrafast tomographic measurements of right ventricular stroke volume were remarkably precise (Fig. 33–12). It has also been demonstrated that measurements of right ventricular stroke volume with ultrafast computed tomography are highly reproducible (Fig. 33–12).

Another approach to determining the accuracy with which ultrafast computed tomography can assess right and left ventricular stroke volume is to measure both right and left ventricular stroke volumes during suspended respiration in the same animal or patient. This has been done in both dogs[R6] and patients,[S3] and the differences between nearly simultaneous measurements of right ventricular and left ventricular stroke volume have been minimal (Fig. 33–13).

Right Ventricular Mass

Right ventricular mass cannot be accurately measured with ultrafast computed tomography if the C-100 scanner is utilized in the standard cardiac mode, because resolution is not adequate to define the precise thickness of the thin right ventricular free wall. However, in the high-resolution mode, the thickness of the right ventricular free wall can be defined. By obtaining sequential 3-mm tomograms of the right ventricle at end-diastole from apex to base, the mass of the right ventricle can be measured with reasonable accuracy and reproducibility (Fig. 33–14).[H2]

Normal values for right ventricular volume and right ventricular

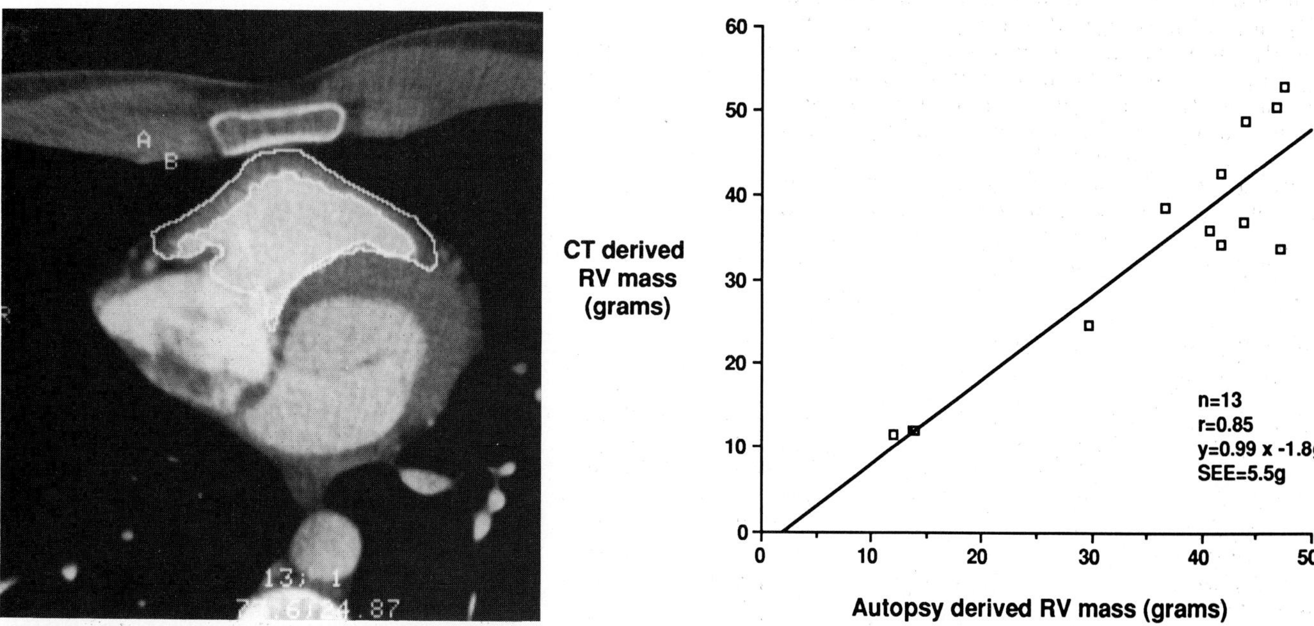

Figure 33–14. *Left panel*—High resolution tomogram taken at the level of the tricuspid and mitral valves in a normal human subject. Regions of interest are drawn for the right ventricular cavity and the right ventricular cavity plus free wall. This allows accurate calculation of right ventricular free wall mass. *Right panel*—Correlation between right ventricular mass as assessed by ultrafast CT when compared with postmortem right ventricular free wall mass. These data were obtained in anesthetized closed-chest dogs. (Adapted from Hajduczok, Z. D., et al.: Determination of right ventricular mass in humans and dogs with ultrafast cardiac computed tomography. Circulation 82:202, 1990, with permission of the American Heart Association.)

free wall mass in young healthy male volunteers have been reported (see Table 33–1). It is notable that in these normal young volunteers, right ventricular end-diastolic volume is invariably larger than left ventricular end-diastolic volume (average = 26 ml or 18 percent) and right ventricular ejection fraction is always less than left ventricular ejection fraction (average difference = 13 ejection fraction units). As expected on the basis of pathologic studies,[G2] the mass of the right ventricular free wall was about one third of the left ventricular mass if the interventricular septum is included as part of the left ventricle.

The studies reviewed with regard to measurements of right ventricular volume and mass with ultrafast computed tomography support the conclusion that precise measurements of right ventricular volume and mass (±5 percent) can be obtained with ultrafast computed tomography. It is emphasized that the evaluation of the right ventricle with two-dimensional echocardiography,[L2] conventional nuclear techniques,[K2, S4] and invasive ventriculography[A3] are far less precise in providing measurements of right ventricular volume and mass, compared with data that can be obtained with ultrafast computed tomography.

RIGHT AND LEFT ATRIAL VOLUMES

Validation studies of atrial volume measurements with ultrafast tomography are less comprehensive than ventricular volume measurements because of a paucity of available standards for comparison. In contrast to the ventricles, in which stroke volume can be measured with an independent standard such as an implanted electromagnetic flowprobe, measurements of atrial volume with an independent in vivo standard are not feasible. Furthermore, the mass of the atrial wall cannot be measured with ultrafast tomography because the resolution is inadequate to assess accurately the dimensions of the very thin atrial walls. Radiopaque casts of the right and left atrial chambers from various animals have been imaged in the computed tomographic scanner and calculated volumes compared with cast volumes measured with water displacement. Measurements of atrial appendage volume and the volume of the body of the atria were separately compared. These static atrial volumes could be accurately assessed with ultrafast computed tomography (R = 0.99, slope = 1.08, SE = 2 ml).[V1]

Normal values for right and left atrial volume in a small group of young healthy male volunteers have been assessed (see Table 33–1). Atrial appendage volume is about 10 percent of total atrial volume for both the right and left atria. Total right atrial volume is uniformly larger than left atrial volume. In addition, the changes in atrial volume throughout the cardiac cycle, based on geometric calculations, are only 34 percent and 45 percent of the respective total stroke volumes. This indicates that the conduit function of the atria accounts for a significant percentage of the flow that passes through the atrial chambers.

Studies at the University of Iowa[V1] have compared various echocardiographic measurements of left atrial volume with measurements of left atrial volume obtained with ultrafast computed tomography.[V1] Because the atrial appendage is not often visualized with transthoracic echocardiographic techniques, comparison of the echocardiographic and tomographic atrial measurements was limited to the body of the left atrium. The commonly employed M-mode index of the atrial size—anterior-posterior left atrial diameter—did not correlate well with left atrial volume.[V1] However, several two-dimensional echocardiographic indices of left atrial volume did correlate reasonably well with left atrial volume measurements obtained with ultrafast computed tomography. The echocardiographic estimates of atrial volume systematically underestimated chamber volume.

The limited studies available suggest that right and left atrial volume and the volume of the atrial appendages can be accurately assessed (±5 percent) with ultrafast computed tomography.

MEASUREMENTS OF CARDIAC OUTPUT

Investigators have examined the utility of two approaches to measuring cardiac output with ultrafast computed tomography. As noted, stroke volume of the right and left ventricles can be accurately measured with ultrafast computed tomography.[R1] Consequently, cardiac output can be easily calculated by multiplying heart rate times stroke volume.

An alternative approach is to apply the Stewart-Hamilton indicator dilution technique to assessing cardiac output, based on contrast clearance curves obtained in the aorta following a bolus injection of intravenous contrast.[R7] This technique works best if the relationship between iodine concentration and Hounsfield (CT) number is calibrated in each study by imaging a series of syringes placed on the chest wall that contain varying known concentrations of iodine. When an independent calibration is utilized, cardiac output can be accurately measured with ultrafast computed tomography with the indicator-dilution principle (Fig. 33–15).

SHUNT CALCULATIONS

Indicator dilution curves from various regions of interest can be utilized to assess both right-to-left and left-to-right shunts from computed tomographic images. Such studies require rapid contrast bolus injection and sequential imaging. With this approach, the site of left-to-right and right-to-left shunts can be identified, and shunt volumes can be calculated. This area is discussed in greater detail in Chapter 37.

EVALUATION OF CARDIAC VALVES

Several inherent problems with ultrafast computed tomography limit the information about valve function and anatomy that can be obtained with this diagnostic modality. Normal valve leaflets are only 1 to 2 mm thick, which is close to the in-plane resolution of ultrafast CT in the cardiac mode. Furthermore, a slice thickness of 8 mm in the cardiac mode produces volume averaging of

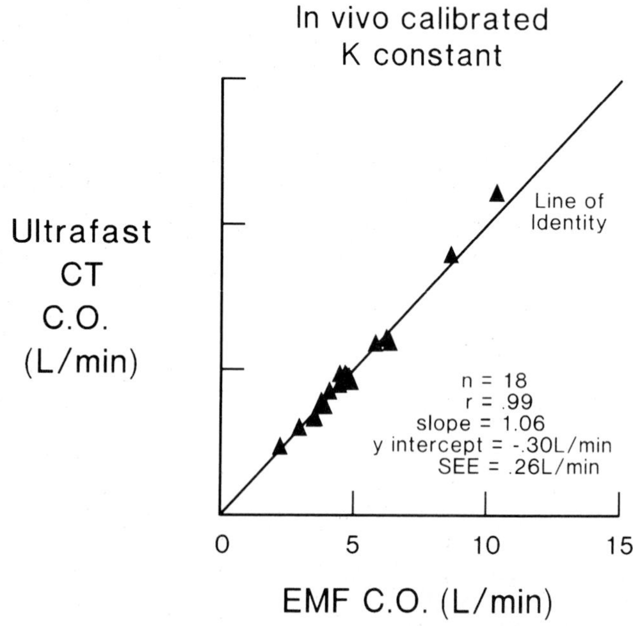

Figure 33–15. Measurements of cardiac output by dye dilution analysis using ultrafast CT compared with actual cardiac output as measured by chronically implanted aortic electromagnetic flowprobe (EMF). These data were obtained in closed-chest anesthetized dogs. (Data from Reiter, S. J., et al.: Precise measurements of contrast clearance curve cardiac outputs using cine computed tomography. J. Am. Coll. Cardiol. 9:161A, 1987.)

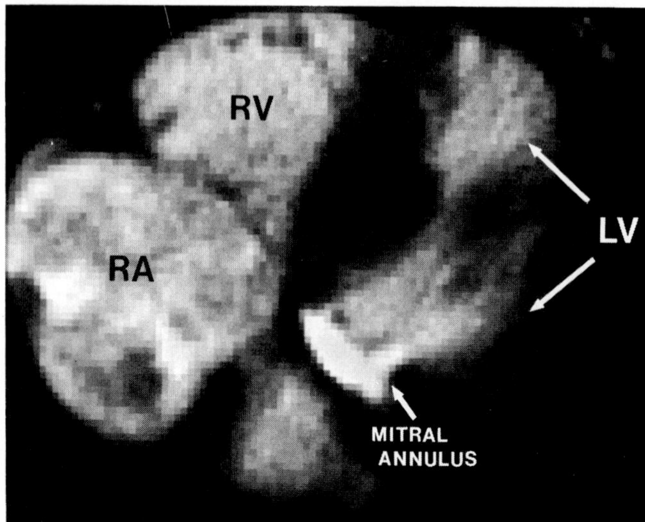

Figure 33–16. Long-axis tomogram in a patient with heavy calcification of the mitral apparatus due to rheumatic disease.

valvular structures that seriously interferes with adequate visualization of valve anatomy. Frequently, the valves are imaged at an angle that is oblique to the valve plane. As a consequence, the surface area of the valves seldom can be measured accurately. These problems are decreased if the valves are imaged in the high-resolution mode (in-plane resolution, 0.7 mm; slice thickness, 3 mm). An additional problem is that intense calcification of valvular structures and some prosthetic valves produces severe artifacts in ultrafast computed tomographic images. In the aggregate, these problems significantly restrict the amount of useful information that can be obtained with ultrafast tomography concerning valvular structure and function.

Despite these problems, all four cardiac valves can be visualized with ultrafast computed tomography. In general, the mitral and aortic valves are better visualized than the tricuspid or pulmonary valves if conventional imaging projections are employed. Annulus and leaflet calcification can be readily separated, and the magnitude of calcification can be determined qualitatively. Occasionally, bicuspid aortic valves can be identified. Restricted valve motion and markedly thickened leaflets can be detected. Rarely, vegetations on valve leaflets can be observed.

A few diseases that affect the cardiac valves can be diagnosed with ultrafast computed tomography. These include the characteristic abnormal mitral valve motion associated with idiopathic hypertrophic subaortic stenosis, the systolic posterior displacement of the mitral valve leaflets in mitral valve prolapse, and the displacement of the tricuspid valve associated with Ebstein's anomaly. In selected patients with mitral stenosis, both annular and valvular abnormalities can be detected (Fig. 33–16). All these findings represent qualitative valvular abnormalities that can occasionally be noted on computed tomographic examinations.

In contrast to these qualitative abnormalities in valvular structure and function, ultrafast computed tomography can be utilized to quantitatively determine the precise amount of valvular regurgitation in patients who have a regular cardiac rate, no intracardiac shunts, and regurgitation of only one valve.[R6] Because right ventricular and left ventricular stroke volume measurements with ultrafast tomography are nearly identical during suspended respiration in normals, the difference between left ventricular and right ventricular stroke volume can provide a precise index of the magnitude of univalvular regurgitation. Studies in animals indicate that, with this approach, the magnitude of valvular regurgitation can be precisely measured with ultrafast computed tomography (Fig. 33–17). Studies in patients utilizing this approach have also been promising.[S3]

Ultrafast computed tomographic examinations can provide additional correlative information in patients with isolated aortic regurgitation. An ultrafast examination can yield information on the structure of the ascending aorta, aortic annulus size, presence and location of valvular and annular calcification, left ventricular function, and left ventricular mass.

In patients with mitral valvular disease, ultrafast computed tomography can provide information about the left atrial size, the presence of left atrial thrombi, the extent and localization of valvular and annular calcification, and the presence or involvement of the subvalvular apparatus, left ventricular volume and function, left ventricular mass, and right ventricular size and function.

In summary, although ultrafast computed tomography is not the examination of choice for the evaluation of the structure and function of cardiac valves, such examinations can provide a great deal of information in the evaluation of selected patients with valvular disease.

INTERVENTIONAL STUDIES OF LEFT VENTRICULAR FUNCTION

Although the great majority of studies with ultrafast computed tomography have been performed under resting conditions, two studies in humans have examined left ventricular function during an intervention. In one study performed in healthy males, ventricular function was assessed at rest and during intravenous dobutamine infusion.[S2] During dobutamine infusion, the left ventricular ejection fraction increased and the heterogeneity of segmental left ventricular function decreased. Thus, during an inotropic stress, the left ventricle contracted in a more homoge-

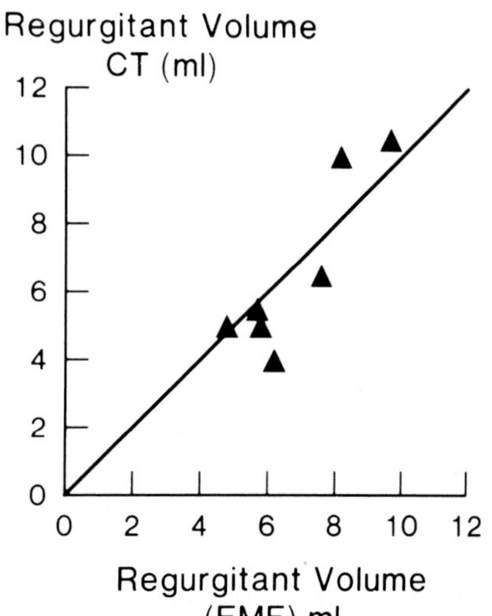

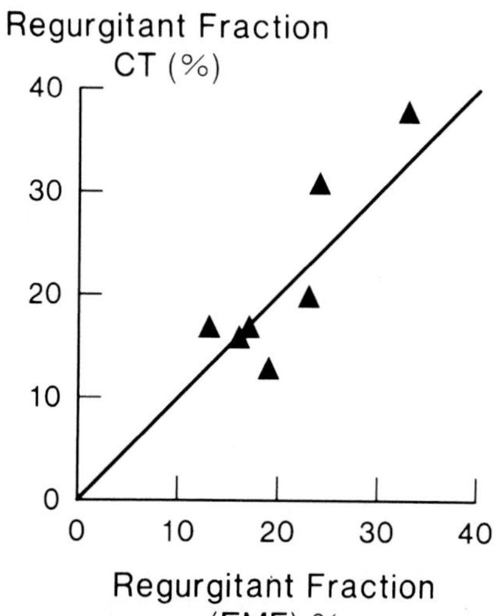

Figure 33–17. Measurement of aortic regurgitant volume (*left panel*) and regurgitant fraction (*right panel*) in an experimental model of isolated aortic regurgitation. Results obtained with ultrafast CT are compared with those obtained by chronically implanted electromagnetic flow meters (EMF). There is a very close correlation between the two methods. These data were obtained in closed-chest anesthetized dogs. (Adapted from Reiter, S. J., et al.: Quantitative determination of aortic regurgitant volumes in dogs by ultrafast computed tomography. Circulation 76:728, 1987, with permission of the American Heart Association.)

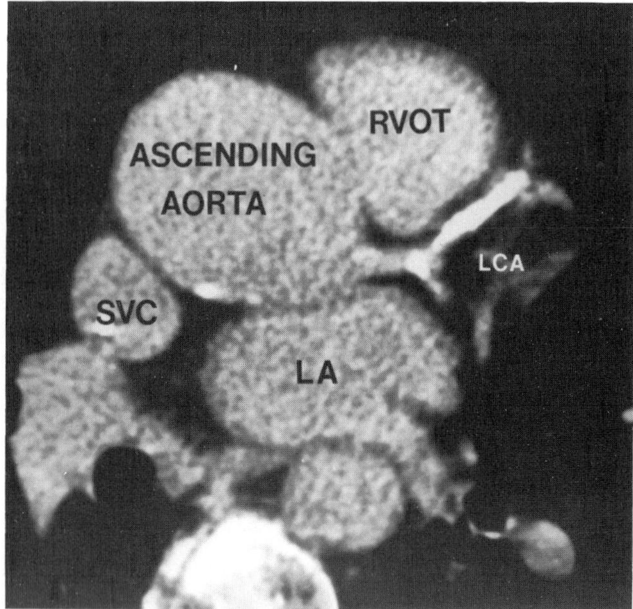

Figure 33–18. High-resolution tomogram of a coronary artery. This image, obtained without the need for iodinated contrast medium, shows dense coronary calcification indicating the presence of atherosclerosis. SVC—superior vena cava; RVOT—right ventricular outflow tract; LA—left atrium; LCA—left coronary artery.

neous manner. In a second study, left ventricular function was assessed at rest and during semi-upright bicycle exercise in patients with and without obstructive coronary disease.[R8] In patients with normal coronary arteries, exercise was associated with an increased left ventricular ejection fraction and a decrease in heterogeneity of left ventricular wall motion. In patients with obstructive coronary lesions, exercise was associated with a variable change in global left ventricular ejection fraction and the prominent development of impaired wall motion in the perfusion field of the diseased vessel or vessels. In this study, the sensitivity and specificity of detecting obstructive coronary disease with exercise ultrafast computed tomography compared favorably with other noninvasive testing modalities.

These interventional studies demonstrate that, like other imaging modalities, ultrafast computed tomographic images can be obtained during various interventions. Further studies of this type should be encouraged.

CORONARY ANATOMY

Calcification in coronary vessels can be readily detected with ultrafast computed tomography without contrast media (Fig. 33–18).[J1, T1] The sensitivity for the detection of coronary calcification is greater with ultrafast tomography than with conventional fluoroscopy.[J1] The value of such information remains to be determined, but conceivably it could be useful in screening patients for the presence of coronary atherosclerosis.

Studies with a Dynamic Spatial Reconstructor by Spyra and associates at the Mayo Clinic[S5] and limited studies with the Imatron C-100 suggest that, with rapid computed tomographic imaging and three-dimensional reconstruction, the anatomy of the proximal coronary arteries and the severity of stenosis may be measurable with sufficient accuracy to be of clinical value. This application of ultrafast computed tomography is in the developmental stage.[N1, W3]

CONCLUSIONS

With ultrafast computed tomography, it is possible to assess cardiac structure and function with impressive precision that in most applications far exceeds what can be accomplished with conventional imaging approaches. Now that many of the standard measurements with ultrafast tomography have been carefully validated against appropriate standards, it will be important to perform studies to determine whether these precise measurements of cardiac structure and function will significantly influence patient management.

References

A

1. Abbott, J. A., Botvinick, E. A., Scheinman, E. D., et al.: Noninvasive localization of accessory pathways. J. Am. Coll. Cardiol. 13:8A, 1989.
2. Azhari, H., Grenadier, E., Dinnar, U., et al.: Quantitative characterization and sorting of three-dimensional geometries: Application to left ventricles *in vivo*. IEEE Trans. Biomed. Eng. 36:322, 1989.
3. Arcilla, R. A., Tsai, P., Thilenius, O., and Ranniger, K.: Angiocardiographic method for volume estimation of right and left ventricles. Chest 60:446, 1971.

B

1. Bove, A. A., Ziskin, M. C., Freeman, E., et al.: Selection of optimum cineradiographic frame rate—relation to accuracy of cardiac measurements. Invest. Radiol. 5:329, 1970.
2. Bacharach, S. L., Auen, M. V., Bores, J. S., et al.: Left ventricular peak ejection rate, filling rate, and ejection fraction—frame rate requirements at rest and exercise. J. Nucl. Med. 20:189, 1979.
3. Bonow, R. O., Vitole, D. F., Bacharich, S. L., et al.: Asynchronous left ventricular regional function in impaired global diastolic filling in patients with coronary artery disease: Reversal after coronary angioplasty. Circulation 71:297, 1985.

C

1. Collins, S. M., Higgs, D. M., Fisher, D. J., et al.: Automated analysis of the sequence of ventricular contraction using ultrafast computed tomography: Initial clinical evaluation. Circulation 80:II-155, 1989.
2. Collins, S. J., Yashodhar, P., Rumberger, J. A., et al.: Three-dimensional reconstruction of the contracting canine heart using cine computed tomography. Proceedings of the IEEE Computers in Cardiology, 1985, p. 67.

F

1. Feiring, A. J., Rumberger, J. A., Reiter, S. J., et al.: Determination of left ventricular mass in dogs with rapid-acquisition cardiac computed tomographic scanning. Circulation 72:1355, 1985.
2. Feiring, A. J., Rumberger, J. A., Reiter, S. J., et al.: Sectional and segmental variability of left ventricular function: Experimental and clinical studies using ultrafast computed tomography. J. Am. Coll. Cardiol. 12:415, 1988.
3. Feiring, A. J., Rumberger, J. A., Collins, S. M., et al.: Regional ventricular function with cine CT. J. Am. Coll. Cardiol. 7:44A, 1986.

G

1. Grenadier, E., Weiss, R. M., Lemmer, J. H., et al.: Surgically resectable left ventricular aneurysm: Specific characteristics by ultrafast computed tomography. J. Am. Coll. Cardiol. 13:47A, 1989.
2. Gould, S. E. (ed.): Gross examination of the heart. *In* Pathology of the Heart and Blood Vessels. Charles C Thomas, Springfield, Ill., 1968, p. 1132.

H

1. Hessel, S. J., Adams, D. F., and Abrams, H. L.: Complications of angiography. Radiology 138:273, 1981.
2. Hajduczok, Z. D., Weiss, R. M., Stanford, W., and Marcus, M. L.: Determination of right ventricular mass in humans and dogs with ultrafast cardiac computed tomography. Circulation 82:202, 1990.

I

1. Iwasaki, T., Sinak, L. J., Hoffman, E. A., et al.: Mass of left ventricular myocardium estimated with dynamic spatial reconstructor. Am. J. Physiol. 246:H138, 1984.

J

1. Janowitz, W. R., Agatston, A. S., Zusmer, N. R., et al.: Comparison of ultrafast CT and fluoroscopy in detecting coronary artery calcification. Circulation 80:II-108, 1989.

K

1. Kantor, H. L., Rzedzion, R. R., Berliner, E., et al.: Detection of coronary stenosis by high speed NMR imaging: The utility of dysprosium-DTPA. J. Am. Coll. Cardiol. 13:48A, 1989.
2. Khaja, F., Alam, M., Goldstein, S., et al.: Diagnostic value of visualization of the right ventricle using thallium-201 myocardial imaging. Circulation 59:182, 1979.

L

1. Lanzer, P., Garrett, J., and Lipton, M. J.: Quantitation of regional myocardial function by cine computed tomography: Pharmacologic changes in wall thickness. J. Am. Coll. Cardiol. 8:682, 1986.
2. Levine, R. A., Gibson, T. C., Zretz, T., et al.: Echocardiographic measurements of right ventricular volume. Circulation 69:497, 1984.

N

1. Napel, S., Rutt, B. K., and Pflugfelder, P.: Three-dimensional images of the coronary arteries from ultrafast computed tomography: Method and comparison with two-dimensional angiography. Am. J. Cardiac Imag. 3:237, 1989.

R

1. Reiter, S. J., Rumberger, J. A., Feiring, A. J., et al.: Precision of measurements of right and left ventricular volume by cine computed tomography. Circulation 74:890, 1986.
2. Reiter, S. J., Rumberger, J. A., Stanford, W., and Marcus, M. L.: Precise stroke volume measurements by cine CT in the presence of abnormal left ventricular shape and size. Circulation 74:122A, 1986.
3. Roig, E., Chomka, E., Lobalbo, C., et al.: Variability of left ventricular mass measurements by ultrafast computed tomography. J. Am. Coll. Cardiol. 11:157A, 1988.
4. Rumberger, J. A., Weiss, R. M., Feiring, A. J., et al.: Patterns of regional diastolic function in the normal human left ventricle: An ultrafast CT study. J. Am. Coll. Cardiol. 14:119, 1989.
5. Rumberger, J. A., Vonk, G. N., Sinak, L. J., et al.: Impaired early diastolic filling in patients with compensated aortic insufficiency. Circulation 78:II-399, 1988.
6. Reiter, S. J., Rumberger, J. A., Stanford, W., and Marcus, M. L.: Quantitative determination of aortic regurgitant volumes in dogs by ultrafast computed tomography. Circulation 76:728, 1987.
7. Reiter, S. J., Feiring, A. J., Stanford, W., et al.: Precise measurements of contrast clearance curve cardiac outputs using cine computed tomography. J. Am. Coll. Cardiol. 9:161A, 1987.
8. Roig, E., Chomka, E. V., Castaner, A., et al.: Exercise ultrafast computed tomography for the detection of coronary artery disease. J. Am. Coll. Cardiol. 13:1073, 1989.

S

1. Slager, C. J., Hooghoudt, T. E. H., Serruys, P. W., et al.: Quantitative assessment of regional left ventricular motion using endocardial landmarks. J. Am. Coll. Cardiol. 7:317, 1986.
2. Stark, C. A., Rumberger, J. A., Stanford, W., and Marcus, M. L.: Dobutamine stress CT. Circulation 74:122A, 1986.
3. Stark, C. A., Rumberger, J. A., Reiter, S. J., and Marcus, M. L.: Use of cine CT in assessing the severity of aortic regurgitation in patients. Circulation 74:II-4, 1986.
4. Slutsky, R., Ashburn, W., and Karliner, J.: A method for the estimation of right ventricular volume by equilibrium radionuclide angiography. Chest 80:471, 1981.
5. Spyra, W. J. T., Bell, M. R., Bove, A. A., et al.: Detection and localization of moderate coronary stenosis by fast CT with a single nonselective angiogram. Circulation 78:II-398, 1988.

T

1. Tannenbaum, S. R., Kondos, G. T., Veselik, K. E., et al.: Detection of calcific deposits in coronary arteries by ultrafast computed tomography and correlation with angiography. Am. J. Cardiol. 63:870, 1989.

V

1. Vandenberg, B. R., Weiss, R., Kienzey, J., et al.: Left atrial volume measurement: Cine computed tomography and echocardiography. J. Am. Coll. Cardiol. 11:217A, 1988.

W

1. Weiss, R. M., Shonka, M., Kinzey, J. E., and Marcus, M. L.: Effects of loading alterations on the pattern of heterogeneity of regional left ventricular function. FASEB J 2:1494A, 1988.
2. Weiss, R. M., Rumberger, J. A., and Marcus, M. L.: Determinants of regional diastolic function assessed with ultrafast computed tomography. Circulation 76:IV-6, 1987.
3. Weiss, R. M., Clothier, J. L., McKay, C. R., et al.: Three-dimensional imaging of coronary arteries with cine computed tomography. Circulation 80:II-155, 1989.

Chapter 34

Determination of Bypass Graft Patency with Ultrafast Computed Tomography

■ *WILLIAM STANFORD, M.D.* ■ *MELVIN L. MARCUS, M.D*

HISTORICAL ASPECTS 682
BYPASS GRAFT PATENCY ASSESSED WITH ULTRAFAST COMPUTED TOMOGRAPHY 684
Procedure 684
Sensitivity, Specificity, and Accuracy of Ultrafast Computed Tomography in Determining Bypass Graft Patency 684
Multicenter Study 684
Sensitivity, Specificity, and Accuracy 684
Assessment of Internal Mammary Artery Versus Vein Bypass Graft Patency With Ultrafast Computed Tomography 684
Assessment of Stenotic Versus Open Bypass Graft Patency With Ultrafast Computed Tomography 684
Effect of the Number of Grafts on Accuracy of Determining Bypass Graft Patency With Ultrafast Computed Tomography 685
Interobserver and Intraobserver Variability 685
Pitfalls Associated With Assessment of Bypass Graft Patency With Ultrafast Computed Tomography 685
BYPASS GRAFT FLOW RATE 686
BYPASS GRAFT FLOW RESERVE 686
ASSESSMENT OF BYPASS GRAFT PATENCY BY ULTRAFAST COMPUTED TOMOGRAPHY VERSUS OTHER IMAGING MODALITIES 686
SUMMARY 686

Coronary bypass surgery was introduced in 1968 by Favaloro.[F1] This procedure gained enormous popularity in the United States because it relieved symptoms of myocardial ischemia. In addition, it decreased morbidity and mortality in selected subgroups of patients.[C1] In 1985, approximately 200,000 patients had coronary bypass surgery.[W1] Since the long-term mortality rate in postoperative patients is low (2 to 5 percent per year) and the operative procedure has been performed for 21 years, it is reasonable to estimate that the number of living patients with coronary bypass grafts in the United States is in excess of 3.5 million. This is an impressive number when compared with the number of new patients with coronary disease who present each year for evaluation by a physician (6.7 million).[M1]

In an adult cardiology practice, many patients have had one or more coronary bypass operations. One of the questions critical to management of patients in this group concerns the status of bypass grafts. Although bypass graft patency can be assessed by invasive diagnostic procedures, the best noninvasive approach to evaluating graft patency is with ultrafast computed tomography.[S1]

This chapter will review the current status of ultrafast computed tomography in the assessment of bypass graft patency and flow reserve.

HISTORICAL ASPECTS

Computed tomography was introduced by Hounsfield in the early 1970's[H1] and was initially used almost exclusively to define intracranial lesions. The first reported use in assessing coronary bypass graft patency was in 1980.[B1] Subsequently, seven large clinical series were reported in which standard computed tomographic assessment of bypass graft patency was compared with coronary angiography (Table 34–1).[D1, F2, G1, K1, K2, M2, W2] In general, for these series high sensitivities (79 to 97 percent) and specificities (77 to 100 percent) in the detection of bypass graft patency were reported. However, only a small percentage of the patients had internal mammary artery implants and no multicenter studies or intraobserver variabilities have been reported.

In view of these excellent results, it is surprising that this diagnostic procedure has never gained significant popularity. The reasons are speculative. One possible explanation is that the results can be obtained only by highly skilled examiners who perform the examinations in a very meticulous manner. Our experiences with conventional computed tomography would tend to support this. Ultrafast computed tomography, on the other hand, has the advantage of being able to visualize the kinetics of the contrast bolus (Figs. 34–1, 34–2). This allows better identification of grafts and decreases the sources of error. The kinetics of the contrast bolus differentiates pulmonary veins, pulmonary arteries, and atrial appendages, which may interfere with the interpretations of graft patency.

At present, very few if any hospitals employ standard computed tomography in the assessment of coronary bypass graft patency.

Table 34–1. CONVENTIONAL COMPUTED TOMOGRAPHY IN CORONARY BYPASS GRAFT PATENCY

Reference	No. of Grafts	Sensitivity* (%)	Specificity* (%)
Daniel et al.[D1]	125	91	88
Brundage et al.[B1]	62	93	95
Godwin et al.[G1]	47	79	77
Wilson et al.[W2]	63	85	100
Kahl et al.[K1]	100	82	69
Kawasuji et al.[K2]	43	97	100
Foster et al.[F2]	65	96	83
Moncada et al.[M2]	33	96	91

*Compared with coronary angiography.

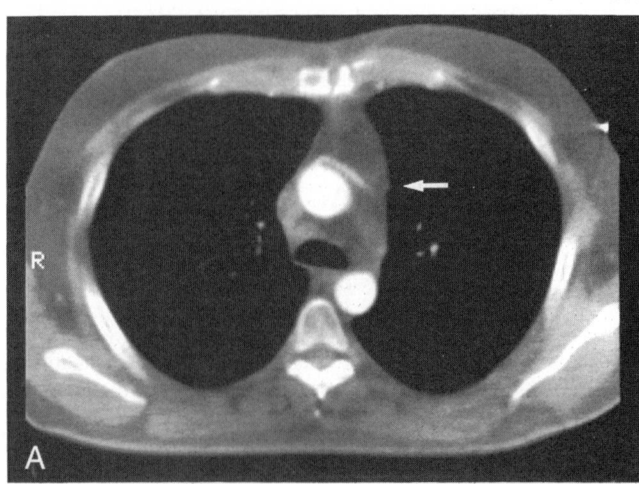

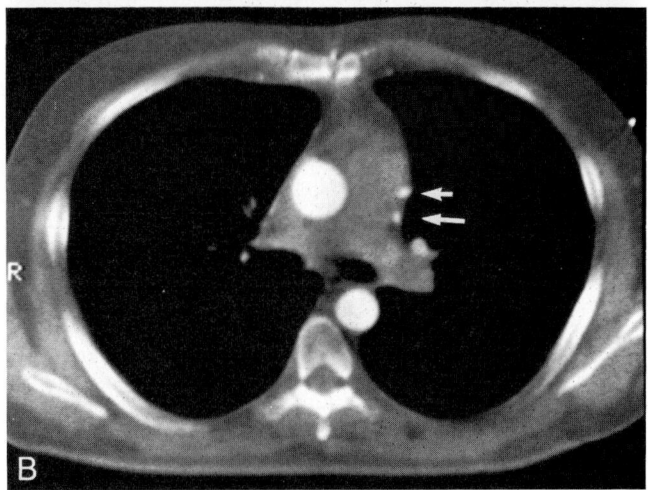

Figure 34–1. Representative tomographic scans. *A*, Patent left anterior descending coronary artery graft is seen tangentially as it exits the aorta *(arrow)*. *B*, Grafts in the left anterior descending coronary artery distribution *(short arrow)* and left circumflex artery distribution *(long arrow)* are seen in cross section. R—right. (Reprinted with permission from the American College of Cardiology Journal of the American College of Cardiology 12:1–7, 1988.)

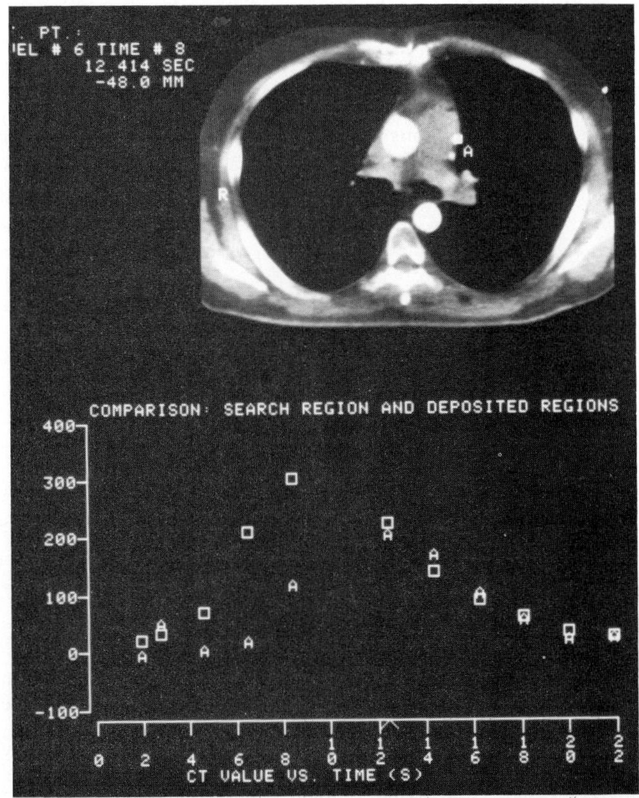

Figure 34–2. Time-density curve from the patent graft in Figure 34–1. The time-density curve shows the height of the contrast bolus (Hounsfield units) within the graft at arrival, peak concentration, and washout. The squares indicate contrast within the aorta; "A" indicates graft contrast.

BYPASS GRAFT PATENCY ASSESSED WITH ULTRAFAST COMPUTED TOMOGRAPHY

Procedure

Before initiating an ultrafast CT examination for bypass graft patency, it is essential to review the patient's operative record to determine the number of grafts placed, the type of grafts (i.e., saphenous vein grafts or internal mammary artery grafts), and whether the grafts were single or sequential. This information is then used to determine the scanning sequence to be employed.

The imaging sequence begins with the patient supine and with the scanner table perpendicular to the scanner gantry. If internal mammary grafts have been placed, it is important to begin image acquisition at the thoracic inlet. If only vein grafts have been placed, imaging can begin at the undersurface of the aortic arch. If grafts are placed to branches of the right coronary circulation, the imaging sequence must include sufficient levels to extend 2 to 3 cm below the takeoff of the native right coronary artery. If grafts are only to the left coronary circulation, imaging can stop 2 to 3 cm below the takeoff of the left main coronary artery. If two contrast injections are needed to encompass all of the necessary tomographic levels, the acquisitions should include sufficient overlap to avoid gaps in the imaging sequence. Occasionally, when graft visualization is indefinite, angulated views or views that are offset by 0.5 cm from the original acquisition may be used to ensure that gaps between the slices do not contain information necessary for a conclusive diagnosis. Motion of the patient between or during image acquisition must be avoided, and ideally images should be obtained during a held inspiration. Rapid inspiration during scan acquisition makes image interpretation more difficult.

To provide sufficient vascular opacification, the contrast medium is injected via a peripheral intravenous site as a bolus of 10 ml per second for 4 seconds. Before the contrast injection, the circulation time is determined with either magnesium sulfate (0.5 % solution) or the Cardio-Green-dye technique.[C2, S2] Image acquisition commences 6 seconds earlier than the patient's recorded circulation time and continues every one to two cardiac cycles until 10 or 13 images are acquired. Because the memory of the Imatron C-100 scanner is limited to 80 images, a 10-frame acquisition can examine eight 8-mm tomographic levels, whereas a 13-frame acquisition would include only six levels. Because the distance from the aortic arch to a point 2 to 3 cm below the takeoff of the right coronary artery is typically 12 to 16 cm, most studies of bypass graft patency require two injections of contrast medium.

Sensitivity, Specificity, and Accuracy of Ultrafast Computed Tomography in Determining Bypass Graft Patency

Four studies[B2, B3, S2, S3] have compared assessment of bypass graft patency by ultrafast computed tomography with that by selective angiography. All four studies concluded that the sensitivity (93 to 96 percent), specificity (86 to 100 percent), and accuracy (92 to 96 percent) of ultrafast computed tomography in assessing bypass graft patency were very high (Table 34–2). The largest was the Multicenter Study,[S2] and since this was the best controlled, these data will be reviewed in some detail.

Multicenter Study

Sensitivity, Specificity, and Accuracy

The Multicenter Study showed 93.4 percent sensitivity, 88.9 percent specificity, and 92.1 percent accuracy in assessing bypass graft patency. It also showed that technically successful examinations could be performed in 94.2 percent of patients for whom the study was requested.

Table 34–2. ULTRAFAST COMPUTED TOMOGRAPHY IN CORONARY BYPASS GRAFT PATENCY

Reference	No. of Grafts	Sensitivity* (%)	Specificity* (%)
Stanford et al.[S2]†	127	93	89
Bateman et al.[B2]	39	95	86
Bateman et al.[B3]‡	80	96	97
Stanford et al.[S3]	21	94	100

*Compared with angiography.
†11 internal mammary artery grafts.
‡15 internal mammary artery grafts.
(From Stanford, W., Brundage, B. H., MacMillan, R., et al.: Sensitivity and specificity of assessing coronary bypass graft patency with ultrafast computed tomography: Results of a multicenter study. J. Am. Coll. Cardiol. 12:1, 1988. Reprinted with permission of the American College of Cardiology.)

When assessment of graft patency by ultrafast computed tomography was evaluated on a per-patient instead of a per-graft basis, the study showed that patency of all grafts was determined correctly in 52 of 62 patients (84 percent). In 9 of 62 patients (14.5 percent) there was one error, and in 1 of 62 patients (1.6 percent) there were two errors.

Assessment of Internal Mammary Artery Versus Vein Bypass Graft Patency With Ultrafast Computed Tomography

Internal mammary artery conduits are smaller in diameter and more likely to be associated with significant numbers of surgical clips, which produce imaging artifacts and obscure patent grafts. For these reasons, it was postulated that the sensitivity, specificity, and accuracy of determining conduit patency with ultrafast computed tomography would not be as high for internal mammary implants as for vein bypass grafts. Clinical studies have not supported this postulate. In the two studies that have addressed this issue[B3, S2] the sensitivity, specificity, and accuracy of ultrafast computed tomography in determining internal mammary and vein graft patency have not been significantly different (Fig. 34–3).

Assessment of Stenotic Versus Open Bypass Graft Patency With Ultrafast Computed Tomography

Grafts with obstructions are sometimes less well opacified than are open conduits. Hence, it is possible that ultrafast CT detection

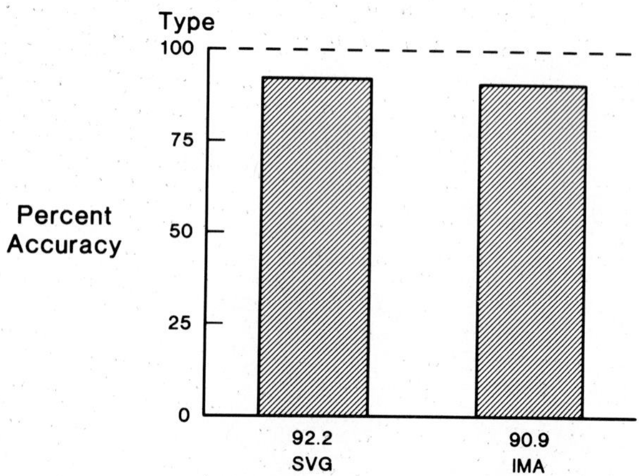

Figure 34–3. Comparison of interpretive accuracies for saphenous vein (SVG) versus internal mammary artery (IMA) grafts. The results were not significantly different. (Data from Stanford, W., Brundage, B. H., MacMillan, R., et al.: Sensitivity and specificity of assessing coronary bypass graft patency with ultrafast computed tomography: results of a multicenter study. J. Am. Coll. Cardiol. 12:1, 1988.)

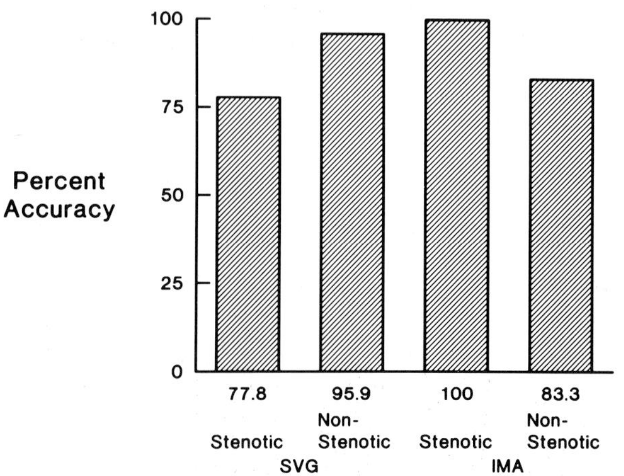

Figure 34–4. Comparison of interpretive accuracies for stenotic versus open saphenous vein grafts (SVG) and internal mammary artery (IMA) grafts. The results were not significantly different. (Data from Stanford, W., Brundage, B. H., MacMillan, R., et al.: Sensitivity and specificity of assessing coronary bypass graft patency with ultrafast computed tomography: results of a multicenter study. J. Am. Coll. Cardiol. 12:1, 1988.)

of patent but partially obstructed grafts would be more difficult than that of widely patent grafts. In a small group of patients,[52] the sensitivities of detecting open grafts with or without obstructive lesions were similar (Fig. 34–4). It is possible, however, that if a larger group of patients were examined and if this population included grafts with very severe obstructions, visualization of such conduits with ultrafast computed tomography might be less successful. Nonetheless, it is important to understand that graft visualization provides no information about the presence of an obstruction or about the distal coronary bed (runoff).

Effect of the Number of Grafts on Accuracy of Determining Bypass Graft Patency With Ultrafast Computed Tomography

One might expect that the detection of patency of all grafts in patients with up to five separate conduits might be more difficult than that in patients with fewer conduits. The data from the Multicenter Study suggest, however, that the number of grafts did not influence the accuracy of the examination (Fig. 34–5).

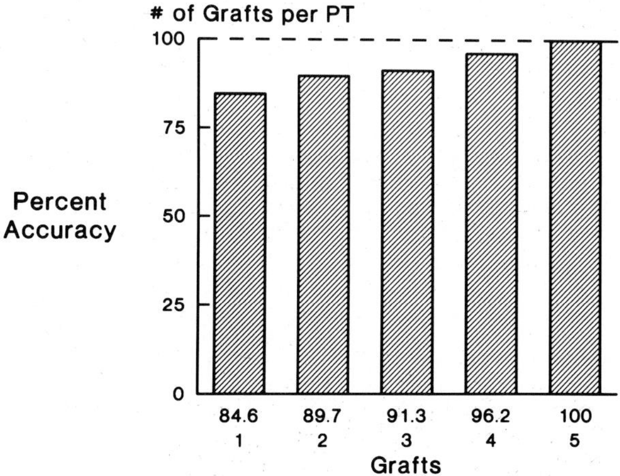

Figure 34–5. Comparison of interpretive accuracy per number of grafts placed. The results were not significantly different. (Data from Stanford, W., Brundage, B. H., MacMillan, R., et al.: Sensitivity and specificity of assessing coronary bypass graft patency with ultrafast computed tomography: results of a multicenter study. J. Am. Coll. Cardiol. 12:1, 1988.)

Interobserver and Intraobserver Variability

One study has examined interobserver and intraobserver variability for determining bypass graft patency in patients studied by ultrafast computed tomography.[52] Interobserver variability was 5.8 percent and intraobserver variability was 8.6 percent. Until interobserver and intraobserver variability are improved, the determination of bypass graft patency with ultrafast computed tomography will remain an imperfect diagnostic procedure.

Pitfalls Associated With Assessment of Bypass Graft Patency With Ultrafast Computed Tomography

Even though determination of bypass graft patency with ultrafast computed tomography is remarkably accurate, there are several patient-related and procedural problems that may result in errors. Fortunately, many of them are avoidable.

Patient-related problems include movement (which often leads to gaps between the tomographic slices), excessive size (greater than 120 kg), and rapid breathing. These all impair image quality. If patients are imaged in the early postoperative period (less than 3 weeks after bypass graft surgery), residual mediastinal hematoma is frequently present and may interfere with graft visualization. Ideally, the definitive studies of bypass graft patency with ultrafast computed tomography should be delayed until 6 weeks postoperatively, at which time the mediastinal hematoma will have resolved and the patients are sufficiently recovered to be able to take a deep breath and to breath-hold during image acquisition.

Other problems that adversely affect ultrafast CT studies of bypass graft patency are limited venous access, which may result in administration of inadequate contrast agent, and prolonged circulation times due to either congestive heart failure or valvular insufficiency. Prolonged circulation times can make timing of the image acquisition less than ideal. Lastly, the "shepherd's crook" deformity of the proximal right coronary artery (Fig. 34–6) and structures such as surgical clips and calcium can foster errors in interpretation. In patients with a shepherd's crook deformity of the right coronary artery, the tomographic image can simulate the cross section of a patent graft adjacent to the right coronary artery when, in fact, both structures are segments of the proximal native right coronary artery that has looped up and out of the imaging plane. Additional interpretive problems include surgical clips and calcium, which can produce artifacts, obscure adjacent opacified bypass grafts, and simulate open grafts as they come in and out of the imaging plane in synchrony with the aortic opacification.

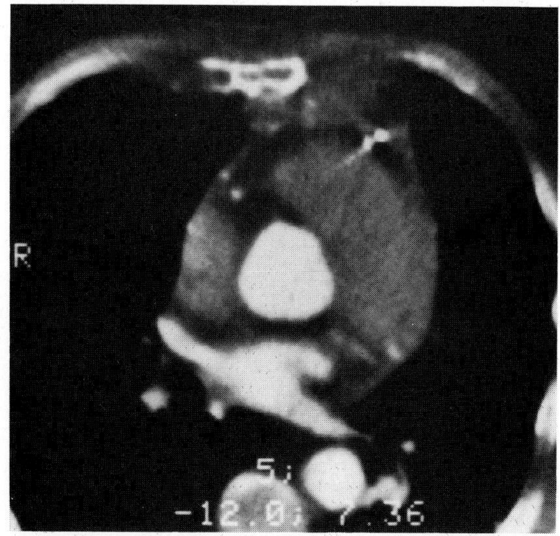

Figure 34–6. "Shepherd's crook" deformity of native right coronary artery simulating a patent saphenous vein graft. For explanation see text.

Procedure-related problems include errors in following established protocols and inadequate knowledge of the details of the operative procedure. These can lead to mistakes in defining the correct imaging protocol. Finally, the quality of the images must be carefully maintained.

This relatively lengthy list of potential pitfalls indicates that best results with this diagnostic procedure, as with all diagnostic tests, will be obtained when a well-trained team of physicians and technologists perform the tests in a very careful, thoughtful manner.

BYPASS GRAFT FLOW RATE

Ultrafast computed tomography, in addition to assessing bypass graft patency, can determine the flow rates of individual grafts if accurate measurements of the conduit diameter and contrast transit times can be obtained. Whiting and associates have suggested this approach.[W3]

There are many problems in interpreting these data even when the procedure is performed accurately. First, the determination of the transit times is limited by the constraints of the image acquisition procedure (typically one frame every one to two cardiac cycles) and by the memory of the C-100 ultrafast computed tomographic scanner (currently 80 frames). As a consequence, flow rates can be obtained only under control conditions and not during maximal coronary dilation. Second, the flow rate in a normal or partially obstructed graft is determined by several variables including the graft perfusion field, viability of the perfused myocardium, metabolic requirements of the myocardium, gain in autoregulation if an obstruction is present, and status of the coronary vasculature distal to the site of graft placement. As a consequence, the range of "normal" graft flow rates is very broad and only extreme deviations may be indicative of graft obstruction.

BYPASS GRAFT FLOW RESERVE

Determination of flow reserve—the difference between control and maximal flow in the conduit system—represents a different approach to assessing the presence of obstruction in a bypass graft or its distal coronary vasculature. Rumberger and associates[R1] suggested an approach to measuring bypass flow reserve that depends on comparison of the arrival time of a bolus of contrast agent in the aorta with the arrival time in a bypass graft. Studies in dogs have shown that there is a close relationship between the ultrafast CT estimates of bypass flow reserve and directly measured flow reserve.[R2] However, when such data are examined across a large number of measurements in many animals, although a significant relationship exists between ultrafast CT and direct measurement flow reserve, there is considerable scatter in the data. Furthermore, attempts to apply this approach to patients have not been extremely successful. Thus, although this approach is potentially promising, additional studies will be necessary before it can be recommended as a useful clinical diagnostic procedure.

ASSESSMENT OF BYPASS GRAFT PATENCY BY ULTRAFAST COMPUTED TOMOGRAPHY VERSUS OTHER IMAGING MODALITIES

At present, assessment with ultrafast computed tomography is the most successful noninvasive procedure for evaluating bypass graft patency. It is far more accurate than conventional noninvasive approaches such as thallium-201 scintigraphy,[S4] electrocardiography during treadmill exercise,[D2] or exercise radionuclide ventriculography.[L1] Magnetic resonance imaging shows considerable promise[W4, W5] in the evaluation of bypass graft patency, but this imaging technique is not currently as accurate as ultrafast computed tomography.

SUMMARY

The assessment of bypass graft patency with ultrafast computed tomography is a significant advance in the noninvasive evaluation of patients after bypass surgery. However, until stenotic and open grafts can be effectively separated on the basis of ultrafast CT flow studies, the interpretation of bypass graft patency with this technique will have to be tempered by the knowledge that both obstructive and open grafts may have a similar appearance. Finally, one must be aware that an open conduit as visualized with ultrafast computed tomography does not provide information about the flow and about the patency of distal anastomoses in cases of sequential grafts.

References

B

1. Brundage, B. H., Lipton, M. J., Herfkens, R. J., et al.: Detection of patent coronary bypass grafts by computed tomography. A preliminary report. Circulation 61:826, 1980.
2. Bateman, T. M., Gray, R. J., Whiting, J. S., et al.: Cine computed tomographic evaluation of aortocoronary bypass graft patency. J. Am. Coll. Cardiol. 8:693, 1986.
3. Bateman, T. M., Gray, R. J., Whiting, J. S., et al.: Prospective evaluation of ultrafast cardiac computed tomography for determination of coronary bypass graft patency. Circulation 75:1018, 1987.

C

1. Califf, R. M., Harrell, F. E., Lee, K. L., et al.: The evaluation of medical and surgical therapy for coronary artery disease. A 15-year perspective. JAMA 261:2077, 1989.
2. Chomka, E. V., Wolfkiel, C. J., and Brundage, B. H.: Indocyanine green ear densitometry to predict left ventricular contrast enhancement during ultrafast computed tomography. (Abstract.) Clin. Res. 34:289, 1986.

D

1. Daniel, W. G., Dohring, W., Stender, H.-S., and Lichtlen, P. R.: Value and limitations of computed tomography in assessing aortocoronary bypass graft patency. Circulation 67:983, 1983.
2. Dodek, A., Kassebaum, D. G., and Griswold, H. E.: Stress electrocardiography in the evaluation of aortocoronary bypass surgery. Am. Heart J. 86:292, 1973.

F

1. Favaloro, R. G.: Saphenous vein autograft replacement of severe segmental coronary artery occlusion. Operative technique. Ann. Thorac. Surg. 5:334, 1968.
2. Foster, C. J., Sekiya, T., Brownlee, W. C., and Isherwood, I.: Computed tomographic assessment of coronary artery bypass grafts. Br. Heart J. 52:24, 1984.

G

1. Godwin, J. D., Califf, R. M., Korobkin, M., et al.: Clinical value of coronary bypass evaluation with CT. AJR 140:649, 1983.

H

1. Hounsfield, G. N.: A method of an apparatus for examination of the body by radiation such as X or gamma radiation. British Patent No. 1283915, 1972. Referenced in: Moss, A. A., Gamsu, G., and Genat, H. K.: Computed Tomography of the Body. W. B. Saunders, Philadelphia, 1983, p. 20.

K

1. Kahl, F. R., Wolfman, N. T., and Watts, L. E.: Evaluation of aortocoronary bypass graft status by computed tomography. Am. J. Cardiol. 48:304, 1981.
2. Kawasuji, M., Aoyama, T., Iwa, T., and Suzuki, M.: Noninvasive evaluation of aortocoronary bypass graft patency by contrast-enhanced computed tomography: Incrementation mode and dynamic mode. Jpn. Circ. J. 48:611, 1984.

L

1. Lewis, R. L., Videll, J. S., Strong, M. D., et al.: Exercise radionuclide assessment of left ventricular function before and after coronary bypass surgery. Angiology 38:601, 1987.

M

1. McLemore, T., and DeLozier, J.: 1985 summary: National ambulatory medical care survey. Natl. Center Health Statistics 128:1, 1987.

2. Moncada, R., Salinas, M., Churchill, R., et al.: Patency of saphenous aortocoronary-bypass grafts demonstrated by computed tomography. N. Engl. J. Med. 303:503, 1980.

R

1. Rumberger, J. A., Feiring, A. J., Hiratzka, L. F., et al.: Quantification of coronary artery bypass flow reserve in dogs using cine-computed tomography. Circ. Res. 61(Suppl. II):117, 1987.
2. Rumberger, J. A., Feiring, A. J., Hiratzka, L. F., et al.: Quantitation of coronary artery bypass graft flow rates in dogs using ultrafast computed tomography: Preliminary observations. Am. J. Cardiac Imag. 2:194, 1988.

S

1. Stanford, W., Skorton, D., Marcus, M., and Behrendt, D.: Newer imaging modalities in evaluating aortocoronary bypass graft patency: MRI, CT, digital subtraction angiography and Doppler ultrasound. (Abstract.) International Congress of Radiology, July 1989.
2. Stanford, W., Brundage, B. H., MacMillan, R., et al.: Sensitivity and specificity of assessing coronary bypass graft patency with ultrafast computed tomography: Results of a multicenter study. J. Am. Coll. Cardiol. 12:1, 1988.
3. Stanford, W., Rooholamini, M., Rumberger, J., and Marcus, M.: Evaluation of coronary bypass graft patency by ultrafast computed tomography. J. Thorac. Imag. 3:52, 1988.
4. Starling, M. R., Walsh, R. A., Dehmer, G. J., et al.: Value of tomographic thallium-201 imaging in patients with chest pain following coronary artery bypass grafting. Clin. Nucl. Med. 12:134, 1987.

W

1. Winslow, C. M., Kosecoff, J. B., Chassin, M., et al.: The appropriateness of performing coronary artery bypass surgery. JAMA 260:505, 1988.
2. Wilson, P. C., Gutierrez, O., and Moss, A.: Early evaluation of coronary artery bypass grafts: CT or selective angiography. Eur. J. Radiol. 4:22, 1984.
3. Whiting, J. S., Bateman, T. M., Sethna, D. H., and Forrester, J. S.: Quantitation of saphenous vein bypass graft flow using intravenous contrast cine CT. (Abstract.) Circ. Suppl. II 74:II-41, 1986.
4. White, R. D., Caputo, G. R., Mark, A. S., et al.: Coronary artery bypass graft patency: Noninvasive evaluation with MR imaging. Radiology 164:681, 1987.

Chapter 35

Measurement of Myocardial Perfusion Using Fast Computed Tomography

■ *JOHN A. RUMBERGER, M.D., Ph.D.*
■ *MALCOLM R. BELL, M.B.B.S.* ■ *ANDREW J. FEIRING, M.D.*
■ *THOMAS BEHRENBECK, M.D., Ph.D.* ■ *MELVIN L. MARCUS, M.D.*
■ *ERIK L. RITMAN, M.D., Ph.D.*

FAST COMPUTED TOMOGRAPHIC SCANNERS 689
THEORETICAL CONSIDERATIONS 689
Historical Aspects of Indicator Dilution Methods 689
Assumptions of Indicator Dilution Theory as Applied to Computed Tomography 689
Assumption 1: Complete Mixing of the Indicator 689
Assumption 2: The Volume of Indicator Injected Is Negligible 689
Assumption 3: The Indicator Does Not Perturb Hemodynamic and Vascular Equilibrium 690
Assumption 4: No Extravascular Loss of Indicator 690
Assumption 5: Indicator Recirculation Can Be Ignored 690
Assumption 6: Appropriate Coronary Input Function 690
Assumption 7: Contrast Density Can Be Accurately Measured 691
Derivation of Basic Flow Algorithm 691
INITIAL STUDIES USING INTRAVENOUS CONTRAST INJECTION 692
In Vitro Studies 692
In Vivo Studies 692
Studies in Animals 692
Studies in Patients 694
Questions Raised From Initial Intravenous Studies 695
IMAGING AND RECONSTRUCTION ARTIFACTS 695
Scanner-Related and Patient-Related Artifacts 695
Volume-Averaging Artifacts 696
Beam Hardening and Photon Scatter 696
REGIONAL INTRAMYOCARDIAL VASCULAR VOLUME 698
KINETICS OF THE INPUT FUNCTION TO THE MYOCARDIUM 699
REGIONAL TRANSFER FUNCTION 700
SUMMARY AND CONCLUSIONS 700

Routine clinical quantitation of regional myocardial perfusion by a safe, reliable, repeatable, and accurate method should significantly aid in the diagnosis and assessment of therapy in patients with cardiac disease. Perhaps most notable in this regard would be the patient with suspected or known coronary heart disease. In such patients, for instance, the physiological significance of coronary artery stenoses could be quantitated from the regional flow reserve.[M1] This would provide a firm foundation for the need (or lack of need) to identify coronary anatomy via selective angiography or direct future therapeutic options (percutaneous transluminal coronary angioplasty [PTCA], bypass grafting, pharmacologic manipulations) in situations in which coronary anatomy is already known.

Two general methods may be applied to studies of coronary/myocardial blood flow in humans: direct measurement techniques and indicator dilution techniques. Direct techniques are invasive and require either selective cardiac catheterization or coronary flow determination during cardiac surgery. Examples of direct measurement techniques include application of a Doppler ultrasonic probe[M1, W1] and the electromagnetic flowmeter.[M2, M3]

Indicator dilution techniques can be divided into internal and external detection methods. Internal detection techniques include coronary sinus thermodilution[G1]; external techniques include thallium scintigraphy,[R1, R2] two-dimensional echocardiography[F1] (qualitative, at present), inert gas clearance,[C1, K1] digital subtraction angiography,[D1, V1] positron emission tomography (PET),[S1, W2] and high-speed (or fast) computed tomography.[G2, R3, R4, W3–W5] Of these techniques, thallium scintigraphy, positron emission tomography, and fast computed tomography do not require direct cardiac catheterization and thus share the potential for widespread determination of regional myocardial perfusion in outpatients. Thallium scintigraphy is routinely employed for the evaluation of regional myocardial flow distribution in patients with coronary heart disease but offers only a qualitative assessment with limited applicability to patients with triple-vessel disease or extensive prior infarction. Positron emission tomography requires assessment of regional uptake kinetics and partition coefficients for diffusible indicators, and computed tomography assesses flow by classical indicator transit kinetics. Only the latter two techniques promise to quantitate absolute regional myocardial perfusion noninvasively.

Thallium scintigraphy and positron emission tomography are

discussed in detail in other chapters of this book. This chapter explores the application of indicator dilution techniques to fast computed tomography (CT) and discusses studies in which this external detection method has been used to quantitate regional myocardial perfusion. As the technique is discussed, the promise of its application to humans and the potential pitfalls or limitations of this application will be specifically examined.

FAST COMPUTED TOMOGRAPHIC SCANNERS

Most of the studies discussed were performed with the ultrafast CT scanner designed by Boyd and associates.[B1] This fourth-generation instrument has no moving parts aside from the couch for the patient. Tomographic images are obtained by magnetic deflection of an electron beam swept rapidly across one of four semicircular (210 degree) tungsten targets that surround the subject. Tomographic images are 0.8 cm thick and are acquired in 0.050 seconds. Up to 80 scans can be taken in rapid sequence. Electrocardiographic triggering at a designated time during each cardiac cycle (nominally one every other QRS) allows stop-action scans to be obtained as indicator (iodinated contrast agent) traverses the left ventricular cavity, proximal aorta, and myocardium. Sophisticated off-line image analysis software allows evaluation of arterial (input) and myocardial (response) indicator transit curves within any operator-defined tomographic region of interest. The rest of the studies discussed were done with the Dynamic Spatial Reconstructor (DSR) at the Mayo Clinic. This unique high-speed CT instrument allows simultaneous volumetric imaging of the heart, as described elsewhere.[R5]

THEORETICAL CONSIDERATIONS

Historical Aspects of Indicator Dilution Methods

The earliest report of use of an indicator to determine circulation times in vivo was that of Haller (cited in Dow[D1]), who, in 1761, reported injection of a colored liquid into the vena cava of an animal to compare pulmonary circulation times through inflated versus collapsed lungs. However, it is Stewart[52–54] who must be credited with applying the indicator dilution technique to determination of cardiac output and the "central blood volume." In addition, he devised the first method for continuous detection of indicator (hypertonic saline) concentration at the sampling site.

Henriques[H1] in 1913 used sodium thiocyanate as an indicator because it was easily quantitated colorimetrically and was the first to note failure of the downslope of the dilution curve to return to baseline in the systemic circulation and the presence of indicator recirculation. He also devised a method for measuring coronary blood flow by simultaneously injecting different indicators into two different sites in the systemic circulation. Koch[K2] first applied indicator dilution principles to measurements in humans, using fluorescein as an indicator. Blumgart and Yens[B2] in 1927 reported the first application of external detection methods involving radioactive tracers, and their work was considered to be the stimulus[D1] for the numerous studies reported thereafter from Hamilton's laboratory.

Hamilton and associates[H2, M4] extended the original work of Stewart by using a sudden, single injection of indicator. They subsequently increased the overall accuracy of the method for determining cardiac output by extracting the contribution of recirculated indicator through semilogarithmic replotting and linear extrapolation of the downslope of the original curve recorded in the systemic circulation. This landmark contribution cannot be overemphasized and amply justifies the application of the name "Steward-Hamilton technique" to classical indicator dilution theory. However, Meier and Zierler[M5, Z1] must be credited with presenting an organized and mathematically sound theory for the general application of indicator dilution concepts to estimation of physiological flows.

Prinzmetal and associates[P1, P2] were the first to provide for ready application of external detection techniques to measurements of cardiac flow in humans, employing radioactive tracers and a technique termed "angiocardiography." Additional data were obtained with external detection methods at the Mayo Clinic laboratories of E. H. Wood,[K3, W6] who employed an ear oximeter to evaluate continuously the concentration of methylene blue in blood. These studies were the first to describe the systemic patterns of circulation for an indicator in the presence of right-to-left and left-to-right shunting compared with the normal intact circulation. Henley and associates[H3] used iodinated serum albumin to make the first measurements of myocardial blood flow in intact dogs, but Love and Burch[L1] and Nolting and associates[N1] first reported the use of external counting methods for measurements of coronary blood flow with radioactive rubidium. These foundations underlie the future developments of thallium scintigraphy (thallium is a potassium analog with a distribution similar to that of rubidium) and PET. It is apparent from the foregoing discussion that indicator dilution methods were developed and widely applied to the calculation of cardiac flow phenomena 30 to 50 years ago.

A general discussion of computed tomography is beyond the scope of this review; however, the principle of the technique is that the Hounsfield "density"[H4] of any object or field within the tomogram is directly proportional to the true roentgen attenuation coefficient of tissue within that area. Use of iodinated contrast agent as a marker for the passage of blood allows ready discrimination of blood vessels from tissue and of the flow of blood across any designated perfusion field. The magnitude of the change in contrast density and the time course of these changes through a region of interest within the tomogram provide a relative index of blood flow and perfusion through direct application of the indicator dilution methods. Computed tomography, as an external dilution device, can be extended to quantitation of tissue perfusion, as will be discussed subsequently.

Assumptions of Indicator Dilution Theory as Applied to Computed Tomography

The general assumptions of classic indicator dilution theory extended to the application of external detection techniques were first discussed by Newman and associates in 1951.[N2] These assumptions, as modified and discussed below, also bear directly on the application of the CT method to analysis of contrast clearance data from the myocardium. The indicator in this instance is iodinated contrast medium.

Assumption 1: Complete Mixing of the Indicator

When applied to the CT measurement of myocardial blood flow by use of an intravenous injection of contrast medium, the assumption that the indicator is well mixed with the blood is generally true because it will have traversed at least two cardiac mixing chambers (right and left ventricles) prior to entry into the coronary ostia. For central (aortic root) injection, this assumption is less secure, since the contrast medium would not have entered a true mixing chamber; however, external sampling of arterial input from the coronary ostia should provide an accurate characterization of the input to the myocardium. Incomplete mixing will lead to erroneous values for regional myocardial perfusion, but the magnitude of error introduced is unknown. Implicit in the assumption of complete mixing of the indicator with the blood is that the distribution volume of the indicator is identical to the distribution volume of blood.

Assumption 2: The Volume of Indicator Injected Is Negligible

In practice, for intravenous (and presumably systemic) injection routes, the amount of contrast agent required per study is between 0.5 and 1.0 ml/kg.[G2, R3, R4, W5] This volume is negligible compared to the central circulating blood volume (or total volume of distribution). Roughly 5 percent of this injected volume enters the coronary circulation, and this amount (0.025–0.05 ml/kg) can be assumed to be negligible compared to the total intramyocardial vascular volume (see discussion related to intramyocardial vascular blood volume).

Assumption 3: The Indicator Does Not Perturb Hemodynamic and Vascular Equilibrium

Measurements of regional myocardial perfusion with high-speed computed tomography are made by sampling contrast clearance data during the first pass of the indicator through the system; this also requires that the flow be at a steady state at least during the determination. This requirement mandates not only that the baseline hemodynamics remain invariate during the passage of the indicator but also that the volume of distribution of the indicator (vascular or blood volume) remains constant during the measurement.

Intravascular administration of conventional ionic contrast agents such as meglumine sodium diatrizoate is associated with a variety of significant hemodynamic perturbations that may occur within seconds of the injection. Thus, myocardial flow and vascular volume could be dynamically changing during the first pass of such an indicator, violating assumption 3. However, studies in which the newer nonionic contrast agents were compared directly with conventional agents have demonstrated little or no change in coronary flow or systemic hemodynamics following intravenous administration, as shown in Figure 35–1.[R3, R6] In this canine study, left ventricular pressure, coronary flow velocity (Doppler velocimetry[M1]), and the first derivative of the left ventricular pressure (dP/dt) were measured following rapid intravenous administration of an ionic contrast agent (meglumine sodium diatrizoate, Renografin-76, 370 mg I/ml) and a nonionic contrast agent (Iohexol, 350 mg I/ml) (1 ml/kg over 3 seconds). Significant changes in systemic and coronary hemodynamics were seen within a few seconds after injection of the ionic agent but not after injection of the nonionic agent. Nonionic contrast agents are the indicators of choice for studies of regional myocardial perfusion with high-speed computed tomography.

Assumption 4: No Extravascular Loss of Indicator

It is known that iodinated contrast medium has both an intravascular and an extravascular volume of distribution. However, several studies have shown that during the first pass the contrast agent remains primarily (95 percent) intravascular.[N3, N4] Since first-pass regional indicator contrast clearance curves are used in the determination of regional myocardial perfusion by high-speed computed tomography, the minimal extravascular loss of contrast agent during this time does not appear to be a significant problem.

Assumption 5: Indicator Recirculation Can Be Ignored

Recirculation of indicator occurs in the intact, closed circulation and is routinely observed in contrast clearance data for both the central circulation and the myocardium obtained with fast computed tomography. However, in most cases the "recirculation" peak can be eliminated directly from the final analysis either by semilogarithmic extrapolation of the wash-out portion of the curve or by application of a gamma variate curve fit[T1] to the rising, peak, and initial falling portions of the measured regional indicator dilution curve.

Assumption 6: Appropriate Coronary Input Function

This assumption is related to the overall shape and character of the indicator input function to the coronary ostia. The nature of this assumption has far-reaching implications and may underlie one of the pitfalls of the CT technique with respect to application across the entire physiologic range of values for myocardial perfusion.

Intravenous contrast agent cannot be administered as an ideal bolus (or impulse function) input. The contrast agent must be given sufficiently rapidly to avoid overlap with recirculation but at a rate that does not alter the subsequent characteristics of the coronary (aortic root) input function. Burbank and associates[B3] have shown that characteristics of intra-aortic digital subtraction contrast clearance curves (such as mean transit time and peak

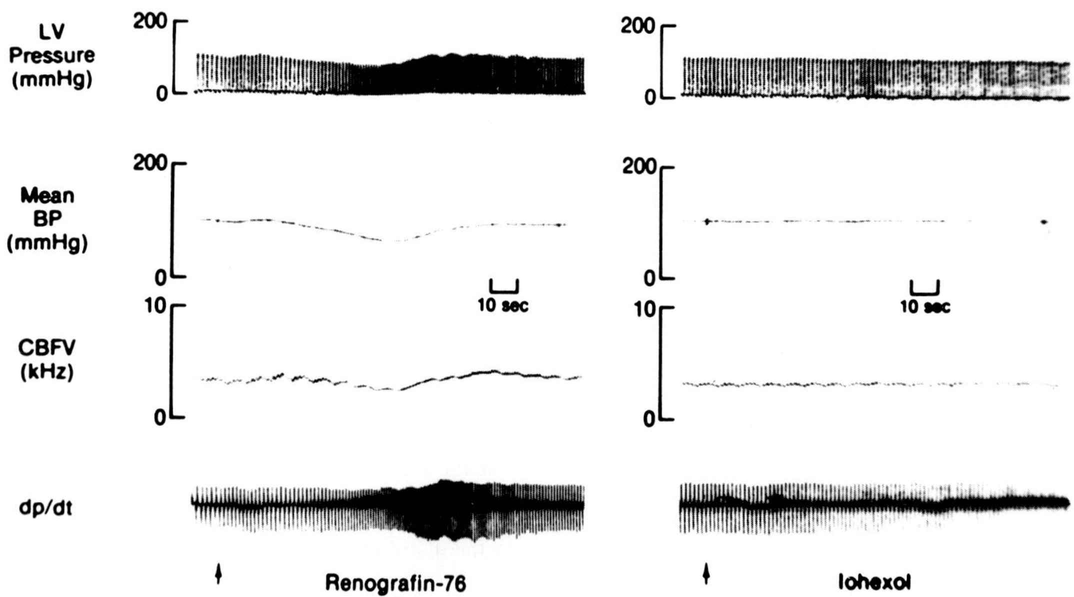

Figure 35–1. Canine study demonstrating high-fidelity left ventricular (LV) pressure, mean aortic pressure, coronary blood flow velocity (CBFV, Doppler probe), and dP/dt following injection of iodinated contrast agent into the inferior vena cava (1 ml/kg over 3 seconds). *(Left)* Results after injection of conventional ionic contrast agent (Renografin-76); *(right)* results after injection of nonionic contrast agent (Iohexol-350). Note the significant changes seen following injection of ionic contrast agent, whereas no change in systemic hemodynamics is noted following injection of nonionic contrast agent. (From Rumberger, J. A., Feiring, A. J., and Lipton, M. J.: Use of ultrafast computed tomography to quantitate regional myocardial perfusion: A preliminary report. J. Am. Coll. Cardiol. 9:59, 1987. Reprinted with permission of the American College of Cardiology.)

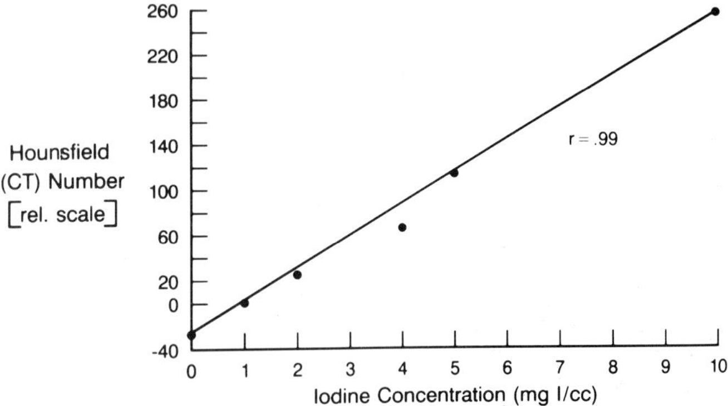

Figure 35–2. Study in a phantom with fast computed tomography comparing iodine concentration with Hounsfield (CT) number above baseline. This demonstrates the linear system response and the use of CT values (relative scale *above* baseline) to substitute for videodensitometric values to define flow phenomena following injection of iodinated contrast agent.

opacification) following intravenous administration of contrast agent are not altered, provided that the injection time is less than one-half the subsequent aortic mean transit time. Contrast injection times of 3 seconds or less in the central venous circulation in the dog probably satisfy this requirement (see later). Tacit in this assumption, however, for application to studies of myocardial perfusion, is that the mean transit time of the indicator through the vascular or tissue volume is greater than the mean transit time for the indicator input function to that vascular or tissue space. The potential limitations of the intravenous injection method for this application are discussed in a later section.

Assumption 7: Contrast Density Can Be Accurately Measured

This assumption requires that the CT device (acting as an external videodensitometer) accurately record the time-dependent contrast densities from baseline across a defined dynamic range. The assumption mandates that the system response be known and that imaging artifacts be minimal. Under certain conditions, this assumption may not be completely satisfied (see later section on imaging artifacts), although in most instances fast computed tomography provides a reliable and linear system response for subsequent CT density values across the range of contrast concentrations generally used in vivo (Fig. 35–2).

Derivation of the Basic Flow Algorithm

Classical indicator dilution theory (Stewart-Hamilton principle), as elegantly described by Meier and Zierler,[M5, Z1] denotes the absolute flow rate in the central systemic circulation (or forward cardiac output from the left ventricle), F_{LV}, as the ratio of the absolute amount of indicator injected into that vascular volume, q, to the area under the indicator clearance curve in the systemic circulation, A_{LV} (the subscript LV designates the left ventricular cavity, but the same concept holds true for the central aorta). Thus:

$$F_{LV} = q/A_{LV} \tag{1}$$

Figure 35–3 is a schematic of the left ventricular cavity/aorta/coronary artery system. Here K = a + b + c, where K is the *fraction* of total indicator injected, q, that enters the coronary system from the input (left ventricular cavity). Thus q*a, q*b, and q*c represent the amounts of indicator delivered to the three major coronary branches individually, as illustrated. However, the amount of indicator delivered to the coronary system (K*q) remains small compared to q itself—that is, the fraction of total indicator delivered to the coronary system is much less than the amount of indicator remaining in the aorta (i.e., $q - K^*q) \simeq q$).

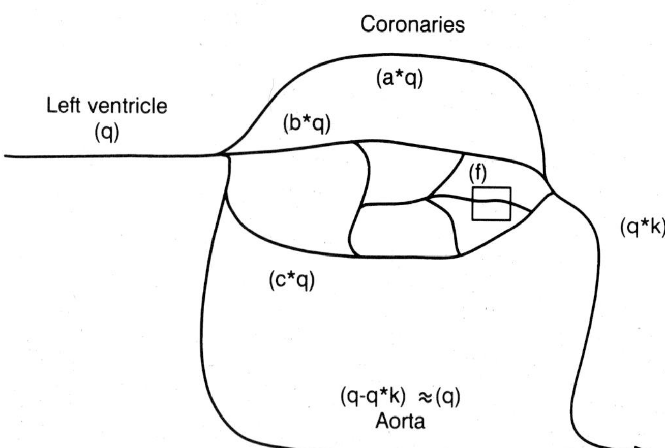

Figure 35–3. Schematic illustration of coronary artery/aorta system. Note that the portion of contrast entering the coronary system (k) is only a small portion of the total amount injected at the source (q). The portions (fractions of k) that enter each coronary artery are designated as a, b, and c. The portion that enters a given myocardial region is designated as f. (From Rumberger, J. A., Feiring, A. J., and Lipton, M. J.: Use of ultrafast computed tomography to quantitate regional myocardial perfusion: A preliminary report. J. Am. Coll. Cardiol. 9:59, 1987. Reprinted with permission of the American College of Cardiology.)

The absolute flow through any coronary artery (or region) is directly proportional to the fraction of total indicator delivered to that region. This underlies the principle initially proposed by Sapirstein[S5] for organ flow and is the basis for the radiolabeled-microsphere technique used experimentally to determine regional organ flow. Therefore,

$$F_a = a^*F_{LV}, \quad F_b = b^*F_{LV}, \quad F_c = c^*F_{LV}$$

By analogy, this should hold true for any "myocardial" region, f. Thus,

$$F_f = f^*F_{LV} \tag{2}$$

where f represents the fraction of total indicator injected (intravenously or systemically) that enters that myocardial region. However, the question remains: What is the value of f?

Figure 35–4 is a schematic of an indicator dilution curve recorded in the systemic circulation after intravenous injection of indicator. For such a curve as recorded, for example, in the left ventricular cavity, the area under the curve can be approximated as[M5]

$$A_{LV} = C_{PH}^*t_A \tag{3}$$

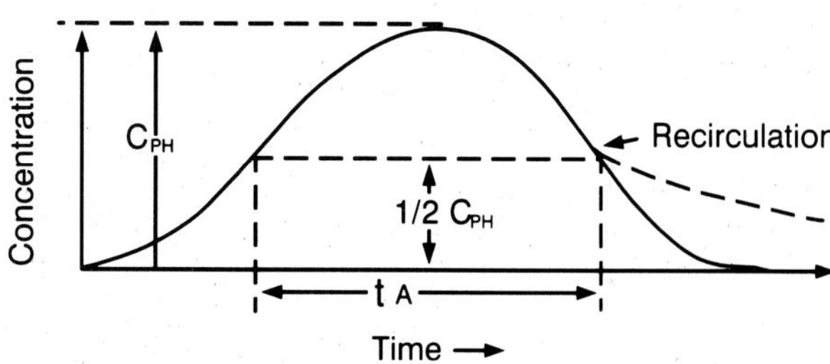

Figure 35–4. Schematic of an indicator dilution curve as recorded in the systemic circulation following an intravenous injection of indicator (iodinated contrast agent). C_{PH}—peak concentration (height) above baseline; t—full width at half-maximum time (see text for details); A—area under the curve. (From Rumberger, J. A., Feiring, A. J., and Lipton, M. J.: Use of ultrafast computed tomography to quantitate regional myocardial perfusion: A preliminary report. J. Am. Coll. Cardiol. 9:59, 1987. Reprinted with permission of the American College of Cardiology.)

Here C_{PH} is the peak indicator concentration (or density above baseline) and t_A is the "full width at half-maximum time" (a characteristic of the time spread of the curve). Both of these parameters are easily and rapidly determined from the curve.

From classical indicator dilution theory,[M5] the following equation is valid:

$$F_{LV}/V_{LV} = 1/MTT_A \quad (4)$$

Here, V_{LV} is the central blood volume (volume of distribution of the indicator) and MTT_A is the "mean transit time" of the indicator dilution curve for an impulse-type input function. The mean transit time is equal to the centroid or first moment of the indicator curve if appearance time and injection time are considered to be simultaneous (i.e., impulse injection at time t = 0). Equation (4) then simply states that the cardiac output per unit distribution (blood) volume is inversely proportional to mean transit time.

Now consider t_A and MTT_A (both of which describe the time spread of the clearance curve) to be related by the nondefined parameter, E_A, as

$$t_A = E_A{*}MTT_A \quad (5)$$

For a true bolus (impulse) type of input function (satisfying assumption 6), t_A is exactly equal to MTT_A.[M5, Z1]

Combining equations (1), (3), (4), and (5):

$$q = C_{PH}{*}V_{LV}{*}E_A \quad (6)$$

By direct analogy, the contrast clearance curve in the myocardium, f, can be described as

$$A_f = C_f{*}t_f \quad (7)$$

Again, by analogy with the equations that describe the indicator kinetics in the systemic circulation and equation (2),

$$f{*}q = C_f{*}V_f{*}E_f \quad (8)$$

Therefore,

$$f = E_f{*}C_f{*}V_f/q \quad (9)$$

Here A_f is the area under the myocardial indicator clearance curve, C_f is a "characteristic" concentration (density above baseline) for the clearance curve (e.g., the "peak concentration" by analogy with the systemic circulation), t_f is the full width at half-maximum time for the myocardial indicator curve, E_f is analogous to E_A but remains undefined at present, and MTT_f is the myocardial (tissue) mean transit time. As before, V_f is the volume of distribution of the indicator in the region (in this case, the myocardium—i.e., the regional myocardial volume), which is unknown a priori.

The flow (absolute) in the myocardial region, f, is given by direct substitution into equation (2) as

$$F_f = C_f{*}E_f{*}V_f{*}F_{LV}/q \quad (10)$$

Combining equation (10) and equation (1),

$$F_f = C_f{*}V_f{*}E_f/A_{LV} \quad (11)$$

Although V_f is not known a priori, the flow per unit volume of myocardium can be given as

$$F_f/V_f = C_f{*}E_f/A_{LV} \quad (12)$$

From the previous discussion, there are two obvious values for C_f (setting E_f = 1.0, i.e., satisfying assumption 6):

$$C_f = A_f/t_f \quad (13)$$

or

$$F_f/V_f = (A_f/A_{LV}){*}1/t_f \quad (14)$$

and

$$C_f = C_{PH} \quad (15)$$

or

$$F_f/V_f = C_{PH}/A_{LV} \quad (16)$$

Here C_{PH} refers to the peak concentration (CT density above baseline) of the indicator dilution curve within the myocardial region f. Equation (14) is the equation put forward by Axel[A1] for studies of regional cerebral perfusion by computed tomography, and equation (14) was employed by Mullani and Gould[M6] for analysis of regional myocardial perfusion with ^{82}Rb.

INITIAL STUDIES USING INTRAVENOUS CONTRAST INJECTION

In Vitro Studies

Limited in vitro (phantom) studies have been performed to evaluate the application of computed tomography to studies of vascular flow. Investigations involving models of the circulation serve several purposes: to test theoretical constructs, to evaluate the dynamic range of the measuring device, and to reveal limitations of the method that are seen even under ideal conditions.

Tonge and associates[T2] and Guthaner and associates[G3] used conventional CT devices (1- to 3-second scan acquisition) for studies of cardiac output and direct application of the Stewart-Hamilton principle; however, the only in vitro (phantom) study of tissue perfusion with fast computed tomography was that of Jaschke and associates.[J1] The flow phantom consisted of a system of tubes used to simulate vessels and a central cylinder packed with small, irregularly shaped plastic parts used to simulate tissue. Saline was pumped into the cylinder via a single tube downstream of a mixing chamber to which the indicator (iodinated contrast agent) was added as a bolus (1 to 3 seconds in duration to simulate intravenous injection techniques). Recirculation of contrast agent was avoided by directing the outflow into a collecting tank. The total volume of the "central" input tubing and the "tissue" equivalent cylinder was fixed and known.

With this injection technique, the mean transit time of the "input" to the tissue equivalent ranged from 6 to 20 seconds. CT scans were performed in the flow mode, and flow within the cylinder (timed collections) ranged from 0.4 to 1.45 L/min. Calculations of regional tissue flow were made with equation (16). The distribution volume, V_f, was known, so absolute flow through the tissue equivalent could be calculated. Results of this study are shown in Figure 35–5. Note that the calculation of flow is very linear over a range of flows that could be expected in vivo in a system such as the coronary arteries. However, the investigators were aware of assumption 6 and therefore kept the input flow rate sufficiently high to allow no outflow of contrast medium from the sampled region prior to complete entry of the indicator from the input.

In Vivo Studies

Studies in Animals

The potential of ultrafast computed tomography to measure regional myocardial perfusion was first reported by Rumberger

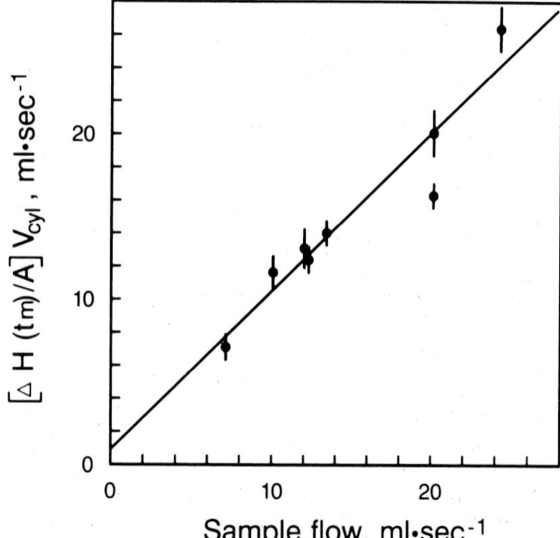

Figure 35–5. Comparison of flow per unit volume in a flow phantom compared to metered flow measurement. This study by Jaschke and associates demonstrates a very linear relationship across an expected physiologic range. In this study the volume of distribution (analogous to vascular volume) was fixed and known. (From Jaschke, W., Gould, R. G., Assimakopoulos, P. A., and Lipton, M. J.: Flow measurements with a high-speed computed tomography scanner. Med. Phys. 14:238, 1987. Reproduced by permission of the American Institute of Physics.)

and associates.[R3] In this study of six dogs, serial CT scans were taken during rapid injection of nonionic contrast agent into the inferior vena cava under resting conditions and various states of myocardial vasodilation (intravenous injection of adenosine). For comparison, regional myocardial perfusion per unit mass was quantitated during simultaneous injection of radiolabeled microspheres via the left atrium.

Figure 35–6 shows a representative example of the time-dependent contrast density data obtained from the left ventricular cavity and myocardium at a resting flow state (left panel) and following coronary vasodilation (right panel). Note that the peak opacification of the left ventricular cavity is significantly greater than that of the adjacent myocardium and that the peak myocardial opacification occurs well after that observed in the left ventricular cavity (left panel). In the right panel, quantitative differences are readily apparent in the peak opacification above baseline, area inscribed by the myocardial time-density curve, and overall contrast transit time of the curves when the high myocardial perfusion state is compared to the resting perfusion state. These observations are consistent with the theoretical considerations previously stated, which indicated that, for values of flow per unit volume above baseline compared to control values, the peak concentration above baseline increases and the mean transit time decreases (equation 16).

A total of 13 scan and microsphere pairs were judged technically adequate for analysis. Absolute regional myocardial perfusion values as assessed by the microsphere technique ranged from 30 to 450 ml/min/100 g (mean 167 ± 125). Regional myocardial flow per unit mass by ultrafast computed tomography was calculated by multiplying the flow per unit by the density of the myocardium (1.05 g/cm³). Individual time-density (contrast clearance) data were displayed simultaneously from the left ventricular cavity and the region of the posterior myocardium for each flow state in each animal. Parameters were derived from the CT studies by use of a gamma variate fit to the data for the left ventricular cavity and myocardium,[T1] calculation of the peak concentrations (CT densities) above baseline, areas under the curves, and the full width at half-maximum transit time for the myocardium.

Calculated myocardial flow per unit mass ranged from 30 to 390 ml/min/100 g (mean 150 ± 140, not significantly different from the microsphere data). A comparison of the regional myocardial flow per unit mass assessed with microspheres (abscissa) and with fast computed tomography (ordinate) is shown in Figure 35–7 as calculated using equation 16. The correlation was statistically significant (r = 0.72, standard error of the estimate = 65 ml/min/100 g, $P < 0.01$).

Wolfkiel and associates[W5] performed a similar study with a group of 16 dogs in which ionic contrast agent was administered from the femoral vein and not the inferior vena cava, but the

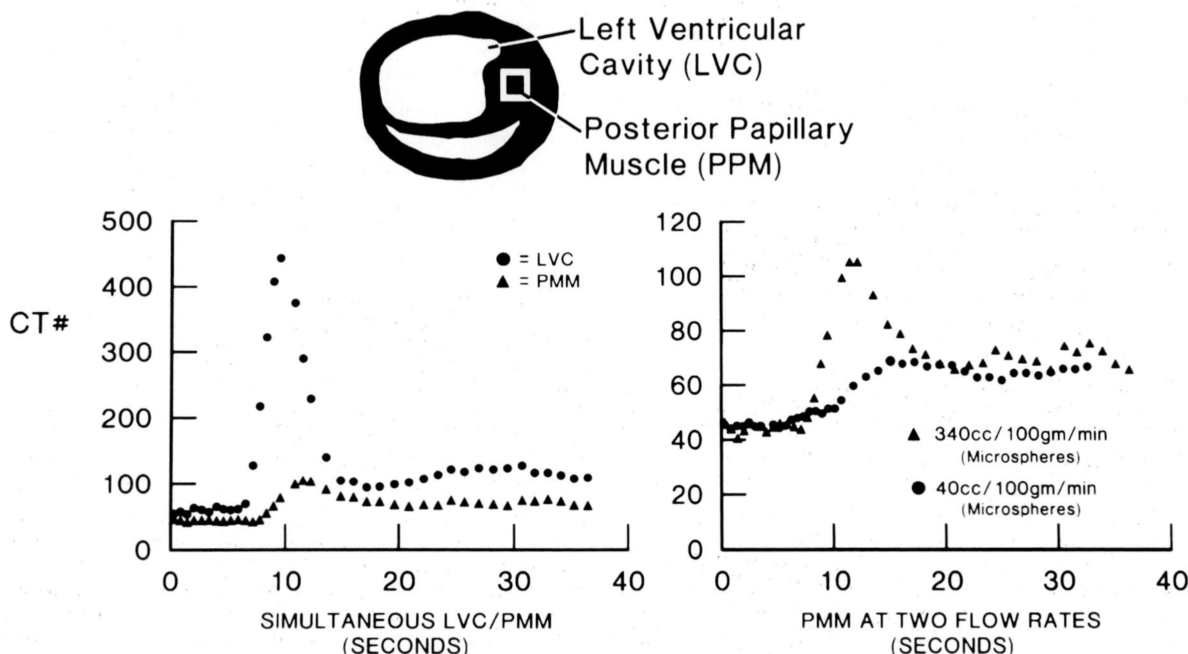

Figure 35–6. *(Top)* Schematic illustration of a cardiac short-axis tomogram in the dog at the posterior papillary muscle area in the mid-left ventricle. *(Left)* Simultaneous indicator (contrast) clearance versus time within the left ventricular cavity (LVC) and posterior myocardial muscle (PPM) regions after bolus inferior vena cava injection of nonionic contrast. *(Right)* Posterior myocardial muscle contrast density versus time from a dog at a high regional myocardial perfusion rate (340 ml/100 g/min) and a low resting perfusion state (40 ml/100 g/min). See text for details. (From Rumberger, J. A., Feiring, A. J., and Lipton, M. J.: Use of ultrafast computed tomography to quantitate regional myocardial perfusion: A preliminary report. J. Am. Coll. Cardiol. 9:59, 1987. Reprinted with permission of the American College of Cardiology.)

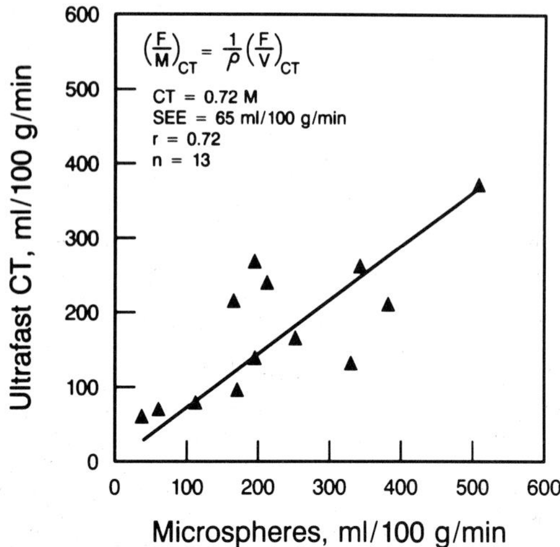

Figure 35–7. Comparison of myocardial perfusion in the posterior papillary muscle region of the dog as assessed with radiolabeled microspheres and fast computed tomography using equation (16); see text for details. A_f—area under contrast clearance curve in the myocardium; A_{LV}—area under contrast clearance curve in the left ventricular cavity; t_f—mean transit time of the contrast clearance curve in the myocardium (full width at half-maximum time, assuming E_f = 1.0; see text).

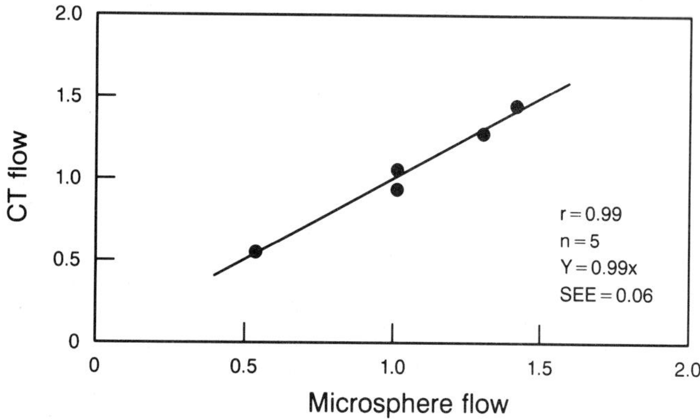

Figure 35–9. Regional myocardial perfusion (flow per unit mass) versus regional perfusion as measured with radiolabeled microspheres in a single dog. Data are from Wolfkiel and associates.[W5] Note the relative linear relationship within a given animal across the range of perfusion values studied. (From Wolfkiel, C. J., Ferguson, J. L., Chomka, E. V., et al.: Measurement of myocardial blood flow by ultrafast computed tomography. Circulation 76:1262, 1987. Reproduced by permission of the American Heart Association, Inc.)

data analysis was performed in a fashion similar to that noted above. Intravenous chromonar was administered to produce variable degrees of coronary vasodilation in 10 dogs, and temporary occlusion of the left anterior descending coronary artery was done prior to scanning in a separate group of 6 dogs. Radiolabeled microspheres again were employed to allow comparison with flow rates calculated from CT results. In this study three separate flow algorithms were evaluated, but the best fit to the microsphere data was obtained with the formulation given by equation (16).

The composite data from this study are shown in Figure 35–8. Note that the calculation of regional flow per unit mass with ultrafast computed tomography is nearly linear from zero up to approximately 150 ml/min/100 g. Above this range, CT estimates of flow significantly underestimated microsphere estimates; in fact, the calculation reached a plateau at the higher flow rates. Data from a single experiment (Fig. 35–9) demonstrated significant accuracy of the technique when applied to an individual; however, in this case the actual flows evaluated were well within the normal resting range (nominally 100 ml/min/100 g) and not above 150 ml/min/100 g.

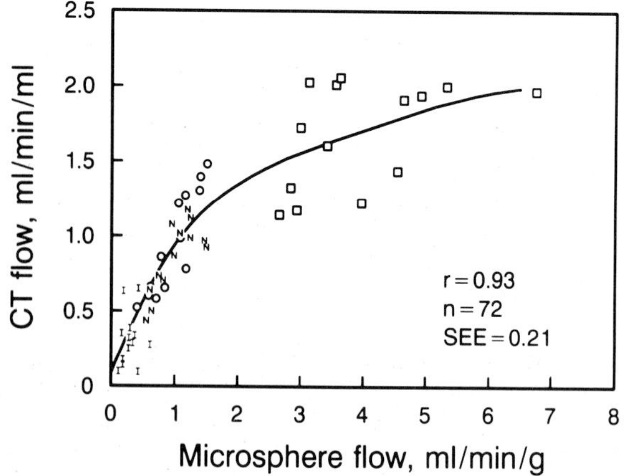

Figure 35–8. Regional myocardial perfusion (flow per unit mass) versus regional perfusion as measured with radiolabeled microspheres in a series of canine experiments. Data are from Wolfkiel and associates.[W5] Femoral vein injection of contrast agent was used. Note the plateau in the relationship at approximately 1.3 ml/g/min (130 ml/100 g/min). The CT calculations were made using equation (14). (From Wolfkiel, C. J., Ferguson, J. L., Chomka, E. V., et al.: Measurement of myocardial blood flow by ultrafast computed tomography. Circulation 76:1262, 1987, with permission of the American Heart Association, Inc.)

Gould and associates[G2] have reported additional studies of regional myocardial perfusion with fast computed tomography in the canine model. The animal model and methods of contrast injection were similar to those in the two previous in vivo studies; however, in this study, they modified the basic flow algorithm (equation 16) after noting some difficulties with the linearity of the standard calculation at high flow rates. The modification consisted of adding an empiric term to account for the difference between the time of peak contrast opacification in the left ventricle and that in the myocardium. A parameter related to the "effective" mean transit time from the input (aorta) to the myocardium was added. Addition of this factor allows for a first-order estimate for deconvolution (see later) between the input and the (tissue) response contrast clearance curves. However, their approach was empiric, and the results, although suggesting that this algorithm might allow extension of the ultrafast-CT calculation to high flow rates, were very inconclusive.

Studies in Patients

Limited clinical data have been obtained with fast computed tomography. Rumberger and associates[R4] presented preliminary data for six normal individuals before and after intravenous injection of dipyridamole, a powerful coronary artery vasodilating agent that has been used to assess flow reserve in patients undergoing selective coronary angiography.[W7]

Nonionic contrast agent (0.33 ml/kg) was injected as a rapid bolus into an antecubital vein just prior to CT scanning in the baseline (resting) state and following dipyridamole injection (0.56 mg/kg over 4 minutes with maximum effect at 9 minutes post-infusion). Data analysis was performed on the subsequent images from the mid-left ventricle in a fashion identical to that described for the animal studies.

Figure 35–10 shows simultaneous left ventricular cavity and regional myocardial time-density curves for the same subject at rest (left) and following intravenous infusion of dipyridamole (right). The myocardial curve during maximum vasodilation demonstrated a greater peak concentration (density above baseline) and a shorter contrast transit time compared to the data for the control state. These qualitative observations with respect to the shape and character of the indicator dilution curves in humans are in accord with the observations in animals (see Fig. 35–6).

For each patient, the areas under the left ventricular cavity and regional myocardial contrast clearance curves were determined. The mean contrast transit times through the myocardial region of interest were calculated and the values of flow per unit mass determined using equation (14). Individual resting regional

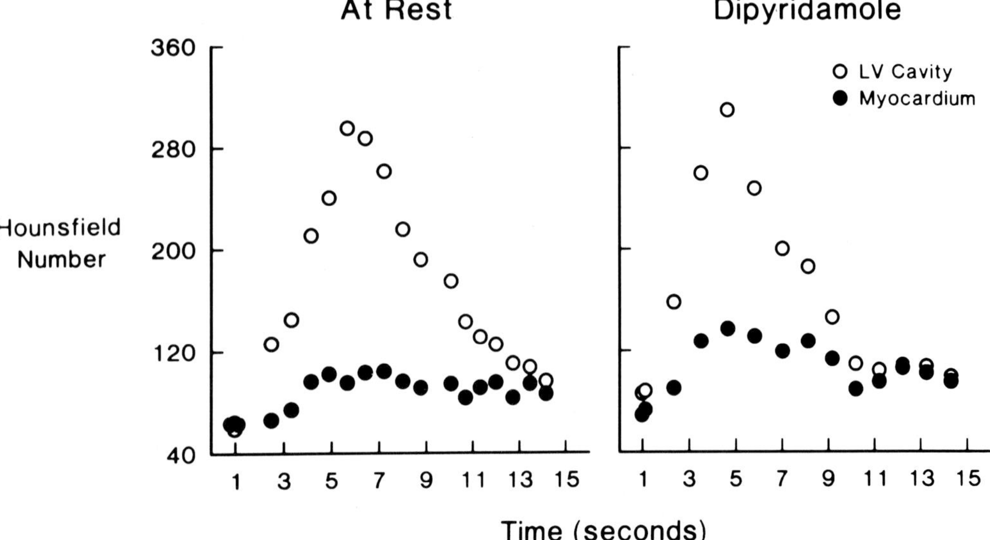

Figure 35–10. Simultaneous left ventricular cavity and regional myocardial time-density curves from the same patient at rest *(left)* and following intravenous injection of dipyridamole *(right)* (0.56 mg/kg). Note that these data resemble the data for the dog as shown in Figure 35–7. (From Rumberger, J. A., Stanford, W., and Marcus, M. L.: Quantitation of regional myocardial perfusion by ultrafast-CT: Promises and pitfalls. Am. J. Card. Imag. 1:336, 1987. Reproduced by permission of the American Journal of Cardiac Imaging.)

myocardial flow ranged from 55 to 141 ml/min/100 g (104 ± 30), while perfusion rates following dipyridamole infusion ranged from 128 to 389 ml/min/100 g (277 ± 88, $P < 0.01$ compared to baseline). Regional flow reserve was calculated for each subject as the ratio of flow per unit mass during maximum vasodilation to that at baseline. This parameter ranged from 2.23 to 3.5 (2.67 ± 0.50) (Fig. 35–11).

Questions Raised From Initial Intravenous Studies

Studies by Wolfkiel and associates,[W8] Garrett and associates,[G4] and Reiter and associates[R7] have demonstrated that absolute cardiac output can be quantitated by using fast computed tomography after intravenous injection of contrast agent by direct application of classic indicator dilution theory. Similarly, the studies discussed above indicate that fast computed tomography can be employed to evaluate regional myocardial perfusion, but there remain shortcomings with respect to scatter of the data and potential limitations of the theory at flow rates much above the normal resting values. The studies in normal patients aptly point out the later problem. The calculated values of regional myocardial flow per unit mass in the resting or baseline state totally agree with data available from other sources for normal patients;[C1, G1, I1] however, the calculated maximum flow reserve was found to be on the order of 2.67:1. This flow reserve calculation in normal individuals falls significantly short of the expected value of 5:1 to

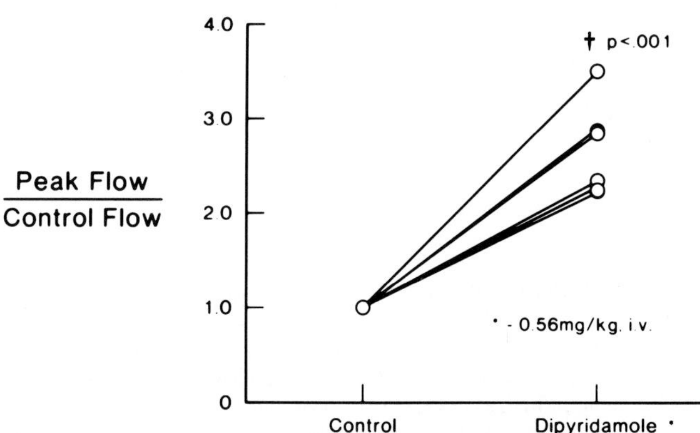

Figure 35–11. Regional myocardial flow reserve in the posterior myocardium as assessed by fast computed tomography in normal patients (n = 6). The average flow reserve calculated in this group was 2.67. (From Rumberger, J. A., Stanford, W., and Marcus, M. L.: Quantitation of regional myocardial perfusion by ultrafast-CT: Promises and pitfalls. Am. J. Card. Imag. 1:336, 1987. Reproduced by permission of the American Journal of Cardiac Imaging.)

7:1 from direct Doppler coronary artery flow measurements reported by Wilson and associates.[W1, W7] The causes for these errors as well as for other errors noted in the animal studies are multifactorial but can be divided into three categories:

1. Imaging or reconstruction artifacts.
2. Failure to account for changes in intramyocardial vascular volume during vasodilation.
3. Failure to characterize or completely understand the limitations related to the input function to the myocardium when contrast agent is administered intravenously.

These problems and limitations are discussed more fully in the following sections.

IMAGING AND RECONSTRUCTION ARTIFACTS

Scanner-Related and Patient-Related Artifacts

Significant image artifacts may result from the CT system or from the patient. Artifacts from the system may arise secondary to instability, imbalance, and misalignment of the detector/x-ray system. However, developments in scanner tuning and digital evaluation of the systems on a regular basis make basic alignment and hardware problems minimal and predictable; thus, these potential sources of artifacts are not expected to contribute significantly to the scanning process with fast computed tomography.

Patient-related artifacts arise from motion during scanning and include peristaltic, muscular, respiratory, and cardiac movements. Of these potential sources of artifacts, respiratory and cardiac motions during scanning are of the most importance for fast-CT images. Scanning in patients for analysis of regional myocardial perfusion takes about 20 seconds. Subjects are asked to suspend respiration during scanning at approximately one-half tidal volume.[R4] Except in unusual circumstances, most patients can hold their breath for this period of time without difficulty; thus, artifacts due to respiratory motion may be kept to a minimum during fast-CT scanning. Cardiac motion is complex and represents three-dimensional conformational changes that occur with each cardiac cycle. There is no agreement as to which portion of the cardiac cycle is best for scans intended to evaluate regional myocardial perfusion; however, consistency in maintaining a stable position for the region of interest during data analysis is of paramount concern. Ultrafast-CT images are acquired within 50 milliseconds, that is, 1/20 of a second. Dynamic Spatial Reconstruction studies are acquired in only 1/60 of a second. During this short acquisition, very little cardiac motion occurs except during the most rapid phases of ejection and early diastolic filling. Imaging confined to either end-diastole or end-systole should avoid confounding problems related to cardiac motion during scanning. The authors prefer to scan at end-diastole to ensure a more reliable time index (peak of the R wave on the electrocardiogram) and anatomic location for the region of interest; however, a variable region of interest can be employed for each image to allow for changes in anatomic position of the region of interest between scans acquired during end-systole, as has been used by Wolfkiel and associates.[W5]

Volume-Averaging Artifacts

A CT image is a composite or grid (matrix) of picture elements (pixels) displayed on a video monitor. During reconstruction of the x-ray data, each pixel is assigned an x-ray attenuation (or density) value compared, by convention, to the attenuation coefficient of water; generally, this represents 2000 gray levels or densities (10-bit data) with scaling as follows: bone = 1000, water = 0, and air = −1000. Although one evaluates the image as a two-dimensional data set, the tomogram has a finite thickness and thus the CT densities are actually representative of volume elements (voxels). Averaging of the density across the voxel may produce a "partial volume" artifact.

A partial volume artifact can be a problem with fast computed tomography by falsely altering the actual CT tissue density; however, by carefully examining the region chosen for data analysis (both within the myocardium and within the left ventricular cavity/aorta), viewing the voxel above and below the tomographic region of interest, and avoiding analysis near the border of the cavity or lung with the myocardium, one can, in practice, substantially reduce or virtually eliminate this problem.

Beam Hardening and Photon Scatter

Subtle artifacts may result from alterations of the x-ray beam not dependent on the configuration of the scanning device. The CT density (or Hounsfield unit) for a given material (regardless of the partial volume effect) may be highly variable, depending on what structures surround that material. For instance, it was originally thought that one could determine the benignity of a pulmonary nodule if its Hounsfield number was above a certain value[S6] (presumably indicating the presence of calcium); however, it has been shown subsequently that the density of pulmonary nodules is highly variable between patients. This variability is an artifact of the variable beam energy as the beam traverses patients of different physiognomy. This artifact arises because the beam energy spectrum is polychromatic rather than the ideal monochromatic.

As this polychromatic x-ray beam traverses the body, the lower energies attenuate preferentially so that the effective beam energy increases (or the beam "hardens"). These spectral or beam-hardening changes then artificially reduce the density of the object on which the beam is incident.[H5] All manufacturers of CT devices are aware of these problems, and specific reconstruction algorithms have been designed to account for them;[H6] however, the subsequent effect on the final images has not been totally eliminated.

Photon scatter is also a problem. Ideally, the detector should receive only x-ray information directly in line with the incident beam on the object; however, scatter of photons through an object will alter the beam path, and the detector may receive x-ray information from nonparallel sources. For CT imaging and for random geometry of the object evaluated, the effect of photon scatter is to reduce the density of a given object, analogously to beam hardening. Manufacturers of CT devices install collimators external to the detectors to reduce substantially x-ray information from scattered photons not directly parallel with the incident beam/detector pair.

Artifacts due to beam hardening and/or photon scatter are apparent on fast-CT images and may specifically affect the calculations of regional myocardial perfusion. Regional blood flow within the normal myocardium (and thus indicator clearance data) should be relatively uniform in character.[C2] Figure 35–12 shows time-density data from the dog myocardium following rapid intravenous injection of nonionic contrast agent at a dose of 1 ml/kg. This example demonstrates a significant degree of nonuniformity of the indicator clearance curve, depending on the position of the operator-defined region of interest within the myocardium (anterior, lateral, ventricular septum, or posterior myocardium, as indicated). These data show the mean regional CT density and standard deviation of that density within the region as a function of time. The most striking differences between data are seen in the anterior wall, where a distinct "dip" is seen in the data prior to maximal opacification of the myocardium from the influx of contrast agent; surprisingly, these appar-

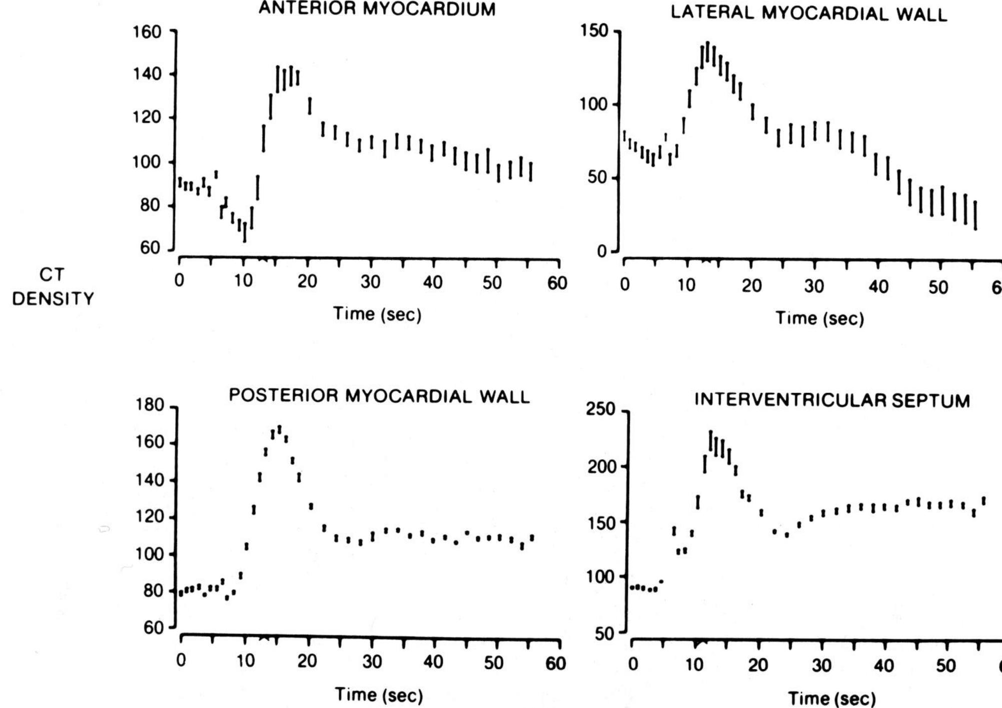

Figure 35–12. Simultaneous CT density versus time in a dog within four separate myocardial regions (anterior, lateral, posterior, and interventricular septal walls). Each data point represents a mean CT density ± standard deviation. Note the significant nonuniformity of the curves. These data were derived following an injection into the inferior vena cava of nonionic contrast agent at a dose of 1 ml/kg. (From Rumberger, J. A., Feiring, A. J., and Lipton, M. J.: Use of ultrafast computed tomography to quantitate regional myocardial perfusion: A preliminary report. J. Am. Coll. Cardiol. 9:59, 1987. Reprinted with permission of the American College of Cardiology.)

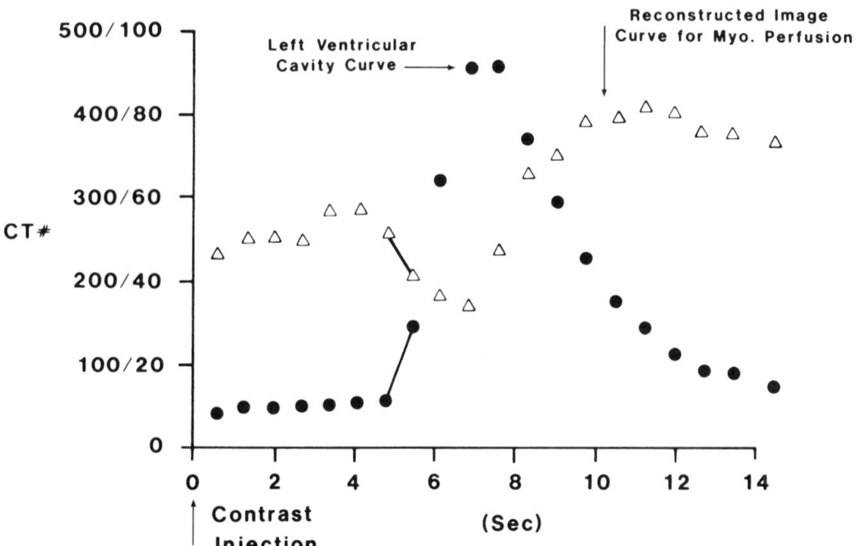

Figure 35–13. Simultaneous left ventricular cavity and anterior myocardial time density curves from a dog following intravenous bolus contrast administration (1 ml/dg). Note the significant "dip" in the myocardial contrast density data coincident with the appearance of the iodinated contrast into the adjacent left ventricular cavity ("shadow phenomenon," see text for details). As the contrast enters the myocardium the positive deflection in the myocardial contrast density is subsequently observed. (Reproduced by permission of the American Journal of Cardiac Imaging.) (From Rumberger, J. A., Stanford, W., and Marcus, M. L.: Quantitation of regional myocardial perfusion by ultrafast-CT: Promises and pitfalls. Am. J. Card. Imag. 1:336, 1987. Reproduced by permission of the American Journal of Cardiac Imaging.)

ent artifacts are not seen in the posterior myocardium, where the corresponding deviations from the mean are quite minimal. This posterior myocardial region was the area from which the data presented in Figure 35–7 were derived (data from Rumberger and associates[R3]).

It may be anticipated theoretically[J2] that artificial (artifactual) reduction of the myocardial CT densities would occur in proportion to the changing CT density within the adjacent left ventricular cavity during the first passage of the contrast bolus. This "shadow phenomenon" (which may result from beam hardening, photon scatter, and undefined reconstruction artifacts) results in the artificial reduction of peak tissue contrast density and an artificial prolongation of the true contrast transit time. For example, Figure 35–13 shows contrast clearance curves from the anterior myocardium in a dog simultaneous with the contrast clearance curve within the left ventricular cavity following bolus intravenous injection of indicator. Note that the previously noted dip in CT density within the myocardium is simultaneous with the initial rise of CT density within the adjacent left ventricular cavity. As more contrast agent enters the myocardium from the aortic input, a more positive (above baseline) density deflection is observed.

Figure 35–14 demonstrates a method used to account for the artifacts noted above and also suggests a way to reduce (but not necessarily eliminate) the problem when employing intravenous injections. If one considers the situation in which there is no regional distribution of indicator within the myocardium adjacent to the left ventricular cavity, then the CT density-time curve within that myocardial region will reflect only the artifactual shadow phenomenon. The "no-perfusion" curve shows a decrease and subsequent return to baseline of the CT densities in direct proportion to the increasing and then decreasing CT density in the adjacent left ventricular cavity. As a first-order approximation, the actual reconstructed curve within the myocardium is a combination of the "artifact" and the "true" change in density reflective of the regional flow. A convolution of the CT reconstructed curve with the no-perfusion curve yields the final (true) curve shown. This curve resembles the one noted in the posterior myocardium of Figure 35–6. Using this new myocardial curve, the ventricular input curve and equation (14) yield an estimation of regional flow by computed tomography of 173 ml/min/100 g; the actual flow per unit mass from regional microsphere data was 190 ml/min/100 g, representing a subsequent error of only about 10 percent.

The theoretical construct above implies that a reduction in the CT density within the left ventricular cavity following intravenous injection of contrast agent will reduce the myocardial shadow artifacts. Reducing the amount of indicator administered intravenously (i.e., total iodine load) will reduce the concentration in the left ventricular cavity and the subsequent imaging artifact seen within the adjacent myocardium. This assumption has been validated in vivo in our laboratory and is probably the reason

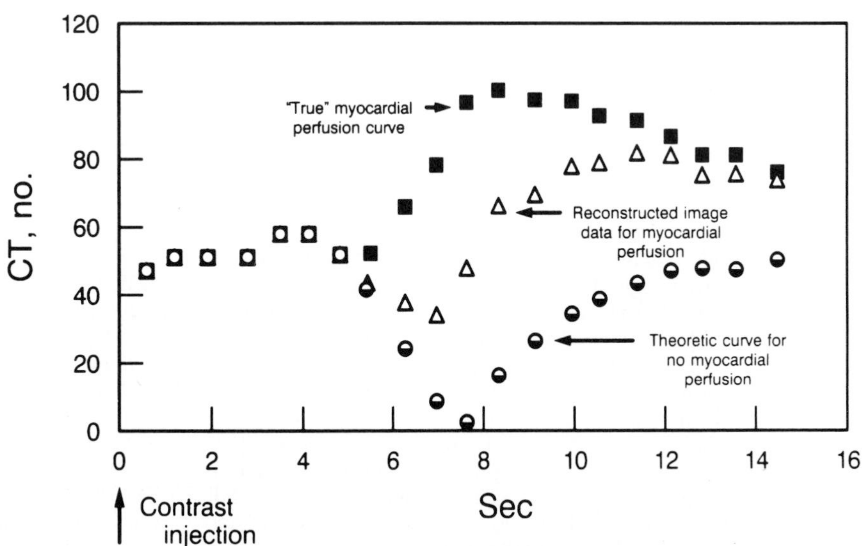

Figure 35–14. Construct of a possible method (first-order approximation) for eliminating the "dip" in the myocardial contrast curve noted in the myocardium as a result of increasing contrast density within the adjacent left ventricular cavity following intravenous injection of iodinated contrast agent. Here the "true" myocardial perfusion curve is the sum of the reconstructed (raw) contrast clearance curve and the "no-perfusion" curve (which characterizes the extent of the artifact over time). Imaging artifacts (see text for details) alter the shape and character of the contrast clearance data within the myocardium.

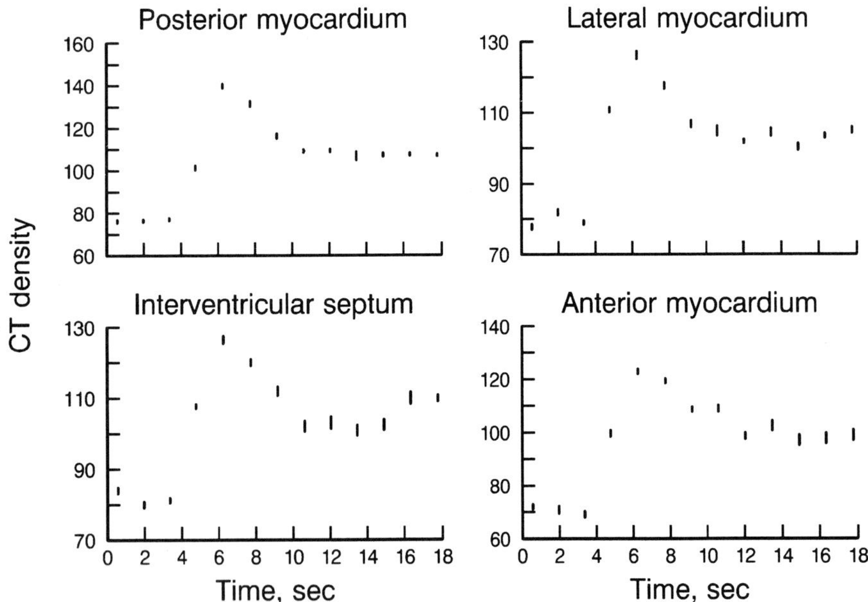

Figure 35–15. Simultaneous contrast density (clearance) data in the dog from four separate myocardial regions (anterior, lateral, posterior, and interventricular septal walls) following aortic root injection of iodinated contrast agent. Note here, as compared with the data in Figure 35–13, that the contrast clearance data are relatively uniform across all fields examined. Values are means ± standard deviation.

why Wolfkiel and associates[W5] failed to note the shadow artifacts (the dose of contrast agent given was 0.33 ml/kg, versus 1.0 ml/kg as reported by Rumberger and associates[R3]).

A final way to reduce shadow artifacts in the myocardium is to inject contrast agent into the aortic root. This approach avoids several problems. Aortic root injections eliminate overlapping opacification of the left ventricular cavity and myocardium that occurs with intravenous injections. Figure 35–15 shows simultaneously acquired fast-CT data from the four myocardial areas noted in Figure 35–12; however, these data were derived following an aortic root injection of contrast agent. Note here that there is little regional variability of the myocardial time-density curves.

REGIONAL INTRAMYOCARDIAL VASCULAR VOLUME

The prior in vivo studies noted[G3, R3, R4, W5] assumed that the "distribution" volume, V, for the contrast agent within the myocardium was the ratio of muscle density, ρ, and the muscle mass, m (i.e., $V = m/\rho$). One could use this simple relationship to compare flow per unit mass determined by computed tomography to flow per unit mass determined with microspheres. However, fast computed tomography actually measures flow per unit volume, as suggested by the studies of Wang and Ritman[W4]; microsphere determinations are made in exsanguinated tissue; and CT determinations are made in vivo. One must then account for the additional volume of the vasculature, b, separately from the volume of the muscle mass present in vivo. Thus, the volume (V) to be used in equations (14) and (16) is not m/ρ but is $m/\rho + b$.

The physiologic determinants of regional myocardial perfusion are multifactorial. Classical theory, as noted previously, defines flow as directly proportional to vascular blood volume and inversely proportional to mean transit time (equation 4); however, regional vascular volume is not a static parameter but changes in response to physiologic demand for increased regional flow. On the other hand, little is known about its relationship to regional flow, and the literature is confusing in this regard.

Spaan,[S7] in his review of coronary pressure flow relationships, quoted a value of 1.6 ml per 100 g of myocardium for the entire volume of the coronary arterial tree at baseline (normal, resting) flow (vessels larger than 200 μm, at a perfusion pressure of 100 mm Hg). Studies from Schaper's laboratory,[W9] using postmortem barium angiography, noted an average vascular volume of the left ventricular free wall of 3.6 ml/100 g under control conditions. This is roughly twice the value quoted by Spaan.

No direct measurements of myocardial or venous vascular volumes have been reported. However, Weiss and associates[W10] examined the volume of blood in the small (<100 μm) vessels. They found the small-vessel vascular volume to be approximately 7 ml/100 g at rest and 14 ml/100 g during asphyxia. Unfortunately, although they assumed that maximum coronary flow was achieved during asphyxia, no direct comparison was made between regional small-vessel vascular volume and absolute regional flow.

Total intramyocardial vascular volume has been examined by several investigators. Eliasen and associates[E1] calculated total red cell and plasma volume within regions of canine left ventricle by using radioactive tracers at basal levels of regional myocardial flow (70–95 ml/min/100 g). Corresponding values for vascular volume ranged from 3.6 to 4.9 ml per 100 g of myocardium. Both Ziegler and Goresky[Z2] and Morgenstern and associates[M7] evaluated total regional myocardial volume in relation to regional values for myocardial flow per unit mass. Both groups indicated a linear relationship between vascular volume and perfusion. Ziegler and Goresky noted a value of 8 ml/100 g at baseline and an increase to 12 ml/100 g at 220 ml/min/100 g. Morgenstern and associates noted a value of 11 ml/100 g at rest, which increased to 14 ml/100 g at a regional value for perfusion of 130 ml/min/100 g. If their data were extrapolated to a maximum myocardial flow of 400 ml/100 g/min (normal flow reserve of at least 4:1), estimates of regional intramyocardial vascular volume at maximum vasodilation would range from 20 to 29 ml/100 g. Although the shape of the vascular volume versus regional flow relationship is more likely curvilinear, as will be suggested subsequently, it is apparent that regional vascular volume is not necessarily inconsequential, especially at high values for regional myocardial flow.

Substituting $V = m/\rho + b$ into equation (16) and rearranging yields

$$F_r/m_r = (1/\rho + b/m)*C_{PH}/A_{LV} \quad (17)$$

The question remaining is how to calculate b/m.

Wang and Ritman,[W3] in their initial studies evaluating regional myocardial perfusion with the Dynamic Spatial Reconstructor at the Mayo Clinic, noted the need to account for changes in regional intramyocardial vascular volume as regional myocardial perfusion increased from baseline and added a nonlinear factor to equation (16), assuming theoretically that b/m was proportional to the ratio of the areas under the regional myocardial and aortic input contrast clearance curves. However, b/m can be estimated directly from the indicator "concentration" data derived from the myocardium and a purely vascular segment such as the aorta or left ventricular cavity.

The CT densities of myocardium and blood are nearly identical, as are the specific gravities. Therefore, iodinated contrast agent must be used to separate structures of similar densities. Consider, for example, two regions within a CT image in which the CT densities were noted before and after administration of contrast agent: one that is totally vascular (e.g., the aorta or ventricular cavity) and another that is exactly one-half nonvascular and one-half vascular. The ratio of the mean concentration (or CT density) in the mixed region above baseline to that within the purely vascular region, again above baseline, should be 0.5—that is, exactly, one-half vascular and one-half avascular. In the limit that the mixed region becomes totally vascular, the ratio approaches 1.0. In the limit that the mixed region becomes less and less vascular, the ratio becomes very small. The ratio of the densities (above baseline) within the mixed region compared to a purely vascular region then defines the ratio of tissue vascular volume per unit total volume (i.e., b/V). This may be more easily thought of as a "partial volume parameter" that reflects the dilution of the purely vascular region by nonopacified tissue within the region of interest.

The paradigm discussed above is analogous to determining the activity of combined red cell and plasma markers (total vascular volume) within the myocardium compared to the activity within the aorta, as defined by Eliasen and associates[E1] to calculate the microvascular blood content in the canine myocardium. The same principle has also been used by Iida and associates[I1] to define the partitioning of $H_2{}^{15}O$ within the myocardial vasculature as applied to quantitation of regional myocardial perfusion by positron emission tomography.

The parameter b/V may be defined as the ratio of mean CT density (above baseline) in the myocardium ($\bar{C}_t$) to the mean CT density (above baseline) in the ventricular cavity ($\bar{C}_{LV}$) determined by ultrafast computed tomography following intravascular contrast administration (one could also use the density in the aorta in place of that in the ventricular cavity). Assuming no extravasation of contrast agent during the first pass, homogeneous mixing of indicator with the blood, and no perturbation of the vascular volume by the contrast agent (assumptions 1–4), then

$$b/V = \bar{C}_t/\bar{C}_{LV} \tag{18}$$

However,

$$V = m/\rho + b \tag{19}$$

Therefore,

$$\frac{b}{m} = \frac{1}{\rho}\left[\frac{(\bar{C}_t/\bar{C}_{LV})}{(1 - (\bar{C}_t/\bar{C}_{LV}))}\right] \tag{20}$$

The original data[R3] were reanalyzed in light of significant changes in region intramyocardial vascular volume during pharmacologic vasodilation. In this model, b/V was calculated directly from the contrast clearance data in the left ventricular cavity and posterior myocardium by determining the mean (time-averaged) density above baseline noted during the passage of the contrast agent through each region.

Figure 35–16 shows a comparison of b/V versus regional flow per unit mass (defined, as before, directly from the regional microsphere data). Values of regional intramyocardial vascular volume at baseline (normal regional flow of 100 ml/min/100 g) are on the order of 0.05 (i.e., 4.9 ml/100 g myocardium, using a density of 1.05 g/ml). These results are in general agreement with data reported by others; however, note that as regional perfusion increases, regional intramyocardial vascular volume increases rapidly but asymptotically approaches a maximum toward the end of the usual physiologic range.

The maximum value for regional intramyocardial vascular volume as estimated by fast computed tomography may be on the order of 0.20 (24 ml/100 g), as noted in Figure 35–17, and this value is not inconsequential. Figure 35–17 is based on the same CT data as presented in Figure 35–7, but the flow algorithm

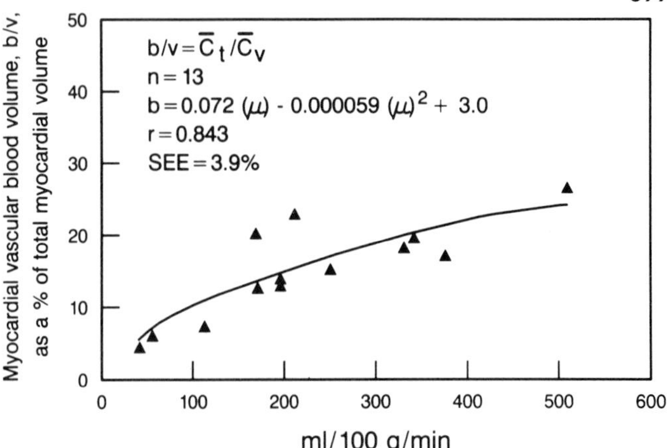

Figure 35–16. Myocardial vascular blood volume, b/V, as a percentage of total myocardial volume within a region of the myocardium. Data were obtained by reanalysis of the data from Figure 35–8. See text for details.

employed was equation (17). Note that, although computed tomography still underestimates flow per unit mass at the higher values for regional perfusion, the slope of the regression line across the range of flows examined now approaches unity. Failure to account for changes in regional intramyocardial vascular volume during vasodilation results in artifactual underestimation of regional myocardial perfusion by computed tomography. This principle is not confined to fast computed tomography but must apply to other methods that use vascular indicators (digital subtraction angiography, echocardiography, positron emission tomography, and myocardial scintigraphy).

KINETICS OF THE INPUT FUNCTION TO THE MYOCARDIUM

Assumption 6, related to the application of classical indicator dilution theory to ultrafast computed tomography, required that the mean transit time of the indicator from the input to the coronary ostia be less than the mean time for that indicator to traverse the vascular/tissue space within the myocardium. This concept is not new but was initially applied to an external detection system by Mullani and associates[M6] for studies with the positron emitter ^{82}Ru. Although the analogy of ^{82}Ru to iodinated

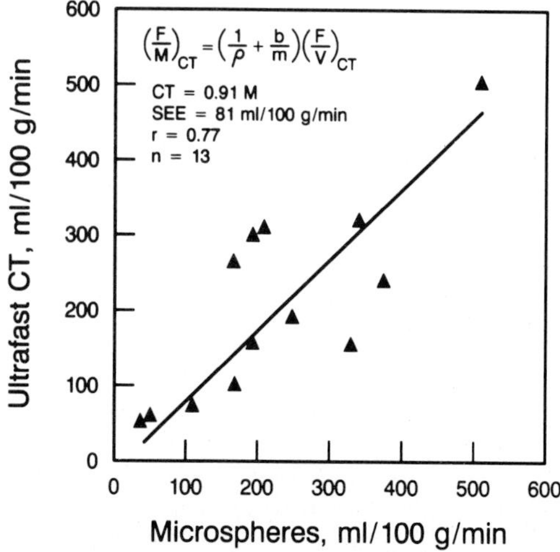

Figure 35–17. Regional myocardial perfusion (flow per unit mass) versus radiolabeled microspheres as calculated by using fast computed tomography and the modified algorithm in equation (17). The data were obtained by reanalysis of the data shown in Figure 35–8. Here the algorithm incorporates the concept of changes in regional intramyocardial vascular volume during vasodilation. See text for details.

contrast agent is not direct, the "extraction" of rubidium by the myocardium may be likened to the subsequent appearance of contrast agent in the coronary sinus. The appearance of contrast agent within the coronary sinus before the entry of all the input to that region from the source could account for the curvilinear relationship between calculated myocardial flow and microsphere flow noted by Mullani when the extraction fraction was underestimated. This is also part of the reason for the underestimations of myocardial flow made by Wolfkiel and associates[W5] with fast computed tomography, because the contrast input function to the coronary ostia was severely splayed following femoral vein injection.

Figure 35–18 shows a schematic whereby the quantitation of regional myocardial perfusion, given satisfaction of all other assumptions, is limited by the injection site of the contrast agent. As contrast agent is administered closer to the coronary ostia, the dynamic range of quantitation or regional flow by computed tomography is expanded. The characterization of the transit of the bolus to the input is then a function of the actual initial injection time and the site of injection.

The data set defined by Wolfkiel and associates,[W5] using femoral vein injection of contrast agent (see Fig. 35–8), demonstrated a plateau above 200 ml/min/100 g, where the data set defined by Rumberger and associates,[R3] using an injection into the inferior vena cava (see Figs. 35–7 and 35–17), suggests a significant underestimation above 300 to 350 ml/min/100 g. Wang and associates,[W4] employing aortic root injection of contrast agent, suggested that regional myocardial perfusion can be quantitated by CT techniques at flow rates up to 1000 ml/min/100 g. This study also included a flow algorithm accounting for changes in regional myocardial blood volume during vasodilation. An additional CT study that evaluated the usefulness of systemic (aortic root) injection of indicator for analysis of regional myocardial perfusion has been reported by Weiss and associates.[W11] In this study, they employed a square wave-type input function of contrast agent delivered over 6 to 8 seconds. An empirically derived flow algorithm was developed from analysis of the subsequent regional myocardial wash-in kinetics (absolute values above baseline and slope of CT density curve). Myocardial vascular blood volume was also accounted for in a manner similar to that previously described. Regional perfusion rates from 26 to 613 ml/100 g/min were evaluated, where the slope of the regression line and coefficient of correlation were both nearly unity. They concluded that this approach allowed a calculation of regional myocardial perfusion by high-speed computed tomography over the physiologic range. These results are comparable to those previously reported by Wang and Ritman.[W3] Thus it may be possible to quantitate resting and ischemic myocardial flow by fast computed tomography with intravenous injection of contrast agent; however, examination of the full dynamic range of possible values for perfusion may require an aortic root injection.

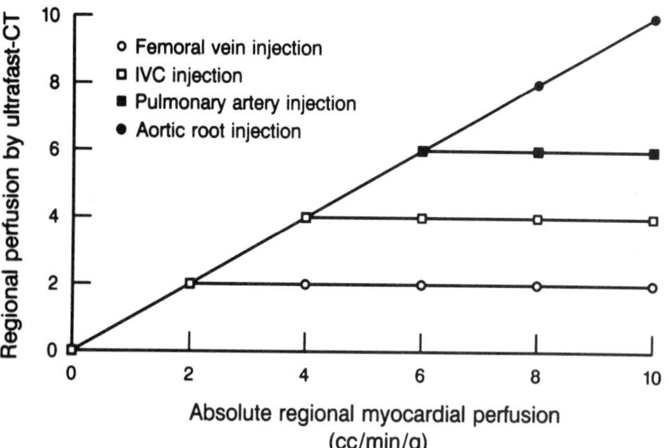

Figure 35–18. Theoretical construct relating the absolute value of regional myocardial perfusion and that determined by using fast computed tomography for various contrast injection sites. Note that as contrast agent is administered closer and closer to the systemic circulation, the plateau reached by the calculations extends farther into the physiologic range of known myocardial perfusion values. (Reproduced by permission of the American Journal of Cardiac Imaging.) (From Rumberger, J. A., Stanford, W., and Marcus, M. L.: Quantitation of regional myocardial perfusion by ultrafast-CT: Promises and pitfalls. Am. J. Card. Imag. 1:336, 1987. Reproduced by permission of American Journal of Cardiac Imaging.)

REGIONAL TRANSFER FUNCTION

High-speed CT scanning may also be useful in providing data related to the fractional distribution of myocardial flow in various physiologic, pathologic, or pharmacologically altered flow states. Segmental, spatial, and temporal nonuniformity of regional perfusion has been described in the normal mammalian heart.[Y1] Nonuniformity of flow may be important if one is attempting to quantitate accurately the transport of nondiffusible substrates or metabolites through the myocardium or to assess the efficacy of therapeutic interventions aimed at normalizing flow distribution.

If one assumes a steady-state flow situation during the first pass of contrast agent, the studies presented have demonstrated the potential of high-speed computed tomography to determine segmental differences in myocardial perfusion. However, the fractional distribution of that regional blood flow among microvessels of different path lengths is not apparent from the analysis of the regional contrast clearance data. This is because the "response" curve in the myocardium depends on the input bolus kinetics of the indicator (e.g., intravenous versus aortic root injection), the intravascular dispersion due to velocity gradients between microvessels, and the spatial uniformity (or nonuniformity) of the microvasculature.

With a hypothetical instantaneous (impulse) input function, the response (output function) would reflect the inherent impulse response of the regional vasculature and describe any spatial nonuniformity within the system. The relationship between input and output is referred to as the "transfer function"[B5] and is derived by deconvolving the recorded input and response functions (contrast clearance or time-density data) to yield an idealized response for that system based on an idealized step input.

Such a deconvolution model has been described for the canine heart by Knopp and associates,[K4] who attempted to define a transcoronary transfer function by analysis of indocyanine green dye injected into the left atrium and sampled in the coronary sinus. More recently, Bell and associates,[B4] using the Dynamic Spatial Reconstructor, employed the same deconvolution method and were able to evaluate the regional transfer function of the myocardium at rest and following maximum vasodilation. Eigler and associates[E2] measured the myocardial transfer function in dogs, using direct coronary contrast injections and digital angiography. They found the transfer function to be independent of bolus kinetics and superior to conventional contrast clearance analysis for determination of coronary flow and flow reserve.

Transfer function or deconvolution analysis with high-speed computed tomography may be helpful in characterizing the microvasculature in a variety of conditions known to alter small vessels (e.g., left ventricular hypertrophy[W12] and aortic stenosis[M8]) and may allow further insight into the functional significance of coronary collateral vessels.

SUMMARY AND CONCLUSIONS

Clinical quantitation of regional myocardial perfusion using a minimally invasive and easily applied technique could allow ready quantitation of the physiologic significance of coronary disease, allow further understanding of flow reserve in various cardiomyopathic and overload (pressure versus volume) conditions, and possibly provide firm concepts regarding the development and clinical significance of coronary collateral vessels. Perhaps one of the most laudable aims for quantitation of myocardial perfusion would be to follow, characterize, and then alter if necessary the pharmacologic therapy of a variety of cardiac ailments. For instance, the objective of anti-anginal therapy is to reduce myocardial oxygen demand during exertion (i.e., to limit the need to increase regional perfusion above a maximum threshold). This threshold is determined by the physiologic significance of any given coronary lesion. Quantitation of appropriate flow redistribution or limitation of myocardial flow during provocative testing may provide foundations for the required pharmacologic therapy of a patient or serve to assess the efficacy of a pharmacologic agent. The studies discussed here suggest that fast computed tomography may ultimately provide such a vehicle for quantitation of regional myocardial perfusion.

This chapter has demonstrated the development of the concept of classical indicator techniques for use with an external detection system such as fast computed tomography. Initial and preliminary studies in vitro and in vivo have been presented, and the potential limitations of the techniques as applied to humans have been discussed. These potential limitations, which are not insurmountable, require further investigation into the physics of fast computed tomography and better understanding of indicator transit kinetics and regional intramyocardial vascular volume.

Significant attenuation of imaging artifacts can be accomplished via a reduction in total amount of contrast agent administered for intravenous injection techniques or implementation of appropriate CT hardware and software modifications developed to address this issue. An approach to account for changes in regional intramyocardial vascular volume has been demonstrated, and a more general theoretical approach that incorporates this concept is presented.

A limitation remains regarding input function kinetics if the entire dynamic range of possible regional myocardial perfusion is to be studied. However, use of a less invasive central venous injection for contrast injection, as compared to the more invasive aortic root injection, may depend on the question posed for a given subject. The data presented from the original study using inferior vena cava injection,[R3] after accounting for changes in regional vascular volume, suggest that absolute regional myocardial perfusion can be quantitated up to about 400 ml/min/100 g. If normal resting flow is approximately 100 ml/min/100 g, this would imply that studies could be done with intravenous injection methods for characterization of regional myocardial perfusion up to 4:1. Flow reserve above this value would, however, be underestimated. However, studies by Wilson and associates,[W1, W7] using a unique intracoronary Doppler catheter, have shown that "normal" flow reserve (in the absence of hypertrophy) is 3.7:1 or greater and that patients with physiologically significant coronary artery disease have reserve usually less than 3:1. Ultrafast computed tomography in patients with coronary artery disease may then be adequate to separate significant from insignificant coronary lesions. In a practical sense, therefore, an aortic root contrast injection may be necessary only for research purposes when more precision regarding the total range of flow reserve in a subject is required. Even then, a 5 Fr. catheter/sheath system (as currently used for coronary angiography) may be all that is required and the study may be completed on an outpatient basis.

Fast computed tomography offers a unique approach to quantitating regional myocardial perfusion in both the clinical and the research setting.

References

A

1. Axel, L.: Cerebral blood flow determination by rapid-sequence computed tomography: Theoretical analysis. Radiology 137:679, 1980.

B

1. Boyd, D. B.: Computerized transmission tomography of the heart using scanning electron beams. *In* Higgins, C. H. (ed.): Computed Tomography of the Heart and Great Vessels. Futura Publishing, New York, 1983, p. 45.
2. Blumgart, H. L., and Yens, O. C.: Studies on the velocity of blood flow. I. The method utilized. J. Clin. Invest. 4:1, 1927.
3. Burbank, F. H., Brody, W. R., and Bradley, B. R.: Effective volume and rate of contrast medium injection on intravenous digital subtraction angiographic contrast median curves. J. Am. Coll. Cardiol. 4:308, 1984.
4. Bell, M. R., Spyra, W. J. T., Thomas, P. J., and Ritman, E. L.: A method for characterizing the spatial distribution of regional transcoronary transfer-function using fast-CT. Physiology 31:A64, 1988.
5. Bassingthwaighte, J. B.: Circulatory transport and the convolution integral. Mayo Clin. Proc. 42:137, 1967.

C

1. Canon, P. J.: Measurement of coronary blood flow in evaluation of regional myocardial perfusion by intracoronary injection techniques. *In* Donath, A., and Righetti, A. (eds.): Cardiovascular Nuclear Medicine (Progress in Nuclear Medicine, Vol. 6). Karger, New York, 1980, p. 85.
2. Cobb, F. R., Bache, R. J., and Greenfield, J. C., Jr.: Regional myocardial blood flow in awake dogs. J. Clin. Invest. 53:H1618, 1974.

D

1. Dow, P.: Estimations of cardiac output in central blood volume by dye dilution. Physiol. Overview 36:77, 1956.

E

1. Eliasen, P., Amtorp, O., Tondevold, E., and Haunso, S.: Regional blood flow, microvascular blood content, and tissue hematocrit in canine myocardium. Circ. Res. 16:593, 1982.
2. Eigler, N., Zeiher, A., Pfaff, J. M., et al.: Digital angiographic transfer function analogies of myocardial flow and coronary reserve: Comparison with conventional time-density curve parameters. (Abstract.) J. Am. Coll. Cardiol. 9:44A, 1987.

F

1. Feinstein, S. B.: Myocardial perfusion imaging: Contrast echocardiography today and tomorrow. J. Am. Coll. Cardiol. 8:251, 1986.

G

1. Ganz, W., Tamura, K., Marcus, H. S., et al.: Measurement of coronary sinus blood flow using continuous thermodilution in man. Circulation 44:181, 1971.
2. Gould, R. G., Lipton, M. J., McNamara, M. T., et al.: Measurement of regional myocardial blood flow in dogs by ultrafast-CT. Invest. Radiol. 23:348, 1988.
3. Guthaner, D. F., Nassi, M., and Bradley, B.: Validation of a CT method for flow determination. Radiology 151:429, 1984.
4. Garrett, J. S., Lanzer, P., Janchke, W., and Lipton, M. J.: Measurement of cardiac output by cine computed tomography. Am. J. Cardiol. 56:657, 1985.

H

1. Henriques, V.: Uber die Verteilung des, Blutes vom, linken, Herzen zwischen dem Herzen und dem ubrigen Organismus. Biochem. Z. 56:230, 1913.
2. Hamilton, W. F., Moore, J. W., Kinsman, J. M., and Spurling, R. G.: Studies on the circulation. IV. Further analysis of the injection method and of changes in hemodynamics under physiological and pathological conditions. Am. J. Physiol. 99:534, 1932.
3. Henley, W. S., Creech, O., Couves, C. M., et al.: Determination of myocardial blood flow utilizing iodinated (I^{131}) human serum albumin. Surg. Forum 8:237, 1957.
4. Hounsfield, G. N.: Picture quality of computed tomography. AJR 127:3, 1976.
5. Herman, G. T.: Correction for a beam hardening in computed tomography. Phys. Med. Biol. 24:81, 1979.
6. Herman, G. T.: Demonstration of beam hardening correction in computed tomography of the head. J. Comput. Assist. Tomogr. 3:373, 1979.

I

1. Iida, H., Kanno, I., Takahashi, A., et al.: Measurement of absolute myocardial blood flow with H_2O^{15} and dynamic positron-emission tomography: Strategy for quantification in relation to the partial-volume effect. Circulation 78:104, 1988.

J

1. Jaschke, W., Gould, R. G., Assimakopoulos, P. A., and Lipton, M. J.: Flow measurements with a high-speed computed tomography scanner. Med. Phys. 14:238, 1987.
2. Joseph, B. M.: Artefacts in computed tomography. *In* Newton, P. M., and Potts, D. G. (eds.): Radiology of the Skull and Brain, Technical Aspects of Computed Tomography. C. B. Mosby, St. Louis, 1980, p. 3980.

K

1. Klocke, F. J., Bunnell, I. L., Green, E. D. G., et al.: Average coronary blood flow per unit weight of the left ventricle in patients with and without coronary artery disease. Circulation 50:547, 1974.
2. Koch, E.: Die Stromgeschwindigkeit des Blutes: Ein Beitrag Zur Arbeitsprufung des Kreislaufes. Arch. Klin. Med. 140:39, 1922.
3. Knutson, J. R. B., Taylor, B. E., Ellis, E. J., and Wood, E. H.: Studies on circulation time with the aid of the oximeter. Mayo Clin. Proc. 25:405, 1950.
4. Knopp, T. J., Dobbs, W. A., Greenleaf, J. F., and Bassingthwaighte, J. B.: Transcoronary intravascular transport functions obtained via a stable deconvolution technique. Ann. Biomed. Eng. 4:44, 1976.

L

1. Love, W. D., and Burch, G. E.: A study in dogs of methods suitable for estimating the rate of myocardial uptake of Rb^{86} in man and the effect of L-norepinephrine and pitressin on Rb^{86} uptake. J. Clin. Invest. 36:468, 1957.

M

1. Marcus, M., Wright, C., Doty, D., et al.: Measurements of coronary velocity in reactive hyperemia in the coronary circulation of humans. Circ. Res. 49:877, 1981.
2. Marston, E. L., Barefoot, C. A., and Spencer, M. P.: Non-cannulating measurements of coronary blood flow. Surg. Forum 10:636, 1959.
3. Mills, C. J.: Measurement of pulsatile flow and flow velocity. *In* Bergel, D. H. (ed.): Cardiovascular Fluid Dynamics, Vol. 1, Chap. 3. Academic Press, London, 1970, p. 71.
4. Moore, J. W., Kinsman, J. M., Hamilton, W. F., and Spurling, R. G.: Studies on the circulation. II. Cardiac output determinations: Comparison of the injection method with the direct Fick procedure. Am. J. Physiol. 89:331, 1929.
5. Meier, P., and Zierler, K. L.: On theory of indicator-dilution method for measurement of blood flow and volume. J. Appl. Physiol. 6:731, 1954.
6. Mullani, N., Goldstein, R. A., Gould, K. L., et al.: Myocardial perfusion with rubidium-82. I. Measurements of extraction fraction and flow with external detectors. J. Nucl. Med. 24:898, 1983.
7. Morgenstern, C., Holjes, U., Arnold, G., and Lochner, W.: The influence of coronary pressure and coronary flow on intracoronary blood volume angiometry of the left ventricle. Pfluegers Arch. 340:101, 1973.
8. Marcus, M. L., Doty, D. B., Hiratzka, L. F., et al.: Decreased coronary reserve—a mechanism for angina pectoris in patients with aortic stenosis and normal coronary arteries. N. Engl. J. Med. 307:1362, 1982.

N

1. Nolting, D., Mack, R., Luthy, E., et al.: Measurement of coronary blood flow and myocardial rubidium uptake with Rb^{86}. (Abstract.) J. Clin. Invest. 37:921, 1958.
2. Newman, E. V., Merrell, M., Genecin, A., et al.: The dye dilution method for describing the central circulation: An analysis of factors shaping the time-concentration curves. Circulation 4:735, 1951.
3. Newhouse, J. H.: Fluid compartment distribution of intravenous iothallamate in the dog. Invest. Radiol. 12:346, 1977.
4. Newhouse, J. H., and Murphy, R. X.: Tissue distribution of soluble contrast: Effective dose variation and changes with time. AJR 136:436, 1981.

O

1. O'Neill, W. W., Vogel, R. A., and LeFree, M. P.: Digital coronary radiographic assessment of relative regional coronary blood flow. Circ. Suppl. II 66:II-229, 1982.

P

1. Prinzmetal, M., Corday, E., Bergman, H. C., et al.: Radiocardiography: A new method for studying blood flow through the chambers of the heart in human beings. Science 108:340, 1948.
2. Prinzmetal, M., Corday, E., Spritzler, R. J., and Flieg, W.: Radiocardiograhy and its clinical applications. JAMA 139:617, 1949.

R

1. Rigo, P., Baley, I. K., Griffith, L. S. C., et al.: Value and limitations of segmental analysis of stress thallium myocardial imaging for localization of coronary artery disease. Circulation 61:973, 1980.
2. Ritchie, J. L.: Myocardial perfusion imaging. Am. J. Cardiol. 49:1341, 1982.
3. Rumberger, J. A., Feiring, A. J., and Lipton, M. J.: Use of ultrafast computed tomography to quantitate regional myocardial perfusion: A preliminary report. J. Am. Coll. Cardiol. 9:59, 1987.
4. Rumberger, J. A., Stanford, W., and Marcus, M. L.: Quantitation of regional myocardial perfusion by ultrafast-CT: Promises and pitfalls. Am. J. Card. Imag. 1:336, 1987.
5. Ritman, E. L., Kinsey, J. H., Robb, R. A., et al.: Physics and technical considerations in the design of the DSR: A high-temporal resolution volume scanner. AJR 134:369, 1980.
6. Reiter, S. J., Rumberger, J. A., Feiring, A. J., et al.: Precision of measurements of right and left ventricular volumes by cine computed tomography. Circulation 74:890, 1986.
7. Reiter, S. J., Feiring, A. J., Stanford, W., et al.: Precise measurement of contrast clearance curve cardiac outputs using cine computed tomography. J. Am. Coll. Cardiol. 9:161A, 1987.

S

1. Shah, A., Shelbert, H., and Schwaiger, M.: Measurement of regional myocardial blood flow with N-13 ammonia and positron emission tomography in intact dogs. J. Am. Coll. Cardiol. 5:92, 1985.
2. Stewart, G. N.: Researches on the circulation time in organs and on the influences which affect it. I. Preliminary paper. II. The time of the lesser circulation. III. The circulation time in the thyroid gland and the effect of secretion and stimulation of nerves upon it. J. Physiol. (London) 15:1, 1893.
3. Stewart, G. N.: Researches on the circulation time and on the influences which affect it. IV. The output of the heart. J. Physiol. (London) 22:159, 1897.
4. Stewart, G. N.: Researches on the circulation time and on the influences which affect it. Circulation time of the spleen, kidney, intestine, heart (coronary circulation), and retina, with observations on time of lesser circulation. Am. J. Physiol. 58:278, 1921.
5. Sapirstein, L. A.: Regional blood flow by fractional distribution of indicators. Am. J. Physiol. 193:161, 1958.
6. Siegelman, S. S., Zerhouni, E. A., Leo, F. P., et al.: CT of the solid solitary pulmonary nodule. AJR 135:1, 1980.
7. Spaan, J. A. E.: Coronary diastolic pressure-flow relation in 0 flow pressure explained on the basis of intramyocardial compliance. Circ. Res. 56:293, 1985.

T

1. Thompson, H. K., Starmer, C. F., Waylon, R. F., and Macintosh, H. D.: Indicator transit time considered as a gamma variate. Circ. Res. 14:502, 1964.
2. Tonge, K. A., Wright, C. H., Mathew, J., et al.: Flow rate determination using computed tomography. Br. J. Radiol. 53:946, 1980.

V

1. Vogel, R., LeFree, M., and Bates, E.: Application of digital techniques to selective coronary arteriography: Use of myocardial contrast clearance time to measure coronary flow reserve. Am. Heart J. 107:153, 1984.

W

1. Wilson, R. F., Laughlin, D. E., and Ackell, P. H.: Transluminal subselective measurement of coronary artery blood flow velocity and vasodilator reserve in man. Circulation 72:82, 1985.
2. Weisenberg, G., Shelbert, H. R., and Hoffman, E. J.: In-vivo quantitation of regional myocardial blood flow by positron emission computed tomography. Circulation 63:1248, 1981.
3. Wang, T., and Ritman, E. L.: Myocardial perfusion estimated with multi-slice high-speed CT. Clin. Res. 34:942A, 1986.
4. Wang, T., Wu, X., Chung, N., and Ritman, E. L.: Myocardial blood flow quantitated by synchronous, multi-slice, high-speed computer tomography. IEEE Trans. Med. Imag. 8:70, 1989.
5. Wolfkiel, C. J., Ferguson, J. L., Chomka, E. V., et al.: Measurement of myocardial blood flow by ultrafast computed tomography. Circulation 76:1262, 1987.
6. Wood, E. H., and Geraci, J. E.: Photoelectric determination of arterial oxygen saturation in man. J. Lab. Clin. Med. 34:387, 1949.
7. Wilson, R. F., Laughlin, D. E., Hartley, C. G., et al.: Selective measurements of coronary blood flow velocity and vasodilator reserve in man. J. Am. Coll. Cardiol. 3:529, 1984.
8. Wolfkiel, C. J., Ferguson, J. L., Chomka, E. V., and Brundage, B.: Determination of cardiac output by ultrafast computed tomography. Am. J. Cardiac Imag. 1:117, 1986.
9. Wusten, B., Buss, D. D., Deist, H., and Schaper, W.: Dilatory capacity of the coronary circulation and its correlation to the arterial vasculature in the canine left ventricle. Basic Res. Cardiol. 72:636, 1977.
10. Weiss, H. R., and Winbury, M. M.: Nitroglycerin and chromonar on small-vessel blood content of the ventricular wall. Am. J. Physiol. 226:838, 1974.
11. Weiss, R. M., Hajduczok, Z. D., and Marcus, M. L.: A new algorithm for quantitation of myocardial perfusion with cine computed tomography. Clin. Res. 36:832A, 1988.
12. Wangler, R. D., Peters, K. G., Marcus, M. L., and Tomanek, R. J.: Effects of duration and severity of arterial hypertension in cardiac hypertrophy and coronary vasodilator reserve. Circ. Res. 51:10, 1982.

Y

1. Yipintsoi, T., Dobbs, W. A., Jr., Scanlon, P. D., et al.: Regional distribution of diffusible tracers and carbonized microspheres in the left ventricle of isolated dog hearts. Circ. Res. 33:573, 1973.

Z

1. Zierler, K. R.: A simplified explanation of the theory of indicator-dilution for measurement of fluid flow and volume and other distributive phenomena. Bull. Johns-Hopkins Hosp. 103:199, 1958.
2. Ziegler, W. H., and Goresky, C. A.: Transcapillary exchange in the working left ventricle of the dog. Circ. Res. 24:181, 1971.

Chapter 36

Assessment of Intracardiac Masses and Extracardiac Abnormalities by Ultrafast Computed Tomography

WILLIAM STANFORD, M.D. ▪ SEYED A. ROOHOLAMINI, M.D. ▪ JEFFREY R. GALVIN, M.D.

INTRACARDIAC TUMORS 703
Atrial Myxomas 703
Ultrafast CT Appearance of Atrial Myxomas 703
Imaging Sequences 704
Less Common Primary Cardiac Tumors 704
Metastatic Tumors and Intracardiac Extensions of Infradiaphragmatic Tumors 704
Summary 705
INTRACARDIAC AND PULMONARY ARTERY THROMBI 705
Ultrafast CT Appearance of Thrombi 705
Indications for Ultrafast CT Imaging in Suspected Thrombi 706
Scanning Sequences 706
Accuracy of Ultrafast Computed Tomography in Detecting Intracavity Thrombi 706
Ultrafast Computed Tomography in Imaging Pulmonary Emboli 706
Summary 707
PERICARDIUM 707
Pericardial CT Anatomy 707
Pericardial Imaging Techniques and Protocols 708
Pericardial Effusions 708
Pericardial Thickening 708
Malignant Disease 709
Constrictive Pericarditis 709
Less Common Pericardial Lesions 709
Advantages and Disadvantages of Ultrafast Computed Tomography in Pericardial Disease 709
Summary 710
THORACIC AORTIC ANEURYSMS AND DISSECTIONS 710
Thoracic Aneurysms 710
Experience 710
CT Appearance of Aneurysms 710
Imaging Protocols 710
CT Criteria for Leak 710
Thoracic Dissections 710
Scanner Protocols 711
Decision Making in Imaging Aortic Dissection 711
Advantages and Disadvantages of Ultrafast Computed Tomography in Imaging Aortic Aneurysms and Dissections 711
Summary 712
MEDIASTINAL MASSES 712
Scanner Protocols 713
Other Mediastinal Lesions 713
Advantages and Disadvantages of Ultrafast Computed Tomography in Mediastinal Disease 713
Summary 713
CONCLUSION 713

Ultrafast computed tomography (ultrafast CT) shows significant promise in imaging intracardiac masses and extracardiac abnormalities of the chest. The 1- to 2-mm resolution, superb vessel opacification, reduced motion artifact, and decreased radiation dosage make the Imatron C-100 ultrafast CT scanner ideal for cardiac, pericardial, and mediastinal imaging. In this chapter we discuss the use of the ultrafast CT scanner in the imaging of intracardiac masses and extracardiac abnormalities. The comments that follow are based on a 3-year experience in scanning over 1000 cardiac patients.

INTRACARDIAC TUMORS

Atrial Myxomas

Atrial myxomas account for 50 percent of primary cardiac tumors. They generally arise within the left atrium in the area in and around the limbus of the fossa ovalis, average 4 to 8 cm in diameter,[H1] and are often pedunculated. The pedunculation allows the myxoma to prolapse through the mitral valve in diastole; in systole the tumor usually lies within the atrium. The second most common site of origin is the right atrium. Here myxomas tend to be more solid and have a flat or sessile configuration. The third site is within the right ventricle. The size, location, attachment, and configuration of the myxoma can be demonstrated by ultrafast CT imaging, as can any movement occurring during the cardiac cycle. Computed tomography, with its axial orientation, does not have the superimposition of other tissues and therefore is very useful for defining multiple myxomas.

Ultrafast CT Appearance of Atrial Myxomas

Intracavitary tumor masses appear as filling defects within the opacified cardiac chambers. The myxoma configuration may be

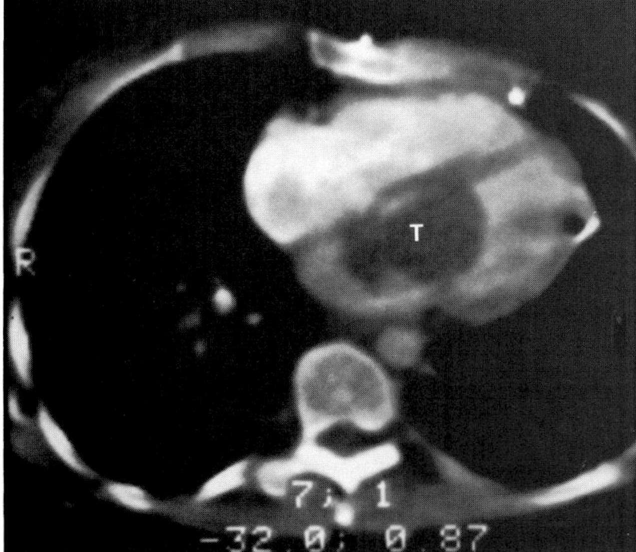

Figure 36–1. Long-axis view of a left atrial myxoma (T) prolapsing through the mitral valve in diastole. The tumor often abuts the anterior leaflet of the mitral valve. A left atrial myxoma was found at operation. R = right. (From Scholtz, T. D., Boskis, M., Roust, L., et al.: Noninvasive diagnosis of recurrent familial left atrial myxoma: Observations with echocardiography, ultrafast computed tomography, nuclear magnetic resonance imaging and in vitro relaxometry. Am. J. Cardiac Imag. 3:142, 1989, with permission.)

sessile but more often is pedunculated. The pedunculation allows the tumor to prolapse through the mitral valve. If this occurs, the tumor may abut the anterior leaflet of the mitral valve and thicken or deform the valve (Fig. 36–1). Sessile tumors are more commonly located on the right side of the interatrial septum and appear on CT images as a thickening of the septum. Right ventricular myxomas are usually located within the right ventricular chamber and have a more rounded appearance. They are usually attached to the right ventricular free wall, interventricular septum, or a papillary muscle of the tricuspid valve (Fig. 36–2).

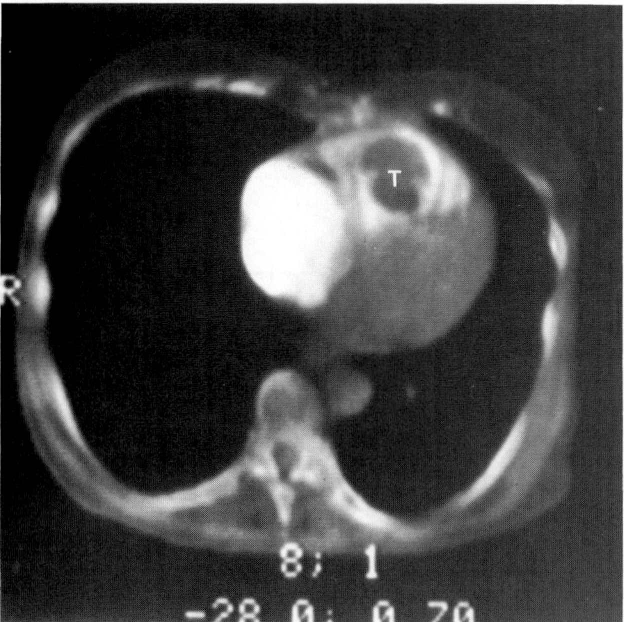

Figure 36–2. Right ventricular myxoma (T) arising from a papillary muscle of the tricuspid valve. This was confirmed at operation. (From Stanford, W., and Galvin, J. R.: The radiology of right heart dysfunction: Chest roentgenogram and computed tomography. Reprinted from the Journal of Thoracic Imaging, Vol. 4, No. 3, p. 7, with permission of Aspen Publishers, Inc., © July 1989.)

The Hounsfield numbers approximate those of the myocardium, but this does not usually interfere with the diagnosis. The tumors may be multiple.

Imaging Sequences

When an examination is ordered primarily as a screening procedure, flow mode may be the best initial imaging sequence. In the flow mode sequence, eight 8-mm slice thicknesses of the heart are taken in 224 msec. This sequence is repeated with triggering on every heartbeat or every other heartbeat. Contrast material is administered as a 40-ml bolus given via a power injection at 10 ml/sec. As the contrast material sequentially defines the cardiac chambers, the location of the lesion(s) is readily appreciated. Since opacification is usually greater in the flow mode and since the structures are stationary, the definition of the tumor margin is often better than in the movie mode. The flow mode also has the advantage of showing arrival times of the contrast bolus within the chambers, and by determining this arrival time, the amount of contrast material required on subsequent runs can be reduced. It is preferable to take these images with the patient in the neutral position.

The flow mode, however, does not show movement relationships, and since these are particularly important in myxomas, scanning in the movie mode is commonly added. In the movie mode sequence, images at one level are taken at a rate of 17 images per second. This rate is sufficient to image cardiac contraction in near real time. During the sequence, chamber opacification is provided by a continuous infusion of 70 ml of contrast material at 1.5 to 1.8 ml/sec. If the myxoma is known to lie within the left atrium, we would initially position the patient in the long-axis projection, since this provides superior definition of the mitral valve. The reasoning is that if the scanning has to be discontinued, the scan sequence best showing the lesion would be the first accomplished, and since myxomas commonly lie in approximation to the mitral valve, the long-axis movie images would be preferred. Because the contrast administration is via a peripheral vein, a catheter does not have to be manipulated in the vicinity of a possible right-sided myxoma.

Less Common Primary Cardiac Tumors

Rhabdomyomas, fibromas, and lipomas comprise a group of less common benign cardiac tumors. Rhabdomyomas usually occur in children and are associated with tuberous sclerosis.[S1] They frequently arise within the ventricular free wall or septum and are seen as deformities of the contrast-filled ventricular cavity. Fibromas may present a similar appearance. The tumor densities in both instances are the same as that of the myocardium, and this may preclude separation of the tumor from normal myocardium. Fibromas, however, may calcify. Lipomas tend to arise within the atrial septum and cause deformity of the septum on CT images. Their density is less than that of the myocardium.

The imaging sequences used for the less common primary cardiac tumors are similar to those used for myxomas.

Metastatic Tumors and Intracardiac Extensions of Infradiaphragmatic Tumors

Melanomas and lung and breast carcinomas are the most frequent tumors to metastasize to the heart.[N1, R1] They appear either as mass lesions within the cardiac chambers or as nodules on the epicardial surface. Lymphomas and renal carcinomas may grow intraluminally within the inferior vena cava and, at times, may extend into the right atrium and ventricle (Fig. 36–3). If an intracavitary extension is suspected, the flow mode is the better sequence since it can both define tumor location and show the route of contrast material as it passes around the tumor. A movie sequence may also be helpful to show tumor movement and define wall motion irregularities. Both modes show the extent of tumor involvement and define the presence of tumor outside the atrial or ventricular cavities. Conventional CT images similarly

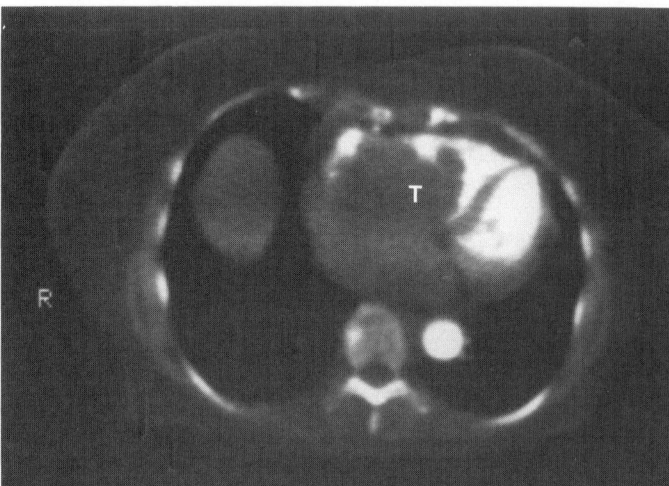

Figure 36–3. Histiocystic lymphoma (T) arising from the liver and growing up the inferior vena cava into the right atrium and ventricle. The tumor was infiltrating the wall of the right atrium. (From Stanford, W., and Galvin, J. R.: The radiology of right heart dysfunction: Chest roentgenogram and computed tomography. Reprinted from the Journal of Thoracic Imaging, Vol. 4, No. 3, p. 7, with permission of Aspen Publishers, Inc., © July 1989.)

show the extent of the tumor, but movement artifact and poor opacification may detract from the images. Conventional computed tomography does not show flow characteristics or wall motion abnormalities.

Summary

Ultrafast computed tomography is a useful, minimally invasive imaging technique for evaluating intracardiac tumors. Both the anatomy and tumor movement occurring during the cardiac contraction can be readily defined.

INTRACARDIAC AND PULMONARY ARTERY THROMBI

Thrombi may be solitary or multiple and occur within the cardiac chambers or the pulmonary artery. We have seen many examples of both. Thrombi within the heart are seen as filling defects within the opacified cardiac chambers (Fig. 36–4). The thrombi may be sessile or pedunculated. In the ventricle they usually lie adjacent to areas of myocardial infarction or otherwise diseased and poorly contractile myocardium. Because thrombus identification may be difficult, it is our practice to image patients with both short-axis and long-axis projections. This allows viewing in different orientations and helps to identify and differentiate structures such as aberrant muscle bands and papillary muscles. Axial images allow excellent visualization of the left atrial appendage and of the entrance of the pulmonary veins.

Ultrafast CT Appearance of Thrombi

Sessile or flat thrombi are more difficult to diagnose. Characteristically, they present as curvilinear filling defects along the wall of a contrast-opacified ventricle. Alternatively, they may present as an oval-shaped filling defect projecting into the ventricular cavity. There is usually an associated wall motion abnormality, and if this is not seen one should be cautious in diagnosing thrombus. Occasionally, we have seen cases in which thrombi projected a considerable distance into the ventricle. However, in these cases, the thrombus can often be seen moving or swirling within the ventricular chamber during cardiac contraction (Fig. 36–5).

The differentiation of thrombus from papillary muscle may be difficult. It is best done by knowledge of the location and configuration of the papillary muscles. In the left ventricle the anterior papillary muscle arises from the anterior wall lateral to the apex and away from the interventricular septum. The location of the posterior papillary muscle is somewhat more variable. It is usually seen along the posterolateral aspect of the ventricle on both the long-axis and short-axis images. Both muscles appear as smooth, oval filling defects approximately 1 cm in diameter. A problem arises when the papillary muscles are prominent and there is thickening or conglutination of the subchordal structures, as is often the case in mitral stenosis. In these instances, the thickening may extend almost to the valve leaflet. Thrombi, on the other hand, often lie adjacent to the apex of the left ventricle and septum. They are commonly associated with abnormalities of wall motion. An alternative site is the inferior aspect of the left ventricle. Inferior thrombi are best seen on short-axis views, whereas apical thrombi are best seen on long-axis views.

Atrial thrombi may be present in patients with mitral stenosis, especially if there is associated atrial fibrillation. The tip of the

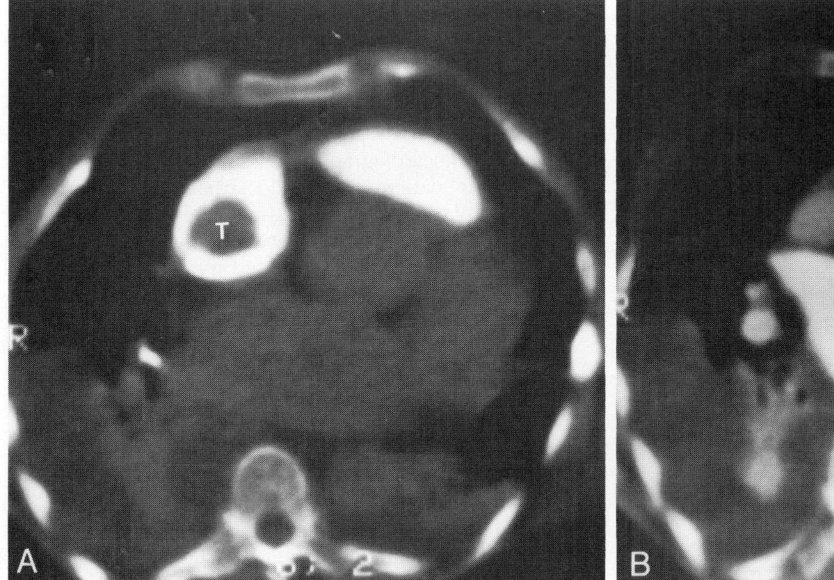

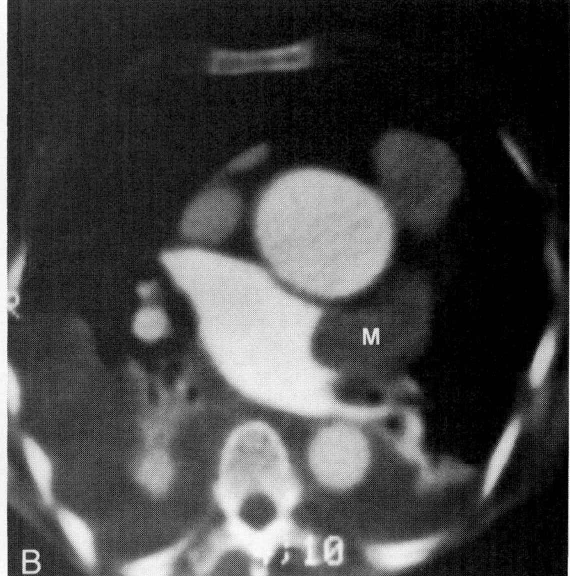

Figure 36–4. *A*, Right atrial (T) and *B*, left atrial appendage (M) thrombi in a patient with breast carcinoma. The patient was anticoagulated but lost to follow-up. Metastatic tumor could not be completely excluded.

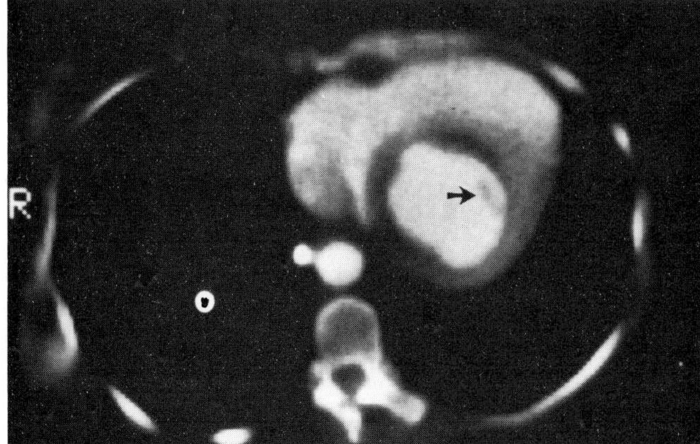

Figure 36–5. Long flame-shaped ventricular thrombus *(arrow)* arising from an area of posterior myocardial infarction. In the movie mode sequences the thrombus could be seen swirling within the ventricular cavity.

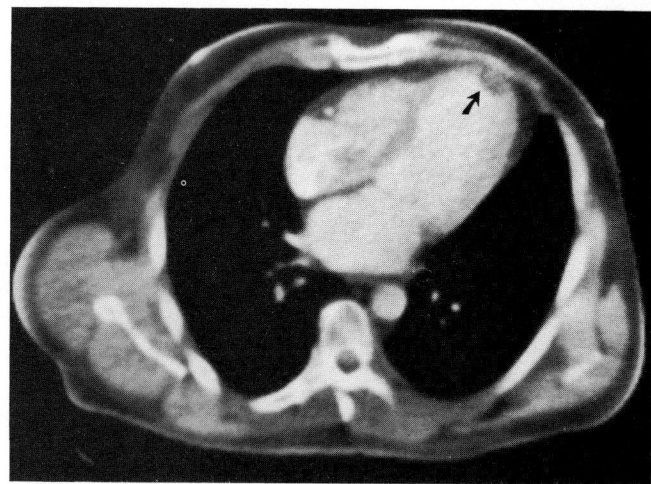

Figure 36–7. Thrombus *(arrow)* in the apex of the left ventricle in a patient with syncopal attacks. The patient had a history of myocardial infarction.

left atrial appendage has the highest incidence of thrombus formation.[H1] Ultrafast computed tomography shows the left atrial appendage in cross section, and this often provides better information than echocardiography. Fibrous tissue ingrowth can occur in long-standing thrombi, as can calcification. Calcifications are readily seen on ultrafast computed tomography (Fig. 36–6). Since the density of thrombus is similar to that of myocardium, Hounsfield numbers may not help differentiate thrombus from normal myocardium or from papillary muscle.

Indications for Ultrafast CT Imaging in Suspected Thrombi

Patients with recent cerebrovascular accidents and/or pulmonary emboli are candidates for scanning; however, we have scanned a number of patients in whom thrombus was an unexpected finding (Fig. 36–7). In the evaluation of intracavitary thrombi, it is our usual practice to scan in both the short-axis and long-axis projections. If a thrombus is identified, anticoagulation therapy is often instituted and ultrafast CT is a useful technique for following the results of the anticoagulation treatment (Fig. 36–8).

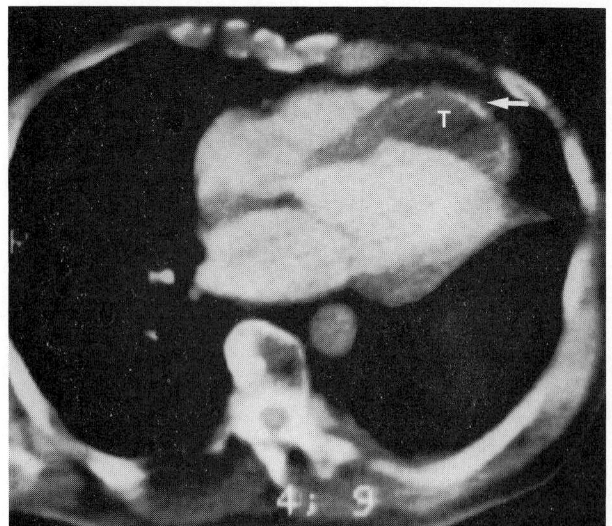

Figure 36–6. Calcification in the wall of the left ventricle *(arrow)* in a patient with a previous myocardial infarction. There is a large thrombus (T) adjacent to the infarct.

Scanning Sequences

In suspected thrombi, the movie mode is the most informative sequence, since the images show associated abnormalities of wall motion. If the examination is done for screening and the probability of thrombus is low, we sometimes do a single 10- or 12-level movie sequence with the patient positioned in the neutral axis. This sequence encompasses the heart with one injection of contrast material but gives only six to eight images at each level. The sequence is sufficient to identify thrombi but not sufficient to evaluate wall motion thoroughly. For these reasons we commonly do complete short-axis and long-axis movie sequences. This allows imaging of the cardiac chambers in two projections and gives excellent visualization of ventricular movement throughout a full cardiac contraction. These sequences require only slightly more scan time and only a small amount of additional contrast material (60 ml).

Accuracy of Ultrafast Computed Tomography in Detecting Intracavitary Thrombi

In a study comparing ultrafast computed tomography with two-dimensional echocardiography in the detection of intracardiac thrombi in 41 stroke patients, Beattie and associates[B1] found agreement between the techniques in 86 percent of patients (both were negative in 76 percent, both positive in 10 percent). In the six patients (14 percent) for whom there was disagreement, echocardiography was positive and tomography equivocal in four patients, echocardiography was equivocal and tomography negative in one patient, and echocardiography was equivocal and tomography positive in one patient (the latter patient had autopsy confirmation of left ventricular thrombus). Beattie and associates concluded that ultrafast computed tomography was an important imaging technique for detecting intracardiac thrombi, especially in patients for whom two-dimensional echocardiography was difficult or equivocal.

Ultrafast Computed Tomography in Imaging Pulmonary Emboli

Pulmonary emboli can be visualized on ultrafast CT images if the emboli are proximal and do not lodge beyond the second division of the pulmonary arteries (Figs. 36–9 and 36–10). Distal thrombi may be missed. No definitive studies have yet been done to determine the accuracy of this technique in detecting pulmonary emboli.

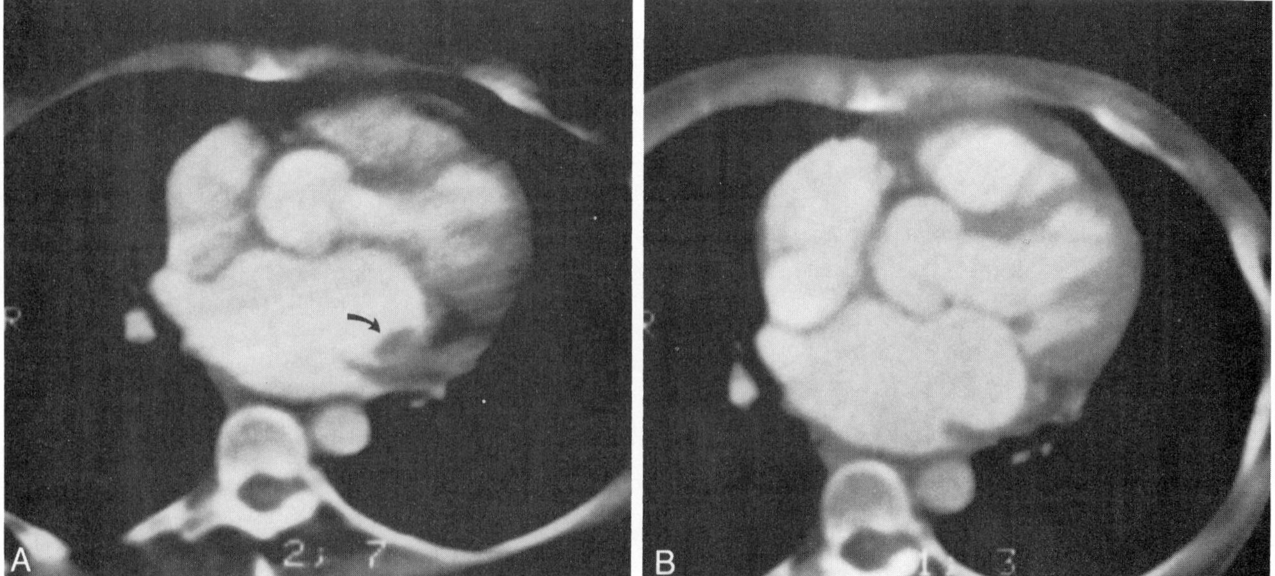

Figure 36–8. Images from a patient with mitral stenosis and a normal atrial echo examination. *A*, On ultrafast computed tomography there was a small thrombus *(arrow)* attached to the lateral wall of the left atrium just below the orifice of the superior pulmonary vein. *B*, Six weeks later, after the patient had been treated with anticoagulants, the thrombus had disappeared.

Summary

The identification of intracardiac thrombi is a major indication for ultrafast CT imaging. The technique is rapid, requires only peripheral injections of contrast materials, and readily identifies intracavitary thrombi and proximal pulmonary emboli. In addition, it can define associated ventricular aneurysms and wall motion abnormalities. It is useful in identifying pathologic conditions that predispose to thrombus formation, such as mitral valve stenosis, and in following patients with known thrombi.

PERICARDIUM

Our experience consists of imaging of 83 patients for suspected pericardial disease. The ultrafast CT images provide excellent detail, especially when 3-mm, high-resolution axial images are taken. These images consistently show pericardial thickening, calcification, intrapericardial tumors, and fluid collections. The scanner has the additional capability to evaluate chamber volumes and define wall motion.

Pericardial CT Anatomy

The pericardium is a fibrous sac that surrounds the heart. It attaches to the great vessels at the level of the aortic and pulmonary valves and to the central tendon of the left hemidiaphragm.[N1] It has two layers, parietal and visceral, which are separated by a potential space containing approximately 25 ml of serous fluid.[C1, H2] The parietal pericardium is usually separated from the sternum by mediastinal fat and from the myocardium by a layer of epicardial fat. This makes the pericardium visible on computed tomography, especially in the area ventral to the right ventricle.

The pericardium is seen as a 1- to 2-mm line of soft-tissue density lying between mediastinal fat ventrally and epicardial fat dorsally (Fig. 36–11). Inferiorly at its insertion into the diaphragm, it thickens to 3 to 4 mm.[M1] Although the ventral pericardium is usually visualized, the dorsal pericardium is seen only about 25 percent of the time. There is little fat superiorly, so the pericardium is often not seen in this view. Only if the pericardial cavity is distended by air, fluid, or mass lesions is the dorsal pericardium visualized by computed tomography.[M1]

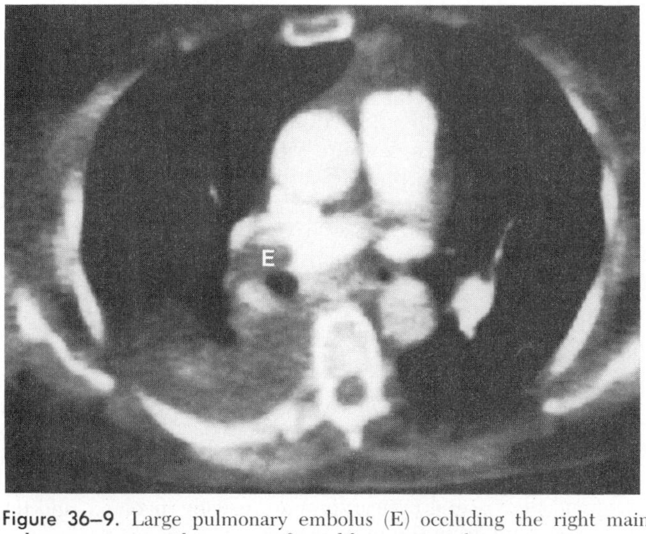

Figure 36–9. Large pulmonary embolus (E) occluding the right main pulmonary artery. This was confirmed by angiography.

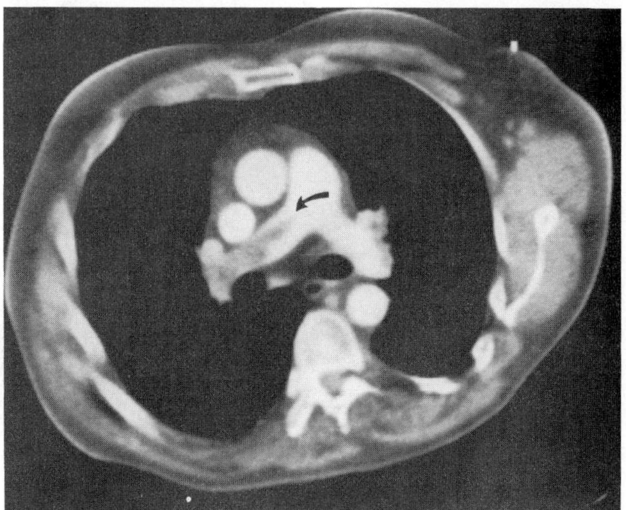

Figure 36–10. Flame-shaped pulmonary embolus *(arrow)* in a patient presenting with syncopal attacks. The embolus was an unexpected finding.

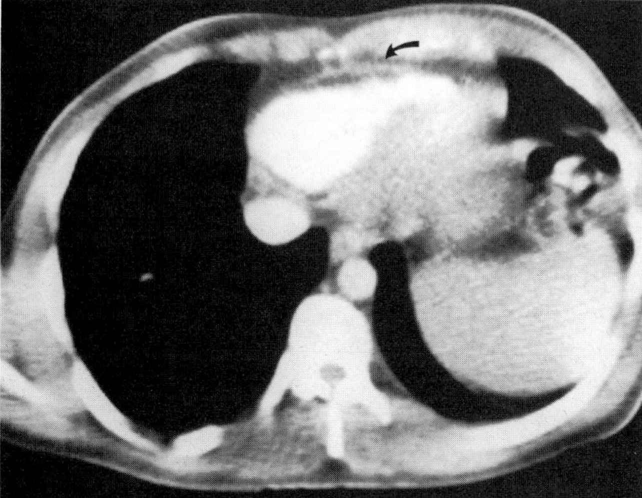

Figure 36–11. Neutral axis image of a patient with a normal pericardium. The pericardium is seen as a 2-mm linear soft tissue density *(arrow)* lying between the anterior mediastinal and epicardial fat.

There can be problems in imaging the pericardium. Thickening at the attachment to the diaphragm is commonly seen and should not be confused with an infiltrative process. Similarly, nodular thickenings over the right atrium and ventricle are common. Superoposteriorly, at its attachment to the aorta, there is a recess that can sometimes be mistaken for adenopathy.[A1]

Pericardial Imaging Techniques and Protocols

Ultrafast CT imaging sequences vary. Our most frequently used sequence consists of movie mode images in the short axis and then the long axis. Several 3-mm cuts with the patient in the neutral position are often added to better define anatomy.

Examinations can be done either with or without contrast material. If there is a moderate or excessive amount of epicardial and mediastinal fat, the non-contrast images will show the anatomy with great clarity. Low-density cysts, effusions, and pericardial calcification can be visualized without contrast, and Hounsfield numbers can be used to characterize the composition of any fluid collections.

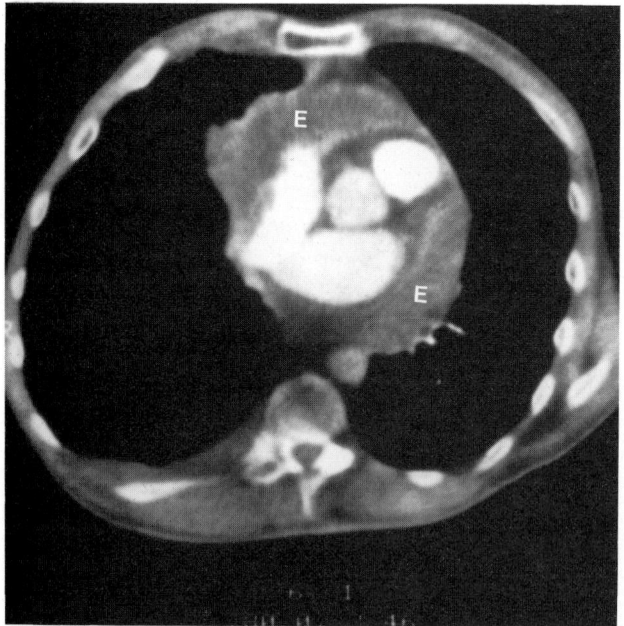

Figure 36–12. Loculated pericardial effusions (E) lying anteriorly to the right atrium and posterior to the left atrium. (From Stanford, W., and Galvin, J. R.: The radiology of right heart dysfunction: Chest roentgenogram and computed tomography. Reprinted from the Journal of Thoracic Imaging, Vol. 4, No. 3, p. 7, with permission of Aspen Publishers, Inc., © July 1989.)

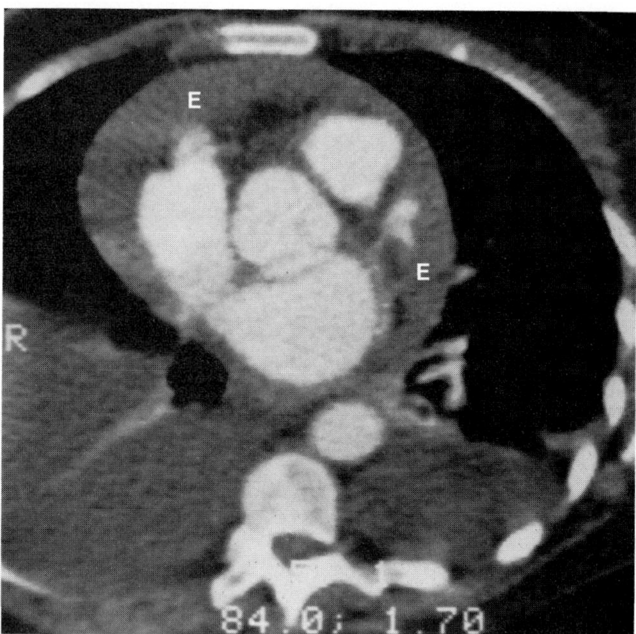

Figure 36–13. Large pericardial effusion (E) surrounding the heart and great vessels.

Contrast enhancement is useful in delineating cardiac chambers, assessing wall motion abnormalities, defining inflammatory and vascular lesions, and differentiating pericardial thickening from adjacent atelectatic lung.

Pericardial Effusions

The pericardium reacts to injury by fluid production, fibrin formation, and cellular proliferation.[R2] These may occur together or independently. If fluid is present, it initially accumulates in the caudal portion of the pericardium and appears as a thin elliptical density lying dorsal to the left ventricular myocardium. As the effusion increases, it extends up and over the ventral surface of the right atrium and ventricle (Fig. 36–12) and may even surround the origins of the great vessels (Fig. 36–13).[L1] Localized small effusions are more commonly seen inferiorly and dorsolaterally to the left ventricle and in pericardial recesses such as the transverse sinus, the area surrounding the ascending aorta and pulmonary trunk, the oblique sinus, and the pulmonic recess.[L2]

The amount of fluid and its physiologic effects vary. A normal pericardium may become significantly distended yet produce little hemodynamic alteration. Conversely, if the fluid accumulates rapidly or in an area where a thickened pericardium limits its distensibility, it may produce cardiac tamponade (Fig. 36–14).

Fluid composition may be serous or proteinaceous. Effusions with a high protein content may have CT numbers that approach those of soft tissue and hence may be difficult to distinguish from thickened pericardium.

Pericardial Thickening

Pericardial thickening is seen as a response to trauma, inflammation, or tumor and as a sequela of pericardiotomy incisions and radiation injury. The thickening may be localized or generalized and may extend beyond 6 cm. Both the parietal pericardium and the visceral pericardium are usually involved, and the process may infiltrate the myocardium.

If identification of the effusion is difficult, placing the patient

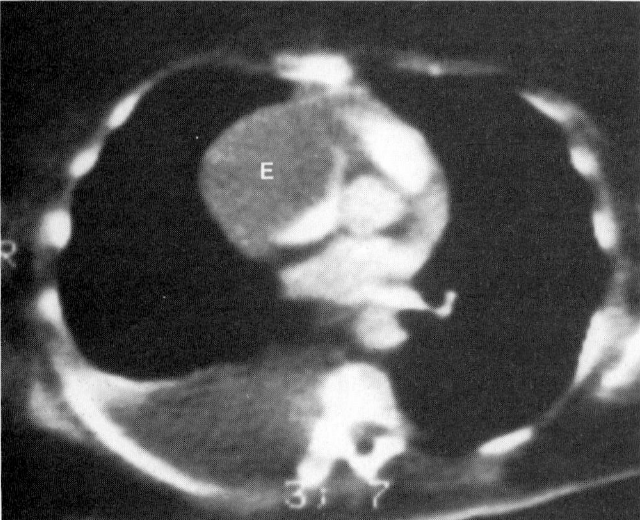

Figure 36–14. Loculated effusion (E) compressing the right atrium in a postoperative coronary artery bypass patient. The patient presented with low cardiac output. After the collection was drained, her cardiac output immediately returned to normal. (From Stanford, W., and Galvin, J. R.: The radiology of right heart dysfunction: Chest roentgenogram and computed tomography. Reprinted from the Journal of Thoracic Imaging, Vol. 4, No. 3, p. 7, with permission of Aspen Publishers, Inc., © July 1989.)

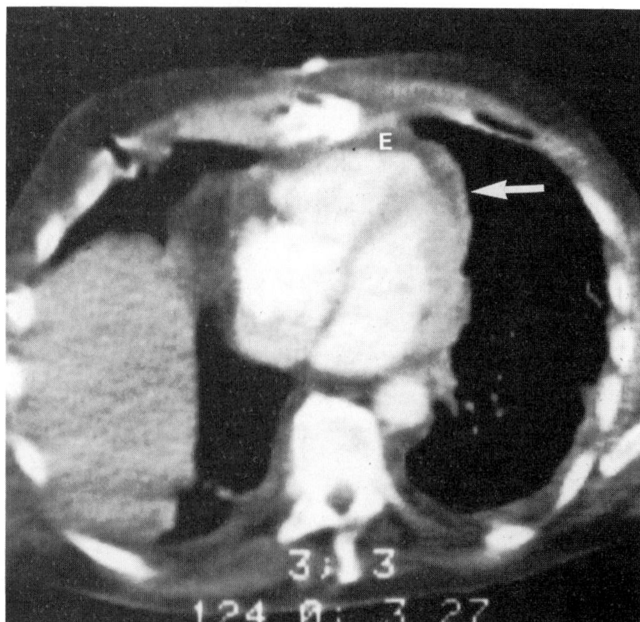

Figure 36–16. Image from a postoperative coronary artery bypass patient with thickened pericardium *(arrow)* and loculated effusions (E). The patient exhibited constrictive physiology. The cardiac output returned to normal after pericardiectomy.

in a decubitus position may change the configuration of the effusion and help define its location. This change does not occur in fibrous thickening, and this difference may be useful in differentiating fluid from thickening. Atelectatic lung usually enhances with contrast, and this may help differentiate this entity from pericardial thickening.

Malignant Disease

Breast and lung carcinomas commonly metastasize to the pericardium. Malignant mesothelioma may also invade the pericardium. The latter tumor may present as a solitary mass or form diffuse plaques that encase the parietal pericardium (Fig. 36–15). Lymphoma may present as a diffuse infiltration.

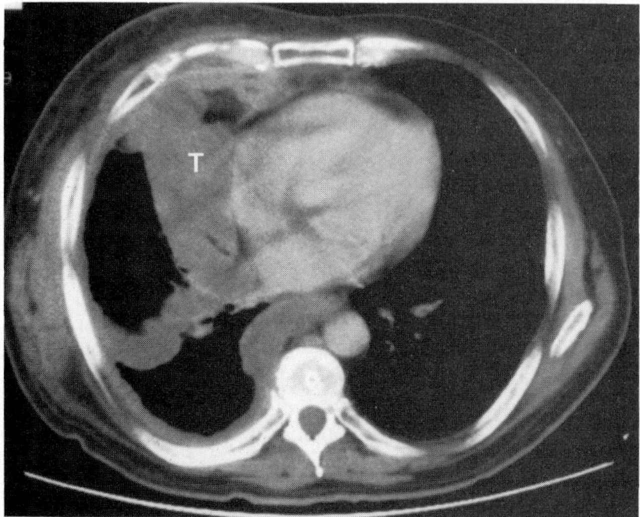

Figure 36–15. A mesothelioma (T) involving the parietal pericardium. (From Stanford, W., and Galvin, J. R.: The radiology of right heart dysfunction: Chest roentgenogram and computed tomography. Reprinted from the Journal of Thoracic Imaging, Vol. 4, No. 3, p. 7, with permission of Aspen Publishers, Inc., © July 1989.)

Constrictive Pericarditis

Tuberculosis, mediastinal fibrosis, tumor infiltration, and infection may result in pericardial fibrosis and constriction. The fibrosis may prevent diastolic filling and result in a low cardiac output. The extent of pericardial involvement can be identified with ultrafast computed tomography (Fig. 36–16).

Ultrafast computed tomography can also differentiate cardiomyopathy from constrictive pericarditis. In cardiomyopathy, the pericardium is normal in thickness but the ventricle contracts poorly. In constrictive pericarditis, the pericardium is thickened and the ventricle may show impaired diastolic filling.

Less Common Pericardial Lesions

Pericardial cysts are less common pericardial lesions; however, they are readily identifiable by computed tomography. This lesion appears as a mass in the right or occasionally the left pericardiophrenic angle. The cysts are filled with a clear, low-density fluid and have Hounsfield numbers approaching that of water density (Fig. 36–17).[M1]

Congenital absence of the pericardium often presents as a lack of pericardial continuity in association with herniation of the left atrial appendage through the defect.[N2] If the entire left hemipericardium is absent, one may see direct apposition between the heart and the lung tissue.

Benign tumors of the pericardium include teratomas, bronchogenic cysts, leiomyomas, hemangiomas, and lipomas.[L3] Lipomas have densities ranging from −55 to −120 Hounsfield units and are readily identifiable. Hemangiomas may be enhanced significantly with contrast material and are easy to identify. High-protein bronchogenic cysts and leiomyomas of the esophagus have CT numbers similar to those of soft tissue, and malignancy often cannot be excluded. In teratomas, both fat and tooth calcifications are readily seen.

Advantages and Disadvantages of Ultrafast Computed Tomography in Pericardial Disease

Ultrafast computed tomography is a useful adjunct to echocardiography. The CT images show loculations and thickening better

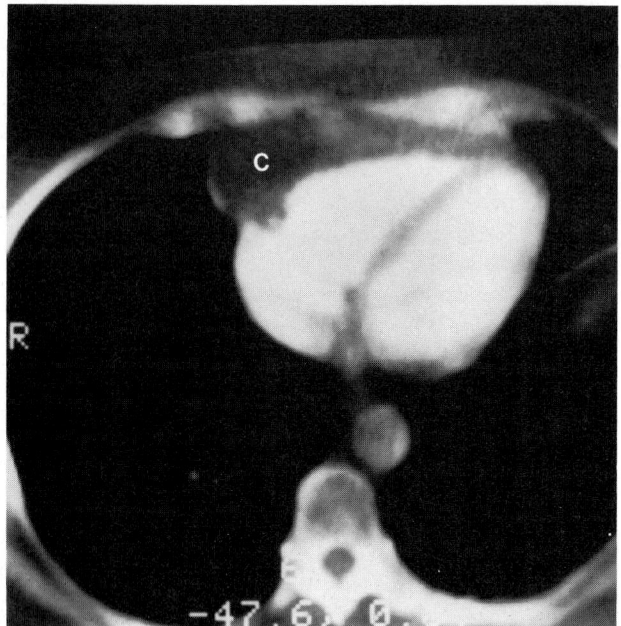

Figure 36–17. Pericardial cyst (C) located in the right pericardiophrenic angle. The cyst contents had Hounsfield numbers similar to that of water.

than echocardiography. In addition, the images are reproducible and allow the assessment of ventricular function and assessment of the composition of the effusion. The ability to calculate functional parameters is an additional advantage. The technique is particularly useful in assessing loculated effusions and compressive hematomas as causes of postoperative low cardiac output.

Ultrafast computed tomography is not suitable for use in the agitated patient who cannot lie supine or who is too ill to be transported to the imaging suite. It cannot be used in patients with renal compromise or contrast allergies. However, it is suitable for patients who cannot hold their breath.

Summary

Ultrafast CT retains the advantages of conventional CT in showing pericardial anatomy and, by virtue of its ability to assess wall motion, is especially helpful in the evaluation of pericardial disease. The ability to determine left and right ventricular end-diastolic and end-systolic volumes, stroke volume, ejection fraction, left ventricular mass, and cardiac output is important in patients suspected of having constrictive physiology.

THORACIC AORTIC ANEURYSMS AND DISSECTIONS

Thoracic Aneurysms

Experience

Our experience in aortic aneurysmal disease encompasses more than 50 patients with suspected aneurysm. In this group, there were 14 ascending aortic aneurysms, 8 descending aortic aneurysms, 13 thoracoabdominal aneurysms, and 7 abdominal aneurysms. No aneurysms were found in 8 patients. Correlation with angiography or surgery was possible in 26 of these patients. Except for one false-positive examination, there was excellent correlation between the ultrafast CT findings and the findings at angiography or surgery.

CT Appearance of Aneurysms

The most significant radiologic sign in aneurysmal disease of the aorta is an increased aortic diameter. Because of the changes that occur with aging, no definitive number can be placed on the aortic diameter, but approximately 4 cm is the norm. Clots or irregular wall thickenings are present in a significant percentage of arteriosclerotic aneurysms. Conversely, in cases of Marfan's disease or aneurysmal involvement due to syphilis, only a thin-walled dilated aorta is seen. Calcification may be present and, if seen, should lie within the outer wall. This is best appreciated on unenhanced images.

Aneurysms may take several forms. They may be fusiform with gradual enlargement and then a tapering back to a normal-sized vessel, or they may be saccular outpouchings from a specific area of the aortic wall. A nonleaking aneurysm should have a distinguishable wall and definitive adjacent fat planes. At times, adjacent lung atelectasis may be mistaken for extravasation. In thin individuals, the surrounding fat planes may be absent and it may appear as if the aneurysm is leaking. A problem often seen in the aging patient is obliquity of the aorta. In these cases, the axial slices may cut the aorta in an oblique fashion, and this gives an elongated or saccular appearance to the images. This too should be recognized, and in these cases a diagnosis of aneurysm should not be made.

Aneurysms resulting from trauma have a different CT appearance. They are classically in the area of the ligamentum arteriosum and are seen primarily in patients with lateral translation injuries, such as those occurring in motor vehicle accidents. The trauma frequently is associated with hematomas, which widen the mediastinum on the plain chest film. Computed tomography is especially helpful in demonstrating the presence of an aneurysm and defining its size and location. The CT images may also show associated injury, the extent of the hematoma, and the presence of effusion or atelectasis.

Imaging Protocols

The initial imaging sequence used to evaluate aneurysmal disease of the aorta is a volume study of the chest. This is done with 10-mm contiguous slices and should encompass a field extending from above the aortic arch to below the level of the suspected involvement. Scanning is usually done during continuous infusion of about 60 ml of 76 percent contrast material injected at a rate of 1.4 to 1.8 ml/sec. Prior to the injection it is often helpful to take a series of non-contrast images to encompass the area of concern. These non-contrast images provide a background with which to judge calcification.

In areas where leak is suspected or where branch vessel occlusion may be a problem, the addition of a flow sequence is helpful. Flow sequences will better delineate atelectatic lung as well as show differential contrast arrival times at sites within the aorta or periaortic tissues. The flow sequences also show perfusion delays in cases of retrograde flow occurring secondary to branch vessel occlusion.

The timing of the bolus may be a problem, especially in aneurysmal disease of the lower thoracic aorta. In most patients, the estimation of contrast bolus arrival time is based on the magnesium sulfate circulation time. In difficult or unresponsive patients, the use of Cardio-Green dye or a small bolus (20 ml) of contrast material with scanning in flow mode is helpful in determining the optimal scan delay.

CT Criteria for Leak

Extravasation of contrast material beyond the confines of the aortic wall is the definitive sign of rupture (Fig. 36–18). The obliteration of periaortic tissue planes is suggestive of a leak. Signs suggestive of expansion are adjacent atelectatic lung, new fluid collections or pleural effusions, and, in the case of posterior aneurysms, bony erosions. In spite of these criteria, the diagnosis of a leak may still be problematic. We have found previous images extremely helpful in that they allow the identification of changes in aneurysmal size as well as changes in the periaortic tissue planes.

Thoracic Dissections

Aortic dissections are especially well imaged by computed tomography. As with aneurysms, initial imaging without contrast

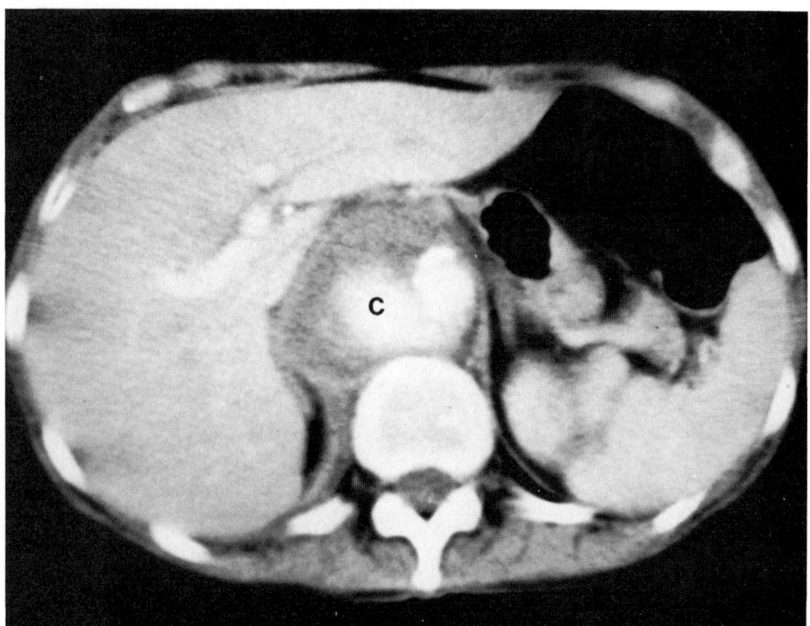

Figure 36–18. Periaortic leak in a patient with a mycotic aneurysm involving the thoracic aorta. Contrast material (C) can be seen outside the aortic lumen.

material is often desirable. Calcifications within the wall of the aorta are frequently present, and displacement of calcifications from the outer vessel wall by more than 5 mm is diagnostic for dissection (Fig. 36–19). In dissection, the tissues around the aorta often exhibit a loss of tissue planes, secondary to the periaortic inflammation. Associated atelectasis and pleural effusion may indicate dissection activity and require early recognition.

In dissection, aortic branch vessel occlusion and differential flow within the aortic lumina may be important. Branch vessel occlusion may be determined by time-density analyses. This is not always required, but in some cases it may be helpful, particularly in patients with retrograde fill. This information is important for the surgeon. The displacement of structures within the mediastinum is better appreciated on the axial CT sections, and this is another advantage.

Associated findings in dissection may be cardiomegaly, especially in patients with aortic insufficiency; compression of the esophagus and left atrium by the aneurysm; and lack of organ perfusion.

Occasionally, contrast material may appear outside the aortic lumen in the absence of leak or dissection. This occurs in saccular or mushroom-type aneurysms with narrow necks. When the neck of the aneurysm is reached on the axial slices, a single column of contrast material is seen extending into the periaortic tissue. These configurations can be appreciated on the sagittally reconstructed images (Fig. 36–20).

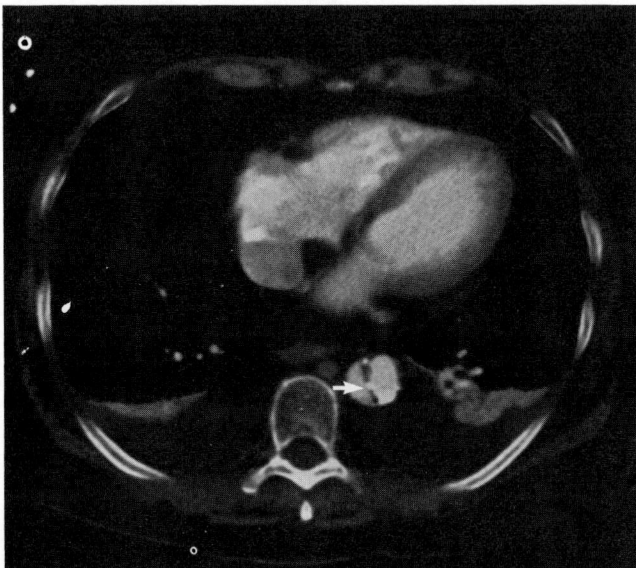

Figure 36–19. Aortic dissection beginning at the level of the mid-descending aorta. Calcification *(arrow)* is displaced medially.

Dissection flaps are best seen on cross-sectional images, and this is one of the main advantages of computed tomography. The flaps often spiral down the aorta and produce significant changes in the width of the aortic lumina. It is relatively easy with ultrafast computed tomography to see the origin of the branch vessels as they arise from the lumina (Fig. 36–21). This is helpful information that may not be provided by other imaging techniques.

In the flow mode sequences the dissection flap does not move, since each image is taken at the same instant in the cardiac cycle. If one wishes to see the actual movement of the flap, a movie mode could be used, and in difficult cases this may help delineate the dissection flap.

Scanner Protocols

Dissection is imaged with the same protocols as used for aortic aneurysms. The flow mode protocols may be of additional help in evaluating branch vessel occlusion. Delay in perfusion or lack of perfusion in branch vessels can be determined by placing time-density cursors over specific vessels. The arrival time of contrast material within the vessel is then compared with arrival time within the aorta. Delays signify proximal occlusion with or without retrograde flow.

Decision Making in Imaging Aortic Dissection

In screening patients with abnormal radiographs, in nonoperable patients, in stable symptomatic patients, in the follow-up of known dissection, and in postoperative patients, ultrafast computed tomography is the imaging technique of choice. This is also true in the acute trauma patient who is nonoperable or in whom there is a low probability of aneurysm. If, on the other hand, there is a high probability of aneurysm and the patient is a candidate for operation, most centers would prefer that the patient go directly to angiography. This is especially true if the aneurysm is associated with chest pain, appears to be enlarging, or is associated with a left pleural effusion. These all may indicate progressive dissection.

Advantages and Disadvantages of Ultrafast Computed Tomography in Imaging Aortic Aneurysms and Dissections

Ultrafast computed tomography provides a reasonable imaging alternative to angiography. The high-resolution images, excellent

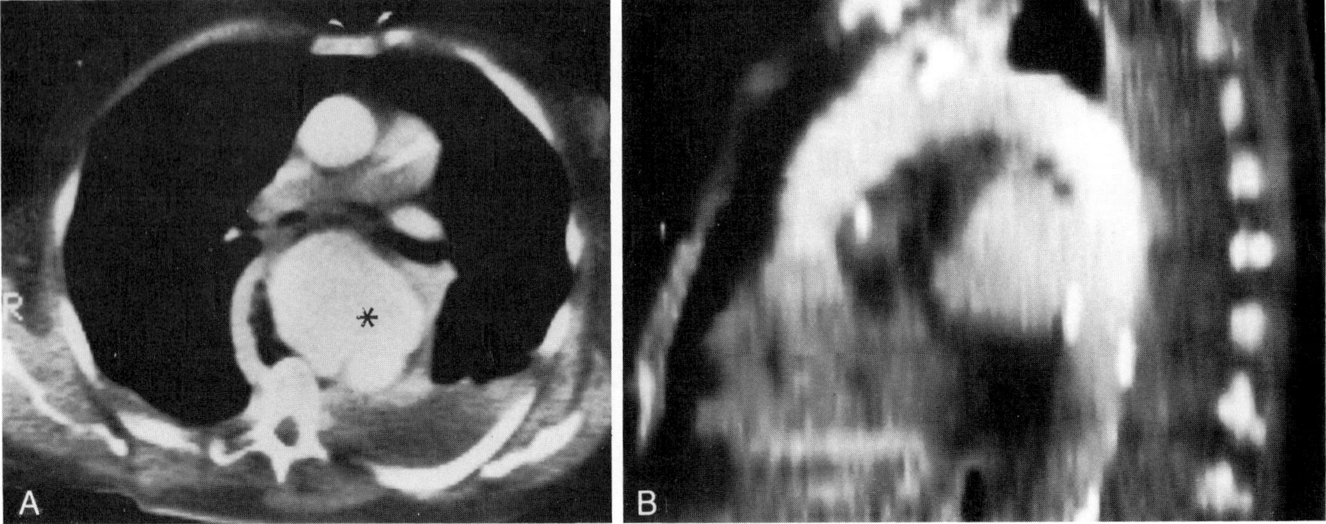

Figure 36–20. *A*, Axial image of a saccular aneurysm of the descending aorta. Note the contrast material extending beyond the aortic lumen in the plane of the aneurysm neck (asterisk). *B*, The reformatted image shows the saccular configuration.

vessel opacification, decreased radiation, and minimal motion artifact allow a high degree of interpretive accuracy. In addition, the axial images define anatomy that might otherwise be obscured by superimposed structures. The technique has the advantage of defining associated mediastinal disease processes such as lymphoma, carcinoma, and abscess. Calcifications are exquisitely appreciated and fat and tissue planes are well demonstrated. Breath holding is not required. In instances of uncertainty, reconstructions can be done to define the longitudinal orientation of the aneurysm. Ultrafast computed tomography has the capability of allowing flow studies to define organ perfusion and branch vessel occlusion. The technique requires only a peripheral intravenous injection of contrast material, and hospitalization is unnecessary. In our series, ten patients were operated on without the necessity for angiography.

The disadvantages are the lack of longitudinal images and poorer resolution than angiography. Additional interventional procedures cannot be performed. Renal compromise and contrast allergies may be problems, and the patients must be transportable to the imaging suite.

Summary

In summary, the current role of ultrafast CT is in the screening of patients with a low probability of dissection, the exclusion of aneurysmal involvement in asymptomatic or minimally symptomatic patients with mass lesions, and the follow-up of known aneurysms and dissection.

MEDIASTINAL MASSES

Computed tomography is the imaging technique of choice in evaluating the mediastinum and in staging patients with lung carcinoma (Fig. 36–22). It provides information about tumor anatomy, location, and composition. It also demonstrates vascular displacement and invasion. We do approximately 20 to 30 CT examinations per day, and because of its speed, improved vascular opacification, and excellent resolution, ultrafast computed tomography is our primary scanner for evaluating chest disease. Studies by Stanford and associates[52] have shown that ultrafast CT images

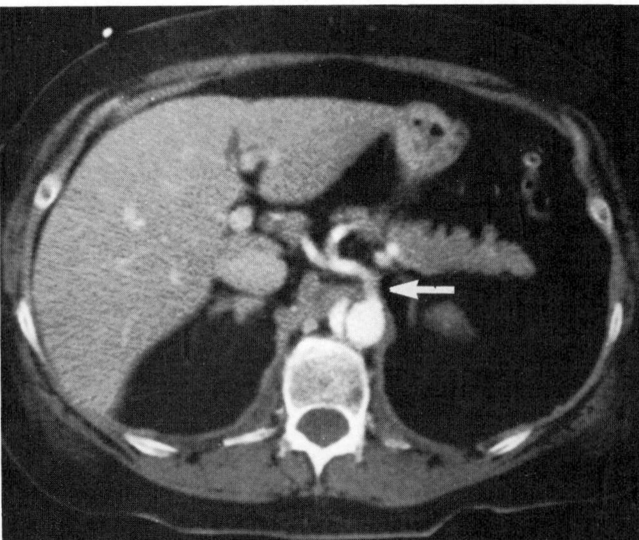

Figure 36–21. Celiac axis *(arrow)* coming off the lateral lumen in a patient with aortic dissection.

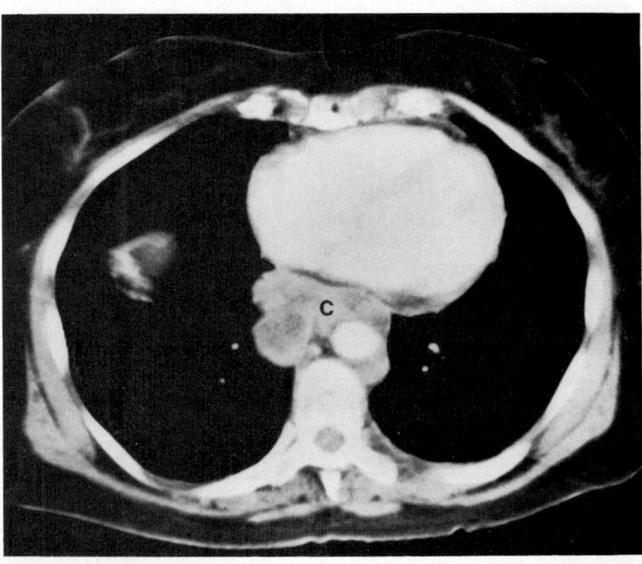

Figure 36–22. Large lung carcinoma (C) growing into the mediastinum.

provide diagnostic information that is equal to or better than that available from conventional computed tomography.

Tumors originating in the mediastinum or beneath the diaphragm may grow upward and involve the cardiac chambers. Ultrafast computed tomography has the ability to show both intracardiac and extracardiac involvement as well as intracavitary invasion (see Fig. 36–3). It plays a significant role in the evaluation of these patients.

Scanner Protocols

For investigation of mediastinal disease, the volume mode with 10-mm contiguous slices is used. Imaging is from lung apex to adrenals. In selected cases, the flow mode may be used to define lesion vascularity or to differentiate arteriovenous malformations. Three-millimeter-thick images can be taken at the time of maximal vessel opacification, and this will improve image quality and provide greater anatomic detail.

Other Mediastinal Lesions

Diaphragmatic lesions, foramen of Morgagni hernias, and eventrations of the diaphragm may present as parasternal and retrosternal masses. They are easily differentiated from pericardial or cardiac disease by ultrafast computed tomography.

Advantages and Disadvantages of Ultrafast Computed Tomography in Mediastinal Disease

Fast scan times, decrease in motion unsharpness, and imaging during peak vascular opacification are important advantages. The scanner can routinely show mediastinal masses as small as 5 mm. It can also image patients who cannot hold their breath. All of the studies can be accomplished with a peripheral injection of contrast material.

The disadvantages are those associated with transporting patients to the scanner, contrast allergies, renal compromise, and occasionally poor-quality images in obese patients.

Summary

Ultrafast computed tomography plays an important role in the assessment of mediastinal lesions. Axial imaging, excellent vascular opacification, and decreased motion unsharpness are useful in evaluating tumor invasion and in showing great-vessel displacement from mediastinal mass lesions.

CONCLUSION

Ultrafast computed tomography is ideally suited for imaging intracardiac masses and extracardiac abnormalities. There are limitations, as with any scanning method, but this should be considered one of the primary imaging techniques for the evaluation of chest and mediastinal disease.

References

A

1. Aronberg, D. J., Peterson, R. R., Glazer, H. S., and Sagel, S. S.: The superior sinus of the pericardium: CT appearance. Radiology 153:489, 1984.

B

1. Beattie, B. A., Struck, L., Stanford, W., et al.: Two dimensional echocardiography and ultrafast cardiac computed tomography for the detection of intracardiac thrombi in cerebral ischemia. Ann. Neurol. 24:155A, 1988.

C

1. Clemente, C. D., ed.: Grays Anatomy, 30th ed. Lea & Febiger, Philadelphia, 1985, p. 622.

H

1. Harrison, T. R.: Principles of Internal Medicine, 11th ed. McGraw-Hill, New York, 1987, p. 957 and p. 1004.
2. Holt, J. P.: The normal pericardium. Am. J. Cardiol. 26:455, 1970.

L

1. Lee, J. K., Sagel, S. S., and Stanley, R. J.: Computed Body Tomography. Raven Press, New York, 1983, p. 122.
2. Levy-Ravetch, M., Auh, Y. H., Rubenstein, W. A., et al.: CT of pericardial recesses. AJR 144:707, 1985.
3. Lipton, M. J., Herfkens, R. J., and Gamsu, G.: Computed tomography of the heart and pericardium. *In* Moss, A. A., Gamsu, G., and Gerot, H. K. (eds.): Computed Tomography of the Body. W. B. Saunders, Philadelphia, 1983, p. 414.

M

1. Moncada, R., Demos, T. C., Posniak, H. V., and Hammer, R.: Computed tomography of pericardial heart disease. *In* Taveras, J. M., and Ferrucci, J. T. (eds.): Radiology: Diagnosis-Imaging-Intervention. Lippincott, Philadelphia, 1988, Vol. 2, Ch. 43, p. 1.

N

1. Naidich, D. P., Zerhouni, E. A., and Siegelman, S. S.: Computerized Tomography of the Thorax. Raven Press, New York, 1984, p. 269.
2. Nasser, W. K.: Congenital absence of the left pericardium. Am. J. Cardiol. 26:466, 1970.

R

1. Roberts, W. C.: *In*: Taveras, J. M., and Ferruci, J. T. (eds.): Radiology: Diagnosis-Imaging-Intervention. Lippincott, Philadelphia, 1988, Vol. 2, Ch. 55, p. 1.
2. Roberts, W. C., and Spray, T. L.: Pericardial heart disease: A study of its causes, consequences and morphologic features. Cardiovasc. Clin. 7:11, 1976.

S

1. Stanford, W., Abu-Yousef, M., and Smith, W.: Intrauterine rhabdomyoma diagnosed by in utero ultrasound: A case report. J. Clin. Ultrasound 15:337, 1987.
2. Stanford, W., Hemann, L., Rooholamini, S., et al.: Ultrafast computed tomography in noncardiac thoracic imaging: Comparison with conventional computed tomography. Presented at the Society of Thoracic Radiology Meeting, Washington, D.C., 1988.

Chapter 37

Comprehensive Evaluation of Congenital Heart Disease Using Ultrafast Computed Tomography

■ *W. JAY ELDREDGE, M.D.*

CLINICAL EXPERIENCE 715
SCANNING TECHNIQUES FOR CONGENITAL CARDIAC DEFECTS 715
ANALYSIS OF CARDIAC ANATOMY 715
Abnormalities of Visceral Situs 715
Abnormalities Involving the Atria 715
Abnormalities of Venous Return 715
Abnormalities of the Atrioventricular Valves 716
Abnormalities Involving the Ventricles 717
Abnormalities of the Semilunar Valves 725
Abnormalities of the Great Vessels 725
BLOOD FLOW DETERMINATIONS 725
MEASUREMENT OF VENTRICULAR VOLUME AND MASS 728
POSTOPERATIVE EVALUATION 728
CONCLUSIONS 730

Accurate evaluation of the many complex anatomic abnormalities found in patients with congenital heart disease remains one of the most interesting and challenging problems facing the cardiologist. To date, all imaging modalities that have been utilized in this field have acquired their information in a one-dimensional or at best two-dimensional format. Cardiac catheterization with axial cineangiography[B1] has become the standard against which all other diagnostic methods are compared. However, it remains ultimately invasive and expensive and in most cases requires hospitalization. In the present era of cost containment and decreasing utilization of inpatient diagnostic services, increasing emphasis is being placed on alternative noninvasive means of obtaining the same information with a similar degree of accuracy. Any new imaging modality that can noninvasively describe complex anatomic malformations as well as provide important physiologic information regarding blood flow and cardiac function deserves serious consideration and evaluation.

Computed tomography (CT) offers many significant advantages that appear to make it an ideal imaging modality for the definition of complex cardiac anatomy. When sufficient contiguous cross-sectional tomographic slices are obtained, the entire heart and great vessels may be encompassed within a volume of CT data. Review of the resulting volumetric information in a variety of available formats permits a true three-dimensional analysis of cardiac anatomy. The high spatial resolution offered by computed tomography permits accurate delineation of most of the important cardiac structures. High density resolution not only allows discrimination of various tissue densities but also permits the use of small doses of contrast material when opacification of the blood pool is necessary. When scanning the thorax, not only the various cardiac structures but also the surrounding pulmonary and mediastinal structures within that specific tomographic section can be seen. Such a wide field of view greatly facilitates the important task of defining the complex spatial relationships encountered in patients with congenital heart disease. In addition, the single greatest imaging problem experienced with cineangiography or any other projection imaging technique—the loss of important anatomic information due to overlapping structures—is overcome.

Despite these recognized advantages, conventional computed tomography has never enjoyed widespread use as a cardiac imaging modality, predominantly because of the low temporal resolution associated with current CT equipment. Such long data acquisition times resulted in images with serious motion artifacts that were considered unacceptable for cardiac imaging. A unique multislice rapid-acquisition CT scanner (Imatron C-100 ultrafast CT, Imatron, Inc., South San Francisco, California) based on a magnetically defected electron beam has been in clinical use for over 4 years. Details of the ultrafast CT scanner have been described.[B2–B4] Certain aspects of the geometry of the scanner as well as the modes of data acquisition appear to make it an ideal imaging tool for the analysis of congenital heart disease. With each pass of the electron beam over one of the four available tungsten target rings, two side-by-side 8-mm-thick tomographic slices are obtained in 50 msec. By serially scanning each of the four target rings in rapid sequence, eight contiguous cross-sectional images are produced in 224 msec (8 msec interscan delay time between each sweep of the beam). When sufficient contiguous cross-sectional slices are obtained, the entire heart and great vessels will be encompassed within the CT scan volume, thereby creating a true three-dimensional imaging modality that is available for the analysis of complex cardiac anatomy.

CLINICAL EXPERIENCE

Since conventional CT has been used only sporadically for cardiac evaluation, little information has been available on the cross-sectional anatomy of congenital heart disease.[F1, L1] Our initial experience with 42 patients with congenital heart disease suggested that ultrafast computed tomography represented an accurate and potentially valuable new imaging technique.[E1] These early observations were confirmed by other users of this technique.[B5, D1, G1, M1, M2, S1] Our subsequent experience with more than

500 patients with a wide variety of congenital cardiac defects has resulted in further improvement of the sensitivity of the modality.[E2, E3] Our total experience with these patients forms the basis of this chapter.

SCANNING TECHNIQUES FOR CONGENITAL CARDIAC DEFECTS

All patients undergoing ultrafast CT scanning for cardiac evaluation require the injection of a small amount of an iodinated contrast medium. Contrast injection protocols vary according to the type of information to be obtained and the scanning mode to be utilized. In general, however, a dose of only 0.3 to 0.5 ml/kg is sufficient to ensure adequate contrast enhancement of the blood pool. Patients with very large intracardiac shunts may require up to 1 ml/kg per injection to overcome the dilutional effect of the large shunt volume. Our experience suggests that a peripheral injection site such as an antecubital vein is entirely adequate and permits the injection of a satisfactory contrast bolus when a power injector is used. Because of the short acquisition times associated with ultrafast CT scanning, sedation of patients is rarely necessary. This gives ultrafast computed tomography a distinct advantage over other currently available imaging modalities, which have a much lower temporal resolution.

Three different scanning modes are available. Each mode acquires data in a different manner and therefore provides distinctly different information. In the flow mode, the scanner is triggered by the patient's electrocardiogram following the bolus injection of contrast material. Continuous contrast-enhanced scans in the same phase of the cardiac cycle may be obtained in up to eight levels. The wash-in and wash-out of contrast material through any desired region of interest can then be observed. The flow mode remains our primary mode of data acquisition, since it may be used to define cardiac anatomy as well as to calculate flow parameters such as cardiac output and shunt ratios.

In the cine mode, the scanner is fired as rapidly as possible. Sufficient 50-msec scans are obtained so that one entire heartbeat is covered. The primary use of the cine mode is to evaluate cardiac function. Replaying the images in a "closed-loop" movie mode provides the viewer with a real-time demonstration of segmental cardiac function. All studies that are performed to calculate ejection fractions, ventricular volumes, or ventricular mass or to evaluate regional wall motion are performed in the cine mode. Images obtained in the cine mode have also proved useful for defining various dynamic features of cardiac anatomy.

The volume mode is similar to the dynamic scanning mode utilized in conventional CT scanning. Following the injection of contrast material, continuous cross-sectional images are obtained during table incrementation. Sufficient images are obtained to cover the region of interest. The volume mode is used predominantly to evaluate cardiac anatomy and has proved particularly useful in defining abnormalities of the aorta and pulmonary arteries.

Our initial studies were all performed in the conventional transaxial CT position (0-degree table slew, 0-degree table tilt). The scanner is, however, equipped with a unique table that can be slewed 20 to 25 degrees in either direction as well as tilted downward 20 to 25 degrees. With more experience, it has become increasingly apparent that proper positioning of the patient within the scanner is extremely important for obtaining optimal images of the region of interest. In addition to the transaxial position, two additional table positions have been described, which generally approximate their echocardiographic or cineangiographic counterparts.[D1, R1] The long-axis position is achieved by slewing the table 20 to 25 degrees counterclockwise with no table tilt. This position is used for optimal visualization of the atrial and ventricular septa as well as the left ventricular outflow tract. The short-axis position is used for all studies in which the calculation of ventricular volume or mass is contemplated. The aortic valve and frequently the pulmonary valve are seen well with this view. It is achieved by slewing the table 15 to 20 degrees clockwise and tilting the table 15 to 20 degrees downward. We have also described a "cranial-caudal" position (20-degree downward table tilt, 0-degree slew).[E3] This position was developed predominantly for evaluating the pulmonary valve and right ventricular outflow tract and has proved particularly useful in tetralogy of Fallot. The transaxial position remains our position of choice when defining complex spatial relationships such as those involving the great vessels and their underlying ventricles.

ANALYSIS OF CARDIAC ANATOMY

Segmental analysis has long been advocated as an orderly, logical method for accurately describing the complex anatomic problems encountered in patients with congenital heart disease.[A1, V1] Volumetric imaging with ultrafast computed tomography is ideal for implementing this process. During the acquisition of data, all attempts are made to incorporate the entire heart and great vessels into the matrix of CT data. When questions of visceral situs arise, the study may be continued to include the upper abdomen. The system of segmental image analysis begins by evaluating the most superior slice and then progressing inferiorly in a sequential fashion. In this manner, all cardiac segments may be identified and localized, their connections defined, and any associated abnormalities described.

Abnormalities of Visceral Situs

The ability of conventional computed tomography to image accurately the abdominal viscera is well known. The technique has also been used to describe the situs of the abdominal viscera in patients with complex forms of congenital heart disease.[T1] Since visceral and atrial situs correspond in nearly all patients, this determination becomes important in many cases of complex congenital heart disease.

Abnormalities Involving the Atria

Atrial septal defects of three types have been imaged successfully to date. Not only can the presence of a shunt at the atrial level be determined and the pulmonary-to-systemic flow ratio calculated,[M3, S1] but also the precise location of the defect within the septum can be identified (Fig. 37–1). Atrial septal defects of the secundum variety are readily visualized in the middle or fossa ovalis portion of the atrial septum. The less common atrial septal defects of the primum type are located in the lower portion of the septum and are closely related to the mitral valve. Mild foreshortening of the ventricular septum is also noted in this incomplete form of atrioventricular canal defect. Although the position of the mitral valve can be seen well in this abnormality, the finer details of valve anatomy such as chordal attachments and clefts have not been successfully imaged.

Atrial septal defects located in the high sinus venosus portion of the atrial septum have also been successfully imaged with ultrafast computed tomography (Fig. 37–2). When this type of atrial septal defect is suspected, care must be taken to begin the imaging sequence with the most superior slice localized above the junction of the superior vena cava and the right atrium. The presence of any associated partial anomalous pulmonary venous drainage can also be determined in these patients. Our experience suggests that ultrafast computed tomography is the most accurate noninvasive method for identification of this type of atrial septal defect.

Abnormalities of Venous Return

Abnormalities of both systemic and pulmonary venous return have been identified with ultrafast computed tomography. Although these anatomic problems may appear to be of little interest, accurate determination of the various sites of venous connection is of critical importance when planning the surgical repair of complex malformations. The presence of a persistent left superior vena cava can be identified following the injection

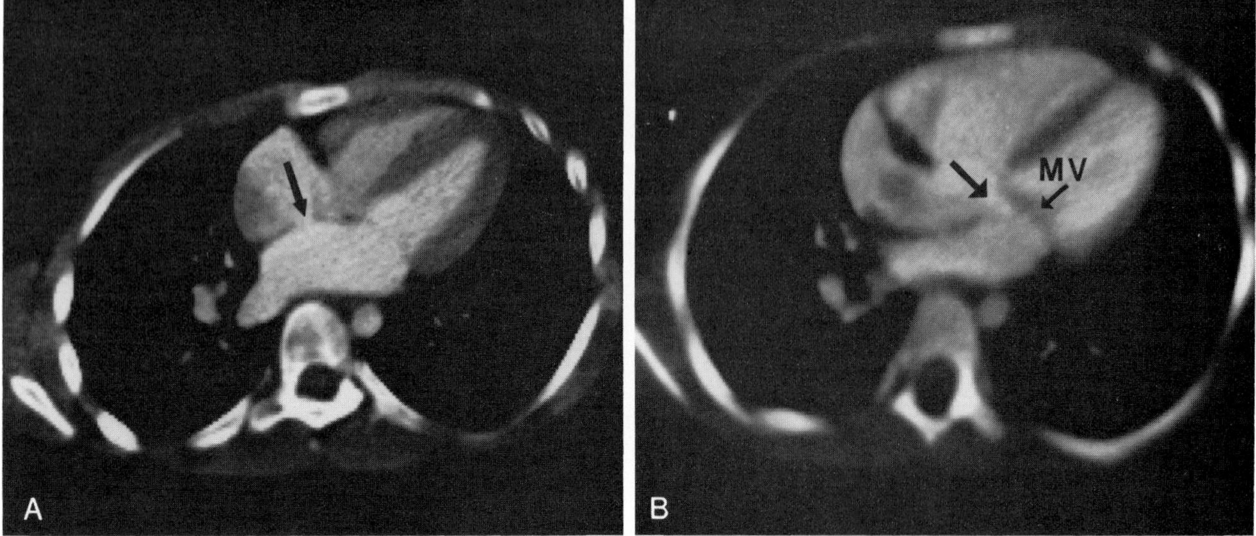

Figure 37–1. Atrial septal defects. Selected frames from the flow studies of two patients with different types of atrial septal defects. *A*, A defect is demonstrated in the mid or secundum portion of the atrial septum *(arrow)*. A primum atrial septal defect is seen in *B (large arrow)*. This defect can be differentiated from the more common secundum type by its more inferior position and close relationship to the mitral valve (MV).

of contrast material through a left arm vein. The site of entry of the persistent cava and the presence or absence of any communication with the right cava can be determined from the same injection (Fig. 37–3).

Normal pulmonary veins are readily imaged with ultrafast computed tomography. Determination of the exact site of pulmonary venous drainage in patients with complex congenital heart disease is often difficult with the other currently available imaging techniques. Although we have not had occasion to study any patients with total anomalous pulmonary venous drainage, several types of partial anomalous drainage have been identified. As previously noted, anomalies of pulmonary venous drainage involving right upper lobe pulmonary veins in association with sinus venosus atrial septal defects have been successfully identified. Enhancement of the pulmonary venous phase of a CT flow study by using the subtraction techniques available in the computer software further increases the ability of this modality to define these abnormalities (see Fig. 37–2). One patient with severe rheumatic mitral stenosis had the presence of a left-to-right shunt into the superior vena cava identified with oxygen saturations obtained during cardiac catheterization. The site of the shunt, however, could not be adequately visualized with cineangiography. Following a single intravenous injection of contrast material, an ultrafast CT study correctly localized the site of the partial anomalous drainage, which was high in the superior vena cava at the level of the left pulmonary artery (Fig. 37–4). The presence of an intact atrial septum was also documented. A volumetric imaging technique incorporating multiple contiguous cross-sectional tomographic slices should prove to be the imaging method of choice for defining abnormalities of pulmonary venous return, since the sites of drainage are not obscured from view by any other overlapping structures and can be clearly identified.

Abnormalities of the Atrioventricular Valves

The mitral and tricuspid valves are readily imaged with ultrafast computed tomography. The valve leaflets are well seen and their

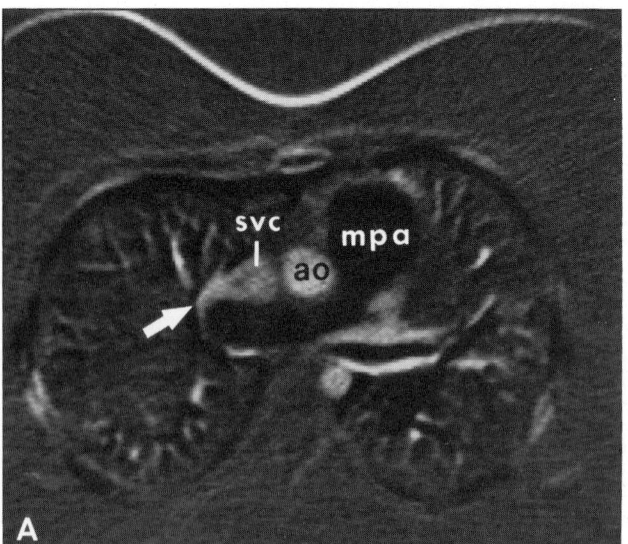

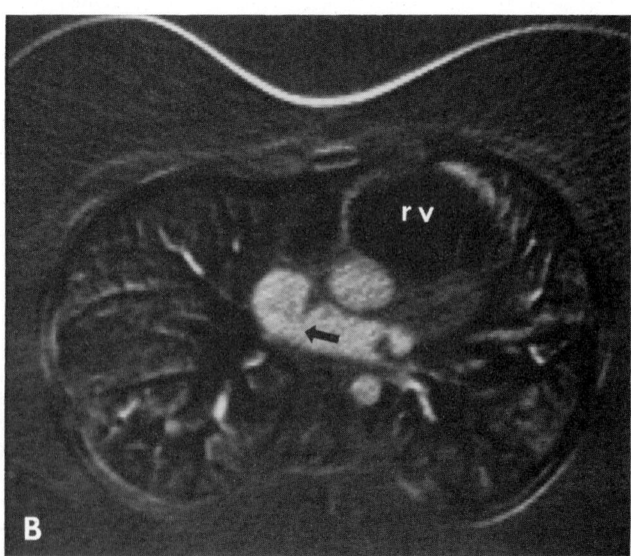

Figure 37–2. Sinus venosus atrial septal defect. Two subtraction images created from the flow study of a patient with a sinus venosus-type atrial septal defect and partial anomalous pulmonary venous return are shown. The computer subtraction process was performed to enhance the pulmonary veins and left heart structures and remove contrast material from the pulmonary arteries. The two cross-sectional images are immediately adjacent. *A*, A pulmonary vein *(arrow)* can be seen draining into the superior vena cava (SVC). The SVC has been reopacified by the left-to-right shunt. *B*, The defect in the sinus venosus portion of the atrial septum is well demonstrated *(arrow)*. ao—aorta; mpa—main pulmonary artery; rv—right ventricle.

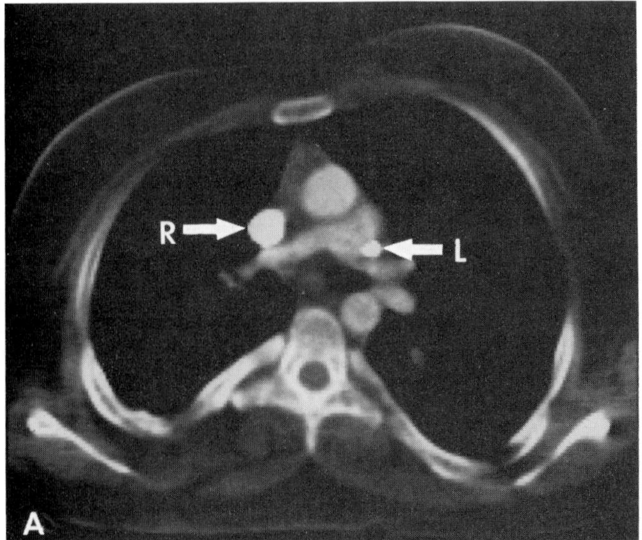

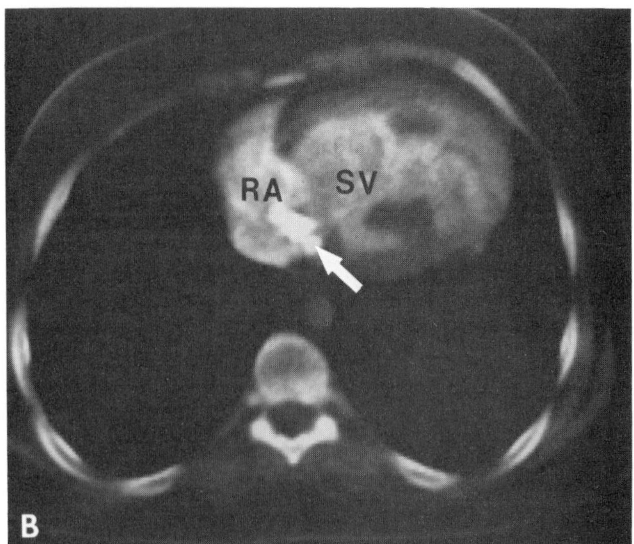

Figure 37–3. Persistent left superior vena cava. These two frames are taken from the flow study of a patient with a single ventricle (SV) and a persistent left superior vena cava. *A*, Opacification of a normal right cava (R) and smaller left cava (L) can been seen following an injection of contrast material into a left arm vein. Near-simultaneous opacification of both cavae following the injection confirms the presence of communication between the two structures. *B*, The left cava can be seen draining into the right atrium (RA) via the coronary sinus *(arrow)*.

motion may be analyzed with the cine mode.[R2] The current resolution of the scanner, however, prevents consistent imaging of the chordae, especially in infants and small children. Although an atrioventricular valve may appear to "override" a ventricular septal defect, the diagnosis of "straddling" of the valve cannot be made using this technique. At present, the important issue of chordal attachments is best defined by using two-dimensional echocardiography.

The volumetric nature of ultrafast CT imaging makes it an ideal method for detecting the presence and exact location of the atrioventricular valves. Since the entire heart is contained in the imaging matrix, the absence of one valve can be easily determined. Patients with both mitral and tricuspid atresia have been successfully imaged using this technique. In patients with tricuspid atresia the spatial relationships of the great vessels and the size of the right ventricle can be defined (Fig. 37–5). The size of an associated ventricular septal defect can also be assessed.

Ultrafast computed tomography has proved useful in patients with Ebstein's anomaly of the tricuspid valve. Evaluation of the degree of downward displacement of the abnormal tricuspid leaflets has been possible in all of the cases studied. The presence of an associated atrial septal defect can also be determined, and evaluation of both the degree and direction of atrial shunting is possible.

A common atrioventricular (AV) valve is most often encountered in patients with the complete form of atrioventricular canal defect or common ventricle. In complete defects, the common atrioventricular valve leaflets can be seen sweeping across a large defect in the endocardial cushion portion of the atrial and ventricular septa (Fig. 37–6*A*). Evaluation of ventricular size in the same study will also readily detect the presence of a dominant right or left form of complete atrioventricular canal, which will alter the surgical management of the patient (Fig. 37–6*B*).

Abnormalities Involving the Ventricles

More than 150 cases of isolated ventricular septal defect have been successfully imaged to date. These patients are best imaged in the long-axis position so that the most cephalad slice of the study will traverse the level of the aortic root. Progressing inferiorly, the outlet, perimembranous, muscular, and inlet portions of the septum will be imaged sequentially (Fig. 37–7). By

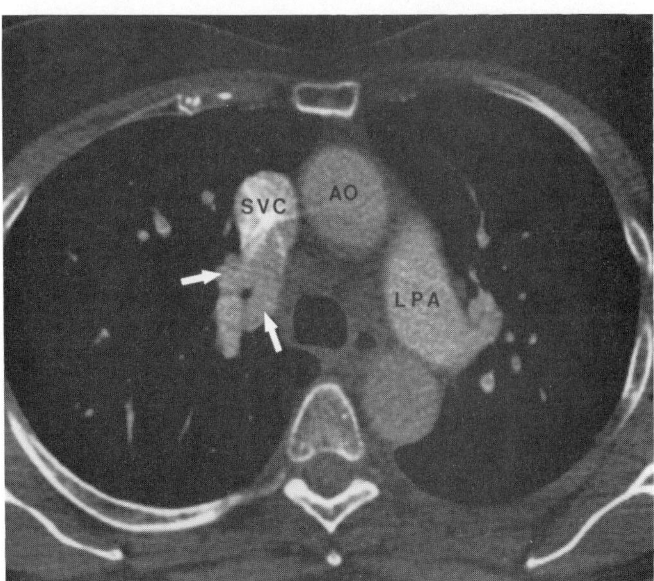

Figure 37–4. Partial anomalous pulmonary venous drainage. Two pulmonary veins *(arrows)* are seen draining into the high superior vena cava (SVC) at the level of the left pulmonary artery (LPA). This patient did not have an associated atrial septal defect. AO—aorta.

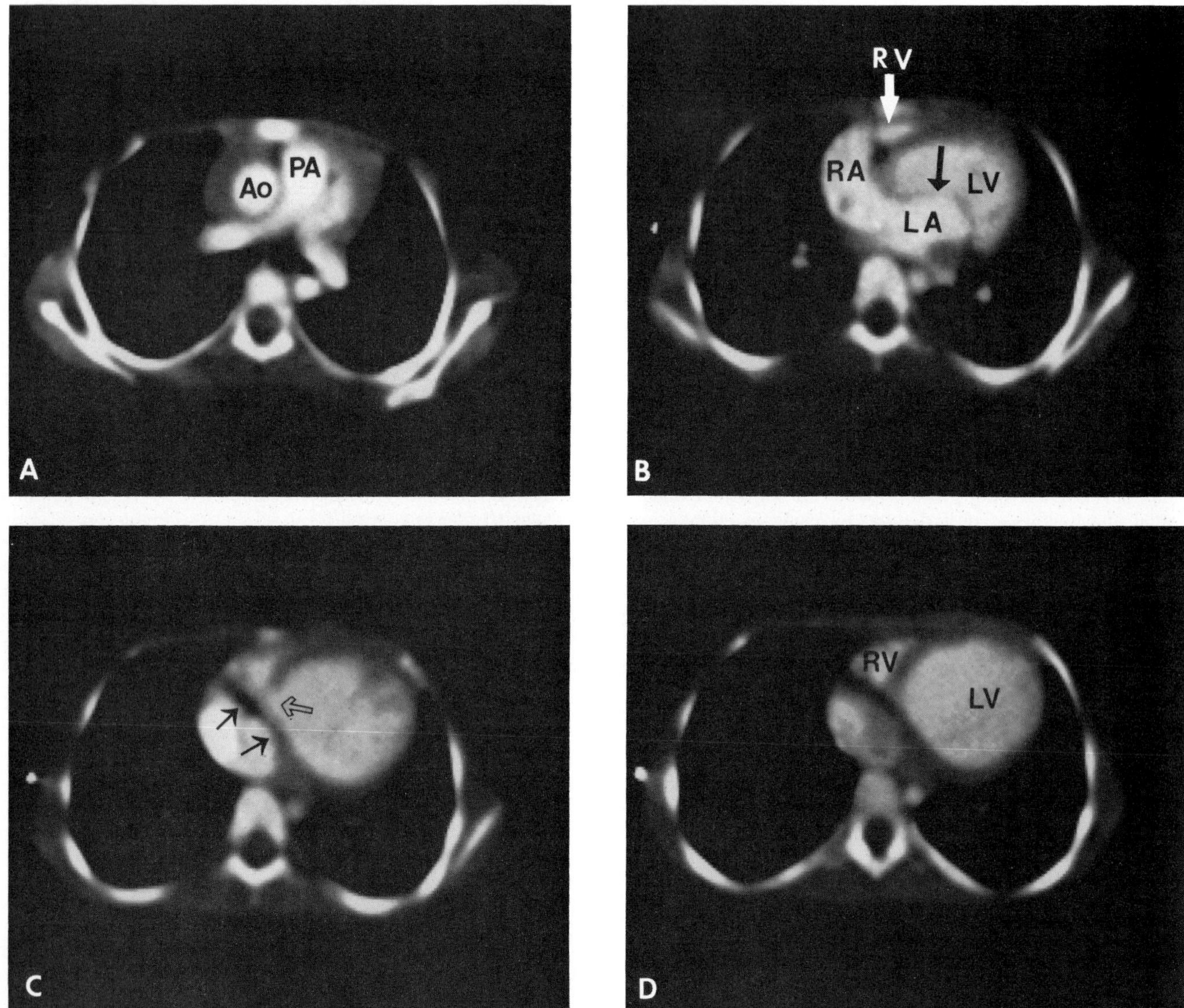

Figure 37–5. Tricuspid atresia. Four selected images from the flow study of a patient with tricuspid atresia are shown. *A*, A normal relationship between the anterior and leftward pulmonary artery (PA) and the posterior, rightward aorta (Ao). Progressing inferiorly, a diminutive right ventricle (RV) is seen in *B*. This small chamber lies directly beneath the PA, while the left ventricle (LV) is directly beneath the Ao. Wide-open communication between the right atrium (RA) and left atrium (LA) can easily be seen. One atrioventricular valve is present between the LA and LV *(black arrow)*. A ventricular septal defect *(hollow arrow)* is imaged in *C*. Also note the absence of a normal tricuspid valve *(black arrows)*. *D*, The relative sizes of the two ventricles can be immediately appreciated. (From Eldredge, W. J., Diethelm, N. E., and Lipton, M. J.: Ultrafast computed tomography in the diagnosis of congenital heart disease. *In* Imaging for Pediatric Disorders. W. B. Saunders, Philadelphia, to be published, with permission.)

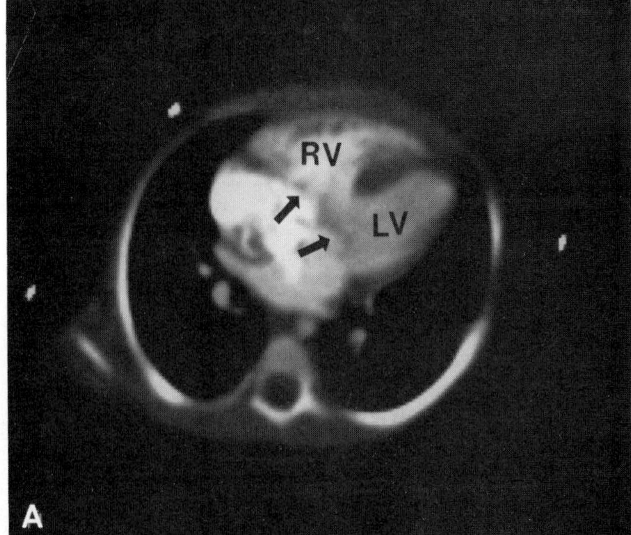

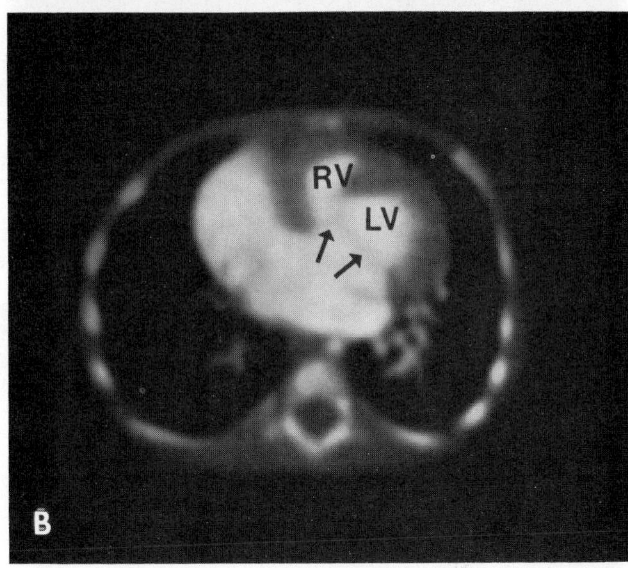

Figure 37–6. Common atrioventricular canal. Single frames from studies of two patients with varying forms of complete atrioventricular canal (AVC) are shown. *A*, A balanced type of AVC in which both ventricles appear to be of normal size. A single common atrioventricular valve leaflet *(arrows)* can be seen stretching across the large central defect in the endocardial cushion. *B*, Frame from a patient with a dominant left form of AVC. The right ventricle (RV) is smaller than the left ventricle (LV). The common atrioventricular valve *(arrows)* is predominantly committed to the LV. The anatomic differences between these two types of AVC can be readily appreciated by using cross-sectional imaging.

relating the position of the defect to the aortic root, precise localization of the defect within the septum is possible.[E4] Our recent experience suggests that ultrafast computed tomography is the most consistently accurate technique for the detection of multiple ventricular septal defects. It also appears to be more sensitive for the noninvasive identification of very small defects than two-dimensional echocardiography studies employing either Doppler or color flow methods.

Obstructive lesions within the outflow tract of either ventricle can be readily evaluated using ultrafast computed tomography. Hypertrophy of the right ventricular outflow tract or infundibulum occurs most often in association with valvular pulmonic stenosis or in tetralogy of Fallot but may also develop in certain patients with isolated ventricular septal defects. This area can be best evaluated by studying the patient in the cranial-caudal position with the cine mode. In this manner, the severity of the dynamic right ventricular outflow tract narrowing can be accurately assessed throughout the entire cardiac cycle.

Tetralogy of Fallot represents abnormal development of the outflow septum resulting in a malalignment defect in the ventricular septum, narrowing of the right ventricular outflow tract, and overriding of the aorta over the ventricular septal defect to varying degrees. The diagnosis of tetralogy of Fallot can be established by ultrafast computed tomography (Fig. 37–8*A*, *B*). Imaging in the cranial-caudal position using the cine mode clearly demonstrates the pathology of the right ventricular outflow tract as well as stenosis of the pulmonary valve, when present. The ventricular septal defect is also seen in this view, but its relationship to the aorta is often better seen in the transaxial position. An abnormal origin of the left anterior descending coronary from the right coronary artery has been successfully imaged in one patient with tetralogy of Fallot. Since the proximal one-third of the coronary arteries are well visualized with this technique, it is possible that this may offer a simple noninvasive approach to the preoperative identification of this particular problem.

Evaluation of the left ventricular outflow tract is best performed with the patient in the long-axis position. Using this technique, it has been possible to visualize a discrete subaortic membrane in three out of five patients imaged. Although the actual membrane was not seen in every patient, the secondary left ventricular hypertrophy, which can be present to a severe degree, was well documented in each case.

Hypertrophic cardiomyopathies are frequent causes of obstruction to outflow from either ventricle. The volumetric imaging method of ultrafast computed tomography is particularly well suited to evaluation of such problems. Since the entire ventricle may be scanned, both the severity and extent of the pathologic involvement can be assessed. Localized forms of the disease can be readily distinguished from cases with more extensive involvement.[E5] Since the endocardial and epicardial borders of the myocardium can easily be identified, measurements of myocardial thickness and calculation of ventricular mass are possible with a computer-assisted technique. Serial measurement of left ventricular mass appears to be an excellent method of determining

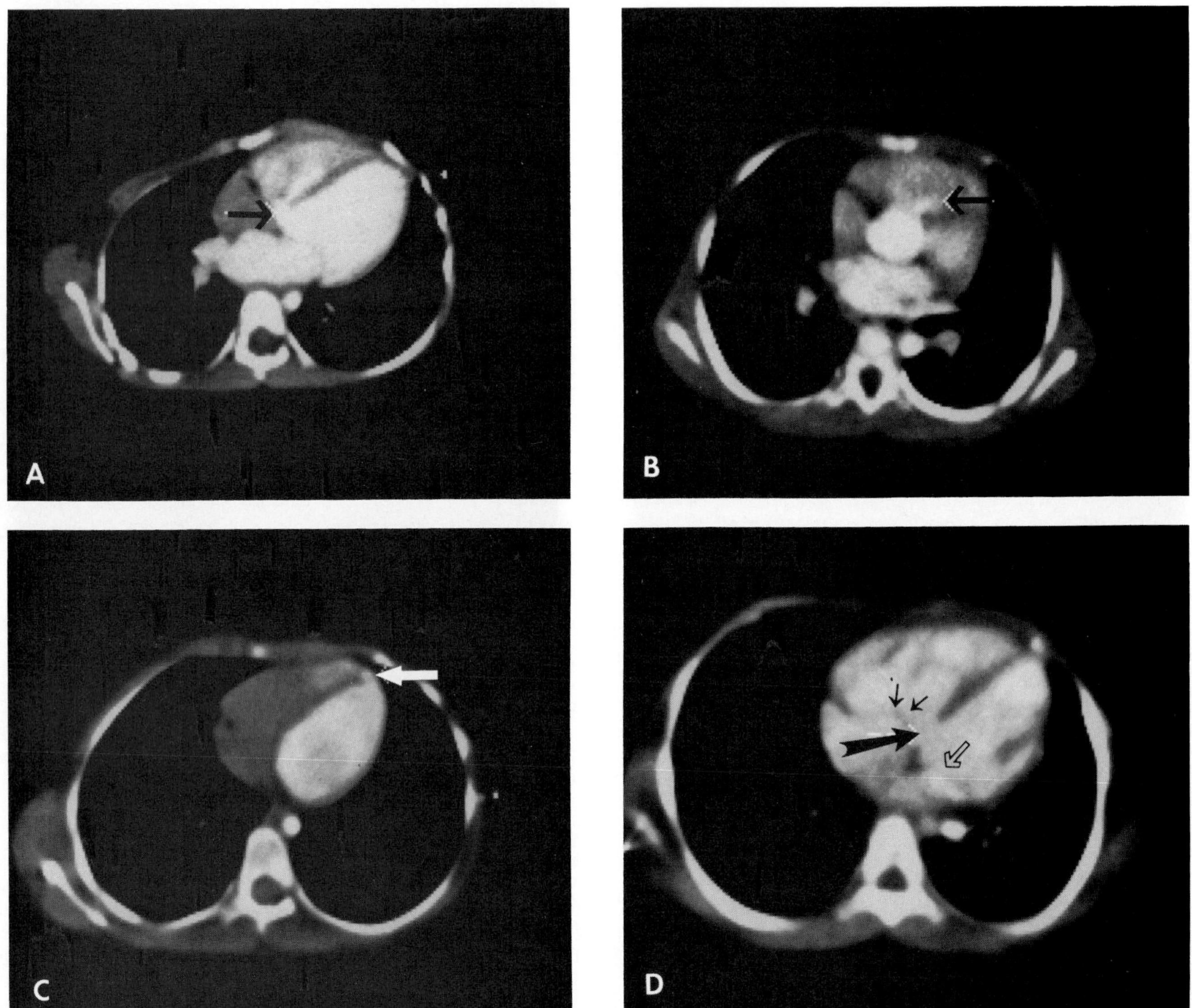

Figure 37–7. Ventricular septal defects. Single frames from studies of four patients with ventricular septal defects (VSD) in different locations are shown. *A*, The VSD is located in the perimembranous septum and is imaged immediately below the aortic valve. The associated aneurysm of the perimembranous septum can be readily appreciated *(arrow)*. The tomographic slice seen in *B* is slightly higher than the one shown in the previous frame. A supracristal or subarterial VSD *(arrow)* is imaged in the same plane as the aortic valve. *C*, Frame beautifully demonstrating a small muscular VSD at the apex of the left ventricle *(arrow)*. This defect was not detected with color flow Doppler and two-dimensional echocardiography. A large, low defect in the inlet portion of the ventricular septum *(large black arrow)* is demonstrated in *D*. Portions of both the mitral *(hollow arrow)* and tricuspid *(small black arrows)* are imaged in the same plane as the VSD. (From Eldredge, W. J., Diethelm, N. E., and Lipton, M. J.: Ultrafast computed tomography in the diagnosis of congenital heart disease. *In* Imaging for Pediatric Disorders. W. B. Saunders, Philadelphia, to be published, with permission.)

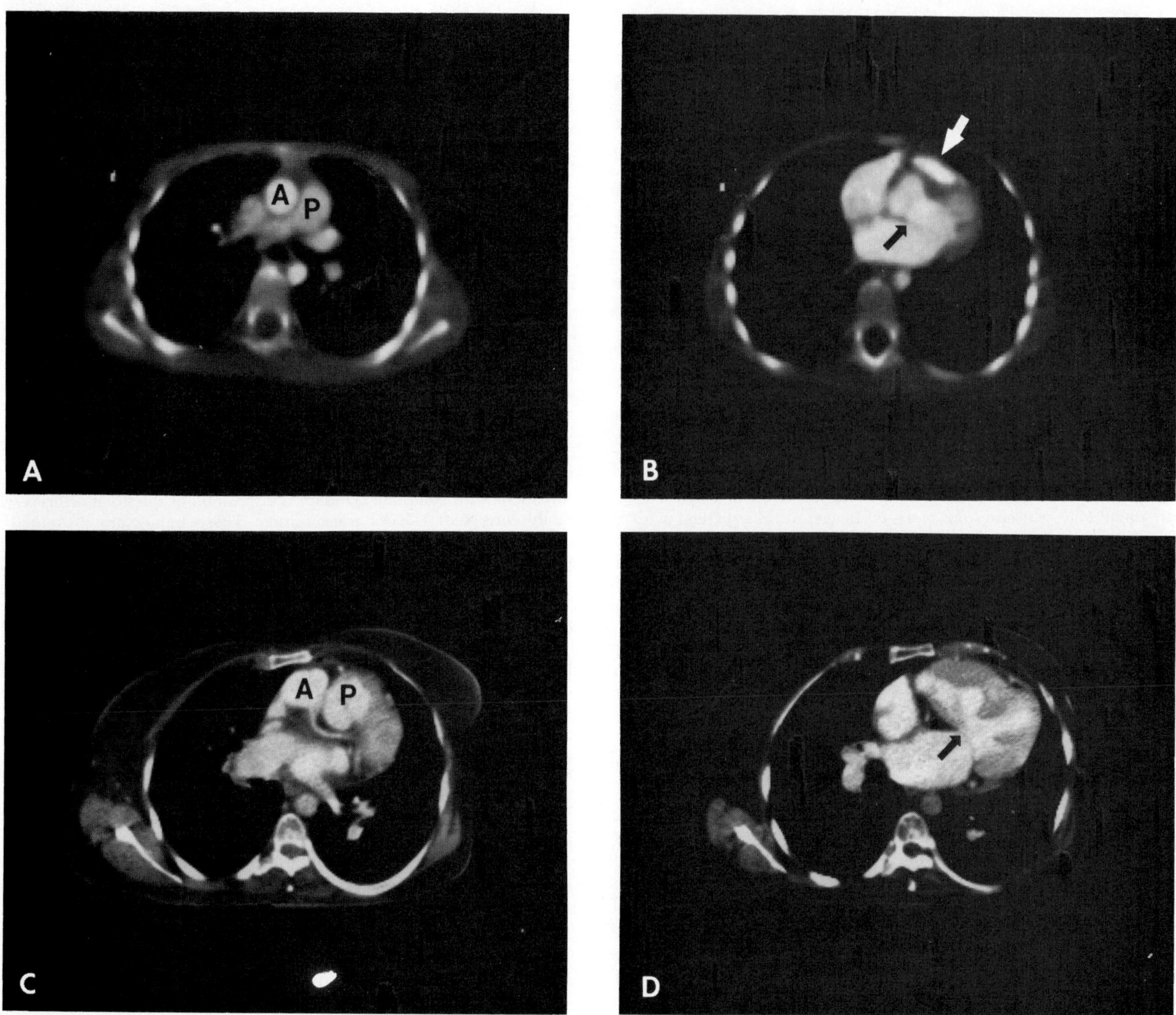

Figure 37–8. Tetralogy of Fallot versus double-outlet right ventricle. *A* and *B*, Frames taken from the study of a patient with tetralogy of Fallot. *A*, The relationship of the great vessels, with the aorta (A) located slightly more anterior than normal. *B*, Continuity between the aortic and mitral valves *(black arrow)*. The *white arrow* points to the narrowed right ventricular outflow tract. *C* and *D*, Frames from a study of a patient with double-outlet right ventricle. Marked anterior displacement of the aorta is seen in *C*. Frame *D* beautifully demonstrates the complete loss of continuity between the anteriorly displaced aorta and the more inferior mitral valve *(black arrow)*.

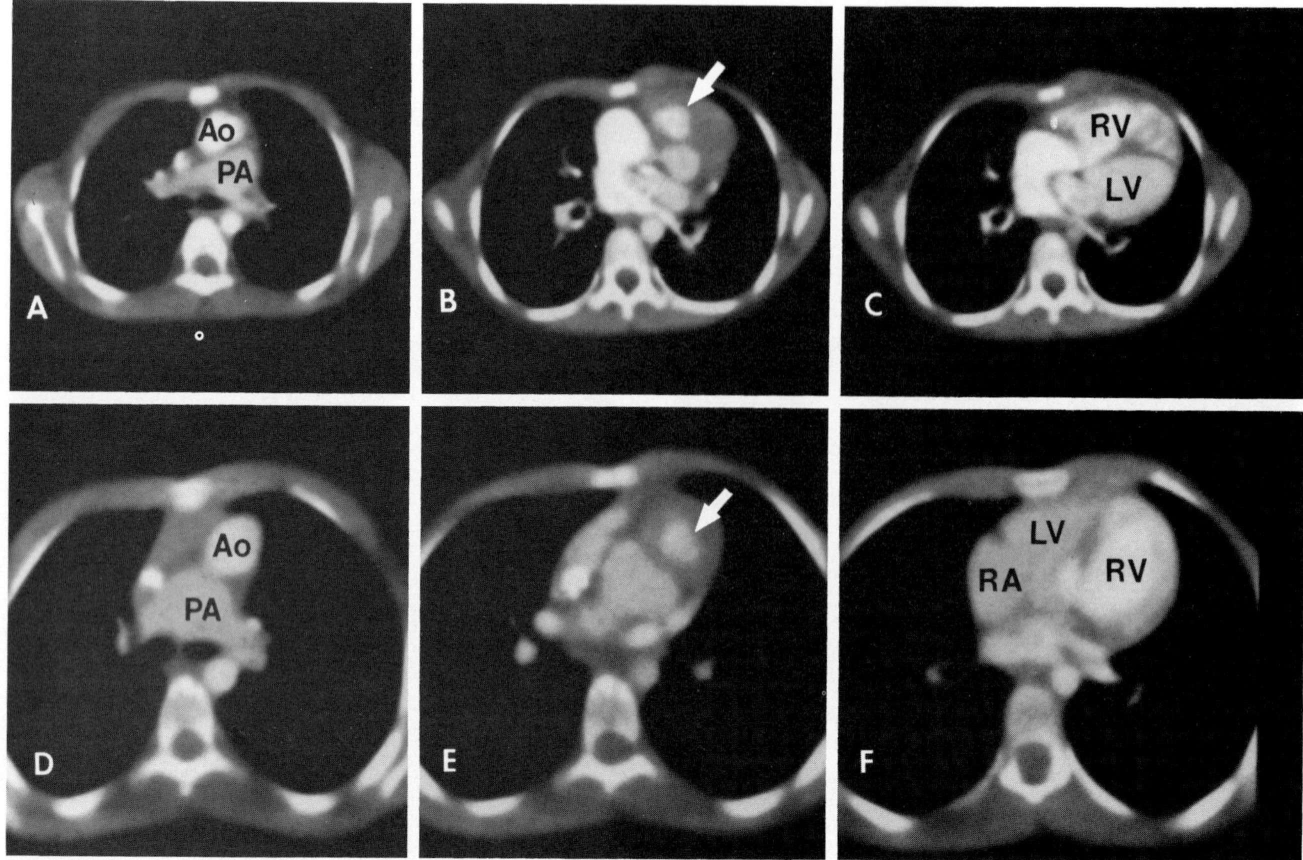

Figure 37–9. Transposition of the great arteries. *A–C*, Selected images from a patient with complete (D-loop) transposition of the great arteries who had undergone Mustard repair. *D–F*, Images from a patient with congenitally corrected (L-loop) transposition. These frames are presented to demonstrate the ability of ultrafast computed tomography to define the spatial relationships of the great vessels to each other and to their underlying ventricles. In *A*, the great vessels are seen in the classic position for complete transposition with the aorta (Ao) anterior and to the right of the posterior, leftward pulmonary artery (PA). The subaortic ventricle *(B)* is anterior and has an infundibulum *(arrow)* as well as the morphologic characteristics of a right ventricle *(C)*. In *D*, the great vessels are in the classic L-loop position as seen in patients with congenitally corrected transposition (Ao) anterior and to the left of the posterior, rightward PA. The subaortic ventricle *(E)* has an infundibulum *(arrow)* as well as the morphologic characteristics of an RV *(F)*. In contradistinction to the previous case, however, the ventricle is in a posterior location. The anterior ventricle has the smooth-walled characteristics of a morphologic left ventricle (LV) and connects to the right atrium (RA) across an atrioventricular valve (atrioventricular discordance, ventriculoarterial discordance).

progression of the disease in any patient with a hypertrophic cardiomyopathy.

The right and left ventricles have certain anatomic characteristics as seen with ultrafast imaging that appear to allow anatomic differentiation between them. The coarse internal trabecular pattern of the right ventricle, especially in its apical region, is readily distinguishable from the smoother pattern of the left ventricle. The moderator band that passes between the ventricular septum and the anterior wall of the right ventricle near its apex is nearly always imaged and may be considered a CT hallmark of the morphologic right ventricle. The morphologic left ventricle is usually identifiable by its smooth trabecular pattern, the lack of a subvalvular infundibulum, and the presence of its typical papillary muscles. The ability to distinguish ventricular morphology becomes important when analyzing more complex forms of congenital heart disease. For example, the diagnosis of ventricular inversion as seen in patients with congenitally corrected (L loop) transposition of the great vessels requires such morphologic identification of the ventricles in order to establish the presence of ventriculoarterial discordance (Fig. 37–9).

Many forms of single ventricle have been imaged with ultrafast computed tomography. Using segmental analysis, it has been possible to describe accurately all of our cases of single ventricle, often with more precise anatomic information than had been obtained with other imaging modalities (Fig. 37–10). The presence of a single ventricle, its relationship to a rudimentary outlet chamber, the status of its atrioventricular valves, the sites of pulmonary and systemic venous drainage, and the position of the great vessels can all be defined from a single study with contrast medium injected through a peripheral venous site (Fig. 37–11).

Figure 37–10. Single ventricle. Six frames from the flow study of a patient with a complex univentricular heart are shown to demonstrate the unique ability of ultrafast computed tomography to define difficult anatomic problems precisely. The plain chest x-ray in this patient showed situs solitus with the apex of the heart to the right. The patient had previously undergone both cardiac catheterization and two-dimensional echocardiography. Although the presence of a gradient between the aorta and single ventricle had been documented, the exact anatomic site of the obstruction could not be identified with either imaging modality. In *A*, the relationship of the great vessels is clearly defined. The aorta (Ao) is anterior and slightly to the right of the posterior pulmonary artery (PA). Progressing inferiorly, a left superior vena cava *(white arrow)* is seen in *B*. A tricuspid aortic valve is imaged anterior and to the left of a small, stenotic bicuspid pulmonary valve *(black arrow)*. In *C*, a narrowed subaortic chamber *(arrow)* can be seen. Proceeding inferiorly, this small subaortic tunnel (white arrows) becomes progressively narrower *(D, E)*. In *F*, the subaortic chamber communicates with the single ventricle through a small ventricular septal defect *(black arrow)*. This long, narrow subaortic chamber represented the site of the severe obstruction documented during catheterization. The single ventricle has the morphologic characteristics of a left ventricle (LV). Two discrete atrioventricular valves *(hollow arrows)* communicate with this chamber *(D, F)*. In *E* and *F*, a very dilated, partially obstructed coronary sinus (cs) is imaged.

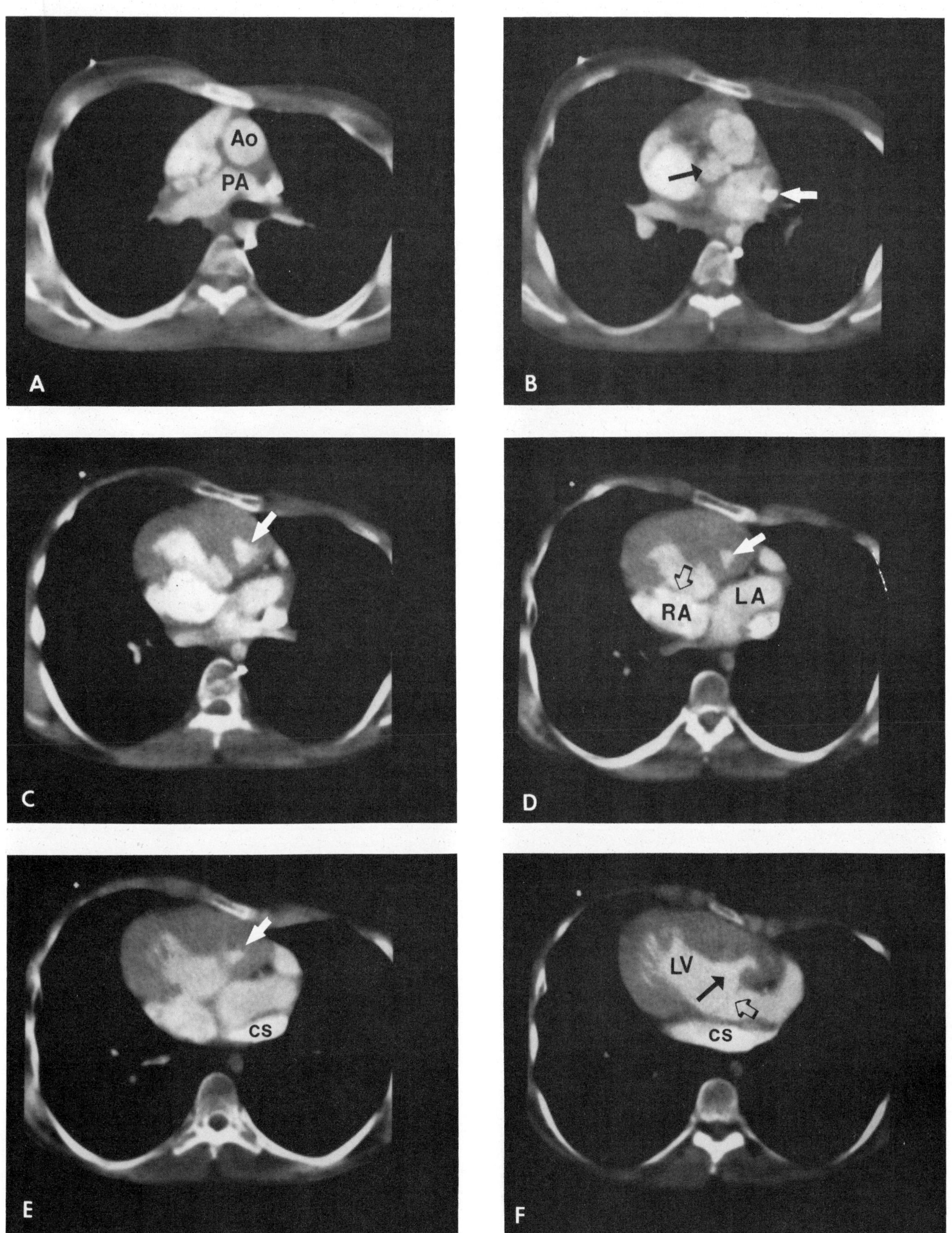

Figure 37–10 *See legend on opposite page*

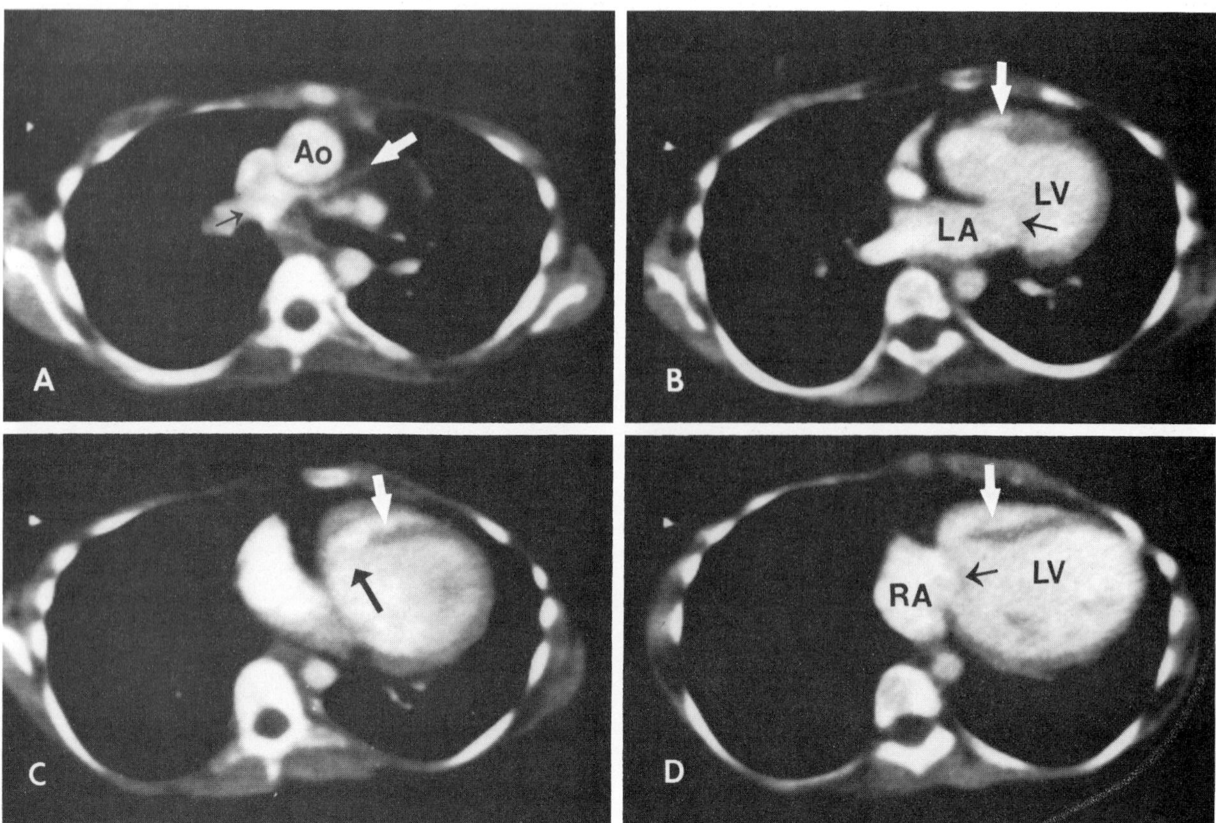

Figure 37–11. Single ventricle. Four selected images from a study in a patient with a single ventricle are shown. In *A*, the relationship between the great arteries is demonstrated. A severely hypoplastic main pulmonary artery *(white arrow)* is faintly visualized arising to the left of the aorta (Ao). The right pulmonary artery is small proximal to a Waterston anastomosis but becomes larger distal to the shunt *(black arrow)*. A slit-like right ventricle *(white arrow)* from which the pulmonary artery arises is seen in *B*. The mitral valve *(black arrow)* is imaged in the same frame. In *C*, the hypoplastic anterior right ventricle *(white arrow)* can be seen communicating with the left ventricle through a ventricular septal defect *(black arrow)*. The tricuspid valve *(black arrow)* is imaged in *D*. This valve appears to be primarily committed to the larger left ventricle. The hypoplastic right ventricle *(white arrow)* is again seen.

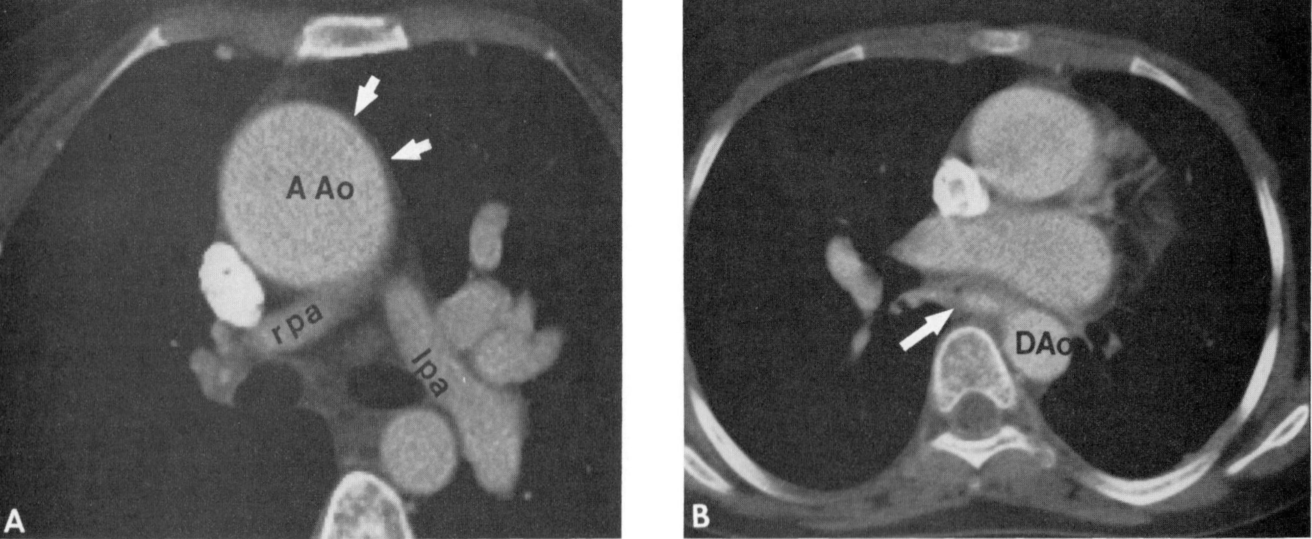

Figure 37–12. Pulmonary atresia. Single frames from the studies of two patients with ventricular septal defect and pulmonary atresia are shown. In *A*, both the right pulmonary artery (rpa) and left pulmonary artery (lpa) are imaged. The right ventricular outflow tract, which is normally seen anterior to the ascending aorta (AAo) at this level, is absent *(arrows)*. In *B*, a large bronchial collateral vessel *(arrow)* can be seen arising from the descending aorta (DAo) to supply a portion of the right pulmonary blood flow.

Abnormalities of the Semilunar Valves

Our initial experience suggested that imaging of the semilunar valves was more problematic and inconsistent than that of the atrioventricular valves. This was most likely due to the plane of the particular valve with respect to the plane of the scanning beam. With further experience it has been possible to determine the proper position of the patient that will allow consistent visualization of both the aortic and pulmonary valves.

The pulmonary valve is best seen when the patient is placed in the cranial-caudal position. Pulmonary valve stenosis can readily be seen with ultrafast computed tomography (Fig. 37–10*B*). The severity of the obstruction, however, can only be indirectly inferred from the presence and degree of severity of any associated right ventricular hypertrophy. Although this has been helpful in some extremely complex conditions in which the pulmonary valve could not be visualized by any other currently available technique, ultrafast computed tomography does not allow a quantitative measurement of the valve gradient.

Many patients with pulmonary valve atresia have been studied. The cross-sectional imaging hallmark of pulmonary atresia is the absence of the distal right ventricular outflow tract, which can normally be seen anterior to the aortic root (Fig. 37–12*A*). The primary benefit of ultrafast CT imaging in patients with pulmonary atresia is its ability to visualize clearly the pulmonary arteries, determine the presence or absence of confluence between the branches, and precisely measure the vessel size. The sites of abnormal pulmonary blood supply such as bronchial collateral vessels can also be identified with this noninvasive technique (Fig. 37–12*B*). Precise definition of these difficult anatomic problems has been possible even in those instances in which the pulmonary blood is severely restricted. The extremely high density resolution of computed tomography compared to cineangiography permits adequate visualization of the pulmonary artery anatomy despite relatively poor enhancement of the pulmonary blood pool.

The aortic valve is more easily imaged than the pulmonary valve, and although it can be seen in any position, the short-axis position is preferable for visualization of the valve leaflets. Although pathologic aortic valves have been imaged on a routine basis, ultrafast computed tomography cannot quantitate the severity of the obstruction.[M4] As with pulmonic stenosis, the secondary hypertrophy of the left ventricle can be precisely quantitated and serve as an indirect evaluation of the severity of the valve obstruction. This technique may ultimately prove useful for serially evaluating patients before and after surgical relief of the obstruction.[K1]

Abnormalities of the Great Vessels

The cross-sectional imaging approach employed in computed tomography offers great advantages when studying abnormalities of anatomy and spatial orientation of the great vessels.[B6] Defining the precise position of the great vessels with respect to each other as well as describing the relationship to their underlying structures is vitally important when analyzing complex congenital cardiac anomalies. Since there is no superimposition of structures to interfere with adequate visualization, the relationship of the great vessels to each other can easily be described and any associated congenital or acquired abnormalities readily detected.

Various forms of transposition of the great arteries have been studied with ultrafast computed tomography. A segmental approach to the diagnosis of the various forms of transposition of the great arteries begins with a description of the position of the aorta relative to the pulmonary artery. In the complete transposition of the great arteries (D loop), the aorta is positioned anterior and to the right of the posterior, leftward pulmonary artery (Fig. 37–9). In the less common congenitally corrected (L loop) transposition, the aorta is located anterior and to the left of the posterior, rightward pulmonary artery. These great vessel positions are easily determined. The diagnosis of transposition of the great arteries, however, is not complete with only a description of the spatial relationships of the great vessels. The ventriculoarterial connections must then be described, followed by analysis of the atrioventricular connections. Finally, the presence of any anatomic abnormalities within any of the cardiac structures can be determined. Defects that are commonly associated with complete transposition of the great arteries and have been detected by ultrafast computed tomography include atrial and ventricular defects and isolated pulmonary valve stenosis.

Two forms of double-outlet right ventricle have been studied using ultrafast computed tomography. The cross-sectional imaging format permits precise localization of the origin of the great vessels from the right ventricle. It has been possible to differentiate the less common Taussig-Bing variety, in which the pulmonary artery straddles a ventricular septal defect, from the more common type in which the aorta is directly related to the septal defect. Accurate definition of these relationships is frequently difficult with the more conventional imaging techniques. Double-outlet right ventricle that is associated with pulmonary stenosis and a ventricular septal defect related to the aorta must be distinguished from tetralogy of Fallot, which it closely resembles. Using ultrafast computed tomography, it has been possible to make this distinction accurately by demonstrating the presence or absence of aortomitral continuity (Fig. 37–8).

The pulmonary arteries are, as previously mentioned, particularly well visualized by using a cross-sectional imaging format. Abnormalities of the pulmonary arteries such as hypoplasia, peripheral coarctations, and congenital absence have all been identified (Fig. 37–13). Two patients with surgical banding of the pulmonary artery have been evaluated with this technique. In one patient with truncus arteriosus, distal migration of the band causing obstruction of the left pulmonary artery was clearly identified. One of the most important uses of the technique in our experience is related to its unique ability to measure pulmonary artery size precisely by use of a computerized "measure-distance" program. At present, any potential surgical patient in whom there is a question of the pulmonary artery anatomy or size will undergo a volume study for complete evaluation.

Patent ductus arteriosus, although extremely common, has proved to be particularly difficult to image with ultrafast computed tomography. Although the presence of a left-to-right shunt at the pulmonary artery level can be documented and the pulmonary-to-systemic flow ratio calculated, it has been possible to visualize the actual ductus structure in only 28 percent of the cases studied. Further refinements in positioning of the patient may improve our ability to image a patent ductus arteriosus consistently, but at present ultrafast computed tomography does not appear to play any significant role in its primary diagnosis.

Computed tomography has been utilized for many years to study disease of the aorta.[B6, G2] Coarctation of the aorta has proved to be particularly amenable to cross-sectional imaging using multiple contiguous slices obtained in a volume mode protocol. The ability to reconstruct these images in any operator-determined off-axis plane has provided an exquisite method for comprehensive evaluation of aortic pathology (Fig. 37–14). The resulting images provide excellent anatomic detail and have permitted patients to undergo surgical repair without the need for invasive angiography. Other aortic anomalies that have been successfully evaluated with this technique include Marfan's syndrome with aortic dissection, double aortic arch, and diffuse supravalvular aortic stenosis.

BLOOD FLOW DETERMINATIONS

In addition to the unique ability of ultrafast computed tomography to define complex cardiac anatomy accurately, this innovative technology allows direct quantitation of certain parameters of blood flow and cardiac function at the same time.[S2, S3] Short scan times permit an injected bolus of contrast material to be followed in and out of a given region of interest. By using an on-line time-density program, the computer can plot the mean CT number of the injectate against time to generate a contrast clearance curve. Following a gamma variate fit, the area under

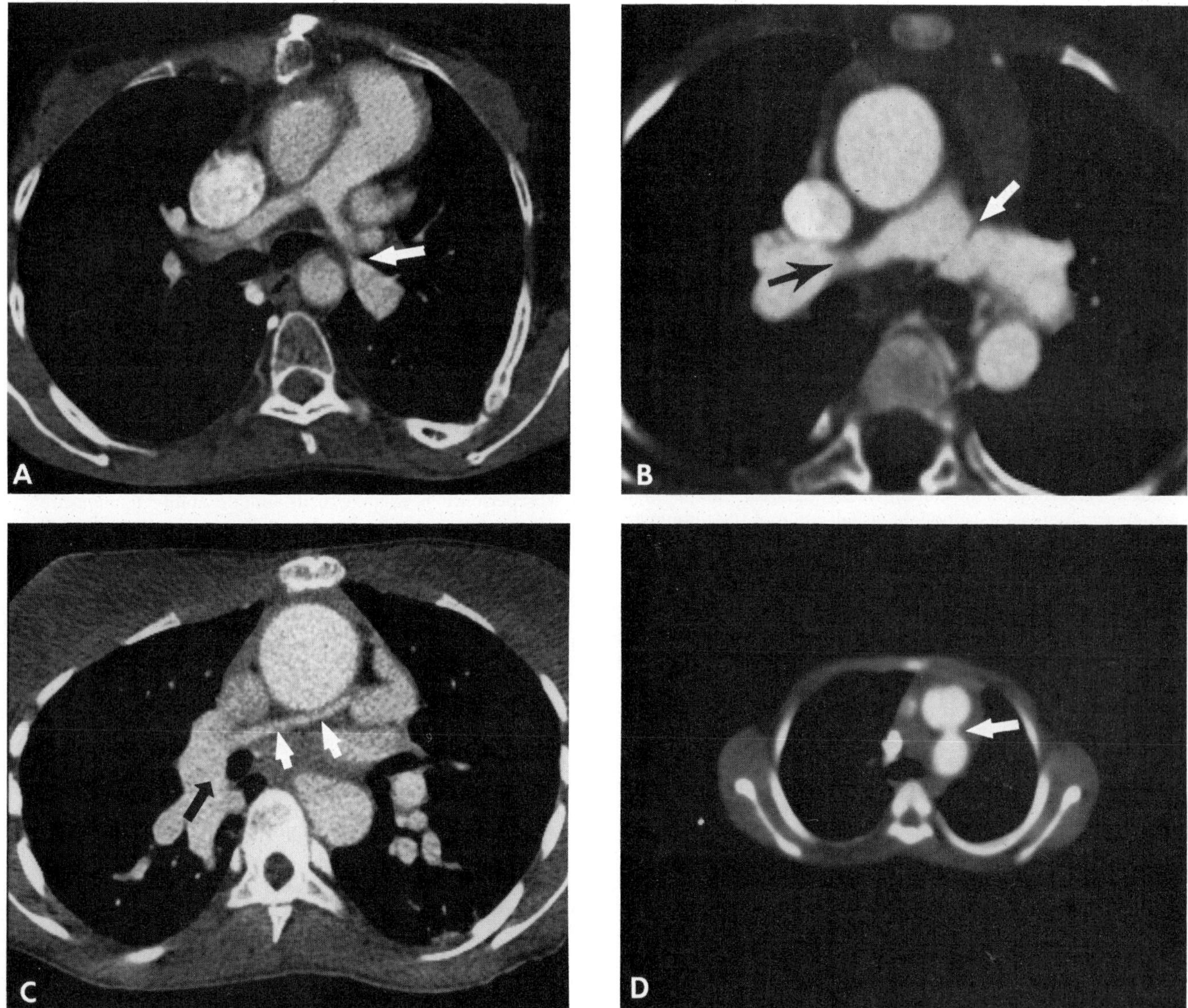

Figure 37–13. Pulmonary artery abnormalities. *A*, A single slice from a volume study in a patient with rubella syndrome. Both the right and left pulmonary arteries are hypoplastic beginning at the bifurcation. A coarctation in seen in the midportion of the left pulmonary artery *(arrow)*. Note the poststenotic dilatation distal to the coarctation site. *B*, Two different pulmonary artery abnormalities in a patient with pulmonary artresia. The right pulmonary artery is narrowed *(black arrow)* near the site of an anastomosis with a Blalock-Taussig shunt (see also Fig. 37–17A). A discrete membrane-like obstruction was also seen within the left pulmonary artery *(white arrow)* just beyond the bifurcation of the main pulmonary artery. Neither abnormality could be seen on angiography. Frame *C* is also from a patient with pulmonary atresia and severely hypoplastic pulmonary arteries. The right pulmonary artery distal to a Blalock-Taussig shunt *(black arrow)* has enlarged, while its proximal portion *(white arrows)* has remained diminutive. *D*, Narrowing and distortion of the main pulmonary artery at the site of a pulmonary artery banding.

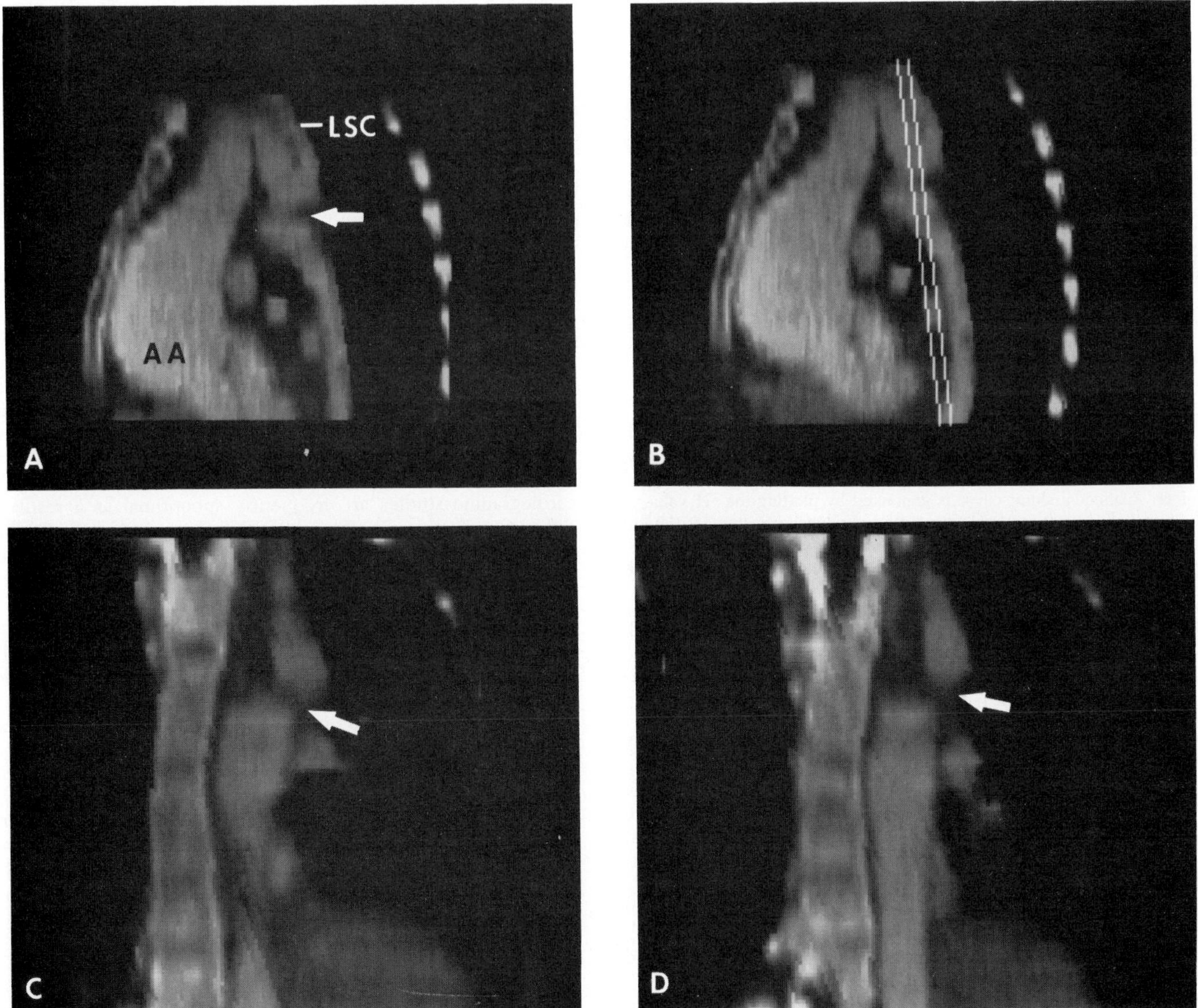

Figure 37–14. Coarctation of the aorta. Four reconstructed images from a volume study of a patient with coarctation of the aorta are shown. *A*, A sagittal reconstruction of the contiguous cross-sectional slices. The site of the coarctation *(arrow)* and its relation to the left subclavian artery (LSC) are beautifully demonstrated. The ascending aorta (AA) is markedly dilated, while the descending aorta below the coarctation site is normal in size. To further delineate the anatomy of the coarctation, two additional operator-determined planes *(B)* are selected for further reconstruction. The resulting images, seen in *C* and *D*, help to clarify further the anatomy of the coarctation *(arrows)*. These images demonstrate the unique ability of ultrafast computed tomography to provide exquisite tomographic definition of aortic anatomy by reformatting previously reconstructed images in any desired plane.

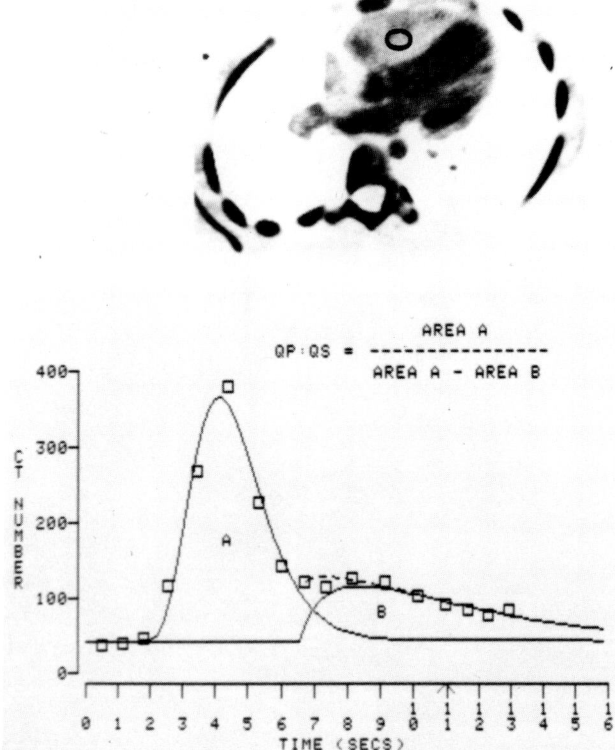

Figure 37–15. Shunt calculation. A region-of-interest marker is placed over the right ventricle in this patient with a small ventricular septal defect. A bimodal shunt curve is generated by plotting the CT value of the injected contrast material against time. Following a gamma variate fit to the two portions of the curve, the areas under the primary (A) and secondary (B) curves are calculated and the pulmonary-to-systemic flow ratio (Qp:Qs) is calculated. (From Eldredge, W. J., Diethelm, N. E., and Lipton, M. J.: Ultrafast computed tomography in the diagnosis of congenital heart disease. *In* Imaging for Pediatric Disorders. W. B. Saunders, Philadelphia, to be published, with permission.)

the flow curve is measured. Cardiac output can then be accurately calculated using the standard Stewart-Hamilton equation.[G3]

Of far more interest in patients with congenital heart disease is the ability to evaluate shunts noninvasively. Following the injection of a bolus of contrast material, a region-of-interest marker is placed over any chamber or vessel distal to the shunt. A bimodal time-density curve is then generated (Fig. 37–15). The pulmonary-to-systemic flow ratio is then calculated by an algorithm that is in use in many nuclear medicine laboratories.[T2] The feasibility of calculating shunt flows with ultrafast computed tomography has been validated by use of flow phantoms.[G4] Retrospective analysis of our own experience suggests that within the range of flow ratios between 1.3:1 and 2.5:1, these CT measurements correlate well with the values calculated from oxygen data by standard Fick methods.

MEASUREMENT OF VENTRICULAR VOLUME AND MASS

Precise measurements of ventricular volumes are assuming an increasingly important role in both the preoperative and postoperative evaluation of patients with complex congenital heart disease. All currently available methods for measuring volumes require geometric assumptions, which, in the presence of abnormalities of ventricular size, location, and shape, are subject to great error. Computed tomography has been shown to be a highly accurate method for measuring ventricular volumes irrespective of the shape or orientation of the chamber.[L2, L3, R3] Reports from several centers indicated that highly accurate measurements of right and left ventricular volume as well as left atrial volume can be obtained with ultrafast computed tomography.[L4, R4, V2] Following the injection of contrast material, a multilevel short-axis cine study encompassing the entire volume of both ventricles is obtained. During image analysis, the endocardial borders of the ventricular cavities are traced with a computer-assisted edge detection program and the cavity area for each slice is measured.[W1] The total volume of each respective ventricle is calculated by summing the volumes of the individual tomographic levels by using a modified Simpson's rule. The ability to obtain accurate measurements of right ventricular volume in a simple, noninvasive manner represents a major addition to the imaging capabilities available to cardiologists interested in evaluation of patients with congenital heart disease.

Ventricular mass may be precisely measured using the same apex-to-base cine studies used to calculate ventricular volume.[F2, F3] After outlining both the epicardial and endocardial borders of the left ventricle in each tomographic slice, the computer calculates the ventricular mass, stroke volume, end-diastolic volume, and ejection fraction for each level as well as for the entire ventricle. This permits both regional and global evaluation of ejection fraction[R5] as well as calculation of stroke volume[R6, R7] and regurgitant volume.[R8, R9]

POSTOPERATIVE EVALUATION

In the immediate postoperative period, ultrafast computed tomography has been used successfully to evaluate the adequacy of surgical repair, determine the presence of any significant residual defects, calculate cardiac output, and quantitate ventricular function. Other imaging modalities have been used extensively for the same purposes but are often associated with considerable limitations and problems. Two-dimensional echocardiographic studies are frequently suboptimal as a result of difficulties in obtaining an adequate acoustic window. Cardiac catheterization presents an additional risk and can often be difficult or impossible to perform due to problems in finding additional venous or arterial access for catheter insertion. With ultrafast computed tomography, however, a comprehensive cardiac evaluation of anatomy, flow, and function can be very rapidly obtained from a single study regardless of the presence of life-support equipment or surgical dressings covering the region of interest. Since only small doses of contrast material are required, the injections can be administered through monitoring lines or intravenous catheters that are already in place. Because the cross-sectional images obtained with computed tomography offer such a wide field of view, additional postoperative problems involving the pulmonary parenchyma, pleural spaces, upper airway, pericardium, or chest wall can also be evaluated in the same study.

At present, there is great interest in determining the long-

Table 37–1. POSTSURGICAL EVALUATION OF CONGENITAL HEART DISEASE USING ULTRAFAST COMPUTED TOMOGRAPHY

Diagnosis	Number of Cases
Anomalous coronary artery origin	1
Aortic stenosis	23
Atrial septal defects	13
Atrioventricular canal	4
Coarctation of the aorta	15
Complete transposition of the great vessels	10
Cor triatriatum	2
Double-outlet right ventricle	2
Marfan's syndrome	4
Pulmonic stenosis	3
Single ventricle	5
Systemic-to-pulmonary artery shunts	11
Tetralogy of Fallot	26
Tricuspid atresia	6
Vascular ring	1
Ventricular septal defect	11
Ventricular septal defect with pulmonary atresia	2

term outcome of patients who have undergone surgical procedures for repair or palliation of complex congenital cardiac anomalies. Factors that are important in this regard include documentation of the adequacy of the surgical repair as well as serial evaluation of myocardial function. In no other area does ultrafast CT imaging offer greater potential benefit than in the evaluation of this group of patients. The ability to evaluate noninvasively anatomy, flow, and myocardial function with one single imaging modality should significantly increase our ability to better define these complex long-term issues. To date, our own experience in postoperative evaluation is small and has been limited to resting studies (Table 37–1). This experience, however, has allowed us to define certain distinct uses for ultrafast computed tomography in long-term postoperative evaluation.

Postoperative anatomy, which can often be significantly altered from its presurgical appearance, has been accurately defined and the adequacy of the surgical repair evaluated (Fig. 37–16). The presence of residual shunts following closure of atrial or ventricular septal defects has been documented and their exact location identified. Various sites of residual or surgically created obstruction to blood flow have also been correctly identified. Unsuspected baffle obstruction was accurately identified in three asymptomatic patients who had previously undergone Mustard repair of complete transposition of the great arteries. Subsequent cardiac catheterization confirmed the CT findings, and two of the three patients underwent subsequent successful surgical repair. Postsurgical evaluation of repair of coarctation of the aorta has proved particularly successful. Ultrafast computed tomography is now used routinely as a noninvasive method for documentation of satisfactory surgical results or for the identification of residual or recurrent obstruction.

Evaluation of the postoperative anatomy of the pulmonary arteries with ultrafast computed tomography has been highly successful. In several patients it has been possible to detect significant distortion of a pulmonary artery near the site of a Waterston anastomosis. The severity of the distortion could not be well seen with cineangiography, since the area of interest was hidden from view by a large, contrast-filled aorta anterior to it.

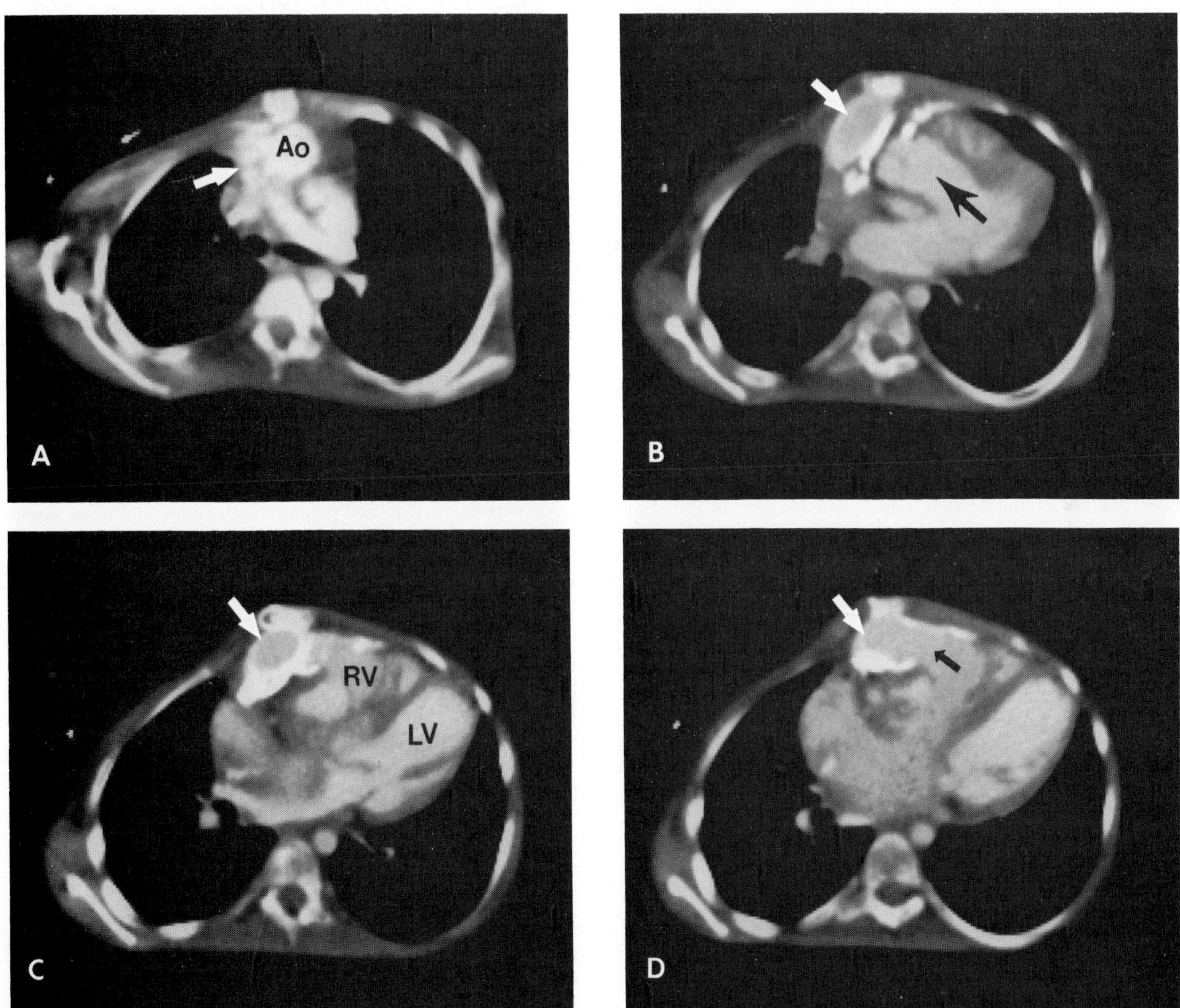

Figure 37–16. Postoperative evaluation. Four selected frames from a flow study of a patient with complete transposition of the great vessels, ventricular septal defect, and pulmonary stenosis are shown. The patient had previously undergone a Rastelli repair with a valved homograft conduit between the anterior right ventricle and the posterior pulmonary artery. In *A*, the aorta (Ao) is seen anterior to the site of the anastomosis of the conduit to the pulmonary artery *(arrow)*. Progressing inferiorly, a densely calcified substernal conduit *(white arrows)* can be identified in *B*, *C*, and *D*. The surgically created outlet between the posterior left ventricle and the anterior aorta is beautifully demonstrated in *B (black arrow)*. The connection is widely patent. Frame *D* shows a wide anastomosis *(black arrow)* between the heavily trabeculated, anterior right ventricle and the conduit *(white arrow)*. The patient had an excellent surgical result at the time of this ultrafast CT study but subsequently developed calcification and severe stenosis of the homograft valve leaflets.

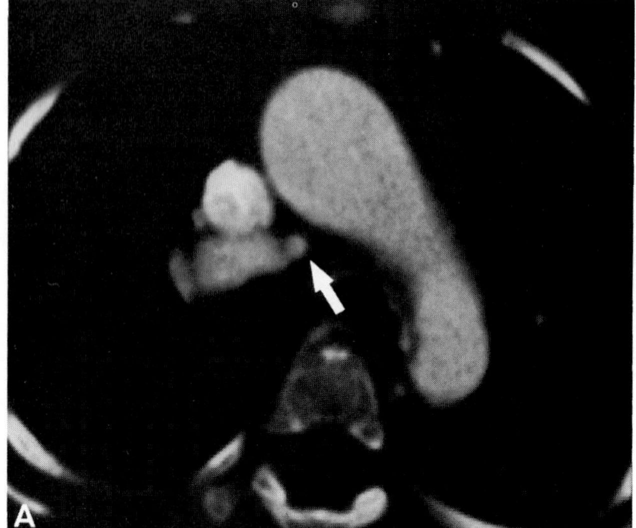

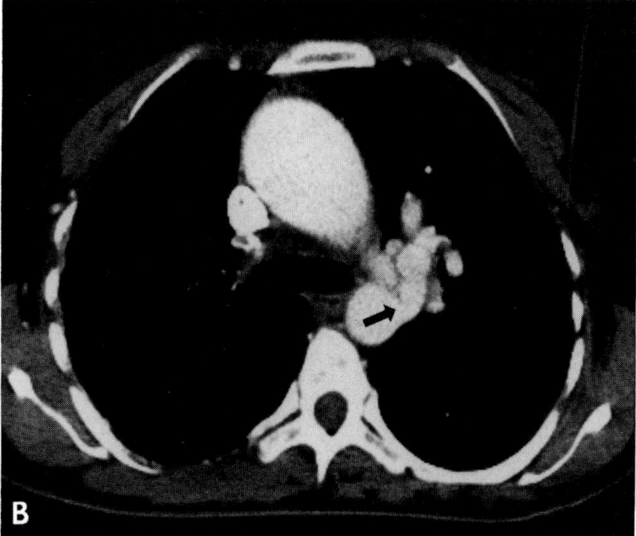

Figure 37–17. Surgical shunts. Frame *A* is from the study of a patient with ventricular septal defect and pulmonary atresia. A patent right Blalock-Taussig shunt *(arrow)* is seen just above its anastomosis point with the right pulmonary artery. In Figure 37–13B the next contiguous slice from the same study is shown, demonstrating narrowing of the pulmonary artery at the site of anastomosis. In *B*, a patent Potts shunt *(arrow)* can be seen between the left pulmonary artery and the descending aorta.

Measurement of pulmonary artery growth in patients with small pulmonary arteries who have undergone a surgical procedure designed to increase pulmonary blood flow has also been possible. Currently, all patients undergoing such a procedure will have preoperative and serial postoperative CT studies of the pulmonary arteries to measure pulmonary artery size precisely.

Long-term flow-related issues in postoperative cardiac patients include the determination of surgical shunt patency and the quantitation of the pulmonary-to-systemic ratio in patients with residual shunts. Using the flow mode studies, it has been possible to visualize various systemic-to-pulmonary artery shunts (Blalock-Taussig, Waterston, Glenn and Potts) and determine their patency (Fig. 37–17). This modality may eventually prove to be an accurate noninvasive alternative to cardiac catheterization for the determination of shunt patency, but further validation studies are necessary. In patients with suspected residual shunts following surgical closure, the presence and exact site of the residual shunt can be accurately determined and the size of the shunt quantitated.

The capability of ultrafast computed tomography to evaluate cardiac function and accurately measure the effects of exercise or drug intervention on myocardial performance is of major clinical importance.[C1, R10, S4] Some of the most important unanswered issues regarding the long-term fate of patients with operated congenital cardiac defects are related to questions of cardiac function. The long-term effects on cardiac function of cardiopulmonary bypass, ventriculotomy, and insertion of large prosthetic outflow tract patches remain to be completely defined. As an example, it is becoming increasingly apparent that certain patients who have undergone repair of tetralogy of Fallot do not tolerate the inevitable pulmonary valve regurgitation as well as expected. This is particularly true for patients who have associated left ventricular dysfunction. Many such questions regarding the long-term fate of the myocardium and its performance remain unanswered, and ultrafast computed tomography offers a unique imaging modality capable of obtaining this type of information.

CONCLUSIONS

A wide variety of imaging modalities are currently available to the cardiac diagnostician. Our initial experience with ultrafast computed tomography suggests that it offers certain advantages not currently available with other imaging modalities. The major advantage to those interested in congenital heart disease is its ability to provide accurate three-dimensional volumetric information about cardiac anatomy, even in its most complex presentations. In addition, quantitative information regarding blood flow and myocardial performance can be obtained from the same studies. Of great advantage is the fact that this information can be obtained in a resting state or following stress or drug intervention. No other one imaging modality can provide such a wide range of precisely accurate anatomic and functional information from a single study.

Currently, there is a movement in the direction of more noninvasive approaches to cardiac imaging and diagnosis. This is partially due to major improvements in noninvasive imaging technology but is also an important result of the nationwide trends toward improving cost containment and achieving greater utilization of outpatient diagnostic and treatment facilities. Ultrafast computed tomography offers many important advantages in this context. The exact role that this exciting new modality will eventually play in the entire scheme of imaging techniques remains to be determined. However, based on our early experience with more than 500 patients with congenital heart disease, it is apparent that this cross-sectional imaging modality can, through its unique combination of high density and temporal resolution, provide much important new diagnostic information in a safe, rapid, accurate, noninvasive way.

References

A

1. Anderson, R. H., Becker, A. E., Lucchese, F. A., et al.: Sequential segmental analysis. *In* Anderson, R. H., Becker, A. E., Lucchese, F. A., et al. (Eds.): Morphology of Congenital Heart Disease. University Park Press, Baltimore, 1983, p. 1.

B

1. Bargeron, L. W., Jr., Elliot, L. P., Soto, B., et al.: Axial cineangiography in congenital heart disease. 1. Concept, technical and anatomic considerations. Circulation 56:1075, 1977.
2. Boyd, D. P.: Computerized transmission tomography of the heart using scanning electron beams. *In* Higgins, C. B. (ed.): CT of the Heart and Great Vessels: Experimental Evaluation and Clinical Evaluation. Future Publishing, Mt. Kisko, 1983, p. 46.
3. Boyd, D. P., Couch, J. L., Napel, S. A., et al.: Ultra Cine-CT for cardiac imaging: Where have we been? What lies ahead? Am. J. Cardiac Imag. 1:175, 1987.
4. Boyd, D. P., and Lipton, M. J.: Cardiac computed tomography. Proc. IEEE 7:289, 1983.
5. Bali, C., Chomka, E. V., Fisher, E. A., and Brundage, B.: Ultra-fast computed tomography in congenital heart disease. (Abstract.) Circ. Suppl. III 72:28, 1985.
6. Baron, R. L., Butierrez, F. R., and McKnight, R. C.: Computed tomographic (CT) evaluation of the great arteries and aortic arch malformations. *In*

Friedman, W. F., and Higgins, C. B. (eds.): Pediatric Cardiac Imaging. W. B. Saunders, Philadelphia, 1984, p. 135.

C

1. Chomka, E. V., Fletcher, M., Stein, M., and Brundage, B.: Ultrafast computed tomography during exercise bicycle ergometry. (Abstract.) J. Am. Coll. Cardiol. 7:154A, 1986.

D

1. Dery, R., Lipton, M. J., Garrett, J. S., et al.: Cine-computed tomography of arrythmogenic right ventricular dysplasia. J. Comput. Assist. Tomogr. 10:120, 1986.

E

1. Eldredge, W. J., Bharati, S., Flicker, S., et al.: Cine CT scanning in the diagnosis of congenital heart disease: Analysis of the first 42 cases. *In* Doyle, E. F., et al. (eds.): Pediatric Cardiology. Springer-Verlag, New York, 1985, p. 404.
2. Eldredge, W. J., Flicker, S., and Steiner, R. M.: Cine-CT in the anatomical evaluation of congenital heart disease. *In* Pohost, G. M., Higgins, C. B., Morganroth, J., et al. (eds.): New Concepts in Cardiac Imaging 1987. Year Book Medical Publishers, Chicago, 1987, p. 256.
3. Eldredge, W. J., and Flicker, S.: Evaluation of congenital heart disease using cine-CT. Am. J. Cardiac Imag. 1:38, 1987.
4. Eldredge, W. J., Rees, M. R., Flicker, S., and Clark, D. L.: Cine-CT scanning of the ventricular septum for the diagnosis of ventricular septal defect. (Abstract.) Circ. Suppl. III 72:27, 1985.
5. Eldredge, W. J., Rees, M. R., and Flicker, S.: Diagnosis and evaluation of hypertrophic obstructive cardiomyopathy in adolescents and young adults using cine computed tomography. Presented at the Annual Meeting of the American Roentgen Ray Society, Washington, D.C., April 1986.

F

1. Farmer, D. W., Lipton, M. J., Webb, W. R., et al.: Computed tomography in congenital heart disease. J. Comput. Assist. Tomogr. 8:677, 1984.
2. Feiring, A. J., Rumberger, J. A., Higgins, C. B., et al.: Determination of left ventricular mass by rapid acquisition computed tomography. (Abstract.) Circ. Suppl. II 70:250, 1984.
3. Feiring, A. J., Rumberger, J. A., Reiter, S. J., et al.: Determination of left ventricular mass in dogs with rapid-acquisition cardiac computed tomographic scanning. Circulation 72:1355, 1985.

G

1. Garrett, J. S., Schiller, N. B., Botvinick, E. H., et al.: Cine-computed tomography of Ebstein anomaly. J. Comput. Assist. Tomogr. 10:664, 1986.
2. Godwin, J. D.: Computerized transmission tomography of diseases of the thoracic aorta. *In* Higgins, C. B. (ed.): CT of the Heart and Great Vessels: Experimental Evaluation and Clinical Evaluation. Future Publishing, Mt. Kisko, 1983, p. 353.
3. Garrett, J. S., Lanzer, P., Jaschke, W., et al.: Noninvasive measurement of cardiac output by cine-CT. Am. J. Cardiol. 56:657, 1985.
4. Garrett, J. S., Jaschke, W., Aherne, T., et al.: Quantitation of intracardiac shunts by cine-CT. J. Comput. Assist. Tomogr. 12:82, 1988.

K

1. Kurnik, P. B., Wachspress, J. D., Innerfield, M., et al.: Wall mass regression after aortic valve replacement measured by cine computed tomography. (Abstract.) J. Am. Coll. Cardiol. 11:157A, 1988.

L

1. Lipton, M. J., and Higgins, C. B.: Computed tomography—the technique and its use for the evaluation of cardiocirculatory anatomy and function. *In* Friedman, W. F., and Higgins, C. B. (eds.): Pediatric Cardiac Imaging. W. B. Saunders, Philadelphia, 1984, p. 120.
2. Lipton, M. J., Hayashi, T. T., Davis, P. L., and Carlsson, E.: The effects of orientation on volume measurements of human left ventricular casts. Invest. Radiol. 15:469, 1980.
3. Lipton, M. J., Hayashi, T. T., Boyd, D. P., and Carlsson, E.: Measurement of left ventricular cast volume by computed tomography. Radiology 127:419, 1978.
4. Lipton, M. J.: Quantitation of cardiac function by cine-CT. Radiol. Clin. North Am. 23:613, 1985.

M

1. MacMillan, R. M., Rees, M. R., Maranhao, V., and Clark, D. L.: Cine-computed tomography of cor triatriatum. J. Comput. Assist. Tomogr. 10:124, 1986.
2. MacMillan, R. M., Shahriari, A., Sumithisena, et al.: Contrast-enhanced cine computed tomography for diagnosis of right coronary artery to coronary sinus arteriovenous fistula. Am. J. Cardiol. 56:997, 1985.
3. MacMillan, R. M., Rees, M. R., Eldredge, W. J., et al.: Quantitation of shunting at the atrial level utilizing rapid acquisition computed tomography with comparison with cardiac catheterization. J. Am. Coll. Cardiol. 7:946, 1986.
4. MacMillan, R. M., Rees, M. R., Lumia, F. J., and Maranhao, V.: Preliminary experience in the use of ultrafast computed tomography to diagnose aortic valve stenosis. Am. Heart J. 115:665, 1988.
5. Mahoney, L. T., Smith, W., Noel, M. P., et al.: Measurement of right ventricular volume using cine computed tomography. (Abstract.) Circ. Suppl. III 72:28, 1985.

R

1. Rees, M. R., Feiring, A. J., Rumberger, J. A., et al.: Heart evaluation by cine CT: Use of two new oblique views. Radiology 159:804, 1986.
2. Rees, M. R., MacMillan, R. M., Lopez, M., et al.: Demonstration of mitral valve function by cine computed tomography using a new long axis view. Angiology 37:79, 1986.
3. Ringertz, H. G., Rodgers, B., Lipton, M. J., et al.: Assessment of human right ventricular cast volume by CT and angiocardiography. Invest. Radiol. 20:29, 1985.
4. Reiter, S. J., Rumberger, J. A., Feiring, A. J., et al.: Precision of measurements of right and left ventricular volume by cine computed tomography. Circulation 74:890, 1986.
5. Rich, S., Chomka, E. V., Stagl, R., et al.: Determination of left ventricular ejection fraction using ultrafast computed tomography. Am. Heart J. 112:392, 1986.
6. Reiter, S. J., Rumberger, J. A., Feiring, A. J., et al.: Precise determination of left and right ventricular stroke volume with cine computed tomography. (Abstract.) Circ. Suppl. III 72:179, 1985.
7. Reiter, S. J., Rumberger, J. A., Stanford, W., and Marcus, M. L.: Precise stroke volume measurements by cine-CT in the presence of abnormal left ventricular shape and size. (Abstract.) Circ. Suppl. II 74:122, 1986.
8. Reiter, S. J., Rumberger, J. A., Feiring, A. J., et al.: Measurement of aortic regurgitation with cine-CT. (Abstract.) J. Am. Coll. Cardiol. 7:154A, 1986.
9. Reiter, S. J., Rumberger, J. A., Stanford, W., and Marcus, M. L.: Quantitative determination of aortic regurgitant volume in dogs by ultrafast computed tomography. Circulation 76:728, 1987.
10. Rees, M. R., MacMillan, R. M., Fender, B., and Clark, D. L.: Cine-CT technique for evaluation of left ventricular function during supine exercise. AJR 147:916, 1986.

S

1. Skotnicki, R., MacMillan, R. M., Rees, M. R., et al.: Detection of atrial septal defect by contrast-enhanced ultrafast computed tomography. Cathet. Cardiovasc. Diagn. 12:103, 1986.
2. Sethna, D. H., Bateman, T. M., Whiting, J. S., and Forrester, J. S.: Comprehensive and quantitative cardiac assessment using cine-CT: Description of a new clinical diagnostic modality. Am. J. Cardiac Imag. 1:18, 1987.
3. Steiner, R. M., Flicker, S., Eldredge, W. J., et al.: The functional and anatomic evaluation of the cardiovascular system with rapid-acquisition computed tomography (cine CT). Radiol. Clin. North Am. 24:503, 1986.
4. Stark, C. A., Rumberger, J. A., Stanford, W., and Marcus, M. L.: Dobutamine stress cine-CT. (Abstract.) Circ. Suppl. II 74:122, 1986.

T

1. Tonkin, I. L. D.: The definition of cardiac malpositions with echocardiography and computed tomography. *In* Friedman, W. F., and Higgins, C. B. (eds.): Pediatric Cardiac Imaging. W. B. Saunders, Philadelphia, 1984, p. 157.
2. Treves, S., and Kurac, A.: Radionuclide evaluation of circulatory shunts. Cardiol. Clin. 1:427, 1983.

V

1. Van Praagh, R.: The segmental approach to understanding complex cardiac lesions. *In* Eldredge, W. J., et al. (eds.): Current Problems in Congenital Heart Disease. Spectrum Publications, New York, 1979, p. 1.
2. Vandenberg, B. F., Weiss, R., Kinzey, J., et al.: Left atrial volume measurement: Cine computed tomography and echocardiography. (Abstract.) J. Am. Coll. Cardiol. 11:217A, 1988.

W

1. Whiting, J. S., Bateman, T. M., Pfaff, M., et al.: Semi-automated method for quantitating LV mass and chamber volume from cine-CT scans. (Abstract.) Circ. Suppl. III 72:180, 1985.

Part VII

Cardiac Nuclear Magnetic Resonance Imaging

Chapter 38

Principles of Nuclear Magnetic Resonance

S. L. TALAGALA, Ph.D. ▪ G. L. WOLF, M.D., Ph.D.

FUNDAMENTAL CONCEPTS OF NUCLEAR MAGNETIC RESONANCE 732
Nuclear Spin 732
Behavior of Nuclei in a Magnetic Field 733
Resonance Phenomenon and the NMR Spectrum 734
PULSE FOURIER TRANSFORM NUCLEAR MAGNETIC RESONANCE 735
Semiclassical Vector Description 735
Free Induction Decay and the Fourier Transform 736
Signal-to-Noise Ratio and Signal Averaging 737
Relaxation 737
Rotating-Frame Concept 738
MULTIPULSE NUCLEAR MAGNETIC RESONANCE 740
Inversion-Recovery Sequence 740
Spin-Echo Sequence 741
CONCLUSION 743

The nuclear magnetic resonance (NMR) phenomenon in bulk matter was first demonstrated by Bloch and associates[B1, B2] and Purcell and associates[P1] in 1946. Since then, nuclear magnetic resonance has developed into a sophisticated technique with applications in a wide variety of disciplines that now include physics, chemistry, biology, and medicine. Over the years, NMR has proved to be an invaluable tool for molecular structure determination and investigation of molecular dynamics in solids and liquids. In its latest development, application of NMR to studies of living systems has attracted considerable attention from biochemists and clinicians alike. These studies have progressed along two parallel and perhaps complementary paths. First, NMR is used as a spectroscopic method to provide chemical information from selected regions within an object; such information from a localized area in living tissue provides valuable metabolic data that are directly related to the state of health of the tissue and, in principle, can be used to monitor tissue response to therapy. In the second area of application, NMR is used as an imaging tool to provide anatomic and pathologic information.

The rapid progress of NMR to diverse fields of study can be attributed to the development of pulse Fourier transform techniques in the late 1960's.[E1] Additional impetus was provided by the development of fast Fourier transform algorithms, advances in computer technology, and the advent of high-field superconducting magnets. More recently, introduction of new experimental concepts such as two-dimensional NMR has further broadened its applications.

This chapter focuses on the basic principles and practice of pulse Fourier transform NMR. Our objectives are to present the subject as simply as possible so that the essential concepts can be grasped by the novice. Hence, mathematical rigor is sacrificed in favor of descriptiveness. Proton NMR is stressed for simplicity and its direct relevance to NMR imaging. Material from a variety of sources has been extracted for this account, and the reader is encouraged to consult texts on the subject[C1, F1, F2, G1, M1, S1] for more detailed discussions.

FUNDAMENTAL CONCEPTS OF NUCLEAR MAGNETIC RESONANCE

Nuclear Spin

The basis of NMR lies in a property possessed by certain nuclei, called the spin angular momentum (p). The spin angular momentum of the nucleus can be considered as an outcome of the rotational or spinning motion of the nucleus about its own axis. For this reason, nuclei having spin angular momentum are often referred to as nuclear spins. The spin angular momentum of a nucleus is defined by the nuclear spin quantum number (I) and is given by the relationship

$$p = \frac{h}{2\pi}[I(I + 1)]^{1/2} \tag{1}$$

where h denotes a constant value called the Planck constant. The value of spin quantum number depends on the structure of the nucleus—the number of protons and neutrons—and can be an integer, half-integer, or zero. The spin quantum numbers of

Table 38–1. NMR PROPERTIES OF SOME SELECTED NUCLEI

Nucleus	Nuclear Spin	Gyromagnetic Ratio (MHz/T)	Larmor Frequency (MHz) at 2.3 T	Natural Abundance (%)	Relative Sensitivity*
^{1}H	½	42.58	100.0	99.98	1
^{13}C	½	10.71	25.14	1.11	1.7×10^{-4}
^{19}F	½	40.05	94.07	100	0.83
^{23}Na	3⁄2	11.26	26.45	100	9.2×10^{-2}
^{31}P	½	17.23	40.48	100	6.6×10^{-2}

*Includes correction for natural abundance.

some selected nuclei are given in Table 38–1. Hydrogen (^{1}H) (I = 1/2), the most abundant element in nature and in the body, is most receptive to NMR experiments. On the other hand, the most common isotopes of carbon (^{12}C) and oxygen (^{16}O) have nuclei with I = 0 and hence cannot be observed by magnetic resonance experiments.

Since the nucleus is a charged particle, spin angular momentum is accompanied by a magnetic moment (μ) given by $\mu = \gamma p$, where γ is called the magnetogyric ratio of the nucleus. Note that both μ and p are vector quantities having magnitude and direction. The magnetogyric ratio is characteristic of a particular nucleus (see Table 38–1) and is proportional to the charge-to-mass ratio of the nucleus. The parameter γ can be positive or negative, and hence the nuclear magnetic moment may point either in the same direction as the angular momentum (positive γ) or in the opposite direction (negative γ).

From the discussion so far, an analogy between a nucleus having spin angular momentum and a bar magnet can be drawn. A spinning charged body, such as a nucleus, can be considered equivalent to an electric current through a small loop of wire, which in turn has an associated magnetic field surrounding it similar to that of a bar magnet. The strength of this bar magnet is expressed in terms of its magnetic moment.

Behavior of Nuclei in a Magnetic Field

In magnetic resonance experiments, we are concerned with the behavior of nuclei placed in an external magnetic field. In the case of a bar magnet, application of an external magnetic field would cause the magnet simply to align with or against the direction of the field. However, a nucleus possesses angular momentum and, consequently, precesses about the direction of the applied field just as a spinning top precesses in the earth's gravitational field. This precessional motion is indicated in Figure 38–1 as a rotation of the magnetic moment vector about the direction of the external magnetic field (B_0) in addition to the nuclear spin about its own axis. The frequency of precession, ν_0 (rate at which μ rotates about B_0), called the Larmor frequency, is given by the relationship

$$\nu_0 = \frac{\gamma}{2\pi} B_0 \qquad (2)$$

This result can be deduced from the laws of classical physics. However, in order to obtain a complete description of the behavior of nuclei in a magnetic field, quantum mechanical theory must be considered.

Quantum mechanical analysis shows that the orientation of the spin angular momentum vector, and hence the magnetic moment, of the nucleus with respect to the direction of B_0 cannot be arbitrary and is subjected to certain restrictions. The allowed orientations are governed by the rule that the component of the angular momentum along a given direction (e.g., the *z* direction) be expressed by

$$p_z = m_I \frac{h}{2\pi} \qquad (3)$$

where m_I is the magnetic quantum number. The allowed values for m_I are determined by the spin quantum number I of the nucleus such that $m_I = -I, -I + 1, \ldots, I - 1, I$. Therefore, in general, a magnetic moment can assume any one of 2I + 1 orientations with respect to the field B_0, and in the case of hydrogen nuclei (I = 1/2) two orientations are allowed (Fig. 38–2*A*). These two orientations are similar to the two directions in which a bar magnet may orient in a magnetic field and are consequently called the parallel or spin-up (m = +1/2 state) and the antiparallel or spin-down (m = −1/2 state) orientations. In the discussions to follow, nuclei with I = 1/2 are considered.

As a result of the interaction with the field B_0, the magnetic moments in these two possible states acquire different energies; hence, they can be represented by a corresponding energy diagram with two levels (Fig. 38–2*B*). These allowed orientations or the energy levels are also referred to as spin states of the

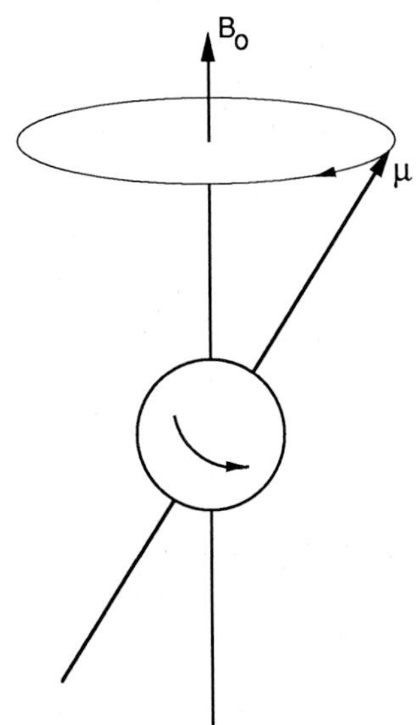

Figure 38–1. Precession of nuclear magnetic moment μ about the external magnetic field B_0.

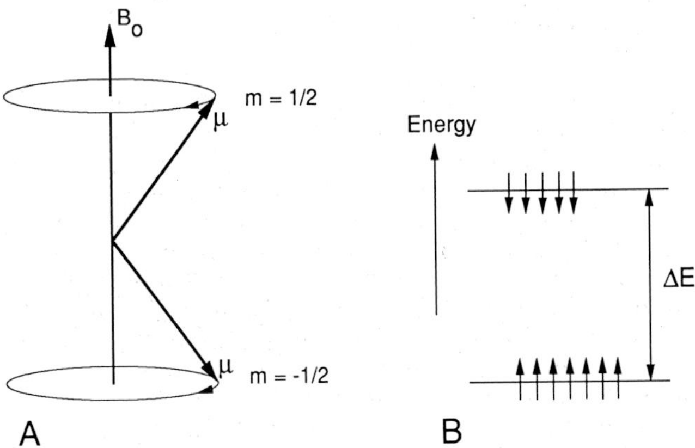

Figure 38–2. Allowed orientations of μ (*A*) and corresponding energy levels (*B*) for a nucleus with I = 1/2 in a magnetic field. Arrows in (*B*) represent nuclei in each energy level.

nucleus. The energy difference between the two spin states, ΔE, is proportional to the magnetogyric ratio of the nucleus and the external field strength and is given by

$$\Delta E = \frac{h}{2\pi}\gamma B_0 \tag{4}$$

So far, the behavior of a single isolated nucleus has been considered. However, in practice, the mean result due to a large number of similar nuclei is observed. When an ensemble of nuclei is subjected to an external magnetic field, nuclei distribute themselves between the allowed orientations. At equilibrium, the population of nuclei in the parallel orientation (lower energy state) exceeds that in the antiparallel orientation (higher energy state) by a small amount, as governed by Boltzmann statistics. The excess population in the lower energy state (Δn) is dependent on the energy difference between the spin states and the absolute temperature (T):

$$\Delta n \simeq n_0 \frac{\Delta E}{2kT} \tag{5}$$

where n_0 is the total number of nuclei in the sample and k is the Boltzmann constant. The fractional excess of population ($\Delta n/n_0$) in the lower energy state is extremely small; for example, for hydrogen nuclei at body temperature (310 K) in a magnetic field of 1 tesla (10,000 gauss), $\Delta n/n_0 = 3.295 \times 10^{-6}$.

Consider the case of a water sample placed in an external magnetic field. Before the introduction of the sample into the field, the magnetic moment vectors of hydrogen nuclei are oriented randomly in space without any preferred direction, since the external field is zero. Once the sample is placed in the field, the hydrogen nuclei begin to align themselves in either one of the allowed orientations. This process continues for a time determined by the spin-lattice relaxation time (see Relaxation) until an equilibrium situation is reached with a slight excess of nuclei in the parallel orientation.

Resonance Phenomenon and the NMR Spectrum

It is possible to induce transitions of nuclei between the two orientations and hence between the allowed energy levels. This can be accomplished by the application of a second magnetic field (B_1) that rotates in a plane perpendicular to the B_0 field (Fig. 38–3). The magnitude of the applied B_1 field is much smaller than that of the B_0 field. It can be appreciated that the B_1 field should rotate at the same frequency as the Larmor frequency of spins to exert a significant torque on the magnetic moment and to cause it to change its orientation. Induction of nuclear transitions by matching the frequency of the "driving" B_1 field to the "natural" Larmor frequency of nuclei is called resonance. Thus, the resonance frequency, the frequency of the B_1 field required to cause resonance, is equal to the Larmor frequency.

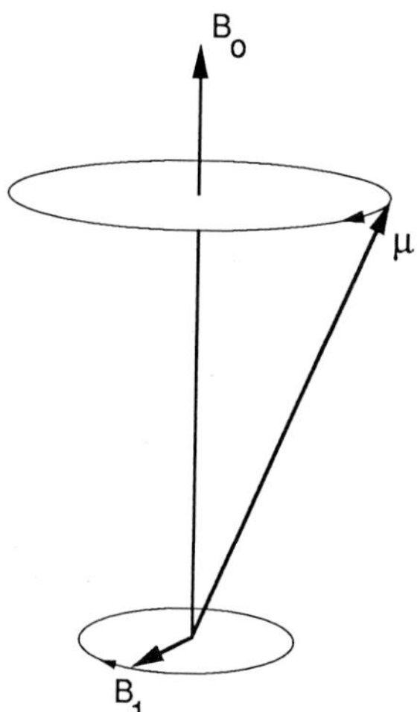

Figure 38–3. Relative orientation of B_0 and B_1 fields required to induce transitions of nuclei between the two spin states.

Alternatively, the resonance phenomenon can be viewed in energy terms. Transition of nuclei between the energy levels is stimulated only when the energy of the B_1 field is made equal to the energy difference between the two nuclear spin states (ΔE). Thus, if a B_1 field of frequency ν is considered as a carrier of photons (packets of energy) with energy equal to $h\nu$, the condition for resonance is given by $\Delta E = h\nu$, and substituting for ΔE from equation (4), it is seen that the frequency of the B_1 field needed to cause resonance is equal to the Larmor frequency. It should be noted that electromagnetic radiation is not required for stimulation of nuclear transitions between the energy levels. This has been discussed in a recent publication.[H1]

In practice, the rotating B_1 field required to cause resonance is generated by establishing an alternating electric current of appropriate frequency in a coil of wire. At the magnetic field strengths currently used in NMR, the resonance frequency of nuclei falls in the range of millions of cycles per second (megahertz, MHz). This corresponds to the frequency range encompassed by "radio waves" in the electromagnetic spectrum. Therefore, the B_1 field needed to cause resonance is frequently referred to as a radio-frequency field.

Since the Larmor frequency is dependent on the magnetogyric ratio (see equation 2), different nuclear species (e.g., ^1H and ^{31}P) require radio-frequency fields of different frequencies to achieve resonance when placed in the same B_0 field. For example, in a B_0 field of 1.0 tesla, the ^1H resonance frequency is 42.57 MHz whereas that of ^{31}P is 17.23 MHz. This provides a means of studying a particular nucleus (either ^1H or ^{31}P, for example) without undue interference from other nuclear species.

Fundamentally, an NMR experiment involves the measurement of the Larmor frequency by detecting the resonance condition. The most common method of detecting NMR resonance is that of nuclear induction, in which the resonance condition is indicated by a sharp increase in voltage induced in a receiver coil. A simple experimental procedure for determining the Larmor frequency of an ensemble of nuclei placed in a magnetic field is to subject the sample to a rotating B_1 field of continuously changing frequency—that is, to sweep B_1 from one frequency to another. If the Larmor frequency of the nuclei falls within the scanned frequency range, it will be indicated by the voltage signal induced in the receiver coil. The result of this experiment is generally shown as a plot of signal strength versus frequency, and such a presentation is referred to as the NMR spectrum. The particular experimental method described above is referred to as the continuous-wave method. However, the pulse method described in the next section offers several advantages over the continuous-wave method and therefore is predominantly used.

In the case of a sample of water, the NMR spectrum due to ^1H consists of a single peak at the resonance frequency of hydrogen nuclei. More often the NMR spectra of other substances consist of several peaks within a narrow range of frequencies. For example, the ^1H NMR spectrum of ethanol consists of at least three different peaks (or more, depending on the resolution of the instrument used) as shown in Figure 38–4. The molecular structure of ethanol shows three groups of hydrogen nuclei in different chemical environments. Due to the variation in electron density, nuclei in different chemical environments experience slightly different magnetic fields compared to B_0. The differences in the field caused by the changes in electron density are extremely small compared to the value of B_0. Since the Larmor frequency is proportional to the local magnetic field experienced by the nuclei, nuclei in different environments have different resonance frequencies. This phenomenon is called the chemical shift effect. Large organic molecules (e.g., enzymes, proteins) contain a large number of ^1H nuclei in slightly different environ-

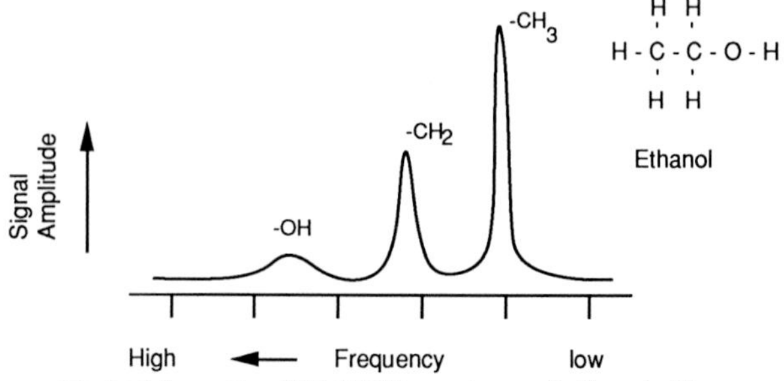

Figure 38–4. Schematic of ^1H NMR spectrum of ethanol. The group of ^1H nuclei corresponding to each signal is also shown.

ments and thus give rise to ^1H NMR spectra of great complexity. However, the ^1H NMR spectrum of a human arm shows only two predominant peaks: one due to ^1H in mobile water in tissue and the other due to ^1H nuclei in lipids.

The differences in resonance frequencies exhibited in an NMR spectrum (chemical shift frequencies) provide information about the molecular structure or, in the case of a sample mixture, about the chemical composition of the mixture. Therefore, it is the relative differences between the resonance frequencies that are of interest and not the absolute values of resonance frequencies in megahertz. Furthermore, the relative differences between resonance frequencies are dependent on the magnitude of B_0 used. Therefore the horizontal axis of the spectrum is usually expressed as a relative scale in dimensionless units of parts per million (ppm) with respect to the resonance frequency of a chosen reference compound. Another important feature of the NMR spectrum is that the intensities of the peaks, as measured from their areas, are proportional to the number of nuclei that contribute to them. However, the signal intensities can be altered by factors such as spin-lattice and spin-spin relaxation times (see Relaxation), depending on the experimental conditions.

PULSE FOURIER TRANSFORM NUCLEAR MAGNETIC RESONANCE

In the pulse Fourier transform NMR technique, the B_1 radio-frequency field is applied as a short burst (a radio-frequency pulse) typically of 20 to 100 μsec or longer, depending on the type of experiment being performed. Application of the radio-frequency pulse disturbs the equilibrium population distribution of the nuclei and hence creates an excited state. Following the radio-frequency pulse, the nuclei return to the equilibrium state (relaxation) in a time determined by the spin-lattice relaxation time. During the relaxation period, a voltage signal is induced in a receiver coil. This initial NMR signal, obtained in the form of a curve of voltage versus time, is subsequently subjected to frequency conversion, sampling (digitization), and mathematical analysis (Fourier transform) to produce the NMR spectrum. Thus the simplest pulse NMR experiment is composed of two separate time periods, excitation and then detection (Fig. 38–5).

Semiclassical Vector Description

The events during a pulse Fourier transform experiment can be most easily comprehended by considering the net macroscopic magnetization rather than its individual components, using the vector model described below.

As described previously, an ensemble of I = 1/2 nuclei placed in an external magnetic field B_0, at equilibrium, is distributed between two orientations with a slight excess of nuclei in the parallel orientation. This is depicted in Figure 38–6*A*, where the direction of B_0 is taken to define the z axis of the xyz Cartesian coordinate system and the arrows represent the magnetic moment vectors μ of the individual nuclei. The nuclei in the two orientations are shown distributed randomly over the surface of the double cone traced out by the precession of magnetic moment

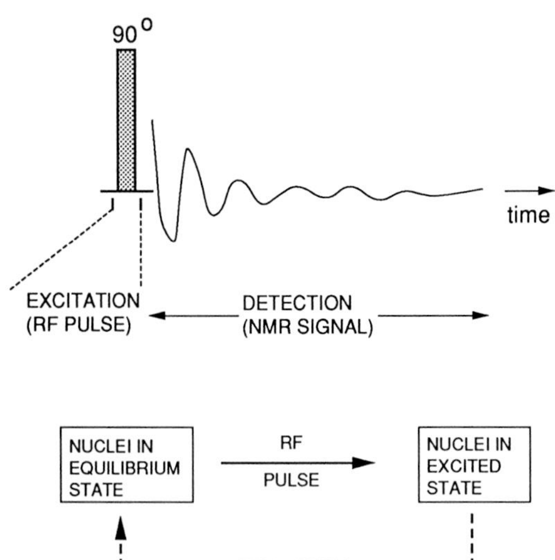

Figure 38–5. Illustration of separate time periods and the state of the nuclei during a pulse nuclear magnetic resonance experiment.

vectors, since there is no preferred direction in the transverse xy plane (the plane perpendicular to B_0). The net effect of the individual moments aligned as such is equivalent to having a single magnetic moment oriented along the B_0 direction (z axis). This resultant moment (Fig. 38–6*B*), referred to as the equilibrium magnetization, M_0, is a macroscopic property of the sample, and its magnitude is determined by the excess of population in the parallel orientation. It can be shown that this net magnetization behaves similarly to individual magnetic moments; that is, if displaced from its equilibrium position along B_0, it precesses about the B_0 axis at the Larmor frequency. As will be discussed shortly, the net magnetization is responsible for the observed NMR signal, so any perturbation that increases or decreases the population difference of nuclei between the orientations directly influences the magnitude of the observed signal.

Application of a radio-frequency pulse, a rotating B_1 magnetic field perpendicular to B_0, exerts a torque on M_0 and causes it to be displaced from the z axis towards the xy plane (Fig. 38–7). The effect of B_1 on the magnetization is dependent on the frequency difference ($\Delta\nu$) between the rotation of B_1 and the Larmor frequency and is greatest when $\Delta\nu$ is zero (on-resonance condition). The effect of B_1 decreases as $\Delta\nu$ increases, and at

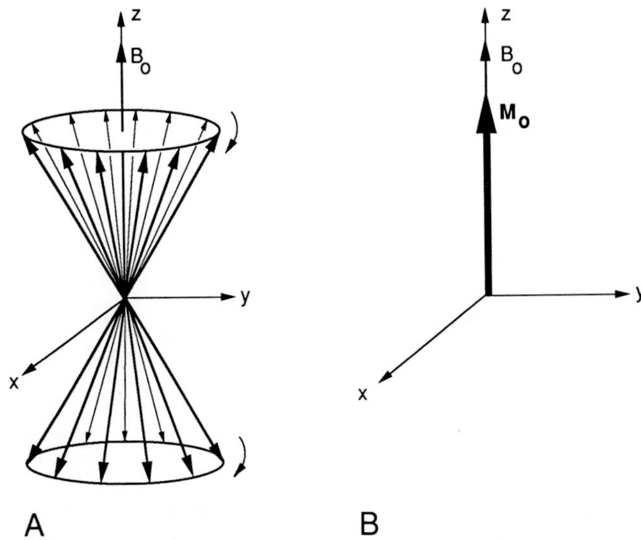

Figure 38–6. (*A*) Precession of individual magnetic vectors about B_0 at equilibrium. (*B*) Resultant equilibrium magnetization M_0.

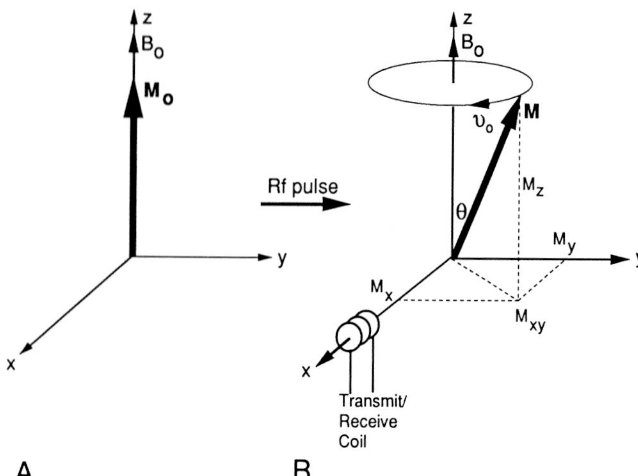

Figure 38–7. Creation of nonequilibrium magnetization M by application of a radio-frequency pulse to the equilibrium magnetization M_0 *(A)*. Possible orientation of M immediately after the pulse is shown in *(B)*. Following the pulse, M precesses at the Larmor frequency ν_0 in the stationary *xyz* frame. Orientation of a solenoidal coil that could be used to produce the required B_1 field as well as to receive the signal is also indicated.

sufficiently large values of $\Delta\nu$, B_1 has no effect on the magnetization. The angle of displacement of the magnetization from the *z* axis (flip angle, Θ) depends on the strength of the B_1 field and its duration (t_p) according to

$$\Theta = \gamma B_1 t_p \tag{6}$$

Equation (6) is appropriate for magnetization on-resonance. In general, a radio-frequency pulse that affords a flip angle of Θ for the on-resonance magnetization is called a Θ pulse. For example, a radio-frequency pulse of appropriate amplitude B_1 and duration t_p that causes the magnetization to be displaced by 90 degrees from the *z* axis is referred to as a 90-degree pulse.

Once displaced from the *z* axis by the radio-frequency pulse, the net magnetization is no longer at equilibrium. In the discussion to follow, this nonequilibrium magnetization vector will be denoted by M and the magnitudes of its components along the *x*, *y*, and *z* axes will be denoted by M_x, M_y, and M_z, respectively. The magnitude of the component of M in the transverse *xy* plane (i.e., the resultant of M_x and M_y) will be denoted by M_{xy} (Fig. 38–7*B*). The equilibrium magnetization M_0 represents the situation in which M is aligned along the *z* axis corresponding to the case of $M_z = M_0$ and $M_{xy} = M_x = M_y = 0$.

During the period following the pulse, M experiences a torque due to the B_0 field and thus precesses about the B_0 field at the Larmor frequency. The effect of the precessing magnetization is similar to that of a rotating bar magnet and hence is equivalent to producing a periodically changing magnetic field in the transverse plane. Now, if the sample being investigated is surrounded by a suitably oriented coil of wire, an alternating voltage will be induced in the coil according to Faraday's law of induction. The coil used to receive the signal can be the same as or different from that used to produce the B_1 field.

In terms of the components of M, precession of M corresponds to reorientation of M_{xy} in the *xy* plane at a rate equal to the Larmor frequency while M_z is unchanged. This translates to the fact that M_x and M_y are oscillatory with time at a frequency equal to the Larmor frequency.

It can be shown that the amplitude of the alternating voltage induced in the receiver coil is proportional to the transverse magnetization component M_{xy} created by the radio-frequency pulse. Hence a maximum-amplitude voltage signal is obtained following a 90-degree pulse, since such a pulse creates maximum M_{xy} component equal to M_0. In general, for radio-frequency pulse of flip angle Θ, the amplitude of the alternating voltage is proportional to $M_0 \sin \Theta$. The frequency of the induced alternating voltage is equal to the Larmor frequency, that is, the rate of reorientation of M_{xy}. Closer examination reveals that the voltage induced in the receiver coil at any instant is proportional to the transverse magnetization component perpendicular to the coil axis; if the coil (e.g., a solenoid) axis is along the *x* axis, the voltage induced follows the time dependence of M_y (Fig. 38–7). To reiterate, reorientation of the transverse magnetization M_{xy} is solely responsible for the NMR signal induced in the receiver coil.

As a result of relaxation, M_{xy} (i.e., the amplitudes of oscillation of M_x and M_y) decays to zero exponentially with time constant T_2, the spin-spin relaxation time (see Relaxation). Thus the voltage signal observed in practice corresponds to an oscillating signal at the Larmor frequency with exponentially decaying (time constant T_2) signal amplitude. It should be noted that such a signal is observed only when a single group of equivalent nuclei are studied in a uniform magnetic field. In practice, nonuniformity of the magnetic field causes the signal to decay faster than the rate dictated by T_2.

Free Induction Decay and the Fourier Transform

The NMR signal induced in the receiver coil is extremely weak and has a frequency in the radio-frequency range (radio-frequency signal). Very high frequency signal information cannot easily be stored in a computer, and direct amplification of the same to the required level without introducing distortions is a difficult task. Therefore, following low-level amplification of the initial NMR signal at the Larmor frequency, it is converted to a low-frequency signal by subtracting a frequency component equal to the frequency of a chosen reference signal (radio-frequency detection). The frequency of the reference signal is commonly chosen to be equal to that of B_1, and thus the low-frequency signal following radio-frequency detection has a frequency of $\Delta\nu$ in the hertz-kilohertz range (audio signal) (Fig. 38–8). This signal is amplified again to the required level. The audio signal contains all the information (which was previously present in the radio-frequency signal) required to generate the NMR spectrum.

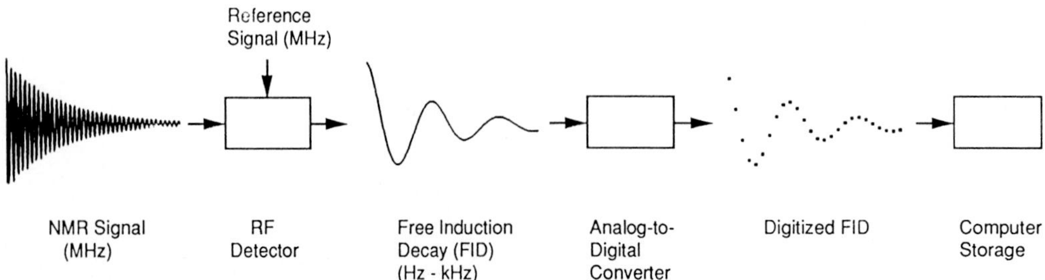

Figure 38–8. Block diagram of the NMR signal detection and storage scheme (signal amplification stages are not shown). Here the NMR signal is shown to be detected with respect to a single reference frequency (single-phase detection). The frequency of the reference signal is generally set equal to the frequency of B_1. More commonly, the NMR signal is detected with respect to two reference signals of the same frequency but 90 degrees out of phase (quadrature phase detection).

The initial radio-frequency signal is called a free induction decay (FID) because it was induced in the receiver coil during a period free of any external influences (e.g., radio-frequency pulses) and because of its decaying nature. However, the term FID is also used to refer to the audio signal that is derived from the radio-frequency signal. In this discussion, the term FID will refer exclusively to the audio signal.

It is clear that the frequency of the observed FID depends on the frequency of B_1 used to create the nonequilibrium magnetization. If a B_1 frequency exactly equal to the Larmor frequency is used (on-resonance condition, $\Delta\nu = 0$), the FID will represent a continuously decaying signal. Otherwise, an alternating and exponentially decaying signal of frequency $\Delta\nu$ will be observed as the FID.

Like the initial radio-frequency signal, the FID represents a continuously varying voltage with time (analog signal). In order to store this information in a computer, the analog FID signal is sampled at specific times (analog-to-digital conversion) and an array of numbers representing the sampled voltages are stored in the computer memory (Fig. 38–8). The process of analog signal sampling must be performed in accordance with the Nyquist sampling theorem (see Chapter 39) to ensure that the analog signal is correctly represented in digital form. The time duration in which the FID is sampled is referred to as the acquisition or read-out time.

In the discussion so far, a single group of equivalent nuclei has been considered. In such a situation (e.g., ^1H in a water sample), the FID represents a simple decaying oscillation at a particular frequency. This frequency can be determined simply by measuring the period of the oscillation, T_p, and calculating the value of $1/T_p$. However, if the sample being examined contains different chemical shift frequencies, the observed FID represents the composite of several individual FID signals with slightly different frequencies. In this case, the FID is too complicated for simple analysis. The individual frequency components of any FID are most conveniently identified by subjecting the FID to Fourier transformation.

Fourier transformation is a general mathematical process. In the analysis of time-dependent signals, it provides the link between the time and frequency variables. Data collected as a function of time (i.e., the time domain signals, such as FID) can be converted to a function of frequency (i.e., the frequency domain, such as the NMR spectrum) by Fourier transformation of the time domain data. Further, the data in the frequency domain can be converted to the time domain by inverse Fourier transformation.

The Fourier relationship between the FID and the NMR spectrum is shown in Figure 38–9. It should be noted that all the characteristics of the FID are represented in the spectrum, but now in a different format. The frequency of oscillation of the FID is indicated by the horizontal scale of the spectrum. The rate of decay of the FID is inversely related to the width of the spectral line at its half-maximum. Further, the height (amplitude) of the spectral line is directly proportional to initial amplitude of the FID and, more precisely, can be shown to be equal to the area under the FID envelope. Hence a more slowly decaying FID gives rise to a narrower and higher-amplitude spectral line.

The Fourier transform can be efficiently computed by a digital computer if the time domain function is represented by N discrete data points, with N being a power of 2. Thus, the analog FID signal is digitized appropriately and the data are subjected to Fourier transformation to obtain the NMR spectrum (Fig. 38–9).

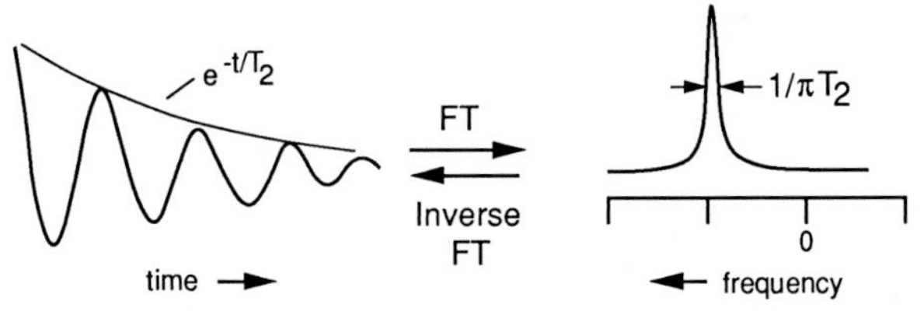

Figure 38–9. Fourier transform relationship between time domain and frequency domain data.

Signal-to-Noise Ratio and Signal Averaging

Noise is an integral part of any electrical or electronic system and represents the random fluctuations of the intended signal. The parameter known as the signal-to-noise ratio (the ratio of the amplitude of the signal to that of its random fluctuations) indicates the degree to which the desired signal can be distinguished from unwanted noise and hence is a measure of the quality of the signal received.

As mentioned previously, the maximum free induction signal is received following a 90-degree pulse. Hence, in a given experimental situation, the signal-to-noise ratio of the NMR spectrum can be maximized by using the appropriate radio-frequency pulse parameters (B_1 and t_p) so that a flip angle of 90 degrees is achieved.

However, the signal-to-noise ratio of an NMR spectrum generated by a single free induction decay can be inadequate. In such a situation, the simplest way to obtain a further improvement in the signal-to-noise ratio is by the procedure known as signal averaging. In this method, the pulse sequence is repeated several times and the resulting FID signals are summed to produce a single FID. If n FID signals are summed, the signal component of the FID increases by a factor of n while the noise amplitude increases only by a factor of $n^{1/2}$ due to its random nature. Thus, the signal-to-noise ratio of the FID obtained by summation of n individual signals will be increased by $n^{1/2}$. Fourier transformation of this summed FID produces a spectrum with a correspondingly higher signal-to-noise ratio than that produced by a single FID. It should be noted that the improvement so obtained is not without penalty. Acquisition of n FID signals increases the experimental time by a factor of n, since the experiment must be repeated n times. If the pulse repetition time is denoted by TR (i.e., TR is the time between successive radio-frequency pulses), the total experimental time needed to obtain a signal-to-noise enhancement by a factor of $n^{1/2}$ is given by $n \cdot TR$. When signal averaging, the signal-to-noise ratio obtained in given total experimental time can be maximized by using radio-frequency pulses with flip angles less than 90 degrees. The optimum flip angle, Θ_{opt} (Ernst angle), to be used is determined by the spin-lattice relaxation time T_1 and the pulse repetition time TR according to $\cos \Theta_{opt} = \exp(-TR/T_1)$.

Relaxation

Following the perturbation by the radio-frequency pulse, the spin system returns to the equilibrium population distribution between the energy levels by releasing excess energy into the surroundings. In the classical vector model, this corresponds to the return of the nonequilibrium magnetization M to the equilibrium position along the *z* axis. Thus, during the relaxation period, any transverse magnetization component (M_{xy}) created by the radio-frequency pulse decays to zero, and at the same time the longitudinal magnetization component (M_z) recovers to the equilibrium value of M_0. The decay of M_{xy} and the recovery of M_z are two distinct processes, and they are referred to as spin-spin and spin-lattice relaxation, respectively. Both relaxation processes are generally first-order (i.e., exponential) processes, with respective time constants.

Molecules in solution are in random translational and rotational motion due to their thermal energy. As a result of this random motion, the magnetic nuclei in molecules experience fluctuating local magnetic fields. The microscopic fluctuating fields experienced by a particular nucleus can originate from several sources, the most important being the presence of other magnetic nuclei in close proximity. Any fluctuating magnetic field with a component in the *xy* plane that oscillates at the Larmor frequency is

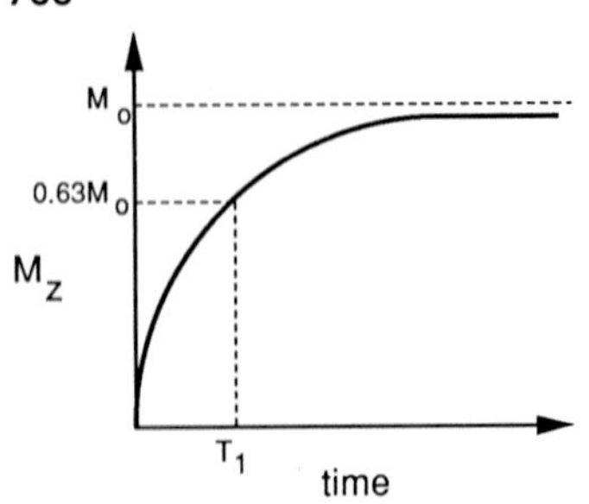

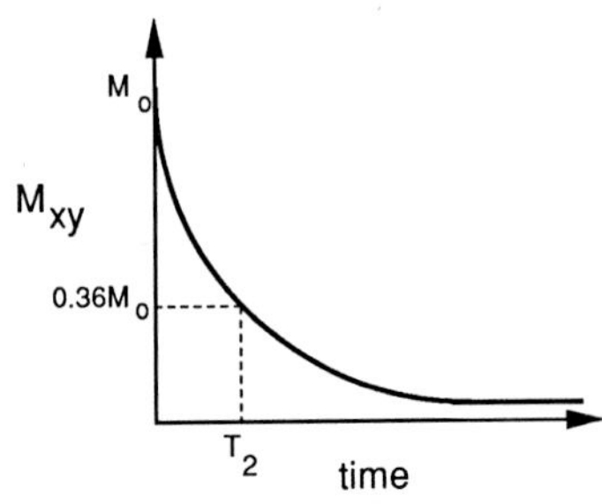

Figure 38–10. *(A)* Exponential growth of longitudinal magnetization and *(B)* exponential decay of transverse magnetization following a 90-degree pulse.

able to induce transitions between the spin states of the nuclei. This is analogous to the effects of an oscillating B_1 field discussed earlier. These transitions, which are stimulated by molecular motion, are responsible for restoring the equilibrium population distribution during the relaxation period. More detailed accounts on relaxation processes can be found in the cited texts.

The growth of longitudinal magnetization following a 90-degree pulse due to spin-lattice relaxation is described by

$$M_z = M_0[1 - \exp(-t/T_1)] \qquad (7)$$

where M_z is the magnitude of longitudinal magnetization at time t following the pulse (Fig. 38–10*A*). The time constant T_1 of this recovery curve, referred to as the spin-lattice relaxation time, represents the time interval needed for the longitudinal magnetization to recover to a value of 63.2 percent of the equilibrium value M_0. From equation (7), it can be deduced that the recovery of M_z to 99.3 percent of its final value M_0 requires a time equal to $5T_1$.

If several FID signals are collected by repetitive application of radio-frequency pulses (for signal-to-noise improvement or otherwise), T_1 determines the pulse repetition rate that should be used in order to obtain the maximum signal. For a series of 90-degree pulses applied to magnetization at equilibrium, if the pulse repetition time (TR) is greater than $5T_1$, each FID will be of maximum possible initial amplitude proportional to M_0, since the magnetization would recover almost to the equilibrium value between the pulses. If $TR < 5T_1$, the amplitude of the first FID will still be proportional to M_0, while the second and successive FID signals will be of reduced amplitude proportional to $M_0[1 - \exp(-TR/T_1)]$.

The decay of the transverse magnetization following a 90-degree pulse due to spin-spin relaxation is described by

$$M_{xy} = M_0 \exp(-t/T_2) \qquad (8)$$

where M_{xy} is the magnitude of the transverse magnetization at time t following the pulse (Fig. 38–10*B*). The time constant T_2, called the spin-spin relaxation time, represents the time interval required for the transverse magnetization to decay to 36.7 percent of its initial value.

Since T_2 determines the decay rate of M_{xy}, it also determines the rate of decay of the FID when the whole sample experiences a uniform B_0 field, that is, a homogeneous field. Thus, the half-height line width of the NMR spectrum obtained in a homogeneous field is a measure of T_2 (see Fig. 38–9). However, in practice, the B_0 field is inhomogeneous; that is, the magnetic fields at different spatial locations within the magnet are slightly above or below the nominal value B_0 to different extents. This causes the nuclei in different regions of the sample to experience slightly different magnetic fields and hence to precess at different Larmor frequencies. The FID obtained in such a field is seen to decay faster (time constant T_2^*) than that determined by T_2 ($T_2^* < T_2$). Consequently, the spectral line width obtained is broader and related to T_2^* rather than T_2.

As commented earlier, the relaxation times T_1 and T_2 are determined by the molecular environment and thus are dependent on the sample. If the sample contains chemically shifted resonances, the nuclei in different chemical environments exhibit T_1 and T_2 values characteristic of the particular environment. Knowledge of T_1 and T_2 values is obtained experimentally by perturbing the equilibrium magnetization in an appropriate manner (see Multipulse Nuclear Magnetic Resonance). For pure liquids $T_1 = T_2$, and for biological samples $T_2 < T_1$. Molecules in a mobile liquid environment have T_1 and T_2 values in the range of tens to hundreds of milliseconds. In the solid state, T_2 values become very short (less than 1 msec) and T_1 values can become very long (greater than 1 minute). Therefore, signals from molecules in the solid state decay very rapidly and are not generally observed unless solid-state NMR techniques are used.

Rotating-Frame Concept

In the analysis of NMR experiments, the rotating-frame concept is frequently used to simplify the motion of the magnetization in the presence of a B_1 field. In order to introduce this concept, consider the trajectory of M as it is nutated away from the *z* axis by the B_1 field. In the presence of the B_1 field (during the radio-frequency pulse), M experiences two magnetic fields: the static B_0 field and the rotating B_1 field perpendicular to B_0. Under the influence of the torques exerted by these fields, the motion of M corresponds to a simultaneous precession about two orthogonal directions (one static and the other rotating) with respective precessional frequencies depending on the strength of each field. For a magnetization on-resonance ($\Delta\nu = 0$) with the B_1 field, the motion M during the pulse is shown in Figure 38–11. However, the motion of an off-resonance ($\Delta\nu \neq 0$) magnetization is more complicated.

The complex motion of M as seen in the *xyz* stationary frame can be simplified by viewing its motion in a frame that rotates

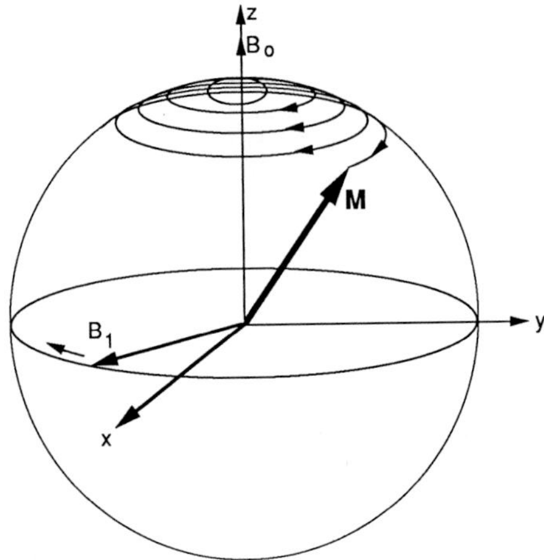

Figure 38–11. Motion of on-resonance M under the influence of B_0 and rotating B_1 fields as viewed in the *xyz* stationary frame. The position of the magnetization, assumed initially to be at equilibrium, is shown after an arbitrary time period.

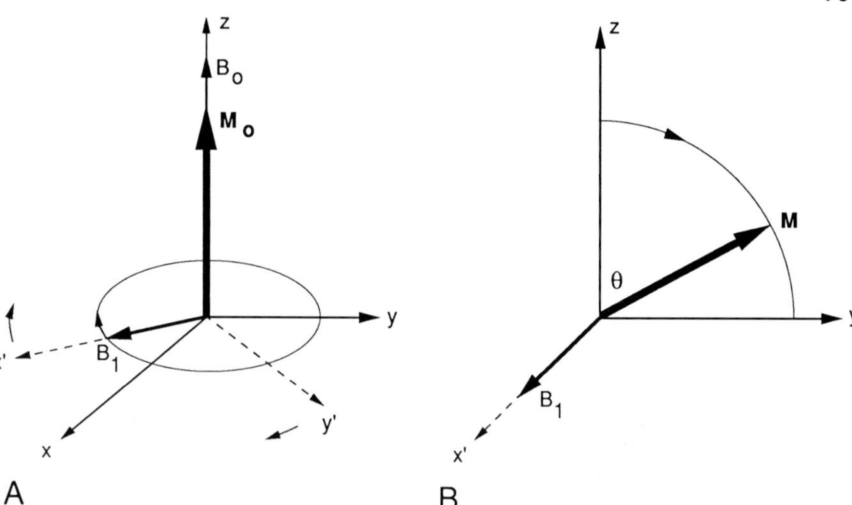

Figure 38–12. *(A)* The *xyz* stationary frame view of the x' and y' axes that rotates synchronously with the B_1 field. The rotating axes have been chosen so that B_1 lies along the x' axis. *(B)* $x'y'z$ rotating frame view of the motion of on-resonance M in the presence of B_1.

synchronously with the B_1 field. Such a frame of reference is referred to as a rotating reference frame, and its axes will be denoted by $x'y'z$ (Fig. 38–12*A*). In relation to the *xyz* stationary coordinate frame, the x' and y' axes rotate at a frequency equal to that of B_1, and the *z* coordinate is common to both frames of reference.

When viewed from the rotating reference frame, the B_1 field appears static, and the motion of an on-resonance magnetization is seen as a simple precession about B_1 (Fig. 38–12*B*). The angle of precession (flip angle) is given by equation (6). If the rotating-frame axes are chosen so that B_1 lies along the x' axis, the motion of on-resonance magnetization is then in the zy' plane, and following a 90-degree pulse M will be aligned along the y' axis. In retrospect, it can be stated that, when viewed in the rotating frame, the effect of B_0 is nullified for the on-resonance magnetization.

When considering an off-resonance magnetization in the rotating frame (Fig. 38–13), the effect of B_0 is not completely canceled, and hence a residual static field along the *z* axis, ΔB, also must be taken into account; for the on-resonance case discussed earlier, ΔB is zero. ΔB is determined by Δν according to $\gamma\ \Delta B = 2\pi\ \Delta\nu$. Therefore, when $\Delta\nu \neq 0$, the motion of M in the rotating frame is governed by two static fields (B_1 and ΔB) perpendicular to each other. The direction of the effective resultant field (B_{1eff}) of B_1 and ΔB, which lies in the zx' plane, defines the axis of precession, and the angle α between the direction of B_{1eff} and the x' axis is given by $\tan \alpha = \Delta B/B_1$ (see Fig. 38–13). The effective flip angle Θ_{eff} for an off-resonance magnetization is given by $\Theta_{eff} = \gamma B_{1eff} t_p$, where $B_{1eff} = [B_1^2 + (\Delta B)^2]^{1/2}$.

As mentioned previously, once the radio-frequency pulse is terminated, M precesses about B_0 at the Larmor frequency when viewed from the *xyz* stationary frame. In the rotating frame, this precession appears to be of frequency Δν, that is, proportional to the residual field ΔB (Fig. 38–14). For the on-resonance case, M would appear to be stationary in the rotating frame since Δν is zero.

In summary, in the rotating-frame view for the case of a 90-degree pulse applied to a magnetization close to the on-resonance condition, the excitation and detection periods correspond to precession of M in nearly orthogonal planes in the two successive time periods—that is, precession in a plane near the zy' plane (excitation period) followed by precession in the $x'y'$ plane (detection period).

In an earlier section, precession of M in the *xyz* stationary frame was described by the time evolution of the components of M along the *x*, *y*, and *z* axes. Similarly, precession of M when viewed in the rotating frame can be described by the time variation of the components of M along the rotating-frame axes. In the discussions to follow, the components of M along the rotating-frame axes x' and y' will be denoted by $M_{x'}$ and $M_{y'}$, respectively, and the net component in the transverse $x'y'$ plane (the resultant of $M_{x'}$ and $M_{y'}$) will be denoted as $M_{x'y'}$ (Fig. 38–14). Precession of M in the rotating frame corresponds to reorientation of $M_{x'y'}$ in the $x'y'$ plane or, equivalently, to oscillation of $M_{x'}$ and $M_{y'}$ at a frequency of Δν. In a homogeneous B_0 field, $M_{x'y'}$ (i.e., amplitudes of oscillations of $M_{x'}$ and $M_{y'}$) decay exponentially with a time constant T_2.

The orientation of $M_{x'y'}$ in the transverse plane at a particular instant is also an important consideration in many situations. The orientation of $M_{x'y'}$ can be specified by the angle ϕ (see Fig. 38–

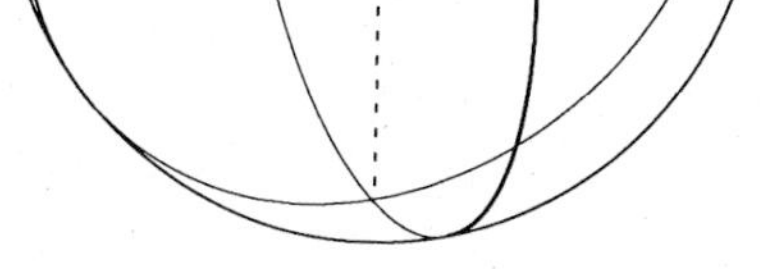

Figure 38–13. Trajectory of off-resonance M in the rotating frame (line *za*) during a radio-frequency pulse. Direction of B_{1eff} represents the axis of the trajectory *za*.

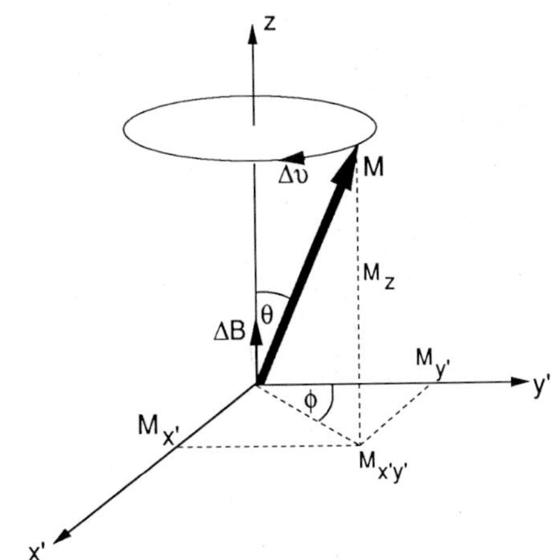

Figure 38–14. Precession of M following a Θ pulse as viewed in the rotating frame. The precessional frequency is equal to Δν. An on-resonance magnetization will appear to be stationary, since $\Delta\nu = 0$. The direction of precession depends on whether Δν is positive or negative.

14) between the direction of $M_{x'y'}$ and a chosen reference axis (e.g., y' axis). The angular position (ϕ) of $M_{x'y'}$, referred to as the phase angle, is related to $M_{x'}$ and $M_{y'}$ components via $\tan \phi = M_{x'}/M_{y'}$. The continuous change of direction of $M_{x'y'}$ implies that its phase angle is time dependent, and the frequency of reorientation of $M_{x'y'}$ corresponds to the rate at which the phase angle is varied. Hence the phase angle of $M_{x'y'}$ at any instant t is given by the expression

$$\phi = 2\pi \Delta\nu t + \phi_0 \quad (9)$$

where ϕ_0 represents the phase angle at the chosen initial time (t = 0).

In addition to simplification of the motion of M, the utility of the rotating-frame concept is enhanced by the fact that it represents the frame of signal detection. The process of subtraction of the B_1 frequency component from the initial NMR signal to produce the free induction decay (see Free Induction Decay and the Fourier Transform) is conceptually equivalent to viewing the precessing magnetization following the pulse from a frame rotating at a frequency equal to that of B_1. This can be appreciated by noticing that the frequency of the FID and the frequency of precession of M in the rotating frame are both equal to $\Delta\nu$. Therefore, the FID represents the time evolution of M in the rotating frame, and it can be shown that the amplitude of the FID at any instant is directly proportional to the transverse components of the magnetization ($M_{x'}$ or $M_{y'}$) in the rotating frame. This result provides an easy mechanism by which the FID can be predicted and, as will become apparent, can be used in the analysis and design of more complicated NMR experiments.

In practice, two FID signals, one corresponding to $M_{x'}$ and the other corresponding to $M_{y'}$, can be detected (quadrature detection). Among other advantages, quadrature detection enables the sense of precession of the magnetization in the rotating frame to be determined; that is, whether the Larmor frequency is greater or less than the B_1 frequency can be ascertained by quadrature detection of the FID.

The initial amplitudes of the FID signals corresponding to $M_{x'}$ and $M_{y'}$ contain information on the initial phase angle ϕ_0 of the magnetization. This information is preserved during Fourier transformation of the FID and is present in the NMR spectrum in a more subtle form. Exploitation of the phase information is best demonstrated in NMR imaging experiments (see Chapter 39) and other two-dimensional NMR techniques.

As mentioned previously, the NMR spectrum of a sample can consist of several chemical shift frequencies. In this case, the magnetization corresponding to each chemical shift frequency can be considered separately and the off-resonance frequency $\Delta\nu$ for each magnetization will be different. In order to obtain an undistorted spectrum, upon application of a 90-degree radiofrequency pulse it is necessary that all chemically shifted magnetizations be excited (rotated to the transverse plane) so that they all lie close to the y' axis of the rotating frame at the end of the pulse. Figure 38–13 indicates that the trajectory of a magnetization is dependent on the direction of B_{1eff} and hence the relative magnitudes of B_1 and ΔB. If the applied pulse is such that $B_1 >> \Delta B$, then $B_{1eff} \simeq B_1$, and the direction of B_{1eff} lies essentially along the x' axis. Therefore, if a strong pulse is used (i.e., a large B_1), then the effect of the off-resonance field ΔB can be neglected. In such a situation all the chemically shifted magnetization will precess about the x' axis during the pulse and, following a 90-degree rotation, will be aligned along the y' axis. Use of a strong radio-frequency pulse requires the duration for which it is applied, t_p, to be reduced accordingly to maintain a flip angle of 90 degrees (see equation 6). Therefore, uniform excitation of magnetization within a broad range of Larmor frequencies requires a short and intense radio-frequency pulse. Such pulses are commonly referred to as nonselective pulses. On the other hand, a pulse with opposite characteristics, a long weak pulse, is able to excite predominantly magnetization within a narrow range of frequency while the magnetization outside this range is unaffected. Pulses of this nature, called selective pulses, are utilized for slice selection in magnetic resonance imaging.

MULTIPULSE NUCLEAR MAGNETIC RESONANCE

Previous sections concentrated on the effects of a single radiofrequency pulse and subsequent detection of the free induction decay (one-pulse experiment). In this section effects of multiple pulses on the magnetization are examined. Interrogation of the nuclear spin system with multiple pulses provides information that is not accessible via a one-pulse experiment. Simple multipulse experiments such as inversion-recovery and spin-echo sequences enable experimental determination of T_1 and T_2, respectively. Further, the spin-echo sequence forms the basis of the most widely used imaging method (see Chapter 39).

Inversion-Recovery Sequence

In the inversion-recovery sequence the equilibrium magnetization is initially perturbed by a 180-degree pulse. Following a short time period τ, a second perturbation is introduced in the form of a 90-degree pulse. This can be written as a 180°-τ-90°-FID sequence or indicated in a pulse sequence diagram as shown in Figure 38–15A.

In order to examine the effects of this pulse sequence, assume that the radio-frequency pulses (B_1) are applied along the x' axis of the rotating frame and are on-resonance. Prior to the 180-

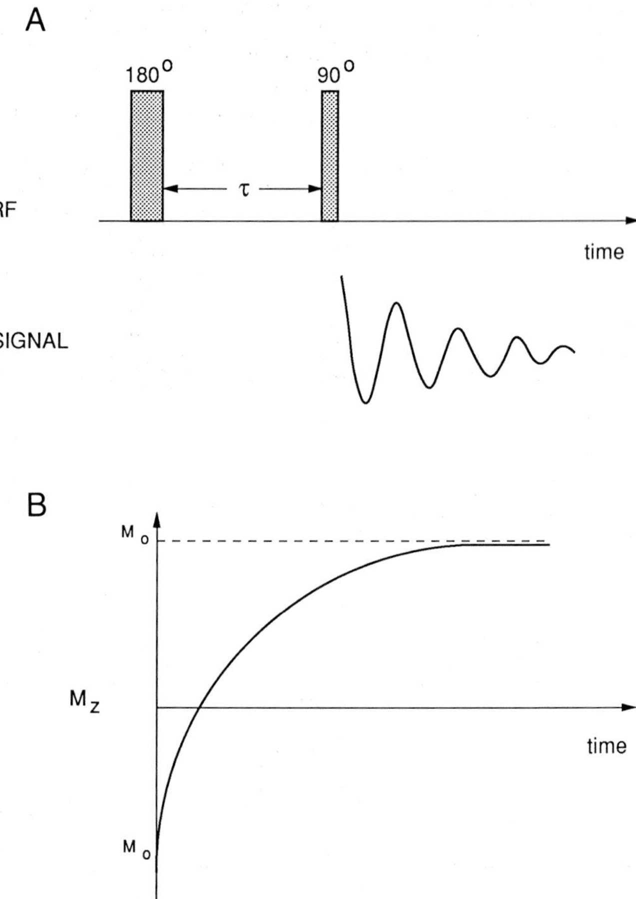

Figure 38–15. *(A)* Inversion-recovery pulse sequence diagram. Shaded areas represent the times at which radio-frequency pulses are applied. The flip angle afforded by each pulse is indicated in the diagram. Signal trace shows the time period during which the free induction decay is observed. *(B)* Exponential recovery of M_z following a 180-degree pulse.

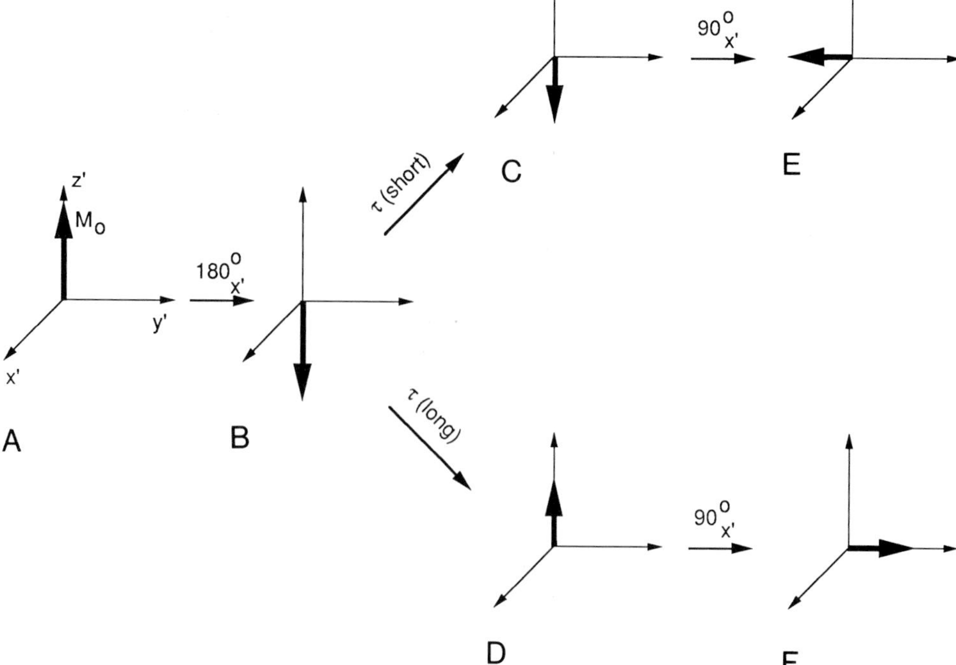

Figure 38–16. Rotating frame view of a magnetization subjected to an inversion-recovery sequence. *(A)* Magnetization at equilibrium. *(B)* Magnetization immediately following a $180°_{x'}$ inversion pulse. The subscript x' in $180°_{x'}$ indicates the orientation of the B_1 field in the rotating frame and thus the axis of rotation of the magnetization during the pulse. *(C and D)* Partially relaxed magnetization after different τ periods following the $180°_{x'}$ pulse. *(E and F)* Corresponding magnetization following a $90°_{x'}$ read pulse.

degree pulse, the magnetization is at equilibrium (Fig. 38–16*A*). The 180-degree pulse causes the magnetization to rotate by 180-degrees about the x' axis, and at the end of the pulse it will be oriented along the negative z axis (Fig. 38–16*B*). Since in this case the 180-degree pulse inverts the magnetization from positive z axis to negative z axis, it is sometimes referred to as an inversion pulse. During the period τ, magnetization relaxes exponentially to the equilibrium position at a rate determined by T_1 (see Fig. 38–15*B*). The magnitude of magnetization along the z axis (M_z) at a time τ after the 180-degree pulse is given by

$$M_z = M_0[1 - 2\exp(-\tau/T_1)] \qquad (10)$$

Hence, the magnetization present at the end of the period τ is dependent on the ratio τ/T_1. The magnetization following relatively short and long τ periods are shown in Figure 38–16*C* and *D*, respectively. During the period τ, the magnetization, though not at equilibrium, is completely oriented along the z axis (i.e., $M_{x'} = M_{y'} = 0$); hence an NMR signal cannot be observed during this delay.

Application of a 90-degree pulse causes the magnetization present at that time to rotate by 90 degrees about the x' axis. Thus, at the end of the 90-degree pulse, the magnetization will be directed along the negative y' axis or the positive y' axis, depending on the value chosen value for τ (Fig. 38–16*E* and *F*). In the subsequent time period, the transverse magnetization generated by the 90-degree pulse allows an FID to be observed. The initial amplitude of the FID will be proportional to M_z remaining at the end of the delay period τ. Consequently, the amplitude of the spectral peak produced by the Fourier transform of this FID will also be proportional to M_z. It is seen that the 90-degree pulse in this case is used to determine the M_z magnetization at a chosen time; a pulse that serves this purpose is sometimes referred to as a read pulse.

In order to obtain the T_1 value, this sequence is repeated with different τ values. The FID corresponding to each τ value is recorded and Fourier-transformed. For short τ values, M_z remains negative and an inverted peak is observed following the Fourier transform. For longer τ values the peak becomes increasingly positive. The peak heights obtained at different τ values represent the recovery of M_z following the 180-degree pulse. Therefore the value of T_1 can be obtained by fitting the experimental data (peak height versus τ) to the theoretical equation (equation 10). For accurate results it is necessary that the magnetization be allowed to recover completely between measurements. This is accomplished by waiting an adequate time ($\sim 5T_1$) after the acquisition of each FID before the next measurement is initiated.

Spin-Echo Sequence

The spin-echo pulse sequence consists of an initial 90-degree pulse followed by a 180-degree pulse after a period τ, that is, a 90°-τ-180°-echo sequence. The pulse sequence diagram is shown in Figure 38–17.

The rotating-frame view of an on-resonance magnetization subjected to this sequence is shown in Figure 38–18. The initial 90-degree pulse rotates the equilibrium magnetization by 90 degrees about the x' axis, creating transverse magnetization oriented along the y' axis (Fig. 38–18A). During the following

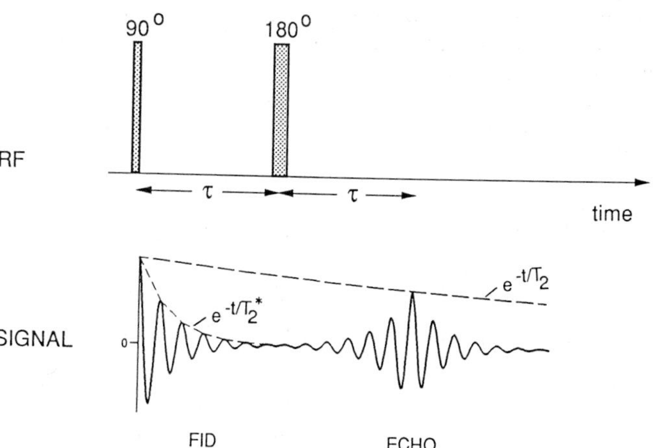

Figure 38–17. Spin-echo pulse sequence diagram. The maximum amplitude of the echo is governed only by the decay due to spin-spin relaxation. The decay of the free induction decay and the echo after its maximum is governed by the field inhomogeneity and spin-spin relaxation.

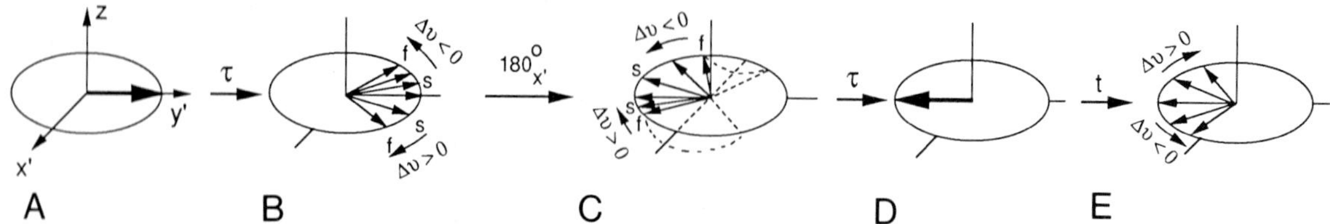

Figure 38–18. Rotating frame view of the magnetization subjected to a spin-echo sequence. *(A)* Magnetization immediately after the intial $90°_{x'}$ pulse. *(B)* Dephasing of isochromats following the $90°_{x'}$ pulse. f (for fast) and s (for slow) indicate the relative rates of precession of the isochromats. *(C)* Position of the isochromats immediately following a $180°_{x'}$ pulse. *(D)* Refocused magnetization after a period τ following $180°_{x'}$. *(E)* Dephasing of isochromats following the refocusing.

period τ, this transverse magnetization decays due to spin-spin relaxation and the inhomogeneity of the B_0 magnetic field. Decay due to spin-spin relaxation can be visualized simply as shortening of the length of the vector representing the magnetization during the period τ.

As mentioned previously, inhomogeneity of the field causes the nuclei in different regions of the sample to have different Larmor frequencies. To understand the effects of this in detail, consider the sample to be composed of a large number of extremely small regions within which the field inhomogeneity is negligible. Hence, the nuclei within any one of the small regions have the same Larmor frequency. The nuclear spin magnetization of a small region is called a spin isochromat. The net magnetization from the whole sample represents the sum of all individual isochromats. Because of the field inhomogeneity across the sample, the individual isochromats possess slightly different Larmor frequencies. This means that the isochromats are off-resonance from the B_1 field to different extents and hence will precess in the $x'y'$ plane at slightly different frequencies. Therefore, individual isochromats will be seen to fan out (dephase) in the $x'y'$ plane following the 90-degree pulse. The position of few isochromats at a time τ after the pulse is shown in Figure 38–18*B*. The isochromats are shown spread out on both sides of the y' axis, since the Larmor frequency of some isochromats will be greater than the nominal value ($\Delta\nu > 0$) while that of others will be lower ($\Delta\nu < 0$). Consequently, isochromats with $\Delta\nu$ greater and less than zero will be seen to precess in opposite directions in the rotating frame. At sufficiently long τ values, isochromats will be completely dephased in the $x'y'$ plane and the net transverse magnetization will be reduced to zero. Hence, in addition to spin-spin relaxation, inhomogeneity of the field contributes to the gradual reduction of net magnetization along the y' axis. However, the additional decay of the magnetization due to field inhomogeneity can be reversed by applying a 180-degree pulse.

Application of a 180-degree pulse at time τ following the initial 90-degree pulse causes all the isochromats (see Fig. 38–18*B*) to rotate by 180 degrees about the x' axis. This brings the isochromats to their mirror-image positions with reference to the x' axis, as shown in Figure 38–18*C*. Following the 180-degree pulse, the frequency and direction of precession of the isochromats in the $x'y'$ plane remain as prior to the 180-degree pulse, since the Larmor frequency of each isochromat is unchanged. Hence, immediately after the 180-degree pulse, the isochromats processing faster are seen to lag behind the slower ones (see Fig. 38–18*C*). Precession of isochromats for a period τ after the 180-degree pulse allows the faster isochromats to catch up (rephase) with the slower ones, and at this instant all the isochromats will be refocused along the negative y' axis (see Fig. 38–18*D*). Further precession of isochromats following refocusing causes them to dephase again in the $x'y'$ plane (see Fig. 38–18*E*). Therefore, following the 180-degree pulse, the net magnetization along the y' axis increases (in the negative direction) until a maximum is reached at time τ. After reaching the maximum, the magnetization decreases in a similar manner to the decay following the initial 90-degree pulse. The NMR signal obtained following the 180-degree pulse follows the same time dependence as the magnetization along the y' axis and is referred to as a spin-echo. The 180-degree pulse in this sequence is also referred to as a refocusing pulse because it serves to refocus the otherwise dephasing isochromats.

The importance of the spin-echo sequence lies in the fact that at the time all the isochromats are refocused, the contribution from the magnetic field inhomogeneity is completely eliminated. The net magnetization along the y' axis ($M_{y'}$) at this time is determined by the decay due to spin-spin relaxation only and is given by

$$M_{y'} = M_0 \exp(-2\tau/T_2) \qquad (11)$$

Hence, the maximum amplitude of the echo and the amplitude of the spectral peak produced by Fourier transformation of the echo will be proportional to $M_{y'}$ given by equation (11). Note that the echo signal can be regarded as two back-to-back FID signals, and either the whole echo or one-half of it (usually the second half) can be acquired and Fourier-transformed to produce the spectrum. Equation 11 is applicable when the effect of molecular diffusion is negligible. For complete refocusing of isochromats, each nucleus must experience the same field during period 2τ. Movement of nuclei in an inhomogeneous field due to diffusion causes the echo amplitude to be reduced.

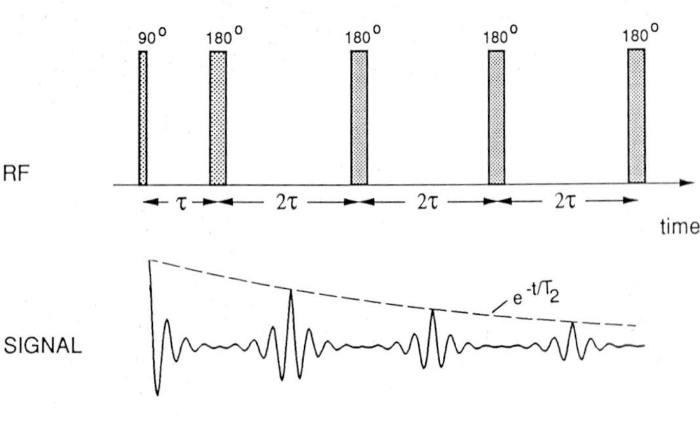

Figure 38–19. The Carr-Purcell pulse sequence. The maximum echo amplitude decay due only to spin-spin relaxation.

An important modification of the spin-echo experiment is the Carr-Purcell sequence. In this method the initial 90-degree pulse is followed by a series of 180-degree pulses separated by a time delay 2τ, where τ is the time between the 90-degree pulse and the first 180-degree pulse (Fig. 38–19). It can easily be seen that successive 180-degree pulses serve to create additional spin-echoes by repeated refocusing of the isochromats. The maximum amplitudes of the echoes are influenced only by spin-spin relaxation and decay at the rate determined by T_2. Hence the maximum amplitude of the nth echo is proportional to $\exp(-t_n/T_2)$, where t_n is the total time between the initial 90-degree pulse and the time at which the nth echo becomes a maximum.

The basic spin-echo sequence of Figure 38–17 can be employed to determine the T_2 value by repeating the sequence with different τ values. The echo signal corresponding to each τ value is recorded and Fourier-transformed, and the experimental data (peak height versus τ) are fitted to equation (11) to obtain the T_2 value. However, more accurate results can be obtained by employing a modified Carr-Purcell sequence, details of which can be found in the texts cited.

CONCLUSION

In this chapter we have reviewed the basic principles of the NMR phenomenon. The NMR signals are generated by perturbing the equilibrium state of the nuclei placed in a magnetic field with radio-frequency pulses. The response of the spin system to the radio-frequency pulses is Fourier-transformed to produce the NMR spectrum.

It is hoped that the basic concepts discussed here will serve as a foundation for more advanced study of the subject. Utilization of basic NMR principles to obtain cross-sectional images is described in detail in the following chapter. An account of the use of NMR as a spectroscopic tool is given in Chapter 46 by Ösbakken.

Acknowledgments

We wish to thank Drs. P. D. Davis, V. Rajanayagam, and E. Kanal for their comments and criticism of the manuscript.

References

B

1. Bloch, F., Hansen, W. W., and Packard, M.: Nuclear induction. Phys. Rev. 69:127, 1946.
2. Bloch, F.: Nuclear induction. Phys. Rev. 70:460, 1946.

C

1. Chen, C.-N., and Hoult, D. I.: Biomedical Magnetic Resonance Technology. New York, Adam Hilger, 1989.

E

1. Ernst, R. R., and Anderson, W. A.: Application of Fourier transform spectroscopy to magnetic resonance. Rev. Sci. Instrum. 37:93, 1966.

F

1. Farrar, T. C., and Becker, E. D.: Pulse and Fourier Transform NMR. Academic Press, New York, 1971.
2. Farrar, T. C.: Introduction to Pulse NMR Spectroscopy. Madison, Wis., Farragut Press, 1989.

G

1. Gadian, D. G.: Nuclear Magnetic Resonance and Its Applications to Living Systems. Oxford University Press, New York, 1982.

H

1. Hoult, D. I.: The magnetic resonance myth of radio waves. Concepts Magn. Reson. 1:1, 1989.

M

1. Martin, M. L., Deulpuech, J.-J., and Martin, G. J.: Practical NMR Spectroscopy. Heyden and Son, Philadelphia, 1980.

P

1. Purcell, E. M., Torrey, H. C., and Pound, R. V.: Resonance absorption by nuclear magnetic moments in a solid. Phys. Rev. 69:37, 1946.

S

1. Shaw, D.: Fourier Transform NMR Spectroscopy, 2nd ed. Elsevier, New York, 1984.

Chapter 39

Principles of Magnetic Resonance Imaging

■ S. L. TALAGALA, Ph.D. ■ G. L. WOLF, Ph.D., M.D.

LINEAR MAGNETIC FIELD GRADIENTS 744
Characteristics and Production 744
Nuclear Magnetic Resonance Projections 745
Evolution of Magnetization in Field Gradients .. 746
SLICE SELECTION 748
IMAGE FORMATION IN TWO DIMENSIONS 750
Concepts of Spin-Warp Imaging 750
Practical Aspects of Spin-Warp Imaging 752
Image Parameters 753
Multislice Imaging 754
RAPID IMAGING TECHNIQUES 754
CONCLUSION 757

As with any other imaging modality, the goal of magnetic resonance imaging (MRI) is to generate a map of a heterogeneous object showing its three-dimensional structure. To this end, MRI exploits the spatial variation of the nuclear magnetic resonance (NMR) signal intensity in the sample of interest. In the medical context, use of the word nuclear is avoided for better public acceptance.

As a simple illustration of how NMR could be used as an imaging method, consider the task of generating a cross-sectional image of two tubes of water. A straightforward approach to attaining this objective is to first obtain the ^{1}H NMR spectrum from a small group of nuclei (volume element) in the sample without any interference from the rest of the sample. If a volume element within the cross-sectional area of one of the tubes is observed, the ^{1}H NMR spectrum will consist of a single resonance peak. The amplitude of the peak will be proportional to the number of ^{1}H nuclei in the volume element. In contrast, the NMR spectrum from a volume element outside the cross-sectional area of the tubes will show zero signal intensity due to absence of ^{1}H nuclei. Hence, the NMR spectra obtained by sequential observation of all the volume elements within a cross-sectional plane represent the spatial distribution of water in the chosen plane. The display of signal intensities of the NMR spectra according to the spatial coordinates of the corresponding volume elements produces an image of the sample. This approach to image formation, though conceptually simple, suffers from disadvantages that can be overcome by other methods.

A more efficient approach to image formation involves observation of the NMR signal from the entire object. In this case the conventional ^{1}H NMR spectrum of our test object (two tubes of water) would consist of a single resonance peak and would be devoid of any information regarding the physical shape of the object. The solution to this problem lies in identifying a suitable method for discriminating the NMR signal produced by each volume element in the object. This is accomplished by making a particular parameter (e.g., frequency and/or phase) of the NMR signal produced by a volume element dependent on its position. Since the NMR phenomenon depends on the interaction of nuclei placed in a static external magnetic field (B_0) with the radio-frequency magnetic field (B_1), spatial information can be encoded into the NMR signal by suitable manipulation of either the static field or the radio-frequency field. This can be achieved by the use of static or radio-frequency fields that vary in magnitude with position, that is, field gradients. For example, if two tubes of water are placed in an external magnetic field so that they experience different field strengths, the resonance frequency of the nuclei in the two tubes will be different. Hence, the NMR spectrum of the two tubes will consist of two resonance peaks indicating the presence of separate compartments of nuclei. This concept is expanded on in sections to follow, leading to construction of cross-sectional images. The use of static field gradients is straightforward and is more easily implemented; the use of radio-frequency field gradients is more complicated and will not be discussed further.

Clinical MRI utilizes the nuclear magnetic resonance signal generated by the hydrogen (^{1}H) nuclei. High natural abundance in the body (as water and fat) and high NMR sensitivity make ^{1}H nuclei an ideal candidate for diagnostic imaging.

The idea of MRI was first demonstrated by Lauterbur in 1973.[L1] Since then, several different approaches for image construction with NMR have been proposed. Currently, clinical MRI is largely performed by the so-called spin-warp method.[E1, K1] Therefore, this chapter concentrates on this technique, and the interested reader is referred to the reviews on the subject for discussions on other methods.[B1, E2, M1, M2]

LINEAR MAGNETIC FIELD GRADIENTS

In NMR spectroscopy, where chemical shift information is of interest, a magnetic field of high homogeneity (at least 1 part in 10^8) is essential. High homogeneity of the field ensures that all the chemically equivalent nuclei in different regions of the sample resonate in a narrow frequency range without obscuring the frequency shifts due to chemical shift effects. In contrast, nonuniformity of the field in the form of a linear gradient is deliberately introduced in MRI experiments. This generally obscures the chemical shift information present in a conventional NMR spectrum but provides information on the spatial distribution of the resonating nuclei.

Characteristics and Production

A magnetic field gradient[M1, M2] designates a variation of the magnetic field strength with position. In MRI, linear magnetic field gradients of the static external field B_0 are used. A linear field gradient represents a constant increment or decrement of the field when equal steps are taken along a particular direction. Since, by convention (see Chapter 38), the external B_0 field is taken to be directed along the z axis of an xyz Cartesian coordinate

A

B_z

B_o ΔB Δd

G = slope = $\frac{\Delta B}{\Delta d}$

0 distance

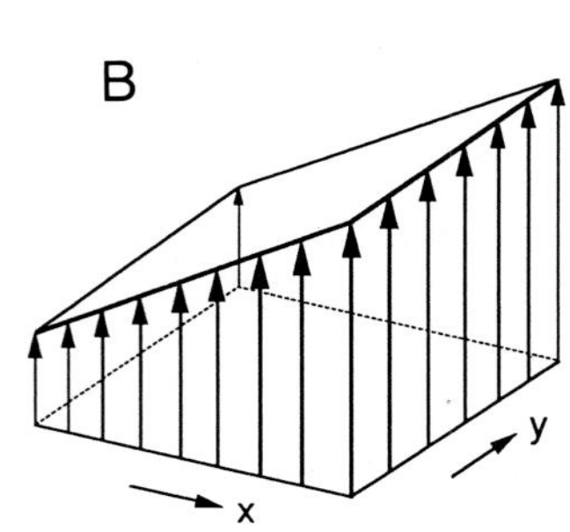

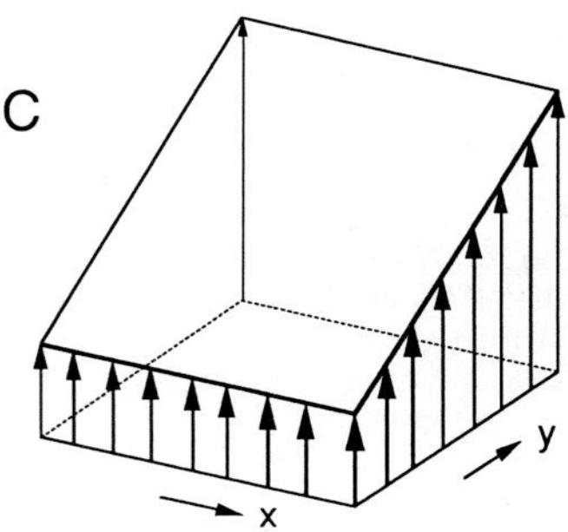

Figure 39–1. Linear field gradient representations. *(A)* Plot of field strength (B_z) versus distance. *(B* and *C)* Diagrammatic representations of linear gradient fields along the *x* axis and *y* axis, respectively. The length of each arrow indicates the field strength at the corresponding position. In a gradient field directed along the *x* axis, the arrow lengths vary along the *x* axis but not along the *y* and *z* axes. In a homogeneous field, the arrows at all points are of equal length.

system, a linear gradient of the B_0 field represents a linear variation of the strength of the field directed along the *z* axis (B_z) with position; that is, a plot of B_z versus distance corresponds to a straight line (Fig. 39–1*A*). The origin of the coordinate system from which the distance is measured is normally chosen to be the position at which the magnetic field strength is of the nominal value B_0.

A linear gradient field is characterized by two parameters, its magnitude and its direction. The magnitude of the gradient, G, represents the change in field strength per unit change in distance and corresponds to the slope of the line in Figure 39–1*A*. The direction of the field gradient corresponds to the direction along which the distance is measured. The magnitudes of the gradient fields along the principal axes are indicated by G_x, G_y, and G_z, and diagrammatic representations of G_x and G_y are shown in Figure 39–1*B* and *C*.

The magnetic field (B_z) at a certain location P in the presence of a linear gradient field G_x is given by

$$B_z = B_0 + G_x X \qquad (1)$$

where X is the *x* coordinate of the point P. Note that in the presence of G_x, the magnetic field strengths at all points having the same *x* coordinate but different *y* and *z* coordinates are equal. Consequently, in a linear gradient field, planes perpendicular to the direction of the gradient represent planes of constant field strength. If the magnitude of the gradient is zero (i.e., $G_x = 0$), the field at all the points, irrespective of their coordinates, is equal to B_0; that is, the field is homogeneous. Relationships similar to equation (1) also hold for G_y and G_z gradients.

The magnitude of the field contributed by the gradient ($G_x X$ in equation 1) is much smaller than the B_0 field. In a whole-body imaging system operating at a B_0 field of 1.5 tesla (15,000 gauss), the typical maximum gradient strength (G) used is 1.0 gauss/cm. Hence the field contributed by the gradient 20 cm away from the origin is only 0.13 percent of the main field.

Magnetic field gradients as shown in Figure 39–1*A* are produced by combining the magnetic fields from two sources. A main homogeneous B_0 field is provided by a large magnet with a bore size appropriate for the intended application. This homogeneous field is transformed into a gradient field with the aid of current-carrying coils (gradient coils) that produce a small magnetic field directed primarily along the *z* axis. However, the design of a gradient coil is such that the strength of the magnetic field produced by it varies linearly along a certain direction (i.e., a linear gradient field). When such a field is superimposed on the homogeneous field B_0, it either reinforces or opposes B_0 to a different degree, depending on the spatial coordinate. This results in a field gradient that is centered on B_0 (see Fig. 39–1*A*).

The location at which the homogeneous B_0 field is unaffected by the field contributed by the gradient coils is called the isocenter and corresponds to the origin of the coordinate system defined earlier. Furthermore, the gradient coils are positioned in the magnet so that the isocenter coincides with the center of the region in which the B_0 field is most homogeneous. Three different sets of gradient coils are required to generate gradients along the principal axes. The strength of the steady current through the gradient coils determines the magnitude (G) of the gradient produced. In MRI, gradient fields are applied in different directions and strengths at different times during the experiment. This is accomplished simply by establishing a suitable current in the appropriate set of coils for the desired time duration. A gradient field along any arbitrary direction can be generated by suitable combination of the three principal gradients.

Nuclear Magnetic Resonance Projections

To understand how magnetic field gradients are utilized in MRI, consider a large sample of water placed in such a field. As discussed in Chapter 38, the Larmor frequency depends on the strength of the local magnetic field experienced by the nuclei. Therefore, if the sample is subjected to a G_x gradient, ^1H nuclei at different *x* coordinates possess different Larmor frequencies. The Larmor frequency of nuclei with coordinate X (ν_X) is given by

$$\nu_X = \frac{\gamma}{2\pi}(B_0 + G_x X)$$

$$= \nu_0 + \frac{\gamma}{2\pi} G_x X \qquad (2)$$

where ν_0 is the Larmor frequency of the nuclei in a homogeneous B_0 field (see Chapter 38, equation 2) and γ is the magnetogyric

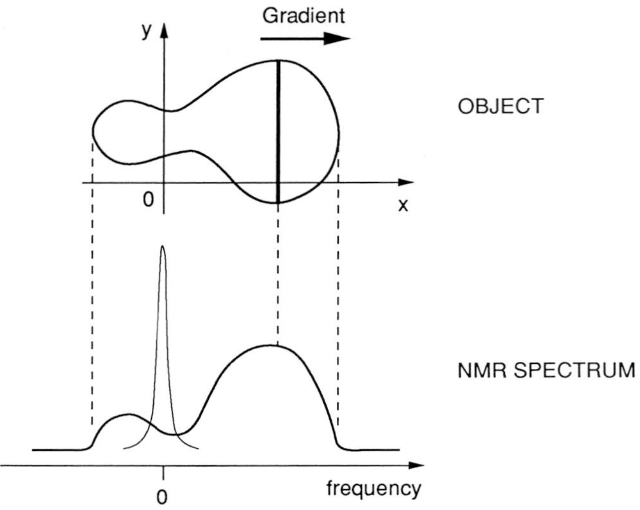

Figure 39–2. Relationship between the spatial extent of the object and the NMR spectrum. In a homogeneous field, the NMR spectrum consists of a single line (narrow line); in the presence of a gradient the NMR spectrum (bold line) corresponds to the projection of the object onto the gradient direction.

ratio. Hence, in the presence of G_x, planes of constant field strength also become planes of constant resonance frequency. Equation (2) shows that a relationship between the position and the resonance frequency can be established by application of a magnetic field gradient.

It follows that the ^{1}H NMR spectrum obtained from the water sample subjected to a gradient magnetic field will show a distribution of resonance frequencies (Fig. 39–2). This is in contrast to the NMR spectrum, consisting of a single resonance frequency, that would be obtained in the absence of the gradient (i.e., in a homogeneous field). The amplitude profile of the spectrum obtained in the presence of a gradient can be rationalized by recalling that the amplitude of the NMR spectrum is proportional to the number of contributing nuclei. Thus the spectral amplitude at a particular frequency is proportional to the number of nuclei in the given constant-frequency plane. Hence it can be seen that the NMR spectrum of an object placed in linear magnetic field gradient corresponds to the projection of the object onto the gradient direction.

Nuclear magnetic resonance projections of an object provide spatial information along a single direction (defined by the direction of the gradient used) and therefore can be regarded as one-dimensional images. The manner in which the gradients were utilized in the preceding discussion encodes the spatial information into the NMR signal by making the frequency of the signal due to a plane of nuclei within the object dependent on the spatial coordinate. Therefore, this process is referred to as frequency encoding.

The use of magnetic field gradients to produce projections of the object under investigation is a key concept in NMR imaging, and, as will be seen later, manipulation of gradients in all three directions provides three-dimensional structural information of the object.

Evolution of Magnetization in Field Gradients

As will become apparent, an understanding of the effects of linear gradients on the sample magnetization (see Chapter 38) is necessary for the analysis of imaging experiments. Therefore basic radio-frequency pulse and gradient sequences are described in this section. It will be seen that the evolution of magnetization in a gradient field can be readily visualized in the $x'y'z$ rotating reference frame (see Chapter 38).

Consider a radio-frequency pulse and gradient sequence consisting of a 90-degree pulse followed by application of a gradient field along the x axis (Fig. 39–3*A*). Ideally, such a sequence can be used to obtain an NMR spectrum that corresponds to the projection of the object onto the x axis. In this analysis it will be assumed that the frequency of the radio-frequency pulse and that of the rotating frame are both equal to the Larmor frequency υ_0 of the nuclei in a homogeneous B_0 field.

The total sample magnetization, which is composed of individual magnetization components that correspond to different planes of nuclei within the sample, is initially aligned along the z axis (Fig. 39–3*B*). The 90-degree pulse along the x' axis causes the total magnetization to be oriented along the y' axis of the rotating frame (Fig. 39–3*C*). Following the pulse, the magnetization is subjected to the G_x gradient. Under the influence of G_x, the individual magnetization components that correspond to different planes perpendicular to the x axis precess at different frequencies, since they now experience different fields; from equation (2), the precessional frequency of a magnetization component at coordinate X when viewed in the rotating frame is equal to $\gamma G_x X/2\pi$. Thus, following the 90-degree pulse the individual magnetization

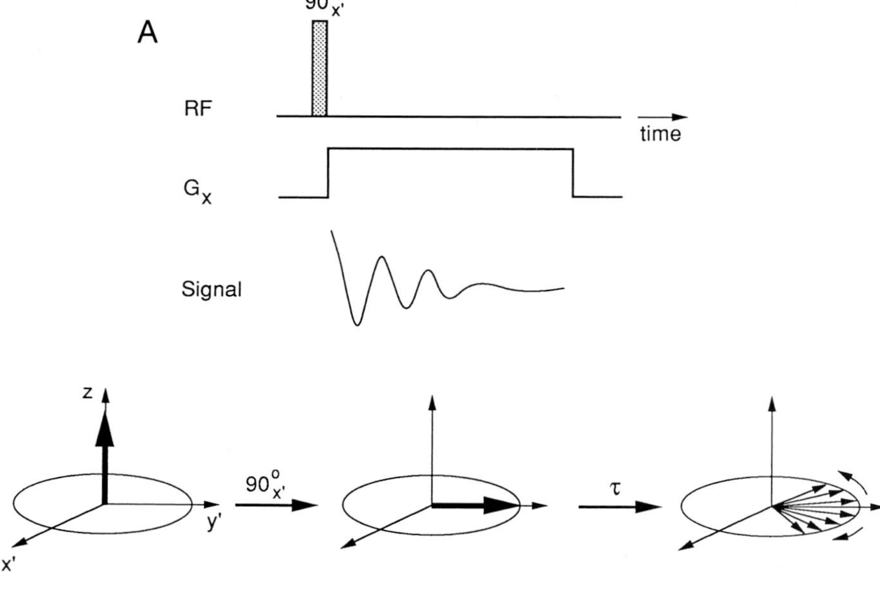

Figure 39–3. *(A)* The basic radio-frequency pulse and gradient sequence that can be used to obtain an NMR spectral projection of an object. *(B–D)* Rotating frame view of the magnetization during the sequence shown in *(A)*. *(B)* Magnetization before the radio-frequency pulse. *(C)* Magnetization immediately after the $90°_{x'}$ pulse. *(D)* Dephased magnetization after an arbitrary time τ following the pulse.

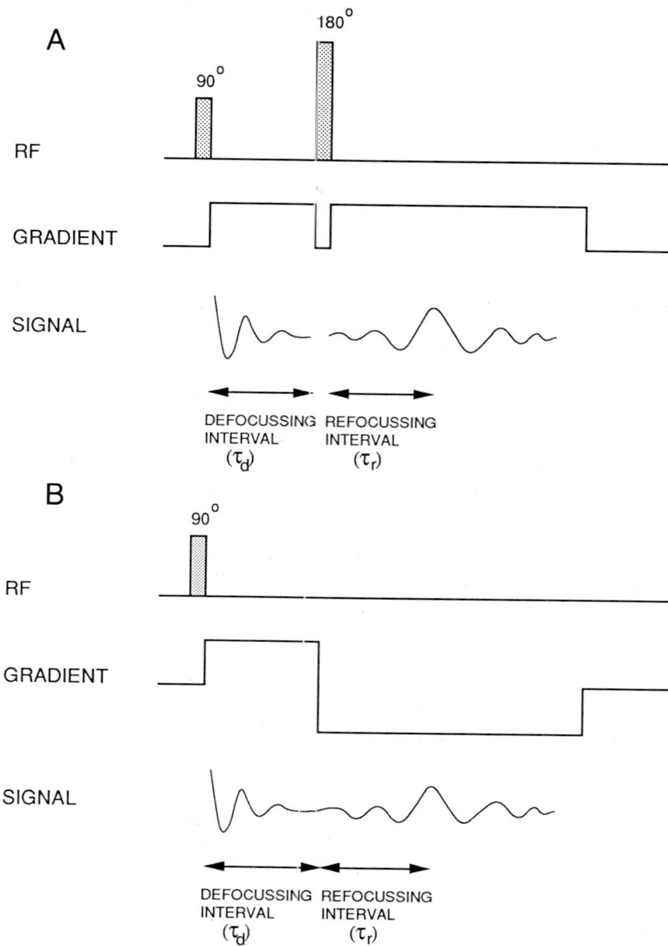

Figure 39–4. Signal refocusing methods. *(A)* Creation of a spin echo in the presence of a gradient. *(B)* Creation of a gradient echo by reversing the gradient direction, that is, by applying a negative gradient.

components will be seen to fan out (dephase) about the y' axis of the rotating frame (Fig. 39–3*D*). This dephasing of magnetization in the transverse $x'y'$ plane is similar to the dephasing effects caused by static B_0 field inhomogeneity (see Chapter 38). In practice, dephasing of magnetization after the 90-degree pulse will be due to the combined effects of both the gradient and the inhomogeneity of the B_0 field.

In the presence of a gradient, the free induction decay (FID) signal (see Chapter 38) that follows the radio-frequency pulse represents a sum of signals at different frequencies that are due to different magnetization components. Consequently, the FID signal will be seen to decay faster than would be observed in the absence of a gradient. The information on the frequencies contained in the FID is recovered by subjecting the FID to Fourier transformation. In the example considered, the spectrum generated by Fourier transformation will correspond to the projection of the object onto the x axis.

At this point it is appropriate to consider possible ways of bringing the dephased magnetization components back into focus. Magnetization refocusing methods are commonly employed in imaging pulse sequences as a means of obtaining the signal at a desired time when the gradient fields are stable (discussed later). Refocusing of dephased magnetization can be accomplished either by applying a 180-degree pulse (Fig. 39–4*A*) or by reversing the direction of the gradient (Fig. 39–4*B*) at a suitable time τ_d after the 90-degree pulse.

The 180-degree pulse refocusing method is the same as the spin-echo technique described in Chapter 38 and is illustrated in Figure 39–5*A–D*. The transverse magnetization generated by the 90-degree pulse (Fig. 39–5*A*) is first allowed to dephase for period τ_d (Fig. 39–5*B*). Application of a 180-degree pulse along the y' axis rotates the dephased magnetization components about the y' axis to their mirror-image positions (Fig. 39–5*C*). If the same gradient that initially dephased the magnetization is applied following the 180-degree pulse, at a time τ_r ($\tau_r = \tau_d$) later, all the magnetization components will be refocused along the y' axis (Fig. 39–5*D*), leading to a signal in the form of an echo. It should be noted that at time τ_r following the 180-degree pulse, the dephasing due to inhomogeneities of the static magnetic field is also refocused.

In the second method of refocusing, reversing the gradient direction has the effect of changing the sign of the precessional frequencies relative to that of the rotating frame; that is, the magnetization components previously precessing clockwise in the rotating frame will begin to precess anticlockwise following gradient reversal (Fig. 39–5*B* and *E*). Therefore, provided that the same gradient magnitude is maintained following the reversal of direction, the magnetization is refocused at time τ_r ($\tau_r = \tau_d$) following the change of gradient polarity (Fig. 39–5*F*). However, unlike the 180-degree pulse, gradient reversal is unable to refocus the dephasing caused by magnetic field inhomogeneities, and the amplitude of the echo signal obtained is therefore reduced. The echo signal obtained by gradient reversal is referred to as a gradient echo to distinguish it from the spin echo obtained following a 180-degree pulse.

With both methods, gradients of unequal magnitudes can be applied during the defocusing and refocusing intervals. In these cases, τ_r will not be equal to τ_d, and refocusing of magnetization will occur when the area (magnitude × time) under the gradient pulse during the refocusing interval equals that during the defocusing interval. However, dephasing due to magnetic field inhomogeneity is refocused only following a 180-degree pulse at a time equal to the defocusing interval.

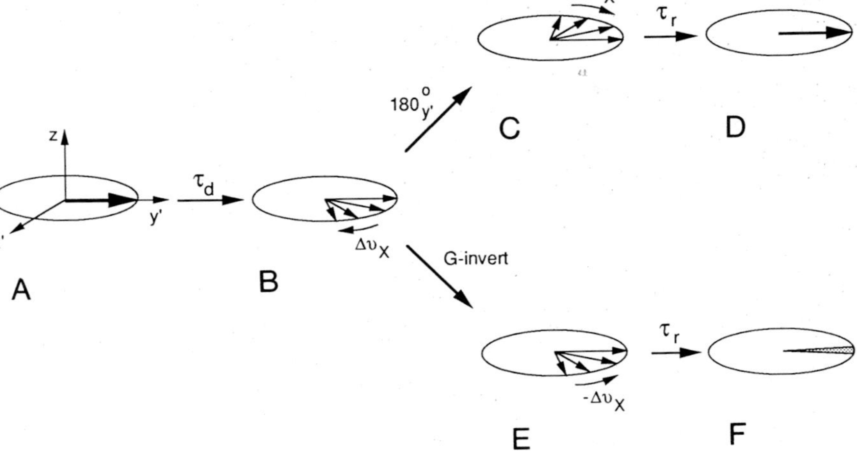

Figure 39–5. *(A)* Rotating frame view of spin echo and gradient echo formation. For clarity, the magnetization is shown to be dephased only on one side of the y' axis *(B)*. The frequency $\Delta\nu_X$ represents the precessional frequency of an arbitrary magnetization in the rotating frame. Following the $180^\circ_{y'}$ pulse *(C)*, the frequency $\Delta\nu_X$ is unchanged and the magnetization continues to rotate in the same direction with respect to the rotating frame. Gradient inversion changes the frequency to $-\Delta\nu_X$, causing the magnetization to rotate in the opposite direction *(E)*. The magnetization is shown slightly dephased at the time of the gradient echo *(F)* to indicate the effect of field inhomogeneities.

SLICE SELECTION

Current practice of clinical magnetic resonance imaging relies on defining an imaging plane or a slice in a three-dimensional object by restricting the NMR response to a particular slice of the object.

In the commonly used method of slice selection,[M1, M2] referred to as selective excitation, the equilibrium magnetization that corresponds to a thin slice of the object is selectively excited toward the transverse plane. Then the NMR signal received corresponds exclusively to this plane. The magnetization from the rest of the object, unaffected by the radio-frequency pulse, is left along the z axis and does not contribute to the signal.

In order to discuss the method used to attain such an excitation scheme, consider a sample placed in a linear magnetic field gradient G_z and subjected to a B_1 radio-frequency magnetic field pulse. Following the discussion in the previous section, under the influence of G_z, each plane of nuclei perpendicular to the z axis is associated with a unique Larmor frequency depending on the z coordinate of the plane (equation 2), and hence the sample magnetization consists of a broad range of Larmor frequencies. The problem of slice selection thus reduces to excitation of magnetization within a narrow frequency range without perturbing the magnetization outside a selected range. Selective excitation of magnetization within a narrow band of frequencies can be achieved by the application of a long, weak (small B_1) pulse, that is, a selective pulse (see also Chapter 38).

The effect of a selective radio-frequency pulse can be explained by considering the motion of the magnetization during the pulse in the rotating frame. As discussed in Chapter 38, the excitation trajectory of a magnetization is governed by the direction of the B_{1eff} field, which in turn is defined by the off-resonance frequency $\Delta\nu$ (the frequency difference between the radio-frequency pulse and the Larmor frequency). Provided that the frequency of the radio-frequency pulse is equal to ν_0, from equation (2), the off-resonance frequency of magnetization due to a plane of nuclei at coordinate Z is equal to $\gamma G_z Z/2\pi$. Therefore, magnetization due to different planes of nuclei perpendicular to the applied gradient correspond to different off-resonance frequencies, hence they will be excited along different trajectories in the rotating frame. Figure 39–6 shows the trajectories of magnetizations from three different planes of nuclei within the object. The magnetization corresponding to a plane of spins at isocenter ($z = 0$ and $\Delta\nu = 0$) will precess in the zy' plane (Fig. 39–6, path a) during the pulse, since for $\Delta\nu = 0$, $B_{1eff} = B_1$, and thus the B_{1eff} field is directed along the x' axis. A 90-degree pulse would cause this magnetization to be oriented along the y' axis at the end of the pulse.

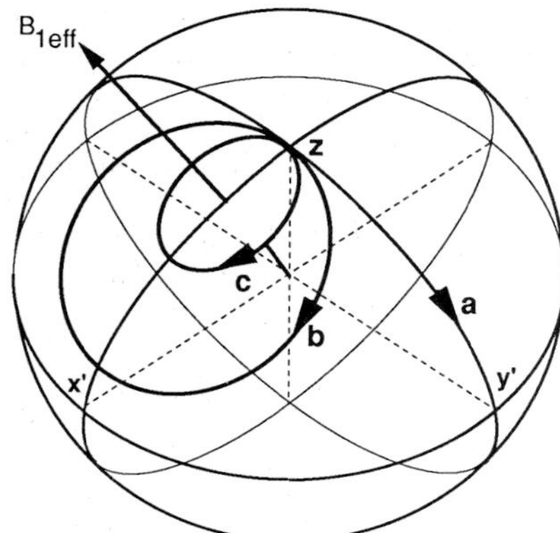

Figure 39–6. Trajectories of magnetizations corresponding to three different planes of nuclei during a selective radio-frequency pulse as viewed in the rotating frame. The different paths are indicated as a, b, and c. The direction of the B_{1eff} that corresponds to path c is shown.

Magnetization from planes other than $z = 0$ are seen to be off-resonance ($\Delta\nu \neq 0$) and the relevant B_{1eff} field is tilted away from the x' axis. Hence, paths labeled b and c (Fig. 39–6) correspond to trajectories of magnetization from planes with nonzero z coordinates (i.e., off-isocenter). It is seen that the magnetization from sufficiently large z coordinates remains close to the z axis (e.g., path c). Hence, the magnetization component in the transverse plane ($M_{x'y'}$) created by excitation of off-resonance magnetization is correspondingly smaller. A plot of $M_{x'y'}$, following a 90-degree pulse, as a function of off-resonance frequency $\Delta\nu$ is shown in Figure 39–7*B*. This indicates that magnetization with a Larmor frequency close to the frequency of the applied B_1 pulse is most efficiently excited toward the transverse plane. Magnetization with a Larmor frequency that differs significantly from that of the pulse suffers less perturbation.

The excitation profile shown in Figure 39–7*B*, however, is not entirely suitable for imaging applications, since the magnetization outside the desired slice also contributes significantly to the received signal. This is evident from the secondary $M_{x'y'}$ lobes appearing at higher frequencies in Figure 39–7*B*. For accurate selection of a slice, uniform excitation of magnetization within the slice and negligible (or zero) excitation outside the slice is needed. This requires a radio-frequency pulse that generates a rectangular excitation profile.

The excitation profile of Figure 39–7*B* was obtained by a radio-frequency magnetic field that was held at constant amplitude B_1 for the duration for which it was applied, that is, a rectangular pulse (Fig. 39–7*A*). Analysis shows that a more rectangular excitation profile can be obtained by the use of a B_1 field that varies in amplitude in a form known as the "sinc" function (Fig. 39–7*C*). Such pulses are generically referred to as amplitude-modulated pulses or more specifically called after the form of the modulation—sinc pulses.

Unfortunately, the rotating-frame view discussed earlier may not be employed to advantage to analyze the effects of a sinc pulse. The time dependence of B_1 causes the direction of B_{1eff} to be variable, and it is difficult to visualize the precession of magnetization about such a field. However, improved selectivity of sinc pulses stems from the fact that the magnetization outside a particular frequency range is returned to a point very close to the z axis at the end of the pulse, leaving a negligible component in the transverse plane.

The principal frequency range excited by a radio-frequency pulse is referred to as the bandwidth (ΔF) of the pulse. The bandwidth of a pulse is equal to $2/t_p$, where t_p represents the duration of the rectangular pulse or, in the case of a sinc pulse, the duration of the main lobe of the sinc function. Hence the frequency selectivity of a pulse can be improved by increasing the pulse duration.

The spatial distance that represents the frequency range ΔF corresponds to the thickness of the selected slice (ΔZ), and from equation (2) its relationship to other parameters is given by

$$\Delta Z = \frac{2\pi\Delta F}{\gamma G_z} \tag{3}$$

Equation (3) shows that the slice thickness is dependent on both the radio-frequency pulse bandwidth and the magnitude of the gradient used.

By now it should be clear that the orientation of the selected slice is perpendicular to the direction of the gradient applied during the pulse. Hence slices of any desired orientation can be selected by imposing a gradient along the appropriate direction.

The spatial location of the selected slice along the z axis (assuming G_z is used for slice selection) is determined by the frequency about which ΔF is disposed, which in this discussion is the same as the frequency of the radio-frequency pulse. Hence, if the frequency of the radio-frequency pulse is chosen to be equal to the Larmor frequency ν_0 of the nuclei in a homogeneous field, the selected slice will be located at isocenter ($z = 0$). Slices away from isocenter can be selected simply by offsetting the

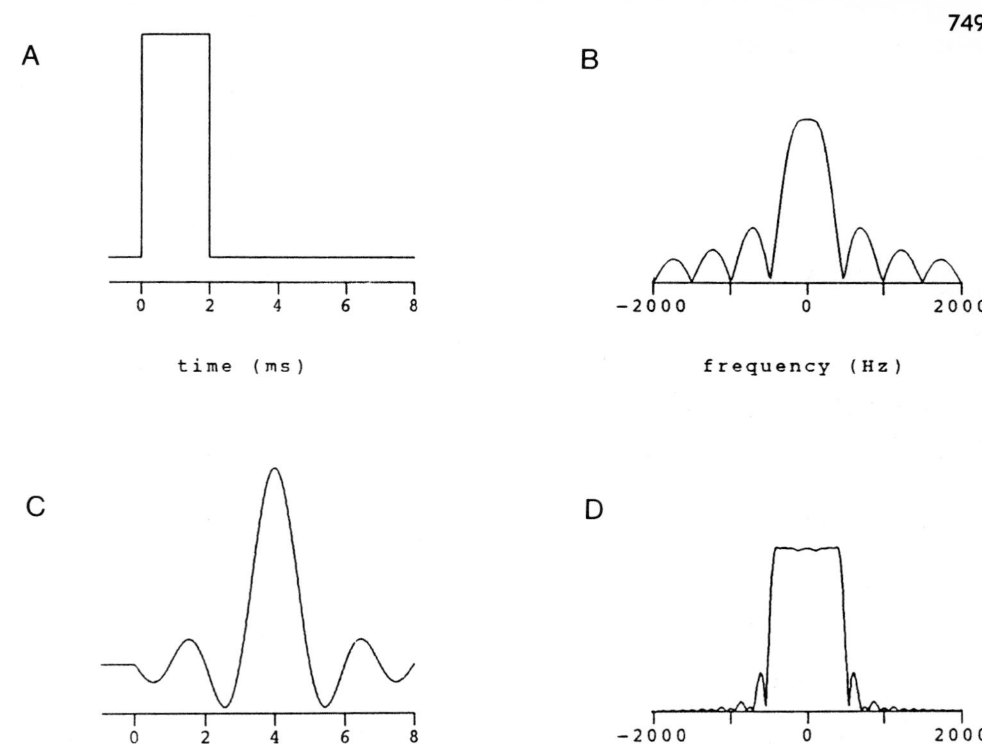

Figure 39–7. Radio-frequency pulse modulation forms and their excitation profiles. *(A* and *B)* Rectangular radio-frequency pulse and its excitation profile. *(C* and *D)* Sinc modulated radio-frequency pulse and its excitation profile. The frequency axes in *(B)* and *(D)* represent the off-resonance frequency relative to the frequency of the radio-frequency pulse.

frequency of the pulse from ν_0. The frequency offset ΔF_1 required to excite a slice at coordinate $z = Z_1$ is given by

$$\Delta F_1 = \frac{\gamma}{2\pi} G_z Z_1 \tag{4}$$

If different slices are to be excited in rapid succession, as in multislice imaging (see Multislice Imaging), the method of changing the frequency of the radio-frequency pulse to obtain different slices is not suitable. In those instances, off-center slice locations are excited by introducing another modulation function to the radio-frequency pulse amplitude in addition to the sinc form.

Before leaving this topic, it is necessary to point out a subtle but important characteristic of selective radio-frequency pulses. Analysis and experiments show that following a sinc pulse, the magnetization corresponding to different planes (perpendicular to the gradient) within the selected slice lies predominantly in the transverse $x'y'$ plane, as desired, but is oriented in different directions (dephased) in the $x'y'$ plane. This is not desirable, since the signals from different planes within the slice interfere destructively with each other. This situation is remedied by reversing the direction of the gradient (i.e., a negative gradient) following the radio-frequency pulse for a short period. Application of a negative gradient serves to rephase the magnetization within the slice and allows an FID or an echo to be detected at a desired time. Representations of the slice selection process and the rotating-frame view of magnetization are shown in Figure 39–8.

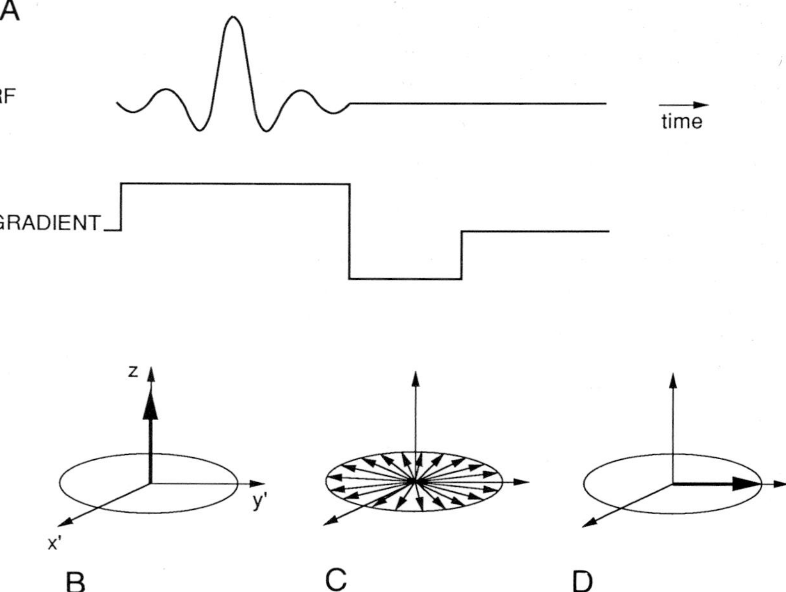

Figure 39–8. *(A)* Radio-frequency pulse and gradient timing diagram for slice selection. *(B–D)* Rotating frame view of the magnetization within the selected slice during the sequence. *(B)* Before the radio-frequency pulse; *(C)* dephased magnetization at the end of the radio-frequency pulse; *(D)* refocused magnetization at the end of negative gradient lobe.

IMAGE FORMATION IN TWO DIMENSIONS

The slice selection procedure restricts the nuclei contributing to the signal to a plane within a three-dimensional object. Once this has been accomplished, the task of image formation[E1, K1, M2] involves discrimination of the NMR response from volume elements that span only two dimensions. The manner in which two-dimensional spatial information is encoded using the spin-warp method is described below.

Concepts of Spin-Warp Imaging

The main concepts of the spin-warp method are most easily understood by concentrating initially on its characteristic features. The pulse sequence shown in Figure 39–9*A* represents the essential aspects of the spin-warp technique used to encode two spatial axes such as x and y. From the outset, the experiment comprises three separate time periods: preparation, evolution, and detection. The preparation period consists of a time duration in which the nuclei are allowed to relax toward the equilibrium condition, followed by excitation of magnetization using a radio-frequency pulse. When imaging a three-dimensional object, the radio-frequency pulse will take the form of a slice-selective pulse applied in the presence of an appropriate gradient, as discussed in the previous section; otherwise a simple nonselective pulse will suffice. During the evolution period, the transverse magnetization created by the radio-frequency pulse is allowed to precess under the influence of a gradient (e.g., G_x) applied along one of the spatial directions to be encoded. The evolution period is commonly referred to as the phase-encoding time, for reasons that will become clear in the course of this discussion. Finally, the detection period, also called the frequency-encoding time, represents the time interval during which the NMR signal is collected in the presence of a gradient (e.g., G_y) applied along the second axis.

Analysis of this sequence by considering the rotating-frame behavior of magnetization due to a single volume element located at spatial coordinates X, Y provides good insight to the technique (Fig. 39–9*B–E*). The frequency of the radio-frequency pulse and that of the rotating frame will be assumed to be equal to the Larmor frequency ν_0 of the nuclei in a homogeneous field. Immediately following the 90-degree pulse, magnetization will be oriented along the y' axis of the rotating frame (Fig. 39–9*B*). Presence of G_x during the evolution period causes the Larmor frequency of the nuclei in the volume element to be $\nu_0 + \gamma G_x X/2\pi$ (see equation 2) and, consequently, the frequency of precession of the magnetization in the rotating frame to be equal to $\gamma G_x X/2\pi$ (Fig. 39–9*C*). Evolution of magnetization under these conditions for a time t_x (see Fig. 39–9*A*) causes it to be oriented at an angle ϕ_X (Fig. 39–9*D*) with respect to the y' axis given by

$$\phi_X = \gamma G_x X t_x \qquad (5)$$

The angle ϕ_X corresponds to the phase of the magnetization at the end of the evolution time.

During the detection period, since G_x is turned off, the magnetization evolves under the influence of G_y only. Hence the precessional frequency of the magnetization in the rotating frame is now changed to $\gamma G_y Y/2\pi$ (Fig. 39–9*E*), and this frequency is reflected in the FID obtained during this period. Fourier transformation of this FID generates a spectrum in which the resonance line is located at frequency $\gamma G_y Y/2\pi$. Note that the position of the resonance line in the spectrum is proportional to the y coordinate of the volume element.

Equation (5) indicates that the information on the x coordinate of the volume element is contained in the phase angle ϕ_X acquired by the magnetization prior to detection. Since the FID signal represents the time variation of the magnetization component along the y' axis, ϕ_X determines the starting amplitude (phase) of the FID. Even though this information is preserved during

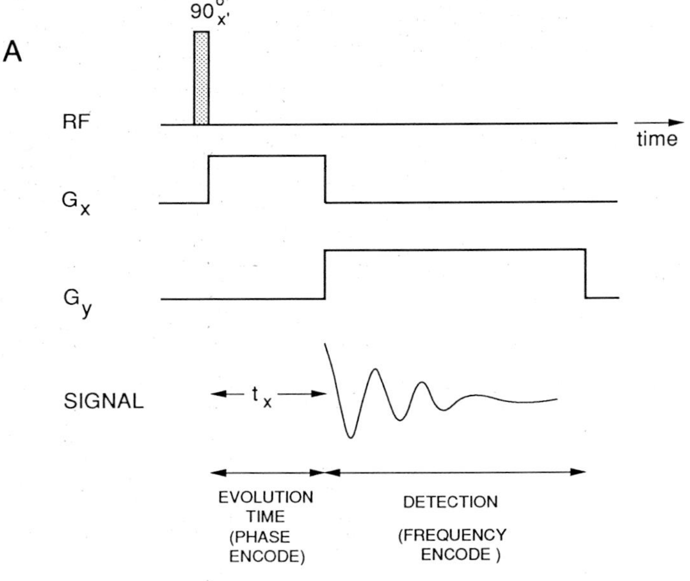

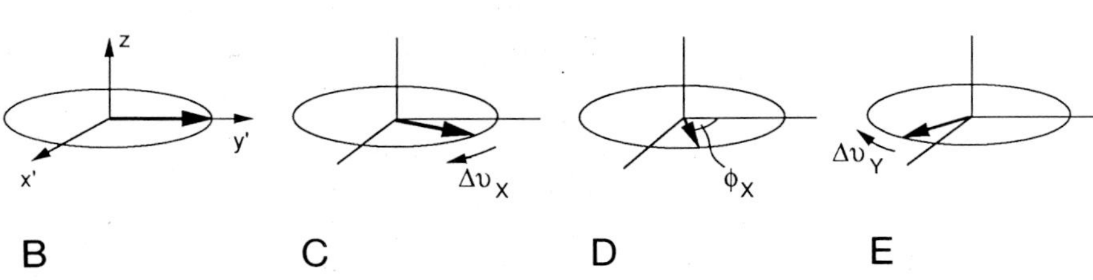

Figure 39–9. *(A)* The basic spin-warp imaging sequence for two-dimensional imaging. *(B–E)* The rotating frame view of the magnetization due to a single volume element at different times during the sequence. *(B)* Immediately after the 90-degree pulse. *(C)* Short period after the application of G_x. *(D)* At the end of the evolution time. *(E)* Short period after the application of G_y. $\Delta\nu_X$ and $\Delta\nu_Y$ represent the precessional frequencies of the magnetization during the evolution and detection periods, respectively.

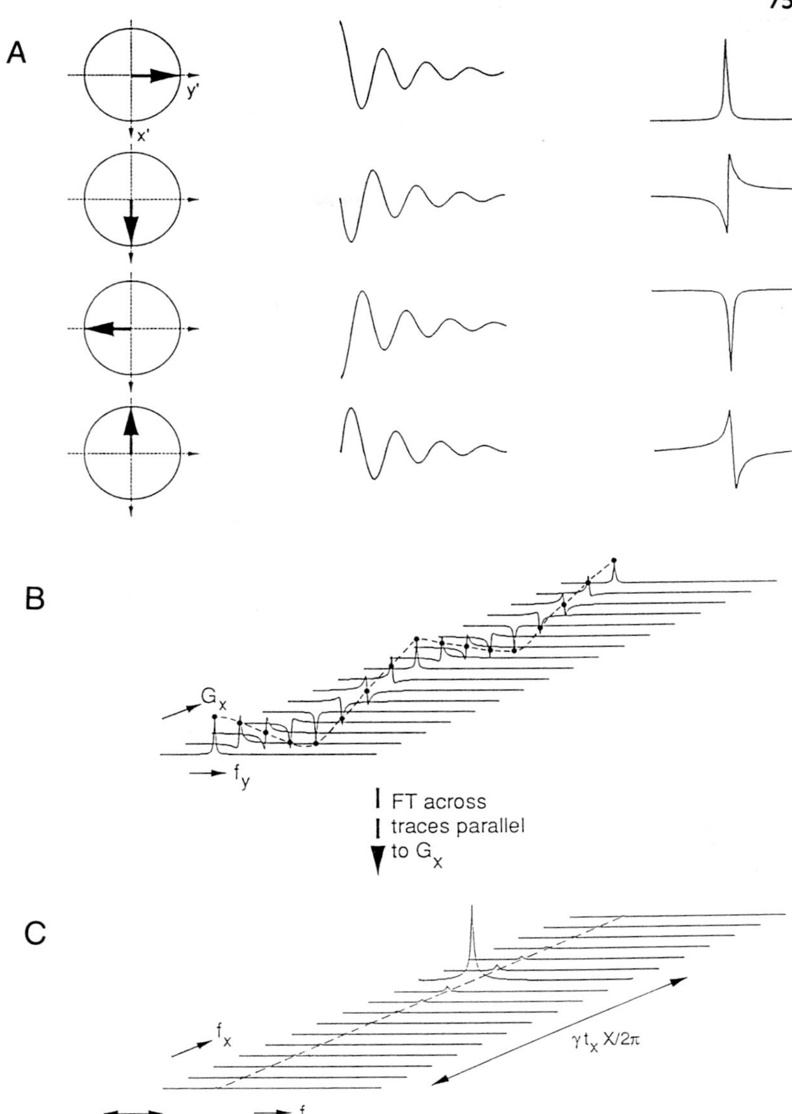

Figure 39–10. *(A)* Dependence of the free induction decay (FID) signal (middle column) and the corresponding spectrum (right column) on the phase angle ϕ_X of the magnetization (left column). The FID signals and spectra that correspond to phase angles of 0, 90, 180, and 270 degrees are shown. *(B)* Series of phase-modulated spectra obtained by repetitive use of the sequence shown in Figure 39–9*A* with an incremented G_x gradient at each pass. The spectra are assumed to originate from a single volume element. *(C)* Data matrix obtained by Fourier-transforming the data traces parallel to G_x in *(B)*.

Fourier transformation, exploitation of the same for imaging purposes is accomplished in an indirect manner.

In order to explain this procedure, the effect of ϕ_X on the FID and the corresponding spectrum obtained by Fourier transformation must be considered. The FID signals and spectra corresponding to selected values of ϕ_X are shown in Figure 39–10*A*. It can be seen that a change in ϕ_X is accompanied by a corresponding change in the shape (phase) of the spectral line while its frequency is unchanged. Such a set of spectra that is modulated by phase can be generated experimentally by repeating the sequence in Figure 39–9*A* so that each FID collected corresponds to a different value of ϕ_X. Examination of equation (5) indicates that this can be achieved by changing either G_x or t_X. In the spin-warp method, G_x is incremented by a chosen constant value (ΔG_x) in successive experiments. A series of phase-modulated spectra that would be obtained by incrementing G_x by a small value in successive experiments is shown in Figure 39–10*B*. The periodic nature of phase variation as G_x is made variable is evident from Figure 39–10*B*, and it is best illustrated by tracing the amplitude of each spectrum in the series at a given frequency (Fig. 39–10*B*, dotted line). The periodicity (frequency) of the indicated trace corresponds to the rate of change of phase ϕ_X as G_x is varied and, from equation (5), can be derived to be $\gamma t_x X/2\pi$. Hence, determination of the periodicity of the trace across the spectra enables the x coordinate of the volume element to be ascertained. The periodicity of the trace can be determined simply by Fourier transformation of the data trace, and the "spectrum" generated will consist of a peak at "frequency" $\gamma t_x X/2\pi$ indicating the position of the volume element along the x axis. The similarity of this process to the method of determining the y coordinate of the volume element is recognized by noting that the data trace indicated in Figure 39–10*B* is analogous to a digitized FID except for the fact that the data are now a function of gradient magnitude rather than time. It can be appreciated that in the case of a spatially unrestricted sample, Fourier transformation of all the data traces perpendicular to the frequency axis f_y (see Fig. 39–10*B*) would be necessary. Fourier transformation of all the traces in Figure 39–10B yields a data matrix (Fig. 39–10*C*) in which both axes now represent frequency, and the resonance peak in the example considered will be located at frequency coordinates $\gamma G_y Y/2\pi$, $\gamma t_x X/2\pi$.

From the above discussion it is clear that the position and the amplitude of the resonance line in the final data matrix are uniquely related to the spatial coordinates and the nuclear spin density of the volume element. Thus, a similar data matrix derived from all the volume elements within a plane corresponds to an image of the plane. The presence of the G_y gradient during signal detection enables the volume elements to be distinguished along the y axis, while the presence of the G_x gradient during evolution helps to identify the volume elements along the x axis.

It should be noted that x and y spatial coordinates were encoded into the FID signal by making the phase and frequency of the signal dependent on the respective coordinates. Consequently, the respective gradients used for these functions are called phase-encoding and frequency-encoding gradients. A similar naming convention is used to refer to the time periods during which these functions are performed.

The close relationship between the frequency-encoding and phase-encoding processes was noted earlier. However, it is emphasized that the frequency-encoding procedure is a single-step process, while phase encoding requires multiple experiments. The final data matrix that corresponds to the image can be described as a two-dimensional spectrum, since it contains two frequency axes. One of the frequency axes in the image matrix is analogous to the frequency axis of a conventional one-dimensional spectrum, and the other was generated via successive experiments. Application of gradients during the imaging sequence causes the frequency axes in the two-dimensional spectrum to be directly proportional to the appropriate spatial dimensions. The final data matrix is a result of two successive sets of Fourier transforms; first, each FID is Fourier-transformed to produce a series of phase-modulated spectra, and second, each data trace across the generated spectra is Fourier-transformed to produce the image. This process is referred to as a two-dimensional Fourier transform.

Practical Aspects of Spin-Warp Imaging

In practice, modified versions of the sequence shown in Figure 39–9A are usually employed to avoid distortions in the FID due to nonideal gradient behavior. Imperfect gradient behavior stems from the fact that it requires a finite time to establish a gradient field. Hence, pulse sequence modifications are introduced to cause the signal to be delayed and occur at a time when the frequency-encoding gradient is stabilized. This is accomplished by formation of an echo signal (see Evolution of Magnetization); either the echo signal that follows a 180-degree pulse or the signal that accompanies a gradient reversal scheme can be utilized. Examples of spin-warp sequences based on both methods of echo formation are frequently used in practice and are discussed in this section.

The radio-frequency pulse and gradient timing diagram for two-dimensional slice imaging based on the observation of a spin-echo signal is shown in Figure 39–11. In this figure, the gradients and the different time periods have been named according to their functions during the sequence. The actual direction of G-slice is chosen to be perpendicular to the desired image plane, and the directions of G-frequency and G-phase correspond to those defining the imaged plane.

The sequence is initiated with a 90-degree frequency-selective radio-frequency pulse applied in the presence of a gradient (G-slice). This serves to excite the magnetization corresponding to a slice in a three-dimensional object as discussed under Slice Selection. Immediately following the 90-degree pulse, the G-slice gradient is inverted for an appropriate period to rephase the transverse magnetization across the slice. Detection of a spin echo is facilitated by the application of a frequency-selective 180-degree radio-frequency pulse in the presence of the G-slice gradient. Application of the frequency-encoding gradient (G-frequency) before and after the 180-degree pulse causes the magnetization along the frequency-encoding direction initially to dephase and then to rephase, forming a spin echo, as described earlier. Since the spin echo is formed under the influence of G-frequency, it contains the spatial information along the direction of G-frequency similar to the FID in the more basic sequence discussed earlier. The phase-encoding gradient (G-phase) is applied at different strengths in successive experiments for a selected time period before the 180-degree pulse to encode the spatial information along the remaining direction. It can be seen that prior to the 180-degree pulse the excited magnetization is dephased by the action of two gradients, G-phase and G-frequency. The dephasing due to the latter is refocused in the subsequent period while that of the former is retained. The presence of G-slice during the 180-degree pulse ensures that only the slice excited by the 90-degree pulse is perturbed, and this enables multiple slices to be imaged in an efficient manner (see Multislice Imaging).

As in the example considered previously, image formation requires the sequence mentioned above to be repeated (typically 128 or 256 times) with a different magnitude of the G-phase

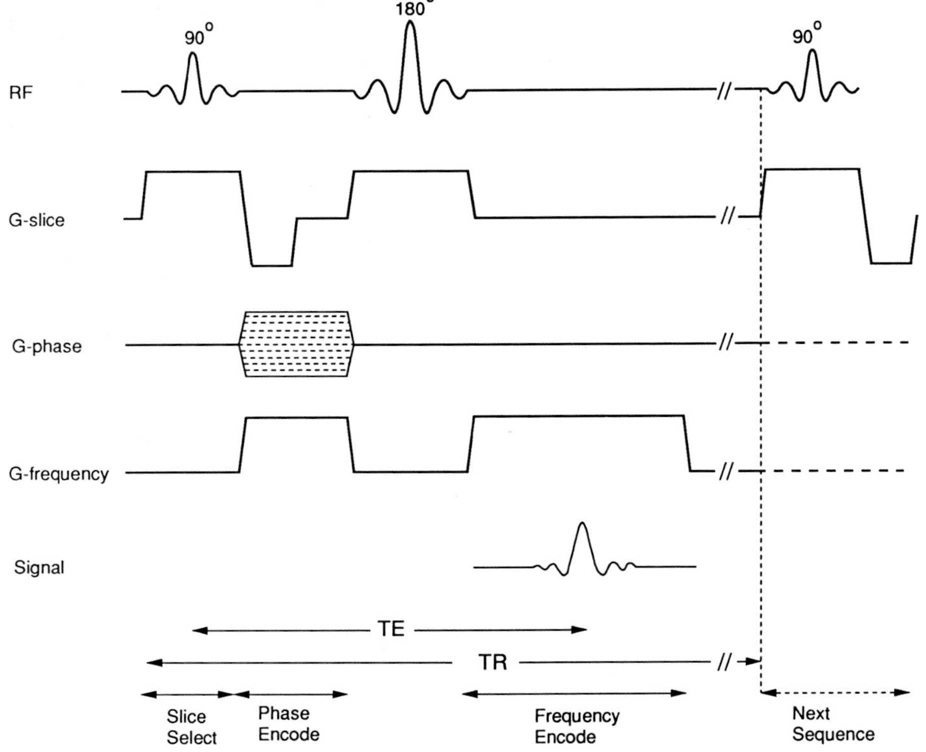

Figure 39–11. Two-dimensional slice spin-warp imaging sequence based on the observation of a spin-echo signal. Representation of G-phase indicates that its magnitude is varied each time the sequence is repeated. TR (repetition time) denotes the time between successive sequences. TE (echo time) denotes the time between the 90-degree pulse and the center of the spin echo.

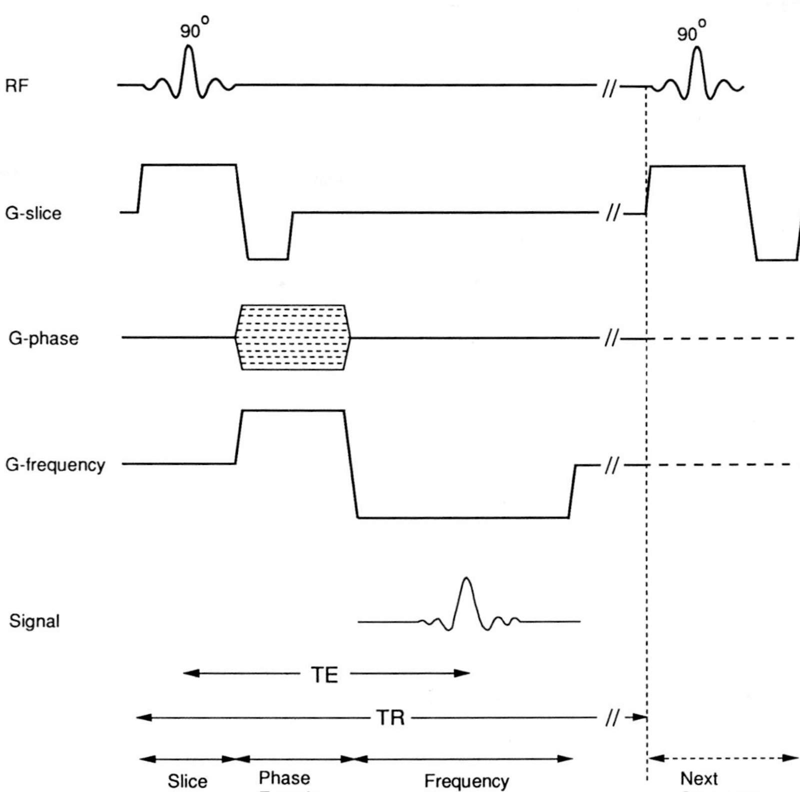

Figure 39–12. Radio-frequency pulse and gradient timing diagram for two-dimensional spin-warp imaging based on the observation of a gradient echo.

gradient at each pass. The magnitude of G-phase is initially set to a high negative value and is incremented by a constant value through zero to a high positive value in successive experiments. Progressive decrease of the gradient from a positive to a negative value is also possible. It is necessary that adequate time delay be inserted between the sequences to permit recovery of magnetization toward the equilibrium condition. The series of spin echoes obtained is then subjected to two-dimensional Fourier transformation to produce the image.

The radio-frequency pulse and gradient sequence for spin-warp imaging based on the observation of a gradient echo is shown in Figure 39–12. Here the frequency-encoding gradient is reversed, leading to the formation of a gradient echo. The other aspects of sequence remain identical to that of the spin echo-based sequence described earlier.

In general, the intensity of the image obtained is dependent on the maximum amplitude of the echo signal. The maximum echo amplitude observed is determined by two experimental parameters: the sequence repetition time, TR (time between the 90-degree pulse in one sequence and that of the immediately following sequence), and the echo time, TE (time from the center of the 90-degree pulse to the top of the echo signal) (see Fig. 39–11). Long TR values permit greater recovery of magnetization between the sequences via spin-lattice relaxation and contribute to enhanced signal intensity. On the other hand, long TE values cause reduced signal intensity due to decay of magnetization between excitation and detection by spin-spin relaxation. The degree of recovery and decay of the magnetization is determined by the relaxation properties—spin-lattice (T_1) and spin-spin (T_2) relaxation times—of the sample, and the differences in relaxation characteristics between tissues provide the necessary contrast in clinical images.

Spin-warp imaging based on the observation of a spin echo is most commonly used for several reasons. Since the 180-degree pulse refocuses the dephasing effects due to magnetic field inhomogeneities, spin-echo images are more tolerant of nonuniformities of the magnetic field than are gradient-echo images. This permits acquisition of undistorted spin-echo images with long TE values showing higher contrast due to differences in T_2. Use of a 180-degree pulse also allows multiple echoes to be generated following a single 90-degree pulse by repeated application of 180-degree pulses as in a Carr-Purcell sequence (see Chapter 38). Multiple echoes obtained in this manner decay by spin-spin relaxation, and images corresponding to each echo show increased contrast due to increased T_2 weighting.

Increased sensitivity of gradient echo-based spin-warp imaging to field inhomogeneities makes it more suitable for short-TE studies. Gradient echo imaging can also be easily adapted for fast imaging (see Rapid Imaging Techniques).

Image Parameters

Control and adjustment of the spatial distance represented in the final image (field of view) play an important role in clinical MRI. The field of view of a magnetic resonance image is determined by the experimental parameters selected, and it can easily be varied to suit the spatial extent of the object being imaged. Furthermore, the fields of view along frequency-encoding and phase-encoding directions are independently variable.

The relationship between the field of view and the relevant parameters arises from consideration of the signal-sampling process. As mentioned in Chapter 38, the analog signal (FID or spin-echo) information is converted into digital form for storage in a computer by sampling the signal voltage at specific time intervals (analog-to-digital conversion). Correct representation of a periodic signal in digital form requires that it be sampled at least twice per cycle. This is known as the Nyquist sampling theorem. Hence, the maximum signal frequency, f_{max}, that can be faithfully represented in digital form is determined by the time interval between adjacent samples (sampling interval or dwell time), Δt_S, and they are related by $f_{max} = 1/(2\Delta t_S)$; f_{max} is known as the Nyquist frequency. Since the FID is usually a composite of several frequencies, the sampling theorem should be satisfied for the maximum frequency present in the signal. If the signal contains frequency components greater than the Nyquist frequency determined by the chosen sampling interval, these frequencies will not be sampled adequately and will be misrepresented (aliased) in the spectrum following Fourier transformation. All the frequency components below the Nyquist frequency will be correctly represented. In addition, since the NMR signal is commonly detected in the quadrature mode (see Chapter 38), both the positive and negative frequencies with respect to a reference frequency can be distinguished. Hence the total range of frequencies unambiguously represented in the digital signal is equal to $2f_{max}$ or $1/\Delta t_S$. This frequency range is referred to as the receiver bandwidth.

From equation (2), the range of precessional frequencies in the spin-echo signal during frequency encoding is given by $\gamma G_f L/2\pi$, where L is the spatial extent of the object along the frequency-encoding dimension and G_f is the magnitude of the frequency-encoding gradient. From the preceding discussion it is clear that this frequency range should not be larger than the receiver bandwidth. Hence the maximum value of L that satisfies this condition corresponds to the field of view (FOV) along the frequency-encoding (FE) dimension and is given by

$$(FOV)_{FE} = \frac{2\pi}{\gamma G_f \Delta t_s} \quad (6)$$

Similar reasoning can be applied for the phase-encoding (PE) dimension. Since each signal trace along the phase-encoded axis is a function of the magnitude of the phase-encoding gradient, the quantity analogous to the sampling interval is the amount by which the phase-encoding gradient is incremented in successive experiments (ΔG_p). Hence the field of view along the phase-encoding dimension can be derived as

$$(FOV)_{PE} = \frac{2\pi}{\gamma \Delta G_p t_p} \quad (7)$$

where t_p is the duration of the phase-encoding gradient. Note that equation (7) applies when the phase-encoding gradient is held constant for the entire time duration t_p (i.e., a rectangular gradient pulse).

An important consideration in any digital image is the number of picture elements (pixels) spanning the image. In MRI this is determined by two independent parameters. The number of pixels in the frequency-encoded image axis is governed by the number of times (N_f) the analog echo signal is sampled during analog-to-digital conversion. If the echo signal is detected in the quadrature mode (which generates two echo signals 90 degrees out of phase), each echo signal will be defined by N_f data points. In this case, following Fourier transformation, the frequency-encoded image axis will be represented by N_f data points, each of which corresponds to a pixel in the displayed image. Hence the image pixel resolution, defined as the spatial distance corresponding to each pixel, along the frequency-encoded axis is given by $(FOV)_{FE}/N_f$. Parenthetically, it is noted that if the sampling interval is Δt_S, then the total time (t_{acq}) during which each echo is sampled (readout time or acquisition time) is equal to $N_f \Delta t_S$. In practice, signal sampling is timed so that both sides of the echo are symmetrically sampled; that is, maximum echo signal occurs at the center of the readout time.

The number of pixels along the phase-encoded image axis is equal to the number of times (N_p) the phase-encoded gradient is incremented, that is, the number of echo signals obtained with different gradient strengths. Therefore the image pixel resolution along the phase-encoded image axis is given by $(FOV)_{PE}/N_p$. Together, N_p and ΔG_p determine the maximum phase-encoding gradient strength ($N_p \Delta G_p/2$) required. The factor of 2 in the denominator accounts for the fact that both positive and negative gradients can be employed.

The values of N_f and N_p are chosen to be a power of 2 to obtain the maximum efficiency in Fourier transform calculations, and values of 128 and 256 are commonly used in generation of clinical images.

The total time (T_{tot}) required to produce an image is determined almost entirely by the time needed to acquire the required number of echo signals, since the data processing time is much smaller. Hence T_{tot} is equal to $N_p TR$, where TR is the time between successive sequences. If each echo signal with a given magnitude of the phase-encoding gradient is acquired multiple times (n) for signal-to-noise improvement (see Chapter 38), then T_{tot} is given by $nN_p TR$.

Multislice Imaging

So far, imaging a single slice has been considered. Multiple slices can be imaged by repeating the entire imaging sequence with suitable changes in the frequency or the modulation of the radio-frequency pulse to excite different slices. Sequential acquisition of N_s slices (Fig. 39–13*A*) increases the total imaging time in direct proportion to the number of slices imaged. The imaging time for N_s slices is equal to $N_s(nN_p TR)$.

More efficient use of time can be devised by considering the time scale of a single experimental sequence in Figure 39–11. Each of the processes—slice selection, phase encoding, and 180-degree refocusing—is generally accomplished in a time less than 5 msec. The frequency-encoding period lasts for approximately 10 msec. Then the time (t_{seq}) from the start of the 90-degree pulse to the end of the frequency-encoding gradient is approximately 25 msec. However, it should be noted that the time required to observe the echo depends on the TE selected. For example, if a TE value of 80 msec is required, the additional time delays are incorporated into the sequence at appropriate places. The time from the end of the frequency-encoding gradient to the next 90-degree pulse (in the following sequence) is determined by the value selected for TR, which is in the range of 400 to 2000 msec. Thus, the dead time between the successive sequences is several times (may be as high as 20, depending on the TR and TE selected) longer than the minimum time required to observe the echo. Hence a major portion of the time taken to generate an image of a single slice is expended on waiting for the magnetization in that slice to recover before it can be stimulated again.

When images of several different slices are required, the dead time between sequences can be used to gather data from other slices.[C1] Since each slice can be stimulated only at an interval of TR, the dead time can be used to excite and detect signals from as many different slices as possible until it is time to return to the first slice. This process, called interleaved multislice mode, is illustrated in Figure 39–13*B*. Note that gradient echo-based multislice imaging is also possible.

Assuming that TR is sufficiently long so that data from N_s slices can be acquired within a single TR time span, the total imaging time in the interleaved mode becomes independent of the number of slices; that is, the time required to image N_s slices is the same as the time ($nN_p TR$) required to image a single slice. Hence the interleaved acquisition mode reduces the imaging time by a factor of N_s compared to the sequential mode.

The number of different slices that can be interrogated in a single TR period is equal to TR/t_{seq}. If $N_s > TR/t_{seq}$, the efficiency factor of the interleaved mode is reduced.

Substantial saving in time offered by the interleaved multislice mode makes it the preferred method in a clinical environment.

RAPID IMAGING TECHNIQUES

Rapid imaging techniques are often desired for several reasons. Techniques requiring long imaging times are more susceptible to motions of the object during the imaging procedure. In clinical MRI, imaging times on the order of minutes cause undesirable image artifacts due to physiologic motions of the body and blood flow. Fast imaging techniques also allow the examination time to be reduced, minimizing patient discomfort and maximizing the throughput. Finally, study of fast physiologic processes requires imaging methods that can be completed in short time periods.

Several fast imaging methods have been suggested and dem-

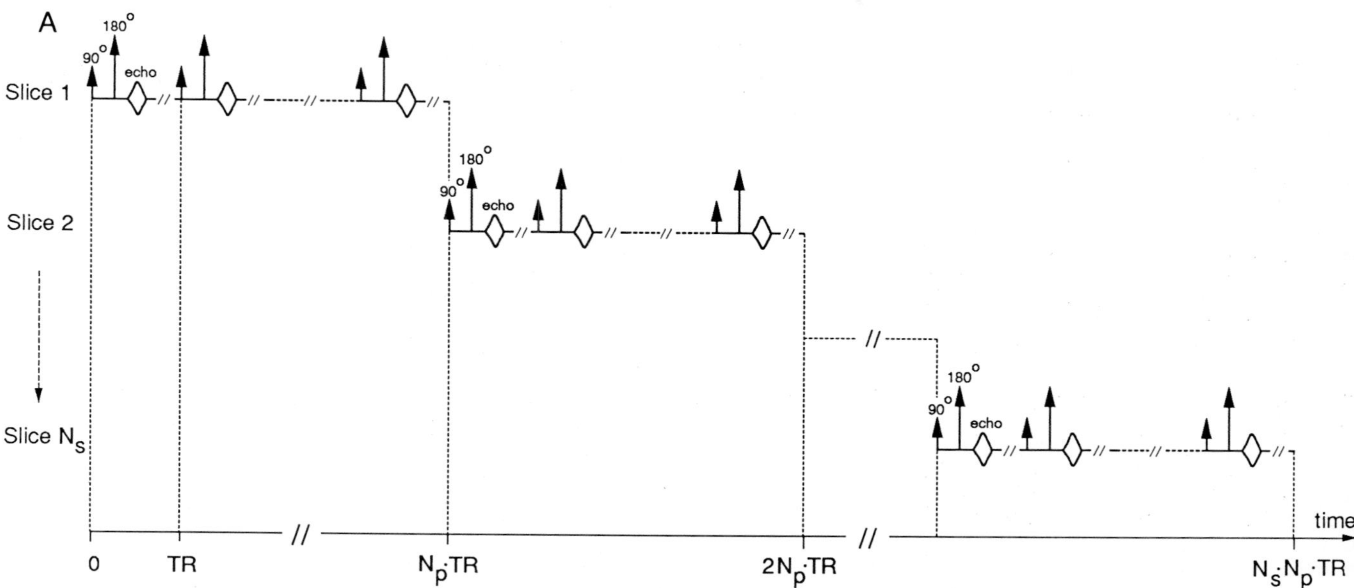

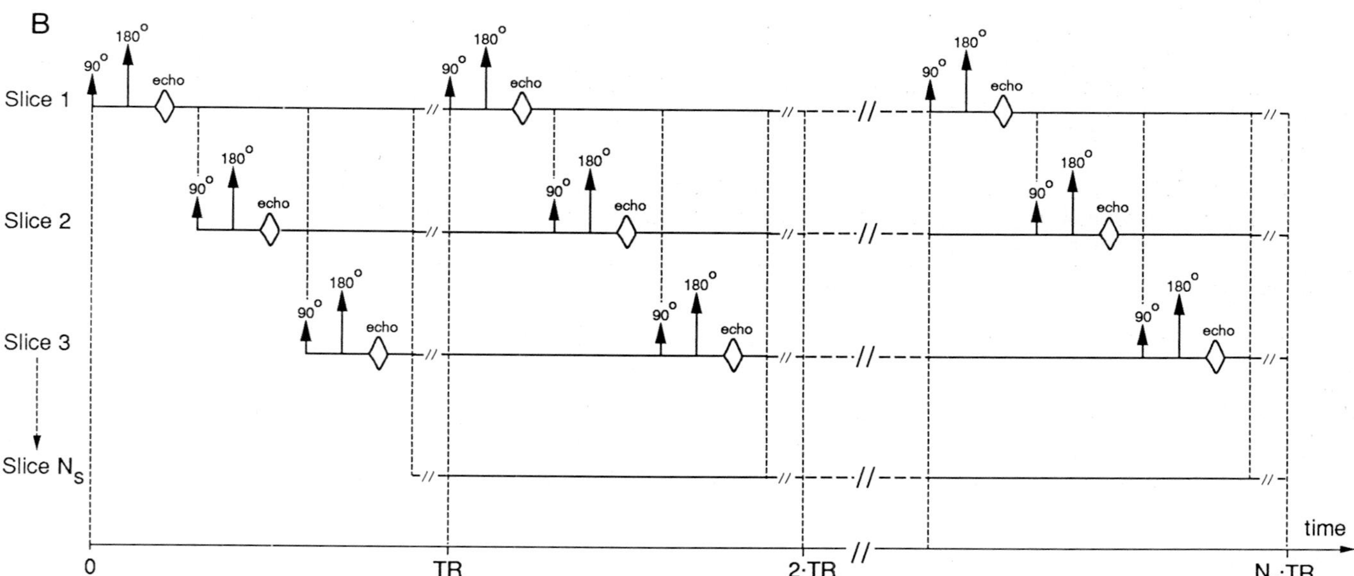

Figure 39–13. Sequential *(A)* and interleaved *(B)* multislice acquisition modes. Note the change in scale of the time axis between *(A)* and *(B)*.

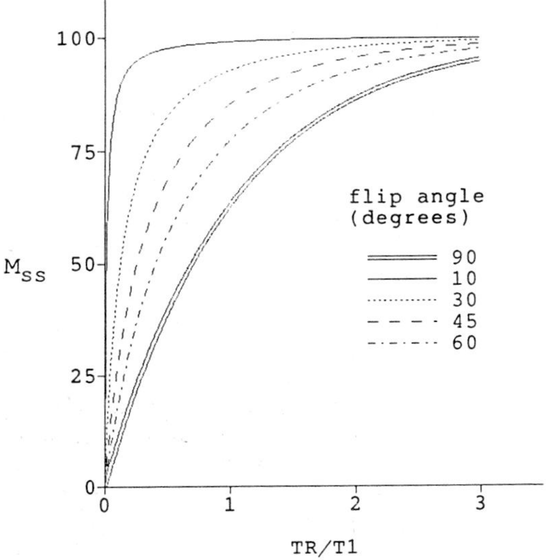

Figure 39–14. Plot of steady-state longitudinal magnetization as a function of the TR/T_1 ratio (equation 8) for various flip angles.

onstrated in recent years. Of these, the most commonly used method, called the fast low-angle shot method (FLASH),[F1, H1] derives directly from the gradient echo-based spin-warp technique. Assuming that no signal averaging is required (n = 1), the imaging time (N_pTR) for spin-warp imaging is determined by the number of phase-encoding gradient increments (N_p) and the sequence repetition time (TR). In the FLASH method a shorter imaging time is sought by decreasing the TR to a minimum possible value. For a gradient echo-based sequence, TR can be as low as 20 msec. This means that successive sequences are initiated without any dead time between sequences and the magnetization is allowed to recover (via spin-lattice relaxation) only for a short time. With a repetition time of 20 msec, a FLASH image can be acquired in approximately 2.5 seconds (N_p = 128).

The consequences of using very short TR values in a gradient-echo spin-warp sequence can be analyzed by considering the magnetization subjected to a train of radio-frequency pulses separated by a time delay TR. Under these conditions, following a few pulses the magnetization achieves a steady state in which the longitudinal magnetization component (M_z) immediately prior to each radio-frequency pulse is constant. This state is attained when the fractional loss in M_z due to the pulse (which causes

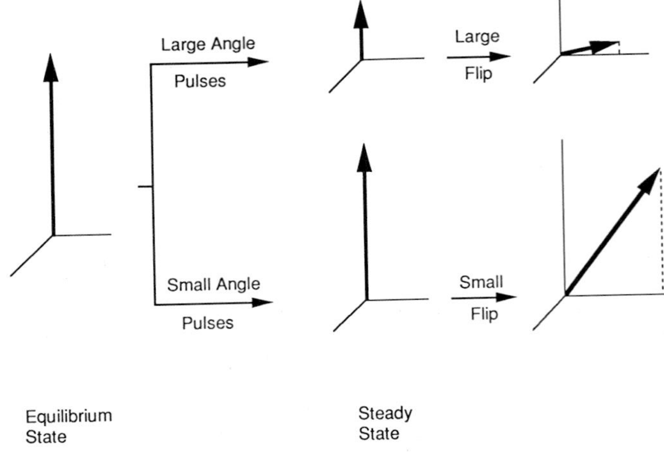

Figure 39–16. Illustration of compensation of signal loss due to short TR/T_1 ratios by the use of low flip angles.

nutation of the magnetization away from the z axis) is compensated by the recovery of M_z (due to spin-lattice relaxation) before the subsequent pulse. The steady-state longitudinal magnetization (M_{ss}) due to a train of radio-frequency pulses of flip angle Θ and separation TR is given by

$$M_{ss} = M_o \frac{1 - \exp(-TR/T_1)}{1 - \cos\Theta \exp(-TR/T_1)} \quad (8)$$

Equation (8) is appropriate when the transverse magnetization caused by the radio-frequency pulse either decays completely or is dephased by gradients before the subsequent pulse. Equation (8) is plotted in Figure 39–14 for various flip angles.

Figure 39–14 indicates that for a given TR/T_1 ratio, a greater steady-state longitudinal magnetization is achieved by using a smaller flip angle. This result is intuitive, since pulses of low flip angle cause a smaller loss in longitudinal magnetization in the first place.

At the steady state, the NMR signal following each radio-frequency pulse is proportional to M_{ss} sin Θ, and its dependence on TR/T_1 is shown in Figure 39–15. The figure indicates that the maximum signal is obtained by using 90 degrees and long TR values (i.e., TR/T_1 > 3). As TR is decreased, with a given flip angle the signal decreases because the steady-state magnetization is reduced. Therefore, use of short TR values in spin-warp imaging causes the image signal-to-noise ratio to be correspond-

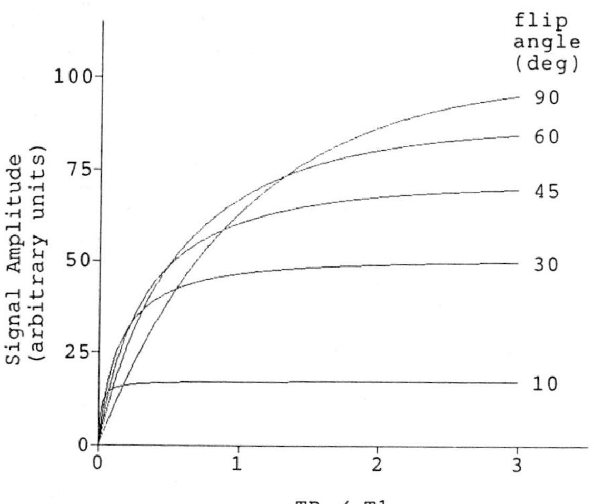

Figure 39–15. Plot of steady-state signal as a function of the TR/T_1 ratio for various flip angles.

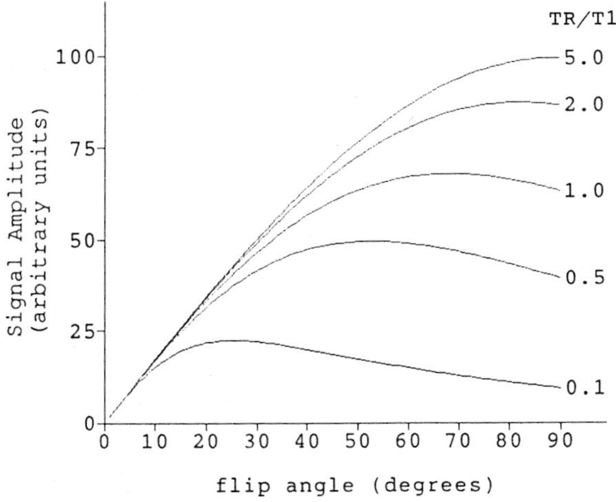

Figure 39–17. Plot of steady-state signal as a function of flip angle for various TR/T_1 ratios. Note that there is an optimum flip angle that gives the maximum signal depending on the TR/T_1 ratio.

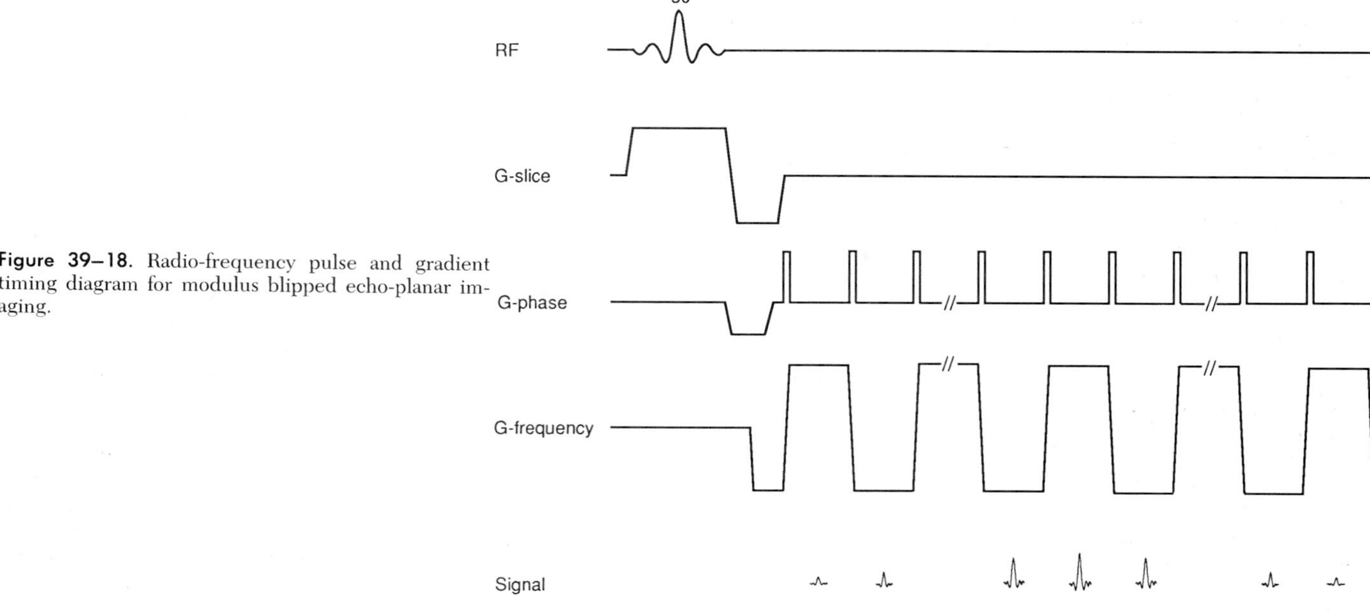

Figure 39–18. Radio-frequency pulse and gradient timing diagram for modulus blipped echo-planar imaging.

ingly lowered. However, Figure 39–15 also indicates that at very small TR/T_1 ratios the loss in signal amplitude can be partially compensated by using flip angles less than 90 degrees. This situation arises when a large steady-state longitudinal magnetization rotated by a small angle (i.e., use of low-flip-angle pulses) creates a transverse magnetization component that is larger than that produced by a small steady-state magnetization rotated by a large angle (i.e., use of high-flip-angle pulses) (see Fig. 39–16).

The signal gained by making the flip angle less than 90 degrees is better illustrated by plotting the data in Figure 39–15 as a function of flip angle for different TR/T_1 ratios (Fig. 39–17). Figure 39–17 indicates that when TR is reduced compared to T_1, the maximum signal is obtained at an optimum flip angle that is determined by the TR/T_1 ratio. Hence, in the FLASH rapid imaging method, low-flip-angle pulses are employed to obtain the maximum possible signal. This ensures that images are obtained with optimum signal-to-noise ratio for the particular TR/T_1 ratio used. Since the signal enhancement provided by the use of a low flip angle does not fully compensate for the signal loss due to reduction in TR, FLASH images show reduced signal-to-noise ratios compared to their long-TR, large-flip-angle counterparts. Hence, in FLASH imaging the signal-to-noise ratio is traded in favor of reduced imaging time.

Several versions of fast imaging based on gradient echoes, short TR times, and reduced flip angles have emerged in the last few years. An overview of these methods can be found in a recent article.[V1]

An imaging technique that is capable of producing images in a fraction of a second is the echo-planar method.[M1] In this method, the NMR signal is recalled several times following a single radio-frequency pulse in the form of an echo train. Each echo in the train is encoded differently so that all the information necessary to reconstruct the image is obtained in a single sequence. This is in contrast to the spin-warp technique, where the echoes are induced by successive application of radio-frequency pulses. Hence in the echo-planar method the total imaging time is reduced to the time required to obtain the echo train, which is on the order of 50 to 100 msec.

One variation of the echo-planar technique, referred to as the modulus blipped echo-planar method,[S1] is shown in Figure 39–18. Here, following slice selection, a rapidly inverted gradient is used to create a series of gradient echoes. Since the echoes are formed under the influence of G-frequency, the frequency content in each echo represents the spatial information along the direction of G-frequency. Spatial information along a second axis is incorporated into the phase of the echoes by sudden application of G-phase for a short time whenever G-frequency is reversed. Successive echoes are phase-encoded differently, since the action of G-phase blips is cumulative. Thus the echo train obtained is analogous to the series of phase-modulated echoes produced in the spin-warp method, and the desired image can be reconstructed by two-dimensional Fourier transformation.

Echo-planar imaging places considerable demands on gradient hardware, but recent developments in gradient coil designs have helped to alleviate some problems. The ultrahigh imaging speed offered by the echo-planar method effectively "freezes" the motion during imaging. This makes the method suitable for cardiac studies, and its successful application to produce "movie" images of the heart with adequate resolution has been demonstrated recently.[R1, S1]

CONCLUSION

In this chapter we have reviewed the basic principles of magnetic resonance imaging. It is clear that numerous parameters can be varied to emphasize the biologic properties of interest. There are innumerable trade-offs; for instance, the strongest magnetic resonance signals are obtained with minimal relaxation effects but differences between tissues are more dependent on relaxation times than nuclear spin density, image resolution is best when the temporal resolution is poorest, and so forth. No other imaging technology offers the choices and consequences of parameter selection. Thus it is necessary for the skilled investigator to combine instrumentation with applied biology in order to pose and answer the questions about the role of MRI in cardiac imaging.

Acknowledgment

We wish to thank Dr. V. Rajanayagam for his comments and criticism of the manuscript.

References

B

1. Bottemley, P. A.: NMR imaging techniques and applications. Rev. Sci. Instrum. 53:1319, 1982.

C

1. Crooks, L. E., Arakawa, M., Hoenninger, J., et al.: NMR whole body imager operating at 3.5 kgauss. Radiology 143:169, 1982.

E

1. Edelstein, W. A., Hutchison, J. M. S., Johnson, G., and Redpath, T. W.: Spin warp NMR imaging and applications to human whole-body imaging. Phys. Med. Biol. 25:751, 1980.
2. Ernst, R. R.: A survey of MRI techniques. *In* Partain, C. L., Price, R. R., Patton, J. A., et al. (eds.): MR Imaging. Volume I—Clinical Principles, 2nd ed., Chap. 3. W. B. Saunders, Philadelphia, 1988.

F

1. Frahm, J., Hanicke, W., and Merboldt, K.-D.: Transverse coherence in rapid FLASH NMR imaging. J. Magn. Reson. 72:307, 1987.

H

1. Hasse, A., Frahm, J., Matthaei, D., et al.: FLASH imaging. Rapid NMR imaging using low-angle pulses. J. Magn. Reson. 67:258, 1986.

K

1. Kumar, A., Welti, D., and Ernst, R. R.: NMR Fourier zeugmatography. J. Magn. Reson. 18:69, 1975.

L

1. Lauterbur, P. C.: Image formation by induced local interactions: Examples employing nuclear magnetic resonance. Nature (London) 242:190, 1973.

M

1. Mansfield, P., and Morris, P. G.: NMR Imaging in Biomedicine. Academic Press, New York, 1982.
2. Morris, P. G.: Nuclear Magnetic Resonance Imaging in Medicine and Biology. Oxford University Press, New York, 1986.

R

1. Rzedzian, R. R., and Pykett, I. L.: Instant images of the human heart using a new, whole body MR imaging system. Am. J. Roentgenol. 149:245, 1987.

S

1. Stehling, M. J., Howseman, A. M., Ordidge, R. J., et al.: Whole-body echo-planar MR imaging at 0.5 T. Radiology 170:257, 1989.

V

1. Van der Meulen, P., Groen, J. P., Tinus, A. M. C., and Bruntink, G.: Fast field echo imaging: An overview and contrast calculations. Magn. Reson. Imaging 6:355, 1988.

Chapter 40

Biologic Basis of Proton Relaxation

GERALD L. WOLF, Ph.D., M.D.

MR PHENOMENOLOGY 759
Proton Relaxation 759
In Vivo vs. in Vitro Measurements 760
MECHANISMS OF PROTON RELAXATION 761
The View of Koenig and Brown 761
The View of Gore 761
The View of Bottomley 761
The View of Fullerton 762
The View of Mathur-DeVre 762
MRI AND MYOCARDIAL ISCHEMIA 764
Reversible Ischemia 764
Irreversible Ischemia 764
Reperfusion 766
Early Repair 766
Late Repair 766

Nuclear magnetic resonance (NMR) techniques are assuming a steadily increasing role in clinical and investigative cardiovascular medicine. The potential applications are broad and include morphologic imaging, tissue characterization, and assessment of perfusion and metabolism. With the exception of metabolic assessment by spectroscopy, the other applications of magnetic resonance imaging to the heart are based on qualitative or quantitative assessment of regional image intensities or the calculation of estimated NMR relaxation times of myocardium. The assessment of intensity and the evaluation of relaxation times are closely related, since among the several factors affecting intensity of gated cardiac magnetic resonance images, spin-lattice (T1) and spin-spin (T2) relaxation times are of paramount importance. The factors affecting T1 and T2 in the normal and abnormal heart are not fully understood, but a literature, mainly based on in vitro NMR experiments, is beginning to explore mechanisms of proton relaxation in biologic tissue. It is probably apparent to the reader that some understanding of the concepts of the biologic mechanisms of proton relaxation are important in the knowledgeable use of magnetic resonance image intensity data in assessing the normal and abnormal heart.

MR PHENOMENOLOGY

It is simple to place myocardial tissue in a homogeneous magnetic field and perturb its macroscopic magnetization with radiofrequency (RF) pulses while recording the tissue's return to magnetic equilibrium in the form of a free induction decay, a spin-echo, or a gradient echo MR signal. The resultant signals are well-behaved mathematically, and we can apply the Bloch equations to describe the rate of nuclear relaxations. We can also use the rates, e.g., proton T1 and T2, to characterize the myocardial wall. However, the Bloch equations are purely phenomenologic and make no reference to the mechanisms of relaxation.[K1]

Tissues have been studied both in vivo and in vitro. There is extensive literature on the measurement of proton T1 and T2 under diverse conditions. Some of the observations conflict, but we should first review the relevant effects about which there is general agreement. Then we will survey valuable hypotheses about the mechanisms of proton relaxation in vivo.

Proton Relaxation

In pure water, T1 and T2 are long and equal, with a value of about 3600 mS at 37°C, and the relaxation rate is not dependent upon the field strength or Larmor frequency of the MR instrument. As the sample temperature is reduced, its protons relax more rapidly, i.e., 1/T1 or R1 increase. As the liquid begins to freeze, T1 becomes very long (>10,000 mS) and T2 becomes very short (<20 mS). Scientists have many arguments about whether water in tissue is different from pure water in its behavior, and the same argument extends to interpretation of proton relaxation in tissue.

In biologic tissues with temperatures of 25 to 37°C, the measured proton signal comes primarily from liquid water and fat, and we find that T1 is shorter and T2 is much shorter than in pure water. Table 40–1 gives representative proton relaxation properties for structures comprising the heart. In general, proton relaxation times are tissue specific. This is what provides MRI with its striking tissue contrast. There is surprisingly little variation across species.[B1] Embryonal tissues or those with less anatomic structure on histologic specimens will usually have a longer T1 and T2 than more differentiated or more histologically complicated tissues.

Tissue water proton T1 varies with the strength of the magnetic field and the Larmor frequency, with relaxation time longer and relaxation rate slower at higher field. Proton T2 for tissue water and both proton relaxation rates for fat are only weakly dependent upon field. The variation of T1 with field is called dispersion, and the general form of this dispersion for tissues of interest is shown in Figure 40–1.

In all tissues, there is a tendency for water content, T1, and T2 to be correlated and to change in the same direction when the tissues are altered, but the changes are not proportional and often the relation differs between tissues.[B2, F3,4, I1, M1, R1] Thus, one cannot predict T1 or T2 from water content unless the tissue type is known, and even then accuracy is poor. The tissue component that affects relaxation most is protein (or other hydrophilic macromolecules with lots of protons), but the amounts of all proteins and their individual effects upon proton relaxation do not appear to account for much more than 50 percent of the observed relaxation.

Table 40–1. PROTON RELAXATION PROPERTIES OF CARDIAC STRUCTURES*

	T1	T2
Myocardium	870	57
Adipose	260	84
Blood	830	160
Valves and fibrous pericardium	200	22

*Approximate mean value at 60 MHz and 37°C.

T1 of water protons is usually found to be a single exponential, indicating that proton relaxation is averaged over typical T1 times. If water mixes only by diffusion, then the distance a water molecule can travel in the time equal to T1 (where T1 = 700 mS) is about 22 microns ($r = \sqrt{6Dt}$), where r is the radius of the sphere explored by a diffusing water molecule, D is the self-diffusion coefficient, and t is the diffusion time; in tissue, D is about 1.1×10^5 cm/sec). As most cells have a radius of 4 to 10 microns, water can diffuse through several cells in one T1.

When appropriate techniques are used, T2 often has more than one exponential relaxation, with an average T2 in myocardium of about 60 mS. The same calculation yields a diffusion radius of about 3 microns and a sphere of influence somewhat smaller than most cells. In vivo, perfusion adds to mixing, and the magnitude of this effect is similar to diffusion. Each myocardial cell abuts 2 to 4 capillaries, and perfusion rate varies with functional requirements; thus perfusion mixes protons best in the capillary, less in the extracellular fluid, and has not yet been measured inside the cell.

Fat protons have a different resonant frequency (chemical shift) than water protons and there is little exchange of protons between water and the hydrophobic lipids. Proton exchange with hydrophilic substances, especially proteins, is much more common. In the process of proton exchange, the spins are also exchanged. This provides the nucleus with an opportunity to transfer its spin within the molecule to other nuclei and facilitates cross-relaxation.

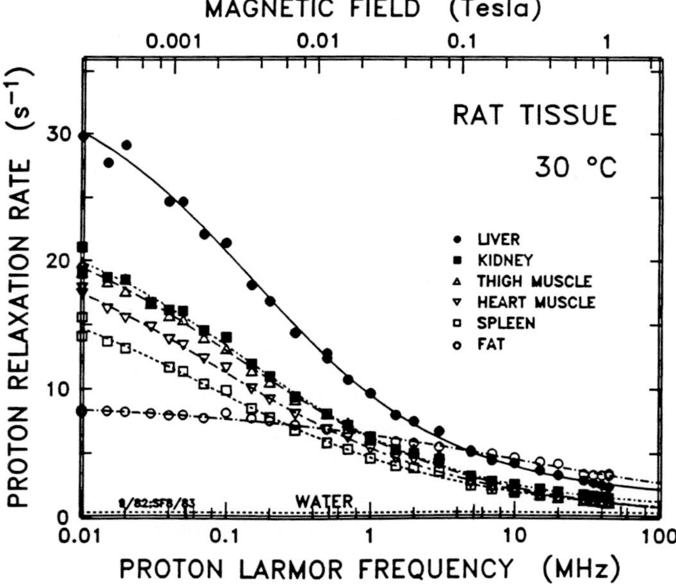

Figure 40–1. Change of proton relaxation rate with frequency; the dispersion of relaxation rate (1/T1) versus the Larmor frequency of the proton in fresh rat tissue studied at 30°C. Imaging frequencies range from 5 to 85 MHz with magnetic field strengths of 0.12 to 2.0 Tesla. The relaxation of fat slows minimally as field increases, but macromolecular-water proton interactions cause other soft tissue to have a stronger field dependent relaxation. (Courtesy of S. Koenig and R. D. Brown, III.)

In Vivo Versus in Vitro Measurements

Tissue samples can be placed in small-bore magnets where homogeneity is high, the coil has better geometry and faster response times, and the amplifiers that produce and detect RF signals have fewer limitations. Thus, in vitro it is possible to use many more pulses, carefully tune the resonance and flip angles, utilize a wide spectrum of interpulse times, and obtain many more data points to derive the value of the T1 and T2 exponents.[B1, D1, E2, F1, M1] In vitro measurements are usually made more accurately, especially if done at physiologic temperature. The very short interpulse times obtained on instruments available for in vitro measurements may report different relaxation values if there is more than one relaxation exponent owing to different relaxation processes or tissue compartments. The biologic problems of in vitro analysis could also be important.[B3, E2] Clearly, metabolism is affected early, along with macromolecular synthesis; this could cause tissue breakdown and cell swelling in vitro, and each process could have a different time course. Studies to date suggest that T1 is not rapidly altered, and, because T1 averages over regions greater than cells, it is not likely to be responsive to water movements between cell compartments. Thus, in vitro T1 measurements, when properly performed, probably accurately reflect in vivo T1. T2 changes could happen earlier and can be more severe, but fewer studies are available. There is evidence for multicomponent T2 relaxation, and the shorter T2 provides less time for averaging and more sensitivity to proton compartmentalization in vivo. For the most part, tissue localization is not used in vitro except by selecting the tissue sample of interest. Finally, in vitro tissue lacks macroscopic motion that may significantly alter MR signal intensity in vivo. For the myocardium, in vivo motion includes tissue perfusion and the effects of contraction, respiration, and complicated blood motion in large vessels.

In vivo measures of proton relaxation are of greater interest to clinicians and applied biologists. If accurate, the advantages would be enormous. The MR signal is obtained noninvasively and nondestructively so patient acceptance is high, and the incredible variety of clinical disease provides a large range of tissue variation. Since the measurements can be made from images, localization methods allow for heterogeneous processes, and the natural response or effects of intervention can be serially studied. However, MR signal is quite sensitive to motion, and the influence of motion is at times the parameter of interest. In order for T1 or T2 to be calculated in vivo, the motion effect must be measured, estimated, or eliminated.

Thus, there are also major technical problems with accurate measurement of tissue relaxation in vivo.[B2, C1, G1, H1, K5, M1,4,5, R2, W1,2, Y1,2] Imaging magnets are very large and usually less homogeneous than in vitro spectrometers. Their RF power requirements for perturbing the protons are huge, field gradients are produced both intentionally and unintentionally, and the detection of a complete free induction decay (FID) is impossible. Signal must be obtained with gradient echos or spin-echos. The former are affected by the inhomogeneous distribution of magnetic susceptibility in tissue. Spin-echos require very precise 90° and 180° pulses, and the flip angles actually achieved are neither accurate nor perfect within any voxel. Thus, one tissue slice often receives an attenuated pulse from the one intended for an adjacent slice. This clearly would excite some protons and alter their measured relaxation time.

Many fewer pulses are used for in vivo relaxation measurement and thus fitting the exponential relaxations is usually done with only two points for T1 and two to four points for T2. The actual input information is signal intensity, which is inherently noisy. The relation between signal intensity and relaxation has numerous parameters, and some are unmeasured (see equation 43–7). The influence of motion is usually not measured and must appear as an altered value for either T1 or T2. Many hundreds of pulses—usually two sequences with 128 pulse sets each—and many minutes of magnet time are required, but the equation assumes that none of the variables change over this time, i.e., motion, proton density, T1, T2, TR, TE, and flip angle, and that each different tissue continues to be in the same voxel. To reduce cardiac motion and control cycle-dependent perfusion, the data collection can be gated to heart rate, but this usually leads to variable repetition times with potentially large effects that are erroneously attributed to T1 or T2 by the "image algebra": when one solves the equation relating image intensity to T1, T2, TR, and TE (see Chapter 43).

Many of these problems can be reduced by normalizing the data, comparing relative changes, or using standards within the imaging field to compensate for machine variables.

In vivo methods remain frequency- and temperature-dependent and are very sensitive to the actual implementation on a particular device. These many problems are increasingly recognized, and recent reports of in vivo measurements of tissue T1 and T2 are much more credible. Careful readers need to pay attention to the methods that are used, and investigators need to report more details about the accuracy and limitation of their estimates of T1 and T2. Currently, in vitro values of T1 and T2 are probably more accurate when performed on fresh tissues with proper preparation and precautions.

MECHANISMS OF PROTON RELAXATION

A single proton in the high energy spin state precessing with its magnetic moment antiparallel to a strong magnetic field would have a relaxation time measured in years. This state is thus fairly stable unless an effective perturbation "stimulates" relaxation. In liquids, the perturbing influence is the magnetic field of another nucleus. The magnetic fields must "couple"—this requires that the two nuclear dipoles are close together and have the same frequency (Table 40–2). At imaging fields of 0.15 to 1.5 T, proton magnetic fields are weak, and the two nuclei must be within a few angstroms of each other. The fields interact more effectively if they have the same (or a multiple) frequency, and this interaction must occur over several thousand cycles of rotation for there to be a finite probability of an effective perturbation.

In water, the protons are precessing at the Larmor frequency but also tumbling rapidly. This causes the protons to move relative to each other and, when directly aligned with the B^o field, the small magnetic fields add (for one proton on water) or subtract (for the other proton) from the other. At all other angles the effect is intermediate. As the water molecules are tumbling randomly over all frequencies up to a maximum (determined by the sample temperature), the proton is experiencing a perturbing magnetic field from its water partner (usually the closest adjacent proton), but only a few are tumbling at the Larmor frequency at which magnetic field coupling is efficient. Further, in periods as short as a picosecond, the tumbling rate can change. Thus, despite the presence of large numbers of closely adjacent protons in water—11 percent protons by weight, 50 M in concentration—the close encounters don't last long enough or have the right frequency, so both T1 and T2 are relatively slow, about 3600 mS.

In ice, the water molecules are fixed and the effect of rotation goes away, causing T1 to become long because the perturbations are not sufficient to allow the proton to give up its antiparallel orientation and return to the base or equilibrium state. However, even fixed protons can get out of phase with each other. This would first happen if the main magnetic field or tissue inhomogeneities were as large as 10 gauss in a 10,000 gauss (1 Tesla) field. Under these conditions, one proton would get out of phase with another within 12 microseconds. As the protons move, they would actually average the inhomogeneities, and T2 would approach T1, in the absence of any other dephasing mechanisms.

Table 40–2. REQUIREMENTS FOR STIMULATED NUCLEAR RELAXATION

- Close encounter with another magnetic field
  (< 10 Å for another proton)
- Right magnetic field
  (same frequency or a multiple)
- Adequate time for effective interaction
  (microseconds at body temperature)

When protein is added to the water, T1 shortens and T2 shortens still more. Cellular structures are more effective than protein and add tissue specificity. The mechanisms for these effects are still speculative, but it is useful to summarize major schools of thought.

The View of Koenig and Brown[K1–4]

In a time interval comparable to a relaxation time, a typical water molecule explores the intracellular and extracellular region over several cell diameters; its relaxation behavior derives from an average of millions of its encounters with tissue substance within this region. The rotation of proteins (which vary with molecular weight, shape, solvent viscosity, temperature, and protein-protein interactions) and protein concentration account for increased 1/T1 of protein solutions as well as their frequency dependence (see Figure 40–1). Some of T2 is due to the same process, but the rest is spin-spin exchanges that do not dissipate energy but do result in loss of phase coherence between spins. The former shows field dependence, but the latter does not. Spins can be exchanged with protons on protein, facilitating cross-relaxation. Spins transferred to the protein are probably relaxed by efficient magnetic field interactions with other protons or other nuclei. Protein enhancement of relaxation is also due to protons slowing their motion to rotate with proteins or by proton exchange. The protons may not spend very long in rotating with the protein, but with millions of encounters the effect is cumulative and averaged. Dr. Koenig is quick to point out that he is *describing* relaxation rather than attributing causation.

The View of Gore and Associates[G1,2]

Detailed interactions governing relaxation in heterogeneous tissues are either not well understood or are quantified with poor precision. It is clear that T1 and T2 are dependent on the percentage composition of water and protein, with cross-relaxation being the dominant process. Within normal tissues, no significant correlations are found between the changes in mean water content and the mean T1, although in heart the water content was correlated with T2. Significant alterations can occur in relaxation without changes in the water content. There is no correlation between relaxation and molecular weight for nine proteins from 10,000 to 150,000 molecular weight, and the value of relaxivity for protein solutions is too low to account for all tissue relaxation. Gore's opinion is that a myriad of small independent factors may each contribute to the overall relaxation process in tissue.

The View of Bottomley and Associates[B1]

All the semiempirical models relating the change in T1 to frequency are multiparametric; usually more than five variables are used to describe a relation that is apparently continuous, monotonic, and slowly varying. Given enough variables, any relation can be fitted with numerous equations. However, an excellent fit does not imply that all or some of the variables have biologic equivalents. The data are also well fit by a simple equation:

$$T1 = AD^B$$

where A and B are tissue specific and D is frequency in Hz.

Estimates of the relative importance of intramolecular and intermolecular interactions to theories of bound water are ambiguous. Effective interaction between macromolecules and water is influenced by the rates of translational and rotational motion and this interaction occurs in the first hydration layer, but the two processes have similar magnitudes and could be indistinguishable.

Like T1, T2 relaxation processes arise from fluctuations in the transverse field that occur at the resonance frequency and at twice this frequency, but T2 also is responsive to static changes in the longitudinal field. Where T2 is much less than T1, this factor also reduces the frequency dependence of T2. T2 is especially sensitive to the local static field inhomogeneity at the exchange interface whereas T1 is much less sensitive to this influence. Thus, microscopic field inhomogeneity adjacent to macromolecules is a likely explanation why T2 is less than T1 in tissue. The evidence for multicomponent relaxation times for T2 is more compelling than for T1. Nonetheless, tissue samples containing mixtures of adipose and nonfat soft tissue will have multicomponent T1 and T2 relaxations as each proton environment behaves independently.

Bottomley tentatively models the biologic case as shown in Figure 40–2. This model behaves as though water had two states, loosely described as bound and free, with fast exchange between the two states: FETS (fast exchange, two-state). In the free phase, water interactions are too fast to cause frequency dependence, and T1 is long (more than 1700 mS). The bound phase is a single layer of water with very brief residence time (about 10 μsec), but faster relaxation of both T1 and T2 is facilitated by intermolecular reactions involving mainly macromolecular hydrogen. This relaxation becomes frequency-dependent owing to the slower motion of the macromolecule. As the water crosses the exchange boundary between free and bound, the low frequency and static components encountered cause dephasing, i.e., a nonenergetic spin-spin process that shortens T2. As the macromolecular environment of each tissue is tissue-specific, so also are T1 and T2. However, the T1 process is averaged over a few cells, whereas T2 has components that reflect a short-range structure of tissue.

The View of Fullerton and Associates[F1–3]

It is clear that widely varying water and macromolecular contents exist in different cell compartments with different inherent relaxations in each location. T1 (spin-lattice relaxation) is a complex reflection of the motional properties of all molecules in solution that contain proton magnetic dipoles. There is an additional term in the expression for T2 (spin-spin relaxation), owing to the anisotropic motion (asymmetric tumbling) that shortens T2 relative to T1.

Dr. Fullerton prefers a three-state hydration model:

1. bulk water	T1 = T2 and long
2. structured water	T1 > T2 and intermediate
3. bound water	T1 and T2 very short

Structured water is influenced by the motion of macromolecules but lacks the hydrogen bonds that allow cross-relaxation of bound water (Fig. 40–3). This model creates five independent parameters: the ratio of each water fraction and the two exchange rates: bulk ↔ structured ↔ bound. In addition, each protein class could have different effects upon relaxation of structured water and bound water and the exchange rate between the two.

Fullerton summarizes the fundamental MRI contrast parameters on a molecular level as:

1. *Water content.* Relaxation rates are generally a linear function of the solute/water ratio, and this is a primary factor for differences between tissue.
2. *Perturbed water motion.* Varying ability of substituent macromolecules to bind and structure water is the second most important tissue characteristic.
3. *Macromolecular motion.* In tissues, slow motion that is most effective at imaging fields is controlled by pH, electrolyte concentrations, other solutes, and macromolecular hydration and aggregation.
4. *Lipid content.* This fraction does not exchange and does not influence water relaxation but does contribute to measurements of overall tissue relaxation unless special techniques are used.
5. *Paramagnetic species.* Tissues may have paramagnetic elements that alter relaxation. This is the least important general mechanism, but may be important in some tissues, especially during oxidation of hemoglobin.

The View of Mathur-DeVre[M1–3]

Most biologic systems contain 70 to 90 percent of water, distributed as intra- or extracellular water. Usually the fraction

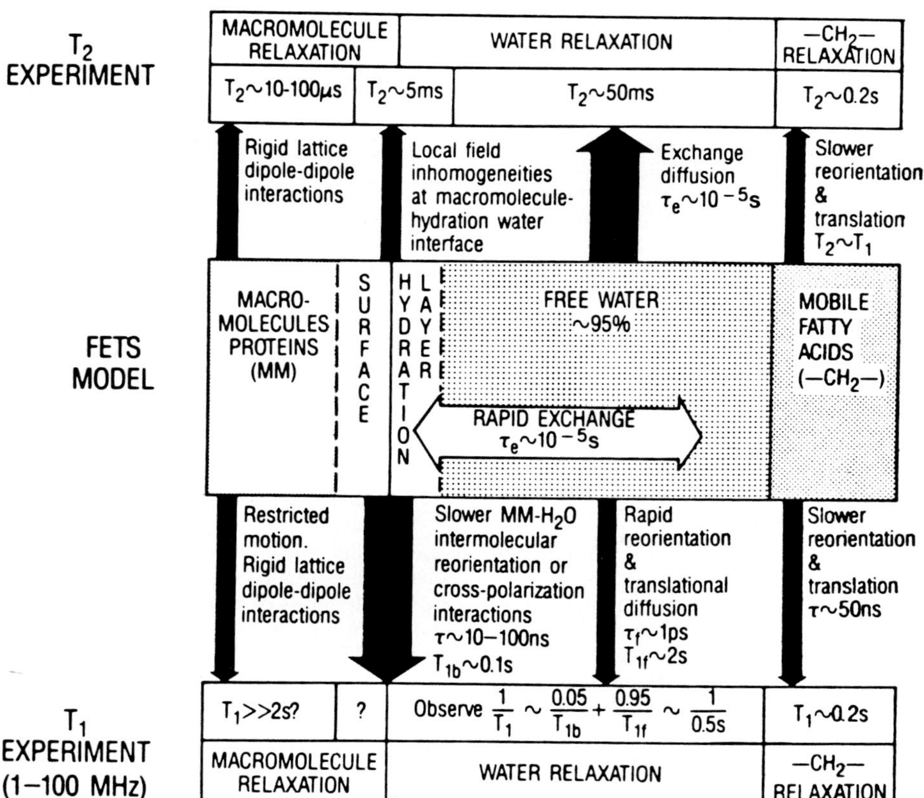

Figure 40–2. The mechanism of proton relaxation in tissue as perceived by Bottomley. The FETS model is assumed. Three chemically different proton species are identified horizontally: macromolecular protons excluding mobile fatty acids, water protons, and mobile fatty acids, denoted –CH_2–. These protons exist in up to five phases, depicted at center. The relaxation in each phase is represented by solid arrows, with the relative effectiveness indicated by the width of the arrows. (From Bottomley, P. A.: Frequency dependence of tissue relaxation times. *In* Partain, C. L., Price, R. R., Patton, J. A., et al. (eds.): Magnetic Resonance Imaging. W. B. Saunders, Philadelphia, 1988, p. 1075.)

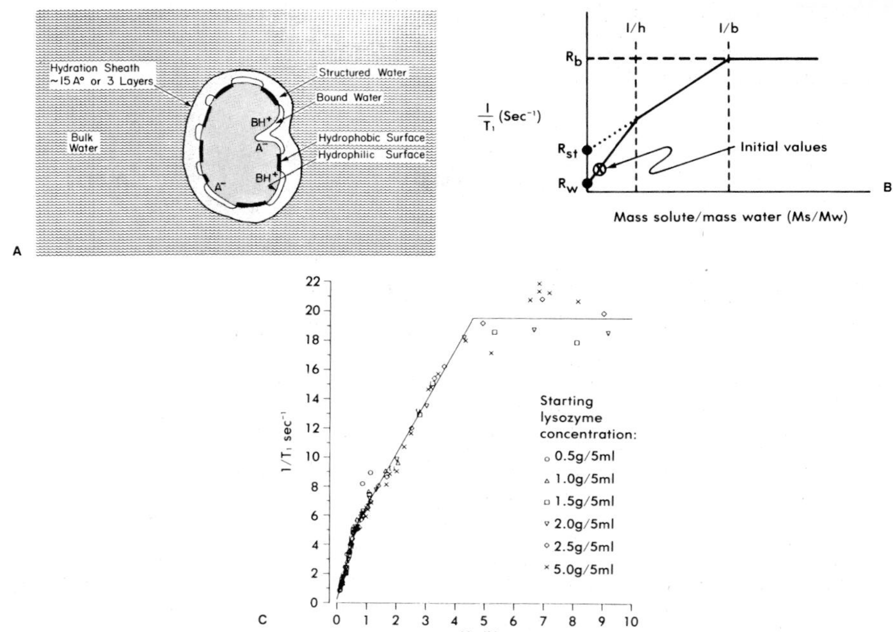

Figure 40–3. The states of water in tissue and the T1 relaxation in the various compartments, as viewed by Fullerton. *A*, Schematic representation of bound, structured, and bulk phase water on a globular protein. *B*, The change in relaxation rate (1/T1) as water is removed from a hypothetic tissue by dehydration. The water is first removed from bulk water, then from structured water, and last from bound water fractions. The slow relaxation of bulk water is extrapolated to the intercept; the break points are assumed to define the relaxation of structured water (1/h) and bound water (1/b). *C*, An actual titration of lysozyme in which concentration and percentage of water are varied. (From Fullerton, G. E.: Physiological basis of magnetic relaxation. *In* Stark, D. D., and Bradley, W. G. Jr. (eds.): Magnetic Resonance Imaging. C. V. Mosby, St. Louis, 1988, p. 36.)

of extracellular water is higher for neonates than for adults, probably because maturation increases cellular macromolecules at the expense of tissue water. Tissue relaxation properties are largely due to specific interactions between water and various charged and polar groups of biologic macromolecules. These interactions result in a dynamically structured water that extends over one to three layers. The hydration water maintains the structural and conformational integrity of the biostructure and represents a substantial part of intracellular water.

Individual soft tissues have a unique protein water composition, giving rise to local macroscopic heterogeneity. The state of water in cells and tissues is readily but nonselectively perturbed by many normal and abnormal biologic processes. Large variations in T1 are observed for tissues exhibiting small changes in water content, but this has little effect on T2 values. The NMR parameters obtained in vivo are likely to be more tissue-specific since they reflect the living state, but in vitro measures provide more reliable T1 and T2 in practice, and similar trends are observed although in vivo relaxation times are higher. This investigator stresses the artifacts that may alter relaxation times in vitro (Fig. 40–4).

SUMMARY. There is general agreement that protons relax faster in biologic tissues with T1 greater than T2 but shorter than that of water. Nearly all agree that this difference is due to an interaction between macromolecules and water and that the tissue specificity comes from the tissue differences in macromolecular composition and organization. Some expect that T2 changes will be most indicative of tissue alteration,[B2] whereas others predict that T1 will be more sensitive.[M1] There is clear conflict between Gore and Koenig about the quantitative influence of macromolecular size. Most are quick to admit that their models are speculative. The limitations of data from normal myocardium and myocardial ischemia derived from in vitro and in vivo experiments are a continuing concern.

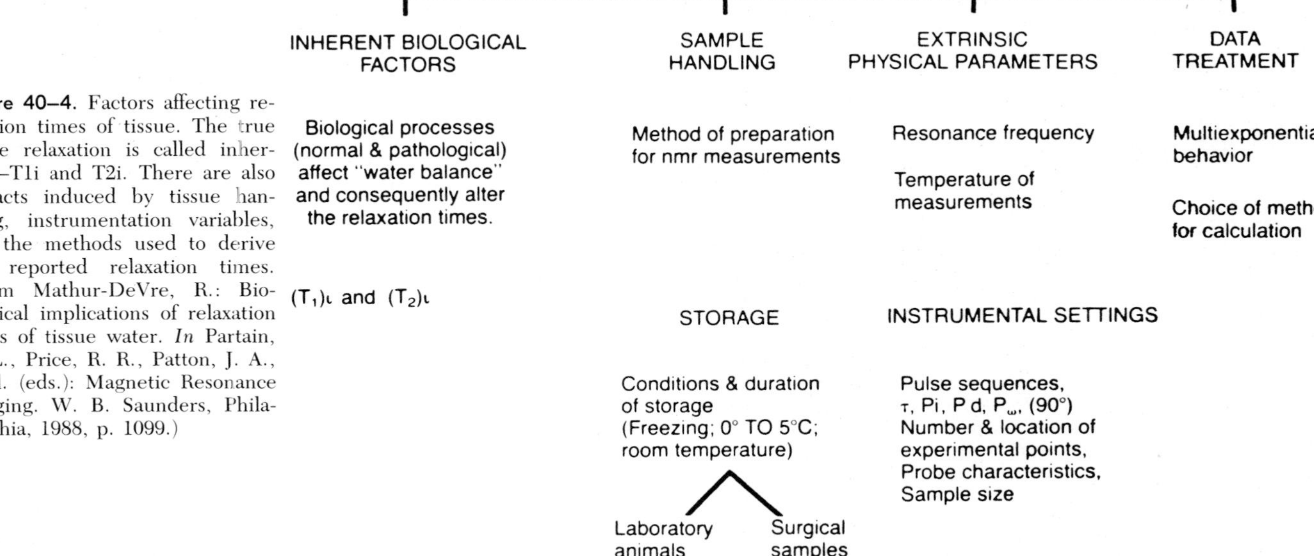

Figure 40–4. Factors affecting relaxation times of tissue. The true tissue relaxation is called inherent—T1i and T2i. There are also artifacts induced by tissue handling, instrumentation variables, and the methods used to derive the reported relaxation times. (From Mathur-DeVre, R.: Biomedical implications of relaxation times of tissue water. *In* Partain, C. L., Price, R. R., Patton, J. A., et al. (eds.): Magnetic Resonance Imaging. W. B. Saunders, Philadelphia, 1988, p. 1099.)

Table 40–3. SUMMARY OF EXPECTED CHANGES IN CARDIAC IMAGES BY STAGE OF MYOCARDIAL ISCHEMIA

	Myocardial Cells	Perfusion	Contractility	Net Imaging Effect
Reversible Ischemia	Mild swelling p ↑, T2 ↑	1. Decreased T2 ↑ 2. Deoxy HB T2 ↓	Decreased T2 ↑ S/N ↑	I slightly ↑
Irreversible Ischemia	1. More swelling p ↑ ↑, T1 ↑, T2 ↑ ↑ 2. Molecular breakdown and release T1 ↓, T2 ↓		Absent T2 ↑ S/N ↑	I ↑ ↑
Reperfusion	Explosive cell swelling p ↑ ↑ ↑, T1 ↑, T2 ↑ ↑ ↑	1. Hypoperfusion T2 ↑ 2. Hyperperfusion T2 ↓	Variable	I ↑ ↑ ↑
Repair				
Early	Granulation tissue p ↑, T1 ↑, T2 sl ↑	Subacute hemorrhage T1 ↓ ↓, T2 ↓	Hypokinetic	I ↑
Late	Scar p ↓, T1 sl ↓, T2 ↓	± Hemosiderin T2 ↓ ↓ ↓		I ↓

p = proton density; I = image intensity; S/N = signal/noise.

MRI AND MYOCARDIAL ISCHEMIA

Given the range of opinion among physicists about methods and measured T1 and T2 values, there should be great caution in biologic interpretations of experimental data. Nonetheless, it is difficult to avoid forming working hypotheses for heuristic purposes, and thus I will offer my own view of the changes in myocardial image intensity in response to ischemia. The histopathologic scheme of Jennings and colleagues has been used to derive the material summarized in Table 40–3 and Figure 40–5.[J1] The reader is duly warned that the actual model and experimental methods used to create myocardial pathology will probably strongly influence the NMR result.

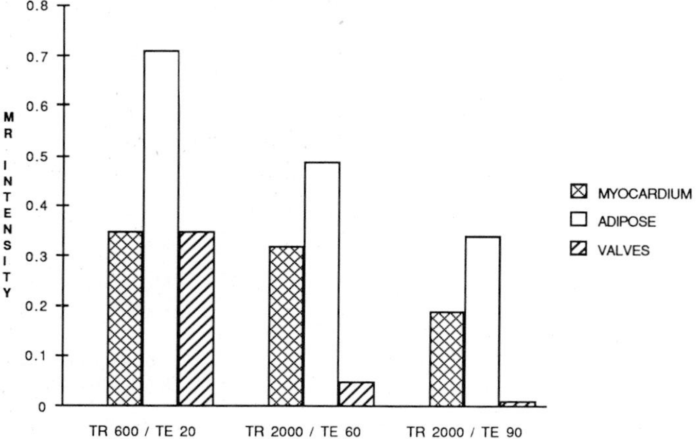

Figure 40–5. Relative MR signal intensity of cardiac structures. To illustrate the interaction of tissue T1 and T2 with the instrument variables TR and TE, we ignore the influence of motion and utilize equation 42–7. For a T1-weighted spin-echo image, we use TR600, TE20; for a mildly T2-weighted image, TR2000, TE60; and for a heavily T2-weighted image, TR2000, TE90. The relaxation values shown in Table 40–2 are utilized. Note that all signals decrease as TE becomes longer, but fat is affected least and tissues such as cardiac valves and the fibrous pericardium are affected most. The relative signal differences for these three structures are greatest on the TR2000, TE90 image, but absolute signal intensity is poorest.

Reversible Ischemia

Early in ischemia there is mild swelling of cells, reduced tissue perfusion, and reduced contractility (Fig. 40–6 *A* and *B*). These cellular changes are expected to cause minor increases in proton density and lengthen T2; both these effects would increase regional MR signal intensity—especially with T2-weighted images. However, rapid deoxygenation would reduce T2 in the tissue blood spaces,[G4] while reduced perfusion would tend to increase T2 owing to reduced motion within the imaging gradients. Reduced contractility should reduce signal artifact and may also reduce the motion-induced shortening of apparent T2 (Table 40–3). The latter will be affected by the use of gating and special pulses to eliminate signal artifacts from flow and out of slice motion. With gated images, the irregular TR times must be taken into account if there are changes in cardiac rhythm. This is because each actual TR influences image intensity in a nonlinear fashion that precludes the use of average TR for image estimation.

Without an MR contrast agent, it seems unlikely that changes observed in reversible ischemia can be assigned to the minimal alteration in relaxation times of myocardial cells. However, most calculations force all the foregoing changes in regional signal intensity to be attributed to T1 and/or T2.

Irreversible Ischemia

This process is signaled by more swelling and the breakdown of macromolecules, along with release of enzymes and increased permeability of the cell membrane (Fig. 40–6*C*). The necrosis occurs as a wave, with considerable spatial, temporal, and species variation. In humans, the pre-existing coronary collateral circulation, the presence of hypertrophy, and adaptation to earlier ischemic events will have an effect. Perfusion and contractility effects are predicted to be similar to the previous stage, but irregular heart beat and therapeutic intervention are more likely to be confounding influences.

In careful studies, this pathologic process should be detectable in myocardial relaxation times or relative signal intensities.[H2] There is a danger that myocardial edema will produce the same signal change over a region larger than the actual zone of irreversible ischemia (Table 40–3). Myocardial wall motion studies, serial MRI studies, and MR contrast agents could be helpful in this setting. Although the change in cell permeability per se

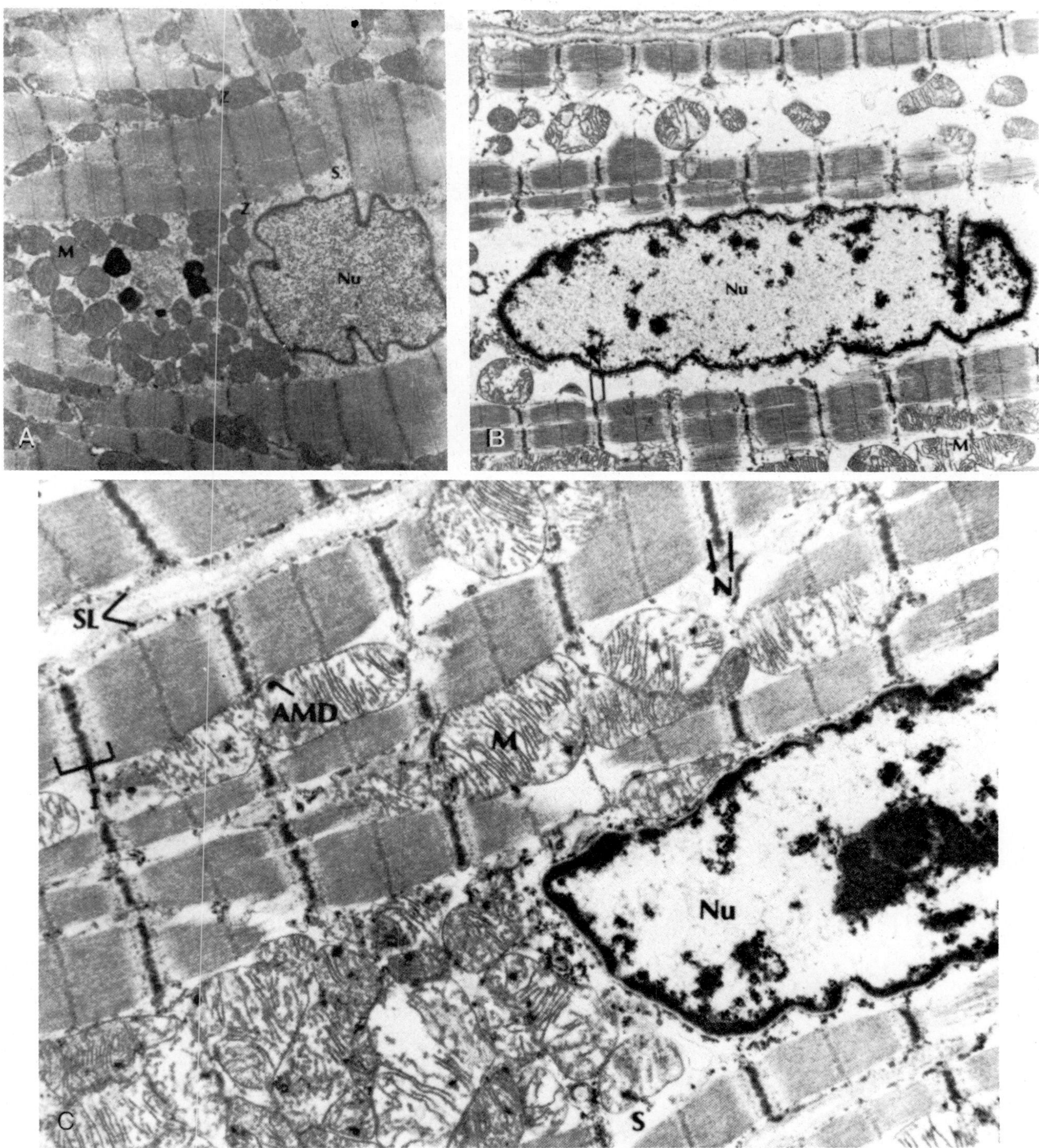

Figure 40–6. Change in myocyte ultrastructure with myocardial ischemia. *A*, Normal structure, where the nucleus (Nu) is finely granular and mitochondria (M) have a consistent size. *B*, After 15 minutes of ischemia, the myocytes are reversibly injured. Nuclear chromatin is marginated and the mitochondrion is swollen. The sarcoplasm is clearer because of cellular edema and the loss of glycogen. *C*, At 40 minutes of ischemia, the damage is irreversible. All mitochondria are greatly swollen, and the sarcoplasm is clear. The plasma membrane of the sarcolemma (SL) is intact here but occasionally disrupted in other sections.

Illustration continued on following page

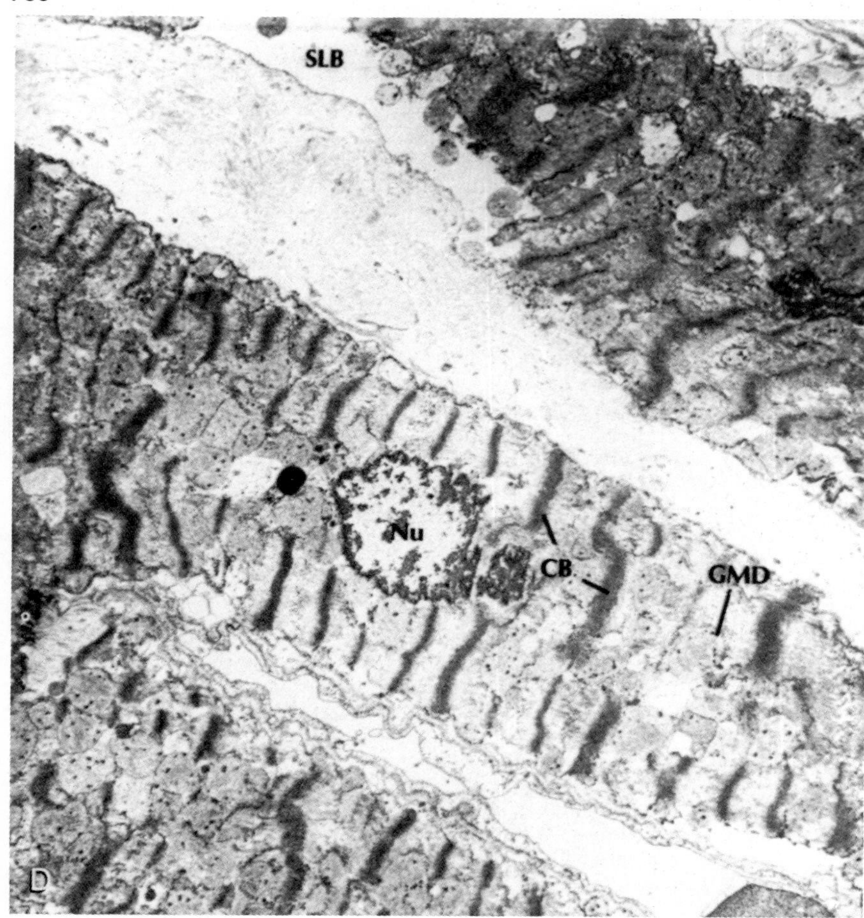

Figure 40–6 *Continued D,* Reperfusion of myocardium accelerates ultrastructural disintegration of myocytes. The myocytes swell explosively; subsarcolemmal blebs (SLB) of edema fluid are a striking feature, and damage to the plasma membrane is severe. (From Jennings, R. B., and Reimer, K. A.: Pathobiology of acute myocardial ischemia. Hosp. Pract. Jan, 15:89, 1989.)

will not affect either T1 (water is already moving freely through this region) or T2 (responsive to macromolecular breakdown and increased water content due to osmotic factors), extracellular contrast agents will now have a larger distribution volume, as does inulin[J2] and this will change washin and washout pharmacokinetics.

Reperfusion

The explosive cell swelling upon reperfusion[S1] (Fig. 40–6*D*; Table 40–3) is expected to lead to large changes in proton spin density, T2, and T1. However, the first two increase MR signal intensity and the last decreases it. The relative effect of the changes in the two relaxation parameters will be sensitive to the actual imaging sequence used. Some tissues may have a further reduction in perfusion because of myocardial edema, while other tissue zones may have hyperperfusion. The contractility response is variable and may not be immediate. Arrhythmias are more likely to impair the relation between MR signal and myocardial relaxation times.

MR signal intensity should increase still further on reperfusion, but the difference between irreversible ischemia and reperfused myocardium may be small or nonspecific, unless serial studies are available to document a change within a particular region.

Early Repair

At the cellular level, granulation tissue has more intracellular and extracellular water and less macromolecular content than normal cells. On T2-weighted images, signal intensity will probably scale as normal < early repair < irreversible ischemia < reperfusion. For T1-weighted images, the differentiation could be much less clear. Biologic variability is the enemy, and serial imaging with careful clinical correlation is a partial defense. In this setting of early repair, the influence of hemorrhage is an important variable since methemoglobin[G4] is a paramagnetic product and a good relaxing agent for protons (Fig. 40–7).

Late Repair

As the edema resolves, the three NMR proton parameters also decline. Scar tissue has low proton density and short T2, which reduces expected myocardial MR signal intensity still further. MR signal returns toward normal levels and may, in dense scar, become hypointense. If hemorrhage has occurred in the acute period, it may now be in the stage of hemosiderin with very short T2.[G4]

SUMMARY. Actual experiments performed in one or more of these abnormal states are extensively reported by Wisenberg in Chapter 50. Given the complicated pathophysiology of myocardial ischemia, reperfusion, and repair, and its imperfect reflection by even skilled imaging, there is strong impetus for further study of new MR imaging techniques, as well as a need for MR contrast agents that provide new information. Both advances may work together to better characterize myocardial ischemia. When experiments on other tissues define the basic mechanisms of proton relaxation in tissues, these will also help. There may be changes in myocardial lipid or metabolites that are detectable with MR spectroscopy, and there is interest in imaging of other nuclei as well.

Despite its relatively high cost, the noninvasive, nondestructive nature of MR and its tantalizing glimpses of unique soft tissue information assure further serious study of its role in cardiac imaging.

Figure 40–7. Comparison of MRI ex vivo canine myocardial infarcts with and without hemorrhage. *A*, Twenty-four hours after an ischemic infarct without hemorrhage, the inversion recovery image shows the infarct as hypointense while the heavily T2-weighted image shows hyperintense signals. These findings principally reflect edema of the infarct with long T1 and T2. *B*, Hemorrhagic canine myocardial infarct. Now the infarct is hyperintense on the T1-weighted inversion recovery image and hypointense on the T2-weighted spin-echo image. This is due to the paramagnetic effects of subacute hemorrhage and methemoglobin formation, which decreases both T1 and T2 relative to normal myocardium. *C*, Light microscopy of hemorrhagic infarct demonstrating loss of muscle fibers with zones of hemorrhage visualized as darker areas within muscle tissue. (This figure appears in color in the color plate at the front of the text.) *D*, Three-dimensional representation of the infarct and normal myocardium, using images where the hemorrhagic infarct has stronger MR signal. (Courtesy of E. S. Goldstein, G. L. Wolf, and G. Herman.)

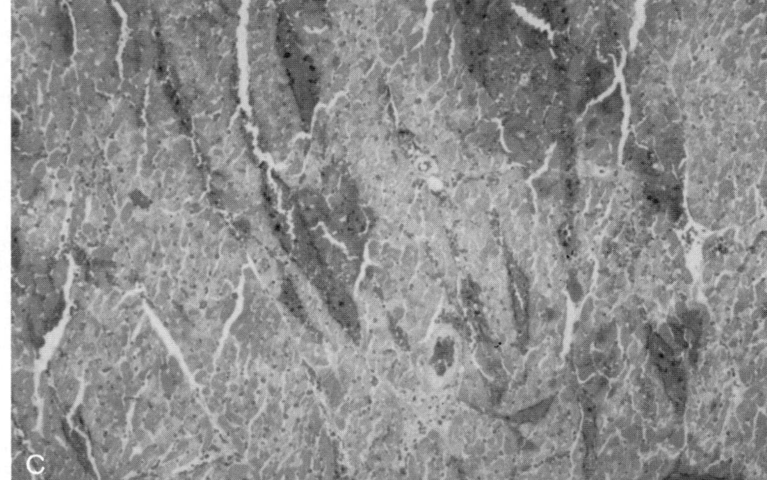

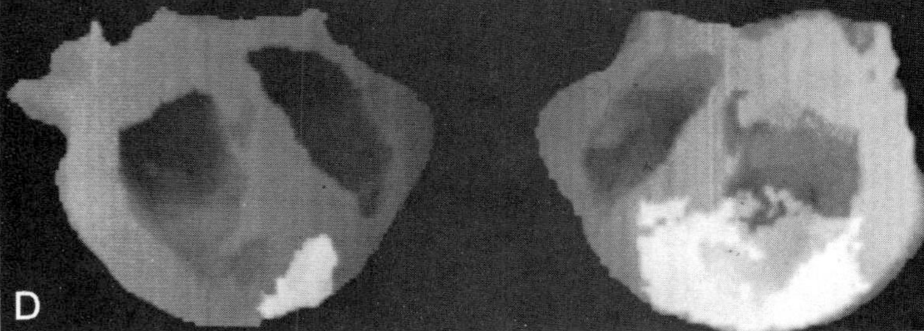

References

B

1. Bottomley, P. A., Foster, T. H., Argersinger, R. E., et al.: A review of normal tissue hydrogen NMR relaxation times and relaxation mechanisms for 1–100 MHz: Dependence on tissue type, NMR frequency, temperature, species, excision, and age. Med. Phys. 11:425, 1984.
2. Bottomley, P. A.: Frequency dependence of tissue relaxation times. *In* Partain, C. L., Price, R. R., Patton, J. A., et al. (eds.): Magnetic Resonance Imaging. W. B. Saunders, Philadelphia, 1988, p. 1075.
3. Beal, P. T.: Practical methods for biological NMR sample handling. Magn. Reson. Imag. 1:165, 1982.
4. Burnett, K. R., Wolf, G. L., and Goldstein, E. J.: NMR in vitro measurements: A quality control study of the RADX table-top spectrometer. Phys. Chem. Phys. Med. NMR 17:123, 1985.
5. Baker, D. G., Schumacher, H. R., Jr., and Wolf, G. L.: Nuclear magnetic resonance evaluation of synovial fluid and articular tissue. J. Rheumatol. 12:1062, 1985.

C

1. Crawley, A. P., and Heckleman, R. M.: Errors in T2 estimation using multislice multiple-echo imaging. Magn. Reson. Med. 4:34, 1987.
2. Conturo, T. E., Price, R. R., Beth, A. H., et al.: Improved determination of spin density, T1 and T2 from a three-parameter fit to multiple-delay–multiple-echo (MDME) NMR images. Phys. Med. Biol. 31:1361, 1986.
3. Campbell, C. F., Pearson, G. A., Collins, S. M., et al.: Myocardial proton spin lattice relaxation times in vitro: Effect of elapsed time after excision. Magn. Reson. Imag. 4:473, 1986.

D

1. Davis, P. L., Sheldon, P., Kaufman, L., et al.: Nuclear magnetic resonance imaging of mammary adenocarcinomas in the rat. Cancer 51:433, 1983.

E

1. Edzes, H. T., and Samulski, E. T.: Cross-relaxation and spin diffusion in proton NMR of hydrated collagen. Nature (Lond.) 265:221, 1977.
2. EEC Concerted Research Project: II. A protocol for in vitro proton relaxation studies. Magn. Reson. Imag. 6:179, 1988.
3. Escange, J. M., Canet, D., and Robert, J.: Frequency dependence of water proton longitudinal nuclear magnetic relaxation times in mouse tissue at 20 degrees C. Biochim. Biophys. Acta 721:30, 1982.

F

1. Fullerton, G. E.: Physiological basis of magnetic relaxation. *In* Stark, D. D., Bradley, W. G., Jr. (eds.): Magnetic Resonance Imaging. C. V. Mosby, St. Louis, 1988, p. 36.

2. Fullerton, G. D., Ord, V. A., and Cameron, I. C.: An evaluation of the hydration of lysozyme by an NMR titration method. Biochim. Biophys. Acta 869:230, 1986.
3. Fullerton, G. D., Potter, J. L., Dornbluth, N. C.: NMR relaxation of protons in tissues and other macromolecular water solutions. Magn. Reson. Imag. 1:20, 1982.
4. Fung, B. M.: Proton and deuteron relaxation of muscle over wide ranges of resonance frequencies. Biophys. J. 18:235, 1977.
5. Fung, B. M., Durham, D. L., and Wassil, D. A.: The state of water in biological systems as studied by proton and deuterium relaxation. Biochim. Biophys. Acta 300:191, 1975.
6. Fried, R., Jolesc, F. A., Lorenzo, A. V., et al.: Developmental changes in proton magnetic resonance relaxation times of cardiac and skeletal muscle. Invest. Radiol. 23:209, 1988.

G

1. Gore, J. C., Doyle, F. H., and Pennock, J. M.: Relaxation rate and enhancement observed in vivo by NMR imaging. *In* Partain, C. L., James, A. E., Rollo, F. D., and Price, R. R. (eds.): Nuclear Magnetic Resonance Imaging. W. B. Saunders, Philadelphia, 1983, p. 94.
2. Gore, J. C., and Brown, M. S.: Pathophysiological significance of relaxation. *In* Partain, C. L., Price, R. R., Patton, J. A., et al. (eds.): Magnetic Resonance Imaging. W. B. Saunders, Philadelphia, 1988, p. 1070.
3. Gillis, P., and Koenig, S. H.: Transverse relaxation of solvent protons induced by magnetized spheres: Application to ferritin, erythrocytes, and magnetite. Magn. Reson. Med. 5:323, 1987.
4. Gomori, J. M., Grossman, R. I., Hackney, D. B., et al.: Variable appearances of subacute intracranial hematomas on high-field spin-echo MR. Am. J. Neuroradiol. 8:1019, 1987.

H

1. Haacke, E. M., Tkach, J. A., and Parrish, T. B.: Reduction of T2 dephasing in gradient field-echo imaging. Radiology 170:457, 1989.
2. Higgins, C. B., Herfkens, R., Lipton, M. J., et al.: Nuclear magnetic resonance imaging of acute myocardial infarction in dogs: Alterations in magnetic relaxation times. Am. J. Cardiol. 52:184, 1983.

I

1. Inch, M. R., McCredie, J. A., Knispel, R. R., et al.: Water content and proton spin relaxation time for neoplastic and non-neoplastic tissues from mice and humans. J. Natl. Cancer Inst. 52:353, 1974.

J

1. Jennings, R. B., Reimer, K. A., and Steenbergen, C.: Myocardial ischemia revisited. The osmolar load, membrane damage, and reperfusion. J. Mol. Cell. Cardiol. 18:769, 1986.
2. Jennings, R. B., and Reimer, K. A.: Pathobiology of acute myocardial ischemia. Hosp. Pract. Jan, 15:89, 1989.
3. Johnston, D. L., Homma, S., Liu, P., et al.: Serial changes in nuclear magnetic relaxation times after myocardial infarction in the rabbit: Relationship to water content, severity of ischemia, and histopathology over a six-month period. Magn. Reson. Med. 4:363, 1988.

K

1. Koenig, S., and Brown, R. D., III: Relaxometry of solvent and tissue protons: Diamagnetic contributions. *In* Partain, C. L., Price, R. R., Patton, J. A., et al. (eds.): Magnetic Resonance Imaging. W. B. Saunders, Philadelphia, 1988, p. 1035.
2. Koenig, S. H., Bryant, R. G., Hullenga, K., et al.: Magnetic cross-relaxation among protons in protein solution. Biochemistry 17:4348, 1978.
3. Koenig, S. H., Brown, R. D., III: Determinants of proton relaxation in tissue. Magn. Reson. Med. 1:437, 1984.
4. Koenig, S. H., and Brown, R. D., III: The importance of the motion of water for magnetic resonance imaging. Invest. Radiol. 20:297, 1985.
5. Kurland, R. J.: Strategies and tactics in NMR imaging relaxation time measurements. I. Minimizing relaxation time errors due to image noise: The ideal case. Magn. Reson. Med. 2:136, 1985.

M

1. Mathur-DeVre, R.: Biomedical implications of relaxation times of tissue water. *In* Partain, C. L., Price, R. R., Patton, J. A., et al. (eds.): Magnetic Resonance Imaging. W. B. Saunders, Philadelphia, 1988, p. 1099.
2. Mathur-DeVre, R.: Biomedical implications of the relaxation behavior of water related to NMR imaging. Br. J. Radiol. 57:955, 1984.
3. Mathur-DeVre, R.: The NMR studies of water in biological systems. Proc. Biophys. Mol. Biol. 35:103, 1979.
4. Majumdar, S., and Gore, J. C.: Effects of selective pulses on the measurement of T2 and apparent diffusion in multiecho MRI. Magn. Reson. Med. 4:120, 1987.
5. MacFall, J. R., Wehrli, F. W., Breger, R. K., et al.: Methodology for the measurement and analysis of relaxation time in proton imaging. Magn. Reson. Imag. 5:209, 1987.

R

1. Rorschach, H. E., Hazelwood, C. F.: Protein dynamics and the NMR relaxation time T1 of water in biological systems. J. Magn. Reson. 70:79, 1986.
2. Rupp, N., Reiser, M., and Stetter, E.: The diagnostic value of morphology and relaxation times in NMR imaging of the body. Eur. J. Radiol. 3:68, 1983.

S

1. Schaper, J., Schwarz, F., Kittstein, H., et al.: The effects of global ischemia and reperfusion on human myocardium: Quantitative evaluation by electron microscopic morphometry. Ann. Thorac. Surg. 33:116, 1982.

W

1. Wong, S. T. S., and Roos, M. S.: Effects of slice selection and diffusion on T2 measurement. Magn. Reson. Med. 5:358, 1987.
2. Wolf, G. L.: Contrast enhancement in biomedical NMR. Phys. Chem. Phys. Med. NMR 16:93, 1984.
3. Wolf, G. L.: Vitalism and proton relaxation. Invest. Radiol. 21:427, 1986.

Y

1. Young, I. R., Bryant, D. J., and Payne, J. A.: Variations in slice shape and absorption as artifacts in determination of tissue parameters in NMR imaging. Magn. Reson. Med. 2:355, 1985.
2. Young, I. R., Hall, A. S., and Bydder, G. M.: The design of a multiple inversion recovery sequence for T1 measurement. Magn. Reson. Med. 5:99, 1987.

Chapter 41

Flow Phenomena in MRI

LEON AXEL, Ph.D., M.D.

NORMAL MR APPEARANCE OF FLOWING BLOOD 769
Flow Enhancement 769
Flow Void 769
Turbulence 769
Artifacts 769
ORIGIN OF GRADIENT-ECHO IMAGING FLOW EFFECTS 773
Washout of Saturated Spins 773
Phase Shifts 773
ORIGIN OF SPIN-ECHO IMAGING FLOW EFFECTS 773
Washout of Excited Spins 773
FLOW ARTIFACT SUPPRESSION 773
Cardiac Gating 773
Saturation 773
Phase Compensation 774
FLOW MEASUREMENT TECHNIQUES 774
Time-of-Flight 774
Phase Shifts 774
FLOW IMAGING TECHNIQUES 774
CONCLUSION 775

It was noticed soon after the discovery of the phenomenon of nuclear magnetic resonance that motion, particularly fluid flow, could significantly affect the nuclear magnetic resonance (NMR) signal,[H1, S1, C1] increasing or decreasing its strength depending on the speed of the motion and the particular NMR technique being used. With the introduction of magnetic resonance imaging (MRI), these signal effects of flow could be seen in the images, along with other effects unique to imaging. Although potentially the source of troublesome artifacts, these flow effects can produce useful image contrast between flowing blood and adjacent blood vessels or cardiac chamber walls, enabling MR imaging of the cardiovascular system without the need for injected contrast agents. These effects also offer the potential for qualitatively or quantitatively evaluating blood flow, although this potential has still not been fully realized. We will here survey some of the commonly encountered effects of blood flow in MRI, describing their appearance and origin and ways to control image artifacts they may produce, and will consider some of their proposed applications to measurement of blood flow.

NORMAL MR APPEARANCE OF FLOWING BLOOD

Flow Enhancement

One striking effect of flow that may be seen in MRI is an increase in the signal of flowing blood relative to the signal of adjacent stationary structures ("bright blood"). This is most commonly seen in gradient-echo imaging, particularly with relatively rapidly repeated excitations (short repetition time, TR) (Fig. 41–1). It can also be seen with spin-echo imaging, particularly with relatively slower flow rates. As some of the early investigators of spin-echo imaging techniques had become accustomed to blood flow usually lowering signal intensity, they initially called this increased signal "paradoxic enhancement." As we shall see, however, there is nothing paradoxic about it, as it can be understood as the effect of washing out saturated spins between excitations.

Flow Void

As mentioned, with some imaging techniques, particularly spin-echo imaging, fast blood flow can lead to a loss of signal ("dark blood") (Fig. 41–2). This void can be inconsistent at times, even in images with overall dark blood, if there are regions of much slower flow, e.g., in aneurysms or within the heart in certain phases of the cardiac cycle (Fig. 41–3), or if the normal pulsatile nature of flow happens to be closely synchronized with the timing of the imaging cycle ("diastolic pseudogating"), so that the blood is consistently flowing slowly whenever certain slices are imaged. This dark signal will be seen to be due to washout of excited spins from the slice being imaged before they can be refocused for the spin echo.

A different sort of flow void is related to the production of phase shifts in excited spins moving along magnetic field gradients. One way these phase shifts can be manifested in conventional imaging, which displays only the magnitude of the signal, is as a loss of signal from regions of large velocity shear, as at the periphery of a vessel lumen or within the aortic root during early systole (Fig. 41–4). This can also be seen in vessels lying within the plane of the image. Such signal loss may be restored on the even-numbered echoes of multiple echo imaging sequences.

Turbulence

One of the more striking MRI flow effects is the loss of signal that can be seen with turbulent jets—for example, those associated with cardiac valve stenosis or regurgitation (Fig. 41–5). When imaging with a gradient echo technique that normally shows blood as bright, this signal loss results in a clear depiction of the jets as dark regions within the surrounding bright blood. The MRI-visualized jets correlate well with the corresponding regions of turbulent flow as mapped with Doppler ultrasound.[S2] However, studies of controlled flows in phantoms have shown that the presence of microscopic turbulence alone may not be enough to induce the loss of signal.[E1]

Artifacts

As the effects leading to changes in MR signal depend on the velocity of the blood, the variations in signal resulting from the pulsatile nature of blood flow can lead to artifacts in the image, similar to those due to motion, with propagation of displaced signal along the phase-encoded direction within the image (Fig. 41–6). This smearing of the signal can obscure the images of other underlying structures.

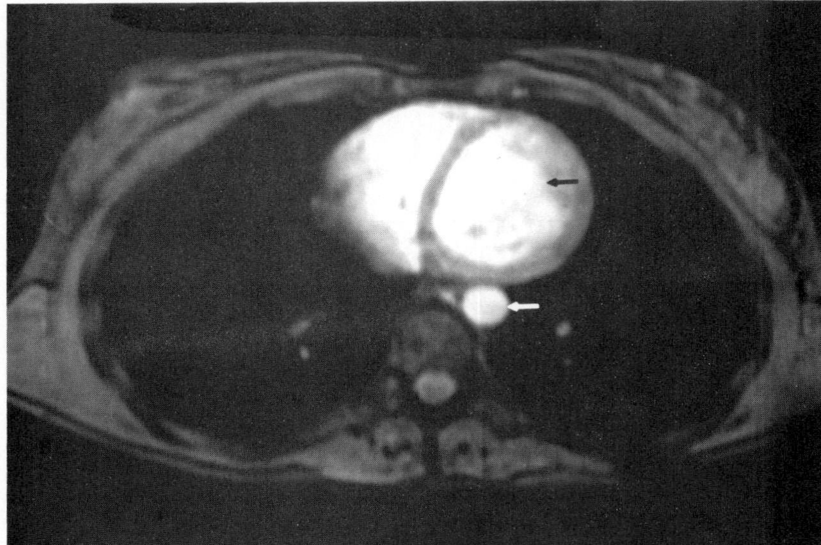

Figure 41–1. Cardiac-synchronized rapid gradient echo imaging of heart, showing strong signal from blood *(arrows)*, due to washout of saturated spins by flow between excitations.

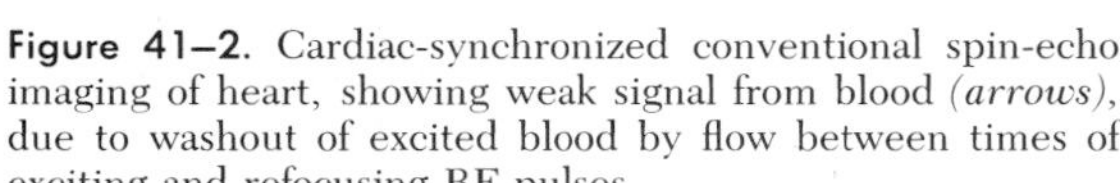

Figure 41–2. Cardiac-synchronized conventional spin-echo imaging of heart, showing weak signal from blood *(arrows)*, due to washout of excited blood by flow between times of exciting and refocusing RF pulses.

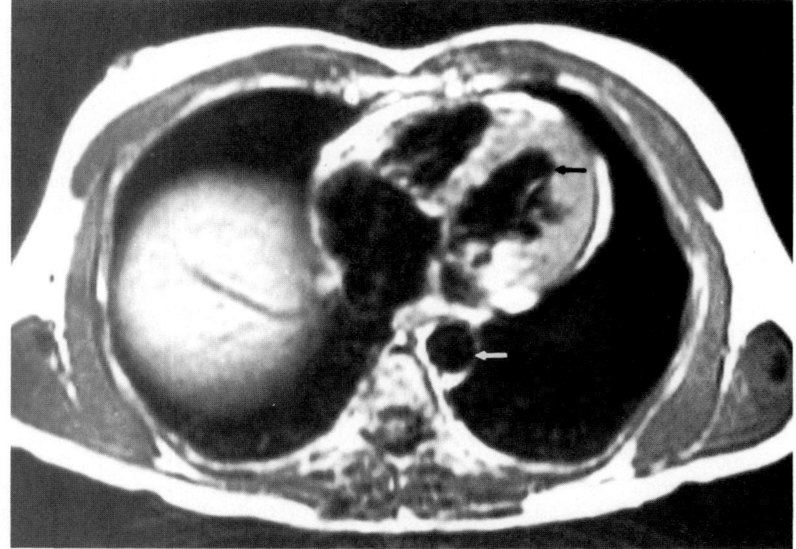

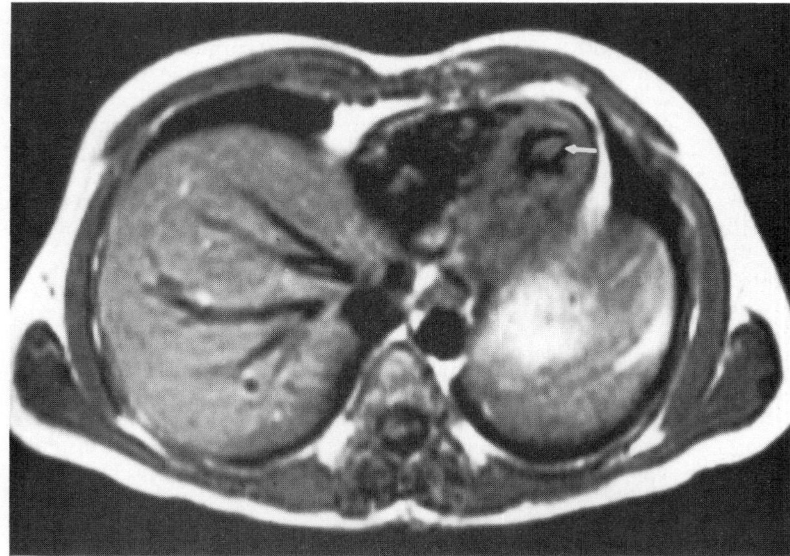

Figure 41–3. Similar to Figure 41–2, but near cardiac apex, showing stronger signal from blood *(arrow)*, due to slower flow.

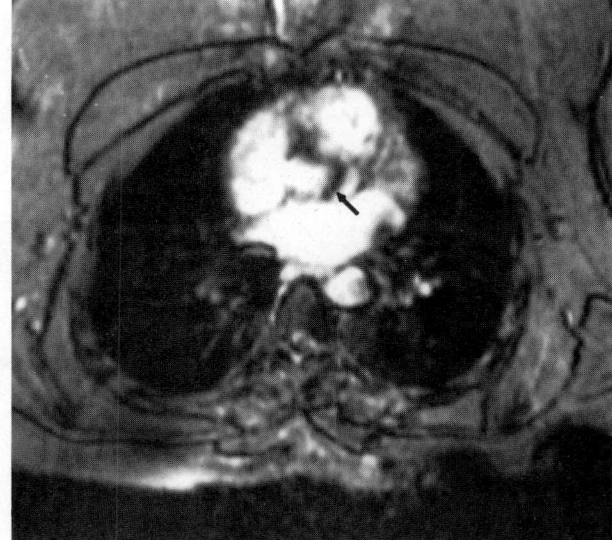

Figure 41–4. Similar to Figure 41–1, but showing loss of signal in left ventricular outflow tract *(arrow)* in normal subject, due to rapid shearing flow in systole.

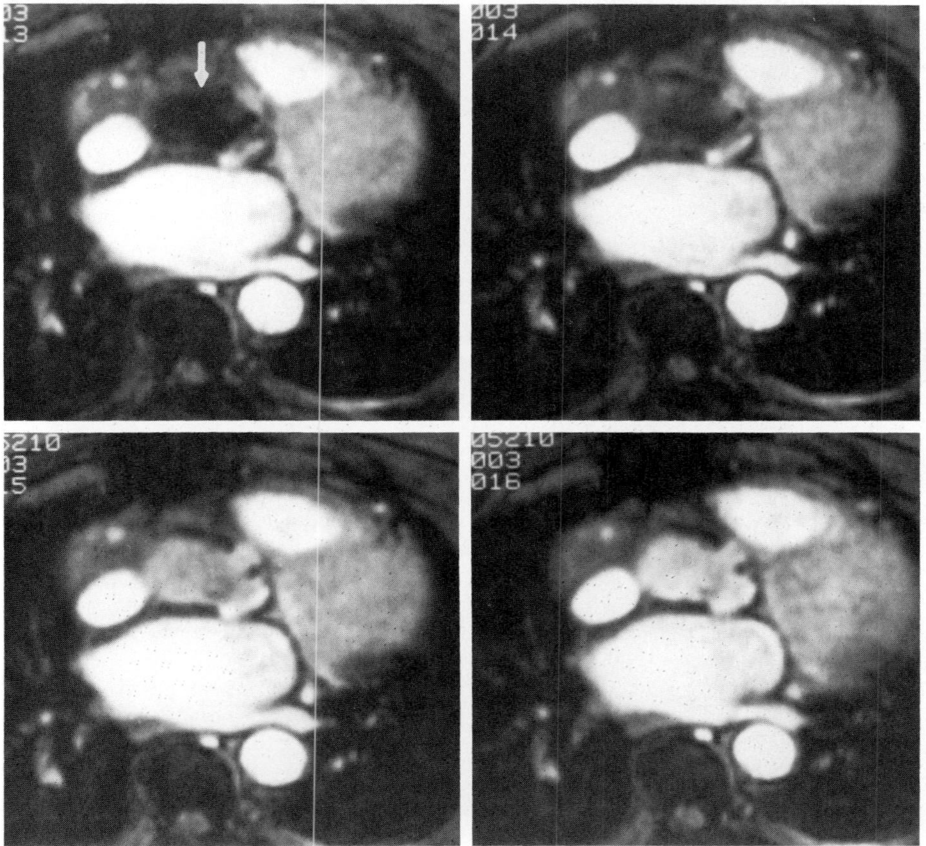

Figure 41–5. Composite image similar to Figure 41–4, but showing much more extensive area of signal loss in aortic root *(arrow)* during systole *(upper left)* in patient with turbulent jet due to aortic stenosis; signal returns during diastole *(lower right)*.

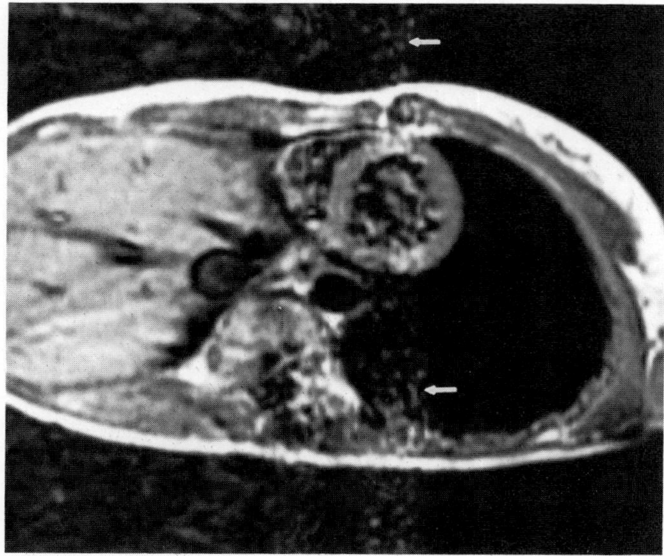

Figure 41–6. Image artifacts *(arrows)* propagating along phase-encoded direction from images of vascular structures, due to inconsistency in flow-related signal.

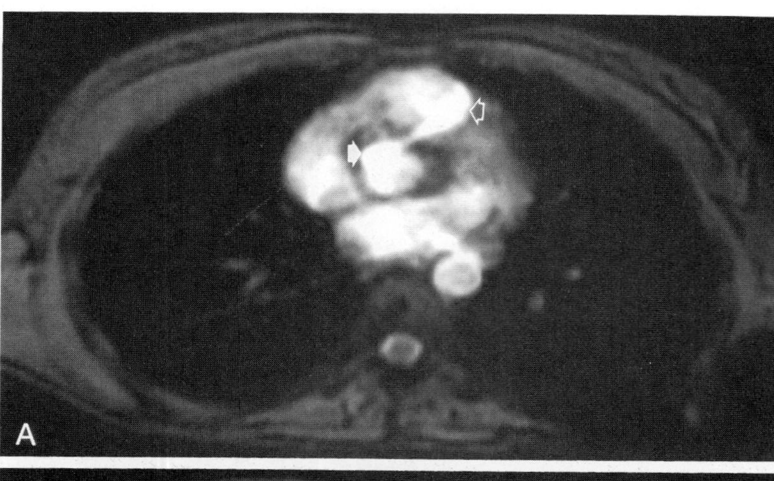

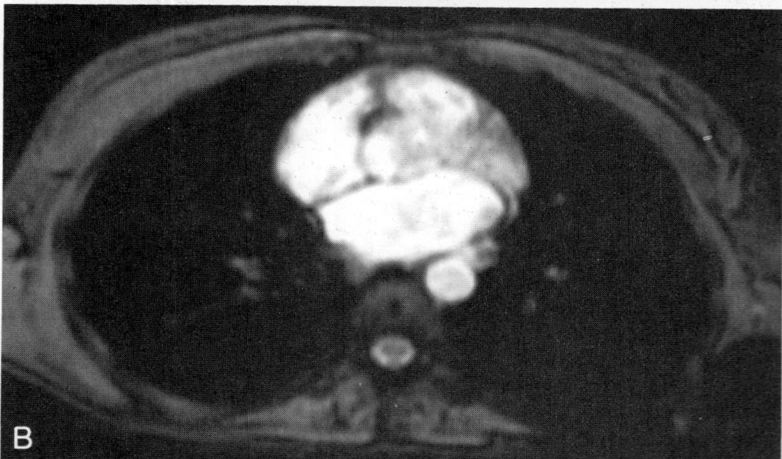

Figure 41–7. Displacement time-of-flight artifact. *A*, Systolic image at base of heart showing apparent displacement of blood image to right in aortic root *(closed arrow)* and to left in pulmonary artery *(open arrow)*. *B*, Diastolic image for comparison.

A different kind of artifact may be seen with motion of the blood within the plane of the imaged slice, where the signal from the blood may appear to be displaced relative to the position of the vessel lumen, owing to motion between the time of initial excitation and subsequent position encoding or between the times of encoding the horizontal and vertical position in the image (Fig. 41–7).

ORIGIN OF GRADIENT-ECHO IMAGING FLOW EFFECTS

Washout of Saturated Spins

The range of different flow appearances that can be seen in MRI can be understood as arising from relatively few basic effects.[A1] The most straightforward effect of blood flow in MRI to understand is the washout of saturated spins, which can lead to increased signal from the moving blood. This is most consistently seen with gradient-echo imaging. In MR imaging, slice selection is achieved by selective excitation of the region to be imaged. It usually takes many repeated excitations of the slice, with different position-encoding magnetic field gradient ("gradient") pulses, before enough data are available to reconstruct an image. If the repetition time between consecutive excitations, TR, is short compared with the longitudinal relaxation time of the tissue, there will be persistent partial saturation of the longitudinal magnetization at the time of the next excitation. This will result in decreased signal from stationary tissue. The signal from blood also would be decreased owing to partial saturation if it were stationary (or nearly so, as in a capillary hemangioma). However, with flow sufficiently rapid to wash the saturated blood out of the slice between the excitations, if the blood being washed into the slice is fully magnetized, it will give a full-strength signal. In the simple case of blood flow perpendicular to the slice with velocity v, if the slice thickness is d, the minimum time TR for blood in the slice to be fully washed out between excitations is d/v. For example, for a TR of 1 second and a 1-cm slice thickness, the blood would be fully washed out between excitations for velocities greater than 1 cm/sec.

In many practical imaging sequences, multiple slice locations are excited in an interleaved manner so that any "dead time" while waiting for magnetization to recover at one location can be usefully spent acquiring imaging data at another. If a particular slice is located in the middle of a stack of slices being acquired in such an interleaved manner, the blood being washed in may have been previously excited at another level upstream and may not be fully magnetized, leading to a potentially more complicated signal behavior with blood flow.

Phase Shifts

The phases of excited spins are normally synchronized at the time of initial excitation, and subsequent radio frequency and gradient pulses usually are adjusted so as to bring them back into synchronization at the time of signal detection (aside from effects of position-encoding magnetic field gradients). The series of magnetic field gradient pulses experienced by a given stationary region in the tissue produce a corresponding position-dependent variation in the local magnetic field; the resulting changes in local resonance frequency produce a position-dependent phase variation. Phase shifts induced by some of the gradient pulses will be compensated for by opposite phase shifts induced by other gradient pulses, so that the net gradient-induced phase shift is zero. However, motion of excited spins along magnetic field gradients can lead to phase shifts relative to adjacent stationary spins.[H2] This can be understood as a result of applying compensating gradient pulses that are appropriate for stationary spins in a given region, but inappropriate for spins that have moved there from regions with a different magnetic field history. For the case of gradient echoes, the phase ϕ of spins at position r is given by:

$$\phi = \int \omega dt = \gamma \int \Delta B dt = \gamma \int \vec{G}(t) \cdot \vec{r}(t) dt$$

where γ is the gyromagnetic ratio, ΔB is the change of field strength; and G is the gradient field strength. For r considered as a Taylor series:

$$r = r_o + vt + at^2/2 + \ldots,$$

where v is velocity and a is acceleration, we have

$$\phi = \gamma[\vec{r}_o \cdot \int \vec{G}(t)\, dt + \vec{v} \cdot \int \vec{G}(t)\, t dt + \vec{a} \cdot \int \vec{G}(t)\, t^2\, dt/2 + \ldots]$$

Thus, by adjusting the successively higher "moments" of the form of the dependence of the gradients on time, we can successively correct for velocity, acceleration, and so on.[P1] Alternatively, we could selectively sensitize the signal phase to any desired motion variables by appropriate adjustments of the gradients.[M1]

ORIGIN OF SPIN-ECHO IMAGING FLOW EFFECTS

Washout of Excited Spins

The washout of excited spins from the region being selectively excited between the times of application of the initial excitation RF pulse and a subsequent refocusing RF pulse can result in signal loss. In this case, the relevant washout condition for full signal loss is when the velocity approaches two times the ratio of the slice thickness to the echo time. This signal loss is not seen in gradient echo imaging, since no refocusing pulse is required to produce the echo, and the signal from excited blood that leaves the slice being imaged can still be picked up by the receiving coil.[W1]

A related effect that can also be seen with gradient-echo imaging is an apparent displacement of the position of excited spins owing to motion between the time of excitation and position encoding. This can be particularly noticeable if there is a long time between the times of phase encoding and frequency encoding, leading to an asymmetry in the apparent motion along the corresponding directions.

FLOW ARTIFACT SUPPRESSION

Cardiac Gating

The origin of the artifacts that can be seen arising from the images of flowing blood is the variation of the signal (magnitude and/or phase) from the blood due to the variation of blood velocity during the cardiac cycle. This signal variation can be controlled by synchronizing the imaging sequence with the cardiac cycle, so that the signal is always acquired at a consistent phase of the cardiac cycle. Although an adequate trigger signal for this synchronization for general vascular imaging can often be obtained from a peripheral pulse, such as with finger photoplethysmography, an electrocardiogram-derived trigger is generally necessary for high-quality cardiac imaging.

Saturation

An alternative way to suppress artifacts from variably moving blood is to ensure that the signal is consistently low. This can be done by applying selective saturation pulses to the blood upstream from the imaging region in order to effectively destroy its magnetization, so that when it flows into the region being imaged, it will not produce a signal.[F1] As long as the total blood signal can be suppressed, any phase variation will not produce a significant artifact. Limitations to this approach can be seen in cardiac imaging, where, due to the intermittent motion of blood through the heart, the region being imaged may not consistently be flushed out with blood from the regions of selective saturation so that the blood may not have a consistently low signal.

Phase Compensation

Variation of signal phase due to motion of excited blood is a major source of flow artifacts. This is particularly true with signals detected as gradient echoes, in which motion of excited spins may not reduce the amplitude of the signal. One means of controlling this source of artifacts is to control the phase shifts acquired by the moving blood. This can be achieved by applying additional pulsed magnetic field gradients between the times of initial excitation and signal detection. These additional pulses are adjusted so that they will have no net effect on stationary tissue but will produce phase shifts opposite to those induced by the original imaging sequence; the final result is a cancellation, and no net phase shift for moving blood. In practice, the unsteady nature of blood flow makes it difficult to completely eliminate phase shift effects from moving blood, but it still makes possible a dramatic improvement in the images.[P1]

FLOW MEASUREMENT TECHNIQUES

Time-of-Flight

One major class of flow measurement techniques uses the aforementioned time-of-flight effects. These rely on the ability to "tag" blood by locally altering its magnetization and then detecting its motion by the displacement of the altered magnetization. The local alteration can be either of the longitudinal magnetization (degree of saturation) or of the transverse magnetization (excitation); the altered magnetization will persist for times on the order of the T1 or T2 relaxation times, respectively. The motion can be detected either indirectly as a replacement of the tagged blood within the region being imaged by untagged blood from upstream (washout) or directly, as a displacement downstream of the tagged blood (time-of-flight).

Washout of tagged blood will be reflected in a change in the signal from the image of blood within the slice being imaged, typically an increase in signal with saturation tagging[S3] and a decrease with excitation tagging.[M2] To calculate the velocity (or the component perpendicular to the image plane), the dependence of the signal on the time between tagging and imaging must be measured, which may require obtaining several images. Measurement of time-of-flight effects will require creating separate tagging (excitation or saturation) and "detection" regions, typically with tagging by excitation or saturation of a thin slab and subsequent imaging of a region oriented at right angles to the tagged slab, in order to show movement of the tagged blood away from the initial tagging region; displacement divided by time between tagging and detection directly yields velocity.[A2, S4, E2] Alternatively, parallel tagging and imaging regions can be employed, with the separation of the regions divided by the time of appearance in the image of the upstream-tagged blood yielding velocity. For example, spin-echo imaging can be employed, with initial selective excitation and subsequent selective refocusing pulses applied to separated regions.[F2, M3] Again, determination of this time may require obtaining several images.

Limitations to time-of-flight flow measurement techniques include difficulties in producing sharply defined tagging regions and the need to include effects of curved and branching vessel geometries in the analysis.

Phase Shifts

The phase shifts that excited spins can acquire by moving along magnetic field gradients can also be used to measure blood flow. We discussed earlier the use of supplementary magnetic field gradient pulses to cancel out these phase shifts to reduce flow artifacts. Similarly, we can use other supplementary gradient magnetic field pulses to produce a controlled dependence of phase shift on velocity. If we then use a phase-sensitive image reconstruction technique, we can directly calculate the corresponding velocities from the phases of the blood images.[M1, F2, O1, N1]

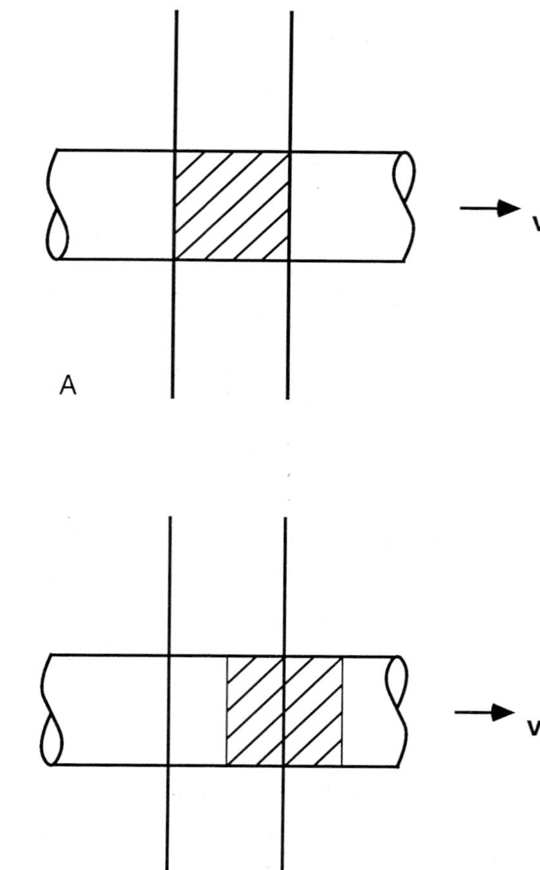

Figure 41–8. Diagrammatic representation of washout of tagged spins in blood vessel (horizontal tube) passing through imaging region (vertical lines), with uniform blood velocity, v. *A*, Initial tagging by selective RF pulse, producing saturation or excitation (diagonal lines). *B*, At a later time (e.g., time of subsequent application of selective excitation or refocusing RF pulses), tagged spins have been carried downstream by flow and partially replaced in the imaging region by spins from upstream.

Potential problems with this technique include the need to correct for possible nonzero base line phases (typically by subtracting two images with different phase sensitivity to motion), and the possibility that the phase shifts may exceed 180 degrees, thereby becoming ambiguous.[O1, A3]

FLOW IMAGING TECHNIQUES

The same techniques that can be applied to the measurement of flow can be adapted to the display of flowing blood for angiographic imaging. Again, the basic effects that are exploited are washout or time-of-flight and phase shifts (Fig. 41–8). "Conventional" projection images can be produced either directly in a projection-type of image acquisition mode, or indirectly by postprocessing a stack of thin cross-sectional images.

Washout effects are used most directly for flow imaging by acquiring a stack of thin images (either sequentially or in a "3-D" mode), using rapidly repeated, small flip angle, gradient-echo imaging to generate "bright blood" images. Postprocessing can then be used to create synthetic projection images in any desired orientation, with the increased signal from moving blood being used to pick out blood vessels and display them above the background of stationary tissues.[L1]

An alternative way to use washout effects is to tag upstream spins, e.g., with a selective inversion pulse, image the desired region downstream after a delay to allow the tagged blood to enter the imaging volume, and then subtract the resulting in from an otherwise identical image acquired without the preliminary upstream tagging.[N2] Similarly, upstream saturation on the appropriate side of the imaged volume can be used in conjunction with the aforementioned washout technique to selectively suppress the signal from arterial or venous blood.

Phase shift effects can also be used to produce MR angiograms by acquiring otherwise identical images with and without phase sensitization to motion and then subtracting them (in a phase-sensitive way) to cancel out the signal from stationary tissues.[A4, D1]

CONCLUSION

The sensitivity of the magnetic resonance signal to motion makes possible the clear separation of heart wall and chamber. Although the appearance of blood in MRI can be very variable, the basic effects that produce these appearances, washout (or time-of-flight) and phase shifts, are fairly simple. Understanding these basic effects of blood flow helps us understand and interpret the appearance of the blood in images; it also helps us devise ways to suppress image artifacts that may result from the pulsatile nature of blood flow. Finally, these basic MR flow effects can be used to design imaging methods for the qualitative (and possibly quantitative) imaging of blood flow.

References

A

1. Axel, L.: Blood flow effects in magnetic resonance imaging. AJR 143:1157, 1984.
2. Axel, L., Shimakawa, A., and MacFall, J. R.: A time-of-flight method of measuring flow velocity by magnetic resonance imaging. Magn. Reson. Imag. 4:199, 1986.
3. Axel, L., and Morton, D.: Correction of phase wrapping in MR imaging. Med. Physics 16:284, 1989.
4. Axel, L., and Morton, D.: MR flow imaging by velocity-compensated/uncompensated difference images. J. Comput. Assist. Tomogr. 11:31, 1987.

C

1. Carr, H. Y., and Purcell, E. M.: Effects of diffusion on free precession in nuclear magnetic resonance experiments. Phys. Rev. 94:630, 1954.

D

1. Dumoulin, C. L., and Hart, H. R.: Magnetic resonance angiography. Radiology 161:717, 1986.

E

1. Evans, A. J., Blinder, R. A., Herfkens, R. J., et al.: Effects of turbulence on signal intensity in gradient echo images. Invest. Radiol. 23:512, 1988.
2. Edelmann, R. R., Mattle, H. P., Kleefield, J., and Silver, M. S.: Quantification of blood flow with dynamic MR imaging and presaturation bolus tracking. Radiology 171:551, 1989.

F

1. Felmlee, J. P., and Ehman, R. L.: Spatial presaturation: A method for suppressing flow artifacts and improving depiction of vascular anatomy in MR imaging. Radiology 166:231, 1988.
2. Feinberg, D. A., Crooks, L. E., Hoenninger, J., et al.: Pulsatile blood velocity in human arteries displayed by magnetic resonance imaging. Radiology 153:177, 1984.

H

1. Hahn, E. L.: Spin echoes. Phys. Rev. 80:580, 1950.
2. Hahn, E. L.: Detection of seawater motion by nuclear precession. J. Geophys. Res. 65:776, 1960.

L

1. Laub, G. A., and Kaiser, W. A.: MR angiography with gradient motion refocusing. J. Comput. Assist. Tomogr. 12:377, 1988.

M

1. Moran, P. R.: A flow velocity zeugmatographic interlace for NMR imaging in humans. Magn. Reson. Imag. 1:197, 1982.
2. Mueller, E., Deimling, M., and Reinhardt, E. R.: Quantification of pulsatile flow in MRI by an analysis of T2 changes in ECG-gated multiecho experiments. Magn. Reson. Med. 3:331, 1986.
3. Merboldt, K. D., Haenicke, W., and Frahm, J.: Flow NMR imaging using stimulated echoes. J. Magn. Reson. 67:336, 1986.

N

1. Nayler, G. L., Firmin, D. N., and Longmore, D. B.: Blood flow imaging by cine magnetic resonance. J. Comput. Assist. Tomogr. 10:715, 1986.
2. Nishimura, D. G., Macovski, A., Pauly, J. M., and Conolly, S. M.: MR angiography by selective inversion recovery. Magn. Reson. Med. 4:193, 1987.

O

1. O'Donnell, M.: NMR blood flow imaging using multi-echo phase contrast sequence. Med. Phys. 12:59, 1985.

P

1. Pattany, P. M., Phillips, J. J., Chiu, L. C., et al.: Motion artifact suppression technique (MAST) for MR imaging. J. Comput. Assist. Tomogr. 11:369, 1987.

S

1. Suryan, G.: Nuclear resonance in flowing liquids. Proc. Indian Acad. Sci. [A] 33:107, 1951.
2. Schiebler, M., Axel, L., Reichek, N., et al.: Correlation of cine MR imaging with two-dimensional pulsed Doppler echocardiography in valvular insufficiency. J. Comput. Assist. Tomogr. 11:627, 1987.
3. Singer, J. R., and Crooks, L. E.: Nuclear magnetic resonance blood flow measurements in the human brain. Science 221:654, 1983.
4. Shimizu, K., Matsuda, T., Sakurai, T., et al.: Visualization of moving fluid: Quantitative analysis of blood flow velocity using MR imaging. Radiology 59:195, 1986.

W

1. Wehrli, F. W., Shimakawa, A., Gullberg, G. T., and MacFall, J. R.: Time-of-flight flow imaging: Selective saturation recovery with gradient refocusing. Radiology 160:781, 1986.

Chapter 42

Optimizing MR Image Quality: Artifact Causes and Cures

■ *PAUL WOZNEY, M.D.* ■ *RICHARD PROROK, R.T.*
■ *RONALD PETCHENY, R.T.(R.)*

WHY STUDY ARTIFACTS? 776
REVIEW OF MR IMAGE CREATION 776
System Tuning and Preparation 777
Scanning (Data Acquisition) 777
Data Transfer and Computer Image Creation 778
PATIENT-RELATED MOTION ARTIFACTS 779
Gross Motion and Sedation 779
Cardiac Motion 781
Triggering: Electrocardiogram and Pulse 781
Retrospective Gating 783
High-Speed MR Imaging 783
Cine-Magnetic Resonance Imaging 783
Respiratory Motion 783
Averaging 783
Triggering and Sorting 783
Gradient Moment Nulling 784
Blood Flow 785
High-Velocity Signal Loss 785
Flow-Related Enhancement 785
Spatial Presaturation 785
Phase Ghost Artifacts 786
Gradient Moment Nulling 786
Pulsatile Flow 787
Magnetic Resonance Angiography and Phase Imaging 787
MRI SYSTEM-RELATED ARTIFACTS AND SOLUTIONS 787
Aliasing (Wraparound) 787
Local Field Inhomogeneity 788
Artifacts from Metal 788
Engineering-Related System Artifacts 788
SUMMARY 788

WHY STUDY ARTIFACTS?

Why do artifacts in magnetic resonance imaging (MRI) deserve more than a perfunctory comment? With most imaging modalities, artifacts can be relegated to a few footnotes. However, because of the mechanism of image formation in MRI, artifacts have a major impact on image quality, and occasionally mimic pathology. Many of the causes can be addressed by the user with an understanding of a few basic principles. This understanding can make the difference between a successful study and total frustration on the part of physician, patient, and technologist. Some artifacts can provide important diagnostic information, such as the "black jet" of flow seen in stenosis and regurgitation. Blood within the heart can be made dark or bright by adjusting image parameters.

This chapter summarizes the current understanding of artifacts in cardiac MRI, with a focus on solutions to optimize image quality. We shall define the term *artifact* to mean anything in the final MR image that does not correspond to actual tissues in the patient at the location being imaged. This discussion is not intended to be an exhaustive list of every MRI artifact that has been described, but rather to focus on those artifacts of particular interest in cardiac imaging. There are several excellent comprehensive summaries of artifacts in magnetic resonance.[C1, H1–3, P1] It is important to understand that clinical MR imaging is still developing, especially imaging at high field strengths (1.0 to 1.5 Tesla). The understanding of MRI artifacts and their correction is also still evolving.

The images in this chapter were all obtained on 1.5 Tesla (T) commercial units (General Electric Medical Systems, Milwaukee, WI), but the variety of artifacts is similar to that observed at lower field strengths, such as 0.15 T and 0.35 T.[H3, P1] The relationship of artifacts to the main magnetic field strength is difficult to isolate from other components of the MRI system. It is well established that the signal-to-noise ratio in the MR image is approximately proportional to field strength: the signal-to-noise from a 1.5 T system is approximately three times the signal-to-noise from a 0.5 T system.[E1] In theory, at higher field strengths there should be more signal from structures we are interested in, and also more motion-related artifactual signal. However, there are no good studies evaluating the effect of magnet strength and image quality in the chest, for two major reasons. First, MRI systems at different field strengths differ markedly in software and hardware, even when made by the same manufacturer. There is an even greater difference between systems made by different manufacturers. Second, the tissue relaxation time known as T1, a major determining factor of the MRI signal, is itself a function of the field strength.[K1] To further complicate matters, we shall see that many artifacts are addressed with computer processing of the information, which usually results in loss of signal, and at higher field strengths there is more signal to "spend" in correcting artifacts. Diagnostic cardiac images have been obtained at many field strengths.[C2, D1, S1, W1]

We first review the creation of the MR image. Artifacts will then be discussed in two major categories: those resulting from patient motion, and those related to the MR imaging equipment.

REVIEW OF MR IMAGE CREATION

It cannot be emphasized enough that MRI is quite different from other imaging modalities. Conventional x-ray, radionuclides,

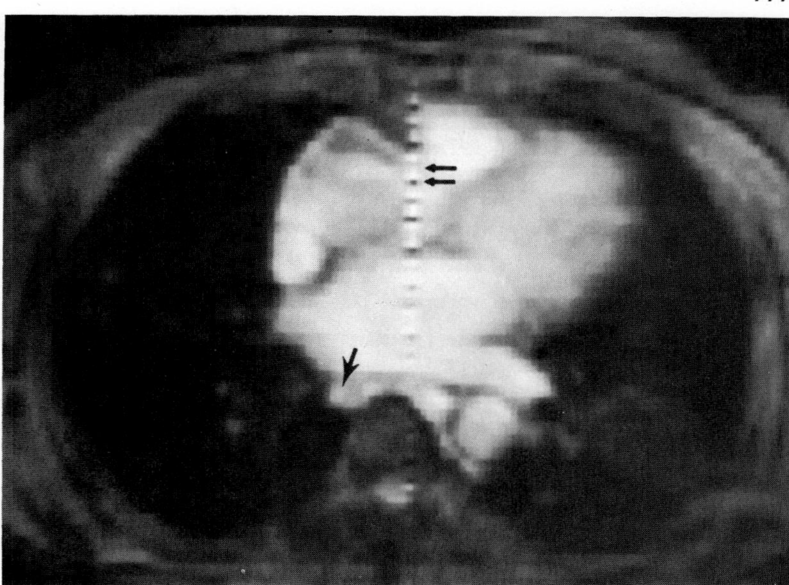

Figure 42–1. The MR image is composed of pixels (arrow), which have depth (the slice thickness) and represent voxels in the patient. The composition of the MR image is evident on this greatly magnified axial image of the heart. The center line artifact (double arrow) probably results from a stray radiofrequency signal from a power line. (MRI parameters: repetition time (TR) = 25 milliseconds, echo time (TE) = 13 milliseconds, gradient-echo with gradient moment nulling, flip angle = 20°. Unless stated otherwise, all images are: 256 frequency × 128 phase acquisition matrix, 10-millimeter slice thickness, 2 excitations, imaged with a body transmit/receive coil and triggered with ECG leads placed on the thorax.)

computed tomography, and ultrasound all produce an image from a beam that is sent in a direct line toward the anatomy of interest. The anatomy then either attenuates the beam (x-ray) or reflects the beam (ultrasound), and this distorted beam is recorded (by x-ray film, computed tomography detector, nuclear medicine camera, or sonographic crystal) and an image created. There is no beam in MRI. Instead, a radio wave is sent by an antenna into the patient (while the patient is in a strong magnetic field), and certain hydrogen nuclei are excited in the patient. An antenna then receives signals from those same excited hydrogen nuclei on water and fat molecules. To create an image, the source of the signal must be localized to the anatomy of interest by "tuning" this anatomy to a certain radio frequency. This is analogous to selecting channels on a two-way radio. A slice low in the heart might be channel 1, a slice higher in the heart, channel 2, and a slice yet higher in the heart, channel 3. A radio wave sent out on channel 1 will excite only a slice low in the heart, whereas a radio transmission on channel 3 will excite only a slice high in the heart.[B1, F1,2, S2, W2]

The final MR image is a computer creation. It is composed of rectangles (or squares) called pixels (picture element). Each pixel represents a voxel (volume element) in the patient: the pixels are arranged in a matrix of rows and columns. For example, an MR image with a 256 × 128 matrix is made up of 256 × 128 = 32,768 pixels. The computer assigns a level of grayness to each pixel, reflecting the strength of the signal received from that voxel in the patient: lighter shades represent stronger signal (Fig. 42–1).

There are four basic steps in creating an MR image: (1) tuning the radio transceiver and antenna to match the patient, (2) transmitting the radiofrequency (RF) signal into the patient, (3) receiving the signal from the patient, and (4) converting the signal into numbers and computer processing to create an image. Artifacts can result from abnormalities at any one of these four stages. A detailed description of each step is necessary to understand causes of artifacts and how to address them. First some terminology. An MRI study consists of several different sets of images: each set is called a *series*. The parameters for a particular series are selected by the operator, and the system then acquires the information and produces a number of images based on those parameters. Images are not usually created one at a time, as in other imaging modalities: a set of images (the series) is created in a batch. A series may rarely consist of only one slice but usually includes from 10 to over 100 images. A single series may take as little as 3 seconds or require over 20 minutes; in general, more images are created during the longer times. The steps in creation of one single MR image in a series are described next (Table 42–1).

System Tuning and Preparation

At the beginning of each series, the equipment must be tuned to the patient. With hydrogen imaging, only the hydrogen protons on fat and water produce enough signal for imaging. The spatial location in the image is determined by the frequency and phase of the returning signals.[S2, W2] *Since the frequency of fat is slightly higher than that of water, it will be "seen" by the equipment at a slightly different place than it actually is: this is known as chemical shift.*[H2, K2] The different frequencies of fat and water can be helpful. By carefully selecting imaging parameters, the fat and water signals within a voxel can be made to cancel, and the fat-water interface will appear as an artifactual dark line.[W3] This dark line may outline the heart and mediastinum to advantage (Fig. 42–2).

The second step in tuning is to adjust the transmitted power to produce the maximal returned signal. Because of the physics,[F1, 2, S2, W2] this is also known as setting the 90° radiofrequency (RF) flip angle. The energy needed to produce a 180° pulse is exactly twice the energy for a 90° pulse, so any error in setting the 90° pulse will be magnified, and rephasing will be incomplete. After the power for the 90° pulse is determined, any other flip angle is determined by setting the power proportionately lower. Flip angles of less than 90° are commonly employed in gradient-echo imaging.[H4, G1, S2, U1, W4]

Scanning (Data Acquisition)

The next step in MR image creation is scanning. Since there are three spatial dimensions, there are three steps to localize each voxel within the patient. These will be illustrated for a conventional 90° to 180° spin-echo (SE) sequence. These three steps are called slice-selection, phase-encoding, and readout (or frequency-encoding) and are all variations of the same technique.

Table 42–1. STEPS IN SPIN-ECHO MR IMAGE CREATION

1. Tune to frequency of hydrogen
2. Adjust transmitted power to determine 90° flip angle
3. 90° radio frequency pulse (<90° for gradient-echo) + slice-select gradient
4. Phase-encoding gradient
5. 180° radio frequency pulse (omit for gradient-echo)
6. Receive echo signal + readout gradient
7. Repeat steps 3 to 6 multiple times to increase spatial resolution in the phase direction (typically 128 or more)
8. Process received signals with computers and make image

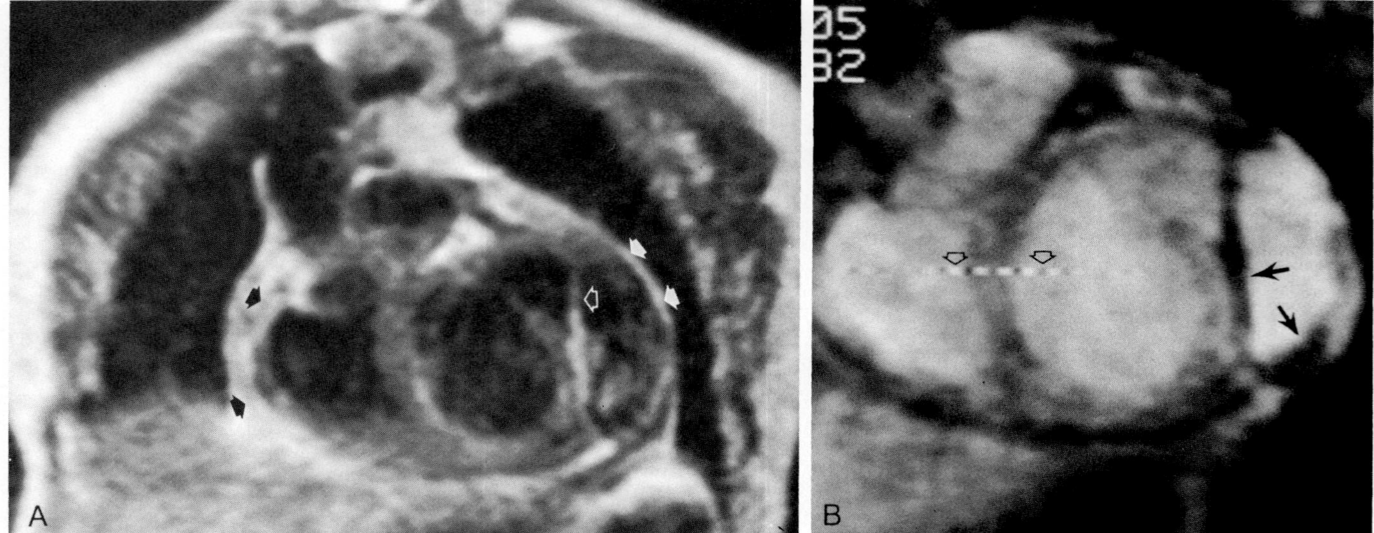

Figure 42–2. Demonstration of differing frequencies for water and fat, and variable appearance of flowing blood. *A*, Coronal spin-echo (SE) chest MRI of a 63-year-old man, 12 days after an acute anterior wall myocardial infarct. The left ventricular pseudoaneurysm is outlined by bright epipericardial fat (solid white arrows) and epicardial fat (open white arrow). The right atrial pericardium (black arrows) is also outlined by fat. With the spin-echo technique, blood in the cardiac chambers is dark, and in the pseudoaneurysm is dark gray. *B*, Gradient-echo cine image of the same slice with technique selected to result in signal cancellation at fat-muscle interfaces, resulting in dark borders to the pseudoaneurysm (solid arrows). With the gradient-echo technique, blood in the cardiac chambers and pseudoaneurysm is bright. Notice also a radiofrequency center line artifact (open arrows) similar to Figure 42–1.

A small additional magnetic field (called a gradient), which gradually increases in strength across the patient, is added to the constant main magnetic field. Since the frequency of protons is directly related to the field strength, protons in the lower portion of the field will have a slightly lower frequency than protons in a higher region of the field. When the system receives a signal that is low in frequency, it knows that the tissue generating the signal is on one side rather than the other side.[B1, F1,2, W2] For example, in our system at 1.5 T, the resonance frequency of protons is 63,700 kilohertz. A typical gradient field applied across the patient results in a frequency range of about 32 kilohertz (63,684 to 63,716 kilohertz). Therefore, the difference in frequency from one side of the patient to the other side is only 0.05 percent.

To localize a voxel in three dimensions, the gradient magnetic field must be applied sequentially at three different times in three different directions (Fig. 42–3).[B1, S3, W2] First, the slice-select gradient is applied, and at the same time the radiofrequency pulse is transmitted. These are tuned together so that only a certain slice of tissue in the patient is excited. The slice-select gradient and the 90° radio frequency pulse are typically applied for only a few milliseconds (msec) and then are turned off. A phase-encoding gradient is then applied orthogonal to the slice-select gradient. During the short time (a few milliseconds) that this gradient is on, protons in a region of higher field will move faster and accumulate phase relative to protons in a lower strength region. They will retain their accumulated phase differences when the phase-encoding gradient is turned off after a few milliseconds. The third step is to apply a readout gradient orthogonal to the first two gradients while listening for the signal ("echo") from the patient. (This gradient is commonly called the "frequency gradient," although the other two gradients also determine position by frequency.) The entire time for these three steps is quite short (9 to 100 milliseconds).

This information, however, will result only in a one-dimensional image. This sequence must be repeated multiple times (typically 128 or more), each time with a slight change in the phase-encoding gradient strength, to resolve the image in the phase-encoding dimension (Fig. 42–4). The time to create the MR image, therefore, is equal to: (repetition time [TR] between each phase-encoding pulse) × (number of phase-encoding pulse steps). For example, when the repetition time (TR) equals 500 milliseconds and 128 phase-encoding pulses, the imaging time is 64 seconds. Each phase pulse step can be repeated (number of excitations) to improve the signal-to-noise ratio and to average motion, but this requires a proportionate increase in imaging time. *Since information in the slice-select and readout directions is acquired in a few milliseconds, there is little effect of motion in these directions. However, the phase-encoding information takes seconds to minutes to acquire, and any motion during this time will appear in the image. Therefore, most motion artifacts are seen in the phase-encoding direction* (Fig. 42–4G).

Careful inspection of Figure 42–3 will show that we have ignored a second 180° radio frequency pulse that is transmitted simultaneously with a second application of the slice-select gradient. This is necessary to refocus the echo signal so that it can be detected. Therefore this pulse sequence, which is the most widely employed, is called a 90° to 180° spin-echo (SE) technique. The echo signal, however, can be refocused in a different way, by reversing the readout gradient,[S2, W2, V4] resulting in a gradient echo. The 180° radio frequency pulse (and corresponding slice-select gradient) is unnecessary, and the echo time (TE) can be shorter. The lack of the second slice-select gradient has important consequences for flow imaging, as shall be discussed. In cardiac imaging, the gradient-echo frequently employs a lower radiofrequency flip angle of 5° to 40° (rather than 90°), and therefore signal from stationary tissues will be less on a gradient-echo image than on a spin-echo image.[K2]

Data Transfer and Computer Image Creation

The radio signal received from the patient is very high frequency (63,700 kilohertz), but the useful signal differences between tissues are of much lower frequency, so the signal is demodulated to under 10 kilohertz and then converted into raw data numbers (digitized) for storage and computation. The computers take the raw data and perform two Fourier transforms to create the final display image data. The signal received is only a few microwatts, similar to that generated by a phonograph needle, and any spurious radio frequency signal can result in severe artifact; therefore the MR equipment must be well shielded from stray radio waves. These can arise from radio or television broadcasts (63,700 kilohertz corresponds to television channel 3).

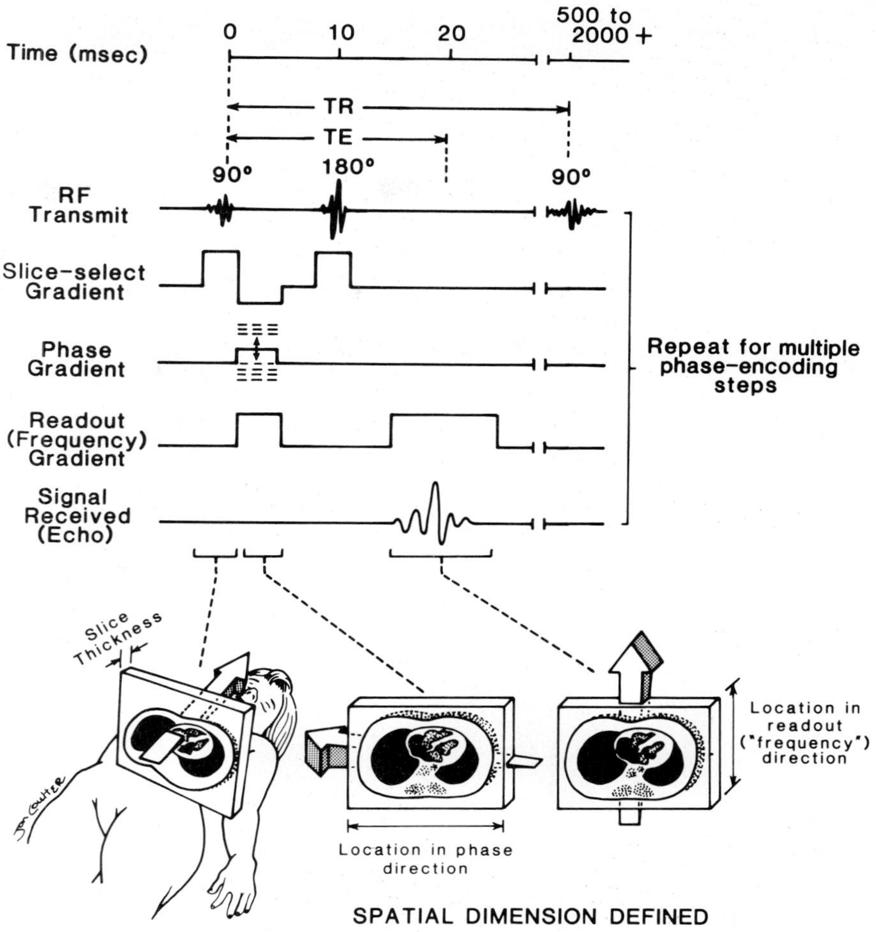

Figure 42–3. MRI signal localization with standard 90° to 180° spin-echo sequence. The times shown are approximate. Three gradients are applied sequentially in three orthogonal spatial directions. Although the illustration shows an axial slice, the slices may be obtained in any oblique plane by gradient adjustment. Time is in milliseconds (msec). The time from transmission of one 90° radiofrequency (RF) excitation pulse to the next one is the repetition time (TR). The time from the radiofrequency pulse to the echo signal is the echo time (TE). The basic steps of excitation and localization with three gradients are common to all pulse sequences, although the details may vary. For example, in a gradient-echo sequence the radiofrequency pulse is usually less than 90° and the 180° pulse is omitted.

After demodulation, stray electronic noise from motors and power lines can appear in the image as a "zipper" artifact (Figs. 42–1 and 42–2*B*) near the center of the image.

For a single image, typically over 65,000 raw data points (256 × 128 × 2) are collected as serial compressed lines from the three-dimensional object. Significant errors in one data collection can translate into significant image degradation as a "corduroy artifact."[H1, 3] The intensity, width, and spacing of the artifactual lines are related to the intensity and location of the data errors in the raw data. If the errors are in a critical location, the image may be unreadable. The artifact is different from that seen in computed tomography, since the mathematical process of image creation is somewhat different. In computed tomography, there is only a one-dimensional Fourier transform, and back-projection is used to create the image.[M1] Therefore, artifacts have a "star" appearance.[J1, S4] In MRI, there is a two-dimensional Fourier transform of phase and frequency-encoded information, and artifacts are propagated throughout the image.[H3, S2]

PATIENT-RELATED MOTION ARTIFACTS

Artifacts may be broadly divided into those related to the patient, those arising from the inherent physics of MR, and those resulting from system malfunction. Despite different origins, the final image degradation can appear superficially similar (Fig. 42–5). A general guideline, however, is that system-related artifact will have no relation to actual patient anatomy (Fig. 42–5*B*), whereas patient-related artifacts usually can be ascribed to structures in the patient, as will become evident. Caution should be exercised in dogmatically explaining an artifact in any individual image. Exact analysis frequently requires examination of the raw data, which is rarely available, since it is not routinely retained after image creation. The best evidence of artifact cause may be a change that corrects the artifact.

Gross Motion and Sedation

Gross movement of the patient is a greater problem in MRI than in other modalities. Since each series of images typically requires several minutes, any motion during this time will translate into image blur (Fig. 42–5*A*). In addition, patient movement between different imaging sequences makes it difficult to correlate anatomy in different planes. It is therefore valuable to invest time in patient comfort. We have found that 15 to 30 minutes of patient orientation relieves anxiety and translates into a greater likelihood that the patient will lie still during the 60- to 90-minute examination. Occasionally the size of the magnet bore causes claustrophobic anxiety, but in our experience this occurs in less than 1 percent of patients. During the first few minutes of the study a patient may be anxious, but the noise that accompanies the gradient pulsing during scanning is monotonous and rather soothing. Most patients relax after a few minutes, and many fall asleep. It is often desirable to have the patient's arms over the head, to reduce aliasing ("wraparound") artifact from the arms. This is tiring for a long time but is easily alleviated by bringing the patient out of the magnet bore (but still on the table) between each series (every 10 to 15 minutes). This also reduces anxiety in those patients who are claustrophobic.

When adult sedation is necessary, a small quantity of oral benzodiazepine, such as triazolam (Halcion, 0.125 milligram), is ideal. The onset of action is 15 to 30 minutes, peak action is 1 to 3 hours, and total duration is usually much less than 24 hours.[R1] Other benzodiazepines, such as diazepam (Valium), are adequate but have a much longer duration of action.[A1]

With children under the age of 5 or 6 years, sedation is necessary. The most common agent for infants under 6 months of age is oral chloral hydrate. For children over 1 year old, the most common regimen is Demerol-Phenergan-Thorazine,[D1, F1, H5] via intramuscular injection. Excellent success has been reported

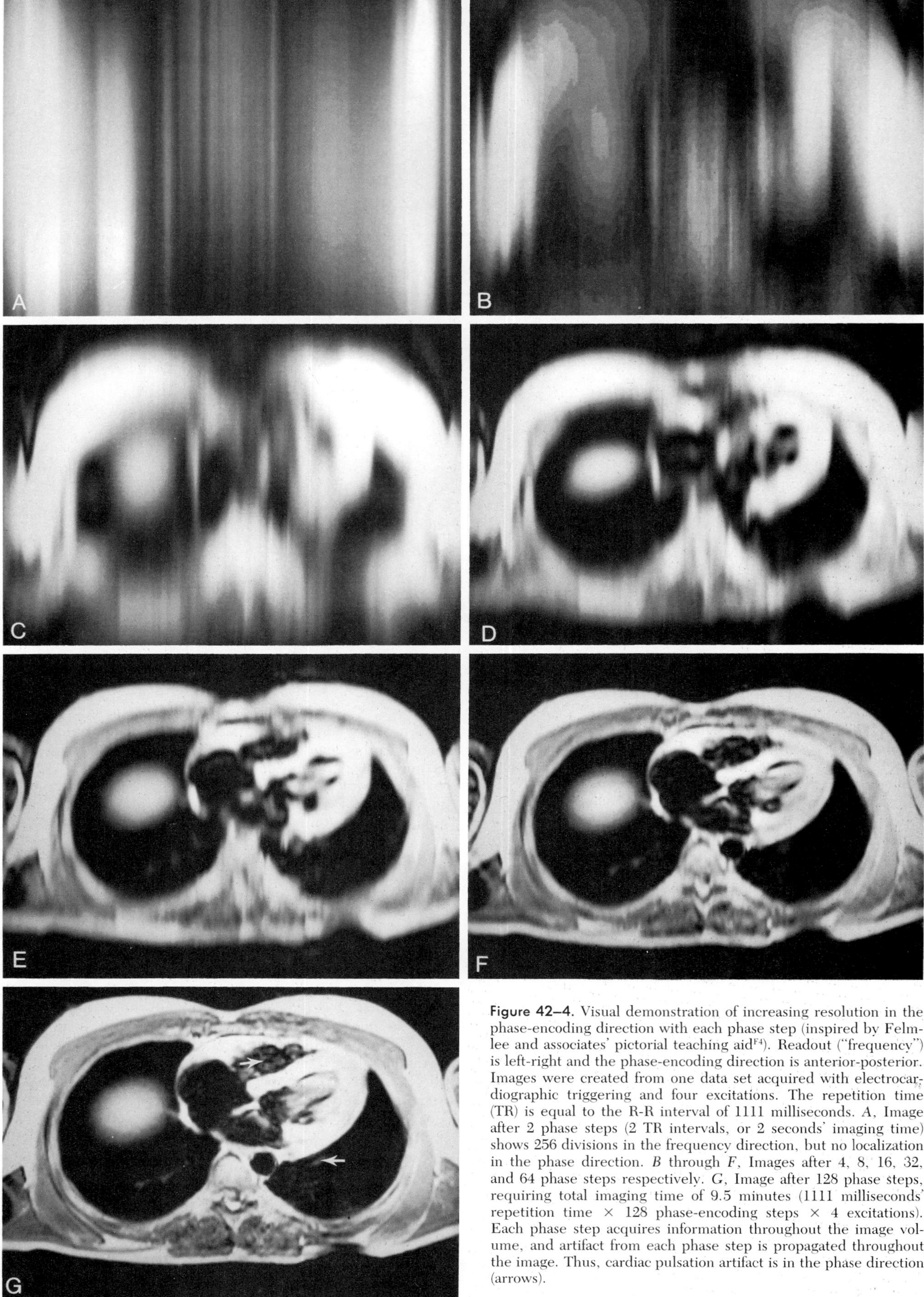

Figure 42–4. Visual demonstration of increasing resolution in the phase-encoding direction with each phase step (inspired by Felmlee and associates' pictorial teaching aid[F4]). Readout ("frequency") is left-right and the phase-encoding direction is anterior-posterior. Images were created from one data set acquired with electrocardiographic triggering and four excitations. The repetition time (TR) is equal to the R-R interval of 1111 milliseconds. *A*, Image after 2 phase steps (2 TR intervals, or 2 seconds' imaging time) shows 256 divisions in the frequency direction, but no localization in the phase direction. *B* through *F*, Images after 4, 8, 16, 32, and 64 phase steps respectively. *G*, Image after 128 phase steps, requiring total imaging time of 9.5 minutes (1111 milliseconds' repetition time × 128 phase-encoding steps × 4 excitations). Each phase step acquires information throughout the image volume, and artifact from each phase step is propagated throughout the image. Thus, cardiac pulsation artifact is in the phase direction (arrows).

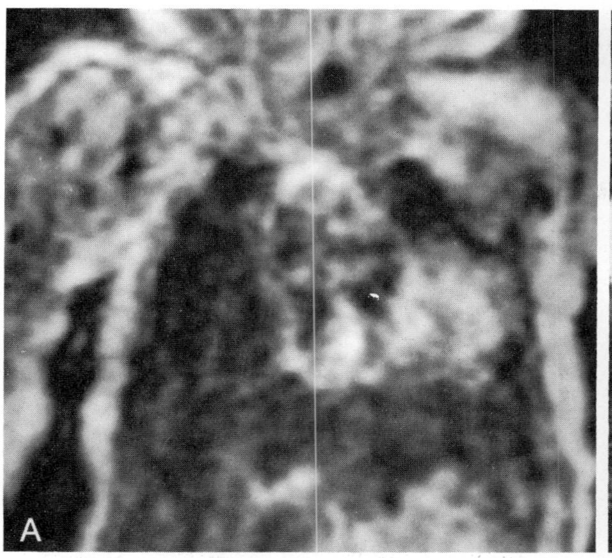

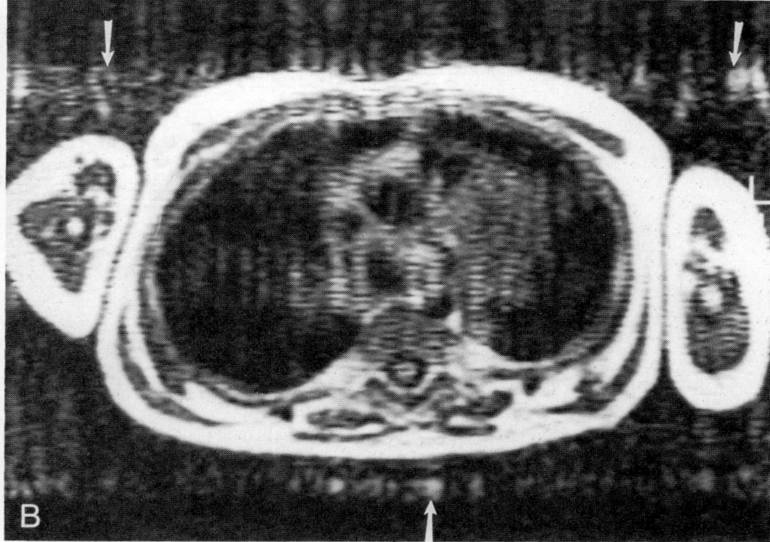

Figure 42–5. Comparison of artifacts from patient motion and system malfunction. *A*, Gross patient motion results in blur severely degrading images of this infant. *B*, System-related artifact is distinguished from patient motion since artifacts (arrows) do not relate to anatomy. Many different component failures may result in a similar result in the image, and isolation of the malfunction is frequently tedious.

with intravenous pentobarbital (Nembutal),[S5,6] which we have increasingly employed. One center reported success with rectal thiopental.[G2] Adequate pulse oximeter monitoring is vital when using deep sedation. General anesthesia has been employed at our center for neurologic studies but not for cardiac imaging.

In a living patient, the organs in the chest are in constant motion. Since it takes at least seconds, and typically minutes, for each series of MR images, it is at first surprising that the heart and great vessels are not a complete blur. In addition to cardiac motion and transmitted pulsations, there is respiration and constantly flowing blood. Each of these entities contributes different artifacts. Since motion artifacts are expressed in the phase direction, by exchanging the phase and frequency directions motion artifacts sometimes may be directed away from the anatomy of interest.[H2]

Cardiac Motion

The motion of the heart is complex, both in time and in space. The heart rate varies with respiration, level of patient relaxation, medication, and pathology.[K3, M2, O1] Not only do the atria and ventricles contract at different times, but also the planes of contraction are oriented differently and obliquely in space. When this motion of the heart is combined with motion of the diaphragm and chest wall from respiration, the result is complex and obviates the use of multiaveraging alone. A variety of techniques, however, have proved valuable in addressing cardiac motion (Table 42–2).

Triggering: Electrocardiogram and Pulse

The most widely employed and effective solution to cardiac motion is known as cardiac triggering or gating. This is analogous to using a strobe to "freeze" motion. The R-wave of the electrocardiogram (ECG) signal (or the peak pressure wave of the peripheral pulse) is continuously monitored and triggers the phase-encoding pulse for each slice at the same time in the cardiac cycle.[H5, L1, U1] Images at different locations in the heart, therefore, are also obtained at different periods or phases in the cardiac cycle.[S1, W1]

The key to successful ECG gating is lead placement. In the magnet, high velocity blood flowing in the aorta induces current that is detected in the ECG leads. This current is directed perpendicular to the aorta and has maximal components in the same direction as conventional limb leads I, II, and III. The resultant ECG deflections may be as large as the R-wave and tend to fill the S-T interval with large oscillations.[P2, S1] The system may then trigger on both the R and T waves. To reduce this effect, leads are usually placed on the back, and a filter is added to the ECG line.[D2]

There are several software subtleties regarding cardiac triggering. Since each slice is excited only once during an R-R interval, the repetition time (TR) is equal to the R-R interval. In children, who have higher heart rates, the repetition time will be shorter than in an adult with a slower heart rate. For example, a child with a rate of 120 beats per minute will have an R-R interval of 500 milliseconds. Images can be collected in 500 milliseconds × 128 phase-encoding steps × 2 excitations = 2.1 minutes. An adult with a rate of 60 beats per minute will have an R-R interval (and also a repetition time TR) of 1000 milliseconds and require 4.3 minutes for the same study. The importance of R-wave detection becomes obvious: if even a few R-waves are missed, the study becomes lengthy. The difference between accurate triggering and poor triggering is readily apparent (Fig. 42–6).

With conventional spin-echo imaging, an ECG signal from central electrodes will usually produce better images in the chest than a peripheral pulse trigger (Fig. 42–7). There are at least two obvious reasons for this. First, the delay from the electrical R-wave until the peripheral pulse varies from 150 to 500 milliseconds.[K3, O2, M2] Second, the R-wave is most closely related to the contraction of the heart, whereas the pulse may not only be delayed but also modified in transit to the periphery. Peripheral gating is entirely adequate when imaging anatomy outside the heart; if an adequate ECG wave cannot be detected, peripheral gating can be used for cardiac imaging. In fact, if the peripheral pulse signal is clearer and results in a more accurate trigger, pulse gating may produce better images. A possible advantage is

Table 42–2. TECHNIQUES TO ADDRESS CARDIAC MOTION

Technique	Effectiveness	Tradeoffs
ECG triggering	Excellent	Need good trace Scan time depends on rate Cannot image near R-wave
Pulse triggering	Fair to good	Inferior to ECG gating but may be easier in some patients
Retrospective gating	Fair to excellent	Easy to image near R-wave Quality variable
Echo-planar imaging	Unknown	Research technique

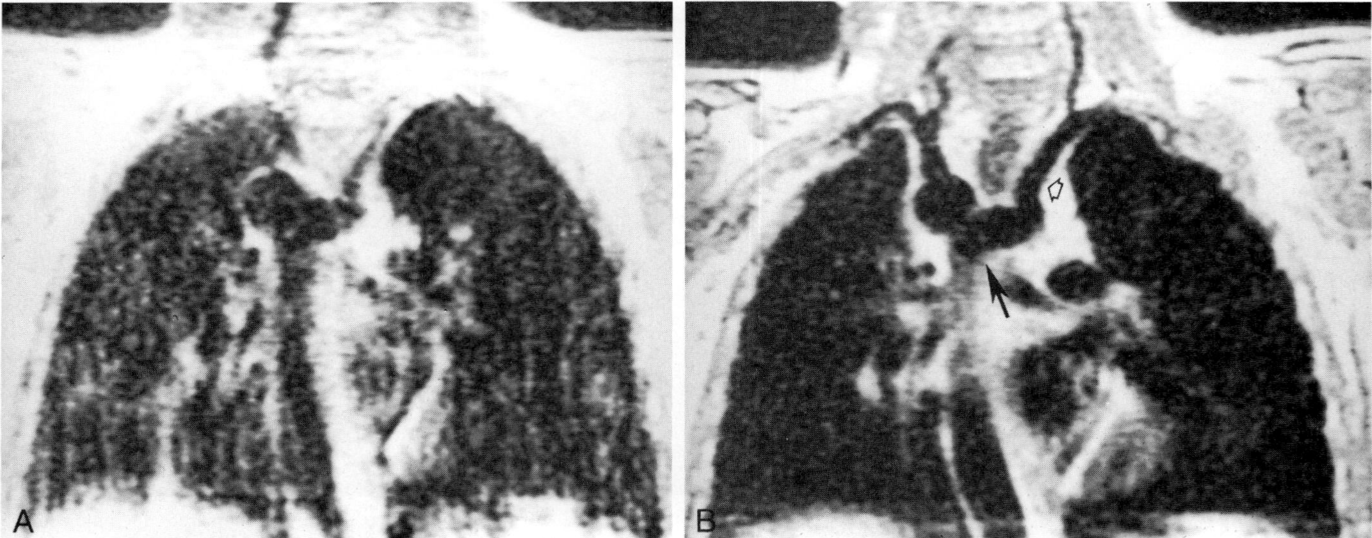

Figure 42–6. Importance of accurate electrocardiographic (ECG) triggering. Coronal spin-echo images of right aortic arch and aberrant left subclavian artery in an 8-year-old boy. *A*, Irregular ECG trigger results in poor image, despite four excitations requiring 6 minutes imaging time. *B*, Identical location and similar parameters with accurate ECG triggering results in markedly improved image quality with only 2 excitations, in half the imaging time (3 minutes). The right aortic arch (arrow) and aberrant left subclavian artery (open arrow) are clearly defined.

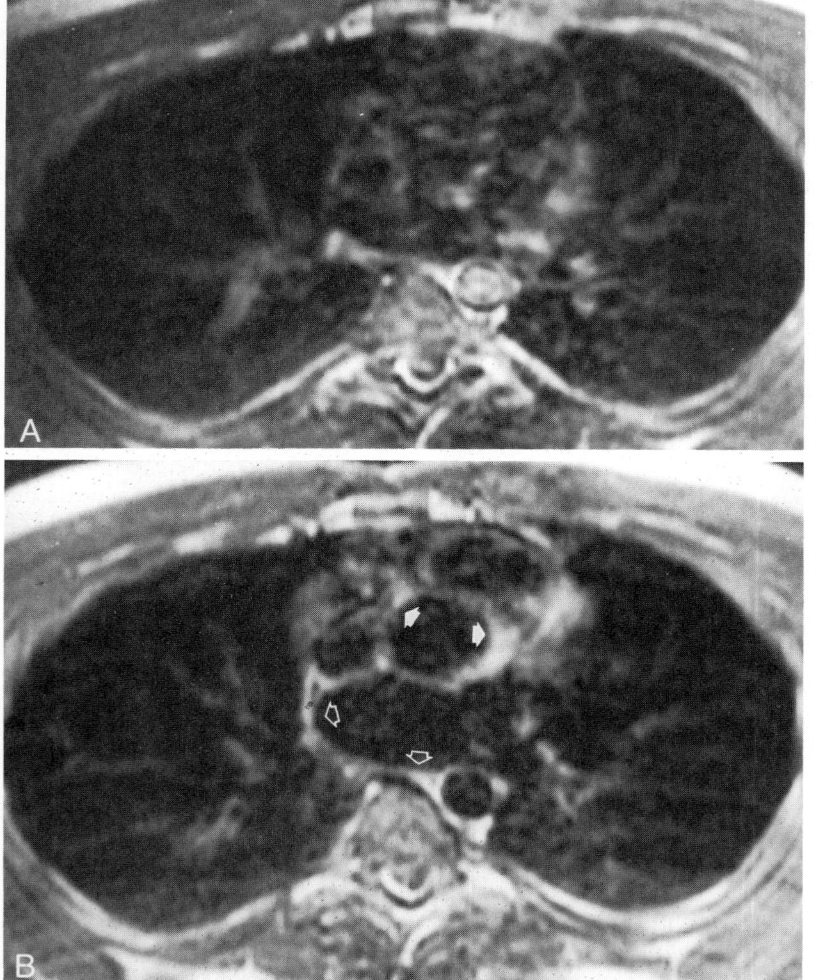

Figure 42–7. Comparison of pulse (peripheral) triggering and electrocardiographic (ECG) triggering. Spin-echo axial images through the upper heart in diastole with identical parameters. *A*, With pulse triggering, artifacts from motion of the heart and blood flow obscure anatomy. *B*, With ECG triggering, definition is improved, and the aortic root (solid arrows) and left atrial wall (open arrows) are clearly visible.

that since there is a 200- to 500-millisecond delay between the R-wave of the ECG and the peripheral pulse,[M2, O1,2] pulse triggering would image during late diastole when flow is slower. Imaging during diastole has been advocated to reduce artifacts.[G2] Our experience suggests that despite this, ECG triggering in general provides better spin-echo images (Fig. 42–7). Cardiac triggering may be employed either with conventional 90° to 180° spin-echo imaging or with gradient-echo imaging.

Retrospective Gating

A second solution to cardiac motion is retrospective gating, similar to a cardiac-gated radionuclide angiocardiogram. Images are acquired continuously throughout many R-R intervals while the ECG is recorded. The computer then retrospectively sorts the data with respect to the R-wave and creates images corresponding to different times in an "ideal" R-R interval.[G1] Since the ECG is not triggering the scan, this method may be less sensitive to arrhythmia. In addition, retrospective gating based on the pulse yields almost identical images to central (ECG) gating, when the pulse is regular (unpublished data). Retrospective gating has the advantage of imaging near the R-wave, which cannot be accomplished with ECG triggering, since the imaging signal obscures the ECG signal. Since retrospective gating requires the acquisition of multiple data points in a short time, gradient-echo imaging is employed. The final images may be displayed rapidly, providing the illusion of cardiac contraction similar to a conventional cineangiocardiogram.[G1]

High-Speed MR Imaging

A potentially exciting direct solution to cardiac motion is the use of echo-planar MR imaging, currently undergoing advanced research and development.[O3, R2,3] With this technique, the human heart has been imaged at a rate of 40 milliseconds per image. This provides a time resolution only slightly less than conventional cineangiography and should eliminate the need for retrospective gating, prospective triggering, and respiratory compensation. Much development will be necessary before this can become routine clinical reality.

Cine-Magnetic Resonance Imaging

Images obtained during different portions of the cardiac cycle (but at the same location) may be displayed rapidly by the computer as the frames of a movie, producing a visual impression of cardiac motion. Images obtained with any of the methods described earlier may be employed to create the movie, including *spin-echo*, prospective *gradient-echo*, retrospective gradient-echo, and *echo-planar* techniques. When a gradient-echo sequence with gradient moment nulling is employed, the blood in the cardiac chambers is bright, and the appearance is similar to a conventional cineangiocardiogram, hence the name cine-MRI. However, if the signal from blood remains displaced from the chambers, the chambers will appear dark, and the resultant movie will appear similar to an echocardiogram. The cine-MRI display is commonly recorded on videotape.

Respiratory Motion

Respiratory motion is relatively simple but difficult to entirely compensate for. With each breath, the chest volume increases with expansion of the chest wall laterally, anteriorly, and posteriorly. There is also movement inferiorly as the diaphragm moves down. This results in motion within the axial and coronal planes, and also motion in and out of these planes. The greatest excursion is at the diaphragm, which frequently appears blurred.

Averaging

There are several methods to address breathing motion (Table 42–3), with varying success in each patient. The simplest solution is to repeat each phase-encoding excitation step multiple times and average them together. This is a remarkably effective technique and is commonly employed (Fig. 42–8). The major tradeoff is time: the study time increases linearly with the number of averages. However, the longer the study, the greater the likelihood of gross patient motion and image degradation. Occasionally breath-holding during a very short scan (less than 20 seconds) is possible.[P3] This addresses chest wall and diaphragmatic motion, but cardiac motion and transmitted pulsation into the mediastinal structures remain. Occasionally, placing the patient prone rather than supine is helpful, so that the posterior chest moves with respiration. This may be employed to evaluate the anterior chest wall. In our experience, it is considerably less comfortable for the patient and does not result in significant image quality improvement. Anterior chest motion, however, can be reduced with a binder around the chest, which encourages the patient to ventilate with diaphragmatic motion. We commonly employ such a binder.

Table 42–3. TECHNIQUES TO ADDRESS RESPIRATORY MOTION

Technique	Effectiveness	Tradeoffs
Averaging	Good to excellent	Linear scan time increase Requires even breathing
Breath-holding	Impractical	Scan times too long to be practical
Triggering	Good	Requires too long scan times
Sorting	Fair to excellent	Interaction between rates of breathing, pulse repetitions, and heart beat determines quality Not useful with infants
Gradient moment nulling	Fair to excellent	Usually makes vessels bright Increases echo time (unimportant) Often better than sorting Excellent with infants Limits slice thickness and size of imaged anatomy Decreases number of slices obtainable within a given time
Chest wall fat suppression	Unknown	Spatial presaturation shows more promise than inversion-recovery

Triggering and Sorting

Respiratory triggering similar to cardiac triggering is an attractive method in theory to address breathing motion. *Breathing is monitored, and scanning performed only while there is no breathing motion: between the end of expiration and the beginning of the next inspiration.*[E2, R4] The difficulty, however, is the respiratory rate. With a typical respiratory rate of 15 breaths per minute and 128 phase-encoding steps, one series of images would require over 8 minutes. With 4 excitations, the study lengthens to 34 minutes. Respiratory triggering is seldom employed clinically.

A different solution is to *rearrange the phase-encoding steps to match breathing*. This has given rise to several acronyms: *respiratory-sorted phase-encoding* (RSPE), *respiratory-ordered phase-encoding* (ROPE), or *respiratory compensation* (RC).[H1,3] As currently implemented on our systems, breathing is sensed with a bellows placed around the chest, and the system selects the phase-encoding steps with respect to respiration. When this works well, there is considerable image quality improvement (Fig. 42–9). It is important that the bellows correctly sense the breathing pattern. Since patients may breathe predominantly with the chest or with the diaphragm, different patients may require different placement of the bellows; sometimes a "bandolier" configuration works well. Even with perfect monitoring, a different problem may arise. The phase-encoding steps must occur in synchrony with the power line frequency of 60 Hertz (or 50 Hertz) to avoid artifact in the images. If respiration is in synchrony with the line frequency, the phase-encoding can occur at a repetitive portion of the cycle. However, if the patient's respiration is not synchronous with the line frequency, the system cannot phase-encode at the appropriate time, and image quality

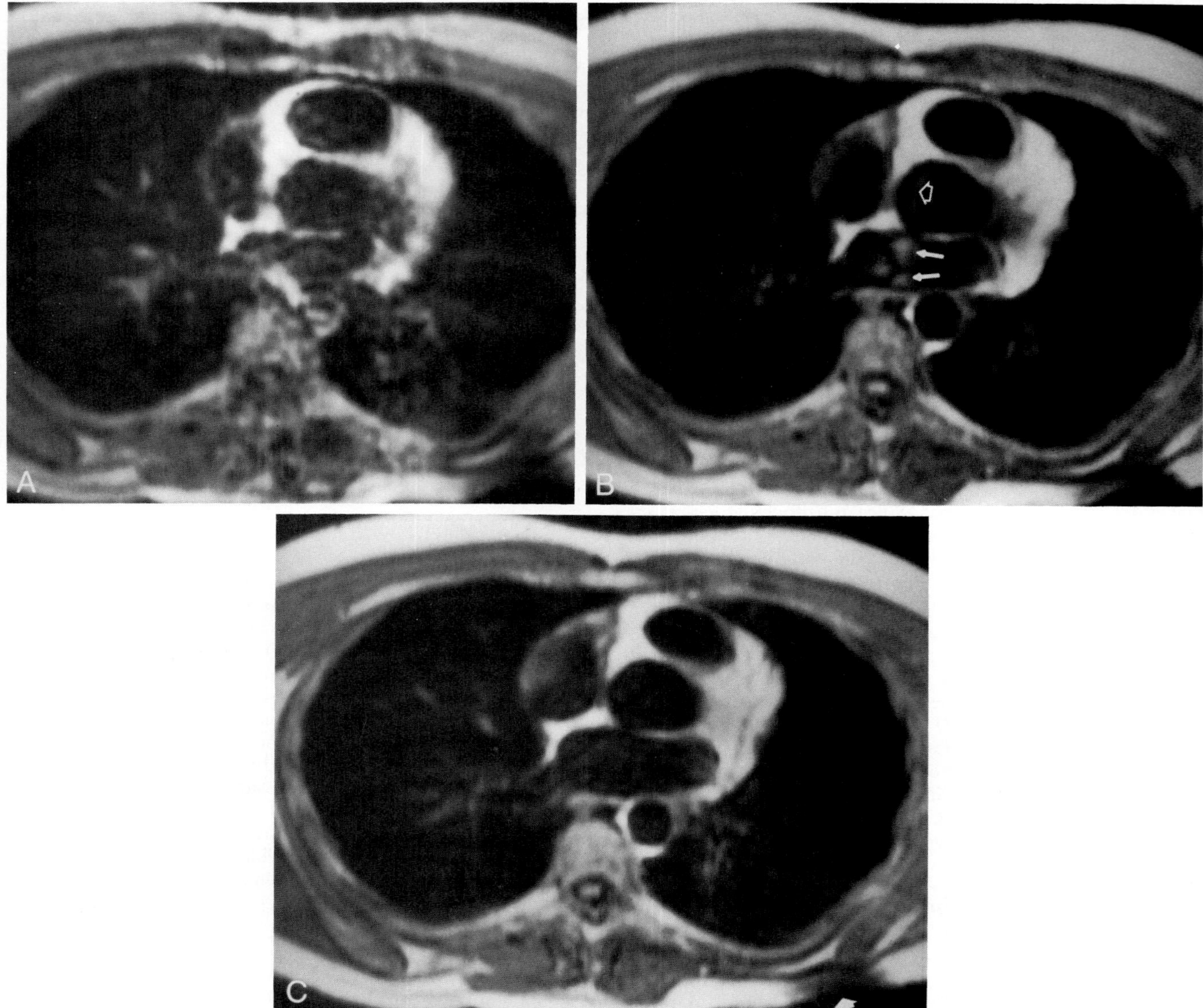

Figure 42–8. Averaging to reduce motion artifacts and spatial presaturation to reduce flow-related enhancement. *A*, Axial spin-echo image through the upper heart with one excitation, requiring 2 minutes' imaging time. Signals from flowing blood, respiration, and heart motion obscure anatomy. *B*, Axial image at the same location with four excitations requiring 7 minutes' imaging time. Resolution is improved, but artifactual signal from phase-displaced flow-related enhancement mimics masses in the left atrium (solid arrows) and dissection of the medial wall of the aortic root (open arrow). *C*, Addition of spatial presaturation reduces the flow artifacts. Note the dark artifact on the posterior left chest wall from the ECG electrode (arrow).

will suffer (Gary Glover, personal communication). If the repetition time (TR) is a multiple of 16.7 milliseconds (1/60 Hertz), the opportunity for the system and the power line to be in synchrony is maximized.[S7]

Cardiac gating, previously discussed, appears frequently to address respiratory motion well, albeit indirectly. Images are collected at multiple points during the cardiac cycle, and since the heart rate is much faster than respiration, the respiratory cycle is divided into many parts. In addition, the heart rate varies with respiration,[M2] and cardiac gating therefore provides an element of respiratory gating.

Gradient Moment Nulling

A different technique to reduce respiratory motion is gradient moment nulling, discussed in more detail with flow artifacts. It is a powerful technique, especially when imaging infants, in whom chest wall motion is too shallow to be sensed with the bellows. In some patients, it may produce a greater improvement in image quality than respiratory-sorted phase-encoding.[M3] The two techniques together can result in marked improvement in image quality.

Fat signal from the moving chest wall causes much of the respiratory artifact, and techniques that selectively decrease fat signal show promise in improving image quality. The inversion recovery sequence can result in nearly complete suppression of fat signal in the abdomen,[H4] but the relatively long imaging times (5 to 10 minutes or more) make this less attractive for chest imaging. Selection of the appropriate parameters with gradient-echo imaging can also result in decrease in fat signal, as previously discussed (see Fig. 42–2). A different technique is spatial presaturation of the anterior chest wall. By repeatedly pulsing at the chest wall location, protons are not allowed to relax and contribute little to signal.[E3, G3] A variation of this technique has been applied to produce dark bands in the myocardium to evaluate ventricular contraction.[Z1]

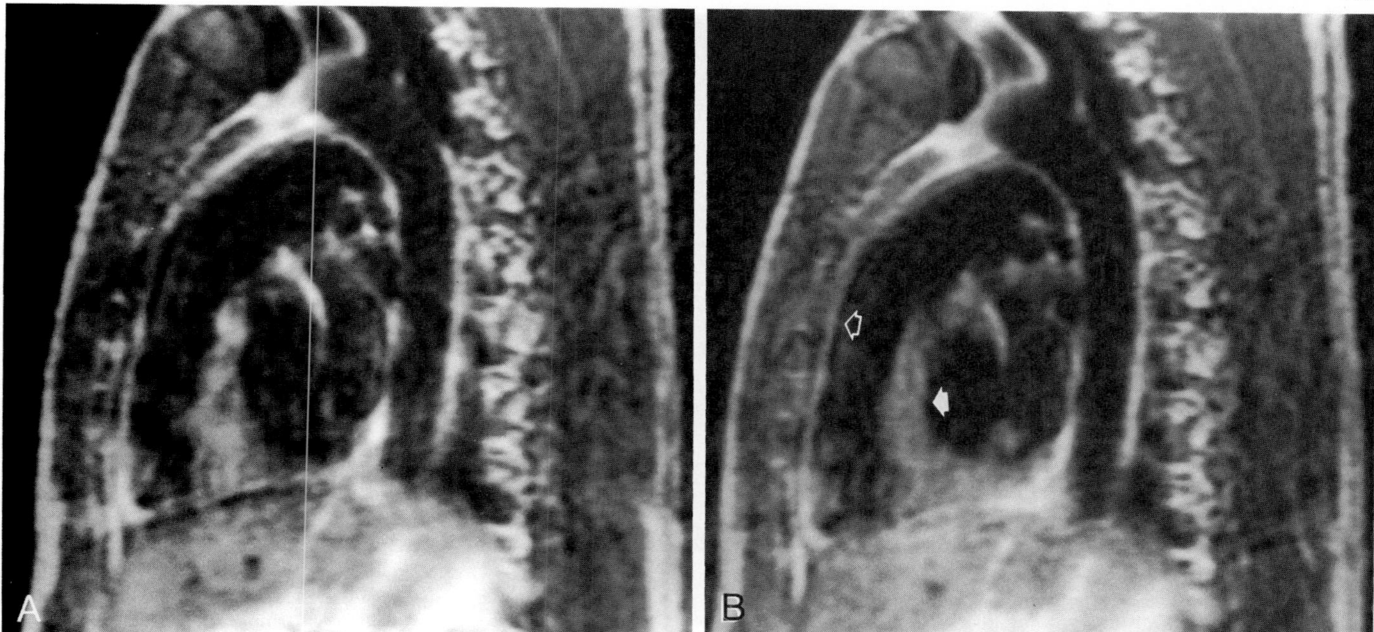

Figure 42–9. Respiratory motion and respiratory-sorted phase encoding in sagittal spin-echo images. *A*, Without, and *B*, with respiratory-sorted phase-encoding. Definition of right ventricular outflow tract (open arrow) and interventricular septum (closed arrow) is improved.

Blood Flow

Flowing blood has a complex appearance on MRI, which is far from completely understood. Blood flow has both constant velocity and pulsatile components. Pure constant velocity flow is rarely present in the chest, due to cardiac pulsations and variations in thoracic pressure during breathing. There are at least three simultaneous effects of blood flow during MR imaging: high-velocity signal loss, flow-related enhancement, and displacement in space from phase error accumulation (the last resulting in phase ghost artifacts). The appearance of flowing blood in the MR image is a function of the interaction of these effects with the imaging sequence and can be either dark or bright in the same patient (see Fig. 42–2). Several techniques have been developed to address blood flow artifacts (Table 42–4).

High-Velocity Signal Loss

If blood leaves the slice before its signal can be detected, the signal will decrease and flowing blood will be dark: this is called *high-velocity signal loss* and has been invoked to explain why vessels and the cardiac chambers are typically dark on spin-echo images.[B2, W5,6] This effect is probably a major cause of the signal void from high-velocity flow seen during the normal phase of cardiac ejection and at areas of stenosis and regurgitation.[E4, M3,4, S8]

Table 42–4. TECHNIQUES TO ADDRESS BLOOD FLOW ARTIFACTS

Technique	Effectiveness	Tradeoffs
Spatial presaturation	Poor to excellent	Makes vessels dark Good for vessels perpendicular to slice plane; poor to good for vessels within slice plane Poor to fair for complex flow in cardiac chambers
Gradient moment nulling	Fair to excellent	Usually makes vessels bright Good to excellent for detection of masses as "filling defects" Limits slice thickness and size of imaged anatomy Decreases number of slices obtainable within a given time
ECG triggering	Poor to good	Fair to good (heart and arteries) Poor to fair (veins)
Pulse triggering	Poor to good	Fair (heart and great vessels) Fair to good (arteries) Poor to fair (veins)

Flow-Related Enhancement

Flow-related enhancement occurs when blood that previously has not been excited enters the imaging volume and is excited with a radio frequency pulse. Most of the tissues in an MR slice have been excited multiple times and never become fully relaxed. However, if unsaturated blood moves into the slice, it has not had an opportunity to be excited previously (i.e., is fully relaxed), and the radio frequency pulse will produce maximal signal[B2, G4, W5–7] (see Fig. 42–8). The effect is commonly present on the first and last slices in a series and is also called the *entry-slice phenomenon*. Up to a point, the faster the flow, the more relaxed blood that enters the slice and the brighter the blood.[W6] This enhancement, however, can be visualized only if the flow is slow enough that the enhanced signal can be detected. If the flow is too fast, high-velocity signal loss will predominate, and the blood will appear dark. The competing effects of high-velocity signal loss and flow-related enhancement thus can make flowing blood have any shade of gray, from very dark to very bright.[W5]

The technique of imaging dramatically alters the ability to detect flow-related enhancement. With the conventional 90° to 180° spin-echo technique, a slice-select gradient is applied during both the 90° and 180° pulses. To be imaged, blood must be in the imaging slice during both the 90° and 180° pulses, which are separated by several milliseconds. At typical flow velocities, signal loss predominates, and the vessels appear dark.[B2, W6,7] Gradient-echo imaging, however, does not employ a second slice-select gradient and detects signal from all excited blood, even if it has left the slice. Flowing blood, therefore, usually is bright on gradient-echo images.[E5, N1, W5,7]

Spatial Presaturation

Flow-related enhancement is a major problem in cardiac imaging, since blood flows in multiple directions at widely varying velocities during the cardiac cycle. The spurious gray signal from flow-related enhancement is commonly present in the cardiac chambers and great vessels and may mimic intracardiac masses

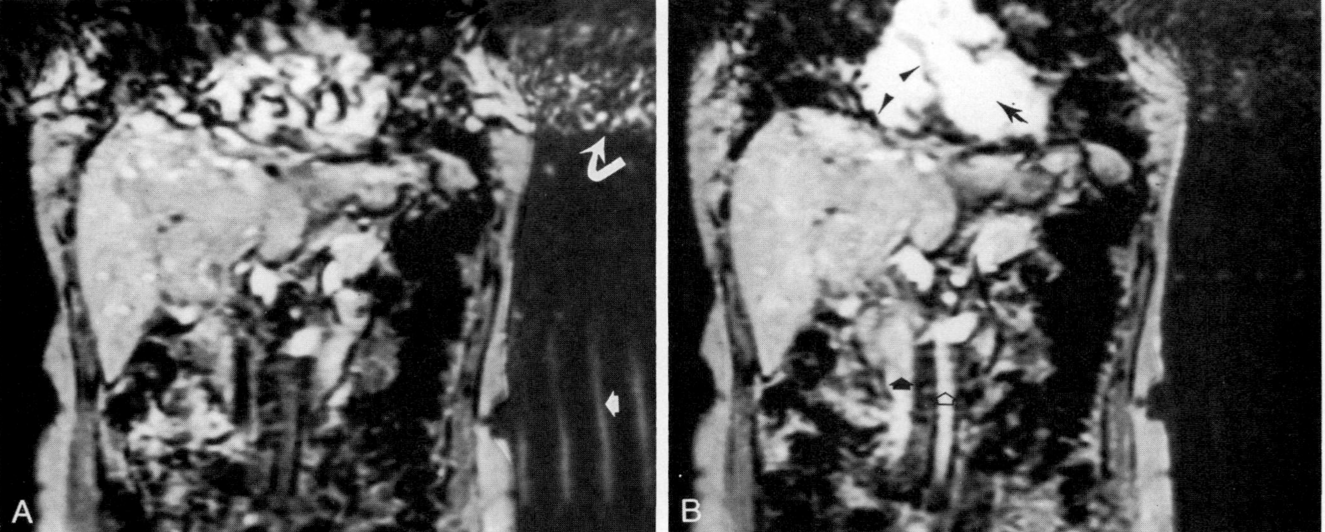

Figure 42–10. Flowing blood produces both flow-related enhancement and phase ghost artifacts. Coronal gradient-echo images obtained during patient breathholding (6 seconds' imaging time). *A*, Coronal image shows bright signal from blood in the cardiac chambers (curved arrow); aorta and inferior vena cava (solid arrow) misplaced in the phase direction as ghosts. *B*, The phase ghosts are corrected in position with application of gradient moment nulling, and the flowing blood in the left ventricle (arrow), right atrium (arrowheads), aorta (open arrow), and vena cava (short solid arrow) is better visualized.

(Fig. 42–8*B*).[H2] This artifact may be substantially reduced by the use of spatial presaturation. This technique typically excites volumes on either side of the slice volume being imaged and in theory eliminates "entry slices."[E3, F3] The success of the spatial presaturation technique varies directly with velocity: if blood is flowing rapidly enough that it traverses the presaturation volume, increased signal will still result. In addition, the effect on flow within the plane is different from flow perpendicular to the plane.[F3] We have found that spatial presaturation applied in a slice-select direction improves spin-echo cardiac images (Fig. 42–8), although frequently some spurious gray signal remains present. Spatial presaturation pulses may be applied within the image plane, producing dark bands in the myocardium, which allows dynamic study of myocardial contraction.[Z1]

Phase Ghost Artifacts

The velocity-induced phase ghost artifact is more difficult to understand, but it results in profound alteration in images. When blood flows from one part of a magnetic field gradient to another, the phase will change.[B2, D3, W5] This phase change is identical to the phase change of nonmoving structures at different locations in the phase-encoding direction. The MR system translates this phase change from flow into ghost images displaced in the phase-encoding direction (Figs. 42–10 and 42–11). The faster the flow, the greater the displacement, until high-velocity signal loss predominates.

Gradient Moment Nulling

The ghost images caused by flow artifact can be minimized with gradient moment nulling. Acronyms include gradient moment reduction (GMR), motion artifact suppression technique (MAST), and flow compensation (FC). Extra gradients are applied that partially correct these phase errors from motion but have no effect on nonmoving structures.[H6, P4, W5] The effect in the image is dramatic: the ghosts are "pushed back" into the correct location (Figs. 42–10 and 42–11). This compensation has limits: if the flow

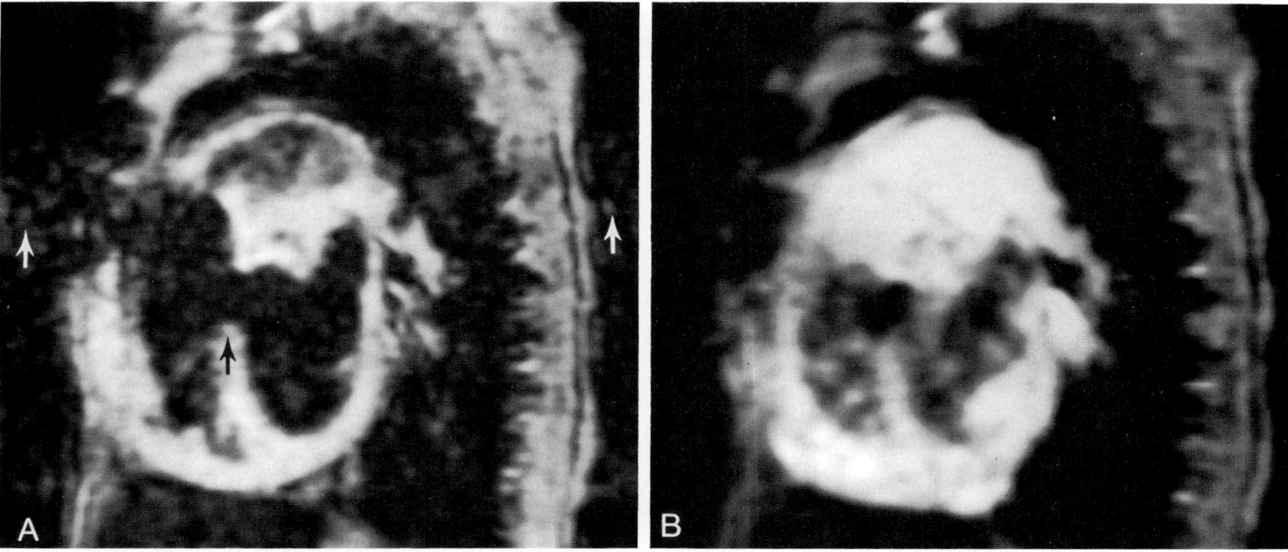

Figure 42–11. Practical application of phase ghosts and gradient moment nulling. Six-week-old girl with ventricular septal defect (VSD) imaged in the head coil with gradient-echo cine technique (5-millimeter slice thickness, 2 minutes' imaging time). *A*, Sagittal image shows the VSD (black arrow) clearly, with flow signal displaced from the cardiac chambers (white arrows). *B*, The addition of gradient moment nulling results in the blood signal being replaced and obscuring the VSD.

is too fast, the system cannot respond rapidly enough or with sufficient power to compensate entirely. Thus, in very fast flow such as during normal systolic ejection, or at sites of regurgitation or stenosis, the flow will be so fast that the signal remains displaced, and there is a flow void (Fig. 42–12). This may be identical to high-velocity signal loss.

It occasionally is desirable to image without gradient moment nulling, to displace blood signal out of the cardiac chambers and better outline anatomy (see Fig. 42–11). In principle, this information may be employed to quantify flow velocity, stenosis, and regurgitation.[D3, G2, H7, M3,4, P5, S8] Flow-induced phase errors may be serendipitously corrected with the application of the second 180° pulse in spin-echo imaging. This effect can be seen on uniformly spaced multiple spin-echoes. On the even echoes, the 180° pulse may correct previous flow dephasing, producing artifactual "even echo rephasing" signal in a vessel.[B2, W2]

Gradient moment nulling involves significant tradeoffs, since the technique employs gradients. The gradients are employed to define the imaging volume, that is, the slice thickness, field of view, and slice plane obliquity. Gradient moment nulling imposes additional stress on the gradients, and therefore there must be a tradeoff between the field-of-view, slice thickness, obliquity, and pulse repetition time (TR). Furthermore, the additional gradients require additional time, and therefore the echo time (TE) must lengthen. For "first order" gradient moment nulling (velocity compensation), the minimum echo time (TE) typically increases by 30 to 50 percent. On our General Electric Signa systems, this translates into the echo time lengthening from 20 to 30 milliseconds for a conventional spin-echo sequence and from 9 to 13 milliseconds for gradient-echo imaging. A longer echo time will result in less signal from stationary structures. However, for moving structures, the decrease in signal from lengthening the echo time is more than compensated for by increase in signal as a result of signal being replaced in its correct location. Clinically, the increase in echo time from gradient moment nulling rarely has a negative impact on image quality. Gradient moment nulling is a powerful technique, which compensates for any motion that has a significant constant velocity component. Therefore, it is applicable not only to venous flow but also arterial flow (see Fig. 42–10) and breathing.[M3] It is of particular value in infants in whom adult respiratory sensors are ineffective.

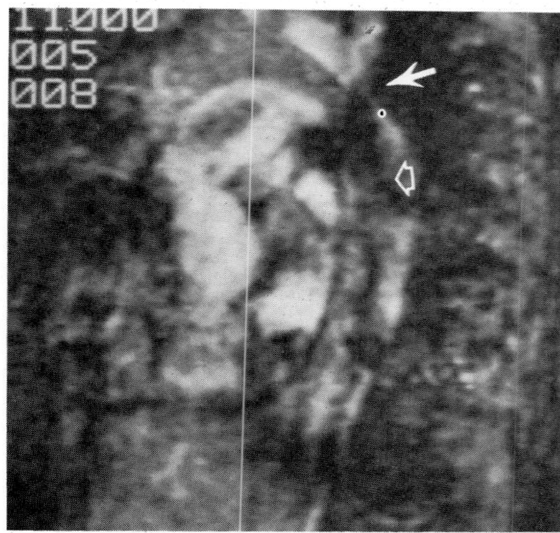

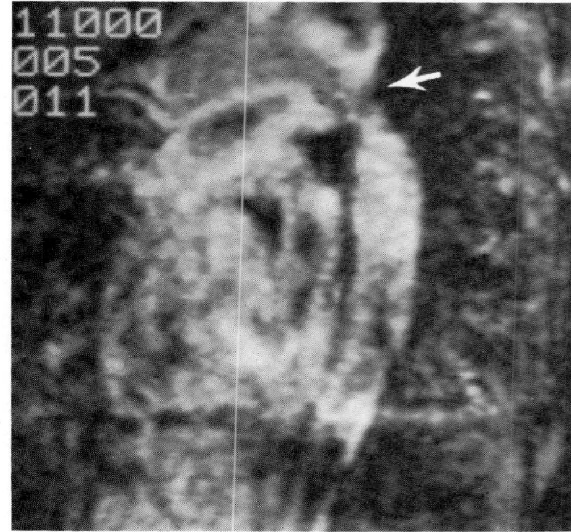

Figure 42–12. Flow-related enhancement and high-velocity signal loss predominate at different times as aortic flow velocity changes during the cardiac cycle. Four-year-old girl with coarctation of aorta evaluated with gradient-echo cine technique (5-millimeter slice thickness, gradient moment nulling, 3 minute imaging time). On the upper image, obtained during rapid systolic flow, high-velocity signal loss results in a poststenotic jet (open arrow) at coarctation (solid arrow). Turbulence also may contribute to signal loss.[E4] On the lower image, obtained during late diastole, the flow is slower, and flow-related enhancement predominates, resulting in bright signal throughout the descending aorta, including the coarctation site (solid arrow).

Pulsatile Flow

Pulsatile flow is a major factor within the chest. All pulsatile flow has a component of constant velocity, and thus correction of constant velocity flow artifact will to a large extent improve artifact from pulsatile flow. A common artifact resulting from pulsatile flow is diastolic pseudogating.[B1] During the diastolic portion of the cardiac cycle, blood is relatively stationary.[K3, M2, O1] This stationary blood with its long relaxation time contributes signal similar to that of any stationary structure and will appear brighter on images acquired during diastole, because the usual high-velocity signal loss does not occur. This knowledge can be utilized clinically by imaging later in the cardiac cycle.[G2]

Magnetic Resonance Angiography and Phase Imaging

These flow artifacts may contribute valuable information. The identification of stenosis and regurgitation relies on the flow void of phase artifact[M3,4, P5, S8] seen in gradient-echo imaging (see Chapter 41). The contribution of turbulent flow to this artifact is unclear, but it at least occasionally contributes to the loss of signal.[E4] It is also possible to image only the signal effects of flow. This is the basis for MR angiography, currently in clinical research evaluation.[D4, 5]

MRI SYSTEM–RELATED ARTIFACTS AND SOLUTIONS

Numerous artifacts are related to the physics and engineering of the MRI system. We will first discuss artifacts inherent in the physics of MRI, and then briefly discuss artifacts related to the current state of equipment development.

Aliasing (Wraparound)

With any form of digital imaging, it is axiomatic that sufficient data must be acquired to uniquely describe a portion of the anatomy. Unfortunately, there are always tradeoffs of time and expense. When the data sampling rate is insufficient to determine an image uniquely, *aliasing* occurs. This term arises from the Fourier transform, in which higher frequencies are incorrectly represented ("aliased") as lower frequencies.[H1,2, K2, S2] There are several manifestations of aliasing in MRI. Aliasing, commonly called *wraparound*, can occur in either the phase (Figs. 42–13*A* and 42–14*A*) or the frequency directions.[H3, P1] If only the heart and mediastinum are of interest, one solution is to center the heart within the magnet and ignore the artifacts on the chest walls. Wraparound aliasing in the left-right direction often results when the patient's arms are at the side. If the arms are held over the head during scanning, this will be eliminated. Alternatively, this can be addressed by expanding the field of view while simultaneously increasing the matrix to maintain resolution (Figs. 42–13*B* and 42–14*B*). The images are then displayed using only

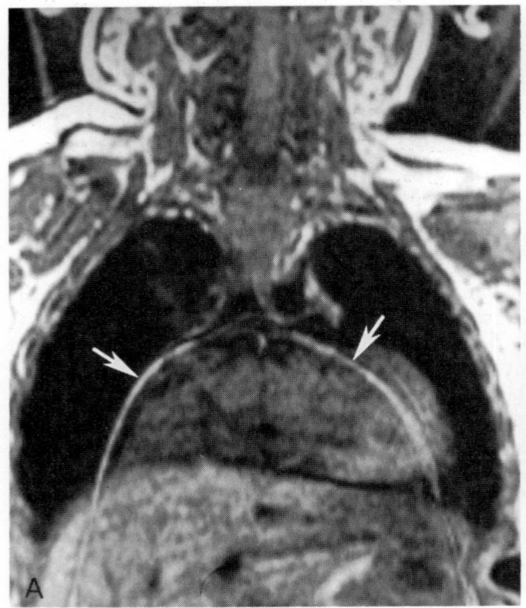

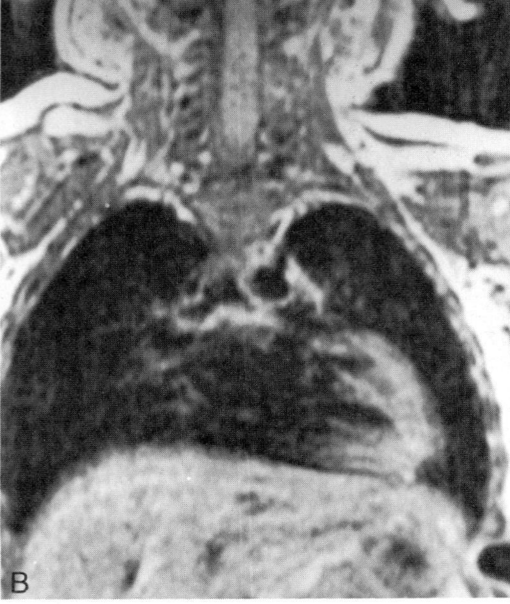

Figure 42–13. Aliasing ("wrap-around") in the phase direction. Readout (frequency direction) aliasing has a similar appearance. Coronal spin-echo images of an 8-month-old boy imaged in the head coil (3-mm slice thickness, 2 minutes' imaging time). *A*, The head is outside the field of view, and its signal is aliased into the chest (arrows). *B*, When the field of view is doubled, the artifact is eliminated.

the center of the expanded matrix. This has been called *no-phase-wrap* or *no-frequency-wrap*.

Local Field Inhomogeneity

Local field inhomogeneity produces localized loss of signal and is easily recognizable. One cause is a local change in magnetic susceptibility, i.e., the degree to which a substance can distort the magnetic field. If two substances next to each other are similar in susceptibility, there is a smooth transition in the magnetic field lines and no image effect. However, when two tissues are very different in susceptibility, there is a sudden change in the field density and contour that causes distortion in the image. In the chest, this commonly occurs where air within the tracheobronchial tree is seen adjacent to soft tissue and is most evident with gradient-echo imaging. This is annoying, since the left main stem bronchus is near the most common aortic coarctation site (Fig. 42–15). Susceptibility artifact also can arise from the air-muscle-fat interfaces of the chest wall. If this lies outside the field of view, it may be aliased on gradient-echo images as a moiré pattern that does not resemble anatomy (see Fig. 42–14). This has also been termed *susceptibility flowering*[H2] and is not observed unless a susceptibility interface exists outside the field of view (Todd Reinke, unpublished data).

Artifacts from Metal

A second cause of local field distortion arises from currents induced in metal objects by the changing gradient fields. This field distortion results in a localized loss of signal (Fig. 42–16). This occurs with all metal, even if it is nonmagnetic. Indeed, nearly all surgical metal in the chest, such as sternal wires, skin staples, and cardiac valves are stainless steel and either nonmagnetic or minimally magnetic.[S9–11] It is striking that even with the large mobile mass of a mitral ball-cage valve, the signal loss is localized, even with gradient-echo imaging. (Fig. 42–16) ECG surface electrodes contain sufficient metal to produce a small artifact; it is desirable to place these so that they are not included in the image plane.

The magnetic field is frequently distorted intentionally to smooth out irregularities. The importance of maintaining a uniform steady field (shimming) cannot be underestimated. There are two general shimming techniques: active and passive, and both can be employed together for optimum field homogeneity. Passive shimming is accomplished by placing large pieces of ferrous metal within the field, whereas active shimming is performed with extramagnetic field coils. When coupled with an aggressive quality control program, image quality can be significantly improved.[H2]

Engineering-Related System Artifacts

Many artifacts are related to the current state of engineering development, and an exhaustive list is impossible. As the causes are identified, they are addressed by the manufacturers, and new artifacts are identified in a continual process. Several artifacts are related to the radio frequencies employed in imaging. The "zipper" artifact from a stray radiofrequency signal has previously been discussed (see Figs. 42–1 and 42–2*B*). An unusual artifact, known as a "transmit ghost," can occur if the radio frequency pulse is not correctly tuned (Fig. 42–17). This will appear symmetrically within slices on either side of the center slice. A significant error in only one data collection of the 65,000 or more raw data points can result in a "corduroy artifact" (see Fig. 42–15*B*).[H1, 3]

SUMMARY

At present, the majority of artifacts in cardiac MRI result from blood flow, cardiac motion, and respiratory motion. A variety of techniques exist for addressing these motion artifacts, which are listed in Table 42–5 in the approximate order of effectiveness. The relative value of these techniques in MRI of the heart differs from their relative value in MRI of the abdomen, head, and spine.

The most important artifact correction techniques are averaging and ECG triggering. In general, good-to-excellent images will be the rule with four excitations and reliable ECG triggering. The next most important technique is gradient moment nulling, which improves artifacts from respiratory motion, pulsatile motion, and flow. This is especially valuable in addressing flow artifact from vessels after the MRI contrast agent gadopentetate dimeglumine (Magnevist, Berlex) has been administered. An added advantage is that blood in vessels and cardiac chambers is bright, providing contrast to dark lungs, bronchi, and relatively dark myocardium.

The anti-aliasing techniques to address frequency wrap and

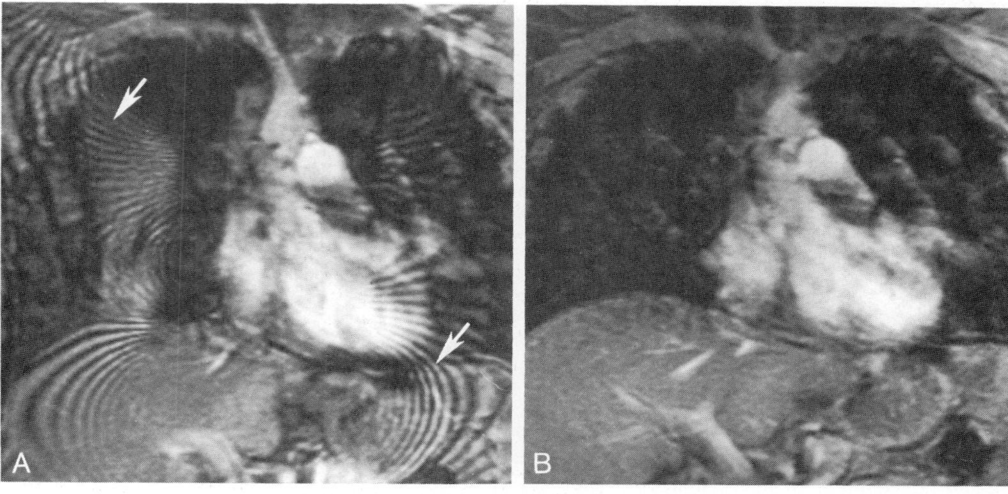

Figure 42–14. Aliasing in the phase direction on gradient-echo images often appears different from spin-echo aliasing and is related to the greater sensitivity of the gradient-echo to field inhomogeneities.[H2] *A*, Coronal gradient-echo image with imaging field smaller than the chest shows moiré lines (arrows) representing wraparound of the chest wall; it is not recognizable as anatomy. *B*, After correcting for wraparound, the artifact is eliminated.

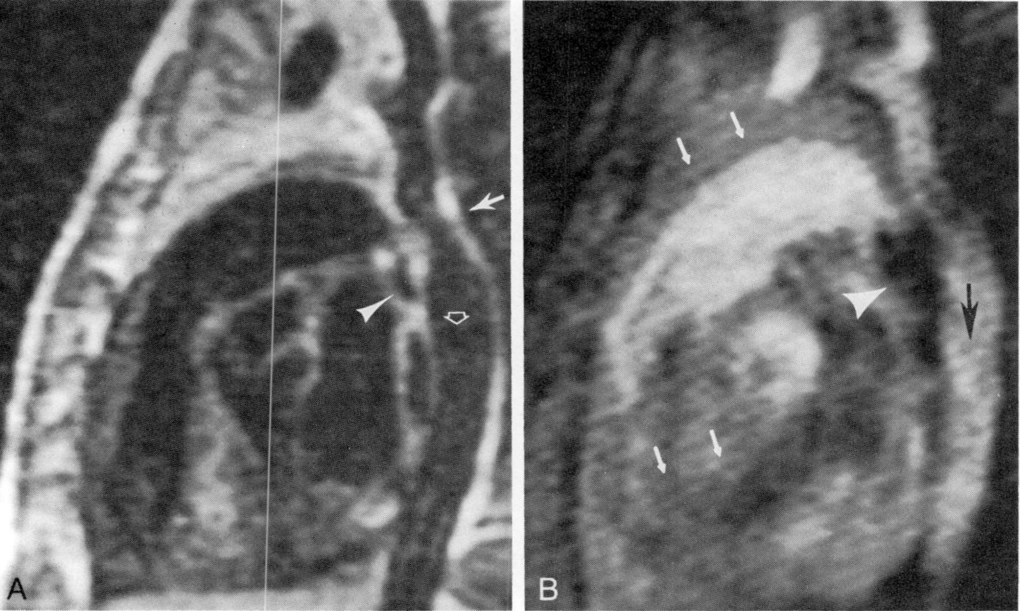

Figure 42–15. Artifacts related to susceptibility, flow, and single raw data collection error. *A*, Sagittal spin-echo image (3-millimeter slice thickness) of focal coarctation of aorta (solid arrow), adjacent to left main stem bronchus (arrowhead). Note that blood in aorta (open arrow) is dark from high-velocity signal loss. *B*, Gradient-echo image (5-millimeter slice thickness) at same location shows dark susceptibility artifact (white arrowhead) from interface of bronchial air with adjacent tissue. Compare also the appearance of blood in the aorta (black arrow): it is bright, since flow-related enhancement usually predominates over high-velocity signal loss on gradient-echo images. The diagonal lines (white arrows) or "corduroy artifact" result from a single data collection error, which is propagated throughout the image.

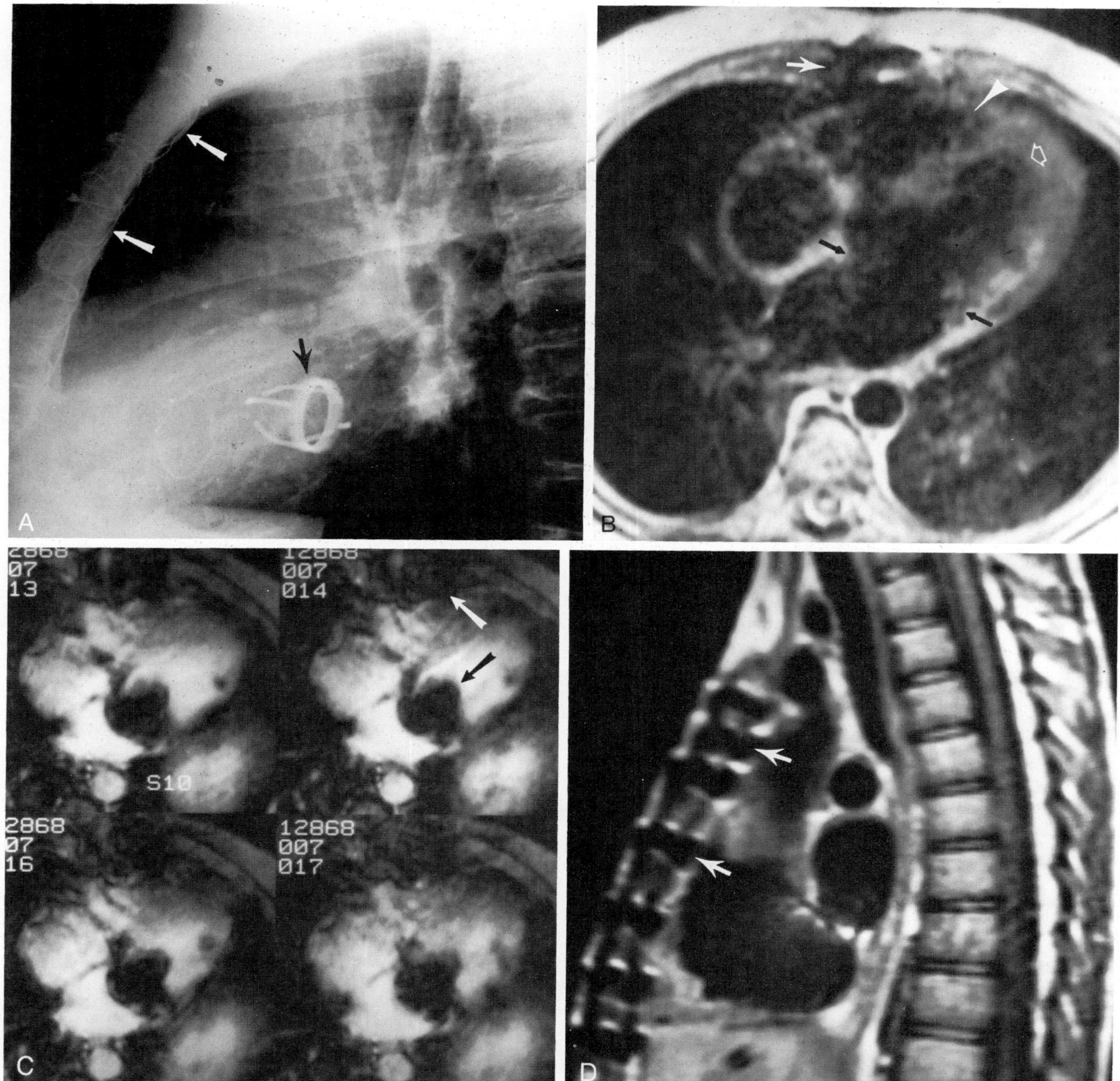

Figure 42–16. Metal artifacts from mitral valve and sternal wire. *A*, Lateral chest radiograph shows mitral valve (black arrow) and sternal wires (white arrows). *B*, Axial spin-echo image shows signal voids in the sternum (white arrow) and in the region of the mitral valve (black arrows). The artifact region is limited, and the majority of the left ventricle including the apex (open white arrow) and right ventricle (white arrowhead) are visible. *C*, Gradient-echo cine-MRI images at the same location show that the artifacts are larger, since the gradient-echo is more sensitive to magnetic field inhomogeneities. However, the artifacts from the sternal wires (white arrow) and prosthetic mitral valve (black arrow) are still relatively localized, and the majority of the left atrium and left ventricle can be evaluated for a mass such as a hematoma. *D*, Sagittal spin-echo image of a different patient demonstrates localized sternal wire artifacts (arrows).

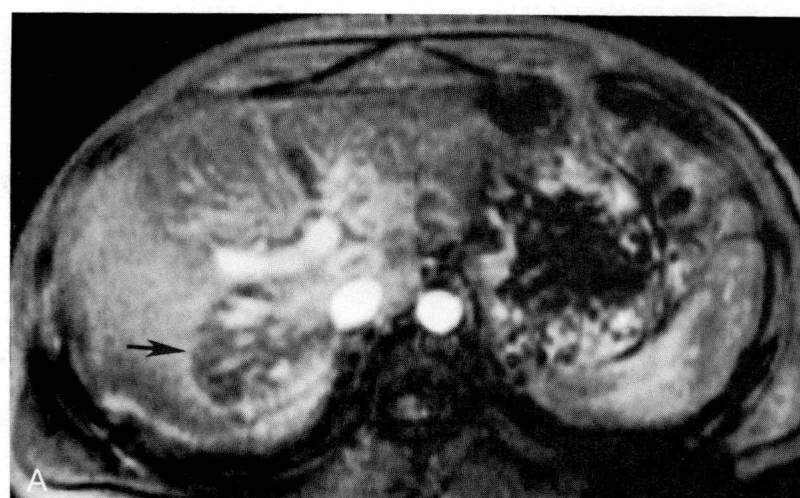

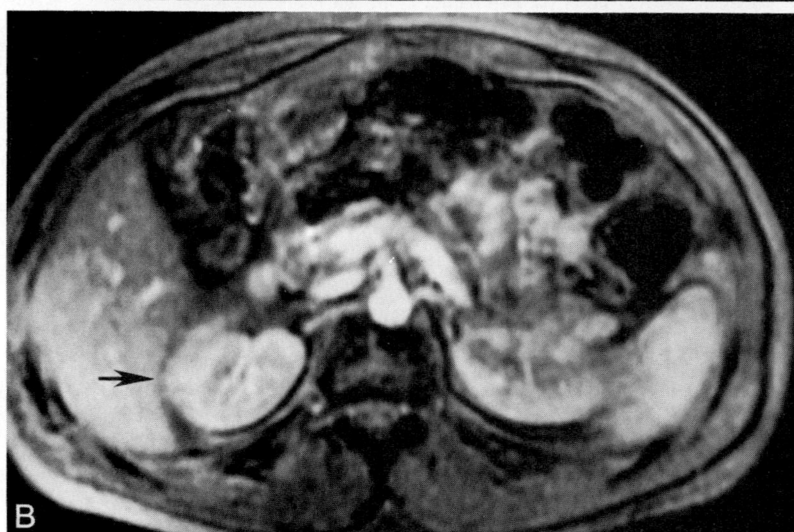

Figure 42–17. Radiofrequency transmit ghost from incorrect pulse tuning on axial gradient-echo images. *A*, The image of the kidney is placed in the liver as a dark shadow (arrow). *B*, The actual kidney location creating the signal is 3 centimeters caudad (arrow).

phase wrap are important, enabling "prospective magnification" of anatomy with improved spatial resolution. The value of retrospective gating is evolving, but preliminary studies suggest that this provides significant clinical information.[P5, S12, 13]

Techniques that are helpful but less important include respiratory-sorted phase-encoding, spatial presaturation, and peripheral pulse triggering. These techniques are extremely valuable in MRI of the abdomen and central nervous system but are less important in MRI of the chest, in part because they offer limited incremental improvement in image quality over the combination of ECG triggering, four excitations, and gradient moment nulling. When the patient is comfortable and lies still, and cardiac and respiratory motion compensation techniques function well, excellent images of the heart are the result. However, the understanding of the appropriate choice of optimal imaging parameters during a particular patient study is still evolving.

Table 42–5. SUMMARY OF TECHNIQUES TO ADDRESS CARDIAC MRI ARTIFACTS

Very Important	Important	Helpful
ECG triggering Averaging	Gradient moment nulling No-frequency-wrap No-phase-wrap Retrospective gating (evolving)	Respiratory sorting Spatial presaturation Peripheral triggering

Potentially Important (Research)	Little or Limited Value
Echo-planar imaging Spatial presaturation of myocardium MR angiography and phase imaging	Respiratory triggering Breath-holding Prone positioning Inversion-recovery for fat suppression

Acknowledgments

We thank the Coulter brothers, Jon and Robert, for artwork and photography; Joseph Gillen, for creation of the images in Fig. 42–4; and Lalith Talagala, Ph.D., Peter Davis, M.D., and Todd Reinke for advice and review. We also extend our appreciation for installation and product support of the research (now production) retrospective-gated cardiac cine package to Rob Newman and Ann Shimakawa of the General Electric Company. Special thanks go to Giselle McClelland and Kathy Frazier for typing multiple revisions of the manuscript.

References

A

1. Abramowicz, M. (ed.): Choice of benzodiazepines. Med. Lett. 30:26, 1988.

B

1. Bottomley, P. A.: MR imaging technique and applications: A review. Rev. Sci. Instrum. 53:1319, 1982.
2. Bradley, W. G.: Flow phenomena. *In* Stark, D. D., and Bradley, W. G. (eds.): Magnetic Resonance Imaging. C. V. Mosby, St. Louis, 1988, p. 108.

C

1. Clark, J. A. II, and Kelly, W. M.: Common artifacts encountered in magnetic resonance imaging. Radiol. Clin. North Am. 26:893, 1988.

2. Choyke, P. L., Kressel, H. Y., Reichek, N., et al.: Nongated cardiac magnetic resonance imaging: Preliminary experience at 0.12 T. AJR 6:1143, 1984.

D

1. Dietrich, R. B., and Kangarloo, H.: Pediatric body imaging. *In* Stark, D. D., and Bradley, W. G. (eds.): Magnetic Resonance Imaging. C. V. Mosby, St. Louis, 1988, p. 1434.
2. Dimick, R. N., Hedlund, L. W., Herfkens, R. J., et al.: Optimizing electrocardiography electrode placement for cardiac-gated magnetic resonance imaging. Invest. Radiol. 22:17, 1987.
3. Dinsmore, R. E., Wedeen, V., Rosen, B., et al.: Phase-offset technique to distinguish slow blood flow and thrombus on MR images. AJR 148:634, 1987.
4. Dumoulin, C. L., and Hart, H. R.: Magnetic resonance angiography. Radiology 161:717, 1986.
5. Dumoulin, C. L., Souza, S. P., and Feng, H.: Multi-echo magnetic resonance angiography. Magn. Reson. Med. 4:47, 1987.

E

1. Edelstein, W. A., Glover, G. H., Hardy, C. J., and Redington, R. W.: The intrinsic signal-to-noise in NMR imaging. Mag. Reson. Med. 3:604, 1986.
2. Ehman, R. L., McNamara, M. T., Pallack, M., et al.: Magnetic resonance imaging with respiratory gating: Techniques and advantages. AJR 143:1175, 1984.
3. Edelman, R. R., Atkinson, D. J., Silver, M. S., et al.: FRODO pulse sequences: A new means of eliminating motion, flow, and wraparound artifacts. Radiology 166:231, 1988.
4. Evans, A. J., Blinder, R. A., Herfkens, R. T., et al.: Effects of turbulence on signal intensity in gradient echo images. Invest. Radiol. 23:512, 1988.
5. Evans, A. J., Hedlund, L. W., Herfkens, R. J., et al.: Evaluation of steady and pulsatile flow with dynamic MRI using limited flip angles and gradient echo. Magn. Reson. Imag. 5:475, 1987.

F

1. Fletcher, B. D., and Jacobstein, M. D.: General principles and imaging techniques. *In* Fletcher, B. D., and Jacobstein, M. D. (eds.): Magnetic Resonance Imaging in Congenital Heart Disease. C. V. Mosby, St. Louis, 1988, p. 9.
2. Fullerton, G. D.: Basic concepts for nuclear magnetic resonance imaging. Magn. Reson. Imag. 1:39, 1982.
3. Felmlee, J. P., and Ehman, R. L.: Spatial presaturation: A method for suppressing flow artifacts and improving depiction of vascular anatomy in MR imaging. Radiology 164:559, 1987.
4. Felmlee, J. P., Morin, R. L., Salutz, J. R., and Lund, G. B.: MR imaging phase encoding: Pictorial teaching aid. Scientific exhibit at the 74th Scientific Assembly and Annual Meeting of the Radiological Society of North America, Chicago, Nov. 27–Dec. 2, 1988.

G

1. Glover, G. H., and Pelk, N. J.: A rapid-gated cine MRI technique. *In* Kressel, H. Y. (ed.): Magnetic Resonance Annual 1988. Raven Press, New York, 1988, p. 299.
2. Gomes, A. S., and Fisher, M. R.: MR imaging of the cardiovascular system. Abstracts of the 74th Annual Meeting of the Radiologic Society of North America, Nov. 28, 1988, p. 119.
3. Gomori, J. M., Holland, G. A., Grossman, R. I., et al.: Fat suppression by section-select gradient reversal on spin-echo MR imaging. Radiology 168:493, 1988.
4. Gullberg, G. T., Simons, M. A., and Wehrli, F. W.: A mathematical model for signal from spins flowing during application of spin echo pulse sequences. Magn. Reson. Imag. 6:437, 1988.

H

1. Haacke, E. M., and Bellon, E. M.: Artifacts. *In* Stark, D. D., and Bradley, W. G. (eds.): Magnetic Resonance Imaging. C. V. Mosby, St Louis, 1988, p. 72.
2. Harris, R., and Wesbey, G.: Artifacts in magnetic resonance imaging. *In* Kressel, H. Y. (ed.): Magnetic Resonance Annual 1988. Raven Press, New York, 1988, p. 71.
3. Henkelman, R. M., and Bronskill, M. J.: Artifacts in magnetic resonance imaging. Rev. Magn. Reson. Med. 2:1, 1987.
4. Hendrick, R. E.: Image contrast and noise. *In* Stark, D. D., and Bradley, W. G. (eds.): Magnetic Resonance Imaging. C. V. Mosby, St. Louis, 1988, p. 72.
5. Higgins, C. B.: The heart: Congenital disease. *In* Higgins, C. B., and Hricak, H. (eds.): Magnetic Resonance Imaging of the Body. Raven Press, New York, 1987, p. 267.
6. Haacke, E. M., and Lenz, G. W.: Improving MR image quality in the presence of motion by using rephasing gradients. AJR 148:1251, 1987.
7. Higgins, C. B.: The heart: Acquired disease. *In* Higgins, C. B., and Hricak, H. (eds.): Magnetic Resonance Imaging of the Body. Raven Press, New York, 1987, p. 239.

J

1. Joseph, P. M.: Artifacts in computed tomography. *In* Newton, T. H., and Potts, D. G. (eds.): Radiology of the Skull and Brain. Vol. 5: Technical Aspects of Computed Tomography. C. V. Mosby, St. Louis, 1981, p. 3877.

K

1. Koenig, S. H., Brown, R. D., Adams, D., et al.: Magnetic field dependence of 1/T1 of protons in tissue. Invest. Radiol. 2:76, 1984.
2. Kanal, E., and Wehrli, F. W.: Signal-to-noise ratio, resolution, and contrast. *In* Wehrli, F. W., Shaw, D., and Kneeland, B. (eds.): Biomedical Magnetic Resonance Imaging. VCH Publishers, New York, 1988, p. 47.
3. Krocker, E. J., and Wood, E. H.: Comparison of simultaneously recorded central and peripheral arterial pressure pulses during rest, exercise and tilted position in man. Circ. Res. 3:623, 1955.

L

1. Lanzer, P., Barta, C., Botvinick, E. H., et al.: ECG-synchronized cardiac MR imaging; Method and evaluation. Radiology 3:681, 1985.

M

1. Macovski, A.: Basic principles of reconstruction algorithms. *In* Newton, T. H., and Potts, D. G. (eds.): Radiology of the Skull and Brain. Vol. 5: Technical Aspects of Computed Tomography. C. V. Mosby, St. Louis, 1981, p. 3877.
2. Marx, H. J., and Yu, P. N.: Clinical examination of the arterial pulse. Prog. Cardiovasc. Dis. 10:207, 1967.
3. Mitchell, D. G., Vinitski, S., Burk, D. L., et al.: Motion artifact reduction in MR imaging of the abdomen: Gradient moment nulling versus respiratory-sorted phase encoding. Radiology 169:155, 1988.
4. Maddahi, J., Osgrzega, E., Crues, J., et al.: Rapid dynamic cardiac magnetic resonance imaging for evaluation of cardiac insufficiency. Dynamic Cardiovasc. Imag. 1:55, 1987.

N

1. Naylor, G. L., Firmin, D. N., and Longmore, D. B.: Blood flow imaging by cine magnetic resonance. J. Comput. Axial Tomogr. 10:715, 1986.

O

1. O'Rourke, M. F.: The arterial pulse in health and disease. Am. Heart J. 82:687, 1971.
2. O'Rourke, R. A.: Physical examination of the arteries and veins. *In* Hurst, J. W. (ed.): The Heart. McGraw-Hill, New York, 1986, p. 141.
3. Ordidge, R. J., Howseman, A., Coxon, R., et al.: Snapshot imaging at 0.5 T using echo-planar techniques. Magn. Reson. Med. 10:227, 1989.

P

1. Porter, B. A., Hastrup, W., Richardson, M. L., et al.: Classification and investigation of artifacts in magnetic resonance imaging. Radiographics 7:261, 1987.
2. Peshock, R. M.: Heart and great vessels. *In* Stark, D. D., and Bradley, W. G. (eds.): Magnetic Resonance Imaging. C. V. Mosby, St. Louis, 1988, p. 887.
3. Paling, M. R., and Brookman, J. R.: Respiration artifacts in MR imaging: Reduction by breath holding. J. Comput. Axial Tomogr. 10:1080, 1986.
4. Pattany, P. M., Phillips, J. J., Chiu, L. C., et al.: Motion artifact suppression technique (MAST) for MR imaging. J. Comput. Axial Tomogr. 11:369, 1987.
5. Pettigrew, R. I., Ziffer, J. A., Churchwell, A. L., et al.: Fast gradient echo imaging at 0.5 T: Assessment of cardiac function and valvular dysfunction. Dynamic Cardiovasc. Imag. 1:220, 1987.

R

1. Roth, T., Roehrs, T. A., and Zorick, F. J.: Pharmacology and hypnotic efficacy of triazolam. Pharmacotherapy 3:137, 1983.
2. Rzedzian, R., Chapman, B., Mansfield, P., et al.: Real-time nuclear magnetic resonance clinical imaging in pediatrics. Lancet 2:1281, 1983.
3. Rzedzian, R. R., and Pykett, I. L.: Instant images of the human heart using a new, whole-body MR imaging system. AJR 149:245, 1987.
4. Runge, V. M., Clanton, J. A., Partain, C. L., and James, A. E.: Respiratory gating in magnetic resonance imaging at 0.5 Tesla. Radiology 151:521, 1984.

S

1. Spritzer, C. E., and Herfkens, R. J.: Magnetic resonance imaging of the heart. *In* Kressel, H. Y. (ed.): Magnetic Resonance Annual 1988. Raven Press, New York, 1988, p. 217.
2. Shaw, D.: Fundamental principles of nuclear magnetic resonance. *In* Wehrli, F. W., Shaw, D., and Kneeland, B. (eds.): Biomedical Magnetic Resonance Imaging. VCH Publishers, New York, 1988, p. 47.
3. Sprawls, P.: Spatial characteristics of the MR image. *In* Stark, D. D., and Bradley, W. G. (eds.): Magnetic Resonance Imaging. C. V. Mosby, St. Louis, 1988, p. 24.
4. Schultz, C. L., Alfidi, R. J., Nelson, A. D., et al.: The effect of motion on two-dimensional Fourier transformation magnetic resonance images. Radiology 152:117, 1984.

5. Strain, J. D., Harvey, L. A., Foley, L. C., and Campbell, J. B.: Intraveneously administered pentobarbital sodium for sedation in pediatric CT. Radiology 161:105, 1986.
6. Strain, J. D., Campbell, J. B., Harvey, L. A., and Foley, L. C.: IV nembutal: Safe sedation for children undergoing CT. AJR 151:975, 1988.
7. Steen, P.: Line gating. MR Sun:Signa Users Newsletter 4:7, 1988.
8. Sechtem, U., Pflugfelder, P. W., and Cassidy, M. M.: Mitral or aortic regurgitation: Quantification of regurgitant volumes with cine MR imaging. Radiology 167:425, 1988.
9. Shellock, F. G., and Crues, J. V.: High-field-strength MR imaging and metallic biomedical implants. AJR 151:389, 1988.
10. Soulen, R. L.: Magnetic resonance imaging of prosthetic heart valves. Radiology 158:279, 1986.
11. Soulen, R. L., Budinger, T. F., and Higgins, C. B.: Magnetic resonance imaging of prosthetic heart valves. Radiology 153:705, 1985.
12. Shoemaker, D. W., Wozney, P., Wolf, G. L., and Petcheny, R.: Cine cardiac MRI in the evaluation of pediatric heart disease. Abstracts of the Eighty-Ninth Annual Meeting of the American Roentgen Ray Society, New Orleans, May 7–12, 1989, p. 149.
13. Simpson, I. A., Chung, K. J., Glass, R. F., et al.: Cine magnetic resonance imaging for evaluation of anatomy and flow relations in infants and children with coarctation of the aorta. Circulation 78:142, 1988.

U

1. Utz, J. A., and Herfkens, R. J.: Dynamic and physiologic cardiac MR. *In* Stark, D. D., and Bradley, W. G. (eds.): Magnetic Resonance Imaging. C. V. Mosby, St. Louis, 1988, p. 921.

W

1. Wesby, G. E.: Cardiovascular and pulmonary magnetic resonance imaging. *In* Wehrli, F. W., Shaw, D., and Kneeland, B. (eds.): Biomedical Magnetic Resonance Imaging. VCH Publishers, New York, 1988, p. 279.
2. Wehrli, F.: Principles of magnetic resonance. *In* Stark, D. D., and Bradley, W. G. (eds.): Magnetic Resonance Imaging. C. V. Mosby, St. Louis, 1988, p. 3.
3. Wehrli, F. W., Perkins, T. G., Shimakawa, A., and Roberts, F.: Chemical shift-induced amplitude modulations in images obtained with gradient refocusing. Magn. Reson. Imag. 5:157, 1987.
4. Wehrli, F. W.: Fast-scan imaging: Principles and contrast phenomenology. *In* Higgins, C. B., and Hricak, H. (eds.): Magnetic Resonance Imaging of the Body. Raven Press, New York, 1987, p. 23.
5. Wehrli, F. W., and Bradley, W. G.: Magnetic resonance flow phenomena and flow imaging. *In* Wehrli, F. W., Shaw, D., and Kneeland, B. (eds.): Biomedical Magnetic Resonance Imaging. VCH Publishers, New York, 1988, p. 459.
6. Williams, D. M., Meyer, C. R., and Schreiner, R. J.: Flow effects in multi-slice, spin-echo magnetic resonance imaging. Invest. Radiol. 22:642, 1987.
7. Wozney, P., Davis, P., Tobben, P. J., and White, R.: Abdominal vascular anatomy and patency: Clinical utility of two new MRI pulse techniques. Abstracts of the 88th Annual Meeting of the American Roentgen Society, San Francisco, May 3–13, 1988, p. 143.

Z

1. Zerhouni, E. A., Parish, D. A., Rogers, W. J., et al.: Human heart: Tagging with MR imaging—a method for noninvasive assessment of myocardial motion. Radiology 169:59, 1988.

Chapter 43

Contrast Agents for Cardiac MRI

GERALD L. WOLF, PH.D., M.D.

INHERENT AND ENHANCED RELAXATION 794
Paramagnetic Agents 794
Superparamagnetic or Ferromagnetic Agents ... 797
MR CONTRAST AGENTS FOR THE HEART 798
Magnetic Resonance Signal and Contrast Agent: The Complex Relation 798
Interaction of Paramagnetic Contrast Agents and the Spin-Echo Pulse Sequence 799
An Illustrative Simulation of the Dynamic Case 799
Available Paramagnetic Agents 804
SUMMARY 808

Early magnetic resonance images provided striking soft tissue contrast that was qualitatively different from x-ray, computed tomography, or ultrasound. Magnetic resonance imaging pioneers made many confident predictions about the impact of this new technology upon medical imaging. Subsequent experience suggests that these pioneeers also promulgated some prominent myths (Table 43–1). They believed that no contrast agents would be required, and that MR imaging techniques always would be slow. Neither assertion is currently true. Of course, MRI is a rapidly evolving technology, and methods may yet be found that eliminate contrast agents. However, I believe such agents always will be useful in cardiac imaging to identify myocardial wall abnormalities or quantify tissue perfusion.

When the nuclear magnetic resonance (NMR) phenomenon was initially described, instrumentation was poor, and it required thousands of signal averages in tedious, often overnight experiments to obtain a single usable measurement. Bloch and colleagues realized that the slow relaxation of water was responsible for the long duration of many experiments and added ferric nitrate (a paramagnetic agent) to increase the proton relaxation rate for the convenience of the experimenters.[B1] Succeeding physicists used paramagnetic ions extensively to study basic relaxation processes.[B2, 3] By 1971, the use of paramagnetic chelates in the chemistry and physics of NMR was sufficiently widespread to justify a review by Horrocks and Sipe.[H3]

Biologic uses have followed a similar pattern. Paramagnetic ions, such as $MnCl_2$, were initially employed to enhance proton relaxation in liver,[L1] and this agent was also used in early cardiac studies.[B4, G1, W1] Soon the paramagnetic chelates were adopted for biologic experiments to avoid the toxicity of paramagnetic ions. Independently, in 1982 Runge and associates began studying the paramagnetic chelate CrEDTA,[R1] while GdDTPA was investigated by two teams: Weinmann and colleagues[B5, W2] and our laboratory.[F1, W3,4]

Table 43–1. EARLY MAGNETIC RESONANCE MYTHS

Signals too weak for imaging
Long wavelengths preclude anatomic resolution
RF penetration inadequate above 15 MHz
MRI will always be slow
MRI will never need contrast agents
No tissue contrast above 100 MHz

INHERENT AND ENHANCED RELAXATION

As noted in Chapter 40, water and tissues have inherent relaxation processes. As there are only two energy states for the proton, all relaxation mechanisms achieve the same end point, and any return to the lower energy state will eliminate further relaxing influences upon that proton. Thus, all proton relaxation processes are additive and competitive.

We utilize two interchangeable designations for relaxation effects: 1/T1 or R1 for the longitudinal rate with units of inverse time, usually in seconds, and 1/T2 or R2 for the transverse process. When contrast agents are present and effective, the observed relaxation is due to inherent relaxation plus the contrast agent effects, as follows:

$$1/T1_{obs} = 1/T1_{Tiss} + 1/T1_{CA} \quad (1)$$

$$R1_{obs} = R1_{Tiss} + R1_{CA} \quad (2)$$

where $T1_{obs}$ = relaxation time measured for the enhanced tissue
$T1_{Tiss}$ = relaxation time of the tissue without the agent
$T1_{CA}$ = relaxation time effects of the contrast agent
$R1_{obs}$ = relaxation rate of the enhanced tissue
$R1_{Tiss}$ = relaxation rate of the tissue without the agent
$R1_{CA}$ = relaxation rate due to the contrast agent

Similar expressions hold for 1/T2 and its equivalent R2.

The relation between T1 and the concentration of an effective paramagnetic agent is thus inverse and curvilinear, whereas the relation between R1 and concentration is direct and linear (Fig. 43–1). The latter is more convenient to use but traditionally relaxation times are reported rather than relaxation rates. For an effective relaxing agent, its *relaxivity* can be calculated from the slope of R1 versus concentration and usually has the units of $mM^{-1}\,sec^{-1}$. This measure of effectiveness is analogous to potency in pharmacologic terms.

Paramagnetic Relaxing Agents

Just as the spin of nuclear particles tends to pair and cancel, so also do the spin or magnetic moments of electrons tend to have equal representation of parallel and antiparallel moments that create no *net* magnetic moment. Some chemical elements

Figure 43–1. Effect of paramagnetics upon proton relaxation: three dose-response relations. Upper left: the change in serum T1 relaxation time (mS) and rate (mS^{-1}) as paramagnetic agent concentration is increased. Upper right: these same data are plotted as T1 versus mM of paramagnetic agent; the result is a curvilinear inverse relation. Bottom right: the direct linear relation between R1 and paramagnetic concentration represents inherent relaxation of the tissue (serum), and the slope is relaxivity. Bottom right: the percent change versus the log of the dose is plotted and again shows an inverse curvilinear relationship.

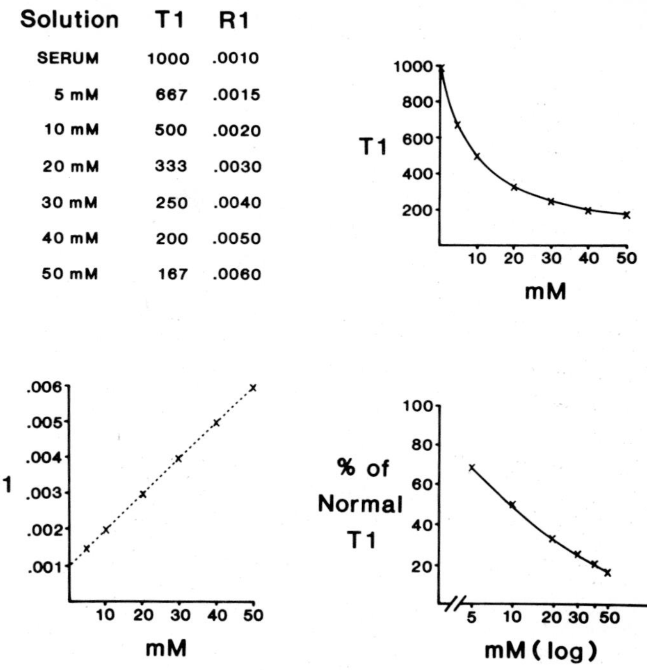

Solution	T1	R1
SERUM	1000	.0010
5 mM	667	.0015
10 mM	500	.0020
20 mM	333	.0030
30 mM	250	.0040
40 mM	200	.0050
50 mM	167	.0060

do have one or more electrons that are unpaired with respect to their spin, and such elements are classed as paramagnetic. In a magnetic field, unpaired electrons generate much larger fluctuation in local fields (about 700 times as large) than that caused by protons (Fig. 43–2). These large fields allow a water proton to remain affected by another magnetic field for a much longer time, and paramagnetic agents can be very potent relaxers: e.g., 0.1 nM/ml of Gd_2Cl_3 will double 1/T1 of water.

The influence of individual electron-proton interactions is characterized by complicated theoretic equations. See Equations 3 and 4 at the bottom of this page.

These formulas are too complicated for intuitive understanding, and the interested reader is referred to our more complete discussions elsewhere.[E1, W4] However, I emphasize that the effectiveness of relaxation is inversely proportional to the distance between the paramagnetic electron and the nucleus raised to the *sixth* power, and it is the numerous frequency (ω) and collision (τ) terms in the descriptive equations that make the process sensitive to the magnetic field, temperature, and macromolecular effects.

The number of unpaired electrons directly influences potency of the agent. In addition, water must rapidly approach and leave the vicinity of the paramagnetic field (about 100 angstroms) if a few micromoles of paramagnetic are to relax large fractions of the huge pools of protons available in tissue (50 to 100 molar). Additional important complexities have an impact upon the design of useful relaxing agents. In general, paramagnetic *ions* have the highest relaxivities (Fig. 43–3), because the many paramagnetic electrons have ready access to water.[G2, K1] However, paramagnetic ions are somewhat toxic and may not have desirable biodistribution properties. $MnCl_2$ may be an exception for the heart because it is very potent and has specific cellular transport properties.[H1] It may have been prematurely discarded from consideration as a useful clinical agent.

CHELATION. Most current paramagnetic contrast agents of clinical interest are not ions but metal chelates of manganese, iron, or gadolinium. Chelation is used to reduce toxicity and obtain useful tissue biodistributions and pharmacokinetics, but chelation decreases the potency, i.e., less relaxation effect per quantity of paramagnetic metal. Each particular metal-chelate complex has its own chemical stability. Stable chelates must trap the paramagnetic metal in a molecular cavity of the right size and shape and also form bonds with the electrons of the metal (Fig. 43–4). These bonds reduce the magnetic moment and field of the paramagnetic's electrons while the very bulk of the chelate reduces close access of the solvent protons to any remaining magnetic field. The chelating molecule also changes the molecular tumbling rate of the complex. All these effects reduce the potency (relaxivity) of the paramagnetic chelate and also alter the field-dependent relaxation effects (dispersion) as shown in Figure 43–3. However, the toxicity of the paramagnetic chelate is often reduced by orders of magnitude compared to the paramagnetic ion, and the tissue biodistribution is determined by the properties of the chelate rather than the metal. Thus, the benefits of chelation outweigh the reduced potency of the paramagnetic aquoion.[E1, K1, W4,5] Many of the useful chelates were initially developed to alter the biodistribution of radioisotopes, such as ^{99m}Tc or ^{111}In. Thus, nuclear medicine studies with these agents can be used to predict the in vivo behavior of paramagnetic chelates.

Paramagnetic centers also can be attached to larger molecules. Such methods often use chelates to trap the metal and chemical

$$\frac{1}{T1} = \underbrace{\frac{2}{15}\frac{S(S+1)\gamma^2 g^2 \beta^2}{r^6}\left(\frac{3\tau_c}{1+\omega_I^2\tau_c^2} + \frac{7\tau_c}{1+\omega_s^2\tau_c^2}\right)}_{\text{Dipole-dipole term}} + \underbrace{\frac{2}{3}\frac{S(S+1)A^2}{\hbar^2}\left(\frac{\tau_c}{1+\omega_s^2\tau_c^2}\right)}_{\text{Scalar term}} \tag{3}$$

$$\frac{1}{T2} = \overbrace{\frac{1}{15}\frac{S(S+1)\gamma^2 g^2 \beta^2}{r^6}\left(4\tau_c + \frac{3\tau_c}{1+\omega_I^2\tau_c^2} + \frac{13\tau_c}{1+\omega_s^2\tau_c^2}\right)} + \overbrace{\frac{1}{3}\frac{S(S+1)A^2}{\hbar^2}\left(\tau_c + \frac{\tau_c}{1+\omega_s^2\tau_c^2}\right)} \tag{4}$$

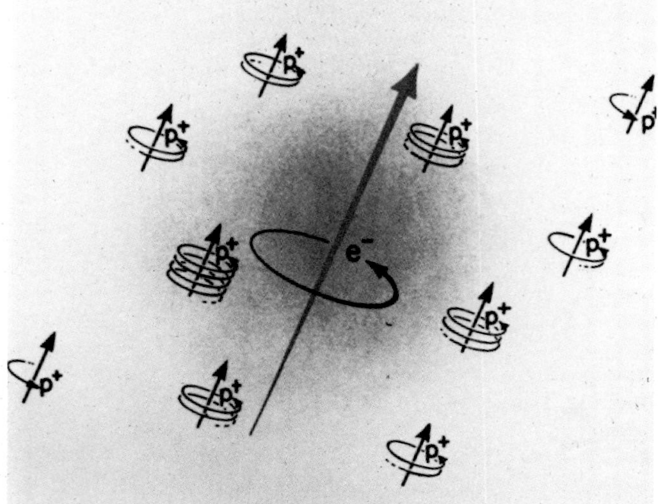

Figure 43–2. Schematic depiction of the magnetic fields around protons and unpaired electrons. The protons have smaller fields (arrow) and a spectrum of tumbling rates (number of spirals around each proton). The electron has a much larger field of influence (large arrow and cloud). The small proton fields are less likely to couple for a long enough time, even though there are many more protons. The protons are more likely to remain under the influence of the large magnetic field of the electron. In actuality, the disparity in local field is much larger for electrons and protons (×657). (Courtesy of R. Brasch.)

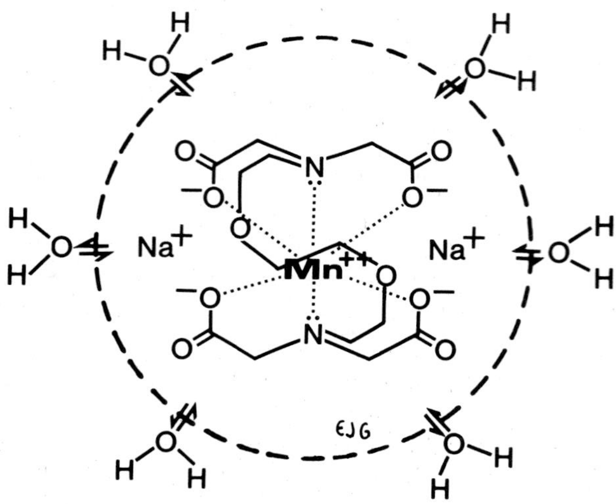

Figure 43–4. Schematic representation of a paramagnetic metal and ligand complex. The Mn^{2+} forms coordination bonds to several of the side chains of the chelate EGTA [ethylene glycol-bis (β-aminoethyleth-ertetra-acetate)]. The diagram helps visualize the paramagnetic lying in a molecular cavity of the ligand, which binds some of the unpaired electrons and partially shields the paramagnetic electrons from solvent water protons. (Courtesy of E. Goldstein.)

linkers to attach the chelate to a larger molecule, such as albumin,[S1] dextran,[G3] or a special protein like concanavalin A (Fig. 43–5). Such large molecules tumble more slowly, and this alters their dispersion and may significantly increase their potency in the fields used for imaging. Tissue biodistribution is affected as well.

Organic nitroxide compounds also have an unpaired electron and are paramagnetic. These compounds can be incorporated into larger molecules that cannot be tagged with paramagnetic metals. With only a single electron spin, they are less potent. The body may also reduce the nitroxide bond and inactivate the relaxation effect. A few nitroxide compounds have been produced that act as extracellular fluid indicators,[B6] but they have few advantages over paramagnetic metal chelates at present.

DECHELATION. If the purpose of chelation is to reduce

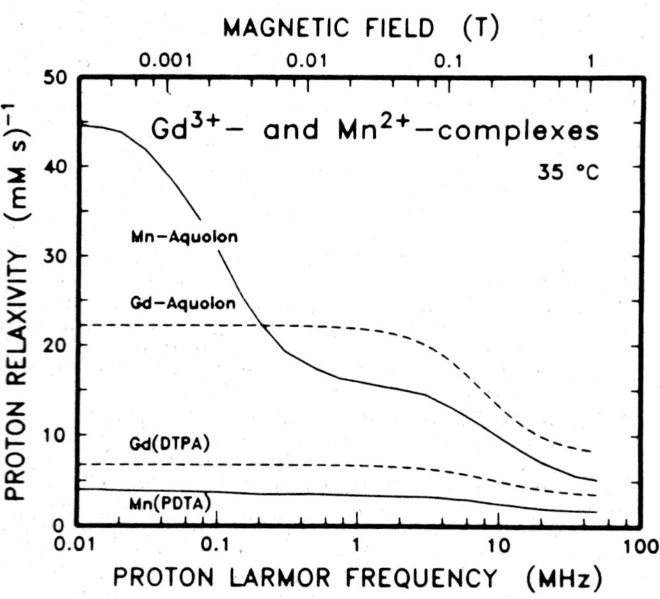

Figure 43–3. Influence of chelation upon relaxivity dispersion. This is the usual form of nuclear magnetic relaxation dispersion where relaxivity is plotted versus proton Larmor frequency. Aquoions (ions in dilute water solutions) have greater relaxivity because water exchange is facilitated, and all the unpaired electrons are effective. The dispersions are qualitatively and quantitatively different for each paramagnetic aquoion. Chelation reduces water exchange and binds many unpaired electrons. Most simple paramagnetic chelates have similar profiles with moderate differences in relaxivity. (Courtesy of S. Koenig.)

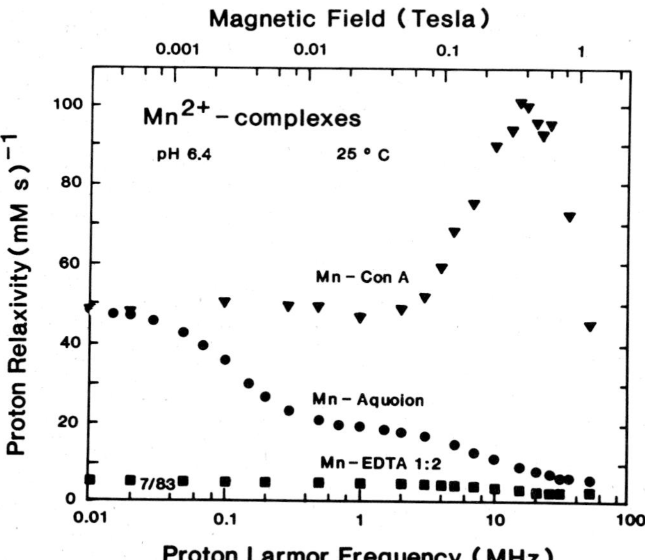

Figure 43–5. Change in relaxivity dispersion of aquoion upon chelation and binding to a macromolecule. The decrease in relaxivity as the aquoion is chelated is identical to Figure 43–3, but the slow tumbling rate of manganese bound to a large protein, concanavalin A, and the slower water movement near the paramagnetic due to hydration effects of the protein cause a dramatic increase in relaxivity and a very prominent high field peak. As most cardiac imaging is done of proton frequencies of 10 to 65 MHz, this enhanced potency is of great interest. (Courtesy of S. Koenig.)

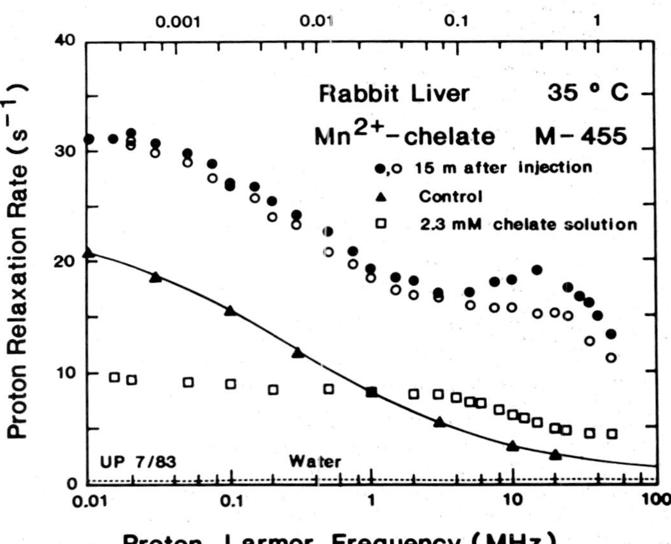

Figure 43–6. Change in relaxation dispersion due to in vivo metabolism. The usual inherent relaxation profile of normal liver (filled triangles) and Mn chelate (open squares) is shown. As relaxation effects are additive, the in vivo appearance of a high field peak in liver plus Mn-chelate (filled and open circles) reveals that either Mn-chelate or stripped Mn has become associated with a liver macromolecule in vivo. (Courtesy of S. Koenig.)

toxicity and control biodistribution, then the paramagnetic metal should not be removed from the chelate in vivo. Many metals have similar size and charge and can compete for the chelation locus. This would displace the paramagnetic metal, often releasing a toxic ion in exchange for chelation of a physiologic metal. The extraordinary stability constants reported for paramagnetic chelates in water may be misleading in biologic circumstances in which the paramagnetic metal may be displaced by another metal. For example, two copper ions can displace one gadolinium ion in the DTPA complex,[T1] and the released gadolinium would then be free to react with protein. Fortunately, usual serum copper levels are low and the reaction rate is quite slow, so this process may have no clinical significance. However, both manganese and iron are essential trace metals and have efficient biologic chelators of high avidity in plasma and tissues. In this case, the endogenous chelator can remove the paramagnetic metal from the chelate in which it was administered. For example, manganese is removed from exogenous chelators following administration (Fig. 43–6), and this alters the observed pharmacokinetics, biodistribution, and relaxivity in tissue of the manganese, as well as its toxicity.[K2] As manganese is of special interest to myocardial cell imaging, this biotransformation potential could become important in experimental studies.

Superparamagnetic or Ferromagnetic Relaxing Agents

Paramagnetic chelates are usually water-soluble and distribute widely, so their magnetic moments are dispersed and they behave as individual centers of relaxation enhancement. However, another class of agents can also be used to alter tissue relaxation. These agents are called superparamagnetic or ferromagnetic, and they are physically different (particles rather than chelates) and magnetically different. Insoluble particles with large numbers of unpaired electrons may align their magnetic moments cooperatively in the magnetic field and actually become a tiny magnet. Some comparisons of these agents versus paramagnetic chelates are shown in Figure 43–7. Superparamagnetic particles significantly disturb the local magnetic field, and protons rapidly lose their coherent precession after the RF pulse that is applied to rotate their magnetic vector into the transverse plane. Thus, these superparamagnetic and ferromagnetic agents cause very rapid T2 relaxation.[G4, M1,3, R2, W4] Of course, the local field perturbation can also facilitate T1 relaxation, but this effect is somewhat weaker and less important because the MR imager is so dependent upon transverse fields for its signal, and because most biologic tissues have much shorter T2 than T1 (the additive effect).

As is evident in Figure 43–7, superparamagnetic agents are huge relative to paramagnetic chelates, and ferromagnetic agents are even larger. Only certain metal states are capable of being magnetic. In the magnetic field, both superparamagnetic and

	Paramagnetic Chelate	Superparamagnetic Particles	Ferromagnetic Particles
T1	↓	—	—
T2	↓	↓ ↓ ↓	↓ ↓ ↓ ↓
Physical Form	Chelates dissolved in solution	Fe aggregates as small particles	Fe aggregates as large particles
Number of paramagnetic atoms per molecule	1	10^{10}	10^{12}
Examples	Iron EDTA Manganese EDTA Gadolinium DTPA	Dextran Plus magnetite	Microspheres plus magnetite

Figure 43–7. Comparison of paramagnetic chelates, superparamagnetic particles and ferromagnetic particles as MR contrast agents. The paramagnetic effect decreases both T1 and T2 in target tissues whereas the particles have a much more powerful effect upon tissue T2. Chelates are dissolved in body fluids while the particles are insoluble; thus, the paramagnetic metals act individually while the ferromagnetic spins act synergistically. In general, superparamagnetic particles are smaller and lose their magnetism quickly outside the magnet whereas larger ferromagnetic particles may maintain their magnetism longer (remnance).

ferromagnetic agents behave similarly. When the patient is removed from the magnetic field, the magnetic field of the smaller superparamagnetic agents will rapidly disappear, because the brownian motion in cells will cause them to lose magnetic alignment with other superparamagnetic particles. Larger ferromagnetic particles remain aligned longer and are said to have a remnant magnetic field. As this persistent magnetic field has no impact upon biologic tissues and imaging is not being performed, the distinction between superparamagnetic or ferromagnetic assignment of particle has little meaning. However, the difference is important in the magnet, because larger particles are more potent and often have different biodistribution properties.

Paramagnetic agents increase their relaxivity slightly in stronger magnetic fields, but ferromagnetic agents are much more dependent upon external magnetic field strength (Fig. 43–8). Paramagnetic agents have a very short range relaxation effect and require rapid exchange of nuclei through their small effective radius for relaxation efficacy. Superparamagnetics may cause relaxation for up to 50 times their diameter.[L2] As their size is often in the micron range, a single particle may increase T2 relaxation within several cells and over a range that far exceeds the diffusion of water within a few tens of milliseconds. The relation between properties of the particle (size, ferromagnetic metal content) and its relaxivity in vivo are hotly disputed. Some claim that these particles are only a special case of paramagnetism due to their dense packing and the resultant change in magnetic field homogeneity,[G4, R2] while others claim that they require new terms to describe their effects mathematically.[H4, M3]

It is clear that such particles are very potent, because their magnetic fields extend much farther into the sample. The motion of the proton within the magnetic field gradient created by the particle is also more important than for paramagnetic chelates. For biologists, the latter means that diffusion and perfusion are variables in addition to location (biodistribution) of the relaxing agent, whereas the imaging specialists relate to the special importance of magnetic susceptibility and gradient details. Both are interested that gradient echo techniques are as much as five times more sensitive to superparamagnetic particles than are spin-echo techniques.[H5]

Experimental measurements show that a magnetic particle of

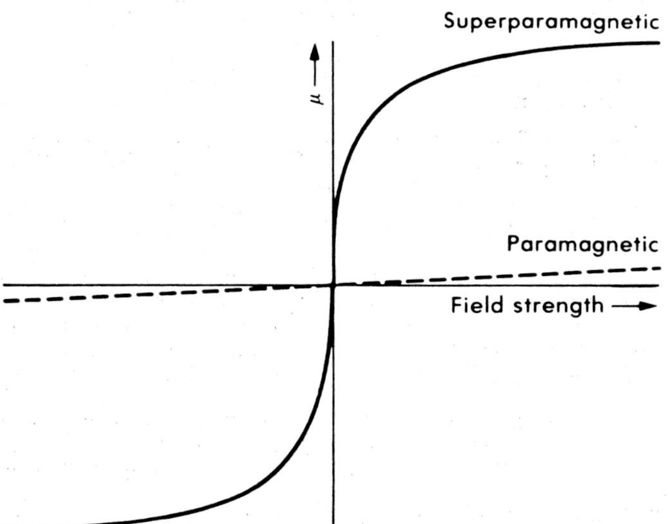

Figure 43–8. Relationship between applied field and induced magnetization μ for paramagnetic and superparamagnetic materials. Paramagnetic materials (dashed line) have susceptibilities that are proportional to field strength and do not saturate. Superparamagnetic materials (solid line) have higher susceptibilities that saturate or maximize at sufficiently high fields. (Courtesy of D. Stark.)

Table 43–2. CHANGE IN LONGITUDINAL RELAXIVITY (R1) AND TRANSVERSE RELAXIVITY (R2) IN TISSUE PHANTOMS

Material	ΔR1*	ΔR2*	R2/R1
Superparamagnetic particle	637.71	3233.47	5.1
Aqueous $FeCl_3$	149.86	229.19	1.5

*Relaxivity (s^{-1} mg Fe/g gel) at 20 MHz.

Modified from Majumdar, S., et al.: A quantitative study of relaxation rate enhancement produced by iron oxide particles in polyacrylamide gels and tissue. Magn. Reson. Med. 9:185, 1989.

micron size will have R2 relaxivity of 100 to 300 $mM^{-1}s^{-1}$ in the 0.5 T range of field strength, whereas GdDTPA under the same conditions has an R2 relaxivity of about 5 $mM^{-1}s^{-1}$. A recent quantitative comparison of relaxivities of paramagnetic iron ($FeCl_3$) and superparamagnetic magnetite particles is shown in Table 43–2. The particle is clearly more potent and has much more T2 effect than the same amount of paramagnetic *ion*. The main magnetic compounds used to prepare superparamagnetic or ferromagnetic contrast agents are magnetite (Fe_3O_4), γ-ferric oxide (γ-Fe_2O_3), or mixed ferrites ($MeOFe_2O_3$). Other magnetic particle compositions are possible but use metals that may not have physiologic clearance pathways in the event of in vivo dissolution.

MAGNETIC RESONANCE CONTRAST AGENTS FOR THE HEART

At velocities above a few centimeters per second, the relative signal intensity of blood is determined more by motion than by the proton relaxation rates of the blood itself. Furthermore, rapidly moving blood can be easily contrasted with other tissues simply by changing the imaging parameters (see Chapter 41). Thus, an administered agent may not be required to alter the appearance of blood in the cardiac chambers or great vessels. However, the washin and washout of a magnetic resonance contrast agent from the myocardial wall can be imaged, and such images indicate local pathophysiology. As we will see, there are potentially effective indicators of tissue perfusion, the extracellular space, the regional blood volume and capillary permeability, and cell membrane transport. The relation between the detected magnetic resonance signal and local tissue concentration of the paramagnetic agent or indicator is more complex than, for example, that of x-ray contrast agents and cine computed tomography (Chapter 35) or ^{201}Th and SPECT (Chapter 60). In part, this is because the x-ray and isotope agents are directly detected whereas proton magnetic resonance signal is used to report the *effects* of the relaxing agent.

Magnetic Resonance Signal and Contrast Agent: The Complex Relation

We next examine the relation between magnetic resonance signal intensity and contrast agent concentration in more detail. The first consideration is the relation between signal intensity and tissue nuclear magnetic resonance properties, neglecting the effects of motion. For spin-echo imaging, this relation has the following form:

$$S_{SE}(TE,TR) = \underbrace{N(H)}_{\text{Spin-density factor}} \underbrace{[1 - 2e^{-(TR - TE/2)/T1} + e^{-TR/T1}]}_{\text{T1 factor}} \underbrace{e^{-TE/T2}}_{\text{T2 factor}} \quad (5)$$

where S_{SE} equals signal and remaining terms are as previously defined. In the absence of the contrast agent, the inherent tissue properties and the imaging parameters mutually determine the signal from the myocardial wall. In general, tissues with a shorter

T1 will give more signal intensity when both TR and TE are short, but the short TR also leads to less total signal and noisier images. Tissues with a longer T2 will give a stronger signal with a long TR and TE, and these signals also become more specific but noisier as the TE is lengthened. These important tradeoffs have been reviewed in more detail for normal, ischemic, and reperfused myocardium in Chapter 40.

When one is trying to identify differences between tissues with adequate inherent differences in proton density, T1 or T2, it is better to consider the *contrast* between the two tissues than the signal from each tissue, while continuing to disregard the influence of motion and with no added contrast agent. The relation for contrast:noise ratio (CNR) between two tissues has the following form for spin-echo imaging:

$$\text{CNR} \propto \frac{|S(1)_A - S(1)_B|}{\sigma_o}[T_{tot}/(N_{pe}TR)]^{1/2}[TE\text{-}T_c]^{1/2} \quad (6)$$

where S(1), $S(1)_A$, and $S(1)_B$ are signals from a single acquisition per phase-encoding step for a prescribed pulse sequence. Each signal term contains an implicit dependence on spin-density, T1, and T2 values and on interpulse delay times and possibly flip angles, as given previously in the chapter. The denominator σ_o is the noise level per unit time from a single repetition of the pulse sequence. The term $[T_{tot}/(N_{pe}TR)]^{1/2}$ is the square root of the number of acquisitions per phase-encoding step, and the term $[TE\text{-}T_c]^{1/2}$ is the sampling time factor.

Each of the various imaging techniques, such as inversion recovery, gradient echo, or echo planar, has a different relation between signal or contrast:noise ratio and inherent tissue nuclear magnetic resonance properties. Although this alters detection of myocardial wall abnormality, we will develop the argument fully only for the spin-echo case.

Interaction of Paramagnetic Contrast Agents and the Spin-Echo Pulse Sequence

The intensity of a voxel is determined by the magnetic resonance signal in a complicated way. Without enhancement, the earlier formulas apply, and, in general, short T1 and long T2 yield strong signal, as do long TR and short TE. Paramagnetic contrast agents reduce both T1 and T2, and their influence upon signal intensity is in addition to that inherent in the tissue. Thus a formal description of the signal response to added contrast agent contains six terms (assuming that tissue motion and hydrogen density are not changed by the contrast agent). Each of these six terms modifies an exponential term, so the result is not intuitive.

Following the expanded formal treatment of Davis and colleagues,[D1] the resulting equation for the spin-echo case is:

$$I = F_V N_H \left[1 + e^{-TR(R1_{Tiss} + R1_{CA})}\right] - 2e^{-TR - TE/2(R1_{Tiss} + R1_{CA})} e^{TE(R2_{Tiss} + R2_{CA})} \quad (7)$$

where N_H is proton density, F_V is the motion effect, and the other parameters are previously defined.

Davis has solved this complicated equation for four hypothetical tissues (muscle—short T1, short T2; liver—short T1, medium T2; brain—medium T1, medium T2; cerebrospinal fluid—long T1, long T2) and water (very long T1 and T2), with a range of GdDTPA concentrations. A graph of the result for TR 300, TE 10 and for TR 3000, TE 10 is shown in Figure 43–9.

From these simulations, several important generalities are derived.

- *Machine parameters TE and TR.* These have considerable impact. For any paramagnetic concentration, the signal intensity increases inversely with TE and directly but asymptotically with TR. At certain combinations of long TR and long TE, positive enhancement is lost, especially with tissue with inherently short T1.
- *Inherent tissue parameters R1 and R2.* Again the impact is considerable; $R1_{Tiss}$ determines the shape of the curve, and $R2_{Tiss}$ determines the amount of enhancement.
- *Tissue concentration of the paramagnetic agent.* For any tissue there is a particular concentration of agent that causes maximal enhancement, and both above and below this value, enhancement is less.

All these interactions are important and make it difficult to relate tissue intensity to concentration of contrast agent (Fig. 43–10).

The situation is somewhat simplified by considering relative enhancement of tissue when its initial magnetic resonance signal intensity is used to normalize the change owing to a given amount of paramagnetic agent. Relative enhancement is [I-Io]/Io × 100, where Io is original intensity and I is from equation 7.

Under such conditions, simulations show that relative enhancement is greatest with short TR, short TE, and long $R1_{Tiss}$. Further, $R2_{Tiss}$ does not affect relative enhancement or curve shape.

I asked Dr. Davis to compute the case for reasonable values of normal myocardium (T1 = 870, T2 = 57, proton density = 1) and infarcted myocardium (T1 = 900, T2 = 75, proton density = 1.25), using short TR, short TE and long TR, and long TE spin-echo images. The simulations are shown for magnetic resonance signal intensity in Figure 43–11.

These figures reveal the difficulty of using an extracellular indicator to distinguish normal from infarcted myocardium under steady-state conditions. However, ischemic and normal myocardium also have different perfusions and dynamic imaging may offer additional opportunities for detecting ischemia with magnetic resonance contrast agents and magnetic resonance imaging.

An Illustrative Simulation of the Dynamic Case

To aid in the intuitive understanding of the complexity of the dynamic case for magnetic resonance signal differences, the time-intensity response is modeled with the data in Table 43–3 and Figures 43–12 and 43–13. I assume that there are important differences in the pharmacokinetics between normal and infarcted myocardium for an agent that is carried to the tissue by perfusion, rapidly equilibrates in the extracellular fluid, and washes out in proportion to flow and sequestered mass of the indicator.

In Table 43–3, normal myocardium is assumed to have T1 = 870 ms and T2 = 57 ms (values for a 1.5T MRI device) and a nominal spin density. As noted, infarcted tissue will have a slight increase in T1 (900 ms), and a greater increase in T2 (75 ms) and proton density (1.2) owing to tissue edema (mainly extracellular). At this magnetic field (1.5T), a spin echo sequence of TR 600, TE 20 is T1-weighted, and the normal myocardium has *less* signal intensity than the infarct. This is a surprise, but it is due to stronger signal from the extra protons in the infarct and less signal loss due to longer T2. These two factors more than compensate for the faster T1 recovery in the normal myocardium. Prior to the arrival of our paramagnetic contrast agent, the relative signal intensity of the infarct is 28 percent greater than normal myocardium.

These same tissue differences lead to larger differences in signal intensity for TR2000, TE60 sequence that is T2-weighted. In this case, the extra protons and the long T2 of the infarct more than compensate for the slower T1 recovery (Fig. 43–13). The careful reader will note that the infarct has more signal on the T2-weighted image but the normal myocardium has less. This follows from the conditions we have chosen for this simulation.

Now we must model the serial response to the washin and washout of the paramagnetic contrast agent. Intuitively, this process should happen more rapidly in the normal myocardium than in the infarct and the *changes* in the T1-weighted images are straightforward for Table 43–3 and Figure 43–12. For this simulation we assume that the peak concentration is achieved at 20 seconds for the normal myocardium and then slowly washes out. The infarct achieves peak concentration at 40 seconds and washes out more slowly. However, our agent distributes to the extracellular space, which is larger in the infarct, and the inherent relaxation of protons in the infarct is slower; both these factors

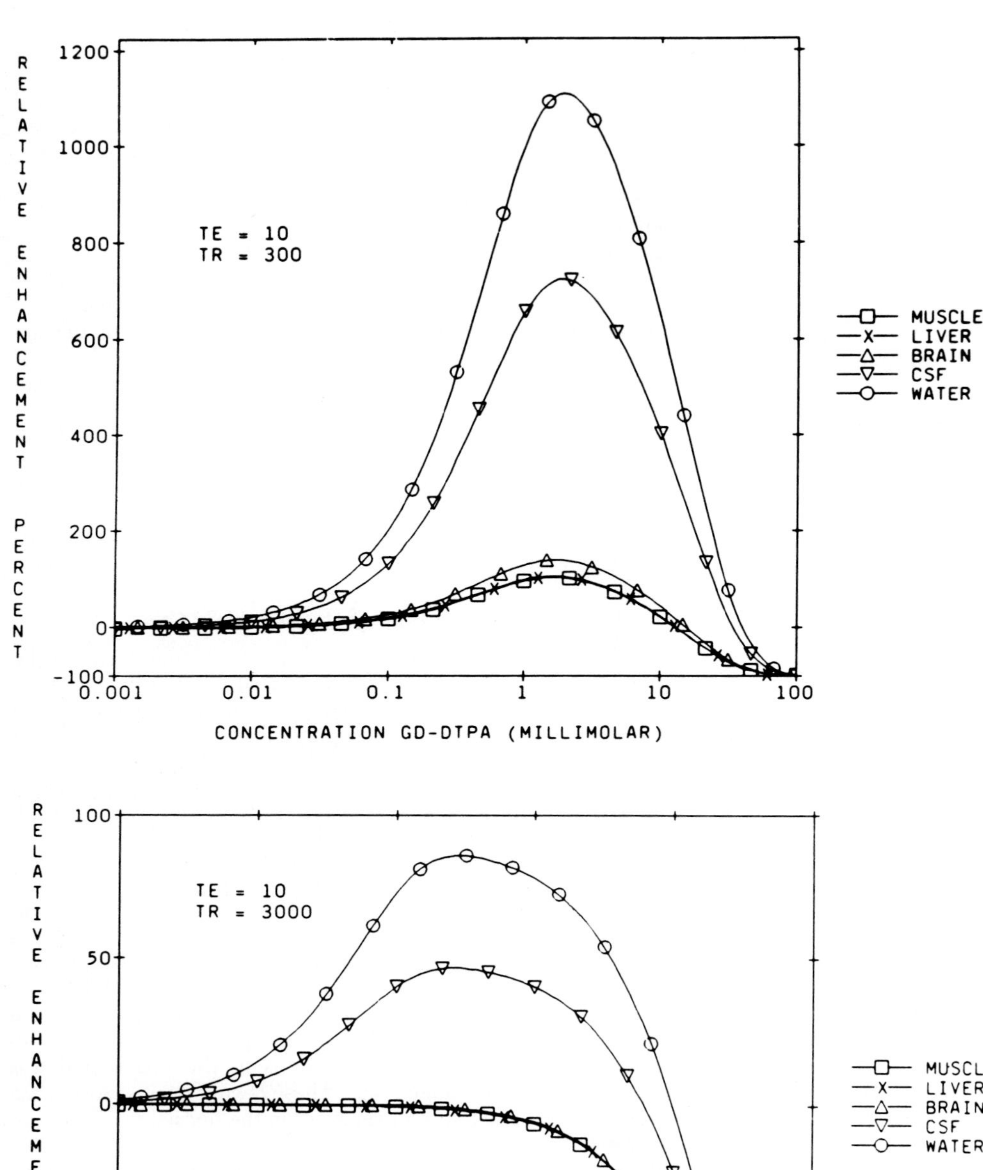

Figure 43–9. Relative enhancement of muscle, liver, brain, CSF, and water resulting from addition of GdDTPA. Top, With strongly T1-weighted images, all tissues increase their signal relative to no GdDTPA to a maxima and then signal is lost as T2 relaxation becomes dominant. Tissues with inherently long T1 and T2 (CSF and water) show greater relative enhancement. Bottom, With long TR and less T1 weighting, only CSF and water show relative enhancement. Note that the GdDTPA concentration required to reach maximal enhancement is higher with short TR/short TE. (From Davis, P. L., et al.: Interactions of paramagnetic contrast agents and the spin echo pulse sequence. Invest. Radiol. 23:381, 1988.)

Figure 43–10. The T1 and T2 effects of GdDTPA and their result upon MR intensity. For this simulation, a tissue with T1 = 652 and T2 = 60 is utilized to show individually the influence of progressive decrease in T1 and T2 due to the paramagnetic agent. The T1 effect is to increase MR intensity to a maximum whereas the T2 effect is to decrease MR intensity to zero. The two effects are inseparable and lead to the complicated interaction shown as the product. (From Davis, P. L., et al.: Interactions of paramagnetic contrast agents and the spin echo pulse sequence. Invest. Radiol. 23:381, 1988.)

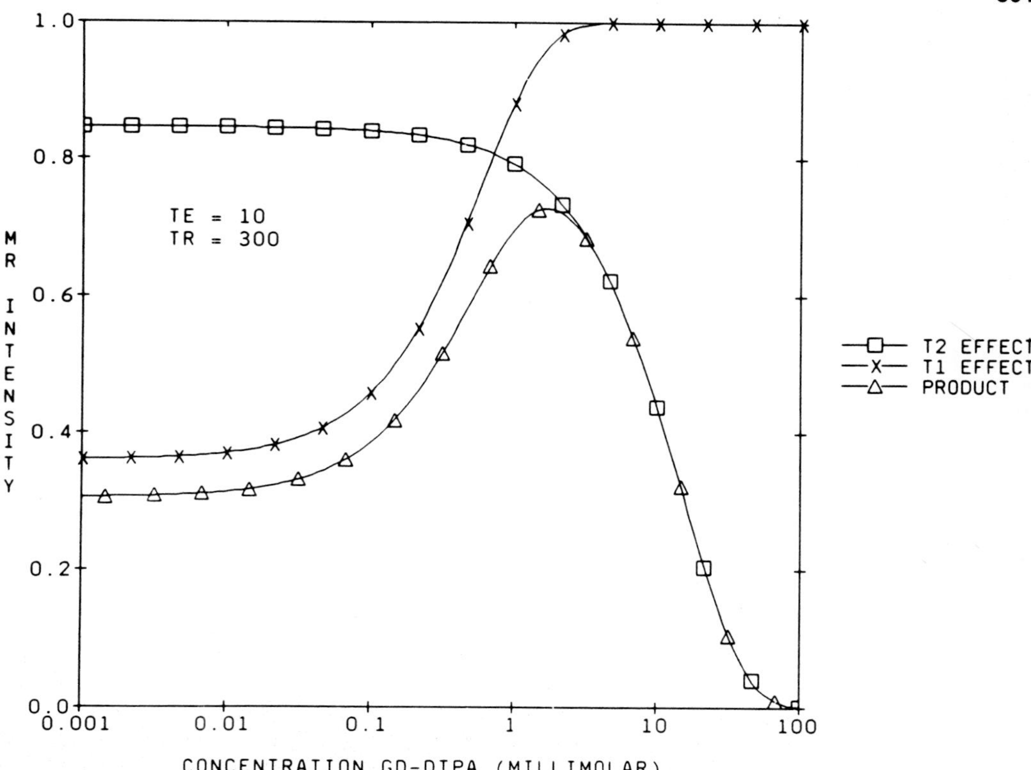

cause a larger *change* of T1 and T2 in the infarct at peak enhancement. The temporal course of both tissues for T1-weighted images is again intuitive, but the relative changes are more variable, as shown in Figure 43–14. The performance of our diagnostic test is best at 40 seconds, and contrast between normal myocardium and infarct at 240 seconds is little improved by our contrast agent. However, this pulse sequence with a single excitation and 128 pulses takes 128 × 0.65 = 77 seconds to perform even without gating. Thus, we would not be able to discern the differences in the time of peak enhancement owing to relative perfusion using spin-echo images because of inadequate temporal resolution. Even optimal "enhanced" images would be only about 77 percent better than our unenhanced images—but the latter are not time dependent. Early investigators solved this timing problem by sacrificing the animal!

The response of our T2-weighted images to the "enhancing" agent is full of surprises. First, both tissues *lose* signal intensity after MR contrast agents "enhancement." The normal myocardium does so more rapidly but with less amplitude. The infarct accumulates more contrast agent (larger extracellular space), but changes less (because the T2 was longer to start with and is still slightly longer at peak enhancement) and changes more slowly. On average, the only benefit of the contrast agent for relative enhancement occurs at 20 seconds. Unfortunately, these T2-weighted images usually require at least two excitations to increase the signal:noise ratio by averaging, and our imaging time now totals 128 × 2.0 sec × 2 averages = 8.5 *minutes*. The 76 percent relative enhancement at 20 seconds is mathematically appealing, but sacrifice of the subject becomes mandatory to achieve it with the spin-echo sequence selected.

It is left as a frustrating exercise for the reader to try different combinations of TR and TE in the hope of finding better results. Indeed, more heavily weighted T1 (shorter TR and TE) and T2 (longer TR and TE) are mathematically attractive but provide unacceptable images (too noisy or technically not achievable) or inappropriate imaging time.

Fortunately, gradient echo or echo planar imaging schemes provide more signal in less time and may enable the potential power of the differential response to an extracellular magnetic resonance contrast agent to be clinically useful. Few investigators have had access to such technology.

The literature, as reviewed by Wisenberg (Chapter 50) and Brown and Higgins,[B7] does record improved clinical detection of infarct with GdDTPA—a proven extracellular agent. This is believable if the difference between infarct and normal myocardium is greater than in our example. If the perfusion mismatch is much larger than we have shown, this would be expected. When the inherent differences in tissue relaxation are larger, often the unenhanced images are anatomically diagnostic as well, and there is less need for a magnetic resonance contrast agent. When the infarct T2 is much larger and the edema more severe,

Table 43–3. RELATIVE CHANGE IN MR SIGNAL INTENSITY ON T1-WEIGHTED OR T2-WEIGHTED STUDIES OF NORMAL AND INFARCTED MYOCARDIUM BEFORE AND AFTER INTRAVENOUS GdDTPA

	MR Signal		Infarct/	MR Signal		Infarct/
Time (*sec*)	***Normal T1W***	***Infarct T1W***	**Normal *T1W***	***Normal T2W***	***Infarct T2W***	**Normal *T2W***
0	0.350	0.447	1.28	0.310	0.480	1.55
20	0.372	0.504	1.35	0.159	0.280	1.76
40	0.367	0.527	1.44	0.196	0.215	1.10
60	0.363	0.512	1.41	0.216	0.280	1.30
90	0.360	0.497	1.38	0.220	0.310	1.41
120	0.358	0.487	1.36	0.257	0.348	1.35
240	0.357	0.467	1.31	0.305	0.440	1.44

PARAMETERS USED

Before Enhancement		Peak Enhanced	
Normal Myocardium	***Infarcted Myocardium***	***Normal Myocardium***	***Infarcted Myocardium***
T1 = 870	T1 = 900	T1 = 522	T1 = 400
T2 = 57	T2 = 75	T2 = 33	T2 = 35
p = 1.0	p = 1.2	p = 1.0	p = 1.2
		T1 ↓ 40%	T1 ↓ 45%
		T2 ↓ 44%	T2 ↓ 47%
		peak at 20 sec	peak at 40 sec

Imaging Values		
T1W	TR = 600	TE = 20
T2W	TR = 2000	TE = 60

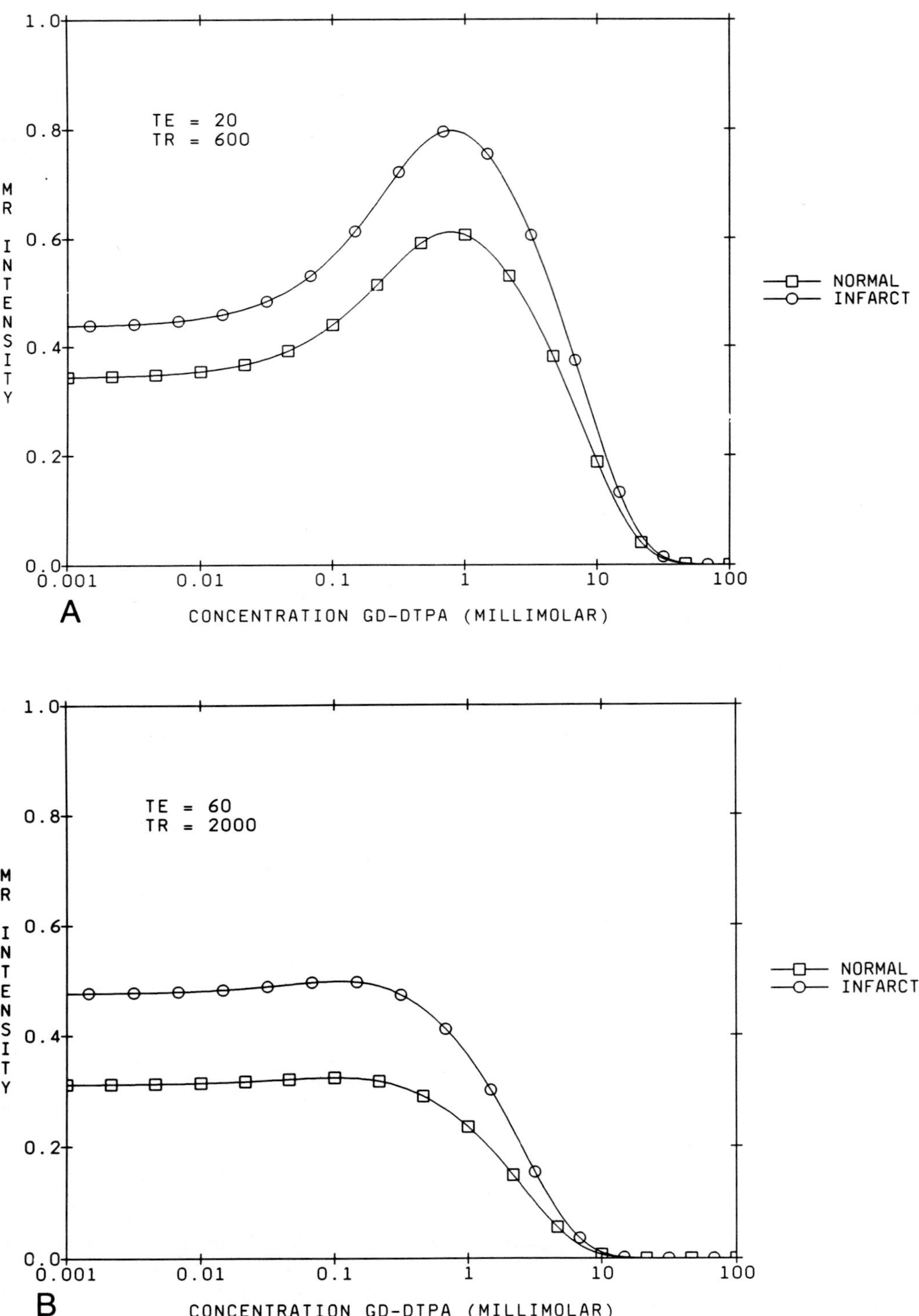

Figure 43–11. Simulations of normal and infarcted myocardial MR intensity versus increasing concentrations of GdDTPA. *A*, With short TR/short TE spin-echo images, the infarcted myocardium has more signal than normal myocardium in the absence of GdDTPA. Each tissue has a similar pattern of response to GdDTPA, although the infarcted myocardium, because of longer T2 and greater proton density, gives more signal at any GdDTPA level.

B, With long TR/long TE, no "enhancement" is seen at any level of GdDTPA, and the tissue contrast between normal and infarcted myocardium is greatest without GdDTPA. (Simulation courtesy of P. Davis.)

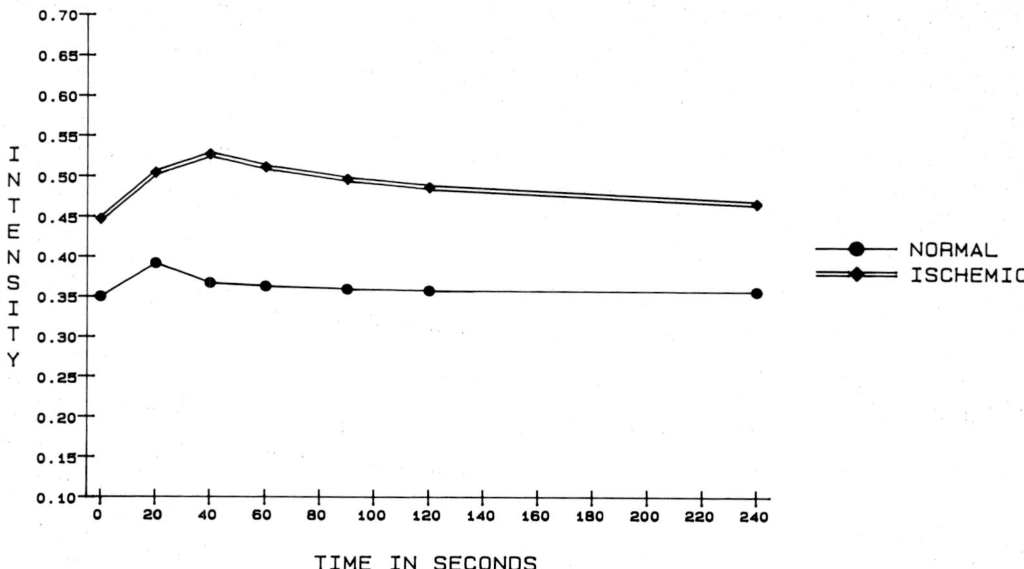

Figure 43–12. Plot of MR signal intensity for TR = 600, TE = 20 (T1-weighted) spin-echo images within normal myocardium and infarct in response to GdDTPA. These data are plotted from Table 43–3 to emphasize the temporal responses. Signal intensity increases in both normal tissue and infarct, but more slowly in the latter owing to slower perfusion. As modeled, the contrast agent is not particularly helpful, and the graph is artifactual because such spin-echo images cannot provide this temporal resolution.

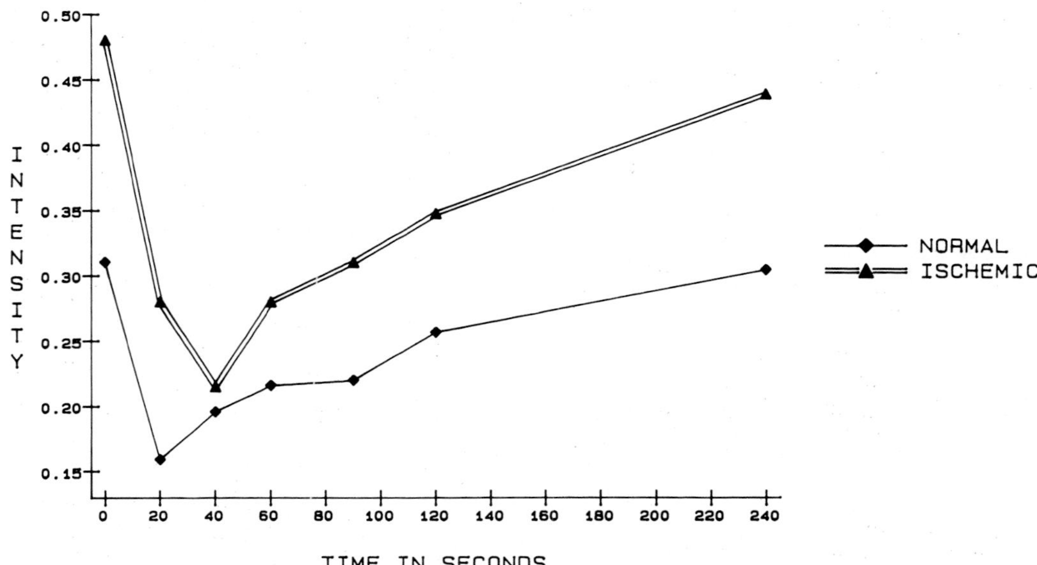

Figure 43–13. MR signal intensity response for TR = 2000, TE = 60 (T2-weighted) spin-echo images. The same tissue T1 and T2 data are used, but now the T2 effects are more prominent. In this case, the GdDTPA causes signal intensity to *fall*. The absolute change is greater in the infarct, and the delay in response is more clearly seen. Unfortunately, temporal resolution for the imaging parameters is many minutes whereas the physiologic differences have a much shorter time scale.

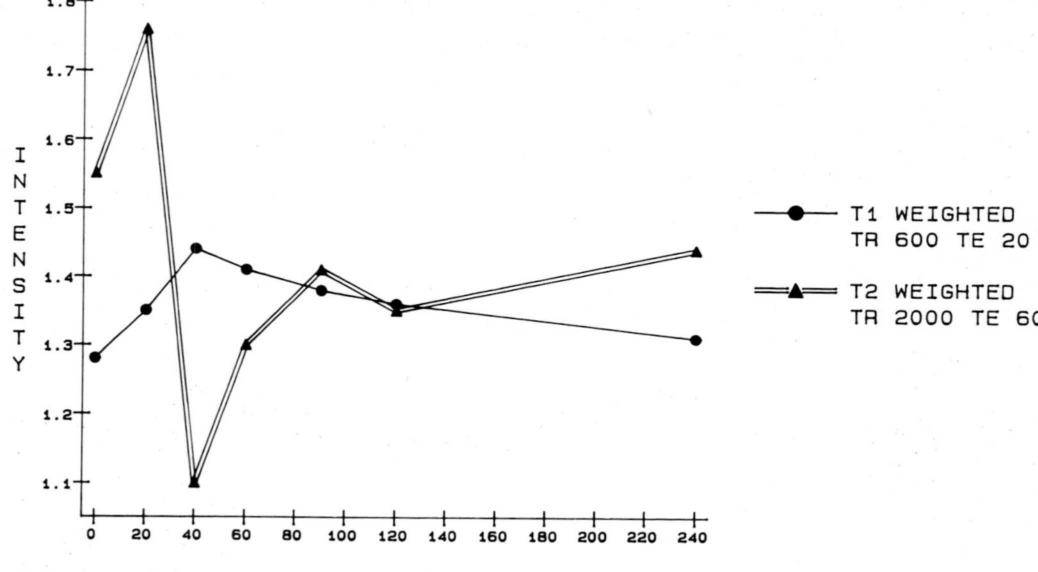

Figure 43–14. The relative change in MR intensity for T1-weighted or T2-weighted MR images in response to GdDTPA. Using the data of Table 43–3, relative changes are depicted. The T1-weighted images show maximal discrimination between normal and infarcted myocardium at 40 seconds. The T2-weighted images are only temporarily better (at 20 seconds) with contrast agent "enhancement" and actually have poorer discrimination at all other times. Different models would lead to large changes in these simulations.

Table 43–4. POTENTIAL INDICATORS (MR CONTRAST AGENTS) FOR CARDIAC IMAGING

Extracellular Agents
GdDTPA
GdDOTA
Nitroxides (TES, etc)
GdDTPA-BMA (S041)
DyDTPA
Blood Pool Agents
GdDTPA-albumin
GdDTPA polysaccharides
Magnetite particles
Intracellular Agents
$MnCl_2$
Mn-TP
Mn-DPDP
Gd-PMP
MnPDTA

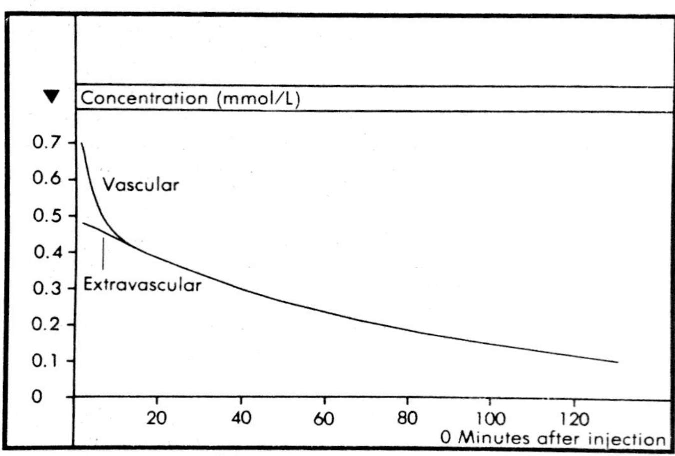

Figure 43–15. Mean plasma concentration of GdDTPA after intravenous injection of 0.1 mM/kg in man. The rapid half-life (vascular) represents dilution in the distribution phase and would be affected by cardiac output and edema but not by renal function. The slower half-life (extravascular) is more consistent with excretion and is little affected by cardiac output but very dependent upon renal function. (From Weinmann, H. J., et al.: GdDTPA and low osmolar Gd chelates. *In* Runge, V. M. (ed.): Enhanced Magnetic Resonance Imaging. C. V. Mosby, St. Louis, 1989, p. 74.)

then somewhat larger doses of contrast agent and later imaging times can be shown to be better. Nonetheless, this model can be a valuable teaching exercise for many cardiologists drawn to this application.

Available Paramagnetic Agents

For experimental purposes, investigators have had access to three different classes of paramagnetic agents to study the pathophysiology of myocardial ichemia or infarction: extracellular agents, blood pool agents, and intracellular agents (Table 43–4). The extracellular agents are small, water-soluble, and diffusable. The blood pool agents are much larger, are usually more potent, and could be useful for detecting increased capillary permeability in the infarction process. Intracellular agents are intended to reflect cellular transport processes and have some tissue specificity that the extracellular fluid and blood pool agents lack.

EXTRACELLULAR AGENTS. The prototype contrast agent in this class is gadolinium diethylenetriamine pentriacetic acid (GdDTPA). This chelate binds gadolinium with exceptional affinity ($K_{sp} \sim 10^{27}$) and good specificity among the numerous other metals that are found in biologic fluids. When chelated, the toxicity of gadolinium is reduced a hundredfold, and its biodistribution is dominated by the DTPA chelate. At physiologic pH, DTPA is anionic and is balanced by two meglumine cations in the FDA-approved formulation (Magnevist, Berlex Corporation, Wayne, N.J.). The molecular size of GdDTPA (590 daltons) is similar to that of many other contrast agents for other modalities, e.g., water-soluble x-ray agents or ^{99m}Tc DTPA for nuclear medicine.

Except for the specialized circulations of the brain and eye, GdDTPA distributes freely in the extracellular fluid space. In the heart, this equilibration between plasma and extracellular fluid is reached during one transit of the capillaries. Although the extracellular fluid volume is larger than the plasma volume, it is distributed as a thin film only a few microns thick around the myocardial syncytium. Each myocardial cell is in contact with about four capillaries, the permeability of the capillaries for GdDTPA is high, the diffusion distance is short, and perfusion velocity is fairly slow. GdDTPA is virtually excluded from normal myocardial cells by the cell membrane.

When GdDTPA is injected intravenously as a bolus, there are two discernible plasma disappearance curves (Fig. 43–15). The fastest process reflects the rapid movement of GdDTPA out of the plasma in each capillary bed during its first transit and is essentially a distribution process. In normal circumstances, this has a half-life of about 10 minutes and varies with the bolus, the cardiac output, the lung extracellular fluid volume, and the distribution volume or entire extracellular fluid volume (minus the small amount in brain and eye). GdDTPA is excreted exclusively by glomerular filtration, and the excretion half-life is 45 to 60 minutes.

A comparison of whole body retention shows the altered biodistribution and clearance of gadolinium when it is effectively chelated (Table 43–5). The finite but low retention in liver probably results from endocytosis. There is no evidence for release of free gadolinium (dechelation) in vivo. Although clearance is delayed by impaired renal function, this is probably without clinical consequences. GdDTPA is dialyzable, but the process is not particularly efficient.

The available Magnevist formulation (Table 43–6) is hypertonic and occasionally may cause transient elevations of serum iron or, less frequently, serum bilirubin. This may reflect a small amount of hemolysis and is said to be absent with low osmolal, nonionic formulations such as GdDTPA bismethylamide.

Chelation reduces the potency of gadolinium and alters its dispersion profile (Fig. 43–16). Only water protons that closely approach the GdDTPA are relaxed, but water diffuses rapidly across the red blood cells and myocardial cell membranes in the time of T1 relaxation. This fast exchange assures that tissue relaxation remains dose-responsive even though the agent has a restricted distribution volume. This relation is quantitative over a huge range of tissue concentrations and can be used to estimate tissue extracellular fluid space.[B1, K3] Unfortunately, the complexity of imaging obscures these simple relations in vivo.

The relaxivity of GdDTPA is excellent and its toxicity is low in the concentrations that are detectable, so its safety is at least as

Table 43–5. URINARY EXCRETION AND WHOLE BODY RETENTION IN MICE FOLLOWING INTRAVENOUS INJECTIONS

	$GdCl_3$	Gd(acetate)	$Gd(DTPA)^{2-}$	$Gd(DOTA)^{-}$
Urine				
5 min	0.92 ± 1.72	2.11 ± 2.32	44.9 ± 14.4	20.6 ± 21.7
60 min	1.38 ± 1.14	4.45 ± 1.14	95.4 ± 12.0	89.5 ± 23.1
Whole Animal				
1 day	93.6 ± 2.13	93.7 ± 8.08	1.26 ± 0.10	1.83 ± 1.60
7 days	72.2 ± 10.7	86.1 ± 14.2	0.35 ± 0.13	0.18 ± 0.06
Liver				
7 days	40.3 ± 12.1	41.0 ± 7.25	0.022 ± 0.004	0.008 ± 0.008

% ID ± 95% confidence limits.

From Tweddle, M. F., et al.: Principles of contrast-enhanced MRI. *In* Partain, L., et al. (eds.): Magnetic Resonance Imaging. W. B. Saunders, Philadelphia, 1983, p. 793.

Table 43–6. FORMULATION OF MAGNEVIST*

Gadopentatate dimeglumine	469.01 mg
Meglumine	0.39 mg
DTPA	0.15 mg
Osmolality	1940 mOsm
Viscosity (37°C)	2.9 cP
Density	1.199 g/ml

*Berlex Corporation, Wayne, N. J.

good as nonionic x-ray contrast agents (and its cost is about the same per dose). The Magnevist formulation has not been shown to have any important effects upon hemodynamics, contractility, or cardiac electrophysiology, although few studies have been performed under rigorous conditions.

Many other gadolinium chelates have been prepared[T1] and have minor chemical differences. Such differences affect patentability but have not been shown to result in a better extracellular agent.

Both Mn and Fe water-soluble chelates have been prepared. Their stability in vivo is much lower, and they are more toxic in the amounts required to achieve the same imaging efficiency. Nitroxide-stable free radicals are also available as extracellular agents but are less potent and subject to in vivo reduction.[B6, G5]

Extracellular agents do not enhance lipid proton relaxation rate, because these protons do not rapidly exchange and are predominately sequestered intracellularly. Extracellular agents can increase relaxation rates of other nuclei (^{19}F, ^{23}Na, ^{31}P, and so on) if the proximity factors and exchange rates are appropriate.

Two pathologic myocardial processes influence the effects of these agents. At some point in the process of irreversible ischemia, the cell membrane becomes permeable to molecules of several hundred to a few thousand molecular weight. This would increase the distribution volume for the agent but would not change the relaxation effect. On the other hand, necrosis, edema, and infarction all increase the diffusion distance for GdDTPA. More time is required for equilibration in both the washin and washout phases following bolus administration. Given the poor temporal resolution of spin-echo imaging, one could still obtain useful images of this process at equilibrium, using infusion techniques and following differential washout rates.[Z1]

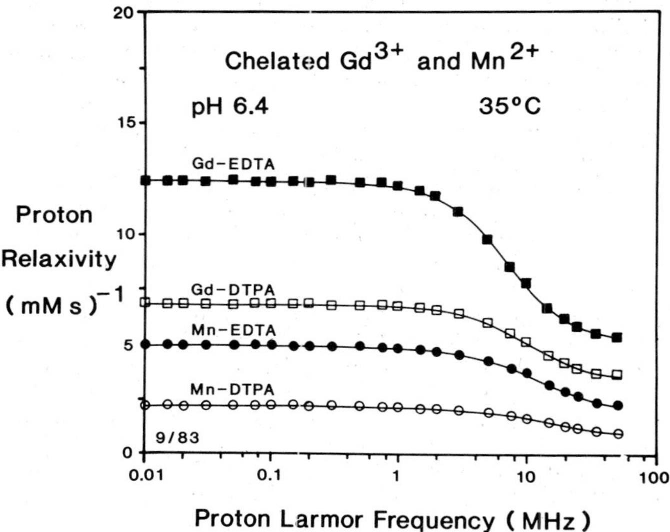

Figure 43–16. Relaxivity dispersion for GdDTPA and other chelates. The many individual measurements at Larmor frequencies from 0.01 to 50 mHz are shown for four chelates. The EDTA ligand binds fewer electrons than DTPA, and its chelates have higher relaxivity. On the other hand, Mn^{2+} has only five unpaired electrons while Gd^{3+} has seven, so GdEDTA is more potent than MnEDTA. Although relaxivity is lower at higher field, inherent relaxation in tissues is declining even more rapidly; thus, GdDTPA is somewhat more effective at 1.0 to 1.5 T than at low imaging fields of 0.06 to 0.12 T. (Courtesy of S. Koenig.)

BLOOD POOL AGENTS. When the size of the MR contrast agent is increased, it eventually becomes too large to escape through the small capillary pores that dominate permeability in normal myocardium. The prototype paramagnetic blood pool agent is GdDTPA-albumin, with a molecular weight of 92,000 daltons. Many such agents can be prepared by covalently binding GdDTPA to the macromolecule (e.g., protein or dextran). Careful preparation is important to avoid damage to the macromolecule. The material must then be meticulously cleared of free GdDTPA and characterized. Each such batch of GdDTPA-albumin can have 17 to 19 GdDTPA per albumin molecule (as prepared by the Contrast Media Laboratory at the University of California, San Francisco).

Because the molecular tumbling of a macromolecule of this size enhances the relaxation processes, the relaxivity of each GdDTPA moiety is increased about threefold while the molecular relaxivities are increased remarkably (R1 ~ 267 mM^{-1} sec^{-1} versus 4.8 for GdDTPA; R2 ~ 304 mM^{-1} sec^{-1} versus 5.2 for GdDTPA). These relaxivities are very field dependent, as shown in Figure 43–5, with much better potency in the 0.5 to 1.5T fields where imaging is also better.

Following intravenous injection by bolus, the blood pool agents and the extracellular agents have about the same transit time to the myocardial wall. Upon reaching the capillaries, however, the distribution volume of the macromolecular agent is about three times smaller than that of the extracellular agent. Relaxation enhancement is still limited to the closely adjacent plasma protons, but the myocardium has a much larger blood pool than other organs such as brain, fat, or skeletal muscle. The rapid diffusion of water in myocardium assures that tissue relaxation rates are appropriately dose-responsive. The different relaxivities and distribution volumes for GdDTPA and GdDTPA albumin make comparison of relative enhancement for a given dose difficult, and the different dispersion profiles make these measurements somewhat device-dependent for the imaging case in vivo or in vitro.

A few studies have compared the dynamic response to the extracellular and blood pool agent in normal myocardium. Using temporal resolution of 5 seconds per image, Schmiedl and associates found maximal myocardial enhancement at 15 seconds following intravenous bolus for each agent.[S2] In theory, the macromolecule should encounter a smaller mixing chamber in the lung and arrive faster and with less dilution. In practice, the injected volumes are larger with the macromolecule, and injection rates are slower, so this subtle difference is not appreciated on images obtained every 5 to 10 seconds.

The blood pool agent with its smaller distribution volume will reach a stable blood level more rapidly than the extracellular agent with a much larger distribution volume. Due to the vagaries of recirculation and relatively slow imaging times, this difference is also difficult to detect. However, the plasma and tissue levels of GdDTPA-albumin are stable for more than 60 minutes while GdDTPA levels in plasma and tissue are rapidly falling due to diffusion and excretion. Fast spin-echo images of rat heart in vivo nicely reflect these physiologic differences (Fig. 43–17).

In normal myocardium, the initial washin reflects tissue perfusion for both GdDTPA and GdDTPA-albumin. This process occurs during the first pass. At plasma *equilibrium*, the contrast agent reflects the distribution volume rather than perfusion, so that GdDTPA indicates relative extracellular volume whereas GdDTPA-albumin identifies relative blood volume. The transition between perfusion-dominated and distribution-dominated information is rapid for normal myocardium.

Myocardial infarction tends to increase microvascular permeability to albumin-sized molecules and the local distribution volume is increased, allowing more GdDTPA-albumin molecules to accumulate per tissue volume in such infarcts. Recall that magnetic resonance imaging reports signal intensity per tissue voxel (volume), and, at equilibrium, this difference could be detectable. The timing for greater MR signal in infarcts than in normal

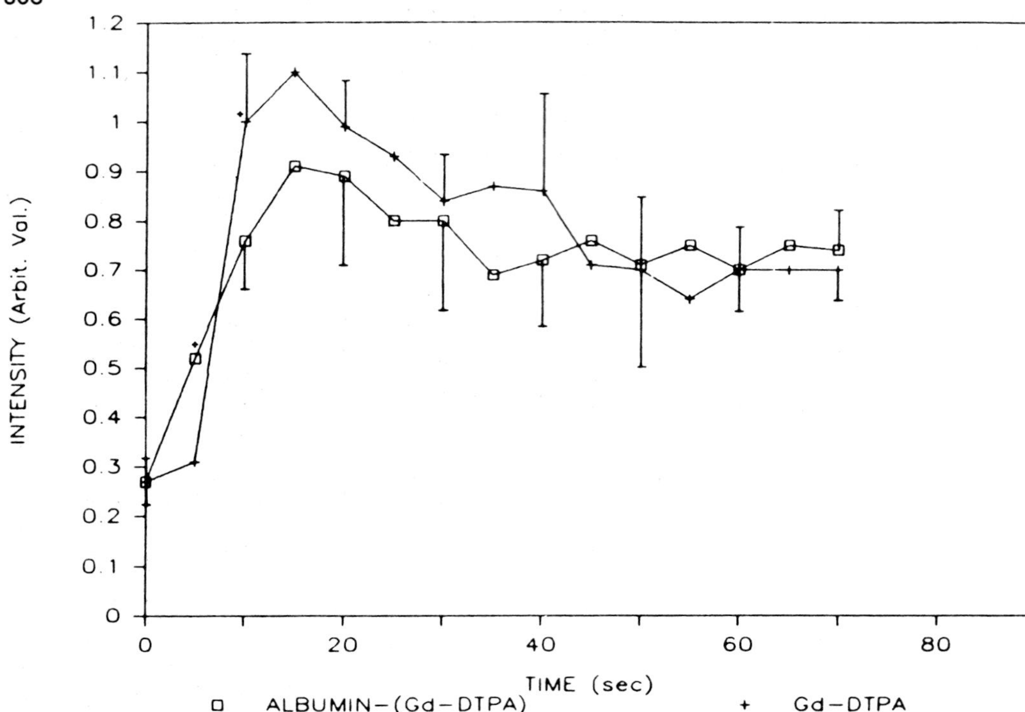

Figure 43–17. Time course of MR intensity change in rat myocardium in response to GdDTPA and Gd-DTPA-albumin. The relative change in signal intensity (arbitrary units) from regions of interest is shown with a temporal resolution of 5 seconds. The two drugs were not given in equivalent doses or with the same injection rate. The washin curves are similar, but GdDTPA has a prominent washout while GdDTPA-albumin is virtually flat after 30 seconds. The values shown are mean ± 1 SD with imaging parameters of 2.0 T; TR = 110, TE = 13. (Courtesy of R. Brasch.)

myocardium depends upon relative perfusion and the microvascular leak rate. It is also possible that local blood volume could increase at the edge of the infarct, but it should be lower within the center of nonhemorrhagic infarcts. In a rat model, Schmiedl and colleagues found significantly increased contrast between normal and infarcted myocardium for 5 to 60 minutes after injection of GdDTPA-albumin. The infarct was created by 6 to 8 hours of coronary occlusion.[S2]

Given the extraordinary range of occlusive and reperfused myocardial ischemia models, it is clear that the relative efficacy of extracellular agents versus blood pool agents requires further study before firm conclusions are reached for the relative preference of a blood pool agent over an extracellular agent in a particular clinical situation. As the equilibrium values for the blood pool agents are stable for longer times, these agents reduce the requirements for high temporal resolution. Spatial resolution and temporal resolution are usually trade-offs for a particular magnetic resonance imaging device, and this becomes an important consideration in the selection of the indicator for myocardial perfusion or infarction.

Unfortunately, albumin is species-specific, and material is tolerated in rats and rabbits but produces anaphylactic shock in dogs. As preparation of these formulations is tedious, their expense to the investigator can be an impediment. Albumin is presumably metabolized, releasing the GdDTPA for rapid renal excretion.

Other macromolecules can be tagged with GdDTPA. A variety of low-to-high molecular weight dextrans have been prepared, but it has been difficult to attach as many GdDTPA moieties to each molecule, and this reduces relaxivity or potency.[G3] Other macromolecules, emulsions, or liposomes are potential blood pool agents as well.

CELLULAR PARAMAGNETIC AGENTS. Manganese chloride was the first myocardial agent for magnetic resonance imaging. Goldman and Brady and their colleagues showed differential uptake between normal and ischemic myocardium.[B4, G1] Manganese is an essential coenzyme for the myocardial cell and has specialized transport systems and possibly a specific intracellular distribution. The metal enters the cell via the same transporter as calcium, but manganese efflux is much slower than calcium extrusion.[H1] This provides very efficient intracellular manganese sequestration in normal cardiac cells, and this process is correlated with myocardial perfusion.[C1] As with thallium, ischemic myocardium does not sequester manganese readily. In the mid 1970s, radioactive manganese was investigated for myocardial imaging, but its imaging properties were suboptimal.[C1]

Excess intracellular manganese interferes with cardiac electrophysiologic processes and cardiac contraction. Wolf and Baum studied the changes in myocardial proton T1 and T2 versus cardiac toxicity in anesthetized dogs and rabbits.[W1] The dose of manganese required to change T1 by 50 percent was less than the toxic dose, but safety ratios were not as good as with GdDTPA. There have been no recent studies using better imaging techniques to evaluate safe imaging of myocardial ischemia with $MnCl_2$. The close correlation between regional myocardial perfusion with microspheres and manganese sequestration in normal and ischemic states justifies further consideration of the benefits and risks of this simple contrast agent.

Manganese can be chelated, but the binding constants are lower than for gadolinium by several orders of magnitude. In vivo, manganese appears to be removed from the chelate and bound to cellular macromolecules, as revealed by a change in the dispersion profile for liver and heart (see Fig. 43–6). Chelation tends to reduce toxicity by keeping the agent extracellular and increasing excretion by liver and kidney. If this process is efficient, it would probably also eliminate specific myocardial uptake. Pflugfelder and associates showed that manganese ethylenediamine tetraphosphonate (Mn-TP) had prolonged retention in normal myocardial cells and differential enhancement between normal and ischemic myocardium.[P1]

Quay and Rutledge developed a manganese pyridoxal analog, Mn-bis pyridoxal ethylenediamine diacetic acid (Mn-DPDP), that also delineated myocardial ischemia after acute coronary occlusion.[P2] The toxicity of these agents and their ability to resist demetallation in vivo requires further study to determine the mechanism of enhancement and safety.

Gadolinium phosphonates have been prepared to be infarct-avid like their radioligands.[C2] However, normal myocardium appears to be more affected for the first hour after administration. A new agent, gadolinium diethyltriamine pentamethylphosphonate (Gd-PMP) appears to have more infarct avidity.[K4]

Iron chelates do not appear to have any advantages for myocardial imaging, and neither do the nitroxide preparations to date.

Receptor agents, or monoclonal antibodies, can be tagged with paramagnetic metals but are not sequestered in the dose (fractions

CAPILLARY

OPEN

OPEN

CLOSED

HYPOPERFUSED
OR
LOW DOSE

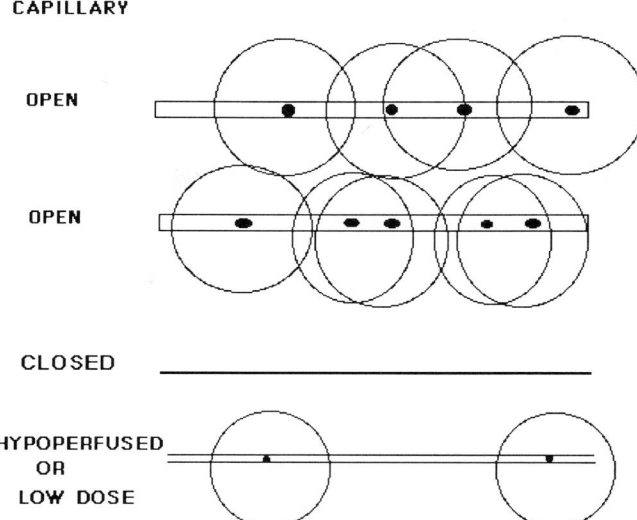

Figure 43–18. Local perfusion patterns: identification with magnetite. Biomag 4125 is a 0.7-micron latex particle containing magnetite. As each particle moves at slow speeds (0.1 mm/sec) through a perfused capillary, it reduces signal from surrounding cells. The particle is depicted as a small dark circle and its effective MR signal change as a large circle. Where the circles overlap sufficiently (high dose or dense capillary perfusion), all tissue MR signal is obliterated at TE's commonly used for imaging. Closed capillaries do not allow entrance of the particle, while hypoperfused or inadequately dosed tissue voxels will have no or less MR signal change.

of micromoles) required for magnetic resonance visibility. Any agent useful for radionuclide imaging would be of interest for MR application because of the excellent spatial resolution of magnetic resonance imaging and its simultaneous depiction of chamber size and myocardial contractility.

An MR contrast agent that accurately depicted myocardial perfusion at the time of its administration and did not redistribute would clearly reduce the use of ^{201}thallium and other cardiac isotope imaging studies.

SUPERPARAMAGNETIC PERFUSION AGENTS. Fairly simple superparamagnetic particles were initially used to image the liver and spleen.[S3, W4] Their size (0.5 to 1 μm) leads to phagocytosis by the reticuloendothelial cells in these two organs. Although the reticuloendothelial cells constitute only about 2 percent of cells in liver, they are dispersed throughout normal liver, and the long-range T2 relaxing effect of the particle could relax protons in surrounding cells nearby. Tumors in liver replace the reticuloendothelial cells, do not accumulate the particles, retain their magnetic resonance signal, and thus are easily contrasted with normal liver where little signal remains following phagocytosis of the particles.

More recently, it has been appreciated that protons losing coherent signal in the vicinity of immobilized particles in tissue also would be affected by slowly moving particles in capillary blood. The same supermagnetic particles that are injected intravenously and slowly removed from blood (half-life of 60 to 90 minutes) will reduce T2 signal for about 50 microns around each capillary. As the oxygen diffusion distance is of the same magnitude for well-perfused tissues, these agents could also be general perfusion agents, as shown in Figure 43–18. Within limits, the

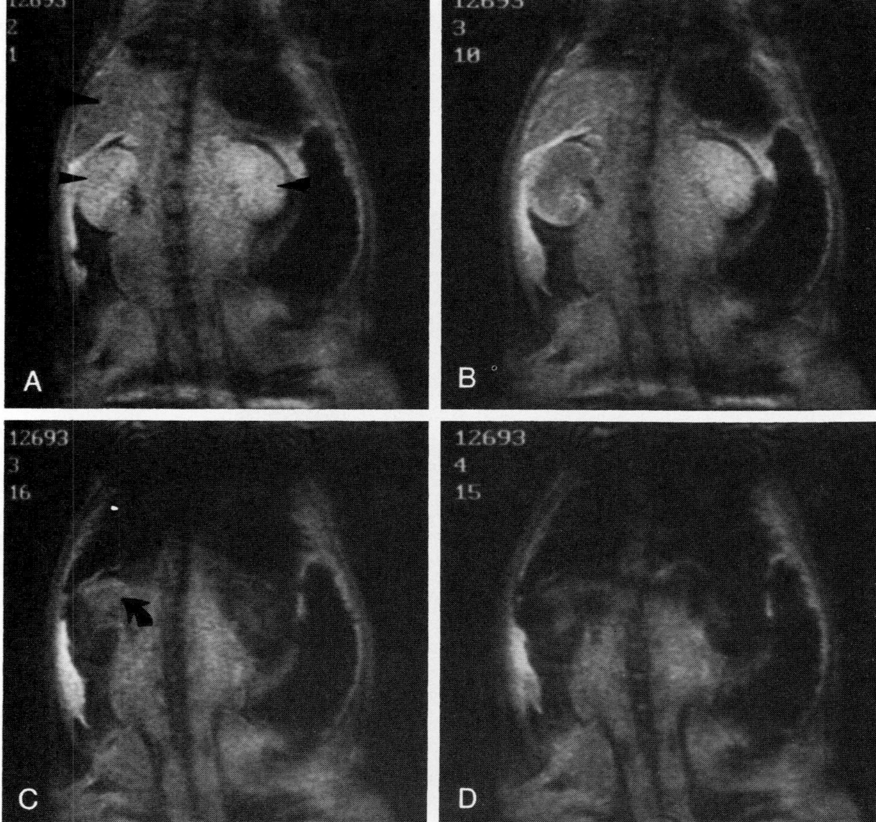

Figure 43–19. Demonstrating tissue perfusion in vivo with magnetite microspheres in a coronal section through the abdomen of a rat. *A*, Before the contrast agent, the liver (large arrowhead) and kidneys (small arrowheads) have strong MR signals. *B*, The artery to the upper pole of the right kidney was ligated and another image obtained. *C*, Thirty seconds after a low dose of magnetite; *D*, 30 seconds after a second dose of magnetite. The liver, left kidney, and lower pole of right kidney lose MR signal owing to the presence of magnetite in well-perfused capillaries. The ischemic upper pole of the right kidney (curved arrow) and poorly perfused tissues such as skeletal muscle, fat, and skin are little altered by the magnetite.

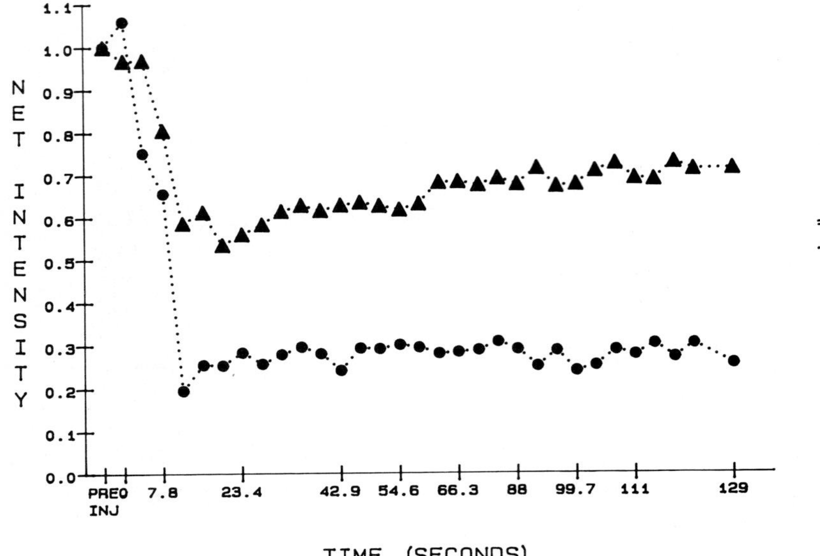

Figure 43–20. Time-intensity curves for normal renal cortex in response to two doses of magnetite microspheres. The MR signal intensity change in two different rats responding to 80 μM Fe/kg (circles) and 400 μM Fe/kg (triangles) of magnetite microspheres as a 1:10 dilution of Biomag 4125. Temporal resolution is 3.9 seconds using a fast gradient echo sequence (TR = 28, TE = 12, 128 phase encoding steps). Faster temporal resolution allows the investigator to obtain 3 to 6 data points on the washin phase for better mathematical analysis. Washout is gradual and minimal.

effect will also be dose-responsive as well as reflecting tissue blood volume at equilibrium.

As the tissue signal decrement would be in proportion to capillary perfusion, this parameter should be responsive to the dynamic state of organ perfusion. For example, capillary dilation or recruitment will result in more particles per tissue voxel whereas reduced perfusion or fewer active capillaries would have the opposite effect. With a fairly long blood half-life, vasoactive challenge or functional testing should be possible for a few hours. Over many hours, the agent would be cleared from blood, allowing repeat studies of the heart.

The superparamagnetic particles are very potent, and the magnetic resonance imager is more sensitive to their effect when gradient echo techniques are utilized than when spin-echo methods are used. Even with spin-echo technique, however, their potent T2 effects reduce MR signal for all selected TR and TE combinations, and this reduces the complexity of interpreting the effects of paramagnetic agents.

Figures 43–19 and 43–20 demonstrate this perfusion effect and dose-responsiveness for kidney cortex. Figure 43–21 shows normally perfused liver adjacent to ischemic liver. Our laboratory has not yet mastered the skills of cardiac-gated magnetic resonance imaging and creating stable myocardial ischemia for small animals such as rabbits or rats, but Figure 43–22 shows the potential for such agents in myocardial perfusion imaging.

SUMMARY

Although the cost is high, magnetic resonance imaging provides exquisite imaging of the cardiac chambers, as shown in the many other chapters of this text. However, it is not possible to confidently image pathologic abnormalities or tissue perfusion within the myocardial wall. Magnetic resonance contrast agents will be helpful when this is the primary purpose of the imaging request. However, a single comprehensive examination that shows chamber size, contractile function, and myocardial perfusion during stress or an intervention would be especially attractive and might replace one or more other imaging options.

Magnetic resonance imaging is certainly capable of providing compelling images with safety and a high degree of patient acceptance. It is a very young discipline that is currently overwhelmed with all the available options for imaging with or without

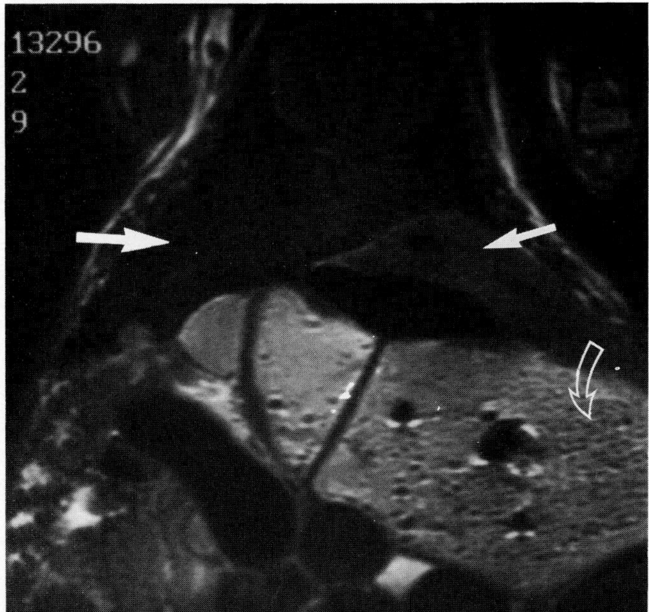

Figure 43–21. Normal and ischemic liver after magnetite. A segmental lobe of rabbit liver was ligated prior to the administration of magnetite microspheres. This image, 30 seconds later, is one of a series obtained with the technique used in the previous figure. The normal liver (large arrow) has virtually no MR signal at this time while the ischemic liver (small arrow) has more intensity. The stomach (open arrow) has a strong signal from ingested food.

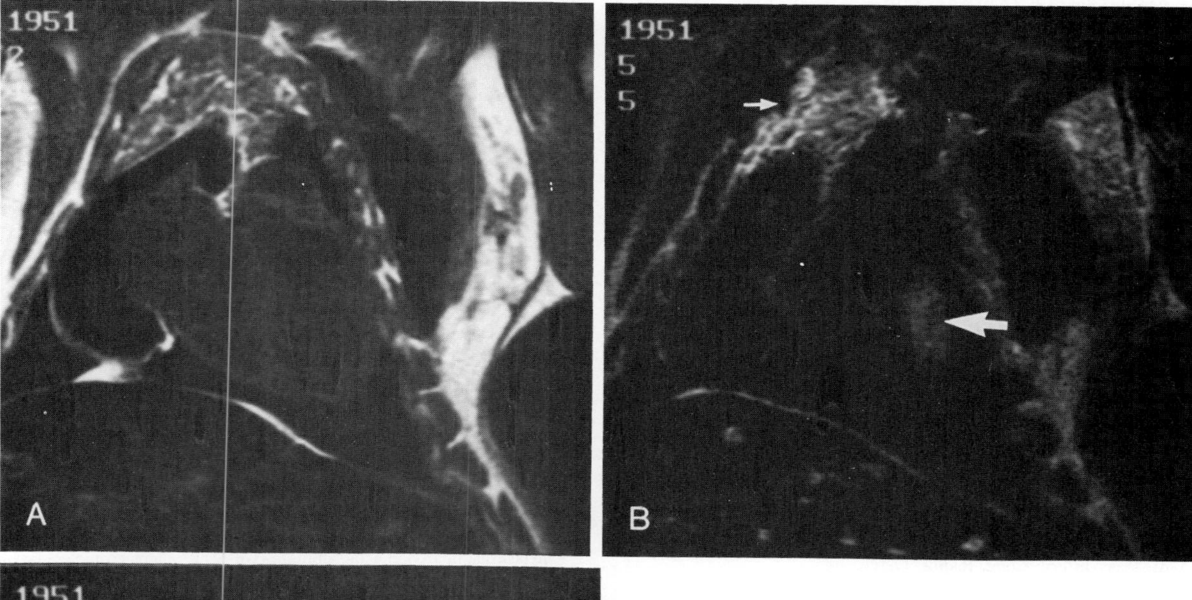

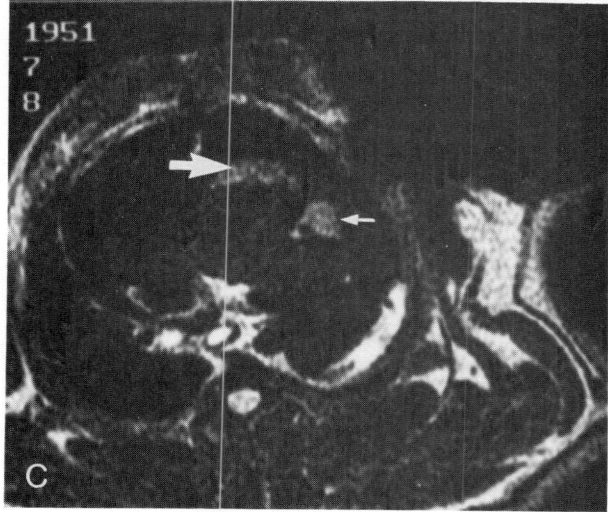

Figure 43–22. Well-perfused and ischemic myocardium delineated by magnetite microsphere perfusion. The left anterior descending artery of a rabbit was ligated in its midportion 20 minutes prior to administering magnetite microspheres. These images were obtained postmortem. *A*, A T1-weighted spin-echo coronal image (TR = 400, TE = 20) and liver and blood have very low signal due to the presence of magnetite. *B* (Coronal), and *C* (axial) are a T2-weighted gradient-echo image (TR = 83, TE = 20, flip angle 10°). The normal myocardium has little signal while the ischemic myocardium (large arrow) and fat (small arrows) have retained signal, reflecting the relative absence of microspheres and blood.

contrast agents. The latter come in nearly as many choices as available for nuclear cardiology but with much improved spatial and temporal resolution. Clearly, there will be a major role for this technology in cardiac imaging, and our opportunity is to define this role amid the challenge of too little time and money.

Acknowledgment

The author is grateful for the support of his research team: Jay Zimmerman, John Canillo, Joe Gillen, Lalith Talagala, Peter Davis, Peter Daly, Janis Gottlieb, and Deborah Bacco.

References

B

1. Bloch, F., Hansen, W. W., and Packard, M.: The nuclear induction experiment. Phys. Reo. 70:474, 1946.
2. Bloembergen, N.: Proton relaxation times in paramagnetic solutions. J. Chem. Phys. 27:572, 1957.
3. Bloembergen, N., and Morgan, L. O.: Proton relaxation times in paramagnetic solutions. Effects of electron spin relaxation. J. Chem. Phys. 34:842, 1961.
4. Brady, T. J., Goldman, M. R., and Pykett, I. L.: Proton nuclear magnetic imaging of regionally ischemic canine hearts: Effects of paramagnetic proton signal enhancement. Radiology 144:343, 1982.
5. Brasch, R. C., Weinman, H. J., and Wesbey, G. E.: Contrast-enhanced NMR imaging: Animal studies using Gd-DTPA. Am. J. Roentgenol. 142:623, 1983.
6. Brasch, R. C., London, D. A., and Wesbey, G. E.: Nuclear magnetic resonance study of a paramagnetic nitroxide contrast agent for enhancement of renal structures in experimental animals. Radiology 147:773, 1983.
7. Brown, J. J., and Higgins, C. B.: Myocardial paramagnetic contrast agents for MR imaging. Am. J. Roentgenol. 151:865, 1988.

C

1. Chauncey, D. M., Jr., Schelbert, H. R., and Halpern, S. E.: Tissue distribution studies with radioactive manganese: A potential agent for myocardial imaging. J. Nucl. Med. 17:933, 1977.
2. Canby, R. C., Elgavish, G. A., Reeves, R. C., and Pohost, G. M.: $Gd(BDP)_2$-induced relaxation rate differentiation between ischemic and non-ischemic myocardium in a transient-ischemia model in ferrets. Proc. Soc. Magn. Reson. Med. 6:844, 1985.

D

1. Davis, P. L., Parker, D. L., Nelson, J. A., et al.: Interactions of paramagnetic contrast agents and the spin echo pulse sequence. Invest. Radiol. 23:381, 1988.

E

1. Engelstad, B. L., and Wolf, G. L.: Contrast agents. *In* Stark, D. D., and Bradley, W. G., Jr. (eds.) Magnetic Resonance Imaging. C. V. Mosby, St. Louis, 1988, p. 161.

F

1. Fobben, E., and Wolf, G. L.: Gadolinium DTPA—a potential NMR contrast agent. Effects upon tissue proton relaxation and cardiovascular function in the rabbit. Invest. Radiol. 18:S5, 1983.

G

1. Goldman, M. R., Brady, T. J., and Pykett, I. L.: Quantification of experimental myocardial infarction using nuclear magnetic resonance imaging and paramagnetic ion contrast enhancement in excised canine hearts. Circulation 66:1012, 1982.
2. Gadian, D. G., Payne, D. J., Bryant, I. R., et al.: Gadolinium-DTPA as a

contrast agent in MR imaging—theoretical projections and practical observations. J. Comput. Assist. Tomogr. 9:242, 1985.
3. Gibby, W. R., Bogdan, A., and Ovitt, T. W.: Cross-linked DTPA polysaccharides for magnetic resonance imaging. Synthesis and relaxation properties. Invest. Radiol. 24:302, 1989.
4. Gillis, P., and Koenig, S. H.: Transverse relaxation of solvent protons induced by magnetized spheres: Application to ferritin, erythrocytes, and magnetite. Magn. Reson. Med. 5:323, 1987.
5. Goldstein, E. J., Wolf, G. L., and Brasch, R. C.: Free radical contrast agents for MRI. *In* Partain, L., Price, R. R., Patton, J. A., et al. (eds.): Magnetic Resonance Imaging. W. B. Saunders, Philadelphia, 1988, p. 838.

H

1. Hunter, D. R., Haworth, R. A., and Berkoff, H. A.: Cellular manganese uptake by the isolated perfused rat heart: A probe for the sarcolemma calcium channel. J. Mal. Cell. Cardiol. 13:823, 1981.
2. Hendrick, R. E.: Image contrast and noise. *In* Stark, D. D., and Bradley, W. G., Jr. (eds.) Magnetic Resonance Imaging. C. V. Mosby, St. Louis, 1988, p. 66.
3. Horrocks, W. D., and Sipe, J. P.: Lanthanide shift reagents: A survey. J. Am. Chem. Soc. 63:6800, 1971.
4. Hardy, P. A., and Henkleman, R. M.: Transverse relaxation rate enhancement caused by magnetic particulates. Magn. Reson. Imag. 7:265, 1989.
5. Hemmingson, A.: Superparamagnetic particles as oral and intravenous contrast agents in MRI. Proc. Intern. Cong. Radiol. 17:120, 1989.

K

1. Koenig, S., Brown, R. D., III: Relaxometry of solvent and tissue protons: Diamagnetic contributions. *In* Partain, C. L., Price, R. R., Patton, J. A., et al. (eds.): Magnetic Resonance Imaging. W. B. Saunders, Philadelphia, 1988, p. 1035.
2. Koenig, S. H., Spiller, M., Brown, R. D., and Wolf, G. L.: Investigation of the biochemical state of paramagnetic ions in vivo using the magnetic field dependence of 1/T1 of tissue protons (NMRD profile): Applications to contrast agents for magnetic resonance imaging. Nuc. Med. Biol. Int. J. Radiat. Appl. Instrum. (Part B) 15:23, 1988.
3. Koenig, S. H., Spiller, M., Brown, R. D., and Wolf, G. L.: Relaxation of water protons in the intra- and extracellular regions of blood containing Gd(DTPA). Magn. Reson. Med. 3:791, 1986.
4. Kulkarni, P. V., Schaeffer, S., Peshock, R. M., et al.: Phosphonate complexes of gadolinium: Potential contrast agents for magnetic resonance imaging of the myocardium. J. Nucl. Med. 28:406, 1987.

L

1. Lauterbur, P. C., Mendonca-Dias, M. H., and Rubin, A. M.: Augmentation of tissue water proton spin-lattice relaxation rates by the in vivo addition of paramagnetic ions. *In* Dulton, P. O., Leigh, J. S., and Scarpa, A. (eds.): Frontiers of Biological Energetics. Academic Press, New York, 1978, p. 752.
2. Lauterbur, P. C., Bernardo, M. C., and Mendonca-Dias, M. H.: Microscopic NMR imaging of the magnetic fields around magnetic particles. Proc. Soc. Magn. Reson. Med. 5:229, 1986.

M

1. Majumdar, S., Zoghbis, S., Pope, C. F., and Gore, J. C.: A quantitative study of relaxation rate enhancement produced by iron oxide particles in polyacrylamide gels and tissue. Magn. Reson. Med. 9:185, 1989.
2. Miller, D. D., Holmuang, G., Gill, J. B., et al.: MRI detection of myocardial perfusion changes by gadolinium-DTPA infusion during dipyridamole hyperemia. Magn. Reson. Med. 10:246, 1989.
3. Majumdar, S., and Gore, J. C.: Studies of diffusion in random fields produced by variation in susceptibility. J. Magn. Res. 77:41, 1988.

N

1. Neindorf, H. P., and Seifert, W.: Serum iron and serum bilirubin after administration of Gd-DTPA dimeglumine: A pharmacologic study in healthy volunteers. Invest. Radiol. 23:S275, 1988.

P

1. Pflugfelder, P. W., Wendland, M. F., and Holt, W. W.: Acute myocardial ischemia: MR imaging with Mn-TP. Radiology 167:129, 1988.
2. Pomeroy, O. H., Holt, W. W., Derugin, N., et al.: Delineation of acute myocardial ischemia on MRI using a new paramagnetic contrast media. Invest. Radiol. 24:531, 1989.

R

1. Runge, V. M., Clanton, J. A., and Lukehart, C. M.: Paramagnetic agents for contrast-enhanced NMR imaging: A review. Am. J. Roentgenol. 141:1209, 1983.
2. Renshaw, P. F., Owen, C. S., McLaughlin, A. C., et al.: Ferromagnetic contrast agents: A new approach. Magn. Reson. Med. 3:217, 1986.

S

1. Schmiedl, U., Moseley, M. E., Ogan, M. D., et al.: Comparison of initial biodistribution patterns of Gd-DTPA and albumin-(Gd-DTPA) using rapid spin echo MR imaging. J. Comput. Assist. Tomogr. 11:306, 1987.
2. Schmiedl, U., Moseley, M. E., and Sievers, R.: Magnetic resonance imaging of myocardial infarction using albumin-(Gd-DTPA), a macromolecular blood-volume contrast agent in a rat model. Invest. Radiol. 22:713, 1987.
3. Stark, D. D., Weislander, R., Elizondo, G., et al.: Superparamagnetic iron oxide: Clinical application as a contrast agent for MR imaging of the liver. Radiology 168:297, 1988.

T

1. Tweddle, M. F., Brittain, H. G., Eckelman, W. C., et al.: Principles of contrast-enhanced MRI. *In* Partain, L., Price, R. R., Patton, J. A., et al. (eds.): Magnetic Resonance Imaging. W. B. Saunders, Philadelphia, 1988, p. 793.

W

1. Wolf, G. L., and Baum, L.: Cardiovascular toxicity and tissue proton T1 response to manganese injection in the dog and rabbit. Am. J. Roentgenol. 141:193, 1983.
2. Weinmann, H. J., Brasch, R. C., Press, W. R., and Wesbey, G. E.: Characteristics of gadolinium-DTPA complex: A potential NMR contrast agent. Am. J. Roentgenol. 142:619, 1984.
3. Wolf, G. L., and Fobben, E.: The tissue proton T1 and T2 response to gadolinium DTPA injection in rabbits: A potential renal contrast agent for NMR imaging. Invest. Radiol. 19:324, 1984.
4. Wolf, G. L., Burnett, K. R., and Goldstein, E. J.: Contrast agents for magnetic resonance imaging. *In* Kressel, H. Y. (ed.): Magnetic Resonance Annual. Raven Press, New York, 1985, p. 231.
5. Wolf, G. L.: Contrast enhancement in biomedical NMR. Phys. Chem. Physics Med. NMR 16:93, 1984.
6. Wesbey, G. E., Higgins, C. B., and McNamara, M. T.: Effect of gadolinium-DTPA on the magnetic relaxation times of normal and infarcted myocardium. Radiology 153:165, 1984.
7. Wolf, G. L., Joseph, P. M., and Goldstein, E. J.: Optimal pulsing sequences for MR contrast agents. Am. J. Roentgenol. 147:367, 1986.
8. Weinmann, H. J., Gries, H., and Speck, U.: GdDTPA and low osmolar Gd chelates. *In* Runge, V. M. (ed.): Enhanced Magnetic Resonance Imaging. C. V. Mosby, St. Louis, 1989, p. 74.

Z

1. Zierler, K. L.: Theoretical basis of indicator-dilution methods for measuring flow and volume. Circ. Res. 10:393, 1962.

Chapter 44

Magnetic Resonance Imaging of the Heart: Quantitation

■ *RONALD M. PESHOCK, M.D.*

TECHNICAL CONCERNS 811
General Approach 811
Technique 812
Orientation 815
MEASUREMENT OF CARDIAC SIZE 815
Conditions for Accurate Measurement 815
Linear Measurements 816
Area Measurements 816
Volume Measurement 816
Wall Thickness and Myocardial Mass 817
ASSESSMENT OF CARDIAC FUNCTION 819
Global Function 819
Segmental Function 819
TISSUE CHARACTERIZATION 820
Relaxation Times 820
Methods for Measurement 820
Limitations 821
Measurement of Infarct Size 821
FLOW QUANTITATION 822
Shunt Calculations 822
Flow Velocity 823
Valvular Regurgitation 823
Myocardial Perfusion 823
FUTURE DEVELOPMENTS 824
High-Speed Imaging 824
Automated Analysis 824
Three-Dimensional Display 824
Magnetic Resonance Spectroscopy 825
SUMMARY 825

Perhaps more than in any other area in medicine, quantitation is an essential element in the practice of cardiology. To evaluate the patient with heart disease completely, the clinician needs answers to a number of critical questions: (1) Are the chambers of normal size? (2) Are global and segmental function normal? (3) Is the myocardial tissue normal or is there evidence of injury? (4) Are blood flow and tissue perfusion normal? and (5) Has the metabolic function of the tissue been altered? As evidenced in this book, a wide variety of approaches have been utilized in attempts to answer these questions.

In attempting to obtain quantitative information regarding the heart and its function, several problems must be addressed. First is the problem of geometry: the heart is a complex, three-dimensional structure. Moreover, its geometry can be significantly altered by common disease processes, such as ischemic heart disease and cardiomyopathy. This point cannot be ignored in attempting to measure the size of chambers. Second, the heart is constantly in motion. Its complex geometry is constantly changing. Methods for evaluation of this motion must deal with this change in geometry. Third, the position and orientation of the heart in the chest are variable from person to person, and from time to time in the same person. Thus, the imaging method must allow measurement with respect to the reference frame of the heart. Fourth, structures of interest in the heart vary in size from millimeters (coronary arteries, valve leaflets) to several centimeters. An ideal imaging method would span this entire range of spatial resolution. Finally, because of the motion of the heart, the images must be obtained at multiple points in time. For this, the temporal resolution, or time between images, must be short to allow accurate evaluation of the multiple events that take place during the cardiac cycle.

The ideal cardiac imaging technique would allow one to address all these clinical questions and problems. Recently, nuclear magnetic resonance (NMR) techniques have emerged as useful tools in the evaluation of the heart. Notably, magnetic resonance imaging (MRI) has several features that make it particularly applicable.

First, magnetic resonance imaging is a remarkably flexible technique. Relatively simple changes in the imaging sequence lead to dramatic changes in image resolution and contrast. This allows one to tailor MRI uniquely to specific problems in the cardiac evaluation. Second, magnetic resonance imaging is fundamentally a three-dimensional imaging technique. In addition, it is not constrained by problems of acoustic window or attenuation. Hence, images can be obtained in virtually any orientation with exact knowledge of the location of the imaging plane. This permits a direct approach to the analysis of the complex shape and motion of the heart. Third, magnetic resonance imaging is inherently sensitive to motion, thus allowing differentiation of chamber lumen and wall without the use of contrast agents. Moreover, this sensitivity to motion can be utilized to directly measure cardiac motion and blood flow.

Thus, the purpose of this chapter is to (1) examine the general problem of cardiac quantitation and the imaging techniques available, (2) review the present status of magnetic resonance imaging in the quantitation of cardiac size and function, and (3) investigate its future potential.

TECHNICAL CONCERNS

General Approach

All approaches to measuring the heart begin with the fundamental problem of attempting to describe a complex, three-dimensional structure, which changes over time, further complicating its evaluation.[F1] In pursuit of the optimal method of imaging the heart, three general approaches have been devised: (1) planar approaches (also termed projection or silhouette approaches), such as contrast ventriculography and planar radionuclide ventriculography; (2) tomographic approaches, such as standard echocardiography, cine computed tomography, single-photon emission computed tomography, and standard magnetic resonance imaging; and (3) direct three-dimensional acquisition with single-photon emission computed tomography and three-dimensional magnetic resonance imaging.

In magnetic resonance imaging, the silhouette or true projection approach has been used extensively in MR angiography[D1] but has been used very little in evaluation of the heart. The tomographic or multislice approach has been the primary method in both standard multislice and cine magnetic resonance imaging. This approach is familiar to most cardiologists and cardiac radiologists from experience with echocardiography and is well suited to most cardiac problems. Most of the discussion in this chapter deals with these tomographic approaches. Direct three-dimensional acquisition is possible with magnetic resonance imaging and allows visualization of the entire three-dimensional volume and, hence, any projection or tomography section. Experience in the use of this method has been limited and acquisition times appear to be lengthy.[C1, G1] However, this approach offers the potential for the most accurate assessments of cardiac structure and geometry and has significant potential for the future.

Technique

Magnetic resonance imaging provides remarkable flexibility for adjusting soft tissue contrast. In the heart, it is possible to alter dramatically the contrast between the blood and myocardium with relatively simple changes in the imaging pulse sequence. Two commonly used approaches are shown in Figure 44–1. The standard spin echo sequence (Fig. 44–1*A*) is generally used to create images in which the blood pool is dark and the myocardium has an intermediate signal intensity. The gradient reversal sequence used in most cine MRI approaches yields an image with high signal intensity from the blood with a lower signal intensity from the myocardium (Fig. 44–1*B*). These two pulse sequences are discussed in more detail later.

SPIN ECHO. The spin echo pulse sequence has been used most widely in the evaluation of cardiac function. Typically, in this sequence, the repetition time, or TR, is gated and, therefore, linked to the patient's heart rate. The time to echo, or TE, is frequently in the range of 20 to 40 msec. In general, the spin echo approach yields high-quality images, and it has been used extensively in evaluation of cardiac structure.[P1] However, in the measurement of chamber size and function, several aspects of the implementation of this approach must be understood and will be addressed in the following sections.

MULTISLICE SPIN ECHO. Generally, the spin echo sequence is implemented in the form of a multislice imaging sequence.[L1] This means that the *images of different slices are acquired at different points in time* (Fig. 44–2). This is not a problem in a stationary organ; however, in the heart it implies that the *different slices are acquired at different points during the cardiac cycle*. As shown in Figure 44–2, if 100 msec are required to image each slice and the first slice is imaged at time 0, then the second slice will be obtained not at that same time but 100 msec later. The third slice will be imaged 200 msec later, and so forth. This is fundamentally different from any other imaging technique presently used in cardiology.

MULTISLICE, MULTIPHASE SPIN ECHO. The fact that standard multislice cardiac MR images are not acquired at the same point in the cardiac cycle means that the timing of the image with respect to the cardiac cycle must be considered in assessing cardiac measurements and function. Multislice, multiphase methods can be used to obtain a complete set of images, in which images of all the slices are available for the same point in the cardiac cycle.[C1] In this approach, the order of slice acquisition is altered during repeated multislice imaging runs, so that each slice is obtained at each point in the cardiac cycle (Fig. 44–3). This approach requires additional scanning time to collect a complete set of data and hence puts a practical limit on the temporal resolution potentially available using this approach.

In summary, gated, multislice spin echo magnetic resonance imaging provides high-quality images of cardiac structure. However, from the standpoint of measurement of chamber size and assessment of function, it is critical to know the point in the cardiac cycle at which each slice is acquired. Multislice, multiphase methods allow one to obtain all slices at similar points in the cardiac cycle, thus facilitating measures of size and function. However, additional time is required to obtain this more complete dataset.

GRADIENT REVERSAL, CINE MAGNETIC RESONANCE IMAGING. In cine MRI (also termed FLASH or GRASS), one typically obtains multiple images in a single slice over time.[F2, G2] As generally implemented, this can be viewed as sacrificing the number of slices obtained for an increased number of images within a given slice. Clearly, however, this is an advantage in the assessment of function in that it allows high temporal resolution within a given slice, particularly if a planar or single tomographic approach is adequate for the measurement. An example of a series of gradient reversal images in a single slice with a time resolution of 33 msec is shown in Figure 44–4. These data were not acquired in real time but instead over a total time of approximately 5 minutes. It, therefore, represents events occurring every 33 msec in the cardiac cycle averaged over a period of 5 minutes. Hence, the images are similar to those obtained in radionuclide ventriculography, in which counts are obtained over a period of minutes, placed into bins representing different points in the cardiac cycle, and then played back to study function and motion. Images acquired using cine magnetic resonance imaging are not acquired in real time and hence are not directly comparable with those obtained in echocardiography.

Finally, it is important to note that all the aforementioned approaches utilize cardiac gating. Pseudogating sometimes allows the acquisition of adequate cardiac images[B1]; however, cardiac gating is required to acquire high-quality images routinely, using

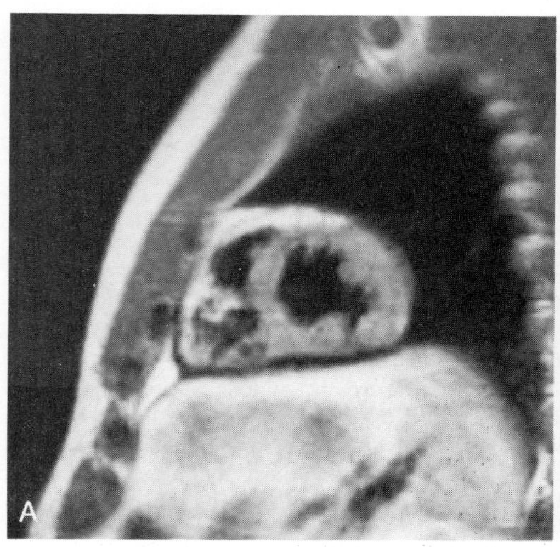

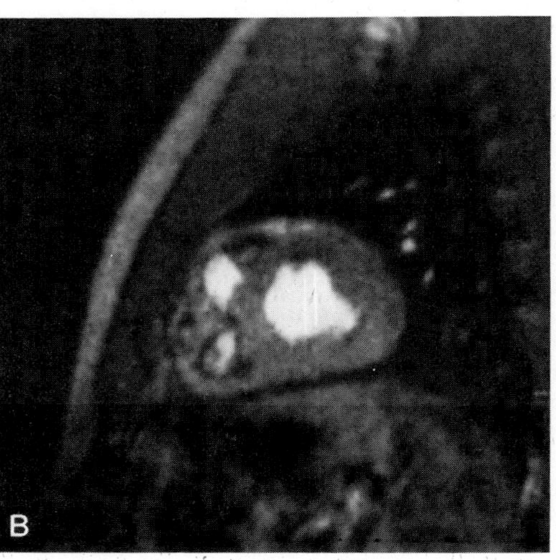

Figure 44–1. Effects of different pulse sequences on blood and myocardial signal intensity. *A*, Image obtained using a standard (TR-gated to every heartbeat, TE-30) spin echo pulse sequence. *B*, The same slice imaged using a cine magnetic resonance imaging gradient reversal pulse sequence (TR-33 msec, TE-17, alpha = 45°).

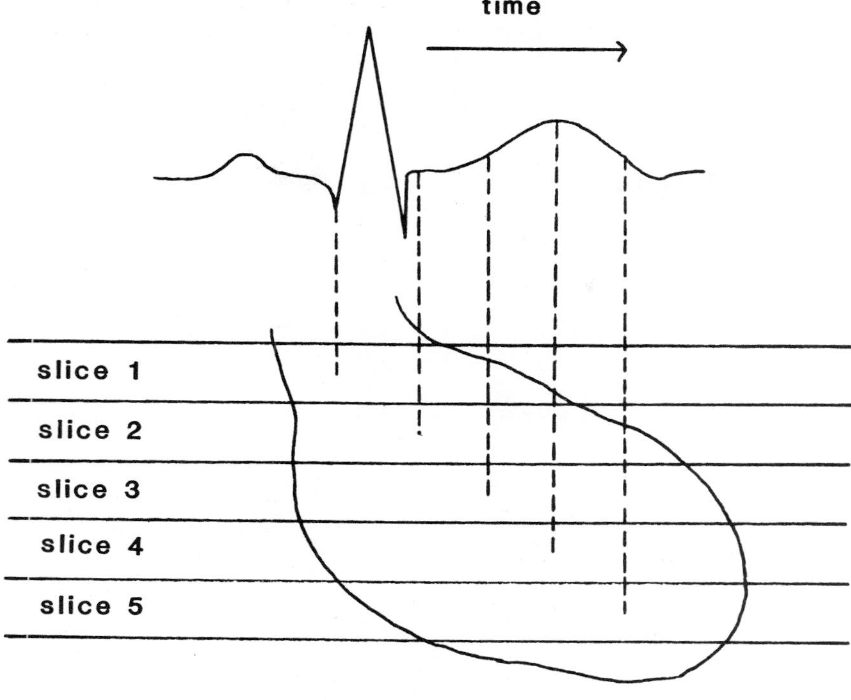

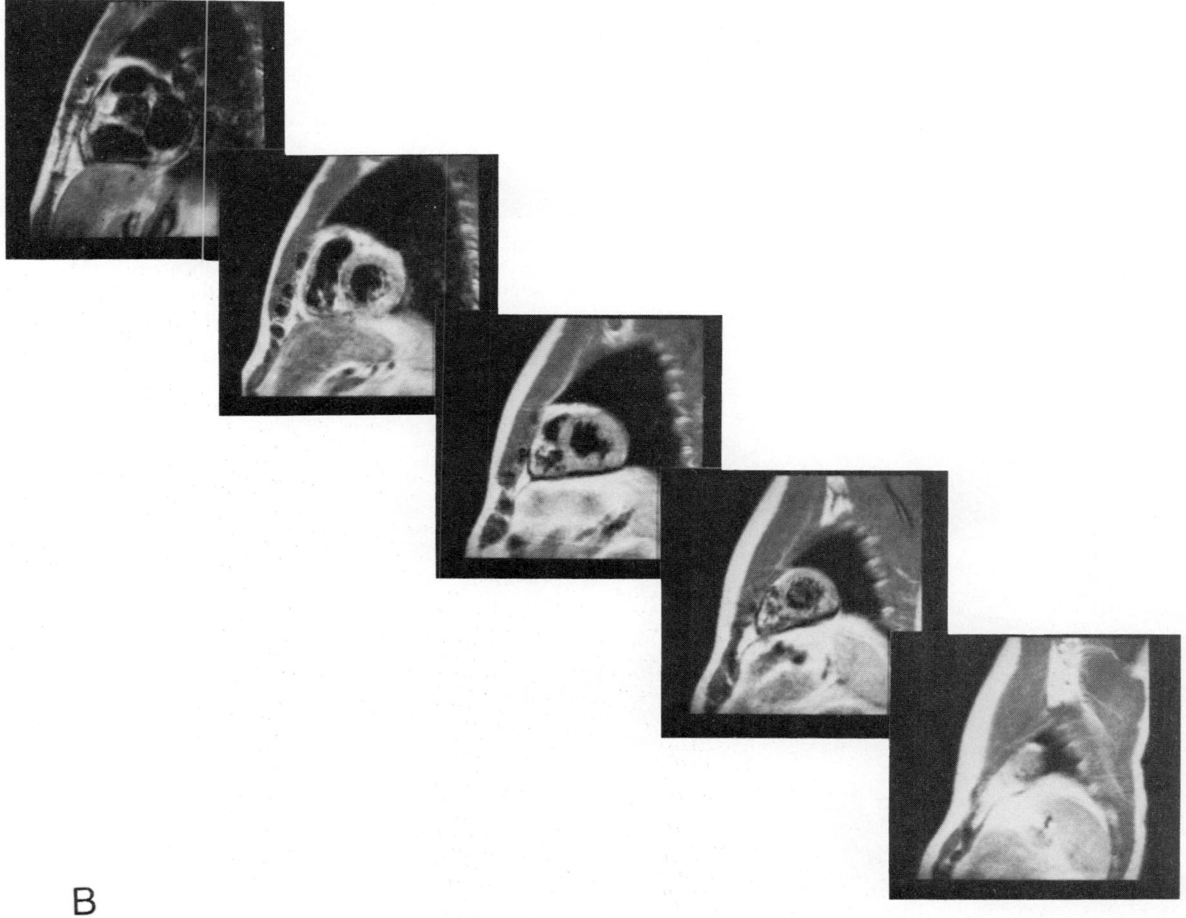

Figure 44–2. Multislice imaging. *A*, As described in the text, multislice images typically are obtained at different points in the cardiac cycle. If the first slice is acquired at the time of QRS, the second is acquired 100 msec later, the third 200 msec later, and so forth. *B*, Images acquired in a standard multislice sequence. The first image is obtained at end-diastole, with subsequent images obtained at later points in the cardiac cycle, as shown.

Time	0	100	200	300	400 msec
Slice 1	X	-	-	-	-
Slice 2	-	X	-	-	-
Slice 3	-	-	X	-	-
Slice 4	-	-	-	X	-
Slice 5	-	-	-	-	X

A

Time	0	100	200	300	400 msec
Slice 1	1	-	-	-	2
Slice 2	2	1	-	-	-
Slice 3	-	2	1	-	-
Slice 4	-	-	2	1	-
Slice 5	-	-	-	2	1

B

Time	0	100	200	300	400 msec
Slice 1	X	X	X	X	X
Slice 2	X	X	X	X	X
Slice 3	X	X	X	X	X
Slice 4	X	X	X	X	X
Slice 5	X	X	X	X	X

C

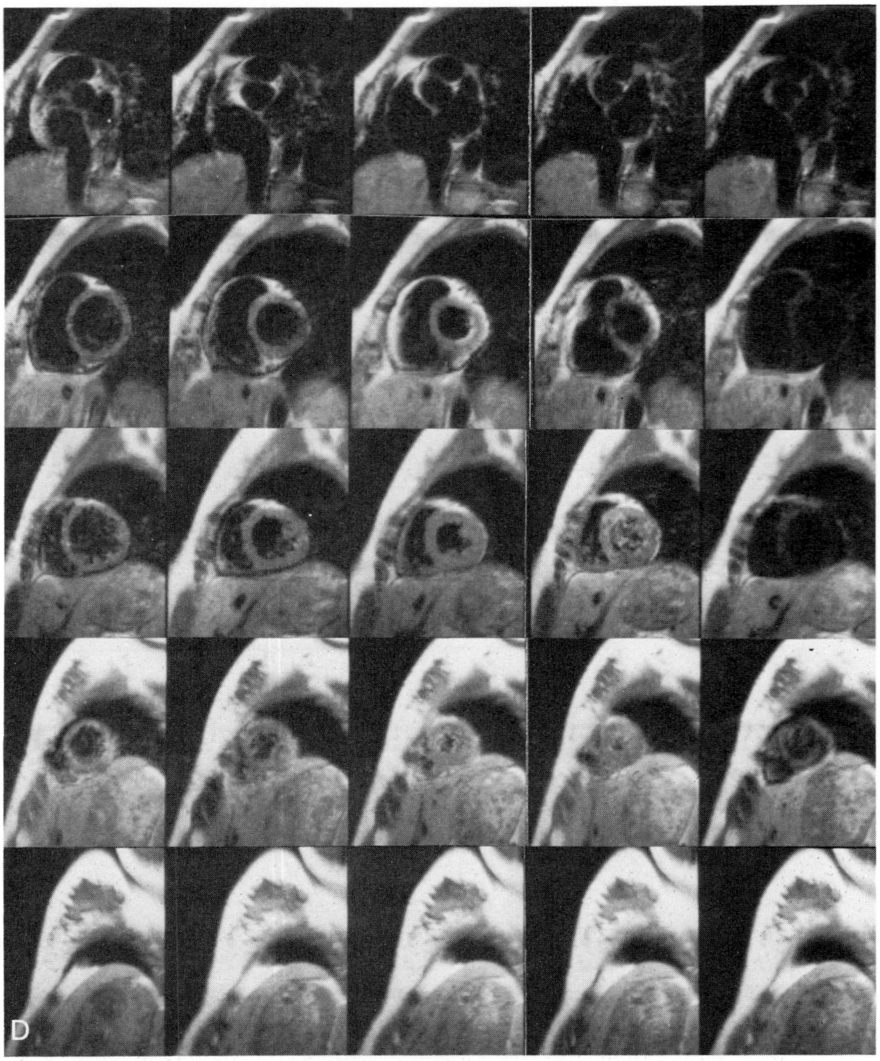

D

Figure 44–3. Multislice, multiphase imaging. *A*, In the first multislice acquisition, the slices are acquired at different points in the cardiac cycle, as described in Figure 44–2. *B*, The first acquisition is now indicated by a "1" at each position. The acquisition is then repeated (indicated by "2" at each position), altering the order of slice acquisition. *C*, The order of slice acquisition is repeatedly altered so that all slices are acquired at all points in time. *D*, A complete multislice, multiphase dataset consisting of five slices obtained at five points in time.

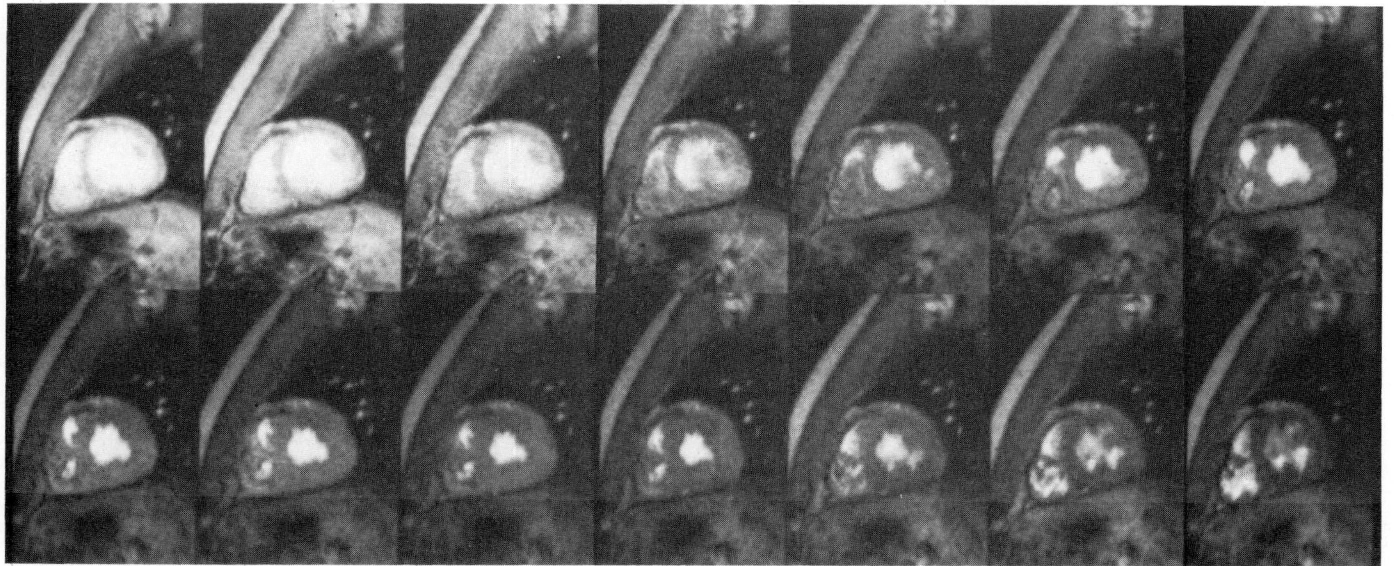

Figure 44–4. Cine magnetic resonance imaging dataset. A series of images obtained beginning at QRS and every 33 msec thereafter.

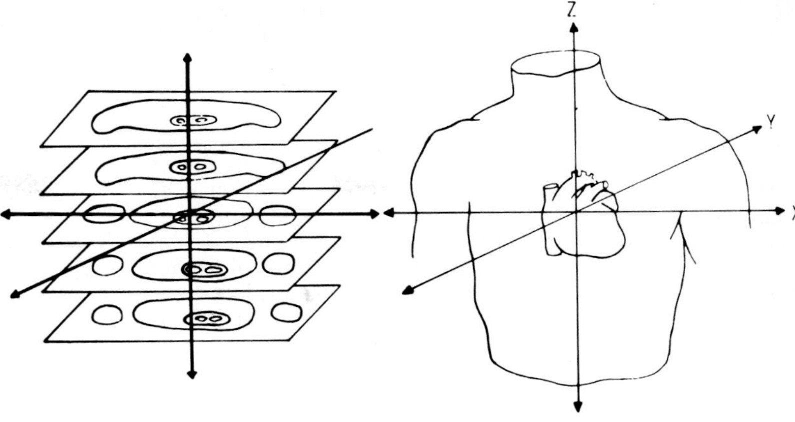

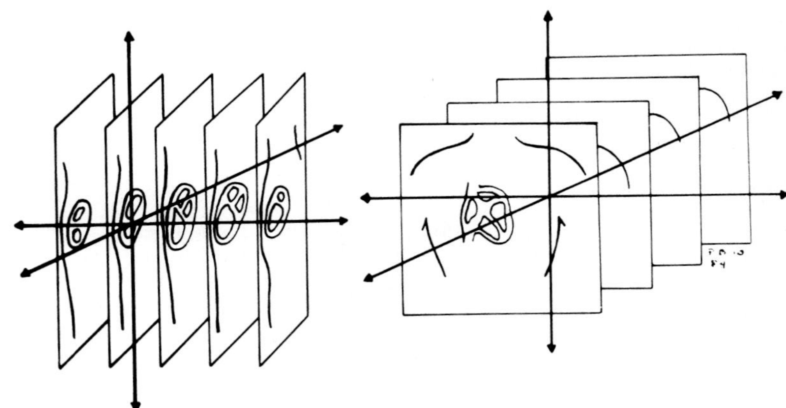

Figure 44–5. Orientation. Positions of standard transaxial, coronal, and sagittal imaging planes relative to the heart.

spin echo and gradient reversal techniques. The technical aspects of gating are discussed in Chapter 42.[P1]

Orientation

An important advantage of magnetic resonance imaging is its ability to electronically obtain images with any orientation. Initially, MR devices were used in evaluation of the central nervous system and typically obtained images only in the reference frame of the body, i.e., standard axial, coronal, and sagittal planes (Fig. 44–5). Hence, early cardiac magnetic resonance imaging studies attempted to use these planes to evaluate cardiac structure and function. Unfortunately, the orientation of the heart relative to these anatomic imaging planes varies from person to person. Because of this, other cardiac imaging techniques almost exclusively obtain images in planes oriented with respect to the functional axes of the heart or the cardiac reference plane.[B2] By use of appropriate patient positioning[M1] and/or electronic rotation of the imaging planes,[F3, P2] it is readily possible to obtain MR images that are oriented in familiar left anterior oblique, right anterior oblique, short-axis, long-axis, and four-chamber views. Although axial, coronal, and sagittal images are useful in determining cardiac structure, the use of oblique views is essential in the evaluation of cardiac function, particularly from the standpoint of correlation with other standard cardiac imaging techniques.

MEASUREMENT OF CARDIAC SIZE

As in other imaging techniques, a variety of simplifying assumptions have been used to assess chamber size using magnetic resonance imaging. These approaches can be grouped into measurements of (1) linear dimension (similar to M-mode echocardiography), (2) area from projections and tomographic sections (as in contrast ventriculography and two-dimensional echocardiography), and (3) direct volume measurement (as in count-based techniques in nuclear medicine and the dynamic spatial constructor.[R1] Results obtained using each approach are reviewed.

Conditions for Accurate Measurement

To make measurements from an MR study, regardless of the approach used, several fundamental requirements must be met. First, the spatial resolution must match the question being addressed. Typically, in-plane resolution in MR images is on the order of 1 to 2 mm. It should be realized, however, that it is possible to obtain different resolutions in different directions in MR images. For example, it is not unusual to obtain cine magnetic resonance images that are acquired with rectangular pixels (e.g., 1.5 by 3.0 mm). This difference in resolution is not necessarily obvious but must be considered in measurements made using magnetic resonance imaging.

Second, the distortion of the images must be small. As described in more detail in Chapter 42, MR uses the local magnetic field to define position in the object; therefore, anything that distorts the magnetic field will distort the image.[Z1] This distortion occurs in the area of sternal wires, prosthetic valves, and vascular clips. In general, the distortion is minimal, but it should be recognized as present. In addition, the effect is more severe for gradient reversal than for spin echo sequences.

Third, the edges for measurement must be well defined. This requires a high contrast-to-noise ratio between the structure of interest and the background. As noted, one of the strengths of MR is its ability to obtain high soft tissue contrast. However, this flexibility also implies that it is possible to have very little soft tissue contrast if the pulse sequence is incorrect.

Last, minimal partial volume effects should be present. Partial volume effects occur because each picture element in an image reflects the average composition of the volume of tissue from which the signal is acquired. If a structure is imaged using large volume elements (i.e., low resolution), then the edges of the structure are blurred because of the averaging of the change in signal intensity across the edge. If the same structure is imaged using small volume elements (i.e., high resolution), then the edge will be less blurred. Unfortunately, in magnetic resonance imaging the signal becomes weaker as the volume elements become smaller, setting a practical limit on the minimum size of volume elements. Typically, MRI of the heart is performed using 5- to 10-mm-thick slices. Given the in-plane resolution described earlier, this means that the typical volume element is approximately 1.7 × 1.7 × 5 to 10 mm. It is clear that the largest dimension of the volume element is defined by the slice thickness, so maximum blurring of the image also occurs in this direction. If the edge is perpendicular to the slice, then the edge will be sharp; however, if the edge is parallel to the slice, then blurring will be prominent. Thus, to minimize partial volume effects, it is important not only to use small volume elements but also to orient them correctly with respect to the structures of interest.

The significance of partial volume effects on the measurement of ventricular volume and mass has been examined.[H1, H2, M2] Both slice thickness and orientation of the slice relative to the structure of interest are important. At present, volume elements on the order of 2 × 2 × 10 mm are believed to be adequate in the evaluation of most adults, whereas thinner slices and smaller volume elements may be necessary in children. The orientation required to minimize partial volume effects depends upon the structure being examined and is discussed in further detail later.

Linear Measurements

In spite of their known limitations,[S1, J1] the use of single linear measurements to describe the size of cardiac chambers is well established in all cardiac imaging techniques. Because of their simplicity and clinical utility, linear measures also have been widely used in magnetic resonance imaging. Reports have shown good correlation with ventriculography[L2] and with echocardiographic measures as long as comparable views are used.[B3, F4, K1] Using MR images obtained in standard two-dimensional echo planes, Kaul and colleagues demonstrated excellent correlations between the two techniques.[K1] Normal values for magnetic resonance imaging linear dimensions for standard two-dimensional echocardiographic positions are reproduced in Table 44–1.[K1] The agreement between echocardiography and magnetic resonance imaging in the evaluation of aortic root size is shown in Figure 44–6.

Area Measurements

Use of area measurements as the basis for estimates of ventricular volumes is also well established in contrast ventriculography and radionuclide ventriculography.[S2] In magnetic resonance imaging, a number of investigators have attempted to use area measurements to assess chamber size and function. Dilworth and associates found that a single transverse plane MR technique

Table 44–1. NORMAL VALUES FOR LEFT VENTRICULAR DIMENSIONS BY MAGNETIC RESONANCE IMAGING

Dimension: Location	Diastole	Systole
Left ventricular cavity diameter (mm):		
Chordal level	46.4 ± 5.5	33.6 ± 3.8
Papillary muscle level	43.4 ± 4.4	29.9 ± 4.8
Septum thickness (mm):		
Chordal level	10.3 ± 0.5	15.5 ± 1.4
Papillary muscle level	10.4 ± 1.8	15.6 ± 2.5
Posterior wall thickness (mm):		
Chordal level	10.2 ± 0.5	15.7 ± 1.0
Papillary muscle level	10.3 ± 1.2	15.4 ± 1.4
Left atrial diameter (mm):		
Anteroposterior	25.6 ± 4.2	

Note: Left ventricular measurements were made at midpapillary muscle level and midway between the aortic valve and papillary muscle (chordal level). Measurements of the same structure from different planes are consolidated in this table. N = 16.

Adapted from Kaul, S., et al.: Measurement of normal left heart dimensions using optimally oriented MR images. AJR 146(1):75, 1986, © by The American Roentgen Ray Society.)

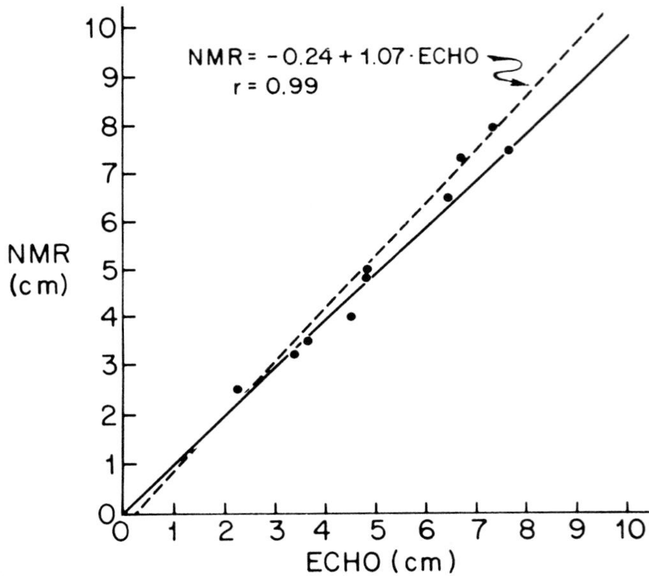

Figure 44–6. Agreement of nuclear magnetic resonance (NMR) imaging and echocardiography in the measurement of aortic root size. (From Schaefer, S., et al.: Nuclear magnetic resonance imaging in Marfan's syndrome. J. Am. Coll. Cardiol. 9:70, 1987. Reprinted with permission from the American College of Cardiology.)

significantly underestimated left ventricular end-diastolic volume and ejection fraction.[D2] Lanzer and associates examined a number of approaches and found that areas measured from MR images obtained in standard right anterior oblique (RAO) ventriculogram orientation yielded good correlation with angiographic volumes.[L3] Van Rossum and colleagues found only a moderate correlation (r = 0.65) between area-length calculations of ejection fraction by magnetic resonance imaging and area-length calculations by single plane angiography.[V1] This was attributed to several factors. First, they had difficulty in defining endocardial borders owing to the presence of intracavitary signal, particularly with shorter echo times. Second, motion of the heart with respect to the fixed tomographic plane used in magnetic resonance imaging contributed to the error, in that systolic and diastolic images were not necessarily obtained through the same portion of the heart. Third, they suggested that the difference could be related to the intrinsic differences between left ventriculography, a projection technique, and MRI, a tomographic technique. In a projection, the largest contour of an object will be displayed, whereas in a tomographic slice only the contour in that slice is available. Hence, if the tomographic slice does not contain the largest contour due to an error in positioning, then the calculated ejection fraction will be in error.

In a preliminary report, Cranney and colleagues have demonstrated that if cine MR images are obtained in standard biplane views (RAO and orthogonal), one can use these data in the Sandler-Dodge equation.[C2] When data are obtained in this way, one obtains good correlation with contrast ventriculography.

Volume Measurement

Magnetic resonance imaging allows the direct measurement of chamber volume through the use of multislice or direct volume acquisition. Using a classic cast technique, and what has been termed the Simpson's rule technique, Rehr and associates showed an excellent correlation between magnetic resonance imaging and cast volume by displacement.[R2] Subsequently, the multislice, Simpson's rule approach has been validated in both animals and humans. Examples of the correlations obtained in the left ventricle are shown in Figure 44–7. A multislice, cine MR technique has been used to measure right and left ventricular outputs for the determination of regurgitant fraction[S3] and shunt size.[S4]

Use of the multislice, Simpson's rule technique is attractive

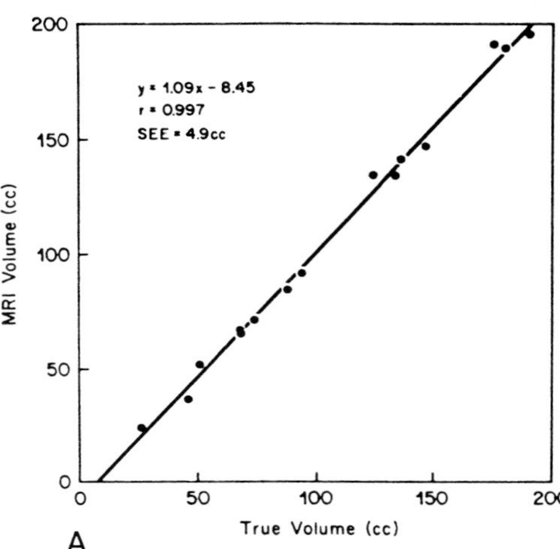

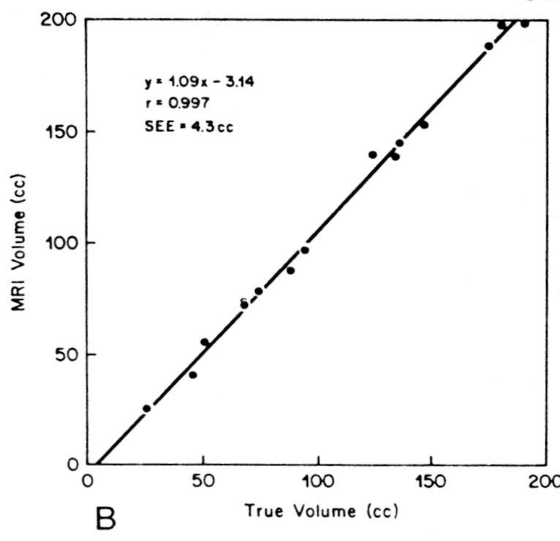

Figure 44–7. Determination of left ventricular volume. There is excellent agreement between calculated volume and actual displacement volume for ventricular casts for both (*A*) low-resolution (1.7 × 1.7 × 10 mm) and (*B*) high-resolution (0.8 × 0.8 × 10 mm) studies. (From Rehr, R. B., et al.: Left ventricular volumes measured by MR imaging. Radiology 156:717, 1985, with permission.)

because it minimizes the geometric assumptions made. However, there are difficulties. First, problems in defining the base of the heart may lead to large errors in volume calculations in Simpson's technique because of the large area at the base of the left ventricle.[C2] Second, these studies presently require long periods for data acquisition, typically about 30 minutes on present MR imaging devices, plus long periods for analysis. These two factors have limited the clinical impact of these approaches. The eventual clinical role of direct volume measurements likely will depend on the degree to which the acquisition time can be reduced and the analysis process automated.

An important issue in the acquisition of complete three-dimensional datasets is the best slice thickness and orientation of the slices.[H1, H2, M2] As mentioned in the discussion of conditions for accurate measurement, volume elements with dimensions of approximately 2 × 2 × 10 mm have been used in most of the studies of ventricular volume and mass. Thinner slices will improve the accuracy of the measurement but at the expense of decreased signal-to-noise or increased acquisition times. Hoffman and Ritman have shown for computed tomography that an acceptable alternative is the use of overlapping thick slices at closer intervals.[H1] This approach in MR can improve the measurement without a decrease in signal-to-noise, but still requires increased acquisition time.

In summary, present data suggest that area measurements can be used to determine reliably left ventricular volumes and ejection fraction if care is taken to ensure that the tomographic plane obtained with MR is comparable to the projection obtained with cine angiography. In a sense this is similar to the problem of errors in echocardiographic measures of volume caused by not including the apex in the tomographic plane. Correspondingly, MR methods that sample the entire volume and use Simpson's rule are highly accurate if care is taken to minimize partial volume effects involving the base.

Wall Thickness and Myocardial Mass

Clearly, if magnetic resonance imaging can be used to measure cardiac volumes, it can be used to estimate myocardial mass. This is done by determining the myocardial wall volume and multiplying by the density of the myocardium. As in the case of determining chamber volume, simplifying assumptions regarding the cardiac geometry can be made to allow estimates from single linear dimensions or area measurements. In echocardiography, simple linear measurements of wall thickness have been used frequently for the estimation of mass, but clearly this fails in cases of deformed ventricles. A variety of other methods have been proposed to deal with these limitations.[W1] In magnetic resonance imaging, it is possible to utilize these same formulas as long as the required measurements are obtained in comparable tomographic planes.

Magnetic resonance imaging can be used to obtain complete three-dimensional datasets spanning the heart without the restrictions of acoustic windows. This makes it particularly useful in making estimates of mass that require more complete measurements of the heart, such as Simpson's rule. Using multiple tomographic slices obtained in the fixed reference frame, it is straightforward to determine myocardial mass. This approach has been verified in animal models and in humans.

Initial validation studies were carried out in animals using both transaxial[C3, F5] and short-axis[K2] imaging planes. Florentine and associates demonstrated an excellent correlation with actual postmortem mass (r = 0.95, standard error of the estimate [SEE] = 13.1 g), using 10-mm-thick transaxial slices.[F5] In addition, intraobserver and interobserver reproducibility were impressive (r = 0.99). Caputo and colleagues obtained a similar correlation and standard error of the estimate for hand-drawn borders. However, automated determination of the borders was somewhat less successful.[C3]

Keller and co-workers used short-axis, end-diastolic images and obtained an additional improvement in the estimation of mass (r = 0.98, SEE = 6.1).[K2] Magnetic resonance imaging slightly overestimated left ventricular mass, which was attributed to partial volume effects and difficulties in proper border definition owing to signal from slowly moving blood in the ventricular cavity.

In extensive studies, Maddahi and co-workers examined the effects of slice orientation and corrections for partial volume effects on determination of myocardial mass, using Simpson's rule, in the dog model.[M2] These studies indicated that in vivo estimates of left ventricular myocardial mass are most accurate when the images are obtained in the short-axis plane of the heart. Correction for partial volume effects at the apex when using the short-axis plane for imaging led to only a small improvement in the correlation coefficient and standard error of the estimate (uncorrected: r = 0.989, SEE = 4.93 versus corrected: r = 0.996, SEE = 3.14). Images obtained in the transaxial and vertical long-axis planes were associated with larger errors regardless of the method used to correct for partial volume effects. Hence, the optimal approach on the basis of animal studies appears to utilize short-axis images.

This approach has been used in the measurement of hearts with infarction[S5] (Fig. 44–8). Gated magnetic resonance imaging was performed in dogs before and after infarction. There was excellent correlation between actual mass and mass after infarction estimated from end-diastolic images (r = 0.94, SEE = 8.7 g) and end-systolic images (r = 0.97, SEE = 6.6 g). It is interesting that in these studies there was also a good correlation (r = 0.95, SEE = 6.5 g) when a standard multislice rather than a multislice, multiphase acquisition was used in the calculation (as noted earlier, in a standard multislice acquisition, the slices are obtained at different points in the cardiac cycle). The investigators suggest that this unexpected finding may be related to the minimal base-to-apex motion in the dog as compared to the human.

Human studies also have demonstrated an excellent correla-

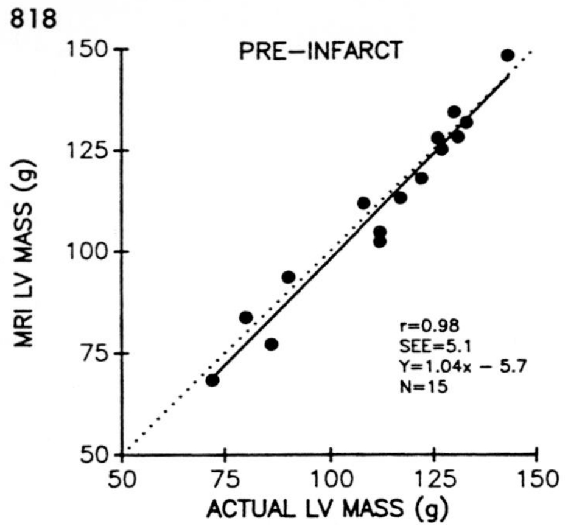

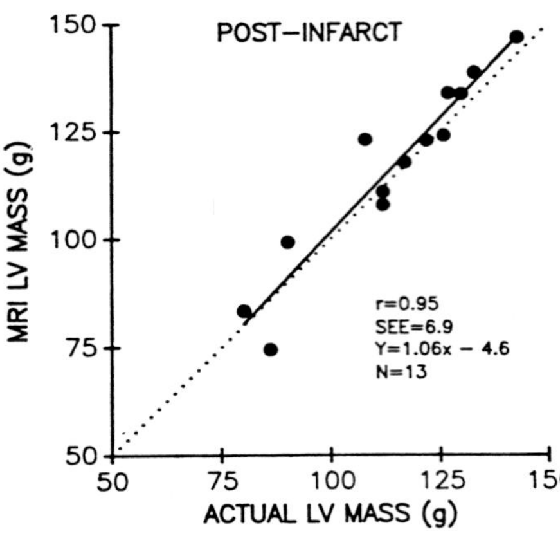

Figure 44–8. Myocardial mass before and after infarction. There is good agreement between magnetic resonance imaging estimates of left ventricular (LV) mass and actual left ventricular mass, even in the setting of infarction. (From Shapiro, E. P., et al.: Determination of left ventricular mass by magnetic resonance imaging in hearts deformed by acute infarction. Circulation 79:706, 1989, by permission of the American Heart Association, Inc.)

tion. Katz and colleagues performed imaging of cadaver hearts and examined intraobserver and interobserver variability in volunteers (Fig. 44–9).[K3] The cadaver studies were used to establish a linear regression equation for human hearts: True left ventricular weight (grams) = 7.14 + 0.91 × MR mass estimate (in grams). The correlation coefficient was 0.99 with a standard error of the estimate of 6.8 grams. Given a representative MR mass estimate of 200 grams, this yields a predicted left ventricular weight of 189 grams, with 95 percent confidence limits of 174.8 to 205.5 grams. Using ten short-axis slices through the heart obtained at end-diastole, the intraobserver variability (r = 0.96, SEE = 11.1 g) and the interobserver variability (r = 0.91, SEE = 17.8 g) were excellent.[K3] Moreover, the reproducibility of the methods on two separate imaging sessions was very good. Subsequent studies have demonstrated good correlation between estimates of myocardial mass in humans and classic autopsy studies that relate heart mass to body weight[O1] (Fig. 44–10). This study also demonstrated excellent interobserver variability. Sub-

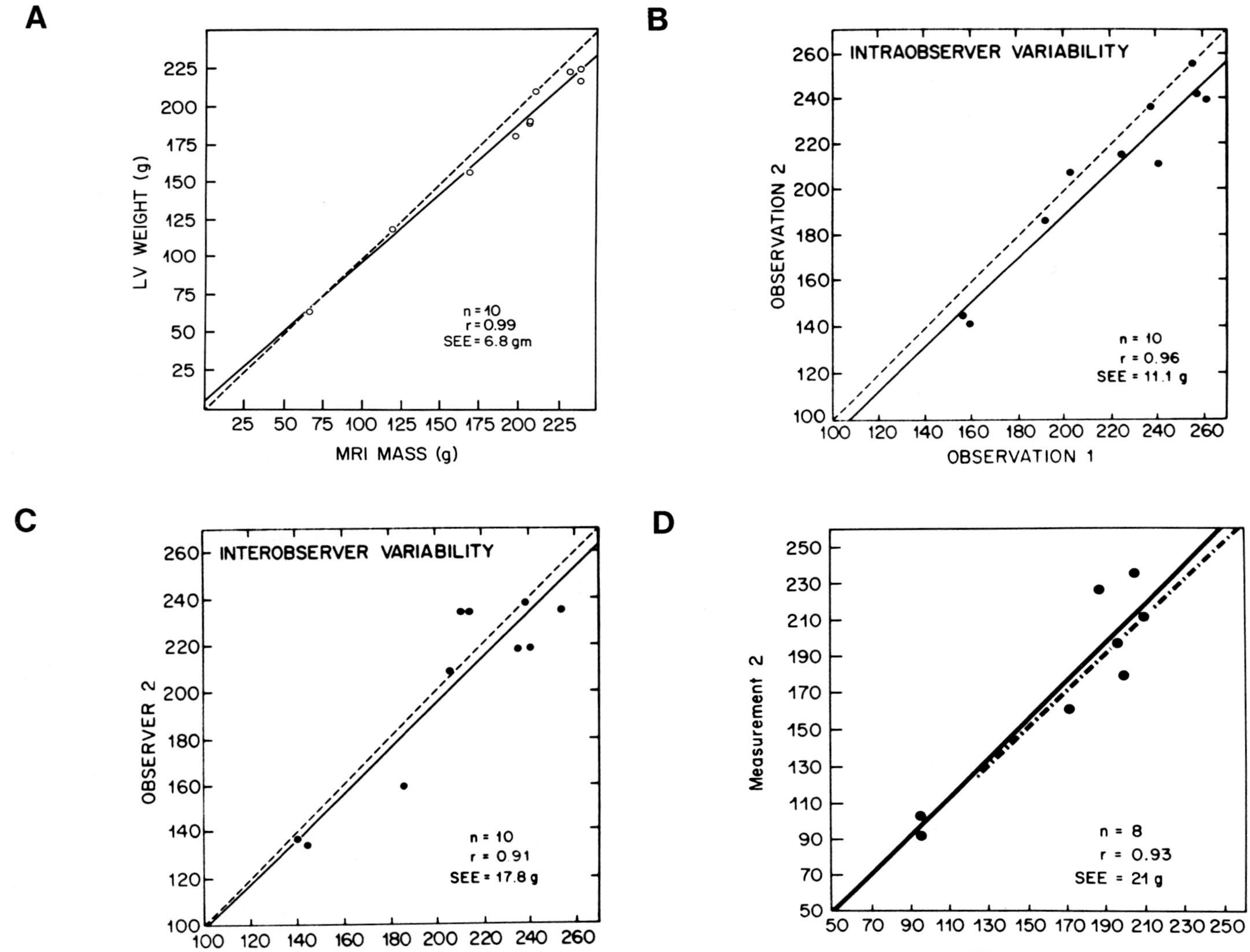

Figure 44–9. Left ventricular (LV) mass in a man. *A*, Shows excellent correlation between the mass as estimated by magnetic resonance imaging and the true left ventricular weight. *B*, *C*, and *D*, The intraobserver, interobserver, and successive measurement differences are small. (From Katz, J., et al.: Estimation of myocardial mass in man using magnetic resonance imaging. Radiology 169:495, 1988, with permission.)

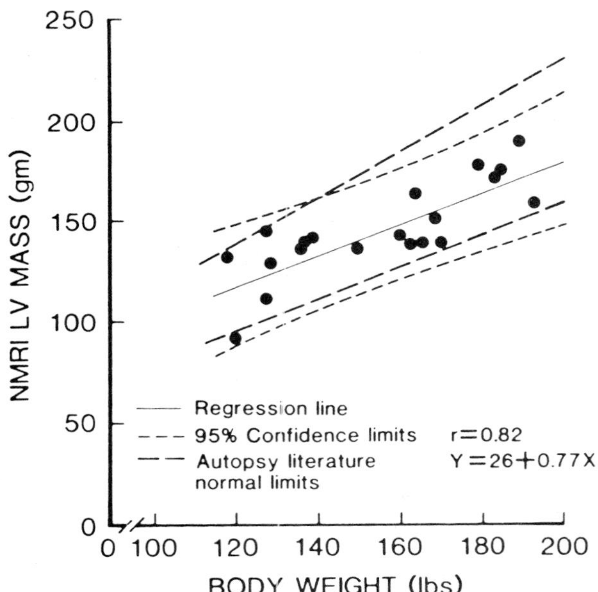

Figure 44–10. Magnetic resonance imaging estimation of left ventricular (LV) mass versus body weight. Estimates of left ventricular mass show good agreement with prior autopsy studies. (From Ostrzega, E., et al.: Quantification of left ventricular myocardial mass in humans using nuclear magnetic resonance imaging. Am. Heart J. 117:444, 1989, with permission.)

sequently, magnetic resonance imaging has been utilized in the estimation of mass in clinical studies.[M3, R3]

All the aforementioned studies have utilized spin echo sequences. Preliminary work suggests that comparable accuracy can be obtained using gradient reversal, cine magnetic resonance imaging sequences.[O2] In addition, presaturating pulses that have been described reduce signal from intracavitary blood[F6] and may remove one potential source of error.

In summary, magnetic resonance imaging using short-axis images and a Simpson's rule approach allows a very accurate and reproducible estimation of myocardial mass in both animal models and humans.

ASSESSMENT OF CARDIAC FUNCTION

Global Function

More than any other aspect of clinical medicine, clinical cardiology depends on the assessment of function. In particular, the left ventricular ejection fraction has become a major determinant in management. A variety of approaches have utilized MR in the calculation of ejection fraction.

Ejection Fraction. A number of groups have demonstrated methods for the calculation of ejection fraction by magnetic resonance imaging. A single-plane approach using an area-length method showed excellent correlation (r = 0.88 to 0.95) with contrast ventriculography.[S6, U1] As has been pointed out by Van Rossum and associates,[V1] contrast ventriculography is a projection technique whereas MR is typically tomographic. Hence, if the motion of the heart carries it out of the tomographic plane, then the ejection fraction will be incorrect. If a projection or thick-slice MR technique is used, then the errors will be similar to those obtained using projection contrast ventriculography.

The most general approach involves the use of multiple tomographic or a three-dimensional dataset. At present, the acquisition of such datasets is lengthy, and the analysis is laborious. However, excellent results have been reported (Fig. 44–11).[C4, S7] The widespread clinical application of these methods will likely require reducing the study time and automating the analysis of the images.

Cardiac Output. Given the ability to determine cardiac volume, it is straightforward to determine stroke volume and cardiac

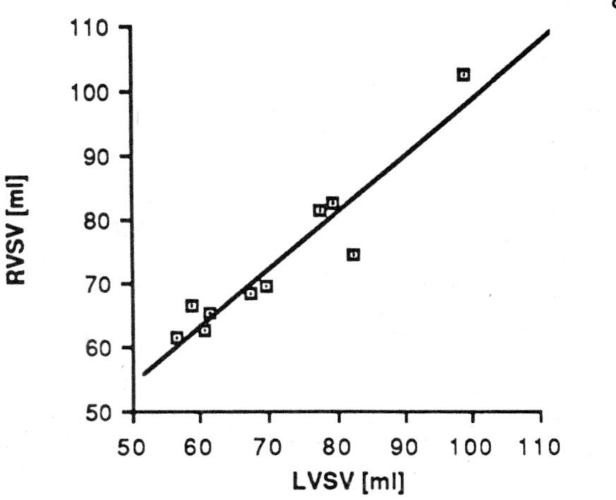

Figure 44–11. Correlation between left (LVSV) and right ventricular stroke volume (RVSV). There is good agreement between right and left ventricular stroke volumes over a wide range in the absence of shunting. (From Sechtem, U., et al.: Measurement of right and left ventricular volumes in healthy individuals with cine MR imaging. Radiology 163:697, 1987, with permission.)

output. Culham and Vince calculated end-diastolic and end-systolic left and right ventricular volumes, using magnetic resonance imaging with a Simpson's rule technique.[C4] Thermodilution cardiac output was determined before and after MR imaging. Results are shown in Figure 44–12.[C4] Although the number of measurements is small, MR appears to provide accurate measures of both right and left ventricular cardiac output, as compared with thermodilution.

Segmental Function

Segmental wall motion is readily evaluated by magnetic resonance imaging, using both multislice, multiphase, and cine MRI.

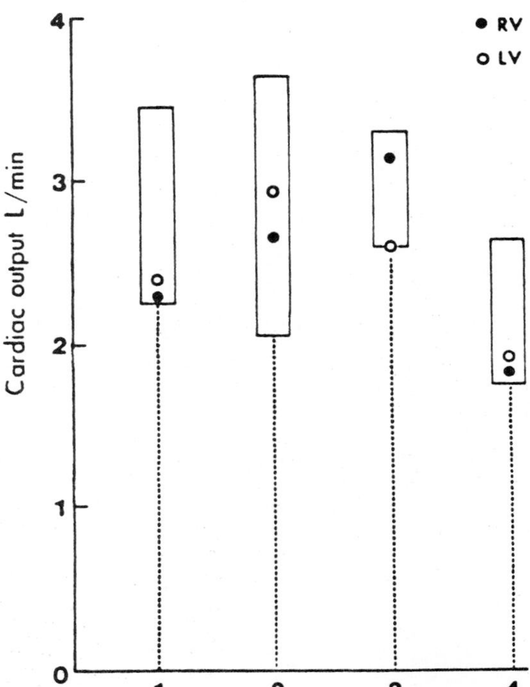

Figure 44–12. Determination of cardiac output. There is good agreement between estimates of right ventricular (RV) and left ventricular (LV) output, by thermodilution, and cardiac output determined by magnetic resonance imaging. (From Culham, J. A. G., and Vince, D. J.: Cardiac output by MR imaging: An experimental study comparing right ventricle and left ventricle with thermodilution. J. Can. Assoc. Radiol. 39:247, 1988, with permission.)

Wall Motion. Again, using analyses similar to those employed in echocardiography, it is possible to determine wall motion. An important fact is that MR allows one to follow the motion of segments in the fixed reference frame and without the limitations of the acoustic window. One can then perform translations and rotations similar to those used in echocardiography in interpreting the motion of the segments.[L4] Clearly, these tomographic approaches have the same limitations as echocardiography or cine computed tomography in that segments move in all three dimensions during contraction, and, hence, move out of the imaging plane. This effect has been shown to account for some of the heterogeneity of wall motion and thickening seen in echocardiography.[L4]

However, these approaches are fundamentally limited, in that one assumes that a segment can be determined uniquely from frame to frame to track its motion. In other words, one cannot prove that the same segment is being examined in two different frames. The classic approach to this problem has been to attach markers, such clips or beads, to the epicardium.[M4] This, of course, requires surgery and hence has limited applicability in patients.

MYOCARDIAL TAGGING. Recently, it has become possible "magnetically" to tag regions of the myocardium noninvasively using MR, thus allowing one to follow the actual trajectory of a region of the myocardium.[Z2] Briefly, this method utilizes an additional pulse to saturate or reduce the signal from the region of interest. This region then can be followed through the contraction. An example of this approach is seen in Figure 44–13. This method allows one to noninvasively determine absolute cardiac wall motion in the fixed reference frame. Additional variations in this approach allow "tagging" of multiple small regions.[A1] This method likely will become the reference standard for assessments of wall motion.

WALL THICKENING. Assessments of wall thickening are also possible using MR. Using multislice, multiphase techniques, Fisher and colleagues examined wall thickening in transverse images and found significant heterogeneity.[F7] With images obtained in the short-axis view, good correspondence was found between the MR assessment of abnormal thickening and contrast ventriculography in the identification of abnormal segments[P3] (Fig. 44–14). Studies using cine MR also allow determination of wall thickening.[H3] Subsequent studies have shown that cine MR obtains measurements of wall thickening comparable with those obtained using echocardiography.[R4]

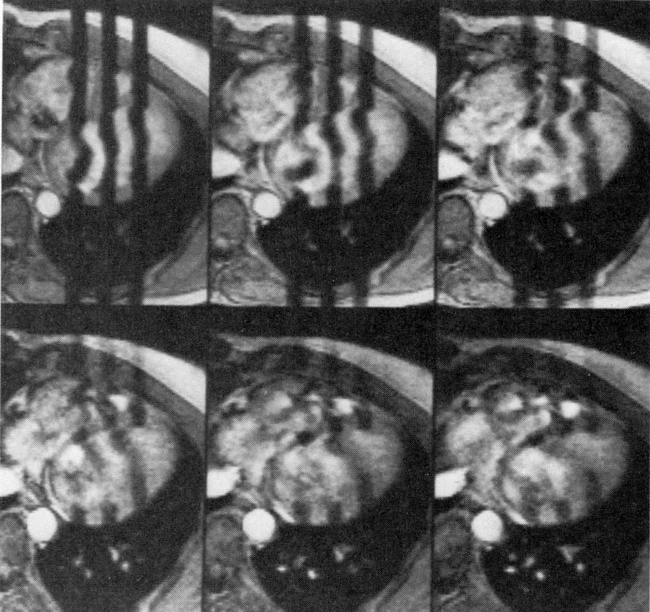

Figure 44–13. Myocardial tagging. Frames from a cine-MRI sequence in which saturating pulses have been applied along three lines, making the tissue dark. With cardiac motion, the dark tagging is seen to be carried with the heart, allowing the unambiguous determination of the exact motion of these segments.

TISSUE CHARACTERIZATION

Relaxation Times

Although the preceding discussion has concentrated on the assessment of structure, one of the great strengths of MR is its soft tissue contrast. As discussed in Chapter 40, soft tissue contrast in MR depends on intrinsic properties of the tissue, such as the proton density and tissue relaxation times T1 and T2, and the pulsing conditions (i.e., the pulse sequence, TR, TE, flip angle) used to acquire the images. In the setting of infarction and other pathologic processes, changes are seen in the tissue relaxation times and other determinants of image intensity.[P4] (This is discussed in more detail in Chapter 50. These changes form the basis for the determination of the extent of infarction.

Methods for Measurement

Estimates of tissue relaxation times can be made from images obtained under different imaging conditions and a mathematical model for the imaging sequence.[O3] A typical mathematical model that is used is shown below for a single echo, spin echo sequence using a 90-degree excitation pulse:

$$I = N_H f(v)[1-e^{-TR/T1}]e^{-TE/T2} \quad (1)$$

where
I = Signal intensity
N_H = Proton density
$f(v)$ = Flow function
T1 = Longitudinal relaxation time
T2 = Transverse relaxation time
TR = Repetition time
TE = Time to echo.

It is essential to realize that use of any such mathematical model requires that certain assumptions be made. These assumptions must then be empirically tested, i.e., do the relaxation times determined by the formula allow the prediction of image intensity under different pulsing conditions? If this is true, then the model, the formula, and the image-derived relaxation times are consistent and predictive.

As can be seen from the formula, the T2 relaxation leads to an exponential loss of signal intensity over time. Hence, measurements of signal intensity at different echo times allow the determination of the T2 relaxation time. This value is classically determined by measuring the intensity at many different echo times using the Carr-Purcell-Meiboom-Gill technique.[F8] Estimates of T2 relaxation time have been used extensively in the evaluation of cardiac disease and require obtaining images with at least two different echo times. Using these data, one can calculate a map of the estimated T2 values of the tissue. Normal human T2 values have been reported by a number of investigators and range from 30 to 45 msec.[L5] Infarcted myocardium analyzed in a similar fashion yields values frequently in the range of greater than 50 msec.[W2]

The use of T2 estimates is attractive in cardiac magnetic resonance imaging because one gated, double-spin echo sequence can be used to obtain the necessary data for the calculation. Problems in the measurement of T2 in cardiac images relate to the limited number of points used to define the exponential decay and motion of the heart between the two echoes.

The estimation of T1 typically requires measurement of signal intensity using sequences with different TR times. This approach has been used to detect and follow infarction in both animals and humans[M5, P5] but requires additional sequences and has been more involved than estimations of T2. Typical normal T1 values in animals have been reported in the range of 550 to 700 at 0.35 to 0.5 Tesla.[A2]

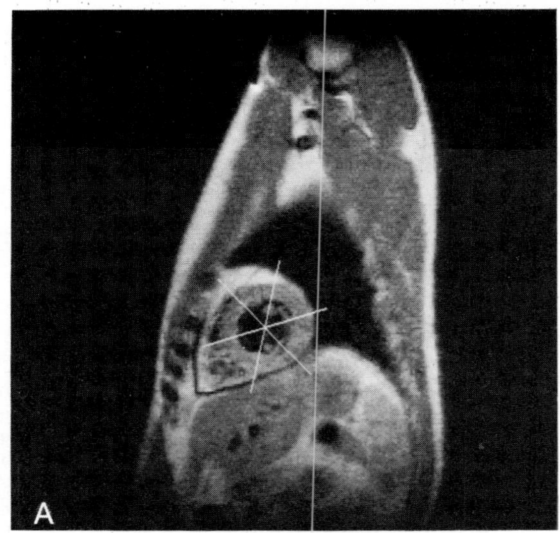

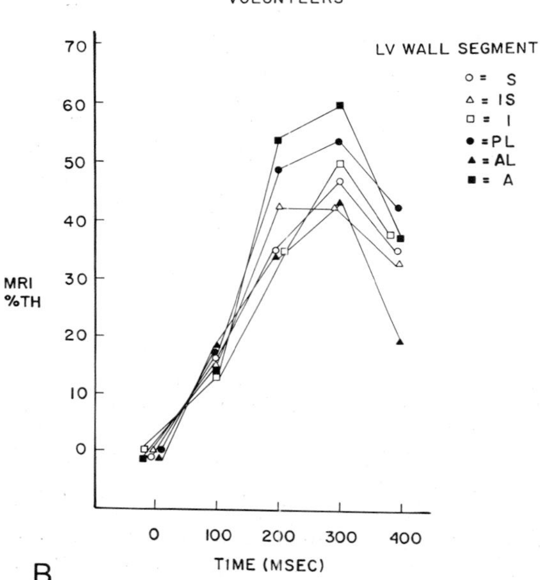

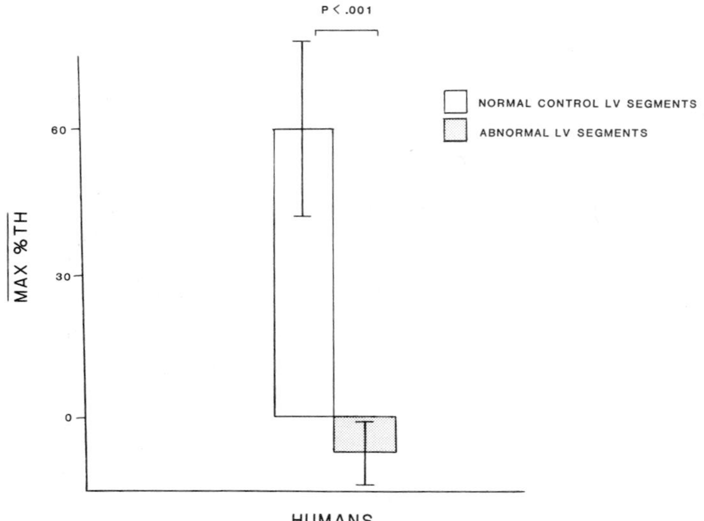

Figure 44–14. Regional left ventricular wall motion. *A*, Short-axis image at the papillary muscle level. Overlying lines define segments for analysis of thickening. *B*, Percent wall thickening for different myocardial segments (S—septal, IS—inferoseptal, I—inferior, PL—posterolateral, AL—anterolateral, and A—anterior). *C*, Maximal percent thickening in a set for normal volunteers and in patients with infarction. (From Peshock, R. M., et al.: Assessment of myocardial systolic wall thickening by nuclear magnetic resonance imaging. J. Am. Coll. Cardiol., 14:653, 1989. Reprinted with permission from the American College of Cardiology.)

Limitations

A discussion of the potential errors in the estimate of relaxation times from images is beyond the scope of this chapter; however, a wide variety of sources of errors have been well described.[B4] *It is important to realize that these estimates are based on the intensity in the image.* If flow artifacts or partial volume effects contribute to the signal in a region, then the estimated T2 or T1 values will be wrong. In addition, the increase in T2 or T1 is a nonspecific response and has been reported in the setting of rejection[L5] and in myocarditis.

Measurement of Infarct Size

Both intensity differences[B5] and tissue relaxation time maps[C5] have been used to estimate infarct size. In excised hearts studied at 6 hours after infarction, Rokey and associates found an excellent correlation (r = 0.98) between infarct size, as determined by magnetic resonance imaging, and anatomic infarct size as determined using triphenyl-tetrazolium-chloride staining (Fig. 44–15).[R5] In an in vivo animal model imaged at 1 week after infarction (Fig. 44–16), there was good agreement (r = 0.88) between infarct mass and percentage of left ventricular mass infarcted (r = 0.97), as determined by pathology and in vivo magnetic resonance imaging.[B6] However, for both measures, MRI tended to overestimate the size of the infarction. In this same study, using multiple regression analysis, there was a better correlation

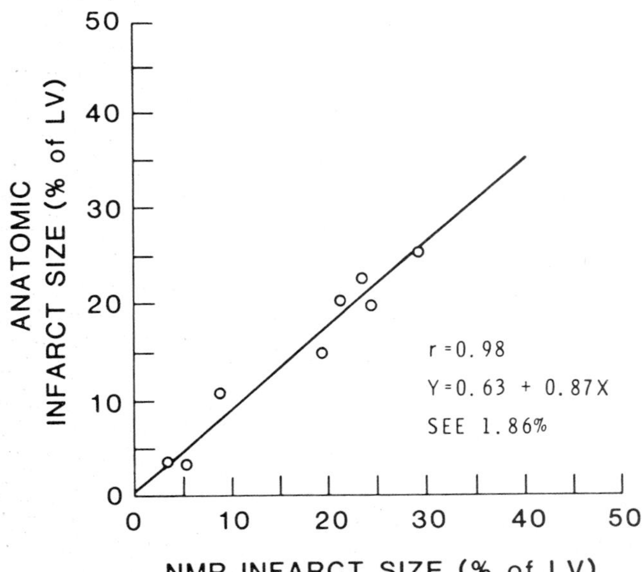

Figure 44–15. Estimation of infarct size in excised hearts. A good correlation of infarct size is seen upon magnetic resonance imaging and triphenyl-tetrazolium-chloride staining. LV—left ventricle. (From Rokey, R., et al.: Myocardial infarct size quantitation after coronary artery occlusion in dogs. Radiology 158:771, 1986, with permission.)

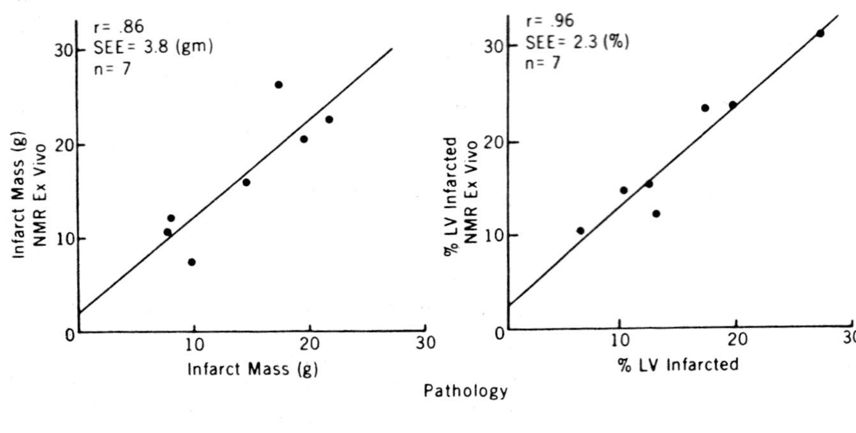

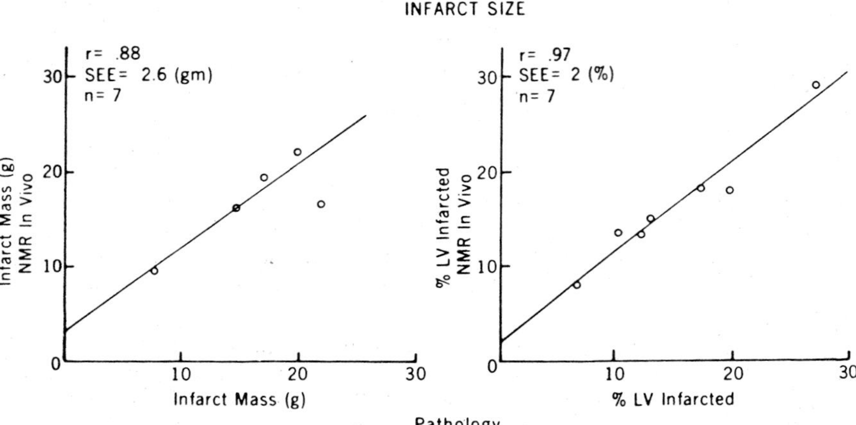

Figure 44–16. Estimation of infarct size in vivo. There is good agreement between magnetic resonance imaging and pathology for both infarct mass and percent left ventricle (LV) infarcted. However, infarct size is overestimated. (From Bouchard, A., et al.: Assessment of myocardial infarct size by means of T2-weighted 1H nuclear magnetic resonance imaging. Am. Heart J. 117:281, 1989, with permission.)

between in vivo MR imaging and microsphere-determined hypoperfused myocardium than with pathology-determined infarct size. This overestimation of the region of injury also appears to be present early in the course of infarction[S8] (Fig. 44–17).

FLOW QUANTITATION

Another critical element of cardiac evaluation relates to the determination of flow, on both a macroscopic and a microscopic level. In this respect, MR offers significant potential because of its fundamental sensitivity to motion. The details of flow and motion effects in MR images are discussed in Chapter 41. From the standpoint of quantitation, both phase shift and time of flight effects can be used. However, as in Doppler ultrasound techniques, only a certain range of velocities can be examined using a given technique. Given the wide range of velocities in the cardiovascular system (Table 44–2), it is not surprising that a variety of methods have been described to evaluate flow. It is also important to note that this is an area of intense investigation at the present time. Hence, the following discussion will concentrate on general approaches and results with the knowledge that the detailed methods are likely to change rapidly over the next few years.

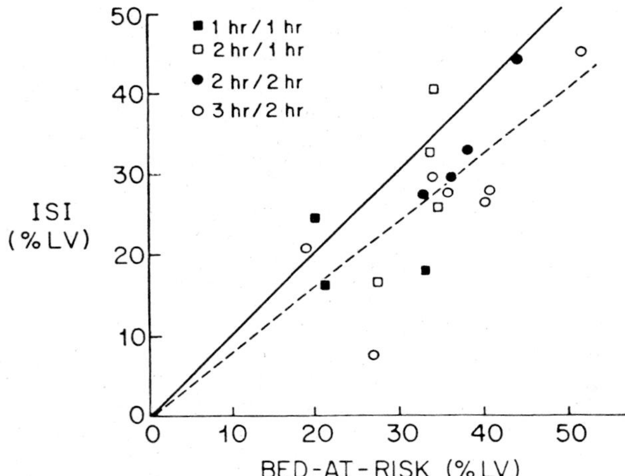

Figure 44–17. Measurement of bed-at-risk. Using Gd-DTPA, there is a good correlation between the volume of tissue with increased signal and the ischemic bed-at-risk as determined by double dye perfusion. LV—left ventricle, ISI—increased signal intensity. (From Schaefer, S., et al. In-vivo identification of reperfused myocardium with nuclear magnetic resonance: Gadolinium-DTPA as a marker of the bed-at-risk. J. Am. Coll. Cardiol. 12:1063, 1988. Reprinted with permission of the American College of Cardiology.)

Shunt Calculations

As described, it is possible to use Simpson's rule techniques to determine left and right ventricular volumes at end-diastole and end-systole. Stroke volume is then calculated and multiplied by heart rate to determine cardiac output. Differences between left and right ventricular stroke volume have been used to do shunt calculations.[S4]

Table 44–2. TYPICAL VELOCITIES IN THE ARTERIAL SYSTEM

Vessel	Diameter *(cm)*	Velocity *(cm/sec)*
Ascending aorta	2.30–4.35	21.3–87.4 (mean systolic)
Main pulmonary artery	2.32–3.50	33.1–63.5 (mean systolic)
Thoracic inferior vena cava	2.0	10.7–16.0 (mean)
Small arteriole	0.01	1.0 (mean)
Capillary	0.0005	0.02–0.17

From Milnor, W. M.: Hemodynamics. Williams and Wilkins, Baltimore, 1989.

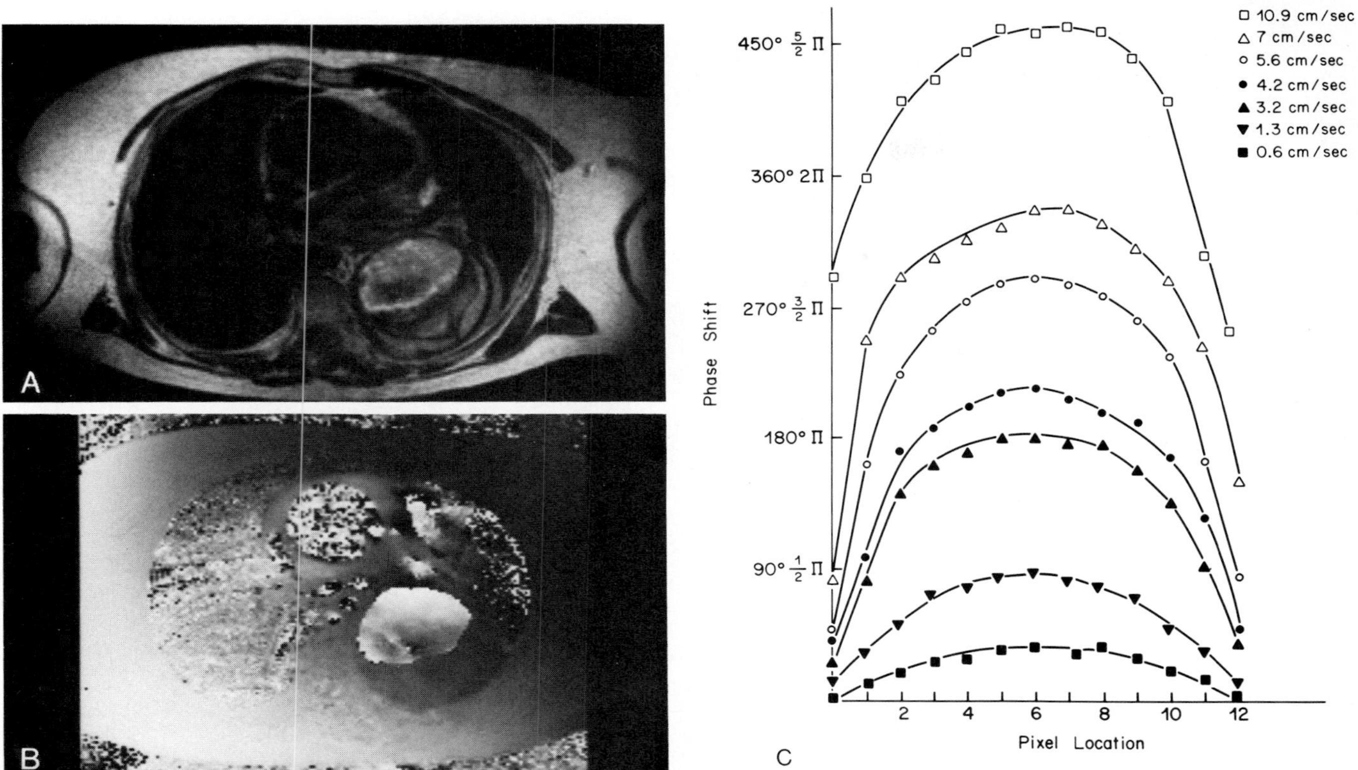

Figure 44–18. Velocity-induced phase shifts. *A*, Magnitude reconstruction of an image. Increased signal intensity in the descending aorta from slowly moving blood can be seen. *B*, Phase reconstruction of the same image, demonstrating a phase shift of moving blood relative to stationary tissue. *C*, Phase shifts demonstrating their use to examine the velocity profile across a tube at different mean velocities.

Flow Velocity

Phase shift and time-of-flight effects can be used to calculate velocity and flow in a variety of ways. Phase shifts have been used extensively to measure flow velocity (Fig. 44–18). Compared with Doppler techniques, MR phase shift methods allow calculation of the velocity across the entire cross-section of a vessel. Flow velocities have been used to estimate cardiac output in the ascending aorta.[F9] It is interesting that phase shifts associated with cardiac wall motion have been used to calculate the direction and magnitude of the velocity of cardiac wall motion.[B7, K4, V2]

Valvular Regurgitation

Another area of recent interest has been in the quantitation of valvular regurgitation (Fig. 44–19) on the basis of turbulence on cine magnetic resonance imaging.[E1, S3] Although correlations with measures of regurgitation by color flow Doppler have been good, it has also been noted that the size of the region of decreased signal intensity is dependent on the voxel size, timing, and other details of the pulse sequence.[H4]

Myocardial Perfusion

A particular area of interest has been the assessment of myocardial perfusion using MR. Two basic methods have been proposed: (1) paramagnetic contrast agents, and (2) diffusion/perfusion imaging. Each has advantages and disadvantages.

Paramagnetic contrast agents are materials that alter the relaxation times of tissue. If such an agent distributes on the basis of blood flow, then it will alter the relaxation times in those areas that are well perfused and not in areas of hypoperfusion. A number of potential perfusion markers for magnetic resonance imaging have been examined.

Gadolinium diethylenetriamine penta-acetic acid (Gd-DTPA) has been examined as a potential agent for the assessment of perfusion but is limited because of its rapid redistribution relative to the time required for standard magnetic resonance imaging.[M6] Miller and co-workers reported using a Gd-DTPA infusion during dipyridamole-induced hyperemia in an animal model of partial coronary occlusion.[M7] In these studies they were able to demonstrate a significant correlation between percent change in signal intensity and microsphere-determined myocardial blood flow.

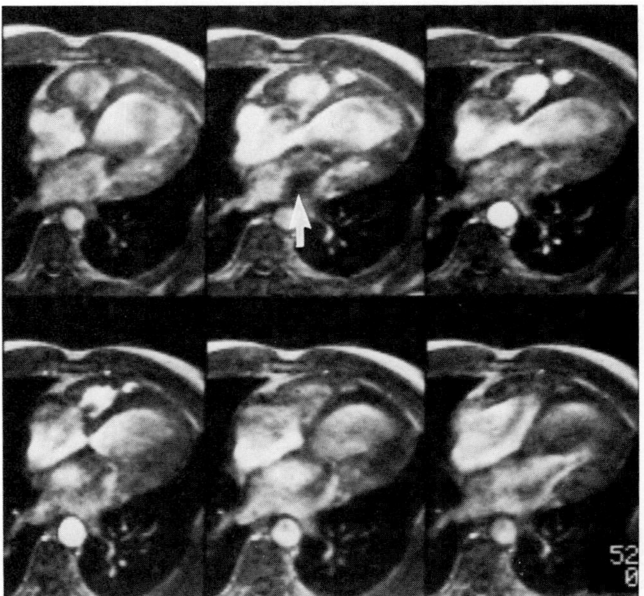

Figure 44–19. Quantitation of regurgitation. Mitral regurgitation in a gradient reversal, cine MRI image demonstrating signal loss in the region of regurgitation (*arrow*).

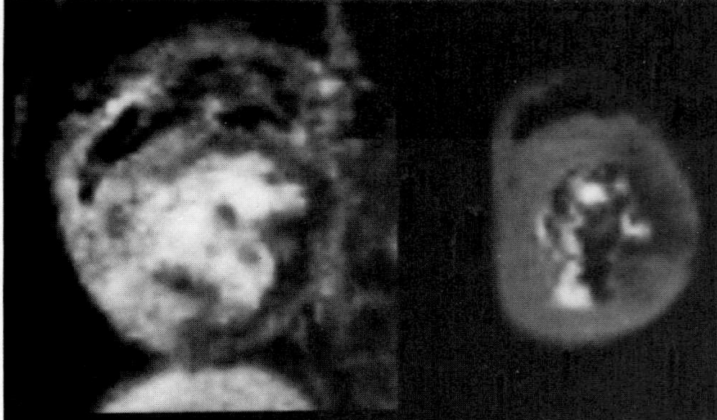

Figure 44–20. Regional hypoperfusion is demonstrated, using a manganese-containing contrast agent. Gradient reversal, cine magnetic resonance imaging in an animal model with coronary occlusion. *Left,* The heart after acute left anterior coronary artery occlusion following administration of a paramagnetic contrast agent. *Right,* The heart after excision. The normal myocardium is seen to increase in intensity, whereas the hypoperfused myocardium remains dark. (From Schaefer, S., et al.: In-vivo nuclear magnetic resonance imaging of myocardial perfusion using the paramagnetic contrast agent manganese gluconate. J. Am. Coll. Cardiol. 14:472, 1989. Reprinted with permission from the American College of Cardiology.)

Manganese compounds have been shown to localize in the heart but present problems with potential toxicity[G3, S9, W3] (Fig. 44–20). Recently, dysprosium compounds have been suggested as potential markers[K5] (Fig. 44–21).

FUTURE DEVELOPMENTS

At present, at least four areas of intense research may have significant impact on the general use of MR in quantitating cardiac size and function.

High-Speed Imaging

The first area is the development of echo planar imaging. This technique (discussed in more detail in Chapter 39) allows the acquisition of images of the heart in a fraction of a second instead of minutes as is now required.[D3, P6, R6] Typical images obtained using this method are shown in Figure 44–22. Echo planar MR allows one to obtain complete three-dimensional datasets in a fraction of the time now presently required. This speed will make analysis of three-dimensional wall motion more clinically acceptable.

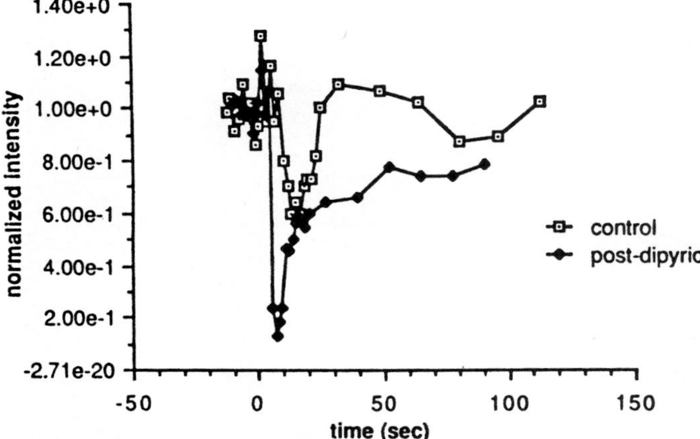

Figure 44–21. Regional hypoperfusion demonstrated, using dysprosium-DTPA. Image intensity over time following the administration of dysprosium-DTPA in the setting of regional hypoperfusion. (From Kantor, H. L., et al.: A new NMR marker of coronary stenosis: The utility of dysprosium-DTPA in high speed cardiac imaging. (Abstract.) Society of Magnetic Resonance in Medicine, San Francisco, 1988, p. 803, with permission.)

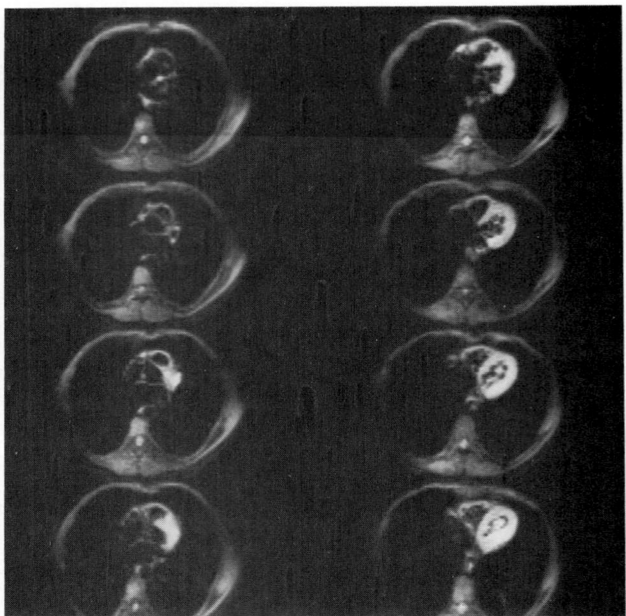

Figure 44–22. Echo-planar magnetic resonance images. A series of images of the heart, with each image obtained in a single heartbeat. (Obtained in collaboration with Drs. Ian Pykett, Richard Rzedzian, Craig Malloy, and James Fleckenstein.)

Automated Analysis

The second area is the further development of methods for the automated analysis of cardiac images. A number of advances are being made in the areas of machine vision and artificial intelligence that may allow the operator independent analysis of cardiac MR images.[S10] These approaches are being applied to the evaluation of tagged myocardial segments.[L6] In addition, methods for the automated determination of myocardial volumes have demonstrated a good correlation with operator-determined borders.[F10]

Three-Dimensional Display

The third area is the development of better methods for the display of the voluminous amounts of data that can be obtained using magnetic resonance imaging. A number of investigators have described three-dimensional displays of cardiac MR data[A3, F11, L7] (Fig. 44–23). With improvements in computer hardware and software, these methods eventually may have substantial clinical impact.

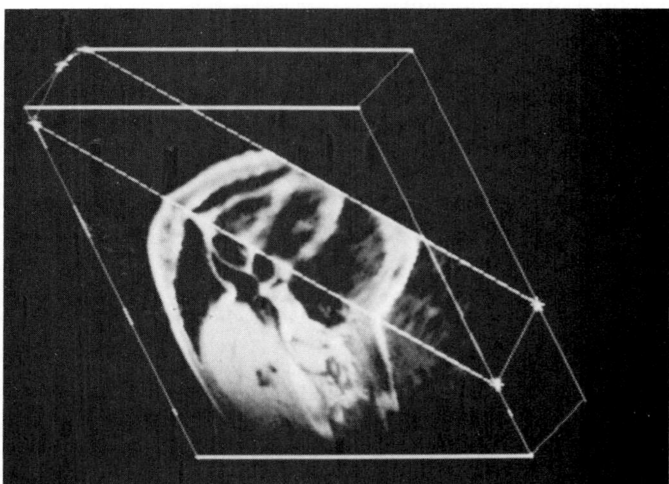

Figure 44–23. Arbitrary oblique reconstruction. From the three-dimensional data obtained with magnetic resonance imaging, it is possible to obtain images at any arbitrary angle through the heart. (Provided by Dr. Tracy Faber.)

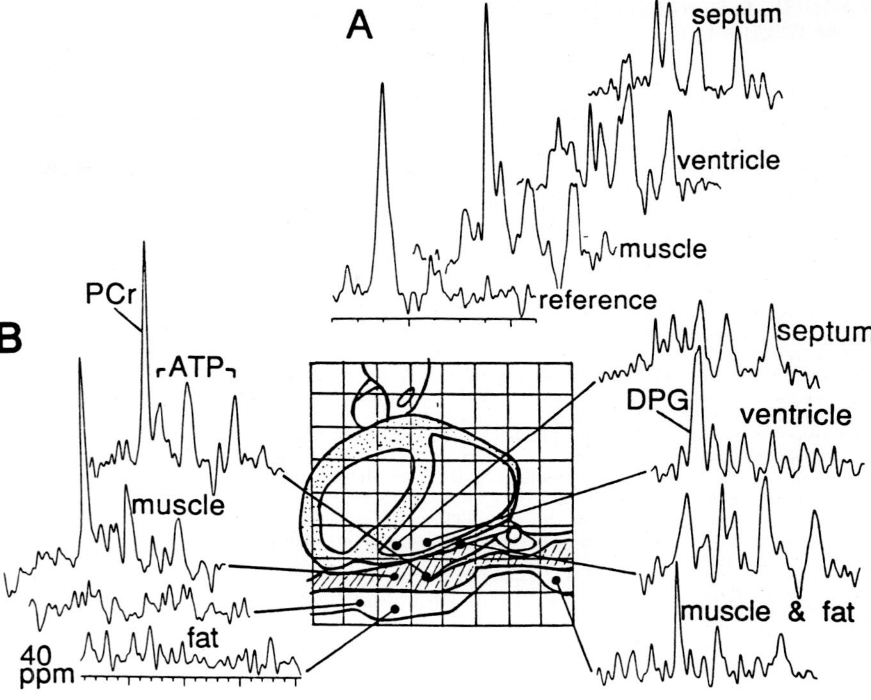

Figure 44–24. Localized spectroscopy. Diagram illustrating the variation in phosphorus spectra obtained at different positions relative to cardiac structures. ppm—parts per million, DPG—diphosphoglycerate, PCr—phosphocreatine, ATP—adenosine triphosphate. (From Bottomley, P. A., and Hardy, C. J.: ^{31}P spectroscopic imaging of the heart. (Abstract.) Society of Magnetic Resonance in Medicine, San Francisco, 1988, p. 832, with permission.)

Magnetic Resonance Spectroscopy

The final area of development is in the area of phosphorus-31 and other forms of magnetic resonance spectroscopy. Spectroscopy (discussed in Chapter 45) allows one to obtain information regarding metabolic function in the heart.[G4] Ideally, this eventually will provide integrated imaging and spectroscopic data (Fig. 44–24).

SUMMARY

The need for quantitation in cardiology has led to the development of a variety of techniques to assess cardiac size and function. In attempting to answer these clinical questions, magnetic resonance imaging brings several important strengths: extraordinary flexibility; powerful contrast mechanisms; sensitivity to flow and motion; and freedom from ionizing radiation, iodinated contrast agents, and acoustic windows. In particular, the flexibility of MR allows it potentially to address all the critical questions in cardiac quantitation: chamber size, global and segmental function, tissue characterization, blood flow, and metabolism. Given this flexibility and strength, it is likely that MR methods will play an increasing role in the evaluation of cardiac structure and function.

References

A

1. Axel, L., and Dougherty, L.: MR imaging of motion with spatial modulation of magnetization. Radiology 171:841, 1989.
2. Aisen, A. M., Buda, A. J., Zotz, R. J., and Buckwalter, K. A.: Visualization of myocardial infarction and subsequent coronary reperfusion with MRI using a dog model. Magn. Res. Imaging 5:399, 1987.
3. Axel, L., Herman, G. T., Udupa, J. K., et al.: Three-dimensional display of nuclear magnetic resonance (NMR) cardiovascular images. J. Comput. Assist. Tomogr. 7:172, 1983.

B

1. Bradley, W. G., Jr., Waluch, V., Lai, K.-S., et al.: The appearance of rapidly flowing blood on magnetic images. AJR 143:1167, 1984.
2. Burbank, F., Parish, D., and Wexler, L.: Echocardiographic-like angled view of the heart obtained by MR imaging. J. Comput. Assist. Tomogr. 12:181, 1988.
3. Byrd, B. F., Schiller, N. B., Botvinick, E. H., and Higgins, C. B.: Normal cardiac dimensions by magnetic resonance imaging. Am. J. Cardiol. 55:1440, 1985.
4. Bakker, C. J. G., and de Graaf, C. N.: Precision in calculated rho, T1, T2 images as a function of data analysis method. Magn. Res. Imaging 6:3, 1988.
5. Buda, A. J., Aisen, A. M., Juni, J. E., et al.: Detection and sizing of myocardial ischemia and infarction by nuclear magnetic resonance imaging in the canine heart. Am. Heart J. 110:1284, 1985.
6. Bouchard, A., Reeves, R. C., Cranney, G., et al.: Assessment of myocardial infarct size by means of T2-weighted 1H nuclear magnetic resonance imaging. Am. Heart J. 117:281, 1989.
7. Bachus, R., Mueller, E., Koenig, H., et al.: Functional imaging using NMR. *In* McCready, V. R., Leach, M., and Ell, P. J. (eds.): Functional Studies Using NMR. Springer-Verlag, New York, 1987.
8. Bottomley, P. A., and Hardy, C. J.: 31P spectroscopic imaging of the heart. (Abstract.) Society of Magnetic Resonance in Medicine, San Francisco, 1988, p. 832.

C

1. Crooks, L. E., Barker, B., Chang, H., et al.: Magnetic resonance imaging strategies for heart studies. Radiology 153:459, 1984.
2. Cranney, G. B., Lotan, C., Dean, L., et al.: Left ventricular volume estimation using NMR—validation of a practical biplane long axis method. (Abstract.) Society of Magnetic Resonance in Medicine, San Francisco, 1988.
3. Caputo, G. R., Tscholakoff, D., Sechtem, U., and Higgins, C. B.: Measurement of canine left ventricular mass using MR imaging. A.J.R. 148:33, 1987.
4. Culham, J. A. G., and Vince, D. J.: Cardiac output by MR imaging: An experimental study comparing right ventricle and left ventricle with thermodilution. J. Can. Assoc. Radiol. 39:247, 1988.
5. Caputo, G. R., Sechtem, U., Tscholakoff, D., and Higgins, C. B.: Measurement of myocardial infarct size at early and late time intervals using MR imaging: An experimental study in dogs. AJR 149:237, 1987.

D

1. Dumoulin, C. L.: Flow imaging. In Budinger, T. F., and Margulis, A. R. (eds.): Medical Magnetic Resonance: A Primer—1988. Society of Magnetic Resonance in Medicine, San Francisco, 1988.
2. Dilworth, L. R., Aisen, A. M., Mancinci, J., et al.: Determination of left ventricular volumes and ejection fraction by nuclear magnetic resonance imaging. Am. Heart J. 113:24, 1987.
3. Doyle, M., Chapman, B., Turner, R., et al.: Real-time cardiac imaging of adults at video frame rates by magnetic resonance imaging. Lancet 2:682, 1986.

E

1. Evans, A. J., Blinder, R. A., Herfkens, R. J., et al.: Effects of turbulence on signal intensity in gradient echo images. Invest. Radiol. 23:512, 1988.

F

1. Falsetti, H. L., Marcus, M. L., Kerber, R. E., and Skorton, D. J.: Quantification of myocardial ischemia and infarction by left ventricular imaging. Circulation 63:747, 1981.

2. Frahm, J., Haase, A., and Matthaei, D.: Rapid NMR imaging of dynamic processes using the FLASH technique. Magn. Reson. Med. 3(2):321, 1986.
3. Feiglin, D. H., George, C. R., MacIntyre, W. J., et al.: Gated cardiac magnetic resonance structural imaging: Optimization by electronic axial rotation. Radiology 154:129, 1985.
4. Friedman, B. J., Waters, J., Kwan, O. L., and DiMaria, A. N.: Comparison of nuclear magnetic resonance and echocardiography in determination of cardiac dimensions in normal subjects. J. Am. Coll. Cardiol. 5:1369, 1985.
5. Florentine, M. S., Grosskreutz, C. L., Chang, W., et al.: Measurement of left ventricular mass in vivo using gated nuclear magnetic resonance imaging. J. Am. Coll. Cardiol. 8:107, 1986.
6. Felmlee, J. P., and Ehman, R. L.: Spatial presaturation: A method for suppressing flow artifacts and improving depiction of vascular anatomy in MR imaging. Radiology 164:559, 1987.
7. Fisher, M. R., von Schulthess, G. K., and Higgins, C. B.: Multiphase cardiac magnetic resonance imaging: Normal regional left ventricular wall thickening. AJR 145:27, 1985.
8. Farrar, T. C., and Becker, E. D.: Pulse and Fourier Transform NMR. Academic Press, New York, 1971.
9. Firmin, D. N., Nayler, G. L., Klipstein, R. H., et al.: In vivo validation of MR velocity imaging. J. Comput. Assist. Tomogr. 11(5):751, 1987.
10. Faber, T., Moore, D., Opperman, R., et al.: Left ventricular surface detection in cardiac MR images. Society of Magnetic Resonance in Medicine, San Francisco, 1989.
11. Faber, T. L., and Stokely, E. M.: Orientation of 3D structure in medical images. IEEE Trans. Pattern Anal. Machine Intell. 10:626, 1988.

G

1. Go, R. T., MacIntyre, W. J., Yeung, H. N., et al.: Volume and planar gated cardiac magnetic resonance imaging: A correlative study of normal anatomy with thallium-201 SPECT and cadaver sections. Radiology 150:129, 1984.
2. Glover, G. H., and Pelc, N. J.: A rapid-gated cine MRI technique. *In* Kressel, H. Y. (ed.): Magnetic Resonance Annual. Raven Press, New York, 1988.
3. Goldman, M. R., Brady, T. J., Pykett, I. L., et al.: Quantification of experimental myocardial infarction using nuclear magnetic resonance imaging and paramagnetic ion contrast enhancement in excised canine hearts. Circulation 66(5):1012, 1982.
4. Gadian, D. G.: Nuclear Magnetic Resonance and Its Application to Living Systems. Clarendon Press, New York, 1982.

H

1. Hoffman, E. A., and Ritman, E. L.: Shape and dimensions of cardiac chambers: Importance of CT section thickness and orientation. Radiology 155:739, 1985.
2. Harris, L. D.: Identification of the optimal orientation of oblique sections through multiple parallel CT image. J. Comput. Assist. Tomogr. 5:881, 1981.
3. Higgins, C. B., Holt, W., Pflugfelder, P., and Sechtem, U.: Functional evaluation of the heart with magnetic resonance imaging. Magn. Reson. Med. 6:121, 1988.
4. Holmvang, G., Edelman, R., Pearlman, J. D., et al.: Study of valvular regurgitation by cine-NMR: Comparison to color Doppler flow maps. Circulation 76(Suppl. IV):30, 1987.

J

1. Jacicki, J. S., Weber, K. T., Gochman, R. F., et al.: Three-dimensional myocardial and ventricular shape: A surface representation. Am. J. Physiol. 10:H1, 1981.

K

1. Kaul, S., Wismer, G. L., Brady, T. J., et al.: Measurement of normal left heart dimensions using optimally oriented MR images. AJR 146(1):75, 1986.
2. Keller, A. M., Peshock, R. M., Malloy, C. R., et al.: In vivo measurement of myocardial mass using nuclear magnetic resonance imaging. J. Am. Coll. Cardiol. 8:113, 1986.
3. Katz, J., Milliken, M. C., Stray-Gundersen, J., et al.: Estimation of myocardial mass in man using magnetic resonance imaging. Radiology 169:495, 1988.
4. Katz, J., Peshock, R., McNamee, P., et al.: Phase reconstruction of magnetic resonance images in the determination of cardiac wall and blood velocity and the possible effects of acceleration. Magn. Reson. Imaging 5:50, 1987.
5. Kantor, H. L., Rzedzian, R. R., Berliner, E., et al.: A new NMR marker of coronary stenosis: The utility of dysprosium-DTPA in high speed cardiac imaging. (Abstract.) Society of Magnetic Resonance in Medicine, San Francisco, 1988.

L

1. Lanzer, P., Barta, C., Botvinick, E. H., et al.: ECG-synchronized cardiac MR imaging: Method and evaluation. Radiology 155:681, 1985.
2. Longmore, D. B., Underwood, S. R., Hounsfield, G. M., et al.: Dimensional accuracy of magnetic resonance studies of the heart. Lancet 1:1360, 1985.
3. Lanzer, P., Cranney, G., and Pohost, G.: Measurements of right and left ventricular volumes: Is angulated cardiac NMR imaging important? (Abstract.) Society of Magnetic Resonance in Medicine, San Francisco, 1988.
4. Levine, R. A., Gillam, L. D., and Weyman, A.: Echocardiography in cardiac research. *In* Fozzard, H. A., Jennings, R. B., Haber, E., and Katz, A. M. (eds.): The Heart and Cardiovascular System: Scientific Foundations. Raven Press, New York, 1986.
5. Lund, G., Morin, R. L., Olivari, M. T., and Ring, W. S.: Serial T2 relaxation time measurements in normal subjects and heart transplant recipients. J. Heart Transpl. 7:274, 1988.
6. Losh, J., Chwialkowski, M., Pfeifer, D., et al.: Detection and description of magnetically tagged heart muscle from MR images. Conference proceedings, IEEE Engineering in Medicine and Biology Society 11th Annual International Conference, Seattle, Washington, 1989.
7. Laschinger, J. C., Vannier, M. W., Gronemeyer, S., et al.: Noninvasive three-dimensional reconstruction of the heart and great vessels by ECG-gated magnetic resonance imaging: A new diagnostic modality. Ann. Thorac. Surg. 45:505, 1988.

M

1. Murphy, W. A., Gutierrez, F. R., Levitt, R. G., et al.: Oblique views of the heart by magnetic resonance imaging. Radiology 154:225, 1985.
2. Maddahi, J., Crues, J., Berman, D. S., et al.: Noninvasive quantitation of left ventricular mass by gated proton magnetic resonance imaging. J. Am. Coll. Cardiol. 10:682, 1987.
3. Milliken, M., Stray-Gundersen, J., Peshock, R. M., et al.: Left ventricular mass as determined by magnetic resonance imaging in male endurance athletes. Am. J. Cardiol. 62:301, 1988.
4. Mitchell, J. H., Wildenthal, K., and Mullins, C. B.: Geometrical studies of the left ventricle using biplane cinefluorography. Fed. Proc. 28:1334, 1969.
5. Been, M., Smith, M. A., Ridgway, J. P., et al.: Serial changes in the T1 magnetic relaxation parameter after myocardial infarction in man. Br. Heart J. 59:1, 1988.
6. McNamara, M. T., Higgins, C. B., Ehman, R. L., et al.: Acute myocardial ischemia: Magnetic resonance contrast enhancement with gadolinium-DTPA. Radiology 153:157, 1984.
7. Miller, D. M., Holmvang, G., Gill, J. B., et al.: MRI detection of myocardial perfusion changes by gadolinium-DTPA infusion during dipyridamole hyperemia. Magn. Reson. Med. 10:246, 1989.
8. Milnor, W. M.: Hemodynamics. Williams and Wilkins, Baltimore, 1989.
9. Mills, C. J., Gabe, I. T., Gault, J. H., et al.: Pressure-flow relationships and vascular impedance in man. Cardiovasc. Res. 4:405, 1970.

O

1. Ostrzega, E., Maddahi, J., Honma, H., et al.: Quantification of left ventricular myocardial mass in humans using nuclear magnetic resonance imaging. Am. Heart J. 117:444, 1989.
2. Ostrzega, E., Crues, J., Honma, H., et al.: Determination of left ventricular mass in man: Cine versus gated spin echo NMR imaging techniques. (Abstract.) Clin. Nucl. Med. 12:22(B), 1987.
3. Ortendahl, D. A., Hylton, N., Kaufman, L., et al.: Analytical tools for magnetic resonance imaging. Radiology 153:479, 1984.

P

1. Peshock, R. M., Stark, D. D., and Bradley, W. G. (eds.): Heart and Great Vessels in Magnetic Resonance Imaging. C. V. Mosby, St. Louis, 1988.
2. Pettigrew, R. I., and Dannels, W.: Use of standard gradients with compound oblique angulation for optimal quantitative MR flow imaging in oblique vessels. A.J.R. 148:405, 1987.
3. Peshock, R. M., Rokey, R., Malloy, C. M., et al.: Assessment of myocardial systolic wall thickening by nuclear magnetic resonance imaging. J. Am. Coll. Cardiol. 14:653, 1989.
4. Peshock, R. M.: Magnetic resonance in the estimation of infarct size. Circulation (in press).
5. Prato, F. S., Drost, D. J., King, M., et al.: Cardiac T1 calculations from MR spin-echo images. Magn. Reson. Med. 4:227, 1987.
6. Pykett, I. L., and Rzedzian, R. R.: Instant images of the body by magnetic resonance. Magn. Reson. Med. 5:563, 1987.

R

1. Robb, R. A., Ritman, E. L., and Harris, L. D.: Digital image processing in x-ray computed tomography: High-speed volume imaging with the DSR. *In* Collins, S. M., and Skorton, D. J. (eds.): Cardiac Imaging and Image Processing. McGraw-Hill, New York, 1986.
2. Rehr, R. B., Malloy, C. R., Filipchuk, N. G., and Peshock, R. M.: Left ventricular volumes measured by MR imaging. Radiology 156:717, 1985.
3. Riley-Hagan, M., Peshock, R. M., Stray-Gundersen, J., et al.: Left ventricular dimensions and mass in female endurance athletes. (Abstract.) Med. Sci. Sports Exerc. 19(2):547, 1987.
4. Rokey, R., Johnston, D. L., Nitz, W., et al.: Assessment of left ventricular wall motion abnormalities by cine magnetic resonance imaging: A comparison with two-dimensional echocardiography. (Abstract.) Society of Magnetic Resonance in Medicine, San Francisco, 1988.
5. Rokey, R., Verani, M. S., Bolli, R., et al.: Myocardial infarct size quantitation after coronary artery occlusion in dogs. Radiology 158:771, 1986.
6. Rzedzian, R. R., and Pykett, I. L.: Instant images of the human heart using a new, whole body MR imaging system. A.J.R. 149:245, 1987.

S

1. Sandler, H.: Dimensional analysis of the heart: A review. Am. J. Med. Sci. 260:56, 1970.
2. Sandler, H., and Dodge, H. T.: The use of single plane angiocardiograms for the calculation of left ventricular volume in man. Am. Heart J. 75:325, 1968.
3. Sechtem, U., Pflugfelder, P. W., Cassidy, M. M., et al.: Mitral and aortic regurgitant volumes with cine MR imaging. Radiology 167:425, 1988.
4. Sechtem, U., Plugfelder, P., Cassidy, M. C., et al.: Ventricular septal defect: Visualization of shunt flow and determination of shunt size by cine MR imaging. AJR 149:689, 1987.
5. Shapiro, E. P., Rogers, W. J., Beyer, R., et al.: Determination of left ventricular mass by magnetic resonance imaging in hearts deformed by acute infarction. Circulation 79:706, 1989.
6. Stratemeier, E. J., Thompson, R., Brady, T. J., et al.: Ejection fraction determination by MR imaging: Comparison with left ventricular angiography. Radiology 158:775, 1986.
7. Sechtem, U., Pflugfelder, P. W., Gould, R. G., et al.: Measurement of right and left ventricular volumes in healthy individuals with cine MR imaging. Radiology 163:697, 1987.
8. Schaefer, S., Peshock, R. M., Malloy, C. R., et al.: In-vivo identification of reperfused myocardium with nuclear magnetic resonance: Gadolinium-DTPA as a marker of the bed-at-risk. J. Am. Coll. Cardiol. 12:1063, 1988.
9. Schaefer, S., Lange, R., Kulkarni, P. V., et al.: In-vivo nuclear magnetic resonance imaging of myocardial perfusion using the paramagnetic contrast agent manganese gluconate. J. Am. Coll. Cardiol. 14:472, 1989.
10. Shile, P., Chwialkowski, M., Pfeifer, D., et al.: Automated identification of the spine in magnetic resonance images: A reference point for automated processing. Comput Assist Radiol. Proceedings of the International Symposium. Springer-Verlag, Berlin, 1989.
11. Schaefer, S., Peshock, R. M., Malloy, C. R., et al.: Nuclear magnetic resonance imaging in Marfan's syndrome. J. Am. Coll. Cardiol. 9:70, 1987.

U

1. Utz, J. A., Herfkens, R. J., and Heinsimer, J. A.: Cine MRI determination of left ventricular ejection fraction. AJR 148:839, 1987.

V

1. Van Rossum, A. C., Visser, F. C., van Eenige, M. J., et al.: Magnetic resonance imaging of the heart for determination of ejection fraction. Int. J. Cardiol. 18:53, 1988.
2. Van Dijk, P.: Direct cardiac NMR imaging of heart wall and blood flow velocity. J. Comput. Assist. Tomogr. 8:429, 1984.

W

1. Wyatt, H. L., Heng, M. K., Meerbaum, S., et al.: Cross-sectional echocardiography. I. Analysis of mathematical models for quantifying mass of the left ventricle in dogs. Circulation 60:1104, 1979.
2. Wesby, G., Higgins, C. B., Lanzer, P., et al.: Imaging and characterization of acute myocardial infarction in vivo by gated nuclear magnetic resonance. Circulation 69(1):125, 1984.
3. Wolf, G. L., and Baum, L.: Cardiovascular toxicity and tissue proton T1 response to manganese injection in the dog and rabbit. AJR 141:193, 1983.

Z

1. Zhu, X. P., Checkley, D. R., Hickley, D. S., and Isherwood, I.: Accuracy of area measurements made from MR images compared with computed tomography. J. Comput. Assist. Tomogr. 10:96, 1986.
2. Zerhouni, E. A., Parish, D. M., Rogers, W. J., et al.: Human heart: Tagging with MR imaging—a method for noninvasive assessment of myocardial motion. Radiology 169:59, 1988.

Chapter 45

Use of Sodium-23 for Cardiac Magnetic Resonance Imaging and Spectroscopy

JOSE KATZ, M.D., Ph.D. ▪ *PAUL J. CANNON, M.D.*

PHYSIOLOGIC PROPERTIES OF SODIUM 828
NUCLEAR CHARACTERISTICS OF SODIUM 828
MAGNETIC RESONANCE SPECTRA OF SODIUM 830
Extreme Narrowing Spectra 830
Crystal-Like Spectra 830
Inhomogeneous Powder Spectra and Homogeneous Spectra 830
SODIUM MR SENSITIVITY AND CONTRAST 831
Relative Magnetic Resonance Sensitivity 831
Sodium Density in Tissue 831
Tissue Sodium "Invisibility" 831
OBSERVING INTRACELLULAR SODIUM 831
Sodium Relaxation Times 831
Paramagnetic Shift Reagents 832
Multiple Quantum Filter Techniques 832
MAGNETIC RESONANCE IMAGING OF SODIUM 833
Sodium Imaging of the Heart 833
Use of Contrast Agents 837
SUMMARY 838

Many elements have at least one naturally occurring isotope with nuclear spin and a nonvanishing magnetic moment. In theory, all such isotopes could be utilized for magnetic resonance (MR) imaging or spectroscopy. In practice, however, only a few elements, such as hydrogen-1, sodium-23, or fluorine-19, yield enough MR signal for imaging or spectroscopy with current equipment. In this chapter, we discuss the use of sodium-23 for cardiac imaging. Sodium-23 does not generate as strong an MR signal as hydrogen-1. However, in spite of this, sodium-23 is the element with the highest MR sensitivity following hydrogen-1. Factors that contribute to the high MR sensitivity of sodium-23 include its natural isotopic abundance (which is 100 percent), its spin of 3/2, and its concentration in living tissue which, although much lower than that of protons, is still on the order of tens of millimoles.

PHYSIOLOGIC PROPERTIES OF SODIUM

The sodium ion is the predominant cation in the extracellular fluid (approximately 135 to 150 mmol/L). The intracellular concentration of sodium is much lower (approximately 5 to 12 mmol/L), because it is actively transported out of cells by the sodium/potassium adenosine triphosphatase (Na/K ATPase).[F1, M1, N1, S1, S2] This enzyme, located in the cell membrane, transports sodium out of cells and potassium into cells against their electrochemical gradients.[F1, M1, N1, S1, S2] It also binds cardiac glycosides via a site localized on the exterior surface of the cell membranes. Other membrane constituents that influence the intracellular sodium concentration to a lesser extent in cells such as cardiac myocytes include (1) a fast sodium channel,[C1, F1, H1, N1, N2, S2, T1] which is voltage sensitive and mediates the upstroke of the cardiac action potential; (2) a sodium-calcium exchanger,[C1, C2, H1, N2, R1, R2, T1, Z1] which is also voltage sensitive and mediates bidirectional exchange of sodium for calcium; and (3) a sodium-hydrogen exchanger,[C1, C2, H1, N1, N2, R1, R2, S1, S2, T1, Z1] which mediates exchange of sodium for hydrogen and which is inhibited by the drug amiloride.

The concentration gradient of sodium across the external membranes of the cardiac myocyte is important in the maintenance of its state of excitability. Disturbances of this gradient can result in the generation of abnormal electrical activity and arrhythmias.[F1, M2, Z1] Because the mechanisms that control sodium flux and content in myocytes are coupled to mechanisms that influence the intracellular calcium and hydrogen content, these mechanisms also influence the contractility of the heart cells. Thus, the positive inotropic effects of digitalis glycosides result indirectly from the effect of these substances to inhibit the Na/K ATPase. Similarly, ischemia and hypoxia have been demonstrated to have major effects upon the trans-sarcolemmal concentration gradients of sodium in cardiac and brain cells and indirectly upon the function of these cells. For example, in cardiac tissue, myocardial intracellular sodium increases significantly in response to ischemia followed by reperfusion, and the contractile state of the ventricle may become impaired—the phenomenon referred to as myocardial "stunning."[B1] In addition, it has been observed that the intracellular concentration of sodium is significantly increased in many neoplasms.[C3–C7] Furthermore, the sodium content in the extracellular compartment of a tissue rises when it becomes edematous. Development of methods to image sodium in vivo using nuclear magnetic resonance may facilitate the detection and analysis of these abnormalities.

NUCLEAR CHARACTERISTICS OF SODIUM

Sodium-23 is the only natural isotope of sodium. Thus, sodium always has spin = 3/2 and a nonvanishing magnetic moment. The gyromagnetic ratio of sodium is approximately 3.76 times smaller than that of the proton. Hence, its Larmor frequency is 11.26 MHz/T, while that of the proton is 42.57 MHz/T.

All nuclei with a spin quantum number 3/2 have four different possible energy levels in the presence of an external static magnetic field. Since sodium-23 has spin = 3/2, it thus follows that there are four possible orientations of the sodium nucleus relative to the applied magnetic field, each characterized by a

Figure 45–1. *A*, Energy level diagram for a spin 3/2 nucleus if the quadrupole interaction vanishes at each instant in time or averages out to zero. Note that the energy difference between any two levels is the same (and denoted here by E_O). *B*, Energy level diagram for spin 3/2 nucleus in the presence of a nonvanishing quadrupole interaction. Note that the energy level difference between any two levels now depends on the levels considered and may also depend on the electric quadrupole moment of the sodium nucleus. (The additional contribution to the energy level splitting due to the quadrupole interaction is here denoted by E_Q.)

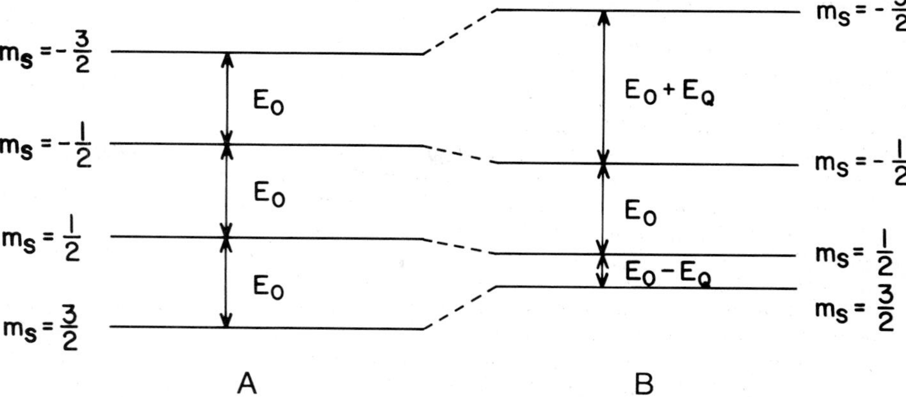

different spin component along the magnetic field axis (z − axis). Each of these orientations corresponds to a possible energy level, which may be distinguished from one another by the spin quantum number m_s, with possible values of −3/2, −1/2, 1/2, and 3/2, respectively. In the absence of a magnetic field, these levels all have the same energy. However, in the presence of a magnetic field, each of the four energy levels has a different energy.

Sodium-23 and, quite generally, all nuclei with spin equal to or greater than 1 have an electric quadrupole moment that arises because they have a spherically nonsymmetric nuclear charge distribution. The relaxation properties of sodium nuclei are determined primarily by the quadrupolar interaction. The quadrupolar interaction is primarily determined by the electric quadrupole moment of the sodium nucleus and local electric field gradients created by surrounding solvent molecules and other macromolecules in the immediate environment of the nucleus.[B2, E1, R3, S3] The local electric field gradients at the nucleus are set up by an asymmetric distribution of dipoles caused by molecules surrounding the nucleus. A typical energy level diagram for a spin 3/2 nucleus in the presence of a magnetic field is shown in Figure 45–1A if the quadrupolar interaction vanishes at each instant in time or averages out to zero. Note that the energy level difference between any two consecutive levels is the same for all levels. In contrast, the energy level diagram when the quadrupolar interaction does not vanish is shown in Figure 45–1*B*. It can be seen from this figure that the energy level difference between any two consecutive levels now depends on the particular levels considered and may also depend on the electric quadrupole moment of the sodium nucleus.

It should be emphasized again at this point that under certain conditions the quadrupolar interaction may vanish at each instant in time or average out to zero. In such cases, the energy difference between any two levels would be the same as that expected if the sodium nucleus did not have a quadrupole moment (Fig. 45–1A). The significance of the conditions required in order for this to occur will be discussed in detail in the section on "Magnetic Resonance Spectra of Sodium." However, it may be noted here that three possible physical situations lead to vanishing of the quadrupolar interaction at each instant in time or to its averaging out to zero.

- The first arises when an axially symmetric electric field gradient is oriented with respect to the magnetic field at an angle such that the quadrupole interaction vanishes. For example, for a single crystal sample, such as in the case of sodium pyrophosphate or for sodium in hydrated oriented deoxyribonucleic acid (Na-DNA), this occurs when the angle between the electric field gradient and the magnetic field axis is 55°.
- The second situation occurs in tissue samples when the sodium nucleus is in a completely unordered environment, with rapidly fluctuating electric field gradients whose axes have random orientations with respect to the magnetic field and in which the transverse magnetization decays multiexponentially. In this situation, the quadrupolar interaction does not vanish at each instant in time but, nevertheless, still averages out to zero.
- Finally, in the extreme narrowing approximation, i.e., in a system with rapid molecular motion and monoexponential decay of the transverse magnetization, such as sodium in dilute aqueous solutions, the quadrupolar interaction is once again present at each instant in time but, nevertheless, averages out to zero.[B2, E1, R3, S3]

A transition between any two consecutive energy levels, i.e., a transition for which $\Delta m_s = \pm 1$, is usually referred to as a single quantum transition. Thus, sodium-23 may undergo three single quantum transitions: −3/2 to −1/2 (transition 1), −1/2 to 1/2 (transition 2), and 1/2 to 3/2 (transition 3). The frequency corresponding to a single quantum transition may be obtained by dividing the energy difference corresponding to the two levels between which the transition occurs by h, where h = Planck's constant.

In an ordered environment with only one or a limited range of possible orientations of the electric field gradients relative to the magnetic field, it follows that each of the single quantum transitions, 1, 2, or 3, will occur at a different transition freqquency.[B2, E1, R3, S3] Thus, three different peaks will be observed in nuclear magnetic resonance spectra under this condition. Quantum mechanical calculations show that the intensity of the central peak is 40 percent of the total intensity while that of each of the outer peaks corresponds to 30 percent of the total intensity.[B2, E1, R3, S3]

In addition to single quantum transitions, defined by $\Delta m_s = \pm 1$, the sodium-23 nucleus, as well as any other spin 3/2 nuclei, may also undergo double and triple quantum transitions.[B3, H2, J1, R3, W1] A double quantum transition, defined by $\Delta m_s = \pm 2$, corresponds to a transition between energy levels with $m_s = -3/2$ and $m_s = 1/2$ or with $m_s = -1/2$ and $m_s = 3/2$. A triple quantum transition, defined by $\Delta m_s = \pm 3$, corresponds to a transition between the energy level with $m_s = -3/2$ and the energy level with $m_s = 3/2$. Double and triple quantum transitions may collectively be referred to as multiple quantum transitions in order to distinguish them from single quantum transitions.*

Recently, MR spectroscopic techniques have been developed to monitor multiple quantum transitions that may be applicable to both MR imaging and spectroscopy.[B4, B5, C8, G1, G2, J1–J4, K1–K5, L1, P1–P3, S4–S6]

---

*The resonance frequency of a single quantum transition ($\Delta m_s = \pm 1$) is usually determined by the difference in energy between the two energy levels divided by h (Planck's constant). For a double quantum transition ($\Delta m_s = \pm 2$), the resonance frequency may be shown to be equal to the energy level difference between the two levels considered divided by 2h. This relationship may be explained by assuming that the spin system actually absorbs two quanta from the radiofrequency field. Finally, for a triple quantum transition the resonance frequency may be explained by assuming that the spin system actually absorbs three quanta from the radiofrequency field, i.e., it is given by the energy difference between the two levels considered divided by 3h.[B3, J1, R3]

MAGNETIC RESONANCE SPECTRA OF SODIUM

We next discuss the possible types of spectra and behavior of tissue relaxation times for spin = 3/2 nuclei, such as sodium-23.[B2, E1, R3, S3] This is useful in order to determine when the decay terms corresponding to transverse magnetization are multiexponential in nature and to understand the conditions under which multiple quantum transitions may occur. Nearly all other nuclei used for cardiac imaging have spin = 1/2 and relatively simple relaxation and spectra, i.e., 1-H, 19-F, and 31-P.

Four possible types of fundamental spectra may be distinguished for spin = 3/2 nuclei. These are the extreme narrowing spectrum, the crystal-like spectrum, the inhomogeneous powder spectrum, and the homogeneous spectrum. Of course, composite spectra that are superpositions of any of these fundamental spectra may also occur in nature.

Extreme Narrowing Spectra

The extreme narrowing spectrum describes the behavior of sodium in solution and is characterized by $\omega_o\tau_c << 1$, where ω_o is the Larmor frequency and τ_c the correlation time (defined as the duration of time in which a nucleus remains in a given position and orientation within an electric field gradient). The spectrum corresponding to the extreme narrowing approximation (Fig. 45–2*A*) consists of a single, narrow line with 100 percent of the total expected intensity, since the average quadrupole interaction here averages out to zero.[A1]

Quite generally, for metal ion nuclei in biologic systems (such as, for example, for metal ion nuclei in solution with a protein possessing a tight metal ion binding site), the values obtained for τ_c are usually rather large and the extreme narrowing approximation is not generally valid. However, for metal ions in low molecular weight complexes, the values obtained for τ_c are much smaller, so that the condition $\omega_o\tau_c << 1$ (i.e., the extreme narrowing approximation) holds.

The transverse magnetization in the extreme narrowing spectrum decays monoexponentially and satisfies the relation $T_1 = T_2$ (where T_1 and T_2 denote the longitudinal and transverse relaxation time, respectively).

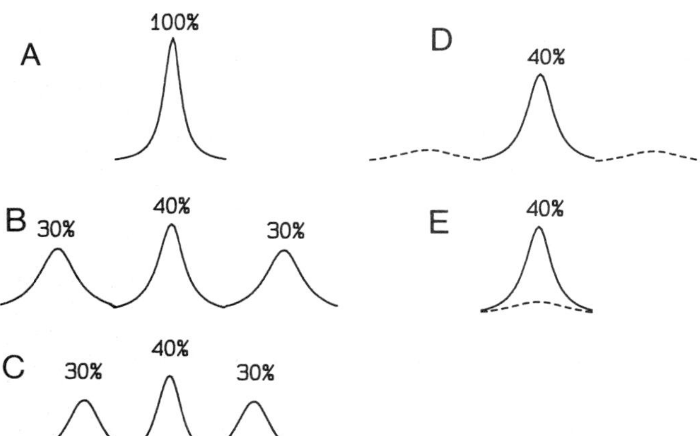

Figure 45–2. *A*, Extreme narrowing spectrum. The spectrum consists of a single, narrow line with 100 percent of the total expected intensity. *B*, Crystal-like spectrum with complete symmetry. The spectrum generally consists of a central peak with 40 percent of the total signal intensity and two broader outer peaks that each account for 30 percent of the total signal intensity. *C*, Crystal-like spectrum without complete symmetry. The spectrum consists of a central peak with 40 percent of the total signal intensity and two broader outer peaks that each account for 30 percent of the total signal intensity. The separation between the outer peaks and the central peak is here typically much smaller than that in the crystal-like spectrum with complete symmetry. *D*, Inhomogeneous powder spectrum. The spectrum consists of a central peak with 40 percent of the possible total signal intensity (*solid curve*). The outer peaks (*dashed curves*) are broadened beyond detection and, hence, do not contribute to the nuclear magnetic resonance spectrum. E, Homogeneous powder spectrum. The spectrum consists of a central peak with 40 percent of the possible total signal intensity (*solid curve*). The two additional peaks (*dashed curves*) occur here at the same frequency as the central peak. However, the relaxation times of these two additional peaks are so shortened as to broaden them beyond detection.

Crystal-Like Spectra

The crystal-like spectrum describes the behavior of 23-sodium in an ordered environment. Typical examples for this situation are sodium pyrophosphate crystals, as well as liquid crystals or oriented samples of hydrated macromolecules.

In the crystal-like spectrum corresponding to sodium pyrophosphate (perfectly symmetric crystal-like spectrum), the axes of the electric field gradients assume only one or a limited range of possible orientations with respect to the magnetic field. Hence, the nuclear MR spectrum here consists of three different frequency peaks.[B2, E1, R3, S3] The intensity of the central peak is 40 percent of the total signal intensity, while each of the outer peaks is broader than the central peak and accounts for 30 percent of the total signal intensity (Fig. 45–2*B*). Depending on the binding between the sodium and pyrophosphate ions and their orientation relative to the applied magnetic field, the maximal separation between the center of any of the outer peaks and the center frequency of the central peak may change from a few kHz to several MHz.

In the crystal-like spectrum corresponding to oriented hydrated macromolecules or liquid crystals (crystal-like spectrum without complete symmetry), one can still observe three frequency peaks. Although partial averaging of the quadrupole interaction occurs, its time-averaged value does not vanish. Thus, the separation between the center frequency of any of the outer peaks and the center frequency of the central peak persists. However, this separation is here typically much smaller than in sodium pyrophosphate (Fig. 45–2*C*).

The transverse magnetization in the crystalline spectrum exhibits multiexponential relaxation. Furthermore, both single and multiple quantum transitions may occur here.

Inhomogeneous Powder Spectra and Homogeneous Spectra

Finally, whenever the effective field gradients have random orientations with respect to the magnetic field, two different types of sodium-23 spectra may be distinguished: the so-called inhomogeneous powder spectrum and the homogeneous spectrum.[B2, E1, R3, S3] These are the typical spectra of most tissue samples in view of the random orientations between the electric field gradients in tissue and the applied magnetic field. The inhomogeneous powder spectrum, furthermore, may also be seen in powdered crystalline samples or unoriented samples of hydrated molecules or liquid crystals.

In the inhomogeneous powder spectrum, the frequencies of transitions 1 and 3 vary over the entire range of possible orientations. Since the area under the outer frequency peaks is a constant (30 percent of the total intensity for each peak), a frequency spread in their positions implies a reduction in peak height. Furthermore, since in an inhomogeneous environment the electric field gradients are also time dependent, the outer frequency peaks are broadened even further. Under these circumstances, the outer peaks are broadened beyond detection and hence only the central frequency peak, whose intensity is 40 percent of the possible total signal intensity, contributes to the nuclear MR signal (Fig. 45–2*D*).

In the homogeneous spectrum, the electric field gradient axes have random orientations with respect to the magnetic field, and the molecular motions are such that fast fluctuations of the electric field gradients occur. In this case, the quadrupole energy splitting averages to zero, and a single frequency peak is observed even though a quadrupolar interaction is present. However, the electric field gradient fluctuations also affect the relaxation times of transitions 1 and 3, so that although these transitions occur at the same frequency as the central frequency peak, their relaxation times are so shortened as to broaden beyond detection the peaks corresponding to these two transitions (Fig. 45–2*E*). Hence, once again, only 40 percent of the possible total signal intensity survives and contributes to the nuclear magnetic resonance signal (central frequency peak).

In both the inhomogeneous powder spectrum and the homogeneous spectrum, the transverse magnetization is multiexponential in nature. Furthermore, it may also be shown that both single and multiple quantum transitions may occur in either of these two spectra.

SODIUM MAGNETIC RESONANCE SENSITIVITY AND CONTRAST

The MR sensitivity (IS) of a nuclear species is simply the maximal signal it can generate during a magnetic resonance experiment. It is frequently referenced to a standard, usually the proton, which is defined as 100 percent. The formula for MR sensitivity at constant magnetic field is

$$IS = C\gamma^{11/4}S\,(S + 1) \times (\text{isotopic abundance}) \times (\text{tissue concentration})$$

where C is a parameter that depends on the MR equipment under discussion, as well as sample volume and temperature; S is the nuclear spin; and γ the gyromagnetic ratio.[H3]

Relative Magnetic Resonance Sensitivity

For an equal number of nuclei, sodium has about one eighth the sensitivity of the proton at constant magnetic field (largely because its gyromagnetic ratio is 11.26 MHz/T compared with 42.58 MHz/T for the proton). Total sensitivity decreases further whenever tissue concentration is taken into account, since the tissue concentration of sodium is much smaller than that of the proton. For example, the typical sodium content of the heart of a 70-kg man is about 0.43 g versus a corresponding proton content of about 34 g. Hence, the MR sensitivity at constant magnetic field in the heart is about 1/1000 the MR sensitivity of the proton when tissue concentration is also taken into account. The lower sensitivity of sodium MR necessitates the use of special imaging equipment and data acquisition techniques.

Sodium Density in Tissue

Another important consideration for sodium MR and, in particular, for cardiac MR, is that of tissue contrast. Proton concentration in blood is comparable to that in myocardium. Thus, there is only a minimal contribution of proton density to tissue contrast between blood and myocardium in proton MR imaging of the heart. On the other hand, sodium concentration in blood is much higher than that in myocardium. Hence, the contribution of sodium density to tissue contrast between these structures is significant whenever MR imaging of the heart is performed using this element.

Tissue Sodium "Invisibility"

A final, somewhat confusing consideration to magnetic resonance spectroscopy (MRS) or imaging (MRI) is the question of sodium "invisibility."* It has been observed experimentally that the sodium content of certain tissues measured by magnetic resonance spectroscopy is only a fraction of that measured chemically by independent techniques. This phenomenon—namely, that some of the sodium appeared to be "invisible" to MR approaches—has been the subject of many papers. Invisibility of a nucleus results from the presence of a very short component of T_2 (broad frequency peak), which effectively makes observation of the corresponding frequency peak impossible under the conditions of the particular experiment being considered. The magnitude of both the short and long components of T_2 depends on the correlation time (degree of ordering of the sodium environment). In particular, if the correlation time is in the range of 10^{-12} sec to 10^{-9} sec, which is typical for biologic systems, then both the short and long components of T_2 decrease as the correlation time lengthens. Some studies reported that 100 percent of sodium was "visible," and others reported that a significant component of the sodium (about 60 percent) was "invisible" to MR approaches. It appears that much of the variability in these reports may be due to different intricacies of each experiment, the MR equipment used and its resolution characteristics, differences in magnetic field strength, temperature, tissues considered, and tissue preparation.

Originally, it was proposed that "invisible" sodium was sodium bound to proteins and phospholipids in tissue.[C9, C11, C15] More recent experiments suggest that the sodium signal from any tissue reflects the quadrupolar interactions between sodium-23 and its molecular environment, which produce spectral patterns that include spectral components with sufficient broadening to render a certain percentage of the total signal unobservable under the conditions of the experiment.[B2, C14, E1, R3, S3, S7]

The observed sodium spectrum for a given tissue is actually a superposition of spectra from various biologic compartments (which, for example, include intracellular cytoplasmic space, mitochondria, interstitium, intravascular space, and so on). Thus, even if the visibility factor for each compartment were constant, the average visibility factor for all the tissue considered may actually differ from these individual values.

Finally, it should also be mentioned here that conditions that produce sodium invisibility using conventional single quantum techniques may exhibit a totally opposite effect when acquisitions are made with a double quantum filter. (A double quantum filter is an MR pulse sequence that allows selection of a double quantum transition.) As the sodium environment becomes more ordered, i.e., the correlation time lengthens, sodium may be invisible when single quantum acquisitions are employed. However, if visualized with a double quantum filter, an increase in signal intensity is observed instead.[K3] Thus, invisibility not only depends on the correlation time (degree of ordering of the sodium environment) but also on the type of acquisition employed.

OBSERVING INTRACELLULAR SODIUM

Since the Larmor frequency of sodium is the same in both the intracellular and the extracellular space, it is not possible to distinguish the sodium ions in these compartments on the basis of their resonant frequencies. However, three alternative approaches may be employed in MR imaging to aid in the discrimination of the intracellular signal from that caused by the extracellular compartment. These include making use of the different relaxation times between intracellular and extracellular sodium, the use of paramagnetic shift reagents and the use of special multiple quantum filter techniques.

Sodium Relaxation Times

The first approach is based on the observation that the tissue transverse relaxation time for the intracellular space is smaller than that for the extracellular compartment (Table 45–1). Hence, magnetic resonance imaging of the intracellular space may be performed by shortening the spin-echo time so that the signal intensity due to the intracellular space proportionally increases.[H4, H5]

Typical mean results for the short (T_{2s}) and long (T_{2l}) compo-

*B2, B5, C9–C15, E1, G3, J5, K3, M3, M4, O1, O2, P4–P6, R3–R5, S3, S7–S10, Y1, W2.

Table 45–1. SODIUM RELAXATION TIMES IN NUCLEAR MAGNETIC RESONANCE IMAGING

	Intracellular Sodium (msec)			Extracellular Sodium (msec)			
	T_{2s}	T_{2l}	T_1	T_{2s}	T_{2l}	T_1	Ref.
Perfused (frog) heart (myocytes)	2	17	23	—	—	—	B5
Skeletal muscle							
Rat	0.9	14	12	–	—	—	C11
	1.59	16.1	18.3	—	—	—	C13
	0.7	10	11	—	—	—	B2
Porcine	3.5	24	—	—	—	—	J5
Frog	2.9	13.7	24.4	—	—	—	S8
Brain							
Rat	0.75	10	15	—	—	—	B2
Cat	5	20	—	—	—	—	J5
Erythrocytes	6.3	27.2	—	—	—	—	P7
	—	—	30	—	—	—	P5
Blood serum	—	—	—	—	24	39	S9
				12	49.5	—	P7
Blood plasma	—	—	—	—	17*	30	P5

*Authors of this reference assumed the validity of the extreme narrowing approximation for tissue.
—Not applicable or not determined.

nents of the transverse relaxation time (T_2), as well as the longitudinal relaxation time (T_1), are given in Table 45–1 for perfused hearts, skeletal muscle, erythrocytes, and blood serum and plasma.[B2–B5, C11–C13, J5, P5, P7, S8] Note that the sodium transverse relaxation time is biexponential when sodium is in an environment of negatively charged macromolecules, such as the one that exists in the intracellular compartment. Theoretically, it would also be expected that T_1 for the intracellular space is biexponential. However, the decay terms corresponding to T_1 are well fitted experimentally with a single exponential for both the intracellular and the extracellular compartment.

Paramagnetic Shift Reagents

An alternative approach to separate the signal arising from sodium in the intracellular compartment from sodium in the extracellular compartment makes use of paramagnetic shift reagents. Paramagnetic shift reagents are chelates of paramagnetic lanthanide ions with anionic complexes. They were first developed to distinguish intracellular from extracellular sodium by MR spectroscopy.[G4, P6, P8] These substances do not cross intact cell membranes. By interacting with sodium in the extracellular fluid, they introduce a frequency shift in the resonance frequency of the extracellular sodium, so that the sodium spectrum consists of separate peaks arising from the intracellular and the extracellular sodium. Lanthanide ions used for this purpose include Dy3+ (dysprosium), Tm3+ (thulium), and Gd3+ (gadolinium); the anions include PPP5− (tripolyphosphate) and TTHA6− (tetraethylene triaminehexacetic acid). It is also possible, using perfused organs, to use paramagnetic shift reagents to discriminate the signal from intracellular sodium for imaging by use of chemical shift techniques.[B6] However, disadvantages of these substances for in vivo studies relate to the fact that they form calcium complexes and thus disturb normal physiology, and that they do possess some toxicity.[C16, C17, G4, P6, P8]

Multiple Quantum Filter Techniques

Another approach that could be useful in the study of intracellular sodium under certain conditions is the use of a multiple quantum filter, such as, for example, a double quantum filter.[B3, B4, G1, G2, H2, J1, K1–K5, P1–P3, S4, S5] A multiple quantum filter is an MR pulse sequence that allows direct observation of a multiple quantum transition. Thus, for example, a double quantum filter allows selection of a double quantum transition.* Intracellular sodium exhibits biexponential transverse relaxation, with short and long components of the transverse relaxation time. On the other hand, dilute crystalline solutions decay monoexponentially, since the extreme narrowing approximation is then valid.[A1, R3] Hence, one might expect that the MR sodium signal obtained using a double quantum filter for erythrocytes in dilute crystalline solutions or for isolated perfused hearts could arise solely from the intracellular sodium. Preliminary reports, however, suggest that the signal obtained in these cases does not only arise from the intracellular compartment but also contains a component arising from extracellular sodium interaction with membrane sites on the cell surface causing biexponential relaxation.[G1, G2, J2–J4] Nevertheless, by use of paramagnetic shift reagents in doses lower than when they are solely employed, the extracellular component to the double quantum signal may be quenched (i.e., made to disappear).[J2–J4] Hence, use of double quantum–filter techniques at least reduces the amount of shift reagents required to only detect intracellular sodium.[J2–J4] Furthermore, changes in the intracellular sodium concentration in a given system also usually alters the double quantum–filtered signal.

Application of double quantum filters for the study of intracellular sodium in intact animals generally also requires additional techniques for spatial interrogation. One such technique, for example, could be the application of double quantum filters through a surface coil. This technique may be shown to have the very useful property of further increasing the spatial selectivity of the surface coil employed.[K2] In fact, the localization characteristics of a double quantum filter are superior to those of other pulse sequences usually employed to increase the spatial selec-

*Multiple quantum filters may usually be constructed by phase cycling manipulations on the pulse sequence 90–J/2–180–J/2–90–S–90-acquire, where J is the creation time and S is the evolution, or by use of pulsed field gradients.[B3, B4] Characteristically, the filters constructed by phase cycling manipulations are relatively insensitive to minor alterations in the phase cycling.[S5] Thus, their filtering characteristics are preserved for variations in the phase cycles of up to about 5 degrees.[S5] On the other hand, multiple quantum filters constructed by the pulsed field gradient techniques are very sensitive to magnetic field inhomogeneities and this may affect the filtering properties of the so-constructed filters.

tivity.[K2] Feasibility studies using double quantum filters in MR imaging and spectroscopy are presently under way in our own and in several other institutions.[C8, G1–G2, K1–K6, P1–P3, S4–S5] In particular, in collaboration with L. Jelinski's group at Bell Laboratories, we have recently succeeded in imaging double quantum transitions containing biologically relevant sodium concentrations in phantoms by use of a double quantum filter.[C8] Two other groups have been successful in performing multiple quantum–filtered sodium imaging for triple quantum transitions. Thus, the group in New Mexico[G1–G2] has carried out triple quantum imaging in a study of tumors implanted in a nude rat model. The group at the National Institutes of Health (NIH),[P3] on the other hand, has performed triple quantum imaging of phantoms at high sodium concentrations (2 molar). At present, we are investigating the potential for imaging double quantum transitions in sodium for the study of cardiac pathology in the rat model. In contrast to nonmoving phantoms or structures at rest, the heart is always beating and blood is always flowing in vivo. However, motion-insensitive pulsed field gradient multiple quantum filters that could be helpful in imaging of the cardiovascular system may be constructed.[K4–K5]

MAGNETIC RESONANCE IMAGING OF SODIUM

There are two main difficulties with the MR imaging of sodium: relatively short tissue relaxation time and relatively low signal-to-noise ratio. Imaging sequences employed in sodium imaging, therefore, should have short spin-echo and repetition times. In order to increase the signal-to-noise ratio, echo generation for signal readout may be carried out by use of 180° radiofrequency pulses or gradient reversal refocusing. However, the spin-echo times obtainable by use of radiofrequency pulses are usually longer than those available using gradient reversal techniques. This is especially important in view of the short relaxation times for sodium in tissue.

To increase the signal-to-noise ratio further, several imaging techniques may be employed: three-dimensional Fourier imaging techniques, prolongation of imaging time, use of surface coils, coherent signal summation of different spin echoes, increase in main magnetic field strength, and decrease of spatial resolution.

Sodium Imaging of the Heart

Techniques employed in the MR imaging of sodium include projection-reconstruction methods, three-dimensional Fourier imaging, hybrid spin-echo pulse sequences for short T_2 imaging, and rotating frame imaging. We next briefly discuss these techniques and their application to sodium imaging in the order in which they were first employed historically for this purpose. Throughout this section cardiac imaging will be emphasized.

PROJECTION-RECONSTRUCTION METHODS. The mathematical foundation of projection-reconstruction methods was first developed by Radon in 1917 in the study of gravitational theory and later employed in MR imaging by Lauterbur in 1973.[M5] It is essentially based on Fourier transformation of the FID (free induction decay) signals that are obtained by rotating a magnetic field gradient with subsequent back projection to determine the spin-density function.[M6]

By use of projection-reconstruction technique, sodium imaging of an isolated perfused beating (rat) heart was first performed in a modified wide-bore spectrometer at 8.45T.[D1] Signals were gated to the heart rate to reduce motion artifacts and were reconstructed from 12 projections, each of which was obtained by averaging 320 free induction decay signals. The image acquisition matrix was 64 × 64, and the data acquisition time for each image was approximately 15 min. Figure 45–3*A* is a diagram of an isolated perfused heart at the midventricular level. The corresponding diastolic sodium image for a perfused beating (rat) heart at the same level is shown in Figure 45–3*B*. The equivalent image in systole is shown in Figure 45–3*C*. Note that the myocardium appears as a negative image, since sodium in the perfusate is actually being visualized.

THREE-DIMENSIONAL FOURIER TECHNIQUES. In three-dimensional Fourier transform techniques, one usually phase-encodes along two orthogonal directions and uses a fixed gradient along the third direction (readout gradient). A frequently employed pulse sequence diagram for three-dimensional sodium imaging is shown in Figure 45–4.[L2] The number of phase-encoding steps may vary but, typically, 40 phase-encoding steps along each phase-encoding direction were performed. Frequently, two echo signals (for example, at spin-echo times of 14 msec and 28 msec) were obtained and coherently added to improve the signal-to-noise ratio. Three-dimensional Fourier transform techniques were first employed for brain imaging in the intact cat[H4] and subsequently performed in humans.[H5]

Three-dimensional Fourier transform techniques also have been employed for sodium nuclear MR imaging ex vivo of myocardial tissue of dogs after coronary artery occlusion and reperfusion.[C18] Data were acquired using 40 phase-encoding steps and 3D Fourier reconstruction on a three-dimensional imager

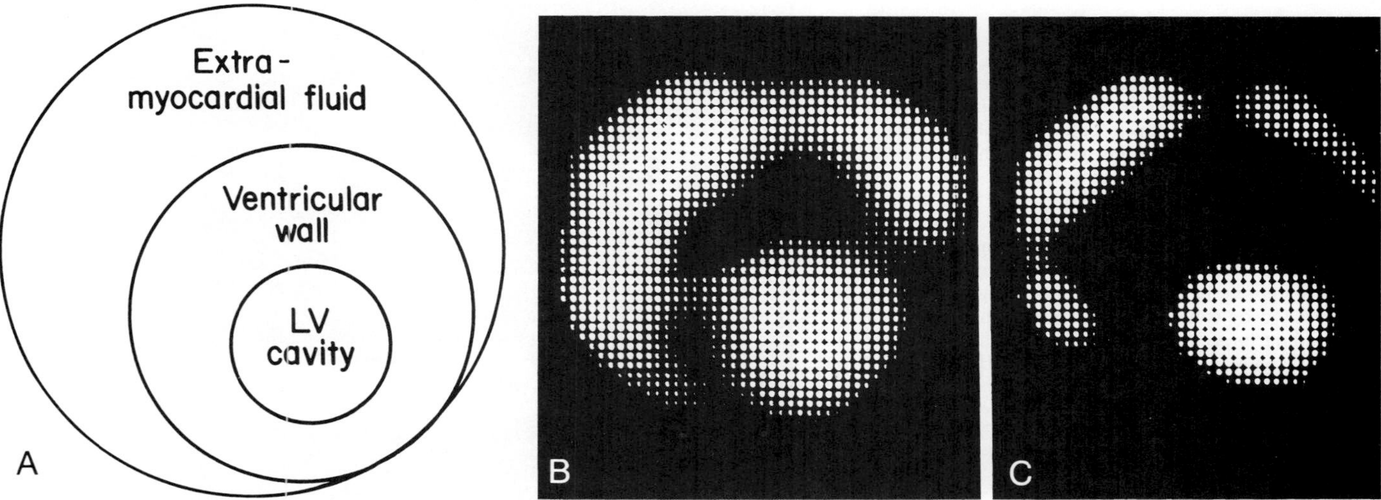

Figure 45–3. *A*, Diagrammatic representation at the midventricular level of an isolated perfused heart. LV—left ventricle. *B*, Gated sodium image at the midventricular level of an isolated perfused rat heart in diastole. *C*, Gated sodium image at the midventricular level of an isolated perfused rat heart in systole. Data in B and C were acquired at 8.45 T. The image acquisition matrix employed was 64 × 64, and the slice thickness was approximately 1.5 mm. Images were reconstructed from 12 projections, and each projection was obtained by averaging 320 free-induction decays. The perfused rat heart is off-center in the sample tube, with the wall of the right ventricle in contact with the wall of the sample tube. (From De Layre, J. L., Ingwall, J. S., Malloy, C., and Fossel, E. T.: Gated sodium-23 nuclear magnetic resonance images of an isolated perfused working rat heart. Science 212:935, 1981.)

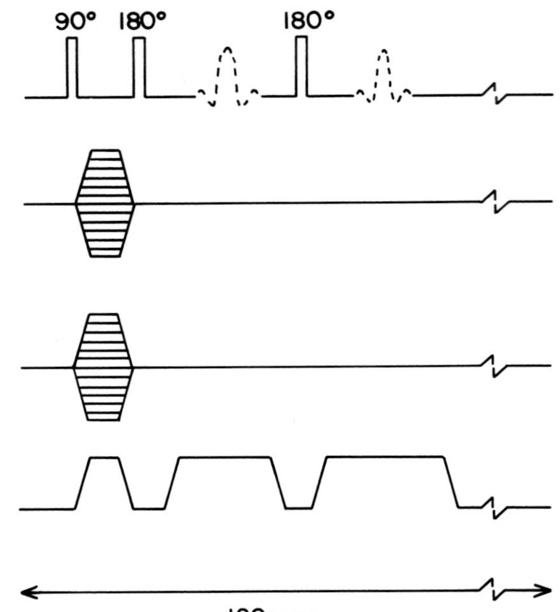

Figure 45–4. Typical pulse sequence diagram for sodium imaging with a three-dimensional Fourier imaging scheme. The numbers of phase encoding steps and signals averaged may vary but frequently are 40 × 40 with 8 averaged signals. The first and second echo times are here chosen at 14 msec and 28 msec, and the repetition time is 120 msec. (From Lee, S. W., Hilal, S. K., and Cho, S. H.: A multinuclear magnetic resonance imaging technique—simultaneous proton and sodium imaging. Magn. Reson. Imaging 4:343, 1986.)

operating at 2.7T. To increase imaging sensitivity, short repetition times of about 100 msec were used. Data acquisition time for each image was 3 to 4 hours. Signals for the first two spin echoes at echo times of 14 and 28 msec were employed and coherently added. Note, however, that for imaging in vivo using this approach, care must be exerted if signals corresponding to different spin echoes are to be added, in view of the different dephasing/rephasing properties between spin echoes in the presence of acceleration.[K7, K8, T2]

Figure 45–5 shows 16 cross-sectional slices of the three-dimensional sodium image of the excised heart of a normal dog. An enlarged transaxial sodium image of a section midway between apex and base is shown in Figure 45–6. Sodium images obtained from a dog subjected to left anterior descending coronary artery occlusion, followed by reperfusion, are shown in Figure 45–7. Note that the sodium signal was significantly greater in tissue in the distribution of the left anterior descending coronary artery distal to the site of occlusion and reperfusion. In Figure 45–8, sodium images of a heart with occlusion and reperfusion of the circumflex coronary artery are shown. Note that the signal intensity was appreciably increased in the posterior and lateral aspects of the myocardium in the distribution of the occluded and subsequently reperfused circumflex coronary artery. Tissue sampling from the hearts verified that the sodium content of tissues in the distribution of the circumflex coronary artery was higher than that in nonischemic tissue perfused by the unoccluded left anterior descending coronary artery.

HYBRID SPIN-ECHO TECHNIQUES. Since intracellular sodium has a transverse relaxation time shorter than that of the extracellular compartment (see Table 45–1), other imaging algorithms have been developed to allow observation of shorter transverse relaxation times. For example, a hybrid spin-echo pulse sequence for imaging shorter transverse relaxation times has been employed.[R6] In this scheme, both projection-reconstruction and Fourier encoding schemes are combined. Slice selection is performed by use of Fourier analysis, and projection-reconstruction is employed for the remaining two orthogonal directions. This technique was first used for the in vivo imaging of the short T_2 component of sodium in the human head.[R6] One of the main advantages of this technique, when compared with usual three-dimensional methods, is the time gain due to Fourier encoding along only one axis. This technique has been used to implement echo times as short as 3.6 msec.

An alternative technique for sodium imaging in vivo and short

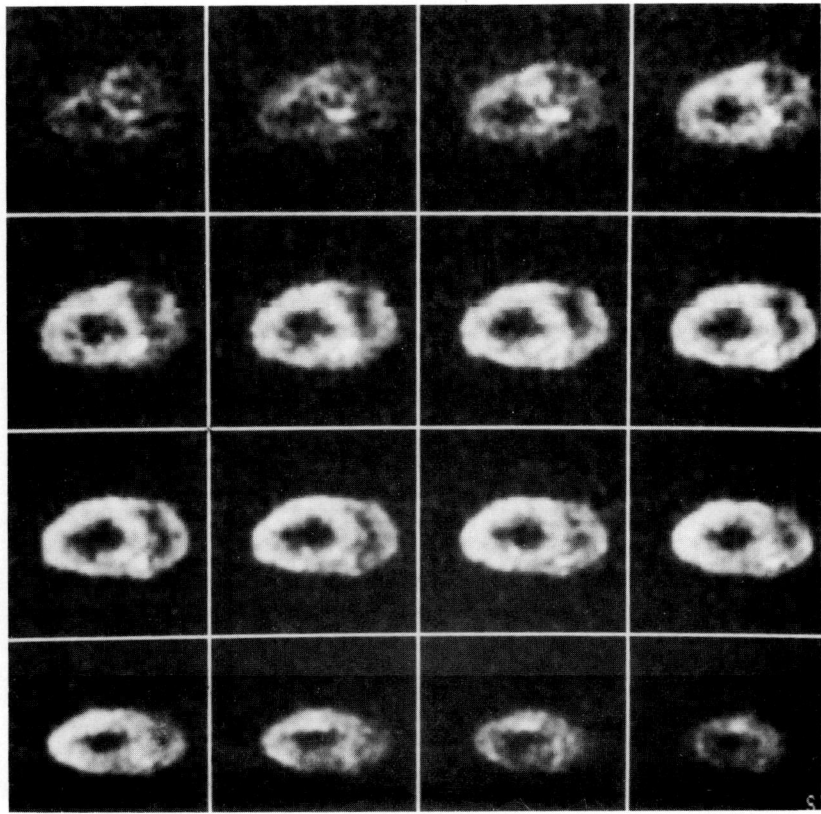

Figure 45–5. Sixteen cross-sectional slices of the three-dimensional sodium image of the excised heart of a normal dog. The frames are arranged sequentially from left to right and from top to bottom so that the base of the heart is in the upper left panel and the apex in the lower right panel. Signals were collected at 2.7T using the pulse sequence cited in Figure 45–4, with first and second spin-echo times of 14 and 28 msec, respectively, a repetition time of about 100 msec, an image acquisition matrix of 40 × 40, increased by zero filling to 64 × 64, and a voxel size of 3 × 3 × 5 mm. Images were then constructed by coherent summation of the signals corresponding to each of the two spin echoes considered. (From Cannon, P. J., Maudsley, A. A., Hilal, S. K., et al.: Sodium nuclear magnetic resonance imaging of myocardial tissue of dogs after coronary artery occlusion and reperfusion. J. Am. Coll. Cardiol. 7:573, 1986.)

Normal Heart

Figure 45–6. Transaxial sodium image at the midventricular level of a normal dog heart. Signals were collected at 2.7T, using the pulse sequence cited in Figure 45–4, with first and second spin-echo times of 14 and 28 msec, respectively, a repetition time of about 100 msec, an image acquisition matrix of 40 × 40 (increased by zero filling to 64 × 64), and a voxel size of 3 × 3 × 5 mm. Images were then constructed by coherent summation of the signals corresponding to each of the two spin echoes considered. (From Cannon, P. J., Maudsley, A. A., Hilal, S. K., et al.: Sodium nuclear magnetic resonance imaging of myocardial tissue of dogs after coronary artery occlusion and reperfusion. J. Am. Coll. Cardiol. 7:573, 1986.)

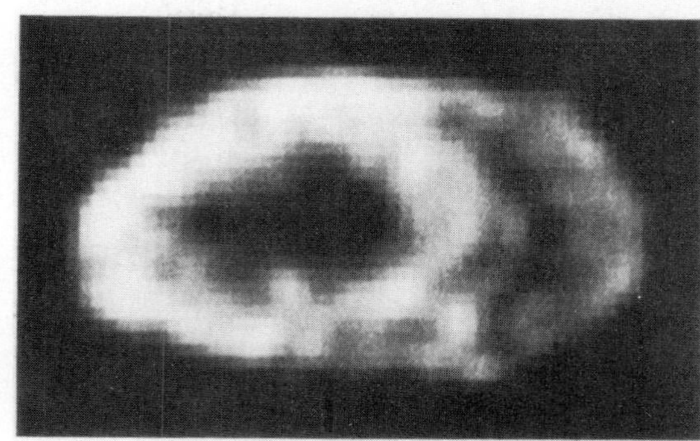

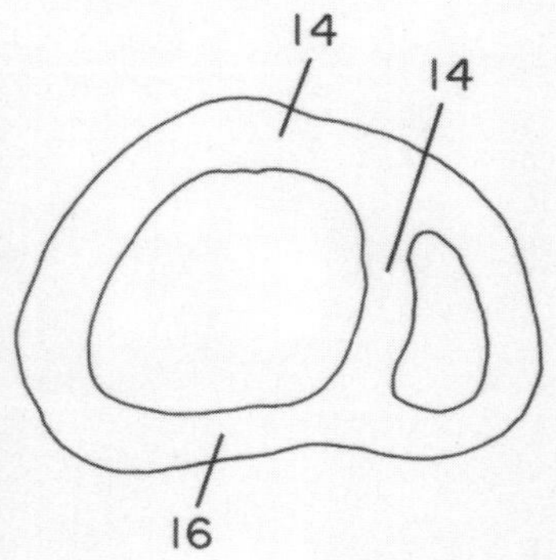

echo times has also been recently developed. It makes use of three-dimensional projection-reconstruction techniques at 1.5T, with a modified head coil and a gradient refocused sequence. In this manner, echo times as short as 2.8 msec have been generated.[S11]

SURFACE COIL TECHNIQUES. Another possible technique for imaging of a short T_2 makes use of three-dimensional projection-reconstruction techniques (assuming as is usually the case that the spin-density distribution function is real) and a specialized radiofrequency coil focused to the region of interest so as to further improve the signal-to-noise ratio. Furthermore, the duration of the applied nonselective 90° radiofrequency pulse (as in Fig. 45–3) and the saturation time of the preamplifier were minimized to decrease the effects of magnetic field inhomogeneity on the free induction decay (FID) image.[R7] In this manner, detection of the short T_2 of sodium was possible. Furthermore, this technique also may be used for the in vivo magnetic resonance imaging of sodium in the human body. Thus, heart, liver, gallbladder, kidney, and spine have also in this manner been successfully imaged in vivo.[R7]

In vivo sodium imaging of the heart in humans by use of the technique described in the preceding paragraph has been per-

Figure 45–7. Sodium images of a dog heart after occlusion and reperfusion of the left anterior descending coronary artery. The frames are arranged sequentially from left to right and from top to bottom with the apex of the heart in the upper left panel and the base in the lower right panel. Signals were collected at 2.7 T using the pulse sequence cited in Figure 45–4, with first and second spin-echo times of 14 and 28 msec respectively, a repetition time of about 100 msec, an image acquisition matrix of 40 × 40 (increased by zero filling to 64 × 64), and a voxel size of 3 mm × 3 mm × 5 mm. Images were then constructed by coherent summation of the signals corresponding to each of the two spin echoes considered. (From Cannon, P. J., Maudsley, A. A., Hilal, S. K., et al.: Sodium nuclear magnetic resonance imaging of myocardial tissue of dogs after coronary artery occlusion and reperfusion. J. Am. Coll. Cardiol. 7:573, 1986.)

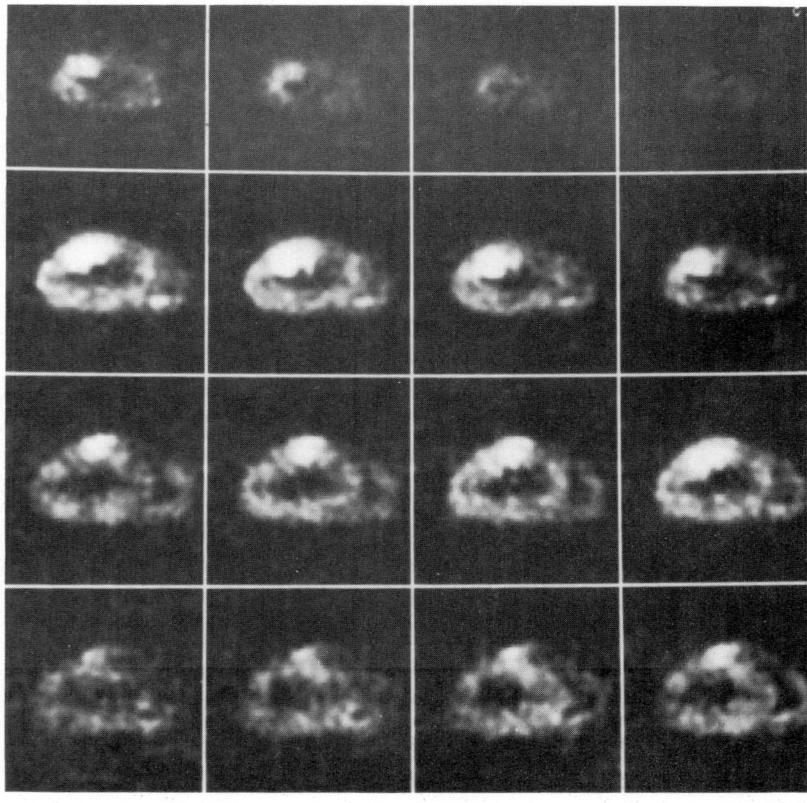

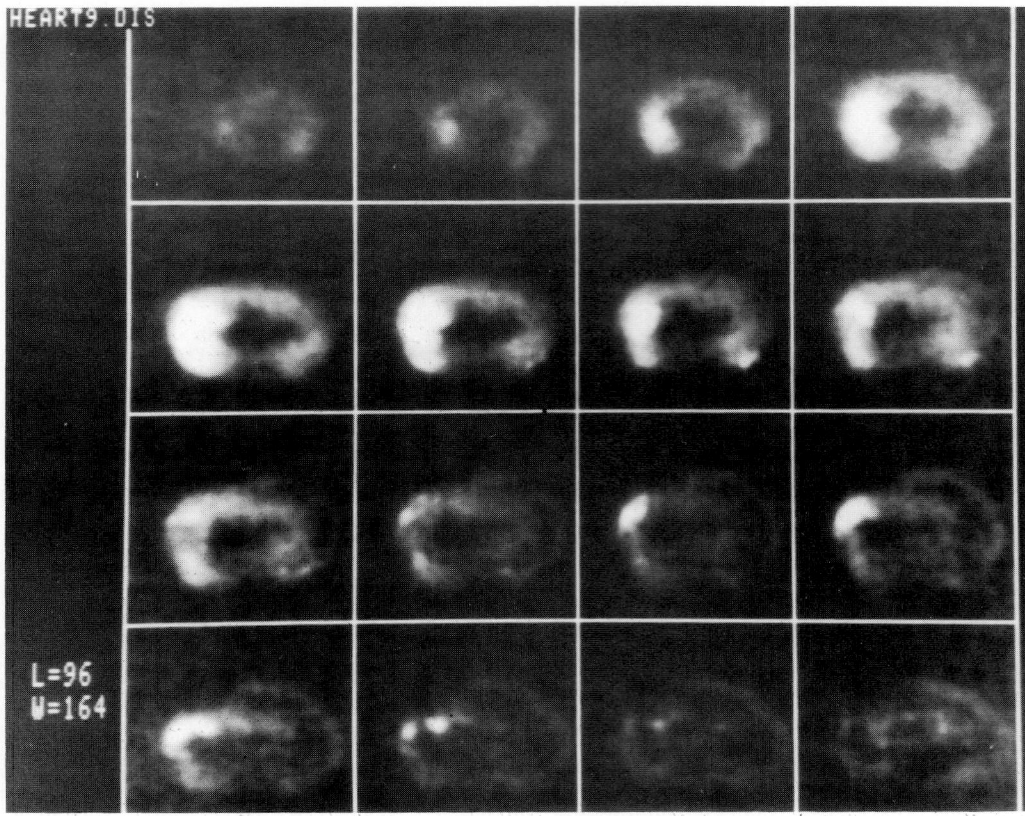

Figure 45–8. Sodium images of a dog heart after occlusion and reperfusion of the circumflex coronary artery. The frames are arranged sequentially from left to right and from top to bottom with the apex in the upper left panel and the base in the lower right panel. Signals were collected at 2.7T using the pulse sequence cited in Figure 45–4, with first and second spin-echo times of 14 and 28 msec, respectively, a repetition time of about 100 msec, an image acquisition matrix of 40 × 40 (increased by zero filling to 64 × 64), and a voxel size of 3 mm × 3 mm × 5 mm. Images were then constructed by coherent summation of the signals corresponding to each of the two spin echoes considered. (From Cannon, P. J., Maudsley, A. A., Hilal, S. K., et al.: Sodium nuclear magnetic resonance imaging of myocardial tissue of dogs after coronary artery occlusion and reperfusion. J. Am. Coll. Cardiol. 7:573, 1986.)

formed on a 1.5T MR imager. Two data acquisition pulses separated from one another by 95 msec on every electrocardiographic beat were employed, and a delay time of 100 msec was used between the R wave and the data acquisition triggering point. Total scanning time was about 70 min. Figure 45–9*A* and 9*B* shows in vivo heart free induction decay axial images of a subject. The corresponding spin-echo images for the same slices at an echo time of 14 msec are shown in Figure 45–9*C* and *D* respectively. The coronal images reconstructed from the same data set are shown in Figure 45–10*A* to *D*.

ROTATING FRAME TECHNIQUE. In principle, sodium imaging may also be performed by use of the rotating frame Fourier technique.[M7] This imaging technique was first proposed in 1979 by Hoult. It is essentially based on superimposing a magnetic field gradient on the excitation field Bl rather than on the main magnetic field Bo. Thus, spatial localization occurs only during the excitation period and is very fast.[M8] Hence, the short time required for spatial encoding in this technique is accomplished with minimal signal intensity losses due to relaxation processes.

Rotating frame imaging of sodium was employed for the one-dimensional spatial localization of sodium absorption in the perfused (rabbit) heart.[M7] A stacked plot of a sodium rotating frame imaging experiment of an isolated perfused rabbit heart is shown

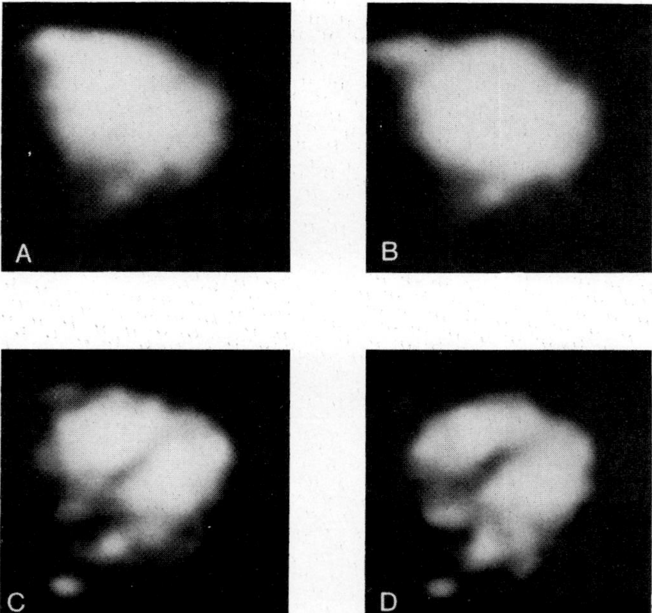

Figure 45–9. *A*, and *B*, In vivo gated transaxial free-induction decay (FID) sodium images of a human heart at two different levels. *C* and *D*, In vivo gated spin-echo images of the human heart in *A* and *B*, corresponding to the same levels as in *A* and *B*. The spin-echo time employed was 14 msec. The images were all acquired at 1.5T, using a projection reconstruction algorithm with a specialized radiofrequency coil focused to the heart. The image matrix was 128 × 128, the time interval between applied pulses on every electrocardiographic beat was 95 msec, and a delay time of 100 msec between R wave and data acquisition triggering point was employed. (From Ra, J. B., Hilal, S. K., and Cho, Z. H.: A method for in vivo MR imaging of the short T_2 component of sodium-23. Magn. Reson. Med. 3:296, 1986.)

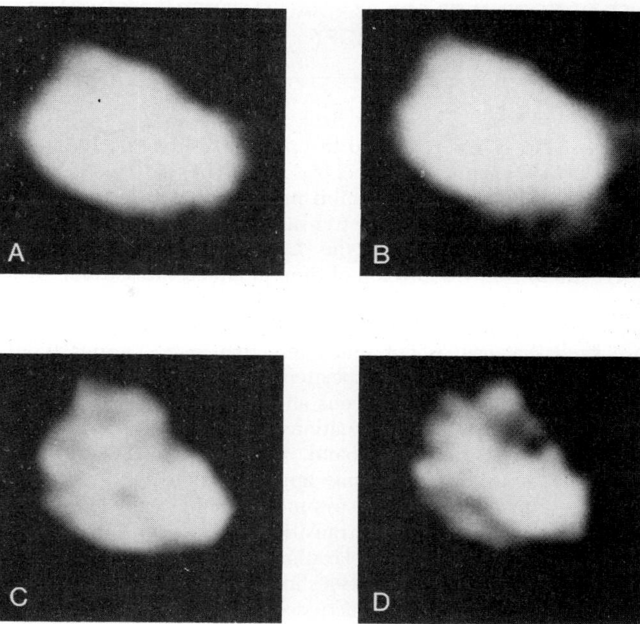

Figure 45–10. *A* and *B*, In vivo gated coronal free-induction decay (FID) sodium images of a human heart at two different levels. *C* and *D*, In vivo gated coronal spin-echo images of the human heart in *A* and *B*, corresponding to the same levels. The spin-echo time employed was 14 msec. Images were acquired at 1.5T, making use of a specialized radiofrequency coil focused to the heart and a projection reconstruction algorithm. The image matrix was 128 × 128, the time interval between applied pulses on every electrocardiographic beat was 95 msec, and a delay time of 100 msec between R wave and data acquisition triggering point was employed.

in Figure 45–11. The data were acquired as 16 datasets, using an increment of 80 msec and a total acquisition time of 12 msec. The spatial resolution used was about 2 mm.

Use of Contrast Agents

To increase the sensitivity and specificity of sodium magnetic resonance imaging, one would expect that contrast agents might also be helpful for this purpose, just as for proton imaging. The use of contrast agents in the study of sodium imaging of rat tumors has, in fact, been investigated.[S12] Although one might also expect that contrast agents could be valuable in sodium imaging of myocardial ischemia, this problem has not yet been addressed.

One approach to the study of contrast agents in proton imaging has been the use of paramagnetic substances, such as gadolinium.[B7, B8, R8, W3] Although Gd-DTPA (gadolinium-diethylene-triamine-penta-acetic acid) is a useful contrast agent in proton imaging, much larger doses are necessary to produce useful contrast in sodium imaging.[S12] Furthermore, the half-life of Gd-DTPA is about 20 minutes, so that continuous infusion during a scan is necessary.

On the other hand, from proton nuclear MR it is known that ferromagnetic and superparamagnetic materials have a strong effect on transverse tissue relaxation times, even when small doses are used.[R9, S13, S14] One superparamagnetic agent, dextran-magnetite, has been investigated in sodium imaging and found to decrease transverse tissue relaxation times much more than paramagnetic compounds like Gd-DTPA.[S12] In addition, it has also been found that dextran-magnetite had a longer half-life in blood than Gd-DTPA. Thus, continuous infusion of the dextran-magnetite during a scan was unnecessary. Just as for proton imaging, dextran-magnetite also increased the contrast between tumor and surrounding soft tissue in the sodium images, since magnetic particles are taken up mostly by the reticuloendothelial system and only slightly by tumors. Hence, contrast agents, and in particular dextran-magnetite, also may be useful in sodium imaging for tumor detection and, perhaps, for a variety of other pathophysiologic problems in which contrast between tissues with different characteristics needs to be highlighted.[S12] Furthermore, as mentioned at the beginning of this section, contrast agents also may be helpful in the study of sodium imaging of myocardial ischemia, although this problem has not yet been investigated.

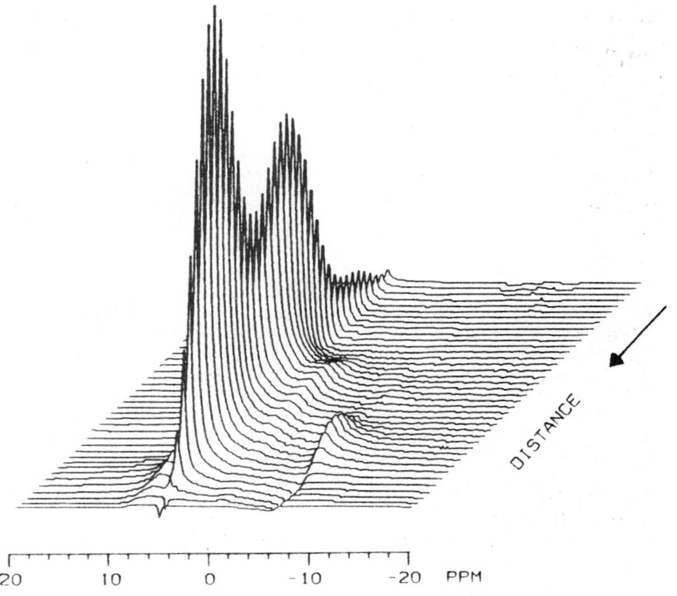

Figure 45–11. Stacked plot of a sodium rotating frame imaging experiment of a perfused rabbit heart after 1 hour of hypoxic, potassium-free perfusion. The x axis shows the chemical shift in parts per million (ppm). The orthogonal axis, labeled distance, shows the spatial dimension. The excised rabbit heart was perfused in a regular 25-mm NMR tube while centered in the receiver coil along the axis of the surface coil. The heart was oriented with its septum nearly parallel to the plane of the surface coil, with the left ventricle nearest to this coil. Data were acquired at 4.7T as 16 datasets using an increment of 80 sec. Resolution in the spatial dimension is about 2 mm. (From Moonen, C. T. W., Anderson, S. E., and Unger, S.: Na rotating frame imaging in the perfused rabbit heart using separate transmitter and receiver coils. Magn. Reson. Med. 5:296, 1987.)

SUMMARY

This chapter has reviewed the present status of sodium-23 for cardiac MR imaging and spectroscopy. The sodium nucleus, in view of its 3/2 spin, may exhibit multiple quantum transitions in addition to single quantum transitions. Multiple quantum transitions may occur only if the Larmor frequency ω_o and the correlation time τ_c (duration of time in which the sodium nucleus remains in a given position and orientation within an electric field gradient, i.e., degree of ordering of the sodium environment) are such that $\omega_o\tau_c$ is not much less than one. Various types of sodium spectra may be associated with this condition, namely crystal-like and inhomogeneous and homogeneous powder spectra. Thus, in any of these situations multiple quantum transitions may occur. On the other hand, for sodium in dilute aqueous solutions (extreme narrowing approximation), $\omega_o\tau_c << 1$, the transverse magnetization decays monoexponentially and, furthermore, only single quantum transitions may occur.

The transverse tissue relaxation time of sodium is usually multiexponential and exhibits a short component. Hence, sodium may be invisible to MR spectroscopy under certain conditions. Possible factors that could account for the enormous variability in the available data regarding the precise amount of invisibility include the MR equipment employed and its resolution characteristics, differences in magnetic field strength, temperature, tissues considered, and tissue preparation. Furthermore, invisibility depends not only on the correlation time but also on the type of MR acquisition employed, i.e., sodium that is invisible to single quantum acquisitions may become visible when double quantum acquisitions are used.

Previously employed techniques for sodium imaging of the heart both ex vivo and in vivo have been presented. These include projection reconstruction methods as well as three-dimensional Fourier, hybrid spin echo, surface coil, and rotating frame techniques. Approaches for imaging intracellular sodium, such as the use of paramagnetic shift reagents along with their potential toxicity, have been reviewed. An alternative approach for the study of image intracellular sodium currently under investigation has also been reviewed, i.e., the use of double quantum filters.

It is apparent that sodium MR imaging is still in its embryonic stages, not yet at the same level as proton MR imaging. Nevertheless, definite progress is being made in the development of sodium MR imaging to allow us to quantify the global and regional intracellular concentration of sodium in the heart and other organs.

References

A

1. Abragam, A.: Principles of Nuclear Magnetism. Clarendon Press, Oxford, England, 1961.

B

1. Braunwald, E., and Kloner, R. A.: The stunned myocardium: Prolonged postischemic ventricular dysfunction. Circulation 66:1146, 1982.
2. Berendsen, H. J. C., and Edzes, H. T.: The observation and general interpretation of sodium magnetic resonance in biological material. Ann. N.Y. Acad. Sci. 204:459, 1973.
3. Bodenhausen, G., Vold, R. L., and Vold, R. R.: Multiple quantum spin-echo spectroscopy. J. Magn. Reson. 37:93, 1980.
4. Bax, A., DeJong, P. G., Mehlkopf, A. F., and Smidt, J.: Separation of the different orders of NMR multiple-quantum transitions by the use of pulsed field gradients. Chem. Phys. Lett. 69:567, 1980.
5. Burstein, D., and Fossel, E. T.: Intracellular sodium and lithium NMR relaxation times in the perfused frog heart. Magn. Reson. Med. 4:261, 1987.
6. Burstein, D., and Mattingly, M.: Magnetic resonance imaging of intracellular sodium. J. Magn. Reson. 83:197, 1989.
7. Brasch, R. C. H., Weinmann, H. J., and Wesley, G. E.: Contrast-enhanced NMR imaging: Animal studies using gadolinium-DTPA complex. A.J.R. 142:625, 1984.
8. Brown, J. J., and Higgins, C. B.: Myocardial paramagnetic contrast agents for MR imaging. A.J.R. 151:865, 1988.

C

1. Carmeliet, E., and Vereecke, S.: Electrogenesis of the action potential and automaticity. *In* Berne, R. M., Sperelakis, N., and Geiger, S. R. (eds.): Handbook of Physiology, Section 2. The Cardiovascular System, Vol. 1. Williams and Wilkins, Baltimore, 1979, p. 269.
2. Cranefield, P. F.: The Conduction of the Cardiac Impulse; The Slow Response and Cardiac Arrhythmias. Futura Publishing Company, Mt. Kisco, N.Y., 1975.
3. Cameron, I. L., Smith, N. K. R., Pool, T. B., and Sparks, R. L.: Intracellular concentration of sodium and other elements as related to mitogenesis and oncogenesis in vivo. Cancer Res. 40:1493, 1980.
4. Cone, C. D., Jr.: Maintenance of mitotic homeostasis in somatic cell populations. J. Theoret. Biol. 30:183, 1971.
5. Cone, C. D., Jr.: The role of the surface electrical transmembrane potential in normal and malignant mitogenesis. Ann. N.Y. Acad. Sci. 238:420, 1971.
6. Cone, C. D., Jr., and Cone, C. M.: Evidence of normal mitosis with complete cytokinesis in central nervous system neurons during sustained depolarization with ouabain. Exp. Neurol. 60:41, 1978.
7. Cone, C. D., Jr., and Tongier, M., Jr.: Control of somatic cell mitosis by simulated changes in the transmembrane potential level. Oncology (Basel) 25:168, 1971.
8. Cockman, M. D., Jelinski, L. W., Katz, J., et al.: Double-quantum-filtered sodium imaging. J. Magn. Reson. 1990 (in press).
9. Cope, F. W.: NMR evidence for complexing of Na^+ in muscle, kidney, and brain, and by actomyosin. The relation of cellular complexing of Na^+ to water structure and to transport kinetics. J. Gen. Physiol. 50:1353, 1967.
10. Czeisler, J. L., Fritz, O. G., Jr., and Swift, T. J.: Direct evidence from nuclear magnetic resonance studies for bound sodium in frog skeletal muscle. Biophys. J. 10:260, 1970.
11. Cope, F. W.: Spin-echo nuclear magnetic resonance evidence for complexing of sodium ions in muscle, brain, and kidney. Biophys. J. 10:843, 1970.
12. Civan, M. M., Degani, H., Margalit, Y., and Shporer, M.: Observations of ^{23}Na in frog skin by NMR. Am. J. Physiol. 245:C213, 1985.
13. Chang, D. C., and Woessner, D. E.: Spin-echo study of ^{23}Na relaxation in skeletal muscle. Evidence of sodium ion binding inside a biological cell. J. Magnet. Reson. 30:185, 1978.
14. Civan, M. M., and Shporer, M.: NMR of sodium-23 and potassium-39 in biological systems. *In* Berliner, L. J., and Rensen, J. (eds.): Biological Magnetic Resonance, Vol. 1. Plenum Publishing Corporation, New York, 1978, p 1.
15. Cope, F. W.: Nuclear magnetic resonance evidence for complexing of sodium ions in muscle. Proc. Natl. Acad. Sci. USA 54:225, 1965.
16. Chu, S. C., Pike, M. M., Fossel, E. T., et al.: Aqueous shift reagents for high-resolution cationic nuclear magnetic resonance. III. Dy $(TTHA)^{3-}$, $Tm(TTHA)^{3-}$, and Tm $(PPP)_2^{7-}$. J. Magn. Reson. 56:33, 1984.
17. Chapman, R. A.: Control of cardiac contractility at the cellular level. Am. J. Physiol. 245:M535, 1983.
18. Cannon, P. J., Maudsley, A. A., Hilal, S. K., et al.: Sodium nuclear magnetic resonance imaging of myocardial tissue of dogs after coronary artery occlusion and reperfusion. J. Am. Coll. Cardiol. 7:573, 1986.

D

1. De Layre, J. L., Ingwall, J. S., Malloy, C., and Fossel, E. T.: Gated sodium-23 nuclear magnetic resonance images of an isolated perfused working rat heart. Science 212:935, 1981.

E

1. Edzes, H. T., and Berendsen, H. J. C.: The physical state of diffusible ions in cells. Annu. Rev. Biophys. Bioeng. 4:265, 1975.

F

1. Fozzard, H. A.: Cardiac muscle: Excitability and passive electrical properties. Prog. Cardiovasc. Dis. 19:343, 1977.

G

1. Griffey, R. H., Griffey, B., Berghmans, K., et al.: Sodium multiple quantum spectroscopy and imaging of tumor cells implanted in nude rats and in cell suspensions. Abstr. Soc. Magnet. Reson. Med. 1:213, 1988.
2. Griffey, R. H., Griffey, B. V., and Matwiyoff, N. A.: Triple-quantum-coherence-filtered imaging of sodium ions in vivo at 4.7 Tesla. Magn. Reson. Med. 13:305, 1990.
3. Gullans, S. R., Avison, M. J., Ogino, T., et al.: NMR measurements of intracellular sodium in the rabbit proximal tubule. Am. J. Physiol. 249:F160, 1985.
4. Gupta, R. K., and Gupta, P.: Direct observation of resolved resonances from intra- and extracellular sodium-23 ions in NMR studies of intact cells using dysprosium (III) tripolyphosphate as paramagnetic shift reagent. J. Magn. Reson. 47:344, 1982.

H

1. Hodgkin, A. L.: The ionic basis of electrical activity in nerve and muscle. Biol. Rev. 26:339, 1951.
2. Hoatson, G. L., and Packer, K. J.: The creation, interconversion and observation of states of zero, single- and double quantum order in the NMR

spectroscopy of spin-1 nuclei using non-selective r.f. pulses. Mol. Phys. 40:1153, 1980.

3. Hoult, D. I., and Richards, R. E.: The signal-to-noise ratio of the nuclear magnetic resonance experiment. J. Magnet. Reson. 24:71, 1976.
4. Hilal, S. K., Maudsley, A. A., Simon, H. E., et al.: In vivo NMR imaging of tissue sodium in the intact cat before and after acute cerebral stroke. Am. J. Neuroradiol. 4:245, 1983.
5. Hilal, S. K., Maudsley, A. A., Ra, J. B., et al.: In vivo NMR imaging of sodium 23 in the human head. J. Comput. Assist. Tomogr. (1):1–7, 1985.
6. Hilal, S. K., Maudsley, A. A., Ra, J. B., et al.: In vivo NMR imaging of sodium-23 in the human head. J. Comput. Assist. Tomog. 9:1, 1985.

J

1. Jaccard, G., Wimperis, S., and Bodenhausen, G.: Multiple-quantum NMR spectroscopy of S = 3/2 spin in isotropic phase. A new probe for multiexponential relaxation. J. Chem. Phys. 85:6282, 1986.
2. Jelichs, L. A., and Gupta, R. K.: Double-quantum NMR of sodium ions in cells and tissues. Paramagnetic quenching of extracellular coherence. J. Magn. Reson. 81:586, 1989.
3. Jelichs, L. A., and Gupta, R. K. Observation of intracellular sodium ions by double-quantum filtered ^{23}Na NMR with paramagnetic quenching of extracellular coherence by gadolinium triphosphate. J. Magn. Reson. 83:146, 1989.
4. Joseph, P. M., and Summers, R. M.: The flip-angle effect: A method for detection of sodium-23 quadrupole splitting in tissue. Magn. Reson. Med. 4:67, 1987.

K

1. Keller, A. M., Sorce, D. J., and Cannon, P. J.: Monitoring myocardial intracellular sodium without a shift reagent using double quantum magnetic resonance spectroscopy. Circulation 78(II):495, 1988.
2. Katz, J., Keller, A. M., Sciacca, R. R., et al.: Flip angle dependence of double quantum filters: The potential for enhanced spatial selectivity and localization. Abstr Soc. Magn. Reson. Med. 2:625, 1989.
3. Keller, A. M., Sorce, D. J., Katz, J., et al.: Sodium invisibility in magnetic resonance spectroscopy: Significant differences between single and double quantum filtered acquisitions. Abstr. Soc. Magn. Reson. Med. 2:502, 1989.
4. Katz, J., Sorce, D. J., Boxt, L. M., et al.: Abstr. Soc. Magn. Reson. Imaging 40, 1990 (in press).
5. Katz, J., Score, D. J., Boxt, L. M., et al.: Abstr. Soc. Magn. Reson. Med. 1990 (in press).
6. Kennedy, D. N., Pearlman, J. D., and Rosen, B. R.: Nth order multiple quantum imaging. Abstr. Soc. Magn. Reson. Med. 2:940, 1988.
7. Katz, J., Peshock, R. M., McNamee, P. M., et al.: Analysis of spin echo rephasing with pulsatile flow in 2DFT magnetic resonance imaging. Magn. Reson. Med. 4:307, 1987.
8. Katz, J., Peshock, R. M., Malloy, C. R., et al.: Even-echo rephasing and constant velocity flow. Magn. Reson. Med. 4:422, 1987.

L

1. Lyon, R. C., Pekar, J., Moonen, C. T. W., et al.: Double-quantum surface-coil NMR studies of sodium and potassium in the rat brain. Magn. Reson. Med., 1990 (in press).
2. Lee, S. W., Hilal, S. K., and Cho, Z. H.: A multinuclear magnetic resonance imaging technique—simultaneous proton and sodium imaging. Magnet. Reson. Imag. 4:343, 1986.

M

1. Mullins, L. J.: Ion Transport in Heart. Raven Press, New York, 1981.
2. Mandel, W. J. (ed.): Cardiac Arrhythmias: Their Mechanisms, Diagnosis, and Management. J. B. Lippincott, Philadelphia, 1987, p. 199.
3. Magnuson, H. S., and Magnuson, J. A.: $^{23}Na^+$ interaction with bacterial surfaces: A comment on nuclear magnetic resonance invisible signals. Biophys. J. 13:1117, 1973.
4. Martinez, D., Silvidi, A. A., and Stokes, R. M.: Nuclear magnetic resonance studies of sodium ions in isolated frog muscle and liver. Biophys. J. 9:1256, 1969.
5. Morris, P. G.: Nuclear Magnetic Resonance Imaging in Medicine and Biology. Clarendon Press, Oxford, England, 1986, p. 123.
6. Ibid., p 122.
7. Moonen, C. T. W., Anderson, S. E., and Unger, S.: Na rotating frame imaging in the perfused rabbit heart using separate transmitter and receiver coils. Magn. Reson. Med. 5:296, 1987.
8. Morris, P. G.: Nuclear Magnetic Resonance Imaging in Medicine and Biology. Clarendon Press, Oxford, England, 1986, p. 174.

N

1. Noble, D.: The Initiation of the Heart Beat. Oxford, Clarendon Press, 1979.
2. Noble, D.: The surprising heart: A review of recent progress in cardiac electrophysiology. J. Physiol. 353:1, 1984.

O

1. Ogino, T., Shulman, G. I., Avison, M. J., et al.: ^{23}Na and ^{39}K NMR studies of ion transport in human erythrocytes. Proc. Natl. Acad. Sci. USA 82:1099, 1985.
2. Ogino, T., den Hollander, J. A., and Schulman, R. G.: ^{39}K, ^{23}Na, and ^{31}P NMR studies of ion transport in *Saccharomyces cerevisiae*. Proc. Natl. Acad. Sci. USA 80:5185, 1983.

P

1. Pekar, J., and Leigh, J. S., Jr.: Detection of biexponential relaxation in sodium-23 facilitated by double-quantum filtering. J. Magn. Reson. 69:582, 1986.
2. Pekar, J., Renshaw, P. F., and Leigh, J. S.: Selective detection of intracellular sodium by coherence-transfer NMR. J. Magn. Reson. 72:159, 1987.
3. Pekar, J., Moonen, C. T. W., and Hoult, D. I.: Three-quantum imaging of sodium-23. Abstr. Soc. Magn. Reson. Med. 2:670, 1989.
4. Pike, M. M., Frazer, J. C., Dedrick, D. F., et al.: ^{23}Na and ^{39}K nuclear magnetic resonance studies of perfused rat hearts. Discrimination of intra- and extracellular ions using a shift reagent. Biophys. J. 48:159, 1985.
5. Pettegrew, J. W., Waessner, D. E., Minshew, N. J., and Glonek, T.: Sodium-23 NMR analysis of human whole blood, erythrocytes, and plasma. Chemical shift, spin relaxation, and intracellular sodium concentration studies. J. Magn. Reson. 57:185, 1984.
6. Pike, M. M., Fossel, E. T., Smith, T. W., and Springer, C. S., Jr.: High-resolution Na-NMR studies of human erythrocytes. Use of aqueous shift reagents. Am. J. Physiol. 246:C528, 1984.
7. Perman, W. H., Turski, P. A., Houston, L. W., et al.: Methodology of in vivo human sodium MR imaging at 1.5T. Radiology 160:811, 1986.
8. Pike, M. M., and Springer, C. S.: Aqueous shift reagents for high-resolution cationic nuclear magnetic resonance. J. Magn. Reson. 46:348, 1982.

R

1. Reuter, H.: The dependence of slow inward current in Purkinje fibers on the extracellular calcium concentration. J. Physiol. 192:479, 1967.
2. Reuter, H.: Properties of two inward membrane currents. Annu. Rev. Physiol. 41:413, 1979.
3. Rooney, W. D., Barbara, T. M., and Springer, C. S., Jr.: Two-dimensional double-quantum NMR spectroscopy of isolated spin 3/2 systems: ^{23}Na examples. J. Am. Chem. Soc. 110:674, 1988.
4. Reisin, L. L., Rotunno, C. A., Corchs, L., et al.: The state of sodium in epithelial tissues as studied by nuclear magnetic resonance. Physiol. Chem. Phys. 2:171, 1970.
5. Rotunno, C. A., Kowalewski, V., and Cereijido, M.: Nuclear spin resonance evidence for complexing of sodium in frog skin. Biochim. Biophys. Acta 135:170, 1967.
6. Ra, J. B., Hilal, S. K., and Cho, Z. H.: A method for in vivo MR imaging of the short T_2 component of sodium-23. Magn. Reson. Med. 3:296, 1986.
7. Ra, J. B., Hilal, S. K., Oh, C. H., and Mun, I. K.: In vivo magnetic resonance imaging of sodium in the human body. Magn. Reson. Med. 7:11, 1988.
8. Runge, V. M., Clauton, J. A., Lukehart, C. M., et al.: Paramagnetic agents for contrast-enhanced NMR imaging: A review. A.J.R. 141:1209, 1983.
9. Renshaw, P. F., Owen, C. S., McLaughlin, A. C., et al.: Ferromagnetic contrast agents: A new approach. Magn. Reson. Med. 3:217, 1986.

S

1. Sperelakis, N.: Origin of the cardiac resting potential. *In* Berne, R. M., Sperelakis, N., and Geiger, S. R. (eds.): Handbook of Physiology, Section 2. The Cardiovascular System, Vol. 1. Williams and Wilkins, Baltimore, 1979, p. 187.
2. Sperelakis, N.: Electrical properties of cells at rest and maintenance of the ion distribution. *In* Sperelakis, N. (ed.): Physiology and Pathophysiology of the Heart. Martinus Nijhoff, Boston, 1984, p. 59.
3. Springer, C. S., Jr.: Measurement of metal cation compartmentalization in tissue by high-resolution metal cation NMR. Annu. Rev. Biophys. Bioeng. 16:375, 1987.
4. Sorce, D. J., Keller, A. M., and Cannon, P. J.: Monitoring myocardial intracellular sodium using double quantum magnetic resonance spectroscopy without the use of shift reagent. Abstr. Soc. Magn. Reson. Med. (works in progress), 162, 1988.
5. Sorce, D. J., Katz, J., Sciacca, R. R., et al.: Characteristics of multiple quantum filters for arbitrary phase angles. Abstr. Soc. Magn. Reson. Med., 1990 (in press).
6. Sanctuary, B. C., Halstead, T. K., and Osment, P. A.: Multipole NMR. IV. Dynamics of single spins. Molec. Phys. 49:753, 1983.
7. Shporer, M., and Civan, M. M.: The state of water and alkali cations within the intracellular fluids: The contribution of NMR spectroscopy. Curr. Topics Membr. Transp. 9:1, 1977.
8. Shporer, M., and Civan, M. M.: Effects of temperature and field strength on the NMR relaxation times of ^{23}Na in frog striated muscle. Biochim. Biophys. Acta 354:291, 1974.
9. Shinar, H., and Navon, G.: Sodium-23 NMR relaxation time in body fluids. Magnet. Reson. Med. 3:927, 1986.
10. Shinar, H., and Navon, G.: Relaxation time measurements of alkali metal ions in red blood cells, serum and plasma. Abstr. Soc. Magn. Reson. Med. 2:333, 1986.
11. Simon, H. E., Roschman, P., and Saner, M.: Sodium imaging with short echo times at 1.5 T with a modified head coil. Abstr. Soc. Magn. Reson. Med. 2:593, 1988.
12. Summers, R. M., Joseph, P. M., Renshaw, P. F., and Kundel, H. L.: Dextran-magnetite: A contrast agent for sodium-23 MRI. Magn. Reson. Med. 8:427, 1988.
13. Saini, S., Stark, D. D., Hahn, P. F., et al.: Ferrite particles: A superparamagnetic MR contrast agent for the reticulo-endothelial system. Radiology 162:211, 1987.

14. Saini, S., Stark, D. D., Hahn, P. F., et al.: Ferrite particles: A superparamagnetic MR contrast agent for enhanced detection of liver carcinoma. Radiology 167:217, 1987.

T

1. Trautwein, W.: Membrane currents in cardiac muscle fibers. Physiol. Rev. 53:793, 1973.
2. Twieg, D., Katz, J., and Peshock, R. M.: A general treatment of imaging with chemical shifts and motion. Magn. Reson. Med. 5:32, 1987.

W

1. Wokaun, A., and Ernst, R. R.: Selective detection of multiple quantum transitions in NMR by two-dimensional spectroscopy. Chem. Phys. Lett. 52:407, 1977.
2. Wittenberg, B. A., and Gupta, R. K.: NMR studies of intracellular sodium ions in mammalian cardiac myocytes. J. Biol. Chem. 260:2031, 1985.
3. Weinmann, H. J., Brasch, R. C., Press, W. R., and Wesley, G. E.: Characteristics of gadolinium-DTPA complex: A potential NMR contrast agent. A.J.R. 142:619, 1984.

Y

1. Yeh, H. J. C., Brinley, F. J., Jr., and Becker, E. D.: Nuclear magnetic resonance studies on intracellular sodium in human erythrocytes and frog muscle. Biophys. J. 13:56, 1973.

Z

1. Zipes, D. P., Bailey, J. C., and Elharrar, V. (eds.): The Slow Inward Current and Cardiac Arrhythmias. Martinus Nijhoff, Boston, 1980.

Chapter 46

Magnetic Resonance Spectroscopy to Study Myocardial Metabolism and Cellular Function

- *MARY D. OSBAKKEN, M.D., Ph.D.*
- *MATTHEW D. MITCHELL, B.A.*

WHAT IS MAGNETIC RESONANCE SPECTROSCOPY? 841
METHODS FOR DATA COLLECTION AND QUANTIFICATION OF MYOCARDIAL METABOLITES 843
THE MAGNETIC RESONANCE SPECTROSCOPY SURFACE COIL 843
BACKGROUND AND RATIONALE FOR USE OF IN VIVO MAGNETIC RESONANCE SPECTROSCOPY TECHNIQUES 844
METHODS USED TO OBTAIN IN VIVO MAGNETIC RESONANCE SPECTROSCOPY DATA 844
NUCLEI OF INTEREST 845
^{31}P Magnetic Resonance Spectroscopy: General Information 845
Use of ^{31}P Magnetic Resonance Spectroscopy to Study Potential Myocardial Metabolic Regulators 845
Correlation of Cardiac Work with Myocardial Metabolism 846
Review of Types of Studies with ^{31}P Magnetic Resonance Spectroscopy 846
Carbon (^{13}C) Magnetic Resonance Spectroscopy 851
Proton (^{1}H) Magnetic Resonance Spectroscopy 854
Sodium (^{23}Na) and Potassium (^{39}K) Magnetic Resonance Spectroscopy 856
Pathology as Seen by Abnormalities in Sodium Metabolism 856
Sodium (^{23}Na) Magnetic Resonance Spectroscopy 856
Shift Reagent Techniques 856
Shift Reagent Applications 857
Relaxation Deconvolution 857
Multiple Quantum Spectroscopy 858
Potassium (^{39}K) Magnetic Resonance Spectroscopy 858
Fluorine (^{19}F) Magnetic Resonance Spectroscopy 858
Deuterium (^{2}H) Magnetic Resonance Spectroscopy 858
POTENTIAL CLINICAL USES 858
CONCLUSION 859

The body has many magnetic properties, including movement of charged particles in flowing blood, movement of ions across membranes, and different chemical compounds based on intrinsic nuclear spin or electron spin magnetism. Recently, scientists have begun to use these magnetic properties to investigate physiologic and biochemical phenomena. Electromagnetic flow meters are used to measure blood flow to different organs. The magnetic properties of the hydrogen nucleus of water are used for imaging (magnetic resonance imaging, MRI). Magnetic resonance spectroscopy (MRS), which measures the magnetic properties of the nuclei of various elements, has been used to investigate and measure biochemical (bioenergetics) and cellular (ion transport across membranes) functions in intact organs and organisms.

To date, several nuclear species have been used in this regard: phosphorus (^{31}P) MRS has been used to measure pH and to study high-energy phosphate bioenergetics. Carbon (^{13}C) MRS has been used to study flux through the citric acid cycle. Proton (^{1}H) MRS has been used to study redox state and metabolite changes under different physiologic conditions. Fluorine (^{19}F) MRS has been used as a marker of blood flow and calcium ion movement in the cellular milieu; sodium and potassium (^{23}Na and ^{39}K) MRS have been used to measure ion movement across membranes; deuterium (^{2}H) MRS has been used to measure blood flow; and lithium (^{6}Li and ^{7}Li) MRS has been used to study brain concentration and location of this element, which is used to treat patients with manic-depressive episodes. All these techniques depend on the measurement of the magnetic properties of the nucleus of the respective element, which vary with its chemical environment. This chapter discusses basic magnetic resonance spectroscopy principles and its uses and potential uses in modern biology and clinical medicine.

WHAT IS MAGNETIC RESONANCE SPECTROSCOPY?

Nuclei of some elements possess magnetic moments that result from the motion of charged subnuclear particles as the nucleus spins around its axis.[D1, G1, H1, O1, P1, S1] Only nuclei that have uneven numbers of protons or neutrons have a net nuclear spin. The magnetic field caused by nearby electrons influences the nuclear magnetism, and thus the magnetic properties of the nucleus provide information concerning the surrounding chemical environment (contribution to chemical shift, which will be discussed later).

From an external microscopic viewpoint, each volume of tissue in a magnetic field possesses a magnetic dipole of magnitude $\mathbf{M_0}$, which is a net vector sum of all the component nuclei. In their natural environment, the individual nuclear magnetic moments have a random direction, and the resultant vector is zero. Placement of nuclei with nuclear magnetic moments into a homogeneous magnetic field causes them to be polarized, with production of a nuclear magnetization aligned along the direction of the external field. When the system is at equilibrium, the net magnetic moment of each volume of tissue is proportional to the applied magnetic field and to the total number of nuclei present. This phenomenon can be described as follows:

$$M = M_z = k\ N\ B_0,$$

where $\mathbf{B_0}$ is the size of the applied field; **M** is the total magnetic moment; M_z is the net component along Z, which by convention is the direction of $\mathbf{B_0}$; N is the total number of spins; and k is a constant. If the equilibrium is disturbed, or when the field is first applied, the spins regain the equilibrium condition exponentially: the system is said to "relax." Following an intervention that makes $M_z \neq M_z(0)$, the system relaxation can be described by:

$$M_z(t) = M_z(0)\ (1\text{-}\exp\ (t/T_1)),$$

where $M_z(t)$ is the Z component of magnetization at time t and T_1 is the time constant of the relaxation process and is called the longitudinal (or spin lattice) relaxation time.

At equilibrium, the net magnetic moment **M** lies along Z. If **M** can be induced to vary from the Z direction, it will precess about the direction of the field $\mathbf{B_0}$. (This is analogous to the movement of an off-vertical gyroscope as it precesses about a vertical axis.) The precession frequency is proportional to the applied field and to an intrinsic property of the nuclear species in question called the gyromagnetic ratio (γ) and is described by an equation $\omega = \gamma\ B_0$, where ω is the frequency at which the spinning nucleus precesses, also termed the Larmor frequency.

Each nucleus with magnetic properties has its own characteristic gyromagnetic ratio (Table 46–1). For example, ^{31}P has a γ of 17.235 MHz/Tesla. Thus, the frequency of ^{31}P at 2.1 Tesla is 35.8 MHz, and at 11.8 Tesla is 202.5 MHz. Application of radiofrequency (RF) energy (an oscillating magnetic field $\mathbf{B_1}$ perpendicular to $\mathbf{B_0}$) at the Larmor frequency of a selected nuclear species can induce the magnetic moment **M** of the selected nuclear species to tilt from the Z axis. As **M** deviates from the Z axis, it also precesses around Z at the Larmor frequency. The rate of rotation away from the Z axis is proportional to the applied field $\mathbf{B_1}$ ($\omega_1 = \gamma\ \mathbf{B_1}$, where ω_1 is the frequency at which **M** rotates about $\mathbf{B_1}$) and continues while $\mathbf{B_1}$ (RF) is applied.

In practice, the effect of the applied RF pulse is more important than its absolute strength and duration; thus RF pulses are described in terms of the angle through which they rotate the vector **M**. For example, a 90° pulse will displace the vector **M** by 90° into the XY plane. The 90° pulse is applied to a biologic system with a surface coil. When a surface coil (transmitter/receiver coil) is placed close to the sample, it can transmit energy to the sample. When the radiofrequency transmission is turned off, the receiver perceives a magnetic dipole of strength M rotating at the Larmor frequency of the selected nuclear species. This small signal (or induced electromotive force, emf) can be amplified, recorded, and digitized for computer analysis. The signal detected is the form of a decaying sine wave, oscillating at the Larmor frequency of the nuclear species in question, and can be described by the following equation:

$$S(t) = S(0)\ \sin(\omega t + \phi)\ \exp(-t/T_2),$$

where S(t) is the signal detected at time t, S(0) is the signal at zero time, ω is the Larmor frequency, ϕ is the phase of the sine wave, and T_2 is the decay constant describing the observed loss of signal (termed the transverse or spin-spin relaxation time).

The signal observed following a pulse is termed the free induction decay (FID). Signal decay after removal of the radiofrequency stimulation is due to the decrease in the size of the component **M** in the XY plane. Eventually, the system regains its equilibrium state with the magnetic moment aligned with the field. It is important to point out that it is not physically possible to regain the original state faster than the excited state is lost. Thus T_1 is always greater than or equal to T_2 (T_2 approaches T_1 in aqueous solutions).

Interpretation of free induction decay signal can be done only if frequency information can be obtained from the time domain.

Table 46–1. CHARACTERISTICS OF SELECTED NMR NUCLEI

Nucleus	Spin	Gyromagnetic Ratio MHZ/Tesla	Magnetic Moment	Percent Abundance	Relative Sensitivity at Constant Field	In Vivo Compounds	Chemical Shift-ppm	Concentration	Net Sensitivity
Phosphorus (^{31}P)	1/2	17.235	+1.131	100.00	1.000	PCr	0	8–10 mM	1
						alpha-ATP	2.4	3–5 mM	0.3–0.5
						beta-ATP	7.8	3–5 mM	0.3–0.5
						gamma-ATP	16.6	3–5 mM	0.3–0.5
						Pi	−5	1–2 mM	0.1–0.2
						Phosphodiesters	−2	1–2 mM	0.1–0.2
						Phosphomonoesters	−7	1–2 mM	0.1–0.2
						2,3-DPG	−5	3–5 mM	0.3–0.5
Protons (^{1}H)	1/2	42.576	+2.793	99.99	15.083	water	−4.5	110 M	166,000
						lactate	−1.3	10 mM	15.1
Deuterium (^{2}H)	1	6.536	+0.857	0.02	0.146	water (natural abundance ^{2}H)	−4.5	110 M	0.8
Carbon (^{13}C)	1/2	10.705	+0.702	1.11	0.240				
Fluorine (^{19}F)	1/2	40.054	+2.627	100.00	12.564				
Sodium (^{23}Na)	3/2	11.262	+2.216	100.00	1.395	Na^+ intracellular		15 mM	2.09
						Na^+ extracellular		140 mM	19.5
Potassium (^{39}K)	3/2	3.491	+0.391	93.10	0.008	K^+ intracellular		150 mM	0.11
						K^+ extracellular		5 mM	0.004

Fourier transformation of the FID is done to produce a spectrum with a peak at the precession frequency, a line width (full width at half maximum height) that is inversely proportional to the transverse relaxation time, and a peak intensity (area under peaks) proportional to the value of M_{xy} immediately following the RF pulse. Since the magnetic moment M is proportional to the number of nuclei, measurement of the integrated peak in the spectrum is a measure of the total number of the particular nuclei excited within the region of study.

The two relaxation times, T_1 and T_2, depend critically on the milieu of the observed nuclei in the tissue and can be used to differentiate tissues and potentially to characterize disease processes.

Nuclear magnetic resonance spectroscopy exploits the fact that nuclei of a given element situated at different positions within molecules will exhibit slightly different precession frequencies. Electron motion around the nucleus of an atom produces small local magnetic fields that modify the effect of the applied field $\mathbf{B_0}$ at the nucleus. Thus the field at the nucleus can be described as:

$$B_{nucleus} = B_0(1 - \sigma),$$

where sigma (σ) is a small fraction that will depend on the local chemical environment. Typically, σ ranges over values of $\pm\ 10^{-7}$ to 10^{-4}. Since the precession frequency is proportional to the field experienced at the nucleus, the chemical environment causes a slight shift in the precession frequency described by:

$$\Delta\omega = \sigma\ \gamma\ B_0$$

This effect is called the chemical shift, and its magnitude depends on the applied field B_0 and the chemical environment. A useful measure of the chemical shift, independent of B_0, is obtained by expressing the frequency shift as a fraction of the basic Larmor frequency. Thus, the position of a particular peak in a spectrum (the chemical shift δ) will be expressed in parts per million (ppm) of the Larmor frequency upfield or downfield from a defined reference peak.

For a sample with several components, the free induction decay signal will consist of the sum of signals from each component, and Fourier transformation of the FID will generate a spectrum with different resonances at different frequencies. The intensity of each resonance, as measured by its integral, is proportional to the number of nuclei with that chemical shift in the sample.

Most spectroscopic signals in nuclear magnetic resonance are very weak. Signal-to-noise (S:N) of a single free induction decay may be only 1:1. Therefore, a certain amount of signal averaging is necessary. A typical ^{31}P spectrum from the heart is presented in Figure 46–1, in which the S:N following 100 summed signal acquisitions (100 FIDs) is still only 20:1. Reduction of high-frequency noise from the spectrum can be done using a filtering process, in which the FID is multiplied by a decaying exponential curve: this process, termed apodization, has the effect of increasing the width and decreasing the height of spectral peaks, so it must be performed with care.

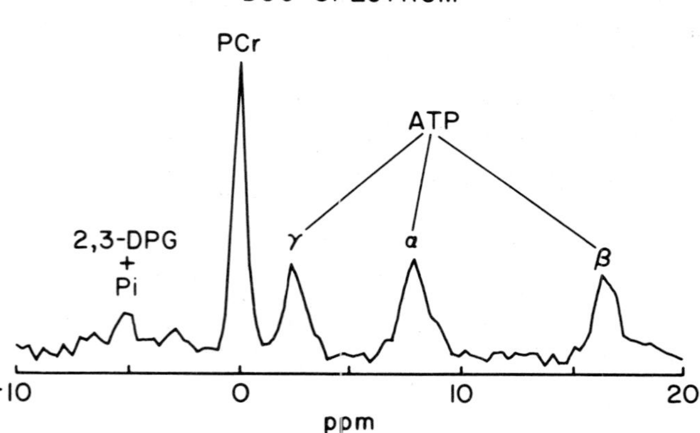

Figure 46–1. Spectrum from dog heart. Note that there is some overlap between the Pi and 2,3-DPG peaks. Pi—inorganic phosphate, 2,3-DPG—2-3 diphosphoglyceric acid, PCr—phosphocreatine, ATP—γ, α, β, adenosine triphosphate, ppm—parts per million.

METHODS FOR DATA COLLECTION AND QUANTIFICATION OF MYOCARDIAL METABOLITES

A major goal of spectroscopy is the quantitative assessment of component peaks, i.e., the number of nuclei with a particular chemical shift per sampled volume. At present there is no entirely satisfactory method of analysis. Three factors interfere with quantification of the peaks. Noise is present in all spectra; it can be reduced by improvements to spectrometer hardware or by signal averaging. A second problem is incomplete resolution of the peaks. A related problem is interference by broad underlying peaks. Spectral editing tools attempt to correct this by fitting a sum of calculated peaks to the real data. This requires sophisticated computer algorithms and assumptions concerning some of the characteristics of the peaks, and is far from a perfected technique. Finally, if nuclear T_1 or T_2 relaxation is not completed between pulses, then the measured peak may not be equal to nuclear concentration for that species.

Manual assessment of peak areas gives results that are in the expected range, with reproducibility commensurate with the S:N. Manual assessment is undesirable in consideration of the effort involved in the analysis and the user bias introduced into the final results. Therefore, considerable efforts are being made to automate this process. Three main approaches are being used at present: (1) curve fitting, by which a computer is directed to simulate a real spectrum[H2]; (2) linear prediction techniques, which analyze the FID directly in terms of decaying sinusoidal components[B1]; and (3) maximum entropy techniques, which use both the FID and the spectrum during the analysis.[L1, N1]

Collection and processing of magnetic resonance spectroscopy data is impossible without sophisticated computer algorithms. A number of investigators have developed algorithms that can be used for data collection and analysis.[B1, C1, L1, N1, T1] Other investigators have developed methods to quantify MRS data from spectral data.[C2, W2, W3] Most are based on using an external sample of known concentration to compare with signals from high-energy phosphorus spectra obtained from the heart.[W1] Another method uses an internal standard, the ^1H signal from water and fat (a concentration that can be easily estimated) as a reference for the phosphorus signal.[W1] When data obtained with most of these methods were compared with data obtained with routine analytical biochemical techniques, the results with both techniques were comparable for many biologically important chemicals (an important exception is adenosine diphosphate [ADP]).

THE MAGNETIC RESONANCE SPECTROSCOPY SURFACE COIL

To generate a magnetic resonance spectroscopy signal, radiofrequency energy must be applied to and measured from the organ of interest. To do this, an MRS probe containing a radiofrequency coil is used.[B2, H3, S2] This coil or inductive structure is tuned by a radiofrequency circuit to the oscillating magnetic field of interest in the sample. The MRS probe coil can be a simple loop of wire or a very complicated array of conductors that form a resonant circuit. The MRS probe functions as both a transmitter (creates a B_1 field) and a receiver (receives or listens to the radiofrequency signals generated by precessing magnetic moments in the organ or sample under the coil). Generally, a single coil is used for both procedures, but there are occasions when separate transmit and receive coils are needed. Both the transmit and receive function are considered later.

For the coil to interact efficiently with the magnetic field, it must be tuned to the Larmor frequency of the nucleus in question. Tuning the coil circuit rejects noise outside of a narrow band containing the specific Larmor frequency. Matching the circuit to the same impedance as the transmitter and cables maximizes the power dissipated in the probe.

Radiofrequency transmission induces spins that are polarized along the Z axis of the static field $\mathbf{B}_0$ to be excited, thus producing a $\mathbf{B}_1$ (magnitude of the RF magnetic field) field perpendicular to the initial axis of polarization produced by $\mathbf{B}_0$ (main magnetic field). The surface coil consists of a conductor through which current can pass to create the $\mathbf{B}_1$ field, which can be described by

$$B_1 = \int I \, dl \times r/r^3,$$

where **r** is the vector from the element of the coil **dl** to the point in space at which the field is being calculated, I is the current which is assumed to be constant throughout the probe, and × is a vector product. The integral is obtained over the entire conductor length. The $\mathbf{B}_1$ field is proportional to the current I. The integral is a function of the coil wire geometry and thus determines the $\mathbf{B}_1$ distribution in space. Different experiments may require a different $\mathbf{B}_1$ distribution and thus different coil geometries. The flip angle imparted to the spin system by the application of a radiofrequency pulse can be defined by:

$$\theta = 360° \cdot \gamma \, B_1 \, t,$$

where θ is the flip angle, B_1 is magnitude of the radiofrequency field, γ is the gyromagnetic ratio of the nuclear species under interrogation, and t is the time the radiofrequency application is on. Application of a 45°, 60°, or 90° pulse over an entire sample requires the generation of a $\mathbf{B}_1$ field that is homogeneous throughout. Different coil geometries have been used in this regard: some examples are the Helmholtz, solenoid, and saddle coils.

To measure radiofrequency signal generated by the sample (organ) under interrogation with application of the initial $\mathbf{B}_1$ field, the MRS coil must also act as a receiver; i.e., the second function of the MRS coil is to detect the transverse magnetization that was created during radiofrequency transmission. The transverse magnetization precessing at a point x within the sample space creates a time-varying magnetic field $\mathbf{B}_m$ which can be described as $\mathbf{B}_m$ (x′, x, t), where x is the position at which the field is being evaluated.[S2] A voltage (electromotive force or emf) is developed by the changing magnetic flux through the surface coil and can be calculated using Faraday's induction law:

$$\text{emf}(x') = -\frac{\delta}{\partial t}\int_{probe} B_m(x', x, t) \cdot n \, dS_{probe},$$

where $\mathbf{B}_m$ is the time-varying magnetic field, x is the position at which the magnetic field is being evaluated, x′ is the area from which the emf is calculated, n is the unit vector perpendicular to the plane of the coil, and dS is an element of area. The integral is obtained over the entire surface enclosed by the coil.

The optimal function of a surface coil as both a transmitter and receiver relies on the efficiency of the inductor. The inductor efficiency depends on the amount of resistance in the circuit. For a coil to obtain optimal signal (or possess an optimal Q value), an efficient resonant circuit is necessary. This is accomplished with an impedance matching network.[S2]

Understanding of the generation of signal and noise (signal:noise ratio) is quite important in design of an MRS probe.[H3] Since most of the noise is generated by the probe, it is important to understand the principles of its generation. Sample loading of an MRS coil may be significant and is due to the sample interaction with the magnetic and electric fields produced by the coil. Living tissue is conductive and also has measurable magnetic susceptibility. Thus, eddy currents can be induced into the tissue sample by the $\mathbf{B}_1$ field of the MRS probe. Power will be dissipated because these eddy currents are passed through a resistive medium. Another deleterious effect is that the induced eddy currents create a $\mathbf{B}_1$ field of their own that can distort the $\mathbf{B}_1$ field of the coil. The electric field generated by the coil interaction with tissue also dissipates energy, and results from the voltage applied across the probe to produce current in it. This energy dissipation results because different electrical potentials exist in different parts of the probe, and thus inhomogeneous electrical potentials are induced in different parts of the sample. The resulting current that can flow through the capacitance between these structures produces a lossy dielectric that dissipates power. It is difficult to remove the effects of magnetically dissipated power, because the magnetic field is necessary for generation of the MRS signal. However, the electrical interactions of the coil and sample are not necessary to generate an MRS signal and can be reduced by shielding the sample from the electric field of the coil. This can be done by using a Faraday shield or by the use of a balanced capacitive drive on the MRS probe.[S2]

BACKGROUND AND RATIONALE FOR USE OF IN VIVO MAGNETIC RESONANCE SPECTROSCOPY TECHNIQUES

Metabolic correlates of mechanical function of the heart have been of interest to cardiovascular physiologists for decades. Many studies have been done on mitochondrial extracts and biopsy samples of hearts from experimental animal models before and after application of various external stimuli. In addition, perfused heart preparations have been used to obtain information concerning the interaction of biochemical and mechanical function in the intact organ. Although some studies have been done to investigate the interaction of metabolic and mechanical function in the intact organism, these studies have been limited by difficulty in obtaining biochemical information from the in vivo organism and generally involve chemical analysis of blood samples obtained from the coronary sinus during various stimuli that cause ischemia or increase the workload of the heart. With the introduction of magnetic resonance spectroscopy, it has become possible to study biochemistry in the intact organ and organism. In the following sections, applications of different MRS techniques to study cardiac metabolism and cellular function are presented.

METHODS USED TO OBTAIN IN VIVO MAGNETIC RESONANCE SPECTROSCOPY DATA

Most early work using MRS to study biologic systems was done in vitro in superfused or perfused cell or organ preparations placed in glass tubes, which were then placed in small-bore high-field magnets. This work was governed by physical constraints of equipment; only small-bore magnets (5 to 20 mm) were available. However, as magnet size increased (20 to 100 cm), studying in vivo cellular function and metabolism became possible. With respect to the heart, both open and closed chest preparations could be studied. Initial in vivo work was done in the open chest organism with a surface coil placed on the exposed heart.

Although this technique provides much interesting metabolic data, hemodynamics and cardiovascular physiology can be different in open chest compared with closed chest organisms. Thus, techniques have been developed to study cardiovascular function in intact closed chest organisms. Some early work was done using intravascular coils placed into the right and left ventricles via peripheral veins and arteries.[B3] Although cardiac data generated with this technique were interesting, they were confounded somewhat by signal from the blood, which contributes 2,3-diphosphoglyceric acid (2,3-DPG) signal to the overall phosphorus spectra (since blood completely surrounded the coil).

Other early work was done with chronically implanted coils.[K1] This technique required a thoracotomy, surgical placement of the coil on the heart, and subsequent closure of the chest wall.

Chronically implanted coils could provide interesting MRS data from intact animals, but this technique had two disadvantages: (1) the polyurethane coil coating, constantly subjected to body fluids, eventually became leaky, resulting in degraded S:N; (2) this technique can be used in animal models but not in patients.

Another technique, developed in animal models, involved placement of a cardiac window in the left thorax.[O2] Two or three ribs and accompanying skeletal muscle were removed, Marlex mesh was sutured between the two exposed ribs, and fascia and skin were sutured closed. After the animal recovered, MR spectra could be obtained from the heart by placing the animal in the left lateral decubitus position over a surface coil. Thus, MRS data could be obtained sequentially in a chronic animal model with simple surface coil techniques. This technique also had the disadvantage that it could be used in animal models but not in humans.

To obtain MRS data from intact humans, a completely noninvasive, nondestructive method of data acquisition is needed. This need inspired the development of depth-resolved and imaging techniques to acquire MRS data.[A1, B4–B8, O3, O4, R1, S3] At present, these techniques are being explored intensively for use in clinical conditions and are discussed in Chapter 54.

NUCLEI OF INTEREST: ^{31}P, ^{13}C, ^{23}Na, ^{39}K, ^{1}H, ^{19}F, AND ^{2}H

A number of nuclei that are involved in important biologic processes have physical properties that allow them to be effectively and efficiently studied in the intact organism with in vivo MRS techniques; these include ^{31}P, ^{13}C, ^{23}Na, ^{39}K, and ^{1}H.[O5] Phosphorus-containing compounds are involved in bioenergetics and can be studied with ^{31}P MRS; carbon-containing compounds are involved in intermediary metabolism (glycolysis, glycogen synthesis, citric acid cycle), which can be studied with ^{13}C MRS; sodium and potassium are involved in the maintenance of the electrical function of the heart's conduction and contractile systems and can be studied with ^{23}Na and ^{39}K MRS. Proton-containing compounds are ubiquitous in biologic systems and are involved in all the aforementioned biologic functions; they can be studied using ^{1}H MRS.

Another nuclear species, ^{19}F, which is not normally observed in the body, can be administered as fluorinated tracers for use in delineation of calcium and magnesium concentration and pH (^{19}F MRS). Deuterium (^{2}H) also can be administered as a tracer for studies of organ perfusion.

Although it is possible to use all these nuclear species to delineate biologic mechanisms, the majority of work in this area has been done with ^{31}P MRS. This may be because phosphorus compounds exist in sufficiently high concentrations and cover a wide range of chemical shifts, so they can be studied with good resolution and good signal:noise. This is fortuitous, because high-energy phosphate bioenergetics are important to normal function of all body systems. Because of the wealth of information in this area, the emphasis in the remainder of this chapter is on the use of ^{31}P MRS in the study of myocardial metabolic function. However, information concerning the use of other nuclear species (^{13}C, ^{23}Na, ^{39}K, ^{1}H, ^{19}F, and ^{2}H) also will be discussed.

^{31}P Magnetic Resonance Spectroscopy: General Information

Most work using MRS techniques to study in vivo biochemistry of the heart has been done with ^{31}P MRS to evaluate the bioenergetic state of the heart under various conditions.[O5] Several ^{31}P spectral peaks are of interest: phosphomonoesters (PM), inorganic phosphate (Pi), phosphocreatine (PCr), and the three phosphate peaks of adenosine triphosphate (ATP): γ, α, and β (see Fig. 46–1). Changes in these peaks (heights or areas), which measure changes in concentration of metabolites, can be followed during physiologic intervention to determine changes in metabolism as they relate to physiologic state. Only mobile phosphorus moieties (and not those bound to membranes or to large macromolecules) can be detected with in vivo MRS.

Because it may not always be easy to calibrate a MRS signal in terms of concentration (using an acceptable internal standard), the ratio of any two MRS peak heights and/or areas (e.g., PCr/Pi, PCr/total phosphate, PCr/ATP), which are proportional to the ratio of the concentrations of these compounds, is often used. These phosphorus data can be used in combination with data obtained from other analytical biochemistry techniques to determine changes in ADP concentration and phosphorylation potential, both potential regulators of cardiac metabolic function. In addition, pH changes, which may also regulate metabolic function, can be measured from the chemical shift in the Pi peak. Determination and use of these regulators in biologic processes are discussed next.

Use of ^{31}P *Magnetic Resonance Spectroscopy to Study Potential Myocardial Metabolic Regulators*

Because ADP concentration in tissue is quite low, it is considered to be a metabolic regulator under some conditions.[M1, T2] ^{31}P MRS techniques can be used to determine in vivo ADP concentrations and thus provide information concerning metabolic regulation. If the creatine kinase reaction is assumed to be at equilibrium (which may not always be the case), and the equilibrium constant (K_{ck}) and creatine (Cr) concentration are obtained from routine analytical biochemical techniques,[V1] ADP concentration can be calculated from cardiac tissue using MRS-determined ATP, PCr, and H^+ concentrations:

$$[ADP] = ([ATP] \bullet [Cr]) / ([PCr] \bullet K_{ck} \bullet [H^+])$$

If Cr concentration is constant and K_{ck} is assumed to be at near-equilibrium, [ADP] can be estimated from the ATP/PCr ratio.

Another potential metabolic regulator, phosphorylation potential, also can be determined from ^{31}P MRS data.[M1] Again the system must be assumed to be in equilibrium and the equilibrium constant for creatine kinase (K_{ck}) and creatine concentration [Cr] must be known. The phosphorylation potential, [ATP]/([ADP])([Pi]), can be calculated using the following equation and ^{31}P-determined PCr, Pi, and H^+:

$$[ATP]/([ADP]\ [Pi]) = [PCr]/[Pi] \times (K_{ck} \bullet [H^+])/[Cr]$$

In addition, phosphorylation potential can be estimated using the PCr/Pi ratio if Cr concentration is assumed to be constant and the K_{ck} is assumed to be at near-equilibrium.

^{31}P MRS data can be used to obtain tissue pH in the following manner. The chemical shift of PCr is stable at all pHs compatible with life (pH between 6 and 8). The chemical shift of Pi changes as pH changes, because of the charge on the phosphorus nucleus. The relationship of Pi chemical shift to PCr chemical shift can be used to determine in vivo pH using the following formula:

$$pH = 6.75 + \log\frac{(\sigma - 3.27)}{(5.69 - \sigma)}$$

where 6.75 is the pK of phosphoric acid, σ is the chemical shift difference between Pi and PCr peaks, and 3.27 and 5.69 are constants determined empirically.[B9, P2, S4] When pH determined with MRS techniques is compared with that obtained with more conventional means, the correlation is good.[B9, S4] It may be possible also to detect the difference between intracellular and extracellular pH with ^{31}P MRS techniques. This can be done when two Pi peaks are resolved.[G2]

Thus, three potential regulators of myocardial metabolism: [ADP], phosphorylation potential, and pH, can be determined from intact organs and organisms with ^{31}P MRS. These parameters can be simply estimated using ATP/PCr and PCr/Pi ratios (provided the assumptions concerning Cr and K_{ck} discussed earlier hold true) and the chemical shift of Pi with respect to PCr (pH or [H^+]), respectively. The use of these data obtained from in vivo systems has the advantage that they can be obtained without the need for absolute quantification in terms of metabolite concentration. In addition, they have direct relevance in expressing MRS data in terms of basic metabolic events.

Correlation of Cardiac Work with Myocardial Metabolism

In vivo correlation of chemical energy expenditure to external myocardial work production can be done in the intact organism[C3, C4] with MRS data and can be described by simple Michaelis-Menten kinetics, as expressed in the following equation:

$$V/V_{max} = 1/(1 + K_{eq}/[S]),$$

where V is the observed velocity of the enzyme reaction, V_{max} is maximum velocity, K_{eq} is the equilibrium constant, and [S] is substrate concentration. If K_{eq} (equilibrium constant) of creatine kinase is measured with routine analytical biochemical techniques, substrate concentration is estimated from ^{31}P MRS data (ADP concentration is considered to be a substrate that can be estimated from ATP/Pcr or PCr/Pi ratios obtained from in vivo ^{31}P MRS), and these values are substituted into the Michaelis-Menten equation, the following equation that describes the interaction of mechanical work with metabolism results:

$$V/V_{max} = 1/(1 + 0.53/\text{ATP/PCr or PCr/Pi})$$

where 0.53 is the K_{eq} calculated from in vitro data and V_{max} measures the maximum velocity of the enzymes of oxidative phosphorylation. This equation, termed a "transfer function," has been used by Chance and colleagues[C3, C4] and others[O5] to estimate the stability of skeletal and cardiac muscle function. If the heart is working at no more than one half V_{max}, there is considerable room for metabolic and mechanical recruitment, and heart function is stable with minimal change in PCr/Pi with increased workloads. If the heart is working close to V_{max}, there is much less room for recruitment, and heart function becomes unstable and may fail (as indicated by large decreases in PCr/Pi) with increased workloads.

Review of Types of Studies with ^{31}P Magnetic Resonance Spectroscopy

Perfused Heart Preparations

The majority of ^{31}P MRS studies have been done in isolated perfused Langendorff or working heart preparations. Most early work involved feasibility studies,[F1, G3, G4, H4, I1, J1, J2, S4] whereas later work was done to investigate the use of ^{31}P MRS techniques to evaluate metabolic regulatory mechanisms[F2, G5, K2–K4, M2, U1] and enzyme kinetics,[B11–B14, H5, K5, K6, N3, N4, P4, S5] the effects of protective agents on myocardial ischemia[D2, E1, H6, K7, L2, L3, N5, O6, P5, S6, S7] and other pathologic conditions,[C2, C5, T3] and the effects of various disease states on myocardial metabolism.[B10, N2, P3] Some specific examples of work done to obtain information during physiologic and pathophysiologic intervention in the perfused heart are presented later.

REGULATION OF MYOCARDIAL METABOLISM. Regulation of bioenergetic processes of the heart is a complex process. Until recently, investigation of this process was limited to the study of cellular and subcellular (mitochondrial) preparations using routine analytic biochemical techniques. Much early work indicated that different regulators were important and active under different physiologic conditions.[G5] Some proposed regulators of myocardial metabolism are ADP concentration, phosphorylation potential, ATP/ADP ratio, pH, Pi concentration, NADH/NAD redox state, oxygen availability, and carbon substrate availability (citric acid cycle intermediates).

With the introduction of MRS techniques, the roles of many of these potential regulators can be studied in intact organs and organisms. ^{31}P MRS has been used to evaluate the role of ATP/ADP, Pi, ADP concentration, phosphorylation potential, and pH in the regulation of myocardial metabolism.[C6, U1] Most of these studies confirm earlier studies that indicate that different regulators are effective under different conditions. For example, increasing workloads are generally associated with an increase in oxygen consumption. However, the increase in rate of oxygen consumption can be affected by different metabolic regulators under different conditions. In the nonischemic, nonhypoxic heart, increases in workload are associated with relatively stable pH and ATP, ADP, and Pi concentrations.[K2] Data obtained from combined ^{31}P MRS and NADH fluorometry experiments indicate that NADH/NAD redox state may be a regulator under these conditions.[K2, U1]

The availability of different substrates during increasing workloads also influences the regulatory process.[F2, K3, U1] In a perfused beating heart model, several investigators have demonstrated that increasing workloads in glucose and/or glucose and insulin perfused hearts were associated with stable ADP, ATP, PCr, Pi, phosphorylation potential, and ATP/ADP ratios.[K4, U1] Therefore, none of these chemicals acted as regulators under the aforementioned conditions. However, when pyruvate was added to the perfusate, ADP concentration varied directly with oxygen consumption, indicating that under these conditions, ADP could be a regulator.

In one study that related aortic pressure, coronary flow rate, oxygen consumption, and contractile function to MRS-determined phosphorylation potential, there was a positive correlation between cytosolic phosphorylation potential and contractile function at low flow rates (below 7.2 ml/min/100 g) but no direct correlation between these parameters at higher flow rate.[C7] In the first case it is likely that the hearts had a limited oxygen supply and thus were relatively ischemic. In the second case, the hearts were normoxic (nonischemic). Results from this study indicate that when oxygen limits myocardial oxidative phosphorylation, there are other bioenergetic controls (ADP, phosphorylation potential, redox state) of contractile function. However, when oxygen supply is adequate, other as yet undefined regulators may link workload with mitochondrial respiration. Another study using ^{31}P MRS suggests that changes in phosphorylation potential regulate the release of adenosine from the smooth muscle of the coronary vessels.[M2]

Thus, although there are many potential metabolic regulators, many of which are not MRS observable, in some conditions metabolic function may be influenced or controlled by changes in high-energy phosphate metabolism. ^{31}P MRS can be used to study these conditions in intact organs and organisms and thus provide a better understanding of in vivo regulatory mechanisms.

STUDIES OF ENZYME KINETICS. Enzyme kinetics of important biochemical reactions in biologic systems have routinely been studied in tissue extracts in the test tube using analytic biochemical techniques. In the past, it has not been possible to directly verify that these biochemical activities are the same or different for in vivo systems. With the introduction of MRS techniques, it is now possible to investigate enzymatic mechanisms in intact organs and organisms.

The MRS technique that allows this in vivo enzymatic evaluation uses magnetic labeling (i.e., saturation or obliteration of one phosphorus moiety such as γ ATP, while observing changes in the PCr peak) of certain magnetically susceptible chemicals and measures chemical exchange between them; this technique is termed *magnetization transfer*. Although a number of enzyme systems can be studied via this technique, at present most work has been done for the creatine kinase system, which catalyzes the exchange between PCr and ATP gamma phosphate (γP):

$$\text{PCr} \underset{K_{rev}}{\overset{K_{for}}{\rightleftharpoons}} \text{ATP}$$

where K is a pseudo-first-order unidirectional rate constant for a forward or reverse creatine kinase reaction. A magnetic label (saturation pulse) is applied to either the PCr or the ATP (γP) resonance. Transfer of the labeled spin to the reciprocal chemical sites occurs at a rate that depends on two processes: the rate of the chemical reaction (given by the unidirectional rate constant) and the rate of disappearance of label (given by T_1 for a simple saturation transfer experiment).[B11] The process of magnetization transfer is illustrated under different physiologic conditions in Figure 46–2.

Magnetization transfer studies can provide information concerning chemical reaction rates such as occur during ATP synthesis and can also be used to estimate the P/O (ATP phosphorylation to oxygen use) ratio in biologic systems. Even though this technique has added a new dimension to our understanding of in vivo enzyme kinetics, it is not without problems. The chemical exchange in intact systems is very complex due to the fact that multiple reactions may use the same substrate. In addition, there may be partitioning of enzyme and/or substrate into different cellular organelles (cytosol versus mitochondria); this compartmentation is associated with some free enzyme which is in solution and some which is bound to macromolecules and membranes. Thus the reaction rates depend on many factors that may be difficult to isolate in the living system. To address this type of problem, multiple saturation transfer techniques, which magnetically label (saturate) a number of important chemical intermediates, can be used.[K3, U1] However, this variation of magnetization transfer technique can be used effectively only if there is no overlap between the spectral peaks of interest.

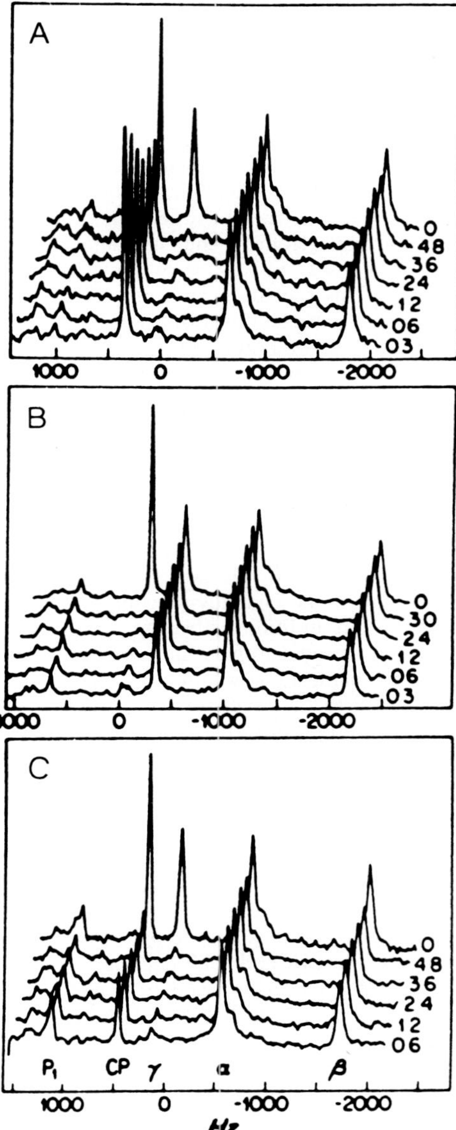

Figure 46–2. Magnetic resonance spectroscopy spectra during three magnetization transfer experiments. *A*, Saturation of γ ATP for different times during KCl cardiac arrest to follow the kinetic exchange between CrP and γ ATP (K_{for}). *B*, Saturation of PCr for different times during KCl cardiac arrest to follow the kinetic exchange between γ ATP and CrP (K_{rev}). *C*, Saturation of γ ATP during imposition of an increased workload to follow kinetic exchange between CrP and γ ATP (K_{for}). ATP—adenosine triphosphate, CrP—creatine phosphate, K_{for}—forward rate constant; K_{rev}—reverse rate constant. In the illustration 0—control; 0.3, 0.6, 1.2, 2.4, 3.6, and 4.8 are saturation times in seconds. (From Bittl, J. A., and Ingwall, J. W.: NMR studies of ATP synthesis reactions in the isolated heart. *In* Osbakken, M. D., and Haselgrove, J. (eds.): NMR Techniques in the Study of Cardiovascular Structure and Function. Futura Publishing Company, Mt. Kisco, N.Y., 1988, p. 239, with permission.)

A number of investigators have used variations of these techniques to investigate ATP synthesis and turnover.* The results of these studies depend on the type of magnetization transfer technique used. Forward rate constants for ATP synthesis may not always equal reverse rate constants for ATP hydrolysis. This inconsistency, which occurs in a system that is supposedly in equilibrium (creatine kinase catalyzed, ATP $\rightleftharpoons$ PCr) is explained by the effects of compartmentation and the effects of multiple reactions using the same substrate on the overall reaction rates determined by magnetization transfer techniques. Even with these complexities in mind, it is now possible to begin extensive study of enzyme mechanisms under in vivo conditions. If used carefully and thoughtfully this type of study will lead to a better understanding of biochemical reaction rates in living systems.

The effects of various conditions, such as age,[P4] hypertrophy,[B13] and ischemia,[N4] on enzyme kinetics have been studied recently. These studies indicate that it may be difficult to identify differences in enzyme function under physiologic conditions but that there are distinct differences during some pathologic conditions (pathologic hypertrophy and ischemia). The extent that the changes in enzyme kinetics are either a cause or an effect of the existing pathophysiologic condition remains to be answered.

CYCLIC CHANGES IN HIGH-ENERGY PHOSPHATES. Several studies have investigated the possibility of change in bioenergetics at different phases in the cardiac cycle—i.e., cyclic changes in energy metabolism related to changes in wall tension and workload.[F3, K9, T4] Several studies in perfused hearts have demonstrated that there may be metabolic cycling, with a decrease in PCr and ATP and an increase in Pi and ADP during various stages of systole, which are reversed during diastole. However, in vivo studies of the same phenomenon did not validate the findings of the in vitro perfused heart studies. An explanation for the discrepancy of these observations may be that perfused hearts are always relatively ischemic (even in the most optimal conditions), and the increased mechanical function during systole may increase this relative ischemia so differences in bioenergetics appear. In the in vivo studies, when hearts are nonischemic and nonhypoxic, it is unlikely that a period of relative ischemia would exist during systole; therefore, the heart would maintain normal metabolic function throughout the cardiac cycle.

EFFECTS OF SUBSTRATES AND IONS ON BIOENERGETICS. Availability of different substrates also may affect generation and use of high-energy phosphates.[S8] Glucose, lactate, and acetate administration is associated with change in both ATP and PCr concentrations during similar heart rates and coronary flow states.[B19, M5] ATP is higher and PCr is lower during glucose administration than during administration of other substrates. Glycogen availability has been demonstrated to affect myocardial tolerance of ischemia; ischemia is better tolerated in glycogen-depleted hearts (possibly because lactic acid does not build up)[B17, B18, G6] which are associated with higher levels of PCr and ATP.

Ion concentrations in perfusate also appear to influence myocardial bioenergetics.[H8, R2] Some early work using perfusion fluid containing low sodium or calcium concentration indicated a protective effect in ischemic hearts when one or both ions were lowered.[B19, M5] These hearts appeared to have better recovery of mechanical function (developed pressure) and faster return of

*(B11–B16, D3, H5, H7, K5, K6, K8, M3, M4, N3, N4, N6, P4, S5, U1, U2).

PCr and ATP to baseline levels. Later work in nonischemic heart demonstrated that the ionic effect was concentration dependent; lower ion concentrations were associated with decreased developed pressure and PCr and ATP concentration and an increase in diastolic pressure,[R3, R4] whereas higher concentrations were associated with opposite changes. In addition, these changes were suppressed if calcium and sodium ions were decreased simultaneously. In another study in which the sodium-potassium pump was inhibited by reduction of perfusate potassium or by ouabain, there was an increase in oxygen consumption and a decrease in ATP and PCr associated with a decrease in systolic pressure and an increase in diastolic pressure.[H8] In addition, there was acidosis and an increase in intracellular calcium and sodium. Similar metabolic and mechanical effects were observed when cellular calcium was increased after a reduction in perfusate sodium.[H8, K10] These effects could be prevented by decreasing calcium in the perfusate. These studies were used to demonstrate the importance of calcium as a metabolic regulator of the interaction of bioenergetics and mechanical function.

POTENTIAL DISEASE STATES

Myocardial Ischemia. Both global and regional ischemia have been studied extensively in perfused hearts with ^{31}P MRS techniques. Initially, ischemia is associated with a decrease in PCr, an increase in Pi, and a decrease in pH. If ischemia is severe enough (or lasts long enough), ATP also decreases.[B17, B18, G3, G4, H4, I1, J2, R5, S4, S9] The increase in Pi generally parallels the decrease in pH.[B20, L4, R5] However, contractile function can be markedly depressed when pH and high-energy phosphate are only minimally decreased, indicating that factors other than phosphate bioenergetics are intrinsically related to mechanical function and may also be due to compartmentation of the PCr and ATP.[B21, J3] However, recovery of mechanical function does appear to be related to ATP content at the end of ischemia.[W4, W5]

An interesting MRS observation that the acidosis that occurs with ischemia is less in hearts which are glycogen depleted or in which glycogenolysis and thus glycolysis are inhibited[B17, B18, G6] indicates that metabolic state is quite important in determination of the adverse effects of myocardial ischemia. Insulin administration prior to induction of ischemia also appears to protect the heart from the effects of ischemia,[R6] with more rapid recovery of mechanical function after ischemia in insulin-perfused hearts. This phenomenon is associated with smaller decreases in ATP during ischemia. The glycogen-sparing effect of glucose-insulin-potassium (GIK) solutions has also been demonstrated to protect the heart from onset of ischemic damage by prolonging the availability of substrate necessary for production of high-energy phosphates.[H6]

Many ^{31}P MRS studies have been done to evaluate the protective effects of different pharmacologic agents on high-energy phosphate metabolism during myocardial ischemia. Beta-blockers,[L2, O6] calcium antagonists,[K7] antianginal agents,[L3, N5] and prostacyclin analogues[P5] have been demonstrated to decrease the deleterious effects of ischemia on oxidative phosphorylation. Propranolol[N7, P8] and acebutolol[L2, N8] administration prior to ischemia attenuate the decrease in pH and high-energy phosphate metabolites. These drugs also enhance normalization of pH in the postischemic period. Administration of verapamil[N8] and nifedipine[R7] prior to ischemia was associated with more stable concentrations of high-energy phosphate metabolites, possibly due to combined effects of vasodilation and protection of mitochondrial oxidative phosphorylation. Adenosine deaminase inhibitors administered prior to ischemia preserved ATP levels during ischemia and promoted more rapid recovery of mechanical function during reperfusion.[D4] Several naturally occurring metabolites, PCr,[S7] inosine,[D2] and branched-chain amino acids[S6] have also been demonstrated to have protective effects on oxidative phosphorylation during ischemia (i.e., delay of the mechanical consequences and enhanced recovery of high-energy phosphates and mechanical function after ischemia).

A number of ^{31}P MRS studies have been done to evaluate the effects of various cardioplegic solutions on prevention of the detrimental effects of myocardial ischemia on bioenergetics.[B7, B22, B23, E1, F4–F6, H9, P6, P7, W6, W7] The benefits and risks of using various combinations of potassium chloride (KCl), hypothermia, calcium, magnesium, perfluorocarbons, and calcium antagonists were demonstrated, using changes in pH and ATP after ischemia and the rates of return to baseline metabolic status after reperfusion. Postischemic ventricular function correlated inversely with the magnitude of intracellular acidosis and the increase in Pi. pH fell less and Pi increased less in combined KCl-hypothermia than with either technique of preservation alone. Addition of calcium to the cardioplegic regimen caused greater decreases in pH and increases in Pi, whereas addition of magnesium helped maintain pH and Pi at more normal levels. Use of perfluorocarbons augmented recovery of high-energy phosphates and ventricular mechanical function.[B22, F6] When calcium antagonists were added to the cardioplegic solutions, high-energy phosphates were maintained at more normal levels, but mechanical function was not improved (this may be due to compartmentation of ATP and PCr).[B7]

Intracellular Acidosis. It has long been accepted that the depression in mechanical function associated with ischemia and hypoxia is secondary to intracellular acidosis. In a working perfused heart model of intracellular acidosis, under nonhypoxic, nonischemic conditions, Jeffrey and associates found that contractile performance was indeed very sensitive to changes in intracellular pH.[J4] This sensitivity was not related to changes in high-energy phosphate metabolism but was associated with alterations in excitation-contraction coupling. There were large changes in aortic flow with only small changes in pressure development, which indicates that the resultant effect of acidosis was due to changes in rates of contraction/relaxation. These data are consistent with the observation that ischemia-induced impairment of diastolic function may be secondary to intracellular acidosis without a change in bioenergetics.

In another study, using different workload conditions during the production of intracellular acidosis, Watters and colleagues found that increased workloads were associated with greater mechanical and metabolic changes (decompensation) than were lower workloads.[W2] In addition, substrate composition and vasodilator-induced increased coronary flow prevented some of the metabolic and mechanical dysfunction. Recovery of mechanical function was related to the levels of ATP, pH, and was directly related to the log of the phosphorylation potential at the end of the acidemic period.

Hypoxia. The ultimate effects of hypoxia on myocardial metabolism are similar to those of ischemia.[A2, B10, N2] However, because initially blood flow is generally not depressed (actually reflexly increased initially), H^+ does not build up in tissue as rapidly. Changes in PCr, Pi, and ATP occur later because glycolysis is not inhibited by early acidosis. However, when reflex mechanisms that maintain blood flow are exhausted, pH does decrease and Pi increases while PCr and ATP decrease.

Diabetes. ^{31}P MRS has been used to evaluate the effects of various substrates on myocardial metabolism in the diabetic heart.[P3, P9] Administration of L-carnitine has a protective effect in that it prevents the loss of ATP during increased workloads. Palmitate infusion was associated with a reduction in ATP, with minimal change in PCr. These studies indicate that different lipid substrates may allow the heart to tolerate increased workloads and thus protect the heart from metabolic decompensation.

Hypertension. Hypertensive heart disease is a common cause of heart failure. An understanding of the metabolic correlates of mechanical dysfunction associated with this disease process may aid in development of therapeutic regimens. One study using ^{31}P MRS has demonstrated that some metabolic sequelae of hypertensive cardiac hypertrophy are lower PCr and ATP levels and a lower metabolic tolerance to hypoxic episodes.[C5] Another study demonstrated that hypertensive hearts have decreased creatine kinase activity,[B13] and that this decrease in metabolic function was associated with a decrease in mechanical function.

Cardiomyopathy. Several studies have been done to evaluate the effects of cardiomyopathic states on myocardial metabolism.

Two recent studies of a congenital cardiomyopathy in Syrian hamsters indicate that these hearts have lower PCr/ATP ratios than age-matched controls.[C2, T3] When these hearts were treated with isoproterenol, the phosphorylation potential estimated by PCr/Pi ratios was improved, as was the developed pressure.[C2] These studies demonstrate the potential use of ^{31}P MRS techniques to investigate metabolic correlates of disease processes and to demonstrate the effectiveness of therapeutic regimens.

EFFECTS OF TOXIC SUBSTANCES. ^{31}P MRS studies demonstrate that administration of doxorubicin (Adriamycin), a chemotherapeutic agent that is cardiotoxic, causes marked decrease in ATP and PCr with an associated severe acidosis.[K12, N9] Maintenance of normal metabolic parameters was improved if an antioxidant was administered prior to Adriamycin administration.[K12] Another study, which compared the effects of acute and chronic Adriamycin administration, demonstrated a significant decrease in the PCr/ATP ratio in acute exposure to the drug, while chronic exposure was associated with near-normal PCr/ATP ratios.[K11] The investigators concluded that the mechanism of development of chronic cardiomyopathy after exposure to this drug was not related to bioenergetic phenomena.

The effects of other commonly used chemicals that can be cardiotoxic have also been studied with ^{31}P MRS. In an alcoholic hamster model, chronic exposure to alcohol has been demonstrated to increase the Pi levels and decrease the ATP levels.[W1] Intracellular pH, PCr, and creatine were within normal limits. These metabolic abnormalities were associated with a significant depression in mechanical function. Verapamil treatment during chronic alcohol exposure prevented the adverse effects on both metabolic and mechanical function.

Another study (using both ^{31}P and ^{1}H MRS) of acute alcohol exposure demonstrated that there were no changes in energetics, but that myocardial cells were dehydrated owing to alcohol exposure.[A3] The cellular dehydration was associated with the myocardial depression.

Halothane, a commonly used anesthetic agent, is known to depress myocardial mechanical function. The etiology of this depressed function may be associated with metabolic decompensation. To investigate this hypothesis, Murray and colleagues used ^{31}P MRS to evaluate the effects of acute halothane exposure on high-energy phosphate metabolism.[M6] These investigators found minimal change in pH and high-energy phosphate metabolites (PCr, ATP, Pi) during acute exposure. Magnetization transfer study of the creatine kinase reaction demonstrated a 32 percent reduction in the forward rate constant, which suggests that depressed enzyme function may be related to the decrease in mechanical function observed with halothane myocardial depression.

Exposure to different heavy metals can be associated with myocardial depression.[K12] The effects of several heavy metals (cadmium and arsenic) on myocardial metabolism and mechanical function have been studied with ^{31}P MRS and indicate that negative inotropic actions are associated with marked loss of ATP and an increase in Pi.

SUMMARY. It can be seen that much basic investigation into metabolic mechanisms under a variety of conditions has been done in perfused heart preparations with ^{31}P MRS techniques. Although studies such as these presented are necessary to lay the foundation for potential use of ^{31}P MRS under in vivo conditions, additional work in animal models under in vivo conditions is necessary before these techniques can be used effectively in the clinic. The next section presents some in vivo investigations using ^{31}P MRS.

In Vivo Metabolic Studies

Study of in vivo myocardial metabolism is an extension of perfused heart studies. However, in vivo studies are somewhat more complicated in that they require methods of signal localization not necessary in perfused heart preparations, in which the entire heart is placed inside a Helmholtz, solenoid, or saddle coil, thus acquiring signal from the entire organ. For in vivo studies, signal is obtained with a surface coil placed directly on the heart (open chest preparations) or with a combination of an imaging coil placed around the organism and a surface coil placed on the chest wall (closed chest preparation). In addition, because signal may not be acquired from the entire heart, and because the heart is generally moving with respect to the surface coil, signal:noise may not be as good as in the perfused heart preparation. This problem can be partially resolved by physiologic gating: i.e., gating the signal acquisition to the cardiac and respiratory cycles.[O7] This increases the amount of time required for data acquisition.

OPEN CHEST PREPARATIONS. A number of studies have been done using ^{31}P MRS to evaluate myocardial metabolism in open chest organisms (dogs, cats).[G8] Studies have been done to evaluate the effects of ischemia,[G7, K1, N8, R8, S9] acidemia,[B24, K15] and various mechanical loading conditions[B3, K13, K14, L6, O7, O8, P10] on myocardial metabolism as it relates to mechanical function. Generally, in vivo data confirm data obtained using perfused heart preparations. However, because blood flow and tissue oxygenation are better maintained under in vivo conditions, the heart is stable for longer periods of time, and more detailed study of myocardial metabolism can be done in a single animal. Most studies support the hypothesis that nonischemic, nonhypoxic hearts are quite stable metabolically. Generally, there are minimal changes in bioenergetics (as measured by ^{31}P MRS) under various loading conditions.[B3, K13, K14, K16, O9] However, these observations are often species-specific and therefore must be interpreted accordingly. For example, dog hearts are more stable than cat hearts during increased heart rate, blood pressure, and/or volume workloads.[L6, O7, O8]

Studies done in our laboratory to evaluate the effects of acute volume loading on cat and dog myocardium demonstrate differences in myocardial metabolic stability.[O7, O8] Acute volume loading in cats can cause an increased or decreased heart rate × systolic blood pressure (HR × SBP) product; increased heart work was associated with a decrease in PCr/ATP, while decreased work was associated with no change in this ratio. Figure 46–3 illustrates the point that different workloads can be associated with different metabolic responses. When HR × SBP was correlated with PCr/ATP to create cardiac transfer functions,[C8] all hearts appeared to be relatively stable with respect to the interaction of mechanical work and metabolism; that is, even though there were individual changes in Pi and PCr/ATP during loading, generally there were minimal overall changes in bioenergetics during continued loading (Fig. 46–4). Similar observations from volume-loaded dogs are shown in Figures 46–5, 46–6, and 46–7.

These findings concerning myocardial metabolic stability are not at all surprising, when one considers that the heart is continually active throughout the lifetime of the organism. Metabolic safeguards must be built in to protect the heart from exhaustion and from adverse effects that might occur during different loading conditions. Some of these adaptive mechanisms can be ascribed to the rate of critical enzyme reactions (ATPases, creatine kinase), which in the heart are very fast. This can be interpreted as very efficient kinetic control. Mechanisms such as these can now be studied in the intact organism with MRS techniques.

CLOSED CHEST PREPARATIONS. Although much information concerning myocardial metabolism can be obtained from open chest organism preparations, a better understanding of cardiac function would be obtained if similar studies could be done in the closed chest organism, where the intrathoracic pressures and cardiac circulation are maintained under normal physiologic conditions. In addition, development of satisfactory closed chest methods would lay the foundation for use of MRS techniques to study cardiac metabolism in humans, with eventual use in the clinic.

Some early studies in closed chest organisms were done with surface coils implanted on the heart,[K1] intravascular coils[B3, K13, K14] placed within the right and/or left ventricle, and surgically created cardiac windows,[O2, O9–O12] which allow data acquisition from a closed chest organism with surface coils placed on the chest wall. These techniques have been used to study both acute and chronic disease processes and loading conditions in animal models.

In our laboratory, we have used the cardiac window model (Fig. 46–8) to follow progressive changes in chronic volume

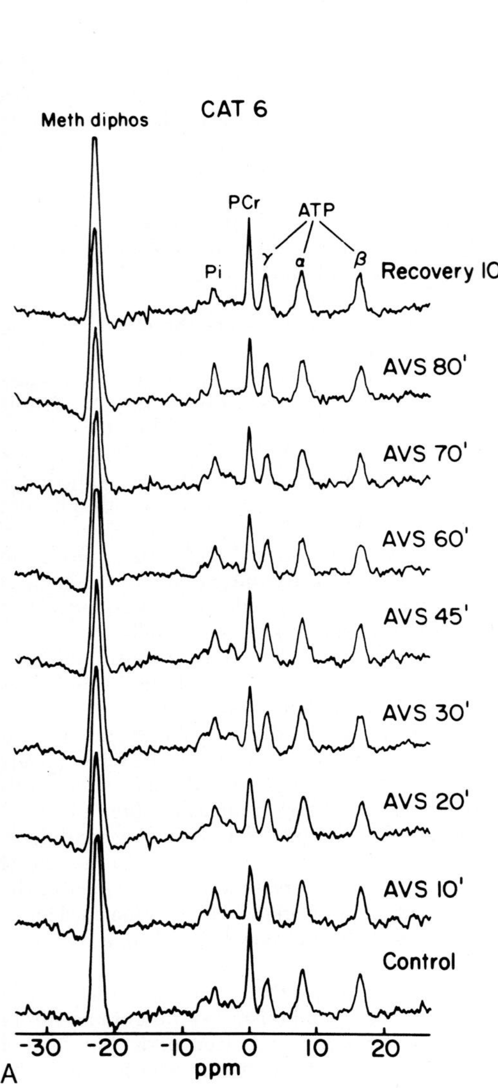

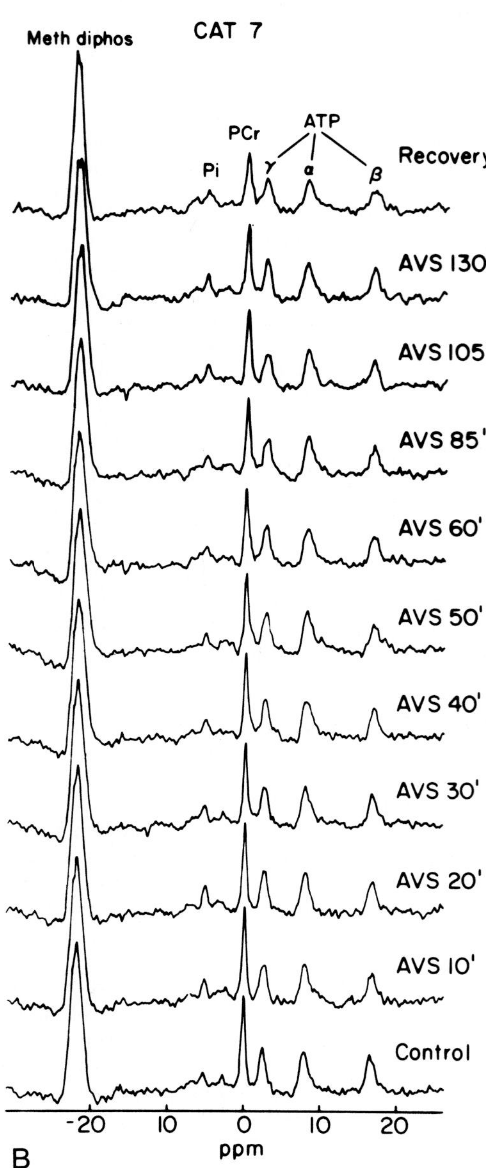

Figure 46–3. *A* and *B*, Spectra from two cats during imposition of acute volume loads. Volume loading in cat 6 produced an increase in heart rate × systolic blood pressure (HR × SBP) with associated increase in inorganic phosphate (Pi) and decrease in phosphocreatine (PCr). In cat 6, there was no change in adenosine triphosphate (ATP). In cat 7, there was no change in HR × SBP and thus little change in bioenergetic parameters. Methylene diphosphonate (Meth diphos) was used as a standard. AVS—abdominal aorta–vena cava shunt.

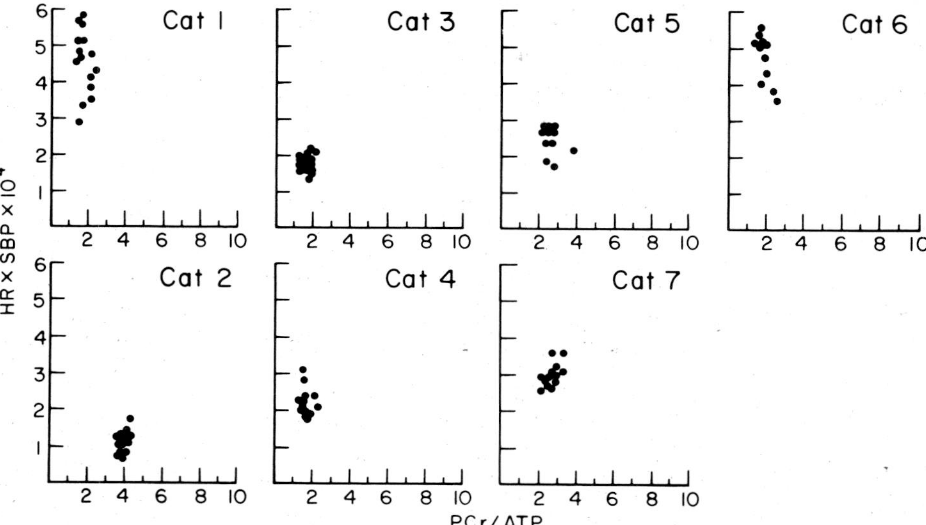

Figure 46–4. Relationship of PCr/ATP and HR × SBP in 7 cats, demonstrating that there are only small changes in PCr/ATP for a large range of HR × SBP responses. This demonstrates the hearts' metabolic stability. PCr/ATP—phosphocreatine/adenosine triphosphate. HR × SBP—heart rate × systolic blood pressure.

loading in dogs. Spectra from closed chest control and chronically loaded dog hearts are presented in Figure 46–9. Note that the volume loaded dogs had an increase in the 2,3-DPG plus Pi (TP) peaks at rest. This may be because of an increase in either or both of these phosphorus-containing compounds, one due to the increased chamber volume (2,3-DPG is in the red blood cell) and one due to a slight shift from oxidative to glycolytic mechanisms in the myocardium. When control and volume loaded dogs were evaluated over 17 months with ^{31}P MRS, there were no differences in the PCr/TP or PCr/ATP ratios at rest and during acute pressure loading with norepinephrine between the control and chronically volume loaded dogs (Fig. 46–10). This demonstrates the metabolic stability of the heart under extreme chronic loading conditions.

Thus, data obtained using these techniques again support the relative stability of myocardial metabolism under various loading conditions in the nonischemic, nonhypoxic heart. Although each of the aforementioned techniques can be used in animal models to delineate metabolic mechanisms under near physiologic conditions, they cannot be used in humans. Thus, the development of depth pulsing and imaging techniques to obtain localized spectra from the heart in the intact closed chest condition was welcomed by the medical community.[A1, B5, B6, B8, B25, B26, L7, O3, O4, R1, S3] These techniques allow acquisition of MR spectra from the heart without invasive methods and with minimal contamination of signal from surrounding tissue. Early studies using these techniques have been done to evaluate myocardial bioenergetics in normal subjects[B4, B25] and in patients with cardiomyopathy[R1, W8] and ischemic heart disease.[B6] These initial studies indicate that it may be possible to characterize myocardial pathology with metabolic measurements and thus gain insight into basic mechanisms of metabolic and mechanical decompensation during disease processes. See Chapter 54 for more details concerning these techniques.

ALLOGRAFT REJECTION. A clinically relevant problem that has been studied in animal models with ^{31}P MRS techniques is the process of allograft rejection. A number of studies in rat and dog allograft models have demonstrated the ability of ^{31}P MRS to diagnose rejection before histologic or mechanical function changes occur. Rejection was characterized by an increase in Pi and a decrease in PCr, and in one study by an increase in phosphodiesters.[F7] Early changes in the PCr/Pi ratio can be used as diagnostic criteria for onset of rejection and can be used to indicate when immunosuppressive therapy should be started, should be increased, or is not working.[C8, H10–H12, S10]

Carbon (^{13}C) Magnetic Resonance Spectroscopy

Many metabolic substrates and metabolites cannot be studied with ^{31}P MRS. Because of this, and because most biologically active chemicals contain carbon, the use of ^{13}C MRS was proposed as a method to delve further into the mysteries of intermediary

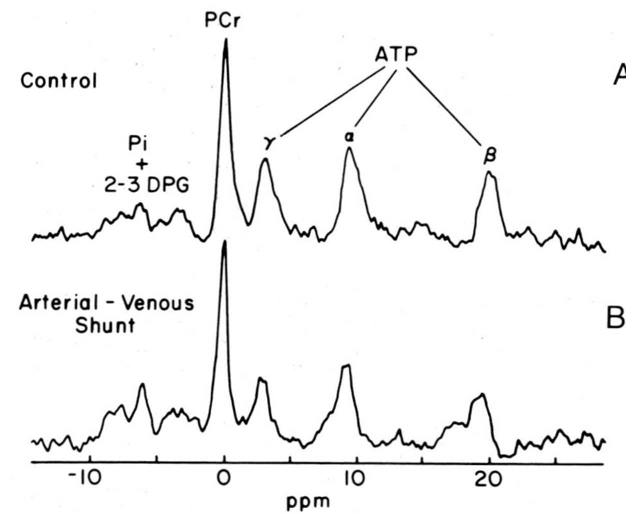

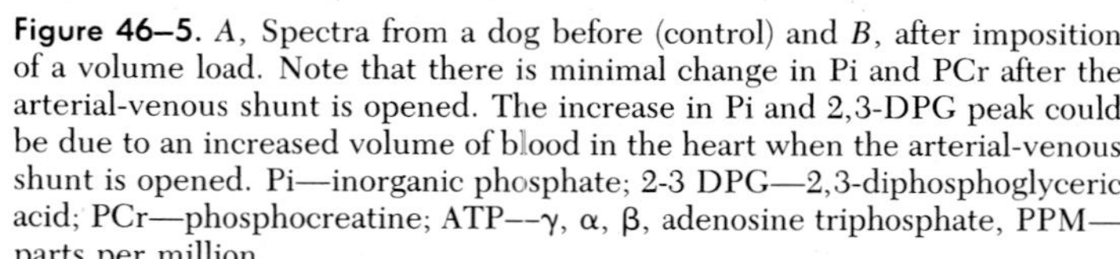
Figure 46–5. *A*, Spectra from a dog before (control) and *B*, after imposition of a volume load. Note that there is minimal change in Pi and PCr after the arterial-venous shunt is opened. The increase in Pi and 2,3-DPG peak could be due to an increased volume of blood in the heart when the arterial-venous shunt is opened. Pi—inorganic phosphate; 2-3 DPG—2,3-diphosphoglyceric acid; PCr—phosphocreatine; ATP—γ, α, β, adenosine triphosphate, PPM—parts per million.

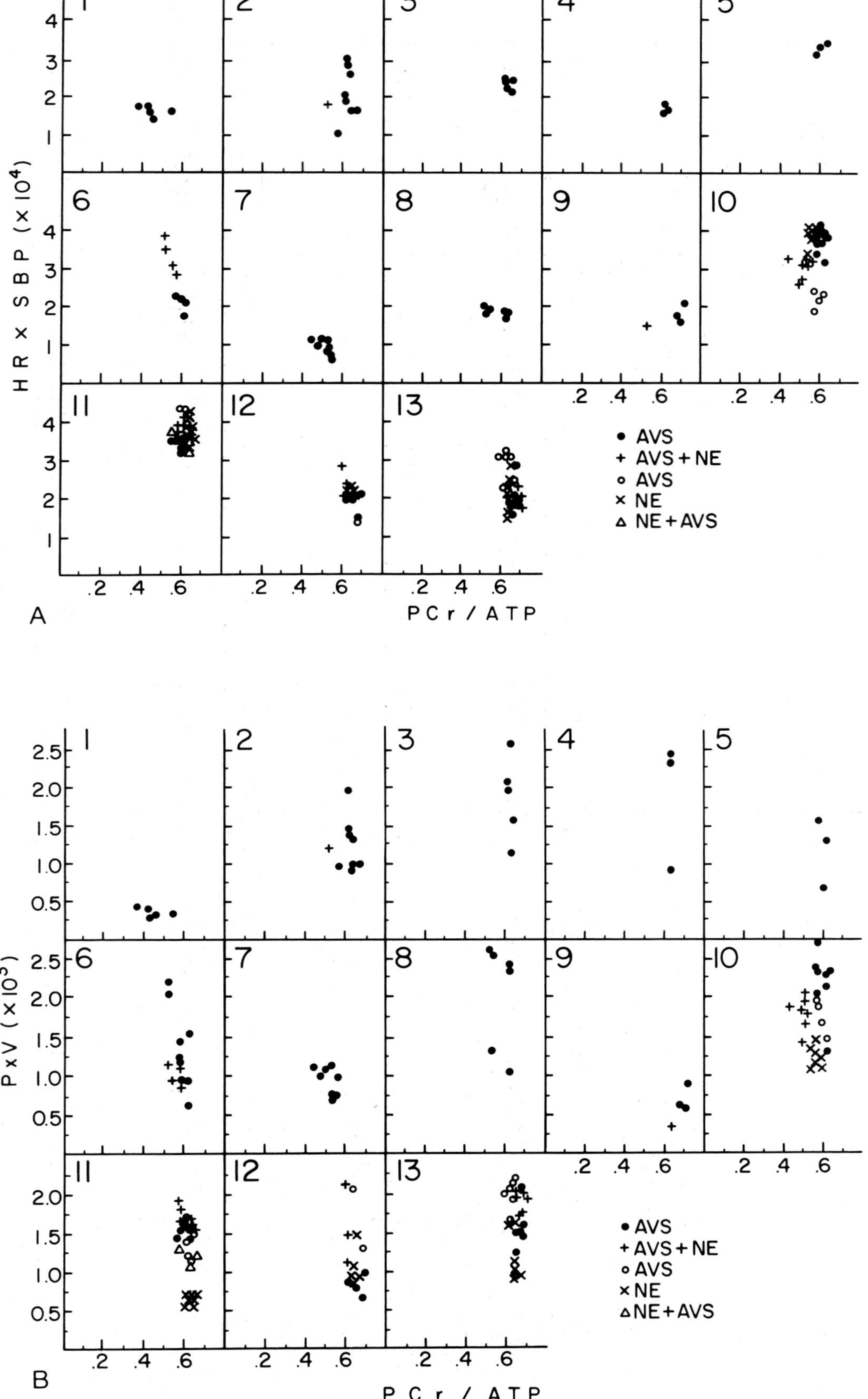

Figure 46–6. *A*, Correlation of heart rate × systolic blood pressure (HR × SBP) work with phosphocreatine/adenosine triphosphate (PCr/ATP) during acute volume and/or pressure loading in a dog. *B*, correlation of pressure × stroke volume (P × V) work with PCr/ATP during acute volume and/or pressure loading in a dog. Note that for both sets of data, widely varying workloads are associated with minimal changes in PCr/ATP, which indicates that metabolic function is quite stable. AVS—abdominal aorta–vena cava anastomosis, NE—norepinephrine, 1 μg/kg/min.

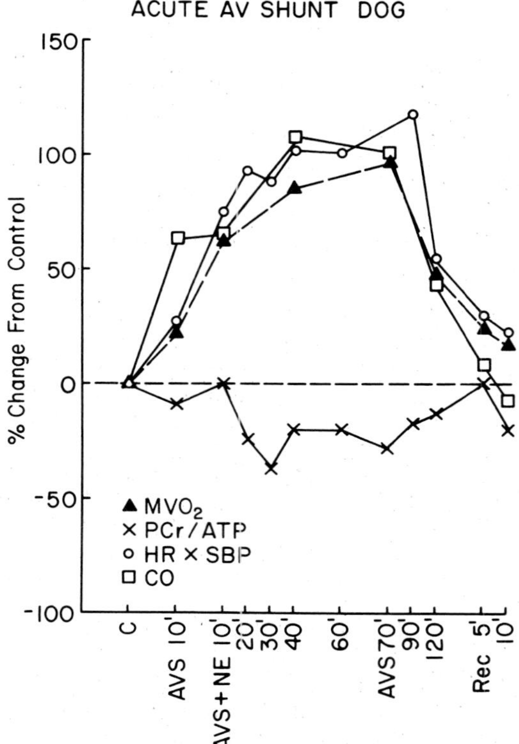

Figure 46–7. Graphic presentation of percent change of mechanical (HR × SBP, CO, and MVO_2) and metabolic (PCr/ATP) function parameters with time after imposition of acute volume (abdominal aorta–vena cava shunt—AVS) and pressure (norepinephrine—NE) loads to dog heart. Note that changes in both mechanical and metabolic functions are less in volume loading alone than in combined pressure plus volume loading. In addition, note that large changes in mechanical function are associated with only minimal to moderate changes in metabolic function. MVO_2—O_2 consumption, PCr/ATP—phosphocreatine/adenosine triphosphate; HR × SBP—heart rate × systolic blood pressure, CO—cardiac output, Rec—recovery.

metabolism in intact organs. However, even though the natural abundance of carbon atoms is high, the natural abundance of the MRS-sensitive carbon (^{13}C) is low (1.2 percent). Therefore, ^{13}C-labeled substrate must be added in order to measure ^{13}C compounds in an intact organ. In addition, the MRS sensitivity of ^{13}C is only 1.6 percent of proton sensitivity (see Table 46–1). Therefore, adequate signal from ^{13}C-containing compounds can be best obtained using high-field systems (4.7 to 11.8 Tesla) or by using long scan times in lower field systems. One advantage of ^{13}C MRS is that it is characterized by a reasonably wide chemical shift range and therefore permits resolution of ^{13}C resonances in molecules that are similar in structure,[S12] which is not possible with proton MRS because of overlap of peaks.

^{13}C MRS experiments generally use two radiofrequency (RF) fields: the observe $\mathbf{B}_1$ field for ^{13}C and a saturating $\mathbf{B}_1$ field at proton (^1H) Larmor frequency used to decouple proton nuclei from carbon nuclei, improving S:N by collapse of multiple lines into a single line. The ^1H radiofrequency field also increases the ^{13}C signal by the nuclear Overhauser effect (NOE)—i.e., as a result of relaxation between ^{13}C and the saturated protons, the population of the nuclear energy levels changes when the proton resonances are saturated.

A number of early studies demonstrated the feasibility of using ^{13}C to investigate metabolic mechanisms in the intact heart.[B27, N10] These studies indicated that amino acid metabolism of the heart could be followed with ^{13}C MRS.[B27] In addition, the effects of pathophysiologic interventions such as hypoxia and anoxia on glycogen metabolism could be studied by following changes in glutamate isotopomers with ^{13}C MRS.[N10] Additional studies following glycogen metabolism (both synthesis and degradation) in perfused hearts[L8] and in hearts in vivo[L9, N11, N12] have been done.

The possibility of measuring the flux of metabolites through the citric acid cycle (intermediary metabolism) has also been explored by a number of laboratories.[C9, L9, M7, M8, S13] The effects of use of different starting ^{13}C-labeled substrates (acetate, pyruvate, glucose, propionate, and lactate) on the metabolic intermediates of the citric acid cycle have been studied using this technique. Mathematical models have been developed to follow and quantify flux of metabolic intermediates through different pathways.[C9, M7, M8] The flux through anapleurotic versus oxidative pathways, as measured using ^{13}C MRS, changes depending on the starting substrates and the physiologic conditions.[M7, M8, S11, S13]

The metabolic consequences of hypoxia and anoxia have also been explored with ^{13}C MRS.[B28] During hypoxia, glutamate and aspartate decrease and succinate increases. This suggests that amino acid metabolism may be an important supplement to glycolytic metabolism during hypoxic and ischemic conditions. If this is the case in vivo, some protection against the effects of ischemia may result from administration of amino acids (glutamate, fumarate, malate, oxaloacetate, 2-oxoglutarate) during and after ischemic events.

Another use of ^{13}C MRS might be to study the effects of different loading conditions and use of different substrates during loading on myocardial intermediary metabolism. We have begun to use ^{13}C MRS to evaluate the effects of exhaustive exercise on the cardiac intermediary metabolism. Preliminary results indicate that exhaustive exercise depletes intrinsic amino acids and other intermediary metabolites and increases the flux through citrate synthetase rather than through anapleurotic pathways. This is especially evident when exhaustively exercised hearts are further stimulated with dobutamine during $^{13}C2$-acetate infusions.

Figure 46–11 presents some ^{13}C data obtained from exhaustively exercised trained and untrained rat hearts during $^{13}C2$-acetate and $^{13}C3$-lactate perfusion and from an extract from a

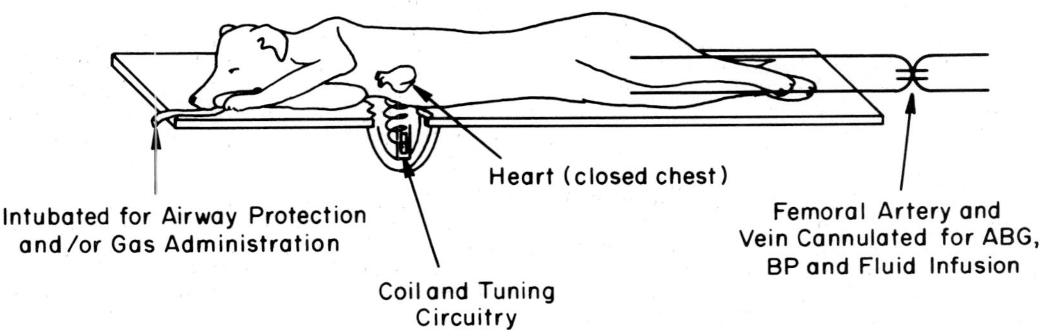

Figure 46–8. Illustration of a setup to obtain MRS data from a closed chest cardiac window dog using a surface coil placed directly under the heart. MRS signal is obtained from the heart using simple saturation recovery pulsing without the use of localization routines because the heart in effect lays directly on the surface coil when the animal is placed in the left lateral decubitus position. (This is possible because two ribs and surrounding skeletal muscle have been removed and replaced by a thin layer of Marlex mesh. When the skin is sutured over the mesh, there is only a 2- to 3-mm distance between the heart and the surface coil.)

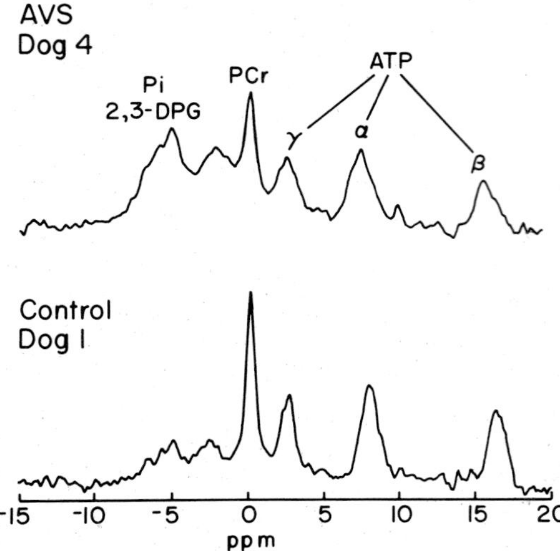

Figure 46–9. Spectra from two dogs with chronic "cardiac windows"; one dog is a control and the other had surgical creation of an abdominal aorta–vena cava shunt (AVS). Both dogs were followed in parallel over 17 months to evaluate the effects of progressive chronic volume loading on the heart. Note that the Pi plus 2,3-DPG peak was larger in the AVS dog than in the control dog. This may be due to an increase in 2,3-DPG (due to increased chamber volume) and/or an increase in Pi due to an increase in glycolysis in the volume overload condition. Pi—inorganic phosphate, 2,3-DPG—2,3 diphosphoglyceric acid, PCr—phosphocreatine, ATP—γ, α, β, adenosine triphosphate, ppm—parts per million.

heart perfused with ^{13}C2-acetate. The peaks of interest are due to glutamate C2, C4, and C3, which are used to estimate flux through the citric acid cycle. These kinds of data can be used to evaluate substrate preference during extremes in myocardial loading.

Thus, although techniques to acquire ^{13}C MRS data are more difficult than acquisition of ^{31}P MRS data, much potential basic biochemical information can be obtained from the intact heart using this technique. Further investigation is necessary to delineate just what the value of ^{13}C MRS may be in the clinical situation.

Proton Magnetic Resonance Spectroscopy

Proton MRS potentially can measure the concentration of many metabolically significant compounds (Fig. 46–12).[P11] However, obtaining localization of proton signal from the heart while retaining spectral resolution sufficient to isolate specific metabolites is difficult, especially in the moving heart. To extract usable chemical information from living systems, sophisticated pulsing methods that suppress the very large water and fat signals are necessary.

Initial work using perfused heart preparations in conjunction with coils that surround the heart, which maximize spectral resolution, has been done in small-bore, high-field magnets. Some of this work has been done to measure changes in lactate during and after ischemia.[D5, K17, R10] One group was able to obtain lactate spectra with reasonable resolution in one minute[K17] (Fig. 46–13). Another group demonstrated that the adverse effects of lower temperature during ischemia (1°C vs. 12°C) were not due to increase in glycolysis and production of lactate because there was less lactate in the hearts maintained at 1°C than at 12°C.[D5]

Other investigators have been able to measure changes in taurine, carnitine, creatine, and glycerides under different physiologic conditions in perfused heart preparations.[U3] In all these studies, there has been a problem of resolution of overlapping peaks and of obtaining sufficient signal for identification of individual peaks.

Some groups have dealt with the problem of signal resolution by evaluating extracts of normal and injured myocardium.[E2, R9] Infarcted tissue could be characterized by specific changes in its chemical composition, i.e., infarcted tissue was found to have an abnormal lipid profile compared with normal tissue.[R11] Proton MRS also has been used to acquire a "spectral signature" of lipid peaks in human atheroma.[P12]

Other work using proton MRS has been done to characterize T_1 and T_2 relaxation times under pathologic conditions (see Chapter 50).[F8, R9, T3] T_2s have been found to be prolonged in hypertrophic and cardiomyopathic states. Lipid/water ratios have been found to be decreased in cardiomyopathy.[T3] Both T_1 and T_2 have been found to be prolonged in infarcted tissue.

Another application of proton MRS to the heart is in the determination of the relative volumes of the intracellular and extracellular water in the cardiac tissue.[N13] This is done with the same shift reagent, dysprosium triethylene tetramine hexaacetate (Dy-TTHA^{-3}), as is used in evaluation of intracellular and extracellular sodium or potassium. Since the concentration of water in both compartments is the same, the ratio of the areas of the two peaks reacts to the change in relative volumes during a pathophysiologic intervention.

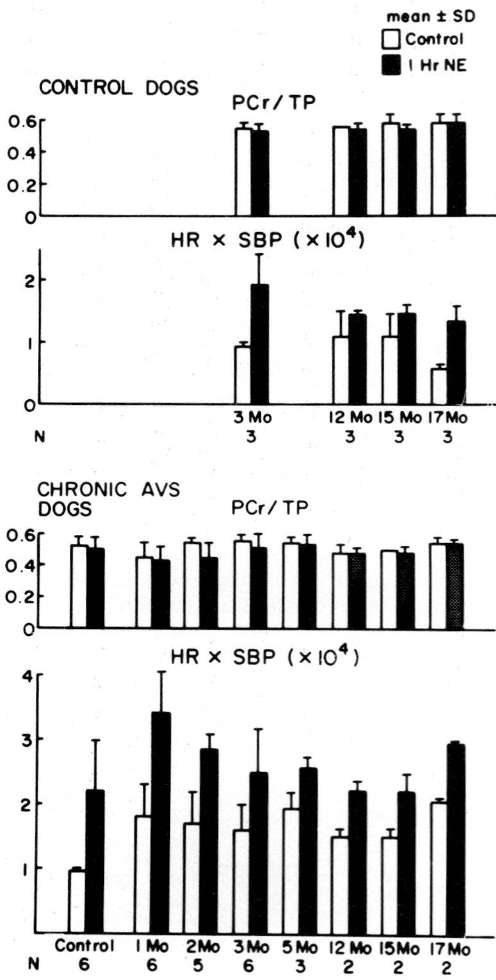

Figure 46–10. Metabolic function (PCr/ATP) and mechanical work (HR × SBP) data in control and chronic AVS dogs. Note that the response to application of acute increases in workload (administration of norepinephrine [NE]) was associated with similar responses in PCr/ATP in both control and AVS dogs; i.e., there was no significant change in PCr/ATP during NE-induced hypertension at any time during the progression of chronic volume loading when compared with control. This demonstrates myocardial metabolic stability during chronic volume loading. PCr/ATP—phosphocreatine/adenosine triphosphate, AVS—abdominal aorta–vena cava anastomosis.

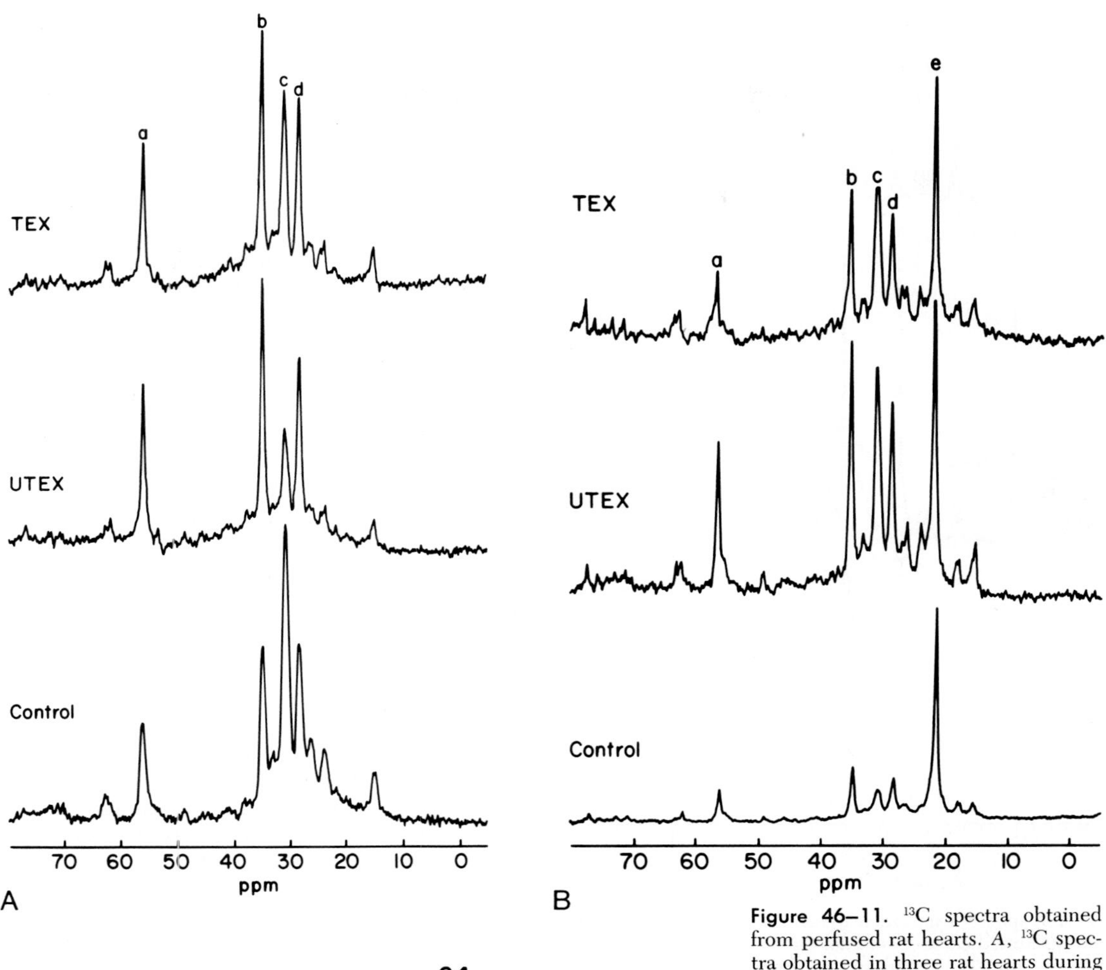

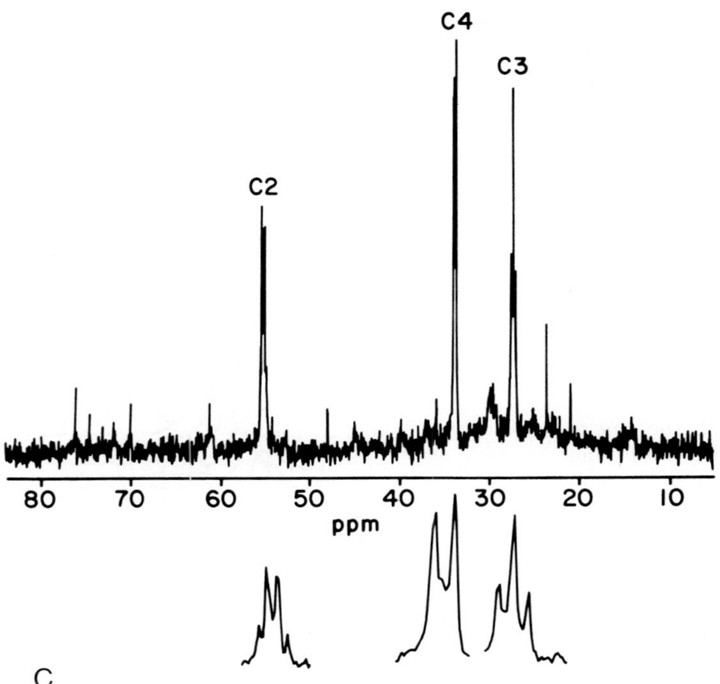

Figure 46–11. ^{13}C spectra obtained from perfused rat hearts. *A*, ^{13}C spectra obtained in three rat hearts during perfusion to steady state with $^{13}C2$-acetate. The peaks of interest are a = glutamate C2, b = glutamate C4, and d = glutamate C3. The ratio of the areas under these peaks can be used to estimate flux through the citric acid cycle using a mathematical algorithm of Malloy and associates.[M7] Note the difference in the peak intensities in control, compared with untrained, exercised to exhaustion (UTEX), and trained, exercised to exhaustion (TEX) rat hearts. Peak c is natural abundance fatty acids. *B*, ^{13}C spectra obtained in three rat hearts during perfusion with $^{13}C2$-lactate to steady state. Note the difference in the C2 glutamate peak intensity and similarity of the C4 and C3 peak ratios when lactate was used as a metabolic substrate. *C*, ^{13}C spectra from an extract of a $^{13}C2$-acetate perfused heart which was perfused to steady state. The small insets correspond to C2, C4, and C3 peaks of glutamate. The individual peaks of each glutamate (C2,C4,C3) can be used with a more sophisticated algorithm[M8] to calculate flux through the citric acid cycle.

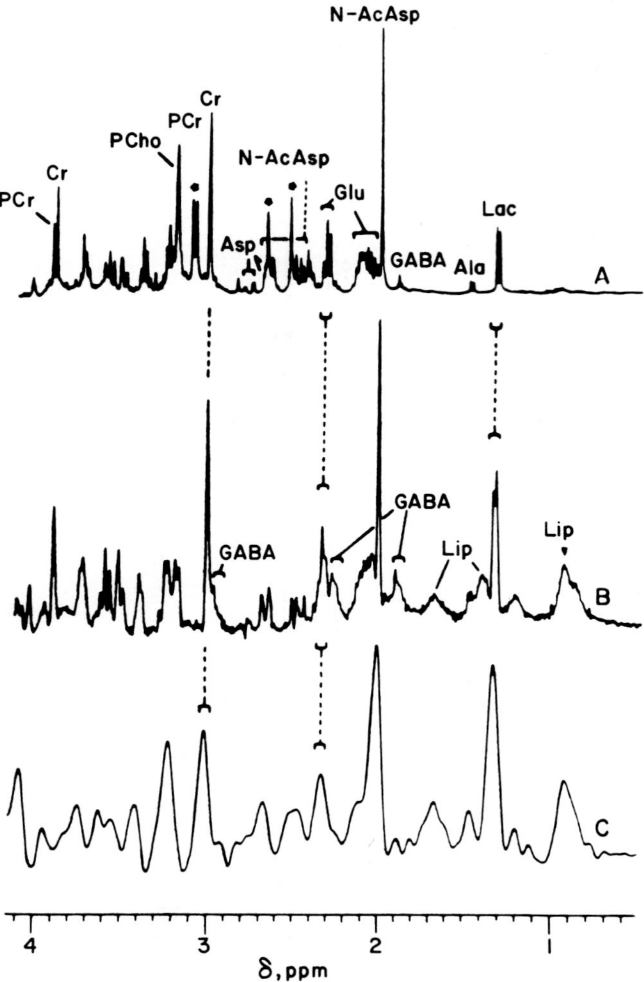

Figure 46–12. Proton spectra from brain tissue obtained under different conditions, demonstrating the variety of information that can be obtained with proton spectroscopy. *A*, Proton spectra from a brain extract; *B*, Proton spectra from excised intact cerebrum; *C*, Proton spectra obtained from an in vivo brain with a surface coil placed over the skull. Note the similarity of the three sets of spectra obtained using different techniques. The potential for acquisition of proton spectra from the heart is equally as exciting but will be more difficult because of artifacts associated with cardiac motion. PCr—phosphocreatine, Cr—creatine, PCho—phosphorylcholine, Asp—aspartate, N-Ac-Asp—N-acetyl aspartate, Glu—glutamate, GABA—gamma aminobutyric acid, Ala—alanine, Lac—lactate, Lip—lipid. (From Behar, K. L., et al.: High-resolution ^{1}H nuclear magnetic resonance study of cerebral hypoxia in vivo. Proc. Natl. Acad. Sci. USA 80:4945, Fig 1, 1983, with permission.)

Sodium (^{23}Na) and Potassium (^{39}K) Magnetic Resonance Spectroscopy

Sodium and potassium flux across membranes is the key to maintenance of electrical membrane potentials in the myocardium and myocardial conduction system. Evaluation of these fluxes in a nondestructive manner can be done with ^{23}Na and ^{39}K MRS.[F9, P13, S14, S15, W9] Early studies were done with paramagnetic shift agents to allow evaluation of intracellular and extracellular ion concentrations. However, the shift reagents can be toxic. More recently developed techniques use pulse editing techniques to obtain similar data with less disruption of the system.[B29, K18, P14, R1, S16, W9] These techniques can be applied in the intact living organism, without destruction of tissue.

Pathology as Seen by Abnormalities in Sodium Metabolism

All cells maintain ionic gradients across their membranes as an energy store to provide energy for some enzymatic reactions and to regulate others. Na^{+} concentration is maintained at low intracellular and high extracellular levels (1 to 20) via an active pump process. Some pathologic conditions manifest themselves in a disruption of the sodium ionic gradient. Ischemia is the most common physiologic condition that results in disruption of active sodium transport out of the cell. Measurement of the changes in intracellular and extracellular sodium under experimental conditions has led to better understanding of some of these reactions.[C10, L10, P15, S17]

Sodium (^{23}Na) Magnetic Resonance Spectroscopy

Sodium-23 is a quadrupolar nucleus of spin 3/2. Its gyromagnetic ratio is 11.262 MHz/Tesla, about two thirds that of phosphorus-31 and one quarter that of protons. Sodium-23 has natural abundance of 100 percent. The nucleus has a high magnetic moment, so its net sensitivity is good. The resulting net sensitivity of ^{23}Na is slightly better than that of ^{31}P (see Table 46–1).

The 3/2 spin results in three single-quantum transitions for ^{23}Na. These occur at slightly shifted frequencies in the solid state. In the liquid state normally found in biologic systems, random tumbling motion averages these orientation-dependent splittings into a single broad peak.[C10] The quadrupolar term dominates the relaxation of ^{23}Na, resulting in short T_1 and T_2.

MRS investigations of sodium in biologic systems began over 20 years ago.[C11, J1, S18] Cope investigated the binding of sodium by actomyosin, sparking a debate over the discrepancy between the levels of intracellular sodium measured by MRS and other techniques.[C11] Many investigators postulated a pool of "MRS-invisible" sodium, but this was ultimately recognized as a relaxation phenomenon.[B30, C10, C12]

Shift Reagent Techniques

To measure the ratio of intracellular to extracellular sodium, one must be able to resolve the sodium MRS signals from the two compartments, which occur naturally at the same chemical shift. The first method used to resolve the ^{23}Na signal from the two compartments involved the use of a shift reagent placed in the extracellular compartment.[B31, P16]

Shift reagents were initially introduced to MRS as a means of resolving overlapping peaks in the proton spectra of complex chemical compounds. The shift reagent is a highly paramagnetic compound that changes the chemical shift of nuclei with which it is coordinated. The rare earth elements of the lanthanide series have the highest paramagnetic moments of any naturally occurring elements, so they are obvious choices for development as

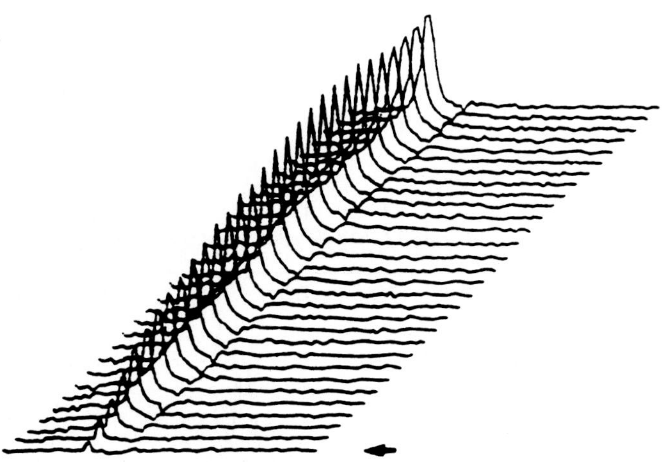

Figure 46–13. Proton spectra of lactate accumulation during myocardial ischemia in a perfused rat heart. Each spectrum was accumulated over 1 minute. These data demonstrate the temporal resolution of metabolic phenomena during a physiologic intervention. (From Keller, A. M., et al.: Very rapid lactate measurement in ischemic perfused hearts using ^{1}H MRS continuous negative echo acquisition during steady-state frequency selective excitation. Magn. Reson. Med. 7:65, 1988, with permission.)

shift reagents. Shift reagent studies in biologic sodium MRS have centered around complexes of dysprosium and gadolinium. The complexes cannot cross the cell membrane, so they only shift the resonance of the sodium ions in the extracellular compartment.

A commonly used complex is dysprosium bis-tripolyphosphate ($Dy(PPP)_2^{-7}$), which causes a downfield shift (to lower frequency) of the extracellular peak.[S14] Gupta and Gupta introduced this reagent,[G9] and it has found broad acceptance. Matwiyoff and associates investigated the stability of this complex, finding that the complex is a substrate for pyrophosphatase, which cleaves the tripolyphosphate into inorganic phosphate in a reaction that can be monitored with ^{31}P MRS.[M9]

The paramagnetic shift of the extracellular sodium resonance in muscle or brain preparations is greatest from 5 to 15 minutes after addition of this shift reagent. As the shift reagent is decomposed, the shift grows smaller, and after 3 hours, the two compartment peaks can no longer be resolved. In erythrocyte suspensions, which have low pyrophosphatase levels, the shift reagent is stable. Intracellular and extracellular resonances remain resolvable for 36 hours or more.[M9]

Szklaruk and co-workers have linked the dissociation of $Dy(PPP)_2^{-7}$ to toxicity.[S19] Other metal ions can compete with dysprosium for the tripolyphosphate and precipitate it. The free Dy^{+3} ions then bind to biologic macromolecules, which can destroy them or make them nonfunctional. It is thus suggested that the toxicity of the shift reagent can be limited by limiting its dissociation.[S19]

The next most commonly used shift reagent, $Dy\text{-}TTHA^{-3}$, is less toxic than $Dy(PPP)_2^{-7}$ but less effective in resolving the two compartments.[F9] Larger quantities of $Dy\text{-}TTHA^{-3}$ are needed to get a shift of even 1 ppm.

Other complexes of dysprosium are being tested in vitro for shifting efficacy and for their effects on biologic systems. Dysprosium tetra(methylenephosphonate) ($DyDOTP^{-5}$) has a strong effect on the chemical shift, but it also has a high affinity for calcium ions and thus interferes with intercellular signaling.[S20] Sherry and co-workers attempt to avoid this complication by substituting terbium for dysprosium. The shifting effects of $TmDOTP^{-5}$ are not affected by the calcium concentrations in the heart.[S20] The terbium complex gives a useful upfield shift of 2.5 ppm.

Szklaruk and colleagues tried to block the degradation of tripolyphosphate by bonding it to a benzene ring in dysprosium o-bis-(tripolyphosphatopropyloxy) benzene ($Dy\text{-}bPPPpob^{-5}$).[S19] This compound is hydrolyzed only slowly in the heart and resolves a third sodium peak, which is believed to represent the interstitial sodium. In an ex vivo test, $Dy\text{-}bPPPpob^{-5}$ caused only minor changes in heart rate and blood pressure while shifting the extracellular resonance upfield by 4 ppm. A comparative study of the shifting effects of various dysprosium and gadolinium complexes was made by Brown and colleagues.[B29]

Shift Reagent Applications

Application of these shift reagent techniques to cardiac MRS has centered on perfused hearts in high-resolution narrow-bore magnets. Some experiments also have been performed on excised pieces of myocardium.

Springer demonstrated the intracellular influx of sodium during ischemic insult[S14] (Fig. 46–14). These data demonstrate the loss of active transport mechanisms during ischemia and the resulting increase in the intracellular sodium concentration. This type of data may be used to diagnose potential reversibility of ischemic episodes.

Fossel and Hoefeler obtained quantitative results from the shift reagent MRS method by comparing peak areas found in the heart with those of a balloon phantom.[F9] A linear relationship between peak area and sodium concentration was found as well. The intracellular concentration of sodium as measured by shift reagent MRS compared well with microelectrode measurement of sodium ions.[F9]

In the perfused heart, decomposed shift reagent is an effective chelator of calcium ions. The chelation process is likely to perturb the physiologic system. Fossel and Hoefeler needed to supplement the perfusate with calcium, even at low shift reagent concentration.[F9]

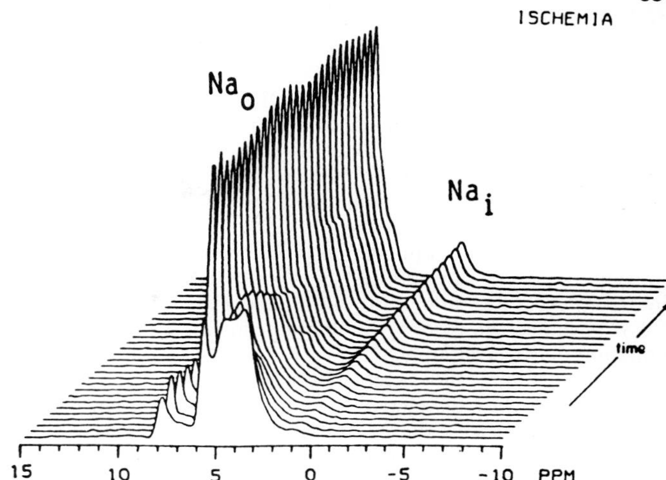

Figure 46–14. ^{23}Na spectra from perfused heart during the development of ischemia. Note that intracellular Na^+ (Na_i) increases with time during ischemia. Na_o—extracellular sodium. (From Springer, C. S.: ^{23}Na and ^{39}K NMR spectroscopic studies of the intact beating heart. *In* Osbakken, M. D., and Haselgrove, J. (eds.): NMR Techniques in the Study of Cardiovascular Structure and Function. Futura Publishing Company, Mt. Kisco, N.Y., 1988, p. 289, with permission.)

Stewart and colleagues used shift reagent ^{23}Na MRS to correlate sodium and ATP concentrations in the perfused guinea pig heart.[S17] The data suggested two ATP pools, one the product of glycolysis and one the product of oxidative phosphorylation. When one source of ATP was inhibited, the other supplied sufficient energy to maintain the sodium gradient. In experiments during the application of hypoxia, glucose administration slowed ATP depletion and sodium accumulation.

Two recent studies using ^{23}Na MRS to investigate the effects of ouabain on the perfused heart appeared simultaneously. Powell and associates found that the effects of ouabain could be counteracted with calcium.[P15] By reducing calcium or potassium or both, intracellular sodium levels could be increased reversibly, and independent of ouabain. The dysprosium tripolyphosphate shift reagent enabled Powell to presaturate the extracellular sodium compartment and get signal only from intracellular sodium.

Using similar techniques, Lotan and co-workers perfused rat hearts with ouabain and compared intracellular sodium in those hearts that fibrillated with those that did not.[L10] The sodium increase was significantly higher in the fibrillating group: 11.56 percent per minute compared with 3.93 percent per minute in the nonfibrillating hearts. Amiloride eliminated this effect of the ouabain and prevented fibrillation. The sodium increase with ouabain and amiloride was only 5.18 percent per minute. However, amiloride increased the acidification rate of the heart from −0.0016 pH units per minute to −0.0045 pH units per minute. Lotan and co-workers concluded that ouabain causes acidification of the heart whereas amiloride inhibits the exchange of intracellular H^+ for extracellular Na^+, which counteracts the acidification.[L10]

Relaxation Deconvolution

Burstein and Fossel's work presaturating the shifted extracellular sodium resonance led to their measuring relaxation times separately in the two compartments.[B32, B33] T_1 and T_2 were both 56 msec in Ringer's solution and were comparably long in the extracellular compartment. Intracellular T_1 was 23 μsec, while T_2 was biexponential with time constants of 2 and 17 μsec. This difference in relaxation between the compartments causes the resulting Fourier transformed NMR spectra to consist of a sharp intracellular peak superimposed over a broad extracellular peak.

This suggests that deconvolution of the sodium peak could be used to resolve the intracellular and extracellular compartments and thus could be used instead of shift reagents, which can adversely affect the physiologic system. Burstein and Fossel were able to isolate the intracellular and extracellular signals and perform further analysis on the unshifted intracellular signal.[B32] Success with this technique depends on having a large difference between the decay rates of the two exponentials representing the different T_1s. If the ratio of the times is less than 3:1 to 5:1, then it is very difficult to resolve the double-exponential fit to the free induction decay accurately.

Renshaw, Blum, and Leigh took a novel approach to solving this problem. They developed a contrast agent, dextran magnetite, which enhances the relaxation of only the extracellular sodium.[R12] The enhancement of the difference in relaxation rates increases the ability to distinguish the two sodium pools. Furthermore, this contrast agent is less toxic than the paramagnetic shift reagents.

Brown and colleagues introduced a combination approach, using a shift reagent and relaxation effects in a model system analysis.[B29] Rather than deconvolve the free induction decay into two relaxation components, they used an inversion-recovery sequence to provide relaxation contrast between the two sodium compartments. A simplified version of this experiment is the null-point technique used by Seo and Kuki and associates to resolve intracellular and extracellular potassium.[K18, S16]

Multiple Quantum Spectroscopy

The double-quantum filter is yet another tool for separation of the slow- and fast-relaxing components of the ^{23}Na signal. It is especially useful when the difference in relaxation rates is relatively small. With sodium, the relaxation of the two outer transitions ($-3/2$ to $-1/2$ and $1/2$ to $3/2$) is faster than the inner ($-1/2$ to $1/2$) transition.[P14, W9] The double-quantum filter inverts the phase of the outer transitions, making it easier to resolve them, though at a cost of increased data acquisition time.[P14, W9]

Potassium (^{39}K) Magnetic Resonance Spectroscopy

The cells of the heart maintain a potassium gradient across their membranes, just as they maintain a sodium gradient. In this case, intracellular potassium is maintained at much higher levels than extracellular. Potassium-39 is a MRS nucleus (spin 3/2 like ^{23}Na) of high natural abundance, but its net sensitivity is 200 times less than that of ^{23}Na (see Table 46–1). Despite this disadvantage, investigators are studying myocardial potassium levels with ^{39}K MRS, using many of the same techniques that are applied to sodium.[W10]

Fossel and Hoefeler shifted the extracellular component of the potassium resonance upfield with Dy-TTHA^{-3} and obtained an intracellular potassium concentration of 31 mmol, which is one fourth of the potassium measured by other techniques.[F9] They theorize that the large NMR-invisible component of potassium is immobilized, so the strong quadrupolar relaxation of potassium can render those nuclei invisible.[F9] The exchange between these nuclei and the NMR-visible free potassium is slow compared with the relaxation time.

A variation of the relaxation deconvolution method previously described for sodium has also been applied to potassium.[K18, S16] If the T_1 of the potassium of either compartment is known, then the resonance of that compartment can be selectively suppressed. This is done with an inversion-recovery pulse sequence ($180° - \tau - 90°$) with the time τ between pulses equal to 0.69 times T_1, at which time the z component of magnetization has relaxed to zero.

Fluorine (^{19}F) Magnetic Resonance Spectroscopy

Fluorine-19, an MRS-sensitive nucleus that has a low intrinsic concentration in biologic tissue and a high MRS sensitivity, has potential for use as an exogenous marker of biologic function. A number of studies have been done, using this tracer to evaluate calcium (Ca^{+2}) and magnesium (Mg^{+2}) concentration and movement in cells.[L11, M10–M12, S21] A fluorinated Ca^{+2} indicator, 5,5′-$^{19}F_2$-BAPTA, has been used to determine cyclical changes in intracellular free Ca^{+2} concentration that are associated with contraction in the intact heart.[M10, M11] During diastole, Ca^{+2} concentration was found to be 200 nM, and during systole Ca^{+2} concentration was found to increase to 1 μM. In these studies, alteration of coronary perfusion was associated with changes in Ca^{+2} transients even when high-energy phosphate concentrations did not change, which indicate that regulatory effects of Ca^{+2} transients can protect bioenergetic function of the heart.[P17]

Other studies have been done to measure progressive changes in ^{19}F-containing tracer levels with ^{19}F MRS to determine organ perfusion.[E3, N14] In these studies, ^{19}F spectra are obtained over time to measure washout of tracer from the heart in a manner similar to the Kety-Schmidt technique.

Deuterium (^{2}H) Magnetic Resonance Spectroscopy

Despite its very low net sensitivity, deuterium (^{2}H) MRS has found use in the heart as a probe of myocardial perfusion. In this technique introduced by Ackerman and associates,[A4, E4] a bolus of heavy water (D_2O) is injected upstream from the organ whose perfusion is being measured. The tracer is taken up rapidly, then washes out more slowly. The exponential washout of tracer fits the Kety-Schmidt model, yielding a direct measure of tissue perfusion. Kim and Ackerman have solved the differential equations of several possible flow models and applied them to several types of tissue.[K19]

In vivo deuterium NMR measurement of perfusion has been extended to the heart by Mitchell and co-workers. They have obtained sufficient time resolution of the deuterium spectra to accurately measure flow rates of 100 ml/min/100 g of tissue or greater.[O13] These perfusion measurements also have been integrated with ^{31}P MRS and other physiologic measurements.[M13, O13] Increases and decreases in cardiac perfusion have been documented.[O13] True perfusion images of the brain have recently been acquired by this group,[D6] but it is unlikely that the heart can ever be imaged in this way.

POTENTIAL CLINICAL USES

Although MRS has potential for clinical use, only a few clinical studies have been done to date.[B4, B25, R1, W8] The reason is that acquisition of clinical ^{31}P magnetic resonance spectra require sophisticated techniques that are not routinely available. Spatial localization is important to obtain signal from the heart without contamination from the surrounding tissue. In addition, because of motion artifacts, cardiac and respiratory gating are necessary. In animal models, cardiac gating is easily done using arterial blood pressure pulses obtained from an indwelling catheter. In humans, however, placement of an arterial line is usually contraindicated. This necessitates the use of another mode of physiologic gating, most often the electrocardiogram. However, the magnetic field can distort the electrocardiographic signal and make it difficult for use in gating. Therefore, sophisticated computer algorithms are often necessary to filter the noise from the electrocardiographic signal, so it can be used for gating. Initial solutions to these problems have been found and some MRS data have been obtained from the heart in humans.[B26]

Use of these data in conjunction with other measurements of metabolic and mechanical function may allow determination of myocardial regulators under different conditions. It may also be possible to develop a metabolic stress test (for use in a similar manner to the electrocardiographic stress test) that will allow determination of myocardial metabolic reserve. Metabolism may be followed during progressively increased workloads to determine metabolic stability. Metabolic decompensation, as evidenced by changes in the high-energy phosphates, pH, flux through the citric acid cycle, and sodium and potassium membrane potentials, may indicate impending mechanical decompensation and may exist before evidence of mechanical decompensation exists. These data may be used to define progression of subclinical and clinically evident disease processes.

CONCLUSION

Considerable progress has been made over the past few years in the use of MRS to study cardiac function in health and disease, with the majority of data generated from animal models of disease. Although much of the information is not entirely new (confirming previous analytical biochemical data), for the first time it is possible to study, in vivo, the sequential progression of disease in one animal. In addition, myocardial metabolism can be simultaneously correlated with mechanical function. Further development of depth pulsing and imaging techniques to obtain localized spectra in humans will permit the more routine use of these techniques in the clinic. See Chapter 50 for more details concerning these techniques.

Acknowledgment

The authors thank Jeannette Forte for her excellent secretarial assistance in the preparation of this manuscript and Dr. Mildred Cohn for her helpful comments concerning NMR theory.

References

A

1. Aue, W. P., Muller, S., Cross, T. A., and Seelig, J.: Volume-selective excitation. A novel approach to topical NMR. J. Magn. Reson. 56:350, 1984.
2. Allen, D. G., Morris, P. G., Orchard, C. H., and Pirolo, J. S.: A nuclear magnetic resonance study of metabolism in the ferret heart during hypoxia and inhibition of glycolysis. J. Physiol. (Lond.) 361:185, 1985.
3. Aufferman, W., Camacho, S. A., Wu, S., et al.: ^{31}P and ^{1}H magnetic resonance spectroscopy of acute alcohol cardiac depression in rats. Magn. Reson. Med. 8:58, 1988.
4. Ackerman, J. J. H., Ewy, C. S., Kim, S. G., and Shalwitz, R. A.: Deuterium magnetic resonance in vivo: The measurement of blood flow and tissue perfusion. Ann. N.Y. Acad. Sci. 508:89, 1986.

B

1. Barkhuijsen, H., DeBeer, R., Bovee, W. M. M. J., and Van Ormondt, D.: Retrieval of frequencies, amplitudes, damping factors and phases from time domain signals using a linear least-squares procedure. J. Magn. Reson. 61:465, 1985.
2. Bottomley, P. A., and Andrew, R. A.: RF magnetic field penetration, phase shift and power dissipation in biological tissue: Implications for NMR imaging. Phys. Med. Biol. 23:630, 1978.
3. Balaban, R. S., Kantor, J. L., Katz, L. A., and Briggs, R. W.: Relation between work and phosphate metabolite in the in vivo paced mammalian heart. Science 232:1121, 1986.
4. Bottomley, P. A.: Noninvasive study of high-energy phosphate metabolism in human heart by depth-resolved ^{31}P NMR spectroscopy. Science 229:769, 1985.
5. Bottomley, P. A., Smith, L. S., Leue, W. M., and Charles, C.: Slice-interleaved depth-resolved surface-coil spectroscopy (SLIT DRESS) for rapid ^{31}P NMR in vivo. J. Magn. Reson. 64:347, 1985.
6. Bottomley, P. A., Herfkens, R. J., Smith, L. S., et al.: Non-invasive detection and monitoring of regional myocardial ischemia in situ using depth-resolved ^{31}P NMR spectroscopy. Proc. Natl. Acad. Sci. USA 82:8747, 1985.
7. Bernard, M., Menasche, P., Fontanarova, E., et al.: Effect of nifedipine in hypothermic cardioplegia: A phosphorus-31 nuclear magnetic resonance study. Clin. Chim. Acta 152:43, 1985.
8. Bolinger, L., Shinnar, M., and Leigh, J. S.: Hadamard spectroscopic imaging for multi-volume localization. Proc. Soc. Magn. Reson. Med. 7:750, 1988.
9. Brooks, W. M., and Willis, R. J.: Determination of intracellular pH in the Langendorff-perfused guinea-pig heart by ^{31}P nuclear magnetic resonance spectroscopy. J. Mol. Cell. Cardiol. 17:747, 1985.
10. Barbour, R. L., Sotak, C. H., Levy, G. C., and Chan, S. H. P.: Use of gated perfusion to study early effects of anoxia on cardiac energy metabolism: A new ^{31}P NMR method. Biochemistry 23:6052, 1984.
11. Bittl, J. A., and Ingwall, J. W.: NMR studies of ATP synthesis reactions in the isolated heart. *In* Osbakken, M. D., and Haselgrove, J. (eds.): NMR Techniques in the Study of Cardiovascular Structure and Function. Futura Publishing Company, Mt. Kisco, N.Y., 1988, p. 239.
12. Brindle, K. M., and Radda, G. K.: ^{31}P-NMR saturation transfer measurements of exchange between Pi and ATP in the reactions catalysed by glyceraldehyde-3-phosphate dehydrogenase and phosphoglycerate kinase in vitro. Biochim. Biophys. Acta 298:45, 1987.
13. Bittl, J. A., and Ingwall, J. S.: Intracellular high-energy phosphate transfer in normal and hypertrophied myocardium. Circulation 75(Suppl. I):I96, 1987.
14. Bittl, J. A., DeLayre, J., and Ingwall, J. S.: Rate equation for creatine kinase predicts the in vivo reaction velocity: ^{31}P NMR surface coil studies in brain, heart, and skeletal muscle of the living rat. Biochemistry 26:6083, 1987.
15. Bittl, J. A., and Ingwall, J. S.: Reaction rates of creatine kinase and ATP synthesis in this isolated rat heart. J. Biol. Chem. 260:3512, 1985.
16. Brindle, K. M., Porteous, R., and Radda, G. K.: A comparison of ^{31}P-NMR saturation transfer and isotope-exchange measurements of creatine kinase kinetics in vitro. Biochim. Biophys. Acta 786:18, 1984.
17. Bailey, I. A., Williams, S. R., Radda, G. K., and Gadian, D. G.: Activity of phosphorylase in total global ischemia in the rat heart. Biochemistry 196:171, 1981.
18. Brooks, W. M., Haseler, L. J., Clark, K., and Willis, R. J.: Relation between the phosphocreatine to ATP ratio determined by ^{31}P nuclear magnetic resonance spectroscopy and left ventricular function in underperfused guinea-pig heart. J. Mol. Cell. Cardiol. 18:149, 1986.
19. Bailey, I. A., Radda, G. K., Seymour, A. M. L., and Williams, S. R.: The effects of insulin on myocardial metabolism and acidosis in normoxia and ischemia. Biochim. Biophys. Acta 720:17, 1982.
20. Bailey, I. A., Seymour, A. M. L., and Radda, G. K.: A ^{31}P-NMR study of the effects of reflow on the ischemic rat heart. Biochim. Biophys. Acta 637:1, 1981.
21. Brooks, W. M., and Willis, R. J.: ^{31}P nuclear magnetic resonance study of the recovery characteristics of high energy phosphate compounds and intracellular pH after global ischemia in the perfused guinea pig heart. J. Mol. Cell. Cardiol. 15:495, 1983.
22. Bernard, M., Menasche, P., Canioni, P., et al.: Enhanced cardioplegic protection by a fluorocarbon-oxygenated reperfusate: A phosphorus-31 nuclear magnetic resonance study. J. Surg. Res. 39:216, 1985.
23. Borchgrevink, P. C., Bergen, A. S., Bakøy, O. E., and Jynge, A. P.: Magnesium and reperfusion of ischemic rat heart as assessed by ^{31}P-NMR. Am. J. Physiol. 256 (Heart Circ. Physiol. 25): H195, 1989.
24. Brindle, K. M., Rajagopalan, B., Williams, D. S., et al.: ^{31}P NMR measurements of myocardial pH in vivo. Biochem. Biophys. Res. Comm. 151:70, 1988.
25. Blackledge, M. J., Rajagopalan, B., Oberhaensli, R. D., et al.: Quantitative studies of human cardiac metabolism by ^{31}P rotating-frame NMR. Proc. Natl. Acad. Sci. USA 84:4283, 1987.
26. Bottomly, P. A., Hardy, C. J., and Roemer, P. B.: Phosphate metabolite imaging and concentration measurements in human heart by nuclear magnetic resonance. Magn. Res. Med. 14:425, 1990.
27. Bailey, I. A., Gadian, D. G., Matthews, P. M., et al.: Studies of metabolism in the isolated perfused rat heart using ^{13}C NMR. FEBS Lett. 123:315, 1981.
28. Brainard, J. R., Hoekenga, D. E., and Hutson, J. Y.: Metabolic consequence of anoxia in the isolated, perfused guinea pig heart: Anaerobic metabolism of endogenous amino acids. Magn. Reson. Med. 3:673, 1986.
29. Brown, M. A., Stenzel, T. T., Ribero, A. A., et al.: NMR studies of combined lanthanide shift and relaxation agents for differential characterization of ^{23}Na in a two-component model system. Magn. Reson. Med. 3:289, 1986.
30. Berendson, H. J., and Edzes, H. T.: The observation and general interpretation of sodium magnetic resonance in biological material. Ann. N.Y. Acad. Sci. 204:459, 1973.
31. Balschi, J. A., Cirillo, V. P., and Springer, C. S.: Direct high resolution nuclear magnetic resonance studies of cation transport in vivo. Na^+ transport in yeast cells. Biophys. J. 38:323, 1982.
32. Burstein, D., and Fossel, E. T.: Intracellular sodium and lithium relaxation times in the perfused frog heart. Magn. Reson. Med. 4:261, 1987.
33. Burstein, D., and Fossel, E. T.: Nuclear magnetic resonance studies of intracellular ions in perfused frog heart. Am. J. Physiol. 252:H1138, 1987.

C

1. Chow, J. L., Olson, D. R., Anderson, S. E., et al.: A microcomputer-based system for processing phosphorus-31 nuclear magnetic resonance spectra from studies of cardiac metabolism in immature hearts. Comp. Methods Prog. Biomed. 25:39, 1987.
2. Camacho, S. A., Wikman-Coffelt, J., Wu, S. T., et al.: Improvement in myocardial performance without a decrease in high-energy phosphate metabolites after isoproterenol in Syrian cardiomyopathic hamsters. Circulation 77:712, 1988.
3. Chance, B., Leigh, J. S., Clark, B. J., et al.: Control of oxidative metabolism and oxygen delivery in human skeletal muscle: A steady-state analysis of the work/energy cost transfer function. Proc. Natl. Acad. Sci. USA 82:8384, 1985.
4. Chance, B., Leigh, J. S., Kent, J., et al.: Multiple controls of oxidative metabolism in living tissues as studied by phosphorus magnetic resonance. Proc. Natl. Acad. Sci. USA 83:9458, 1986.
5. Carlier, P. G., Jacobstein, M. D., Portman, M. A., et al.: Alterations of energy metabolism in the spontaneously hypertensive rat: A ^{31}P nuclear magnetic resonance study. J. Hypertens. 4(Suppl. 6):S95, 1986.
6. Clarke, K., and Willis, R. J.: Energy metabolism and contractile function in rat heart during graded, isovolumic perfusion using nuclear magnetic resonance spectroscopy. J. Mol. Cell. Cardiol. 19:1153, 1987.
7. Camacho, S. A., Parmley, W. W., James, T. L., et al.: Substrate regulation of the nucleotide pool during regional ischemia and reperfusion in an isolated rat heart preparation: A phosphorus-31 magnetic resonance spectroscopy analysis. Cardiovasc. Res. 22:193, 1988.
8. Canby, R. C., Evanochko, W. T., Barrett, L. V., et al.: Monitoring the bioenergetics of cardiac allograft rejection using an in vivo P-31 nuclear magnetic resonance spectroscopy. J. Am. Coll. Cardiol. 9:1067, 1987.
9. Chance, E. M., Seeholzer, S. H., Kobayashi, K., and Williamson, J. R.: Mathematical analysis of isotope labelling in the citric acid cycle with applications to ^{13}C NMR studies in perfused rat hearts. J. Biol. Chem. 258(22):13785, 1983.
10. Civan, M. M., and Shporer, M.: NMR of ^{23}Na and ^{39}K in biological systems. *In* Berliner, L. J., and Reuben, J. (eds.): Biological Magnetic Resonance. Plenum, New York, 1978, p. 1.

11. Cope, F. W.: Nuclear magnetic resonance evidence for complexing of sodium ions in muscle. Proc. Natl. Acad. Sci. USA 54:225, 1965.
12. Cope, F. W.: Spin-echo nuclear magnetic resonance evidence for complexing of sodium ions in muscle, brain, and kidney. Biophys. J. 10:843, 1970.

D

1. Dwek, R. A.: Spin-echo nuclear magnetic resonance evidence for complexing of sodium ions in muscle, brain and kidney. *In* Magnetic Resonance in Biochemistry: Applications to Enzyme Systems. Clarendon Press, Oxford, England, 1975.
2. Devous, M. D., and Lewandowski, E. D.: Inosine preserves ATP during ischemia and enhances recovery during reperfusion. Am. J. Physiol. 252(Heart Circ. Physiol. 21):H1224, 1987.
3. Degani, H., Laughlin, M., Campbell, S., and Shulman, R. G.: Kinetics of creatine kinase in heart: A ^{31}P NMR saturation and inversion-transfer study. Biochemistry 24:5510, 1985.
4. Dhasmana, J. P., Diguiness, S. B., Geckle, J. M., et al.: Effect of adenosine deaminase inhibitors on the heart's functional and biochemical recovery from ischemia: A study utilizing the isolated rat heart adapted to ^{31}P nuclear magnetic resonance. J. Cardiovasc. Pharmacol. 5:1040, 1983.
5. Deslauriers, R., Keon, W. J., Lareau, S., et al.: Cardiac hypothermia ^{31}P and ^{1}H NMR studies of human myocardial tissue. Proc. Soc. Magn. Reson. Med. 7:829, 1988.
6. Detre, J.A., Subramanian, V. H., Mitchell, M. D., et al.: Measurement of regional cerebral blood flow in cat brain using intracarotid D_2O and ^{2}H NMR imaging. Magn. Res. Med. 14:389, 1990.

E

1. English, T. A., Foreman, J., Gadian, D. G., et al.: Three solutions for preservation of the rabbit heart at 0° C. J. Thorac. Cardiovasc. Surg. 96:54, 1988.
2. Evanochko, W. T., Reeves, R. C., Sakai, T. T., et al.: Proton NMR spectroscopy in myocardial ischemic insult. Magn. Reson. Med. 5:23, 1987.
3. Eleff, S. M., Schnall, M. D., Ligeti, L., et al.: Concurrent measurements of cerebral blood flow, sodium, lactate, and high-energy phosphate metabolism using ^{19}F, ^{23}Na, ^{1}H, and ^{31}P nuclear magnetic resonance spectroscopy. Magn. Reson. Med. 7:412, 1988.
4. Ewy, C. S., Bennett, D. L., Ackerman, J. J., and Shalwitz, R. A.: Deuterium NMR measurements of blood flow in normal and tumor tissue. Proc. Soc. Magn. Reson. Med. 5:86, 1986.

F

1. Freeman, D., Mayr, H., Schmidt, P., et al.: Advantages of perfluorochemical perfusion in the isolated working rabbit heart preparation using ^{31}P-NMR. Biochim. Biophys. Acta 927:350, 1987.
2. From, A. H. L., Petein, M. A., Michurski, S. P., et al.: ^{31}P-NMR studies of respiratory regulation in the intact myocardium. FEBS Lett. 206:257, 1986.
3. Fossel, E. T., Morgan, H. E., and Ingwall, J. S.: Measurement of changes in high-energy phosphates in the cardiac cycle by using gated ^{31}P nuclear magnetic resonance. Proc. Natl. Acad. Sci. USA 77:3654, 1980.
4. Flaherty, J. T., Weisfeldt, M. L., Hollis, D. P., et al.: Mass spectrometry and phosphorus-31 nuclear magnetic resonance demonstrate additive myocardial protection by potassium cardioplegia and hypothermia during global ischemia. Adv. Myocardiol. 2:487, 1980.
5. Flaherty, J. T., Weisfelt, M. L., Buckley, B. H., et al.: Mechanisms of ischemic myocardial cell damage assessed by phosphorus-31 nuclear magnetic resonance. Circulation 65:561, 1982.
6. Flaherty, J. R. J., Jaffin, J. H., Magoven, G. J., et al.: Maintenance of aerobic metabolism during global ischemia with perfluorocarbon cardioplegia improves myocardial preservation. Circulation 69:585, 1984.
7. Fraser, D. C., Chacko, V. P., Jacobus, W. E., et al.: Metabolic changes preceding functional and morphological indices of rejection in heterotrophic cardiac allografts. A ^{31}P NMR study. Transplantation 46:346, 1988.
8. Fried, R., Boxt, L. M., Miller, R. H., III, et al.: Nuclear magnetic resonance spectroscopy of rat ventricles following supravalvular aortic banding: A model of left ventricular hypertrophy. Invest. Radiol. 21:622, 1986.
9. Fossel, E. T., and Hoefeler, H.: Observation of intracellular potassium and sodium in the heart by NMR: A major fraction of potassium is invisible. Magn. Reson. Med. 3:534, 1986.

G

1. Gadian, D. G. (ed.): The theoretical basis of the NMR experiment. *In* Nuclear Magnetic Resonance and Its Application to Living Systems. Oxford University Press, Oxford, England, 1982, pp. 77–98.
2. Garlick, P. B., Brown, T. R., Sullivan, R. H., and Ugurbil, K.: Observation of a second phosphate pool in the perfused heart by ^{31}P NMR: Is this the mitochondrial phosphate? J. Mol. Cell. Cardiol. 15:855, 1983.
3. Gadian, D. G., Hoult, D. I., Radda, G. H., et al.: Phosphorus nuclear magnetic resonance studies on normoxic and ischemic cardiac tissue. Proc. Natl. Acad. Sci. USA 73:4446, 1976.
4. Garlick, P. B., Radda, G., Seeley, P. J., and Chance, B.: Phosphorus NMR studies on perfused heart. Biochem. Biophysiol. Res. Commun. 74:1256, 1977.
5. Gyulai, L., Roth, Z., Leigh, J. S., and Chance, B.: Bioenergetic studies of mitochondrial oxidative phosphorylation using ^{31}P NMR. Proc. Natl. Acad. Sci. USA 78:6714, 1981.
6. Garlick, P. B., Radda, G., and Seeley, P. J.: Studies of acidosis in the ischemic heart by phosphorus nuclear magnetic resonance. Biochem. J. 184:547, 1979.
7. Guth, B. D., Martin, J. F., Heusch, G., and Ross, J.: Regional myocardial blood flow, function and metabolism using phosphorus-31 nuclear magnetic resonance spectroscopy during ischemia and reperfusion in dogs. J. Am. Coll. Cardiol. 10:673, 1987.
8. Grove, T. H., Ackerman, J. J. H., Radda, G. K., and Bore, P. J.: Analysis of rat heart in vivo by phosphorus nuclear magnetic resonance. Proc. Natl. Acad. Sci. USA 77:299, 1980.
9. Gupta, R. K., and Gupta, P.: Direct observation of resolved resonances from intra- and extracellular sodium-23 ions in NMR studies of intact cells and tissues using dysprosium (III) tripolyphosphate as paramagnetic shift reagent. J. Magn. Reson. 47:344, 1982.

H

1. Hoult, D. I.: An overview of NMR in medicine. Monograph of National Center of Health Care Technology, Bethesda, Md., 1981, pp. 1–13.
2. Hilberman, M., Subramanian, V. H., Haselgrove, J. C., et al.: In vivo time-resolved brain phosphorus nuclear magnetic resonance. J. Cereb. Blood Flow Metab. 4:334, 1984.
3. Hoult, D. I., and Richards, R. E.: The signal-to-noise ratio of the nuclear magnetic resonance experiment. J. Magn. Reson. 24:71, 1976.
4. Hollis, D. P., Nunnally, F. L., Jacobus, W. E., and Taylor, G. J.: Detection of regional ischemia in perfused beating hearts by phosphorus nuclear magnetic resonance. Biochem. Biophys. Res. Commun. 75:1086, 1977.
5. Hsieh, P. S., and Balaban, R. S.: ^{31}P imaging in vivo creatine kinase reaction rates. J. Magn. Reson. 74:574, 1987.
6. Hoekenga, D. E., Brainard, J. R., and Hutson, J. Y.: Rates of glycolysis and glycogenolysis during ischemia in glucose-insulin-potassium-treated perfused hearts: A ^{13}C, ^{31}P nuclear magnetic resonance study. Circ. Res. 62:1065, 1988.
7. Hollis, D. P., and Nunnally, R. L.: Recent ^{31}P NMR studies of myocardium. Philos. Trans. R. Soc. Lond. 289:437, 1980.
8. Hoerter, J. A., Miceli, M. V., Renlund, D. G., et al.: A phosphorus-31 nuclear magnetic resonance study of the metabolic contractile and ionic consequences of induced calcium alterations in the isovolumic rat heart. Circ. Res. 58:539, 1986.
9. Hollis, D. P., Nunnally, R. L., Taylor, G. J., et al.: Effects of regional ischemia and KCl arrest on the ^{31}P NMR of perfused hearts. Molecular dynamics and structure of tissues and whole cells. *In* Agris, P. F., Laeppky, R. N., and Sykes, B. (ed.); Biomolecular Structure and Function. Academic Press, New York, 1977, p. 217.
10. Hall, T. S., Baumgartner, W. A., Borkon, A. M., et al.: Diagnosis of acute cardiac rejection with antimyosin monoclonal antibody, phosphorous nuclear magnetic resonance imaging, two-dimensional echocardiography, and endocardial biopsy. J. Heart Transplant 5:419, 1986.
11. Haug, C. E., Shapiro, J. I., Chan, L., and Weil, R.: P-31 nuclear magnetic resonance spectroscopic evaluation of heterotopic cardiac allograft rejection in the rat. Transplantation 44(2):175, 1987.
12. Haug, C. E., Shapiro, J. I., Cosby, R. L., et al.: ^{31}P nuclear magnetic resonance spectroscopy of heart, heart-lung, and kidney allograft rejection in the rat. Transplant Proc. 20(Suppl.):848, 1988.

I

1. Ingwall, J. S.: Phosphorus nuclear magnetic resonance spectroscopy of cardiac and skeletal muscles. Am. J. Physiol. 242(Heart Circ. Physiol. 11):H729, 1982.

J

1. Jacobus, W. E., Taylor, G. J., Hollis, D. P., and Nunnally, R. L.: Phosphorus nuclear magnetic resonance of perfused working rat hearts. Nature 265:756, 1977.
2. Jacobus, W. E., Taylor, G. J., Weisfeldt, M. L., et al.: Rapid ^{31}P nuclear magnetic resonance of perfused hearts. Proc. Natl. Acad. Sci. USA 74:207, 1977.
3. Jacobus, W. E., Pores, I. H., Lucas, S. K., et al.: Intracellular acidosis and contractility in the normal and ischemic heart as examined by ^{31}P NMR. J. Mol. Cell. Cardiol. 14:13, 1982.
4. Jeffrey, F. M. H., Malloy, C. R., and Radda, G. K.: Influence of intracellular acidosis on contractile function in the working rat heart. Am. J. Physiol. 253(Heart Circ. Physiol. 22): H1499, 1987.
5. Jardetsky, O., and Wertz, J. E.: Detection of sodium complexes by nuclear spin resonance. Am. J. Physiol. 187:608, 1956.

K

1. Koretsky, A. P., Wang, S., Murphy-Boesch, J., et al.: ^{31}P NMR spectroscopy of rat organs, in situ, using chronically implanted radiofrequency coils. Proc. Natl. Acad. Sci. USA 80:7491, 1983.
2. Koretsky, A. P., and Balaban, R. S.: Changes in pyridine nucleotide levels alter oxygen consumption and extra-mitochondrial phosphates in isolated mitochondria: A ^{31}P-NMR and NAD(P)H fluorescence study. Biochim. Biophys. Acta 893:398, 1987.
3. Kingsley-Hickman, P. B., Sako, E. Y., Mohanakrishnan, P., et al.: ^{31}P NMR studies of ATP synthesis and hydrolysis kinetics in the intact myocardium. Biochemistry 26:7501, 1987.
4. Katz, L. A., Koretsky, A. P., and Balaban, R. S.: Activation of dehydrogenase

activity and cardiac respiration: A ^{31}P-NMR study. Am. J. Physiol. 255(Heart Circ. Physiol. 25):H185, 1988.

5. Kingsley-Hickman, P., Sako, E. Y., Andreone, P. A., et al.: NMR measurement of ATP synthesis rate in perfused intact rat hearts. FEBS Lett. 198(1):159, 1986.
6. Koretsky, A. P., Wang, S., Klein, M. P., et al.: ^{31}P NMR saturation transfer measurements of phosphorus exchange reactions in rat heart and kidney in situ. Biochemistry 25:77, 1986.
7. Kirkels, J. H., Ruigrok, T. J. C., Van Echteld, C. J. A., and Meijler F. L.: Protective effect of pretreatment with the calcium antagonist anipamil on the ischemic-reperfused rat myocardium: A phosphorus-31 nuclear magnetic resonance study. J. Am. Coll. Cardiol. 11(5):1087, 1988.
8. Kupriyanov, V. V., Steinschneider, A. Y., Ruuge, E. K., et al.: Regulation of energy flux through the creatine kinase reaction in vitro and in perfused rat heart. Biochim. Biophys. Acta 805:319, 1984.
9. Kusouka, H., Inoue, M., Tsuneoka, Y., et al.: Augmented energy consumption during early systole as a mechanism of cyclical changes in high-energy phosphates in myocardium assessed by phosphorus nuclear magnetic resonance. Jpn. Circ. J. 49:1099, 1985.
10. Kitakaze, M., Weisman, H. F., and Marban, E.: Contractile dysfunction and ATP depletion after transient calcium overload in perfused ferret hearts. Circulation 77:685, 1988.
11. Keller, A. M., Jackson, J. A., Peshock, R. M., et al.: Nuclear magnetic resonance study of high-energy phosphate stores in models of Adriamycin cardiotoxicity. Magn. Reson. Med. 3:834, 1986.
12. Kopp, S. J., Daar, A. A., Prentice, R. C., et al.: ^{31}P NMR studies of the intact perfused rat heart. A novel analytical approach for determining functional-metabolic correlates, temporal relationships and intracellular actions of cardiotoxic chemicals nondestructively in an intact organ model. Toxicol. Appl. Pharmacol. 82:200, 1986.
13. Kantor, H. L., Briggs, R. W., and Balaban, R. S.: In vivo ^{31}P nuclear magnetic resonance measurements in canine heart using a catheter-coil. Circ. Res. 55:261, 1984.
14. Kantor, H. C., Briggs, R. W., Metz, K. R., and Balaban, R. S.: Gated in vivo examination of cardiac metabolites with ^{31}P nuclear magnetic resonance. Am. J. Physiol. 251(Heart Circ. Physiol. 20):H171, 1986.
15. Katz, L. A., Swain, J. A., Portman, M. A., and Balaban, R. S.: Intracellular pH and inorganic phosphate content of heart in vivo: A ^{31}P-NMR study. Am. J. Physiol. 255(Heart Circ. Physiol. 24):H189, 1988.
16. Katz, L. A., Swain, J. A., Portman, M. A., and Balaban, R. S.: Relation between phosphate metabolites and oxygen consumption of heart in vivo. Am. J. Physiol. 256(Heart Circ. Physiol. 25):H265, 1989.
17. Keller, A. M., Sorce, D. J., Sciacca, R. R., et al.: Very rapid lactate measurement in ischemic perfused hearts using ^{1}H MRS continuous negative echo acquisition during steady-state frequency selective excitation. Magn. Reson. Med. 7:65, 1988.
18. Kuki, S., Suzuki, E., Seo Y., et al.: A new ^{39}K NMR approach to measure myocardial intracellular potassium without shift reagent. Proc. Soc. Magn. Reson. Med. 7:417, 1988.
19. Kim, S. G., and Ackerman, J. J. H.: Multicompartment analysis of blood flow and tissue perfusion employing D_2O as a freely diffusible tracer: A novel deuterium technique demonstrated via application with murine RIF-1 tumors. Magn. Reson. Med. 8:410, 1988.

L

1. Laue, E. D., Skilling, J., Staunton, J., et al.: Maximum entropy method in NMR spectroscopy. J. Magn. Reson. 62:437, 1985.
2. Lavancy, N., Martin, J., Glacomelli, M., and Rossi, A.: Evaluation by ^{31}P NMR of the effects of acebutolol on the ischemic isolated rat heart. Eur. J. Pharmacol. 123:341, 1986.
3. Lavancy, N., Martin, J., and Rossi A.: Anti-ischemic effects of trimetazidine: ^{31}P-NMR spectroscopy in the isolated rat heart. Arch. Int. Pharmacodyn. Ther. 286:97, 1987.
4. Lavancy, N., Martin, J., and Rossi, A.: Graded global ischemia and reperfusion of the isolated perfused rat heart: Characterization by ^{31}P NMR spectroscopy of the extent of energy metabolism damage. Cardiovasc. Res. 18:573, 1984.
5. Lewandowski, E. D., Devous, M. D., and Nunnally, R. L.: High-energy phosphates and function in isolated, working rabbit hearts. Am. J. Physiol. 253(Heart Circ. Physiol. 22):H1215, 1987.
6. Ligeti, L., Osbakken, M., Clark, B. J., et al.: Cardiac transfer function relating energy metabolism to work load in different species as studied with ^{31}P NMR. Magn. Reson. Med. 4:112, 1986.
7. Luyten, P. R., Marien, J. H., Sijtsma, B., and Den Hollander, J. A.: Solvent-suppressed spatially resolved spectroscopy. An approach to high-resolution NMR on a whole-body MR system. J. Magn. Reson. 67:148, 1986.
8. Lavanchy, N., Martin, J., and Rossi A.: Glycogen metabolism: A ^{13}C-NMR study on the isolated perfused rat heart. FEBS Lett. 178:34, 1984.
9. Laughlin, M. R., Petit, W. A., Dizon, J. M., et al.: NMR measurements of in vivo myocardial glycogen metabolism. J. Biol. Chem. 263:2285, 1988.
10. Lotan, C., Miller, S. K., Pohost, G. M., and Elgovish G. A.: The role of Na-H exchange in ouabain-induced intracellular acidification. A ^{23}Na and ^{31}P study in isolated perfused rat hearts. Proc. Soc. Magn. Reson. Med. 7:271, 1988.
11. Levy, L. A., Murphy, E., Raju, B., and London R. E.: Measurement of cytosolic free magnesium ion concentration by ^{19}F NMR. Biochemistry 27:4041, 1988.

M

1. Morgan, H. E., and Neely, J. R.: Metabolic regulation and myocardial function in the heart. *In* Hurst, J. W., Logue, R. B., Rackley, C. I., Schlant, R. C., Sonnenblick, E. H., Wallace, A. G., and Wenger, N. K. (eds): The Heart, 6th ed., McGraw Hill, New York, N.Y., 1986, pp.85–100.
2. Mio-Xiang, H., Wangler, R. D., Dillon, P. F., et al.: Phosphorylation potential and adenosine release during norepinephrine infusion in guinea pig heart. Am. J. Physiol. 253(Heart Circ. Physiol. 22):H1184, 1987.
3. Matthews, P. M., Bland, J. L., Gadian, D. G., and Radda G. K.: The steady-state rate of ATP synthesis in the perfused rat heart measured by ^{31}P NMR saturation transfer. Biochem. Biophys. Res. Commun. 103:1052, 1981.
4. Matthews, P. M., Bland, J. L., Gadian, D. G., and Radda G. K.: A ^{31}P-NMR saturation transfer study of the regulation of creatine kinase in the rat heart. Biochem. Biophys. Acta 721:312, 1982.
5. Matthews, P. M., Williams, S. R., Seymour, A. M., et al.: A ^{31}P-NMR study of some metabolic and functional effects of the inotropic agents epinephrine and ouabain, and the ionophore R02-2985 (X537A) in the isolated, perfused rat heart. Biochim. Biophys. Acta 720:163, 1982.
6. Murray, P. A., Blanck, T. J. J., Rogers, M. C., and Jacobus W. E.: Effects of halothane on myocardial high-energy phosphate metabolism and intracellular pH utilizing ^{31}P NMR spectroscopy. Anesthesiology 67:649, 1987.
7. Malloy, C. R., Sherry, A. D., and Jeffrey, F. M. H.: Carbon flux through citric acid cycle pathways in perfused heart by ^{13}C NMR spectroscopy. FEBS Lett. 212:58, 1987.
8. Malloy, C. R., Sherry, A. D., and Jeffrey, F. M. H.: Evaluation of carbon flux and substrate selection through alternate pathways involving the citric acid cycle of the heart by ^{13}C NMR spectroscopy. J. Biol. Chem. 263(15):6964, 1988.
9. Matwiyoff, N. A., Gasparovic, C., Wenk, R., et al.: ^{31}P and 2^{23}Na NMR studies of the structure and lability of the sodium shift reagent, bis (tripolyphosphate) dysprosium(III) ($[Dy(P_3O_{10})]7-$) ion and its decomposition in the presence of rat muscle. Magn. Reson. Med. 3:164, 1986.
10. Marban, E., Kitakaze, M., Kusuoka, H., et al.: Intracellular free calcium concentration measured with ^{19}F NMR spectroscopy in intact ferret hearts. Proc. Natl. Acad. Sci. USA 84:6005, 1987.
11. Marban, E., Kitakaze, M., Chacko, V. P., and Pike, M. M.: Ca^{2+} transients in perfused hearts revealed by gated ^{19}F NMR spectroscopy. Circ. Res. 63:673, 1988.
12. Metcalfe, J. C., Hesketh, T. R., and Smith, G. A.: Free cytosolic Ca^{2+} measurements with fluorine-labeled indicators using ^{19}F NMR. Cell Calcium 6:183, 1985.
13. Mitchell, M. D., Clark, B. J., and Leigh, J. S.: Simultaneous *in-vivo* phosphorus metabolic spectroscopy and deuterium perfusion measurement. Proc. Soc. Magn. Reson. Med. 6:427, 1987.

N

1. Ni, F., Levy, G., and Scheraga, H. A.: Simultaneous resolution and noise suppression in NMR signal processing by combined use of maximum entropy and Fourier self-deconvolution methods. J. Magn. Reson. 66:385, 1986.
2. Neurohr, K. J., Gallin, G., Barrett, E. J., and Shulman R. G.: In vivo ^{31}P-NMR studies of myocardial high energy phosphate metabolism during anoxia and recovery. FEBS Lett. 159:207, 1983.
3. Nunnally, R. L., and Hollis, D. P.: Adenosine triphosphate compartmentation in living hearts: A phosphorus nuclear magnetic resonance saturation transfer study. Biochemistry 18(16):3642, 1979.
4. Neubauer, S., Hamman, B. L., Perry, S. B., et al.: Velocity of the creatine kinase reaction decreases in postischemic myocardium: A ^{31}P-NMR magnetization transfer study of the isolated ferret heart. Circ. Res. 63:1, 1988.
5. Nokin, P., Jungbluth, L., and Mouton, J.: Protective effects of amiodarone pretreatment on mitochondrial function and high energy phosphates in ischemic rat heart. J. Mol. Cell. Cardiol. 19:603, 1987.
6. Newbauer, S., Hamman, B. L., Perry, S. B., et al.: Velocity of the creatine kinase reaction decreases in post ischemic myocardium: A ^{31}P NMR magnetization transfer study of the isolated ferret heart. Circ. Res. 63:1, 1988.
7. Nakazawa, M., Katano, Y., Imai, S., et al.: Effect of D-propranolol on the ischemic myocardial metabolism of the isolated guinea pig heart as studied by ^{31}P-NMR. J. Cardiovasc. Pharmacol. 4:700, 1982.
8. Nunnally, R. L., and Bottomley, P. A.: Assessment of pharmacological treatment of myocardial infarction by phosphorus-31 NMR with surface coils. Science 211:177, 1981.
9. Ng, T. C., Daugherty, J. P., Evanchko, W. T., et al.: Detection of antineoplastic agent induced cardiotoxicity by ^{31}P NMR of perfused rat hearts. Biochem. Biophys. Res. Commun. 110:339, 1983.
10. Neurohr, K. J., Barrett, E. J., and Shulman, R. G.: In vivo carbon-13 nuclear magnetic resonance studies of heart metabolism. Proc. Natl. Acad. Sci. USA 80:1603, 1983.
11. Neurohr, K. J., Gallin, G., Neurohr, J. M., et al.: Carbon-13 nuclear magnetic resonance studies of myocardial glycogen metabolism in live guinea pigs. Biochemistry 23:5029, 1984.
12. Neurohr, K. J., and Shulman, R. G.: ^{13}C and ^{31}P NMR studies of myocardiol metabolism in live guinea pigs. Adv. Myocardiol. 6:185, 1985.
13. Naritomi, H., Sasaki, M., Kanashiro, M., et al.: In vivo estimation of ischemic cellular swelling in the brain by ^{1}H NMR spectroscopy with shift reagents. Proc. Soc. Magn. Reson. Med. 7:374, 1988.
14. Nunnally, R. L., Babcock, E. E., Horner, S. D., and Peshock, R. M.: Fluorine-19 NMR spectroscopy and imaging investigations of myocardial perfusion and cardiac function. Magn. Reson. Imaging 3:399, 1985.

O

1. Osbakken, M., Haselgrove, J., and Ligeti, L.: Introduction to NMR techniques. *In* Osbakken, M., and Haselgrove, J. (eds.): NMR Techniques in the Study

of Cardiovascular Structure and Function. Futura Publishing Company, Mt. Kisco, N.Y., 1988, pp. 3–34.
2. Osbakken, M. D., Ligeti, L., Clark, B. J., et al.: Myocardial high energy phosphate metabolism in closed chest dog: Creation of an animal model. Magn. Reson. Med. 3:801, 1986.
3. Ordridge, R. J., Connelly, A., and Lohman, J. A. B.: Image-selected in vivo spectroscopy (ISIS). A new technique for spatially selective NMR spectroscopy. J. Magn. Reson. 66:283, 1986.
4. Ordridge, R. J., and Bowley, R. M.: Selection of multiple cubic volume elements using the ISIS technique. Proc. Soc. Magn. Reson. Med 7:751, 1988.
5. Osbakken, M.: Can cardiovascular disease be effectively evaluated with NMR spectroscopy? *In* Osbakken, M., and Haselgrove, J. (eds.): NMR Techniques in the Study of Cardiovascular Structure and Function. Futura Publishing Company, Mt. Kisco, N.Y., 1988, pp. 207–237.
6. Ochi, S., Ogawa, Y., Imai, H., et al.: Effects of beta-blockers on the fall of pH in the early phase of ischemia in the isolated perfused rat heart: A nuclear magnetic resonance study. J. Cardiovasc. Pharmacol. 11:326, 1988.
7. Osbakken, M. D., Young, M., Huddell, J., et al.: Acute volume loading studied in cat myocardium with ^{31}P nuclear magnetic resonance. Magn. Reson. Med. 7:143, 1988.
8. Osbakken, M. D., Ligeti, L., Young, M., et al.: Myocardial bioenergetics during acute arterial venous shunts in a canine model studied with ^{31}P NMR. Magn. Reson. Med. 7:143, 1988.
9. Osbakken, M. D., Ligeti, L., Clark, B. J., et al.: Effects of hypoxia on the myocardium measured in closed chest dogs. Proc. Soc. Magn. Reson. Med. 1:522, 1985.
10. Osbakken, M., Ligeti, L., Subramanian, H., et al.: Myocardial metabolism during acute episodes of hypertension studied in closed chest dogs with ^{31}P NMR. J. Appl. Cardiol. 1:143, 1986.
11. Osbakken, M., Ligeti, L., Pigott, J., et al.: Myocardial metabolism in chronic volume overload studied with ^{31}P NMR. Proc. Magn. Reson. Med. 5:885, 1986.
12. Osbakken, M. D., Pigott, J., Ligeti, L., et al.: Myocardial bioenergetics of chronic volume overload studied with ^{31}P MRS. J. Appl. Cardiol. 5(1):39, 1990.
13. Osbakken, M. D., Mitchell, M. D., Duska, C., et al.: Correlation of myocardial perfusion, metabolism, and mechanical function during increased cardiac work. FASEB Proc. 3:1041, 1989.

P

1. Pykett, I. L.: NMR imaging in medicine. Sci. Am. 246:78, 1982.
2. Pettroff, O. A. C., Prichard, J. W., Behar, K. L., and Alger J. R.: The mean cytosolic pH of normal rodent brain by ^{31}P NMR. Magn. Reson. Med. 1:589, 1984.
3. Pieper, G. M., Murray, W. J., Salhany, J. M., et al.: Salient effects of L-carnitine on adenine-nucleotide loss and coenzyme A acylation in the diabetic heart perfused with excess palmitic acid. A phosphorus-31 NMR and chemical extract study. Biochim. Biophys. Acta 803:241, 1984.
4. Perry, S. B., McAuliffe, J., Balschi, J. A., et al.: Velocity of the creatine kinase reaction in the neonatal rabbit heart: Role of mitochondrial creatine kinase. Biochemistry 27:2165, 1988.
5. Pissarek, M., Grunder, W., and Keller, T.: ^{31}P-NMR spectroscopy on ischemic and reperfused rat hearts: Effects of iloprost. Biomed. Biochim. Acta 46:S564, 1987.
6. Pernot, A. C., Ingwall, J. S., Menasche, P., et al.: Limitations of potassium cardioplegia during cardiac ischemic arrest: A phosphorus-31 nuclear magnetic resonance study. Ann. Thorac. Surg. 32:536, 1981.
7. Pernot, A. C., Ingwall, J. S., Menasche, P., et al.: Evaluation of high-energy phosphate metabolism during cardioplegic arrest and reperfusion: A phosphorus-31 nuclear magnetic resonance study. Circulation 67:1296, 1983.
8. Pieper, G. M., Todd, G. L., Wu, S. T., et al.: Attenuation of myocardial acidosis by propranolol during ischemic arrest and reperfusion: Evidence with ^{31}P nuclear magnetic resonance. Cardiovasc. Res. 14:646, 1980.
9. Pieper, G. M., Salhany, J. M., Murrary, W. J., et al.: Lipid-mediated impairment of normal energy metabolism in the isolated perfused diabetic rat heart studied by phosphorus-31 NMR and chemical extraction. Biochim. Biophys. Acta 803:229, 1984.
10. Portman, M. A., James, S., Heineman, F. W., and Balaban R. S.: Simultaneous monitoring of coronary blood flow and ^{31}P NMR detected myocardial metabolites. Magn. Reson. Med. 7:243, 1988.
11. Petroff, O. A. C.: Biological NMR spectroscopy. Comp. Biochem. Physiol. 90(B):249, 1988.
12. Pearlman, J. D., Zajicek, J., Merickel, M. B., et al.: High-resolution ^{1}H NMR spectral signature from human atheroma. Magn. Reson. Med. 7:262, 1988.
13. Pike, M. M., Frazier, J. C., Dedrick, D. F., et al.: ^{23}Na and ^{39}Ka nuclear magnetic resonance studies of perfused rat hearts: Discrimination of intra- and extracellular ions using a shift reagent. Biophys. J. 48:159, 1985.
14. Pekar, J., and Leigh, J. S.: Detection of biexponential relaxation in sodium-23 facilitated by double quantum filtering. J. Magn. Reson. 69:582, 1986.
15. Powell, D., Burstein, D., and Fossel, E. T.: Studies of intracellular sodium in isolated perfused intact frog hearts: Evidence for sodium-calcium exchange. Proc. Soc. Magn. Reson. Med. 7:281, 1988.
16. Pike, M. M., and Springer, C. S.: Aqueous shift reagents for high-resolution cationic nuclear magnetic resonance. J. Magn. Reson. 46:348, 1982.
17. Pike, M. M., Kitikaze, M., Chacko, V. P., and Marban, E.: Changes in free Ca^{++} during the cardiac cycle revealed by gated ^{19}F NMR spectroscopy in ferret hearts loaded with 5F-BAPTA. Proc. Soc. Magn. Reson. Med. 7:284, 1988.

R

1. Rajagopalan, B., Blackledge, M. J., McKenna, W. J., et al.: Measurement of phosphocreatine to ATP ratio in normal and diseased human heart by ^{31}P magnetic resonance spectroscopy using the rotating frame-depth selection technique. Ann. N.Y. Acad. Sci. 508:321, 1987.
2. Renlund, D. G., Gerstenblith, G., Lakatta, E. G., et al.: Perfusate sodium during ischemia modifies post-ischemic functional and metabolic recovery in rabbit heart. J. Mol. Cell. Cardiol. 16:795, 1984.
3. Renlund, D. G., Lakatta, E. G., Mellits, E. D., and Gerstenblith, G.: Calcium-dependent enhancement of myocardial diastolic tone and energy utilization dissociates systolic work and oxygen consumption during low sodium perfusion. Circ. Res. 57:876, 1985.
4. Rumsey, W. L., Wilson, D. F., and Erecinska, M.: Relationship of myocardial metabolism and coronary flow: Dependence on extracellular calcium. Am. J. Physiol. 253(Heart Circ. Physiol. 22):H1098, 1987.
5. Rossis, A., Martin, J., and deLeires, J.: Phosphorus nuclear magnetic resonance studies of the energetic state and the intracellular pH of the isolated rat heart in the course of ischemia. J. Physiol. (Paris) 76:902, 1980.
6. Radda, G. K., Gadian, D. G., and Ross, B. D.: Energy metabolism and cellular pH in normal and pathological conditions. A new look through ^{31}phosphorus nuclear magnetic resonance. CIBA Found. Sympos. 87:36, 1982.
7. Ruegrok, T. J. C., Van Echteld, C. J. A., Dekrujiff, B., et al.: Protective effect of nifedipine on myocardial ischemia assessed by phosphorus-31 nuclear magnetic resonance. Eur. Heart J. 4(Suppl. C):109, 1983.
8. Rehr, R. B., Tatum, J. L., Hirsch, J. I., et al.: Effective separation of normal, acutely ischemic, and reperfused myocardium with ^{31}P MR spectroscopy. Radiology 168:81, 1988.
9. Richards, T., Tscholokoff, D., and Higgins, C. B.: Proton NMR spectroscopy in canine myocardial infarction. Magn. Reson. Med. 4:555, 1987.
10. Richards, T., Terrier, F., Sievers, R., et al.: Lactate accumulation in ischemic and anoxic-isolated rat hearts assessed by H-1 spectroscopy. Invest. Radiol. 22:638, 1987.
11. Reeves, R. C., Evanochko, W. T., Bittner, V., et al.: Increased myocardial lipid content by proton NMR spectroscopy in post-ischemic dysfunction or "stunning." Proc. Soc. Magn. Reson. Med. 7:834, 1988.
12. Renshaw, P. F., Blum, H., and Leigh, J. S.: Applications of dextran-magnetite as a sodium relaxation enhancer in biological systems. J. Magn. Reson. 69:523, 1986.

S

1. Shaw, D.: In vivo biochemistry. *In* Kaufman, L., et al. (eds.): Nuclear Magnetic Resonance Imaging in Medicine. Igaku-Shoin, New York, 1981, pp. 1–22.
2. Schnall, M. D.: Theory of NMR probe design. *In* Osbakken, M., and Haselgrove, J. (eds.): NMR Techniques in the Study of Cardiovascular Structure and Function. Futura Publishing Company, Mt. Kisco, N.Y., 1988, pp. 35–57.
3. Sharp, J. C., and Leach, M. O.: Conformal ISIS applicable to heart. Royal Marsden Hospital, Sutton England. Proc. Soc. Magn. Reson. Med. 7:705, 1988.
4. Salhany, J. M., Pieper, G. M., Wu, S., et al.: ^{31}P nuclear magnetic resonance measurement of cardiac pH in perfused guinea-pig hearts. J. Mol. Cell. Cardiol. 11:601, 1979.
5. Sako, E. Y., Kingsley-Hickman, P. B., From, A. H. L., et al.: ATP synthesis kinetics and mitochondrial function in the postischemic myocardium as studied by ^{31}P NMR. J. Biol. Chem. 263(22):10600, 1987.
6. Schwalb, H., Kushnir, T., Navon, G., et al.: The protective effect of enriched branched chain amino acid formulation in the ischemic heart: A phosphorus-31 nuclear magnetic resonance study. J. Mol. Cell. Cardiol. 19:991, 1987.
7. Sharov, V. F., Saks, V. A., Kuprijanov, V. V., et al.: Protection of ischemic myocardium by exogenous phosphocreatine. J. Thorac. Cardiovasc. Surg. 94:749, 1987.
8. Seymour, A. M. L., Bailey, I. A., and Radda, G. K.: A protective effect of insulin on reperfusing the ischemic rat heart shown using ^{31}P NMR. Biochim. Biophys. Acta 762:525, 1983.
9. Stein, P. D., Goldstein, S., Sabbah, H. N., et al.: In vivo evaluation of intracellular pH and high-energy phosphate metabolites during regional myocardial ischemia in cats using ^{31}P nuclear magnetic resonance. Magn. Reson. Med. 3:262, 1986.
10. Suzuki, S., Kanashiro, M., and Amemiya, H.: Immunosuppressive effect of a new drug, 15-deoxyspergualin, in heterotopic rat heart transplantation: In vivo energy metabolic studies by ^{31}P-NMR spectroscopy. Transplant Proc. 19:3982, 1987.
11. Sherry, A. D., Nunnally, R. L., and Peshock, R. M.: Metabolic studies of pyruvate and lactate-perfused guinea pig hearts by ^{13}C NMR. J. Biol. Chem. 260:9272, 1985.
12. Sherry, A. D., and Malloy, C. R.: Studies of intermediary metabolism in the heart by ^{13}C NMR spectroscopy. *In* Osbakken, M., and Haselgrove, J. (eds.): NMR Techniques in the Study of Cardiovascular Structure and Function. Futura Publishing Company, Mt. Kisco, N.Y., 1988.
13. Sherry, A. D., Malloy, C. R., Roby, R. E., et al.: Propionate metabolism in the rat heart by ^{13}C NMR spectroscopy. Biochem. J. 254:593, 1988.
14. Springer, C. S.: ^{23}Na and ^{39}K NMR spectroscopic studies of the intact beating

heart. *In* Osbakken, M. D., and Haselgrove, J. C. (eds.): NMR Techniques in the Study of Cardiovascular Structure and Function. Futura Publishing Company, Mt. Kisco, N.Y., 1988, p. 35.

15. Springer, C. S., Pike, M. M., Balschi, J. A., et al.: Use of shift reagents for nuclear magnetic resonance studies of the kinetics of ion transfer in cells and perused hearts. Circulation 72:89, 1985.
16. Seo, Y., Murakami, M., Suzuki, E., and Watari, H.: A new method to discriminate intracellular and extracellular K by ^{39}K NMR without chemical shift reagents. J. Magn. Reson. 75:529, 1987.
17. Stewart, L. C., Van der Elst, L., and Ingwall, J. S.: Does glycolytic ATP support the Na^+, K^+-ATPase? A ^{31}P and ^{23}Na NMR study of isolated perfused guinea pig hearts. Proc. Soc. Magn. Reson. Med. 7:161, 1988.
18. Shporer, M., and Civan, M. M.: Nuclear magnetic resonance of sodium-23 inoleate-water. Basis for an alternative interpretation of sodium-23 spectra within cells. Biophys. J. 12:114, 1972.
19. Szklaruk, J., Clarke, K., Marecek, J. F., et al.: ^{23}Na NMR studies of perfused, beating rat hearts using a new shift reagent: Dy bPPPpob5−. Proc. Soc. Magn. Reson. Med. 7:273, 1988.
20. Sherry, A. D., Geraldes, C. F. G. C., Castro, M. M. C. A., et al.: A new $^{23}Na^+$ shift agent for Ca^{2+} sensitive tissues: Studies of the perfused rat heart. Proc. Soc. Magn. Reson. Med. 7:287, 1988.
21. Smith, G. A., Hesketh, R. T., Metcalfe, J. C., et al.: Intracellular calcium measurements by ^{19}F NMR of fluorine-labeled chelators. Proc. Natl. Acad. Sci. USA 80:7178, 1983.

T

1. Tofts, P. S., and Wray, S.: A critical assessment of methods of measuring metabolite concentrations by NMR spectroscopy. NMR Biomed. 1:1, 1988.
2. Taylor, D. J., Styles, P., Matthews, P. M., et al.: Energetics of human muscle: Exercise-induced ATP depletion. Magn. Reson. Med. 3:44, 1986.
3. Toyo-oka, T., and Nagayama, K.: Noninvasive tissue characterization of myocardium by topical ^{1}H- and ^{31}P-nuclear magnetic resonance spectroscopy. Heart Vessels (Suppl. 1): Spectroscopy, 1985, pp. 50–53.
4. Toyo-oka, T., Najayama, K., Umeda, M., et al.: Rhythmic change of myocardial phosphate metabolite content in cardiac cycle observed by depth-selected and ECG-gated in vivo ^{31}P-NMR spectroscopy in a whole animal. Biochem. Biophys. Res. Commun. 135(3):808, 1986.

U

1. Ugurbil, K., Kingsley-Hickman, P. B., Sako, E. Y., et al.: ^{31}P NMR studies of the kinetics and regulation of oxidative phosphorylation in the intact myocardium. Ann. N.Y. Acad. Sci. 508:265, 1987.
2. Ugurbil, K.: Magnetization transfer measurements of individual rate constants in the presence of multiple reactions. J. Magn. Reson. 64:207, 1985.
3. Ugurbil, K., Petein, M., Maiden, R., et al.: High resolution proton NMR studies of perfused rat hearts. FEBS Lett. 167:73, 1984.

V

1. Veech, R. L., Lawson, J. W. R., Cornell, J. W., and Krebs, R. A.: Cytosolic phosphorylation potential. J. Biochem. 234:6537, 1979.

W

1. Wu, S., White, R., Wikman-Coffelt, J., et al.: The preventive effect of verapamil on ethanol-induced cardiac depression: Phosphorus-31 nuclear magnetic resonance and high-pressure liquid chromatographic studies of hamsters. Circulation 75(5):1058, 1987.
2. Watters, T. A., Wendland, M. J., Parmley, W. W., et al.: Factors influencing myocardial response to metabolic acidosis in isolated rat hearts. Am. J. Physiol. 253(Heart Circ. Physiol. 22):H1261, 1987.
3. Wray, S., and Tofts, P. S.: Direct in vivo measurement of absolute metabolite concentrations using nuclear magnetic resonance spectroscopy. Biochim. Biophys. Acta 886:339, 1986.
4. Whitman, G. J. R., Kieval, R. S., Seeholzer, S., et al.: Recovery of left ventricular function after graded cardiac ischemia as predicted by myocardial ^{31}P nuclear magnetic resonance. Surgery 97:428, 1985.
5. Whitman, G., Kieval, R., Wetstein, L., et al.: The relationship between global ischemia, left ventricular function, myocardial redox state and high energy phosphate profile. J. Surg. Res. 35:332, 1983.
6. Whitman, G. J. R., Roth, R. A., Kieval, R. S., and Harken, A. H.: Evaluation of myocardial preservation using ^{31}P NMR. J. Surg. Res. 38:154, 1985.
7. Walpoth, B., Zhao, H., Jardetzky, N., et al.: Time resolved assessment of ischemic myocardial tolerance in normothermia and hypothermia by ^{31}P nuclear magnetic resonance. Curr. Surg. 42:198, 1985.
8. Whitman, G. J. R., Chance, B., Bode, H., et al.: Diagnoses and therapeutic evaluation of a pediatric case of cardiomyopathy using phosphorus-31 nuclear magnetic resonance spectroscopy. J. Am. Coll. Cardiol. 5:745, 1985.
9. Wittenberg, B. A., and Gupta, R. K.: NMR studies of intracellular sodium ions in mammalian myocytes. J. Biol. Chem. 260:2031, 1985.
10. Wang, Z., Wicklund, S., Subramanian, V. H., and Leigh, J. S.: Potassium-39 NMR in vivo studies of humans. Proc. Soc. Magn. Reson. Med. 7:340, 1988.

Chapter 47

NMR Imaging of the Great Vessels

RONALD M. PESHOCK, M.D.

TECHNICAL CONSIDERATIONS 864
Pulse Sequences 864
Flow Effects 864
Metallic Prostheses 865
AORTA 867
Congenital Abnormalities 867
Acquired Abnormalities 871
PULMONARY ARTERY 876
Congenital Abnormalities 876
Acquired Abnormalities 876
SYSTEMIC VENOUS ABNORMALITIES 879
PULMONARY VENOUS ABNORMALITIES 881
NEW DEVELOPMENTS 881
CONCLUSION 883

Congenital and acquired abnormalities of the great vessels present a variety of important clinical problems.[E1] The potentially lethal nature of many of these processes makes rapid, accurate diagnosis critical in patient management.[A1] This has led to the use of a wide spectrum of imaging techniques in the evaluation of great vessel disease.

Recently, magnetic resonance imaging (MRI) has emerged as an important tool in the evaluation of cardiovascular pathology, particularly in the area of great vessel disease.[C1, K1, M1, R1, R2] The combination of high spatial resolution, intrinsic contrast between vessel lumen and wall, and lack of ionizing radiation makes MRI attractive for evaluation. Moreover, the flexibility and inherent sensitivity of MRI to flow and motion have led to the development of magnetic resonance angiographic techniques that may have substantial application in the evaluation of vascular disease.[D1]

This chapter briefly reviews several technical considerations relevant to the interpretation of magnetic resonance images of the great vessels and summarizes the present state of the clinical application of magnetic resonance imaging in the evaluation of these patients.

TECHNICAL CONSIDERATIONS

Pulse Sequences

An almost endless variety of pulse sequences can be used for imaging the heart and great vessels. A detailed description of these is beyond the scope of this discussion. However, two general approaches are in standard clinical use at present: the spin echo sequence and the gradient reversal sequence.

From the standpoint of imaging the great vessels, spin echo sequences typically have longer echo times (TE 20 to 40 msec), which are generally characterized by low signal intensity from cardiac chambers and the lumen of vessels. In comparison, gradient reversal, cine MRI sequences typically have short echo times (TE 5 to 15 msec) and high intensity from blood in cardiac chambers and vessel lumens.[F1] An example of the change in contrast that occurs just by altering the type of sequence used is shown in Figure 47–1.

At present, the general impression is that spin echo images provide better anatomic definition, whereas gradient reversal, cine MRI sequences allow better evaluation of structures in motion. For this reason, magnetic resonance examinations of the great vessels frequently include both spin echo and gradient reversal sequences.

A second important consideration in choosing pulse sequences relates to the need for gating. Although some have suggested in the past that ungated studies may be adequate to study the great vessels,[C2] the majority of studies have utilized gated sequences.[E3, M3] The improvement in image quality with gating is illustra ted in Figure 47–2. Hence, today it is essential that both spin echo and gradient reversal images of the great vessels be obtained using gated sequences.

Flow Effects

As described in Chapter 41, magnetic resonance imaging is inherently sensitive to motion and, therefore, the flow of blood. For this reason, the appearance of blood on magnetic resonance images depends highly on the velocity and direction of blood flow in the vessel under consideration and the exact pulsing sequence used to obtain the image.[B1] This dependence on motion and pulse sequence explains the marked differences in image contrast between the spin echo and gradient reversal images seen in Figure 47–1. A complete discussion of flow effects is beyond the scope of this section; however, a basic understanding is necessary to allow one to interpret correctly the effects of blood motion in images. Accordingly, the two major groups of flow effects—time-of-flight effects and spin phase effects—will be summarized.

TIME-OF-FLIGHT EFFECTS. Moving blood carries a history of the varying magnetic fields to which it has been exposed in the magnetic resonance imaging process. Because of its motion, blood may be exposed to a different history or series of pulses as compared with stationary tissue. This means that the blood can be bright or dark relative to the surrounding tissue, depending on the exact pulses, the path of the blood through the imaging volume, and the speed with which the blood has moved through the imaging pulses. An example is shown in Figure 47–3. Here the intensity of the blood signal is seen to depend on its velocity and history of exposure to additional pulses.

Time-of-flight effects are frequently manifest in images in two ways. First, in many cases the rapid motion of blood means that it can move through the imaging slice before it sees all the necessary pulses involved in imaging so that no signal is obtained from the blood (termed high-velocity signal loss, Fig. 47–3A). This mechanism plays an important role in the contrast seen in many magnetic resonance images of the great vessels. Second, if the velocity is low or if the series of pulses is carried out rapidly (so that the blood has less time to move), one can obtain increased

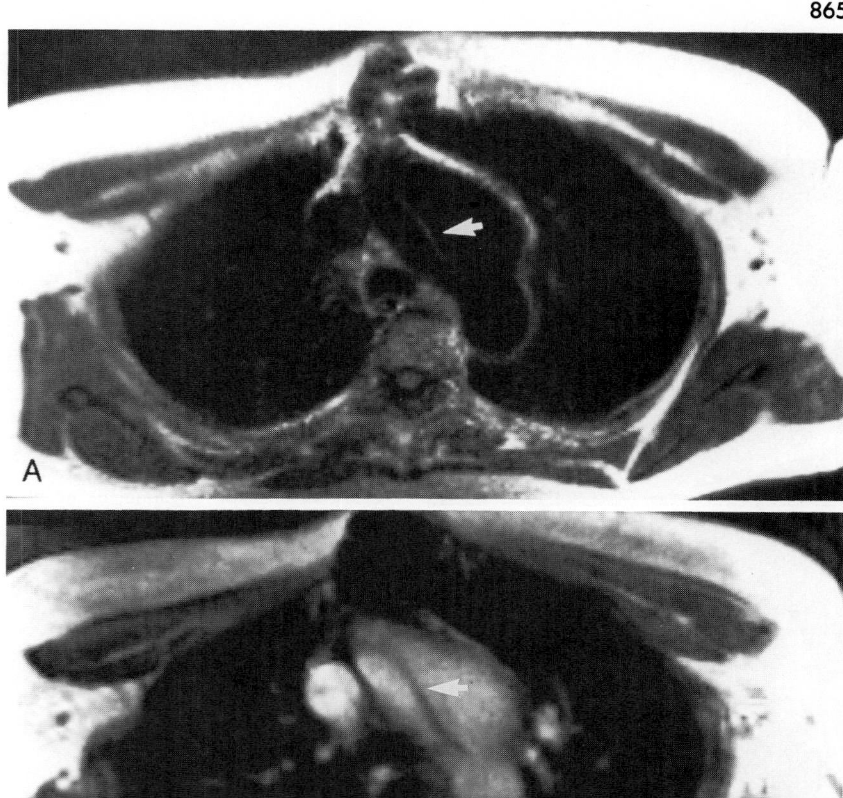

Figure 47–1. Spin echo vs. gradient reversal. Images obtained in a patient with aortic dissection. *A*, An image obtained using a spin echo technique; *B*, the same slice imaged using a gradient reversal technique. The intimal flap is visualized using either method (arrows).

signal in a vessel (termed flow-related enhancement,[M2] Fig. 47–3*B*). This effect is frequently encountered in images of the great vessels obtained in diastole or early in systole in the case of sequences with relatively long echo times and throughout the cardiac cycle for sequence with very short echo times.

This increased signal must be differentiated from thrombus. A number of factors may be helpful in making this distinction: First, flow-related enhancement depends on the exact timing and spatial location of pulses relative to the direction of blood flow. Hence, changing the imaging plane orientation or other aspects of the pulse sequence will make the signal disappear if it is not thrombus. Second, one can apply additional pulses upstream and downstream from the region of interest to reduce the signal from moving blood (so-called out-of-plane presaturation[F2]). Third, the use of properties of the signal, such as even-echo rephasing[B2, K2] and phase shifts,[W1] can be useful. Finally, the interpretation of signal as due to thrombus should make clinical sense, i.e., it should fit with the clinical situation. Chapter 41 discusses these approaches further.

SPIN PHASE EFFECTS. Motion of blood in the presence of the magnetic field gradients used in magnetic resonance imaging results in spin phase effects. These effects frequently lead to a loss in signal intensity in magnetic resonance images,[S1] unless measures are taken to compensate for them.[P1] Of particular importance is the concept of spin dephasing leading to a loss of signal intensity.[S2] Briefly, if the range of velocities in a given picture element or volume element of the image is large, then there will be a wide range of spin phases leading to cancelation of the signal. Thus, in regions of blood flow where there is a wide range of velocities, such as near the walls of vessels or in regions of turbulence, there is potential for significant signal cancellation.

Typical examples of this phenomenon are shown in Figure 47–4. These effects can be both a help and a hindrance. Spin dephasing at vessel borders can actually help define the lumen of vessels[S1] and can be used to define regions of turbulence, as seen in valvular regurgitation.[P2] This same sensitivity to turbulence, however, can also be a disadvantage in magnetic resonance angiographic techniques in that it can lead to loss of signal and an overestimation of the degree of stenosis present.[E2]

Spin phase effects lead to many of the so-called "motion artifacts" (phase-encoding artifacts) associated with blood and organ motion in magnetic resonance imaging. For this reason, several methods for reducing motion artifacts have been developed. One approach is to make the TE or time to echo as short as possible to limit the time available for dephasing.[S3] A second approach involves the use of motion compensating gradients.[Q1] By adjusting the gradient waveforms, it is possible to suppress the effects of velocity, acceleration, and higher moments of motion on the spin phase. The approach has been referred to by a number of terms, including motion compensation, velocity compensation, motion artifact suppression, and others. It has been widely applied in cine MRI to reduce motion artifacts.[G1]

Metallic Prostheses

A variety of metallic prostheses are encountered in patients referred for magnetic resonance imaging. These include pacemakers, vascular clips, and prosthetic heart valves. Pacemakers are considered an absolute contraindication to magnetic resonance imaging for reasons discussed elsewhere. Cerebral aneurysm clips are also a contraindication. However, the clips used in coronary artery bypass surgery and other surgical procedures are not.

Prosthetic heart valves have been evaluated in a number of studies, both with regard to the forces generated on the valve[S4]

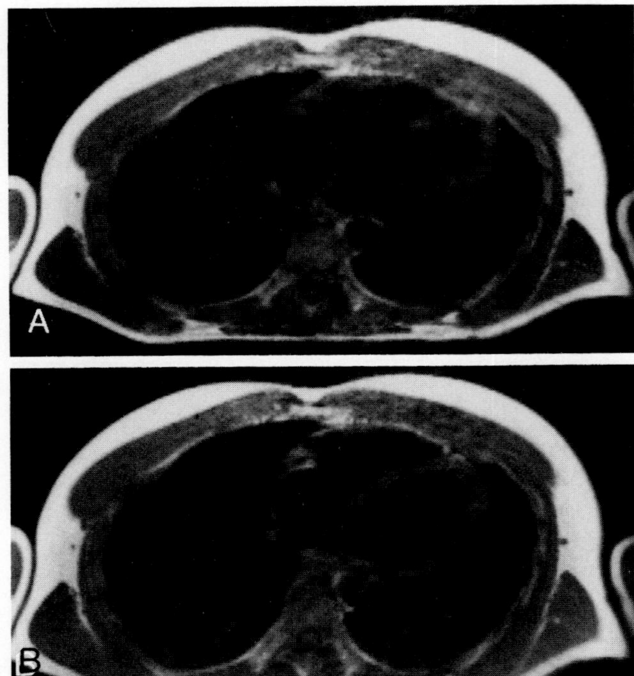

Figure 47–2. Ungated versus gated images. *A*, An image obtained without gating; *B*, an image obtained at the same level with gating, demonstrating a clear improvement in image quality.

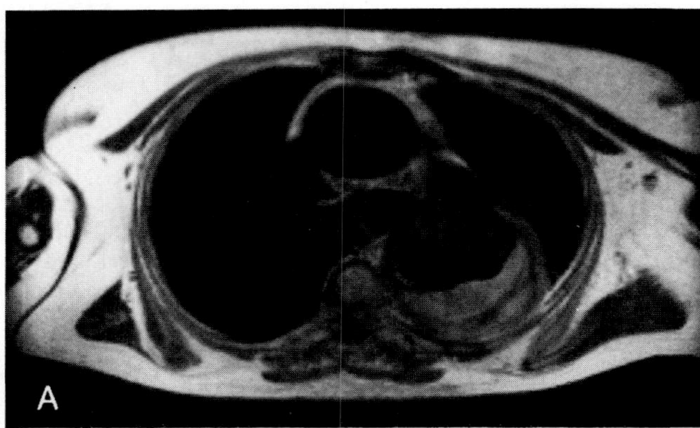

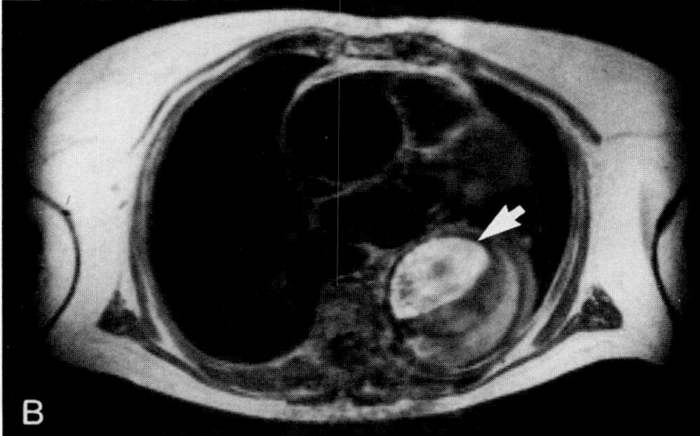

Figure 47–3. Time of flight effects. Transaxial images in a patient with a thoracic aneurysm. *A*, An image obtained during systole, when rapid blood flow leads to loss of signal in both the ascending and descending aorta. A mural thrombus is also present in the descending aorta. *B*, An image obtained in early systole, in which the motion of blood in the ascending aorta leads to loss of signal. The blood in the descending aorta is moving more slowly, leading to intraluminal signal (arrow).

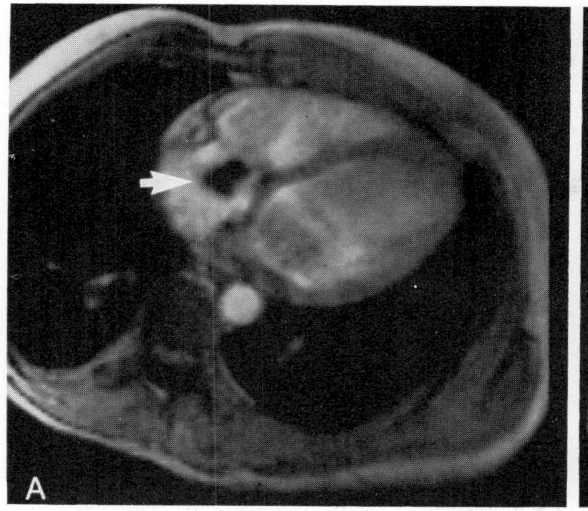

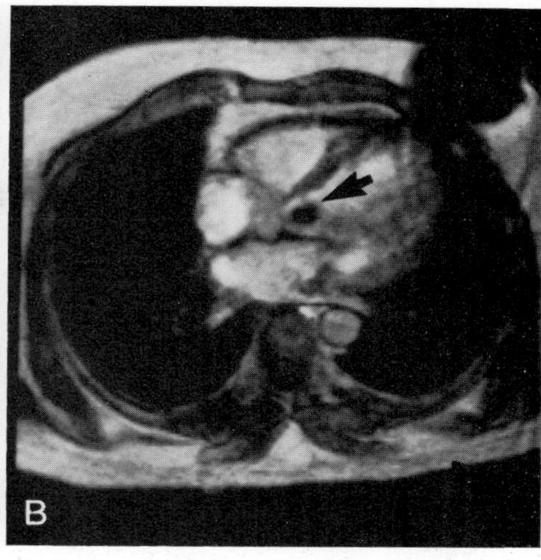

Figure 47–4. Spin dephasing effects. *A*, Signal loss in the right atrium due to tricuspid regurgitation (white arrow). *B*, Loss of signal in a region of turbulence in the setting of aortic insufficiency (black arrow).

and in terms of degradation of the magnetic resonance image due to metal artifact.[R3] It appears that the forces generated on a prosthetic heart valve during cardiac contraction far exceed those generated by a magnetic field, so the probability of the magnetic field altering the position or orientation of the valve appears to be small. However, the presence of a prosthetic valve (Fig. 47–5) does lead to some image degradation in the immediate area of the valve, complicating the interpretation of the image.[R3] It is of note that this degradation will be more severe for gradient echo, cine-MRI sequences, which are more sensitive to differences in magnetic susceptibility than spin echo pulse sequences.

AORTA

Clearly, the widest application of magnetic resonance imaging in the evaluation of the great vessels has been in the area of aortic disease.[A1, A2, C3, E1, F3, S5] MRI has been shown to be useful in the evaluation of both congenital and acquired abnormalities of the aorta.

Congenital Abnormalities

COARCTATION. Coarctation of the aorta was demonstrated early in the development of MRI.[A3, B5] The intrinsic contrast between flowing blood and the aortic wall and the ability to perform imaging in the sagittal plane make it possible to determine directly the extent and degree of coarctation both before and after intervention.[B3, F3] Examples of a discrete postductal coarctation and aortic arch hypoplasia are shown in Figure 47–6. In addition, as shown in Figure 47–7, one can easily evaluate patients in whom there is a question of the adequacy of repair. Magnetic resonance imaging also has been shown to be of use in the evaluation of vascular conduits used in the management of some patients with coarctation.[P3]

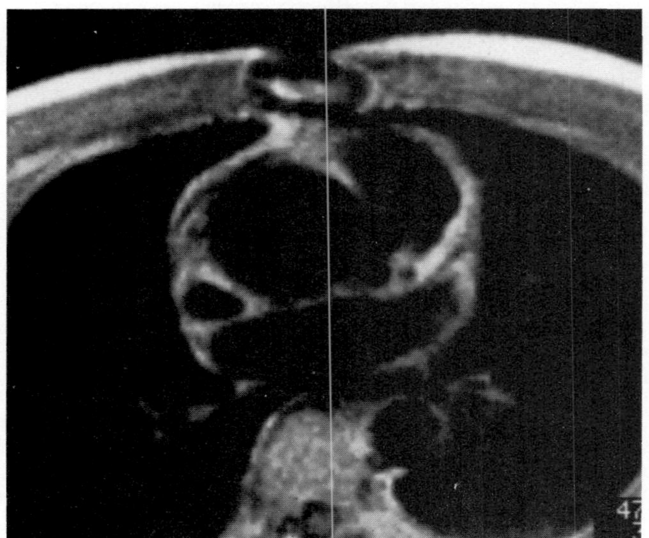

Figure 47–5. Prosthetic heart valve. Image obtained in a patient with a prosthetic heart valve in the aortic position, using a spin echo pulse sequence.

Recently, cine MRI has been used to evaluate patients with coarctation of the aorta.[S6] In those studies, Simpson and colleagues demonstrated an excellent correlation between magnetic resonance and angiographic measures of minimum aortic diameter (r = 0.90) and extensive regions of turbulence whose length correlated with the angiographic severity of the narrowing (r = 0.81) (Fig. 47–8).

One important potential problem in the diagnosis of coarctation is that of artifactual coarctation.[D2, P4] The aorta does not lie in one tomographic plane, hence it is possible to produce a factitious narrowing if the aorta passes in and out of the imaging plane. In general, this problem can be avoided by obtaining images in multiple orientations, i.e., sagittal and axial, for conformation. Artifactual coarctation is to be differentiated from pseudocoarctation, a rare congenital condition associated with kinking of the aorta at the level of the ligamentum arteriosum.[E1, L1, S7]

VASCULAR RING. The presence of a vascular ring is an important consideration in infants with stridor and dysphagia. The vascular ring results from persistence of some portion of the duplicated brachial arches present during embryogenesis.[B4, D5, F4, J1, S8] The basic anatomy associated with a vascular ring is diagrammed in Figure 47–9. An example of magnetic resonance images obtained in a patient with a vascular ring are shown in Figure 47–10. Pulmonary artery sling, in which an aberrant left pulmonary artery arises from the right pulmonary artery, has also been visualized using magnetic resonance imaging.[M4]

MARFAN'S SYNDROME. The severity of aortic involvement is an important consideration in patients with Marfan's syndrome. Examples of aortic abnormalities are demonstrated in Figure 47–11. Several groups have reported the use of MRI in the routine follow-up of aortic root size in patients with Marfan's syndrome.[B5, K3, S9] Schaefer demonstrated an excellent correlation between echo measurements of aortic root size by magnetic resonance and echocardiography (r = 0.99).[S9] Moreover, compared with echocardiography, magnetic resonance imaging can be performed in patients with severe thoracic deformities, such as pectus excavatum and scoliosis, and allows evaluation of the entire aortic root.[K3] A comparable evaluation using computed tomography would require the use of ionizing radiation and a contrast agent. In view of the lack of ionizing radiation, MRI is particularly attractive in the evaluation of pregnant women with Marfan's syndrome in

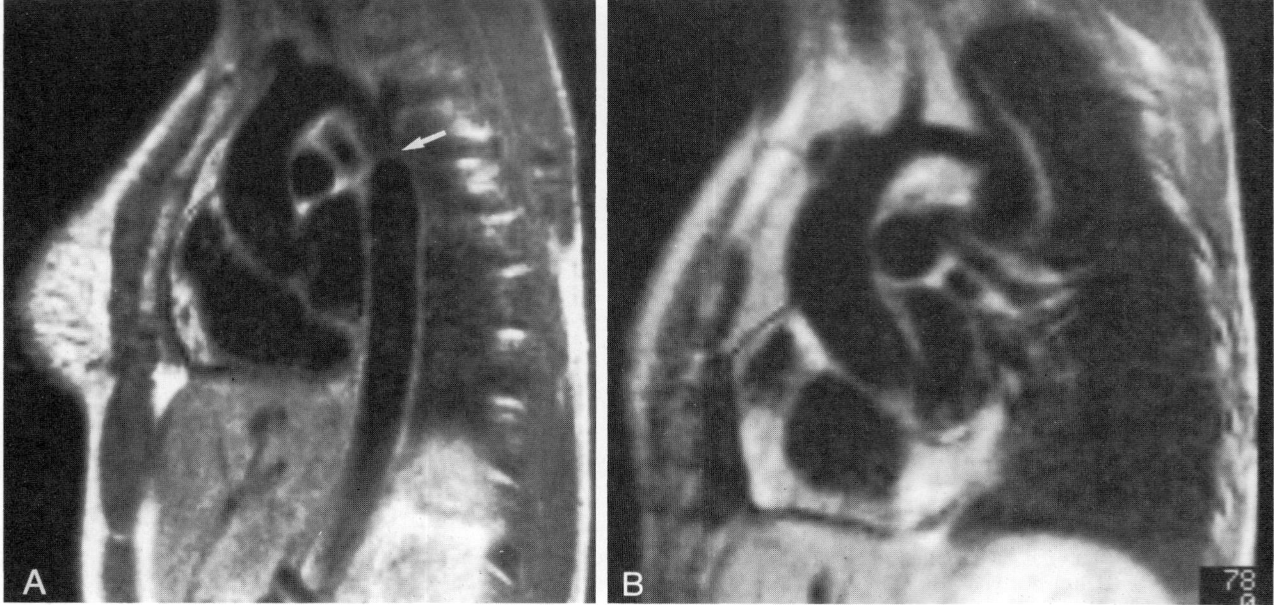

Figure 47–6. Coarctation of the aorta. *A*, Postductal coarctation of the aorta (arrow). *B*, More extensive hypoplasia of the aortic arch in a second patient.

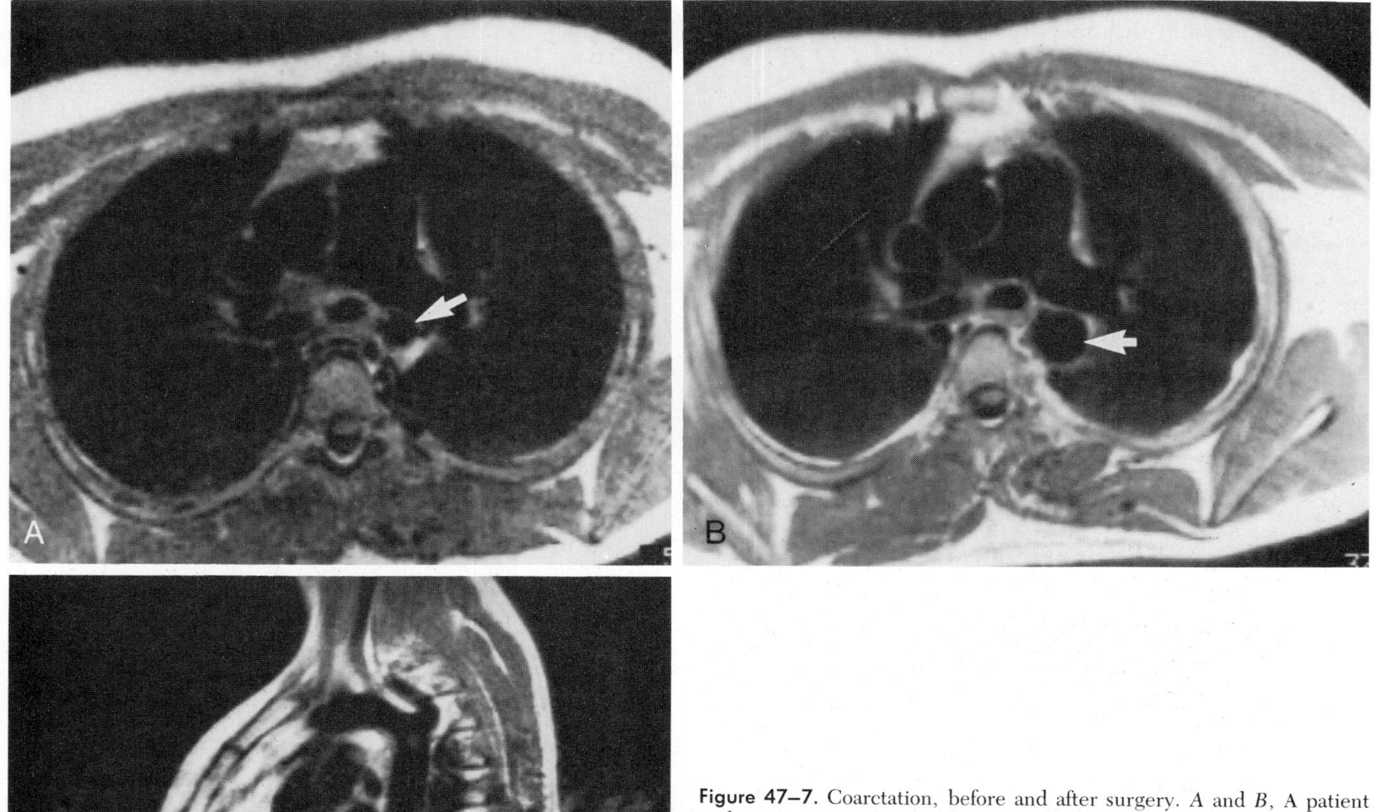

Figure 47–7. Coarctation, before and after surgery. *A* and *B*, A patient with a coarctation (arrows) before and after surgery. *C*, The descending aorta following repair.

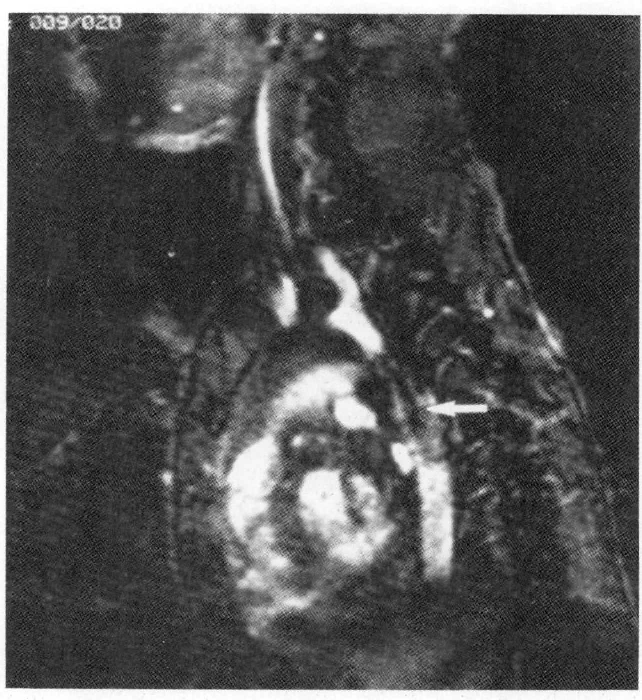

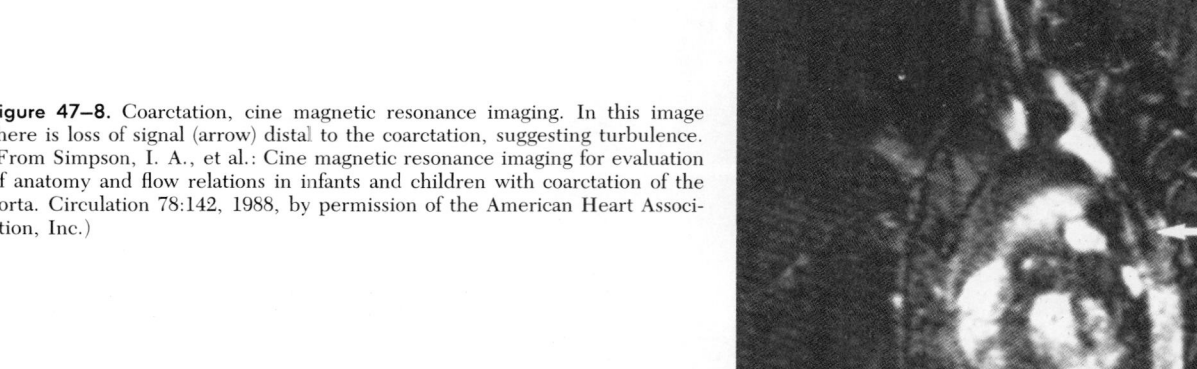

Figure 47–8. Coarctation, cine magnetic resonance imaging. In this image there is loss of signal (arrow) distal to the coarctation, suggesting turbulence. (From Simpson, I. A., et al.: Cine magnetic resonance imaging for evaluation of anatomy and flow relations in infants and children with coarctation of the aorta. Circulation 78:142, 1988, by permission of the American Heart Association, Inc.)

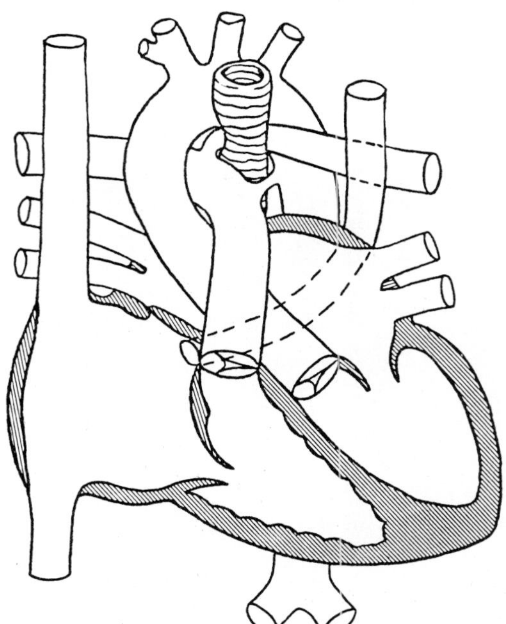

Figure 47–9. Vascular ring. Diagram of the embryologic basis for vascular rings. (From Mullins, C. E., and Mayer, D. C.: Congenital Heart Disease: A Diagrammatic Atlas. Alan R. Liss, Inc., New York, 1988, p. 27, with permission.)

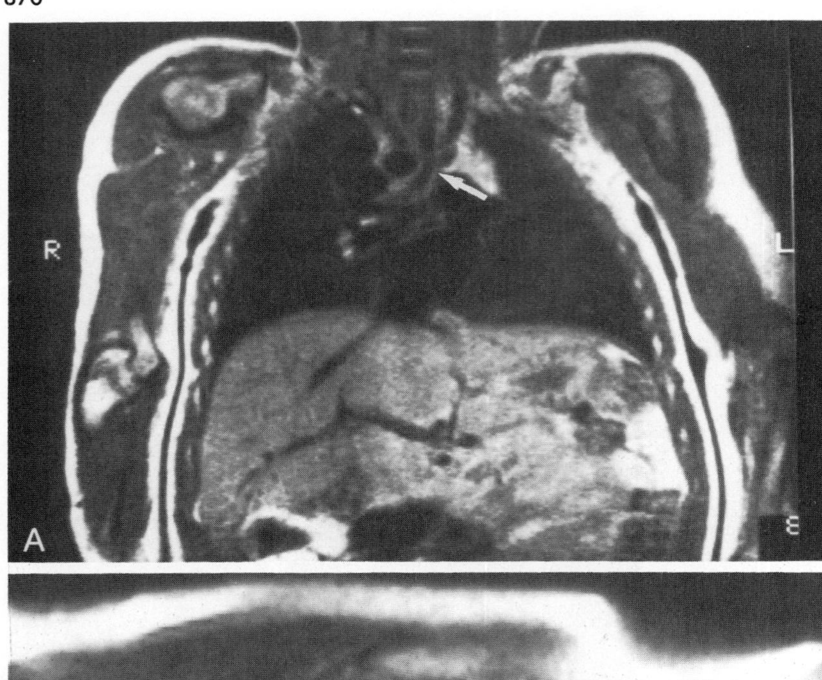

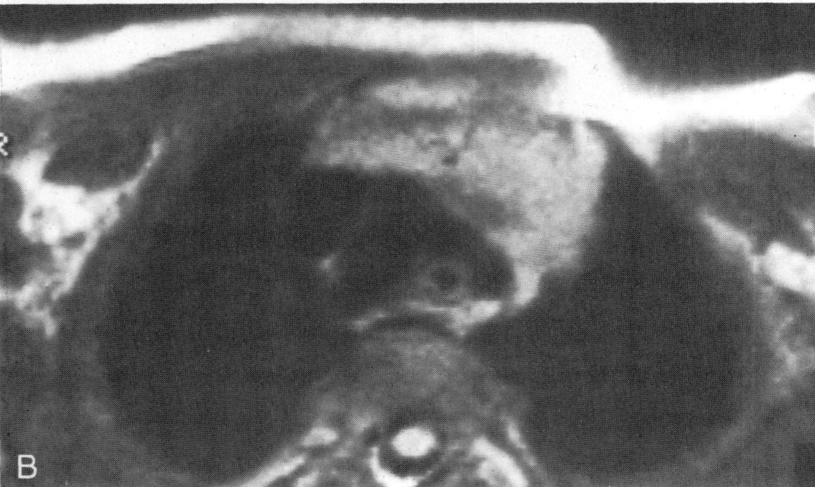

Figure 47–10. Vascular ring. *A*, A coronal image in an 18-month-old infant with stridor, demonstrating a right aortic arch with compression of the trachea by an aberrant left subclavian artery (arrow). *B*, A transverse image at the level of the compression demonstrating the positions of the vessels and the presence of an atretic left aortic arch that completes the ring around the trachea (From Peshock, R. M., and Rollins, N.: Recurrent respiratory difficulty, stridor, and dysphagia in a 15 month old. Curr. Concepts Magn. Reson. Imag. 2(2):22, 1988, with permission.)

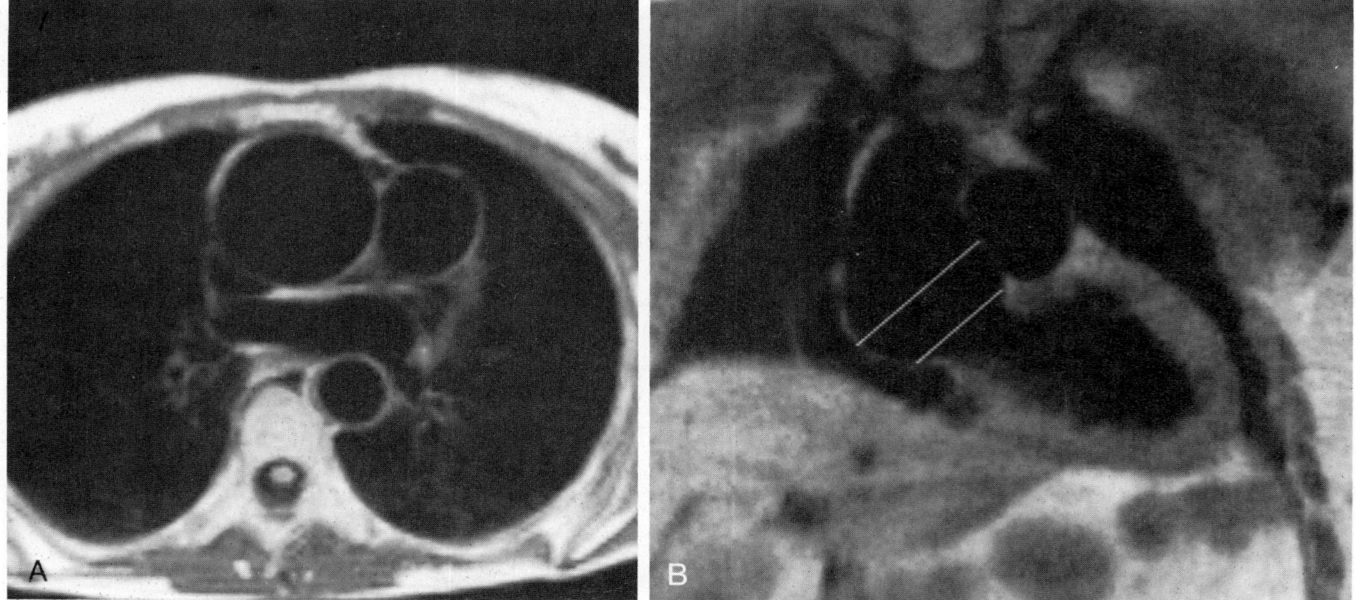

Figure 47–11. Marfan's syndrome. *A*, A transverse image in a patient with marked proximal aortic dilatation (annuloaortic ectasia). *B*, A coronal view obtained in another patient. The lines indicate positions for the measurement of aortic root size.

whom dissection of the aorta is an important potential complication.

SUPRAVALVULAR AORTIC STENOSIS. An uncommon abnormality of the aorta that can be detected with magnetic resonance imaging is the presence of supravalvular aortic stenosis,[B6, F3] as shown in Figure 47–12.

Acquired Abnormalities

AORTIC DISSECTION. In the evaluation of patients with suspected aortic dissection, a number of critical questions need to be addressed: (1) Is a dissection present? (2) Where are the entrance and exit sites? (3) Is there continued flow in the false channel? (4) Are the coronary ostia involved? (5) What is the status of the aortic valve and, in particular, is aortic insufficiency present? A variety of imaging techniques have been used in the evaluation of these patients, including aortography, computed tomography, and echocardiography. However, each of these requires contrast material or is limited in its ability to evaluate all the critical questions.

Magnetic resonance imaging, with its wide field of view and sensitivity to flow, would appear to have significant potential in the evaluation of patients with suspected dissection. This has led to a large number of studies utilizing a variety of magnetic resonance techniques to examine patients with dissection.[A4, A5, B7, D3, K4, G2–G4, L2] In particular, it has been found to be useful in patients with complicated aortic disease, such as dissection in the presence of a coexisting or previously repaired atherosclerotic aneurysm.[C4] It has also been used in patients after surgery for aortic dissection to evaluate the status of the false lumen.[W4]

The appearance of aortic dissection on magnetic resonance MR depends on the velocity of blood flow in the false and true channels and on the exact pulse sequence used. Standard, gated spin echo images obtained in patients with aortic dissection are shown in Figures 47–13 and 47–14. If the velocity of blood flow is rapid in both the true and false channels, there is high-velocity signal loss in both channels, and the flap is seen as an intermediate gray color. Thus, the contrast depends on the rapid flow of blood in both the true and the false lumens. Figures 47–15 and 47–16 show patients in whom there is relatively slow blood flow in the false channel. This leads to increased signal in the false channel. This signal can be assigned to flowing blood and not thrombus because of the presence of even-echo rephasing[D4, W8] or phase shift relative to stationary tissue on phase-reconstructed images (not shown).[R4] However, these techniques cannot distinguish thrombosed blood in a dissection from thrombosed blood in an aneurysm.[G4]

A series of gradient reversal, cine MRI images in a patient with dissection are shown in Figure 47–17. View *A* is an image obtained at end diastole. The intimal flap is seen as a dark line at the level of the transverse arch. View *B* is another frame in the cine sequence at the same level during systole. Rapid flow and turbulence reduce the signal intensity in the true lumen, while the false channel remains bright owing to slower blood flow. Review of all images in a cine loop allows one to determine that there is rapid flow in the true channel with continued, but reduced, flow in the false channel.

Compared with computed tomography, magnetic resonance imaging is not degraded by streak artifacts.[G5, T1] Compared with echocardiography, it allows evaluation of the complete aorta in essentially all patients. Aortography is the established standard but is known to have significant potential complications, and it has a demonstrated incidence of false-negative studies.[G3, S10]

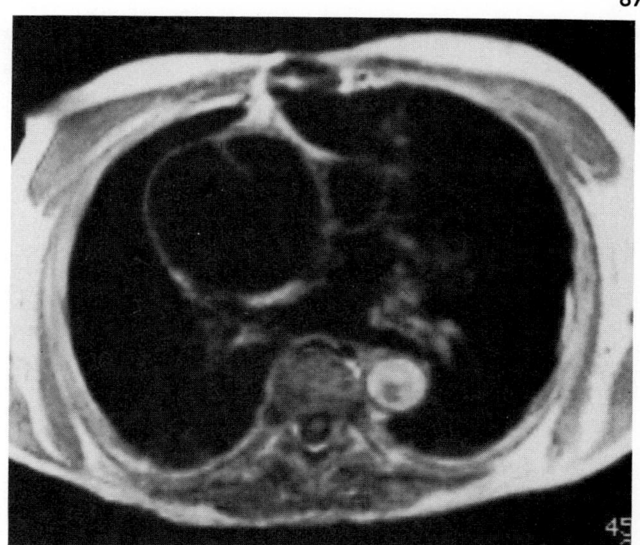

Figure 47–13. Aortic dissection, spin echo image. The ascending aorta is markedly dilated, with an intimal flap visible anteriorly.

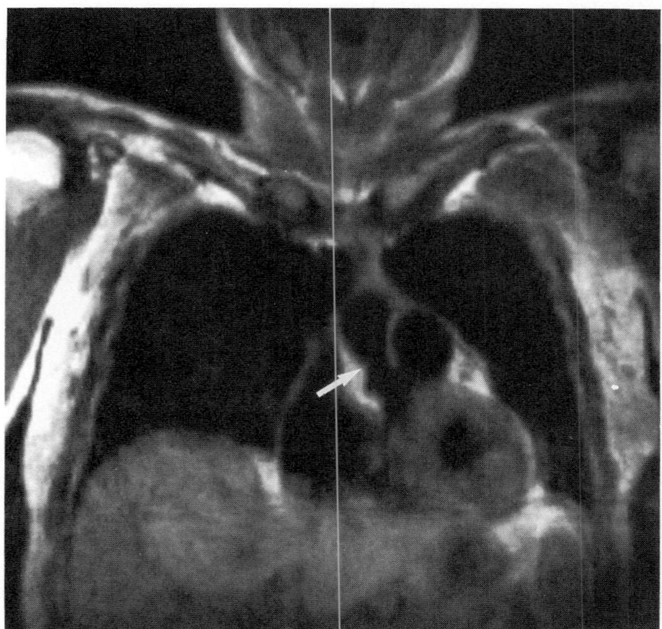

Figure 47–12. Supravalvular aortic stenosis. The region of supravalvular narrowing is indicated by the arrow.

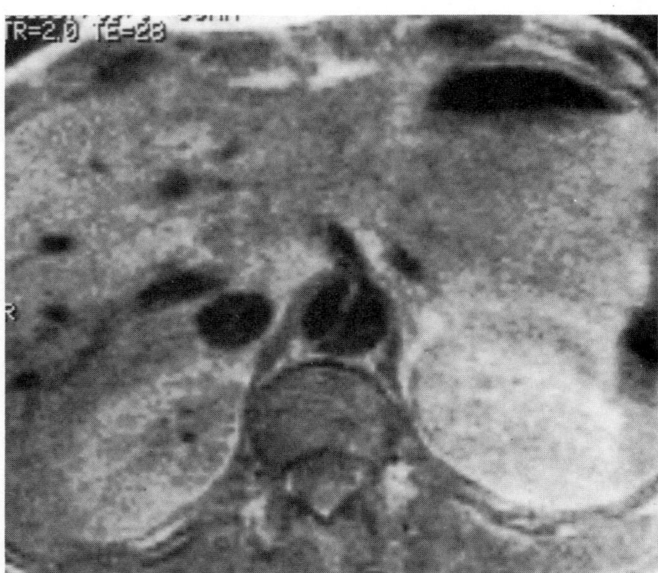

Figure 47–14. Aortic dissection, spin echo image. The intimal flap is clearly seen because of rapid flow in both the true and false channels.

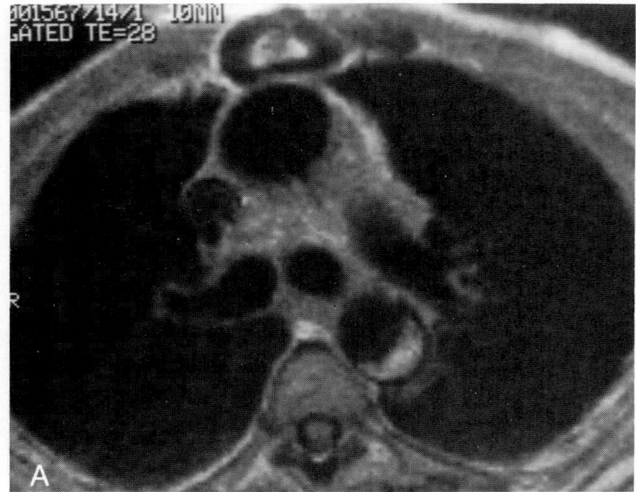

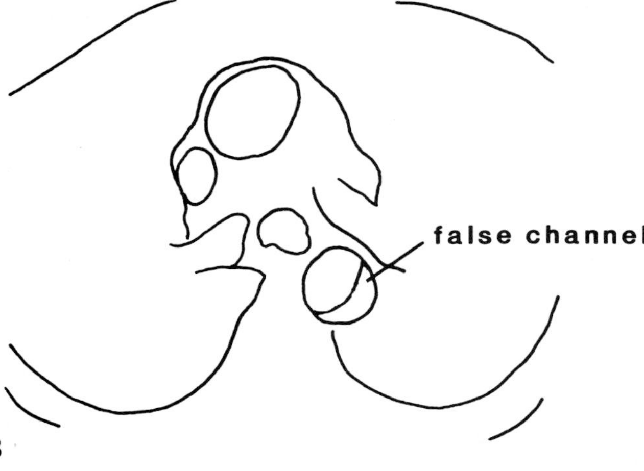

Figure 47–15. Aortic dissection. *A*, A spin echo image in which there is increased signal due to slow blood flow in the false channel. *B* identifies the false channel.

Hence, magnetic resonance imaging would appear to offer significant potential advantages over other available methods. However, three general types of artifacts can complicate the magnetic resonance diagnosis of dissection: anatomic variants, flow artifacts, and chemical shift artifact.

The first important anatomic variant is the extension of the pericardial space over the anterior and posterior aorta (Fig. 47–17). This variant was first observed in computed tomography and can be demonstrated on 49 percent of routine chest CT studies.[A7] It is clear that this space is evident in even a higher percentage of MR studies. McMurdo and associates found evidence of the superior pericardial recesses in over 85 percent of gated transverse MR studies.[M5] It is generally manifest as a dark space on relatively T1-weighted spin echo images, presumably due to the long T1 or motion of normal pericardial fluid. It is interesting that the superior pericardial recesses frequently are well demonstrated in the absence of other evidence of pericardial effusion. This extension of the pericardial space is frequently seen on MR and can be mistaken for dissection involving the ascending aorta (Fig. 47–18), a calcified atherosclerotic plaque, or another vascular structure. In general, an intimal flap is more linear than the normal aortic wall (see Figs. 47–13, 47–14 and 47–18), whereas the superior pericardial recess tends to follow the curve of the aortic wall. However, it is critical to be aware of the presence of this space since at present there is no absolute means of differentiating it from a region of dissection.

A second anatomic pitfall in the evaluation of dissection by magnetic resonance imaging relates to the presence of the innominate vein anterior to the aorta (Fig. 47–19). However, in general this is readily identified by following the vessel across multiple tomographic slices.

The next major concern is the presence of flow artifacts or regions of intraluminal signal due to relatively slow flow in the absence of dissection. This frequently occurs, as mentioned, in images obtained early in the cardiac cycle when blood velocity in the aorta is low. These effects are pulse sequence–dependent and often machine-dependent. In general, the use of multiple sequence types, phase reconstructions,[A3, B7] and presaturation,[F1] as described, allow this distinction. A thorough knowledge of typical flow effects on a given imaging machine must be gained through experience. Because of the complexity of flow effects, it is generally unwise to make the diagnosis of dissection on the basis of the intraluminal signal alone. *Regardless of the pulse*

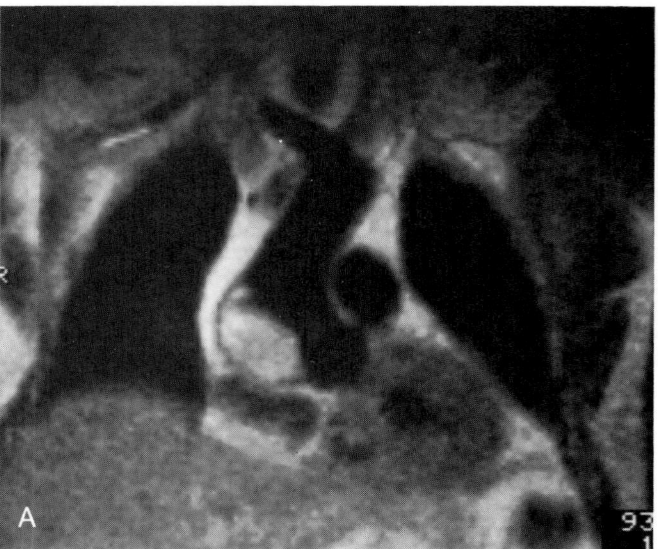

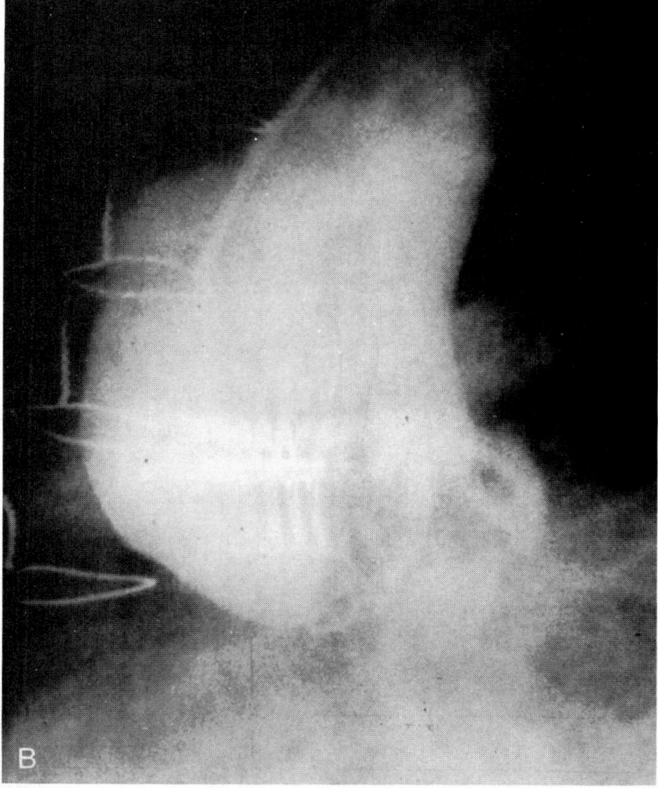

Figure 47–16. Aortic dissection, spin echo image. *A*, A region of increased signal intensity is seen next to the aorta. *B*, This region seen on magnetic resonance imaging corresponds to the location of the false channel in the aortogram (catheter).

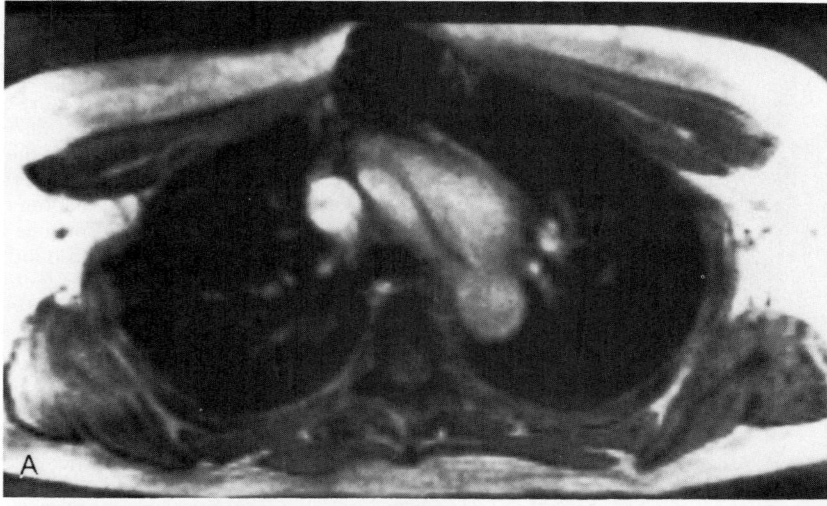

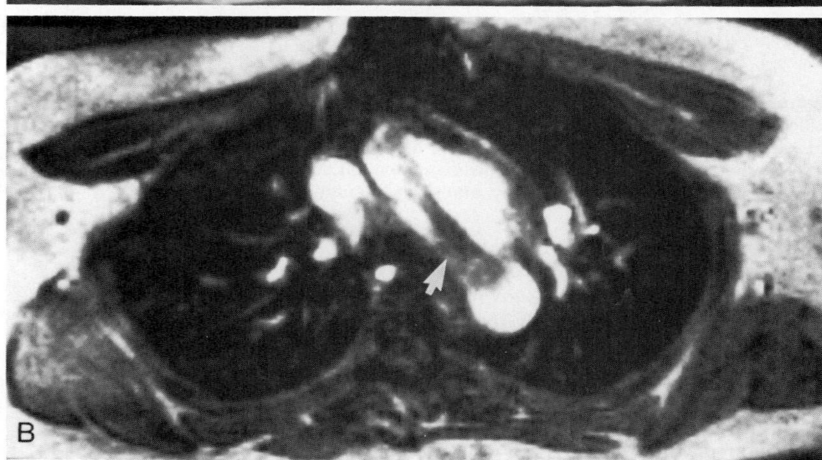

Figure 47–17. Aortic dissection, cine magnetic resonance images. (See text.)

sequence used, the diagnosis of dissection by magnetic resonance imaging rests on the demonstration of the intimal flap.

Recently, the chemical shift artifact has been demonstrated to be a potential pitfall, particularly on high field (1.5 Tesla and above) MRI units[L3] (Fig. 47–20). Chemical shift artifact arises from the fact that hydrogen nuclei in fat experience a slightly different local magnetic field than hydrogen nuclei in water. Because of the methods used to determine the source of signal in the image, this difference leads to a displacement of signal from fat relative to the signal from water. This artifact can be differentiated from a flap by altering the imaging conditions.[L3]

An additional potential limitation of magnetic resonance imaging is the detection of the extension of dissection into branch vessels. Although the involvement of the subclavian and other vessels has been described,[A5] other investigators have found problems with resolution in the evaluation of these smaller vessels.[M6]

In spite of these concerns, early studies reported that the intimal flap was identified in a very high proportion of cases.[A3, G2, G3] Recently, the sensitivity and specificity of magnetic reso-

Figure 47–18. Superior pericardial space. Transverse image demonstrating the superior pericardial space both anterior and posterior to the ascending aorta.

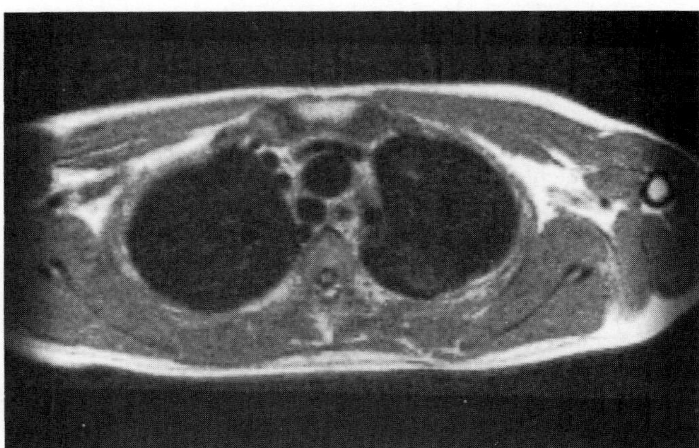

Figure 47–19. Innominate vein. The innominate vein is seen to pass anterior to the ascending aorta in this transverse image.

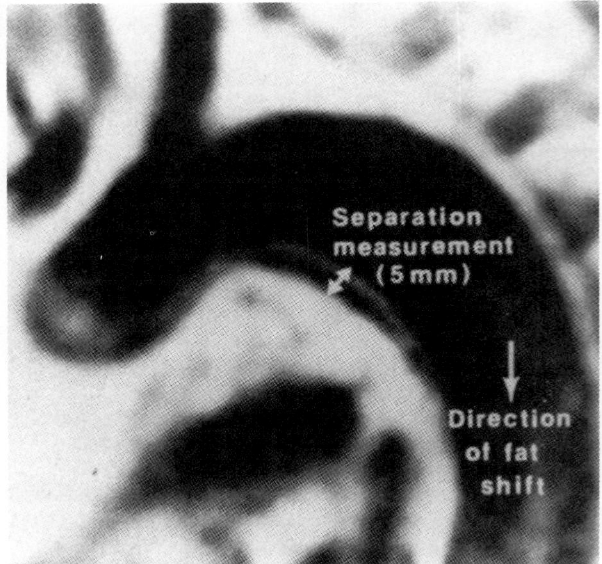

Figure 47–20. Chemical shift artifact simulating dissection. The arrow indicates the position of signal from extravascular fat, which has been shifted into the aorta, simulating an intimal flap. (From Lotan, C. S., et al.: Fat-shift artifact simulating aortic dissection on MR images. AJR 152:385, 1989, with permission. © by American Roentgen Ray Society.)

nance in the diagnosis of dissection have been examined.[K4] Fifty-four studies in patients with known or suspected aortic dissection were examined retrospectively by three reviewers with differing levels of experience in interpreting cardiac magnetic resonance studies. The only criterion for a definite diagnosis was the identification of an intimal flap, although slow flow in false channel was interpreted as highly suggestive. They found a significant difference in the sensitivity of the different observers in the detection of dissection. Using receiver operating characteristic curves, they found that for a specificity level of 90 percent, the most experienced observer (5 years' experience) had the best sensitivity (100 percent). Observers with 2 years of experience and limited experience demonstrated lower sensitivity (96 percent and 83 percent) in the detection of dissection. The difference in sensitivity was felt to be related to experience gained in the interpretation of flow artifacts.[K4]

Thus, the data indicate that magnetic resonance imaging is a sensitive and specific tool in the evaluation of dissection, particularly in the hands of experienced users. It can provide information regarding the presence of dissection, can define the entrance and exit sites, can demonstrate the presence of continued flow in the false channel, and may establish whether aortic insufficiency is present. At present, it cannot establish whether the coronary ostia are involved; this requires selective coronary angiography. The lack of need for iodinated contrast material makes it particularly attractive in patients with compromised renal function. In the hands of experienced users, it appears at present that the major limitation of magnetic resonance imaging relative to computed tomography is that the magnetic environment complicates the observation and monitoring of potentially unstable patients. The patient is typically positioned out of sight in the center of a long tube. Monitoring and support lines must also run out of the magnet. Thus, CT may be simpler than MR in some unstable patients. Recent changes in magnet design[M7] and the development of ultra low field magnets, which are more open with a less demanding magnetic environment,[W5] may allow easier scanning of these unstable patients.

AORTIC ANEURYSM. The same properties that make magnetic resonance useful in the evaluation of aortic dissection make it useful in the assessment of aortic aneurysms.[A8, D5, F5, L4] Detection of post-traumatic false aneurysm of the aorta following deceleration injury has also been reported.[M8] Infectious pseudoaneurysms[W6] and infections of prosthetic aortic grafts have also been detected using magnetic resonance imaging.[A6, O1] Measurements of aortic diameter by MR are comparable to those obtained by computed tomography.[A9, G4] A typical descending thoracic aneurysm is shown in Figure 47–21. A typical abdominal aortic aneurysm is shown in Figure 47–22. In an early study, Lee and associates found magnetic resonance to more reliable than sonography in determining the relationship between the aneurysm and the renal and illiac arteries.[L4] They recommended that ultrasound remain the screening examination because of its lower cost, and that magnetic resonance be reserved for patients with inadequate or equivocal ultrasound examinations.

Magnetic resonance has also been reported to be useful in the examination of patients with complications of aortic surgery, including graft occlusion, infection, pseudoaneurysm formation, perigraft hemorrhage, and aortoenteric fistulas.[A6]

CORONARY ARTERIES AND BYPASS GRAFTS. Although they are not great vessels, the coronary arteries and coronary bypass grafts are important considerations in many patients with aortic disease. Although the coronary arteries are frequently demonstrated on magnetic resonance studies of the heart, the resolution is not adequate for the direct assessment of coronary stenoses at the present time.[P6] MR has been used to demonstrate

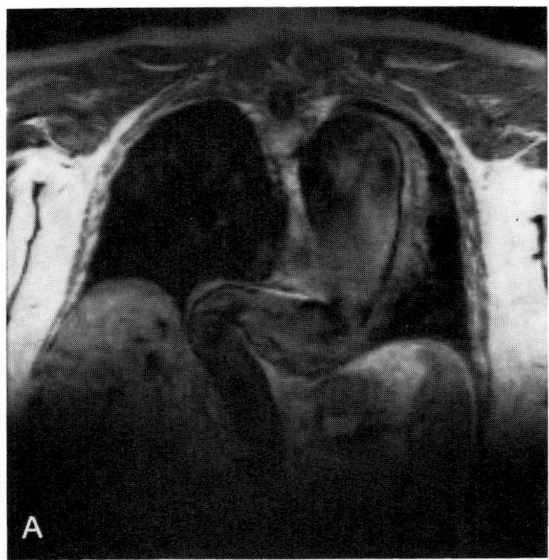

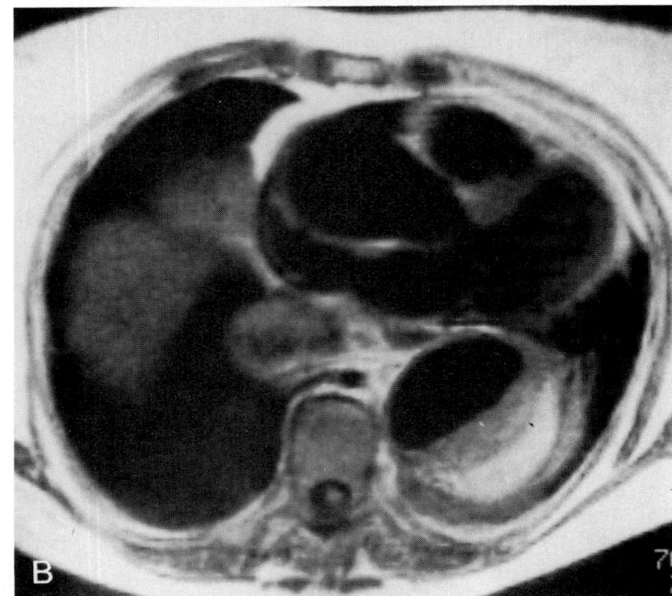

Figure 47–21. Descending thoracic aneurysm. *A*, A coronal image demonstrating a dilated, tortuous descending aorta with increased signal intensity due to slowly moving blood in the lumen. *B*, A transaxial image showing a large descending thoracic aneurysm with layered thrombus.

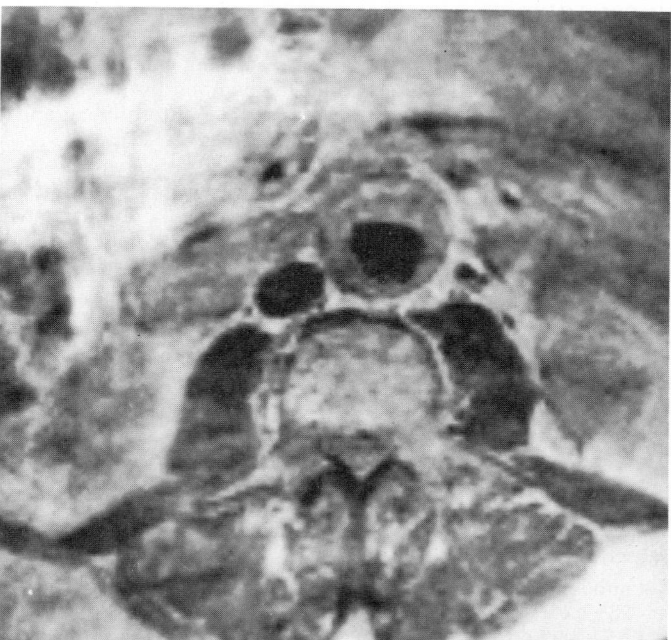

Figure 47–22. Abdominal aortic aneurysm. An aortic aneurysm with thrombus/plaque is demonstrated.

aberrant coronaries and to demonstrate coronary artery aneurysms in Kawasaki disease.[B8] In addition, both spin echo and gradient reversal, cine MR imaging have been used to demonstrate coronary bypass graft patency. Rubinstein and co-workers examined 20 patients with 47 grafts and found an overall sensitivity of 90 percent and a specificity of 72 percent in the detection of graft patency.[R6] In that study, the presence of vascular clips and other graft markers did not interfere with the detection of grafts. Comparable results were obtained by White and associates in 25 patients with 72 grafts.[W2] Using gradient reversal, cine MRI, the sensitivity was 93 percent with a specificity of 86 percent, yielding a predictive accuracy of 89 percent in a group

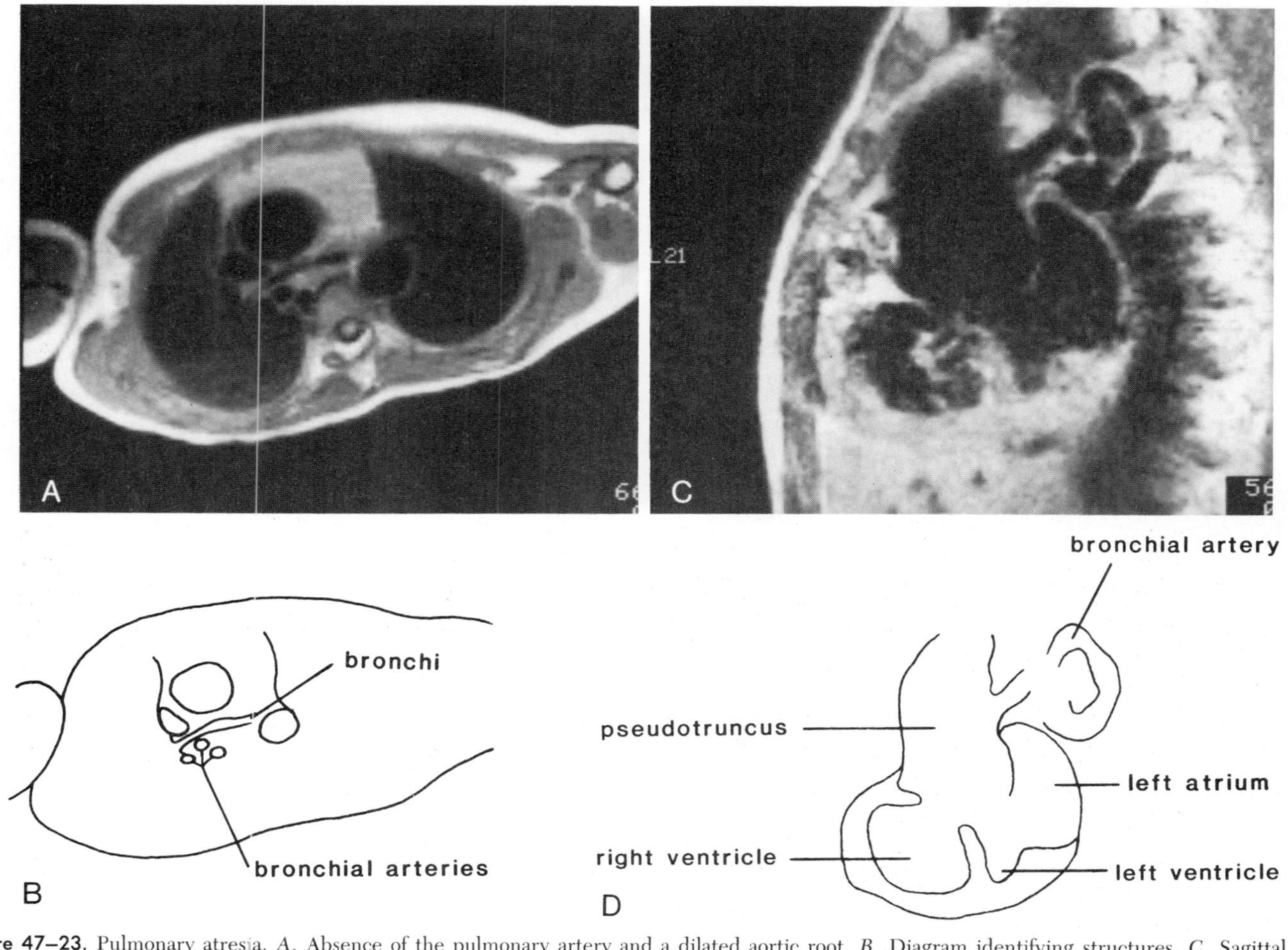

A

C

B

bronchi

bronchial arteries

D

bronchial artery

pseudotruncus

left atrium

right ventricle

left ventricle

Figure 47–23. Pulmonary atresia. *A*, Absence of the pulmonary artery and a dilated aortic root. *B*, Diagram identifying structures. *C*, Sagittal view demonstrating dilated bronchial arteries. *D*, Diagram identifying structures.

of 10 patients with 28 grafts.[W3] These results are comparable with those obtained with standard gated tomography but are slightly worse than those obtained with ultrafast computed tomography (96 percent specificity and 96 percent predictive accuracy[B9]).

TAKAYASU'S ARTERITIS. Takayasu's arteritis is a condition of unknown etiology that predominantly involves the aorta and branches. Although magnetic resonance would be an attractive means of following these patients,[A2] it appears to have limited sensitivity and specificity in the detection of lesions.[M6]

PULMONARY ARTERY

Congenital Abnormalties

PULMONARY ATRESIA. Magnetic resonance imaging has been shown to be helpful in establishing the presence or absence of pulmonary arteries in patients with pulmonary atresia.[F3, H1] Its primary advantage is its ability to scan the entire chest for remnants of the pulmonary arterial tree when it may be impossible to place a catheter into these vessels. Typical images obtained in a patient with pulmonary atresia are shown in Figure 47–23.

PATENT DUCTUS ARTERIOSUS. The ductus arteriosus, when patent, can be readily demonstrated, as is shown in Figure 47–24. It connects the descending aorta to the left main pulmonary artery just past the bifurcation. It can also be visualized in the sagittal view, as shown in Figure 47–25.

MALROTATIONS. A third area in which magnetic resonance has proved useful is in the evaluation of patients with complex congenital heart disease.[F6, G6, R7, S8] The ability to obtain views in multiple orientations without the restrictions of acoustic window allow one to define the exact relationships between the great vessels. In particular, transaxial images can be used to determine the position of the pulmonary valve relative to the aortic valve. Sagittal images around the midsagittal plane are also helpful in establishing the origin and relation of the great vessels.[G6] Moreover, the ability to image the entire heart and other structures in the chest and abdomen aid in establishing atrial situs and the type of atrioventricular and ventriculoarterial connections.[G6] Examples of malrotation are shown in Figure 47–26.

Acquired Abnormalities

PULMONARY EMBOLISM. Pulmonary embolism was first demonstrated by magnetic resonance imaging several years ago.[M9] More recently, there has been considerable interest in this area.[E4, P7, S11] An example of MRI in a patient with a large proximal pulmonary embolism is shown in Figure 47–27. Although magnetic resonance imaging cannot be considered a primary tool for the diagnosis of pulmonary embolism at present, improvements in imaging speed and magnetic resonance angiography techniques may lead to its wider use in this area.

PULMONARY ARTERY ALTERATIONS (BANDING, CONDUITS, AND SHUNTS). Magnetic resonance imaging can be used to gauge the anatomic degree of pulmonary artery banding (Fig. 47–28) and the status of conduits in patients with pulmonary

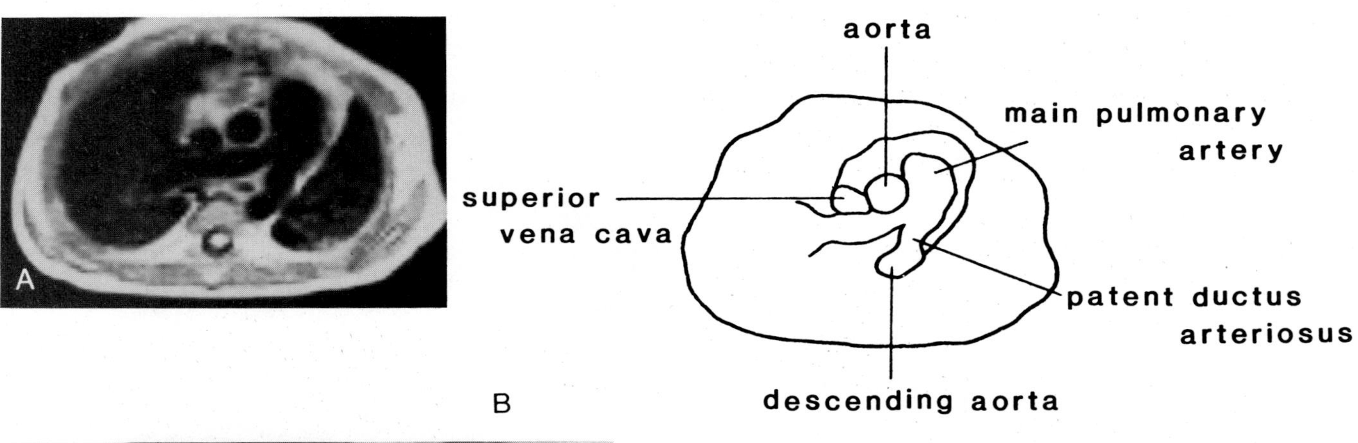

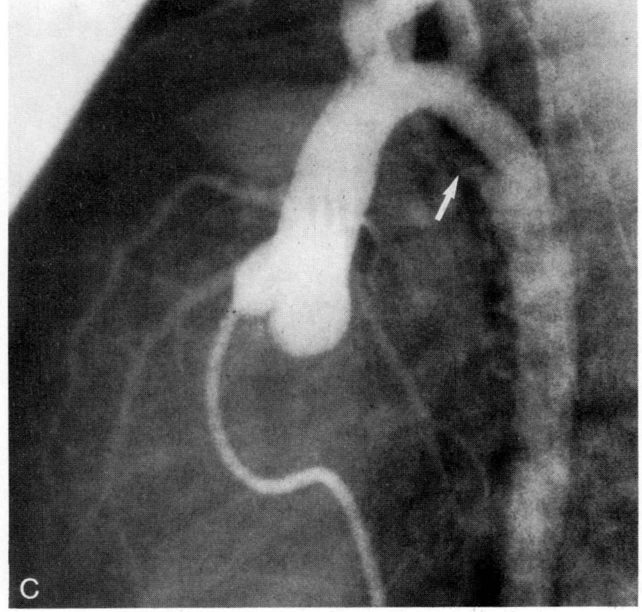

Figure 47–24. Patent ductus arteriosus. *A*, A transaxial magnetic resonance image showing the ductus connecting the left main pulmonary artery and the descending aorta. *B*, Diagram of structures in the magnetic resonance image. *C*, A frame from a cineangiogram in the same patient, demonstrating a patent ductus arteriosus (arrow).

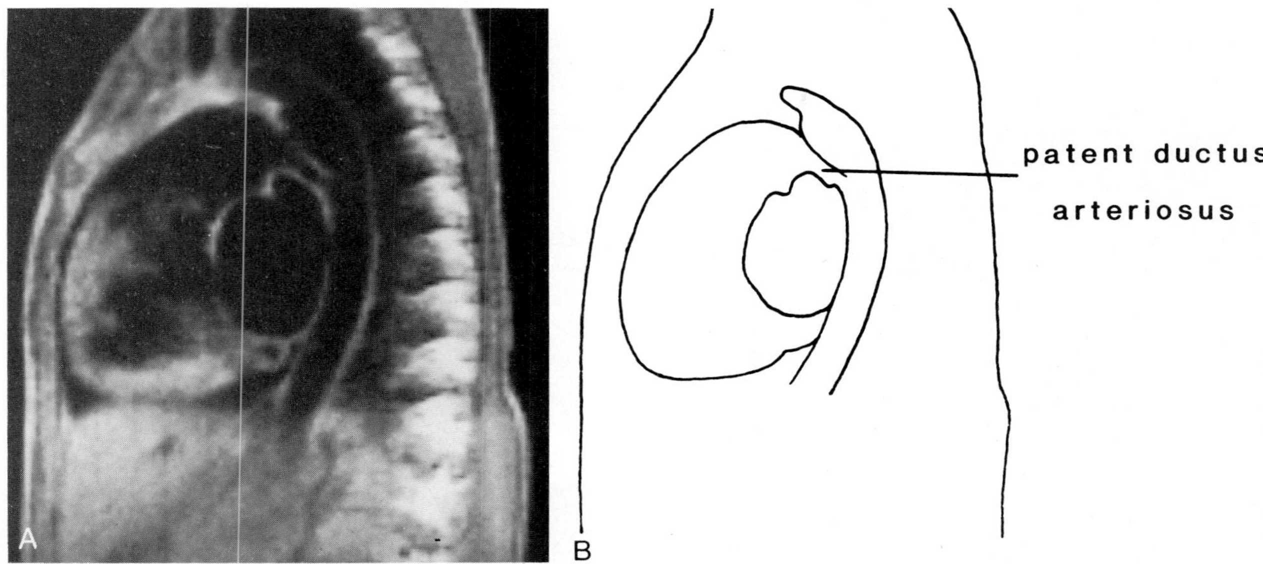

Figure 47–25. Patent ductus arteriosus. *A*, Sagittal image in a patient with a smaller patent ductus. *B*, Diagram indicating the location of the ductus.

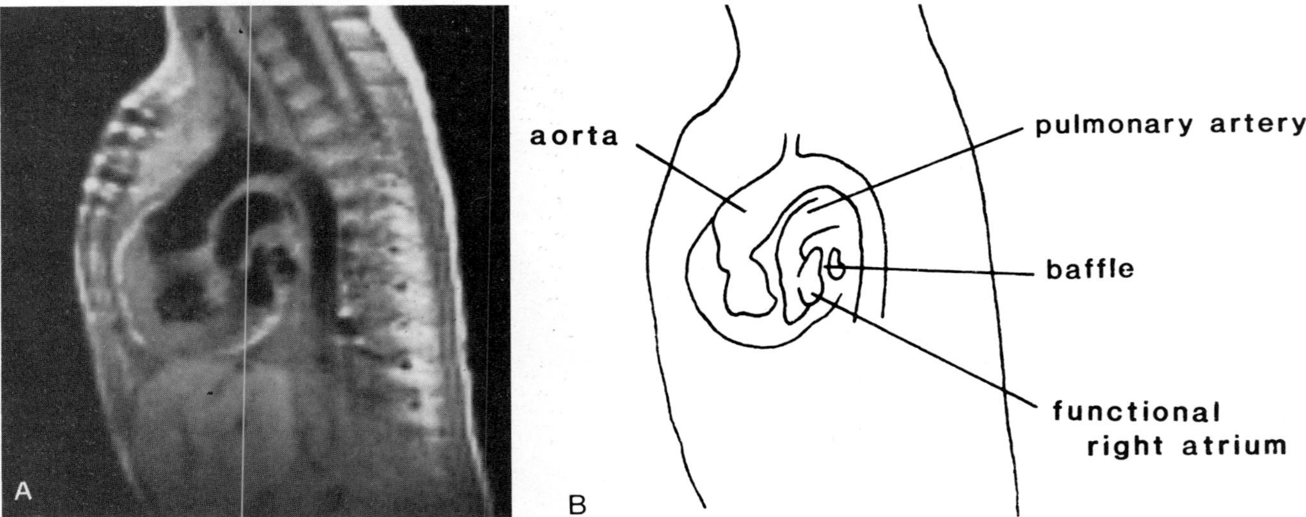

Figure 47–26. Transposition of the great vessels. *A*, Sagittal image in a child with transposition of the great vessels. The aorta is seen to arise anterior to the pulmonary artery. *B*, Diagram identifying major structures.

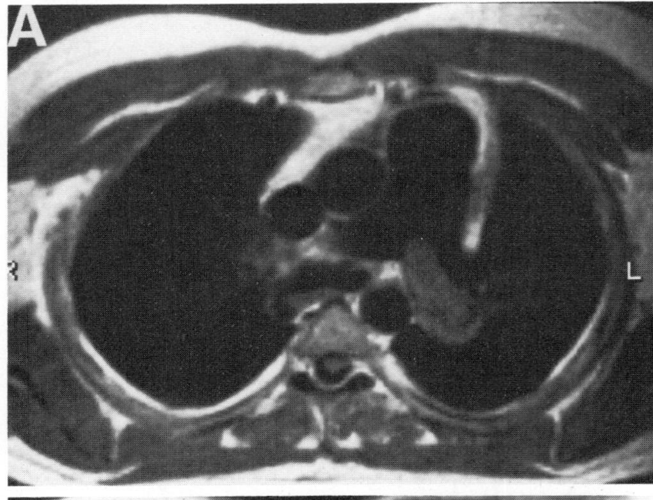

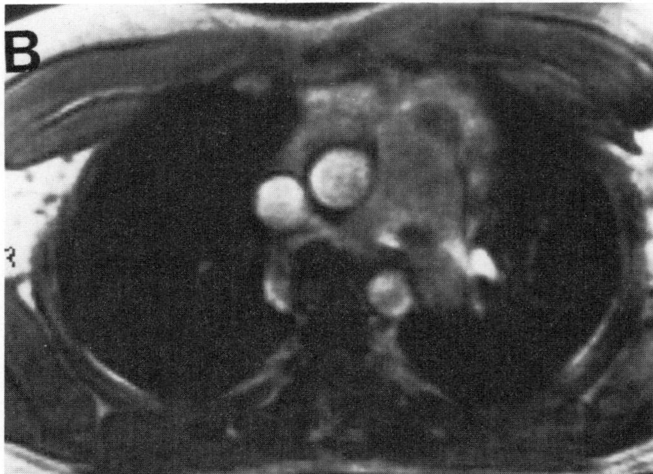

Figure 47–27. Pulmonary embolism. *A*, A standard spin echo image obtained in a patient with a large pulmonary embolism involving the left main pulmonary artery. *B*, A gradient reversal image obtained at the same level.

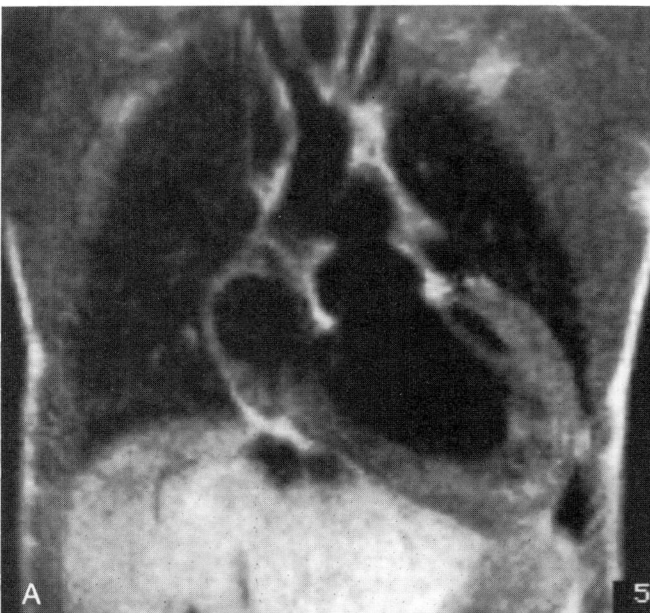

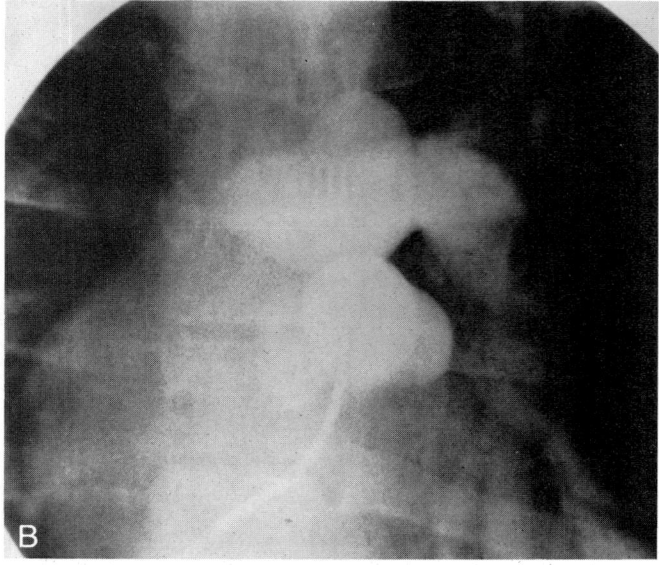

Figure 47–28. Pulmonary artery banding. *A*, A coronal spin echo image demonstrating a narrowing in the proximal main pulmonary artery. *B*, A cineangiogram obtained in the same patient.

atresia (Fig. 47–29).[J2] It may also be useful in evaluation of the size and patency of palliative systemic-to–pulmonary artery shunts, including Blalock-Taussig, Glenn, and Waterston shunts.[F6, J2] An example of a Blalock-Taussig (subclavian-to–right pulmonary artery shunt) is shown in Figure 47–30.

Lastly, it has been suggested that alterations in signal intensity in the pulmonary arteries may be useful in estimating pulmonary vascular resistance.[D6] Given the complex interactions between the direction of blood flow and signal intensity in magnetic resonance, particularly in the setting of pulsatile flow,[K5] it is likely that the validity of such estimates will dependent greatly on the details of the imaging sequences used.

SYSTEMIC VENOUS ABNORMALITIES

DEVELOPMENTAL ANOMALIES. A variety of abnormalities of both systemic and pulmonary venous return can develop during embryogenesis, including complete or partial anomalous pulmonary venous drainage.[B10] Magnetic resonance imaging can readily establish the presence and nature of abnormalities of systemic and pulmonary venous return.[F8, J3] Figure 47–31 shows a relatively common developmental venous abnormality: persistent left superior vena cava draining into the coronary sinus.

SUPERIOR VENA CAVA OBSTRUCTION. Magnetic resonance imaging has been demonstrated to be of use in the

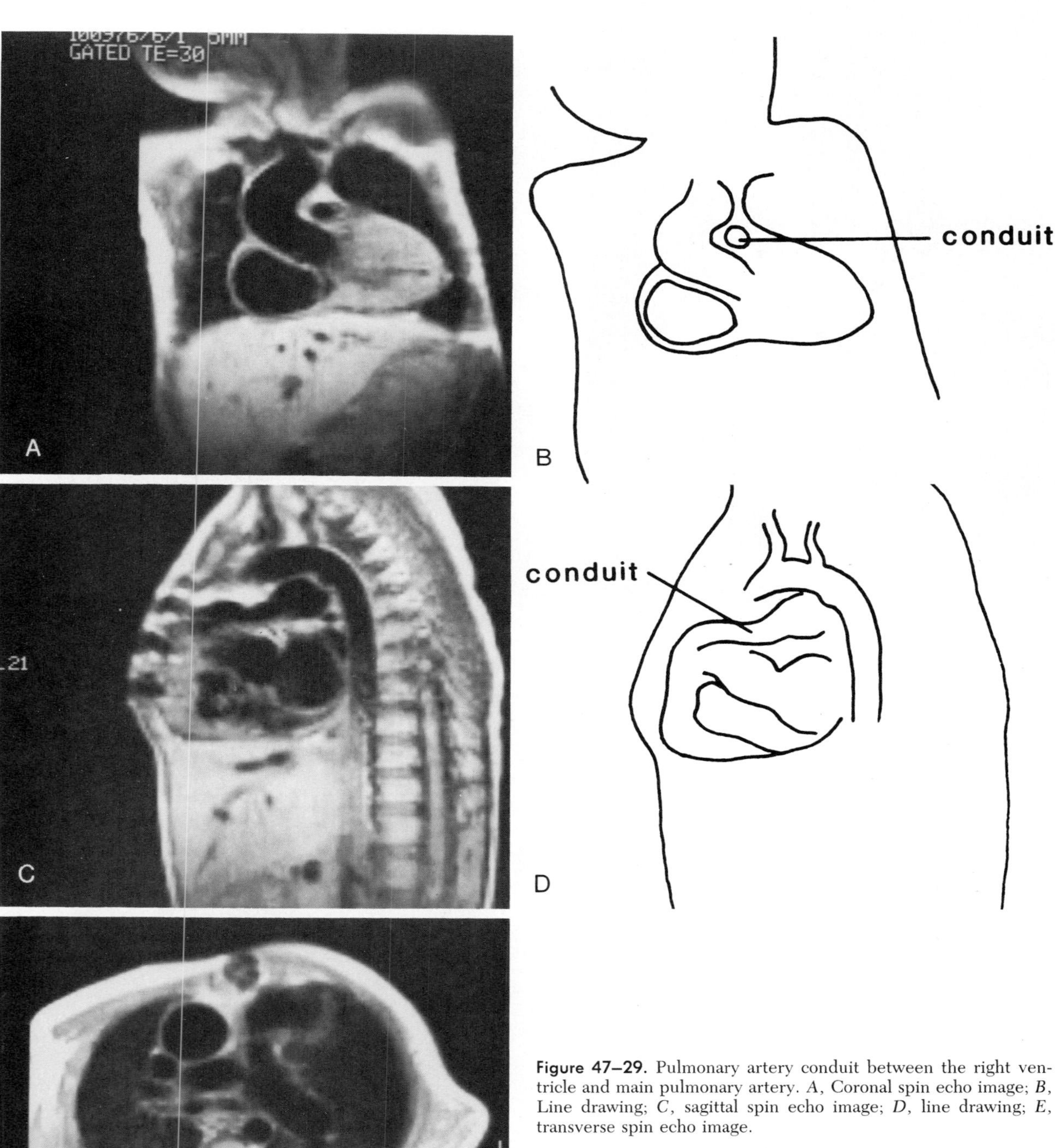

Figure 47–29. Pulmonary artery conduit between the right ventricle and main pulmonary artery. *A*, Coronal spin echo image; *B*, Line drawing; *C*, sagittal spin echo image; *D*, line drawing; *E*, transverse spin echo image.

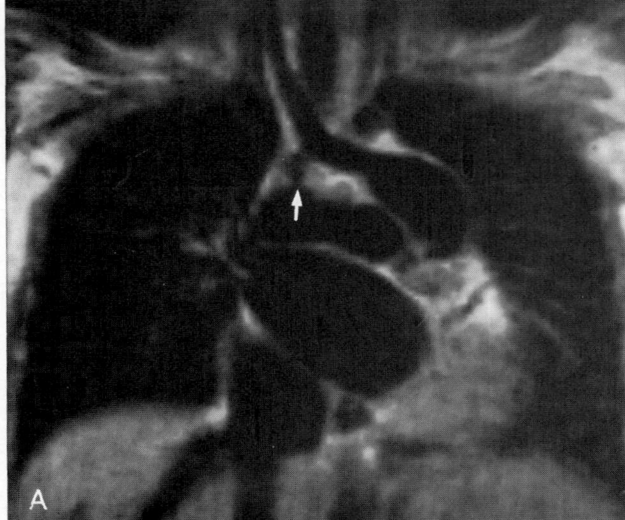

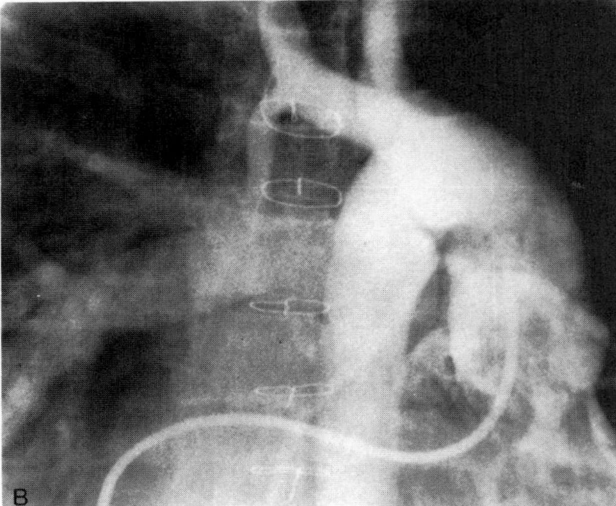

Figure 47–30. Blalock-Taussig shunt. *A*, A coronal image demonstrating a small Blalock-Taussig shunt (arrow) connecting to the right main pulmonary artery. *B*, the corresponding frame from the cineangiogram for comparison.

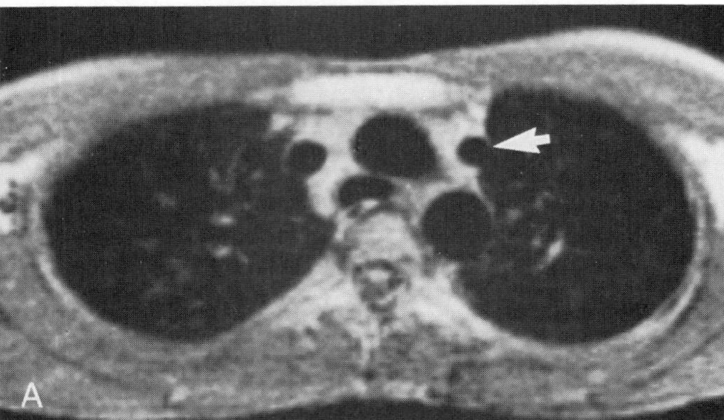

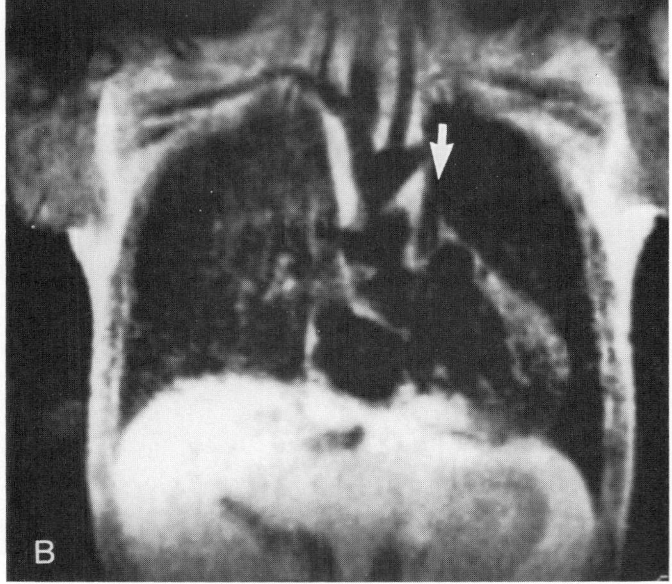

Figure 47–31. Persistent left superior vena cava. In this patient with a single ventricle, there is a persistent left superior vena cava (arrows) to the left of the left atrium on transaxial (*A*) and coronal (*B*) views.

evaluation of superior vena cava syndrome.[W7] An example is shown in Figure 47–32. A primary advantage of magnetic resonance in the evaluation of this problem is the ability to obtain images in multiple orientations. However, care must be exercised in excluding flow effects.[D7]

INFERIOR VENA CAVA OBSTRUCTION. Another area in which magnetic resonance imaging has been used is in the diagnosis of inferior vena cava thrombosis, particularly in the setting of renal cell carcinoma.[P8] A typical study is shown in Figure 47–33. Several studies indicate that magnetic resonance can be an effective tool in determining the extension of renal cell carcinoma into the inferior vena cava. One important concern is that the degree of extension into the right atrium is often not well depicted, even in gated studies, due to the chaotic motion of the tumor/thrombus in the right atrium.[E4]

PULMONARY VENOUS ABNORMALITIES

Pulmonary venous obstruction has also been demonstrated by magnetic resonance imaging.[F7]

NEW DEVELOPMENTS

A number of recent developments have substantial impact on the use of magnetic resonance in the evaluation of the great vessels. In general, these involve enhancements in the sensitivity of imaging to flow, tissue differences, and improvements in speed and display.

Considerable effort is now underway in the area of magnetic resonance angiography.[D8, S12] Most of this effort has involved the evaluation of cerebral[S13] and peripheral circulations,[S12] but many of the techniques can be applied to the great vessels. The details of these approaches are beyond the scope of this presentation; however, these approaches fundamentally take advantage of the same flow effects mentioned earlier. Hence, the same basic principles are potentially applicable to the evaluation of the great vessels.

One method that has been investigated is that of examining the velocity profile in the ascending aorta.[K6, U1, V1] This approach may allow the determination of the actual, complete spatial distribution of velocities in the aorta or other vessel (Fig. 47–34). At this point such information can be obtained noninvasively only by using magnetic resonance imaging. At present these measurements are very time consuming, so their eventual clinical application is not clear.

The second major area of development is in the detection and characterization of atherosclerotic plaque. A number of investigators have examined the potential of magnetic resonance imaging in the detection and characterization of atherosclerotic plaque in the aorta.[H2, K7, W8] It has been suggested that it might be possible to determine the lipid content of plaque using chemical shift imaging techniques.[M10] However, achieving this goal has been complicated by three factors: (1) the lipids in plaque, particularly cholesterol, appear to have very short T2 relaxation times, which complicate imaging;[P9, S14] (2) plaque may have a very heterogeneous structure, including fibroblasts and other cellular elements, lipid deposits, calcification, and hemorrhage, all of which have different MRI characteristics; and (3) the cellular elements in plaque contribute significantly to the MRI signal. However, preliminary results in excised specimens and in animal models have been encouraging.[K8, M11, M12]

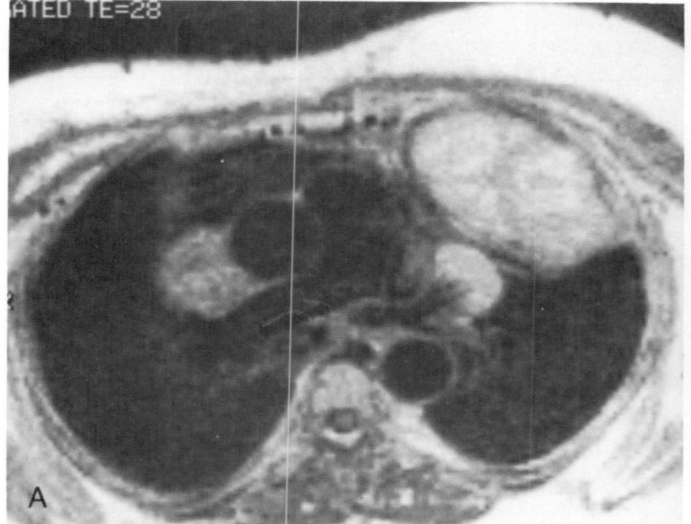

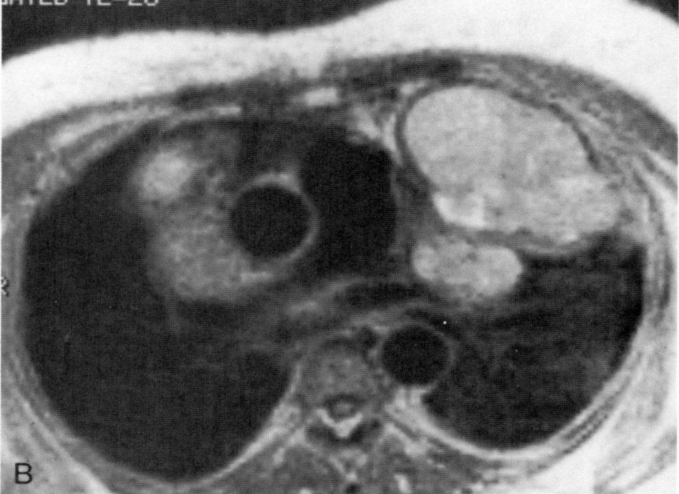

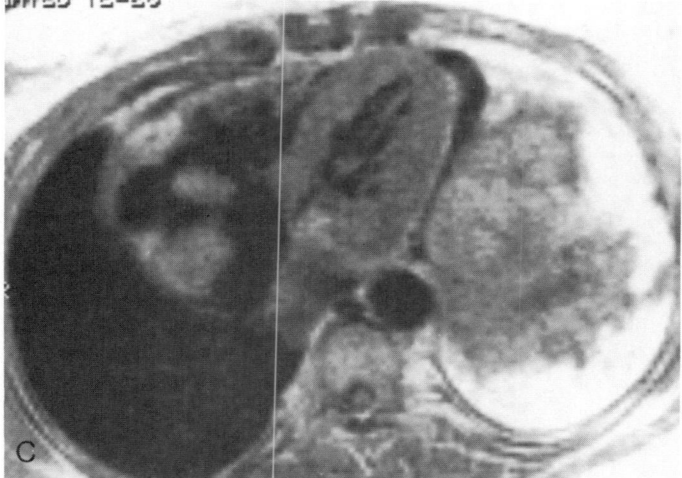

Figure 47–32. Superior vena cava syndrome. *A*, *B*, and *C*, Transaxial images in a patient with malignant thymoma invading the superior vena cava. The tumor is seen to fill the superior vena cava and extend into the right atrium.

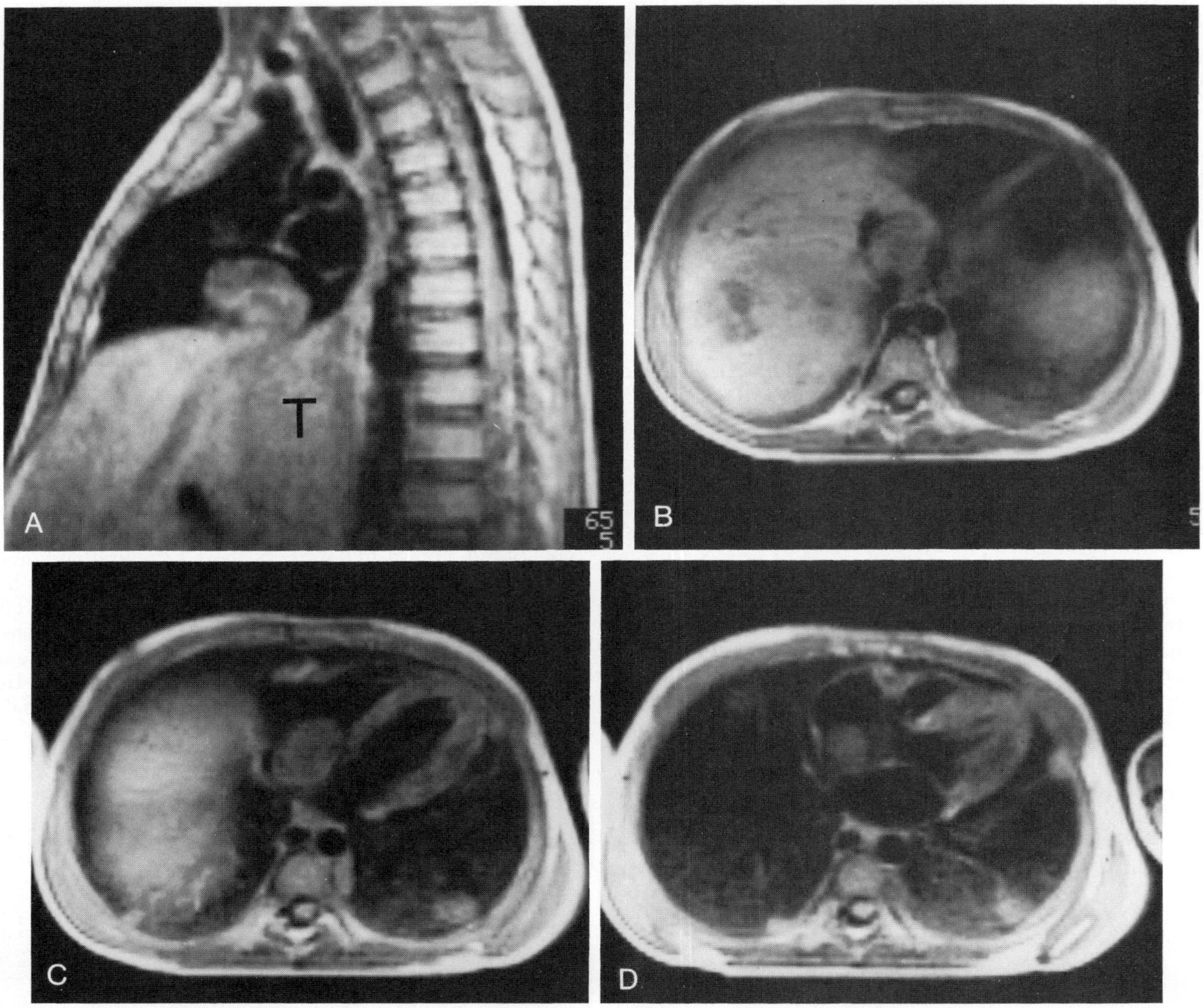

Figure 47–33. Renal cell carcinoma. *A*, Sagittal image demonstrating extension of the tumor/thrombus (T) from the inferior vena into the right atrium. *B*, *C*, and *D* are transaxial slices showing the tumor/thrombus in the inferior vena cava and right atrium.

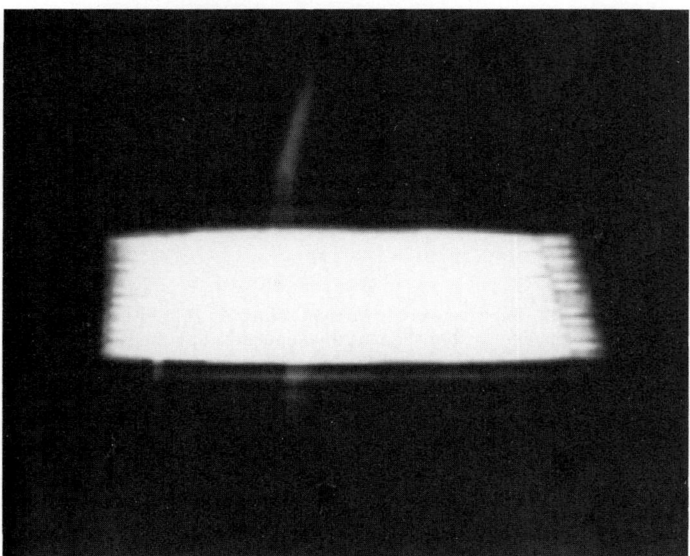

Figure 47–34. Femoral artery velocity profile. Image obtained using a time-of-flight magnetic resonance angiography technique. The parabolic flow profile of laminar flow is apparent.

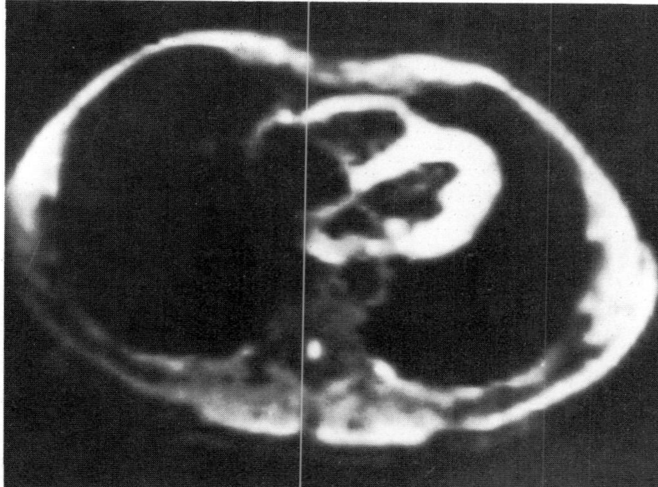

Figure 47–35. Echo planar magnetic resonance imaging. Image of the heart and descending aorta obtained in 30 msec. (Obtained in collaboration with Drs. I. Pykett and R. Rzedzian of Advanced NMR Systems.)

The third area of recent research has been in the development of high-speed imaging techniques, such as echo-planar magnetic resonance imaging.[C5, O2, R8] This approach allows one to obtain images in a fraction of a second, compared with seconds to minutes in the case of conventional magnetic resonance imaging. At present, this method is associated with some loss in spatial resolution (Fig. 47–35). However, this method has significant potential for the evaluation of patients who cannot cooperate for more lengthy examinations and for the evaluation of transient alterations in blood flow.

Finally, improved display approaches are being evaluated.[B9] The tortuous course of many vessels often complicates the interpretation of tomographic images obtained using any current technique. This has made the use of projection techniques like angiography popular (Chapter 44). However, projection techniques are associated with superposition of structures and loss of three-dimensional information. Three-dimensional display techniques may prove useful in dealing with these problems. Although these approaches have been suggested in the past,[C6, V2, V3] they have not gained wide clinical use. With improvements in imaging techniques and speed of display, these methods may find wider application.

CONCLUSION

Magnetic resonance imaging is an effective tool in the evaluation of a variety of abnormalities of the great vessels. With continued improvements in magnetic resonance angiography, tissue characterization, and imaging speed and display, it is anticipated that magnetic resonance will play an ever-increasing role in the evaluation of great vessel disease.

References

A

1. Anagnostopoulos, C. E.: Lethal Diseases of the Ascending Aorta. University Park Press, Baltimore, 1976.
2. Amparo, E. G., Higgins, C. B., Hoddick, W., et al.: Magnetic resonance imaging of aortic disease: Preliminary results. AJR 143:1203, 1984.
3. Amparo, E. G., Higgins, C. B., and Shafton, E. P.: Demonstration of coarctation of the aorta by magnetic resonance imaging. AJR 143:1192, 1984.
4. Akins, E. W., Carmichael, M. J., Hill, J. A., and Mancuso, A. A.: Preoperative evaluation of the thoracic aorta using MRI and angiography. Ann. Thorac. Surg. 44:499, 1987.
5. Amparo, E. G., Higgins, C. B., and Hricak, H.: Aortic dissection: Magnetic resonance imaging. Radiology 155:399, 1985.
6. Auffermann, W., Olofsson, P., Stoney, R., and Higgins, C. B.: MR imaging of complications of aortic surgery. J. Comput. Assist. Tomogr. 11:982, 1987.
7. Aronberg, D. J., Peterson, R. R., Glazer, H. S., and Sagel, S. S.: The superior sinus of the pericardium: CT appearance. Radiology 153:489, 1984.
8. Amparo, E. G., Hoddick, W. K., Hricak, H., et al.: Comparison of magnetic resonance imaging and ultrasonography in the evaluation of abdominal aortic aneurysms. Radiology 154:451, 1985.
9. Aronberg, D. J., Glazer, H. S., Madsen, K., and Sagel, S. S.: Normal thoracic aortic diameters by computed tomography. J. Comput. Assist. Tomogr. 8:247, 1984.

B

1. Bradley, W. G.: Flow phenomena in MR imaging. AJR 150:983, 1988.
2. Bradley, W. G., Waluch, V., and Lai, K. S.: The appearance of rapidly flowing blood on magnetic resonance images. AJR 143:1167, 1984.
3. Boxer, R. A., LaCorte, M. A., Singh, S., et al.: Nuclear magnetic resonance imaging in evaluation and follow-up of children treated for coarctation of the aorta. J. Am. Coll. Cardiol. 7:1095, 1986.
4. Bisset, G. S., Strife, J. L., Kirks, D. R., and Bailey, W. W.: Vascular rings: MR imaging. AJR 149:251, 1987.
5. Boxer, R. A., LaCorte, M. A., Singh, S., et al.: Evaluation of the aorta in the Marfan syndrome by magnetic resonance imaging. Am. Heart J 11:1001, 1986.
6. Boxer, R. A., Fishman, M. C., LaCorte, M. A., et al.: Diagnosis and postoperative evaluation of supravalvular aortic stenosis by magnetic resonance imaging. Am. J. Cardiol. 58:367, 1986.
7. Bogren, H. G., Underwood, S. R., Firmin, D. N., et al.: Magnetic resonance velocity mapping in aortic dissection. Br. J. Radiol. 61:456, 1988.
8. Bisset, G. S., Strife, J. L., and McCloskey, J.: MR imaging of coronary artery aneurysms in a child with Kawasaki disease. AJR 152:805, 1989.
9. Bateman, T. M., Gray, G. R., Whiting, J. S., et al.: Prospective evaluation of ultrafast cardiac computed tomography for determination of coronary bypass graft patency. Circulation 75:1018, 1987.
10. Braunwald, E. (ed.): Heart Disease: A Textbook of Cardiovascular Medicine, (3rd ed.). Vol. 1. W. B. Saunders Company, Philadelphia, 1988, pp. 369, 379.

C

1. Council on Scientific Affairs, Report of the Magnetic Resonance Imaging Panel: Magnetic resonance imaging of the cardiovascular system. JAMA 259:253, 1988.
2. Choyke, P. L., Kressel, H. Y., Reichek, N., et al.: Nongated cardiac magnetic resonance imaging: Preliminary experience at 0.12 T. AJR 143:1143, 1984.
3. Crawford, E. S., and Crawford, J. L.: Diseases of the Aorta. Williams and Wilkins, Baltimore, 1984.
4. Cambria, R. P., Brewster, D. C., Moncure, A. C., et al.: Spontaneous aortic dissection in the presence of coexistent or previously repaired atherosclerotic aortic aneurysm. Ann. Surg. 208:619, 1988.
5. Chapman, B., Turner, R., Ordidge, R. J., et al.: Real-time movie imaging from a single cardiac cycle by NMR. Magn. Reson. Med. 5:246, 1987.
6. Cline, H. E., Lorensen, W. E., Herfkens, R. J., et al.: Vascular morphology by three-dimensional magnetic resonance imaging. Magn. Reson. Imag. 7:45, 1989.

D

1. Dumoulin, C. L.: Flow imaging. *In* Budinger, T. F., and Margulis, A. R. (eds.): Medical Magnetic Resonance: A Primer—1988. Society of Magnetic Resonance in Medicine, San Francisco, 1988.
2. Dinsmore, R. E., Wisner, G. L., Levine, R. A., et al.: Magnetic resonance imaging of the heart: Positioning and gradient angle selection for optimal imaging planes. AJR 143:1135, 1984.
3. Dinsmore, R. E., Wedeen, V. J., Miller, S. W., et al.: MRI of dissection of the aorta: Recognition of the intimal tear and differential flow velocities. AJR 146:1286, 1986.
4. DeBrux, J. L., Grenier, P., Pernes, J. M., and Desbleds, M. T.: Anatomy of the thoracic aorta: Magnetic resonance imaging and interpretation of flow phenomena. Surg. Radiol. Anat. 9:141, 1987.
5. Dinsmore, R. E., Liberthson, R. R., and Wismer, G. L.: Magnetic resonance imaging of thoracic aortic aneurysms: Comparisons with other imaging methods. AJR 146:309, 1986.
6. Didier, D., and Higgins, C. B.: Estimation of pulmonary vascular resistance by MRI in patients with congenital cardiovascular shunt lesions. AJR 146:919, 1986.
7. Dinsmore, R. E., Wedeen, V., Rosen, B., et al.: Phase-offset technique to distinguish slow blood flow and thrombus on MR images. AJR 148:634, 1987.
8. Dumoulin, C. L., and Hart, H. R.: Magnetic resonance angiography. Radiology 161:717, 1986.

E

1. Eagle, K. A., and DeSanctis, R. W.: Diseases of the aorta. *In* Braunwald, E. (ed.): Heart Disease: A Textbook of Cardiovascular Medicine. W. B. Saunders, Philadelphia, 1988, p. 1546.
2. Evans, A. J., Blinder, R. A., Herfkens, R. J., et al.: Effects of turbulence on signal intensity in gradient echo images. Invest. Radiol. 23:512, 1988.
3. Ehman, R. L., McNamara, M. T., Pallack, M., et al.: Magnetic resonance imaging with respiratory gating: Techniques and advantages. AJR 143:1175, 1984.
4. Erdman, W. A., Peshock, R. M., Miller, G., Jayson, H., and Redman, H.: Rate of MR imaging in the patient with an intermediate probability lung scan. Radiology 169:201, 1988.

F

1. Frahm, J., Haase, A., and Matthaei, D.: Rapid NMR imaging of dynamic processes using the FLASH technique. Magn. Reson. Med. 3:321, 1986.
2. Felmlee, J. P., and Ehman, R. L.: Spatial presaturation: A method for suppressing flow artifacts and improving depiction of vascular anatomy in MR imaging. Radiology 164:559, 1987.
3. Fletcher, B. D., and Jacobstein, M. D.: MRI of congenital abnormalities of the great arteries. AJR 146:941, 1986.
4. Fletcher, B. D., and Cohn, R. C.: Tracheal compression and the innominate artery: MR evaluation in infants. Radiology 170:103, 1989.
5. Flak, B., Li, D. K. B., Ho, B. Y. B., et al.: Magnetic resonance imaging of aneurysms of the abdominal aorta. AJR 144:991, 1985.
6. Fletcher, B. D., and Jacobstein, M. D.: Magnetic Resonance Imaging of Congenital Heart Disease. C. V. Mosby, St. Louis, 1988.
7. Farmer, D. W., Moore, E., Amparo, E., et al.: Calcific fibrosing mediastinitis: Demonstration of pulmonary vascular obstruction by magnetic resonance imaging. AJR 143:1189, 1984.
8. Fisher, M. R., Hricak, H., and Higgins, C. B.: Magnetic resonance imaging of developmental venous abnormalities. AJR 145:705, 1985.
9. Faber, T. L., and Stokely, E. M.: Orientation of 3D structure in medical images. IEEE Trans. Pattern Anal. Machine Intell. 10:626, 1988.

G

1. Glover, G. H., and Pelc, N. J.: A rapid-gated cine MRI technique. *In* Kressel, H. Y. (ed.): Magnetic Resonance Annual. Raven Press, New York, 1988, p. 299.
2. Geisinger, M. A., Risius, B., O'Donnell, J. A., et al.: Thoracic aortic dissections: Magnetic resonance imaging. Radiology 155:407, 1985.
3. Goldman, A. P., Kotler, M. N., Scanlon, M. H., et al.: The complementary role of magnetic resonance imaging, Doppler echocardiography, and computed tomography in the diagnosis of dissecting thoracic aneurysms. Am. Heart J. 111:970, 1986.
4. Grenier, P., Pernes, J. M., Desbleds, M. T., and DeBrux, J. L.: Magnetic resonance imaging of aneurysms and chronic dissections of the thoracic aorta. Ann. Vasc. Surg. 1:534, 1987.
5. Gallagher, S., and Dixon, A. K.: Streak artifacts of the thoracic aorta: Pseudodissection. J. Comput. Assist. Tomogr. 8:688, 1984.
6. Guit, G. L., Bluemm, R., Rohmer, J., et al.: Levotransposition of the aorta: Identification of segmental cardiac anatomy using MR imaging. Radiology 161:673, 1986.

H

1. Higgins, C. B., Byrd, B. F., Farmer, D. W., et al.: Magnetic resonance imaging in patients with congenital heart disease. Circulation 70:851, 1984.
2. Herfkens, R. J., Higgins, C. B., Hricak, H. H., et al.: Nuclear magnetic resonance imaging of atherosclerotic disease. Radiology 148:161, 1983.

J

1. Julsrud, P. R., and Ehrman, R. L.: Magnetic resonance imaging of vascular rings. Mayo Clin. Proc. 61:181, 1986.
2. Jacobstein, M. D., Fletcher, B. D., Nelson, A. D., et al.: Magnetic resonance imaging: Evaluation of palliative systemic-pulmonary artery shunts. Circulation 70:650, 1984.
3. Julsrud, P. R., and Ehman, R. L.: The "broken ring" sign in magnetic resonance imaging of partial anomalous pulmonary venous connection to the superior vena cava. Mayo Clin. Proc. 60:874, 1985.

K

1. Kaufman, L., Crooks, L. E., Sheldon, P. E., et al.: The potential impact of nuclear magnetic resonance imaging on cardiovascular diagnosis. Circulation 67:251, 1983.
2. Katz, J., Peshock, R. M., Malloy, C. R., et al.: Even-echo rephasing and constant velocity flow. Magn. Reson. Med. 5:422, 1987.
3. Kersting-Sommerhoff, B. A., Sechtem, U. P., Schiller, N. B., et al.: MR imaging of the thoracic aorta in Marfan patients. J. Comput. Assist. Tomogr. 11:633, 1987.
4. Kersting-Sommerhoff, B. A., Higgins, C. B., White, R. D., et al.: Aortic dissection: Sensitivity and specificity of MR imaging. Radiology 166:651, 1988.
5. Katz, J., Peshock, R. M., McNamee, P. M., et al.: Analysis of spin echo rephasing with pulsatile flow in 2DFT magnetic resonance imaging. Magn. Reson. Med. 4:307, 1987.
6. Klipstein, R. H., Firmin, D. N., Underwood, S. R., et al.: Blood flow patterns in the human aorta studied by magnetic resonance. Br. Heart J. 58:316, 1987.
7. Kaufman, L., Crooks, L. E., Sheldon, P. E., et al.: Evaluation of NMR imaging for detection and quantification of obstructions in vessels. Invest. Radiol. 17:554, 1982.
8. Katz, J., Ma, P., Romig, R., et al.: In-vivo magnetic resonance imaging of atherosclerotic plaque in small arteries. Circulation 76:637, 1987.

L

1. LePage, J. R., Szechenyl, E., and Ross-Dugan, J. W.: Pseudo-coarctation of the aorta. Magn. Reson. Imag. 6:65, 1988.
2. Lin, A. E., Lippe, B. M., Geffner, M. E., et al.: Aortic dilation, dissection, and rupture in patients with Turner syndrome. J. Pediatr. 109:820, 1986.
3. Lotan, C. S., Cranney, G. B., Doyle, M., and Pohost, G. M.: Fat-shift artifact simulating aortic dissection on MR images. AJR 152:385, 1989.
4. Lee, J. K. T., Ling, D., Heiken, J. P., et al.: Magnetic resonance imaging of abdominal aortic aneurysms. AJR 143:1197, 1984.

M

1. Miller, S. W., Brady, T. J., Dinsmore, R. E., et al.: Cardiac magnetic resonance imaging: The Massachusetts General Hospital experience. Radiol. Clin. North Am. 23:745, 1985.
2. Mills, C. M., Brant-Zawadzki, M., Crooks, L. E., et al.: Nuclear magnetic resonance: Principles of blood flow imaging. AJR 142:165, 1984.
3. Mark, A. S., Winkler, M. L., Peltzer, M., et al.: Gated acquisition of MR images of the thorax: Advantages for the study of the hila and mediastinum. Magn. Reson. Imag. 5:57, 1987.
4. Malmgren, N., Laurin, S., and Lundstrom, N. R.: Pulmonary artery sling: Diagnosis by magnetic resonance imaging. Acta Radiol. 29:7, 1988.
5. McMurdo, K. K., Webb, W. R., von Schulthess, G. K., and Gamsu, G.: Magnetic resonance imaging of the superior pericardial recesses. AJR 145:985, 1985.
6. Miller, D. L., Reining, J. W., and Volkman, D. J.: Vascular imaging with MRI: Inadequacy in Takayasu's arteritis compared with angiography. AJR 146:949, 1986.
7. Maas, W. R. A.: A new approach to MR system design. Medicamundi 33:148, 1988.
8. Moore, E. H., Webb, W. R., Verrier, E. D., et al.: MRI of chronic posttraumatic false aneurysms of the thoracic aorta. AJR 143:1195, 1984.
9. Moore, E. H., Gamsu, G., Webb, W. R., and Stulbarg, M. S.: Pulmonary embolus: Detection and follow-up using magnetic resonance. Radiology 253:471, 1984.
10. Majors, A. W., Czerski, L., Takeyama, Y., et al.: MRI and MRS studies of lipid deposits in hyperlipidemic animal model. (Abstract.) Society of Magnetic Resonance in Medicine, San Francisco, 1988.
11. Merickel, M. B., Carman, C. S., Brookeman, J. R., et al.: Identification and 3-D quantification of atherosclerosis using magnetic resonance imaging. Comput. Biol. Med. 18:89, 1988.
12. Moore, D. M., Peshock, R. M., Clubb, F. J., and Willerson, J. T.: The detection and quantitation in vivo of atherosclerosis by magnetic resonance imaging. Circulation 80:II-589, 1989.
13. Mullins, C. E., and Mayer, D. C.: Congenital Heart Disease: A Diagrammatic Atlas. Alan R. Liss, Inc., New York, 1988, p. 27.

O

1. Olofsson, P. A., Aufferman, W., Higgins, C. B., et al.: Diagnosis of prosthetic aortic graft infection by magnetic resonance imaging. J. Vasc. Surg. 8:99, 1988.
2. Ordidge, R. J., Howseman, A., Coxon, R., et al.: Snapshot imaging at 0.5T using echo-planar techniques. Magn. Reson. Med. 10:227, 1989.

P

1. Pattany, P. M., Phillips, J. J., Chiu, L. C., et al.: Motion artifact suppression technique (MAST) for MR imaging. J. Comput. Assist. Tomogr. 11:369, 1987.
2. Pflugfelder, P. W., Landzberg, J. S., Cassidy, M. M., et al.: Comparison of cine MR imaging with Doppler echocardiography for the evaluation of aortic regurgitation. AJR 152:729, 1989.
3. Pucillo, A. L., Schechter, A. G., Kay, R. H., and Herman, M. V.: Magnetic resonance imaging of vascular conduits in coarctation of the aorta. Am. Heart J. 117:482, 1989.
4. Pettigrew, R. I., and Dannels, W.: Use of standard gradients with compound oblique angulation for optimal quantitative MR flow imaging in oblique vessels. AJR 148:405, 1987.
5. Peshock, R. M., and Rollins, N.: Recurrent respiratory difficulty, stridor, and dysphagia in a 15 month old. Curr. Concepts Magn. Reson. Imag. 2:22, 1988.
6. Paulin, S., von Schulthess, G. K., Fossel, E., and Krayenbuehl, H. P.: MR imaging of the aortic root and proximal coronary arteries. AJR 148:665, 1987.
7. Pope, C. F., Sostman, D., Carbo, P., et al.: The detection of pulmonary emboli by magnetic resonance imaging. Evaluation of imaging parameters. Invest. Radiol. 22:937, 1987.
8. Patel, S. K., Stack, C. M., and Turner, D. A.: Magnetic resonance imaging in staging of renal cell carcinoma. Radiographics 7:703, 1987.
9. Pearlman, J. D., Zajicek, J., Merickel, M. B., et al.: High-resolution ^{1}H NMR spectral signature from human atheroma. Magn. Reson. Med. 7:262, 1988.

Q

1. Quencer, R. M., Hinks, R. S., Pattany, P. H., et al.: Improved MR imaging of the brain using compensating gradients to suppress motion-induced artifacts. AJR 151:163, 1988.

R

1. Reed, J. D., Jr., and Soulen, R. L.: Cardiovascular MRI: Current role in patient management. Radiol. Clin. North Am. 26:589, 1988.
2. Reeves, R. C., Evanochko, W. T., and Pohost, G. M.: Potential approaches to evaluating the cardiovascular system using NMR. Prog. Cardiovasc. Dis. 29:53, 1986.

3. Randall, P. A., Kohman, L. J., Scalzette, E. M., et al.: Magnetic resonance imaging of prosthetic cardiac valves in vitro and in vivo. Am. J. Cardiol. 62:973, 1988.
4. Rumancik, W. M., Naidich, D. P., Chandra, R., et al.: Cardiovascular disease: Evaluation with MR phase imaging. Radiology 166:63, 1988.
5. Rehr, R. B., Filipchuk, N. G., Malloy, C. R., and Peshock, R. M.: Magnetic resonance imaging of aortic pathology. Am. J. Cardiol. 55:1243, 1985.
6. Rubinstein, R. I., Askenase, A. D., Thickman, D., et al.: Magnetic resonance imaging to evaluate patency of aortocoronary bypass grafts. Circulation 76:786, 1987.
7. Rees, S., Somerville, J., Warnes, C., et al.: Comparison of magnetic resonance imaging with echocardiography and radionuclide angiography in assessing cardiac function and anatomy following Mustard's operation for transposition of the great arteries. Am. J. Cardiol. 61:1316, 1988.
8. Rzedzian, R. R., and Pykett, I. L.: Instant images of the human heart using a new, whole body MR imaging system. AJR 149:245, 1987.
9. Robb, R. A., Ritman, E. L., and Harris, L. D.: Digital image processing in x-ray computed tomography: High-speed volume imaging with the DSR. *In* Collins, S. M., and Skorton, D. J. (eds.): Cardiac Imaging and Image Processing. McGraw-Hill Book Company, New York 1986, p. 361.

S

1. Schulthess, G. K., von, and Higgins, C. B.: Blood flow imaging with MR: Spin-phase phenomena. Radiology 157:687, 1985.
2. Singer, J. R.: NMR diffusion and flow measurements and an introduction to spin phase graphing. J. Phys. E. Sci. Instrum. 11:281, 1978.
3. Sayre, J., and Wright, A.: Short gradient cine imaging of the heart. (Abstract.) Society of Magnetic Resonance in Medicine, San Francisco, 1988, p. 770.
4. Soulen, R. L., Budinger, T. F., and Higgins, C. B.: Magnetic resonance imaging of prosthetic heart valves. Radiology 154:705, 1985.
5. Soulen, R. L., and Donner, R. M.: Advances in noninvasive evaluation of congenital anomalies of the thoracic aorta. Radiol. Clin. North Am. 23:727, 1985.
6. Simpson, I. A., Chung, K. J., Glass, R. F., et al.: Cine magnetic resonance imaging for evaluation of anatomy and flow relations in infants and children with coarctation of the aorta. Circulation 78:142, 1988.
7. Steinberg, I.: Anomalies (pseudocoarctation) of the arch of the aorta—report of 8 new and review of 8 previously published cases. AJR 88:73, 1962.
8. Swischuk, L. E., and Sapire, D. W.: Basic Imaging in Congenital Heart Disease. Williams and Wilkins, Baltimore, 1986, p. 258.
9. Schaefer, S., Peshock, R. M., Malloy, C. R., et al.: Nuclear magnetic resonance imaging in Marfan's syndrome. J. Am. Coll. Cardiol. 9:70, 1987.
10. St. Amour, T. E., Gutierrez, F. R., Levitt, R. G., and McKnight, R. C.: CT diagnosis of Type A aortic dissections not demonstrated by aortography. J. Comput. Assist. Tomogr. 12:963, 1988.
11. Szucs, R. A., Rehr, R. B., and Tatum, J. L.: Pulmonary artery thrombus detection by magnetic resonance imaging. Chest 95:232, 1989.
12. Society of Magnetic Resonance in Medicine: Syllabus. Berkeley, Cal., Society of Magnetic Resonance in Medicine, 1989.
13. Singer, J. R., and Crooks, L. E.: Nuclear magnetic resonance blood flow measurements in the human brain. Science 221:654, 1983.
14. Soila, K., Nummi, P., Ekfors, T., et al.: Proton relaxation times in arterial wall and atheromatous lesion in man. Invest. Radiol. 20:411, 1986.

T

1. Thorsen, M. K., Sandretto, M. A., Lawson, T. L., et al.: Dissecting aortic aneurysms: Accuracy of computed tomographic diagnosis. Radiology 148:773, 1983.

U

1. Underwood, S. R., Firman, D. N., Klipstein, R. H., et al.: Magnetic resonance velocity mapping: Clinical application of a new technique. Br. Heart J. 57:404, 1987.

V

1. Valk, P. E., Hale, J. D., Crooks, L. E., et al.: MRI of blood flow: Correlation of image appearance with spin-echo phase shift and image intensity. AJR 146:931, 1986.
2. Valk, P. E., Hale, J. D., Crooks, L. E., et al.: MR imaging of aortoiliac atherosclerosis with 3D image reconstruction. J. Comput. Assist. Tomogr. 10:439, 1986.
3. Valk, P. E., Hale, J. D., Kaufman, L., et al.: MR imaging of the aorta with three-dimensional vessel reconstruction: Validation by angiography. Radiology 157:721, 1985.

W

1. Wendt, R. E., III, Murphy, P. H., Ford, J. J., et al.: Phase alterations of spin echoes by motion along magnetic field gradients. Magn. Reson. Med. 2:527, 1985.
2. White, R. D., Caputo, G. R., Mark, A. S., et al.: Coronary artery bypass graft patency: Noninvasive evaluation with MR imaging. Radiology 164:681, 1987.
3. White, R. D., Pflugfelder, P. W., Lipton, M. J., and Higgins, C. B.: Coronary artery bypass grafts: Evaluation of patency with cine MR imaging. AJR 150:1271, 1988.
4. White, R. D., Ullyot, D. J., and Higgins, C. B.: MR imaging of the aorta after surgery for aortic dissection. AJR 150:87, 1988.
5. Winkler, M., Kaufman, L., Hale, J., et al.: Low field (0.064T) MRI of the spine. (Abstract.) Society of Magnetic Resonance in Medicine, San Francisco, 1988.
6. Winkler, M. L., and Higgins, C. B.: Magnetic resonance imaging of perivalvular infectious pseudoaneurysms. AJR 147:253, 1986.
7. Weinreb, J. C., Mootz, A., and Cohen, J. M.: MRI evaluation of mediastinal and thoracic inlet venous obstruction. AJR 146:679, 1986.
8. Wesbey, G. E., Higgins, C. B., Hale, J. D., and Valk, P. E.: Magnetic resonance application in atherosclerotic vascular disease. Cardiovasc. Intervent. Radiol. 2:342, 1986.

Chapter 48

Assessment of Congenital Heart Disease by Nuclear Magnetic Resonance Imaging

■ *WILBUR L. SMITH, JR., M.D.* ■ *WILLIAM STANFORD, M.D.*
■ *DAVID J. SKORTON, M.D.* ■ *GERALD L. WOLF, M.D., Ph.D.*

CLASSIFICATION OF CONGENITAL HEART DISEASE 887
TYPES OF OPERATIVE PROCEDURES ENCOUNTERED 887
Corrective Procedures 887
Palliative Procedures 887
ACYANOTIC CONGENITAL HEART DISEASE 887
Semilunar Valve Disease and Ventricular Outflow Anomalies 887
Atrioventricular Valve Disease 887
Shunt Lesions 888
CYANOTIC CONGENITAL HEART DISEASE 888
Pulmonary Oligemic States 888
Eisenmenger's Physiology 892
Admixture Lesions 892
ANOMALIES OF THE GREAT VESSELS 892
General Considerations 892
Aortic Disease 893
Vascular Rings 893
Truncus Arteriosus 894
Extracardiac Shunts 894
Pulmonary Artery Anomalies 894
Collateral Circulation and Surgical Shunts 894
Venous Anomalies 894
SUMMARY 894

The population of patients with congenital heart disease is steadily increasing. Thus, these patients are becoming an increasingly important part of cardiovascular practice, not only for pediatric cardiologists but also for adult cardiologists and cardiovascular surgeons.[P1, R1, S1] The increase in numbers of patients with congenital heart disease is due to a variety of factors including (1) dramatic advances in palliative and corrective cardiac surgical procedures; (2) the development of catheter interventions for a variety of congenital anomalies; (3) improved medical management of the ill neonate with congenital heart disease; and (4) the fact that more women with congenital heart disease are reaching childbearing age sufficiently healthy to bear children themselves. Since the incidence of congenital heart disease is as much as 10-fold higher in the offspring of mothers with congenital heart disease, compared with the general population,[W1] this will also eventually increase the numbers of patients with congenital heart disease who present for care.

The definitive evaluation of a patient with congenital heart disease requires delineation of the anatomy of the heart and great vessels, the function of the chambers and valves, the identification of abnormal communications between the chambers or great vessels, and the hemodynamic assessment of the effects of these disorders on pressure and flow throughout the cardiovascular system. With the advent of high-quality two-dimensional echocardiography and Doppler methods, accurate noninvasive assessment of congenital heart disease in the fetus, neonate, child, adolescent, and adult has become the accepted standard of practice (see Chapter 24). Catheterization and angiography are seldom required for initial diagnosis; this is increasingly becoming the domain of echocardiographic imaging.

The role of other high-resolution tomographic techniques, including magnetic resonance imaging (MRI), must be assessed against this background of the success of echocardiography in the noninvasive assessment of congenital heart disease. Although echocardiography supplies excellent anatomic information in most patients, MRI has several potential advantages as an adjunct or complementary imaging technique.[C1, J1, L1, S2] First, the field of view of the MRI scan is generally wider than that of the echocardiogram, and this wider field of view may be useful in assessing structures adjacent to the heart. In fact, the entire thorax can be imaged in sequential, parallel high-resolution tomograms utilizing MRI techniques. Second, the anatomic information obtained during an MRI examination is inherently three-dimensional. Using data from several tomographic views, realistic reconstructions of complex anatomy are possible.[L2, V1] Further, high-resolution images of the heart in planes different from those permitted by echocardiography can be obtained with MRI. This may be especially useful in the postoperative evaluation of patients whose anatomy may be particularly complex.[C1, L1] Finally, the breadth of potential information available in an MRI examination is much greater than that of many other imaging techniques. Thus, MRI techniques have the potential to delineate not only cardiac anatomy and flow dynamics but tissue characteristics and some details of cardiac biochemistry as well. These attributes have produced an increasing interest in the use of MRI in congenital heart disease.[B1, D1, H1]

Relative disadvantages of MRI in congenital heart disease should also be noted. These include the need for sedation in young children, the requirement for relatively long scan times, the frequent presence of dysrhythmias that may interfere with cardiac gating, and artifacts from prosthetic devices placed at surgery. The long scan times of current MRI systems may eventually be obviated by recently developed rapid scan acquisition methods.[C2]

In this chapter, we briefly review some of the uses of magnetic resonance imaging in patients with congenital heart disease, concentrating on those defects in which MRI appears to have particular clinical utility.

CLASSIFICATION OF CONGENITAL HEART DISEASE

Although many excellent comprehensive pathoanatomic and functional classifications of congenital heart disease exist, we have chosen a simplified approach to classifying congenital heart disease. We have divided the disorders into acyanotic defects (including disorders of semilunar valves and ventricular outflow, atrioventricular valves, and shunt lesions); cyanotic defects (including those characterized by decreased pulmonary blood flow, those characterized by increased pulmonary vascular resistance, and those characterized by admixture lesions); and anomalies of the great vessels (including disorders of the aorta and pulmonary arteries as well as anomalies of the systemic and pulmonary veins).

TYPES OF OPERATIVE PROCEDURES ENCOUNTERED

Recent strides in the surgical treatment of congenital heart disease have presented clinicians with a bewildering variety of surgical procedures that must be understood to delineate the complex anatomy of the postoperative patient who presents for evaluation in the imaging laboratory. There are two main categories of operative procedures: corrective and palliative.

Corrective Procedures

An increasing number of cardiac surgical procedures are oriented toward complete correction of the abnormal circulation. In some cases, complete or nearly complete anatomic correction is accomplished. Examples of procedures aimed at anatomic correction include closure of atrial septal defects, ventricular septal defects, or patent ductus arteriosus. In assessing the outcome of these procedures, MRI shares with echocardiography the ability to delineate chamber size and shape in response to the alteration in load produced by the operative procedure. Assessment of the details of valvular anatomy are, at present, inferior to those accomplished using ultrasound techniques. However, the strengths of MRI appear to be in the assessment of the presence and extent of valvular regurgitation and of the presence of septal defects and their successful or unsuccessful correction by surgical approaches.

A particularly difficult type of operative procedure to assess in a noninvasive fashion includes those operations in which extra- or intracardiac conduits, tunnels, or baffles are created for redirection of blood flow.[D2, C1] These procedures attempt to make a physiologic correction; the anatomy remains abnormal and frequently is more complex owing to the addition of prosthetic material. Examples are the Fontan procedure (connecting the right atrium to pulmonary artery in patients with tricuspid atresia and other disorders), the Rastelli procedure (redirection of blood flow at the ventricular and great artery levels via conduits in patients with the combination of complete transposition of the great arteries, ventricular septal defect, and pulmonic stenosis), and the Mustard or Senning atrial baffle procedure (redirecting venous inflow within the atria in patients with complete transposition of the great arteries). These and other conduit or baffle procedures require careful serial follow-up because of the eventual development of conduit obstruction or infection in some patients. Assessment of conduits may be difficult using ultrasound. However, MRI may be used in the assessment of these cases, which is another example of the advantages of MRI in the evaluation of postoperative congenital heart defects.

Palliative Procedures

A broad variety of palliative procedures have been developed toward improving the state of the circulation, with or without the future expectation of complete correction[S1] Examples of palliative procedures are the several types of systemic to pulmonary artery shunts used in patients with tetralogy of Fallot and other anomalies characterized by insufficient pulmonary blood flow. Thus, the Blalock-Taussig (subclavian artery to pulmonary artery), Waterston and Potts (aorta to pulmonary artery) shunts and Glenn (superior vena cava to pulmonary artery) anastomosis are procedures directed at increasing pulmonary blood flow. Magnetic resonance imaging can play an important role in the postoperative assessment of patients who have undergone these procedures.

ACYANOTIC CONGENITAL HEART DISEASE

The most common congenital heart diseases are acyanotic lesions, including disorders of the semilunar and atrioventricular valves, and abnormal communications producing left-to-right shunts at atrial, ventricular, or great artery level.

Semilunar Valve Disease and Ventricular Outflow Anomalies

MRI methods using spin-echo techniques are not optimal for direct visualization of anatomic abnormalities of the aortic or pulmonic valves. The thin structure of the valve leaflets, along with the rapid mobility of the valves, preclude reliable visualization using standard spin-echo techniques. In a study of the sensitivity and specificity of spin-echo MRI in a variety of congenital heart defects (with analyses performed using receiver-operating characteristic curve analysis), Kersting-Sommerhoff and colleagues[K1] noted that the poorest sensitivity was in the detection of lesions of the aortic valve (52 percent sensitivity at the 90 percent specificity level).

On the other hand, cine MRI methods using gradient-refocused echoes reliably visualize blood flow disturbances associated with abnormalities of the semilunar valves. Thus, turbulent flow through a stenotic aortic or pulmonic valve, as well as flow disturbances associated with valvular regurgitation, are quite easily seen using cine MRI methods.[S2] Aortic regurgitation may be well visualized using axial scans or "four-chamber" oblique image orientations in which the image plane is perpendicular to the plane of the atrial and ventricular septa (see Chapter 53, Fig. 53–11 and 53–12). Pulmonic regurgitation is often better appreciated using sagittal, coronal or oblique image orientations.

Contrary to the difficulties encountered in visualizing the semilunar valves themselves, abnormalities of the ventricular outflow tracts are superbly shown using both spin-echo and cine MRI methods. In the above-mentioned study by Kersting-Sommerhoff and colleagues, the sensitivity for detection of right ventricular outflow obstructions was 95 percent at a 90 percent specificity.[K1] Other investigators have also shown the ability of MRI to define ventricular outflow tract abnormalities.[B1, C1]

Atrioventricular Valve Disease

As was the case with semilunar valve lesions, anatomic disorders of the atrioventricular valves may be difficult to visualize directly using spin-echo MRI methods.[C1] Kersting-Sommerhoff and colleagues noted sensitivities of 62 percent for mitral valve disease and 76 percent for tricuspid valve disease at a specificity of 90 percent.[K1] However, cine MRI methods permit the accurate evaluation of flow disturbances through the atrioventricular valves. For example, the presence of mitral or tricuspid regurgitation can be established by visualizing low-intensity turbulent retrograde flow "jets" on cine MRI images. These are best seen in axial or four-chamber orientations (see Chapter 49, Fig. 49–5). Cine MRI methods may also be used to quantitate the severity of atrioventricular valve regurgitation. In a recent study, Glogar and coworkers evaluated the ability of cine MRI to assess the degree of mitral regurgitation in a cohort of patients encompassing a variety of etiologies of mitral regurgitation.[G2] These authors found that MRI data correlated well with semiquantitative Doppler ultrasound and angiographic grades as well as with angiographic regurgitant fraction.

Shunt Lesions

Magnetic resonance imaging can be used in two ways to evaluate communications between the right and left sides of the heart at the atrial, ventricular, or great artery level. First, spin-echo imaging methods may be employed to directly identify atrial or ventricular septal defects (Figs. 48–1 and 48–2). In their receiver-operating characteristic curve study, Kersting-Sommerhoff and colleagues found that, at 90 percent specificity, spin-echo MRI exhibited sensitivities of 91 percent for atrial septal defects and 100 percent for ventricular septal defects.[K1] Other authors have also noted excellent sensitivity and specificity of MRI spin-echo imaging for directly imaging septal defects. Dinsmore and associates[D3] noted no false negative examinations and only 9 percent false positive examinations in studies of six patients with atrial septal defects and 33 normal subjects.

A second method of identifying septal defects is by visualizing the shunt as a jet of low intensity flow signal on cine MRI images (Figs. 48–3 and 48–4). Sechtem and coworkers[S3] used cine MRI methods to visualize shunt flow and to measure the cross-sectional area of a defect in patients with ventricular septal defects.

In addition to identifying the presence, location, and anatomic size of septal defects, the physiologic significance of the shunt may also be determined by using MRI. Calculation of pulmonary-to-systemic shunt ratios has been accomplished by comparison of stroke volumes of the right and left ventricles[S3] In addition, attempts have been made to calculate shunt flow based on phase analyses of gradient-refocused echo images to measure volume flow in the pulmonary artery and aorta.[N1]

In summary, magnetic resonance imaging has been shown to be useful in the evaluation of acyanotic congenital heart defects, both by direct imaging of structural anomalies as well as by functional imaging of the shunt using cine MRI gradient-refocused echo methods.

CYANOTIC CONGENITAL HEART DISEASE

Cyanotic congenital heart disease may be divided into three broad categories, depending on the mechanism causing cyanosis: obligate right-to-left shunts (pulmonary oligemic states), pulmonary arterial vascular disease (elevated pulmonary vascular resistance or Eisenmenger's physiology), and admixture lesions (pulmonary blood flow variably affected). The role of MRI in the assessment of cyanotic disease principally involves delineation of ventricular outflow tract anatomy, documentation of pulmonary arterial anatomy, depiction of pulmonary blood supply, and definition of atrioventricular valve anatomy. For convenience, we shall consider the cyanotic lesions according to the above classification.

Pulmonary Oligemic States

The most common of the pulmonary oligemic states is tetralogy of Fallot and its variants. The classical four components of tetralogy include a perimembranous ventricular septal defect, positioning of the aorta so that it "overrides" the interventricular septum, infundibular and/or valvular pulmonic stenosis, and right ventricular hypertrophy. A defect with physiologic effects similar to those of tetralogy is the so-called pseudotruncus, the combination of pulmonary atresia and a ventricular septal defect. Patients with pseudotruncus present earlier in life than those with classical tetralogy and often require urgent palliative surgery to re-establish pulmonary blood supply.

In all forms of tetralogy of Fallot, it is vital to image the pulmonary arteries to establish their size and patency, since surgical palliation and later repair depend on re-establishing normal pulmonary arterial supply. In our hands and those of others, T1-weighted spin-echo images in the axial plane are often the most useful in defining the origin of the right and left pulmonary arteries.[C3] When compared with angiography, Canter and coworkers found an excellent correlation between MRI and angiographic estimates of size of the main, right, and left pulmonary arteries.[C3] Although the ability to localize focal pulmonary stenosis is less precise, MRI is still accurate enough to be valuable. Sagittal plane images are useful for defining the size of the main pulmonary artery, and they yield important surgical information regarding the degree of narrowing of the right ventricular outflow tract.[M1] The choices of technique for surgical repair of tetralogy of Fallot are dependent on reconstruction of pulmonary outflow. If severe muscular hypertrophy obstructs the outflow tract (Fig. 48–5), a pulmonary artery conduit may be preferable to an extensive ventriculotomy.

The aortic anatomy in tetralogy of Fallot also needs to be examined with great care. There is a 25 percent incidence of mirror-image branching right aortic arch in these patients. Approximately 5 percent of patients with tetralogy of Fallot have

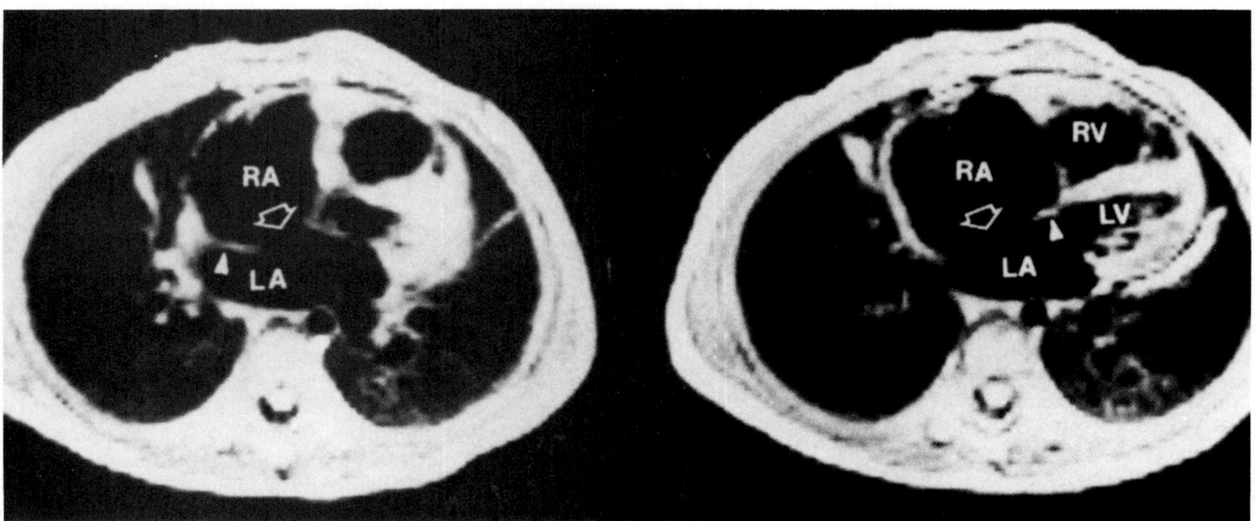

Figure 48–1. Ostium secundum atrial septal defect. Axial MRI scans at two levels are shown. The large open arrow in both images shows the position of the secundum atrial septal defect. In the *left panel,* the white arrowhead indicates the sinus venosus portion of the atrial septum, and in the *right panel,* the white arrowhead indicates the primum portion of the atrial septum. The presence of these portions of the atrial septum indicates that the septal defect is of the secundum variety. RA—right atrium; LA—left atrium; RV—right ventricle; LV—left ventricle. (From Bank, E. R., and Hernandez, R. J.: CT and MR of congenital heart disease. Radiol. Clin. North Am. 26:241–262, 1988, with permission.)

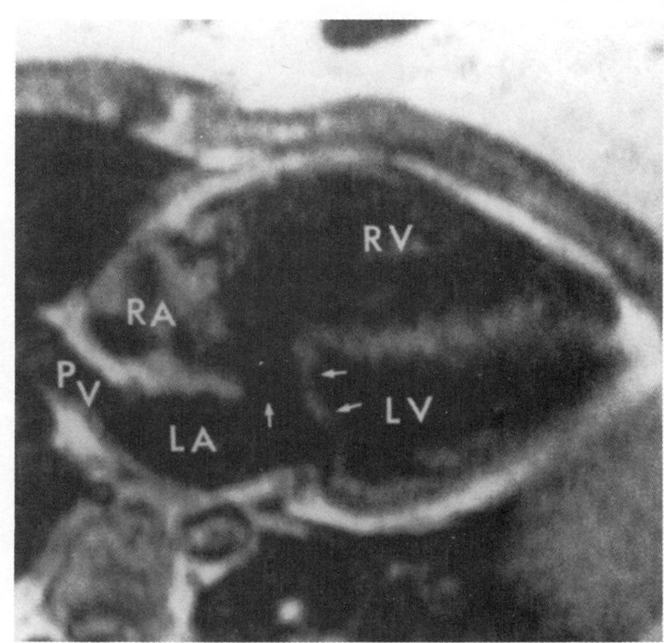

Figure 48–2. Ostium primum atrial septal defect. This oblique (four-chamber) image is oriented perpendicular to the atrial and ventricular septa and shows right and left atria (RA, LA), right and left ventricles (RV, LV) and a pulmonary vein (PV). An ostium primum atrial septal defect is indicated by the single vertical arrow. The two horizontal arrows indicate the anterior leaflet of the mitral valve. (From Dinsmore, R. E., Wisner, G. L., Guyer, D., et al.: Magnetic resonance imaging of the interatrial septum and atrial septal defects. AJR 145:697–703, 1985, © by the American Roentgen Ray Society.)

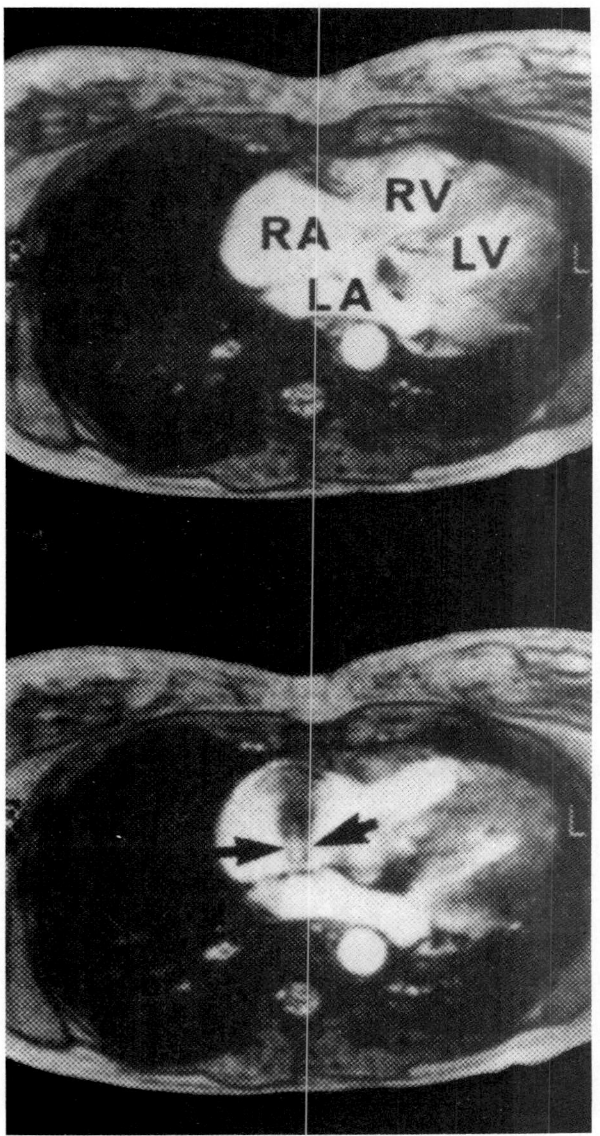

Figure 48–3. Gradient-echo image of a secundum atrial septal defect. The upper panel shows a diastolic axial image demonstrating the right and left atria (RA, LA) and right and left ventricles (RV, LV). Note that the atrial septum is not well visualized. In the lower panel, a systolic image clearly demonstrates the flow disturbance associated with the interatrial left-to-right shunt as an area of decreased image intensity between the black arrows. (From Sechtem, U, and Higgins, C. B.: Cine MRI in acquired and congenital heart disease. *In* Zipes, D. P., and Rowlands, D. J. (eds.): Progress in Cardiology. Lea & Febiger, Philadelphia, 1990, p. 47, with permission.)

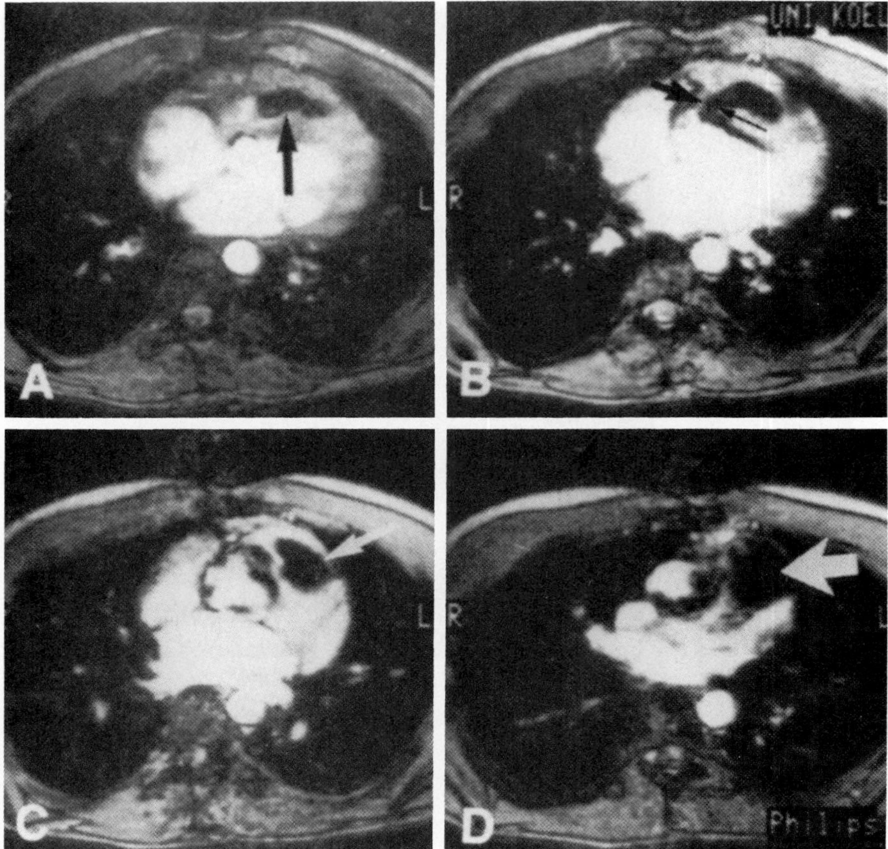

Figure 48–4. Ventricular septal defect. Four axial, gradient-echo images at different levels are shown, demonstrating a supracristal ventricular septal defect. In *Panel A*, the flow disturbance associated with the ventricular septal defect is indicated by the large black arrow in the right ventricle. At a higher anatomic level (*Panel B*) further details of the flow disturbance are shown. In *Panels C* and *D* the flow disturbance is shown in the right ventricular outflow tract and pulmonary artery, respectively (*white arrows*). (From Sechtem, U., and Higgins, C. B.: Cine MRI in acquired and congenital heart disease. *In* Zipes, D. P., and Rowlands, D. J. (eds.): Progress in Cardiology. Lea & Febiger, Philadelphia, 1990, p. 47, with permission.)

anomalous origin or branching of the coronary arteries. The coronary artery anomaly of most importance is origin of the anterior descending artery from the proximal right coronary artery. The anomalous artery traverses the pulmonary outflow area and, therefore, lies in the surgical field when repair is undertaken. Attention to coronary artery origin in the axial plane at the level of the aortic root is necessary to detect this abnormality. Patients who have had previous surgery on the right ventricular outflow tract are at increased risk, since the scar tissue and adhesions may make the artery inconspicuous to the surgeon.

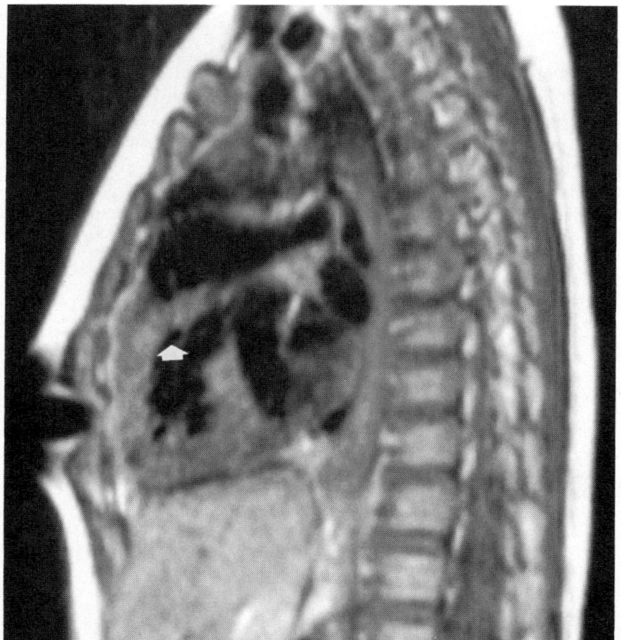

Figure 48–5. A 6-year-old girl with severe cyanosis after attempted repair of tetralogy of Fallot. The sagittal spin-echo image of the right ventricular outflow area shows a muscle bar (*arrow*) separating the right ventricle and pulmonary artery.

Palliation of tetralogy of Fallot patients consists of creating systemic-to-pulmonary arterial shunts, as mentioned earlier. The Blalock-Taussig shunt is the predominant palliative operation, and definition of subclavian and innominate artery anatomy is important for successful shunt construction. The Waterston shunt may be performed in infants, in whom the size of the subclavian artery makes surgical anastomosis difficult. In either case, detailed information concerning aortic arch and pulmonary artery anatomy is invaluable. The presence of large bronchial arterial branches also must be documented prior to repair of tetralogy of Fallot, especially in the case of pseudotruncus. Persistence of high-flow and high-pressure bronchial-to-pulmonary artery anastomoses may elevate pulmonary artery resistance to the point of limiting lung perfusion. Large bronchial arteries, therefore, must often be ligated prior to attempting definitive tetralogy repair. These collaterals are best seen on coronal, T1-weighted spin-echo images of the descending aorta.

MRI is very valuable in evaluating pulmonary artery anatomy after repair of tetralogy of Fallot. Occlusion of either pulmonary artery by the surgical outflow patch or thrombus may be demonstrated by axial plane spin-echo imaging (Fig. 48–6). Inspection of the ventricular septum for residual shunt and right ventricular outflow tract for residual stenosis may also be performed employing spin-echo imaging techniques. Future possibilities for the use of MRI include documenting and quantitating pulmonary artery flow patterns by measurement of signals within the pulmonary arteries.[B2]

Tricuspid atresia is usually associated with hypoplasia of the right ventricle and pulmonary outflow tract. Fletcher and associates[F1] have described the MRI findings of tricuspid atresia in detail, noting that the presence of a bar of fatty tissue projecting

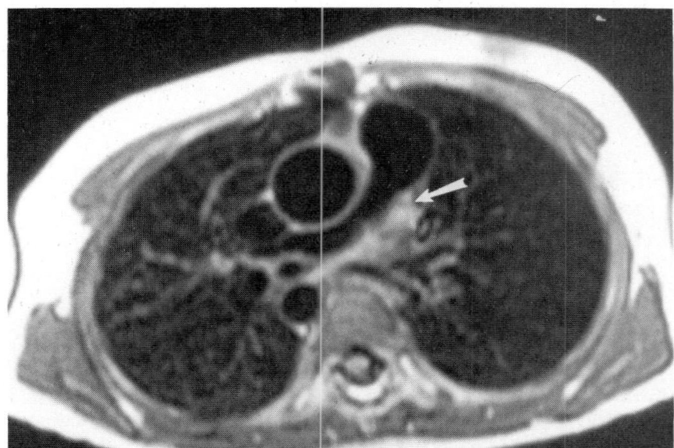

Figure 48–6. A 7-year-old patient who had prior pulmonary artery augmentation for hypoplasia of the main pulmonary artery associated with tetralogy of Fallot. Axial spin-echo image documents that the left pulmonary artery is occluded at the level of the patch graft (*arrow*). Small peripheral segments of the left pulmonary artery are visible near the hilum.

across the atrioventricular sulcus at the bottom of the right atrium is a characteristic finding (Fig. 48–7). From the clinical perspective, evaluation of the size of the pulmonary arteries and of the right ventricular outflow tract are necessary prior to palliative surgery. Imaging of these structures by employing axial spin-echo views appears to be the most valuable. It is important to define the right atrial and extracardiac vascular anatomy,[J2] since many patients with this condition can undergo a Fontan procedure (right atrium to pulmonary artery anastomosis) for physiologic correction. Palliative procedures for these patients are similar to those employed for tetralogy of Fallot, and the same imaging concerns are germane.

In Ebstein's malformation of the tricuspid valve, there is displacement of a portion of tricuspid valve tissue into the right ventricle, creating variable degrees of tricuspid regurgitation and right ventricular failure. The area of the right ventricle proximal to the displaced valve leaflet becomes smooth walled and acts as a reservoir of venous blood (atrialized portion), whereas the portion distal to the valve leaflet acts as a small and obstructed

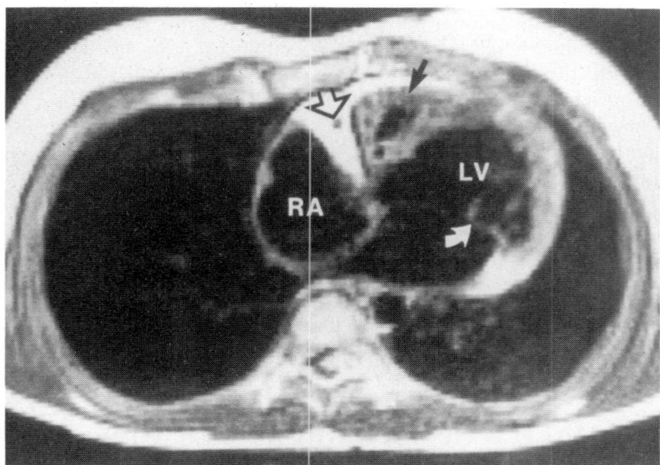

Figure 48–7. Tricuspid atresia. Axial spin-echo image documents fat filling the atrioventricular valve plane (*open arrow*) in a patient with tricuspid atresia. The right ventricle is hypoplastic (*black arrow*). The left atrioventricular valve is partially visualized (*curved white arrow*). RA—right atrium; LV—left ventricle. (Courtesy of B. D. Fletcher; from Fletcher, B. D., Jacobstein, M. D., Abramowsky, C. R., et al.: Right atrioventricular valve atresia: Anatomic evaluation with MR imaging. AJR 148:671–674, 1987, © by The American Roentgen Ray Society.)

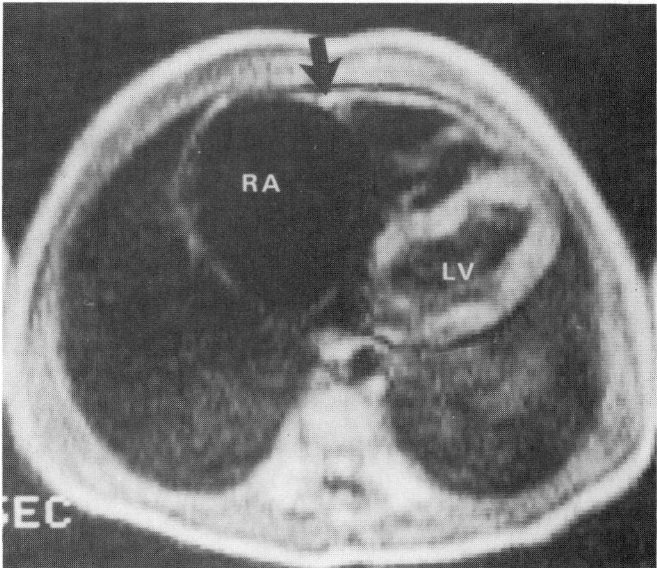

Figure 48–8. Axial spin-echo image of a patient with Ebstein's anomaly. Note the large right atrium (RA) and the tricuspid valve apparatus. The black arrow shows a shallow atrioventricular sulcus in contrast to tricuspid atresia (Fig. 48–7). LV—left ventricle. (Courtesy of B. D. Fletcher; from Fletcher, B. D., Jacobstein, M. D., Abramowsky, C. R., et al.: Right atrioventricular valve atresia: Anatomic evaluation with MR imaging. AJR 148:671–674, 1987, © by The American Roentgen Ray Society.)

right ventricle. Cyanosis supervenes owing to right-to-left shunting via an associated atrial septal defect. Patients of varied ages present with the lesion depending on the degree of valvular and ventricular abnormalities. Axial spin-echo MRI images can show the dilated right atrium and characteristic deformity of the valve apparatus (Fig. 48–8). The "atrialized" segment of the right ventricle proximal to the displaced valve leaflet is easily defined, as are the size and patency of the main pulmonary artery.[L3]

Double-outlet right ventricle is another cyanotic lesion that may be evaluated by MRI. When there is associated pulmonary outflow obstruction, the considerations for surgical palliation and repair are similar to those in tetralogy of Fallot, and imaging strategies should be essentially the same as those noted above. Double-outlet right ventricle may be associated with a subpulmonic ventricular septal defect, in which case the complex is referred to as the Taussig-Bing anomaly (Fig. 48–9). In this case, definition of the anatomy is necessary, with particular attention

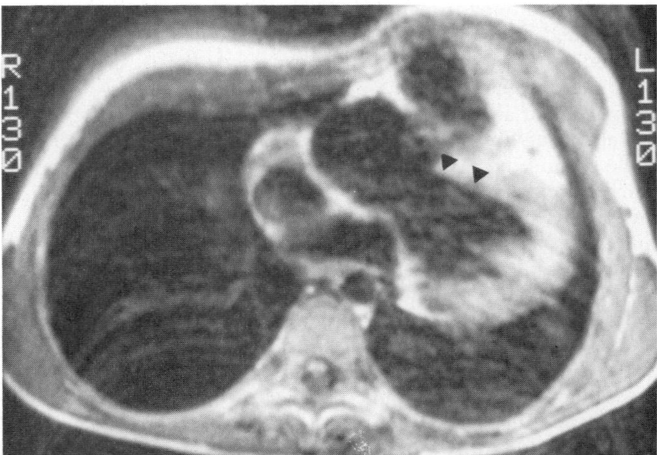

Figure 48–9. Double-outlet right ventricle repaired using a modified Rastelli procedure. The left-ventricle–to–aortic baffle used to close the ventricular septal defect is well demonstrated (*arrowheads*).

directed toward ventricular outflow. Other cases of double-outlet right ventricle may be associated with atresia of the right atrioventricular valve, and it is critical to identify both atrioventricular valves in the axial plane because the size and patency of the valves critically affect the choices for surgical repair.

Eisenmenger's Physiology

Disorders with fixed, elevated pulmonary vascular resistance cause cyanosis because of pulmonary oligemia. This condition is usually seen in a patient with a left-to-right shunt whose pulmonary vascular resistance becomes elevated. As pulmonary artery resistance rises, shunting changes from left-to-right to right-to-left and cyanosis supervenes. Fortunately, in most patients this sequence is preventable with prompt detection and repair. Magnetic resonance–based estimates of pulmonary artery flow and resistance hold great promise for the noninvasive evaluation of patients with this condition.[B2] At present, such methods are under development, but it is anticipated that they may soon become more widely available.

Admixture Lesions

The admixture lesions are those in which cyanosis occurs owing to abnormal mixing of oxygenated and desaturated blood within the systemic circulation. Complete (D) transposition of the great arteries is the prototype of an admixture lesion in that survival is dependent on the existence of a communication between the pulmonary and systemic circuits. Although MRI is capable of aiding the physician to make the initial diagnosis (Fig. 48–10), most patients with transposition of the great arteries are too ill on initial presentation to tolerate MRI and the correct diagnosis should be made by other means, usually echocardiography. The major role of MRI appears to be in the follow-up of patients after palliation or failed repair.[S4] The conventional operative approaches for transposition of the great arteries consist of the creation of Mustard or Senning baffles at the atrial level to conduct systemic venous and pulmonary venous blood to the proper atrioventricular valves. Systemic venous blood is conducted via a baffle to the mitral valve, while pulmonary venous blood is shunted to the tricuspid valve. The anatomic left ventricle remains the pulmonary ventricle, while the right ventricle assumes the role of systemic ventricle. Recently, the "arterial switch" surgical approach has been employed. In this procedure, the aorta and pulmonary arteries are transected and reattached so that they are associated with the proper ventricles. This procedure has a number of theoretical advantages; however, long-term experience with the procedure is just becoming available. An additional repair strategy in patients with transposition of the great arteries with associated ventricular septal defect and pulmonic stenosis is the Rastelli procedure (see Fig. 48–9). In this type of repair, a pulmonary-to-systemic baffle is constructed at ventricular level by directional patch closure of a ventricular septal defect. In imaging postoperative patients with both atrial baffle repairs and conduits, MRI imaging employing T1-weighted, low flip angle coronal and axial scans has been helpful in defining the patency of the systemic venous baffle. Similar strategies using cine MRI can document atrioventricular valve (tricuspid) insufficiency or pulmonary (left) ventricular outflow obstruction that may occasionally occur in patients with this condition.[C4]

Severely ill infants in congestive failure may present with total anomalous venous return below the diaphragm. This type of patient is not often a candidate for MRI. Supracardiac total anomalous pulmonary venous return, on the other hand, is an admixture lesion dependent on the size of an interatrial communication for the timing of its clinical presentation. Magnetic resonance imaging in the transaxial plane[F2] defines the anomalous vein and its point of connection to the systemic venous circulation. In cases of supracardiac total anomalous pulmonary venous return, the insertion of the common pulmonary vein may be variable, with sites at the left brachiocephalic vein, superior vena cava, coronary sinus, and right atrium. Imaging fields of view must be designed so as to include all of these sites. The size of the left heart is critical in these cases, since repair strategies depend on connecting the pulmonary veins to the left atrium. Axial MRI estimates of left atrial size and left ventricular volume and function are invaluable in the surgical planning for infants with this condition.

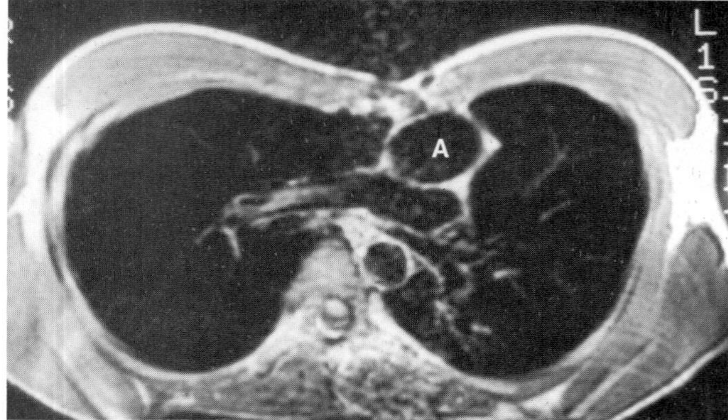

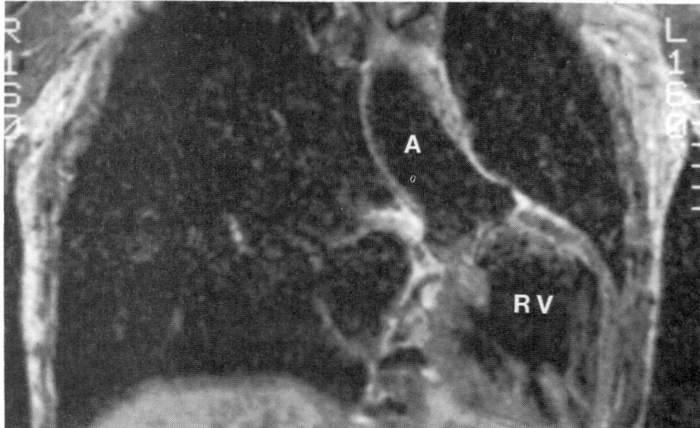

Figure 48–10. D-transposition of the great arteries in a 4-year old who had a Mustard repair. Axial spin-echo image (*upper panel*) demonstrates the large aorta (A) arising as the anterior great artery. Coronal MRI (*lower panel*) confirms origin of the aorta from the right ventricle (RV).

Abnormalities of cardiac or visceral situs often have associated cyanotic heart disease. MRI is especially valuable in that it can provide three-dimensional information regarding chamber anatomy, location, and associated great vessel abnormalities. In general, cyanotic children with situs abnormalities have some combination of transposition of the great arteries (usually congenitally corrected (L) transposition), pulmonary obstruction, ventricular shunting, and absence of the inferior vena cava. Two syndromes in which situs abnormalities are consistently identified are asplenia and polysplenia. Asplenia is frequently associated with severe cyanotic heart disease, whereas cardiac lesions of polysplenia are more variable in nature and may range from venous anomalies or an isolated, congenitally corrected transposition to severe cyanotic congenital heart disease.

ANOMALIES OF THE GREAT VESSELS

General Considerations

MRI is an important imaging modality in evaluating congenital anomalies of the great vessels. Spin-echo sequences, in which flowing blood is seen as a signal void,[F3] and gradient-refocused echo images, in which blood is seen with enhanced signal, delineate the great vessels extremely well and allow the diagnosis and evaluation of congenital anomalies of the great vessels without the need for the administration of contrast medium or exposure to radiation.[S5] Additional advantages of MRI in the assessment of congenital great vessel disease include the ability to image in axial, coronal, sagittal and oblique axes; to reconstruct complex anatomy in three dimensions; and to image with wide fields of view.

Congenital arterial anomalies that lend themselves to MRI evaluation include aneurysmal, stenotic, and positional abnormalities of the aortic arch; various types of truncus arteriosus; and patent ductus arteriosus. Pulmonary arterial abnormalities that lend themselves to MRI evaluation are pulmonary artery stenoses, aneurysms, and shunts. Additional conditions in which evaluation with MRI is useful include abnormalities of the superior and inferior vena cavae and in systemic and venous collateral vessels.

Aortic disease

The thoracic aorta is best imaged in the axial and left anterior oblique planes.[D4] Axial images show the cross-sectional anatomy of the aorta and details of its relationship with the ventricles and with surrounding structures. Axial images will also delineate dissection flaps. Cine MRI can demonstrate aortic valve incompetence, show turbulence at sites of stenoses, and may differentiate slow flow from thrombus.[B3] In order to visualize the entire thoracic aorta, the left anterior oblique view is best; however, if the aorta is very tortuous, combinations of images employing sagittal, coronal, and oblique projections may be necessary.[D4] In patients with aneurysmal dilatation of the ascending aorta, as in the Marfan syndrome, the degree of aortic enlargement and its distal extent are well illustrated on the left anterior oblique images (Fig. 48–11). The relationships of the aortic valve and the sinuses of valsalva can also be seen in this view. Axial images (Fig. 48–12) delineate the cross-sectional diameter of the aorta, and this measurement correlates very well with measurements obtained by angiography, computed tomography, and echocardiography. In evaluating the cross-sectional diameter of the ascending aorta, a ratio of greater than 1.5 to 1 as compared with the descending aorta is considered abnormal.[D5, S6]

The use of gradient-refocused echo imaging in the left anterior oblique or coronal projections demonstrates turbulence and signal drop-out if aortic regurgitation is present. Localized post-stenotic dilatations of the supravalvular aorta can be present in congenital aortic stenosis and with bicuspid aortic valves. These are well delineated with MRI. A hypoplastic arch is also easily seen.[G3]

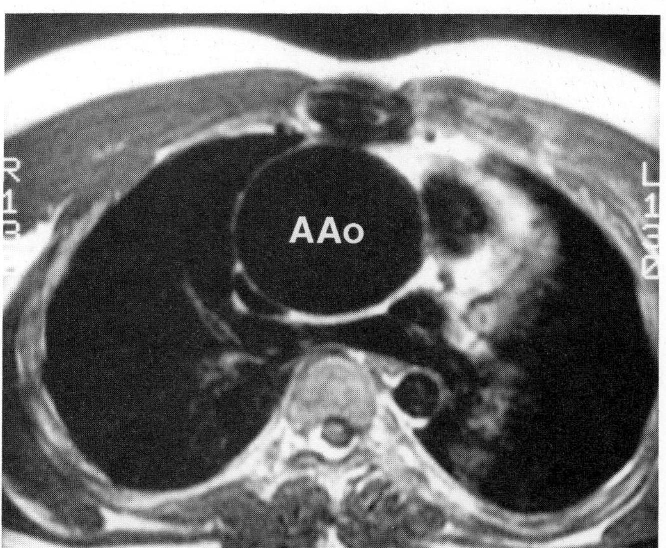

Figure 48–12. Axial spin-echo MRI image of the patient in Figure 48–11. The image was taken at a level 2 cm above the aortic valve. The diameter of the ascending aorta (AAo) at this level was 6.6 cm. There was no evidence of dissection.

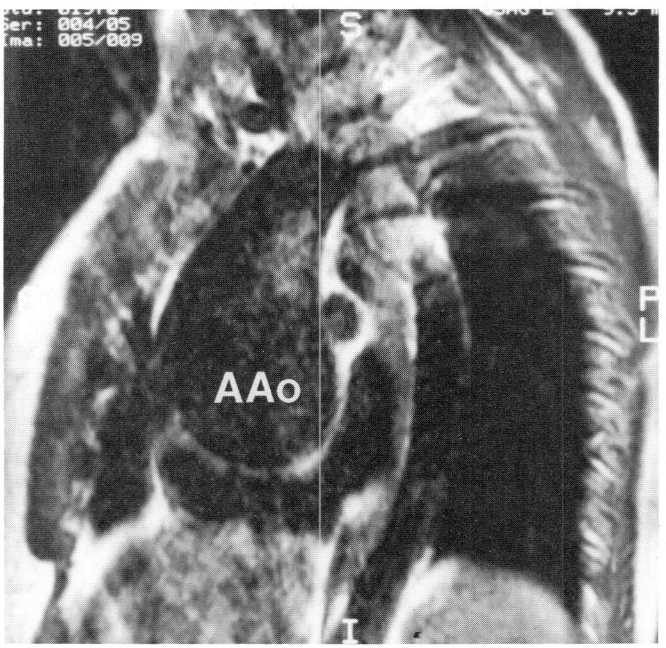

Figure 48–11. Ascending aortic aneurysm in a 26-year-old male studied 4 years after aortic valvulotomy. The sagittal spin-echo image shows a widened ascending aorta (AAo) with dilatation extending from the sinuses of Valsalva to the origin of the right innominate artery.

Aneurysms and dissections are relatively rare occurrences in children but have a higher incidence in such predisposing conditions as the Marfan or Ehlers-Danlos syndromes, bicuspid aortic valve, coarctation of the aorta, systemic hypertension, and Turner syndrome.[L4] They are also seen following inflammatory processes such as Takayasu aortitis or infective endocarditis.[B4] In cases of dissection, the MRI signal intensity within the false lumen on a T2-weighted spin-echo image may be increased secondary to slower blood flow, or may stay the same or be decreased secondary to thrombosis.[G4]

Aneurysms of the sinuses of Valsalva may be congenital or acquired. Their extent is best seen on axial sections, but they can also be identified on sagittal or oblique views.

Supravalvular aortic stenosis can be evaluated very well with MRI. Oblique projections, which show the stenosis along longitudinal orientations, appear to be the better views.

Coarctation of the aorta is seen as a discrete narrowing of the aorta and most commonly occurs just distal to the left subclavian artery (Fig. 48–13). Additionally, there may be associated hypoplasia of the aortic arch. Magnetic resonance imaging is not only useful in assessing the degree and extent of stenosis but also in determining the presence, size, and number of any collateral vessels. However, vessel tortuosities in this area may make assessment difficult.[B5, G5] Magnetic resonance imaging is useful in evaluating postoperative patients; however, mild degrees of narrowing may be difficult to assess. Aneurysms occurring in the postoperative patient are also well evaluated using MRI techniques.[B4]

Vascular Rings

Vascular rings, such as double aortic arch, right aortic arch with an aberrant left subclavian artery, left aortic arch with aberrant right subclavian artery, and pulmonary slings, lend themselves to MRI evaluation. Both axial and coronal images are useful in this regard. In double aortic arch, the arches are seen to encircle the esophagus and trachea. In these instances, the right-sided arch is usually slightly larger and higher than the left and courses to the left and behind the trachea and esophagus as it descends in the thorax. In a right aortic arch with an aberrant left subclavian artery, the vascular ring is completed by a left

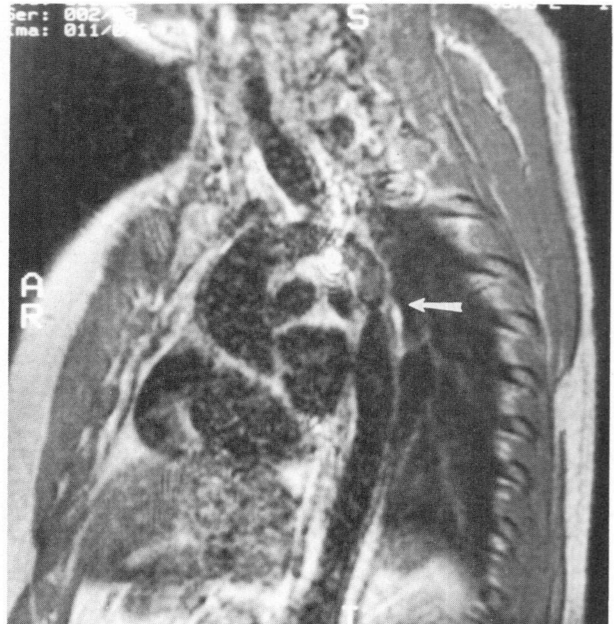

Figure 48–13. Coarctation of the aorta in a 23-year-old male. The oblique spin-echo MRI image shows a localized narrowing of the aorta (arrow) just distal to the origin of the left subclavian artery.

ductus. In pulmonary sling, an anomalous left pulmonary artery arises from the right pulmonary artery and courses posterior to the left main stem broncus and may compress it.

Truncus Arteriosus

In truncus arteriosus, the pulmonary arteries arise from the aorta either from a common trunk or from individual orifices. Additionally, stenosis may be present. MRI can define both the anatomy of the aorta and also the origins of pulmonary arteries.[F4, G3] These appear as flow voids in spin-echo images or as areas of bright signal in cine MRI images. If stenosis or hypoplasia of one or both pulmonary arteries is present, there may be increased signal secondary to turbulence (spin-echo) or signal dropout (cine mode). Evaluation of this anatomy is important because the size of the vessels is crucial to considerations for surgical correction.

Extracardiac Shunts

Aortopulmonary window and patent ductus arteriosus lend themselves to MRI evaluation. Axial, coronal, or left anterior oblique views appear to be the optimal projections.[G3] Complications of repair, such as aneurysms of the pulmonary outflow tract, can also be adequately evaluated with MRI.

Pulmonary Artery Anomalies

MRI is highly accurate in assessing pulmonary artery diameters and exhibits excellent correlations when compared with angiography.[R2] Stenoses in the peripheral pulmonary arteries, however, do not visualize as well,[C3, R2] primarily because of the juxtaposition with the air-filled lung. The size and locations of the main, left, and right pulmonary arteries are best visualized in the axial plane. The same is true for the central pulmonary veins.[C3, G3]

Collateral Circulation and Surgical Shunts

In instances of cyanotic heart disease, the pulmonary circulation is often supplied by collaterals that arise from the systemic circulation. These may be fairly large and may require ligation at the time of the corrective procedure. In this regard, MRI may be helpful and both axial and coronal images may be required. Difficulties in imaging the collateral circulation can occur due to slow flow and vessel tortuosity. In addition, stenoses may not be visualized and depiction of small collateral vessels may be impaired by partial volume averaging effects. In the absence of flow, MRI may not be reliable and the proximity of the air-filled lung to the hilum may preclude identification of these small vessels. Gating is usually needed and cyanotic infants, especially those in respiratory distress and those with rapid or irregular heart beats, often prove difficult to image with gated methods.

Waterston, Blalock-Taussig, Glenn, and Potts shunts can all be visualized with MRI.[C3] As in the previous instances, the axial and coronal image orientations appear to be most useful. Tortuosity and juxtaposition of the air-filled lung, and respiratory and ECG gating problems may compromise the quality of the scans. Surgical conduits from the right ventricle to the pulmonary artery also lend themselves to MRI assessment.

Venous Anomalies

The systemic and pulmonary venous relationships are well delineated using MRI.[F3] Transverse and coronal images appear to be the most reliable, but oblique views are often needed. Aberrant left superior and inferior vena cava and azygous anomalies can usually be seen because these vessels traverse the mediastinum where the mediastinal tissues and fat delineate their position. Total and partial anomalous venous return patterns are less well visualized because they lie in juxtaposition to the low signals of the surrounding lung.[S5]

MRI has established itself as a major imaging modality in the evaluation of congenital anomalies of the great vessels. It has important applications in imaging aortic disease, pulmonary artery anomalies, and venous abnormalities. It can delineate extracardiac and postoperative shunts as well as collateral vessels, and may do so with high degrees of accuracy. Increasing numbers of physicians now believe MRI is the preferred noninvasive imaging modality for monitoring aortic enlargement or hypoplasia.[F4, K2, L5]

SUMMARY

MRI is proving to be a very useful noninvasive diagnostic technique for evaluating the anatomy and physiology of congenital heart disease. MRI methods to date have proved most useful in the assessment of anatomy of the great vessels and ventricular outflow tract. Using both spin-echo and cine MRI approaches is also useful in identifying the presence of atrial and ventricular septal defects. MRI techniques are particularly useful in determining the status of the postoperative patient, particularly when extracardiac conduits or intracardiac baffles have been placed. Poor visualization of cardiac valves is a relative shortcoming of the method, but cine MRI methods permit identification of flow disturbances and, to some extent, quantification of shunts and valvular regurgitation. Because of its unique capabilities in aiding in the assessment of anatomy, physiology, and biochemistry, the use of MRI will continue to grow in the evaluation of the patient with congenital heart disease.

Acknowledgments

The authors acknowledge Larry Mahoney, M.D., for his thoughtful review of the chapter and Ruth Lillie and Carolyn Frisbie for their expert preparation of the manuscript.

References

B

1. Boxer, R. A., Singh, S., LaCorte, M. A., et al.: Cardiac magnetic resonance imaging in children with congenital heart disease. J. Pediatr. 109:460, 1986.
2. Bogren, H. G., Klipstein, R. H., Mohiaddin, R. H., et al.: Pulmonary artery distensibility and blood flow patterns: A magnetic resonance study of normal subjects and of patients with pulmonary arterial hypertension. Am. Heart J. 118:990, 1989.
3. Bittner, V., Cranney, G. B., Lotan, C. S., and Pohost, G. M.: Overview of nuclear magnetic resonance imaging. Cardiol. Clinics 7:631, 1989.

4. Bank, E. R., and Hernandez, R. J. CT and MR of congenital heart disease. Radiol. Clin. North. Am. 26:241, 1988.
5. Bank, E. R., Aisen, A. M., Rocchini, A. P., and Hernandez, R. J.: Coarctation of the aorta in children undergoing angioplasty; pretreatment and posttreatment MR imaging. Radiology 162:235, 1987.

C

1. Chung, K. J., Simpson, I. A., Newman, R., et al.: Cine magnetic resonance imaging for evaluation of congenital heart disease: Role in pediatric cardiology compared with echocardiography and angiography. J. Pediatr. 113:1028, 1988.
2. Chrispin, A., Small, P., Rutter, N., et al.: Transectional echo planar imaging of the heart in cyanotic congenital heart disease. Pediatr. Radiol. 16:293–297, 1986.
3. Canter, C. E., Gutierrez, F. R., Mirowitz, S. A., et al.: Evaluation of pulmonary arterial morphology in cyanotic congenital heart disease by magnetic resonance imaging. Am. Heart J. 118:347, 1989.
4. Chung, K. J., Simpson, I. A., Glass, R., et al.: Cine magnetic resonance imaging after surgical repair in patients with transposition of the great arteries. Circulation 77:104, 1988.

D

1. Didier, D., Higgins, C. B., Fisher, M. R., et al.: Congenital heart disease: Gated MR imaging in 72 patients. Radiology 158:227, 1986.
2. Danielson, G. K., and McGoon, D. C.: Surgical therapy and results. *In* Roberts, W. C. (ed.): Adult Congenital Heart Disease. FA Davis Company, Philadelphia, 1987, pp. 695–715.
3. Dinsmore, R. E., Wisner, G. L., Guyer, D., et al.: Magnetic resonance imaging of the interatrial septum and atrial septal defects. AJR 145:697, 1985.
4. Dinsmore, R. E., Liberthson, R. R., Wisner, G. L., et al.: Magnetic resonance imaging of thoracic aortic aneurysms: Comparison with other imaging methods. AJR 146:309, 1986.
5. Dotter, C. T., and Steinberg, I.: The angiocardiographic measurement of the normal great vessels. Radiol. 52:353, 1949.

F

1. Fletcher, B. D., Jacobstein, M. D., Abramowsky, C. R., and Anderson, R. H.: Right atrioventricular valve atresia: Anatomic evaluation with MR imaging. AJR 148:671, 1987.
2. Fisher, M. R., Hricak, H., and Higgins, C. B.: Magnetic resonance imaging of developmental venous abnormalities. AJR 145:705, 1985.
3. Fisher, M. R., Lipton, M. J., and Higgins, C. B.: Magnetic resonance imaging and computed tomography in congenital heart disease. Semin. Roentgenol. 20:272, 1985.
4. Fletcher, B. D., and Jacobstein, M. D.: MRI of congenital abnormalities of the great arteries. AJR 146:941, 1986.

G

1. Graham, T. P., Jr., and Friesinger, G. C.: Complex cyanotic congenital heart disease. *In* Roberts, W. C. (ed.): Adult Congenital Heart Disease. FA Davis Company, Philadelphia, 1987, pp. 541–566.
2. Glogar, D., Globits, S., Neuhold, A., and Mayr, H.: Assessment of mitral regurgitation by magnetic resonance imaging. Magn. Reson. Imag. 7:611, 1989.
3. Gomes, A.: MR imaging of congenital anomalies of the thoracic aorta and pulmonary arteries. Radiol. Clin. North. Am. 27:1171, 1989.
4. Geisinger, M. A., Risius, B., and Odonnel, J. A.: Thoracic aorta dissections: Magnetic resonance imaging. Radiology 155:407, 1985.
5. Glazer, H. S., Gutierrez, F. R., Levitt, R. G., et al.: The thoracic aorta studied by MR imaging. Radiology 157:149, 1985.

H

1. Higgins, C. B., Byrd, B. F., Farmer, D. W., et al.: Magnetic resonance imaging in patients with congenital heart disease. Circulation 70:851, 1984.

J

1. Jacobstein, M. D.: Magnetic resonance imaging and positron emission tomography. *In* Adams, F. H., Emmanouilides, G. C., and Riemenschneider, T. A. (eds.): Moss' Heart Disease in Infants, Children, and Adolescents. 4th ed. Williams & Wilkins, Baltimore, 1989, p. 114.
2. Julsrud, P. R., Ehman, R. L., Hagler, D. J., and Ilstrup, D. M., Extracardiac vasculature in candidates for Fontan surgery: MR imaging. Radiology 173:503, 1989.

K

1. Kersting-Sommerhoff, B. A., Diethelm, L., Teitel, D. F., et al.: Magnetic resonance imaging of congenital heart disease: Sensitivity and specificity using receiver operating characteristic curve analysis. Am. Heart J. 118:155, 1989.
2. Kersting-Summerhoff, B. A., Sechtem, U. P., Schiller, N. B., et al.: MR imaging of the thoracic aorta in Marfan patients. J. Comput. Assist. Tomogr. 11:63, 1987.

L

1. Link, K. M., Formanek, A. G.: MR imaging in congenital heart disease: Where is the leading edge? Ann. Radiol. 32:15, 1989.
2. Laschinger, J. C., Vannier, M. W., Gutierrez, F., et al.: Preoperative three-dimensional reconstruction of the heart and great vessels in patients with congenital heart disease. J. Thorac. Cardiovasc. Surg. 96:464, 1988.
3. Link, K. M., Herrera, M. A., D'Souza, V. J., and Formanek, A. G.: MR imaging of Ebstein anomaly: Results in four cases. AJR 150:363, 1988.
4. Lin, A. E., Lippe, B. M., Geffner, M. E., et al.: Aortic dilatation, dissection, and rupture in patients with Turner syndrome. J. Pediatr. 109:820, 1986.
5. Lois, J. F., Gomes, A. S., Brown, K., et al.: Magnetic resonance imaging of the thoracic aorta. Am. J. Cardiol. 60:358, 1987.

M

1. Mirowitz, S. A., Gutierrez, F. R., Canter, C. E., Vannier, M. W. Tetralogy of Fallot: MR findings. Radiology 171:207, 1989.

N

1. Nayler, G. L., Firmin, D. N., and Longmore, D. B. Blood flow imaging by cine magnetic resonance. J. Comput. Assist. Tomogr. 10:715, 1986.

P

1. Perloff, J. K.: The Clinical Recognition of Congenital Heart Disease. 3rd ed. WB Saunders, Philadelphia, 1987.

R

1. Roberts, W. C.: Adult Congenital Heart Disease. FA Davis Company, Philadelphia, 1987.
2. Rees, R. S. O., Somerville, J., Underwood, S. R., et al.: Magnetic resonance imaging of the pulmonary arteries and their systemic connections in pulmonary atresia: Comparison with angiographic and surgical findings. Br. Heart J. 58:621, 1987.

S

1. Skorton, D. J., and Mahoney, L. T.: Congenital heart disease in adolescents and adults. Cardio July:68, 1988.
2. Sechtem, U., and Higgins, C. B. Cine MRI in acquired and congenital heart disease. *In* Zipes, D. P., and Rowlands, D. J. (eds.): Progress in Cardiology. Lea & Febiger, Philadelphia, 1990, p. 47.
3. Sechtem, U., Pflugfelder, P., Cassidy, M. C., et al.: Ventricular septal defect: Visualization of shunt flow and determination of shunt size by cine MR imaging. AJR 149:689, 1987.
4. Soulen, R. L., Donner, R. M., and Capitanio, M.: Postoperative evaluation of complex congenital heart disease by magnetic resonance imaging. Radiographics 7:975, 1987.
5. Sandler, M. P., Graham, T. P., Mazer, M. J., et al.: Magnetic resonance imaging of congenital cardiac abnormalities. *In* Freeman, L. M., Weissman, H. S. (eds.): Nuclear Medicine Annual. Raven Press, New York, 1986.
6. Snider, A. R., Enderlein, M. A., and Teitel, D. F.: Two-dimensional echocardiographic determination of aortic and pulmonary artery sizes from infancy to adulthood in normal subjects. Am. J. Cardiol. 53:218, 1984.

V

1. Vannier, M. W., Gutierrez, F. R., Laschinger, J. C., et al.: Three-dimensional magnetic resonance imaging of congenital heart disease. RadioGraphics 8:857, 1988.

W

1. Whittemore, R., Hobbins, J. C., and Engle, M. A.: Pregnancy and its outcome in women with and without surgical treatment of congenital heart disease. Am. J. Cardiol. 50:641, 1982.

Chapter 49

Nuclear Magnetic Resonance Assessment of Valvular Disease

■ *ROBERT J. HERFKENS, M.D.* ■ *JOSEPH A. UTZ, M.D.*

BASIC CONTRAST MECHANISMS 896
T1, T2, and Water 896
Flow 897
BASIC TECHNIQUES 897
Anatomy—Spin Echo Imaging 897
Function—Cine and Velocity Imaging 898
VALVULAR REGURGITANCY 898
VALVULAR STENOSIS 903
COMBINED LESIONS 909
SUMMARY 909

The usefulness of magnetic resonance imaging for evaluation of central nervous system pathology was recognized early in its development. The application to body imaging lagged significantly behind because of a number of technical issues. The most significant of these issues is the relationship of the MR imaging process to motion. In the evaluation of cardiac disease, and most important, valvular disease of the heart, the sensitivity to flow and motion becomes the greatest strength of magnetic resonance imaging.

The basic criteria in any imaging test that determine its usefulness rest upon three different kinds of resolution. Most imagers think spatial resolution is the key element in the success of an imaging test. In the evaluation of cardiac processes, other elements of resolution become increasingly important. Thus, contrast resolution—the ability to resolve two different structures based on some physical property—and temporal resolution—the ability to resolve dynamic events—become the principal predictors of the success of an imaging test for valvular disease.

The development of spin echo techniques provided high-contrast resolution images, but without cardiac gating, limited information was available about the heart. Following the combination of spin echo imaging and consistent gating, or cardiac-triggering techniques, high-spatial and high-contrast images of cardiac and thoracic structures could be obtained in any anatomic orientation. Although these techniques provided accurate measurements of volumetric data, such as ventricular volumes and myocardial mass, a key element remained lacking for the effective evaluation of valvular disease. The temporal resolution of these techniques was quite poor. To evaluate all levels of the heart at all parts of the cardiac cycle, extremely long acquisition times were necessary. These long acquisition times were poorly tolerated by severely ill cardiac patients and required long periods of expensive imager time.

The development of gradient-recalled imaging techniques, coupled to the cardiac cycle, cine MRI, added the necessary temporal resolution for effective functional evaluation of the heart. Of even greater importance, these techniques are sensitive to flow and allow the display of dynamic data throughout the cardiac cycle, which is not only sensitive to flow velocities but allows the identification of "turbulent" flow. This technique, when combined with spin echo imaging, allows for the comprehensive evaluation of patients with valvular disease.[H1, H2]

BASIC CONTRAST MECHANISMS

T1, T2, and Water

The major success of magnetic resonance imaging has been related to the sensitivity of the images to relaxation times (T1 and T2) and water content. This multifactorial relationship to intrinsic tissue differences, accentuated by varying imaging parameters (TR and TE) in spin echo imaging, has accounted for the tremendous contrast differences seen most dramatically in the central nervous system. These factors also play an important role in the evaluation of mediastinal disease and the evaluation of ischemic and neoplastic disease of the heart. In the evaluation of valvular disease, however, the strong relationship to flow is the dominant signal effect that determines the ability to provide a comprehensive examination.[S1, U1, U3]

In gated spin echo imaging, there is a *loss* of signal from moving protons. Spin echo images utilize a slice-selective radiofrequency pulse of 90°, followed by a slice-selective pulse of 180° at a time of TE/2 in order to generate a spin echo at time TE. In order for spins to return signal effectively and contribute to the image, these events must occur in a coordinated fashion. Spins that receive their 90° pulse and have moved outside the imaging plane essentially have a disrupted sequence and do not contribute useful data to the image. In some circumstances these spins will significantly degrade the image.[H1] Methods to decrease the signal from moving spins are routinely used to improve image quality, as discussed elsewhere in this text.

This flow void phenomenon allows for the precise definition of the endocardial borders in spin echo imaging. By precise definition of the endocardial and epicardial borders, accurate measurements of ventricular volumes and myocardial mass are possible (also see Chapter 44).[S1] The expected flow void may not be seen when flow is very slow and spins remain in the imaging slice long enough to contribute to the image. In the case of valvular disease, this slow flow signal can be confused with left atrial thrombus in large, poorly contracting atria.[C1]

Because of their relatively high spatial and contrast resolution, spin echo images are important for the anatomic evaluation of patients with valvular disease. Valve leaflets frequently can be seen during portions of the cardiac cycle. For instance, the aortic valve is best seen during diastole, whereas the mitral and tricuspid valves are best seen during systole. The spatial resolution is insufficient to consistently detect subtle lesions of the leaflets themselves. Spin echo images are also insensitive to detection of calcification because of the lack of contrast. Calcifications have virtually no water content and therefore little MRI signal; contrasted with the signal void from flowing blood, they are virtually invisible on spin echo images[H3] (Fig. 49–1).

Flow

Cine MRI is a technique that combines gradient-recalled echoes, which utilize limited flip angle excitation, with cardiac triggering. This technique differs from spin echo acquisitions in that a single slice-selective radiofrequency pulse is utilized and refocused by a nonslice-selective gradient. This basic process makes flowing blood bright on magnetic resonance images images. By triggering the scanner with a physiologic cardiac trigger, such as the electrocardiogram or a pulse trigger, the data can be acquired prospectively and images can be acquired at multiple parts of the cardiac cycle with a great sensitivity to flow. The images from a single slice can then be displayed in a continuous loop for evaluation of flow phenomena and other dynamic events, such as wall motion or valvular motion. The imaging sequence can acquire up to 4 anatomic levels and be reconstructed into as many as 32 images in a cardiac cycle. The basic acquisition is acquired over as few as 128 cardiac cycles or, more typically, 256 cardiac cycles[U2] (Fig. 49–2).

The inflow of fresh spins or previously unexcited spins increases the signal from flowing blood. The faster the flow, the brighter the signal obtained from flowing or moving spins. This signal enhancement occurs until the volume of the slice is replaced by these fresh spins. An additional factor in cine gradient-recalled imaging is essential for the evaluation of patients with valvular disease: The MRI processes require that the spins have a constant velocity relationship within an imaging voxel. When there is a mixing of velocities within a voxel, there is a lack of so-called phase coherence, resulting in signal loss. Therefore, in areas of turbulence where the velocity vectors are quite chaotic, there is a significant loss of signal contrasted against the normally high signal from coherent flow. This phenomenon also occurs in areas of significant shear, such as the boundary layer of major vessels. These are the processes responsible for a major portion of the utility of cine magnetic resonance imaging in the evaluation of valvular disease.[P1, P2]

BASIC TECHNIQUES

Anatomy—Spin Echo Imaging

The anatomic evaluation of the heart in valvular disease is best accomplished utilizing spin echo imaging. The high contrast from the signal void of flowing blood and relatively strong signal from the myocardium provide an excellent contrast situation for the definition of endocardial and epicardial borders. The multislice capability allows images to be acquired through the entire cardiac volume in a reasonable period of time. The principal limitation is that each anatomic level is at a different part of the cardiac cycle. To cover all parts of the cardiac cycle at all levels, one must repeat the sequence *N* times for *N* parts of the cardiac cycle. This is the multicycle-multigated technique described in Chapter 44.

The measurement of some important data, such as myocardial mass, can be made accurately without this time-consuming acquisition, which does not change throughout the cardiac cycle. Other data such as ventricular volumes require measurements at least at end-systole and end-diastole. One of the major strengths of magnetic resonance imaging volume data is that no geometric assumptions are made. The slices can be essentially contiguous and encompass the entire cardiac volume. By simply summing the areas of the structure of interest on each slice, multiplied by slice thickness, accurate measurements of volumes and mass can be obtained.

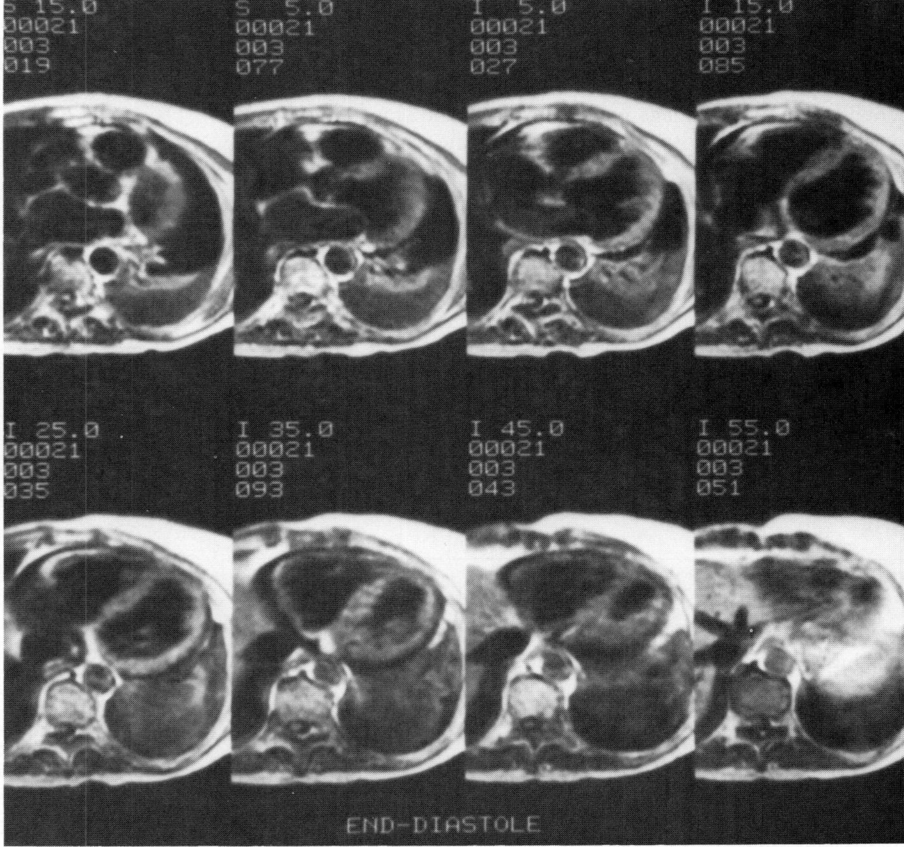

Figure 49–1. A series of eight spin echo images, gated to every heart beat with a TE of 20 msec. This series is extracted from a multicycle, multigated sequence in order to obtain images at the same period of the cardiac cycle, diastole. Note visualization of the aortic valve during diastole; the mitral leaflets are barely visible but are better seen during systolic imaging. From this type of spin echo series, accurate measurements of ventricular volumes, mass, and ejection fraction can be made. Note the large left pleural effusion and atelectatic lung segment.

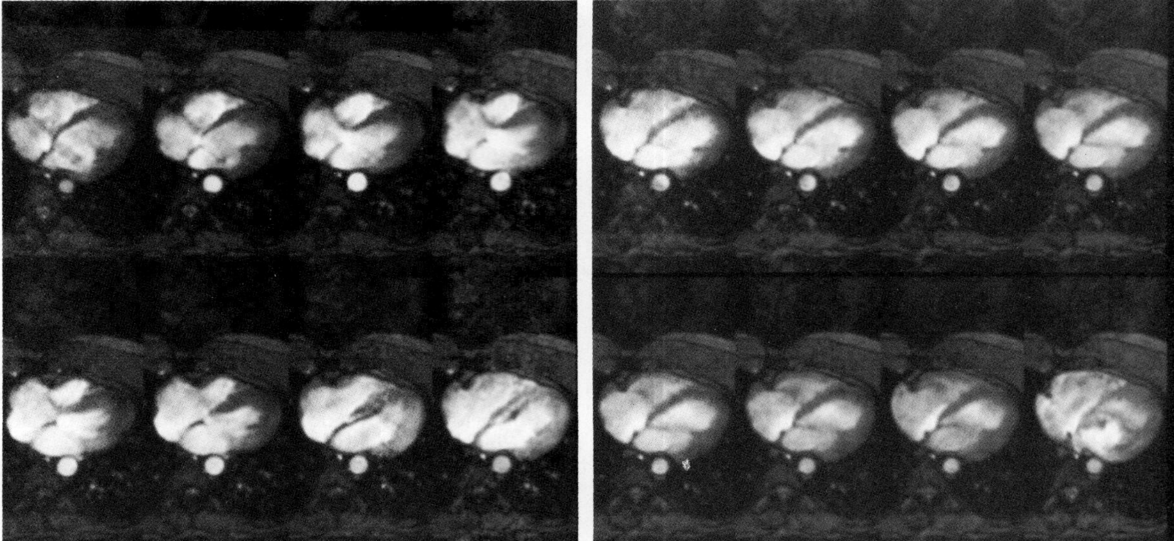

Figure 49–2. Sixteen transaxial cine gradient-recalled images throughout the cardiac cycle, beginning at the QRS. Note minor changes in the relatively bright flow signal within the cardiac chambers. The mitral valve can be seen as a negative defect against the bright blood background. Note the systolic thickening of the left ventricular myocardium. (From Utz, J. A., Herfkens, R. J., Heinsimer, J. A., et al: Valvular regurgitation: Dynamic MR imaging. Radiology 168:91, 1988.)

Function—Cine and Velocity Imaging

The functional evaluation of the heart is best accomplished with cine MRI techniques. Cine MRI techniques have the same intrinsic geometric relationship and can be acquired in much shorter periods of time. They offer the advantage of significantly improved temporal resolution, with images representing up to every 20 msec of the cardiac cycle.[B1]

One of the most important features of cine MRI techniques is the relationship to turbulent flow. The loss of signal with turbulence has been used as a method for relative quantification of valve lesions, as will be discussed later. It must be pointed out, though, that this loss of signal is sensitive to the acquisition parameters, such as TR, TE, and voxel size and orientation to the flow.[B2, P1]

Magnetic resonance imaging has the significant advantage of the ability to obtain contiguous images in any anatomic plane. In general, it is best to image perpendicular to the object of interest in any tomographic technique, but in the case of a three-dimensional structure like the heart, this is impossible to accomplish at all times, and it is impractical to acquire orthogonal images in all patients.[B1, U5] (Fig. 49–3). The advantages of complex oblique angles are obvious; however, they are difficult to reproduce and in general sacrifice image quality.

All the techniques described involve some form of physiologic triggering. The overall quality of any triggered magnetic resonance imaging technique depends on the quality of the trigger. The quality of the images and data obtained from them also depends on the regularity of the heart beat, because cine MRI averages many heart cycles for each image frame. Although images can be obtained in patients with atrial fibrillation, the overall quality depends on the standard deviation of the RR interval during each individual acquisition.[U1]

VALVULAR REGURGITANCY

The hallmark of regurgitant lesions on magnetic resonance imaging in cine MRI is the dynamic loss of signal during the appropriate part of the cycle in a chamber through a valve which during that part of the cycle should normally be closed (Fig. 49–4). The mitral valve that is incompetent will show a triangular loss of signal in the left atrium during systole. Studies comparing the dimensions, duration, and area of this signal loss compare favorably with the findings on echocardiagraphy and angiography.[U3] At present, only relative grading of these lesions is possible.[S4] (Fig. 49–5).

The relative grading of the severity of mitral regurgitation, coupled with the other quantitative data from magnetic resonance imaging may provide the necessary data for improved patient management. Magnetic resonance imaging provides accurate ventricular volumes, stroke volumes, ejection fractions, and cardiac output. It also allows for the comparison of right ventricular and left ventricular stroke volumes accurately obtained without any geometric assumptions. End-diastolic volume appears as a more accurate predictor of surgical success than ejection fraction.[B3] Measurements of wall stress can be calculated from MRI

Text continued on page 903

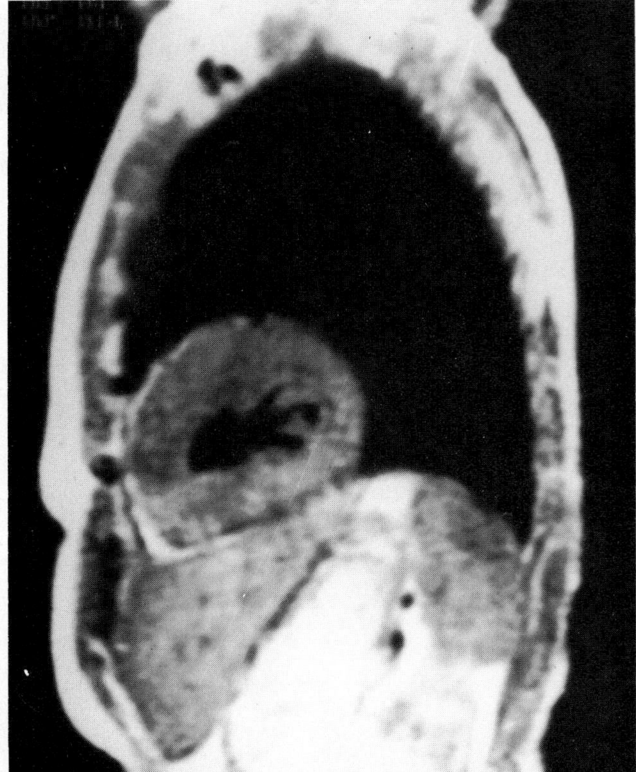

Figure 49–3. A sagittal gated spin echo image through the body of the left ventricle in a patient with left ventricle hypertrophy. Note the excellent definition of endocardial and epicardial walls when imaging perpendicular to the chamber.

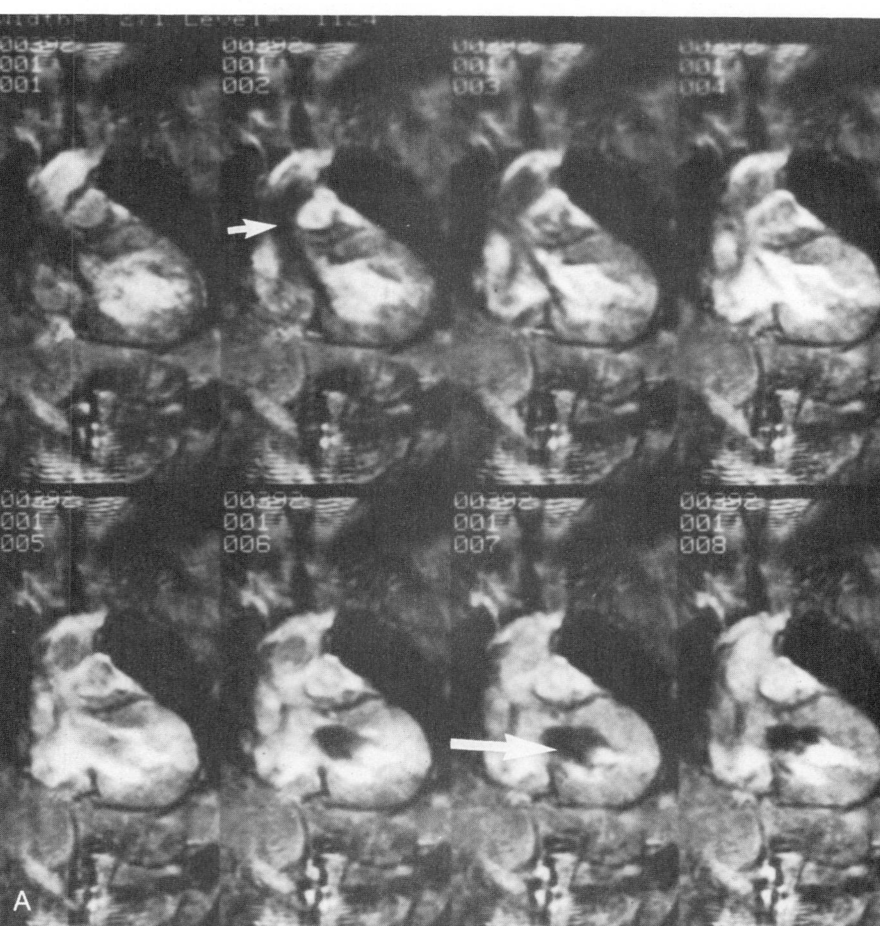

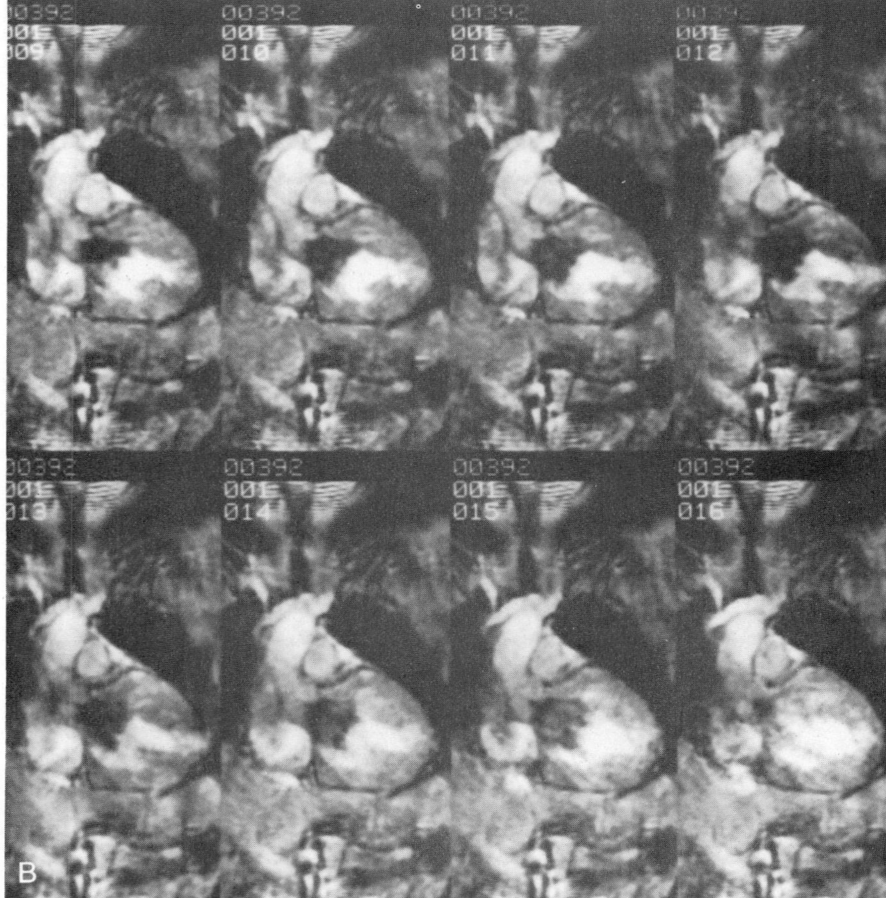

Figure 49–4. *A* and *B* are a series of 16 cine gradient-recalled coronal images through the aortic valve and left ventricle, beginning at the QRS. Note the loss of signal during systole seen in the ascending aorta (small arrow) from relative aortic stenosis. The dominant lesion is aortic insufficiency, causing a diastolic loss of signal (large arrow) originating from the aortic valve and extending into the left ventricular cavity.

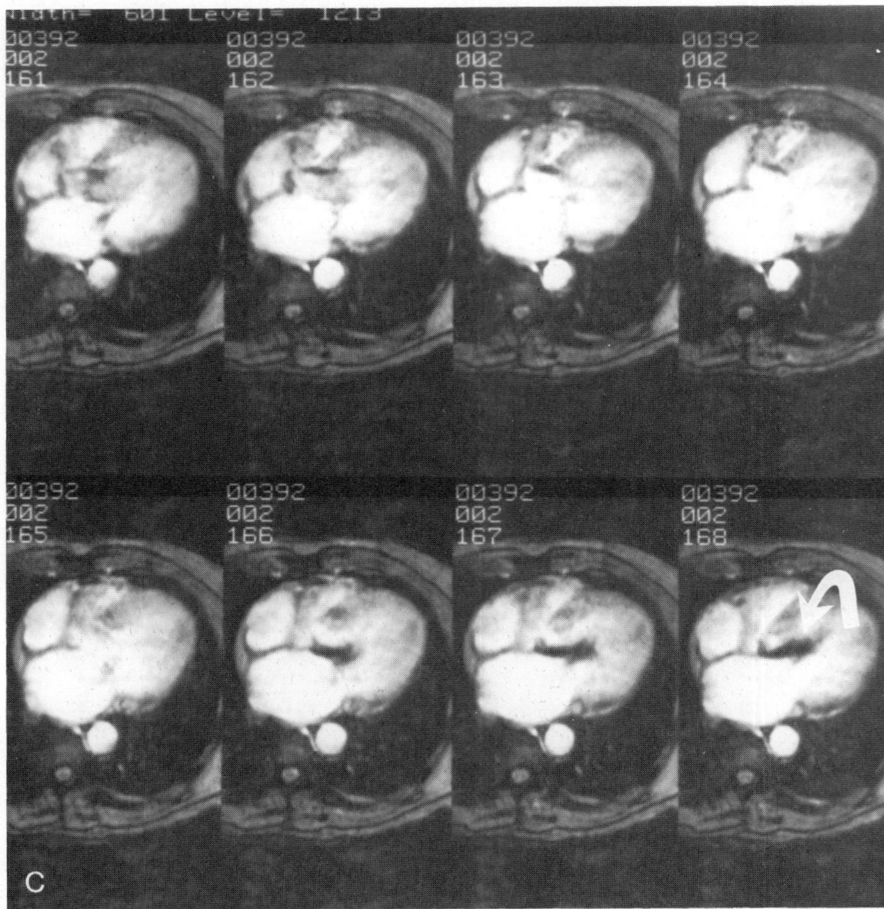

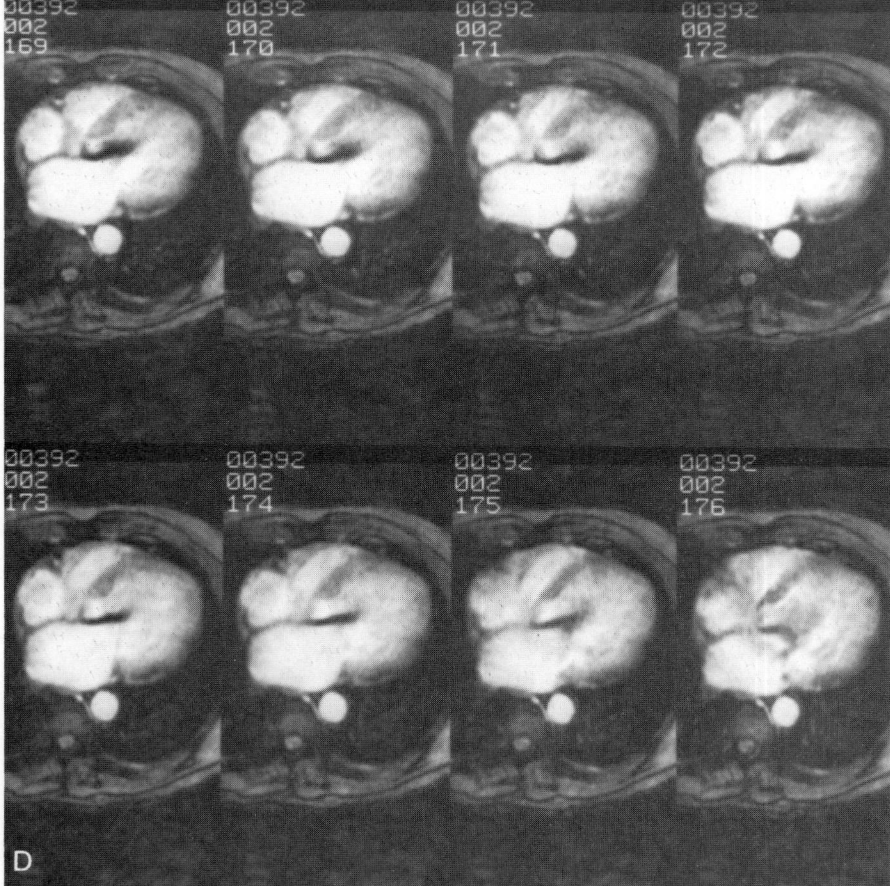

Figure 49–4 *Continued* *C* and *D* are a series of 16 cine gradient-recalled axial images through the left ventricle beginning at the QRS. Note the diastolic loss of signal medial to the anterior leaflet of the mitral valve (curved arrow).

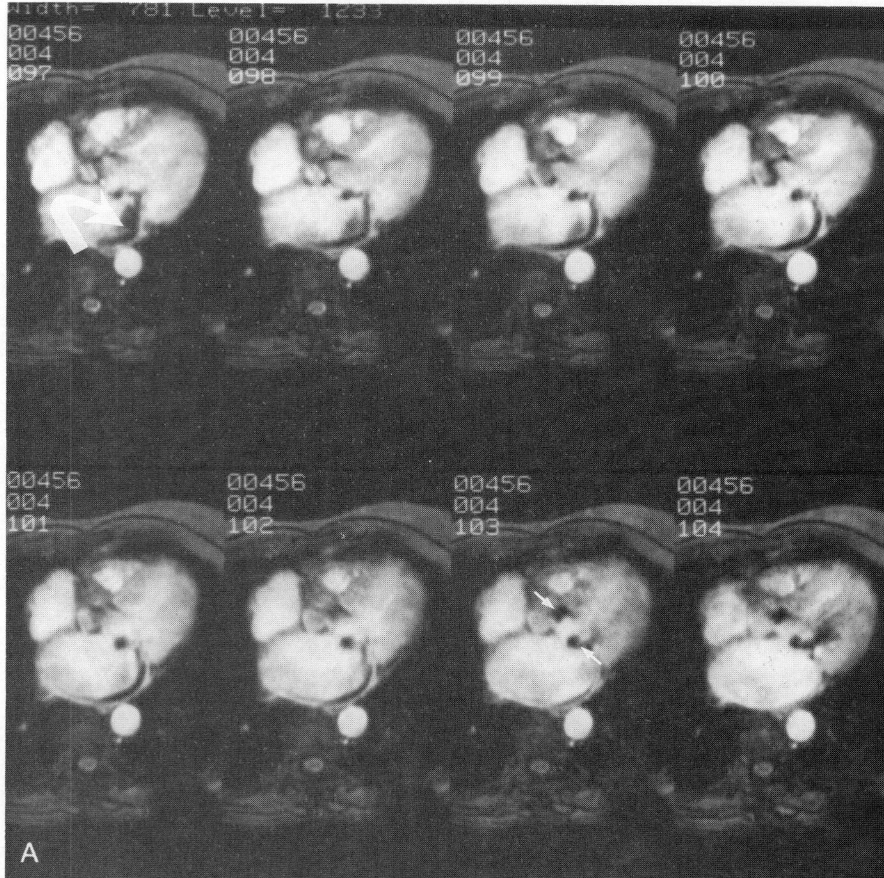

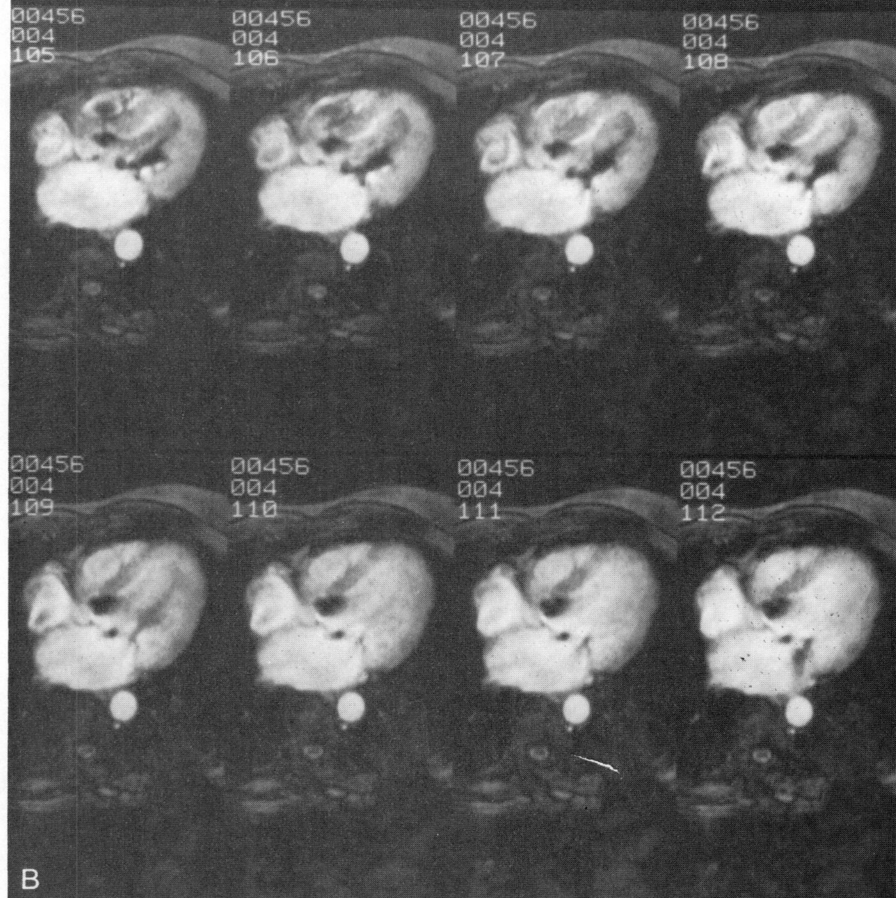

Figure 49–5. *A* and *B* are a series of 16 cine gradient-recalled axial images through the aortic valve, top of mitral valve, and left ventricle, beginning at the QRS. Note the prominent signal loss at the valve leaflets, which does not change throughout the cardiac cycle, secondary to valve thickening and calcification (small arrows). A systolic loss of signal, originating at the mitral valve and wrapping around the posterior aspect of the left atrium, indicates mitral regurgitation (curved arrow). Note the diastolic loss of signal along the interventricular septum, indicative of aortic regurgitation.

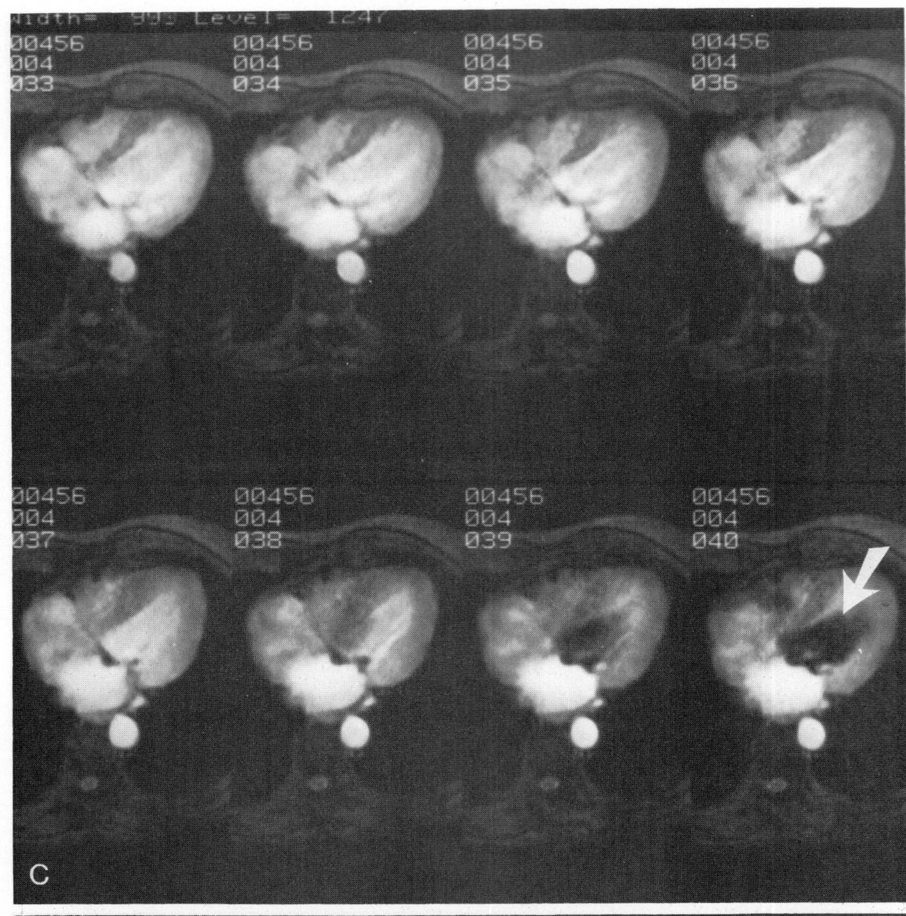

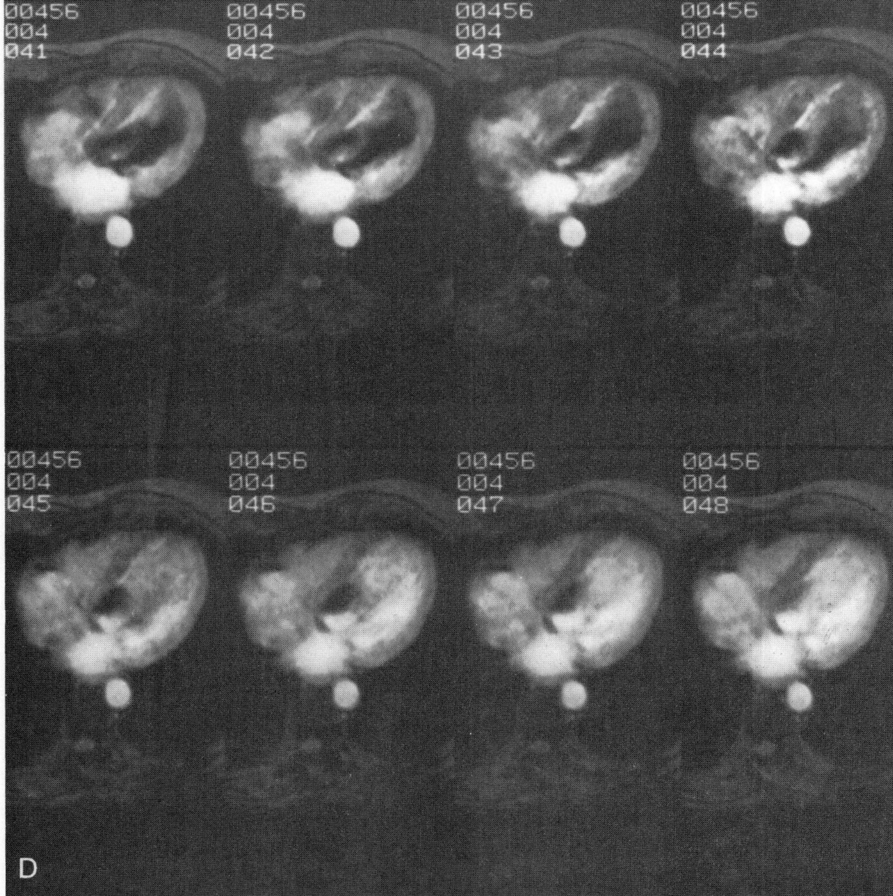

Figure 49–5 *Continued* *C* and *D* are an axial cine series at a level below *A* and *B*. The dramatic signal loss from the aortic insufficiency and mitral stenosis can clearly be seen and separated in the diastolic images (arrow).

data when coupled to peripheral pulse and pressure monitoring. The reproducibility of cine MRI allows a noninvasive functional evaluation to improve the monitoring of medical therapy and for potential prediction of appropriate surgical intervention.[H2]

Magnetic resonance imaging methods also provide important data in the differential diagnosis and evaluation of potential complications. The excellent contrast and large field of view facilitate the evaluation of interventional complications. Magnetic resonance imaging is an extremely sensitive method for evaluation of thrombosis in the left atrium. Typically, chronic thrombus will be of intermediate signal intensity and is less likely to result in thromboembolism. Acute thrombus, because of the paramagnetic effects of some hemoglobin degradation products, will be relatively high in signal on T1-weighted images and dark on gradient-recalled sequences due to its iron content (Fig. 49–6).

Acute mitral valve insufficiency is difficult for magnetic resonance imaging evaluation because of the critical status of the majority of these patients; however, infarctions involving the papillary muscles have been identified.

The identification of aortic insufficiency is made by the presence of a diastolic loss of signal in the left ventricle that originates from the aortic valve coursing apically along the interventricular septum medial to the anterior leaflet of the mitral valve. The severity of the lesion is also crudely evaluated by the size, duration, and dimensions of this signal loss. As in mitral regurgitation, the regurgitant fraction can be reproducibly calculated from differences of the right and left ventricular stroke volumes. In the management of aortic insufficiency, magnetic resonance imaging provides reproducible measurements of ventricular volumes and mass. As with other modalities, it is often difficult to separate fused leaflets from true bicuspid valves.[P3]

The most common cause of tricuspid regurgitation is right atrial enlargement, usually associated with pulmonary hypertension. The characteristic finding on cine MRI is the triangular loss of signal originating from the tricuspid valve into an enlarged right atrium, best seen on transaxial projections. As with two-dimensional echocardiography, it is not unusual to see a small reversal of flow at the valve in early systolic closure in normal individuals.[M1] Magnetic resonance imaging can help exclude potential treatable causes of tricuspid regurgitation, such as chronic pulmonary emboli, pulmonary obstructive lesions, or cardiac tumors.

Although the pulmonic valve may be involved by rheumatic disease or carcinoid, most commonly pulmonic insufficiency is secondary to pulmonary hypertension. The most prominent role of magnetic resonance imaging may be to exclude other, treatable causes. As pulmonary transplantation increases, the sensitive evaluation of pulmonic insufficiency may become increasingly important.[S5]

VALVULAR STENOSIS

Valvular stenosis is identified by the loss of signal generated by the valvular lesion. Also, the immobility of the valve can be identified on cine MRI imaging. It has been stated that magnetic resonance imaging cannot visualize calcification; however, calcification is visible as a negative defect against the bright blood background of cine MRI imaging. Mitral stenosis is characterized by a diastolic loss of signal originating from the mitral valve. Mitral valve motion can be easily identified in normal individuals. In mitral stenosis the motion is clearly restricted, and frequently calcification can be identified in the immobile mitral leaflets. This is best seen in the transaxial or apical four-chamber views. The presence of left atrial thrombus occurs in as many as 20 percent of mitral stenosis patients and represents a potential serious complication to mitral commisurotomy or balloon valvuloplasty. Magnetic resonance imaging is the most sensitive technique in this population for left atrial thrombus detection.

Magnetic resonance imaging provides for the exclusion of other potential causes of mitral stenosis–like symptoms, including tumors involving the pulmonary veins or cardiac tumors such as left atrial myxomas.

Aortic stenosis is easily identified by cine MRI techniques. The mobility of the valve leaflets and associated turbulence during systole are characteristic of aortic stenosis (Fig. 49–7). Magnetic resonance imaging is relatively poor at quantifying the degree of stenosis. Recent improvements in image quality may allow direct images parallel to the valve for extremely accurate valve areas. Velocity maps may allow more accurate calculations of gradients in the future.

The reproducible measurements of end-diastolic volumes, stroke volume, and wall stress may prove to be the optimal method for following aortic stenosis patients preoperatively. Prosthetic valves are in general not a contraindication for imaging, although they will distort the image immediately adjacent to the valve. Older Starr-Edwards valves with metal balls are considered a relative contraindication. Additionally, pacemakers are considered a contraindication. Some individuals also believe that implanted pacemaker wires are a relative contraindication to exposure to an MRI device.

Text continued on page 909

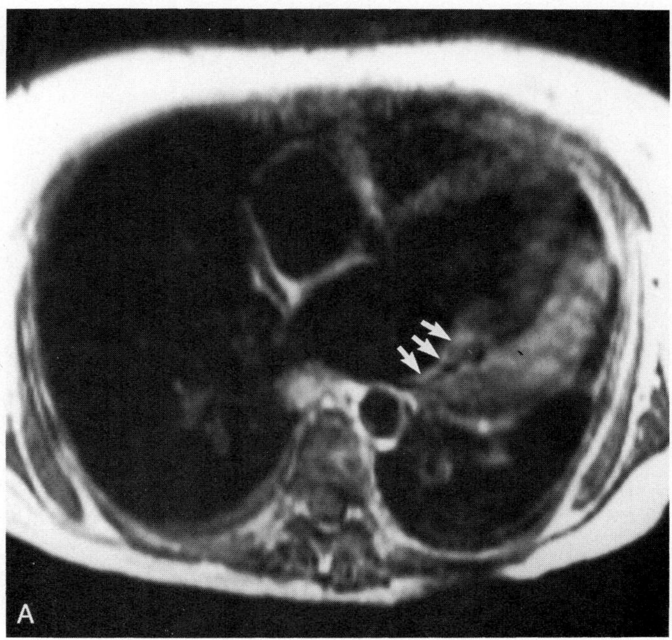

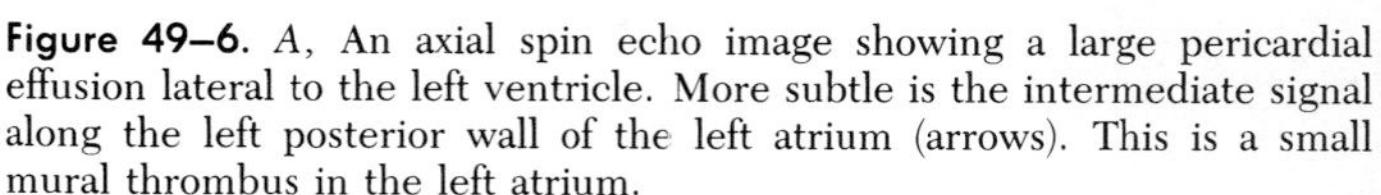

Figure 49–6. *A*, An axial spin echo image showing a large pericardial effusion lateral to the left ventricle. More subtle is the intermediate signal along the left posterior wall of the left atrium (arrows). This is a small mural thrombus in the left atrium.

Illustration continued on following page

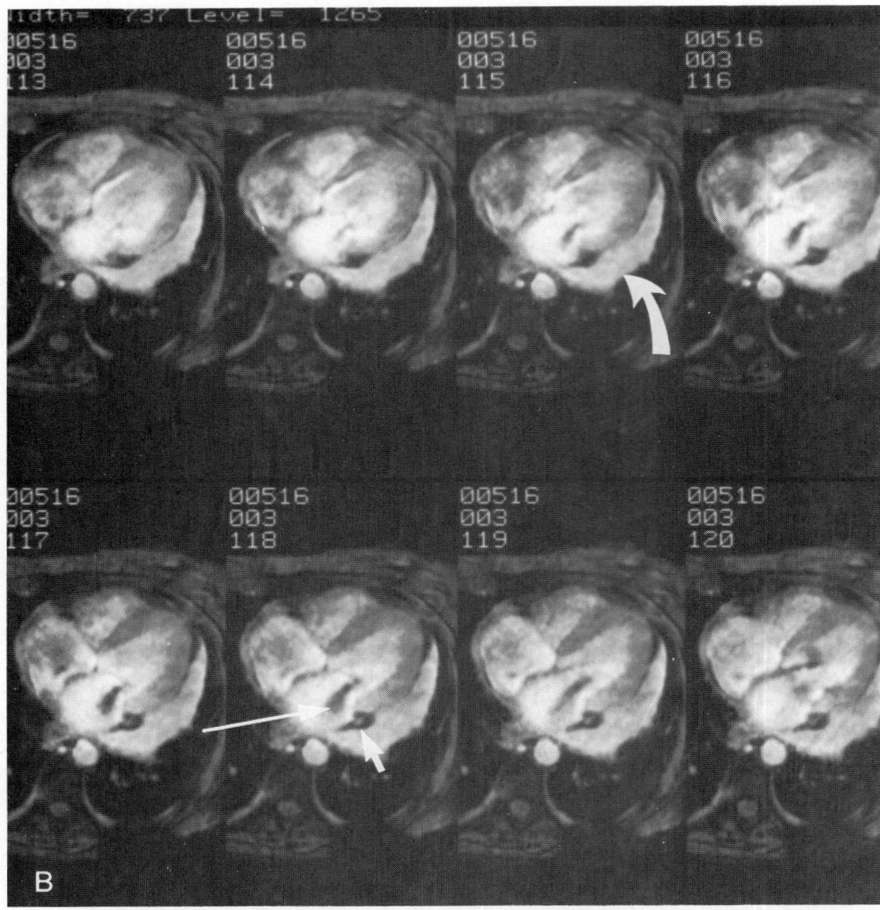

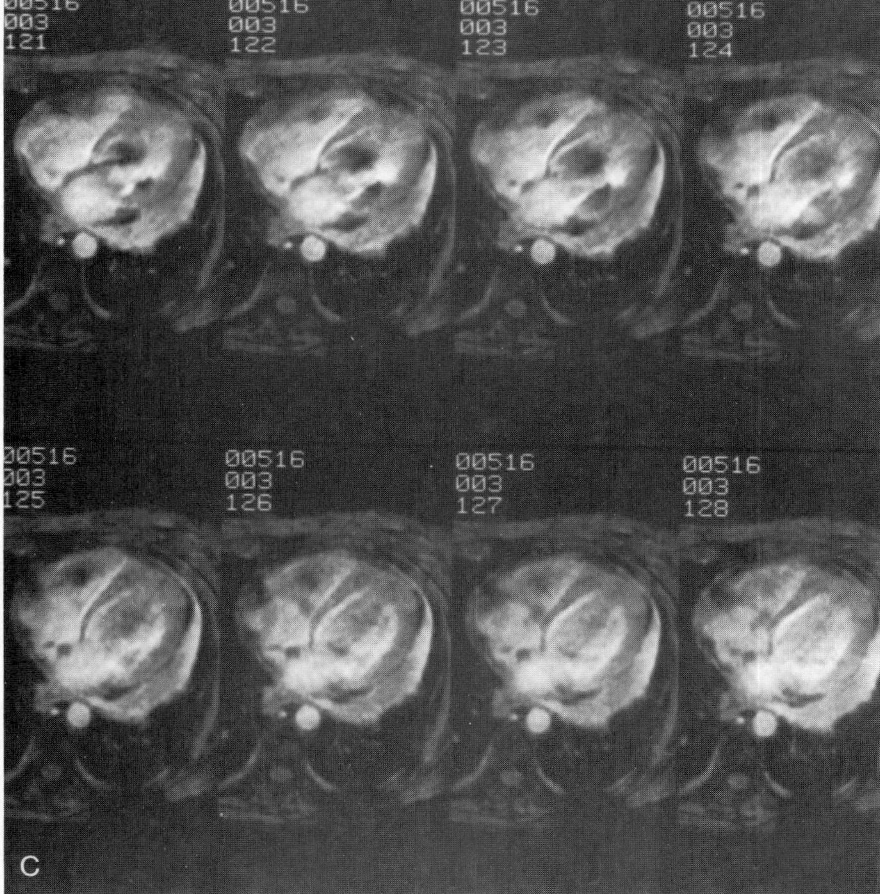

Figure 49–6 *Continued* *B* and *C* are axial cine gradient-recalled images through the same levels as *A*. Note the increased signal from the flowing fluid in the pericardial effusion (curved arrow). There are two areas of signal loss in the left atrium. One area is unchanged throughout the cardiac cycle, posteriorly on the left, corresponding to the signal in *A*—a recent left atrial thrombus (small arrow). The second area of signal loss corresponds to the systolic turbulence of mild mitral regurgitation (long arrow).

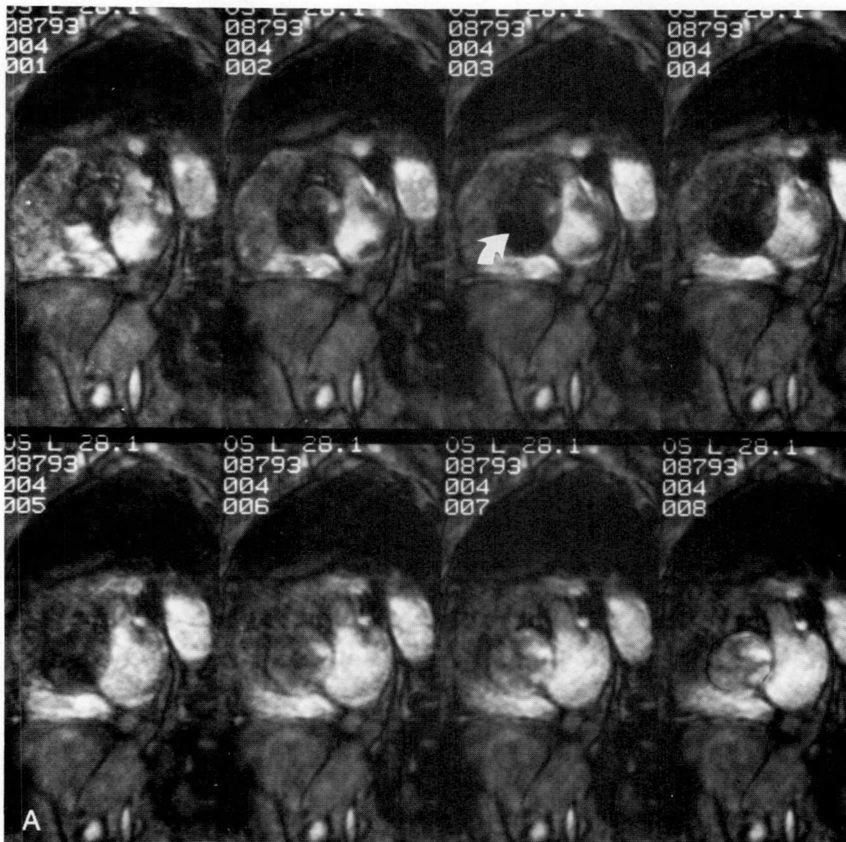

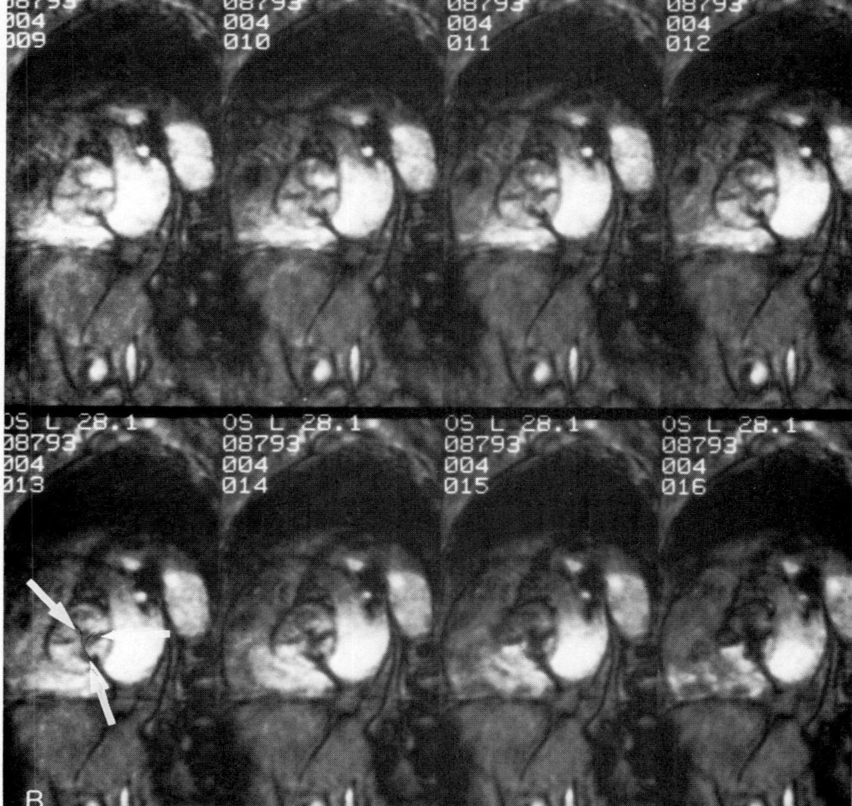

Figure 49–7. *A* and *B* are a series of 16 cine gradient-recalled coronal images through the aortic valve and left ventricle, beginning at the QRS. Note the loss of signal during systole seen in the ascending aorta (curved arrow), from aortic stenosis. Note the markedly dilated ascending aorta. The persistent loss of signal in the region of the aortic valve is consistent with aortic valve calcification (three arrows).

Illustration continued on following page

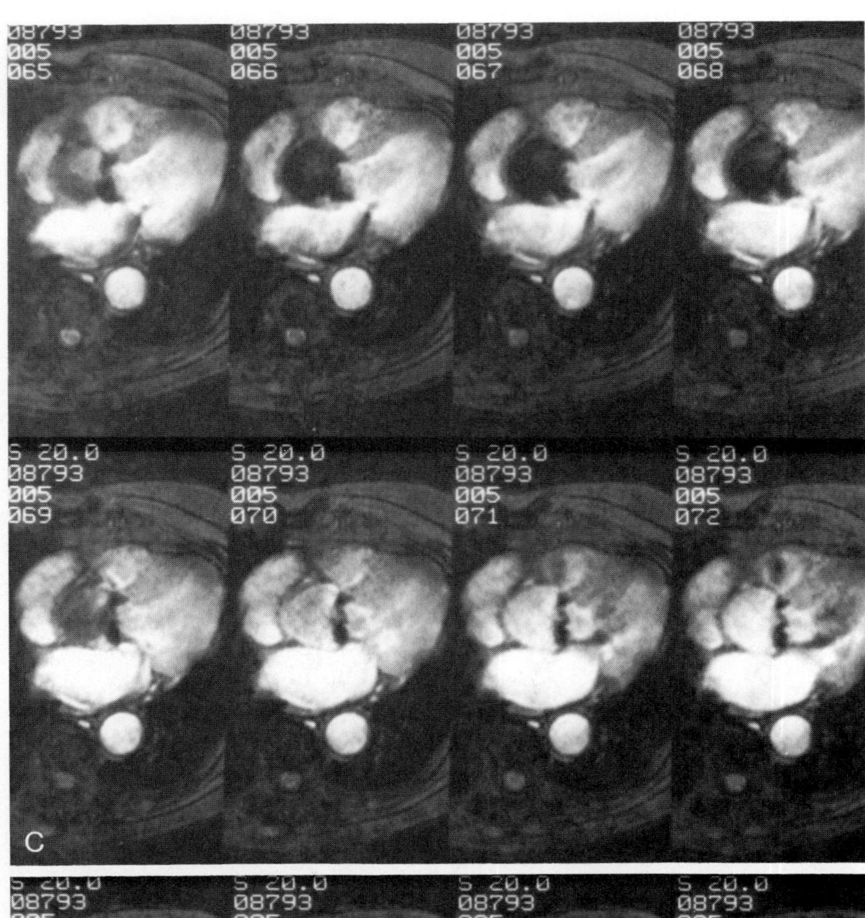

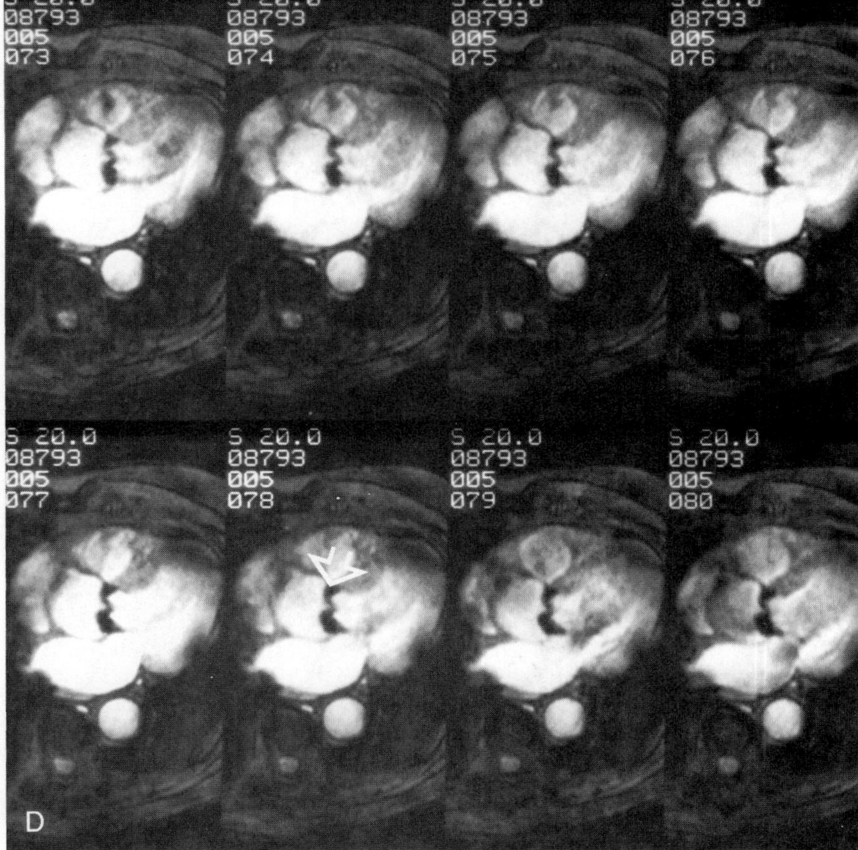

Figure 49–7 *Continued* *C* and *D* are axial cine images through the aortic valve in the same patient. Note the enlarged calcified aortic valve (open arrow) and thickened left ventricle.

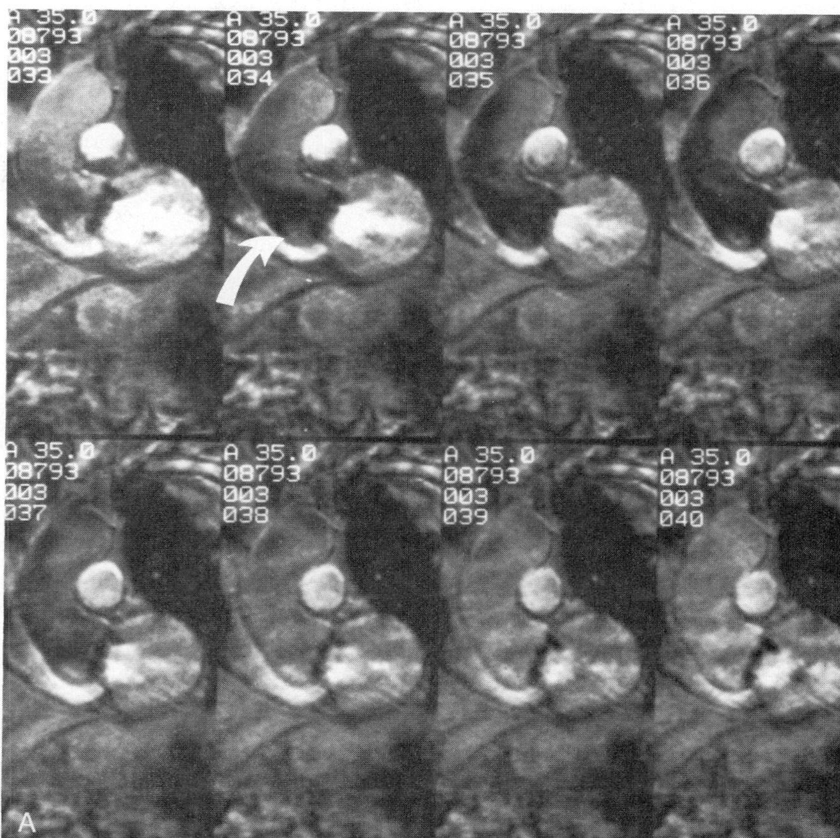

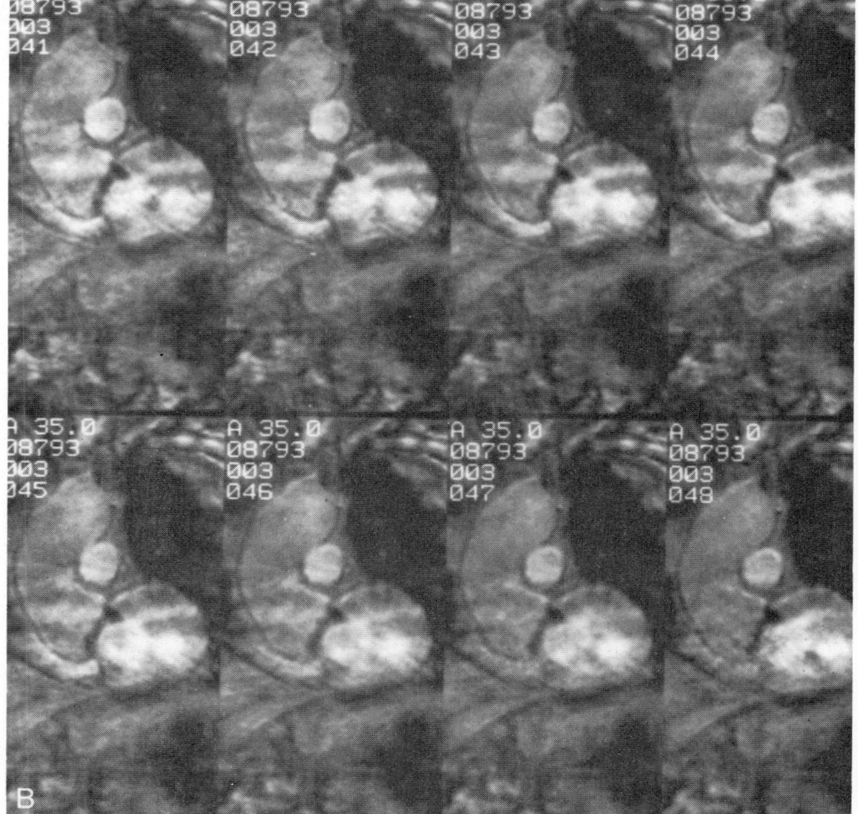

Figure 49–8. *A* and *B*, Double oblique angle imaging through the aortic valve in the same patient as in Figure 49–7. Note the calcified aortic valve leaflet and turbulence (curved arrow) from the aortic stenosis.

Illustration continued on following page

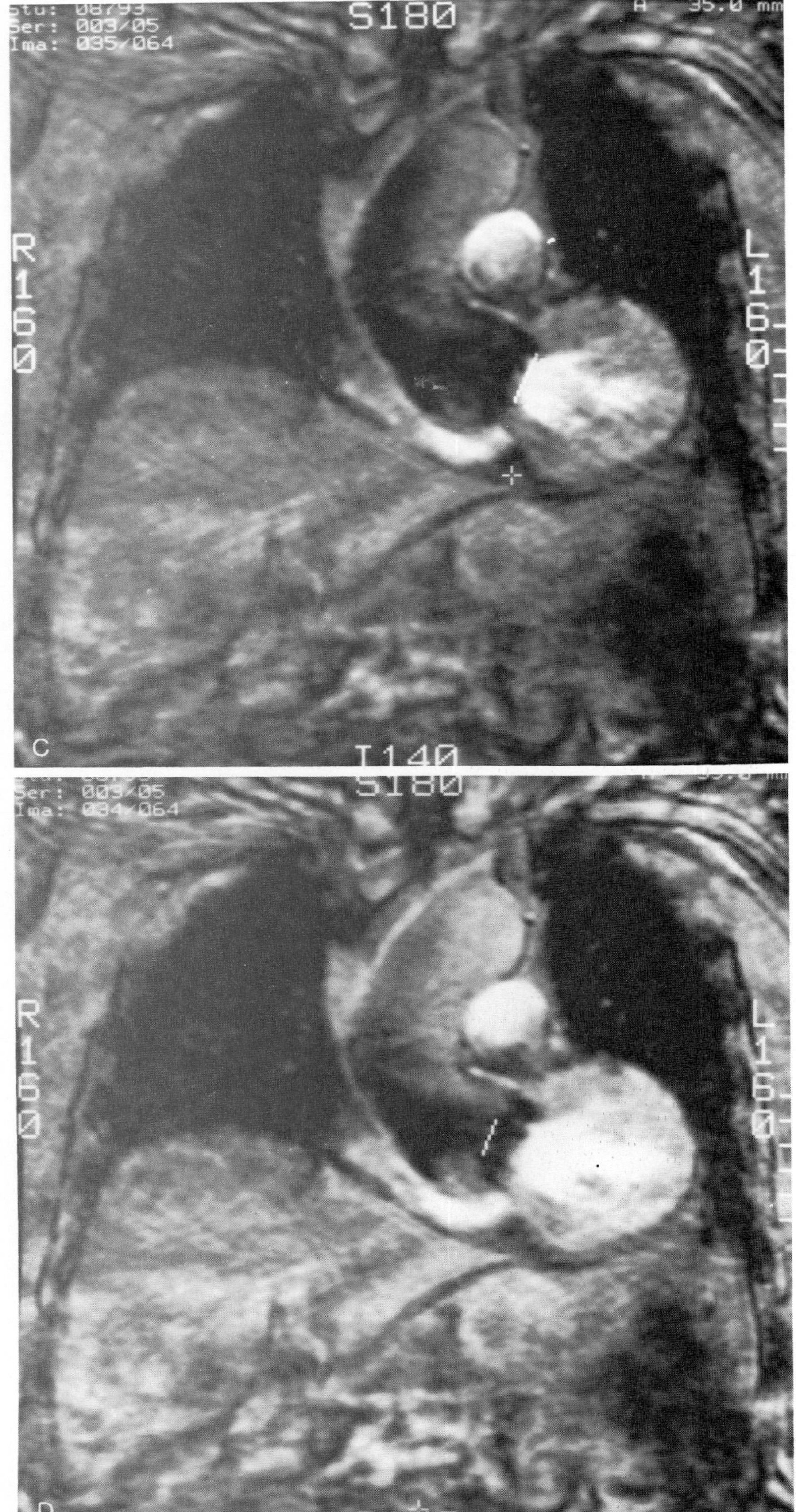

Figure 49–8 *Continued* *C* and *D* are two separate cine frames from which aortic dimensions can be calculated for preoperative planning.

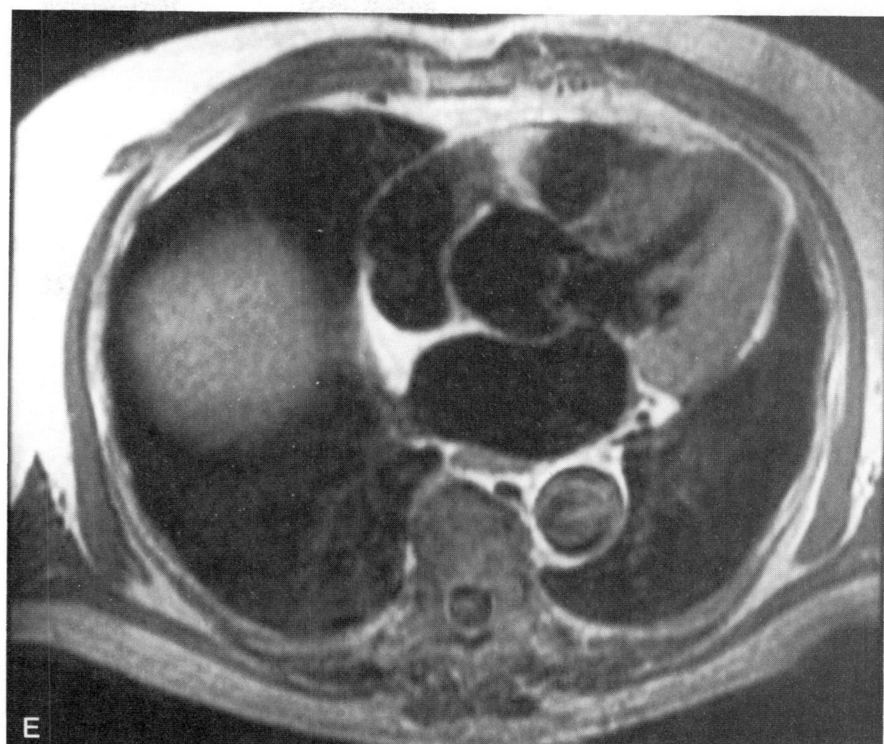

Figure 49–8 *Continued E*, A spin echo image showing the aortic outflow and left venticular wall thickness.

COMBINED LESIONS

The evaluation of combined valvular lesions is similar to that of the individual lesions described earlier. The characteristics by which management decisions are made may in some ways need to modified. The calculation of regurgitant volumes remains accurate, but in the presence of both aortic and mitral regurgitant lesions, the amount attributable to each individual lesion is impossible to determine with these methods. The mainstays of management remain the sensitive, reproducible anatomic and functional measurements, including myocardial mass and volume. If both left-sided and right-sided regurgitant lesions are present, the regurgitant fraction becomes relatively meaningless.[S2]

Aortic insufficiency associated with aortic dissections may require valve replacement at the time of repair. Use of tissue grafts in this surgical therapy may require significant preparation and prior knowledge of the size of the aortic annulus and the aorta itself. When this is performed in the presence of rheumatic disease and significant aortic calcification, estimation of the proper graft size may be difficult preoperatively, even using magnetic resonance imaging performed in the plane parallel to the valve and proximal aorta. However, oblique coronal images through the aorta may provide an accurate measure of the extent of aortic disease or involvement of the great vessels (Fig. 49–8).

SUMMARY

MRI represents a new noninvasive modality for the evaluation of valvular heart disease. When spin echo and cine MRI methods are combined, magnetic resonance imaging provides a relatively comprehensive evaluation of both anatomic and functional parameters necessary for the characterization and reproducible follow-up of patients. The major limitations of magnetic resonance imaging techniques are the relative cost and limited availability. Its use is handicapped in critically ill patients. The overall sensitivity and specificity and wealth of information available may prove to be a major tool in the evaluation and decision process. The recent development of accurate and reproducible velocity maps in any location or projection may improve further our ability to care for valvular disease.

References

B

1. Buser, P. T., Auffermann, W., Holt, W. W., et al.: Noninvasive evaluation of global left ventricular function with use of cine nuclear magnetic resonance. J. Am. Coll. Cardiol. 13:1294, 1989.
2. Bryant, D. J., Payne, J. A., Firmin, D. N., and Longmore, D. B.: Measurement of flow with NMR imaging using a gradient pulse and phase difference technique. J. Comput. Assist. Tomogr. 8:588, 1984.
3. Borrow, K., Green, L. H., Mann, T., et al.: End-systolic volume as a predictor of postoperative left ventricular performance in volume overload from valvular regurgitation. Am. J. Med. 68:655, 1980.

C

1. Chung, K. J., Simpson, I. A., Newman, R., et al.: Cine magnetic resonance imaging for evaluation of congenital heart disease: Role in pediatric cardiology compared with echocardiography and angiography. J. Pediatr. 113:1028, 1988.

H

1. Herfkens, R. J.: Magnetic resonance imaging of the cardiovascular system. *In* Putman, C., and Ravin, C. (eds.): Textbook of Diagnostic Imaging. Vol. 3. W. B. Saunders, Philadelphia, 1988, pp. 1764–1771.
2. Higgins, C. B., Holt, W., Pflugfelder, P., and Sechtem, U.: Functional evaluation of the heart with magnetic resonance imaging. Magn. Reson. Med. 321:121, 1988.
3. Hill, J. A., Akins, E. W., Fitzsimmons, J. R., and Conti, C. R.: Mitral stenosis: Imaging by nuclear magnetic resonance. Am. J. Cardiol. 57:352, 1986.

M

1. Miyatake, K., Okamoto, M., Kinoshita, N., et al.: Evaluation of tricuspid regurgitation by pulsed Doppler and two-dimensional echocardiography. Circulation 66:777, 1982.

P

1. Podolak, M. J., Hedlund, L. W., Evans, A. J., and Herfkens, R. J.: Evaluation of flow through simulated vascular stenoses with gradient echo magnetic resonance imaging. Invest. Radiol. 24:184, 1989.
2. Pfugfelder, P. W., Sechtem, U. P., White, R. D., et al.: Noninvasive evaluation of mitral regurgitation by analysis of left atrial signal loss in cine magnetic resonance. Am. Heart J. 117:1113, 1989.
3. Pflugfelder, P. W., Landzberg, J. S., Cassidy, M. M., et al.: Comparison of cine MR imaging with Doppler echocardiography for the evaluation of aortic regurgitation. AJR 152:729, 1989.

NUCLEAR MAGNETIC RESONANCE ASSESSMENT OF VALVULAR DISEASE

R

1. Rehr, R. B., Filipchuk, N. G., Malloy, C. R., and Peshock, R. M.: Magnetic resonance imaging in aortic valve, ascending aortic and isthmic aortic disease. Am. J. Cardiol. 55:1243, 1985.
2. Roberts, W. C.: Morphologic features of the normal and abnormal mitral valve. Am. J. Cardiol. 51:1005, 1983.
3. Rumancik, W. M.: Cardiovascular disease: Evaluation with MR phase imaging. Radiology 166:63, 1988.

S

1. Sechtem, U., Pflugfelder, P. W., and Higgins, C. B.: Quantification of cardiac function by conventional and cine magnetic resonance imaging. Cardiovasc. Intervent. Radiol. 10:365, 1987.
2. Sechtem, U., Pflugfelder, P. W., Cassidy, M. M., et al.: Mitral aortic regurgitation: Quantification of regurgitant volumes with cine MR imaging. Radiology 167:425, 1988.
3. Sechtem, U., Pflugfelder, P. W., White, R. D., et al.: Cine MR imaging: Potential for the evaluation of cardiovascular function. AJR 148:239, 1987.
4. Schiebbler, M., Axel, L., Reichek, N., et al.: Correlation of cine MR imaging with two-dimensional pulsed Doppler echocardiography in valvular insufficiency. J. Comput. Assist. Tomogr. 11:627, 1987.
5. Slone, R. M., Hill, J. A., Atkins, E. W., and Conti, C. R.: Magnetic resonance imaging late after tricuspid valvulectomy. Am. J. Cardiol. 59:1426, 1987.

U

1. Utz, J. A., Herfkens, R. J., Heinsimer, J. A., et al.: Cine MR determination of left ventricular ejection fraction. AJR 148:839, 1987.
2. Underwood, S. R., Gill, C. R. W., Firmin, D. N., et al.: Left ventricular volume measured rapidly by oblique magnetic resonance imaging. Br. Heart J. 60:188, 1988.
3. Underwood, S. R., Firmin, D. N., Klipstein, R. H., et al.: Magnetic resonance velocity mapping: Clinical application of a new technique. Br. Heart J. 57:404, 1987.
4. Utz, J. A., Herfkens, R. J., Heinsimer, J. A., et al.: Valvular regurgitation: Dynamic MR imaging. Radiology 168:91, 1988.
5. Underwood, S. R., Klipstein, R. H., Firmin, D. N., et al.: Magnetic resonance assessment of aortic and mitral regurgitation. Br. Heart J. 56:455, 1986.

V

1. Van Rossum, A. C., Visser, F. C., Sprenger, M., et al.: Evaluation of magnetic resonance imaging for determination of left ventricular ejection fraction and comparison with angiography. Am. J. Cardiol. 62:628, 1988.

Chapter 50

Evaluation of Ischemic Heart Disease by Nuclear Magnetic Resonance

GERALD WISENBERG, M.D., F.R.C.P.C.

DETECTION OF ACUTE MYOCARDIAL ISCHEMIA ... 911
Changes in Inherent Tissue Properties ... 911
Use of Paramagnetic Agents ... 911
DETECTION OF ACUTE MYOCARDIAL INFARCTION ... 913
Changes in Magnetic Resonance Signal Intensity ... 913
Changes in Myocardial Relaxation Times ... 914
Summary ... 915
DETECTION OF REPERFUSED INFARCTION ... 918
Changes in Inherent Tissue Properties ... 918
Use of Nonproton Nuclei ... 919
Summary ... 919
ESTIMATION OF MYOCARDIAL INFARCT SIZE ... 919
Using Unenhanced Methods ... 920
Use of Paramagnetic Contrast Agents ... 921
ASSESSMENT OF LEFT VENTRICULAR FUNCTION IN ISCHEMIC HEART DISEASE ... 923
Clinical Studies of Contraction ... 923
CLINICAL STUDIES OF THE MYOCARDIUM IN ISCHEMIC DISEASE ... 925
Changes in Magnetic Resonance Signal Intensity and Relaxation Times ... 925
Use of Gd-DTPA ... 925
SUMMARY ... 926

Nuclear magnetic resonance has evolved as a unique, noninvasive tool capable of assessing many aspects of ischemic heart disease. The detection of recent myocardial infarction with and without the use of parenterally administered contrast agents has been consistently demonstrated. In addition, the changes that occur on nuclear magnetic resonance images following myocardial reperfusion potentially may allow the use of this technique for monitoring the effectiveness of revascularization therapy. Further, the use of paramagnetic contrast agents ultimately may allow nuclear magnetic resonance to be used for the quantitation of regional myocardial blood flow, using image-derived T1 and T2 relaxation measurements. Concurrently, using sophisticated pulse sequences, images of ventricular function, presented as an endless loop cine display, provide useful details of global and regional left and right ventricular function, both in terms of changes in cavitary dimensions and systolic wall thickening. Spectroscopy, capable of supplying important metabolic data, may allow the use of nuclear magnetic resonance as a comprehensive, noninvasive modality for assessing acute and chronic ischemic/infarcted myocardial tissue in an unparalleled fashion that no other noninvasive technique can achieve. In this chapter, the capabilities of nuclear magnetic resonance (NMR) for evaluation of ischemic heart disease are discussed, and also the further investigations that are needed and their potential. Cardiac spectroscopy is covered in chapters 46 and 54.

DETECTION OF ACUTE MYOCARDIAL ISCHEMIA

Changes in Inherent Tissue Properties

The factors affecting the ability of nuclear magnetic resonance to demonstrate regional differences in myocardial signal on images are the density or concentration of the nucleus being imaged, and the chemical interactions occurring between the species containing the particular nucleus and the surrounding molecules. In most commercially available instruments, the hydrogen proton is the imaged nucleus. The process of acute myocardial infarction, which, after a period of several hours, produces edema and an increase in tissue proton concentration, would be expected to lead to regional changes in nuclear magnetic resonance relaxation times, T1 and T2. These changes should cause abnormal signal intensity at the site of infarction on NMR images. However, with brief periods of acute ischemia, significant changes in tissue water content or relaxation rates may not evolve for 1 or more hours, although Williams and associates demonstrated an increase in T1 relaxation time within 30 minutes of occlusion.[W3] Nevertheless, significant alterations in relaxation times were not observed by Brown and colleagues at 40 minutes following coronary occlusion when myocardial values were measured ex vivo by spectroscopy.[B3]

Use of Paramagnetic Agents

If inherent tissue properties require a period of time to change in response to acute ischemia, it is possible that a contrast agent could detect physiologic processes earlier. McNamara and associates were the first to demonstrate that the intravenous administration of a paramagnetic contrast agent, gadolinium-DTPA, could be useful for the demonstration of acute ischemia.[M2] In this canine study, dogs underwent coronary ligation. Three of nine received a saline (sham) infusion, while six received Gd-DTPA, 0.5 mmol/kg. Gd-DTPA was given 1 minute after the occlusion of the left anterior descending artery; the animals were sacrificed 1 minute later; and the hearts were excised. The excised hearts were then imaged and samples subsequently removed for T1 and T2 value measurement by spectroscopy (Figs. 50–1 and 50–2). In the sham treated animals, as expected, there was no difference in either T1 or T2 values or percent of water content between regionally ischemic and normal myocardium after only a total of 2 minutes of ischemic insult. However, in the six treated animals,

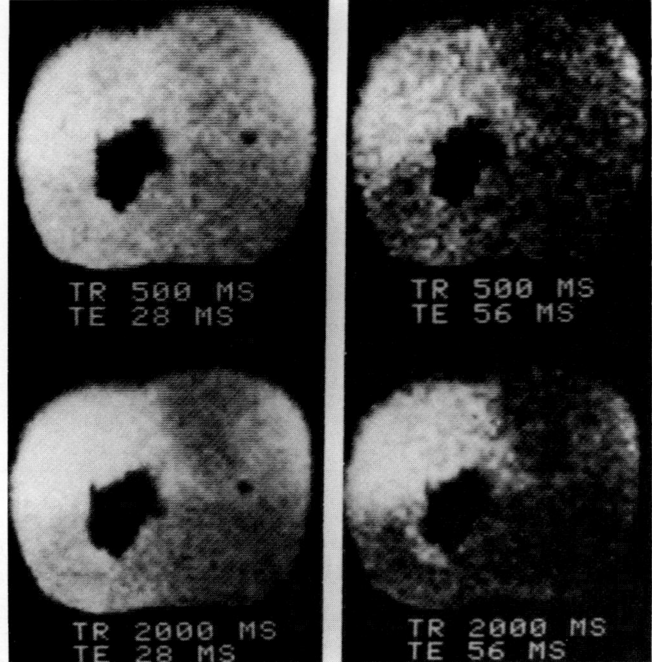

Figure 50–1. Cross-sectional spin-echo images through the mid-portion of the left ventricle of a dog that received Gd-DTPA one minute after acute occlusion of the left anterior descending coronary artery. The TR and TE imaging parameters are shown with each image. The ischemic anterior wall of the left ventricle appears as a high-intensity region owing to negative enhancement of adjacent normal myocardium by Gd-DTPA. Contrast between normal and ischemic myocardium is greatest on the SE 2000/56 image *(lower right)*. (From McNamara, M. T., Higgins, C. B., Ehman, R. L., et al.: Acute myocardial ischemia:magnetic resonance contrast enhancement with Gadolinium-DTPA. Radiology 153:157–163, 1984, with permission.)

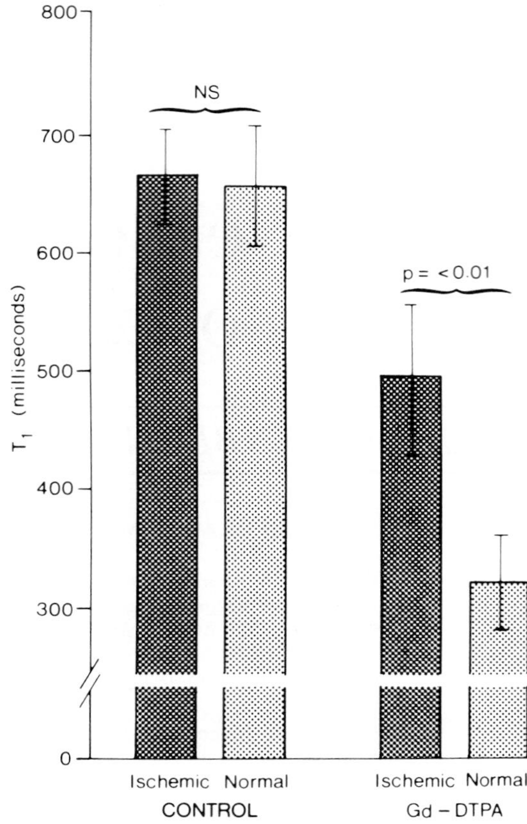

Figure 50–2. Block diagram showing the mean ± standard deviation for T1 relaxation times determined from image intensity for normal myocardial (Normal) and ischemic myocardium (Ischemic) of saline-injected (Control) dogs and of dogs that received intravenous Gd-DTPA (Gd-DTPA) during acute ischemia. There was no significant difference (p = NS) in T1 between ischemic and normal myocardium in the control group. T1 was significantly ($p < 0.01$) shorter in normal myocardium compared with ischemic myocardium in the Gd-DTPA dogs. (From McNamara, M. T., Higgins, C. B., Ehman, R. L., et al.: Acute myocardial ischemia: Magnetic resonance contrast enhancement with Gadolinium-DTPA. Radiology 153:157–163, 1984, with permission.)

there was a significantly greater reduction in nonischemic myocardium versus ischemic myocardium T1 (323 versus 496 msec, respectively) and T2 (31 versus 38 msec).

Runge and co-workers performed in vivo imaging in an attempt to demonstrate acute ischemia both prior to and subsequent to Gd-DTPA injection in dogs.[R5] Before contrast injection, the region of myocardial ischemia produced by 1 hour of occlusion was visualized using multiecho spin echo pulse sequences in only two of the six dogs studied. However, the area of ischemia was consistently observed on spin echo images (TE 30, 60, 90, and 120 msec) obtained 10 minutes after a bolus injection of 0.25 mmol/kg of Gd-DTPA.

Johnston and Liu, in addition to a Gd-DTPA infusion to enhance contrast, used dipyridamole to increase the disparity in regional myocardial blood flows during acute ischemia.[J3, J5] In excised canine heart studies with dipyridamole, the severity of ischemia could readily be characterized, particularly if the reduction in resting blood flow was marked—i.e., less than 0.5 ml/min/g. In this range, there was a significant correlation between regional myocardial blood flow and 1/T1. However, with subocclusive stenoses, it was not possible to demonstrate regional flow differences with acute ischemia using the same vasodilator and paramagnetic agent (Fig. 50–3). The investigators speculated that the use of a constant infusion of Gd-DTPA reduced the rate of

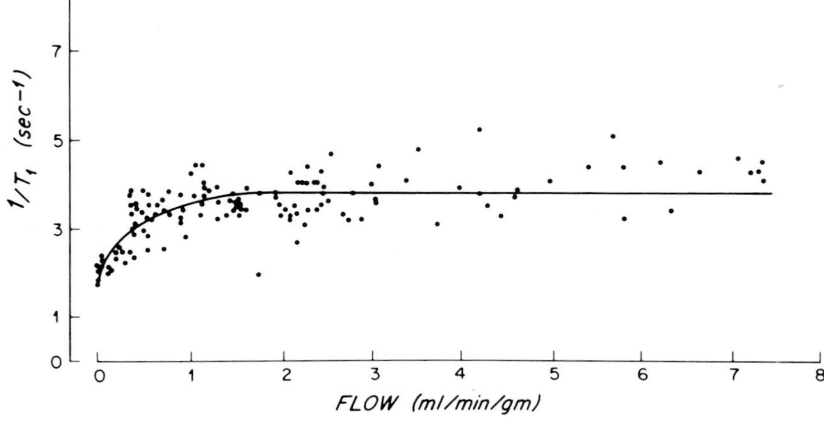

Figure 50–3. Relationship between 1/T1 and regional myocardial flow; r = 0.51, $p < 0.001$. Note that there is little correlation between flow and 1/T1 when flow is > 1 ml/min/g, i.e., hyperemic flow. (From Johnston, D. L., Liu, P., Lauffer, R. B., et al.: Acute myocardial ischemia: Magnetic resonance contrast enhancement with Gadolinium-DTPA. J. Nucl. Med. 28:871, 1987, with permission.)

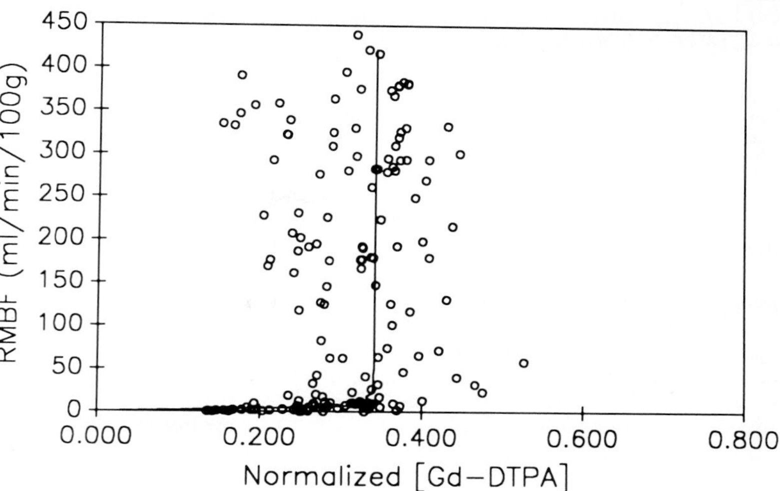

Figure 50–4. Flow versus normalized [Gd-DTPA]: acute, immediate sacrifice. Regional myocardial blood flow (RMBF) versus normalized [Gd-DTPA] following 25-minute constant infusion in acutely ischemic dogs. There is no relationship between flow and [Gd-DTPA], with the differences in concentration occurring over a very narrow range.

washout of Gd-DTPA from the hyperemic normal myocardium, thus decreasing the potential for equalization with the concentrations of material in the stenotic regions.

In our laboratory, we have determined that a constant infusion tends to deliver material not so much in a flow-dependent fashion but rather in a manner dependent on regional extracellular water content[D2] (Fig. 50–4). In acute ischemia of less than 30 minutes' duration, when insufficient time has elapsed for regional edema to develop, no regional differences in Gd-DTPA concentration were observed in excised heart tissue after a 25-minute infusion. However, in subacute infarction (3 to 5 days postocclusion), in which total water content was increased by 6 percent and extracellular volume presumably increased correspondingly, sequestration of Gd-DTPA in infarcted tissue is observed with progressively lower concentrations in the higher flow regions, both during and 2 minutes following the discontinuation of a 25-minute constant infusion.

The quantitative evaluation of acute ischemia across a broad range of flows from near 0 to 300 to 400 ml/min/100 g would require a paramagnetic agent that distributes to myocardium in a direct linear relationship to regional myocardial blood flow, and which has a prolonged residual time in myocardium to allow in vivo imaging for quantitation of regional T1 and T2 values. Such an agent has as yet not been developed.

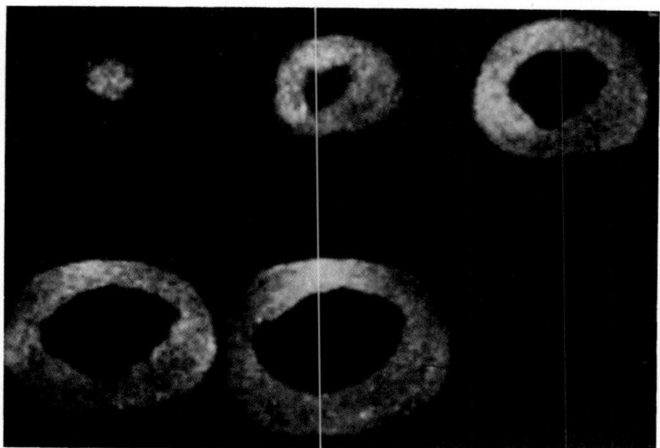

Figure 50–5. Sequential cross-section nuclear magnetic resonance images extending from the apex to the mid-portion of the left ventricle in a dog at 24 hours after ligation of the left anterior descending coronary artery. The high-intensity area (increased brightness) involves almost the entire cross-sectional area *(left upper slices)* in the two caudal sections. On the most cranial slice the high-intensity region is confined to the anterior wall. Images are viewed from above. (From Higgins, C. B., Herfkens, R., Lipton, M. J., et al.: Nuclear magnetic resonance imaging of acute myocardial infarction in dogs: Alterations in magnetic relaxation times. Am. J. Cardiol. 52:184, 1983, with permission.)

DETECTION OF ACUTE MYOCARDIAL INFARCTION

Changes in Magnetic Resonance Signal Intensity

Although brief reversible ischemia is unlikely to lead to detectable tissue changes, the tissue edema that occurs within infarcted tissue following coronary occlusion would be expected to produce changes in regional nuclear magnetic resonance image signal intensity and relaxation values. Higgins and associates were the first to demonstrate that this was true without the need for contrast enhancement[H4] (Fig. 50–5) (Table 50–1). When excised canine hearts were imaged 24 hours after acute coronary occlusion, all demonstrated a regional increase in signal intensity in the infarcted territory; T1 increased from 650 msec control myocardium to 728 msec in infarcted tissue, and T2 increased from 42 to 48 msec. Tissue water content was increased from 76.2 to 78.6 percent. Subsequently, Wesbey and colleagues were the first to demonstrate the ability to visualize infarction in vivo.[W1] Signal intensity in regionally infarcted myocardium was 66 ± 27 percent greater than in normal myocardium in dogs studied 2 to 7 days after ligation of the left anterior descending coronary artery. In vivo images, using two spin echo images from a multiecho sequence, were used to calculate T2 values, and these were found to be 69 ± 3 percent greater in infarcted versus normal myocardium.

Pflugfelder and co-workers, using a 0.15 T instrument in 15 dogs with acute infarction, was able to identify infarction regions

Table 50–1. INDIVIDUAL VALUES FOR T1, T2, AND PERCENT WATER CONTENT

	Infarcted Myocardium			Normal Myocardium		
Dog	*T1 (msec)*	*T2 (msec)*	*Water (%)*	*T1 (msec)*	*T2 (msec)*	*Water (%)*
1	694	45.4	78.4	620	42.8	76.7
2	640	45.7	77.5	549	40.8	76.3
3	599	48.8	78.5	538	43.0	75.2
4	803	52.0	79.2	710	40.2	75.9
5	876	49.2	78.2	771	42.3	75.9
6	758	50.5	78.6	713	43.5	77.3
Mean	728.3	48.4	78.6	650.2	42.1	76.2
SD	94.8	2.4	0.7	87.4	1.2	0.6

SD—standard deviation.

(From Higgins, C. B., et al.: Nuclear magnetic resonance imaging of acute myocardial infarction in dogs: Alterations in magnetic relaxation times. Am. J. Cardiol. 52:184, 1983, with permission.)

by increases in regional signal intensity on in vivo imaging on both early (TE 30 msec), and, to a greater extent, on later spin echo (TE 60 msec) images, within 4 hours of acute coronary occlusion[P3] (Fig. 50–6). Signal intensity in ischemic regions, in comparison with remote, nonischemic myocardium, increased progressively over the 4-hour period from 23 ± 13 percent in the first hour to 36 ± 20 percent in the fourth hour following occlusion on spin echo (TE 30 msec) images, and from 35 ± 34 percent to 116 ± 100 percent on the spin echo (TE 60 msec) images. In a study performed by Peshock and group, regional increases in signal intensity in infarcted territories were not observed in 10 dogs in which imaging of excised hearts was performed after 3 hours of occlusion.[P1] The relative signal intensity observed for a variety of pulse sequences was no greater than 1.16; this was found with a TR value of 1 second on the spin echo 56 msec image, using a 0.35 T system.

It is possible that the variable and apparently conflicting results between studies are related to the different models of coronary occlusion and to the differences between in vitro or in vivo experiments and important magnetic resonance instrument parameters. In addition, despite synchronization of the pulse sequences to the cardiac cycle, there is a significant effect of myocardial motion to decrease signal intensity in areas of normal contractile function, with a much lesser effect to decrease signal intensity in hypo- or akinetic regions of infarction, thus increasing contrast on in vivo imaging, in comparison with ex vivo imaging in which motion effects are absent.

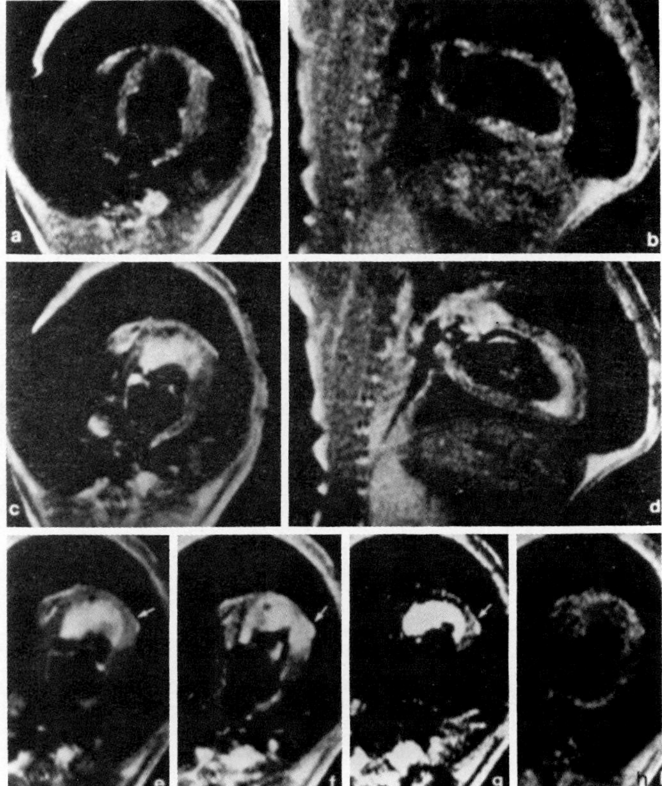

Figure 50–6. Transverse *(a)* and sagittal *(b)* TE 30-msec images obtained before occlusion of the anterior descending artery. *c* and *d*, TE 30-msec images in the same planes showing apical dilatation, thinning, and intracavitary signal suggestive of static blood post occlusion. TE 30-msec images *e* and *f* show progressive signal enhancement in the infarct zone 30 and 150 minutes after coronary artery occlusion. *g*, TE 60-msec image at 1 hr. *h*, The inversion recovery image 4 hours after occlusion. (From Pflugfelder, P. W., Wisenberg, G., Prato, F. S., et al.: Early detection of canine myocardial infarction by magnetic resonance in vivo. Circulation 71[3]:587, by permission of the American Heart Association, Inc.)

Regarding ongoing changes in acute infarction over the initial week, the data suggest that evolving edema in the infarct and peri-infarct regions has played a significant role in producing regional changes in T1 and T2 relaxation times, and thus signal intensity on nuclear magnetic resonance images. Pflugfelder and co-workers performed in vivo imaging on 8 dogs serially over the first 3 weeks following coronary occlusion, using single echo (TE 30, 45, and 60 msec) and gated pulse sequences[P2] (Figs. 50–7 and 50–8). On the day of infarction, mean signal intensity in the infarct region was 30 percent greater than normal myocardium in the 30-msec spin echo images, and 49 percent greater in the 60-msec images.

Imaging was subsequently performed (1) 4 to 6 days, (2) 13 days, and (3) 20 days following coronary occlusion. Signal intensity in the infarct rose to a peak value (62 ± 24 percent higher than normal myocardium) on the second or third imaging day in seven or eight animals in the 30-msec spin echo images. On the 60-msec spin echo images, the signal intensity changes were more variable, with a mean peak of 136 ± 81 percent, although this was not statistically different from day one. Subsequently, there was a trend for signal intensity in the infarct to decline. At 3 weeks postinfarction, on spin echo 30-msec images, mean signal intensity had decreased to 12 ± 19% greater than in normal myocardium and, on spin echo 60-msec images, to 61 ± 67%.

This pattern of signal intensity changes was corroborated by Tscholakoff and colleagues.[T3] In 12 dogs, they found an approximate 10 percent increase in regional signal intensity in infarcted versus normal myocardium on spin echo 30-msec images over the first 5 hours following coronary occlusion, using a TR value equal to a single R-R interval (600 to 900 msec). When dogs were subsequently imaged 4 to 14 days later, this value had increased to 25 ± 8 percent. For 60-msec images (TR = 1 × R-R interval), the magnetic resonance signal increase averaged approximately 25 percent over the first 4 hours, increased to 43 percent in the fifth hour, and still further to 47 percent at 4 to 14 days. When longer TR values (TR = 2 × R-R interval) were used (1200 to 1800 msec), the main effect was for a much larger relative difference in signal intensity on the spin echo 60-msec images at 4 hours (78 percent), 5 hours (92 percent), and 4 to 14 days (104 percent). Similar results on early in vivo imaging within 5 hours postocclusion also were demonstrated in another study by Tscholakoff and associates comparing signal intensities pre- and post-contrast administration,[T2] and by Johnston and colleagues,[J1] who imaged nonreperfused infarcts after 3 hours of occlusion.

Rehr and group studied 10 dogs in vivo at 24 to 48 hours and 4 to 5 days after infarction on a 0.35 T instrument.[R1] The signal:intensity ratio (ischemic:normal myocardium) was 1.4 ± 0.2 in four dogs at 24 to 48 hours, and 1.5 ± 0.3 in six dogs at 4 to 5 days after occlusion. These experiments show a slight increase in signal intensity peaking toward the end of the first week following occlusion, when edema in response to the acute ischemic insult is presumably greatest.

In addition to the changes in myocardial signal intensity, other observations have been noted to occur in acute myocardial infarction. Normally, fast-moving ventricular cavitary blood adjacent to normally contractile myocardium produces little or no signal on magnetic resonance images. Subsequent to coronary occlusion, cavitary blood adjacent to hypokinetic myocardium produces a more intense signal similar to that of stationary blood.[H1, J1] This produces, therefore, a functional representation of the extent of regional dysfunction secondary to coronary occlusion. As well, regional myocardial thinning and impaired systolic thickening have been considered indications of regional infarction.[H1] These will be discussed further in the section on evaluation of left ventricular function.

Changes in Myocardial Relaxation Times

In the data presented to this point, we have seen considerable variation in the changes in signal intensity observed by different investigators following myocardial infarction. As noted earlier, some of these differences may be explained by the different

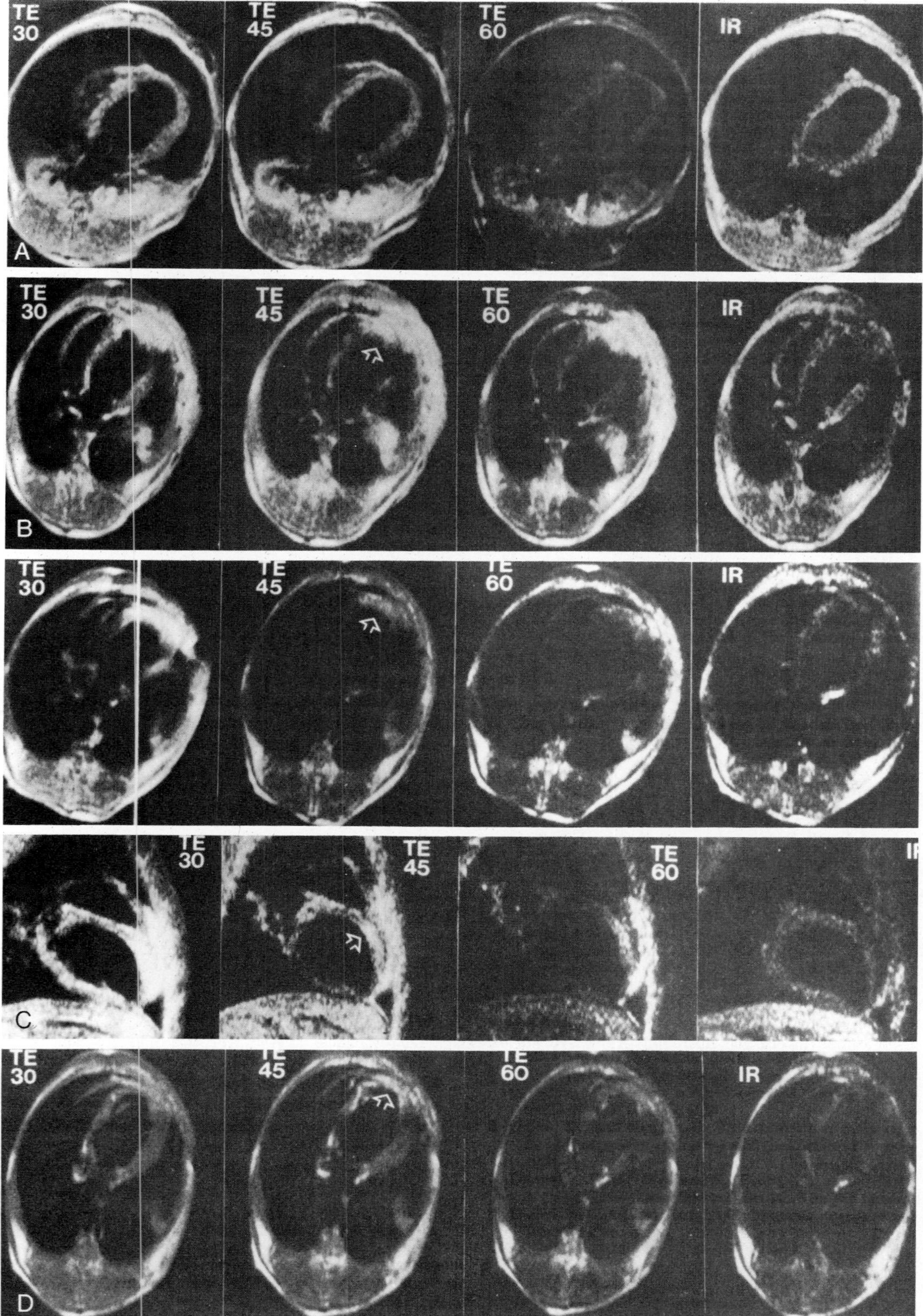

Figure 50–7. The evolution of the intensity and area of magnetic signal changes within the infarct zone with each of the pulse sequences used. *a*, Images from day 1, in which marked cardiac dilation but no observable inhomogeneity in myocardial signal was seen. *b*, The area of infarction *(arrow)* on day 6. *c*, The infarction *(arrow)* on day 13 in two planes, transverse *(upper panel)* and saggital *(lower panel)*. *d*, The infarction *(arrow)* on day 20. (From Pflugfelder, P. W., Wisenberg, G., Prato, F. S., et al.: Serial imaging of canine myocardial infarction by in vivo nuclear magnetic resonance. J. Am. Coll. Cardiol. 7[4]:843, 1986. Reprinted with permission from the American College of Cardiology.)

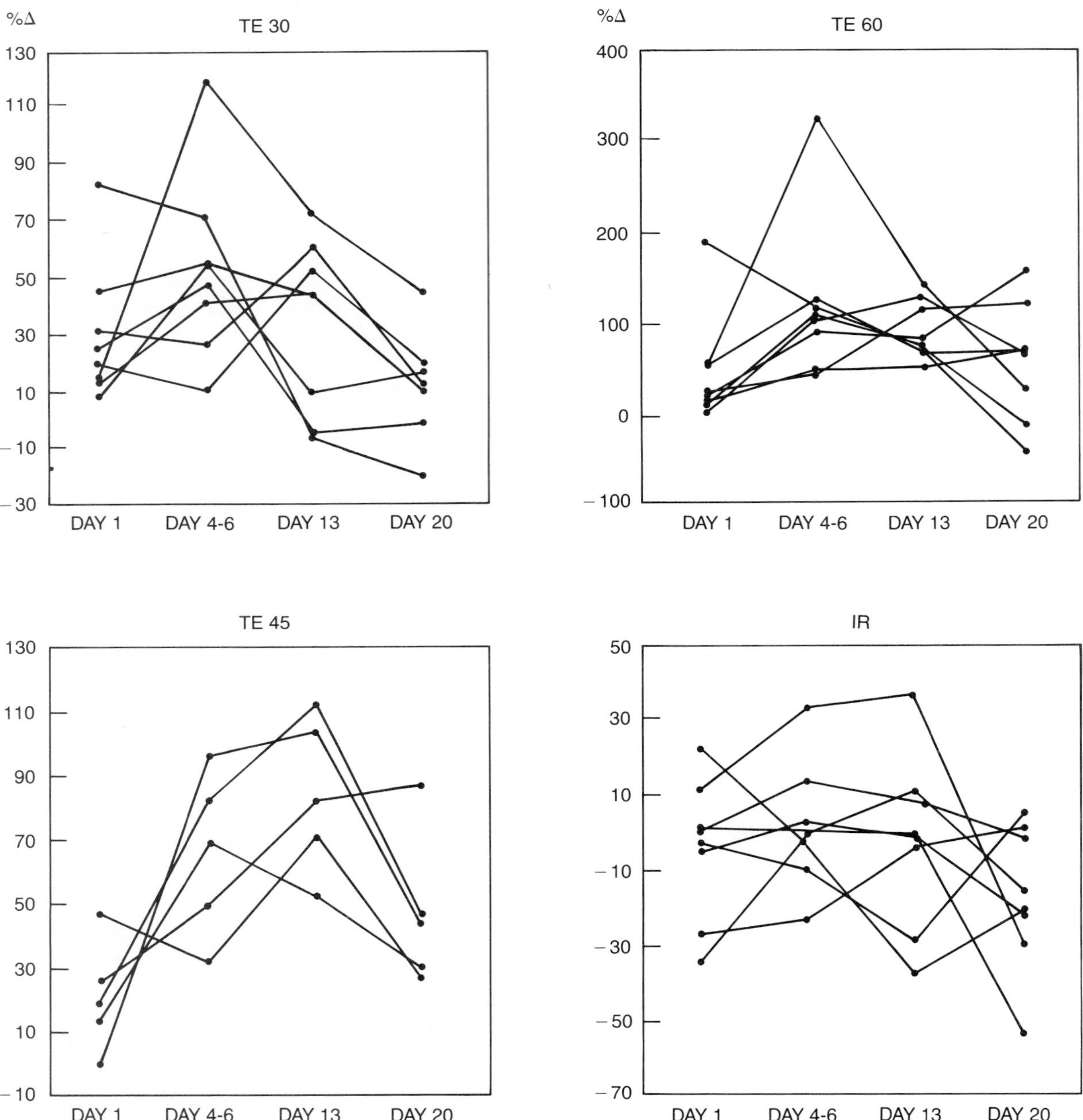

Figure 50–8. Percent signal intensity change (%Δ) in the infarct zone compared with normal myocardial. Data for eight individual animals are given for each imaging day (from day 1 to day 20). IR = inversion recovery; TE = echo time. (From Pflugfelder, P. W., Wisenberg, G., Prato, F. S., et al.: Serial imaging of canine myocardial infarction by in vivo nuclear magnetic resonance. J. Am. Coll. Cardiol. 7[4]:843, 1986. Reprinted with permission from the American College of Cardiology.)

models used, i.e., in vivo versus ex vivo imaging. However, it should be appreciated that signal intensity in spin echo images is influenced by many factors in a given image, as reviewed by Talagala and Wolf in Chapter 39, including the tissue factors of motion, proton density, and T1 and T2 and their interaction with numerous imaging variables.

Although T1 and T2 are important contributors to signal intensity, the specific pulse sequences, with varying TE and TR, also affect signal intensity and increase or decrease regional contrast between infarcted and normal myocardium. Thus, even if the echo times were standardized, the TR value, influenced by the heart rate of the subject, would produce significant intersubject variability in signal intensity. Another confounding problem is the multitude of magnetic field strengths available on commercial instruments. T1 values for a particular tissue depend upon the actual magnetic field of the instrument, increasing in a nonlinear fashion as field strength increases. This occurs to a lesser extent with T2.

Brown and colleagues evaluated T1 values in four groups of dogs, from 3 hours to 56 days after coronary artery occlusion[B4] (Fig. 50–9). In this study, myocardial tissue was obtained at the time of sacrifice, and T1 values were measured in vitro, using a 10.7 MHz (0.26T) spectrometer. Tissue water content was also evaluated. The maximal increase in regional T1 values was at 3 hours, to 626 ± 85 msec versus 512 ± 59 msec in normal myocardium. Subsequently, there was a progressive decrease in T1 values, to 575 ± 22 msec at 4 days, 510 ± 42 msec at 21 days, and to less than control, 451 ± 31 msec, at 56 days. Correlating with these T1 changes were changes in regional tissue water content of +9.5 percent versus normal myocardium at 3 hours, +11.9 percent at 4 days, +1.7 percent at 21 days, and −1.0 percent at 56 days. Such changes would have an impact upon relative signal intensities obtained with magnetic resonance imaging.

Johnston and associates carefully sectioned myocardial tissue into endocardial and epicardial segments in the central ischemic

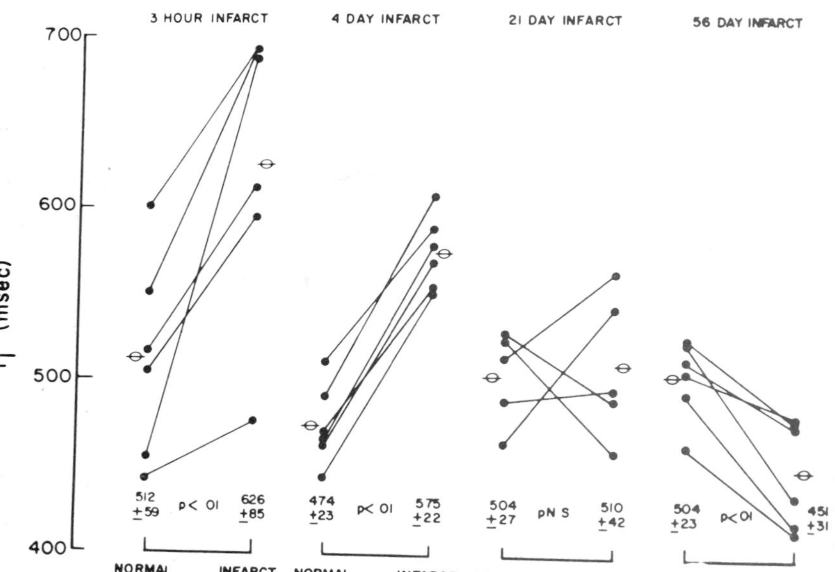

Figure 50–9. T1 response to acute and chronic ischemic myocardial injury. T1 values increased for 3-hour-old and 4-day-old infarcts, showed a variable response to 21-day-old infarcts, and decreased for 56-day-old infarcts. (From Brown, J. J., Peck, W. W., Gerber, K. H., et al.: Nuclear magnetic resonance analysis of acute and chronic myocardial infarction in dogs: alterations in spin lattice relaxation times. Am. Heart J. 108:1292, 1984, with permission.)

zone of 3-hour-old infarcts and measured T1 and T2 in a spectrometer, in vitro, using a 20-MHz (0.48 T) magnet[J4] (Fig. 50–10). The epicardial T1 values did not differ significantly. However, for endocardial segments, T1 increased significantly. The same pattern was also observed for T2.

Brown and associates performed T1 measurements in vitro in tissue obtained 40 minutes, 1 hour, and 2 hours postocclusion, in a 0.26 T spectrometer.[B3] They demonstrated an insignificant change from control values at 40 minutes, 491 ± 27 msec (control) versus 497 ± 34 msec (ischemic), which then rose to 533 ± 37 msec at 1 hour and 561 ± 39 msec at 2 hours. Water content, which averaged 77 percent in normal myocardium, rose slightly to 78 percent at 40 minutes, 79.1 percent at 1 hour, and 80.4 percent at 2 hours, again indicating a strong correlation between water content and regional T1 values, with an r value of 0.80.

Tscholakoff and colleagues were the first to perform serial in vivo T1 and T2 measurements in nonreperfused infarcts, in a 0.35 T system (Tables 50–2 and 50–3). They found large variability in T1 measurements from control values, of 681 ± 230 msec to 831 ± 367 msec 5 minutes postocclusion, with a gradual trend toward a decrease in T1 values over the subsequent 5 hours to 573 ± 133 msec, but then a rise to 705 ± 221 msec at 4 to 14 days.[T3] These results are not consistent with those demonstrated by any of the in vitro spectrometer measurements to date. However, T2 values appeared much more consistent, with less interanimal variability. From control values of 34 ± 4 msec, T2 rose progressively to 58 ± 14 msec at 5 hours and 59 ± 13 msec at 4 to 14 days postocclusion.

The variability in measured T1 times may have been caused by beat-to-beat variations in pulse repetition times. Further, we have found that if the pulse repetition time for the shortest of the two pulse sequences required for T1 measurements is significantly greater than the T1 of the tissue being assessed, then errors as large as 30 percent in T1 may be produced.[P5] This may necessitate the use of additional 90°–180° spin echo pulses, placed between successive QRS triggers, to alter the effective TR value. The resultant signal occurring following these extra pulses would not be incorporated into the image to minimize the blurring effect of data obtained in different portions of the cardiac cycle.

Fisher and co-workers presented data on regional T2 changes observed in patients 3 to 17 days following infarction.[F2] The T2 of the infarcted segments, 79.0 ± 22.1 msec, was significantly longer than that of normal myocardium, 43.9 ± 9.0 msec, on

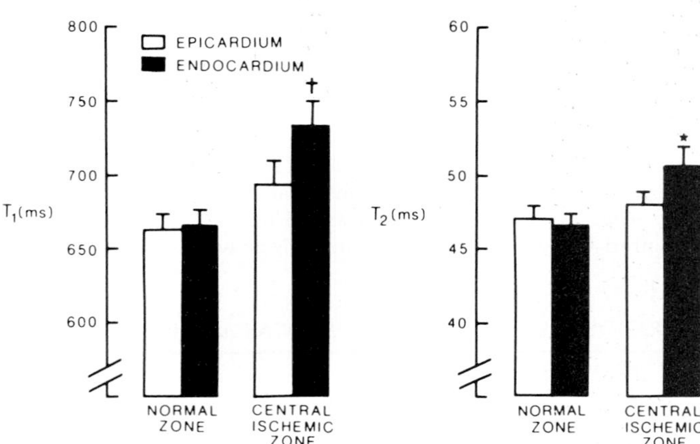

Figure 50–10. Regional myocardial T1 and T2 values. Values are mean ± SEM. *p <.05; †p<.01 versus normal zone. (From Johnston, D. L., Brady, T. J., Ratner, A. V., et al.: Assessment of myocardial ischemia with proton magnetic resonance: effect of a three hour coronary occlusion with and without reperfusion. Circulation 1985, 71[3]:595, by permission of the American Heart Association, Inc.)

Table 50–2. T1 RELAXATION TIMES (MSEC) OF INFARCTED MYOCARDIUM (ANTERIOR) AND NORMAL MYOCARDIUM (POSTERIOR)

Time After Occlusion	Anterior		Posterior	
	Mean	*SD*	*Mean*	*SD*
Preocclusion	613.5	165.9	681.5	237.2
5 min	831.2	367.1	703.2	254.1
30 min	790.5	366.8	746.2	492.2
1 hr	771.8	437.9	689.1	219.6
2 hr	617.7	250.5	631.8	285.2
3 hr	632.1	342.4	650.0	308.1
4 hr	649.3	192.5	565.0	143.0
5 hr	573.0	133.1	613.7	296.4
4–14 days	704.7	220.8	751.5	163.0

SD—standard deviation.

(From Tscholakoff, D., et al.: Early-phase myocardial infarction evaluation by MR imaging. Radiology 159:667, 1986, with permission.)

Table 50–3. T2 RELAXATION TIMES (MSEC) OF INFARCTED MYOCARDIUM (ANTERIOR) AND NORMAL MYOCARDIUM (POSTERIOR)

Time After Occlusion	Anterior		Posterior	
	Mean	*SD*	*Mean*	*SD*
Preocclusion	33.3	4.6	34.1	3.8
5 min	42.3	6.9	35.2	5.0
30 min	43.2	5.6	35.4	3.5
1 hr	44.0	9.8	34.0	3.3
2 hr	48.3	11.8	34.3	6.8
3 hr*	49.2	9.9	33.6	3.7
4 hr*	57.1	11.6	37.1	3.3
5 hr*	58.8	13.6	35.0	4.4
4–14 days*	59.0	13.1	36.0	3.6

SD—standard deviation.
$^{*}P < .01$.
(From Tscholakoff, D., et al.: Early-phase myocardial infarction evaluation by MR imaging. Radiology 159:667, 1986, with permission.)

their 0.35 T system. T1 values were not measured because only one multiecho spin echo sequence was used to image each slice in these subjects.

Canby and group published an interesting study on relaxation times in 4-hour-old infarcts with markedly reduced flow, less than 5 percent of control[C1] (Table 50–4). The greatest T1 and T2 elevations, by spectrometer, were found in regions where flow was between 5 and 50 percent of control, on both 20-MHz and 200-MHz systems. However, in regions served by flow of less than 5 percent of control, neither T1 nor T2 was significantly different than control, although a significant increase in water content, as indicated by the wet to dry weight ratio was present in both tissues with reduced flow. This implies that although total water content is an important contributor to T1 and T2 times, it is not the sole determinant. Other factors include compartmentation of water, concentration and type of lipid present, the macromolecular environment, temperature, and alterations in the chemical milieu, including electrolyte concentration.

In a dog study, we recently obtained serial T1 and T2 measurements in vivo, using the extra pulses alluded to earlier to increase the reliability of T1 measurements[W4] (Table 50–5). Dogs were studied between 1 and 2 hours and 2 and 3 hours postocclusion, and then 5 days and 21 days later. T1 values were already increased in the second hour to 448 ± 51 msec in comparison with control, which was 351 ± 11 msec, and did not change significantly at 2 to 3 hours. T1 of ischemic myocardium peaked at 5 days (490 ± 64 msec), and then fell to 427 ± 43 msec at 21 days. T2 increased in a similar pattern, to 51 ± 8 msec in the second hour, 54 ± 10 msec in the 3rd hour, 63 ± 9 msec on day 5, and 55 ± 11 msec on day 21, in comparison with control T2 values of 40 ± 2 msec on our 0.15 T system.

Summary

Thus, the data presented strongly suggest a progressive rise in T1 and T2 values in nonreperfused infarcts in the early hours following infarction, except in the extreme low flow regions of an infarct, peaking at about 1 week after infarction and subsequently tending to decrease and, in vitro, falling below control values at 56 days. Tissue edema, which occurs early in the postinfarction period, leads to the increased T1 and T2 values. As myocardial tissue is replaced by fibrotic scar, T1 and T2 drop below control values.

For all the reasons cited, it will become increasingly important for investigators to obtain accurate T1 and T2 values, specifying all magnetic resonance parameters used, in order for meaningful comparisons of data to be made between results of different investigators, using different imaging instruments and different animal models. For determination of T1 values from in vivo images, it is necessary to obtain at least two separate images at different TR values, and there are numerous causes of experimental error.

To date, unfortunately, most of the studies in infarction have been performed using ex vivo images or in vitro spectrometer measurements to derive T1 and T2 values. Higgins and colleagues were the first to publish results of T1 and T2 changes in acute canine myocardial infarction in hearts imaged ex vivo[H4] (see Table 50–1). Wesbey and associates, however, were the first to obtain T2 values from in vivo imaging.[W1] Using a 0.35 T system, T2 in normal myocardium was 30 ± 3 msec, and it was 52 ± 4 msec in 2- to 7-day-old infarcted canine myocardium, a 69 ± 3 percent increase.

DETECTION OF REPERFUSED INFARCTION

The introduction of thrombolytic agents for the treatment of acute myocardial infarction has greatly revolutionized the therapy of acute coronary disease. In many cases, clinical indices may clearly indicate the success of reperfusion, with prompt relief of ischemic chest pain and normalization of elevated ST segments on the electrocardiogram. However, often the issue of successful reperfusion is in doubt, and many investigators have examined whether magnetic resonance will help in identifying reperfusion by changes either in the MR image signal intensity or derived regional T1 or T2 values.

Changes in Inherent Tissue Properties

Johnston and co-workers reported on T1 and T2 changes measured in vitro following 3 hours of occlusion and 1 hour of reperfusion, in a 0.48 T spectrometer.[J4] Although the values in nine dogs tended to be higher in the reperfused versus nonreperfused group, they were not statistically different. However, Brown and group documented different results, using a somewhat different model of reperfusion.[B3] Following 40 minutes, 1 hour, and 2 hours of occlusion, animals were reperfused for 3 hours and then sacrificed, with tissue T1 values measured in vitro. As in nonreperfused infarcts, there was little difference between the T1 of normal myocardium, 498 ± 20 msec, versus ischemic myocardium, 506 ± 43 msec, after 40 minutes of ischemia plus 3 hours of reperfusion. After one hour of ischemia plus 3 hours of reperfusion, however, the T1 had increased to 578 ± 57 msec, in comparison with 533 ± 37 msec after 2 hours of ischemia only. After 2 hours of occlusion and 3 hours of reperfusion, T1 measured 603 ± 35 msec, in comparison with 561 ± 39 msec

Table 50–4. RELAXATION TIMES (T1 AND T2) AND WET TO DRY WEIGHT RATIOS FOR THREE REGIONAL MYOCARDIAL FLOW GROUPS

Flow Group	20 MHz (Bulk Proton)		200 MHz (Water Proton)		W/D
	T1 (sec)	*T2 (msec)*	*T1 (sec)*	*T2 (msec)*	
≤5%	0.70 ± 0.02	56.1 ± 2.9	1.78 ± 0.06	42.4 ± 3.1	4.74 ± 0.29
5 to 50%	0.78 ± 0.05	58.3 ± 3.6	1.91 ± 0.12	45.1 ± 4.9	4.92 ± 0.17
>50%	0.69 ± 0.02	52.8 ± 2.7	1.75 ± 0.07	38.6 ± 2.8	4.44 ± 0.17

W/D—wet to dry weight ratio.
(From Canby, R. C., et al.: Proton nuclear magnetic resonance relaxation times in severe myocardial ischemia. J. Am. Coll. Cardiol. 10:412, 1987. Reprinted with permission from the American College of Cardiology.)

Table 50–5. T1 AND T2 VALUES (MSEC)

Occlusion	Reperfusion (n = 7) T1 Infarct	T1 Control	T2 Infarct	T2 Control	Nonreperfusion (n = 7) T1 Infarct	T1 Control	T2 Infarct	T2 Control
1–2 hr	*445 ± 32	350 ± 11	*52 ± 5	40 ± 2	*448 ± 51	351 ± 11	*51 ± 8	41 ± 2
2–3 hr	†555 ± 65‡	348 ± 12	†65 ± 8	39 ± 2	*460 ± 49	349 ± 12	*54 ± 10‡	40 ± 2
Day 5	*512 ± 55	349 ± 11	39 ± 8§	39 ± 2	†490 ± 64	350 ± 11	†63 ± 9§	39 ± 2
Day 21	*450 ± 47	351 ± 11	35 ± 7§	41 ± 2	*427 ± 43	349 ± 1	*55 ± 11§	40 ± 2

*$p < 0.05$
vs. control.
†$p < 0.01$
‡$p < 0.01$
reperfusion vs. nonreperfusion.
§$p < 0.0025$
(From Wisenberg, G., et al.: Serial nuclear magnetic resonance imaging of acute myocardial infarction with and without reperfusion. Am. Heart J. 115:510, 1988, with permission.)

for ischemic tissue without reperfusion. Thus, a more pronounced increase in T1 occurred following reperfusion in these studies. Edema presumably plays an important role, as a greater increase in regional tissue water content occurs in reperfused versus nonreperfused hearts.

Tscholakoff and colleagues found somewhat different results with still another animal model of 1 hour of ischemia followed by 5 hours of reperfusion.[T2] Using only signal intensity changes, they found no difference in either spin echo (TE 30 or 60 msec) in vivo images between reperfused hearts and hearts subject to 5 hours of occlusion. In another in vivo imaging study, Tscholakoff and associates found that changes in T2 relaxation parameters occurred almost immediately with reperfusion after a 1-hour occlusion. Measured T2 remained relatively stable for the subsequent 5 hours and even tended to rise still further at 3 to 5 days[T4] (Table 50–6). However, Peshock and colleagues, who presented only signal intensity ratios between ischemic and normal myocardium on excised hearts, found no difference between hearts exposed to 3 hours of occlusion, and those reperfused for 1 hour after 2 hours of occlusion, except when inversion recovery, as opposed to spin echo pulse sequences, was used.[P1] Johnston and associates, again using different reperfusion models (3 hours of occlusion versus 3 hours of occlusion plus 1 hour of reperfusion) found that T1 and T2 values measured in vitro increased, particularly in the endocardial regions.[J1]

Using extra pulse sequences to improve the accuracy of T1 estimation, we found that different patterns in T1 and T2 evolve over the weeks following reperfusion[W4] (see Table 50–5). In nonreperfused infarcts, T1 and T2 rose gradually, peaked at day 5 following occlusion, and had begun to return to normal by day 21. However, with reperfusion, an abrupt increase in T1 and T2 occurred within the first hour, with T1 increasing to 555 ± 65 msec from the T1 of 445 ± 32 msec measured during the 2 hours of occlusion, and T2 from 52 ± 5 msec during occlusion to 65 ± 8 msec after reperfusion. However, T2 had normalized by days 5 and 21, whereas T1 remained elevated, although tending toward normal. These divergent responses produced a decrease in signal intensity in reperfused areas on spin echo images. The results of this study suggest that serial imaging would allow differentiation of reperfused from nonreperfused infarcts.

Table 50–6. T2 RELAXATION TIMES OF JEOPARDIZED (ANTERIOR) AND NORMAL (POSTERIOR) MYOCARDIUM IN SEVEN DOGS WITH REPERFUSED INFARCTS AND IN THREE DOGS WITHOUT INFARCTS

Time*	T2—Infarct (msec) Anterior	T2—Infarct (msec) Posterior	T2—No Infarct (msec) Anterior	T2—No Infarct (msec) Posterior
Preocclusion	37 ± 4	38.6 ± 5.3	36.5 ± 3.5	39 ± 2.7
Occlusion	46.4 ± 19.2	40.7 ± 3.3	42.5 ± 6.3	37.5 ± 2.8
5	62.6 ± 27.2	41.1 ± 5.7	43.5 ± 4.7	36 ± 4.2
30	59.6 ± 13.1†	42.9 ± 3.1	35.4 ± 4.9	39.5 ± 5.9
60	56.3 ± 7.7†	39 ± 7.5	37.5 ± 2.9	41 ± 4.8
120	64.6 ± 10.1§	41.1 ± 4.6	36.9 ± 6.1	38.7 ± 4.1
180	66.6 ± 12.1‡	38.4 ± 4.3	40.3 ± 5.7	39 ± 8.4
240	67.9 ± 14.2†	40.6 ± 4.5	41.6 ± 6.3	40.8 ± 3.9
300	62.6 ± 12.0‡	41 ± 6.1	38.4 ± 4.9	38.8 ± 5.0
3–5 days	69.2 ± 11.3‡	42.6 ± 6.2	41.2 ± 5.2	40.6 ± 3.7

*Time after reperfusion in minutes unless otherwise indicated. Occlusion—30 minutes postocclusion.
†$p < 0.01$.
‡$p < 0.02$.
§$p < 0.05$.
(From Tscholakoff, D., et al.: MRI of reperfused myocardial infarct in dogs. Am. J. Radiol. 146:925, 1986, with permission.)

Use of Nonproton Nuclei

Although proton imaging is the standard, commercially available procedure, other elements have been used in an attempt to image reperfused infarction. In particular, sodium imaging may offer important additional information about tissue sodium and thus presumably extracellular water content. (See Chapter 45.)

Summary

It is clear that tremendous differences exist in the data reported to date, confounded by (1) the different reperfusion models, (2) the differences in in vivo versus ex vivo image or spectrometer measurements, and (3) the use of signal intensity data versus relaxation parameter measurements by some investigators. However, it does seem that if sufficient time elapses before reperfusion occurs, reperfusion will produce significant increases in both relaxation parameters and signal intensity beyond those that have evolved secondary to the ischemic insult alone.

ESTIMATION OF MYOCARDIAL INFARCT SIZE

Although the confirmation of infarction in most cases has not been a difficult task using clinical, electrocardiographic, and enzymatic criteria, the precise assessment of the extent of myocardial necrosis has been elusive. The use of thrombolytic agents may render both electrocardiographic and enzymatic estimates unreliable, the latter because of acceleration of creatine kinase washout kinetics. Evaluation of ventricular function may lead to an erroneous overestimate of infarction extent as contractile abnormalities observed may be secondary to either chronically ischemic or severely stunned myocardium in the process of recovery. Similarly, perfusion markers, such as thallium-201, may not be taken up by viable myocardial cells whose metabolic integrity has been disrupted by those same processes causing abnormalities of ventricular function.

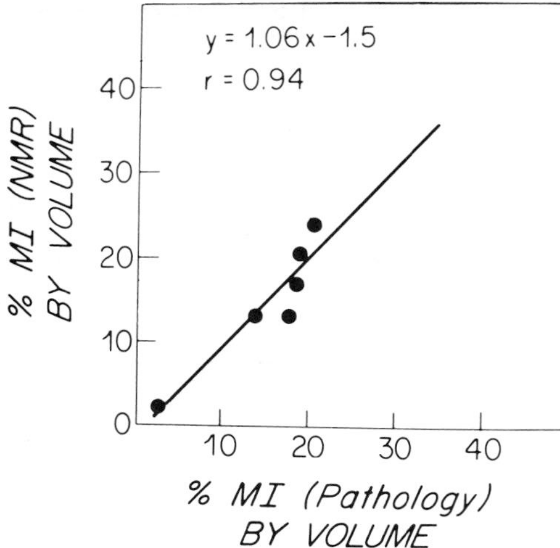

Figure 50–11. Infarct size determined by nuclear magnetic resonance (NMR) (ordinate) plotted against infarct size as determined by pathology (abscissa). % MI—percentage of left ventricular volume occupied by infarct. The data are from six hearts. (From Goldman, M. R., Brady, T. J., Pykett, I. L., et al.: Quantification of experimental myocardial infarction using magnetic resonance imaging and paramagnetic ion contrast enhancement in excised canine hearts. Circulation 66[5]:1012, 1982, by permission of the American Heart Association, Inc.)

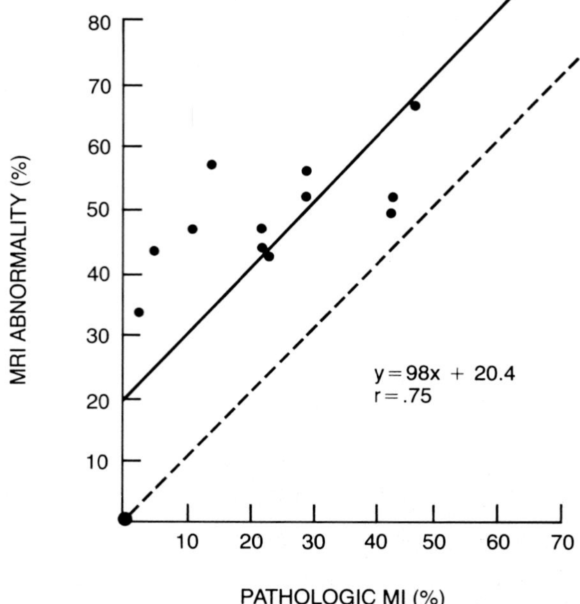

Figure 50–12. Relationship between the pathologic myocardial infarction and the MRI abnormality. The line of identity is indicated by the dashed line. MI—myocardial infarction; MRI—magnetic resonance imaging. (From Buda, A. J., Aisen, A. M., Juni, J. E., et al.: Detection and sizing of myocardial ischemia and infarction by nuclear resonance imaging in the canine heart. Am. Heart J. 110:1294, 1985, with permission.)

Using Unenhanced Methods

Nuclear magnetic resonance, with the potential to characterize tissue, has been investigated with regard to its ability to assess accurately the extent of infarction. Goldman and associates, in 1982, were the first to report on the use of NMR to assess infarct extent.[G1] Six dogs underwent circumflex occlusion. After 24 hours, the animals were given manganese chloride, a paramagnetic agent, were sacrificed, and the hearts were imaged. Compared with measurements of infarct size using triphenyl tetrazolium chloride (TTC), the images correlated well with an r value of 0.94 and a regression line slope of 1.06 and intercept of −1.5 (Fig. 50–11). However, Buda and colleagues found that nuclear magnetic resonance imaging without a contrast agent significantly overestimated infarct size in three dogs subject to a mean of 4.3 ± 1.2 hours of occlusion and in ten dogs that underwent 2.3 ± 1.6 hours of occlusion followed by 2.0 ± 0.6 hours of reperfusion[B5] (Figs. 50–12 and 50–13). In these ex vivo imaging studies, the regression equation between extent of NMR signal abnormality (y) and infarct size (x) was y = 0.98x + 20.4 with an r value of 0.75. There was a much better correlation between NMR signal abnormalities and hypoperfused myocardium (zone at risk) with a regression equation of y = 1.2x + 3.1 and r = 0.95.

Rokey and associates also performed ex vivo imaging in hearts removed 6 hours after coronary artery occlusion.[R4] Calculated T2 images were produced using Carr-Purcell-Meiboom-Gill pulse sequences, and areas of visually increased signal intensity on these images were used to outline the presumed area of infarction. Here again, overestimation of infarct size was observed despite a high r value of 0.98, where y (pathologic infarct size) = 0.87x (magnetic resonance infarct size) + 0.63.

It is interesting that Caputo and group found just the opposite results, on in vivo imaging of anterior infarcts at 3 days and 21 days postocclusion.[C3] At 3 days, the correlation was r = 0.97, with a regression equation of y (NMR infarct size) = 0.67x + 1.8, and at 21 days, r = 0.95, y = 0.76x + 0.77, thus indicating that at both times nuclear magnetic resonance underestimated TTC infarct size, using objective criteria for NMR abnormality (pixels with T2 between 50 and 150 msec). The reasons for this consistent underestimation, and the difference between these results and those of previous investigators, are not clear but are a cause for concern, as the methods used for T2 measurements have been well validated in the investigator's laboratory.

We performed serial in vivo imaging on dogs on the day of occlusion and at 5 days and 21 days postocclusion[W4] (Table 50–7). T1 and T2 values were determined on a pixel by pixel basis for each image. Pixels with relaxation parameters that differed by more than 2 standard deviations from normal tissue were identified by computer as infarct regions. Using this method, nuclear magnetic resonance consistently overestimated light microscopic

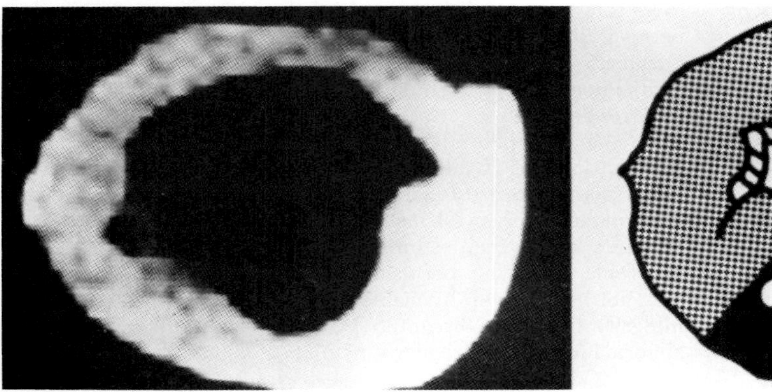

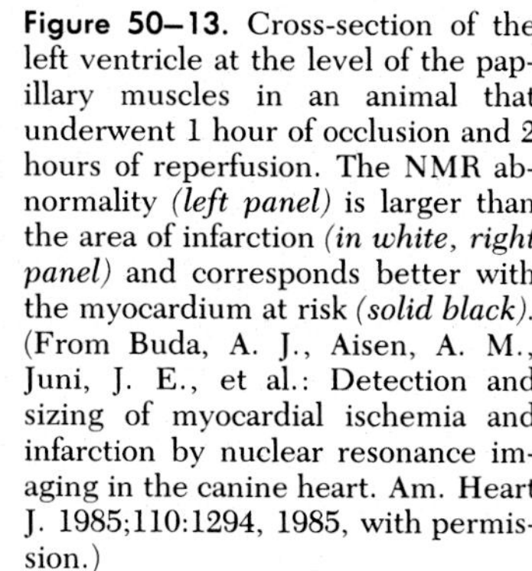

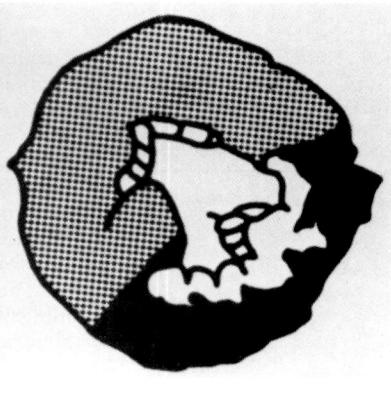

Figure 50–13. Cross-section of the left ventricle at the level of the papillary muscles in an animal that underwent 1 hour of occlusion and 2 hours of reperfusion. The NMR abnormality *(left panel)* is larger than the area of infarction *(in white, right panel)* and corresponds better with the myocardium at risk *(solid black)*. (From Buda, A. J., Aisen, A. M., Juni, J. E., et al.: Detection and sizing of myocardial ischemia and infarction by nuclear resonance imaging in the canine heart. Am. Heart J. 1985;110:1294, 1985, with permission.)

Table 50–7. EXTENT OF SIGNAL ABNORMALITY (PERCENT OF LEFT VENTRICLE)

	Reperfusion (n = 7)	Nonreperfusion (n = 7)
Occlusion		
1–2 hr	‡14 ± 8*	20 ± 11*
2–3 hr	†22 ± 11	22 ± 11
Day 5	13 ± 6*	‡25 ± 12*
Day 21	11 ± 5*	18 ± 11*
Pathology	10 ± 6*	18 ± 9*

*$p < 0.05$ reperfusion vs. nonreperfusion.
†$p < 0.01$
vs. pathology.
‡$p < 0.05$
(From Wisenberg, G., et al.: Serial nuclear magnetic resonance imaging of acute myocardial infarction with and without reperfusion. Am. Heart J. 115:510, 1988, with permission.)

Table 50–8. MAGNETIC RESONANCE CONTRAST AND SPECTROMETER RELAXATION TIMES 90 SECONDS POST-Gd-DTPA

	T1 (msec)		T2 (msec)		MR Contrast (%)
Dog Number	*Normal Myocardium*	*Infarct*	*Normal Myocardium*	*Infarct*	*(SE 500/56)*
4	149.9	226.1	34.1	41.9	45
5	139.0	330.0	33.5	53.3	36
6	112.1	165.7	35.1	41.7	58
Mean	133.6	241.0	34.2	45.6	46
S.D.	19.4	83.0	0.8	6.6	11

(From Wesbey, G., et al.: Effect of gadolinium-DTPA on the magnetic relaxation times of normal and infarcted myocardium. Radiology 153:165, 1984, with permission.)

evaluations of infarct size on all images prior to 21 days postocclusion, in both reperfused and nonreperfused hearts. At 21 days, however, the correlation was good in both models: r = 0.87, y (NMR) = 1.03 + 0.9x for nonreperfusion and r = 0.89, y = 1.06 + 0.4x for reperfusion.

From the available data, it seems that NMR would not be helpful in the early evaluation of infarct size as overestimation often occurs, presumably because of the extension of edema beyond the infarct zone into the reversibly ischemic, peri-infarct territory. This edema leads to changes in signal intensity and T1 and T2 values, inseparable from those in the true infarct zone. Once this peri-infarct edema has resolved into the infarct area only, more accurate estimation of infarct size is possible, but this must be corroborated by other investigations using similar methods.

Use of Paramagnetic Contrast Agents

Although intrinsic changes in myocardial tissue have been shown to produce abnormalities in T1 and T2 values and thus allow identification of acute myocardial infarction by nuclear magnetic resonance imaging, paramagnetic agents potentially may allow improved contrast and delineation between normal and infarcted/ischemic myocardium. Basic properties of paramagnetic agents are reviewed in Chapter 43.

Several paramagnetic agents have been evaluated for the potential of improved definition of regionally infarcted/ischemic tissue, and work has begun to determine whether these agents can be used for the quantitation, in absolute terms, of regional myocardial blood flow.

Manganese chloride was the first paramagnetic agent used to study ischemic heart disease. Shortly after bolus administration intravenously, infarct regions had significantly less reduction in T1 and T2 than did surrounding normal myocardium.[M6] Goldman and associates used manganese chloride to prove excellent visualization of acute infarction in dog hearts excised 10 minutes after a 5-minute injection of 0.05 mmol/kg[G1] (Fig. 50–11). There was a good correlation between the extent of persistently elevated nuclear magnetic resonance signal and TTC staining of these 24-hour-old infarcts. However, serious concerns about the toxicity of manganese limited further investigation and clinical application of this compound.

McNamara and co-workers reported on results with another paramagnetic agent, the nitroxyl spin label PCA (2,2,5,5-tetramethylpyrrolidine–1-oxyl–3-carboxylic acid). Excised infarcted hearts were imaged and T1 and T2 values derived from images.[M5] Hearts were obtained at 5 minutes and 15 minutes postinjection. An interesting differential effect on T1 and T2 was observed. T1 values in the infarct region were lower than in normal myocardium, whereas T2 values were higher, in both the 5- and 15-minute groups. This is unexpected, as paramagnetic agents reduce both T1 and T2. The differential results may be explained by the methods used to calculate T1 and T2, which unfortunately were not presented in the referenced manuscript.

The compound that has undergone the most investigation has been gadolinium-DTPA. Gadolinium, a rare earth element, is highly paramagnetic but is highly toxic. When chelated to DTPA, the element is much safer, and, in fact, this agent is approved for human use. A brief review of the results with this compound to date is presented.

In dogs with 24-hour coronary occlusions, both T1 and T2 were lowered significantly in normal myocardium at 90 seconds following a bolus of 0.35 mmol/kg of Gd-DTPA. Infarcted myocardium changed much less[W2] (Tables 50–8 and 50–9). However, at 5 minutes, the pattern was reversed, with lower values in the infarct regions, presumably because of greater washout of the agent in the well-perfused regions.

In vivo imaging using Gd-DTPA was reported initially by Runge and associates[R5] and Rehr and associates.[R1] Runge found considerably improved definition on in vivo spin echo images of regionally ischemic myocardium when a bolus of 0.25 mmol of Gd-DTPA was administered 1 to 3 hours postcoronary ligation. Contrast increased considerably between normal and ischemic zones and remained elevated for 60 to 100 minutes following injection. This was found for spin echo (TE 30, 60, 90, and 120 msec) images. Rehr observed that greater contrast enhancement occurred with Gd-DTPA injection 4 to 5 days postligation versus 24 to 48 hours, perhaps because of a further increase in edema. Gd-DTPA has been shown to distribute primarily to the extracellular space, and the edema may account for the greater sequestration of Gd-DTPA and associated contrast enhancement.

Tscholakoff and colleagues, who also performed in vivo imaging, found no improvement in infarct contrast, in comparison with pre-Gd-DTPA images, at 5 minutes following a bolus of either 0.5 or 0.1 mmol/kg in 5-hour-old infarcts, using T2-

Table 50–9. MAGNETIC RESONANCE CONTRAST AND SPECTROMETER RELAXATION TIMES 5 MINUTES POST-Gd-DTPA

	T1 (msec)		T2 (msec)		MR Contrast (%)
Dog Number	*Normal Myocardium*	*Infarct*	*Normal Myocardium*	*Infarct*	*(SE 500/56)*
7	212.7	135.5	39.6	38.7	23
8	222.3	139.4	38.1	41.2	33
9	181.6	153.6	37.1	40.2	23
10	220.2	139.4	38.4	40.8	40
11	216.4	167.4	40.5	42.5	31
Mean	210.6	147.1	38.7	40.7	30
S.D.	16.6	13.3	1.33	1.40	7.30

(From Wesbey, G., et al.: Effect of gadolinium-DTPA on the magnetic relaxation times of normal and infarcted myocardium. Radiology 1984, 153:165, with permission.)

weighted imaging sequences (spin echo TE 60 msec, TR varying between 1200 and 1800 msec), although improved contrast was observed on relatively more T1-weighted spin echo images (TE 30 msec, TR 600 to 900 msec).[T2] The data demonstrate the importance of measuring T1 and T2 for accurate objective quantitation rather than relying on increased signal intensity, which is influenced by the particular pulse sequences used. In further experiments, they studied six animals reperfused for 5 hours after 1 hour of occlusion and administered 0.1 mmol/kg of Gd-DTPA (Fig. 50–14). On the relatively T1-weighted images, there was a marked increase in the difference in signal intensity between infarcted and normal myocardium, from 14 ± 8.9 percent to 69.7 ± 22.7 percent.

Peschock and associates also observed a marked improvement in the contrast between reperfused infarcted myocardium with Gd-DTPA, as compared with both nonreperfused hearts and reperfused hearts not given Gd-DTPA.[P1] This influence on contrast was most pronounced on the more T1-weighted inversion recovery sequences, in which the ratio of signal intensity in the ischemic versus normal myocardium increased from 0.91 ± 0.09 to 1.45 ± 0.17, producing a difference in signal in the infarct regions. Similar changes, smaller in degree, were observed on spin echo sequences. In this study, hearts were obtained 55 minutes after Gd-DTPA administration and imaged in vitro.

Eichstaedt and co-workers reported a clinical study in which Gd-DTPA was administered to 11 patients within 7 days of infarction, to 3 patients at 3 weeks, and to 12 patients more than 3 weeks after infarction.[E1] Patients were imaged on a 0.35 or 0.5 T system, with spin echo TE values of 35, 70, and 105 msec and TR values ranging between 400 and 1000 msec, depending on heart rate. Images were obtained immediately after injection of 0.1 to 0.2 mmol/kg, and after 10, 25, and 45 minutes. Signal intensity ratios pre- and post-Gd-DTPA administration only changed significantly in the acute infarction group, to 1.69 ± 0.21. The subacute group did have an increased ratio of 1.31 ± 0.06, but in only 3 patients, and this value was not statistically significant. In chronic infarctions, no enhancement was observed with a ratio equal to 0.97 ± 0.16. These data again suggest that the contrast-enhancing effect is due to the increased extracellular volume associated with edema in acute infarcts, sequestering Gd-DTPA. As edema decreases, particularly in the chronic infarcts in which edema is replaced by fibrous scar, contrast enhancement does not occur.

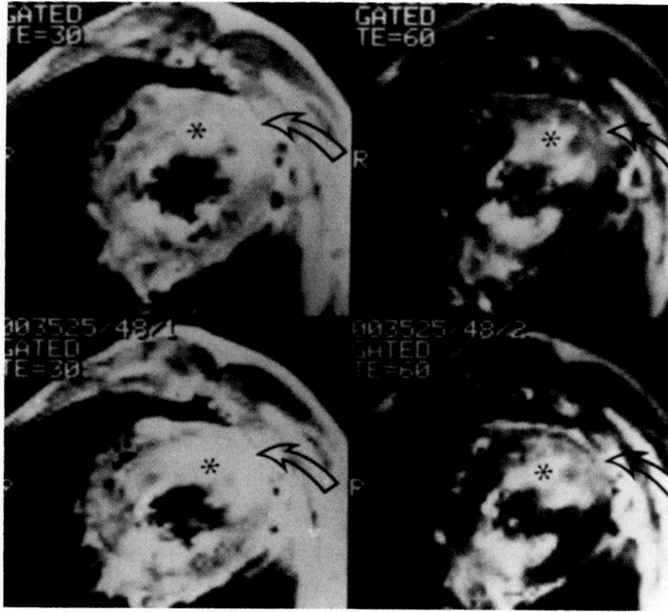

Figure 50–14. Transverse SE images through a canine heart with an acute, reperfused infarct. All four images were acquired with short TR (gated to every heart beat). *Upper images* were obtained prior to Gd-DTPA administration; *lower images* were obtained after administration of 0.1 mmol/kg. Note the marked enhancement of the reperfused infarct *(arrows)* located in the anterior left ventricular wall. *—intracavitary flow signal. (From Tscholakoff, D., Higgins, C. B., Sechtem, U., et al.: Occlusion and reperfused myocardial infarcts: effect of Gd-DTPA on ECG-aged MR imaging. Radiology 160:515–519, 1986, with permission.)

As is clear from the preceding data, Gd-DTPA has rapid clearance from tissues, leading to varying results depending on the time of imaging and whether signal intensity alone is assessed or T1 and T2 are measured. In an attempt to minimize the rapid clearance of Gd-DTPA, Schmiedl and group studied Gd-DTPA labeled to albumin, which reduces the distribution volume to the vascular space.[S1] After early rapid changes associated with achievement of equilibrium, little change in blood, brain, heart, and lung T1 occurred over 90 minutes following injection. They proposed that the agent might prove useful ultimately for the quantitation of regional myocardial flow, as the binding to albumin would reduce the effect of capillary permeability as a determinant of contrast agent accumulation. Further studies of this agent are required.

In our laboratory, we have tried to explore the distribution and clearance kinetics of Gd-DTPA to better understand its potential, particularly for quantitative flow imaging. Studies have been performed following a bolus injection of 0.5 mmol/kg and following a bolus plus constant infusion of 0.01 to 0.02 mmol/kg/min, a regimen which we have found produces constant blood levels and also a significant myocardial tissue paramagnetic effect. In animals sacrificed immediately after a bolus injection, there was a direct linear relationship of Gd-DTPA concentration and regional myocardial blood flow, both in 3- to 5-day-old infarction, and in hearts acutely ischemic, i.e., sacrificed within 30 minutes of coronary ligation. At 5 minutes after a bolus injection, we found that a linear relationship was maintained in acutely ischemic infarcts, albeit at reduced Gd-DTPA tissue concentrations. However, there was little difference between Gd-DTPA concentration in 3- to 5-day-old infarcts and normal myocardium, presumably because at 5 minutes the concentrations were falling in normal myocardium and were stable or slightly rising in infarcted myocardium.

As steady state concentrations are not maintained following a bolus injection, it would be unlikely that a bolus injection technique alone could be used for quantitative flow imaging unless ultrafast imaging becomes feasible. With a 25-minute constant infusion in acutely ischemic animals, there was little relationship of Gd-DTPA concentration to flow (see Fig. 50–4). In fact, most values for contrast agent concentration were in a narrow range, totally independent of flow except at very reduced flows (<50 ml/min/100 g).

The same picture was observed 2 minutes after the end of the constant infusion, an experiment performed to examine washout kinetics. Using the same methods in 3- to 5-day-old infarcts, an inverse curvilinear relationship is found, with lower Gd-DTPA concentrations at higher flows and higher concentrations at moderately reduced flows in the infarct zone (Fig. 50–15). In the center of large infarcts, where flow is severely reduced, Gd-DTPA concentration is minimal; this is presumably because of reduced delivery of the compound despite an increased extracellular volume similar to that of the surrounding infarcted myocardium.

It is obvious from the results to date that a great deal of further investigation is required to clarify the optimal time for imaging following Gd-DTPA injection for contrast enhancement and to determine the true potential for quantitative evaluation of flow with the agent. This is because of the very rapid, dynamic changes in tissue concentration of Gd-DTPA over time. Normal myocardium has rapid washin and washout of material following a bolus injection, ischemic tissue responds at slower rates, and areas with increased extracellular space (edema) serve as reservoirs for the contrast agent.

As mentioned in the earlier section on acute ischemia, the ideal paramagnetic agent would have a linear distribution to

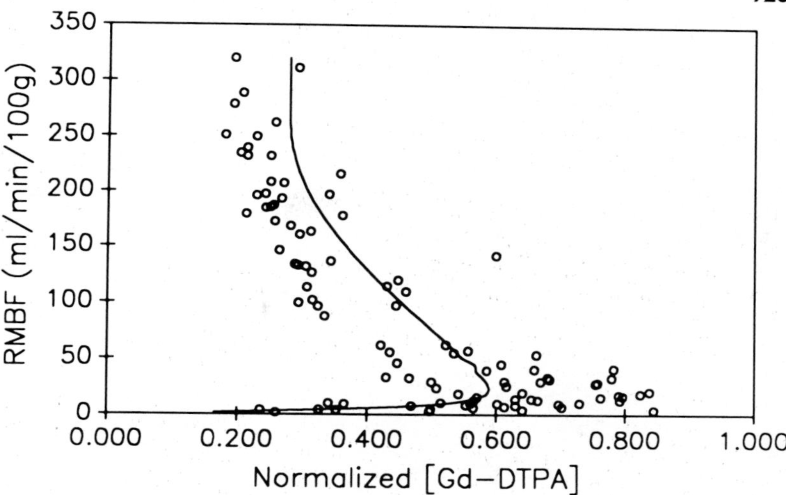

Figure 50–15. Flow versus [Gd-DTPA] chronic; 2-minute delayed sacrifice. Two minutes after the end of the constant infusion in subacute infarction (3–5 days), an inverse curvilinear relationship is observed with the highest [Gd-DTPA] in infarct regions with a 6% increase in total water content. However, in the center of the infarct zones, with greatly reduced flow, [Gd-DTPA] is reduced to the same degree as in the high-flow regions.

myocardium in proportion to flow, prolonged stable retention in myocardium, and minimal-to-no toxicity. As yet, no such agent is available.

ASSESSMENT OF LEFT VENTRICULAR FUNCTION IN ISCHEMIC HEART DISEASE

We have seen how nuclear magnetic resonance imaging may be applicable for characterization of myocardial tissue in the settings of acute ischemia, infarction, and reperfused infarction, with and without the use of contrast agents. Magnetic resonance imaging can also provide functional information about ventricular performance. Because of the superb spatial resolution provided, MRI may be uniquely capable of a comprehensive evaluation of many aspects of myocardial activity.

Clinical Studies of Contraction

Nishikawa and associates reported on the evaluation of left ventricular function in 16 patients with a variety of cardiac diagnoses: normal, cardiomyopathy, pericarditis, and myocardial infarction.[N1] Inversion recovery pulse sequences synchronized to cardiac activity were obtained at end-diastole and end-systole for single slices and ejection fractions calculated and compared with values obtained by equilibrium radionuclide angiography. Although an r value of 0.85 was obtained, the calculated ejection fractions were consistently lower than those obtained by the radionuclide technique. Unfortunately, the regression equation was not provided. Regional wall motion abnormalities did correlate well between the techniques.

Higgins and associates described wall thinning in synchronized multislice images in 23 patients with histories of remote or chronic myocardial infarction [H2] (Fig. 50–16). Mural thrombus was easily detected in 5 patients, correlating with echocardiographic findings. Also, relative stasis of blood in regions of hypokinesis or aneurysm was identified as abnormally increased signal intensity in cavitary blood on the second echo (56 msec) of a multiecho spin echo technique. Similar findings were noted by von Schulthess and colleagues.[V1] Tscholakoff and co-workers used synchronized magnetic resonance images to quantitate the percentage of wall thickening normally observed from diastole to systole.[T1] The anterior wall thickness increased by 70 percent, the lateral wall, by 60 percent, and by 40 percent for the septum. However, no attempt was made to align the imaged slices perpendicular to the long axis of the ventricle, and therefore these values may overestimate the true values. It is possible on most commercially available systems at present to align the slice profiles so as to minimize this error.

Underwood and associates compared regional wall motion analysis between synchronized end-diastolic and end-systolic magnetic resonance images versus contrast ventriculography in 18 patients: 13 with coronary disease, 1 with a congestive cardiomyopathy, 1 with mitral stenosis, 1 with an atrial septal defect, and 2 normal subjects.[U1] Wall motion assessment by the two methods agreed in 68 of 105 segments analyzed, but it differed by one class in 32 segments and by two classes in 5 segments. Sechtem and associates, using similar criteria, claimed 93 per cent sensitivity and specificity in detecting regional wall motion abnormalities in 17 patients with coronary disease.[S2]

All the studies presented thus far have relied on end-diastolic and end-systolic frames being acquired separately. However, a much better technique, imaging all phases of the cardiac cycle concurrently, with up to 24 frames per cardiac cycle, has been developed with acceptable imaging times. Sechtem and colleagues have acquired 10 to 12 levels, covering the entire left ventricle, at up to 24 frames per cycle, requiring an imaging time of 30 minutes, that can be performed even in patients with irregularities of heart rhythm, including atrial fibrillation[S3] (Figs. 50–17 and 50–18). This technique has a variety of names but

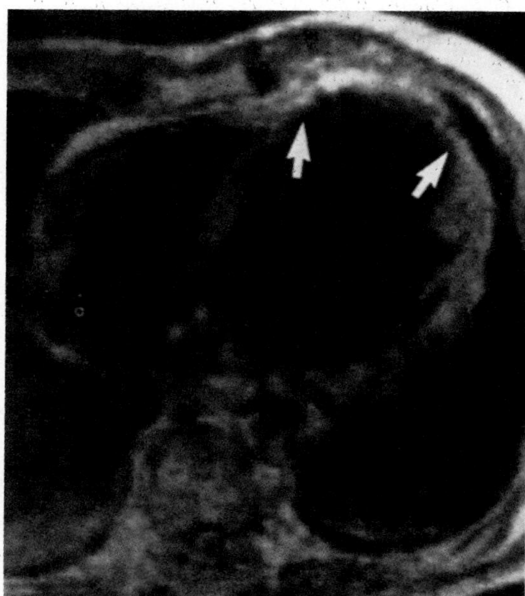

Figure 50–16. Transverse MR image (TE = 28 msec) of a patient who had remote anteroseptal myocardial infarction shows regional thinning of the anterior wall of the left ventricle *(arrows)*. (From Higgins, C. B., Byrd, B. F., McNamara, M. T., et al.: Magnetic resonance imaging of the hearts: a review of the experience in 172 subjects. Radiology 155:671–679, 1985, with permission.)

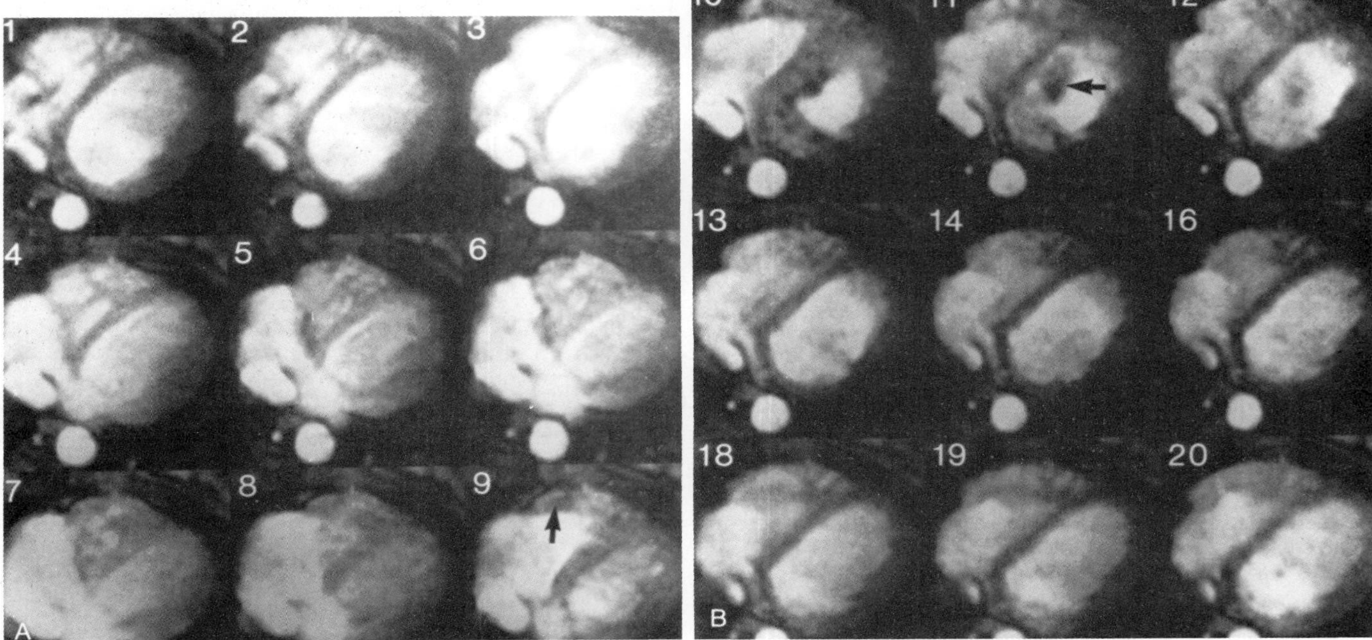

Figure 50–17. Transverse cine MR images in a normal subject with a heart rate of 60 beats/min. Time resolution was 42 msec. Twenty time frames acquired at the same level are shown in *A* and *B*. *A*, Midventricular level of left ventricle. Image 1 was obtained 20 msec after the R wave and subsequent images at 42 msec intervals thereafter. Note area of low signal intensity within right atrium close to tricuspid valve in first three systolic frames. Wall thickening at end systole (image 8) is uniform over circumference of left ventricle. Areas of low signal intensity on ventricular aspect of opened valve leaflet (*arrow*, image 9) likely are related to turbulence caused by rapid diastolic influx of atrial blood. *B*, Diastolic frames at same level as *A*. During early diastole, there is some low-intensity signal within the left ventricle, possibly related to ventricular filling (*arrow*, image 11). Note closing of tricuspid valve in mid-diastole (image 16) and reopening with atrial contraction at end diastole (images 18 and 19). (From Sechtem, U., Pflugfelder, P. W., White, R. D., et al.: Cine MR imaging: potential for the evaluation of cardiovascular function. Am. J. Radiol. 148:239, 1987, © by American Roentgen Ray Society.)

these investigators termed it GRASS (gradient-recalled acquisition in steady state). It uses low flip angles of 30° (as opposed to 90° often used in spin echo imaging), short echo times of 12 msec or less, and pulse repetition times of 15 to 21 msec. When reconstructed, the images are displayed in a cine endless loop format, similar to that used for radionuclide ventriculograms. However, the irregular heartbeat causes some cardiac cycles to be excluded from the data, and this makes functional interpretation hazardous if the rejected beats are common. Using this technique, global left and right ventricular function are readily quantified, as well as regional contraction abnormalities and decreased or absent systolic wall thickening. If concurrent mitral valvular incompetence was present, it was detected as an area of signal *loss* in cavitary blood which now does have signal, extending from the incompetent valve toward the posterior wall of the atrium. This technique, which can be performed within an

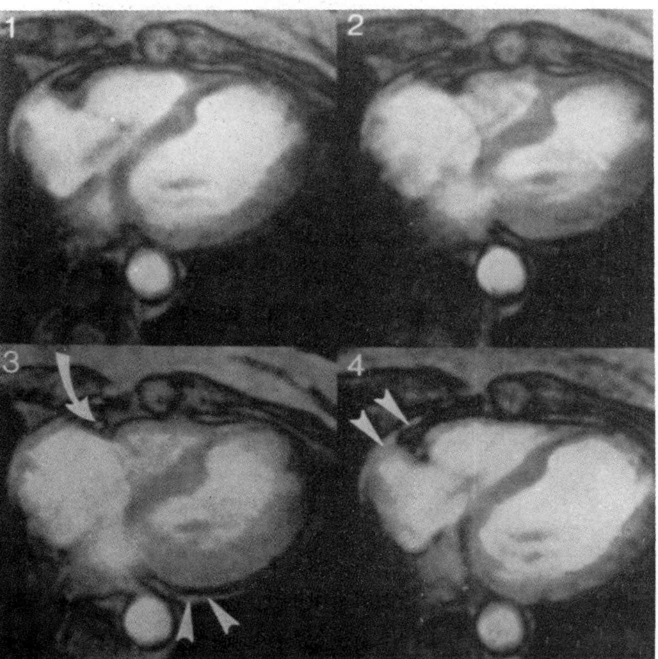

Figure 50–18. Transverse cine MR images through heart of patient with 3-month-old anteroseptal myocardial infarction. Image 1 was obtained in early systole, image 2 further into systole, and image 3 at end systole. Image 4 represents late diastole. Note absence of wall thickening in anteroseptal region and localized hypertrophy of mid-septal area. Damaged myocardium is sharply demarcated from normal myocardium. A small pericardial effusion with high signal intensity is visible over right atrium and behind left ventricle (*arrowheads*, images 3 and 4). Note right coronary artery within right atrioventricular groove (*curved arrow*). (From Sechtem, U., Pflugfelder, P. W., White, R. D., et al.: Cine MR imaging: potential for the evaluation of cardiovascular function. Am. J. Radiol. 148:(2)239–246, 1987, © by American Roentgen Ray Society.)

acceptable time period, will add a great deal to the information that can be derived from the tissue-characterizing spin echo and inversion recovery pulse sequences.

CLINICAL STUDIES OF THE MYOCARDIUM IN ISCHEMIC DISEASE

A great deal of necessary work has been performed in animals thus far to ascertain the limits of magnetic resonance imaging and to help in appropriately interpreting regional signal intensity differences. MRI is being used increasingly in the evaluation of patients with ischemic heart disease, and the results have corroborated the earlier studies in animals in the main.

Changes in Magnetic Resonance Signal Intensity and Relaxation Times

Liebermann and associates reported their findings in patients with subacute and chronic myocardial infarction.[L1] Using only spin echo TE 30-msec images on a 0.30 T system, no observable signal differences were observed in 8-, 10-, and 21-day-old infarctions. Only two of six early infarct patients and four of seven with 21-day-old infarcts had myocardial thinning. Similar findings were reported by Higgins and associates,[H2] and McNamara and Higgins[M3] (Fig. 50–19).

The first report of imaging of more acute infarctions (5 to 12 days) in nine patients reported a mean percent difference in signal intensity between normal and infarcted myocardium of 70.2 ± 21.3 per cent in spin echo TE 56-msec images, with less pronounced differences of 27.1 ± 13.6 percent in spin echo TE 28-msec images.[M4] T2 was also increased to 78.3 ± 30.5 msec in infarcted myocardium versus 42.1 ± 8.4 in normal myocardium. These values are similar to those reported by the same group in canine myocardial infarction and also were confirmed by a later report in six patients imaged 4 to 10 days after infarction,[H3] and in 25 patients 3 to 17 days after infarction.[F2]

However, Johnston and colleagues noted a regional increase in signal intensity on spin echo TE 30/60 msec images in 34 patients studied 3 to 30 days postinfarction, with the area of increased signal corresponding to the electrocardiographic site of abnormality in all cases.[J2, J3]

Been and colleagues measured T1 values in 13 patients with 2- to 12-day-old infarctions.[B1] T1 images were obtained by an interlaced saturation recovery and inversion recovery sequence. In the investigators' 0.08 T system, T1 was increased to a mean of 329 ± 60 msec versus 305 ± 25 in seven normal volunteers and to 307 ± 27 msec in five patients with chronic infarction (more than 2 months). However, in a separate study of chronic infarcts 9 months to 16 years old, signal intensity and T2 were found to be decreased to a mean of 28.7 versus 45.4 in normal myocardium[M1] (Fig. 50–19). Presumably, the replacement of myocardium by fibrous scar is responsible for these changes.

Filipchuk and colleagues looked at the sensitivity and specificity for a variety of nuclear magnetic resonance criteria for infarction in 27 patients at a mean of 15 days after acute myocardial infarction and in 18 asymptomatic volunteers.[F1] NMR detected increased myocardial signal intensity in 88 percent, cavitary signal in 74 percent, and regional wall thinning in 67 percent. However, increased myocardial signal was observed in 83 percent of normal volunteers, cavitary signal in 94 percent, and wall thinning in 11 percent of cases. It is interesting that wall thinning in this group was the most predictive of and specific for acute myocardial infarction.

Akins and associates confirmed the reliability of looking at regional wall thickness for infarctions 10 days to 6 years old.[A1] In 16 patients, the ratio of the thickness of the infarct region in relationship to adjacent normal myocardium averaged 0.40. Further, detection of these subacute and chronic infarctions was facilitated by appropriate imaging plane selection. Anterolateral, apical, and inferior infarctions were best seen using a long axis projection parallel to the septum, i.e., slightly angulated coronal sections. Septal, apical, and posterior infarcts were best seen using the long axis projection perpendicular to the septum, i.e., sagittal.

Dilworth and colleagues reported serial magnetic resonance imaging changes that occur in humans, and the results again parallel those observed in experimental canine infarction.[D1] Nine patients were imaged 3 to 5 days after acute infarction and restudied 10 to 14 days after the acute event prior to hospital discharge. Normalized regional myocardial signal intensity values on the first echo of a two-echo sequence were increased to 37 ± 13 percent on initial study and increased to 51 ± 17 percent on the predischarge study. On the second echo, the respective values were 89 ± 33 percent decreasing to 53 ± 17 percent. The second echo sequence, being a more T2-weighted sequence, more closely indicates T2 changes, and this is corroborated by the normalized T2 relaxation time increases of 51 ± 22 percent on initial study and 33 ± 39 percent on the predischarge study.

Use of Gd-DTPA

As mentioned in the section on contrast agents, Gd-DTPA has been used with varying results in different aged infarctions: acute (5 to 10 days), subacute (10 to 21 days), and chronic (over 21 days)[E1] (Fig. 50–20). Enhancement of delineation of the infarct region by signal intensity changes occurred only in the acute infarct group, for only that group had sufficient alterations in tissue extracellular volume to affect regional clearance kinetics of Gd-DTPA.

We have used magnetic resonance imaging to assess the effectiveness of thrombolytic therapy in reducing infarct size in

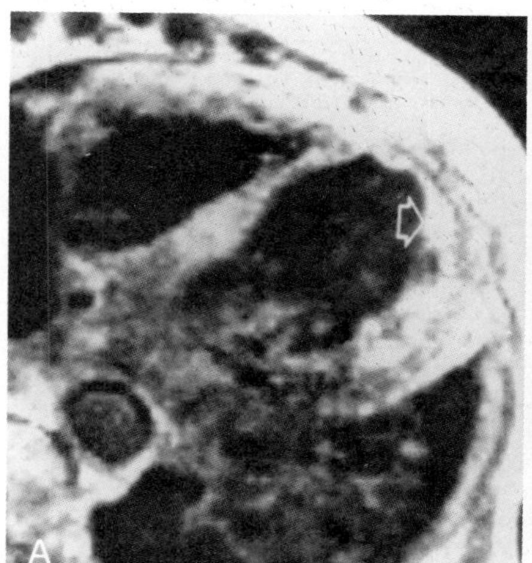

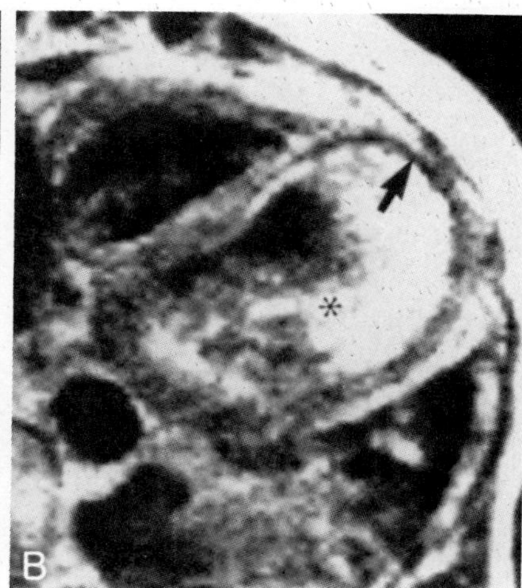

Figure 50–19. Old anteroseptal myocardial infarction. ECG-gated SE images at 28 msec TE *(A)* and 56 msec TE *(B)*: anterior wall thinning and adherent mural thrombus within left ventricle *(open arrow)*. Thinned myocardium *(solid arrow)* is characterized by relatively low signal intensity. Intracavitary flow signal *(asterisk)* appears on second-echo image. (From McNamara, M. T., Higgins, C. B. Magnetic resonance imaging of chronic myocardial infarcts in man. Am. J. Radiol. 146:(2)315–320, 1986, © by American Roentgen Ray Society.)

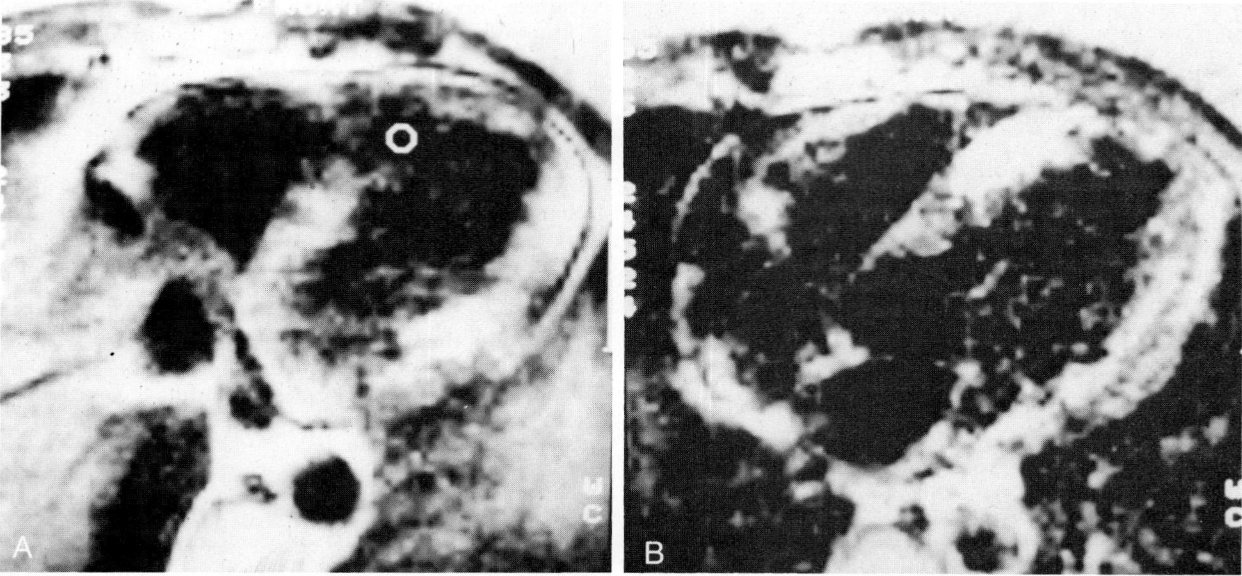

Figure 50–20. *A*, Image of infarction in the inferior septum in transversal MR plane. The signal decrease is quantified in three circular regions in the area of interest. *B*, After application of gadolinium, a significant increase of signals may be measured in the same regions of infarcted area. The signal contrast is artificially enhanced by later echoes. (From Eichstaedt, H. W., Felix, R., Dougherty, F. C., et al.: Magnetic resonance imaging (MRI) in different stages of myocardial infarction using the contrast agent gadolinium-DTPA. Clin. Cardiol. 9[11]:527–535, 1986. Copyrighted and reprinted with the permission of CLINICAL CARDIOLOGY PUBLISHING CO., INC./FACM, INC., The JBI Building, Box 832, Mahwah, New Jersey 07430, USA.)

66 patients randomized to placebo or streptokinase therapy[W5] (Table 50–10). Spin echo TE 30 and 60 msec images, using pulse repetition times equal to twice the R-R interval, 1200 to 2000 msec, were used. Areas of abnormal signal intensity of greater than 2 standard deviations from nonischemic myocardium were determined at 3 weeks after infarction. This was the time we had found MRI to be most accurate for infarct size estimation in canine infarction in both reperfused and nonreperfused hearts. Despite comparable values for resting left ventricular function by radionuclide angiography, streptokinase-treated patients had abnormal NMR signal in only 3 ± 2 percent of left ventricular volume, as opposed to 10 ± 4 percent for the placebo-treated group, $p < 0.05$. It is likely that these values underestimated the true extent of infarction, for T1 and T2 values, which were calculated in the canine study, were not used in this clinical study.

Table 50–10. COMPARISON OF MEAN VALUES OF PLACEBO AND STREPTOKINASE THERAPY

	Streptokinase	p Value	Placebo
Peak CK (IU/liter)	2367 ± 1486	NS	2637 ± 1305
Percent LV	3 ± 2	$p < 0.05$	10 ± 4
Global function			
REF (%)	54 ± 11	NS	47 ± 10
EEF (%)	53 ± 12	NS	49 ± 11
NEF (%)	61 ± 13	$p < 0.05$	48 ± 10
ΔEF (%)	7 ± 7	NS	1 ± 2
Regional function			
Infarct segments			
Rest	1.2 ± 0.6	NS	1.7 ± 0.8
Exercise	1.4 ± 0.8	NS	1.6 ± 0.8
Nitroglycerin	0.5 ± 0.7	$p < 0.025$	1.7 ± 0.8

CK—creatine kinase; ΔEF—change in ejection fraction from rest to postnitroglycerin image; EEF—exercise ejection fraction; NEF—after nitroglycerin ejection fraction; REF—resting ejection fraction.

(From Wisenberg, G., et al.: Nuclear magnetic resonance and radionuclide angiographic assessment of acute myocardial infarction in a randomized trial of intravenous streptokinase. Am. J. Cardiol. 62:1011, 1988, modified with permission.)

SUMMARY

Nuclear magnetic resonance imaging has undergone a period of active animal and clinical investigation to determine the potential role for this technique. It appears that in many areas considerable further work is required.

In the assessment of acute ischemia with occlusion periods of less than one hour, imaging will prove sensitive to reduced flow only upon the addition of paramagnetic agents. These agents would have to remain in myocardium in proportion to flow for a sufficiently long period for imaging to be performed—approximately 2 to 3 minutes.

With nonreperfused infarction, unenhanced magnetic resonance imaging relies a great deal on the evolution of changes in regional tissue water content to produce alterations in signal intensities and/or T1 and T2 values. These changes appear to peak within the first 1 to 2 weeks and then decline. As edema is replaced by fibrous scar tissue formation, the ability to detect infarction depends more on regional wall thinning and contraction abnormalities.

Reperfusion remains an area in which considerable controversy remains in the literature as to whether magnetic resonance imaging will allow the distinction between reperfused and nonreperfused infarcts. When reperfusion causes a large influx of edema fluid, this process could be detectable but would require serial imaging. The edema of infarction and reperfusion probably produce similar changes in tissue NMR properties.

Because tissue edema extends beyond the infarct zone in the early weeks after coronary occlusion, nuclear magnetic resonance does not estimate accurately the true extent of tissue necrosis. However, with resolution of edema by 3 weeks, infarct estimation appears to be accurate.

Paramagnetic contrast agents, in particular Gd-DTPA because of its extracellular distribution, may provide images that reflect local tissue extracellular water content. Thus, early infarcts, with and without reperfusion, show considerable enhancement with Gd-DTPA that is not observed in the chronic state.

For evaluation of ventricular function, the recently developed gradient focused pulse sequences will greatly add to the ability of NMR to provide quantitative information.

Finally, published clinical studies have corroborated the results in animal experiments and have been extended to study the effect of interventions on infarct size when nuclear magnetic resonance imaging is performed at the appropriate time after infarction.

References

A

1. Akins, E. W., Hill, J. A., Sievers, K. W., and Conti, C. R.: Assessment of left ventricular wall thickness in healed myocardial infarction by magnetic resonance imaging. Am. J. Cardiol. 59:24, 1987.

B

1. Been, M., Ridgeway, J. P., Douglas, R. H. B., et al.: Characterisation of acute myocardial infarction by gated magnetic resonance imaging. Lancet 2:348, 1985.
2. Brady, T. J., Goldman, M. R., Pykett, L., et al.: Proton nuclear magnetic resonance imaging of regionally ischemic canine hearts: Effect of paramagnetic proton signal enhancement. Radiology 144:343, 1982.
3. Brown, J. J., Strich, G., Higgins, C. B., et al.: Nuclear magnetic resonance analysis of acute myocardial infarction in dogs: The effects of transient coronary ischemia at varying duration and reperfusion on spin lattice relaxation times. Am. Heart J. 109:486, 1984.
4. Brown, J. J., Peck, W. W., Gerber, K. H., et al.: Nuclear magnetic resonance analysis of acute and chronic myocardial infarction in dogs: Alterations in spin lattice relaxation times. Am. Heart J. 108:1292, 1984.
5. Buda, A. J., Aise, A. M., Juni, J. E., et al.: Detection and sizing of myocardial ischemia and infarction by nuclear resonance imaging in the canine heart. Am. Heart J. 110:1294, 1985.

C

1. Canby, R. C., Reeves, R. C., Evanochko, W. T., et al.: Proton nuclear magnetic resonance relaxation times in severe myocardial ischemia. J. Am. Coll. Cardiol. 10:412, 1987.
2. Cannon, P. J., Maudsley, A. A., Hilal, S. K., et al.: Sodium nuclear magnetic resonance imaging of myocardial tissue of dogs after coronary artery occlusion and reperfusion. J. Am. Coll. Cardiol. 7:573, 1986.
3. Caputo, G. R., Sechtem, U., Tscholakoff, D., and Higgins, C. B.: Measurement of myocardial infarct size at early and late time intervals using MR imaging: An experimental study in dogs. Am. J. Radiol. 149:237, 1987.

D

1. Dilworth, L. R., Aisen, A. M., Mancini, G. B. G., and Buda, A. J.: Serial nuclear magnetic resonance imaging in acute myocardial infarction. Am. J. Cardiol. 59:1203, 1987.
2. Diesbourg, L. D., Wisenberg, W., Prato, F. S., et al.: Relationship of Gd-DTPA concentration to NMR relaxation times and blood flow in ischemic canine myocardium following a constant infusion of GD-DTPA. (Submitted to Magnetic Resonance in Medicine.)

E

1. Eichstaedt, H. W., Felix, R., Dougherty, F. C., et al.: Magnetic resonance imaging (MRI) in different stages of myocardial infarction using contrast agent gadolinium/DTPA. Clin. Cardiol. 9:527, 1986.

F

1. Filipchuk, N. G., Peshock, R. N., Malloy, C. R., et al.: Detection and localization of recent myocardial infarction by magnetic resonance imaging. Am. J. Cardiol. 58:214, 1986.
2. Fisher, M. R., McNamara, M. T., and Higgins, C. B.: Acute myocardial infarction: MR evaluation in 29 patients. AJR 148:247, 1986.

G

1. Goldman, M. R., Brady, T. J., Pykett, I. L., et al.: Quantification of experimental myocardial infarction using magnetic resonance imaging and paramagnetic ion contrast enhancement in excised canine hearts. Circulation 66:1012, 1982.

H

1. Higgins, C. B., and McNamara, M. T.: Magnetic resonance imaging of ischemic heart disease. Prog. Cardiovasc. Dis. 28:257, 1986.
2. Higgins, C. B., Lunzer, P., Stark, D., et al.: Imaging by nuclear magnetic resonance in patients with chronic ischemic heart disease. Diagn. Meth. 69:523, 1984.
3. Higgins, C. B., Byrd, B. F., McNamara, M. T., et al.: Magnetic resonance imaging of the heart: A review of the experience in 172 subjects. Radiology 155:671, 1985.
4. Higgins, C. B., Herfkens, R., Lipton, M. J., et al.: Nuclear magnetic resonance imaging of acute myocardial infarction in dogs.: Alterations in magnetic relaxation times. Am. J. Cardiol. 52:184, 1983.

J

1. Johnston, D. L., Liu, P., Rosen, B. R., et al.: In vivo detection of reperfused myocardium by nuclear magnetic resonance imaging. J. Am. Coll. Cardiol. 9:127, 1987.
2. Johnston, D. L., Thompson, R. C., Liu, P., et al.: Magnetic resonance imaging during acute myocardial infarction. Am. J. Cardiol. 57:1059, 1986.
3. Johnston, D. L., and Liu, P.: Evaluation of myocardial ischemia and infarction by nuclear magnetic resonance techniques. Can. J. Cardiol. 4:116, 1988.
4. Johnston, D. L., Brady, T. J., Ratner, A. V., et al.: Assessment of myocardial ischemia with proton magnetic resonance: Effect of a three hour coronary occlusion with and without reperfusion. Circulation 71:595, 1985.
5. Johnston, D. L., Liu, P., Lauffer, R. B., et al.: Use of gadolinium-DTPA as a myocardial perfusion agent: Potential applications and limitations for magnetic resonance imaging. J. Nucl. Med. 28:871, 1987.

L

1. Liebermann, J. M., Alfidi, R. J., Nelson, D. A., et al.: Gated magnetic resonance imaging of the normal and diseased heart. Radiology 152:465, 1984.

M

1. McNamara, M. T., and Higgins, C. B.: Magnetic resonance imaging of chronic myocardial infarcts in man. AJR 146:315, 1986.
2. McNamara, M. T., Higgins, C. B., Ehman, R. L., et al.: Acute myocardial ischemia magnetic resonance contrast enhancement with Gadolinium-DTPA. Radiology 153:157, 1984.
3. McNamara, M. T., and Higgins, C. B.: Cardiovascular applications of magnetic resonance imaging. Magn. Reson. Imag. 2:167, 1984.
4. McNamara, M. T., Higgins, C. B.: Schechtmann, N., et al.: Detection and characterization of acute myocardial infarction in man with use of gated magnetic resonance. Circulation 71:717, 1985.
5. McNamara, M. T., Wesbey, G. E., Brasch, R. C., et al.: Magnetic resonance imaging of acute myocardial infarction using an nitroxyl spin label (PCA). Radiology 20:591, 1985.
6. Mendonca-Dias, H. M., Gaggelli, E., and Lauterbur, P. C.: Paramagnetic contrast agents in nuclear magnetic resonance medical imaging. Semin. Nucl. Med. XIII 13:364, 1983.

N

1. Nishikawa, J., Machida, K., Lio, M., et al.: ECG-gated NMR-CT for cardiovascular disease. Radiat. Med. 1:274, 1983.

P

1. Peshock, R. M., Malloy, C. R., Maximilian, B., et al.: Magnetic resonance imaging of acute myocardial infarction: Gadolinium diethylenetetramine pentaacetic acid as a marker of reperfusion. Circulation 74:1434, 1986.
2. Pflugfelder, P. W., Wisenberg, G., Prato, F. S., et al.: Serial imaging of canine myocardial infarction by in vivo nuclear magnetic resonance. J. Am. Coll. Cardiol. 7:843, 1986.
3. Pflugfelder, P. W., Wisenberg, G., Prato, F. S., et al.: Early detection of canine myocardial infarction by magnetic resonance in vivo. Circulation 71:587, 1985.
4. Pohost, G. M., and Canby, M. E. E.: Nuclear magnetic resonance imaging: Current applications and future prospects. Circulation 75:88, 1987.
5. Prato, F. S., Drost, D. J., King, M., et al.: Cardiac T1 calculations from MR spin-echo images. Magn. Reson. Med. 4:227, 1987.

R

1. Rehr, R. B., Peshock, R. M., Malloy, C. R., et al.: Improved in vivo magnetic resonance imaging of acute myocardial infarction after intravenous paramagnetic contrast agent administration. Am. J. Cardiol. 57:864, 1986.
2. Revel, D., Higgins, C. B.: Magnetic resonance imaging of ischemic heart disease. Radiol. Clin. North Am. 23:719, 1985.
3. Rokey, R., Wendt, R. E., and Johnston, D. L.: Monitoring of acutely ill patients during nuclear magnetic resonance imaging: Use of a time-varying filter electrocardiographic gating device to reduce gradient artifacts. Magn. Reson. Med. 6:240, 1988.
4. Rokey, R, Verani, M. S., Bolli, R., et al.: Myocardial infarct size quantification by NMR imaging early after coronary artery occlusion in dogs. Radiology 158:771, 1986.
5. Runge, V. M., Clanton, J. A., Wehr, C. J., et al.: Gated magnetic resonance imaging of acute myocardial ischemia in dogs: Applications of multi-echo techniques and contrast enhancement with Gd-DTPA. Magn. Reson. Imag. 3:255, 1985.

S

1. Schmiedl, U., Ogan, M., Paajanen, H., et al.: Albumin labelled with Gd-DTPA as an intravascular blood pool-enhancing agent for MR imaging: Biodistribution and imaging studies. Radiology 162:205, 1987.
2. Sechtem, U., Sommerhoff, B. A., Markiewicz, W., et al.: Regional left ventricular wall thickening by magnetic resonance imaging: Evaluation in normal persons and patients with global and regional dysfunction. Am. J. Cardiol. 59:145, 1987.
3. Sechtem, U., Pflugfelder, P. W., White, R. D., et al.: Cine MR imaging: Potential for the evaluation of cardiovascular function. Am. J. Radiol. 148:239, 1987.

EVALUATION OF ISCHEMIC HEART DISEASE BY NUCLEAR MAGNETIC RESONANCE

T

1. Tscholakoff, D., and Higgins, C. B.: Gated magnetic resonance imaging for assessment of cardiac function in myocardial infarction. Radiol. Clin. North Am. 23:449, 1985.
2. Tscholakoff, D., Higgins, C. B., Sechtem, U., and McNamara, M. T.: Occlusion and reperfused myocardial infarcts: Effect of Gd-DTPA on ECG-gated MR imaging. Radiology 160:515, 1986.
3. Tscholakoff, D., Higgins, C. B., McNamara, M. T., and Derugin, N.: Early-phase myocardial infarction evaluation by MR imaging. Radiology 159:667, 1986.
4. Tscholakoff, D., Higgins, C. B., Sechtem, U., et al.: MRI of reperfused myocardial infarct in dogs. Am. J. Radiol. 146:925, 1986.

U

1. Underwood, S., Rees, R. S. O., Savage, P. E., et al.: Assessment of regional left ventricular function by magnetic resonance. Br. Heart J. 56:334, 1986.

V

1. von Schulthess, G. K., Fisher, M., Crooks, L. E., and Higgins, C. B.: Gated MR imaging of the heart: Intracardiac signals in patients and healthy subjects. Radiology 156:125, 1985.

W

1. Wesbey, G., Higgins, C. B., Lanzer, P., et al.: Imaging and characterization of acute myocardial infarction in vivo by gated nuclear magnetic resonance. Circulation 69:125, 1984.
2. Wesbey, G, Higgins, CB, McNamara, M. T., et al.: Effect of Gadolinium-DTPA on the magnetic relaxation times of normal and infarcted myocardium. Radiology 153:165, 1984.
3. Williams, E. S., Kaplan, J. J., Thatcher, F., et al.: Prolongation of proton spin lattice relaxation times in regionally ischemic tissue from dog hearts. J. Nucl. Med. 2:449, 1980.
4. Wisenberg, G., Prato, F. S., Carroll, S. E., et al.: Serial nuclear magnetic resonance imaging of acute myocardial infarction with and without reperfusion. Am. Heart J. 115:510, 1988.
5. Wisenberg, G., Finnie, K. J., Jablonsky, G., et al.: Nuclear magnetic resonance in radionuclide angiographic assessment of acute myocardial infarction in a randomized trial of intravenous streptokinase. Am. J. Cardiol. 62:1011, 1988.

Chapter 51

Cardiomyopathy: Assessment by Magnetic Resonance

PETER T. BUSER, M.D. ▪ CHARLES B. HIGGINS, M.D.

HYPERTROPHIC CARDIOMYOPATHY 929
Morphology 929
Function 931
Tissue Characterization 931
DILATED CARDIOMYOPATHY 931
Morphology 931
Function 931
Tissue Characterization 932
MYOCARDIAL METABOLISM IN CARDIOMYOPATHY 932
Animal Studies 932
Clinical Studies 933
RESTRICTIVE AND INFILTRATIVE CARDIOMYOPATHIES 933

According to the definition and classification agreed upon by the World Health Organization and the International Society and Federation for Cardiology in 1980,[W1] the term cardiomyopathy should be limited to disease of unknown origin of the myocardium. This means that this diagnosis can be established only after exclusion of specific heart diseases such as coronary artery disease, valvular heart disease, or rheumatic heart disease. Often this goal cannot be reached by means of clinical examination, electrocardiography, or noninvasive imaging studies but may require angiography to exclude coronary arterial disease as well as endomyocardial biopsy to demonstrate myofibrillar loss and fibrosis.

Magnetic resonance imaging (MRI), a totally noninvasive technique, is one of the newer imaging modalities for the diagnosis of cardiovascular diseases. The technique provides high contrast resolution, good spatial resolution, a three-dimensional data set, and natural contrast between the blood pool and myocardium. The latter attribute results in excellent delineation of the endocardial border of the myocardium and therefore clear depiction of intracardiac anatomy. Aside from the capability of displaying cardiovascular anatomy in a completely noninvasive manner and in a variety of imaging planes, other attributes of the technique render it attractive for the assessment of cardiomyopathies. Magnetic resonance provides four potential diagnostic insights: morphology, function, tissue characterization, and metabolism. Whereas initial techniques were applicable only for achieving morphologic assessment of cardiac disease, more recent fast imaging techniques can be used to quantitate ventricular function. Cine MRI has now provided images corresponding to 21-msec segments of the cardiac cycle at a frequency greater than 30 per cardiac cycle. This technique achieves a temporal resolution adequate for the evaluation of the cardiac function and blood flow. Tissue characterization with MRI involves measurements of signal intensity, relaxation times (T_1 and T_2), proton density, and magnetic susceptibility in order to differentiate normal and abnormal tissue in an organ. It has now become clear that in vivo measurements of such parameters are fraught with inaccuracies that make them very limited for the description of myocardial diseases.

Phosphorus–31 magnetic resonance spectroscopy (MRS) provides information about the high-energy phosphate compounds within the myocardium, such as phosphocreatine, ATP, and inorganic phosphate, and can estimate intracellular pH. There is currently very little experience with the use of MRS in patients with myocardial disease, but it is intriguing to consider the possibility of monitoring the high-energy phosphate stores and fluxes of such compounds, especially in response to therapeutic interventions.

The cardiomyopathies are usually divided into three major groups: hypertrophic, dilated, and restrictive. This classification will be followed and the experience and potential role of magnetic resonance in each of the three groups will be considered. However, since magnetic resonance is such a new technique, there may be no current experience with some MRI options that are available at a few research sites.

HYPERTROPHIC CARDIOMYOPATHY

Morphology

The electrocardiographically gated spin-echo technique has been used to depict morphologic abnormalities in hypertrophic cardiomyopathy. Images are acquired with gating to every R wave with TE = 25 to 30 msec for T_1-weighted images and gated to every second or third R wave with TE = 60 to 90 msec for T_2-weighted images. Electrocardiographically gated MRI has identified the presence and the extent of the hypertrophy in a group of patients in whom the disease had already been established by two-dimensional echocardiography and/or angiography.[H1] The distribution of the hypertrophy in the left ventricle was demonstrated because of the wide field of view and the acquisition of sequential tomograms that encompassed the entire heart (Figs. 51–1 and 51–2). Hypertrophic cardiomyopathy has been demonstrated in images acquired in the transverse plane, but this may not be the ideal imaging plane for the assessment of this disease. Since this plane sections the myocardial wall obliquely, it may overestimate wall thickness. Measurement of wall thickness and wall thickening during the cardiac cycle requires acquisition of images in the cardiac short-axis plane.

Magnetic resonance imaging has had its major role in identifying the variant forms of hypertrophic cardiomyopathy, such as the apical and the midventricular forms. It has also demonstrated a more extensive distribution of hypertrophy in some patients considered to have hypertrophy confined to the septum based on two-dimensional echocardiography (Fig. 51–2). An interesting observation from magnetic resonance has also been the prominent hypertrophy of the free wall of the right ventricle in some patients with hypertrophic cardiomyopathy (Fig. 51–3).

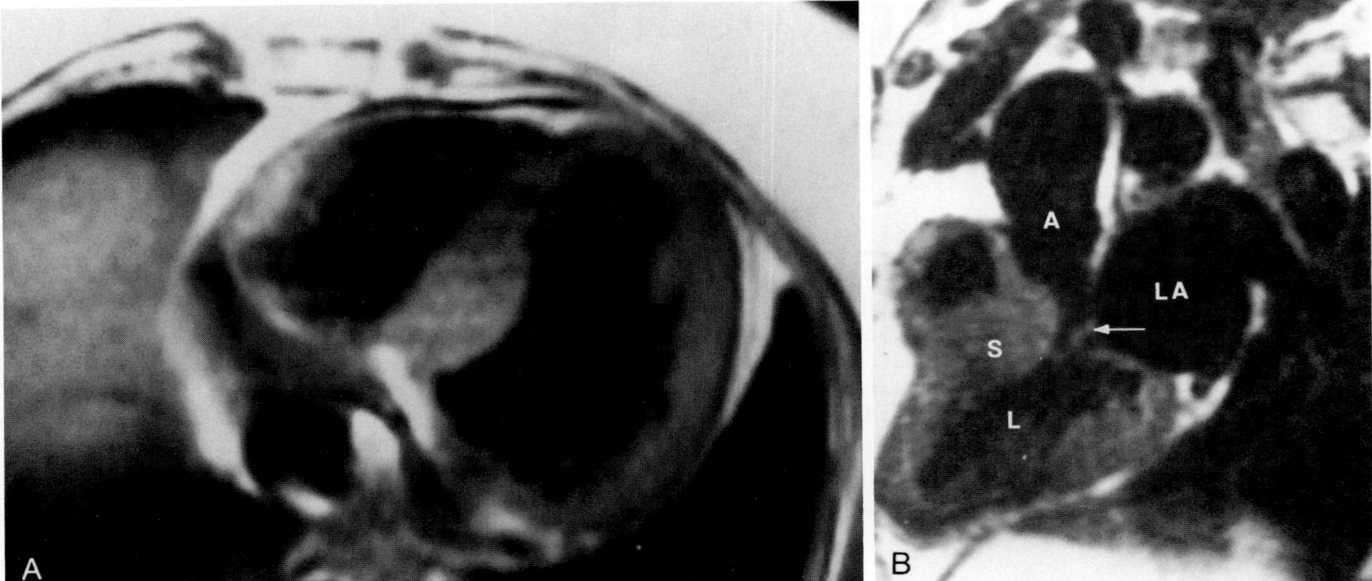

Figure 51–1. Transverse *(A)* and oblique sagittal *(B)* ECG gated images of a patient with hypertrophic cardiomyopathy. There is asymmetric thickening of the ventricular septum. Note apposition of the anterior leaflet of the mitral valve with the septum *(arrow)* in systole. A—aorta; L—left ventricle; LA—left atrium; S—ventricular septum. (Reprinted with permission from Higgins, C. B.: MR of the Heart: Anatomy, physiology and metabolism. AJR 151:239–248, 1988, © by The American Roentgen Ray Society.)

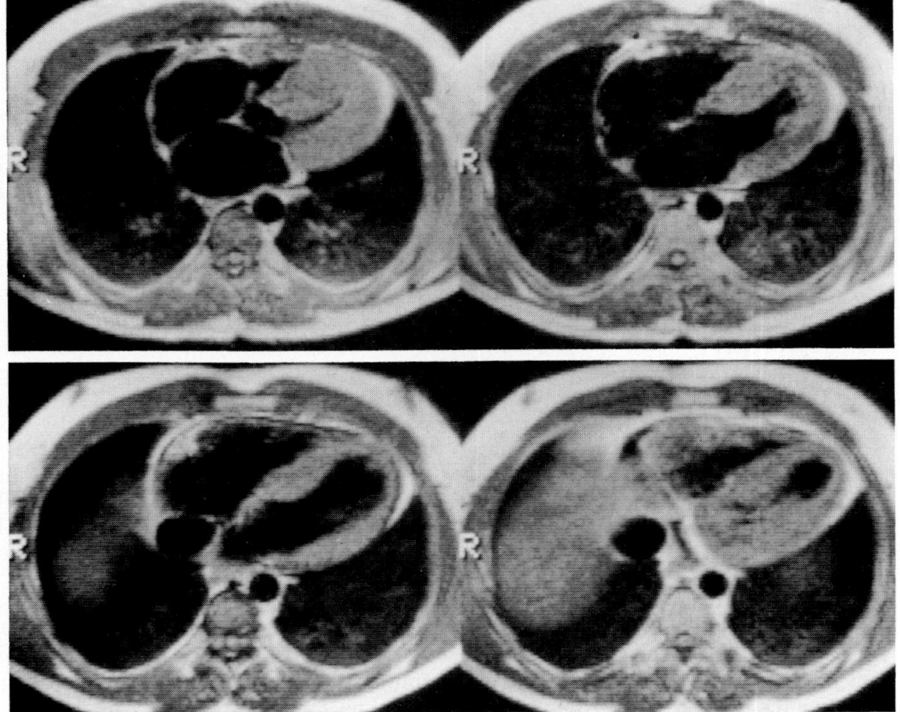

Figure 51–2. Multiple adjacent ECG gated spin-echo images extending from the base (upper left) of the left ventricle toward the apex (lower right). There is marked hypertrophy of the septal (upper left) and lateral walls of the left ventricular outflow region. (Reprinted with permission from Higgins, C. B., et al.: MRI in hypertrophic cardiomyopathy. Am. J. Cardiol. 55:1121, 1985.)

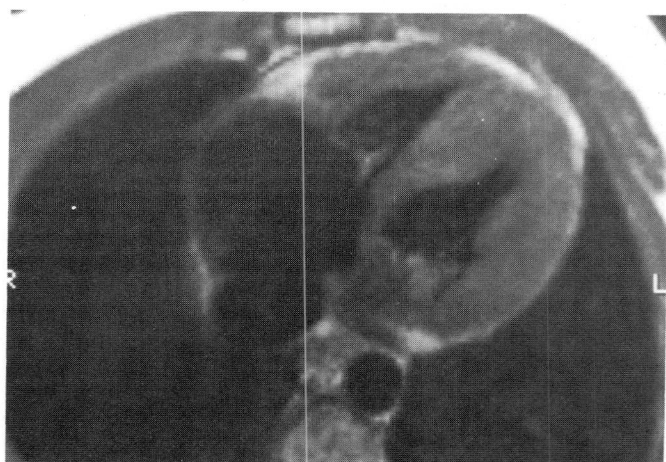

Figure 51–3. ECG gated transverse image of the heart in a patient with hypertrophic cardiomyopathy. There is marked hypertrophy of the ventricular septum. Note also the marked thickening of the free wall of the right ventricle.

Function

Wall-thickening dynamics have been assessed by MRI. Systolic wall thickening was found to be within normal limits in patients with hypertrophic cardiomyopathy compared to normal volunteers, but percent systolic wall thickening of hypertrophic septal segments was significantly lower than that of nonhypertrophied segments.[S1] The assessment of wall thickness by MRI correlated highly with measurements obtained by two-dimensional echocardiography, and a good correlation was found between ejection fraction measured by MRI and left ventricular angiography.[T1]

Mitral regurgitation frequently is a component of hypertrophic cardiomyopathy, especially the obstructive form. Cine MRI has been found to be sensitive and specific for the identification of mitral regurgitation.[S2] The regurgitation is displayed as a signal void emanating from the closed aortic valve and projecting into the left atrium. The severity of regurgitation has been measured as the difference in stroke volume between the two ventricles and also by measurement of the flow void itself on the sequential tomograms encompassing the left atrium.[S2]

By using short-axis cardiac tomograms obtained by MRI, cardiac mass in patients with hypertrophic cardiomyopathy was measured.[L1] There was a good correlation with mass calculated by two-dimensional echocardiography.[L1] Diastolic filling parameters, such as time to peak filling, were assessed and correlated well with measurements obtained by radionuclide techniques.[L1]

Tissue Characterization

The myocardium in most patients with hypertrophic cardiomyopathy exhibits homogeneous signal intensity on high-quality magnetic resonance images. In patients with a variant form of hypertrophic cardiomyopathy who developed a region of apical dyskinesis, MRI demonstrated regions of both high and low signal intensity, probably indicating ischemic injury (high signal intensity) and fibrosis (low signal intensity).[F1] By using a low field strength system (0.08 tesla), the T_1 relaxation time of the septal and left ventricular free wall myocardium was shown not to be different in hypertrophic cardiomyopathy compared with normal hearts, but the T_1 of the septal myocardium was consistently higher than that of the free wall myocardium.[B1] Signal intensity of the myocardium was analyzed by using a spin-echo pulse sequence in 14 patients with hypertrophic cardiomyopathy and 15 normal subjects during systole and diastole. Slight variance of the signal intensity during the cardiac cycle occurred in the normal myocardium but the intensity remained constant in hypertrophic cardiomyopathy.[W2] These two reports[B1, W2] suggest the possibility that relaxation times measured from magnetic resonance images might define the abnormal myocardial regions in hypertrophic cardiomyopathy. However, the sensitivity and specificity of such differential measurements have not been tested.

Alterations in magnetic resonance signal intensity and T_2 relaxation time have been shown in regions of abnormal myocardium in a patient with hypertrophic cardiomyopathy. Increases of intensity and T_2 were correlated with edematous myocardium at sites of nonocclusive coronary ischemia, apparently caused by disproportion between oxygen supply and the increased oxygen demands of the hypertrophied myocardium. Regions with low intensity in the left ventricle were correlated with fibrosis.[F1]

Magnetic resonance imaging has shown potential efficacy for noninvasive assessment of the distribution and extent of the hypertrophic process in hypertrophic cardiomyopathy (see Fig. 51–2). It may be able to characterize regional tissue alterations such as ischemic injury and abnormal tissue composition of the region of hypertrophy. Functional valvular abnormalities such as mitral regurgitation, volumes of left heart chambers, and myocardial mass can be assessed with cine MRI. Because MRI is an investigator-independent modality, it may be sufficiently reproducible among repeated studies for long-term monitoring of these patients.

DILATED CARDIOMYOPATHY

Morphology

The morphologic features of dilated cardiomyopathy displayed on electrocardiographically gated magnetic resonance images consist of enlarged left ventricular cavity with normal wall thickness or thin myocardial walls. In most cases wall thickness is nearly homogeneous throughout the left ventricle.

In patients with dilated cardiomyopathy, MRI demonstrated dilatation of the left ventricle; left atrial and right ventricular enlargements were observed less frequently[H2] In addition, a disproportionate thinning of the ventricular septum was observed in four patients with idiopathic dilated cardiomyopathy in whom coronary arteriography showed no obstructive disease. Generally, left ventricular wall thickness in these patients was normal or mildly reduced.[H2]

Function

Cine MRI in a short-axis view, a plane perpendicular to the intrinsic left ventricular long axis, may be used to demonstrate left ventricular wall thickness and regional wall thickening more accurately than images in planes oblique to the intrinsic heart axis, because the left ventricular myocardium is transected perpendicularly.[B2] By using contiguous tomograms encompassing the left ventricle from apex to base, left ventricular end-systolic and end-diastolic volumes, stroke volume, ejection fraction, and left ventricular mass can be measured in order to define the severity of the dilated cardiomyopathy.[B2] Cine MRI can also be used to detect and estimate the severity of mitral regurgitation or tricuspid regurgitation which may accompany dilated cardiomyopathy.

Cine MRI was used to compare the functional characteristics of 10 normal volunteers and 10 patients with dilated cardiomypathy.[B2] Left ventricular end-systolic and end-diastolic volumes and left ventricular mass were shown to be significantly larger and ejection fraction significantly diminished in dilated cardiomyopathy.[B2] The left ventricular mass-to-volume ratio, as well as the ejection fraction, distinguished the patients from the normal subjects (Fig. 51–4). Left ventricular systolic wall thickening was shown to be more heterogeneous in the patients. Figure 51–5 shows frames at end-diastole, mid-systole, and end-systole from cine magnetic resonance studies of a normal subject and a patient with dilated cardiomyopathy. In the normal subject there is nearly homogeneous wall thickening during the cardiac cycle, whereas in the patient, wall thickening is greatly reduced, especially in the septal region. The patterns of systolic wall thickening throughout the normal and the dilated left ventricle were different. Percent left ventricular systolic wall thickening

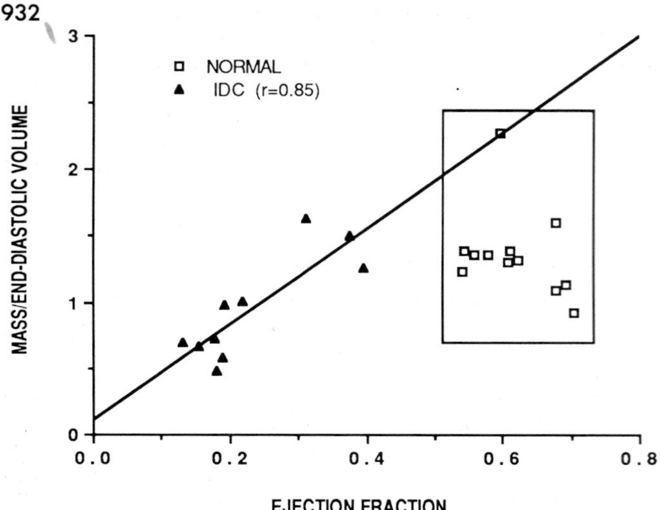

Figure 51–4. Plot of the ratio of left ventricular mass to end-diastolic volume versus ejection fraction for normal individuals and patients with idiopathic dilated cardiomyopathy (IDC). Parameters were calculated from cine magnetic resonance imaging studies. These parameters distinguish between the two groups.

increased from base to apex in normal hearts, whereas this gradient was absent in cardiomyopathic hearts (Fig. 51–6). Wall thickness in the cardiomyopathic left ventricle was normal, but left ventricular mass was nearly twice as large as in the normal subjects.

A more sophisticated parameter of left ventricular function and loading condition is meridional wall stress. This can be calculated from cine magnetic resonance images when blood pressure is recorded continuously and the cardiac events are monitored with simultaneous carotid pulse tracing. The variables needed for the assessment of meridional wall stress, such as end-systolic pressure, left ventricular end-systolic diameter, and end-systolic wall thickness, are thereby provided noninvasively. A recent study has demonstrated a marked increase in end-systolic wall stress in hearts with dilated cardiomyopathy compared to normal hearts.[H3] This measurement may provide a useful, reproducible parameter for monitoring the evolution of myocardial diseases and the response of myocardial function to therapeutic interventions.

Tissue Characterization

Relaxation times of tissues measured in vitro have indicated differences in normal myocardium compared with that in doxorubicin (Adriamycin) cardiomyopathy[T2] or viral myocarditis.[L2] However, it is not clear that the small differences in relaxation times will be detectable on images of the heart in situ.

Cardiac transplant rejection, characterized by generalized inflammation and tissue edema, has been differentiated from normal myocardium in non-immunosuppressed animal models by a significant increase in T_2 relaxation time and intensity values as early as 1 week after transplantation.[A1] There was a significant correlation between histologic grading of severity of rejection and T_2 relaxation times. On the other hand, there was no significant difference in T_1, T_2, or intensity values in cyclosporine-treated allografts and native hearts without histologic evidence of rejection. In patients who had undergone cardiac transplantation, late cardiac allograft rejection was assessed by means of elevated T_1 and T_2 relaxation times and an increase in myocardial wall thickness on magnetic resonance images.[W3] Within the initial 4 weeks following transplant surgery, grafts with rejection exhibited an increase in T_1 and T_2 relaxation times that was apparently related to the surgical procedure, and differentiation from acute rejection was difficult in this time frame.[W3] After the initial 4 weeks, increase in T_1 and T_2 was indicative of rejection. Thus, MRI may have the potential for noninvasively monitoring rejection in patients after cardiac transplantation. Phosphorus–31 MRS may have the potential to differentiate grafts with acute rejection from nonrejected grafts even within the early days following cardiac transplantation by showing a reduction of the phosphocreatine peak and a decrease in the phosphocreatine/ATP ratio in grafts with rejection.[S3]

The potential of MRI in the diagnosis and therapeutic monitoring of other types of cardiomyopathy that may present with cavity dilation and impaired ventricular function has been demonstrated. In cardiomyopathy due to idiopathic hemochromatosis, an enlargement of the left ventricle with normal wall thickness was found. Signal intensity in T_1-weighted images was diminished, and T_2 relaxation time was significantly shorter.[S4] Because of the paramagnetic properties of iron, the myocardial signal intensity is markedly diminished compared with that of normal hearts. From the absolute T_2 values, not only may the excessive iron deposition be diagnosed but also it may be possible to monitor the changes in tissue iron content during therapy.[S4]

MYOCARDIAL METABOLISM IN CARDIOMYOPATHY

Animal Studies

Phosphorus–31 MRS has been shown to provide important information about the levels of high-energy phosphate compounds such as phosphocreatine (PCr) and β adenosine triphosphate (ATP), as well as inorganic phosphate (Pi) and intracellular pH (pH_i) in cardiomyopathic hamsters.[S5] During an increase of the heart rate from 170 to 220 beats per minute, Pi increased and ATP, Pi/PCr, and ATP/Pi decreased significantly in normal hamster hearts as well as in cardiomyopathic hamster hearts. However, the alterations in cardiomyopathic hamsters were significantly more pronounced than in normal hamsters and pH_i also

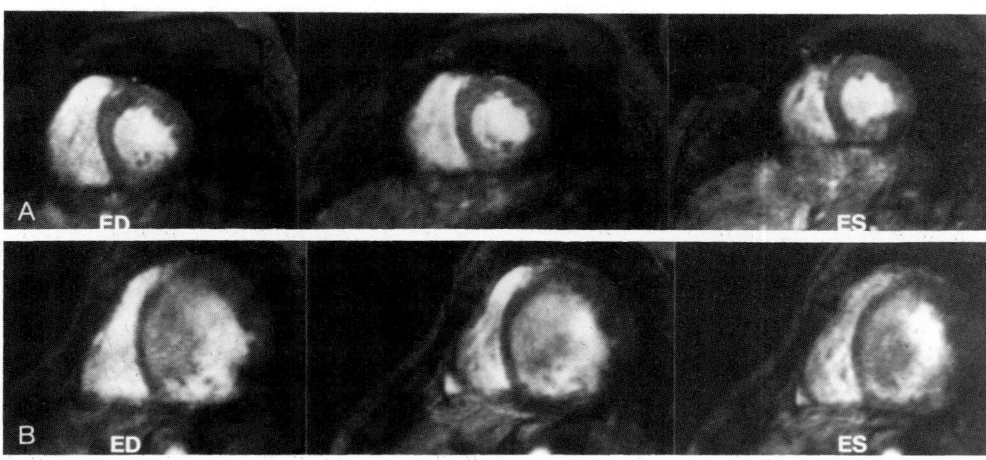

Figure 51–5. Cine magnetic resonance images from a normal subject *(A)* and a patient with dilated (congestive) cardiomyopathy *(B)*. Images were acquired at end-diastole (left), mid-systole (middle), and end-systole (right). There is homogeneous wall thickening in the normal subject during the cardiac cyle. In the patient with cardiomyopathy, wall thickening is reduced, especially in the septal region.

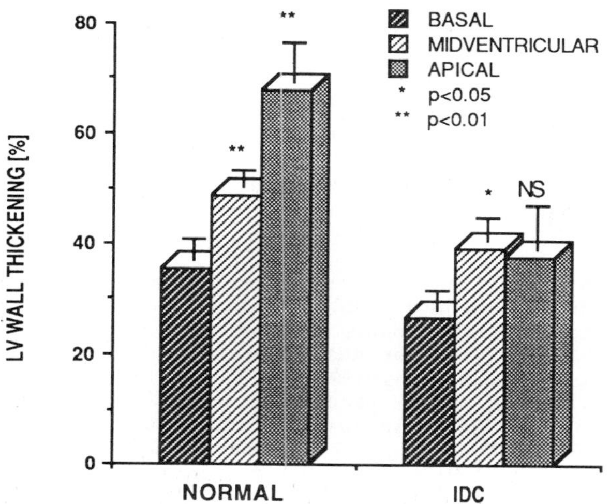

Figure 51–6. Block diagram of percent systolic wall thickening for various layers extending from base to apex of the left ventricle in normal subjects (n = 10) and patients with idiopathic dilated cardiomyopathy (IDC) (n = 10). In normal subjects, there is a gradient in wall thickening from base to apex. The gradient is not evident for the left ventricle in the patients with IDC. (Reprinted with permission from Buser, P. T., et al.: Noninvasive Evaluation of Global Left Ventricular Function with Use of Cine Nuclear Magnetic Resonance J. Am. Coll. Cardiol. 13(6):1294, 1989. Reprinted with permission of the American College of Cardiology.)

decreased significantly in the former group,[M1] indicating that the requirements for energy-rich phosphate compounds exceeded synthesis during rapid increase in heart rate of the isolated heart. These abnormalities in the ^{31}P magnetic resonance spectra were more pronounced in cardiomyopathic hearts. The influence of therapeutic interventions on high-energy phosphate compounds in cardiomyopathic hearts of Syrian hamsters has been studied with ^{31}P MRS. Compared to hearts of age-matched normal hamsters, cardiomyopathic hearts were characterized by significantly higher levels of Pi; lower levels of PCr, PCr/Pi, and ATP/Pi; and regions of decreased pH. Following acute administration of verapamil to the cardiomyopathic heart, ^{31}P MRS showed increases in PCr and PCr/Pi consistent with a salutory action of the drug on function.[M2] In cardiomyopathic hearts of Syrian hamsters at an age at which severe heart failure ensues, isoproterenol improved myocardial performance without any significant change in high-energy phosphate metabolites.[C1] On the other hand, administration of dobutamine in cardiomyopathic hamster hearts in a moderate stage of congestive heart failure had similar effects, whereas in an advanced stage of heart failure no beneficial effect of the drug on mechanical performance or high-energy phosphate metabolism could be demonstrated.[B3] Administration of amrinone and the combination of amrinone plus dobutamine was shown to be more effective than dobutamine alone in the treatment of moderate heart failure, since the phosphorylation potential, calculated from Pi, PCr, ATP, and pH_i levels obtained from ^{31}P measurements, and the mechanical performance improved. The same effect was observed for amrinone alone in the treatment of advanced heart failure.[B4] These experiments demonstrate the great potential of ^{31}P MRS for monitoring alterations of high-energy phosphate metabolites under different therapeutic conditions in congestive heart failure caused by cardiomyopathy.

Clinical Studies

Recent advances in magnetic resonance technology have made possible ^{31}P MRS in vivo studies of human myocardium. For the evaluation of myocardial disease, it is important to monitor simultaneously and correlate the hemodynamic and metabolic information. Initial studies have also been done using electrocardiographically gated MRI to guide surface coil ^{31}P MRS in patients with congestive cardiomyopathy. In these studies, left ventricular functional parameters are assessed with cine MRI performed at the same time as the acquisition of ^{31}P MRS. The two were combined in order to measure myocardial functional and metabolic parameters in normal subjects and patients with congestive (dilated) cardiomyopathy. Cine MRI showed severe reduction in ejection fraction and extent of wall thickening and increase in end-systolic wall stress in comparison with normal subjects. Prominent peaks representing phosphodiesters and phosphomonoesters were observed in the ^{31}P magnetic resonance spectra of the cardiomyopathic patients compared with the normal subjects (Fig. 51–7). The PCr and ATP levels were not different between the two groups. Thus, preliminary results suggest that localized gated ^{31}P MRS combined with cine MRI can identify both abnormal myocardial phosphate metabolism and abnormal ventricular function, which might be useful in characterizing patients with cardiomyopathy and in monitoring the course of the disease.

RESTRICTIVE AND INFILTRATIVE CARDIOMYOPATHIES

There has been very little experience with MRS for the diagnosis of these rare types of cardiomyopathy. The most im-

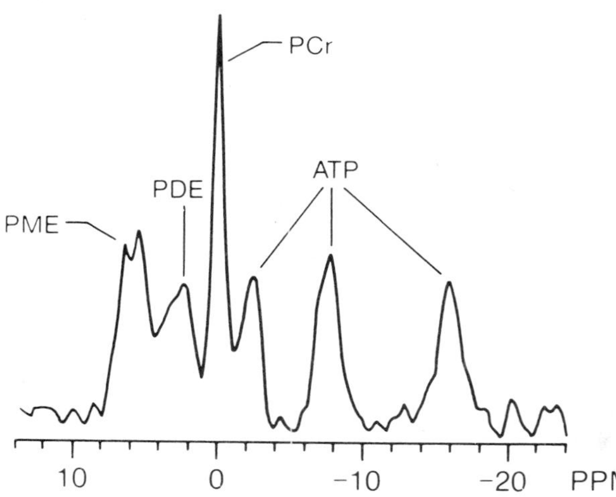

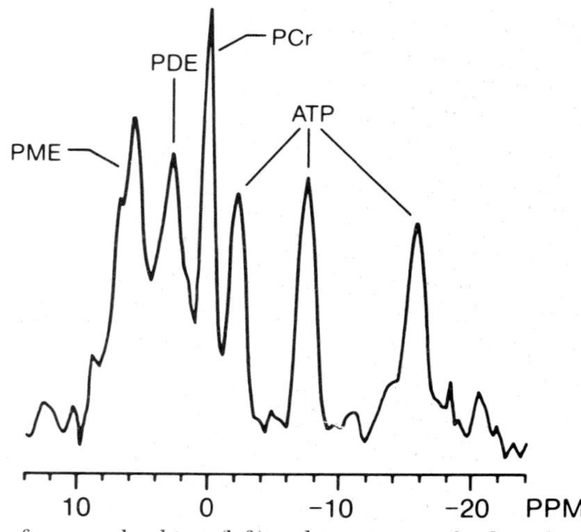

Figure 51–7. Localized phosphorus-31 magnetic resonance spectra from the heart of a normal subject (left) and a patient with idiopathic dilated cardiomyopathy (IDC). Localization was done using one-dimensional chemical shift imaging with a surface coil for signal reception. Compared to the spectrum for the normal subject, the spectrum in IDC shows large phosphomonoester (PME) and phosphodiester (PDE) peaks. The phosphocreatine (PCr) and adenosine triphosphate (ATP) peaks were not significantly different between the two groups.

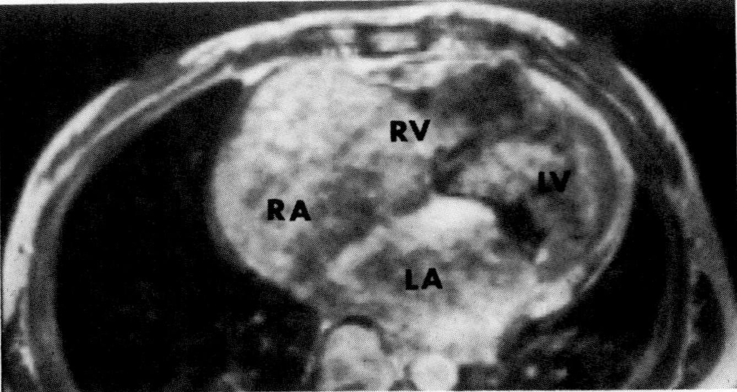

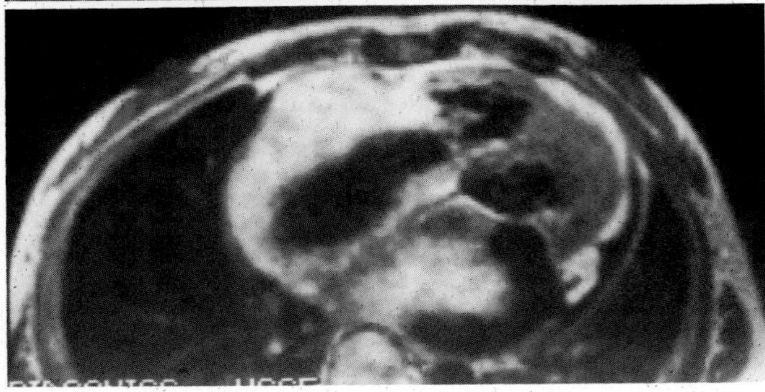

Figure 51–8. ECG gated spin-echo images of the four cardiac chambers of a patient with restrictive cardiomyopathy: second echo (above) and first echo (below) images. Restrictive cardiomyopathy is characterized by prominent dilatation of the atria and nearly normal-sized ventricles. Presumably, because of the resistance to filling of the ventricles in this disease, there is stasis of blood in the atria, causing a prominent intracavitary signal. Intensity of signal from the slowly flowing blood increases from the first to the second echo. LA—left atrium; LV—left ventricle; RA—right atrium; RV—right ventricle.

portant role of MRI in restrictive cardiomyopathy is to demonstrate the pericardial thickness in order to exclude the diagnosis of constrictive pericardial disease.[S6]

Magnetic resonance imaging demonstrates the anatomical changes of infiltrative myocardial diseases and also may indicate stasis of blood in the atria (Fig. 51–8). The characteristic features are dilated atria with relatively normal-sized ventricles and prominent intracavitary signal in the cardiac chambers, especially the atria, due to stasis of blood in these chambers. Magnetic resonance imaging therefore provides important information to distinguish various restrictive from dilated cardiomyopathies.[S7] A thickened pericardium, together with right ventricular narrowing resulting in a tubular-shaped chamber of modest size, and a disproportionately dilated right atrium, inferior vena cava, and hepatic veins are diagnostic features of constrictive pericardial disease on MRI. They permit the differentiation of constrictive pericarditis from restrictive cardiomyopathy,[B5] a distinction that is sometimes difficult even with invasive studies but that is critical because the treatment of the former is surgical and of the latter, medical. In one patient with restrictive cardiomyopathy due to amyloidosis, left ventricular wall thickness was increased in a concentric pattern, but systolic wall thickening was normal.[S1] In a patient with Pompe's disease (a glycogen-storage disease), alterations of the heart were described by using MRI.[B5] The left and right ventricular walls, as well as the interventricular septum, were thickened and appeared irregular and inhomogeneous. Information on other diseases, such as endomyocardial fibrosis or sarcoidosis, is currently lacking. However, the potential of MRI to provide tissue characterization suggests that this technique may be a useful imaging modality for suspected restrictive cardiomyopathies.

References

A

1. Aheme, T., Tschokaloff, D., Finkbeiner, W., et al.: Magnetic resonance imaging of cardiac transplants: The evaluation of rejection of cardiac allografts with and without immunosuppression. Circulation 74:145, 1986.

B

1. Been, M., Kean, D., Smith, M. A., et al.: Nuclear magnetic resonance in hypertrophic cardiomyopathy. Br. Heart J. 54:48, 1985.
2. Buser, P. T., Auffermann, W., Holt, W. W., et al.: Noninvasive evaluation of the global left ventricular function using cine MR imaging. J. Am. Coll. Cardiol. 13:1294, 1989.
3. Buser, P. T., Camacho, S. A., Wu, S. T., et al.: The effect of dobutamine on myocardial performance and high energy phosphate metabolism at different stages of heart failure in cardiomyopathic hamsters: A^{31}P MRS study. Am. Heart J. 117:86, 1989.
4. Buser, P. T., Auffermann, W., Wu, S. T., Dobutamine potentiates amrinone's beneficial effects in moderate but not in advanced heart failure: ^{31}P NMR in isolated hamster hearts. Circ. Res. 66:747, 1990.
5. Boxer, R. A., Fishman, M., La Corte, M. A., et al.: Cardiac MR imaging in Pompe disease. J. Comput. Assist. Tomogr. 10:857, 1986.

C

1. Camacho, S. A., Wikman-Coffelt, J., Wu, S. T., et al.: Improvement in myocardial performance without a decrease in high-energy phosphate metabolites after isoproterenol in Syrian cardiomyopathic hamsters. Circulation 77:712, 1988.

F

1. Farmer, D., Higgins, C. B., Yee, E., et al.: Tissue characterization by magnetic resonance imaging in hypertrophic cardiomyopathy. Am. J. Cardiol. 55:230, 1985.

H

1. Higgins, C. B., Byrd, B. F., Stark, D., et al.: Magnetic resonance imaging in hypertrophic cardiomyopathy. Am. J. Cardiol. 55:1121, 1985.
2. Higgins, C. B., Byrd, B. F., McNamara, M. T., et al.: Magnetic resonance imaging of the heart: A review of the experience in 172 subjects. Radiology 155:671, 1985.
3. Holt, W. W., Wolfe, C., Pflugfelder, P., et al.: Quantitation of left ventricular wall stress measurement in normal and cardiomyopathic subjects. The Society of Magnetic Resonance in Medicine Book of Abstracts, 1988, p. 136.

L

1. Liu, P., Wilansky, S., Poon, P., et al.: Myocardial mass quantitation by magnetic resonance imaging in hypertrophic cardiomyopathy. Circ. Suppl. III 74:226, 1986.
2. Liu, P., Matsumori, A., Abelman, W. H., et al.: Changes of NMR relaxation parameters in myocarditis. Circ. Suppl. II 70:342, 1984.

M

1. Markiewicz, W., Wu, S. T., Sievers, R., et al.: Influence of the heart rate on metabolic and hemodynamic parameters in the Syrian hamster cardiomyopathy. Am. Heart J. 114:362, 1987.
2. Markiewicz, W., Wu, S.T., Parmley, W. W., et al.: Evaluation of the hereditary Syrian hamster cardiomyopathy by ^{31}P nuclear magnetic resonance spectroscopy: Improvement after acute verapamil therapy. Circ. Res. 59:597, 1986.

S

1. Sechtem, U., Sommerhoff, B. A., Markiewicz, W., et al.: Regional left ventricular wall thickening by magnetic resonance imaging: Evaluation in normal

persons and patients with global and regional dysfunction. Am. J. Cardiol. 59:145, 1987.
2. Sechtem, U., Pflugfelder, P. W., Cassidy, M. M., et. al.: Mitral or aortic regurgitation: Quantification of regurgitant volumes with cine MR imaging. Radiology 167:425, 1988.
3. Shorr, L. D., Thompson, A. A., Morell, D. T., et al.: Early noninvasive detection of rejection in heterotopic heart transplants using ^{31}P-NMR spectroscopy. Transpl. Proc. 1(Suppl. 1):842, 1988.
4. Streudel, A., Krahe, T., Becher, H., and Streudel, H.: Kardiomyopathie bei idiopathischer Hămochromatose. Diagnostische Mŏglichkeiten mit der Kernspintomographie. Dtsch. Med. Wschr. 112:590, 1987.
5. Sievers, R., Parmley, W. W., James, T., and Wikman-Coffelt, J.: Energy levels at systole vs diastole in normal hamster hearts vs myopathic hamster hearts. Circ. Res. 53:759, 1983.
6. Soulen, R. L., Stark, D. D., and Higgins, C. B.: Magnetic resonance imaging of constrictive pericardial disease. Am. J. Cardiol. 55:480, 1985.
7. Sechtem, U., Higgins, C. B., Sommerhoff, B. A., et al.: Magnetic resonance imaging of restrictive cardiomyopathy. Am. J. Cardiol. 59:480, 1987.

T

1. Thompson, R. C., Levine, R. A., Mille, S., and Dinsmore, R. E.: Magnetic resonance imaging along the left ventricular axes in hypertrophic heart disease: Accurate characterization of cardiac hypertrophy. Circ. Suppl. III 72:122, 1985.
2. Thompson, R. C., Lojeski, E. W., Ratner, A. V., et al.: Detection of Adriamycin cardiotoxicity using proton NMR techniques. Circ. Suppl. III 68:387, 1983.

W

1. Report of the WHO/IFSC task force on the definition and classification of the cardiomyopathies. Br. Heart J. 44:672, 1980.
2. Waters, J. S., Elion, J. L., and Friedman, B. J.: Analysis of magnetic resonance imaging (MRI) of hypertrophic cardiomyopathy. Circ. Suppl. III 72:122, 1985.
3. Wisenberg, G., Pflugfelder, P. W., Kostuk, W. J., et al.: Diagnostic applicability of magnetic resonance imaging in assessing human cardiac allograft rejection. Am. J. Cardiol. 60:130, 1987.

Chapter 52

Nuclear Magnetic Resonance Assessment of Pericardial Disease

■ *DAVID A. BLUEMKE, M.D., Ph.D.* ■ *JEFFREY T. LUND, M.D.*
■ *MARTIN J. LIPTON, M.D., F.R.C.P.C., F.A.C.C.*

ANATOMY ... 937
IMAGE ACQUISITION ... 937
NORMAL PERICARDIUM ... 938
Magnetic Resonance Visualization of the Pericardium ... 938
Origin of the Pericardial Signal ... 939
CONGENITAL ANOMALIES ... 940
Congenital Absence and Defects of the Pericardium ... 940
Pericardial Cysts ... 940
Pericardial Diverticula ... 940
Developmental Masses of the Pericardium ... 941
PERICARDIAL EFFUSION ... 941
PERICARDIAL THICKENING ... 942
POST-PERICARDIOTOMY SYNDROME AND POST-MYOCARDIAL-INFARCTION PERICARDITIS (DRESSLER'S SYNDROME) ... 942
CONSTRICTIVE PERICARDITIS ... 943
POSTOPERATIVE PERICARDIUM ... 944
PERICARDIAL NEOPLASM ... 944
Primary Pericardial Neoplasm ... 944
Pericardial Metastasis ... 944
SUMMARY ... 945

"There are few diseases attended by more symptoms and more difficult diagnosis than this."

—Laennec, on pericardial disease

Our ability to diagnose disease of the pericardium has grown remarkably over a relatively short period of time. Particularly with the development of echocardiography in the 1960's, the prevalence of pericardial involvement in a variety of disease processes began to be more widely appreciated. Also beginning about this time, fundamental advances in understanding normal pericardial physiology as well as that of tamponade and constriction were accomplished.[M1, R1, S1] The development of computed tomography (CT) and, most recently, magnetic resonance imaging continues to expand the spectrum of pericardial diseases that may be studied by noninvasive imaging techniques.
tomography (CT) and, most recently, magnetic resonance imaging continues to expand the spectrum of pericardial diseases that may be studied by noninvasive imaging techniques.

With the development of cardiac gating techniques, routine magnetic resonance evaluation of pericardial disease has become possible.[A1, L1] In this method, pulse sequences are synchronized to the R-wave peaks of the patient's electrocardiogram. The hundreds of radiofrequency signals that must be acquired to form a single magnetic resonance image can thus be obtained from an operator-specified portion of the cardiac cycle. Without gating, induced artifacts dominate the final images with unacceptable motion degradation of the pericardial and myocardial signal.

Portions of the pericardium can be visualized in up to 100 percent of images by using cardiac gating techniques.[S2] An important advantage of magnetic resonance compared with computed tomography is that excellent contrast is inherent in magnetic resonance, without the need for additional contrast agents within the cardiac pool. For commonly applied pulse sequences, the dark-appearing pericardium is outlined by much higher intensity fat and myocardial signal, which is further contrasted by black-appearing flowing blood. Magnetic resonance, however, is less successful than computed tomography in identifying pericardial calcification—often an important sign of pericardial disease.

Although significant progress has been achieved with gated imaging, further advances must be made in understanding the images that are acquired. For example, as discussed below, considerable disagreement remains regarding the origin of the pericardial signal itself. In addition, for pericardial disease, the "promise" of magnetic resonance to characterize not only anatomy but also pathologic tissue has not yet been realized. Although these current limitations must be acknowledged, even at its present stage of development, magnetic resonance is a most effective technique for detecting almost the entire spectrum of pericardial disease.

The indications for magnetic resonance evaluation of the pericardium are dictated primarily by the need for efficient use of expensive medical technology. Echocardiography continues to be the simplest, least expensive, and most widely applied method for imaging the pericardium. In most cases of suspected pericardial disease, it is the screening tool that will determine whether more sophisticated imaging methods are required. Often, no further characterization of the pericardium will be necessary. Magnetic resonance is justified in three situations: (1) when clinical symptoms are not consistent with the echocardiographic diagnosis, (2) when the echocardiographic examination is inadequate due to technical limitations (e.g., intervening pleural fluid), and (3) when more precise characterization of lesions is required (e.g., planning the extent of a surgical resection).

When further evaluation of the echocardiographic findings is indicated, the cardiologist and cardiovascular radiologist must decide whether computed tomography or magnetic resonance is more appropriate. Optimally, this decision would be simply a judgment based on the "best" available imaging modality. In reality, additional factors, including cost and scan time availability, play important roles. Although no controlled studies are yet available, magnetic resonance appears to be equal or superior to computed tomography in detecting the majority of pericardial lesions, with the exception of calcific pericarditis. Although comparisons with ultrafast computed tomography are not yet available, it is likely that ultrafast computed tomography would be much better than conventional computed tomography for defining a variety of pericardial abnormalities. A number of factors may preclude gated magnetic resonance studies but are not directly related to pericardial disease. These contraindications include cardiac pacemakers, irregular cardiac rhythm, unstable condition of the patient, metallic brain implants, and excessive motion of the patient.

In this chapter, anatomic considerations and imaging strategies relevant to magnetic resonance of the pericardium will first be reviewed. Visualization of the normal pericardium is then presented, followed by consideration of the pathological pericardial lesions that have been studied thus far by this technique. Although the material in this chapter is intended to be comprehensive, clinical experience with magnetic resonance of pericardial disease is still limited and based on a relatively small number of studies; these limitations of our current understanding are noted as appropriate in the text.

ANATOMY

The pericardium is a flask-shaped sac that envelops all four cardiac chambers and extends to the origin of the great vessels. It is composed of an outer fibrocollagenous layer and an inner serous membrane consisting of a monolayer of mesothelial cells.[S1] The inner serosal layer is closely applied to the epicardial surface of the heart and is termed the *visceral* pericardium. The serous mesothelial cells have microvilli that act as friction-bearing surfaces and increase the area for fluid transport.[I2] The serosal layer reflects back on itself to become the inner lining of the outer fibrous layer. Together, these layers form the *parietal* pericardium. The outer fibrous layer blends with the adventitia of the great vessels close to their origin, forming a closed sac around the heart.[S10]

The base of the pericardium is attached to the central tendon of the diaphragm. Anteriorly, ligaments attach the pericardium to the sternum extending from the manubrium to the xiphoid process. Additional ligaments extend posteriorly to the dorsal spine.[H12] These sites of attachment limit the extent of displacement of the heart associated with changes in posture and may limit the motion of the parietal pericardium during cardiac ejection. This reduced motion may contribute to better visualization of the anterior portions of the pericardium with CT or MR imaging.[S2]

The pericardium contains two major serosal tunnels. Knowledge of these is important so that they are not mistaken for other pathological structures. The *oblique sinus* lies behind the left atrium so that the posterior wall of the left atrium is actually separated from the pericardial space. This sinus accounts for the echocardiographic observation that posterior pericardial effusions behind the left ventricle are seen behind the left atrium only when they are very large. The *transverse sinus* is the connection between two tubes of pericardium that envelop the great vessels. Anterosuperiorly, the aorta and pulmonary artery are enclosed in one tube, and the superior and inferior vena cava and pulmonary veins are enclosed by a second posterior tube. On the right side, the transverse sinus communicates with the right pericardial space anterior to the superior vena cava. On the left it merges with the pericardial space lateral to the left atrial appendage.

The potential space between the parietal and visceral pericardium normally contains between 15 and 50 ml of fluid.[R5] Pericardial fluid is an ultrafiltrate of plasma. Protein concentrations are about one-third those of plasma, with albumin present in a higher ratio compared to that of total plasma proteins.[G1] The visceral pericardium is believed to be the source of normal pericardial fluid. Drainage of the pericardial space is probably via multiple efferent lymphatics forming a plexus by way of both the right lymphatic duct and the thoracic duct.[R3]

IMAGE ACQUISITION

Imaging of the fine anatomic details of the pericardium is complicated by cardiac and respiratory motion as well as motion of the patient. In general, electrocardiographically (ECG)-gated imaging is necessary to image the normal pericardium.[S9] Nongated scans may potentially require less scan time but are adequate only for the demonstration of fixed pericardial masses or large pericardial effusions. Nongated magnetic resonance is not used for characterization of pericardial wall thickness. In the ECG-gated technique, the TR interval for successive pulse sequences is determined by the R-R interval of each heartbeat.[L1] Although slight beat-to-beat variations in the heart rate lead to some variation in TR intervals during a study, these changes are on the order of 5 percent of TR[L2] and the error introduced is much less than that involved in sampling and averaging different portions of the cardiac cycle in nongated techniques. If longer TR intervals are desired, gating to every second or third heartbeat is possible. Whereas longer TR intervals will generally emphasize fluids and describe anatomy, short TR times will improve contrast between mediastinal fat and pathology. Cardiac gating may not be possible for patients with irregular rhythms, since incorrect triggering of the pulse signal may result. In addition, gating difficulties may be encountered with patients presenting with low ECG voltages or severe tachycardia.

Optimal pericardial visualization is a function of magnetic field strength, pulse sequence, number of image averages, slice thickness, slice gap, and the nature of the pathologic lesion being studied. Although few comparative studies have been made of the effect of these parameters on the appearance of the pericardium, general recommendations can be made regarding parameters that have been successful in defining pericardial lesions. Pericardial anatomy has been studied most closely at field strengths of 0.3 to 0.6 tesla (T); the effect of higher field strengths (1 to 1.5 T) on the pericardial signal has not been systematically compared with lower-strength images. Single-slice techniques are rarely used; multislice spin-echo techniques[C5] are able to acquire between 5 and 10 anatomic levels in the same time interval. In the multislice technique, a pulse sequence would typically be generated 5 msec following an R wave of the patient's electrocardiogram. Following a 100-msec delay, a second sequence would be generated at an anatomic level caudal to the first. For a heart rate of 100 beats per minute, five slices spanning the level of the aortic root to the apex of the left ventricle could be acquired during the 600-msec R-R interval. Note that each successive anatomic level is 100 msec further into the cardiac cycle. Variation in the contractile state of the heart and its attendant effect on pericardial fluid may account for slight changes in the thickness of the pericardial signal with myocardial contraction.[S9]

Both first and second echo times are sampled in multiecho, multislice imaging. TE values on the order of 30 and 60 msec in duration for first and second echos have been successful in depicting pericardial anatomy. Shorter TE values of 10 to 20 msec have been applied [C2] but result in more signal (and therefore less contrast) from intracardiac blood[W2] and potentially from pericardial fluid. Anatomic detail is greatest on first echo images, while second echo images may provide information regarding the nature of the lesion (cystic versus solid, fat). However, since the acquisition time for the second echo is twice that for the first, increased motion artifact may cause slight degradation of the image.[H9] Slice thicknesses of 0.7 to 1.0 cm with interslice gaps of 0 to 0.3 cm have been used. Generally, two to four signals are averaged to improve the signal-to-noise ratio.

A rotating-gated multislice technique or *permutation-gated* technique is useful for evaluation of the pericardium. In this method, typically five anatomic levels are sampled at five different times in the cardiac cycle.[C6] The disadvantage is that scan times therefore increase by a factor of 5. Permutation gating is generally reserved for cases in which the variation in pericardial fluid or mass must be identified to characterize a pathologic lesion.[S3]

A disadvantage of ECG-gated magnetic resonance is that TR values are restricted to multiples of the R-to-R time interval. The TE values must also be chosen to accommodate a specified number of anatomic slices compatible with a range of heart rates. Typically, the combination of TR and TE values used are categorized as partial saturation sequences. These sequences are not optimal for contrast separation of nonfatty soft tissues. Nevertheless, experience indicates that available contrast is adequate for identification of pericardial morphology.

Total imaging time (T_i) for spin-echo gated imaging may be calculated as[S2]

$$T_i\ (\text{min}) = 60\ \text{TR (sec)} \times N_{\text{averages}} \times N_{\text{phase-encoding signals}} \times N_{\text{cycles}} \qquad 52\text{–}1$$

For a heart rate of 60 beats per minute, two signal averages, a scan array of 256 pixels, and only one portion of the cardiac cycle, the imaging time is $(1 \times 2 \times 256 \times 1)/60 = 8.5$ minutes. For five permutation-gated portions of the cardiac cycle ($N_{\text{cycles}} = 5$), imaging time increases by a factor of 5 to about 43 minutes. Experience dictates that the total time required per patient is two to five times the imaging time.

New fast imaging techniques have recently been developed and have been used thus far primarily in evaluation of cardiac function.[H8, L8] Their role in depicting pericardial disease has not yet been defined.

Magnetic resonance signal intensities are discussed qualitatively in the following sections in reference to the myocardial signal as imaged by the standard pulse sequences stated above. A *medium*-intensity signal is of the same intensity as the myocardium. *High*-intensity and *low*-intensity signals are greater and less than that of the myocardium, respectively.

NORMAL PERICARDIUM

The stiff, fibrous pericardium has a thickness of 0.8 to 1 mm in anatomic studies.[F2] By computed tomography, the pericardium is visualized as a pencil-thin curvilinear line averaging 1 to 2 mm in thickness.[D1, H14, M9] It is best visualized in the caudal and ventral areas adjacent to mediastinal and subepicardial fat. The ventral portion of the pericardium can be visualized in nearly 100 percent of patients by computed tomography, but at the level of the left ventricle, the dorsal aspect of the normal pericardium is seen in less than 25 percent of cases. Focal areas of thickening of up to 5 mm may be identified by computed tomography adjacent to the right ventricle and caudally at the region of ligamentous insertions onto the central tendon of the diaphragm. This thickening is thought to be the normal response to the stress induced by pulsations of the right ventricle.[M10]

Magnetic Resonance Visualization of the Pericardium

On magnetic resonance images, *the normal pericardium appears as a low-intensity signal between the high-intensity mediastinal and subepicardial fat or medium-intensity epicardium.* Figure 52–1 shows transaxial and sagittal cardiac gated magnetic resonance images that depict the normal pericardial anatomy. Table 52–1 shows a comparison of the normal and abnormal pericardial signals. Normal pericardium is consistently visualized only on gated MRI scans. In a series of normal subjects, Stark and associates[S9] were unable to identify pericardium in 20 individuals with nongated spin-echo scans by using TR values ranging from 0.5 to 1.5 seconds and TE times of 28 and 56 msec. In another series, by decreasing the TR intervals to 143 msec and using TE times from 10 to 20 msec, cardiac motion artifacts were found to be significantly reduced.[C2] The images obtained were thought to be diagnostic of a variety of cardiac lesions. Normal pericardium, however, was identified in only 2 of 33 patients.

In gated studies, the low-intensity pericardial signal is best observed about 200 msec into systole following the ECG-recorded R-wave.[S2] The visibility of the pericardial line is enhanced by increased subepicardial or mediastinal fat. In areas adjacent to the lung, such as the posterolateral aspect of the left ventricle,

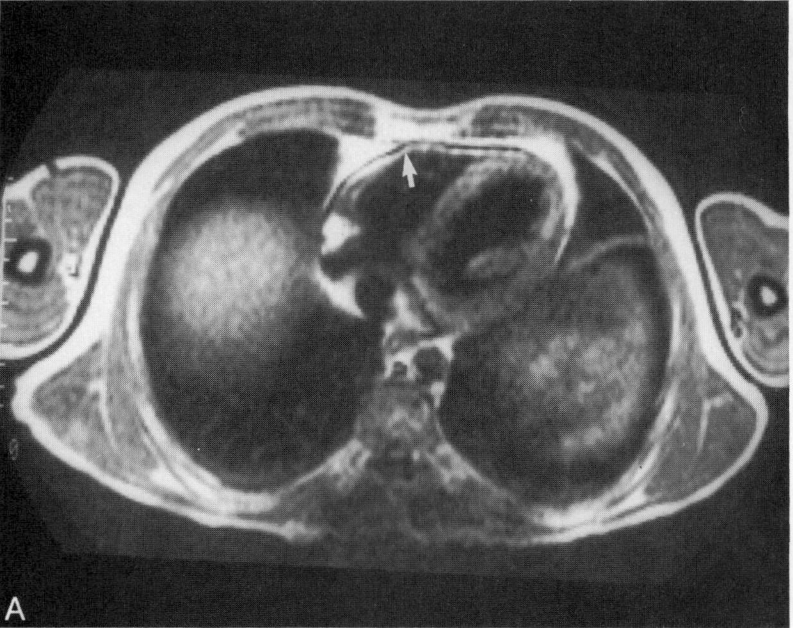

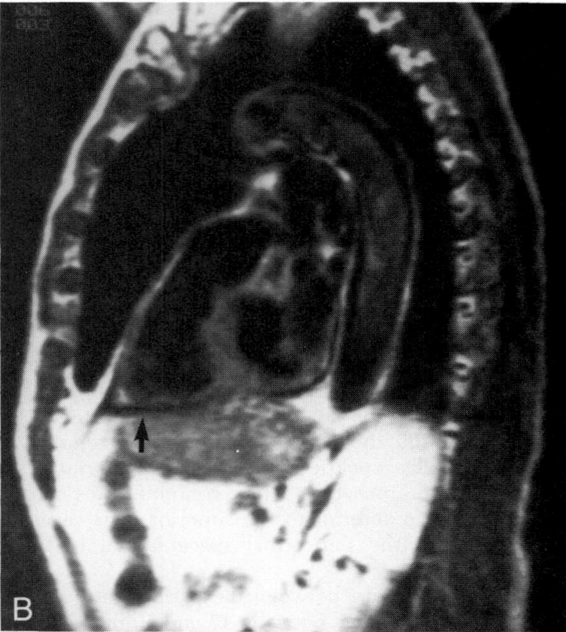

Figure 52–1. Normal pericardium. Transaxial *(A)* and sagittal *(B)* cardiac gated magnetic resonance images (TE = 35 msec) demonstrate the hypointense signal of the normal pericardium *(arrow)* in these two patients.

Table 52–1. NORMAL AND ABNORMAL MR SIGNAL CHARACTERISTICS OF THE PERICARDIUM*

Classification	Signal Intensity† First SE Image	Signal Intensity† Second SE Image	Other Features
Normal pericardium	low	low	1.4 mm average thickness
Cysts and diverticula	low to medium	increased	smooth contour
Pericardial effusion			
Serous	low	low	
Inflammatory	low to medium	increased	
Loculated	low to medium	increased	visible adhesions
Bloody	medium to high	medium to high	thickening
Thickening			
Fibrous	low	low	
Inflammatory	low to medium	medium to high	associated effusion
Calcification	low	low	
Constriction			
Chronic	low	low	
Subacute	medium to high	medium to high	focal or diffuse and ≥5 mm thickness
Postoperative change	medium	increased	
Neoplasm			
Benign	variable	variable	intact pericardial line
Malignant	variable	variable	associated effusion absent pericardial line

*Typical features with gated spin echo (SE) imaging, first and second SE images at 30 and 60 msec. See text for further explanation.

†Signal intensities are relative to myocardial intensity. "Medium" intensity is the same as that of myocardium, "low" and "high" are less and greater than that of myocardium, respectively. "Increased" indicates greater intensity than the first SE signal.

the pericardium is poorly visualized against the low-intensity lung parenchyma (see Fig. 52–1A). The sensitivity for visualization of the pericardium over five anatomic regions as determined by Sechtem and associates[S2] is given in Table 52–2. In their studies, the sensitivity of magnetic resonance for the pericardial signal was 100 percent over the region of the right ventricle. The average pericardial thickness was 1.2 mm in diastole and 1.7 mm in systole. The maximum thickness of normal pericardium was 2.6 mm. In agreement with CT observations,[M2] the pericardial thickness seen by magnetic resonance is a function of anatomic level. Caudal sections of the heart showed considerable increases in pericardial thickness (up to 7 mm). This increased thickness is due to diaphragmatic ligamentous insertions of the pericardium at caudal levels. Also, the observed thickness may reflect tangential sectioning of the caudal border of the heart, since transverse image slices are approximately parallel to the inferior heart wall and associated pericardium at this level. For these reasons, *the thickness of the pericardium should be measured on sections at an anatomic level that displays the right atrium, right ventricle, and left ventricle.*

The transverse sinus of the pericardium is much more readily visualized on MR images than on CT images.[I1, L4] The sensitivity of magnetic resonance for imaging the transverse sinus is about 80 percent in transverse and sagittal planes on gated images and about 50 percent without cardiac gating. Its low-intensity signal is visualized in these planes as the inferior extension of the retroaortic segment of the sinus. On coronal images, the sensitivity of magnetic resonance is about 70 percent, with the infrapulmonary segment visualized most frequently. The sensitivity of magnetic resonance for the preaortic and retroaortic recesses of the pericardium ranges from 67 to 100 percent,[M5] compared to 24 to 49 percent of normal subjects by computed tomography. The highest sensitivities are achieved with ECG-permutation-gated acquired images in the transverse plane. Unfamiliarity with the normal pericardial anatomy in this region may lead to misinterpretation of the superpericardial recesses as mediastinal vessels, lymph nodes, or possibly aortic dissection.[A4, M5]

Table 52–2. SENSITIVITY OF GATED MR IN VISUALIZING THE PERICARDIUM AT VARIOUS REGIONS OF THE HEART

Region	Sensitivity* (%)
Right atrium	78
Right ventricle—right of sternum	100
Right ventricle—left of sternum	100
Left ventricle—apex	83
Left ventricle—lateral wall	61

*Number visualized divided by total number of subjects; N = 18 subjects.

Modified from Sechtem, U., Tscholakoff, D., and Higgins, C. B.: MRI of the normal pericardium. AJR 147:239, 1986, © by the American Roentgen Ray Society.

Visualization of the pericardium is a function of the phase of the cardiac cycle. In general, the pericardial signal is more clearly discerned in systole and the width of the pericardial line has been observed to increase slightly during cardiac contraction.[S2] During systole, the parietal pericardium over the right ventricle is largely fixed in place by the pericardiosternal ligaments. The visceral pericardium is applied to the contracted ventricle, perhaps resulting in an increased pericardial space during cardiac ejection. Similar observations obtained with M-mode echocardiography of an echo-free space present only during systole support this explanation of the magnetic resonance findings.[H13] Angiographic observations of increased thickness of pericardial effusion during systole are also consistent with magnetic resonance observations of variations in pericardial thickness as a function of cardiac contraction.[B4]

The pericardial signal is better visualized on first than on second echo images (at 28 and 56 msec, respectively).[S2] Blurring of the pericardial line may be present on second echo images, contributing to small increases in the observed pericardial thickness. Occasionally, the pericardial line is not visualized at all on second echo images when it is clearly identified on the first echo. Finally, the normal pericardial signal may be slightly increased on second compared to first echo images. These findings suggest that *first echo images should be utilized in characterizing anatomic relationships of the pericardium,* whereas second echo images may help differentiate and classify pathology.[S3]

Origin of the Pericardial Signal

Having discussed the appearance of the pericardial line in the magnetic resonance image, the origin of that signal will now be considered. The average pericardial thickness measured is slightly greater than that determined from anatomic studies (averaging 1.4 mm by magnetic resonance versus 0.8 to 1 mm anatomically).

This discrepancy can be evaluated by considering the *expected* appearance of the pericardial signal. Under ideal imaging conditions without motion or reconstruction artifact, there are three potential sources of signal: the parietal pericardium, the pericardial fluid, and the visceral pericardium. The visceral pericardium consists of a single layer of mesothelial cells and, as in computed tomography, will not be imaged in normal subjects.[M10, S2] The parietal pericardium is a stiff sheath of fibrous tissue. Fibrous tissue has low intensity on magnetic resonance images[K3] due to long longitudinal relaxation times (T_1) and short transverse relaxation times (T_2).[H15, P2] In addition, the spin density is reported to be low compared to that of fat tissue.[T3] Thus, the parietal pericardium is expected to display low intensity on both T_1-weighted and T_2-weighted images.[S2]

The parietal pericardium thus accounts for most of the observed low-intensity magnetic resonance signal. *An additional contribution may result from pericardial fluid surrounding the heart.* Based on an average pericardial fluid volume of 20 ml, the thickness of an evenly distributed fluid layer around the heart is estimated to range from 0.4 to 1.3 mm, inversely related to heart diameter.[S2] Since the fluid layer is not necessarily distributed evenly around the heart, the fluid thickness could be essentially zero in some regions and more than 1.3 mm in others. It has been postulated that fluid within the pericardial sac is subjected to forces resulting in nonlaminar flow as a result of cardiac motion.[I1, S2] This would result in loss of signal intensity on first echo and second echo images due to effects caused by changes in spin phase.[V1, V2] The resulting signal intensity would thus be low, contributing to the measured thickness of the apparent pericardial line. This line of reasoning is supported by three observations: (1) variation of the thickness of the pericardial signal during the cardiac cycle as pericardial fluid is redistributed, (2) lower than expected intensity of pericardial effusion,[S3] and (3) cadaver studies showing increased pericardial signal compared to that with cardiac motion.[I1] It is therefore possible that the *apparent* pericardial line arises not only from the low-intensity pericardial signal but also from motion-induced signal loss of pericardial fluid.

Having considered the possible morphological sources of pericardial signal, the possibility of motion-induced artifact must also be acknowledged. The visceral pericardium is closely applied to the surface of the heart, while the parietal pericardium is largely fixed by ligamentous attachments. A phase-continuity artifact may arise from the local velocity gradient between the two pericardial surfaces.[M11, V3] This could contribute to a reduction in signal intensity for volume elements that span the pericardium. The relative magnitude of this effect on the observed pericardial line remains to be determined.

CONGENITAL ANOMALIES

Congenital anomalies of the pericardium are uncommon. They are classified as (1) congenital absence or defects of the pericardium and (2) pericardial cysts, diverticula, and benign teratomas.[G3] The origin of embryologic abnormalities is obscure, but they may be secondary to abnormalities in the vascular supply of the pericardium. Such congenital anomalies may mimic other lesions such as mediastinal, cardiac, or pericardial tumors; anterior mediastinal or costophrenic angle masses; or a dilated pulmonary artery.

Congenital Absence and Defects of the Pericardium

Absence of the pericardium is rarely complete. The most common site of involvement is the left pericardium (70 percent of cases).[N2] In about half of these, the entire left side of the pericardium is absent, and in the remainder, partial defects occur.[N1, S4] Of the cases, 17 percent represent diaphragmatic defects and 4 percent are partial defects of the right pericardium. The incidence of pericardial absence is approximately 1 in 10,000 at autopsy, with a 3:1 male-to-female ratio. In one-third of cases, pericardial defects are associated with other anomalies such as tetralogy, atrial septal defect, patent ductus arteriosus, bicuspid aortic valve, hiatus hernia, or bronchogenic cyst.[B2] Partial defects may result in cardiac herniation or compression of the coronary vasculature.

Total absence of the pericardium is generally asymptomatic. It is suggested on chest film by an abnormal left cardiac contour, with better definition and separation of the segments that comprise the cardiac border.[G2] The medial and lateral border of the pulmonary artery may be seen as a result of absence of the anterior pericardial reflection between the aorta and pulmonary artery. Echocardiographic findings include exaggerated cardiac motion without bright pericardiac echo, but are not diagnostic.[N3] Computed tomography displays the pericardial defect and may show direct contact between lung and cardiac chambers.[B1, M8]

Like computed tomography, magnetic resonance evaluation of pericardial defects provides a definitive diagnosis and allows determination of the extent of the lesion. Since coronal, axial, or sagittal sections may be acquired, otherwise confusing or atypical cases may be diagnosed by direct visualization of the pericardial anatomy.[G4] Associated leftward shift of the heart may be visualized with herniation of lung in the region of the base of the left ventricle, inferior vena cava, and left hemidiaphragm. In one case, absence of the left portion of parietal pericardium was accompanied by significant blurring of the posterior left ventricular border by magnetic resonance imaging.[S5] The reason for this blurring is not clear; the authors postulated an artifact secondary to irregular cardiac motion in the absence of containment of the left ventricle by the pericardium. Herniation of the left ventricle through a pericardial window has been diagnosed by using nongated magnetic resonance.[R6] Coronal sections were of particular value in demonstrating cardiac anatomy, precluding the need for cardiac catheterization. Magnetic resonance and computed tomography are the procedures of choice in the diagnosis of congenital pericardial defect.

Pericardial Cysts

Pericardial cysts are congenital in origin, arising from embryologically separated lacunae of pericardial tissue.[L5] True cysts are encapsulated and should not communicate with the pericardial cavity.[N1] The majority (70 percent) are right-sided lesions, and 90 percent are located in either the right or left costophrenic sulcus. In this location, they may easily be confused with pericardial fat pads or diaphragmatic hernias, but they usually have more sharply defined borders. If they are located in positions other than these, differentiation from other mediastinal masses such as lymphoma, thymoma, teratoma, and pericardial-based lesions is more difficult. Computed tomographic examination depicts cysts as homogeneous fluid-filled cavities with smooth walls and densities of 0 to 20 Hounsfield units (HU).[L7]

Magnetic resonance provides a diagnosis as specific as that based on computed tomography in the case of pericardial cysts. They are visualized as paracardiac masses with long T_1 and T_2 values.[S3] Low signal intensity is observed on first echo images, with increased intensity on second echo images. A line of low intensity surrounding the cyst consistent with pericardium has been observed. Since magnetic resonance is superior to computed tomography in depicting the anatomic structures of the mediastinum, it may be preferred to computed tomography in the evaluation of an unknown mediastinal soft tissue mass.[A1, W2]

Pericardial Diverticula

Pericardial diverticula may be congenital in origin or acquired as the result of herniation through a defect in the parietal pericardium.[N1] They contain all layers of pericardium and communicate with the pericardial space, so that their volume varies with the total volume of pericardial fluid. The appearance would be expected to be similar to that of simple cysts with low-intensity first echo images followed by increased second echo intensity.[B6]

Developmental Masses of the Pericardium

Intrapericardial teratomas and bronchogenic cysts are the most common causes of the very rare benign primary pericardial neoplasm.[A5] An enlarged cardiac silhouette and a pericardial effusion may be present, the latter particularly in association with teratoma.[A5, Z1] Echocardiography will allow initial detection of the mass and will display its degree of homogeneity. Computed tomography may be more specific, since the various densities in the mass may be identified as fat, fluid levels, or calcification.[M7] Magnetic resonance may be of utility in characterizing the anatomic relations of the mass, particularly for an intrapericardial mass, since excellent contrast resolution is achieved without requiring contrast agents as in computed tomography.[M10, W3] Additional information regarding magnetic resonance tissue relaxation parameters to distinguish different histologic types of masses has not yet been reported.

PERICARDIAL EFFUSION

Normal pericardial fluid is a serous ultrafiltrate of plasma, normally containing 1.7 to 3.5 g/dl protein.[H12] Pericardial effusions develop as a response to acute injury of the pericardium. They are classified as serous, bloody, and lymphatic or chylous in nature. The common etiologies of pericardial effusion are listed in Table 52–3, along with associated morphologic pericardial changes that may occur acutely or chronically. The development of clinical symptoms of pericardial effusion depends on (1) the nature of the effusion, (2) the absolute volume of the effusion, and (3) the rapidity of fluid accumulation.[B2]

The diagnosis of pericardial effusion is best accomplished by echocardiography.[J1] There are well-known instances, however, in which echocardiographic findings are nondiagnostic or easily misinterpreted.[H13, Y1] Limitations in the accuracy of echocardiographic diagnosis include (1) false-positive scans in which adjacent pleural effusion, atelectasis, or mediastinal lesions mimic pericardial effusions; (2) distinguishing fluid from epicardial fat in the anterior and posterior recesses; (3) loculated fluid and hemopericardium; and (4) differentiation of pericardial thickening from fluid.[C3, I3, K2, W1]

Table 52–3. ETIOLOGY OF PERICARDIAL EFFUSION

Classification	Associated Morphologic Changes*
Serous	
Congestive heart failure	
Hypoalbuminemia	c, d, e
Irradiation	a, b
Infectious	
Viral pericarditis	a, b
Tuberculous pericarditis	a, b, c, d, e
Bacterial pericarditis	a, b, d
Parasitic	a, b, c, d
Fungal	a, b, c, d
Idiopathic	a, b, d, e
Blood (hematocrit >10%)	
Iatrogenic	
Cardiac surgery	a, b
Cardiac catheterization	a
Trauma	a, b, e
Anticoagulant agents	a, b
Chemotherapeutic agents	a
Neoplasm	a, b
Trauma	a, b, d, e
Acute myocardial infarction	a, b
Cardiac or great vessel rupture	a, b
Coagulopathy	a, b
Uremia	a, b
Lymph or Chyle	
Neoplasm	a, b, e
Iatrogenic (surgery)	a, b, e
Congenital	a, b, e
Idiopathic ("primary chylopericardium")	a, b, e
Nonneoplastic obstruction of thoracic duct	a, b, e

*a, fibrous; b, fibrinous; c, granulomatous; d, calcific; e, cholesterol

Modified from Roberts, W. C., and Ferrans, V. J.: A survey of the causes and consequences of pericardial heart disease. *In* Reddy, P. S., Leon, D. F., and Shaver, J. A. (eds.): Pericardial Disease. Raven Press, New York, 1982, p. 56.

Computed tomographic scanning accurately detects as little as 50 ml of pericardial effusion in dogs, which is similar to the sensitivity of echocardiography.[W4] In addition, the false-positive rate of diagnosis is considerably reduced relative to that of echocardiography because of superior detection of anatomic boundaries between intracardiac, pericardial, plural, and mediastinal structures.[M8] An additional advantage is possible diagnosis of the etiology of the effusion. For example, hemorrhagic and myxedemic effusions are associated with increased density compared to those associated with heart failure or renal failure.[T2] Because of its high sensitivity and low false-positive and false-negative rate, computed tomography has been recommended as the imaging method of choice for stable patients following surgery or trauma, in whom pulmonary or mediastinal pathology is suspected in addition to pericardial disease.[Y1]

The capabilities of magnetic resonance in detecting pericardial effusion appear to be equal to those of echocardiography, and detection of fluid collections as small as 30 ml has been reported.[S3] Furthermore, magnetic resonance has similar advantages to computed tomography in that the nature of the effusion in many cases may be identified. Prospective trials comparing the sensitivity and specificity of echocardiography, computed tomography, and magnetic resonance in the detection and characterization of pericardial effusion have not yet been performed.

As discussed previously, the apparent pericardial signal observed by magnetic resonance consists of contributions from both parietal pericardium and pericardial fluid. Pericardial effusions generally show an increased protein content and, depending on the nature of the effusion, may have a higher cellular content than normal pericardial fluid.[F1] Stark and associates[S9] compared the intensity of pericardial fluid under in vitro and in vivo conditions and found them to be equal for an effusion resulting from myxedema with a protein content of 5.5 g/dl. The effect of cellular content on the relaxation parameters T_1 and T_2 determined in vitro are given by Levine and associates[L3] as

$$\text{cells/mm}^3 = 2.04 \times 10^7 e^{-0.0028T_1} \quad (52\text{–}2)$$

$$\text{cells/mm}^3 = 1.42 \times 10^7 e^{-0.0081T_2} \quad (52\text{–}3)$$

for T_1 and T_2 in milliseconds. No effect of routine chemistries on T_1 or T_2 values was found. The value of these predictions in the analysis of in vivo disease has not yet been determined but is crucial to the utilization of magnetic resonance in characterizing the nature of effusions noninvasively.

The average width of the normal pericardial signal is 1.4 mm, with an upper limit of 2.6 mm. Regions in which the pericardial dimensions exceed 4 mm are regarded as abnormal.[S3] Effusions appear on first spin-echo images as an area of low intensity that displaces the parietal pericardium and associated fat away from the myocardial wall. They may be distinguished from thickened pericardium by the elliptical shape of the effusion seen posterolaterally to the left ventricle (discussed further below). The appearance of pericardial effusion varies depending on the etiology, but all reported cases have shown *low intensity (i.e., less than myocardium) on first spin-echo images. Intensity on second spin-echo images varies according to the nature of the effusion.* This is in contrast to thickened pericardium, which is often of medium or high signal intensity. Effusions resulting from congestive heart failure are primarily of low intensity on second echo images. Uremic effusions have been observed to be of either high (i.e., greater than myocardium) or low intensity. Figure 52–2 shows an example of a large pericardial effusion secondary to uremia as depicted by cardiac gated magnetic resonance with TE = 28 msec. Examples of the characteristics of effusions in other disorders are shown in Table 52–4.

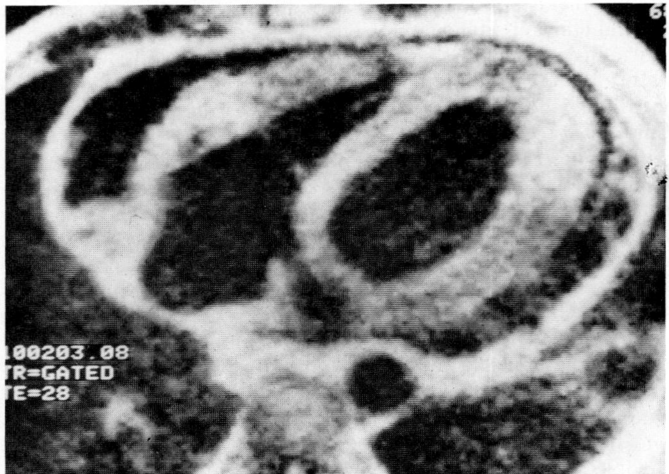

Figure 52–2. Uremic pericardial effusion. Gated cardiac magnetic resonance (TE = 28 msec). Adhesions are apparent between the visceral and parietal pericardium. The parietal pericardium is abnormally thick and of high intensity.

The distribution of pericardial fluid imaged by MR shows considerable variation. In a series of 23 patients, the maximum fluid collection appeared posterolaterally to the left ventricle in 17 (74 percent).[S3] Significant amounts of fluid were also observed posterolaterally to the right atrium in 16 cases (70 percent). Another common site of fluid collection was the anterosuperior recess. Because of the focal accumulations of fluid, the relationship between the measured width of the pericardial space and total fluid volume is not linear. The magnitude of pericardial effusion instead may be quantitatively assessed by image analysis techniques. By outlining the regions of effusion on each MR slice, the total fluid volume is calculated by multiplying the number of pixels in the identified regions by the slice thickness and an appropriate magnification factor. Comparison with echocardiographic estimations of total fluid shows good agreement between the two techniques.[M3, S3] Effusions that are semiquantitatively classified by echocardiography as *moderate* contain between 100 and 500 ml of fluid. By magnetic resonance, moderate effusions are associated with a greater than 5 mm pericardial space anterior to the right ventricle. Several cases have been reported in which small effusions have been more easily detected by magnetic resonance than by echocardiography.[C2, S3]

By using gated magnetic resonance, loculated effusions may be diagnosed when adhesions are visualized between the visceral and parietal pericardium. Associated pericardial inflammation may be separately recognized as thickened pericardium with higher signal intensity.[S9] Both adhesions and pericardial inflammation are observed in the case of uremic effusion shown in Figure 52–2. An inflammatory exudate resulting in adhesions has an abnormally high protein content. Such effusions should have a shortened T_1 relaxation time[L3] and thus appear with increased intensity relative to a normal pericardial signal. Cardiac motion, however, induces the flow of pericardial fluid, and in the general case a signal *loss* may result due to spin phase changes. For loculated effusion or inflammatory exudate adhering to the pericardium, such fluid motion is reduced and localized regions of higher-intensity signal are observed.[M6, S3, S9]

Using MR imaging, hemopericardium is recognized by a markedly increased pericardial signal.[H5] The hematoma displays two different intensity components in a manner similar to chronic hematomas in other parts of the body.[B3] The clot portion is associated with a lower intensity than the serum component of the hematoma.

Table 52–4. SECOND ECHO MR SIGNAL INTENSITY* OF PERICARDIAL EFFUSION

Clinical Disorder	Number of Patients	Low	High
Congestive heart failure	10	9	1
Uremia	5	2	3
Myocardial infarction	2	2	0
Radiation therapy	2	2	0
Previous resuscitation	1	0	1
Lupus erythematosis	1	1	0
Tuberculosis	1	1	0
Idiopathic pericarditis	1	1	0

*Low intensity is less than myocardial signal, high intensity is greater than myocardial signal.

Modified from Sechtem, U., Tscholakoff, D., and Higgins, C. B.: MRI of the abnormal pericardium. AJR 147:245, 1986, © by the American Roentgen Ray Society.

PERICARDIAL THICKENING

Thickening of the pericardium is a radiologic description of focal or diffuse increases in the width of the pericardium greater than that which is considered normal. In both computed tomography and magnetic resonance, a pericardial thickness of more than 4 mm is considered to be abnormal.[S3] Thickening is a common pathologic end point resulting from a wide variety of injuries to the pericardium. Pericardial thickening may be associated with, but is not synonymous with, constriction of the pericardium.[L7, S6, S11]

Morphologically, pericardial thickening is a manifestation of fibrous pericarditis.[R4] Pericardial thickening may involve either the parietal or visceral surfaces and may be associated with adhesions between them. Disorders that may result in fibrous pericarditis are indicated in Table 52–3. Etiologies include systemic disease such as renal disease, rheumatoid arthritis, systemic lupus erythematosus, and scleroderma; infection; irradiation; or healing of hemopericardium in response to surgery or trauma.

By magnetic resonance, thickening of the pericardium appears as a widened pericardial line with low intensity on the first spin-echo signal. This is also the case for pericardial effusion and calcific pericarditis, and an attempt must therefore be made to distinguish between these entities. Three features help identify and differentiate thickening from other pericardial lesions. First, thickening that is inflammatory in nature is accompanied by changes in normal low-intensity pericardial signal to medium or high intensity. This is consistent with a lengthened T_2 relaxation time.[S3] Second, calcifications are often associated with fibrous pericarditis. Calcifications appear as focal areas of decreased signal intensity with irregular borders. Third, the distribution of focal or diffuse thickening is not similar to the elliptically shaped accumulation of pericardial fluid that is typically seen posterolaterally to the left ventricle. Also, an enlarged anterosuperior pericardial recess is reported to be associated with effusion but not with thickening.[S3] With effusions that are not loculated, comparison of images from different portions of the cardiac cycle will display variations in thickness of the pericardial signal. This is consistent with redistribution of fluid resulting from cardiac contraction. The thickened, fibrotic pericardium has a constant appearance throughout the cardiac cycle.

POST-PERICARDIOTOMY SYNDROME AND POST–MYOCARDIAL-INFARCTION PERICARDITIS (DRESSLER'S SYNDROME)

Post-pericardiotomy syndrome is characterized by fever and chest pain beginning 2 to 4 weeks following surgical or traumatic injury to the pericardium. There is usually clinical evidence of pericarditis and, often, pleuritis. Post-pericardiotomy syndrome is distinct from the pericarditis and low-grade fever that occur in the first few days following cardiac surgery. The incidence ranges from 10 to 30 percent following open-heart surgery.[F4, K1] Post–myocardial-infarction pericarditis[D2] is a similar syndrome occurring 10 days to 2 months after an acute myocardial infarction.

The incidence of Dressler's syndrome was originally estimated as 1 to 3 percent but is probably decreasing.[F4] Both syndromes seem to be the result of a common pathologic mechanism that may be autoimmune in nature.[E1] The majority of cases resolve spontaneously, but, infrequently, constrictive pericardial disease may complicate recovery. In Figure 52–3, the thinned anterior wall of the left ventricle is consistent with previous myocardial infarction, but normal pericardial anatomy is preserved anterior to the thinned ventricle.

The most common finding in these syndromes is pericardial thickening,[I7] which may be either focal or diffuse. Associated pericardial effusion has been shown in 25 percent of cases by computed tomography.[M10] In contrast to mild thickening and small effusions, which normally resolve completely following cardiac surgery, post-pericardiotomy syndrome is associated with persistent and progressive pericardial thickening. In their series, Sechtem and associates[S3] noted 13 of 16 patients with postoperative thickening of the pericardium; six had associated effusions. Thickened pericardium appeared as a medium-intensity signal similar to that of myocardium, but separated from it by the interposition of epicardial fat with high signal intensity. No serial examinations of postoperative patients by magnetic resonance have been reported to date.

CONSTRICTIVE PERICARDITIS

Constrictive pericardial disease results from progressive pericardial fibrosis leading to restriction of the cardiac ventricles during diastole. The disease progresses over a period of years, leading to increased systemic and pulmonary venous pressures. Symptoms include fatigue, dyspnea, and chest pain accompanied by ascites, hepatomegaly, and peripheral edema. Atrial fibrillation is present in one-fourth of patients. Pathologic findings include calcium deposition in a symmetrically scarred and fibrotic pericardium that is adherent to the myocardium. Exceptional cases of localized constriction in the atrioventricular groove, aortic groove, or pulmonary outflow tract or circumferentially around the semilunar valves have been reported.[C1, M4]

Constrictive pericarditis may follow any injury to the pericardium that evokes an inflammatory response. Early descriptions considered tuberculosis to be the most common cause,[W5] but this now accounts for less than 20 percent of cases.[R5] The cause in most cases is unknown.[H11] Identified etiologies include infectious pericarditis, connective tissue disease (rheumatoid arthritis, lupus erythematosis), neoplasm, or trauma. Constriction is a recognized complication of long-term treatment of chronic renal failure by dialysis,[L6] cardiac surgery,[K4] and radiation therapy of more than 4000 rads to the mediastinum.[A2]

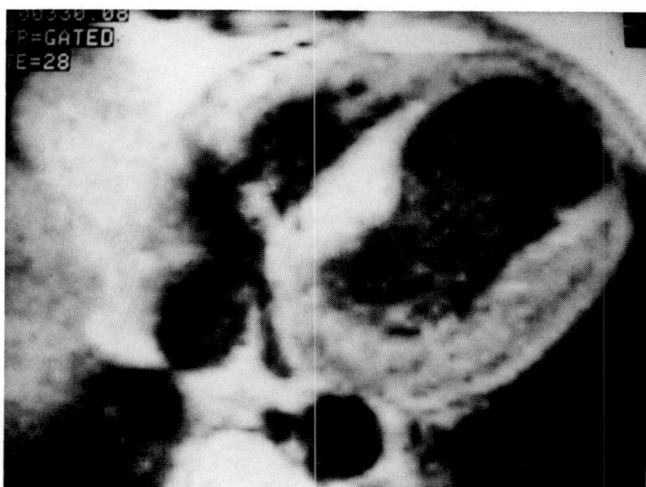

Figure 52–3. Normal pericardium in a patient with an old anterior wall myocardial infarct. Gated cardiac magnetic resonance (TE = 28 msec). Thinning of the anterior wall of the left ventricle is present with a normal low-intensity pericardial signal.

Effusive-constrictive pericarditis is the presence of pericardial effusion and constriction not relieved by reduction of intrapericardial pressure to zero.[H1, H3] This condition may represent an early stage of chronic constrictive pericarditis. *Occult constrictive pericarditis* is a variant of constrictive pericarditis with symptoms of chest pain, fatigue, and dyspnea but without overt evidence of cardiac constriction.[B5] Histologic evidence of fibrosis and adhesions are present in grossly normal-appearing pericardium.

The major dilemma in diagnosing pericardial constriction is distinguishing it from restrictive cardiomyopathy (e.g., amyloid heart disease).[B2, I3, N4, S7] A number of cardiac lesions may present with symptoms of right-sided cardiac failure, fatigue, and dyspnea. Echocardiography, however, will rule out conditions such as pericardial effusion or tamponade, valvular dysfunction, and dilated cardiomyopathy mimicking constrictive pericarditis. Findings that suggest constriction such as early pulmonic valve opening, abnormal septal wall motion, and diastolic posterior wall flattening may also be seen with restrictive disease. Cardiac catheterization shows equalization of diastolic left and right ventricular pressures in both conditions. Other hemodynamic differences between constrictive pericarditis and restrictive cardiomyopathy are subtle and nonspecific.[R2] Despite these difficulties, distinguishing between pericardial constriction and restrictive cardiomyopathy is critical since the treatment of constriction is surgical (pericardiectomy) and has a long-term success rate of 75 percent.[B2] If a regimen of medical management is applied instead (appropriate for cardiomyopathy), the patient will continue to deteriorate progressively.

Examination of the pericardium by computed tomography has been valuable in diagnosing constrictive pericarditis.[D1, L7] The entire cardiac perimeter is visualized with excellent identification of pericaridal calcifications. In the presence of clinical symptoms, a pericardial thickness of more than 2 mm supports the diagnosis of constriction rather than restrictive cardiomyopathy.[I3, I4, M8] Diagnostic difficulties may occasionally arise in using computed tomography in distinguishing pericardial thickening from effusion.[I3] The limited criterion of thickening may also be insufficient in the case of local constriction near the right ventricular outflow tract.

Early evidence suggests that magnetic resonance may be superior to computed tomography in the evaluation of constrictive pericarditis.[J1, S3, S8] The finding of an abnormally thickened pericardium in a patient with clinically suspected constriction is supportive of that diagnosis. All reported cases of patients examined by magnetic resonance and with proven constrictive pericarditis have had associated pericardial thickening of greater than 5 mm. In *chronic* constriction, the thickened pericardium is of lower intensity than pericarditis-associated thickening due to other causes because of the low-intensity signal of fibrous tissue. Thickening in *subacute* forms of constrictive pericarditis resulting from uremia, cardiac surgery, or irradiation has moderate to high intensity.[H6] Differentiation of low-intensity effusion from fibrotic thickening and calcification has been extensively discussed in an earlier section.

A disadvantage of magnetic resonance is that calcifications of the pericardium are not easily identified. Their presence may be indirectly inferred by the presence of signal voids. Computed tomography, however, readily depicts regions of calcified pericardium. It also provides fast scan times and in many cases allows the patient to be imaged in a semierect position. This may be critical for the patient's comfort if dyspnea associated with cardiac failure is accentuated in the horizontal position. A disadvantage is that contrast agents must be utilized to visualize the internal structure of the heart. An alternative to either method may be the application of ultrafast CT imaging.[L8] This technique allows direct assessment of myocardial wall thickness as well as pericardial calcifications. Determination of myocardial wall thickness may determine prognosis and help in determining the surgical approach to pericardectomy.

Additional structural abnormalities are observed in association with constriction.[H5, H6] Typically a small, tubular-shaped right ventricle is seen on MR images. Further abnormalities include dilatation of the right atrium, inferior and superior vena cava, and hepatic veins. These changes, together with thickening and the presence of symptoms of constriction, strongly suggest the diagnosis of constrictive pericarditis. The precise sensitivity and specificity of magnetic resonance remain to be established.

POSTOPERATIVE PERICARDIUM

Following pericardial fenestration or resection, magnetic resonance can be used to define the postsurgical anatomy of the pericardium, such as the size of the pericardial window or extent of pericardiectomy. Acute pericardial changes following surgery include thickening, effusion, hematoma, and cardiac tamponade. Chronic sequelae include fibrosis and pericardial constriction with a reported incidence of 0.2 percent.[K4] Thickening and constrictive disease of the pericardium have been discussed in previous sections.

Magnetic resonance is well suited for postoperative follow-up because of its excellent differentiation between hematoma and effusion. Surgical clips that may cause significant distortions in CT images appear as localized voids in MR images. Unfortunately, immediate postoperative monitoring with MR is complicated by several factors. First, cardiac pacemakers are an absolute contraindication to MR imaging. In addition, because of the relatively long scan times that are currently used, patients must be in stable condition. They must also be capable of remaining motionless and breathing quietly during image acquisition to avoid excessive scan artifacts.

PERICARDIAL NEOPLASM

Magnetic resonance evaluation of pericardial neoplasm in most cases involves identification of abnormal anatomic structures and boundaries rather than characterization of relative tissue intensities. A few notable exceptions to this are included in the differential diagnosis of mediastinal masses; examples include fibroma, lipoma, and pericardial cyst. Each of these has a distinct intensity profile.[A1, S9] The value of magnetic resonance for evaluation of potential neoplasm lies largely in treatment planning and particularly preoperative assessment.[C4]

The loss of normal anatomic boundaries is an important sign of neoplasm. *Neoplastic involvement of the pericardium results in focal or diffuse obliteration of the normal pericardial signal.* In the case of malignancy adjacent to cardiac structures, visualization of the pericaridal line is an indication that pericardial invasion has not occurred. Examples of this include congenital cyst in which pericardial signal is visible at the perimeter of the cyst[S9] and lymphoma, which was clearly identified invading from the lung through the pericardium into the right atrium.[S3]

Primary Pericardial Neoplasm

Primary malignancies of the pericardium are much less frequent than metastatic disease. Primary tumors include malignant fibrosarcoma, angiosarcoma, and benign and malignant teratoma. Hemorrhagic effusions result from erosion into intrapericardiac vessels or myocardial wall, with possible acute or subacute tamponade. Paracardiac tumors include entities such as pheochromocytoma and lipoma. Lipoma and pericardial fat pad are easily distinguished by the high-intensity signal of fat tissue.[A1, H4]

Pericardial Metastasis

The involvement of the pericardium by metastatic disease at autopsy is much higher than clinically suspected, ranging from 1.5 to 22 percent in incidence.[M10] The recognized incidence of pericardial involvement in metastasis has increased partly because of the prolonged survival of patients with surgical and chemotherapeutic palliation.[F4] Of malignant pericardial disease, 80 percent is associated with lung or breast carcinoma, leukemia, and lymphoma.[A2, H2, T1] Metastatic involvement of the pericardium is characterized by large effusions out of proportion to the amount of tumor present; this occurs to the extent that neoplasm is the most frequent cause of tamponade. Focal or diffuse plaque-like thickening may occur, obliterating the pericardial space. In the past, pericardiocentesis of neoplastic effusions was followed by introduction of air into the pericardium in an attempt to identify tumor by chest radiography. The development of computed tomography has significantly improved diagnostic capabilities and detection of pericardial metastasis.[J2, M10]

Radiation-induced heart disease arises 1 to 3 years following irradiation of the mediastinum.[H2] This is most often associated with the treatment of Hodgkin's disease, particularly with doses of more than 4000 rads.[A3] Forms of radiation-induced disease include acute pericarditis with self-limited effusion, asymptomatic chronic pericardial effusion, and effusive-constrictive pericarditis syndrome. Sechtem and associates reported a case of radiation-induced pericarditis in a patient with Hodgkin's disease.[S3] Pericardial effusion and pericardial adhesions were identified by magnetic resonance. The adhesions could not be identified specifically as either inflammatory or metastatic in nature.

Magnetic resonance evaluation of metastatic disease of the pericardium has two potential advantages. It provides excellent anatomic detail and may eventually yield information regarding the nature of the neoplasm.[F3] In comparison to computed tomography, metastatic implant on or invasion of the pericardium is more clearly distinguished from associated effusion by magnetic resonance.[P1, S3, W2] The additional anatomic detail obtained with

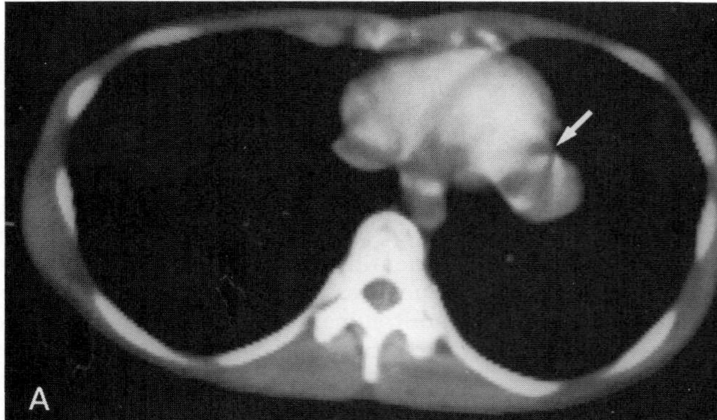

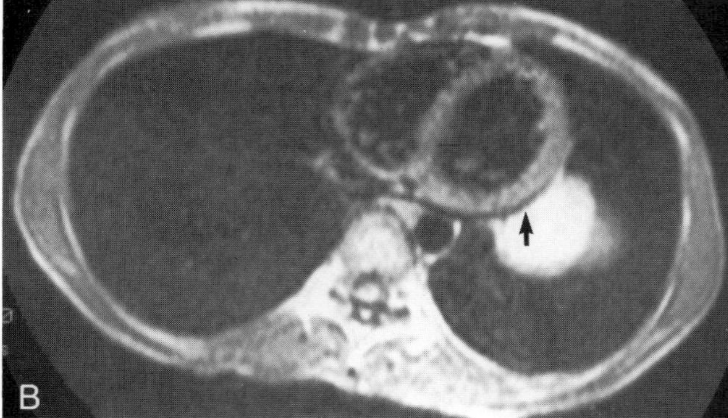

Figure 52–4. Primary lung spindle cell sarcoma. Preoperative assessment by cardiac gated magnetic resonance imaging of the lack of pericardial involvement altered the surgical approach. *A*, Computed tomography image demonstrates mass *(arrow)* adjacent to the left ventricle. Accurate assessment of pericardial involvement is difficult because of the artifact. *B*, Cardiac gated magnetic resonance image (TE = 25 msec) at a level similar to the CT image clearly shows the normal thin low-intensity pericardial line *(arrow)*. Based on this, a left thoracotomy rather than a median sternotomy was performed. No pericardial involvement by the lung spindle cell sarcoma was found at surgery in this 35-year-old woman.

magnetic resonance compared to computed tomography has altered the surgical management of patients with paracardiac masses.[L9] In Figure 52–4, the low-intensity pericardial signal is intact, indicating that the spindle cell sarcoma has not invaded the pericardial tissue. In contrast, Figures 52–5 and 52–6 demonstrate focal absence of the pericardial line in patients with fibrosarcoma and recurrent osteogenic sarcoma, respectively. Regions in which the pericardial line is absent are those that have been invaded by tumor. Because of its superior delineation of pericardium, myocardial walls, and heart chambers, magnetic resonance is the procedure of choice in general for assessment of mediastinal masses.[A1, H6, S9]

SUMMARY

The development of gated-MR techniques allows routine evaluation of patients with suspected pericardial disease, although the indications for these examinations are still being evaluated. Compared with computed tomography and echocardiography, magnetic resonance offers superior anatomic visualization of the pericardium and adjacent structures. Factors such as pleural effusions and obesity, which may degrade echocardiographic studies, do not limit the effectiveness of the MR scan. Contrast agents, which are needed in computed tomography, are not necessary with magnetic resonance to delineate intracardiac structures. Several difficulties, however, may limit the application of magnetic resonance, particularly for patients with cardiac disease. For patients who are critically ill or who have severe orthopnea, the prolonged scan times, ranging from 30 to 60 minutes, may be intolerable. Image quality will be degraded for patients with premature ventricular contractions or other arrhythmias. Severe tachycardia or low-voltage electrocardiograms may also present difficulties in gating the pulse sequences to the cardiac cycle.

For the evaluation of paracardiac masses, magnetic resonance offers advantages over computed tomography and echocardiographic studies. In the case of suspected malignancy, the visualization of an intact pericardial line strongly suggests that invasion of cardiac structures has not occurred. The anatomic detail gained by magnetic resonance may directly affect the surgical management of such patients. For a mass with calcified components, such as a teratoma, comparison with CT images would be of obvious benefit in characterization.

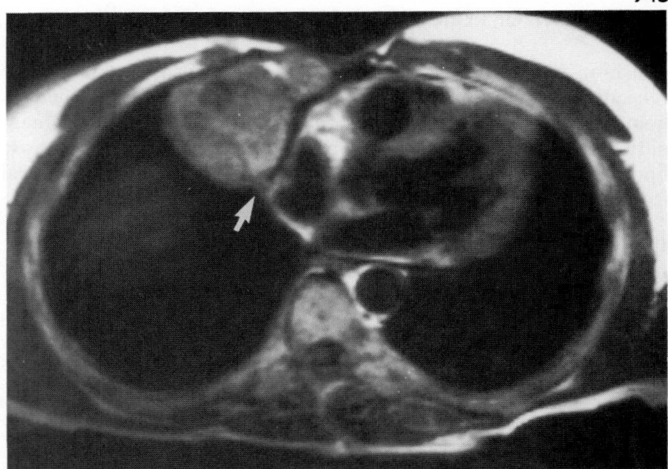

Figure 52–5. Focal pericardial invasion by fibrosarcoma. Fibrosarcoma developed 25 years after this 48-year-old man underwent radiation therapy for Hodgkin's lymphoma. Cardiac gated magnetic resonance image (TE = 25 msec) demonstrated focal absence *(arrow)* of the low signal intensity pericardial line lateral to the right atrium indicative of tumor invasion. This was confirmed at surgery.

The diagnosis of constrictive pericarditis using noninvasive methods is difficult. Magnetic resonance offers an advantage over echocardiography in this regard again by virtue of obtaining outstanding delineation of cardiac anatomy over all regions of the heart. Thickening of the pericardium associated with constriction can be reliably assessed. In the correct clinical setting, its absence can largely rule out constriction in favor of a restrictive cardiomyopathy. However, calcification of the pericardium, another important sign of constriction, is better detected by CT than by MR methods.

Magnetic resonance can detect pericardial effusions with accuracy equal to that of echocardiography and computed tomography, yet echocardiography remains the procedure of choice because of its simplicity and low cost. Magnetic resonance may offer other potential advantages such as identification of loculated effusions and, potentially, characterization of etiology of the

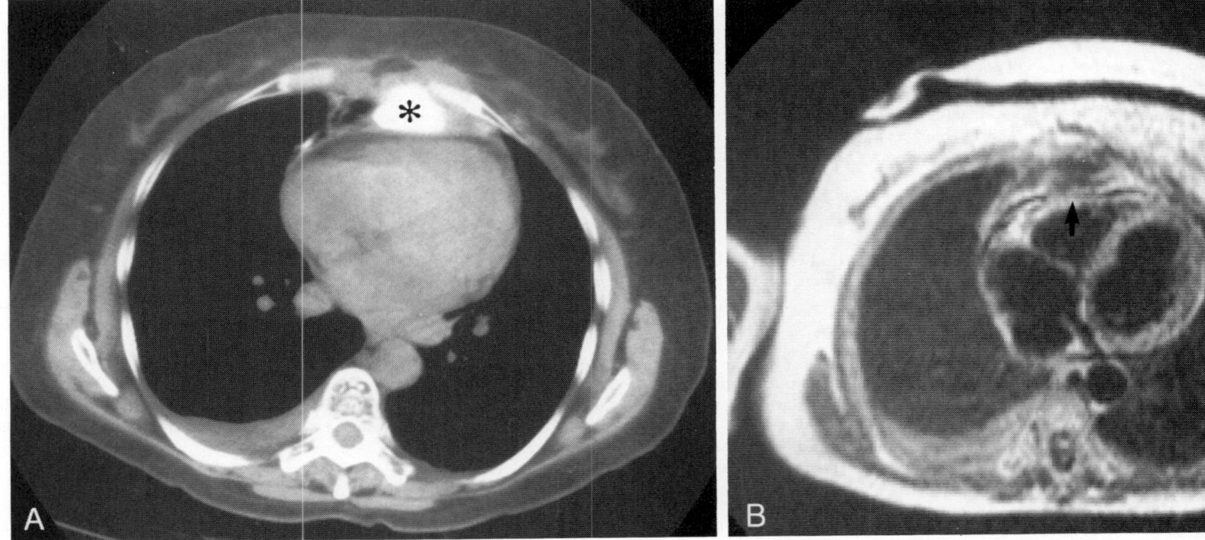

Figure 52–6. Recurrent osteogenic sarcoma of the sternum in a 54-year-old woman 10 years after initial radiation therapy. *A*, Computed tomography demonstrates the ossified recurrent osteogenic sarcoma of the sternum (asterisk) but not pericardial involvement. *B*, Cardiac gated magnetic resonance image (TE = 25 msec), while not displaying the recurrent osteogenic sarcoma ossification as well as computed tomography, clearly demonstrates the focal absence of the low signal intensity pericardial line *(arrow)*. This is indicative of tumor invasion, which was surgically confirmed.

effusion. At present, the etiology of effusions based on tissue relaxation parameters is clear only in selected cases, such as hemopericardium. For evaluation of pericardial effusion, magnetic resonance is appropriate in instances in which diagnostic findings are inconsistent with clinical presentation or technical factors limit the quality of the echocardiographic study.

References

A

1. Amparo, E. G, Higgins, C. B., Farmer, D., et al.: Gated MRI of cardiac and paracardiac masses: Initial experience. AJR 143:1151, 1984.
2. Applefeld, M. M., and Pollock, S. H.: Cardiac disease in patients who have malignancies. Curr. Probl. Cardiol. 4:1, 1980.
3. Applefeld, M. M., Cole, J. F., and Pollock, S. H.: The late appearance of chronic pericardial disease in patients treated by radiotherapy for Hodgkin's disease. Ann. Intern. Med. 94:338, 1981.
4. Aronberg, D. J., Peterson, R. R., Glazer, H. S., and Sagel, S. S.: The superior sinus of the pericardium: CT appearance. Radiology 153:489, 1984.
5. Arciniegas, E., Hakimi, M., Favooki, Z. Q., and Green, E. W.: Intrapericardial teratoma in infancy. J. Thorac. Cardiovasc. Surg. 79:306, 1980.

B

1. Baim, R. S., Macdonald, I. L., Wise, D. J., and Kenkei, S. C.: Computed tomography of absent left pericardium. Radiology 135:127, 1980.
2. Braunwald, E., and Lorell, B. H.: Pericardial disease. *In* Braunwald, E. (ed.): Heart Disease. A Textbook of Cardiovascular Medicine. Saunders, 1984, p. 1470.
3. Brown, J. J., van Sonnenberg, E., Gerber, K. H., et al.: Magnetic resonance relaxation times of percutaneously obtained normal and abnormal body fluids. Radiology 154:727, 1985.
4. Bryk, D., Kroop, I. G., and Budow, J.: The effect of heart size, cardiac tamponade and phase of the cardiac cycle on the distribution of pericardial fluid. Radiology 93:273, 1969.
5. Bush, C. A. Stang, J. M., Wooley, C. F., and Kilman, J. W.: Occult constrictive pericardial disease. Diagnosis by rapid volume expansion and correction by pericardiectomy. Circulation 56:924, 1977.
6. Boisserie-La Croix, M., Martigne, C. H., Laurent, T., et al.: A pleuro-pericardial cyst in an unusual location: The value of magnetic resonance. Comput. Med. Imag. Graphics 12:277, 1988.

C

1. Chesler, E., Matha, A. S., Matisonn, R. E., and Rogers, M. N. A.: Subpulmonic stenosis as a result of noncalcific pericarditis. Chest 69:245, 1976.
2. Choyke, P. L., Kressel, H. Y., Reichek, N., et al.: Nongated cardiac magnetic resonance imaging. Preliminary experience at 0.12 T. AJR 143:1143, 1984.
3. Come, P. C., Riley, M. F., and Fortuin, N. J.: Echocardiography mimicry of pericardial effusion. Am. J. Cardiol. 47:365, 1981.
4. Conti, V. R., Saydjari, R., and Amparo, E. G.: Paraganglioma of the heart: The value of magnetic resonance imaging in preoperative evaluation. Chest 90:604, 1986.
5. Crooks, L. E., Arakawa, M., Hoenninger, J., et al.: Nuclear magnetic resonance whole body imager operating at 3.5 gauss. Radiology 143:169, 1982.
6. Crooks, L. E., Barker, B., Chang, H., et al.: Magnetic resonance imaging strategies for heart studies. Radiology 153:459, 1984.

D

1. Doppman, J. L., Reinmuller, R., Lissner, J., et al.: Computed tomography in constrictive pericarditis. J. Comput. Assist. Tomogr. 5:1, 1981.
2. Dressler, W. H.: The post-myocardial infarction syndrome. Arch. Intern. Med. 103:28, 1959.

E

1. Engle, M. A.: Postpericardiotomy and allied syndromes. *In* Reddy, P. S., Leon, D. F., and Shaver, J. (eds.): Pericardial Disease. Raven Press, New York, 1982, p. 313.

F

1. Ferrans, V. J., and Roberts, W. C.: Pathology of pericardial effusion. *In* Reddy, P. S., Leon, D. F., and Shaver, J. (eds.): Pericardial Disease. Raven Press, New York, 1982, p. 77.
2. Ferrans, V. J., Isihara, T., and Roberts, W. C.: Anatomy of the pericardium. *In* Reddy, P. S., Leon, D. F, and Shaver, J. A. (eds.): Pericardial Disease. Raven Press, New York, 1982, p. 31.
3. Fisher, M. R., Higgins, C. B., and Andereck, W.: MR imaging of an intrapericardial pheochromocytoma. J. Comput. Assist. Tomogr. 9:1103, 1985.
4. Fowler, N. O., ed.: The Pericardium in Health and Disease. Futura, Mount Kisco, N.Y., 1985, p. 301.

G

1. Gibson, A. T., and Segal, M. B.: A study of the composition of pericardial fluid, with special reference to the probable mechanism of fluid formation. J. Physiol. (London) 277:367, 1978.
2. Glover, L. B., Barcia, A., and Reeves, T. J.: Congenital absence of the pericardium. AJR 106:542, 1969.
3. Gould, S. E. *In* Edwards, J. (ed.): Pathology of the Heart and Blood Vessels. 3rd ed. Charles Thomas, Springfield, Ill., 1968.
4. Gutierrez, F. R., Shackelford, G. D., McKnight, R. C., et al.: Diagnosis of congenital absence of left pericardium by MR imaging. J. Comput. Assist. Tomogr. 9:551, 1985.

H

1. Hanock, E. W.: On the rigid and elastic forms of constrictive pericarditis. Am. Heart J. 100:917, 1980.
2. Hanock, E. W.: Pericardial disease in patients with neoplasm. *In* Reddy, P. S., Leon, D. F., and Shaver, J. A. (eds.): Pericardial Disease. Raven Press, New York, 1982, p. 325.
3. Hanock, E. W.: Subacute effusive-constrictive pericarditis. Circulation 43:183, 1971.
4. Herfkens, R., Davis, P., Crooks, L., et al.: Nuclear magnetic resonance imaging of the abnormal live rat and correlations with tissue characteristics. Radiology 141:211, 1981.
5. Higgins, C. B.: MRI of heart disease. Int. J. Cardiac Imag. 2:259, 1987.
6. Higgins, C. B.: Overview of MR of the heart—1986. AJR 146:907, 1986.
7. Higgins, C. B., Byrd, B. F., McNamara, M. T., et al.: Magnetic resonance imaging of the heart: A review of the experience in 172 subjects. Radiology 155:671, 1985.
8. Higgins, C. B., Holt, W., Pflugfelder, P., and Sechtem, U.: Functional evaluation of the heart with magnetic resonance imaging. Magn. Res. Med. 6:121, 1988.
9. Higgins, C. B., Kaufman, L., and Crooks, L. E.: Magnetic resonance imaging of the cardiovascular system. Am. Heart J. 109:136, 1985.
10. Higgins, C. B., Lanzer, P., and Stark, D.: Assessment of cardiac anatomy using nuclear magnetic resonance imaging. J. Am. Coll. Cardiol. 5:77S, 1985.
11. Hirschmann, J. V.: Pericardial constriction. Am. Heart J. 96:110, 1978.
12. Holt, J. P.: The normal pericardium. Am J. Cardiol. 26:455, 1970.
13. Horowitz, M. S., Schultz, C. S., and Stinson, E. R.: Sensitivity and specificity of echocardiographic diagnosis of pericardial fluid. Circulation 50:239, 1974.
14. Houang, M. T. W., Arozena, X., and Shaw, E. G.: Demonstration of the pericardium and pericardial effusion by computed tomography. J. Comput. Assist. Tomogr. 3:601, 1979.
15. Hricak, H., Higgins, C. B., and Williams, R. D.: Nuclear magnetic resonance imaging in retroperitoneal fibrosis. AJR 141:35, 1983.

I

1. Im, J-G., Rosen, A., Webb, W. R., and Gamsu, G.: MR imaging of the transverse sinus of the pericardium. AJR 150:79, 1988.
2. Ishihara, T., Ferrans, V. J., and Jones, M.: Histologic and ultrastructural features of the human parietal pericardium. Am. J. Cardiol. 46:744, 1980.
3. Isner, J. M., Carter, B. L., and Bankoff, M. S.: Computed tomography in the diagnosis of pericardial heart disease. Ann. Intern. Med. 97:473, 1982.
4. Isner, J. M., Carter, B. L., and Bankoff, M. S.: Differentiation of constrictive pericarditis from restrictive cardiomyopathy by computed tomographic imaging. Am. Heart J. 105:1019, 1983.
5. Isner, J. M., Carter, B. L., Roberts, W. C., and Bankoff, M. S.: Subepicardial adipose tissue producing echocardiographic appearance of pericardial effusion. Am. J. Cardiol. 51:565, 1983.

J

1. Jacobson, H. G., ed.: Magnetic resonance imaging of the cardiovascular system. Present state of the art and future potential. Council on Scientific Affairs. Report of the Magnetic Resonance Imaging Panel. JAMA 259:253, 1988.
2. Jochelson, M. S., Balikain, J. P., Mauch, P., and Liebman, H.: Peri- and paracardial involvement in lymphoma. AJR 140:483, 1983.

K

1. Kaminsky, M. E., Rodan, B. A., Osborne, D. R., et al.: Postpericardiotomy syndrome. AJR 138:503, 1982.
2. Kerber, R. E., and Payvandi, M. N.: Echocardiography in acute hemopericardium. Production of false-negative echocardiograms by clots. Circulation 55–56:III–24, 1977.
3. King, C. L., Henkelman, M., Poon, P. Y., and Rubenstein, J.: MR imaging of the knee. J. Comput. Assist. Tomogr. 8:1147, 1984.
4. Kutcher, M. A., King, S. B., Alimurung, B. N., et al.: Constrictive pericarditis as a complication of cardiac surgery: Recognition of an entity. Am J. Cardiol. 50:742, 1982.

L

1. Lanzer, P., Barta, C., Botvinick, H., et al.: ECG-synchronized cardiac imaging: method and evaluation. Radiology 155:681, 1985.
2. Lanzer, P., Botvinick, E. H., Schiller, N. B., et al.: Cardiac imaging using gated magnetic resonance. Radiology 150:121, 1984.

3. Levine, R. A., Thompson, R. C., Brady, T. J., and Okada, R. D.: Proton relaxation parameters of pericardial fluid as predictors of cellular content. Circ. Suppl. III 72:124, 1985.
4. Levy-Ravetch, M., Auh, Y. H., Rubenstein, W. A., et al.: CT of the pericardial recesses. AJR 144:707, 1985.
5. Lilley, W. I., McDonald, J. R., and Clagett, O. T.: Pericardial celomic cysts and pericardial diverticula: A concept of etiology and reports of cases. J. Thorac. Surg. 20:494, 1950.
6. Lindsay, J. Jr., Crawley, I. S., and Callaway, G. M., Jr.: Chronic constrictive pericarditis following uremic hemopericardium. Am Heart J. 79:390, 1970.
7. Lipton, M. J.: Computed tomography of the heart and pericardium. *In* Moss, A. A., Gamsu, G., and Genant, H. K. (eds.): Computed Tomography of the Body. W. B. Saunders, Philadelphia, 1983, p. 414.
8. Lipton, M. J., and Higgins, C. B.: Ultrafast CT and dynamic MRI. Dynamic Cardiovasc. Imag. 1:40, 1987.
9. Lund, J. T., Ehman, R. L., Julsrud, P. R., et al.: Cardiac masses: Assessment by MR imaging. AJR 152:469, 1989.

M

1. Mangano, D. T.: The effect of the pericardium on ventricular systolic function in man. Circulation 6:352, 1980.
2. Mark, A. S., Winkler, M. L., Peltzer, M., et al.: Gated acquisition of MR images of the thorax: Advantages for the study of the hila and mediastinum. Magn. Reson. Imag. 5:57, 1987.
3. Martin, R. P., Rakowski, H., French, J., and Popp, R. L.: Localization of pericardial effusion with wide angle phased array echocardiography. Am. J. Cardiol. 42:904, 1978.
4. McGaff, R. J., Haller, J. A., Leight, L., and Towery, B. T: Subvalvular pulmonic stenosis due to constriction of the right ventricular outflow tract by a pericardial band. Am. J. Med. 34:142, 1963.
5. McMurdo, K. K., Webb, W. R., von Schulthess, G. K., and Gamsu, G.: Magnetic resonance imaging of the superior pericardial recesses. AJR 145:985, 1985.
6. Miller, S. W., Brady, T. J., Dinsmore, R. E., et al.: Cardiac magnetic resonance imaging: The Massachusetts General Hospital experience. Radiol. Clin. North Am. 23:745, 1985.
7. Moncada, B., Baliga, K., Moguillansky, S. J., et al.: CT diagnosis of congenital intrapericardial masses. J. Comput. Assist. Tomogr. 9:56, 1985.
8. Moncada, R., Baker, M., Salinas, M., et al.: Diagnostic role of computed tomography in pericardial heart disease: Congenital defects, thickening, neoplasms and effusions. Am Heart J. 103:263, 1982.
9. Moncada, R., Demos, T. C., Posniak, H. V., and Hammer, R.: Computed tomography of pericardial heart disease. *In* Taveras, J. M., and Ferrucci, J. T. (eds.): Radiology. Diagnosis-Imaging-Intervention, Vol II. Cardiac and Vascular Radiology. Lippincott, Philadelphia, 1987, Chap. 43, p. 1.
10. Moncada, R., Kotler, M. N., Churchill, R. J., et al.: Multimodality approach to pericardial imaging. Cardiovasc. Clin. 17:409, 1986.
11. Moran, P. R., Moran, R. A., and Karstaedt., N.: Verification and evaluation of internal flow and motion. Radiology 154:433, 1985.

N

1. Nassar, W. K.: Congenital defects of the pericardium. *In* Fowler, N. O. (ed.): The Pericardium in Health and Disease. Futura, Mount Kisco, N.Y., 1985, p. 51.
2. Nasser, W. K., Helmen, C., Tavel, M. E., Congenital absence of the left pericardium: Clinical, electrocardiographic, radiographic, hemodynamic and angiographic findings in six cases. Circulation 41:469, 1970.
3. Nicolosi, G. L., Borgioni, L., and Alberti, E.: M-mode and two-dimensional echocardiography in congenital absence of the pericardium. Chest 81:610, 1982.
4. Nishimura, R. A., Connolly, D. C., Parkin, T. W., and Stanson, A. W.: Constrictive pericarditis: Assessment of current diagnostic procedures. Mayo Clin. Proc. 60:397, 1985.

P

1. Pizzarello, R. A., Goldberg, S. M., Goldman, M. A., et al.: Tumor of the heart diagnosed by magnetic resonance imaging. J. Am. Coll. Cardiol. 5:989, 1985.
2. Pope, C. F., Gore, J. C., Sostman, D., et al.: The apparent pericardium on cardiac NMR images. Circ. Suppl. III 72:124, 1985.

R

1. Reddy, P. S., Cutriss, E. I., O'Toole, J. D., and Shaver, J. A.: Cardiac tamponade: Hemodynamic observations in man. Circulation 58:265, 1978.
2. Reddy, P. S.: The hemodynamics of constrictive pericarditis. *In* Reddy, P. S., Leon, D. F., and Shaver, J. A. (eds.): Pericardial Disease. Raven Press, New York, 1982, p. 275.
3. Rhode, E. A.: Physiology of the normal pericardium. *In* Reddy, P. S., Leon, D. F., and Shaver, J. A. (eds.): Pericardial Disease. Raven Press, New York, 1982, p. 31.
4. Roberts, W. C., and Ferrans, V. J.: A survey of the causes and consequences of pericardial heart disease. *In* Reddy, P. S., Leon, D. F., and Shaver, J. (eds.): Pericardial Disease. Raven Press, New York, 1982, p. 49.
5. Roberts, W. C., and Spray, T. L.: Pericardial heart disease: A study of its causes, consequences and morphologic features. *In* Spodick, D. (ed.): Pericardial Diseases. Davis, Philadelphia, 1976, p. 17.
6. Rothchild, P. A., Tarver, R. D., Boyko, O. B., and Conces, D. J.: MR diagnosis of herniation of the left ventricle through a pericardial window. Comput. Radiol. 11:15, 1987.

S

1. Shabetai, R.: Function of the pericardium. *In* Fowler, N. O. (ed.): The Pericardium in Health and Disease. Futura, Mount Kisco, N.Y., 1985, p. 19.
2. Sechtem, U., Tscholakoff, D., and Higgins, C. B.: MRI of the normal pericardium. AJR 147:239, 1986.
3. Sechtem, U., Tscholakoff, D., and Higgins, C. B.: MRI of the abnormal pericardium. AJR 147:245, 1986.
4. Saint Pierre, A., and Froement, R.: Absences totales et partielees du pericarde. Arch. Mal. Coeur. 63:638, 1970.
5. Schiavone, W. A., and O'Donnell, J. K.: Congenital absence of the left portion of parietal pericardium demonstrated by nuclear magnetic resonance imaging. Am. J. Cardiol. 55:1439, 1985.
6. Schnittger, I., Bowden, R. E., Abrams, J., and Popp, R. L.: Echocardiographic diagnosis of pericardial disease. Am. Heart J. 97:420, 1979.
7. Scully, R. E., ed.: Case Records of the Massachusetts General Hospital. Weekly clinicopathological exercises. Case 22—1987. A 58-yr-old woman with progressive pericardial disease. N. Engl. J. Med. 316:1394, 1987.
8. Soulen, R. L., Stark, D. D., and Higgins, C. B.: Magnetic resonance imaging of constrictive pericardial disease. Am. J. Cardiol. 55:480, 1985.
9. Stark, D. D., Higgins, C. B., Lanzer, P., et al.: Magnetic resonance imaging of the pericardium: Normal and pathologic findings. Radiology 150:469, 1984.
10. Steiner, R. M., and Rao, V. M.: The pericardium. *In* Grainger, R. G., and Allison, D. J. (eds.): Diagnostic Radiology. Churchill Livingston, New York, 1986, p. 675.
11. Sutton, F. J., Whitley, N. O., and Applefeld, M. M.: The role of echocardiography and computed tomography in the evaluation of constrictive pericarditis. Am. Heart J. 109:350, 1985.

T

1. Theoligides, A.: Neoplastic cardiac tamponade. Semin. Oncol. 5:181, 1978.
2. Tomoda, H., Hoshiai, M., Furuya, H., et al.: Evaluation of pericardial effusion with computed tomography. Am. Heart J. 99:701, 1980.
3. Turner, D. A., Prodromos, C. C., Petasnick, J. P., and Clark, J. W.: Acute injury of the ligaments of the knee: Magnetic resonance evaluation. Radiology 154:717, 1985.

V

1. von Schulthess, G. K., Fisher, M., Crooks, L. E., and Higgins, C. B.: Gated MR imaging of the heart: Intracardiac signals in patients and healthy subjects. Radiology 156:125, 1985.
2. von Schulthess, G. K., and Higgins, C. B.: Blood flow imaging with MR: Spin phase phenomena. Radiology 157:687, 1985.
3. van Dijk, P.: Direct NMR imaging of heart wall and blood velocity. J. Comput. Assist. Tomogr. 8:429, 1984.

W

1. Walinsky, P.: Pitfalls in the diagnosis of pericardial effusion. Cardiovasc. Clin. 9:111, 1978.
2. Westcott, J. L., and Steiner, R. M.: Clinical applications of magnetic resonance imaging (MRI) of the heart. Cardiovasc. Clin. 17:323, 1986.
3. Winsett, M. Z., Amparo, E. G., Fagan, C. J., et al.: MR imaging of mediastinal pseudocyst. J. Comput. Assist. Tomogr. 12:320, 1988.
4. Wong, B. Y. S., Lee, K. R., and MacArthur, R. I.: Diagnosis of pericardial effusion by computed tomography. Chest 81:177, 1982.
5. Wood, P.: Chronic constrictive pericarditis. Am. J. Cardiol. 7:48, 1961.

Y

1. Yousem, D., Traill, T. T., Wheller, P. S., and Fishman, E. K.: Illustrative cases of pericardial effusion misdetection: Correlation of echocardiography and CT. Cardiovasc. Intervent. Radiol. 10:162, 1987.

Z

1. Zerella, J. T., and Halpe, D. C.: Intrapericardial teratoma: Neonatal cardiorespiratory distress amenable to surgery. J. Pediatr. Surg. 15:961, 1980.

Chapter 53

Dynamic Imaging: Principles of Cine Magnetic Resonance Imaging

▪ *NATHANIEL REICHEK, M.D.* ▪ *LEON AXEL, M.D., Ph.D.*

PHYSICAL PRINCIPLES 948
TECHNICAL IMPLEMENTATION 949
ADVANTAGES 949
LIMITATIONS 949
EFFECTS OF LAMINAR AND TURBULENT FLOW 950
EVALUATION OF CARDIAC CHAMBER SIZE AND FUNCTION 951
EVALUATION OF GREAT VESSELS 953
The Aorta 953
Pulmonary Circulation 954
Pulmonary Embolism 954
Pulmonary Hypertension 954
Pulmonary Veins 955
VALVULAR HEART DISEASE 955
Regurgitant Lesions 955
Mitral Regurgitation 955
Aortic Regurgitation 957
Tricuspid Regurgitation 958
Pulmonic Regurgitation 959
Stenotic Lesions 959
Aortic Stenosis 961
Mitral Stenosis 962
Tricuspid Stenosis 962
CONGENITAL HEART DISEASE 962
CORONARY ARTERY DISEASE 962
Evaluation of Segmental Myocardial Function 963
Coronary Bypass Graft Imaging 963
INTRACARDIAC MASSES 964
FLOW QUANTITATION 965
FUTURE DIRECTIONS 965

Cine magnetic resonance imaging (cine MRI) is one of a number of cardiovascular applications of MRI methods in which gradient echoes are used.[G1] Such methods are relatively fast and can provide much useful dynamic information regarding cardiovascular structure and function and intracardiac and great vessel flow. Consequently, much of the early effort in development of cardiovascular applications of MRI has been directed at these approaches. A number of potentially important uses have been identified. Although implementations vary considerably, all such methods have in common certain general principles, advantages, limitations, and applications. In this chapter, we seek to provide a balanced overview of the current state of the field and a perspective on directions for further development. More extensive discussions of MRI physics in general and of flow effects in MRI can be found in Chapters 38, 39, and 41.

Cine MRI is relatively new, and it is developing rapidly. Much of the technology is proprietary, and clinical research using the method is in an early phase. Much interesting work has been presented in preliminary reports only. Thus, when the published literature has fallen short of the full extent of relevant information at the time of this writing, we have been obliged to refer to preliminary reports or, in some instances, unpublished data.

PHYSICAL PRINCIPLES

In conventional spin-echo cardiac-gated MRI of the heart, images are acquired at set delays after detection of a trigger pulse derived from the electrocardiogram (ECG). If images of multiple levels are recorded in an interleaved manner, the delay differs at each level in relation to the ECG. To acquire images of a given level at multiple phases of the cardiac cycle (e.g., for studying dynamic events such as regional wall motion), or to acquire images at multiple levels in the same phase of the cardiac cycle (e.g., for measurement of global properties such as myocardial mass or chamber volumes), one can make repeated passes through the stack of slices to be imaged, permuting the order of slice acquisition so that each slice is acquired at a different phase of the cardiac cycle each time. Such a process requires an extended time for all these images to be acquired, however, which increases the possibility of patient motion during the acquisition period and could produce errors in analysis.

An alternative approach to acquiring images of a given level at multiple phases of the heart cycle involves excitation of that level multiple times during the heart cycle. If detection of an ECG-derived trigger is used to initiate the excitation sequence, variations in the dead time between cycles due to R-R interval variation can lead to artifacts in the first image. Also, if conventional spin-echo imaging is used with a pulse repetition time (TR) short enough to give reasonable time resolution of the cardiac cycle, incomplete magnetic relaxation between excitations results in a weak magnetic resonance signal and noisy images. The key differences of the "cine" MRI techniques from conventional cardiac MRI as described previously are (1) the use of a free-running sequence of radiofrequency (RF) excitation at a constant pulse-repetition rate, with retrospective processing to create images representing specific phases of the cardiac cycle, and (2) the use of a limited flip angle and of gradient echoes to maintain a reasonable signal-to-noise ratio even with rapid repetition of RF excitations. A full description of the principles of the cine MRI technique is given by Glover and Pelc.[G1]

Use of a constant interpulse interval results in the asynchronous acquisition of magnetic resonance signals relative to the heart cycle. If the timing information is recorded for each signal acquisition in relation to the ECG-derived trigger, however, the raw data can be retrospectively processed with sorting and interpolation to generate synthetic data corresponding to particular phases of the cardiac cycle. Images can then be reconstructed with the Fourier transform in the usual fashion. The phase-encoding gradient can be incremented with the ECG-derived trigger to help ensure a full set of raw data to use in the retrospective processing. The minimum data-acquisition time (for no signal averaging) is then given by the product of the R-R interval and the number of phase-encoding steps to be employed. Multiple levels can be acquired in an interleaved mode, at the cost of a coarser effective temporal sampling of the cardiac cycle at each level. The large number of images that cine imaging generates can be viewed most easily with a dynamic display as an endless "movie loop."

The intensity contrast in the rapidly repeated, small flip-angle images generated with this technique is largely due to flow phenomena. The principal source of flow contrast is the signal from the blood, resulting from wash-out/wash-in effects, which is relatively strong overall. Even with the reduced flip angle, the signal from relatively stationary structures such as the heart wall is somewhat weakened, owing to partial saturation of the magnetization. Because the exciting RF pulses are spatially selective, however, blood flowing into the imaging region from upstream may be fully magnetized and generally produces a full-strength signal. Thus, a strong signal from blood is typically seen in cine MRI.

The phase shifts that excited spins can acquire while moving along magnetic field gradients are another important source of flow contrast. Although the conventional magnetic resonance image reconstruction does not directly display phase, the presence of a range of phases in the signals contributing to a given picture element in the final image can result in destructive interference and a decrease in the net signal, with a corresponding decrease in the image brightness at that location. Similarly, highly disordered flow, resulting in an inconsistent phase in consecutive signal acquisitions, can result in a loss of brightness in the final image. In practice, this phenomenon can result in a striking demonstration of turbulence, as in jets flowing across stenotic or regurgitant cardiac valves. It can also produce apparent signal loss in normal flows with a high degree of shear, such as in parts of the aortic root and left ventricular outflow tract during systole. Such normal areas of transient signal loss are usually readily distinguished from the areas of signal loss caused by abnormal flow patterns.

TECHNICAL IMPLEMENTATION

Details of implementation of cine MRI methods vary widely. In general, retrospective ECG gating has been found to be more effective than prospective gating, in which the steady state produced by short repetition times and shallow flip angles is interrupted periodically. With retrospective gating, the timing of the QRS complex on the ECG, typically detected using simple peak-detection algorithms, is stored along with the signal acquired by the free-running pulse sequence. Typically, a 128 × 256 pixel matrix is used. Because the phase-encoding gradient is advanced with each QRS complex detected, 128 cardiac cycles are required to obtain data throughout the slice imaged. Frequently, the signal-to-noise ratio is further improved by signal averaging, so that 256 or 512 cardiac cycles may be used.

A single acquisition in a patient with a heart rate of 60 beats per minute may take 2, 4, or 8 minutes, depending on the amount of signal averaging used. After completion of signal acquisition, data must then be sorted by their temporal relationship to the QRS peak. Repetition times in the 20- to 30-msec range are widely used for cardiac imaging, with echo times ranging from 12 to 20 msec. The number of temporal samples obtained is the cardiac cycle length divided by the repetition time of the system. Thus, with a cycle length of 1000 msec and repetition time of 25 msec, 40 temporal samples are obtained. If only one slice location is imaged, temporal resolution is relatively high, and signal-to-noise is relatively good, even without signal averaging. If multiple slices are imaged simultaneously, however, the 40 temporal samples are evenly allocated among the slice locations, reducing temporal fidelity. Further, the signal-to-noise ratio is reduced on multi-slice imaging as compared with single-slice imaging. Signal averaging is more often required, therefore.

Cine imaging can be performed in any standard or oblique plane. In some implementations, however, axial-plane imaging produces superior image quality and freedom from artifact. Compound oblique imaging causes the greatest problems with artifact and also increases available repetition and echo times significantly, resulting in further diminution of temporal fidelity. Although the technique has been most commonly implemented on high-field (≥ 1 tesla) systems, it can be applied at much lower magnetic field strengths.

ADVANTAGES

Like other magnetic resonance imaging methods, cine MRI is free of ionizing radiation, is totally noninvasive, requires no contrast injection, and has no known biologic hazards. Another major advantage of cine MRI is its relative speed. Although some major qualitative structural cardiovascular abnormalities can be diagnosed with relatively few images, obtained at any time in the cardiac cycle, functional analyses are either highly desirable or essential for many other cardiovascular applications. For such purposes, images must be obtained at many points in the cardiac cycle on each slice imaged. Further, much of the rationale for development of cardiac MRI is based on its ability to image all slices through the cardiac volume in a reasonable amount of time. Imaging of many slices through the thorax at multiple points in the cardiac cycle is quite time-consuming when conventional spin-echo gated multi-slice imaging protocols are used. In contrast, cine MRI permits acquisition of many slices at many points in the cardiac cycle with imaging and reconstruction times that are typically 20 to 30 percent of comparable spin-echo imaging times. Thus, performing volumetric studies of even the largest left ventricle, for example, becomes practical.

With the anticipated introduction of "ultrafast" cardiac MRI implementations for commercially available systems, the time advantage of cine MRI may disappear in the next 3 to 5 years; however, echo planar methods using gradient echo signal, and resulting in images similar to cine MRI images, already exist and are likely to become a mainstay of cardiac MRI.

Another major advantage of the cine technique is its depiction of flowing blood. Laminar blood flow produces a bright signal that is qualitatively similar (Fig. 53–1), but may vary in amplitude with velocity and various technical factors.[F1] This feature gives the method enormous power in depicting vascular and intracardiac flow. Moreover, abnormal flow regions of several types are readily recognized on cine images as signal voids.[S1] This property permits application of cine MRI to assessment of valvular dysfunction, nonvalvular obstruction to flow, and some central shunts. Use of these signal properties in conjunction with image acquisition through an entire cardiac or chamber volume permits, for the first time, three-dimensional depiction of flow dynamics over the cardiac cycle. It also may permit more accurate noninvasive quantitation of valvular dysfunction, including direct determination of the size of regurgitant and stenotic valve orifices.[R1]

In addition, one can extract directional and absolute flow velocity information from cardiac gated gradient echo images.[U1] Although this potential is not currently realized in most existing commercial software packages, it is likely to become more widely available in the future. Thus, the approach has the potential to provide quantitation of cardiac output, shunt flow ratios, and even flow in individual coronary arteries.

LIMITATIONS

Cine MRI also has some significant disadvantages. As with any gated, temporally averaged technique for producing MRI images, each image represents information obtained over many cardiac

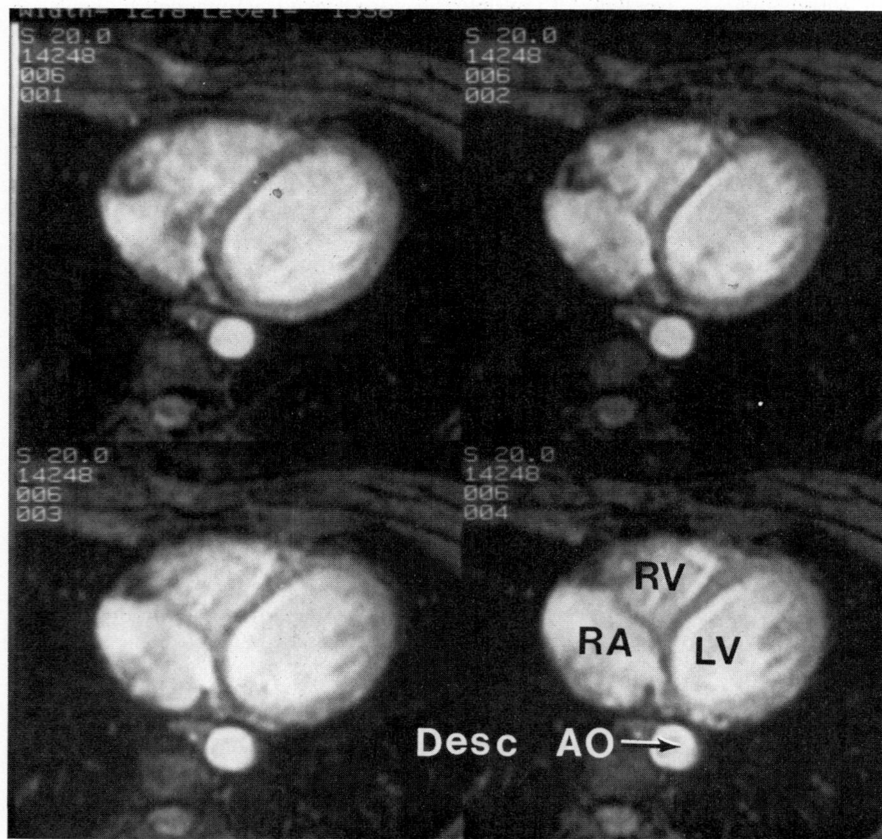

Figure 53–1. Four serial systolic frames (50-msec intervals) of an axial cine slice in a normal volunteer at the level of the mid–left ventricle (LV), right atrium (RA), right ventricle (RV), and descending thoracic aorta (Desc. AO). In these images, the chest wall is located anteriorly, and the spine is located posteriorly.

cycles and is not an accurate depiction of the heart at any single instant in time. With existing hardware and software, primary data can be obtained either on a few slices at many points in the cardiac cycle or on more slices at fewer points. Moreover, distributing information over several slices can diminish the signal obtained on each slice. Thus, signal properties can vary with the number of slices simultaneously imaged. Temporal interpolation methods can provide a smoother depiction of the cardiac cycle and can lessen effects of limited temporal sampling. Such limitations can result in lengthy imaging times, however, or potentially, in errors in determining the full range of cardiac chamber sizes throughout the cardiac cycle. In addition, while cine MRI offers excellent depiction of flow disturbances due to valvular heart disease, partial volume effects limit imaging of thin structures such as valve leaflets at currently available pixel sizes.

Another important limitation of current versions of cine MRI is that the images rarely match spin-echo images in resolution, clarity, and detail. Furthermore, motion-related variations in signal amplitude in pixels representing similar tissue, particularly myocardium, are common. Such variations further complicate the already formidable problem of developing successful automatic segmentation strategies for MRI images. Both of these problems are mainly consequences of the effects of respiratory motion and of the limitations of the usual flow compensation routines used for cine imaging. Such routines are essential for appropriate spatial display of signal from moving blood. Many commercial implementations provide only velocity compensation, however, not acceleration compensation. Often, flow compensation is performed only along one axis in space, whereas flow actually occurs along multiple axes.

Finally, available pixel sizes and slice thicknesses for cine imaging may result in significant partial volume effects. Although techniques to compensate for phase wrap and frequency wrap effects are widely available for spin-echo imaging and permit the use of small fields of view and, hence, small pixel sizes, similar pixel sizes are not yet available for cine imaging. Thus, for studies in adult humans, pixel sizes commonly exceed 4 mm^2 before interpolation. Slice thicknesses of 3 mm are now available. Both minimal pixel size and minimal slice thickness depend on the magnitude of the magnetic field gradients that can be obtained with existing gradient amplifiers. Given the short TR of cine sequences as compared with spin-echo sequences, the demands placed on gradient amplifiers by small-pixel, thin-slice cine imaging are great; further improvements in gradient amplifiers are important to the future development of the technology. The practical importance of these considerations results from the fact that partial volume effects at an interface between bright blood signal and either myocardium or a turbulent flow signal void can produce gradations in signal that may greatly complicate image interpretation and analysis.

Despite these limitations, cine MRI is an exceptionally powerful method for cardiovascular imaging. Rapid, ongoing improvement of hardware and software will enhance its value in the future. In particular, wider implementation of echo planar techniques similar to cine and flow quantitation methods are likely to make it a dominant noninvasive flow imaging method in the 1990's.

EFFECTS OF LAMINAR AND TURBULENT FLOW

Laminar blood flow produces bright signal in cardiac chambers and in systemic and pulmonary arteries and veins (see Fig. 53–1). If TR and echo time (TE) are held constant in vitro, signal amplitude in laminar flow varies with flow velocity.[F1] In images obtained in vitro, signal tends to rise from 5 cm/sec to more than 70 cm/sec and tends to plateau thereafter, possibly declining at velocities greater than 1 m/sec. Images obtained in vivo, however, do not show such a simple, orderly set of relationships. For example, systolic signal is not systematically greater in amplitude in the left ventricle than in the left atrium, even though flow velocities are substantially greater. Whether this finding reflects nonlaminar flow, limitations of flow compensation methods, or other factors is uncertain at this time.

Turbulent flow results in coexistence of many different velocities and, hence, many different signal phases within a single pixel. Cancellation of signal occurs, resulting in a signal void (Fig. 53–2). Signal voids are of three principal types. First, shear effects between rapidly moving laminar flow and adjacent cardiac tissue can result in a small region of disturbed flow and a resultant signal void. Thus, in the normal heart during systolic ejection, shear between rapidly moving blood that is leaving the left ventricle and the adjacent left side of the interventricular septum is sufficient to produce a small signal void, which propagates into the aortic root. One can similarly demonstrate a small region of aliasing in the same location using color flow Doppler echocardiography, although maximal velocities on pulsed Doppler ultrasonography rarely exceed 110 cm/sec.

A second pattern of signal void that can occur in the normal heart is produced by apparent turbulence in high-velocity flow streams in the absence of structural disease. For example, high systolic ejection velocities can produce an ejection signal void in either aortic root or proximal pulmonary artery. Similarly, rapid diastolic inflow from left atrium to left ventricle, or rapid inflow from pulmonary veins into left atrium, can be associated with signal void.

The third common pattern of signal void is generated during flow through a restricted orifice, such as a stenotic or regurgitant valve (Fig. 53–3). In this setting, the signal void phenomenon has three distinct components. Pre-orificial convergence and acceleration of flow proximal to the orifice often result in a signal void, presumably owing to phase cancellation, and corresponding in general location to the color flow Doppler phenomenon of pre-orificial aliasing. At the orifice, high flow velocities are generated in the jet through the valve, often in the range of 400 to 600 cm/sec. Here, mechanisms other than phase cancellation may dominate. In vitro studies of cine signal and velocity have not systematically explored this velocity domain, but cine signal does begin to diminish above 100 cm/sec and may well be absent at significantly higher velocities.[F1] Downstream from an orifice, turbulent flow dissipates the kinetic energy of high-velocity jet flow, and a volume of disturbed flow is generated, which results in another signal-void region. All three signal-void regions—pre-orifice, orifice jet, and post-orifice—are in continuity, and in general, the jet signal void forms a narrow waist linking pre-orificial and post-orificial flow regions.

The size of a signal void may depend on many factors. Technical factors, including TR, TE, and the number of slices imaged in an acquisition, may influence cine signal.[F1] Furthermore, the particular location of a given slice in relation to other slices excited in the acquisition, as well as the direction of flow, can influence the signal void size. Lastly, partial volume effects related to pixel size and slice thickness (see the previous section, "Limitations") may be important.

Many physiologic variables also contribute to downstream signal voids. For a given orifice size, the size of the downstream signal void varies with the volume of flow. If flow is held constant, the size of the signal void varies inversely with the size of the orifice. Mixing of turbulent and laminar flow streams, as occurs when normal antegrade and turbulent retrograde flow enter a chamber simultaneously, may have complex effects, which depend on the spatial relationship of the two flow streams. Finally, the damping properties of the receiving chamber may significantly modulate the size of turbulent flow domains.

EVALUATION OF CARDIAC CHAMBER SIZE AND FUNCTION

Because of its relative speed, cine MRI is a promising method for quantitative evaluation of cardiac chamber size, systolic and diastolic function, and myocardial mass. To date, only a limited number of validation studies have been performed, and they often rely on other imaging methods, such as two-dimensional echocardiography and contrast ventriculography, which have their own limitations. Much additional work is required, including the use of either pathologic validation (e.g., for left ventricular mass quantification) or well-validated, precise imaging methods such as cine computed tomography (CT).[R2] Most work has been devoted to evaluation of the left ventricle. In principle, however, applications to the right ventricle and to both atria are equally feasible.

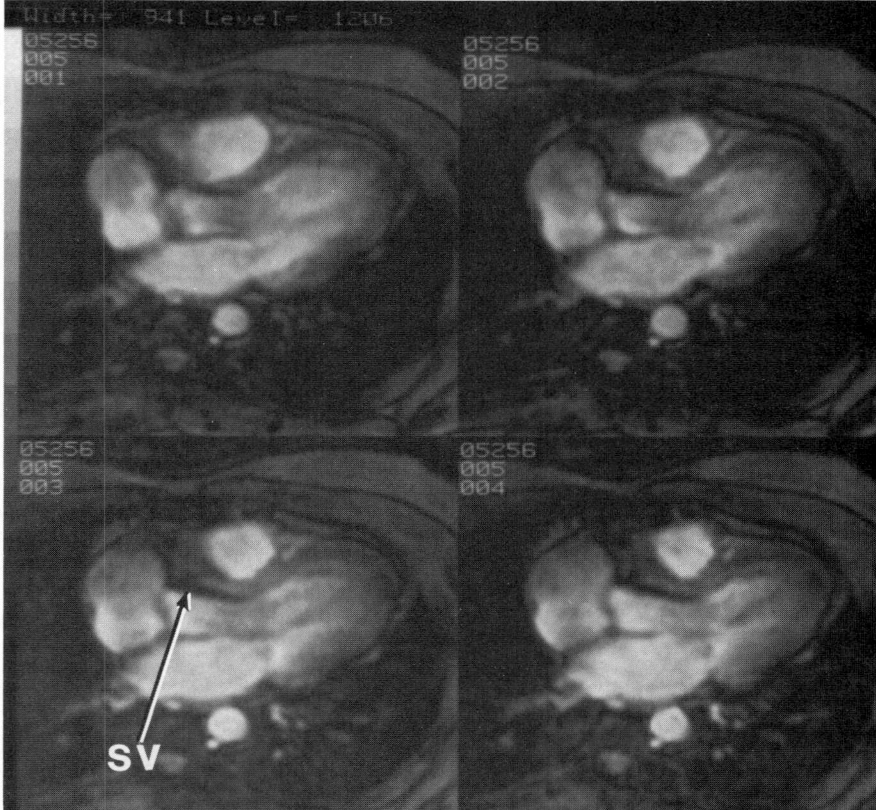

Figure 53–2. Four serial axial systolic images in a normal volunteer show a signal void (SV) in the aortic root due to shear effects with rapid normal ejection.

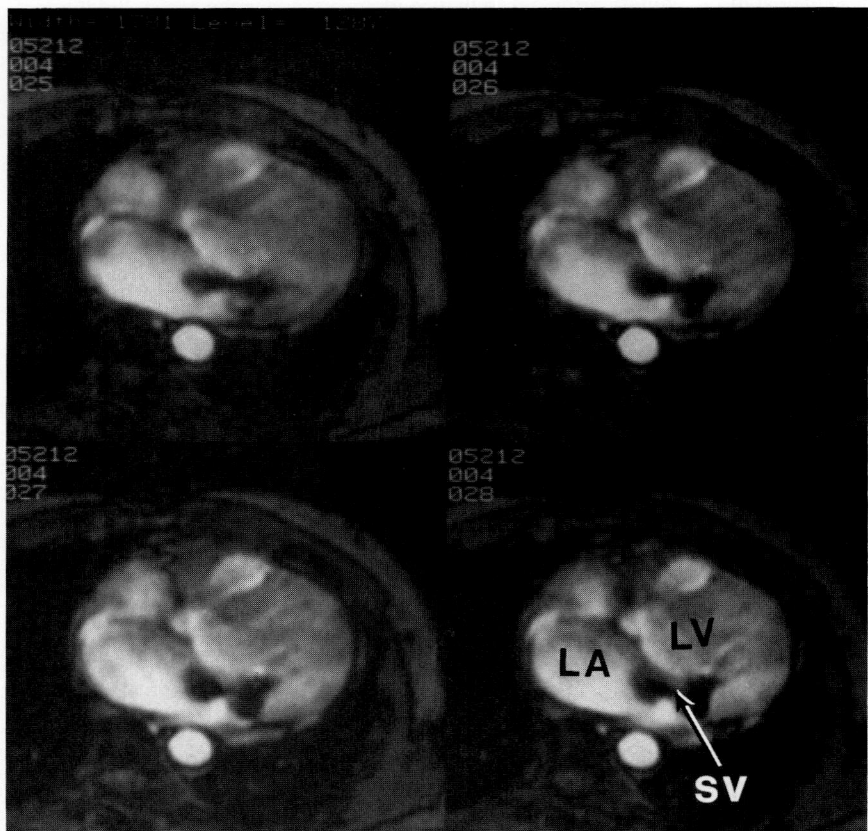

Figure 53–3. Serial systolic images of the left atrium (LA) and left ventricle (LV) in a patient with mitral regurgitation. A dumbbell-shaped three-component signal void (SV) across the mitral valve plane is shown to consist of a zone of accleration in the left ventricle, a narrow jet across the valve plane, and a region of downstream turbulence in the left atrium.

Two alternative approaches to evaluation of the left ventricle have been proposed.[B1, C1] The first approach exploits the ability of cine MRI to acquire all slices through the left ventricle at many points in the cardiac cycle. Quantitation is performed by summing the products of slice thickness and cross-section area for each slice. Images are preferably obtained in the short-axis projection (Fig. 53–4), as prescribed from a localizing coronal series that is used to define the compound oblique orientation of the left ventricular long axis in three-dimensional space.

This approach involves important trade-offs regarding slice thickness, temporal fidelity, and imaging times. With cine MRI, primary data are obtained at many points in the cardiac cycle, with the number determined by dividing cycle length by TR. Thus, for a heart rate of 60 (1000-msec cycle length) and a typical TR of 25 msec, 40 temporal samples are obtained. If all these samples are applied to a single slice, the frame rate is 40 frames/sec without temporal interpolation. On the other hand, if one is seeking to obtain 20 short-axis slices that are each 5 mm thick through a left ventricle that is 10 cm long, 20 acquisitions are required to complete a quantitative study. Imaging would take 113 minutes. Clearly, time considerations are prohibitive.

The use of multislice image acquisitions greatly reduces imaging and reconstruction time, at the cost of reduced temporal fidelity, and it requires the use of signal averaging to generate adequate signal, so that time savings are slightly less than proportional. Use of seven acquisitions—each of three slices, with one signal average—reduces frame rate to 13 frames per cycle reduces frame rate to 13 frames per second and imaging time to 54 minutes. For most purposes other than determination of peak left ventricular ejection and filling rates, such a reduction in temporal fidelity would be acceptable. Use of 1-cm slice thickness would further reduce imaging time. Use of thicker slices is probably acceptable because cine CT uses 8-mm slice thickness with 4-mm skips between pairs, whereas effective slice thickness with echocardiography probably exceeds 1 cm in many applications, particularly in the far field. Using each of 3-cm-thick slices would reduce imaging time to 31 minutes. Clearly, at this point, the method becomes quite competitive with alternative noninvasive methods. Wide availability of echo planar cine-like gradient-echo techniques obviates this problem because acquisition times should drop by more than 80 percent.

Using this approach, several investigators have demonstrated that estimates of left ventricular end-diastolic and end-systolic volume, ejection fraction, and stroke volume and mass can be obtained.[B1, P1, S1] Volumetric results correlated closely with high-quality biplane two-dimensional echocardiography. Similarly, Utz and colleagues compared cine MRI left ventricular ejection fraction with biplane angiographic left ventricular volumes and ejection fraction in 11 patients and found an excellent correlation (r = 0.88).[U2]

The second approach currently taken to volumetric quantitation involves the use of selected orthogonal imaging planes, which are usually equivalent to the echocardiographer's four-chamber and two-chamber views. The geometric assumption is made that the structure of interest can be treated as a solid of revolution using a Simpson's rule approximation.[C1] The approach is analogous to biplane contrast ventriculography or echocardiography. Imaging time is reduced to 15 minutes or less, including a localizing series. Temporal fidelity is good, with frame rates of 30 or more per cycle usually achieved. Thus, even at present, the method is highly competitive with other noninvasive methods that use similar principles. Because of its speed, this second approach is likely to prevail as the norm for routine applications of cine imaging to cardiac pump function. One can predict, however, that marked asymmetric abnormalities of cardiac chamber shape are likely to result in significant errors in volumetric estimation when this approach is used, as is the case for other imaging techniques that use similar principles.

Selected orthogonal long-axis planes have been used extensively by several investigators.[C1, L1] They have demonstrated that left ventricular volume and ejection fraction results compare favorably with biplane cine angiography and with the use of multiple cine MRI short-axis slices. In 17 patients, end-diastolic volume obtained by orthogonal long-axis cine MRI correlated well (r = 0.97; SEE = 22 ml) with that obtained by angiography and with short-axis cine MRI (r = 0.96; SEE = 25 ml). End-systolic volume correlations were r = 0.98 and SEE = 16 ml for angiography, and r = 0.98 and SEE = 15 ml for short-axis cine MRI, respectively. Ejection fraction correlations were r = 0.90 and SEE = 8%, and r = 0.92 and SEE = 7%, respectively.[C1] If these promising results could be confirmed in multiple centers and validated with more reliable reference standards for misshapen ventricles, such as cine CT, the biplane long-axis method would clearly be the method of choice for cine MRI quantification of left ventricular size and function.

A principal limitation on the ease of application of volumetric cine MRI analyses has been the paucity of software to support the required image analysis. Flexible, sophisticated analytic software has been only slowly incorporated into commercial MRI systems; cardiac applications now constitute a small proportion of the demand for MRI. This problem is receding in importance and can be addressed with a variety of approaches to off-line image analysis, which are analogous to those used for many other cardiac imaging techniques.

A more challenging problem, although it is not unique to cine MRI, is that of automating image segmentation. At present, segmentation is performed by a skilled observer, using a manual interface such as a mouse or track ball. This approach, similar to that used for echocardiography or, in most centers, for contrast ventriculography, makes data analysis laborious and subject to additional variation due to observer factors. Automated segmentation is relatively straightforward for CT, but for MRI, individual pixel values do not have an absolute physical significance, unlike Hounsfield's numbers. The problem is particularly severe for cine MRI, in which many technical variables and many sources of artifact can influence pixel values. Practical solutions are likely to emerge over time. Perhaps they will be based on the directional and velocity information inherent in the signal properties, but as is true for echocardiography and contrast ventriculography, lack of automated segmentation is an important limitation at present.

EVALUATION OF GREAT VESSELS

The Aorta

Because cine MRI allows depiction of both structure and flow, it is quite useful in diseases of the thoracic aorta, including Marfan's syndrome, suspected aortic dissection, atherosclerotic aneurysm, and coarctation.

In patients with Marfan's syndrome and in patients with cystic medial necrosis of the aorta of other types, cine MRI permits periodic determination of aortic size (Fig. 53–5), as does spin-echo MRI. Both methods offer better sampling of the aorta than is possible with echocardiography, so that both the topographic extent of dilation and the site of maximal dilation are readily determined. Spin-echo MRI is preferable for image quality, but cine MRI permits simultaneous assessment of the presence or absence of aortic regurgitation, an important covariable (see later discussion).

Spin-echo MRI is proving to be a powerful method for evaluation of aortic dissection. Like CT, MRI offers comprehensive sampling of the thoracic aorta in suspected dissection. MRI, with its ability to image any plane of interest, however, offers distinct advantages over CT, which is largely confined to the axial plane. Thus, the imaging plane for each portion of the aorta can be tailored to offer optimal information relative to location, size, and shape of the false lumen and involvement of branch vessels.

Spin-echo imaging is often sufficient for evaluation of dissection; however, cine MRI offers significant additional information in several respects. First, patterns of pulsation and flow in true and false lumens are depicted. Indeed, quantitation of velocity maps in true and false lumens is feasible.[B2] Partial obstruction of the true lumen, the false lumen, the arch vessels, or in extreme cases, the pulmonary artery branches may result in signal voids. Stagnant flow in a patent false lumen is particularly well demonstrated. When contrast methods are used, such conditions

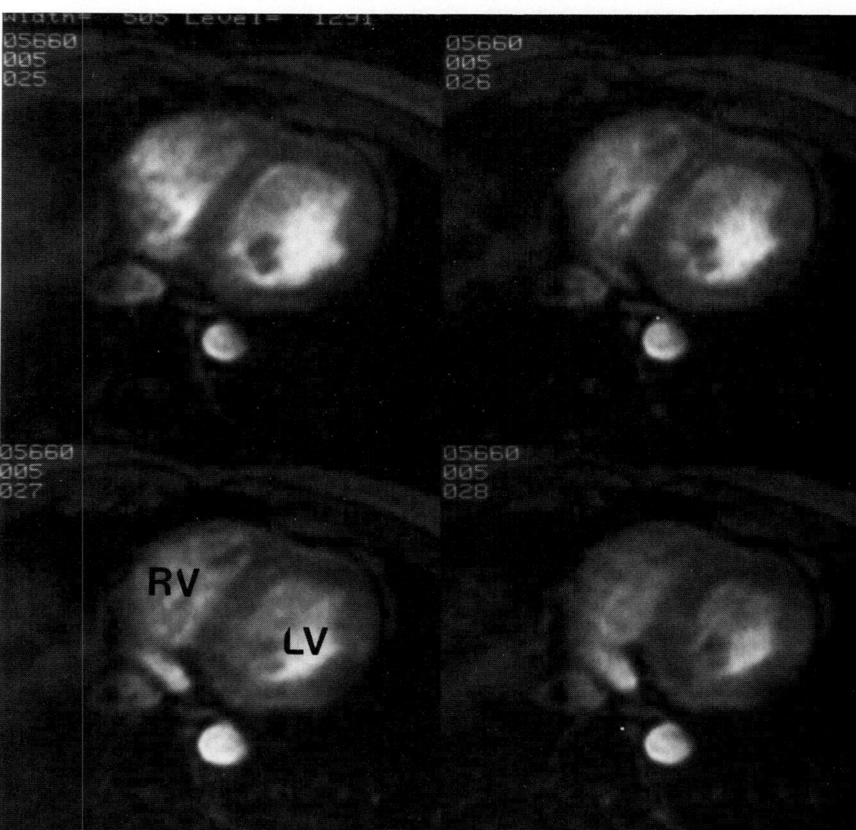

Figure 53–4. Serial systolic short-axis images of the right (RV) and left (LV) ventricles in a normal volunteer.

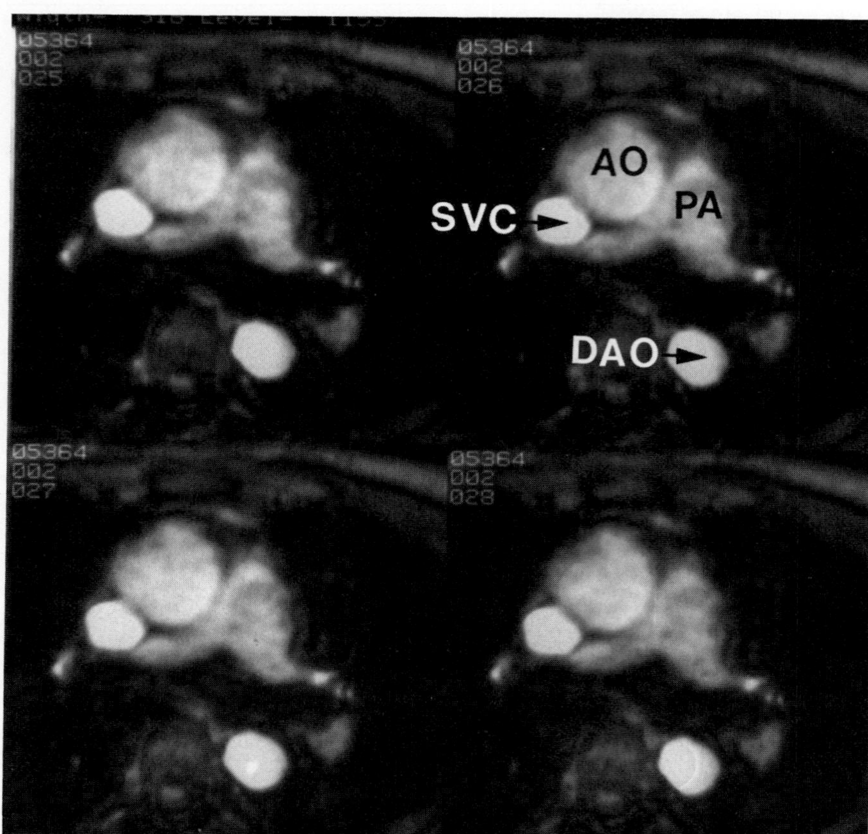

Figure 53–5. Serial images at the levels of the aortic root (AO), pulmonary arteries (PA), superior vena cava (SVC), and descending aorta (DAO) in a patient with cystic medial necrosis and marked dilation of the aortic root.

often result in nonopacification, while with spin-echo MRI, slow flow may result in high signal levels from blood in the false lumen, which may mimic thrombosis or soft tissue thickening. In contrast, cine MRI shows bright signal at flow velocities as low as 10 cm/sec. In one comparative study of 18 patients with dissection, with results validated at surgery or angiographically, cine MRI permitted correct diagnoses in all cases, including one in which neither spin-echo MRI nor CT demonstrated the lesion.[S2] Thus, the optimal approach to evaluation of dissection often consists of the use of spin-echo imaging for speed and morphology, with selective use of cine MRI to evaluate pertinent flow conditions in selected regions.

The use of MRI in patients with dissection raises particular problems regarding patient safety. Because monitoring capability and access to patients for emergency care are less in the magnetic resonance scanner than in an angiographic laboratory or CT scanner, great care must be taken to assure patient stability and safety. Hemodynamically unstable patients are best evaluated with other methods, whereas more stable patients are best monitored by personnel in the scanning room, as well as with conventional ECG and respiratory monitoring and continuous use of a two-way intercom.

Cine MRI provides dramatic images in patients with atherosclerotic aneurysm of the thoracic aorta. No inherent advantage is obtained, however, in relation to spin-echo imaging. Findings in studies of coarctation of the aorta are discussed in a later section (see "Congenital Heart Disease").

Pulmonary Circulation

Pulmonary Embolism

In principle, cine MRI should be an effective method for evaluation of pulmonary embolism, because it easily provides images of proximal and peripheral pulmonary artery branches (Fig. 53–6; see Fig. 53–5). Only limited empiric data are available to document its utility, however. In one reported study, cine MRI detected pulmonary emboli in all 11 patients studied, and its results corresponded well with angiographic and scintigraphic data.[P2] Nonetheless, any tomographic imaging method has inherent limitations when applied to an intricate branching vascular pattern, such as the pulmonary arterial tree. For this application, magnetic resonance angiography, which produces projection images but also uses cine-like gradient echo signal, is likely to be the preferred approach. Such techniques have already been used effectively outside the thorax to image the carotid, intracranial, and lower extremity vessels.[D1] Within the thorax, however, respiratory and cardiac motion pose formidable problems for existing MRI angiographic methods. Thus, further development of software may be necessary before a gradient echo approach to acute pulmonary embolism proves suitable for clinical use.

Cine MRI has already proved to be helpful, however, in evaluation of patients with chronic large-branch pulmonary embolism, in whom surgical therapy may be of dramatic benefit if a correct diagnosis is made. Angiographic recognition of this disorder is complicated by dilation of the central pulmonary vessels, so that lumen size may appear normal even when a thick layer of thrombus is present. Spin-echo MRI can display the increased thickness of the vessel wall, leading to correct diagnosis. Slow flow velocities in the right and left pulmonary arteries, however, are common in severe pulmonary hypertension and can produce sufficient blood signal within a patent vessel to suggest thrombus (Fig. 53–7*A*). In contrast, cine MRI readily demonstrates bright flow signal even at the low flow velocities found in this setting (see Fig. 53–7*B*). Thus, use of cine MRI may be essential to avoid false-positive diagnoses due to chronic pulmonary emboli in the evaluation of surgically correctable pulmonary hypertension.

Pulmonary Hypertension

Cine MRI shows promise for evaluation of pulmonary hypertension regardless of the cause. Preliminary studies indicate that with the use of surface coils, high-quality images down to fourth-order branches can be obtained.[G2] The physical motion of pulmonary arterial branches shows arterial pulsation in a distinctive manner that permits ready differentiation from pulmonary veins. Marked dilation of central pulmonary arterial branches is readily demonstrated (see Fig. 53–7*B*). Moreover, phasic pulmonary arterial branch pulsations in both large and small branches are altered in pulmonary hypertension, with reductions in pulsatile change in lumen diameter and with altered patterns of phasic change in signal amplitude. Investigators should soon be able to complement such qualitative findings with quantitative analysis of flow velocity patterns in pulmonary arterial branches.[U1]

Pulmonary Veins

Cine MRI is likely to become the method of choice for assessment of pulmonary veins, which are readily depicted on cine images. In part, this choice reflects the inadequacy of alternative methods. Chest wall echocardiography rarely provides extensive depiction of even the pulmonary vein orifices in adults. Radionuclide methods are of little value, and angiographic contrast-based methods are often limited in obtaining pulmonary vein opacification or in correctly timing imaging for depiction of pulmonary veins. In contrast, cine MRI readily depicts both central and peripheral pulmonary veins. Their multiphasic patterns of pulsation and signal amplitude change make them readily distinguishable from pulmonary arterial branches.[G2] Moreover, alterations in physical pulsation and phasic signal amplitude changes are readily demonstrated in mitral regurgitation. Central pulmonary venous obstruction, including partial obstruction with resultant turbulent flow, is also readily demonstrated (Fig. 53–8). Addition of quantitative velocity determination to assessment of pulmonary venous pathophysiology should further enhance the utility of cine MRI in this setting.

VALVULAR HEART DISEASE

Regurgitant Lesions

Mitral Regurgitation

Application of cine magnetic resonance imaging to evaluation of mitral regurgitation began relatively early, largely because the disorder is common and the images are dramatic (Fig. 53–9).[A1, P3, S3] The general pattern of flow abnormality follows the schema outlined in the earlier section "Effects of Laminar and Turbulent Flow." Pre-orifice acceleration produces a small signal void on the left ventricular aspect of the mitral apparatus, which extends into the high-velocity jet at the regurgitant orifice and then propagates as a turbulent downstream flow volume, producing a larger signal void within the left atrium. Specificity of a signal void within the left atrium for the diagnosis of mitral regurgitation is conferred by demonstration that the signal void originates at the mitral valve plane and propagates away from the valve plane in progressive fashion.

Streams of mitral regurgitant flow are usually better demarcated on cine MRI images than on color flow Doppler images in the same patient. The shape of the signal void is often complex and multilobar, at times producing jets propagating along different planes within the left atrium. The size and shape of the jet vary, often dramatically, during the regurgitant period. Localization of the site of the regurgitant orifice is relatively easy and may be useful in patients considered for surgical mitral valvuloplasty. Visualization of multiple jets is common. Although jets are often directed at the center of the left atrium, signal void may be absent from the center of the atrium, and be found tracking along the lateral atrial wall or atrial septum to the posterior dome of the left atrium (Fig. 53–10). In this setting, pulsed Doppler imaging or even color flow Doppler imaging could underestimate severity of mitral regurgitation.

In general, however, planar analysis of cine MRI imaging of the regurgitant signal void in mitral regurgitation is closely analogous to Doppler flow mapping in its sensitivity, specificity, and quantitation.[P3] Our own studies have compared cine MRI to pulsed Doppler flow mapping in 30 subjects and to color flow mapping in 20 subjects.[A1] Sensitivity and specificity were 94 and 100 percent, respectively, with Doppler flow mapping used as a reference standard. As with pulsed or color flow Doppler imaging, a useful rough guide to the severity of mitral regurgitation using cine MRI is the absolute or relative size of the signal void. Despite differences in imaging plane and the physical basis of imaging, the ratio of mitral regurgitant jet area (JA) to left atrial

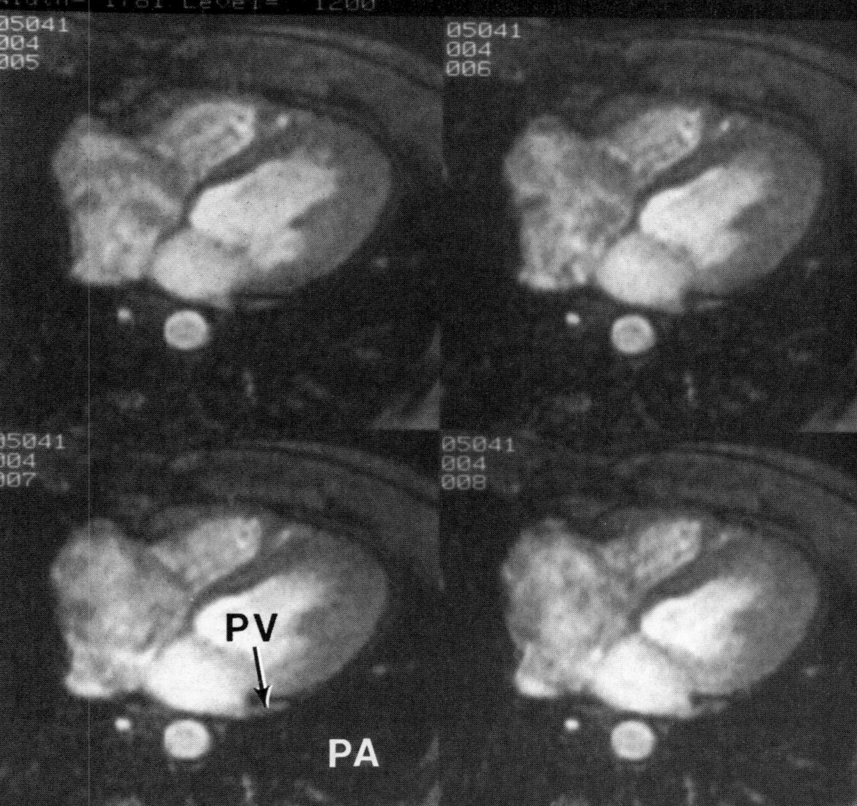

Figure 53–6. Serial axial images in a normal volunteer show a central pulmonary vein (PV) and peripheral pulmonary artery branches (PA). With dynamic cine-loop display, contrasting patterns of motion and signal variation in pulmonary arteries and veins facilitate identification.

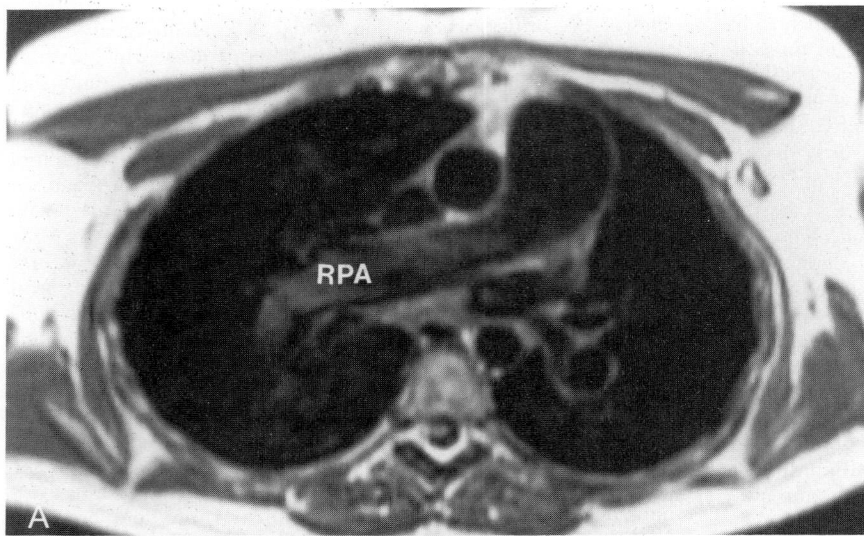

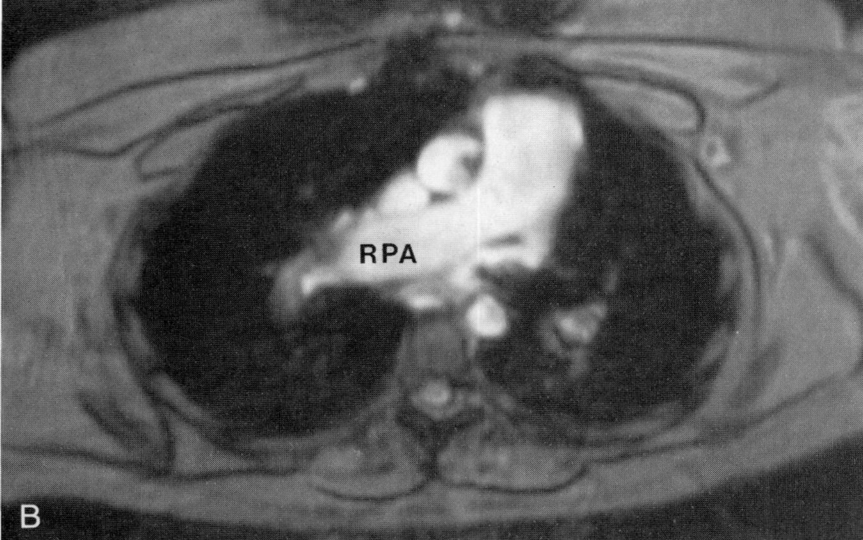

Figure 53–7. *A*, Axial spin-echo image at the great-vessel level in a patient with primary pulmonary hypertension. There is marked dilation of the right pulmonary artery (RPA), in which intravascular signal due to slow flow is seen. (Courtesy of Dr. Warren Gefter.) *B*, Cine image of the same patient. Bright signal in right pulmonary artery (RPA) despite slow flow demonstrates that no thrombus is present. (Courtesy of Dr. Warren Gefter).

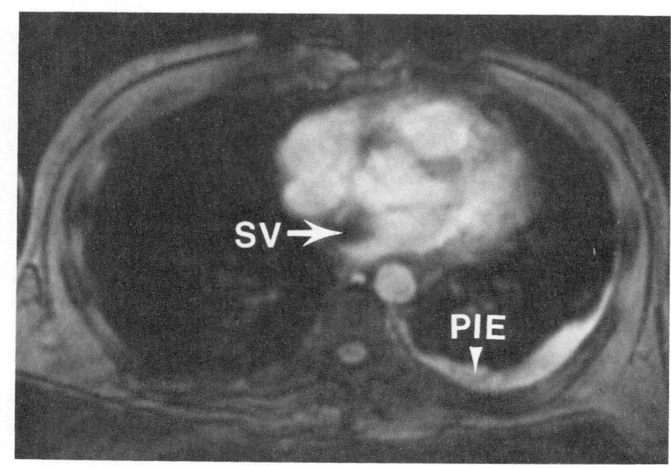

Figure 53–8. Axial image in a patient with fibrosing mediastinitis. A large signal void (SV) is seen in the left atrium as a result of partial obstruction of the right superior pulmonary vein, which causes turbulent flow into the left atrium. A left pleural effusion (Pl. E) is also present.

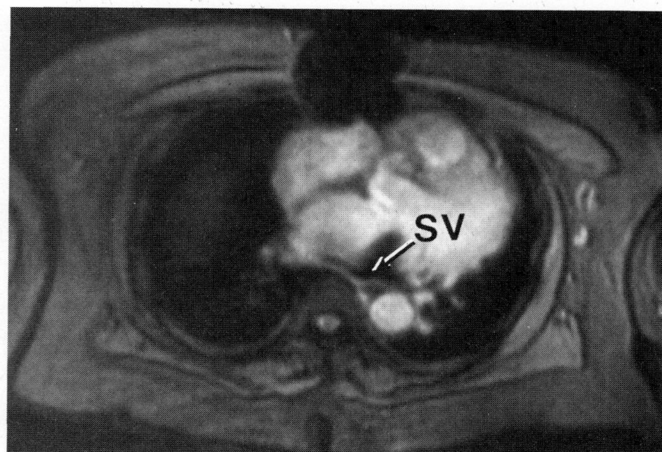

Figure 53–9. Large signal void (SV) in left atrium in systole results from mitral regurgitation. Connection to the valve plane does not appear in this section. The signal void diverges as it extends toward the posterior left atrium. The large signal void appearing anteriorly in the chest wall is an artifact due to sternal wire sutures from a prior median sternotomy.

area (LA) by cine MRI correlates well with pulsed and color flow Doppler imaging results, and semiquantitative grading of severity as proposed by Helmcke and colleagues (JA/LA < 20% = mild; 20 to 40% = moderate; > 40% = severe) is also comparable.[H1]

A second approach to quantitation of mitral regurgitation using cine MRI may be planimetric determination of right and left ventricular stroke volume, in which all slices obtainable through right and left ventricles are used.[A1] Although this method is time-consuming, the resultant stroke-volume ratio and stroke-volume difference appear to be useful measures of severity of regurgitation. This approach has not been evaluated as rigorously for cine MRI, however, as it has been for cine CT, which has been shown to provide extremely precise estimates of right and left ventricular stroke volumes and regurgitant fraction.[R2] Cine MRI evaluation of mitral regurgitation by both flow mapping and stroke volume quantitation requires further validation studies using quantitative "gold standards" such as cine CT.

Other consequences of mitral regurgitation that are readily demonstrated using cine MRI include changes in left atrial and ventricular size. If desired, volumetric determinations of chamber size and left ventricular ejection fraction can be made. The method also depicts altered pulmonary venous pulsations (see the previous section, "Pulmonary Veins"), right heart remodeling due to pulmonary hypertension, and increased left ventricular inflow velocities, which results in a diastolic transmitral signal void. While cine MRI is an excellent method for localization of the regurgitant orifice, it is generally less useful than echocardiography for evaluation of valvular morphology and motion. An exception is the demonstration of valvular calcification. Because calcified tissue produces no signal, calcium stands out sharply as a signal void that is associated with the valve plane and that persists throughout the cardiac cycle and generally has limited mobility. Mitral annular calcification is also readily demonstrated.

When one considers only planar imaging results, cine MRI imaging in mitral regurgitation appears to offer limited advantages over alternative imaging approaches. A unique potential of cine MRI imaging of valvular dysfunction, however, is three-dimensional display and analysis of the results.[C2, R1] This approach has not yet been applied to mitral regurgitation, but initial results in aortic valve disease indicate that it may have considerable value, permitting volumetric assessment of the flow disturbance, as well as depiction and quantitation of the regurgitant valve orifice (see the following section). Nonetheless, at this writing, the ultimate clinical role of cine MRI for evaluation of valvular regurgitation remains to be defined.

Aortic Regurgitation

In aortic regurgitation, cine MRI is an excellent method for qualitative recognition and a promising method for quantitation of severity. Several approaches are used. The diastolic flow disturbance in aortic regurgitation results in a signal void, which begins above the aortic valve plane in the zone of pre-orifice acceleration. The signal void continues through the high-velocity jet within the regurgitant orifice and then propagates more widely within the left ventricle (Fig. 53–11). In systole, a large stroke volume, ejected rapidly, commonly results in an exaggerated ejection signal void that propagates up the aorta in rough proportion to the severity of the volume load. Specificity of diagnosis depends on demonstration of the combination of appropriate diastolic timing of appearance of the regurgitant signal void, connection of the signal void region within the left ventricle to the aortic valve plane, and serial propagation of the signal void from the valve plane. If these features are not demonstrated, one may mistake a diastolic signal void due to turbulent mitral inflow in mitral regurgitation or mitral stenosis, or both, for aortic regurgitation.

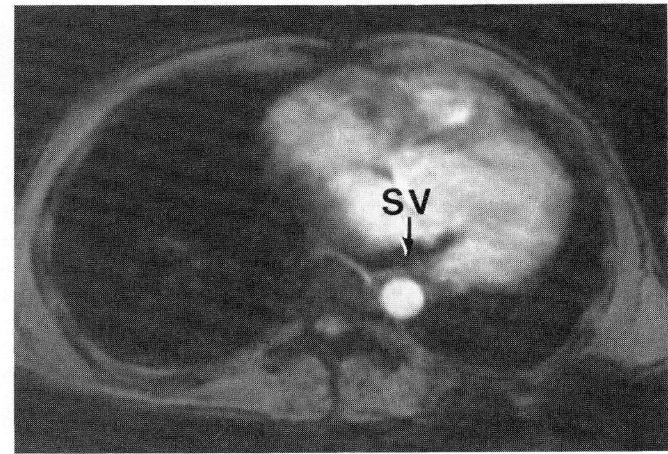

Figure 53–10. Axial systolic image in a patient with mitral regurgitation shows a signal void (SV) originating in the left ventricle, crossing the valve plane at its narrowest point, and tracking laterally and posteriorly along the left atrial wall before expanding into a broader grayer zone that reaches the interatrial septum.

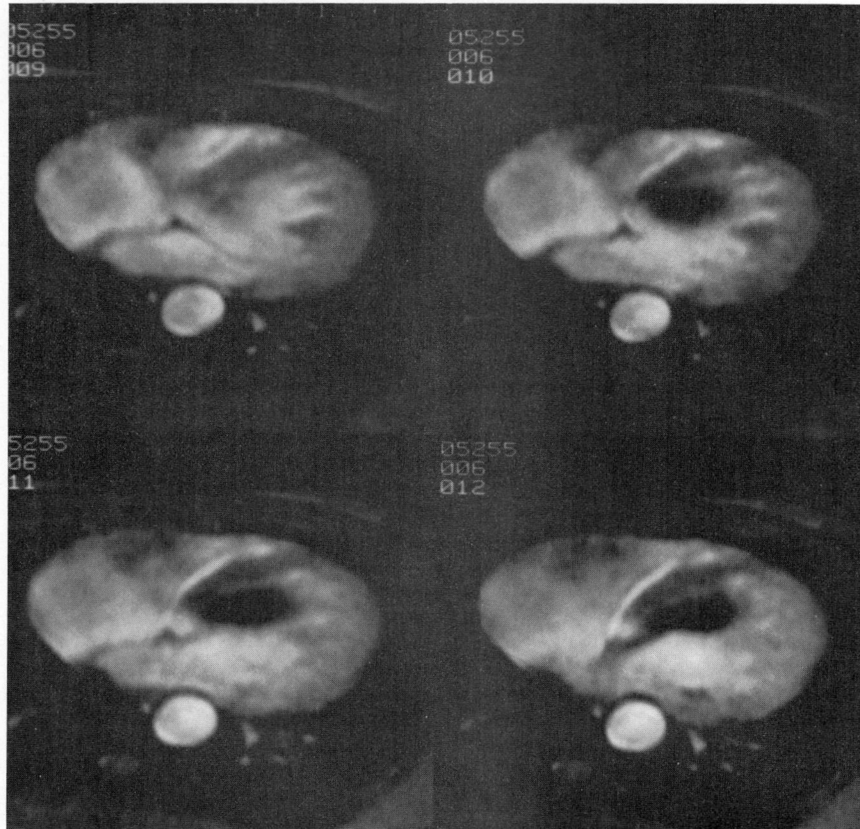

Figure 53–11. Serial diastolic images in a patient with aortic regurgitation show a large signal void of elliptic shape in the left ventricular outflow tract at a level just below the aortic valve. The signal void expands as it extends into the left ventricle.

Within the left ventricle, the signal void of aortic regurgitation typically has a complex, multilobar, time-varying shape, so that no single imaging plane or image at a single point in diastole is representative of the whole. Multiple jets emanating from the valve plane are common. Turbulent flow tends to track along the left ventricular surface of the anterior mitral leaflet or the left side of the interventricular septum, or along both. In a study of 50 subjects, we have found that cine MRI sensitivity and specificity are both 95 percent or greater if color flow or pulsed Doppler echocardiography is used as a reference standard. Similarly, results of semiquantitative or quantitative estimation of severity based on the area of the signal void are comparable to Doppler mapping. Pflugfelder and co-workers studied 25 patients with aortic regurgitation and 10 normal individuals, and they found that cine MRI was 100 percent sensitive in comparison with Doppler echocardiography.[P1] They were readily able to distinguish mild, moderate, and severe aortic regurgitation by determining the area of the regurgitant signal void.

As is generally true in valvular disease, cine MRI is likely to demonstrate the shape and size of the turbulent flow region in a given patient more clearly than color flow Doppler imaging. Thus, the width of the aortic regurgitation jet near the valve plane, which has been suggested as a more reliable index of severity with color flow Doppler imaging, is more readily determined by cine MRI than by Doppler imaging in many patients. With correct oblique orientation of the image plane, even direct imaging of the regurgitant orifice is possible (Fig. 53–12).

The value of cine MRI for assessment of the diastolic signal void of aortic regurgitation can be enhanced by imaging all slices through the region of interest. This method permits volumetric assessment of the flow disturbance region. In addition, using advanced computer graphic methods one can create a three-dimensional surface display of the signal-void region and evaluate its dynamic change in volume and shape throughout the cardiac cycle from any perspective of interest (Fig. 53–13).[C2, R1] Furthermore, the actual gray-scale image volume can be resectioned to depict the regurgitant valve orifice, even if that orifice lies oblique to the original imaging plane (Fig. 53–14). Early work suggests close relationships between the cine MRI size of the regurgitant orifice, the size of the regurgitant flow signal void volume, and other measures of severity of aortic regurgitation.

In addition to appraisal of the diastolic flow disturbance in aortic regurgitation, cine MRI can provide other qualitative and quantitative information of value. Alterations in left ventricular size and function can be evaluated volumetrically.[B1] Estimates of regurgitant volume and fraction can be derived from volumetric analysis of right and left ventricle, and as described by Pflugfelder and co-workers, they can readily distinguish mild, moderate, and severe aortic regurgitation.[P1] These investigators found that cine MRI regurgitant fraction was 4 ± 7 percent for normal individuals, 31 ± 8 percent in mild aortic regurgitations, 45 ± 11 percent in moderate aortic regurgitation, and and 56 ± 9 percent in severe aortic regurgitation.

Phasic analysis of systolic forward and diastolic retrograde aortic root flow using cine MRI should also be feasible.[U2] Aortic root disease is readily depicted. Although aortic valve leaflets are not ordinarily well visualized, a bicuspid aortic valve can be delineated by the shape of the signal void at the valve plane. Because calcified tissue does not generate signal, aortic valve calcifications appear as signal voids at the valve plane that persist throughout the cardiac cycle and typically show little motion. Using thin sections through the valve plane, one usually can easily distinguish these from the signal voids produced by turbulent systolic or diastolic flow.

Tricuspid Regurgitation

Cine MRI manifestations of tricuspid regurgitation are closely analogous to those found in mitral regurgitation (see earlier discussion). A signal void initiated in the pre-orifice zone of acceleration extends through the high-velocity jet and propagates in the region of turbulence in the right atrium (Fig. 53–15). With cine MRI, mild tricuspid regurgitation is commonly demonstrated in normal individuals, as is true with Doppler methods. No definitive data are available, but sensitivity, specificity, and

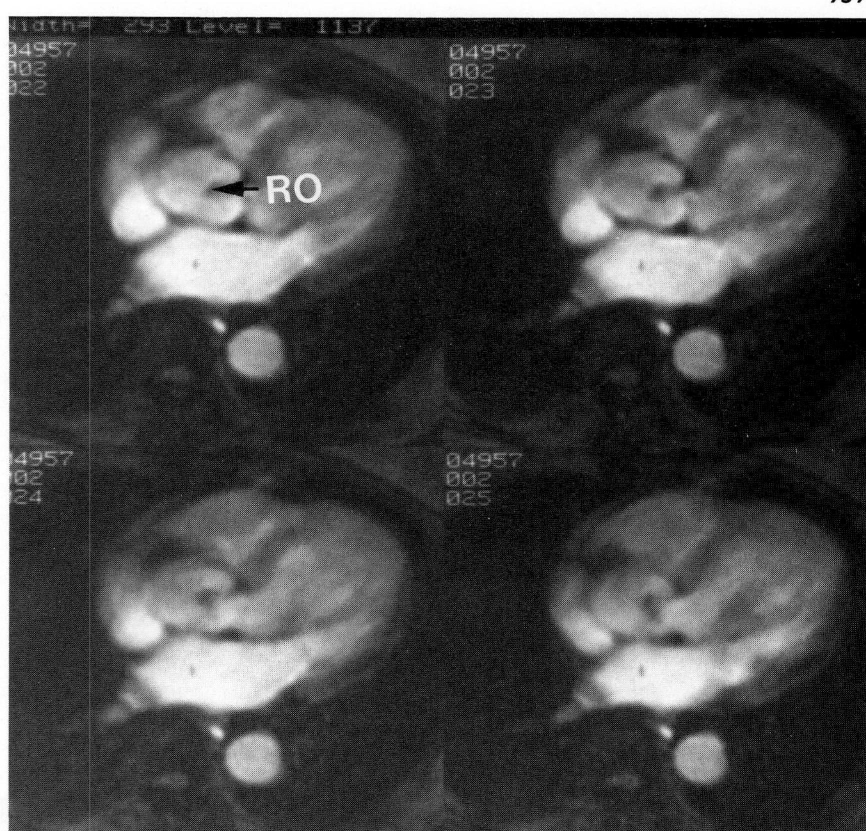

Figure 53–12. Diastolic images in a patient with aortic regurgitation. A section at the valve plane is shown, and a small central signal void within the aorta depicts the regurgitant orifice (RO).

quantitation by Doppler and by cine MRI are likely to be similar for tricuspid regurgitation, as is true for mitral and aortic regurgitation. Rarely, cine MRI demonstrates that tricuspid regurgitation is severe when it appears to be milder by Doppler methods. This situation can occur if jet direction results in the bulk of the signal void being found in a plane that cannot be accessed from the chest wall by Doppler methods (Fig. 53-16).

Pulmonic Regurgitation

Pulmonic regurgitation results in a diastolic signal void within the right ventricular outflow tract (Fig. 53–17). A small signal void due to pulmonic regurgitation is found in many normal individuals, which is analogous to Doppler findings.

Stenotic Lesions

The utility of cine MRI for assessment of stenotic valve lesions has been less widely explored than for assessment of regurgitant lesions. As in regurgitation, a signal void begins in the zone of acceleration of flow proximal to the valve orifice, extends through the high-velocity orifice jet, and propagates as a larger zone of turbulent flow downstream of the valve orifice. Because stenotic

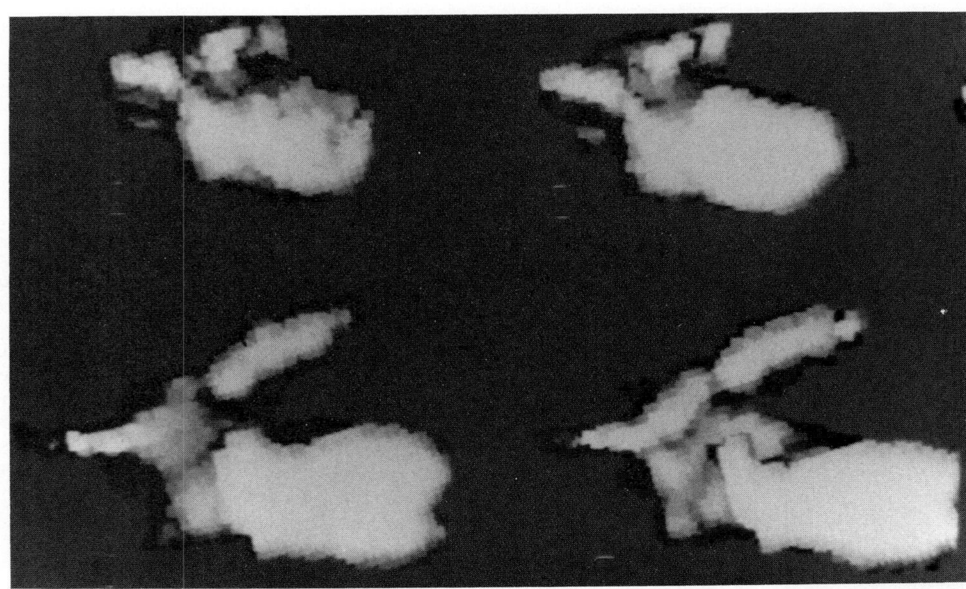

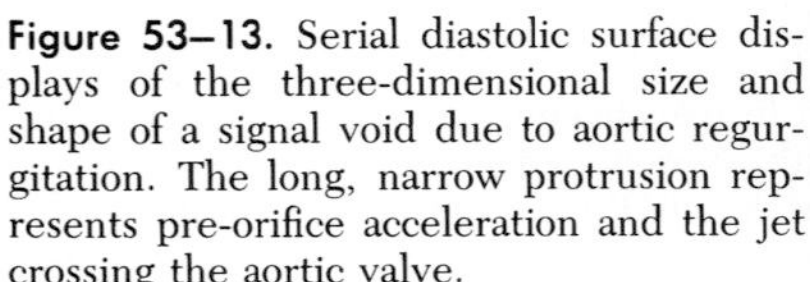

Figure 53–13. Serial diastolic surface displays of the three-dimensional size and shape of a signal void due to aortic regurgitation. The long, narrow protrusion represents pre-orifice acceleration and the jet crossing the aortic valve.

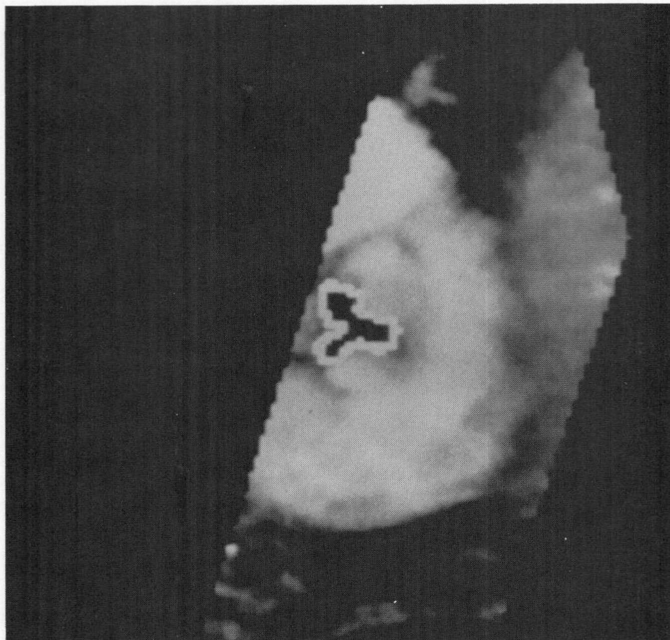

Figure 53–14. The gray-scale volume of the signal void due to aortic regurgitation has been resectioned at the valve plane to depict the valve orifice.

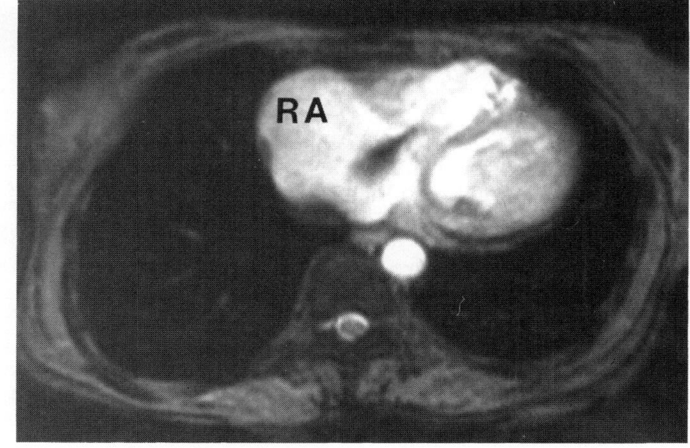

Figure 53–15. Systolic image showing a dilated right atrium (RA) in a patient with rheumatic valvular disease. A signal void due to tricuspid regurgitation diverges after crossing the tricuspid valve plane.

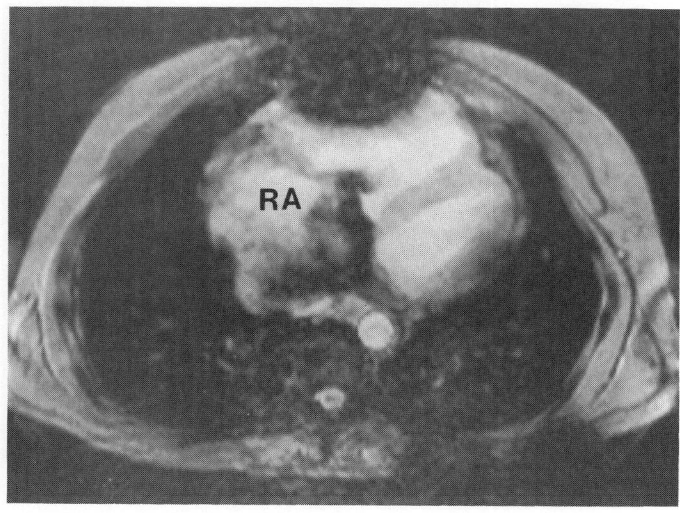

Figure 53–16. Axial systolic image obtained through the inferior right atrium (RA) in a patient with a prior median sternotomy for repair of tetralogy of Fallot, which has resulted in a large signal void in the chest wall due to sternal wire sutures. In the right atrium, one can see a large signal void due to severe tricuspid regurgitation; the signal void runs posteromedially toward the interatrial septum. Color-flow Doppler echocardiography could not access the site of the bulk of the signal void, so that the severity was mistakenly judged to be mild. Angiographic and hemodynamic confirmation of severe tricuspid regurgitation was obtained.

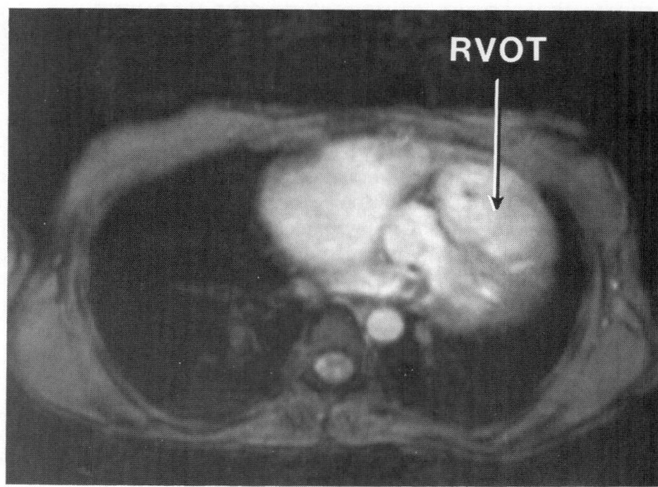

Figure 53–17. Diastolic frame through dilated right atrium and right ventricular outflow tract (RVOT) in a patient with primary pulmonary hypertension shows a small signal void in the RVOT produced by mild pulmonic regurgitation. Similar findings are often obtained in normal individuals.

valves in adults often calcify, and calcified material produces no signal on cine MRI, distinction between valvular calcification and signal void due to flow is an important consideration. Persistence of the signal void due to calcification throughout the cardiac cycle, combined with the general immobility of most calcified valves, permits such differentiation.

Aortic Stenosis

Aortic stenosis has several principal features that permit qualitative recognition with cine MRI. The presence of a pre-orifice acceleration signal void that is more prominent than the normal ejection signal void, a large signal void in the ascending aorta (Fig. 53–18), and persistent signal voids due to calcification within the valve leaflets are common. In general, the length of the signal void within the thoracic aorta indicates severity if cardiac output is normal; however, data have not been obtained to support quantitative use of this finding. Ancillary findings such as severity of left ventricular hypertrophy and assessment of left ventricular size and performance may all be useful in the individual patient with aortic stenosis.

Visualization of the stenotic valve orifice with cine MRI is feasible, but suitable methods are in an early stage of development. An important problem in imaging the aortic valve orifice in aortic stenosis is the complex variation encountered in the spatial orientation of the orifice. Thus, specification of the appropriate imaging plane is usually impossible without extensive trial-and-error imaging runs.

An attractive alternative approach involves use of advanced three-dimensional graphics software, such as the Mayo Clinic's Analyze package,[R3] to stack consecutive slices taken at a single point in systole into a three-dimensional gray-scale volume. The volume can then be resliced in varying planes until the valve orifice is found. The orifice itself forms a narrow waist connecting the pre-acceleration signal void and the turbulent flow region signal void, so that the minimal cross-sectional area at the valve plane provides a good working estimate of the valve orifice. Preliminary experience with this approach suggests that it provides valve orifice area values that closely approximate those obtained with invasive hemodynamic assessment.[R1] High spatial resolution—an uninterpolated pixel size of 1.8 × 0.9 mm and slice thicknesses of 3 mm or less is currently available—is a requirement for obtaining optimal results with this approach. Further technologic enhancements, particularly in gradient amplifiers, should permit thinner slices and smaller pixel sizes.

Distinguishing the jet through the orifice from calcification of the valve leaflets is essential. The persistence of calcific signal voids throughout the cardiac cycle and their immobility are helpful. In general, one can steer the image plane to a point just above the leaflet calcifications where only the cross section of the jet is displayed.

The ultimate role of cine MRI in assessment of aortic stenosis is far from clear. In particular, the excellent results often obtained with Doppler echocardiography may limit the impact of cine MRI. Doppler estimates of aortic valve area are critically dependent, however, on the quality of both Doppler velocimetric recordings of the aortic stenosis jet and the left ventricular outflow tract velocities during ejection, as well as on the quality of images of the left ventricular outflow tract. Thus, one commonly encounters patients in whom either technically satisfactory velocity recordings or good estimates of the cross-sectional area of the outflow tract cannot be obtained. In such settings, cine MRI aortic valve area could play an important role.

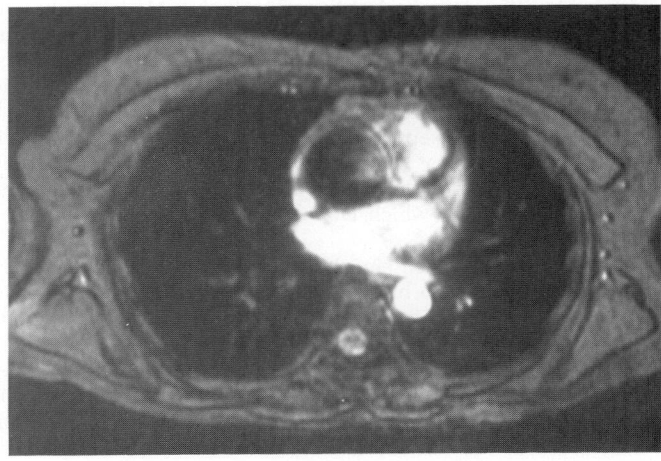

Figure 53–18. Axial systolic image in a patient with severe aortic stenosis shows a large signal void in the aortic root.

Mitral Stenosis

In mitral stenosis, cine MRI can feasibly depict the turbulent flow into the left ventricle, the calcified valve leaflets, the abnormal leaflet motion, and the stenotic orifice, as well as any coexistent mitral regurgitation or other valvular disorder. Chamber size estimates for all four cardiac chambers can also be readily performed. Limited experience suggests that recognition of left atrial thrombus, an area of limited sensitivity for chest-wall echocardiography, may be performed more satisfactorily with cine MRI used in conjunction with spin-echo MRI. In particular, the atrial appendage is readily visualized; such visualization with echocardiography is usually not possible in adults. Nonetheless, the superb results ordinarily obtained with echocardiographic and Doppler techniques in mitral stenosis limit the need to apply cine MRI to this problem. In addition, the frequent occurrence of atrial fibrillation in this patient population requires use of "instant" MRI gradient-echo imaging rather than the retrospectively gated cine technique currently in widespread use.

Tricuspid Stenosis

Although experience is quite limited, cine MRI readily demonstrates the qualitative effects of tricuspid stenosis, and three-dimensional image analysis to depict the valve orifice should be quite feasible. In tricuspid stenosis, echocardiography has not fully met the need for quantitation of severity. Pressure gradients are relatively small, even with severe stenosis; thus, Doppler gradient estimation has more pitfalls. Moreover, velocity half-time estimation of valve area is not well validated, and direct imaging of the valve orifice is usually not feasible with echocardiography. Cine MRI may therefore have appreciable impact.

In summary, cine MRI shows promise for assessment of both flow disturbance regions and quantitation of flow and cardiac chamber volumes in many types of valvular heart disease. In a variety of settings, it may uniquely provide three-dimensional depiction of the flow disturbance and reconstructed planar depiction of the valve orifice. Work with the method is at an early stage, however. Rigorous quantitative validation of most applications has not been completed. Until such data are available, justification of the routine use of cine MRI for evaluation of patients with valvular heart disease will be difficult, because planar depiction is, in most instances, readily performed with far simpler, cheaper Doppler echocardiographic techniques.

CONGENITAL HEART DISEASE

The flexibility of imaging planes available with MRI, and the possibility of imaging the entire mediastinum and great vessels comprehensively, promise to make MRI a valuable technique for evaluation of congenital heart disease. At present, however, optimal morphologic detail for anatomic diagnosis is usually obtained with spin-echo imaging. Thus, cine MRI usually plays an adjunctive role, clarifying the location and severity of intracardiac flow disturbances. As it does for acquired heart disease, cine MRI excels in depicting valvular regurgitation, obstruction to antegrade flow, and turbulent flow of any cause, as may be seen in left-to-right septal defects. Given the ease of applicability of color flow Doppler imaging in young patients with congenital heart disease, cine MRI can contribute unique information mainly in circumstances for which Doppler methods are inapplicable or unsuccessful.

One setting in which cine MRI excels is the demonstration of sites of obstruction to blood flow in the cardiac chambers or the great vessels, including the central pulmonary and systemic veins. On the right side, obstruction to pulmonary flow at levels ranging from the inlet of the infundibulum to the pulmonary artery branches is readily demonstrated (Fig. 53–19). When pulmonic atresia has interrupted antegrade flow, the combination of spin-echo and cine MRI has unique capabilities for evaluating the size of branch pulmonary arteries and their sources of flow. On the left side, subvalvular aortic stenosis, valvular and supravalvular stenosis, and aortic coarctation are readily demonstrated.[S4]

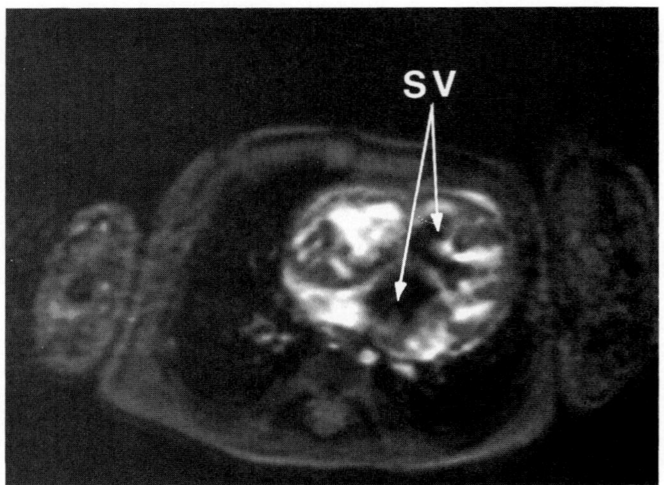

Figure 53–19. Systolic image in an infant with single ventricle, infundibular pulmonic stenosis, and mitral regurgitation shows a posterior signal void (SV) due to atrioventricular valve regurgitation and an anterior signal void due to acceleration of flow proximal to the narrowest portion of the infundibulum.

In patients with uncomplicated left-to-right central shunts, cine MRI may be helpful in shunt quantitation, using either right and left ventricular stroke-volume ratios or phase velocity mapping.[C3] In one preliminary report, nine normal individuals and five patients with left-to-right shunts were studied with a phase velocity method. Normal individuals had values ranging from 0.86 to 1.08, and aortic and pulmonary flow were well correlated ($r = 0.91$), whereas in the shunt patients, the MRI estimate of the pulmonary-to-systemic flow ratio (Qp/Qs) correlated with invasive or radionuclide first-pass measurements ($r = 0.96$, SEE = 0.2, range = 0.95 to 2.3)[C3] Similarly, shunt fractions in atrial septal defect in 12 patients, obtained by comparison of right and left ventricular stroke volumes by ventricular planimetry, correlated well with invasive data ($r = 0.98$).[S5] Furthermore, preliminary results suggest the possibility of actually depicting the cross-sectional area of ventricular septal defects with suitably oriented oblique image planes.[S6] Cine MRI should also prove useful in demonstrating multiple ventricular septal defects.

An area in which cine MRI may be particularly helpful is assessment of intracardiac repairs in which prosthetic material has been used, particularly in the form of conduits. In that setting, neither angiographic evaluation nor color flow echocardiography may provide clear depiction of flow dynamics. Similarly, slow flow can produce sufficient blood signal on spin-echo MRI to render interpretation difficult. In this setting, Chung and associates have described excellent results, with angiographic confirmation, in 14 patients.[C4] Cine MRI can be the most effective way to demonstrate patency and obstruction to flow, because most prosthetic materials do not preclude satisfactory imaging with the technique. Initial studies in patients with pulmonary artery bands, for example, suggest that the severity of obstruction to flow can be determined both from measurement of the diameter of the stream and from measurement of the size of the preband region of acceleration of flow.[S7] Obstruction to venous return, either systemic or pulmonary, in patients who have undergone prior surgery is another area in which cine MRI appears to excel.

Application of cine MRI to congenital heart disease is in an early phase. Thus, many more applications are likely to be described in the near future.

CORONARY ARTERY DISEASE

Current applications of cine MRI to coronary artery disease include assessment of segmental myocardial dysfunction; assessment of complications of myocardial infarction, including left ventricular thrombus, mitral regurgitation, and ventricular septal defect; and evaluation of coronary bypass grafts.

Evaluation of Segmental Myocardial Function

Cine MRI appears to be an effective method for assessment of segmental myocardial function (Fig. 53–20).[P4] The optimal approach involves obtaining all short-axis slices through the left ventricle. Both endocardial excursion and segmental wall thickening can be evaluated. As is true in echocardiography, wall thickening is likely to prove to be a more sensitive index of segmental function than endocardial excursion.

In an initial study of 13 normal subjects and 15 patients with ischemic heart disease, Pflugfelder and colleagues demonstrated normal regional heterogeneity of wall thickening in normal subjects and detected abormal wall motion in patients. Their results correlated well with results of contrast ventriculography and echocardiography for recognition of normal, hypokinetic, akinetic, and dyskinetic segments.[P1] Similarly, Meese and associates studied 15 patients and compared cine MRI with biplane angiography. They found that angiography and cine MRI showed 85 percent concordance in identifying regional wall motion abnormalities and strong agreement for global ejection fraction ($r = 0.86$).[M1] In addition, in myocardial segments showing reduced regional ejection fraction on contrast ventriculography in 10 patients, Chow and associates found significant reductions in short-axis cine MRI endocardial radius change and wall thickening in systole.[C5] Clearly, larger validation studies with better reference methods are required to complete validation of this promising approach.

A second approach that has been shown to be effective is the use of orthogonal long-axis planes to depict a single section each through the anterior and inferior walls, the septum, and the lateral wall, respectively. Preliminary reports suggest that results obtained from this approach compare favorably with those obtained from biplane angiography. Thus, Lotan and colleagues compared cine MRI two-chamber (or "RAO equivalent") and four-chamber (or "LAO equivalent") views with those from invasive contrast ventriculography in 43 patients. They found cine MRI to be 93 percent sensitive and 87 percent specific in comparison with ventriculography in which a 5-segment point score system was used, with differences of more than one grade occurring in only 13 of 318 segments.[L1] Similarly, Askenase and associates have described promising preliminary results, with validation by sonomicrometry, in an experimental model of acute infarction, using three orthogonal image planes.[A3]

Considerable further experience is required to determine the relative value of cine MRI for evaluation of segmental myocardial function, particularly in light of recently developed methods for "tagging" the myocardium using modified spin-echo techniques.[A4] Similar "tagging" is feasible using gradient-echo methods. Like all quantitative methods using cine MRI, analysis of segmental wall motion is limited by the large numbers of images generated and the dependence on operator segmentation of each image into left ventricular cavity and myocardium. Development of effective automated methods for such tasks depends both on substantial improvement in the consistency of myocardial signal on cine images and on creative new approaches to computerized image analysis, which are likely to include the use of expert systems.

Coronary Bypass Graft Imaging

Current cine MRI implementations are inadequate for morphologic evaluation of the native coronary circulation, although approaches to evaluation of coronary flow have been described (see the later section "Flow Quantitation").[U2] Several major advances in cardiac gated gradient-echo methodology are required to permit noninvasive coronary artery imaging with the use of this approach. First, any tomographic imaging approach is unlikely to be effective given the complex geometry of the coronary arterial tree. Cine-like MRI gradient-echo projection angiographic methods have been developed and applied successfully outside the thorax,[D1] but successful strategies managing both cardiac gating and respiratory motion during angiographic acqui-

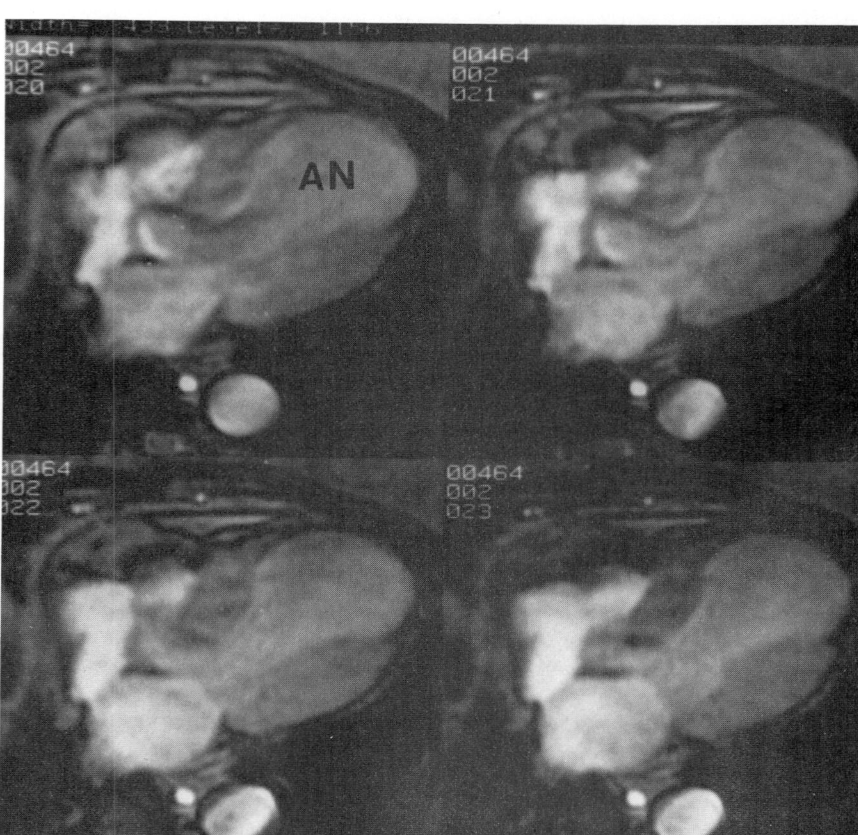

Figure 53–20. Serial systolic images of a thin-walled apical left ventricular aneurysm (AN) in a patient with underlying left ventricular hypertrophy.

sitions are required. Furthermore, practical pixel sizes would need to be reduced from the current 1.8 mm^2 by a factor of at least 10. Given the rate of recent progress in cardiac MRI imaging techniques, further progress can be anticipated in this area, but success in coronary imaging is likely to come slowly.

Even at present, however, cine MRI is an effective method for noninvasive imaging of coronary bypass grafts.[A5, W1] A successful approach involves imaging of an entire volume of the thorax, encompassing most of the length of the graft, from near its aortic insertion to the epicardial surface of the heart, near the receiving vessel. Such imaging can typically be achieved with three interleaved acquisitions, each of three 1-cm-thick slices spaced 2 cm apart. Imaging time for such a study, using one signal average, ranges from 22 to 35 minutes. Bypass grafts are depicted as vascular channels showing bright signal (Fig. 53–21 and 53–22) that do not correspond in course and location to normal vessels.

Cine-loop review of all contiguous slices is often required to make correct determination of graft patency. Signal-void artifacts are produced by sternal wire sutures and by graft clips. Unless vascular clips have been placed all along the course of a graft, however, adequate images for diagnosis are readily obtained. Internal mammary artery grafts are visualized as well as saphenous vein bypass grafts. Occluded grafts show no flow signal whatsoever, because they usually thrombose proximally. Stenotic grafts and grafts to stenotic receiving vessels show flow signal that is qualitatively similar to that found in normal grafts to normal receiving vessels. Application of phase velocity methods to bypass grafts, however, should permit functional appraisal of graft flow and flow reserve.[U2]

Although published studies of series of cases are small, the sensitivity and specificity of cine MRI for graft patency have both exceeded 90 percent.[A5, W1] In our own blinded study of 22 patients with 49 grafts (of which 35 were patent), we found a sensitivity of 89 percent and specificity of 100 percent.[A5] All false-negative results occurred in the first seven subjects studied before the imaging protocol was optimized. Similarly, White and colleagues, in a study of 28 grafts in 10 patients, found a sensitivity of 93 percent, a specificity of 86 percent, and an overall predictive accuracy of 89 percent.[W1] The method has several potential advantages in comparison with other noninvasive methods. Unlike spin-echo MRI, it produces positive flow signal and appears to be relatively free of false-positive results.[F2, R4]

Moreover, quantitation of flow and flow reserve is feasible. As compared with ultrafast roentgen CT or cine CT, cine MRI requires neither radiation nor contrast injection, and it appears to have comparable sensitivity and specificity.[S8]

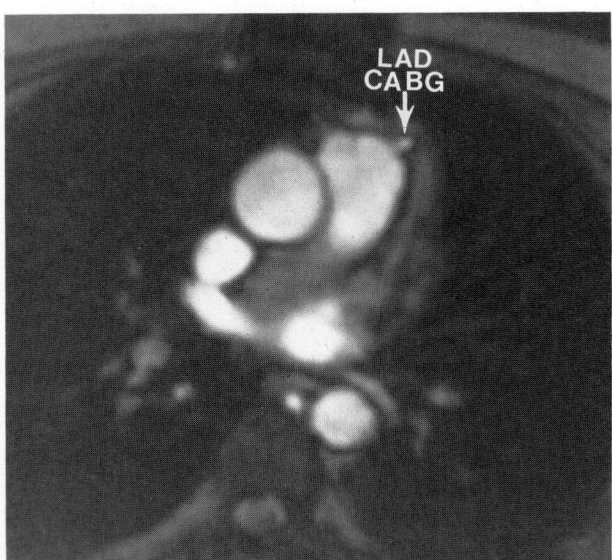

Figure 53–21. A saphenous vein graft (LAD CABG) is draped over the pulmonary artery en route to the left anterior descending coronary artery. (From Aurigemma, G. P., Reichek, N., Axel, L., et al.: Noninvasive determination of coronary artery bypass graft patency by cine magnetic resonance imaging. Circulation 80:1595, 1989. Reprinted by permission of the American Heart Association.)

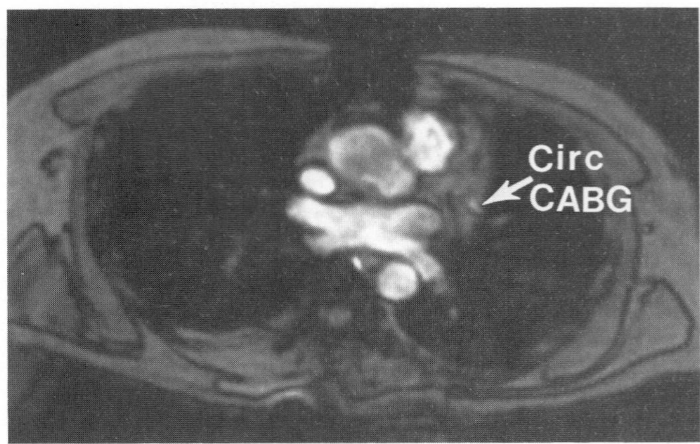

Figure 53–22. A saphenous vein graft abutting the left atrial appendage is imaged en route to the circumflex coronary artery bypass graft (Circ. CABG). (From Aurigemma, G. P., Reichek, N., Axel, L., et al.: Noninvasive determination of coronary artery bypass graft patency by cine magnetic imaging. Circulation 80:1595, 1989. Reprinted by permission of the American Heart Association.)

INTRACARDIAC MASSES

Cardiac MRI lends itself to assessment of intracardiac masses (Fig. 53–23). Spin-echo imaging alone is often sufficient for diagnosis. Cine MRI has important additive value, however, when a mass lesion shows dynamic motion, or when abnormal flow patterns in conjunction with a mass lesion require evaluation. Soft tissue masses within the blood pool are depicted as lower signal-filling defects within the bright flow signal. In patients with mobile tumors, such as atrial myxoma, either left atrial, right atrial, or biatrial motion of the tumor delineated by dynamic imaging helps to clarify its point of attachment to the heart and the presence and severity of atrioventricular valve obstruction or regurgitation. When echocardiographic images are technically of good quality, the use of cine MRI may be redundant; however,

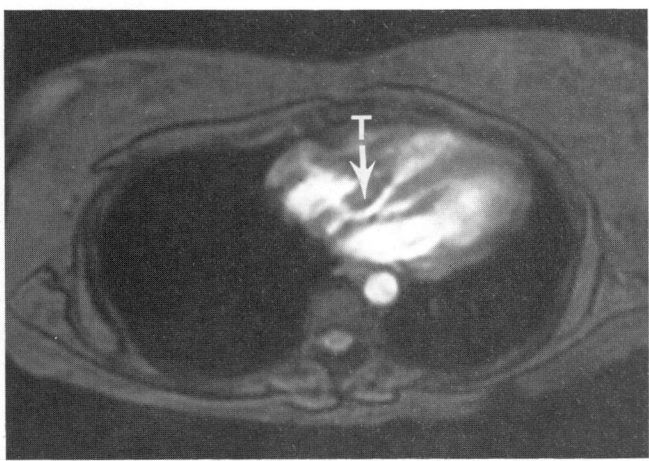

Figure 53–23. Mobile thrombus (T) in tricuspid valve orifice in diastole in a patient with a coagulopathy due to a lupus anticoagulant. The thrombus was multilobed and had formed on Chiari's network, a normal filamentous network found within the right atrium.

chest-wall echo may be technically limited in such patients. In addition, the ability to depict multiple contiguous slices with cine MRI can clarify size, shape, and motion of such masses even when echocardiography is of good quality. Moreover, in adults, mass lesions in the central systemic or pulmonary veins are difficult to demonstrate with echo Doppler techniques but are readily evaluated with cine MRI.

In patients with intracardiac thrombus, cine MRI is of particular value when slow blood flow results in increased intracavitary blood signal in the region of the suspected thrombus. Such an occurrence is likely in patients with apical left ventricular aneurysm or infarction with suspected apical thrombus. In this setting, spin-echo images may not definitively demonstrate presence or absence of thrombus, even when multiple echo times are used. Cine MRI continues to show bright signal in slowly moving blood, however, and a thrombus, if present, has lower signal intensity and is seen as a filling defect.

FLOW QUANTITATION

Gradient-echo techniques like cine MRI capture phase information that can be used to depict both qualitative direction and absolute velocity of flow.[U2] Velocity information can be obtained along all three spatial axes and can be used to depict velocity profiles within vessels and to calculate volume flow within a vessel.[F3, U2] These applications are at an early stage, but the method compares favorably with conventional invasive methods for determination of cardiac output and left-to-right shunt flow in atrial septal defect. Changes in velocity in coronary arteries downstream of a stenosis have been demonstrated. Wider availability of software for these applications may greatly expand the utility of cine MRI.

FUTURE DIRECTIONS

Cine MRI is a young technique undergoing rapid development. The coming years are likely to bring many further enhancements of the utility of the method. Ultrafast imaging,[S9] reduced flow artifacts, smaller pixel sizes, shorter repetition and echo times resulting in improved signal-to-noise and signal acquisition at higher velocities, as well as viable strategies for intrathoracic projection angiography gated to cardiac and respiratory motion are all likely to result. When combined with continuing advances in computer hardware and software for three-dimensional depiction and analysis of cardiac structure and flow, such advances are likely to make cine MRI a major cardiac imaging method in the coming decade.

References

A

1. Aurigemma, G., Reichek, N., Schiebler, M., and Axel, L.: Evaluation of mitral regurgitation by cine magnetic resonance imaging. Am. J. Cardiol. (in press) 1990.
2. Aurigemma, G., Reichek, N., Schiebler, M., et al.: Evaluation of aortic regurgitation by cine magnetic resonance imaging. J. Am. Coll. Cardiol. 11(Suppl. A):155A, 1988.
3. Askenase, A. D., Chen, G., Heo, J., et al.: Cine MRI evaluation of regional asynergy after experimental coronary occlusion. Am. J. Cardiac Imag. 3:2, 1989.
4. Axel, L., and Dougherty, L.: MR imaging of motion with spatial modulation of magnetization. Radiology 171:841, 1989.
5. Aurigemma, G. P., Reichek, N., Axel, L., et al.: Noninvasive determination of coronary artery bypass graft patency by cine magnetic resonance imaging. Circulation 80:1595, 1989.

B

1. Buser, P. T., Auffermann, W., Holt, W. W., et al.: Noninvasive evaluation of global left ventricular function with use of cine nuclear magnetic resonance. J. Am. Coll. Cardiol. 13:6, 1989.
2. Bogren, H. C., Underwood, S. P., Firmin, D. N., et al.: Magnetic resonance velocity mapping in aortic dissection. Br. J. Radiol. 61:726, 1988.

C

1. Cranney, G. B., Lotan, C. S., Dean, L., et al.: Left ventricular volume estimation using intrinsic axis cine NMR—validation by calibrated ventricular angiography. (Abstract.) Circulation 78 (Suppl. II):1717, 1988.
2. Clark, N., Reichek, N., Axel, L., and Hoffman, E. A.: Three-dimensional evaluation of regurgitant orifices and jet volumes in aortic regurgitation by cine magnetic resonance imaging. Clin. Res. 37:245A, 1989.
3. Cranney, G. B., Lotan, C. S., Reeves, R. C., et al.: Cardiac shunt quantitation using nuclear magnetic resonance phase velocity mapping. (Abstract.) Circulation 78 (Suppl. II):2350, 1988.
4. Chung, K. J., Simpson, I. A., Glass, R. F., and Hesselink, J. R.: Cine magnetic resonance imaging in children after surgical repair of cyanotic cardiac defects. (Abstract.) Circulation 76(Suppl. IV):0118, 1987.
5. Chow, L. C., Dittrich, H. C., Bhargava, V., et al.: Quantitative assessment of regional left ventricular wall motion and thickening by cine-MRI: Comparison with contrast ventriculography. (Abstract.) Circulation 78(Suppl. II):2359, 1988.

D

1. Dumoulin, C. L., Souza, S. P., Walker, M. F., and Yoshitome, E.: Time-resolved magnetic resonance angiography. Magn. Res. Med. 6:275, 1988.

F

1. Fram, E., Hedlund, L., Dimick, R., et al.: Parameters determining the signal of flowing fluid in gradient refocused imaging: Flow velocity, TR, and flip angle. Proceedings of the Vth Annual Meeting, Society of Magnetic Resonance Imaging 1:84, 1986.
2. Frija, G., Schouman-Claeys, T., Lacombe, P., Bismuth, V., Ollivier, J. P.: A study of coronary artery bypass graft patency using MR imaging. J. Comput. Assist. Tomogr. 13:2, 1989.
3. Firmin, D. N., Nayler, G. L., Klipstein, R. H., et al.: In vivo validation of MR velocity imaging. J. Comput. Assist. Tomogr. 11:5, 1987.

G

1. Glover, G. H., and Pelc, N. J.: A rapid-gated cine MRI technique. *In* Kressel, H. Y. (ed.): Magnetic Resonance Annual 1988. Raven Press, New York, 1988.
2. Gefter, W. B., Hatabu, H., Kressel, H. Y., et al.: Cine magnetic resonance imaging of the pulmonary circulation. (Abstract.) Circulation 76(Suppl. IV):0117, 1987.

H

1. Helmcke, F., Nanda, N., and Hsiung, M.: Color Doppler assessment of MR with orthogonal planes. Circulation 75:1, 1987.

L

1. Lotan, C., Cranney, G. B., Bouchard, A., et al.: Regional wall motion assessment by cine NMR: New approach using intrinsic long axis planes. (Abstract.) Circulation 78(Suppl. II):1716, 1988.

M

1. Meese, R. B., Herfkens, R. J., Negro-Vilar, R., et al.: Rapid dynamic magnetic resonance images of the heart in evaluation of acute myocardial infarction. Circulation 76(Suppl. IV):0123, 1987.

P

1. Pflugfelder, P. W., Sechtem, U. P., White, R. D., and Higgins, C. B.: Quantification of regional myocardial function by rapid cine MR imaging. AJR 150:3, 1988.
2. Posteraro, R. H., Sostamn, H. D., Spritzer, C. E., and Herfkens, R. J.: Cine-gradient–refocused MR imaging of central pulmonary emboli. AJR 152:3, 1989.
3. Pflugfelder, P. W., Sechtem, U. P., White, R. D., et al.: Noninvasive evaluation of mitral regurgitation by analysis of left atrial signal loss in cine magnetic resonance. Am. Heart J. 117:5, 1989.
4. Pflugfelder, P. W., Landzberg, J. S., Cassidy, M. M., et al.: Comparison of cine MR imaging with Doppler echocardiography for the evaluation of aortic regurgitation. AJR 152:4, 1989.

R

1. Reichek, N., Hoffman, E. A., Gnanaprakasam, D., and Axel, L.: Three-dimensional evaluation of aortic valvular jets throughout the cardiac cycle. (Abstract.) Circulation 78(Suppl. II):2348, 1988.
2. Reiter, S. J., Rumberger, J. A., Feiring, A. J., et al.: Precision of measurements of right and left ventricular volume by cine computed tomography. Circulation 74:4, 1986.
3. Robb, R. A., Heffernan, P. B., Camp, J. H., and Hanson, D. P.: A workstation for multidimensional display and analysis of biomedical images. Comput. Methods Programs Biomed. 25:169, 1987.
4. Rubinstein, R. I., Askenase, A. D., Thickman, D., et al.: Magnetic resonance imaging to evaluate patency of aortocoronary bypass grafts. Circulation 76:4, 1987.

S

1. Sechtem, U., Pflugfelder, P. W., Gould, R. G., et al.: Measurement of right and left ventricular volumes in healthy individuals with cine MR imaging. Radiology 163:3, 1987.
2. Sechtem, U., Theissen, P., Deider, S., et al.: Assessment of aortic dissection

and aortic rupture by gradient echo magnetic resonance imaging. (Abstract.) Circulation 78(Suppl. II):2352, 1988.
3. Schiebler, M., Axel, L., Reichek, N., et al.: Correlation of cine MR imaging with two-dimensional pulsed Doppler echocardiography in valvular insufficiency. J. Comput. Assist. Tomogr. 11:4, 1987.
4. Simpson, I. A., Glass, R. F., Sherman, F. S., et al.: New methods for evaluation of anatomic and flow relationships in coarctation of the aorta by cine magnetic resonance imaging. Circulation 76(Suppl. IV):0119, 1987.
5. Sechtem, U., Theissen, P., Mennicken, U., et al.: Comprehensive noninvasive evaluation of atrial septal defects and anomalous pulmonary venous connection by magnetic resonance imaging. (Abstract.) Circulation 78(Suppl. II):2356, 1988.
6. Sechtem, U., Pflugfelder, P., Cassidy, M. C., et al.: Ventricular septal defect: Visualization of shunt flow and determination of shunt size by cine MR imaging. AJR 149:4, 1987.
7. Simpson, I. A., Chung, K. J., Powell, J. B., et al.: Cine magnetic resonance imaging for the evaluation of pulmonary artery binding in infants and children. J. Am. Coll. Cardiol. 11:2, 1988.
8. Stanford, W., Brundage, B. H., McMillan, R., et al.: Sensitivity and specificity of assessing bypass graft patency with cine computed tomography: Results of a multicenter study. Circulation 74(Suppl. II):162, 1986.
9. Stehling, M. J., Howseman, A. M., Ordidge, R. J., et al.: Whole body echoplanar MR imaging. Radiology 170:257, 1989.

U

1. Underwood, S. P., Firmin, D. N., Klipstein, R. H., et al.: Magnetic resonance velocity mapping: Clinical application of a new technique. Br. Heart J. 57:5, 1987.
2. Utz, J. A., Herfkens, R. J., Heinsimer, J. A., et al.: Cine MR determination of left ventricular ejection fraction. AJR 148:839, 1987.

W

1. White, R. D., Pflugfelder, P. W., Lipton, M. J., and Higgins, C. B.: Coronary artery bypass grafts: Evaluation of patency with cine MR imaging. AJR 150:6, 1988.

Chapter 54

Clinical Applications of Cardiac Spectroscopy

▪ *SAUL SCHAEFER, M.D.* ▪ *MICHAEL W. WEINER, M.D.*
▪ *BARRY M. MASSIE, M.D.*

METHODOLOGY FOR CLINICAL STUDIES 967
LOCALIZATION TECHNIQUES 967
Rotating Frame 968
Depth-Resolved Surface Coil Spectroscopy (DRESS) 968
Image-Selected In Vivo Spectroscopy (ISIS) 968
Spectroscopic Imaging 968
NORMAL MYOCARDIUM 969
MYOCARDIAL ISCHEMIA 970
DILATED CARDIOMYOPATHIES 970
HYPERTROPHIC CARDIOMYOPATHY 971
CARDIAC TRANSPLANTATION 971
SKELETAL MUSCLE METABOLISM IN HEART DISEASE 972
WORKS IN PROGRESS 974
SUMMARY 975

Nuclear magnetic resonance spectroscopy (MRS) has great potential for defining metabolic alterations in the human myocardium under conditions of stress and disease. As noted in Chapter 46, this technique allows nondestructive and serial examination of high-energy phosphates, including creatine phosphate (PCr) and adenosine triphosphate (ATP), and determination of intracellular pH using phosphorus-31 spectroscopy.[N1] In addition, the feasibility of measuring lactate (with ^{1}H MRS) and the fate of carbon compounds in the tricarboxcylic acid cycle (with ^{13}C MRS) is being established in animal studies.[M1] However, the ultimate application of these measurements to human studies remains to be determined. Important considerations in the implementation of these techniques in human studies will be the technical requirements for magnetic resonance spectroscopy and the value of these measurements in the diagnosis and assessment of disease. The purpose of this chapter is to review the experimental basis for human cardiac spectroscopy, describe the current methodology, summarize the available human results, and consider potential developments and applications. The reader is referred to Chapter 46 for a thorough discussion of the basic principles of magnetic resonance spectroscopy and a complete discussion of investigations in animals.

METHODOLOGY FOR CLINICAL STUDIES

The successful implementation of spectroscopy for human studies requires the resolution of several issues. The first issue is that of the sensitivity of the ^{31}P MRS experiment. At current field strengths (1.5 to 2.0 tesla), spectra with adequate signal-to-noise ratio can be achieved only from volumes in the order of 25 to 50 ml within 10 to 20 minutes. Although applicable to rest studies, these volume and time requirements may limit the feasibility of interventional studies that require multiple sequential acquisitions of spectra. In addition, this problem of sensitivity is exacerbated in the study of other nuclei (such as ^{13}C) with lower tissue concentrations. Sensitivity may be increased by increasing the volume of interest and/or by increasing the field strength of the magnet.

Second, accurate localization techniques that sample a defined volume of tissue must be utilized. As described below, several techniques have been developed for localization to a rectangular or discoid volume. This localization is required to avoid contamination of the signal from tissues outside the heart, such as the chest wall, that may alter the metabolite concentrations observed in the spectra. Localization within the heart will also be important, since accurate sampling of specified volumes will allow the investigation of regional as well as global metabolic changes.

Third, since the heart is a moving structure, due to its contractile motion and its movement with respiration, techniques for coping with this motion are necessary. Electrocardiographic gating is usually employed in spectroscopic studies to reduce contamination, but compensation for the motion due to respiration is not currently used because of the amount of time it would add to the study.

Fourth, identification and resolution of the inorganic phosphate (Pi) peak in the spectra are often complicated by the signal from the 2,3-diphosphoglycerate in chamber blood, which often overlies the Pi signal. Therefore, resolution and quantitation of the Pi peak, as well as determination of pH (which is based on the position of the Pi peak relative to the PCr peak), is often impossible. Since the PCr/Pi ratio has been a sensitive indicator of ischemia experimentally,[S1] this is an important goal. Enhanced resolution of the Pi peak by precise shimming of the magnetic field to improve its homogeneity and the use of proton decoupling has been demonstrated by one group of investigators.[L1] Other methods that reduce the signal from chamber blood have been utilized in animals[G1, Z1] but have not been applied in human studies.

LOCALIZATION TECHNIQUES

Although many schemes exist to provide anatomic localization, the following four have been successfully applied to studies of the human heart. They all use a surface coil on the chest for signal transmission and reception and provide localization by spatially encoding nuclei using either the varying magnetic field produced by a surface coil (termed the B_1 field, Fig. 54–1) or magnetic fields along the axes of the magnet produced by gradient coils in the magnet. These latter fields are called B_0 fields and are the same fields used for spatial encoding of protons in routine magnetic resonance imaging.

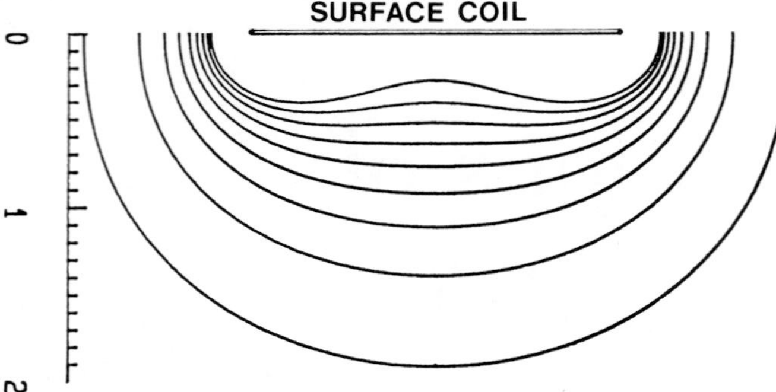

Figure 54–1. Schematic of the B_1 field isocontour lines produced by a surface coil. The known variation of the magnetic field strength as the distance from the coil increases is used in localization techniques (such as the rotating-frame experiment) to define discoid volumes.

Rotating Frame

This technique utilizes the changes in the radio-frequency (B_1) field produced by the surface coil.[G2] With increasing distance from the coil along its axis, the B_1 field produced by the coil decreases in intensity at a known rate. Thus, each set of nuclei at a given isocontour from the coil receives a radio-frequency pulse and rotates at a rate dependent on its distance from the coil. Increasing the radio-frequency pulse length (and, thus, power) will excite nuclei in an isocontour that is farther away from the coil. If the coil excitation pulses are lengthened for each successive data acquisition, a series of spectra are acquired that correspond to varying distances from the coil (Fig. 54–2). Since the lines of constant B_1 field, or isocontours, are convex, the spectra correspond to convex anatomic sections parallel to the coil and may include tissues that are not of interest. Although this technique is simple in that no gradients from the magnet are required for localization, it lacks the flexibility to choose more anatomically or clinically appropriate volumes. Furthermore, the localization of the spectra must be inferred from their appearance, rather than from an independent indicator such as imaging.

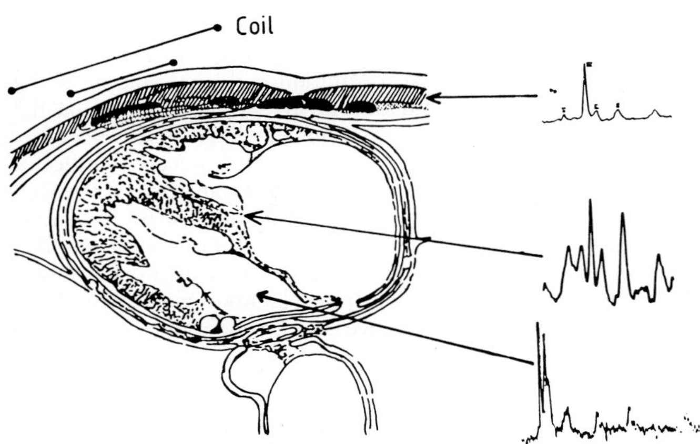

Figure 54–2. Schematic of the spectra obtained with the rotating-frame technique. The coil is placed on the chest and spectra are obtained from discoid volumes corresponding to the chest wall muscle (top), the myocardium (middle), and the chamber blood (bottom). Note that the PCr/ATP ratio is much higher in skeletal muscle than myocardium and that the primary signal from the chamber is that of 2,3-diphosphoglycerate of blood. (From Rajagopalan, B., Blackledge, M. J., McKenna, W. J., et al.: Measurement of phosphocreatine to ATP ratio in normal and diseased human heart by ^{31}P magnetic resonance spectroscopy using the rotating frame–depth selection technique. Ann. N.Y. Acad. Sci. 508:321, 1987, with permission.)

Depth-Resolved Surface Coil Spectroscopy (DRESS)

This technique uses the sensitivity profile of the surface coil, as well as the B_0 field gradients produced by the magnet, to provide localization.[B1] The nuclei in one or more slices parallel to the surface coil are first selected by the B_0 gradients, which are then excited and detected by a surface coil. Each volume for signal acquisition is a flat plane whose lateral dimensions are defined by the surface coil B_1 field. This technique has been used for both phosphorus and proton spectroscopy in humans (see below). DRESS has the advantage of selecting a plane from the magnetic resonance image prior to spectroscopy, but it cannot localize the volume of interest in the lateral dimensions parallel to the surface coil. Thus, there is a potential for significant signal contamination from undesired tissues (such as skeletal muscle) and potential loss of sensitivity from a gradient refocusing pulse required before acquisition of the signal.

Image-Selected in Vivo Spectroscopy (ISIS)

ISIS is a B_0 technique that allows selection of a three-dimensional volume of interest.[M1, O1] This volume is typically chosen from a magnetic resonance image of the subject obtained immediately before the spectroscopy examination (Fig. 54–3). A series of magnetic field gradients and radio-frequency pulses are used to select this volume of interest in space, which is relatively independent of the position or sensitivity profile of the surface coil. Signals outside the volume of interest are canceled by subtraction over eight data acquisitions. This technique is attractive in its flexibility to choose a volume with relatively sharp boundaries from an image of the subject. Also, its spatial precision allows the calculation of absolute metabolite concentrations from the volume of interest.[R1] However, its requirement for adding signals from multiple acquisitions makes it more sensitive to degradation of the signal due to either cardiac or respiratory motion, and it allows the acquisition of signals from only one volume of interest.

Spectroscopic Imaging

Spectroscopic imaging employs phase-encoding gradients in three dimensions to define an array of voxels in a manner similar

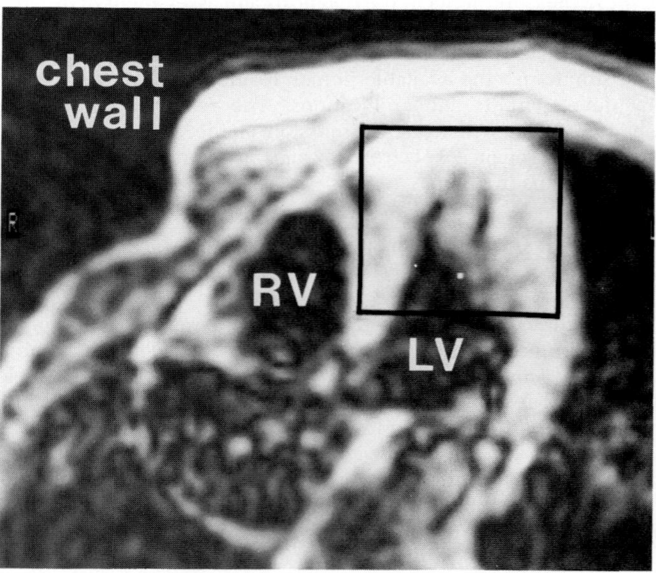

Figure 54–3. Transverse magnetic resonance proton image of a normal subject prior to an ISIS spectroscopic study. The box outlines the volume of interest used to acquire the phosphorus–31 spectrum from the left ventricle (LV). The surface coil is on the chest wall *(top)*. RV—right ventricle.

to that used in conventional proton imaging.[B2] By using either a surface coil or a volume coil, spectra are obtained from voxels over the entire sensitive volume of the coil. These voxels can, in some variations of the method, be defined at any point in the volume. In contrast to ISIS, in which the volume of interest must be defined before data acquisition, spectroscopic imaging allows the selection of voxel positions from a corresponding proton image *after* data acquisition (Fig. 54–4). Thus, spectra can be reconstructed from multiple volumes of interest chosen to correspond to selected anatomic regions. Spectra can also be summed from multiple volumes (to approximate a nonrectangular region) or displayed as a metabolic map similar to the display of proton density in conventional magnetic resonance imaging. This technique also has the advantage of providing relative insensitivity to motion, since it does not depend on cancellation of signals to provide localization. However, its pulse profile, and hence spatial selectivity, is not as good as that of ISIS, which translates into theoretically more contamination from tissues outside the chosen volume.

NORMAL MYOCARDIUM

The study of myocardial energetics has been pursued with isolated perfused heart and in vivo animal preparations with both surface coils and catheter coils.[B3, B4, K1, K2] These studies have dealt with the response of high-energy phosphate concentrations and kinetics under conditions of increased or decreased myocardial oxygen demand. In general, the response of the myocardium with adequate physiologic substrate (either pyruvate-perfused isolated hearts or in vivo hearts) has been to maintain concentrations and kinetics at baseline values with moderate stresses (such as atrial pacing). However, in situations with greatly increased demand (such as with catecholamine stimulation) or dependence on less physiologic substrates such as glucose, or in preparations where the heart is potentially ischemic (such as in the Langendorff preparation), phosphocreatine concentrations have decreased and creatine kinase fluxes have increased in order to maintain ATP concentrations under steady-state conditions. Increasing the ADP level under these conditions may serve a regulatory function by enhancing oxidative phosphorylation to maintain energy equilibrium.

The techniques used in these experiments, including magnetization transfer methods for measurement of creatine kinase flux, have not been applied to human studies. Rather, initial human studies have focused on the acquisition of resting spectra from normal subjects by a variety of techniques. The first localized human cardiac spectra were obtained by Bottomley using DRESS,[B5] followed by studies by Blackledge and associates using the rotating-frame technique[B6] and Schaefer and associates using both ISIS and spectroscopic imaging.[S2, S3] All of these studies defined normal values of PCr/ATP (approximately 1.3 to 1.5) under conditions in which the MR signal from ^{31}P was partially saturated—that is, with pulse repetition times less than five times the longitudinal relaxation time (T_1). These repetition times were usually on the order of one to two cardiac cycle lengths (1 to 2 seconds), compared to T_1 values of approximately 4 seconds for PCr and 2 seconds for ATP in animal hearts.[B4] Thus, when relatively short repetition times were used, less signal was obtained from PCr than from ATP and their ratio was altered. Although these data are useful for intergroup comparisons, the T_1 for phosphate compounds in the human heart must be determined to define PCr/ATP accurately.

Figure 54–5 shows a typical spectrum acquired with spectroscopic imaging and demonstrates the resonances of the three phosphates of ATP, as well as resonances of PCr, phosphodiesters (PDE), and a combined resonance from phosphomonoesters (PME) and inorganic phosphate (Pi). The phosphomonoester in this resonance is primarily the 2,3-diphosphoglycerate (2,3-DPG) of chamber blood. Unfortunately, as noted earlier, its presence precludes the exact determination of myocardial Pi, and therefore pH, under most circumstances.

Spectra acquired with these different localization techniques have different characteristics, although all are equally valid for determination of the tissue contents of most high-energy phosphates. Since exact determination of metabolite concentrations requires knowledge of the volume being studied, only ISIS and spectroscopic imaging can be used for these calculations. An algorithm for the calculation of metabolite concentrations has been developed for spectra acquired with ISIS and has been applied to studies of human brain.[H1] Recently, metabolite concentrations of the human heart have been calculated for spectra acquired by spectroscopic imaging[B7] with a simplified method using reference standards.

Stressing the human heart, in both health and disease, has been done only in preliminary studies. Exercise devices for use in whole-body magnets have been developed by Schaefer and associates[S4] and Conway and associates.[C1] As in animal studies, no changes in high-energy phosphate concentrations have been demonstrated in normal subjects with low levels of exercise. A potential drawback of exercise as a modality for stressing the heart is the length of time required for the acquisition of spectra, currently on the order of 15 to 20 minutes. Thus, a subject must ideally maintain a constant level of exercise for this length of time.

This concern has led investigators to consider other modalities for increasing myocardial oxygen consumption. Efforts in this laboratory have concentrated on using transesophageal atrial

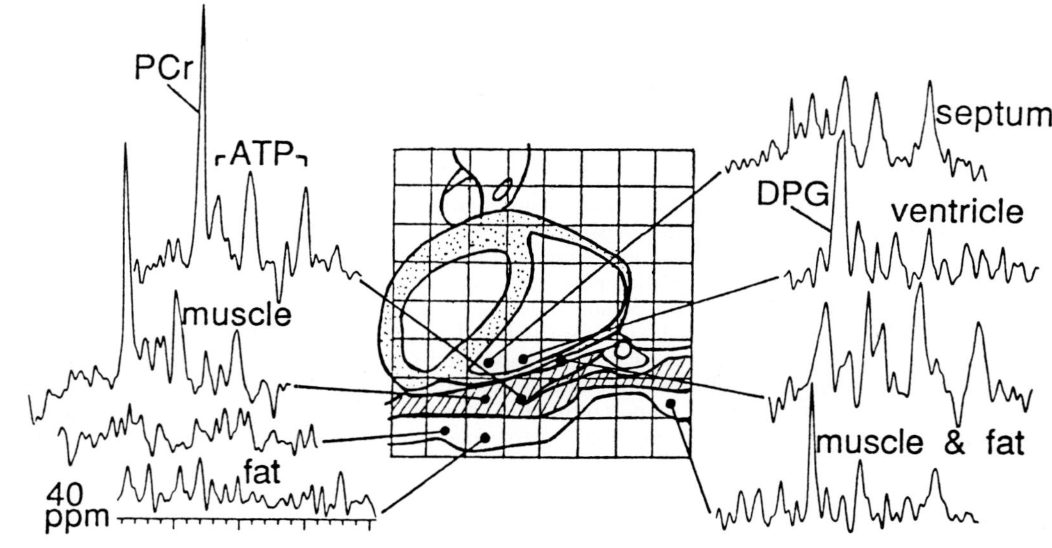

Figure 54–4. Illustration of an array of spectra acquired with spectroscopic imaging. The simultaneous acquisition of spectra from multiple sites enables measurement of the metabolic profiles of different structures. Although the array is spatially fixed in this experiment, other spectroscopic imaging techniques allow the selection of voxels in any location. (From Bottomley, P. A., and Hardy, C. J.: ^{31}P spectroscopic imaging of the human heart. Society of Magnetic Resonance in Medicine, Seventh Annual Meeting, San Francisco, 1988, p. 832, with permission.)

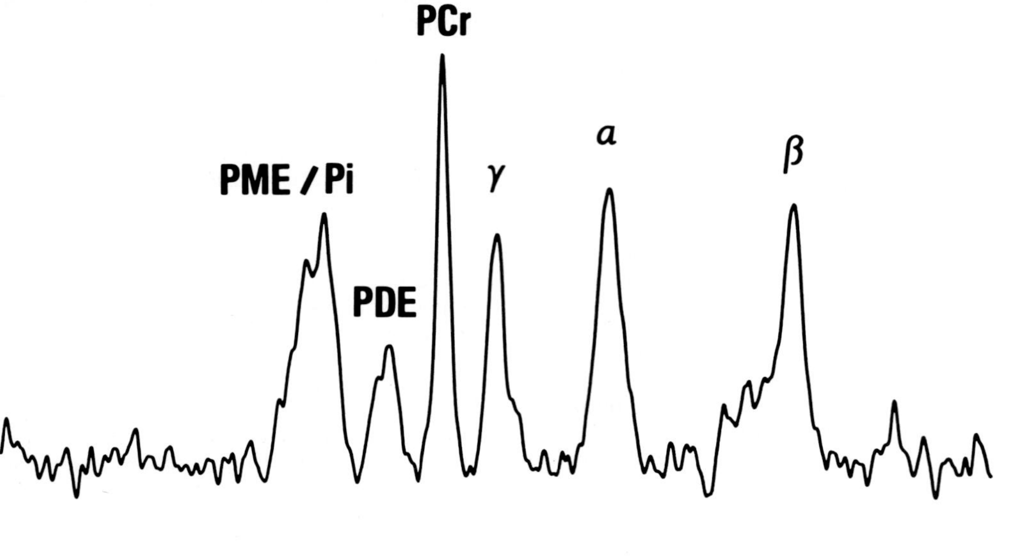

Figure 54–5. A cardiac phosphorus–31 spectrum acquired from a normal subject by spectroscopic imaging. The resonances of adenosine triphosphate (γ,α,β), phosphocreatine (PCr), and phosphodiesters (PDE) are seen, along with a combined peak due to myocardial inorganic phosphate (Pi) and the 2,3-diphosphoglycerate (PME) of chamber blood.

pacing to increase the heart rate, and the safety of this method has been established in animals and normal subjects. Whether this method or others, including inotropic stimulation, will be successful in maintaining a sufficiently elevated oxygen consumption for diagnostic studies remains to be determined.

MYOCARDIAL ISCHEMIA

The changes in high-energy phosphate levels during myocardial ischemia have been well characterized in animal studies. Following total occlusion of a coronary artery, there is a rapid decline of PCr and a concomitant increase in Pi without a significant change in ATP.[C2] With prolonged ischemia, ATP falls and intracellular pH decreases. These values return to baseline if reperfusion occurs in a timely manner. However, if the myocardial cells are irreversibly damaged, ATP continues to fall and Pi remains elevated.[R2] Thus, normal, ischemic, and infarcted myocardium can be recognized by using these patterns of changes in high-energy phosphates.

The use of ^{31}P MRS in the diagnosis of myocardial ischemia in the presence of chronic coronary artery disease is currently limited by questions of the sensitivity of the metabolic changes to ischemia as well as the issues of localization. If ^{31}P MRS is to be useful diagnostically, it must be able to detect changes in high-energy phosphates resulting from reductions in myocardial blood flow distal to a partial stenosis of a coronary artery. To address this question, Schaefer and associates[S1] performed a study with an open-chest porcine model of graded myocardial ischemia. By using a surface coil over the ischemic region and acquiring blood flow and ^{31}P MRS data at multiple steady-state degrees of coronary artery stenosis, a relationship between relative blood flow in the subendocardium of the ischemic region and the PCr/Pi ratio (an indicator of the phosphorylation potential) was established. This relationship (Fig. 54–6A) demonstrated the close relationship of PCr/Pi to reductions in myocardial blood flow. The potential diagnostic application of ^{31}P MRS is supported by the apparent high sensitivity of these metabolic changes to relatively small reductions in flow. Importantly, the PCr/ATP ratio, which currently is the most accessible measurement in human studies, did not fall until subendocardial blood flow was reduced by at least 50 percent (Fig. 54–6B).

Because myocardial blood flow, and hence ischemia, is generally more pronounced in the subendocardium,[H2] several investigators have employed the rotating-frame experiment (or modifications thereof, such as the Fourier series window experiment) to examine changes in the subendocardium and subepicardium during ischemia.[C2, R3, R4] Spectra acquired under conditions of graded ischemia in the pig by the Fourier series window experiment (Fig. 54–7) demonstrate the differences in the PCr and Pi resonances between the subendocardium and subepicardium. These differences also reflected differences in myocardial blood flow between these layers, thus providing hope that subendocardially localized spectra may be acquired in humans.

To date, the only human cardiac spectroscopy studies of ischemic heart disease are those of Bottomley and associates.[B8] Employing DRESS to examine five patients following myocardial infarction, they found abnormal PCr/Pi ratios in several of them, with some evidence that the abnormal metabolism was primarily localized in the subendocardium of some patients (Fig. 54–8). Further studies of high-energy phosphate metabolism under conditions of acute ischemia in humans need to be performed to determine the role of this method in the diagnosis and therapy of coronary artery disease.

DILATED CARDIOMYOPATHIES

The changes in high-energy phosphate metabolism with cardiomyopathies are less well defined than with ischemia and depend on the type and severity of cardiomyopathy being investigated. Markiewicz and associates[M3] showed abnormalities of high-energy phosphates in a cardiomyopathic Syrian hamster, and changes in high-energy phosphates have also been observed in an experimental model of alcoholic cardiomyopathy.[W1]

An important issue in clinical cardiology is the diagnosis of early doxorubicin (Adriamycin) toxicity, which currently limits the dose of this agent in cancer chemotherapy. Available techniques require the detection of functional abnormalities by nuclear wall motion studies. Attempts have been made to utilize ^{31}P MRS to detect early biochemical abnormalities in animal models of this toxicity.[B9, K3] These efforts have given mixed results, with some studies indicating sensitivity of the technique to the toxicity of this agent, while other studies have shown biochemical changes occuring with acute, but not chronic, drug administration. To date, no human studies of this problem have been reported.

The first investigation of a cardiomyopathy in a human was

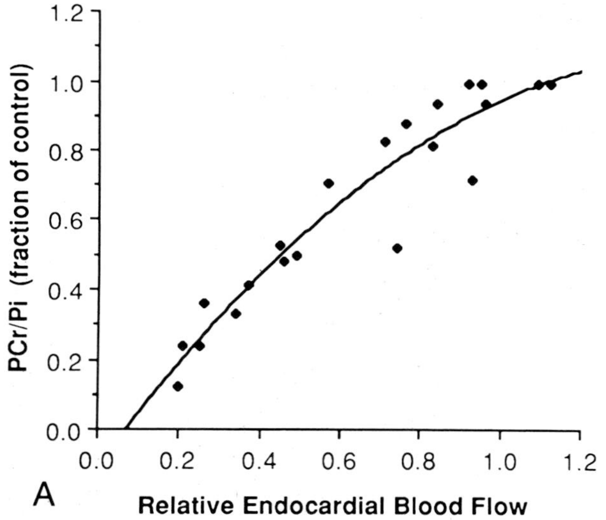

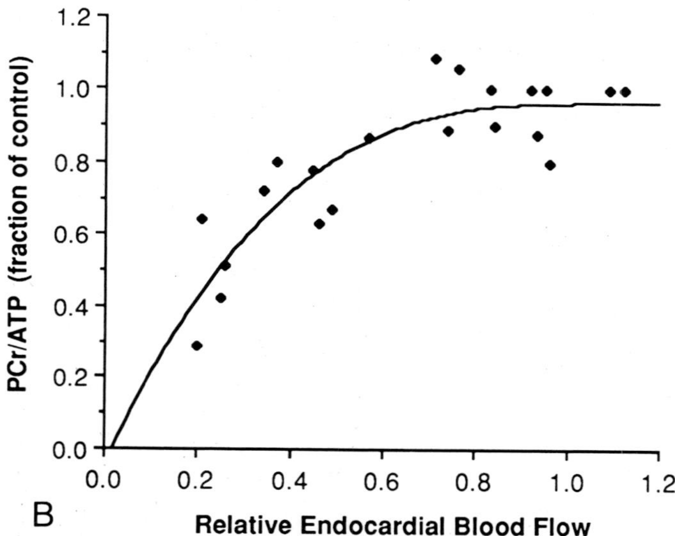

Figure 54–6. The ratio of PCr/Pi *(A)* and PCr/ATP *(B)* as a function of relative endocardial blood flow (ischemic/normal myocardium) under steady-state conditions of graded myocardial ischemia in five pigs. PCr/Pi is reduced with blood flow reductions as low as 20 percent, indicating the potential of metabolic changes as markers of ischemia. However, PCr/ATP is reduced only when blood flow is less than 50 percent of normal. (Adapted from Schaefer, S., Camacho, S. A., Gober, J., et al.: Response of myocardial metabolites to graded regional ischemia: ^{31}PNMR studies of porcine myocardium in vivo. Circ. Res. 64:968, 1989.)

performed by Whitman and associates[W2] on an 8-month-old female child with massive cardiomegaly. Using only a surface coil for localization, they found her PCr/Pi ratio to be 1.0, a value half that of a normal control. Furthermore, glucose or carbohydrate loading raised this ratio to 1.8, suggesting that magnetic resonance spectroscopy could guide therapy in selected cardiac disorders. This investigation was feasible without specialized localization techniques because of the child's poorly developed musculature and massive cardiomegaly, which heavily weighted the cardiac muscle component of the signal.

HYPERTROPHIC CARDIOMYOPATHY

Hypertrophic cardiomyopathy is a congenital disorder resulting in myocardial fiber disarray and hypertrophy.[B10] In studies of hemodynamically compensated patients, Rajagopalan and associates[R5] and Schaefer and associates[S3] did not find any abnormalities in the PCr/ATP ratio. However, two patients in each group did have abnormally large resonances in the phosphodiester region corresponding to abnormalities in the membrane constituents glycerophosphoryl choline (GPC) and glycerophosphoryl ethanolamine (GPE) (Fig. 54–9). These preliminary data suggest that membrane abnormalities due to the myopathic process may be detectable by ^{31}P MRS.

Similar findings have not been seen in patients with left ventricular hypertrophy due to pressure overload from hypertension. Abnormalities in enzyme fluxes (but not metabolite concentrations) have been noted in an animal model of hypertrophy.[B11] In the examination of a small number of patients with left ventricular hypertrophy due to hypertension or aortic stenosis,[S3] no differences were found in either the PCr/ATP or the phosphodiester/PCr ratio between the patients and control subjects. Thus, it appears that the hypertrophic process in hypertrophic cardiomyopathy is sufficiently different from that seen in hypertension (either in quality or severity) to produce changes not seen with pressure overload. Since the evaluation of hypertrophy currently relies on anatomic measures that may not accurately predict the risk or severity of disease, the ability of ^{31}P MRS to provide an independent measure of disordered metabolism may provide additional diagnostic information. Further studies of patients are under way to furnish these answers.

CARDIAC TRANSPLANTATION

Monitoring the rejection of transplanted hearts currently requires invasive endomyocardial biopsy. Because animal studies have demonstrated alterations in the high-energy phosphate

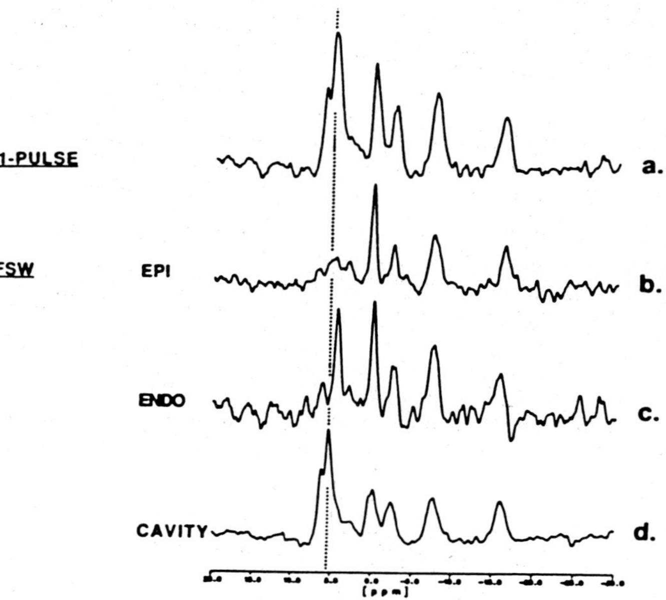

Figure 54–7. Spectra acquired with the standard one-pulse (a) and Fourier series window (FSW) experiments (b–d) in a pig with regional myocardial ischemia. As in Figure 54–5, the one-pulse spectrum shows a combined resonance from inorganic phosphate (Pi) and blood 2,3-diphosphoglycerate (2,3-DPG). The FSW spectrum (b), localized to the subendocardium, shows a relatively normal-appearing spectrum without significant contribution from Pi or 2,3-DPG. In contrast, spectrum (c), localized to the subendocardium, has a large resonance that is shifted upfield (to the right) of the 2,3-DPG peak. This resonance is due to elevated myocardial Pi during ischemia, and its shift results from intracellular acidosis. Spectrum (d) is localized to the chamber and is similar to (a), but with lower PCr and ATP. (Adapted from Gober, J., Schaefer, S., Camacho, S. A., et al.: Epicardial and endocardial localized ^{31}P magnetic resonance spectroscopy: evidence for metabolic heterogeneity during regional ischemia. Magn. Reson. Med. 13:204, 1990.)

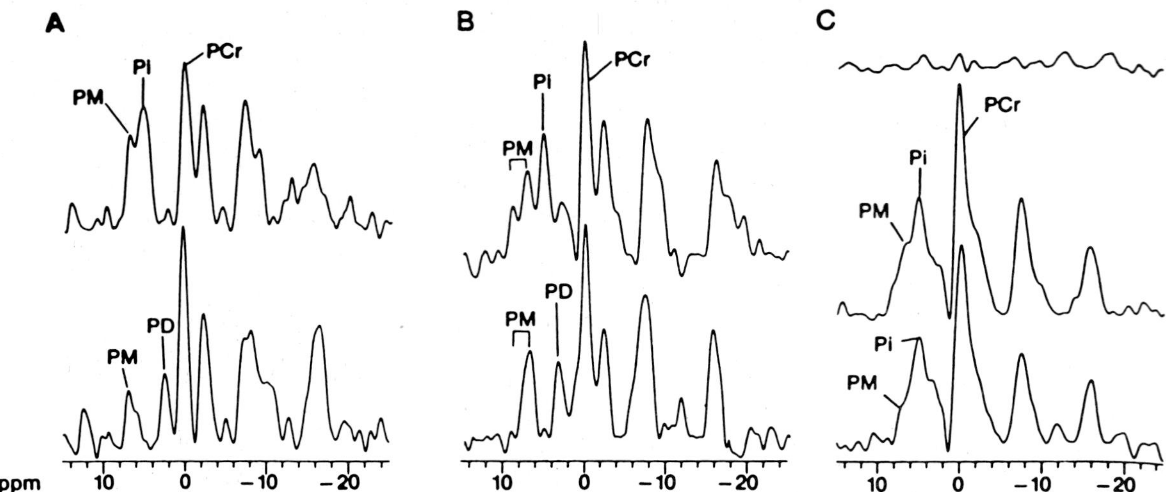

Figure 54–8. Spectra acquired from three patients following myocardial infarction, using the DRESS technique for localization. In these patients, there is an abnormal peak in the spectra at 5 ppm that indicates elevated myocardial inorganic phosphate (Pi). (From Bottomley, P. A., Herfkens, R. J., Smith, L. S., and Bashore, T. M.: Altered phosphate metabolism in myocardial infarction: P–31 MR spectroscopy. Radiology 165:703–707, 1987, with permission.)

metabolism of rejecting hearts that temporally correspond to the degree of rejection,[C3, W3] attention has been given to the evaluation of transplant rejection in humans. Using one-dimensional spectroscopic imaging, Herfkens and associates[H4] studied eight patients following cardiac transplantation. Compared with biopsy results, there was an association (albeit not statistically significant) between increasing Pi and decreasing PCr with the degree of rejection. As before, further studies need to be performed to determine the sensitivity of this technique in this group of patients.

SKELETAL MUSCLE METABOLISM IN HEART DISEASE

Although magnetic resonance spectroscopy of the human heart is a technically difficult and evolving technique, ^{31}P MRS of skeletal muscle is a straightforward procedure and has revealed interesting information about patients with congestive heart failure. Spectra can be obtained at rest and during exercise by utilizing a surface coil over the muscle of interest. This technique has been used to evaluate muscle bioenergetics in normal subjects and in patients with a variety of myopathic diseases.[C4, T2]

The primary symptom in most patients with mild to moderate heart failure is limitation of exercise or activity, often due to fatigue. Many investigators have found that, surprisingly, exercise capacity correlates poorly with indices of cardiac function, suggesting that part of this limitation may be in the periphery.[M4] Two groups have employed ^{31}P MRS to examine muscle bioenergetics in patients with heart failure.[M5, W4] Both found that PCr decreases and Pi rises at lower work rates in the patients than in controls, even when work rates are normalized for the lower maximum capacity in the patients. Massie and associates found a greater tendency in the patients to acidify at low and moderate work rates.[M6] Figure 54–10 illustrates characteristic resting and exercise spectra from a patient and an age-matched control.

These findings indicate that, compared to normal subjects, patients with heart failure are unable to produce ATP in proportion to its utilization by oxidative phosphorylation and depend more on glycolytic metabolism. Since data from a number of laboratories indicate that intracellular pH or the concentration of H_2PO_4, which increases as pH declines, may be responsible for muscle fatigue,[M7, N2, W5] these findings suggest a possible explanation for easy fatigability in heart failure. Most studies have examined forearm muscles rather than lower-extremity muscle groups, which are involved in most forms of exercise and fatiguing activity. Nonetheless, it is intriguing that patients with more severe symptoms and greater limitation of exercise tolerance have the most prominent abnormalities of muscle bioenergetics (Fig. 54–11).[M5]

These changes can be explained either by impaired blood flow and oxygen delivery to exercising muscle or by intrinsic changes in muscle bioenergetics. In support of at least a partial role for the latter are measurements performed during ischemic exercise with the brachial artery occluded.[M8] These indicate that patients

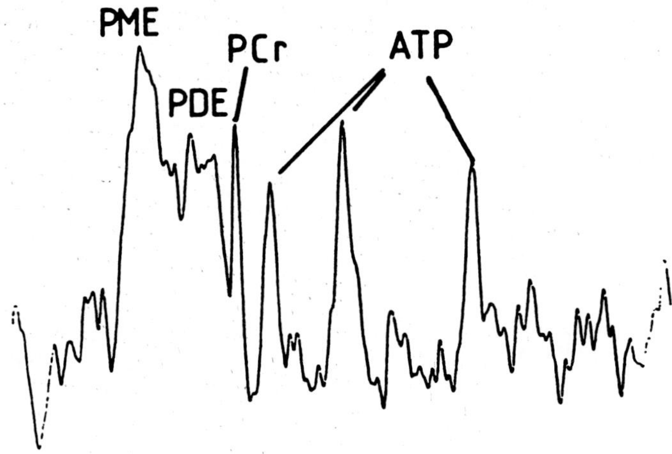

Figure 54–9. Spectrum acquired with the rotating-frame technique from a patient with hypertrophic cardiomyopathy and compensated congestive heart failure. The elevated phosphodiester (PDE) peak may reflect membrane abnormalities during disease but is also seen in normal patients. (From Rajagopalan, B., Blackledge, M. J., McKenna, W. J., et al.: Measurement of phosphocreatine to ATP ratio in normal and diseased human heart by ^{31}P magnetic resonance spectroscopy using the rotating frame–depth selection technique. Ann. N.Y. Acad. Sci. 508:321, 1987, with permission.)

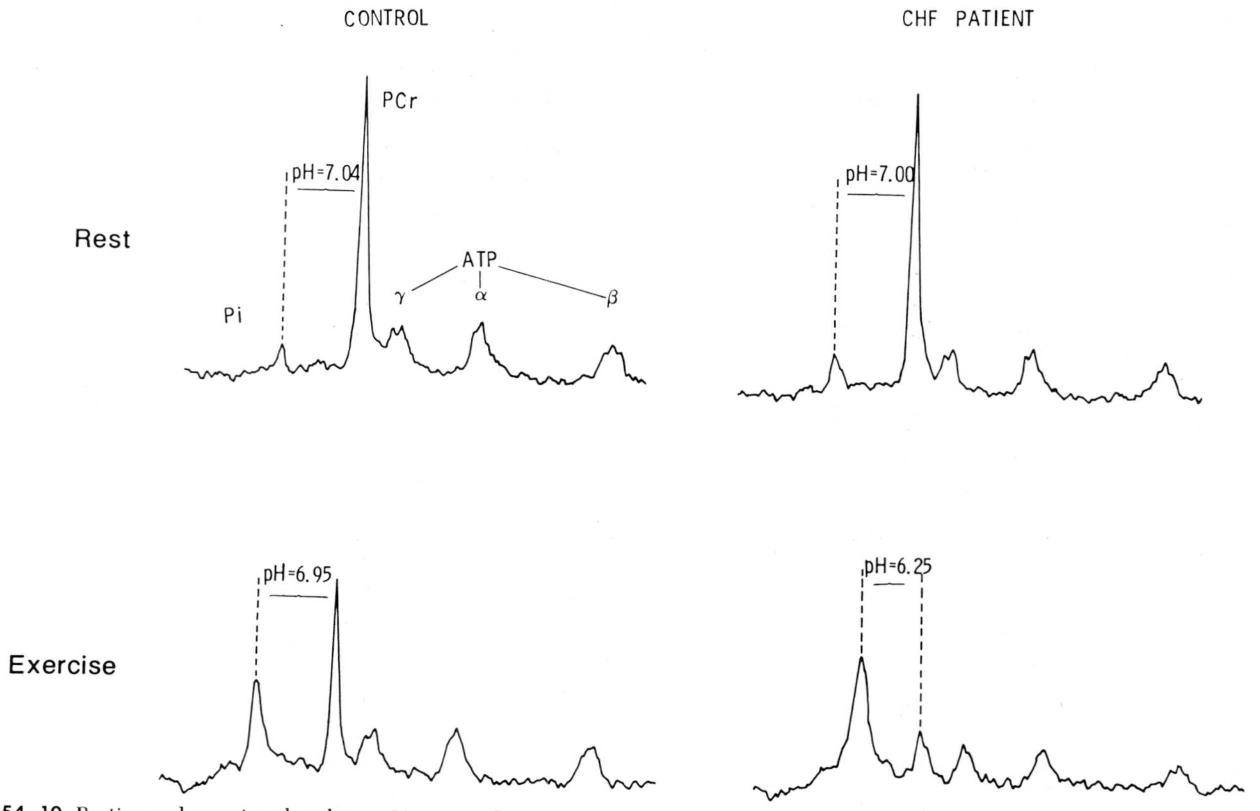

Figure 54–10. Resting and exercise phosphorus–31 spectra from a control subject and a patient with moderately severe congestive heart failure. The phosphocreatine (PCr), adenosine triphosphate (ATP), and inorganic phosphate (Pi) peaks are identified, and the pH values determined by the chemical shift of the Pi peak are shown. The spectrum from the patient and the control spectrum were similar at rest. However, with exercise, PCr declined to a greater extent and pH fell faster and to a lower value in the patient. (From Massie, B., Conway, M., Yonge, R., et al.: Skeletal muscle metabolism in patients with congestive heart failure: Relation to clinical severity and blood flow. Circulation 76:1009, 1987, by permission of the American Heart Association, Inc.)

Figure 54–11. Difference in intracellular pH in the forearm flexors at submaximal (50 percent) exercise in patients with New York Heart Association Class I and II versus Class III and IV heart failure (left) and in those with relatively preserved exercise capacity (>100 watts) versus those with more limitations (right). Although there is some overlap, it is noteworthy that the more symptomatic and impaired patients developed more acidosis. Some of the overlap may reflect differences between the forearm muscle and the larger muscle groups, which are more important in limiting ordinary activities. (From Massie, B., Conway, M., Yonge, R., et al.: Skeletal muscle metabolism in patients with congestive heart failure: Relation to clinical severity and blood flow. Circulation 76:1009, 1987, by permission of the American Heart Association, Inc.)

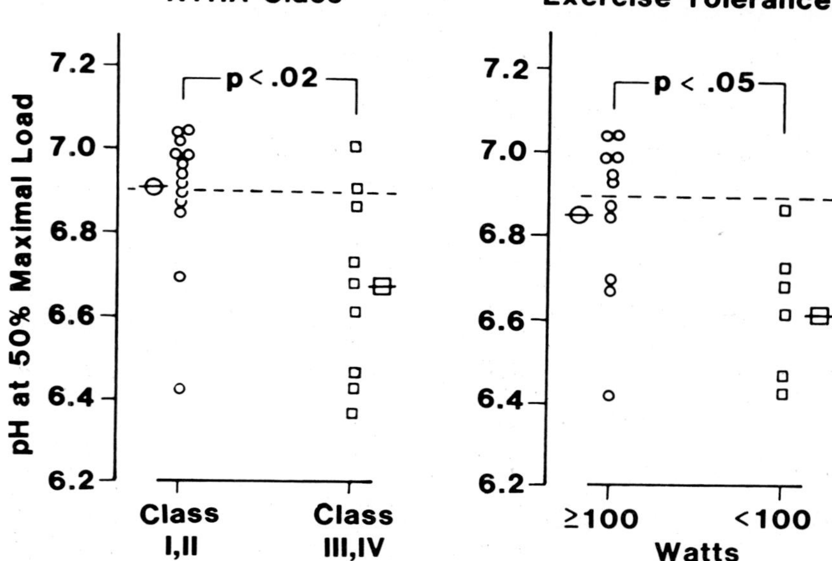

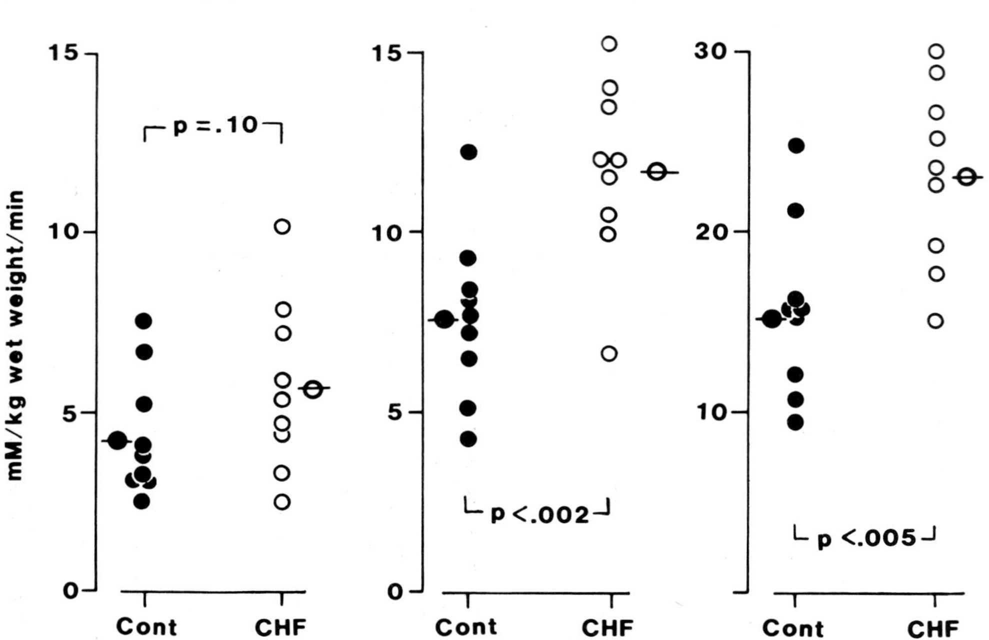

Figure 54–12. Rates of phosphocreatine (PCr) utilization, lactate production, and adenosine triphosphate (ATP) consumption during a period of ischemic exercise. The patients with heart failure (CHF) had higher rates than age-matched controls (Cont), indicating intrinsic differences in muscle metabolism that are not explained by differences in blood flow. (From Massie, B. M., Conway, M., Rajagopalan, B., et al.: Skeletal muscle metabolism during exercise under ischemic conditions in congestive heart failure. Evidence for abnormalities unrelated to blood flow. Circulation 78:320, 1988, by permission of the American Heart Association, Inc.)

produce more lactate and consume more ATP than normal individuals at matched work rates (Fig. 54–12).

Thus, ^{31}P MRS of muscle has been useful in evaluating the pathophysiology of heart failure. A number of laboratories are now investigating the effect of treatment and exercise programs on skeletal muscle metabolism in patients with heart failure.

WORKS IN PROGRESS

The success and ultimate utility of cardiac spectroscopy clearly depend on the evolution of technical developments that will allow the study of patients in less time and with greater spatial and spectral resolution. Currently, a localized examination requires approximately 20 minutes for spectral acquisition and another 40 minutes for imaging and setup. Reduction of this time will be important for the comfort of patients and for the acquisition of multiple spectra under differing conditions.

One solution for this problem is the use of higher-field magnets, which improve sensitivity and enhance spectral resolution. Most whole-body magnets in use today operate at 1.5 or 2.0 tesla, but there are a few 4.0-tesla magnets in corporate research settings. These larger magnets provide the potential for improved phosphorus-31 spectroscopy as well as the ability to perform ^{1}H MRS and ^{13}C MRS.[B12]

Proton (^{1}H) spectroscopy of the heart may have the potential to detect "stunned" or ischemic myocardium, since preliminary studies have demonstrated elevated lipids in presumably ischemic myocardium surrounding an infarct zone[M9, R6, R7] as well as in tissue following 15 minutes of regional ischemia.[E1] In addition, the detection of lactate is possible with ^{1}H MRS, although current techniques have demonstrated detection of lactate only with surface coils in open-chest preparations or on skeletal muscle.[H3] That in vivo proton spectroscopy of the human heart is feasible at commonly used field strengths was demonstrated by Barany and associates[B13] using a 1.5-tesla system. They employed a dual surface coil and DRESS to acquire water-suppressed proton spectra in six normal subjects. These spectra demonstrated resonances from phosphocreatine/creatine and taurine, as well as resonances from saturated and unsaturated fatty acids. Higher-field magnets should make these measurements more feasible by

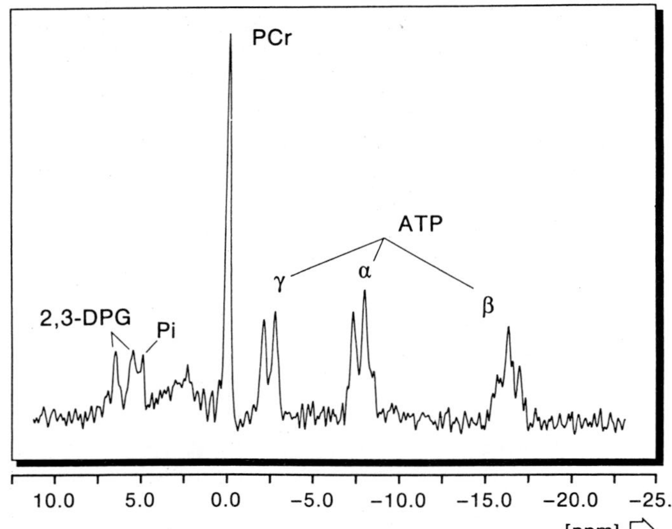

Figure 54–13. A spectrum acquired from a normal subject by using localized shimming and proton decoupling. The resolution of the spectrum is enhanced by these techniques and allows the identification and separation of peaks due to inorganic phosphate (Pi) and 2,3-diphosphoglycerate (2,3-DPG). (From Luyten, P. R., Bruntink, G., Sloff, F. M., et al.: Broadband proton decoupling in human ^{31}P NMR spectroscopy. NMR Biomed. 1:177, 1989, with permission.)

increasing the sensitivity of the experiment and providing clearer separation of closely spaced resonances.

The use of ^{13}C MRS could give insight into cardiac metabolism, especially into metabolic pathways of oxidative metabolism[M2] and utilization of glycogen (see Chapter 46).[N3] While higher-field magnets make these measurements less difficult, these studies are still limited by spectral overlap (that is, many resonances in a small frequency range), the low concentrations of lactate seen in ischemic tissue, the low natural abundance of ^{13}C, the expense of exogenously administered ^{13}C, and the previously noted problems of spatial localization.

Efforts to improve the ability of current systems to acquire diagnostic spectra have resulted in promising advances in two technical areas of cardiac ^{31}P MRS. First, localized shimming[L1] has enabled investigators to enhance the homogeneity of the magnetic field in the region of the heart, thus improving spectral resolution and the accuracy of the measurements. Second, the use of proton decoupling has allowed the detection of the resonance of inorganic phosphate separate from the blood 2,3-diphosphoglycerate resonance (Fig. 54–13). Proton decoupling, although requiring the use of a second transmission channel in the system, reduces line width by decoupling the phosphorus and hydrogen nuclei in the compounds of interest. Implementation of these techniques should aid in the diagnostic utility of ^{31}P MRS, since the PCr/Pi ratio appears to be an important indicator of metabolic dysfunction in disease.

The study of regional, rather than global, metabolic abnormalities has spurred the development of techniques to quantify and map local abnormalities in high-energy phosphates over the myocardium. An example of these efforts was demonstrated by Bottomley and Hardy[B8] using spectroscopic imaging and self-shielded gradient coils in a 1.5-tesla system. Acquiring data from 20-cm^3 voxels in less than 15 minutes and using a reference standard on the surface coil, they were able to acquire quantitative information over the myocardium. Using a similar spectroscopic imaging technique, this laboratory has developed techniques for displaying spectral information as two-dimensional gray maps similar to those for standard proton imaging. It is expected that display of the metabolic information in this format, as well as accurate quantification of metabolite concentrations, will increase the ease and utility of this technique for cardiac diagnosis.

SUMMARY

It should be clear to the reader that human cardiac magnetic resonance spectroscopy is a field in rapid technical evolution with a promising, but uncertain future. Its role in the diagnosis of cardiac disease will depend on the demonstration of sensitivity and specificity for disease states and correlation between metabolic abnormalities and the severity of the pathologic process. With the exception of a few patients studied following myocardial infarction or cardiac transplantation, demonstration of diagnostic changes in high-energy phosphate concentrations in humans has not yet been accomplished. However, animal studies suggest that in ischemia and other pathologies, ^{31}P magnetic resonance spectroscopy is sensitive to abnormalities in myocardial blood flow and that changes in high-energy phosphates correlate with functional abnormalities. Hence, with further technical development, there is significant potential for magnetic resonance spectroscopy to detect and quantify metabolic abnormalities and assess the response to therapy in a variety of cardiac diseases.

References

B

1. Bottomley, P. A., Foster, T. H., and Darrow, R. D.: Depth resolved surface coil spectroscopy (DRESS) for in vivo ^1H, ^{31}P, and ^{13}C NMR. J. Magn. Reson. 59:338, 1984.
2. Brown, T. R., Kincaid, B. M., and Ugurbil, K.: NMR chemical shift imaging in three dimensions. Proc. Natl. Acad. Sci. USA 79:3523, 1982.
3. Bittl, J. A., Balschi, J. A., and Ingwall, J. S.: Effects of norepinephrine infusion on myocardial high-energy phosphate content and turnover in the living rat. J. Clin. Invest. 79:1852, 1987.
4. Balaban, R. S., Kantor, H. L., Katz, L. A., and Briggs, R. W.: Relation between work and phosphate metabolite in the in vivo paced mammalian heart. Science 232:1121, 1986.
5. Bottomley, P. A.: Noninvasive study of high-energy phosphate metabolism in human heart by depth-resolved ^{31}P NMR spectroscopy. Science 229:769, 1985.
6. Blackledge, M. J., Rajagopalan, B., Oberhaensli, R. D., et al.: Quantitative studies of human cardiac metabolism by ^{31}P rotating-frame NMR. Proc. Natl. Acad. Sci. USA 84:4283, 1987.
7. Bottomley, P. A., and Hardy, C. J.: ^{31}P spectroscopic imaging of the human heart. Society of Magnetic Resonance in Medicine, Seventh Annual Meeting, San Francisco, 1988, p. 832.
8. Bottomley, P. A., Herfkens, R. J., Smith, L. S., and Bashore, T. M.: Altered phosphate metabolism in myocardial infarction: P–31 MR spectroscopy. Radiology 165:703, 1987.
9. Bittner, V., Reeves, R. C., Digerness, S. B., et al.: Myocardial phosphocreatine depletion after chronic Adriamycin exposure. (Abstract.) Society of Magnetic Resonance in Medicine, Seventh Annual Meeting, 1988, p. 275.
10. Braunwald, E., Lambrew, C. T., Rockoff, S. D., et al.: Idiopathic hypertrophic subaortic stenosis. I. A description of the disease based upon analysis of 64 patients. Circ. Suppl IV 30: 3, 1964.
11. Bittl, J. A., and Ingwall, J. S.: Intracellular high-energy phosphate transfer in normal and hypertrophied myocardium. Circ. (Suppl) 75: 1–96, 1987.
12. Bomsdorf, H., Helzel, T., Kunz, D., et al.: In vivo natural abundance ^{13}C spectroscopy with a 4 tesla whole-body MR system. Society of Magnetic Resonance in Medicine, Seventh Annual Meeting, San Francisco, 1988, p. 22.
13. Barany, M., Langer, B. G., Glick, R. P., et al.: In vivo H–1 spectroscopy in humans at 1.5T. Radiology 167:839, 1988.

C

1. Conway, M. A., Bristow, J. D., Blackledge, M. A., et al.: Human cardiac metabolism during exercise by ^{31}P magnetic resonance spectroscopy. (Abstract.) Society of Magnetic Resonance in Medicine, Seventh Annual Meeting, San Francisco, 1988, p. 84.
2. Camacho, S. A., Lanzer, P., Toy, B. J.., et al.: In vivo alterations of high energy phosphates and intrcellular pH during reversible regional ischemia: A ^{31}P magnetic resonance spectroscopy study. Am. Heart J. 116:701, 1988.
3. Canby, R. C., Evanochko, W. T., Barrett, L. V., et al.: Monitoring the bioenergetics of cardiac allograft rejection using in vivo P–31 nuclear magnetic resonance spectroscopy. J. Am. Coll. Cardiol. 9:1067, 1987.
4. Chance, B., Eleff, S., Leigh, J. S., et al.: Mitochondrial regulation of phosphocreatine/inorganic phosphate ratios in exercising human muscle: A gated ^{31}P NMR study. Proc. Natl. Acad. Sci. USA 78:6714, 1981.

E

1. Evanochko, W. T., Reeves, R. C., Sakai, T. T., et al.: Proton NMR spectroscopy in myocardial ischemic insult. Magn. Reson. Med. 5:23, 1987.

G

1. Garwood, M., Schleich, T., Matson, G. B., and Acosta, G.: Spatial localization of tissue metabolites by phosphorus–31 NMR rotating frame zeugmatography. J. Magn. Reson. 60:268, 1984.
2. Gober, J., Schaefer, S., Camacho, A., et al.: Epicardial and endocardial localized ^{31}P magnetic resonance spectroscopy: Evidence for metabolic heterogeneity during regional ischemia. Magn. Reson. Med. 13:204, 1990.

H

1. Hubesch, B., Sappey Marinier, D., Roth, K., et al.: ^{31}P spectroscopy of normal human brain and brain tumors. Radiology 174:401, 1990.
2. Hofmann, J. I. E.: Transmural myocardial perfusion. Prog. Cardiovasc. Dis. 29:429, 1987.
3. Hetherington, H. P., Hamm, J. R., Pan, J. W., et al.: Fully localized homonuclear edited ^1H NMR spectra of lactate in the human arm after aerobic exercise. J. Magn. Reson. 82:86, 1989.
4. Herfkens, R. J., Charles, H. C., Negro-Vilar, R., and Van Trigt, P.: In vivo phosphorus–31 NMR spectroscopy of human heart transplants. (Abstract.) Society of Magnetic Resonance in Medicine, 1988, p. 827.

K

1. Koretsky, A. P., Wang, S., Murphy-Boesch, J., et al.: ^{31}P NMR spectroscopy of rat organs, in situ, using chronically implanted radiofrequency coils. Proc. Natl. Acad. Sci. USA 80:7491, 1983.
2. Kantor, H. L., Briggs, R. W., Metz, K. R., and Balaban, R. S.: Gated in vivo examination of cardiac metabolites with ^{31}P nuclear magnetic resonance. Am. J. Physiol. 251:H171, 1986.
3. Keller, A. M., Jackson, J. A., Peshock, R. M., et al.: Nuclear magnetic resonance study of high-energy phosphate stores in models of Adriamycin cardiotoxicity. Magn. Res. Med. 3:834, 1986.

L

1. Luyten, P. R., Bruntink, G., Sloff, F. M., et al.: Broadband proton decoupling in human ^{31}P NMR spectroscopy. NMR Biomed. 1:177, 1989.

M

1. Matson, G. B., Tweig, D. B., Karczmar, G. S., et al.: Image-guided surface coil ^{31}P MRS of human liver, heart, and kidney. Radiology 169:541, 1988.
2. Malloy, C. R., Sherry, A. D., and Jeffrey, F. M.: Carbon flux through citric acid cycle pathways in perfused heart by ^{13}C NMR spectroscopy. FEBS Lett. 212:58, 1987.
3. Markiewicz, W., Wu, S. S., and Parmley, W. W.: Evaluation of the hereditary Syrian hamster cardiomyopathy by ^{31}P nuclear magnetic resonance spectroscopy: Improvement after acute verapamil therapy. Circ. Res. 59:597, 1986.
4. Massie, B. M.: Exercise tolerance in congestive heart failure: Role of cardiac function, peripheral blood flow, and muscle metabolism and effect of treatment. Am. J. Med. 84(Suppl. 3A):75, 1988.
5. Massie, B., Conway, M., Yonge, R., et al.: ^{31}P nuclear magnetic resonance evidence of abnormal skeletal muscle metabolism in patients with congestive heart failure. Am. J. Cardiol. 60:309, 1987.
6. Massie, B., Conway, M., Yonge, R., et al.: Skeletal muscle metabolism in patients with congestive heart failure: Relation to clinical severity and blood flow. Circulation 76:1009, 1987.
7. Miller, R. G., Boska, M. D., Moussani, R. S., et al.: ^{31}P nuclear magnetic resonance studies of high energy phosphates and pH in human muscle fatigue. J. Clin. Invest. 81:1190, 1988.
8. Massie, B. M., Conway, M., Rajagopalan, B., et al.: Skeletal muscle metabolism during exercise under ischemic conditions in congestive heart failure. Evidence for abnormalities unrelated to blood flow. Circulation 78:320, 1988.
9. Miller, D. D., Rosen, B. R., Dragotakes, D., et al.: Nuclear magnetic resonance detection of increased lipid in the ischemic border of reperfused myocardial infarction by 3-dimensional chemical shift imaging. (Abstract.) Clin. Res. 35:306A, 1987.

N

1. Nunnally, R. L., and Hollis, D. P.: Adenosine triphosphate compartmentation in living hearts: A phosphorus nuclear magnetic resonance saturation transfer study. Biochemistry 18: 3642, 1979.
2. Noseli, T. M., Fender, K. Y., and Godt, R. E.: It is the diprotonated form of inorganic phosphate that causes force depression in skinned skeletal muscle fibers. Science 236:1191, 1987.
3. Neurohr, K. J., Gollin, G., Neurohr, J. M., et al.: Carbon–13 nuclear magnetic resonance studies of myocardial glycogen metabolism in live guinea pigs. Biochemistry 23:5029, 1984.

O

1. Oridge, R. J., Connelly, A., and Lohman, J. A. B.: Image-selected in vivo spectroscopy (ISIS). A new technique for spatially selective NMR spectroscopy. J. Magn. Reson. 66:283, 1985.

R

1. Roth, K., Hubesch, B., Meyerhoff, D. J., et al.: Noninvasive quantitation of phosphorus metabolites in human tissue by NMR spectroscopy. J. Magn. Reson. 81:299, 1988.
2. Rehr, R. B., Tatum, J. L., Hirsch, J. I., et al.: Effective separation of normal, acutely ischemic, and reperfused myocardium with P–31 MR spectroscopy. Radiology 168:81, 1988.
3. Rajagopalan, B., Bristow, J. D., and Radda, G.: Phosphorus magnetic resonance spectroscopic imaging of the transmural distribution of metabolites in the pig heart. Circulation (Abstract.) 78:11496, 1988.
4. Robitaille, P. M., Merkle, H., Sublett, E., et al.: Spectroscopic imaging and spatial localization using adiabatic pulses and detection of transmural metabolite distributions in the canine heart. (Abstract.) Society of Magnetic Resonance in Medicine, Seventh Annual Meeting, 1988, p. 664.
5. Rajagopalan, B., Blackledge, M. J., McKenna, W. J., et al.: Measurement of phosphocreatine to ATP ratio in normal and diseased human heart by ^{31}P magnetic resonance spectroscopy using the rotating frame-depth selection technique. Ann. N.Y. Acad. Sci. 508:321, 1987.
6. Reeves, R. C., Evanochko, W. T., Canby, R. C., et al.: H–1 NMR spectroscopic detection of increased myocardial lipids in post-ischemic "stunned" myocardium. (Abstract.) Society of Magnetic Resonance in Medicine, Fifth Annual Meeting, 1986.
7. Richards, T., Tscholakoff, D., and Higgins, C. B.: Proton NMR spectroscopy in canine myocardial infarction. Magn. Reson. Med. 4:555, 1987.

S

1. Schaefer, S., Camacho, S. A., Gober, J., et al.: Response of myocardial metabolites to graded regional ischemia: ^{31}P NMR studies of porcine myocardium in vivo. Circ. Res. 64:968, 1989.
2. Schaefer, S., Gober, J., Valenza, M., et al.: Magnetic resonance imaging guided phosphorus–31 spectroscopy of the human heart. J. Am. Coll. Cardiol. 12:1449, 1988.
3. Schaefer, S., Gober, J., Camacho, S. A., et al.: ^{31}P MRS of normal and diseased human myocardium: Localization with ISIS and MRSI. (Abstract.) Society of Magnetic Resonance in Medicine, 1988, p. 296.
4. Schaefer, S., Peshock, R. M., Parkey, R. W., and Willerson, J. T.: A new device for exercise magnetic resonance imaging. AJR 147:1289, 1986.

T

1. Thompson, R. C., Canby, R. C., Lojeski, E. W., et al.: Adriamycin cardiotoxicity and proton nuclear magnetic resonance relaxation properties. Am. Heart J. 113:1444, 1987.
2. Taylor, D. J., Styles, P., Matthews, P. M., et al.: Bioenergetics of intact human muscle. A ^{31}P magnetic resonance study. Mol. Biol. Med. 1:77, 1983.

W

1. Wu, S., White, R., Wikman-Coffelt, J., et al.: The preventive effect of verapamil on ethanol-induced cardiac depression: Phosphorus–31 nuclear magnetic resonance and high-pressure liquid chromatographic studies of hamsters. Circulation 75:1058, 1987.
2. Whitman, G. J. R., Chance, B., Bode, H., et al.: Diagnosis and therapeutic evaluation of a pediatric case of cardiomyopathy using phosphorus–31 nuclear magnetic resonance spectroscopy. J. Am. Coll. Cardiol. 5:745, 1985.
3. Wisenberg, G., Pflugfelder, P. W., Kostuk, W. J., et al.: Diagnostic applicability of magnetic resonance imaging in assessing human cardiac allograft rejection. Am. J. Cardiol. 60:130, 1987.
4. Wilson, J. R., Fink, L., Maris, J., et al.: Evaluation of energy metabolism in skeletal muscle in patients with heart failure with gated phosphorus–31 nuclear magnetic resonance. Circulation 71:57, 1985.
5. Wilke, D. R.: Muscular fatigue: Effects of hydrogen ions and inorganic phosphate. Fed. Proc. 45:2921, 1986.

Z

1. Zahler, R., Majumdar, S., Fredrick, B., et al.: NMR determination of myocardial pH in vivo: Separation of tissue inorganic phosphate from blood 2,3 DPG. (Abstract.) Circulation 78:II-495, 1988.

Part VIII

Conventional Radionuclide Imaging

Chapter 55

Physics and Instrumentation of Radionuclide Imaging

ERNEST V. GARCIA, Ph.D.

PRINCIPLES OF RADIATION DETECTION 977
Scintillation Counter 977
IMAGING INSTRUMENTATION 978
Single-Crystal Gamma Camera 978
Multicrystal Gamma Camera 980
Multiwire Gamma Camera 981
NONIMAGING DEVICES FOR THE DETECTION OF RADIATION 981
Nuclear Stethoscope 981
VEST 981
ACQUISITION OF SCINTIGRAPHIC IMAGES 982
Planar Imaging in Frame Mode 982
Static Imaging 982
Dynamic Imaging 983
Planar Imaging in List Mode 984
Equilibrium Studies 984
First-Pass Studies 984
TOMOGRAPHIC IMAGING 984
Acquisition of Projections 985
Image Reconstruction 985
Factors Influencing Clinical Interpretation 986
Multiple-Gated SPECT 988
TECHNICAL ASPECTS OF QUANTIFYING CARDIAC PARAMETERS 988
Quantification of Myocardial Perfusion 989
Planar Methods 989
Tomographic Methods 992
Three-Dimensional Display 995
Quantification of Radionuclide Ventriculograms 996
Image Processing 996
Global Function Calculations 997
Regional Function Calculations 998
FUTURE DEVELOPMENTS 1002
SPECT Instrumentation 1002
Artificial Intelligence and Expert Systems 1002

PRINCIPLES OF RADIATION DETECTION

Radionuclide imaging of the heart is based on the ability to detect electromagnetic radiation emitted from an injected radioactive tracer, which is taken up by the myocardium or is mixed in the cardiac blood pool. The electromagnetic radiation used is in the form of a γ-ray or an x-ray, depending on whether it originates in the nucleus or from transitions of the orbital electrons. Ideally, this radiation should not interact with the patient, and it should be totally absorbed by the detector, which is usually a sodium iodide (NaI) crystal. The main interactions of γ-rays (or x-rays) with matter are photoelectric absorption and Compton scatter. These interactions cause an attenuation and scatter of the beam of γ-rays in the patient from which the radiation was emitted. These interactions lead to tissue ionization and ultimately contribute to a small radiation absorbed dose (rad) deposited in the patient, roughly equivalent to that from a standard chest x-ray. The γ-rays that are not absorbed by the patient can potentially be detected by scintigraphic devices.

This work was supported in part by grant RO1 HL42052 from the National Heart, Lung, and Blood Institutes, NIH and by grant R29-LM 04692 from the National Library of Medicine.

Scintillation Counter

The fundamental principles that govern how scintigraphic devices detect radiation can be explained using the basic detector unit called the scintillation counter. This device operates on the basis of two principles: scintillation and photodetection.

SCINTILLATION. A suitable material such as a sodium iodide thallium–activated [NaI(Tl)] crystal is used to stop the radiation to be measured. The γ-ray interacts with the crystal in the same manner as with the patient (i.e., photoelectric absorption and Compton scatter). The result of this interaction is the ejection of a high-speed electron from an atom in the crystal. This energetic electron disturbs other atoms in its path and creates pairs of ions in numbers proportional to its total kinetic energy. In the NaI(Tl) crystal, an additional phenomenon takes place. The ion pairs migrate in the crystal until trapped by an impurity (such as thallium), causing the emission of a photon of light per ion pair. Thus, a large number of visible photons are emitted per γ-ray absorbed, in direct proportion to the energy of the γ-ray. This large number of visible photons emitted per γ-ray absorbed gives rise to a burst of visible light, known as a scintillation.

PHOTODETECTION. Although many visible photons are emitted per scintillation, their number is still not high enough to be seen by the naked eye. This burst of visible light (photons) is converted into an electrical pulse through the use of a light-sensitive device known as a photomultiplier tube (Fig. 55–1). To gather as many of the visible photons as possible, this device is coupled optically to the crystal. The photomultiplier detects the visible photons by means of a thin plate known as the photocathode, which releases electrons in proportion to the photons striking it. This signal is then amplified by acceleration of these released electrons through a series of plates known as dynodes, which multiply the number of electrons striking them in proportion to the voltage difference between the plates. As this interaction is repeated through 10 plates and a voltage difference of hundreds of volts, the original number of electrons is amplified by a factor of approximately 1 million. The electrons are collected by a plate known as the anode and shaped by a preamplifier to generate an electrical pulse. The voltage (height) of this pulse, which is created by a single scintillation, is directly proportional to the amount of light released by the crystal, which in turn is directly proportional to the energy of the γ-ray absorbed by the crystal. Each of these pulses could be counted by a scaler to measure the number of γ-rays absorbed by the crystal without regard for its energy.

Discriminating the energy of the γ-ray absorbed by the crystal is important because it allows the selection of different radionuclides with different energies or the elimination of less energetic scattered photons from the patient. A pulse height analyzer is used to preselect from the distribution of available energies (energy spectrum) the range of energies to be counted (energy window) (Fig. 55–2). Pulses corresponding to γ-rays of energies outside this window are rejected. The combination of a NaI(Tl) crystal, a photomultiplier, a pulse height analyzer, and a scaler make up the scintillation counter, which may be used to count radioactive samples in vitro (well counter) or in vivo (probe) (see Fig. 55–1).

The use of a pulse height analyzer is particularly important for imaging with radiation because a basic assumption of scintigraphy is that the γ-rays interacting with the crystal travel in a straight line from the emitting source. Therefore, the pulse height analyzer, by rejecting energies below a certain threshold, eliminates γ-rays that could have lost their original energy and direction during a Compton scatter event in the patient and that continue on to strike the crystal. Unfortunately, the pulses generated by unscattered γ-rays that strike the crystal are not all of the exact same amplitude, but are spread around the amplitude corresponding to the exact characteristic energy of the radionuclide (photopeak). The less the spread of energies around the photopeak, the better the *energy resolution* of the system, and the better the inherent counting and imaging characteristics of the device.

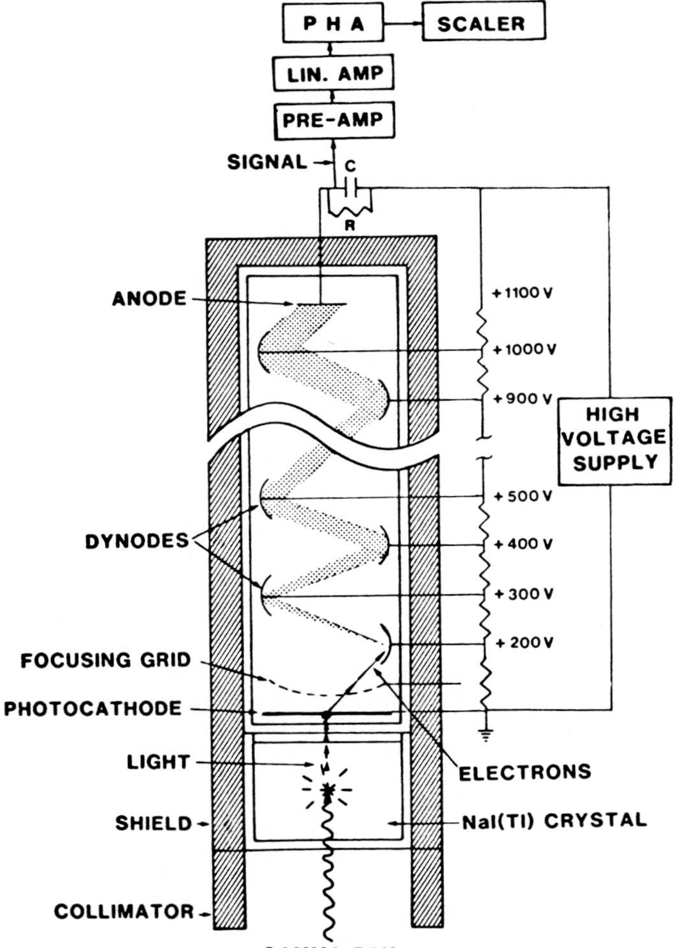

Figure 55–1. Schematic diagram of a sodium iodide thallium (NaI [Tl]) detector. PHA—pulse height analyzer. (From Patton, J. A., et al. (eds.): Clinical Radionuclide Imaging. Grune and Stratton, Orlando, 1984, p. 48, with permission.)

IMAGING INSTRUMENTATION

Single-Crystal Gamma Camera

The most significant breakthrough in nuclear medicine instrumentation occurred in 1958, when Hal Anger invented the conventional analog scintillation camera.[A1] This device is able both to detect and to localize the scintillation event, thus providing the potential for imaging a radionuclide distribution using a stationary detector without the necessity for scanning.

The scintillation camera uses a large (~300- to 500-mm), flat (0.25- to 0.5-inch) NaI(Tl) crystal and an array of photomultipliers (19 to 91). The photomultipliers are arranged in a specific array covering the area of the crystal face (Fig. 55–3). The γ-rays are first collimated to preselect a desired direction from which to strike the crystal. The γ-rays that pass through the holes of the lead collimator are usually absorbed by the crystal, giving rise to a scintillation. The light (visible photons) from the scintillation is detected by all photomultipliers. Those photomultiplier tubes closer to the event gather more light than those farther away. All tubes feed their output into the electronic computer circuitry (positional analyzer), where it is analyzed. The point at which each scintillation occurs, beneath the array of photomultipliers, is determined, and an x coordinate and a y coordinate are assigned to each such event. In addition, the output of all tubes is summed to form an energy or z pulse.

ELECTRONIC PROCESSING. For each γ-ray that interacts with the sodium iodide crystal, the scintillation camera generates three information pulses. Two of these pulses correspond to the Cartesian coordinates of the scintillation, and the third is the z pulse, representing the total energy of the γ-ray that interacted with the crystal (Fig. 55–4*A*). The z pulse is sent to the pulse height analyzer, which has been set to accept a preselected range of energies. Once the z pulse has been accepted by the pulse height analyzer, it becomes a trigger pulse, also known as a signal (s) pulse, which signals a scintillation event to be counted. The x, y, and z pulses are in analog format and are meant to be used in conjunction with a cathode ray tube (CRT) scope. The word *analog* signifies that the information of these pulses is coded as a continuously variable voltage; in other words, a small deflection in the voltage implies a small change in the position of the scintillation.

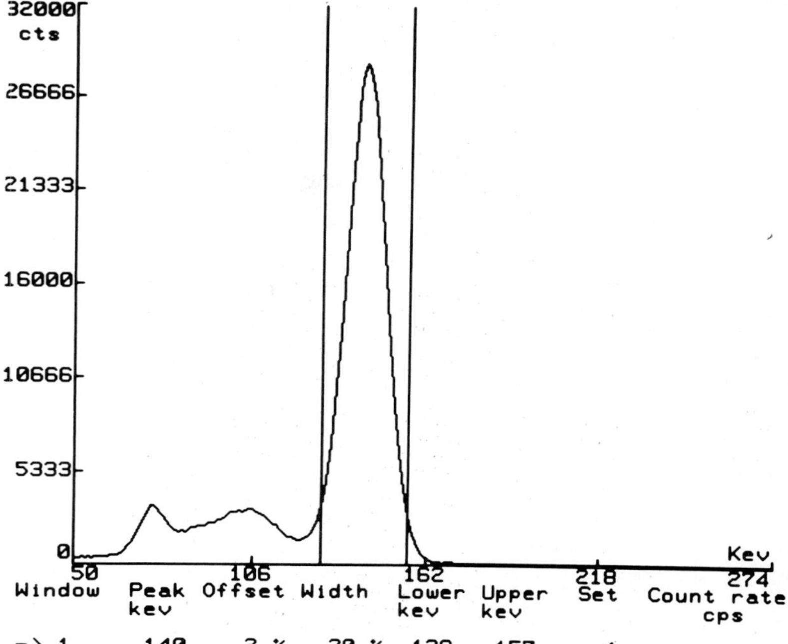

Figure 55–2. Technetium–99m (^{99m}Tc) energy spectrum with superimposed energy window *(vertical lines)* around the 140-keV photopeak (cts—counts; cps—counts per second).

The *z* pulse, or trigger pulse, is also known as the unblank signal when it is used to control a CRT. Each time this trigger pulse comes in, it allows the emission of electrons from the electron gun. The *x* and *y* positional pulses are fed to the horizontal and vertical plates, which create a deflection in the path of the electrons corresponding to the scintillation coordinates (see Fig. 55–4*A*).

The electrons then hit the phosphor screen of the CRT, creating a small scintillation that can be recorded on a photographic film as a dot. The analog nuclear medicine image is a collection of these dots, which are distributed according to the radioactivity in the patient.

ADVANCED ELECTRONICS. The basic electronic scheme developed by Anger to position the scintillation event has been improved by correction circuitry implemented as part of most state-of-the-art cameras. These cameras are able to perform signal processing in real time, which corrects the position of the scintillation event before the event is recorded on film or on a digital matrix. In general, real-time correction electronics are of three different types. These are corrections for tube drift, energy variations, and spatial nonlinearity.

The tube drift correction is used to calibrate or "tune" the photomultipliers automatically so that each tube generates the same pulse voltage when it gathers the same light from reference

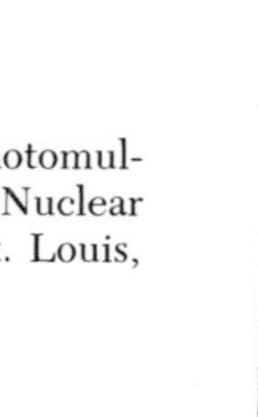

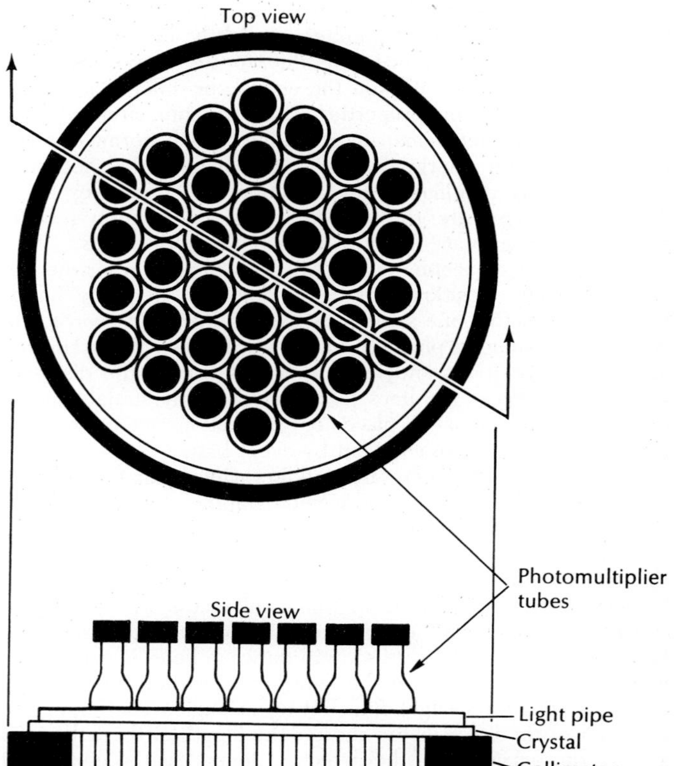

Figure 55–3. Diagram showing the relative placement of the photomultiplier tubes in a scintillation camera. (From Rollo, F. D. (ed.): Nuclear Medicine Physics, Instrumentation, and Agents. C. V. Mosby, St. Louis, 1977, p. 234, with permission.)

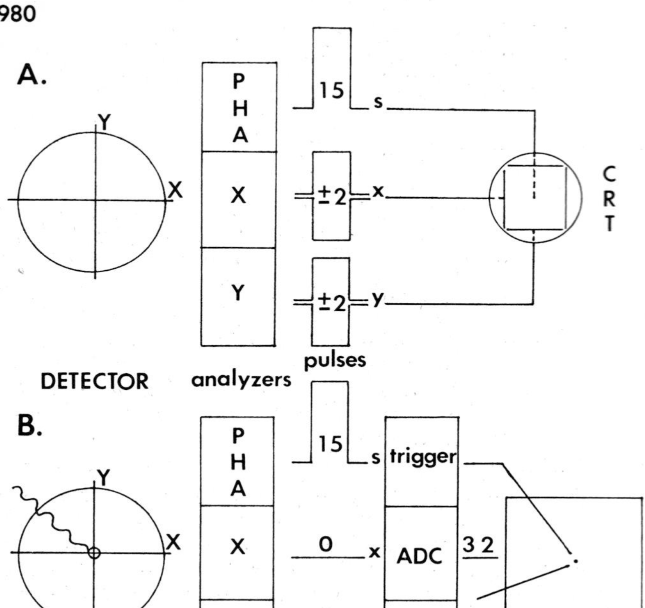

Figure 55–4. Block diagram of a scintillation camera. *A*, Diagram shows generation of the *x* and *y* positional pulses and the *s* (or *z*) trigger pulse to control the cathode ray tube (CRT). *B*, Block diagram of a computer interface illustrating how the *x*, *y*, and *s* (or *z*) pulses, which are generated by the camera when the scintillation occurs in the center of the sodium iodide crystal, are used to update the digital image. PHA—pulse height analyzer; ADC—analog to digital converter.

light sources, which flash up to 1000 times per second during acquisition. This type of correction is particularly needed for rotational tomography to provide correction for differences in photomultiplier output as a function of angle resulting from the influence of the earth's magnetic field. Placement of Mu metal shields around each photomultiplier tube has also been used to reduce this effect.[W1]

The energy correction circuit provides correction for the fact that each photomultiplier, even after being automatically tuned for its light sensitivity, generates a slightly different energy spectrum. These differences are due to the response of the photomultiplier, differences in the crystal, or differences in the regional light-gathering properties. This correction circuit applies a premeasured energy map in real time, which normalizes the relationship of the energy window to the shape of the spectrum, thus effectively eliminating the variations in energy response. This correction requires the periodic acquisition of energy-specific field floods to generate the time-dependent energy maps.

The linearity correction circuit provides correction for the fact that the Anger positioning scheme does not perfectly image straight radioactive line sources as straight lines. The correction consists of imaging a phantom of straight lines in the horizontal and vertical positions and measuring and storing the displacement, which forces the lines to appear perfectly straight in the image. These regional displacement correction factors are then applied in real time on an event-by-event basis.

COLLIMATION. There are no known lenses that can gather and refract (bend) γ-rays, as can photographic cameras. Instead, a collimator or lead disk with multiple holes is used to cause *selective interference* or blocking of those γ-rays not traveling in the selected direction. The most commonly used collimator in nuclear cardiology is the parallel-hole collimator. This collimator consists of a large number of parallel holes perpendicular to the face of the crystal. The lead septum between holes is made thick enough to absorb most of the γ-rays of a preselected energy, which travel in a straight line but at an angle. The larger the diameter of the holes or the shorter the length of the holes, the greater the *sensitivity* of the detector, defined as the number of γ-rays counted per unit of time (per γ-ray emitted). Improvements in sensitivity are usually accompanied by a deterioration of the *spatial resolution* of the system—that is, the ability to discern in the image two distinct radioactive objects. Although the parallel-hole collimator is by far the most widely used, several other collimators are available that may out perform the parallel-hole collimator for a specific application. Available collimators include the pinhole, converging, diverging, and parallel-hole slant collimators.

COMPUTER INTERFACE USED BY ANALOG CAMERAS. The same *x*, *y*, and *z* analog pulses that are sent to the cathode ray tube in analog cameras are also routed to the computer interface input. The term *interface* is defined as the coupling between two instruments (anything needed to make one system understand the other). The computer cannot handle these analog pulses in their natural format. Before these pulses can have meaning within the computer, they must be converted into digital information. The term *digital* refers to a discrete number or a countable number, such as an integer. Therefore, the computer must be equipped with an analog-to-digital converter (ADC). The ADC converts the pulse height into discrete numbers. The *x* and *y* pulses each have an ADC. The *z* pulse acts as a trigger, signaling the ADCs to convert the analog pulses into digital numbers (see Fig. 55–4*B*). Most computers have a direct memory access (DMA). This is a hardware device that updates the memory without any software or CPU intervention, thus freeing up the computer while it is acquiring. How the memory is updated depends on the preselected acquisition format, which is the topic of the section on ACQUISITION in this chapter.

DIGITAL CAMERA. When the computer hardware is an integral part of the scintillation camera system and it is used for processing the scintillation event, the computer/camera system is called a digital camera. In reality, there is no commercial system that is totally analog or totally digital, so it is a confusing term. In general, manufacturers use the term to mean that systems use advanced digital circuits that provide correction for the photomultiplier output, energy, and position of the scintillation event. A more strict definition is a scintillation camera that only generates digital images in a matrix format without generating an analog image. As implemented by one manufacturer, one advantage of the digital camera is that it can effectively reduce the dead time of the system by utilizing distributed processing with multiple microprocessors and temporary memory storage (buffers) of the pulses. This type of digital camera implementation has allowed the possibility of acquiring count rates close to those of the multicrystal camera but using a single large crystal and Anger-type positioning. The manufacturers of one digital camera system claim that their detector has a count-rate capability of 200,000 cps at a 10-percent loss.[R1]

Multicrystal Gamma Camera

In addition to the popular, single-crystal gamma camera, another camera design, known as the multicrystal or autofluoroscope camera, has been also used in nuclear cardiology. This camera, which was originally developed by Bender and Blau,[B1] consists of a mosaic pattern of 294 (1 cm by 1 cm by 1 inch) sodium chloride crystals arranged in an array of 14 rows by 21 columns and 35 photomultipliers (one for each row and one for each column). Each crystal is coupled to two photomultiplier tubes (one for the row position and one for the column position) by means of fiber optics. The light from the scintillation emitted for each γ-ray absorbed by the crystal is detected by the corresponding horizontal and vertical photomultipliers, quickly identifying the crystal position. Because of the simplicity of the electronics, the *deadtime* that it takes to process the necessary pulses, during which the system cannot respond to new events, is much shorter than in the conventional Anger camera. This shorter deadtime implies that, for an intense radioactive source emitting a high count rate (~200,000 cps), the system is able to observe a count rate much closer to the true rate than the conventional Anger camera.

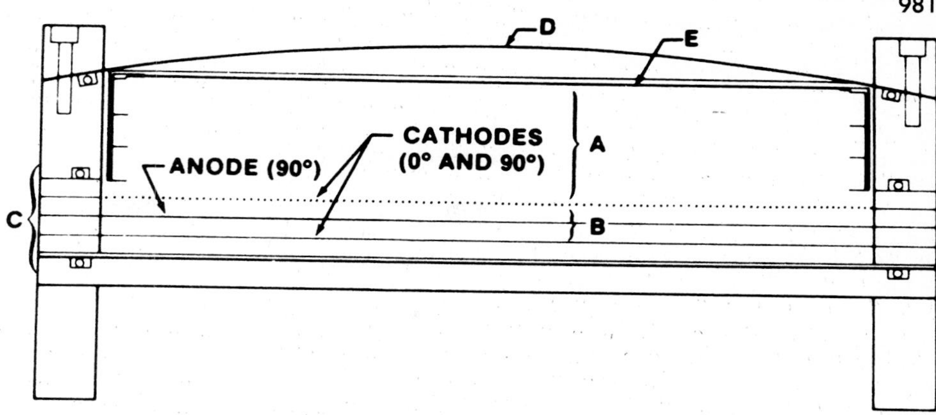

Figure 55–5. Longitudinal diagram of multiwire proportional counter gamma camera. Diagram shows the following: drift region *(A)*, detection region *(B)*, detection region *(B)*, aluminum pressure vessel *(C)*, aluminum entrance window *(D)*, and negative high-voltage collection electrode (E). (From Lacey, J. L., et al.: A gamma camera for medical applications, using a multiwire proportional counter. J. Nucl. Med. 25:1004, 1984, with permission from The Society of Nuclear Medicine.)

Because its potential for fast counting, the multicrystal camera became the instrument of choice at many institutions for imaging the transit of the first pass of a radiotracer through the heart chambers. The ability to count fast has been exploited by many specialists through the use of collimators with holes close to the dimensions of the crystals, thus allowing a higher γ-ray flux incident on the crystals. Thus, a 25-mCi dose of ^{99m}Tc imaged with a high sensitivity collimator (1-inch thick) results in over 400,000 cps in the overall image.[B2] A newer version of this design with improved fiber optics and updated electronics performs even better.

Multiwire Gamma Camera

Single-photon imaging detectors based on multiwire proportional counters (MWPC) have been developed. One group in particular[L1] has developed a multiwire gamma camera with both high count rate capability and spatial resolution and has used it in first-pass radionuclide angiography.[L2] The detector seen in Figure 55–5 consists of a drift region and a detection region contained within an aluminum pressure vessel that has a thin aluminum entrance window of spherical shape. Photons entering through the aluminum window interact with the xenon gas that is moderately pressurized in the drift region. The interaction causes the creation of ions that are drifted to the detection region. The detection region consists of three parallel wire planes, a central anode plane, and the two outer cathode planes. The drifted ionization is collected at the anode, where the charge is amplified by a gas avalanche. Position determination of the anode avalanche is obtained by detection of the signals induced in the two cathode grids, which are oriented perpendicular to each other. This detector is very compact, lightweight, and portable.

Because the stopping power of the pressurized xenon gas is low compared with sodium iodide crystals, detection efficiency limits the application of the multiwire camera to energies below 100 keV. Tantalum–178(^{178}Ta), a generator-produced tracer with low energy (60 keV) and a short half-life (9.3 minutes), has been shown to be ideal[L2] when used in the performance of first-pass angiography with this camera. Since the duration of the signal in the MWPC detector is one tenth that of sodium iodide detectors, these devices can be designed for high count rates, similar to those of the multicrystal cameras. In particular, the multiwire gamma camera described earlier has an intrinsic peak count rate of 850,000 cps with an intrinsic spatial resolution of 2.5 mm.[L1]

NONIMAGING DEVICES FOR THE DETECTION OF RADIATION

Nonimaging probes are being used to monitor radioactivity in the heart. In contrast to gamma cameras, these probes do not produce an image of the heart but are used specifically to record count changes within its field of view. Since no image is generated by the system, detector design is as simple as that described for the scintillation counter. This simplicity in detector configuration makes the system portable and less expensive and more count efficient compared with gamma cameras.

Nuclear Stethoscope

The most popular nonimaging probe is the nuclear stethoscope, which is used for measuring and monitoring left ventricular global function following labeling of the cardiac blood pool with ^{99m}Tc. The detector for this probe consists of a sodium iodide crystal, 2 inches in diameter and 1 1/2-inch thick, a photomultiplier, and a single-bore, flat-field converging collimator.[W2] This detector is mounted on a 50-inch arm with 2 degrees of freedom and is interfaced to a dedicated microprocessor. The microprocessor simultaneously samples and, in real-time, records counts emanating within the field of view and the patient's electrocardiogram. The microprocessor is also used to assist in the positioning of the detector for measuring counts from the region of the left ventricle and a background region. The detector position for the left ventricular region is identified by the microprocessor as the highest ratio of stroke counts to average counts. The position of the detector for the background region is identified by the microprocessor as that position immediately inferolateral of the left ventricular region that yields minimal stroke counts and where the average counts initially decrease.

After positioning the probe, beat-to-beat left ventricular time-activity curves are displayed. After filtering the time-activity curves, left ventricular ejection fraction may be calculated on a beat-to-beat basis, or the cardiac cycle time-activity data may be averaged over any length of time, usually ranging from 30 seconds to 2 minutes. This averaging significantly improves the statistical accuracy of the data, yielding high temporal resolution volume curves from which parameters of left ventricular function may be automatically calculated, such as ejection fraction and filling and emptying rates.

Although the positioning of the detector is based on algorithms, accurate measurements still require considerable expertise in positioning the detector. Because of this limitation, this probe is most useful in monitoring changes in cardiac performance over an acquisition session with the detector placed in the same relative position. If relative detector-to-heart geometry is carefully recorded and reproduced, this device is also useful in studying changes in cardiac performance from separate acquisition sessions.

VEST

More recently, new nonimaging probe systems have been made smaller so that the entire system can be worn, like a vest. This device, known as the VEST, allows for continuous, ambulatory monitoring of left ventricular performance during normal day-to-day activities that may cause ischemic events different from those found during exercise testing. Similar to the nuclear stethoscope, the VEST simultaneously and continuously records the electrocardiogram and the counts from the detector's field of view.

The VEST consists of a radionuclide detector, a molded plastic garment to hold the detector in place, and electronic devices to count the scintillations and record the events. In addition, the recorder contains an event marker and a real-time clock. The entire device weighs 3.1 kg. Positioning of the device is done with the assistance of a gamma camera. After injection of 15 to 25 mCi of ^{99m}Tc-radiolabeled red blood cells, the best septal left anterior oblique view of the left ventricle is identified. The VEST's detector is then positioned in place over the left ventricle by using the shadow casted on the gamma camera display by the lead shield around the detector as a guide. Once the VEST is fixed in place, monitoring of left ventricular function is performed while the patient is mentally or physically challenged or while the patient goes on with his or her regular daily activities. Recording of cardiac performance may be carried out for up to 6 hours.

After the data recording session is ended, the stored data are replayed into a computer system for analysis and graphic display. Background activity is currently determined as 70 percent of the end-diastolic counts. A patient's beat-to-beat, background-corrected time-activity curve of the left ventricle and corresponding electrocardiogram are available for display. The beat-to-beat time-activity curves may be added and filtered to yield high-resolution time-activity curves of the left ventricle. A decrease of ejection fraction of greater than 6 percent units lasting greater than or equal to 1 minute is considered significant.[T1] Preliminary validation[W3] has shown the ability of the VEST to measure ejection fraction at rest with the same degree of accuracy obtained from gated blood pool imaging.

ACQUISITION OF SCINTIGRAPHIC IMAGES

Three basic considerations determine the format in which scintigraphic data should be collected. Of prime importance is appropriate matching of the speed of the physiologic event to that of the acquisition of the image, which determines the temporal resolution. A second important consideration is matrix resolution, which is based on matching the spatial resolution of the imaging system to the number of pixels per frame. The third is information density, which determines whether the number of counts per pixel is appropriate for the information intended to be extracted from the images. The temporal resolution, matrix resolution, and information density needed varies with the specific cardiac study being acquired and the type of information being extracted. For example, for cardiac blood pool imaging, the variables associated with these respective acquisition formats are the number of frames per cardiac cycle, the number of pixels per frame, and the number of bits per pixel. The formats also differ in how the incoming scintillation and physiologic events are handled by the computer. This section describes the options that most nuclear medicine computer systems provide for handling these data-acquisition requirements.

Planar Imaging in Frame Mode

Almost all planar studies are acquired in frame (histogram) mode, in which a portion of computer memory is used to represent an image that has been acquired for either a predefined time or a total number of scintillations or counts. Each memory location allocated to this frame represents a digital counter of how many scintillations occurred at each picture element (pixel) location during acquisition. In the preset time mode, when the time of acquisition for that frame has elapsed, the frame is transferred to a peripheral device such as a disk for longer term storage. In the preset counts mode, the computer also updates a counter that keeps track of the total number of counts; after this counter reaches a preset number, the frame is transferred. The frame mode can be subdivided into static and dynamic forms of acquisition.

Static Imaging

Static image acquisition, either non-gated or gated, is used when the radionuclide distribution is assumed not to change for a period of time. This applies to myocardial perfusion imaging with ^{201}Tl, acute myocardial infarction imaging with ^{99m}Tc-PYP, and in a variation, to cardiac blood pool imaging.

NON-GATED STATIC ACQUISITION. ^{201}Tl myocardial scintigrams of stress/redistribution or rest/redistribution are usually acquired for a preset time, such as 6 to 10 minutes per view. Optimally, following the injection of ^{201}Tl, sequential imaging begins within 5 to 6 minutes, in the anterior, mid–left anterior oblique (LAO), and steep LAO views, respectively. The same views are repeated 3 to 6 hours later to aid in the study of both washout and reversibility. A matrix format of 128 by 128 pixels is normally used as a trade-off between spatial resolution and adequate information density per pixel. The field of view is usually about 8 inches by 8 inches to allow an ample number of pixels to define the heart and to give an accurate representation of the background surrounding the heart. A 10-minute acquisition session yields between 300,000 and 800,000 total counts in the image from a 2-mCi dose of ^{201}Tl.[B3]

MULTIPLE-GATED ACQUISITION. Multiple-gated acquisition employs 14 to 100 frames, using a physiologic marker (R wave) as a synchronizing signal.[G1] Corresponding frames are added together over a pre-set time or number of counts, thus making this a form of static imaging. Scintigraphic data from the camera are channeled to a series of image frames located in the computer memory. Count allocations to particular frames are governed by the time-delay between the R wave and the count event (Fig. 55–6). Immediately after the trigger, counts are placed in frame 1 for a fixed duration of time. When the desired R–R sampling interval has elapsed, scintigraphic data are channeled to frame 2, and the process continues up to the last frame (N). When the time interval for the last frame has elapsed, the remaining data from the camera are discarded until the next trigger signal arrives. Data from successive beats are added into the appropriate frames until the desired total count is achieved or the preset time is reached.

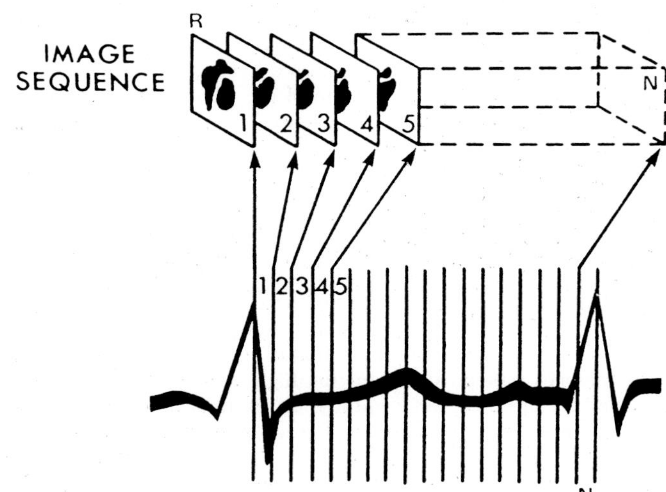

Figure 55–6. The method by which the computer generates multiple-gated images. The cardiac cycle is divided into a preselected number of frames of equal duration. Scintigraphic data from successive beats are placed into separate parts of the computer memory, depending on the temporal relation of the scintigrahic data to the R wave marker (R). For each frame (1 … N), scintigraphic data from successive beats are accumulated until either a preset time is reached (e.g., 2 minutes for exercise scintigraphy) or the average cardiac image contains a predetermined number of counts (e.g., 200,000 counts for typical resting studies).

The time interval of each frame can be shortened or lengthened according to the application and the number of frames available to represent the cardiac cycle. Approximately 20 frames per cycle are required for accurate measurement of left ventricular ejection fraction (LVEF).[H1] If a system is limited to a few frames, these should be divided over the initial two thirds of the cardiac cycle to maintain high accuracy of ejection fraction. For detailed analysis of the activity versus the time curve, as for accurate assessment of ejection and filling velocities, more frames are required for each cardiac cycle (e.g., 64 to 100 frames).[H2]

An important aspect of multiple-gated acquisition is that the gating signal accurately represents the onset of systole (truly end-diastole). Potential problems with achieving this accurate representation include the following: gating on noise, which results from a faulty electrode connection or electrical interference, rather than on the R wave; gating on the P or T wave, which may be of larger amplitude than the R wave in some disease states; gating on an atrial pacing spike; and delayed onset of mechanical systole caused by left bundle branch block (LBBB). These problems can usually be prevented by evaluating the resting ECG and the relationship of the R wave to the gating signal prior to commencing with the acquisition procedure.

Constancy of the interval between gating signals is important for high temporal resolution. This requires that either the cardiac rhythm is regular or that the computer compensates for fluctuations in the R–R interval. At least two computer techniques can compensate for rhythm or rate changes. The first is directed toward the problem of changing heart rates as seen during exercise. With this method, the time per frame automatically changes as a function of the average heart rate of the last few beats.[B4] The second technique, which requires a much larger computer memory and greater sophistication than the first, is designed to solve the problem of arrhythmia. In this method, part of the computer memory is used for transitory storage of the counts from only the last cardiac cycle. If the R–R interval of this cycle is not within a preselected range, the counts are discarded. If it is within this interval, the counts are used to update the images recorded from previous beats.[B5] A recent development in this technique has been the use of multiple R–R windows for each study. This allows a narrow window to be used for providing images with optimal temporal resolution at the same time that a broad window can be used to provide images with the maximum number of counts. This technique also permits reconstruction of the cardiac cycles of arrhythmic and compensating beats as well as that of the standard beat.[K1] Another development that helps to maintain correct temporal sampling is to synchronize the acquisition of scintigraphic data not only from the R wave forward in time, as explained earlier, but also from the R wave backward in time (Fig. 55–7). Some form of beat rejection or backward gating is needed for accurately synchronizing the last third of the cardiac cycle, required for the measurement of diastolic events.[B6]

Attention to the potential problems of gating is an important aspect of quality control for multiple-gated equilibrium scintigraphy. For assessment of R–R interval constancy, a computer program that provides a beat-length histogram (plot of the number of beats versus their cycle length) should be used. In this histogram, an ideal study is represented by a single narrow spike centered on the patient's cycle length, indicating little variation in the R–R interval (Fig. 55–8).

Proper selection of matrix type and size is another major consideration for acquisition and storage of multiple-gated equilibrium scintigraphic studies. In order to assess regional wall motion, the highest possible digital resolution with adequate counts per pixel should be achieved. Nevertheless, the greater the number of pixels, the less the counts per pixel. As a general rule, a minimum matrix size of 64 by 64 pixels is recommended for the accurate assessment of regional wall motion, whereas a matrix size of 32 by 32 pixels may suffice for ejection fraction and other parameters derived from activity-versus-time curves.

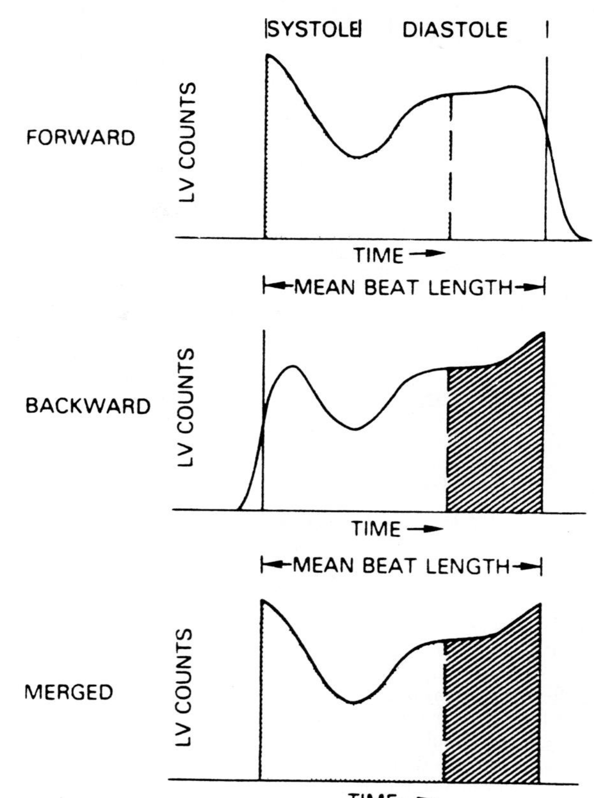

Figure 55–7. Reconstruction of cardiac cycle by framing acquired count events both forward and backward in time from the R wave. *Top panel* illustrates a left ventricular (LV) volume-time curve created by forward gating, exhibiting a trailing off in late diastole caused by fluctuations in cardiac cycle length. *Middle panel* illustrates a volume-time curve created by backward gating, exhibiting a trailing off in the systolic region. *Bottom panel* illustrates a curve in which the first two thirds of the top curve has been merged to the last one third of the middle curve, yielding a complete cardiac cycle with improved registration of the late-diastolic counts compared with the standard forward gating alone. (From Bacharach, S., et al.: Instrumentation and data processing in cardiovascular nuclear medicine: Evaluation of ventricular function. Sem. Nucl. Med. IX(4):269, 1979, with permission.)

Dynamic Imaging

FIRST-PASS ACQUISITION. Dynamic frame mode acquisition is similar to filming a movie of the heart. It is used when the radionuclide distribution is rapidly changing. The frame rate for this acquisition depends on the speed of this change and the frequency of the information that needs to be extracted. Thus, to analyze beat-to-beat changes from a first-pass study of a bolus of ^{99m}Tc, a fast frame rate is required. To analyze a change that takes place at a lower frequency, such as the transit time of the same bolus of ^{99m}Tc between cardiac chambers, a slow frame rate can be employed.

The number of frames per second is pre-selected. For example, acquisition of the first pass of a radionuclide bolus through the heart for assessing biventricular function should be acquired at a minimum of 20 frames/sec for 25 seconds and, ideally, 25 to 100 frames/sec for 60 seconds. This type of acquisition requires storage of at least 500 separate frames, necessitating a storage device other than computer memory. Magnetic disks can hold thousands of frames and can store the information efficiently, making them the storage media of choice. If the acquisition is being performed at 20 frames/sec, a frame is transferred to a disk every 50 msec.

After acquisition, the study is formatted into images of representative cardiac cycles for the right and left ventricles. The images of the two ventricles are distinguished by identifying the anatomic configuration and temporal appearance of the bolus as it passes through the central circulation. Regions of interest are assigned for each ventricle. Preliminary time-activity curves are generated from each ventricular region of interest. These time-activity curves consist of multiple peaks and valleys that correspond to end-diastolic and end-systolic frames of individual beats. These time-activity curves are used to generate representative

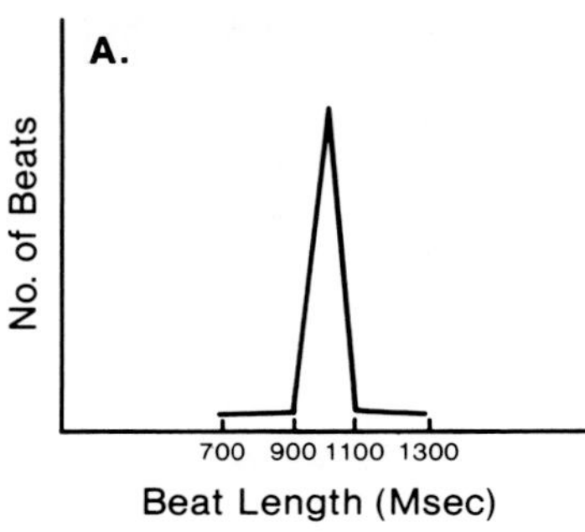

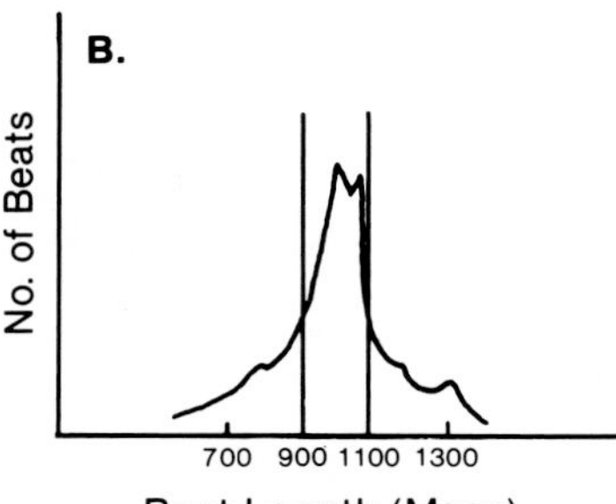

Figure 55–8. Examples of R-R histograms. Graph *A* is an example of an ideal R-R histogram of a patient with a stable heart rate (approximately 1 beat per second). Graph *B* is an example of a patient exhibiting significant beat-to-beat variations (between 800 and 1300 msec), which give rise to a poorly registered volume-time curve (*not shown*). The vertical lines through histogram *B* illustrate the potential in some systems of limiting the length of the beats accepted, thus resulting in a better registered (more accurate) volume-time curve at the cost of rejecting a significant number of beats.

cardiac cycles by utilizing the frames with the highest peaks as the starting points, summing all of them together, then summing together the next 50-msec frames of each cardiac cycle and then the next, and so on until end-diastole is again reached. This is done for the time-activity curve from the right ventricle and the left ventricle separately, which generates representative cardiac cycles for both the right and left hearts.

Another technique that aids in generating a representative cardiac cycle is to use the maximum of the first derivative of the time-activity curves as points of alignment.

First-pass studies can also be acquired at a slower frame rate of 2 frames/sec for adults in order to evaluate events that take place at a lower frequency. Such studies can be obtained either by acquiring the counts at that rate or by combining the frames from a study obtained at a higher frame rate. Thus a first-pass study used in assessing ventricular function obtained at 20 frames/sec can be converted to a study obtained at 2 frames/sec by combining every 10 frames into a single composite frame until an entire sequence of these 0.5-sec composite frames is created.

Using regions of interest over the different cardiac chambers, low-frequency time-activity curves are extracted. These low-frequency time-activity curves have a purpose in measuring transit times between the different chambers and in indicating the relative volume and flow of blood from each chamber. When combined with measurements of blood volume, these curves can approximate cardiac output. In addition, quantification of left to right shunts and regurgitant fractions is possible.

FIRST-PASS MULTIPLE-GATED ACQUISITION. The most common cardiac function study is multiple-gated equilibrium blood pool scintigraphy, in which the imaging is performed over several minutes. However, the same hardware and software can be applied to multiple-gated first-pass studies.[G2] In this approach, a bolus of radionuclide is injected intravenously. The computer is manually started when the bolus enters the right atrium and is stopped when the tracer clears the right ventricle (RV). A similar process is repeated for the phase that images the left ventricle. During the time of imaging, changes of tracer concentration are ignored; thus, this process, too, is a form of static imaging. Because the right atrium overlaps the right ventricle in equilibrium studies, a first-pass study is the method of choice for measurement of right ventricular ejection fraction.[B7]

Planar Imaging in List Mode

The list (serial) mode is the alternative to frame mode acquisition. The principle here is that a portion of computer memory is reserved to keep a temporal list of each event that takes place. The list usually consists of one computer word (memory location) for each event describing the x,y coordinates of each scintillation, physiologic markers indicating each occurrence of an R wave trigger, and time markers every 1 to 10 msec as appropriate for the particular study. These data are reconstructed after acquisition, allowing the operator to have a choice of frame rate and matrix size and dynamic or static format. The main advantage is the flexibility of what can be done with the data after acquisition, whereas the main disadvantages are the large storage requirements and the time needed for reconstructing the cardiac images before a display is available or an analysis can be performed.

Equilibrium Studies

The list mode can be used to reconstruct cardiac images similar to those obtained from multiple-gated equilibrium acquisition.[B5] The reconstruction software program is similar to that of the acquisition program, which formats the multiple-gated images. The operator selects the number of frames per cardiac cycle, and the reconstruction program divides the calculated R–R interval by the number of frames to obtain the time per frame. Each R wave marker informs the program to incorporate the following counts on the first frame until enough time markers have been counted corresponding to the calculated time per frame. The subsequent scintigraphic data are then channeled to frame 2, and the process continues until the last time interval has elapsed or until the next R wave is encountered in the list.

An advantage of this approach is that R–R tolerance intervals can be easily assigned so that counts from ectopic beats outside of this window are not added to the cardiac cycle. This technique also allows for reconstruction of the cardiac cycle from the R wave both forward and backward in time. This option produces increased temporal resolution to the last third of the cardiac cycle, improving the calculations of diastolic events.

Because of these advantages, list mode acquisition with real-time reconstruction has been incorporated in some multiple-gated acquisitions.[B5] In this combined mode, counts from the last heart beat are acquired in list mode. These counts are examined in real-time to see if the last beat fell outside the preselected R–R interval. If it did, the beat is rejected; if it fell inside the preselected interval, the list mode buffer is formatted into frames using both forward and backward gating and the formatted frames are added to the composite images of the cardiac cycle.

First-Pass Studies

The list mode can also be used to acquire first-pass studies.[J1] The incorporation of R wave triggers, if acquired, enhances the temporal resolution of the reconstructed image of the representative cardiac cycle. This method is theoretically superior to using the ventricular time-activity curves themselves to synchronize the different beats, since these curves are contaminated by background interference and are affected by camera and computer performance. List mode acquisition of first-pass studies also allows the reformatting of the scintillation data into fast dynamic, slow dynamic, or gated first-pass studies.

TOMOGRAPHIC IMAGING

Tomographic imaging, or single-photon emission computed tomography (SPECT), in contrast to conventional planar imaging, yields slices of the heart without overlapping counts from radioactivity of neighboring slices or background tissue. This attribute results in an increase in *contrast resolution,* i.e., the ability to discern differences in tracer concentration in neighboring tissue. This increase in contrast resolution is advantageous in thallium imaging in which ischemic hypoperfused areas need to be separated from normally perfused myocardium. In circular rotational tomography, since the detector is forced to orbit far away from the patient at times, the increase in contrast resolution is accompanied by a decrease in spatial resolution. Figure 55–9 illustrates the difference between contrast and spatial resolution. In myocardial perfusion imaging, the increase in contrast resolution yielded by tomographic imaging is preferred over the higher spatial resolution yielded by planar imaging. Clinically, this improvement in contrast resolution translates into improved detection of perfusion defects that are less ischemic. This improvement is realized at the expense of an increase in technical difficulty, which requires, among other things, that the center of rotation of the camera's mechanical axis of rotation is aligned to the electronic axis representing the acquired projection and that the plane defined by the camera's crystal remains parallel to the axis of rotation during scanning.[W1]

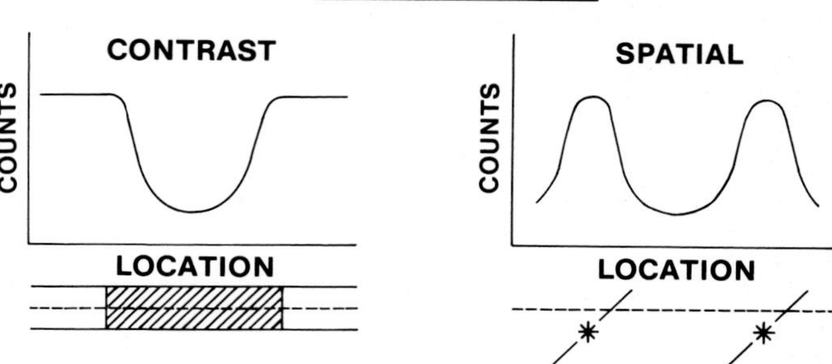

Figure 55–9. Diagram illustrating the differences in the definition of contrast resolution (resolution of differences in tracer concentration of neighboring myocardial walls) versus spatial resolution (resolution of two separate radioactive line sources). Curves represent count profiles extracted from corresponding radioactive distributions.

Acquisition of Projections

Most nuclear medicine single-photon emission computed tomography (SPECT) is performed with one gamma camera mounted on a gantry. This gantry allows rotation of the detector around the patient up to a full 360-degree angular sampling. The orbit of the detector can be either circular or elliptical. Elliptical orbits have the advantage of keeping the detector closer to the patient during rotation and, thus, preserving the spatial resolution lost by circular orbits when the detector occasionally is forced to image far from the patient.

The most widely used mode of tomographic acquisition is the step-and-shoot method. In this approach, the detector stops at pre-selected angles (32 to 128 times per 360 degrees). The detector acquires γ-rays (shoots) while it is stationary for a preselected period of time. When the time allotted for each projection is elapsed, it steps to the next angular position. While it is stepping, it is not recording events. This process is repeated until the total number of preselected projections is acquired.

The angular range that should be used in tomographic scanning of cardiac studies remains a source of disagreement. Some investigators insist that accurate, artifact-free reconstruction necessitates acquiring images from a full 360-degree orbit.[G3] Nevertheless, most of the groups using SPECT in clinical settings point out that 180-degree orbits (45° RAO to 45° LPO) yield, in half the acquisition time, higher contrast resolution than the 360-degree orbits that are contaminated by noise from a significant amount of attenuation for the projections acquired through the patient's back.[G4] This is particularly true for the low energy (80 keV) photons emitted by ^{201}Tl that are acquired using a single gamma camera system.

Image Reconstruction

BACK-PROJECTION. As discussed earlier, tomographic projections are a series of planar images taken at different angles around the patient. These images are then back-projected into transverse axial (or transaxial) images, which are slices that are inherently oriented perpendicular to the axis of rotation, which usually corresponds to the long axis of the patient. The transaxial images can then be re-oriented to produce sagittal, coronal, or oblique angle images. The back-projection algorithm is based on the fact that any photon that interacted with the camera crystal must have passed through one of the collimator holes, thus defining its direction. Since parallel hole collimators usually are used, the reconstruction algorithm back-projects or "sends back" the counts from their recorded location in the crystal, along a line perpendicular to the face of the crystal. These back-projected lines are recorded in the computer memory, which represents the three-dimensional space occupied by the object being imaged. Since the location where the emissions took place along this back-projected line is not included in the algorithm, the algorithm deposits the counts in each pixel traversed by the line. Tomograms are generated, since the back-projected lines cross at the locations where the radiation originated. Unfortunately, the parts of the lines that do not cross at the correct locations give rise to a star pattern, which blurs the image and reduces its contrast (Fig. 55–10).

FILTERED BACK-PROJECTION. The goal of tomographic reconstruction is to provide a blur-corrected transaxial tomogram from processed planar projections. The solution to this problem in frequency space involves the application of a Ramp filter (Fig. 55–11) to the frequency components of each projection. The reader is directed to reference G5 for an in-depth description of filtering in frequency space. Once filtered, each projection is

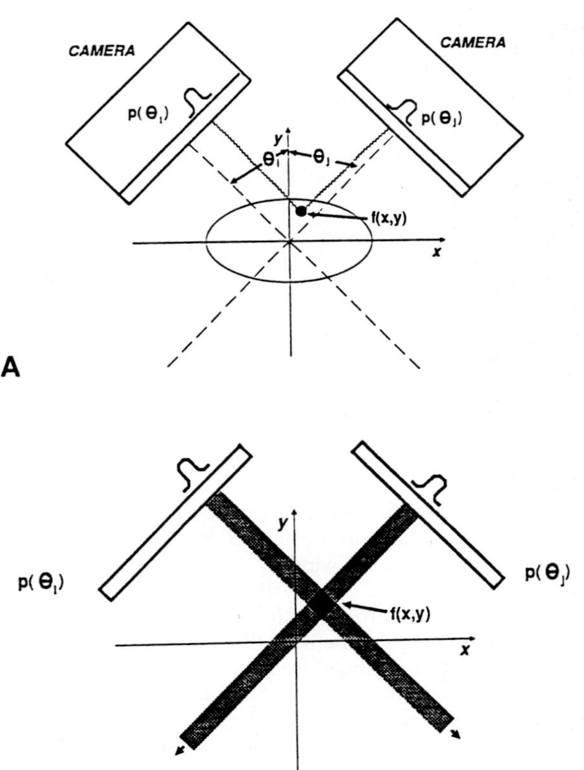

Figure 55–10. Principle of back-projection. *A,* The acquisition of two planar projections of a point source (f(x,y)) of radioactivity. *B,* The back-projection of these images. The back-projected counts are summed at the original source of activity, but counts are left in other parts of the image, resulting in star artifact. (Diagram courtesy of James Galt).

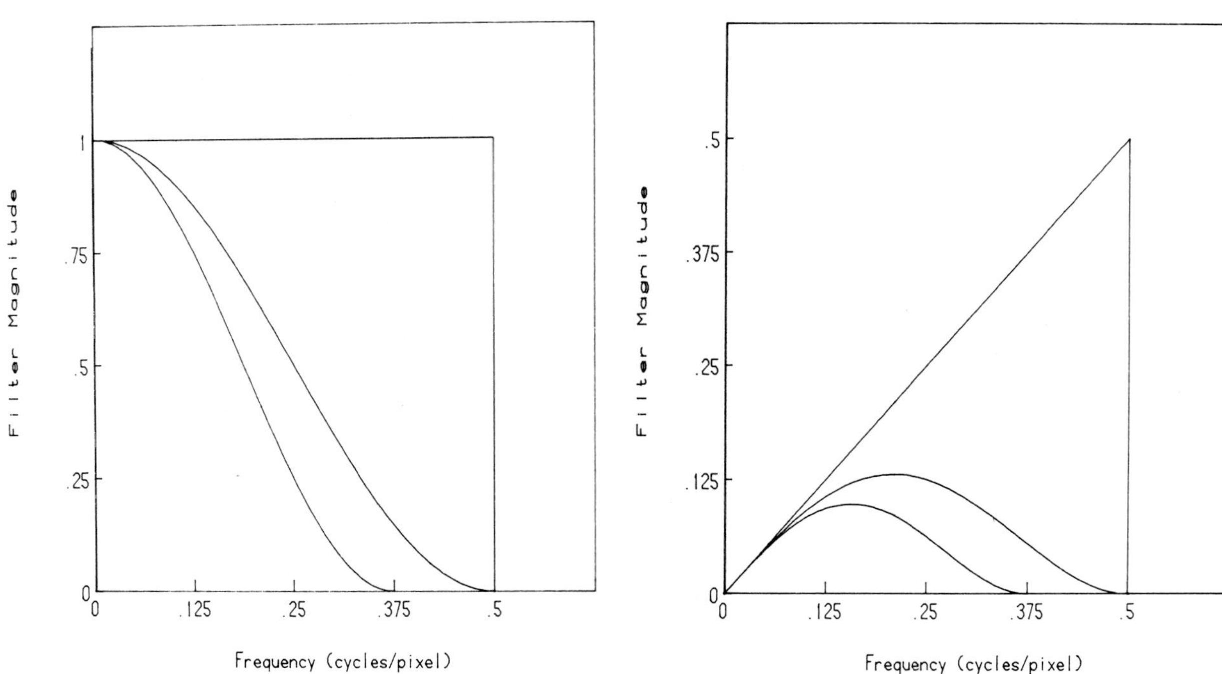

Figure 55–11. Curve representation of commonly used filters. *A*, Plot of filter amplitude versus frequency for a rectangular window, a Hanning filter with cutoff of 0.5 cycles per pixel, and a Hanning filter with cutoff of 0.375 cycles per pixel, filter windows. The same filters *(B)* were then multiplied by a Ramp filter and plotted as magnitude versus frequency.

transformed back into the conventional spatial domain and then back-projected to form the blur-corrected transaxial tomograms.

The Ramp filter, as shown in Figure 55–11, is a high-pass filter that enhances the edges of the radioactive distribution in the image. As its name suggests, the reconstruction process known as filtered back-projection may be thought of as, first, extracting the edges of a three-dimensional radioactive source from different angles and, second, back-projecting the edges from the different angles to generate the count distribution in a transaxial tomogram. Since it is a high-pass filter that linearly enhances higher frequencies, the Ramp filter yields the highest resolution possible in a reconstruction but also propagates, along the back-projected lines, the high-frequency noise associated with low-count statistics. This propagation of noise often results in clinically uninterpretable images.

FILTERING. The Ramp filter must be modified to compensate for the undesirable noise. This is done by combining the Ramp characteristics with those of a low-pass (smoothing) filter or window. Hanning and Butterworth filters are two commonly used windows that can be combined with a Ramp filter to yield different degrees of trade-off between reduction of statistical noise versus degradation of spatial and contrast resolution.

Figure 55–11*A* illustrates examples of a Rectangular filter, a Hanning filter with the cutoff frequency of 0.5 cycles per pixel and a Hanning filter with the cutoff frequency of .375, which may be used to modify or "window" the Ramp filter. When these windows are multiplied by the Ramp, the filter function then becomes those in Figure 55–11*B*. When this is done, the filter is referred to as a Ramp-Hanning filter for clarification.

Noise can also be removed from the final tomograms either by applying the smoothing filters to the planar projections prior to back-projection or afterward by filtering the transaxial slices. It is argued that filtering prior to back-projection is more desirable for two reasons. First, it reduces the propagation of noise at an earlier stage in the image formation process, and second, it promotes the implementation of a filter symmetric in three-dimensions (same resolution in the X, Y, and Z directions). Proponents of post-processing would argue that the same results could be obtained by careful selection of filters applied to the transaxial tomograms.

Factors Influencing Clinical Interpretation

It is generally assumed by clinicians interpreting tomograms from SPECT imaging procedures that the distribution of intensities (counts) that they observe is directly proportional to the radionuclide concentration. Thus, in interpreting a ^{201}Tl myocardial short-axis slice, it may be naively assumed that if the intensity of the septum is twice as bright as the lateral wall, then the septum has twice the concentration. Although this ability of extracting counts (brightness) directly proportional to the concentration of tracer is the ultimate goal of SPECT imaging, there are several limiting physical and technical factors. These factors not only affect the quantitative aspects of the reconstructed tomograms but also degrade the overall quality of the image. Methods of correction exist that compensate for these effects, some of which are commercially available and some which are being tested in experimental settings.

SCATTER CORRECTION. Scatter correction is the ability to compensate for photons that have undergone a Compton scattering event in the patient and have continued on to be recorded by the detector. These accepted scattered photons significantly degrade the image during the reconstruction process since they are back-projected along lines different from their original path.

There are two main approaches currently being investigated for determining the amount of scatter present: (1) determination of a scatter mask calculated from the projections or tomograms,[A2] and (2) determination of a scatter mask from counts acquired using a second (or more) pulse height analyzer (PHA) window.[J2] In the first approach, the scatter characteristics are measured a priori and are used to predict the scatter contribution. In the second approach, two PHA windows are used, one on the photopeak and another below it, defining the Compton scatter component of the photopeak. Once the scatter image mask is generated, it is then subtracted from the photopeak image, thus compensating for scattered photons.

The two above-mentioned methods have been shown to provide improvements in image contrast and quantification.[A2, J2] Nevertheless, to date, they remain largely investigational. The correction method used, although seldomly in cardiac studies, is one that assumes a lower than actual linear attenuation coefficient during attenuation correction so that the events that are scattered but not absorbed are not overcompensated.

ATTENUATION CORRECTION. Attenuation correction is the ability to compensate for photons that have been absorbed in the patient, never reaching the detector. Since activity located deeper in the body is attenuated more than activity near the surface, attenuation manifests itself in a transaxial slice by artifactually decreasing the counts near the center of the body. Moreover, in SPECT thallium tomograms, photon attenuation is responsible for generating artifactual defects in the anterior wall of women with large breasts or in the inferior wall of men with elevated diaphragms.

Currently, only methods that correct radionuclide distributions in a constant attenuation medium (such as the liver) are available clinically. The two methods most commonly used consist of the Sorenson pre-processing method and the Chang post-processing method.

In Sorenson's method, the length of the attenuating tissue traversed by each projection is either assumed or determined from the patient's transaxial body contour. A hyperbolic sine function of this attenuating length is then multiplied by the mean count value of the corresponding pixel of the 180-degree opposing projections.[S1] Some groups have reported the use of this approach for correcting ^{201}Tl SPECT studies,[G3] which necessitates acquisition of a 360-degree angular range.

In Chang's method, the patient's transaxial body contour is used to define the length of medium that attenuates each pixel in each projection. Each voxel (volume element) from the transaxial slice is corrected for attenuation by multiplying its reconstructed count value by the inverse of the average attenuation from all projections, measured from the voxel location to the body contour at each projection.[C1] As stated above, a linear attenuation coefficient lower than actual is routinely used to help compensate for scatter. The original method proposed by Chang was an iterative process in which the attenuation-corrected reconstructions are re-projected into planar projections. The differences between these re-projected planar projections and the originally acquired projections are used as error calculations to improve the previous estimation.

Unfortunately, these methods do not work well in the thorax since the heart is surrounded by tissue of varying density and, thus, of different attenuation coefficients such as found in the lung, the blood, and the spine. Accurate attenuation compensation in cardiac imaging requires that the methods used allow for the variable attenuation distribution surrounding the heart. Recently, investigators have shown that multiplicative methods inspired by the Chang approach may incorporate a map of the variable attenuation distribution surrounding the heart to significantly improve the quantitative estimation of regional tracer concentration.[G6, M1] To date, these approaches necessitate the use of an additional transmission scan in order to obtain the required variable attenuation distribution.

OBJECT SIZE CORRECTION. It has been shown for SPECT that even after scatter and attenuation correction, the pixel brightness (counts) recovered from reconstructed tomograms are dependent on the size of the object for objects smaller than two resolution elements (full width at half maximum) in any of its three dimensions.[G7, H2] This dependence limits the accuracy with which regional radionuclide distributions are derived from these objects. For example, in a ^{201}Tl myocardial short axis slice, if the septal wall is significantly thicker than the lateral wall and the tracer is uniformly distributed, the septum in the image appears hot in relation to the lateral wall. This may cause the clinician to interpret that the patient has a perfusion defect in the lateral wall.

To date, correction methods remain experimental and depend on either measuring or calculating a recovery coefficient as a function of object size. The object size is then independently estimated. Correction consists of multiplying the voxel count value by the appropriate recovery coefficient.[G7, H2]

UNIFORMITY CORRECTION. Most state of the art gamma cameras correct for differences in energy response from the different photomultipliers and for nonlinearities. Although these corrections are important in reducing field uniformity errors in planar projections, uniformity requirements for SPECT are more stringent and require further correction. The greatest sources of image nonuniformities in SPECT imaging are imperfect collimators. A local nonuniformity from a collimator is propagated in the reconstructed transaxial slice in the form of a circular or "ring" artifact since the same nonuniformity is back-projected at each angle of acquisition. The higher the number of acquired counts for that slice, the more prominent the artifact, since it rides above the random noise error. Thus, this correction is less important in SPECT that uses thallium, in which the number of counts per slice is low as compared with blood pool imaging. Also, the closer the local nonuniformity is to the axis of rotation, the higher the amplitude of the artifact, since the back-projected lines are closer together and there is more overlapping of the count values.

Uniformity correction for SPECT usually requires imaging a cobalt–57 (^{57}Co) flood source for 30 million counts in order to reduce the error due to nonuniformity to less than 1 percent.[R2] For this reason, it is important that the flood source used have a variation of radionuclide concentration of less than 1 percent. Normalization factors are determined from this image and applied to each of the projection views. Importantly, the 30 million count rule assumes that a matrix of 64 by 64 pixels is used to reconstruct a 1 million count slice. A matrix of 128 by 128 pixels requires four times the 30 million count flood in order to maintain the same variation. It is generally suggested that these floods be acquired to generate new normalization matrices once a week, as well as any time a different collimator is used, although actual need may vary according to the stability of the specific detector.

PATIENT MOTION DETECTION AND CORRECTION. Patient motion as small as half a voxel (3 mm) has been reported[E1, F1] to create ^{201}Tl SPECT image artifacts mimicking perfusion defects. The larger the motion, the greater the defect, particularly if it is abrupt and occurs halfway through the scan. Another type of motion artifact that has been reported is "diaphragmatic creep."[F1] This phenomenon occurs in patients after stress whose breathing patterns change drastically from deep to shallow during acquisition, allowing the heart to gradually "creep" upward in the chest. Because this motion is gradual and of small magnitude, it seldom leads to significant artifacts. It is also easily circumvented by delaying the start of acquisition for approximately 10 to 15 minutes after peak stress.

Patient motion of 3 mm is easily detected by inspection of the planar projections that are dynamically displayed in a movie format. Recently, computer algorithms have been developed that automatically detect and correct for patient motion, particularly vertical motion.[E1] These algorithms usually track either the entire myocardium or the center of mass of the myocardium from projection to projection. The shifts in the position of the heart are then reported to the operator on a projection-by-projection basis. The operator then decides whether or not to allow the computer to translate the image projections back to a fixed frame of reference. Although the motion detection algorithms are useful in flagging potential artifacts, the value of the methods of motion correction in eliminating artifacts is yet to be established.

TECHNETIUM–99m VERSUS THALLIUM–201. Another factor that influences image quality and thus image interpretation is the choice of radionuclide. Recently, ^{99m}Tc myocardial perfusion agents have been developed, most notably ^{99m}Tc Methoxy-IsoButil Isonitrile (sestamibi). A technetium perfusion agent has several imaging advantages over an agent containing ^{201}Tl. Compensation for variable attenuation correction in the thorax is more feasible with a monoenergetic, higher energy, technetium agent. Compensation for the myocardial ^{201}Tl distribution is difficult for two reasons: First, the 80-keV photopeak of ^{201}Tl, which is the most commonly used because of its high relative abundance compared with the other peaks, is associated with greater scattering, greater attenuation, and greater variability of attenuation coefficients across the thorax. Second, the ^{201}Tl spectrum exhibits several photopeaks, including 135 and 167 keV, and down-scattered photons from these peaks that fall in the pulse height analyzer window corresponding to the 80-keV photopeak make the atten-

Table 55–1. SPECT MYOCARDIAL IMAGING CHARACTERISTICS OF ^{201}Tl VERSUS ^{99M}TC MIBI

	^{201}Tl (3.5 mCi)	^{99m}Tc (15 mCi)
Spatial resolution (mm)	19	15
Relative sensitivity		
Stress	1.0	1.6
Delayed/rest	.5	1.5
% Scattered counts	40	22
Average attenuation	4.9	3.8
Correction factor		

uation compensation problem even more difficult. In addition, the ideal energy of ^{99m}Tc for imaging yields both a higher spatial resolution and a more favorable radiation dosimetry. The higher spatial resolution not only improves image quality but also reduces the effects produced by object size, which is a function of finite spatial resolution. The favorable radiation dosimetry, which in part is due to a shorter half-life (6 hours versus 73 hours for ^{201}Tl) allows the administration of up to 30 mCi of ^{99m}Tc sestamibi compared with the maximum dose of ^{201}Tl of 3.5 mCi. This higher dose leads to more counts per image and thus reduced statistical image noise. Table 55–1 illustrates the imaging superiority of the ^{99m}Tc sestamibi perfusion agent over ^{201}Tl. Figure 55–12 shows the superior image quality of ^{99m}Tc sestamibi versus ^{201}Tl tomograms in the same patient.

Multiple-Gated SPECT

Many commercial nuclear medicine computer systems now have the capability of acquiring and reconstructing multiple-gated tomographic studies. This feature has promoted studies investigating the use of SPECT for assessing cardiac global and regional function, including the assessment of myocardial wall thickening. These assessments have been primarily investigated using ^{99m}Tc red blood cell blood pool tomographic imaging,[M2] and using tomographic imaging of the ^{99m}Tc-Sestamibi perfused myocardial wall.[C1]

ACQUISITION AND RECONSTRUCTION. Acquisition consists of performing multiple-gated acquisition at each of the planar projections for the same total time in each projection. These acquisitions are usually obtained at 1 minute or less per projection so as to confine the entire study to within 30 minutes to an hour. Because of both the short amount of time for acquisition per projection and the consideration of reconstruction times, the number of frames per cardiac cycle are kept to a minimum, i.e., between 8 and 16 frames. The reconstruction process is the same as that for non-gated SPECT except that each of the frames per cardiac cycle have to be shuffled so that individual projection sets are created for each frame of the cardiac cycle. Thus, for example, if a multiple-gated SPECT study is acquired at eight frames per cardiac cycle, eight individual sets of projections are created and subsequently individually reconstructed. Once reconstructed into transaxial slices, each set is reconstructed along the same oblique angles in order to generate vertical, horizontal, and short-axis slices that have the same orientation from frame to frame. Once these oblique slices are generated, the program reshuffles each of the slices from each of the eight individual tomographic sets into sets of eight frames, which are multiple-gated tomographic slices that may be displayed in a closed-loop cine format for assessment of cardiac function. This same procedure is performed for either blood pool imaging or for imaging of the perfused myocardial walls (Fig. 55–13).

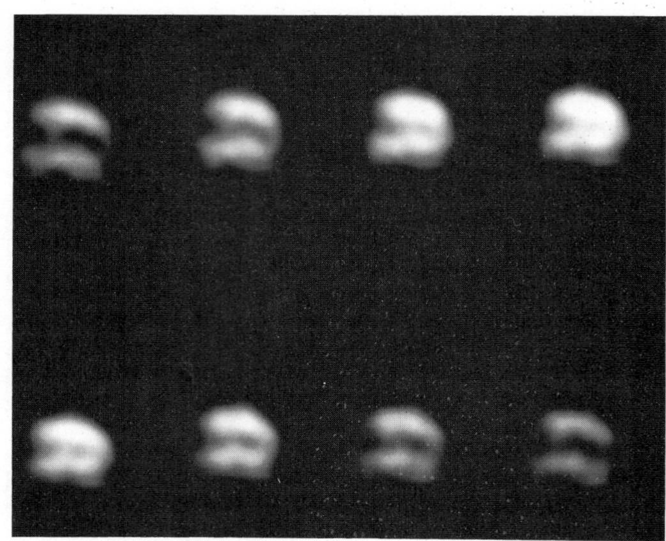

Figure 55–13. Technetium–99m MIBI multiple-gated myocardial SPECT mid–vertical long-axis slice. Eight frames are displayed throughout the cardiac cycle from end-diastole *(top left)* to end-systole *(top right)* back to end-diastole *(bottom left)*. Note that apical perfusion defect, which is obvious at end-diastole, disappears at end-systole. Also note that walls become brighter as the myocardium contracts and thickens.

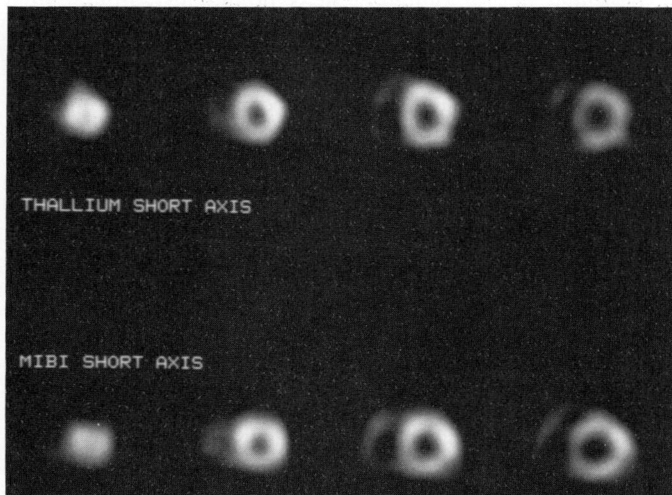

Figure 55–12. Comparison of thallium–201 (^{201}Tl) myocardial short-axis slices *(top)* and corresponding technetium–99m (^{99m}Tc) MIBI slices *(bottom)* in the same normal patient. Note the superior image quality of the ^{99m}Tc MIBI tomograms. These four representative short-axis slices are arranged from apex (left) to base.

TECHNICAL ASPECTS OF QUANTIFYING CARDIAC PARAMETERS

Assessment of cardiac performance is markedly enhanced by a quantitative description of the specific physiologic parameters evaluated by scintigraphic images. Quantification enables objective interpersonal comparison and objective assessment of cardiac status in a single patient over time or as a result of intervention. Furthermore, computer algorithms that enhance the images, extract parameters of cardiac performance, and define criteria for normality and abnormality have the potential to be precisely described. These algorithms can then be widely disseminated to promote standardization of image interpretation. More importantly, these algorithms can stand as a foundation from which specific criticisms can be assessed and into which improvements can be readily incorporated.

Cardiovasuclar nuclear medicine techniques are inherently quantitative. This is because the pixel count value from within a cardiac region is related to some parameter of cardiac performance. In the case of planar equilibrium blood pool studies, in which the radionuclide concentration is assumed to be constant, the pixel count value from a region within the heart is related to chamber volume. In case of myocardial perfusion imaging, in which the volume is assumed to be constant, the pixel count value from a region is related to the concentration of the radionuclide and, thus, blood flow.

In this section, digital image processing techniques developed for quantifying myocardial perfusion and ventricular function are reviewed. Many of the techniques illustrated reflect computer methods developed either at Cedars-Sinai Medical Center or at Emory University.

Quantification of Myocardial Perfusion

Sequential ^{201}Tl scintigraphy following injection at peak exercise is a useful noninvasive method for detecting and evaluating patients with significant coronary artery disease (CAD). Visual interpretation of analog ^{201}Tl images is subject to substantial variability, even when performed by experienced observers.[T2] This approach is further limited by the interpreter's dependence on the quality of the hard copy output and inability to accurately compensate for background activity or attenuation. Finally although the myocardial ^{201}Tl regional washout characteristics contain important diagnostic information, these can be difficult to detect by visual inspection.

Several approaches have provided significant contributions to the quantitation of the initial distribution and washout of myocardial ^{201}Tl both from planar scintigraphic projections[B8, G8, M3, W4] and tomographic sections.[C3, D1, G4, V2] The purpose of this section is to discuss the steps involved in quantitation of stress-redistribution ^{201}Tl planar and tomographic studies.

Planar Methods

BACKGROUND SUBTRACTION. Background is an important consideration because it degrades the contrast of perfusion defects and contaminates the measurement of the washout of ^{201}Tl from the myocardium with the clearance from overlapping tissue.[G9, G10, W4] Interpolative background subtraction provides the most satisfactory approach, since it compensates for nonuniformity in background distribution, which changes spatially and as a function of time in the delayed images. Therefore, methods that do not correct for "tissue crosstalk"[B8, V2] or those that use the subtraction of a constant background[V1] appear to be inadequate.

In the approach used by the Cedars-Sinai Quantitative Thallium Programs (Cedars-Sinai Medical Center), each image is compensated for tissue crosstalk by performing bilinear interpolative background subtraction, as described by Goris and coworkers.[G9] For this purpose, a rectangular boundary enclosing the heart is positioned by the computer operator approximately four pixels away from the myocardium. The pixels defining the rectangle are used as the origin of background. Each pixel outside the rectangle is set to 0, and each pixel inside the rectangle is corrected by subtracting from it the weighted average of the four pixels falling in the rectangle with a common Cartesian coordinate of the point being modified. The average is weighted in relation to how close to each of these four pixels the point being corrected is located. Thus if it is exactly equidistant it is a simple average. The program at Cedars-Sinai Medical Center uses a modification of this proximity weighting function, first described by Watson and associates,[W4] which produces a more rapid fall-off of the computed tissue crosstalk. Without this more rapid fall-off (and sometimes even with it), interpolative background subtraction tends to over-subtract in myocardial regions close to where the rectangle crosses areas of high uptake, such as the liver. This over-subtraction may result in artifactual perfusion defects or washout measurements.

More recently, several investigators have reported on the use of different methods of interpolative background subtraction,[D2, L3] designed for use mostly in blood pool studies. There is no consensus that any one method is better than another.[D2] Nichols[N1] reported on the use of irregular rather than rectangular regions as the source of background. Leidholdt and coworkers[L3] reported on the use of polygonal matrices of 12 vertices surrounding the heart. Chesler[O1] used all of the pixels outside a user-defined ellipse to correct each of the points inside the ellipse. All of these irregular region approaches are important improvements in cases in which a rectangle is forced to cross a high-count background away from the heart. This is particularly true when correcting for tissue crosstalk in resting ^{201}Tl studies, in which the background counts are considerably higher than in stress studies.

SMOOTHING FILTERING. Smoothing serves two purposes. First, it improves statistical accuracy, which varies in low information density scintigraphic studies. Second, the algorithm, which searches radially for the myocardial sample, looks for one pixel with the maximum counts. In order that this pixel be more representative of a larger segment of the myocardium, smoothing is necessary. The approach used at Cedars-Sinai Medical Center employs simple spatial smoothing by a 9-point weighted average that uses a 3×3 convolving kernel with weights of 4 in the center, 1 in the diagonals, and 2 elsewhere. Other investigators have also used unweighted 5-point smoothing. Although the 9-point weighted smoothing has been found to be effective when applied to stress-redistribution images, it might not be enough for resting studies, which have even lower count densities. In such cases, the application of Fourier filtering[M3] could offer better image enhancement.

GENERATION OF CIRCUMFERENTIAL PROFILES. Several methods have been developed for extracting the regional count distribution from ^{201}Tl images. The program at Cedars-Sinai Medical Center employs maximum-count circumferential profiles. For this purpose, profiles are generated of the maximum counts per pixel along each of 60 radii spaced 6 degrees apart and plotted clockwise. These profiles quantitate the segmental activity as an angular function referenced from the visually located center of the LV cavity (Fig. 55–14). This also could be located by automatic determination of the geometric center of the myocardium.[R3] The operator also assigns the maximum and minimum radius to which the computer is to search, to prevent the algorithm from searching outside the myocardium.

The choice of maximal rather than average or total counts was

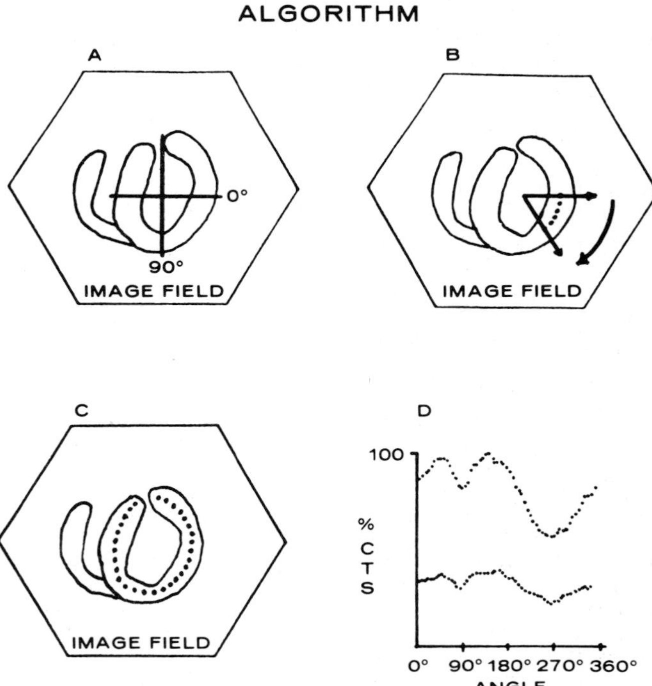

Figure 55–14. Method for obtaining circumferential profiles of the myocardium. Coordinate reference axis is shown in *A*. Image pixels for circumferential profile analysis are found by performing radial search for maximum count (cts) value at 6 degree intervals (*B*) through 360 degree intervals. Maximal values shown as black dots in *B* and *C* are then plotted in *D* for each angle as a percentage of the maximum value for the circumferential profile. *Top curve* in *D* represents circumferential profile from stress ^{201}Tl image; *bottom curve* represents that from the 4-hour delayed image.

based on the work of Vogel and associates,[V3] who determined that maximal count circumferential profiles provided the most accurate measure of abnormality. Furthermore, the use of average counts in circumferential profile analysis has been found to be less sensitive than visual interpretation.[B8] Several available algorithms allow the user to choose different methods of assigning counts to the circumferential profile. Chesler used the mean counts in three (or more) pixels that define the myocardial regions.[O1] These regions are defined as the area between an inner and an outer ellipse surrounding the myocardium.

The profiles are aligned so that the apex in each view is assigned to 90 degrees. Apex alignment is valuable[B8] for partially correcting for a variation in the position of the heart. This alignment is particularly important, since the lower limits or normal profiles vary for the different angular locations in each view. For example, if in a normal study the apex was misaligned, this region, which characteristically has the fewest counts, might fall below the lower limits of normal, causing a false abnormality. Therefore, methods that use lower limits of normal without proper alignment are limited. Apex alignment is also important when performing washout or reversibility calculations in which one curve is operated by another curve and each angle has to correspond region by region.

In the approach used at Cedars-Sinai Medical Center, the computer automatically shifts that point in the circumferential profile identified as the apex to coincide with 90 degrees. Profiles are subsequently plotted for each view at each time interval. These distribution curves are normalized to the maximum pixel value found in either the stress or delayed profile (see Fig. 55–14D). Watson and colleagues[W4] and Chesler[O1] aligned the stress and redistribution images themselves rather than the count profiles. This is done by an iterative translation of the position of the delayed images until the cross-correlation coefficient between the two images is maximized.

GENERATION OF WASHOUT RATE PROFILES. Different methods have been developed to quantitatively assess regional myocardial ^{201}Tl content change over time. The approach used at Cedars-Sinai Medical Center employs washout circumferential profiles, calculated as percentage washout from stress to the approximately 4-hour redistribution time. Figure 55–15 demonstrates the manner in which each point on the washout rate profile is calculated. As shown, despite regional count variation at the time of stress and 4-hour redistribution, percentage of regional washout rate of ^{201}Tl is fairly uniform from all myocardial regions.

The mean effective half-life of ^{201}Tl in the myocardium for stress-redistribution studies by this technique, assuming a monoexponential net washout (3.97 $\pm$ 1.3 hour), was in excellent agreement with the values reported by Watson and associates.[W5] The main difference between these methods is that the approach discussed here recommends imaging at 4 hours instead of 2 hours after injection, allowing for a greater degree of washout to occur, and that the algorithm automatically calculates washout for each 6-degree location in each view, as opposed to automatically sampling a limited number of preselected myocardial locations.

By assuming a monoexponential washout, difficulty was encountered in extrapolating the 4-hour percentage washout normal limit profile to less than 2.5 hours or greater than 6 hours. Patients with imaging delay of less than 2.5 hours tended to have falsely normal washout, and those with greater than 6 hours tended to have falsely abnormal washout. It has been shown that the normal patient population behaves as though it exhibited a multiexponential washout. These results indicate that, between 3 and 7 hours, the mean half-life is 12.2 hours.

The amount of washout that takes place in patients injected at rest has also been studied. These preliminary results suggest that regional myocardial percentage of washout of ^{201}Tl is much slower than that observed after injection at peak exercise.[M4]

Reversibility analysis is an additional technique that offers promise for better differentiation between infarcted and ischemic regions. Patients with significant CAD but no myocardial infarction usually demonstrate the pattern of reversible relative hypoperfusion (redistribution). In this phenomenon, a perfusion defect seen in the immediate post-stress images "fills in" and disappears by the time of delayed imaging. Vogel and coworkers[V2] implemented a quantitative method for analyzing reversibility. They normalized the highest point in each of the stress and delayed maximal count circumferential profiles. The patient showed reversibility if a profile that showed a defect at stress, below normal limits, significantly improved during delayed imaging. We further developed this technique for planar analysis[A3] by scaling the stress distribution to the delay profile so that the normal areas, defined by the stress distribution and washout, were superimposed. Watson and associates[W4] and Chesler[O1] also displayed functional images that help to visually assess reversibility. In Chesler's approach, normal segments that show no change between initial and delayed images are displayed in red. Abnormal segments that exhibit redistribution are shown in green and infarcted segments are shown in black.

Washout and reversibility occur for the same physiologic reason: the amount of thallium leaving the myocardium compared with the amount entering it (net washout) is less in an ischemic than in a normal myocardial segment. Nevertheless, the mechanisms for detection are technically quite different. Washout analysis is an absolute (spatially nonrelative) measurement that does not require a normal reference segment in the view to detect an abnormality. Since it is an absolute measurement, it is associated with a wide variation of normal responses and, thus, a large standard deviation around the mean normal response. Reversibility analysis is a relative measurement that does require a normal reference segment in the view to detect an abnormality. Because it is a relative measurement, it is associated with less of a variation in the normal response and, thus, less error. Wackers and coworkers have pointed out that localized drops in the washout rate profiles are an indication of a reversible segment.[W6] The incorporation of reversibility analysis to differentiate ischemic from infarcted myocardial segments may provide an improvement in such assessments.

ESTABLISHMENT OF NORMAL LIMITS. Once stress-

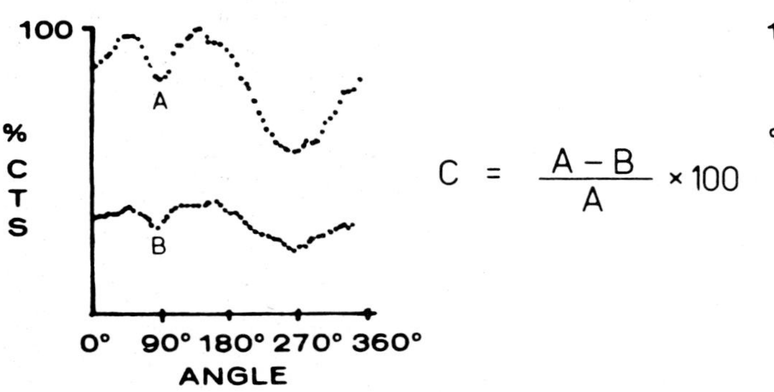

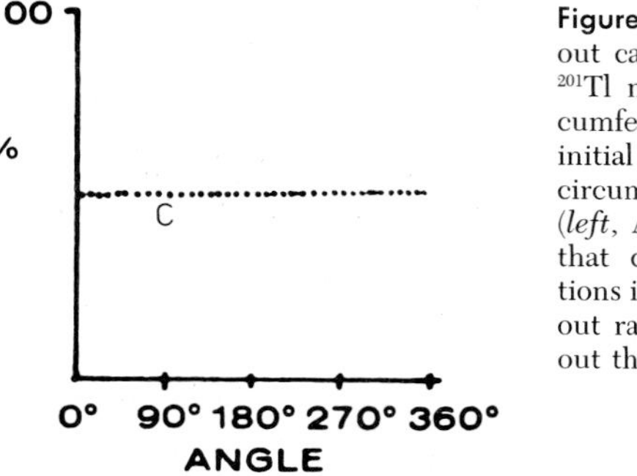

Figure 55–15. Percentage of washout calculation. Generation of the ^{201}Tl myocardial washout rate circumferential profile (*right*, C) from initial and 4-hour redistribution circumferential count (cts) profiles (*left*, A and B, respectively). Note that despite inter-regional variations in thallium counts, ^{201}Tl washout rate is fairly uniform throughout the myocardium.

redistribution regional count and washout profiles have been generated, some method of determining whether they are normal or abnormal must be employed. The approach used at Cedars-Sinai Medical Center incorporates lower limits of normal circumferential profiles generated from patients with a less than 1 percent pretest likelihood of having CAD.[G8] This approach avoids the pitfalls of using patients with normal coronary arteriograms who may have nonatherosclerotic ischemic disease.[M5, P1] Furthermore, it allows the use of age-matched controls, which if attempted with normal volunteers may result in inclusion of an unacceptable proportion of patients with occult coronary disease. The mean value and standard deviations were established from the pooled data of these patients for each of the 60 angular locations in the anterior, 45-degree, LAO, and steep LAO images for each time interval. The time between the stress and redistribution imaging, if other than the 4-hour limit, was used to extrapolate the washout profile to exactly 4 hours.[G8] The lower limits of normal for the stress and washout profile were established as the profile 2.5 standard deviations below the mean observed profiles. Alternative approaches have used a threshold for detection of perfusion defects and the range of regional normal values as lower limit profiles.[W4]

DEVELOPMENT OF QUANTITATIVE CRITERIA FOR ABNORMALITY. The next step in the development of a quantitative method is to determine which type of mechanism is significant in detecting an abnormality and the extent to which this mechanism (profile) should fall below normal limits before the patient is considered abnormal. In the Cedars-Sinai Medical Center approach, a pilot group of normal and CAD patients was used to establish these criteria.[G8] This algorithm compared each patient's stress and washout profiles against the lower limits of normal. The program identified any arc of the profile that fell below normal limits. Different quantitative criteria for type and magnitude of abnormality were assessed in all patients in this pilot group for their ability to best differentiate between normal and CAD patients. The following criteria best distinguish each population:

1. A "stress defect" was defined for any 18-degree segment (three contiguous radii) of this stress profile falling below normal limits.
2. A "slow-washout" abnormality was defined by any 18-degree segment of the washout profile falling below normal limits.
3. To be considered abnormal, the patient needed at least two abnormal 18-degree arcs in the combined stress and washout rate profiles in three views.

COMPUTERIZED DISPLAY OF RESULTS. Once the patient's study has been analyzed, it is important that the results be displayed in a concise but comprehensive report. Figure 55–16 demonstrates an example of the computerized quantitative display of the results that have recently been developed by Van Train and associates.[V4] The stress and washout profiles in this patient with CAD were compared with the established normal limits. Using the above-mentioned criteria, myocardial regions with a stress-perfusion defect or a slow-washout abnormality were identified. Findings were then displayed on concentric ellipses in all three planar views. In each view, the inner ellipse is the diagrammatic representation of the myocardium in that view, the border of different myocardial regions being shown as small break points on this ellipse. The missing portions of the middle ellipse demonstrate the presence of stress-perfusion defects. The missing portions of the outer ellipse indicate the presence of a slow-washout abnormality. These abnormalities are listed according to view and location in the lower right of the written report. The concentric ellipse display not only facilitates interpretation of a given case as normal or abnormal but also aids in assignment of abnormalities to specific myocardial regions.

Another method for displaying quantitative results has been described by Reiber and coworkers.[R3] With this method, the location, extent, and type of abnormality is presented in a functional image. To this end, for each radial line, it is determined whether the stress, redistribution, and washout profile values are normal or abnormal. The outcomes are then compared with the entries of a decision table to define the type of abnormality for that particular radial line.

Comprehensive computerized quantitative approaches to the analysis of the regional stress myocardial distribution and washout

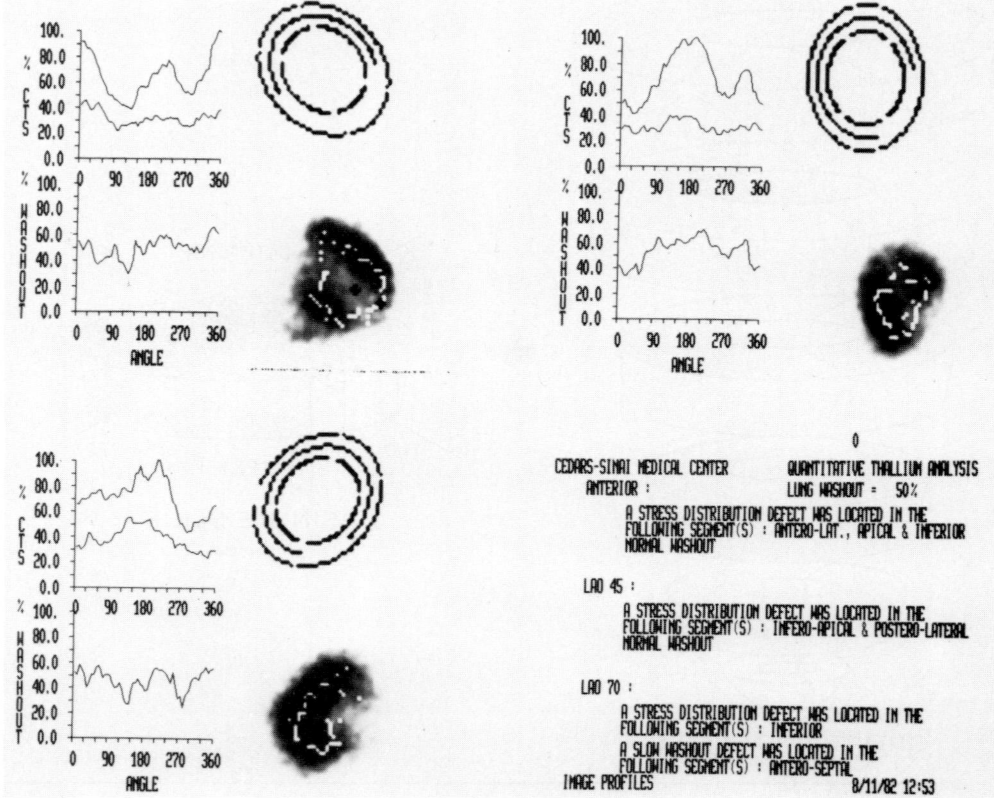

Figure 55–16. Computerized display of the quantitative, planar, stress-washout ^{201}Tl interpretation in a patient with coronary artery disease, exhibiting multiple regions with perfusion defects and slow-washout abnormalities. LAO—left anterior oblique projection. *Top left panel*: Anterior results. *Top right panel*: Mid (45-degree) LAO results. *Bottom left panel*: Steep (70-degree) LAO results. *Bottom right panel*: English report.

rate of ^{201}Tl have been developed. These methods minimize many of the problems associated with the subjectivity of visual analysis of ^{201}Tl scintigrams. In addition, the quantitative techniques have been shown to be more accurate than visual interpretation of images for detection and localization of coronary artery disease.[M6]

Tomographic Methods

Preliminary investigations have suggested that rotational myocardial tomography following injection of ^{201}Tl at peak exercise offers significant improvement over planar scintigraphy for the detection and localization of myocardial ischemia.[G11, M7] Rotational ^{201}Tl tomography at rest has also been reported to be better than planar imaging for detection and localization of myocardial infarction and for estimating the extent of infarcted myocardium.[R4, T3] Several investigators[D1, G4, T4] have used extensions of the planar quantitation concept to quantify the three-dimensional distribution of ^{201}Tl in the myocardium at stress and redistribution from rotational tomograms. These algorithms express the percentage of the myocardium that is involved with perfusion defect, washout abnormality, and reversible abnormality.

PROTOCOL. In the approach implemented at Emory University,[D1] the patient undergoes the same exercise protocol described for planar imaging, with the exception that a thallium dose of 3.5 mCi is used. Acquisition consists of obtaining 32 projections for 40 seconds, each over the 180-degree arc extending from the 45-degree right anterior oblique to the 45-degree left posterior oblique projection. Each of the 32 projections are corrected for field nonuniformity and for misalignment of the mechanical center of rotation with respect to the reconstruction matrix. The projections are prefiltered prior to back-projection by using a Hanning filter with a cutoff frequency of 0.82 cycles/cm. Filtered back projection is then performed to reconstruct the transverse axial tomograms (of 6.25 mm each) encompassing the entire heart. Oblique tomograms parallel to the vertical and horizontal long axis and the short axis of the left ventricle are extracted from the filtered transaxial tomograms by performing a coordinate transformation with appropriate interpolation.[B10] The tomograms are reconstructed without scatter or attenuation correction owing to the difficulties involved in correcting for the variable attenuation of ^{201}Tl 80-KeV x-rays through the thorax. These effects are accounted for in part by a comparison of each patient's thallium distribution with distribution files of normal patients who exhibit similar effects.

THREE-DIMENSIONAL QUANTIFICATION—EMORY UNIVERSITY APPROACH. The short slices to be quantified are selected by an operator following a strict protocol. Using the long-axis slice with the longest cavity length, the operator selects the short-axis cuts for quantification to extend from the base of the left ventricle (LV) to the apical cap. On the short-axis cut, falling halfway between the apex and base, the operator then defines the center of the LV cavity and the radius of search (Fig. 55–17*B*). The maximal count circumferential profiles (CPs) for each short-axis cut are then generated automatically from the most apical to the most basal cut, as shown in Figure 55–18*A*. The actual raw counts are extracted and used without normalization. This procedure is performed for each stress and each delayed tomographic study. Percent washout CPs are also calculated, using the profiles of the corresponding anatomic cut at stress and delayed tomography, respectively.

In Figure 55–17*A*, alternating short-axis slices of the left ventricle are displayed from base to apex. Approximately 12 slices are obtained from a normal-sized heart. In this example, there is a defect in the septum, which is highlighted in the middle slice. In Figure 55–17*B*, this slice has been divided into 40 sectors of 9 degrees each. The septum is represented by the sectors from 90 degrees to 180 degrees. The maximal counts per pixel (mcp) within each sector is determined. In Figure 55–18*A*, these 40 values have been plotted as a circumferential profile of the mcp versus angular location. A similar profile is constructed for each slice, except for the first two containing the apex, which are represented by a single value representing the mcp within the entire slice. To take into account variations in the number of slices per study these curves are interpolated to produce a total

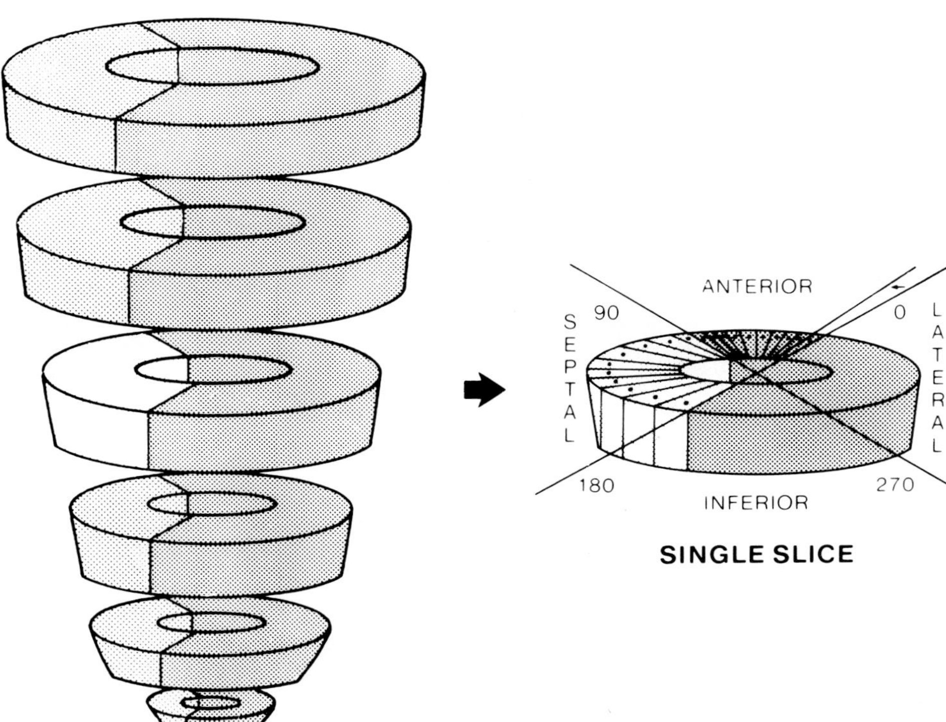

Figure 55–17. Method for obtaining circumferential profiles from tomographic slices. *A*, Alternating short-axis slices of the left ventricle are displayed. A septal defect is present from base to apex. *B*, The highlighted middle slice is divided into 40 sectors, each 9 degrees.

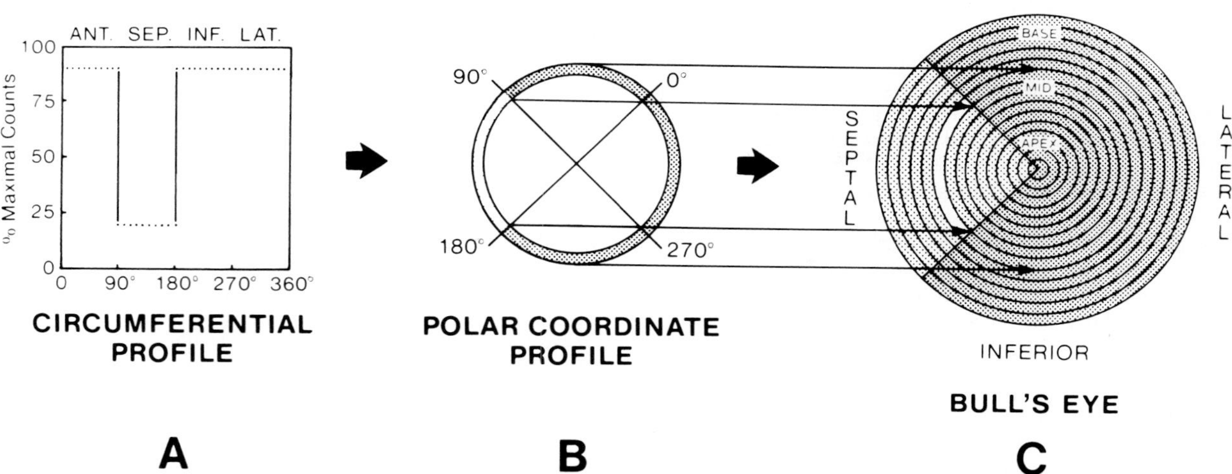

Figure 55–18. Method for obtaining bull's eye polar maps. *A*, The maximal counts per pixel for each sector are plotted as a circumferential profile. Similar profiles are constructed for each slice. *B*, The rectangular coordinate profiles are converted into a polar coordinate profile, which displays the curve as a circle composed of 40 pixels. *C*, The polar coordinate profiles are displayed as a polar map (bull's eye) with the apex at the center and the base at the periphery.

of 15 profiles. Each of the rectangular coordinate profiles is translated into a polar coordinate profile (see Fig. 55–18*B*), which displays the curve as a circle composed of 40 pixels. In Figure 55–18*C*, these data are displayed as a polar map called a bull's eye plot, which consists of a series of 15 concentric circles with the apex at the center and the base at the periphery. Individual bull's eyes are constructed for the stress and delayed images as well as for percent washout. The bull's eyes from a patient with myocardial hypoperfusion in the inferior and inferolateral walls are displayed in Figure 55–19. In this display format, the stress and delay bull's eyes have been adjusted by multiplying each pixel in the delayed bull's eye by the ratio of the mcp in the stress bull's eye to the mcp in the delay bull's eye. Note the large anteroseptal defect at stress, which demonstrates marked redistribution in the delay bull's eye.

Figure 55–19. See Color Plate 14.

Normalization occurred only when the profiles were compared with the gender-matched normal files developed from the low probability of the disease group, in which the mean values and standard deviations (SD) were established from the pooled data for each of the angular locations in each of the 15 profiles.[E2] This was accomplished by dividing each bull's eye into four regions of 90 degrees each (anterior, septal, inferior, and lateral) from profiles 4 through 12 and determining the ratio of the average counts per pixel in each region of the patient's bull's eye to the same region in the appropriate normal file. The region with the highest ratio was assumed to be normal and each pixel in the patient's bull's eye was multiplied by the reciprocal of this ratio. The comparison of each individual patient's bull's eye to a gender-matched normal file resulted in the conversion of the bull's eye into a standard deviation map displaying pixels that were color coded to correlate with the number of SDs below normal (see Fig. 55–19). The pixels that fell below these limits were submitted to an analysis using clustering criteria that eliminated pixels without two adjacent abnormal neighbors from being displayed. These quantitative images were compared with the angiographic data of a pilot group of patients to determine the best criteria for identifying the presence and location of a significant coronary stenosis. This analysis resulted in establishing the profile curves representing 2.5 SD below the mean normal responses as the threshold for defect detection. The clustered profile points falling below this established normal limit are plotted in a "blackout bull's eye," in which the black region within the bull's eye plot defines the extent of the perfusion abnormality. The location, size, and shape of these blackout regions are used in conjunction with heuristic rules developed from a pilot group to identify the stenosed coronary artery associated with specific patterns of perfusion abnormality. Figure 55–20 illustrates the approximate location on a bull's eye plot of the regions perfused by specific coronary arteries.

Washout and reversibility bull's eyes are also generated. Similar to planar quantification, washout profiles are determined for each short-axis slice as the counts percent change from stress to delayed imaging. Before comparing the washout profiles with the corresponding normal profiles, the normal curves were adjusted to correspond to the same acquisition interval as the patient's study by moving the values in the normal curves along a monoexponential curve. Reversibility bull's eyes are generated by subtracting the stress profiles from the corresponding delayed profiles after normalizing to a 5-by-5 pixel maximal count reference area in the stress study. In addition to this reversibility bull's eye polar plot and the reversibility standard deviation bull's eye, a third polar plot is generated to easily display the application of the best single cutoff criterion determined (1.5 standard

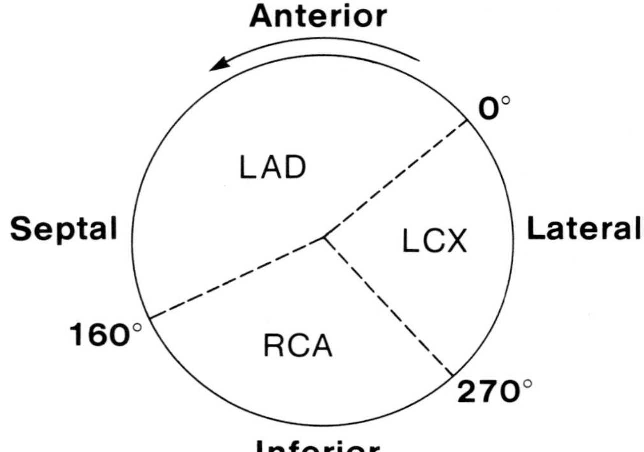

Figure 55–20. Coronary vascular territories corresponding to the bull's eye polar map. LAD—left anterior descending artery; LCX—left circumflex artery; RCA—right coronary artery.

deviations). This plot duplicates the stress blackout bull's eye plot but also includes the region that has reversed, by the time of delayed imaging, to a whiteout region, as determined from the application of normal limits and criteria for reversibility that have been developed (see Fig. 55–19).[K2, L4]

A numerical report accompanies this reversibility whiteout bull's eye map, which includes, for each defect, the extent (number of pixels) of both the stress-perfusion defect (blackout area) and the subregion (whiteout area) within the defect that reverses by 4 hours. A severity score is also reported as the sum of the number of SDs from the mean of the pixels in the stress map that have been blacked out and those in the reversibility map that have been whited out. These scores are determined for each defect. A reversal of 15 percent or more of the original stress defect has been determined to be a significant degree of reversibility.[K2]

OTHER APPROACHES. Other investigators have also used circumferential profiles to extract the initial ^{201}Tl myocardial distribution and washout rate. Tamaki and associates[T4] assessed the myocardium by using circumferential profiles from three short-axis sections and one middle RAO long-axis section. Other approaches differ in how the the CPs are normalized. Caldwell and coworkers[C3] scaled the CPs to a percentage of maximal counts in the entire left ventricular region of interest. In the method developed at Cedars-Sinai Medical Center,[G4] each profile is normalized to the maximum pixel value for that profile.

In the approach used at Cedars-Sinai Medical Center, the CP arcs between 60 and 120 degrees of each ventricle long-axis cut are mapped into the central region of the display to depict the apical ^{201}Tl distribution. Immediately surrounding the apical region, the entire CP corresponding to the most apical short-axis slice is mapped, with all the following short-axis CPs being mapped in increasingly larger circles until the most basal CP is reached. This approach helps to circumvent the partial volume effect at the apex inherent in the Emory approach. In the two-dimensional polar map used at Cedars-Sinai Medical Center, the size of the display always remains the same so the size of the LV is reflected by the number of CPs that are mapped. Thus in larger LVs, the band representing each slice is thinner compared with smaller LVs.

ASSESSMENT OF CORONARY ARTERY DISEASE. The severity of a perfusion defect in a thallium tomographic study may be judged objectively when patient data are compared with gender-matched normal files. Through clinical experience and comparison with coronary angiography,[D1] the investigators at Emory University have realized optimum accuracy in the diagnosis of coronary artery disease if only those bull's eye abnormalities that are 2.5 SD or more below normal limits are judged abnormal.

A number of important limitations and potential errors of this quantitative method must be emphasized. The bull's eye plot is dependent on an observer's correct selection of the apex and the base of the LV from oblique tomographic slices. If the slices extend too far past the actual base or apex, there is a rim of apparently decreased tracer concentration at the periphery of the bull's eye or a localized central defect near the apex, respectively. Recalling that the basal portion of the ventricle is relatively magnified in the bull's eye plot and that regions near the apex are extremely reduced in size, basal perfusion abnormalities appear larger than equivalent defects in the middle and distal portions of the LV. Furthermore, image artifacts resulting in decreased count density, such as attenuation by unusually large breasts or an elevated left hemidiaphragm, patient motion, and center of rotation errors, appear as defects in the bull's eye and are represented as abnormalities in the thallium score. Alterations in myocardial anatomy and symmetry also create relative abnormalities in patient data as compared with normal gender-matched files. An artifact of this type is commonly encountered in patients with hypertrophic cardiomyopathy in whom there is a disproportionate increase in thickness of the septum in addition to concentric myocardial hypertrophy. Since the highest count density is in the septum, the remainder of the ventricle appears relatively decreased in intensity and is judged to be abnormal when compared with normal files. Relative septal hypertrophy causes a marked abnormality to appear in the thallium score in all regions of the myocardium, with the exception of the septum.

With due consideration of the limitations in the quantitative analysis of thallium bull's eye plots, this method serves as a valuable tool for the determination of the severity of myocardial ischemia and the amount of myocardium at jeopardy in patients with CAD. In the experience at Emory University, a thallium score greater than 40 SDs represents a true perfusion defect. Patients with more severe and extensive CAD demonstrate more markedly abnormal thallium scores.

Applying the Emory University bull's eye quantitative technique to a prospective group of 210 patients (179 with and 31 without CAD) resulted in an overall sensitivity of 95 percent, a specificity of 74 percent, and an accuracy of 92 percent for detecting the presence or absence of CAD. The ability of this analysis to identify individual coronary stenoses is displayed in Figure 55–21 for each major coronary artery and for the left circumflex and right coronary arteries combined. The results of this prospective evaluation of the method demonstrate a high sensitivity and specificity for the detection of CAD in patients and in individual coronary stenoses.[D1] Although these results are encouraging, they are based on the manual measurement of percent diameter stenosis using digital electronic calipers on the coronary arteriogram as a gold standard and they include patients taking anti-anginal medications and do not specifically exclude patients with prior myocardial infarction, left ventricular hypertrophy, and coronary artery collaterals, which could significantly interfere with the sensitivity and specificity of the procedure. In particular, the use of percent diameter stenosis as a gold standard for assessing the physiologic significance of a region of coronary obstruction has been heavily criticized.[M8] As a consequence of these problems, additional studies that use more sophisticated gold standards and more carefully defined patient populations are necessary to further define the specificity and sensitivity of SPECT thallium perfusion images.

PRESENT LIMITATIONS OF SIZING. It is possible to approximate the percentage of the myocardium that is abnormal by using the methods described above. Of major prognostic importance is how accurately these calculations reflect the amount of myocardium that is in jeopardy or infarcted. Accuracy of sizing the percentage of abnormal myocardium is somewhat affected by cardiac and thoracic motion. This motion has been reported to account for overestimation of defect activity when quantifying infarct size[K3] or myocardial blood flow.[C4] This motion has also been reported by Kirsch and coworkers[K4] to be responsible for false-negative results in patients with small hearts and high ejection fractions or hypertrophy. Kirsch and associates also reported cardiac motion to result in false-positive findings in large hypertrophic hearts and in patients with cardiomyopathy. This distortion caused by motion nevertheless is considered to be small when compared with that caused by attenuation and scatter. As pointed out in previous sections, accuracy for sizing the percentage of abnormal myocardium is also affected by spatial resolution. It is likely that this dependence on the system's spatial resolution would tend to mask small nontransmural perfusion defects while it overestimates the size of transmural defects.

With respect to sizing of perfusion defects, Tamaki and colleagues[T3] used manual computer planimetry of the normal and infarcted regions applied to tomographic cross-sections to measure the infarct volume. Measurements obtained by this approach were compared with similar measurements using ^{201}Tl tomography for its ability to correlate with the accumulated creatinine kinase-MB (CK-MB) isoenzyme release. In spite of the limitations of ^{201}Tl tomography described above, the researchers found a better correlation with CK-MB release using manual computer planimetry of the reconstructed tomograms than with planar measurements. Although they are encouraging, these results need further verification with gold standards that have less problems than those of CK-MB in predicting infarct size.

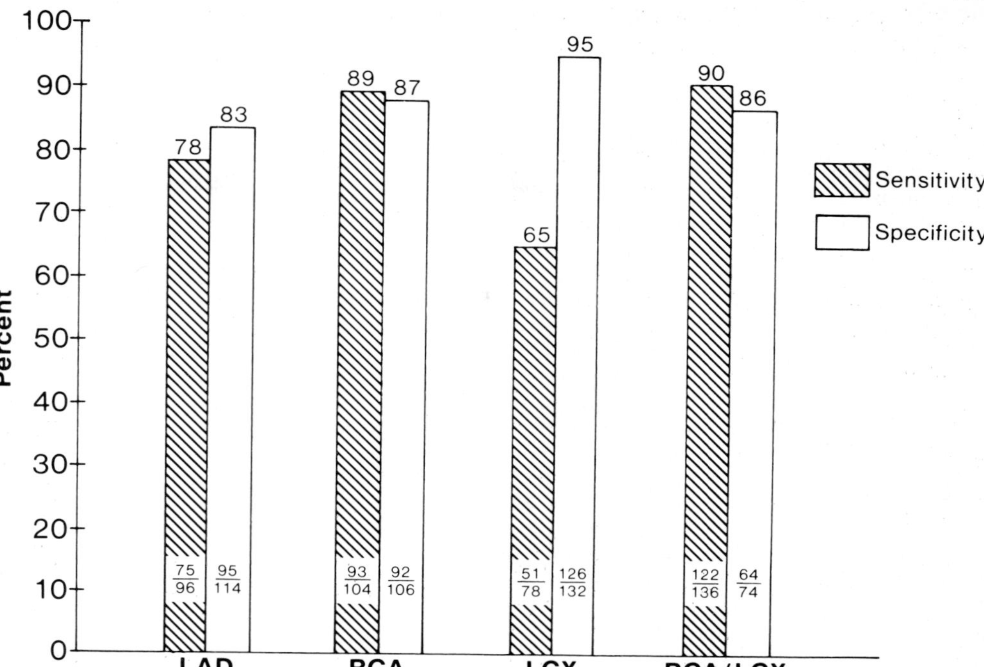

Figure 55–21. Sensitivity and specificity of quantitative ^{201}Tl tomography for detection of individual coronary artery stenoses. LAD—left anterior descending artery; LCX—left circumflex artery; RCA—right coronary artery.

Although the polar map approach offers the important attribute of objectivity over manual or visual assessment methods, some limitations in defect sizing are worthy of note. The polar map approach gives equal weight to the contribution of small and large slices. Accurate measurement of the size of perfusion defects, therefore, necessitates the development of methods that account for differences in myocardial mass contributed by slices of different sizes and different endocardial-to-epicardial thickness.[P2] Methods of calculating the severity of an abnormality also become increasingly significant with the incorporation of true LV mass. Nevertheless, without corrections for scattering, attenuation, finite resolution, heart motion, and myocardial thickness, the error of measuring infarct size of perfusion defect size could be considerable.

Three-Dimensional Display

Methods are being developed to extend the functional two-dimensional polar map approaches to a three-dimensional format. Three-dimensional representations of myocardial perfusion SPECT studies will aid physicians in the visualization and determination of the extent and severity of perfusion defects. At present, the investigated methods that render three-dimensional images code the myocardial perfusion information on a three-dimensional surface. These approaches that use a three-dimensional surface display either render a surface that approximates the actual myocardial shape[M9, N2] or a surface that models the shape of the myocardium, such as an ellipsoid.[E3, P4]

SURFACE RENDERING. Methods that render the actual myocardial shape have similar processing steps that originate in methods developed for the three-dimensional display of bony surfaces from CT imaging.[H3] The input is usually a set of contiguous two-dimensional tomographic slices. Each slice is composed of a matrix of "voxels" or volume elements. From these sets of voxels, an algorithm generates a binary representation of the myocardium by determining whether a voxel is part of the myocardium (setting that voxel to 1) or outside the myocardium (setting that voxel to 0). Often a single count threshold is used to determine this classification. Once all the voxels have been classified as 0 or 1, another computer algorithm performs surface tracking as the boundaries between zeros and ones. For representing the myocardium, an outside (epicardium) and an inside surface (endocardium) may be generated, although current methods use a single surface to code the myocardial perfusion information.

Once a three-dimensional surface is generated in the memory of the computer, it can be used to generate a set of multiple projections that may be animated in cinematic form in order to give the illusion of a moving three-dimensional surface. A number of common processing tricks are used to shade the surfaces of the image in order to create a sense of realism. Each projection is coded so that the surfaces that are to appear farther from the viewer are shaded dimmer and the ones that are to appear closer are brighter. If a far surface falls behind a front surface along the viewer's line-of-sight, it is hidden from the display at that projection. A light source is assumed in generating these projections so that if a surface is perpendicular to the "rays" from the light source, it is shaded brighter, and if it is parallel, it is dimmer. Figure 55–22 illustrates the application of this methodology by Nowak.[N2]

Figure 55–22. See Color Plate 14.

Figure 55–23. See Color Plate 14.

SURFACE MODELING. A more direct approach to extend the two-dimensional polar maps (bull's eye displays) to a three dimensional format is being developed in a joint project between Emory University and the Georgia Institute of Technology.[C5, E3, P4] In this approach, the myocardial surface is modeled as a three-dimensional ellipsoid, covered by small tiles of equal dimensions. The same maximal count circumferential profiles that are mapped onto the so-called bull's eye displays are now mapped onto the three-dimensional ellipsoidal surface, with length and width relative to actual myocardial dimensions. Each circumferential profile count value that is used to assign a color to the bull's eye map is also used to assign the same color to a tile on the ellipsoidal surface representative of the ^{201}Tl concentration in that region of the myocardium. In addition to this color coding, each tile is further shaded for each generated two-dimensional projection to give the illusion of a three-dimensional display, as described in the section on surface rendering. These projections are then animated to give the illusion of a left ventricular myocardium rotating about the patient's long axis. Figure 55–23*B* shows an example of this display.

Ideally, accurate assessment of the extent and severity of CAD requires the integration of physiologic information, derived from thallium SPECT images, and anatomic information, derived from coronary arteriography. In order to accomplish this goal, the above-mentioned method that uses a surface model for representing myocardial perfusion is currently being enhanced by superimposing the patient's own coronary arterial tree. The patient-specific coronary arterial tree is obtained from a three-dimensional geometric reconstruction performed on simultaneously acquired, digital, biplane angiographic projections.[C5] The coronary arterial tree is approximated by successive conical segments. After the arterial tree is reconstructed in a three-dimensional image, it is scaled, transformed (warped), and rotated to fit onto the myocardial ellipsoidal surface. The left and right coronary arteries are fixed onto the myocardial perfusion ellipsoidal model by registering the proximal left anterior descending coronary artery onto the region corresponding to the anterior interventricular groove and the posterior descending artery onto the inferior interventricular groove. Figure 55–23 illustrates this unified display. Although the use of these three-dimensional images offers potential for a better understanding of coronary artery disease, they represent very preliminary results. Several years of development and evaluation are needed to determine the true validity of this approach.

Quantification of Radionuclide Ventriculograms

Radionuclide ventriculography is important for the assessment of ventricular function at rest and during exercise. Background-corrected total counts extracted from a LV region of interest provides a measurement of the relative volume of the ventricle at that instant of the cardiac cycle. To date, measurement of EF remains, for the most part, dependent on the operator. Moreover, assessment of regional function is usually performed by visual evaluation of closed-loop cine displays of the beating heart.

Manual assignment of regions of interest to calculate ejection fraction as well as the visual assessment of regional wall motion are imprecise because of observer variability. This imprecision results in the need to have expert observers perform these subjective tasks in order to obtain acceptable levels of interobserver and intraobserver variability. Moreover, the operator time involved in preparing studies for visual evaluation and for the determination of EF is extensive. These limitations have prompted the development of quantitative techniques for the automatic (or semiautomatic) determination of global and regional LV function from either multiple-gated equilibrium or first-pass studies. In general, these quantitative techniques involve the following: preprocessing or filtering of the scintigraphic images, isolation of the LV chamber, determination of background, edge detection of the LV throughout the cardiac cycle, quantification of the parameter of regional function, establishment of normal limits, and development of a quantitative criterion for the definition of an abnormality. This section explains each of these steps as applied to multiple-gated equilibrium scintigraphic (MGES) studies.

Image Processing

PREPROCESSING OF IMAGES. Preprocessing is applied to the digital images of the cardiac cycle before any analysis is undertaken. It consists of space-time smoothing of the images in either the spatial or the frequency domain, as explained earlier. It is mainly performed to minimize the statistical count fluctuations, which are random in space and time. This image enhancement is obtained at the expense of both spatial and temporal resolution. Degradation of resolution gives rise to a blurred cardiac cycle. Nevertheless, because the counts at the edge of the ventricle determine the accuracy of the assessment of regional wall motion[C6] as well as the accuracy of defining the LV edge, it is imperative that preprocessing be performed before any quantitative or visual analysis of wall motion is attempted.

LEFT VENTRICULAR ISOLATION. The next step in the quantitative process is to localize the LV chamber using image segmentation techniques. An early implementation of this technique suggested by Burow and associates[B10] consisted of a manually assigned box around the left ventricle.

Other investigators locate the LV by first identifying a pixel somewhere close to the center of the chamber. Douglass and colleagues[D3] and Reiber[R5] use properties of profiles representing the column and row sums either of the difference image (end-diastolic minus end-systolic) or of the first frame of the study.

Nelson and associates[N3] developed a novel approach by using a minimum pixel image to separate the atria from the ventricles. In this approach, for each pixel's Cartesian coordinate, the computer searches throughout the cardiac cycle and the minimum value of each coordinate is assigned to a minimum image. This image is then subtracted from each frame. Subtraction eliminates the structures that are not moving and results in stroke images with the isolated ventricles at end-diastole (ED) and the isolated atria at end-systole (ES). The LV is then found from the frame of the isolated ventricles as the counts left of the center of gravity of the entire cycle of stroke images. Links and coworkers[L5] and the Cedars-Sinai Medical Center group[A4, A5, G12, G13] have used variations of the methods described earlier.

In the approach used at Cedars-Sinai Medical Center, stroke images defined as described earlier are used to simplify identification of the moving structures. The four stroke images with the lowest center of mass (closest to the bottom) are summed to create a composite of ventricular ED. The four images with the highest center of mass are summed to create a composite of ventricular ES. After subtracting the atrial image from the ventricular image to minimize problems with overlapping structures, thresholding of the column and row profiles is used to determine the location and size of a rectangle, enclosing only the ventricles. The interventricular septum is located by scanning each horizontal profile inside the rectangle for a local minimum between two maxima.

BACKGROUND DETERMINATION. In order to truly isolate the counts coming from the left ventricle, the computer algorithm must subtract the counts that fall in the region of the LV from radioactivity in tissues in front of and behind the ventricle as well as from radiation that is scattered into the region of the LV from surrounding tissues. This type of background is also known as tissue crosstalk. Moreover, in order to isolate the LV, the counts in the background that define the RV, the atria, the great vessels, and the lungs need to be eliminated.

Both of the above-mentioned types of elimination of background counts can be simultaneously performed using interpolative background subtraction techniques. The approach used at Cedars-Sinai Medical Center uses a rectangle around the LV to define the origin of the background to be subtracted by using the same interpolative background scheme described for the analysis of planar ^{201}Tl scintigrams. The pixels outside the rectangle are set at 0. This subtraction is performed on a frame-by-frame basis. This technique not only is effective in eliminating the background counts but also serves to increase the image contrast, thus preparing the image for subsequent edge enhancement and detection. Several investigators[A4, G12, G13, L3] have reported on the usefulness of applying interpolative background subtraction to MGES studies and on the improvements in this technique. In particular, Stamm and associates[S2] showed that wall motion from interpolative background-subtracted gated blood pool images compared well with contrast angiographic results; Leidholdt and colleagues[L3] have reported that EFs calculated by subtracting polygonal matrices of 12 vertices from the entire heart in MGES data showed good correlation to the standard measurement of EF. The Cedars-Sinai Medical Center approach differs from these techniques in that the LV alone is identified as the matrix to be subtracted. Nichols[N1] reported on the use of irregular regions and weights without arbitrary roll-off constants as improvements in the method, thus more accurately approximating true ventricular background.

Other approaches require that the LV edges be defined before the background is determined. One of the methods for semiautomated background determination was first suggested by Burow and coworkers.[B11] In their approach, a background region of interest is assigned a set distance to the left of the LV. The region is defined as a set number of pixels wide and extending from the apex to two-thirds of the length of the LV vertical axis. The method requires that the time-activity curve extracted from this region be confirmed by the operator to be flat or that the region be moved away from blood pool structures.

In another approach, described by Almasi and associates,[A6] background activity is also automatically subtracted on a pixel-by-pixel basis by using two perimeters or edges. The inner perimeter corresponds to the LV edge. The outer perimeter corresponds to the septal border of the right ventricle to right of the LV, whereas it may correspond to the edge of the liver or lung elsewhere. The pixels outside of the outer perimeter are set at 0. The global background is determined from the pixels with the lowest count rate located around the 45-degree sector between the outer and inner perimeters. In addition to subtracting global background, the counts extracted from the pixels in the region between the inner and outer perimeter also compensate for the contribution of tissue crosstalk from the LV and surrounding chambers. This compensation is done regionally by interpolating the counts between the inner and outer perimeters.

EDGE DETECTION. Edge detection is needed to define the borders of the LV throughout the cardiac cycle. These borders are used to define regions of interest from which counts are extracted for calculation of global or regional EF. The radial change of these edges is also used to assess regional wall motion. The process of edge detection includes edge enhancement, boundary recognition, and edge tracking in both space and time. These techniques were covered in detail in the section on image processing.

An example of edge detection methodology used by the Cedars-Sinai Medical Center group is described here. A 3-by-3 Laplacian operator is applied to obtain nondirectional, second derivative images that are termed Laplacian images. These images are then smoothed in space and time. From the smoothed Laplacian images, the program searches radially out from the center for the highest pixel value, which is defined as the ventricular edge. These edge points are then connected, subject to threshold analysis with respect to radial length so as not to allow any one edge point to be too far away from its neighbors. After thresholding, the edge points are smoothed in space and time. This approach had a success rate of 100 percent in detecting the LV edges from a training set of 80 2-minute MGES studies acquired in the best septal LAO projection (approximately 100,000 counts/frame).[G13] Goris and colleagues[G14] have also reported on their successful use of Laplacian algorithms for edge detection. Although there are other edge enhancement operators, such as the Sobel operator, that are less sensitive to noise and could work with MGES data, the implementation of those more sophisticated operators could considerably slow down execution time.

Global Function Calculations

Two parameters of global function that can be evaluated from radionuclide ventriculographic studies are EF and absolute chamber volume.

EJECTION FRACTION. In the approach implemented at Cedars-Sinai Medical Center,[A5] the regions of interest generated from edge detection of the LV throughout the cardiac cycle are applied to the images of the MGES study. The total counts within each region are plotted against the frame number to create a volume curve (time-activity curve), from which ejection fraction is calculated. The point in the volume curve that has the highest value corresponds to the global ED frame, and the point that has the minimum value corresponds to the global ES frame. As suggested by Burow and coworkers,[B11] the outline of the ES region is used to create a paraventricular background region that is located to the left of the LV edge and follows the edge contour. An average background value in counts per pixel is calculated by summing the counts in the background region and dividing the sum by the number of pixels in that region. This background value is used to correct the LV volume curve after normalization for the number of pixels within the LV region. Ejection fraction is then calculated in the standard manner, i.e., the background-corrected ED counts minus the ES counts divided by the ED counts.

This automatic approach yielded a success rate of 100 percent in detecting the LV edges from a training set of 80 MGES studies applied to 20 patients, and resulted in a good correlation coefficient for LVEF measurements compared with manual techniques. Figure 55–24 illustrates an example of a global function report generated from this type of automatic analysis.

Other investigators have also reported on the accuracy of automatic methods. Links and colleagues,[L5] processing only the ED and the ES frame, reported a 90-percent operating success rate in 40 patients, with a correlation coefficient of 0.95 for LVEF by manual techniques. Almasi and associates,[A6] processing all frames of the cardiac cycle in 69 patients at rest, reported an 84-percent success rate and a 0.91 correlation coefficient for manual LVEF. Yuille and coworkers[Y1] reported on the use of a space-time smoothing algorithm followed by a high-emphasis filter to improve edge definition. These methods are significantly more successful in measuring LVEF when they are applied to high-count density, high-resolution resting MGES, compared with low-count, low-resolution exercise MGES.

VOLUME DETERMINATIONS. Automatic measurement of absolute LV volume from MGES has not been described to date, but several manual approaches exist for geometric and nongeometric determination of LV volume.

Geometric techniques, first described by Dodge and associates[D4] for application in contrast ventriculography, have been applied to gated blood pool studies by Strauss and colleagues.[S3] This method assumes the LV to be either an ellipsoid or a prolate spheroid, which is not an accurate assumption for hearts with regional dysfunction. Geometric determination of absolute LV volume from MGES studies have been shown to give good correlation with angiographically determined volumes.[P5, V2]

Nongeometric radionuclide techniques for the measurement of LV volume were first described for tracer dilution curves[I1, V5] and more recently for MGES studies.[L6, S4, S5] In another method,[S4] the count rate from the LV is converted to arbitrary volume units by using the activity measured from a small sample of the patient's

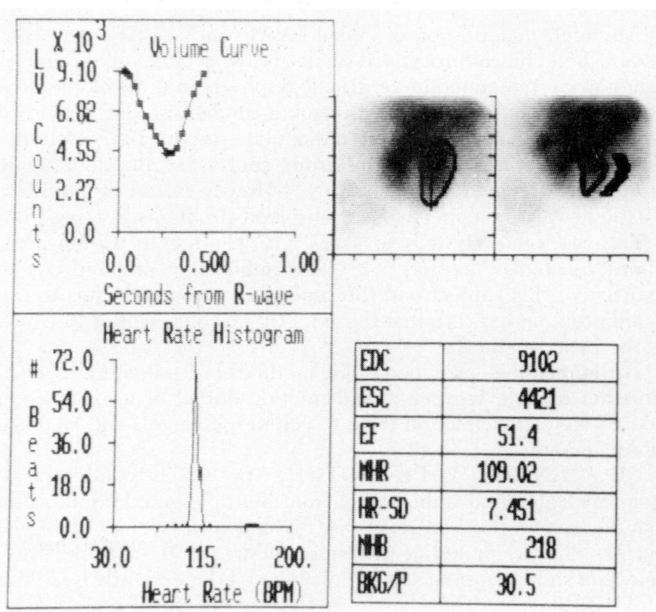

EDC	9102
ESC	4421
EF	51.4
MHR	109.02
HR-SD	7.451
NHB	218
BKG/P	30.5

Figure 55–24. Global function report. Global function report generated from a totally automatic analysis of a peak exercise MGES study from a patient with triple-vessel CAD. Shown are the left ventricular (LV) volume curve *(top left)*, the heart rate histogram *(bottom left)*, the automatically chosen end-diastolic (ED), end-systolic (ES), and background regions *(top right)*, and the measured parameters *(bottom right)*. (EDC—end-diastolic counts; EDS—end-systolic counts; EF—ejection fraction; MHR—mean heart rate; HR-SD—heart rate ejection fraction; NHB—number of heart beats; BKG/p—background counts per pixel.)

blood. This approach, which does not account for photon attenuation through the chest wall, yielded only an index rather than an absolute measurement of LV volume. In nongeometric methods, a blood sample is withdrawn during imaging of the LAO view and counted on the collimator face after completion of the acquisition session. Left ventricular volume at ED is calculated as the ratio of the attenuation-corrected count rate in the LAO view to the count rate per milliliter from the blood sample. The left ventricular ED count rate is given by dividing the total background-corrected counts in the LVED region of interest by the product of time per ED frame and the number of cardiac cycles acquired.

Other investigators such as Links and colleagues[L6] and Schwaiger and associates[S5] have pointed out the need to correct for attenuation and have developed preliminary methods for this correction. In the approach used by Schwaiger, the attenuation factor is calculated as the ratio of the deadtime-corrected counts obtained from the image of the bolus in the RV and the counts derived from a reference activity image close to the collimator surface. In the approach used by Links, attenuation correction is made by dividing the LVED count rate by e^{-ud}. In this equation, u is the linear attenuation coefficient for water (0.15/cm) and d is the distance from a skin marker (placed on the skin over the LV in the LAO view, and imaged during the anterior view) to the center of the LV in the anterior view divided by the sine of 40 degrees to yield the depth of the LV in the LAO view. Although both techniques have been reported to have excellent correlations for LVED volume with angiography, in our experience both are cumbersome and prone to error. Schwaiger's approach requires a very tight bolus and the additional effort of acquiring and processing a first-pass study. Links' method, in addition to requiring additional acquisition and processing, uses a simple exponential equation assuming the ventricle is a point source. This assumption tends to overcorrect for the attenuation from large ventricles and to undercorrect for the attenuation from small ventricles.

Regional Function Calculations

Although quantitation of global LVEFs and RVEFs is a well-established clinical procedure, quantitative evaluation of regional function by radionuclide ventriculography is in a developmental stage, as it is for all cardiac imaging modalities. Extraction of regional myocardial function indices started in 1967 with the work on hemiaxis shortening from contrast ventriculographic studies by Herman and associates.[H4] However, the literature in this field reveals a spectrum of unsolved problems ranging from which coordinate system to use[C7, I2] to whether to use an area, chord, or radial method.[D5, G15] The publication of hundreds of articles on this subject and the multiplicity of approaches to the same problem indicate that there is still no consensus as to which is the best approach.

Radionuclide ventriculographic methods for evaluating regional function include segmental wall motion (radial or area change), regional ejection fraction (count [volume] change), and regional phase analysis.

SEGMENTAL WALL MOTION. In an early attempt to quantify segmental wall motion from multiple-gated equilibrium scintigrams,[G16] the ventricle was divided into twelve 30-degree sectors that originated at the center of area of the ES mid-LAO image (a similar approach was developed independently by Silber and associates[S6]). The change in the area of these sectors from ED to ES was expressed as a contraction fraction and compared with lower limits of normal values obtained from normal volunteers. The limitations were that the sectors were too large and masked either small regional abnormalities or abnormalities at boundaries between sectors. Lack of an alignment system led to improper comparison with normal limits in some cases. Further limitations were (1) even though LV edge detection was semiautomatic, there were disagreements between operators on what the correct edges should be; and (2) quantifying the regional area change gave no information regarding the walls when motion was perpendicular to the plane of the detector in this view.

The last-mentioned limitation was partially circumvented by the work on regional EF originating from the John Hopkins Medical Institutions and reported separately by Burow and colleagues[B11] and Douglass and associates.[D3] In their approach, the ventricle was divided into 45-degree sectors, each constructed from the ED region of interest about its geometric center. The EF from each of these eight regions is calculated from the background-corrected counts (volume) versus the time curve. Since the counts are proportional to volume disregarding attenuation, then the regional EF reflects the function of all of the walls contained within it, thus providing information regarding the motion of all ventricular segments from a single view. Burow and colleagues[B12] and Douglass and associates[D3, D6] have independently reported that regional EF is more accurate than global EF for the detection of CAD. Preliminary results from Cedars-Sinai Medical Center suggest that this approach is more sensitive than the contraction fraction technique.[G13]

In the most recent approach used by Cedars-Sinai Medical Center to quantitate regional wall motion and ejection fraction, 60 6-degree arcs are evaluated, letting observed data dictate the criterion for abnormality, that is, how many contiguous areas represent a significant abnormality. In addition, this approach has a major advantage over arbitrary segmental division of the LV in that no matter how large the combined sector deemed the criterion for abnormal is, it can move at 6-degree increments. This approach circumvents the problems inherent in undersampling.[F2]

CEDARS-SINAI MEDICAL CENTER APPROACH. Segmental parameters are based on two composite edges rather than the actual edge determined for any one frame (Fig. 55–25).[A4, G16] A composite ED edge represents the greatest relaxation of each angular position not only in the global ED frame but also in the frame before and the frame after. Likewise, a composite ES edge represents the greatest contraction of each segment within one frame of global ES. The reason for the composite edge is the fact that all segments do not reach ED and ES at the same point in time. On the other hand, constraining the definition of edges to be close to the global state precludes misinterpreting dyskinesis as normal motion.

The contraction fraction is used as a measure of regional wall motion. It is based solely on the composite ED and ES edges. For each angular position the contraction fraction is defined as ED minus ES divided by ED, where ED is the end-diastolic

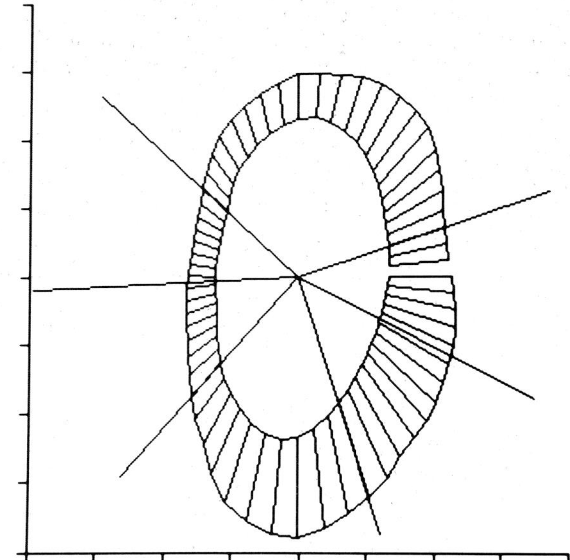

Figure 55–25. Segmental wall motion in resting MGES study. Graphical representation of segmental wall motion of a resting MGES study from a normal patient. Outer border corresponds to end-diastole and inner one to end-systole. Zero degrees is aligned at 3 o'clock and proceeds clockwise.

length of that segment and ES is the end-systolic length and is plotted as a CP (Fig. 55–26).

The regional EF is based on the measured activity in small regions of the ventricular cavity. The ED length of a segment is divided in half, the inner half representing a volume that moves perpendicular to the detector face. The outer region is affected primarily by walls that move parallel to the detector face. A region representing the entire segment is also used (Fig. 55–27). For each segment, a search is made for the largest volume near ED and the smaller volume near ES. In order to mitigate the effect of such small regions, the regions of interest used in these calculations are interpolated to 128 by 128 pixel resolution. After the raw curves are created, they are smoothed to reduce the effect of low-counting statistics (Fig. 55–28). Vitale and coworkers have also reported on a similar method of separating the LV into an inner and outer regional EF.[V6]

Burow and colleagues initially demonstrated,[B8] and the Cedars-Sinai Medical Center group implemented in their work in planar thallium and regional function, the alignment of the regional CPs to an anatomic landmark (the cardiac apex). This alignment is needed for two reasons: First, since the lower limits of normal exhibit regional variations, alignment of the apex to the 90-degree sector ensures that the correct segment will be compared with the lower normal limits. Second, when comparing a change in response (i.e., between rest and exercise) of a segment, this approach compensates for changes in the orientation of the heart that could create miscalculation of the difference profiles.

The system used by Cedars-Sinai Medical Center since 1979 employs polar coordinates centered at the geometric center of ES in a fixed frame of reference (see Fig. 55–25). The ES geometric centroid was chosen because, in the mid-LAO view at peak exercise, contraction of the normal ventricle often is such that the ES silhouette lies outside the ED centroid. Thus, using the ES centroid in this case would result in calculations of regional parameters that are more closely aligned to the intuitive visual observation of the motion. Choosing the ED centroid should result in similar accuracy but in less intuitive findings. This hypothesis needs further testing. Ingels and coworkers[I2] reported that using an ES point would be the optimum position for the polar origin of a fixed external reference system. Because of the low-resolution matrices used in MGES studies, a fixed reference system is mandatory. The error that would result from trying to align the different frames of the cardiac cycle to anatomic landmarks would greatly outweight any benefits. In regard to the choice of using polar coordinates, Steckley and associates[S7] have reported that there was a higher correlation coefficient for polar area reduction techniques compared with rectangular areas.

PHASE ANALYSIS. In radionuclide ventriculographic studies, the combined time-activity curves derived from pixels within the LV represent volume changes over time.[B13, L7] The counts contributed by each pixel within the LV represent the volume change behind their projected data. The volume-time curve from each pixel, since it resembles a sinusoidal wave, can be reasonably well approximated using a single cosine component with the frequency of the heart rate. Since this frequency is the lowest frequency extracted from the volume-time curve, it is known as the fundamental frequency; the cosine component of that frequency multiplied by the extracted amplitude is the first harmonic. The cosine component with the next higher frequency is known as the second harmonic. Each pixel within the heart region can then be expressed as a cosine wave with the frequency of the heart rate times an amplitude, and aligned by a phase angle such that

$$\text{Counts}\ (x,y,t) = A_0 + \text{Amplitude}\ (x,y)\cos[\text{heart rate}\ (t) + \text{phase}\ (x,y)]$$

The constant A_0, known as the zero harmonic (divided by two) or DC term, is given by the average value of counts at that pixel

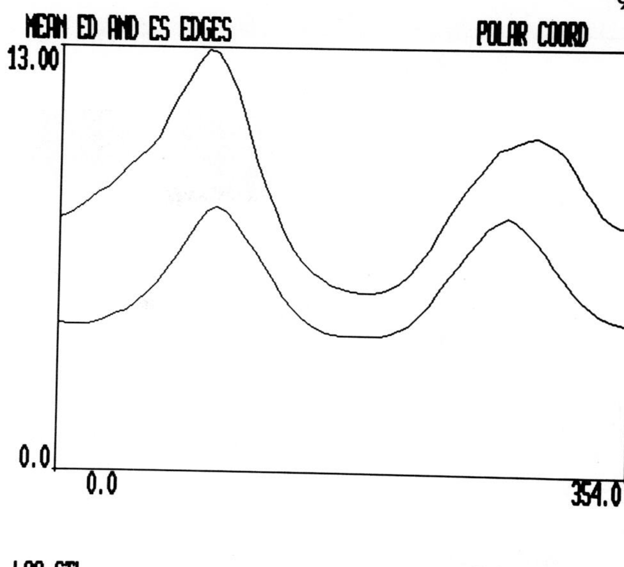

Figure 55–26. Circumferential profile of segmental wall motion. Circumferential profile representation corresponding to the segmental wall motion of the patient in Figure 55–25. Graph shows distance versus angle for each of 60 end-diastolic (ED) *(top curve)* and end-systolic (ES) *(bottom curve)* circumferential profile points. The first peak is the point chosen to represent the apex, which is then used to align the circumferential profiles to 90°. The contraction fraction profile is then determined from these two profiles on a point-by-point basis as the percent change of ES from ED, similar to the determination of the myocardial ^{201}Tl washout profile shown in Figure 55–15. Polar Coord.—Polar coordinates, i.e., angle versus radius.

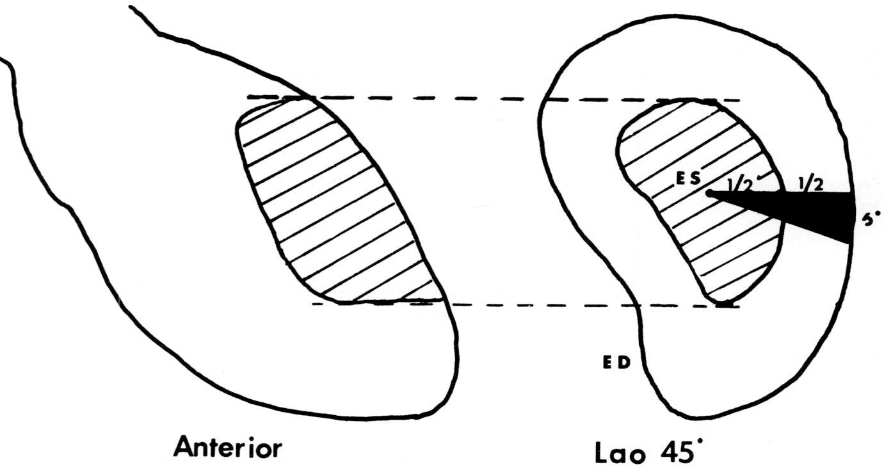

Figure 55–27. Schematic representation of division of a lateral region into inner, outer, and combined sectors for regional ejection fraction. The inner and outer regions are arbitrarily defined as half the distance to the end-diastolic (ED) edge from the end-systolic (ES) center of mass. Note that the inner region corresponds mostly to anterior wall function. LAO—left anterior oblique.

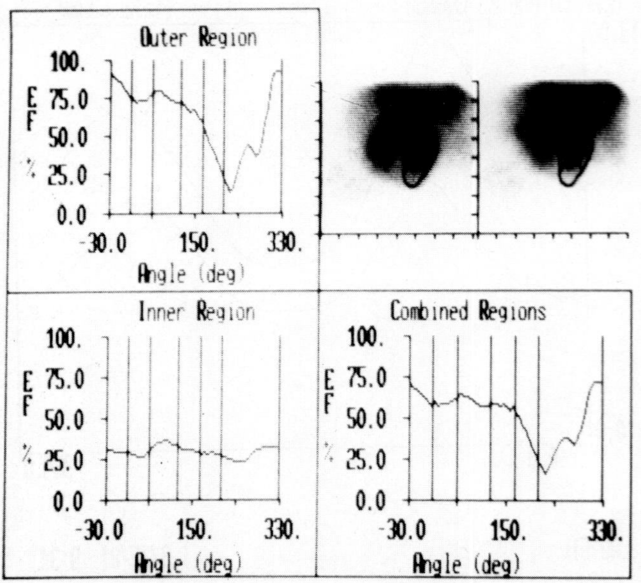

Figure 55–28. Regional ejection fraction (EF) report of a peak exercise MGES study in the same patient as in Figure 55–24. Comparison of the patient's regional ejection fraction profiles with normal limits profiles predicted abnormality of the posterolateral and inferoapical areas from the outer EF and the anterior wall from the inner EF, consistent with triple-vessel disease, which was documented by subsequent cardiac catheterization.

location. To a first approximation, the amplitude of the fundamental frequency is proportional to stroke volume, and the phase is related to the time in the cardiac cycle at which emptying begins (Fig. 55–29).[L7] If two of the pixels defining the heart reach a maximum (end-diastole) or a minimum (end-systole) at the same time, then there is no phase difference between the two; otherwise the difference in time at which the two reach a maximum is given by the phase angle difference between them (Fig. 55–30). Given that a cycle is represented by 360 degrees, since the normal ventricle reaches a maximum at the same time that the atrium reaches a minimum, the two are said to be 180 degrees out of phase. Functional cardiac images can be generated that display the values for the temporal average, stroke counts, and phase shift on a pixel-by-pixel basis (Fig. 55–31). Studying the differences in phase between one part of the ventricle and another, or one chamber of the heart and another, gives information as to the pattern that the wave of contraction follows. This type of information extraction is helpful in studying the pattern of electrical activity of the heart and regional wall motion contraction patterns.

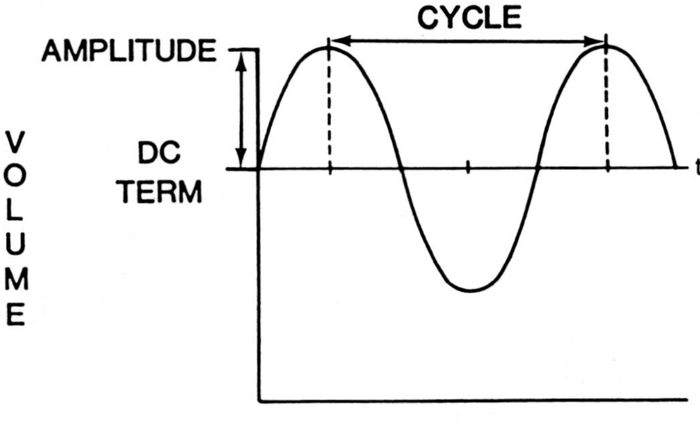

Figure 55–29. Cosine wave and phase analysis. Diagram illustrating relationships between a cosine wave and the definitions associated with phase analysis discussed in the text. The cosine function is used to approximate the volume-time curve of the cardiac cycle. (See text for definition of DC term.)

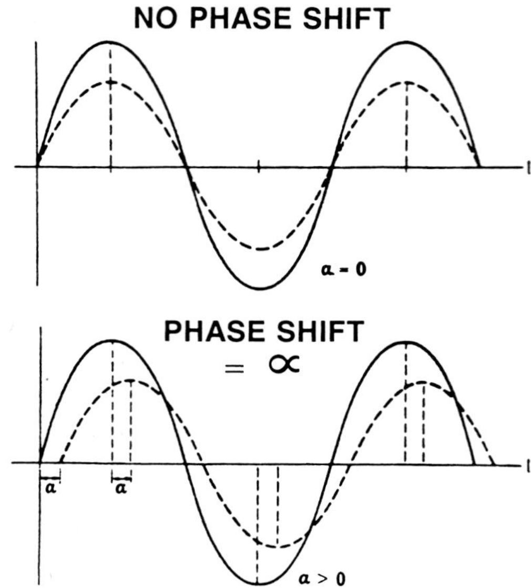

Figure 55–30. Diagram illustrating two sets of cosine waveforms with ($\alpha > 0$) and without ($\alpha = 0$) phase shifts.

Figure 55–31. See Color Plate 14.

The accuracy of determining phase shifts has been reported[B14] to improve when the first harmonic analysis is generalized to include the first three harmonics. This improvement is due to a better representation of the volume-time curve while still maintaining a marked degree of temporal filtering.

Phase analysis can aid in the evaluation of the temporal sequence of systolic ventricular wall motion from MGES studies in the modified LAO view.[A7, B13, L7] In the preliminary approaches, the computer was used to perform Fourier transform of the pixel's time-activity curve on a pixel-by-pixel basis, and only the first Fourier coefficients were used.

There are two major limitations to the method as reported. First, as has been pointed out by Bacharach,[B5] using only the first Fourier coefficient results in significant errors in determination of the phase. Second, the current approach to assessing regional wall motion from this analysis is to visually assess the display of the wave of contraction in color or in black and white. This visual assessment is again subjective, cumbersome, and imprecise. A method for overcoming this subjectivity was reported by Ratib and colleagues,[R6] who studied wall motion abnormalities due to stress-induced ischemia by assessing histograms of the entire LV phase distribution. In this method, the standard deviation from the mean of this distribution was calculated and the change between rest and exercise was compared with that of a group of normal patients. Although this was a significant contribution to quantifying phase distributions for the detection of regional wall motion abnormality, the method does not predict where the regional abnormality can be found and thus cannot be used for localizing disease.

It has also been demonstrated that the LV phase histograms of patients with wall motion abnormalities exhibit asymmetries. Gerber and associates[G17] suggested analyzing the skewness of the distribution to detect disease. This asymmetry of the LV histogram is likely due to the superimposition of the phase distribution from normally contracting segments on abnormally contracting segments. In another approach, Yaron and colleagues[Y2] divided the ventricle into four regions (posterolateral wall, septum, inferoapical wall, and midventricular wall) and quantified the standard deviation of the phase in each of the regions. This method further proposed to differentiate the abnormal from the normal phase distribution by measuring the difference in angle between the onset of the contraction (emptying) of the entire LV and the mean of the regional phase histogram in each of the four regions. One limitation of this method of dividing the ventricle into four regions is statistics. Because the regions are smaller, there are fewer pixels to form the phase distribution, thus creating a source of statistical error in the calculation.

NORMAL LIMITS AND ABNORMALITY CRITERIA. Previous work[G4, G8] has demonstrated the value of defining lower limits of normal for each mechanism of detecting disease (e.g., stress defect and washout abnormality with ^{201}Tl) and of comparing prospective patients against these normal limits for detecting regional abnormalities. Similarly, the mean value and standard deviation can be established from the pooled data of low-likelihood normal patients for each of the 60 angular locations. In the approach used at Cedars-Sinai Medical Center, this was done for the contraction fraction profile and the inner, outer, and combined regional EF profiles in the control and at maximum stress, as well as for the difference of each corresponding profile between one state and another (see Fig. 55–28). For all these profiles, normal limits are defined as the curves representing two standard deviations below the mean, and are used as a threshold for detection of wall motion abnormalities. These curves are obtained by averaging the profile for each view, point by point, around the circumference of the left ventricle and calculating the standard deviation from each point (Fig. 55–32).

The criterion for an abnormality was developed for rest-exercise studies in a group of 20 CAD patients and 20 normal subjects.[G13] The criterion for abnormality that best differentiated jeopardized regions from normal regions was defined as five contiguous 6-degree arcs (30 degrees) of the inner and/or outer regional EF that falls below the normal limits.

Of 42 jeopardized regions in the CAD patients, 36 were detected by quantitative analysis and 35 by visual analysis. Of the 11 nonjeopardized regions, four were abnormal by combined quantitative analysis. The remaining seven regions were apical and could not be ascribed to a specific vessel in this view alone. Among the 20 normal subjects, all 60 regions were normal by visual analysis, as were 56 by quantitative analysis. Furthermore, when the mechanism for detection of disease was assessed in the 36 regions found by visual analysis, regional EF of the inner region or the outer region or both regions was present in all 36. No additional regions were identified by analysis of regional contraction fraction or by analysis of the combined EF (the inner plus the outer regions). Thus, this preliminary experience suggests that quantitative assessment is as accurate as the visual method for detecting regional dysfunction, that this accurate detection is primarily made by regional EF measurement, and that no additional information appears to be gained through the automated assessment of contraction fraction. These data suggest that the approach described results in accurate objective assessment of regional function.

Preliminary results regarding regional phase analysis in 30 patients undergoing exercise radionuclide ventriculography have also been reported.[Y2] This population included 15 patients undergoing clinically indicated cardiac catheterization. Patients with prior myocardial infarction as well as conduction abnormalities were excluded. All of the catheterized patients had CAD. For the entire LV, the rest-exercise variation of the standard deviation and of the onset-mean (O-M) interval was significantly different between the normal and CAD populations. Additionally, there was a significant difference between the normal subjects and the patients with CAD in the corresponding vessels for both the variation of the standard deviation and the regional O-M interval between rest and exercise, except for the O-M interval of the posterolateral wall. With the small amount of data in this report, however, there was a significant overlap between patients with and without coronary disease as well as in regions with and

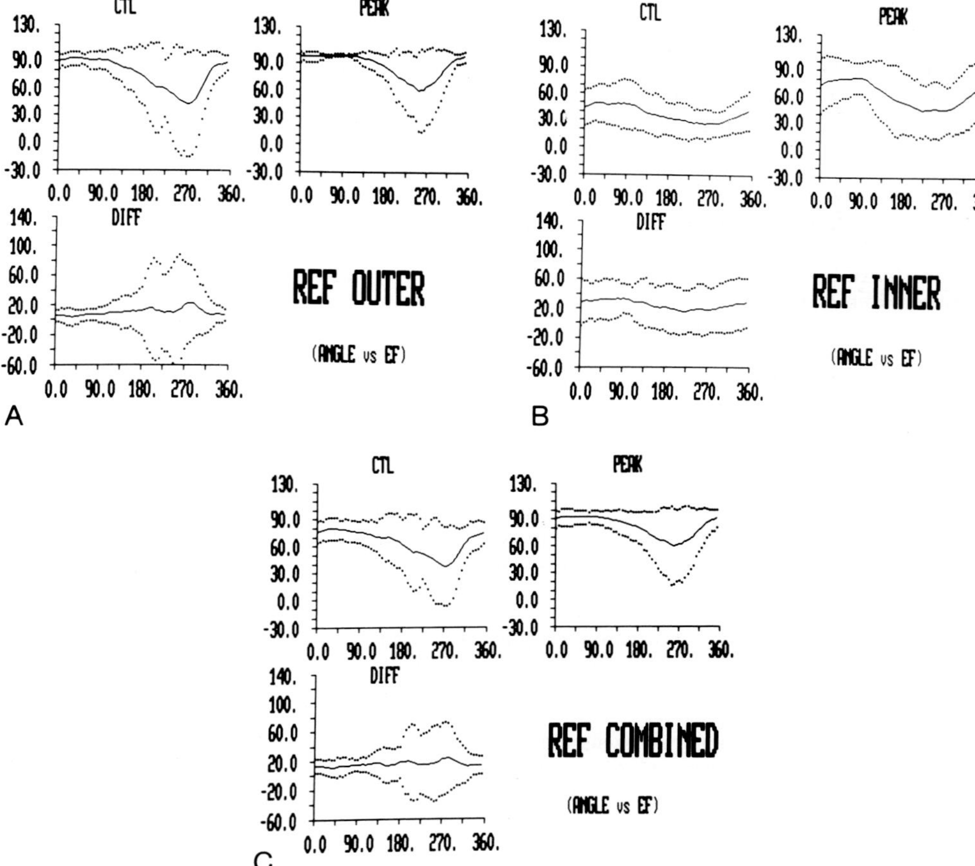

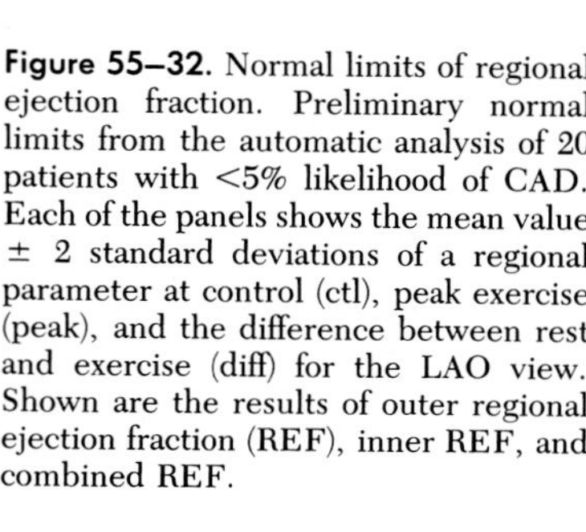

Figure 55–32. Normal limits of regional ejection fraction. Preliminary normal limits from the automatic analysis of 20 patients with <5% likelihood of CAD. Each of the panels shows the mean value ± 2 standard deviations of a regional parameter at control (ctl), peak exercise (peak), and the difference between rest and exercise (diff) for the LAO view. Shown are the results of outer regional ejection fraction (REF), inner REF, and combined REF.

without coronary disease, thus limiting the value of this analysis in the assessment of individual patients. Of note, however, analysis was performed with only the first Fourier harmonic. Additionally, skewness was not evaluated in this population. The question as to whether analysis of phase significantly adds to the other regional analysis described (regional EF, outer and inner regions; regional wall motion), has not yet been evaluated.

FUTURE DEVELOPMENTS

SPECT Instrumentation

As nuclear diagnosticians continue to switch from planar scintigraphy to SPECT imaging, the demand for dedicated tomographic devices is increasing. These dedicated SPECT devices have, to date, taken the form of multiple detector systems or ring configurations similar to PET scanners. The most innovative multiple detector system uses three detectors separated 120 degrees apart, giving the field of view a triangular appearance.[L8] Of the SPECT ring systems, the SPRINT developed by Rogers and coworkers[R7] appears to be promising. In this system, rings of NaI crystals and photomultiplier tubes surround the cylindrical field of view. A rotating cylindrical lead drum with multiple slits takes on the role of collimator. The main advantage of these new systems is increased absolute sensitivity while maintaining or improving spatial resolution. The main disadvantage is that their costs begin to approximate those of PET scanners.

Another expected development that should significantly enhance SPECT quantification in the thorax is the clinical implementation of algorithms for Compton scatter, variable attenuation, and object size correction. This implementation, particularly when applied to new imaging agents such as ^{99m}Tc sestamibi, should help bridge the gap between the type of absolute quantification being done on PET scanners versus that being done on SPECT scanners. This also implies that the degree of technical sophistication expected for routine SPECT studies will increase. This increase will also be accompanied by a need for faster computers and larger storage media, such as optical disks, to be able to process and store the large amounts of information available. This increase also points to the need for implementing data compression techniques.

Artificial Intelligence and Expert Systems

In the next few years, most progress in applying powerful computers to the analysis of cardiovascular disease is expected to be in the area of image interpretation and decision making. This advancement will entail the implementation of artificial intelligence techniques. Artificial intelligence is concerned with designing systems that exhibit the characteristics of human behavior in interpreting images, learning, reasoning, solving problems, and so on. Expert systems use artificial intelligence techniques to allow the collection of knowledge from human experts, which can then be used by the computer at a later time. Other important attributes of expert systems are their ability to handle incomplete or noisy data, justify their results in English, and use certainty factors to assert their conclusions. Already, preliminary expert systems have been developed to automatically interpret tomographic thallium studies from processed polar maps.[G18] Artificial intelligence techniques have also been used to help automate edge detection from ^{99m}Tc multiple-gated equilibrium studies[D7, N4] and to quantify wall motion.

It should be evident from this discussion that powerful computers with large, well-organized data bases that can handle sophisticated image processing algorithms will soon play a significant role in aiding the physician in image interpretation and in day-to-day clinical decision making.

Acknowledgments

The author gratefully acknowledges the collaboration in the development of many of the described methods by Kenneth Van Train, David Cooke, Joseph Areeda, Robert Eisner, Norberto Ezquerra, John Peifer, Gordon DePuey, Jamshid Maddahi, Timothy Bateman, Alan Rosanski, and Daniel Berman.

References

A

1. Anger, H. O.: Scintillation camera. Rev. Sci. Instrument 29:27, 1958.
2. Axelsson, B., Msaki, P., and Israelsson, A.: Subtraction of scattered photons in single photon computerized tomography. J. Nucl. Med. 25:490, 1984.
3. Areeda, J., Van Train, K., Garcia, E., et al.: Improved analysis of segmental thallium myocardial scintigrams: Quantitation of distribution, washout, and redistribution. *In* Esser, P. (ed.): Digital Imaging. Society of Nuclear Medicine, New York, 1982, p. 257.
4. Areeda, J., Garcia, E., Van Train, K., et al.: Comprehensive analysis of rest/exercise segmental left ventricular function from radionuclide ventriculograms. *In* Computers in Cardiology. IEEE Computer Society, Long Beach, CA, 1982, p. 109.
5. Areeda, J., Garcia, E., Van Train, K., et al.: A comprehensive method for automatic analysis of rest/exercise ventricular function from radionuclide ventriculography. *In* Esser, P. (ed.): Digital Imaging. Society of Nuclear Medicine, New York, 1982, p. 241.
6. Almasi, J. J., DePuey, E. G., Eisner, R. L., et al.: Totally automated computer processing of gated blood pool studies. (Abstract.) J. Nucl. Med. 23:42, 1982.
7. Adam, W. E., Tarkowski, A., Bitter, F., et al.: Equilibrium (gated) radionuclide ventriculography. Cardiovasc. Radiol. 2:161, 1979.

B

1. Bender, M. A., and Blau, M.: The autofluoroscope. *In* Kniseley, R. M., et al. (eds.): Progress in Medical Radioisotope Scanning. TID–7673, USAEC, 1963, p. 151.
2. Berger, H. J., and Zaret, B. L.: Radionuclide assessment of cardiovascular performance. *In* Freeman, L. M. (ed.): Freeman and Johnson's Clinical Radionuclide Imaging. Grune & Stratton, Orlando, FL, 1984, p. 418.
3. Berman, D. S., Garcia, E. V., and Maddahi, J.: Thallium–201 myocardial scintigraphy in the detection and evaluation of coronary artery disease. *In* Berman, D. S., and Mason, D. T. (eds.): Clinical Nuclear Cardiology. Grune & Stratton, New York, 1981, p. 49.
4. Bell, G. B., Spade, B. W., and Scheibe, P. O.: Cyclically gated cardiac studies with R-R interval dependent window widths. Nuclear cardiology: Selected computer aspects. 1978 Symposium Proceedings sponsored by the Computer Council of the Society of Nuclear Medicine, Atlanta, January 22–23, 1978, p. 63.
5. Bacharach, S. L., Green, M. V., and Borer, J. S.: Instrumentation and data processing in cardiovascular nuclear medicine: Evaluation of ventricular function. Semin. Nucl. Med. 9:257, 1979.
6. Bacharach, S. L., Green, M. V., Borer, J. S., et al.: ECG-gated scintillation probe measurement of left ventricular function. J. Nucl. Med. 18:1176, 1977.
7. Berger, H. J., Matthay, R. A., Loke, J., et al.: Assessment of cardiac performance with quantitative radionuclide angiocardiography: Right ventricular ejection fraction with reference to findings in chronic obstructive pulmonary disease. Am. J. Cardiol. 41:897, 1978.
8. Burow, R. D., Pond, M., Schafer, A. W., and Becker, L.: "Circumferential profiles": A new method for computer analysis of thallium–201 myocardial perfusion images. J. Nucl. Med. 20:771, 1979.
9. Borello, J. A., Clinthorne, N. H., Rogers, W. L., et al.: Oblique-angle tomography: A restructuring algorithm for transaxial tomographic data. J. Nucl. Med. 22:471, 1981.
10. Burow, R., Pond, M., Rehn, T., et al.: A semiautomatic edge detection program for the analysis of multiple-gated acquisition cardiac blood pool images. J. Nucl. Med. 18:608, 1977.
11. Burow, R. D., Strauss, W. H., Singleton, R., et al.: Analysis of left ventricular function from multiple-gated acquisition cardiac blood pool imaging: Comparison to contrast angiography. Circulation 56:1024, 1977.
12. Burow, R. D., Wilson, M. F., Allen, E. W., and Schechter, E.: Regional left ventricular time-activity curves from multiple-gated equilibrium scintigraphy: Correlation with contrast angiography. (Abstract.) J. Nucl. Med. 22:61, 1981.
13. Bacharach, S. L., de Graaf, C. N., Van Rijk, P., et al.: Fourier distribution maps: Toward an understanding of what they mean. *In* Esser, P. D. (ed.): Functional Mapping of Organ Systems and Other Computer Topics. Society of Nuclear Medicine, New York, 1981, p. 139.
14. Bacharach, S. L., Green, M. V., Vitale, D., et al.: Optimum number of harmonics for fitting cardiac volume curves. (Abstract.) J. Nucl. Med. 24:17, 1983.

C

1. Chang, L. T.: A method for attenuation correction in radionuclide computed tomography. IEEE Trans. Nucl. Sci. NS–25:638, 1978.
2. Corbett, J. R., Henderson, E. B., Akers, M. S., et al.: Gated tomography with technetium–99m RP–30A in patients with myocardial infarcts: Assessment of myocardial perfusion and function. (Abstract.) Circulation 76(Suppl. IV):217, 1987.

3. Caldwell, J., Williams, D., Harp, G., et al.: Quantitation of size of relative myocardial perfusion defect by single-photon emission computed tomography. Circulation 70:1048, 1984.
4. Caldwell, J. H., Williams, D. L., Hamilton, G. W., et al.: Regional distribution of myocardial blood flow measured by single-photon tomography: Comparison with in vitro counting. J. Nucl. Med. 23:490, 1982.
5. Cooke, C., Jofre, L., Klein, L., et al.: Three-dimensional reconstruction of arterial structure from biplane angiography. Proceedings of IEEE Technicon '87 Conference, Miami, Catalog No. 87–82761, 1987, p. 31.
6. Chapman, D. R., Garcia, E. V., Berman, D. S., et al.: Detection of 1-mm motion under conditions simulating equilibrium blood pool scintigraphy. J. Nucl. Med. 23:42, 1982.
7. Chaitman, B. R., Bristow, J. D., and Rahimtoola, S. H.: Left ventricular wall motion assessed using fixed external reference systems. Circulation 48:1043, 1973.

D

1. DePasquale, E., Nody, A., DePuey, G., et al.: Quantitative rotational thallium–201 tomography for identifying and localizing coronary artery disease. Circulation 77:316, 1988.
2. Douglass, K. H., Links, M. J., Gedra, T., and Wagner, H.: A comparison of interpolative background subtraction algorithms using analytical surfaces. *In* Esser, P. D. (ed.): Functional Mapping of Organ Systems and Other Computer Topics. Society of Nuclear Medicine, New York, 1981, p. 83.
3. Douglass, K., Links, J., and Wagner, H. N.: Fully automated measurement of regional left ventricular ejection fraction. (Abstract.) J. Nucl. Med. 23:024, 1982.
4. Dodge, H. T., Sandler, H., Ballew, D. W., and Lord, J. D.: The use of biplane angiocardiography for the measurement of left ventricular volume in man. Am. Heart J. 60:762, 1960.
5. Daughters, G. T., Schwarzkopf, A., Merd, C. W., et al.: A clinical evaluation of five techniques for left ventricular wall motion assessment. *In* Computers in Cardiology. IEEE Computer Society, Long Beach, CA, 1981, p. 249.
6. Douglass, F. H., Chen, D. C. P., Wond, D. F., et al.: Relative accuracy of automated analysis of regional wall motion in diagnosis of CAD. (Abstract.) J. Nucl. Med. 24:P91, 1983.
7. Duncan, J. S.: Intelligent determination of left ventricular wall motion from multiple-view, nuclear medicine image sequences. *In* Proceedings of the International Symposium on Medical Images and Icons. IEEE, New York, 1984, p. 265.

E

1. Eisner, R. L., Noever, T., Nowak, D., et al.: Use of cross-correlation function to detect patient motion during SPECT imaging. J. Nucl. Med. 28:97, 1987.
2. Eisner, R. L., Gober, A., Cerqueira, M., et al.: Quantitative analysis of normal thallium–201 tomographic studies. (Abstract.) J. Nucl. Med. 26:p49, 1984.
3. Ezquerra, N. F., Zerbi, M., Cooke, C. D., and Garcia, E.: A method of 3D display of arterial structure superimposed on myocardial perfusion distribution. (Abstract.) J. Nucl. Med. 28:675, 1987.

F

1. Friedman, J., Berman, D. S., Van Train, K., et al.: Patient motion in thallium–201 myocardial SPECT imaging: An easily identified frequent source artifactual defect. Clin. Nucl. Med. 13(5):321–324, 1988.
2. Freeman, M., Garcia, E., Berman, D., et al.: An objective and quantitative method for assessment of regional left ventricular wall motion using multiple-gated equilibrium scintigraphy. (Abstract.) J. Nucl. Med. 21:P62, 1980.

G

1. Green, M. V., Ostrow, H. G., Douglas, M. A., et al.: High temporal resolution ECG gated scintigraphic angiocardiography. J. Nucl. Med. 16:95, 1975.
2. Garcia, E. V., Sardi, E., Hammer, S., et al.: A method for isolating the left ventricle in the right anterior oblique projection from equilibrium gated blood pool radionuclide imaging. Circulation 56:11–52, 1977.
3. Go, R. T., MacIntyre, W. J., Houser, T. S., et al.: Clinical evaluation of 360° and 180° data sampling techniques for transaxial SPECT thallium–201 myocardial perfusion imaging. J. Nucl. Med. 26:695–706, 1985.
4. Garcia, E. V., Van Train, K., Maddahi, J., et al.: Quantification of rotational thallium–201 myocardial tomography. J. Nucl. Med. 26:17–26, 1985.
5. Galt, J. R., Hise, L. H., Garcia, E. V., and Nowak, D. J.: Filtering in frequency space. J. Nucl. Med. Tech. 14:152–162, 1986.
6. Galt, J. R.: Reconstruction of the absolute radionuclide distribution in a scattering medium from scintillation camera projections. (Doctoral dissertation.) University microfilms, Ann Arbor, MI, 237 pages.
7. Galt, J. R., Garcia, E. V., and Robbins, W. L.: SPECT quantitation: Dependence of radionuclide concentration on object size. (Abstract.) J. Nucl. Med. 27:1799, 1986.
8. Garcia, E. V., Maddahi, J., Berman, D. S., and Waxman, A.: Space-time quantitation of thallium–201 myocardial scintigraphy. J. Nucl. Med. 22:309–317, 1981.
9. Goris, M. L., Daspit, S. G., McLaughlin, P., and Kriss, J.: Interpolative background subtraction. J. Nucl. Med. 17:744–747, 1976.
10. Goris, M. L.: Nontarget activities: Can we correct for them? J. Nucl. Med. 20:1312–1314, 1979.
11. Go, R. T., Cook, S. A., MacIntyre, W. J., et al.: Comparative accuracy of stress and redistribution thallium–201 cardiac single photon emission transaxial tomography and planar imaging in the diagnosis of myocardial ischemia. (Abstract.) J. Nucl. Med. 23:24–25, 1982.
12. Garcia, E., Areeda, J., Van Train, K., et al.: A comprehensive method for quantitative analysis of rest/exercise ventricular function from radionuclide ventriculography. (Abstract.) Circulation 66 (Suppl. II): II–127, 1982.
13. Garcia, E., Areeda, J., Rozanski, A., et al.: Clinical validation of a totally automated method for assessing regional left ventricular function from rest/exercise radionuclide ventriculography. (Abstract.) J. Nucl. Med. 24:53, 1983.
14. Goris, M. L., McKillop, J. H., Fawcett, H. D. S., and Briandet, P. A.: Edge tracing for the determination of the left ventricular projection area. J. Nucl. Med. 21:60, 1980.
15. Gelberg, H. J., Brundage, B. H., Glantz, S., and Parmley, W. W.: Quantitation of left ventricular wall motion analysis: A comparison of area, chord, and radial methods. Circulation 59:991–1000, 1979.
16. Garcia, E. V., Sardi, E., Hammer, S., et al.: A method for isolating the left ventricle in the right anterior oblique projection from equilibrium gated blood pool radionuclide imaging. (Abstract.) Circulation 56 (Suppl. III):III–52, 1977.
17. Gerber, K. H., Norris, S. L., Slutsky, R. A., et al.: Quantitative phase analysis of exercise radionuclide left ventriculography in normals and patients with coronary artery disease. Comput. Biomed. Res. 16:88–98, 1983.
18. Garcia, E., Ezquerra, N., DePuey, E. G., et al.: Artificial intelligence interpretation of thallium–201 myocardial tomograms: Method and pilot study. (Abstract.) Circulation 74(Suppl. II): II–295, 1986.

H

1. Hamilton, G. W., Williams, D. L., and Caldwell, J. H.: Frame-rate requirements for recording time-activity curves by radionuclide angiocardiography. Nuclear cardiology: Selected computer aspects. 1978 Symposium Proceedings sponsored by the Computer Council of the Society of Nuclear Medicine, Atlanta, Georgia, January 22–23, 1978, pp. 75–83.
2. Hoffman, E. J., Huang, S. C., and Phelps, M. E.: Quantitation in positron emission computed tomography: 1. Effect of object size. J. Comput. Assist. Tomogr. 3:299–308, 1979.
3. Herman, G. T.: Computerized reconstruction and 3-D imaging in medicine. Ann. Rev. Comput. Sci. 1:153–179, 1986.
4. Herman, M. V., Heinie, R. A., Lein, M. D., and Gorlin, R.: Localized disorders in myocardial contraction. N. Engl. J. Med. 227:222, 1967.

I

1. Ishii, Y., and MacIntyre, W. I.: Measurement of heart chamber volumes by analysis of dilution curves simultaneously recorded by scintillation camera. Circulation 44:37, 1971.
2. Ingels, N. B., Daughters, G. T., Stinson, E. B., and Alderman, E. L.: Evaluation of methods for quantitating left ventricular segmental wall motion in man using myocardial markers as a standard. Circulation 60:966–972, 1980.

J

1. Jengo, J. A., Mena, I., Blaufuss, A., and Cliley, J. M.: Evaluation of left ventricular function (ejection fraction and segmental wall motion) by single-pass radioisotope angiography. Circulation 57:326, 1978.
2. Jaszczak, R. J., Floyd, C. E., and Coleman, R. E.: Scatter compensation techniques for SPECT. IEEE Trans. Nucl. Sci. NS–32:786–793, 1985.

K

1. Kalff, V., Chan, W., Rabinovitch, M., O'Neill, W., et al.: Radionuclide evaluation of post extrasystolic potentiation of left ventricular function induced by atrial and ventricular stimulation. Am. J. Cardiol. 50:106–111, 1982.
2. Klein, L., Garcia, E., DePuey, E. G., et al.: Reversibility of stress induced SPECT T1–201 myocardial perfusion defects. (Abstract.) J. Nucl. Med. 28 (4):642, 1987.
3. Keyes, J. W., Leionard, P. F., Brody, S. L., et al.: Myocardial infarct quantification in the dog by single photon emission computed tomography. Circulation 58:227–232, 1978.
4. Kirsch, C. M., Doliwa, R., Buell, U., and Roedler, D.: Detection of severe coronary heart disease with Tl–201: Comparison of resting single photon emission tomography with invasive arteriography. J. Nucl. Med. 24:761–767, 1983.

L

1. Lacy, J. L., LeBlanc, A. D., Babich, J. W., et al.: A gamma camera for medical applications, using a multiwire proportional counter. J. Nucl. Med. 25:1003–1012, 1984.
2. Lacy, J. L., Verani, M. S., Ball, M. E., et al.: Improved first-pass radionuclide angiography in man using a new multiwire gamma camera and short-lived tantalum–178. J. Nucl. Med. 29:293–301, 1988.
3. Leidholdt, E. M., Watson, D. D., Read, M. E., et al.: Interpolative background subtraction using polygonal boundary regions for gated blood pool imaging. *In* Esser, P. D. (ed.): Functional Mapping of Organ Systems and Other Computer Topics. Society of Nuclear Medicine, New York, 1981, pp. 91–101.
4. Luna, E., Klein, L., and Garcia, E., Reversibility bullseye polar map: Accuracy in detecting myocardial ischemia. J. Nucl. Med. 29(5), 1987.

5. Links, J., Brown, G., Hau, D., et al.: A new method of fully automatic processing of gated blood pool studies. (Abstract.) J. Nucl. Med. 23:85, 1982.
6. Links, J. M., Becker, L. C., Shindledecker, J. C., et al.: Measurement of absolute left ventricular volume from gated blood pool studies. Circulation 65:82–90, 1982.
7. Links, J. M., Douglas, K. H., and Wagner, H. N.: Patterns of ventricular emptying by Fourier analysis of gated blood-pool studies. J. Nucl. Med. 21:978–982, 1980.
8. Lim, C. B., Walker, R., and Pinkstaff, C., et al.: Triangular SPECT system for 3-D organ volume imaging: Clinical prototype and dynamic imaging potential. (Abstract.) J. Nucl. Med. 26:5–11, 1985.

M

1. Manglos, S. H., Jaszczak, R. J., Floyd, C. E., et al.: Non-isotropic attenuation in SPECT: Quantitative tests of effects and compensation techniques. J. Nucl. Med. 28:1884, 1987.
2. Moore, M. L., Murphy, P. H., and Burdine, J. A.: ECG-gated emission computed tomography of the cardiac blood pool. Radiology 134:233–235, 1980.
3. Meade, R. C., Bamrah, V. S., Horgan, J. D., et al.: Quantitative methods in the evaluation of thallium–201 myocardial perfusion images. J. Nucl. Med. 19:1175, 1978.
4. Murphy, F. L., Maddahi, J., Van Train, K., et al.: Thallium–201 uptake and washout of rest vs exercise in patients without coronary artery disease—implications for quantitation. (Abstract.) J. Am. Coll. Cardiol. 1:601, 1983.
5. McKillop, J. H., Murray, R. G., Truner, J. G., et al.: Can the extent of coronary artery disease be predicted from thallium–201 myocardial images? J. Nucl. Med. 20:715, 1979.
6. Maddahi, J., Garcia, E. V., Berman, D. S., et al.: Improved noninvasive assessment of coronary artery disease by quantitative analysis of regional stress myocardial distribution and washout of thallium–201. Circulation 64:924, 1981.
7. Maddahi, J., Van Train, K. F., Wong, C., et al.: Comparison of thallium–201 SPECT and planar imaging for evaluation of coronary artery disease. (Abstract.) J. Nucl. Med. 27:999, 1986.
8. Marcus, M. L., Skorton, D. J., Johnson, M. R., et al.: Visual estimates of percent diameter coronary stenosis: "A battered gold standard." J. Am. Coll. Cardiol. 11: 882–885, 1988.
9. Miller, T. R., Starren, J. B., and Grothe, R. A.: Three-dimensional display of positron emission tomography of the heart. J. Nucl. Med. 29:530–537, 1988.

N

1. Nichols, K.: Interpolative background corrections for gated blood pool studies on low signal-to-noise ratios. *In* Esser, P. (ed.): Digital Imaging. Society of Nuclear Medicine, New York, 1982, pp. 227–240.
2. Nowak, D. J.: Three dimensional surface display of nuclear medicine images. (Course Summary.) J. Nucl. Med. 29:967, 1988.
3. Nelson, T. R., Perkins, G. C., Slutsky, R. A., and Verba, J. W.: Automated on-line analysis of all four cardiac chambers for rapid setup, data acquisition, and reduction. (Abstract.) J. Nucl. Med. 22:P63, 1981.
4. Niemann, H., Bunke, H., Hofman, I., et al.: A knowledge based system for analysis of gated blood pool studies, IEEE Trans. Patt. An. Mach. Int., Vol. PAMI–7, 3:246–258, 1985.

O

1. Okada, R. D., Lim, Y. L., Boucher, C. A., et al.: Clinical, angiographic, hemodynamic, perfusional, and functional changes after one-vessel left anterior descending coronary angioplasty. Am. J. Cardiol. 55:347–356, 1985.

P

1. Pohost, G. M., O'Keefe, D. D., Gewirtz, H., et al.: Thallium redistribution in the presence of severe fixed coronary stenosis. (Abstract.) Clin. Res. 26:260A, 1978.
2. Prigent, F., Maddahi, J., Garcia, E., et al.: Comparative methods for quantifying myocardial infarct size by thallium–201 SPECT. J. Nucl. Med. 28:325–333, 1987.
3. Prigent, F., Maddahi, J., Garcia, E., et al.: Quantification of myocardial infarct size by thallium–201 single photon emission computerized tomography: Experimental validation in the dog. Circulation 74:852–861, 1986.
4. Peifer, J. W., Cooke, C. D., Skelton, J. P., et al.: 3D visualization of coronary arterial tree superimposed on myocardial perfusion distribution. (Abstract.) J. Nucl. Med. 29:810, 1988.
5. Pantaleo, N., Freeman, M., Van Train, K., et al.: A simple, objective method for measurement of absolute left ventricular end-diastolic volume with multiple-gated equilibrium scintigraphy. Clin. Nucl. Med. 5:S29, 1980.
6. Pavel, D., Pietras, R., Lam, W., et al.: Quantification of regional wall motion abnormalities (RWMA) detected by phase analysis of gated cardiac studies. J. Nucl. Med. 21:62, 1980.

R

1. Rollo, F. D., and Patton, J. A.: Instrumentation and information portrayal. *In* Freeman, L. M. (ed.): Freeman and Johnson's Clinical Radionuclide Imaging. Grune and Stratton, Orlando, FL, 1984, p. 241.
2. Rogers, W. L., Clinthorne, H. N., Harkness, B. A., et al. FField-flood requirements for emission computed tomography with an Anger camera. J. Nucl. Med. 23:162–168, 1982.
3. Reiber, J. H. C., Lie, S. P., Simoons, M. L., et al.: Computer quantitation of location, extent, and type of thallium–201 myocardial perfusion abnormalities. *In* Proceedings of the 1st International Symposium on Medical Imaging and Image Interpretation (ISMIII), IEEE Cat. No. CH 1804–4/82. New York Institute of Electrical and Electronics Engineers, New York, 1982, pp. 123–128.
4. Ritchie, J. L., Williams, D. L., Harp, G., et al.: Transaxial tomography with thallium–201 for detecting remote myocardial infarction. Am. J. Cardiol. 50:1236–1241, 1982.
5. Reiber, J. N. C.: Review of methods for computer analysis of global and regional left ventricular function from equilibrium gated blood pool scintigrams. *In* Simon, M. L., and Reiber, J. N. C. (eds.): Nuclear Imaging in Clinical Cardiology. Martinus Nijhoff, Boston, 1984, p. 172.
6. Ratib, O., Henze, E., Schon, H., and Schelbert, H. R.: Phase analysis of radionuclide ventriculograms for the detection of coronary artery disease. Am. Heart J. 104:1–12, 1982.
7. Rogers, W. L., Clinthorne, N. H., Stamos, J. A., et al.: Performance evaluation of SPRINT, a single photon ring tomograph for brain imaging. J. Nucl. Med. 25:1013–1018, 1984.

S

1. Sorenson, J. A.; Methods for quantitative measurement of radioactivity in vivo by whole body counting. *In* Hine, G. J., and Sorenson, J. A. (eds.): Instrumentation in Nuclear Science. Vol. 2. Academic Press, New York, 1974, pp. 311–348.
2. Stamm, R. B., Watson, D. D., and Taylor, G.: Comparison of two-dimensional echocardiography, gated heart pool scan, and left ventriculography in the detection of regional wall motion abnormalities. Am. J. Cardiol. 45:403, 1980.
3. Strauss, H. W., Zaret, B. L., Hurley, P. J., et al.: A scintiphotographic method for measuring left ventricular ejection fraction in man without cardiac catherization. Am. J. Cardiol. 28:575, 1971.
4. Slutsky, R., Karliner, J., and Ricci, D.: Left ventricular volume by gated equilibrum radionuclide angiography: A new method. Circulation 60:556, 1979.
5. Schwaiger, M., Henze, E., Ratib, O., et al.: Accurate determination of left ventricular volumes with gated blood pool studies using a direct measurement of photon attenuation. (Abstract.) J. Nucl. Med. 23:P70, 1982.
6. Silber, S., Schwaiger, M., Klein, U., and Rudolph, W.: Quantitative Beurteilung der linkensventrikularen Funktion mit der Radionuklid-ventrikulographie. Herz 5:146–158, 1980.
7. Steckley, R. A., Kronenbert, M. W., Born M. L., et al.: Radionuclide ventriculography: Evaluation of automated and visual methods for regional wall motion analysis. Radiology 142:179–185, 1982.

T

1. Tamaki, N., Yasuda, T., Moore, R. H., et al.: Continuous monitoring of left ventricular function by an ambulatory radionuclide detector in patients with coronary artery disease. J. Am. Coll. Cardiol. 12:669–79, 1988.
2. Trobaugh, G. V., Wackers, F. J. Th., Sokole, E. B., Thallium–201 myocardial imaging: An interinstitutional study of observer variability. J. Nucl. Med. 19:395, 1978.
3. Tamaki, S., Nakajima, H., Murakami, T., et al.: Estimation of infarct size by myocardial emission computed tomography with thallium–201 and its relation to creatine kinase-MB release after myocardial infarction in man. Circulation 66:994–1001, 1982.
4. Tamaki, N., Yonekura, Y., Kadaa, S., et al.: Value of quantitative stress thallium–201 emission CT for localization of coronary artery disease: Comparison with qualitative analysis. J. Nucl. Med. 25:61, 1984.

U

1. Uhl, G. S., and Kay, T. D.: Computer analysis of thallium–201 myocardial perfusion scintigraphy: Circumferential mapping. (Abstract.) Am. J. Cardiol. 45:481, 1980.
2. Uren, R. F., Newman, H. N., Hutton, B. F., et al.: Geometric determination of left ventricular volume from gated blood-pool studies using a slant-hole collimator. Radiology 147:541–545, 1983.

V

1. Verba, J. W., Bornstein, I., Alazraki, N. P., et al.: A new computer program for the extraction of global and regional behavior of all four cardiac chambers from gated radionuclide data. (Abstract.) J. Nucl. Med. 20:665, 1979.
2. Vogel, R. A., Kirch, D. L., LeFree, M. T., et al.: Thallium–201 myocardial perfusion scintigraphy: Results of standard and multi-pinhole tomographic techniques. Am. J. Cardiol. 43:787, 1979.
3. Vogel, R. A., Kirch, K. L., LeFree, M. T., and Steele P.: Improved diagnostic results of myocardial perfusion tomography using a new rapid inexpensive technique. (Abstract.) J. Nucl. Med. 19:P730–P731, 1978.

4. Van Train, K., Garcia, E., Maddahi, J., et al.: Improved space-time quantitation of segmental thallium–201 myocardial scintigrams. Clin. Nucl. Med. 6:449, 1981.
5. Van Kyke, D., Anger, H. O., Sullivan, H. W., et al.: Cardiac evaluation from radioisotope dynamics. J. Nucl. Med. 13:585, 1972.
6. Vitale, D., Bacharach, S., Bonow, R., et al.: Assessment of regional left ventricular function by sector analysis: A method for objective evaluation of radionuclide blood pool studies. Am. J. Cardiol. 52:1112–1119, 1983.

W

1. Williams, D. L., Ritchie, J. L., Harp, G. D., et al.: Preliminary characterization of the properties of a transaxial whole-body single-photon tomograph: Emphasis on future application to cardiac imaging. *In* Esser, P. D. (ed.): Functional Mapping of Organ Systems. Society of Nuclear Medicine, New York, 1981, p. 149.
2. Wagner, H. N., Jr., Wake, R., Nickoloff, E., and Natarajan, T. K.: The nuclear stethoscope: A simple device for generation of left ventricular volume curves. Am. J. Cardiol. 38:747, 1976.
3. Wilson, R. A., Sullivan, P. J., Moore, R. H., et al.: An ambulatory ventricular function monitor: Validation and preliminary results. Am. J. Cardiol. 52:601–606, 1983.
4. Watson, D. D., Campbell, N. P., Read, E. K., et al.: Spatial and temporal quantitation of plane thallium myocardial images. J. Nucl. Med. 22:577–584, 1981.
5. Watson, D. D., Campbell, N. P., Berger, B. C., and Beller, G.: Quantitation of thallium–201 myocardial distribution and washout: Normal standards for graded exercise studies. (Abstract.) Am. J. Cardiol. 45:480, 1980.
6. Wackers, F. J., Bales, D., Fetterman, R. C., et al.: Nonuniform washout of thallium–201 (within normal range): Criterion for improved detection of single vessel coronary disease. (Abstract.) J. Nucl. Med. 24:P46, 1983.

Y

1. Yuille, D. L.: Analysis of stress or nitroglycerin gated heart studies utilizing dimensional filtering and MUGG: A new program for automatic analysis of gated heart studies. (Abstract.) J. Nucl. Med. 21:47, 1980.
2. Yaron, M., Garcia, E., Friedman, J., et al.: A new objective approach assessing regional left ventricular (LV) function at rest and exercise (R/Ex) using phase analysis of radionuclide ventriculography (RNV). (Abstract.) Circulation 66(Suppl. II):II–353, 1982.

Chapter 56

Radionuclide Angiocardiography

ROBERT H. JONES, M.D.

HISTORY 1006
INSTRUMENTATION FOR RADIONUCLIDE ANGIOCARDIOGRAPHY 1006
RADIOPHARMACEUTICALS 1010
DATA ACQUISITION 1010
PROCESSING RADIONUCLIDE ANGIOCARDIOGRAM DATA 1011
Acquisition and Filtering 1011
Curve Generation 1012
Use of Low-Frequency Curve Data 1014
Hemodynamic Measurements Derived from Pulsatile Radionuclide Angiocardiogram Data 1016
Accuracy and Reproducibility 1018
RADIONUCLIDE ANGIOCARDIOGRAPHY IN NORMAL SUBJECTS 1018
RADIONUCLIDE ANGIOCARDIOGRAPHY IN PATIENTS WITH CONGENITAL HEART DISEASE 1021
APPLICATIONS OF RADIONUCLIDE ANGIOCARDIOGRAPHY IN PATIENTS WITH VALVULAR CARDIAC DISORDERS 1021
APPLICATIONS IN PATIENTS WITH CORONARY ARTERY DISEASE 1021
RADIONUCLIDE ANGIOCARDIOGRAPHY FOR EVALUATION OF MYOCARDIAL REVASCULARIZATION 1024
THE FUTURE OF RADIONUCLIDE ANGIOCARDIOGRAPHY 1024

HISTORY

Herrman Blumgart first grappled with approaches to assessing blood flow in patients with pulmonary congestion while a medical student in the laboratory of Walter Cannon at Harvard Medical School. After a medical internship and a traveling fellowship in London, Blumgart entered the Thorndyke Memorial Laboratory at the Beth Israel Hospital in 1924 and began an unusally productive four years of research. In a remarkable series of 11 papers published between 1926 and 1928 in the Journal of Clinical Investigation, Blumgart and his colleagues described the first use of radioactive tracers in humans and outlined all the basic principles underlying modern nuclear medicine (Fig. 56–1). Radon gas obtained from spent radium seeds was injected intravenously, and its course through the circulation was mapped using a Wilson cloud chamber that recycled every second.[B1] In later experiments, he used a modification of the Hewitt electroscope built by General Electric to measure central cardiac and pulmonary transit times in a large number of normal subjects and patients with a variety of cardiac diseases.[B2] Cardiac transit times measured with modern technology have confirmed the accuracy of Blumgart's original results (Fig. 56–2).

The crude technology then available for detecting radiation and the lack of apparent clinical use for these measurements caused the early insightful work of Blumgart to lapse into obscurity for two decades. In 1948, Prinzmetal and colleagues used a Geiger-Müller tube to quantitate passage of a tracer bolus of radioactive sodium through the heart and named this rediscovered procedure radiocardiography.[P1] Radionuclide angiocardiography is a better name for a procedure that aquires real-time data depicting the passage of a radionuclide bolus through the heart and great vessels. Redundant nomenclature, such as first pass, is not necessary to differentiate radionuclide angiocardiography from radionuclide ventriculography obtained by gated acquisition of counts at tracer equilibrium.

The first radionuclide studies undertaken to measure shunts and cardiac output acquired data using the output of a scintillation probe and recorder.[M1, P2] These inexpensive devices offered advantages of simplicity and portability but imposed the disadvantage of a single, fixed field of view. As early as 1962, single-probe data were recorded with sufficient temporal resolution to identify phasic count changes during a cardiac cycle (Fig. 56–3).[F1] Attempts to calculate ejection fraction proved unsuccessful because of the difficulty in isolating left ventricular counts from activity in adjacent sites.

In 1963, gamma cameras were first used to image individual cardiac chambers as tracer flowed through the heart (Fig. 56–4).[B3] In 1972, gamma cameras interfaced with computers provided data with sufficient anatomic resolution to construct indicator dilution curves from individual cardiac chambers.[J1] Radionuclide angiocardiography has subsequently evolved as a clinical modality used primarily to measure left ventricular function. Full realization of the potential of this procedure for characterization of cardiac physiology in individual patients conceived more than 60 years ago by Blumgart still awaits further refinement of technology. The final chapter in the history of radionuclide angiocardiography has not yet been written.

INSTRUMENTATION FOR RADIONUCLIDE ANGIOCARDIOGRAPHY

Cardiac anatomy and physiology dictate design characteristics of instruments to be used for radionuclide angiocardiography. The projected silhouette of the heart can be encompassed by a 20×20 cm^2 detector surface. A cardiac image with 2 mm resolution and a 10-level gray scale requires an information density of $100 \times 100 \times 10$ or 100,000 events. Static gamma camera images begin to appear coherent after 50,000 counts are acquired and progressively add resolution up to the level of 500,000 counts, after which little further information accrues from additional counts. Most gamma cameras achieve maximum

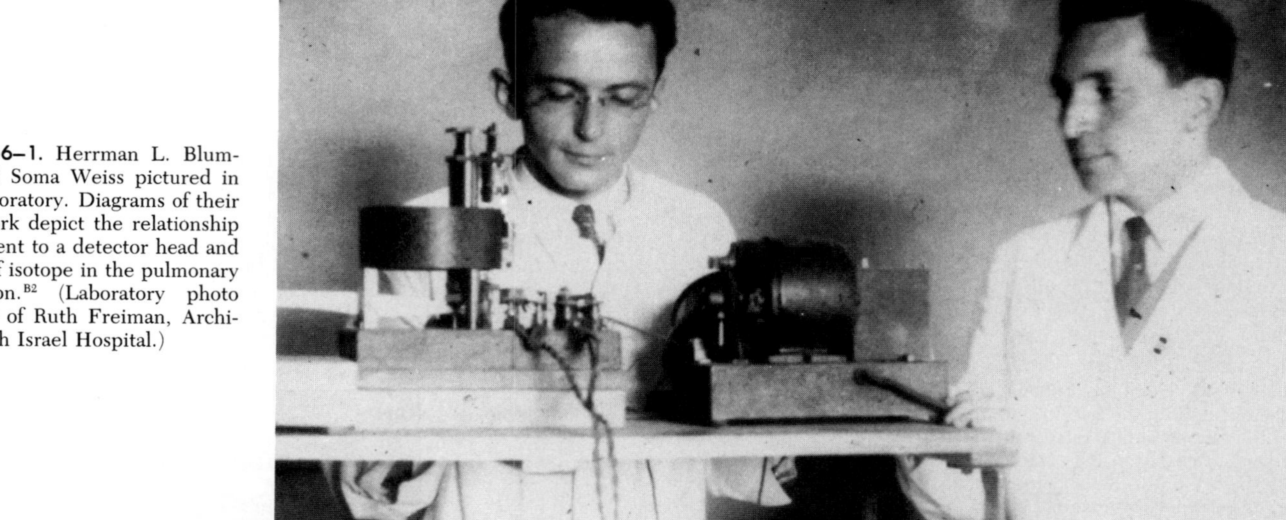

Figure 56–1. Herrman L. Blumgart and Soma Weiss pictured in their laboratory. Diagrams of their early work depict the relationship of a patient to a detector head and transit of isotope in the pulmonary circulation.[B2] (Laboratory photo courtesy of Ruth Freiman, Archivist, Beth Israel Hospital.)

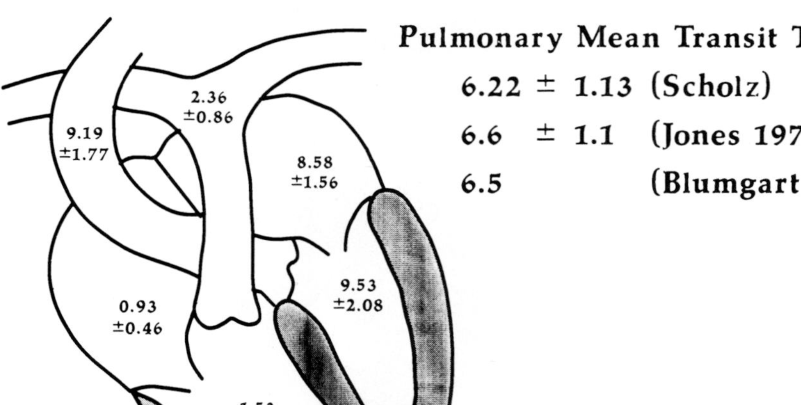

Figure 56–2. Individual cardiac chamber times in normal subjects defined by Scholz.[S1] The pulmonary mean transit time is essentially the same as that reported earlier by Blumgart in 1927 and Jones in 1972.[B2, J1]

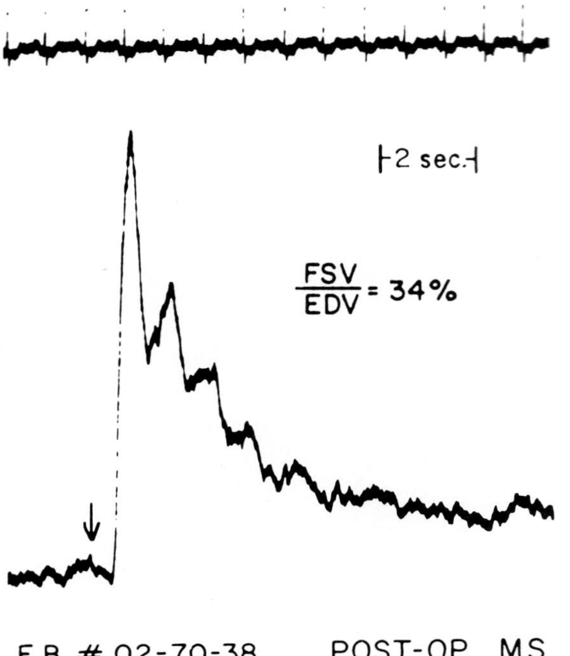

Figure 56–3. These data, obtained with a single probe after injection of radionuclide into the left atrium, are the first to demonstrate pulsatility resulting from individual cardiac contractions and represent the first attempt to calculate left ventricular ejection fraction from radionuclide data. (From Folse, R., and Braunwald, E.: Pulmonary vascular dilution curves recorded by external detection in the diagnosis of left-to-right shunts. Br. Heart J. 24:166, 1962.)

counting rates of at least 50,000 counts per second, suggesting a theoretic imaging time of 10 seconds. In reality, *static* cardiac imaging time is determined more by the number of photons presented to the detector by the radiopharmaceutical dose administered and the collimator selected than by the intrinsic sensitivity of the gamma camera.

Radionuclide angiocardiography requires *dynamic* cardiac imaging intervals to be as brief as 25 msec to avoid temporal blurring of counts at end systole and early diastole.[B4] Standard radiopharmaceutical doses provide photon fluxes adequate to provide 25-msec radionuclide angiocardiogram images containing 100,000 counts. Unfortunately, the maximal counting rate of even the most sensitive gamma cameras provides 25-msec images with about one-fifth of the desired counts. Therefore, the count rate characteristic of the detecting instrument is an important determinant of the quality of the radionuclide angiocardiogram study.

A gamma ray interaction in the thallium-activated sodium iodide crystal used as a scintillator in a gamma camera causes a light pulse with a 1-μsec decay. This decay time limits the absolute maximum counting rate of an individual sodium iodide crystal to 1 million counts per second. Single-crystal gamma cameras electronically vector signals from three adjacent phototubes to locate an interaction. The spatial accuracy of event positioning is influenced by the time devoted to electronic processing and to the energy limits set for event rejection. Broad energy window settings reduce electronic processing time and increase maximal counting rates but degrade spatial resolution. Single-crystal gamma cameras with the most advanced electronics typically saturate at a maximal counting rate of 300,000 per second with a 30 percent energy window setting.

A gamma camera constructed from multiple individual crystals should attain maximal counting rates equal to the multiple of the number of crystals used. Miniaturization of components necessary to construct a camera with multiple independent single crystals is feasible but costly. A less expensive approach was used to construct a multiple-crystal detector, marketed by Scinticor, Inc. A single block of sodium iodide partially divided into 400 crystal units of 1 cm per side is coupled to a matrix of 121 phototubes (Fig. 56–5). Events are rapidly assigned to only one of the 1-cm detector regions, resulting in lower spatial resolution but a maximal counting rate approaching 1 million counts per second (Fig. 56–6). The 1-cm intrinsic spatial resolution of this multicrystal camera represents a significant limitation for static imaging of a small perfusion defect against a background of radioactivity. However, radionuclide angiocardiography relies on the accurate regional quantitation of rapidly changing counts to define the border of a moving bolus, and this task requires an interplay of spatial and temporal discrimination.

The relationship between spatial and temporal resolution is illustrated by imaging a flask containing radioactivity at 10 measured positions 1 mm apart and three counting intervals to provide identical spatial data with different information densities (Fig. 56–7). The first image is subtracted from each successive image to illustrate the relationship between motion and counting intervals in producing a coherent crescent difference image. High-count-density images obtained from a multicrystal gamma camera with 1 cm resolution depict 1 mm of motion, but low-count-density data lose coherence at 5 mm of motion. Radionuclide angiocardiography requires both spatial and temporal resolution, and instruments that balance both domains produce the best clinical studies. As clinical use of radionuclide angiocardiography increases the demand for high-sensitivity and high-resolution

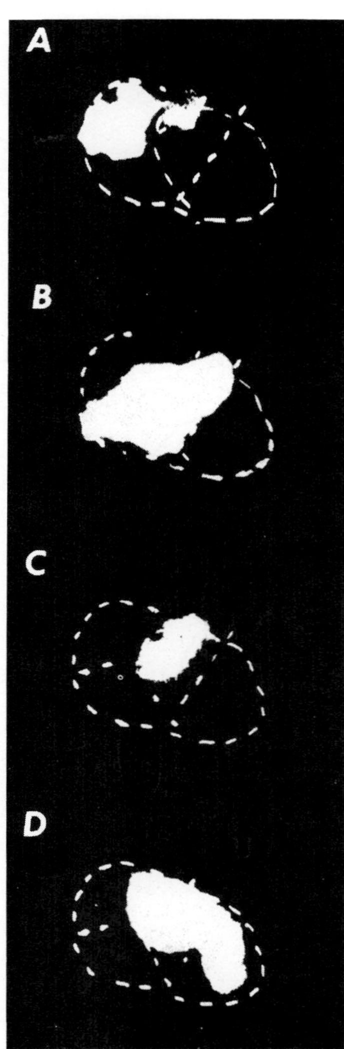

Figure 56–4. The first published radionuclide angiocardiogram images, which were obtained with the autofluoroscope after injection of 25 mCi of barium-137m.

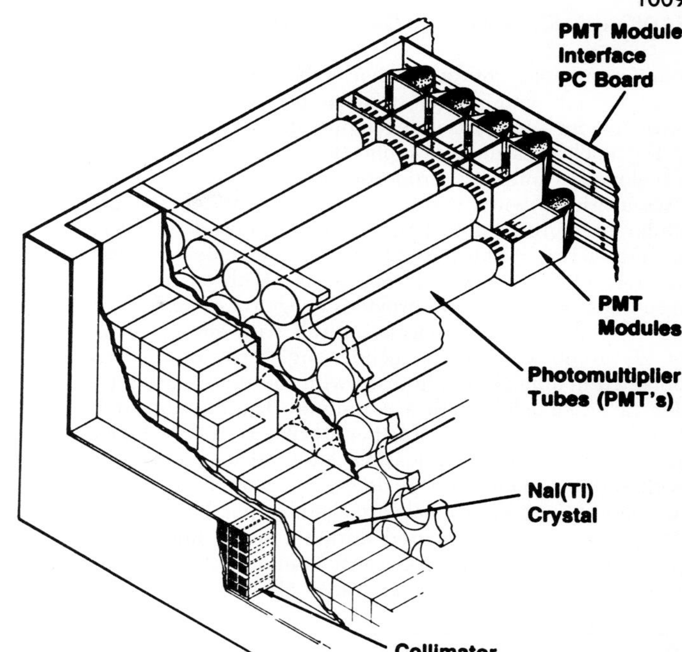

Figure 56–5. This schematic of the Scinticor detector illustrates the configuration used to achieve high counting rates.

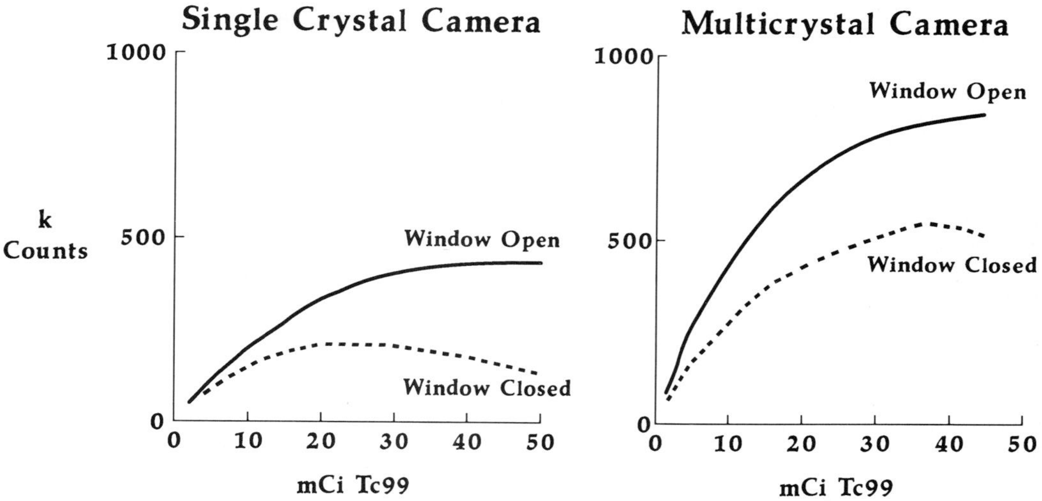

Single Crystal Camera

Multicrystal Camera

k Counts

Window Open

Window Closed

mCi Tc99

Figure 56–6. Comparison of counting rates achieved with a single-crystal camera (Elscint) and with a multicrystal camera (Scinticor) with open and closed windows, showing the total counting rates attained by using technetium–99m pertechnetate.

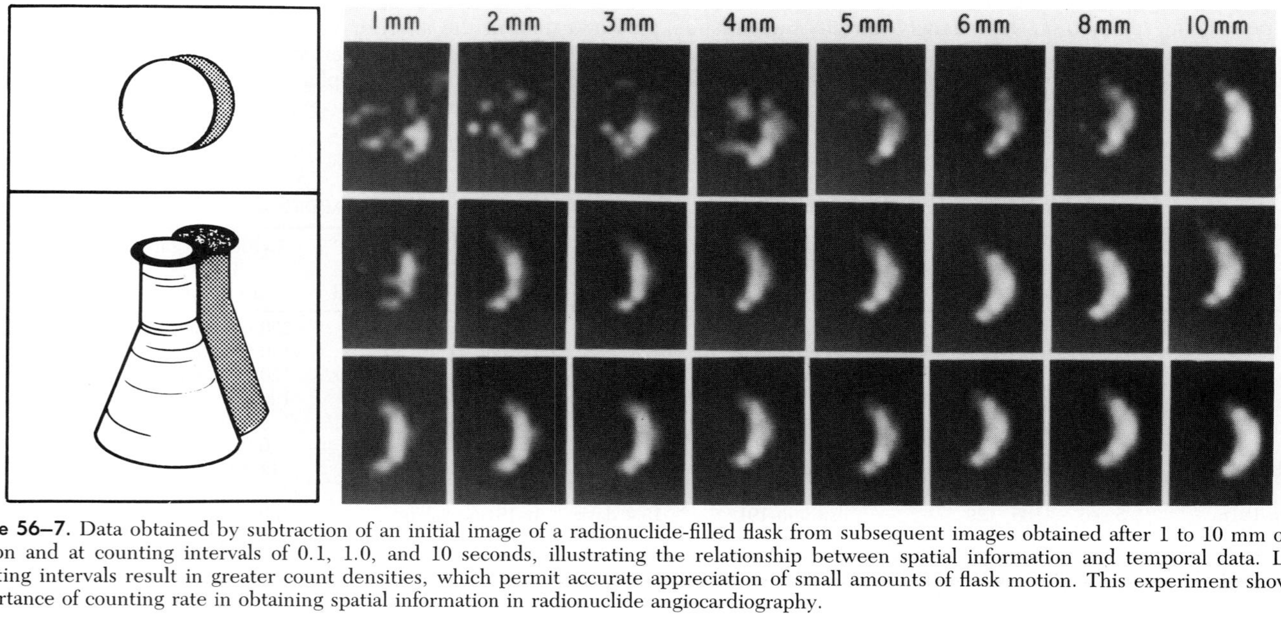

1 mm 2 mm 3 mm 4 mm 5 mm 6 mm 8 mm 10 mm

Figure 56–7. Data obtained by subtraction of an initial image of a radionuclide-filled flask from subsequent images obtained after 1 to 10 mm of flask motion and at counting intervals of 0.1, 1.0, and 10 seconds, illustrating the relationship between spatial information and temporal data. Longer counting intervals result in greater count densities, which permit accurate appreciation of small amounts of flask motion. This experiment shows the importance of counting rate in obtaining spatial information in radionuclide angiocardiography.

gamma cameras, improved devices that use multiple small solid-state crystals and do not require phototubes should become attractive for commercial development.

For nuclear cardiology applications, Lacy and colleagues have developed a multiwire proportional counter gamma camera that uses a grid of wires within a chamber containing stable xenon under pressure to detect the ion drift induced by each gamma ray interaction.[L1] This portable instrument achieves a peak counting rate of 850,000 counts per second with an intrinsic spatial resolution of 2.5 mm and provides images of excellent uniformity when used with radiopharmaceuticals with energy in the range of 20 to 80 keV. Radionuclide angiocardiograms have been obtained in animals and humans with this device using tantalum-178, a radionuclide with a 9.3-minute half-life obtained from a tungsten-178 generator. Further work with this technology may provide a commercially feasible alternative to gamma cameras with sodium iodide crystal detectors. Moreover, the relatively low cost of the proportional wire chamber would appear to permit several detectors to be used during a single injection, thereby providing radionuclide angiocardiograms from multiple simultaneous views during the initial transit of a radioactive bolus.

RADIOPHARMACEUTICALS

The physical characteristics and dosimetry are summarized for several radiopharmaceuticals that have been used for radionuclide angiocardiography (Table 56–1). An ideal radiopharmaceutical would inflict a negligible radiation burden when administered in a dose sufficient to approach the saturation counting rate of the detecting instrument as it passes through the central circulation and then rapidly disappears. Technetium–99m pertechnetate, the agent used most commonly for radionuclide angiocardiography, is available and inexpensive and emits photons with a 140-keV energy ideal for gamma cameras. The 6-hour half-life of technetium-99m is longer than ideal, and it is commonly complexed to DTPA to use rapid renal clearance to shorten the biologic half-life of the radiopharmaceutical.

Radionuclide angiocardiograms can be obtained by monitoring the injection of a technetium-99m–labeled radiopharmaceutical administered for any purpose. For example, a single dose of technetium–99m-labeled red blood cells may provide both a radionuclide angiocardiogram during injection and subsequent equilibrium gated images. Injection of technetium-labeled, bone-scanning radiopharmaceuticals in patients without cardiac disease can provide data useful for establishing normal ranges of radionuclide angiocardiogram variables specific to individual laboratories. More recently, technetium-99m–labeled radiopharmaceuticals that have a high myocardial extraction fraction have been developed.[H1] The technetium-99m activity permits radionuclide angiocardiograms to be recorded during initial bolus transit.[B5] The myocardial distribution of tracer on subsequent cardiac images indexes regional blood flow.[W1]

Development of generators that produce radionuclides with short half-lives has the potential to decrease the radiation burden of individual studies and thereby permit multiple serial studies in individual patients. Tantalum-178, with a 9.3-minute half-life and a 60-keV energy, is produced from a tungsten-178 parent.[L2] This tracer can be used with the proportional wire chamber as well as with a standard scintillation camera. Gold-195m has a 30.6-second half-life and an energy of 262 keV, which makes this agent well suited for radionuclide angiocardiography.[W2] Unfortunately, the generator is expensive because of the 41.6-hour half-life of its parent, mercury–195m. The short-lived tracer that is now receiving the most attention for commercial development is iridium-191m, which is produced from an osmium-191 generator.[P3] The half-life of 5 seconds and the energy of 129 keV make this tracer ideal for radionuclide angiocardiography.[H2, H3] The short half-lives of gold-195m and iridium-191m demand that these tracers be injected directly from the generator into the patient. The theoretic, but unlikely, possibility of accidental injection of a large amount of the long-lived parent has hindered commercial development of these generators. The many advantages of short-lived tracers for radionuclide angiocardiography justify continued developmental efforts.

DATA ACQUISITION

The discrete tracer bolus mandatory for radionuclide angiocardiography is most consistently obtained by injection into either a medial antecubital or an external jugular vein. The external jugular route has the added advantage of not being influenced by shoulder girdle tension during exercise, which may impede bolus inflow from arm veins. The venipuncture site may be anesthetized prior to insertion of a short 20-gauge intravascular cannula (Fig. 56–8). The cannula is secured by tape and connected to a saline-filled tubing, stopcock, and syringe. The radiopharmaceutical is loaded into the tubing, and the stopcock is positioned for flow from the syringe to the vein. A brisk, but not forceful, injection consistently introduces a discrete tracer bolus into the circulation.

The heart can be imaged from any orientation, but posterior views include more scatter than anterior views because of the greater bone and muscle mass posteriorly. The partial spatial separation of the right and left ventricles achieved with a straight anterior view simplifies data processing. Moreover, pressing the detector firmly against the anterior chest reduces artifactual motion during exercise and offers the most reproducible positioning for serial studies. Right anterior oblique angulation provides images that correspond to standard contrast angiographic views and orients the heart in its true long axis. Left anterior oblique views provide images with the greatest anatomic separation of the right and left ventricles.[D1] Resolution is less in both oblique views than in the anterior view because of the greater distance between the heart and the crystal.

Dividing the total radiopharmaceutical dose makes feasible acquisition of as many as six separate studies on the same patient

Table 56–1. RADIOPHARMACEUTICALS USED FOR RADIONUCLIDE ANGIOCARDIOGRAPHY

Radionuclide	Half-Life	Primary Energy (keV)	Parent	Half-Life	Radiopharmaceutical	Critical Organ Dose (mrad/mCi)	Total Body Dose (mrad/mCi)
Technetium-99m	6.0 hr	140	molybdenum-99	2.8 days	Tc-99m pertechnetate	250 (stomach)	14
					Tc-99m DTPA	140 (bladder)	7.5
					Tc-99m red blood cells	120 (bladder)	16
					Tc-99m hexamibi isonitrile	190 (large intestine)	16
Tantalum-178	9.3 min	55–65	tungsten-178	21.7 days	Ta-178 chloride	6 (bladder)	0.53
Gold-195	30.6 sec	262	mercury-195m	41.6 hr	Au-195m sodium thiosulfate	12 (kidney)	0.35
Iridium-191m	5 sec	65, 129	osmium-191	15.4 days	Ir-191m oxalate	100 (vein at injection site)	.018

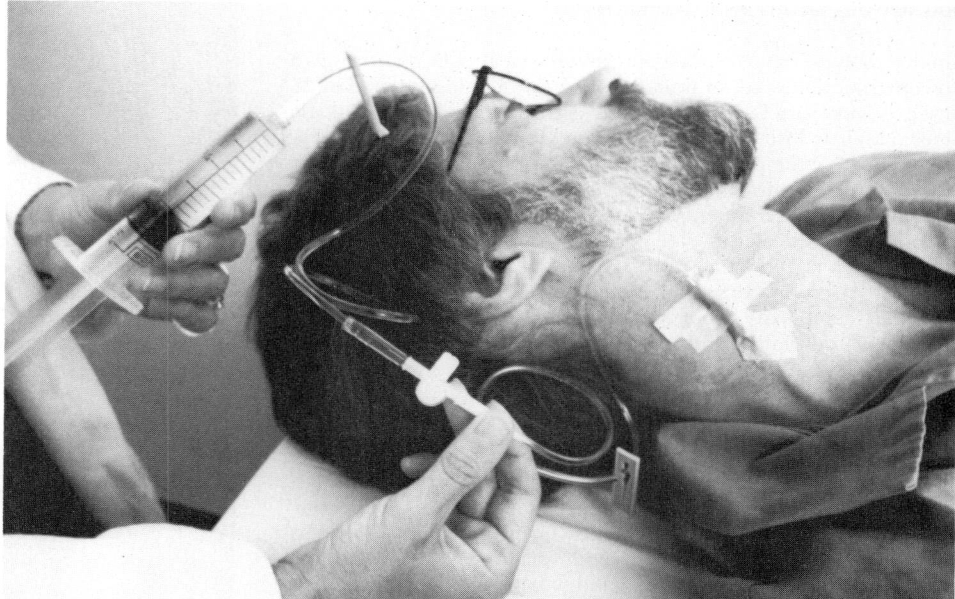

Figure 56–8. Careful injection technique is required for radionuclide angiocardiography. Placement of a catheter in the external jugular vein with tubing connected to a stopcock and a syringe provides a reservoir for the injectate and permits injection of a discrete tracer bolus.

during a single study interval. Therefore, multiple studies can be obtained on the same day from different projections or at different physiologic states as required by the clinical indication. Hemodynamic measurements are influenced by body orientation to gravity, but in most patients the magnitude of difference in hemodynamic parameters measured in the erect and supine positions is sufficiently small to be of little clinical significance. However, this influence can be substantial in patients who are hypovolemic or who have depressed cardiac function. Resting studies on very ill patients are commonly performed with the patients supine. Exercise studies in all patients and resting studies in most patients are easier to perform in the erect position.

Both bicycles and treadmills have been used to induce exercise stress for radionuclide angiocardiography. The advantage of the bicycle is that vigorous leg exercise evokes little artifactual chest movement. However, bicycle exercise stresses specific leg muscles that often fatigue readily in patients, especially those with peripheral vascular disease. Some patients with poor coordination cannot reach high levels of stress on the bicycle. An important advantage of the treadmill over the bicycle for stress testing of cardiac patients is the extensive clinical familiarity with use of treadmill results for management of patients. Gamma cameras with compact detectors suspended on partially flexible arms to absorb motion permit patients to grasp the detector firmly against the chest for imaging during maximal treadmill exercise (Fig. 56–9).

PROCESSING RADIONUCLIDE ANGIOCARDIOGRAM DATA

Acquisition and Filtering

Radionuclide angiocardiogram instrumentation incorporates one or more computers for acquisition, processing, and archiving of data. Data acquisition requires recording a series of frames of digital data containing spatially oriented counts at each accumulation interval. The optimal counting interval is determined by the heart rate of the patient and the sensitivity of the gamma camera.[B4] When high-count-rate gamma cameras are used to perform studies at high heart rates, acquisition intervals of 25 msec for 30 seconds are reasonable times and result in studies with 1200 frames of data. In patients with normal hemodynamics, only about 600 of these frames contain the entire initial transit of the bolus. The series of frames constituting an individual study is corrected for field nonuniformity, electronic dead-time count losses, and persistent background radioactivity from prior injections. Modern instruments perform data corrections and simultaneously incorporate other biologic signals, such as digitized pressures or electrocardiograms during initial data acquisition.

Processing of corrected data begins with temporal filtering to minimize noise without altering the signal reflecting biologic information. The rationale used in designing temporal filters is that count changes caused by cardiac events occur in rhythm with the heart, whereas noise in the data is erratic.[J2] The most simple temporal filter adds one-half of the preceding and following

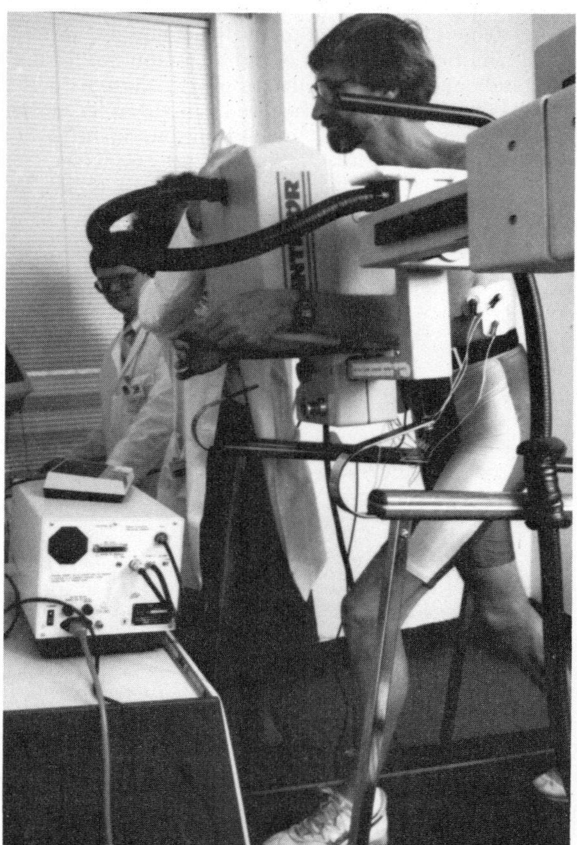

Figure 56–9. The flexible arm and small detector size of the Scinticor permit use of treadmill exercise for exercise radionuclide angiocardiography. The up-and-down motion resulting from walking on the treadmill is absorbed by the detector arm as the detector is grasped firmly against the chest of the exercising subject.

frames to each frame of data and divides each data point by two to construct a new set of frames. Since the framing interval of 25 msec is very brief relative to the cardiac cycle, little biologic information is lost but a great amount of noise is eliminated. A more effective temporal filter utilizes Fourier analysis to describe the data of the entire initial transit by the relative contribution of each harmonic frequency. Data can be eliminated at frequencies that add little to the signal and those that do not correspond to multiples of the heart rate or exceed biologically meaningful levels.[K1] Appropriate spatial filters enhance image quality and range in complexity from simple interpolations of data into a finer-resolution image to complex spatial Fourier filters.

Curve Generation

Real-time cine displays of the bolus passing sequentially through individual cardiac chambers permit a quick visual assessment of the study quality by attention to sharpness of injection and amount of motion of the patient during the study (Fig. 56–10). Moreover, these images provide anatomic orientation and an initial estimate of cardiac chamber size and flow, which is essential for further processing of data for patients with congenital heart disorders and useful for many other patients. Images selected at times of maximal bolus concentration are used to define borders of detector zones to generate time-activity curves corresponding to individual cardiac chambers (Fig. 56–11). These radionuclide indicator dilution curves from individual cardiac chambers appear similar to those one would expect if catheters could be inserted into each chamber for indicator sampling. However, radionuclide angiocardiogram curves differ from curves obtained from other indicators in three important characteristics. Blood sampling quantitates tracer *concentration* as a function of time, whereas radionuclide curves represent the *total quantity* of injected tracer during its catenary movement through the circulation. The total amount of radionuclide in any cardiac chamber at any time is the sum of the total input minus the total output. If radionuclide curves that approach the purity of those theoretically possible could be recorded in practice, instantaneous chamber volumes and flows, including abnormalities of flow associated with valvular regurgitation and intracardiac shunting, would be accurately reflected. The second major difference between radionuclide data and other indicator dilution curves is the high temporal resolution reflecting cardiac volume changes during individual cardiac beats. Unlike the prior two differences, which offer potential advantages, the third difference—difficulty in obtaining radionuclide curves containing counts from only one

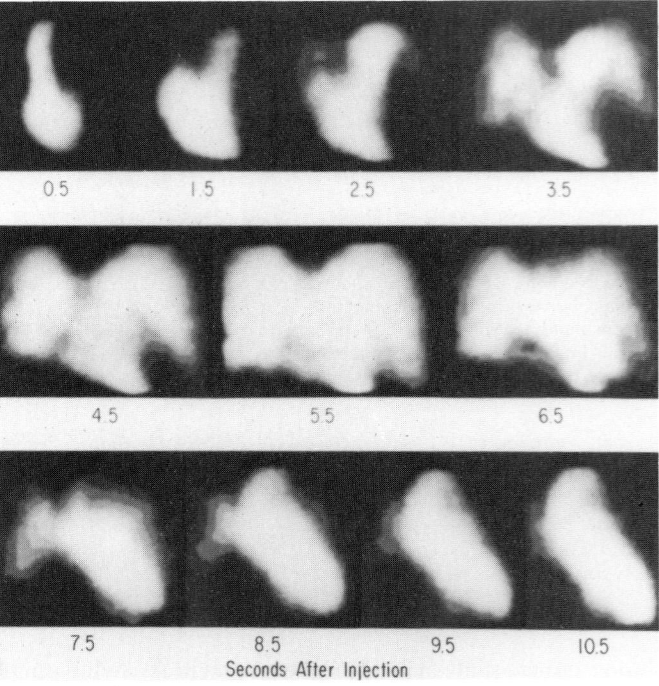

Figure 56–10. Serial 1-second images, each composed of twenty 0.05-second data frames, depict the progression of the tracer bolus through the central circulation in the anterior view. The rapid transit through the heart is apparent by the almost complete clearance of counts from the right ventricle during the time when count rates are maximal in the left ventricle.

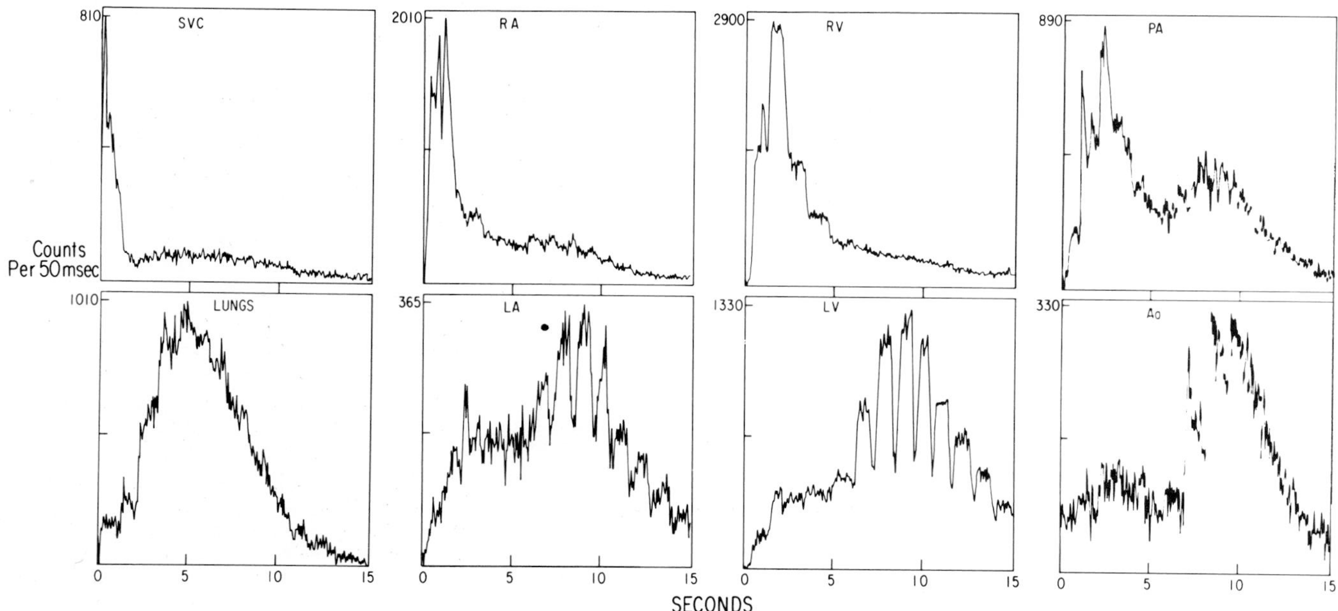

Figure 56–11. These indicator dilution curves obtained from a radionuclide angiocardiogram of a normal 18-year-old girl quantitate transit of the tracer bolus through individual cardiac regions. The curve obtained from the lung regions devoid of overlapping adjacent cardiac structures shows a single exponential clearance of tracer. Because of the anatomic overlap of adjacent structures in the area of the pulmonary artery as well as both ventricles, the indicator dilution curves have several components. Individual cardiac contractions are apparent in the time-activity curve obtained from the region of the left ventricle.

cardiac chamber—represents a major limitation of radionuclide techniques.

All indicator dilution curves are contaminated by normal recirculation of tracer, and extrapolation of early portions of the curves effectively corrects the later data, which contain a progressively increasing amount of recirculation. Recirculation is also apparent in the radionuclide data except for studies done with tracers with a very brief half-life, such as iridium-191m. However, a more troublesome source of contamination of radionuclide data results from including counts from adjacent structures obtained from individual cardiac chambers because of the complex geometry of the heart, which cannot be unraveled by a single detector in any precordial position. Any detector position that optimally divides two cardiac chambers, such as the right and left ventricles, increases the overlap of other chambers, such as the two atria, with corresponding ventricles and the aorta and pulmonary outflow tracts. This contamination from anatomic overlap can be reduced but not eliminated by careful selection of the region of interest. In addition to using the unprocessed flow images for region selection, functional images are quite useful in border delineation. Early work identified the time of peak count in each pixel to represent a simple but effective functional image for separating right heart from left heart structures.[J3] However, separation of adjacent cardiac chambers with similar times of peak tracer activity proved impossible with this simplistic approach.

A more promising technique uses a three-step automated computer model to delineate cardiac chamber borders using characteristics of the radionuclide data itself. The first step in data processing uses Fourier analysis to separate the mean and pulsatile components of data corresponding to each cardiac chamber derived from regions of interest identified by the operator (Fig. 56–12). The second step applies Fourier analysis to individual pixel data throughout the study and matches mean and pulsatile characteristics of individual pixel data with those from regions preselected to correspond to individual cardiac chambers. The third modeling step groups the appropriate temporal and intensity components of individual pixel data into a new set of curves representing individual cardiac chambers. The model iterates by using these new curves to recompare the individual pixel data and generate new sets of curves repetitively until minimal change occurs, which stops the iteration. This approach to curve definition may assign observed counts from any individual pixel to one of three regions, such as right atrium, left atrium, or aorta, in different amounts at different points in time during the study. Moreover, the number of pixels contributing to a specific chamber changes dynamically as the tracer bolus moves in space as well as in time. The resulting curves are free of anatomic contamination, scattered background counts, and recirculation (Fig. 56–13). This effective, but rather complicated, approach to radionuclide data analysis is useful for laboratory investigation but has not been sufficiently developed to merit routine use for clinical studies. However, most available programs are structured using a similar logic of relying on mean and phasic

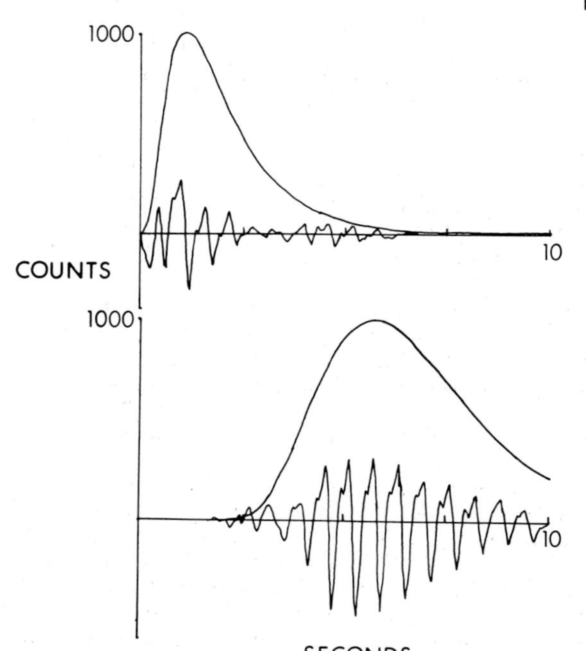

Figure 56–12. Typical characteristic curve components for the right ventricle and the left ventricle.

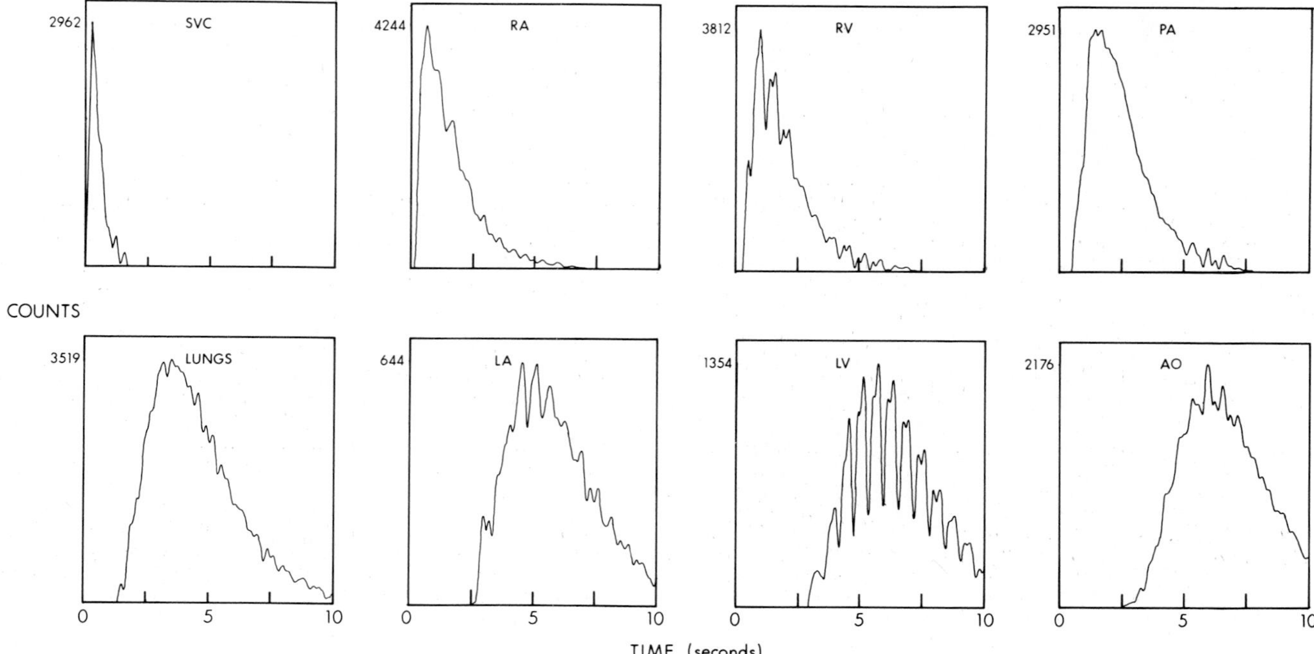

Figure 56–13. Characteristic curves that result from the decontamination sequence. The characteristic curves preserve the appropriate mean flow and pulsatile components expected for the chambers and show the correct sequence of peak concentration times and first moments expected in the catenary system.

changes in the counts to delineate limits of cardiac borders. Continued refinements of data processing techniques promise to enhance greatly the purity of radionuclide angiocardiogram data available for quantitative analysis.

Use of Low-Frequency Curve Data

The low-frequency component of radionuclide indicator dilution curves can be used to measure hemodynamic events that occur over several heartbeats, such as cardiac output, intracardiac shunt, and transit time measurement.[D2] Data necessary for these measurements can be acquired with low-counting-rate instrumentation and were the first clinical measurements made in nuclear cardiology. Cardiac output derived from an indicator dilution curve is linearly related to the amount of injected tracer and inversely related to the area of the curve. Use of a radionuclide tracer for calculation of cardiac output requires a way to relate counts from the dose administered to those from the curve recorded. However, if a constant amount of radionuclide was injected into different patients with identical cardiac outputs, the area of curve observed from precordial counting would differ because of individual variation in count attentuation and detector geometry. Therefore, radionuclide use as an indicator for cardiac output measurement requires an additional step to relate counts of the intravascular tracer measured by blood sampling to those obtained by precordial counting. To perform a radionuclide cardiac output determination, a measured dose of a blood pool tracer is injected and the area under the combined right and left heart curves is calculated after extrapolation. After an intervening period of 5 or 10 minutes, which is sufficient to permit equilibration within the blood pool, an equilibrium count is recorded from the identical detector zone utilized to generate the indicator dilution curve. A simultaneous blood sample is withdrawn and counted in the same instrument used to calibrate the injected dose. Although many workers have demonstrated that radionuclide indicator dilution curves provide accurate cardiac output measurements, the technique is sufficiently clumsy that it is not routinely used clinically. Moreover, volumetric cardiac outputs are available from alternative methods of analysis, which further reduces the demand for measurements that require equilibrium blood sampling and determination of the area of indicator dilution curves.

Another early use of mean data from radionuclide curves was for quantitation of intracardiac shunts. It is important to avoid biphasic injections of the tracer bolus in shunt quantitation studies that demand separation of counts reflecting the initial transit from those resulting from left-to-right intracardiac shunt flow. Large right-to-left intracardiac shunts are apparent on radionuclide angiocardiogram images, but accurate recognition of small shunts requires quantitative analysis of curves generated from the heart and aorta (Fig. 56–14). Counts detected in the aorta soon after tracer appearance in the right heart confirm the presence of right-to-left shunting. Data used to quantitate the shunt must be recorded from a site peripheral to the heart, such as the carotid arteries, because data recorded from more central sites, such as the ascending aorta, may include counts scattered from the adjacent pulmonary artery. Systemic radionuclide curves in patients with right-to-left shunting have configurations similar to those obtained with dye indicator dilution methodology (Fig. 56–15). Scattered radiation causes an early, relatively constant counting rate prior to the actual levophase in patients without a right-to-left shunt. In children with a right-to-left shunt, the early plateau is replaced by a definite increase in carotid counts, and the magnitude of this increase is greatest in the child with the

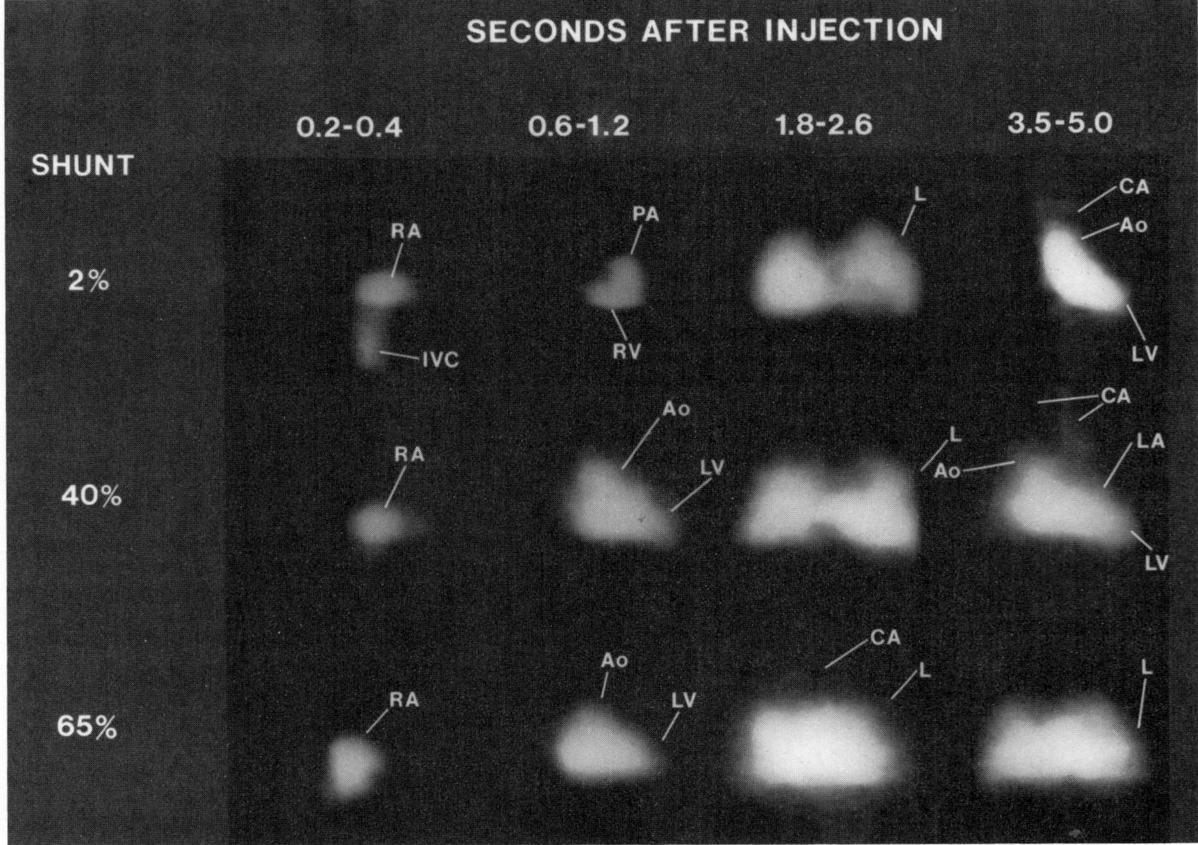

Figure 56–14. These images depict tracer transit through the right heart, lung (L), and left heart in three children. The child with a 2 percent right-to-left shunt had a small ventricular septal defect. The 3-year-old boy with a 40 percent right-to-left shunt had tetralogy of Fallot. The child with a 65 percent right-to-left shunt was a 9-month-old boy with transposition of the great vessels. RA—right atrium; IVC—inferior vena cava; PA—pulmonary artery; RV—right ventricle; CA—carotid artery; Ao—aorta; LV—left ventricle; LA—left atrium.

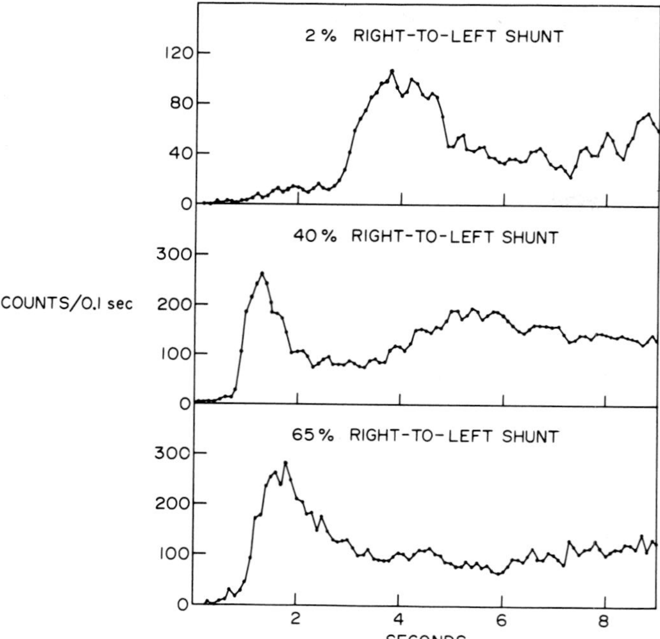

Figure 56–15. Carotid artery time-activity curves recorded in three children. The ratio of the first to the second component reflects the size of the right-to-left shunt.

largest shunt. In 20 children with cyanotic heart disease studied by Peter and associates, right-to-left shunts calculated from Fick data obtained at time of cardiac catheterization correlated well with shunt values calculated from radionuclide data.[P4]

Left-to-right intracardiac shunts greater than 30 percent of the systemic blood flow can be consistently recognized on serial images by a more brisk than normal transit of tracer through the lungs and by reappearance of tracer in right heart chambers distal to the site of shunt. Shunts of smaller magnitude return less tracer to the right heart and, therefore, prove more difficult to recognize by images alone. The most proximal site of left-to-right shunting can usually be located unless shunt flow is trivial. Further improvement in data processing techniques should permit localization of multiple sites of left-to-right shunting.

The curve configuration typical of left-to-right shunting shows an initial transit of tracer through sites distal to the shunt followed by an early reappearance of tracer returned by the shunt flow. Shunted tracer interrupts the exponential decline of counts and may actually increase counts sufficiently to cause a second curve peak. More commonly, the recirculated counts blend with the initial counts and the multiple rapid recirculations cause the curve to break from an exponential decline and remain relatively flat with a high background. Curves over the right and left heart chambers may show typical alterations, with tracer entering the right heart chambers prior to transit through the lungs and again shortly following left heart appearance. However, this typical curve configuration may also be erroneously produced by including counts from the left cardiac chambers within regions of interest designated as right atrium and right ventricle. Therefore, data recorded over the lung at a site remote from the heart provide the most accurate quantitation of shunt flow (Fig. 56–16). All approaches to quantitation of left-to-right shunts using these curves require separation of the first passage of tracer from the subsequent transit of tracer through the lungs. Shunt calculation by radionuclide methods has been found to be accurate even in very young children.[A1]

Radionuclide angiocardiogram data have been used to calculate valvular regurgitation. The most simple approach utilizes a forward measurement of cardiac output to subtract from a volumetric cardiac output to determine the quantity of regurgitant flow. An alternative approach views the regurgitant flow as similar to that of intracardiac shunt between the ventricle and atria and quantitates the break in clearance of the curve resulting from bidirectional motion of the tracer bolus.[P5] These techniques appear to provide reasonably accurate quantitation of valvular regurgitation but have not found widespread clinical use. Lack of a clinical need for this measurement and the complexity of curve analysis for patients with severe multiple hemodynamic abnormalities, for whom these measurements might provide the greatest clinical benefit, have been the greatest deterrents to their use.

Quantitation of cardiac transit times represents another application of mean radionuclide data. Appearance and peak times for counts recorded from each individual cardiac chamber provide a useful index of the speed of tracer passage through the central circulation. However, the mean transit time is the most useful time parameter. The mean transit time, which represents the average time necessary for a tracer unit to traverse two points, is calculated as the sum of counts multiplied by time divided by the summed counts. Therefore, very early or very late counts exert a greater influence on transit time measurements than that which occur near the time of mean transit. Curves must be carefully constructed to avoid contamination from adjacent cardiac chambers and recirculation, which can introduce significant error into transit time measurements. By a similar mechanism, the mean transit time recorded over the left ventricle always appears longer than that recorded over the aorta because of the influence of coronary blood flow, which artificially prolongs the tracer clearance late in left ventricular curve data. Despite limited clinical use at present, accurately quantitated mean transit times

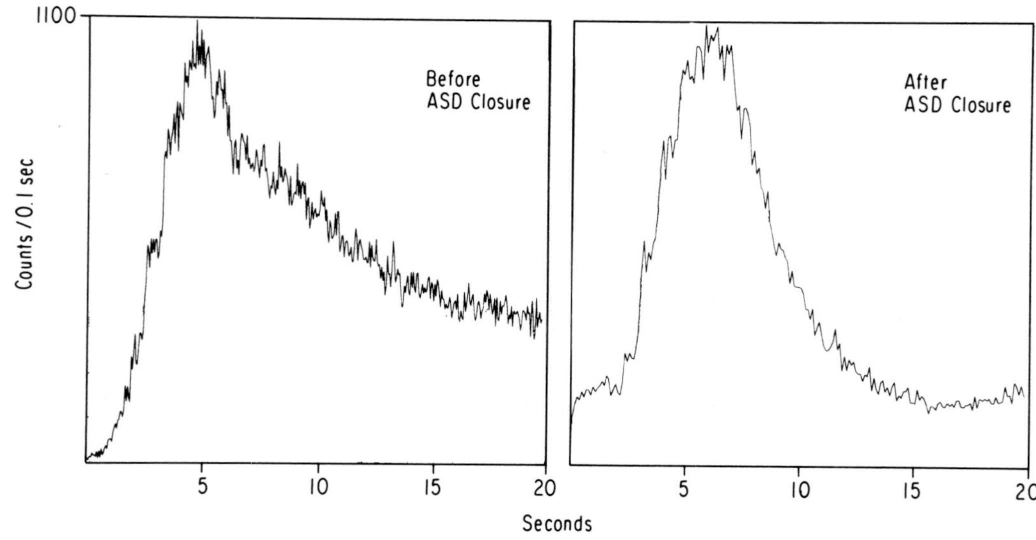

Figure 56–16. These lung curves obtained before (left) and after (right) closure of an atrial septal defect (ASD) document change from a pattern typical of left-to-right shunting, with early reappearance of tracer in the lung interrupting the expected exponential decline of counts. The study performed after closure of the atrial septal defect provides a normal lung curve documenting absence of shunting.

are useful hemodynamic indices, especially for serial assessments of hemodynamics in patients with valvular heart disease.

Mean transit time values depend on the rate of blood flow and the volume of blood included between the sites of measurement. The site of injection and the configuration of tracer bolus influence uncorrected mean transit times calculated from data from individual cardiac regions. Injection directly into the vena cava causes a shorter observed mean transit time through the central circulation than injection into a peripheral vein. However, the mean transit time between points within the circulation remains independent of these variables and can be determined by the difference in mean transit times of data observed from individual areas.[J1] A convenient normalization of observed mean transit times among patients results from subtraction of the observed mean transit time to the right atrium from the mean transit times to other cardiac chambers to remove variation caused by injection timing and by the different blood volumes between the injection site and the right atrium. The difference in mean transit time values of the main pulmonary artery and the left atrium provides the pulmonary mean transit time. Absolute pulmonary blood volumes can be calculated from cardiac output in milliliters per second multiplied by pulmonary mean transit time in seconds.

Hemodynamic Measurements Derived from Pulsatile Radionuclide Angiocardiogram Data

The major use of radionuclide angiocardiogram data has been in construction of right and left ventriculograms, which can then be used for calculation of volumetric data and ejection fraction. The rationale for data processing is similar for both ventricles, but techniques are more standardized for processing left ventricular data.[S1] Indicator dilution curves with high temporal resolution representing counts in the region of the left ventricle during the initial transit of tracer provide data for calculation of left ventricular volumes and ejection fraction. The number of individual contractions apparent in left ventricular data depends on the compactness of tracer bolus presenting to the left heart and usually ranges from 5 to 10 individual beats for a normal patient (Fig. 56–17). Tracer concentration in the left ventricle does not change during individual systoles, and the decrease in count rate during systole reflects volume changes. Diastolic count changes reflect variations in tracer concentration, as well as an increase in left ventricular volume. Data recorded from animal experimentation using multiple thermisters implanted in the endocardium and an injected bolus of cold saline have shown the assumption of instantaneously even tracer mixing within the ventricle to be erroneous.[C1] As a tracer bolus traverses a cardiac chamber, a period of ascending tracer concentration is followed by progressive tracer washout. Entry of blood into the ventricle while the tracer concentration is increasing results in the blood at the base of the heart containing more tracer per unit volume than blood at the apex of the heart. During the period of descending tracer concentration, this effect is reversed and blood that enters the base of the ventricle at end diastole has less tracer than the residual blood in the apex of the ventricle. Incomplete mixing introduces a relatively small amount of error in measurements of ventricular function. This source of inaccuracy can be eliminated by averaging beats on both the ascending and descending phases of the curve, which begin and end at times of similar tracer concentrations.

Definition of the area of the left ventricle is enhanced by interrogation of the spatial distribution of counts at end diastole and end systole. Since the only change that occurs during systole is a loss of counts from the ventricle, subtraction of the end-systolic count distribution from the end-diastolic count distribution results in significant residual counts only in the region of the left ventricle (Fig. 56–18). The more accurately defined left ventricular area that results is used to generate a second left ventricular curve from the original unprocessed data, which is interrogated for similarity in the timing of diastole and systole in each beat with that of the curve from the previously defined area. This iterative process is continued until a constant time of end diastole and end systole is defined for each beat. This process results in a left ventricular curve from an area reproducibly and objectively outlined by a computer algorithm. Summation of the individual beats from this curve into a single curve requires interpolation of data to an identical time for systole and diastole.

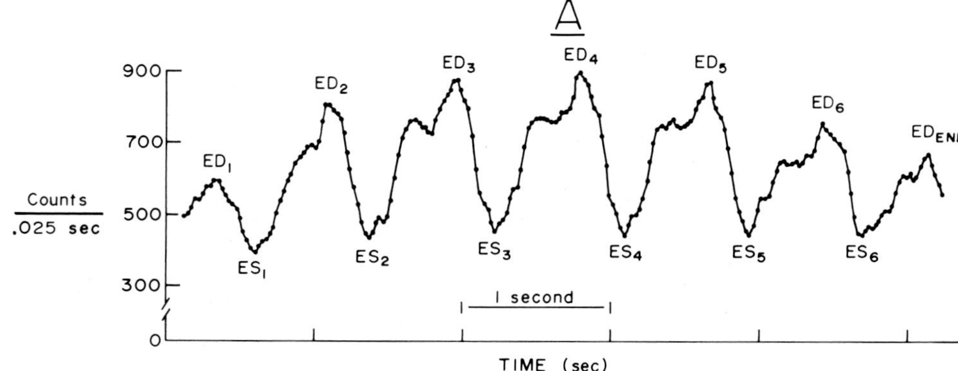

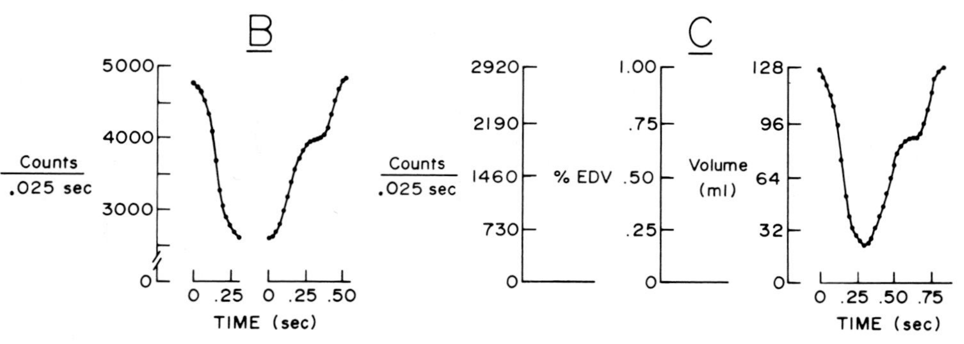

Figure 56–17. Construction of left ventricular volume curve from initial transit radionuclide angiocardiography. *A*, Uncorrected counts measured within the left ventricular region of interest during the levophase. *B*, Summed systolic and diastolic segments. *C*, Final volume curve after normalization and background correction. ED—end diastole; ES—end systole; EDV—end-diastolic volume.

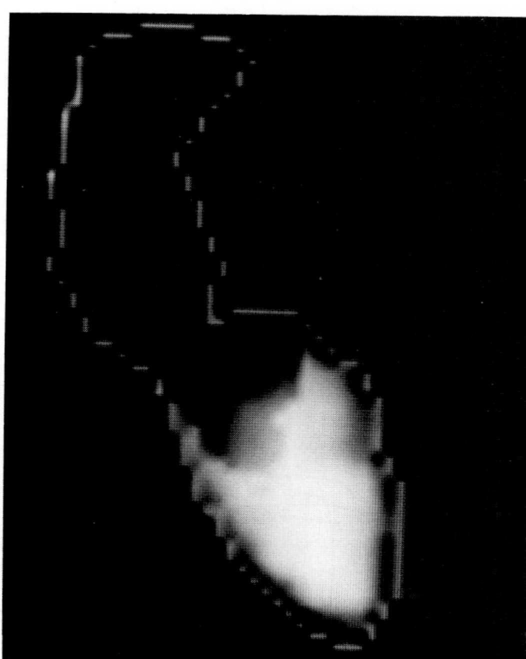

Figure 56–18. This image of stroke counts derived by subtracting end systole from end diastole accentuates the border of the left ventricular chamber and aids in selecting the left ventricular region of interest by automated computer algorithms.

In patients with severe arrhythmias, beats corresponding to the most frequent R-R interval are chosen for inclusion. This representative cardiac cycle constructed by using the identified end diastoles and end systoles retains the appropriate phasic relationship of data from each 25-msec accumulation interval throughout the entire cardiac cycle.

Data recorded from the left ventricle during the levophase contain few counts from the right ventricle because of tracer clearance from the right heart. However, images and the volume curves of the representative cardiac cycle include large amounts of tracer from other cardiac structures adjacent to the left ventricle, particularly the pulmonary veins and left atrium. Subtraction of these background counts is necessary for accurate determination of left ventricular ejection fraction. Furthermore, the linear relationship between counts and left ventricular volume demands data from which all background counts have been excluded.

All methods of determination of background are somewhat empiric and do not fully describe all complex changes of tracer as the bolus moves through the left heart. The left atrium represents the primary source of background contamination, but the pulmonary veins, lungs, right ventricle, aorta, and coronary circulation also contain counts that may be included in the left ventricular region of interest. Moreover, scatter of counts within the body represents another potential source of background counts. The technique more commonly used for background subtraction defines the spatial distribution of counts that coincides with the appearance of the tracer bolus in the left atrium but that occurs prior to entry of tracer into the left ventricle. The relative intensity of this spatial background remains unchanged, but the magnitude of actual background counts subtracted from each frame of the cycle varies as a function of change in counts over the entire detector in the area outside the border of the left atrium, left ventricle, and aorta. The ratio of total counts outside this left heart silhouette in the spatial background frame and uncorrected end-diastolic frame of the representative cycle defines a constant for altering the intensity of counts in each element of the spatial background, which is subtracted from each image of the representative cycle. Therefore, true background count intensity is estimated by multiplying the spatial background matrix by a constant that reflects the changing absolute count intensity during tracer transit through the left heart. Background correction provides left ventricular volume curves that linearly reflect volume changes and dynamic images of the left ventricle and aorta, which permits assessment of the left ventricular wall motion from the radionuclide ventriculograms.[A2]

Functional images, such as the stroke volume and phasic images, are useful for definition of the left ventricular border and aortic valve plane (Fig. 56–19). The area (A) of the left ventricular silhouette and the length of the major axis (L) are used to calculate the end-diastolic volume from the equation for an ellipsoid of revolution modified for the single anterior plane projection, which is $EDV = 0.85A^2/L$.[S2] Since the background corrected volume curve changes linearly with the left ventricular volume during the cardiac cycle, determination of the actual end-diastolic volume also described the chamber volume in milliliters throughout the entire cycle. Multiplication of the corrected end-diastolic volume by the radionuclide ejection fraction provides the stroke volume. The cardiac output is obtained by multiplying the stroke volume by the heart rate determined from the left ventricular beats observed on the radionuclide curve from this chamber. In addition to calculation of the left ventricular ejection fraction and end-diastolic, end-systolic, and stroke volumes, this curve may prove useful for deriving other indices of contractility from the rate of volume change.

Left ventricular wall motion may be assessed from static images of the left ventricle, or each static image of the representative cardiac cycle may be displayed on the black-and-white or color video as a real-time, continuous-loop cine, which appears similar to contrast left ventriculograms. In addition, derived functional images describing changes in left ventricular counts may prove useful for assessment of left ventricular function.[S3] An image of the difference in counts between end systole and end diastole, when divided by the end-diastolic counts, provides an image reflecting regional ejection fraction over the left ventricle. This two-dimensional image reflects changes within the entire volume of the left ventricular chamber and provides more information

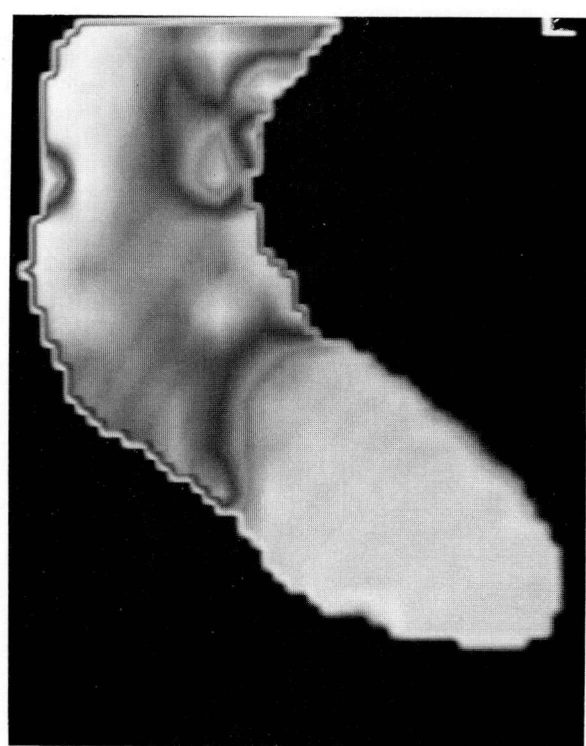

Figure 56–19. This phase image demonstrates the aortic valve plane by identifying the zone demarcating region where counts increase at alternate times of the cardiac cycle.

than assessment of the amount of excursion of the left ventricular silhouette during systole.

A more recent application of radionuclide volume curves has been for generation of pressure-volume loops in patients when it is feasible to insert a high-fidelity micromanometer catheter into the left ventricle.[P6] Stroke volume and stroke work derived from radionuclide pressure-volume curves compare favorably with those derived from cardiac catheterization data.[H4] Determination of pressure-volume loops at different levels of filling provides an excellent characterization of myocardial performance, and it is especially useful during periods of interventions, such as at the time of cardiac surgery (Fig. 56–20).

Processing of right ventricular data to characterize function is done with techniques similar to those applied to left ventricular data.[B6] Right ventricular curve background consists primarily of the right atrium, and this structure is difficult to separate accurately from the right ventricle because of tricuspid motion during each cardiac cycle and the angular orientation of the tricuspid valve relative to the anterior projection. Programs that use phase analysis to track the location of the tricuspid valve throughout individual cardiac cycles provide the most accurate assessment of right ventricular function. Geometric formulas have been applied to right ventricular end-diastolic images obtained by cardiac catheterization, but the less predictable shape of the right ventricle limits the accuracy of any geometric approach to volume determination. In the absence of intracardiac shunting, the volumetric left ventricular output obtained from radionuclide data can be used to calculate right ventricular stroke volume. Right ventricular end-diastolic volume can be calculated from this stroke volume and the radionuclide ejection fraction of the right ventricle. Validation of the accuracy of right ventricular volume and ejection fraction measurements is difficult by any methodology, but radionuclide measurements appear sufficiently accurate to be of clinical value.

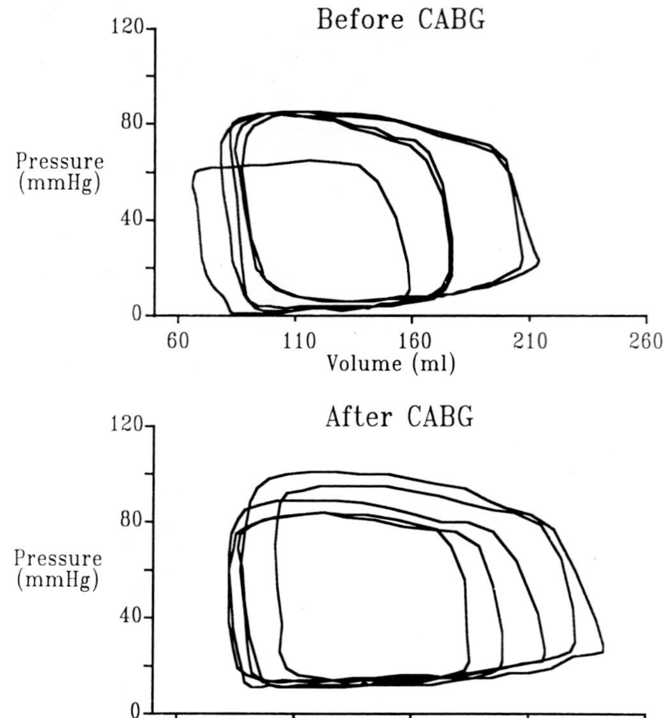

Figure 56–20. Pressure-volume loops before *(top)* and after *(bottom)* coronary artery bypass grafting.

Accuracy and Reproducibility

Many different laboratories have documented reasonable correlations between radionuclide angiocardiogram and cardiac catheterization measurements of hemodynamic variables. Moreover, phantom and experimental studies in animals with implanted ultrasonic crystals showed good correlation with radionuclide measurement of cardiac volumes.[A3] Hemodynamic values obtained in asymptomatic subjects at rest and exercise showed reasonable standard deviations in groups of patients as well as a close range of reproducibility for measurements done on subsequent days (Table 56–2).[U1] The high level of reproducibility is important to provide validity for serial radionuclide tests. The greatest testimony to the accuracy of radionuclide techniques is their general acceptance and widespread clinical use. Radionuclide measurements of cardiac function probably more accurately reflect baseline physiologic state than do catheterization measurements, which are often obtained in stressed or medicated patients.

RADIONUCLIDE ANGIOCARDIOGRAPHY IN NORMAL SUBJECTS

The heart must adapt to a changing demand for total blood flow to the body throughout each day. Cardiac output can be

Table 56–2. NORMAL LIMITS OF RADIONUCLIDE ANGIOCARDIOGRAM VARIABLES

	Rest			Exercise		
Variable	*Mean*	*Standard Deviation*	*95% Level of Reproducibility*	*Mean*	*Standard Deviation*	*95% Level of Reproducibility**
Heart rate (beats/min)	75	±15	57–93	159	±10	149–169
Blood pressure (mm Hg)	97	±11	87–107	118	±10	108–128
Ejection fraction	0.61	±.07	0.53–0.69	0.76	±9	0.71–0.81
End-diastolic volume (ml)	158	±29	148–168	172	±42	168–184
End-systolic volume (ml)	63	±22	52–74	41	±19	31–52
Cardiac output (L/min)	7.1	±1.7	4.7–9.5	21.0	±3.4	19.7–27.3
Pulmonary transit time (sec)	6.0	1.4	4.7–7.3	2.4	±0.4	1.9–2.9
Pulmonary blood volume (ml)	687	176	561–813	861	296	665–1057

*95% level of reproducibility is the range within which 95 of 100 measurements would fall on subsequent measurements if the initial results were the mean volumes.

altered by changes in heart rate, contractility, preload, or afterload. Using strict cardiac physiology definitions, only heart rate can be accurately measured by radionuclide angiocardiography. However, from the practical perspective of clinical cardiology, parameters related to the more basic physiologic variables can be derived from the radionuclide angiocardiogram. The systolic blood pressure is a clinically important influence on left ventricular afterload. Left ventricular ejection fraction reflects intrinsic myocardial contractility, although pressure-volume loops measured at different levels of cardiac filling are necessary to fully define contractility in patients. Left ventricular end-diastolic volume represents a good index of preload.

As long as limitations of interpretation are understood, it is useful to conceptulize hemodynamic adaptations of individual patients in terms of change in heart rate, blood pressure, ejection fraction, and end-diastolic volume. The sudden startle response, which everyone has experienced, testifies to the rapid and effective heart rate-related increase in cardiac output achieved by sympathetic stimulation. Both myocardial oxygen utilization and cardiac output tend to increase linearly as a function of heart rate. Many physiologic stimuli that increase heart rate also increase left ventricular ejection fraction. Cardiac contractility is influenced by the sympathetic nervous system and, therefore, can be increased rapidly. Myocardial ischemia and infarction usually depress myocardial contractility. Systolic blood pressure represents the major component of afterload that can be altered clinically. Systemic blood pressure must be maintained at a level adequate to support organ perfusion. However, systemic vascular resistance can often be lowered in patients to maintain adequate blood pressure and yet significantly reduce the afterload to the left ventricle. Cardiac function in patients with diseases associated with abnormally high afterload to the left ventricle, such as systemic hypertension and aortic stenosis, often improves greatly when afterload is appropriately treated. Within the physiologic range, an increase in end-diastolic volume is converted to an increase in stroke volume by the heart. The heart works more efficiently at high preloads, since as the preload increases the oxygen required does not increase as much as the work performed. Preload changes involve the entire circulatory system and cannot be activated as rapidly as heart rate changes but tend to be evoked as the heart approaches levels of maximal function.

Infants and young children have a dynamic resting circulation and very brief central circulation times.[J4] Older normal subjects show few age-related differences in resting cardiac function.[P7] However, cardiac function during maximal exercise progressively declines in subjects after age 25, with lower levels of ejection fraction and cardiac output. This age-related decline in cardiac function is probably related to both the aging processes in the myocardium and the greater amount of asymptomatic coronary artery disease in older subjects. Interpretation of radionuclide angiocardiogram studies in patients must compare results with normal values derived from normal subjects similar in age.

A number of other environmental factors influence hemodynamic measurements obtained by radionuclide angiocardiography (Fig. 56–21). Changes of body position appear to alter cardiac function primarily by change in preload. Normal subjects exhibit a lower end-diastolic volume in the erect than in the supine position. Head-down inversion greatly increases end-diastolic volume. Stress that suddenly increases afterload or preload, such as ventilatory alterations or handgrip, usually evokes compensatory changes that maintain a constant cardiac output. Chronic exercise conditioning slows the heart rate and increases end-diastolic volume at rest.[R1] Exercise conditioning increases the end-diastolic volume attained during maximal exertion. Populations of patients with different levels of exercise conditioning will show a wide range of end-diastolic volumes at rest and during

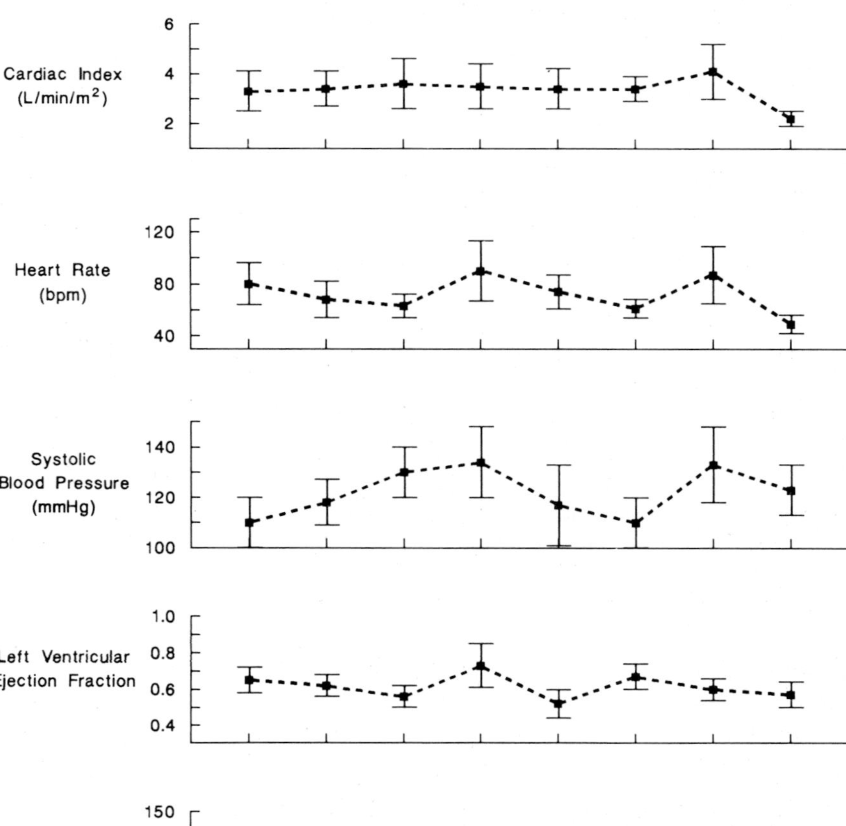

Figure 56–21. These data illustrate cardiovascular adaptations to common environmental changes observed in normal subjects. Data were obtained in different groups of volunteers and normalized to the same baseline to illustrate the direction of change evoked by these environmental influences.

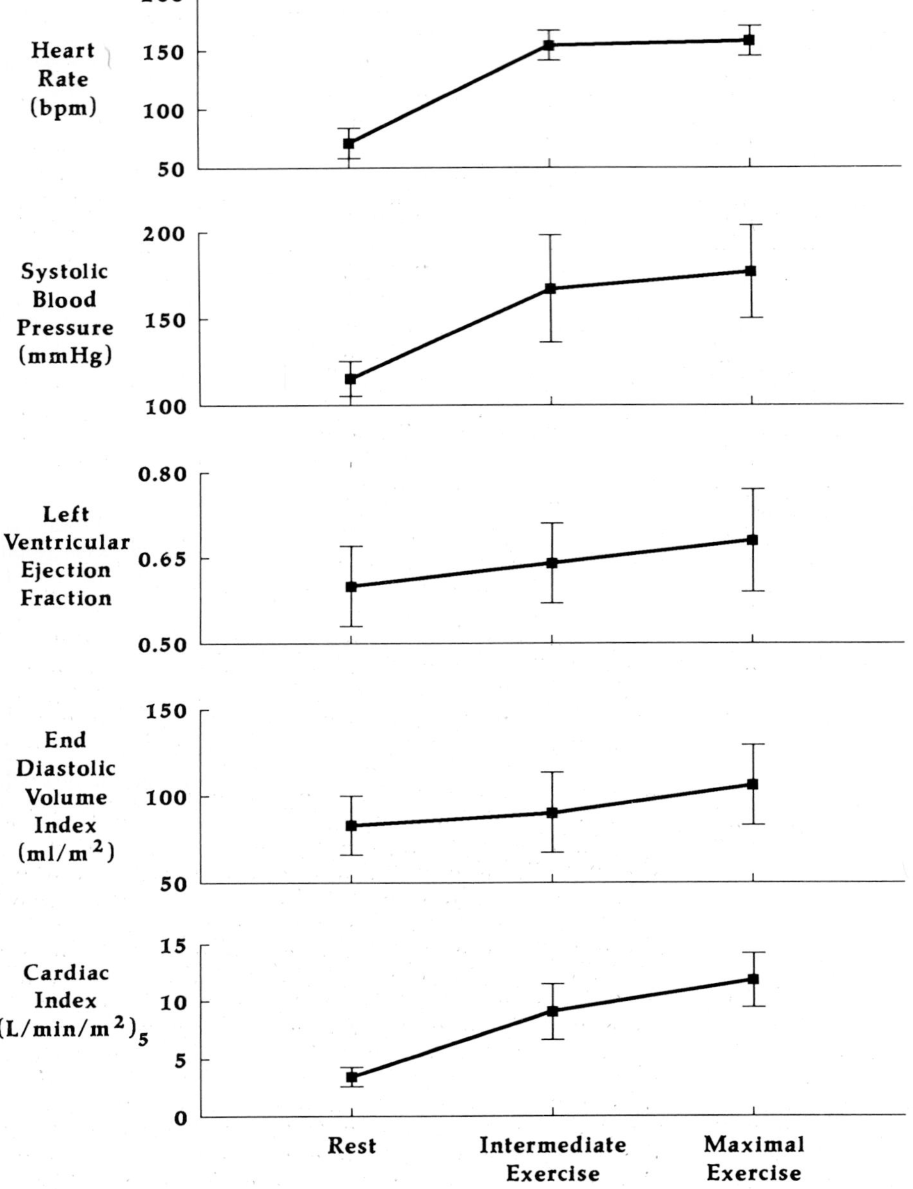

Figure 56–22. These data adapted from Christopher describe the cardiovascular response of trained athletes to sudden intense exercise.[C2] Intermittent levels of increased cardiac output increase the heart rate, systolic blood pressure, and left ventricular ejection fraction. At the highest level of cardiac output, end-diastolic volume increases.

exercise. Beta-blocking agents influence cardiac function by depressing heart rate and blunting the heart rate response to stress.[P8] Radionuclide angiocardiography provides an ideal method for study of changes in cardiac function evoked by specific drugs in normal subjects and patients with cardiac disease.

Exercise is the most common stress imposed on the cardiovascular system in life and is that used most consistently for evaluation of cardiac disease. During dynamic exercise the heart evokes all mechanisms at its disposal for increasing cardiac output, and the magnitude of increase can often approach dramatic levels. Cardiac outputs in excess of 50 L/min have been measured in trained athletes during the several seconds of most intense performance.[R1] Moreover, the cardiac output may increase severalfold within a few seconds of the onset of exercise.[C2] An increase in heart rate and ejection fraction occurs early after the onset of exercise (Fig. 56–22). Later in exercise, end-diastolic volumes increase to further augment cardiac output by the Frank-Starling mechanism.

Older patients who undergo cardiac catheterization for chest pain and are found to have normal coronary arteries demonstrate less vigorous cardiac responses to exercise (Table 56–3).[J5] However, the direction of change is similar to that seen in younger asymptomatic individuals. The ejection fraction response to exercise is a complex response influenced by multiple physiologic variables. In any large population of normal subjects, the magnitude of change in ejection fraction will vary as a function of the resting ejection fraction, peak work load, age, sex, body surface area, and change in diastolic volume with exercise.[G1] The most

Table 56–3. RESPONSE TO EXERCISE IN PATIENTS WITH NORMAL CORONARY ARTERIOGRAMS

	28 Men		28 Women	
Variable	*Rest*	*Exercise*	*Rest*	*Exercise*
Heart rate (beats/min)	81 ± 18	154 ± 18	90 ± 18	151 ± 14
Blood pressure (mm Hg)	120 ± 25	164 ± 28	126 ± 22	164 ± 26
Cardiac output (L/min)	6.1 ± 1.5	16.7 ± 4.6	5.8 ± 22	11 ± 4.2
Ejection fraction	63 ± 9	73 ± 7	63 ± 12	65 ± 11
End-diastolic volume (ml)	122 ± 31	144 ± 38	105 ± 34	118 ± 49
End-systolic volume (ml)	44 ± 17	38 ± 16	40 ± 20	43 ± 28

significant independent variables that determine the change in exercise ejection fraction are the resting ejection fraction, the change in end-diastolic volume index during exercise, and the sex. The normal amount of increase in ejection fraction expected during exercise can be predicted from the following equations:

(males)
$$\text{EXREF} = 45.0 - (0.52 \times \text{resting EF}) - (0.19 \times \text{EXREDVI})$$
(females)
$$\text{EXREF} = 38.5 - (0.52 \times \text{resting EF}) - (0.19 \times \text{EXREDVI})$$

Definition of normal from abnormal responses in cardiac performance during exercise represents a complex physiologic undertaking involving a large number of individual variables in the patient.

RADIONUCLIDE ANGIOCARDIOGRAPHY IN PATIENTS WITH CONGENITAL HEART DISEASE

Much of the early work with radionuclide angiocardiography was devoted to characterization of congenital heart disease in children. These studies to evaluate intracardiac shunting and assess ventricular function commonly influence clinical management and are performed with less risk and discomfort than cardiac catheterization.[J6] The recent introduction of high-resolution cardiac ultrasound with color flow Doppler has resulted in decreased use of radionuclide angiocardiography for diagnosis of congenital heart disorders. Concern about radiation in children has been one of the major reasons for decreased use of radionuclide studies. With the development of short-lived radionuclides, the dramatic decrease in radiation dose should again prompt more widespread use of tracer modalities, which are ideally suited for characterization of blood flow and evaluation of left ventricular function.

Definition of the path of blood flow through the central circulation represents an important use of radionuclide angiocardiography in patients with congenital heart disorders. Examples of these uses include demonstration of a persistent left superior vena cava in a patient with an atrial septal defect, evaluation of vena cava flow after Mustard repair of transposition of the great vessels, and definition of relative flow to each lung after Fontan correction of tricuspid atresia. In these and similar situations in which answers to simple questions about blood flow may influence management decisions, radionuclide angiocardiography offers a quantitative assessment of hemodynamics with less anatomic definition, but also less risk, than cardiac catheterization.

Radionuclide assessment of shunts is a simple outpatient procedure that can confirm the presence or absence of a left-to-right shunt without the risk and discomfort of cardiac catheterization. Functional cardiac murmurs are common in children and often raise the consideration of congenital heart disease. Even when the diagnosis of cardiac pathology appears highly unlikely in many of these patients, objective documentation of the normal blood flow may provide worthwhile information to reassure the patient and his family. Moreover, many intracardiac defects associated with left-to-right shunting are not repaired surgically when the diagnosis is first recognized, and radionuclide angiocardiography can document the magnitude of shunting. In addition, postoperative studies may provide documentation of complete closure of septal defects.

Surgical treatment of congenital heart disorders has progressed so that a majority of patients with these diseases who previously would have died now survive. Therefore, therapy is no longer evaluated in terms of survival alone, and attention has recently been focused on forms of treatment that minimize myocardial tissue loss and optimally preserve cardiac function. Studies in adults with cardiac disease have documented that many patients with normal resting ventricular function have depressed ejection fractions during exercise. Much of this change appears to be related to exercise-induced myocardial ischemia, but these changes have also been observed in patients with long-standing ventricular volume overload resulting from valvular regurgitation. Therefore, the definition of cardiovascular function should, ideally, describe heart performance both at rest and during the maximum level of activity typical in the daily routine of individual patients. Children studied after Fontan and Mustard operations increased cardiac output during exercise as much as normal children.[P9, P10] However, cardiac volume changes were abnormal during exercise in both groups, reflecting chronic adaptations to abnormal anatomy of the congenital abnormality altered surgically. These measurements of ventricular function during exercise provide valuable insight into myocardial reserve in children with surgically corrected congenital heart disorders.

APPLICATIONS OF RADIONUCLIDE ANGIOCARDIOGRAPHY IN PATIENTS WITH VALVULAR CARDIAC DISORDERS

Cardiac valvular abnormalities may alter left ventricular function either by the direct effect of the valve disorder on ventricular filling and emptying or by chronic myocardial changes in response to the long-standing hemodynamic alteration. Patients with mitral stenosis have restriction of left ventricular filling that becomes more prominent during exercise and limits forward cardiac output. Mitral valvulotomy or replacement eliminates the restriction to filling and returns cardiac function toward normal during both rest and exercise.[N1] Aortic stenosis restricts left ventricular emptying, and the decrease in left ventricular ejection fraction during exercise that occurs in these patients may result from the very large afterload imposed by the stenosis. Also, myocardial ischemia may occur during exercise when myocardial work increases oxygen utilization above that supplied by the coronary blood flow, which is limited by the stenosis. Early in the course of aortic stenosis, left ventricular hypertrophy decreases the end-diastolic volume and results in an abnormally high left ventricular ejection fraction. Later in the natural history of aortic stenosis, the ejection fraction during exercise decreases, and ultimately the resting ejection fraction is also abnormally low. Patients with aortic stenosis who are permitted to progress to resting left ventricular dysfunction have a less favorable prognosis following aortic valve replacement.

Aortic and mitral valve regurgitations increase left ventricular end-diastolic and stroke volumes, and patients with incompetent left-sided valves commonly eject a normal forward cardiac output in addition to the amount of regurgitant blood. An ideal management strategy for patients with aortic and mitral regurgitation would be to withhold valve replacement until the time in the natural history of disease when the ultimate prognosis of the patient would be adversely affected by further nonoperative therapy. Signs or symptoms of cardiac failure in these patients are a frequently used, but inconsistent, index of cardiac deterioration. The appearance of moderate resting left ventricular dysfunction identifies patients who have greater operative risk if operation is further delayed.[P11] Moreover, patients with clinical cardiac failure or left ventricular dysfunction before replacement or repair of an insufficient valve may not regain normal exercise tolerance or cardiac function following valve replacement. Serial measurements of left ventricular function during rest and exercise by radionuclide angiocardiography define the time of onset of exercise-induced left ventricular dysfunction, which consistently appears before resting dysfunction.[P12] Patients with mild exercise-induced left ventricular dysfunction may be safely continued on medical treatment. Those with more severe dysfunction should be carefully considered for valve replacement.

APPLICATIONS IN PATIENTS WITH CORONARY ARTERY DISEASE

Pathologic studies in war or accident victims and patients with noncardiac causes of death demonstrate a high prevalence of atherosclerotic change in coronary arteries, which is more common in men than women and more prevalent and severe with increasing age. This information combined with the known annual mortality rate of only 3 to 5 percent in medically treated patients with documented coronary artery disease characterizes coronary atherosclerosis as a chronic disease with a slowly progressive course spanning several decades in most patients. However, the sudden clinical symptoms that can acutely interrupt the chronic course of this disease preclude a leisurely attitude toward its management. Data from the Framingham study suggest that approximately 13 percent of newly symptomatic patients with coronary artery disease have death as their first symptom.[O1] The other newly symptomatic patients are evenly divided between those with a myocardial infarction and those with onset of angina pectoris.

Cardiologists have largely ignored the large number of asymptomatic individuals who would probably have benefited from myocardial revascularization if they could have been identified before their sudden death from coronary occlusion. Moreover, the patients with end-stage complications of coronary artery disease, such as severe left ventricular dysfunction, left ventricular aneurysm with arrhythmias, or ventricular septal defects, who with much effort survive operation, may be appropriately viewed as surgical triumphs but actually represent failures in the present ability of medical technology to recognize patients prior to these untoward events. Clinical studies are sorely needed to assess approaches to detect and treat the high-risk asymptomatic patient with coronary artery disease. It is reasonable to remain optimistic about the likely effectiveness of myocardial revascularization in this setting and eager for any approach that enhances the capability of predicting the future course of this disease in an individual patient.

Patients in whom coronary artery disease becomes apparent with myocardial infarction or angina continuously join the pool of about 6 million patients in this country who receive medical treatment for this disorder. Even though the annual death rate is relatively low in this group, the population at risk is large, so that a majority of patients who die each year with coronary artery disease will have interacted with a physician. The group of about 500,000 patients with coronary artery disease treated annually in this country with bypass surgery or angioplasty represent a small subset of those for whom these therapies must be considered.

The major challenge in current management of symptomatic patients known to have coronary artery disease is a problem of risk stratification. The large group of low-risk patients must be separated from the smaller subset of patients with a sufficiently high probability of a cardiac event in the near future to warrant evaluation for interventional therapy. Prior clinical studies of treatment of coronary artery disease have emphasized the anatomic severity and extensiveness of coronary atherosclerosis as one of the most important predictors of natural history of the disease in an individual patient. Patients with more, more severe, and more proximal stenoses in coronary arteries have a greater amount of myocardium at jeopardy for ischemic events and a higher incidence of myocardial infarction and cardiac death than other patients with less extensive disease. Patients with the most extensive forms of disease, such as left main coronary artery stenosis, derive the greatest benefit from revascularization procedures. Despite the prognostic importance of coronary angiographic definition of extensiveness of disease, this single parameter does not contain all the information needed for risk stratification. For example, even in patients with left main stenosis treated medically, 70 percent will survive at least 5 years, so even this very strong predictor of risk contains much uncertainty when applied to an individual patient.

Radionuclide tests appear particularly well suited for screening large groups of patients, and individuals with the most severe abnormalities can be selected for cardiac catheterization and possible further intervention, whereas those defined to be at very low risk would require catheterization only in special circumstances. Myocardial ischemia can be detected clinically by angina pectoris, electrocardiographically by ST segment depression, and functionally by regional perfusion abnormalities and segmental contraction abnormalities with associated hemodynamic alterations. Exercise-induced left ventricular dysfunction is a very sensitive marker of ischemia that commonly occurs prior to electrocardiographic abnormality as ischemia progressively increases in an individual patient.[U2] Radionuclide techniques measuring ventricular function and myocardial perfusion reflect similar biologic processes because of the close link between myocardial integrity and blood flow. Myocardial infarction with subsequent fibrosis decreases resting regional and global ventricular function and also results in a resting perfusion defect because of loss of myocardial mass and the lower tissue blood flow rate of fibrotic myocardium.

Reversible left ventricular dysfunction as an indicator of ischemia was first demonstrated in humans by Herman and associates, who studied patients with unstable angina during and after periods of spontaneous pain.[H5] Sharma and associates in 1976 used contrast angiography to demonstrate reversible alterations of regional left ventricular function induced by exercise and cardiac pacing.[S4] Radionuclide measurements of ventricular function obtained at rest and during exercise in patients with coronary artery disease were first reported by Borer and associates.[B7] In 1978, Rerych and associates measured cardiac volumes with rest and exercise radionuclide angiocardiography in 30 normal subjects and 30 patients with coronary artery disease.[R2] These data were the first that conclusively characterized the functional ischemic response to exercise. High levels of exercise stress decreased pulmonary transit time and increased pulmonary blood volume and left ventricular stroke volume in normal subjects and patients with coronary artery disease. However, patients with coronary artery disease demonstrated very large increases in end-diastolic volume and pulmonary blood volume as the Starling mechanism was used to maintain stroke volume. In contrast to a normal decrease in exercise end-systolic volume, patients with coronary artery disease significantly increased end-systolic volume. Left ventricular ejection fraction decreased with exercise-induced ischemia, and diminished wall excursion was apparent on dynamic ventriculograms. Moreover, the magnitude of these exercise-induced ischemic functional abnormalities was related to the anatomic extensiveness of coronary artery disease, with the most severe exercise dysfunction observed in patients with three-vessel and left main coronary artery disease.

The dramatic decreases observed in left ventricular ejection fraction during exercise in patients with coronary artery disease focused attention on use of this single parameter for diagnosis of coronary artery disease. Many early reports contained small numbers of studies of patients with very severe coronary artery disease and even smaller numbers of normal controls, who were often asymptomatic young volunteers. The dramatic separation observed between those with and those without disease led to overenthusiastic reports of the diagnostic perfection of a drop in ejection fraction for identification of patients with coronary artery disease. Growing experience with carefully performed measurements of cardiac function during exercise in a large consecutive group of patients referred for cardiac catheterization showed that the exercise ejection fraction response is a complex physiologic variable influenced by a number of factors. In a group of 150 patients with coronary artery disease, Port and associates found the magnitude of resting left ventricular ejection fraction to be a significant predictor of the change in ejection fraction during exercise even after adjustment for the influence of extensiveness of coronary artery disease.[P13] Patients with normal resting ejection fractions showed the most profound decreases in ejection fraction during exercise. In contrast, patients with low resting ejection fractions had a lower incidence and magnitude of decrease in ejection fraction during exercise (Fig. 56–23). Subsequent studies of larger numbers of patients with low resting ejection fractions have shown a higher incidence of decrease in ejection fraction during exercise in patients with coronary artery disease than in those with idiopathic dilated cardiomyopathy.[H6]

In 281 patients with chest pain, significant coronary artery disease, and normal resting ventricular function, Gibbons and associates found that the change in ejection fraction during exercise appeared to be a complex response influenced by a number of pathophysiologic variables. The resting pulse pressure, the level of exercise, the magnitude of resting ejection fraction, the change in end-diastolic volume index with exercise, and a

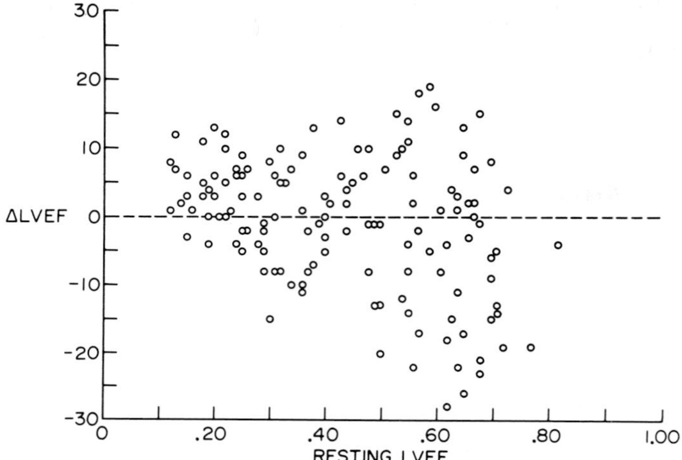

Figure 56–23. Left ventricular ejection fraction response to exercise (ΔLVEF) versus resting LVEF. Patients with normal resting LVEF show the greatest variability as well as the most profound decreases in LVEF with exercise. As resting LVEF decreases, the magnitude of the decrease with exercise also diminishes. Patients with resting LVEF less than 0.25 rarely have decreased LVEF with exercise.

positive electrocardiogram were related to the magnitude of change in exercise ejection fraction in addition to the number of diseased vessels.[G2] Therefore, optimal diagnostic information cannot be obtained from the application of an arbitrary threshold to a single parameter, such as the change in ejection fraction during exercise.

Criteria optimal for diagnosis were developed on the basis of 486 patients studied by radionuclide angiocardiography and catheterized for the diagnosis of coronary artery disease.[J5] Prospective application of these criteria to a new consecutive series of 221 similar patients identified a sensitivity of 0.87 and a specificity of 0.54 for the entire group.[A4] The test demonstrated more diagnostic accuracy in patients with multivessel disease than those with minimal coronary artery stenosis. Application of a continuous Bayesian model further enhanced the diagnostic usefulness of exercise measurements of cardiac function by permitting probability calculations for the presence of disease in individual patients based on the magnitude of abnormality observed.[C3] Logistic regression analysis in a group of 736 patients identified the absolute exercise ejection fraction, the exercise heart rate, and the ischemia score during exercise (defined by angina and electrocardiogram changes) as the most useful parameters for recognition of disease.[C3] Proper application of these variables enhanced the diagnostic information derived from clinical characteristics of patients. The observation that the absolute ejection fraction provided more diagnostic information than the change in ejection fraction was confirmed in a large group of patients assembled from several centers.[R3] In these patients, an exercise ejection fraction threshold of 0.62 provided the best diagnostic discrimination between patients with and without coronary artery disease.

Two studies have compared thallium-201 perfusion scans and measurements of ventricular function for diagnosis of coronary artery disease. In a group of 120 patients with coronary artery disease, accurate diagnosis by planar thallium-201 images and left ventricular function appeared equivalent.[O2] A marked difference was not observed in the diagnostic usefulness of these tests in subgroups differing in gender, level of exercise, history of angina or myocardial infarction, number of diseased vessels, or extent of coronary artery obstruction. Another study compared tomographic thallium-201 imaging and radionuclide angiocardiography in 46 patients with single coronary artery stenosis. Thallium-201 myocardial perfusion imaging proved more diagnostic for coronary artery disease than exercise radionuclide angiocardiography.[P14] For most populations of patients, both tests offer similar diagnostic accuracy. However, both radionuclide tests contribute only a modest increase in diagnostic information over that available from a clinical history and a treadmill examination. The cost of neither radionuclide test is probably justified simply for diagnosis. The cardiac catheterization remains the best procedure for determining definitively whether a coronary artery is anatomically obstructed or not in an individual patient.

Groups of patients demonstrate a consistent relationship between the extent of coronary stenosis and the magnitude of exercise-induced dysfunction, but this relationship is less apparent in individual patients. Even the most sophisticated approaches to radionuclide measurements of exercise left ventricular function identify some patients with dysfunction who have no recognizable coronary artery disease by arteriography and other patients with anatomically significant coronary artery stenosis in whom function remains normal during exercise. The small number of patients with normal coronary arteries and exercise dysfunction usually demonstrate borderline abnormalities that are probably related to small-vessel disease, prior myocarditis, or individual variation in myocardial metabolism. Patients with anatomically significant coronary artery disease and normal cardiac function during exercise probably maintain adequate myocardial perfusion by vasodilation and enhancement of collateral flow. Discrepancies between coronary anatomy and myocardial function negatively influence diagnostic uses of radionuclide angiocardiography, but the independence of these variables suggests that they might be complementary for prognostic assessment.

Pryor and associates used multivariate analysis of radionuclide variables to identify those which were related to later myocardial infarction or cardiovascular death in 386 medically treated patients.[P15] The exercise ejection fraction was the most important radionuclide variable providing prognostic information in patients with coronary artery disease. This simple variable contained over 70 percent of the prognostic information provided by combination of other important variables such as the coronary anatomy on arteriogram. The relationship between cardiac event and exercise ejection fraction was not linear, and patients with an exercise ejection fraction above 0.50 had very few myocardial infarctions or cardiac deaths for 2 years after study (Fig. 56–24). In groups of patients with progressively lower ejection fractions, the number of cardiac events increased dramatically. Recent observations in over 2000 patients confirm that measurement of variables such as the exercise ejection fraction, which is related to the magnitude of ischemia, can be used to stratify risk for individual patients with coronary artery disease. Moreover, measurement of left ventricular function during exercise provided as much prognostic information as cardiac catheterization in patients with coronary artery disease.

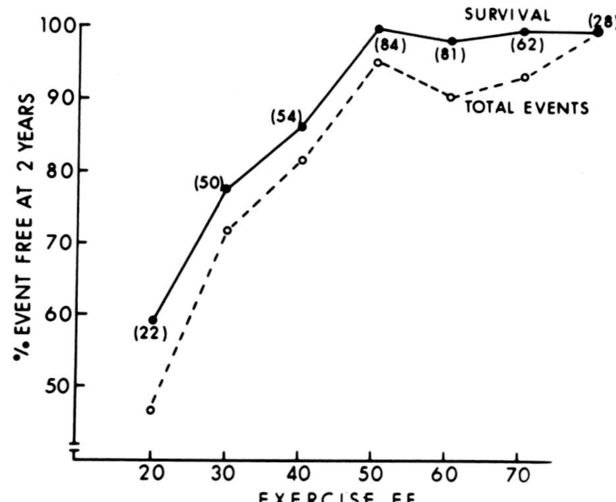

Figure 56–24. Two-year survival and total cardiac event-free rates as a function of the exercise ejection fraction (EF) rounded to the nearest 10. Numbers in parentheses show the number of patients within each exercise EF subgroup. (Five patients with an exercise EF less than 15 or greater than 85 are not included.)

Measurement of cardiac function during exercise, and especially documentation of the exercise ejection fraction, appears to provide a very sensitive index of the magnitude of myocardial ischemia. The amount of potential myocardial ischemia is the main determinant of survival in individual patients with coronary artery disease. Patients recognized to have a low risk of cardiac event should receive medical treatment. Patients identified as having a high likelihood of myocardial infarction or death benefit most from bypass surgery or other interventional therapy. Interventional therapy that is devised to reverse ischemia can be expected to benefit only patients with a significant amount of ischemic potential. Definition of the pathologic anatomy of the coronary arterial tree by angiography is indispensable for planning interventional procedures and provides some insight into the magnitude of myocardium at potential risk. However, radionuclide measurements of ventricular function during exercise provide one of the most useful independent sources of prognostic information for identifying patients likely to benefit from interventional therapy (Fig. 56–25).[J7] The simplicity and low cost of this radionuclide measurement also make it ideally suited as one of the first procedures to be performed in patients evaluated for stable chronic coronary artery disease.

RADIONUCLIDE ANGIOCARDIOGRAPHY FOR EVALUATION OF MYOCARDIAL REVASCULARIZATION

Not every patient who survives myocardial revascularization has an optimal functional result. Even the absence of angina after a procedure cannot be used as a valid end point, since either a placebo effect or a procedure-related infarction of myocardium previously ischemic may decrease or obliterate anginal pain. Patients with good anatomic results documented by angiography after coronary bypass grafting usually show resolution of exercise-induced myocardial dysfunction and perfusion deficits after successful revascularization. However, the potential for augmentation of coronary blood flow during exercise cannot always be predicted from the coronary angiogram, and vessel patency on arteriogram is not always correlated with improvements in regional function and perfusion. Therefore, as before operation, radionuclide tests provide important data that complement but do not always duplicate the information obtained from coronary angiography. Radionuclide procedures appear useful for objectively documenting improvement in myocardial perfusion and function, judging the effectiveness of operative outcome, and predicting the future clinical course of individual patients.

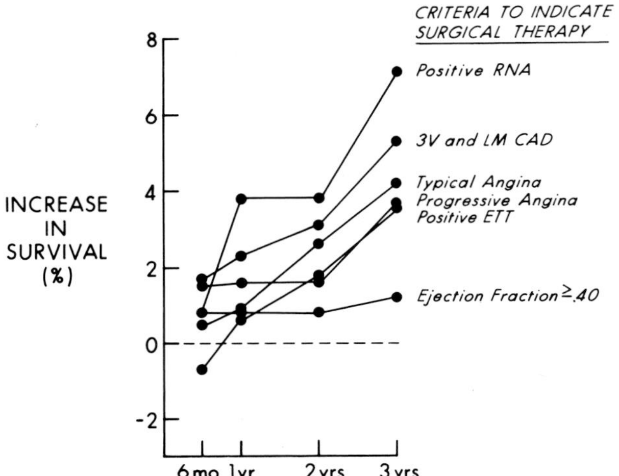

Figure 56–25. Data documenting the maximal percent increase in survival of the total population that could be achieved at each time interval by using specific criteria to indicate surgical therapy and absence of the criteria to indicate medical therapy.

Radionuclide measurements of resting left ventricular function before and after bypass operation show that 10 to 20 percent of patients have a significant decrease in left ventricular function.[F2] This documented loss in function is permanent and often occurs without clinical symptoms or changes suggestive of infarction on the electrocardiogram. A prospective study of 104 patients showed a surprising lack of relationship between QRS change on the electrocardiogram and left ventricular function after coronary artery bypass grafting.[F3] Loss of left ventricular function was not related to the duration of hypothermic cardioplegic arrest, and the etiology of this functional result is probably related to multiple causative factors that are now poorly understood. About 10 to 20 percent of patients will have significantly improved resting function after myocardial revascularization, suggesting that reversible resting ischemic dysfunction was present before operation in the absence of resting pain. Although resting improvement in left ventricular function is modest in most patients, in some patients quite abnormal function observed before operation dramatically normalized after revascularization.

Physiologic improvement after myocardial revascularization is most consistently documented by radionuclide studies of myocardial function and perfusion during exercise. As early as 8 days after surgery, patients have been shown to greatly improve exercise left ventricular ejection fraction, and this improvement has persisted in later studies.[A5] This early documentation of reversal of myocardial ischemia provides a useful baseline for patients who later become symptomatic. Subsequent radionuclide studies can quantify the amount of return of ischemia associated with disease progression or graft occlusion and provide a rational basis for selection of patients who might profit from repeat catheterization and consideration of another revascularization procedure.

THE FUTURE OF RADIONUCLIDE ANGIOCARDIOGRAPHY

Radionuclide angiocardiography remains a partially developed technique despite its position as the first nuclear medicine procedure used in humans and a total life span of more than 60 years. All past major advances have resulted from improvements in technology, and future progress will also depend on the development of new technologies. Interrelated improvements in instrumentation, radiopharmaceuticals, and data processing will amplify their usefulness.

The major instrumentation need is for enhanced sensitivity and resolution of detectors that can be placed in arrays around the chest for acquisition of data in multiple simultaneous views during transit of a single radionuclide bolus. Because frames of radionuclide data contain information about the intensity and distribution of counts, three-dimensional reconstruction of data can become meaningful with as few as three simultaneously acquired views. The enhanced spatial resolution resulting from three-dimensional imaging should greatly facilitate anatomic characterization of cardiac structures. It should prove feasible to separate overlying myocardial counts from those within cardiac chambers.

Development of short-lived radionuclide generators promises to lower the radiation burden and permit administration of high amounts of activity to capitalize on improved counting rates of newer instrumentation. In addition, serial studies could be performed frequently because of the lower radiation dose and the decrease in background. Except for technetium–99m-labeled perfusion agents, radionuclides now used for radionuclide angiocardiography are not selected for any specific biologic activity. Led by clinical applications of metabolic measurements made by position emission tomography scanning, radiopharmaceuticals labeled with short-lived gamma-emitting tracers might be developed to assess myocardial integrity and metabolism. If it proves possible to differentiate myocardial activity from that of the underlying blood pool, the first-pass kinetics of biologically specific tracers could also be used to reflect regional myocardial integrity and metabolism.

Improvement in instrumentation and radiopharmaceuticals would produce data with enhanced spatial and temporal integrity and thereby simplify data analysis. Completely automated computer algorithms should calculate and display images of real-time flow and volume from all cardiac chambers viewed from any desired orientation. Cost savings resulting from more widespread use of radionuclide angiocardiography and increased automation of data processing should greatly decrease the intrinsic cost of the study. Radionuclide measurements of cardiac function, perfusion, and metabolism may cost little more than an electrocardiogram in the future. Much has been done over the past six decades, yet much more work remains to improve radionuclide angiocardiography in the decades ahead.

References

A

1. Anderson, P. A. W., Bowyer, K. W., and Jones, R. H.: Effects of age on radionuclide angiographic detection and quantitation of left-to-right shunts. Am. J. Cardiol. 53:879, 1984.
2. Austin, E. H., and Jones, R. H.: Radionuclide left ventricular volume curves in angiographically proved normal subjects and patients with three-vessel coronary disease. Am. Heart J. 106:1357, 1983.
3. Anderson, P. A. W., Rerych, S. K., Moore, T. E., and Jones, R. H.: Accuracy of left ventricular end-diastolic dimension determinations obtained by radionuclide angiocardiography. J. Nucl. Med. 22:500, 1981.
4. Austin, E. H., Cobb, F. R., Coleman, R. E., and Jones, R. H.: Prospective evaluation of radionuclide angiocardiography for the diagnosis of coronary artery disease. Am. J. Cardiol. 50:1212, 1982.
5. Austin, E. H., Oldham, H. N., Jr., Sabiston, D. C., Jr., and Jones, R. H.: Early assessment of rest and exercise left ventricular function following coronary artery surgery. Ann. Thorac. Surg. 35:159, 1983.

B

1. Blumgart, H. L., and Yens, O. C.: Velocity of blood flow. The method utilized. J. Clin. Invest. 4:1, 1926.
2. Blumgart, H. L., and Weiss, S.: Clinical studies on the velocity of blood flow. The pulmonary circulation time, the velocity of venous blood flow to the heart and related aspects of the circulation in patients with cardiovascular disease. J. Clin. Invest. 5:343, 1927.
3. Bender, M. A., and Blau, M.: The autofluoroscope. Nucleonics 21:52, 1963.
4. Bowyer, K. W., Konstantinow, G., Jr., Rerych, S. K., and Jones, R. H.: Optimum counting intervals in radionuclide cardiac studies. *In* Nuclear Cardiology: Selected Computer Aspects. Society of Nuclear Medicine, New York, 1978, p. 85.
5. Baillet, G. Y., Mena, I. G., Kuperus, J. H., et al.: Simultaneous technetium–99m MIBI angiography and myocardial perfusion imaging. J. Nucl. Med. 30:38, 1989.
6. Berger, H. J., Matthay, R. A., Loke, J., et al.: Assessment of cardiac performance with quantitative radionuclide angiocardiography: Right ventricular ejection fraction with reference to findings in chronic obstructive pulmonary disease. Am. J. Cardiol. 41:897, 1978.
7. Borer, J. S., Bacharach, S. L., Green, M. V., et al.: Real-time radionuclide cineangiography in the noninvasive evaluation of global and regional left ventricular function at rest and during exercise in patients with coronary artery disease. N. Engl. J. Med. 296:839, 1977.

C

1. Castellana, F. S., Snapinn, S. M., Tam, S. Y., and Case, R. B.: Inlet and intrachamber concentration distributions in tracer studies of the canine central circulation and their relation to the isotope dilution residue function. Circ. Res. 47:10, 1980.
2. Christopher, T. D., Fagraeus, L., and Jones, R. H.: Cardiovascular adaptations to sudden strenuous exercise in normal subjects. Am. J. Noninvas. Cardiol. 2:347, 1988.
3. Christopher, T. D., Konstantinow, G., Jones, R. H.: Bayesian analysis of data from radionuclide angiocardiograms for diagnosis of coronary artery disease. Circulation 69:65, 1984.

D

1. Dymond, D. S., Elliott, A., Stone, D., et al.: Factors that affect the reproducibility of measurements of left ventricular function from first-pass radionuclide ventriculograms. Circulation 65:311, 1982.
2. Donato, L.: Basic concepts of radiocardiography. Semin. Nucl. Med. 3:111, 1973.

F

1. Folse, R., and Braunwald, E.: Pulmonary vascular dilution curves recorded by external detection in the diagnosis of left-to-right shunts. Br. Heart J. 24:166, 1962.
2. Floyd, R. D., Sabiston, D. C., Jr., Lee, K. L., and Jones, R. H.: The effect of duration of hypothermic cardioplegia on ventricular function. J. Thorac. Cardiovasc. Surg. 85:606, 1983.
3. Floyd, R. D., Wagner, G. S., Austin, E. H., et al.: Relation between QRS changes and left ventricular function after coronary artery bypass grafting. Am. J. Cardiol. 52:943, 1983.

G

1. Gibbons, R. J., Lee, K. L., Cobb, F. R., and Jones, R. H.: Ejection fraction response to exercise in patients with chest pain and normal coronary arteriograms. Circulation 64:952, 1981.
2. Gibbons, R. J., Lee, K. L., Cobb, F. R., et al.: Ejection fraction response to exercise in patients with chest pain, coronary artery disease and normal resting ventricular function. Circulation 66:643, 1982.
3. Gibbons, R. J., Lee, K. L., Pryor, D. B., et al.: The use of radionuclide angiography in the diagnosis of coronary artery disease—a logistic regression analysis. Circulation 68:740, 1983.

H

1. Holman, B. L., Jones, A. G. A., Lister-James, J., et al.: A new Tc–99m-labeled myocardial imaging agent, hexakis (*t*-butylisonitrile)-technetium(I) [Tc–99m TBI]: Initial experience in the human. J. Nucl. Med. 25:1350, 1984.
2. Heller, G. V., Treves, S. T., Parker, J. A., et al.: Comparison of ultrashort-lived iridium–191m with technetium–99m for first pass radionuclide angiocardiographic evaluation of right and left ventricular function in adults. J. Am. Coll. Cardiol. 7:1295, 1986.
3. Hellman, C., Zafrir, N., Shimoni, A., et al.: Evaluation of ventricular function with first-pass iridium–191m radionuclide angiocardiography. J. Nucl. Med. 30:450, 1989.
4. Harpole, D. H., Skelton, T. N., Davidson, C. J., et al.: Validation of pressure-volume data obtained in patients by initial transit radionuclide angiocardiography. Am. Heart J. 118:983, 1989.
5. Herman, M. V., Heinle, R. A., Klein, M. D., et al.: Localized disorders in myocardial contraction: Asynergy and its role in congestive heart failure. N. Engl. J. Med. 277:222, 1967.
6. Higginbotham, M. B., Coleman, R. E., Jones, R. H., and Cobb, F. R.: Mechanism and significance of a decrease in ejection fraction during exercise in patients with coronary artery disease and left ventricular dysfunction at rest. J. Am. Coll. Cardiol. 3:88, 1984.

J

1. Jones, R. H., Sabiston, D. C., Jr., Bates, B. B., et al.: Quantitative radionuclide angiocardiography for determination of chamber to chamber cardiac transit times. Am. J. Cardiol. 30:855, 1972.
2. Jones, R. H., Klaphaak, R. B., and Sabiston, D. C., Jr.: Anatomic resolution in dynamic radionuclide studies by computer identification of radioactivity fluctuation with time. Symposium on Sharing of Computer Programs and Technology in Nuclear Medicine. Atomic Energy Commission, Oak Ridge, Tenn., 1972, p. 151.
3. Jones, R. H., and Scholz, P. M.: Data enhancement techniques for radionuclide cardiac studies. *In* Medical Radionuclide Imaging, Vol. 2. International Atomic Energy Agency, Vienna, 1977, p. 255.
4. Jones, R. H., Scholz, P. M., and Anderson, P. A. W.: Radionuclide studies in patients with congenital heart disease. *In* Willerson, J. T. (ed.): Cardiovascular Clinics. Davis, Philadelphia, 1979, p. 225.
5. Jones, R. H., McEwan, P., Newman, G. E., et al.: Accuracy of diagnosis of coronary artery disease by radionuclide measurement of left ventricular function during rest and exercise. Circulation 64:586, 1981.
6. Jones, R. H., Austin, E. H., Peter, C. A., and Sabiston, D. C., Jr.: Radionuclide angiocardiography in the diagnosis of congenital heart disorders. Ann. Surg. 193:710, 1981.
7. Jones, R. H., Floyd, R. D., Austin, E. H., and Sabiston, D. C., Jr.: The role of radionuclide angiocardiography in the preoperative prediction of pain relief and prolonged survival following coronary artery bypass grafting. Ann. Surg. 197:743, 1983.

K

1. Konstantinow, G., Pizer, S. M., and Jones, R. H.: Decontamination of time-activity curves in first-pass radionuclide angiocardiography. Proceedings of the Society of Nuclear Medicine Computer and Instrumentation Councils—Emission Computer Tomography and Medical Data Processing Symposium, San Francisco, 1983, p. 251.

L

1. Lacy, J. L., LeBlanc, A. D., Babich, J. W., et al.: A gamma camera for medical applications using a multiwire proportional counter. J. Nucl. Med. 25:1003, 1984.
2. Lacy, J. L., Ball, M. E., Verani, M. S., et al.: An improved tungsten–178/tantalum–178 generator system for high volume clinical applications. J. Nucl. Med. 29:1526, 1988.

M

1. MacIntyre, W. J., Pritchard, W. H., Eckstein, R. W., and Friedell, H. L.: The determination of cardiac output by a continuous recording system utilizing iodinated (I–131) human serum albumin. I. Animal studies. Circulation 4:552, 1951.

N

1. Newman, G. E., Rerych, S. K., Bounous, E. P., et al.: Noninvasive assessment of hemodynamic effects of mitral valve commissurotomy during rest and exercise in patients with mitral stenosis. J. Thorac. Cardiovasc. Surg. 78:750, 1979.

O

1. Oberman, A., Kouchoukos, N. T., Holt, J. H., Jr., and Russell, R. O., Jr.: Long-term results of the medical treatment of coronary artery disease. Angiology 28:160, 1977.
2. Osbakken, M. D., Okada, R. D., Boucher, C. A., et al.: Comparison of exercise perfusion and ventricular function imaging: an analysis of factors affecting the diagnostic accuracy of each technique. J. Am. Coll. Cardiol. 3:272, 1984.

P

1. Prinzmetal, M., Corday, E., Bergman, H. C., et al.: Radiocardiography: A new method for studying the blood flow through the chambers of the heart in human beings. Science 108:340, 1948.
2. Prinzmetal, M., Corday, E., Spritzler, R. J., and Flieg, W.: Radiocardiography and its clinical applications. JAMA 139:617, 1949.
3. Packard, A. B., Treves, S. T., O'Brien, G. M., and Lim, K. S.: An osmium–191/iridium–191m radionuclide generator using an oxalato osmate parent complex. J. Nucl. Med. 28:1571, 1987.
4. Peter, C. A., Armstrong, B. E., and Jones, R. H.: Radionuclide quantitation of right-to-left intracardiac shunts in children. Circulation 64:572, 1981.
5. Philippe, L., Mena, I., Darcourt, J., and French, W. J.: Evaluation of valvular regurgitation by factor analysis of first-pass angiography. J. Nucl. Med. 29:159, 1988.
6. Purut, C. M., Sell, T. L., and Jones, R. H.: A new method to determine left ventricular pressure-volume loops in the clinical setting. J. Nucl. Med. 29:1492, 1988.
7. Port, S., Cobb, F. R., Coleman, R. E., and Jones, R. H.: Effect of age on the response of the left ventricular ejection fraction to exercise. N. Engl. J. Med. 303:1133, 1980.
8. Port, S., Cobb, F. R., and Jones, R. H.: Effects of propranolol on left ventricular function in normal men. Circulation 61:358, 1980.
9. Peterson, R. J., Franch, R. H., Fajman, W. A., et al.: Noninvasive determination of exercise cardiac function following Fontan operation. J. Thorac. Cardiovasc. Surg. 88:263, 1984.
10. Peterson, R. J., Franch, R. H., Fajman, W. A., and Jones, R. H.: Comparison of cardiac function in surgically corrected and congenitally corrected transposition of the great arteries. J. Thorac. Cardiovasc. Surg. 96:227, 1988.
11. Peter, C. A., and Jones, R. H.: Cardiac response to exercise in patients with chronic aortic regurgitation. Am. Heart J. 104:85, 1982.
12. Peter, C. A., and Jones, R. H.: Radionuclide measurements of left ventricular function. Arch. Surg. 115:1348, 1980.
13. Port, S., McEwan, P., Cobb, F. R., and Jones, R. H.: Influence of resting left ventricular function on the left ventricular response to exercise in patients with coronary artery disease. Circulation 63:856, 1981.
14. Port, S. C., Oshima, M., Ray, G., et al.: Assessment of single vessel coronary artery disease: Results of exercise electrocardiography, thallium–201 myocardial perfusion imaging and radionuclide angiography. J. Am. Coll. Cardiol. 6:75, 1985.
15. Pryor, D. B., Harrell, F. E., Jr., Lee, K. L., et al.: An improving prognosis over time in medically treated patients with coronary artery disease. Am. J. Cardiol. 52:444, 1983.

R

1. Rerych, S. K., Scholz, P. M., Sabiston, D. C., Jr., and Jones, R. H.: Effects of exercise training on left ventricular function in normal subjects: A longitudinal study by radionuclide angiography. Am. J. Cardiol. 45:244, 1980.
2. Rerych, S. K., Scholz, P. M., Newman, G. E., et al.: Cardiac function at rest and during exercise in normals and in patients with coronary heart disease: Evaluation by radionuclide angiocardiography. Ann. Surg. 187:449, 1978.
3. Rozanski, A., Diamond, G. A., Forrester, J. S., et al.: Should the intent of testing influence its interpretation? J. Am. Coll. Cardiol. 7:17, 1986.

S

1. Scholz, P. M., Rerych, S. K., Moran, J. M., et al.: Quantitative radionuclide angiocardiography. Cathet. Cardiovasc. Diagn. 6:265, 1980.
2. Sandler, H., and Dodge, H. T.: Use of single plane cine angiocardiograms for the calculation of left ventricular volume in man. Am. Heart J. 75:325, 1968.
3. Schad, N., Andrews, E. J., Fleming, J. W.: Colour Atlas of First Pass Functional Imaging of the Heart. MTP Press, Lancaster, Pa., 1985.
4. Sharma, B., Goodwin, J. F., Raphael, M. J., et al: Left ventricular angiography on exercise. A new method of assessing left ventricular function in ischaemic heart disease. Br. Heart J. 38:59, 1976.

U

1. Upton, M. T., Rerych, S. K., Newman, G. E., et al.: The reproducibility of radionuclide angiographic measurements of left ventricular function in normal subjects at rest and during exercise. Circulation 62:126, 1980.
2. Upton, M. T., Rerych, S. K., Newman, G. E., et al.: Detecting abnormalities in left ventricular function during exercise before angina and ST-segment depression. Circulation 62:341, 1980.

W

1. Wackers, F. J., Berman, D. S., Maddahi, J., et al.: Technetium–99m hexakis 2-methoxyisobutyl isonitrile: Human biodistribution, dosimetry, safety, and preliminary comparison to thallium–201 for myocardial perfusion imaging. J. Nucl. Med. 30:301, 1989.
2. Wackers, F. J., Giles, R. W., Hoffer, P. B., et al.: Gold–195m, a new generator-produced short-lived radionuclide for sequential assessment of ventricular performance by first pass radionuclide angiocardiography. Am. J. Cardiol. 50:89, 1982.

Chapter 57

Equilibrium Radionuclide Angiography

RAYMOND J. GIBBONS, M.D.

TECHNICAL ASPECTS ... 1027
Red Blood Cell Labeling ... 1027
Exercise Equipment and Techniques ... 1028
Arrhythmias ... 1029
MEASUREMENTS FROM EQUILIBRIUM RADIONUCLIDE ANGIOGRAPHY ... 1029
Left Ventricular Ejection Fraction ... 1029
Regional Wall Motion ... 1029
Left Ventricular Volumes ... 1030
Regurgitant Fraction ... 1031
Right Ventricular Ejection Fraction ... 1031
Pulmonary Blood Volume ... 1031
Left Ventricular Output ... 1031
Diastolic Parameters ... 1031
Tomography ... 1032
CLINICAL APPLICATIONS ... 1032
Diagnosis of Chest Pain ... 1032
Identification of Severe Coronary Artery Disease ... 1034
Prognostic Implications ... 1035
Functional Assessment and Patient Management ... 1037
Myocardial Infarction ... 1038
Cardiomyopathy ... 1039
Valvular Heart Disease ... 1040
Other Indications ... 1042
CONCLUSION ... 1042

Equilibrium radionuclide angiography, also known as radionuclide ventriculography or gated blood pool imaging, is a well established noninvasive technique for the assessment of ventricular function. Albumin or red blood cells are labeled with technetium-99m, allowed to distribute uniformly throughout the blood volume, and then imaged using a standard single-crystal gamma camera. The earliest studies with this technique employed human serum albumin that was labeled with technetium-99m before it reached the patient and was then injected intravenously. The labeled albumin that remained within the blood volume was then imaged. In recent years, this method has been replaced by technetium-99m–labeled red blood cells, because red blood cells remain in the blood pool for a longer period than does albumin.[T1]

This chapter reviews the technical aspects of equilibrium radionuclide angiography, the measurements that can be made using this modality, and its application to a variety of clinical situations.

TECHNICAL ASPECTS

Red Blood Cell Labeling

The *in vitro*[E1, S1] method of red blood cell labeling requires withdrawal of a small quantity (less than 10 ml) of blood from the patient. The blood is mixed with stannous citrate and gently agitated for approximately 5 minutes. After centrifugation, the red blood cells are mixed with technetium-99m and incubated for 5 minutes. The red blood cells are then reinjected into the patient and allowed to distribute throughout the blood volume. This method is time consuming and technically demanding. In contrast, the *in vivo* method,[P1, S2] which is carried out completely within the patient, is rapid and technically simple. Several milligrams of stannous pyrophosphate are injected intravenously and allowed to circulate for approximately 30 minutes. During this time, the stannous ion binds to the red blood cells. A separate intravenous injection of 20 to 30 mCi of technetium-99m pertechnetate is then performed. The technetium-99m will label red blood cells over the following 5 minutes. Since technetium-99m is injected separately as an intravenous bolus, first-pass measurements of right ventricular function can be performed during the same study. The major disadvantage of this method is that a significant portion of the injected radionuclide dose will distribute to the thyroid gland, the stomach, and the kidneys before binding to the red blood cells. The activity in noncardiac organs will therefore be considerable. The activity in the stomach may contribute significantly to the background counts within the cardiac image. In addition, this method will have a reduced labeling efficiency in some patients, presumably because technetium-99m has not remained within the blood pool long enough to permit satisfactory labeling.

The third method employed to label red blood cells is the *modified in vivo* method, which was first described by Callahan and associates.[C1] This approach combines the speed of the in vivo method with the labeling efficiency of the in vitro method. The first step of the labeling procedure is an intravenous injection of stannous pyrophosphate identical to that performed in the in vivo method. Thirty minutes later, 30 to 50 ml of the patient's blood are withdrawn into a heparinized syringe through a three-way stopcock. Technetium-99m pertechnetate, which is attached to the other port of the stopcock, is then injected into the syringe containing the patient's blood. The mixture is gently agitated for 5 minutes and then reinjected into the patient. Although this method is somewhat more time consuming and technically demanding than the in vivo method, it does result in a uniformly high labeling efficiency and virtually eliminates the background activity in the stomach that occurs with in vivo labeling. Because rapid injection of the labeled red blood cells is generally not possible without significant red blood cell damage, first-pass studies of the right ventricle are not possible using this labeling method.

Once the red blood cells have been labeled by any of these methods, the major determinant of blood pool activity is the 6-hour half-life of technetium-99m, as the biologic half-life of the labeled red blood cells is approximately 20 hours.[B1] Depending on the body size of the patient, high-quality images are generally feasible for at least 3 to 5 hours, permitting the assessment of ventricular function at multiple different levels of exercise, during different exercise protocols, and before and after drug interventions. Occasional difficulties with adequate labeling do occur. The majority of these are due to improper technique, including extravasation of the stannous pyrophosphate, improper preservation of the stannous pyrophosphate (which requires refrigeration), and injection of an inadequate quantity of technetium-99m.

Rarely, technically suboptimal labeling can occur even with meticulous technique. Concurrent intravenous administration of heparin is recognized to reduce labeling efficiency.[R1] Although multiple other drugs have been shown to interfere with labeling,[H1, L1] usually through the formation of drug–antibody complexes, they do not usually prevent adequate clinical studies. In our experience, the modified in vivo labeling procedure will fail rarely (approximately once every 1000 patients), usually because of the use of multiple drugs that are known to interfere with the labeling process.

Exercise Equipment and Techniques

In addition to the aforementioned standard single-crystal gamma camera, the performance of equilibrium radionuclide angiography requires an electrocardiographic monitoring device capable of generating a signal triggered by the R-wave of the electrocardiogram, and a computer system to acquire, organize, analyze, and display the data. Acquisition of the data occurs over many different cardiac cycles. The most common acquisition utilizes *frame mode,* in which counts recorded during the same time interval of successive cycles are added together to create an image of the great vessels and cardiac chambers. The R-wave trigger indicates the timing of each new cardiac cycle. The computer divides each cardiac cycle into a predetermined number of frames, which may range in number from 16 to 64. Each frame represents a predetermined time interval occurring at a specified time after the R-wave. Data collected during the same frame of several hundred successive cardiac cycles are then added together (Fig. 57–1). The result is a sequence of 16 to 64 images, each representing a particular time interval in the cardiac cycle. These images may be displayed individually or in an endless-loop motion picture format for purposes of review and analysis. Less commonly utilized is *list-mode* acquisition, in which all image data are recorded as a single list, along with frequent time markers and R-wave markers. The data are subsequently reformatted for image analysis. Although technically superior, this method is more time consuming and requires more sophisticated computer hardware and software.

Multiple views of the heart at rest can be obtained from different angles to assess wall motion. The most commonly employed views to assess resting wall motion are an anterior view, a left anterior oblique view that is adjusted to optimally visualize the interventricular septum, and a steeper left anterior oblique or left lateral view.[K1] Quantitative measurements are generally only performed on the "best septal" left anterior oblique view. Time constraints and the desire to perform quantitation generally restrict exercise studies to only this view. In selected patients who are able to exercise for a sufficiently long period, an anterior view may also be obtained at peak exercise. Occasionally, the additional information derived from an anterior view may justify a second exercise study.[B2]

Exercise studies are performed with use of a bicycle ergometer. Before the introduction of exercise tables that could tilt to a semi-upright position, supine bicycle exercise was most often employed as a means of minimizing patient motion during the radionuclide acquisitions. There are some clear physiologic differences between supine and semi-upright exercise.[M1, P2, S3] Patients who exercise in the supine position generally start with larger end-diastolic volumes, have less increase in heart rate and end-diastolic volume with exercise, and show a greater increase in systolic blood pressure with exercise. Although these differences are important for physiologic and drug intervention studies, they

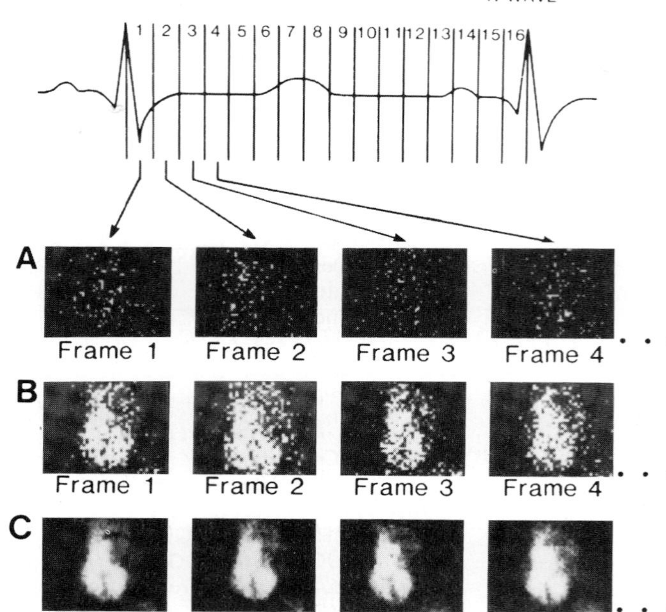

Figure 57–1. The cardiac cycle is divided into equal intervals (16 in this example). Counts recorded during each interval are stored in different computer frames. After a single cardiac cycle (row *A*), there are no recognizable images. After 20 cardiac cycles (row *B*), the images begin to be recognizable. After 400 cardiac cycles (300,000 counts per frame), image quality has improved considerably in row *C*. (From Parker, D. A., et al.: Radionuclide ventriculography: Methods. *In* Gerson, M. C. [ed.]: Cardiac Nuclear Medicine. McGraw-Hill, New York, 1987, p. 68, with permission.)

do not appear to have a major impact on the general clinical use of equilibrium radionuclide angiography for diagnostic and prognostic purposes.[F1] Despite the lower exercise heart rates achieved in the supine position, electrocardiographic ST segment changes are somewhat more frequent with supine exercise, presumably because of greater ventricular wall tension.[C2]

Exercise is performed in stages, each of which typically lasts for 3 minutes. During the first minute of each new exercise workload, the subject's heart rate and blood pressure will increase to a near steady-state condition. The radionuclide acquisition is then performed during the last 2 minutes of the stage, when a reasonably steady hemodynamic state exists. There is a wide variation in the actual sequence of exercise bicycle workloads employed. Some evidence suggests that a sudden, severe workload will lead to spurious results.[F2] With this exception, no clear evidence exists to support the use of one protocol rather than another. The most commonly employed protocols begin at workloads of 200 or 300 kg-m/min (37 to 50 watts) and increase in increments of 200 to 300 kg-m/min (37 to 50 watts).

One of the advantages of equilibrium radionuclide angiography is that multiple acquisitions can be performed during exercise at different exercise workloads. One of the disadvantages of this modality is that the patient must be able to exercise for a minimum of 3 minutes to acquire any reasonable exercise data. Although cold pressure testing and dipyridamole infusions have been employed with equilibrium radionuclide angiography,[H2, M2] these techniques are poor alternatives to exercise. Since many successive cardiac cycles are added together to produce a composite image in equilibrium radionuclide angiography, the maintenance of a near steady state during exercise is critical. If the patient is not allowed sufficient time to reach a near steady state before the acquisition begins, considerable increases in heart rate and blood pressure may occur during the acquisition period, which may adversely affect the data. Similarly, reductions in bicycle workload during the 2-minute acquisition should be avoided, as the changes in hemodynamics that they create may lead to spurious results.[S4]

Arrhythmias

Arrhythmias during exercise will clearly degrade the data. Sustained supraventricular or ventricular tachycardia is a clear cause for termination of an equilibrium radionuclide angiogram, since data from periods of different rhythm cannot be combined. Frequent premature ventricular contractions will lead to degradation of the data. If more than 10 percent of the cardiac cycles recorded are premature ventricular contractions, the data will be less accurate but usable.[B3] If more than 20 percent of the cardiac cycles are premature ventricular contractions, it is generally advisable not to analyze or report the data. A change in the ventricular conduction pattern during the acquisition is also a cause for concern. Fixed left bundle branch block[G1, R2] and rate-dependent left bundle branch block[B4] have been clearly demonstrated to alter mechanical function. Should left bundle branch block appear during an acquisition, the acquisition should either be aborted at that time or restarted so that it consists entirely of that conduction pattern.

The presence of atrial fibrillation will cause a wide variation in R-R interval in most patients. Although this variation will decrease somewhat during exercise, it will still influence the acquisition. The results, which represent an unusual "average" over many cardiac cycles of varying length, will provide a reasonable approximation of ventricular function, but with less accuracy than an acquisition performed in sinus rhythm.

Two approaches are available to try to address the problem of arrhythmias during exercise. The first is pharmacologic. Intravenous lidocaine may be administered in an attempt to reduce the frequency of premature ventricular contractions. To the degree that this therapy is effective, it will improve the accuracy of the data. A second approach relies on computer processing. The most comprehensive computer method employed is that of list-mode acquisition, which will permit the retrospective identification and elimination of all premature beats and other arrhythmias from the acquired data. This approach, however, is very time-consuming and very demanding from the standpoint of computer memory. As a result, it is fairly impractical for most busy clinical laboratories. More recent computer systems have permitted the "on the fly" identification of premature beats during the acquisition, which has permitted their elimination from the data. However, these identification programs are not perfect, and the degree to which they correct the problem is not well documented.

MEASUREMENTS FROM EQUILIBRIUM RADIONUCLIDE ANGIOGRAPHY

Left Ventricular Ejection Fraction

The parameters that can be measured by equilibrium radionuclide angiography are listed in Table 57–1. The most important measurement made from these studies is left ventricular ejection fraction. The best-validated approach to the measurement of ejection fraction utilizes a semiautomated, operator-assisted method that identifies the border of the left ventricle throughout the cardiac cycle from the left anterior oblique view. The ejection fraction is computed from the formula:

$$\frac{(\text{end-diastolic counts} - \text{end-systolic counts})}{\text{end-diastolic counts}}$$

where both end-diastolic and end-systolic counts are corrected for background. The region of interest employed to calculate background is usually placed along the left lateral edge of the end-systolic border. It is emphasized that this approach does not rely on any assumptions regarding the geometry of the left ventricle, which is a major strength of the technique. Although some investigators have employed a single, or fixed, region-of-interest method, in which the left ventricular border is identified only on the initial frame (which is assumed to represent end-diastole), the most commonly employed technique utilizes a variable region-of-interest in which the left ventricular border is outlined in every frame throughout the cardiac cycle. Multiple studies from different institutions have found that the left ventricular ejection fraction obtained in this fashion by equilibrium radionuclide angiography correlates very well with that obtained by contrast ventriculography over a wide range[B5, B6, F3, G2, P3, S5] (Table 57–2). In addition, the technique has an acceptable intraobserver and interobserver variability, which is not surprising, as most of the analysis is done by computer with little modification by the operator.[P4, W1] However, most of the validation studies were performed using a particular computer system and a particular generation of software. Other computer systems and software programs should not be assumed to yield identical results unless they have been similarly validated. It is therefore vital that every laboratory validate its own method and thereafter maintain a consistent technique. The radionuclide angiographic measurement of ejection fraction may be more accurate than that by other modalities, as it does not rely on any assumption regarding left ventricular geometry. However, the variation in attenuation with distance from the camera may occasionally lead to systematic errors, particularly in the presence of localized dyskinesia.[S6]

Table 57–1. MEASUREMENTS OBTAINED FROM EQUILIBRIUM RADIONUCLIDE ANGIOGRAPHY

Left ventricle—ejection fraction
—regional wall motion
—volumes
Right ventricle—ejection fraction
—regional wall motion
—volumes
Phase analysis
Left ventricular output
Regurgitant fraction
Pulmonary blood volume
Diastolic filling measurements

Regional Wall Motion

Equilibrium radionuclide angiography also permits an accurate assessment of regional wall motion. Regional wall motion is usually judged visually from a video display of all the images throughout the cardiac cycle in an endless-loop motion picture format. As mentioned, multiple different views of the heart are obtained at rest, while exercise studies are usually restricted to a single left anterior oblique view. Regional wall motion assessed by this technique has been demonstrated to correlate well with the subjective assessment of regional wall motion by contrast ventriculography.[O1, O2] Furthermore, the interobserver variability of this technique is comparable with the interobserver variability of biplane contrast ventriculography[O1] (Fig. 57–2). Right ventricular overlap makes the assessment of inferior wall motion on the anterior view difficult; for that reason a steep left anterior oblique or left lateral view is required.[K1] During exercise, the interobserver variability of the technique for regional wall motion is greater than that at rest, as a result of the shorter imaging period

Table 57–2. STUDIES COMPARING LEFT VENTRICULAR EJECTION FRACTION BY CONTRAST VENTRICULOGRAPHY AND RADIONUCLIDE ANGIOGRAPHY

First Author	Reference	Number of Subjects	r
Berman	B6	27	0.93
Burow	B5	17	0.93
Folland	F3	30	0.84
Green	G2	39	0.92
Pfisterer	P3	24	0.92
Secker-Walker	S5	16	0.87
Wackers	W1	26	0.84

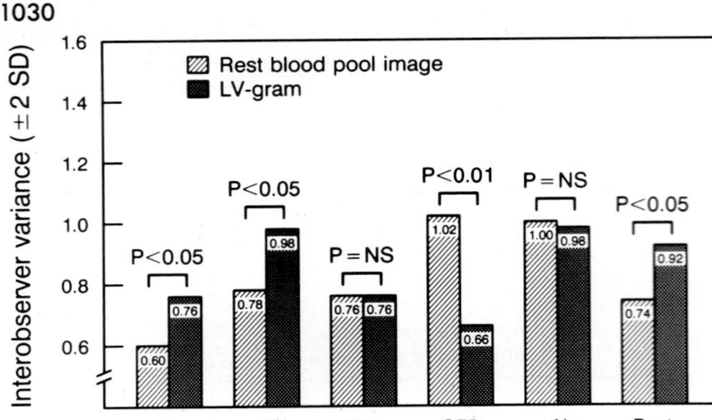

Figure 57–2. Left ventricular regional wall motion was judged on a five-point scale by equilibrium radionuclide angiography (rest blood pool image) and contrast ventriculography (LV-gram). The segments are anterolateral (AL), apical (AP), inferior (INF), septal (SEP), apical-inferior (AI), and posterior (POST). The two modalities have a comparable interobserver variance. (From Okada, R. D., et al.: Observer variance in the qualitative evaluation of left ventricular wall motion and the quantitation of left ventricular ejection fraction using rest and exercise multigated blood pool imaging. Circulation 61:128, 1980, by permission of the American Heart Association, Inc.)

and lower resolution images obtained during exercise. The assessment of regional wall motion change in the interventricular septum during exercise is generally more difficult than the assessment of the inferoapical or lateral walls.

Several different methods have been reported for the quantitative assessment of regional wall motion.[G3, M3, P5, S7] In each of these methods, the left ventricular end-diastolic frame in the left anterior oblique view is divided into several different regions. The change in counts during the cardiac cycle within each region is then employed to calculate a regional ejection fraction. Such measurements have been shown to correlate well with quantitative measurements on contrast ventriculography, although there is clearly an inherent difference between these two measurements. The count change measured by equilibrium radionuclide angiography represents a change in ventricular volume. It is, therefore, influenced by the wall motion along surfaces that are tangential to the imaging plane. On the other hand, contrast ventriculography measures wall motion in those segments that are perpendicular to the imaging plane. Two small studies have reported the application of quantitative regional ejection fractions to exercise studies and suggested that they are superior to the subjective assessment of wall motion.[D1, G3] However, no quantitative method for the assessment of regional wall motion has achieved broad acceptance. Most clinical laboratories currently employ a subjective assessment of regional wall motion by one or more observers.

An alternative approach to the assessment of regional wall motion employs Fourier phase analysis of individual computer pixels.[B7, M4, N1, R3, S8] Various phase parameters that are derived from the first Fourier harmonic will permit the detection of abnormal regional function. Although some reports have suggested that this technique is superior to the visual assessment of regional wall motion,[R3] other studies have not found it to be as helpful,[M4, N1] particularly in patients with abnormal wall motion at rest.[S8] This technique has provided insights into a broad spectrum of ventricular conduction disturbances, as well as ventricular arrhythmias.[B7]

Left Ventricular Volumes

Left ventricular volumes also can be assessed by equilibrium radionuclide angiography. The first method described, which continues in common clinical use because of its simplicity, was a count-based method without any geometric assumptions.[C3, D2] The formula used in this method is:

$$\text{Volume} = K \frac{\text{Left ventricular activity}}{\text{Number of cardiac cycles} \times \dfrac{\text{time}}{\text{frame}} \times \text{blood activity}}$$

where K is an attenuation correction factor.

The counts recorded from the ventricular region of interest in a particular frame are corrected for the time of acquisition for that frame and the activity of a blood sample of known volume (which can be determined in a well counter or by counting a sample placed directly on the camera face). The volume "units" determined by the equation are then related to volumes measured by contrast ventriculography. The constant K is determined from the resulting regression equation and represents an average attenuation correction. Ideally, every nuclear cardiology laboratory should develop its own regression equation and its own constant K to account for differences in equipment and technique. The particular volume measurements obtained by radionuclide angiography in this fashion have correlated well with those obtained from contrast ventriculography. The correlation coefficient reported by Dehmer and associates was 0.98, with an average error of the estimate of 16 ml for end-diastolic volume and 15 ml for end-systolic volume (Fig. 57–3). However, since the constant represents an "average" attenuation correction, and since chest wall attenuation will clearly vary with body geometry, more substantial errors can be expected from this method in very thin and very obese patients. More substantial errors also can be expected in patients with very large ventricular volumes, as counts within the regions of the left ventricle that are farthest from the camera will be attenuated.

Despite these limitations, this methodology remains very useful for making sequential measurements in the same patient, since attenuation can be assumed to be relatively constant unless body weight changes substantially. Thus, changes in ventricular volume between rest and different levels of exercise can be estimated using this method, as well as changes in resting left ventricular volume over time in the same patient.[B8, G4, W2] It has been demonstrated that the blood activity employed in the equation to measure left ventricular volume will change during exercise if the patient is labeled by the in vivo method.[K2] As a result, multiple blood samples must be obtained during exercise when this labeling method is employed. However, the modified in vivo method does not result in changes in blood activity during exercise.[V2] As a result, a single blood sample can be employed to measure blood activity, which is a significant advantage for this labeling method.

Many extensive efforts have been made to develop methods that calculate attenuation in individual patients to eliminate the

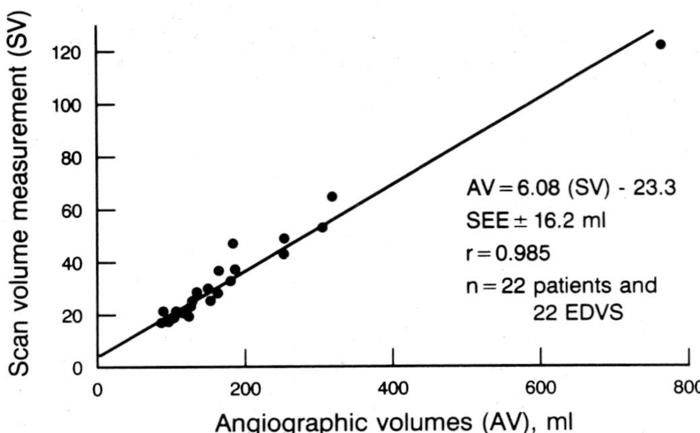

Figure 57–3. Left ventricular end-diastolic volumes (EDVS) measured by equilibrium radionuclide angiography (SV) and contrast ventriculography (AV). The results for end-systolic volume were comparable. (From Dehmer, G. J., et al.: Nongeometric determination of left ventricular volumes from equilibrium blood pool scans. Am. J. Cardiol. 45:293, 1980, with permission.)

problem of variable attenuation.[L2, P6, S9] The actual distance from the gamma camera detector to the center of the left ventricle can be estimated in individual patients.[L2] However, even when this distance can be judged accurately, the actual attenuation coefficient may still vary from individual to individual. Thus, these more detailed methods, which clearly require additional time and effort compared with the simple count-based method, still will have some systematic error in the determination of absolute left ventricular volumes. In clinical situations when the determination of absolute left ventricular volumes is of importance, these measurement techniques may be worthwhile. However, in general clinical practice, in which relative volume changes are probably sufficient, the count-based volume method without attenuation correction provides important information with a modest amount of time and effort.

Similar count-based techniques have been applied to the determination of right ventricular volume.[D3] Unfortunately, it is quite difficult to validate these measurements, as there is no generally accepted ventriculographic "gold standard" for the measurement of right ventricular volume. The right ventricular stroke volume measured by a count-based method appears to agree closely with the stroke volume derived from thermodilution cardiac output measurements.[D3] Thus, on the basis of this indirect validation, these measurements appear to be reasonably accurate.

Regurgitant Fraction

A variety of other measurements can be made from equilibrium radionuclide angiography. Although they are generally not employed on a routine clinical basis, they may be of great interest in particular clinical settings. One such measurement is the regurgitant fraction, a noninvasive determination of the severity of mitral or aortic regurgitation. Equilibrium radionuclide angiography is employed to calculate the stroke counts from the right ventricle and the left ventricle.[G5, M5, N2, R4, S10] The stroke counts from the right ventricle are generally best measured from a left anterior oblique view that employs significant caudal-cranial angulation to minimize overlap between the right atrium and the right ventricle. Further processing of this image, including phase and amplitude images, may help delineate the tricuspid valve plane.[S11] The ratio of left-to-right ventricular stroke counts or the difference between left ventricular and right ventricular stroke counts as a percentage of left ventricular stroke counts can be employed to estimate the severity of regurgitation. The ratio of stroke counts will be near unity in patients without evidence of left-sided regurgitation. This ratio will considerably exceed unity, and occasionally be as high as 5, in patients with mitral or aortic regurgitation. The stroke-count ratio has been shown to agree well with the qualitative angiographic assessment of regurgitation. The regurgitant fraction that can be calculated from this ratio correlates well with the regurgitant fraction obtained from the difference of angiographic and Fick cardiac output measurements.[S10] The major limitation of this approach is the presence of some right atrial and right ventricular overlap in most patients. As a result, there is a systematic error in this calculation, which can produce a regurgitant fraction as high as 20 percent and a stroke-count ratio as high as 1.25 in normal patients without regurgitation. This systematic error reduces the ability of this parameter to detect minor degrees of regurgitation and causes an overestimation of the regurgitant fraction. For example, a calculated regurgitant fraction of 30 percent indicates, at most, mild left-sided regurgitation.

Right Ventricular Ejection Fraction

Right ventricular ejection fraction can be determined from equilibrium radionuclide angiography using a variety of different methods.[H3, K4, M6] One is similar to that employed for the determination of left ventricular ejection fraction, in which a region of interest is drawn manually around the right ventricle in end-diastole and end-systole.[M4] The major technical limitation of this technique is the determination of the tricuspid and pulmonic valve planes. Phase and amplitude images, as well as stroke-volume images, can be employed to help locate these valve planes. However, as noted, right atrial and right ventricular overlap is unavoidable in many patients and is due in part to the motion of the tricuspid valve plane throughout the cardiac cycle, which is difficult to characterize on the left anterior oblique view. Despite these technical limitations, the right ventricular ejection fraction determined in this fashion agrees well with other methods and has acceptable interobserver and intraobserver variability.[H3, K4, M5]

An alternative approach to the measurement of right ventricular ejection fraction is to acquire a gated, first-pass study during the initial injection of technetium-99m. This technique, which requires use of the in vivo labeling method, allows visual determination of the motion of the tricuspid valve plane. However, the counting statistics are generally inferior to a first-pass study obtained with a multicrystal camera (see chapter 56). Right ventricular ejection fraction determined by this method has been validated against contrast ventriculography.[M7]

Pulmonary Blood Volume

It is also possible to measure changes in pulmonary blood volume during exercise using equilibrium radionuclide angiography.[O3] This measurement has been demonstrated to be a valid noninvasive indicator of the changes that occur in pulmonary capillary wedge pressure with exercise.[O4] Although the initial report describing this measurement suggested that it might be superior to the ejection fraction in detecting exercise-induced ischemia, this has yet to be confirmed. Recent work in our laboratory has suggested that the change in pulmonary blood volume is not superior to ejection fraction and is more difficult to measure.[H4]

Left Ventricular Output

Equilibrium radionuclide angiography also can estimate left ventricular output. This output is derived from the product of heart rate, ejection fraction, and end-diastolic volume. The methodology for the determination of ejection fraction and end-diastolic volume has already been described. The major source of error in the measurement of left ventricular output is the potential error in the measurement of end-diastolic volume due to variable attenuation. Left ventricular output determined in this fashion correlates surprisingly well ($r = 0.97$) with thermodilution measurement of cardiac output in patients without significant left-sided regurgitation.[D4, M8, S12] On the other hand, in the presence of aortic or mitral regurgitation, left ventricular outputs determined in this fashion will consistently exceed the Fick cardiac output. As a result, these outputs can be used to calculate a regurgitant fraction, which correlates with the severity of regurgitation assessed angiographically.[K3]

Diastolic Parameters

All the measurements described thus far are derived from the systolic phase of the cardiac cycle. In recent years, there has been increasing interest in the use of equilibrium radionuclide angiography to make diastolic measurements as well. Methodologic details are generally much more important for these measurements, as they are clearly more technically demanding. Higher temporal resolution is required, requiring higher framing rates and longer acquisition times. Statistical fluctuations in counts within the ventricular region of interest impose a need for curve fitting, which can influence the results. The duration of diastole clearly depends on cardiac cycle length; minor variations in R-R interval, therefore, will significantly influence diastolic filling parameters. Such variations in R-R interval add greatly to the technical difficulty of performing diastolic measurements by equilibrium radionuclide angiography, because of the difficulty of superimposing many different cardiac cycles of slightly different length. Atrial pacing will eliminate these variations and permit highly accurate measurements, but this step clearly complicates the procedure from a practical standpoint.

A variety of different methods have been utilized to make diastolic measurements by equilibrium radionuclide angiography.[A1, B9–B11, C4, J1, M9–M11, P7] List-mode acquisition, the most accurate method, is the most technically demanding from the standpoint of time, computer software, and computer storage.[B9, B10] Using this method, the cardiac cycle can be reconstructed in forward or backward fashion from the R-wave. Cardiac cycles that are too long or too short can be eliminated from consideration. An alternative is to employ the same standard gating procedure that is utilized for systolic measurements but to increase the framing rate to 32 or 64 frames per cardiac cycle and increase the acquisition time to permit adequate counting statistics in each frame.[A1, M9, P7] This method will avoid the technical demands of list-mode acquisition, but its accuracy will be greatly affected by any variability in R-R interval.[J1] As a result, measurements in late diastole, including the atrial filling phase, will be virtually impossible. A third alternative, which is technically simple but permits late diastolic measurements, is alternative R-wave gating.[C4] This method employs a simple filter that allows every other R-wave trigger signal to reach the computer. As a result, the cardiac "cycle" constructed by the computer actually consists of two successive cardiac cycles. This technically simple method permits measurements in both early diastole and late diastole, including the entire atrial filling phase. However, these measurements will still be affected by variability in the R-R interval.

A variety of different diastolic parameters have been measured, including the peak filling rate, the time to peak filling, the first one third and first one half filling fraction, and the atrial filling fraction. These parameters generally contain a great deal of overlapping information. When one parameter is abnormal, all other parameters will frequently be abnormal as well. The exact significance of these parameters, and their relationship to left ventricular compliance, is a subject of ongoing research. Measurements of volume, or of rates of change in volume, by equilibrium radionuclide angiography, or by any other technique, are at best indirect indicators of left ventricular compliance in the absence of simultaneous pressure measurements. Simultaneous measurements of ventricular volume by radionuclide angiography and pressure by micromanometer have been reported.[M10]

Tomography

Several centers have now utilized single photon emission computed tomography in association with equilibrium radionuclide angiography.[C5, G6, M13, T2] The tomographic imaging systems used in these studies are similar to those employed with thallium-201 myocardial scintigraphy. Modifications of the acquisition software are required to permit gating. The required acquisition time is too long to permit acquisitions during exercise. For resting studies, however, tomographic studies offer the advantages of less chamber overlap and more accurate localization. Initial studies have suggested that tomography will provide more accurate measurements of left ventricular volume and more sensitive detection of regional wall motion abnormalities.[C5, G6]

CLINICAL APPLICATIONS

Diagnosis of Chest Pain

Equilibrium radionuclide angiography is one of several different exercise modalities that is frequently employed to help establish the diagnosis of chest pain. The ultimate goal of clinical evaluation and noninvasive exercise testing is to establish the likelihood that an individual patient has significant coronary artery disease. To the statistician, this is what is known as the *post-test probability*. Ideally, one would like to separate all patients into two groups—in one group, no patient would have coronary artery disease and in the other group, all the patients would have coronary artery disease. Such a separation, however, is not possible with our current testing modalities. One must be satisfied, therefore, with a characterization of a patient as "likely" or "unlikely" to have coronary artery disease.

The determination of the post-test probability requires a knowledge of the *pretest probability*, the performance characteristics of the test employed, and the test results.[D5, D6] Detailed discussions of the proper application of Bayes' theorem to such a determination have been published elsewhere.[G7, G8] The pretest probability is simply the likelihood that a patient has coronary artery disease on the basis of clinical characteristics before any test is performed. Age, sex, and the patient's description of chest pain are the most important characteristics.[D5] Published estimates of the pretest probability of disease on the basis of these three characteristics are shown in Tables 57–3 and 57–4. It is obvious there is a very wide range of pretest probability, ranging from 1 percent for a woman in her thirties with nonanginal chest pain to 94 percent for a man in his sixties with typical angina.

Table 57–3. PRETEST PROBABILITY OF CORONARY ARTERY DISEASE IN MEN

Age (Years)	Pretest Probability (%) Nonanginal Chest Pain	Atypical Angina	Typical Angina
30–39	5	22	70
40–49	14	46	87
50–59	22	59	82
60–69	28	67	94

(From Diamond, G. A., and Forrester, J. S.: Analysis of probability as an aid in the clinical diagnosis of coronary-artery disease. N. Engl. J. Med. 300:1350, 1979. Reprinted with permission from the New England Journal of Medicine.)

A number of other noninvasive characteristics are important in the determination of pretest probability. A detailed, statistical analysis in 3627 patients from the Duke University Medical Center data bank[P8] found that evidence for previous myocardial infarction by history and/or electrocardiogram, smoking, hyperlipidemia, ST-T wave changes on the resting electrocardiogram, and diabetes are all highly significant predictors ($P < 0.001$) of the presence of coronary artery disease, in addition to age, sex, and chest pain description.

In addition to the pretest probability of disease, the ability of the test to distinguish normal from abnormal, i.e., its performance characteristics, is important in determining post-test probability. The statistical parameters that have been most widely used to assess test performance are sensitivity and specificity. The sensitivity of the test is defined as the percentage of people *with disease* who have a positive test. The specificity of the test is the percentage of patients *without disease* who have a negative test.

Many different studies have compared equilibrium radionuclide angiography and first-pass radionuclide angiography with exercise thallium-201 scintigraphy and exercise electrocardiographic testing for the diagnosis of coronary artery disease.[B12–B14, C6, G7, G8, J2–J5] Equilibrium radionuclide angiography generally has been found to have a higher sensitivity and a lower specificity

Table 57–4. PRETEST PROBABILITY OF CORONARY ARTERY DISEASE IN WOMEN

Age (Years)	Pretest Probability (%) Nonanginal Chest Pain	Atypical Angina	Typical Angina
30–39	1	4	26
40–49	3	13	55
50–59	8	32	79
60–69	19	54	91

(From Diamond, G. A., and Forrester, J. S.: Analysis of probability as an aid in the clinical diagnosis of coronary-artery disease. N. Engl. J. Med. 300:1350, 1979. Reprinted with permission from the New England Journal of Medicine.)

than exercise electrocardiographic testing. However, it is important to note that these comparisons have often omitted patients whose treadmill tests were felt to be "inadequate" or "uninterpretable." If such treadmills were counted as negative, the difference in sensitivity between equilibrium radionuclide angiography and treadmill tests would widen considerably.

The exact specificity of equilibrium radionuclide angiography has been a subject of some controversy. The first large reported series described a specificity of 100 percent.[B10] This, and similar early series, reported high values for specificity that were probably clinically unrealistic, since they were based on normal volunteers rather than on patients with chest pain. These normal volunteers were generally not representative of clinical patient populations with respect to age, sex, or exercise capacity. As a result, they tended to perform better on these tests; they were "supernormals." Later series suggested that the specificity of radionuclide angiography was as low as 50 percent.[G9] However, these estimates were probably falsely low, as the decision to send these patients to cardiac catheterization was influenced by the abnormal results of their radionuclide angiograms. As a result, there were many patients with normal radionuclide angiograms who did not undergo cardiac catheterization and, therefore, were not included in the calculation of specificity. This "post-test referral bias"[R5] has resulted in declining estimates of specificity that are incorrectly low. The calculated level of specificity obviously will depend on the criteria required to label a test as abnormal, since a higher specificity can always be achieved by more stringent criteria, at a cost of a lower sensitivity.[M14]

The criteria employed to label an equilibrium radionuclide angiogram as abnormal have varied considerably among different reports. The earliest series used a combination of the peak exercise ejection fraction and the presence or absence of regional wall motion abnormalities.[B10] Later workers tended to focus on the change in ejection fraction from rest to exercise and suggested that an increase in ejection fraction of 0.05 from rest to exercise was necessary for a "normal" response.[B12, C6, J4, J5] The change in ejection fraction from rest to exercise is clearly a complex response that is influenced by many physiologic and pathologic variables, including the rest ejection fraction, the gender of the patient, the change in end-diastolic volume index from rest to exercise, the rest pulse pressure, the presence of electrocardiographic changes with exercise, and the extent of coronary artery disease.[G9, G10] It is not surprising that patients with higher resting ejection fractions tend to have a lesser increase in ejection fraction with exercise. Thus, a patient with a resting ejection fraction of 0.70 and an exercise fraction of 0.70 has a normal functional response to exercise, not an abnormal one as was once thought.[G9, R6]

The peak exercise ejection fraction combines information about both prior ventricular damage (as reflected in the resting ejection fraction) and the presence of exercise-induced ischemia (as reflected in the change in ejection fraction). Thus, this parameter is an indicator of the "maximal performance" of the heart and is less subject to influence by resting conditions. A detailed analysis of 736 patients comparing the change in ejection fraction and the peak exercise ejection fraction for diagnostic purposes found that the latter was a better parameter for the detection of coronary artery disease.[G11] Other series have confirmed the superiority of the peak exercise ejection fraction, not only for diagnosis[G12] but also for the identification of severe disease[D7, D8, G13] and prognosis.[P9, T3] When the peak exercise ejection is analyzed, equilibrium radionuclide angiography will have a specificity of 80 percent and a sensitivity of 70 to 80 percent.[G12] Thus, it is clearly more sensitive than a treadmill exercise test, but less specific.

The difference between men and women in the left ventricular response to exercise must be considered in the evaluation of both specificity and test criteria. The largest reported series of patients with chest pain and normal coronary arteriograms found that many patients had abnormal ejection fraction responses to exercise without evidence of other cardiovascular abnormality, and that such responses were clearly more common in women than in men.[G9] Using equilibrium radionuclide angiography and upright exercise in a small series of normal volunteers, Higgenbotham and associates demonstrated that there was a clear gender

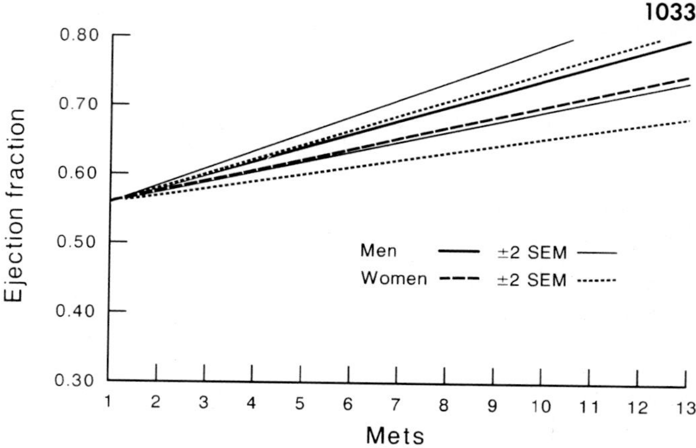

Figure 57–4. Relationship between ejection fraction and metabolic equivalents (METS) of exercise for 192 men and 67 women with a low probability of coronary artery disease. Shown are the mean slopes ± two standard errors of the mean. Men had greater increases in ejection fraction with exercise. (From Hanley, P. C., et al.: Sex-related differences in cardiac response to supine exercise assessed by radionuclide angiography. J. Am. Coll. Cardiol. 13:624, 1989. Reprinted with permission from the American College of Cardiology.)

difference in the response of the left ventricle to exercise.[H5] The women in their series tended to have less increase in ejection fraction with exercise and a greater increase in end-diastolic volume index with exercise. Hanley and associates have subsequently confirmed these findings in a much larger series of 259 patients with a low likelihood of coronary artery disease.[H6] They identified a large number of gender differences in ejection fraction and end-diastolic volume index at rest and exercise. More important, when the exercise response of ejection fraction and end-diastolic volume index were plotted versus exercise intensity in METS, there was a clear gender difference in the slope of this response between men and women (Figs. 57–4 and 57–5). Women tended to have more left ventricular dilatation with exercise and less increase in ejection fraction than men. This gender difference may be related to the long-standing observation that women tend to have smaller hearts than men, even after adjustment for body size.[S13] This difference, which is not explained by differences in exercise capacity, clearly will affect the interpretation of the results of equilibrium radionuclide angiography in women.

The proper interpretation of the results of equilibrium radionuclide angiography requires careful consideration of all the

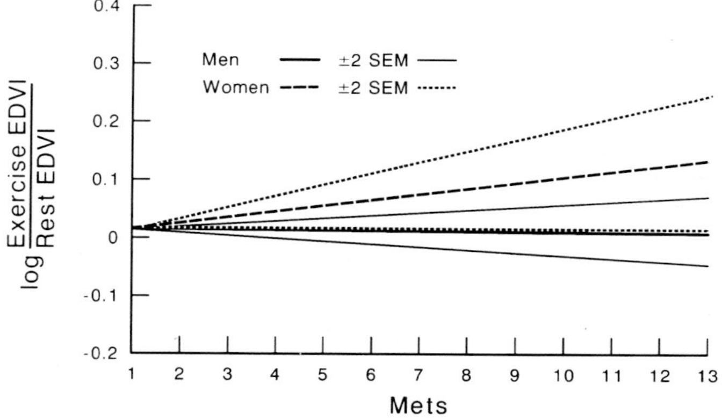

Figure 57–5. Relationship between end-diastolic volume index and metabolic equivalents (METS) of exercise for 192 men and 67 women with a low probability of coronary artery disease. Shown are mean slopes ± two standard errors of the mean. Women have greater increases in end-diastolic volume index with exercise. (From Hanley, P. C., et al.: Sex-related differences in cardiac response to supine exercise assessed by radionuclide angiography. J. Am. Coll. Cardiol. 13:624, 1989. Reprinted with permission from the American College of Cardiology.)

information from the test, including the hemodynamics,[G14] the symptoms,[G11] and electrocardiographic changes during exercise.[C7, G11, G13] The magnitude of myocardial oxygen demand achieved (as reflected in the exercise heart rate and blood pressure) and the presence or absence of symptomatic and/or electrocardiographic evidence of ischemia have each been demonstrated to be complementary to radionuclide parameters for diagnostic and prognostic purposes. Thus, all the information from the test should be considered, and the results should be considered as a continuous variable rather than as a dichotomous one.

The choice of which exercise modality to employ in an individual patient is often dictated by the particular clinical circumstances and the particular expertise present in a given medical center. In addition to diagnostic information, equilibrium radionuclide angiography provides valuable additional information regarding ventricular function and prognosis. In the absence of left bundle branch block, frequent premature ventricular complexes, or other known exercise-induced arrhythmias, it is a valuable diagnostic tool, particularly in men.

Identification of Severe Coronary Artery Disease

Equilibrium radionuclide angiography may be employed noninvasively to identify patients who are likely to have severe anatomic coronary artery disease. The rationale for noninvasive screening of patients with chest pain and known or suspected coronary artery disease is based on two premises: (1) coronary artery bypass surgery is known to improve survival in certain patient subgroups, and (2) coronary angiography is expensive, not available in every community, and has a finite risk. Large randomized trials[C8, E2, T4] have demonstrated that patients with significant left main coronary artery disease or three-vessel disease and abnormal resting left ventricular function have an improved survival when treated with initial surgical management rather than initial medical management. The impact of surgery on survival in patients with three-vessel disease and normal resting function is more controversial. The potential role of exercise radionuclide angiography in the identification of patients with three-vessel disease and normal left ventricular function who are most likely to benefit from coronary revascularization will be addressed in a later section.

Equilibrium radionuclide angiography can identify patients subsets who are likely to have left main and/or three-vessel coronary artery disease. Initial studies using first-pass radionuclide angiography[D7, D8] suggested that the exercise ejection fraction might be the most important variable in the identification of severe coronary artery disease. Subsequent studies using first-pass radionuclide angiography were generally promising, but either failed to consider all the available data[C9] or required the impractical calculation of multiple discriminant functions.[W3]

Our laboratory attempted to provide clinically useful noninvasive predictions of the likelihood of left main or three-vessel coronary artery disease, using supine equilibrium radionuclide angiography.[G13] The study group consisted of 681 patients who underwent equilibrium radionuclide angiography and coronary angiography within 6 months. Patients with significant valvular heart disease or previous coronary revascularization were excluded. Logistic regression analysis identified seven different variables that were independently predictive of the presence of left main or three-vessel coronary disease (Table 57–5). The first four variables were the most significant and provided most of the predictive power of the model. In order of importance, these were the magnitude of ST segment depression with exercise, the peak exercise ejection fraction, the peak exercise heart rate–systolic blood pressure product, and the gender of the patient. Patients could be separated into high-probability, intermediate-probability, and low-probability subgroups on the basis of their predicted likelihood of left main or three-vessel coronary artery disease (Table 57–6). Of the 216 patients predicted to be at low probability, 20 (9 percent) had left main or three-vessel disease.

Table 57–5. VARIABLES INDEPENDENTLY PREDICTIVE OF THE PRESENCE OF LEFT MAIN OR THREE-VESSEL CORONARY ARTERY DISEASE

Variable	p
Magnitude of ST segment depression	<0.0001
Exercise ejection fraction	<0.0001
Exercise heart rate × systolic blood pressure product	<0.0001
Patient gender	0.0001
Exercise end-systolic volume index	0.001
Exercise pressure/volume ratio/rest pressure/volume ratio	0.01
METS of exercise	0.02

Variables are listed in order of importance. (From Gibbons, R. J., et al.: Noninvasive identification of severe coronary artery disease using exercise radionuclide angiography. J. Am. Coll. Cardiol. 11:28, 1988. Reprinted with permission from the American College of Cardiology.)

In contrast, of the 258 patients predicted to have a high-probability, 144 (56 percent) had left main or three-vessel disease.[G13]

These same four variables were employed to provide practical estimates of the risk of left main or three-vessel disease using six simple graphs (Figs. 57–6 and 57–7). Each graph displays the probability of left main or three-vessel disease as a function of exercise ejection fraction and exercise heart rate–systolic blood pressure product for a given degree of ST segment depression in a man or a woman. For example (Fig. 57–7), a man with less than 1 mm of ST segment depression, an exercise ejection fraction of 0.60, and an exercise heart-rate systolic blood pressure product of 20,000 would have a low probability of left main or three-vessel disease. In contrast (Fig. 57–7), a man with 1 mm of ST segment depression, an exercise ejection fraction of less than 0.60, and a heart rate–systolic blood pressure product of less than 18,000 would have a high probability of left main or three-vessel disease. As indicated in Figure 57–7, for a given level of ST segment depression, exercise heart-rate systolic blood pressure product, and exercise ejection fraction, men generally have a greater probability of left main or three-vessel disease.[G13]

From the standpoint of clinical management, the prevalence of left main or three-vessel disease in patients judged to be at low probability appears to be sufficiently low that the decision to proceed with coronary angiography should be based primarily on the severity of symptoms. On the other hand, the prevalence of left main or three-vessel disease in those patients judged to be at high probability exceeds 50 percent, and early coronary angiography appears to be warranted in this group. The management of those patients judged to be at intermediate probability remains a matter of clinical judgment. Thus, it appears that equilibrium radionuclide angiography can easily separate patients into low probability, intermediate probability, and high probability groups using the four simple variables described.[G13]

Table 57–6. SEPARATION OF PATIENTS ACCORDING TO THE PROBABILITY OF LEFT MAIN OR THREE-VESSEL CORONARY ARTERY DISEASE

Group	Total Patients	Patients with Left Main or Three-Vessel CAD *Number*	*%*
Low probability	216	20	9
Intermediate probability	207	51	25
High probability	258	144	56
TOTAL	681	215	32

(From Gibbons, R. J., et al.: Noninvasive identification of severe coronary artery disease using exercise radionuclide angiography. J. Am. Coll. Cardiol. 11:28, 1988. Reprinted with permission from the American College of Cardiology.)

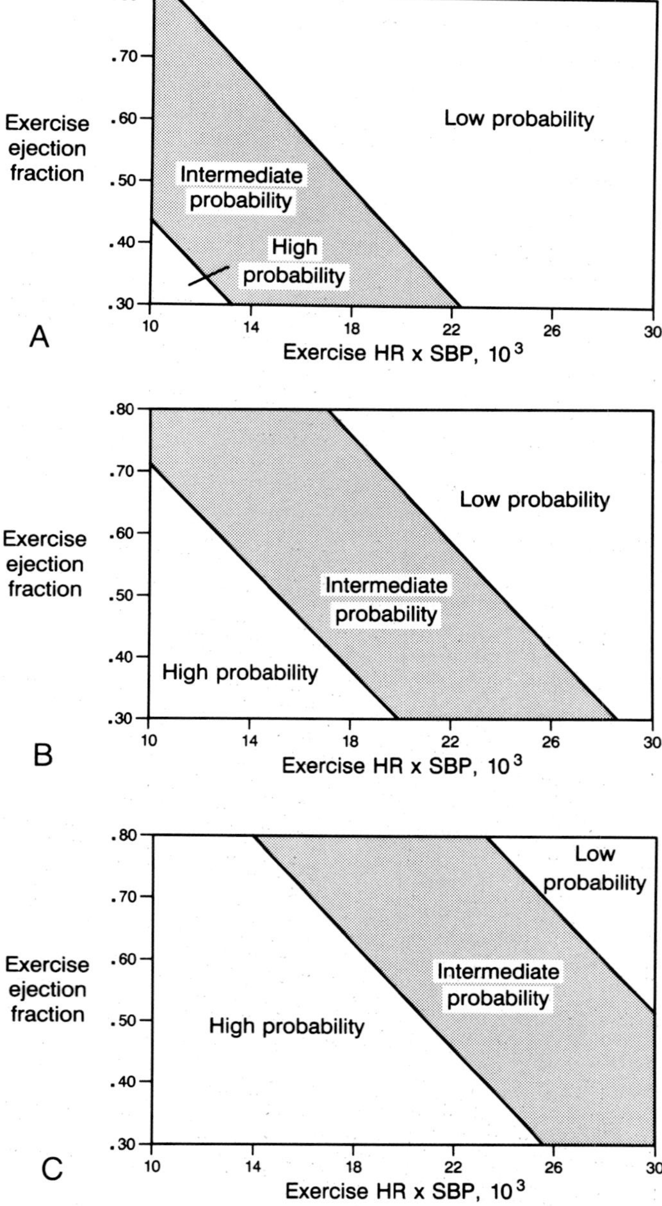

Figure 57–6. Estimated probability of left main or three-vessel coronary artery disease for women with *(A)* less than 1-mm ST segment depression, *(B)* 1.0-mm ST segment depression, and *(C)* 2.0-mm ST segment depression. Zones of different probability are shown. Exercise heart rate (HR) × systolic blood pressure (SBP) = exercise heart rate–systolic blood pressure product. (From Gibbons, R. J., et al.: Noninvasive identification of severe coronary artery disease using exercise radionuclide angiography. J. Am. Coll. Cardiol. 11:28, 1988. Reprinted with permission from the American College of Cardiology.)

Prognostic Implications

The ultimate goal of the evaluation of patients with chest pain is to identify those patients who are most likely to benefit from subsequent coronary revascularization because they will have cardiac events if treated initially with medical therapy. Multiple large studies have demonstrated that both the number of diseased vessels and the state of resting left ventricular function are the most important determinants of subsequent patient outcome.[H7, H8, M15] However, even when these parameters are known, the subsequent outcome of an individual patient cannot be predicted with great certainty, a point that is obvious but often overlooked. For example (Fig. 57–8), the cumulative event rate for nonfatal infarction and death in patients with three-vessel disease and moderate left ventricular function is approximately 50 percent over 5 years of follow-up.[H9] If these data were used to predict whether or not an individual patient would need revascularization to prevent an event within the next 5 years, the likelihood that this prediction would be correct is only 50 percent.

At least part of this prognostic uncertainty can be attributed to widely recognized limitations of coronary angiography.[H10, W4] It is now clear that the angiographic, or anatomic, assessment of the degree of coronary stenosis does not always correlate well with the physiologic significance of the stenosis. These limitations of angiography for the assessment of physiologic significance and the estimation of subsequent patient outcome have led to the evaluation of the potential complementary role of exercise testing modalities, including equilibrium radionuclide angiography.

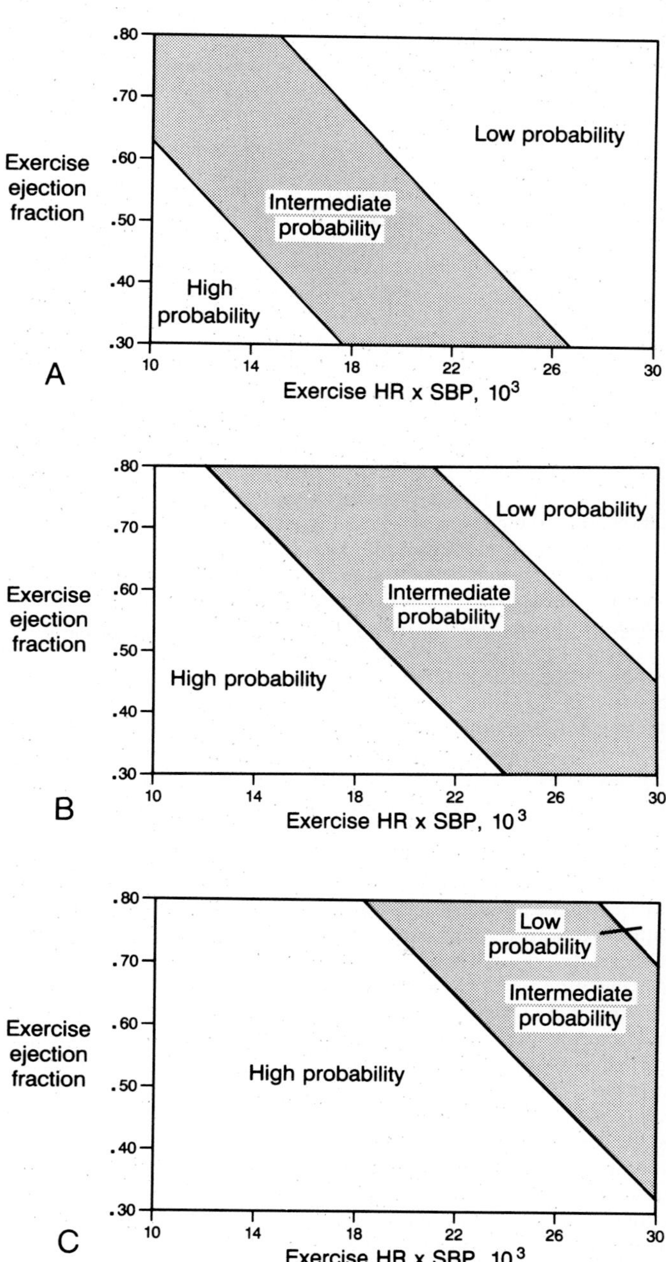

Figure 57–7. Estimated probability of left main or three-vessel coronary artery disease for men with *(A)* less than 1-mm ST segment depression, *(B)* 1.0-mm ST segment depression, and *(C)* 2.0-mm ST segment depression. Zones of different probability are shown. Exercise heart rate (HR) × systolic blood pressure (SBP) = exercise heart rate–systolic blood pressure product. (From Gibbons, R. J., et al.: Noninvasive identification of severe coronary artery disease using exercise radionuclide angiography. J. Am. Coll. Cardiol. 11:28, 1988. Reprinted with permission from the American College of Cardiology.)

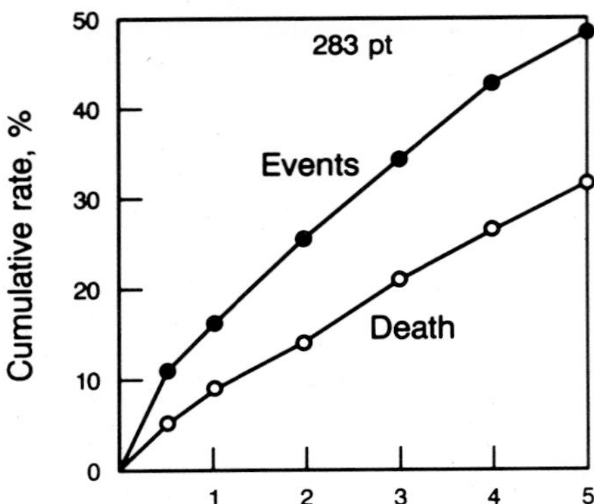

Figure 57–8. Five-year follow-up of 283 medically treated patients with three-vessel disease and moderate left ventricular dysfunction. Events consisted of death and nonfatal myocardial infarction. (From Harris, P. J., et al.: Survival in medically tested coronary artery disease. Circulation 60:1259, 1979, by permission of the American Heart Association, Inc.)

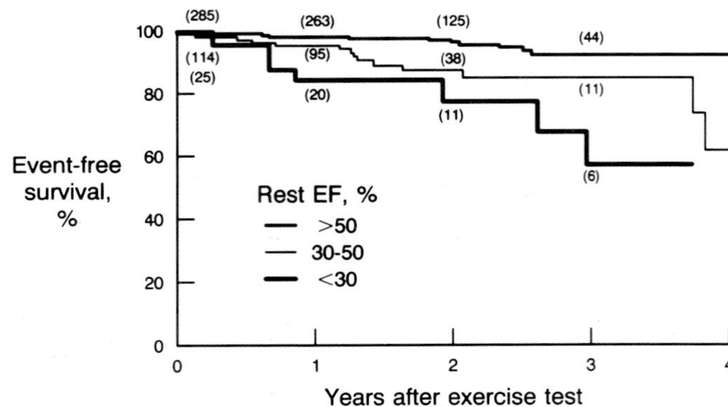

Figure 57–9. Event-free survival as a function of resting ejection fraction (EF) in 424 medically treated patients with known or suspected coronary artery disease. Events consisted of death, nonfatal myocardial infarction, and nonfatal out-of-hospital cardiac arrest. (From Taliercio, C. P., Clements, I. P., Zinsmeister, A. R., and Gibbons, R. J.: Prognostic value and limitations of exercise radionuclide angiography. Mayo Clin. Proc. 63:573, 1988, with permission.)

Considered alone as a noninvasive prognostic tool, exercise radionuclide angiography is very powerful.[I1, P9] The initial published data, which employed first-pass radionuclide angiography, demonstrated that exercise ejection fraction was the single most important variable for predicting subsequent cardiovascular death or nonfatal myocardial infarction. Similar findings have been demonstrated with equilibrium radionuclide angiography.[T2] Both rest ejection fraction (Fig. 57–9) and exercise ejection fraction (Fig. 57–10) can be employed to identify subsets of patients who are more likely to have cardiac events over the next 4 years. An exercise ejection fraction of less than 0.30 is associated with a cardiac event rate of almost 50 percent over the next 4 years.

These findings, based on patients undergoing cardiac catheterization in tertiary referral centers, recently have been confirmed in a community population.[G15] Among 526 residents of Olmsted County, Minnesota, who were followed for a median of 42 months, there were 71 cardiac events (26 deaths and 45 nonfatal myocardial infarctions). There were four independent predictors of outcome: exercise ejection fraction, exercise heart rate, age, and evidence of prior myocardial infarction (by history or electrocardiogram). Using the two most powerful variables (exercise ejection fraction and exercise heart rate), the patients could be divided into various prognostic groups (Fig. 57–11). One hundred fifty-seven patients in this community-based population (30 percent of the total group) had an exercise ejection fraction of less than 0.60 and an exercise heart rate of less than 120 beats per minute. This high-risk subgroup had a 4-year event-free survival of only 68 percent. These results clearly suggest that the noninvasive prognostic value of equilibrium radionuclide angiography applies to both tertiary care center patient populations as well as community populations.[G15]

A more important issue is whether equilibrium exercise radionuclide angiography contributes prognostic information that is independent of the information (number of diseased vessels and resting ejection fraction) that can be obtained by cardiac catheterization. Does exercise radionuclide angiography add to our ability to predict outcome in an individual patient once his or her coronary anatomy and resting ejection fraction are known? Bonow and associates examined the outcome of medically treated, mildly symptomatic patients with three-vessel disease and normal or near-normal resting left ventricular function.[B15] The presence of severe exercise-induced ischemia on equilibrium exercise radionuclide angiography identified a subset of patients who were at high risk for subsequent death (Fig. 57–12). The 18-month survival of the 19 patients with a decline in ejection fraction with exercise, ST segment depression, and a limited exercise capacity was less than 80 percent. In contrast, 24 patients with three-vessel disease who did not have severe exercise-induced ischemia had a 4-year survival of 100 percent. This study clearly suggested that equilibrium radionuclide angiography provides prognostic information that is independent of the number of diseased vessels and resting left ventricular ejection fraction, and that this modality could be utilized to identify patients with three-vessel disease and normal or near-normal resting function who were likely to benefit from coronary revascularization.

Taliercio and associates sought to confirm these findings in a group of 424 medically treated patients followed for a median of 21.7 months.[T3] Univariate analysis demonstrated that multiple individual parameters were associated with subsequent cardiac death and nonfatal myocardial infarction, including both the exercise ejection fraction and the resting ejection fraction. However, as assessed by multivariate analysis, only three variables were independently associated with subsequent cardiac events: the number of diseased vessels, the resting ejection fraction, and patient age. Thus, exercise-induced ischemia did not contribute independent prognostic information in this study, even when a subgroup similar to that of Bonow and associates was analyzed (Fig. 57–13). The potential reasons for these apparently conflicting data have been well reviewed in detail elsewhere.[B16]

Other studies have tended to confirm the independent prognostic value of exercise-induced ischemia assessed by equilibrium exercise radionuclide angiography. In a study of 53 mildly symptomatic patients with one-vessel or two-vessel coronary artery disease and abnormal resting left ventricular function (resting ejection fraction < 0.40), Mazzotta and associates found that the exercise ejection fraction and the change in ejection fraction from rest to exercise were highly predictive of subsequent events (Fig. 57–14).[M16] In the 17 patients with an exercise ejection fraction of

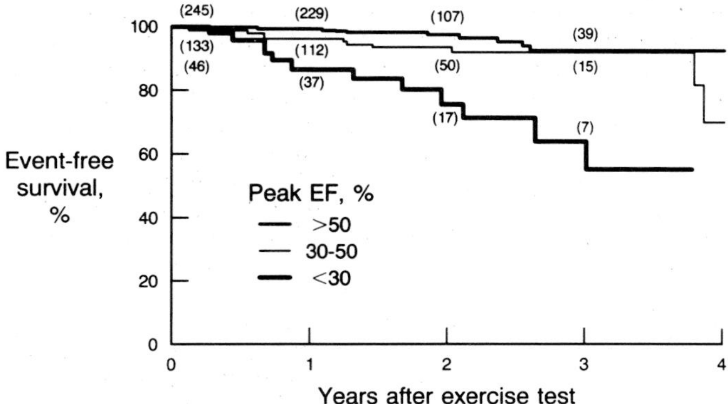

Figure 57–10. Event-free survival as a function of peak exercise ejection fraction (EF) in 424 medically treated patients with known or suspected coronary artery disease. Events as defined for Figure 57–9. (From Taliercio, C. P., Clements, I. P., Zinsmeister, A. R., and Gibbons, R. J.: Prognostic value and limitations of exercise radionuclide angiography. Mayo Clin. Proc. 63:573, 1988, with permission.)

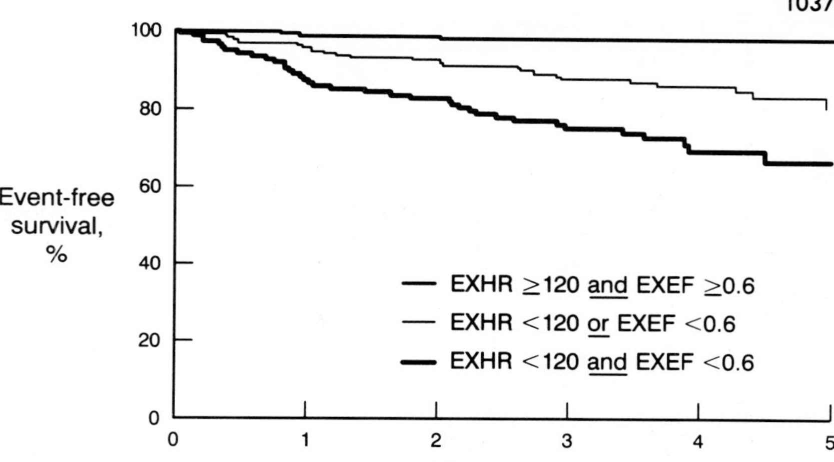

Figure 57–11. Event-free survival as a function of exercise ejection fraction (EF) and heart rate (HR) in 526 medically treated patients from a community-based population with known or suspected coronary artery disease. Events were defined as in Figure 57–9.

less than 0.30, the 5-year survival was only 61 percent, compared with a 97 percent 5-year survival in the 36 patients with an exercise ejection fraction of greater than 0.30.

Miller and associates confirmed these findings in 68 patients with one-vessel or two-vessel disease and a resting left ventricular ejection fraction of less than 0.50.[M17] The presence of ischemia on equilibrium exercise radionuclide angiography, defined as a decrease in ejection fraction with exercise, a peak workload of ≤ 600 kg-m/min, and ≥ 1.0 mm ST segment depression, was a significant ($P < 0.001$) predictor of subsequent patient outcome (Fig. 57–15). The 12 patients with ischemia had a 33 percent event rate within 1 year, compared with only 2 percent in the 56 patients without ischemia. Thus, both these studies confirmed the earlier findings of Bonow and colleagues, suggesting that equilibrium exercise radionuclide angiography provides prognostic information that is complementary to cardiac catheterization in predicting patient outcome. However, the extent of coronary disease (as reflected by the number of diseased vessels and the presence or absence of left main disease) and resting left ventricular function (as reflected by the resting ejection fraction) remain the two most important determinants of outcome in most long-term follow-up studies.

Functional Assessment and Patient Management

Equilibrium radionuclide angiography may also be utilized to guide patient management in patients with chronic angina. Most often, this involves the assessment of the physiologic importance of anatomic coronary artery disease. For the reasons already outlined, such an assessment is often complementary to the information provided by coronary arteriography. Functional information is particularly important for clinical patient management when coronary arteriography has demonstrated arterial obstructions that are likely to be of borderline hemodynamic significance. The presence or absence of exercise-induced ischemia in such patients will help determine the physiologic significance of the lesion and greatly influence the management of the patient. In addition, there may be situations when the symptomatology appears to be out of proportion to the coronary anatomy. Functional testing with equilibrium radionuclide angiography may help provide evidence that the patient's symptomatology is in fact due to myocardial ischemia. The ability of equilibrium radionuclide angiography to assess ventricular performance at multiple levels of exercise and thereby determine whether functional evidence of ischemia is present at low levels of exercise (and presumably low levels of myocardial oxygen demand) is particularly helpful in these circumstances.

Equilibrium radionuclide angiography may also be employed to assess the results of coronary revascularization. Such testing can be employed to provide objective confirmation of the relief

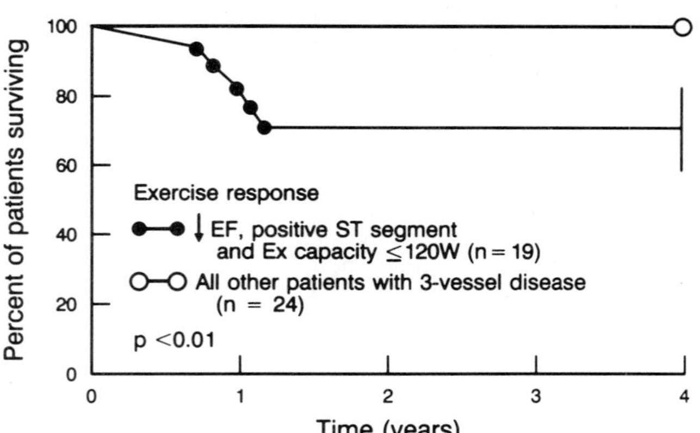

Figure 57–12. Survival in 43 patients from the National Institutes of Health with three-vessel disease and a resting ejection fraction of more than 0.40, as a function of the presence of a markedly abnormal exercise response. Patients with marked ischemia had a poor prognosis. (From Bonow, R. O., et al.: Exercise-induced ischemia in mildly symptomatic patients with coronary artery disease and preserved left ventricular function: Identification of subgroups at risk of death during medical therapy. N. Engl. J. Med. 311:1339, 1984. Reprinted with permission from the New England Journal of Medicine.)

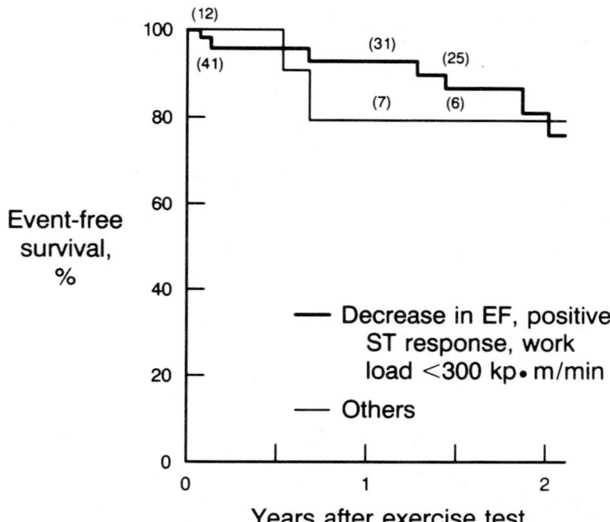

Figure 57–13. Event-free survivals in 53 patients from the Mayo Clinic with three-vessel disease and an ejection fraction (EF) of more than 0.40, as a function of the presence of a markedly abnormal exercise response. There was no significant difference between the two groups. (From Taliercio, C. P., Clements, I. P., Zinsmeister, A. R., and Gibbons, R. J.: Prognostic value and limitations of exercise radionuclide angiography. Mayo Clin. Proc. 63:573, 1988, with permission.)

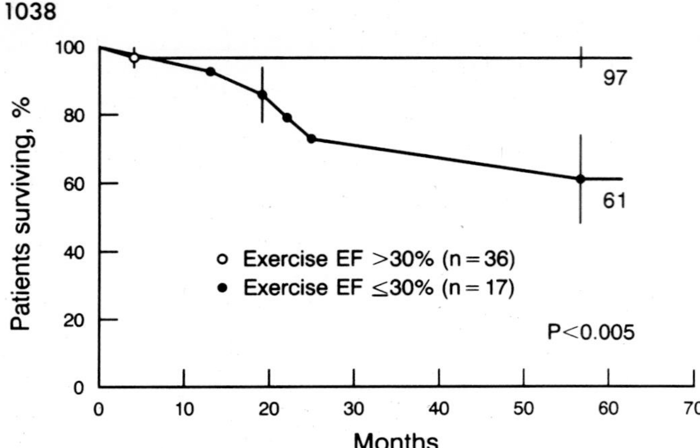

Figure 57–14. Survival in 53 patients from the National Institutes of Health with one- or two-vessel disease and a resting ejection fraction of less than 0.40. The exercise ejection fraction was highly predictive of survival. (From Mazzotta, G., et al.: Relation between exertional ischemia and prognosis in mildly symptomatic patients with single or double vessel coronary artery disease and left ventricular dysfunction at rest. J. Am. Coll. Cardiol. 13:567, 1989. Reprinted with permission of the American College of Cardiology.)

of exercise-induced ischemia, to evaluate the physiologic importance of nonrevascularized lesions, to reassure the patient, and to provide a baseline for subsequent follow-up. Several studies have employed equilibrium radionuclide angiography to assess the impact of coronary artery bypass grafting on left ventricular function.[F4, K5, K6, L3] Many factors influence the result, including patient selection, coronary anatomy, perioperative infarction, graft patency, ventricular loading conditions, drug therapy, and the timing of the postoperative study. The findings in individual patients, therefore, may be highly variable. In groups of patients, the most consistent finding is an improvement in exercise left ventricular function, particularly in those patients who had the most exercise-induced ischemia preoperatively.[K6] Recent evidence suggests that resting function may also improve postoperatively in selected patients.[D9, R7]

Equilibrium radionuclide angiography early after successful percutaneous transluminal coronary angioplasty appears to predict the presence or absence of restenosis on coronary angiography months later. DePuey and colleagues found that severe degrees of restenosis were present in 43 percent of patients with positive radionuclide angiograms early after percutaneous transluminal coronary angioplasty.[D10] In contrast, only 7 percent of those with a negative early radionuclide angiogram developed severe late restenosis. O'Keefe and colleagues confirmed the ability of early radionuclide angiography to predict subsequent restenosis.[O5] In those patients with normal radionuclide angiograms within 1 month after percutaneous transluminal coronary angioplasty, no patient developed late restenosis. In those patients with abnormal early radionuclide angiograms, the incidence of subsequent restenosis was 42 percent. Thus, early exercise radionuclide angiography identifies subgroups of patients who are at low risk and high risk for restenosis after percutaneous transluminal coronary angioplasty.

Myocardial Infarction

Equilibrium radionuclide angiography is useful for the evaluation of patients following acute myocardial infarction. Approximately one of four patients who are discharged from the hospital following an acute myocardial infarction will suffer a recurrent infarction or die during the following year. A great variety of different modalities to predict patient outcome following acute myocardial infarction are reported in the medical literature. Two factors are consistently noted to relate to patient outcome—the extent of myocardial damage and the extent of exercise-induced ischemia.

The extent of myocardial damage clearly can be assessed by the resting ejection fraction. This measurement provides information that is complementary to clinical data and is predictive of short-term prognosis.[N3, R8, S14, S15] In addition, the resting ejection fraction is a very important determinant of survival during the next year. The Multicenter Post-infarction Research Group identified four independent predictors of survival following acute myocardial infarction in a large group of 799 patients.[M18] One of these was a resting ejection fraction of less than 0.40, a cut-off value selected for analysis before the study. However, a review of the data from that study clearly indicates that 1-year cardiac mortality is inversely related to the ejection fraction in a continuous fashion (Fig. 57–16). Of note is the fact that the 1-year cardiac mortality approaches 50 percent in those patients with a resting ejection fraction of less than 20 percent.

Equilibrium radionuclide angiography is one of several noninvasive exercise testing modalities that have been employed prior to a patient's hospital discharge in an attempt to determine the presence and extent of exercise-induced ischemia. Corbett and

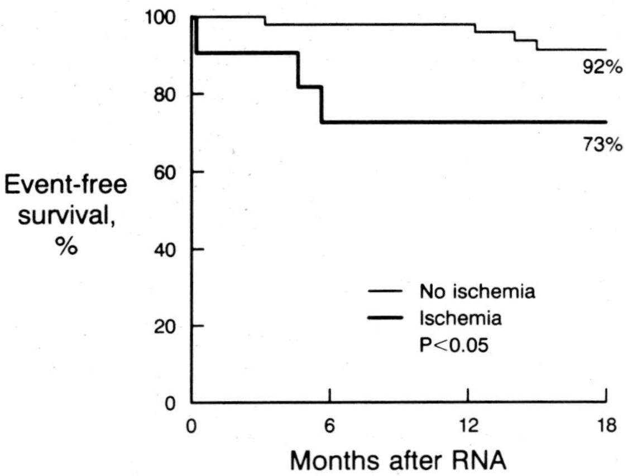

Figure 57–15. Event-free survival in 68 patients from the Mayo Clinic with one- or two-vessel disease and a resting ejection fraction of less than 0.50, as a function of the presence of a markedly abnormal exercise response. Patient outcome was significantly different in the two groups. (From Miller, T. D., et al.: Risk stratification of single or double vessel coronary artery disease and impaired left ventricular function using exercise radionuclide angiography. Am. J. Cardiol. 65:1317, 1990, with permission.)

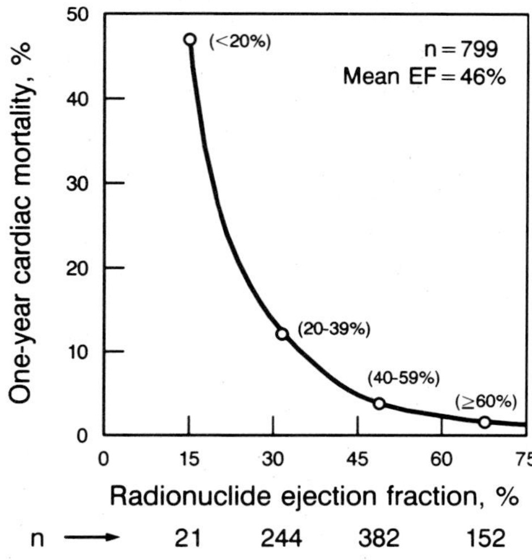

Figure 57–16. One-year cardiac mortality in 799 patients following acute myocardial infarction as a function of the resting ejection fraction (EF) on predischarge radionuclide angiography. N = number of patients in each category and the total population. (From Multicenter Post-infarction Research Group: Risk stratification and survival after myocardial infarction. N. Engl. J. Med. 309:331, 1983. Reprinted with permission from The New England Journal of Medicine.)

colleagues examined the results of exercise radionuclide angiography in 117 patients with uncomplicated myocardial infarction, who were then followed for at least 6 months.[C10, C11] The change in ejection fraction with submaximal exercise was the most useful parameter for predicting subsequent patient outcome. Seventy-four patients failed to increase their ejection fraction with exercise; of these, 70 (95 percent) had events within 6 months. In contrast, of the 43 patients who increased their ejection fraction with exercise, only four (9 percent) had events. However, it should be noted that congestive heart failure, medically refractory angina, and limiting angina were all considered events in this analysis.

Dewhurst and Muir studied 100 consecutive patients who underwent exercise radionuclide angiography 1 month after infarction.[D11] A resting ejection fraction of less than 0.35 identified a high-risk group with a very poor prognosis. In those patients with a resting ejection fraction of greater than 0.35, a decrease in ejection fraction of at least 0.05 with exercise identified patients who were at high risk for postinfarction angina. Their study is one of the few true "natural history" studies in the literature, as coronary revascularization was not undertaken in any of the patients.

Hung and associates compared the prognostic value of the treadmill exercise test, exercise thallium-201 scintigraphy, and equilibrium exercise radionuclide angiography in 117 men who received all three tests within 3 weeks after myocardial infarction.[H11] They compared the ability of a large number of parameters from each of these modalities to predict the subsequent development of death, recurrent myocardial infarction, or ventricular fibrillation. The single best predictor of outcome was the change in ejection fraction at an exercise workload of 450 kg-m/min. The only other variable that provided additional prognostic information was the peak treadmill workload. Thus, on the basis of their study, equilibrium exercise radionuclide angiography appears to be the preferred technique for the assessment of prognosis following acute myocardial infarction. However, there is a clear variation in patient population across the various studies in the literature, suggesting the use of different selection criteria for testing. It is particularly difficult to relate the previously published studies to current populations, now that percutaneous transluminal coronary angioplasty, acute thrombolytic therapy, and early beta-blockade are commonly used. In fact, one recent study demonstrated significant changes over time in multiple clinical and exercise parameters in those patients undergoing exercise radionuclide angiography early after myocardial infarction.[G16] The applicability of previously published results to current patient populations, therefore, is in question.

Equilibrium radionuclide angiography is also frequently employed to assess the efficacy of acute intervention with thrombolytic therapy or percutaneous transluminal coronary angioplasty in patients with myocardial infarction. Such interventions are presumed to limit the extent of myocardial damage. The resting ejection fraction after infarction has been employed as an end-point in many investigations of therapeutic efficacy.[A2, G16, K8, L4, O6, R9, R10, S16] Other studies have utilized the change in the resting ejection fraction measured during and after infarction as an end-point to assess efficacy in an attempt to adjust for the variable amount of myocardium that is "at risk." The change in ejection fraction measured during and after infarction has generally demonstrated a more significant treatment effect than the ejection fraction measured only after infarction.[G17, O6] However, it should be noted that the resting ejection fraction measured during infarction is influenced by many factors other than the amount of hypoperfused myocardium, including preload, afterload, the duration of myocardial ischemia, and hyperkinesia in normal segments. These factors may contribute to the large spontaneous changes that occur in ejection fraction during the first 24 hours of acute myocardial infarction.[W5] Early studies with technetium-99m-sestamibi suggest that this radiopharmaceutical agent will be able to assess the amount of myocardium "at risk" in acute infarction without any delay in therapy, and that the change in myocardial perfusion determined by this radiopharmaceutical agent before and after therapy may be a superior measurement tool for the assessment of the efficacy of acute interventions.[G18]

LIMITATIONS OF EXERCISE RADIONUCLIDE ANGIOGRAPHY. Like any other sophisticated medical procedure, radionuclide angiography has both strengths and weaknesses. Although the limitations of this procedure have been mentioned previously, it is important to summarize and re-emphasize them here. *First* and foremost, the test must be performed carefully and correctly, with a great deal of attention to quality control. As with many other sophisticated procedures, exercise radionuclide angiography can be useful when performed and interpreted by experts, but it also can be misleading in the hands of unskilled practitioners. *Second*, the test requires approximately 2 minutes of a steady state during exercise for adequate exercise images. For a variety of cardiac and noncardiac reasons, many patients cannot sustain exercise for this period of time. In other individuals who are able to exercise, left ventricular dysfunction may occur for only a very brief period at the peak of exercise and will therefore be missed by this technology. *Third*, left ventricular response to exercise is a complex phenomenon dependent upon patient gender, age, medications, exercise workload, ventricular loading, and exercise position. *Fourth*, the assessment of regional dysfunction by this technique is limited because of the nontomographic format and the usual use of only one projection during exercise. *Fifth*, significant arrhythmias, including atrial fibrillation, interfere with the gating required for accurate studies. Depending on their prevalence, arrhythmias will reduce the accuracy of the data or totally invalidate it. *Finally*, the previous validation studies mentioned throughout the chapter have often relied on comparison with coronary anatomy, as assessed by subjective estimates of percent diameter stenosis on coronary arteriography. The limitations of subjective assessment by coronary arteriography have now been well demonstrated.[H10, W4] Further studies comparing exercise radionuclide angiography with more sophisticated angiographic assessment, including quantitative angiography and direct measurements of coronary flow reserve, are needed to determine the true accuracy of radionuclide angiography. Such angiographic comparisons, however, are of importance primarily because of the demonstrated relationship of coronary anatomy to patient outcome. As previously mentioned, the prognostic significance of exercise radionuclide angiography is already well demonstrated.

Cardiomyopathy

Equilibrium radionuclide angiography is useful in the evaluation of patients with known or suspected congestive cardiomyopathies. Measurement of resting ejection fraction and resting left ventricular volume can provide objective documentation of left ventricular size and function. Those patients with a possible restrictive physiology may be identified. Radionuclide angiography may provide potential clues to the underlying etiology. A combination of radionuclide angiography and thallium-201 perfusion imaging can help identify those patients with end-stage ischemic heart disease rather than a true cardiomyopathy.[B17]

The presence and importance of diastolic dysfunction in patients with hypertrophic cardiomyopathy and restrictive cardiomyopathy is now well established. Abnormalities of diastolic filling in such patients can be objectively documented by equilibrium radionuclide angiography.[B18, B19] The potential response to medical therapy, including calcium channel blockers, can be evaluated using diastolic filling measurements on equilibrium radionuclide angiography as an end-point.[B19]

Radionuclide angiography can help guide the medical management and follow-up of patients with congestive cardiomyopathy as well. Since the clinical course of these patients is frequently variable, this modality may be employed as an objective means of assessing any temporal change in left ventricular size or function. The stability of equilibrium radionuclide angiography left ventricular volume measurements over time has been examined[B8] and an end-diastolic volume index change of greater than 36 ml/m^2 is necessary to indicate a true change between two serial examinations. The response of the left ventricle to therapeutic interventions, including vasodilator therapy and abstention from alcohol, may be assessed objectively in this fashion.[H12, O7] Such information clearly may be important in the clinical management of these patients.

Valvular Heart Disease

Equilibrium radionuclide angiography has little place at this time in the assessment of stenotic valvular lesions. Its principal role in valvular heart disease is in the assessment of left-sided regurgitant lesions, i.e., mitral and aortic insufficiency, although it has been utilized to assess tricuspid insufficiency as well.[H13]

In patients with mitral or aortic insufficiency, equilibrium radionuclide angiography may be employed to measure resting left ventricular size and resting left ventricular ejection fraction. As mentioned previously, the estimates of the volume of the left ventricle obtained by radionuclide angiography in this setting are subject to greater error than usual because of the attenuation of counts from the portions of the ventricle that are farthest away from the gamma camera. In addition, relatively few patients with very large hearts have been included in many of the previous studies validating methods for the assessment of volume. Despite these potential limitations with respect to absolute volumes, measurements of relative volume changes in the same patient remain highly accurate and, therefore, have been employed to assess the response to exercise[B20, B21, D12, H14, J6, S17] and the long-term response to medical therapy.[G4]

Measurements of resting ejection fraction in patients with aortic insufficiency are highly accurate by equilibrium radionuclide angiography. Although the measurement of ejection fraction by contrast ventriculography may become difficult in the presence of severe left ventricular enlargement, the presence of such enlargement improves the accuracy of equilibrium radionuclide angiography by increasing the counts within the left ventricle and thereby reducing statistical fluctuation. In patients with mitral insufficiency, the increase in accuracy due to statistical considerations may be offset by the increasing degree of overlap between the left atrium and left ventricle. This overlap can be reduced by increasing the caudal-cranial angulation of the gamma camera; in the presence of severe left atrial enlargement, it usually cannot be eliminated.

As described earlier, the magnitude of left-sided regurgitation can be quantified by using the regurgitant fraction and left ventricular output. Such measurements are useful when the magnitude of regurgitation is not evident from clinical examination. This is particularly true in cases of severe left ventricular enlargement with mitral regurgitation, when the magnitude of mitral regurgitation and the issue of whether it is a primary or secondary phenomenon often are not readily apparent from clinical examination.

Equilibrium radionuclide angiography potentially can make an important contribution to the timing of valve replacement in patients with severe left-sided regurgitation. This issue has been best studied in patients with aortic regurgitation. Despite substantial volume overload of the left ventricle, patients with aortic regurgitation may remain asymptomatic for many years. Once symptoms occur, the downhill course of patients treated medically is often quite rapid. Therefore, there is general agreement that patients with aortic insufficiency and significant symptoms should undergo aortic valve replacement.[B22] The treatment of the asymptomatic or minimally symptomatic patient is a much more controversial issue. The long-term survival of patients who undergo aortic valve replacement for chronic aortic insufficiency is somewhat disappointing. Many of the late postoperative deaths in such patients have been related to chronic congestive heart failure.[B23] The long-standing volume overload in these patients apparently has led to irreversible left ventricular dysfunction. Thus there has been considerable interest in identifying such patients earlier in their natural history, so that aortic valve replacement can be undertaken before irreversible left ventricular dysfunction occurs.

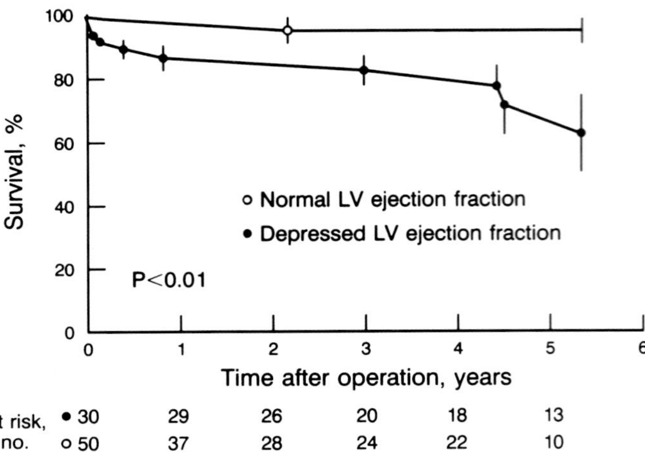

Figure 57–17. Survival of patients with aortic insufficiency after aortic valve replacement. Preoperative resting left ventricular (LV) ejection fraction is a determinant of postoperative survival. (From Bonow, R. O., et al.: Survival and functional results after valve replacement for aortic regurgitation from 1976 to 1983: Impact of preoperative left ventricular function. Circulation 72:1244, 1985, by permission of the American Heart Association, Inc.)

However, the benefit of performing early aortic valve replacement must be weighed against the risks of the surgery as well as the subsequent morbidity and mortality because of presence of a prosthetic heart valve.

The issue of the timing of aortic valve replacement has been addressed in a series of published studies from Bonow et al at the National Institutes of Health.[B22–B26] Preoperative left ventricular function, as assessed by the rest ejection fraction by equilibrium radionuclide angiography, is a major determinant of postoperative survival (Fig. 57–17). Survival at 5.5 years was 96 percent in patients with a normal preoperative ejection fraction, compared with 63 percent in patients with an abnormal preoperative ejection fraction.[B23] Further analysis demonstrated that the risk of postoperative death in patients with an abnormal preoperative ejection fraction depended on two other factors—preoperative exercise tolerance and the duration of resting left ventricular dysfunction. Postoperative survival was poor in patients with a poor exercise tolerance or resting left ventricular

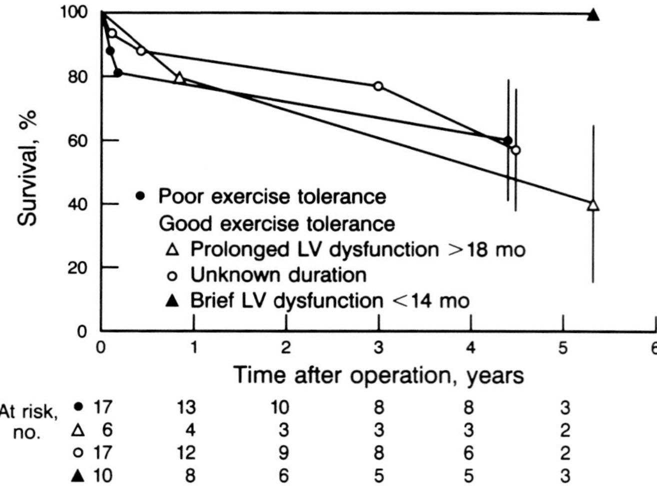

Figure 57–18. Postoperative survival of patients with aortic insufficiency and abnormal preoperative resting left ventricular (LV) ejection fraction. Exercise tolerance and the duration of left ventricular dysfunction are determinants of survival. (From Bonow, R. O., et al.: Survival and functional results after valve replacement for aortic regurgitation from 1976 to 1983: Impact of preoperative left ventricular function. Circulation 72:1244, 1985, by permission of the American Heart Association, Inc.)

dysfunction of either unknown duration or known to have been present for greater than 18 months (Fig. 57–18). In contrast, postoperative survival was excellent in patients with a good exercise tolerance and an abnormal resting left ventricular ejection fraction for less than 14 months (Fig. 57–18). These findings strongly suggest that patients with asymptomatic or minimally symptomatic aortic insufficiency should have their resting ejection fraction assessed by equilibrium radionuclide angiography at regular intervals. Surgery can be safely postponed until symptoms develop or until the resting ejection fraction becomes abnormal.

Bonow and associates have demonstrated that death is rare when this strategy is utilized in asymptomatic patients with aortic insufficiency and normal left ventricular function, and less than 4 percent of the patients require aortic valve replacement each year.[B26] More important, when this strategy is followed postoperative survival is excellent, and left ventricular size (Fig. 57–19) and resting function (Fig. 57–20) both improve postoperatively.[B24]

Earlier studies had suggested that exercise-induced left ventricular dysfunction might be an early sign of impending irreversible left ventricular failure in patients with aortic insufficiency.[B21] Exercise-induced changes in ejection fraction correlate with the end-systolic pressure-volume ratio[S18] and with the resting systolic wall stress,[G19, L5] but not with left ventricular filling pressure.[B27] Changes in regurgitant volume, end-diastolic volume, and stroke volume during exercise are variable, depending on when patients are studied during the natural history of the disease.[H14, J6, S14] The ejection fraction response to exercise is clearly influenced by the marked changes in ventricular loading that occur in patients with aortic insufficiency. Patients with an increase in ejection fraction during exercise are unlikely to develop symptoms or left ventricular dysfunction during subsequent follow-up[B24] (Fig. 57–21). However, in patients with a decrease in ejection fraction with exercise, the magnitude of the decrease does not appear to predict subsequent clinical course.[B26] Thus, exercise radionuclide angiography can identify a subgroup of patients who are apparently earlier in the natural history of disease (and therefore unlikely to develop symptoms or resting left ventricular dysfunction over the next 4 years), but its routine use for follow-up purposes does not appear to be justified.

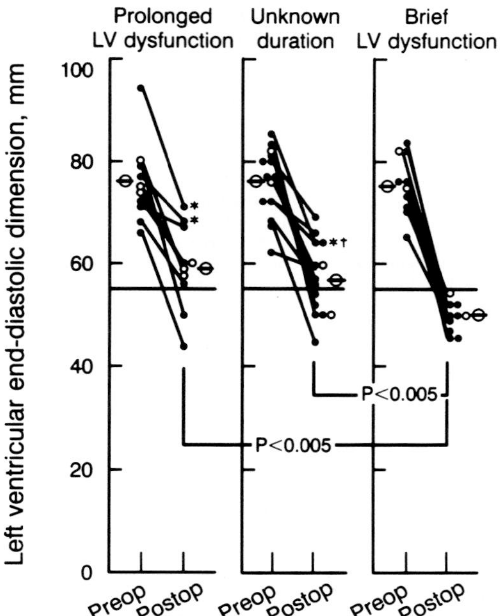

Figure 57–19. Change in echocardiographic left ventricular (LV) end-diastolic dimension from before (preoperation) to 6 months after (postoperation) aortic valve replacement. Open symbols, asymptomatic patients; asterisks, patients who subsequently died with symptoms of heart failure; cross, one patient who subsequently died with prosthetic valve dysfunction; slashed circles, mean values. The horizontal solid line at 55 mm indicates upper limit of normal. (From Bonow, R. O., et al.: Reversal of left ventricular dysfunction after aortic valve replacement for chronic aortic regurgitation: Influence of duration of preoperative left ventricular dysfunction. Circulation 70:570, 1984, by permission of the American Heart Association, Inc.)

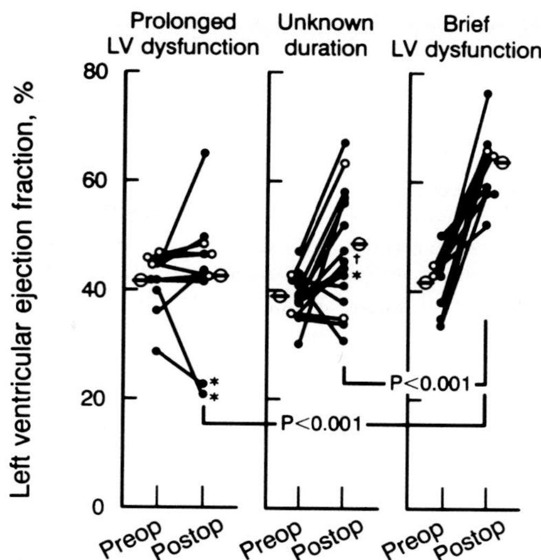

Figure 57–20. Change in radionuclide angiographic resting left ventricular (LV) ejection fraction from before to after aortic valve replacement. Symbols as defined for Figure 57–19. (From Bonow, R. O., et al.: Reversal of left ventricular dysfunction after aortic valve replacement for chronic aortic regurgitation: Influence of duration of preoperative left ventricular dysfunction. Circulation 70:570, 1984, by permission of the American Heart Association, Inc.)

Radionuclide angiography also can assess the effects of aortic valve replacement on left ventricular size, left ventricular function, and exercise performance.[B28] Such an assessment can be particularly important in postoperative patients with vague symptoms that may or may not be due to myocardial dysfunction, and it may identify patients who have suffered perioperative myocardial damage despite optimal preservation techniques. However, an early postoperative decrease in resting ejection fraction may be seen in the presence of an altered loading condition and does not necessarily imply a decline in ventricular contractility.[B29]

Published data regarding patients with severe mitral regurgitation are far fewer.[H15, S19] Right ventricular ejection fraction is clearly important, as its resting value is correlated with exercise tolerance.[H15] Resting right ventricular ejection fraction and resting left ventricular ejection fraction both predict survival in medically treated patients. Further studies are needed in this area.

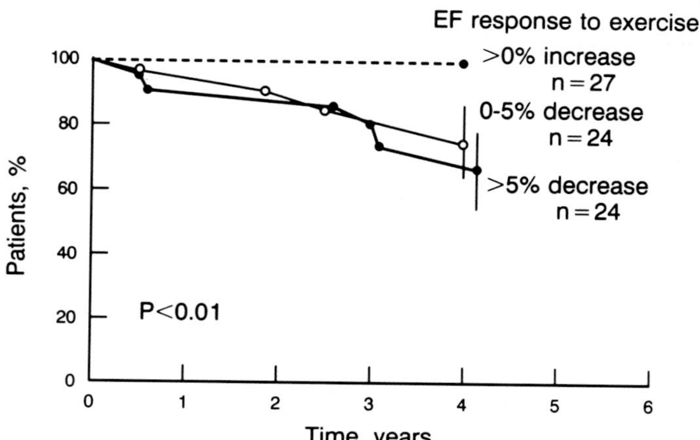

Figure 57–21. Influence of left ventricular ejection fraction (EF) response to exercise on the subsequent course of patients with asymptomatic aortic insufficiency. The onset of symptoms or the onset of resting left ventricular dysfunction was taken as an end point. (From Bonow, R. O., et al.: The natural history of asymptomatic patients with aortic regurgitation and normal left ventricular function. Circulation 68:509, 1983, by permission of the American Heart Association, Inc.)

Other Indications

Equilibrium radionuclide angiography may be employed in a wide variety of other clinical situations. A few of these miscellaneous indications will be briefly highlighted in this section.

The early diagnosis of cor pulmonale in patients with severe chronic obstructive pulmonary disease is often difficult. A measurement of right ventricular ejection fraction by radionuclide angiography, both at rest and with exercise, may assist in this diagnosis. Patients with known chronic obstructive pulmonary disease may have depressed right ventricular function in the absence of clinical evidence of cor pulmonale. Recognition of this dysfunction at an earlier stage may permit the institution of intensive therapy when the dysfunction is more likely to be reversible.[B30, M19]

Patients with a presenting complaint of dyspnea frequently may have known co-existing cardiac and pulmonary disease. The identification of the primary problem is often difficult on clinical grounds. Rest and exercise radionuclide angiography may provide an objective assessment of cardiac function to clarify the situation. The experience in our laboratory has been that cardiac dysfunction in such patients is often much greater than anticipated.

The potential cardiotoxic effects of antitumor drugs such as doxorubicin may be monitored by radionuclide angiography.[A3, G20] Although one early study reported the use of exercise radionuclide angiography for this purpose, resting radionuclide angiography is usually sufficient. Serial measurements of resting ejection fraction can provide evidence of impending cardiac dysfunction before there is any overt evidence of congestive failure. Discontinuation of the drug in these early stages can prevent irreversible cardiac dysfunction.

Finally, a wide variety of pathophysiologic and pharmacologic studies have employed rest and exercise radionuclide angiography as a measurement tool. The effects of drug intervention[B31, D13, R11, T5] and exercise training[C12, J7] on coronary artery disease has been well studied using this approach. Other studies have examined the effects of the aging process.[A1, B32]

CONCLUSION

In the past 15 years, equilibrium radionuclide angiography has progressed from its first description as a research tool to a common clinical test that is widely utilized in the community. Although the technical aspects of this technique have changed little in recent years, our understanding of its proper utilization in clinical patient management continues to evolve.

References

A

1. Arora, R. R., Machac, J., Goldman, M. E., et al.: Atrial kinetics and left ventricular diastolic filling in the healthy elderly. J. Am. Coll. Cardiol. 9:1255, 1987.
2. Anderson, J. L., Marshall, H. W., Bray, B. E., et al.: A randomized trial of intracoronary streptokinase in the treatment of acute myocardial infarction. N. Engl. J. Med. 308:1312, 1983.
3. Alexander, J, Dainiak, N., Berger, H. J., et al.: Serial assessment of doxorubicin cardiotoxicity with quantitative radionuclide angiocardiography N. Engl. J. Med. 300:278, 1979.

B

1. Berger, H. J., and Zaret, B. L.: Nuclear cardiology. N. Engl. J. Med. 305:855, 1981.
2. Berman, D. S., Maddahi, J., Garcia, E. V., et al.: Assessment of left and right ventricular function with multiple gated equilibrium cardiac blood pool imaging. *In* Berman, D. S., and Mason, D. T. (eds.): Clinical Nuclear Cardiology. Grune and Stratton, New York, 1981, pp. 224–284.
3. Brash, H. M., Wraith, P. K., Hannan, W. J., et al.: The influence of ectopic heart beats in gated ventricular blood pool studies. J. Nucl. Med. 21:391, 1980.
4. Bramlet, D. A., Mooris, K. G., Coleman, R. E., et al.: Effects of rate-dependent left bundle branch block on global and regional left ventricular function. Circulation 67:1059, 1983.
5. Burow, R. D., Strauss, H. W., Singleton, R., et al.: Analysis of left ventricular function from multiple gated acquisition cardiac blood pool imaging: Comparison to contrast angiography. Circulation 56:1024, 1977.
6. Berman, D. S., Salel, A. F., DeNardo, G. L., et al.: Clinical assessment of left ventricular regional contraction patterns and ejection fraction by high-resolution gated scintigraphy. J. Nucl. Med. 16:865, 1975.
7. Botvinick, E. H., Dae, M. W., O'Connell, J. W., et al.: First harmonic Fourier (phase) analysis of blood pool scintigrams for the analysis of cardiac contraction and conduction. *In* Gerson, M. C.: Cardiac Nuclear Medicine. McGraw-Hill, New York, 1987, pp. 109–148.
8. Brown, M. L., Vaqueiro, M., Clements, I. P., et al.: Stability of radionuclide left ventricular volume measurements. Nucl. Med. Commun. 9:117, 1988.
9. Bacharach, S. L., Green, M. V., Borer, J. S., et al.: Left ventricular peak ejection rate, filling rate, and ejection fraction-frame rate requirements at rest and exercise: Concise communication. J. Nucl. Med. 20:189, 1979.
10. Bonow, R. O., Bacharach, S. L., Green, M. V., et al.: Impaired left ventricular diastolic filling in patients with coronary artery disease: Assessment with radionuclide angiography. Circulation 64:315, 1981.
11. Bowman, L. K., Lee, F. A., Jaffe, C. C., et al.: Peak filling rate normalized to mitral stroke volume: A new Doppler echocardiographic filling index validated by radionuclide angiographic techniques. J. Am. Coll. Cardiol. 12:937, 1988.
12. Berger, H. J., Reduto, L. A., Johnstone, D. E., et al.: Global and regional left ventricular response to bicycle exercise in coronary artery disease: Assessment by quantitative radionuclide angiocardiography. Am. J. Med. 66:13, 1979.
13. Bodenheimer, M. M., Banka, V. S., Fooshee, C. M., and Helfant, R. H.: Comparative sensitivity of the exercise electrocardiogram, thallium imaging and stress radionuclide angiography to detect the presence and severity of coronary heart disease. Circulation 60:1270, 1979.
14. Borer, J. S., Kent, K. M., Bacharach, S. L., et al.: Sensitivity, specificity and predictive accuracy of radionuclide cineangiography during exercise in patients with coronary artery disease: Comparison with exercise electrocardiography. Circulation. 60:572, 1979.
15. Bonow, R. O., Kent, K. M., Rosing, D. R., et al.: Exercise-induced ischemia in mildly symptomatic patients with coronary artery disease and preserved left ventricular function: Identification of subgroups at risk of death during medical therapy. N. Engl. J. Med. 311:1339, 1984.
16. Bonow, R. O.: Prognostic implications of exercise radionuclide angiography in patients with coronary artery disease. Mayo Clin. Proc. 63:630, 1988.
17. Bulkley, B. H., Hutchins, G. M., Bailey, I., et al.: Thallium-201 imaging and gated cardiac blood pool scans in patients with ischemic and idiopathic congestive cardiomyopathy: A clinical and pathologic study. Circulation 55:753, 1977.
18. Betocchi, S., Bonow, R. O., Bacharach, S. L., et al.: Isovolumic relaxation period in hypertrophic cardiomyopathy: Assessment by radionuclide angiography. J. Am. Coll. Cardiol. 7:74, 1986.
19. Bonow, R. O., Rosing, D. R., Bacharach, S. L., et al.: Effects of verapamil on left ventricular systolic function and diastolic filling in patients with hypertrophic cardiomyopathy. Circulation 64:787, 1981.
20. Boucher, C. A., Kanarek, D. J., Okada, R. D., et al.: Exercise testing in aortic regurgitation: Comparison of radionuclide left ventricular ejection fraction with exercise performance at the anaerobic threshold and peak exercise. Am. J. Cardiol. 52:801, 1983.
21. Borer, J. S., Bacharach, S. L., Green, M. V., et al.: Exercise-induced left ventricular dysfunction in symptomatic and asymptomatic patients with aortic regurgitation: Assessment with radionuclide cineangiography. Am. J. Cardiol. 42:351, 1978.
22. Bonow, R. O., Rosing, D. R., Kent, D. M., and Epstein, S. E.: Timing of operation for chronic aortic regurgitation. Am. J. Cardiol. 50:325, 1982.
23. Bonow, R. O., Picone, A. L., McIntosh, C. L., et al.: Survival and functional results after valve replacement for aortic regurgitation from 1976 to 1983: Impact of preoperative left ventricular function. Circulation 72:1244, 1985.
24. Bonow, R. O., Rosing, D. R., Maron, B. J., et al.: Reversal of left ventricular dysfunction after aortic valve replacement for chronic aortic regurgitation: Influence of duration of preoperative left ventricular dysfunction. Circulation 70:570, 1984.
25. Bonow, R. O., Borer, J. S., Rosing, D. R., et al.: Preoperative exercise capacity in symptomatic patients with aortic regurgitation as a predictor of postoperative left ventricular function and long-term prognosis. Circulation 62:1280, 1980.
26. Bonow, R. O., Rosing, D. R., McIntosh, C. L., et al.: The natural history of asymptomatic patients with aortic regurgitation and normal left ventricular function. Circulation 68:509, 1983.
27. Boucher, C. A., Wilson, R. A., Kanarek, D. J., et al.: Exercise testing in asymptomatic or minimally symptomatic aortic regurgitation: Relationship of left ventricular ejection fraction of left ventricular pressure during exercise. Circulation 67:1091, 1983.
28. Borer, J. S., Rosing, D. R., Kent, K. M., et al.: Left ventricular function at rest and during exercise after aortic valve replacement in patients with aortic regurgitation. Am. J. Cardiol. 44:1297, 1979.
29. Boucher, C. A., Bingham, J.B., Osbakken, M. D., et al.: Early changes in left ventricular size and function after correction of left ventricular volume overload. Am. J. Cardiol. 47:991, 1981.
30. Berger, H. J., Matthay, R. A., Loke, J., et al.: Assessment of cardiac performance with quantitative radionuclide angiocardiography: Right ventricular ejection fraction with reference to findings in chronic obstructive pulmonary disease. Am. J. Cardiol. 41:897, 1978.
31. Borer, J. S., Bacharach, S. L., Green, M. V., et al.: Effect of nitroglycerin on exercise-induced abnormalities of left ventricular regional function and ejection fraction in coronary artery disease. Assessment by radionuclide cineangiography in symptomatic and asymptomatic patients. Circulation 57:314, 1978.

32. Bonow, R. O., Vitale, D. F., Bacharach, S. L., et al.: Effects of aging on asynchronous left ventricular regional function and global ventricular filling in normal human subjects. J. Am. Coll. Cardiol. 11:50, 1988.

C

1. Callahan, R. J., Froelich, J. W., McKusick, K. A., et al.: A modified method for the in vivo labeling of red blood cells with Tc-99m: Concise communication. J. Nucl. Med. 23:315, 1982.
2. Currie, P. J., Kelly, M. J., and Pitt, A.: Comparison of supine and erect bicycle exercise electrocardiography in coronary heart disease: Accentuation of exercise-induced ischemic ST depression by supine posture. Am. J. Cardiol. 52:1167, 1983.
3. Clements, I. P., Brown, M.L., and Smith, H. C.: Radionuclide measurement of left ventricular volume. Mayo Clin. Proc. 56:733, 1981.
4. Clements, I. P., Nelson, M. A., O'Connor, M. K., et al.: Diastolic measurements from alternate R-wave gating. Am. Heart J. 116:113, 1988.
5. Corbett, J. R., Jansen, D. E., Lewis, S. E., et al.: Tomographic gated blood pool radionuclide ventriculography: Analysis of wall motion and left ventricular volumes in patients with coronary artery disease. J. Am. Coll. Cardiol. 6:349, 1985.
6. Caldwell, J. H., Hamilton, G. W., Sorensen, S. G., et al.: The detection of coronary artery disease with radionuclide techniques: A comparison of rest-exercise thallium imaging and ejection fraction response. Circulation 61:610, 1980.
7. Currie, P. J., Kelly, M. J., Harper, R. W., et al.: Incremental value of clinical assessment, supine exercise electrocardiography, and biplane exercise radionuclide ventriculography in the prediction of coronary artery disease in men with chest pain. Am. J. Cardiol. 52:927, 1983.
8. CASS Principal Investigators and Associates: Coronary Artery Surgery Study (CASS): A randomized trial of coronary artery bypass surgery: Survival data. Circulation 68:939, 1983.
9. Campos, C. T., Chu, H. W., D'Agostino, H. J., Jr., and Jones, R. H.: Comparison of rest and exercise radionuclide angiography and exercise treadmill testing for diagnosis of anatomically extensive coronary artery disease. Circulation 67:1204, 1983.
10. Corbett, J. R., Nicod, P. H., Huxley, R. L., et al.: Left ventricular functional alterations at rest and during submaximal exercise in patients with recent myocardial infarction. Am. J. Med. 74:577, 1983.
11. Corbett, J. R., Nicod, P., Lewis, S. E., et al.: Prognostic value of submaximal exercise radionuclide ventriculography after myocardial infarction. Am. J. Cardiol. 52:82, 1983.

D

1. Douglas, K. H., Links, J. M., Chen, D. C. P., et al.: Linear discriminant analysis of regional ejection fractions in the diagnosis of coronary artery disease. Eur. J. Nucl. Med. 12:602, 1987.
2. Dehmer, G. J., Lewis, S. E., Hillis, L. D., et al.: Nongeometric determination of left ventricular volumes from equilibrium blood pool scans. Am. J. Cardiol. 45:293, 1980.
3. Dehmer, G. J., Firth, B. G., Hillis, L. D., et al.: Nongeometric determination of right ventricular volumes from equilibrium blood pool scans. Am. J. Cardiol. 49:78, 1982.
4. Dehmer, G. J., Firth, B. G., Lewis, S. E., et al.: Direct measurement of cardiac output by gated equilibrium blood pool scintigraphy: Validation of scintigraphic volume measurements by a nongeometric technique. Am. J. Cardiol. 47:1061, 1981.
5. Diamond, G. A., and Forrester, J. S.: Analysis of probability as an aid in the clinical diagnosis of coronary-artery disease. N. Engl. J. Med. 300:1350, 1979.
6. Diamond, G. A., Forrester, J. S., Hirsch, M., et al.: Application of conditional probability analysis to the clinical diagnosis of coronary artery disease. J. Clin. Invest. 65:1210, 1980.
7. DePace, N. L., Iskandrian, A. S., Hakki, A. H., et al.: Value of left ventricular function during exercise in predicting the extent of coronary artery disease. J. Am. Coll. Cardiol. 1:1002, 1983.
8. DePace, N. L., Hakki, A. H., Weinreich, D. J., and Iskandrian, A. S.: Noninvasive assessment of coronary artery disease. Am. J. Cardiol. 52:715, 1983.
9. Dilsizian, V., Bonow, R. O., Cannon, R. O., et al.: The effect of coronary artery bypass grafting on left ventricular systolic function at rest: Evidence for preoperative subclinical myocardial ischemia. Am. J. Cardiol. 61:1248, 1988.
10. DePuey, E. G., Leatherman, L. L., Leachman, R. D., et al.: Restenosis after transluminal coronary angioplasty detected with exercise gated radionuclide ventriculography. J. Am. Coll. Cardiol. 4:1103, 1984.
11. Dewhurst, N. G., and Muir, A. L.: Comparative prognostic value of radionuclide ventriculography at rest and during exercise in 100 patients after first myocardial infarction. Br. Heart J. 49:111, 1983.
12. Dehmer, G. J., Firth, B. G., Hillis, L. D., et al.: Alterations in left ventricular volumes and ejection fraction at rest and during exercise in patients with aortic regurgitation. Am. J. Cardiol. 48:17, 1981.
13. Dehmer, G. J., Falkoff, M., Lewis, S. E., et al.: Effect of oral propranolol on rest and exercise left ventricular ejection fraction, volumes, and segmental wall motion in patients with angina pectoris. Assessment with equilibrium gated blood pool imaging. Br. Heart J. 45:656, 1981.

E

1. Eckelman, W., Richards, P., Hauser, W., and Atkins, H.: Technetium-labeled red blood cells. J. Nucl. Med. 12:22, 1971.
2. European Coronary Surgery Study Group: Long-term results of prospective randomized study of coronary artery bypass surgery in stable angina pectoris. Lancet 2:1173, 1982.

F

1. Freeman, M. R., Berman, D. S., Staniloff, H., et al.: Comparison of upright and supine bicycle exercise in the detection and evaluation of extent of coronary artery disease by equilibrium radionuclide ventriculography. Am. Heart J. 102:182, 1981.
2. Foster, C., Dymond, D. S., Auholm, J. D., et al.: Effect of exercise protocol on the left ventricular response to exercise. Am. J. Cardiol. 51:859, 1983.
3. Folland, E. D., Hamilton, G. W., Larson, S. M., et al.: The radionuclide ejection fraction: A comparison of three radionuclide techniques with contrast angiography. J. Nucl. Med. 18:1159, 1977.
4. Freeman, M. R., Gray, R. J., Berman, D. S., et al.: Improvement in global and segmental left ventricular function after coronary bypass surgery. Circulation (Suppl. II)II–64:34, 1981.

G

1. Gibbons, R. J., and Essandoh, L. K.: Exercise radionuclide angiography in left bundle branch block. Dynam. Cardiovasc. Imag. 1:206, 1987.
2. Green, M. V., Brody, W. R., Douglas, M. A., et al.: Ejection fraction by count rate from gated images. J. Nucl. Med. 19:880, 1978.
3. Gibbons, R. J., Morris, K. G., Lee, K., et al.: Assessment of regional left ventricular function using gated radionuclide angiography. Am. J. Cardiol. 54:294, 1984.
4. Greenberg, B., Massie, B., Bristow, J. D., et al.: Long-term vasodilator therapy of chronic aortic insufficiency. Circulation 78:98, 1988.
5. Gobert, P., Kremer, R., Rigot, P., et al.: Value, sensitivity and specificity of stroke volume ratio in routine equilibrium gated scintigraphy. Eur. Heart J. 8:(Suppl. C):77, 1987.
6. Gill, J. B., Moore, R. H., Tamaki, N., et al.: Multigated blood-pool tomography: New method for the assessment of left ventricular function. J. Nucl. Med. 27: 1916, 1986.
7. Gibbons, R. J.: Noninvasive exercise testing in cardiac disease. *In* Spittell, J. A. (ed.): Clinical Medicine. Harper & Row, Philadelphia, 1985.
8. Gibbons, R. J.: Nuclear cardiology. *In* Brandenburg, R., Fuster, V., Giuliani, E., and McGoon, D. C. (eds.): Cardiology: Fundamentals and Practice. Year Book Medical Publishers, Chicago, 1987.
9. Gibbons, R. J., Lee, K. L., Cobb, F., and Jones, R. H.: Ejection fraction response to exercise in patients with chest pain and normal coronary arteriograms. Circulation 64:952, 1981.
10. Gibbons, R. J., Lee, K. L., Cobb, F. R., et al.: Ejection fraction response to exercise in patients with chest pain, coronary artery disease, and normal resting ventricular function. Circulation 66:643, 1982.
11. Gibbons, R. J., Lee, K. L., Pryor, D., et al.: The use of radionuclide angiography in the diagnosis of coronary artery disease—a logistic regression analysis. Circulation 68:740, 1983.
12. Gibbons, R. J., Clements, I. P., Zinsmeister, A. R., and Brown, M. L.: Exercise response of the systolic pressure to end systolic volume ratio in patients with coronary artery disease. J. Am. Coll. Cardiol. 10:33, 1987.
13. Gibbons, R. J., Fyke, F. E., III, Clements, I. P., et al.: Noninvasive identification of severe coronary artery disease using exercise radionuclide angiography. J. Am. Coll. Cardiol. 11:28, 1988.
14. Gibbons, R. J., Hu, D. C., Clements, I. P., et al.: Anatomic and functional significance of a hypotensive response during supine exercise radionuclide ventriculography. Am. J. Cardiol. 60:1, 1987.
15. Gibbons, R. J., Zinsmeister, A. R., Ballard, D. J., and Mock, M. B.: Prognostic value of exercise radionuclide angiography in community population. Circulation 78(Suppl. II):II423, 1988.
16. Gibbons, R. J., Lavie, C. L., Zinsmeister, A. R., and Gersh, B. J.: Exercise assessment after myocardial infarction—long-term changes in patient selection. J. Am. Coll. Cardiol. 11:122A, 1988.
17. Guerci, A. D., Gerstenbligh, G., Brinker, J. A., et al.: A randomized trial of intravenous tissue plasminogen activator for acute myocardial infarction with subsequent randomization to elective coronary angioplasty. N. Engl. J. Med. 317:1613, 1987.
18. Gibbons, R. J., Verani, M. S., Behrenbeck T., et al.: Feasibility of tomographic technetium-99m-hexakis-2-methoxy-2-methylpropyl-isonitrile imaging for the assessment of myocardial area at risk and efficacy of thrombolytic therapy in acute myocardial infarction. Circulation 80:1277, 1989.
19. Goldman, M. E., Packer, M., Horowitz, S. F., et al.: Relation between exercise-induced changes in ejection fraction and systolic loading conditions at rest in aortic regurgitation. J. Am. Coll. Cardiol. 3:924, 1984.
20. Gottdiener, J. S., Mathisen, D. J., Borer, J. S., et al.: Doxorubicin cardiotoxicity: Assessment of late left ventricular dysfunction by radionuclide cineangiography. Ann. Intern. Med. 94:430, 1981.

H

1. Hladik, W. B., Nigg, K. N., and Rhodes, B. A.: Drug induced changes in biologic distribution of radiopharmaceuticals. Semin. Nucl. Med. 12:184, 1982.
2. Harris, D., Taylor, D., Condon, B., et al.: Myocardial imaging with dipyridamole: Comparison of the sensitivity and specificity of ^{201}Tl versus MUGA. Eur. J. Nucl. Med. 7:1, 1982.
3. Holman, B. L., Wynne, J., Zielonka, J. S., and Idoine, J. D.: A simplified technique for measuring right ventricular ejection fraction using the equilibrium radionuclide angiocardiogram and the slant-hold collimator. Radiology 138:429, 1981.

4. Hanley, P. C., and Gibbons, R. J.: The value of radionuclide determined changes in pulmonary blood volume for the detection of coronary artery disease. Chest 97:7, 1990.
5. Higgenbotham, M. B., Morris, K. G., Coleman, E., and Cobb, F. R.: Sex-related differences in normal cardiac response to upright exercise. Circulation 70:357, 1984.
6. Hanley, P. C., Gibbons, R. J., Zinsmeister, A. R., et al.: Sex-related differences in cardiac response to supine exercise assessed by radionuclide angiography. J. Am. Coll. Cardiol. 13:624, 1989.
7. Harris, P. J., Lee, K. L., Harrell, F. E., et al.: Survival in medically tested coronary artery disease. Circulation 60:1259, 1979.
8. Hammermeister, K. E., DeRouen, T. A., and Dodge, H. T.: Variables predictive of survival in patients with coronary artery disease: Selection by univariate and multivariate analysis from the clinical, electrocardiographic, exercise, arteriographic, and quantitative angiographic evaluations. Circulation 59:421, 1979.
9. Harris, P. J., Lee, K. L., Hurrell, F. E., et al.: Outcome in medically treated coronary artery disease. Circulation 62:718, 1980.
10. Harrison, D. G., White, C. W., Hiratzka, L. F., et al.: The value of lesion cross-sectional area determined by quantitative coronary angiography in assessing the physiologic significance of proximal left anterior descending coronary arterial stenoses. Circulation 69:1111, 1984.
11. Hung, J., Goris, M. L., Nash, E., et al.: Comparative value of maximal treadmill testing, exercise thallium myocardial perfusion scintigraphy and exercise radionuclide ventriculography for distinguishing high- and low-risk patients soon after acute myocardial infarction. Am. J. Cardiol. 53:1221, 1984.
12. Hindman, M. C., Slosky, D. A., Peter, R. H., et al.: Rest and exercise hemodynamic effects of oral hydralazine in patients with coronary artery disease and left ventricular dysfunction. Circulation 61:751, 1980.
13. Handler, B., Pavel, D. G., Pietras, R., et al.: Equilibrium radionuclide gated angiography in patients with tricuspid regurgitation. Am. J. Cardiol. 51:305, 1983.
14. Huxley, R. L., Gaffney, F. A., Corbett, J. R., et al.: Early detection of left ventricular dysfunction in chronic aortic regurgitation as assessed by contrast angiography, echocardiography, and rest and exercise scintigraphy. Am. J. Cardiol. 51:1542, 1983.
15. Hochtreiter, C., Niles, N., Devereux, R. B., et al.: Mitral regurgitation: Relationship of noninvasive descriptors of right and left ventricular performance to clinical and hemodynamic findings and to prognosis in medically and surgically treated patients. Circulation 73:900, 1986.

I

1. Iskandrian, A. S.: Prognostic implications at rest and exercise radionuclide ventriculography in patients with suspected or proven coronary heart disease. Int. J. Cardiol. 6:707, 1984.

J

1. Juni, J. E., and Chen, C. C.: Effects of gating modes on the analysis of left ventricular function in the presence of heart rate variation. J. Nucl. Med. 29:1272, 1988.
2. Jengo, J. A., Oren, V., Conant, R., et al.: Effects of maximal exercise stress on left ventricular function in patients with coronary artery disease using first pass radionuclide angiocardiography: A rapid, noninvasive technique for determining ejection fraction and segmental wall motion. Circulation 59:60, 1979.
3. Jones, R. H., McEwan, P., Newman, G. E., et al.: Accuracy of diagnosis of coronary artery disease by radionuclide measurement of left ventricular function during rest and exercise. Circulation 64:586, 1981.
4. Johnstone, D. E., Sands, M. J., Berger, H. J., et al.: Comparison of exercise radionuclide angiocardiography and thallium-201 myocardial perfusion imaging in coronary artery disease. Am. J. Cardiol. 45:1113, 1980.
5. Jengo, J. A., Freman, R., Brizendine, M., and Mena, I.: Detection of coronary artery disease: Comparison of exercise stress radionuclide angiocardiography and thallium stress perfusion scanning. Am. J. Cardiol. 45:535, 1980.
6. Johnson, L. L., Powers, E. R., Tzall, W. R., et al.: Left ventricular volume and ejection fraction response to exercise in aortic regurgitation. Am. J. Cardiol. 51:1379, 1983.
7. Jensen, D., Atwood, J. E., Froelicher, V., et al.: Improvement in ventricular function during exercise studied with radionuclide ventriculography after cardiac rehabilitation. Am. J. Cardiol. 46:770, 1980.

K

1. Kelly, M. J., Giles, R. W., Simon, T. R., et al.: Multigated equilibrium radionuclide angiocardiography: Improved detection of left ventricular wall motion abnormalities and aneurysms by the addition of the left lateral view. Radiology 139:167, 1981.
2. Konstam, M. A., Tumeh, S., Wynne, J., et al.: Effect of exercise on erythrocyte count and blood activity concentration after technetium-99m in vivo red blood cell labeling. Circulation 66:638, 1982.
3. Konstam, M. A., Wynne, J., Holman, B. L., et al.: Use of equilibrium (gated) radionuclide ventriculography to quantitate left ventricular output in patients with and without left-sided valvular regurgitation. Circulation 64:578, 1981.
4. Korr, K. S., Gandsman, E. J., Winkler, M. L., et al.: Hemodynamic correlates of right ventricular ejection fraction measured with gated radionuclide angiography. Am. J. Cardiol. 49:71, 1982.
5. Kent, K. M., Borer, J. S., Green, M. B., et al.: Effects of coronary artery bypass on global and regional left ventricular function during exercise. N. Engl. J. Med. 298:1434, 1978.
6. Kronenberg, M. W., Pederson, R. W., Harston, W. E., et al.: Left ventricular performance after coronary artery bypass surgery. Ann. Intern. Med. 99:305, 1983.
7. Kennedy, J. W., Martin, G. V., Davis, K. B., et al.: The Western Washington Intravenous Streptokinase in Acute Myocardial Infarction Randomized Trial. Circulation 77:345, 1988.
8. Khaja, F., Walton, J. A., Jr., Brymer, J. F., et al.: Intracoronary fibrinolytic therapy in acute myocardial infarction: Report of a prospective randomized trial. N. Engl. J. Med. 308:1305, 1983.

L

1. Lee, H. B., Wexler, J. P., Scarf, S. C., and Blaufox, M. D.: Pharmacologic alterations in Tc-99m binding by red blood cells. J. Nucl. Med. 24:397, 1983.
2. Links, J. M., Becker, L. C., Shindledecker, J. G., et al.: Measurements of absolute left ventricular volume from gated blood pool studies. Circulation 65:82, 1982.
3. Lim, Y. L., Kalff, V., Kelly, M. J., et al.: Radionuclide angiographic assessment of global and segmental left ventricular function at rest and during exercise after coronary artery bypass graft surgery. Circulation 66:972, 1982.
4. Leiboff, R. H., Katz, R. J., Wasserman, A. G., et al.: A randomized, angiographically controlled trial of intracoronary streptokinase in acute myocardial infarction. Am. J. Cardiol. 53:404, 1984.
5. Lewis, S. M., Riba, A. L., Berger, H. J., et al.: Radionuclide angiographic exercise left ventricular performance in chronic aortic regurgitation. Relationship to resting echographic ventricular dimensions and systolic wall stress index. Am. Heart J. 103:498, 1982.

M

1. Manyari, D. E., and Kostuk, W. J.: Left and right ventricular function at rest and during bicycle exercise in the supine and sitting positions in normal subjects and patients with coronary artery disease. Am. J. Cardiol. 51:36, 1983.
2. Manyari, D. E., Nolewajka, A. J. Purves, P., et al.: Comparative value of the cold-pressor test and supine bicycle exercise to detect subjects with coronary artery disease using radionuclide ventriculography. Circulation 65:571, 1982.
3. Maddox, D. E., Wynne, J., Uren, R., et al.: Regional ejection fraction: A quantitative radionuclide index of regional left ventricular performance. Circulation 59:1001, 1979.
4. Mancini, G. B. J., Peck, W. W., and Slutsky, R. A.: Analysis of phase-angle histograms from equilibrium radionuclide studies: Correlation with semi-quantitative grading of wall motion. Am. J. Cardiol. 55:535, 1985.
5. Melchior, J. P., Chevigne, M., Righetti, A., et al.: Quantification of valvular regurgitation by cardiac blood pool scintigraphy: Correlation with catheterization. Eur. Heart J. 8(Suppl. C):71, 1987.
6. Maddahi, J., Berman, D. S., Matsuoka, D. T., et al.: A new technique for assessing right ventricular ejection fraction using rapid multiple-gated equilibrium cardiac blood pool scintigraphy. Circulation 60:581, 1979.
7. Morrison, D. A., Turgeon, J., and Ovitt, T.: Right ventricular ejection fraction measurement: Contrast ventriculography versus gated blood pool and gated first-pass radionuclide methods. Am. J. Cardiol. 54:651, 1984.
8. Melin, J. A., Wijns, W., Robert, A., et al.: Validation of radionuclide cardiac output measurements during exercise. J. Nucl. Med. 26:1386, 1985.
9. Miller, T. R., Grossman, S. J., Schechtman, K. B., et al.: Left ventricular diastolic filling and its association with age. Am. J. Cardiol. 58:531, 1986.
10. Miller, T. R., Fountos, A., Biello, D. R., and Ludbrook, P. A.: Detection of coronary artery disease by analysis of ventricular filling. J. Nucl. Med. 28:837, 1987.
11. Mancini, G. B. J., Slutsky, R. A., Norris, S. L., et al.: Radionuclide analysis of peak filling rate, filling fraction, and time to peak filling rate: Response to supine bicycle exercise in normal subjects and patients with coronary disease. Am. J. Cardiol. 51:43, 1983.
12. Magorien, D. J., Shaffer, P., Bush, C. A., et al.: Assessment of left ventricular pressure-volume relations using gated radionuclide angiography, echocardiography, and micromanometer pressure recordings: A new method for serial measurements of systolic and diastolic function in man. Circulation 67:844, 1983.
13. Maublant, J., Bailly, P., Mestas, D., et al.: Feasibility of gated single-photon emission transaxial tomography of the cardiac blood pool. Radiology 146:837, 1983.
14. Metz, C. E.: Principles of ROC analysis. Semin. Nucl. Med. 8:283, 1978.
15. Mock, M. B., Ringqvist, I., Fisher, L. D., et al.: Survival of medically treated patients in the Coronary Artery Surgery Study (CASS) registry. Circulation 66:562, 1982.
16. Mazzotta, G., Bonow, R. O., Pace, L., et al.: Exertional ischemia and prognosis in mildly symptomatic patients with single or double vessel coronary artery disease and left ventricular dysfunction at rest. (Abstract.) J. Am. Coll. Cardiol. 11:153, 1988.
17. Miller, T. D., Taliercio, C. P., Zinsmeister, A. R., and Gibbons, R. J.: Risk stratification of patients with single or double vessel disease and impaired left ventricular function using exercise radionuclide angiography. Am. J. Cardiol. 65:1317, 1990.
18. Multicenter Post-infarction Research Group: Risk stratification and survival after myocardial infarction. N. Engl. J. Med. 309:331, 1983.
19. Matthay, R. A., Berger, H. J., Loke, J., et al.: Effects of aminophylline upon right and left ventricular performance in chronic obstructive pulmonary disease: Noninvasive assessment by radionuclide angiocardiography. Am. J. Med. 65:903, 1978.

N

1. Norris, S. L., Slutsky, R. A., Gerber, K. H., et al.: Sensitivity and specificity of nuclear phase analysis versus ejection fraction in coronary artery disease. Am. J. Cardiol. 53:1547, 1984.
2. Nicod, P., Corbett, J. R., Firth, B. G., et al.: Radionuclide techniques for valvular regurgitant index: Comparison in patients with normal and depressed ventricular function. J. Nucl. Med. 23:763, 1982.
3. Nicod, P., Corbett, J. R., Sanford, C. F., et al.: Comparison of the influence of acute transmural and nontransumural myocardial infarction on ventricular function. Am. Heart J. 107:28, 1984.

O

1. Okada, R. D., Kirshenbaum, H. D., Kushner, F. G., et al.: Observer variance in the qualitative evaluation of left ventricular wall motion and the quantitation of left ventricular ejection fraction using rest and exercise multigated blood pool imaging. Circulation 61:128, 1980.
2. Okada, R. D., Pohost, G. M., Nichols, A. B., et al.: Left ventricular regional wall motion assessment by multigated and end-diastolic, end-systolic gated radionuclide left ventriculography. Am. J. Cardiol. 45:1211, 1980.
3. Okada, R. D., Pohost, G. M., Kirshenbaum, H. D., et al.: Radionuclide-determined change in pulmonary blood volume with exercise: Improved sensitivity of multigated blood-pool scanning in detecting coronary artery disease. N. Engl. J. Med. 301:569, 1979.
4. Okada, R. D., Osbakken, M. D., Boucher, C. A., et al.: Pulmonary blood volume ratio response to exercise: A noninvasive determination of exercise-induced changes in pulmonary capillary wedge pressure. Circulation 65:126, 1982.
5. O'Keefe, J. H., Lapeyre, A. C., Holmes, D. R., and Gibbons, R. J.: Early radionuclide angiography identifies low risk patients for late restenosis after transluminal coronary angioplasty. Am. J. Cardiol. 61:51, 1988.
6. O'Rourke, M., Baron, D., Keogh, A., et al.: Limitation of myocardial infarction by early infusion of recombinant tissue-type plasminogen activator. Circulation 77:1311, 1988.
7. O'Connell, J. B., Robinson, J. A., Henkin, R. E., and Gunnar, R. M.: Immunosuppressive therapy in patients with congestive cardiomyopathy and myocardial uptake of gallium-67. Circulation 64:780, 1981.

P

1. Pavel, D. G., Zimmer, A. M., and Patterson, V. N.: In vivo labeling of red blood cells with ^{99m}Tc: A new approach to blood pool visualization. J. Nucl. Med. 18:305, 1977.
2. Poliner, L. R., Dehmer, G. J., Lewis, S. E., et al.: Left ventricular performance in normal subjects: A comparison of the responses to exercise in the upright and supine position. Circulation 62:528, 1980.
3. Pfisterer, M. E., Ricci, D. R., Schuler, G., et al.: Validity of left-ventricular ejection fractions measured at rest and peak exercise by equilibrium radionuclide angiography using short acquisition times. J. Nucl. Med. 20:484, 1979.
4. Pfisterer, M. E., Battler, A., Swanson, S. M., et al.: Reproducibility of ejection fraction determinations by equilibrium radionuclide angiography in response to supine bicycle exercise: Concise communication. J. Nucl. Med. 20:491, 1979.
5. Papapietro, S. E., Yester, M. V., Logic, J. R., et al.: Method for quantitative analysis of regional left ventricular function with first pass and gated blood pool scintigraphy. Am. J. Cardiol. 47:618, 1981.
6. Petru, M. A., Sorenson, S. G., Chandhuri, T. K., et al.: Attenuation correction of equilibrium radionuclide angiography for noninvasive quantitation of cardiac output and ventricular volumes. Am. Heart J. 107:1221, 1984.
7. Poliner, L. R., Farber, S. H., Glaeser, D. H., et al.: Alterations of diastolic filling rate during exercise radionuclide angiography: A highly sensitive technique for detection of coronary artery disease. Circulation 70:942, 1984.
8. Pryor, D. B., Harrell, F. E., Jr., Lee, K. L., et al.: Estimating the likelihood of significant coronary artery disease. Am. J. Med. 75:771, 1983.
9. Pryor, D. B., Harrell, F. E., Lee K. L., et al.: Prognostic indicators for radionuclide angiography in medically treated patients with coronary artery disease. Am. J. Cardiol. 53:18, 1984.
10. Port, S., Cobb, F. R., Coleman, R. E., and Jones, R. H.: The effects of age on the response of the left ventricular ejection fraction to exercise. N. Engl. J. Med. 303:1133, 1980.

R

1. Rao, S. A., Knobel, J., Collier, B. D., and Isitmon, A. T.: Effect of Sn(II) ion concentration and heparin on technetium-99m red blood cell labelling. J. Nucl. Med. 27:1202, 1986.
2. Rowe, D. W., DePuey, E. G., Sonnemaker, R. E., et al.: Left ventricular performance during exercise in patients with left bundle branch block: Evaluation by gated radionuclide ventriculography. Am. Heart J. 105:66, 1983.
3. Ratib, O., Henze, E., Schon, H., and Schelbert, H. R.: Phase analysis of radionuclide ventriculograms for the detection of coronary artery disease. Am. Heart J. 104:1, 1982.
4. Rigo, P., Alderson, P. O., Robertson, R. M., et al.: Measurement of aortic and mitral regurgitation by gated cardiac blood pool scans. Circulation 60:306, 1979.
5. Rozanski, A., Diamond, G. A., Berman, D., et al.: The declining specificity of exercise radionuclide ventriculography. N. Engl. J. Med. 3409:518, 1983.
6. Rozanski, A., Diamond, G. A., Jones, R., et al.: A format for integrating the interpretation of exercise ejection fraction and wall motion and its application in identifying equivocal responses. J. Am. Coll. Cardiol. 5:2388, 1985.
7. Rozanski, A., Berman, D., Gray, R., et al.: Preoperative prediction of reversible myocardial asynergy by postexercise radionuclide ventriculography. N. Engl. J. Med. 307:212, 1982.
8. Reduto, L. A., Berger, H. J., Cohen, L. S., et al.: Sequential radionuclide assessment of left and right ventricular performance after acute transmural myocardial infarction. Ann. Intern. Med. 89:441, 1978.
9. Rentrop, K. P., Feit, F., Blanke, H., et al.: Effects of intracoronary streptokinase and intracoronary nitroglycerin infusion on coronary angiographic patterns and mortality in patients with acute myocardial infarction. N. Engl. J. Med. 311:1457, 1984.
10. Ritchie, J. L., Davis, K. B., Williams, D. L., et al.: Global and regional left ventricular function and tomographic radionuclide perfusion: The Western Washington Intracoronary Streptokinase in Myocardial Infarction Trial. Circulation 70:867, 1984.
11. Ritchie, J. L., Sorensen, S. G., Kennedy, J. W., and Hamilton, G. W.: Radionuclide angiography: Noninvasive assessment of hemodynamic changes after administration of nitroglycerin. Am. J. Cardiol. 43:278, 1979.

S

1. Smith, T. D., and Richards, P.: A simple kit for the preparation of Tc-99m-labeled red blood cells. J. Nucl. Med. 17:126, 1976.
2. Stokley, E. M., Parkey, R. W., Bonte, F. J., et al.: Gated blood pool imaging following Tc-99m stannous pyrophosphate imaging. Radiology 120:433, 1976.
3. Stengart, R. M., Wexler, J., Slagle, S., and Scheuer, J.: Radionuclide ventriculographic responses to graded supine and upright exercise: Critical role of the Frank-Starling mechanism at submaximal exercise. Am. J. Cardiol. 53:1671, 1984.
4. Seaworth, J. F., Higginbotham, M. B., Coleman, R. E., and Cobb, F. R.: Effect of partial decreases in exercise workload on radionuclide indices of ischemia. J. Am. Coll. Cardiol. 2:522, 1983.
5. Secker-Walker, R. H., Resnick, L., Kunz, H., et al.: Measurement of left ventricular ejection fraction. J. Nucl. Med. 14:798, 1973.
6. Schneider, R. M., Jaszczak, R. J., Coleman, R. E., and Cobb, F. R.: Disproportionate effects of regional hypokinesis on radionuclide ejection fraction: Compensation using attenuation-corrected ventricular volumes. J. Nucl. Med. 25:747, 1984.
7. Steckley, R. A., Kronenberg, M. W., Born, M. L., et al.: Radionuclide ventriculography: Evaluation of automated and visual methods for regional wall motion analysis. Radiology 142:179, 1982.
8. Schwaiger, M., Ratib, V., Henze, E., and Schelbert, H. R.: Limitations of quantitative phase analysis of radionuclide angiograms for detecting coronary artery disease in patients with impaired left ventricular function. Am. Heart J. 108:942, 1984.
9. Starling, M. R., Dell'Italia, L. J., Walsh, R. A., et al.: Accurate estimates of absolute left ventricular volumes from equilibrium radionuclide angiographic count data using a simple geometric attenuation correction. J. Am. Coll. Cardiol. 3:789, 1984.
10. Sorensen, S. G., O'Rourke, R. A., and Chaudhuri, T. K.: Noninvasive quantitation of valvular regurgitation by gated equilibrium radionuclide angiography. Circulation 62:1089, 1980.
11. Sciagra, R., Voth, E., Tebbe, U., et al.: Evaluation of three methods for quantifying valvular regurgitation using gated equilibrium radionuclide ventriculography. Eur. Heart J. 8:1109, 1987.
12. Sorensen, S. G., Ritchie, J. L., Caldwell, J. H., et al.: Serial exercise radionuclide angiography: Validation of count-derived changes in cardiac output and quantitation of maximal exercise ventricular volume change after nitroglycerin and propranolol in normal men. Circulation 61:600, 1980.
13. Smith, H. L.: The relation of the weight of the heart to the weight of the body and of the weight of the heart to age. Am. Heart J. 4:79, 1928.
14. Sanford, C. F., Corbett, J., Nicod, P., et al.: Value of radionuclide ventriculography in the immediate characterization of patients with acute myocardial infarction. Am. J. Cardiol. 49:637, 1982.
15. Shah, P. K., Pichler, M., Berman, D. S., et al.: Left ventricular ejection emmefraction determined by radionuclide ventriculography in early stages of first transmural myocardial infarction: Relation to short-term prognosis. Am. J. Cardiol. 45:542, 1980.
16. Simoons, M. L., Serruys, P. W., van den Brand, M., et al.: Early thrombolysis in acute myocardial infarction: Limitation of infarct size and improved survival. J. Am. Coll. Cardiol. 7:717, 1986.
17. Steingart, R. M., Yee, C., Weinstein, L., and Scheuer, J.: Radionuclide ventriculographic study of adaptations to exercise in aortic regurgitation. Am. J. Cardiol. 51:488, 1983.
18. Schuler, G., von Olshausen, K., Schwarz, F., et al.: Noninvasive assessment of myocardial contractility in asymptomatic patients with severe aortic regurgitation and normal left ventricular ejection fraction at rest. Am. J. Cardiol. 50:45, 1982.
19. Schuler, G., Peterson, K. L., Johnson, A., et al.: Temporal response of left ventricular performance to mitral valve surgery. Circulation 59: 1218, 1979.

T

1. Thrall, J. H., Freitas, J. E., Swanson, D., et al.: Clinical comparison of cardiac blood pool visualization with technetium-99m red blood cells labeled in vivo and with technetium-99m human serum albumin. J. Nucl. Med. 19:796, 1978.
2. Tamaki, N., Mukai, T., Ishii, Y., et al.: Multiaxial tomography of heart chambers by gated blood-pool emission computed tomography using a rotating gamma camera. Radiology 147:547, 1983.

3. Taliercio, C. P., Clements, I. P., Zinsmeister, A. R., and Gibbons, R. J.: Prognostic value and limitations of exercise radionuclide angiography. Mayo Clin. Proc. 63:573, 1988.
4. Takaro, T., Hultgren, H. N., Lipton, M. J., and Detre, K. M.: VA Cooperative Randomized Study for coronary artery occlusive disease: II. Left main disease. Circulation 54 (Suppl. 3):III–107, 1976.
5. Tan, A. T., Sadick, N., Kelly, D. T., et al.: Verapamil in stable effort angina: Effects on left ventricular function evaluated with exercise radionuclide ventriculography. Am. J. Cardiol. 49:425, 1982.

V

1. Vitale, D. F., Green, M. V., Bacharach, S. L., et al.: Assessment of regional left ventricular function by sector analysis: A method for objective evaluation of radionuclide blood pool studies. Am. J. Cardiol. 52: 1112, 1983.
2. Vatterott, P. J., Gibbons, R. J., Hu, D. C., et al.: Assessment of left ventricular volume changes during exercise radionuclide angiography in coronary artery disease. Am. J. Cardiol. 61:912, 1988.

W

1. Wackers, F. J. T., Berger, H. J., Johnstone, D. E., et al.: Multiple gated cardiac blood pool imaging for left ventricular ejection fraction: Validation of the technique and assessment of variability. Am. J. Cardiol. 43:1159, 1979.
2. Warren, S. E., Royal, H. D., Markis, J. E., et al.: Time course of left ventricular dilation after myocardial infarction: Influence of infarct-related artery and success of coronary thrombolysis. J. Am. Coll. Cardiol. 11:21, 1988.
3. Weintraub, W. S., Schneider, R. M., Seelaus, P. A., et al.: Prospective evaluation of the severity of coronary artery disease with exercise raidonuclide angiography and electrocardiography. Am. Heart J. 111:537, 1986.
4. White, C. W., Wright, C. B., Doty, D. B., et al.: Does visual interpretation of the coronary arteriogram predict the physiologic importance of a coronary stenosis? N. Engl. J. Med. 310:819, 1984.
5. Wackers, F. J., Berger, H. J., Weinberg, M. A., and Zaret, B. L.: Spontaneous changes in left ventricular function over the first 24 hours of acute myocardial infarction: Implications for evaluating early therapeutic interventions. Circulation 66:748, 1982.

Chapter 58

Myocardial Perfusion Imaging with Thallium-201

GEORGE A. BELLER, M.D.

HISTORICAL PERSPECTIVE 1047
TISSUE TRACER KINETICS OF THALLIUM-201 1047
Thallium Uptake Kinetics 1047
Delayed Thallium-201 Redistribution 1048
Persistent Thallium-201 Defects 1050
Reverse Thallium-201 Redistribution 1051
Lung Thallium-201 Uptake 1051
TECHNETIUM-99m ISONITRILES 1053
STRESS AND REST IMAGING 1053
Exercise 1053
Dipyridamole 1055
Rest Imaging 1056
IMAGE DISPLAY AND ANALYSIS 1057
Planar Methods 1057
Single Photon Emission Computed Tomography (SPECT) 1057
CLINICAL APPLICATIONS 1057
Thallium-201 Scintigraphy in the Asymptomatic Patient 1057
Thallium-201 Scintigraphy in Patients with Chest Pain 1058
Prognostic Applications 1060
Thallium-201 Scintigraphy After Myocardial Infarction 1063
Thallium-201 Scintigraphy for Assessment of Myocardial Revascularization 1064
Thallium-201 Scintigraphy After Thrombolytic Therapy 1064
SPECT Thallium-201 Scintigraphy 1065
Dipyridamole Thallium-201 Scintigraphy 1065
THALLIUM-201 SCINTIGRAPHY IN NONCORONARY HEART DISEASE 1066
LIMITATIONS OF THALLIUM-201 SCINTIGRAPHY 1067
CLINICAL APPLICATION OF TECHNETIUM-99m ISONITRILE IMAGING 1067
SUMMARY 1068

HISTORICAL PERSPECTIVE

Accumulation of basic information concerning active and passive transport mechanisms for concentrating monovalent cations in myocardial tissue led to the exploration of the use of radioisotopes of potassium, rubidium, cesium, ammonia, and thallium for evaluation of regional myocardial perfusion employing radionuclide imaging technology. The uptake of these cations in the myocardium is in proportion to blood flow, cellular integrity, and the size of the regional potassium pool. When administered intravenously, their uptake by heart muscle approximates the fraction of the cardiac output perfusing the heart. These cations must first traverse the capillary wall, interstitial space, and sarcolemmal membrane before equilibrating in the intracellular monovalent cation pool. Both passive and active transport mechanisms appear to be operative in this intracellular sequestration. The active transport system involves the adenosine triphosphate (ATP)–dependent sodium-potassium exchange mechanism. An abnormal reduction in regional myocardial blood flow, a functional or anatomic alteration in cell membrane transport activity, a lack of appropriate energy production, or a defect in energy utilization by the cell results in diminished uptake of radionuclide monovalent cations.

Recently, a new class of radiopharmaceutical agents for assessment of myocardial perfusion has emerged, and these agents are presently undergoing clinical testing.[H1] They are the technetium-99m (^{99m}Tc)-labeled isonitriles, which are cationic complexes and do not require the active sodium pump for myocardial uptake.

The first radionuclide monovalent cations applied clinically were ^{43}K and ^{81}Rb. Potassium-43 was limited by its relatively long half-life (22.4 hours), by highly energetic photons with a peak keV of 373—making imaging with the gamma scintillation camera difficult—and by beta emission that resulted in a high absorbed dose to the patient. Despite these limitations, imaging with this agent was shown to localize regions of transmural myocardial infarction and exercise-induced hypoperfusion accurately.[Z1]

Myocardial imaging with ^{81}Rb was also successfully carried out with gamma camera imaging technology and was shown to have an 88 percent sensitivity for coronary artery disease (CAD) detection.[B1, B2] Although initially promising, ^{81}Rb imaging could not be easily performed, since a pinhole collimator was required. Imaging interpretation using such a collimator is difficult if the heart is not well centered within the camera field of view. When thallium-201 (^{201}Tl) emerged as a perfusion agent more suitable for the gamma scintillation camera, clinical studies with ^{43}K and ^{81}Rb terminated. However, the knowledge acquired during this early period of radionuclide imaging paved the way for the diagnostic and prognostic applications now well established for thallium-201 scintigraphy. Presently, ^{82}Rb scintigraphy is being performed in conjunction with dipyridamole infusion and positron emission tomography methodology for assessment of nutrient myocardial blood flow, and it has emerged as the major alternative to single photon emission computed tomography (SPECT) with ^{201}Tl and ^{99m}Tc isonitriles for tomographic imaging of the heart. $^{13}NH_4^+$ is an alternative to ^{82}Rb for positron imaging of regional myocardial perfusion but requires a cyclotron for its production.

TISSUE TRACER KINETICS OF THALLIUM-201

Thallium Uptake Kinetics

Of all the radionuclide monovalent cations evaluated for clinical use, thallium-201 has emerged as the most widely used agent.

The knowledge of thallium-201 uptake and washout kinetics under normal, ischemic, and necrotic conditions is required for its optimal utilization as a perfusion imaging agent. This is particularly true when computer-assisted quantitative imaging algorithms are applied to myocardial scintigrams in order to detect an abnormal response. Thallium-201 is a metallic element in group III-a of the periodic table. It decays by electron capture with a 73-hour half-life. Its principal photo peaks are at 135 and 167 keV, and it emits mercury x-rays of 69 to 83 keV with 98 percent abundance. The 80 keV mercury x-ray is at the low end of the energy spectrum for resolution with a scintillation camera. Thus, imaging can be undertaken with a high-resolution, low-energy collimator and a gamma scintillation camera.

Because it is a monovalent cation, thallium-201 behaves similarly to ^{43}K and ^{81}Rb biologically, although the percentage dose of thallium concentrated in the myocardium after intravenous injection is greater with thallium than with other potassium analogs.[L1] There also appears to be a somewhat lower hepatic and gastric uptake of thallium-201 compared with the other two monovalent cation tracers. After intravenous injection, the early myocardial uptake of thallium-201 is directly proportional to regional myocardial blood flow and the extraction fraction of thallium-201 by the myocardium.[S1, W1] The extraction fraction is defined as the percentage of the dose of thallium entering the coronary circulation that is extracted on the first pass through the heart, and it ranges from 85 to 90 percent. At high myocardial blood flows, the extraction of thallium-201 diminishes.[M1]

A slight diminution in thallium-201 extraction fraction is seen with acidosis and hypoxemia, whereas drugs such as propranolol and digitalis have little effect on extraction.[F1, W1] Some controversy still persists with respect to the effect of hypoxia on thallium extraction. In a more recent study, the extraction and permeability × surface area (PS) product for thallium were not affected by cellular hypoxia, which caused severe cardiac hemodynamic dysfunction.[L2] In another study by the same group, myocardial uptake of thallium during a constant infusion into an isolated rabbit heart was unaffected by hypoxia when coronary flow was held constant.[L3] First-pass extraction of thallium-201 is normal in stunned myocardium characterized by postischemic dysfunction following repetitive brief periods of flow reduction.[M2] Similarly, when coronary perfusion pressure is transiently lowered, the extraction fraction is not altered as long as cellular necrosis has not developed.[G1] Finally, myocardial thallium-201 uptake was not impaired out of proportion to the flow diminution in a model of a sustained reduction in perfusion resulting in systolic dysfunction.[S16] Thus, intracellular extraction of thallium-201 via transport across the sarcolemmal membrane is not altered unless irreversible membrane injury is present.

The uptake of thallium-201 in the canine heart is significantly correlated with regional flow as determined by the radioactive microsphere technique.[N1, P1] Figure 58–1 illustrates this excellent relationship between uptake of thallium-201 and microsphere-determined blood flow in the myocardium in conscious dogs undergoing treadmill exercise.[N1] Irreversibly damaged myocardial tissue cannot concentrate thallium-201 intracellularly. In a flow-independent model in which myocardial accumulation of thallium-201 in response to ischemia-like myocardial injury was assessed in a cultured fetal mouse heart preparation, accumulation of the radionuclide within injured hearts was related in a decreasing fashion to the loss of lactic dehydrogenase.[G2]

Delayed Thallium-201 Redistribution

Following the initial myocardial uptake phase after intravenous injection, there is a continuous exchange of myocardial thallium-201 and thallium-201 in the blood pool that recirculates from the systemic compartment (Fig. 58–2). Thallium-201 is continually washing out of normally perfused myocardium and replaced by

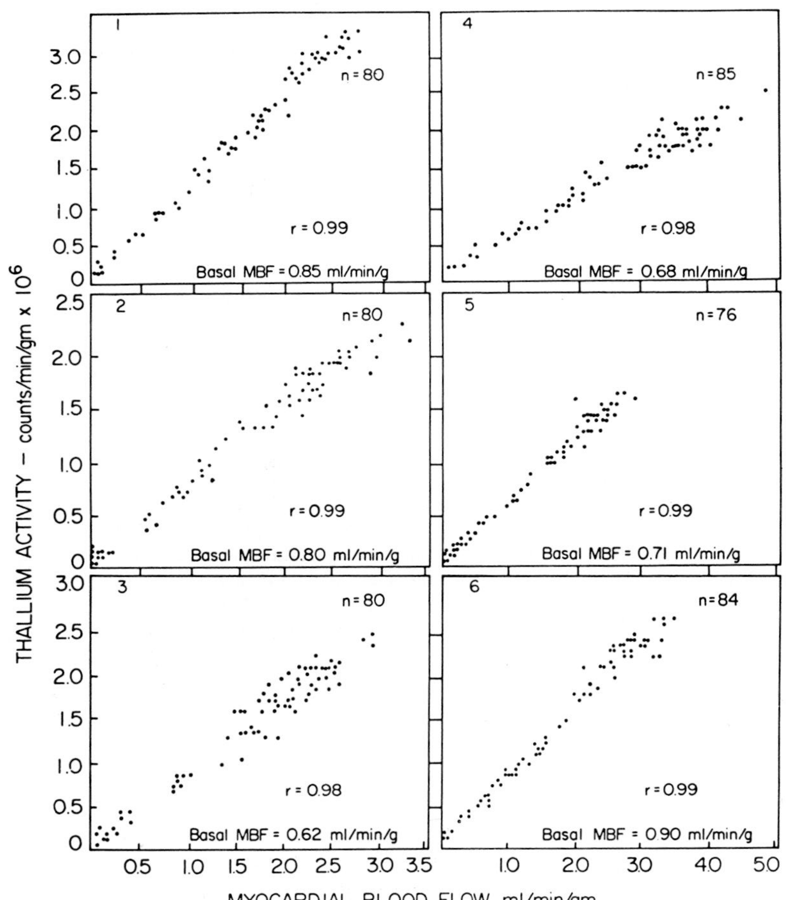

Figure 58–1. The relationship between thallium-201 activity and myocardial blood flow in six dogs during exercise and ischemia. n = number of samples analyzed. (From Nielson, A. T., et al.: Linear relationship between the distribution of thallium-201 and blood flow in ischemic and non-ischemic myocardium during exercise. Circulation 61:797, 1980, by permission of the American Heart Association, Inc.)

recirculating thallium-201 from residual activity in the blood pool. This process of continuous exchange forms the basis of the phenomenon of thallium-201 "redistribution" that is observed when the radionuclide is administered during transient underperfusion of the myocardium, or even when there is a chronic reduction in myocardial blood flow (rest redistribution).* With respect to myocardial imaging, redistribution is defined as the total or partial resolution of initial defects as assessed by repeat imaging at 2.5 to 4 hours after thallium-201 administration. The degree of resolution of an ischemic defect over several hours reflects the amount of redistribution. For example, when thallium-201 is injected during peak exercise, the disparity of flow will be marked if one compares radionuclide uptake between normal myocardium with tissue that is relatively underperfused. After rest has resulted in a restoration of relatively homogeneous flow to normal myocardium and to the region perfused by a stenotic artery, delayed redistribution occurs as the thallium-201 rapidly washes out of the normal region and exhibits late accumulation or flat washout, in the ischemic segment perfused by the stenotic artery.

Delayed redistribution is also observed when inhomogeneity of myocardial blood flow is produced by intravenous dipyridamole or adenosine infusion.[B5] The vasodilator markedly enhances flow in normally perfused myocardium but causes an attenuated flow increase or, actually, an absolute decrease (coronary steal) in regions perfused by stenotic vessels.[B5]

The redistribution phenomenon has been studied extensively in various animal models. In one study, thallium-201 was injected during transient total occlusion. During the occlusion phase, the uptake of thallium-201 was markedly diminished in the myocardial zone supplied by the obstructed artery.[G1] When flow was restored 20 minutes later, continuous delayed extraction of thallium via the systemic recirculation of the tracer resulted in delayed redistribution, with a narrowing of the gradient in thallium-201 activity between normal and previously ischemic myocardial zones (Fig. 58–3). The defect completely resolved in 360 minutes. As long as sarcolemmal membrane function is not physiologically or structurally altered, restored perfusion will permit the myocardial cells initially deprived of thallium-201 at the time of tracer administration to continue to extract the radionuclide as it recirculates through the myocardium. Eventually, the intracellular thallium-201 concentration will normalize, and a new equilibrium distribution between nonischemic and previously ischemic myocardium will be achieved. When this occurs, all viable myocardial cells will reach a stable value of intracellular thallium-201 concentration.

Thallium-201 clearance from nonischemic myocardium becomes monoexponential 5 minutes after intracoronary injection of the radionuclide and is directly related to the rate of thallium clearance from the blood and the myocardial-to-blood thallium-201 concentration ratio. There is an early rapid clearance component with a half-life of approximately 2.5 minutes, which represents washout of unextracted thallium-201 from the interstitial space. Peak exercise heart rate significantly influences thallium-201 clearance.[K1] It has been shown that for each heart rate reduction by 1 beat per minute, normal clearance slows by 0.05 hour in terms of half-life of thallium-201 in the myocardium.[K1] This may be due to the fact that with increasing heart rates, particularly during exercise stress, there is increased flow of blood to the myocardium, resulting in a higher initial uptake of thallium with a subsequent faster clearance. In the presence of a high-grade coronary narrowing, there is "slow late" thallium-201 clearance from the abnormally perfused segment, compared with the rate of thallium clearance from normally perfused zones. When thallium-201 is injected during peak exercise, the early clearance of the tracer from normally perfused myocardium is

*References B3, B4, G1, G3, L4, N2, O1–3, P1, P2, S2–4, W2–4.

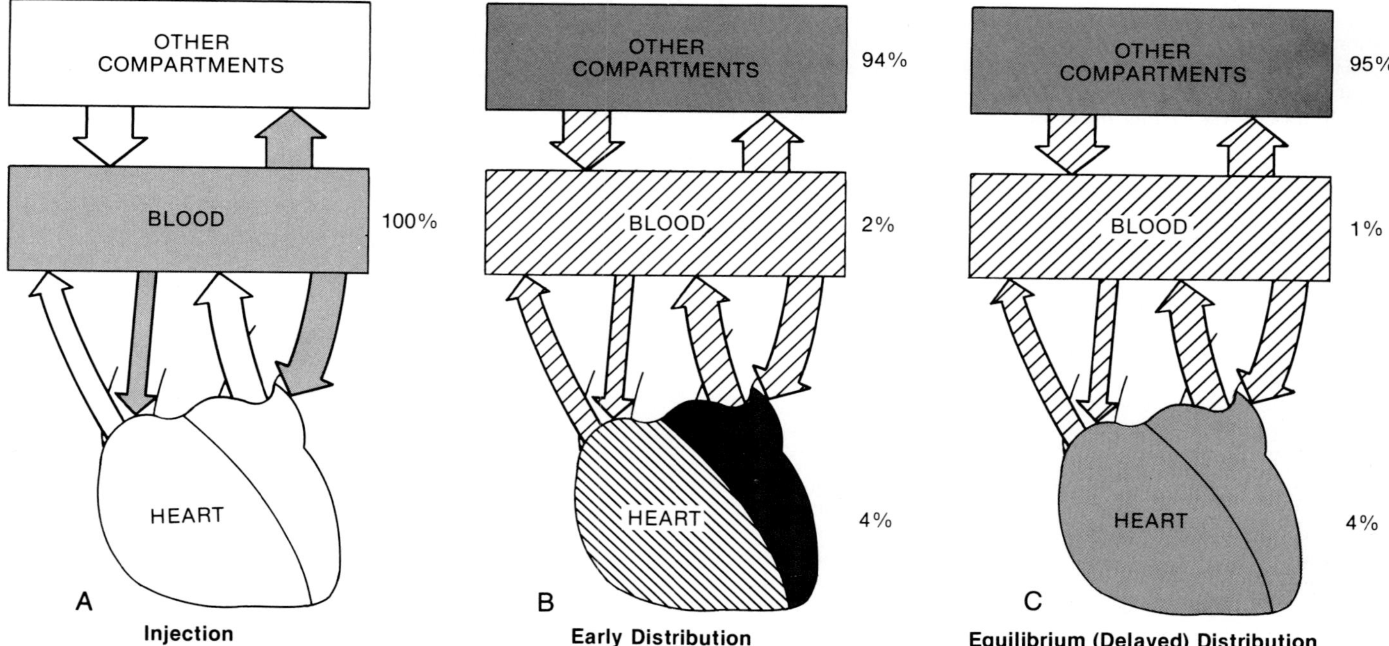

Figure 58–2. Diagrammatic representation of Tl-201 uptake washout kinetics. *A*, Immediately after intravenous administration, 100 percent of the thallium activity is in the blood pool. It is rapidly taken up by myocardial tissue and other systemic organs in proportion to blood flow. The small cross-hatched arrow indicates diminished uptake of thallium in a regional myocardial zone, compared with a normal area depicted by the larger arrow pointing to the myocardium. *B*, After initial distribution only 2 percent of the injected dose of thallium-201 remains in the blood pool, with 4 percent taken up by the myocardium and 94 percent by other compartments. This distribution pattern reflects the fraction of cardiac output delivered to the heart versus "other compartments." The lightly cross-hatched region represents diminished uptake, compared with the darker cross-hatched region in the myocardium. *C*, The equilibrium, or delayed distribution, phase several hours after intravenous thallium administration is depicted by uniform uptake of thallium in the myocardium secondary to redistribution. One percent of the activity now remains in the blood pool secondary to renal clearance of the tracer. The uniform thallium-201 uptake in the delayed redistribution phase is due to washout of thallium from normally perfused zones with delayed accumulation or slow thallium-201 washout from the hypoperfused zone.

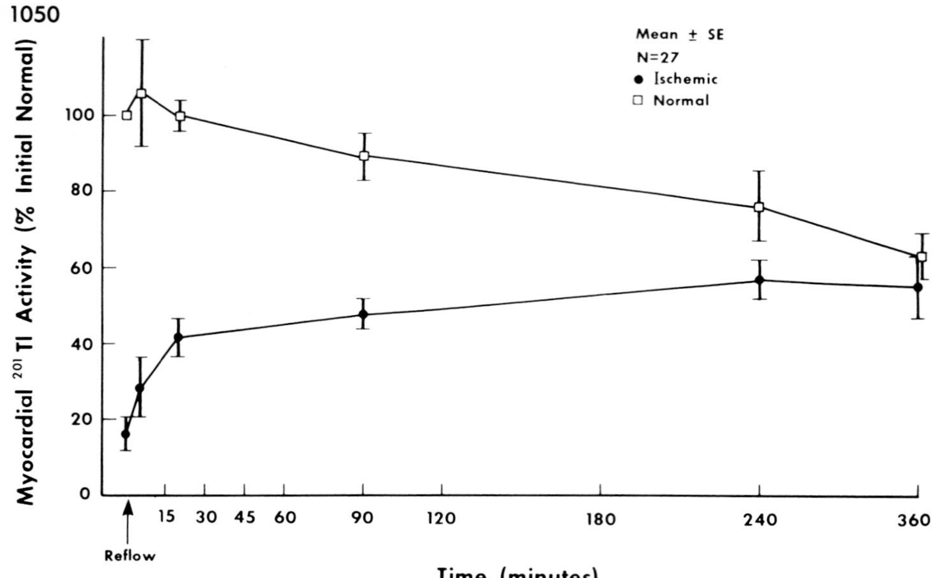

Figure 58–3. Serial changes in myocardial thallium-201 activity (percent of initial normal activity depicted as 100 percent) from ischemic and normal zones in 27 dogs undergoing 20 minutes of left anterior descending coronary artery occlusion followed by reflow. Note the narrowing of the gradient of activity between normal and ischemic zones over time, attributed to washout of thallium from the normal region and delayed accumulation of thallium in the transiently ischemic region. At 360 minutes there is near total redistribution. (From Beller, G. A., et al.: Time course of thallium-201 redistribution after transient myocardial ischemia. Circulation 61:791, 1980, with permission.)

more rapid than the clearance from the blood. This relationship between ischemia and abnormal thallium-201 clearance is important, since the phenomenon has diagnostic utility in the detection of coronary lesions in patients.

In clinical imaging studies, some patients may not demonstrate substantial delayed redistribution until 12 to 24 hours after thallium-201 injection.[C6, K2] Potential mechanisms for this delayed redistribution could include low thallium-201 blood levels, a high-grade coronary stenosis limiting the influx of thallium during the recirculation phase, thus delaying achievement of equilibrium relative to regions supplied by normal vessels, or a possibility of a functional impairment in monovalent cation transport consequent to ischemia. Many patients with apparent "late redistribution" that is only detected at 18 to 24 hours do demonstrate abnormal thallium-201 kinetics by quantitative analysis of thallium activity on earlier images.

Thallium-201 redistribution over time when the tracer is injected in the resting state can be observed under conditions of a chronic reduction in regional flow, as with a severe coronary stenosis.[P2] The mechanism for this rest redistribution during chronic ischemia is both a diminution in the initial uptake of thallium-201 and a decrease in the intrinsic efflux rate of thallium-201.[G1] There is substantially slower washout of thallium-201 over time from the stenosis region, compared with washout from the nonischemic region. These disparate washout rates from hypoperfused and normal myocardium result in ultimate normalization of thallium-201 activity between nonischemic and stenotic regions by 3 to 4 hours. Serial imaging at rest has been used to evaluate myocardial perfusion and viability in patients with severe angina or after myocardial infarction.[B6, B7, F2, G4] Patients with severe ischemia but without necrosis often demonstrate resting defects showing delayed redistribution. Many of these segments are associated with hypokinetic wall motion on ventriculography and are characteristic of a phenomenon now referred to as "hibernating myocardium." However, failure to demonstrate delayed thallium-201 uptake at rest or with exercise does not preclude the presence of viable myocardium. Brunken and associates reported that 58 percent of myocardial segments with no demonstrable thallium-201 redistribution demonstrated residual glucose utilization as assessed by positron emission tomography.[B28] Thus, a potential limitation of thallium-201 scintigraphy is the failure accurately to detect myocardial viability.

If thallium-201 is injected during a hyperemic phase following resolution of spontaneous ischemia, a defect may not be demonstrated. This may occur if thallium-201 is injected immediately following resolution of coronary vasospasm, when hyperemia may exist for the period of time during the initial rapid uptake phase of the tracer.[K3] A similar phenomenon occurs when thallium-201 is administered soon after coronary reperfusion preceded by varying periods of coronary occlusion.[G17] In fact, a "hot spot" of thallium-201 activity may be observed in an infarct region if thallium-201 is injected immediately following reflow before the hyperemic phase has resolved. This phenomenon is shown in Figure 58–4. Similarly, if myocardial hemorrhage or interstitial edema occurs consequent to reperfusion injury, thallium-201 administered during this phase of injury will be trapped in myocardial tissue, yielding a scintigraphic pattern that might overestimate the amount of myocardial salvage.

Persistent Thallium-201 Defects

When thallium-201 is administered intravenously under conditions of a total occlusion of a coronary vessel or in the presence of a myocardial scar, a "persistent" defect in the coronary supply

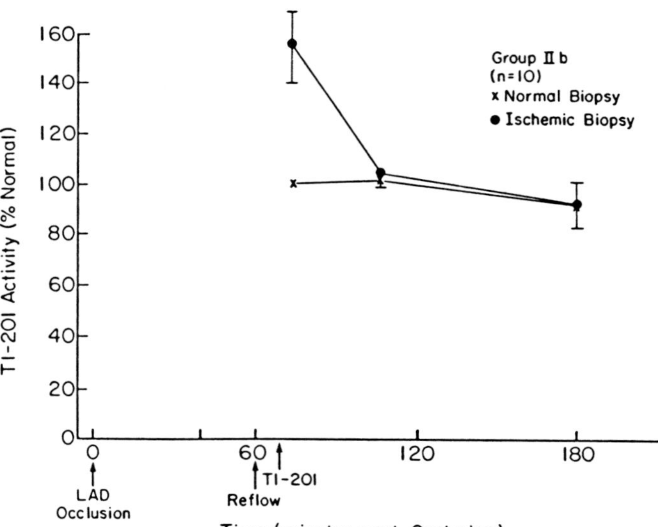

Figure 58–4. Myocardial thallium-201 time activity curves in ten dogs undergoing 1 hour of coronary occlusion followed by rapid reperfusion through a totally patent vessel. Thallium-201 was administered at peak reflow. Note that initial thallium-201 activity in the ischemic region is higher than nonischemic activity, reflecting "excess" uptake from hyperemia consequent to reperfusion. (From Granato, G. E., et al.: Myocardial thallium-201 kinetics during coronary occlusion and reperfusion: Influence of method of reflow and timing of thallium-201 administration. Circulation 73:150, 1986, by permission of the American Heart Association, Inc.)

region of the irreversibly damaged area is observed. In the presence of infarction or scar, a defect is noted both soon after thallium-201 administration and several hours later when repeat imaging is performed. In this situation, no delayed redistribution can be detected. Partial redistribution is observed if there is physiologically significant collateral flow to viable myocardium in the distribution of the occluded artery, or if some antegrade flow is preserved. Partial redistribution indicates the presence of viable myocardium. As expected, persistent thallium defects can be observed over time after injections made during exercise, during dipyridamole infusion, or in the resting state, and these correlate with Q-waves on the electrocardiogram and akinetic or dyskinetic wall motion. In an animal infarct model, persistent thallium-201 defects correlated with irreversibly damaged myocardium, as assessed by radiolabeled antimyosin antibody uptake.[K4] There was an inverse relationship between the amount of thallium-201 redistribution and the magnitude of radiolabeled antibody uptake. For the most part, redistribution-type defects represent hypoperfused but viable areas of myocardium, whereas persistent defects indicate infarction or scar.[P1] Some mild, persistent defects may represent significant ischemia rather than scar.[G5] These defects usually show no more than a 25 to 50 percent reduction in thallium-201 counts relative to the normally perfused zone.

Figure 58–5 illustrates the relationship between preoperative thallium-201 defect patterns and postoperative improvement in myocardial perfusion in patients who underwent coronary bypass surgery. If such defects are observed in the presence of intact regional wall motion, then viability may be present. Often after revascularization, these mild, persistent defects resolve. Some have advocated repeat imaging at 8 to 24 hours to detect late redistribution in such mild, persistent defects, which is proposed to separate better areas of severe ischemia from myocardial scar.[C6, K2] Others have advocated reinjection of a second dose of thallium-201 at rest if the 2- to 4-hour delayed redistribution images show a persistent defect.[D10] Enhanced thallium uptake after reinjection is observed in a substantial number of defects that appear persistent on the redistribution images, suggesting the presence of viable myocardium. As mentioned previously, some persistent defects identified in clinical thallium-201 scintigrams, particularly by visual scan analysis, may not represent irreversible cellular injury.[B28, G5]

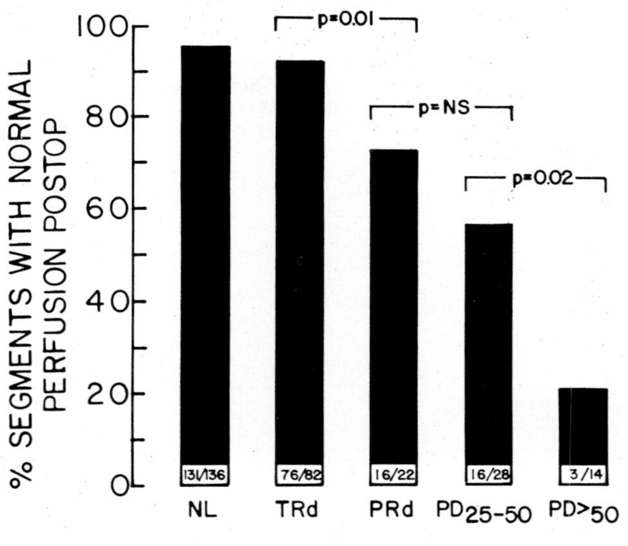

Figure 58–5. Relationship between preoperative thallium-201 defect patterns and postoperative improvement in myocardial perfusion in patients with coronary artery disease who underwent coronary bypass surgery. (NL—normal; TRd—total redistribution; PRd—partial redistribution; PD_{25-50}—persistent defects of 25 to 50 percent reduction in thallium activity; $PD_{>50}$—persistent defects of greater than 50 percent thallium-201 reduction.) Note that the majority of segments showing preoperative thallium-201 redistribution show improvement in myocardial perfusion on postoperative thallium-201 exercise scintigrams. However, more than 50 percent of the mild persistent defects also show improvement. Few of the severe persistent defects show postoperative improvement in perfusion. (From Gibson, R. S., Prospective assessment of regional myocardial perfusion before and after coronary revascularization surgery by quantitative thallium-201 scintigraphy. J. Am. Coll. Cardiol. 1:804, 1983. Reprinted with permission from the American College of Cardiology.)

Reverse Thallium-201 Redistribution

Reverse redistribution is defined as the appearance of a defect for the first time on delayed images obtained 2 to 3 hours after thallium-201 injection. The early initial images appear to be normal, with no significant focal defects. At least three explantions for reverse redistribution have been suggested. First, this phenomenon is observed now most frequently after thrombolytic therapy, with or without coronary angioplasty, in which reperfusion has been successful, resulting in salvage of myocardium in the distribution of the infarct-related vessel.[W5] When thallium-201 is injected during exercise testing in a patient who previously underwent successful reperfusion with a thrombolytic agent or after angioplasty, there may be significant exercise-induced hyperemia in the subepicardial viable regions of the infarct zone. The increased thallium-201 uptake in subepicardial layers prevents the appreciation of the zone of subendocardial necrosis. Thus, the early postexercise images do not demonstrate a relative defect when compared with the contralateral, presumably normal, zone. However, there is faster thallium-201 washout from the region of subendocardial infarction compared with normal zone washout, yielding a numerically significant defect for the first time on the delayed scintigrams.

A second mechanism for reverse redistribution is delayed accumulation of thallium-201 uptake in a zone of ischemia with thallium-201 washout from an area that is a mixture of scar and viable myocardium. The initial images might show "balanced" thallium-201 distribution in the ischemic and partially scarred zones. The delayed images show the appearance of a new defect because of the relative inhomogeneity between the ischemic zone, which accumulated thallium-201 over time, compared with the partially infarcted zone, which demonstrated a normal washout pattern from residual viable cells. Thus, the myocardial scar would show a defect only on the delayed image.

Third, reverse redistribution can be observed as an artifact produced by oversubtraction of background activity, utilizing the interpolative background subtraction algorithm.[L5] Some observers have noted that the presence of reverse redistribution as an artifact is more prevalent on SPECT than planar thallium-201 images. If reverse redistribution is seen in a patient with a low pretest likelihood of coronary artery disease with no other evidence of exercise-induced ischemia (e.g., ST segment depression, anginal chest pain), then the finding is most likely artifactual. When observed on exercise scintigrams in patients who previously had reperfusion therapy for an acute infarction, reverse redistribution is a mark of viability in the infarct zone and is associated with enhanced regional systolic function compared with the prethrombolytic regional wall motion.[T8] It does not represent an ischemic response, as does an initial defect with delayed redistribution.

Lung Thallium-201 Uptake

Abnormally increased lung thallium-201 uptake (Fig. 58–6) can be observed in certain patients on the initial anterior view image obtained 5 to 10 minutes after cessation of exercise.[B8–10, G6, H3, K5, L6, L7, R1, W6] At times, abnormal lung thallium-201 uptake is seen on resting images. This abnormality represents thallium-201 that is transiently sequestered in the pulmonary interstitial fluid space because of an elevated pulmonary capillary wedge pressure and consequent pulmonary edema. This pulmonary edema could develop as a result of severe, exercise-induced left ventricular

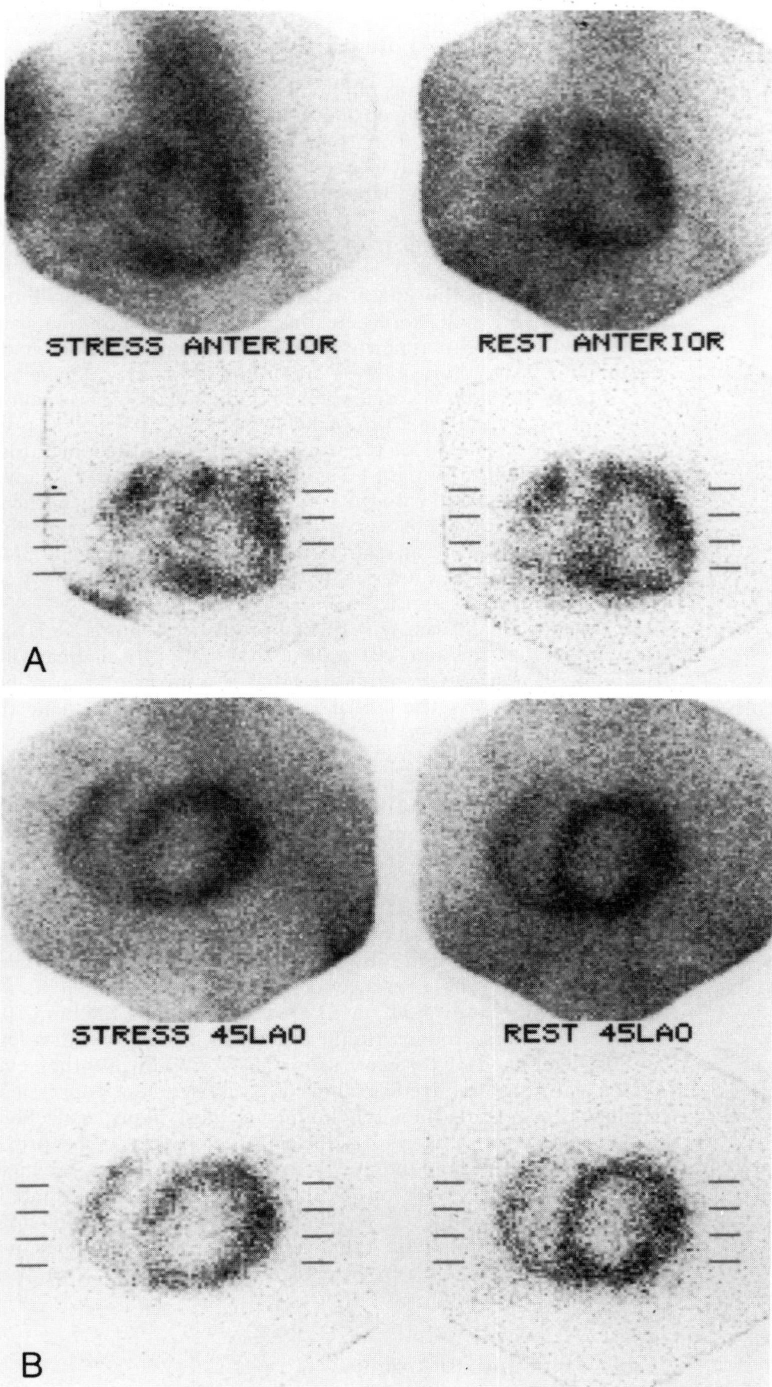

Figure 58–6. *A*, Initial postexercise (stress) anterior and delayed rest anterior thallium-201 scintigrams demonstrating abnormal lung thallium-201 uptake that resolves over time. There are also postexercise defects in the anterolateral wall, apex, and inferior wall that demonstrate delayed redistribution. Background subtracted images are shown below the unprocessed scintiphotos. *B*, Initial and delayed postexercise (stress) 45° left anterior oblique (LAO) thallium-201 scintigrams in the same patient. Septal and inferoapical defects show delayed redistribution.

dysfunction, with a sudden rise in the left ventricular filling pressure, or it could be present in the resting state, usually in conjunction with myocardial infarction and diastolic dysfunction. Since thallium-201 is injected intravenously and must traverse the lungs during the initial transit through the circulation, a portion of the dose will equilibrate with interstitial edema fluid in the lung parenchyma. When the filling pressure falls to normal levels with reversal of ischemia, the pulmonary thallium-201 concentration decreases as the radionuclide clears the lungs into the pulmonary capillary blood pool.

Pulmonary thallium uptake can be quantified on the initial anterior view scintigram, and quantitative pulmonary-to-heart thallium-201 ratios can be derived. The number of diseased coronary vessels has been reported to be the best discriminator between patients with increased ratios, compared with those with normal ratios.[H3] Double product at peak exercise, number of segments with abnormal wall motion, patient gender, and duration of exercise were also significant discriminators. Although abnormal left ventricular ejection fraction at rest had a negative correlation with lung/heart ratio of thallium-201, it did not discriminate between normal and increased ratios. Abnormally increased lung thallium-201 activity also has been reported on dipyridamole thallium-201 scans in patients with coronary artery disease compared with normal control subjects.[O9, V6]

Unless an initial anterior view planar image is acquired, performing thallium-201 scintigraphy using only the SPECT technique will result in failure to assess lung thallium-201 activity. This may significantly diminish the prognostic worth of thallium imaging in coronary artery disease. In one study, the unprocessed set of SPECT projection images (16 of 60) that corresponded to the anterior position was analyzed for pulmonary thallium-201 activity with lung/heart ratios derived.[K16] Lung thallium-201 uptake was elevated in 67 percent of 70 patients with coronary artery disease, compared with normal subjects, but patients with increased lung thallium-201 uptake did not differ from patients with coronary artery disease who had normal lung thallium-201 ratios, with respect to extent of angiographic coronary artery disease, left ventricular function, or severity of myocardial ischemia as assessed from exercise and redistribution thallium-201 SPECT images.

TECHNETIUM-99m ISONITRILES

Technetium-99m isonitriles have been proposed as potentially better agents for the assessment of myocardial perfusion at rest and under conditions of stress than thallium-201.[H1, K6, O4] The initial myocardial distribution of one of these agents, technetium-99m hexakis 2-methoxyisobutyl isonitrile (^{99m}Tc sestamibi), is proportional to blood flow, as is thallium-201. Technetium-99m sestamibi, unlike thallium-201, does not redistribute after transient ischemia and requires separate injections of the radionuclide during stress and rest to distinguish between reversible and irreversible myocardial injury. In dogs undergoing left circumflex coronary artery stenosis, the 4-hour fractional technetium-99m sestamibi clearances from the normal and ischemic zones were minimal and equivalent (0.15).[O4]

During the first 60 minutes after a resting injection of technetium-99m sestamibi, marked accumulation of the tracer is present in liver and spleen. Nevertheless, the heart is well visualized. After an exercise injection, there is significantly less uptake in the splanchnic organs, and excellent visualization of the heart is attained. There is substantial excretion of technetium-99m sestamibi in the gallbladder after administration at either rest or exercise, which reaches a maximum approximately 1 hour after injection.

In studies in human volunteers, blood technetium-99m sestamibi decreases to 9 percent of the injected dose at 5 minutes after tracer administration.[W7] By 30 minutes, blood pool activity decreases even further, to 1.3 percent. Inspection of blood decay corrective clearance curves yields an approximate dual exponential curve with an initial fast component, with a half-life at rest of approximately 2.18 minutes and a later slow component.

Although the first-pass myocardial extraction of technetium-99m sestamibi is less efficient than that of thallium, the relative uptake of both tracers is identical under physiologic flow conditions.[L8] Preliminary in vitro studies suggest that technetium-99m sestamibi may be more influenced by metabolic disturbances than thallium-201.[K7] In isolated perfused heart preparations, the myocardial uptake of technetium-99m sestamibi may be more influenced by hypoxia than thallium-201 under conditions of comparable flow. However, in recent studies in intact dogs, severe resting myocardial ischemia or postischemic dysfunction ("stunning") did not appear to affect technetium-99m sestamibi uptake, which was comparable to thallium-201 uptake in the same model.[S16]

The absence of redistribution and the relatively slow myocardial clearance are favorable characteristics for SPECT studies, in which data acquisition requires 30 minutes. Postexercise imaging is performed as late as 1 hour after injection, when liver activity has cleared sufficiently for improved visualization of the inferior wall on myocardial scans. Since no myocardial redistribution occurs, the pattern of technetium-99m sestamibi uptake at 1 hour is comparable to what it would be soon after tracer injection. Figure 58–7 shows an example of SPECT images from a normal subject receiving an intravenous dose of technetium-99 sestamibi administered at peak exercise.

The precise mechanism of cellular uptake and sequestration of the technetium-99m isonitriles is unknown. Preincubation with ouabain has no effect on isonitrile uptake, suggesting that the uptake mechanism is unrelated to Na^+, K^+, and ATPase.[M3]

STRESS AND REST IMAGING

Exercise

Thallium-201 scintigraphy has been primarily undertaken in conjunction with conventional exercise treadmill testing or bicycle ergometry in order to detect the presence of underlying coronary artery stenoses in patients with known or suspected coronary artery disease.* The dose of 2 to 3 mCi of thallium-201 is administered through a freely flowing intravenous cannula at symptom-limited end-points, such as angina pectoris, dyspnea, fatigue, lower extremity claudication, or achieving a predefined exercise level (e.g., 90 percent of maximal predicted heart rate for age). Often, the thallium-201 dose might be injected at the appearance of more than 4.0 mm of ST depression, although symptoms are absent. After intravenous administration, the patient is encouraged to exercise for another 30 to 45 seconds to ensure that the initial myocardial uptake phase will reflect the perfusion pattern that was present at peak stress. Within 8 minutes after cessation of exercise, the patient is positioned under the collimator of a gamma scintillation camera to obtain anterior and several left anterior oblique (LAO) projection images (ideally, 45° and 70° LAO projections). Each image is collected for a preset time, rather than for preset counts, and, with currently available instrumentation, typically 400,000 counts are collected over a period of 8 minutes. Delayed images in the same views are obtained from 2.5 to 4 hours later to assess presence or absence of redistribution.

For normal individuals without coronary artery disease, the myocardial distribution of thallium-201 on initial postexercise images is relatively homogeneous. There is some relative diminution of thallium-201 uptake at the apex of the left ventricle, since this region is thinner than other myocardial zones. There is also a relative diminution of thallium-201 at the base of the heart in the areas of the outflow and inflow tracts. This will be observed as apparent thinning of the upper septum and upper posterolateral wall, particularly on the 45° LAO view, which could be misconstrued as representing abnormal perfusion. Overreading defects at the base of the heart is a frequent cause of false-positive interpretations.

---

*References B11–15, C1–3, D1, D2, F3, G7–9, H2, I1, K8, M4–8, N3, R2–4, S5, V1, V2, W8, W9.

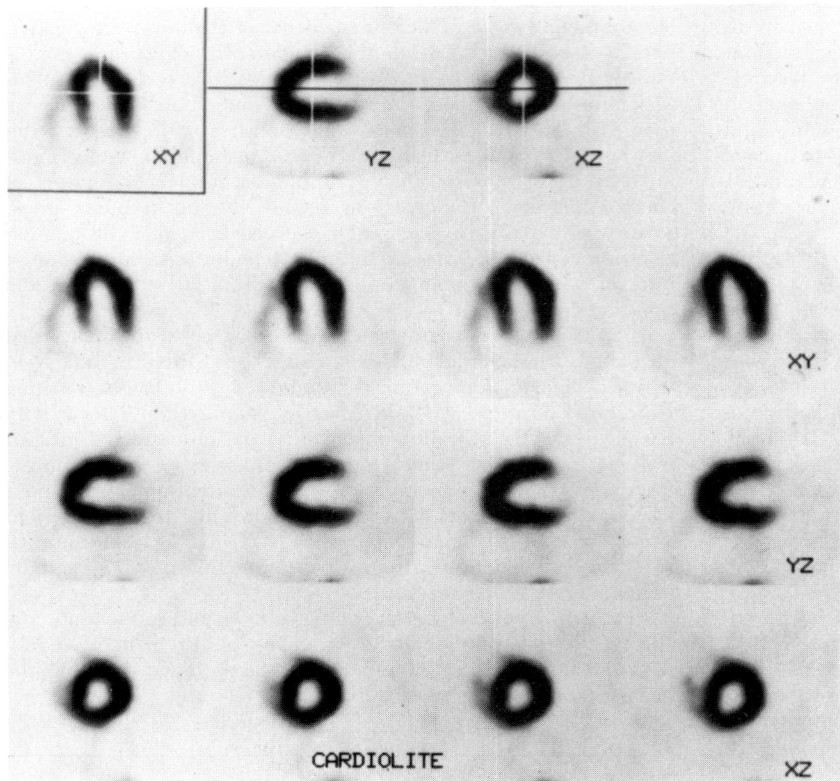

Figure 58–7. Representative vertical long-axis *(second row)*, horizontal long-axis *(middle row)*, and short-axis *(bottom row)* slices from a technetium-99m sestimibi (cardiolite) SPECT scintigraphic study from a normal patient. Note the excellent quality of these reconstructed tomographic images.

Fifty percent of thallium-201 photons will be absorbed in 4 cm of tissue. Because of this attenuation, a relative diminution of thallium-201 will be appreciated because of overlying bone and soft tissue, even when myocardial cellular uptake is entirely uniform. This will vary in male and female patients, with body size and chest wall configuration, with the orientation of the long axis of the heart, with the configuration and size of the right ventricular chamber and overlying right ventricular outflow track, and with the position of mitral and aortic valve planes. Breast tissue interposed between the camera head and the chest wall may give the appearance of a perfusion defect in the septum on the 45° LAO view because of the absorption effect resulting in attenuation of thallium-201 activity. A large right ventricular blood pool overlying the inferior wall and the anterior view image also may cause an attenuation artifact. A high left hemidiaphragm overlying the posterior wall on the 70° LAO view can cause an attenuation artifact that could be misconstrued as a posterior wall scar. Figure 58–8 shows examples of attenuation artifacts secondary to breast tissue. However, no false-positive defects are observed.

Acute cardiac dilatation secondary to ischemia may produce a relative defect in the apex. When interpreting myocardial thallium-201 scintigrams, these anatomic variants should be taken into account. This is a matter of pattern recognition by experienced observers, one that cannot be performed automatically by computer processing. Failure to recognize anatomic variants of the normal will result in a high false-positive interpretation rate. An example is the female breast shadow, which often is interpreted as a septal defect. Attenuation of technetium-99m sestamibi is less than that of thallium-201 but is still appreciable. Breast tissue attenuation artifacts have been observed on clinical isonitrile images.

To optimally employ myocardial perfusion imaging with either thallium-201 or technetium-99m sestamibi, quantitation of regional activity over time must be used to confirm the presence or absence of thallium-201 redistribution by measuring the magnitude of a defect and the change in this magnitude in the delayed images.[B13, W9] Gray-scale images alone, which are a nonlinear representation of count density, do not provide a reliable estimate either of redistribution or of the time dependence of thallium-201 uptake and washout. Figure 58–9 depicts examples of redistribution and persistent defects in three representative patients with underlying coronary artery disease.

Some have advocated arm exercise thallium-201 imaging for detection of coronary artery disease in patients who have lower limb impairment.[B16] In one report, an exercise bicycle equipped with an electronic braking system was adapted for arm ergometry by replacing the pedals with rubber handles.[B16] Exercise was

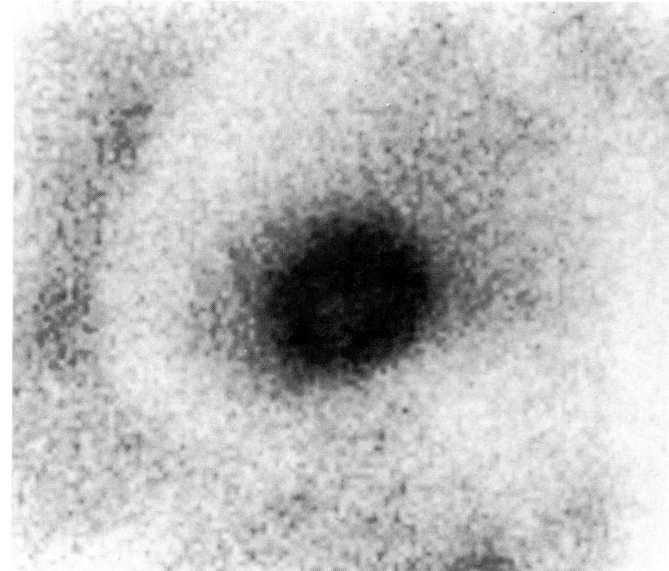

Figure 58–8. A 45° left anterior oblique myocardial thallium-201 scintigram in a woman with no coronary artery disease. Note the curved attenuation artifact adjacent to the myocardium with localized diminution of thallium-201 photons. This is an attenuation artifact secondary to breast tissue interposed between the gamma camera and the chest wall. The breasts have been positioned as to not result in attenuation artifacts over the myocardial zones.

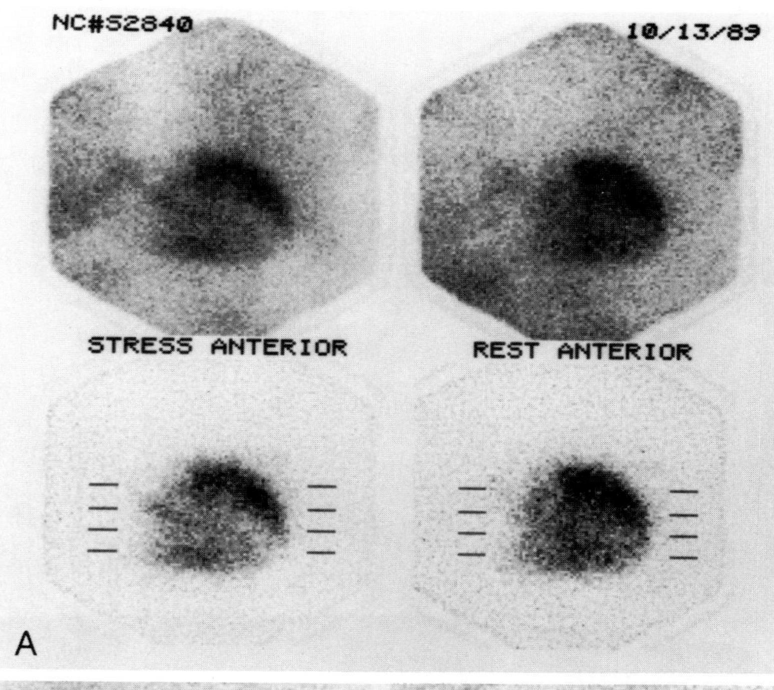

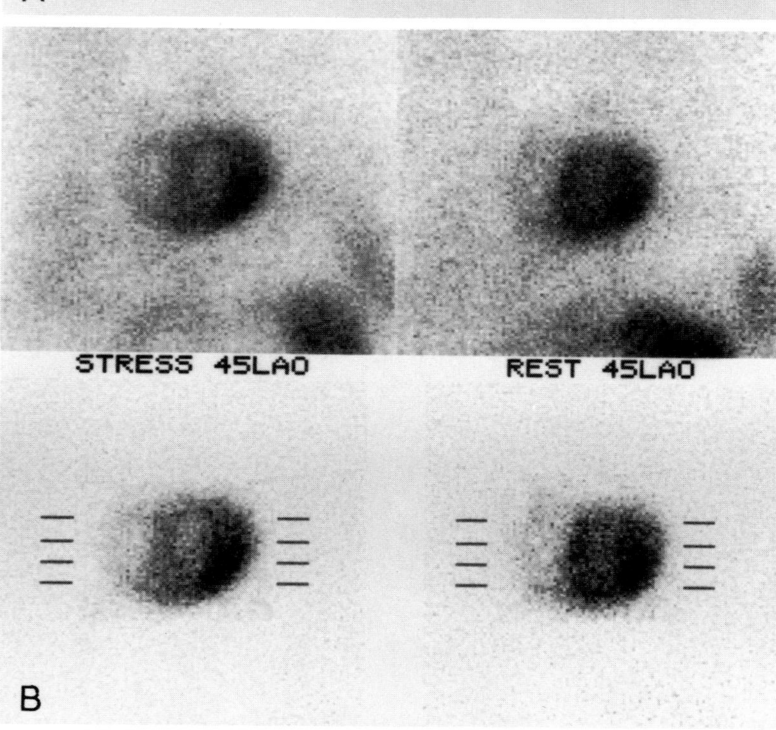

Figure 58–9. *A*, Postexercise (stress) anterior and delayed rest anterior thallium-201 scintigrams in a patient with an initial inferior wall defect that shows delayed redistribution. *B*, Postexercise (stress) and delayed rest 45° left anterior oblique (LAO) thallium-201 scintigrams in a patient with an initial anteroseptal defect showing delayed redistribution.

begun at a workload of 10 W for 2 minutes, followed by 10 W increments every 2 minutes until the test was terminated. Subjects were encouraged to maintain a handle speed of 75 to 80 revolutions per minute in order to maximize the dynamic component of exercise. As with treadmill exercise, at peak stress 2 mCi of thallium-201 was injected intravenously and the patient encouraged to continue exercise for an additional minute. In this study, there was an 83 percent sensitivity and 78 percent specificity for detecting coronary artery disease, compared with a sensitivity and specificity of 54 percent and 67 percent, respectively, for exercise electrocardiography. The difference in sensitivity was statistically significant.

Dipyridamole

Intravenous infusion of dipyridamole is an acceptable alternative to exercise stress for detecting coronary artery disease by thallium-201 myocardial perfusion imaging. The pronounced coronary vasodilating effect of dipyridamole enhances regional myocardial perfusion to zones supplied by nonobstructed coronary arteries but not in zones supplied by stenotic vessels.[B17, B18] This inhomogeneity of flow is detected by abnormal thallium-201 uptake when the radionuclide is administered intravenously during peak vasodilation. Redistribution occurs with dipyridamole thallium-201 scintigraphy similar to that observed with exercise stress.[B18] The test is performed in the following manner: First, no caffeinated beverages or teas are permitted for 12 hours prior to dipyridamole imaging. Patients receiving theophylline-type compounds cannot be considered for testing. An intravenous cannula is inserted intravenously and kept patent by an infusion of dextrose/saline. Heart rate and blood pressure are determined every minute with continuous electrocardiographic monitoring. After baseline hemodynamics are acquired, 0.56 mg per kg of dipyridamole is infused over a period of 4 minutes. Thallium-201 is injected at 9 minutes, and imaging commences 7 minutes later

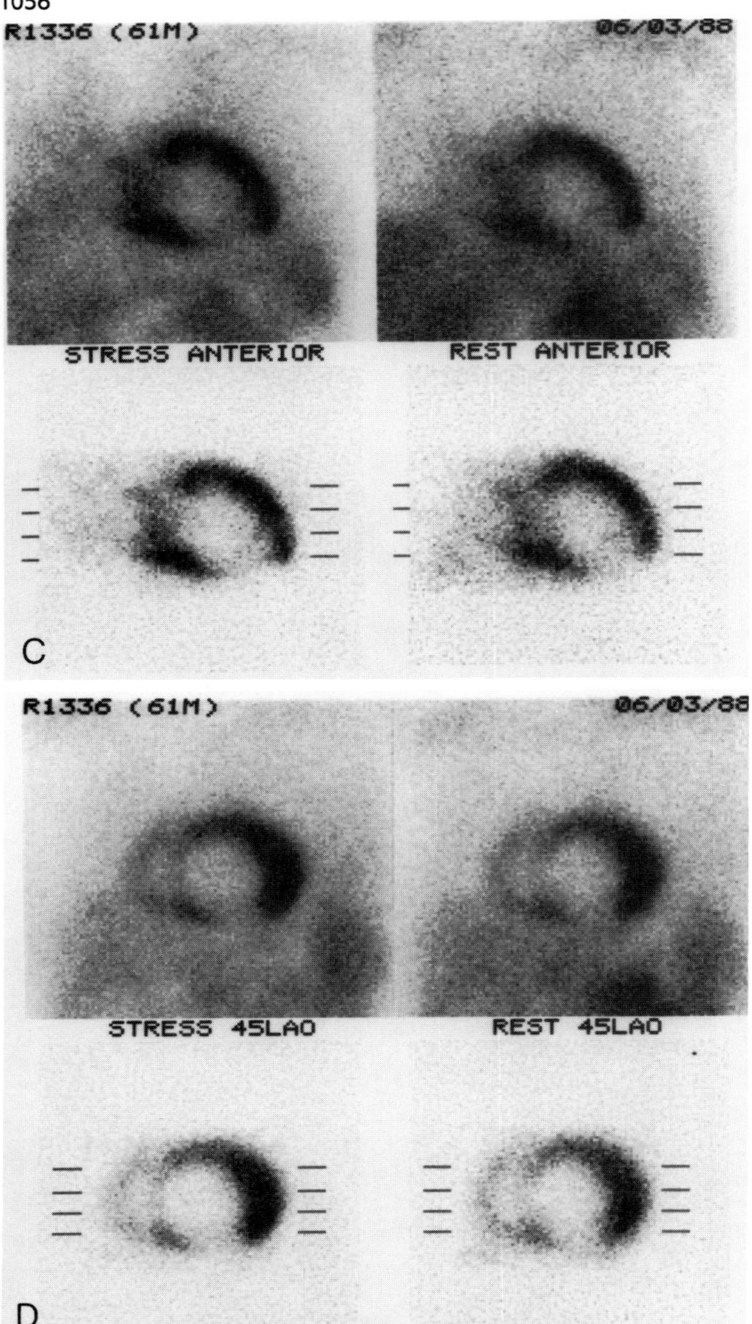

Figure 58–9 *Continued C*, Postexercise (stress) and delayed rest anterior thallium-201 scintigrams in a patient with cardiac dilatation and a persistent inferoapical defect. *D*, Postexercise (stress) and delayed rest 45° LAO images in the same patient whose anterior images are shown in *C*. There is a persistent inferoapical defect and some slight partial redistribution in the septal region.

in the three views described previously. As with exercise scintigraphy, delayed images are obtained 2.5 to 4 hours later. It has been estimated that from 10 to 25 percent of patients do not achieve maximal coronary dilation when dipyridamole is administered.

Some reports in the medical literature describe the use of oral dipyridamole for thallium-201 imaging.[T1] With this approach, a patient is given a 30-ml suspension of four 75-mg tablets (sugar-free base) of dipyridamole. Blood pressure, heart rate, and electrocardiogram are monitored in the supine position for 45 minutes. At the end of that time period, 2.0 mCi of thallium-201 is injected intravenously and serial images obtained as described.

Dipyridamole exerts its vasodilating effect by elevating myocardial tissue adenosine levels. Thus, the antagonist to dipyridamole is aminophylline, which is an adenosine receptor antagonist. A dose of 75 to 125 mg of aminophylline is administered intravenously to patients exhibiting significant side effects from the dipyridamole infusion. These will include systemic hypotension, chest pain, significant ST depression, and nausea. A more detailed description of dipyridamole is presented in Chapter 66 on myocardial perfusion.

Rest Imaging

Thallium-201 scintigraphy also can be performed in the resting state without any preceding interventions.[B6, G4] The technique for acquiring and interpreting serial images is similar to that described when imaging is performed in conjunction with a stress state. Regional thallium-201 clearance from the myocardium is significantly slower at rest than following exercise. Thus, it is difficult to interpret isolated washout abnormalities as reflective of resting myocardial ischemia. Many normal subjects can show a flat washout or even prolonged delayed accumulation despite the absence of any significant coronary obstructive lesions. Thus, mere demonstration of diffuse slow washout of thallium-201 after a resting injection does not necessarily imply abnormal resting perfusion. The major clinical indications for rest thallium-201 imaging are detecting and localizing infarction, assessing myocardial viability after myocardial infarction treated with reperfusion, and identifying myocardial regions demonstrating hypoperfusion at rest in patients with unstable or severe stable angina.

IMAGE DISPLAY AND ANALYSIS

Planar Methods

As previously described, anterior, 45° left anterior oblique, and steep LAO (70°) images are obtained approximately 8 minutes after thallium-201 administration. For computer quantification of segmental thallium-201 activity, all images are stored by a computer using either a 64 × 64 or 128 × 128 matrix. These images are then processed by first compensating for background activity, next registering automatically the early and delayed images, then smoothing images to attenuate Poisson noise, and, finally, determining the regional thallium-201 uptake and washout from the myocardium. In thallium-201 myocardial images, a significant fraction of the total counts within a myocardial target region arise from "background" or, more correctly, "tissue cross talk." The distribution of this cross talk is nonuniform and can be adequately treated as a constant. It also changes with time. An interpolative background subtraction algorithm provides the most satisfactory approach, since it takes into account this background nonuniformity. The most commonly used method is an adaptation of a technique described by Goris and associates,[G23] utilizing a nonuniform background reference plane but one that produces a more rapid fall-off of the computer tissue cross talk.[W9] Several methods have been described to display count profiles from the smoothed, processed images that represent regional thallium-201 distribution. These count profiles can be displayed in a horizontal[W9] or circumferential manner.[M8] Residual myocardial counts above the background reference plane can be quantified from the profiles on the early and delayed images. Thallium-201 clearance curves also can be calculated from sequential images. Changes in counts/pixel with time can be measured using the same profiles for each sequential image.

A lung:heart ratio of thallium can be measured on the initial anterior view planar image.[H3] The operator identifies an area over the lung on the initial image, and activity per pixel in that area is measured. An area is then chosen over the most active segment of the myocardium in the same image, and lung activity is expressed as a percent of myocardial activity.

Computer programs have developed that express the clearance of thallium-201 from the myocardium as the half-life of thallium-201. This is accomplished by fitting a monoexponential curve between the average segmental activity in the initial and delayed images.

Single Photon Emission Computed Tomography (SPECT)

Single photon emission computerized tomography (SPECT) has recently enjoyed greater popularity for imaging of myocardial thallium-201 distribution.[D3, F4, G10, T2] This approach offers higher contrast resolution and better separation of overlapping myocardial segments than does the planar approach. For SPECT imaging, the thallium-201 dose is increased to 3 to 3.5 mCi. A higher dose is required because of the poor counting statistics of single detector tomography. Acquisition consists of obtaining 30 to 32 projections, each for 40 seconds, over a 180° rotation starting from the 45° right anterior oblique to the 45° left posterior oblique projections. Each of these 30 to 32 projections is corrected for field nonuniformity, and the mechanical center of rotation is determined from the projection data, to align detector data with respect to the reconstruction matrix. After smoothing of the raw data, a filtered-back projection technique is performed to reconstruct the transverse tomograms encompassing the entire heart. Each short-axis slice is approximately 6 mm thick.

Quantification of thallium-201 SPECT can be undertaken from apex to base. In one quantification scheme, maximal count circumferential profiles for each short-axis cut are generated automatically, and this procedure is performed for each stress and each delayed tomographic study. Percent washout from the circumferential profiles can also be calculated. SPECT thallium-201 results can also be mapped onto a two-dimensional polar display (bullseye) that depicts thallium-201 activity throughout the left ventricular muscle. The center of this display represents the left ventricular apex, and the periphery represents the base of the left ventricle. The display is coded so that all regions 5 percent above the normal limits are white, and points more than 5 percent below the normal limit are gray or black, depending on the severity of hypoperfusion.

CLINICAL APPLICATIONS

The various clinical applications of myocardial perfusion are summarized in Table 58–1.

Thallium-201 Scintigraphy in the Asymptomatic Patient

It has been proposed that a significant number of totally asymptomatic patients with multiple risk factors for coronary artery disease manifest painless ischemia and, therefore, are subject to subsequent cardiac events without premonitory warning signs. Diamond and Forrester provided an approach that employs analysis of probability as an aid in the clinical diagnosis of coronary artery disease.[D9] The exercise electrocardiogram alone generally is not useful when it is applied to a patient population with a low pretest likelihood of coronary artery disease. The predictive accuracy of any test for coronary artery disease detection, such as the exercise electrocardiogram, is based not only on sensitivity and specificity values but also on the prevalence of the disease in the population under study. This is recognized as Bayes' theorem. For example, in a patient with only a 10 percent pretest likelihood of coronary artery disease, 1.0 mm of ST segment depression at peak exercise will increase the likelihood of CAD after testing to only 35 percent, because the false-positive rate is quite high for the mildly positive exercise ST response in this type of patient. On the other hand, if an exercise-induced thallium-201 defect showing delayed redistribution were observed in conjunction with this ST depression, the post-test likelihood of coronary artery disease would increase to nearly 85 percent. Therefore, in patients with a low-to-intermediate pretest likelihood of coronary artery disease, multiple tests might be required to enhance the predicted value of noninvasive stress testing for detection of myocardial ischemia. Concordant positive findings indicative of ischemia would result in a high probability of coronary artery disease despite the asymptomatic state.

In one study of asymptomatic siblings of patients with premature coronary artery disease, both planar and tomographic thallium-201 scintigraphy identified more patients with silent ischemia than the exercise electrocardiographic stress test alone.[B19] In a study of 138 asymptomatic Air Force pilots referred for catheterization because of coronary risk factors or a positive stress electrocardiogram, 22 had at least one stenosis of 50 or more percent. All 22 had an abnormal thallium-201 scan.[U1] There were few false-positive thallium-201 scintigraphic results in the asymptomatic patients with a normal coronary arteriogram. In a subsequent study by Uhl and associates in 191 flight crewmen with an abnormal ST segment response to exercise, the predictive value of the exercise electrocardiogram was 21 percent, versus 74 percent for thallium-201 scintigraphy for detection of coronary artery disease.[U2] The specificity of the computer-processed scans was 90 percent. In that study, Uhl and colleagues pointed out that if both an abnormal exercise electrocardiogram and abnormal thallium-201 scintigram had been required before angiography was performed, 136 subjects with ST depression and no underlying coronary artery disease would have been spared angiography.

Table 58–1. CLINICAL APPLICATIONS OF THALLIUM-201 PERFUSION IMAGING

1. Detect CAD in the totally asymptomatic patient
   a. Subjects with multiple risk factors and/or strong family history
   b. Siblings of patients with premature coronary deaths
   c. Airline pilots ≥ 50 years of age with CAD risk factors
2. Differential diagnosis of chest pain
   a. Atypical chest pain syndrome (intermediate pretest likelihood of CAD)
   b. Nondiagnostic electrocardiographic exercise stress test (e.g., failure to reach more than 85% of maximum predicted heart rate)
   c. Equivocal exercise-induced ST segment response (e.g., slow upsloping ST depression; 0.5- to 1.0-mm horizontal ST depression)
   d. Suspected false-positive exercise ST segment depression
   e. Resting ECG abnormalities (e.g., WPW syndrome, bundle branch blocks, left ventricular hypertrophy, digitalis effect, hyperventilation ST-T changes)
3. Assess functional significance of known CAD
   a. Detect left main or multivessel CAD (multiple Tl-201 defects in more than one vascular scan segment)
   b. Identify "culprit" stenosis in multivessel CAD
   c. Identify left ventricular dysfunction indirectly exercise-induced (abnormal lung Tl-201 uptake)
   d. Determine functional significance of angiographic collaterals
   e. Detect residual ischemia (redistribution) within a zone of prior infarction, particularly in non-Q infarction
4. Risk stratification and assessing prognosis
   a. Separate high- and low-risk patients by extent of Tl-201 perfusion abnormalities and presence or absence of increased lung Tl-201 uptake
   b. Prognostication after uncomplicated myocardial infarction
   c. Selection of patients for revascularization
      1) Localization of regional ischemia
      2) Determine size of risk area distal to a known stenosis
      3) Assess myocardial viability by demonstrating normal thallium uptake or redistribution in zone of asynergy)
      4) Identify high-risk CAD patients (multiple segments demonstrating redistribution, abnormal lung thallium uptake, exercise-induced LV dilatation)
5. Evaluate results of therapy
   a. Assess improvement in exercise perfusion after PTCA or CABG
   b. Determine etiology of recurrent chest pain after CABG or PTCA
   c. Assess adequacy of graft flow after CABG
   d. Detect restenosis after PTCA
   e. Follow progression of native CAD after PTCA or CABG
   f. Assess changes in perfusion during exercise after medical therapy
6. Rest Tl-201 imaging
   a. Localize and size myocardial infarction
   b. Assess changes in perfusion after thrombolytic therapy
   c. Differential ischemia from necrosis after myocardial infarction
7. Dipyridamole Tl-201 imaging
   a. Detect CAD in patients unable to exercise
   b. Risk stratification prior to vascular surgery in patients with peripheral vascular disease
   c. Risk stratification after uncomplicated myocardial infarction
8. Tl-201 scintigraphy in noncoronary artery disease
   a. Differentiate ischemic from nonischemic cardiomyopathy
   b. Assess myocardial perfusion in progressive systemic sclerosis, myocardial sarcoidosis, and so on
   c. Assess right ventricular systolic overload

Thallium-201 scintigraphy has been employed to differentiate true from false-positive ST segment responses in certain patient populations (Fig. 58–10).[G11] Also, the test can be employed in those patients who have baseline electrocardiographic abnormalities caused by hypertension, mitral valve prolapse, Wolff-Parkinson-White syndrome, digitalis effect, or pathologic Q-waves. In such individuals the electrocardiographic response to exercise stress will be nondiagnostic. Thallium-201 scintigraphy may not be very useful in detecting occult coronary artery disease in patients with left bundle branch block. Many such patients will exhibit thallium-201 defects in the interventricular septum despite having angiographically normal coronary arteries. Similarly, some patients with hypertensive cardiomyopathy may have perfusion abnormalities on thallium-201 scintigraphy without demonstrable coronary artery disease.

The issue of screening high-risk asymptomatic patients for functionally important silent myocardial ischemia has not yet been resolved. The cost-effectiveness of such an approach in selected patient populations (e.g., siblings of patients with premature cardiac death or infarction or those who have multiple risk factors) has yet to be carefully assessed.

Thallium-201 Scintigraphy in Patients with Chest Pain

Planar or SPECT Tl-201 scintigraphy performed in conjunction with symptom-limited exercise stress testing has enhanced both the sensitivity and specificity for coronary artery disease detection.[G8] Results of studies published in the literature have revealed that the predictive value of a negative stress electrocardiogram in a patient with chest pain is in the range of 60 to 65 percent. This is because the sensitivity of the ST segment response is suboptimum. When only visual analysis of thallium-201 scintigrams is performed, sensitivity and specificity for coronary artery disease detection are approximately 80 to 85 percent and 85 to 90 percent, respectively.* Kotler and Diamond, in their review of the literature, found an average sensitivity of 84 percent and a specificity of 87 percent when data from 33 published studies were pooled,[K14] utilizing visual assessment of thallium-201 scintigrams. Gerson reviewed 30 studies published from 1976 to 1981 and found an average 83.6 percent sensitivity and 88.4 percent specificity for thallium-201 scintigraphy.[G22] Only one of these 30 studies employed quantitative analysis of serial thallium-201 images. Both sensitivity and specificity have been increased to the 90 percent range when early and delayed exercise scintigrams are assessed quantitatively using computer-assisted approaches for image analysis (Table 58–2).[B14, G7, K11, M8, M18, W8] Stenosis detection rate in certain patients with coronary artery disease is enhanced by demonstrating abnormal segmental washout of thallium-201 by quantitative criteria, in addition to defects elsewhere, when a comparison of exercise and delayed images is made.[B14] In this instance, abnormal segmental thallium-201 clearance has the same significance as redistribution and represents ischemic response.

Several published clinical studies have shown the superiority of quantitative scintigraphy when compared with visual analysis of scintigrams obtained in the same patients.[B14, W8] One major advantage of quantitative imaging is the increased detection rate of patients with multivessel coronary artery disease. Certain variables affect the sensitivity of exercise thallium-201 scintigraphy for coronary artery disease detection in patients presenting with chest pain. These are summarized in Table 58–3. The location of coronary artery lesions appears to affect the sensitivity of thallium-201 scintigraphy for appropriately assessing the extent of coronary artery disease. With both planar and SPECT imaging, it is more difficult to detect lesions in the left circumflex coronary artery compared with the left anterior descending or right coronary artery.[B14, F4] Branch stenoses of the left anterior descending and circumflex vessels are more difficult to identify than the more proximal lesions in the major coronary vessels.[I4] Perfusion abnormalities are more often present in the distribution of vessels with severe (over 90 percent) stenoses than in those with more moderate (50 to 90 percent) stenosis.[F4]

The sensitivity of thallium-201 scintigraphy is slightly lower in patients with single-vessel disease than in patients with multivessel disease. In their review, Kotler and Diamond found a 78 percent sensitivity of thallium-201 scintigraphy for detecting single-vessel coronary artery disease, compared with 89 percent for detecting double-vessel disease.[K14] Utilizing quantitative image analysis enhances the detection rate for single-vessel disease.[B14] In one study, a 90 percent sensitivity for quantitative thallium-201 scintigraphy for detecting single-vessel coronary

*References B11–13, C1–3, H2, I1, M4–6, N3, P5, R2–4, S5, V1, V2.

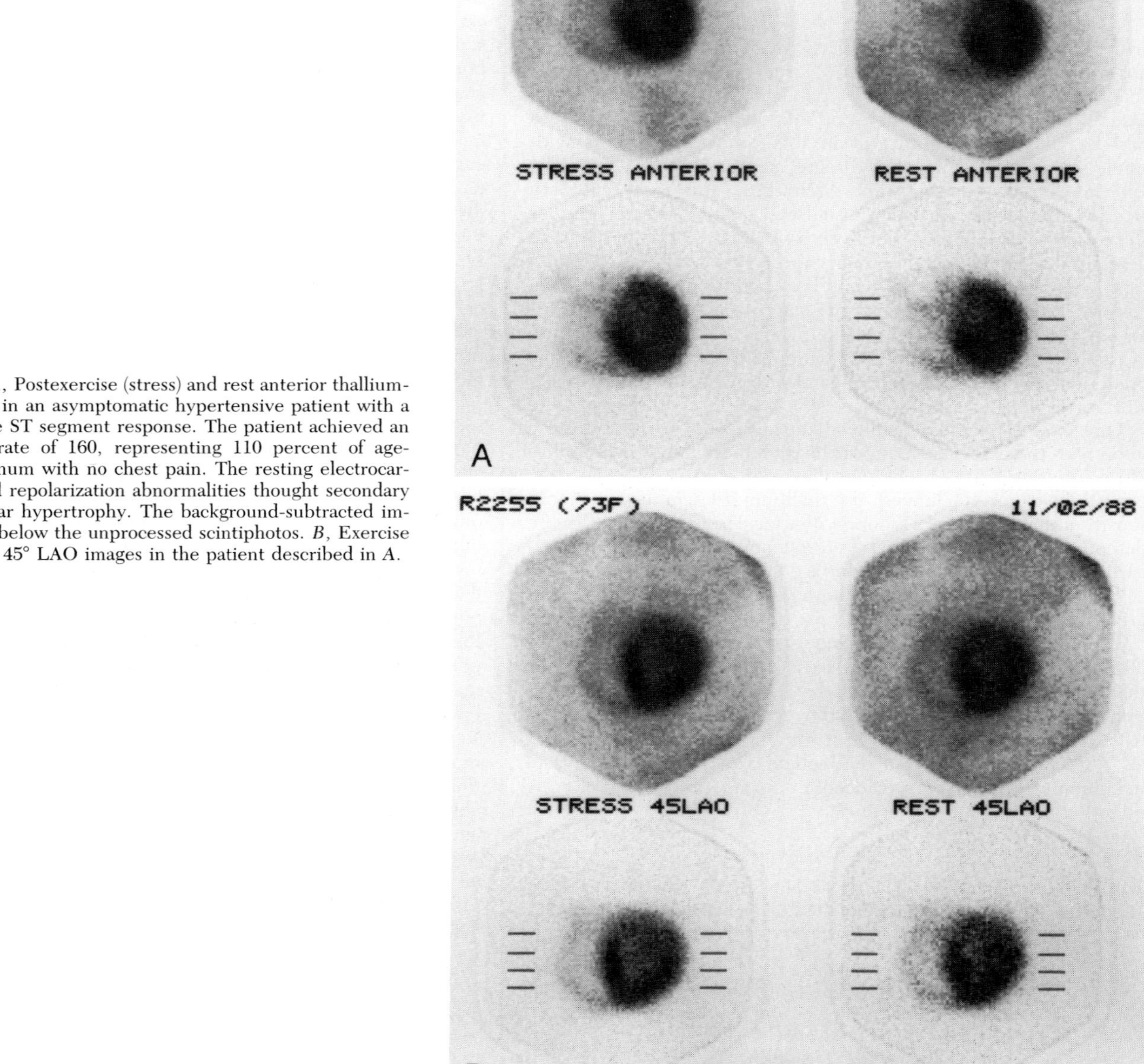

Figure 58–10. *A*, Postexercise (stress) and rest anterior thallium-201 scintigrams in an asymptomatic hypertensive patient with a positive exercise ST segment response. The patient achieved an exercise heart rate of 160, representing 110 percent of age-predicted maximum with no chest pain. The resting electrocardiogram showed repolarization abnormalities thought secondary to left ventricular hypertrophy. The background-subtracted images are shown below the unprocessed scintiphotos. *B*, Exercise (stress) and rest 45° LAO images in the patient described in *A*.

Table 58–2. SENSITIVITY AND SPECIFICITY OF CORONARY ARTERY DISEASE DETECTION BY QUANTITATIVE THALLIUM-201 SCINTIGRAPHY

Study	Year	Number of Patients	Sensitivity (%)	Specificity (%)
Berger	1981	140	91	90
Maddahi	1981	67	93	91
Wackers	1985	150	89	95
Kaul	1986	325	90	80
Van Train	1986	157	84	88
	TOTAL	839	89.4	88.8

artery disease was found.[B14] Similarly, in another study employing quantitative analysis of thallium-201 scintigrams, a sensitivity of 92 percent was reported in 124 patients with single-vessel disease.[K11] In patients without prior infarction, sensitivity was 78 percent. It is interesting that in this cohort of patients with single-vessel coronary artery disease, sensitivity was similar for left anterior descending, left circumflex, and right coronary arteries. In a study in which visual and quantitative techniques were directly compared, there was a sensitivity of 55 percent for detection of single-vessel coronary artery disease by visual analysis, compared with 84 percent by quantitative analysis.[W8] In contrast, another study found the same sensitivity (86 percent) for visual and quantitative techniques in patients with single-vessel disease.[M8] As expected, patients with prior myocardial infarction have a higher frequency of positive scans than patients without prior myocardial damage.[S16]

The level of exercise achieved during exercise stress testing influences the exercise electrocardiogram more than the thallium-201 scintigram.[B15, M5] Throughout the range of exercise workloads, or peak heart rates achieved, the thallium-201 scintigram is more sensitive than exercise ST depression for coronary artery disease detection.[E1] It may be that heterogeneity of flow is induced earlier during the course of exercise stress than the myocardial cellular changes that mediate the ST segment response or generate ischemic pain.

The influence of collateral vessels on sensitivity of thallium-201 scintigraphy remains controversial. One group has reported that perfusion abnormalities are frequently noted in the distribution of occluded arteries not fed by collateral vessels, compared with occluded arteries filled in a retrograde fashion by collaterals.[R5] Others have reported that collaterals are not protective in maintaining normal or enhanced perfusion during exercise by quantitative thallium-201 criteria.[B20, F5, V1]

Table 58–3. VARIABLES AFFECTING SENSITIVITY OF THALLIUM-201 SCINTIGRAPHY FOR DETECTION OF CORONARY ARTERY DISEASE

Enhancing Sensitivity
- Prior myocardial infarction
- Achieving high exercise heart rate
- Advanced age
- Left main and/or multivessel CAD
- High-grade coronary stenoses
- Proximal location of stenoses
- Associated ST segment depression

Diminishing Sensitivity
- Circumflex coronary stenoses
- Branch (e.g., diagonal) or distal stenoses
- Single-vessel CAD
- Nonjeopardized coronary collaterals
- Lesser degrees of coronary narrowing
- Low exercise workload without symptoms
- Antianginal drug therapy during testing
- Visual analysis of scintigrams

Certain drugs affect the accuracy of thallium-201 scintigraphy. Pretreatment with isosorbide dinitrate improves thallium-201 uptake on exercise scintigraphy and thus diminishes sensitivity.[T3] Reports on the influence of beta-blockers on sensitivity and specificity of thallium-201 scintigraphy are conflicting. Some have reported that propranolol therapy decreases the specificity of thallium-201 scintigraphy,[O5] whereas other investigators have shown no influence of the drug on either sensitivity or specificity.[B14] In most nuclear cardiology laboratories, beta-blockers are not discontinued prior to exercise thallium-201 scintigraphy.

SPECT Tl-201 imaging may improve sensitivity for coronary artery disease detection compared with planar imaging,[D3, F4, G10, T2] although no prospective studies comparing SPECT with quantitative planar imaging have been undertaken in a large number of patients. The detection of circumflex coronary artery disease can be improved by SPECT Tl-201 imaging without loss of specificity.[T2] In another study of 112 patients undergoing cardiac catheterization and 23 normal volunteers performing symptom-limited exercise testing and redistribution imaging by both SPECT and planar techniques, paired receiver operating characteristic curves revealed that SPECT was more accurate than planar imaging over the entire range of decision thresholds for the overall detection and exclusion of coronary artery disease.[F4] SPECT offered relatively greater advantages in male patients and in patients with milder forms of coronary artery disease. It is interesting that although visual SPECT Tl-201 imaging was more accurate than visual planar imaging for detection of coronary artery disease and localizing individual diseased arteries, the diagnostic improvement was not evident in women or in the detection of right coronary artery disease.

Virtually all the studies that have involved the determination of sensitivity and specificity of thallium-201 imaging techniques for coronary artery disease detection either have not employed quantitative coronary angiography or have not employed direct measurements of flow reserve with a precise technique like the Doppler catheter. The standard for determining presence or absence of coronary artery disease in prior studies has most often been qualitative assessment of the coronary angiogram. In one quantitative angiographic study, alterations in myocardial thallium-201 uptake and washout kinetics correlated better with minimal lumen diameter and area stenosis than with percent diameter stenosis.[H12] Certain patients classified as showing a false-positive response when an abnormal thallium-201 scan is seen in the presence of coronary lesions that demonstrate a 25 to 50 percent reduction in lumen diameter by visual inspection actually may be "true positive" responders.[B30] In this instance, there could have been an underestimation of the physiologic severity of the stenosis, which would have been documented better by techniques in which coronary flow reserve is evaluated. Conversely, thallium-201 scintigrams could be normal in patients exhibiting abnormal flow reserve by the Doppler catheter or by quantitative angiographic techniques. These patients would be "false-negative" responders. Hence, the true sensitivity and specificity of all exercise radionuclide imaging techniques for coronary artery disease detection have not been definitively ascertained. A truly valid standard for functionally important coronary artery disease has been lacking.

Prognostic Applications

Exercise thallium-201 scintigraphy may be useful for identifying patients with high-risk coronary anatomy (e.g., left main coronary artery disease) and for risk stratification and prognostication.* Thus, myocardial thallium-201 imaging may be clinically useful even after coronary angiographic findings are known. As summarized in Table 58–4, high-risk thallium-201 scan findings include (1) multiple perfusion defects or washout abnormalities or both in more than one coronary supply region; (2) thallium-201 redistribution in multiple myocardial segments; (3) increased

*References A1, A2, B21, B29, C4, G12, I2, I3, K9, K10, K15, L9, N4, P3, R6, W10, W11.

Table 58–4. HIGH-RISK EXERCISE THALLIUM-201 STRESS TEST VARIABLES

Left main Tl-201 scan pattern
Multivessel CAD scan pattern with multiple perfusion defects or washout abnormalities in more than one vascular supply region
Tl-201 redistribution in multiple segments
Abnormal lung Tl-201 uptake
Exercise-induced left ventricular cavity dilatation
Tl-201 redistribution defects remote from a zone of infarction
Tl-201 redistribution within infarct zone in non-Q myocardial infarction

lung thallium-201 uptake; and (4) apparent left ventricular cavity dilatation on the initial postexercise images. Most patients with left main coronary artery disease have an abnormal thallium-201 scintigram, and nearly two thirds of patients with a 50 or more percent stenosis of the left main coronary artery have perfusion defects in more than one coronary supply region.[N4] Slightly greater than 40 percent of patients with a significant left main stenosis demonstrate increased lung thallium-201 uptake as the initial postexercise anterior view scintigram.[N4] Similarly, approximately 50 to 60 percent of patients with proximal three-vessel disease exhibit redistribution defects in the territory of at least two of the coronary vessels that are narrowed.[N4] In patients with multivessel disease, it is the circumflex stenosis that often goes undetected on the perfusion scan. Figure 58–11 is an example of a patient with underlying multivessel coronary artery disease and a high-risk thallium-201 scintigram.

Thallium-201 scintigraphic findings have prognostic value. In one of the first published studies evaluating the prognostic utility of exercise thallium-201 scintigraphy from the Massachusetts General Hospital, it was reported that the number of thallium-201 redistribution defects was the only independent significant predictor of future cardiac events employing a logistic regression analysis.[B21] In that study, neither the exercise electrocardiographic findings nor the angiographic extent of disease (no quantitative angiography) added significant prognostic information to the thallium-201 scintigraphic data. In another study from Cedars-Sinai in Los Angeles, the ability of exercise thallium-201 scintigraphy to predict future cardiac events was evaluated in 1689 patients with symptoms consistent with coronary artery disease without prior infarction.[L9] Stepwise logistic regression identified the number of myocardial regions with redistribution defects, the maximum magnitude of hypoperfusion on the post-exercise scintigram, and the achieved exercise heart rate as the only independent predictors of subsequent cardiac events. Both extent and severity of hypoperfusion were exponentially correlated with event rate.

In a similar study, the best predictor of future cardiac events was the number of myocardial scan segments with perfusion defects, whether of the redistribution or persistent types.[I2] More recently, Kaul and associates from the University of Virginia reported a 4- to 8-year follow-up study of 383 patients who

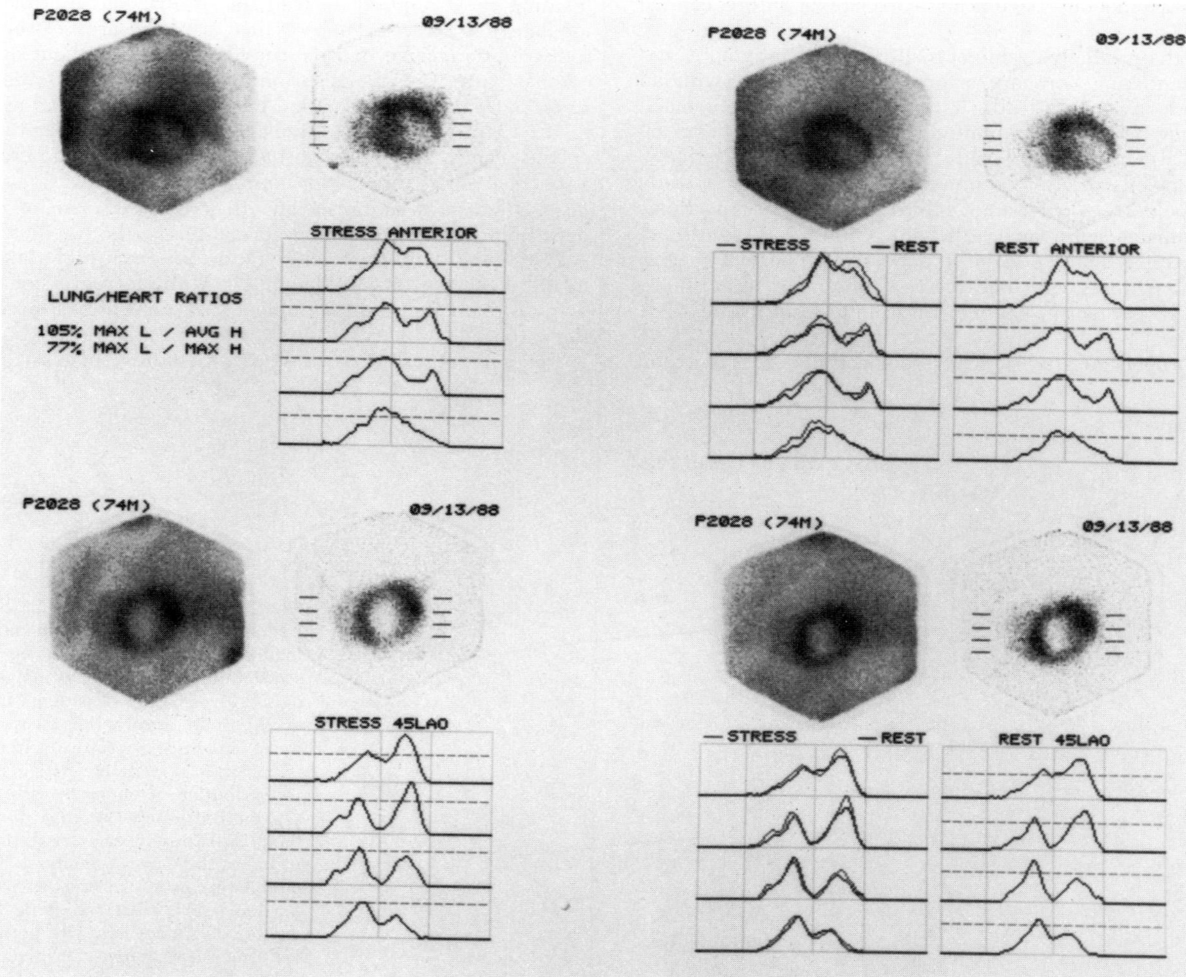

Figure 58–11. Unprocessed and background-subtracted exercise (stress) and rest anterior scintigrams *(upper two panels)* and exercise (stress) and rest 45° left anterior oblique (LAO) scintigrams *(lower panels)* in a patient with multivessel coronary artery disease and a prior anterior infarction. The quantitative count profiles are shown below each background-subtracted image. The overlap of the stress and rest profiles is shown under the unprocessed rest scintiphotos. Abnormal lung thallium uptake and initial defects involving the anterolateral wall, apex, inferior wall, septum, and inferoapical regions are seen. The delayed images show partial redistribution in all but the apical defect, which remains persistent.

underwent both exercise thallium-201 exercise testing and cardiac catheterization.[K9] One patient was lost to follow-up. Eighty-three patients had a revascularization procedure performed within 3 months of thallium-201 testing and were excluded from the prognostic analysis. Of the remaining 299 patients, 210 had no events and 89 had events (41 deaths, 9 nonfatal myocardial infarctions, and 39 late revascularization procedures performed 3 months or later after testing) during follow-up. When all clinical, exercise, thallium-201 scintigraphic and catheterization variables were analyzed by Cox regression analysis, the number of diseased vessels was the single most important predictor of future cardiac events, followed by the number of segments demonstrating thallium-201 redistribution. Other variables independently found to predict future events included the change in heart rate from rest to exercise, presence of exercise ST depression, occurrence of ventricular arrhythmias on exercise, and beta-blocker therapy. The combination of both catheterization and exercise thallium-201 data was superior to either alone for determining future events. Figure 58–12 shows the cardiac event rate during the period of follow-up in patients with and without thallium-201 redistribution on exercise scintigraphy in this study.

In a recent study by Bairey and colleagues, the 1-year cardiac event rate in 190 patients with typical angina but negative exercise electrocardiograms was related to clinical and thallium-201 imaging variables.[B29] The event rates were 4 percent in the normal scan group versus 15 percent in the abnormal scan group. Multivariate analysis revealed that an abnormal thallium-201 scintigram was the only significant correlate of future cardiac events.

Although the predictive value of thallium-201 scintigraphy was good for identifying coronary artery disease patients with an increased risk of cardiac death, its predictive value for nonfatal infarction may be somewhat limited.[K15] Elderly patients over 60 years of age also can be successfully stratified into high- and low-risk subgroups by exercise thallium-201 scintigraphy.[13] In a study of this more elderly population of 449 patients, the risk of cardiac death or nonfatal acute myocardial infarction at 25 months of follow-up was less than 1 percent in patients with normal images, 5 percent in patients with one-vessel thallium-201 scan abnormality, and 13 percent in patients with multivessel thallium-201 scan patterns.

Several prognostic studies have demonstrated the powerful predictive value of increased lung thallium-201 uptake for identifying high-risk coronary artery disease patients. In one recent study, increased thallium-201 lung uptake, a marker of left ventricular dysfunction and pulmonary congestion during exercise, was identified as the best predictor of a future cardiac event (relative risk ratio = 3.5).[G12] In another report from the Massachusetts General Hospital group, the lung : heart ratio by quantitative image analysis was the most important predictor of future cardiac events in 293 patients who underwent both exercise thallium-201 scintigraphy and coronary angiography and were followed up to 4 to 9 years (Fig. 58–13).[K11] In that study, although the number of diseased vessels was an important independent predictor of cardiac events, it did not add to the overall ability of exercise thallium-201 scintigraphy to predict future cardiac events. This prognostic index (lung : heart ratio) may be lost with SPECT imaging unless an initial anterior view planar image is first obtained.

Patients who have a normal perfusion scan have been found to have an excellent short-term prognosis with an extremely low mortality (less than 0.5 percent per year) and nonfatal infarction rate.[P3, W10, W16] In one study, patients with a normal myocardial perfusion scan and a peak exercise heart rate of less than 85 percent of maximal predicted heart rate for age had a prognosis equally as good as patients with a normal perfusion scan who achieved greater than 85 percent of maximal predicted heart rate during stress testing.

A postexercise transient increase in left ventricular cavity size on thallium-201 images is a marker of high-risk coronary artery disease.[W11] A "transient dilatation ratio" can be determined by dividing the computer-derived left ventricular area of the immediate postexercise anterior image by the area of the 4-hour redistribution image. In this study,[W11] patients without significant coronary artery disease seen on angiography had a ratio of 1:02 ± 0.05. A transient dilatation ratio was then defined as greater than 1:12 (mean ± 2 SD). Transient dilatation of the left ventricle on the scan by this criterion had a sensitivity of 60 percent and a specificity of 95 percent for identifying patients with multivessel disease and was more specific than the presence of multiple perfusion defects, washout abnormalities, or both.

Thallium-201 exercise scintigraphy has been undertaken early in the course of unstable angina.[F9] Multiple regression analysis demonstrated that thallium defect size was the best predictor of the extent of coronary artery disease.

Taken together, these and other studies suggest that even

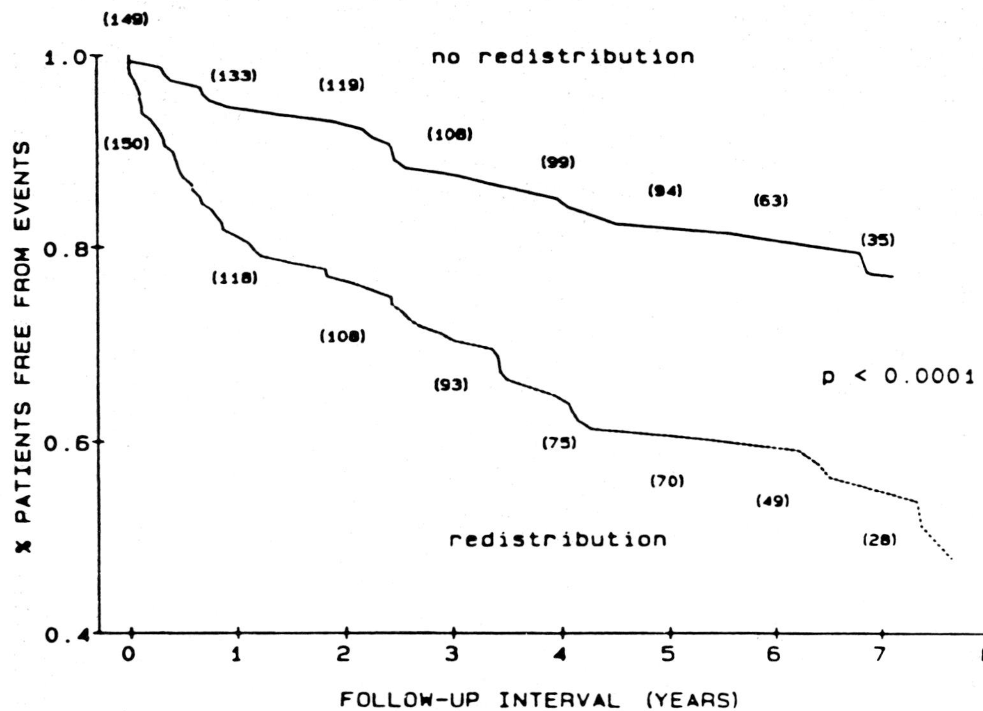

Figure 58–12. Difference in the event-free survival of patients with and without thallium-201 redistribution on exercise scintigraphy. The numbers in parentheses denote the number of patients still at risk at the time during the follow-up. The mean ± 1 SEM 5-year event-free survival is 82 ± 3 percent for patients with no redistribution, compared with 60 ± 4 percent for those with redistribution ($P < 0.0001$). (From Kaul, S., et al.: Prognostic utility of the exercise thallium-201 test in ambulatory patients with chest pain: Comparison with cardiac catheterization. Circulation 77:745, 1988, with permission of the American Heart Association, Inc.)

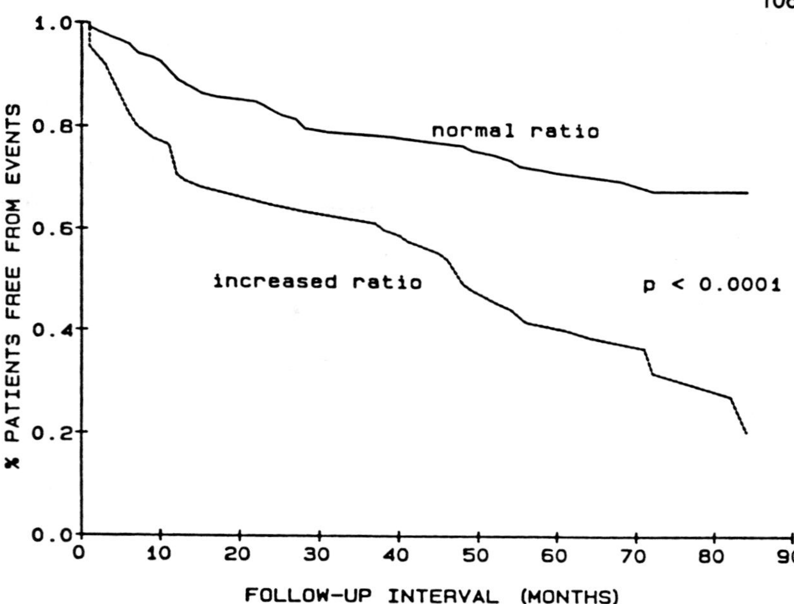

Figure 58–13. The difference in the event-free survival in 118 patients with a normal lung/heart ratio of thallium-201 activity (≤ 0.52) versus 86 patients with an increased ratio (> 0.52). (From Kaul, S., Finkelstein D M, Homma S, Leavitt M, Okada R D, Boucher CA: Superiority of quantitative exercise thallium-201 variables in determining long-term prognosis in ambulatory patients with chest pain: A comparison with cardiac catheterization. J. Am. Coll. Cardiol. 12:25, 1988. Reprinted with permission from the American College of Cardiology.)

when cardiac catheterization findings are known, thallium-201 scintigraphic information is additive in identifying coronary artery disease patients at increased risk for subsequent events. The extent of myocardial ischemia, as reflected by the number of thallium-201 scan segments showing redistribution coupled with abnormal lung thallium-201 uptake, appears to be the most important variable in predicting future cardiac events in patients presenting with chest pain. Most of these patients will exhibit underlying multivessel coronary artery disease. Perhaps when more physiologic information, such as coronary flow reserve, can be obtained from coronary angiography, the prognostic value of the invasive test for predicting future cardiac events will be enhanced.

Thallium-201 Scintigraphy After Myocardial Infarction

Thallium-201 scintigraphy is a useful approach to risk stratification after acute myocardial infarction.* Those patients who have experienced an uncomplicated clinical course during hospitalization with acute myocardial infarction and demonstrate no evidence of clinical heart failure, serious ventricular arrhythmias, or recurrent angina will be eligible for predischarge submaximal exercise testing for further risk stratification. Alternatively, it has been shown that symptom-limited testing is safe at 3 weeks following infarction. Approximately 75 percent of all infarct survivors will be eligible for exercise testing during the recovery phase after infarction. Certain high-risk variables have been identified on exercise electrocardiographic stress testing that are associated with an increased risk of mortality in the first year after discharge following an uncomplicated infarction. These variables include poor exercise tolerance characterized by failure to reach at least 4 METs or attain a target heart rate of 120 to 130 beats per minute, failure to increase systolic blood pressure by 10 or more mm Hg, exercise-induced ventricular arrhythmias, and exercise-induced ST segment shifts.

Myocardial perfusion imaging performed in conjunction with exercise testing has been shown to separate high- and low-risk survivors of uncomplicated infarction better than exercise electrocardiographic testing alone. High-risk thallium-201 scan variables after uncomplicated myocardial infarction include multiple defects in more than one coronary supply region, the presence of thallium-201 redistribution within or remote from the infarct zone, an abnormal increase in lung thallium-201 uptake, and exercise-induced left ventricular cavity dilatation. In one study, the ability of predischarge quantitative thallium-201 scintigraphy to predict future cardiac events was evaluated prospectively in 140 consecutive patients under 65 years of age who experienced an uncomplicated myocardial infarction.[G14] Exercise electrocardiography and coronary angiography were also performed in this group. By a mean of 15 months, 50 patients had experienced a cardiac event; 7 died, 9 developed recurrent infarction and 34 were rehospitalized with severe angina. Thallium-201 scintigraphy separated high- from low-risk status better than exercise electrocardiographic stress testing or coronary angiographic variables. Fifteen of the sixteen patients who either died or experienced a reinfarction demonstrated one of the high-risk scintigraphic findings.

One explanation for the superiority of exercise thallium-201 scintigraphy over exercise electrocardiographic stress testing alone in stratifying survivors after myocardial infarction relates to its capacity for enhanced sensitivity and specificity for identifying postinfarction patients with multivessel coronary artery disease.[G13] It has been shown that multivessel coronary artery disease is the angiographic substrate for the high-risk thallium-201 perfusion variables that predict subsequent mortality and reinfarction.[G14] Data from several studies have shown that multiple defects in more than one coronary supply region were present in approximately 70 percent of patients with underlying multivessel coronary artery disease who underwent exercise scintigraphy after infarction.[A3, B22, D4, G13] On the other hand, only about 10 percent of postinfarction patients with underlying single-vessel disease had multiple defects in more than one vascular supply region.

High-risk non-Q-wave infarction patients also can be identified by demonstration of thallium-201 redistribution within the zone of infarction on predischarge exercise scintigraphy.[G15] As depicted in Figure 58–14, the prevalence and extent of thallium-201 redistribution within the zone of infarction were greater in patients with non-Q-wave infarction, compared with those with Q-wave infarction (60 percent versus 36 percent).[G15] Patients with non-Q infarction who subsequently experience cardiac events had a higher incidence of infarct zone redistribution, compared with nonevent patients. This is not surprising since patients with non-Q-wave infarction have less myocardial necrosis and therefore more myocardium still jeopardized in the risk area of the infarct-related vessel.

Exercise-induced lung thallium-201 uptake is a particularly important predictor of an adverse outcome after uncomplicated myocardial infarction.[A4, G14] Patients with an abnormal resting ejection fraction have a higher lung : heart thallium-201 uptake ratio than do patients with a normal ejection fraction. Abnormal

*References A3, A4, B22, D4, E2, G13–15, H4, P4, S6, S7, T4, W12.

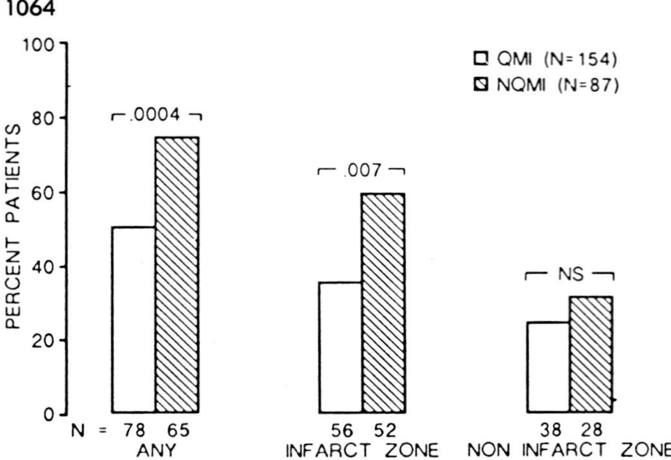

Figure 58–14. Percentage of patients with Q-wave MI and non-Q-wave MI demonstrating any Tl-201 redistribution, infarct zone redistribution and noninfarct redistribution on predischarge quantitative exercise Tl-201 scintigraphy. Note the increased prevalence of redistribution in non-Q-wave MI (NQMI) patients. (From Gibson, R. S.: Clinical, functional, and angiographic distinctions between Q wave and non-Q wave myocardial infarction: Evidence of spontaneous reperfusion and implications for intervention trials. Circulation 75(6 Pt. 2):V128, 1987, with permission of the American Heart Association, Inc.)

lung thallium uptake had a 70 percent sensitivity and a 72 percent specificity for detecting multivessel coronary artery disease after acute infarction in one study.[A4] Patients with abnormal lung thallium-201 uptake had more reversible ischemia than patients with less lung uptake. Thus, it is not surprising that the presence of increased lung thallium-201 uptake should be a good predictor of a poor prognosis. It reflects abnormal resting left ventricular function, underlying multivessel disease, and exercise-induced ischemia, all variables that have been demonstrated to be associated with an adverse prognosis.

Thallium-201 Scintigraphy for Assessment of Myocardial Revascularization

Exercise thallium-201 scintigraphy has been utilized for evaluating regional myocardial perfusion and viability in patients undergoing coronary artery bypass graft surgery or percutaneous transluminal coronary angioplasty (PTCA).* Preprocedure thallium-201 scintigraphy is useful for predicting the functional response to revascularization.[G5] Myocardial zones demonstrating thallium-201 redistribution before surgery or percutaneous transluminal coronary angioplasty (PTCA) are most often associated with preserved wall motion and demonstrate improvement in both perfusion and function postoperatively. In contrast, most persistent thallium-201 defects are associated with akinetic or dyskinetic wall motion preoperatively and do not show improved function following revascularization. Most of these regions represent nonviable myocardium. However, as cited previously, a certain percentage of mild persistent defects do show significant improvement in perfusion and function after revascularization.[G5] These areas may represent zones of severe ischemia perfused by high-grade stenosis or zones of very slow redistribution. Some of these persistent defects demonstrate increased glucose uptake by positron tomography.[B28] Rarely do severe persistent defects, characterized by a greater than 50 percent reduction in thallium-201 counts, show improved thallium-201 uptake after revascularization.

Postoperative or post-PTCA perfusion imaging can be used for evaluating the functional patency of bypass grafts[G16, H5, R7, R8, S8, V3] and dilated coronary vessels,[H6, S10, W13, W14] respectively. Patients with patent grafts[H5] or successful coronary angioplasty demonstrate improved perfusion at higher exercise heart rates when tested after the procedure. On the other hand, patients with obstructed grafts or restenosis at the site of balloon dilatation will show reappearance of ischemia, as evidenced by the presence of thallium-201 redistribution with or without ST depression. Thallium-201 redistribution on symptom-limited exercise testing may precede the development of angina and restenosis by several months.[B31, S10]

Exercise thallium-201 scintigraphy may be particularly useful in patients who develop atypical chest pain after successful angioplasty by angiographic criteria. A normal perfusion scan at a high exercise heart rate or workload should exclude the presence of significant restenosis.

In one recent study, quantitative exercise thallium-201 scintigraphy was performed approximately 2 weeks after successful percutaneous transluminal coronary angioplasty in 68 asymptomatic patients, 94 percent of whom had class III or IV angina before the procedure.[S10] At a mean of 10 months of follow-up, 23 patients (34 percent) developed recurrent angina. Multivariate analysis of 22 clinical, angiographic, and exercise test variables revealed that thallium-201 redistribution, any thallium-201 scan abnormality, the presence of a distal stenosis, and treadmill time were the only significant predictors of recurrent angina after PTCA. Using a stepwise discriminate function model, thallium-201 redistribution was the only significant independent predictor of recurrent angina. Only 9 percent of the patients who remained asymptomatic throughout the follow-up period demonstrated thallium-201 redistribution at the time of exercise testing 2 weeks after the procedure. However, despite its prognostic value relative to other variables as a predictor of recurrent angina after PTCA, thallium-201 redistribution was observed in only 9 of the 23 patients (39 percent) who subsequently developed recurrent angina at this early time point (2 weeks). In another study, the predictive accuracy of thallium-201 imaging for the diagnosis of restenosis after angioplasty was evaluated in 121 patients who had undergone a successful procedure.[B31] Of 104 asymptomatic patients at 4 to 6 weeks after angioplasty, 26 (25 percent) had thallium-201 redistribution on scintigraphy. Evidence of restenosis was present by 6 months in 22 (85 percent) of these 26 patients and by 1 year in 25 (96 percent). In this study, thallium-201 scintigraphy was superior to exercise electrocrdiography in detecting restenosis.

The combination of an abnormal thallium-201 scan showing redistribution, together with a postangioplasty gradient of 20 mm Hg or greater, identified patients at 1 year with a fourfold greater risk for restenosis and recurrent angina or myocardial infarction.[M10]

Continued improvement in exercise myocardial perfusion has been reported to occur up to 7 months after PTCA, as assessed by serial thallium-201 scintigraphy (Fig. 58–15).[M9] These investigators concluded that since thallium-201 scans after percutaneous transluminal coronary angioplasty often show this delay in improvement, an abnormal scan soon after PTCA does not necessarily reflect significant coronary restenosis. Exercise thallium-201 scintigraphy can be utilized for identification of a "culprit lesion" in patients with multivessel coronary disease and symptoms of angina. In one report, approximately 50 percent of patients who underwent successful dilatation of a culprit lesion in the presence of multivessel coronary artery disease had evidence of ischemia in a second vascular distribution on repeat thallium-201 imaging.[B23] In the group with no evidence of ischemia on repeat testing, only 13 percent required dilatation of a second vessel at 1 year of follow-up. There is no doubt that myocardial perfusion imaging performed in conjunction with exercise stress testing is the most sensitive and specific approach to detecting restenosis noninvasively. However, the cost-effectiveness of routine post-PTCA exercise scintigraphy in asymptomatic patients who experienced a good angiographic result has not yet been ascertained.

Thallium-201 Scintigraphy After Thrombolytic Therapy

Thallium-201 scintigraphy may be useful in evaluating the efficacy of coronary reperfusion after acute myocardial infarction.[B24, D5, G17, G18, H7, M11–13, S11]

---

*References B23, G16, H5, H6, K12, M9, M10, R7, R8, R13, S8–10, V3, V4, W13, W14.

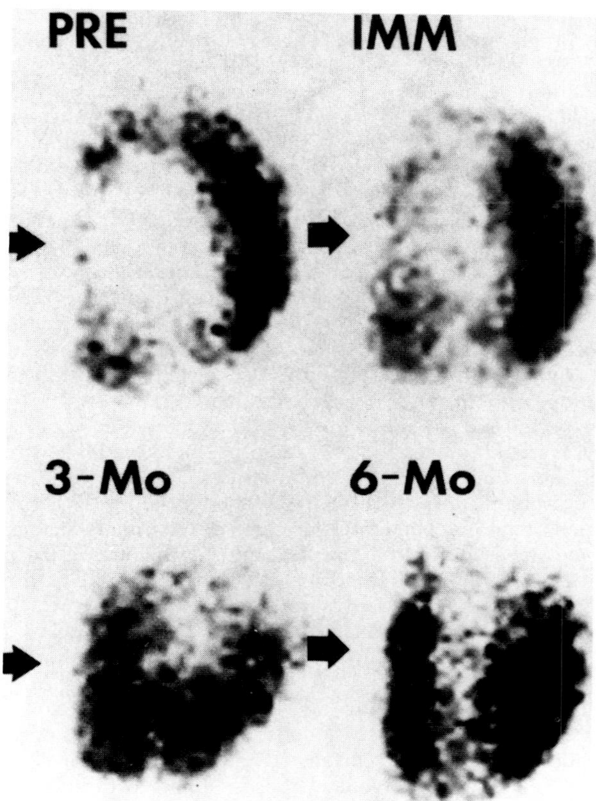

Figure 58–15. Serial thallium-201 exercise scintigrams in the 45° left anterior oblique projection before PTCA (PRE), at 5 days after PTCA (IMM), and 3 and 6 months after PTCA in a patient who had an angiographically successful dilatation of a 90 percent proximal left anterior descending coronary artery stenosis. Note the progressive improvement in septal thallium uptake *(arrows)*. (From Manyari, D. E., et al.: Sequential thallium-201 myocardial perfusion studies after successful percutaneous transluminal coronary artery angioplasty: Delayed resolution of exercise-induced scintigraphic abnormalities. Circulation 77:86, 1988, with permission of the American Heart Association, Inc.)

Serial thallium-201 imaging in the resting state in patients undergoing thrombolytic therapy for acute myocardial infarction has shown that patients with a patent infarct-related vessel have more thallium-201 redistribution on delayed images obtained several hours after thrombolysis, compared with patients who have persistently occluded arteries. There is a continued improvement in thallium-201 uptake over months after thrombolytic therapy, suggesting further improvement in perfusion or reversal of membrane transport abnormalities.[D5] With achievement of myocardial salvage, a significant improvement in thallium-201 uptake should be observed when comparing the pre-treatment and post-treatment serial images. With no salvage occurring as a result of reperfusion therapy, the resting thallium-201 defect size should not show a significant change.

Patients with acute infarction who have been successfully treated with thrombolytic agents and remain asymptomatic during hospitalization are candidates for a predischarge exercise thallium-201 scintigraphy. In one interesting study reported from the University of Michigan, tomographic SPECT thallium imaging was performed 3 days after admission in uncomplicated myocardial infarction patients who received thrombolytic therapy on admission in order to separate high- from low-risk patients.[T5] In 132 such patients, 93 (65 percent) constituted a low-risk group with a negative thallium perfusion scan for ischemia. These patients were randomized to discharge at 72 hours or late discharge. At 7 months of follow-up after discharge, there were no deaths in either subgroup of patients with a normal scan. Patients with a positive scan for residual ischemia were managed more aggressively with delayed discharge.

A word of caution should be expressed with respect to the interpretation of thallium-201 scintigrams obtained in the early phase following reperfusion. When thallium-201 is injected for the first time intravenously immediately after reperfusion, an overestimation of myocardial salvage may occur because of "excess" thallium-201 uptake in the infarct zone consequent to significant hyperemia.

SPECT Thallium-201 Scintigraphy

As previously suggested, the technique of SPECT Tl-201 imaging is gaining increased popularity for imaging of regional myocardial perfusion. SPECT offers higher contrast resolution and better separation of overlying myocardial segments. The extent of perfusion abnormalities can be expressed as a percentage of the entire myocardium by use of the polar maps.[M14] Using quantitative criteria for determining the presence of a significant defect on SPECT imaging, an 89 percent sensitivity and 92 percent specificity for coronary artery disease detection has been reported.[G10] In another study, the sensitivity of SPECT thallium imaging was 78 percent for detecting left anterior descending stenoses, 89 percent for detecting right coronary lesions, and 65 percent for identifying narrowings in the left circumflex artery.[D3] The sensitivity for detecting individual coronary stenoses is approximately 10 percent greater when quantitative analysis of SPECT images is employed, compared with merely visual evaluation of the tomographic studies.[T2]

Dipyridamole Thallium-201 Scintigraphy

Intravenous infusion of dipyridamole is an acceptable alternative to physical exercise for myocardial imaging with thallium-201 or ^{82}Rb.* The coronary dilating effect of dipyridamole results in a marked increase in regional blood flow to areas supplied by normal coronary vessels, but abnormal flow reserve is observed in regions supplied by stenotic arteries. This inhomogeneity of flow is detected by abnormal thallium-201 uptake when the radionuclide is administered during the peak vasodilatory effect of the drug. Redistribution occurs in areas of viable but underperfused myocardial regions, comparable to what is observed with exercise scintigraphy.[B17, B18] As shown in Table 58–5, the sensitivity and specificity for dipyridamole imaging are in the range of 80 to 90 percent and are comparable to what is achieved with exercise scintigraphy. Approximately 15 to 20 percent of patients undergoing dipyridamole thallium-201 imaging will manifest ischemia by ST-segment depression. Some patients will develop chest pain without associated ST depression with dipyridamole infusion, even in the presence of normal coronary arteries.[P6]

Because the sensitivity for detecting underlying coronary artery disease with dipyridamole thallium-201 scintigraphy is comparable to exercise scintigraphy,[V7] the pharmacologic test should be

*References C5, D6, F6, H8, H9, L10, L11, O6, O7, R9, R10, W15.

Table 58–5. SENSITIVITY AND SPECIFICITY FOR DIPYRIDAMOLE THALLIUM-201 SCINTIGRAPHY

Study	Year	Number of Patients	Sensitivity (%)	Specificity (%)
Albro	1978	62	67	91
Francisco	1982	75	80	67
Leppo	1982	60	93	80
Okada	1983	30	91	100
Sochor	1984	194	92	81
Taillefer	1986	50	82	91
Walker	1986	87	88	87
Ruddy	1987	80	85	93
Lam	1988	142	84	71
TOTAL		780	84.7	84.5

considered in patients who have normal exercise perfusion scans at suboptimal heart rate responses, or in patients who are deemed unable to exercise because of noncardiac abnormalities such as arthritis, cerebrovascular disease, and orthopedic abnormalities. Dipyridamole thallium-201 scintigraphy has been shown to provide important prognostic information in patients with peripheral vascular disease who are scheduled for major vascular surgery.[B25, E3, L12] In this group of patients, the cost-effectiveness of dipyridamole thallium-201 scintigraphy was greater when certain clinical variables were present, such as a history of angina or prior infarction, presence of diabetes mellitus, signs of congestive heart failure, or Q-waves on an electrocardiogram.[E3] Similarly, dipyridamole thallium-201 imaging has been shown to be useful for risk stratification after uncomplicated myocardial infarction.[L11]

THALLIUM-201 SCINTIGRAPHY IN NONCORONARY HEART DISEASE

Table 58–6 lists some of the noncoronary conditions in which thallium-201 scintigraphy has been performed. Thallium-201 scintigraphy occasionally can assist in the detection of septal hypertrophy in patients with presumed idiopathic hypertrophic subaortic stenosis.[B26] Asymmetric hypertrophy is characterized by a ratio of septum to left ventricular free wall thickness of 1:7. In normal volunteers and in patients with concentric left ventricular hypertrophy, this ratio is approximately 1:0. Approximately one half of patients with hypertrophic cardiomyopathy will demonstrate regional myocardial perfusion defects on symptom-limited thallium-201 SPECT imaging. In one study, perfusion abnormalities were observed in all regions of the left ventricle, although persistent defects were predominantly observed in segments of the left ventricular wall that were normal or showed only mildly increased thickness.[O8] In contrast, a great proportion of the redistribution defects in patients with hypertrophic cardiomyopathy were detected in areas of moderate-to-marked wall thickness. Patients who had only perfusion defects showing complete redistribution had either normal or hyperdynamic left ventricular systolic function. Of those patients who had persistent defects or demonstrated only partial redistribution, more than 80 percent had a subnormal left ventricular ejection fraction. The investigators concluded that myocardial perfusion abnormalities are common among patients with hypertrophic cardiomyopathy.

The configuration of hypertrophied myocardium has been evaluated by thallium-201 SPECT. When thallium-201 images are reconstructed into multiple 12-mm-thick slices in three planes, the ventricular septal wall thickness has been observed to be increased, with a septal to posterior wall ratio of 1:45 in patients with obstructive hypertrophic myopathy.[S12] In this latter study, in patients with nonobstructed hypertrophied cardiomyopathy with large negative T-waves or in those with concentric left ventricular hypertrophy, the ratio employing SPECT imaging was 1:03 and 0:98, respectively.

Table 58–6. ABNORMAL THALLIUM-201 SCINTIGRAMS IN NONCORONARY CARDIAC DISEASE

Hypertrophic cardiomyopathy with normal epicardial coronary arteries
Progressive systemic sclerosis with diffuse scleroderma
Hypertensive heart disease
Diabetic heart disease with normal coronary arteries
Duchenne-type muscular dystrophy
Myocarditis
Nonischemic dilated cardiomyopathy
Left bundle branch block with normal coronary arteries
Anomalous left coronary artery arising from the pulmonary artery
Myocardial sarcoidosis
Cardiac lymphoma
Sickle cell anemia
Thickened interventricular septum on 45° left anterior oblique view in hypertrophic subaortic stenosis
Increased right ventricular Tl-201 activity in pulmonary hypertension

Myocardial perfusion abnormalities are common in patients with progressive systemic sclerosis with diffuse scleroderma.[A5, F7, K13] Nearly 50 percent of patients with scleroderma have redistribution-type defects on exercise scintigraphy, with a majority also demonstrating fixed defects.[F7] Usually, coronary angiography is normal. It is hypothesized that myocardial perfusion abnormalities in patients with progressive systemic sclerosis with diffuse scleroderma are due to a disturbance of the myocardial microcirculation. Both right and left ventricular dysfunction also has been reported in this disease, suggesting ischemic-induced injury. Some patients with systemic sclerosis and scleroderma show reversible cold-induced abnormalities in myocardial perfusion and function.[A5] Cold exposure may result in reflex coronary vasoconstriction in these patients, resulting in reversible myocardial ischemia. Resting thallium-201 defects also have been reported in patients with myocardial sarcoidosis.[M15]

Hypertensive patients with a low likelihood of coronary artery disease are more likely to have abnormal thallium-201 test results than their normotensive counterparts.[S13] It was speculated by these investigators that these findings might indicate that hypertension may independently produce myocardial changes and changes in perfusion that are detected by thallium-201 exercise scintigraphy. The scan abnormalities consisted of redistribution defects or abnormal washout as assessed quantitatively. It was further suggested that abnormal coronary vascular reserve in the hypertensive patients may have played a role in the abnormalities observed.

Results of a recent study have shown that thallium-201 scintigraphic perfusion defects were observed in 20 percent of asymptomatic patients with hypertension and left ventricular hypertrophy.[T9] Seventy-five percent of those patients with an abnormal scan or an abnormal computerized treadmill exercise score developed typical angina during follow-up. Thus, there were not a substantial number of false-positive thallium-201 scintigrams in these patients with hypertension and left ventricular hypertrophy.

Similarly, certain diabetic patients may demonstrate abnormal myocardial perfusion on thallium-201 scintigrams without significant large vessel coronary artery disease.[G19, N5] The explanation for abnormal thallium-201 scintigrams in these diabetic patients was a pathologic change in the microcirculation.[G19] Diabetic patients with coronary artery disease have a higher prevalence of painless abnormal thallium scintigrams consistent with ischemia than do nondiabetics.[N5] Patients with the Duchenne type of muscular dystrophy have been reported to demonstrate abnormalities in SPECT Tl-201 scintigrams frequently. In one recent study, SPECT thallium scintigraphy showed hypoperfusion in 90 percent of boys with Duchenne-type dystrophy and in 61 percent of patients with either fascioscapulo-humeral, limb-girdle, or myotonic dystrophies.[Y1] Multifocal thallium-201 defects have been observed in patients presenting with clinically documented myocarditis, characterized by electrocardiographic abnormalities and elevation of serum cardiac enzymes.[T6] These defects were observed at rest in the presence of angiographically normal coronary arteries.[T6]

Thallium-201 imaging has been undertaken in conjunction with resting radionuclide angiography or echocardiography in assessment of patients with severe congestive heart failure.[B27, D7, Y2] The combined approach is useful for distinguishing ischemic from idiopathic dilated cardiomyopathy. Thallium-201 scintigrams in patients with ischemic cardiomyopathy most often have defects involving greater than 40 percent of the circumference of the left ventricular image, which corresponds well to the segmental asynergy noted on the radionuclide angiogram or echocardiogram. In contrast, patients with dilated congestive cardiomyopathy show relatively homogeneous thallium-201 uptake in a thinned wall ventricle or have defects of less than 20 percent of the image circumference. Some patients with dilated cardiomyopathy have more focal redistribution-type defects and normal coronary arteries.

Certain patients with chest pain and left bundle branch block are evaluated by thallium-201 scintigraphy for detection of possible underlying coronary artery disease.[D8, H10, H11, R11] It is apparent that the exercise electrocardiogram is not diagnostic in such patients. It is interesting that certain asymptomatic patients with left bundle branch block and angiographically normal coronary arteries may demonstrate abnormal myocardial perfusion on exercise scintigraphy. Most often, the perfusion defects are localized to the intraventricular septum. The significance of this finding is still undetermined. In one recently reported study, electrical induction of left bundle branch block in dogs resulted, in most instances, in a comparable reduction in septal thallium-201 uptake.[H10] The investigators suggested that these septal defects in the presence of left bundle branch block may reflect functional ischemia caused by asynchronous septal contraction.

Marked perfusion abnormalities can be found in the anterolateral wall in patients with anomalous origin of the left coronary artery arising from the pulmonary artery.[G20, M16] After surgery, there may be improvement in these anterior wall defects,[M17] but most often persistent defects are observed that do not improve since they represent myocardial fibrosis. Postoperative thallium-201 imaging can also be useful in assessing the results of surgical repair of hemodynamically significant coronary artery anomalies.[R12] Imaging of the right ventricular myocardium can be accomplished with thallium-201 scintigraphy. Several groups have shown exercise-induced transient defects in the right ventricle on serial redistribution imaging. This has been associated with the presence of a high-grade right coronary stenosis.[B31, L13] Right ventricular overloading has been successfully detected by thallium-201 scintigraphy. With pressure overload, the degree of right ventricular visualization of thallium-201 correlates with elevation of right ventricular systolic pressure.[O10] Normally, the right ventricular free wall is not visualized at rest with thallium-201. If pulmonary hypertension is present, the right ventricular free wall is most often visualized on perfusion images.[C7]

Abnormal thallium-201 scans also have been reported in myocardial sarcoidosis,[M19] sickle-cell anemia,[M20] postoperative coarctation patients,[K17] and cardiac lymphoma.[M13] Patients with mitral valve prolapse and absence of coronary artery disease should have normal thallium-201 scintigrams.

LIMITATIONS OF THALLIUM-201 SCINTIGRAPHY

Certain problems are encountered with thallium-201 scintigraphy that could adversely affect scintigraphic results. Many of these have already been discussed in other sections of this chapter. Unfortunately, clinical results with myocardial perfusion imaging in the community hospital setting are not yet optimal when compared with data accumulated in the university hospital setting. These limitations are summarized in Table 58–7.

First, visual interpretation of unprocessed thallium-201 scintiscans can be difficult if one is not knowledgeable regarding attenuation artifacts or variants of normal. Such knowledge, as well as personal experience with correlating imaging results with coronary angiography, is required in order to decrease false-positive interpretations. As previously mentioned, an overlying breast shadow, an altered position of either the inflow or outflow tracts of the left ventricle, a greater than normal degree of apical thinning, an enlarged right ventricular blood pool overlying the inferior wall on the anterior image, or a high diaphragm overlying the posterior wall on a steep left anterior oblique image can result in false-positive interpretations. In certain patients, the upper septum and upper posterolateral wall (basal portions of the left ventricle) may be thin, which could be misinterpreted as defects or even a left main coronary pattern. In markedly obese individuals, thallium-201 images of the heart may be of such poor quality because of attenuation as to make the studies uninterpretable. Subtle degrees of redistribution are not detected by visual scan analysis, nor is the extent of redistribution well estimated.[D2]

Table 58–7. FACTORS CONTRIBUTING TO FALSE-POSITIVE THALLIUM-201 SCINTIGRAMS

Defects due to attenuation artifacts from overlying breast shadow (anterior and septal), overlying right ventricular blood pool (inferior), and high diaphragm (inferior)
Exaggerated apical thinning
Upper septal and upper posterolateral wall thinning
Poor quality images from marked obesity
Oversubtraction of background activity on quantitative imaging
Infiltration of Tl-201 in subcutaneous tissue
Patient motion on SPECT imaging—"upward creep"
Suboptimal technical quality
Lack of experience of interpreters

False-positive washout abnormalities will be produced if oversubtraction of background on the initial image occurs. This seems to occur when increased lung uptake is present. Isolated washout abnormalities without concomitant numerically significant defects elsewhere are more often than not artifactual and a cause of false-positive interpretation. In contrast to positron imaging techniques, absolute quantitation of myocardial blood flow in ml/min/g of myocardium cannot be obtained with thallium-201 scintigraphy and gamma scintillation techniques. The resolution and sensitivity of the gamma scintillation camera depend on the depth of distribution of thallium activity within the patient, as well as on absorption of radiation within the body.

Other limitations of thallium scintigraphy are interobserver variability with visual scan interpretations, the long imaging time required to obtain serial postexercise images, and the rather high cost of the procedure.

It has been proposed that SPECT thallium imaging should enhance both sensitivity and specificity of the myocardial perfusion technique. Unfortunately, SPECT imaging is also associated with certain problems that result in poor specificity in certain laboratories. With SPECT imaging, patient motion is more likely to occur than with planar imaging, since the patient remains in an awkward position for a rather lengthy period of time. Patient motion is a source of artifactual defects on tomographic reconstruction. A phenomenon encountered with SPECT imaging is called "upward creep" of the heart.[F8] In normal individuals, an upward creep of 2 or more pixels' shift is associated with a high incidence of reversible inferior or septal perfusion defects in the absence of coronary artery disease. This phenomenon is observed in patients who exercise longer and achieve a higher heart rate, raising the possibility that upward creep is related to persistent hyperventilation following exhaustive stress.

Although one recent study found that visual SPECT stress redistribution thallium imaging was more accurate than the visual planar method for detection of coronary artery disease and localization of individual diseased arteries, this diagnostic improvement was not evident in women and in detection of right coronary disease.[F4] The lack of diagnostic improvement in women may be related to the fact that breast attenuation artifacts also are present in SPECT images. The problem with the right coronary artery could be related to inferior wall attenuation or the upward creep artifact.

CLINICAL APPLICATION OF TECHNETIUM-99m ISONITRILE IMAGING

Several clinical studies have been reported describing the preliminary clinical experience with technetium-99m isonitriles in evaluating patients with suspected or known coronary artery disease.[K6, S14, W7] The clinical efficacy of technetium-99m sestamibi planar stress and rest imaging was evaluated in a multicenter phase II clinical trial involving 38 patients.[W7] Of 36 patients with significant coronary artery disease, 35 (97 percent) had abnormal thallium-201 stress images, and 32 (89 percent) had abnormal technetium-99m sestamibi stress images. These differences were not statistically significant. Technetium-99m sestamibi images correlated in 31 of 35 patients (86 percent), who had either scar or ischemia on thallium-201 images. By segmental myocardial analysis, precise concordance between the two tests was obtained in 463 of 570 myocardial segments (81 percent).

In another study, stress-rest technetium-99m sestamibi scans were compared with thallium-201 perfusion imaging in 36 patients who were studied by both the SPECT and planar methods.[K6] For

SPECT, overall sensitivities for identification of patients with coronary artery disease were 93 percent by technetium-99m sestamibi and 80 percent by thallium-201 (P = NS). For planar methods, overall sensitivities were 73 percent by both thallium-201 and technetium-99m sestamibi. Specificity, as assessed in patients with a low likelihood of coronary artery disease, was comparable for both tracers. Some preliminary data are available concerning the utility of performing the rest and exercise technetium-99m sestamibi studies on the same day several hours apart.[T7] It was shown that injection of a low dose (10 mCi) of technetium-99m sestamibi at rest, followed 1 hour later with a higher dose (25 to 30 mCi) at stress, may be a useful alternative to performing exercise stress and rest studies 24 hours apart as is presently required. The short protocol yielded the same number of ischemic segments and fixed defects as the 24-hour interval protocol in one reported study.

An exciting clinical application of technetium-99m sestamibi is the evaluation of reperfusion following thrombolytic therapy in patients with acute myocardial infarction.[V5] In this setting, an initial dose of technetium-99m sestamibi is administered intravenously just prior to infusion of a thrombolytic agent. Since the tracer does not redistribute, images can be acquired up to several hours after technetium-99m sestamibi injection, which would demonstrate the perfusion pattern present at the time of initiation of thrombolytic therapy. A second injection of technetium-99m sestamibi is then administered at some time later (e.g., 24 hours), demonstrating the perfusion pattern achieved following thrombolysis. Preliminary results from a multi-center trial demonstrate that patients with patent infarct vessels after thrombolytic therapy show a significant reduction in defect size on both planar and SPECT images, compared with patients with persistently occluded vessels.[G21] The final defect size derived from analysis of the post-thrombolysis images correlated inversely with the left ventricular ejection fraction at the time of hospital discharge.

One advantage of technetium-99m isonitriles for myocardial scintigraphy is that because of higher count rates than with thallium-201, the images can be ECG-gated, permitting simultaneous assessment of perfusion and function. A first-pass ejection fraction of the left and right ventricles also can be derived from the transit of the bolus of technetium-99m sestamibi after intravenous administration.

Many of the limitations of technetium-99m sestamibi are similar to those for thallium-201. For example, although attenuation is somewhat less than with thallium-201, image artifacts owing to attenuation (breast tissue interposed between the gamma camera and the heart) will still be observed. Occasionally, on rest images, the high activity in the liver, spleen, and gallbladder may affect optimal visualization of the inferior wall. Modification of the existing interpolative background subtraction algorithm has been performed on technetium-99m sestamibi images to account for this higher activity beneath the rim of the heart on the technetium-99m sestamibi scans.[S15] Quantification of images can be undertaken similar to that undertaken for thallium-201 stress/rest scintigrams.

SUMMARY

The addition of myocardial perfusion imaging to exercise stress testing has provided the clinician with the means of improving sensitivity and specificity of coronary artery disease detection among patients with undiagnosed chest pain. It can noninvasively determine the extent and severity of functionally significant coronary artery stenoses and separate high- and low-risk subsets. Myocardial perfusion imaging with either thallium-201 or the technetium-99m isonitriles can be employed for evaluating the efficacy of revascularization in patients undergoing coronary bypass surgery or percutaneous transluminal coronary angioplasty. More recently, this imaging approach has been utilized to assess the degree of myocardial salvage and improvement in myocardial blood flow after thrombolytic therapy. To maximize the diagnostic and prognostic worth of myocardial perfusion imaging techniques, computer-assisted quantitative scan analysis of myocardial thallium-201 uptake and washout is required.

Thallium-201 scintigraphy is helpful in detecting residual myocardial viability in regions of abnormal systolic function. The predictive value of a normal or abnormal scintigraphic study depends on the prevalence of coronary artery disease in the population studies. Knowledge of principles of Bayesian analysis is crucial to the application of all radionuclide imaging techniques employed for coronary artery disease detection. As outlined in this chapter, some important limitations of thallium-201 scintigraphy have to be acknowledged and appreciated in order to optimize imaging results.

New radiopharmaceutical agents and technical advances in instrumentation and imaging methodology should enhance the clinical usefulness of perfusion imaging. The new technetium-99m–labeled isonitriles employed with gated quantitative SPECT imaging are undergoing investigation and show promise for the future.

References

A

1. Ascoop, C., Klein, B., Niemeyer, M., et al.: On the clinical value of thallium-201 washout analysis in the detection of multiple jeopardized myocardial regions. Int. J. Cardiol. 11:305, 1986.
2. Abdulla, A., Maddahi, J., Garcia, E., et al.: Slow regional clearance of myocardial thallium-201 in the absence of perfusion defect: Contribution to detection of individual coronary artery stenoses and mechanism for occurrence. Circulation 71:72, 1985.
3. Abraham, R. D., Freedman, S. B., Dunn, R. F., et al.: Prediction of multivessel coronary artery disease and prognosis early after acute myocardial infarction by exercise electrocardiography and thallium-201 myocardial perfusion scanning. Am. J. Cardiol. 58:423, 1986.
4. Al-Khawaja, I. M., Lahiri, A., Rodrigues, E. A., et al.: Clinical significance of exercise-induced pulmonary uptake of thallium-201 in uncomplicated myocardial infarction. Am. J. Card. Imag. 2:135, 1988.
5. Alexander, E. L., Firestein, G. S., Weiss, J. L., et al.: Reversible cold-induced abnormalities in myocardial perfusion and function in systemic sclerosis. Ann. Intern. Med. 105:661, 1986.

B

1. Berman, D. S., Salel, A. F., DeNardo, G. L., and Mason, D. T.: Noninvasive detection of regional myocardial ischemia using rubidium-81 and the scintillation camera. Circulation 52:619, 1975.
2. Botvinick, E. H., Shames, D. M., Gerschengorn, K. M., et al.: Myocardial stress perfusion scintigraphy with rubidium-81 versus stress electrocardiography. Am. J. Cardiol. 39:364, 1977.
3. Beller, G. A., Watson, D. D., Ackell, P., and Pohost, G. M.: Time course of thallium-201 redistribution after transient myocardial ischemia. Circulation 61:791, 1980.
4. Bergman, S. R., Hack, S. N., and Sobel, B. E.: "Redistribution" of myocardial thallium-201 without reperfusion: Implications regarding absolute quantification of perfusion. Am. J. Cardiol. 49:1691, 1982.
5. Beller, G. A., Holzgrefe, H. H., and Watson, D. D.: Effects of dipyridamole-induced vasodilation on myocardial uptake and clearance kinetics of thallium-201. Circulation 68:1328, 1983.
6. Berger, B. C., Watson, D. D., Burwell, L. R., et al.: Redistribution of thallium at rest in patients with stable and unstable angina and the effect of coronary artery bypass graft surgery. Circulation 60:1114, 1979.
7. Brown, K. A., Okada, R. D., Boucher, C. A., et al.: Serial thallium-201 imaging at rest in patients with stable and unstable angina pectoris: Relationship of myocardial perfusions at rest to presenting clinical syndrome. Am. Heart J. 106:70, 1983.
8. Bingham, J. B., Mckusick, K. A., Strauss, H. W., et al.: Influence of coronary artery disease on pulmonary uptake of thallium-201. Am. J. Cardiol. 46:821, 1980.
9. Boucher, C. A., Zir, L. M., Beller, G. A., et al.: Increased lung uptake of thallium-201 during exercise myocardial imaging: Clinical, hemodynamic and angiographic implications in patients with coronary artery disease. Am. J. Cardiol. 46:189, 1980.
10. Brown, K. A., Boucher, C. A., Okada, R. D., et al.: Quantification of pulmonary thallium-201 activity after upright exercise in normal persons: Importance of peak heart rate and propranolol usage in defining normal values. Am. J. Cardiol. 53:1678, 1984.
11. Bailey, I. K., Griffith, L. S. C., Rouleau, J., et al.: Thallium-201 myocardial perfusion imaging at rest and during exercise: Comparative sensitivity to electrocardiography in coronary artery disease. Circulation 55:79, 1977.
12. Blood, D. K., McCarthy, D. M., Sciacca, R. R., and Cannon, P. J.: Comparison of single-dose and double-dose thallium-201 myocardial perfusion scintigraphy for the detection of coronary artery disease in prior myocardial infarction. Circulation 58:777, 1978.
13. Botvinick, E. H., Taradash, M. R., Shames, D. M., and Parmley, W.: Thallium-201 myocardial perfusion scintigraphy for the clinical clarification of normal, abnormal and equivocal electrocardiographic stress test. Am. J. Cardiol. 41:43, 1978.

14. Berger, B. C., Watson, D. D., Taylor, G. J., et al.: Quantitative thallium-201 exercise scintigraphy for detection of coronary artery disease. J. Nucl. Med. 22:585, 1981.
15. Bateman, T. M., Maddahi, J., Gray, R. J., et al.: Diffuse slow washout of myocardial thallium-201: A new scintigraphic indicator of extensive coronary artery disease. J. Am. Coll. Cardiol. 4:55, 1984.
16. Blady, G. J., Weiner, D. A., Rothendler, J. A., and Ryan, T. J.: Arm exercise-thallium imaging testing for the detection of coronary artery disease. J. Am. Coll. Cardiol. 9:84, 1987.
17. Beller, G. A., Holzgrefe, H. H., and Watson, D. D.: Effects of dipyridamole-induced vasodilation on myocardial uptake and clearance kinetics of thallium-201. Circulation 68:1328, 1983.
18. Beller, G. A., Holzgrefe, H. H., and Watson, D. D.: Intrinsic washout rates of thallium-201 in normal and ischemic myocardium after dipyridamole-induced vasodilation. Circulation 71:378, 1985.
19. Becker, L. C., Becker, D. M., Pearson, T. A., et al.: Screening of asymptomatic siblings of patients with premature coronary artery disease. Circulation 75(Suppl. II):14, 1987.
20. Berger, B. C., Watson, D. D., Taylor, G. J., et al.: Effect of coronary collaterals on regional myocardial perfusion using thallium-201 scintigraphy. Am. J. Cardiol. 46:365, 1980.
21. Brown, K. A., Boucher, C. A., Okada, R. D., et al.: Prognostic value of exercise thallium-201 imaging in patients presenting for evaluation of chest pain. J. Am. Coll. Cardiol. 1:994, 1983.
22. Brown, K. A., Weiss, R. M., Clements, J. P., and Wackers, F. J.: Usefulness of residual ischemic myocardium within prior infarct zone for identifying patients at high risk late after acute myocardial infarction. Am. J. Cardiol. 60:15, 1987.
23. Breisblatt, W. M., Barnes, J. V., Weiland, F., and Spaccavento, L. J.: Incomplete revascularization in multivessel percutaneous transluminal coronary angioplasty: The role for stress thallium-201 imaging. J. Am. Coll. Cardiol. 11:1183, 1988.
24. Beller, G. A.: Role of myocardial perfusion imaging in evaluating thrombolytic therapy for acute myocardial infarction. J. Am. Coll. Cardiol. 9:661, 1987.
25. Boucher, C. A., Brewster, D. C., Darling, R. C., et al.: Determination of cardiac risk by dipyridamole-thallium imaging before peripheral vascular surgery. N. Engl. J. Med. 312:389, 1985.
26. Bulkley, B. H., Rouleau, J., Stauss, H. W., and Pitt, B.: Idiopathic hypertrophic subaortic stenosis: Detection by thallium-201 myocardial perfusion imaging. N. Engl. J. Med. 293:1113, 1975.
27. Bulkley, B. H., Hutchins, G. M., Bailey, I., et al.: Thallium-201 imaging and gated cardiac blood pool scans in patients with ischemic and idiopathic congestive cardiomyopathy. A clinical and pathologic study. Circulation 55:753, 1977.
28. Brunken, R., Schwaiger, M., Grover-McKay, M., et al.: Positron emission tomography detects tissue metabolic activity in myocardial segments with persistent thallium perfusion defects. J. Am. Coll. Cardiol. 10:557, 1987.
29. Bairey, C. N., Rozanski, A., Maddahi, J., et al.: Exercise thallium-201 scintigraphy and prognosis in typical angina pectoris and negative exercise electrocardiography. Am. J. Cardiol. 64:282, 1989.
30. Brown, K. A., Osbakken, M., Boucher, C. A., et al.: Positive exercise thallium-201 test responses in patients with less than 50% maximal coronary stenosis: Angiographic and clinical predictors. Am. J. Cardiol. 55:54, 1985.
31. Breisblatt, W. M., Weiland, F. L., and Spaccavento, L. J.: Stress thallium-201 imaging after coronary angioplasty predicts restenosis and recurrent symptoms. J. Am. Coll. Cardiol. 12:1199, 1988.
32. Brown, K. A., Boucher, C. A., Okada, R. D., et al.: Serial right ventricular thallium-201 imaging after exercise: Relation to anatomy of the right coronary artery. Am. J. Cardiol. 50:1217, 1982.

C

1. Carrillo, A. P., Marks, D. S., Pickard, S. D., et al.: Correlation of exercise 201-thallium myocardial scan with coronary arteriograms and the maximal exercise test. Chest 73:321, 1978.
2. Corne, R. A., Gotsman, M. S., Weiss, A., et al.: Thallium-201 scintigraphy in diagnosis of coronary stenosis: Comparison with electrocardiography and coronary arteriography. Br. Heart J. 41:575, 1979.
3. Caralis, D. G., Bailey, I., Kennedy, H. L., and Pitt, B.: Thallium-201 myocardial imaging in evaluation of asymptomatic individuals with ischaemic ST segment depression on exercise electrocardiogram. Br. Heart J. 42:562, 1979.
4. Canhasi, B., Dae, M., Botvinick, E., et al.: Interaction of "supplementary" scintigraphic indicators of ischemia and stress electrocardiography in the diagnosis of multi-vessel coronary disease. J. Am. Coll. Cardiol. 6:581, 1985.
5. Chambers, C. E., and Brown, K. A.: Dipyridamole-induced ST segment depression during thallium-201 imaging in patients with coronary artery disease: Angiographic and hemodynamic determinants. J. Am. Coll. Cardiol. 12:37, 1988.
6. Cloninger, K. G., GePuey, E. G., Garcia, E. V., et al.: Incomplete redistribution in delayed thallium-201 single photon emission computed tomographic (SPECT) images: An overestimation of myocardial scarring. J. Am. Coll. Cardiol. 12:955, 1988.
7. Cohen, H., Baird, M. G., Rouleau, J. R., et al.: Thallium-201 myocardial imaging in patients with pulmonary hypertension. Circulation 54:790, 1976.

D

1. Dunn, R. F., Freedman, B., Bailey, I. K., et al.: Localization of coronary artery disease in exercise electrocardiography: Correlation with thallium-201 myocardial perfusion scanning. Am. J. Cardiol. 48:837, 1981.
2. DiCola, J., Moore, M., Shearer, D., et al.: Limitations of visual assessment of redistribution in thallium images. Am. Heart J. 108:926, 1984.
3. DePasquale, E. E., Nody, A. C., DePuey, E. G., et al.: Quantitative rotational thallium-201 tomography for identifying and localizing coronary artery disease. Circulation 77:316, 1988.
4. Dunn, R. F., Freedman, B., Bailey, I. K., et al.: Non-invasive prediction of multivessel disease after myocardial infarction. Circulation 62:726, 1980.
5. De Coster, P. M., Melin, J. A., Detry, J.-M. R., et al.: Coronary artery reperfusion in acute myocardial infarction: Assessment by pre- and postintervention thallium-201 myocardial perfusion imaging. Am. J. Cardiol. 55:889, 1985.
6. Deambroggi, L., Barbieri, P., DeBiase, A. M., et al.: Assessment of diagnostic value of dipyridamole testing in angina pectoris. Clin. Cardiol. 5:269, 1982.
7. Dunn, R. F., Uren, R. F., Sadick, N., et al.: Comparison of thallium-201 scanning in idiopathic dilated cardiomyopathy and severe coronary artery disease. Circulation 66:804, 1982.
8. DePuey, E. G., Guertler-Krawczynska, E., and Robbins, W. L.: Thallium-201 SPECT in coronary artery disease patients with left bundle branch block. J. Nucl. Med. 29:1479, 1988.
9. Diamond, G. A., and Forrester, J. S.: Analysis of probability as an aid in the clinical diagnosis of coronary artery disease. N. Engl. J. Med. 300:1350, 1979.
10. Dilsizian, V., Rocco, T. P., Freedman, N., et al.: Thallium reinjection after stress-redistribution imaging improves detection of ischemic myocardium: A qualitative and quantitative SPECT study. (Abstract.) J. Am. Coll. Cardiol. 15:147A, 1990.

E

1. Esquivel, L., Pollock, S. G., Beller, G. A., et al.: Effect of the degree of effort on the sensitivity of the exercise thallium-201 stress test in symptomatic coronary artery disease. Am. J. Cardiol. 63:160, 1989.
2. Ericsson, C.-G., Hamsten, A., Granath, A., et al.: Repeated exercise and redistribution thallium-201 scintigrams in patients with myocardial infarction treated with timolol or placebo. Am. Heart J. 111:916, 1986.
3. Eagle, K. A., Singer, D. E., Brewster, D. C., et al.: Dipyridamole-thallium scanning in patients undergoing vascular surgery: Optimizing pre-operative evaluation of cardiac risk. JAMA 25:2185, 1987.

F

1. Fredman, B. J., Beihn, R., and Friedman, J. P.: The effect of hypoxia on thallium kinetics and cultured chick myocardial cells. J. Nucl. Med. 28:1453, 1987.
2. Freeman, M. R., Williams, A. E., Chisholm, R. J., et al.: Role of resting $thallium^{201}$ perfusion in predicting coronary anatomy, left ventricular wall motion, and hospital outcome in unstable angina pectoris. Am. Heart J. 117:306, 1989.
3. Faris, J. V., Burt, R. W., Graham, M. C., and Knoebel, S. B.: Thallium-201 myocardial scintigraphy: Improved sensitivity, specificity and predictive accuracy by application of a statistical image analysis algorithm. Am. J. Cardiol. 49:733, 1982.
4. Fintel, D. J., Links, J. M., Brinker, J. A., et al.: Improved diagnostic performance of exercise thallium-201 single photon emission computed tomography over planar imaging in the diagnosis of coronary artery disease: A receiver operating characteristic analysis. J. Am. Coll. Cardiol. 13:600, 1989.
5. Freedman, S. B., Dunn, R. D., Bernstein, L., et al.: Influence of coronary collateral blood flow on the development of exertional ischemia and Q wave infarction in patients with severe single-vessel disease. Circulation 71:681, 1985.
6. Francisco, D. A., Collins, S. M., Go, R. T., et al.: Tomographic thallium-201 myocardial perfusion scintigrams after maximal coronary artery vasodilation with intravenous dipyridamole: Comparison of qualitative and quantitative approaches. Circulation 66:370, 1982.
7. Follansbee, W. P., Curtiss, E. I., Medsger, T. A., Jr., et al.: Physiologic abnormalities of cardiac function in progressive systemic sclerosis with diffuse scleroderma. N. Engl. J. Med. 310:142, 1984.
8. Friedman, J., Van Train, K., Maddahi, J., et al.: "Upward creep" of the heart: A frequent source of false-positive reversible defects on Tl-201 stress-redistribution SPECT. (Abstract.) J. Nucl. Med. 27:899, 1986.
9. Freeman, M. R., Chisholm, R. J., and Armstrong, P. W.: Usefulness of exercise electrocardiography and thallium scintigraphy in unstable angina pectoris in predicting the extent and severity of coronary artery disease. Am. J. Cardiol. 62:1164, 1988.

G

1. Grunwald, A. M., Watson, D. D., Holzgrefe, H. H., Jr., et al.: Myocardial thallium-201 kinetics in normal and ischemic myocardium. Circulation 64:610, 1981.
2. Goldhaber, S. Z., Newell, J. B., Alpert, N. M., et al.: Effects of ischemic-like insult on myocardial thallium-201 accumulation. Circulation 67:778, 1983.
3. Gerry, J. L., Becker, L. C., Flaherty, J. T., and Weisfeldt, M. L.: Evidence for a flow-independent contribution to the phenomenon of thallium redistribution. Am. J. Cardiol. 45:58, 1980.
4. Gewirtz, H., Beller, G. A., Strauss, H. W., et al.: Transient defects of resting thallium scans in patients with coronary artery disease. Circulation 59:707, 1979.
5. Gibson, R. S., Watson, D. D., Taylor, G. J., et al.: Prospective assessment of

regional myocardial perfusion before and after coronary revascularization surgery by quantitative thallium-201 scintigraphy. J. Am. Coll. Cardiol. 1(3):804, 1983.
6. Gibson, R. S., Watson, D. D., Carabello, B. A., et al.: Clinical implications of increased lung uptake of thallium-201 during exercise scintigraphy two weeks after myocardial infarction. Am. J. Cardiol. 49:1586, 1982.
7. Garcia, E., Maddahi, J., Berman, D. S., and Waxman A: Space/time quantitation of thallium-201 myocardial scintigraphy. J. Nucl. Med. 22:309, 1981.
8. Gibson, R. S., and Beller, G. A.: Should exercise electrocardiographic testing be replaced by radioisotope methods? *In* Rahimtoola, S. H., Brest, A. N. (eds.): Controversies in Coronary Artery Disease. F. A. Davis, Philadelphia, 1982, pp. 1–31.
9. Gewirtz, H., Paladino, W., Sullivan, M., and Most, A. S.: Value and limitations of myocardial thallium washout rate in the noninvasive diagnosis of patients with triple-vessel coronary artery disease. Am. Heart J. 106:681, 1983.
10. Garcia, E. V., Van Train, K., Maddahi, J., et al.: Quantification of rotational thallium-201 myocardial tomography. J. Nucl. Med. 26:17, 1985.
11. Guiney, T. E., Pohost, G. M., McKusick, K. A., and Beller, G. A.: Differentiation of false- from true-positive ECG responses to exercise stress by thallium-201 perfusion imaging. Chest 80:4, 1981.
12. Gill, J. B., Ruddy, T. D., Newell, J. B., et al.: Prognostic importance of thallium uptake by the lungs during exercise in coronary artery disease. N. Engl. J. Med. 317:1485, 1987.
13. Gibson, R. S., Taylor, G. J., Watson, D. D., et al.: Predicting the extent and location of coronary artery disease during the early post-infarction period by quantitative thallium-201 scintigraphy. Am. J. Cardiol. 47:1010, 1981.
14. Gibson, R. S., Watson, D. D., Craddock, G. B., et al.: Prediction of cardiac events after uncomplicated myocardial infarction: A prospective study comparing predischarge exercise thallium-201 scintigraphy and coronary angiography. Circulation 68:321, 1983.
15. Gibson, R. S., Beller, G. A., Gheorghiade, M., et al.: The prevalence and clinical significance of residual myocardial ischemia 2 weeks after uncomplicated non-Q wave infarction: A prospective natural history study. Circulation 73:1186, 1986.
16. Greenberg, B. H., Hart, R., Botvinick, E. H., et al.: Thallium-201 myocardial perfusion scintigraphy to evaluate patients after coronary bypass surgery. Am. J. Cardiol. 42:167, 1978.
17. Granato, J. E., Watson, D. D., Flanagan, T. L., et al.: Myocardial thallium-201 kinetics during coronary occlusion and reperfusion: Influence of method of reflow and timing of thallium-201 administration. Circulation 73:150, 1986.
18. Granato, J. E., Watson, D. D., Flanagan, T. L., and Beller, G. A.: Myocardial thallium-201 kinetics and regional flow alterations with 3 hours of coronary occlusion and either rapid reperfusion through a totally patent vessel or slow reperfusion through a critical stenosis. J. Am. Coll. Cardiol. 9:109, 1987.
19. Genda, A., Mizuno, S., Nunoda, S., et al.: Clinical studies on diabetic myocardial disease using exercise testing with myocardial scintigraphy and endomyocardial biopsy. Clin. Cardiol. 9:375, 1986.
20. Gutgesell, H. P., Pinsky, W. W., and DePuey, E. G.: Thallium-201 myocardial perfusion imaging in infants and children. Value in distinguishing anomalous left coronary artery from congestive cardiomyopathy. Circulation 61:596, 1980.
21. Gibbons, R. J., Verani, M. S., Pellikka, P. A., et al.: Tomographic assessment of myocardial reperfusion during acute myocardial infarction using Tc-99m methoxy isobutyl isonitrile (MIBI). (Abstract.) J. Am. Coll. Cardiol. 13:153A, 1989.
22. Gerson, M.: Test accuracy, test selection and test result interpretation in chronic coronary artery disease. *In* Gerson, M. C. (ed.): Cardiac Nuclear Medicine. McGraw-Hill, New York, 1987, pp. 309–348.
23. Goris, M. L., Daspit, S. G., McLaughlin, P., et al.: Interpolative background subtraction. J. Nucl. Med. 17:744, 1976.

H

1. Holman, B. L., Jones, A. G., Lister-James, J., et al.: A new Tc-99m–labeled myocardial imaging agent, hexakis (t-butyliso-nitrile)-technetium(I) [Tc-99m TBI]: Initial experience in the human. J. Nucl. Med. 25:1350, 1984.
2. Hamilton, G. W., Trobaugh, G. B., Ritchie, J. L., et al.: Myocardial imaging with intravenously injected thallium-201 in patients with suspected coronary artery disease: Analysis of technique and correlation with electrocardiographic, coronary anatomic and ventriculographic findings. Am. J. Cardiol. 39:347, 1977.
3. Homma, S., Kaul, S., and Boucher, C. A.: Correlates of lung/heart ratio of thallium-201 and coronary artery disease. J. Nucl. Med. 28:1531, 1987.
4. Hung, J., Goris, M. L., Nash, E., et al.: Comparative value of maximal treadmill testing, exercise thallium myocardial perfusion scintigraphy and exercise radionuclide venriculography for distinguishing high- and low-risk patients soon after acute myocardial infarction. Am. J. Cardiol, 53:1221, 1984.
5. Hirzel, H. O., Nuesch, K., Sialer, R. G., et al.: Thallium-201 exercise myocardial imaging to evaluate myocardial perfusion after coronary bypass surgery. Br. Heart J. 43:426, 1980.
6. Hirzel, H. O., Nuesch, K., Gruentzig, A. R., and Luetolf, U. M.: Short- and long-term changes in myocardial perfusion after percutaneous transluminal coronary angioplasty assessed by thallium-201 exercise scintigraphy. Circulation 63:1001, 1981.
7. Heller, G. V., Parker, J. A., Silverman, K. J., et al.: Intracoronary thallium-201 scintigraphy after thrombolytic therapy for acute myocardial infarction compared with 10 and 100 day intravenous thallium-201 scintigraphy. J. Am. Coll. Cardiol. 9:300, 1987.
8. Homma, S., Callahan, R. J., Ameer, B., et al.: Usefulness of oral dipyridamole suspension for stress thallium imaging without exercise in the detection of coronary artery disease. Am. J. Cardiol. 57:503, 1986.
9. Homma, S., Gilliland, Y., Guiney, T. E., et al.: Safety of intravenous dipyridamole for stress testing with thallium imaging. Am. J. Cardiol. 59:152, 1987.
10. Hirzel, H. O., Senn, M., Nuesch, K., et al.: Thallium-201 scintigraphy in complete left bundle branch block. Am. J. Cardiol. 53:764, 1984.
11. Huerta, E. M., Padial, L. R., Beiras, J. M. C., et al.: Thalllium-201 exercise scintigraphy in patients having complete left bundle branch block with normal coronary arteries. Int. J. Cardiol. 16:43, 1987.
12. Hadjimiltiades, S., Watson, R., Hakki, A.-H., et al.: Relation between myocardial thallium-201 kinetics during exercise and quantitative coronary angiography in patients with one-vessel coronary artery disease. J. Am. Coll. Cardiol. 13:1301, 1989.

1. Iskandrian, A. S., Wasserman, L. A., Anderson, G. S., et al.: Merits of stress thallium-201 myocardial perfusion imaging in patients with inconclusive exercise electrocardiograms: Correlation with coronary angiograms. Am. J. Cardiol. 46:553, 1980.
2. Iskandrian, A. S., Hakki, A. H., and Kane-Marsch, S.: Prognostic implications of exercise thallium-201 scintigraphy in patients with suspected or known coronary artery disease. Am. Heart J. 110:135, 1985.
3. Iskandrian, A. S., Heo, J., DeCoskey, D., et al.: Use of exercise thallium-201 imaging for risk stratification of elderly patients with coronary artery disease. Am. J. Cardiol. 61:269, 1988.
4. Iskandrian, A. S., Scherer, H., Croll, M. N., et al.: Exercise ^{201}Thallium myocardial scans in patients with disease limited to the secondary branches of the left coronary system. Clin. Cardiol. 2:121, 1979.

K

1. Kaul, S., Chesler, D. A., Pohost, G. M., et al.: Influence of peak exercise heart rate on normal thallium-201 myocardial clearance. J. Nucl. Med. 27:26, 1986.
2. Kiat, H., Berman, D. S., Maddahi, J., et al.: Late reversibility of tomographic myocardial thallium-201 defects: An accurate marker of myocardial viability. J. Am. Coll. Cardiol. 12:1456, 1988.
3. Kronenberg, M. W., Robertson, R. M., Born, M. L., et al.: Thallium-201 uptake in variant angina: Probable demonstration of myocardial reactive hyperemia in man. Circulation 66:1332, 1982.
4. Khaw, B. A., Strauss, H. W., Pohost, G. M., et al.: Relation of immediate and delayed thallium-201 distribution to localization of iodine-125 antimyosin antibody in acute experimental myocardial infarction. Am. J. Cardiol. 51:1428,1983.
5. Kushner, F. G., Okada, R. D., Kirshenbaum, H. D., et al.: Lung thallium-201 uptake after stress testing in patients with coronary artery disease. Circulation 63:341, 1981.
6. Kiat, H., Maddahi, J., Roy, L. T., et al.: Comparison of technetium-99m methoxy isobutyl isonitrile and thallium-201 for evaluation of coronary artery disease by planar and tomographic methods. Am. Heart J. 117:1, 1989.
7. Kronage, J. F., Piwnica-Worms, D., and Holman, B. L.: Effect of metabolic inhibitors on Tc-MIBI uptake into cultured chick heart cells. (Abstract.) J. Nucl. Med. 29:820, 1988.
8. Kaul, S., Boucher, C. A., Newell, J. B., et al.: Determination of the quantitative thallium ranging variables that optimize detection of coronary artery disease. J. Am. Coll. Cardiol. 7:527, 1986.
9. Kaul, S., Lilly, D. R., Gascho, J. A., et al.: Prognostic utility of the exercise thallium-201 test in ambulatory patients with chest pain: Comparison with cardiac cathetrization. Circulation 77:745, 1988.
10. Kaul, S., Finkelstein, D. M., Homma, S., et al.: Superiority of quantitative exercise thallium-201 variables in determining long-term prognosis in ambulatory patients with chest pain: A comparison with cardiac catheterization. J. Am. Coll. Cardiol. 12:25, 1988.
11. Kaul, S., Keiss, M. C., Liu, P., et al.: Comparison of exercise electrocardiography and quantitative thallium imaging for one-vessel coronary artery disease. Am. J. Cardiol. 56:257, 1985.
12. Kanemoto, N., and Hor, G.: Improvement of regional myocardial perfusion following percutaneous transluminal coronary angioplasty in patients with coronary artery disease. Jap. Heart J. 26:495, 1985.
13. Kahan, A., Devaux, J. Y., Amor, B., et al.: Nifedipine and thallium-201 myocardial perfusion in progressive systemic sclerosis. N. Engl. J. Med. 314:1397, 1986.
14. Kotler, T. S., and Diamond, G. A.: The efficacy of exercise thallium-201 myocardial perfusion scintigraphy in the diagnosis, prognosis, and functional evaluation of coronary artery disease, Ann. Intern. Med. (in press).
15. Koss, J. H., Kobren, S. M., Grunwald, A. W., and Bodenheimer, M. M.: Role of exercise thallium-201 myocardial perfusion scintigraphy in predicting prognosis in suspected coronary artery disease. Am. J. Cardiol. 59:531, 1987.
16. Kahn, J. K., Carry, M. M., McGhie, I., et al.: Quantitation of postexercise lung thallium-201 uptake during single photon emission computed tomography. J. Nucl. Med. 30:288, 1989.
17. Kimball, B. P., Shurvell, B. L., Mildenberger, R. R., et al.: Abnormal thallium kinetics in postoperative coarctation of the aorta: Evidence for diffuse hypertension-induced vascular pathology. J. Am. Coll. Cardiol. 7:538, 1986.

L

1. Lebowitz, E., Greene, M. V., Fairchild, R., et al.: Thallium-201 for medical use. J. Nucl. Med. 16:151, 1975.

2. Leppo, J. A.: Myocardial uptake of thallium and rubidium during alterations in perfusion and oxygenation in isolated rabbit hearts. J. Nucl. Med. 28:878, 1987.
3. Leppo, J. A., MacNeil, P. B., Moring, A. F., and Apstein, C. S.: Separate effects of ischemia, hypoxia and contractility on thallium-201 kinetics in rabbit myocardium. J. Nucl. Med. 27:66, 1986.
4. Leppo, J., Rosenkrantz, J., Rosenthal, R., et al.: Quantitative thallium-201 redistribution with a fixed coronary stenosis in dogs. Circulation 63:632, 1981.
5. Lear, J. L., Raff, U., and Jain, R.: Reverse and pseudo redistribution of thallium-201 in healed myocardial infarction and normal negative thallium-201 washout in ischemia due to background oversubtraction. Am. J. Cardiol. 62:543, 1988.
6. Lahiri, A., O'Hara, M. J., Bowles, M. J., et al.: Influence of left ventricular function and severity of coronary artery disease on exercise-induced pulmonary thallium-201 uptake. Int. J. Cardiol. 5:475, 1984.
7. Levy, R., Rozanski, A., Berman, D. S., et al.: Analysis of the degree of pulmonary thallium washout after exercise in patients with coronary artery disease. J. Am. Coll. Cardiol. 2:719, 1983.
8. Leppo, J. A., and Moring, A. F.: An evaluation of technetium-labeled isonitrile analog as a myocardial imaging agent and comparison to Tl-201. (Abstract.) Circulation 74(Suppl. II):297, 1986.
9. Ladenheim, M. L., Pollock, B. H., Rozanski, A., et al.: Extent and severity of myocardial hypoperfusion as predictors of prognosis in patients with suspected coronary artery disease. J. Am. Coll. Cardiol. 7:464, 1986.
10. Leppo, J., Boucher, C. A., Okada, R. D., et al.: Serial thallium-201 myocardial imaging after dipyridamole infusion: Diagnostic utility in detecting coronary stenoses and relationship to regional wall motion. Circulation 66:649, 1982.
11. Leppo, J. A., O'Brien, J., Rothendler, J. A., et al.: Dipyridamole-thallium-201 scintigraphy in the prediction of future cardiac event after acute myocardial infarction. N. Engl. J. Med. 310:1014, 1984.
12. Leppo, J., Plaja, J., Gionet, M., et al.: Noninvasive evaluation of cardiac risk before elective vascular surgery. J. Am. Coll. Cardiol. 9:269, 1987.
13. Lahiri, A., Carboni, G. P., Crawley, J. W., and Raftery, E. B.: Reversible ischaemia of right ventricle detected by exercise thallium-201 scintigraphy. Br. Heart J. 48:260, 1982.
14. Lam, J. Y. T., Chaitman, B. R., Glaenzer, M., et al.: Safety and diagnostic accuracy of dipyridamole-thallium imaging in the elderly. J. Am. Coll. Cardiol. 11:585, 1988.

M

1. Melin, J. A., and Becker, L. C.: Quantitative relationship between global left ventricular thallium uptake and blood flow: Effects of propranolol, ouabain, dipyridamole and coronary artery occlusion. J. Nucl. Med. 27:641, 1986.
2. Moore, C. A., Cannon, J., Watson, D. D., et al.: Normal thallium-201 extraction despite marked regional left ventricular dysfunction in a canine model of "stunned myocardium." Circulation 81:1622, 1990.
3. Meerdink, D. J., Thurber, M., and Leppo, J.: Effects of ouabain and hypoxia on the myocardial extraction of thallium and a technetium-labeled isonitrile analogue. Circulation 76(Suppl. IV): IV–216, 1987.
4. Massie, D. M., Wisneski, J. A., Hollenberg, M., et al.: Quantitative analysis of seven-pinhole tomographic thallium-201 scintigrams: Improved sensitivity and estimation of the extent of coronary involvement by evaluation of radiotracer uptake and clearance. J. Am. Coll. Cardiol. 3:1178, 1984.
5. McCarthy, D. M., Blood, D. K., Sciacca, R. R, and Cannon, P. J.: Single dose myocardial perfusion imaging with thallium-201: Application in patients with nondiagnostic electrocardiographic stress test. Am. J. Cardiol. 43:899, 1979.
6. Murray, R. G., McKillop, J. H., Bessent, R. G., et al.: Evaluation of thallium-201 exercise scintigraphy in coronary heart disease. Br. Heart J. 41:568, 1979.
7. McCarthy, D. M., Sciacca, R. R., Blood, D. K., and Cannon, P. J.: Discriminant function analysis using thallium-201 scintiscans and exercise stress variables to predict the presence and extent of coronary artery disease. Am. J. Cardiol. 49:1917, 1982.
8. Maddahi, J., Garcia, E., Berman, D. S., et al.: Improved noninvasive assessment of coronary artery disease by quantitative analysis of regional stress myocardial distribution and washout of thallium-201. Circulation 64:924, 1981.
9. Manyari, D. E., Knudtson, M., Kloiber, R., and Roth, D.: Sequential thallium-201 myocardial perfusion studies after successful percutaneous transluminal coronary artery angioplasty: Delayed resolution of exercise-induced scintigraphic abnormalities. Circulation 77:86, 1988.
10. Miller, D. D., Liu, P., Strauss, H. W., et al.: Prognostic value of computer-quantitated exercise thallium imaging early after percutaneous transluminal coronary angioplasty. J. Am. Coll. Cardiol. 10:275, 1987.
11. Maddahi, J., Weiss, A. T., Garcia, E. V., et al.: Split-dose thallium-201 quantitative imaging for immediate post-reperfusion assessment of intravenous coronary thrombolysis. Eur. Heart J. 6:127, 1985 (Suppl. E).
12. Melin, J. A., Wijns, W., Keyeux, A., et al.: Assessment of thallium-201 redistribution versus glucose uptake as predictors of viability after coronary occlusion and reperfusion. Circulation 77:927, 1988.
13. Maddahi, J., Ganz, W., Ninomiya, K., et al.: Myocardial salvage by intracoronary thrombolysis in evolving acute myocardial infarction: Evaluation using intracoronary injection of thallium-201. Am. Heart J. 102:664, 1981.
14. Maddahi, J., Van Train, K. F., Prigent, F., et al.: Utility of Tl-201 myocardial rotational tomography with polar mapping for evaluation of patients without myocardial infarction. (Abstract.) Circulation 74(Suppl. II):42, 1986.
15. Makler, P. T., Lavine, S. J., Denenberg, B. S., et al.: Redistribution on the thallium scan in myocardial sarcoidosis: Concise communication. J. Nucl. Med. 22:428, 1981.
16. Moodie, D. S., Cook, S. A., Gill, C. C., and Napoli, C. A.: Thallium-201 myocardial imaging in young adults with anomalous left coronary artery arising from the pulmonary artery. J. Nucl. Med. 21:1076, 1980.
17. Manier, S. M., Blue, P. W., Abreu, S. H., et al.: Thallium-201 scintigraphy in anomalous origin of the coronary artery from the pulmonary artery: Ischemia masquerading as infarction. Am. J. Card. Imag. 1:267, 1987.
18. Maddahi, J., Abdulla, A., Garcia, E. V., et al.: Noninvasive identification of left main and triple vessel coronary artery disease: Improved accuracy using quantitative analysis of regional myocardial stress distribution and washout of thallium-201. J. Am. Coll. Cardiol. 7:53, 1986.
19. Makler, P. T., Lavine, S. J., Derenberg, B. S., et al.: Redistribution on the thallium scan in myocardial sarcoidosis: Concise communication. J. Nucl. Med. 22:428, 1981.
20. Manno, B. V., Burka, E. R., Hakki, A.-H., et al.: Biventricular function in sickle-cell anemia: Radionuclide angiographic and thallium-201 scintigraphic evaluation. Am. J. Cardiol. 52:584, 1983.
21. McDonnell, P. J., Becker, L. C., and Bulkley, B. H.: Thallium imaging in cardiac lymphoma. Am. Heart J. 101:809, 1981.

N

1. Nielson, A. T., Morris, K. G., Murdock, R., et al.: Linear relationship between the distribution of thallium-201 and blood flow in ischemic and non-ischemic myocardium during exercise. Circulation 61:797, 1980.
2. Nishiyama, H., Adolph, R., Gabel, M., et al.: Effective coronary blood flow on thallium-201 uptake and washout. Circulation 65:534, 1982.
3. Nohara, R., Kambara, H., Suzuki, Y., et al.: Stress scintigraphy using single-photon emission computed tomography in the evaluation of coronary artery disease. Am. J. Cardiol. 53:1250, 1984.
4. Nygaard, T. W., Gibson, R. S., Ryan, J. M., et al.: Prevalence of high risk thallium-201 scintigraphic findings in left main coronary artery stenosis: Comparison with patients with multiple- and single-vessel coronary artery disease. Am. J. Cardiol. 53:462, 1984.
5. Nesto, R. W., Phillips, R. T., Kett, K. G., et al.: Angina and exertional myocardial ischemia in diabetic and nondiabetic patients: Assessment by exercise thallium scintigraphy. Ann. Intern. Med. 108:170, 1988.

O

1. Okada, R. D., Jacobs, M. L., Daggett, W. M., et al.: Thallium-201 kinetics in nonischemic myocardium. Circulation 65:70, 1982.
2. Okada, R. D.: Myocardial kinetics of thallium-201 after stress in normal and perfusion-reduced canine myocardium. Am. J. Cardiol. 56:969, 1985.
3. Okada, R. D., Leppo, J. A., Strauss, H. W., et al.: Mechanisms and time course for the disappearance of thallium-201 defects at rest in dogs: Relation of time to peak activity to myocardial blood flow. Am. J. Cardiol. 49:699, 1982.
4. Okada, R. D., Glover, D., Gaffney, T., and Williams, S.: Myocardial kinetics of technetium-99m-hexakis–2-methoxy-2-methal-propyl-isonitrile. Circulation 77:491, 1988.
5. Osbakken, M. D., Okada, R. D., Boucher, C. A., et al.: Comparison of exercise perfusion and ventricular function imaging: An analysis of factors affecting the diagnostic accuracy of each technique. J. Am. Coll. Cardiol. 3:272, 1984.
6. Okada, R. D., Dai, Y. H., Boucher, C. A., and Pohost, G. M.: Serial thallium-201 imaging after dipyridamole for coronary disease detection: Quantitative analysis using myocardial clearance. Am. Heart J. 107:475, 1984.
7. Okada, R. D., Lim, Y. L., Rothendler, J., et al.: Split dose thallium-201 dipyridamole imaging: A new technique for obtaining thallium images before and immediately after an intervention. J. Am. Coll. Cardiol. 1:1302, 1983.
8. O'Gara, P. T., Bonow, R. O., Maron, B. J., et al.: Myocardial perfusion abnormalities in patients with hypertrophic cardiomyopathy: Assessment with thallium-201 emission computed tomography. Circulation 76:1214, 1987.
9. Okada, R. D., Dai, Y.-H., Boucher, C. A., and Pohost, G. M.: Significance of increased lung thallium-201 activity on serial cardiac images after dipyridamole treatment in coronary artery disease. Am. J. Cardiol. 53:470, 1984.
10. Ohsuzu, F., Handa, S., Kondo, M., et al.: Thallium-201 myocardial imaging to evaluate right ventricular loading. Circulation 61:620, 1980.

P

1. Pohost, G. M., Zir, L. M., Moore, R. H., et al.: Differentiation of transiently ischemic from infarcted myocardium by serial imaging after a single dose of thallium-201. Circulation 55:294, 1977.
2. Pohost, G. M., Okada, R. D., O'Keefe, D. B., et al.: Thallium redistribution in dogs with severe coronary artery stenosis of fixed caliber. Circ. Res. 48:439, 1981.
3. Pamelia, F. X., Gibson, R. S., Watson, D. D., et al.: Prognosis with chest pain and normal thallium-201 exercise scintigrams. Am. J. Cardiol. 55:920, 1985.
4. Patterson, R. E., Horowitz, S. F., Eng, C., et al.: Can noninvasive exercise test criteria identify patients with left main or three-vessel coronary disease after a first myocardial infarction? Am. J. Cardiol. 51:361, 1983.
5. Port, S. C., Oshima, M., Ray, G., et al.: Assessment of single vessel coronary artery disease: Results of exercise electrocardiography, thallium-201 myocardial perfusion imaging and radionuclide angiography. J. Am. Coll. Cardiol. 6:75, 1985.
6. Pearlman, J. D., and Boucher, C. A.: Diagnostic value for coronary artery disease of chest pain during dipyridamole-thallium stress testing. Am. J. Cardiol. 61:43, 1988.

R

1. Rothendler, J. A., Boucher, C. A., Strauss, H. W., et al.: Decrease in the ability to detect elevated lung thallium due to delay in commencing imaging after exercise. Am. Heart J. 110:830, 1985.
2. Ritchie, J. L., Trobaugh, G. B., Hamilton, G. W., et al.: Myocardial imaging with thallium-201 at rest and during exercise: Comparison with coronary arteriography and resting and stress electrocardiography. Circulation 56:66, 1977.
3. Ritchie, J. L., Zaret, D. L., Strauss, H. W., et al.: Myocardial imaging with thallium-201: A multicenter study in patients with angina pectoris or acute myocardial infarction. Am. J. Cardiol. 42:345, 1978.
4. Rigo, P., Bailey, I. K., Griffith, L. S. C., et al.: Stress thallium-201 myocardial scintigraphy for the detection of individual coronary arterial lesions in patients with and without previous myocardial infarction. Am. J. Cardiol. 48:209, 1981.
5. Rigo, P., Becker, L. C., Griffith, L. S. C., et al.: Influence of coronary collateral vessels on the results of thallium-201 myocardial stress imaging. Am. J. Cardiol. 44:452, 1979.
6. Reisman, S., Maddahi, J., Van Train, K., et al.: Quantitation of extent, depth, and severity of planar thallium defects in patients undergoing exercise thallium-201 scintigraphy. J. Nucl. Med. 27:1273, 1986.
7. Robinson, T. S., Williams, B. T., Webb-Peploe, M. M., et al.: Thallium-201 myocardial imaging and assessment of results of aorto-coronary bypass surgery. Br. Heart J. 42:455, 1979.
8. Ritchie, J. L., Narahara, K. A., Trobaugh, J. B., et al.: Thallium-201 myocardial imaging before and after coronary revascularization: Assessment of regional myocardial blood flow and graft patency. Circulation 56:830, 1977.
9. Ruddy, T. D., Gill, J. B., Finkelstein, D. M., et al.: Myocardial uptake and clearance of thallium-201 in normal subjects: Comparison of dipyridamole-induced hyperemia with exercise stress. J. Am. Coll. Cardiol. 10:547, 1987.
10. Ruddy, T. D., Dighero, H. R., Newell, J. B., et al.: Quantitative analysis of dipyridamole-thallium images for the detection of coronary artery disease. J. Am. Coll. Cardiol. 10:142, 1987.
11. Rothbart, R. M., Beller, G. A., Watson, D. D., et al.: Diagnostic accuracy and prognostic significance of quantitative thallium-201 scintigraphy in patients with left bundle branch block. Am. J. Noninvas. Cardiol. 1:197, 1987.
12. Rajfer, S. I., Oetgen, W. J., Weeks, K. D., Jr., et al.: Thallium-201 scintigraphy after surgical repair of hemodynamically significant primary coronary artery anomalies. Chest 81:687, 1982.
13. Reed, D. C., Beller, G. A., Nygaard, T. W., et al.: The clinical efficacy and scintigraphic evaluation of post-coronary bypass patients undergoing percutaneous transluminal coronary angioplasty for recurrent angina pectoris. Am. Heart J. 117:60, 1989.

S

1. Strauss, H. W., Harrison, K., Langan, J. K., et al.: Thallium-201 for myocardial imaging: Relation of thallium-201 to regional myocardial perfusion. Circulation 51:641, 1975.
2. Schwartz, J. S., Ponto, R., Carlyle, P., et al.: Early redistribution of thallium-201 after temporary ischemia. Circulation 57:332, 1982.
3. Schelbert, H. R., Schuler, G., Ashburn, W. L., and Covell, J. W.: Time-course of "redistribution" of thallium-201 administered during transient ischemia. Eur. J. Nucl. Med. 4:351, 1979.
4. Steingart, R. M., Bontemps, R., Scheuer, J., and Yipintsoi, T.: Gamma camera quantitation of thallium-201 redistribution at rest in a dog model. Circulation 65:542, 1982.
5. Sonnemaker, R. E., Floyd, J. L., Nusynowitz, M. L., et al.: Single injection thallium-201 stress and redistribution myocardial perfusion imaging: Comparisons with stress electrocardiography and coronary arteriography. Radiology 131:199, 1979.
6. Smeets, J. P., Rigo, P., Legrand, V., et al.: Prognostic value of thallium-201 stress myocardial scintigraphy with exercise ECG after myocardial infarction. Cardiology 68:67, 1981(Suppl. 2).
7. Smucker, M. L., Beller, G. A., Watson, D. D., and Kaul, S.: Left ventricular dysfunction in excess of the size of infarction: A possible management strategy. Am. Heart J. 115:749, 1988.
8. Sbarbaro, J. A., Karunaratne, H., Cantez, S., et al.: Thallium-201 imaging and assessment of aorto-coronary artery bypass graft patency. Br. Heart J. 42:553, 1979.
9. Scholl, J. M., Chaitman, B. R., David, P. R., et al.: Exercise electrocardiography and myocardial scintigraphy in the serial evaluation of the results of percutaneous transluminal coronary angioplasty. Circulation 66:380, 1982.
10. Stuckey, T. D., Burwell, L. R., Nygaard, T. W., et al.: Value of quantitative exercise thallium-201 scintigraphy for predicting angina recurrence after percutaneous transluminal coronary angioplasty. Am. J. Cardiol. 65:517, 1989.
11. Simoons, M. L., Wijns, W., Balakumaran, K., et al.: The effect of intracoronary thrombolysis with streptokinase on myocardial thallium distribution and left ventricular function assessed by blood-pool scintigraphy. Eur. Heart J. 3:433, 1982.
12. Suzuki, Y., Kadota, K., Nohara, R., et al.: Recognition of regional hypertrophy in hypertrophic cardiomyopathy using thallium-201 emission-computed tomography: Comparison with two-dimensional echocardiography. Am. J. Cardiol. 53:1095, 1984.
13. Schulman, D. S., Francis, C. K., Black, H. R., and Wackers, F. J. T.: Thallium-201 stress imaging in hypertensive patients. Hypertension 10:16, 1987.
14. Seldin, D. W., Johnson, L. L., Blood, D. K., et al.: Myocardial perfusion imaging with technetium-99m SQ30217: Comparison with thallium-201 and coronary anatomy. J. Nucl. Med. 30:312, 1989.
15. Sinusas, A. J., Beller, G. A., Smith, W. H., et al.: Quantitative planar imaging with technetium-99m methoxy-isobutyl isonitrile: Comparison of uptake patterns with thallium-201. J. Nucl. Med. 30:1456, 1989.
16. Sinusas, A. J., Watson, D. D., and Beller, G. A.: Effect of ischemia and post-ischemic dysfunction on myocardial uptake of Tc-99m labeled methoxy-isobutyl isonitrile and thallium-201. J. Am. Coll. Cardiol. 14:1785, 1989.
17. Schicha, H., Rentrop, P., Facorro, L., et al.: Predictive value of thallium scintigraphy in coronary artery disease. Clin. Cardiol. 3:184, 1980.

T

1. Taillefer, R., Lette, J., Phaneuf, D.-C., et al.: Thallium-201 myocardial imaging during pharmacologic coronary vasodilation: Comparison of oral and intravenous administration of dipyridamole. J. Am. Coll. Cardiol. 8:76, 1986.
2. Tamaki, N., Yonekura, Y., Mukai, T., et al.: Stress thallium-201 transaxial emission computed tomography: Quantitative versus qualitative analysis for evaluation of coronary artery disease. J. Am. Coll. Cardiol. 4:1213, 1984.
3. Tono-oka, I., Satoh, S., Kanaya, T., et al.: Alterations in myocardial perfusion during exercise after isosorbide dinitrate infusion in patients with coronary disease: Assessment by thallium-201 scintigraphy. Am. Heart J. 111:525, 1986.
4. Turner, J. D., Schwartz, K. M., Logic, J. R., et al.: Detection of residual jeopardized myocardium 3 weeks after myocardial infarction by exercise testing with thallium-201 myocardial scintigraphy. Circulation 61:729, 1980.
5. Topol, E. J., Burek, K., O'Neill, W. W., et al.: A randomized controlled trial of hospital discharge three days after myocardial infarction in the era of reperfusion. N. Engl. J. Med. 318:1083, 1988.
6. Tamaki, N., Yonekura, Y., Kadota, K., et al.: Thallium-201 myocardial perfusion imaging in myocarditis. Clin. Nucl. Med. 10:562, 1985.
7. Taillefer, R., Laflamme, L., Dupras, G., et al.: Myocardial perfusion imaging with ^{99m}Tc-methoxy-isobutyl-isonitrile (MIBI): Comparison of short and long time intervals between rest and stress injections. Preliminary results. Eur. J. Nucl. Med. 13:515, 1988.
8. Touchstone, D. A., Beller, G. A., Nygaard, T. W., et al.: Functional significance of predischarge exercise thallium-201 findings following intravenous streptokinase therapy during acute myocardial infarction. Am. Heart J. 116:1500, 1988.
9. Tubau, J. F., Szlachcic, J., Hollenberg, M., and Massie, B. M.: Usefulness of thallium-201 scintigraphy in predicting the development of angina pectoris in hypertensive patients with left ventricular hypertrophy. Am. J. Cardiol. 64:45, 1989.

U

1. Uhl, G., Kay, T. N., Hickman, J. R., et al.: Detection of coronary artery disease in asymptomatic aircrew members with thallium-201 scintigraphy. Aviat. Environ. Med. 51:1250, 1980.
2. Uhl, G. S., Kay, T. N., and Hickman, J. R., Jr.: Computer-enhanced thallium scintigrams in asymptomatic men with abnormal exercise tests. Am. J. Cardiol. 48:1077, 1981.

V

1. Verani, M. S., Marcus, M. L., Razzak, M. A., and Ehrhardt, J. C.: Sensitivity and specificity of thallium-201 perfusion scintigrams under exercise and the diagnosis of coronary artery disease. J Nucl Med 19:773, 1978.
2. Verani, M. S., Jhingran, S., Attar, M., et al.: Poststress redistribution of thallium-201 in patients with coronary artery disease, with and without prior myocardial infarction. Am. J. Cardiol. 43:1114, 1979.
3. Verani, M. S., Marcus, M. L., Spoto, G., et al.: Thallium-201 myocardial perfusion scintigrams in the evaluation of aorto-coronary saphenous bypass surgery. J. Nucl. Med. 19:765, 1978.
4. Verani, M. S., Tadros, S., Raizner, A. E., et al.: Quantitative analysis of thallium-201 uptake and washout before and after transluminal coronary angioplasty. Int. J. Cardiol. 13:109, 1986.
5. Verani, M. S., Jeroudi, M. O., Mahmarian, J. J., et al.: Quantification of myocardial infarction during coronary occlusion and myocardial salvage after reperfusion using cardiac imaging with technetium-99m hexakis 2-methoxyisobutyl isonitrile. J. Am. Coll. Cardiol. 12:1573, 1988.
6. Villenueva, F. S., Watson, D. D., Smith, W. H., et al.: Significance of increased lung/heart ratio on dipyridamole thallium-201 scintigraphy. (Abstract.) Circulation 80 (Suppl. II):II–210, 1989.
7. Varma, S. K., Watson, D. D., and Beller, G. A.: Quantitative comparison of thallium-201 scintigraphy following exercise and dipyridamole. Am. J. Cardiol. 64:871, 1989.
8. Van Train, K. F., Berman, D. S., Garcia, E. V., et al.: Quantitative analysis of stress thallium-201 myocardial scintigrams: A multicenter trial. J. Nucl. Med. 27:17, 1986.

W

1. Weich, H. F., Strauss, H. W., and Pitt, B.: The extraction of thallium-201 by the myocardium. Circulation 56:188, 1977.
2. Wharton, T. P., Neill, W. A., Oxendien, J. M., and Painter, L. N.: Effect of duration of regional myocardial ischemia and degree of reactive hyperemia on the magnitude of the initial thallium-201 defect. Circulation 62:516, 1980.
3. Wilson, R. A., Okada, R. D., Barlai-Kovach, M., and Strauss, H. W.: The

effect of glucose-insulin-potassium on thallium-201 myocardial redistribution. Int. J. Nucl. Med. Biol. 12:97, 1985.

4. Wilson, R. A., Okada, R. D., Strauss, H. W., and Pohost, G. M.: Effect of glucose-insulin-potassium infusion on thallium myocardial clearance. Circulation 68:203, 1983.
5. Weiss, A. T., Maddahi, J., Lew, A. S., et al.: Reverse redistribution of thallium-201: A sign of nontransmural myocardial infarction with patency of the infarct-related coronary artery. J. Am. Coll. Cardiol. 7:61, 1986.
6. Wilson, R. A., Okada, R. D., Boucher, C. A., et al.: Radionuclide-determined changes in pulmonary blood volume and thallium lung uptake in patients with coronary artery disease. Am. J. Cardiol. 51:741, 1983.
7. Wackers, F. J. T., Berman, D. S., Maddahi, J., et al.: Technetium-99m hexakis 2-methoxyisobutyl isonitrile: Human biodistribution, dosimetry, safety, and preliminary comparison to thallium-201 myocardial perfusion imaging. J. Nucl. Med. 30:301, 1989.
8. Wackers, F. J. T., Fetterman, R. C., Mattera, J. A., and Clements, J. P.: Quantitative planar thallium-201 stress scintigraphy: A critical evaluation of the method. Semin. Nucl. Med. 15:46, 1985.
9. Watson, D. D., Campbell, N. P., Read, E. K., et al.: Spatial and temporal quantitation of plane thallium myocardial images. J. Nucl. Med. 22:577, 1981.
10. Wackers, F. J.-Th., Russo, D. J., Russo, D., and Clements, J. P.: Prognostic significance of normal quantitative planar thallium-201 stress scintigraphy in patients with chest pain. J. Am. Coll. Cardiol. 6:27, 1985.
11. Weiss, A. T., Berman, D. S., Lew, A. S., et al.: Transient ischemic dilation of the left ventricle on stress thallium-201 scintigraphy: A marker of severe and extensive coronary artery disease. J. Am. Coll. Cardiol. 9:752, 1987.
12. Wilson, W. W., Gibson, R. S., Nygaard, T. W., et al.: Acute myocardial infarction associated with single vessel coronary artery disease: An analysis of clinical outcome and the prognostic importance of vessel patency and residual ischemic myocardium. J. Am. Coll. Cardiol. 11:223, 1988.
13. Wijns, W., Serruys, P. W., Simoons, M. L., et al.: Predictive value of early maximal exercise test and thallium scintigraphy after successful percutaneous transluminal coronary angioplasty. Br. Heart J. 53:194, 1985.
14. Wijns, W., Serruys, P. W., Reiber, J. H., et al.: Early detection of restenosis after successful percutaneous transluminal coronary angioplasty by exercise-redistribution thallium scintigraphy. Am. J. Cardiol. 55:357, 1985.
15. Walker, P. R., James, M. A., Wilde, R. P. H., et al.: Dipyridamole combined with exercise for thallium-201 myocardial imaging. Br. Heart J. 55:321, 1986.
16. Wahl, J. M., Hakki, A. H., and Iskandrian, A. S.: Prognostic implications of normal exercise thallium-201 images. Arch. Intern. Med. 145:253, 1985.

Y

1. Yamamoto, S., Matsushima, H., Suzuki, A., et al.: A comparative study of thallium-201 single-photon emission computed tomography and electrocardiography in Duchenne and other types of muscular dystrophy. Am. J. Cardiol. 61:836, 1988.
2. Yamaguchi, S., Tsuiki, K., Hayasaka, M., and Yasui, S.: Segmental wall motion abnormalities in dilated cardiomyopathy: Hemodynamic characteristics and comparison with thallium-201 myocardial scintigraphy. Am. Heart J. 113:1123, 1987.

Z

1. Zaret, B. L., Strauss, H. W., Martin, N. D., et al.: Noninvasive regional myocardial perfusion with radioactive potassium: Study of patients at rest, exercise and during angina pectoris. N. Engl. J. Med. 288:809, 1973.

Chapter 59

Infarct Avid Imaging

- JAMES T. WILLERSON, M.D. ▪ IAIN McGHIE, M.D.
- ROBERT W. PARKEY, M.D. ▪ FREDERICK J. BONTE, M.D.
- L. MAXIMILIAN BUJA, M.D. ▪ JAMES R. CORBETT, M.D.

CELLULAR ALTERATIONS THAT OCCUR DURING EXPERIMENTAL MYOCARDIAL ISCHEMIA ... 1074
MITOCHONDRIAL INCLUSIONS IN DAMAGED CELLS ... 1074
INTERRELATIONSHIPS BETWEEN CALCIUM DEPOSITION AND Tc-99m-PPi DEPOSITION IN IRREVERSIBLY DAMAGED MYOCARDIAL CELLS ... 1077
Tc-99m-PPi CONCENTRATION IN IRREVERSIBLY DAMAGED MYOCARDIUM ... 1079
SITES AND MECHANISMS OF LOCALIZATION OF Tc-99m-PPi IN ACUTE MYOCARDIAL INFARCTS ... 1079
DETECTION WITH Tc-99m-PPi OF MYOCARDIAL INFARCTION IN PATIENTS ... 1080
SENSITIVITY OF Tc-99m-PPi ... 1080
SIZING OF ACUTE MYOCARDIAL INFARCTS WITH Tc-99m-PPi ... 1080
ESTIMATES OF INFARCT SIZE PRODUCED BY TEMPORARY CORONARY ARTERY OCCLUSION AND REPERFUSION WITH Tc-99m-PPi ... 1083
OTHER INFARCT AVID IMAGING AGENTS ... 1083

Myocardial scintigraphy with the infarct avid tracer, Tc-99m-pyrophosphate (Tc-99m-PPi), has been used widely to detect, localize, and size acute myocardial infarction in patients.[B1, C1, C2, F1, P1, R1, W1] The potential for using Tc-99m-PPi for the noninvasive detection of region(s) of myocardial necrosis was suggested initially by the observations of Shen and Jennings[S1] and D'Agostino.[D1] These investigators demonstrated that calcium is deposited in crystalline and subcrystalline form in irreversibly damaged myocardial cells. These early observations led Bonte and associates to speculate that Tc-99m-PPi might provide a means of identifying myocardial infarct cells, reasoning that pyrophosphate might complex with calcium deposited in crystalline or precrystalline form in irreversibly damaged myocardial cells.[B2] Subsequent experimental animal and extensive clinical studies at our institution and elsewhere have confirmed that Tc-99m-PPi concentrates in regions of irreversible myocardial damage (Figs. 59–1 and 59–2) and, thus, provides a relatively noninvasive means to detect, localize, and estimate the size of acute myocardial infarcts.*

Cellular Alterations That Occur During Experimental Myocardial Ischemia

Fixed experimental coronary artery occlusion and temporary coronary artery occlusion for at least 40 minutes followed by reperfusion are associated with the development of alterations in cell membrane integrity.[B8, C6, C7, J3, J4, K2, K3, L2, T1, W6, W7] Alterations in sarcolemmal and subcellular membrane integrity contribute to the development of cell and mitochondrial swelling (Fig. 59–3), followed by marked myofibrillar hypercontraction and the distortion of cellular architecture, including segmentation of edematous cytoplasm into subsarcolemmal blebs.[B8, C6, C7, J3, J4, K2, K3, L2, T1, W6, W7] With relatively short periods of coronary artery occlusion, only a minority of myocardial cells are altered, but if the period of myocardial ischemia is prolonged, more muscle cells demonstrate these changes. Cell swelling and interstitial edema are most prominent with temporary coronary artery occlusion followed by reperfusion, but cell swelling without interstitial edema also occurs with longer periods of fixed coronary artery occlusion. In most experimental models of myocardial ischemia and in patients, initial cellular alterations occur in subendocardial tissue, with subsequent spread of the damage into subepicardial regions. The development of abnormal myocardial fluid retention and the loss of cell volume regulation appear to precede the development of extensive myocardial necrosis, as judged by both ultrastructural and biochemical criteria.[W7] Direct evidence of altered cell membrane integrity following temporary and permanent coronary artery occlusion for periods lasting up to 1 hour is available from the demonstration of structural breaks in cell membrane integrity, the electron microscopic identification of the development of mitochondrial edema, and the accumulation of various tracers ordinarily excluded from the interior of cells, including lanthanum, various molecular weight proteins, and Tc-99m-PPi.[B8, C7, K3, L2, T1, W6, W7]

Early during the time period following ischemic injury, a minority of muscle cells within the damaged region demonstrates changes indicative of irreversible cellular injury, including flocculent mitochondrial densities, marked mitochondrial calcification, severe myofibrillar disruption, and breaks of plasma membranes. The number of muscle cells showing such changes progressively increases with duration and severity of the ischemic insult. Temporary coronary artery occlusion followed by reperfusion is particularly likely to be associated with multiple structural breaks in the plasma membrane as early as 40 to 60 minutes after coronary artery occlusion.[J4, K3, W6, W7] Although small defects in the plasma membrane have been observed after 40 to 60 minutes of permanent coronary artery occlusion,[J4] longer periods of permanent coronary artery occlusion are necessary to demonstrate prominent structural alterations in cell membrane integrity.[B4, J3, W7]

Mitochondrial Inclusions in Damaged Cells

At least two types of mitochondrial inclusions may be identified in necrotic muscle cells of myocardial infarcts produced by

*References B1, B3–7, C1–5, F1, H1, J1, J2, K1, L1, P1–P4, R1–3, S2, W1–5.

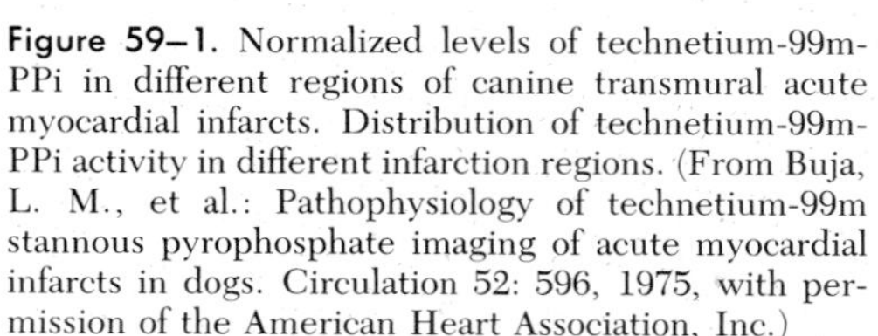

Figure 59–1. Normalized levels of technetium-99m-PPi in different regions of canine transmural acute myocardial infarcts. Distribution of technetium-99m-PPi activity in different infarction regions. (From Buja, L. M., et al.: Pathophysiology of technetium-99m stannous pyrophosphate imaging of acute myocardial infarcts in dogs. Circulation 52: 596, 1975, with permission of the American Heart Association, Inc.)

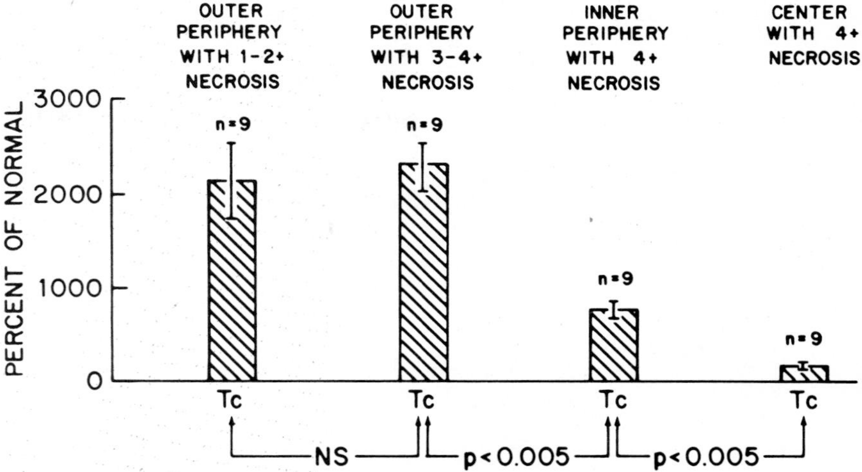

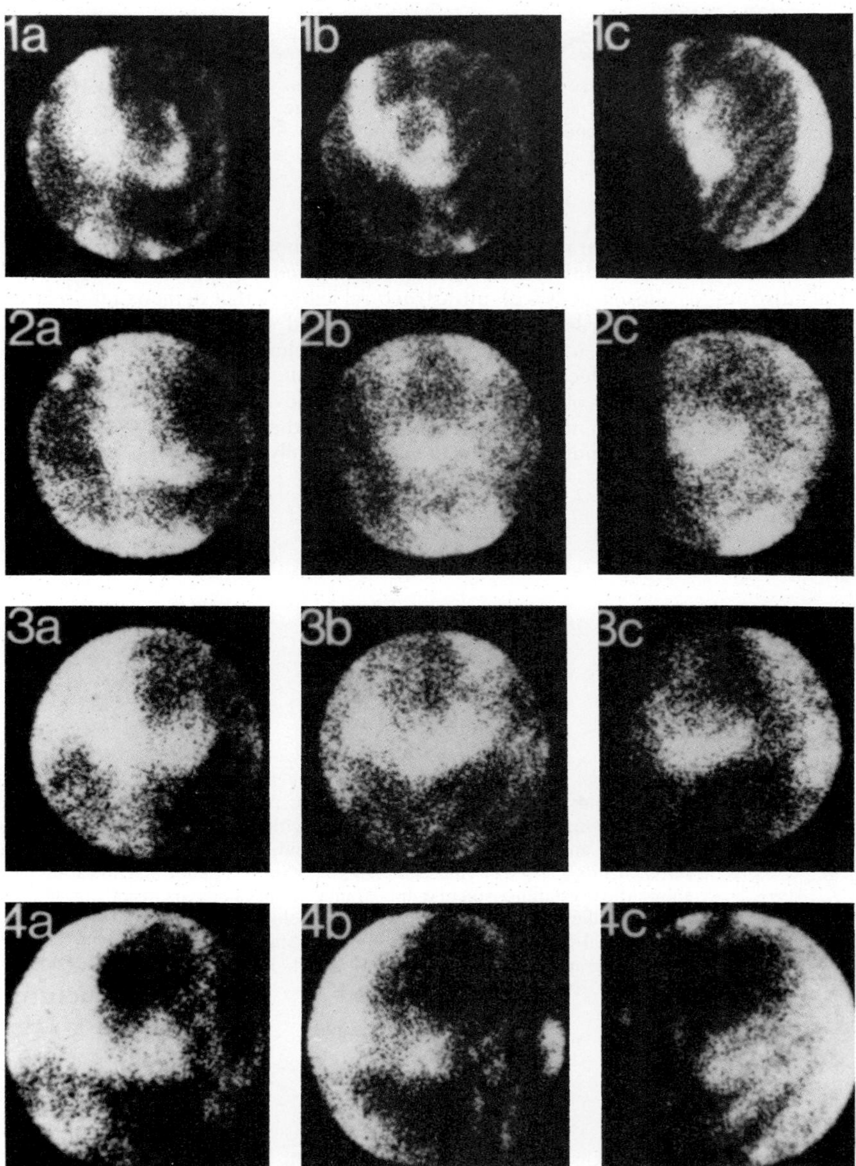

Figure 59–2. The various patterns of Tc-99m-PPi uptake with acute myocardial infarcts in patients. In each set of figures, Panel *A* is an anterior view, Panel *B* a left anterior oblique view, and Panel *C* a left lateral view. Panels 1a, 1b, and 1c demonstrate a large anterolateral myocardial infarct with a "doughnut" pattern; Panels 2a, 2b, and 2c demonstrate an inferior myocardial infarct; Panels 3a, 3b, and 3c demonstrate an inferior lateral and posterior myocardial infarct with some septal uptake; and Panels 4a, 4b, and 4c demonstrate a true posterior myocardial infarct. (From Willerson, J. T., et al.: Circulation 51:1046, 1975. By permission of the American Heart Association, Inc.)

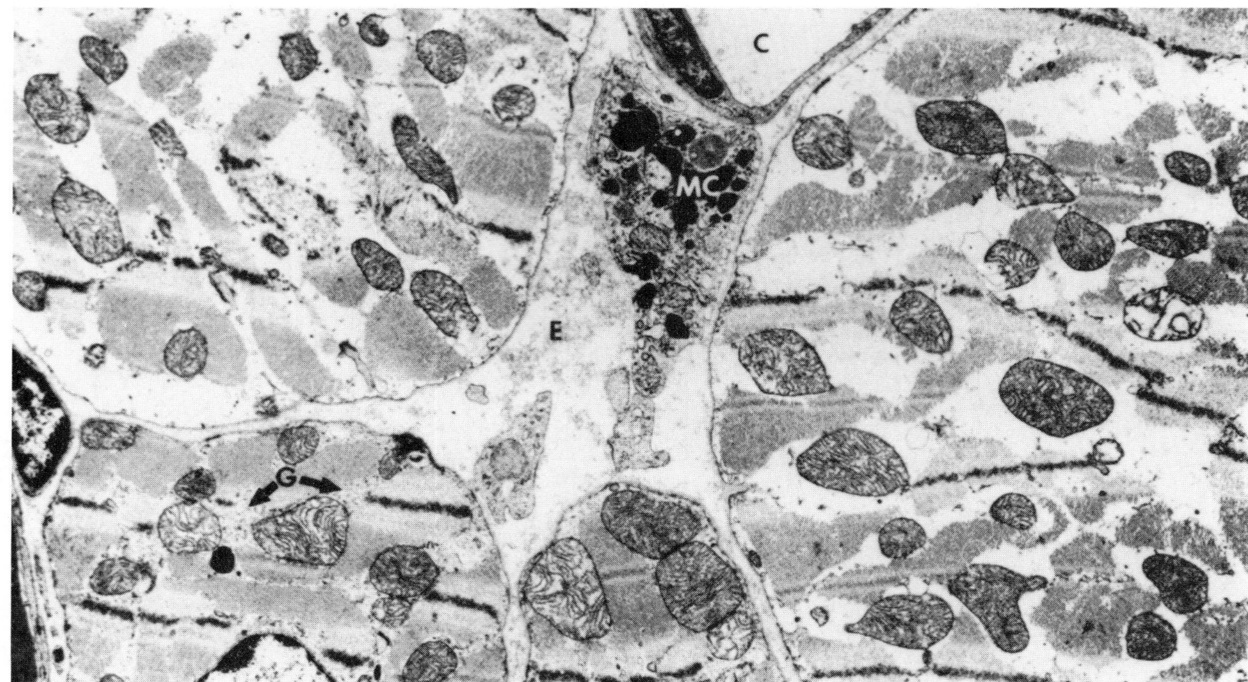

Figure 59–3. Posterior papillary muscle from isolated heart with 40-minute temporary circumflex coronary occlusion and reflow. Two muscle cells exhibit prominent swelling with marked separation of organelles, glycogen depletion, and focal mitochondrial damage. Adjacent muscle cells do not exhibit swelling and contain glycogen deposits *(G)*. The interstitial space is widened and contains precipitated edema fluid *(E)*. The capillary *(C)* and adjacent mast cell *(MC)* are normal. (X6400.) (From Willerson, J. T., et al.: Abnormal myocardial fluid retention as an early manifestation of ischemic injury. Am. J. Pathol. 87:159, 1977, with permission.)

permanent coronary artery occlusion (Fig. 59–4).[B9, H2] Inclusions of the first type are characterized by the presence of variable amounts of very electron-dense material and exhibit a substructure consisting of aggregates of thin spicules (Fig. 59–4). These spicular inclusions range from 500 to 4000 Å in diameter.[B9] The second type of inclusions is composed of moderately electron-dense amorphous material. These are devoid of very electron-dense spicular material (Fig. 59–4). The amorphous inclusions range from 750 to 2000 Å in diameter.[B9]

In the most severely damaged subendocardial regions of myocardial infarcts, there is a homogeneous population of abnormal muscle cells with ultrastructural features that demonstrate relaxed myofibrils, prominent I bands, and swollen mitochondria and contain a uniform population of inclusions composed of moderately electron-dense amorphous material. Muscle cells from the centers of the infarcts are usually devoid of very electron-dense spicular material. Cells containing the spicular as well as amorphous mitochondrial inclusions usually exhibit contracted myofi-

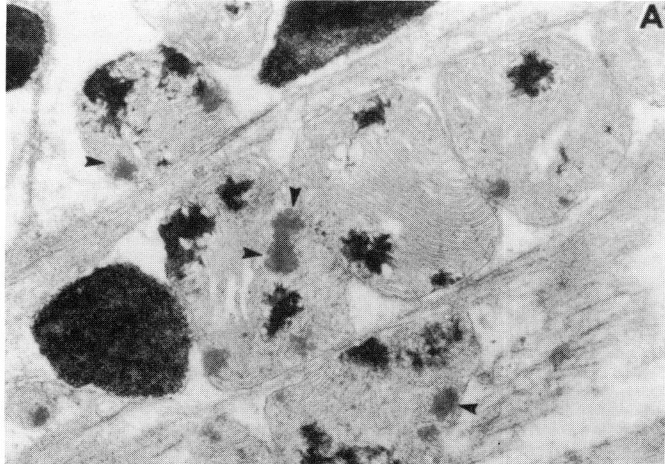

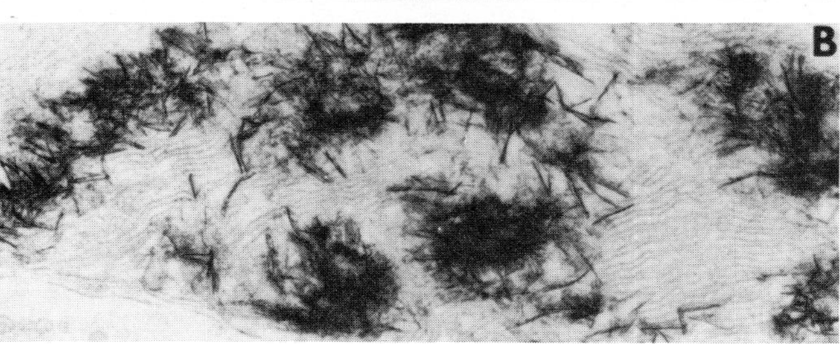

Figure 59–4. *A*, Necrotic muscle cell from periphery of canine infarct has disrupted myofibrils and mitochondria with very electron-dense calcific inclusions and moderately dense flocculent (amorphous matrix) densities *(arrowheads)*. Electron micrograph × 32,500. *B*, Higher magnification view shows the crystalline, spicular appearance of the calcific inclusions. × 65,870. (From Willerson, J. T., et al.: Pathophysiologic considerations and clinicopathological correlates of technetium-99m stannous pyrophosphate myocardial scintigraphy. Semin. Nucl. Med. 10:54, 1980, with permission.)

brils and are primarily located at the peripheries of myocardial infarcts.

Electron microscopic studies have demonstrated that one may differentiate the two types of abnormal mitochondrial inclusions in necrotic muscle cells based on the elemental content of the inclusions.[B9, H2] Calcium and other trace elements are not detectable in moderately electron-dense amorphous inclusions located in mitochondria of muscle cells from the periphery and centers of experimental myocardial infarcts. These amorphous inclusions are similar to those previously described in numerous studies of cell injury and which have been termed "flocculent" or "amorphous matrix" densities.[J3, S1, T1, T2] These mitochondrial inclusions are found in irreversibly injured cells and develop as a consequence of denaturation and precipitation of mitochondrial lipids and protein without mitochondrial calcification.

Mitochondrial inclusions containing very electron-dense spicular material represent relatively advanced stages of mitochondrial calcification in myocardial infarcts (Fig. 59–5). This type of calcification is localized to the peripheries of the infarcts and is most likely explained by the dual requirements of cellular injury and persistent tissue perfusion allowing delivery of serum calcium to damaged myocardial cells.[B9, H2, J3, K2, K3, S1, T, T2, W6] Mitochondrial calcification appears to develop selectively in a subpopulation of calcium-loaded muscle cells with impaired plasma membrane integrity and sufficient mitochondrial function to initiate the accumulation and precipitation of calcium phosphate.[B9, H2, J3, K2, K3, W6] The spicular quality of these mitochondrial inclusions suggests that they represent apatite-crystalline material.[B9–11, D2, H2, T2] Data obtained from our laboratory by means of an electron probe suggest a correlation between calcium content of individual inclusions and the amount of spicular material contributing to the electron density of these deposits.[B9, H2]

Earlier studies have shown that calcium accumulation in tissues may be associated with the formation of two types of very electron-dense mitochondrial inclusions. Inclusions composed of finely granular material have been found in mitochondria obtained from necrotic cells in a variety of conditions,[B10] and they have been described in cardiac muscle cells irreversibly injured by prolonged intervals of temporary coronary artery occlusion followed by reperfusion.[J3, K3, S1] This type of inclusion also has been observed in mildly injured muscle cells with abnormal lipid accumulation in the outermost regions of myocardial infarcts, i.e., the "border zone" regions of myocardial infarcts (Fig. 59–6).[H2, T1] These annular, granular inclusions are usually smaller (less than 1000 Å) than the spicular inclusions.[H2] It has been suggested previously that the granular inclusions represent a readily soluble subcrystalline precursor of a calcium-deficient hydroxyapatite.[B9–11, H2, S1, T1, T2] Mitochondrial inclusions composed of apatite-like, needle-shaped crystals have been found in structurally intact muscle cells subjected to calcium overloading[B10, B11] and in cardiac muscle cells from patients following cardiovascular surgery.[D2] Studies from our laboratory have shown the presence of large granular, finely spicular, and spicular types of calcium-containing precipitates in mitochondria of necrotic muscle cells in experimental canine myocardial infarcts.[B9, H2, T1]

Interrelationships Between Calcium Deposition and Tc-99m-PPi Deposition in Irreversibly Damaged Myocardial Cells

There is a close temporal and topographic relationship between calcium accumulation in acute myocardial infarcts and Tc-99m-PPi deposition responsible for scintigraphic detection of acute myocardial infarcts in experimental animals that have permanent proximal left anterior descending coronary artery occlusion.[B4, B5] In experimental canine myocardial infarcts, central zones of the infarcts are characterized by a virtual absence of neutrophils initially and by the presence of a homogeneous population of muscle cells exhibiting (1) nuclear alterations consisting of pyknosis and pallor; (2) hypereosinophilic cytoplasm with either indistinct or markedly relaxed myofibrils; (3) glycogen depletion; (4) diffuse, diastase-resistant PAS staining that is fainter than that demonstrated by muscle cells in the peripheries of infarcts; and (5) the absence of calcification (Fig. 59–7).

Histologic and ultrastructural studies of experimental infarcts show that discrete calcium deposition occurs initially in the outer regions of the peripheral zones of the infarcts (Fig. 59–7). Early mitochondrial calcification in the form of small, annular, granular calcific deposits occurs in some "border zone" muscle cells with marked lipid accumulation but without cytoplasmic disruption or flocculent mitochondrial densities indicative of advanced irreversible injury.[B4, H2] More advanced mitochondrial calcification, including spicular apatite crystals, appears in muscle cells with

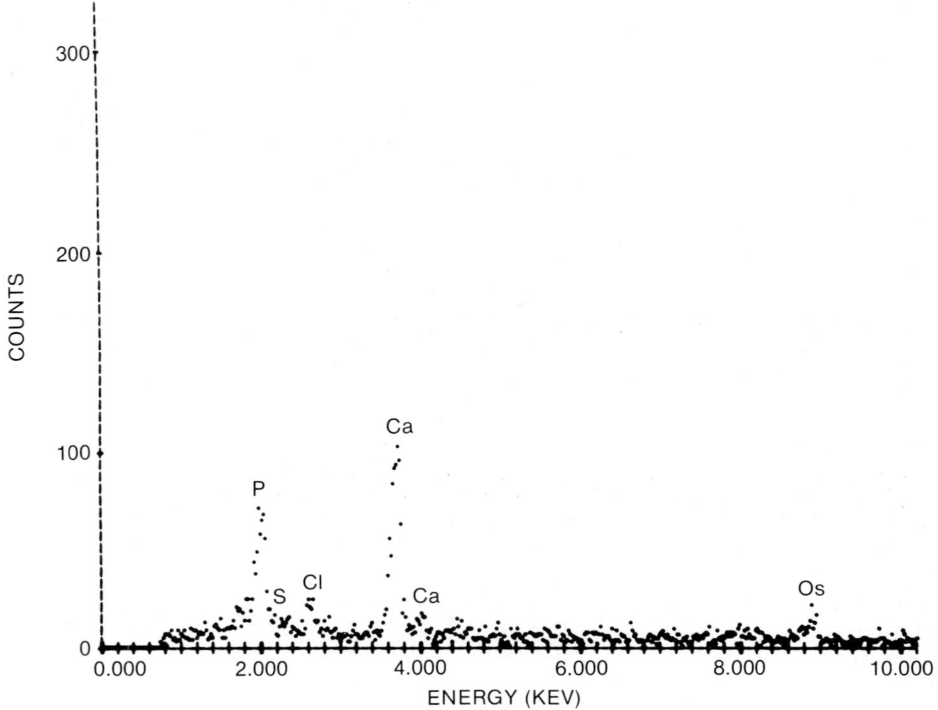

Figure 59–5. X-ray spectrum obtained by analytical electron microscopy from very electron-dense calcific inclusions similar to those shown in Figure 59–4. The inclusions exhibit prominent calcium (Ca) and phosphorus (P) peaks. The small sulfur (S) peak may be from protein-SH groups. The chlorine (Cl) is from the plastic embedding medium and the osmium (Os) from the fixative. For details, see references B9 and H2. (From Willerson, J. T., et al.: Pathophysiologic considerations and clinicopathological correlates of technetium-99m stannous pyrophosphate myocardial scintigraphy. Semin. Nucl. Med. 10:54, 1980, with permission.)

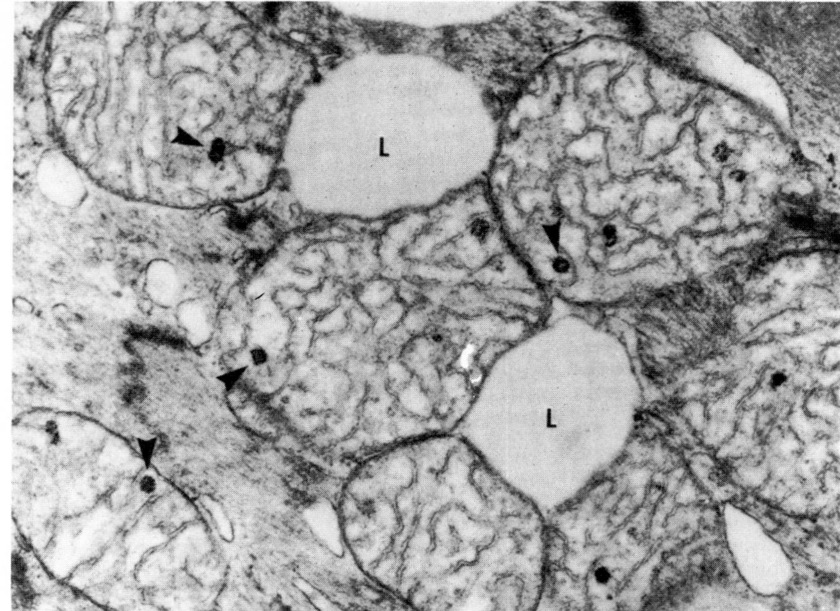

Figure 59–6. Injured muscle cell from outermost region of canine infarct ("border zone" cell) has prominent neutral lipid droplets (L) and mitochondria, with numerous small, granular calcific deposits (arrowheads). Flocculent (amorphous matrix) mitochondrial densities are not present. Electron micrograph, X 28,500. (From Willerson, J. T., et al.: Pathophysiologic considerations and clinicopathological correlates of technetium-99m stannous pyrophosphate myocardial scintigraphy. Semin. Nucl. Med. 10:54, 1980, with permission.)

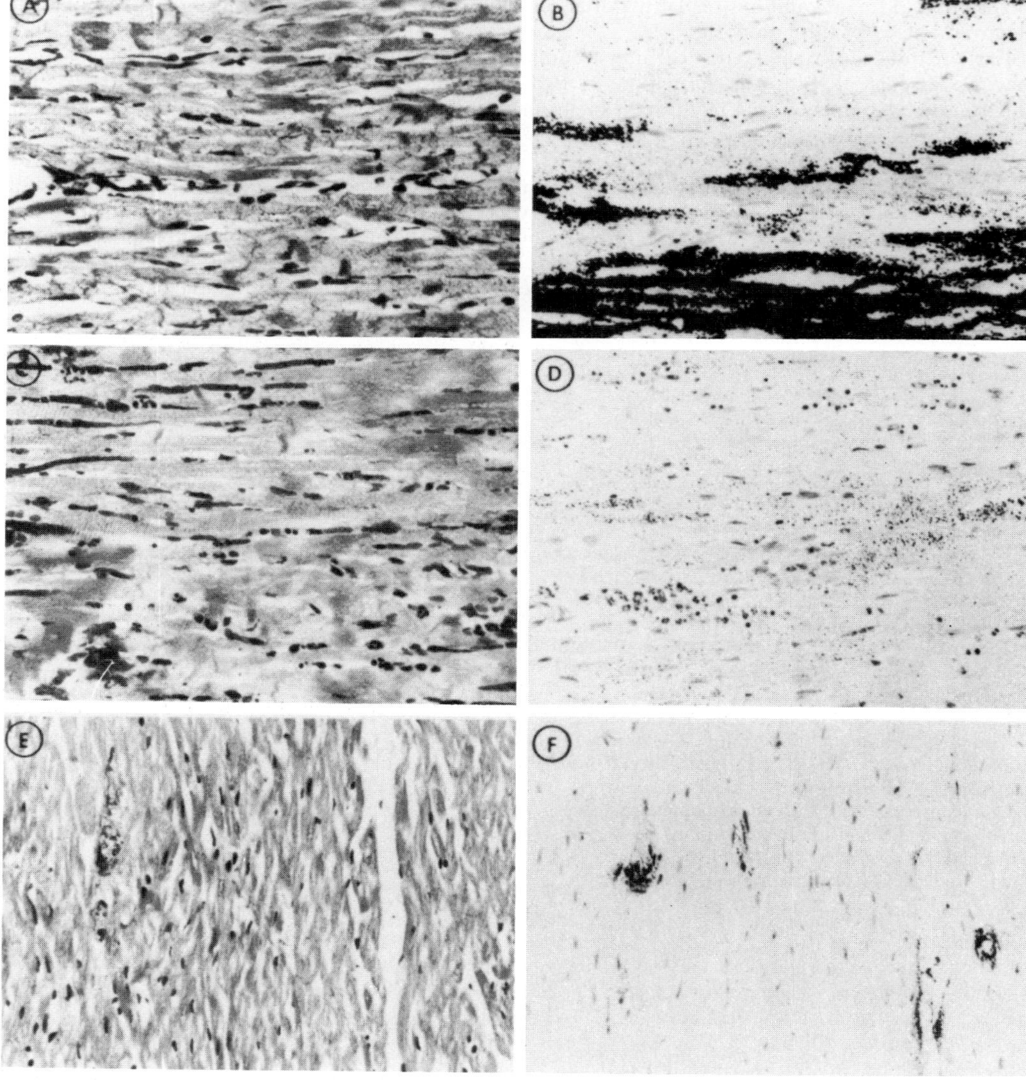

Figure 59–7. Histologic features of 2-day-old canine infarcts. Peripheral infarct regions exhibit necrotic muscle cells with contraction bands (*A–C*) and variable degrees of histologically demonstrable calcification (*D*). Many muscle cells in the outer peripheral zones have disrupted myofibrils and numerous contraction bands and contain variable numbers of discrete granular calcium deposits. Muscle cells in the central zone have indistinct myofibrils and are devoid of calcium deposits. Calcification, however, is present in the walls of small blood vessels and along a tissue space. *A, C,* and *E,* hematoxylin and eosin stain; *B, D,* and *F,* von Kossa stain; all, X 300. (From Buja, L. M., et al.: Morphologic features of technetium-99m stannous pyrophosphate imaging of acute myocardial infarcts in dogs. Circulation 52:596, 1975, with permission of the American Heart Association, Inc.)

features of advanced irreversible injury, including nuclear damage, severe myofibrillar hypercontraction with frequent contraction bands, and flocculent mitochondrial density.[B4, B5, B9, H2] Many muscle cells in the peripheral zones also contain large, very electron-dense structures that appear to represent completely calcified mitochondria. Muscle cells in the centers of experimental canine infarcts exhibit only flocculent mitochondrial densities.[B5, B9, T1]

Older myocardial infarcts demonstrate narrow rims of granulation tissue that replace the outermost portion of the infarcts.[B5] Finely granular calcium deposits in moderate amounts are present in the necrotic muscle cells, macrophages, and degenerating neutrophils in peripheral zones of the lesions. Thirteen-day-old infarcts demonstrate (1) wide zones of dense granulation tissue that replace peripheral zones of the infarcts, and portions of the central zones as well, and (2) central areas of unresorbed necrotic myocardium that contain few inflammatory cells. These infarcts are usually devoid of calcium deposits.[B5]

Tc-99m-PPi Concentration in Irreversibly Damaged Myocardium

There are important differences in the concentration of Tc-99m-PPi in the various infarct regions following experimental myocardial infarction. Maximal Tc-99m-PPi concentration occurs initially in peripheral zones of the infarcts with some collateral blood flow, and later in the central zones with severely reduced blood flow. Tc-99m-PPi uptake in the peripheral infarct zones, with histologic evidence of focal or homogeneous advanced necrosis, is 10 to 50 times that noted in normal muscle; that occurring in the central infarct region varies from being initially less than normal to 2 to 12 times the activity found in normal muscle.[B4–6] Low levels of Tc-99m-PPi are detected in samples obtained from histologically normal muscle immediately adjacent to the peripheries of the infarcts. With reperfusion after temporary coronary artery occlusion, central areas of the infarct demonstrate marked increases in tissue calcification and Tc-99m-PPi uptake.

The time course of the development of abnormal Tc-99m-PPi myocardial scintigrams in experimental canine infarcts includes the scintigrams becoming abnormal within the first 12 to 24 hours after a "permanent" coronary artery occlusion and progressively more abnormal during the initial 24 to 72 hours.[B4, B5] On the other hand, Tc-99m-PPi myocardial scintigrams become abnormal virtually immediately with reperfusion in experimental canine myocardial infarcts with "temporary" coronary artery occlusion artery lasting only 1 to 2 hours, followed by reperfusion (Fig. 59–8).[J1, P3] Tc-99m-PPi scintigrams remain abnormal for up to 6 days after myocardial infarction with permanent coronary artery occlusion, but probably resolve to become normal within 3 to 4 days, in most instances, with temporary coronary artery occlusion followed by reperfusion. Thus, there is a strong temporal and topographic relationship between calcium accumulation in experimental canine myocardial infarcts and Tc-99m-PPi deposition in irreversibly injured myocytes; the rapidity of Tc-99m-PPi concentration in the irreversibly damaged cells depends largely on the rate and extent of calcium deposition, which itself is related to the extent of myocardial perfusion.

Sites and Mechanisms of Localization of Tc-99m-PPi in Acute Myocardial Infarcts

Autoradiographic studies with hydrogen-3 diphosphonate have revealed extensive labeling in the infarct periphery in regions containing necrotic muscle cells. The features of severe calcium overloading include widespread hypercontraction as well as selective formation of mitochondrial calcific deposits.[B4] These same studies have also demonstrated hydrogen-3 diphosphonate labeling in the small population of damaged border zone muscle cells that exhibit prominent accumulation of lipid droplets and focal early mitochondrial calcification. In vitro studies showed that Tc-99m-PPi binds to amorphous calcium phosphate and crystalline

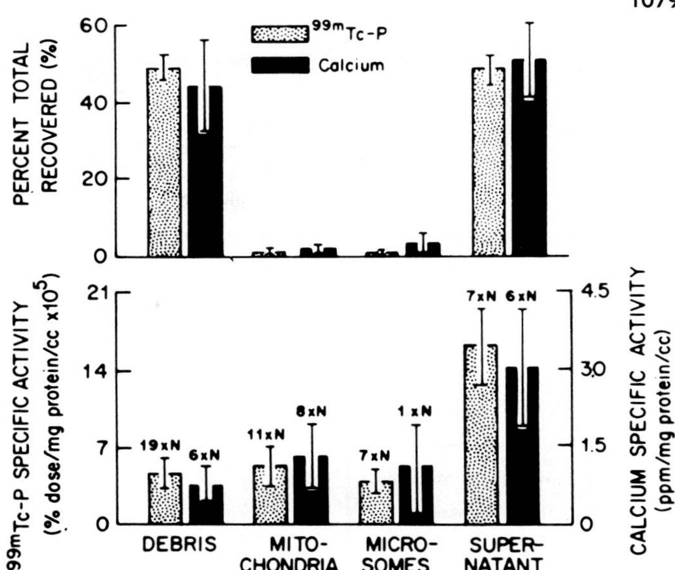

Figure 59–8. Cell fractionation data from three canine myocardial infarcts show a similar distribution of Tc-99m-PPi with calcium in the various fractions, with major localization in the soluble supernatant. The observed distribution is influenced by the marked solubility of some calcium species and by disruption of fragile mitochondria of infarcted tissue. (From Buja, L. M., et al.: J. Clin. Invest. 60:724, 1977.)

hydroxyapatite, but that the Tc-99m-PPi is easily displaced into supernatant and nonmitochondrial fractions during cell fractionation (Fig. 59–8).[B4] The latter data also are consistent with some binding to proteins, such as myofibrils.[B4] There was a general association between tissue Tc-99m-PPi and calcium levels, although the relationship was not linear.[B4]

Therefore, (1) Tc-99m-PPi uptake occurs in experimentally infarcted canine myocardium, and it concentrates selectively in regions of necrosis and in severely injured myocardial cells; (2) concentration of Tc-99m-PPi results from selective adsorption of this agent to various forms of tissue calcium stores, including amorphous calcium phosphate, crystalline hydroxyapatite, and calcium complex with myofibrils and other macromolecules; and (3) the lack of a linear relationship between Tc-99m-PPi concentration and tissue calcium levels is probably the result of local differences in composition and physical chemical properties of tissue calcium stores, as well as local variations in residual blood flow that are responsible for the delivery of Tc-99m-PPi.[B4] The total calcium content of infarcted myocardium results from accumulation of calcium from the onset of injury, whereas the Tc-99m-PPi level results from accumulation of the agent over the relatively brief period following Tc-99m-PPi injection. The scheme that we have proposed to explain the concentration of Tc-99m-PPi in necrotic myocardium is shown in Figures 59–9 and 59–10.

TECHNETIUM 99m

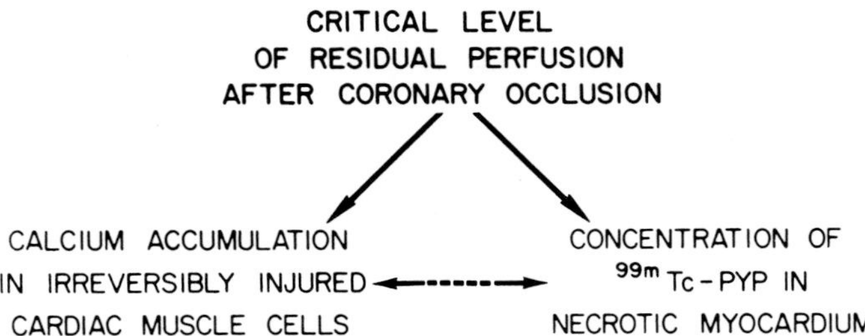

Figure 59–9. Relationship between collateral blood flow, pathologic calcification, and concentration of Tc-99m-PPi in necrotic myocardium.

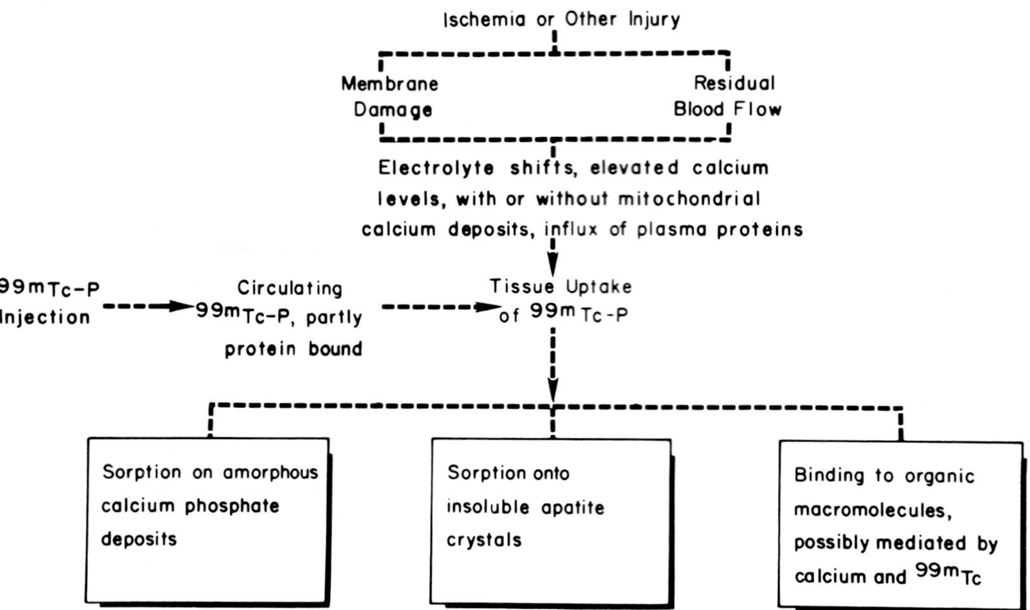

Figure 59–10. Proposed pathophysiologic factors involved in the concentration of Tc-99m-PPi agents in damaged myocardium and other soft tissues. (From Buja, L. M., et al.: Sites and mechanisms of localization of technetium-99m phosphorous radiopharmaceuticals in acute myocardial infarcts and other tissues. J. Clin. Invest. 60:724, 1977, with permission.)

Detection with Tc-99m-PPi of Myocardial Infarction in Patients

It is sometimes difficult to confirm the presence of acute myocardial infarction using traditional techniques.[A1, E1, R4] The recognition of acute non-Q wave (subendocardial) myocardial infarcts is not possible from the electrocardiogram alone. There are also temporal restrictions on enzyme elevations that may limit their usefulness in individual patients who delay their hospital admission following the development of chest pain. In patients with previous myocardial infarcts, in those with intraventricular conduction defects (particularly left bundle branch block), in those receiving cardioversion for life-threatening arrhythmias, and in those during the peri- and postoperative periods after open heart surgery, the clinical recognition of myocardial infarction using traditional techniques may be difficult.

We have demonstrated that Tc-99m-PPi myocardial imaging may be used to identify, localize, and estimate the size of myocardial infarcts.* In clinical studies done at our institution, we have found that Tc-99m-PPi uptake begins approximately 10 to 12 hours after symptom onset with permanent coronary artery occlusion and within 1 to 2 hours following thrombolytic therapy and reperfusion. Tc-99m-PPi myocardial scintigrams become increasingly abnormal during the initial 24 to 72 hours in the absence of thrombolytic therapy (just as occurs in experimental canine models of myocardial infarction), but the scintigrams may evolve to become negative within 2 to 3 days when thrombolytic therapy and reperfusion have occurred. Virtually all acute myocardial infarcts 3 or more gm in weight may be visualized by Tc-99m-PPi myocardial scintigraphy, if serial imaging is used. If single photon emission computed tomography (SPECT) is used, even smaller infarcts may be detected (Figs. 59–11 through 59–19). Occasionally, patients first develop an abnormal scintigram 4 to 5 days after acute myocardial infarction; these patients are among those with the most severe intrinsic coronary artery stenoses and the most severely reduced flow to the area of infarction.[F1] Presumably, the delayed development of collateral flow to the region(s) of damage is responsible for the delayed development of abnormal scintigrams in these patients. Thrombolytic therapy and successful reperfusion of infarcts should result in their detection with Tc-99m-PPi imaging within 2 hours of their occurrence, especially if single photon emission computed tomography is used.

*References B7, C4, C5, J1, L1, P3, P4, R1–3, S2, W4, W5.

Sensitivity of Tc-99m-PPi

Several previous clinical studies and clinicopathologic correlations have demonstrated that Tc-99m-PPi planar (two-dimensional) myocardial scintigraphy has a sensitivity of approximately 90 percent in the detection of acute Q wave and 85 to 90 percent in the detection of non-Q wave myocardial infarcts.[B7, C4, P4, R1, R3, W1, W2] On the other hand, Tc-99m-PPi with single photon emission computed tomography, especially when utilized with blood pool overlay studies, has a sensitivity of over 90 percent in the detection of both Q wave and non-Q wave infarcts (Fig. 59–12).[C4]

Figure 59–12. See Color-Plate 15.

Other causes of acute myocardial necrosis also lead to abnormal Tc-99m-PPi myocardial scintigrams, including structurally damaged heart muscle following repeated cardioversion,[P2] traumatic and penetrating injury to the heart, invasive tumor of the heart, viral injury, and infiltrative cardiomyopathies. Tc-99m-PPi myocardial uptake generally identifies the presence of acute myocardial necrosis or acute myocardial necrosis followed by continuing chronic, severe, multifocal cell injury progressing to necrosis.[B4, B6, B7, P4] Although myocardial infarction and chronic ischemic heart damage are the most common causes of such a process, any other cause of such injury will also result in an abnormal Tc-99m-PPi myocardial scintigram if (1) calcium accumulation in the area of injury occurs, and (2) residual myocardial blood flow is adequate to deliver Tc-99m-PPi during the evolution of the myocyte injury.

Sizing of Acute Myocardial Infarcts with Tc-99m-PPi

Early studies from our laboratory indicated that planar (two-dimensional) myocardial scintigraphy with Tc-99m-PPi provided relatively accurate measurements of acute anterior transmural (Q wave) myocardial infarcts, but this approach failed to estimate the size of inferior, posterior, and nontransmural (non-Q wave) myocardial infarcts with accuracy.[L1, S2, W3] However, single photon emission computed tomography (SPECT) and Tc-99m-PPi have been shown to estimate myocardial infarct size in varying locations accurately in animals (Figs. 59–13 through 59–19).[C5, W5] More recent studies have shown that SPECT with Tc-99m-PPi and blood pool subtraction also allow accurate estimates of the size of

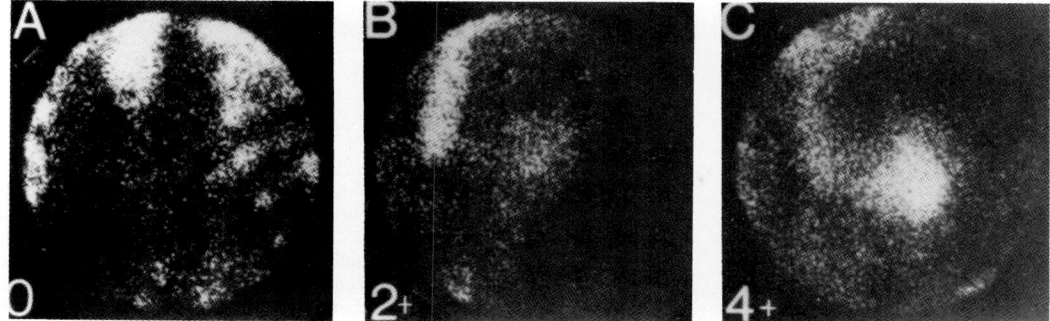

Figure 59–11. The qualitative grading scheme used in the interpretation of Tc-99m-PPi myocardial scintigram. "2+"—"4+" myocardial scintigrams are considered abnormal. 2+ scintigrams represent Tc–99m-PPi myocardial uptake less than adjacent bone structures and are found with non-Q wave or subendocardial infarcts. 3+ uptake is equivalent to adjacent bone, and 4+ uptake is greater than adjacent bone and is usually found with Q wave or transmural myocardial infarcts. (From Willerson, J. T., et al.: Technetium stannous pyrophosphate myocardial scintigrams in patients with chest pain of varying etiology. Circulation 51:1046, 1975, with permission of the American Heart Association, Inc.)

Figure 59–13. Comparison of size of infarction by SPECT and by MB-CK analysis in all patients with myocardial infarctions. (From Jansen, D. E., et al.: Quantification of myocardial infarction: A comparison of single photon emission computed tomography with pyrophosphate to serial plasma MB-CK measurements. Circulation 72:327, 1985, with permission of the American Heart Association, Inc.)

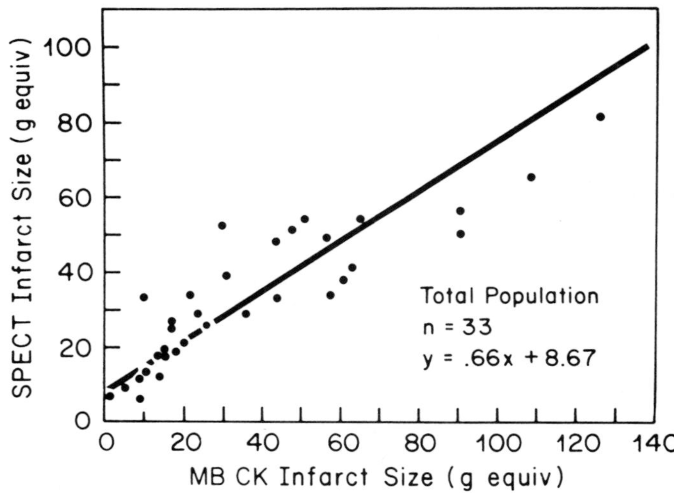

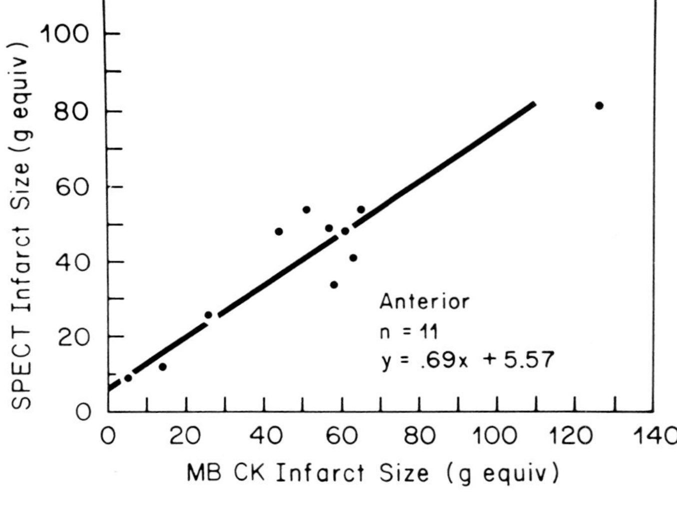

Figure 59–14. Comparison of size of infarction by SPECT and by MB-CK analysis in patients with transmural anterior myocardial infarctions. (From Jansen, D. E., et al.: Quantification of myocardial infarction: A comparison of single photon emission computed tomography with pyrophosphate to serial plasma MB-CK measurements. Circulation 72:327, 1985, with permission of the American Heart Association, Inc.)

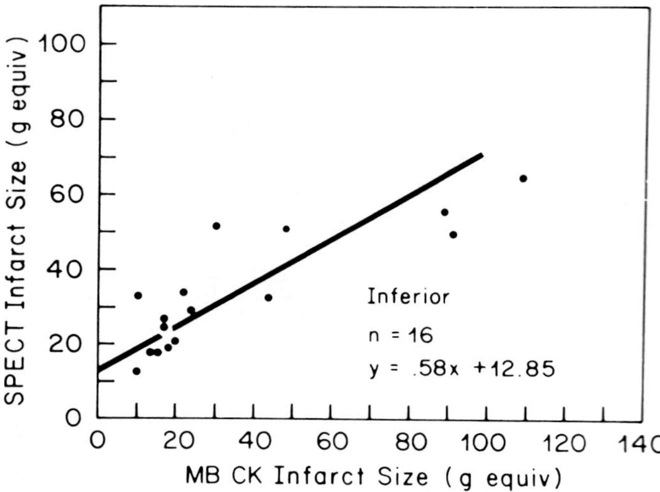

Figure 59–15. Comparison of size of infarction by SPECT and by MB-CK analysis in patients with transmural inferior myocardial infarctions. (From Jansen, D. E., et al.: Quantification of myocardial infarction: A comparison of single photon emission computed tomography with pyrophosphate to serial plasma MB-CK measurements. Circulation 72:327, 1985, with permission of the American Heart Association, Inc.)

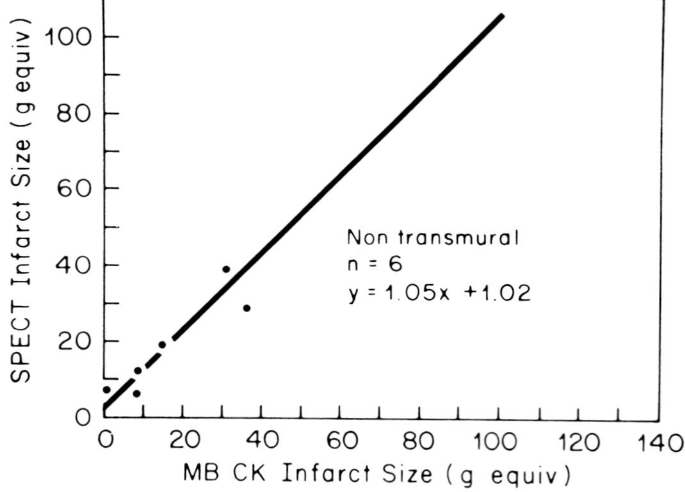

Figure 59–16. Comparison of size of infarction by SPECT and by MB-CK analysis in patients with nontransmural myocardial infarctions. (From Jansen, D. E., et al.: Quantification of myocardial infarction: A comparison of single photon emission computed tomography with pyrophosphate to serial plasma MB-CK measurements. Circulation 72:327, 1985, with permission of the American Heart Association, Inc.)

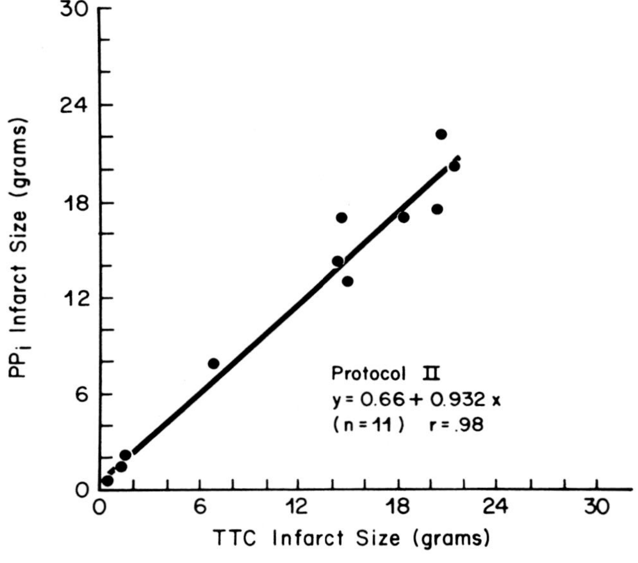

Figure 59–17. Comparison of TTC and Tc-99m-PPi estimates of infarct size for dogs in group B (protocol II). (From Jansen, D. E., et al.: Quantification of myocardial injury produced by temporary coronary artery occlusion and reflow with technetium-99m-pyrophosphate. Circulation 75:611, 1987, with permission of the American Heart Association, Inc.)

Figure 59–18. See Color-Plate 15.

myocardial infarction in patients regardless of the location of the infarcts.[C4, J2] In recent studies, we have demonstrated that SPECT with Tc-99m-PPi accurately sizes infarcts in patients and that these measurements correlate closely with those by an established clinically useful method, i.e., infarct size measurements with serial plasma creatine kinase-MB isoenzyme levels.[J2]

We have also shown in experimental animals that myocardial infarct size may be expressed as myocardial "infarction fraction" by using a combination of SPECT-estimated infarct size from Tc-99m-PPi and identifying left ventricular mass from SPECT measurements of thallium-201 myocardial uptake (Fig. 59–19).[W5] This approach allows an estimation of infarction fraction, i.e., the extent of myocardial infarction compared with total left ventricular muscle mass. This information may be useful in that different infarct sizes may have different implications, depending on the relative extent of the left ventricular myocardium that is infarcted. Instead of thallium-201, other perfusion markers (including technetium-99m isonitrile analogs) could be used.

Estimates of Infarct Size Produced by Temporary Coronary Artery Occlusion and Reperfusion with Tc-99m-PPi

More recently, we have demonstrated in animal models that Tc-99m-PPi may be used to estimate the size of myocardial infarcts in animals after temporary coronary artery occlusion followed by reperfusion (Fig. 59–17).[J1] We have shown previously that myocardial infarction may be detected within 1 to 2 hours following reperfusion after release of a temporary coronary artery occlusion or thrombolytic therapy. In studies done in the canine model, we have found that Tc-99m-PPi injected 90 minutes or later after reperfusion provides an excellent means to identify and size myocardial infarcts produced by temporary coronary artery occlusion and reflow (Fig. 59–17).[J1] If Tc-99m-PPi is injected prior to 90 minutes of reperfusion, some overestimation of infarct size may occur, possibly because of Tc-99m-PPi incorporation into injured but not irreversibly damaged myocardial cells that may be transiently calcium overloaded.[J1] Thus, the ability to estimate infarct size accurately in this model represents a potentially important clinical contribution.

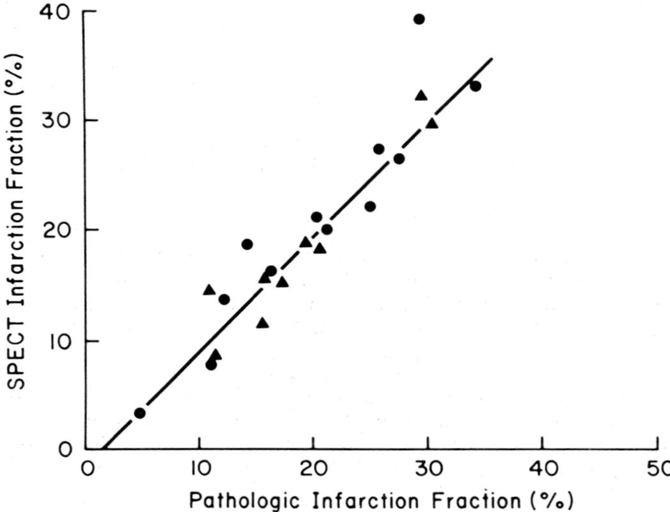

Figure 59–19. Correlation between postmortem and single photon emission computed tomographic (SPECT) determinations of "infarction fraction" in 21 dogs with circumflex (12 dogs) or left anterior descending (LAD) (9 dogs) occlusion. SPECT infarction fraction = 1.09 × pathologic infarct mass − 1.7 (r = 0.94, SEE = 3.1). ●, Circumflex occlusions (r = 0.94); ▲, LAD occlusions (r = 0.95). (From Wolfe, C. L., et al.: Measurement of myocardial infarction fraction using single photon emission computed tomography. J. Am. Coll. Cardiol. 6:145, 1985. Reprinted with permission from the American College of Cardiology.)

Other Infarct Avid Imaging Agents

Haber and colleagues have described the use of monoclonal antibodies to cardiac myosin labeled with iodine-123 or indium-111 as a means to detect myocardial infarcts in experimental animals and patients.[J5, K4–6] This approach allows accurate detection and sizing of experimentally created canine infarcts in the initial few days after their occurrence.[K4, K5] Recent clinical studies using monoclonal antibodies to cardiac myosin have shown good sensitivity in infarct detection in the moderate numbers of patients that have been studied thus far, including those with permanent coronary artery occlusion and those with reperfusion.[J5, K6] Thus far, no important allergic reaction has been described with one or two single injections of the monoclonal antibody against cardiac myosin, but there is concern about the need for serial myocardial imaging or repetitive administrations of the monoclonal antibody in regard to the risk of allergic responses. Nevertheless, this approach is a viable alternative to Tc-99m-PPi myocardial scintigraphy in its ability to detect and size myocardial infarcts.

Acknowledgments

We thank Nancy Dickey for expert secretarial assistance.

References

A

1. Alison, H. W., Moraski, R. E., Mantle, J. A., et al.: Coronary anatomy and arteriography in patients with unstable angina pectoris. Am. J. Cardiol. 35:118, 1975.

B

1. Berman, D. S., Amsterdam, E. A., Hines, H. H., et al.: New approach to interpretation of technetium-99m pyrophosphate scintigraphy in detection of acute myocardial infarction. Clinical assessment of diagnostic accuracy. Am. J. Cardiol. 39:341, 1977.
2. Bonte, F. J., Parkey, R. W., Graham, K. D., et al.: A new method for radionuclide imaging of acute myocardial infarction. Radiology 110:473, 1974.
3. Berman, D. S., Amsterdam, E. A., Hines, H. H., et al.: Problem of diffuse cardiac uptake of technetium-99m pyrophosphate in the diagnosis of acute myocardial infarction: Enhanced scintigraphic accuracy by computerized selective blood pool subtraction. Am. J. Cardiol. 40:768, 1977.
4. Buja, L. M., Tofe, A. J., Kulkarni, P. V., et al.: Sites and mechanisms of localization of technetium-99m phosphorous radiopharmaceuticals in acute myocardial infarcts and other tissues. J. Clin. Invest. 60:724, 1977.
5. Buja, L. M., Parkey, R. W., Dees, J. H., et al.: Morphologic correlates of technetium-99m stannous pyrophosphate imaging of acute myocardial infarcts in dogs. Circulation 52:596, 1975.
6. Buja, L. M., Parkey, R. W., Dees, J., et al.: Pathophysiology of technetium-99m stannous pyrophosphate imaging of acute myocardial infarcts in dogs. Circulation 52:596, 1975.
7. Buja, L. M., Poliner, L. R., Parkey, R. W., et al.: Clinicopathologic studies of persistently positive technetium-99m stannous pyrophosphate myocardial scintigrams and myocytolytic degeneration after acute myocardial infarction. Circulation 56:1016, 1977.
8. Burton, K. P., Hagler, H. K., Templeton, G. H., et al.: Lanthanum probe studies of cellular pathophysiology induced by hypoxia in isolated cardiac muscle. J. Clin. Invest. 60:1289, 1977.
9. Buja, L. M., Dees, J. H., Harling, D. F., and Willerson, J. T.: Analytical electron microscopic study of mitochondrial inclusions in canine myocardial infarcts. J. Histochem. Cytochem. 24:508, 1976.
10. Bonucci, E., Derenzini, M., and Marinozzi, V.: The organic-inorganic relationship in calcified mitochondria. J. Cell Biol. 59:185, 1973.
11. Bonucci, E., and Sadun, R.: Experimental calcification of the myocardium. Ultrastructural and histochemical investigations. Am. J. Pathol. 71:167, 1973.

C

1. Coleman, R. E., Klein, M. S., Roberts, R., and Sobel, B. E.: Improved detection of myocardial infarction with technetium-99m stannous pyrophosphate and serum MB creatine phosphokinase. Am. J. Cardiol. 37:732, 1976.
2. Cowley, M. J., Mantle, J. A., Rogers, W. J., et al.: Technetium–99m stannous pyrophosphate myocardial scintigraphy: Reliability and limitations in assessment of acute myocardial infarction. Circulation 56:192, 1977.
3. Corbett, J. R., Lewis, S. E., Dehmer, G., et al.: Simultaneous display of gated technetium-99m stannous pyrophosphate and gated blood-pool scintigrams. J. Nucl. Med. 22:671, 1981.

4. Corbett, J. R., Lewis, M., Willerson, J. T., et al.: 99m-Tc-pyrophosphate imaging in patients with acute myocardial infarction: Comparison of planar imaging with single-photon tomography with and without blood pool overlay. Circulation 69:1120, 1984.
5. Corbett, J. R., Lewis, S. E., Wolfe, C. L., et al.: Measurement of myocardial infarct size by technetium pyrophosphate single-photon tomography. Am. J. Cardiol. 54:1231, 1984.
6. Csapo, Z., Dusek, J., and Rona, G.: Peculiar myofilament changes near the intercalated disc in isoproterenol-induced cardiac muscle cell injury. J. Molec. Cell. Cardiol. 6:79, 1974.
7. Connors, J. P., West, P. N., Roberts, R., et al.: Loss of functional integrity of the microvasculature in ischemic myocardium. (Abstract.) Clin. Res. 24:213A, 1976.

D

1. D'Agostino, A. N.: An electron microscopic study of cardiac necrosis produced by 9 [-fluorocortisol] and sodium phosphate. Am. J. Pathol. 45:633, 1964.
2. D'Agostino, A. N., and Chiga, M.: Mitochondrial mineralization in human myocardium. Am. J. Clin. Pathol. 58:820, 1970.

E

1. Eliot, R. S., and Edwards, J. E.: Pathology of coronary atherosclerosis and its complications. *In* Hurst, J. W., and Logue, R. B. (eds.): The Heart. McGraw-Hill, New York, 1974, p. 1003.

F

1. Falkoff, M., Parkey, R. W., Bonte, F. J., et al.: Technetium-99m stannous pyrophosphate myocardial scintigraphy: Serial imaging to detect myocardial infarcts in patients. Clin. Cardiol. 1:163, 1978.

H

1. Henning, S. H., Schelbert, H. R., Righetti, A., et al.: Dual myocardial imaging with technetium-99m pyrophosphate and thallium-201 for detecting, localizing, and sizing acute myocardial infarction. Am. J. Cardiol. 40:147, 1977.
2. Hagler, H. K., Sherwin, L., and Buja, L. M.: Effect of different methods of tissue preparation on mitochondrial inclusions of ischemic and infarcted canine myocardium. Transmission and analytic electron microscopic study. Lab. Invest. 40:529, 1979.

J

1. Jansen, D. E., Corbett, J. R., Buja, L. M., et al.: Quantification of myocardial injury produced by temporary coronary artery occlusion and reflow with technetium-99m-pyrophosphate. Circulation 75:611, 1987.
2. Jansen, D. E., Corbett, J. R., Lewis, S. E., et al.: Quantification of myocardial infarction: A comparison of single photon emission computed tomography with pyrophosphate to serial plasma MB-CK measurements. Circulation 72:327, 1985.
3. Jennings, R. B., and Ganote, C. E.: Structural changes in myocardium during acute ischemia. Circ. Res. 34–35 (Suppl. III):III–156, 1974.
4. Jennings, R. B., Hawkins, H. K., Lowe, J. E., et al.: Relationship between high energy phosphate and lethal injury in myocardial ischemia in the dog. Am. J. Pathol. 92:187, 1978.
5. Johnson, L., Seldin, D., Becker, L., et al.: Antimyosin imaging in acute transmural myocardial infarction. J. Am. Coll. Cardiol. 13:27, 1989.

K

1. Keyes, J. W., Jr., Leonard, P. F., Brody, S. L., et al.: Myocardial infarct quantification in the dog by single photon emission computed tomography. Circulation 58:227, 1978.
2. Kloner, R. A., Ganote, C. E., and Jennings, R. B.: The "no reflow" phenomenon after temporary coronary occlusion in the dog. J. Clin. Invest. 54:1496, 1974.
3. Kloner, R. A., Ganote, C. E., and Whalen, D. A., Jr.: Effect of a transient period of ischemia on myocardial cells. II. Fine structure during the first few minutes of reflow. Am. J. Pathol. 74:399, 1974.
4. Khaw, B. A., Fallon, J. T., Beller, G., and Haber, E.: Specificity of localization of myosin-specific antibody fragments in experimental myocardial infarction. Circulation 60:1527, 1979.
5. Khaw, B. A., Scott, J., Fallon, J. T., et al.: Myocardial injury. Quantitation by cell sorting initiated with antimyosin fluorescent spheres. Science 217:1050, 1982.
6. Khaw, B. A., Gold, H. K., Yasuda, T., et al.: Scintigraphic quantification of myocardial necrosis in patients after intravenous injection of myosin specific antibody. Circulation 74:501, 1986.

L

1. Lewis, S. E., Stokely, E. M., DeVous, M. D., Sr., et al.: Quantitation of experimental canine infarct size with multi-pinhole and rotating-slanthole tomography. J. Nucl. Med. 22:1000, 1981.
2. Leaf, A.: Regulation of intracellular fluid volume and disease. Am. J. Med. 49:291, 1970.

P

1. Parkey, R. W., Bonte, F. J., Meyer, S. L., et al.: A new method for radionuclide imaging of acute myocardial infarction in humans. Circulation 50:450, 1974.
2. Pugh, B. R., Buja, L. M., Parkey, R. W., et al.: Cardioversion and "false positive" technetium-99m stannous pyrophosphate myocardial scintigrams. Circulation 54:399, 1976.
3. Parkey, R. W., Kulkarni, P., Lewis, S., et al.: Effect of coronary blood flow and site of injection on Tc-99m-PPi detection of early canine myocardial infarcts. J. Nucl. Med. 22(2):133, 1981.
4. Poliner, L. R., Buja, L. M., Parkey, R. W., et al.: Clinicopathologic findings in 52 patients studied by technetium-99m stannous pyrophosphate myocardial scintigraphy. Circulation 59:257, 1979.

R

1. Rutherford, J. D., Roberts, R., Muller, J. E., et al.: Multicenter Investigation of the Limitation of Infarct Size (MILIS): Comparison of enzymatic, scintigraphic and electrocardiographic methods of detecting acute myocardial infarction. Circulation 64 (Suppl. IV):IV–84, 1981.
2. Rude, R. E., Parkey, R. W., Bonte, F. J., et al.: Clinical implications of the technetium-99m stannous pyrophosphate myocardial scintigraphic "doughnut" pattern in patients with acute myocardial infarcts. Circulation 59:721, 1979.
3. Rude, R. E., Rubin, H. S., Stone, M. J., et al.: Radioimmunoassay of serum creatine kinase B isoenzyme: Correlation with technetium-99m stannous pyrophosphate myocardial scintigraphy in the diagnosis of acute myocardial infarction. Am. J. Med. 68:405, 1980.
4. Roberts, W. C.: The coronary arteries and left ventricle in clinically isolated angina pectoris: A necropsy analysis. Circulation 54:388, 1976.

S

1. Shen, A. C., and Jennings, R. B.: Myocardial calcium and magnesium in acute ischemic injury. Am. J. Pathol. 67:417, 1972.
2. Stokely, E. M., Tipton, D. M., Buja, L. M., et al.: Quantitation of experimental canine infarct size using multi-pinhole single-photon tomography. J. Nucl. Med. 22:55, 1981.

T

1. Trump, B. F., Croker, B. P., Jr., and Mergner, W. J.: The role of energy metabolism, ion, and water shifts in the pathogenesis of cell injury. *In* Richter, G. W., and Scarpelli, D. G. (eds.): Cell Membranes: Biological and Pathological Aspects. Williams & Wilkins Company, Baltimore, 1971, p. 84.
2. Trump, B. F., Strum, J. M., and Bulger, R. E.: Studies on the pathogenesis of ischemic cell injury. I. Relation between ion and water shifts and cell ultrastructure in rat kidney slices during swelling at 0–4° C. Virchows Arch. Abt. B Cell. Pathol. 16:1, 1974.

W

1. Willerson, J. T., Parkey, R. W., Bonte, F. J., et al.: Technetium stannous pyrophosphate myocardial scintigrams in patients with chest pain of varying etiology. Circulation 51:1046, 1975.
2. Willerson, J. T., Parkey, R. W., Bonte, F. J., et al.: Acute subendocardial myocardial infarction in patients. Its detection by technetium-99m stannous pyrophosphate myocardial scintigrams. Circulation 51:436, 1975.
3. Willerson, J. T., Parkey, R. W., Bonte, F. J., et al.: Pathophysiologic considerations and clinicopathological correlates of technetium-99m stannous pyrophosphate myocardial scintigraphy. Semin. Nucl. Med. 10:54, 1980.
4. Wheelan, K., Wolfe, C., Corbett, J. R., et al.: Early positive technetium-99m stannous pyrophosphate images as a marker of reperfusion in patients receiving thrombolytic therapy for acute myocardial infarction. Am. J. Cardiol. 56:252, 1985.
5. Wolfe, C. L., Lewis, S. E., Corbett, J. R., et al.: Measurement of myocardial infarction fraction using single photon emission computed tomography. J. Am. Coll. Cardiol. 6:145, 1985.
6. Whalen, D. A., Jr., Hamilton, D. G., and Ganote, C. E.: Effect of a transient period of ischemia on myocardial cells. I. Effects on cell volume regulation. Am. J. Pathol. 74:381, 1974.
7. Willerson, J. T., Scales, F., Mukherjee, A., et al.: Abnormal myocardial fluid retention as an early manifestation of ischemic injury. Am. J. Pathol. 87:159, 1977.

Chapter 60

Metabolic Imaging with Single-Photon Emitting Tracers

■ *HEINZ SOCHOR, M.D.* ■ *JOHANNES CZERNIN, M.D.*
■ *HEINRICH R. SCHELBERT, M.D.*

HISTORICAL PERSPECTIVE 1085
TRACER TISSUE KINETICS OF IODO FATTY ACID ANALOGS 1086
General Considerations 1086
Iodine-for-Methyl Fatty Acid Analogs 1086
Aromatic Fatty Acid Analogs 1088
Branch-Chain Fatty Acid Analogs 1089
Isosteric Fatty Acid Analogs 1090
Comparison of Fatty Acid Analogs 1090
TECHNICAL ASPECTS OF IODO FATTY ACID IMAGING 1090
CLINICAL EXPERIENCE WITH IODO FATTY ACID ANALOGS 1091
Myocardial Infarction 1091
Chronic Coronary Artery Disease 1093
Cardiomyopathy 1094
SUMMARY AND CONCLUSIONS 1094

Insertion of radioactive isotopes into physiologically active compounds offers the exciting prospect of noninvasive evaluation and quantification of local organ function with radionuclide imaging techniques. These prospects have largely materialized for positron-emitting isotopes of elements, such as carbon, nitrogen, and fluorine, and positron emission tomography but have remained limited with single-photon–emitting isotopes. This is because only a small number of radioisotopes are suitable for imaging with conventional nuclear medicine instrumentation. Furthermore, labeling of physiologic substrates with, for example, technetium-99m or iodine-123, two of the most commonly employed radiotracers, dramatically alters the biologic properties of physiologic compounds so that, in most cases, the resulting radiopharmaceuticals no longer behave like their natural, unlabeled parents. Radioiodination of free fatty acid thus far has been the only exception; here studies of myocardial metabolism indeed appear feasible.

This chapter briefly reviews the historical development of myocardial imaging with radioiodinated fatty acids, then describes the behavior of these radiotracers in myocardium and how it relates to myocardial fatty acid metabolism, and concludes with a review of clinical observations with this radionuclide imaging technique in ischemic heart disease, cardiomyopathy, and left ventricular hypertrophy.

HISTORICAL PERSPECTIVE

Myocardium avidly extracts long chain free fatty acids. Steady state extraction fractions in human myocardium average 45 percent for oleic acid and 32 percent for palmitic acid.[R1] If labeled with radioactive markers, these long chain fatty acids therefore appeared attractive for myocardial scintigraphy because they could serve as vehicles for transport of radiolabel into myocardium. Evans and co-workers in 1965 were the first to demonstrate this possibility.[E1] They radioiodinated the double carbon bond of oleic acid and obtained myocardial scintigrams of adequate diagnostic quality. Limited imaging capabilities at that time and the high radiation burden associated with the available iodine-131, together with an altered biologic behavior of the radioiodinated fatty acid caused by the radioiodination of the carbon double bond, prevented widespread acceptance of this compound for myocardial imaging. To preserve the structural integrity of long chain fatty acids and, consequently, their biologic behavior, Robinson and Lee replaced the methyl group in the terminal (or omega) position with a radioactive iodine atom.[R2, R3] These investigators soon demonstrated that adequate myocardial images could indeed be obtained with this newly synthesized iodo fatty acid.[P1, P2] The biexponential clearance of the radiolabel from myocardium suggested further the possibility that metabolic information could be derived noninvasively with these tracers. Comparative studies with C-14– and C-11–labeled palmitate subsequently demonstrated the correspondence of the biexponential clearance pattern of iodo fatty acid analogs to the known metabolic fate of free fatty acid in myocardium. Serial imaging and construction of regional tissue time activity curves therefore offered the possibility to explore regional myocardial fatty acid metabolism noninvasively. However, limitations remained. Rapid clearance of tracer from myocardium together with liberation of free iodine and high radioiodine blood levels required complicated and error-sensitive corrections. To obviate the need for such corrections, Machulla and associates introduced a new radioiodinated aromatic fatty acid analog. Stabilization of radioiodide on a terminal phenyl ring prevented rapid deiodination. Myocardial uptake and subsequent clearance generally corresponded to those of the iodine-for-methyl group straight chain fatty acid analogs and to those of C-11 palmitate. Unlike earlier fatty acid analogs, the radioiodine was released from myocardium

This work was supported in part by the Director of the Office of Energy Research, Office of Health and Environmental Research, Washington, D.C., by Research Grants #HL 29845 and #HL 33177, National Institutes of Health, Bethesda, Maryland and by an Investigative Group Award by the Greater Los Angeles Affiliate of the American Heart Association, Los Angeles, California. Johannes Czernin is a recipient of a scholarship by the Max Kade Foundation, New York.

in the form of benzoic acid and subsequently cleared from blood via the kidney in the form of hippuric acid. The rapid clearance of this tracer from myocardium continued to present limitations, especially as newly introduced tomographic imaging techniques required longer myocardial residence times in order to record adequate tomographic images. This prompted the search for tracers that would be retained in or clear more slowly from myocardium. The notion that branch-chain fatty acids were less susceptible to β-oxidation led to the synthesis of numerous iodo fatty acids with methyl branches.[G1, G2, K1, K2, L1, L2] Other approaches included insertion of, for example, tellurium into the central position of the long chain fatty acid and resulted in isosteric fatty acid analogs.[G3] The latter two groups of fatty acid analogs are currently still in a developmental stage, and their metabolic fate in myocardium is understood only incompletely.[B1]

We do not disregard the importance of numerous other iodo fatty acid analogs, but a detailed description of their merits and limitations is beyond the scope of this chapter. The following review, therefore, will focus on those iodo fatty acid analogs that have been tested more extensively and have been employed in humans.

TRACER TISSUE KINETICS OF IODO FATTY ACID ANALOGS

General Considerations

The myocardial tissue kinetics of C-11–labeled palmitate serve as a yardstick for determining the quality and type of metabolic information that is available through iodo fatty acid analogs. As detailed in Chapter 65, this tracer most closely approximates the uptake and subsequent metabolic fate of free fatty acids in myocardium. Injected intravenously, the tracer rapidly accumulates in myocardium and subsequently clears from it in a biexponential fashion (Fig. 60–1). The biexponential clearance curve morphology implies distribution of tracer between two functional pools from which it clears at different rates. These two functional pools have been shown to correspond to oxidation of free fatty acid—the rapid clearance curve component, and storage of fatty acid in the endogenous lipid pool—the slow clearance phase. The latter pool includes diglycerides, triglycerides, and phospholipids.

After crossing the capillary and cellular membranes, free fatty acid becomes esterified via an energy-requiring reaction to acyl-CoA. The reaction is largely unidirectional and thus represents effective sequestration of free fatty acid into myocardium. The metabolic fate of acyl-CoA branches thereafter. It can be synthesized to glycerides or phospholipids (the slow functional pool) or transported via the carnitine shuttle to the inner mitochondrial membrane, where β-oxidation metabolizes the acyl-CoA to two carbon units, which then enter the tricarboxylic acid (TCA) cycle for oxidation to carbon dioxide and water (for details, see Chapter 4). Transport into mitochondria, β-oxidation, TCA cycle oxidation, and release of end products from myocardium correspond to the rapid clearance phase on the tissue time activity curve and represent a rapid turnover, functional pool. The relative size of the rapid phase corresponds to the fraction of fatty acid that is immediately oxidized (Fig. 60–1), while its slope is related to the transmembranous transport, oxidation of fatty acid, and release of metabolic end products. The relative size of the slow clearance phase is related to the fraction of fatty acid that is incorporated into the endogenous lipid pool and its slope to its turnover rate.

Physiologic interventions alter the clearance curve morphology in a predictable manner (see Chapter 65 for details). These alterations are important for understanding the tissue clearance kinetics of iodo fatty acid analogs. Higher cardiac workload and, thus, higher oxygen consumption increase the relative size and slope of the rapid clearance phase as a reflection of increased fatty acid oxidation. Conversely, ischemia lowers the relative size and clearance rate of the rapid phase as a reflection of impaired fatty acid oxidation. The relative size of the slow clearance phase increases as an expression of increased incorporation of radiolabel into the endogenous lipid pool. Changes in myocardial substrate utilization similarly affect the clearance curve morphology. The preferential fatty acid oxidation in the fasted state, when plasma fatty acid levels are high and glucose and insulin levels are low, is reflected on the time activity curve by high tracer uptake, a large relative size, and a steep slope of the rapid clearance phase. Increases in plasma glucose and insulin levels in the postprandial state shift substrate oxidation from free fatty acid to glucose or lactate. The time activity curve mirrors this change by a decrease in the relative size and slope of the rapid clearance curve component, together with an increase in the relative size of the slow clearance phase.

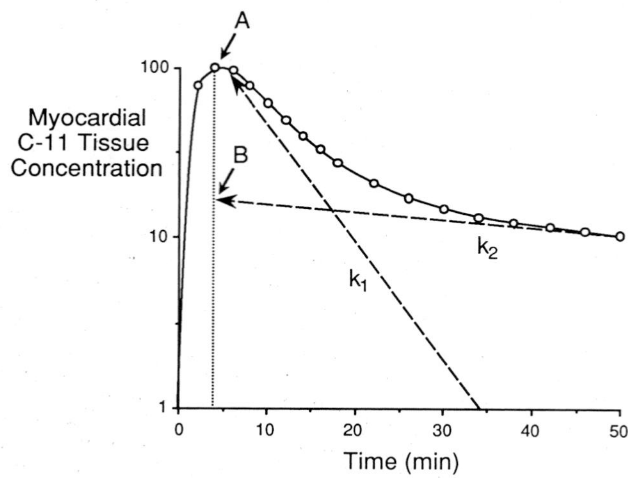

Figure 60–1. Schematic representation of the myocardial uptake and subsequent clearance of C-11 palmitate. The tissue time activity curves are obtained from serially acquired positron emission tomographic images of intravenous injection of C-11 palmitate. Note the rapid accumulation of activity in myocardium. Peak activity concentrations are reached within 4 to 5 minutes. Least square fitting of the subsequent clearance of tracer from myocardium indicates two distinct clearance phases defined by slopes k_1 and k_2 and their intercepts. The relative sizes as an index of the fractional distribution of fatty acid in myocardium are estimated by extrapolation of the slow clearance curve component to the time of peak activity A. The activity concentration B is an estimate of the fraction of tracer incorporated into the slow turnover functional pool. Its relative size is estimated by the ratio of B/A. The relative size of the rapid clearance phase is the difference between A and B divided by A. The clearance rate constants (slopes of the two phases) can be converted into clearance half-times and are expressed in minutes.

The various iodo fatty acid analogs participate to different extents in the overall fatty acid metabolism and its responses to physiologic intervention. They therefore provide different degrees of information on myocardial fatty acid metabolism. As listed in Table 60–1, iodo fatty acid analogs are generally grouped into iodine-for-methyl group analogs, aromatic fatty acid analogs, branch-chain fatty acid analogs, and isosteric fatty acid analogs.

Iodine-for-Methyl Fatty Acid Analogs

In this group of fatty acid analogs, the radioactive iodine replaces a methyl group in the terminal (or omega) position of the long chain fatty acid (see also Figure 60–2).[R2, R3] The two most commonly used fatty acid analogs in this group are 16-[1-123] iodo hexadecanoic acid (IHDA) and 17-[1-123] iodo heptadecanoic acid (IHPA). Both differ in chain length by one carbon but generally exhibit comparable tracer properties. They are therefore reviewed together.

Administered intravenously, both IHDA and IHPA rapidly accumulate in myocardium. Poe and associates reported first-pass extraction fractions of as high as 80 percent following intracoronary injections in dogs.[P1, P2] In both animal experimental studies

Table 60–1. IODO FATTY ACID ANALOGS FOR EVALUATION OF MYOCARDIAL FATTY ACID METABOLISM

Iodine-for-methyl group analogs
17-[p-^{123}I]-heptadecanoic acid (IHPA)
16-[p-^{123}I]-hexadecanoic acid (IHDA)
Aromatic fatty acid analogs
15-(p-[^{123}I]-iodophenyl)-pentadecanoic acid (IPPA)
Isosteric analogs
17-[p-^{123}I]-iodo-9-tellura heptadecanoic acid
15-(p-[^{123}I]-iodophenyl)-6-tellura pentadecanoic acid
Branch-chain fatty acid analogs
14-(p-[^{123}I]-iodophenyl)-beta methyltetradecanoic acid (BMTDA)
15-(p-[^{123}I]-iodophenyl)-3,3-dimethyl pentadecanoic acid (DMIPP)
15-(p-[^{123}I]-iodophenyl)-3-methylpentadecanoic acid (BMIPP)

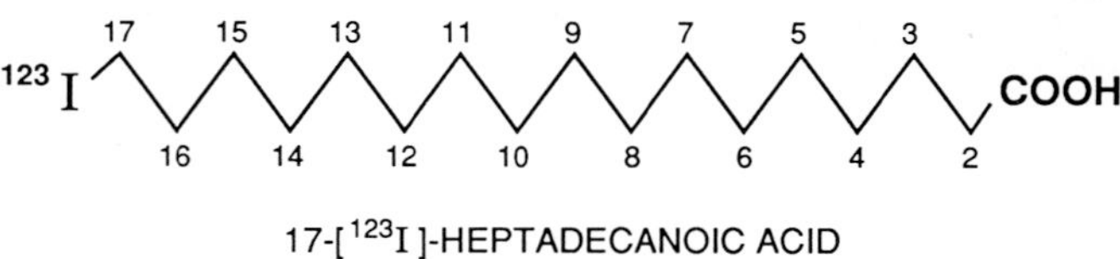

17-[^{123}I]-HEPTADECANOIC ACID

15-(p-[^{123}I]-IODOPHENYL)PENTADECANOIC ACID

15-(p-[^{123}I]-IODOPHENYL)-3,3-DIMETHYLPENTADECANOIC ACID

Figure 60–2. Schematic representation of examples of three different types of radioiodo fatty acid analogs (see text).

and clinical investigations, the radiolabel was found to clear from myocardium in a biexponential manner.[D1, D2, M1] Correlative studies in rabbit myocardium with C-14–labeled palmitate demonstrated comparable clearance characteristics and provided additional support for the utility of these two iodo fatty acid analogs as tracers of fatty acid metabolism.[D3, K3, K4, M1] Further, studies in six patients revealed similar clearance characteristics for C-11 palmitate and IHDA in human myocardium.[N1] For C-11 palmitate, clearance half-times for the early phase averaged 6.0 ± 1.1 minutes and for the slow phase, 157 ± 103 minutes. The corresponding values for IHDA were 9 ± 3 and 43 ± 26 minutes. Discrepancies between both tracers were attributed by the investigators to differences in heart rate and blood pressure products between studies and thus in myocardial oxygen consumption. Consistent with the change in myocardial fatty acid oxidation, the relative size and slope of the clearance curve component of IHDA was found to be decreased in ischemic myocardium.[V1, V2] Global ischemia in isolated rabbit hearts was associated with monoexponential rather than biexponential IHDA clearance, with mean clearance half-times of 60.5 minutes.[K3] It is interesting that a small fraction of the total tissue activity cleared rapidly from myocardium, with an average half-time of 3.8 minutes. The loss of the rapid clearance phase was thought to reflect the impairment of fatty acid oxidation. The residual slow clearance may have been related to some extent to residual fatty acid oxidation or to release of nonmetabolized tracer after hydrolysis of labeled triglycerides. The initial, rapid loss of a small fraction of activity, on the other hand, might have resulted from back diffusion of nonmetabolized iodo fatty acid or from enhanced diffusibility because of a possible increase in the mitochondrial surface area and, consequently, a higher permeability surface product. Either possibility remains unconfirmed because the chemical species containing the radiolabel in the myocardial effluent was not determined. Infusion of glucose and insulin in patients altered the clearance curve morphology in a fashion similar to that of C-11 palmitate (Fig. 60–3). The decrease in the relative size and slope of the rapid clearance phase reflected the known shift in oxidative metabolism from fatty acid to glucose.[D3, D4] The observed changes of the clearance curve morphology in response to physiologic interventions, therefore, confirmed the

●●● CONTROL ○○○ INSULIN + GLUCOSE

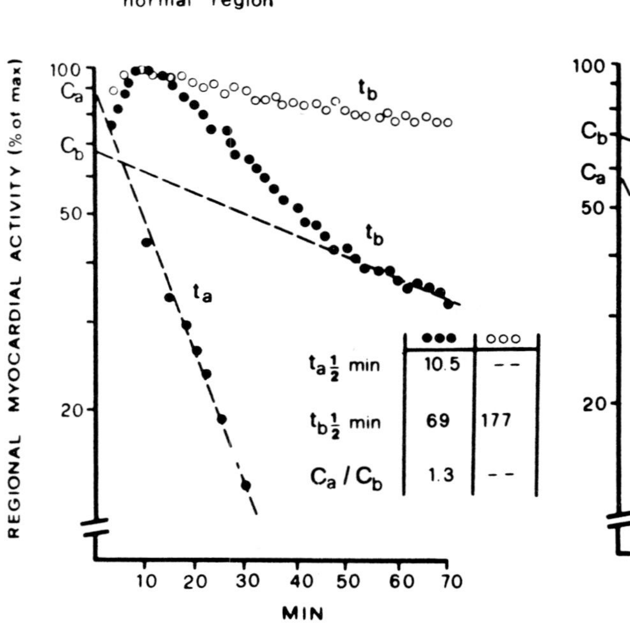

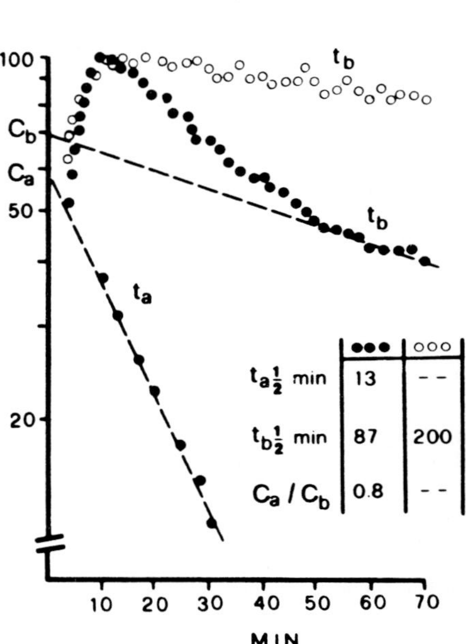

Figure 60–3. Uptake and clearance of IHDA normal (left) and ischemic myocardium (right) in a patient with coronary artery disease studied in the fasted state and again after glucose and insulin infusion. In the fasted state, iodine activity clears biexponentially from both myocardial regions. The relative size and slope of the rapid clearance phase are lower in ischemic than in normal myocardium. Glucose and insulin infusion abolishes the rapid clearance curve component, consistent with a shift from fatty acid to glucose oxidation. (t_a and t_b are the clearance half-times for the rapid and the slow clearance curve component, and C_a and C_b are their relative sizes). (From Dudczak, K., et al.: The use of I-123 heptadecanoic acid (HDA) as a metabolic tracer: Preliminary report. Eur. J. Nucl. Med. 9:81, 1984, with permission.)

utility of this fatty acid analog for the noninvasive evaluation of regional myocardial fatty acid metabolism. However, there were inconsistencies. The failure of the clearance slope to increase with exercise[V2] and accelerated clearance rates in infarcted human myocardium[V3] raised questions as to what extent or how accurately the slope of this rapid clearance phase reflected the rate of fatty acid oxidation.

In addition to the fractional distribution of radiolabel in myocardium, subsequent studies elucidated several factors that determine the slope of the rapid clearance curve component. Tissue assays of myocardium from isolated heart preparations and from dogs demonstrated that the radioiodine label was in fact incorporated into triglycerides and phospholipids (Fig. 60–4).[K3, K5, V4, V5] They also revealed high intracellular concentrations of free iodide early after tracer administration. Ischemia caused a predicted change of the fractional distribution of label. The decline of the ratio of free to lipid-bound radioiodine appears to reflect the reduced oxidation as well as the augmented deposition of fatty acid in the endogenous lipid pool.[V4] Nevertheless, free iodide still represented 41 to 84 percent of the total tissue activity at 5 and 120 minutes. These observations raised two questions. First, was there nonspecific deiodination? And second, was the transfer of free iodine from mitochondria into cytosol and across the cellular membrane into blood the rate-limiting step for clearance of radiotracer from myocardium?

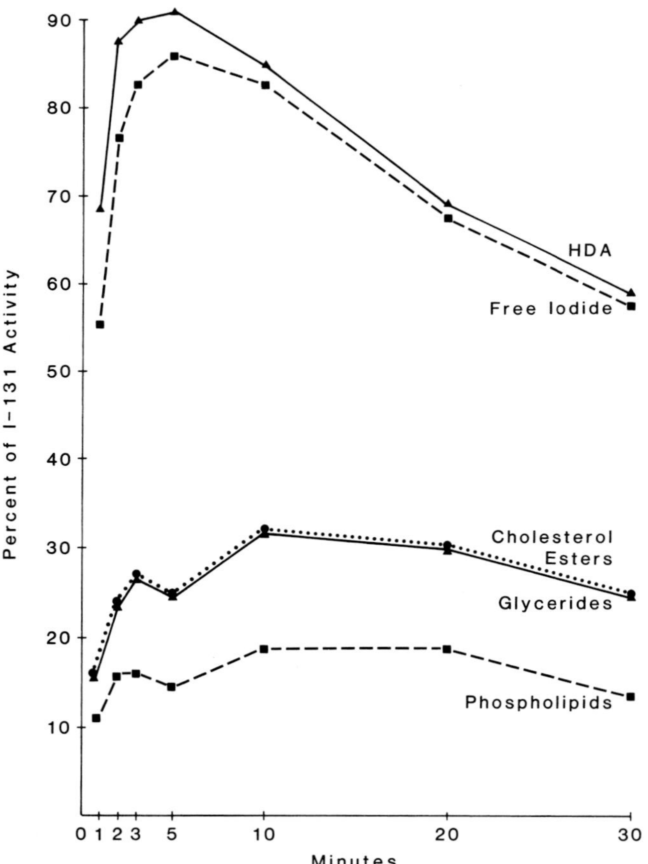

Figure 60–4. Fractional distribution of the radiolabel in myocardium and its changes over time as determined from serial myocardial biopsies and tissue assays in normal canine myocardium after intravenous administration of IHDA. Note the large fraction of free iodine in myocardium. (Adapted from Visser, F., et al.: Metabolic fate of radioiodinated heptadecanoic acid in the normal canine heart. Circulation 72:565, 1985. Reproduced from Schelbert, H.: Current status and prospects of new radionuclides and radiopharmaceuticals for cardiovascular nuclear medicine. Semin. Nucl. Med. 17:145, 1987, with permission.)

Observations in isolated hearts implicated oxidation rather than a nonspecific process as the primary mechanism for the rapid liberation and accumulation of free iodine in the cell.[C1] Depending on the carbon chain length, the radiolabel resides after β-oxidation in either acetic acid or propionic acid and is subsequently released as halide ion.[K4] These observations, together with findings in normal and ischemic myocardium of dogs, suggested that *transmembranous* exchange of iodide rather than rates of oxidation primarily accounted for the rate of tracer clearance from myocardium.[C1, V5, V6] Similar conclusions were reached with "prelabeling" of isolated perfused rabbit hearts with free iodide.[K3] Tissue clearance half-times of free iodide from myocardium averaged 14.3 ± 2.1 minutes and thus were similar to those after IHDA labeling. More recent observations in canine myocardium further supported this possibility.[S1] Comparative studies of IHDA and C-14–labeled palmitate failed to demonstrate a direct relationship between changes in the clearance rates of IHDA and of C-14 palmitate in response to changes in myocardial oxygen consumption. In fact, the slope of the early clearance phase of IHDA declined with higher oxygen consumption. The investigators concluded that the fractional distribution of tracer between the rapid and slow clearance phase or the ratio of the relative sizes reflected changes in fatty acid oxidation rather than the slope of the rapid clearance phase.

In summary, high first-pass extraction fractions indicate that the initial uptake of IHDA and IHPA in myocardium largely depends on regional myocardial blood flow. While the biexponential clearance curve morphology generally corresponds to the fractional distribution of fatty acid between oxidation and incorporation into the endogenous lipid pool, clearance rates of tracer from myocardium may inaccurately reflect rates of fatty acid oxidation. This is because transfer of iodide across the mitochondrial or cellular membranes is the rate-limiting step. On the other hand, the fractional distribution of tracer in myocardium, as reflected by the relative sizes of the two clearance curve components, can provide information on myocardial fatty acid metabolism.

Aromatic Fatty Acid Analogs

Machulla proposed 15-p-iodophenyl pentadecanoic acid (IPPA) as an alternate and potentially useful tracer of myocardial fatty acid metabolism.[M1, M2] As illustrated in Figure 60–2, the radioiodine is stabilized on the terminal phenyl ring on the straight chain fatty acid. The compound undergoes β-oxidation, with release of radioiodine from myocardium in the form of benzoic acid, which the liver metabolizes to its glucuronid and hippuric acid. Both substances clear from blood via the kidney.[R4] Initial investigations in rabbits as well as in patients with coronary artery disease and with cardiomyopathy established the utility of this new compound for myocardial imaging and for the evaluation of regional myocardial fatty acid metabolism.[D1] The biodistribution of this new agent and its subcellular distribution in myocardium have been determined. Within 5 minutes of intravenous administration, its uptake in myocardium averaged 4.4 percent of the total injected dose, compared with only 2.7 percent of co-injected C-14–labeled palmitate.[R4] IPPA subsequently cleared biexponentially from myocardium. Fractional distributions and clearance rates were similar to those of radiolabeled palmitate, although myocardial IPPA concentrations remained higher than those of C-14–labeled palmitate. Furthermore, the fractional distributions of the iodine label between free fatty acid, triglycerides, and phospholipids correlated well with those of the C-14 label originating from palmitate. Other studies[R5] demonstrated the anticipated effects of dietary interventions on the myocardial uptake and fractional distribution of IPPA. Higher incorporation of label into triglycerides and phospholipids in the postprandial state (70 to 80 percent in triglycerides and 6 to 15 percent in phospholipids) than in the fasted state (40 to 57 percent in triglycerides and 17 to 28 percent in phospholipids) suggested that preferential fatty acid utilization resulted in enhanced β-oxidation of IPPA and reduced incorporation into the endogenous lipid pool. Additional studies by the same investigators confirmed the similarity of the fractional distributions of the radioiodine label of IPPA and of radiolabels of oleic acid and palmitic acid in rat myocardium.[R6] In isolated rat heart experiments, the rate of release of iodo benzoic acid as a metabolite of IPPA was found to correlate closely to the rate of C-14 carbon dioxide release as the oxidative end product of co-injected C-14–labeled palmitate.[R6] Isoproterenol-mediated increases and lactate-induced decreases in fatty acid oxidation in these studies were associated with comparable changes in rates of C-14 carbon dioxide and iodo benzoic acid release. DeGrado and colleagues, using isolated working rat hearts, pharmacologically inhibited the carnitine palmitoyl transferase I and observed nearly a 70 percent suppression of oxidation of IPPA, compared with a reduction of about 90 percent of C-14 palmitate oxidation.[D5] These changes were correctly identified by a decline of the relative size of the rapid clearance curve component. Thus, considerable experimental evidence supports the utility of IPPA as a tracer of myocardial fatty acid metabolism. Compared with C-11–labeled palmitate, most studies indicate higher myocardial uptake of IPPA. Altered binding of IPPA to albumin, differences in transmembranous exchange, or differences in metabolic handling may serve as possible explanations.[R7] Regional myocardial clearance rates and changes in the biexponential clearance curve morphology after substrate interventions or during ischemia appear accurately to identify directional changes in myocardial fatty acid oxidation and storage in the endogenous lipid pool.

The rapid accumulation of IPPA in myocardium and its subsequent biexponential clearance pattern has been demonstrated in humans. Using high temporal sampling with serial gamma camera imaging, myocardial activity concentrations reached a plateau phase within 5 to 10 minutes after injection, which lasted from about 8 to 18 minutes and was followed by biexponential clearance of tracer from myocardium (Fig. 60–5).[V7] Tissue clearance half-times, as Dudczak and associates determined by monoexponential curve fitting, were found to average 43.8 ± 6.2 minutes in normal myocardium[D1] (Table 60–2).

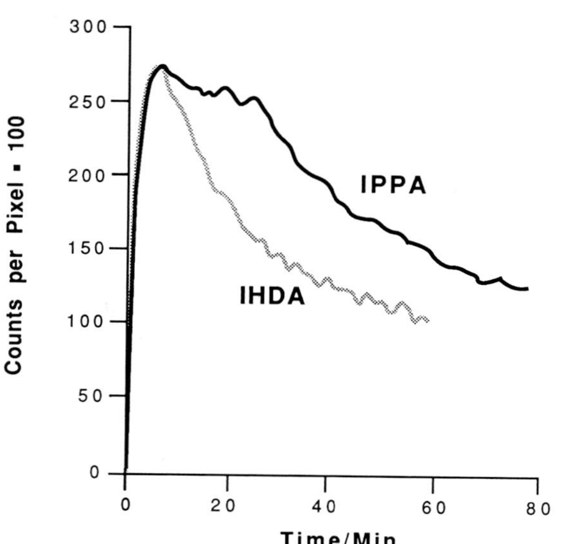

Figure 60–5. Myocardial uptake and clearance of IHDA and IPPA in normal human myocardium after intravenous tracer injection and serial planar gamma camera imaging. The two time activity curves were normalized to the same maximum activity. Note the plateau phase for IPPA that is not present for IHDA. (Adapted from Vyska, K., et al.: Regional myocardial free fatty acid extraction in normal and ischemic myocardium. Circulation 78:1218, 1988, with permission of the American Heart Association, Inc.)

Branch-Chain Fatty Acid Analogs

The search for iodo fatty acid analogs with longer myocardial retention times prompted the development of this class of compounds. As discussed by Otto and co-workers, methyl branching of the fatty acid chain is thought to protect these compounds against metabolism by β-oxidation.[O1] Provided they retained some of the physiologic properties critical for the initial transmembranous exchange and for effective sequestration into myocardium, these modified fatty acid analogs would then be retained in myocardium for longer time periods. They therefore would be more suitable for the lower temporal sampling requirements of single-photon emission computed tomography (SPECT). Based on findings with several newly synthesized fatty acid analogs, Otto and his group concluded that branching of the fatty acid chain significantly lowered the heart-to-blood ratios relative to straight chain analogs but resulted in constant myocardial activity concentrations.[O1] The degree of branching as well as the chain length determined the myocardial uptake of these tracers.

Table 60–2. CLEARANCE HALF-TIMES OF IODO FATTY ACID ANALOGS IN NORMAL AND DISEASED MYOCARDIUM

	Number	Normal Myocardium	Clearance Half-times (Minutes) *Infarcted Myocardium*	*Ischemic Myocardium*	Tracer
Normal Volunteers					
Freundlieb et al. 1980	10	25.5 ± 5.0	—	—	IHDA
Poe et al. 1977		>25	—	—	IHDA
Stoddart et al. 1987	9	18.8 ± 3.3	—	—	IHDA
Van der Wall et al. 1981	6	27.5 ± 3.0	—	—	IHDA
Höck et al. 1983	6	24.7 ± 2.5	—	—	
		24.7 ± 2.0*	—	—	
Coronary Artery Disease					
Freundlieb et al. 1980	10			31.8 ± 19.6	IHDA
Van der Wall et al. 1981	25	34.0 ± 8.4	18.5 ± 2.5	46.7 ± 7.1*	IHDA
		34.8 ± 7.7	16.8 ± 3.5	29.1 ± 4.7	IHPA
Stoddart et al. 1987	10	20.8 ± 4.0	15.5 ± 7.8	35.5 ± 41.5	IHDA
Dudczak et al. 1983	40	43.8 ± 6.2	66.1 ± 15.1	54.5 ± 9.6	IPPA
Kennedy et al. 1986	18			Prolonged‡	IPPA
Cardiomyopathy					
Dudczak et al. 1983	10	68.3 ± 29.6	—	—	IPPA
Rabinovitch et al. 1985	16	15.0–105†	—	—	IHDA
Ugolini et al. 1988	19	accelerated‡	—	—	IPPA
Höck et al. 1983	20	15.1–116.2†	—	—	IHPA

*Studied after exercise; †range of regional clearance values; ‡no absolute values available.
The specific radioiode fatty acid analog used in each study is indicated on the right.

An example of this class of compounds is β-methyl-heptadecanoic acid, which contains a methyl group in the 2-(or β)-carbon position of the straight chain fatty acid. Labeled with iodine or carbon-11 and examined in isolated, arterially perfused hearts and in intact animals,[E2, J1, L1] the compound rapidly accumulated in myocardium but cleared only slowly from it. The agent, therefore, has been employed in several experimental animal studies for delineation of regional differences in myocardial fatty acid uptake.[Y1, Y2] Images obtained with this type of fatty acid analog in normal volunteers and in patients with cardiac disease were of excellent diagnostic quality.[L2]

More information on the biologic properties of this type of iodo fatty acid analog is available for two other side branch aromatic fatty acids, 15-(p-iodophenyl)-3-R,S-methyl pentadecanoic acid (BMIPP) and 15-(p-iodophenyl)-3,3-dimethyl pentadecanoic acid (DMIPP).[G1, G2, G4, K6, K7] As illustrated in Figure 60–2, either one (BMIPP) or two (DMIPP) methyl side branches are attached to the 3-carbon of the straight chain fatty acid with a terminal, radioiodinated phenyl ring. Comparative studies in fasted rat myocardium revealed distinct differences between these two compounds and the earlier described IPPA.[K8] All three compounds rapidly accumulated in myocardium. At 5 minutes, an average of about 4 percent of the total injected dose resided in 1 gram of myocardium (or about 2 percent in the whole heart). As expected, IPPA cleared most rapidly from myocardium. Over the 2-hour observation period, myocardial activity concentrations declined by more than 50 percent. Myocardial concentrations of BMIPP declined more slowly (by only 25 percent) over the same observation period. In contrast, DMIPP exhibited virtually no clearance. These differences in clearance kinetics were associated with differences in heart-to-blood activity ratios. At 30 minutes after administration, they were highest for DMIPP (12 to 1), compared with ratios of 2 to 1 or less for BMIPP and IPPA. The fractional distribution of the radiolabel between the functional and structural compartments in myocardium similarly differed among the three compounds.[A1] Thirty minutes after injection in fasted rats, 65 to 80 percent of the total radioactivity resided in the triglyceride fraction for the three compounds. The fraction of total tissue activity contained in free fatty acid, however, differed markedly among the three compounds when examined early after injection (at 5 minutes). It ranged from 10 to 15 percent for IPPA, was about 20 percent for BMIPP, and amounted to more than 60 percent for DMIPP. Competition of oxidation with lipid incorporation for activated free fatty acid is likely to account for these differences. For example, if oxidation is reduced or impaired, as appears to be true for DMIPP, more tracer is available for esterification to triglycerides. Moreover, 34 and 38 percent of the total activity for DMIPP was associated at 30 minutes with the mitochondrial and microsomal fractions, compared with only 18 percent and 15 percent for IPPA. The same studies further indicated that DMIPP cleared most rapidly from blood, which largely accounted for the high myocardium-to-blood activity ratios.

In summary, experimental data support the notion of a protective effect of the side branch against β-oxidation. However, the clearance of radioactivity from myocardium, as observed for some of these compounds, implies some degree of metabolic degradation. Whether this occurs via β-oxidation or α-oxidation or other metabolic pathways or whether it can be explained, at least in part, by hydrolysis of triglycerides and back-diffusion of nonmetabolized tracer remains uncertain at present. Branch-chain fatty acid analogs with virtually complete trapping, on the other hand, may prove useful for noninvasive measurements of total fatty acid utilization, although some uncertainty remains as to whether these analogs might trace the uptake of only that fraction of fatty acid that is subsequently incorporated into the endogenous lipid pool. Although this class of compound is unlikely to provide comprehensive information on fatty acid metabolism, it offers an opportunity for quantitative measurements of total myocardial fatty acid utilization. The virtually unidirectional transport, together with high myocardium-to-blood activity ratios, analogous to the F-18 2-fluoro-2-deoxyglucose method (described in Chapter 65), permit design of relatively simple tracer kinetic models for the external quantification of myocardial fatty acid utilization.

Isosteric Fatty Acid Analogs

Other attempts to protect fatty acid analogs against degradation via β-oxidation resulted in the development of isosteric fatty acid analogs. The inclusion of a tellurium atom at a central position within the fatty acid chain has been one of such modifications.[G5] Several experimental animal studies have conclusively demonstrated that these isosteric fatty acid analogs continue to be avidly extracted by myocardium but are then, as postulated, retained in myocardium.[G3, G5] Although regional myocardial blood flow has been found to determine the initial distribution of these tracers in myocardium, there is little information on their subsequent metabolic fate.[K2]

Comparison of Fatty Acid Analogs

Independent of structural differences, fatty acid analogs are avidly extracted by myocardium. Their initial uptake in myocardium therefore depends largely on blood flow but may be modified by dietary interventions or by regional myocardial ischemia. Both iodine-for-methyl (IHDA and IHPA) and aromatic fatty acid analogs (IPPA) clear biexponentially from myocardium. Myocardial tissue clearance half-times for IPPA are moderately longer than those for IHDA and IHPA (see Table 60–2). For both groups of fatty acid analogs, the biexponential clearance curve morphology reflects the fractional distribution of tracer between oxidation and storage of free fatty acid. Mitochondrial membranes apparently exert a significant barrier effect to the egress of liberated free iodide. Therefore, the slope of the early clearance phase of IHDA and IHPA inaccurately reflects changes in the rate of β-oxidation of free fatty acid. The same does not pertain to clearance rates of IPPA, in which the radiolabel is released from myocardium in the form of benzoic acid. It appears, therefore, that the fractional distribution of IHDA and IHPA, as reflected by the ratio of the relative sizes of the two clearance phases, offers more accurate information on fatty acid metabolism than determination of individual clearance rates. Higher blood pool and background activity for IHDA and IHPA than for the aromatic fatty acid analog IPPA degrade image quality and require complex corrections for determining regional myocardial tissue clearance rates. Furthermore, the longer myocardial residence time of IPPA renders this compound more suitable for tomographic radionuclide imaging. In terms of image quality, branch-chain and isosteric fatty acid analogs appear to be superior. They are metabolically trapped in myocardium. Blood pool and background activities are low. The metabolic information provided by the latter compounds, however, is limited and pertains largely to the initial uptake by and metabolic sequestration of fatty acid into myocardium.

TECHNICAL ASPECTS OF IODO FATTY ACID IMAGING

The metabolic information obtained noninvasively by imaging of the myocardial uptake and subsequent clearance of radioiodinated fatty acid analogs depends upon several factors.

SPECIFIC TYPE OF FATTY ACID ANALOG. The particular type of fatty acid analog employed largely determines the specific information that can be obtained. Tracers virtually trapped in myocardium provide mostly information on regional myocardial fatty acid utilization and, because of their high first-pass extraction fraction, on regional myocardial blood flow. In contrast, radiotracers that subsequently clear from myocardium offer information on fatty acid oxidation as well as on storage of fatty acid in the endogenous lipid pool. The relative sizes of the two clearance curve components correspond to the fractional distribution of tracer between oxidation and storage of free fatty acid, whereas their slopes or clearance half-times can provide information on rates of fatty acid oxidation and of turnover of the endogenous lipid pool.

IMAGE ACQUISITION. The time of acquisition of serial images is equally important.[V8, V9] As clearance half-times differ significantly among the various iodo fatty acid analogs, sufficiently long acquisition times are required in order to delineate adequately this biexponential clearance pattern. Total image acquisition times, therefore, should be tailored to the characteristics of the fatty acid analog employed. Short image acquisition times will indicate only the initial clearance of tracer from myocardium, which can be approximated by monoexponential least square fitting techniques. Differences in acquisition times are likely to account for differences in reported tissue clearance rate constants. As emphasized by Dudczak and associates, only sufficiently long image acquisition times, for example, 70 minutes, uncover the characteristic biexponential clearance pattern and permit determination of the fractional distribution of tracer and their clearance half-times by appropriate biexponential least square fitting techniques.

DIETARY CONDITIONS. The dietary state must be standardized or at least be monitored. Similar to C-11 palmitate, the relative size and slope of the early clearance curve component as the reflection of fatty acid oxidation depend upon substrate availability and consequently, on substrate utilization. Thus, in the postprandial state, when glucose and insulin plasma levels may be high, myocardium preferentially oxidizes glucose, so less free fatty acid will be oxidized. Therefore, both the size and slope of the rapid clearance curve component are likely to be low, as implied by the findings after infusion of glucose and lactate.[D2, D6]

BACKGROUND ACTIVITY. Correction of myocardial tracer uptake for background activity can be equally important. Obviously, the need for such correction depends on the type of fatty acid analog. It applies especially to iodine-for-methyl group analogs, in which there are high free iodide concentrations in blood. Freundlieb and associates, therefore, have devised a special correction technique.[F1] After acquisition of IHDA images, a separate dose of I-123 sodium iodide is injected intravenously. The resulting step-increase in activity concentrations, determined from a region of interest assigned to myocardium, indicates the magnitude of contamination of myocardial tracer uptake by background activity and serves as a measure for the correction of myocardial activity. Because of an additional injection of radioactive iodine and increases in cost as well as radiation burden to the patient, this approach has not been widely accepted. No such corrections have been developed for or are employed with the aromatic fatty acid analog IPPA.

PLANAR VERSUS TOMOGRAPHIC IMAGING. Another important technical aspect is the mode of image acquisition. Early investigations employed only planar imaging. Studies with limited angle tomography—for example, the seven-pinhole collimator—followed but have now been largely replaced by imaging with single-photon emission computed tomography (SPECT). Emergence of iodo fatty acid analogs—for example, IPPA—with long myocardial residence times has favored the latter approach. The images are of high diagnostic quality with good contrast resolution. Adequate delineation of temporal changes in myocardial tissue activity concentrations, such as intravenous administration of iodine for methyl group fatty acid, appears possible at present only with conventional planar imaging. However, the rate of temporal sampling depends upon the type of fatty acid analog employed. Using IPPA, Hansen and associates were able to detect regional abnormalities in tracer tissue clearance rates from only two SPECT image sets acquired for 20 minutes each with an interval of 40 minutes.[H1] Using the same approach, the investigators succeeded in detecting with a high degree of sensitivity regional impairments of fatty acid metabolism after exercise in patients with coronary artery disease. Therefore, depending on the type of fatty acid analog employed, low temporal sampling may not necessarily limit the detection of metabolic abnormalities. Generally, the superior image quality achievable with SPECT has favored the use of iodo fatty acid tracers with slower myocardial clearance rates.

CLINICAL EXPERIENCE WITH IODO FATTY ACID ANALOGS

The promise of iodo fatty acid analogs for the evaluation of regional myocardial blood flow and, most important, for the evaluation of fatty acid metabolism prompted clinical investigations in patients with acute and chronic coronary artery disease and cardiomyopathies. The utility of fatty acid analogs also has been explored for delineating responses to therapeutic interventions like coronary thrombolysis, coronary angioplasty, and coronary artery bypass grafting.

Myocardial Infarction

Early investigations with IHDA and IHPA and serial planar scintigraphic imaging demonstrated the possibility of accurately localizing acute or recent myocardial infarctions and determining their extent.[V3] Severity and extent of segmental reductions in myocardial iodo fatty acid uptake correlated with defects on thallium-201 scintigraphy (Fig. 60–6) or with the electrocardiographic infarct location (Fig. 60–7). Although ischemia had been expected to prolong the tissue clearance rates of iodo fatty acid significantly, investigations in 30 patients studied within 1 week of onset of acute symptoms demonstrated accelerated clearance

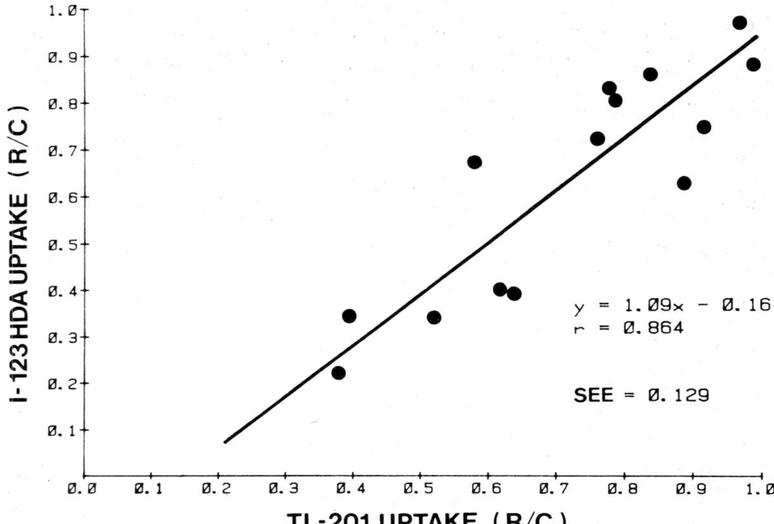

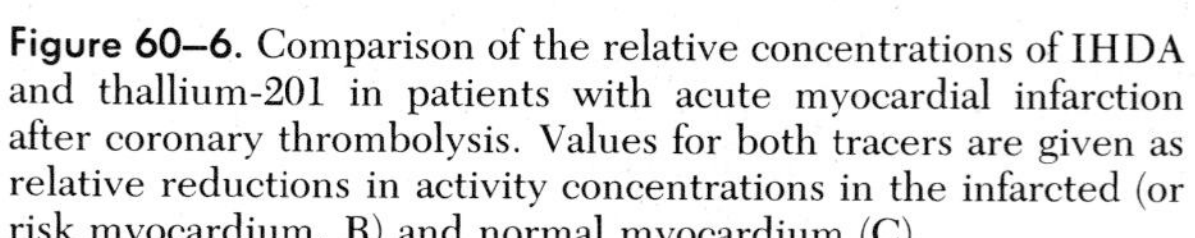
Figure 60–6. Comparison of the relative concentrations of IHDA and thallium-201 in patients with acute myocardial infarction after coronary thrombolysis. Values for both tracers are given as relative reductions in activity concentrations in the infarcted (or risk myocardium, R) and normal myocardium (C).

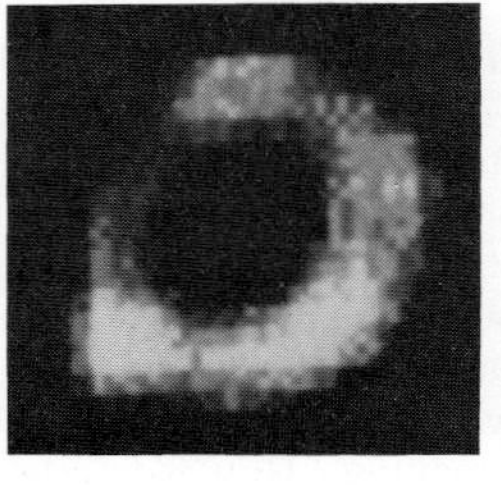

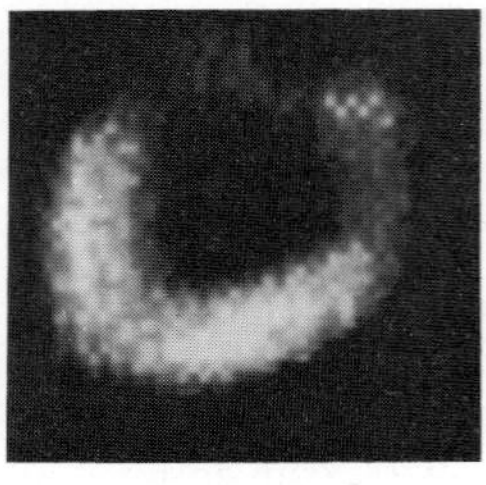

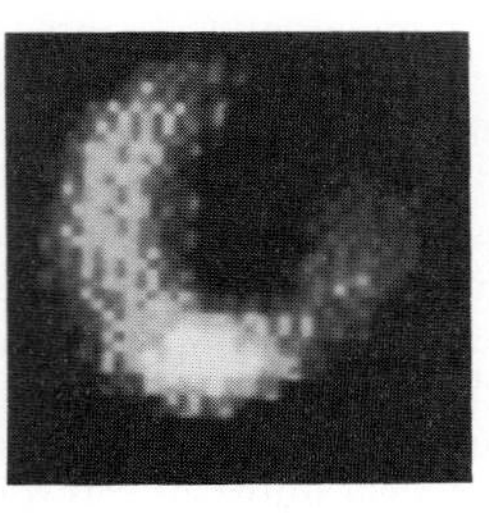

Figure 60–7. Serial planar myocardial scintigrams recorded after intravenous injection of IPPA at rest in a patient with a 70 percent diameter stenosis of the left anterior descending coronary artery. Note the initially decreased tracer uptake in the interventricular septum, which subsequently resolves on the late images. However, tracer is retained, as seen on the 80-minute image, in the interventricular septum but has cleared from myocardium (lateral wall) supplied by normal coronary arteries. (From Dudczak, R., Kletter, K., Angelberger, P., et al.: Imaging with I-23–labelled fatty acids. In Biersack, H. J., and Cox, P. H. [eds.]: Radioisotope Studies in Cardiology. Kluwer Academic Publishers [Martin Nijhoff Publishers], Hingham, MA, 1985, pp. 295–317.)

rates in recently infarcted myocardium.[V3] The rates averaged 18.5 ± 2.5 minutes and, thus, were 46 percent shorter than the clearance half-times in presumably normal myocardium (34.0 ± 8.4 minutes) (see Table 60–2). Stoddart and colleagues more recently confirmed these unexpected findings in a group of 20 patients restudied within 1 week of acute myocardial infarction.[S2] Clearance half-times in myocardial infarct regions averaged 15.5 ± 7.5 minutes, compared with 20.8 ± 4.0 minutes in noninfarcted myocardium (see Table 60–2). Several mechanisms for the shortened rather than prolonged clearance half-times in acutely infarcted myocardium have been proposed. They range from possible contamination of myocardial uptake by blood pool activity to increased contractile work by noninfarcted myocardium in the epicardial layer of the left ventricular wall.[V3] Studies in isolated hearts suggest another possibility. An increase in the mitochondrial surface associated with severe but reversible ischemia may facilitate the rate of exchange of free iodide across the mitochondrial membrane.[K3, K5]

In the study by Stoddart and colleagues in early postinfarction patients, global left ventricular function was found to have improved at 6 months' follow-up in patients with prolonged clearance half-times in infarcted myocardium, whereas shortened tissue clearance half-times in the infarct region were associated with a decline of left ventricular function.[S2] Although the small number of observations precludes definitive conclusions, differences in clearance half-times might be related to the severity of the ischemic injury and thus might be of prognostic significance.

Other investigators observed consistently prolonged regional tissue clearance rates with IPPA in patients with remote myocardial infarction.[D1] These prolonged clearance half-times were observed for both IHDA[F2] and IPPA.[D1] Uptake of IPPA in infarct regions was reduced by 38 percent, and regional tissue clearance half-times were markedly prolonged. They averaged 66.5 ± 15.1 minutes, compared with 43.6 ± 6.2 minutes in myocardium supplied by normal coronary arteries. Fridrich and co-workers reported similar clearance half-times for IHDA for infarcted and normal myocardial segments (29.8 ± 6.2 versus 25.8 ± 4.2 minutes).[F2] However, there was a considerable overlap of tissue clearance half-times between infarcted myocardium and myocardium supplied by stenosed but patent coronary arteries. Nevertheless, the difference in clearance half-times for IPPA between ischemic and infarcted areas was statistically significant (54.4 ± 9.6 minutes versus 66.5 ± 15.1 minutes; $p < 0.025$). It is important to note that tracer clearance rates in both types of myocardial regions were significantly slower than those in myocardium supplied by normal coronary arteries or those with the least stenosed coronary artery. It is interesting that there was a statistically significant positive correlation between clearance half-times of IPPA and the degree of impairment in regional contractile function.[D1] Rösler and colleagues examined 28 patients with limited angle tomography and IHDA within 10 days of acute myocardial infarction and again at 6 months.[R8] Two different infarct patterns were observed: Pattern 1 was associated with low uptake and accelerated washout, whereas pattern 2 was associated with reduced tracer uptake but delayed clearance. Pattern 1 was attributed to scar tissue and pattern 2 to viable but ischemically injured myocardium. For both patterns, the extent and severity of the defect size declined with time, but infarct size remained significantly larger in areas with accelerated washout during the initial study. However, left ventricular performance, as assessed by radionuclide ventriculography, did not correlate with these different patterns, which were further unrelated to the clinical outcome of patients. Thus, it remains unclear as to what extent the impairment of fatty acid oxidation, as evidenced by regional clearance rates, may be directly related to the severity of the ischemic injury, as evidenced by the severity of wall motion abnormality. Conversely, it is possible that reduced energy demand in dysfunctional myocardium could have resulted in a proportionate reduction in fatty acid oxidation. Both explanations also may pertain to recent observations by Vyska and colleagues.[V7] In three patients examined prior to and following an acute myocardial infarction, the location and extent of postinfarction thallium-201 defects corresponded to regions of delayed IPPA clearance rates prior to infarction. The investigators suggest that delayed clearance rates may have identified myocardium at risk, but no information was provided on pre-existing wall motion abnormalities or the severity of coronary artery disease.

The initial uptake of iodo fatty acid analogs in infarcted myocardium is generally reduced in direct proportion to regional myocardial blood flow. This is expected because of the high first-pass extraction fraction of iodo fatty acid and the flow-dependent tracer net extraction. However, discrepancies between blood flow and iodo fatty acid uptake can occur and have been observed in both experimental animal studies and in clinical investigations. Miller and co-workers recently explored the issue in a coronary occlusion-reperfusion dog model in which the utility of BMIPP for identifying viability in reperfused myocardium was examined.[M4] As mentioned, this agent does not undergo β-oxidation and so mostly traces myocardial fatty acid uptake. In these experiments, coronary occlusions were maintained for either 15 minutes ($n = 5$) or 60 minutes ($n = 5$) and were followed by reperfusion for 3 hours. Myocardial blood flow was measured with microspheres, and segmental systolic function was measured with ultrasonomicrometry. Myocardial tissue samples were submitted to triphenyl tetrazolium chloride (TTC) staining and electron microscopy. An additional group of dogs underwent a 60-minute occlusion of the left anterior descending coronary artery, followed by 3 hours of reperfusion. However, the distal portion of the left anterior descending coronary artery remained occluded in these dogs in order to create an anteroapical perfusion defect that could be visualized on SPECT imaging. In this latter group of dogs, dual imaging with thallium-201 and BMIPP was performed.

Iodo fatty acid activity concentrations were 37 percent higher in TTC staining than in non-TTC staining tissue samples, whereas occlusion blood flows and contractile function were similarly depressed during occlusion. After 3 hours of reperfusion, TTC-negative segments remained akinetic while TTC-positive zones had partially recovered systolic function. Furthermore, regional BMIPP activity concentrations in TTC-stained myocardium significantly exceeded myocardial blood flow. Electron microscopy demonstrated ultrastructural changes in these segments that were consistent with reversible injury. In the third group of dogs, SPECT imaging disclosed that uptake of the fatty acid analog exceeded the uptake of thallium-201. Thus, the discordant uptakes of the blood flow and the fatty acid tracer noninvasively identified myocardial segments as viable or ischemically stunned. Because methyl branch fatty acid analogs do not undergo β-oxidation, their metabolic fate in myocardium is relatively limited. Most of the label is incorporated into the triglyceride pool from which it may be released by lipoprotein lipase-mediated hydrolysis and back diffusion of label into blood. Incorporation of the label into the triglyceride pool most likely accounted for the tracer retention in postischemic myocardium. Branch chain fatty acid analogs may thus prove useful for delineating ATP-dependent esterification of free fatty acid and fatty acid storage in the endogenous triglyceride pool as an indicator of myocardial viability.

Clinical observations in patients after coronary thrombolysis also disclosed differences between myocardial blood flow and the initial myocardial uptake of iodo fatty acid analogs. For example, Pachinger and colleagues observed in post-thrombolysis patients segmental defects in myocardial iodo fatty acid analog uptake that were larger and more severe than perfusion defects on thallium-201 scintigrams.[P3] Follow-up studies of such defects in a subset of patients indicated that reperfused myocardium with this blood flow metabolism discrepancy recovered more often than myocardium in which blood flow and fatty acid uptake were concordantly reduced. However, verification of these findings requires studies in larger patient numbers and careful evaluation of wall motion abnormalities and their changes over time.

Chronic Coronary Artery Disease

Initial studies following exercise in patients with chronic coronary artery disease failed to demonstrate the anticipated prolongation of regional clearance half-times of fatty acid analogs. The fact that IHDA was injected after exercise, when the double product and thus fatty acid oxidation might already have returned to normal, most likely accounted for the failure to demonstrate metabolic abnormalities. Planar imaging with IPPA also established the relationship between reduced IPPA uptake and clearance rates in the presence of significant coronary artery disease (Fig. 60–7). Kennedy and colleagues employed SPECT in order to determine whether exercise-induced ischemia in 18 patients with coronary artery disease resulted in identifiable segmental reductions in myocardial IPPA uptake and clearance rates.[K9] The radioiodo fatty acid analog was injected 1 minute prior to the end of exercise, and SPECT images were recorded at 9 and at 40 minutes after tracer injection. Normal values were established in a group of 15 normal volunteers studied in an identical fashion. Overall, early and delayed IPPA imaging detected the presence of coronary artery disease with a sensitivity of 89 percent and a specificity of 67 percent when 1 standard deviation from the mean, as determined in the normal volunteers, was employed as the upper limit of normal. Use of a 2 standard deviation limit lowered the sensitivity to 72 percent but raised the specificity to 100 percent. Abnormal IPPA uptake or washout patterns were observed in 26 of a total of 27 noninfarcted regions. Increased tracer uptake in myocardial regions supplied by significantly stenosed coronary arteries, as seen on the early images, was one of the interesting findings in this study. Differential clearance rates most likely accounted for this observation. Although the tracer rapidly cleared from normal myocardium, it was retained in postischemic segments. The even more prominent relative increase in segmental tracer uptake, as demonstrated in some of the patients on the late images, appears to support this explanation.

Using the same study protocol in 33 patients with stable symptomatic coronary artery disease and with at least one coronary artery with an arteriographically determined diameter stenosis equal to or greater than 70 percent, segmental abnormalities in tracer uptake or clearance or both were found in 27 patients (82 percent) when the aforementioned 2 standard deviation limit was used. A subgroup of 25 patients underwent treadmill exercise testing with both IPPA and thallium-201. Workloads were comparable for the two exercise studies. The thallium-201 images were abnormal in 18 (or 72 percent) and the IPPA images in 21 (or 84 percent) of the 25 patients. Although IPPA tended to detect coronary artery disease with a greater sensitivity than thallium-201 imaging, this difference failed to reach statistical significance.

Reske and associates studied 41 patients with coronary artery disease and 10 normal volunteers after maximal bicycle exercise (Fig. 60–8).[R8] The investigators observed that 65 percent and 89 percent of myocardial segments supplied by coronary arteries with earlier 50 to 75 percent or greater than 75 percent luminal

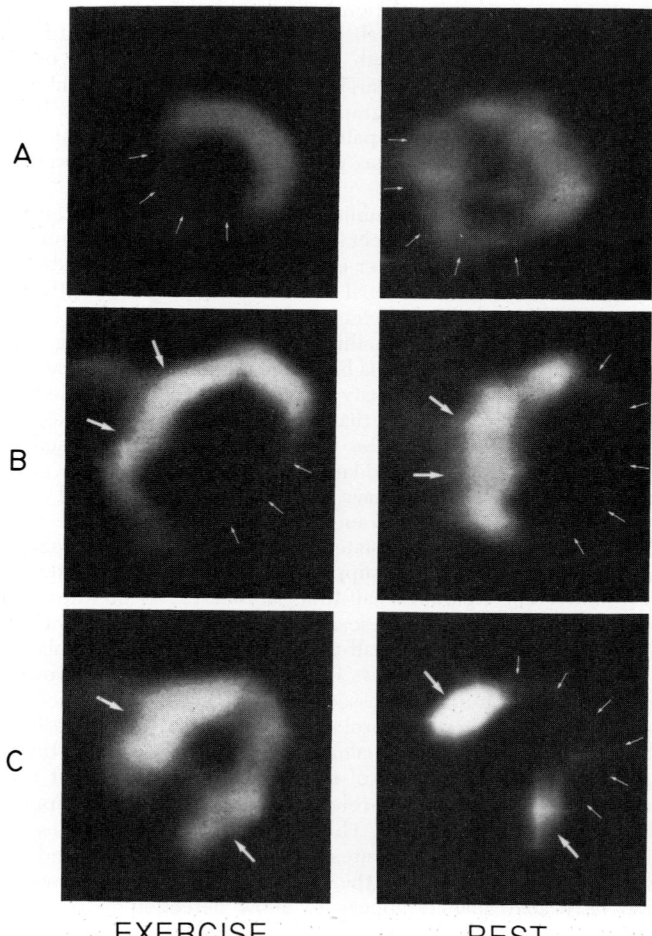

Figure 60–8. SPECT images of the initial myocardial uptake of IPPA in three patients (*A*, *B*, and *C*) early (5 minutes, left) and late (35 minutes) after exercise. Panel *A* represents a short axis cut through the mid-left ventricle, which indicates reduced uptake of IPPA in the interventricular septum and the inferior wall on the early postexercise images, with increased tracer retention on the late images. Angiography in this patient revealed a 95 percent diameter stenosis of the left anterior descending coronary artery. Panel *B*, Long-axis cuts in a patient with a prior myocardial infarction and a complete occlusion of the left circumflex coronary artery, a high-grade stenosis of the left anterior descending coronary artery after bypass grafting. The early postexercise images reveal a large defect in the posterolateral wall, with normal uptake in the interventricular septum and the anterior wall. The late images indicate increased retention of tracer in the interventricular septum. Panel *C*, Horizontal long-axis cuts in a patient with a complete occlusion of the right coronary artery and a 70 percent diameter stenosis of the left circumflex coronary artery. The early images reveal relatively homogeneous uptake of IPPA, whereas the late images indicate increased retention of tracer in the lateral wall. (From Reske, S. N., Nitsch, J., von der Lohe, E., et al.: Eingeschränkte myokardiale Fettsäure–Ultilisation bei koronarer Herzerkrankung nach symptomlimitierter ergometrischer Belastung. Nachweis pathologischer Stoffwechselmuster mit Hilfe von Jod–123–Phenylpentadekansäure und sequentieller SPECT. Z Kardiol 78:262–270, 1989.)

narrowing exhibited reduced uptake at the early image 5 to 7 minutes postinjection and/or increased retention, i.e., delayed washout, at the time of late imaging. It is interesting that segmental metabolic abnormalities persisted for significantly longer time periods than exercise-induced chest pain or electrocardiographic abnormalities. In normal subjects, uptake and clearance of the iodo fatty acid analog were homogeneous, but patients with coronary artery disease revealed retention of tracer in ischemic zones and persistent defects in infarcted territories. In a semiquantitative analysis for three tomographic planes, the investigators found a correlation between severity of stenosis and extent of the uptake abnormality. Thus, the results derived from these studies in patients with exercise-induced ischemia using SPECT and IPPA are comparable to those with C-11 palmitate and positron emission tomography in experimental animals with segmentally reduced C-11 palmitate uptake and washout and enhanced F-18 2-fluoro 2-deoxyglucose uptake in ischemic segments. (See Chapter 67.)

Vyska and colleagues examined the myocardial extraction of IPPA in 18 normal volunteers and in patients with coronary artery disease at rest and after exercise.[V7] A subgroup of patients was studied after interventional revascularization. In 15 of the 20 patients, exercise-induced defects of fatty acid uptake were larger than those seen on the thallium-201 images, suggesting that acute, stress-induced ischemia had reduced the extraction fraction of IPPA. Following angioplasty, stress scintigraphy revealed an improvement in segmental thallium-201 and IPPA uptake, although the extraction fraction of IPPA remained depressed in seven of ten patients. Stoddart and colleagues studied eight patients with chronic coronary artery disease before and after coronary angioplasty.[S3] Clearance half-times for IHDA averaged 35.5 ± 41.5 minutes in poststenotic segments and thus tended to be longer than in regions supplied by normal coronary arteries, with an average clearance half-time of 18.8 ± 3.4 minutes (see Table 60–2). Thus, the researchers failed to demonstrate a significant change in tracer half-times after successful angioplasty.

In summary, exercise stress in patients with chronic coronary artery disease is frequently associated with segmental reductions in myocardial uptake and prolonged myocardial clearance half-times of iodo fatty acid analogs. Segmentally reduced tracer uptake is largely a function of the reduced blood flow but may be modified by an ischemia-related effect on metabolic trapping of fatty acid in myocardium. The longer clearance half-times are likely to reflect abnormal rates of fatty acid oxidation and increased incorporation into the endogenous lipid pool. Lastly, iodo fatty acid analogs appear to allow detection of coronary artery disease with a sensitivity and specificity comparable to those of myocardial perfusion scintigraphy.

Cardiomyopathy

Several clinical investigations have explored the utility of iodo fatty acid analogs for identifying metabolic abnormalities in dilated, congestive cardiomyopathy. Using IHPA, Höck and group studied 20 congestive cardiomyopathy patients with different etiologies after a 3-minute, low level stress test.[H2] In addition to heterogeneous uptake of tracer in myocardium, clearance half-times were markedly prolonged (see Table 60–2). In a subgroup of seven patients with normal left ventricular ejection fractions and normal wall motion but abnormally increased pulmonary wedge pressures during exercise, myocardial clearance half-times averaged 26.8 ± 6.7 minutes and thus did not differ from those of normal volunteers. In contrast, in the remaining 13 patients with reduced left ventricular ejection fractions, clearance half-times were markedly prolonged and averaged 42 ± 13.1 minutes. Values derived from six normal volunteers averaged 21.7 ± 2 minutes after stress and 24 ± 5 minutes after rest. Furthermore, the regional clearance half-times significantly varied between the interventricular septum and the inferior and posterolateral walls. This variability was greater than that observed in normal volunteers. Although an elevated pulmonary wedge pressure alone would appear to be a tenuous indicator of impending dilated cardiomyopathy, the investigators argued that a correlation between the severity of disease and the impairment of myocardial fatty acid metabolism existed. Other recent investigations using IPPA[D1] revealed a similar heterogeneity in myocardial tracer uptake and prolonged clearance half-times (see Table 60–2). They averaged 69.3 ± 29.6 minutes in the ten study patients and thus were significantly longer than in normal and ischemic myocardium of patients with coronary artery disease (43.8 ± 6.2 minutes and 54.4 ± 9.6 minutes). Both uptake and clearance of IPPA were normal in four patients. In the remaining six patients, there were regional abnormalities in uptake and clearance rates, although there was no close correlation between uptake and clearance abnormalities.

The utility of IHDA as a metabolic probe for cardiomyopathy was examined in 16 patients with different types of cardiomyopathies.[R6] These etiologies included idiopathic dilated cardiomyopathy in four patients and myotonic dystrophy in another four patients. The remaining patients had Duchenne's muscular dystrophy, complex congenital heart disease, hypertrophic heart disease, and other types of disease. Mean clearance half-times for the patient group were similar to those observed for normal controls (32.7 ± 7.0 versus 33 ± 7.0). This finding is not surprising in view of the heterogeneous patient population. Only two patients revealed prolonged clearance half-times. One of these patients suffered from carnitine deficiency, which can be associated with cardiomyopathy.

Using IPPA and SPECT imaging, Ugolini and colleagues demonstrated highly heterogeneous myocardial uptake but, unlike other reports, they observed shortened clearance half-times. The degree of heterogeneity of the initial myocardial IPPA uptake was related to the clinical status as classified by the New York Heart Association. Yet there was no significant relationship between the initial uptake and left ventricular ejection fractions as determined by radionuclide ventriculography. The researchers postulate that increased catecholamine levels in their patients might have enhanced rates of β-oxidation and thus accelerated the myocardial clearance of IPPA. They argue further that the degree of heterogeneity in tracer uptake potentially might provide prognostic information.

In summary, the observed heterogeneous uptake is consistent with that observed with C-11 palmitate and positron emission tomography (see Chapter 68). However, the observation of myocardial clearance rates varied, possibly because of heterogeneous patient populations or inadequate standardization of study conditions. The reports also failed to demonstrate convincingly a significant correlation of tracer uptake and clearance half-times with left ventricular function, which might be of predictive value. Finally, the mechanisms remain unexplained that accounted for the delay of tracer tissue clearance as observed in the majority of these studies.

SUMMARY AND CONCLUSIONS

Animal experimental studies and clinical investigations with a variety of radioiodinated fatty acid analogs have demonstrated the possibility of noninvasively deriving metabolic information with single-photon planar and tomographic imaging. The extent of metabolic information obtained with these tracers depends on their specific properties and ranges from myocardial uptake of exogenous fatty acid to incorporation of fatty acid into the endogenous lipid pool, as well as β-oxidation of fatty acid. At present, the fractional distribution of tracer in myocardium, rather than its rates of clearance from myocardium, appears to be an indicator of fatty acid metabolism. Observations in patients with coronary artery disease have demonstrated the known impairment of oxidation of fatty acid and increased incorporation into the endogenous lipid pool as consequences of myocardial ischemia. Findings in patients with cardiomyopathy have been less conclusive and warrant further studies. Quantification of exogenous fatty acid utilization might ultimately become possible with some of the described fatty acid analogs and an appropriate tracer kinetic model. Although this class of metabolic tracers has remained underutilized, possibly because of limited availability, cost, and complexities of tracer synthesis, it nevertheless offers the potential for identifying viable myocardium and for gaining novel insights into the pathophysiology of cardiovascular disease.

Acknowledgments

The authors thank Wendy Wilson and Mary Lee Griswold for preparing the illustrations for this chapter and Kerry Engber for her secretarial assistance in preparing this manuscript.

References

A

1. Ambrose, K. R., Owen, B. A., Goodman, M. M., and Knapp, F. F., Jr.: Evaluation of the metabolism in rat hearts of two new radioiodinated 3-methyl-branched fatty acid myocardial imaging agents. Eur. J. Nucl. Med. 12:486, 1987.

B

1. Bianco, J. A., Pape, L. A., Alpert, J. S., et al.: Accumulation of radioiodinated 15-(p-iodophenyl)-6-tellurapentadecanoic acid in ischemic myocardium during acute coronary occlusion and reperfusion. J. Am. Coll. Cardiol. 4:80, 1984.

C

1. Cuchet, P., Demaison, L., Bontemps, L., et al.: Do iodinated fatty acids undergo a nonspecific deiodination in the myocardium? Eur. J. Nucl. Med. 10:505, 1985.

D

1. Dudczak, R., Schmoliner, R., Kletter, K., et al.: Clinical evaluation of I-123-labeled p-phenyl pentadecanoic acid (p-IPPA) for myocardial scintigraphy. J. Nucl. Med. Allied Sci. 27:267, 1983.
2. Dudczak, K., Kletter, K., Frischauf, H., et al.: The use of I-123 heptadecanoic acid (HDA) as metabolic tracer: Preliminary report. Eur. J. Nucl. Med. 9:81, 1984.
3. Dudczak, R., Kletter, K., Frischauf, H., et al.: Myocardial turnover rates of I-123 heptadecanoic acid (HD): Isopte. Klinik und Forschung 15. Gasteiner Internationale Symposium 685–696, 1982.
4. Dudczak, R., Homan, R., Zanganeh, A., et al.: Myocardial metabolic studies in patients with cardiomyopathy. J. Nucl. Med. 24:P20, 1983.
5. DeGrado, T. R., Holden, J. E., Ng, C. K., et al.: Quantitative analysis of myocardial kinetics of 15-p-[iodine-125] iodophenylpentadecanoic acid. J. Nucl. Med. 30:1211, 1989.
6. Dudczak, R., Schmoliner, R., Angelberger, P., et al.: Structurally modified fatty acids: Clinical potential as tracers of metabolism. Eur. J. Nucl. Med. 12:S45, 1986.
7. Dudczak, R., Kletter, K., Angelberger, P., et al.: Imaging with I-23–labelled fatty acids. In Biersack, H. J., and Cox, P. H. (eds.): Radioisotope Studies in Cardiology. Kluwer Academic Publishers (Martin Nijhoff Publishers), Hingham, MA, 1985, pp. 295–317.

E

1. Evans, J. R., Gunton, R. W., Baker, R. G., et al.: Use of radioiodinated fatty acid for photoscans of the heart. Circ. Res. 16:1, 1965.
2. Elmaleh, D. R., Livni, E., Levy, S., et al.: Comparison of ^{11}C and ^{14}C-labeled fatty acids and their beta-methyl analogs. Int. J. Nucl. Med. 10:181, 1983.

F

1. Freundlieb, C., Höck, A., Vyska, K., et al.: Myocardial imaging and metabolic studies with (17-123) iodoheptadecanoic acid. J. Nucl. Med. 21:1043, 1980.
2. Fridrich, L., Pichler, M., Gassner, A., et al.: Tracer elimination in I-123 heptadecanoic acid: Half-life, component ratio and washout profiles in patients with cardiac disease. Eur. Heart J. 6 (Suppl. B):61, 1985.

G

1. Goodman, M. M., Kirsch, G., and Knapp, F. F., Jr.: Synthesis of radioiodinated ω-(p-iodophenyl)-substituted methyl-branched long-chain fatty acids. J. Lab. Comp. Radiopharm. XIX:1316, 1982.
2. Goodman, M. M., Kirsch, G., and Knapp, F. F., Jr.: Synthesis and evaluation of radioiodinated terminal p-iodophenyl-substituted alpha- and beta-methyl-branched fatty acids. J. Med. Chem. 25:390, 1984.
3. Goodman, M. M., and Knapp, F. F., Jr.: Synthesis of 15-(p-iodo-phenyl)-6-tellurapentadecanoic acid: A new myocardial imaging agent. J. Org. Chem. 47:3004, 1982.
4. Goodman, M. M., Knapp, F. F., Elmaleh, D. R., and Strauss, H. W.: New myocardial imaging agents: Synthesis of 15(p-iodo-phenyl)-3-(R,S)-methyl-pentadecanoic acid by decomposition of a 3,3-(1,5-pentanedyl) triazene precursor. J. Org. Chem. 49:2322, 1984.
5. Goodman, M. M., Knapp, F. F., Jr., and Callahan, A. P.: Synthesis and biological evaluation of 17-[^{131}I]-iodo-9-telluraheptadecanoic acid, a potential imaging agent. J. Med. Chem. 25:613, 1982.

H

1. Hansen, C. L., Corbett, J. R., Pippin, J. J., et al.: Iodine-123 phenylpentadecanoic acid and single photon emission computed tomography in identifying left ventricular regional metabolic abnormalities in patients with coronary heart disease: Comparison with thallium-201 myocardial tomography. J. Am. Coll. Cardiol. 12:78, 1988.
2. Höck, A., Freundlieb, C., Vyska, K., et al.: Myocardial imaging and metabolic studies with (17-I-123) iodoheptadecanoic acid in patients with congestive cardiomyopathy. J. Nucl. Med. 24:22, 1983.

J

1. Jones, G., Livni, E., Strauss, H., et al.: Synthesis and biologic evaluation of 1-[11C]-3, 3-dimethylheptadecanoic acid. J. Nucl. Med. 29:68, 1988.

K

1. Kirsch, G., Goodman, M. M., Knapp, F. F., Jr.: Orano-tellurium compounds of biological interest—unique properties of the *N*-chlorosuccinimide oxidation product of 9-telluraheptadecanoic acid. Organometallics 2:357, 1983.
2. Knapp, F. F., Jr., Ambrose, K. R., Callahan, A. P., et al.: Effects of chain length and tellurium position on the myocardial uptake of Te-123m fatty acids. J. Nucl. Med. 22:988, 1981.
3. Kloster, G., Stöcklin, G., Smith, E., and Schrör, K.: ω-Halofatty acids: A probe for mitochondrial membrane integrity. In vitro investigations in normal and ischaemic myocardium. Eur. J. Nucl. Med. 9:305, 1984.
4. Knust, E. J., Kupfernagel, C. H., and Stöcklin, G.: Long chain F-18 fatty acids for the study of regional metabolism in heart and liver: Odd-even effects of metabolism in mice. J. Nucl. Med. 20:1170, 1979.
5. Kloster, G., and Stoecklin, G.: Determination of the rate-determining step in halofatty acid turnover in the heart. Radioakt. Isotope Klin. Forsch. 15:235, 1982.
6. Knapp, F. F., Jr., Goodman, M. M., Kirsch, G., and Callahan, A. P.: Radioiodinated 15-(p-iodophenyl)-3,3-dimethylpentadecanoic acid (DMIPP): A new agent to evaluate regional myocardial fatty acid uptake. J. Nucl. Med. 26:123, 1985.
7. Knapp, F. F., Jr., Ambrose, K. R., and Goodman, M. M.: New radioiodinated methyl-branched fatty acids for cardiac studies. Eur. J. Nucl. Med. 12:S39, 1986.
8. Knapp, F. F., Jr., Goodman, M. M., Callahan, A. P., and Kirsch, G.: Radioiodinated 15-(p-iodophenyl)-3,3-dimethylpentadecanoic acid: A useful new agent to evaluate myocardial fatty acid uptake. J. Nucl. Med. 27:521, 1986.
9. Kennedy, P. L., Corbett, J. R., Kulkarni, P. V., et al.: Iodine I-123 phenylpentadecanoic acid myocardial scintigraphy: Usefulness in identifying myocardial ischemia. Circulation 74:1007, 1986.

L

1. Livni, E., Elmaleh, D. R., Levy, S., et al.: Beta-methyl (1-C-11)-heptadecanoic acid: A new myocardial metabolic tracer for positron emission tomography. J. Nucl. Med. 23:169, 1982.
2. Livni, E., Elmaleh, D. R., Barlai-Kovach, M. M., et al.: Radioiodinated beta-methyl phenyl fatty acids as potential tracers for myocardial imaging and metabolism. Eur. Heart J. 6: (Suppl. B) 85, 1985.

M

1. Machulla, H., Stöcklin, G., Kupfernagel, C., et al.: Comparative evaluation of fatty acids labeled with C-11, Cl-34m, Br-77, and I-123 for metabolic studies of myocardium: Concise communication. J. Nucl. Med. 19:298, 1978.
2. Machulla, H., Marsmann, M., and Dutschka, K.: Biochemical concept and synthesis of a radioiodinated phenylfatty acid for in vivo metabolic studies of the myocardium. Eur. J. Nucl. Med. 5:171, 1980.
3. Machulla, H. J., Kartje, M., Vyska, K., et al.: Substituent effects on the physiologic behavior of various radioiodinated phenylpentadecanoic acids. J. Nucl. Med. 276:P123, 1985.
4. Miller, D., Gill, J., Elmaleh, D., et al.: Fatty acid analogue accumulation: A marker of myocyte viability in ischemic-reperfused myocardium. Circulation 63:681, 1988.

N

1. Notohamiprodjo, G., Schmid, A., Spohr, G., et al.: Comparison of 11-C-palmitic acid (CPA) and 123-I-heptadecanoic acid (IHA) turnover in human heart. (Abstract.) J. Nucl. Med. 26:P88, 1985

O

1. Otto, C. A., Brown, L. E., and Scott, A. M.: Radioiodinated branched-chain fatty acids: Substrates for beta oxidation? Concise communication. J. Nucl. Med. 25:75, 1985.

P

1. Poe, N., Robinson, G., Graham, L., and MacDonald, N.: Experimental basis for myocardial imaging with I-123-labeled hexadecanoic acid. J. Nucl. Med. 17:1077, 1976.

2. Poe, N., Robinson, G., Zielinski, F., et al.: Myocardial imaging with ^{123}I-hexadecanoic acid. Radiology 124:419, 1977.
3. Pachinger, O., Sochor, H., Ogris, E., et al.: Salvage of ischemic myocardium by intracoronary streptokinase therapy? *In* Faivre, G., Betrand, A., Cherrier, F., et al. (eds.): Non-invasive methods in ischemic heart disease. Specia, Nancy, 1982, pp. 410–414.

R

1. Rothlin, M. E., and Bing, R. J.: Extraction and release of individual free fatty acids by the heat and fat depots. J. Clin. Invest. 40:1380, 1961.
2. Robinson, G. D.: Rapid synthesis of high specific activity, biologically active ^{18}F-fluoroaliphatic analog compounds. J. Nucl. Med. 14:446, 1973.
3. Robinson, G. D., and Lee, A. W.: Radioiodinated fatty acids for heart imaging: Iodine monochloride addition compared with iodide replacement labeling. J. Nucl. Med. 16:17, 1975.
4. Reske, S., Sauer, W., Machulla, H., and Winkler, C.: 15(-[I-123]iodophenyl) pentadecanoic acid as a tracer of lipid metabolism: Comparison with (I-C-14) palmitic acid in murine tissues. J. Nucl. Med. 25:1335, 1984.
5. Reske, S. N., Machulla, H. J., and Winkler, C.: Metabolic turnover of p-I-123 phenylpentadecanoic acid in the hearts of rats. (Abstract.) J. Nucl. Med. 23:P10, 1982.
6. Rabinovitch, M. A., Kalff, V., Allen, R., et al.: ω-^{123}-I-hexadecanoic acid metabolic probe of cardiomyopathy. Eur. J. Nucl. Med. 10:222, 1985.
7. Reske, S. N., Koischwitz, D., Reichmann, K., et al.: Cardiac metabolism of 15(p-I-123)phenylpentadecanoic acid after intracoronary tracer application. Eur. J. Radiol. 4:144, 1984.
8. Rösler, H., Noelpp, U., Toth, T., et al.: On the prognostic potential of the sequential ^{123}I-HDA tomoscintigram after the first MI. Eur. Heart J. 6: (Suppl. B) 49, 1985.
9. Reske, S. N., Nitsch, J., von der Lohe, E., et al.: Eingeschränkte myokardiale Fettsäure–Ultilisation bei koronarer Herzerkrankung nach symptomlimitierter ergometrischer Belastung. Nachweis pathologischer Stoffwechselmuster mit Hilfe von Jod–123–Phenylpentadekansäure und sequentieller SPECT. Z Kardiol 78:262–270, 1989.

S

1. Schön, H. R., Senekowitsch, R., Berg, D., et al.: Measurement of myocardial fatty acid metabolism: Kinetics of iodine-123-heptadecanoic acid in normal dog hearts. J. Nucl. Med. 27:1449, 1986.
2. Stoddart, P., Papouchado, M., and Wilde, P.: Prognostic value of 123-iodo-heptadecanoic acid imaging in patients with acute myocardial infarction. Eur. J. Nucl. Med. 12:525, 1987.
3. Stoddart, P., Papouchado, M., Vann Jones, J., and Wilde, P.: Assessment of percutaneous transluminal coronary angioplasty with ^{123}iodo-heptadecanoic acid. Eur. J. Nucl. Med. 12:605, 1987.
4. Schelbert, H.: Current status and prospects of new radionuclides and radiopharmaceuticals for cardiovascular nuclear medicine. Semin. Nucl. Med. 17:145, 1987.

U

1. Ugolini, V., Hansen, C., Kulkarni, P., et al.: Abnormal myocardial fatty acid metabolism in dilated cardiomyopathy detected by iodine-123 phenyl pentadecanoic acid and tomographic imaging. Am. J. Cardiol. 62:923, 1988.

V

1. van der Wall, E. E., Heidendal, G. A. K., den Hollander, W., et al.: I-123 labeled hexadecanoic acid in comparison with thallium-201 for myocardial imaging in coronary heart disease. A preliminary study. Eur. J. Nucl. Med. 5:401, 1980.
2. van der Wall, E., Heidendal, G., Hollander, W., et al.: Metabolic myocardial imaging with I-123-labeled heptadecanoic acid in patients with angina pectoris. Eur. J. Nucl. Med. 6:391, 1981.
3. van der Wall, E., Hollander, W., Heidendal, G., et al.: Dynamic myocardial scintigraphy with I-123-labeled free fatty acids in patients with myocardial infarction. Eur. J. Nucl. Med. 6:383, 1981.
4. Visser, F., Eenige, M., Westera, G., et al.: Metabolic fate of radioiodinated heptadecanoic acid in the normal canine heart. Circulation 72:565, 1985.
5. Visser, F., Westera, G., van Eenige, M., et al.: The myocardial elimination rate of radioiodinated heptadecanoic acid. Eur. J. Nucl. Med. 10:118, 1985.
6. Visser, F. C., van Eenige, M. J., Duwel, C. M. B., and Roos, J. P.: Radioiodinated free fatty acids; Can we measure myocardial metabolism? Eur. J. Nucl. Med. 12:S20, 1986.
7. Vyska, K., Machulla, H. J., Stremmel, W., et al.: Regional myocardial free fatty acid extraction in normal and ischemic myocardium. Circulation 78:1218, 1988.
8. von Eenige, M., Visser, F., Duwel, C., et al.: Analysis of myocardial time-activity curves of ^{123}I-heptadecanoic acid. II. The acquisition time. Nuklearmedizin 26:248, 1987.
9. von Eenige, M., Visser, F., Duwel, C., et al.: Analysis of myocardial time-activity curves of ^{123}I-heptadecanoic acid. I. Curve fitting. Nuklearmedizin 26:241, 1987.

Y

1. Yamamoto, K., Som, P., Brill, A. B., et al.: Dual tracer autoradiographic study of β-methyl-(1-^{14}C) heptadecanoic acid and 15-p-(^{131}I)-iodophenyl-β-methyl-pentadecanoic acid in normotensive and hypertensive rats. J. Nucl. Med. 27:1178, 1986.
2. Yonekura, Y., Brill, A. B., Som, P., et al.: Regional myocardial substrate uptake in hypertensive rats: A quantitative autoradiographic measurement. Science 227:1494, 1985.

Part IX

New Developments in Cardiac Radionuclide Imaging

Chapter 61

Technetium-99m Myocardial Perfusion Imaging Agents

▪ *DANIEL S. BERMAN, M.D.* ▪ *HOSEN KIAT, M.D.*
▪ *JEFFREY LEPPO, M.D.* ▪ *JAMSHID MADDAHI, M.D.*

PHYSIOLOGIC AND IMAGING PROPERTIES .. 1097
Technetium-99m Isonitriles 1097
Technetium-99m BATO Compounds 1100
Comparison of Single-Photon Perfusion Tracers 1101
TECHNETIUM-99m SESTAMIBI 1102
Results of Clinical Trials 1102
Ischemia Trials 1102
Infarct Trials 1105
Ventricular Function Trials 1106
Future Development 1107
TECHNETIUM-99m TEBOROXIME 1107
Results of Clinical Trials 1107
Future Development 1108
CONCLUSION 1108

Although thallium-201 (Tl-201) has excellent physiologic characteristics for imaging myocardial perfusion and viability, its low energy (68 to 80 KeV) is suboptimal for scintillation camera imaging, and its relatively long half-life (73 hours) results in suboptimal radiation dosimetry. To circumvent these limitations, investigators have attempted for over a decade to develop a myocardial perfusion agent labeled with technetium-99m, a tracer with ideal physical properties for scintillation camera imaging (monoenergetic gamma of 140 KeV and 6-hour half-life). This search for a technetium-99m–labeled myocardial perfusion imaging tracer finally met with success in 1982, when the group at the Peter Bent Bringham Hospital announced the development of technetium-99m isonitriles.[J1] In the experimental animal, the myocardial uptake of these agents was shown to be proportional to the regional myocardial blood flow. More recently, another group of technetium-99m–labeled tracers, called boronic acid adducts of technetium dioximes (BATO compounds), was demonstrated to have high myocardial extraction, with subsequent myocardial concentration also proportional to regional perfusion.[R1] In 1989, radiopharmaceuticals from both these classes were submitted to the Food and Drug Administration for approval; in the near future they are expected to be available for routine clinical use.

This work was supported in part by SCOR Grant 7651 from the National Institutes of Health, Specialized Center of Research, Bethesda, Maryland, and a grant from the American Heart Association, Greater Los Angeles Affiliate, Los Angeles, California.

PHYSIOLOGIC AND IMAGING PROPERTIES

Technetium-99m Isonitriles

A thorough understanding of cellular tracer uptake, distribution, and retention is important in the accurate interpretation of myocardial perfusion images. Three compounds of the technetium-labeled isonitriles have been applied clinically (Fig. 61–1). All three have similarly avid myocardial uptake. The first, technetium-99m-t-butyl isonitrile (TBI), was suboptimal for myocardial imaging because of its prominent hepatic and pulmonary uptake.[H1, H2, M1, S1] Persistent liver uptake of TBI frequently obscured defects in the inferior left ventricular wall. In addition to further obscuring myocardial defects, pulmonary TBI could behave as a reservoir of the tracer. With the subsequent washout of the tracer from the lungs, a significant amount could be delivered to the myocardium and obscure the perfusion pattern resulting from the initial injection and uptake of TBI. The second tracer, technetium-99m carboxyisopropyl isonitrile (CPI), demonstrated progressive hepatic accumulation over time despite excellent myocardial uptake, and also relatively rapid washout from the myocardium.[H3, M1] The third, technetium-99m methoxyisobutyl isonitrile, known generically as Tc-sestamibi, has emerged as the isonitrile with the most favorable biologic characteristics for myocardial perfusion imaging.[O1] Unlike the previously described technetium-99m isonitriles (CPI, TBI), Tc-sestamibi has transient hepatic uptake, with prompt hepatobiliary excretion and minimal lung uptake.[W1]

Although the mechanism of uptake of Tc-sestamibi is unknown, it has been shown to be different from that of thallium-201. Unlike thallium-201, the uptake of Tc-sestamibi is not blocked by ouabain and is thus not dependent on the Na^+-K^+ ATPase transport mechanism.[M2] In addition, whereas nonradioactive Tc-sestamibi decreases the uptake of Tc-sestamibi (suggesting that cellular affinity and saturable binding sites have a role in Tc-sestamibi transport), it has no effect on thallium-201 uptake.[M2] The distribution of Tc-sestamibi in the myocardium is proportional to blood flow in a manner parallel to that observed with thallium-201 (i.e., with a fall-off of extraction at very high flow rates), with somewhat lower overall myocardial extraction fraction.[O1] In a canine coronary artery occlusion and reperfusion ischemic model, Canby and co-workers demonstrated that Tc-sestamibi myocardial activity was significantly correlated with thallium-201 activity following 2 hours of coronary occlusion and at different intervals following reperfusion.[C1] The Tc-sestamibi activity also directly correlated with the microsphere-determined blood flow during ischemic episodes and soon after reperfusion, but a negative linear correlation was observed following prolonged reperfusion (35 minutes). It was postulated that the latter finding was caused by rapid tracer washout in the reperfused zone secondary to reperfusion hyperemia.

Unlike thallium-201, Tc-sestamibi exhibits minimal redistribution over time.[L1, O1] The combination of transient early hepatic uptake and the lack of significant redistribution makes 30 minutes to 1 hour postinjection the ideal imaging time. The earlier imaging time (30 minutes postinjection) may be preferable following stress to reduce overall study time and minimize the contribution of any redistribution of the tracer. Poststress and rest whole body images of the distribution of Tc-sestamibi acquired 5 minutes, 60 minutes, and 240 minutes after tracer injections are shown in Figures 61–2 and 61–3, respectively.

When considering the physiologic properties of myocardial perfusion tracers, it might be helpful to establish the properties of a hypothetic ideal tracer. The capillary transport of a diffusible compound is dominated by its extraction fraction. Microspheres (radiolabeled) have essentially a 100 percent first-pass extraction at any level of blood flow. In contrast, all available diffusible cardiac tracers show an inverse relationship between peak extraction and coronary flow, because at progressively higher flows transcapillary transport is diffusion limited. This fall in extraction does not imply that tissue uptake of the tracer decreases with increasing flow levels. In fact, capillary flux or total permeation across this barrier, which is measured as the permeability–surface area product (PScap), actually increases with higher levels of perfusion because the slight fall in extraction (10 to 20 percent) is compensated for by a 200 to 300 percent increase in blood flow. Therefore, it is crucial to evaluate both the peak extraction and capillary flux for all diffusible perfusion tracers in order to understand their imaging potential. In addition to transcapillary transport, it is important to consider the residual fraction of injected tracer that is in the heart during the actual imaging process. This can be evaluated by a net extraction (Enet) calculation derived from first-pass studies. Since most single photon gamma-emitting tracers require several minutes of clinical imaging time to collect a myocardial perfusion study, it is important to assess peak extraction and capillary flux as well as net retention over time. Therefore, the discussion of transport analysis will focus on all three of these parameters. One might hypothesize that an ideal diffusible blood flow tracer would have a high peak extraction and a direct linear relationship between capillary flux (PScap) and absolute flow, with a slope approaching the line of identity. This ideal tracer also should have stable tissue distribution during the imaging process (high Enet). If a highly diffusible tracer has relatively rapid back-diffusion from the tissue space, then appropriate adjustments in image collection time must be made.

The myocardial transport of thallium-201 and Tc-sestamibi can be compared using indicator-dilution analysis, as previously described by Bassingthwaighte and co-workers.[B1–3] This technique entails a bolus injection of multiple tracers (indicators) into the arterial supply of an organ and collection of the entire venous efflux so as to produce a continuous transport function. This transport function is the fraction of each tracer emerging from the organ per second, normalized to the total injected dose (Fig. 61–4). The different indicators are the perfusion tracers under study and known intravascular tracers (radiolabeled albumin) and interstitial markers (radiolabeled ethylene diamine tetra-acetic acid or sucrose), against which diffusible perfusion tracers can be simultaneously compared. In this type of analysis, a two-barrier, three-compartment model is used to describe the blood-tissue exchange in the heart.

The first barrier represents the endothelial capillary wall, which separates the intravascular from the interstitial compartment. The instantaneous fractional extraction of a diffusible perfusion tracer across this barrier can be calculated by comparing the transport curve of the tracer to that of a nonpermeating tracer (albumin) (Fig. 61–4). The peak value for this extraction curve is called Emax. The rate constant for flux, which represents the total unidirectional permeation of the diffusible tracer across the

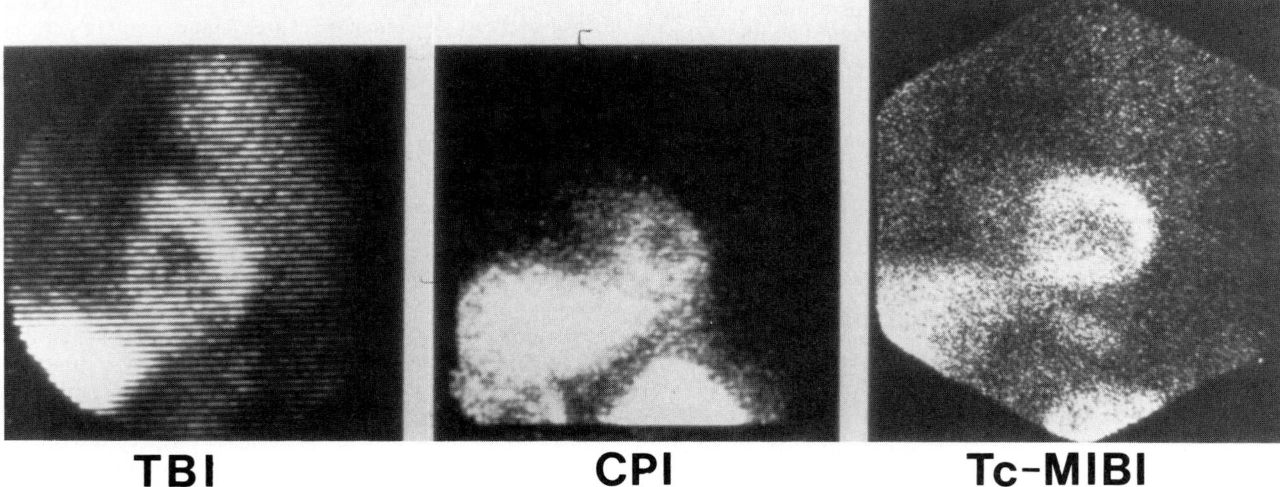

Figure 61–1. Comparative anterior planar images obtained following injection of TBI, CPI, and Tc-sestamibi. Note the more prominent hepatic uptake with TBI and CPI than with Tc-sestamibi, and the prominent pulmonary uptake with TBI.

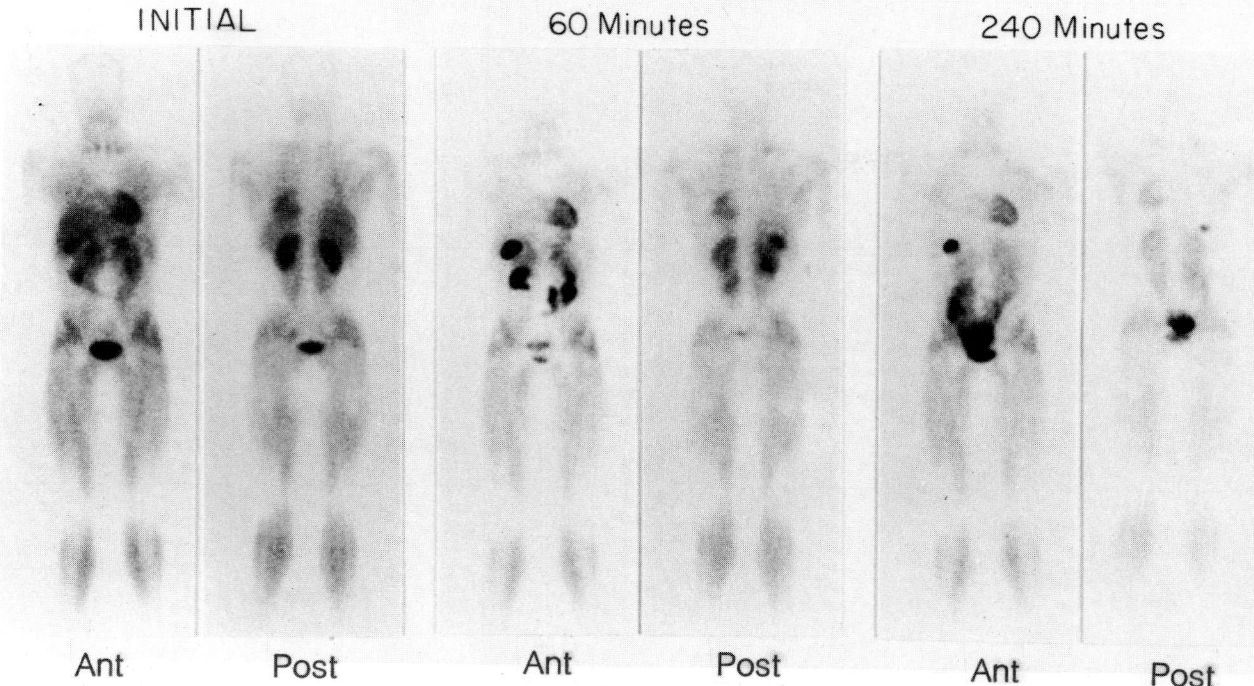

Figure 61–2. Postexercise whole body images of Tc-sestamibi in the first patient studied in the Phase I clinical trials (performed at Cedars-Sinai Medical Center). Shown are images in the anterior (Ant) and posterior (Post) views, obtained beginning 5 to 10 minutes, 60 minutes, and 240 minutes after exercise injection. The images demonstrate that both the liver and kidneys are major excretory pathways for Tc-sestamibi. The visual gallbladder activity noted at 60 and 240 minutes can be eliminated through the administration of milk or a small fatty meal.

capillary wall, can be calculated from the blood flow rate into the organ and the Emax value. This capillary exchange is defined as the permeability–surface area product (PScap).

The second barrier is the parenchymal cell barrier, which is represented by the parenchymal cell membrane, separating the interstitial and intracellular compartments. Computer modeling of the tracer exchange at the parenchymal cell barrier can be used to obtain a rate constant or permeation estimate, as well as the apparent cellular volume distribution of the tracer. An additional analysis involves an estimate of net tissue exchange over time (Enet). This Enet function is the integrated difference between the reference (albumin) transport function and that of the diffusible tracer. Enet values evaluate the ability of the extracted tracer to remain in the cellular compartment and can be considered equivalent to the residual fraction of injected tracer remaining in the heart after a longer interval (2 to 4 minutes). Ideally, for predicting clinical efficacy, this interval should be at least as long as the time required for imaging the agent.

Utilizing nine blood-perfused isolated rabbit hearts, the myocardial kinetics of Tc-sestamibi were recently compared with

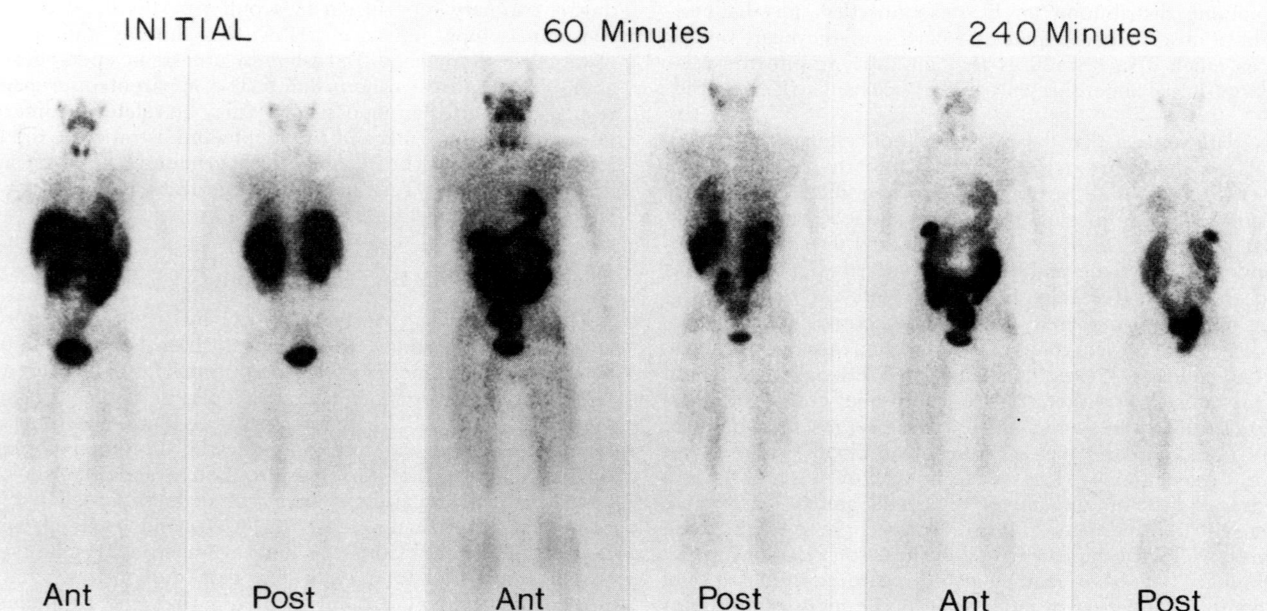

Figure 61–3. Whole body images of the distribution of Tc-sestamibi obtained after rest injection in the same patient as shown in Figure 61–2. Note the relatively lower heart to liver ratios in the initial images obtained following rest injection, and the more prominent hepatobiliary excretion of the tracer into the bowel over time.

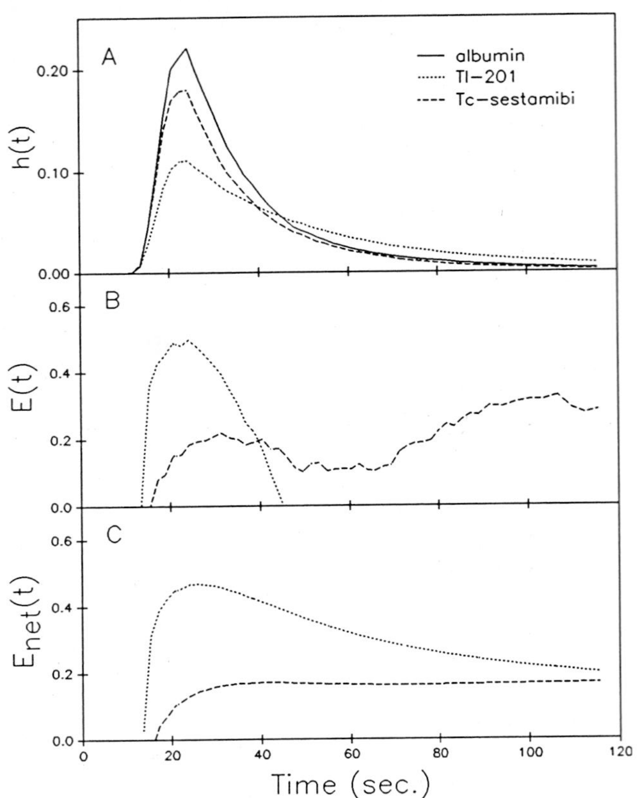

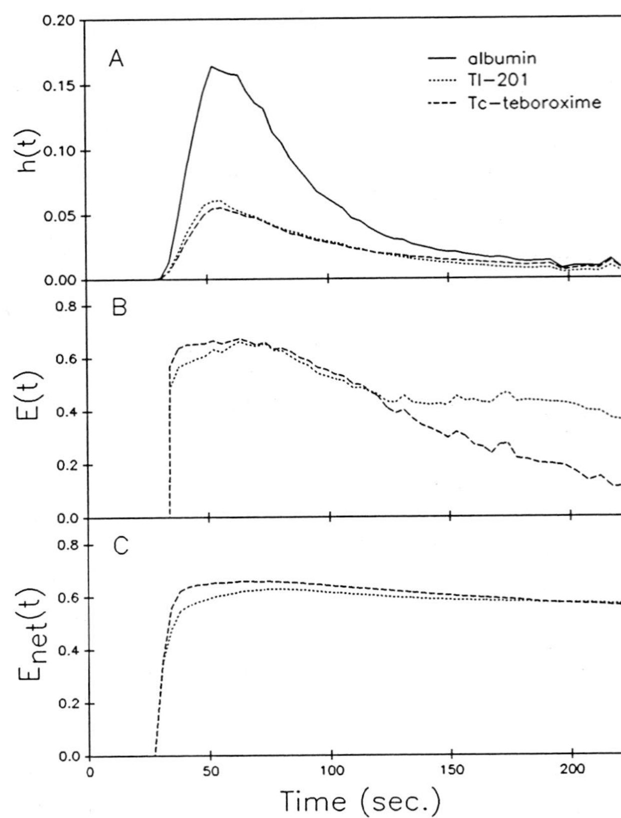

Figure 61–4. *A, B, C*: Examples of transport function [h(t)], instantaneous fractional extraction [E(t)], and instantaneous net extraction [$E_{net}(t)$] curves. In both panels, albumin (solid line) and Tl-201 (dotted line) are plotted with concurrently injected Tc-99m perfusion tracers (dashed line of the left panel: Tc-sestamibi; dashed line of the right panel: Tc-teboroxime). Note that the time illustrated covers only the first 2 minutes and 4 minutes after injection for Tc-sestamibi and Tc-teboroxime, respectively. See text for details.

thallium-201 by Leppo and Meerdink.[L2] They reported that the mean Emax for Tc-sestamibi was 0.39, compared with 0.73 for thallium-201 over an average flow of 1.5 ml/min/g. Capillary flux (PScap) and net retention (Enet) for Tc-sestamibi were both significantly less than the corresponding thallium-201 determinations. However, computer modeling estimates for Tc-sestamibi exchange at the parenchymal cell (PSpc) showed the opposite effect (i.e., greater transport across the parenchymal cell and a larger volume distribution for Tc-sestamibi than for thallium-201). These observations explain, in part, how the heart retains almost as much Tc-sestamibi as thallium-201, despite the relatively large initial difference in capillary exchange (Emax) (Fig. 61–4).

These data suggest that the mechanism of cellular transport is different for these two tracers, and that both have adequate characteristics to permit myocardial perfusion imaging. A similar conclusion has been reported by Marshall and associates, utilizing a similar protocol.[M3] Peak extraction averaged 0.57 for Tc-sestamibi and 0.80 for thallium-201, and myocardial retention was 2.5-fold greater for the technetium compound.

Using miniature implanted radiation-detecting probes in normal and ischemic cardiac zones of an intact dog heart preparation, Okada and colleagues noted no changes in fractional Tc-sestamibi clearance rates from either zone.[O1] The 4-hour fractional clearances for Tc-sestamibi averaged 0.15, which represents a minimal washout rate. Over the same period, mean blood clearance was 0.98 for these animals. This suggests that Tc-sestamibi has a stable tracer distribution and is thus well suited for SPECT imaging with its prolonged acquisition times. In general, these data agree well with the in vitro rabbit heart observations.[L2]

Preliminary data have been collected regarding the kinetics of Tc-sestamibi in reperfusion models. In preliminary experiments performed in isolated rabbit hearts by Meerdink and associates,[M4] transport of Tc-sestamibi and thallium-201 was evaluated at control and after 5 and 30 minutes of reperfusion (following 30 to 60 minutes of zero-flow ischemia). These investigators conclude that, overall, coronary reperfusion at control levels of blood flow results in slightly decreased myocardial transport of thallium-201 but enhanced transport of Tc-sestamibi. This suggests that cellular or metabolic function can affect myocardial tracer uptake of thallium-201 and Tc-sestamibi during coronary reperfusion. Liu and colleagues have also noted enhanced Tc-sestamibi transport during coronary reperfusion in a buffer-perfused rat heart with constant isotope infusion.[L1] However, Sinusas and associates observed a diminished Tc-sestamibi uptake in open-chest dogs after 90 minutes of reperfusion.[S2] The apparent discrepancy in results in reperfusion models[L1, M4, S2] may be related to differences in duration of ischemia and timing of administration of the tracer following reflow. The combined experimental findings suggest that the timing of Tc-sestamibi administration after reflow may have a critical effect on its transport.

Technetium-99m BATO Compounds

The second class of technetium-99m myocardial perfusion agents currently under clinical investigation is neutral lipophilic complexes of boronic acid. The most promising BATO compound, referred to as teboroxime, was developed by Squibb Diagnostics (SQ30217).[M5, R1, S3] Utilizing an isolated blood-perfusion rabbit heart model and the multiple-indicator dilution technique as described earlier for Tc-sestamibi, Leppo and Meerdink compared the myocardial transport of two technetium-labeled BATO compounds and thallium-201 during varying levels of coronary flow[L3] (Fig. 61–4). Coronary flow averaged 1.31 ml/min/g and varied from 0.30 to 2.44. These data demonstrate that each teboroxime extraction point is higher than the simultaneously determined thallium-201 value. Mean teboroxime extraction (Emax) was 0.71 and was 25 percent higher than the mean thallium-201 Emax of 0.57 ($p < 0.001$). The mean capillary flux (PScap) for teboroxime was 1.1 ml/min/g, and this was also higher (46 percent) than the mean thallium-201 PScap of 0.75 ($p < 0.001$). Although the net retention (Enet) for teboroxime was higher than that of thallium-201, this important parameter showed a relatively smaller disparity than might have been expected based on the relatively large initial capillary extraction (Emax) of teboroxime. This implies that cellular retention of teboroxime is much less than that of thallium-201 and that back-diffusion of teboroxime is a prominent kinetic factor. Other preliminary results by Stewart and colleagues, in open-chest dogs, show relatively high extraction of teboroxime after intracoronary injection.[S4] In addition, myocardial washout of technetium-teboroxime appears to be flow-related and quite rapid.

In an experimental cell culture line (neonatal rat cardiac cells), Maublant and colleagues compared uptake and release characteristics of technetium-sestamibi, thallium-201, and technetium-teboroxime.[M6, M7] They showed (Table 61–1) that, of all tracers, teboroxime has the fastest uptake and greatest accumulation (as expressed as the ratio of inner cell concentration to external buffer; Ci/e). Thallium-201 has relatively fast uptake and the quickest release, which results in the lowest net accumulation (after 3 hours). Tc-sestamibi has the slowest uptake and release of any tracer, but shows a greater net accumulation than thallium-201. Maublant and colleagues also reported the results on tracer kinetics of several interventions involving inhibition of membrane transport, glycolysis, and the respiratory chain (cytochrome oxidase). Variable results have been reported, suggesting, in general, that teboroxime is the least and thallium-201 the most sensitive to metabolic inhibition at the cellular level.

In humans, myocardial uptake of teboroxime is rapid, with excellent myocardial visualization at 2 minutes after injection. The myocardial clearance, however, is also rapid, with biexponential clearance half-times of 2 minutes (68 percent) and 78 minutes (32 percent).[N1] Furthermore, Stewart and colleagues have demonstrated in dogs that the clearance rate of Tc-teboroxime from the myocardium is inversely related to myocardial blood flow.[S5] Thus the pattern of distribution of the tracer in the myocardium would be expected to change rapidly over time in the setting of regional myocardial ischemia. Although the myocardium is clearly visualized for approximately 20 minutes after injection, these kinetic properties suggest that initial imaging with Tc-teboroxime must be completed within the first few minutes after injection of the tracer in order to best reflect blood flow distribution at the time of injection. Since tomographic acquisition with the standard single-headed camera typically requires imaging times of approximately 20 to 30 minutes, SPECT imaging with BATO compounds is problematic. Although SPECT image quality may be adequate, due to the rapidly changing tracer concentrations, the SPECT images would represent varying components of initial distribution and clearance, potentially obscuring perfusion defects. In addition, persistent hepatic accumulation of the tracer with a liver residence half-time of approximately 1.5 hours may be a limitation in some patients as this hepatic uptake may interfere with inferior wall visualization.

Both Tc-sestamibi and Tc-teboroxime have been shown to be safe through their respective Phase I and II clinical trials.[S3, W1] Comparative physiologic properties of these two technetium-labeled myocardial perfusion agents are listed in Table 61–2.

Table 61–1. UPTAKE AND RELEASE CHARACTERISTICS OF MYOCARDIAL PERFUSION TRACERS IN NEONATAL RAT CARDIAC CELLS

	Half-Life (Min)		Ci/e
	Uptake	*Release*	*3 Hr Postincubation*
Tc-sestamibi	35	28	155
Thallium-201	5	6	136
Tc-teboroxime	<2	13	585

Ci/e—ratio of myocardial cellular perfusion tracer concentration to external buffer.

Table 61–2. COMPARISON OF THE PHYSIOLOGIC PROPERTIES OF Tc-SESTAMIBI AND Tc-TEBOROXIME

	Tc-Sestamibi	Tc-Teboroxime
Class	Isonitrile	BATO compound
Extraction fraction (peak)	~.65	~.90
Clearance half-time		
Heart	~12 hours	~10–15 minutes
Liver	~0.5 hour	~1.5 hour
Redistribution	minimal	possible
Dose	30 mCi	30 mCi

Overall, all three tracers (Tc-sestamibi, teboroxime, and thallium-201) show a positive, liner relationship between myocardial tissue distribution and myocardial perfusion, determined with microspheres in the resting blood flow range and in the lower range of augmentation of blood flow above resting levels. All tracers show evidence for diffusion limitation at flow levels above 1.5 to 2.0 ml/min/g but possess properties that permit adequate evaluation of myocardial perfusion. Since Tc-sestamibi, Tc-teboroxime, and thallium-201 have very different cardiac transport mechanisms, imaging protocols will need to be optimized for each agent for the various clinical settings in which they are used.

Comparison of Single-Photon Perfusion Tracers

The technetium tracers offer several advantages over thallium-201. Since they are labeled with technetium-99m, these agents can be available from a technetium-99m generator in a nuclear medicine laboratory 24 hours a day, without requiring a special delivery from a commercial radiopharmacy or manufacturer's distribution center. The ideal energy (140 KeV) for standard gamma camera imaging results in improved resolution on a count-by-count basis, owing principally to less scatter and attenuation in the patient and, to a lesser extent, to brighter scintillations within the detector crystal. More importantly, the improved radiation dosimetry of technetium-99m compared with thallium-201 allows injection of ten times as much radioactivity. When coupled with good myocardial tracer extraction, the technetium-99m agents provide images with much higher count rates than does thallium-201. Such high count rates, in turn, make first-pass imaging feasible and provide for the first time the potential of assessing exercise ejection fraction and myocardial perfusion from a single tracer injection.[B4] For Tc-sestamibi, the lack of significant myocardial redistribution leads to increased convenience by permitting the uncoupling of the time of injection and the time of imaging. Such flexibility is of potential importance in busy laboratories or when myocardial perfusion is to be assessed in the acute phase of myocardial infarction, in which imaging often will be delayed so that the patient can be stabilized. The combination of high count rates and lack of redistribution also allows adequate time for gated SPECT acquisition. Following injection with Tc-sestamibi, the gated SPECT study provides information with respect to the state of myocardial perfusion at the time of tracer injection and the myocardial function at the time of imaging.[K1] In addition, gated SPECT acquisition enables the myocardial perfusion to be assessed using the end-diastolic images only. These end-diastolic tomograms may offer a more accurate assessment of perfusion defect extent, since they obviate the problems related to cardiac motion during image acquisition in ventricular systole. Gated tomographic acquisition may become the method of choice for use with Tc-sestamibi.

It is also important to note that the relatively rapid uptake and washout of Tc-teboroxime permits sequential stress and rest myocardial imaging studies over a 1 to 1.5 hour period without need for background subtraction, since residual myocardial activity is fairly low. Tomographic imaging with Tc-teboroxime, earlier noted to be a problem, may be more feasible using a multidetector camera, which will be able to complete the entire acquisition

Table 61–3. COMPARISON OF THE IMAGING PROPERTIES OF Tc-SESTAMIBI AND Tc-TEBOROXIME

	Tc-Sestamibi	Tc-Teboroxime
Begin imaging	1 hour	1 minute
Complete rest-stress	3–4 hours	1–1.5 hours
Total myocardial counts	excellent	transiently good
SPECT	yes	possible (quickly)
Gated SPECT	yes	no
First-pass	yes	yes

within the available 10 to 15 minutes of myocardial tracer residence time. The relatively rapid tracer disappearance from the myocardium probably excludes gated SPECT acquisition as a practical approach to data acquisition. A potential advantage of the differential washout rates of Tc-teboroxime is that a very early image (possibly between 1 and 4 minutes after injection) might be obtained representing the stress myocardial perfusion distribution, and a delayed image might be obtained soon thereafter (approximately 10 to 15 minutes after injection), with viable but ischemic areas demonstrating slower washout of the tracer. This property, theoretically, could result in the equivalent of stress-redistribution thallium-201 imaging being performed in approximately 15 minutes. The clinical imaging characteristics of Tc-sestamibi and Tc-teboroxime are compared in Table 61–3.

TECHNETIUM-99m SESTAMIBI

Results of Clinical Trials

Ischemia Trials

For Tc-sestamibi, three separate phase III clinical application protocols have been completed in the United States. The "ischemia" protocols compared Tc-sestamibi with thallium-201 in patients undergoing coronary angiography. The sensitivity and specificity values for Tc-sestamibi and thallium-201 by SPECT and planar imaging methods, from currently published manuscripts, are summarized in Tables 61–4 and 61–5. In the multicenter phase II trial reported by Wackers and co-workers, Tc-sestamibi stress-rest planar studies were compared with thallium-201 stress-redistribution planar studies in 38 patients and were found to have similar sensitivity and specificity for diagnosis of coronary artery disease (CAD) and detection of individual diseased vessels.[W1] Kiat and associates[K2] compared sensitivities and specificities of Tc-sestamibi and thallium-201 with SPECT and planar imaging in a study of 36 patients (Tables 61–4 and 61–5; Figures 61–5, 61–6, and 61–7 depict a case example). There was no significant difference between Tc-sestamibi and thallium-201 for sensitivity, specificity (findings in patients with normal coronary arteries), and normalcy rate (findings in patients with a low likelihood of CAD) with either planar or SPECT imaging. With both tracers, however, improved sensitivity for diseased vessel identification by SPECT over planar imaging was observed. Taillefer and associates studied 100 consecutive patients, comparing rest-stress Tc-sestamibi and stress-redistribution thallium-201 planar imaging.[T1] In 65 of the patients in whom angiographic correlation was available, no significant difference was noted in detecting vessels with 70 or more percent stenosis. Iskandrian and associates reported the results of SPECT imaging in 28 patients with coronary artery disease (50 percent or more diameter stenosis) and 11 patients with normal or nearly normal arteriograms. Tc-sestamibi had sensitivity for detection of disease equal to that of thallium-201 and a trend toward higher specificity.[I1] Using quantitatively analyzed SPECT studies, Kahn and associates reported the comparison of thallium-201 and Tc-sestamibi imaging in 12 normal subjects and 38 patients with angiographically documented coronary artery disease (50 or more percent diameter stenosis).[K3] These investigators also demonstrated no significant difference in overall detection of coronary artery disease using the two tracers. With respect to individual coronary stenoses, however, Tc-sestamibi identified 59 of 75 (79 percent) significantly stenosed arteries, compared with detection of 45 of 75 (60 percent) by thallium-201 ($p < 0.05$). The increased detection of individual coronary arteries was most marked in the vessels with mild stenosis (50 to 75 percent), with 65 percent of these lesions detected by Tc-sestamibi compared with 35 percent by thallium-201 ($p < 0.05$). Furthermore, Tc-sestamibi rest-stress scintigraphy identified more segments with reversible hypoperfusion than stress-redistribution thallium-201 SPECT (Tc-sestamibi versus thallium-201: 134 versus 104 segments; $p < 0.05$).

Preliminary worldwide data from phase III trials, with studies interpreted at the institution where they were performed, have been analyzed by Du Pont Pharmaceuticals, Incorporated. With respect to planar imaging in 426 patients, sensitivities and specificities for Tc-sestamibi versus thallium-201 were 89 percent versus 91 percent and 79 percent versus 60 percent, respectively. In tomographic studies of 454 patients, sensitivities and specificities of Tc-sestamibi versus thallium-201 were 91 percent versus 93 percent and 51 percent versus 50 percent, respectively (unpublished data). Thus, to date, a large body of data exists suggesting very similar accuracy for detection of coronary artery disease between Tc-sestamibi and thallium-201 exercise studies for both planar and tomographic imaging. Virtually all these studies were acquired using acquisition and processing protocols that had been optimized for thallium-201 and not for Tc-sestamibi.

With respect to the type of defect observed, data from the currently published manuscripts that permit this analysis are summarized in Tables 61–6 and 61–7. When the segment-by-segment comparison between Tc-sestamibi and thallium-201 findings was assessed, each of these manuscripts demonstrated no major difference in the frequency of segments with normal, reversible (ischemic), and nonreversible (myocardial scar) defect for either planar[K2, T1, T2, W1] or SPECT[I1, K2] imaging. Overall, the exact agreement for the type of defect was 88 percent for planar imaging and 92 percent for SPECT. From a theoretical standpoint, it was anticipated that the lack of redistribution of Tc-sestamibi might result in patients with ischemia at rest demonstrating evidence of scar by Tc-sestamibi and of ischemia by thallium-201. Tables 61–6 and 61–7 demonstrate, however, that

Table 61–4. SENSITIVITY AND SPECIFICITY OF THALLIUM-201 AND Tc-SESTAMIBI BY PLANAR IMAGING

	SENSITIVITY				SPECIFICITY					
	OVERALL		*INDIVIDUAL VESSEL*		*OVERALL*				*INDIVIDUAL VESSEL*	
					Normal Arteriogram		*Low Likehood‡*			
	Tc-MIBI	Tl-201	Tc-MIBI	Tl-201	Tc-MIBI	Tl-201	Tc-MIBI	Tl-201	Tc-MIBI	Tl-201
Wackers et al.†[W1]	32/36 (89%)	35/36 (97%)	39/65 (60%)	45/64 (69%)	2/2 (100%)	2/2 (100%)	—	—	38/49 (78%)	40/49 (82%)
Taillefer et al.*[T2]	—	—	68/97 (70%)	72/97 (74%)	—	—	—	—	—	—
Kiat et al.†[K2]	11/15 (73%)	11/15 (73%)	21/35 (60%)	19/35 (54%)	3/4 (75%)	2/4 (50%)	16/17 (94%)	15/17 (88%)	19/22 (80%)	16/22 (73%)
Total:	43/51 (84%)	46/51 (90%)	128/197 (65%)	136/196 (69%)	5/6 (83%)	4/6 (67%)	16/17 (94%)	15/17 (88%)	57/71 (80%)	56/71 (79%)

*Seventy or more percent stenosis as significant coronary artery disease.
†Fifty or more percent stenosis as significant coronary artery disease.
‡Less than 5 percent likelihood of coronary artery disease.

Table 61–5. SENSITIVITY AND SPECIFICITY OF THALLIUM-201 AND Tc-SESTAMIBI BY SPECT IMAGING

	SENSITIVITY				SPECIFICITY					
	OVERALL		*INDIVIDUAL VESSEL*		*OVERALL*				*INDIVIDUAL VESSEL*	
					Normal Arteriogram		*Low Likehood*†			
	Tc-MIBI	Tl-201	Tc-MIBI	Tl-201	Tc-MIBI	Tl-201	Tc-MIBI	Tl-201	Tc-MIBI	Tl-201
Kiat et al.*[K2]	14/15 (93%)	12/15 (80%)	31/35 (87%)	27/35 (77%)	3/4 (75%)	3/4 (75%)	17/17 (100%)	13/17 (77%)	19/22 (86%)	19/22 (86%)
Kahn et al.*[K3]	36/38 (95%)	32/38 (84%)	59/75 (79%)	45/75 (60%)	—	—	—	—	28/39 (72%)	27/39 (69%)
Iskandrian et al.*[I1]	23/28 (82%)	23/28 (82%)	—	—	11/11 (100%)	9/11 (82%)	—	—	—	—
Total:	73/81 (90%)	67/81 (83%)	90/110 (82%)	72/110 (66%)	14/15 (93%)	12/15 (80%)	17/17 (100%)	13/17 (77%)	47/61 (77%)	46/61 (75%)

*Fifty or more percent stenosis as significant coronary artery disease.
†Less than 5 percent likelihood of coronary artery disease.

this discordance was no more common than the reverse (ischemia by Tc-sestamibi and scar by thallium-201). This apparent paradox is likely to be explained by a worsening of perfusion during exercise in patients with resting hypoperfusion, thereby producing evidence of partial reversibility by rest-stress Tc-sestamibi imaging, which is then categorized into the reversible group. The unique capability of thallium-201 studies of rest redistribution to differentiate resting ischemia from scar, however, is unlikely to be afforded by Tc-sestamibi. Which of these tracers would provide the best correlation with other goal standards of myocardial viability, such as glucose metabolism by positron emission tomography, is yet unclear; however, Tc-sestamibi correlations with thallium-201 have been with standard redistribution protocols and not with protocols that utilize 24-hour redistribution imaging[K4] or reinjection of thallium-201 prior to redistribution imaging.[B5]

All the aforementioned Tc-sestamibi results were derived from 2-day protocols in which the rest and exercise studies were separated by at least 24 hours. Taillefer and colleagues demonstrated that rest and stress Tc-sestamibi studies could be performed on a same-day protocol instead of using a 2-day approach.[T3] The rest-stress same-day protocol involves a 7- to 10-

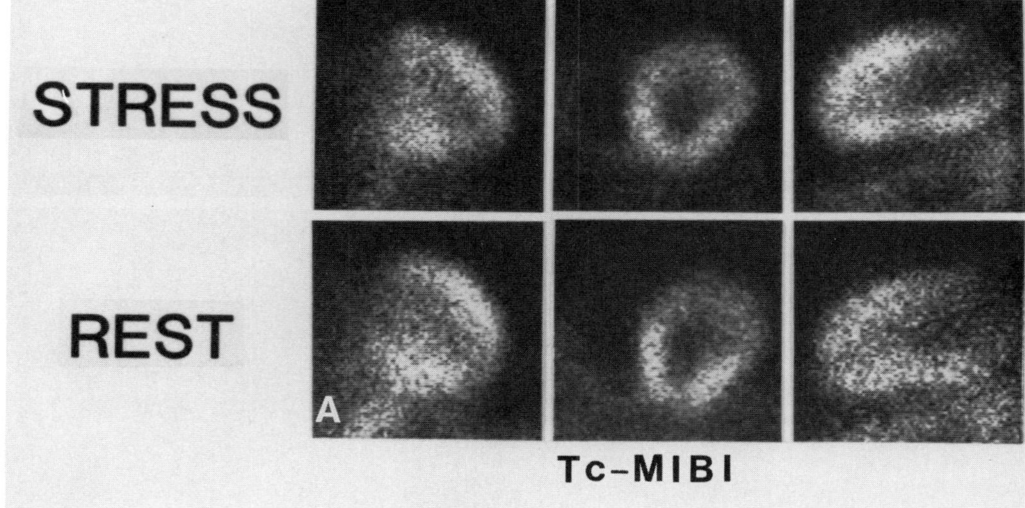

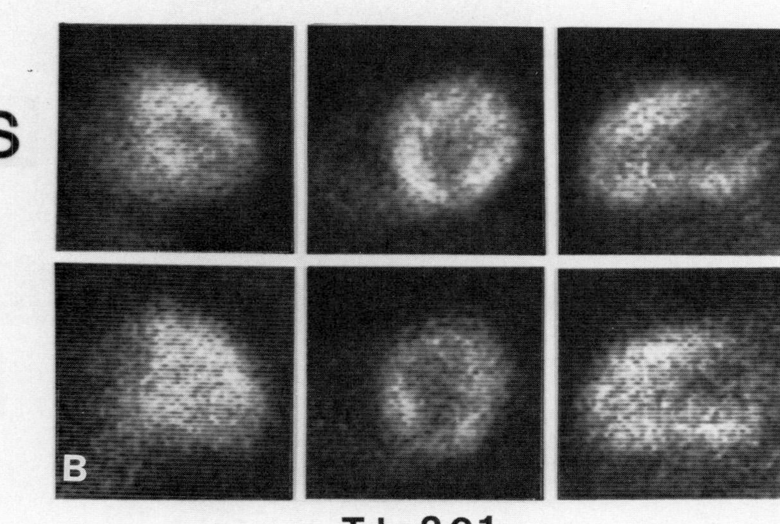

Figure 61–5. Planar images with Tc-sestamibi *(A)* and Tl-201 *(B)* from a patient with triple vessel coronary artery disease. Both tracers demonstrate reversible inferior wall perfusion defects.

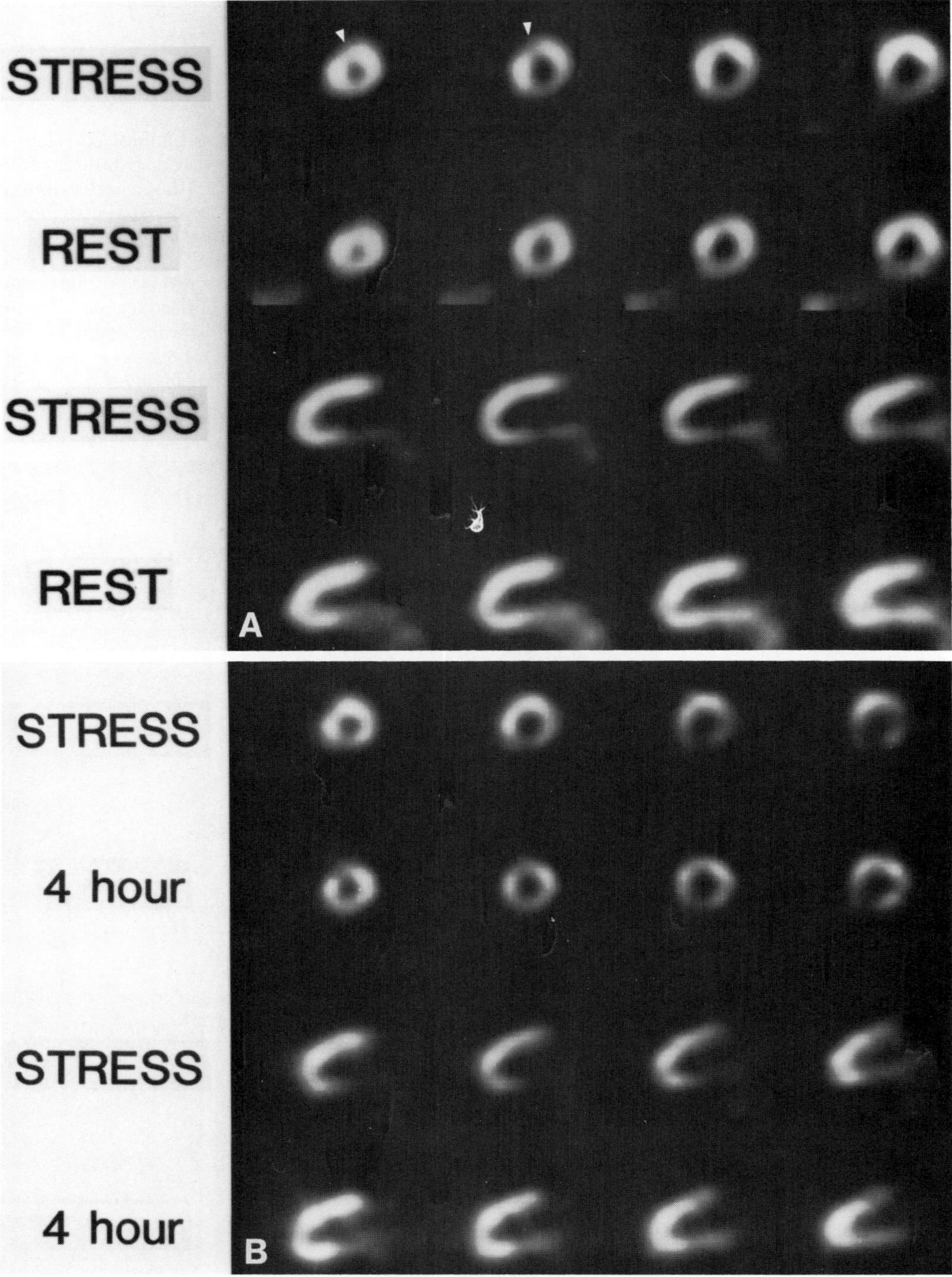

Figure 61–6. SPECT images of the patient shown in Figure 61–5, using Tc-sestamibi *(A)* and Tl-201 *(B)*. Partially reversible defects are seen in the RCA and LCX territories by both tracers, illustrating the superiority of tomographic imaging over planar imaging for detection of left circumflex disease. In addition, the Tc-sestamibi study demonstrates a small distal anterior reversible defect *(arrowheads)*, not seen on the SPECT Tl-201 study, corresponding to a mid-LAD stenosis.

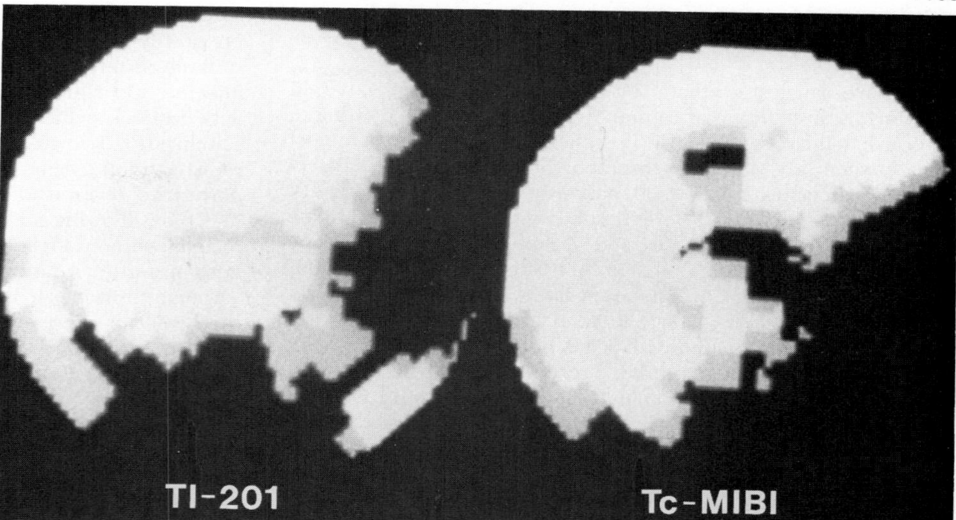

Figure 61–7. Quantitative stress polar maps of Tl-201 and Tc-sestamibi derived from the patient illustrated in Figure 61–6. The quantitative Tc-sestamibi study detected the mid-LAD stenosis as a small defect at 11 o'clock on the polar map, not detected by Tl-201.

Figure 61–8. See Color Plate 15.
Figure 61–9. See Color Plate 15.

mCi injection for the resting study followed by a 25- to 30-mCi Tc-sestamibi injection for the stress study. An example is shown in Figure 61–8. Using this protocol, the group demonstrated excellent agreement for the presence and type of defects between Tc-sestamibi and thallium-201 in planar studies. In a subsequent study using SPECT, 18 patients underwent both same-day rest-stress and stress-rest Tc-sestamibi studies using 7- 10-mCi for the first study and 25 mCi for the second study.[T4] Overall, for the perfusion-defect type (normal, ischemia, or scar), there was good agreement between rest-stress and stress-rest sequences, with 283 of the 324 (87 percent) segments being categorized identically. However, an important outlying group was evident. Although only one segment demonstrated evidence of ischemia by the stress-rest approach and scar by the rest-stress approach, 24 of the 324 (7.4 percent) segments demonstrated evidence of scar by the stress-rest technique but were ischemic by the rest-stress imaging sequence. Thus, the rest-stress sequence appeared to be more effective for defining the presence of reversible abnormalities (Fig. 61–9). It is postulated that with the stress-rest imaging sequence, the residual activity of the stress injection causes an uneven background at the time of performance of the rest study, resulting in an overestimation of the frequency of fixed defects or scar. Overall, the preliminary results from these investigators provide convincing evidence that same-day rest-stress (or stress-rest) protocols are practical with this new tracer.

Taillefer and associates also have reported preliminarily that Tc-sestamibi can be effectively used in dipyridamole myocardial perfusion imaging as an alternative to exercise in patients unable to achieve an adequate level of stress.[T5] In a study of 27 patients with assessment of 243 myocardial segments, dipyridamole Tc-sestamibi and thallium-201 planar imaging were compared. Exact agreement was 82 percent for the type of defects noted, with no particular outlying group. Finally, exercise and dipyridamole Tc-sestamibi studies also have been recently compared.[T6] In 17 patients, the results for detection of ischemic segments and segments with fixed defects were virtually identical. The heart-lung ratio of Tc-sestamibi was significantly higher, and the ischemic-to-normal myocardial wall ratio was significantly lower with dipyridamole than with exercise. Overall, therefore, the available data suggest that Tc-sestamibi will be useful with dipyridamole as a hyperemic stimulus.

Infarct Trials

Several phase III "infarct protocols" have examined the use of Tc-sestamibi in the setting of acute myocardial infarction. High sensitivity has been reported for detecting regional perfusion defect in patients with myocardial infarction documented by abnormal electrocardiographic and radionuclide ventriculographic findings (Du Pont: Data on File). A sensitivity of 94 percent for detecting myocardial infarction was shown, with a normalcy rate of 100 percent found in normal volunteers.

Data from dog experiments have shown that Tc-sestamibi SPECT accurately assesses pathologic infarct size in a reperfusion model.[V1] Preliminary data from multicenter thrombolytic therapy

Table 61–6. COMPARISON OF PLANAR TECHNETIUM-SESTAMIBI AND THALLIUM-201 MYOCARDIAL PERFUSION IMAGING: SEGMENTAL ANALYSIS

	Technetium-Sestamibi		
	Normal (%)	*Reversible* (%)	*Nonreversible* (%)
Thallium-201			
Normal **(%)**	1930 (66)	75 (3)	20 (1)
Reversible **(%)**	120 (4)	410 (14)	37 (1)
Nonreversible **(%)**	46 (2)	51 (2)	218 (7)
Exact segmental agreement:			
Kiat et al.[K2]:		510/540 = 95%	
Taillefer et al.[T2]:		259/297 = 87%	
Taillefer et al.[T3]:		1326/1500 = 88%	
Wackers et al.[W1]:		463/570 = 81%	
TOTAL		2558/2907 = 88%	

Table 61–7. COMPARISON OF SPECT TECHNETIUM-SESTAMIBI AND THALLIUM-201 MYOCARDIAL PERFUSION IMAGING: SEGMENTAL ANALYSIS

	Technetium-Sestamibi		
	Normal (%)	*Reversible* (%)	*Nonreversible* (%)
Thallium-201			
Normal **(%)**	1127 (75)	25 (2)	5 (<1)
Reversible **(%)**	41 (3)	87 (6)	11 (1)
Nonreversible **(%)**	28 (2)	14 (1)	182 (12)
Exact segmental agreement:			
Kiat et al.[K2]:		653/720 = 91%	
Iskandrian et al.[I1]:		723/780 = 93%	
TOTAL		1376/1500 = 92%	

trials have suggested that Tc-sestamibi may be effective in monitoring the efficacy of thrombolytic therapy in the setting of myocardial infarction[G1, W2] by documenting reduction in defect size between pre– and post–thrombolytic therapy images. Wackers and associates studied 30 patients with acute myocardial infarction, of whom 23 were treated with recombinant tissue plasminogen activator (rt-PA) and 7 had conventional therapy without thrombolysis.[W2] Tc-sestamibi was injected before thrombolysis with imaging several hours later. Tc-sestamibi was repeated 18 to 40 hours later and then again 6 to 14 days after infarction. Patients treated with rt-PA demonstrated a significant reduction in quantitative planar Tc-sestamibi defect size between the pre- and early post-thrombolytic studies ($p < 0.001$), whereas patients treated conventionally demonstrated no significant difference in the defect size between the pre- and early postinfarct studies. Additionally, a decrease in defect size of more than 30 percent was strongly predictive of a patent infarct-related artery. In this study there was a trend toward further decrease in defect size by the time of the late (6 to 14 days) postinfarct Tc-sestamibi studies. The investigators concluded that serial planar Tc-sestamibi imaging provides an effective means for assessing the initial risk zone and the presence of reperfusion in patients undergoing thrombolytic therapy.

Gibbons and associates have demonstrated that SPECT imaging with Tc-sestamibi in the setting of acute myocardial infarction provides accurate information with respect to infarct size.[G1] This approach has been indirectly validated in clinical studies by demonstrating a very close relationship between infarct size from a quantitatively analyzed Tc-sestamibi SPECT study and resting ejection fraction measured shortly thereafter. Phantom data obtained by the same investigation also has documented that the quantitative SPECT approach was highly accurate in assessing technetium-99m pertechnetate perfusion defect size in a heart model.[O2] As with the planar study by the Wackers group, the preliminary data obtained from this study, with SPECT Tc-sestamibi performed before and 6 to 14 days after thrombolytic therapy, demonstrated a significant decrease in the extent of hypoperfused myocardium in patients who received thrombolytic therapy, with no significant change in patients who did not receive thrombolytic therapy.[G1] Although similar results were previously demonstrated with thallium-201,[M8, M9] that approach suffered from the problem of potential redistribution of the injected tracer, decreasing the feasibility of performing the study with SPECT, which generally requires transport of a clinically stabilized patient to a nuclear medicine department. Since little redistribution occurs with Tc-sestamibi, the imaging can be performed several hours after the prethrombolysis Tc-sestamibi injection, allowing for clinical stabilization of the patient prior to imaging without loss of imaging information. This approach offers great promise for an objective method to compare the efficacy of various approaches to thrombolytic therapy. Outcome information then could be derived much earlier and using smaller groups of patients than would be required if mortality were the principal end-point.

Ventricular Function Trials

The phase III "global left ventricular function" protocols studied the ability of Tc-sestamibi to measure ejection fraction, compared with standard pertechnetate left ventricular ejection fraction measurements with both using the first-pass technique. A multicenter study of 66 patients (Du Pont: Data on File) demonstrated a close linear correlation ($r = 0.94$) between standard technetium-99m and Tc-sestamibi ejection fraction determinations from first pass studies (Fig. 61–10). In a study reported by Baillet and associates, very high correlation ($r = 0.93$) was also noted in measurements of ejection fraction by standard pertechnetate and Tc-sestamibi first-pass studies.[B4] These investigators also demonstrated that Tc-sestamibi first-pass studies can be used to assess regional left ventricular wall motion.[B4] It may be possible to measure exercise ejection fraction at the peak of treadmill exercise.[B6] Conventionally, ejection fraction studies with exercise have been performed during bicycle exercise. Since there are data suggesting that a greater degree of ischemia is produced with treadmill exercise and it is more commonly used, it would be important to evaluate whether first-pass treadmill exercise studies are feasible. In a preliminary communication, Borges-Neto and colleagues demonstrated the feasibility of treadmill exercise first-pass Tc-sestamibi procedures and showed no significant difference between 1-day and 2-day rest-exercise protocols for the assessment of left or right ventric-

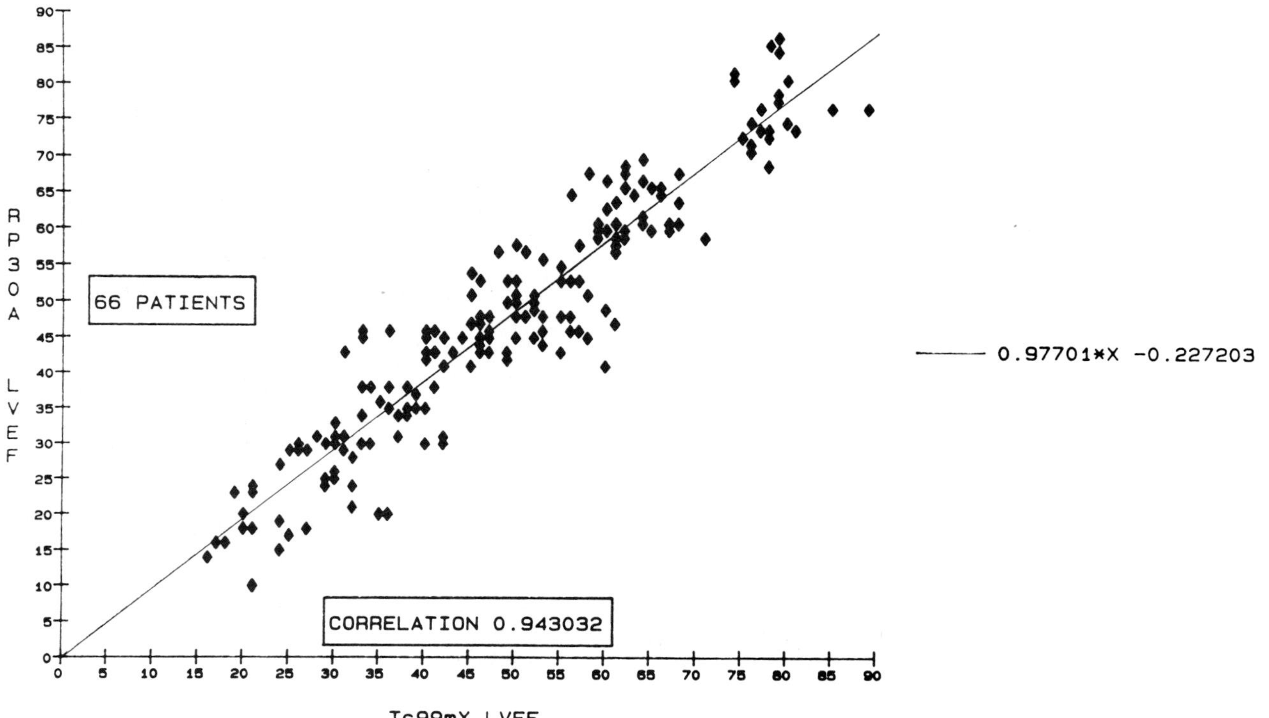

Figure 61–10. Relationship between first-pass measurements of left ventricular ejection fraction, using Tc-sestamibi (RP30A) and technetium-99m pertechnetate or technetium-99m diethylene triamine penta-acetic acid (Tc-99mX). Each patient was studied three times.

ular ejection fraction.[B6] These measurements were obtained using a first-pass scintillation camera especially designed with a small detector head that has the capability of direct imaging during treadmill exercise.

Clinical studies to date with Tc-sestamibi, therefore, indicate that it appears to be equal to thallium-201 for detection of coronary artery disease. It accurately detects and locates myocardial infarction and can assess both left and right ventricular ejection fraction accurately by the first-pass technique. In addition, studies have shown that rest-stress studies can be performed on the same day and that Tc-sestamibi can be used to assess the results of thrombolytic therapy.

Future Development

We predict that use of Tc-sestamibi will eventually replace much of the work currently performed with thallium-201. As noted, the clinical work with Tc-sestamibi has been performed with protocols utilizing acquisition and processing parameters that have been optimized for thallium-201. Even with these initial protocols using either planar or SPECT imaging, investigators have found a general improvement in image quality with Tc-sestamibi, compared with thallium-201. Kahn and associates had two experienced observers rate image quality in their comparative study of thallium-201 and Tc-sestamibi SPECT.[K3] Tc-sestamibi tomograms were rated of superior quality in 88 per cent of studies and were rated comparable in the remaining 12 per cent. Since confidence in image interpretation is related to image quality, this factor alone is likely to cause many users to select Tc-sestamibi over thallium-201.

Important preliminary evidence suggests that further improvement in image quality is likely to evolve when protocols specifically tailored to the physical and biologic characteristics of this new agent are developed. A recent collaborative study[V2] between Cedars-Sinai Medical Center and Emory University, designed to optimize acquisition and processing parameters for Tc-sestamibi, employed a realistic cardiac phantom that mimics the myocardium, myocardial perfusion defects, lungs, and spine, with count rates simulating those encountered in the clinical setting. Various combinations of SPECT acquisition and processing parameters were compared with the all-purpose collimator and 64 × 64 matrix combination, which were previously shown to be optimal for thallium-201. The study showed that a 128 × 128 matrix and high-resolution collimator combination greatly improved defect contrast and the definition of the endocardial and epicardial borders in the phantom. The former approach has been used in most of the clinical data derived to date with SPECT Tc-sestamibi. Our preliminary animal and clinical data have also supported the results of the phantom study with respect to improvement in image quality (unpublished data). Thus, it appears likely that further improvement in image quality using Tc-sestamibi over thallium-201 will be forthcoming, which in turn is likely to be a major factor in guiding the choice of agents utilized. Furthermore, new imaging protocols are likely to be developed that take advantage of the first-pass and gated SPECT acquisition capabilities afforded by the technetium-99m agent, thus providing additional clinical information not provided by static perfusion studies.

TECHNETIUM-99m TEBOROXIME

Results of Clinical Trials

With respect to the other major class of Tc-99m perfusion agents, the BATO compounds, phase I, phase II, and phase III

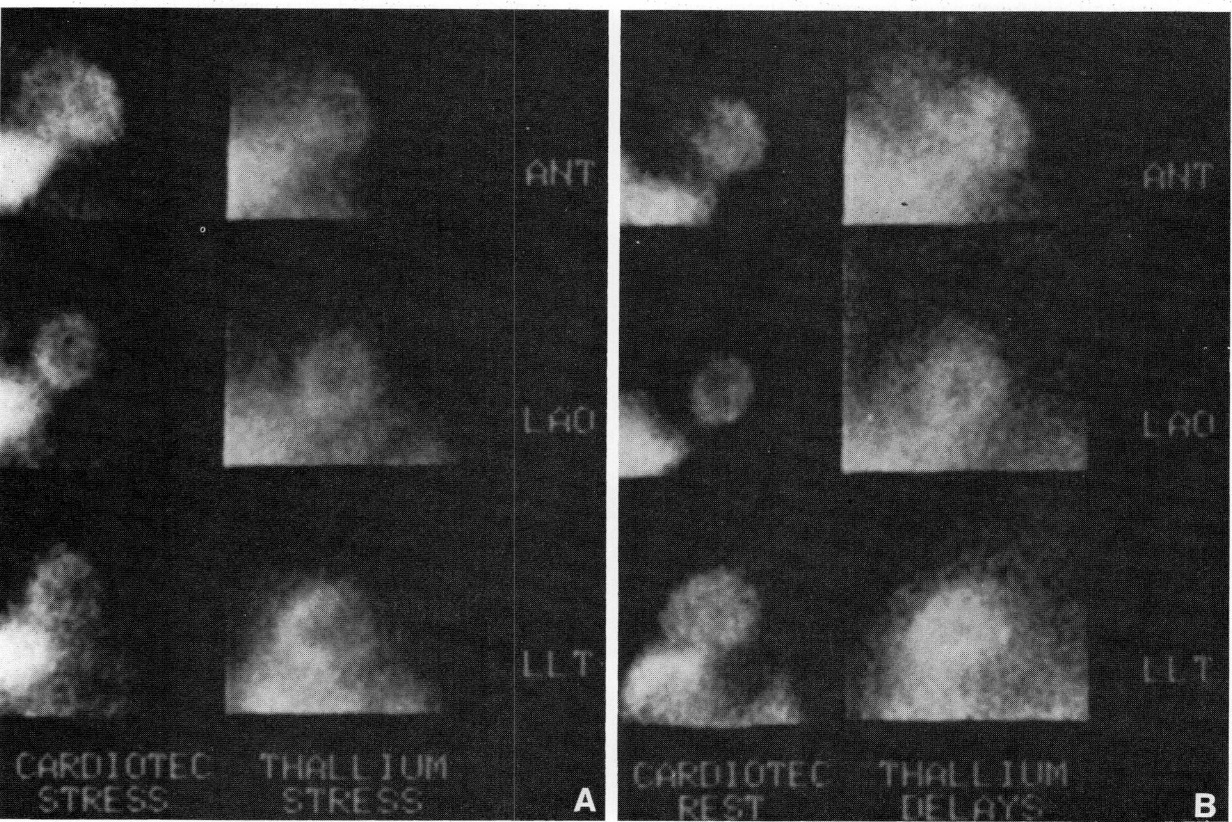

Figure 61–11. Planar images with Tc-teboroxime (termed "Cardiotec" on the figure) and Tl-201 from a patient with left circumflex coronary artery disease. *A*, The post-stress images; *B*, the rest Tc-teboroxime and 4-hour redistribution Tl-201 images. Reversible stress defects in posterolateral wall (LAO view) and posterobasal wall (LLT view) are more clearly visualized by the Tc-teboroxime study. The Tl-201 images are somewhat degraded by backscatter from the simultaneous Tc-teboroxime injection. Of note, stress images were obtained following 10 mCi Tc-teboroxime and 2.8 mCi Tl-201 injection, respectively. Tc-teboroxime image acquisition was 40 seconds/view, starting immediately post-tracer injection. The Tl-201 image acquisition was 6 minutes/view, starting 9 minutes after tracer injection. ANT—anterior, LAO—45° left anterior oblique, LLT—left lateral.

clinical trials have been performed with Tc-teboroxime. These clinical results have suggested that this tracer yields image quality similar to that of thallium-201, provided the images are obtained very rapidly after injection. In 10 normal volunteers and 20 patients with coronary artery disease, Tc-teboroxime stress and rest studies were compared with thallium-201 stress redistribution studies using planar imaging.[S3] For the Tc-teboroxime studies, three-view planar imaging was completed by approximately 16 minutes after injection. Tc-teboroxime detected abnormalities in 16 of the 20 patients with coronary artery disease (80 percent), which was not significantly different from the 17 of 20 (85 percent) detected by thallium-201. Similarly, considering 70 or more per cent as significant stenosis, no significant difference was noted between Tc-teboroxime and thallium-201 for identifying diseased coronary arteries, with 19 of 45 (42 percent) being detected by Tc-teboroxime and 21 of 45 (47 percent) being detected by thallium-201. Both agents were found to be positive in 1 of 15 vessels without significant stenosis. It was reported that hepatic uptake of Tc-teboroxime obscured inferoapical segments in some views in 14 of the 20 coronary artery disease patients, but this did not interfere with abnormal vessel identification. A case example of a stress-rest Tc-teboroxime study is shown in Figure 61–11.

In a large multicenter trial, 177 patients were studied with Tc-teboroxime imaging, using either planar or SPECT methods, and results were compared with cardiac catheterization or thallium-201 imaging or both. In the angiographic correlations, the overall sensitivity for coronary artery disease was 84 percent and specificity was 91 percent. Teboroxime imaging results agreed with thallium-201 interpretations in 91 percent of the cases (data on file with Food and Drug Administration, and Squibb Diagnostics). A preliminary report by Hendel and co-workers showed that rapid planar imaging techniques could be used with the patient in a seated position, to collect complete diagnostic teboroxime studies within 5 minutes of injection.[H4]

Future Development

The ability to do complete rest-stress studies with Tc-teboroxime in a very short period of time appears to be an advantage over thallium-201 or Tc-sestamibi; however, the very rapid myocardial clearance detracts from the ability to obtain images of the high quality possible using Tc-sestamibi. With the advent of three-detector SPECT imaging systems, this agent may be particularly well suited to kinetic SPECT imaging, allowing rapid tomographic assessment of initial uptake and washout of the tracer. Preliminary data employing a single-photon ring detector system have suggested that compartmental modeling of kinetic data with this tracer could permit the quantification of regional myocardial blood flow.[S5] The feasibility of very rapid stress-"redistribution" imaging with a single injection of this tracer deserves further investigation.

CONCLUSION

Two new myocardial perfusion imaging agents labeled with technetium-99m are likely to be routinely available for clinical use in the near future. Both these new agents allow assessment of ejection fraction by the first-pass technique at rest or during exercise, thus providing additional information not available with thallium-201. With Tc-sestamibi, gated SPECT acquisition protocols are feasible. Clinical trials of myocardial perfusion with both tracers have shown results similar to those obtained with thallium-201 for detection of coronary artery disease. With Tc-sestamibi, image quality already has been shown to be superior to that achieved with thallium-201. Further improvement in image quality is likely as acquisition protocols are optimized for this tracer. Because of its slow myocardial clearance and absence of redistribution, Tc-sestamibi allows uncoupling of the time of injection from the time of imaging and thus may be clinically valuable in assessing patients undergoing thrombolytic therapy. Tc-teboroxime has excellent myocardial tracer uptake characteristics but is cleared very rapidly from the myocardium. Although these features make this agent well suited to rapid serial studies, they also reduce the ability to obtain time-intensive SPECT images of high resolution. It is considered likely that these new technetium myocardial perfusion agents will replace thallium-201 in many of its clinical applications.

Acknowledgments

The authors gratefully acknowledge the expert secretarial assistance of Judy Manders in the preparation of the manuscript for this article.

References

B

1. Bassingthwaighte, J.B., and Goresky, C.A.: Modeling in the analysis of solute and water exchange in the microvasculature. *In* Handbook of Physiology. Section 2, The Cardiovascular System. Vol. IV. American Physiological Society, Bethesda, Md., 1984, pp. 549–626.
2. Bassingthwaighte, J.B., Chinard, F.P., Crone, C., et al.: Terminology for mass transport and exchange. Am. J. Physiol. 250:H539, 1986.
3. Bassingthwaighte, J.B.: Physiology and theory of tracer washout techniques for the estimation of myocardial blood flow: Flow estimation from tracer washout. Prog. Cardiovasc. Dis. 20:165, 1977.
4. Baillet, G., Mena, I., Kuperus, J., et al.: Simultaneous Tc-99m-sestamibi angiography and myocardial perfusion imaging. J. Nucl. Med. 30:38, 1989.
5. Bonow, R.O., Bacharach, S.L., Cuocolo, A., and Dilsizian, V.: Myocardial viability in coronary artery disease and left ventricular dysfunction: Thallium-201 reinjection vs. fluorodeoxyglucose. Circulation 80(4):II–377, 1989.
6. Borges-Neto, S., Coleman, R.E., and Jones, R.H.: Comparison of one and two day rest and treadmill Cardiolite tests. J. Nucl. Med. 30:790, 1988.

C

1. Canby, R.C., Silber, S., and Pohost, G.: Relations of the myocardial imaging agents ^{99m}Tc-sestamibi and ^{201}Tl to myocardial blood flow in a canine model of myocardial insult. Circulation 81:289, 1990.

G

1. Gibbons, R.J., Verani, M.S., Behrenbeck, T., et al.: Feasibility of tomographic technetium-99m-hexakis-2-methoxy-2-methylpropyl-isonitrile imaging for the assessment of myocardial area at risk and the effect of acute treatment in myocardial infarction. Circulation 80:1277, 1989.

H

1. Holman, B.L., Jones, A.G., Lister-James, J., et al.: A new Tc-99m–labelled imaging agent, hexakis(t-butylisonitrile)-technetium(I) [Tc-99m TBI]: Initial experience in the human. J. Nucl. Med. 25:1350, 1984.
2. Holman, B.L., Campbell, C.A., Lister-James, J., et al.: Effect of reperfusion and hyperemia on the biodistribution of the myocardial imaging agent Tc-99m TBI. J. Nucl. Med. 27:1172, 1986.
3. Holman, B.L., Sporn, V., Jones, A.G., et al.: Myocardial imaging with technetium-99m CPI: Initial experience in the human. J. Nucl. Med. 28:13, 1987.
4. Hendel, R.C., McSherry, B., Karimeddini, M., and Leppo, J.A.: Diagnostic utility of a new Tc-99m myocardial imaging agent (SQ30217) utilizing a rapid imaging protocol. J. Nucl. Med. 30:730, 1989.

I

1. Iskandrian, A.S., Heo, J., Kong, B., et al.: Use of technetium-99m isonitrile (RP–30A) in assessing left ventricular perfusion and function at rest and during exercise in coronary artery disease, and comparison with coronary arteriography and exercise thallium-201 SPECT imaging. Am. J. Cardiol. 64:270, 1989.

J

1. Jones, A.G., Davison, A., Abrams, M.J., et al.: Biological studies of a new class of technetium complexes: The hexakis(alkylisonitrile) technetium(I) cations. Int. J. Nucl. Med. Biol. 11:225, 1984.

K

1. Kahn, J.K., McGhie, I., Faber, T.L., et al.: Assessment of myocardial viability with technetium-99m-2methoxy isobutyl isonitrile (MIBI) and gated tomography in patients with coronary artery disease. J. Am. Coll. Cardiol. 13(2):31A, 1989.
2. Kiat, H., Maddahi, J., Roy, L., et al.: Comparison of Tc-99m methoxy isobutyl isonitrile with Tl-201 imaging by planar and SPECT techniques for assessment of coronary disease. Am. Heart J. 117(1):1, 1989.

3. Kahn, J., McGhie, I., Akers, M., et al.: Quantitative rotational tomography with Tl-201 and Tc-99m 2-methoxy-isobutyl-isonitrile: A direct comparison in normal individuals and patients with coronary artery disease. Circulation 79: 1282, 1989.
4. Kiat, H., Berman, D.S., Maddahi, J., et al.: Late reversibility of tomographic myocardial thallium-201 defects: An accurate marker of myocardial viability. J. Am. Coll. Cardiol. 12:1456, 1988.

L

1. Liu, P., Houle, S., Mills, L., and Dawood, F.: Kinetics of Tc-99m MIBI in clearance in ischemia-reperfusion: Comparison with Tl-201. Circulation 76:IV–216, 1987.
2. Leppo, J.A., and Meerdink, D.A.: Comparison of the myocardial uptake of a technetium-labeled isonitrile analogue and thallium. Circ. Res. 65:632, 1989.
3. Leppo, J.A., and Meerdink, D.J.: Comparative myocardial extraction of two technetium-labeled BATO derivatives (SQ30217, SQ32014) and thallium. J. Nucl. Med. 31:67, 1990.

M

1. McKusick, K., Holman, B.L., Jones, A.G., et al.: Comparison of three Tc-99m isonitriles for detection of ischemic heart disease in humans. (Abstract.) J. Nucl. Med. 27:878, 1986.
2. Mousa, S.A., Williams, S.J., and Sands, H.: Characterization of in vivo chemistry of cations in the heart. J. Nucl. Med. 28:1351, 1987.
3. Marshall, R.C., Leidholdt, E.M., Jr., and Barnett, C.A.: Single pass myocardial extraction and retention of a Tc-99m isonitrile vs. Tl-201. Circulation 76(Suppl. IV):IV–218, 1987.
4. Meerdink, D.J., Thurber, M., Savage, S., and Leppo, J.A.: Effect of reperfusion on the first-pass myocardial extraction of (RP30) and thallium. J. Nucl. Med. 29:819, 1988.
5. Meerdink, D., Moring, A., and Leppo, J.: Comparative myocardial transport of technetium-labeled SQ30217 (Cardiotec) and Tl-201. J. Am. Coll. Cardiol. 9:137A, 1987.
6. Maublant, J.C., Gachon, P., and Moins, N.: Hexakis (2-methoxy isobutylisonitrile) technetium-99m and thallium-201 chloride: Uptake and release in cultured myocardial cells. J. Nucl. Med. 29:48, 1988.
7. Maublant, J.C., Moins, N., and Gachon, P.: Uptake and release of two new Tc-99m–labeled myocardial blood flow imaging agents in cultured cardiac cells. Eur. J. Nucl. Med. 15:180, 1989.
8. Maddahi, J., Ganz, W., Ninomiya, K., et al.: Myocardial salvage by intracoronary thrombolysis in evolving myocardial infarction: Evaluation using intracoronary injection of thallium-201. Am. Heart J. 102:664, 1981.
9. Maddahi, J., Weiss, T., Geft, I., et al.: Coronary thrombolysis with intravenous streptokinase salvages jeopardized myocardium in evolving myocardial infarction: Assessment by quantitative Tl-201 imaging. Circulation 68:III–120, 1983.

N

1. Narra, R.K., Feld, T., Wedeking, P., et al.: SQ30,217, a technetium-99m–labelled myocardial imaging agent which shows no interspecies differences in uptake. Nuklearmedizin 23(Suppl.):489, 1987.

O

1. Okada, R., Glover, D., Gaffney, T., and Willliams, S.: Myocardial kinetics of Tc-99m-hexakis-2-methoxy-2-methylpropylisonitrile. Circulation 77:491, 1988.
2. O'Conner, M.K., Hammell, T., and Gibbons, R.J.: In vitro validation of a simple tomographic technique for estimation of % myocardium "at risk" using technetium-99m methoxy isobutyl isonitrile (sestamibi). J. Nucl. Med. (in press).

R

1. Rama, K.N., Nunn, A.D., Kuczynski, B.L., et al.: A neutral technetium-99m complex for myocardial imaging. J. Nucl. Med. 30:1830, 1989.

S

1. Sia, S.T.B., Holman, B.L., McKusick, K., et al.: The utilization of Tc-99mTBI as a myocardial perfusion agent in exercise studies: Comparison with Tl-201 thallous chloride and examination of its biodistribution in humans. Eur. J. Nucl. Med. 12:333, 1986.
2. Sinusas, A.J., Weber, K.A., Bergin, J.D., et al.: Correlation of myocardial uptake of technetium-99m methoxy-isobutyl isonitrile with regional flow during coronary occlusion and reperfusion. J. Nucl. Med. 30:756, 1989.
3. Seldin, D.W., Johnson, L.L., Blood, D.K., et al.: Myocardial perfusion imaging with technetium-99m SQ30217: Comparison with thallium-201 and coronary anatomy. J. Nucl. Med. 30:312, 1989.
4. Stewart, R.E., Hutchins, G.D., Brown, D., et al.: Myocardial retention and clearance of the flow tracer Tc-99m Sq30217 in canine heart. J. Nucl. Med. 30:860, 1989.
5. Stewart, R.E., Chiao, P., Rogers, W.L., et al.: Assessment of myocardial blood flow by SPECT based on clearance kinetics of the new technetium-labeled flow tracer SQ30217. Circulation 80(Suppl. 2):II–618, 1989.

T

1. Taillefer, R., Lambert, R., Dupras, G., et al.: Clinical comparison between thallium-201 and Tc-99m-methoxy isobutyl isonitrile (hexamibi) myocardial perfusion imaging for detection of coronary artery disease. Eur. J. Nucl. Med. 15:280, 1989.
2. Taillefer, R., Dupras, G., Sporn, V., et al.: Myocardial perfusion imaging with a new radiotracer, technetium-99m–hexamibi (methoxy isobutyl isonitrile): Comparison with thallium-201 imaging. Clin. Nucl. Med. 14:89, 1989.
3. Taillefer, R., La Flamme, L., Dupras, G., et al.: Myocardial perfusion imaging with Tc-99m (MIBI): Comparison of short- and long-term intervals between rest and stress injections: Preliminary results. Eur. J. Nucl. Med. 13:515, 1988.
4. Taillefer, R., Gagnon, A., La Flamme, L., et al.: Same-day injections of Tc-99m–methoxy isobutyl isonitrile (MIBI) for myocardial tomographic imaging: Comparison between rest-stress and stress-rest injection sequences. Eur. J. Nucl. Med. 15:113, 1989.
5. Taillefer, R., La Flamme, L., Dupras, G., et al.: Myocardial imaging with pharmacologic coronary vasodilator (dipyridamole): Comparison between Tc-99m–methoxy isobutyl isonitrile and thallium-201. J. Nucl. Med. 29:781, 1988.
6. Taillefer, R., Lambert, R., Phaneuf, D.C., et al.: Comparison between treadmill stress test and intravenous dipyridamole for myocardial perfusion imaging with Tc-99m methoxy isobutyl isonitrile (MIBI) in detection of coronary artery disease. J. Nucl. Med. 30:759, 1989.

V

1. Verani, M.S., Jeroudi, M.O., Mahmarian, J.J., et al.: Quantification of myocardial infarction during coronary occlusion and myocardial salvage after reperfusion using cardiac imaging with technetium-99m hexakis 2-methoxyisobutyl isonitrile. J. Am. Coll. Cardiol. 12:1573, 1988.
2. Van Train, K., Folks, R., Wong, C., et al.: Optimization of Tc-sestamibi SPECT acquisition and processing parameters: Collimator, matrix size, and filter evaluation. J. Nucl. Med. 30(5):75, 1989.

W

1. Wackers, F., Berman, D., Maddahi, J., et al.: Technetium-99m hexakis 2-methoxyisobutyl isonitrile: Human biodistribution, dosimetry, safety and preliminary comparison to thallium-201 for myocardial perfusion imaging. J. Nucl. Med. 30:301, 1989.
2. Wackers, F., Gibbons, R., Verani, M., et al.: Serial quantitative planar Tc-99m isonitrile imaging in acute myocardial infarction: Efficacy for non-invasive assessment of thrombolytic therapy. J. Am. Coll. Cardiol. 14:861, 1989.

Chapter 62

Monoclonal Antibody Imaging

■ *PHILIP D. NICOL, M.D.* ■ *BAN AN KHAW, Ph.D.*

PRINCIPLES OF ANTIMYOSIN IMAGING 1110
ANTIBODY FRAGMENTS AND RADIOLABELING OF ANTIMYOSIN ANTIBODIES 1110
Preparation of Monoclonal Antimyosin 1110
Intact Antibody versus Fragments 1111
EXPERIMENTAL GAMMA IMAGING 1112
Myocardial Infarction 1112
Cardiac Allograft Rejection 1114
Myocarditis 1114
ANTIMYOSIN IMAGING IN HUMANS 1114
Myocardial Infarction 1114
Cardiac Allograft Rejection 1115
Myocarditis 1116
Adverse Reactions to Antimyosin 1117
ANTIBODY IMAGING OF BLOOD CLOTS 1118
Antifibrin Imaging 1118

The impetus for ubiquitous application of radiolabeled antibodies in gamma imaging of specific tissues and organs has been hitherto limited by the lack of sufficient quantities of antibodies and the difficulties associated with radiolabels and radiolabeling techniques. Recent advances in the field of radioimmunoscintigraphy have propelled radiolabeled antibody imaging to the forefront of biotechnology. The first successful demonstration of the use of antibodies as potential target-specific localizing reagents was in 1947. Pressman and Keighley showed specific concentration of an ^{131}I-labeled gamma globulin fraction of anti-kidney antiserum in rat kidneys in vivo.[P1] Since this demonstration, numerous studies and refinements in the radiolabeling technology for gamma imaging with antibodies have been reported. Antibodies have been used to image tumors,[S2] myocardial necrosis,[K1–K15, K17–K19] and blood clots.[F1, O2, R1–R2] The most thoroughly studied and reproducible antibody imaging system to date is the use of antimyosin for the detection and visualization of myocardial necrosis.[K1–K15]

PRINCIPLES OF ANTIMYOSIN IMAGING

Cardiac myosin is an intracelluar fibrous contractile protein consisting of two identical heavy chains (200,000 daltons) and two pairs of light chains (19,000 and 27,000 daltons) constituting a molecule of approximately 500,000 daltons.[K21] The heavy chains of myosin are highly insoluble in physiologic fluids, and require high salt concentrations for solubility.[S3] Thus, myosin molecules remain as insoluble myofibrils intracellularly even after disruption of the sarcolemma in necrotic myocardium. Unlike the highly soluble myosin light chain molecules, the heavy chains are not washed out of the damaged myocardium. Therefore, an antibody specific for myosin, when administered in vivo, can bind to its homologous antigen only in necrotic myocardial tissues while the intact cell membranes of normal myocardium prevent the macromolecular antibody from binding with the antigen. If the antibody were radiolabeled with an appropriate isotope, the area and extent of myocardial necrosis could be assessed by imaging the regions of radioisotope accumulation.

Based on this hypothesis, antimyosin antibodies were generated and feasibility studies were performed in acute canine experimental myocardial infarction models.[K1–K3] This was followed by the demonstration of its usefulness in myocardial infarction in clinical trials.[K16–K19] Subsequently, this method has been applied to the diagnosis of myocardial necrosis associated with both acute myocarditis[Y1] and heart transplant rejection.[F2, I1]

ANTIBODY FRAGMENTS AND RADIOLABELING OF ANTIMYOSIN ANTIBODIES

Preparation of Monoclonal Antimyosin

Monoclonal antimyosin antibodies were generated by fusing immune murine spleen cells with murine SP2\OA myeloma cells.[K20] Human ventricular cardiac myosin, which consists mainly of the V3 isoform of myosin, was used to immunize mice.[K1, K2, M4] A murine monoclonal antibody, designated R11D10, was developed that was V3-specific and showed no cross-reactivity with the V1 or atrial isoform of cardiac myosin. This antibody has an apparent affinity (K_a) of 5 × 10^8 L/M. Another monoclonal antimyosin, designated 2G42D7, was not isoenzyme specific and was found to react equally well with both the V1 and V3 forms of cardiac myosin (K_a 1 × 10^8 L/M.)

Both R11D10 and 2G42D7 can be fragmented to give Fab or $(Fab')_2$ after digestion with either papain[P1] or pepsin[E1] respectively. These fragments can be purified from the undigested antibodies and other non-antigen-binding fragments by molecular sieve and affinity column chromatographies. Purity of the antibody fragment preparations can be determined by sodium dodecylsulfate polyacrylamide disk gel electrophoresis,[L1] and by the Ouchterlony method using rabbit antimurine IgG antibody.[O1]

Antimyosin and its fragments can be readily radioiodinated with ^{125}I, ^{123}I, and ^{131}I by various methods such as the lactoperoxidase, chloramine-t, iodogen, and iodobead methods, without affecting the antigen-binding capacity of the antibody preparations.[M1, H1] Although radiolabeling of antibodies with ^{125}I and ^{131}I is relatively easy and has been used successfully to image experimental myocardial infarction (Fig. 62–1), it may not be suited for clinical use. The 60-day half-life (T½) and the low peak energy of emission of ^{125}I make it unsuitable for imaging acute infarction in patients.[S6] Similarly, ^{131}I is not ideal for imaging because of its high peak emission energy and the presence of beta emission.[S6] The radioiodine most suitable for in vivo gamma imaging is ^{123}I with a peak emission energy of 159 keV and a 13-hour T½. Until recently, however, ^{123}I was not available in isotopically pure form for a reasonable cost.

The major disadvantage of radioiodinated antibodies for in vivo gamma imaging is their propensity for dehalogenation at the target organs. However, for myocardial infarct imaging, the differential dehalogenation in various organs may be an advantage. Dehalogenation is greatest in the liver and minimal in the necrotic myocardium. Nonspecific activity that accumulates in the liver is rapidly cleared by dehalogenation, thus resulting in

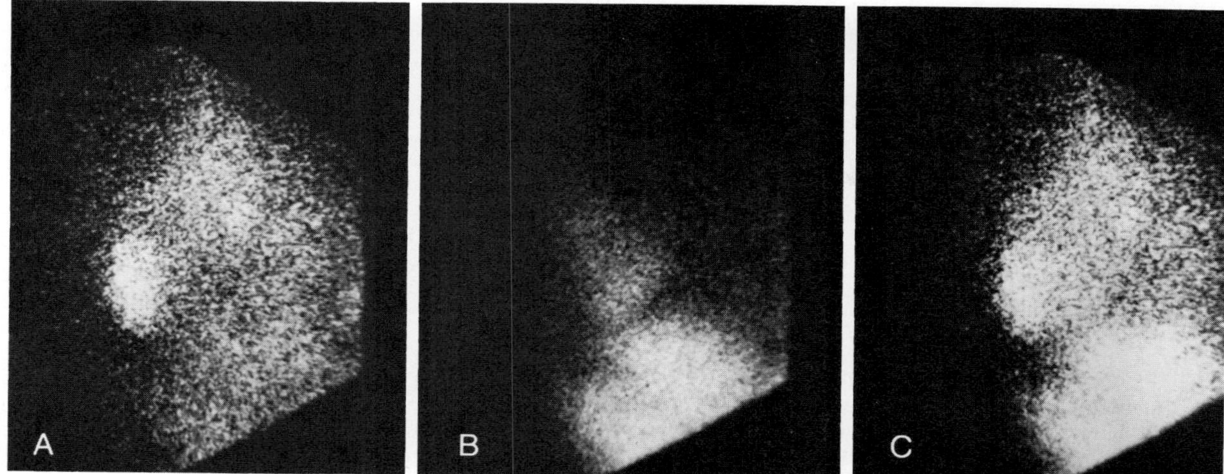

Figure 62–1. In vivo left lateral gamma images obtained after administration of ^{131}I antimyosin (Fab′)$_2$. *A*, ^{131}I antimyosin (Fab′)$_2$. *B*, ^{201}Tl. *C*, Composite of *A* and *B* showing concordance of the antimyosin-delineated infarct region with the ^{201}Tl defect. (From Khaw, B. A., et al.: Early imaging of experimental myocardial infarction by intracoronary administration of ^{131}I-labeled anticardiac myosin (Fab′)$_2$ fragments. Circulation 58:1137, 1978, by permission of the American Heart Association, Inc.)

minimal radioactivity in the liver. Therefore, visualization of even small myocardial infarcts adjacent to the diaphragm is possible (Fig. 62–2).

After our initial experimental studies with ^{125}I- and ^{131}I-labeled antibodies, focus was turned to the use of ^{111}In and ^{99m}Tc radioisotopes for clinical application.[K16, F1] ^{111}In has a dual peak energy emission of 174 and 246 keV, and it is well suited for radiolabeling antibodies via the use of bifunctional chelating agents.[T3] However, ^{111}In requires the use of a medium energy collimator for imaging with a gamma camera. ^{99m}Tc, with a T½ of 6 hours and a peak energy emission of 140 keV, is optimally suited for imaging with a portable gamma camera equipped with an all-purpose collimator. For this reason, ^{99m}Tc was used first in clinical trials even though radiolabeling of antibodies with ^{99m}Tc is technically more difficult.[K8, C1] Radiolabeling of antibodies with ^{99m}Tc is achieved

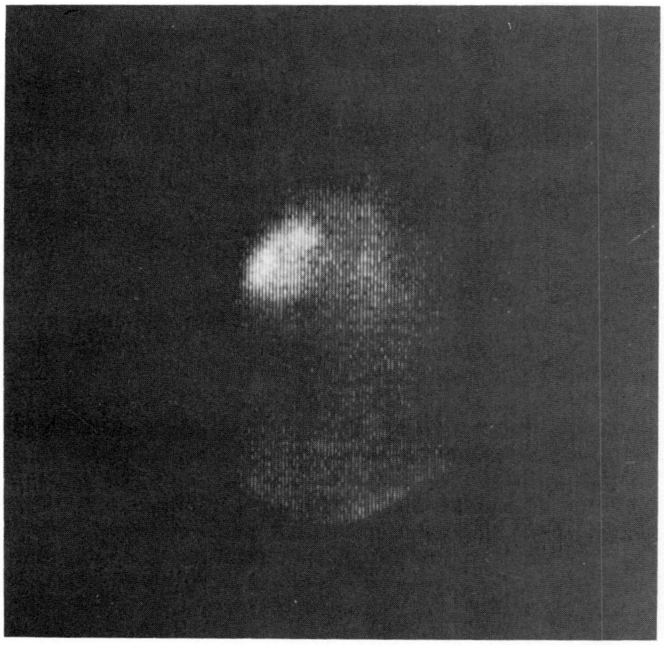

Figure 62–2. In vivo left lateral gamma image of a dog following experimental LAD ligation, at 5 hours following the intravenous administration of ^{123}I antimyosin Fab. Very little radioactivity is seen in the liver. The area of intense uptake delineates the acute anterior infarction.

by a three-step procedure as follows: (1) The antibody is modified with diethylenetriaminepentaacetic acid (DTPA); (2) the generator-eluted ^{99m}Tc pertechnetate ($^{99m}TcO4^-$) is reduced for 10 minutes with solid sodium dithionite; and (3) the DTPA modified antimyosin is added to the reduced ^{99m}Tc. The ^{99m}Tc-labeled antimyosin is separated by column chromatography.[C1, K8, K16]

As discussed above, radiolabeling antibodies with ^{111}In is simpler. The antibody must be modified with a chelator such as DTPA. In the original method,[K16] chelation of ^{111}In by the DTPA-modified protein was achieved in a glycine-HCl (pH 3.5) buffer. However, this acidic pH was observed to cause partial denaturation of the antibody, especially when Fab fragments were labeled.[K5] To overcome this, a transchelation method of radiolabeling-DTPA antibody with ^{111}In at pH 5.5 was developed utilizing citrate as the initial weak chelator.[K13] This method of radiolabeling enabled development of a kit for ^{111}In radiolabeling of antibodies.

Intact Antibody versus Fragments

Immunoreactivity of antimyosin antibody fragments is unchanged by enzymatic fragmentation. However, the in vivo biodistribution characteristics of Fab and (Fab′)$_2$ are very different from that of the intact antibody. The blood clearance of the intact antimyosin has the longest half-life, with (Fab′)$_2$ clearing faster (T½ = 8 hours) and the Fab clearing the fastest (T½ = 4 hours). Both Fab and (Fab′)$_2$ follow a two-compartment clearance system. The initial fast compotent is due to equilibration in vivo in the blood between the intravascular and extravascular space, and the slow component is due to the catabolic and renal excretion mechanisms. In the case of Fab, the fast component has T½ of 0.6 hour and the slow component has a T½ of 12 hours.[B1, K15] This results in an effective clearance of the Fab fragments from the blood by 24 hours. By 48 hours after intravenous administration of the fragments, only about 4 percent of the initial injected dose remains in the circulation (Fig. 62–3).[B1, K15]

The use of antimyosin fragments has also reduced the potential for eliciting the adverse effect of human anti-murine antibody response in patients. The presence of human anti-murine antibody response, which appears to be frequent in both therapeutic and diagnostic oncologic applications of intact antibodies, [P3] has reduced the effectiveness of the reagents. Despite the disadvantages. The use of intact antibody for imaging does have, at least, one advantage. The increased T½ of intact antibodies should allow detection of small lesions while requiring less of the antibody for in vivo administration.

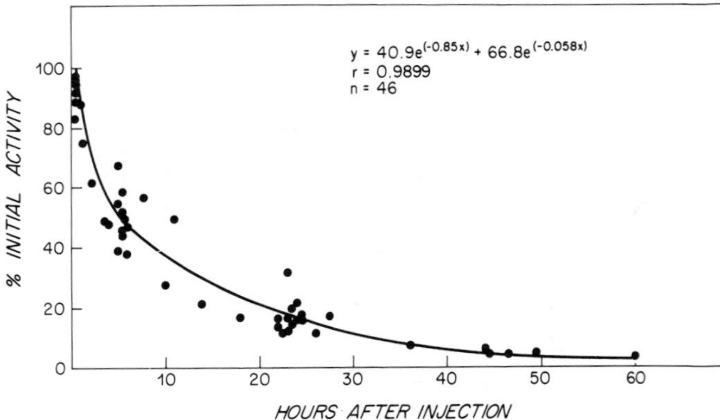

Figure 62–3. The blood clearance of ^{111}In antimyosin Fab in 14 patients was determined from 46 blood samples taken from 1 minute to 58 hours following intravenous injection. The mean clearance of ^{111}In AM Fab has a T½ of 4 hours. Clearance follows a two-compartment model with the initial fast component (T½ = 0.6 h) resulting from distribution within the extracellular compartment. The second slower phase is due to excretion (T½ = 12 h). By 12 to 14 hours blood activity has decreased to 30 percent of injected dose, allowing visualization of the acute infarction. At 48 hours following intravenous injection only 4 percent of the injected dose is present. (From Khaw, B.A., et al.: Acute myocardial infarct imaging with indium-111 labeled monoclonal antimyosin Fab. J Nucl Med 28:1671, 1987, by permission of The Society of Nuclear Medicine.)

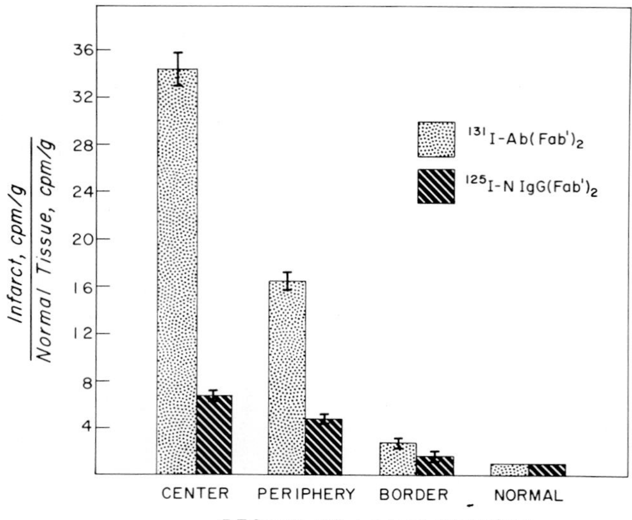

Figure 62–4. Comparison of regional uptake of ^{125}I normal rabbit IgG $(Fab')_2$ and ^{131}I antimyosin $(Fab')_2$ in canine infarction. Antimyosin uptake is greatest at the center of infarction. Nonspecific uptake of normal rabbit IgG $(Fab')_2$ is significantly different from the specific uptake of antimyosin at the center of infarction. (From Khaw, B. A., et al.: Early imaging of experimental myocardial infarction by intracoronary administration of ^{131}I-labeled anticardiac myosin $(Fab')_2$ fragments. Circulation 58:1137, 1978, by permission of the American Heart Association, Inc.)

EXPERIMENTAL GAMMA IMAGING

Myocardial Infarction

The specificity of radiolabeled antimyosin for myocyte necrosis has been demonstrated in several in vivo and in vitro studies. When ^{131}I antimyosin $(Fab')_2$ and control ^{125}I normal IgG $(Fab')_2$ were administered simultaneously into dogs with experimental myocardial infarction, the uptake of both isotopes could be quantitated. The mean ratio of uptake of radioactivity in necrotic versus normal canine myocardium has been shown to be 36:1 in the case of ^{131}I antimyosin $(Fab')_2$ at the center of infarction and 6:1 for ^{125}I normal IgG $(Fab')_2$ in the same tissue samples (Fig. 62–4). Thus, the uptake of radiolabeled antimyosin is due primarily to specific antigen–antibody interaction and is not the result of nonspecific uptake of normal rabbit IgG $(Fab')_2$ at the site of infarction.[K3] Gamma images of the heart slices from canine myocardial infarction folllowing ^{131}I-labeled antimyosin $(Fab')_2$ administration showed good correlation to histochemically delineated infarction using triphenyltetrazolium chloride staining.

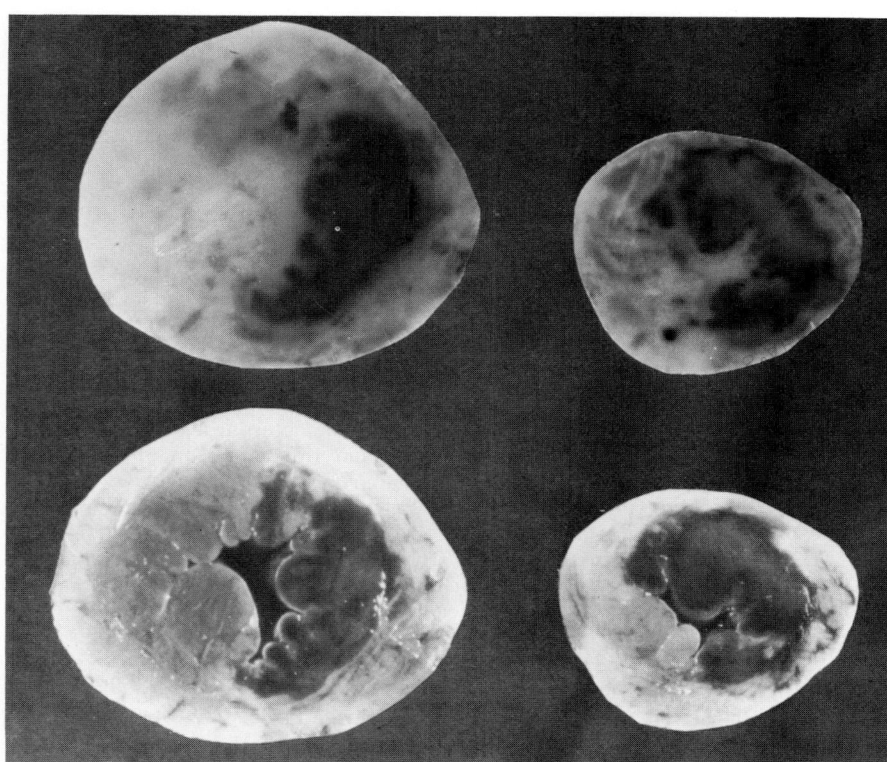

Figure 62–5. Comparison of infarction delineated by triphenyltetrazolium chloride (TTC) and corresponding ^{131}I antimyosin uptake in canine heart slices by macroautoradiography. The lower panels demonstrate the extent and location of the hemorrhagic infarction as delineated by TTC staining (dark areas). The upper panels are the corresponding macroautoradiographs demonstrating the close correlation between the two methods. (From Khaw, B. A., et al.: Specificity of localization of myosin-specific antibody fragments in experimental myocardial infarction: histologic, histochemical, autoradiographic and scintigraphic studies. Circulation 60:1527, 1979, by permission of the American Heart Association, Inc.)

Macroautoradiographic delineation of these sections with ^{131}I-labeled antimyosin showed an almost identical infarct outline to that obtained with triphenyltetrazolium chloride (Fig. 62–5).[K18] Further confirmation of antimyosin specificity for myocyte necrosis and membrane disruption was demonstrated by using antimyosin-coupled fluorescent microspheres and primary neonatal murine myocytes in culture. These antimyosin microspheres were demonstrated by scanning electron microscopy to bind only to necrotic myocytes with cell membrane disruption (Fig. 62–6).[K7, K9]

Antimyosin distribution in the infarct is also dependent on regional myocardial blood flow as measured by the radiolabeled microsphere technique[K1, K10] and early ^{201}Tl distribution.[K10] There is an inverse exponential relationship between antimyosin uptake and regional blood flow. However, antimyosin localization showed an inverse relationship to delayed ^{201}Tl distribution.[K10] These studies showed that antimyosin localization was maximal in regions of maximal myocardial damage assessed by regional blood flow criteria. In contrast, ^{99m}Tc pyrophosphate, which is also an infarct-avid imaging agent, has no simple relationship to regional myocardial blood flow (Fig. 62–7).[B1, K18] Pyrophosphate localization was maximal in myocardial tissues with intermediate regional myocardial blood flow, with decreasing pyrophosphate activity in regions of maximal blood flow reduction.[K18] Furthermore, the regions of myocardial necrosis delineated by antimyosin imaging were observed to be smaller than those delineated by pyrophosphate.[K18] Although there is a good correlation between infarct sizes determined by ^{111}In antimyosin and ^{99m}Tc pyrophosphate (Fig. 62–8), mean pyrophosphate infarct size was approximately 1.5 times larger than mean antimyosin infarct size in dogs with reperfused infarction injected simultaneously with a mixture of the two infarct-avid imaging agents. On the other hand, antimyosin infarct size was not significantly different from histochemical infarct size obtained with triphenyltetrazolium chloride from the same animals. Pyrophosphate infarct size was significantly larger than the triphenyltetrazolium chloride infarct size ($P < 0.01$). Thus, it appears that antimyosin imaging results in delineation of the extent of myocardial necrosis, whereas pyrophosphate may also delineate myocardium that is severely ischemic but that may be reversed.[K18]

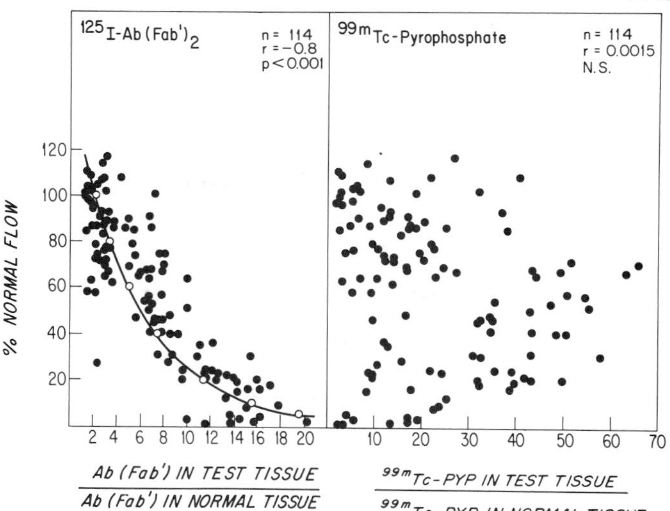

Figure 62–7. The relation of ^{125}I antimyosin $(Fab')_2$ uptake and ^{99m}Tc pyrophosphate uptake to regional blood flow in canine infarcts. Regional flow was determined by the radioactive microsphere technique. ^{125}I antimyosin $(Fab')_2$ and ^{99m}Tc pyrophosphate were administered to the same animal, and the uptake of all three compounds was determined in tissue samples. There is an inverse exponential relation between antimyosin uptake and blood flow. No simple relationship is seen for pyrophosphate uptake in comparison with blood flow. (From Beller, G. A., et al.: Localization of radiolabeled cardiac myosin-specific antibody in myocardial infarcts: Comparison with technetium-99m stannous pyrophosphate. Circulation 55:74, 1977, by permission of the American Heart Association, Inc.)

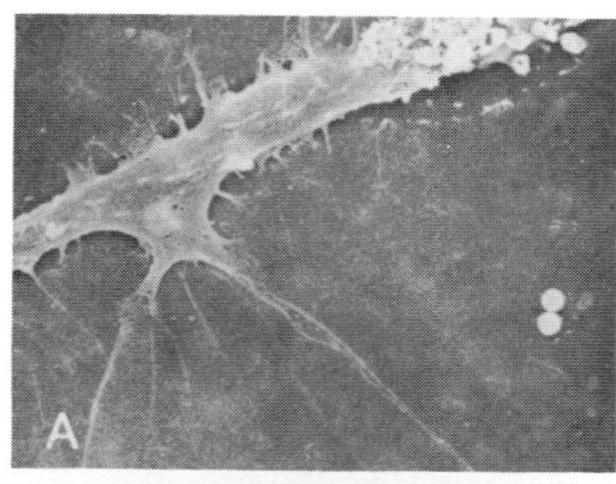

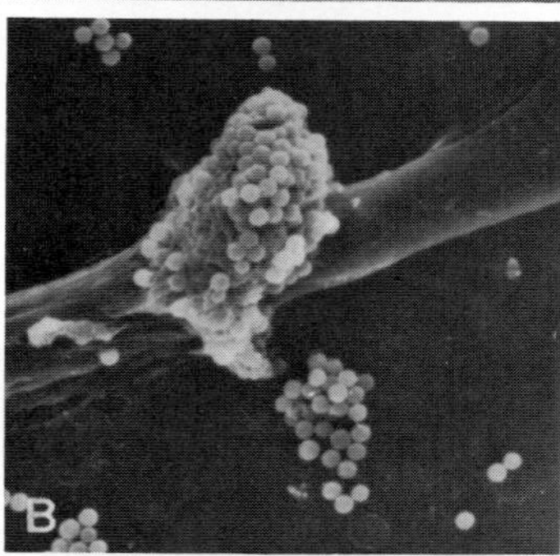

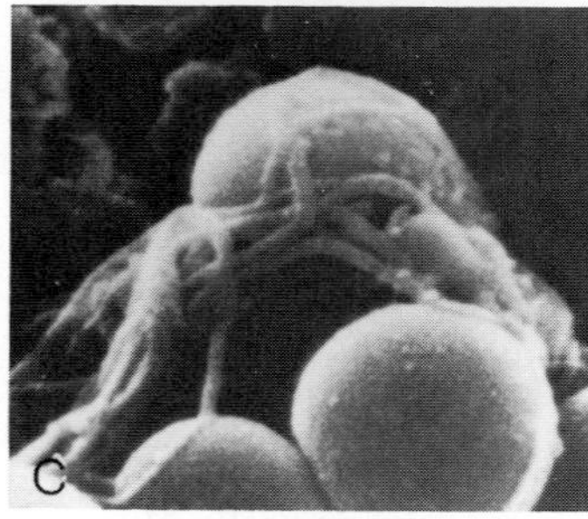

Figure 62–6. Scanning electron micrographs show localization of antimyosin beads (1 μ diameter) in *(A)* normal myocytes, *(B)* necrotic myocytes, and *(C)* a necrotic region demonstrating sarcolemmal disruption and binding of antimyosin beads to the myofibrils that are now exposed (magnification × 100,000). Normal myocytes do not accumulate antimyosin beads *(A)*. (From Khaw, B. A., et al.: Myocardial injury quantitation by cell sorting initiated with antimyosin fluorescent spheres. Science 217:1050, 1982, with permission of the American Association for the Advancement of Science. Copyright 1982 by the AAAS.)

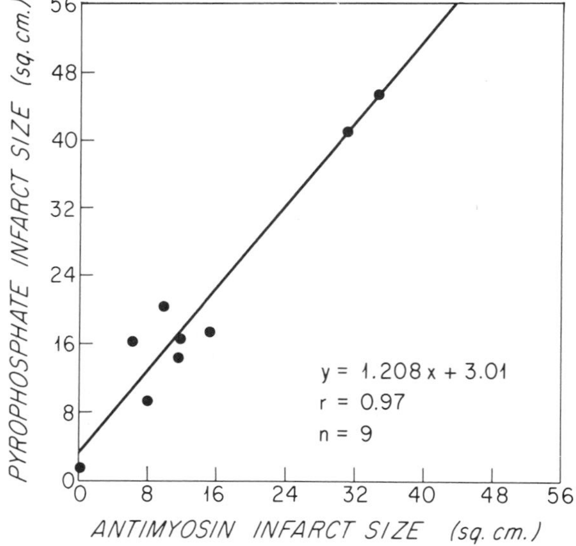

Figure 62–8. Comparison of ^{99m}Tc pyrophosphate infarct size versus ^{111}In antimyosin–delineated infarction in nine canine experimental infarcts. Linear correlation is observed. Antimyosin infarct size, however, is consistently smaller than that calculated from pyrophosphate images.

Cardiac Allograft Rejection

The technique of heterotopic cardiac allograft transplantation has been used to study the usefulness of antimyosin imaging in detecting acute and chronic allograft rejection. Unlike myocardial infarction, allograft rejection is characterized by white blood cell infiltration and patchy myocyte necrosis. In this laboratory, heterotopic cardiac transplantation was performed using B10D2 donor to B6AF1 mice as recipients for allograft rejection studies.[I1] These were compared with isograft controls. In these studies, a monoclonal antimyosin, 2G42D7, that has no isomyosin (V1 or V3) specificity and reacts with all cardiac myosin was used. Since the V1 isomyosin is the predominant isoenzyme form in adult murine myocardium, antimyosin R11D10, which is specific for the V3 isomyosin, cannot be used efficiently to image myocardial necrosis due to murine heart transplant rejection. All animals with allograft rejection showed significant localization of radiolabeled antimyosin in the allografts relative to either the autologous grafts or isografts. Histologic examination of all allografts confirmed the presence of acute rejection, as evidenced by myocyte necrosis and white blood cell infiltration.[I1] This technique has also been used successfully in dogs. Addonizio and coworkers used intrathoracic heterotopic heart allografts in a canine model to demonstrate the utility of antimyosin for diagnosis of acute heart transplant rejection.[A1] Animals were divided into two groups as follows: (1) animals allowed to undergo rejection without treatment, and (2) animals treated with cyclosporine. ^{111}In antimyosin was administered and both planar and single-photon emission computed tomography (SPECT) images were obtained. Uptake of ^{111}In antimyosin in transplanted hearts of dogs not undergoing treatment for rejection was striking. The autologous hearts did not show antimyosin localization. In the second group of animals treated with cyclosporine showing no clinical evidence of rejection, ^{111}In antimyosin localization in transplanted hearts was not observed. Histopathologic examinations confirmed no myocyte necrosis or other evidence of rejection. When immunosuppressive therapy was withdrawn and the animals were allowed to undergo acute rejection, antimyosin scans became positive, thus correlating with the extent of histopathologic rejection. The authors concluded that ^{111}In-labeled antimyosin was useful in the noninvasive diagnosis of transplant rejection.[A1]

Myocarditis

Similar to acute heart transplant rejection, myocarditis is also a disease characterized by the inflammatory response of white blood cell infiltration and myocyte necrosis. A definitive diagnosis of this disease can be made only by histopathologic examination, and it is difficult to diagnose noninvasively. Several good animal models of myocarditis are presently available. The most studied has been the coxsackievirus-induced myocarditis in genetically predisposed mice.[L3] The usefulness of antimyosin imaging in myocarditis was tested in the coxsackievirus B3 murine myocarditis model.[R1] Administration of ^{125}I-labeled 2G42D7 Fab in infected mice, followed by microautoradiography of excised hearts, demonstrated specific localization of antimyosin in necrotic myocytes. This technique was applied to an autoimmune myocarditis model developed by immunizing inbred CD rats with rat heart homogenates. Histologically, this model reveals focal myocyte necrosis and white cell infiltrates characteristic of myocarditis. Imaging of these rats with ^{111}In-labeled 2G42D7 Fab revealed diffuse unequivocal uptake of antimyosin throughout the myocardium.[K25]

Thus, it appears that antimyosin imaging can be used to visualize myocardial necrosis associated with acute experimental myocardial infarcts, heterotopic heart transplant rejection, and experimental acute myocarditis.

ANTIMYOSIN IMAGING IN HUMANS

Myocardial Infarction

Although detailed experimental studies have shown the usefulness of antimyosin for localization and visualization of acute myocardial infarction, the clinical experience of using antimyosin in the evaluation of acute myocardial infarction is limited at the present time. In the initial clinical trial conducted by Khaw and colleagues, 30 patients with definite electrocardiographic and enzymatic evidence of myocardial infarction received 500 μg of

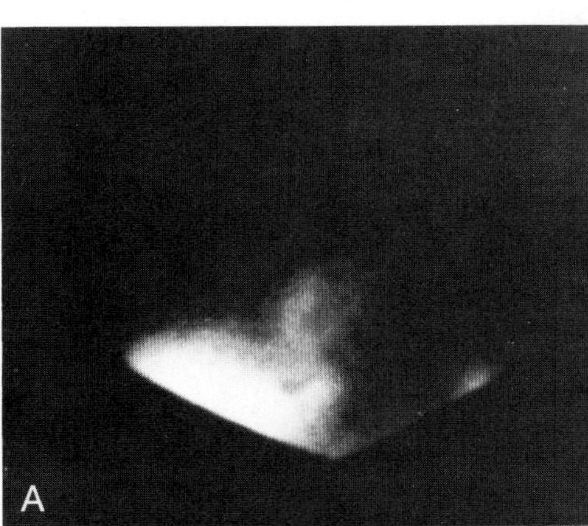

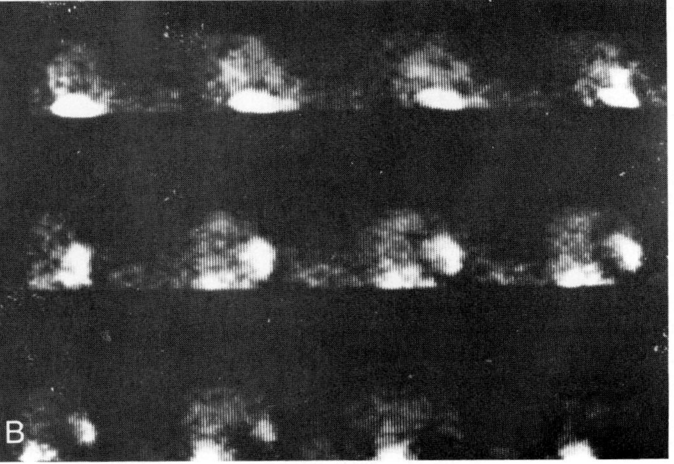

Figure 62–9. *A*, Left anterior oblique gamma scintigraph and *(B)* sagittal tomograms from single-photon emission computed tomography (SPECT) of a patient with an acute myocardial infarction imaged with ^{99m}Tc antimyosin Fab 18 hours after intravenous administration. Both infarct activity and hepatic activity (lower central) can be clearly separated. (From Khaw, B. A., et al.: Scintigraphic quantification of myocardial necrosis in patients after intravenous injection of myosin-specific antibody. Circulation 74:501, 1986, by permission of the American Heart Association, Inc.)

antimyosin Fab labeled with 15 to 25 millicuries of ^{99m}Tc within 24 hours of admission.[K19] All patients underwent planar imaging using standard anterior and 45-degree left anterior oblique views. Sixteen patients also underwent SPECT prior to planar imaging. Planar images were acquired at an average of 18 hours after intravenous antibody administration, and SPECT images were acquired at an average of 15 hours following antimyosin injection. The results of antimyosin imaging were compared with both planar ($n = 23$) and SPECT ($n = 12$) ^{99m}Tc stannous pyrophosphate images obtained 4 hours after injection on the third day of admission. All patients underwent cardiac catheterization and left ventriculography 10 to 14 days following admission. The results of imaging with both agents were compared with peak creatine kinase, creatine kinase-MB, ECG, and catheterization data. Planar imaging showed discrete antimyosin localization in 19 of 19 patients (100 percent) with anterior infarction and 7 of 11 patients (64 percent) with inferior infarction (overall 87 percent). Discrete antimyosin uptake was seen as early as 7 hours and was optimally visualized at 18 hours following antibody injection. Antimyosin infarct location corresponded to electrocardiographic infarct location in all but two cases. SPECT images were positive in all patients with anterior infarction and four of six patients with inferior infarction. Of the two patients with negative findings, one had no angiographic hypokinetic segment and had undergone reperfusion following streptokinase therapy. The combined sensitivity of SPECT and planar antimyosin imaging was 90 percent in this group of patients. Figure 62–9 shows that SPECT delineates the infarct margins in the myocardium more sharply than does planar imaging. Both are clearly positive, however. In comparison, ^{99m}Tc pyrophosphate planar images were positive in all patients with anterior infarction and in seven of nine (78 percent) with inferior infarction. Images were positive in two of three patients with negative findings on planar antimyosin scans and negative in one patient with positive findings on an antimyosin scan. Overall, the sensitivity of ^{99m}Tc pyrophosphate in this group of patients was 91 percent. Twelve of sixteen patients undergoing antimyosin SPECT also underwent pyrophosphate SPECT. Infarct weights calculated from antimyosin and pyrophosphate SPECT differed. Mean infarct weight was 29.2 g ± 28 for antimyosin and 56.5 g ± 52 for pyrophosphate. Pyrophosphate SPECT images were consistently larger than corresponding antimyosin SPECT images by a factor of 1.7 in the same patients. When compared with angiographically determined lengths of hypokinetic segments, SPECT infarct weight in grams was linearly related to both antimyosin ($r = 0.787$) and pyrophosphate ($r = 0.793$) infarct sizes (Fig. 62–10). The slope of the antimyosin SPECT infarct size was approximately half that of the SPECT pyrophosphate infarct size. This difference could not be attributed to differences in target-to-background ratios or to the timing of injections and imaging with the various agents.

In a more recent publication, a newer radiolabeling technique utilizing a transchelation method was used to label ^{111}In to DTPA-antimyosin Fab. This resulted in higher target-to-background ratios and less liver activity. In this study, 54 patients with documented acute myocardial infarction were studied.[K15] All patients received approximately 1.8 mCi of ^{111}In-labeled R11D10 Fab intravenously. Imaging was performed usually 24 hours following antibody injection in the standard anterior and left anterior oblique views. Image analysis was conducted by two observers who were blinded to patient identity and clinical course. Antimyosin images were positive in 52 of 54 patients (96 percent). Of the two patients with negative scans, one underwent reperfusion in association with thrombolytic therapy. The second patient had a small inferior infarction. Although the patient also underwent thrombolytic therapy, recanalization was not evident.

Patterns of antimyosin uptake differ from patient to patient and fall broadly into two categories. The first pattern is shown in Figure 62–11. It is characterized by intense homogeneous uptake of antimyosin with discrete localization in the myocardium. Human postmortem pathologic data are incomplete at this time. However, the same pattern is observed in canine infarction corresponding to homogeneous transmural infarction. The second

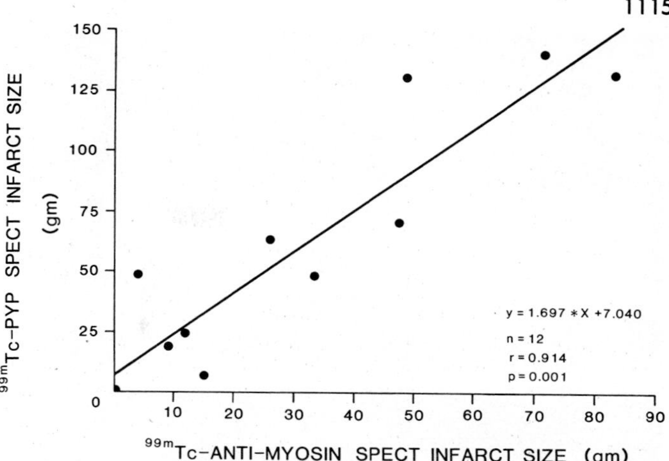

Figure 62–10. The relationship between infarct size calculated in grams using ^{99m}Tc-PYP and ^{99m}Tc-antimyosin SPECT imaging in 12 patients with acute myocardial infarction. Linear correlation is again observed between antimyosin- and pyrophosphate-delineated infarct size. In humans, antimyosin infarct size is again observed to be smaller, confirming previous experimental observations in animals. (From Khaw, B. A., et al.: Scintigraphic quantification of myocardial necrosis in patients after intravenous injection of myosin-specific antibody. Circulation 74:501, 1986, by permission of the American Heart Association, Inc.)

pattern seen in infarction is that of diffuse low intensity uptake shown in Figure 62–12. This pattern corresponds to patchy or subendocardial necrosis. We believe that the pathologic correlates of these patterns are the same in humans. However, definitive evidence is not currently available.

Cardiac Allograft Rejection

The encouraging work in experimental cardiac allograft transplant rejection imaging has been confirmed and extended to humans. Frist and coworkers[F2] reported on the use of ^{111}In antimyosin Fab to diagnose rejection in 18 cardiac transplant patients up to 3215 days following transplantation. All patients underwent routine or emergency right ventricular biopsy, and antimyosin scans were performed either at that time or within 24 hours of biopsy. Histologic evaluation of the three to five biopsy samples obtained from each patient was performed by a pathologist who was blinded to the scintigraphic results. A total of 20 studies were performed in 18 patients. Eight of the 20 studies had biopsy-documented rejection and positive antimyosin scans. Another eight patients had negative biopsies and negative antimyosin scans. Two patients had positive biopsies with negative scans and two patients had positive scans with negative biopsies. The sensitivity and specificity of the antimyosin scan were both determined to be 80 percent. The overall accuracy of 80 percent in the detection of transplant rejection by this noninvasive technique was encouraging (Fig. 62–13). All time points showed baseline cardiac activity at 48 hours after intravenous administration. However, antimyosin localization increased dramatically with acute rejection.

Endomyocardial biopsy allows the evaluation of only a small portion of the ventricle, whereas antimyosin scanning allows the examination of the uptake of radionuclide throughout the whole myocardium wherever there is myocyte necrosis. Degrees of transplant rejection, on the other hand, fall within a spectrum from mild lymphocytic infiltration without myocyte necrosis to full-blown myocyte necrosis with exudate formation, to healing rejection. Although the biopsy is the current gold standard, it is of interest to discuss those patients who had false-negative and false-positive results in the above-mentioned study.

In the first patient with a false-positive scan, acute rejection had been diagnosed 15 days earlier and treatment had been instituted. The biopsy demonstrated resolved rejection. In the

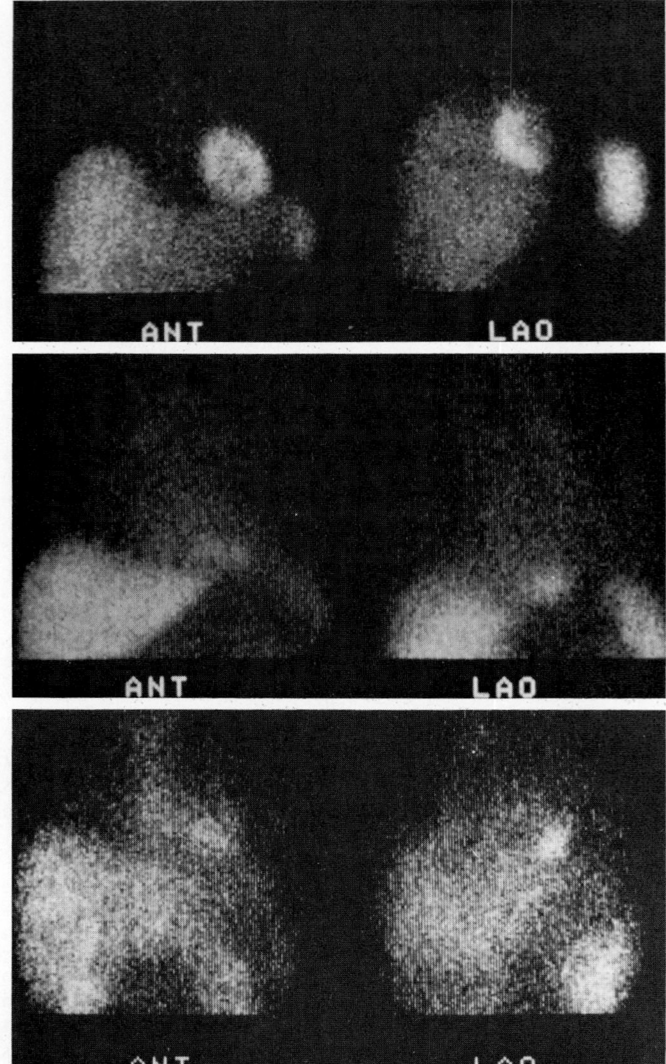

Figure 62–11. Gamma scintigraphic patterns of ^{111}In-labeled antimyosin uptake. The upper panel represents the pattern of discrete antimyosin uptake seen in a patient with an acute anterior infarction. The anterior and left anterior oblique views show striking uptake at the apex and in the anterior wall of the left ventricle. The middle panel was obtained from a patient with an acute inferior infarction. Discrete uptake in the inferior wall of the ventricle is seen just above the left lobe of the liver. The lower panel is from a patient with an acute posterior infarction. Again, discrete uptake of antimyosin is seen above the diaphragm. (From Khaw, B. A., et al.: Diagnosis of acute myocarditis with radiolabeled monoclonal antimyosin antibody: immunoscintigraphic evaluation. *In* Schultheiss, H.-P. (ed.): New Concepts in Viral Heart Disease. Springer-Verlag, Berlin, Heidelberg, 1988, pp. 363–373. Reprinted by permission.)

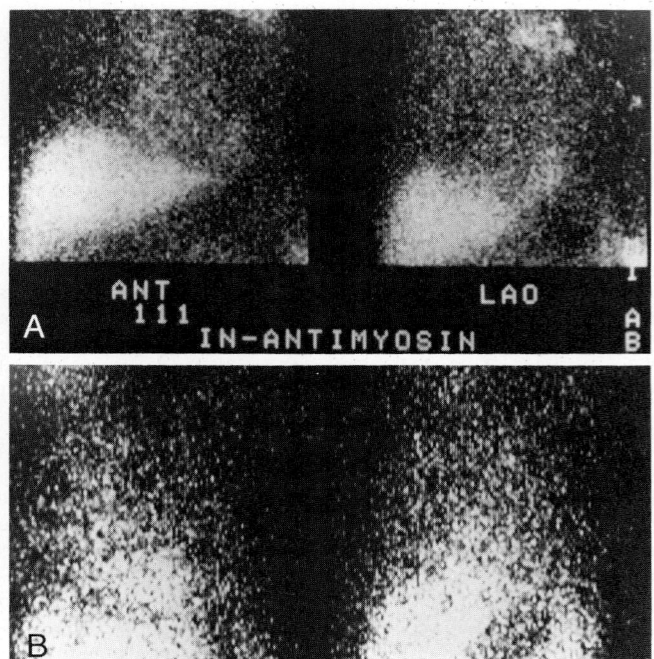

Figure 62–12. Diffused ^{111}In antimyosin uptake in patients with *(A)* inferior myocardial infarction and *(B)* anterior myocardial infarction, which may represent subendocardial or patchy necrosis following successful thrombolysis therapy.

second patient with a false-positive scan, a diagnosis of mild acute rejection had been made by biopsy 21 days prior to antimyosin injection. This patient had not been treated because of the high incidence of spontaneous remission and the biopsy taken at the time of the scan showed healed rejection. It is conceivable then that areas sampled by the biopsy may not have included the area of myocardium containing necrosis. At the present time, we believe that these results warrant further investigation on a larger scale.

Myocarditis

Like cardiac allograft rejection, the diagnosis of myocarditis can be difficult based on clinical grounds. Biopsy evidence of

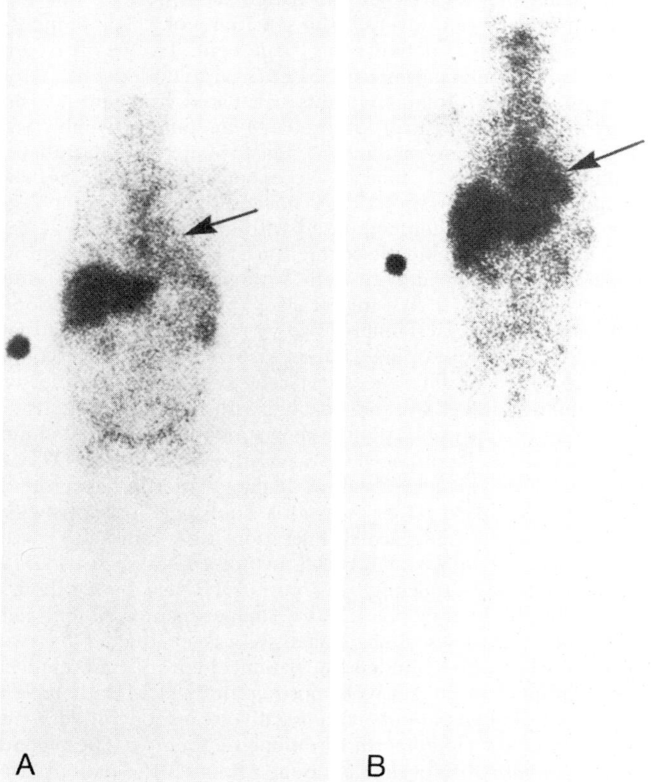

Figure 62–13. Anterior whole body gamma scintigraphs of two patients with cardiac transplants. *Panel A* shows a negative scan. Uptake of antimyosin is seen in the liver and kidneys, and minimal uptake is seen in the region of the heart *(arrow)*. *Panel B* is of a patient in whom rejection was confirmed by biopsy. Global intense uptake of antimyosin is seen, indicating myocyte necrosis. (From Frist W., et al.: Noninvasive detection of human cardiac transplant rejection with indium-111 antimyosin (Fab) imaging. Circulation 76:V81, 1987, by permission of the American Heart Association, Inc.)

white cell infiltration and myocyte necrosis is again the gold standard of diagnosis. Antimyosin imaging was used to study 28 patients at this institution who presented with histories and clinical findings suggestive of myocarditis.[Y1] All patients underwent right and left heart catheterization, right ventricular endomyocardial biopsy, and imaging with ^{111}In antimyosin Fab. All patients had normal coronary arteries angiographically. Twenty-five of these patients presented with global left ventricular dysfunction (LVEF 27 ± 2). The others presented with chest pain, pericardial effusion, or both. All patients underwent right ventricular biopsy, and three to six samples were taken. The results of the biopsy were then compared with ^{111}In antimyosin Fab imaging performed within 24 to 48 hours of biopsy using our standard anterior and 45-degree left anterior oblique views (Fig. 62–14). In these patients, right ventricular biopsy was diagnostic for myocarditis in 9 (32 percent), showed nonspecific changes in 13 (47 percent), and were normal in 6 (21 percent). In contrast, antimyosin images were positive in 17 patients (61 percent) and negative in 11 (39 percent). In all patients with uptake of ^{111}In antimyosin, the pattern of uptake was global, with a few patients showing focal uptake within the left ventricle. All of the patients with biopsy-positive myocarditis had positive scans yielding a sensitivity of 100 percent. Eight patients, however, had positive scans with no evidence of myocarditis on biopsy. Five of these patients were classified as normal on biopsy, and three had nonspecific changes consisting of varying degrees of interstitial fibrosis and myocyte hypertrophy without inflammation. All had depressed left ventricular function. Interestingly, in four of the false positive scan patients, left ventricular dysfunction improved spontaneously. The results could again be attributed to the diffuse nature of myocarditis and the difficulty in obtaining representative biopsy samples containing the necrotic myocardium showing white cell infiltration. Three patients in the same study who had negative biopsies and negative antimyosin scans also showed spontaneous improvement in left ventricular function. The reason for this cannot be explained at the present time.

In spite of this, antimyosin correctly identified all patients with biopsy-proven myocarditis. Although the patient number was small, none of the patients with negative scans (Fig. 62–15) were subsequently shown to have myocarditis. Thus, by these methods a negative scan may negate the need for biopsy. All patients with positive scans, however, should be biopsied to achieve a histopathologic diagnosis.

Adverse Reactions to Antimyosin

The antibodies presently used for antimyosin imaging are purified murine monoclonal antibodies of the IgG2a subclass. Injection of up to 500 μg of Fab are routinely given in human studies. These xeno-antibodies may be immunogenic. To date, injection of the monoclonal antimyosin Fab into humans has not resulted in any adverse effects. Many patients have received multiple injections of antimyosin over the course of myocarditis and transplant follow-up. We examined the sera of myocarditis patients with up to two administrations of antimyosin Fab for the presence of human anti-murine antibodies.[N1] To date, no anti-murine antibody response has been detected in these patients. Although skin testing prior to antimyosin administration is recommended to assess whether or not an immediate type hypersensitivity reaction is elicited as a contraindication, the test itself may increase the possibility of hypersensitization and of eliciting an immune response to the murine monoclonal antibody. Therefore, many centers involved in the clinical trials with antimyosin have elected to forgo the skin test. On the other hand, we routinely test patients who have undergone previous antimyosin imaging for the presence of anti-murine IgG antibodies prior to injection.

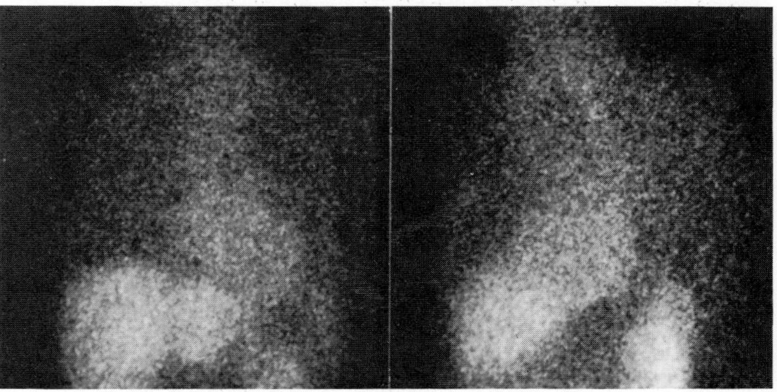

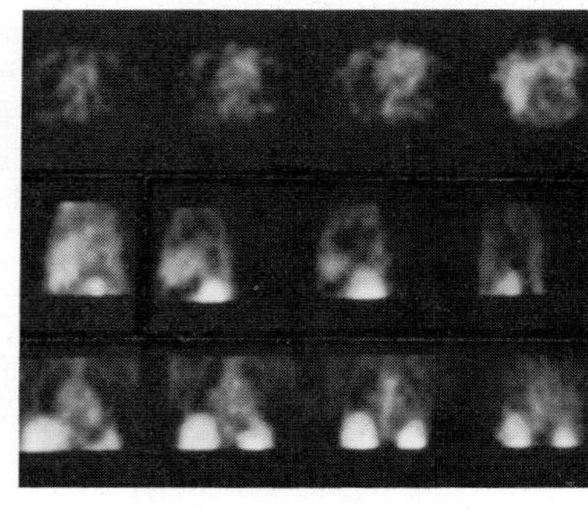

Figure 62–14. The upper panels are anterior and left anterior oblique gamma scintigraphs from a patient with biopsy-proven myocarditis. Diffuse global uptake is seen in the heart, indicating diffuse necrosis. The lower panels are transverse (cephalocaudad), sagittal, and coronal sections taken from the same patient. Uptake of antimyosin is again seen in more detail in the area of the heart. (From Khaw, B. A., et al.: Diagnosis of acute myocarditis with radiolabeled monoclonal antimyosin antibody: immunoscintigraphic evaluation. *In* Schultheiss, H.-P. (ed.): New Concepts in Viral Heart Disease. Springer-Verlag, Berlin, Heidelberg, 1988, pp. 363–373. Reprinted with permission.)

MYOCARDITIS
(NEGATIVE)

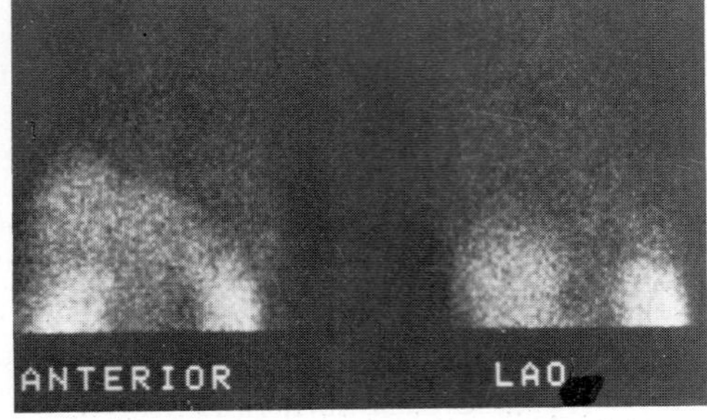

TRANSVERSE

SAGITTAL

CORONAL

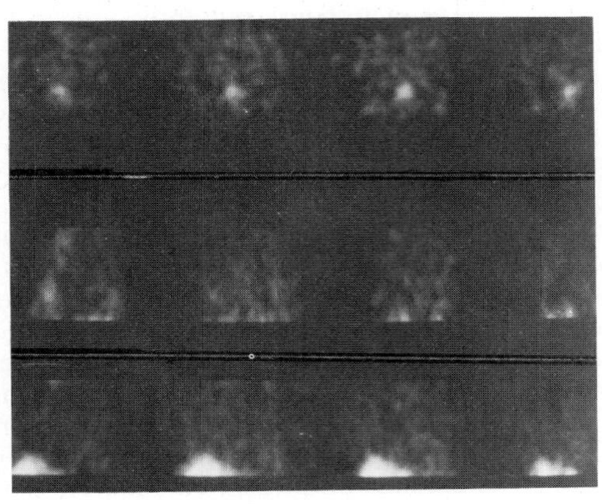

Figure 62–15. The upper panels are anterior and left anterior oblique (LAO) scintigraphs obtained from a patient suspected of having myocarditis and given ^{111}In-antimyosin Fab. Biopsies were negative for myocarditis, and antimyosin uptake was not seen in the region of the heart. Tomographic reconstructions also show cardiac activity in the transverse, sagittal, and coronal sections. (From Khaw, B. A., et al.: Diagnosis of acute myocarditis with radiolabeled monoclonal antimyosin antibody: immunoscintigraphic evaluation. *In* Schultheiss, H.-P. (ed.): New Concepts in Viral Heart Disease. Springer-Verlag, Berlin, Heidelberg, 1988, pp. 363–373. Reprinted with permission.)

ANTIBODY IMAGING OF BLOOD CLOTS

Antifibrin Imaging

The first use of antibody imaging of blood clots took place in 1966 when Spar and associates used ^{131}I-labeled antisera to human fibrinogen.[S4] The resolution of the technique was poor, however, because of a low signal-to-background ratio due to cross-reactivity of the antisera to both clots and circulating fibrinogen. The development of antibodies specific for fibrin but not fibrinogen had generated renewed interest in antibody-directed imaging of thrombi in vivo. Two approaches to the generation of these antibodies have been successful. In 1983, Hui and coworkers described the properties of a fibrin-specific murine monoclonal antibody designated 59D8.[H2] This antibody was generated by immunization of mice with the N-terminal heptapeptide sequence of the beta chain of human fibrin. Antibody 59D8 is fibrin-specific and also binds to native blood clots in vivo. It appears to recognize the same epitope as the antibody T2G1S. The latter antibody was generated using the thrombin-treated N-terminal disulfide knot region of fibrinogen.[K24] Another approach is to use whole blood clots or cross-linked fibrin to induce fibrin-specific antibodies. This approach has also been successful.

Antibody labeling with ^{123}I, ^{125}I, ^{111}In, and ^{99m}Tc is performed, and the labeled antibody is separated as described earlier for antimyosin antibodies. As with antimyosin, whole antibodies or fragments can be labeled equally well.

To date, few data are available on the use of antifibrin antibodies for imaging blood clots in humans. Experimental data have been generated using either rabbit models employing jugular vein ligation and thrombin-induced clot formation, or dog models of pulmonary embolism with femoral vein clots.

The rabbit jugular vein model has demonstrated the binding of antifibrin antibodies in vivo and the ability to image these antibodies using ^{123}I- and ^{99m}Tc-labeled whole antibody.[F1, P4, L2] Rosebrough used ^{131}I-labeled monoclonal antifibrin (T2G1s) to image thrombi generated in canine femoral veins by copper coils.[R1, R2] Knight has investigated the use of an ^{111}In-labeled DTPA-Fab conjugate of the 59D8 antibody in rabbits and dogs.[K23] He has demonstrated faster blood clearance with this fragment as well as higher target-to-background ratios when peripheral thrombi are imaged at 24 hours. Our own experience is with the 59D8 antibody developed at this institution. Using dog models of femoral vein, foreleg thrombi, and pulmonary embolus, we have been able to visualize clots using ^{111}In DTPA $(Fab')_2$ antifibrin.[S4] At our institution, the use of this antibody for detection of peripheral vein thrombosis in dogs has a sensitivity of 100 percent. Interestingly, the presence of heparin appears to markedly decrease the uptake of the antibody by clots. The sensitivity of the technique dropped to 40 percent in the presence of heparin. Although we were successful in imaging pulmonary emboli in these same dogs, the sensitivity of the technique was poor (41 percent) and decreased dramatically in the presence of heparin (13 percent). At the moment, it appears that the technique may be useful in visualizing peripheral thrombi. However, more data are needed in this area.

Initial clinical trials involving small groups of patients have been undertaken to determine the usefulness of the technique. Gupta and colleagues have reported their results using ^{111}In-labeled 59D8 Fab in 18 patients. In this comparison with venography, antifibrin imaging correctly identified 19 of 20 thrombus sites.[G1]

Radiolabeled antimyosin imaging is highly specific for the localization and visualization of myocardial necrosis associated with acute myocardial infarction, heart transplant rejection, and acute myocarditis. It is a noninvasive technique with a high sensitivity and specificity. To date, it appears to have no adverse effects on patients even after repeated administrations of the radiolabeled antimyosin Fab. As a clinical tool, the major contribution of antimyosin imaging may lie in the diagnosis of acute myocarditis, cardiac transplant rejection, and equivocal infarction. Furthermore, in this era of aggressive thrombolytic interventions, antimyosin imaging techniques may provide invaluable information in the immediate assessment of myocardial salvage.

Antifibrin imaging, though currently less refined, demonstrates promise particularly in the area of peripheral clot detection. Its usefulness in the detection of pulmonary emboli and coronary thrombosis in humans remains to be established.

References

A

1. Addonizio, L.J., Michler, R.E., Marboe, C., et al.: Imaging of cardiac allograft rejection in dogs using indium 111 monoclonal antimyosin Fab. J. Am. Coll. Cardiol. 9:555, 1987.

B

1. Beller, G.A., Khaw, B.A., Haber, E., and Smith, T.W.: Localization of radiolabeled cardiac myosin–specific antibody in myocardial infarcts: Comparison with technetium-99m stannous pyrophosphate. Circulation 55:74, 1977.

C

1. Childs, R.L., and Hnatowich, D.J.: Optimum conditions for labeling of DTPA-coupled antibodies with technetium-99m. J. Nucl. Med. 26:293, 1985.

E

1. Edelman, G.M., and Marchalonis, J.J.: Preparation of antigens and antibodies. *In* Williams, C. A., and Chase, M. W. (eds.): Methods in Immunology and Immunochemistry. Vol. 1. Academic Press, New York, 1968, pp. 422–423.

F

1. Feitsma, R.I.J., Block, D., Wasser, M.N.J.M., et al.: A new method for ^{99m}Tc-labeling of proteins with an application to clot detection with an antifibrin monoclonal antibody. Nucl. Med. Commun. 8:771, 1987.
2. Frist, W., Yasuda, T., Segall, G., et al.: Noninvasive detection of human cardiac transplant rejection with indium-111 antimyosin (Fab) imaging. Circulation 76 (Suppl. V):V81, 1987.

G

1. Gupta, N., Alavi, A., Palevski, H., et al.: The detection of deep venous thrombi using indium-111 antifibrin monoclonal antibody. (Abstract.) J. Nucl. Med. 28:1930, 1987.

H

1. Hunter, W.M., and Greenwood, F.C.: Preparation of iodine-131 labelled human growth hormone of high specific activity. Nature (London) 194:495, 1962.
2. Hui, K.Y., Haber, E., and Matsueda, G.R.: Monoclonal antibodies to a synthetic fibrin-like peptide bind to human fibrin but not fibrinogen. Science 222:1129, 1983.

I

1. Isobe, M., Nossiff, N.D., and Chase, C.: Early detection with indium-111 monoclonal antimyosin imaging of cardiac rejection in heterotopic heart transplantation in mice. (Abstract.) J. Nucl. Med. 29:746, 1988.

K

1. Khaw, B.A., Beller, G.A., Haber, E., and Smith, T.W.: Localization of cardiac myosin-specific antibody in myocardial infarction. J. Clin. Invest. 58:439, 1976.
2. Khaw, B.A., Beller, G.A., and Haber, E.: Experimental myocardial infarct imaging following intravenous administration of iodine-131 labeled antibody (Fab′)2 fragments specific for cardiac myosin. Circulation 57:743, 1978.
3. Khaw, B.A., Gold, H.K., Leinbach, R.C., et al.: Early imaging of experimental myocardial infarction by intracoronary adminstration of ^{131}I-labeled anticardiac myosin (Fab′)2 fragments. Circulation 58:1137, 1978.
4. Khaw, B.A., Fallon, J.T., Katus, H., et al.: Positron imaging of experimental myocardial infarction with ^{68}Ga-DTPA-antimyosin antibody. (Abstract.) Circulation 59–60 (Suppl. II):II–135, 1979.
5. Khaw, B.A., Fallon, J.T., Strauss, H.W., and Haber, E.: Myocardial infarct imaging of antibodies to canine cardiac myosin with indium-111-diethylenetriamine penta-acetic acid. Science 209:295, 1980.
6. Khaw, B.A., and Haber, E.: Radioimmunochemical imaging of myocardial infarction: Utilization of anticardiac myosin antibodies. *In* Burchiel, S.W., Rhodes, B.A., and Friedman, B. (eds.): Tumor Imaging: The Radioimmunochemical Detection of Cancer. Masson Publishing, New York, 1982, pp. 189–198.
7. Khaw, B.A., Scott, J., Fallon, J.T., et al.: Myocardial injury: Quantitation by cell sorting initiated with antimyosin fluorescent spheres. Science 217:1050, 1982.
8. Khaw, B.A., Strauss, H.W., and Carvalho, A.: Technetium-99m labeling of antibodies to cardiac myosin Fab and to human fibrinogen. J. Nucl. Med. 23:1011, 1982.
9. Khaw, B.A., Homcy, C.H., Fallon, J.T., et al.: Irreversible ischemic injury in anoxic cultured myocytes: Demonstration by cell sorting with antimyosin fluorescent beads and scanning electron microscopy. *In* Chazov, E.I., Smirnov, V.N., and Oganov, R.G. (eds.): Cardiology. Plenum Press, New York, 1984, pp. 1135–1147.
10. Khaw, B.A., Strauss, H.W., Pohost, G.M., et al.: Relation of immediate and delayed thallium-201 distribution to localization of iodine-125 antimyosin antibody in acute experimental myocardial infarction. Am. J. Cardiol. 51:1428, 1983.
11. Khaw, B.A., Gold, H.K., Moore, R., et al.: Infarct size after reperfusion by simultaneous intracoronary In-111-monoclonal antimyosin and Tc-99m pyrophosphate; comparison by gamma scintigraphy. (Abstract.) J. Nucl. Med. 25:P69, 1984.
12. Khaw, B.A., Mattis, J.A., and Melincoff, G.: Monoclonal antibody to cardiac myosin: Imaging of experimental myocardial infarction. Hybridoma 3:11, 1984.
13. Khaw, B.A., Strauss, H.W., Cahill, S.L., et al.: Sequential imaging of indium-111–labeled monoclonal antibody in human mammary tumours hosted in nude mice. J. Nucl. Med. 25:592, 1984.
14. Khaw, B.A., Yasuda, T., Moore, R., et al.: In-111-monoclonal antimyosin and Tc-99m pyrophosphate imaging in reflowed hearts. (Abstract.) Circulation 70 (Suppl. II):II–273, 1984.
15. Khaw, B.A., Yasuda, T., Gold, H.K., et al.: Acute myocardial infarct imaging with indium-111 labeled monoclonal antimyosin Fab. J. Nucl. Med. 28:1671, 1987.
16. Krejcarek, G.E., and Tucker, K.L.: Covalent attachment of chelating groups to macromolecules. Biochem. Biophys. Res. Commun. 77:581, 1977.
17. Khaw, B.A., Fallon, J.T., Beller, G.A., and Haber, E.: Specificity of localization of myosin-specific antibody fragments in experimental myocardial infarction: Histologic, histochemical, autoradiographic, and scintigraphic studies. Circulation 60:1527, 1979.
18. Khaw, B.A., Strauss, H.W., Moore, R., et al.: Myocardial damage delineated by In-111 antimyosin Fab and Tc-99m pyrophosphate. J. Nucl. Med. 28:76, 1987.
19. Khaw, B.A., Gold, H.K., Yasuda, T., et al.: Scintigraphic quantification of myocardial necrosis in patients after intravenous injection of myosin-specific antibody. Circulation 74:501, 1986.
20. Köhler, G., and Milstein, C.: Continuous cultures of fused cells secreting antibody of predefined specificity. Nature (London) 256:495, 1975.
21. Klotz, C., Aumont, M.C., Leger, J.J., and Swynghedauw, B.: Human cardiac myosin ATPase and light subunits: A comparative study. Biochim Biophys Acta 386:461, 1975.
22. Kanke, M., Khaw, B.A., Matsueda, G., et al.: Comparison of two kinds of monoclonal antibodies to detect clots in pulmonary artery. (Abstract.) J. Nucl. Med. 27:923, 1986.
23. Knight, L.C.: Imaging thrombi with radiolabeled antifibrin monoclonal antibodies. Nucl. Med. Commun. 9:823, 1988.
24. Kudryk, B., Rohoza, A., Ahadi, M., et al.: Specificity of a monoclonal antibody for the NH_2-terminal region of fibrin. Mol. Immunol. 21:89, 1984.
25. Khaw, B.A., Yasuda, T., Palacios, I.F., et al.: Diagnosis of acute myocarditis with radiolabeled monoclonal antimyosin antibody: Immunoscintigraphic evaluation. *In* Schultheiss, H.-P. (ed.): New Concepts in Viral Heart Disease. Springer-Verlag, Berlin, Heidelberg, 1988, pp. 363–373.

L

1. Laemmli, U.K.: Cleavage of structural proteins during the assembly of the head of bacteriophage T4. Nature 227:680, 1970.
2. Liau, C.S., Haber, E., and Matsueda, G.R.: Evaluation of monoclonal antifibrin antibodies by their binding to human blood clots. Thromb. Haemost. 57:49, 1987.
3. Lerner, A.M., and Wilson, F.M.: Virus myocardiopathy. Prog. Med. Virol. 15:63, 1973.

M

1. Marchalonis, J.J.: An enzymic method for the trace iodination of immunoglobulins and other proteins. Biochem. J. 113:299, 1969.
2. Markwell, M.A.K.: A new solid-state reagent to iodinate proteins. I. Conditions for the efficient labeling of antiserum. Anal. Biochem. 125:427, 1982.
3. Moser, K.M., Guisan, M., Bartimmo, E.E., et al.: In vivo and post mortem dissolution rates of pulmonary emboli and venous thrombi in the dog. Circulation 48:170, 1973.
4. Mercadier, J.-J., Bouveret, P., Gorza, L., et al.: Myosin isoenzymes in normal and hypertrophied human. Ventricular myocardium. Circ. Res. 53:52, 1983.

N

1. Nicol, P.D., Yasuda, T., and Locke, E.: Multiple intravenous administration of In-111-labeled antimyosin Fab: Determination of antimurine Fab response in patients with myocarditis. J. Nucl. Med. 29:939,1988.

O

1. Ouchterlony, O.: Diffusion in gel methods for immunological analysis. Prog. Allergy 5:1, 1968.
2. Oster, Z.H., Srivastava, S.C., Som, P., et al.: Thrombus radioimmunoscintigraphy: An approach using monoclonal antiplatelet antibody. Proc. Natl. Acad. Sci. USA 82:3465, 1985.

P

1. Pressman, D., and Keighley, G.: The zone of activity of antibodies as determined by the use of radioactive tracers; the zone of nephrotoxic antibody serum. J. Immunol. 59:141, 1948.
2. Porter, R.R.: The hydrolysis of rabbit γ-globulin and antibodies with crystalline papain. Biochem. J. 73:119, 1959.
3. Pimm, M.V., Perkins, A.C., Armitage, N.C., and Baldwin, R.W.: The characteristics of blood-borne radiolabels and the effect of anti-mouse IgG antibodies on localization of radiolabeled monoclonal antibody in cancer patients. J. Nucl. Med. 26:1011, 1985.
4. Pauwels, E.K.J., Feitsma, R.I.J., Nieuwenhuizen, W., et al.: Imaging of thrombi with Tc-99m labeled fibrin-specific monoclonal antibody, in a rabbit model. (Abstract.) J. Nucl. Med. 27:975, 1986.

R

1. Rosebrough, S.F., Kudryk, B., Grossman, Z.D., et al.: Radioimmunoimaging of venous thrombi using iodine-131 monoclonal antibody. Radiology 156:515, 1985.
2. Rosebrough, S.F., Grossman, Z.D., McAfee, J.G., et al.: Aged venous thrombi: Radioimmunoimaging with fibrin-specific monoclonal antibody. Radiology 162:575, 1987.

S

1. Som, P., Oster, Z.H., Zamora, P.O., et al.: Radioimmunoimaging of experimental thrombi in dogs using technetium-99m-labeled monoclonal antibody fragments reactive with human platelets. J. Nucl. Med. 27:1315, 1986.
2. Soule, H.R., Linder, E., and Edington, T.S.: Membrane 126 kilodalton phosphoglycoprotein associated with human carcinomas identified by a hybridoma antibody to mammary carcinoma cells. Proc. Natl. Acad. Sci. USA 80:1332, 1983.
3. Szent-Gyögyi, A.: The preparation of myosin. *In* Szent-Gyögyi, A. The Chemistry of Muscular Contraction. Academic Press, New York, 1947.
4. Spar, I.L., Goodland, R.L., Schwartz S.I.: Detection of preformed venous thrombi in dogs by means of ^{131}I-labeled antibodies to dog fibrinogen. Circ. Res. 17:322, 1965.
5. Saito, T., Powers, J., Nossiff, N., et al.: Radioimaging of experimental thrombi in dogs using monoclonal antifibrin and antiplatelet antibodies. Effect of heparin on uptake by pulmonary emboli and venous thrombi. J. Nucl. Med. 29(5):825, 1988.

T

1. Thakur, M.L.: Gallium-67 and indium-111 radiopharmaceuticals. Int. J. Appl. Rad. Isot. 28:183, 1977. D.J. Hnatowitch, ibid, p. 169.

Chapter 63

Thrombosis Imaging with Indium-111–Labeled Platelets

JOHN R. STRATTON, M.D.

LABELING, DOSIMETRY, IMAGING, AND QUANTITATIVE METHODS 1121
Platelet-Labeling Techniques 1121
Function of Labeled Platelets—Aggregation, Recovery, Survival 1122
Radiation Dosimetry in Humans 1122
Imaging and Quantitative Techniques 1122
CARDIAC THROMBI 1124
Coronary Artery Thrombi 1124
Left Ventricular Thrombi 1124
Left Atrial Thrombi 1125
VASCULAR THROMBI 1125
Carotid Atherosclerosis 1126
Carotid Endarterectomy 1127
Arterial Aneurysms, Arterial Injury, and Peripheral Angioplasty 1127
Atherosclerosis 1128
VENOUS THROMBOSIS AND PULMONARY EMBOLISM 1128
PROSTHETIC MATERIALS 1129
Natural History of Platelet Deposition on Prosthetic Arterial Grafts 1129
Evaluation of Different Graft Materials 1129
Drug Effects on Platelet Deposition on Grafts 1130
SUMMARY AND CONCLUSIONS 1131

The central role of platelets in cardiovascular diseases has been increasingly apparent. Several lines of evidence indicate that platelets contribute to the genesis of the atherosclerotic lesion, in part by the production and release of growth factors that promote smooth cell hyperplasia. In addition, it has become increasingly clear that intra-arterial platelet-fibrin thrombus formation is the final common pathway leading to the majority of complications that ensue once an atherosclerotic lesion forms, including acute myocardial infarction, unstable angina, stroke, transient cerebral ischemia, and sudden cardiac death. Another important pathophysiologic function of platelets is the platelet thrombus formation that uniformly occurs following implantation of intravascular prosthetic materials, which are increasingly used for the construction of arterial and venous substitutes, heart valves, vascular catheters, and artificial hearts. With virtually all these prosthetic materials, thrombotic and embolic complications caused by platelet thrombus formation are an important long-term side effect. The importance of platelets in causing cardiovascular events is further indicated by the success of platelet inhibitory therapy in reducing mortality or morbidity in a variety of vascular disease states.

Given the great importance of intravascular platelet-fibrin thrombosis in causing cardiovascular diseases, finding a noninvasive in vivo method capable of diagnosing the presence and extent of intravascular thrombi would be of great clinical value. Thrombosis imaging using radionuclide techniques involves the injection of a tracer that accumulates preferentially in areas of thrombosis. Multiple approaches to thrombosis imaging are being explored, including the labeling of monoclonal antibodies directed against platelets or fibrin and the labeling of other compounds, such as tissue plasminogen activator, that also localize in areas of thrombosis (see chapter 62). To date, however, most thrombosis imaging in humans has utilized indium-111–labeled platelets. Thrombosis imaging with indium-111–labeled platelets has shown promise as a technique for studying localized thrombosis as well as for the assessment of therapies in a wide variety of human disease states. The main advantages of indium-111 platelet imaging over previously used techniques for the detection of thrombosis are that it is noninvasive, it can be performed in humans, it can be done serially to assess the effects of time or therapy, and it provides semiquantitative organ-specific information. In addition to defining the presence and location of localized thrombosis, platelet imaging also provides kinetic information regarding thrombus activity, unlike anatomic methods such as angiography or ultrasound.

Indium-111 platelet imaging has proved particularly useful as a research tool in animal studies, since an accurate measurement of the magnitude of platelet thrombus formation can be made by either external in vivo imaging or by ex vivo counting of resected specimens. This chapter, however, will focus on a discussion of platelet imaging findings in humans. In addition to the cardiovascular disorders reviewed in this chapter, platelet imaging has been utilized in humans to assess platelet survival and the sites of platelet destruction in thrombocytopenic syndromes and has been used to aid in the diagnosis of organ rejection. Indium-111 platelet labeling, imaging, and quantitative techniques will first be reviewed, followed by a discussion of findings in patients with intracardiac thrombi, arterial thrombi, venous thrombi, and intravascular prosthetic materials.

LABELING, DOSIMETRY, IMAGING, AND QUANTITATIVE METHODS

Platelet-Labeling Techniques

During indium-111 decay, two gamma rays at 173 and 247 keV are emitted that are responsible for 87 percent of the energy released. Both of these gamma rays can be detected readily by conventional gamma cameras. The 2.8-day half-life of indium-111 corresponds reasonably closely to the 4.5-day half-life of normal circulating platelets, thus allowing the assessment of the dynamics of platelet deposition over several days. Since Thakur and associates[T1] originally described the preparation of indium-111-oxine–labeled platelets in 1976, numerous additional methods of

Supported by the Medical Research Service of the Veterans Administration, by the American Heart Association—Washington Affiliate, and by N.H.L.B.I. grant HL31641.

platelet labeling have been described.* Many of these methods have been reviewed recently.[J1, M2, T2, T6] The described techniques vary widely with regard to the blood volume utilized, the chelate (oxine, tropolone, acetylacetone, mercaptopyridine-*N*-oxide), the centrifugal forces, the medium in which platelets are labeled (acid citrate dextrose, saline, plasma, Tyrode's buffer), the labeling efficiency, the duration of the procedure, and the injected dose of radioactivity. Techniques also vary as to whether the platelets are labeled in an open test tube, using a laminar flow hood to minimize airborne contamination, or in a closed blood bag system, which effectively eliminates the possibility of airborne contamination.

Several steps, however, are common to all labeling techniques. All procedures require the separation of platelets from other blood cells and plasma. Whole blood is drawn into an anticoagulant mixture, and platelet-rich plasma is separated by a "soft" (640 to 2000 g) centrifugation to yield platelet-rich plasma. A platelet pellet is then formed, washed, and resuspended in plasma or another physiologic medium, such as Ringer's citrate dextrose or a modified Tyrode's solution. Indium complexed to oxine or another chelate is then added, and the platelets are incubated for up to 30 minutes. Indium alone will not penetrate the platelet membrane because it is not lipid soluble. The labeled platelets are then typically recentrifuged, washed, and finally resuspended in autologous platelet-poor plasma. The injected dose ranges between 100 and 500 microcuries in human studies. Depending on the technique, labeling requires 30 minutes to 3.5 hours.

Once the indium-111 complex is inside the cell, the oxine or other ligand is probably displaced, with subsequent binding of the indium-111 to intracellular components almost irreversibly. Over 70 percent of the indium-111 is located in the platelet cytosol,[H6, J1] and the remainder is distributed between the alpha and dense granules and the platelet membrane. The mechanism of labeling probably involves an exchange reaction between the oxine carrier and subcellular cytosol platelet components that chelate indium-111 more strongly than oxine.[J2] The components to which indium-111 binds are not involved in the platelet release reaction, since several researchers have demonstrated that less than 5 percent of indium-111 is lost from human platelets following exposure to strong release-inducing agents, including collagen, thrombin, and adenosine diphosphate (ADP).[H1, H2, J1, J2, T3] In addition, minimal release of the indium-111 label from human platelets occurs during incubation in vitro at 37°C.[H1, J1, J2, S2, T1] Because of the long life span of labeled platelets and their relatively small mass, the estimated radiation dose to an individual platelet incubated with 1 mCi of indium-111 is 12,900 rads.[B2]

Function of Labeled Platelets—Aggregation, Recovery, Survival

Although platelets clearly undergo some mechanical, chemical, and radiation-induced trauma as a result of the labeling procedure, multiple lines of evidence suggest that minimal permanent damage is inflicted, since platelets largely retain their normal function. Several studies have demonstrated near-normal aggregation patterns of labeled platelets.[H1, H2, H6, H7, M2, S5, S6, T1, T3] Additionally, Thakur and associates reported no marked change in the ultrastructure of labeled platelets.[T3, T7]

Following injection into humans, we and others have noted that typically less than 5 to 10 percent of the indium-111 present in whole blood is "free" circulating indium-111 unattached to platelets, confirming that indium-111 appears to remain complexed to platelets in vivo. In addition, Peters and colleagues[P1] and Kotze and group[K2] have demonstrated that there is minimal elution of indium-111 once it is taken up by reticuloendothelial cells following platelet senescence. Owing to the minimal redistribution of indium-111 over time, it is well suited for quantifying sites of platelet destruction. Total body indium-111 activity remains nearly 100 percent following isotope injection, indicating minimal loss in the urine or feces.[G2, H7]

Studies of platelet recovery and platelet survival in humans offer more convincing evidence that indium-111–labeled platelets retain normal function following injection. Trauma during the labeling procedure would be expected to decrease recovery and survival, since damaged cells would be removed from the circulation rapidly. Utilizing a variety of platelet-labeling techniques, platelet recoveries with indium-111–labeled platelets have ranged between 52 and 72 percent,[G2, H1, H2, H7, K1, S7] which is similar to that found using autologous chromium-51–labeled platelets (59 ± 4 percent).[S8] Platelet survival is also a measure of the viability of labeled platelets, and several laboratories have demonstrated that indium-111 and chromium-51 survivals are similar in both normal subjects and in patients with reduced survivals.[D5, H8, P2, S9] In our laboratory, in 13 normal subjects the autologous platelet survival using indium-111 was 7.7 ± 1.5 days versus 7.6 ± 1.2 days using chromium-51; in 14 patients with a variety of thrombocytopenic disorders, survival was also similar using indium-111 and chromium-51 (3.9 ± 2.4 versus 3.9 ± 1.9 days). Heaton recently reviewed other available data comparing indium-111 and chromium-51 platelet-labeling and concluded that there was little in vivo difference in terms of either survival or recovery.[H8] Dewanjee and associates noted similar platelet survivals with indium-111-oxine–labeled, indium-111-tropolone–labeled, and chromium-51–labeled platelets; they found no difference between the two indium markers in terms of isotope distribution.[D5] Recently, the International Committee for Standardization in Hematology recommended a specific method of labeling for studies performed to calculate platelet survival.[I1]

Additional evidence that labeled platelets retain viability is the demonstration of labeled platelet uptake in areas of active thrombosis. Thus, despite clear evidence that improper labeling techniques can adversely affect labeled platelet function, multiple in vitro and in vivo tests suggest that labeled platelets can retain viability despite labeling trauma.

Radiation Dosimetry in Humans

For each 1 mCi injected, the estimated spleen dose is 25 to 33 rads, the whole body dose is 0.3 to 0.9 rad, the red marrow dose is 0.5 to 1.1 rads, the liver dose is 0.6 to 4.2 rads, the male gonad dose is 0.1 to 0.5 rad, and the ovarian dose is 0.3 to 0.7 rad.[G2, R1, V2] Because of the splenic dose, although it is well within acceptable limits, we do not perform more than one study in young normal subjects, and we limit the total injected dose to 0.33 mCi. In subjects with vascular diseases, we limit the total injected dose to 1 mCi per year. We do not study women of childbearing potential.

Imaging and Quantitative Techniques

Imaging of labeled platelets can be performed using either conventional planar techniques or single photon emission computed tomography. Owing to the relatively low count rates, simultaneous collection of both 173 and 247 keV photo peaks of indium-111 is desirable. We use a medium-energy parallel hole collimator and 15 to 20 percent energy windows. The low count rates obtained from most vascular structures necessitate relatively long imaging times (15 to 30 minutes per view). Owing to the platelet life span of approximately 8 days in the circulation, there is substantial blood pool background for several days following injection. Therefore, serial imaging over a period of 4 to 5 days is usually necessary to distinguish areas of increased uptake due to thrombosis from circulating blood pool activity. Areas of active thrombosis become more apparent on later images because of continued accumulation of labeled platelets over time, as well as a reduction in the circulating background blood pool as senescent platelets are removed from the circulation. Extended imaging clearly improves lesion detection; in one study of patients with left ventricular thrombi, only one half of the images were positive at 24 hours following injection compared with images obtained

*B1, C1, D1–4, E1, G1, H1–5, J1, K1, M1, S1–4, T2–5, V1, W1.

at 48 or 72 hours.[S10] Static and whole body scanning techniques have been recently reviewed,[B3] as have dual isotope imaging methods.[M3] Despite the low count rates, tomographic imaging of labeled platelets is feasible (Fig. 63–1) and probably improves thrombus detection as well as allowing improved quantification of platelet uptake.[S11, S12]

For planar images of the thorax and heart, we typically obtain 300,000 counts per view. For lower abdominal images that exclude the liver and spleen, we obtain images for 150,000 counts per view. For single photon emission computed tomographic imaging of labeled platelets, the patient is positioned lying supine, and 64 sequential images for 30 seconds each are obtained at 2.8-degree angular intervals over the 180 degrees centered about the region of interest. Tomographic reconstruction is performed in a transaxial projection at increments of 0.6 cm, using filtered back-projection techniques without attenuation correction.

The in vivo quantification of indium-111–labeled platelet uptake in humans has not been standardized, and many approaches have been described. Experimental studies have demonstrated that small areas of deposition, or relatively large changes induced by drugs, cannot be adequately assessed by simple visual analysis of the images,[W3] which emphasizes the need for accurate quantitative techniques. To quantify thrombus activity, localized platelet activity in a region has been compared with a noninvolved area in the same image, with simultaneously collected whole blood activity, with injected indium-111 dose, or with whole body activity. Although no quantitative methods have been validated in human studies, several techniques have been assessed in animal models. For measurement of platelet uptake in large organs like the liver and spleen, a geometric mean method has been developed by van Reenen and Heyns and colleagues,[H9, V3] in which activity in an organ is expressed as a percentage of whole body activity. In studies in baboons, the values obtained in vivo correlated closely with in vitro values. This method is relatively simple and practical, but whether it will offer similar results for smaller regions of platelet uptake remains to be determined.

A background subtraction technique has been developed by Powers and associates, Mathias and Welch, and Allen and colleagues,[A1, M3, P3] in which autologous red blood cells are labeled with technetium–99m, and estimated indium-111 counts contributed by the blood radioactivity are subtracted from an indium-111 image. This technique attempts to compensate for the fact that circulating platelet activity may obscure the detection of platelets incorporated into a thrombus. This dual-isotope technique of quantification correlated closely with in vitro well counting results in animals with prosthetic grafts (r = 0.94) and in animals with arterial thrombi.[A1, P3] A recent report compared the blood pool subtraction technique of quantification to a simpler indium excess ratio, which related counts in the region of interest to a reference region in dogs with vascular prostheses.[W2] The blood pool subtraction method had a very poor correlation to the actual gamma activity of excised grafts, whereas the simpler indium excess ratio, which does not require the injection of a second radioisotope, had a much better correlation with the in vitro results.[W2] In addition, Powers did not find that the blood pool subtraction technique improved the detection of localized platelet deposition compared with simple visual analysis alone in 28 patients.[P4] Thus, the superiority of blood pool subtraction techniques to simpler methods has not been established.

Other in vivo approaches of quantification using planar images have been described by Dewanjee and colleagues,[D6, D7] Goldman

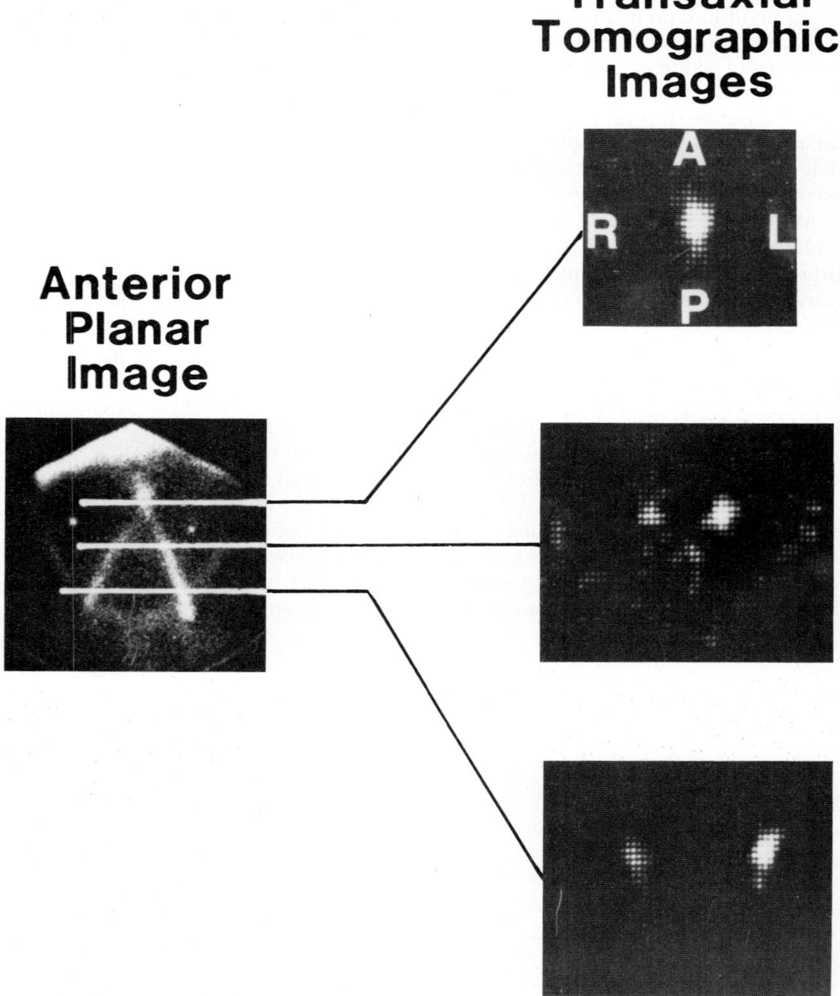

Figure 63–1. Single-photon emission tomographic images of ^{111}In platelet deposition on a Dacron aortic bifurcation graft. The transaxial tomographic images are 1.2 cm thick. The approximate level from which each tomographic image was obtained is depicted on a standard anterior planar image from the same patient on the left. Activity in the upper left of the planar image originates from the liver; the two localized white spots are anatomic markers used for patient positioning. The orientation of the tomographic images is in standard x-ray CT format. A—anterior; P—posterior; R—patient's right; L—patient's left. (From Stratton, J.R., and Ritchie, J.L.: Reduction of indium-111 platelet deposition on Dacron vascular grafts in humans by aspirin plus dipyridamole. Circulation 73:325–330, 1986, with permission.)

and colleagues,[G3, G4] Pumphrey and colleagues,[P5] and Stratton and colleagues,[S13] but without in vitro validation. In addition, we have described methods for quantifying platelet uptake on tomographic images.[S11, S12] Our findings have suggested that the quantification of platelet uptake on grafts was improved by tomographic imaging compared with standard planar imaging, since tomographic quantification was able to detect more subtle changes.[S11] Further studies that will develop and validate accurate methods of quantifying platelet uptake are needed.

CARDIAC THROMBI

(Table 63–1)

Coronary Artery Thrombi

Because of the great importance of coronary artery thrombi in causing acute myocardial infarction, unstable angina, and sudden cardiac death, a noninvasive method of detection that would also allow assessment of thrombolytic therapy would be of immense clinical importance. To date, the only clinically valid method for determining the efficacy of thrombolytic therapy has been invasive contrast angiography; a noninvasive substitute would be very helpful. In animal models of coronary artery thrombosis, labeled platelets have detected thrombi using either unprocessed images[R2] or a blood pool subtraction technique.[B4] However, old (over 24 hours) or small (11 to 17.5 g) thrombi were not detectable externally.

In humans, the evidence that coronary artery thrombi can be externally imaged has been less convincing. Although Fox and colleagues described the possible detection of coronary thrombi in nine patients using a blood pool subtraction technique, no patient had independent confirmation of thrombus, and only one thrombus was visualized on an unprocessed image.[F1] In 27 survivors of sudden cardiac death, we detected no coronary artery thrombi.[S15] In the setting of acute infarction, platelet uptake on left ventricular thrombi or platelet accumulation in reperfused infarcted areas has been documented;[L1, R3] uptake in these areas may be confused with uptake on a coronary artery thrombus and further restricts the ability to diagnose coronary artery thrombi.

Although platelet imaging has detected uptake in experimental models of endocarditis[R4] and in experimental animal models of prosthetic valve placement,[D8] detection of platelet thrombus in humans with endocarditis or with prosthetic heart valves has not been possible.[D6]

Clinical and experimental studies suggest that platelet mechanisms contribute to angioplasty failure as well as to coronary artery vein bypass graft failure. Although platelet accumulation has been demonstrated at coronary angioplasty sites in animal models, preliminary reports in humans have noted no detectable deposition.[C2, T8] Similarly, although animal studies have demonstrated that in vivo imaging of deposition in recently implanted vein grafts is possible,[D7, F2] platelet uptake in 10 patients with recent saphenous vein bypass grafts was not detectable.[D6] Thus, attempts to image platelet deposition in the coronary arteries or in vein bypass grafts in humans following infarction, angioplasty, or coronary bypass grafting have been disappointing. Some contributory factors include the poor intrinsic spatial resolution of gamma imaging systems, attenuation effects, the relatively low injected isotope dose, surrounding background activity, cardiac motion, and the small amounts of deposition that occur in the coronary vasculature.

Table 63–1. STUDIES OF CARDIAC THROMBI IN HUMANS

	References
Coronary artery thrombi	F1, S15
Left ventricular thrombi	B5, B6, E2–6, F3–5, K5, S10, S16, S18, V4
Atrial thrombi	B5, E7, K3, K6, T9
Bacterial endocarditis	D6
Percutaneous transluminal coronary angioplasty	C2
Coronary artery bypass grafts	D6
Prosthetic heart valves	D6

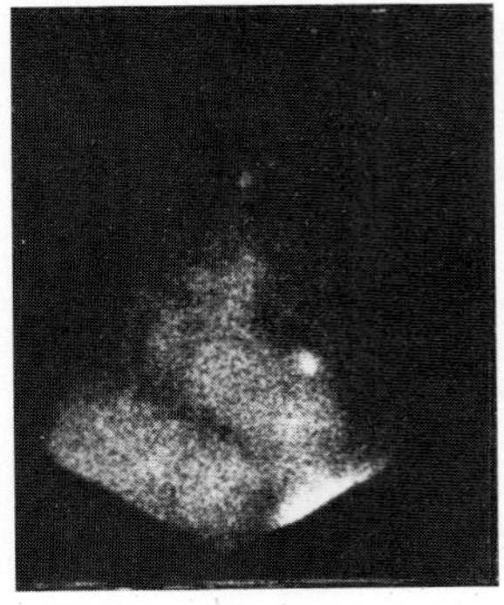

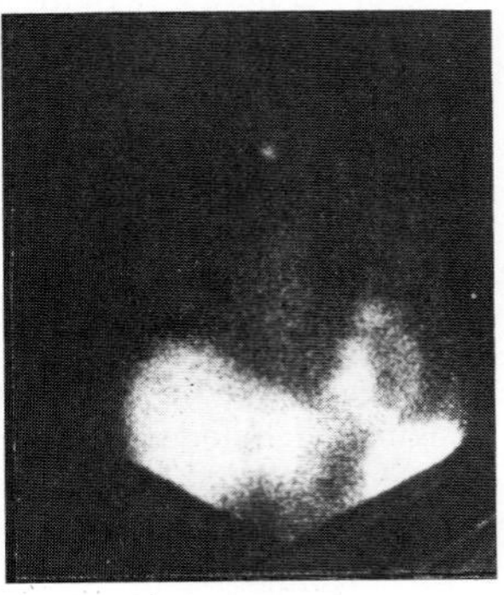

Figure 63–2. Left ventricular thrombus. ^{111}In platelet images in the anterior view obtained at 24 and 96 hours following labeled platelet injection (300,000 counts/view). On the later image, platelet uptake within the thrombus was more apparent. Improved lesion detection at later imaging times is due to continued accretion of labeled platelets onto the thrombus as well as to a reduction in circulating background blood pool activity. The liver is at the lower left and the spleen at the lower right in both images.

Left Ventricular Thrombi

Although the detection of small intracardiac thrombi is not possible, larger thrombi, such as left atrial or left ventricular thrombi, can be imaged using labeled platelets. Left ventricular thrombi occur in approximately one third of patients with either transmural anterior myocardial infarction or idiopathic congestive cardiomyopathy, and left atrial thrombi occur in approximately 10 to 20 percent of patients with atrial fibrillation. Left ventricular and left atrial thrombi are of clinical importance because they lead to embolic events. Overall, it is estimated that left ventricular or left atrial thrombi account for approximately 10 percent of all acute stroke syndromes, while other cardiac thrombotic conditions (prosthetic valves, endocarditis, and so on) account for an additional 5 percent.[S14] Thus, the detection of intracardiac thrombi may be of clinical importance, since it allows the identification of patients at risk for embolism and may permit the selection of optimal drug therapy.

Indium-111 platelet imaging can detect left ventricular thrombi in humans.[B5, E2–6, F3, K3, S10, S16, V4, V5] Positive images for left ventricular thrombi are defined as those demonstrating one or more discrete areas of intracardiac activity present on at least two views (Fig. 63–2). Obtaining late images in multiple views is important for accurate thrombus detection and localization.[E5, S10] Of the 10 patients with thrombi that we initially studied, none were positive at 2 hours after platelet injection, only five were positive at 24 hours, whereas all were positive at 48 or 72 hours after injection.[S10] Similarly, Ezekowitz and associates found that the sensitivity of platelet imaging at 3 to 4 days was two- to threefold greater than at 1 to 2 days.[E5] In surgically excised specimens, the left ventricular thrombus to whole blood radioactivity count ratios have ranged from 10:1 to 355:1 in patients with positive images, and from 0.03:1 to 16:1 in patients with negative images.[E3, S10] Ezekowitz and associates have determined the sensitivity of platelet imaging to range from 65 to 71 percent, and the specificity to be 99 to 100 percent.[E3–5] Thus, only two thirds of left ventricular thrombi have externally detectable platelet uptake by platelet imaging. The risk of a false-positive study, however, is very low. It is possible that tomographic imaging will improve the sensitivity.

In an experimental animal study of left ventricular thrombi, Seabold and colleagues noted that the apparent sensitivity of platelet imaging for the detection of a left ventricular thrombus decreased over time following thrombus formation; among recently formed thrombi, 75 percent (9 of 12) were detected by platelet imaging.[S17] In contrast, among 1-week-old thrombi, only 57 percent (4 of 7) were detected. In a cross-sectional study in patients, Bellotti and associates noted that the hematologic activity of recent thrombi (less than 1 month) was significantly greater than of older thrombi (2 to 14 months).[B6] However, despite the apparent decrease in activity over time, all thrombi continued to be externally detectable.

To determine whether a positive indium-111 platelet image for a left ventricular thrombus, which indicates ongoing thrombogenic activity, predicts an increased risk of systemic embolization, we compared the embolic rate in patients with positive images to the rate in patients with negative images during a mean follow-up of 31 ± 24 months. The groups with positive and negative images were similar with respect to all clinical features, including antithrombotic therapy. During follow-up, embolic events occurred in 12 percent (4 of 33) of patients with positive platelet images for left ventricular thrombi, compared with only 2 percent (1 of 65) of patients with negative images ($p = 0.02$).[S18] By actuarial methods at 5 years of follow-up, only 71 percent of patients with positive images were embolus-free, compared with 98 percent of patients with negative images.

Our data also suggested that platelet imaging offered additional predictive value to two-dimensional echocardiography. In the subset of 53 patients who had evidence of a left ventricular thrombus by echocardiography, 29 had a positive platelet image whereas the remaining 24 patients had a negative platelet image. Among patients with a positive echocardiogram and a positive platelet image, embolic events occurred in 14 percent (4 of 29) versus 0 percent (0 of 24) of patients with a positive echocardiogram but a negative platelet image ($p = 0.06$). These data strongly suggest that a positive platelet image predicts an increased embolic risk even among patients with echocardiographically documented left ventricular thrombi. Platelet imaging stratifies patients into those with a high risk of subsequent embolization and those with a low risk of embolization. These findings suggest that thrombosis imaging may be useful to assess the risk of thromboembolic complications in patients with left ventricular thrombi.

Antithrombotic drug effects on left ventricular thrombi have been assessed in several studies. In two randomized trials of patients with acute myocardial infarction, Funke-Kupper and colleagues found no effect of either low-dose aspirin (100 mg daily) or of sulfinpyrazone (200 mg qid) in preventing the development of left ventricular thrombi or in reducing the activity of established thrombi as studied by platelet imaging.[F4, F5] Similarly, in uncontrolled series, aspirin in variable doses (300 to 2400 mg daily) did not prevent platelet uptake onto the left ventricular thrombus surface in five patients,[E4] nor did subcutaneous heparin.[E6]

In patients with chronic (over 3 months postmyocardial infarction) left ventricular thrombi, we assessed the effects of 2 to 3 weeks of therapy with sulfinpyrazone (200 mg qid), aspirin (325 mg tid) plus dipyridamole (75 mg tid), or full-dose warfarin. To establish the reproducibility of platelet imaging findings, five subjects with thrombi were serially restudied on no medications; all studies remained positive.[S16] Among seven patients treated with sulfinpyrazone, five had evidence of decreased platelet deposition by platelet imaging (three became negative, two equivocal). Among six patients treated with aspirin plus dipyridamole, three had decreased deposition (one became negative, three equivocal). Among four warfarin-treated patients, three became negative and one was unchanged (Fig. 63–3). Of note, despite evidence of reduced or absent platelet uptake in many patients during drug therapy, thrombus resolution by echocardiography was seen in only one patient who received warfarin; the remaining studies showed no change or only a small decrease in estimated thrombus size. These results suggest that platelet-active agents or warfarin diminishes left ventricular thrombus activity in some patients. Furthermore, the results suggest that platelet imaging may be superior to echocardiography as an early indicator of drug effect.

Left Atrial Thrombi

There are only limited data regarding the ability of indium-111 platelet imaging to detect left atrial thrombi.[B5, K3, P5, Y1] Yamada and associates reported findings compatible with left atrial thrombi in 7 of 28 patients with mitral valve disease.[Y1] Only 12 patients had operative or autopsy confirmation of the findings; platelet imaging detected four of five proven thrombi and was negative in all seven patients without thrombi. In case reports, platelet imaging has detected uptake onto a left atrial myxoma[E7] and onto a giant right atrial thrombus.[T9]

The role of platelet imaging in the detection and management of patients with suspected intracardiac thrombi remains unclear. For left ventricular thrombi, the sensitivity is approximately 71 percent while the specificity is close to 100 percent; false-negative studies can occur in patients receiving antithrombotic drugs or in patients with very small or inactive thrombi. In general, echocardiography is preferable as a diagnostic test because it is relatively quick, involves no radiation exposure, is widely available, and has a reasonable diagnostic accuracy with a sensitivity of 80 to 90 percent and a specificity of 90 to 95 percent. However, platelet imaging may have a role in identifying left ventricular thrombi in patients who have technically poor or equivocal echocardiograms. In addition, since thrombosis imaging appears to stratify embolic risk even in patients who have echocardiographically detected thrombi, platelet imaging or some other form of thrombosis imaging may help in making decisions regarding long-term anticoagulation. For left atrial thrombi, additional data are needed, but the preliminary results suggest that platelet imaging may have a reasonably high accuracy. Transthoracic echocardiography, in contrast, has a very poor sensitivity (50 percent or lower) for left atrial thrombi. In a recent study in experimental animals, platelet imaging detected 100 percent (17 of 17) of recently formed left atrial appendage thrombi whereas two-dimensional echocardiography detected only 18 percent (3 of 17). However, platelet imaging had a low sensitivity for "chronic" thrombi that had been present for 4 to 8 days prior to platelet injection.[V6]

VASCULAR THROMBI

Platelet imaging has been used to assess platelet accumulation at sites of atherosclerosis or arterial injury and to evaluate pharmacologic and other interventions. In humans, studies have evaluated carotid artery platelet deposition in patients with

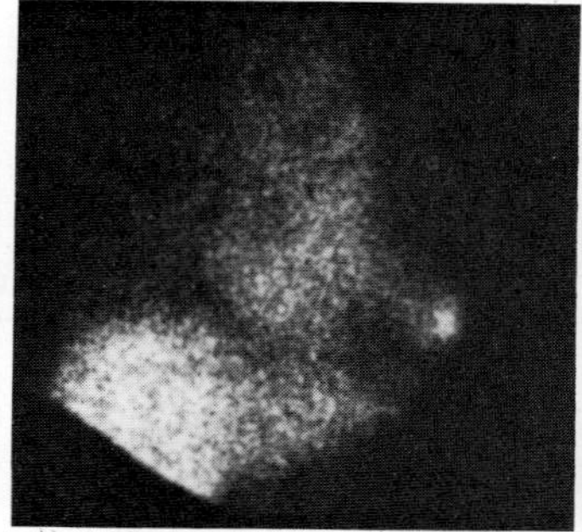

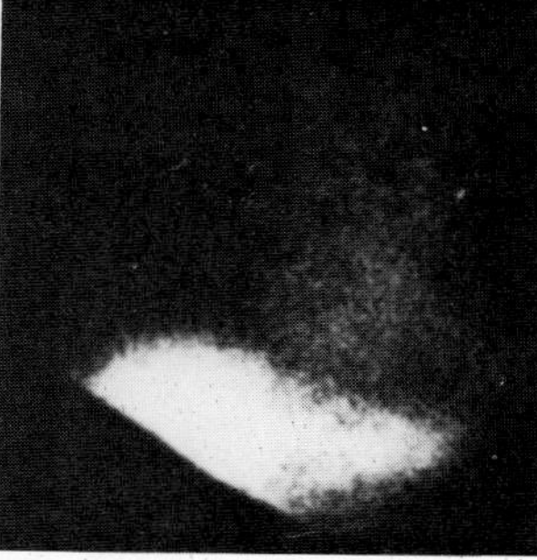

Figure 63–3. Anterior 72-hour images obtained on a patient with a left ventricular thrombus at baseline while receiving no therapy *(left panel)* and then while receiving warfarin *(right panel)*. During warfarin therapy, platelet deposition ceased. (From Stratton, J.R., and Ritchie, J.L.: The effects of antithrombotic drugs in patients with left ventricular thrombi: Assessment with indium-111 platelet imaging and two-dimensional echocardiography. Circulation 69:561–568, 1984, by permission of the American Heart Association, Inc.)

cerebral ischemia, platelet uptake in carotid arteries following endarterectomy, platelet uptake following injury or peripheral angioplasty, and platelet uptake in aneurysms or atherosclerotic plaques (Table 63–2). Experimental studies have demonstrated that maximal platelet accumulation occurs very early following an arterial injury.[F6, G4, W3]

Carotid Atherosclerosis

Atherosclerosis of the internal carotid artery, with associated platelet fibrin thrombus formation, is one mechanism leading to stroke and transient ischemic attacks. Other nonplatelet mechanisms, such as intracranial lesions or interplaque hemorrhage, are also potential causes of ischemic cerebral vascular disease.[P4] Several groups have attempted to determine whether platelet deposition in the region of the carotid artery was externally detectable in patients with known or suspected cerebral vascular disease.[D9, D10, G6, I2, K3, K4, P4, P7, P8] In an early report, labeled platelet uptake was detected in 61 percent of 33 atherosclerotic carotid arteries demonstrated by angiography using unblinded interpretation; however, lesion detection dropped to 36 percent using blinded interpretation.[D10] The largest series are summarized in Table 63–3.

Powers and colleagues studied 100 patients, 54 with clinically suspected carotid artery disease and 46 with a variety of other syndromes, including seizures, syncope, and migraine.[P7] The frequency of positive images was not different between patients with carotid artery symptoms and patients without carotid artery symptoms. Moreover, among patients with symptomatic carotid artery disease, images of the asymptomatic carotid artery were as equally likely to be abnormal as those of the symptomatic carotid artery. Platelet deposition was detected in 13 percent of angiographically normal sites and in 43 percent of stenotic or ulcerative sites detected angiographically. There was no correlation between platelet imaging findings and the subsequent risk of stroke or in the frequency of symptoms. Kessler and colleagues found that among 29 patients with positive carotid images, the frequency of abnormal scans in the clinically affected vessel (79 percent) was greater than in the unaffected vessel (45 percent).[K4] The correlation between angiographic and imaging findings was poor, with 62 percent of angiographically normal or near-normal arteries demonstrating abnormal scans, whereas only 40 percent of angiographically abnormal arteries demonstrated abnormal scans. Similarly, Goldman and group did not find a marked increase in positive images in symptomatic (64 percent) compared with asymptomatic (40 percent) arteries or in arteriographically abnormal (60 percent) compared with arteriographically normal (38 percent) regions.[G6] On 11 resected specimens, indium-111 platelet uptake was present but relatively minor.

More recently, Isaka and colleagues noted that the blood pool subtraction technique appeared to improve the accuracy of the analysis compared with visual techniques.[I2] Upon visual analysis, 31 percent of the arteries had evidence of abnormal platelet uptake, whereas only 6 percent had semiquantitative evidence of abnormal deposition by blood pool subtraction. In 12 subjects with symptomatic carotid artery disease and positive platelet images, Isaka and associates studied the efficacy of aspirin (325 mg bid) or ticlopidine (100 mg tid).[I3] Aspirin reduced platelet uptake in the affected carotid arteries, but there was no significant change following ticlopidine. Additional studies in patients with neurologic syndromes have demonstrated platelet uptake in patients with giant intracranial aneurysms[S19] and in one patient with a superior sagittal sinus thrombosis.[B7]

Approximately 10 to 15 percent of all stroke syndromes are due to a cardiac embolic source. In 27 patients with cerebral ischemic syndromes (stroke: 16, TIA: 11) possibly from a cardiac cause, Kessler and colleagues obtained platelet imaging of the heart within 10 days of the onset of the stroke syndrome.[K3, K5] Associated cardiac diseases were prior myocardial infarction (n = 8), atrial fibrillation (n = 10), cardiomegaly (n = 6), coronary artery disease (n = 7), and rheumatic heart disease (n = 3). Among the 27 patients, 13 had platelet images that were interpreted as positive for an intracardiac source; nine subjects had evidence of a left ventricular thrombus, three of a left atrial thrombus, and one of an aortic valve thrombus. The data suggest that platelet imaging may have some role in detecting embolic sources in patients with clinically suspected embolic strokes, but further confirmation is needed.

In summary, the correlation between platelet imaging findings and clinical symptoms and arteriographic findings in patients with suspected carotid artery disease has been poor. In addition, Powers and associates noted no prognostic value of a positive scan in this patient population in regard to subsequent risk of stroke or transient ischemic attack.[P7] The high rate of positive images obtained in angiographically normal vessels suggests a high rate of false positivity. In addition, observer disagreement in two of the studies was high at 20 percent[I2] and 24 percent.[G6]

Table 63–2. STUDIES OF ARTERIAL AND VENOUS DISEASES IN HUMANS

	References
Carotid artery disease	D9, D10, G2, G6, I2, I3, K4, O1, P4, P7, P8
Suspected embolic stroke	K3, K5
Carotid endarterectomy	F7, L2, S20
Endothelial or arterial injury	D10, K6, O1
Percutaneous peripheral transluminal angioplasty	C3, K6, P9
Arterial thrombosis, aneurysms	D11, H10, R5, S21
Intracranial aneurysm, sagittal sinus thrombosis	B7, S18
Homocystinuria	H12
Atherosclerotic plaques	S22, S28
Deep venous thrombosis	C4, C5, D13, E8, F8, F9, G7, M4, M5, S23, S28, W4, W6
Pulmonary emboli	C4, D13, E9, S25, S28

Table 63–3. PLATELET IMAGING IN CEREBROVASCULAR DISEASE

				% Positive Platelet Scans		Correlation with Arteriography		
							% Positive Platelet Scans	
	Total Patients	Patients with Carotid Symptoms	Type of Analysis	Symptomatic Carotid (%)	Asymptomatic Carotid (%)	Number of Patients	Abnormal Artery (%)	Normal Artery (%)
Powers et al.[P7]	100	54	Visual	"not different"		64	43	13
Kessler et al.[K4]	62	52	Visual	79*	45*	60	40	62
Goldman et al.[G6]	25	25	Visual	64	40	18	60	38
Isaka et al.[I2]	37	25	Blinded visual	—	—	25	54	31
			Semiquantitative	—	—	25	56	6

*Data given only on the 29 patients with a positive scan.

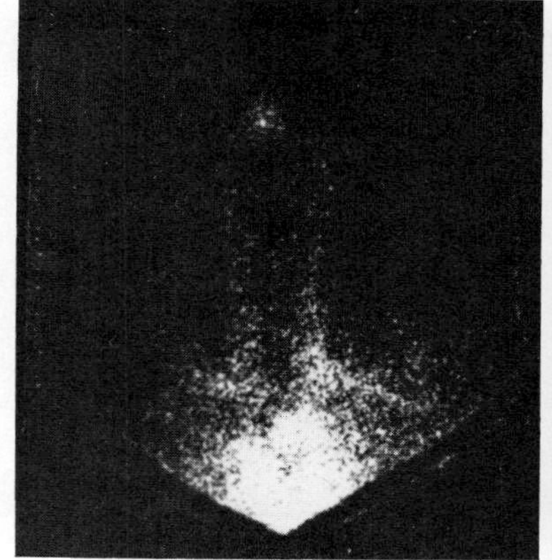
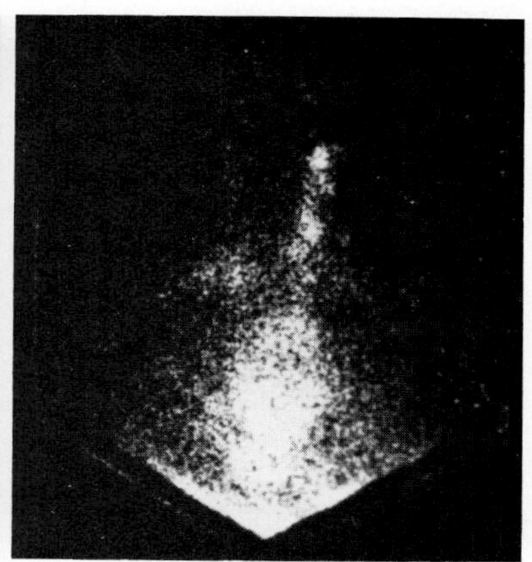

Figure 63–4. Anterior ^{111}In platelet images of the head and neck of a young normal control subject on the left and of a patient with a recent left carotid endarterectomy on the right. In the patient imaged following an endarterectomy, localized platelet accumulation was apparent at the endarterectomy site. Labeled platelets were injected 30 minutes postoperatively and images were obtained 48 hours later. (From Stratton, J.R., Zierler, R.E., and Kazmers, A.: Platelet deposition at carotid endarterectomy sites in man. Stroke 18:722–727, 1987, with permission.)

Carotid Endarterectomy

Endarterectomy involves the removal of atherosclerotic plaque, with substantial exposure of underlying media and adventitia. The complications of carotid endarterectomy include early thrombotic occlusion (approximately 2 percent of vessels) and late recurrent high-grade stenosis (9 to 18 percent of vessels). Both these complications may be related to platelet mechanisms.

In an animal study, Lusby and colleagues demonstrated labeled platelet accumulation at recent endarterectomy sites; deposition decreased by 2 to 3 weeks following surgery owing to re-endothelialization.[L2] Among 17 patients who had platelet injection within 1 hour following endarterectomy, 16 had externally detectable deposition.[L2]

In a study in our laboratory, we injected labeled platelets less than 30 minutes postoperatively following carotid endarterectomy and obtained images 24 to 96 hours later[S20] (Fig. 63–4). Semiquantitative analysis was performed using an index that compared activity in the operated side with the unoperated side. Patients with recent endarterectomy had a mean deposition index of 1.7 ± 0.5, compared with a similarly determined ratio of 1.1 ± 0.1 in normal subjects without surgery (Fig. 63–5). In addition, to determine the amount of uptake caused by surgical dissection in the absence of endarterectomy, we studied a surgical control group composed of six patients with noncarotid surgery. Among the surgical controls, the deposition index ratio was only 1.2 ± 0.1. Twelve patients had follow-up studies 0.5 to 24 months following endarterectomy. The deposition index decreased at follow-up in all subjects to a mean of 1.0 ± 0.1, documenting reduced platelet deposition over time, compatible with re-endothelialization of the endarterectomized surface (Fig. 63–6).

To determine whether aspirin (330 mg tid) plus dipyridamole (75 mg tid) reduces platelet uptake at endarterectomy sites, Findlay and co-workers conducted a randomized double-blind trial in 22 patients.[F7] Treated patients had a significant reduction in labeled platelet accumulation measured at approximately 48 hours following carotid endarterectomy.

These data indicate that the arterial injury of carotid endarterectomy results in predictable early platelet deposition, which decreases late and which may be reduced by pretreatment with platelet inhibitory agents.

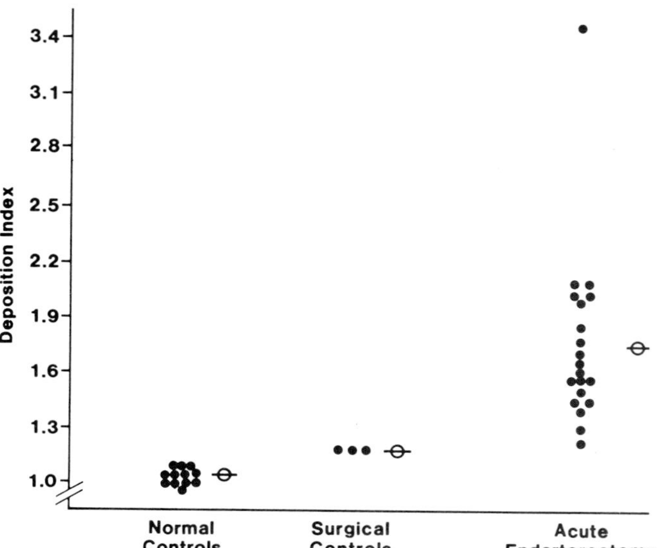

Figure 63–5. The deposition index in patients with a recent carotid endarterectomy was greater than for the normal controls and for the surgical controls ($p \leq 0.05$). Only one subject with a recent endarterectomy overlapped with either control group. (From Stratton, J.R., Zierler, R.E., and Kazmers, A.: Platelet deposition at carotid endarterectomy sites in man. Stroke 18:722–727, 1987, with permission.)

Arterial Aneurysms, Arterial Injury, and Peripheral Angioplasty

Large-vessel aneurysms are frequently associated with mural thrombus. We studied 18 unoperated patients with either abdominal aortic aneurysms (n = 17) or bilateral femoral artery aneurysms (n = 1).[R5] By visual analysis, 12 studies were definitely positive, two equivocal, and four negative (Fig. 63–7). In two resected specimens, the portion of thrombus in contact with flowing blood had 3.4 and 6.0 times more indium-111 activity per gram compared with the outer section of thrombus in contact with the arterial wall. Heyns and colleagues studied the kinetics of accumulation of platelets in abdominal aortic aneurysm thrombi.[H10] Shortly after the injection of labeled platelets, 1.5 ± 1.1 percent of whole body activity was in the aneurysm thrombus,

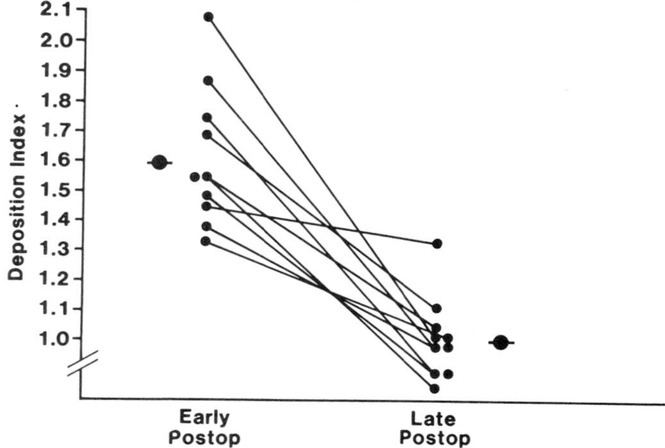

Figure 63–6. The deposition index decreased in all subjects who had both acute and follow-up studies. (From Stratton, J.R., Zierler, R.E., and Kazmers, A.: Platelet deposition at carotid endarterectomy sites in man. Stroke 18:722–727, 1987, with permission.)

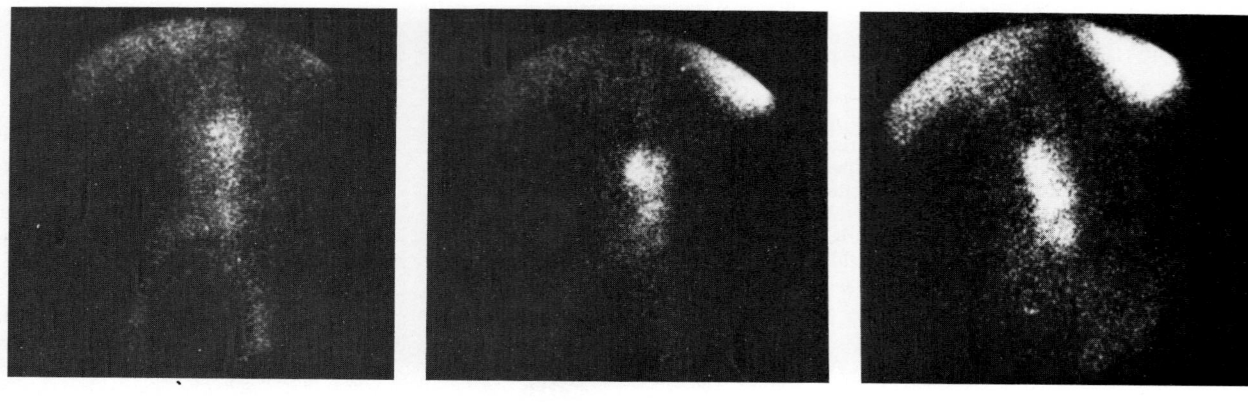

Figure 63–7. Serial anterior abdominal views of a patient with a 6-cm abdominal aortic aneurysm that contained a thrombus at surgery. Over time, platelet deposition in the aneurysm increased relative to the background blood pool in the iliac and femoral arteries. The edge of the liver is at the upper left, the edge of the spleen at the upper right, and the aortic bifurcation in the lower mid-section of each image. (From Ritchie, J.L., Stratton, J.R., Thiele, B., et al.: Indium-111 platelet imaging for detection of platelet deposition in abdominal aneurysms and prosthetic grafts. Am. J. Cardiol. 47:882–889, 1981, with permission.)

which increased to 4.7 ± 3.6 percent at 132 hours. These quantitative data confirm the visual impression that greater platelet uptake occurs at later imaging times.

Asymptomatic aortic aneurysms are not uncommon. Among 860 patients imaged for other reasons, Sinzinger and co-workers detected 21 asymptomatic aneurysms from localized platelet uptake in the aneurysm thrombus.[S21] Prostacyclin infusions (95 ng/kg/min) caused a reduction in platelet uptake in four patients. Arterial injury from puncture causes detectable platelet deposition, as noted by several investigators.[D10, G2, O1] In addition, a femoral artery embolus has been detected.[D11]

In contrast to the negative findings with coronary angioplasty, several investigators have noted detectable uptake at the sites of peripheral percutaneous transluminal angioplasty. Pope and associates detected uptake in 73 percent (11 of 15) of patients undergoing peripheral angioplasty, despite the fact that all subjects received either heparin, warfarin, streptokinase, or platelet inhibitory drugs.[P9] Kadir and colleagues also noted uptake in three subjects despite treatment with aspirin.[K6] In contrast, Cunningham and co-workers detected deposition at 0 of 11 sites in patients pretreated with aspirin versus 6 of 8 sites in patients not pretreated with aspirin.[C3]

Atherosclerosis

Peripheral atherosclerotic plaques are occasionally associated with platelet deposition. Powers and colleagues found evidence of platelet deposition in the abdominal aortas of macaques with diet-induced atherosclerosis using blood pool subtraction techniques, but not with unprocessed, visually interpreted images.[P10] At autopsy, however, the extent of apparent deposition did not correlate with the severity of atherosclerosis.

In 36 patients with angiographically proved femoral artery stenosis, 61 percent had abnormally high platelet uptake in the diseased leg compared with the contralateral leg, documenting increased platelet uptake in atherosclerotic vessels. Patients with ulceration or recent thrombus that was noted subsequently at surgery had particularly high uptake ratios.[S22]

VENOUS THROMBOSIS AND PULMONARY EMBOLISM

In animal models of venous thrombosis, labeled platelets have detected uptake over a several-day period in both the calf and the proximal leg,[M4, M5] and indium-111 platelet imaging has offered superior radioactivity count ratios to iodine-125 fibrinogen.[K7] The age of the thrombus at the time of platelet injection has critically influenced the ability to image thrombus,[D12, G5, K7, M4, M5] with older thrombi either being undetectable or taking longer to visualize. In addition, antithrombotic agents can inhibit labeled platelet uptake and lead to negative images. For example, heparin in high doses blocks platelet incorporation, as does prostacyclin (PGI_2).[M4, M5]

Platelet imaging, in contrast to some other techniques, may be capable of detecting venous thrombi at all sites, including the calf, thigh, and pelvis. In studies in humans, the sensitivity of indium-111 platelet imaging for the detection of deep venous thrombosis has varied widely, with reported sensitivities of between 42 and 100 percent.[C4, E8, F8, G7, S23] Specificity has ranged from 67 to 100 percent. In a study in 31 patients, only two of whom were receiving heparin, the sensitivity of platelet imaging was 100 percent and the specificity 89 percent.[S23] The sensitivity of platelet imaging appears to drop dramatically if patients are receiving heparin. In a study by Ezekowitz and colleagues of patients with deep venous thrombosis documented by prior venography, platelet imaging was positive in 80 percent (4 of 5) of patients not receiving heparin but in only 33 percent (5 of 15) of patients who were receiving heparin at the time of platelet imaging.[E8] Imaging to at least 24 hours following the injection of labeled platelets appears to improve the sensitivity. In one study, the sensitivity improved from 69 percent at 4 hours to 100 percent at 24 hours following platelet injection.[S23]

Platelet imaging has been utilized to monitor patients at high risk for development of deep venous thrombosis, usually because of recent surgery. Clarke-Pearson and co-workers noted positive images (deep vein thrombi or pulmonary emboli) in 30 percent of patients following abdominal or pelvic surgery.[C4] Winter and associates noted positive images for deep venous thrombi in 64 percent of 64 patients with femur fractures[W4] and in 45 percent of 29 patients with respiratory failure.[W5]

Platelet imaging appears to offer little promise in the diagnosis of pulmonary emboli. Although acute pulmonary emboli have been detected by platelet imaging in animal models, older thrombi (more than 24 hours) could not be detected. In addition, heparin blocked the ability to detect pulmonary emboli platelet uptake.[S24] Although isolated case reports[E9, S25] have noted pulmonary emboli in humans, platelet imaging failed to detect platelet uptake in 11 of 12 heparinized patients with pulmonary emboli.[D13] Clarke-Pearson and colleagues detected five asymptomatic pulmonary emboli among 146 patients studied with platelet imaging following abdominal or pelvic surgery.[C4]

To summarize, platelet imaging has demonstrated some promise in the noninvasive diagnosis of deep venous thrombosis, particularly since it may be capable of detecting calf, thigh, and pelvic thrombi. The detection of pulmonary emboli, in contrast, does not appear to be routinely possible. The sensitivity of platelet imaging for the detection of deep venous thrombosis appears to be adversely affected by concomitant heparin therapy or by early imaging times. It is possible that platelet imaging might prove useful in the serial monitoring of patients at high risk for the development of deep venous thrombosis. However, other thrombosis imaging techniques, possibly utilizing antifibrin antibodies, may be able to detect thrombi at earlier imaging times and potentially may be less influenced by heparin therapy.

PROSTHETIC MATERIALS

Intravascular prosthetic materials are increasingly used as arterial and venous substitutes, vascular catheters, membrane oxygenators, heart valves, ventricular assist devices, and even as totally artificial hearts. Owing to improved materials and improved fabrication techniques, mechanical failure of prosthetic devices is now extremely rare. The most common current complications of prosthetic materials are thromboembolic events. There is now abundant evidence that platelet mechanisms play a dominant role in the thrombotic and embolic events caused by intravascular prosthetic materials. Despite improved materials, all currently used prosthetic devices are thrombogenic when placed in humans (Table 63–4). Two strategies have been used to reduce thromboembolic complications. First is the construction of new, less thrombogenic materials. Second is the development of improved, safe antithrombotic drug regimens. Testing of either new materials or new drug regimens prior to widespread clinical use is necessary. However, the assessment of thrombogenicity of prosthetic materials in the past has been limited by the lack of suitable methods. Recently, platelet imaging has been widely utilized in animal studies to measure platelet uptake in vivo or in vitro following sacrifice.[S26] Platelet imaging also has been increasingly utilized in human studies to quantitatively evaluate new materials as well as new drug regimens.

Natural History of Platelet Deposition on Prosthetic Arterial Grafts

Indium-111 platelet deposition is detectable in virtually all recently implanted large-caliber prosthetic arterial grafts in humans by both visual and quantitative analysis.[A2, G3, G4, G8, I4, K8, P5, R5, S26, S27] In contrast, autologous vein grafts typically do not have visually detectable platelet accumulation.[G3]

After implantation, as grafts mature they become less thrombogenic and have less associated platelet deposition.[G8, I4, R6, S27] For example, among 24 patients studied 1 to 2 weeks following Dacron bifurcation graft implantation and again at 6 to 9 months, the graft thrombogenicity index decreased from 0.16 ± 0.02 to 0.08 ± 0.01 (± SEM).[G8] Similarly, we noted a reduction in a graft-to-blood ratio from 4.4 ± 2.1 (± SD) at 1 to 2 weeks postoperatively to 3.0 ± 1.8 at 31 weeks ($p = 0.02$) in patients with Dacron bifurcation grafts. There was no further decrease at 55 weeks (2.8 ± 2.0).[S27] Isaka and group noted a significant negative correlation between their semiquantitative estimate of graft platelet accumulation and graft age ($r = -0.76$).[I4] Goldman and colleagues also found a significant reduction in platelet deposition over time, with the mean thrombogenicity index decreasing from 0.21 to 0.08 between 1 week and 6 to 12 months following Dacron graft implantation.[G4] Similarly, in patients with woven Dacron grafts, the deposition index decreased from 0.19 to 0.06 over the first 6 to 9 months following graft implantation.[G8] Thus, multiple studies have reached a similar conclusion: in humans, platelet uptake onto prosthetic grafts significantly decreases over time following implantation in the absence of therapy.

Platelet imaging done early postoperatively may predict ultimate graft patency in patients with prosthetic femoral popliteal bypass grafts. The mean thrombogenicity index 1 week following surgery in 21 femoral popliteal grafts that eventually occluded within 1 year was 0.19 ± 0.02 (± SEM), compared with 0.07 ± 0.01 in the 36 grafts that remained patent ($p < 0.001$).[G9] When grafts were split into those that had a thrombogenicity index below the median at 1 week following implantation versus those with a higher thrombogenicity index, there was a marked difference in the patency rate at 1 year by life table methods. Among patients with a low index, the patency rate at 1 year was 90 percent, compared with a patency rate of only 39 percent in those with a higher thrombogenicity index.[G9]

Although platelet deposition decreases over time following implantation, substantial data document that deposition does continue, albeit at a lesser rate (Fig. 63–8*A* and *B*). Several studies have noted both visual and quantitative evidence that Dacron grafts have ongoing deposition for indefinite periods of time up to 10 years following implantation[G4, G8, I4, K8, R6, S13, S27, Y2] (Fig. 63–9). In a study of patients with chronically implanted Dacron grafts (9 months to 10 years), 12 of 15 subjects had visually positive evidence of platelet deposition. In contrast, among 12 normal subjects, all had visually negative studies[S13] (Fig. 63–8*A*). The quantitative results more convincingly demonstrate that continued platelet accumulation occurs (Fig. 63–10). In the case of the normal subjects, the graft-to-blood ratio was unchanged at the serial imaging times between 24 and 96 hours following platelet injection (2.0 ± 0.7, 1.8 ± 0.6, 1.7 ± 0.8, and 1.7 ± 0.9, respectively) (Fig. 63–10). In contrast, among 15 patients with chronically implanted prosthetic grafts, there was a significant serial increase in the graft-to-blood ratio over time following platelet injection (3.0 ± 1.6 at 24 hours to 7.8 ± 5.0 at 96 hours).[S13] Most subjects with chronically implanted grafts have evidence of diffuse deposition. However, several also have relatively irregular foci of deposition.[I4, S13]

Evaluation of Different Graft Materials

There are limited data in humans comparing the thrombogenicity of different types of graft materials. Recently implanted Dacron and polytetrafluoroethylene (PTFE) femoropopliteal grafts have significantly higher thrombogenicity indices than autologous vein grafts (0.25, 0.16, and 0.03, respectively). Thus, autologous vein grafts are less thrombogenic than either type of prosthetic material.[G3, G9] In a randomized trial, Goldman and colleagues found no difference in platelet deposition between woven (USCI, DeBakey) Dacron grafts and more porous, double-velour, knitted (Mirovel, Meadox Medical) Dacron grafts in 24 patients studied at 1 week and at 6 to 9 months.[G8] Similarly, we noted no qualitative or quantitative difference in platelet accumulation between knitted DeBakey Dacron ($n = 6$) and knitted Sauvage double-velour Dacron grafts ($n = 8$).[S13] In a uniquely designed study, 20 patients who received aortobifemoral grafts had one limb constructed of knitted Dacron and the other limb constructed of woven Dacron. Patients were then studied at a single time that varied between 1 week to 42 months following implantation. Platelet accumulation was nearly identical in the two graft limbs, documenting no significant difference in thrombogenicity between knitted and woven Dacron arterial grafts.[R6]

Small numbers of patients with vascular access grafts,[R7] cardiopulmonary bypass,[H11] mechanical heart valves,[D6] and indwelling

Table 63–4. STUDIES OF PROSTHETIC GRAFT MATERIALS IN HUMANS

	References
Acutely placed grafts	A2, G3, G8, G9, P5, R5, S27
Grafts implanted longer than 1 month	G4, G8, I4, K8, S13, S27, Y2
Comparison of different graft materials	G3, G8, G9, R6, R7, S13
Drug effects on graft platelet deposition	G9, G10, P4, R7, S11, S12, S29–31
Cardiopulmonary bypass	H11
Mechanical heart valves	D6
Indwelling catheters	S28

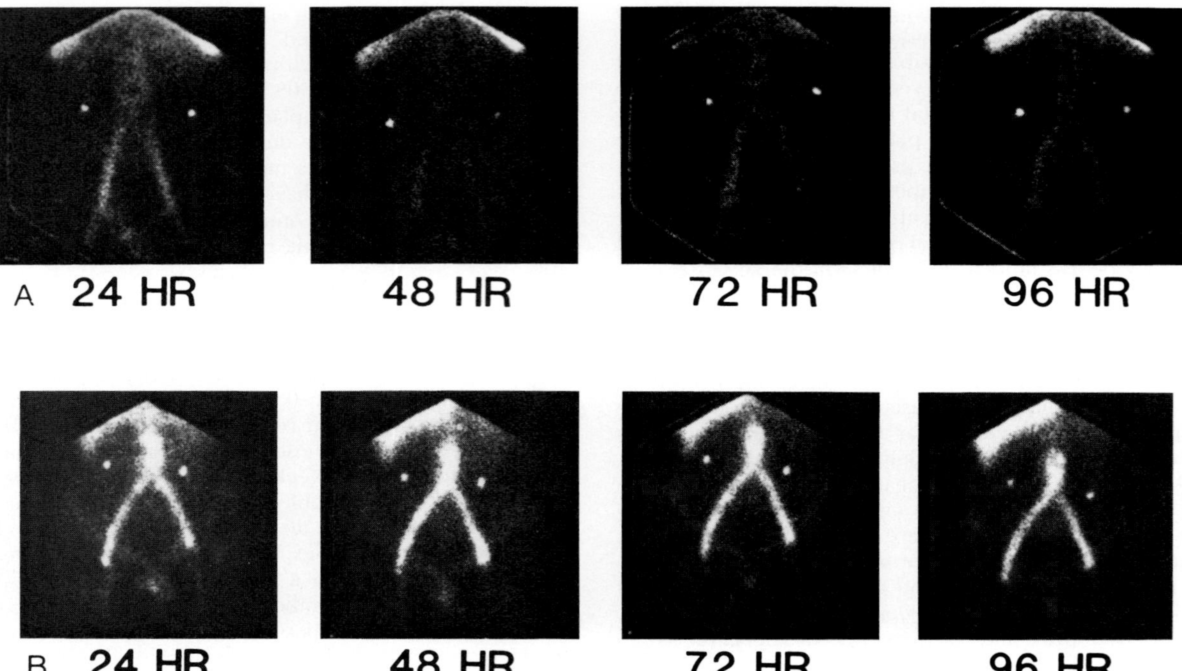

Figure 63–8. *A*, Serial anterior abdominal images in a young normal subject showed only faint circulating platelet activity present in the aortofemoral vessels (150,000 counts). The two white spots are anatomic markers that are placed 8 cm to each side of the umbilicus to aid in patient positioning. *B*, Anterior abdominal images (150,000 counts) of a 13-month-old Dacron aortic graft demonstrating diffuse uptake throughout the graft. (From Stratton, J.R., Thiele, B.L., and Ritchie, J.L.: Platelet deposition on Dacron aortic bifurcation grafts in man: Quantitation with indium-111 platelet imaging. Circulation 66:1287–1293, 1982, by permission of the American Heart Association, Inc.)

catheters[S28] have also been assessed in regard to platelet uptake onto differing prosthetic surfaces.

Drug Effects on Platelet Deposition on Grafts

The combination of aspirin plus dipyridamole has been most extensively studied in patients with both acute and chronically implanted grafts. In eight subjects with recently implanted Dacron aortofemoral grafts, the combination of aspirin (325 mg tid) plus dipyridamole (100 mg qid preoperatively and 75 mg tid postoperatively) decreased platelet uptake in all portions of the graft, compared with eight untreated control patients.[P5] In contrast, the same regimen had no apparent effect in five patients with polytetrafluoroethylene (PTFE) femoropopliteal grafts, compared with controls. In a randomized trial involving 47 patients with recently implanted Dacron, PTFE, or vein grafts, aspirin plus dipyridamole treatment decreased the deposition index in Dacron grafts from 0.25 ± 0.09 to 0.16 ± 0.05 ($p < 0.05$) and in PTFE grafts from 0.16 ± 0.03 to 0.05 ± 0.01 ($p < 0.05$). However, in vein grafts no detectable reduction in deposition was induced by drug therapy (0.03 ± 0.01).[G10] The reduction in early platelet deposition was associated with an improved patency rate in drug-treated patients at 1 year (67 percent), compared with placebo-treated controls (36 percent, $p < 0.05$).[G9] In patients with older Dacron bifurcation grafts (10 to 121 months), short-term therapy with aspirin (325 mg tid) plus dipyridamole (75 mg tid) also reduced platelet accumulation[S12] (Fig. 63–11). The mean drug-induced decrease in a tomographically obtained graft-to-blood ratio was 13 ± 4 percent, and the decrease in a planar imaging graft-to-blood ratio was 12 ± 4 percent.

Prostacyclin (PGI_2) also reduces platelet deposition in both recently implanted and chronically implanted grafts in humans.[S29] The magnitude of the reduction was greater among patients with more recently implanted grafts, compared with patients with chronically implanted grafts. Some evidence suggested that the prostacyclin effect persisted following discontinuation of the infusion.

In general, results of drug therapy in patients with chronically implanted grafts have been much less impressive than in patients with recently implanted prostheses. We have assessed the effects of three agents in patients with chronically implanted grafts (greater than 9 months old). In randomized placebo-controlled crossover studies, the experimental agents suloctidil (200 mg tid) and ticlopidine (250 mg bid) failed to cause a significant reduction in platelet uptake onto the surface of chronic grafts.[S11, S30] Similarly, sulfinpyrazone (200 mg qid) also failed to reduce platelet uptake on chronic grafts.[S31]

To summarize, platelet deposition on prosthetic arterial grafts has been present on all materials studied in humans. Deposition is greatest early following implantation. Despite a reduction in

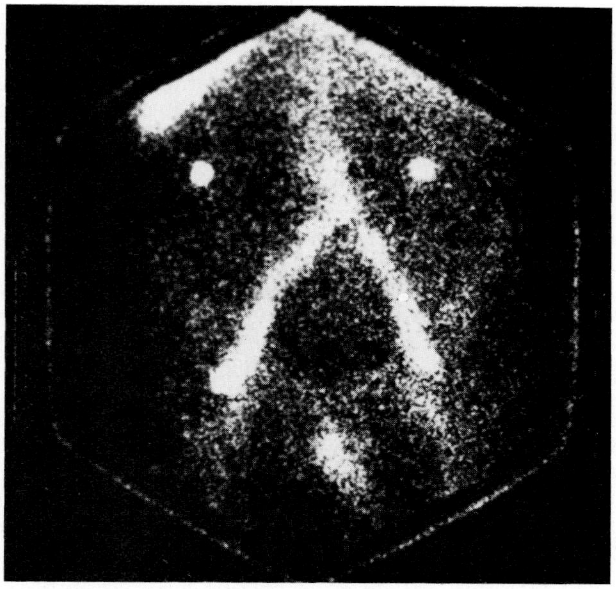

Figure 63–9. Diffuse platelet accumulation was present in this 10-year-old Dacron bifurcation graft (48 hours, 150,000 count image). Deposition appears to continue for indefinite periods following Dacron graft placement in humans.

deposition over the first few months following implantation, detectable deposition appears to remain present indefinitely in most, if not all, patients. Deposition has been decreased on both recently and chronically implanted grafts by aspirin plus dipyridamole, as well as by prostacyclin. On chronically implanted grafts, suloctidil, ticlopidine, and sulfinpyrazone have failed to reduce deposition. Deposition is clearly less on autologous vein grafts, compared with either PTFE or Dacron grafts. The magnitude of platelet uptake detected early on prosthetic materials appears to predict ultimate graft patency.

SUMMARY AND CONCLUSIONS

The ability of indium-111 platelet imaging to localize noninvasively and define platelet kinetics during life already has offered a new window for examining the pathophysiologic role of platelets in a broad range of diseases. Thrombosis imaging using labeled platelets has proved to be a very useful research tool in experimental animal studies and is increasingly utilized to study a variety of diseases in humans. To date, platelet imaging as a method of thrombosis detection, however, has several constraints that have limited its clinical utility. Current labeling and imaging techniques are time consuming and costly, and rapid diagnosis is not possible since delayed imaging is usually necessary. The resolution of platelet imaging has been limited to some extent by the relatively high circulating blood pool activity that occurs, and in part by the inherent limitations of all gamma imaging techniques.[P8] Small arterial thrombi that have great clinical importance, such as coronary artery thrombi, cannot be routinely detected with indium-111 platelet imaging in humans. The lack of simple, validated methods of quantification of platelet uptake in humans is also a limitation, since it is clear that quantitative analysis is necessary to detect small changes in platelet accumulation induced by drugs or by time.

To realize the full potential of thrombosis imaging, improvements in imaging techniques as well as improved thrombosis tracers are needed. It is possible that the development of positron emitters for thrombosis imaging would improve spatial resolution and quantification, but positron production and imaging facilities are unlikely to be widely available because of their cost. It is more likely that superior methods of thrombosis detection using gamma-emitting isotopes tagged to tracers that localize in areas of ongoing thrombosis will be found. Improved thrombosis imaging may be possible with labeling of compounds, such as tissue plasminogen activator or antifibrin or antiplatelet monoclonal antibodies, that are incorporated into thrombus. To be clinically useful, new approaches need to offer thrombus-to-background ratios that exceed those achieved with indium-111–labeled platelets at earlier times following injection. With future improvements, it is likely that thrombosis imaging will play an increasingly important role in detecting localized thrombosis and assessing the effects of therapy in humans.

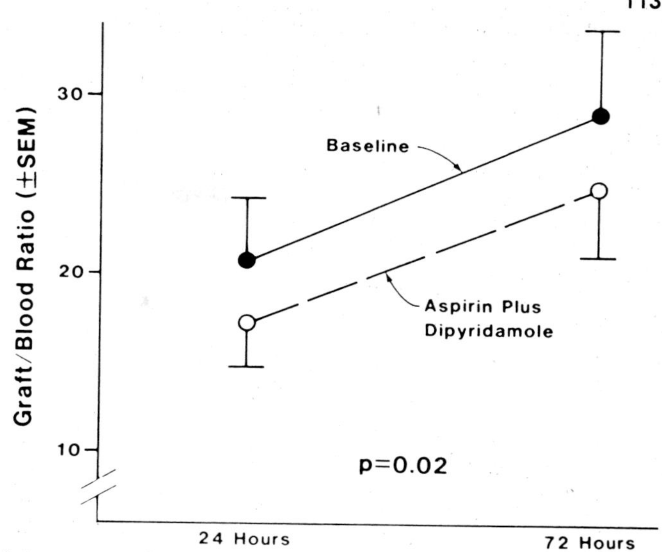

Figure 63–11. The effects of aspirin plus dipyridamole on the tomographic graft/blood ratio are summarized here. The graft-to-blood ratio was significantly reduced by aspirin plus dipyridamole compared with control testing (p = 0.02). (From Stratton, J.R., and Ritchie, J.L.: Reduction of indium-111 platelet deposition on Dacron vascular grafts in humans by aspirin plus dipyridamole. Ciculation 73:325–330, 1986, by permission of the American Heart Association, Inc.)

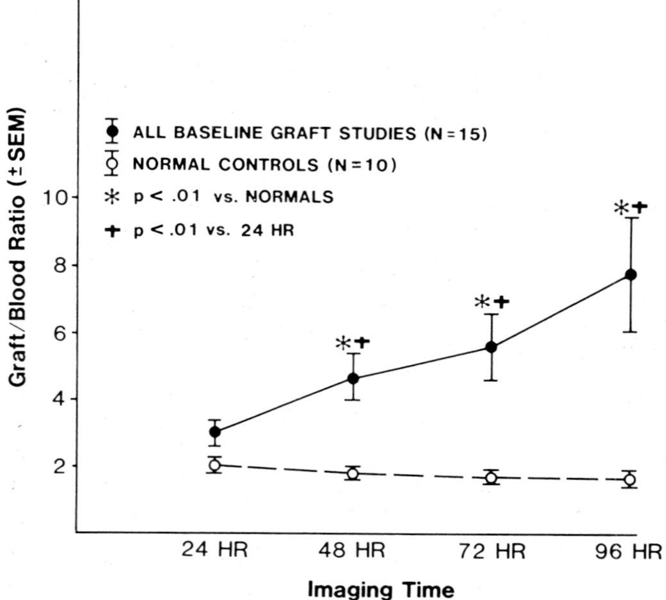

Figure 63–10. The graft-to-blood ratio obtained in 15 patients with grafts that were in place for greater than 9 months, as well as in 10 normal controls without grafts, is displayed here. Patients with grafts had a higher graft-to-blood ratio at all imaging times than did normal subjects. In normal subjects, the ratio represents an aortofemoral blood pool/whole blood ratio. Patients with grafts had an increasing ratio over time in contrast with normal subjects who exhibited no change. By quantitative analysis, later imaging times (72 or 96 hours) better discriminated patients with grafts from normal subjects. (From Stratton, J.R., Thiele, B.L., and Ritchie, J.L.: Platelet deposition on Dacron aortic bifurcation grafts in man: Quantitation with indium-111 platelet imaging. Circulation 66:1287–1293, 1982, by permission of the American Heart Association, Inc.)

References

A

1. Allen, B.T., Sicard, G.A., Welch, M.J., et al.: Platelet deposition on vascular grafts: The accuracy of in vivo quantitation and the significance of in vivo platelet reactivity. Ann. Surg. 203:318, 1986.
2. Agarwal, K.C., Wahner, H.W., Dewanjee, M.K., et al.: Imaging of platelets in right-sided extracardiac conduits in humans. J. Nucl. Med. 2:342, 1982.

B

1. Bunting, R.W., Callahan, R.J., Finkelstein, S., et al.: A modified method for labeling human platelets with indium-111 oxine using albumin density-gradient separation. Radiology 145:219, 1982.
2. Bassano, D.A., and McAfee, J.G.: Cellular radiation doses of labeled neutrophils and labeled platelets. J. Nucl. Med. 20:255, 1979.
3. Badenhorst, P.N., and Pieters, H.: Platelet imaging. *In* Heyns, A. duP., Badenhorst, P.N., and Lotter, M.G. (eds.): Platelet Kinetics and Imaging. Vol. 1. CRC Press, Boca Raton, Fla., 1985, pp. 73–88.
4. Bergmann, S.R., Lerch, R.A., Mathias, C.J., et al.: Noninvasive detection of coronary thrombi with In-111 platelets: Concise communication. J. Nucl. Med. 24:130, 1983.
5. Benichou, M., Bernard, P.J., Sarrat, P., et al.: La detection des caillots intracardiaques par la scintigraphie aux plaquettes marquees a l'indium-111: Confrontation avec l'echographie bidimensionnelle et la scanographie cardiaque. Arch. Mal Cour 9:1054, 1984.
6. Bellotti, P., Claudiani, F., Chiarella, F., et al.: Activity of left ventricular thrombi of differing ages. Assessment with indium-oxine platelet imaging and cross-sectional echocardiography. Eur. Heart J. 8:855, 1987.

7. Bridgers, S.L., Strauss, E., Smith, E.O., et al. Demonstration of superior sagittal sinus thrombosis by indium-111 platelet scintigraphy. Arch. Neurol. 43:1079, 1986.

C

1. Christenson, J.T., Arvidsson, D., Thorne, J., et al.: A comparison of two methods of labelling autologous platelets with ^{111}In-oxine in five different species. Eur. J. Nucl. Med. 8:389, 1983.
2. Callahan, R.J., Bunting, R.W., Block, P.C., et al.: Evaluation of platelet deposition at the site of coronary angioplasty using indium-111 labeled platelets. (Abstract.) J. Nucl. Med. 24:P60, 1983.
3. Cunningham, D.A., Kumar, B., Siegel, B.A., et al.: Aspirin inhibition of platelet deposition at angioplasty sites: Demonstration by platelet scintigraphy. Radiology 151:487, 1984.
4. Clarke-Pearson, D.L., Coleman, R.E., Sigel, R., et al.: Indium-111 platelet imaging for the detection of deep venous thrombosis and pulmonary embolism in patients without symptoms after surgery. Surgery 98:98, 1985.
5. Clarke-Pearson, D.L., Creusman, W.T., Ralston, M., and Coleman, R.E.: Indium-labelled platelet imaging of post-operative pelvic vein thrombi. Obstet. Gynecol. 62:109, 1983.

D

1. Danpure, H.J., Osman, S., and Brady, F.: The labelling of blood cells in plasma with ^{111}In-tropolonate. Br. J. Radiol. 55:247, 1982.
2. Danpure, H.J., and Osman, S.: Cell labelling and cell damage with indium-111 acetylacetone—an alternative to indium-111 oxine. Br. J. Radiol. 54:597, 1981.
3. Dewanjee, M.K., Rao, S.A., Rosemark, J.A., et al.: Indium-111 tropolone, a new tracer for platelet labeling. Radiology 145:149, 1982.
4. Datz, F.L.: Radiolabeled leukocytes and platelets. Invest. Radiol. 21:191, 1986.
5. Dewanjee, M.K., Wahner, H.W., Dunn, W.L., et al.: Comparison of three platelet markers for measurement of platelet survival time in healthy volunteers. Mayo Clin. Proc. 61:327, 1986.
6. Dewanjee, M.K.: Cardiac and vascular imaging with labelled platelets and leukocytes. Semin. Nucl. Med. 3:154, 1984.
7. Dewanjee, M.K., Tago, M., Josa, M., et al.: Quantification of platelet retention in aortocoronary femoral vein bypass graft in dogs treated with dipyridamole and aspirin. Circulation 69:350, 1984.
8. Dewanjee, M.K., Trastek, V.F., Tago, M., and Kaye, M.P.: Radioisotopic techniques for noninvasive detection of platelet deposition in bovine-tissue mitral-valve prostheses and in vitro quantification of visceral microembolism in dogs. Invest. Radiol. 19:535, 1984.
9. Davis, H.H., Siegel, B.A., Joist, J.H., et al.: Scintigraphic detection of atherosclerotic lesions and venous thrombi in man by indium-111-labelled autologous platelets. Lancet 1:1185, 1978.
10. Davis, H.H., Siegel, B.A., Sherman, L.A., et al.: Scintigraphic detection of carotid atherosclerosis with indium-111-labelled autologous platelets. Circulation 61:982, 1980.
11. Davis, H.H., Siegel, B.A., and Welch, M.J.: Scintigraphic detection of an arterial thrombus with In-111-labelled autologous platelets. J. Nucl. Med. 21:548, 1980.
12. Dormehl, I.C., Jacobs, D.J., Pretorius, J.P., et al.: Baboon (*Papio ursinus*) model to study deep vein thrombosis using 111-indium-labeled autologous platelets. J. Med. Primatol. 16:27, 1987.
13. Davis, H.H., Siegel, B.A., Sherman, L.A., et al.: Scintigraphy with ^{111}In-labelled autologous platelets in venous thromboembolism. Radiology 136:203, 1980.

E

1. Ezekowitz, M.D., and Smith, E.O.: Indium-111 labeling of stored platelet concentrates. Transfusion 26:13, 1986.
2. Ezekowitz, M.D., Leonard, J.C., Smith, E.O., et al.: The identification of left ventricular thrombi in man using indium-111 labelled autologous platelets: A preliminary report. Circulation 63:803, 1981.
3. Ezekowitz, M.D., Wilson, D.A., Smith, E.O., et al.: Comparison of indium-111 platelet scintigraphy and two-dimensional echocardiography in the diagnosis of left ventricular thrombi. N. Engl. J. Med. 306:1509, 1982.
4. Ezekowitz, M.D., Smith, E.O., Cox, A.C., and Taylor, F.B.: Failure of aspirin to prevent incorporation of indium-111 labelled platelets into cardiac thrombi in man. Lancet 2:440, 1981.
5. Ezekowitz, M.D., Burrow, R.D., Heath, P.W., et al.: Diagnostic accuracy of indium-111 platelet scintigraphy in identifying left ventricular thrombi. Am. J. Cardiol. 51:1712, 1983.
6. Ezekowitz, M.D., Kellerman, D.J., Smith, E.O., and Streitz, T.M.: Detection of active left ventricular thrombosis during acute myocardial infarction using indium-111 platelet scintigraphy. Chest 86:35, 1984.
7. Ezekowitz, M.D., Smith, E.O., Rankin, R., et al.: Left atrial mass: Diagnostic value of transesophageal 2-dimensional echocardiography and indium-111 platelet scintigraphy. Am. J. Cardiol. 51:1563, 1983.
8. Ezekowitz, M.D., Pope, C.F., Sostman, H.D., et al.: Indium-111 platelet scintigraphy for the diagnosis of acute venous thrombosis. Circulation 73:668, 1986.
9. Ezekowitz, M.D., Eichner, E.R., Scatterday, R., and Elkins, R.C.: Diagnosis of a persistent pulmonary embolus by indium-111 platelet scintigraphy with angiographic and tissue confirmation. Am. J. Med. 72:839, 1982.

F

1. Fox, K.A.A., Bergmann, S.R., Mathias, C.J., et al.: Scintigraphic detection of coronary artery thrombi in patients with acute myocardial infarction. J. Am. Coll. Cardiol. 4:975, 1984.
2. Fuster, V., Dewanjee, M.K., Kaye, M.P., et al.: Noninvasive radioisotopic technique for detection of platelet deposition in coronary artery bypass grafts in dogs and its reduction with platelet inhibitors. Circulation 60:1508, 1979.
3. Funke-Kupper, A.J., Verheugt, F.W.A., Jaarsma, W., et al.: Detection of ventricular thrombosis in acute myocardial infarction: Value of indium-111 platelet scintigraphy in relation to two-dimensional echocardiography and clinical course. Eur. J. Nucl. Med. 12:337, 1986.
4. Funke-Kupper, A.J., Verheugt, F.W.A., Jaarsma, W., et al.: Failure of sulfinpyrazone to prevent left ventricular thrombosis in patients with acute anterior myocardial infarction treated with oral anticoagulants: A randomized trial in 100 patients. Submitted for publication.
5. Funke-Kupper, A.J., Verheugt, F.W.A., Peels, C., et al.: Effect of low-dose acetysalicylic acid on the frequency and hematologic activity of left ventricular thrombus in anterior wall myocardial infarction. Am. J. Cardiol. 63:917, 1989.
6. Finklestein, S., Miller, A., Callahan, R.J., et al.: Imaging of acute arterial injury with ^{111}In-labelled platelets: A comparison with scanning electron micrographs. Radiology 145:155, 1982.
7. Findlay, J.M., Lougheed, W.M., Gentili, F., et al.: Effect of perioperative platelet inhibition on postcarotid endarterectomy mural thrombus formation. J. Neurosurg. 63:693, 1985.
8. Fenech, A., Hussey, J.K., Smith, F.W., et al.: Diagnosis of deep vein thrombosis using autologous indium-111-labelled platelets. Br. Med. J. 282:1020, 1981.
9. Fenech, A., Dendy, P.P., Hussey, J.K., et al.: Indium-111 labelled platelets in diagnosis of leg-vein thrombosis: Preliminary findings. Br. Med. J. 280:1571, 1980.

G

1. Goedemans, W.T., and deJong, M.M.T.: Comparison of several indium-111 ligands in labeling blood cells: Effect of diethylpyrocarbonate and CO_2. J. Nucl. Med. 28:1020, 1987.
2. Goodwin, D.A., Bushberg, J.T., Doherty, P.W., et al.: Indium-111-labelled autologous platelets for location of vascular thrombi in humans. J. Nucl. Med. 19:626, 1978.
3. Goldman, M., Norcott, H.C., Hawker, R.J., et al.: Femoropopliteal bypass grafts—an isotope technique allowing in vivo comparison of thrombogenicity. Br. J. Surg. 69:380, 1982.
4. Goldman, M., Norcott, H.C., Hawker, R.J., et al.: Platelet accumulation on mature Dacron grafts in man. Br. J. Surg. 69(Suppl.):S38, 1982.
5. Grossman, Z.D., Wistow, B.W., McAfee, J.G., et al.: Platelets labelled with oxine complexes of Tc-99m and In-111. Part 2. Localization of experimentally induced vascular lesions. J. Nucl. Med. 19:488, 1978.
6. Goldman, M., Leung, J.O., Aukland, A., et al.: 111-Indium platelet imaging, Doppler spectral analysis and angiography compared in patients with transient cerebral ischaemia. Stroke 14:752, 1983.
7. Grimley, R.P., Rafigi, E., Hawker, R.J., et al.: Imaging of ^{111}In-labelled platelets—a new method for diagnosis of deep vein thrombosis. Br. J. Surg. 68:714, 1981.
8. Goldman, M., McCollum, C.N., Hawker, R.J., et al.: Dacron arterial grafts: The influence of porosity, velour, and maturity on thrombogenicity. Surgery 92:947, 1982.
9. Goldman, M., Hall, C., Dykes, J., et al.: Does ^{111}indium-platelet deposition predict patency in prosthetic arterial grafts? Br. J. Surg. 70:635, 1983.
10. Goldman, M.D., Simpson, D., Hawker, R.J., et al.: Aspirin and dipyridamole reduce platelet deposition on prosthetic femoro-popliteal grafts in man. Ann. Surg. 198:713, 1983.

H

1. Heaton, W.A., Davis, H.H., Welch, M.J., et al.: Indium-111: A new radionuclide label for studying human platelet kinetics. Br. J. Haematol. 42:613, 1979.
2. Hawker, R.J., Hawker, L.M., and Wilkinson, A.R.: Indium (^{111}In)-labelled human platelets: Optimal method. Clin. Sci. 58:243, 1980.
3. Heyns, A. duP., Badenhorst, P.N., Pieters, H., et al.: Preparation of a viable population of indium-111-labelled human blood platelets. Thromb. Haemost. 42:1473, 1980.
4. Heyns, A. duP.: Method for labeling platelets with ^{111}In-oxine. *In* Heyns, A. duP., Badenhorst, P.N., and Lotter, M.G. (eds.): Platelet Kinetics and Imaging. Vol. 1. CRC Press, Boca Raton, Fla., 1985, pp. 153–158.
5. Hill-Zobel, R.L., Gannon, S., McCandless, B., and Tsan, M.-F.: Effects of chelates and incubation media on platelet labeling with indium-111. J. Nucl. Med. 28:223, 1987.
6. Hudson, E.M., Ramsey, R.B., and Evatt, B.L.: Subcellular localization of indium-111 in indium-111-labelled platelets. J. Lab. Clin. Med. 97:577, 1981.
7. Heyns, A. duP., Lotter, M.G., Badenhorst, P.N., et al.: Kinetics, distribution and sites of destruction of ^{111}indium-labelled human platelets. Br. J. Haematol. 44:269, 1980.
8. Heaton, W.A.L.: Indium-111 (^{111}In) and chromium-51 (^{51}Cr) labeling of platelets: Are they comparable? Transfusion 26:16, 1986.
9. Heyns, A. duP., Lotter, M.G., Kotze, H.F., et al.: Quantification of in vivo distribution of platelets labeled with indium-111 oxine. (Letter.) J. Nucl. Med. 23:943, 1982.
10. Heyns, A. duP., Lotter, M.G., Badenhorst, P.N., et al.: Kinetics and fate of

indium-111 oxine-labelled platelets in patients with aortic aneurysms. Arch. Surg. 117:1170, 1982.

11. Hope, A.F., Heyns, A. duP., Lotter, M.G., et al.: Kinetics and sites of sequestration of indium-111-labelled human platelets during cardiopulmonary bypass. J. Thorac. Cardiovasc. Surg. 81:880, 1981.
12. Hill-Zobel, R.L., Pyeritz, R.E., Scheffel, U., et al.: Kinetics and distribution of ^{111}indium-labelled platelets in patients with homocystinuria. N. Engl. J. Med. 307:781, 1982.

I

1. International Committee for Standardization in Hematology: Recommended method for indium-111 platelet survival studies. J. Nucl. Med. 29:564, 1988.
2. Isaka, Y., Kimura, K., Yoneda, S., et al.: Platelet accumulation in carotid atherosclerotic lesions: Semiquantitative analysis with indium-111 platelets and technetium-99m human serum albumin. J. Nucl. Med. 25:556, 1984.
3. Isaka, Y., Kimura, K., Etani, H., et al.: Effect of aspirin and ticlopidine on platelet deposition in carotid atherosclerosis: Assessment by indium-111 platelet scintigraphy. Stroke 17:1215, 1986.
4. Isaka, Y., Kimura, K., Etani, H., et al.: Imaging platelet deposition on Dacron bifurcation grafts in man: Quantification by a dual-tracer method using ^{111}In-labeled platelets and ^{99m}Tc-labeled human serum albumin. Eur. J. Nucl. Med. 11:386, 1986.

J

1. Joist, J.H., Baker, R.K., and Welch, M.J.: Methodologic and basic aspects of indium-111 platelets. Semin. Thromb. Hemost. 9:86, 1983.
2. Joist, J.N., Baker, R.K., Thakur, M.L., and Welch, M.J.: Indium-111-labelled human platelets: Uptake and loss of label and in vitro function of labelled platelets. J. Lab. Clin. Med. 92:829, 1978.

K

1. Klonizakis, I., Peters, A.M., Fitzpatrick, M.L., et al.: Radionuclide distribution following injection of ^{111}indium-labelled platelets. Br. J. Haematol. 46:595, 1980.
2. Kotze, H.F., Lotter, M.G., Heyns, A. duP., et al.: ^{111}In-labelled baboon platelets: The influence of in vivo redistribution and contaminating ^{114m}In on the radiation dose. Nucl. Med. Biol. 14:593, 1987.
3. Kessler, C., Henningsen, H., and Reuther, R.: Der Nachweis intrakardialer Thromben mit der ^{111}In-Plattchenszintigraphie. Nervenarzt 56:311, 1985.
4. Kessler, C., Reuther, R., Berentelg, J., and Kimmig, B.: The clinical use of platelet scintigraphy with 111-In-oxine. J. Neurol. 229:255, 1983.
5. Kessler, C., Henningsen, H., Reuther, R., et al.: Identification of intracardiac thrombi in stroke patients with indium-111 platelet scintigraphy. Stroke 18:63, 1987.
6. Kadir, S., Hill-Zobel, R.L., and Tsan, M.F.: Evaluation of arterial injury due to balloon angioplasty by ^{111}In-labelled platelets. Nucl. Med. 6:324, 1983.
7. Knight, L.C., Primeau, J.L., Siegel, B.A., and Welch, M.J.: Comparison of In-111-labelled platelets and iodinated fibrinogen for the detection of deep vein thrombosis. J. Nucl. Med. 19:891, 1978.
8. Kotze, H.F., Pieters, H., Heyns, A. duP., et al.: Quantification of the thrombogenicity of Dacron aortic prostheses. S. Afr. J. Surg. 24:65, 1986.

L

1. Laws, K.H., Clanton, J.A., Starnes, V.A., et al.: Kinetics and imaging of indium-111-labelled autologous platelets in experimental myocardial infarction. Circulation 67:110, 1983.
2. Lusby, R.J., Ferrell, L.D., Englestad, B.L., et al.: Vessel wall and indium-111 labelled platelet response to carotid endarterectomy. Surgery 93:424, 1983.

M

1. Mortelmans, L., Verbruggen, A., deRoo, M., and Vermylen, J.: Evaluation of three methods of platelet labelling. Nucl. Med. Commun. 7:519, 1986.
2. Mathias, C.J., and Welch, M.J.: Radiolabeling of platelets. Semin. Nucl. Med. 14:118, 1984.
3. Mathias, C.J., and Welch, M.J.: Dual isotope scintigraphy for the detection of platelet deposition. *In* Heyns, A. duP., Badenhorst, P.N., and Lotter, M.G. (eds.): Platelet Kinetics and Imaging. Vol. 1. CRC Press, Boca Raton, Fla., 1985, pp. 89–106.
4. Moser, K.M., and Fedullo, P.F.: Imaging of venous thromboemboli with labelled platelets. Semin. Nucl. Med. 3:188, 1984.
5. Moser, K.M., and Fedullo, P.F.: Imaging of venous thromboemboli with ^{111}In-labeled platelets. *In* Heyns, A. duP., Badenhorst, P.N., and Lotter, M.G. (eds.): Platelet Kinetics and Imaging. Vol. 2. CRC Press, Boca Raton, Fla., 1985, pp. 57–70.

O

1. O'Connor, M.K., Brennan, S.S., and Shanik, D.G.: Indium-111 labeled platelet deposition following transfemoral angiography. Radiology 158:191, 1986.

P

1. Peters, A.M., Klonizakis, I., Lavender, J.P., and Lewis, S.M.: Elution of ^{111}indium from reticuloendothelial cells. J. Clin. Pathol. 35:507, 1982.
2. Peters, A.M., and Lavender, J.P.: Platelet kinetics with indium-111 platelets: Comparison with chromium-51 platelets. Semin. Thromb. Hemost. 9:100, 1983.
3. Powers, W.J., Hopkins, K.T., and Welch, M.J.: Validation of the dual radiotracer method for quantitative In-111 platelet scintigraphy. Thromb. Res. 34:135, 1984.
4. Powers, W.J.: In-111 platelet scintigraphy: Carotid atherosclerosis and stroke. J. Nucl. Med. 25:626, 1984.
5. Pumphrey, C.W., Chesebro, J.H., Dewanjee, M.K., et al.: In vivo quantitation of platelet deposition on human peripheral arterial bypass grafts using indium-111 labelled platelets: Effect of dipyridamole and aspirin. Am. J. Cardiol. 51:796, 1983.
6. Piekarski, A., Drouet, L., Fauchet, M., et al.: Diagnosis of left atrial thrombi using noninvasive techniques: 2D echography and isotopic exploration with indium labelled platelets. *In* Raynaud, C. (ed.): Proceedings of the Third World Congress of Nuclear Medicine and Biology. Pergamon Press, Paris, 1982, pp. 2377–2380.
7. Powers, W.J., Siegel, B.A., Davis, H.H., et al.: Indium-111 platelet scintigraphy in cerebrovascular disease. Neurology 32:938, 1982.
8. Powers, W.J., and Siegel, B.A.: Thrombus imaging with indium-111 platelets. Semin. Thromb. Hemost. 9:115, 1983.
9. Pope, C.F., Ezekowitz, M.D., Smith, E.O., et al.: Detection of platelet deposition at the site of peripheral balloon angioplasty using indium-111 platelet scintigraphy. Am. J. Cardiol. 55:495, 1985.
10. Powers, W.J., Mathias, C.J., Welch, M.J., et al.: Scintigraphic detection of platelet deposition in atherosclerotic macaques: A new technique for investigation of anti-thrombotic drugs. Thromb. Res. 25:137, 1982.

R

1. Robertson, J.S., Dewanjee, M.K., Brown, M.L., et al.: Distribution and dosimetry of ^{111}In-labelled platelets. Radiology 140:169, 1981.
2. Riba, A.L., Thakur, M.L., Gottschalk, A., and Zaret, B.L.: Imaging experimental coronary artery thrombosis with indium-111 platelets. Circulation 60:767, 1979.
3. Romson, J.L., Hook, B.G., Rigot, V.H., et al.: The effect of ibuprofen on accumulation of indium-111-labelled platelets and leukocytes in experimental myocardial infarction. Circulation 66:1002, 1982.
4. Riba, A.L., Thakur, M.L., Gottschalk, A., et al.: Imaging experimental infectious endocarditis with indium-111-labelled blood cellular components. Circulation 59:336, 1979.
5. Ritchie, J.L., Stratton, J.R., Thiele, B., et al.: Indium-111 platelet imaging for detection of platelet deposition in abdominal aneurysms and prosthetic grafts. Am. J. Cardiol. 47:882, 1981.
6. Robicsek, F., Duncan, G.D., Anderson, C.E., et al.: Indium-111-labeled platelet deposition in woven and knitted Dacron bifurcated aortic grafts with the same patient as a clinical model. J. Vasc. Surg. 5:833, 1987.
7. Ritchie, J.L., Lindner, A., Hamilton, G.W., and Harker, L.A.: ^{111}Indium-oxine platelet imaging in hemodialysis patients: Detection of platelet deposition at vascular access sites. Nephron 31:333, 1982.

S

1. Scheffel, U., Tsan, M., and McIntyre, P.A.: Labelling of human platelets with (^{111}In) 8-hydroxyquinoline. J. Nucl. Med. 20:524, 1979.
2. Schmidt, K.G., and Rasmussen, J.W.: Labelling of human and rabbit platelets with ^{111}indium-oxine complex. Scand. J. Haematol. 23:97, 1979.
3. Sinzinger, H., Kolbe, H., Strobl-Jager, E., and Hofer, R.: A simple and safe technique for sterile autologous platelet labeling using "Monovette" vials. Eur. J. Nucl. Med. 9:320, 1984.
4. Sharefkin, J., and Rich, N.M.: Technical considerations in the study of indium-111-oxine labelled platelet survival patterns in dogs. Lab. Anim. Sci. 32:183, 1982.
5. Schmidt, K.G., Rasmussen, J.W., and Arendrup, H.: Function ex vivo of ^{111}In-labelled platelets: Simultaneous aggregation of labelled and unlabelled platelets induced by collagen. Scand. J. Haematol. 29:51, 1982.
6. Schmidt, K.G., Rasmussen, J.W., and Lorentzen, M.: Function and morphology of ^{111}In-labelled platelets: In vitro, in vivo and ex vivo studies. Haemostasis 11:193, 1982.
7. Stratton, J.R., Ballem, P.J., Gernsheimer, T., et al.: Platelet destruction in autoimmune thrombocytopenic purpura: Quantitation of platelet kinetics and sites of clearance using indium-111-labeled autologous platelets. J. Nucl. Med. 30:629, 1989.
8. Slichter, S.J., and Harker, L.A.: Preparation and storage of platelet concentrates. I. Factors influencing the harvest of viable platelets from whole blood. Br. J. Haematol. 34:395, 1976.
9. Schmidt, K.G., Rasmussen, J.W., Rasmussen, A.D., and Arendrup, H.: Comparative studies of the in vivo kinetics of simultaneously injected ^{111}In- and ^{51}Cr-labeled human platelets. Scand. J. Haematol. 30:465, 1983.
10. Stratton, J.R., Ritchie, J.L., Hamilton, G.W., et al.: Left ventricular thrombi: In vivo detection by indium-111 platelet imaging and two-dimensional echocardiography. Am. J. Cardiol. 47:874, 1981.
11. Stratton, J.R., and Ritchie, J.L.: Effect of suloctidil on tomographically quantitated platelet accumulation in Dacron aortic grafts. Am. J. Cardiol. 58:152, 1986.
12. Stratton, J.R., and Ritchie, J.L.: Reduction of indium-111 platelet deposition on Dacron vascular grafts in humans by aspirin plus dipyridamole. Circulation 73:325, 1986.
13. Stratton, J.R., Thiele, B.L., and Ritchie, J.L.: Platelet deposition on Dacron aortic bifurcation grafts in man: Quantitation with indium-111 platelet imaging. Circulation 66:1287, 1982.

14. Sherman, D.G., Dylan, M.L., Fisher, M., et al.: Cerebral embolism. Chest 89:82S, 1986.
15. Stratton, J.R., Ritchie, J.L., Werner, J.A., et al.: Indium-111 platelet imaging for the detection of intracardiac thrombi in survivors of sudden cardiac death. (Abstract.) Clin. Res. 28:68A, 1980.
16. Stratton, J.R., and Ritchie, J.L.: The effects of antithrombotic drugs in patients with left ventricular thrombi: Assessment with indium-111 platelet imaging and two-dimensional echocardiography. Circulation 69:561, 1984.
17. Seabold, J.E., Schroder, E., Conrad, G.R., et al.: Indium-111 platelet scintigraphy and two-dimensional echocardiography for detection of left ventricular thrombus: Influence of clot size and age. J. Am. Coll. Cardiol. 9:1057, 1988.
18. Stratton, J.R., and Ritchie, J.L.: Indium-111 platelet imaging of left ventricular thrombi: Predictive value for systemic emboli. Circulation 81:1182, 1990.
19. Sutherland, G.R., King, M.E., Peerless, S.J., et al.: Platelet interaction within giant intracranial aneurysms. J. Neurosurg. 36:53, 1982.
20. Stratton, J.R., Zierler, R.E., and Kazmers, A.: Platelet deposition at carotid endarterectomy sites in man. Stroke 18:722, 1987.
21. Sinzinger, H., Fitscha, P., O'Grady, J., et al.: Detection of aneurysms by gamma-camera imaging after injection of autologous labelled platelets. Lancet 2:1365, 1984.
22. Sinzinger, H., and Fitscha, P.: Scintigraphic detection of femoral artery atherosclerosis with 111-indium-labelled autologous platelets. Vasa 13:350, 1984.
23. Seabold, J.E., Conrad, G.R., Ponto, J.A., et al.: Deep venous thrombophlebitis: Detection with 4-hour versus 24-hour platelet scintigraphy. Radiology 165:335, 1987.
24. Sostman, H.D., Neumann, R.D., Zoghbi, S.S., et al.: Experimental studies with ^{111}indium-labelled platelets in pulmonary embolism. Invest. Radiol. 17:367, 1982.
25. Sostman, H.D., Neumann, R.D., Loke, J., et al.: Detection of pulmonary embolism in man with ^{111}In-labelled autologous platelets. Am. J. Radiol. 38:945, 1982.
26. Stratton, J.R.: Platelet kinetics and imaging of prosthetic materials. *In* Heyns, A. duP., Badenhorst, P.N., and Lotter, M.G. (eds.): Platelet Kinetics and Imaging. Vol. 2. CRC Press, Boca Raton, Fla., 1985, pp. 21–44.
27. Stratton, J.R., Thiele, B.L., and Ritchie, J.L.: Natural history of platelet deposition on Dacron aortic bifurcation grafts in the first year after implantation. Am. J. Cardiol. 52:371, 1983.
28. Schmidt, K.G., and Rasmussen, J.W.: Scintigraphic visualization of haemostatic and thromboembolic processes using ^{111}indium-labelled platelets. Acta Med. Scand. 215:173, 1984.
29. Sinzinger, H., O'Grady, J., Fitscha, P., and Kaliman, J.: Effect of epoprostenol on platelet deposition on synthetic arterial grafts. (Letter.) Lancet 2:1212, 1984.
30. Stratton, J.R., and Ritchie, J.L.: Failure of ticlopidine to inhibit deposition of indium-111 labeled platelets on Dacron prosthetic surfaces in humans. Circulation 69:677, 1984.
31. Stratton, J.R., Thiele, B.L., and Ritchie, J.L.: The effect of sulfinpyrazone on platelet deposition on Dacron vascular grafts in man. Am. Heart J. 3:453, 1985.

T

1. Thakur, M.L., Welch, M.J., Joist, J.H., and Coleman, R.E.: Indium-111 labelled platelets: Studies on preparation and evaluation of in vitro and in vivo functions. Thromb. Res. 9:345, 1976.
2. Thakur, M.L.: Radioisotopic labelling of platelets: A historical perspective. Semin. Thromb. Hemost. 9:79, 1983.
3. Thakur, M.L., Walsh, L., Malech, H., and Gottschalk, A.: Indium-111-labelled human platelets: Improved method, efficacy, and evaluation. J. Nucl. Med. 22:381, 1981.
4. Thakur, M.L., and McKenney, S.M.: Indium-111-mercaptopyridine *N*-oxide-labeled human leukocytes and platelets: Mechanism of labeling and intracellular location of ^{111}In and mercaptopyridine *N*-oxide. J. Lab. Clin. Med. 107:141, 1986.
5. Thakur, M.L., McKenney, S.L., and Park, C.H.: Simplified and efficient labeling of human platelets in plasma using indium-111-2-mercaptopyridine-*N*-oxide: Preparation and evaluation. J. Nucl. Med. 26:510, 1985.
6. Thakur, M.H.: Radionuclides and chelates used for platelet labeling. *In* Heyns, A. duP., Badenhorst, P.N., and Lotter, M.G. (eds.): Platelet Kinetics and Imaging. Vol. 1. CRC Press, Boca Raton, Fla., 1985, pp. 23–34.
7. Thakur, M.L., and Sedar, A.W.: Ultrastructure of human platelets following indium-111 labeling in plasma. Nucl. Med. Commun. 8:69, 1987.
8. Thakur, M.W.: A look at radiolabeled blood cells. Nucl. Med. Biol. 13:147, 1986.
9. Takeda, T., Ishikawa, N., Sakakibara, Y., et al.: A giant tumor thrombus in the right atrium clearly detected by ^{111}In-oxine labeled platelet scintigraphy. Eur. J. Nucl. Med. 11:49, 1985.

V

1. Vallabhajosula, S., Machac, J., Goldsmith, S.J., et al.: Indium-111 platelet kinetics in normal human subjects: Tropolone versus oxine methods. J. Nucl. Med. 27:1669, 1986.
2. van Reenen, O.R., Lotter, M.G., Minnaar, P.C., et al.: Radiation dose from human platelets labelled with indium-111. Br. J. Radiol. 53:790, 1980.
3. van Reenen, O., Lotter, M.G., Heyns, A. duP., et al.: Quantification of the distribution of ^{111}In-labelled platelets in organs. Eur. J. Nucl. Med. 7:80, 1982.
4. Verheugt, F.W., Lindenfeld, J., Kirch, D.L., and Steele, P.P.: Left ventricular platelet deposition after acute myocardial infarction: An attempt at quantification using blood pool subtracted indium-111 platelet scintigraphy. Br. Heart J. 52:490, 1984.
5. Vandenberg, B.F., Seabold, J.E., Schroder, E., and Kerber, R.E.: Noninvasive imaging of left ventricular thrombi: Two-dimensional echocardiography and indium-111 platelet scintigraphy. Am. J. Cardiac Imag. 1:289, 1987.
6. Vandenberg, B.F., Seabold, J.E., Conrad, G.R., et al.: Indium-111 platelet scintigraphy and two-dimensional echocardiography for the detection of left atrial appendage thrombi: Studies in a new canine model. Circulation 78:1040, 1988.

W

1. Wistow, B.W., Grossman, Z.P., McAfee, J.G., et al.: Labelling of platelets with oxine complexes of Tc-99m and In-111. Part I. In vitro studies and survival in the rabbit. J. Nucl. Med. 19:483, 1978.
2. Wakefield, T.W., Lindblad, B., Graham, L.M., et al.: Nuclide imaging of vascular graft-platelet interactions: Comparison of indium excess and technetium subtraction techniques. J. Surg. Res. 40:388, 1986.
3. Wu, K.K., Chen, Y.-C., Fordham, E., et al.: Differential effects of two doses of aspirin on platelet-vessel wall interaction in vivo. J. Clin. Invest. 68:382, 1981.
4. Winter, J.H., Fenech, A., Bennett, B., and Douglas, A.S.: Preoperative antithrombin-III activities and lipoprotein concentrations as predictors of venous thrombosis in patients with fracture of neck of femur. J. Clin. Pathol. 36:570, 1983.
5. Winter, J.H., Buckler, A.W., Bartista, A.P., et al.: Frequency of venous thrombosis in patients with an exacerbation of chronic obstructive lung disease. Thorax 38:605, 1983.
6. Winter, J.H., Fenech, A., Mackie, M., et al.: Treatment of venous thrombosis in antithrombin III deficient patients with concentrates of antithrombin III. Clin. Lab. Haemat. 4:101, 1982.

Y

1. Yamada, M., Hoki, N., Ishikawa, K., et al.: Detection of left atrial thrombi in man using indium-111 labelled autologous platelets. Br. Heart J. 51:298, 1984.
2. Yui, T., Uchida, T., Matsuda, S., et al.: Detection of platelet consumption in aortic graft with ^{111}In-labelled platelets. Eur. J. Nucl. Med. 7:77, 1982.

Chapter 64

Imaging Cardiac Neurons and Receptors

■ MICHAEL W. DAE, M.D. ■ ELIAS H. BOTVINICK, M.D.

SCINTIGRAPHIC ASSESSMENT OF SYMPATHETIC INNERVATION 1135
Radiolabeled Metaiodobenzylguanidine 1135
Experimental Evidence for Neuronal Localization of Metaiodobenzylguanidine .. 1135
Metaiodobenzylguanidine Uptake After Myocardial Infarction 1136
Initial Clinical Experience 1137
ADRENERGIC AND CHOLINERGIC RECEPTOR IMAGING 1138
CONCLUSION 1139

One of the new areas in conventional radionuclide studies relates to imaging cardiac nerves and receptors. This is a potentially very exciting area of investigation that may eventually have some clinical relevance. In theory, receptors and nerves can be imaged with radionuclide techniques if the appropriate ligands and isotopes can be joined together to form the appropriate nuclide. At the present time, most activity in this area has focused on the imaging of the adrenergic nerves and, hence, this chapter concentrates primarily on this area.

The heart is richly innervated with sympathetic nerves, which are distributed on a regional basis.[R1] The sympathetic nervous system has been implicated in the pathophysiology of numerous clinical disorders of cardiac function.[M2] However, a detailed assessment of myocardial sympathetic nerve innervation, particularly in vivo, has not been practical until recently.

SCINTIGRAPHIC ASSESSMENT OF SYMPATHETIC INNERVATION

In order for observations of animal experiments demonstrating the role of sympathetic innervation on myocardial pathophysiology to be applicable to humans, noninvasive assessment of changes in sympathetic innervation must be possible. The ability of sympathetic nerve endings to take up exogenously administered catecholamines is well established. Axelrod and associates[A1] and Whitby and co-workers[W1] showed rapid accumulation of ^{3}H-norepinephrine and ^{3}H-epinephrine in heart, spleen, and other peripheral tissues in cats and mice. Many subsequent reports have confirmed the existence of a high-affinity, neuronal uptake mechanism confined to postganglionic sympathetic nerves (uptake 1), and a low-affinity, high-capacity extraneuronal uptake mechanism (uptake 2).[I1] Tracer amounts of injected radiolabeled catecholamines are largely distributed to neuronal sites. However, even at low concentrations, extraneuronal uptake has been shown to occur.[L1] Neuronally bound catecholamines are generally sequestered in storage vesicles and retained for long periods of time; whereas, in the case of norepinephrine, the extraneuronal material is rapidly metabolized and washes out of the myocardium at a fairly rapid rate.[LI] ^{11}C–norepinephrine has been used to provide an image of the isolated dog heart.[C1] However, owing to the significant metabolism of the agent, the distribution was not limited to sympathetic nerves.

Radiolabeled Metaiodobenzylguanidine

Previous studies have demonstrated the affinity of radioiodinated metaiodobenzylguanidine (MIBG) (Fig. 64–1), an analog of guanethidine, an adrenergic-blocking agent, for the adrenal medullae and adrenergic nerves.[W2] Myocardial localization has been demonstrated with MIBG in several animal species and in humans.[K1] MIBG is thought to have the same uptake and storage mechanisms as norepinephrine[M2] but is not metabolized by monoamine oxidase or catechol-o-methyl transferase.[W3]

Experimental Evidence for Neuronal Localization of Metaiodobenzylguanidine

A few early reports suggested that MIBG was localized to sympathetic nerves. Reserpine, which blocks the vesicular uptake of norepinephrine in adrenergic neurons, caused a marked decrease in canine myocardial concentration of MIBG.[W3] Nakajo and colleagues[N1] found an inverse relationship between the accumulation of ^{131}-I-MIBG in the heart and the plasma concentration of catecholamines, suggesting competitive uptake of ^{131}-I-MIBG by the heart with circulating catecholamines. Salivary gland uptake of MIBG was blocked by the administration of tricyclic antidepressants, which are known to inhibit neuronal uptake of norepinephrine.[N2]

Several recent studies have more thoroughly evaluated the characteristics of MIBG uptake and distribution. Sisson and associates[S1] assessed the uptake of ^{125}I-MIBG in rat hearts subjected to various interventions to disrupt the sympathetic nerves. They observed reduced MIBG uptake in hearts treated with 6-hydroxydopamine, which has been shown to cause a chemical degeneration of sympathetic nerves. Pretreatment with the uptake I inhibitor desmethylimipramine also leads to a significant inhibition of MIBG uptake. In addition, substantial fractions of MIBG were released from the heart by the sympathomimetic drug phenylpropanolamine. The responses of MIBG to pertubations of sympathetic nerves were qualitatively similar to the responses of ^{3}H-norepinephrine.

To facilitate the assessment of myocardial sympathetic activity, we developed a new method using ^{123}I-labeled MIBG to map the distribution of sympathetic nerve endings, and thallium-201 (^{201}Tl) to map the distribution of myocardial perfusion simultaneously.[D1]

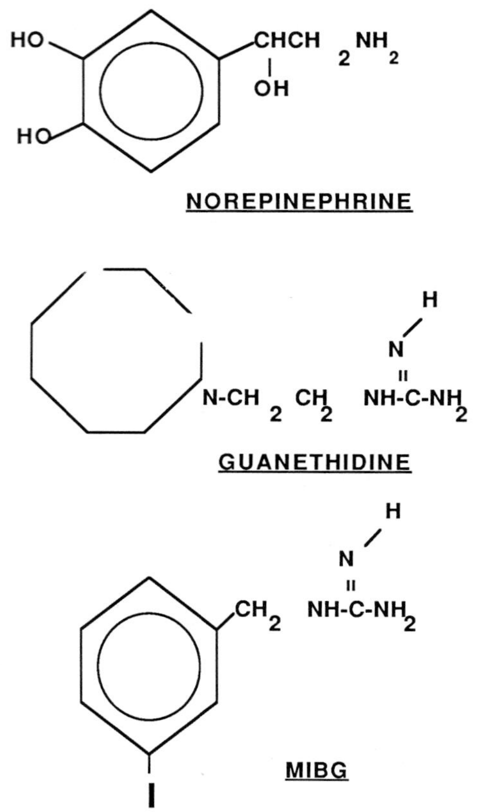

HO CHCH2NH2 OH HO

NOREPINEPHRINE

H N N-CH2CH2 NH-C-NH2

GUANETHIDINE

H N CH2 NH-C-NH2 I

MIBG

Figure 64–1. Shown are the chemical structures for metaiodobenzylguanidine, guanethidine, and norepinephrine.

In a series of in vitro phantom studies, we determined that imaging the two isotopes (^{123}I and ^{201}Tl) simultaneously was feasible owing to the difference in their energy spectra. Thallium has a major photopeak at 80 KeV and ^{123}I has a major peak at 159 KeV. With equal amounts of the two isotopes, the signal-to-noise ratio for imaging thallium in the presence of ^{123}I was $> 10:1$, and for imaging ^{123}I in the presence of thallium, greater than 6:1. We developed a computer-derived functional image that allows the spatial display of two independent variables in a single image using color coding (Fig. 64–2). With this functional map, we are able to display regional changes in MIBG uptake relative to the underlying myocardial perfusion.

Figure 64–2. See Color Plate 16.

To assess the feasibility of detecting altered sympathetic innervation noninvasively, we compared the distribution of ^{123}I-MIBG with myocardial perfusion in normal and regionally denervated dog hearts. Regional denervation was created by removing the left or right stellate ganglion and by application of phenol to the epicardial surface. Images were taken 3 hours after the injection of MIBG to allow washout of the non-neuronally bound radionuclide. Normal hearts showed a homogeneous distribution of MIBG and thallium in the left ventricle (Fig. 64–3). There was a striking decrease of myocardial localization in the posterior left ventricle in left-stellectomized hearts, whereas the distribution of thallium was homogeneous (Fig. 64–4). The anterior left ventricle showed reduced localization of MIBG in right-stellectomized hearts (Figs. 64–5 and 64–6). Phenol-treated hearts showed a broad area of reduced MIBG extending beyond the area of phenol application (Fig. 64–7). Regions of reduced MIBG uptake showed significant reductions in tissue norepinephrine content, confirming denervation. MIBG efflux kinetics were assessed in these same animals by analyzing regional MIBG washout between initial images (5 to 15 minutes after injection), and delayed images (3 hours after injection) with the aid of a color-coded washout map.[D2] Denervated areas showed a large degree of washout, whereas normally innervated regions showed little change in activity, or slight washin. These patterns are consistent with the more rapid efflux of MIBG from non-neuronal compartments, as has been reported for radiolabeled norepinephrine.[P1] Sisson and co-workers have also shown reduced MIBG uptake in regionally denervated dog hearts.[S2]

Figure 64–3. See Color Plate 16.

Figure 64–5. See Color Plate 16.

Figure 64–6. See Color Plate 16.

Figure 64–7. See Color Plate 16.

To further assess the degree of neuronal uptake of MIBG, we studied dogs at baseline and at one week after the intravenous injection of 50 mg/kg of ^{6}OH-dopamine,[D3] which has been shown to cause degeneration of sympathetic nerve endings.[T1] At baseline, there was homogeneous uptake of MIBG on initial images, with retention of MIBG and a homogeneous pattern at 3 hours. All of the globally denervated dog hearts showed homogeneous uptake of MIBG initially but near complete washout of MIBG at three hours, adding further support to the fact that MIBG localization on the delayed images represents accumulation in sympathetic nerve endings.

We assessed the functional implications of MIBG uptake in regionally denervated dog hearts. We measured the contractile response to stellate stimulation, tyramine infusion, and isoproterenol (Isuprel) infusion using implanted ultrasonic crystals in innervated and denervated regions as determined by MIBG distribution.[M3] Studies were done immediately (within 1 to 2 hours) and after an extended period of time (3 to 7 days) after phenol application. The phenolized regions in the later preparations showed a marked decrease in MIBG uptake at the lateral and posterior left ventricle and a significant reduction in norepinephrine content (see Fig. 64–7). There was no augmentation in the contractile response of the phenolized region in response to stellate stimulation or to intracoronary tyramine infusion, whereas the normally innervated anterior left ventricle showed a significant increase in fractional shortening with both interventions. Both the phenolized area and the normal area, however, showed an increase in fractional shortening in response to isoproterenol infusion. These results indicate that the decreased MIBG uptake is associated with functional evidence of sympathetic denervation, and that the postsynaptic responses to β-receptor stimulation by isoproterenol, which is not taken up by nerve endings, is maintained.

The functional responses to sympathetic nerve stimulation in acutely sympathectomized regions, however, were dissociated from the biochemical and uptake responses of sympathetic nerve endings. In dogs studied immediately after application of phenol (1 to 2 hours), the contractile response to stellate stimulation was diminished in the phenolized region, whereas MIBG uptake and tissue norepinephrine were normal. These findings indicate that the metabolic function of sympathetic nerve endings can continue for some time after the acute loss of neurotransmission. The exact time required for nerve degeneration to occur is unknown. However, it is present as early as 3 days after nerve damage. Morphologic confirmation of the absence of sympathetic nerve fluorescence in regions of decreased MIBG uptake has also been obtained (see later section).

Metaiodobenzylguanidine Uptake After Myocardial Infarction

It was recently demonstrated that transmural myocardial infarction produces necrosis of nerves coursing in the epicardium,

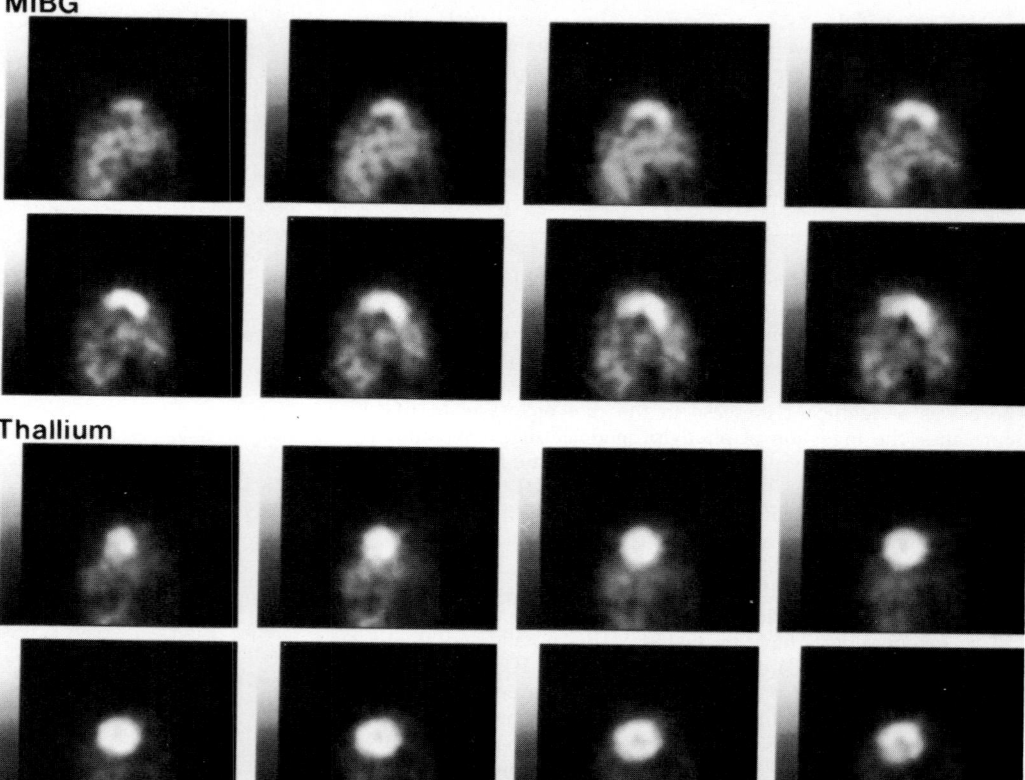

Figure 64–4. Shown here are dual isotope emission computed tomograms from a dog with left stellectomy. MIBG images *(upper rows)* show a region of decreased uptake at the posterior left ventricle, whereas the corresponding thallium images show normal perfusion to this area, indicating regional denervation of the posterior left ventricle. (From Dae, M. W., O'Connell, J. W., Botvinick, E. H., et al.: Scintigraphic assessment of regional cardiac adrenergic innervation. Circulation 79:634–644, 1989, by permission of the American Heart Association, Inc.)

leading to viable but denervated myocardium.[B1] This partial denervation may produce imbalanced sympathetic innervation, which, during enhanced sympathetic tone, may predispose the heart to arrhythmia.[H1] To assess the feasibility of detecting denervated myocardium after transmural infarction, we compared the distribution of MIBG with that of thallium in dogs studied 4 to 7 days after latex injection of either the left anterior descending artery (LAD) or its first diagonal to create a transmural myocardial infarction.[D4] Tissue samples were also assessed for norepinephrine content. All of the infarcted dogs showed reduced MIBG relative to thallium both distal and lateral to the zone of scar, indicating denervated but viable perfused myocardium. Regions proximal to the infarct showed balanced MIBG and thallium uptake as in normal dogs (Fig. 64–8). Norepinephrine content from the region of decreased MIBG relative to thallium was lower (112 ± 139 ng/gm) than that from basal regions (698 ± 66 ng/gm, $p < .002$). The basal regions showed normal-appearing sympathetic nerve fluorescence and normal histology by H & E staining, whereas the denervated regions did not show nerve fluorescence in muscle with normal histology (Fig. 64–9).

Figure 64–8. See Color Plate 17.

Figure 64–9. See Color Plate 17.

Minardo and associates[M4] performed MIBG scintigraphy in dogs at various times after epicardial phenol application and transmural myocardial infarction produced by latex injection into the diagonal coronary artery. They correlated the image patterns with electrophysiologic responses obtained during sympathetic stimulation and norepinephrine infusion. They found apical defects on the MIBG images that were associated with either normal thallium perfusion in the phenol-treated dogs or much smaller thallium defects in the infarcted dogs.

During ansae subclavian stimulation, the apical regions showed less refractory period shortening than regions at normal basal myocardium. However, during norepinephrine infusion, the effective refractory period shortened more at the apex than at the base. These findings were thought to be consistent with apical sympathetic denervation and supersensitivity to norepinephrine. Serial imaging studies in another group of dogs showed normalization after a mean of 14 weeks. During ansae subclavian stimulation in these dogs, the effective refractory period shortened equally at the apex and base. These results were consistent with apical sympathetic reinnervation. An interesting finding, however, was the persistence of the supersensitive response to infused norepinephrine in the apical regions.

Initial Clinical Experience

Few studies have assessed the myocardial localization of MIBG in pathologic situations. In 12 individuals, including five with normal hearts and seven patients studied 2 weeks to 7 years after myocardial infarction, we studied the distribution of MIBG and thallium using functional maps.[D4] The normal human patients showed the homogeneous parallel distribution of MIBG and thallium, as in normal dogs. Patients with infarcts showed reduced MIBG relative to thallium in a zone of myocardium generally apical and lateral to the zone of scar, indicating the presence of viable but denervated myocardium (Fig. 64–10). Six of the seven patients were initially referred for electrophysiologic testing because of a history of sustained ventricular tachycardia, and two patients also had associated ventricular fibrillation. In a preliminary investigation, Tuli and colleagues have also detected denervated myocardium in human subjects after myocardial infarction.[T2] Single-photon emission computed tomography (SPECT) MIBG and thallium imaging was done in eight patients with spontaneous ventricular tachycardia. Areas of reduced MIBG uptake in the presence of thallium uptake were found in seven. Six of the seven had inducible sustained ventricular tachycardia at control electrophysiologic testing and after the intravenous administration of 15 mg of metoprolol. One patient with a large area of denervation developed repetitive nonsustained ventricular tachycardia during exercise testing that was suppressed by metoprolol.

Figure 64–10. See Color Plate 17.

Sisson and associates[S3] studied MIBG uptake 2 to 4 hours after injection in 20 control subjects and assessed the responses to perturbations in autonomic function. They demonstrated a 50 percent reduction in MIBG uptake after the administration of imipramine, a tricyclic antidepressant and uptake 1 inhibitor. There was a significant increase in the rate of loss of MIBG 4 hours after the ingestion of phenylpropanolamine, a sypathomimetic drug that acts by displacing norepinephrine from neurons. Following exercise, the blood levels of both MIBG and norepinephrine increased significantly. Five patients with generalized autonomic neuropathy showed markedly reduced uptake of MIBG in the heart. Nakajo and co-workers[N3] showed rapid washout of MIBG from the heart in three patients with generalized adrenergic dysfunction.

Two recent reports have evaluated MIBG uptake and kinetics in patients with dilated cardiomyopathy. Henderson and associates[H2] studied 16 patients with severe dilated cardiomyopathy and 14 healthy volunteers. Tomographic images were obtained 15 minutes and 85 minutes after injection of ^{123}I-MIBG. There were no significant differences in MIBG concentrations on the initial images between the hearts of patients with dilated cardiomyopathy and controls. Myocardial retention of MIBG was significantly reduced in the patients with cardiomyopathy on the delayed images, however (Fig. 64–11). These results are similar to our findings in globally denervated dog hearts,[D3] raising the possibility of diminished myocardial innervation as a significant factor in explaining the image findings in these patients. Also, patients with congestive cardiomyopathy had significantly greater heterogeneity in the distribution of MIBG, suggesting the possibility of imbalanced innervation. Henderson and colleagues concluded from these studies that because of the significant differences in MIBG distribution and kinetics between normals and patients with dilated cardiomyopathy, MIBG scintigraphy may provide a noninvasive means to evaluate the severity of altered adrenergic innervation in the hearts of these patients.

Schofer and associates studied MIBG uptake patterns in 28 patients with idiopathic dilated cardiomyopathy.[S4] They compared the ratio of myocardial MIBG activity versus mediastinal MIBG activity and found a significant correlation with left ventricular ejection fraction and with myocardial norepinephrine content analyzed from biopsy samples obtained at cardiac catheterization, but not with plasma catecholamine concentrations.

Further studies are needed to evaluate the functional and prognostic significance of MIBG scintigraphic patterns in patients with heart failure, ischemic heart disease, and other conditions that may relate to derangements in sympathetic activity. These initial results are very promising, however.

ADRENERGIC AND CHOLINERGIC RECEPTOR IMAGING

Cardiac β-adrenergic receptors have been studied extensively using radioligand-binding experiments on isolated membrane preparations. Recent studies have indicated the feasibility of imaging β-receptors in vivo.[H3] Hughes and co-workers demonstrated uptake of ^{131}I-pindolol in the heart and lungs of rabbits. This accumulation was blocked by l-propranolol, consistent with localization in β-receptors. A major problem with this agent is the relatively high degree of nonspecific binding, which represents about 50 to 60 percent of total binding.[H3] Hughes and colleagues suggested an approach for correcting for nonspecific binding by labeling the d-stereoisomer, which showed diffuse and nonspecific uptake, and subtracting the nonspecific uptake from total uptake. They proposed the use of ^{123}I-pindolol for nonspecific binding and ^{131}I-l pindolol for total binding.

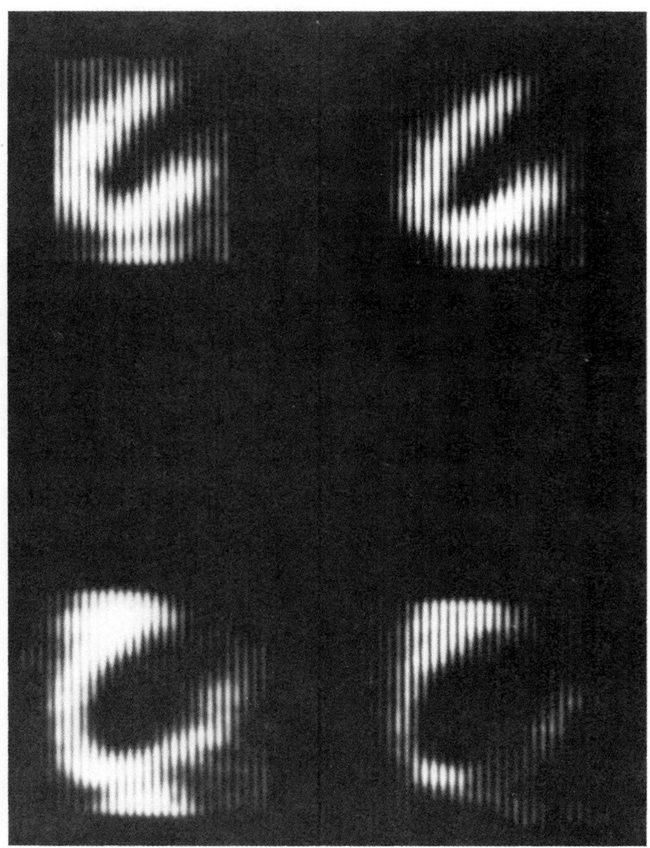

Figure 64–11. Immediate (*left*) and delayed (*right*) vertical long-axis images from a control subject (*top*) and a patient with cardiomyopathy (*bottom*) demonstrate the diminished myocardial retention of MIBG in the patient. The control had a 9 percent washout rate compared with a 33 percent washout rate in the patient. (From Henderson, E. B., Kahn, J. K., Corbett, J. R., et al.: Abnormal I-123 metaiodobenzylguanidine myocardial washout and distribution may reflect myocardial adrenergic derangement in patients with congestive cardiomyopathy. Circulation 78:1192–1199, 1988, by permission of the American Heart Association, Inc.)

A high degree of pulmonary uptake remains a significant limitation to imaging β-receptor density. Sisson and associates recently showed the feasibility of imaging β-receptors in dog hearts using ^{123}I-iodocyanopindolol.[S5] They inhibited the pulmonary uptake of ^{123}I-iodocyanopindolol by injecting a selective β_2 antagonist, ICI 118,551, which blocked uptake in the pulmonary β-receptors, which are primarily β^2-receptors. The doses used did not affect binding of ^{123}I-iodocyanopindolol to cardiac β-receptors, which are primarily β^1-receptors. A twofold increase in the lung-to-heart ratio was achieved.[S6]

Studies demonstrating β-receptor imaging using positron-emitting radioligands have also been very encouraging (see Chapter 69).

Imaging of muscarinic cholinergic receptors with positron agents (^{11}C-MQNB) has been very successful in animal and human studies.[S7] Radioiodinated quinuclidinyl benzilate (QNB) has not resulted in a useful imaging agent for cardiac muscarinic cholinergic receptors, however.[E1]

The iodination of QNB alters the stereospecficity of the compound such that 4-IQNB favors the M_1-subtype of muscarine receptors thought to be located primarily in the central nervous system. Specific binding in the heart is low for 4-IQNB because the heart contains the M_2 muscarinic receptor subtype.[E1] Further investigations to find alternative derivatives of QNB are needed.

CONCLUSION

Recent studies with MIBG are extremely promising. To date, the results have shown that imaging of myocardial sympathetic nerve distribution is feasible and that alterations in innervation in various disease states can be characterized. This new capability may provide clinically useful approaches to enhance the understanding of the pathophysiology of altered adrenergic function in patients and may lead to new diagnostic strategies. Although less well explored, the imaging of β-receptors seems possible and may provide new and important complementary information to allow a more comprehensive assessment of sympathetic influences in the heart. Image characterization of parasympathetic influences remains a major unresolved challenge.

References

A

1. Axelrod, J., Weil-Mahherbe, H., and Tomchick, R.: The physiological disposition of 3H-epinephrine and its metabolite, metanephrine. J. Pharmacol. Exp. Ther. 127:251–256, 1959.

B

1. Barber, M.J., Mueller, T.M., Henry, D.P., et al.: Transmural myocardial infarction in the dog produces sympathectomy in noninfarcted myocardium. Circulation 67:787, 1983.

C

1. Carr, E. A.: The development of radiotracers that are substrates for catecholamine uptake 1 and uptake 2. *In* Lambrecht, R.M., and Eckelman, W.C. (eds): Animals Models in Radiotracer Design. Springer-Verlag, New York, pp 35–59, 1981.

D

1. Dae, M.W., O'Connell, J.W., Botvinick, E.W., et al.: Scintigraphic assessment of regional cardiac adrenergic innervation. Circulation 79:634–644, 1989.
2. Dae, M., Botvinick, E., O'Connell, J., et al.: Regional MIBG washout parallels regional sympathetic innervation. J. Nucl. Med. 28:746, 1987.
3. Dae, M., O'Connell. J., Chin, M., et al.: Scintigraphic assessment of global adrenergic nerve density with MIBG washout maps. J. Am. Coll. Card. 11:214, 1988.
4. Dae, M., Herre, J., Botvinick, E., et al.: Scintigraphic assessment of adrenergic innervation after myocardial infarction. Circulation 74:II297, 1986.

E

1. Exkelman, W.C.: Receptors labeled with gamma-emitting radiotracers. Int. J. Rad. Appl. Instrum. (B) 13:135–139, 1986.

H

1. Herre, J., Wetstein, L., Lin, Y.L., et al.: Effect of transmural versus nontransmural myocardial infarction on inducibility of ventricular arrhythmias during sympathetic stimulation. J. Am. Coll. Cardiol. 11:414–421, 1988.
2. Henderson, E.B., Kahn, J.K., Corbett, J.R., et al.: Abnormal I-123 metaiodobenzylguanidine myocardial washout and distribution may reflect myocardial adrenergic derangement in patients with congestive cardiomyopathy. Circulation 78:1192–1199, 1988.
3. Hughes, B., Marshall, D.R., Sobel, B.E., and Bergmann, S.R.: Characterization of beta-adrenoreceptors in vivo with iodine-131 pindolol and gamma scintigraphy. J. Nucl. Med. 27:660–667, 1986.

I

1. Iversen, L.L.: Role of transmitter uptake mechanisms in synaptic neurotransmission. Br. J. Pharmacol. 41:571–591, 1971.

K

1. Kline, R.C., Swanson, D.P., Wieland, D.M., et al.: Myocardial imaging in man with I-123 meta-iodobenzylguanidine. J. Nucl. Med. 22:129–32, 1981.

L

1. Lightman, S.L., and Iversen, L.L.: The role of uptake in the extraneuronal metabolism of catecholamines in the isolated rat heart. Br. J. Pharmacol. 37:638–649, 1969.

M

1. Manger, W.M.: Adrenergic involvement in cardiac pathophysiology. *In* Manger, W.M. (ed.): Catecholamines in Normal and Abnormal Cardiac Function. Karger Press, New York, 1982.
2. Manger, W.M., and Hoffman, B.B.: Heart imaging in the diagnosis of pheochromocytoma and assessment of catecholamine uptake. Teaching editorial. J. Nucl. Med. 24:1194–1196, 1983, pp 71–107.
3. Mori, H., Pisarri, T., Aldea, G., et al.: Usefulness and limitations of regional cardiac sympathectomy by phenol. Am. J. Physiol. 257:H1523–533, 1989.
4. Minardo, J.D., Tuli, M.M., Mock, B.H., et al.: Scintigraphic and electrophysiologic evidence of canine myocardial sympathetic denervation and reinnervation produced by myocardial infarction or phenol application. Circulation 78:1008–1019, 1988.

N

1. Nakajo, M., Shapiro, B., Glowniak, J., et al.: Inverse relationship between cardiac accumulation of meta (131-I) iodobenzylguanidine (I–131 MIBG) and circulating catecholamines in suspected pheochromocytoma. J Nucl Med 24:1127–1134, 1983.
2. Nakajo, M., Shapiro, B., Sisson, J.C., et al.: Salivary gland accumulation of meta (131I) iodobenzylguanidine. J. Nucl. Med. 25:2–6, 1984.
3. Nakajo, M., Shimabukuro, K., Miyji, N., et al.: Rapid clearance of iodine-131 MIBG from the heart and liver of patients with adrenergic dysfunction and pheochromocytoma. J. Nucl. Med. 26:357–365, 1985.

P

1. Potter, L.T., Copper, T., Willman, V.L., and Wolfe, D.E.: Synthesis, binding, release, and metabolism of norepinephrine in normal and transplanted dog hearts. Circ. Res. 26:468–481, 1965.

R

1. Randall, W.C., Szentivanyi, M., Pace, J.B., et al.: Patterns of sympathetic projections onto the canine heart. Circ. Res. 22:315–323, 1968.

S

1. Sisson, J.C., Wieland, D.M., Sherman, P., et al.: Metaiodobenzylguanidine as an index of the adrenergic nervous system integrity and function. J. Nucl. Med. 28:1620–16124, 1987.
2. Sisson, J.C., Lynch, J.J., Johnson, J., et al.: Scintigraphic detection of regional disruption of adrenergic neurons in the heart. Am. Heart J. 116:67–76, 1988.
3. Sisson, J.C., Shapiro, B., Meyers, L., et al.: Metaiodobenzylguanidine to map scintigraphically the adrenergic nervous system in man. J. Nucl. Med. 28:1625–1636, 1987.
4. Schofer, J, Spielmann, R., Schuchert, A., et al.: Iodine-123 metaiodobenzylguanidine scintigraphy: A noninvasive method to demonstrate myocardial adrenergic nervous system disintegrity in patients with idiopathic dilated cardiomyopathy. J. Am. Coll. Cardiol. 12:1252–1258, 1988.
5. Sisson, J., Wieland, D., Johnson, J., et al.: Portrayal of cardiac beta receptors in living animals. J. Am. Coll. Cardiol. 13:64A, 1989.
6. Sisson, J., Wieland, D., Johnson, J., et al.: Scintigraphy of beta receptors in the heart. Circulation 78:II349, 1988.
7. Syrota, A., Comar, D., Paillotin, G., et al.: Muscarinic cholinergic receptor in the human heart evidenced under physiological conditions by positron emission tomography. Proc. Natl. Acad. Sci. USA 82:584–488, 1985.

T

1. Thoenen, H.: Surgical, immunological and chemical sympathectomy. *In* Buschko and Muschoel (eds.): Catecholamines: Handbook of Experimental Pharmacology. Vol. 2. Springer-Verlag, New York, 1972, pp. 813–844.
2. Tuli, M.M., Stanton, M.S., Mock, B.H., et al.: Comparative SPECT I–123-metaiodobenzyl guanidine (MIBG) and thallium 201 cardiac imaging following myocardial infarction. J. Nucl. Med. 29:840, 1988.

W

1. Whitby, L.G., Axelrod, J., and Weil-Malherbe, H.: The fate of 3H-norepinephrine in animals. J. Pharmacol. Exp. Ther. 132:193–201, 1961.
2. Wieland, D.M., Wu, J.L., Brown, L.E., et al.: Radiolabeled adrenergic neuron-blocking agents: Adrenomedullary imaging with (131-I) iodobenzylguanidine. J. Nucl. Med. 21:349–353, 1980.
3. Wieland, D.M., Brown, L.E., Rogers, W.L., et al.: Myocardial imaging with a radioiodinated norepinephrine storage analog. J. Nucl. Med. 22:22–31, 1981.

Part X

Positron Emission Tomography

Chapter 65

Principles of Positron Emission Tomography

HEINRICH R. SCHELBERT, M.D.

POSITRON-EMITTING TRACERS FOR CARDIAC STUDIES 1141
General Considerations 1141
Tracers of Myocardial Blood Flow 1141
General Principles 1141
Positron-Labeled Albumin Microspheres 1142
Nitrogen-13 Ammonia 1143
Oxygen-15 Water 1143
Rubidium-82 1144
Choice of Flow Tracer 1144
Other Tracers of Blood Flow 1144
Tracers of Myocardial Metabolism 1145
Carbon-11–Labeled Palmitate 1145
Fluorine-18–Labeled 2-Fluoro 2-Deoxyglucose 1147
Carbon-11–Labeled Acetate 1150
Evaluation of Myocardial Substrate Metabolism 1151
Amino Acids Labeled with Nitrogen-13 or Carbon-11 1152
Tracers of Cardiac Innervation and Receptors 1152
Other Tracers 1152
IMAGING WITH POSITRON EMISSION TOMOGRAPHY 1153
General Principles 1153
Image Acquisition 1154
Image Analysis and Tracer Concentration Measurements 1157
TRACER KINETIC MODELS AND APPLICATIONS 1158
NONINVASIVE MEASUREMENT OF FUNCTIONAL PROCESSES 1159
Evaluation and Quantification of Regional Myocardial Blood Flow 1160
The Fractionation Principle 1160
Net Extraction of Tracer 1160
Use of Tracer Kinetic Models 1161
Measurements of Myocardial Glucose Metabolism 1163
SUMMARY AND FUTURE DEVELOPMENTS 1164

Positron emission tomography offers several unique advantages over conventional scintigraphic approaches for the noninvasive study of the human heart. A virtually unlimited number of positron-emitting tracers is available to explore and to define specific aspects of myocardial tissue function. The concentrations of these tracers in blood and in myocardium and their changes over time can be quantified noninvasively by static or by serial imaging with positron emission tomography. Combining the quantitative imaging capabilities with positron-emitting tracers of myocardial tissue function permits the application of tracer kinetic principles in vivo and, consequently, the noninvasive quantification of blood flow and substrate fluxes in human myocardium. With these capabilities, positron emission tomography offers the opportunity to explore and characterize directly in human myocardium biologic processes that to date have been described only in experimental animal systems. In addition, this new capability should provide new insights into the physiology of the normal and diseased human heart and result in more accurate definition and characterization of human myocardial disease.

This chapter describes the major components of positron emission tomography for the noninvasive study of myocardial

This work was supported in part by the Director of the Office of Energy Research, Office of Health and Environmental Research, Washington, D.C., by Research Grants #HL 29845 and #HL 33177, National Institutes of Health, Bethesda, Md., and by an Investigative Group Award by the Greater Los Angeles Affiliate of the American Heart Association, Los Angeles, Cal.

tissue function. It examines currently used tracers as probes for various aspects of myocardial tissue function, describes the technical components of positron emission tomography, reviews concepts of tracer compartmental modeling, and, finally, describes how these various components are combined for the quantitative assessment of regional myocardial tissue function.

POSITRON-EMITTING TRACERS FOR CARDIAC STUDIES

General Considerations

Tracers employed most commonly with positron emission tomography are labeled with positron-emitting isotopes of elements that are abundant in nature (Table 65–1). These radioisotopes can be incorporated into organic compounds, therefore, while maintaining their structural and biologic properties intact. For example, despite insertion of a radioactive carbon-11 atom, radiolabeled palmitate or acetate continues to behave like natural myocardial fuel substrates and is metabolized by myocardium in a fashion identical to that of unlabeled "parents." Other positron-emitting isotopes, for example, nitrogen-13 or oxygen-15, similarly can be inserted into numerous other organic substances. The availability of isotopes like carbon-11, nitrogen-13, and oxygen-15 thus accounts for the large number of potentially useful tracers for positron emission tomography.[F1] Only the rapid physical decay limits their number, because it necessitates synthesis of tracer compounds within one or two physical half-lives and thus within usually less than 1 hour. Rapid synthesis methods for routine production of high specific activity tracers, however, are available for only a limited number of substances.

Generally, positron-emitting substances must meet several criteria to be suitable for positron emission tomography: (1) They must clear from blood and accumulate in myocardium at high concentrations and for sufficiently long time periods to permit external imaging; (2) their specific activity must be high so that they do not exert a mass effect and perturb the very process to be studied; and (3) the externally measured signal, that is, the concentrations of radioactivity in tissues and their changes over time, must closely and predictably correspond to the physiologic process to be examined. The latter requirement is especially important because images of myocardial tracer uptake provide information only on the activity concentrations of the radiolabel but not on the chemical species to which it is bound. Therefore, careful delineation of the relationships between the externally measured signal, the metabolic fate of the label, and the process under study is essential.

Labeled compounds currently used with positron emission tomography generally can be classified into tracers of blood flow, of metabolism, and of pre- and postsynaptic neuron activity (Table 65–2).

Tracers of Myocardial Blood Flow

General Principles

Tracers of blood flow are categorized generally into particulate tracers and diffusible, extractable tracers. An ideal tracer of blood flow accumulates in or clears from myocardium in linear proportion to myocardial blood flow. The relationship between uptake and clearance of the tracer and blood flow should be constant and should be unaffected by blood flow itself, by physiologic and pathophysiologic changes of the myocardial tissue state, and by myocardial metabolism. As discussed below, not all tracers of blood flow fully meet these requirements.

Table 65–1. POSITRON-EMITTING ISOTOPES FOR CARDIAC STUDIES

Isotope	Physical Half-Life	Parent Isotope	Physical Half-Life
Cyclotron-Produced			
Carbon-11	20.4 min	—	—
Fluorine-18	109.7 min	—	—
Nitrogen-13	9.96 min	—	—
Oxygen-15	2.07 min	—	—
Rubidium-81	4.58 hours		
Generator-Produced			
Rubidium-82	1.26 min	Strontium-82	25 days
Gallium-68	68.1 min	Germanium-68	288 days
Copper-62	9.73 min	Zinc-62	9.2 hours

Table 65–2. POSITRON-EMITTING TRACERS FOR CARDIAC EVALUATION

Tracers of Blood Flow	
C-11 or Ga-68 labeled albumin microspheres	
N-13 ammonia	
Rb-82	
O-15 water, O-15 carbon dioxide	
Cu-62 or Cu-64 PTSM	
Tracers of Metabolism	
C-11 palmitate	Fatty acid metabolism
F-18 2-fluoro 2-deoxyglucose	Exogenous glucose utilization
C-11 acetate	Oxidative metabolism
C-11 labeled amino acids	
N-13 labeled amino acids	Amino acid metabolism and protein synthesis
Tracers of Cardiac Innervation and Receptors	
F-18 metaraminol	
C-11 hydroxyephedrine	Adrenergic neuron density
C-11 CGP-12177	Beta-adrenergic receptors
C-11 MQNB	Cholinergic muscarinic receptors
Other Tracers	
Rb-81	Potassium pool
C-11 triphenylmethylphosphonium	Membrane potential
C-11 PK 11195	Peripheral benzodiazepine receptors
F-18 misonidazole	Hypoxic/ischemic tissue
O-15 carbon monoxide	Blood pool

CGP-12177 and PK-11195 are the catalog numbers of these industrial research compounds; PTSM—pyruvaldehyde bis-(N^4-methylthiosemicarbazone); MQNB—methiodide salt of quinuclinidyl benzylate.

Tracers of blood flow share a number of common features. The concentration of a tracer in myocardium (Q_t) at time t after injection depends upon several factors and can be described by

$$Q_t = E \cdot F \int_0^t C_a(t)dt \quad (1)$$

where E is the first-pass unidirectional extraction or (more appropriately) retention fraction of tracer, F is myocardial blood flow, and C_a the tracer concentration in arterial blood. In any given heart, the arterial input function and its integral to time t are the same for all myocardial regions. Regional differences in myocardial tracer concentrations depend therefore only on E and regional blood F. If the extraction fraction E were 1, then regional differences in tracer concentrations would depend solely on blood flow and would be related linearly to regional differences in blood flow.

The first-pass unidirectional extraction fraction E is the fraction of tracer that exchanges across the capillary membrane during a single transit of a tracer bolus through the coronary circulation. For most diffusible tracers, E is less than 1 and declines further as blood flow increases. This is because higher flow velocities in the capillaries reduce the time for exchange of tracer across the capillary membrane. Assuming a model of rigid cylindrical tubes, Renkin[R1] and Crone[C1] described this relationship by

$$E = 1 - e^{-PS/F} \quad (2)$$

where P is the capillary permeability ($cm \cdot min^{-1}$) and S the exchangeable surface ($cm^2 \cdot g^{-1}$). The product of P and S, or the permeability surface product, is unique to each tracer. The term PS/F is defined as the extraction coefficient and reflects the competitive rates between extraction in tissue and clearance by blood.

Experimentally measured first-pass extraction fractions often fail to conform strictly to the relationship described by Equation 2. Experimentally measured extraction fractions exceed at higher flows extraction fractions predicted by the equation, indicating that the PS product is not constant but increases with flow. Recruitment of capillaries may account for a flow-dependent increase in the PS product,[H1, P1, P2] which can be accommodated in the flow extraction fraction relationship by modifying the original Renkin-Crone equation to

$$E = 1 - e^{-(a+b/F)/F} \qquad (3)$$

where a and b are derived from the best fit of the experimentally obtained data. The term (a + b/F) represents the flow-dependent PS product. The single capillary transit extraction fraction must be distinguished from the steady state extraction fraction E_s which, as described by Equation 4, is defined as the ratio of the difference between tracer concentrations in arterial (C_a) and coronary sinus blood (C_{cs}) over the concentration of tracer in arterial blood (C_a):

$$E_s = \frac{C_a - C_{cs}}{C_a} \qquad (4)$$

E_s reflects the bidirectional or forward and reverse transmembranous transport of tracer and is therefore usually lower than the first-pass unidirectional extraction fraction.

The first-pass extraction fraction should further be distinguished from the first-pass retention fraction R, or the fraction of tracer that is effectively retained in myocardium after a transit of a tracer bolus through the coronary circulation. As illustrated in Figure 65–1, E and R may differ significantly. After exchanging across the capillary membrane and entering the interstitial space, further transport of tracer across the sarcolemmal membranes and trapping of tracer in myocytes competes with back-diffusion of tracer into blood. The rate of back-diffusion may depend upon blood flow. At higher flows, a greater fraction of tracer returns from the extravascular space into blood and results in lower retention fractions.

Lastly, different mechanisms account for exchange of tracer across the capillary and sarcolemmal membranes. Tracers can exchange across membranes via passive diffusion along a concentration gradient. The exchange can be facilitated by energy-independent but saturable transport mechanisms. The facilitated transport of glucose across the cell membrane is an example. Conversely, tracers may be actively transported through energy-requiring processes against concentration gradients across the sarcolemmal membranes. The latter mechanism accounts, for example, for the transmembranous exchange of radioactive potassium or its analogs and its retention in myocardium.

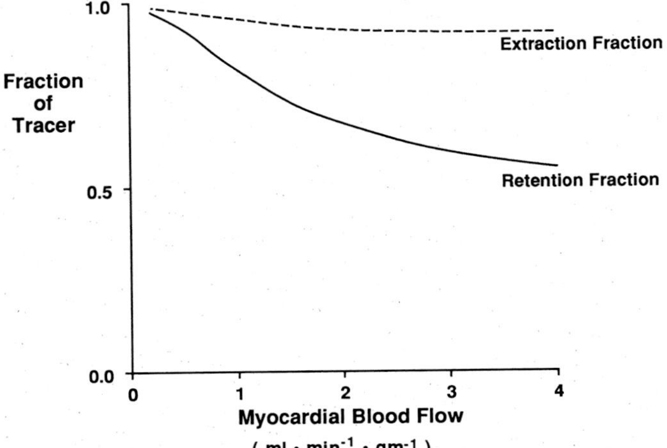

Figure 65–1. First-pass extraction and retention fractions of [^{13}N]ammonia and myocardial blood flow. The extraction fraction denotes the fraction of tracer that exchanges across the capillary and sarcolemmal membranes during a single capillary transit of tracer, whereas the retention fraction denotes the fraction of tracer that is metabolically retained in myocardium. Metabolic trapping competes with flow-dependent back diffusion of tracer, accounting for the progressive decline in retention fractions with increasing blood flow.

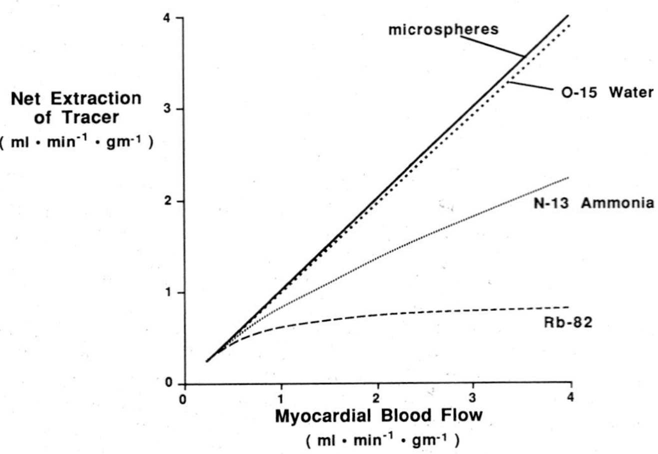

Figure 65–2. Net extraction of flow tracers in myocardium as a function of blood flow. The net extraction is the product of the first-pass extraction (retention) fraction and blood flow. Note the progressively smaller increments in net extractions of [^{13}N]ammonia and ^{82}Rb with higher flows because of the flow-dependent decline in first-pass retention fractions.

Positron-Labeled Albumin Microspheres

Microspheres most closely meet the requirements of an ideal tracer of blood flow. Because their size exceeds the diameter of the myocardial capillaries, microspheres are mechanically trapped in myocardium. Nearly 100 percent of microspheres are retained during a single capillary transit. Their first-pass extraction fraction, therefore, is 1 and is independent of flow and changes in tissue state or in myocardial metabolism. Regional myocardial concentrations of radiolabeled microspheres, therefore, correlate linearly with myocardial blood flow and, as will be discussed, permit the in vivo quantification of regional myocardial blood flow.

For positron emission tomography, biodegradable human serum albumin microspheres with a diameter of from 15 to 20 microns are used. They can be labeled with either gallium-68[H2, H3, Z1] or with carbon-11.[T1] Although gallium-68 is generator produced and thus does not require an on-site cyclotron, the gallium-chelate complex is susceptible to disruption by plasma constituents as demonstrated in animal experiments.[W1] Intravenous administration of gallium-68–labeled microspheres was associated with an initial 10 to 15 percent loss of label from microspheres into blood. Determination of the arterial input function, therefore, requires correction for unbound gallium-68. The carbon-11 label is thus preferable because of its more stable covalent binding to microspheres.[W2] Once trapped in myocardium, tissue activity concentrations have been found to remain constant for both tracers for at least 60 minutes.[W1, W2] The amount of tracer retained in myocardium is a function of its first-pass extraction fraction and blood flow. The product of E and F is also defined as the net tracer uptake. Because the first-pass extraction fraction is 1, the net uptake of microspheres in myocardium is linearly related to blood flow (Fig. 65–2).

Positron-labeled microspheres have been successfully employed for qualitative and quantitative evaluation of regional blood flow.[B1, S1, W1, W2] Quantification is based on Equation 1, in which blood flow is calculated from the microsphere concentrations in myocardium Q_t and the integral of the arterial input function. With positron emission tomography, Q_t can be determined directly from the cross-sectional images instead of by in vitro counting of postmortem-obtained tissue samples. The arterial input function is obtained by withdrawal of arterial blood. In dogs, in vivo estimates of blood flow by this approach were found to correlate closely with simultaneous blood flow measurements by the standard microsphere technique, using in vitro counting of tissue samples.[H4] When employed in humans after retrograde

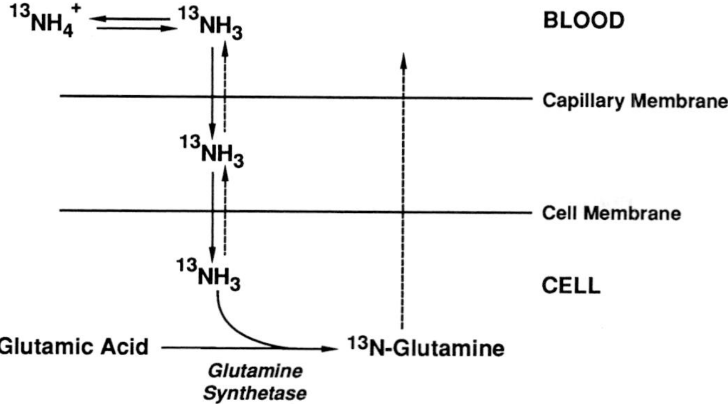

Figure 65–3. Schematic representation of the transmembranous exchange and metabolic trapping of [^{13}N]ammonia in the myocardium (see text).

delivery of carbon-11–labeled microspheres into the left ventricular cavity, the approach predicted average blood flows of 0.8 ± 0.3 ml · min^{-1} · g^{-1} in presumably normal myocardium and ranged from 0 to 0.4 ml · min^{-1} · g^{-1} in previously infarcted myocardial regions.[S1]

Although most accurate, the microsphere approach for measurements of blood flow in humans has been largely abandoned in favor of techniques with diffusible extractable tracers that do not require delivery of tracer into the left ventricular cavity but that can be conveniently administered intravenously or by inhalation.

Nitrogen-13 Ammonia

Use of nitrogen-13 ammonia was first proposed by Hunter and Monahan[H5] and Harper and associates.[H6] Its utility as a tracer of blood flow was subsequently demonstrated in animals[P3, S2] and in clinical investigations.[W3] Figure 65–3 schematically depicts the mechanism of uptake and retention of this tracer in myocardium. In blood, nitrogen-13 ammonia (NH_3) exists primarily in its ionic species, the ammonium ion (NH_4^+). In red blood cells, the ammonium ion can substitute for K^+ on the sodium-potassium transmembranous exchange system.[P4] It thus may be actively transported into myocardium. Another route of exchange, the one which most likely predominates, is that the lipid-soluble N-13 ammonia passively diffuses across the capillary and sarcolemmal membranes, because its first-pass extraction fraction exceeds that of potassium ions.[P5, S3] If the tracer leaves the vascular space in the form of ammonia, it then must be rapidly replenished by conversion of NH_4^+ to NH_3. Equilibrium between both species is achieved within about 19 microseconds,[P5] which is fast enough to permit almost complete extraction of nitrogen-13 ammonia during a 2- to 3-second transit through the coronary circulation.

Several metabolic routes are available to the cell for fixation of nitrogen-13 ammonia. Foremost are the α-ketoglutarate–glutamic acid and the glutamic acid–glutamine reactions. The latter reaction appears to be the predominant trapping mechanism, because inhibition of glutamine synthetase with L-methionine sulfoximine abolishes the retention of tracer in myocardium.[B2, K1, K2, S3] Because of a large intracellular pool of glutamine and its slow turnover rate, the nitrogen-13 label clears only slowly from myocardium (clearance half-times range from 100 to 400 minutes in canine myocardium).[S3] Therefore, for the duration of the study, nitrogen-13 ammonia becomes effectively trapped in myocardium.

Residue function measurements in canine myocardium have demonstrated that as much as 95 to 100 percent of tracer initially exchanges across the capillary membrane (see Fig. 65–1).[S3] Metabolic fixation competes with back-diffusion of tracer into the vascular space. Because back-diffusion depends upon blood flow, the fraction of tracer that is ultimately retained in myocardium declines with higher flows. This relationship, as shown in Figure 65–1, can be described by

$$E_R = 1 - 0.607e^{-1.25/F} \tag{5}$$

where E_R is the first-pass retention fraction and F is blood flow. Equation 5 predicts for a flow of 1 ml · min^{-1} · g^{-1} a first-pass retention fraction of 0.83, which, however, progressively declines with increasing flow and averages 0.60 at flows of 3 ml · min^{-1} · g^{-1}. The net extraction of nitrogen-13 ammonia as the product of first-pass retention fraction and flow and its relationship to blood flow are shown in Figure 65–2 and compared with net extractions of other diffusible tracers. The nonlinear relationship indicates an initial steep rise of the net extractions in response to blood flow. Further increases in the higher flow range, however, are associated with successively smaller increments in net extraction and thus tracer tissue concentrations.

Although trapped metabolically in myocardium, changes in cardiac work and in inotropic state as well as in myocardial metabolism do not significantly perturb the observed relationship between tracer tissue concentrations and blood flow.[S3] Only unphysiologically low plasma pH levels and acute myocardial ischemia reduced moderately but significantly the retention fraction of nitrogen-13 ammonia—without, however, invalidating its utility as a flow tracer.

Nitrogen-13 ammonia is now widely employed for the evaluation of regional myocardial blood flow with positron emission tomography in humans.[B3, S4, T2, T3] Typically, 10 to 20 mCi of nitrogen-13 ammonia are injected intravenously. Imaging commences 4 to 7 minutes later to allow for sufficient clearance of tracer from blood (about 5 percent of peak activity). Whereas uptake of nitrogen-13 ammonia is usually low in lung tissue, it may be high and degrade image quality in patients with severely depressed left ventricular function or pulmonary disease, and in smokers. Because the tracer clears more rapidly from the lungs than from myocardium, longer time intervals between tracer injection and imaging may improve the myocardium-to-background signal ratios.

Oxygen-15 Water

This agent meets most closely the criteria of an ideal tracer of blood flow. Because it is virtually freely diffusible, its first-pass extraction fraction approaches unity, is independent of blood flow, and does not vary with changes in metabolic state.[B4, B5, W4]

Water, labeled with the short-lived positron-emitting oxygen-15 (physical half-life of 75 seconds), readily diffuses across the capillary and sarcolemmal membranes. Based on residue function measurements in dogs, the first-pass extraction fraction approaches unity at flows of 1 ml · min^{-1} · g^{-1}. In contrast to other diffusible flow indicators, the first-pass extraction fraction remains constant despite increases in blood flow. The high first-pass extraction fraction substantiates the notion that the capillary and sarcolemmal membranes exert only little if any resistance to exchange of labeled water. The concentration of oxygen-15 water in myocardium relative to blood flow depends further on the volume of distribution of water in both myocardium and blood.[B4, H1] This relation, frequently defined as the tissue/blood partition coefficient, represents the ratio of the tracer concentrations in myocardium to blood at equilibrium and depends upon the water content in myocardium and in blood. The latter strictly represents the plasma water content and is, therefore, a function of the hematocrit.

The advantages of oxygen-15–labeled water are partly offset by physical and physiologic properties. The rapid physical decay of radioactivity results in low count and often diagnostically unsatisfactory images. Furthermore, the tracer distributes into tissue adjacent to myocardium, as, for example, into arterial blood and lungs. Although this activity can be removed by blood pool imaging and image substraction, it furthers reduces image count statistics. This subtraction is accomplished by labeling of red blood cells with oxygen-15–labeled carbon monoxide.[B4] Inhaled during a single breath, it firmly binds to hemoglobin by forming oxygen-15 carboxyhemoglobin. The carbon monoxide blood pool images are normalized to and then substracted from the oxygen-15 water images.

Oxygen-15 water can be administered either as a short or distributed single intravenous bolus[B4, I1, K4] or by continuous inhalation of oxygen-15–labeled carbon monoxide. Carbonic anhydrase rapidly converts CO_2 to H_2O. Depending upon the performance characteristics of the positron emission tomograph, doses of 0.5 mCi/kg or 15 mCi of oxygen-15 water[I1, W5] are administered intravenously, and imaging commences either immediately[11] or after 2 to 3 minutes. After oxygen-15 has physically decayed, the blood pool is labeled with a single-breath inhalation of oxygen-15 carbon monoxide, imaged and subtracted from the oxygen-15 water images. For the continuous tracer delivery approach, the subject inhales oxygen-15 carbon dioxide for about 3 to 4 minutes, or until labeled water has equilibrated with blood and myocardium.[A1, A2] Serial images are recorded throughout the inhalation phase and for several minutes thereafter. The blood pools are then labeled with oxygen-15 carbon monoxide and subtracted from the equilibrium water images. A more recently described modification utilizes differential clearance rates of tracer from blood and myocardium to correct for blood pool activity and thus eliminates the need for an additional blood pool scan.[B6, H7, L1]

Rubidium-82

This cation substitutes for potassium on the sodium-potassium–dependent transmembranous ion exchange system and is actively transported across the sarcolemmal membranes into the cell. As demonstrated by residue function measurements in arterially perfused isolated hearts, rubidium-82 ions rapidly exchange across the capillary membranes.[H84] Active transport across the sarcolemmal membrane competes then with back-diffusion of tracer from the interstitial to the vascular space. Because the rate of back-diffusion is a function of blood flow, first-pass retention fractions decline in a nonlinear fashion with increasing myocardial blood flows (see Fig. 65–2). In isolated, arterially perfused rabbit myocardium, retention fractions were related to blood flow by $0.84/(F + 0.84)$.[H8] Comparable relationships have been observed in canine myocardium, employing either external scintillation detectors[G1, G2, M1] or dynamic imaging with positron emission tomography.[B7, G3] The relationship of $E = 1-\exp(-0.9/F)$, as reported by Budinger and associates,[B8] predicts an average extraction fraction of 0.59 for flows of 1 $ml \cdot min^{-1} \cdot g^{-1}$, which declines to 0.26 for flows of 3.0 $ml \cdot min^{-1} \cdot g^{-1}$. The same relationship predicts a tracer net extraction of 0.59 $ml \cdot min^{-1} \cdot g^{-1}$ for a flow of 1 $ml \cdot min^{-1} \cdot g^{-1}$, which increases in a nonlinear fashion to further increases in blood flow. Relatively large increments in blood flow, therefore, are associated only with small and successively lower increments in myocardial rubidium-82 concentrations.

Although the energy-requiring active transport of tracer into the cell appears to render myocardial tracer uptake more susceptible to metabolic alterations, Goldstein and associates failed to demonstrate significant effects of hyperglycemia, insulin, digoxin, and propranolol on the first-pass extraction fraction.[G2] Increased plasma pH levels similarly remained without effect on the extraction fraction, whereas acidosis reduced it. The researchers attributed the latter effect to hyperkalemia and competition of potassium for uptake of rubidium-82.[G2] Tracer first-pass extraction fraction in acutely ischemic and postischemic myocardium did not significantly deviate from the flow extraction fraction relationship.[G4] However, rubidium-82 subsequently leaked from irreversibly injured (non-TTC-staining) myocardium but was retained or continued to accumulate in only reversibly injured (TTC-staining) myocardium. The different tracer clearance kinetics may thus prove useful for distinguishing between reversible and irreversible ischemic injury. On the other hand, studies by Wilson and associates suggested that the tracer first-pass extraction fraction may be significantly reduced in post-ischemic, though viable, myocardium.[W6]

One major advantage of rubidium-82 is its availability through a generator infusion system.[B9, B10, G5, G6] Strontium-82 is the parent isotope, has a 23 day physical half-life, and permits the use of a generator system for about 4 to 5 weeks. Furthermore, the only 78-second physical half-life of rubidium-82 affords evaluation or quantification of regional myocardial blood flow at short time intervals—for example, 8 to 10 minutes. Largely automated infusion systems are now available. They are pushbutton operated and automatically deliver a preselected dose of activity at a preselected rate of infusion.[G5] Typically, 40 to 60 mCi are administered intravenously and 60 to 90 seconds are allowed for clearance of tracer from blood before imaging begins.[G7–9, K3] Myocardial rubidium-82 images are generally of good diagnostic quality. Rapid radioactivity decay and increased photon attenuation, particularly in obese patients, may result in low count and diagnostically suboptimal images.

Choice of Flow Tracer

All three tracers of blood flow—nitrogen-13 ammonia, rubidium-82, and oxygen-15 water—yield comparable diagnostic information on regional myocardial blood flow. Specific advantages of one tracer are often offset by limitations and drawbacks. For example, oxygen-15 water is theoretically the most ideal tracer of flow. On the other hand, its use is technically demanding and requires additional image manipulation—for example, in acquisition of a blood pool image and subtraction from oxygen-15 water image. Resulting low count statistics may degrade the image quality. In contrast, imaging of regional myocardial blood flow is more convenient with nitrogen-13 ammonia because the tracer is fixed in myocardium; the longer physical half-life of nitrogen-13 allows a more flexible acquisition schedule. Furthermore, longer acquisition times yield images of higher count densities. Yet, lower and flow-dependent first-pass extraction fractions that are possibly sensitive to metabolic alterations render the tracer less than perfect. Production of both oxygen-15 water and nitrogen-13 ammonia depends on an on site cyclotron. Blood flows studies with either tracer, therefore, need to be coordinated with cyclotron production. In contrast, rubidium-82 is available through a generator/infusion system that largely facilitates the logistics of blood flow imaging. Furthermore, studies can be repeated at short time intervals and their timing can be closely coordinated with responses to interventions, rather than with the cyclotron production schedule. These significant practical advantages must be weighed against the cost and the short physical half-life of rubidium-82. About 50 percent of the activity is lost to physical decay during the interval from tracer injection to the beginning of image acquisition alone. Further decay during image acquisition may result in low count and diagnostically limited image quality. The preference for a given tracer therefore depends often on practical and economic considerations—for example, the availability of a rubidium-82 generator system and multiorgan use of a given tracer, such as sharing the same cyclotron-produced batch of tracer between studies performed simultaneously on two tomographs.

Other Tracers of Blood Flow

Other agents, such as the carbon-11–labeled alcohols like butanol or carbon-11–labeled antipyrine, have been proposed as alternate tracers of blood flow but remain still unexplored.[D1, H9, T5] Potassium-43 similarly has been employed as a cationic tracer of blood flow.[D2]

More recently, a lipophilic copper (II) complex of derivatives of pyruvaldehyde bis (thiosemicarbazone), referred to as PTSM, labeled with a positron-emitting isotope of copper, has been proposed as a potentially useful tracer of flow. In tumors, these complexes are known to diffuse across the same cell membrane and are reduced by sulfhydryl groups with liberation copper, which binds nonspecifically to intracellular macromolecules.[G10] If the same redox process does in fact occur in myocardium, it will account for the retention of radioactive copper as observed by Green and colleagues in hearts of rats, monkeys, and gerbils.[G10] Of the total administered dose of [^{67}Cu] Cu (PTSM), 4.0 percent and 2.2 percent was retained in hearts of monkeys and of rats, respectively. In isolated, arterially perfused rabbit hearts, the first-pass extraction fraction of copper-labeled PTSM averaged 0.45 ± 0.07 at flows of 1.5 ml/min/g.[S5] Hypoxia and ischemia failed to alter significantly the extraction fraction of Cu-PTSM. Most importantly, the radiolabel becomes fixed in myocardium, as evidenced by clearance half-times of greater than 3600 minutes,[S6] whereas it rapidly clears from blood, as demonstrated in preliminary dog studies. Myocardial blood flow images recorded with positron emission tomography were of good diagnostic quality and reflected accurately the regional distribution of blood flow as confirmed by the close correlation between tracer and microsphere concentrations in myocardial tissue samples by in vitro counting.[S6] The compound, therefore, appears particularly attractive as a tracer of myocardial blood flow with positron emission tomography, because it can be labeled with generator-produced positron-emitting isotopes of copper—for example, copper-62 and copper-64.[G10, R2] Its use does not require an on site cyclotron. Furthermore, the microsphere-like retention of fixation of tracer in myocardium affords a more flexible tracer administration schedule, immediately before or several hours before imaging with positron emission tomography. Because of the relatively low first-pass extraction fraction and further flow-dependent decreases with higher blood flows (as predicted by Equation 2), the tracer would appear to be of limited value in the high flow range.

Tracers of Myocardial Metabolism

Several positron-emitting tracers are currently employed for the evaluation and quantification of regional myocardial metabolism. Because free fatty acid has long been considered the heart's preferred fuel substrate, early efforts focused on the evaluation and testing of carbon-11–labeled palmitate as a tracer of myocardial fatty acid metabolism. However, depending on substrate availability or circulating levels of substrates, often as a function of the dietary state or dependent upon physical activity, a greater share in myocardial substrate metabolism may fall to other substrates, such as glucose. Furthermore, utilization of glucose can assume a predominate role under certain conditions, as in ischemia and hypoxia, for example. For the evaluation and quantification of exogenous glucose utilization, fluorine-18 2-fluoro 2-deoxyglucose is available. However, both carbon-11 palmitate and fluorine-18 2-fluoro 2-deoxyglucose fall short of providing sufficient information on overall oxidative metabolism as the sum of all oxidative processes, which has now become possible with carbon-11 acetate.

Carbon-11–Labeled Palmitate

Uptake and subsequent turnover of this tracer in myocardium provide information on regional myocardial fatty acid metabolism. This information is derived from regional tissue time activity curves constructed from serially acquired cross-sectional images. Image acquisition commences at the time of intravenous tracer bolus injection and continues for about 40 to 60 minutes. Images recorded early after tracer injection, as seen in Figure 65–4, depict the initial bolus transit through the central circulation, followed by tracer accumulation in myocardium and clearance from blood.[H10] The late images depict the decrease in myocardial activity concentrations over time.

After regions of interest are assigned to the left ventricular myocardium, tissue time activity curves are constructed and reveal a characteristic biexponential clearance pattern (Fig. 65–5). The clearance curve morphology corresponds to the metabolic fate of carbon-11 palmitate in myocardium and thus provides information on myocardial fatty acid metabolism. The biexponential clearance implies that the tracer enters at least two metabolic pools of different sizes and different turnover rates. Quantitative parameters of the tissue activity curves can be obtained by biexponential least square fitting routines and extrapolation of the slow clearance phase to the time of myocardial peak activity. Both the rapid and slow clearance curve components are then defined by their slopes and relative sizes.

The carbon-11 label is attached to palmitate in the one-position of the 16-carbon fatty acid chain ([1-^{11}C] palmitate). It is suspended in 6 percent albumin and, after intravenous administration into blood, continues to be reversibly bound to albumin. Because of first-pass extraction fractions of about 0.67 at flows of 1 $ml \cdot min^{-1} \cdot gm^{-1}$(as observed in dog experiments),[S7, S8] the initial uptake and regional distribution of tracer in myocardium are largely determined by regional myocardial blood flow. Transmembranous exchange occurs presumably via passive diffusion across a concentration gradient, although several other mechanisms, including a facilitated transport system, have been proposed.[L4] As depicted schematically in Figure 65–6, the radiotracer becomes esterified in cytosol to carbon-11 acyl-CoA. The thiokinase-mediated and energy-dependent reaction is largely unidirectional and is, therefore, thought of as the effective step of tracer sequestration into myocardium.[R4] However, esterification of tracer competes with back-diffusion of nonmetabolized carbon-11 palmitate into the vascular space. Once activated to acyl-CoA, the metabolic fate of carbon-11 palmitate branches thereafter. A fraction of esterified tracer moves via the carnitine shuttle to the

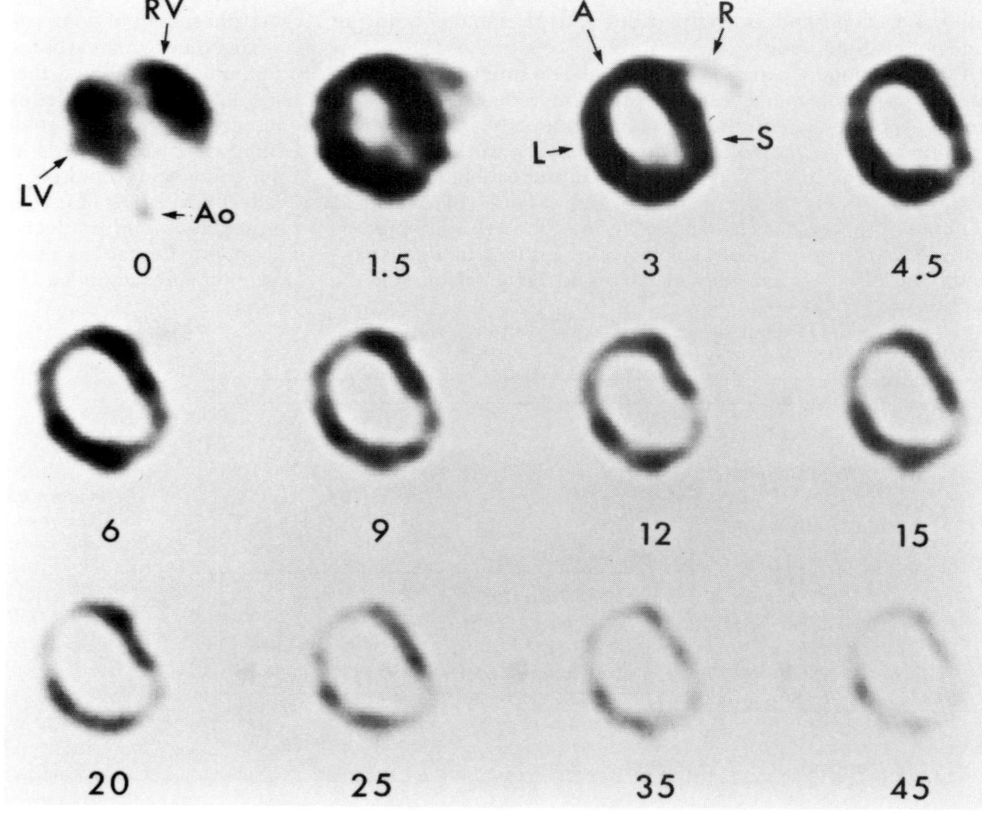

Figure 65–4. Serially acquired cross-sectional images following intravenous ^{11}C-palmitate administration. The images are recorded for a 45-minute period beginning at the time of tracer injection. The numbers under each frame indicate the time of acquisition after tracer injection (in minutes). RV—right ventricle; LV—left ventricle; Ao—aorta; A—anterior; L—lateral; S—septum; R—right ventricular myocardium. The first image reveals most of the activity in the right and left ventricular blood pool. After clearance of activity of ^{11}C-palmitate from blood, the myocardium is optimally visualized at 3 minutes. The decline in intensity of myocardial activity indicates clearance of activity of ^{11}C-palmitate from the myocardium.

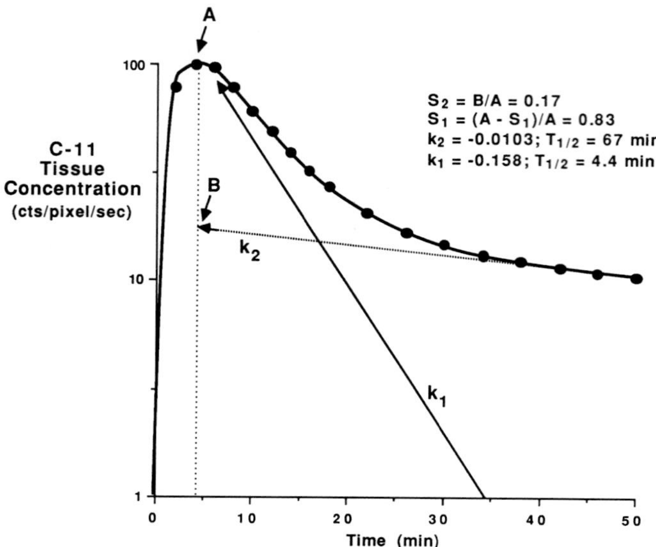

Figure 65–5. Myocardial tissue time activity curves of ^{11}C-palmitate obtained from serially acquired cross-sectional images after intravenous tracer injection. Note the initial rapid increase in myocardial activity concentrations of ^{11}C-palmitate. Maximum activity A occurs at 4 minutes, followed by biexponential clearance of activity of ^{11}C-palmitate from the myocardium. The slopes of the two clearance phases k_1 and k_2 are determined by biexponential least square curve fitting routines. Extrapolation of the slope k_2 to the time of peak activity (A) permits determination of the relative size (S_2) of the slow clearance phase by dividing B by A. The relative size of the rapid clearance phase is obtained from the difference between A and B divided by A. T½ is the tissue clearance halftime expressed in minutes. In this example, 83 percent of tracer enters the rapid clearance phase, whereas the remainder enters the slow clearance phase. The two clearance phases correspond to different metabolic fates of the radiolabel in form of deposition in the endogenous lipid pool and immediate oxidation and release as ^{11}C-CO_2 (as depicted schematically in Fig. 65–6).

inner mitochondrial membrane where β-oxidation cleaves two carbon fragments off the long carbon chain, which enter the tricarboxylic acid (TCA) cycle and are completely oxidized to CO_2 and water. Another fraction of acyl-CoA becomes further esterified and is deposited as triglycerides and phospholipids in the endogenous lipid pool.

A large amount of experimental animal data supports the notion that the rapid clearance curve component reflects oxidation of carbon-11 palmitate and thus corresponds to fatty acid oxidation. Its slope and relative size correlate with cardiac work and oxygen consumption,[G1, K5, L2, S8, W8] as well as with production and release of carbon-11 CO_2 as the oxidative end product of carbon-11 palmitate. Further, the clearance curve morphology appropriately changes in response to physiologic interventions and thus correctly tracks known changes in fatty acid metabolism. For example, increases in plasma glucose and lactate levels associated with a decline in plasma free fatty acid levels induce changes in myocardial substrate selection and oxidation (Fig. 65–7). The resultant decrease in fatty acid oxidation in favor of an increase in carbohydrate oxidation is associated with a proportionate decline of the relative size and slope of the rapid clearance curve component.[S9–11, W7] Changes in the clearance curve morphology in response to inhibition of specific steps in the fatty acid metabolic pathway have further substantiated the nature of the rapid clearance curve component. For example, impairment of fatty acid oxidation by inhibiting the transfer of acyl-CoA units into mitochondria with 2-tetradecylglycidic acid, an inhibitor of the carnitine acyl transferase I, resulted in a marked decline or even disappearance of the rapid clearance component and cessation of carbon-11 CO_2 release.[W7] The known impairment of fatty acid oxidation and the disproportionate increase in fatty acid deposition in the endogenous lipid pool during ischemia/hypoxia are reflected on the clearance curve by a decline in the slope and relative size of the early clearance curve component[F2, L2, L3, S7, W8] and are associated with a proportionate decrease in carbon-11 CO_2 release, as demonstrated in isolated, arterially perfused rat hearts and in dog experiments.[F2, R3, S7, S8]

Biochemical assays of myocardial tissue samples at various times after intracoronary tracer bolus injection have confirmed that the slow tissue clearance phase corresponds to incorporation of carbon-11 label into the endogenous lipid pool.[R3] In control hearts in dogs, about 75 percent of the initially extracted tracer was oxidized to carbon-11 CO_2 and 10 percent was diffused back into the vascular space in nonmetabolized form (Fig. 65–8*A*). The remainder of the carbon-11 label was retained in tissue in the form of diglycerides, triglycerides, and phospholipids and corresponded to the slow clearance phase on the tissue time activity curve. Water-soluble carbon-11 containing such metabolites as CO_2, acyl-CoA and acetyl-CoA was found to account for most of the activity cleared from myocardium in the form of carbon-11 CO_2. As predicted, ischemia dramatically altered the distribution of the radiolabel between metabolic pools (Fig. 65–8*B*). Consistent with an impairment of oxidation of fatty acid, a significantly smaller fraction of label was released as carbon-11 CO_2, and back-diffusion of nonmetabolized carbon-11 palmitate markedly increased. The fraction present in the aqueous pools declined, whereas the fractions of label in the di- and triglyceride and phospholipid pools markedly increased.

Together with earlier established relationships to functional and metabolic indices, the results of the biochemical tissue assays are important for adequate interpretation of the tissue time activity curves. They confirm that the late slow clearance curve component corresponds to incorporation of carbon-11 label into the endogenous lipid pool. The early clearance curve component reflects oxidation of carbon-11 palmitate and the rate of release of metabolic end products from myocardium. The results further point out limitations of the slope of the early clearance curve component as an index of fatty acid oxidation. First, the slope of

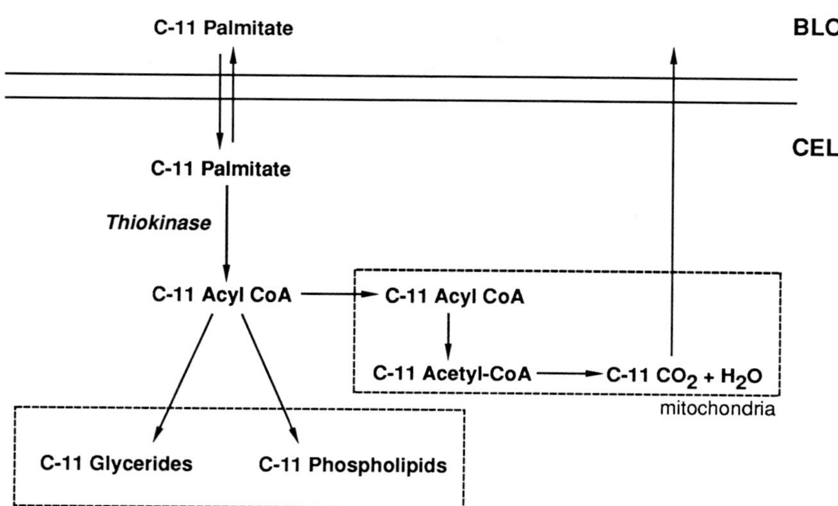

Figure 65–6. The metabolic fate of ^{11}C-palmitate in the myocardium (see text). The two boxes indicate the two major pathways of the ^{11}C label, oxidation of ^{11}C palmitate to ^{11}C-CO_2 and deposition of the ^{11}C label in the endogenous lipid pool as reflected on the biexponential clearance curve as shown in Fig. 65–5.

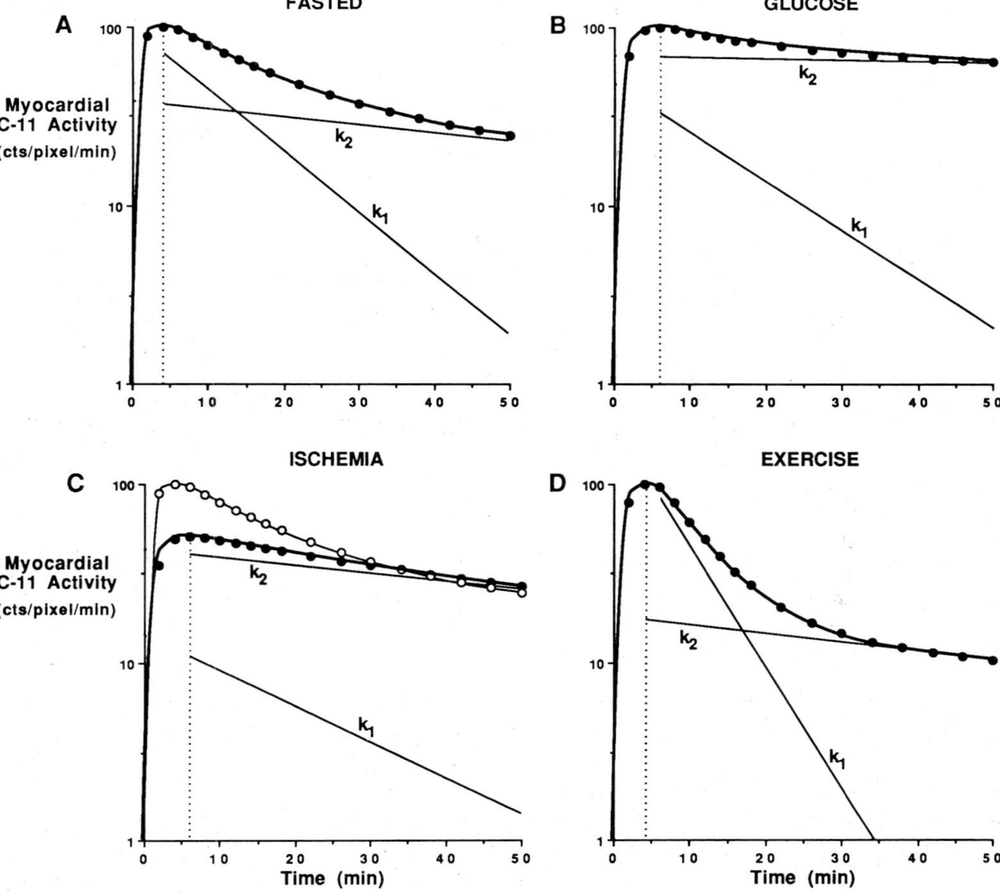

Figure 65–7. Effects of substrate availability, cardiac work and ischemia on the clearance curve morphology of ^{11}C-palmitate. *A*, In the fasted state, when plasma fatty acid levels are high and glucose levels are low, the myocardium meets its energy requirements by oxidizing predominantly free fatty acid. The relative size and slope of the rapid clearance phase are high. *B*, An increase in glucose concentrations in plasma associated with a decline in free fatty acid levels after a carbohydrate-rich meal results in a shift in myocardial substrate selection from free fatty acid to glucose, which is reflected on the tissue clearance curve by a decrease in the relative size and slope of the rapid clearance curve phase, indicating a decrease in the rate of fatty acid oxidation. *C*, Regional myocardial ischemia results in a regional impairment of fatty acid oxidation which the regional time activity curve *(solid circles)* mirrors by a correspondent decline in regional ^{11}C-palmitate uptake and a decrease of both relative size and slope of the rapid clearance curve component. The time activity curve derived from ischemic myocardium is compared with that in normal myocardium *(open circles)*. *D*, The increase in myocardial oxygen consumption in response to exercise and increased cardiac work is reflected by an increase in relative size and slope of the rapid clearance curve component, reflecting augmented fatty acid oxidation.

the clearance curve component may be contaminated by increased back-diffusion of nonmetabolized carbon-11 palmitate. Recent observations have suggested that the rate of back-diffusion exceeds the rate of release of carbon-11 CO_2 from myocardium.[W7] Second, the rate of tissue activity clearance depends on the volume of distribution of metabolites in addition to substrate flux through the oxidative pathways. For example, the increase in the fraction of label present in the aqueous phase, reflecting carbon-11 bound to CO_2, acyl-CoA, and acetyl-CoA, may delay the tissue tracer clearance rate and thus cause the underestimation of the true flux rate through oxidative pathways.

For studies in humans, 15 to 20 mCi of carbon-11 palmitate is injected intravenously. Myocardial uptake of carbon-11 palmitate and its relative distribution can be evaluated from a single image, recorded after tracer clearance from blood in about 5 to 8 minutes following tracer administration.[S12, T4, W9] As mentioned earlier, the initial distribution of tracer in myocardium is largely a function of regional blood flow. Nevertheless, these images of the initial uptake contain some metabolic information because retention or effective trapping of tracer in myocardium requires energy-dependent esterification of tracer to carbon-11 acyl-CoA. More complete evaluation of myocardial fatty acid metabolism requires serial imaging, which commences at the time of tracer administration and continues for about 40 to 60 minutes.[S9–11] Regional myocardial tissue time activity curves are then obtained from regions of interest assigned to the left ventricular myocardium on the serial cross-sectional images. Because of the dependency of fatty acid metabolism and thus of the tissue clearance kinetics of carbon-11 palmitate on myocardial substrate selection, standardization of study conditions, for example, overnight fasting or determination of plasma substrate levels, is critical for adequate interpretation of the time activity curves.

Although a tracer compartmental model for the quantification of regional myocardial fatty acid metabolism has been proposed for carbon-11 palmitate, this model needs further refinement and validation.[H11] Therefore, assessment of myocardial fatty acid metabolism with carbon-11 palmitate remains qualitative or semi-quantitative at present. Regional myocardial tissue time activity curves are analyzed by biexponential least square fitting routines for determination of the relative sizes and slopes of the rapid and slow clearance curve components. Alternatively, the slope of the early clearance curve component is derived by monoexponential least square fitting.

Tissue time activity curves characteristic for different dietary states, exercise, and ischemia are depicted in Figure 61–7. Under conditions of preferential fatty acid utilization as, for example, after an overnight fast, the major fraction of tracer enters the rapid turnover pool and is rapidly oxidized, as indicated by the large relative size and steep slope of the rapid clearance curve component. Under conditions of low plasma fatty acid and high plasma glucose levels, disproportionately more glucose is oxidized, which is reflected on the tissue time activity curves by the decrease in both relative size and slope of the same clearance curve component. Impairment of fatty acid oxidation during ischemia causes a similar decline of both curve parameters but occurs characteristically in a well-defined myocardial region and differs strikingly from the normal appearance of the clearance curve in normally perfused myocardial regions.

Fluorine-18–Labeled 2-Fluoro 2-Deoxyglucose

Among several potentially useful tracers, the glucose analog fluorine-18 2-fluoro 2-deoxyglucose has emerged as the tracer of choice of myocardial glucose metabolism. It traces only one, but well-defined and representative, step of the initial metabolism of exogenous glucose and is amenable to tracer kinetic modeling and thus is more suitable for quantification of glucose metabolic rates with positron emission tomography.[P6, S13] In contrast, glucose

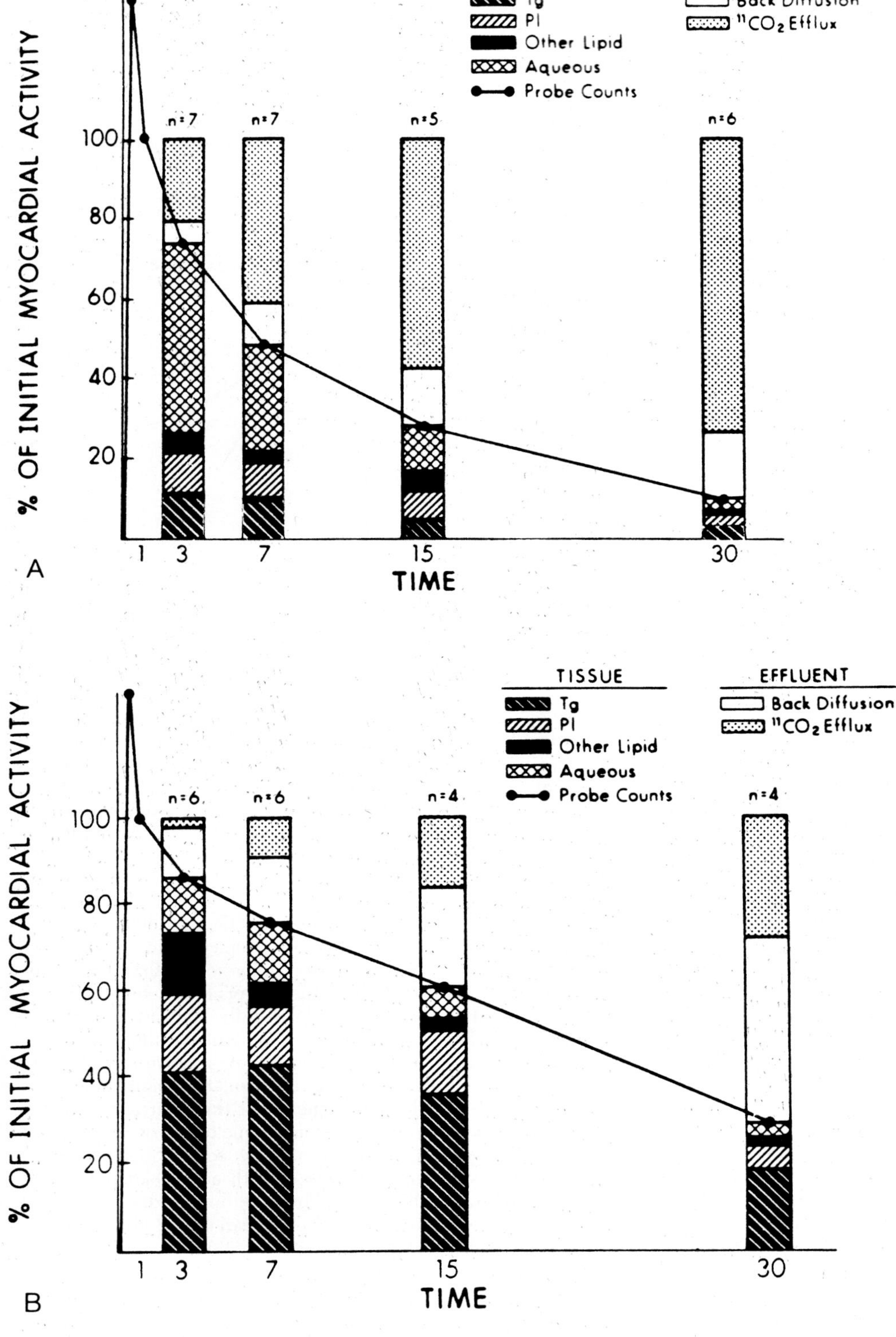

Figure 65–8. Metabolic fate of ^{11}C-palmitate in myocardium and coronary sinus effluent following intracoronary bolus administration of ^{11}C-palmitate in open-chested dog experiments at control *(A)* and low flow ischemia *(B)*. The solid lines depict the tissue residue function and represent the average percentage of initially extracted tracer at each biopsy time point. The values above the curve at each time point indicate the cumulative contributions of ^{11}C-CO_2 and ^{11}C-palmitate efflux to tracer clearance from the myocardium. The values below the curves depict the fractional distribution of the radiolabel between various pools of fatty acid metabolites in the myocardium as determined by tissue assays. As shown in Panel B, ischemia caues an increase in efflux of nonmetabolized ^{11}C-palmitate and a disproportionate increase in the fraction of ^{11}C label deposited in tissue as triglycerides (TG) and phospholipids (PL). (From Rosamond, T.L., Abendschein, D.R., Sobel, B.E., et al.: Metabolic fate of radiolabeled palmitate in ischemic canine myocardium: Implications for positron emission tomography. J. Nucl. Med. 28:1322–1329, 1987, with permission of The Society of Nuclear Medicine.)

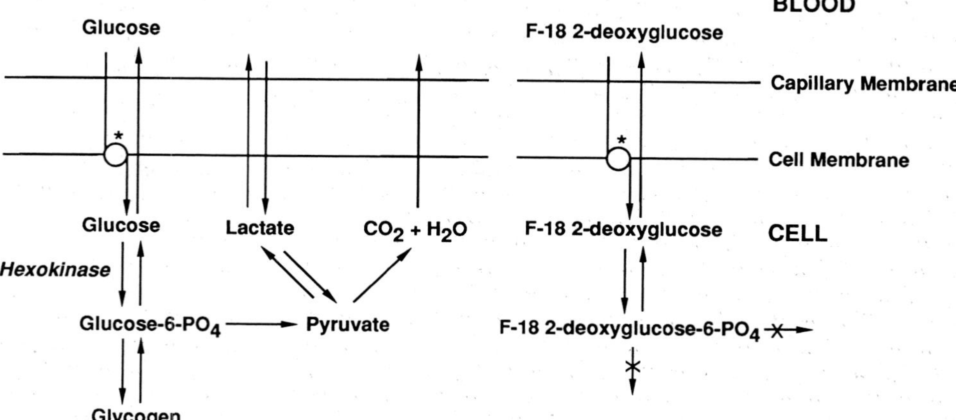

Figure 65–9. Comparison of the transmembranous exchange in the initial metabolic steps of glucose and of ^{18}F-2-fluoro 2-deoxyglucose in the myocardium (asterisks denote the facilitated transport across the sarcolemmal membrane). (See text.)

labeled with carbon-11, which is also available,[W8] participates in the entire metabolic fate of glucose. Distribution of the carbon-11 label into numerous metabolic pools and loss of label during the transit of metabolic intermediates through the glycolytic and final oxidative pathway of glucose pose considerable limitations on adequate interpretation of the externally recorded tissue time activity curve, as well as for tracer kinetic modeling.

Fluorine-18 2-fluoro 2-deoxyglucose, as shown schematically in Figure 65–9, exchanges across the capillary and sarcolemmal membranes in proportion to glucose. In cytosol, it competes with glucose for hexokinase and is phosphorylated to fluorine-18 2-fluoro 2-deoxyglucose-6-phosphate.[S13] Unlike natural glucose-6-phosphate, the phosphorylated glucose analog is a poor substrate for glycogen synthesis, glycolysis, and the fructose-phosphate shunt. It is also relatively impermeable to the sarcolemmal membrane. Because the activity of phosphatase, the enzyme that reverses the initial phosphorylation of glucose, is low in normal myocardium, transport of tracer into the cell is largely unidirectional. The tracer is sequestered into myocardium by the hexokinase reaction in proportion to glucose, so that images of the myocardial fluorine-18 tissue concentrations reflect the relative distribution of exogenous glucose utilization in myocardium.

Following intravenous administration (about 5 to 10 mCi in humans), fluorine-18 2-fluoro 2-deoxyglucose rapidly exchanges across the capillary and cellular membranes. Fluorine-18 concentrations initially rise rapidly in myocardium. Back-diffusion of tracer competes then with phosphorylation and effective sequestration of tracer into myocardium. The rate of rise of myocardial fluorine-18 activity concentrations progressively declines and may finally reach a plateau. This occurs at about 50 to 60 minutes after tracer injection, when tracer concentrations in arterial blood have declined and a relative equilibrium state between phosphorylated tracer, tracer in tissue, and tracer in arterial blood has been attained. At that time, more than 80 percent of the fluorine-18 label in myocardium is contained as fluorine-18 2-fluoro 2-deoxyglucose-6-phosphate.[K6] In normal myocardium, the rate of effective sequestration of fluorine-18 2-deoxyglucose (e.g., transmembranous transport and phosphorylation minus loss due to back-diffusion of tracer) relative to phosphorylation of glucose has been found to be relatively constant.[R5] Studies of in vitro exper-

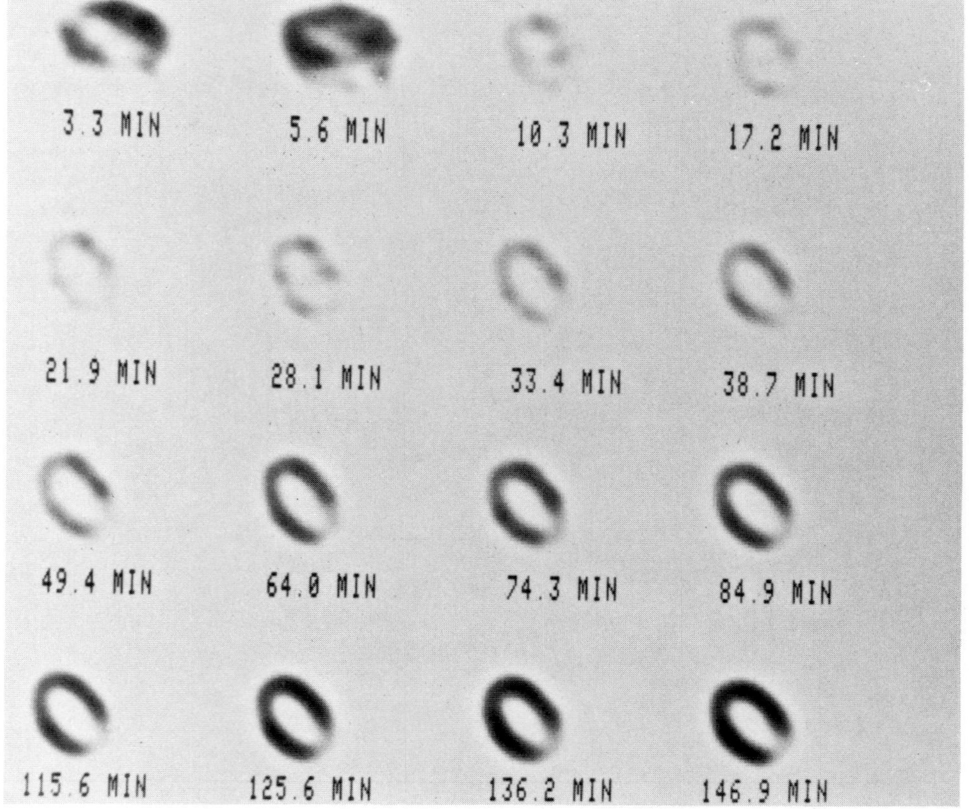

Figure 65–10. Serially acquired cross-sectional images after intravenous injection of ^{18}F-2-fluoro 2-deoxyglucose in a normal volunteer. Note the high activity concentrations in blood early after injection. The subsequent images depict the accumulation of tracer activity in the myocardium and clearance of tracer from the blood. (From Schelbert, H.R., and Schwaiger, M.: PET studies of the heart. *In* Phelps, M., Mazziotta, J., and Schelbert, J. [eds.]: Positron Emission Tomography and Autoradiography: Principles and Applications for the Brain and Heart. Raven Press, New York, 1986, pp. 581–661, with permission.)

imental systems have suggested that this constancy is also maintained during abnormal states such as hypoxia and ischemia.[K7, M2] However, further studies are needed to determine this relationship definitively over a wide range of physiologic and pathophysiologic conditions.

Because fluorine-18 2-fluoro-2-deoxyglucose traces only the initial metabolic steps of exogenous glucose in myocardium, the compound provides only limited information on the metabolic fate of glucose beyond the major branch point between glycolysis and glycogen formation. The tracer does not indicate the fraction of glucose that is subsequently synthesized to glycogen nor the fraction that is directly catabolized through glycolysis. The contribution of endogenous glucose to overall glycolytic flux also remains unknown. However, when employed under strict steady state conditions during which rates of exogenous glucose utilization can be assumed to be at equilibrium with rates of glycogen formation and breakdown through glycolysis, some inferences in overall glycolytic flux should be possible. Furthermore, under extreme conditions, such as during ischemia, when glycogen stores are depleted, the rate of exogenous glucose utilization as determined with this tracer should approach the rate of glycolytic flux.

Qualitative evaluation of the relative distribution of myocardial glucose utilization requires acquisition of a single set of cross-sectional images at about 30 to 50 minutes after tracer injection or at the time of the plateau phase. On these images, regional activity concentrations represent relative rates of regional glucose utilization. If exogenous glucose utilization is to be quantified, acquisition of serial images commences at the time of tracer injection and continues for about 60 minutes (Fig. 65–10). As described later, regions of interest are then assigned to myocardium and arterial blood and rates of glucose utilization derived from the tissue time activity curves.

Carbon-11–Labeled Acetate

This tracer permits the evaluation of flux through the TCA cycle, and because of its close linkage to oxidative phosphorylation, it also permits the evaluation of myocardial oxygen consumption. Its suitability for external imaging and potential utility for the evaluation of myocardial oxidative metabolism were demonstrated in the early 1980s[A3, P7, S14] but only recently were defined more clearly.[A4, A5, B11–14]

Myocardium avidly extracts acetate. First-pass extraction fractions of carbon-11 acetate in canine myocardium average 63 percent at flows of 1 ml · min^{-1} · gm^{-1} and are inversely related to blood flow.[A4] In cytosol, the tracer is activated to acetyl-CoA, which is oxidized in mitochondria by the TCA cycle to carbon-11 CO_2 and H_2O. Following intravenous bolus injection, carbon-11 acetate rapidly clears from blood into myocardium (Fig. 65–11). Serial images reveal subsequent clearance of carbon-11 activity from myocardium. Regional time activity curves as shown in Figure 65–12 indicate a biexponential clearance pattern that implies distribution of tracer between at least two metabolic pools of largely different sizes and turnover rates. The slow clearance phase, although still unexplored, presumably represents deposition of label in a pool (or pools) of amino acids and possibly lipids.[B12, B13] The rapid clearance phase, however, corresponds closely to release of carbon-11 CO_2 from myocardium and thus to the rate of oxidation of carbon-11 acetate to carbon-11 CO_2 in the TCA cycle and release of oxidative end products from myocardium. In both in vitro experimental systems and in intact dogs, the rate of efflux of CO_2 correlated closely and linearly with the externally measured rate of carbon-11 activity clearance from myocardium or with consumption of oxygen.[A4, B10–15] Furthermore, the clearance rate is independent of blood flow and thus appears to depend almost exclusively on the rate of oxygen consumption and flux through the TCA cycle. Although nonmetabolized carbon-11 acetate clears together with carbon-11 CO_2 from myocardium, it represents only about 5 to 10 percent of the total activity released. This fraction remains relatively constant, even during markedly abnormal states, such as ischemia, hypoxia, and postischemia as well as hyperemia, so that the tissue clearance slope of carbon-11 activity reliably and accurately reflects the rate of oxidative turnover of carbon-11 acetate and, consequently, of oxidative metabolism.[A4]

Tissue activity clearance curves of carbon-11 acetate are typically analyzed by biexponential least square fitting routines (Fig. 65–12).[A4, B14] The relative size and slope of the slow clearance phase have been found to remain relatively constant over a wide range of oxygen consumption. In contrast, the slope of the rapid clearance curve component in intact dogs correlated closely and

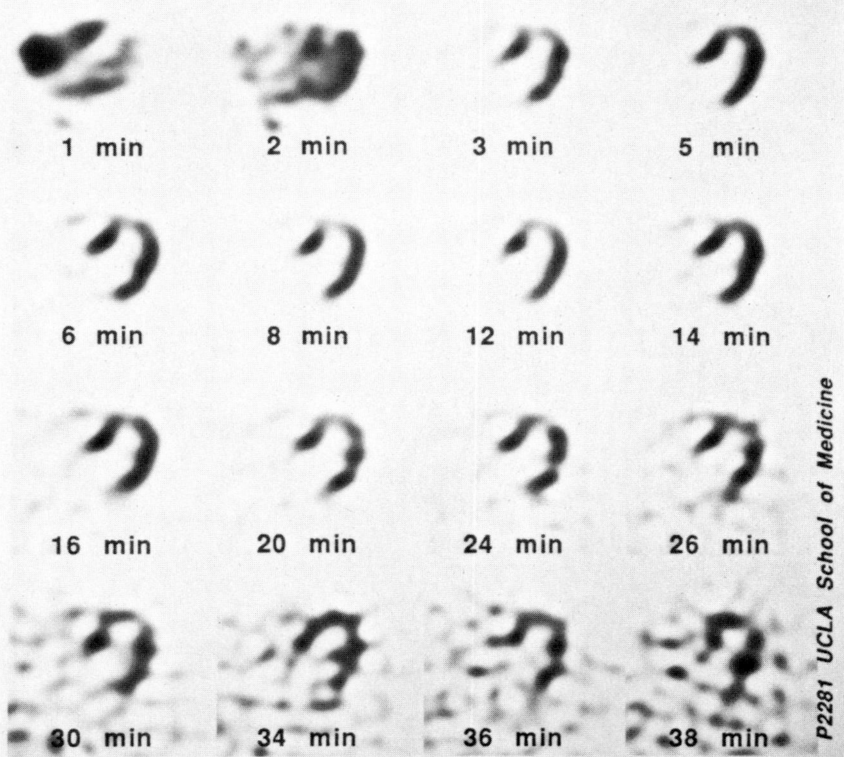

Figure 65–11. Serial cross-sectional images after intravenous ^{11}C-acetate in a normal volunteer. The initial images depict the activity in arterial blood, followed by rapid clearance of tracer from the blood and accumulation of tracer in the myocardium. The subsequent images indicate clearance of tracer from myocardium with decreasing myocardium-to-background activity ratios.

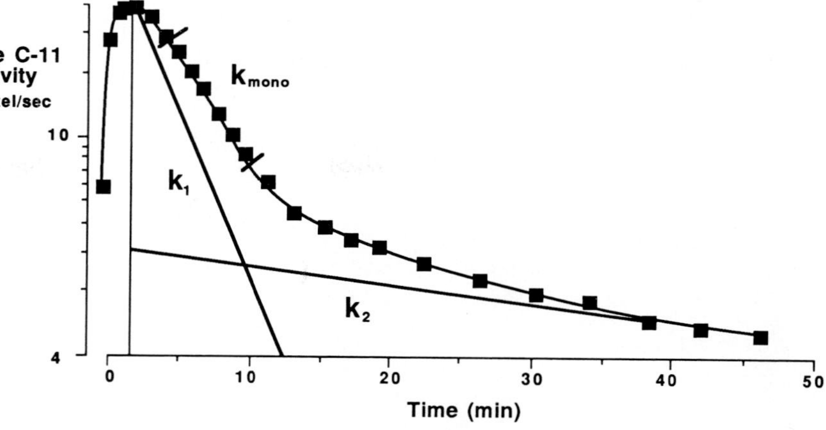

Figure 65–12. Myocardial ^{11}C-acetate tissue time activity curve. Note the biexponential clearance of tracer from the myocardium. The slopes of the two clearance phases are obtained by biexponential least square fitting and are denoted as k_1 and k_2. Monoexponential fitting of the early portion of the clearance phase yields the slope k_{mono}.

linearly with the rate of oxygen consumption,[A4, B12, B14] and in normal human volunteers with the heart rate blood pressure product as an index of cardiac work and oxygen consumption (Fig. 65–13).[A5, H12]

Because the slow clearance phase is not always adequately visualized on the tissue time activity curves, especially when tissue clearance rates are slow, as at rest, biexponential clearance curve fitting often proves to be difficult or impossible. Slopes are then obtained by least square fitting of only the early monoexponential portion of the clearance curve (see Fig. 65–12). These monoexponential slopes are less sensitive to fitting errors due to low count rates and thus statistical noise toward the end of the clearance curve. Slopes by monoexponential fitting correlate well with oxygen consumption in dogs and with the heart rate blood pressure product in humans.[A5, B14]

Both initial uptake of carbon-11 acetate in normal myocardium and its subsequent clearance are homogeneous. Using eight sectorial regions of interest, clearance slopes by monoexponential curve fitting varied between regions by less than 10 percent and by biexponential fitting by 16 percent.[A4] Difficulties in biexponential fitting, as indicated earlier, accounted mostly for the higher variability of the latter clearance slopes. In normal fasted volunteers at rest, the slope of the rapid clearance phase averaged 0.059 ± 0.016 for an average heart rate blood pressure product of 6500 beats mmHg $\cdot$ min^{-1}. This slope corresponds to a clearance half-time of 11.7 min, which is similar to that reported initially by Selwyn and colleagues.[S14] The slope increases in linear relation with higher workloads, as seen in Figure 65–13*B*.

Both uptake and clearance rates of carbon-11 acetate change with regional abnormalities in blood flow and metabolism. In ischemic myocardial regions, the initial uptake of carbon-11 acetate decreases in proportion to myocardial blood flow. High tracer first-pass extraction fractions as observed in canine myocardium[A4] account for the flow dependency of the initial tracer uptake. Regional clearance rates are reduced in proportion to regional reductions in oxidative metabolism.[A4] For example, Selwyn and colleagues observed a 30 percent reduction in regional clearance rates in acutely ischemic myocardium relative to normal myocardium in patients with severe coronary artery disease during supine bicycle exercise.[S14]

Changes in plasma substrate concentrations and, thus, in myocardial substrate selection, hardly affect myocardial tissue clearance rates of carbon-11 acetate. Shifts in substrate selection from predominantly fatty acid to glucose in experimental dogs resulted in a small but statistically significant increase in clearance rates for the same amount of oxygen consumption.[B14] Differences in the proportions of oxygen consumption utilized in tricarboxylic acid oxidation of fatty acid versus glucose may account for this effect. For glucose and lactate, for example, 67 percent of overall myocardial oxygen consumption occurs via the TCA cycle, compared with 70 percent for palmitate and 72 percent for oleate. Nevertheless, this effect is small and is likely to remain undetected on tissue clearance curves obtained in vivo with positron emission tomography in humans.[A5, W4]

Evaluation of Myocardial Substrate Metabolism

Both fluorine-18 2-fluoro-2-deoxyglucose and carbon-11 palmitate afford the evaluation of well-defined segments of myocardial substrate metabolism, whereas carbon-11 acetate traces the overall myocardial oxidative metabolism of myocardium. Information obtainable with fluorine-18 2-deoxyglucose is confined to the initial steps of exogenous glucose utilization, whereas carbon-

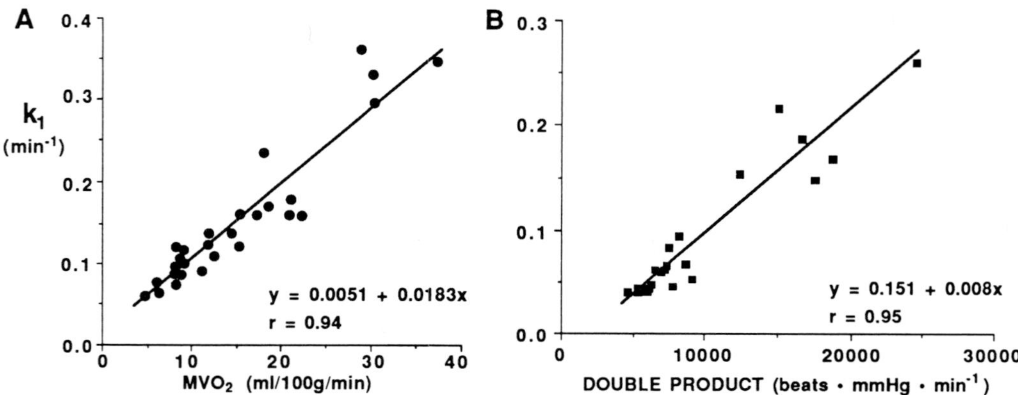

Figure 65–13. Relationship between the slope of the rapid clearance phase k_1 of ^{11}C-acetate by serial PET imaging and myocardial oxygen consumption in dogs (*Panel A*) and the heart rate blood pressure product in normal human volunteers. (Adapted from Buxton, D.B., Nienaber, C.A., Luxen, A., et al.: Noninvasive quantitation of regional myocardial oxygen consumption in vivo with [1-^{11}C] acetate and dynamic positron emission tomography. Circulation 79:134–142, 1989, with permission; and Armbrecht, J.J., Buxton, D.B., Brunken, R.C., et al.: Regional myocardial oxygen consumption determined noninvasively in humans with [1-^{11}C] acetate and dynamic positron tomography. Circulation 80:863, 1989, by permission of the American Heart Association, Inc.)

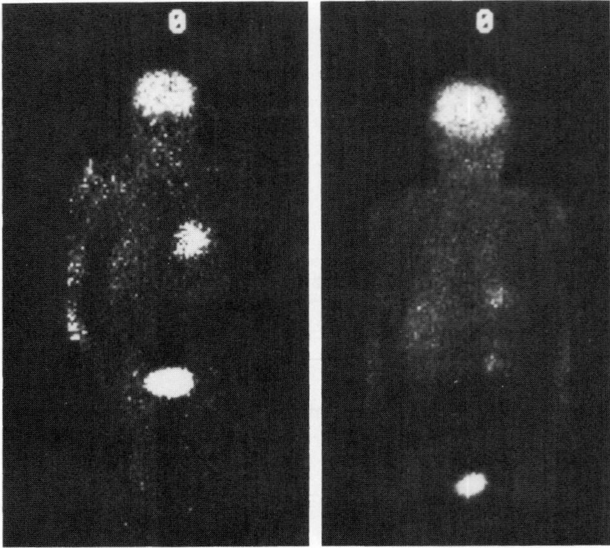

Figure 65–14. Effects of circulating plasma substrate levels on myocardial ^{18}F-2-fluoro-2-deoxyglucose uptake. The two rectilinear (two-dimensional) scans show the body distributions of the tracer in two normal volunteers, one examined after an overnight fast *(left panel)* and the other one after a carbohydrate-rich meal *(right panel)*. The brain utilizes glucose almost exclusively and does not participate in changes of substrate utilization in response to altered substrate availability. Therefore, it reveals, under both fasted and postprandial conditions, uptake of ^{18}F-2-fluoro-2-deoxyglucose. In contrast, the heart predominantly utilizes free fatty acid in the fasted state. The lack of glucose utilization in this condition is reflected by the absence of myocardial tracer uptake. After a carbohydrate load with an increase in plasma glucose and a decline in plasma free fatty acid levels, myocardial substrate selection shifts to glucose, which is demonstrated on the images by enhanced tracer accumulation in the myocardium.

11 palmitate traces the entire metabolic pathway of fatty acid, including deposition of fatty acid in the endogenous lipid pool and oxidation of fatty acid. The latter includes both β-oxidation as well as final oxidation of the two carbon fragments via the TCA cycle. The information derived with these two tracers largely depends, therefore, on the specific state of substrate selection and further on substrate availability and plasma substrate levels. In the fasted state, when plasma fatty acid levels are high and glucose insulin levels are low, and when myocardium preferentially utilizes fatty acid, little if any fluorine-18 2-fluoro 2-deoxyglucose accumulates in myocardium (Fig. 65–14). Conversely, on the tissue clearance curves of carbon-11 palmitate, the relative size of the rapid clearance curve component will be large and its clearance slope steep. Changes in substrate levels, such as a postprandial increase in glucose and decline in fatty acid levels, dramatically alter the clearance kinetics of carbon-11 palmitate and the myocardial uptake of fluorine-18 2-deoxyglucose (see Figs. 65–7 and 65–14). The latter increases in response to augmented myocardial usage of exogenous glucose, whereas the slope and relative size of the rapid carbon-11 palmitate clearance curve component decline, consistent with lesser oxidation of fatty acid in favor of glucose. The effects of substrate availability and of resultant changes in myocardial substrate selection on the uptake and turnover of tracers in myocardium emphasize the need for standardization of study conditions and for monitoring of plasma substrate levels. Changes in tracer tissue kinetics in response to alterations in substrate availability can also be used advantageously to elicit abnormal and normal responses.[S10] Lastly, combined use of metabolic tracers—for example, carbon-11 palmitate and carbon-11 acetate—permits assessment of the contribution of free fatty acid or of glucose to overall oxidative metabolism[B13] or, under conditions of ischemia, an assessment of anaerobic versus oxidative glucose metabolism.

Amino Acids Labeled With Nitrogen-13 or Carbon-11

The use of positron-emitting amino acids for the study of myocardial amino acid metabolism and rates of protein synthesis has remained relatively unexplored. As demonstrated in canine myocardium, the clearance curve morphology of these agents depends upon the specific label.[H13] When labeled with carbon-11, the activity clears from myocardium in three phases, compared with only two phases when amino acids are labeled with nitrogen-13. The rapid clearance phase is thought to represent a pool of amino acids that communicates with the vascular space by back-diffusion, with a slow turnover pool presumably reflecting labeled precursors for protein synthesis, as well as with a third, oxidative pool, presumably representing oxidation via the TCA cycle and release of carbon-11 CO_2 into blood.[B16–18, K2, K7, R6]

Low first-pass retention fractions and, consequently, low myocardial uptake of labeled amino acids in canine myocardium are most likely species related, because amino acids such as nitrogen-13 glutamate avidly accumulate in human myocardium.[G11–13, K8, K9] Comparisons with nitrogen-13 ammonia uptake suggest that the distribution of nitrogen-13 glutamate in human myocardium depends largely upon regional myocardial blood flow.[K8, R7] Nevertheless, Zimmerman and co-workers reported relative or absolute increases in nitrogen-13 glutamate uptake in acutely ischemic human myocardium and suggested the potential utility of nitrogen-13 glutamate for exploring and delineating ischemia-related abnormalities in amino acid metabolism.[Z2] Labeled amino acids further offer the possibility to measure rates of myocardial protein synthesis.[12, 13]

Tracers of Cardiac Innervation and Receptors

There are several positron-emitting tracers for the study of myocardial adrenergic neuron densities and of β-adrenergic and cholinergic muscarinic receptors. The properties of carbon-11–labeled β-receptor antagonists and especially of the carbon-11–labeled experimental drug CGP 12177 as probes for myocardial β-receptors,[D3, S15] as well as of carbon-11–labeled MQNB for the study of myocardial cholinergic muscarinic receptors[M3, M4, S16–18] are described in detail in Chapter 69.

Several other tracers of myocardial adrenergic neuron density have recently become available. Fluorine-18–labeled metaraminol, a norepinephrine analog, accumulates in myocardium in proportion to regional catecholamine concentrations.[S9, W10] The agent traces recapture and uptake of circulating norepinephrine by adrenergic nerve endings and is thought to accumulate in storage granules.[H14] Because fluorine-18 metaraminol can be synthesized in only low specific activity, pharmacologic doses of tracer are required for imaging. Therefore, another agent, carbon-11 hydroxy ephedrine has recently been synthesized and has undergone initial testing in humans.[H15, W11]

Other Tracers

Several other potentially useful tracers for studies of myocardial tissue function with positron emission tomography have recently been described.

Rubidium-81. The 4.6-hour physical half-life of this cation offers the possibility of studying the equilibrium distribution of cations between blood and myocardium rather than only the initial, flow-dependent uptake of the short-lived rubidium-82 in myocardium. When imaged several hours after intravenous administration and after rubidium-81 has equilibrated between blood and myocardium, tracer activity concentrations in myocardium probably reflect the potassium pool.[S20, S21] The regional size of this pool and its variations in disease might prove useful as a reference to which metabolic measurements can be related. Equilibrium rubidium-81 images have also been found useful for assessing partial volume-related, "artifactual" underestimation of regional true tracer tissue concentrations in abnormally contracting myocardial regions.[S20]

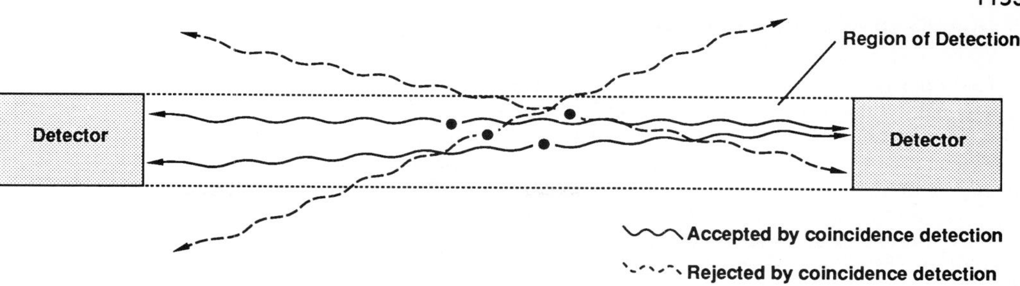

Figure 65–15. Detection of positron decay. Pairs of 511 KeV photons leave the site of the annihilation event in diametrically opposed directions. They are detected by a pair of radiation detectors positioned at an angle of 180 degrees and connected by a coincidence circuitry. The region of detection is defined by the two radiation detectors.

Membrane Function. A carbon-11–labeled lipophilic agent, triphenylmethylphosphonium, binds to myocardium in dogs and humans and can be readily displaced by potassium chloride administration. Preliminary studies with this agent suggested the possibility of calculating membrane potentials from the tracer distribution ratio (or the partition coefficient) between the cellular and plasma water space and to obtain information on the energy state of myocardium.[F3]

Another compound, a peripheral type of benzodiazepine receptor antagonist, referred to as PK 11195 and labeled with carbon-11, has been reported to bind specifically peripheral-type benzodiazepine receptors in canine and human myocardium.[C2] The agent is of potential interest for cardiac studies because the investigators postulated a possible relationship between peripheral-type benzodiazepine receptors and calcium channels in the heart.

Fluorine-18 Misonidazole. Among currently emerging tracer compounds, fluorine-18 misonidazole is perhaps the most attractive because it specifically labels ischemic/hypoxic myocardium. Based on investigations in tumors, the agent appears to diffuse across sarcolemmal membranes. Nitro reduction then results in formation of the RNO_2 radical anion, which, in the presence of oxygen, is oxidized to superoxide and noncharged misonidazole that diffuses back into blood. If oxygen is absent, the RNO_2 radical is reduced to nitrous compounds and, further, to hydroxylamines and other amines that covalently bind to intracellular macromolecules with effective trapping of radiolabel in hypoxic/ischemic cells.[F4, G14, M5, R8, W13] Initial studies in isolated perfused rabbit hearts and in dogs have confirmed the utility of fluorine-18 misonidazole as a marker of hypoxic/ischemic myocardium. During hypoxia or low flow ischemia, isolated perfused hearts retained 40 to 50 percent of the total administered tracer activity, compared with only 16 to 18 percent tracer retention in normal or postischemic hearts.[S22] In dog experiments, 1.5 ± 0.8 percent of the tracer was extracted by normal myocardium, compared with 34 ± 24 percent in ischemic myocardium 75 minutes after coronary ligation.[S23] The magnitude of tracer retention depends upon the time after coronary occlusion. It declines to 12 ± 3 percent at 150 minutes and to only 3 ± 2 percent at 24 hours after coronary ligation. Thus, as ischemia proceeds to necrosis, progressively less tracer accumulates in ischemically injured myocardium, suggesting that the tracer specifically binds to ischemic rather than necrotic tissue. Imaging studies in dog experiments after coronary ligation have demonstrated segmentally enhanced tracer uptake in hypoperfused myocardial regions.[M6, S23]

IMAGING WITH POSITRON EMISSION TOMOGRAPHY

General Principles

The quantitative imaging capability as a feature unique to positron emission tomography enables noninvasive measurements of regional tracer tissue concentrations. Cross-sectional images acquired with positron emission tomography quantitatively represent regional tracer tissue concentrations. The images are therefore comparable to autoradiographs but are acquired in vivo. The quantitative imaging capability derives from two technical aspects of positron emission tomography: a relatively uniform or depth-independent spatial resolution and appropriate correction for photon attenuation. Both are related to physical decay characteristics specific for positrons.

Positrons are particles with a mass equal to that of electrons, but they are charged positively. As they travel through tissue, they lose kinetic energy and combine with an electron. The total mass converts into energy, which is released in the form of two 511 KeV photons that simultaneously leave the site of "annihilation" in diametrically opposed directions (Fig. 65–15). When both photons simultaneously (or near-simultaneously) strike two scintillation detectors connected by a coincidence circuitry, an "annihilation" event is registered.

Because the two photons are given off at an angle of 180 degrees, the site of the annihilation event must have occurred and must therefore be located within the field between the two detectors. The region of detection, as shown in Figure 65–15, is thus defined by the size of the detectors. Multiple detector pairs arranged in circular arrays permit localization of the site of the annihilation events and thus of the geographic distribution of positron-emitting isotopes within the plane described by the detector arrays. When multiple circular detector arrays are joined in series, the location of the annihilation event in space can be determined (Fig. 65–16). Back-projection techniques and reconstruction algorithms locate the distribution of positron-emitting isotopes in space and form images of their concentrations in tissue. A detailed description of image reconstruction techniques is beyond the scope of this chapter but is available elsewhere.[H16, P5]

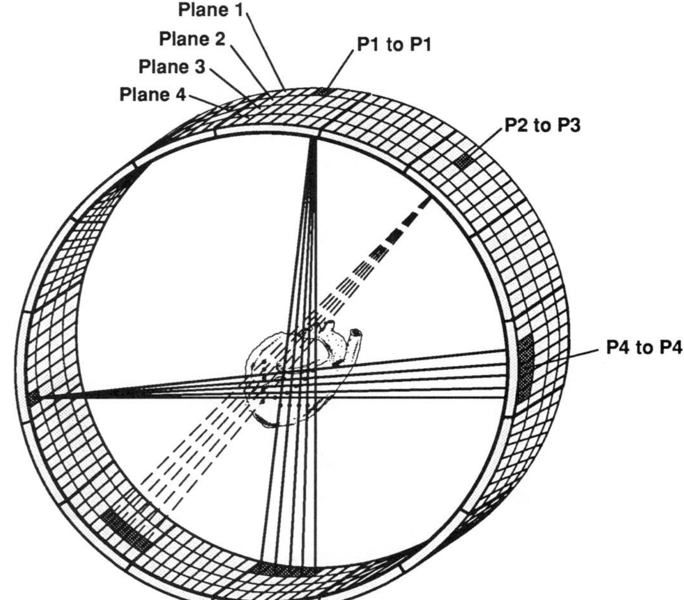

Figure 65–16. Schematics of positron emission tomographic imaging. Four circular arrays of detectors (Plane 1 to Plane 4) in a series are shown. Within each detector ring, detectors are connected with several opposite detectors by coincidence circuitry and result in true plane images. Detectors are also connected by coincidence circuitries with several detectors in the adjacent detector ring and provide cross-plane images. Shaded rectangles indicate detectors in coincidence.

Early positron emission tomographs were equipped with single hexagonal, octagonal, or circular arrays of detector pairs in coincidence and therefore permitted cross-sectional images in only one plane at a time. Modern state-of-the-art tomographs acquire simultaneously 15 to 22 planes with an interplane spacing of 7 mm and an axial field of view of 10 to 15 cm.[H17, H18, 14, M7, M8, S24, S25] Refinements in detector technology have improved spatial resolution from an early 20-mm full-width half-maximum (FWHM) to a current 5- to 6-mm FWHM and, in some instances, even to 2- to 3-mm FWHM.[V1] The physical size of individual detectors or the density of detector packing largely determines the spatial resolution characteristics and counting efficiency and sensitivity of a positron emission tomograph. As a general rule, the smaller the detector, the higher the spatial resolution. The detectors are coupled to photomultiplier tubes. Because they are larger than the detector crystals, the number of photomultiplier tubes that can be coupled to detectors and packed into the detector gantry therefore determines to a large extent the spatial resolution.

The physics of the annihilation process itself imposes additional limitations, which include the positron range and the angle at which the photons leave the annihilation site. The positron range is the distance positrons travel in tissue before they "annihilate." This range is small (less than 1 mm) for most positron emitters but can be as large as 3 to 4 mm for some (e.g., rubidium-82). As a general rule, the positron range is inversely related to the physical half-life of the positron-emitting isotope. The second limitation relates to the fact that not all photon pairs leave the site of an annihilation at an angle of exactly 180 degrees. Therefore, annihilation events outside the region of detection (as shown in Figure 65–16) are registered and placed wrongly into the region of detection. Given these limitations, 2 to 3 mm appears to be the currently attainable spatial resolution of positron emission tomographs.

Image Acquisition

The relatively limited axial field of view mandates careful patient positioning for adequate imaging. Some laboratories rely on a supine chest radiograph and demarcate the upper and lower limits of the cardiac silhouette on the patient's chest. Other laboratories record a rectilinear or two-dimensional transmission scan that resembles a low spatial resolution chest tomograph. Cursors on the computer display are moved to the cardiac silhouette and define the upper and lower imaging planes and thus the available axial field of view. They control the bed position of the tomograph and automatically move the patient into the predefined position.

The imaging procedure itself begins with acquisition of cross-sectional transmission images using a ring source of positron-emitting isotope inserted into the imaging gantry. These transmission images measure the photon attenuation and are used for correction of the emission images. Acquisition times typically range from 10 to 20 minutes. The positron-emitting tracer is then injected intravenously, and sequential or static images are acquired. Static images display the relative distribution of functional processes throughout the left ventricular myocardium and are acquired after accumulation of radiotracer in myocardium and clearance from blood (Fig. 65–17). The time interval between tracer injection and image acquisition depends, therefore, on the type of tracer and may range from 5 to 50 minutes. If regional functional processes are to be determined quantitatively, serial images are recorded (Fig. 65–18). Image acquisition commences at the time of tracer administration and continues, depending on the type of tracer, for 10 to 60 minutes. For short-lived tracers like rubidium-82 or nitrogen-13 ammonia, acquisition of an image set is typically completed within 10 to 15 minutes, whereas definition of the tissue clearance curve morphology of, for example, carbon-11 palmitate or carbon-11 acetate requires acquisition periods of 40 to 50 minutes.

Rapid acquisition of serial images, also referred to as dynamic imaging, visualizes, as seen in Figure 65–18, the transit of the

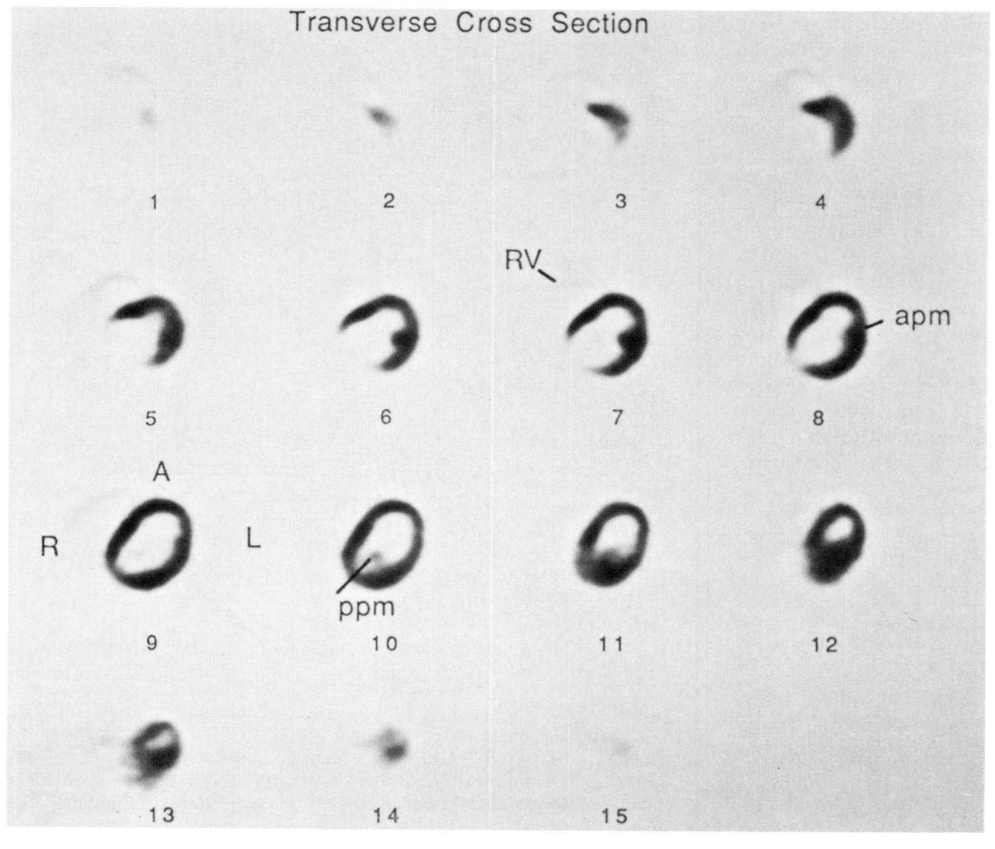

Figure 65–17. Contiguous cross-sectional images of the distribution of a positron emitting tracer in the myocardium of a normal volunteer. The images were acquired with a state-of-the-art multi-slice positron emission tomograph after the administration of intravenous ^{18}F-2-fluoro 2-deoxyglucose and are viewed from the subject's feet. The images begin at the base of the heart (levels 2 to 4) and proceed to the mid-portion (levels 7 to 9) and diaphragmatic (levels 11 to 14) portion of the left ventricle. (A—anterior; L—lateral; S—septum, R—right ventricular myocardium; APM and PPM—anterior and posterior papillary muscle, B—base, and AP—apex of the left ventricle).

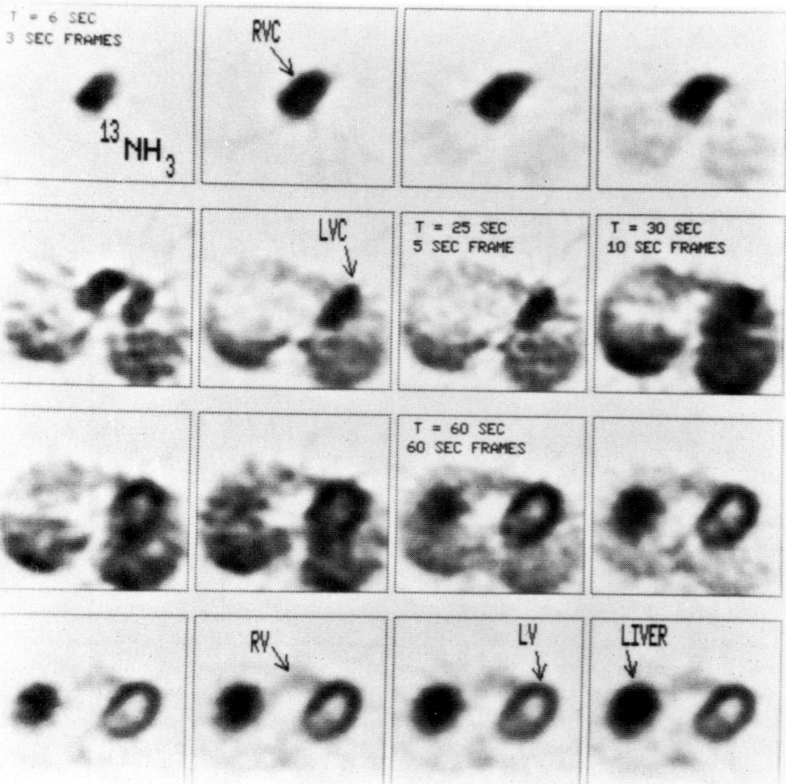

Figure 65–18. Dynamic image acquisition after an intravenous bolus of [^{13}N]ammonia (10 mCi) in a normal volunteer. The initial six 3-second frames depict the transit of radioactivity through the right ventricle, both lungs, and the left ventricle. The last six 60-second frames show accumulation of [^{13}N]ammonia in the left and right ventricular myocardium (From Schelbert, H.R., and Schwaiger, M.: PET studies of the heart. *In* Phelps, M., Mazziotta, J., and Schelbert, J. [eds.]: Positron Emission Tomography and Autoradiography: Principles and Applications for the Brain and Heart. Raven Press, New York, 1986, pp. 581–661, with permission.)

tracer bolus through the central circulation, as well as its subsequent accumulation and clearance in myocardium. From these dynamically acquired images, the arterial input function of tracer and the myocardial tissue response can be determined (Fig. 65–19).

Image acquisition can also be synchronized with the patient's electrocardiogram (Fig. 65–20). As many as 16 to 32 frames per cardiac cycle can be collected and permit the evaluation of

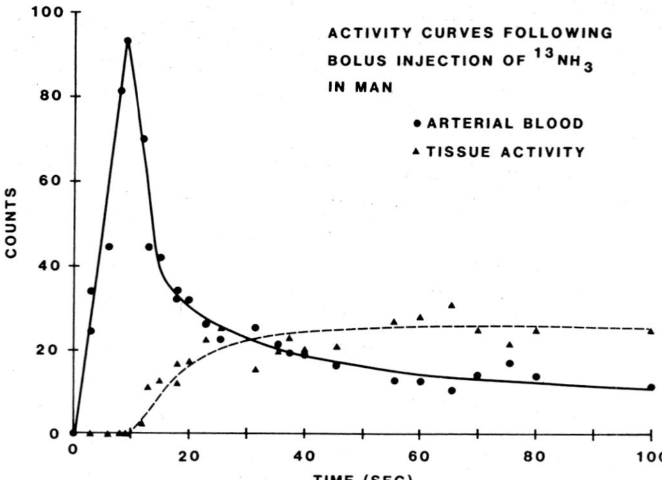

Figure 65–19. Time activity curves of arterial and myocardial ^{13}N activity concentrations derived from dynamically acquired cross-sectional images as shown in Figure 65–17. Determination of the arterial input function from the dynamic PET studies *(solid circle)* agrees well with the arterial input function derived from serial blood samples *(solid line)*. Note also the tissue response *(solid triangles)*, which for better visualization shows the myocardial tissue ^{13}N activities multiplied by a factor of 2. (From Schelbert, H.R., and Schwaiger, M.: PET studies of the heart. *In* Phelps, M., Mazziotta, J., and Schelbert, J. [eds.]: Positron Emission Tomography and Autoradiography: Principles and Applications for the Brain and Heart. Raven Press, New York, 1986, pp. 581–661, with permission.)

regional myocardial wall motion or wall thickening.[H17, H19, N1, W1] Gated image acquisition also has been employed for minimizing motion artifacts and improving accuracy with which regional myocardial tracer concentrations can be determined from the cross-sectional images.[T6, W1]

Identical patient positioning during transmission and emission image acquisition is critical, because positional changes are likely to cause inadequate correction for photon attenuation and, consequently, introduce image artifacts. Most tomographs, therefore, are equipped with low power neon laser beams that facilitate patient positioning as well as permit constant monitoring of patient positioning during image acquisition. Other efforts to minimize changes in patient positioning include measurements of photon attenuation after tracer injection, for example, with the recently proposed[C3, R9] rotating sources of positron-emitting tracers, so that emission and transmission images are recorded in close temporal proximity. An alternate approach entails acquisition of a transmission scan for only a short time period. On these images or on post-tracer injection images as described earlier, the boundaries of the chest and its organs are defined in order to determine the spatial distribution of various tissues, such as chest wall, lungs, and mediastinum. Fixed attenuation coefficients for each tissue-type are then employed for correction of photon attenuation.[H20]

A set of 15 contiguous cross-sectional images obtained with a multislice tomograph in a normal volunteer is shown in Figure 65–17. These images depict the distribution of tracer within the left and right ventricular myocardium. The anterior and posterior papillary muscles are clearly visualized. Due to the transaxial orientation of the image planes, visualization of the diaphragmatic portions of the left ventricular myocardium often remains unsatisfactory and has prompted the development of slice reorientation techniques.[H21, M9, R10, S20] Contiguous images, reoriented perpendicular to the long axis of the left ventricle, are shown in Figure 65–21. The slice reorientation also reduces the partial volume-related variability of apparent regional tracer concentrations owing to regional differences in myocardial wall thickness and the angle between myocardium and image plane. Circumferential activity profiles derived from short axis slices are more homogeneous than those derived from transaxial slices and therefore are

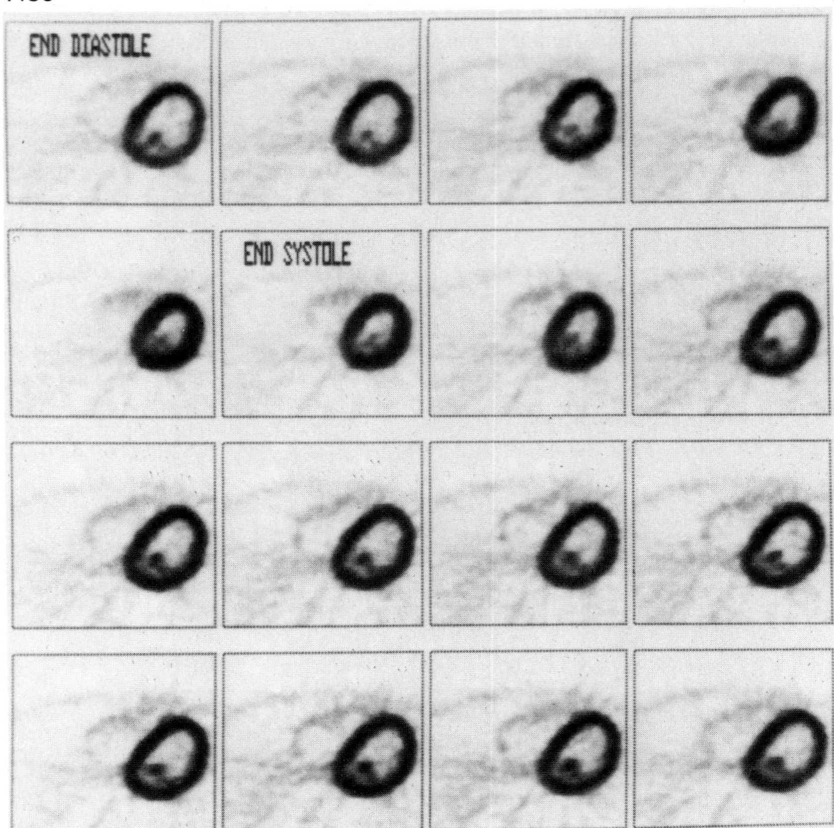

Figure 65–20. Multiple-gated myocardial images acquired with positron emission tomography. The image plane was positioned through the mid–left ventricle and the RR interval divided into 16 frames, each of 50-msec duration. The sequence of images is presented from left to right and proceeds from end-diastole to end-systole and back to end-diastole. Note the corresponding changes in left ventricular size and myocardial wall thickness between diastole and systole. (From Schelbert, H.R., and Schwaiger, M.: PET studies of the heart. *In* Phelps, M., Mazziotta, J., and Schelbert, J. [eds.]: Positron Emission Tomography and Autoradiography: Principles and Applications for the Brain and Heart. Raven Press, New York, 1986, pp. 581–661, with permission.)

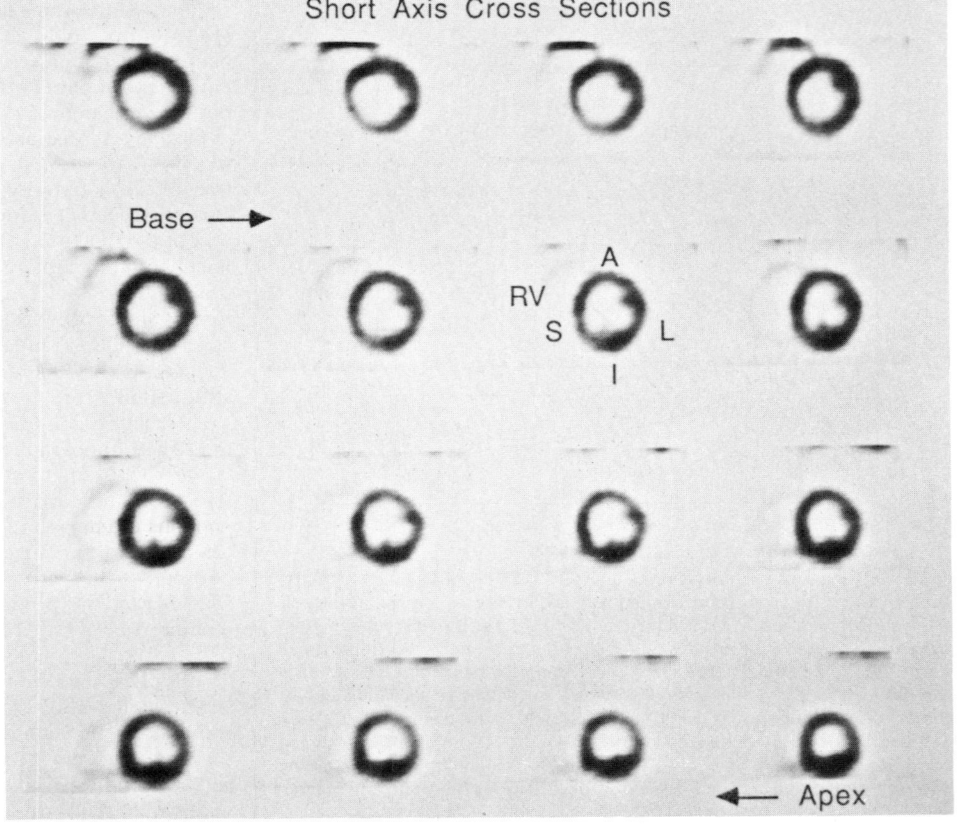

Figure 65–21. Reorientation of cross-sectional images. After reformatting the transaxial images shown in Figure 65–17, the tracer distribution in myocardium is depicted in 16 contiguous short axis cross sections that are oriented perpendicular to the long axis of the left ventricle. The cross sections begin at the base and continue to the apex of the left ventricle (RV—right ventricle; A, L and I—anterior, lateral, and inferior wall; S—septum.)

more suitable for interindividual comparisons. Lastly, the activity profiles derived from contiguous short axis cuts can be displayed in the form of "polar maps" as employed routinely with single photon emission computed tomography.[H21] Thus, the three-dimensional distributions of activity can readily be presented in the form of two-dimensional maps of the left ventricular myocardium. "Surface displays" are an alternative means of presenting the three-dimensional distribution of tracer throughout the left ventricular myocardium. The individual cross-sectional images are reconstructed to form a three-dimensional image of the heart, which is then displayed and rotated on the computer scope of the tomograph for viewing at an angle of 360°.[D4]

Image Analysis and Tracer Concentration Measurements

Positional changes between transmission and emission images and low count statistics can result in erroneous or inaccurate measurements of regional tracer concentrations. Additional errors can result from partial volume effect and activity spillover.

PARTIAL VOLUME EFFECT. Regional tracer concentrations, as visualized on or determined quantitatively from the cross-sectional images, depend upon the size of the object or, in the case of the heart, on the regional myocardial wall thickness. As demonstrated in phantom experiments, apparent tissue concentrations equal true tissue concentrations only if the regional myocardial wall thickness is at least twice the spatial resolution of the imaging device.[H16, H22] Observed tracer tissue concentrations, however, decrease nonlinearly with decreasing object size or regional myocardial wall thickness (Fig. 65–22).[H22, W1] Loss of systolic thickening alone, as during ischemia, as demonstrated in dogs by Parodi and associates,[P8] can result in an apparent further reduction in regional tracer activity on ungated images because the average myocardial wall thickness declines.

Corrections for the partial volume-related underestimation of true tracer tissue concentrations are possible if the regional wall thickness is known.[H22] From the relationship between recovered and true tissue activity concentrations and the object size, a recovery coefficient RF is derived. The recovery coefficient is a nonlinear function of the regional wall thickness. If the wall thickness is known, then the true tracer tissue concentration (C_m) is calculated by

$$C_m = \frac{C_{mo}}{RF} \text{ (cts} \cdot \text{min}^{-1} \cdot \text{ml}^{-1}) \tag{6}$$

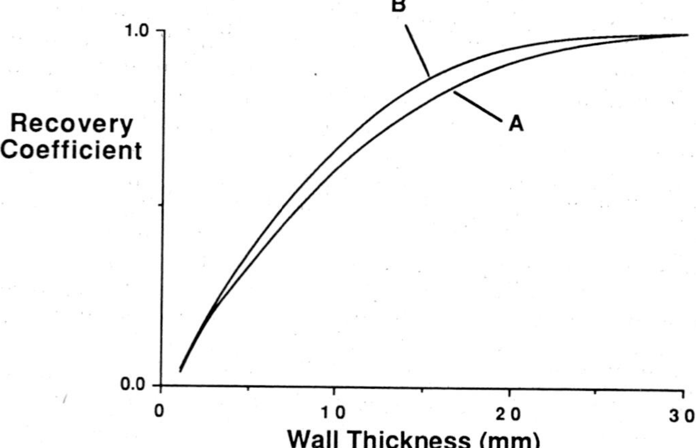

Figure 65–22. Partial volume effect and underestimation of true tracer tissue concentrations as a function of myocardial wall thickness and the tomograph's performance characteristics. The recovery coefficient as the ratio of observed to true tracer tissue concentrations increases with myocardial wall thickness (in mm). Curve A was obtained from bar phantom images reconstructed with an effective spatial resolution of 13.7 mm FWHM and curve B with an effective spatial resolution of 11.9 mm FWHM.

where C_{mo} is the observed tracer tissue concentration as derived from a region of interest. Myocardial wall thickness can be determined by echocardiography[W1] or, as proposed more recently, directly from the positron emission tomographic images.[N1, R11] The magnitude of the partial volume effect and thus the recovery coefficient vary with the performance characteristics of the tomograph and must be determined for each instrument.

ACTIVITY SPILLOVER. This effect results from the imperfect spatial resolution of the imaging device and misplaces activity between adjacent structures or organs. If, for example, the regional myocardial tracer concentration is determined from a region of interest assigned to the left ventricular myocardium, the observed activity is contaminated by spillover of activity from the left ventricular blood pool (as well as by activity in the vascular space of the left ventricular myocardium itself). Correction for activity spillover is especially important for serially acquired images, at a time when tracer concentrations are high in blood but low in myocardium, and conversely, after tracer clearance from blood into myocardium, when activity is high in myocardium but low in blood. Thus, early after tracer injection, activity predominantly spills from blood into myocardium, whereas late after injection, the spillover direction reverses (Fig. 65–23). The degree of activity spillover is defined as the spillover fraction. It is calculated as the ratio of the activity measured in a region of interest outside of but adjacent to the structure to the activity measured in a region of interest assigned directly to the same structure. The spillover fraction is then applied to observed tissue concentrations in order to remove or correct for contamination by "misplaced" activity.

The magnitude of the spillover depends upon the proximity of the organ or measurement regions of interest and the performance characteristics of the tomograph. For an intrinsic resolution of 5 to 6 mm, the spillover fraction from the blood pool into myocardium was found to amount to as much as 40 percent after blood pool labeling with oxygen-15 carbon monoxide in dogs.[N1] "Spillover" of activity from blood into myocardium is caused only in part by instrument-related misplacement of activity, for it also includes activity in the vascular space of the myocardium. The myocardial blood volume amounts to about 10 percent of the myocardial volume but may vary considerably, for example, during hyperemia. Accurate determinations of regional tracer concentrations in myocardium as well as in arterial blood therefore require corrections for activity spillover. Such corrections are possible and are based on the performance characteristics of the tomograph as well as the dimensions of the left ventricular cavity and myocardium.[H23–25]

QUANTIFICATION OF TRACER CONCENTRATIONS. Circumferential activity profile analysis approaches are employed to determine relative tracer concentrations throughout the left ventricular myocardium.[B3, R11, T2, T3] Radii, originating from the center of the left ventricular blood pool at 6° intervals, search for the maximum (or average) activity of the myocardium and plot relative regional tracer concentrations as a function of the angle along the circumference. Individual patient profiles are compared with standard profiles derived from normal volunteers in order to define the extent and magnitude of segmental increases or reductions in tracer uptake.

Quantification of regional tissue concentrations from serially recorded images is facilitated by semiautomated analysis routines.[R11] They define the inner and outer borders of the left ventricular myocardium and divide the myocardium into sectorial regions of interest. Together with an additional region of interest assigned to the left ventricular blood pool, this matrix is then copied to all serial images and regional tissue tracer concentrations, and their changes over time are determined in counts per second per pixel. They are then corrected for physical decay, partial volume effect, and activity spillover and are used for construction of time activity curves for arterial blood and regional myocardium. Measurements of the arterial input function and of myocardial tracer activity concentrations determined in this manner have been validated and were found to correlate well with in vivo counting of tissue samples.[N1, W1, W12] High count rates at the time of the transit of the bolus activity through the central

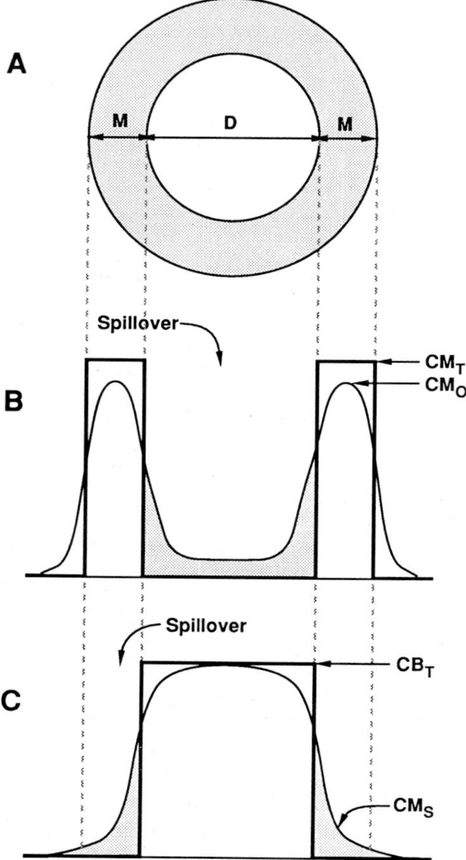

Figure 65–23. Partial volume and activity spillover. *A*, Schematic drawings of a cross section through the left ventricle with a cavity diameter D and a myocardial wall thickness M. *B*, Activity profile through the left ventricular cross section at a time when concentrations are high in the myocardium and low in arterial blood and, *C*, at a time when myocardial concentrations are low or negligible and are high in arterial blood. The bold lines in *B* and *C* reflect the true tissue activity profiles and the fine lines the observed tissue activity profiles. Because myocardial wall thickness (M) is less than twice the spatial resolution of the tomograph, the observed tracer tissue concentration (CM_O) is less than the true tracer tissue concentration (CM_T). CM_O can be corrected for by the recovery coefficient if M is known. In arterial blood, the CM_O approximates the true blood activity concentration (CB_T) because the diameter of the blood pool is greater than twice the spatial resolution. Misplacement of activity from the myocardium to the blood is shown in Panel B and from the blood into the myocardium in Panel C. The spillover fraction can be determined from the blood pool image from the ratio of activity in the myocardium due to spillover (CM_S) and CB_T.

circulation can exceed count rate capabilities of positron emission tomographs and result in losses in counts due to deadtime. Excessive peak activities and thus significant deadtime losses can be avoided by use of a more distributed bolus input function, achieved by spreading out the tracer injection over a longer time period (e.g., 30 seconds) and by lowering tracer activities (e.g., 15 mCi) if the arterial input function is to be determined quantitatively by serial imaging. Correction routines for deadtime losses have also been developed[G15, W1] and are implemented in several commercially available positron emission tomographs.

When the arterial input function cannot be obtained directly from the serially acquired images, activity concentrations in arterial blood can be counted in vitro and then related to the noninvasively derived activity concentrations, e.g., in myocardium. In vitro measurements are normalized to in vivo measurements of tissue concentrations by calibrating the cross-sectional images.[W1] A small sample of the tracer is diluted in water and imaged in a cylindrical, 20-cm diameter phantom. An aliquot of the radioactive solution in the phantom is then submitted to well counting. A calibration factor K is determined by

$$K = \frac{\text{in vitro counts } (\text{gm}^{-1} \cdot \text{sec}^{-1})}{\text{in vivo counts } (\text{ml}^{-1} \cdot \text{sec}^{-1})} \cdot \frac{1}{\sigma} \qquad (7)$$

where the imaged volume in milliliters is a function of the number of picture or volume elements (pixels or voxels) in the region of interest and where σ is the specific gravity ($\text{ml} \cdot \text{gm}^{-1}$). The factor K converts in vivo–derived activity concentrations into activity concentrations per gram tissue per time and thus effectively calibrates the tomograph against in vitro measurements of tissue activity concentrations.

TRACER KINETIC MODELS AND APPLICATIONS

In vivo quantification of concentrations of positron-emitting tracers in blood and in myocardium and determination of their changes over time provide the basis for the in vivo application of tracer kinetic principles. Such models describe the time-dependent distribution of radiolabel between various functional (rather than anatomic) pools or compartments in tissue and the rate of exchange of radiolabel between such pools. They relate the tracer tissue kinetics and thus the externally measured signal to the process to be studied and form the base for an operational equation that serves to derive quantitative estimates of rates of blood flow, biochemical reactions, or mass fluxes through metabolic pathways from externally measured tracer tissue concentrations.

The myocardial tissue response to a tracer input function largely determines the general configuration of a tracer compartmental model. The tissue response depends on the type of tracer as well as on its distribution in arterial blood.[H1] As seen in Figure 65–24*A*, a distributed tracer bolus input function with slow tracer clearance from blood results in slow but continuous tracer accumulation in myocardial tissue. The fact that tracer tissue concentrations continue to rise during the observation period implies that the tracer becomes effectively trapped in myocardium. The tracer compartment model describes the exchange of tracer between blood and tissue accordingly. There is forward and reverse transport between the blood and tissue compartments but unidirectional exchange from the tissue to, for example, a third and metabolic compartment. For the same tracer and the same process, the tissue response markedly changes if the tracer input function is shortened. If, for example, the tracer is administered as a short and well-defined bolus, tissue concentrations rise rapidly and subsequently reach a plateau (Fig. 65–24*B*). An equilibrium state between tracer present in the three compartments has been attained. Analysis of the tissue response alone would indicate a change in the process examined with the tracer. However, because the tracer compartment model includes both tissue response and tracer input function, it adjusts for differences in the tissue response to different input functions. The same distribution of the tracer input function for a different tracer, however, results in an entirely different tissue response. As shown in Figure 65–24*C*, myocardial activity concentrations rapidly rise but subsequently decline again. After initially being transported into myocardium, the tracer label must therefore be released again from myocardium into blood in either nonmetabolized form or bound to metabolites.

The myocardial clearance curve morphology offers additional information for tracer kinetic modeling. For example, monoexponential clearance of activity from myocardium implies distribution of tracer in only one functional pool and clearance from it. In contrast, a biexponential clearance pattern indicates that the tracer label distributes in tissue between at least two functional pools of different sizes and turnover rates. These differences must be sufficiently large to be reflected clearly on the time activity curves. If the pools are of similar size and turnover rate, then the clearance rates will be similar for different pools and

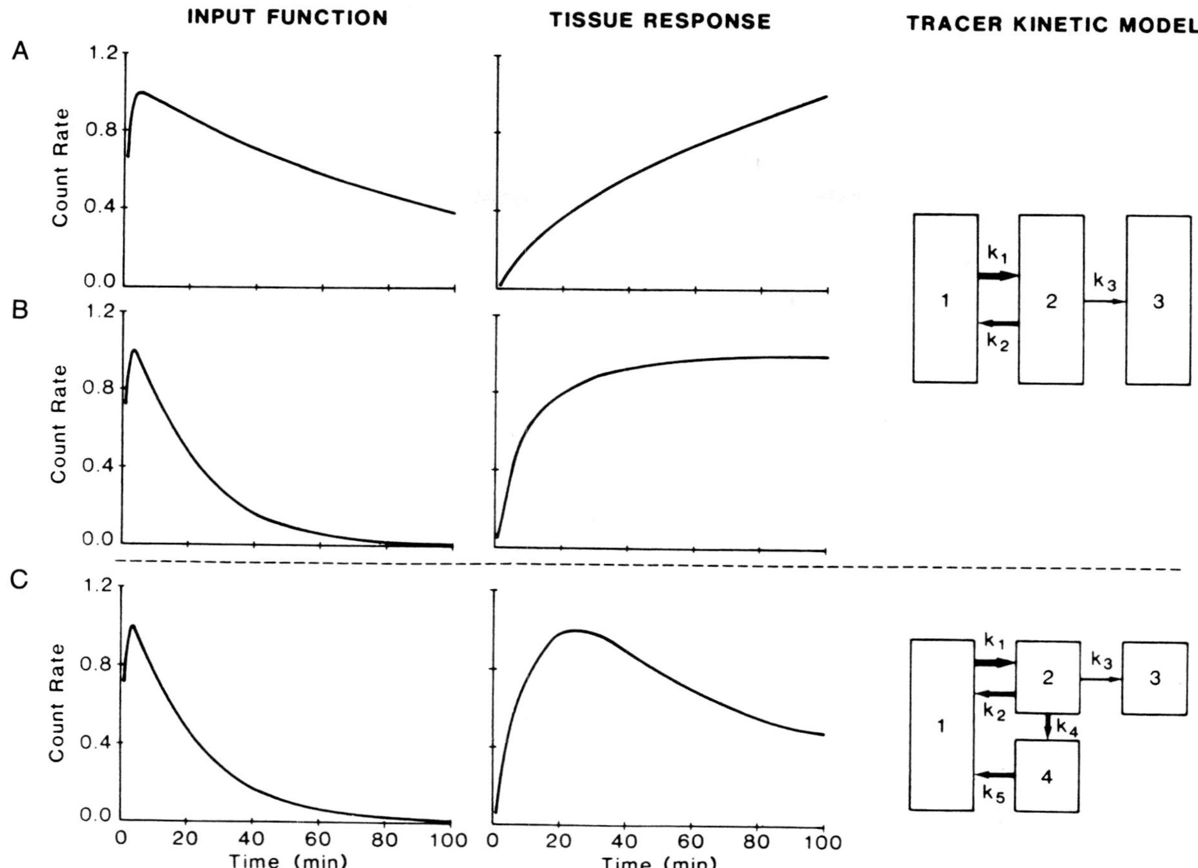

Figure 65–24. Dependency of the tissue response on changes in the distribution of the arterial tracer input function and on the specific tracer itself. *Panels A and B* compare for the same tracer the effects of changes in the tracer input function on the tissue response, and *Panels B and C* compare for the tracer-specific differences in the tissue response to an identical distribution of the tracer input function. The rate of the functional process under study is the same in Panels A and B. In response to the distributed arterial input function as seen in *Panel A*, the tissue concentrations increase over the entire study period. Tracer exchanges from Compartment 1 (blood) to Compartment 2 (tissue). Effective sequestration of tracer from Compartment 2 into Compartment 3 (metabolic pool) competes with reversed transport of tracer from Compartment 2 to 1. The rates of exchange of tracer between the three compartments are identical in the example shown in *Panel B;* however, the arterial input function is shorter. An initial rapid increase in tissue concentrations is followed by a plateau when tracer concentrations in blood have decreased and an equilibrium state is attained. Tracer kinetic models account for the effects of variations in the arterial input function on the tissue response, which, if it were measured alone, would erroneously indicate a change in the functional process. *Panel C* depicts the same arterial input function as in *Panel B*, but for a different tracer. Tissue concentrations rapidly rise but subsequently decline, indicating an exchange of tracer from blood into tissue (Compartments 1 and 2), return of tracer into Compartment 1 as well as unidirectional sequestration into Compartment 3, and movement of tracer into Compartment 4 with release of radiolabel bound to metabolites from the myocardium into the blood (Compartment 1). (From Phelps, M.E., Mazziotta, J.M., and Huang, S.C.: Study of cerebral function with positron computed tomography. J. Cereb. Blood Flow Metab. 2:113–162, 1982, with permission.)

will be difficult to distinguish by examination of the clearance curves.

The error sensitivity of estimates predicted by tracer kinetic models increases with the number of functional pools.[H1] Model approaches, therefore, attempt to reduce the number of compartments while maintaining an acceptable degree of accuracy of predicted measurements. It is recognized that metabolism of tracer compounds results in transfer of the radiolabel to numerous metabolites that may distribute among numerous metabolic pools. Some of these pools may be small and therefore contribute little to the overall tracer tissue kinetics. These pools are then lumped together with other, more dominant pools.

Careful characterization of the metabolic fate of the radiolabel in tissue through biochemical assays is essential for formulating as well as testing tracer kinetic models. An initial model configuration must be examined for its accuracy in predicting the distribution of the radiolabel between various pools and how well estimates of functional processes correlate with actual independent measurements. Adjustments are then made, followed by retesting, until model estimates approximate actual measurements over a wide range of altered conditions.

An important requirement for the application of tracer kinetic models is that conditions be in equilibrium at the time of the study. Unstable study conditions may alter relative pool sizes and rate constants for tracer exchange and thus degrade the accuracy or even invalidate estimates of functional processes. Furthermore, assumptions inherent to a model configuration must be valid over a wide range of physiologic and pathophysiologic conditions.

NONINVASIVE MEASUREMENT OF FUNCTIONAL PROCESSES

The noninvasive quantification of functional processes, e.g., of regional myocardial blood flow and myocardial rates of substrate metabolism, takes advantage of the quantitative imaging capability of positron emission tomography and of the availability of positron-emitting substances that trace a specific process in a well-defined manner and applies tracer kinetic principles in vivo. Because adequate tracer kinetic models have not been developed or validated for all currently employed tracers, evaluation of some functional processes—for example, fatty acid and oxidative metabolism—remains at present only qualitative or semiquantitative.

Evaluation and Quantification of Regional Myocardial Blood Flow

Initial attempts to derive quantitative indices of regional myocardial blood flow relied on either the "fractionation principle" or normalized the myocardial tracer uptake to the arterial input function, which resulted in a quantitative index of blood flow.

The Fractionation Principle

As described by Sapirstein, this principle implies that tracer distributes and is retained in an organ in proportion to the fractional cardiac output it receives.[S27] Applied to positron emission tomography, this relationship can be described by

$$\frac{A_R}{A_T} = \frac{Q_F}{CO} \tag{8}$$

where A_R is the activity concentration in a myocardial region of interest, A_T the total activity administered, Q_F the fraction of flow to the myocardial region of interest, and CO cardiac output. The fractional flow Q_F is then determined by rearranging Equation 8 to

$$Q_F = \frac{A_R}{A_T} \cdot CO = \frac{(ct \cdot min^{-1} \cdot gm^{-1})}{(ct \cdot min^{-1})} \cdot (ml \cdot min^{-1}) = \frac{ml}{gm \cdot min} \tag{9}$$

Changes in regional myocardial blood flow induced by an intervention are then calculated by

$$\frac{Q_F \text{ intervention}}{Q_F \text{ control}} = \frac{A_R \text{ intervention}}{A_R \text{ control}} \times \frac{A_T \text{ control}}{A_T \text{ intervention}} \times \frac{CO \text{ control}}{CO \text{ intervention}} \tag{10}$$

Assuming that cardiac output CO remains unchanged from control to intervention and only flow to the region of interest increases and that the same amount of activity (A_T) is administered at control and during the intervention, the change in blood flow to the region of interest is then estimated by

$$\frac{Q_F \text{ intervention}}{Q_F \text{ control}} = \frac{A_R \text{ intervention}}{A_R \text{ control}} \tag{11}$$

However, changes in regional myocardial blood flow induced pharmacologically with intravenous dipyridamole, estimated by this approach, indicated only a 50 to 100 percent increase in regional myocardial blood flow, which is strikingly less than the previously reported four- to fivefold increase in normal volunteers.[G9, S32] Several factors account for this underestimation. First, myocardial concentrations of diffusible tracers fail to increase linearly with blood flow. As predicted by the Renkin-Crone equation (Equation 2) and as shown in Figure 65–2, the myocardial net extraction for nitrogen-13 ammonia increases by only 220 percent, for a fivefold increase in myocardial blood flow from a control value of 0.9 $ml \cdot min^{-1} \cdot gm^{-1}$. Second, the cardiac output is assumed to be constant. However, changes in heart rate and arterial blood pressure during dipyridamole infusion indicate a systemic effect of this agent and thus a change in cardiac output. If, for example, cardiac output were to increase by 50 percent and blood flow to the myocardial region of interest by 400 percent, then the fractional flow to the region of interest increases only 3.3 instead of 5.0 times. If both the increase in myocardial blood flow and in cardiac output were constant for all patients, then fixed values for correction of the flow-dependent decline of the first-pass extraction fraction and the change in cardiac output could be used, and the actual increase in myocardial blood flow could be predicted more accurately.

Net Extraction of Tracer

An alternative approach for deriving a quantitative index of myocardial blood flow has been the normalization of the myocardial tracer uptake to the measured arterial input function. As seen in Equation 1, the net myocardial tracer uptake is defined as the product of extraction fraction and blood flow and can be calculated from the myocardial tracer concentration Q_t divided by the integral of the arterial input function to that time. Measurements of tracer net extractions have been performed with both nitrogen-13 ammonia and rubidium-82, employing either an equilibrium or tracer bolus approach.

Equilibrium Approach

The equilibrium approach entails constant infusion of rubidium-82 until tracer concentrations in arterial blood reach a plateau, as determined by external scintillation detectors. An equilibrium image is then acquired, tracer infusion is discontinued and 30 seconds are allowed for tracer clearance from blood. A second image, a myocardial image, is then recorded. Myocardial rubidium-82 concentrations are then divided by the concentration of tracer in arterial blood at the time of equilibrium, and this is considered the arterial input function. Values for net extractions of rubidium-82, as reported by Selwyn and associates,[S28] corresponded to those predicted from the blood flow to first-pass extraction relationship, as observed in dogs. Although the same investigators described a linear increase in tracer net extractions with higher blood flows, careful inspection of their data suggests that the observed increase may have been nonlinear and thus consistent with the experimentally observed nonlinear relationship between the product of extraction fraction and flow and blood flow.

Bolus Technique

The tracer bolus approach has been employed more recently and takes advantage of the higher temporal and spatial resolution capabilities of modern positron emission tomographs. The arterial input function is derived from a region of interest assigned to the left ventricular blood pool. The myocardial tracer tissue concentration at time t after tracer injection is then derived by the integral of the arterial tracer concentration to that time t and again yields the tracer net extraction. The approach has been utilized with both rubidium-82 and nitrogen-13 ammonia in experimental animals and in humans.[N2, S29–31]

In dog experiments, net extractions of nitrogen-13 ammonia were estimated from the myocardial nitrogen-13 tissue activity concentrations and the arterial input function initially determined by constant withdrawal of arterial blood[S29] or, more recently, by serial imaging and noninvasive measurements of arterial tracer concentrations.[N2, W12] Net extractions at control and changes in response to increases in myocardial blood flow correlated well with the noninvasively determined relationship between first-pass extraction fractions and blood flow and thus provided a noninvasive but quantitative index of regional myocardial blood flow (Fig. 65–25). In normal volunteers, the tracer net extractions increased 1.38 ± 0.34 times with moderate supine bicycle exercise and about 2.0 times during dipyridamole-induced hyperemia.[K10, K11, S31–33]

As expected, these increases are lower than the true increase in blood flow because of the flow-dependent decline in the first-pass extraction fraction. Moreover, contamination of the arterial input function by nitrogen-13 activity bound to amino acids rather than to ammonia further contributes to the underestimation of the true increase in the tracer net extraction. It results in an overestimation of the input function. In dogs, as much as 75 percent of the total nitrogen-13 activity in arterial blood is bound to amino acids 1 minute after intravenous nitrogen-13 ammonia administration (Schelbert and associates, unpublished data). In humans, the nitrogen-13 label similarly transfers from ammonia to amino acids, although at a slower rate. About 6 percent of the nitrogen-13 activity in arterial blood was found to be bound to amino acids at 2 minutes after tracer injection.[R12] Effects of the contamination of the arterial input function can be avoided by calculating the flow index early after tracer injection (e.g., at 60 seconds in dogs and at 90 seconds in humans), when the degree of contamination is small. On the other hand, the nonlinearity of

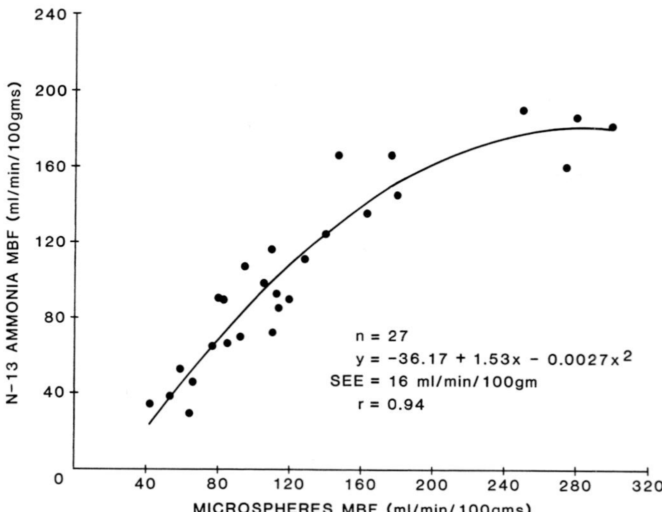

Figure 65–25. Comparison between in vivo measured myocardial net extractions of [^{13}N]ammonia and blood flow by microspheres in dog experiments. In these studies, the myocardial ^{13}N activity was determined from the cross-sectional positron emission tomographic images and divided by the arterial tracer input function obtained by in vitro counting of arterial blood, withdrawn for 2 minutes after tracer injection. (From Shah, A., Schelbert, H.R., Schwaiger, M., et al.: Measurement of regional myocardial blood flow with N-13 ammonia and positron emission tomography in intact dogs. J. Am. Coll. Cardiol. 5:92–100, 1985. Reprinted with permission from the American College of Cardiology.)

the relationship between the tracer net extraction and blood flow remains a major limitation but can be overcome by use of appropriate tracer kinetic models.

Use of Tracer Kinetic Models

Tracer kinetic models differ from the more qualitative or semiquantitative approaches for deriving indices of blood flow. Their use in conjunction with quantitative imaging yields direct estimates of regional myocardial blood flow in milliliters of blood per minute per gram of myocardium. Such models have been developed or are already in use for several tracers of blood flow: for example, rubidium-82, nitrogen-13, and oxygen-15–labeled water.

Rubidium-82 and Nitrogen-13 Ammonia

Measurements of regional myocardial blood flow with either tracer employ comparable model configurations. Consistent with the biexponential clearance curve morphology of the tracer residue function in myocardium, the model describes the tracer tissue kinetics by two communicating functional compartments. As seen in Figure 65–26, a fast exchangeable compartment corresponds to the initial rapid exchange of tracer across the capillary membrane and back-diffusion (see also Fig. 65–3), and a slow exchangeable compartment corresponds to the slow clearance slope of tracer from myocardium. In this model, the fast exchangeable compartment describes the tracer in the vascular and interstitial space, and the slow exchangeable compartment describes retention of tracer in myocardium. For rubidium-82, the slow exchangeable compartment corresponds to the fraction of tracer that has been actively sequestered into myocardium via the sodium-potassium ATPase transmembranous exchange system.[H8] For nitrogen-13 ammonia, the slow exchangeable compartment corresponds to the fraction of tracer that has been metabolically trapped via the glutamine synthetase reaction in myocardium.

In this model, K_1 ($ml \cdot min^{-1} \cdot g^{-1}$) describes the clearance of tracer from the fast to the slow exchangeable compartment and k_2 (min^{-1}) the transport rate constant of tracer from the slow to the fast exchangeable compartment. Further, the volume of distribution of tracer in the fast exchangeable compartment is described by V ($ml \cdot g^{-1}$) and F corresponds to blood flow ($ml \cdot min^{-1} \cdot g^{-1}$).

Estimates of myocardial blood flow obtained with the two-compartment model approach in animal experiments correlated well with independent measurements of blood flow by microspheres. Mullani and colleagues and subsequently Goldstein and associates recorded the myocardial tissue time activity curve in open chest dogs following intravenous rubidium-82 bolus injections with beta-probes.[G2, M1] The initial 40 to 50 seconds of data were then fitted with a Gauss-Newton least square fitting—algorithm in order to decompose the time activity curve into the free rubidium activity and into the trapped rubidium activity (Fig. 65–27). Assuming that venous egress of tracer at the time of the measurement remained negligible, the curve-fitting algorithm estimates the amount of tracer trapped in the slow compartment as the fraction of the total amount of tracer delivered to tissue at the time of peak myocardial activity. The ratio of the fraction of tracer in the slow exchangeable compartment at the time of maximum tissue activity (as extrapolated by the curve-fitting algorithm) to the maximum tissue activity (Fig. 65–27) yields an estimate of the retention fraction that is entered into the Renkin-Crone equation. After correction for the flow-dependent extraction fraction, flow is then calculated from the amount of tracer ultimately retained in myocardium. The derived estimates of blood flow were found to correlate well with those measured independently by the microsphere technique (Fig. 65–27).[M1]

Because the approach relies on a single parameter: the first-pass unidirectional extraction (retention) fraction as determined by deconvolution of the time activity curve, estimates of blood flows are sensitive to statistical noise of the recorded time activity curves and also sensitive to errors. Huang and colleagues proposed a multiparameter approach with nonlinear regression fitting of the time activity curves.[H8] Examination of the model parameters in isolated rabbit myocardium indicated that the volume of distribution of tracer (V) in the fast exchangeable pool and the clearance of tracer from the slow exchange compartment (K_1) were independent of blood flow. Both parameters are therefore fixed in the operational equation, which, after fitting of the tissue time activity curves accurately and reproducibly, yielded a flow estimate that corresponded to actual measured flow. The latter approach appears less sensitive to statistical noise of the data and has been successfully employed with dynamic positron emission tomography imaging to rubidium-82 in both animals and humans.[G3]

A similar two-compartment model has recently been applied to nitrogen-13 ammonia,[S30] and it predicted in dogs estimates of flow that correlated linearly with microsphere measurements. However, flow estimates by the nitrogen-13 ammonia tracer compartmental model consistently underestimated true blood flow by about 40 to 50 percent. Failure to correct for partial volume effect accounted to some extent for this underestimation.

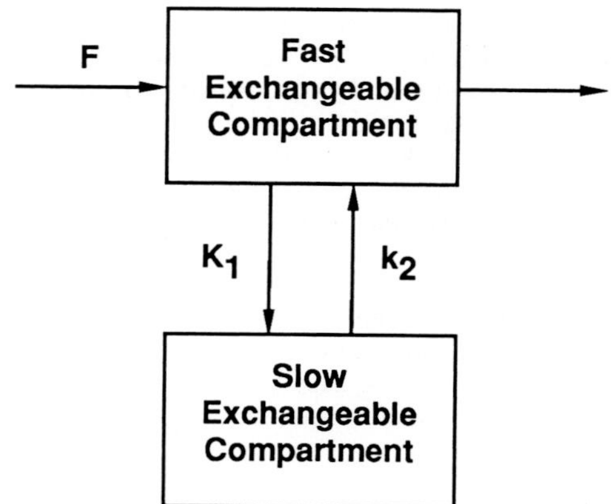

Figure 65–26. Two compartment tracer kinetic model for ^{82}Rb and [^{13}N]ammonia (see text).

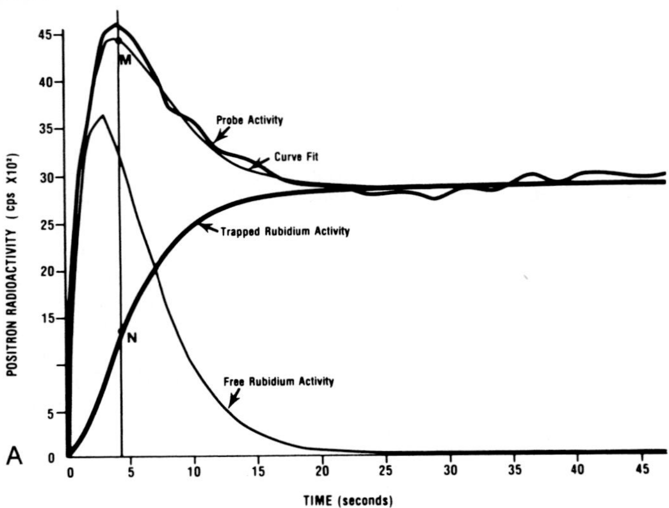

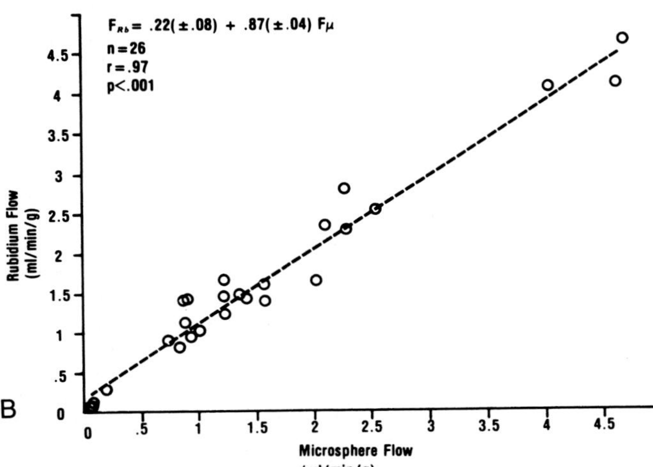

Figure 65–27. Probe measurements of myocardial activity tissue concentrations after intravenous ^{82}Rb injection *(Panel A)* and comparison of estimates of blood flow of ^{82}Rb with microsphere measurements of blood flow in dog experiments *(Panel B)*. The time activity curve in *Panel A* is fitted with the operational equation of the tracer kinetic model and predicts the free and trapped activity ^{82}Rb. The extraction fraction is estimated from the ratio of N over M (see text). (From Goldstein, R.A., Mullani, N.A., Marani, S.K., et al.: Perfusion imaging with rubidium-82: II. Effects of pharmacologic interventions on flow and extraction. J. Nucl. Med. 24:907–915, 1983, with permission of The Society of Nuclear Medicine.)

Contamination of the arterial input function of nitrogen-13 ammonia by transfer of label to amino acids and release of labeled amino acids into blood proved to be the primary reason for this underestimation. A similar transfer of nitrogen-13 label from ammonia to amino acids has been reported in humans, although to a lesser degree.[R12] Correction of the arterial input function for contamination of labeled amino acids raised the slope of the regression line to unity, and flow estimates by the noninvasive nitrogen-13 ammonia approach provided values that equaled those obtained independently by the microsphere technique.

Estimates of regional myocardial blood flow as predicted with this noninvasive approach averaged 0.70 ± 0.17 ml · min^{-1} · g^{-1} in normal volunteers at rest.[K10, K11] Blood flow increased 1.97 ± 0.27 times with moderate supine bicycle exercise and 4.5 times during dipyridamole infusion.[K11, S32, S33] Measurements in humans did not include corrections for contamination of the arterial input function, because they were based on only the initial 90 seconds of data when the degree of contamination is small (approximately 4 to 50 percent).[R12]

Oxygen-15–Labeled Water

Measurements of myocardial blood flow with oxygen-15–labeled water are based largely on a single tracer compartmental model (Fig. 65–28). The model lumps the concentrations of tracer in tissue and blood into a single compartment and assumes that the tracer immediately and completely equilibrates between plasma and tissue. Differences in tracer concentrations between blood and tissue are then a function of the respective distribution volumes that depend, in blood, on the hematocrit and, in tissue, on its water content.[B5] Application of this model to oxygen-15 water assumes (a) that the tracer freely exchanges across the capillary membrane and instantaneously achieves equilibrium, and (b) that the partition coefficient between plasma and myocardium is constant. First-pass extraction fractions of 0.95 or greater, as observed by Bergmann and associates (and as described earlier),[B4] support the first assumption that the capillary and sarcolemmal membranes exert a negligible barrier effect. According to Equation 1, the tracer concentration in myocardium Q at time t is equal to the product of the integral of the arterial tracer concentrations to time t and blood flow corrected for the flow-dependent first-pass extraction fraction E. The latter is assumed to be 1. By rearranging Equation 1, myocardial blood flow F is then obtained by

$$F = \frac{Q_t}{\int_0^t C_a(t)dt \cdot \lambda} \qquad (12)$$

where λ is the partition coefficient and represents the ratio of distribution volumes of water in myocardium and in blood. The volume of distribution in myocardium is assumed to equal the myocardial water content (0.7 g H_2O/g muscle). In blood, the volume of distribution corresponds to the plasma water content and depends upon the hematocrit.

Single intravenous bolus injections of oxygen-15 water and continuous oxygen-15–labeled carbon dioxide administration techniques have been employed. In experimental animals, estimates of blood flow after single bolus tracer injections correlated with independent measurements by the microsphere technique[A1, H24, L1] but underestimated flows slightly to moderately. The observed underestimation may have been related to a lack of correction for partial volume effect and incomplete correction for activity spillover. Employed in human myocardium and incorporating correction techniques for partial volume and activity spillover into the operational equation, Iida and associates recently reported values of 0.95 ± 0.09 ml · min^{-1} · g^{-1} of myocardium in normal subjects and significant reductions of regional flow in patients with severe coronary artery disease with and without prior myocardial infarction.[I1] Bergmann and colleagues further developed a parameter estimation procedure that corrects for partial volume effect, activity spillover, and cardiac motion.[B5] Inclusion of these parameters in the operational equation of the flow model in experimental animals resulted in noninvasively obtained flow values that closely and linearly correlated with independent microsphere measurements over a range of 0.3 to 5.0 ml · min^{-1} · g^{-1}. It is important to note that the slope of the regression line between noninvasive and invasive flow measurements approached unity (1.096; r = 0.95). Used in 11 normal human volunteers at rest, the approach yielded flow values that were uniform throughout the left ventricular myocardium and, like those reported by Iida and associates,[I1] averaged 0.90 ± 0.22

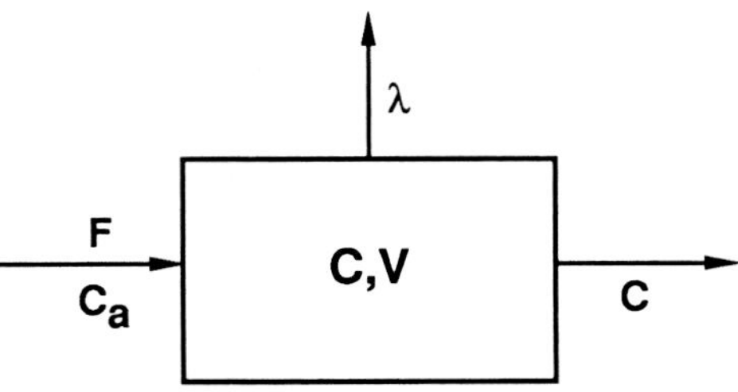

Figure 65–28. One compartmental model for ^{15}O-water (F—blood flow; C_a—tracer concentration in arterial blood, C—tracer concentration in tissue; V—volume of distribution in tissue; λ—physical decay constant of ^{15}O). (See text.)

ml · min^{-1} · g^{-1}. Intravenous dipyridamole in the same normal volunteers raised myocardial blood flow 4.35 times, to 3.55 ± 1.15 ml · min^{-1} · g^{-1}. The continuous oxygen-15 carbon dioxide inhalation approach employed by other investigators yielded comparable values of blood flow.[A2, L1]

The results with both techniques—the two-compartment rubidium-82 or nitrogen-13 ammonia and the single compartment oxygen-15 water technique—have been encouraging. Limitations remain, however. The oxygen-15 water approach assumes a constant value for the blood tissue partition coefficient. Whether this value remains constant for conditions of hyperemia, ischemia, and intrinsic myocardial disease needs further clarification. Furthermore, spillover of activity, partial volume, and substraction of blood pool activity, together with the short physical half-life of oxygen-15 result in images of relatively poor count statistics. Similarly potential limitations exist for the rubidium-82 approach, which, like the oxygen-15 water bolus technique, requires bolus injections of high activity and thus tomographs with high count rate capabilities during the initial tracer transit, as well as high efficiency for imaging the myocardial tracer uptake late after tracer injection. To avoid errors due to contamination of the arterial input function, measurements with the nitrogen-13 ammonia approach are based on only the initial 90 seconds of data and are thus susceptible to statistical noise. On the other hand, the latter approach might prove sensitive to changes in metabolism on the trapping of tracer in myocardium.

Measurements of Myocardial Glucose Metabolism

Quantification of regional rates of glucose utilization in micromoles of glucose per minute per gram of myocardium takes advantage of the unidirectional transport of labeled 2-deoxyglucose and a three-compartment tracer kinetic model proposed initially by Sokoloff and colleagues for autoradiographic measurements of regional cerebral glucose metabolism in cats.[S34] Labeling of the glucose analog with the positron emitter fluorine-18, with substitution of the methyl group by fluorine in the 2 position, permitted the application of the deoxyglucose tracer compartmental model to the in vivo study of regional glucose metabolism in human brain and heart.[G16, H26, P9, R5]

A three-compartment model describes the tissue kinetics of fluorine-18 2-fluoro 2-deoxyglucose. As seen in Figure 65–29,

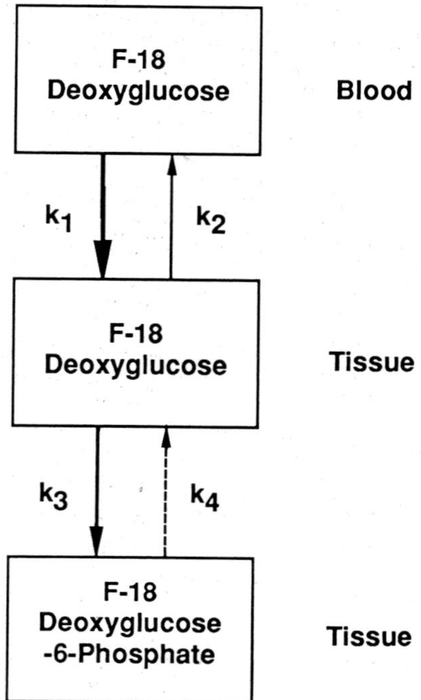

Figure 65–29. Three-compartment model for ^{18}F-2-fluoro 2-deoxyglucose. (See text.)

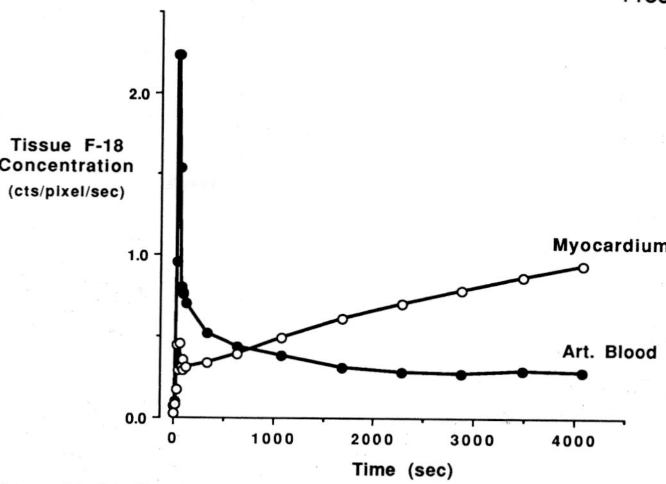

Figure 65–30. ^{18}F activity concentrations in arterial blood and myocardium following intravenous injection of ^{18}F-2-fluoro 2-deoxyglucose in a normal volunteer. The time activity curves were derived from serially acquired cross-sectional positron emission tomographic images.

Compartment 1 represents tracer concentrations in blood, Compartment 2 the tracer concentration in tissue and Compartment 3 the concentration of the phosphorylated compound, fluorine-18 2-deoxyglucose-6-phosphate in myocardium. The linear rate constants k_1 and k_2 describe the forward and reverse transport of tracer between blood and tissue (transmembranous exchange), k_3 the hexokinase-mediated rate of phosphorylation, and k_4 the rate of phosphatase-mediated dephosphorylation. Although activity of phosphatase is very low in myocardium, modifications of Sokoloff's initial tracer kinetic model now accommodate dephosphorylation rates.[G17, H26, P9]

The model relates the rate of exogenous glucose utilization or the myocardial metabolic rate of glucose (MMRGlc) to the measured rate constants for fluorine-18 2-fluoro 2-deoxyglucose by

$$\text{MMRGlc} = \frac{C_p}{LC} \cdot \frac{k_1 k_3}{k_2 + k_3} \ (\mu\text{mol} \cdot \text{min}^{-1} \cdot \text{g}^{-1}) \qquad (13)$$

where $k_1 \cdot k_3/k_2 + k_3$ (also referred to as K) reflects the rate of effective metabolic sequestration or clearance of fluorine-18 2-fluoro 2-deoxyglucose from plasma into myocardium. The term C_p is the concentration of glucose in plasma. The lumped constant LC adjusts for differences in transport and phosphorylation rates between glucose and fluorine-18 2-fluoro 2-deoxyglucose, as both compete for the same transport sites and are competitive substrates for hexokinase.

For measurements of rates of myocardial utilization of exogenous glucose, fluorine-18 2-fluoro 2-deoxyglucose is administered intravenously. Serial images are acquired for 60 to 90 minutes, and regional myocardial tissue time activity curves are obtained. Least square-fitting of the time activity curves (Fig. 65–30) with the operational equation yields the individual rate constants k_1 to k_4, which are then entered, together with the arterial plasma glucose concentrations, into Equation 13. For the lumped constant LC, a fixed value of 0.67 is used, as determined in canine myocardium.[R5] The lumped constant LC links the externally measured tracer tissue kinetics to glucose and thus to metabolism of glucose in myocardium. Estimates of glucose utilization by this approach were found to correlate in dog experiments with glucose consumption rates as determined by the Fick principle (Fig. 65–31)[R5] and predicted glucose utilization rates in normal human subjects that were similar to those reported previously in the literature.[G14, S35]

More recent developments promise to simplify data analysis and facilitate use of the approach in humans. As proposed by Patlak and co-workers[P10, P11] and as shown in Figure 65–32, the rate of glucose consumption can also be estimated graphically.[G2]

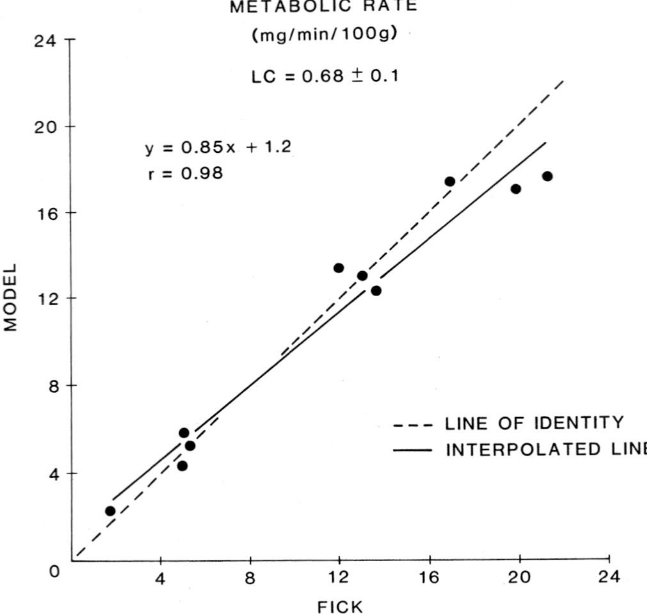

Figure 65–31. Comparison of noninvasively obtained estimates of regional myocardial exogenous glucose utilization rates with the ^{18}F-2-deoxyglucose PET approach and simultaneous invasive measurements by the Fick method in dog experiments. (From Ratib, O., Phelps, M.E., Huang, S.C., et al.: Positron tomography with deoxyglucose for estimating local myocardial glucose metabolism. J. Nucl. Med. 23:577–586, 1982, with permission of The Society of Nuclear Medicine.)

Tracer concentrations at time t in myocardium (A_m) over tracer concentrations in plasma are plotted against the integral of the arterial tracer input function divided by the arterial concentration at time t. The slope of this graph corresponds to $k_1 \cdot k_2/k_2 + k_3$ and thus indicates the fraction of fluorine-18 2-fluoro-2-deoxyglucose in plasma that is phosphorylated and metabolically sequestered into myocardium. The approach, as described recently by Gambhir and group,[G17] includes corrections for bidirectional spillover of activity between myocardium and blood and provides for k_4 or phosphatase activity. The graphic analysis approach provided estimates of glucose metabolism in six normal volunteers that were in close agreement with those obtained by the traditional derivation of individual rate constants by least square fitting of the time activity curve. The graphic approach offers several advantages: it is computationally fast, corrects for activity spillover, and can be performed from only three tissue time points. In addition to reducing sampling requirements (only three myocardial images are required), the approach also appears suitable for development of parametric images with pixel-by-pixel display of regional glucose utilization rates.[C4]

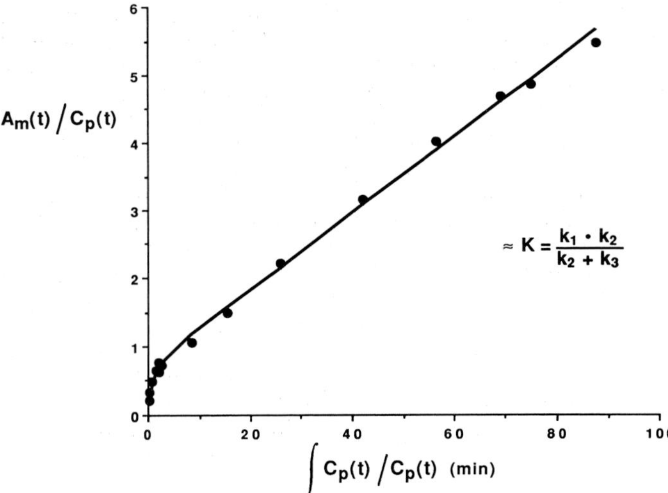

Figure 65–32. Patlak graphical analysis for the noninvasive quantification of myocardial rates of exogenous glucose utilization. (A_m—activity concentrations in myocardium; C_p—tracer concentration in arterial blood.) The slope of the plot corresponds to K or $k_1 \times k_3/k_2 + k_3$.

Although the fluorine-18 2-fluoro 2-deoxyglucose approach has been successfully employed for noninvasive quantification of regional myocardial glucose utilization rates, several issues remain unresolved at present. Foremost is the use of a fixed value for the LC. Although this value has been found relatively constant over a wide range of normal and abnormal conditions in isolated, arterially perfused rat hearts[K7, M2] and in dogs,[R5] other investigations suggest that LC may be affected by such conditions as ischemia. Therefore, careful characterization of the tissue kinetics of this tracer and its relation to glucose is required before accurate and reliable measurements can be obtained in altered and abnormal states of myocardial metabolism.

SUMMARY AND FUTURE DEVELOPMENTS

Initial developments have demonstrated the possibility of quantifying regional functional processes in myocardium. They advantageously combined the unique quantitative imaging capability of positron emission tomography with use of physiologically active positron-emitting tracers of myocardial tissue function. Most advanced at present are the quantification of regional myocardial blood flow and glucose metabolism. Other tracers have permitted the qualitative evaluation of additional aspects of tissue function—for example, fatty and acid metabolism and overall oxidative metabolism. Appropriate tracer kinetic models await development and validation before these functions can be quantified. Furthermore, emergence and characterization of new tracers will expand the scope with which myocardial tissue function can be characterized noninvasively in human myocardium. These new and developed approaches should allow more accurate and complete definition of the human heart's normal and abnormal physiology.

Acknowledgments

The author wishes to thank Wendy Wilson for preparing the illustrations and Kerry Engber for her skillful secretarial assistance in preparing this manuscript. The author is also grateful to Edward J. Hoffman and Sung-Cheng Huang for their helpful comments and suggestions.

References

A

1. Araujo, L.I., McFalls, E.O., Lammertsma, A.A., et al.: PET quantitation of myocardial blood flow using O-15 water in dogs and patients. Circulation 78:II–322, 1988.
2. Araujo, L.I., McFalls, E.O., Lammertsma, A., et al.: Quantitative measurement of myocardial blood flow and coronary flow reserve in patients with CAD employing O-15 water and positron emission tomography (PET). J. Am. Coll. Cardiol. 13:97A, 1989.
3. Allan, R.M., Pike, V.W., Maseri, A., and Selwyn, A.P.: Myocardial metabolism of ^{11}C-acetate: Experimental and patient studies. Circulation 64 (Suppl. IV):IV–75, 1981.
4. Armbrecht, J.J., Buxton, D.B., and Schelbert, H.R.: Validation of [1-^{11}C] acetate as a tracer for noninvasive assessment of oxidative metabolism with positron emission tomography in normal, ischemic, post-ischemic and hyperemic canine myocardium. Circulation 81:1594, 1990.
5. Armbrecht, J.J., Buxton, D.B., Brunken, R.C., et al.: Regional myocardial oxygen consumption determined noninvasively in humans with [1-^{11}C] acetate and dynamic positron tomography. Circulation 80:863, 1989.

B

1. Beller, G.A., Alten, W.J., Cochavi, S., et al.: Assessment of regional myocardial perfusion by positron emission tomography after intracoronary administration of Ga-68 labeled albumin microspheres. J. Comput. Assist. Tomogr. 3:447, 1979.
2. Bergmann, S.T., Hack, S., Tewson, T., et al.: The dependence of accumulation of $^{13}NH_3$ by myocardium on metabolic factors and its implications for the quantitative assessment of perfusion. Circulation 61:34, 1980.

3. Brunken, R., Schwaiger, M., Grover-McKay, M., et al.: Positron emission tomography detects tissue metabolic activity in myocardial segments with persistent thallium perfusion defects. J. Am. Coll. Cardiol. 10:557, 1987.
4. Bergmann, S.R., Fox, K.A.A., Rand, A.L., et al.: Quantification of regional myocardial blood flow in vivo with $H_2{}^{15}O$. Circulation 70:724, 1984.
5. Bergmann, S.R., Herrero, P., Markham, J., et al.: Noninvasive quantitation of myocardial blood flow in human subjects with oxygen-15-labeled water and positron emission tomography. J. Am. Coll. Cardiol. 14:639, 1989.
6. Bacharach, S.L., Cuocolo, A., Bonow, R.O., et al.: PET myocardial bloodflow by H_2O-15 without a bloodpool scan. J. Nucl. Med. 30:807, 1989.
7. Bergmann, S.R., Shelton, M.E., Weinheimer, C.J., and Herrero, P.: Accuracy of quantitative estimates of myocardial blood flow with rubidium-82 and positron emission tomography. J. Nucl. Med. 30:807, 1989.
8. Budinger, T.F., Yano, Y., Moyer, B., et al.: Myocardial extraction of Rb-82 vs. flow determined by positron emission tomography. Circulation 68:III–81, 1983.
9. Budinger, T.F., Yano, Y., Derenzo, S.E., et al.: Rb-82 myocardial positron emission tomography. J. Nucl. Med. 20:P603, 1979.
10. Budinger, T.F., Yano, Y., Derenzo, S.E., et al.: Infarction sizing and myocardial perfusion measurements using rubidium-82 and positron emission tomography. Circulation 45:39, 1980.
11. Brown, M.D., Marshall, R., Burton, B.S., et al.: Delineation of myocardial oxygen utilization with carbon-11-labeled acetate. Circulation 76:687, 1987.
12. Brown, M.A., Myears, D.W., and Bergmann, S.R.: Noninvasive assessment of canine myocardial oxidative metabolism with ^{11}C-acetate and positron emission tomography. J. Am. Coll. Cardiol. 12:1054, 1988.
13. Buxton, D.B., Schwaiger, M., Nguyen, A., et al.: Radiolabeled acetate as a tracer of myocardial tricarboxylic acid cycle flux. Circ. Res. 63:628, 1988.
14. Buxton, D.B., Nienaber, C.A., Luxen, A., et al.: Noninvasive quantitation of regional myocardial oxygen consumption in vivo with [1-^{11}C] acetate and dynamic positron emission tomography. Circulation 79:134, 1989.
15. Brown, M.A., Myears, D.W., and Bergmann, S.R.: Validity of estimates of myocardial oxidative metabolism with carbon-11 acetate and positron emission tomography despite altered patterns of substrate utilization. J. Nucl. Med. 30:187, 1989.
16. Barrio, J.R., Egbert, J.E., Henze, E., et al.: L-[4-^{11}C] aspartic acid: Enzymatic synthesis, myocardial uptake and metabolism. J. Med. Chem. 25:93, 1982.
17. Barrio, J.R., Baumgartner, F.J., Henze, E., et al.: Synthesis and myocardial kinetics of N-13 and C-11 labeled branched chain L-amino acids. J. Nucl. Med. 24:937, 1983.
18. Baumgartner, F.J., Barrio, J.R., Henze, E., et al.: ^{13}N-labeled L-amino acids for in vivo assessment of local myocardial metabolism. J. Med. Chem. 24:764, 1981.

C

1. Crone, C.: Permeability of capillaries in various organs as determined by use of the indicator diffusion method. Acta Physiol. Scand. 58:292, 1963.
2. Charbonneau, P., Syrota, A., Crouzel, C., et al.: Peripheral-type benzodiazepine receptors in the living heart characterized by positron emission tomography. Circulation 73:476, 1986.
3. Carson, R.E., Daube-Witherspoon, M.E., Jacobs, G.I., and Herscovitch, P.: Validation of post-injection transmission measurements for PET. J. Nucl. Med. 30:825, 1989.
4. Choi, Y., Hawkins, R.A., Huang, S.C., et al.: Parametric images of myocardial glucose utilization generated from dynamic cardiac FDG-PET studies. J. Nucl. Med. 30:735, 1989.

D

1. Ducan, C.C., Shiue, C.Y., Wolf, A.P., et al.: ^{18}F-4-fluoroantipyrene for the measurement of cerebral blood flow. J. Cereb. Blood Flow Metabol. (Suppl. 1):S78, 1981.
2. De Landsheere, C.M., Raets, D., Pierard, L.A., et al.: Fibrinolysis and viable myocardium after an acute infarction: A study of regional perfusion and glucose utilization with positron emission tomography. Circulation 72:III–393, 1985.
3. Delforge, K., Nakajima, K., Syrota, A., et al.: PET investigation of β-adrenergic receptors using CGP 12177. J. Nucl. Med. 30:825, 1989.
4. DePasquale EE, Nody AC, DePuey EG, et al.: Quantitative rotational thallium-201 tomography for identifying and localizing coronary artery disease. Circulation 77:316, 1988.

F

1. Fowler, J.S., and Wolf, A.P.: Positron emitter-labeled compounds: Priorities and problems. *In* Phelps, M., Mazziotta, J., and Schelbert, H. (eds.): Positron Emission Tomography and Autoradiography: Principles and Applications for the Brain and Heart. Raven Press, New York, 1986, pp. 391–450.
2. Fox, K.A.A., Abendschein, D.R., Ambos, H.D., et al.: Efflux of metabolized and nonmetabolized fatty acid from canine myocardium. Implications for quantifying myocardial metabolism tomographically. Circ. Res. 57:232, 1985.
3. Fukuda, H., Syrota, A., Charbonneau, P., et al.: Use of ^{11}C-triphenylmethylphosphonium for the evaluation of membrane potential in the heart by positron emission tomography. Eur. J. Nucl. Med. (in press).
4. Franko, A.J.: Misonidazole and other hypoxia markers: Metabolism and applications. J. Radiat. Oncol. Biol. Phys. 12:1195, 1986.

G

1. Goldstein, R.A., Klein, M.S., Welch, M.J., and Sobel, B.E.: External assessment of myocardial metabolism with C-11 palmitate in vivo. J. Nucl. Med. 21:342, 1980.
2. Goldstein, R.A., Mullani, N.A., Marani, S.K., et al.: Perfusion imaging with rubidium-82: II. Effects of pharmacologic interventions on flow and extraction. J. Nucl. Med. 24:907, 1983.
3. Grover-McKay, M., Huang, S.C., Hoffman, E.J., et al.: Noninvasive quantification of myocardial blood flow in dogs with rubidium-82 and PET. J. Nucl. Med. 27:976, 1986.
4. Goldstein, R.A.: Kinetics of rubidium-82 after coronary occlusion and reperfusion. Assessment of patency and viability in open-chested dogs. J. Clin. Invest. 75:1131, 1985.
5. Gennaro, G.P., Neirinckx, R.D., Bergner, B., et al.: A radionuclide generator and infusion system for pharmaceutical quality Rb-82. American Chemical Society, Series #241, Radionuclide Generators: New Systems for Nuclear Medicine Applications. 1984, pp. 135–150.
6. Grant, P.M., Erdal, B.R., and O'Brien, H.A.: A ^{82}Sr-^{82}Rb isotope generator for use in nuclear medicine. J. Nucl. Med. 16:300, 1975.
7. Go, R.T., Marwick, T.H., MacIntyre, W.J., et al.: Initial results of comparative rubidium-82 and thallium-201 myocardial perfusion imaging in diagnosis of CAD. J. Nucl. Med. 30:759, 1989.
8. Goldstein, R.A., Mullani, N.A., Wong, W.H., et al.: Positron imaging of myocardial infarction with Rubidium-82. J. Nucl. Med. 27:1824, 1986.
9. Goldstein, R.A., Kirkeeide, R.L., Smalling, R.W., et al.: Changes in myocardial perfusion reserve after PTCA: Noninvasive assessment with positron tomography. J. Nucl. Med. 28:1262, 1987.
10. Green, M.A., Klippenstein, D.L., and Tennison, J.R.: Copper (II) bis(thiosemicarbazone) complexes as potential tracers for evaluation of cerebral and myocardial blood flow with PET. J. Nucl. Med. 29(9):1549, 1988.
11. Gelbard, A.S., Clarke, L.P., McDonald, J.M., et al.: Enzymatic synthesis and organ distribution studies with ^{13}N-labeled L-glutamine and L-glutamic acid. Radiology 116:127, 1975.
12. Gelbard, A.S., McDonald, J.M., Reiman, R.E., and Laughlin, S.S.: Species differences in myocardial localization of N-13 labeled amino acids. J. Nucl. Med. 16:529, 1975.
13. Gelbard, A.S., Benua, R.S., Reiman, R.E., et al.: Imaging of the human heart after administration of L-[N-13] glutamate. J. Nucl. Med. 21:988, 1980.
14. Grierson, J.R., Link, J.M., Mathis, C.A., et al.: A radiosynthesis of fluorine-18 fluoromisonidazole. J. Nucl. Med. 30:343, 1989.
15. Germano, G., and Hoffman, E.J.: Investigation of count rate capability and deadtime for a high resolution PET system. J. Comput. Assist. Tomogr. 12:836, 1988.
16. Gallagher, B.M., Ansari, A., Atkins, H., et al.: Radiopharmaceuticals XXVII. ^{18}F-labeled 2-deoxy-2-fluoro-D-glucose as a radiopharmaceutical for measuring regional myocardial glucose metabolism in vivo: Tissue distribution and imaging studies in animals. J. Nucl. Med. 18:990, 1977.
17. Gambhir, S.S., Schwaiger, M., Huang, S.C., et al.: Simple noninvasive quantification method for measuring myocardial glucose utilization in humans employing positron emission tomography and Fluorine-18 deoxyglucose. J. Nucl. Med. 30:359, 1989.

H

1. Huang, S.C., and Phelps, M.E.: Principles of tracer kinetic modeling in positron emission tomography and autoradiography. *In* Phelps, M., Mazziotta, J., and Schelbert, H. (eds.): Positron Emission Tomography and Autoradiography: Principles and Applications for the Brain and Heart. Raven Press, New York, 1986, pp. 287–346.
2. Hnatowich, D.J.: A method for the preparation and quality control of Ga-68 radiopharmaceuticals. J. Nucl. Med. 16:764, 1975.
3. Hnatowich, D.J.: Labeling of human albumin microspheres with Ga-68. J. Nucl. Med. 17:57, 1976.
4. Heymann, M.A., Payne, B.D., Hoffman, J.I.E., and Rudolph, A.M.: Blood flow measurements with radionuclide-labeled particles. Prog. Cardiovasc. Dis. 20:55, 1977.
5. Hunter, W., and Monahan, W.G.: A new physiologic radiotracer for nuclear medicine. J. Nucl. Med. 12:368, 1971.
6. Harper, P.V., Lathrop, K.A., Krizek, H., et al.: Clinical feasibility of myocardial imaging with $^{13}NH_3$. J. Nucl. Med. 13:278, 1972.
7. Herrero, P., Markham, J., and Bergmann, S.R.: Error analysis of a novel mathematical approach for measurement of myocardial blood flow with O-15 H_2O and positron emission tomography (PET). J. Nucl. Med. 30:825, 1989.
8. Huang, S.C., Williams, B.A., Krivokapich, J., et al.: Rabbit myocardial ^{82}Rb kinetics and a compartmental model for blood flow estimation. Am. J. Physiol. 256:H1156, 1989.
9. Hack, S.N., Eichling, J.O., Bergmann, S.R., et al.: External quantification of myocardial perfusion by exponential infusion of positron-emitting radionuclides. J. Clin. Invest. 66:918, 1980.
10. Hoffman, E.J., Phelps, M.E., Weiss, E.S., et al.: Transaxial tomographic imaging of canine myocardium with ^{11}C-palmitic acid. J. Nucl. Med. 18:57, 1977.
11. Huang, S.C., Schwaiger, M., Selin, C., et al.: Tracer kinetic model of C-11 palmitate (CPA) for estimating regional free fatty acid (FFA) utilization in myocardium. J. Nucl. Med. 24:P12, 1983.
12. Henes, C.G., Bergmann, S.R., Walsh, M.N., et al.: Noninvasive quantification of myocardial metabolic reserve by positron emission tomography (PET) with C-11 acetate and dobutamine. Circulation 80:II–312, 1989.
13. Henze, E., Schelbert, H.R., Barrio, J.R., et al.: Evaluation of myocardial metabolism with N-13 and C-11 labeled amino acids and positron computed tomography. J. Nucl. Med. 23:671, 1982.
14. Hutchins, G.D., Schwaiger, M., Haka, M.S., et al.: Compartmental analysis of the behavior of catecholamine analogs in myocardial tissue. J. Nucl. Med. 30:735, 1989.
15. Haka, M.S., Rosenspire, K.C., Gildersleeve, D.L., et al.: Synthesis of [C-11]-m-hydroxyephedrine (HED) for neuronal cardiac imaging. J. Nucl. Med. 30:783, 1989.

16. Hoffman, E.J., and Phelps, M.E.: Positron emission tomography: Principles and quantitation. *In* Phelps, M., Mazziotta, J., and Schelbert, H. (eds.): Positron Emission Tomography and Autoradiography: Principles and Applications for the Brain and Heart. Raven Press, New York, 1986, pp. 237–286.
17. Hoffman, E.J., Phelps, M.E., Huang, S.C., et al.: Dynamic, gated and high resolution imaging with the ECAT; III. IEEE Trans. Nucl. Sci. 33:452, 1986.
18. Holte, S., Eriksson, L., Larsson, J.E., et al.: A preliminary evaluation of a positron camera system using weighted decoding of individual crystals. IEEE Trans. Nucl. Sci. 35(1):730, 1988.
19. Hoffman, E.J., Phelps, M.E., Wisenberg, G., et al.: Electrocardiographic gating in positron emission computed tomography. J. Comput. Assist. Tomogr. 3:731, 1979.
20. Huang, S.C., Carson, R.E., Phelps, M.E., et al.: A boundary method for attenuation in positron emission computed tomography. J. Nucl. Med. 22:627, 1981.
21. Hicks, K., Ganti, G., Mullani, N., and Gould, K.L.: Automated quantitation of three dimensional cardiac positron emission tomography for routine clinical use. J. Nucl. Med. 30:775, 1989.
22. Hoffman, E.J., Huang, S.C., and Phelps, M.E.: Quantitation in positron emission computed tomography. J. Comput. Assist. Tomogr. 3:299, 1979.
23. Henze, E., Huang, S.C., Ratib, O., et al.: Measurements of regional tissue and blood pool radiotracer concentrations from serial tomographic images of the heart. J. Nucl. Med. 24:987, 1983.
24. Huang, S.C., Schwaiger, M., Carson, R.E., et al.: Quantitative measurement of myocardial blood flow with oxygen-15 water and positron computed tomography: An assessment of potential and problems. J. Nucl. Med. 26:616, 1985.
25. Huang, S.C., Grover, M., Hoffman, E.J., et al.: Use of temporal information for spillover correction in dynamic PET studies of the heart. J. Nucl. Med. 27:980, 1986.
26. Huang, S.C., Phelps, M.E., Hoffman, E.J., et al.: Non-invasive determination of local cerebral metabolic rate of glucose in man. Am. J. Physiol. 238:E69, 1980.

I

1. Iida, H., Kanno, I., Takahashi, A., et al.: Measurement of absolute myocardial blood flow with $H_2{}^{15}O$ and dynamic positron-emission tomography. Strategy for quantification in relation to the partial-volume effect. Circulation 78:104, 1988.
2. Ishiwata, K., Vaalburg, W., Elsinga, P.H., et al.: Comparison of L-[1-^{11}C] methionine and L-methyl-[^{11}C] methionine for measuring in vivo protein synthesis rates with PET. J. Nucl. Med. 29:1419, 1988.
3. Isiwata, K., Vaalburg, W., Elsinga, P.H., et al.: Metabolic studies with L-[1-^{14}C] tyrosine for the investigation of a kinetic model to measure protein synthesis rates with PET. J. Nucl. Med. 29:524, 1988.
4. Iida, H., Miura, S., Kanno, I., et al.: Design and evaluation of headtome-IV, a whole-body positron emission tomograph. IEEE Trans. Nucl. Sci. 36:1006, 1989.

K

1. Krivokapich, J., Huang, S.C., Phelps, M.E., et al.: Dependence of $^{13}NH_3$ myocardial extraction and clearance on flow and metabolism. Am. J. Physiol. 242:H536, 1982.
2. Krivokapich, J., Barrio, J.R., Phelps, M.E., et al.: Kinetic characterization of $^{13}NH_3$ and ^{13}N-glutamine metabolism in rabbit heart. Am. J. Physiol. 246:H267, 1983.
3. Kalus, M.E., Stewart, R.E., Gacioch, G.M., et al.: Comparison of Rb–82 PET and Tl–201 SPECT for the detection of regional coronary artery disease. J. Nucl. Med. 30:829, 1989.
4. Knabb, R.M., Fox, K.A.A., Sobel, B.E., and Bergmann, S.R.: Characterization of the functional significance of subcritical coronary stenoses with $H_2{}^{15}O$ and positron-emission tomography. Circulation 71:1271, 1985.
5. Klein, M.S., Goldstein, R.A., Welch, M.J., and Sobel, B.E.: External assessment of myocardial metabolism with ^{11}C-palmitate in rabbit hearts. Am. J. Physiol. 237:H51, 1979.
6. Krivokapich, J., Huang, S.C., Phelps, M.E., et al.: Estimation of rabbit myocardial metabolic rate for glucose using fluorodeoxyglucose. Am. J. Physiol. 243:H884, 1982.
7. Keen, R.E., Krivokapich, J., Phelps, M.E., et al.: Nitrogen-13 flux from L-[^{13}N] glutamate in the isolated rabbit heart: Effect of substrates and transaminase inhibition. Biochim. Biophys. Acta 884:531, 1986.
8. Krivokapich, J., Huang, S.C., Hoffman, E.J., et al.: N-13 glutamate as a tracer of blood flow at rest and with exercise in human myocardium. Circulation 76:IV–4, 1987.
9. Knapp, W.H., Helus, F., Ostertag, H., et al.: Uptake and turnover of L-(^{13}N)-glutamate in the normal human heart and patients with coronary artery disease. Eur. J. Nucl. Med. 7:211, 1982.
10. Krivokapich, J., Kobashigawa, J., Stevenson, L.W., et al.: Positron emission tomography reveals decreased coronary flow response to exercise after cardiac transplantation. J. Am. Coll. Cardiol. 13:242A, 1989.
11. Krivokapich, J., Smith, G.T., Huang, S.C., et al.: N-13 ammonia myocardial imaging at rest and with exercise in normal volunteers: Quantification of absolute myocardial perfusion with dynamic positron emission tomography. Circulation 80:1328, 1989.

L

1. Lammertsma, A.A., Araujo, L.I., McFalls, E.O., et al.: A new method to quantitate regional myocardial blood flow. J. Nucl. Med. 30:808, 1989.
2. Lerch, R.A., Ambos, H.D., Bergmann, S.R., et al.: Kinetics of positron emitters; In vivo characterization by a beta-probe. Am. J. Physiol. 11:H62, 1982.
3. Lerch, R.A., Bergmann, S.A., Ambos, H.D., et al.: Effect of flow-independent reduction of metabolism on regional myocardial clearance of ^{11}C palmitate. Circulation 65:731, 1982.
4. Little, S.E., van der Vusse, G.J., Moffett, T.C., and Bassingthwaighte, J.B.: Myocardial transcapillary transport of palmitate. J. Nucl. Med. 27:966, 1986.

M

1. Mullani, N.A., Goldstein, R.A., Gould, K.L., et al.: Perfusion imaging with rubidium-82: I. Measurement of extraction and flow with external detectors. J. Nucl. Med. 24:898, 1983.
2. Marshall, R.C., Huang, S.C., Nash, W.W., and Phelps, M.E.: Investigation of the 18-fluorodeoxyglucose tracer kinetic model to accurately measure the myocardial metabolic rate for glucose during ischemia: Preliminary notes. J. Nucl. Med. 24:1060, 1983.
3. Maziere, M., Comar, D., Godot, J.M., et al.: In vivo characterization of myocardium muscarinic receptors by positron emission tomography. Life Sci. 29:2391, 1981.
4. Mulholland, G.K., Schwaiger, M., Sherman, P.S., et al.: New positron labeled quaternized muscarinic ligand as potential PET imaging agent. Circulation 78:II–598, 1988.
5. Martin, G.V., Caldwell, J.H., McGrath, P.W., et al.: Positron tomographic imaging of the hypoxic cell marker F-18 fluoromisonidazole in ischemic myocardium. Circulation 78:II–598, 1988.
6. Martin, G.V., Caldwell, J.H., Link, J.M., et al.: Detection of viable hypoxic myocardium by positron emission tomography using [F-18] fluoromisonidazole. J. Nucl. Med. 30:846, 1989.
7. Mazoyer, B.M., Schoukroun, C., Verrey, B., et al.: Physical performances and first clinical images of a high spatial resolution time-of-flight positron tomograph. J. Nucl. Med. 30:766, 1989.
8. Mullani, N.A., Wong, W.H., Hartz, R.K., et al.: Design and preliminary results from posicam: A high resolution positron camera. J. Nucl. Med. 27:973, 1986.
9. Miller, T.R., Starren, J.B., Grothe, R., Jr.: Three-dimensional display of positron emission tomography of the heart. J. Nucl. Med. 29:530, 1988.

N

1. Nienaber, C., Ratib, O., Bidaut, L., et al.: Simultaneous measurement of regional myocardial metabolism and function by multi-gated positron emission tomography (PET). J. Am. Coll. Cardiol. 11:38A, 1988.
2. Nienaber, C., Ratib, O., Weinberg, I., et al.: Noninvasive quantification of regional myocardial blood flow with N-13 ammonia and dynamic positron tomography. J. Am. Coll. Cardiol. 11:10A, 1988.

P

1. Phelps, M.E., Huang, S.C., Hoffman, E.J., et al.: Cerebral extraction of N-13 ammonia: Its dependence on cerebral blood flow and capillary permeability surface area product. Stroke 12:607, 1981.
2. Phelps, M.E., Mazziotta, J.M., and Huang, S.C.: Study of cerebral function with positron computed tomography. J. Cereb. Blood Flow Metab. 2:113, 1982.
3. Phelps, M.E., Hoffman, E.J., Coleman, R.E., et al.: Tomographic images of blood pool and perfusion in brain and heart. J. Nucl. Med. 17:603, 1976.
4. Post, R.L., and Jolly, P.C.: The linkage of sodium, potassium and ammonium active transport across the human erythrocyte membrane. Biochim. Biophys. Acta 25:118, 1957.
5. Poe, N.D.: Comparative myocardial uptake and clearance characteristics of potassium and cesium. J. Nucl. Med. 13:557, 1972.
6. Phelps, M.E., Hoffman, E.J., Selin, C.E., et al.: Investigation of [^{18}F] 2-fluoro-2-deoxyglucose for the measure of myocardial glucose metabolism. J. Nucl. Med. 19:1311, 1978.
7. Pike, V.W., Eakins, M.N., Allan, R.M., and Selwyn, A.P.: Preparation of [1-^{11}C] acetate—An agent for the study of myocardial metabolism by positron emission tomography. Int. J. Appl. Radiat. Isot. 33:505, 1982.
8. Parodi, P., Schelbert, H.R., Schwaiger, M., et al.: Cardiac emission computed tomography: Underestimation of regional tracer concentrations due to wall motion abnormalities. J. Comput. Assist. Tomogr. 8:1083, 1984.
9. Phelps, M.E., Huang, S.C., Hoffman, E.J., et al.: Tomographic measurement of local cerebral glucose metabolic rate in humans with (F-18) 2-fluoro-2-deoxy-D-glucose: Validation of method. Ann. Neurol. 6:371, 1979.
10. Patlak, C.S., Blasberg, R.G., and Fenstermacher, J.D.: Graphical evaluation of blood-to-brain transfer constants from multiple-time uptake data. J. Cereb. Blood Flow Metab. 3:1, 1983.
11. Patlak, C.S., and Blasberg, R.G.: Graphical evaluation of blood-to-brain transfer constants from multiple-time uptake data. Generalizations. J. Cereb. Blood Flow Metab. 5:584, 1985.

R

1. Renkin, E.M.: Transport of potassium-42 from blood tissue in isolated mammalian skeletal muscles. Am. J. Physiol. 197:1205, 1959.

2. Robinson, J, G.D., Jr.: Generator systems for positron emitters. *In* Reivich, M., and Alavi, A. (eds.): Positron Emission Tomography. A.R. Liss, New York, 1985, pp. 81–101.
3. Rosamond, T.L., Abendschein, D.R., Sobel, B.E., et al.: Metabolic fate of radiolabeled palmitate in ischemic canine myocardium: Implications for positron emission tomography. J. Nucl. Med. 28:1322, 1987.
4. Rose, C.P., and Goresky, C.A.: Constraints on the uptake of labeled palmitate by the heart. The barriers at the capillary and sarcolemmal surfaces and the control of intracellular sequestration. Circ. Res. 41:534, 1977.
5. Ratib, O., Phelps, M.E., Huang, S.C., et al.: Positron tomography with deoxyglucose for estimating local myocardial glucose metabolism. J. Nucl. Med. 23:577, 1982.
6. Ropchan, J.R., and Barrio, J.R.: Enzymatic synthesis of [1-^{11}C] pyruvic acid, L-[1-^{11}C] lactic acid and L-[1-^{11}C] alanine. J. Nucl. Med. 25:887, 1984.
7. Rigo, P., Beckers, J., De Landsheere, C., et al.: N-13 glutamate as a myocardial imaging agent in man. J. Nucl. Med. 27:891, 1986.
8. Rasey, J.S., Grunbaum, Z., Magee, S., et al.: Characterization of radiolabeled fluoromisonidazole as a probe for hypoxic cells. Radiat. Res. 111:292, 1987.
9. Ranger, N.T., Thompson, C.J., and Evans, A.C.: The application of a masked orbiting transmission source for attenuation correction in PET. J. Nucl. Med. 30:1056, 1989.
10. Raylman, R.R., Hutchins, G.D., Schwaiger, M., and Paradise, A.H.: Axial sampling requirements for 3-dimensional quantification of myocardial function with positron emission tomography. IEEE Trans. Nucl. Sci. 36(1):1030, 1989.
11. Ratib, O., Bidaut, L., Nienaber, C., et al.: Semiautomatic software for quantitative analysis of cardiac positron tomography studies. SPIE 914:412, 1988.
12. Rosenspire, K.C., Schwaiger, M., Mangner, T.J., et al.: Metabolic fate of N-13 ammonia in human and canine blood. J. Nucl. Med. 31:163, 1990.

S

1. Selwyn, A.P., Shea, M.J., Foale, R., et al.: Regional myocardial and organ blood flow after myocardial infarction: Application of the microsphere principle in man. Circulation 73:433, 1986.
2. Schelbert, H.R., Phelps, M.E., Hoffman, E.J., et al.: Regional myocardial perfusion assessed with N-13 labeled ammonia and positron emission computerized axial tomography. Am. J. Cardiol. 43:209, 1979.
3. Schelbert, H.R., Phelps, M.E., Huang, S.C., et al.: N-13 ammonia as an indicator of myocardial blood flow. Circulation 63:1259, 1981.
4. Schelbert, H.R., Wisenberg, G., Phelps, M.E., et al.: Noninvasive assessment of coronary stenoses by myocardial imaging during pharmacologic coronary vasodilation. VI. Detection of coronary artery disease in man with intravenous N-13 ammonia and positron computed tomography. Am. J. Cardiol. 49:1197, 1982.
5. Shelton, M.E., Green, M.A., Mathias, C.J., et al.: Microsphere-like retention in isolated hearts of copper-PTSM: A potential generator produced tracer for measuring blood flow with PET. J. Nucl. Med. 30:768, 1989.
6. Shelton, M.E., Green, M.A., Mathias, C.J., et al.: Measurement of regional blood flow using copper-PTSM and positron emission tomography (PET). J. Nucl. Med. 30:807, 1989.
7. Schön, H.R., Schelbert, H.R., Najafi, A., et al.: C-11 labeled palmitic acid for the noninvasive evaluation of regional myocardial fatty acid metabolism with positron computed tomography. II. Kinetics of C-11 palmitic acid in acutely ischemic myocardium. Am. Heart J. 103:548, 1982.
8. Schön, H.R., Schelbert, H.R., Najafi, A., et al.: C-11 labeled palmitic acid for the noninvasive evaluation of regional myocardial fatty acid metabolism with positron computed tomography. I. Kinetics of C-11 palmitic acid in normal myocardium. Am. Heart J. 103:532, 1982.
9. Schelbert, H.R., Henze, E., Schön, H.R., et al.: C-11 palmitate for the noninvasive evaluation of regional myocardial fatty acid metabolism with positron computed tomography. III. In vivo demonstration of the effects of substrate availability on myocardial metabolism. Am. Heart J. 105:492, 1983.
10. Schelbert, H.R., Henze, E., Sochor, H., et al.: Effects of substrate availability on myocardial C-11 palmitate kinetics by positron emission tomography in normal subjects and patients with ventricular dysfunction. Am. Heart J. 111:1055, 1986.
11. Schelbert, H.R., Henze, E., Schön, H.R., et al.: C-11 palmitic acid for the noninvasive evaluation of regional myocardial fatty acid metabolism with positron computed tomography. IV. In vivo demonstration of impaired fatty acid oxidation in acute myocardial ischemia. Am. Heart J. 106:736, 1983.
12. Sobel, B.E., Weiss, E.S., Welch, M.J., et al.: Detection of remote myocardial infarction in patients with positron emission tomography and intravenous ^{11}C-palmitate. Circulation 55:853, 1977.
13. Schelbert, H.R., and Schwaiger, M.: PET studies of the heart. *In* Phelps, M., Mazziotta, J., and Schelbert, J. (eds.): Positron Emission Tomography and Autoradiography: Principles and Applications for the Brain and Heart. Raven Press, New York, 1986, pp. 581–661.
14. Selwyn, A.P., Allan, R.M., Pike, V., et al.: Positive labeling of ischemic myocardium: A new approach to patients with coronary disease. Am. J. Cardiol. 47:81, 1981.
15. Seto, M., Syrota, A., Crouzel, C., et al.: Beta-adrenergic receptors in the dog heart characterized by ^{11}C-CGP 12177 and PET. J. Nucl. Med. 27:949, 1986.
16. Syrota, A., Maziere, M., Crouzel, M., et al.: Visualization of muscarinic acetylcholine receptors in the human heart using ^{11}C-methyl-QNB and positron emission tomography. *In* Raynaud, J. (ed.): Nuclear Medicine and Biology. Pergamon Press, France, 1982, pp. 2503–2505.
17. Syrota, A., Paillotin, G., Davy, J.M., and Aumont, M.C.: Kinetics of in vivo binding of antagonist to muscarinic cholinergic receptor in the human heart studied by positron emission tomography. Life Sci. 35:937, 1984.
18. Syrota, A., Comar, D., Paillotin, G., et al.: Muscarinic cholinergic receptor in the human heart evidenced under physiological conditions by positron emission tomography. Proc. Natl. Acad. Sci. USA 82:584, 1985.
19. Schwaiger, M., Guibourg, H., Rosenspire, K., et al.: F-18 metaraminol uptake as marker for neuronal function in post-ischemic canine myocardium. J. Am. Coll. Cardiol. 13:64A, 1989.
20. Shea, M.J., Wilson, R.A., de Landsheere, C.M., et al.: A new and independent measure of the volume of viable myocardium: The effects of transient ischemia. J. Am. Coll. Cardiol. 3:475, 1984.
21. Shea, M.J., Wilson, R.A., Delandsheere, C.M., et al.: Use of short- and long-lived rubidium tracers for the study of transient ischemia. J. Nucl. Med. 28:989, 1987.
22. Shelton, M.E., Dence, C.S., Hwang, D.R., et al.: Myocardial kinetics of fluorine-18 misonidazole: A marker of hypoxic myocardium. J. Nucl. Med. 30:351, 1989.
23. Shelton, M.E., Dence, C.S., Hwang, D.-R., et al.: Enhanced extraction of [F-18] fluoromisonidazole by jeopardized myocardium assessed with PET. J. Nucl. Med. 30:730, 1989.
24. Senda, M., Tamaki, N., Yonekura, Y., et al.: Performance characteristics of positologica III: A whole body positron emission tomograph. J. Comput. Assist. Tomogr. 9:940, 1988.
25. Spinks, T.J., Guzzardi, R., Bellina, C.R.: Performance characteristics of a whole-body positron tomograph. J. Nucl. Med. 29:1833, 1988.
26. Senda, M., Yonekura, Y., Tamaki, N., et al.: Interpolating scan and oblique-angle tomograms in myocardial PET using nitrogen-13 ammonia. J. Nucl. Med. 27:1830, 1986.
27. Sapirstein, L.A.: Regional blood flow by fractional distribution of indicators. Am. J. Physiol. 193:161, 1958.
28. Selwyn, A.P., Allan, R.M., L'Abbate, A., et al.: Relation between regional myocardial uptake of rubidium-82 and perfusion: Absolute reduction of cation uptake in ischemia. Am. J. Cardiol. 50:112, 1982.
29. Shah, A., Schelbert, H.R., Schwaiger, M., et al.: Measurement of regional myocardial blood flow with N-13 ammonia and positron emission tomography in intact dogs. J. Am. Coll. Cardiol. 5:92, 1985.
30. Smith, G.T., Huang, S.C., Nienaber, C.A., et al.: Noninvasive quantification of regional myocardial blood flow with N-13 ammonia and dynamic PET. J. Nucl. Med. 29:940, 1988.
31. Schwaiger, M., Krivokapich, J., Ratib, O., et al.: Dipyridamole-induced coronary vasodilation quantitatively assessed by PET and N-13 ammonia in humans. J. Nucl. Med. 29:818, 1988.
32. Schwaiger, M., Krivokapich, J., Ratib, O., et al.: Noninvasive quantification of coronary reserve by N-13 ammonia and positron emission tomography (PET). J. Am. Coll. Cardiol. 11:11A, 1988.
33. Schwaiger, M., Hutchins, G.D., Krivokapich, J., et al.: PET assessment of coronary reserve (CR) in humans using a tracer kinetic model for N-13 ammonia. Circulation 78:II–597, 1988.
34. Sokoloff, L., Reivich, M., Kennedy, C., et al.: The [^{14}C]-deoxyglucose method for the measurement of local cerebral glucose utilization: Theory, procedure and normal values in the conscious and anesthetized albino rat. J. Neurochem. 28:897, 1977.
35. Schwaiger, M., Huang, S.C., Krivokapich, J., et al.: Myocardial glucose utilization measured noninvasively in man by positron tomography. J. Am. Coll. Cardiol. 1:688, 1883.

T

1. Turton, D.R., Brady, F., Pike, V.W., et al.: Preparation of human serum [methyl-^{11}C] methylalbumin microspheres and human serum [methyl-^{11}] methylalbumin for clinical use. Int. J. Appl. Radiat. Isot. 35:337, 1984.
2. Tamaki, N., Yonekura, Y., Senda, M., et al.: Value and limitation of stress thallium-201 single photon emission computed tomography: Comparison with nitrogen-13 ammonia positron tomography. J. Nucl. Med. 29:1181, 1988.
3. Tillisch, J., Brunken, R., Marshall, R., et al.: Reversibility of cardiac wall motion abnormalities predicted by positron tomography. N. Engl. J. Med. 314:884, 1986.
4. Ter-Pogossian, M.M., Klein, M.S., Markham, J., et al.: Regional assessment of myocardial metabolic integrity in vivo by positron-emission tomography with ^{11}C-labeled palmitate. Circulation 61:242, 1980.
5. Tewson, T.J., and Welch, M.: Preparation and preliminary biodistribution of no carrier added ^{18}F fluoroethanol. J. Nucl. Med. 21:559, 1980.
6. Ter-Pogossian, M.M., Bergmann, S.R., and Sobel, B.E.: Influence of cardiac and respiratory motion on tomographic reconstructions of the heart: Implications for quantitative nuclear cardiology. J. Comp. Assist. Tomogr. 6:1148, 1982.

V

1. Valk, P.E., Geyer, A.B., Jagust, W.J., et al.: Clinical efficiency of high-resolution (2.6 MM) positron emission tomography. J. Nucl. Med. 30:765, 1989.

W

1. Wisenberg, G., Schelbert, H.R., Hoffman, E.J., et al.: In vivo quantitation of regional myocardial blood flow by positron emission computed tomography. Circulation 63:1248, 1981.
2. Wilson, R.A., Shea, M.J., De Landsheere, C.H., et al.: Validation of quantitation of regional myocardial blood flow in vivo with ^{11}C-labeled human albumin microspheres and positron emission tomography. Circulation 70:717, 1984.

3. Walsh, W.F., Harper, P.V., Resnekov, L., and Fill, H.: Noninvasive evaluation of regional myocardial perfusion in 112 patients using a mobile scintillation camera and intravenous nitrogen-13 labeled ammonia. Circulation 54:226, 1976.
4. Walsh, M.N., Brown, M.A., Henes, C.G., et al.: Estimation of regional myocardial oxidative metabolism by positron emission tomography with carbon-11-acetate in patients. Circulation 78:II–599, 1988.
5. Walsh, M.N., Bergmann, S.R., Steele, R.L., et al.: Delineation of impaired regional myocardial perfusion by positron emission tomography with $H_2{}^{15}O$. Circulation 78:612, 1988.
6. Wilson, R.A., Shea, M., De Landsheere, C., et al.: Rubidium-82 myocardial uptake and extraction after transient ischemia: PET characteristics. J. Comput. Assist. Tomogr. 11:60, 1987.
7. Wyns, W., Schwaiger, M., Huang, S.C., et al.: Effects of inhibition of fatty acid oxidation on myocardial kinetics of C-11 labeled palmitate. Circ. Res. 65:1787, 1989.
8. Weiss, E.S., Hoffman, E.J., Phelps, M.E., et al.: External detection and visualization of myocardial ischemia with ^{11}C-substrates in vitro and in vivo. Circ. Res. 39:24, 1976.
9. Weiss, E.S., Ahmed, S.A., Welch, M.J., et al.: Quantification of infarction in cross sections of canine myocardium in vivo with positron emission transaxial tomography and ^{11}C-palmitate. Circulation 55:66, 1977.
10. Wieland, D.M., Rosenspire, K.C., Hutchins, G.D., and Schwaiger, M.: Validation of 6-[^{18}F]fluorometaraminol (FMR) for positron tomography. Circulation 78:II–598, 1988.
11. Wieland, D.M., Hutchins, G.D., Rosenspire, K.C., et al.: [C-11] hydroxyephedrine (HED): A high specific activity alternative to 6 -[F-18] fluorometaraminol (FMR) for heart neuronal imaging. J. Nucl. Med. 30:767, 1989.
12. Weinberg, I.N., Huang, S.C., Hoffman, E.J., et al.: Validation of PET-acquired functions for cardiac studies. J. Nucl. Med. 29:241, 1988.
13. Woods, S.D., Rasey, J.S., Graham, M.M., and Krohn, K.A.: A model for fluoromisonidazole retention as a function of local PO_2: In vitro calibration for interpretation of PET images. J. Nucl. Med. 30:735, 1989.

Z

1. Zole, I., Rhodes, B.A., Wagner, H.N., Jr.: Preparation of metabolized radioactive human serum albumin microspheres for studies of the circulation. Int. J. Appl. Radiat. Isot. 21:155, 1970.
2. Zimmerman, R., Tillmanns, H., Knapp, W.H., et al.: Regional myocardial nitrogen-13 glutamate uptake in patients with coronary artery disease: Inverse post-stress relation to thallium-201 uptake in ischemia. J. Am. Coll. Cardiol. 11:549, 1988.

Chapter 66

Evaluation of Myocardial Blood Flow in Cardiac Disease

LINDA L. DEMER, M.D., Ph.D

METHODS ... 1170
Tracers ... 1170
Nitrogen-13 Ammonia ... 1170
Oxygen-15 Water ... 1170
Rubidium-82 ... 1170
Technique ... 1171
Positioning ... 1171
Monitoring ... 1171
Transmission Images ... 1171
Emission Images ... 1171
Display ... 1172
Analysis and Interpretation ... 1172
Circumferential Profile Analysis ... 1173
Myocardial Perfusion Reserve ... 1173
Quantification: Absolute Perfusion Versus Tracer Uptake ... 1173
DETECTION OF CORONARY ARTERY DISEASE 1174
Standards for Comparison ... 1174
Subjective Versus Quantitative Arteriography ... 1174
Percent Narrowing Versus Stenosis Flow Reserve ... 1175
Stenosis Flow Reserve Versus Coronary Flow Reserve ... 1175
Coronary Flow Reserve Versus Myocardial Perfusion Reserve ... 1176
Accuracy of Detection of Coronary Artery Disease ... 1176
Sensitivity and Specificity of Detecting Coronary Artery Disease with Measurements of Perfusion with Positron Emission Tomography ... 1176
Confidence Limits ... 1177
Limitations of Sensitivity and Specificity Analysis ... 1178
Localization of Coronary Artery Disease ... 1178
Comparison with Thallium Scintigraphy ... 1178
Limitations ... 1179
Potential for Screening Asymptomatic Patients ... 1179
QUANTITATIVE ANALYSIS OF TRACER UPTAKE ... 1179
MEASUREMENT OF ABSOLUTE MYOCARDIAL PERFUSION ... 1179
Flow-dependent Extraction ... 1180
Geometric Limitations ... 1180
Models ... 1180
DETECTION OF TRANSIENT AND SILENT ISCHEMIA ... 1182
Mental Stress ... 1182
Smoking ... 1182
Daily Activities ... 1182
EVALUATION FOR MYOCARDIAL INFARCTION ... 1183
RESPONSE TO THERAPY ... 1185
Percutaneous Transluminal Coronary Angioplasty ... 1185
Effect of Dietary Interventions ... 1185
Coronary Collaterals ... 1185
Other ... 1187
SUMMARY ... 1187

Positron emission tomographic imaging of myocardial perfusion has been used for nearly a decade for investigation of cardiovascular physiology. It is now gaining recognition as a useful clinical tool. Over 350 patients with suspected coronary artery disease have been studied by positron emission tomography (PET) for noninvasive assessment of myocardial blood flow. PET perfusion imaging is well suited for the evaluation of coronary artery disease, providing information that is complementary to invasive coronary arteriography, not directly substituting for it. Arteriographic imaging identifies the location and anatomic severity of epicardial coronary artery stenoses. However, the physiologic significance of such lesions may be difficult to assess from angiographic data alone, and perfusion abnormalities may occur in the absence of arteriographically evident stenoses. Noninvasive PET imaging complements arteriography by revealing the effects of the stenosis on blood supply reaching the myocardium. For example, PET perfusion images are useful for identifying physiologic abnormalities of perfusion in the absence of arteriographic abnormalities and for assessing the significance of known stenoses in terms of absolute or relative perfusion or perfusion reserve and the amount of heart wall involved. Conventional noninvasive methods, such as thallium-201 planar imaging or, more recently, single-photon emission computed tomography (SPECT), provide conceptually similar information, but they are theoretically less accurate owing to dependence of tracer attenuation and resolution on the distance of the tracer from the detectors and the lower signal-to-noise ratio.

The three primary clinical applications of PET perfusion imaging are (1) qualitative detection of coronary artery disease with potentially greater accuracy than conventional noninvasive methods, (2) assessment of response to medical and surgical interventions designed to augment perfusion, and (3) quantitative measurement of absolute myocardial perfusion. The first application has undergone the most extensive clinical evaluation, revealing high sensitivity and specificity. Additional research is in progress to compare directly positron emission tomography to thallium-

Table 66–1. CHARACTERISTICS OF COMMON TRACERS IN POSITRON EMISSION TOMOGRAPHY

Tracer	Physical Half-Time	Dose
^{13}N ammonia	10.0 min	10–20 mCi
^{15}O water	2.1 min	30–40 mCi (0.5 mCi/kg)
^{82}Rb	1.25 min	20–50 mCi

201 SPECT imaging, to assess accuracy in asymptomatic patients, and to overcome technical limitations in achieving accurate measurements of absolute myocardial perfusion.

METHODS

Tracers

The three most common tracers used for PET perfusion imaging are nitrogen-13 ammonia, rubidium-82, and oxygen-15 water (Table 66–1). They have been selected for their physical and biochemical properties. None of the tracers tested thus far has all the characteristics required for optimal quantitation: short physical half-life, minimal radiation dose, uptake directly related to flow and independent of metabolic conditions, and availability without a cyclotron. At present, quantification requires sophisticated mathematical analysis, rapid data acquisition free of detector saturation, and concomitant administration of blood pool tracer. Nevertheless, all three tracers allow more flexible protocols than does thallium-201, which has a 73.1-hour physical half-life.

Nitrogen-13 Ammonia

Nitrogen-13 ammonia provides high image contrast because it is rapidly cleared from blood and avidly retained in myocardial tissue. Its extraction and clearance have been described in terms of compartmental analysis.[K1] It has a 10-minute physical half-time, allowing sequential studies. The radiation dose to the patient is approximately 6 to 7 mrad/mCi.[L1] Because it is lipid soluble, it diffuses readily into cells, where most is trapped as glutamine. At physiologic pH, ammonia is primarily in the form of NH_4^+. Its concentration in the myocardium depends not only on flow but also on the amount of nitrogen-13 ammonia administered as a function of time (input function), its extraction at the instantaneous flow, and metabolic state.[B1, S1] This tracer has been used extensively for both experimental and clinical PET imaging.[S2–4, T1, T2] A related tracer, nitrogen-13 glutamate, also has been investigated as a possible flow tracer because its net extraction parallels nitrogen-13 ammonia extraction during exercise and rest in patients with coronary artery disease.[K2]

Oxygen-15 Water

Oxygen-15 water is useful for qualification of myocardial perfusion.[H1] It is essentially freely diffusible in the heart, with minimal effect of flow on uptake and nearly 100 percent extraction.[B2] However, it also remains in the blood pool, contaminating the image with uptake within the ventricular chambers and surrounding structure. To overcome this problem, oxygen-15 carbon monoxide is administered by inhalation after each perfusion scan to label the blood pool. The myocardial activity is then identified by digital subtraction of the blood pool activity. With present techniques, the signal-to-noise ratio is not as high as for nitrogen-13 ammonia or rubidium-82. When faster data acquisition rates are possible, larger tracer doses may be used to overcome this limitation. At present, because of their short physical half-lives, oxygen-15 and nitrogen-13-labeled tracers are used only at major centers with on-site cyclotrons.

Rubidium-82

In contrast, rubidium-82,[B3] a potassium analog, can be eluted from a strontium-82 generator system using normal saline,[Y1] eliminating the need for an on site cyclotron. Rubidium isotopes were first used over 30 years ago to assess myocardial blood flow,[L2] after Knoebel and colleagues[K3] demonstrated the feasibility of external detection of myocardial rubidium uptake. Because of its short, 74-second half-life, rubidium-82 is particularly convenient for frequent sequential examinations under rapidly changing conditions, such as during ischemia or acute myocardial infarction. A dose of 30 to 50 mCi is administered in a 10 to 20-ml saline solution intravenously as a bolus. The radiation dose to the patient is approximately 1.6 to 2 mrad/mCi.[K4]

The predicted flow, derived by correcting rubidium-82 uptake for extraction, is nearly linearly related to microsphere flow (Fig. 66–1), and anticipated effects of acidosis, alkalosis, digoxin, propranolol, and glucose-insulin levels on extraction are minimal.[G1] One inherent difference between the quality of rubidium and nitrogen-13 ammonia scans is that the distance traversed by rubidium-82 positrons in tissue, prior to interaction with electrons and annihilation, is longer than for nitrogen-13, resulting in a lower theoretic limit of resolution.

The rubidium generator contains strontium-85 as a production contaminant, which has a half-life of 65 days. An upper limit of 1 microCurie per liter of strontium-82 and strontium-85 breakthrough has been set. This amount corresponds to a skeleton

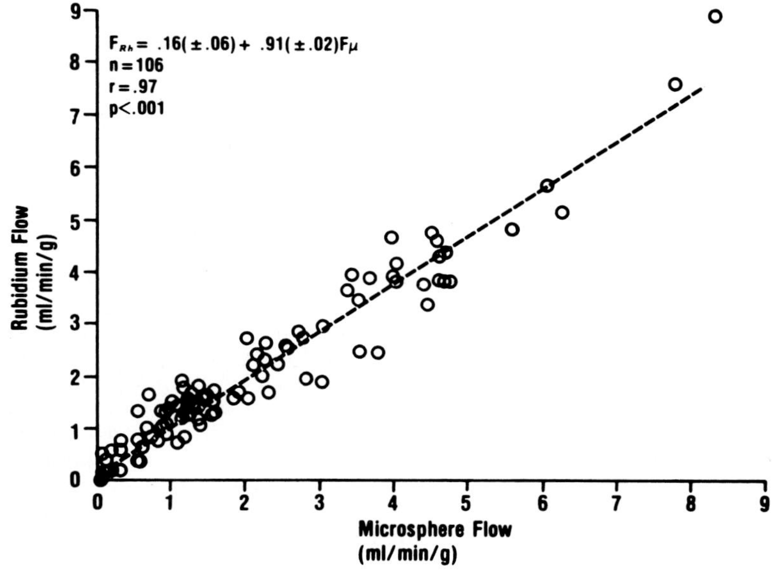

Figure 66–1. Lumped results for flow by ^{82}Rb compared with flow by microspheres. (From Goldstein, R.A., Mullani, N.A., Marani, S.K., et al.: Myocardial perfusion with rubidium-82. II. Effects of metabolic and pharmacologic interventions. J. Nucl. Med. 24:907–915, 1983, with permission of The Society of Nuclear Medicine.)

dose of approximately 8 mrad and 70 mrad, respectively. The output is pumped over a calibrated dosimeter and is passed through a Millipore filter before injection into the intravenous line. Since the parent strontium has a half-life of 25 days, the generator provides sufficient concentration of rubidium-82 for 4 to 6 weeks.

Carbon-11 butanol, with a half-life of 20.3 minutes, also has been proposed as a flow tracer but has not been widely used. Despite their limitations, all three tracers have been shown to have practical utility for qualitative assessment of myocardial perfusion in patients.

Technique

For rest-dipyridamole myocardial perfusion PET imaging, patients are fasted for 4 to 8 hours because of potential side effects of dipyridamole, such as nausea, vomiting, and hypotension. Patients are not allowed to have caffeine or theophylline for 8 hours before imaging, to prevent interference with the hyperemic effect of dipyridamole. An intravenous line is started for injection of radiotracer and infusion of dipyridamole.

Positioning

Positioning within the camera must be accurate to assure that the entire heart is contained within the narrow detector window. One approach is to mark the skin at the locations of the upper and lower borders of the heart as determined by fluoroscopy. Another approach is to assess heart location by early data from the transmission image. In addition, patient position must be maintained at a constant level during the entire series of scans, including the transmission scan, so that all scans superimpose. For some whole-body PET cameras, the patient's arms must be held outside the opening during cardiac imaging (Fig. 66–2), to some extent limiting the scanning time tolerated by patients. False defects may result and true defects may be missed when the emission image is shifted relative to the transmission image. To monitor patient position, appropriate laser light sources may be mounted on the camera frame to illuminate the patient's skin with two orthogonal lines. In this respect, cameras providing multiple simultaneous scans have an advantage over those able to provide only one slice at a time, because the latter require accurate shifting of the patient in the long axis of the camera.

When scans are compared before and after stress or other interventions, it is critical to exclude changes in patient position or of the orientation of the heart within the chest. Such changes may create artifactual defects, especially when only a few slices are obtained. As seen in Figure 66–3, not all tomographic PET slices from a normal heart are ring shaped. When the tomographic plane includes the atrioventricular valves, the image of the left ventricle is C shaped. Thus, a small amount of translational or rotational movement of the patient or change in intrathoracic position of the heart relative to the chest wall after an intervention can create false defects. For example, if a ring-shaped section of the heart were scanned at rest, then the patient moved inferiorly so that the mitral valve orifice shifted into the imaging plane, the repeat scan would show a C-shaped section. Such an image pair, showing a new defect with stress, may be interpreted as indicating posterior wall disease. Translational motion is a particular concern with supine bicycle exercise in which caudal forces against the pedals may cause cephalad shifting of the heart relative to the camera. Most PET cameras also have motorized tables that allow adjustments in axial position.

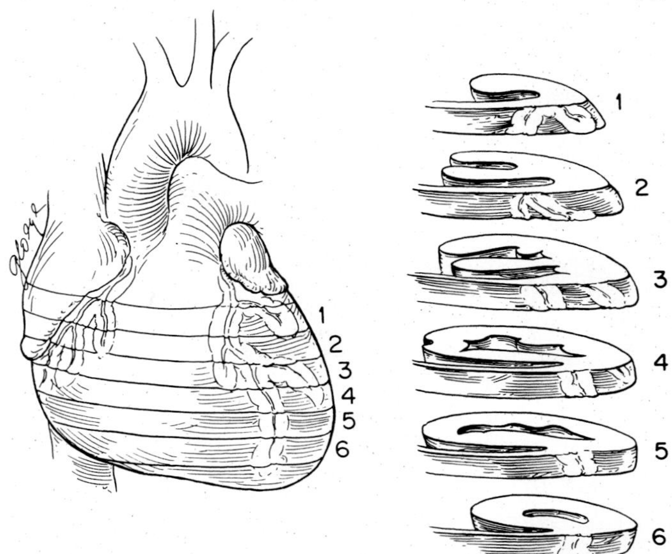

Figure 66–3. Schematic representation of the cross-sectional images through the left and right ventricles. (From Schelbert, H.R., Wisenberg, G., Phelps, M.E., et al.: Non-invasive assessment of coronary stenoses by myocardial imaging during pharmacologic coronary vasodilation. VI. Detection of coronary artery disease in man with intravenous 13-NH_3 and positron computed tomography. Am. J. Cardiol. 49:1197–1207, 1982, with permission.)

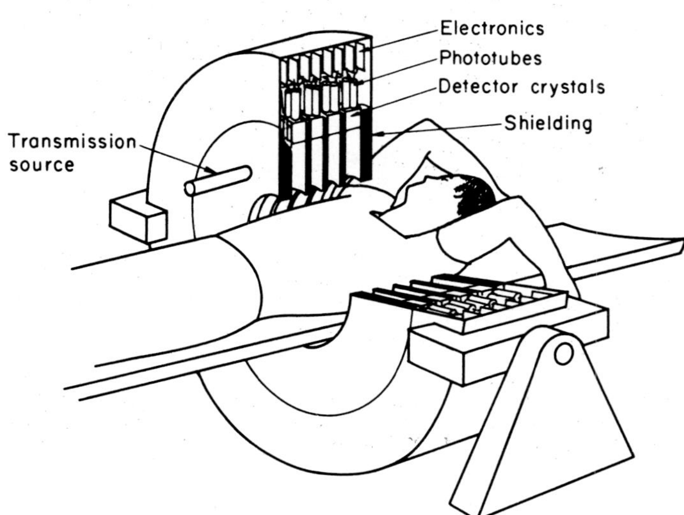

Figure 66–2. Schematic of PET device for imaging the thorax. (From Budinger, T.F., Yano, Y., Huesman, R.H., et al.: Positron emission tomography of the heart. The Physiologist, 26:31, 1983, with permission.)

Monitoring

Vital sign measurements and a 12-lead electrocardiogram are obtained prior to scanning. Vital sign measurements are repeated every 2 minutes after the start of the dipyridamole infusion, and the electrocardiogram is repeated every 5 minutes for a total of 30 minutes, or longer if necessary, for resolution of any ST changes that develop. Vials of aminophylline, 125 mg injectable, and a fully equipped resuscitation cart are kept in the imaging room.

Transmission Images

Transmission images are usually performed using an external ring of positron-emitting isotope, such as gallium-86. Data from this image are used to correct for photon attenuation. The tracer is injected in bolus form through a well-seated intravenous catheter. To allow for blood pool clearance, there is usually a 1-minute delay after rubidium-82 and a 3-minute delay after ammonia administration before the qualitative scan is acquired. Quantitative imaging requires acquisition of this first-pass activity as a function of time.

Emission Images

The resting scan is then obtained for 5 to 8 minutes for rubidium-82 and 15 to 20 minutes for ammonia. Following isotope decay, 10 minutes after administration of the first dose of rubid-

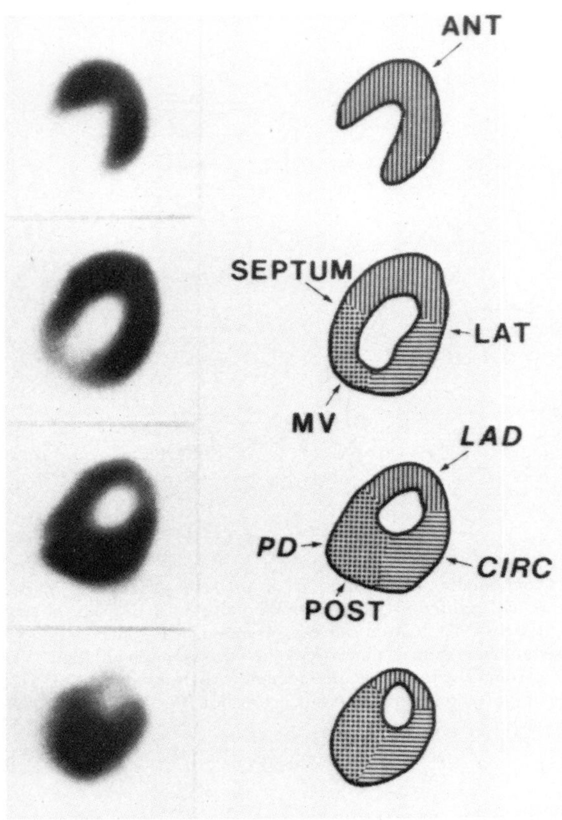

Figure 66–4. Contiguous cross-sectional images of the heart obtained after intravenous administration of [^{13}N] ammonia in a normal volunteer. The cross-sections of the left ventricular myocardium are displayed as if viewed from below. The cross section on the top is through the high anterior wall, whereas the image at the bottom is at an oblique angle through the posterior and inferior wall of the left ventricle. The schematic representation of the cross-sectional images on the right indicates the intraventricular septum and the anterior (ANT), lateral (LAT), and posterior (POST) walls of the left ventricle and mitral valve (MV). The distributions of the left anterior descending (LAD), left circumflex (CIRC), and posterior descending (PD) coronary arteries are indicated by the different shades of gray. (From Schelbert, H.R., Wisenberg, G., Phelps, M.E., et al.: Non-invasive assessment of coronary stenoses by myocardial imaging during pharmacologic coronary vasodilation. VI. Detection of coronary artery disease in man with intravenous 13-NH_3 and positron computed tomography. Am. J. Cardiol. 49:1197–1207, 1982, with permission.)

ium-82 or 40 minutes after nitrogen-13 ammonia, dipyridamole (0.142 mg/kg/min) is infused over 4 minutes. Aminophylline, 125 mg injectable, is kept on hand in case it is needed to reverse potential side effects. At some centers, aminophylline is given routinely at the end of the study. Two minutes after the infusion is completed, 25 percent of the predetermined maximal handgrip is begun. Four minutes after the infusion is completed, a second dose of the same amount of the same tracer is injected, and imaging is repeated. For patients developing significant angina or other side effects of dipyridamole described earlier, aminophylline is given in a dose of 125 mg. This is required for 3 percent of noncardiac side effects and 18 percent of cardiac side effects.[H2] Approximately 20 percent of patients develop ST depression and 19 percent have nonsustained arrhythmias. The most common noncardiac side effects are headache, lightheadedness, dizziness, nausea, flushing, and vomiting. The value of adding handgrip to dipyridamole stress has been questioned recently.[R1]

Display

Rest and stress scan images representing distribution of tracer activity uptake in the myocardium are usually displayed simultaneously as multiple tomographic slices. They may be oriented as seen from below, in accordance with conventional x-ray computed tomographic orientation, or from above, depending on the individual PET center. Black/white intensity or color shades are used to represent the quantity of tracer activity. In a normal scan, the slices have a variety of shapes because the heart is situated in the chest at an angle so that tomographic slices of the heart are not along any of its primary axes. (see Fig. 66–3). A normal scan induces horseshoe-shaped, ring-shaped, and oval sections. The right ventricular wall and valve plane are normally not seen because they are too thin. The regions of myocardium perfused by each major coronary artery cannot be determined with certainty. Assuming typical coronary anatomy, the borders of the myocardial beds may be estimated (Fig. 66–4).

These images may be processed to provide long-axis, short-axis, and other cross-sectional views. Further processing allows a "bulls-eye" display, which consists of a circular map of the three-dimensional activity distribution (Fig. 66–5). At the center is the apical short-axis slice with concentric rings of sequentially more superior short-axis slices. That is, the breadloaf slices are organized concentrically. This method introduces distortion in stretching the most superior slices to fit around the more apical slices. As a result, the area of bull's-eye map is not proportional to the area of myocardium that it represents. Bull's-eye display was first introduced for use in SPECT imaging. Software also has been developed for three-dimensional reconstruction and for displaying the ratio of stress-to-rest tracer uptake (Fig. 66–6). This ratio is not the same as myocardial perfusion reserve, because uptake is not directly related to perfusion, and the input function of tracer may not be identical for the two images. It is also possible to display perfusion images superimposed on metabolic images in different colors to allow visual detection of mismatches between perfusion and metabolism, as in areas of hibernating myocardium.

Figure 66–6. See Color Plate 17.

Analysis and Interpretation

Distribution of perfusion tracer activity may be assessed subjectively or by quantitative criteria. Subjective interpretation is based on recognition of defects, similar to the conventional interpretation of scintigraphic images. A defect on a rest image usually represents myocardial infarction or ischemia at rest, but it also may be due to normal anatomic thinning, such as at the apex. The key finding is a defect that appears only in the hyperemic (dipyridamole or exercise) image, which is evidence of a coronary artery stenosis of sufficient severity to reduce coronary flow reserve.

One method of objective interpretation is measurement of homogeneity, defined as the ratio of counts in a given region to

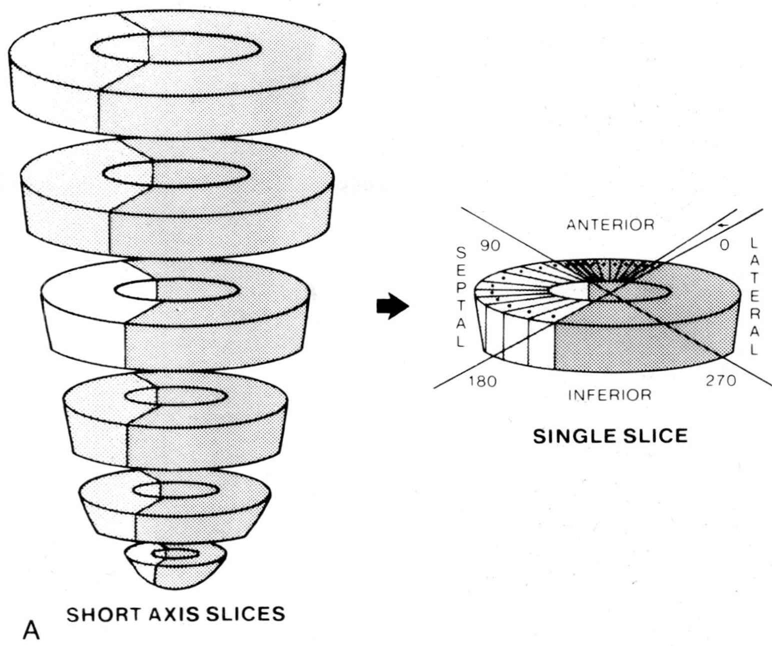

Figure 66–5. *A*, Alternating short axis slices of the left ventricle are displayed with the middle slice highlighted. A septal defect is present from base to apex. *B*, Generation of the bull's eye display is shown. (From DePasquale, E.E., Nody, A.C., DePuey, E.G., et al.: Quantitative rotational thallium-201 tomography for identifying and localizing coronary artery disease. Circulation 77:316, 1988 by permission of the American Heart Association, Inc.)

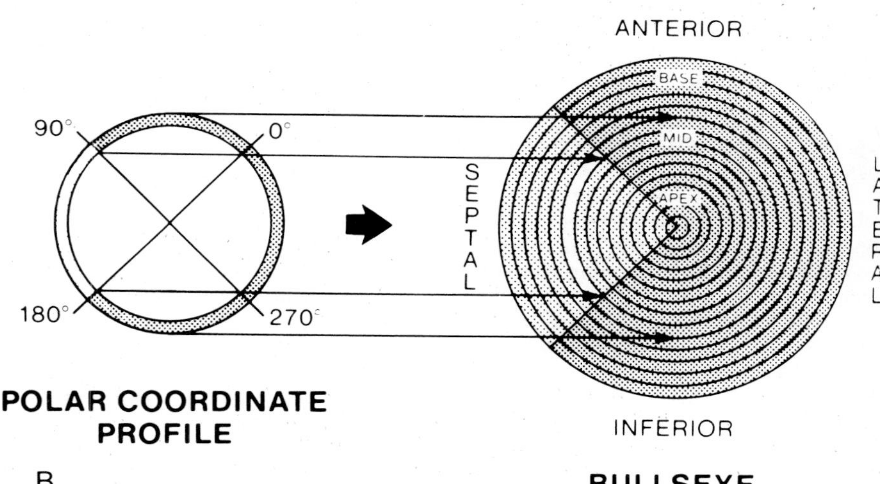

the maximal counts in the entire scan.[D1, G2, W1] Because of statistical variation and noise from pixel to pixel, it is necessary to select regions of interest of consistent and sufficient size to provide a reliable estimate of mean regional activity. Excessively large regions of interest may introduce artifact owing to partial volume and spillover effects.[P1] Small regions of interest may accentuate the effects of statistical noise.

Circumferential Profile Analysis

Another method of objective interpretation of tracer uptake images is the circumferential profile technique, in which the activity along a line passing through the midwall of each ring or C-shaped scan is plotted as a function of angle or distance along the line (Fig. 66–7). Regional defects may be identified as portions of the circumferential activity curve that lie outside the range defined by two standard deviations from the mean profile values for normal subjects.

Myocardial Perfusion Reserve

A third method of quantitative interpretation of tracer uptake images involves the concept of relative myocardial perfusion reserve (MPR). It is analogous to the concept of coronary flow reserve, the ratio of flow at maximal vasodilation to resting flow. Correspondingly, for a given region of myocardium, myocardial perfusion reserve is defined as the ratio of perfusion at maximal vasodilation to resting perfusion of the same region. This ratio is closely related to stenosis flow reserve and coronary flow reserve (Fig. 66–8). However, it may be abnormal despite normal coronary flow reserve, under certain conditions such as in the presence of myocardial hypertrophy, or normal despite abnormal coronary flow reserve in the presence of coronary collaterals.

One limitation of the flow reserve concept is that resting flow and state are not well defined,[K5] especially during the period of time surrounding percutaneous transluminal coronary angioplasty (PTCA). Hoffman has described the limitations of coronary flow reserve in this regard.[H3] In addition, resting flow may vary with time even without intervention. A detailed discussion of flow reserve is provided in Chapter 2.

Quantification: Absolute Perfusion Versus Tracer Uptake

It is important to distinguish measurement of tracer uptake from absolute perfusion measurements. Although uptake is not linearly related to flow, quantitative assessment of tracer uptake is useful for objective assessment of relative perfusion defects. Absolute perfusion measurements in terms of flow per volume of

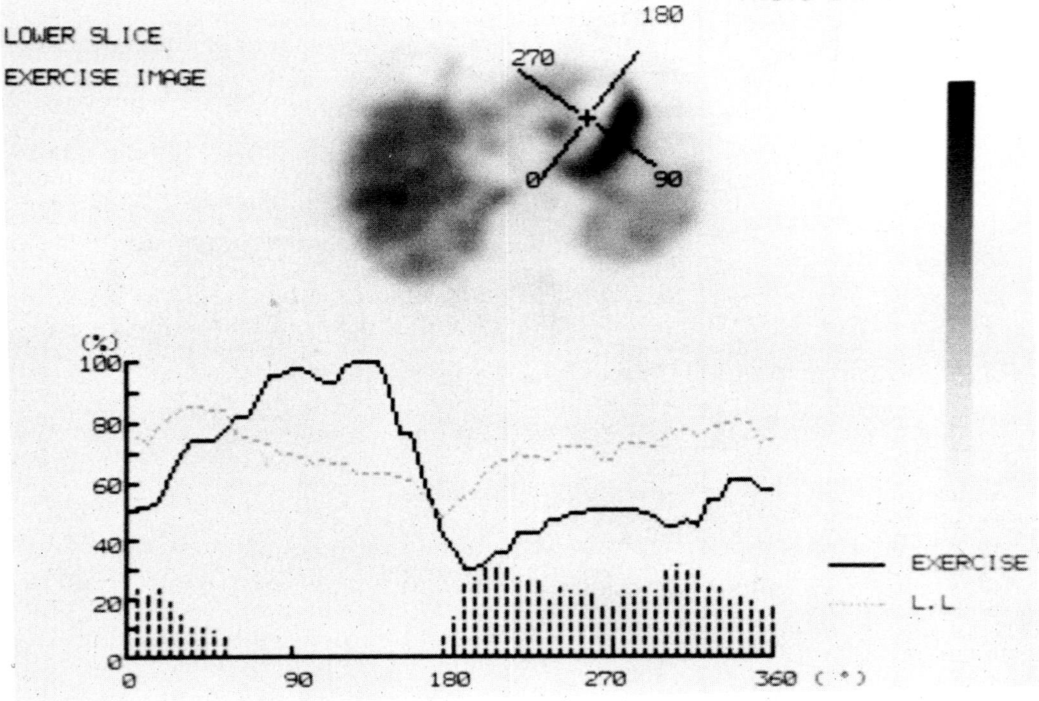

Figure 66–7. Circumferential analysis of lower section of left ventricular myocardium in exercise PET study, indicating involvement of left anterior descending artery and right coronary artery. (From Yonekura, Y., Tamaki, N., Senda, M., et al.: Detection of coronary artery disease with N-13 ammonia and high resolution positron emission computed tomography. Am. Heart J. 113:645–654, 1987, with permission.)

tissue require mathematical models using compartmental analysis to account for variable extraction.

DETECTION OF CORONARY ARTERY DISEASE

Diagnosis of coronary artery disease is currently the primary clinical application of PET perfusion imaging. On theoretic grounds, it promises to be more accurate for detection of coronary disease than exercise electrocardiographic testing and planar or even SPECT thallium-201 imaging. The basis for improved accuracy is that positron emission tomography provides quantitative attenuation correction and a higher signal-to-noise ratio.[B4] PET and SPECT have been directly compared only in patients undergoing exercise treadmill stress rather than pharmacologic coronary vasodilation. With exercise, coronary flow increases indirectly in response to increased myocardial oxygen demand. Pharmacologic stress permits identification of disease without requiring the development of ischemia (Fig. 66–9). Because exercise often shifts the patient away from the position held during the transmission scan, much of the advantage of attenuation correction may be lost. Studies directly comparing PET with SPECT using pharmacologic stress are currently in progress.

Standards for Comparison

Subjective Versus Quantitative Arteriography

Conventionally, results of myocardial perfusion imaging have been tested against visually assessed coronary stenosis severity

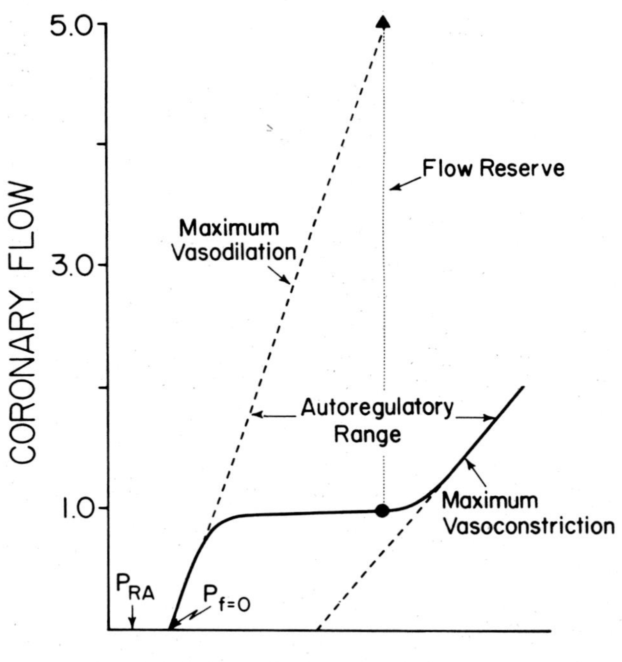

Figure 66–8. Steady-state relationship between coronary flow and coronary arterial pressure in the left ventricle. The solid line depicts the normal relationship. At a constant level of myocardial metabolic demand, coronary flow is maintained constant over a wide range of coronary pressure, between the bounds of maximum coronary vasodilation and constriction (*dashed lines*). (From Klocke, F.J.: Measurements of coronary flow reserve: Defining pathophysiology versus making decisions about patient care. Circulation 76:1183, 1987, by permission of the American Heart Association, Inc.)

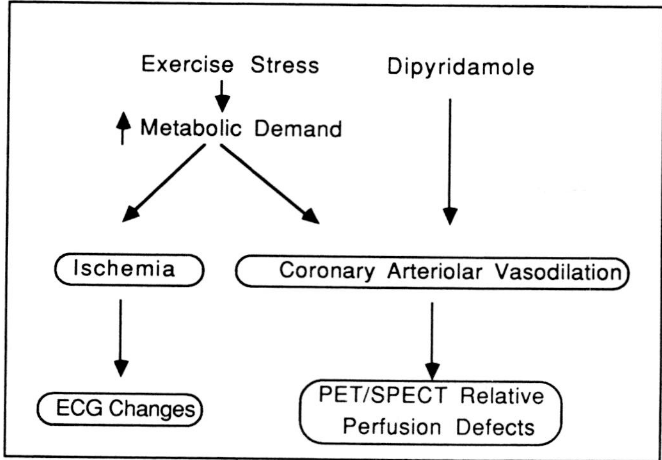

Figure 66–9. Conceptual diagram comparing exercise stress with pharmacologic stress and dipyridamole-induced vasodilation.

in terms of percent diameter reduction estimated from coronary arteriograms. This subjective method is no longer considered acceptable for research purposes because of the unacceptably higher interobserver differences.[D2, D3, G3, M1, W2, Z1] Percent diameter narrowing is also not meaningful in the presence of diffuse disease or following PTCA because there is no appropriate reference diameter.[B5, M2] A more objective approach to assessing stenosis severity is measurement of absolute stenosis diameter and cross-sectional area by quantitative arteriography.[B6] An extensive review of quantitative arteriography and videodensitometry is presented in Chapter 13.

Percent Narrowing Versus Stenosis Flow Reserve

One method of assessing stenosis severity is measurement of its dimensions and calculation of its pressure-flow relation (Fig. 66–10). This method allows comparison of anatomic stenosis severity from patient to patient independent of hemodynamic factors. The pressure-flow relation may be more conveniently described in terms of "stenosis flow reserve," previously termed "x-ray predicted" coronary flow reserve. It is the expected flow reserve of an artery with the given stenosis dimensions under standard hemodynamic conditions.[K6] Stenosis flow reserve may be determined from computed quantitative arteriography. Coronary perfusion pressure distal to each stenosis may be calculated as a function of flow[K6, M3] according to the equation:

$$P_{cor} = P_A - (fQ + sQ^2)$$

where
P_{cor} = distal coronary pressure
P_A = aortic pressure
Q = coronary flow
f = $8\mu \pi L/A_s^2$
s = $\beta [(1/A_s) - (1/A_n)]^2$
A_s = minimum absolute area of stenosis
A_n = absolute area of normal adjacent artery
μ = blood viscosity
β = blood density
L = stenosis length

Under conditions of maximal coronary arteriolar vasodilation, the pressure-flow relation is represented by a straight line intersecting with the above relation. Stenosis flow reserve is identified as the flow at maximal coronary vasodilation, relative to rest flow, under standardized hemodynamic conditions. Graphically, this may be represented by the intersection of the two lines representing the pressure-flow relation at maximal vasodilation with the pressure-flow relation of the stenosis. Predicted stenosis flow reserve correlates (r = 0.91) with direct, electromagnetic flow measurements in animals with artificial stenoses.[K6]

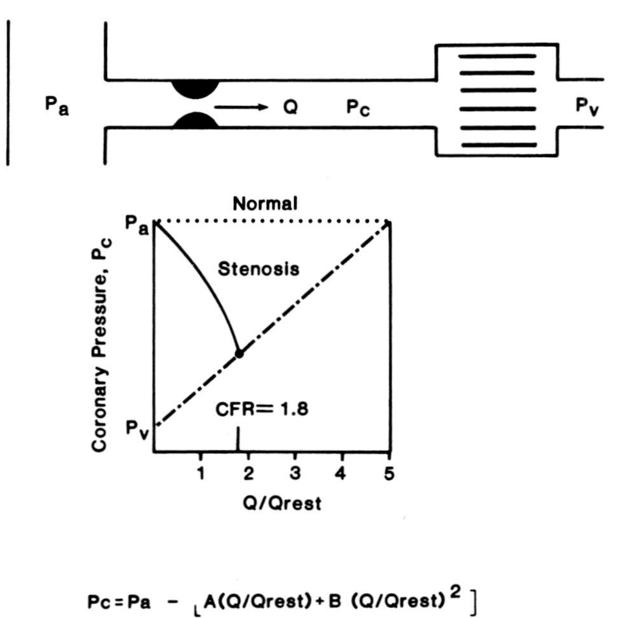

Figure 66–10. Correlation of distal coronary perfusion pressure with coronary flow reserve. For a constant absolute diameter and length, measurement of coronary flow reserve under conditions of maximum coronary vasodilation predicts the distal perfusion pressure as well as percent diameter narrowing. (From Gould, K.L., Mullani, N., and Kirkeeide, R.L.: Coronary circulation. *In* Phelps, M.E., Mazziotta, J.C., and Schelbert, H. (eds.): PET & Autoradiography: Principles and Applications for the Brain and Heart. Raven Press, New York, 1986, p. 133.)

Stenosis Flow Reserve Versus Coronary Flow Reserve

Anatomy alone does not predict the full physiologic consequence of coronary stenoses: physiologic measures of stenosis severity have been developed to incorporate effects of other factors. In previous reports, x-ray-predicted stenosis severity calculated from the fluid dynamic equations described earlier had been termed "coronary flow reserve" without distinction from direct measurement, because the technology for direct measurement of coronary flow velocity in patients had not yet been developed. To avoid confusion with methods now available, the new term "stenosis flow reserve" may be used to distinguish anatomic, x-ray-predicted from physiologic stenosis severity.[D4] The equations for stenosis flow reserve were described earlier.

Stenosis flow reserve provides information different from that for direct measurements of coronary flow reserve, but both are clinically relevant. Stenosis flow reserve is useful for assessing changes in stenosis severity resulting from interventions, such as angioplasty, intracoronary stents, or cholesterol-lowering regimens. The two measures of flow reserve may differ substantially in certain clinical situations, such as left ventricular hypertrophy, hypotension, and the no-reflow phenomenon, when coronary flow reserve is diminished despite normal stenosis flow reserve.

In its original description, coronary flow reserve referred to the ratio of maximal to rest flow in the proximal portion of a coronary artery as measured by a flowmeter. However, circumferential flow probes are not suitable for use in patients. Instead, blood velocity is measured, and "coronary flow reserve" is then calculated with the assumption that arterial cross-sectional area does not change. Since flow is the product of velocity and cross-sectional area, then velocity reserve should equal flow reserve if the cross-sectional area does not change during arteriolar vasodilation.

$$\text{Coronary flow reserve} = \frac{\text{maximal flow}}{\text{rest flow}} = \frac{\text{maximal velocity} \times \text{area}}{\text{rest velocity} \times \text{area}}$$

Blood flow velocity is measured invasively, using an intracoronary Doppler velocity probe on the tip of a 3 Fr. selective coronary

Table 66–2. MEASURES OF MYOCARDIAL BLOOD SUPPLY RESERVE IN PATIENTS

Reserve Measure	Parameter(s)	Device	Hemodynamic Conditions	Interpretation
Stenosis Flow Reserve	Stenosis dimensions	Cineangiogram	Standardized	Anatomic stenosis severity
Coronary Flow Reserve	Blood velocity	Doppler catheter	Instantaneous at time of test	"Physiologic" effect on flow
Myocardial Perfusion Reserve	Tracer uptake	PET camera	Instantaneous at time of scan	Effect of stenosis on perfusion

catheter.[W3] Measurements are obtained at rest and following injection of intracoronary papaverine. The ratio of velocity at rest and during vasodilation is considered coronary flow reserve. Directly measured coronary flow reserve of the same stenosis may be different in different patients or in the same patient at different times, depending on the moment-to-moment hemodynamic conditions. Coronary flow reserve may also be estimated using videodensitometric analysis of digital subtraction coronary arteriography by calculation of contrast arrival time and disappearance.[V1]

Coronary flow reserve depends on perfusion pressure, coronary venous tone, and strength of the hyperemic stimulus; two stenoses of exactly the same geometry (and thus the same *stenosis* flow reserve) may have entirely different values of *coronary* flow reserve in different patients, or even in the same patient at different times under different hemodynamic conditions. In contrast, stenosis flow reserve is independent of hemodynamic conditions, by definition. It indicates the conductance of the stenosis itself as if the arterial segment were excised and studied in vitro under controlled conditions.

The difference between stenosis flow reserve and coronary flow reserve is best described by analogy to the difference between automobile mileage estimated by the industry or the Environmental Protection Agency and actual automobile mileage. The former is obtained under standardized conditions, the same for all makes, for purposes of comparing one car model to another on a uniform scale, allowing objective comparison. Actual mileage depends on the individual driving conditions, such as load and velocity. Two cars of exactly the same make (and thus the same EPA mileage) may have entirely different values of actual mileage with different drivers or even with the same driver at different times under different load conditions. The two measures are likely to differ, but each is useful for its own purpose.

In analogy, stenosis flow reserve is obtained under standardized conditions, the same for all arteries, for purposes of comparing one artery to another on a uniform scale. Stenosis flow reserve differs from the actual coronary flow reserve depending on hemodynamic conditions. The two measures are likely to differ, but each is useful for its own purpose.

Even coronary flow reserve may not be directly comparable to positron emission tomography defect severity because it is measured at the time of cardiac catheterization rather than at the time of PET imaging, and hemodynamic conditions may change. Thus, neither stenosis flow reserve nor coronary flow reserve provides the value of flow reserve at the time of the PET scan (Table 66–2). The choice is between (1) stenosis flow reserve, based on standardized hemodynamic conditions, or (2) coronary flow reserve, based on hemodynamic conditions at the time of cardiac catheterization when anxiety or sedative effects may alter hemodynamics.

Coronary Flow Reserve Versus Myocardial Perfusion Reserve

Even directly measured coronary flow reserve does not always reflect the ultimate physiologic significance of stenoses, which is its effect on myocardial perfusion. A large artery with the same coronary flow reserve as a small artery may have a more profound effect on perfusion. Arteries with the same coronary flow reserve may have different values of perfusion reserve in the presence of collaterals.

Accuracy of Detection of Coronary Artery Disease

The practical limit of detection of flow reserve impairment by positron emission tomography perfusion imaging was first estimated using labeled microspheres, which are virtually 100 percent extracted, and direct gamma-camera imaging of cross-sectional myocardial slices.[G4] The least amount of coronary narrowing detected using this method with submaximal coronary vasodilation in animals was 40 to 50 percent diameter narrowing. Even less severe stenoses may be detectable with improved camera resolution, maximal vasodilatory stimulus, or the addition of handgrip to counterbalance the dipyridamole-induced fall in blood pressure.

A similar detection threshold is achieved in vivo with pharmacologic coronary vasodilation. Dogs instrumented with adjustable stenoses (inflatable cuffs) of the left circumflex artery were imaged using nitrogen-13 ammonia before and after intravenous dipyridamole infusion. Subjective defects were identified during vasodilation with circumflex narrowing of as little as 47 percent diameter narrowing, measured by quantitative arteriography with manually traced borders.[G5]

Sensitivity and Specificity of Detecting Coronary Artery Disease with Measurements of Perfusion with Positron Emission Tomography

Sensitivity and specificity have been remarkably high in patient studies (Table 66–3). Schelbert and co-workers studied 45 patients with $^{13}NH_3$ PET imaging at rest and with dipyridamole stress.[S5] Results were 97 percent sensitive and 100 percent specific for coronary artery disease in 32 patients with arteriographically documented coronary artery disease and 13 healthy subjects. Overall, 52 of 58 stenotic vessels were correctly identified. However, in this study, the standard for definition of coronary artery disease was the visual assessment of 50 percent narrowing by coronary arteriography. Selwyn and associates[S6] found normal homogeneous uptake of rubidium-82 in positron emission tomography scans of 5 normal volunteers, but an approximate 36 percent decrease in regional myocardial rubidium-82 uptake after exercise in 5 patients with coronary artery disease.

Table 66–3. POSITRON EMISSION TOMOGRAPHY DETECTION OF CORONARY ARTERY DISEASE: CORRELATION WITH CORONARY ARTERIOGRAPHY

Study	No. of Patients	Tracer	Sensitivity	Specificity	Correlation
Schelbert et al.[S2]	32	$^{13}NH_3$	97	100	
Tamaki et al.[T1]	25	$^{13}NH_3$	95	100	
Gould et al.[D6, G5, G6]	50	$^{13}NH_3$, ^{82}Rb	95	100	
Demer et al.[D6]	193*	$^{13}NH_3$, ^{82}Rb	94	95	0.77
Yonekura et al.[Y2]	49	$^{13}NH_3$	97	100	
Tamaki et al.[T2]	48	$^{13}NH_3$	98	—	

*Excluding 37 patients with intermediate severity of disease.

Similarly high sensitivity and specificity have been found despite inclusion of patients without angina. In 50 patients undergoing PET perfusion imaging with rubidium-82 or nitrogen-13 ammonia, at rest and with dipyridamole/hand-grip stress, scan results were 98 percent sensitive and 100 percent specific for coronary artery disease defined by quantitative arteriographic criteria of stenosis flow reserve.[G6] When this study group was expanded to 193 patients, accuracy was minimally reduced.[D5, D6] PET perfusion imaging was performed with dipyridamole stress and compared with stenosis flow reserve derived from quantitative arteriographic measurements. To reflect the continuous spectrum of severity of coronary artery disease, a five-point scale was used to describe the subjective PET defect severity, to derive a rank correlation coefficient of 0.77 (Fig. 66–11), which is less dependent on disease distribution and arbitrary cut-off values than is sensitivity/specificity analysis.

When exercise stress is substituted for pharmacologic stress, sensitivity and specificity remain high.[T1–3] Tamaki and colleagues found 95 percent sensitivity and 98 percent specificity for rest and exercise PET imaging with nitrogen-13 ammonia in 25 patients, and 98 percent sensitivity in a group of 48 patients with known coronary artery disease.[T1] Specificity was not assessed because only three normal patients were studied. These results were based on subjective assessment of arteriographic percent diameter narrowing, with coronary disease defined as one or more stenoses of greater than 50 percent diameter narrowing.

Quantitative analysis using circumferential profiles of tracer uptake may enhance detection of exercise-induced ischemia by positron emission tomography. Yonekura and associates studied 40 patients with coronary artery disease and 20 normals using PET with circumferential profile analysis (see Fig. 66–7). At rest, regional PET defects were present in 96 percent of coronary artery disease patients with prior myocardial infarction and in 29 percent without infarction. Exercise scans showed defects in 93 percent with coronary artery disease without myocardial infarction. No exercise defects appeared in normals. Overall, 89 percent of 75 stenosed vessels were identified by exercise PET, where coronary artery disease was defined as 75 percent diameter narrowing.

Other tracers have been found useful for imaging relative perfusion defects in coronary artery disease. Walsh and colleagues recently showed the feasibility of identifying relative perfusion defects using $H_2{}^{15}O$ with dipyridamole stress in 33 subjects.[W1] Uniformity was significantly greater for the nine normal subjects than for the patients with coronary artery disease. The $H_2{}^{15}O$ cardiac images were of lower quality than nitrogen-13 ammonia or rubidium-82 images due to low signal-to-noise ratios. This limitation may be overcome when higher doses can be used in newer cameras. The main advantage of this tracer is its potential for measurement of absolute perfusion. Spontaneous and induced episodes of silent ischemia are also accurately detected by PET perfusion imaging with rubidium-82, [D7] as described later.

Metabolic tracers are also capable of identifying coronary artery disease. For example, carbon-11 palmitate, a metabolic tracer, has been used to distinguish normal and ischemic myocardium because of its greater uptake and more rapid clearance in normal myocardium than in ischemic zones.[G7] However, with severely compromised flow, less tracer arrives in the area of interest, reducing the signal-to-noise ratio of the tracer washout curve beyond the point of clinically reliable identification of ischemia.

Confidence Limits

The studies in Table 66–3 report sensitivity values from 94 to 97 percent and specificity values from 95 to 100 percent. Since such values are merely statistical estimates of the true sensitivity and specificity for a larger population, descriptions of the accuracy for comparison to other imaging methods in terms of sensitivity and specificity should include confidence intervals to indicate the accuracy of the estimate. The accuracy of the estimate depends on the population sizes and consistency. Confidence intervals indicate the accuracy of an estimate as a function of probability. For example, applying standard statistical tables[D8] to data from Schelbert and associates,[S5] the lower limit of the 95 percent confidence interval for sensitivity is 84 percent, and the lower limit for specificity is 75 percent. For Gould and colleagues,[G6] the corresponding lower limits of the 95 percent confidence intervals are 77 percent and 66 percent, respectively. The overlap of these wide confidence intervals with the sensitivity and specificity values reported for planar thallium imaging, and even electrocardiographic exercise testing, indicates the need for larger study populations. In the one large study, coronary artery disease severity was described in terms of three rather than two levels of severity to reduce the effects of binary classification as described later.

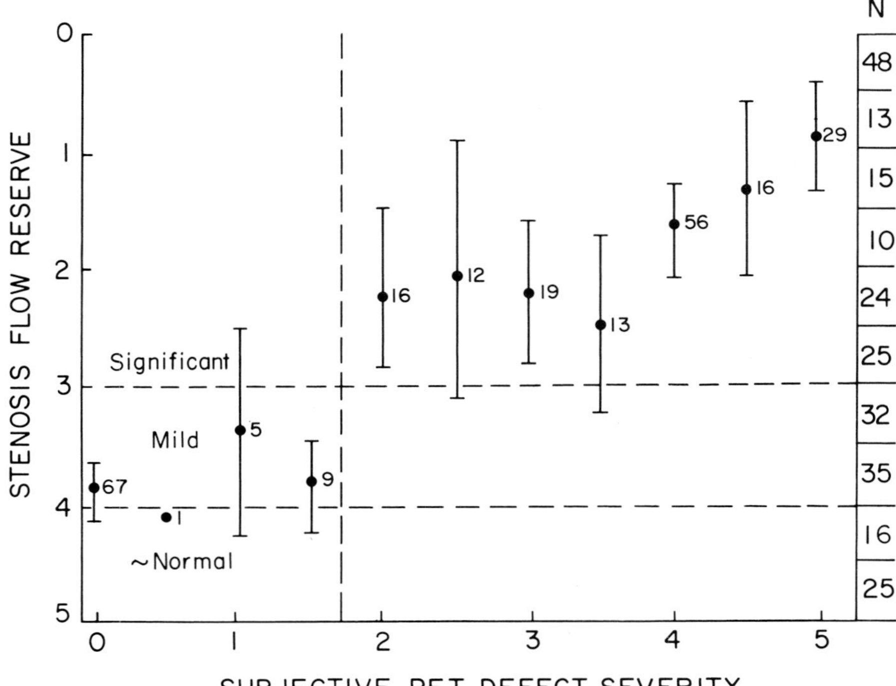

Figure 66–11. Relation between arteriographic stenosis flow reserve and subjective PET defect severity in the corresponding anatomic region of 243 stenoses. Mean value of stenosis flow reserve is plotted as a function of PET defect severity. The horizontal dashed lines identify the ranges of normal, mildly reduced, and significantly reduced stenosis flow reserve. The vertical dashed line indicates that PET defect scores of 2 or greater predict the presence of mild or significant stenoses. The error bars represent 90 percent confidence intervals. The number of patients represented is shown adjacent to each point. (From Demer, L.L., Gould, K.L., Goldstein, R.A., et al.: Diagnosis of coronary artery disease by positron emission tomography: Comparison to quantitative arteriography in 193 patients. Circulation 79:825, 1989, by permission of the American Heart Association, Inc.)

Limitations of Sensitivity and Specificity Analysis

Most reports of the diagnostic accuracy of PET, SPECT, and planar thallium perfusion imaging of the heart are based on sensitivity/specificity analysis.[D9, G6, H4, R2, S5, V2, Z2] Unfortunately, reported sensitivity and specificity values of tests are not comparable if they are based on different patient populations, different criteria for coronary artery disease, different criteria for positive perfusion defects, or different imaging methods.

First, threshold values that yield optimal sensitivity and specificity for one imaging method may yield suboptimal values for another test with a different threshold for detection. For example, a hypothetic test with perfect sensitivity and specificity using a cutoff value of 40 percent diameter narrowing will have falsely low specificity if the cutoff value is defined as 50 percent, particularly if the study population includes many patients with stenosis severity between 40 and 50 percent.

In addition, binary (positive or negative) classification of imaging and arteriographic results does not reflect the continuous nature of coronary artery disease severity. In the past, arteriographic results have been classified by the arbitrary cutoff values of 50, 70, or 75 percent diameter narrowing. Defining a 45 percent stenosis as normal and a 50 percent stenosis as abnormal has questionable meaning. Perfusion scan results also have been classified into a binary scale as normal or abnormal despite a continuous spectrum of defect severity, both in terms of defect intensity and size. However, criteria for distinguishing positive and borderline defects are even more subjective than arteriographic percent diameter narrowing.

A third limitation of sensitivity/specificity analysis is the dependence on distribution of disease severity in the study population.[H5] A sample population with a high frequency of mild disease, near the cutoff points, will tend to have lower sensitivity and specificity for the same amount of scatter. Thus sensitivity and specificity determined for one population may not apply to a different population, as in symptomatic and asymptomatic patients. Use of continuous variables has been proposed to overcome these limitations.[H5] Studies are in progress to re-evaluate the accuracy of PET perfusion imaging with continuous scales over the entire range of disease severity, using direct correlation analysis and quantitative arteriographic flow reserve rather than percent diameter narrowing in larger series of patients.

Localization of Coronary Artery Disease

To assess the accuracy of positron emission tomography imaging in identifying the specific coronary arteries with significant stenoses, it is necessary to assign each myocardial region to a particular artery. However, no one correspondence is applicable to all patients. Anatomic variations in the coronary tree, such as right and left dominant systems, and overlap of perfusion beds greatly limit any algorithm for matching each stenosis to a corresponding defect. With this limitation, most studies have shown a fair relation between the region supplied by a narrowed coronary artery and the location of the PET defect, assuming standard anatomy. Alternatively, case-by-case comparison would allow more accurate assignment of vessels to regions, but it may introduce subjective bias.

Comparison with Thallium Scintigraphy

Few data are available *directly* comparing positron emission tomography to more widely available methods, such as thallium-201 scintigraphy. Theoretically, PET images are expected to have higher accuracy than thallium images[B4] because of three main limitations of single-photon imaging: (1) inability to correct for photon attenuation, (2) superimposition of radioactivity from nonmyocardial structures, and (3) depth-dependent resolution. To determine whether positron emission tomography indeed has greater accuracy in practice, it will be necessary to compare results directly with arteriography in the same group of patients because of the known effects of patient selection and disease distribution on statistical estimation of sensitivity and specificity.

Early studies have compared planar 201-thallium scintigraphy with nitrogen-13 ammonia PET imaging,[K7] but with the availability of tomographic thallium imaging the issue is now comparison of SPECT with PET, because SPECT does not require a cyclotron. Two studies[T2, T3] provide direct comparison between exercise PET and SPECT for several patients. Tamaki and colleagues[T3] compared exercise thallium-SPECT to PET perfusion imaging in conjunction with PET metabolic imaging in 20 patients with coronary artery disease. The tracers with nitrogen-13 ammonia and fluorine-18 fluorodeoxyglucose were used. Results showed similar sensitivity and specificity for PET and SPECT, ranging from 60 to 89 percent sensitivity for identification of the diseased coronary artery. However, in this study, the PET imaging was handicapped. Only three tomographic slices were obtained for each patient, which may have missed small portions of the anterior wall and large portions of the inferior wall. The entire inferior wall may be left out of such a limited-slice image.

These same investigators[T2] later compared bicycle exercise imaging using nitrogen-13 ammonia-PET to thallium-SPECT imaging in 51 patients, including 48 with known coronary artery disease. SPECT detected 96 percent and PET detected 98 percent of patients with greater than 50 percent diameter narrowing of at least one coronary artery, based on subjective interpretation of arteriograms. The apparent lack of improvement with positron emission tomography may have been due to the use of exercise stress, which negates the value of attenuation correction by PET. Repositioning patients in the camera after exercise usually results in misregistration of the transmission and stress emission images, causing faulty attenuation correction. Because there were only two normal subjects, specificity was assessed on an artery-to-artery basis. Values of specificity were much lower than sensitivity for both imaging methods. However, prediction of the diseased artery may be a suboptimal test for accuracy of either imaging method, because there is not a one-to-one correspondence between myocardial regions and coronary arteries. Even with a hypothetically perfect imaging method demonstrating a posterolateral defect, it cannot be predicted with certainty whether the disease is in the circumflex or the right coronary artery.

PET and thallium SPECT perfusion imaging also provide indirect evidence of viability. In thallium imaging, a region with a "fixed defect," in which the tracer does not redistribute over time, is generally considered infarcted. In PET imaging, a region is considered infarcted or ischemic when the defect is present at rest. In many patients, regions with fixed thallium defects show defects only with stress by PET, suggesting that SPECT may underestimate the presence of myocardial ischemia and overestimate infarction.[T2] This effect is confirmed by findings of metabolic PET imaging in patients with fixed thallium defects. Fluorodeoxyglucose uptake, indicating viability, is detected by metabolic PET imaging in regions of myocardium with fixed thallium defects.[B7]

Most studies of the accuracy of thallium scintigraphy have been based on subjective arteriography and not directly compared with positron emission tomography. DePasquale and colleagues reported high sensitivity (97 percent) and moderate specificity (71 percent) for quantitative thallium-SPECT in comparison with subjective arteriographic interpretation.[D9] Such studies must be considered in light of the limitations of subjective arteriography and patient selection. Visual interpretations of coronary arteriograms are marked by such great observer variability that quantitative comparison of arteriograms in different patients, or at different times in the same patient, is essentially invalid. In addition, sensitivity and specificity are highly dependent on the cutoff value of percent diameter stenosis used to define coronary artery disease. With regard to patient selection, these data were obtained in patients with anginal symptoms or known coronary artery disease. As expected, specificity is lower in asymptomatic subjects.[S7]

Two studies have directly compared thallium-201 and PET imaging in the same patients. Schelbert compared PET nitrogen-

imaging in the same patients. Schelbert compared PET nitrogen-13 ammonia imaging to planar thallium-201 scintigraphy in 11 patients having both tests and found slightly greater sensitivity for positron emission tomography than planar thallium imaging (100 percent vs. 91 percent).[S5] Of the 19 stenosed arteries in this subgroup, thallium identified only 11 (58 percent) compared with 17 (89 percent) by PET. Preliminary data from a more recent study[C1] suggest that even a single cross-sectional PET slice provides equal or greater sensitivity than a complete three-dimensional thallium-201 SPECT image in patients.

Limitations

In general, sensitivity and specificity of perfusion imaging for coronary artery disease depend on four factors: (1) the patient population studied (i.e., the pretest probability), (2) the standard of comparison used to define presence and absence of coronary artery disease, (3) the subjective or objective criteria for defining positive and negative scans, and (4) the adequacy of the vasodilator stimulus.

Unfortunately, there is no ideal "gold standard" for assessing accuracy of perfusion imaging in identifying coronary artery disease severity. Perfusion reserve may not correspond to stenosis flow reserve in the presence of altered physiologic conditions, such as very high or low perfusion pressure, marked bradycardia or tachycardia, collateral vessels, increased resting flow, ventricular hypertrophy, abnormal venous pressure, or inadequate vasodilatory stimulus.[K8] Perfusion reserve may not correspond to directly measured coronary flow reserve in the presence of collateral vessels or when hemodynamic conditions change between the time of catheterization and the time of PET imaging.

Potential for Screening Asymptomatic Patients

It is now recognized that angina pectoris is an insensitive marker for transient myocardial ischemia. If dipyridamole-PET imaging is found to have sufficient accuracy, it may ultimately permit screening of high-risk asymptomatic individuals. Asymptomatic coronary artery disease is now appreciated as a significant problem. In the Framingham study population, more than 25 percent of all infarctions were discovered only by routine electrocardiographic testing, and the prognosis for these "unrecognized" infarctions was found to be as serious as that of "recognized" infarctions.[K9] In a Finnish study population, 67 percent of coronary heart disease deaths in men aged 40 to 59 years were in those without a history of symptoms.[R4] Asymptomatic coronary artery disease is found in up to 13 percent of patients undergoing preoperative cardiac catheterization for valvular heart disease.[O1]

When it is sufficiently severe, asymptomatic coronary artery disease also may be detected by thallium-201 SPECT imaging. The two features of positron emission tomography that render it potentially more suitable for screening are (1) its potential for higher specificity and sensitivity of detection, and (2) its potential for early detection of coronary stenoses, as mild as a 47 percent reduction in diameter.[G5]

It is essential to recognize that the specificity for a test depends on the study population—that is, the pretest probability of disease. More false-positives are expected in an asymptomatic population. Even a small likelihood of false-positive tests may result in large numbers of unnecessary invasive procedures when a large population is studied. For this reason, PET accuracy must be established in asymptomatic patients as well as symptomatic patients, and patient selection for clinical applications must be performed with this in mind. At present, it is difficult to measure the accuracy of PET perfusion imaging in a large group of purely asymptomatic individuals without known coronary artery disease or myocardial infarction, because the standard for comparison, coronary arteriography, is rarely warranted in such patients.

QUANTITATIVE ANALYSIS OF TRACER UPTAKE

The main feature that distinguishes positron emission tomography from other myocardial perfusion imaging methods is its unique capability of providing accurate quantitative information. This capacity derives from the dual photon release, which allows emission images to be corrected for the specific photon attenuation pattern of the specific individual being scanned.

In patients with known coronary artery disease, quantitative PET perfusion imaging may clarify the physiologic significance of individual stenoses when severity is difficult to judge arteriographically. Methods of quantitative analysis of perfusion images have been developed already for thallium planar and SPECT imaging, such as circumferential profile analysis and bull's-eye format. In normal segments of myocardium, nitrogen-13 ammonia tracer uptake increases approximately 15 percent with exercise compared with rest, for a 1-minute acquisition time, with normalization for the total dose of ammonia administered. There is less increase, no change, or decrease in areas supplied by stenosed arteries.[T1] By plotting tracer uptake as a function of angular position in each slice, defects may be more easily recognized, and objective criteria may be established based on normal populations. Caution is required in establishing criteria for "normal" tracer uptake. In the past, normal ranges for quantitative tracer uptake have been based on subjects identified as normal on the basis of their arteriograms, which are interpreted subjectively and which do not exclude abnormal perfusion reserve.

Goldstein and colleagues found a correlation between stenosis severity and relative myocardial perfusion reserve, particularly for LAD lesions (Fig. 66–12).[G8] In this study, stenosis flow reserve was determined by quantitative coronary arteriography for 41 stenoses, and results were correlated to myocardial perfusion reserve from PET perfusion imaging. In contrast, percent diameter narrowing and cross-sectional area reduction correlated less well to perfusion reserve. Relative myocardial perfusion reserve remained nearly normal for cross-sectional area reductions approaching 70 percent. A minimal cross-sectional area of 3 mm^2 was associated with normal perfusion reserve.

MEASUREMENT OF ABSOLUTE MYOCARDIAL PERFUSION

Active research is directed at obtaining accurate measurement of absolute myocardial perfusion by positron emission tomography. Certain biologic characteristics of the tracers and physical limitations of the detector systems are being overcome.

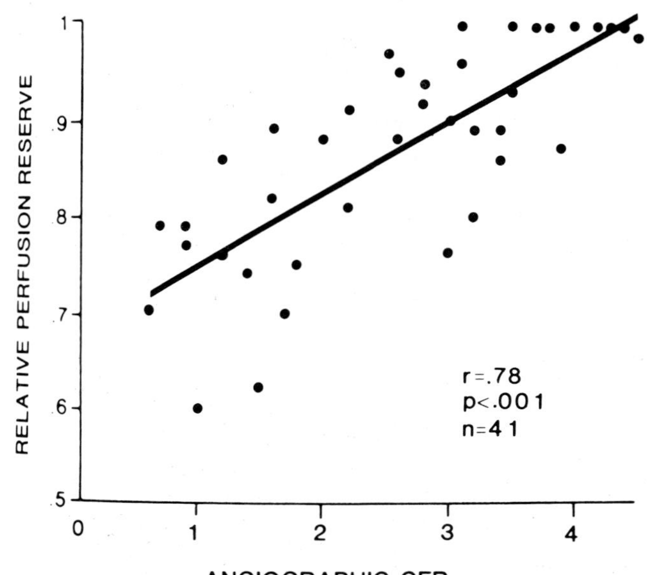

Figure 66–12. Relation of relative myocardial perfusion reserve and stenosis flow reserve derived from quantitative coronary arteriography. (From Goldstein, R.A., Kirkeeide, R.L., Demer, L.L., et al.: Relation between geometric dimensions of coronary artery stenoses and myocardial perfusion reserve in man. Reproduced from the Journal of Clinical Investigation, 1987, 79:1473 by copyright permission of the American Society of Clinical Investigation.)

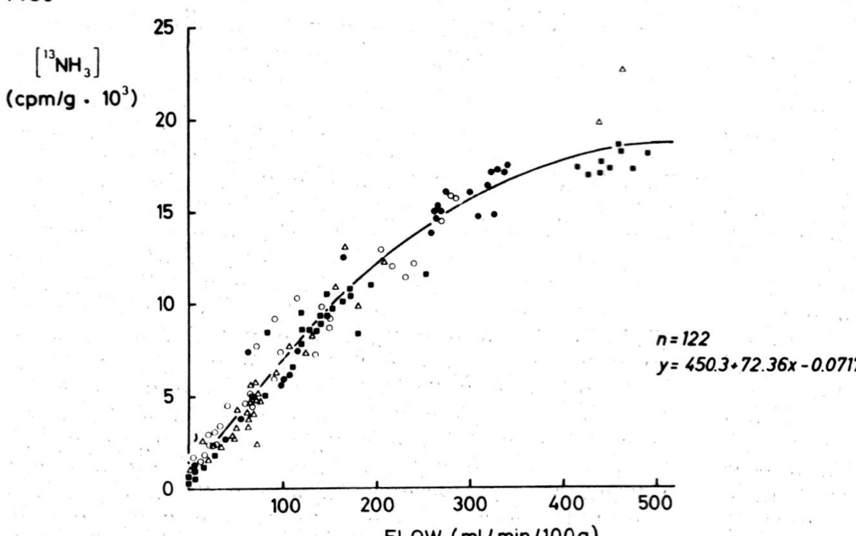

Figure 66–13. Relation between microsphere-determined myocardial blood flow and regional myocardial [^{13}N] ammonia tissue concentration. (From Schelbert, H.R., Phelps, M.E., Hoffman, E.J., et al.: Regional myocardial perfusion assessed with N-13 labeled ammonia and positron emission computerized axial tomography. Am. J. Cardiol. 43:209, 1979 with permission.)

Flow-Dependent Extraction

One property of perfusion tracers that complicates measurement of absolute flow is the nonlinear dependence of extraction on flow for nitrogen-13 ammonia and rubidium-82 (Figs. 66–13 and 66–14). Transmembrane cellular transport of these tracers decreases as the capillary residence time of the tracer decreases. Determination of absolute flow thus requires more sophisticated models to allow for the decreasing first-pass extraction of these tracers with increasing flow. In contrast, qualitative interpretation of perfusion is not distorted; the dependence of extraction on flow simply blunts the changes in uptake. For example, a 50 percent change in coronary flow would be expected to produce only about a 40 percent change in uptake.[L2] Similarly, extraction of ammonia decreases from approximately 82 percent at resting flow to about 60 percent at high flows of 3 ml/min/gm.[S1, S3]

Geometric Limitations

Geometric factors, such as resolution, wall motion, spillover, and the partial volume effect, described in an earlier chapter, also limit the accuracy of absolute flow measurements by both perfusion PET and SPECT imaging. An important advance in quantitative PET has been development of analytic methods to correct for some of these effects.[W4] A deconvolution technique for calculation of spillover fractions derived from geometric measurements of the imaged cross-section and the intrinsic resolution of the tomograph has been developed and validated by direct measurement of tracer concentration in dogs.[H6] More recently, a direct imaging method has been proposed[S8] to quantify these geometric effects and allow correction of perfusion images. This method requires injection of long-lived and short-lived isotopes of the same tracer element, such as rubidium-81 (half-life = 4.6 hr) and rubidium-82 (half-life = 74 sec). After a 4-hour period of equilibrium, the long-lived isotope labels the myocardial tissue mass. The resulting image may be used to correct the rubidium-82 perfusion image for effects of thinning and decreased wall motion in ischemic areas.[S8]

Models

The conceptually simplest approach to measure absolute perfusion is by labeled microspheres or particles that are essentially entirely trapped in the capillary bed.[F1] Radiolabeled microspheres are often used in animal studies. In patients, labeled, macroaggregated albumin particles have been used, because diffuse capillary embolization is prevented by gradual disruption and scavenging of the albumin. However, such particles must be

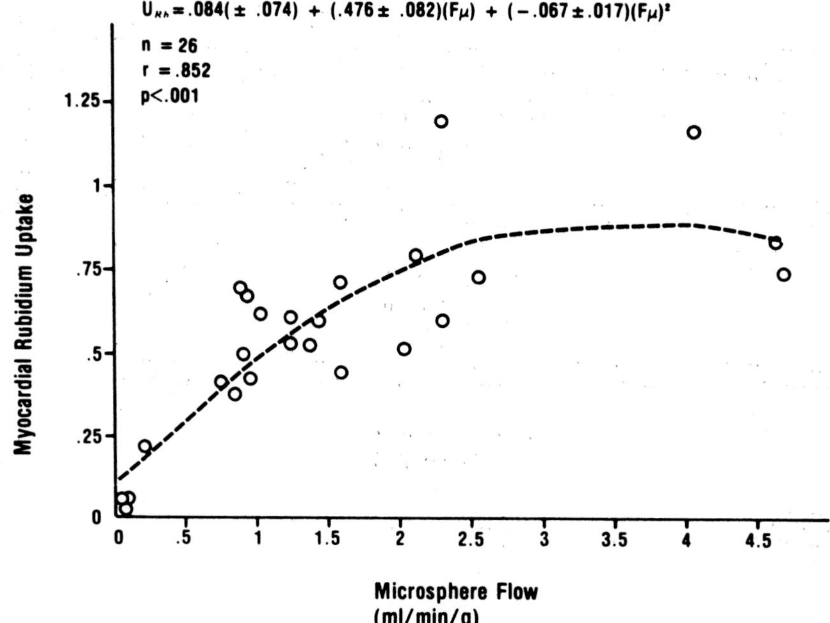

Figure 66–14. Relation between myocardial uptake (normalized for arterial input) of ^{13}Rb and microsphere-determined flow under control conditions. Uptake product of flow and extraction is linearly related to flow up to 2.5 times normal, but it overestimates low flow rates and underestimates high flow rates. (From Goldstein, R.A., Mullani, N.A., Marani, S.K., et al.: Myocardial perfusion with rubidium-82. II. Effects of metabolic and pharmacologic interventions. J. Nucl. Med. 24: 907–915, 1983, with permission of The Society of Nuclear Medicine.)

injected via left heart catheterization; intravenous administration is fruitless because such particles lodge in the pulmonary capillary bed. Regional perfusion can be determined by comparison with microsphere uptake in a reference flow sink, such as a constant rate withdrawal reservoir.[Z3]

Absolute myocardial perfusion has been calculated from the clearance curve of radioactivity from bolus injection of freely diffusible tracers, such as oxygen-15 water or carbon-11 butanol, using equations modified from the Kety-Schmidt[K10, K11] model, which was originally derived for use of nitrous oxide to trace cerebral blood flow:

$$Q = kLM/D$$

where Q = flow in mL/100 g/min
k = rate constant derived from the time-activity curve of isotope clearance
L = partition coefficient of the tracer in tissue and blood
M = myocardial mass
D = density of myocardium (approximately 1.03 to 1.05)

Accurate determination of the rate constant or clearance requires very rapid data acquisition at the limits of current technology, and the statistical methods used for exponential curve fitting are highly sensitive to noise or error.

Regional absolute myocardial blood flow also can be determined with radiotracers that are taken up and released over time, using the fractional distribution approach.[S9] Relative regional perfusion (relative to cardiac output) can be derived by the following proportionality:

$$Q_f/CO = U_f/U_T$$

where Q_f = fractional flow to the region of interest
CO = cardiac output
U_f = radiotracer activity in the region of interest
U_T = total radiotracer administered

This model assumes that the cellular uptake and release kinetics are not dependent on flow or metabolic state. Unfortunately, rubidium-82 and nitrogen-13 ammonia have flow-dependent extraction, and there is evidence that nitrogen-13 ammonia uptake is affected by metabolic factors.[S1]

A mathematical model has been derived to correct for flow-dependent extraction of rubidium.[G9, M4] This model is based on the assumption that the time course of free rubidium is described by the two-compartment model equation:

$$C(t) = bte^{-at}$$

where b and a are coefficients derived by curve-fitting. Total measured tracer uptake is fit by this exponential form to calculate the time course of free rubidium-82 concentration (Fig. 66–15). This value is subtracted from total measured activity to derive the time course of trapped rubidium-82 concentration. The ratio of trapped to total measured activity at peak counts is an estimate of first-pass extraction, which can be applied to the equation for flow:

$$\text{Flow} = \frac{U(T)}{E\int C_a(t)dt}$$

where U = trapped activity
T = the time from the start of the scan
E = extraction
$C_a(t)$ = arterial concentration as a function of time where the integral is taken from 0 to T

This method requires rapid data acquisition or invasive arterial sampling to determine the input function. The high count rates that occur during first-pass of tracer through the heart cause saturation of the data transfer mechanism in some PET camera systems. Recently, a new method of deriving absolute myocardial perfusion from rubidium-82 images has been proposed, based on a similar compartmental model.[H7]

Another approach to quantification of regional myocardial blood flow is the use of a freely diffusible tracer, such as oxygen-15 water. Methods of quantification have been based on a modification of the tissue autoradiographic approach as tested in animals. Bergmann and associates found a close correlation between $H_2{}^{15}O$ uptake and both tomographic and direct measurement of radioactive microsphere distribution (Fig. 66–16).[B2] Huang and associates found a linear correlation to blood flow measured by gamma-emitting radioactive microspheres (r = 0.88), but with a consistent underestimation of flow by positron emission tomography, owing to the partial volume effect.[H8]

The potential and limitations of myocardial perfusion quantification have been evaluated in detail.[H9] Iida and associates have recently modified this approach using the concept of "tissue fraction."[I1] Tissue fraction is defined as the fraction of tissue mass in the volume of the region of interest, which is used to correct for the partial volume effect. Using $H_2{}^{15}O$ with $C^{15}O$ and dynamic

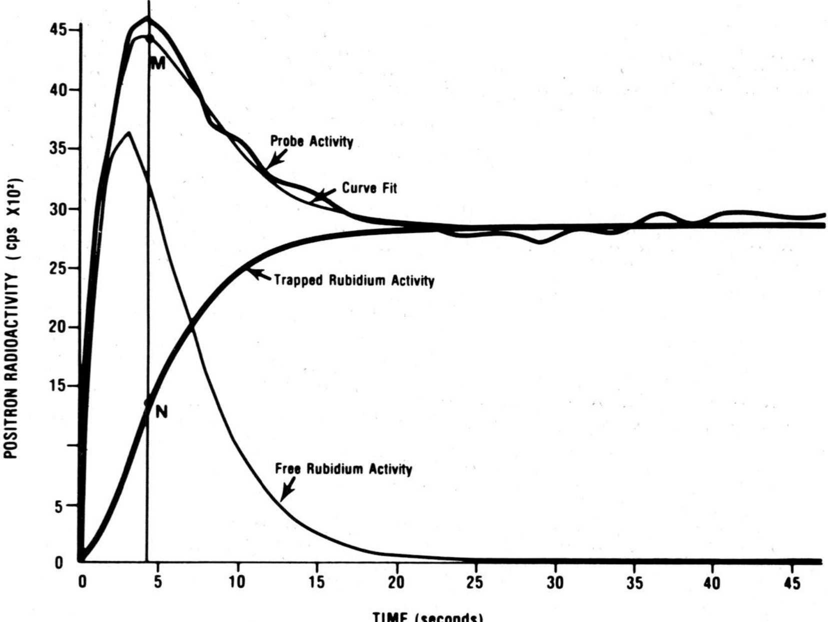

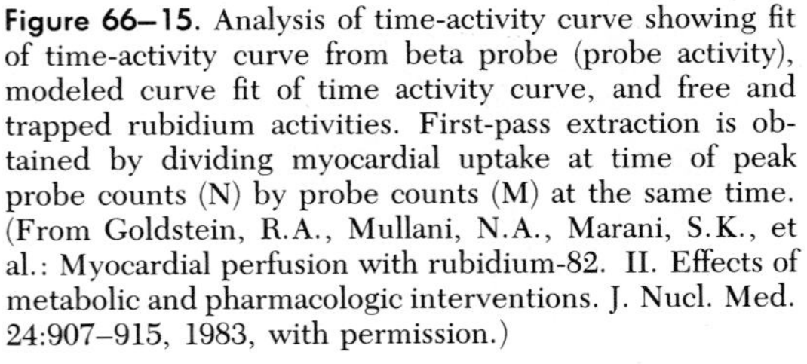
Figure 66–15. Analysis of time-activity curve showing fit of time-activity curve from beta probe (probe activity), modeled curve fit of time activity curve, and free and trapped rubidium activities. First-pass extraction is obtained by dividing myocardial uptake at time of peak probe counts (N) by probe counts (M) at the same time. (From Goldstein, R.A., Mullani, N.A., Marani, S.K., et al.: Myocardial perfusion with rubidium-82. II. Effects of metabolic and pharmacologic interventions. J. Nucl. Med. 24:907–915, 1983, with permission.)

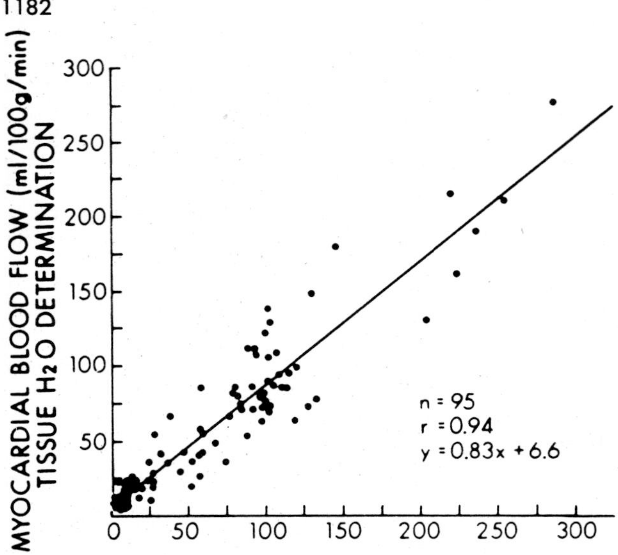

Figure 66–16. The correlation between myocardial blood flow determined with microspheres and that determined with $H_2{}^{15}O$ calculated with the one-compartment model. The results were obtained from nine open-chest dogs after a 60-second intravenous infusion of the tracer and from direct assay of radioactivity in tissue. (From Bergmann, S.R., Fox, K.A.A., Rand, A.L., et al.: Quantification of regional myocardial blood flow in vivo with $H_2{}^{15}O$. Circulation 70:724, 1984, by permission of the American Heart Association, Inc.)

PET imaging, absolute blood flow was measured at 0.95 ml/min/g in normal subjects and 0.55 ml/min/g in patients with three-vessel coronary artery disease.

DETECTION OF TRANSIENT AND SILENT ISCHEMIA

Transient changes in perfusion occurring during spontaneous coronary spasm, smoking, or mental stress cannot be detected by conventional perfusion imaging owing to the long physical half-life of thallium-201. Selwyn, and colleagues[C2, S10, S11] have demonstrated the usefulness of PET perfusion imaging for recognizing the causes of short-term variations in myocardial blood flow.

Mental Stress

Deanfield and colleagues first documented PET perfusion defects occurring during episodes of silent ST-segment depression induced by mental stress.[D7] Abnormal regional rubidium-82 uptake and ST-segment depression developed in patients undergoing a mental arithmetic test consisting of serial subtraction of sevens from 100 (Fig. 66–17). In 12 of 16 patients with chronic stable angina and exercise-induced PET defects, PET defects occurred with mental stress in the same regions as the exercise-related defects. Only half of these patients had S-T changes on electrocardiogram, and two thirds had no associated chest discomfort.

Smoking

Relative perfusion defects as well as absolute reduction in tracer uptake have been documented during smoking (Fig. 66–18) in patients with coronary artery disease.[D1] Abnormal regional uptake of rubidium-82 was found in 6 of 13 chronic smokers with typical stable angina (Fig. 66–19). Patients with smoking-induced perfusion defects also had exercise-induced defects. The degree of heterogeneity of perfusion scans, which indicates the presence of relative perfusion defects, doubled with smoking and tripled with exercise. Regional uptake decreased approximately 30 percent with smoking, without concomitant angina. The mechanism of smoking's effect on myocardial perfusion is not known. However, because absolute reduction in perfusion tracer uptake occurred at lower levels of oxygen consumption than required for exercise-induced defects, the supply-side is implicated, suggesting effects of smoking on neurohumoral, prostaglandin, platelet, and/or vasomotor function.

Daily Activities

Positron emission tomography also has been used to evaluate the importance of ST segment changes seen on ambulatory electrocardiographic monitoring. Deanfield and associates documented temporary impairment of segmental myocardial perfusion

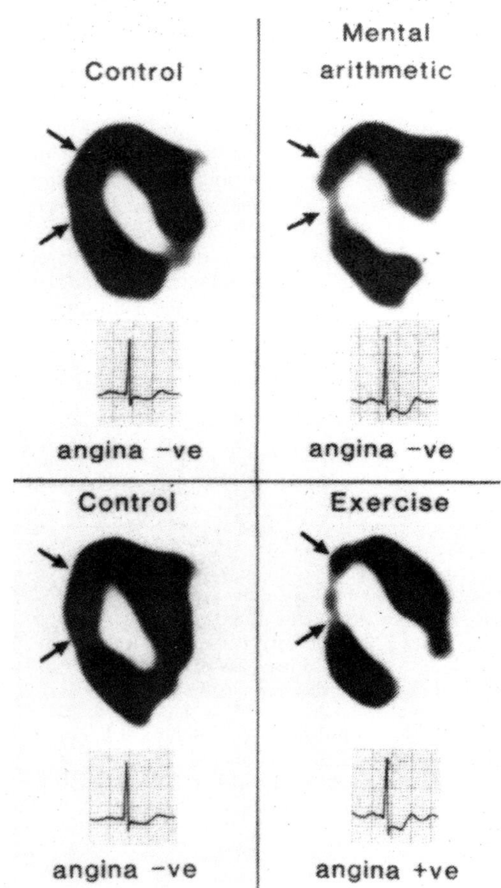

Figure 66–17. Changes in regional myocardial uptake of ^{82}Rb with silent ST-segment depression induced by mental stress: anterior and free wall ischemia. (From Deanfield, J.E., Kensett, M., Wilson, R.A., et al.: Silent myocardial ischemia due to mental stress. Lancet 2:1003, Nov. 3, 1984, with permission.)

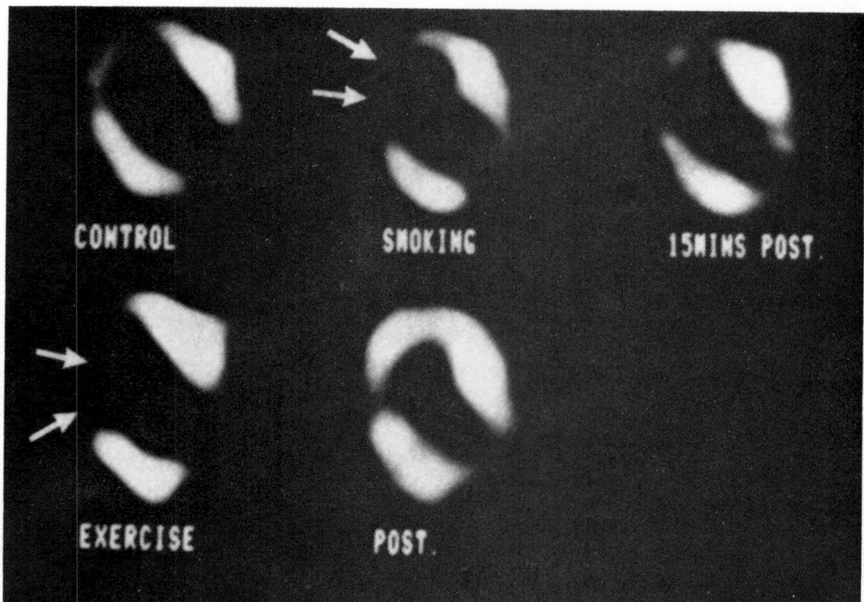

Figure 66–18. Tomograms from a patient showing changes in regional uptake of ^{82}Rb with smoking and exercise. (From Deanfield, J.E., Shea, M.J., Wilson, R.A., et al.: Direct effects of smoking on the heart: Silent ischemic disturbances of coronary flow. Am. J. Cardiol. 57:1007, 1986, with permission.)

coinciding with ST segment depression on electrocardiogram in 30 patients with coronary artery disease.[D10, N1] Transient, segmental reductions of uptake were present in 97 percent of 63 episodes of ST segment depression with angina and all 30 episodes of asymptomatic ST depression at rest and with mental and exercise stress. Perfusion normalized simultaneously with resolution of the electrocardiographic changes (Fig. 66–20). The duration of such defects associated with transient ischemic electrocardiographic changes is shortened by nitrates.

These findings imply that ischemic episodes are more common than previously suspected, and that daily activities, such as mental stress and smoking, may be more common triggers of silent ischemia than is physical exertion.

EVALUATION FOR MYOCARDIAL INFARCTION

Although conventional imaging methods detect and localize myocardial infarction, accurate and quantitative assessment of infarct size is more likely to be achieved by positron coincidence imaging. Knowledge of infarct size is clinically important because of its known relation to prognosis.[S12]

Nitrogen-13 ammonia was first used to detect myocardial infarction in patients with planar scintigraphy rather than coincidence positron emission tomography. Harper and colleagues studied 50 patients using nitrogen-13 ammonia and planar scintigraphy.[H10] Of 22 with definite infarcts, 17 had definite defects, 2 had possible defects, and 3 had no defects. Of 8 patients with possible infarcts, 5 showed definite defects and 3 had possible defects. Using nitrogen-13 ammonia in dogs with ligated coronary arteries, Hoop and colleagues showed a correlation between decreased tracer uptake and decreased flow in the area of infarct.[H11] Using nitrogen-13 ammonia and planar scintigraphy, Walsh and associates found localized uptake defects in 19 of 20 patients with acute myocardial infarction.[W5, W6]

Rubidium-82 is also useful for assessing myocardial infarction. Budinger and colleagues reported visualization of infarcts as small as 0.7 ml in patient studies.[B8] Rubidium-82 uptake defects correlated well with electrocardiographic and coronary arteriographic findings in these 15 patients. Goldstein and colleagues performed rubidium-82 imaging within 96 hours of onset of symptoms in 17 patients with transmural infarction.[G10] The infarct-related artery was correctly diagnosed by positron emission tomography in all patients. Rubidium-82 is well suited for imaging of acute infarct because its short half-life permits sequential studies as frequently as every 10 minutes. There is also evidence that rubidium-82 transfer rate constants derived from a two-compartment model may predict reversible from irreversible injury during acute occlusion with reperfusion in animals (Fig. 66–21). At present, assessment of viability is performed by comparing perfusion and metabolic tracer PET images (Fig. 66–22); this method has also been shown to distinguish Q wave and non-Q wave infarctions.[B7]

Quantification of myocardial infarction size by PET imaging was first performed using carbon-11 palmitate, which is a physiologic substrate of the heart ordinarily used as a metabolic rather than a perfusion tracer. Weiss and associates found a close correlation between estimated infarct size from carbon-11 pal-

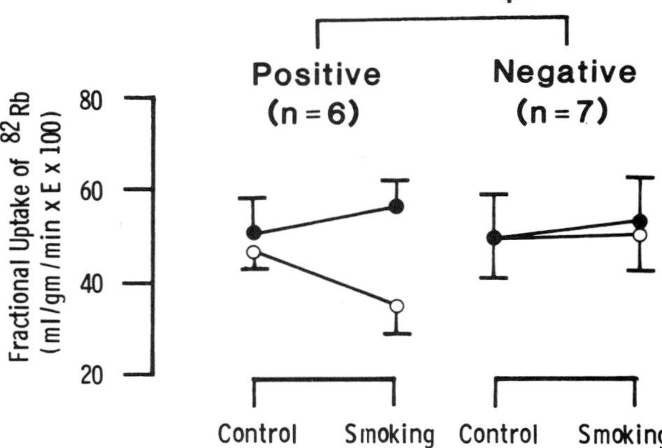

Figure 66–19. Effects of smoking on regional myocardial uptake of ^{82}Rb in 13 patients. Six patients showed a positive response with abnormal inhomogeneity and an absolute reduction in ^{82}Rb uptake in an affected segment, which was always the same segment that developed abnormal uptake after exercise. (From Deanfield, J.E., Shea, M.J., Wilson, R.A., et al.: Direct effects of smoking on the heart: Silent ischemic disturbances of coronary flow. Am. J. Cardiol., 57:1007, 1986, with permission.)

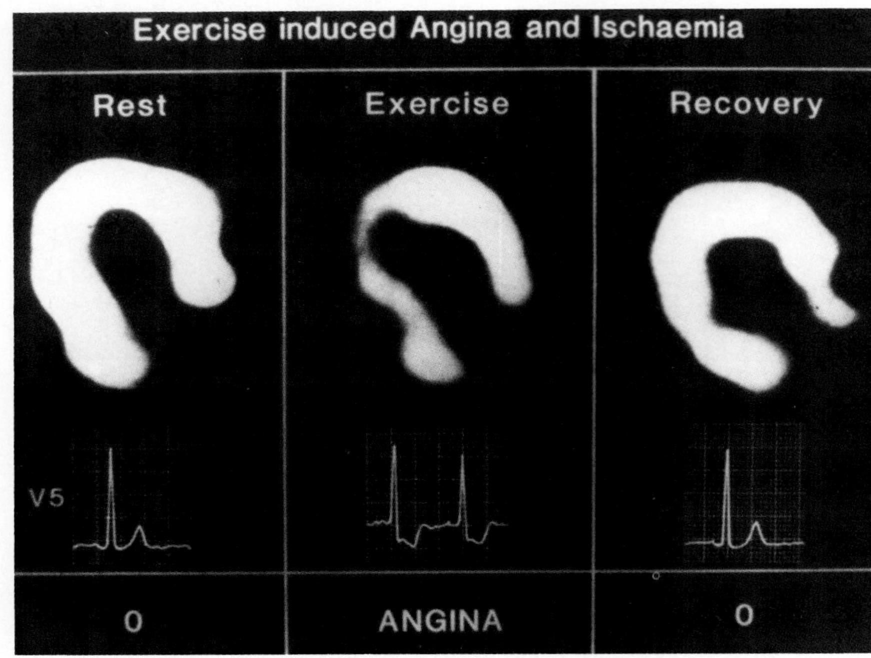

Figure 66–20. Tomograms through the midportion of the left ventricle, recorded in a patient with chronic stable angina and three-vessel coronary artery disease. Under control conditions, the regional myocardial perfusion to the anterior wall of the left ventricle is normal. During exercise, there is a marked decrease in the regional uptake of ^{82}Rb, suggesting a decrease in myocardial perfusion. Simultaneous recordings of a 12-lead electrocardiogram demonstrate isoelectric ST segments during control conditions and ST segment depression during exercise. (From Nabel, E.G., Rocco, M.B., and Selwyn, A.P.: Characteristics and significance of ischemia detected by ambulatory electrocardiographic monitoring. Circulation, 75:V74, 1987, by permission of the American Heart Association, Inc.)

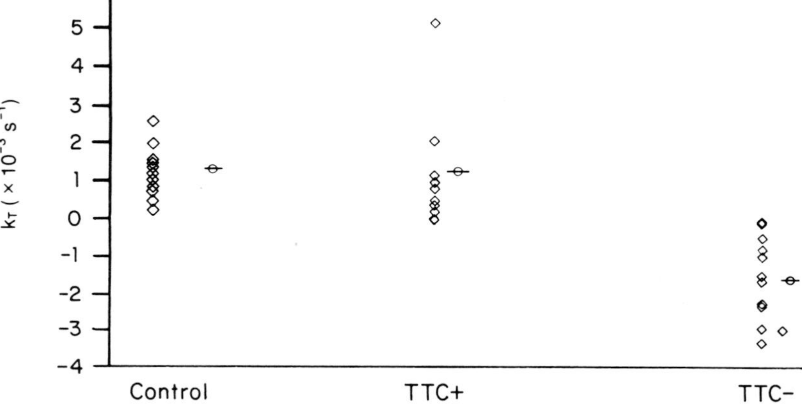

Figure 66–21. ^{82}Rb transfer rate constant at baseline and after reperfusion in viable (TTC+) and irreversibly injured samples (TTC−). (From Goldstein, R.A.: Assessment and patency and viability in open-chest dog. Reproduced from the Journal of Clinical Investigation, 1987, 79:1473 by copyright permission of the American Society of Clinical Investigation.)

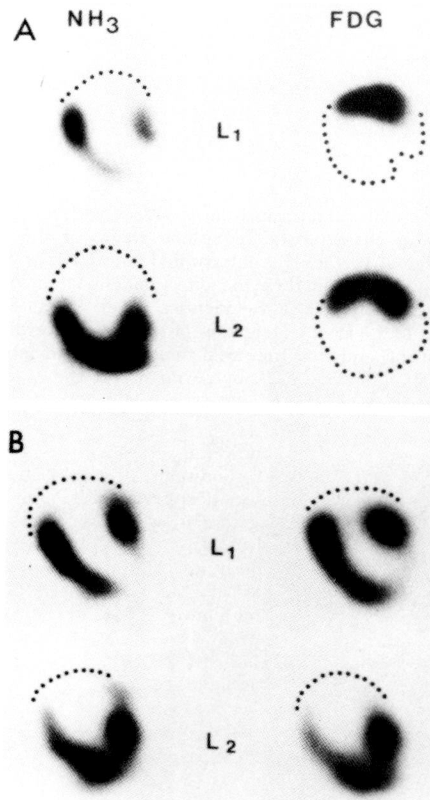

Figure 66–22. Cross-sectional [^{13}N] ammonia (NH_3) and ^{18}F-fluorodeoxyglucose (FDG) images obtained 48 hours after the onset of acute symptoms. In the study, there is a mismatch of FDG and NH_3 uptake, suggesting viable tissue in the segments with decreased flow. (From Schwaiger M., Brunken, R., Grover-McKay, M., et al: Metabolism and flow in acute myocardial infarction. J. Am. Coll. Cardiol. 8:806, 1986. Reprinted with permission from the American College of Cardiology.)

mitate PET images and direct morphometric measurement of infarct size (r = 0.97), as well as enzymatic estimation of infarct size (r = 0.93), 48 hours after occlusion of the left anterior descending coronary arteries in dogs.[W7] Tomographic estimates of infarct size also correlate closely (r = 0.92) to enzymatic estimates of infarct size in patients[T4] with a reproducibility within 1 percent based on four patients having repeat scans.[S13]

Infarct location is also accurately determined by PET images. In normal subjects, carbon-11 palmitate uptake distribution is homogeneous, whereas in patients with documented myocardial infarction, the area of injury is delineated by diminished tracer uptake (Fig. 66–23). PET defect regions correspond to the areas identified by electrocardiographic localization.[S14]

The potential use of positron emission tomography for assessing the progress of thrombolysis during acute myocardial infarction has been suggested by results of studies in animals.[B2]

RESPONSE TO THERAPY

Noninvasive imaging of myocardial perfusion has an important role in follow-up of response to therapy to aid clinical management and to enhance long-term clinical research of prevention and therapy. In the past, clinical cardiology research has relied on difficult end points, such as angina, which is difficult to quantify or on myocardial infarction or death, which are infrequent, especially in prevention trials.

Percutaneous Transluminal Coronary Angioplasty

The effect of percutaneous transluminal coronary angioplasty on relative myocardial perfusion reserve (RMPR) has been evaluated by Goldstein and associates, using quantitative assessment of relative perfusion defects.[G11] Myocardial perfusion reserve (MPR) was estimated as the ratio of stress to rest activity in any given area. Relative myocardial perfusion reserve of a bed supplied by a stenosed artery was defined as the ratio of myocardial perfusion reserve in that area to the myocardial perfusion reserve of an area supplied by an arteriographically normal coronary artery in the same patient.

$$\text{RMPR} = \frac{\text{stress activity/rest activity (area of interest)}}{\text{stress activity/rest activity (normal area)}}$$

Except for very severe stenoses or areas of infarct, rest perfusion is generally not affected by coronary stenoses, so that the rest activity cancels, leaving

$$\text{RMPR} = \frac{\text{stress activity in area of interest}}{\text{stress activity in normal area}}$$

Changes in relative myocardial perfusion reserve corresponded closely to changes in angiographic stenosis flow reserve in 11 patients who underwent dipyridamole PET imaging before and after coronary balloon angioplasty (Fig. 66–24). Walsh and associates found a correspondence between successful coronary balloon angioplasty and results of dipyridamole PET imaging using oxygen-15 water uptake.[W8]

Effect of Dietary Interventions

PET perfusion imaging may aid in serial evaluation of progression and regression of known coronary artery disease. In an ongoing study by Ornish and colleagues of the value of cholesterol-lowering regimens, PET perfusion imaging is being used as one end point, allowing earlier feedback than with alternative end points such as myocardial infarction.[O2] Similar longitudinal clinical trials are needed to test the value of altering other risk factors in halting or possibly reversing the encroachment of coronary lumen by atherosclerotic plaque. Although quantitative coronary arteriography is the standard, it is not practical and often not warranted in study patients. Preliminary data suggest the feasibility of detecting progression/regression by positron emission tomography in comparison with quantitative arteriography. In a preliminary study of 21 patients with known coronary artery disease, dipyridamole perfusion images and cardiac catheterization were repeated approximately 18 months following risk factor interventions.[D11] Changes in PET perfusion defect severity followed the changes in stenosis severity by quantitative arteriography in most cases before and after the interventions.

Coronary Collaterals

Coronary collateral steal is defined as an absolute decrease in collateral-dependent myocardial perfusion following coronary arteriolar vasodilation.[S15] The conditions necessary for occurrence of collateral steal are controversial. The proposed mechanism is as follows: with vasodilation of distal coronary arteriolar beds, such as by dipyridamole, flow increases in the supply artery, causing pressure to fall at the origin of the collaterals. As a result, collateral perfusion pressure falls (Fig. 66–25). Because collateral channels do not appear to have normal vasoregulation,[H12] collateral flow depends primarily on this driving pressure at the arteriolar level of the supply artery. To the extent that collaterals supply a portion or all of resting perfusion to a given region, a corresponding degree of steal occurs in that bed with coronary arteriolar dilation. According to simulation analysis,[D4] the greater the collateral conductance, the greater the decrease in collateral perfusion with vasodilation. Hence, collateral steal may be recognized as a myocardial perfusion reserve of less than 1—that is, perfusion following vasodilation is less than resting perfusion; and the lower the myocardial perfusion reserve, the greater is the functional collateral conductance.

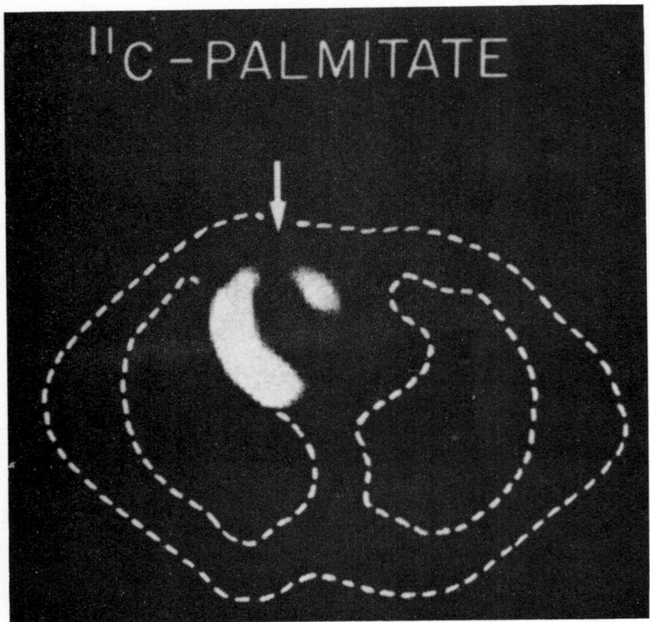

Figure 66–23. ^{11}C-palmitate tomogram from a patient with an anterior myocardial infarction. The characteristic horseshoe shape of the normal left ventricular PET image at this level is interrupted anteriorly by a transmural defect. The dashed lines surrounding the emission tomogram derived from the transmission image obtained at the identical level. (From Sobel, B.E., Weiss, E.S., Welch, M.J., et al.: Detection of remote myocardial infarction in patients with positron emission transaxial tomography and intravenous C-11 palmitate. Circulation 55:853, 1977, by permission of the American Heart Association, Inc.)

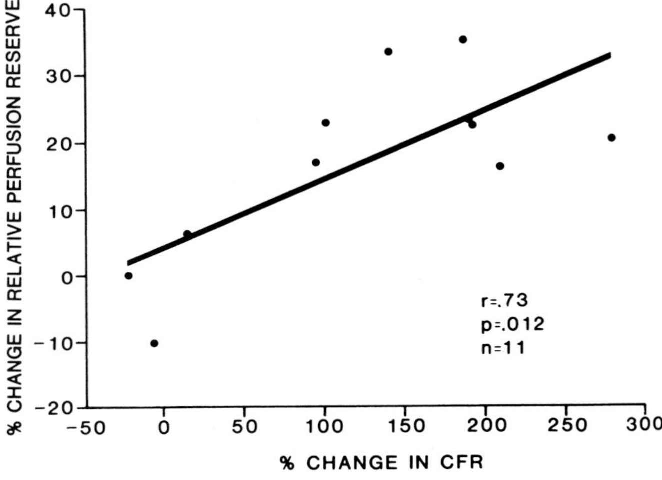

Figure 66–24. Relation between changes in angiographic coronary stenosis flow reserve and changes in relative myocardial perfusion reserve. (From Goldstein, R.A., Kirkeeide, R., Smalling, R.W., et al.: Changes in myocardial perfusion reserve after PTCA: Noninvasive assessment with positron tomography. J. Nucl. Med. 28:1262, 1987, with permission of The Society of Nuclear Medicine.)

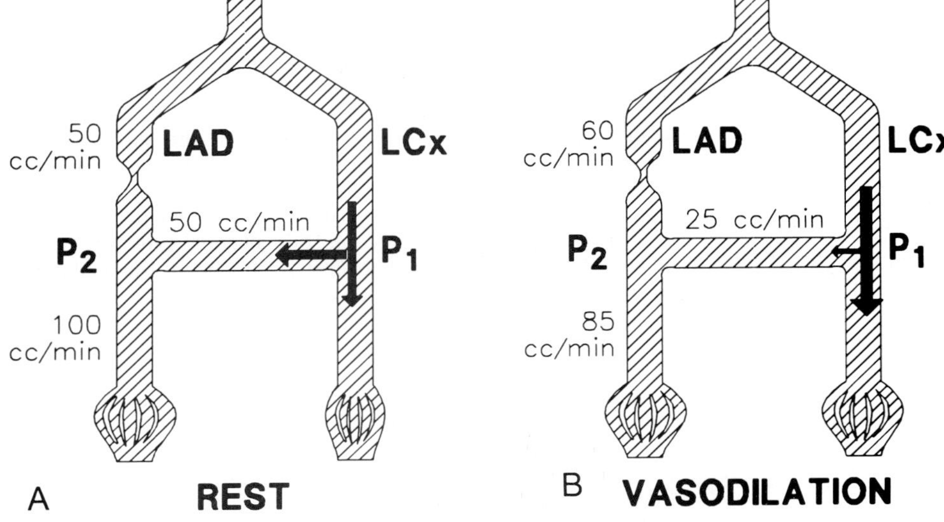

Figure 66–25. Hydraulic model illustrating possible mechanism of coronary steal. For this example, the LCx is the supply artery with the vascular distribution of the LAD being supplied by collaterals from the LCx coronary artery. P_1 is the perfusion pressure at the origin of the collaterals from distal circumflex branches. P_2 is the perfusion pressure of the vascular distribution of the LAD coronary artery, which is severely stenotic. In *A*, recipient bed vasodilates to maintain normal resting perfusion, thus expending its flow reserve. In *B*, with pharmacologic vasodilation, collateral driving pressure falls as LCx flow increases. (From Demer, L.L., Gould, K.L., and Kirkeeide, R.: Assessing stenosis severity: Coronary flow reserve, collateral function, quantitative coronary arteriography, positron imaging, and digital subtraction angiography: A review and analysis. Prog. Cardiovasc. Dis. 30:312, 1988, with permission.)

At present, there is no noninvasive method for assessing the functional significance of coronary collaterals in patients. During coronary arteriolar vasodilation, myocardial perfusion may decrease in areas of collateralization because of decreased driving pressure at the origin of the collaterals as a result of higher flows in the supply artery.[D4] Preliminary studies suggest that this phenomenon may be used to detect collateralization noninvasively by PET perfusion imaging with dipyridamole coronary vasodilation, by observation of a regional absolute decrease in flow following coronary vasodilation by intravenous dipyridamole.[D12, 13]

Other

PET perfusion imaging also has potential use in the noninvasive, serial evaluation of graft patency and myocardial salvage following coronary artery bypass surgery, medical therapy, rehabilitation, and other treatments for coronary artery disease. Perfusion imaging also may be useful for distinguishing cardiomyopathy and ischemic heart disease, described in chapters 67 and 68.

Summary

Technical aspects of positron emission tomographic imaging continue to improve. PET perfusion imaging is now entering the stage of routine clinical application. Quantitative assessment of tracer uptake is readily available, and measurement of absolute regional myocardial perfusion is imminent. Enormous clinical benefit may be derived from appropriate applications of positron emission tomography for noninvasive, quantitative characterization of blood supply to the heart.

References

B

1. Bergmann, S.R., Hack, S., Tewson, T., et al.: The dependence of accumulation of 13-NH_3 by myocardium on metabolic factors and its implications for quantitative assessment of perfusion. Circulation 61:34, 1980.
2. Bergmann, S.R., Fox, K.A.A., Rand, A.L., et al.: Quantification of regional myocardial blood flow in vivo with $H_2{}^{15}O$. Circulation 70:724, 1984.
3. Budinger, T.F., Yano, Y., and Hoop, B.: A comparison of 82Rb+ and $^{13}NH_3$ for myocardial positron scintigraphy. J. Nucl. Med. 16:429, 1975.
4. Budinger, T.F., Derenzo, S.E., Gullbert, G.T., et al.: Emission computer assisted tomography with single-photon and positron annihilation photons. J. Comput. Assist. Tomogr. 1:131, 1977.
5. Beatt, K.J., Luijten, H.E., DeFeyter, P.J., et al.: Change in diameter of coronary artery segments adjacent to stenosis after percutaneous transluminal coronary angioplasty: Failure of percent diameter stenosis measurement to reflect morphologic changes induced by balloon dilation. J. Am. Coll. Cardiol. 12:315, 1988.
6. Brown, B.G., Bolson, E., Frimer, M., and Dodge, H.T.: Quantitative coronary arteriography: Estimation of dimensions, hemodynamic resistance and atheroma mass of coronary artery lesions using the arteriogram and digital computation. Circulation 55:329, 1977.
7. Brunken, R., Tillisch, J., Schwaiger, M., et al.: Regional perfusion, glucose metabolism, and wall motion in patients with chronic electrocardiographic Q wave infarctions: Evidence for persistence of viable tissue in some infarct regions by positron emission tomography. Circulation 73:951, 1986.
8. Budinger, T.F., Yano, Y., Derenzo, S.E., et al.: Infarction sizing and myocardial perfusion measurements using rubidium-82 and positron emission tomography. (Abstract.) Am. J. Cardiol. 45:399, 1980.

C

1. Coyle, J.J., Josephson, M.A., Beyer, R.W., et al.: Comparison of rubidium-82 PET and thallium-201 SPECT for detection and localization of coronary artery disease. J. Nucl. Med. 29:817, 1988.
2. Chierchia, S., Lazzari, M., Freedman, B., et al.: Impairment of myocardial perfusion and function during painless myocardial ischemia. J. Am. Coll. Cardiol. 1:924, 1983.

D

1. Deanfield, J.E., Shea, M.J., Wilson, R.A., et al.: Direct effects of smoking on the heart: Silent ischemic disturbances of coronary flow. Am. J. Cardiol. 57:1005, 1986.
2. DeRouen, T.A., Murray, J.A., and Owen, W.: Variability in the analysis of coronary arteriograms. Circulation 52:979, 1977.
3. Detre, K.M., Wright, E., Murphy, M.L., and Takaro, T.: Observer agreement in evaluating coronary angiograms. Circulation 52:979, 1975.
4. Demer, L.L., Gould, K.L., and Kirkeeide, R.: Assessing stenosis severity: Coronary flow reserve collateral function, quantitative coronary arteriography, positron imaging, and digital subtraction angiography: A review and analysis. Prog. Cardiovasc. Dis. 30:307, 1988.
5. Demer, L.L., Gould, K.L., Goldstein, R.A., et al.: Diagnosis of coronary artery disease by positron emission tomography: Comparison to quantitative arteriography in 193 patients. Circulation 79 (4):825, 1989.
6. Demer, L.L., Gould, K.L., Goldstein, R.A., et al.: Diagnosis of coronary artery disease by positron imaging: Large scale clinical trial. J. Am. Coll. Cardiol. 11:11A, 1988.
7. Deanfield, J.E., Kensett, M., Wilson, R.A., et al.: Silent myocardial ischemia due to mental stress. Lancet 2: 1001, 1984.
8. Documenta Geigy: Scientific Tables (Diem, K. (ed.). 6th ed. Geigy Pharmaceuticals, Ardsley, N.Y., 1962, p. 88.
9. DePasquale, E.E., Nody, A.C., DePuey, E.G., et al.: Quantitative rotational thallium-201 tomography for identifying and localizing coronary artery disease. Circulation 77:316, 1988.
10. Deanfield, J.E., Shea, M., Ribiero, P., et al.: Transient ST segment depression as a marker of myocardial ischemia during daily life. Am. J. Cardiol. 54:1195, 1984.
11. Demer, L.L., Kirkeeide, R.L., Haynie, M.P., et al.: Feasibility of following progression/regression of coronary artery stenosis by positron emission tomography during dipyridamole–hand grip stress. Circulation 76:IV–4, 1988.
12. Demer, L.L., Gould, K.L., Goldstein, R.A., and Kirkeeide, R.L.: Noninvasive assessment of coronary collaterals in man by PET perfusion imaging. J. Nucl. Med. 31:259, 1990.
13. Demer, L.L., Gould, K.L., Goldstein, R.A., and Kirkeeide, R.L.: Identification of significant collateral function in patients with coronary artery disease by positron imaging. Circulation 74:II, 1986.

F

1. Fan, F.C., Schuessler, G.B., Chen, R.Y.Z., and Chien, S.: Determination of blood flood and shunting of 9- and 15-micron spheres in regional beds. Am. J. Physiol. 237:H25, 1979.

G

1. Goldstein, R.A., Mullani, N.A., Marani, S.K., et al.: Myocardial perfusion with rubidium-82. II. Effects of metabolic and pharmacologic interventions. J. Nucl. Med. 24:907, 1983.
2. Geltman, E.M., Smith, J.L., Beecher, D., et al.: Altered regional myocardial metabolism in congestive cardiomyopathy detected by positron tomography. Am. J. Med. 7:773, 1983.
3. Gould, K.L.: Percent coronary stenosis: Battered gold standard, pernicious relic, or clinical practicality? J. Am. Coll. Cardiol. 11:886, 1988.
4. Gould, K.L.: Assessment of coronary stenoses with myocardial perfusion imaging during pharmacologic vasodilation. IV. Limits of detection of stenosis with idealized experimental cross-sectional myocardial imaging. Am. J. Cardiol. 42:761, 1978.
5. Gould, K.L., Schelbert, H.R., Phelps, M.E., and Hoffman, E. J.: Noninvasive assessment of coronary stenoses with myocardial perfusion imaging during pharmacologic coronary vasodilation. V. Detection of 47 percent diameter coronary stenosis with intravenous 13-N ammonia and emission-computed tomography in intact dogs. Am. J. Cardiol. 43:200, 1979.
6. Gould, K.L., Goldstein, R.A., Mullani, N.A., et al.: Noninvasive assessment of coronary stenoses by myocardial perfusion imaging during pharmacologic coronary vasodilation. VIII. Clinical feasibility of positron cardiac imaging without a cyclotron using generator-produced rubidium-82. J. Am. Coll. Cardiol. 7:775, 1986.
7. Grover-McKay, M., Schelbert, H.R., Schwaiger, M., et al.: Identification of impaired metabolic reserve by atrial pacing in patients with significant coronary artery stenosis. Circulation 74:281, 1986.
8. Goldstein, R.A., Kirkeeide, R.L., Demer, L.L., et al.: Relation between geometric dimensions of coronary artery stenoses and myocardial perfusion reserve in man. J. Clin. Invest. 79:1473, 1987.
9. Goldstein, R.A.: Kinetics of rubidium-82 after coronary occlusion and reperfusion. Assessment of patency and viability in open-chest dog. J. Clin. Invest. 75:1131, 1985.
10. Goldstein, R.A., Mullani, N.A., Wong, W.H., et al.: Positron imaging of myocardial infarction with rubidium-82. J. Nucl. Med. 27:1824, 1986.
11. Goldstein, R.A., Kirkeeide, R., Smalling, R.W., et al.: Changes in myocardial perfusion reserve after PTCA: Noninvasive assessment with positron tomography. J. Nucl. Med. 28:1262, 1987.

H

1. Huang, S.C., Schwaiger, M., and Carson, R.E.: Noninvasive quantitation of myocardial blood flow by O-15 water and positron emission tomography. (Abstract.) J. Am. Coll. Cardiol. 1:578, 1983.
2. Homma, S., Gilliand, Y., Guiney, T.E., et al.: Safety of intravenous dipyridamole for stress testing with thallium imaging. Am. J. Cardiol. 59: 152, 1987.
3. Hoffman, J.I.E.: A critical view of coronary reserve. Circulation 75:1, 1987.
4. Hamilton, G.W., Trobaugh, G.B., Ritchie, J.L., et al.: Myocardial imaging with intravenously injected thallium-201 in patients with suspected coronary artery disease: Analysis of technique and correlation with electrocardiographic coronary anatomic and ventriculographic findings. Am. J. Cardiol. 39:347, 1977.
5. Hlatky, M.A., Mark, D.B., Harrell, F.E., et al.: Rethinking sensitivity and specificity. Am. J. Cardiol. 59:1195, 1987.
6. Henze, E., Huang, S.C., Ratib, O., et al.: Measurement of regional tissue and

blood radiotracer concentrations from serial tomographic images of the heart. J. Nucl. Med. 24:987, 1983.

7. Huang, S.C., Williams, B.A., Krivokapich, J., et al.: Rapid myocardial Rb-82 kinetics and a compartmental model for blood flow estimation. Heart Circ. Physiol. 25:H1156, 1989.
8. Huang, S.C., Schwaiger, M., Carson, R.E., et al.: Noninvasive quantitation of myocardial blood flow by O-15 water and positron emission tomography. (Abstract.) J. Am. Coll. Cardiol. 1:578, 1983.
9. Huang, S.C., Schwaiger, M., Carson, R.E., et al.: Quantitative measurement of myocardial blood flow with oxygen-15 water and positron computed tomography: An assessment of potential and problems. J. Nucl. Med. 26:616, 1985.
10. Harper, P.V., Schwartz, J., Beck, R.N., et al.: Clinical myocardial imaging with N-13 ammonia. Radiology 108:613, 1973.
11. Hoop, B., Jr., Smith, T.W., Burnham, C.A., et al.: Myocardial imaging with $13NH^{+}_{4}$ and a multicrystal positron camera. J. Nucl. Med. 14:181, 1973.
12. Harrison, D.G., Chilian, W.M., and Marcus, M.L.: Absence of functioning alpha adrenergic receptors in mature canine coronary collaterals. Circ. Res. 59:133, 1986.

I

1. Iida, H., Kanno, I., Takahashi, A., et al.: Measurement of absolute myocardial blood flow with $H_2{}^{15}O$ and dynamic positron emission tomography. Strategy for quantification in relation to the partial-volume effect. Circulation 78:104–115, 1988.

K

1. Krivokapich, J., Huang, S.C., Phelps, M.E., et al.: Dependence of $13\text{-}NH_3$ myocardial extraction and clearance on flow and metabolism. Am. J. Physiol. 242:H536, 1982.
2. Krivokapich, J., Huang, S.C., Hoffman, E.J., et al.: N-13 glutamate as a tracer of blood flow at rest and with exercise in human myocardium. Circulation 76:(Suppl. IV): IV–4, 1987.
3. Knoebel, S.B., Lowe, D.K., Lovelace, D.E., and Friedman, J.J.: Myocardial blood flow as measured by fractional uptake of rubidium-84 and microspheres. J. Nucl. Med. 19:1020, 1978.
4. Kearfot, K.J.: Radiation absorbed dose estimates for positron emission tomography (PET): K-38, Rb-81, Rb-82, and Cs-130. J. Nucl. Med. 23:1128, 1982
5. Kirkeeide, R.L., Buchi, M., Demer, L.L., and Gould, K.L.: Afterload affects flow reserve of stenotic coronary arteries. Circulation 76(Suppl. IV):IV–386, 1987.
6. Kirkeeide, R.L., Gould, K.L., and Parsel, L: Assessment of coronary stenoses by myocardial perfusion imaging during pharmacologic coronary vasodilation. VII. Validation of coronary flow reserve as a single integrated functional measure of stenosis severity reflecting all its geometric dimensions. J. Am. Coll. Cardiol. 7:103, 1986.
7. Kambara, H., Nohara, R., Kawsai, C., et al.: 201-Thallium myocardial scintigraphy and $13N\text{-}NH_3$ positron computed tomography in evaluating myocardial blood flow. J. Cardiogr. 16:519, 1986.
8. Klocke, F.J.: Measurements of coronary flow reserve: Defining pathophysiology versus making decisions about patient care. Circulation 76:1183, 1987.
9. Kannel, W.B., and Abbott, R.D.: Incidence of unrecognized myocardial infarction. An update on the Framingham study. N. Engl. J. Med. 311:1144, 1984.
10. Kety, S.S.: Measurement of local blood flow by the exchange of an inert, diffusible substance. Meth. Med. Res. 8:228, 1960.
11. Kety, S.S.: Measurement of regional circulation by the local clearance of radioactive sodium. Am. Heart J. 38:321, 1949.

L

1. Lockwood, A.H.: Absorbed doses of radiation after an intravenous injection of N-13 ammonia in man: Concise communication. J. Nucl. Med. 21:276, 1980.
2. Love, W.D., and Burch, G.E.: Influence of rate of coronary plasma flow on the extraction of Rb-86 from coronary blood. Clin. Res. 6:211, 1958.

M

1. Marcus, M.L., Skorton, D.J., Johnson, M.R., et al.: Visual estimates of percent diameter coronary stenosis: "A battered gold standard." J. Am. Coll. Cardiol. 11:882, 1988.
2. Marcus, M.L., Armstrong, M.L., Heistad, D.D., et al.: Comparison of three methods of evaluating coronary obstructive lesions: Postmortem arteriography, pathologic examination and measurement of regional myocardial perfusion during maximal vasodilation. Am. J. Cardiol. 49:1699, 1982.
3. Mates, R.E., Gupta, R.L., Bell, A.C., and Klocke, F.: Fluid dynamics of coronary artery stenosis. Circ. Res. 42:152, 1978.
4. Mullani, N.A., and Gould, K.L.: First-pass measurements of regional blood flow with external detectors. J. Nucl. Med. 24:577, 1983.

N

1. Nabel, E.G., Rocco, M.B., and Selwyn, A.P.: Characteristics and significance of ischemia detected by ambulatory electrocardiographic monitoring. Circulation 75 (Suppl. IV):V–74, 1987.

O

1. Olofsson, B.-O., Bjerle, P., Aberg, T., et al.: Prevalence of coronary artery disease in patients with valvular heart disease. Acta Med. Scand. 218:365, 1985.
2. Ornish, D.M., Scherwitz, L.W., Brown, S.E., et al.: Can lifestyle changes reverse atherosclerosis? Circulation 78:11, 1988.

P

1. Parodi, O., Schelbert, H.R., Schwaiger, M., et al.: Cardiac emission computed tomography: Underestimation of regional tracer concentrations due to wall motion abnormalities. J. Comput. Assist. Tomogr. 8:1083, 1984.

R

1. Rossen, J.D., Simonetti, I., Marcus, M.L., and Winniford, M.D.: Coronary dilation with standard dose dipyridamole combined with handgrip. Circulation 79:566, 1989.
2. Ritchie, J.L., Zaret, B.L., Strauss, H.W., et al.: Myocardial imaging with thallium-201: A multicenter study in patients with angina pectoris or acute myocardial infarction. Am. J. Cardiol. 42:345, 1978.
3. Ritchie, J.L., Trobaugh, G.B., Hamilton, G.W., et al.: Myocardial imaging with thallium-201 at rest and during exercise: Comparison with coronary angiography and resting and stress electrocardiography. Circulation 56:66, 1977.
4. Reunanen, A., Aromaa, A., Pyorala, K., et al.: The Social Insurance Institution's coronary heart disease study: Baseline data and 5-year mortality experience. Acta Med. Scand. (Suppl.)673:67, 1983.

S

1. Schelbert, H.R., Phelps, M.E., Huang, S.C., et al.: N-13 ammonia as an indicator of myocardial blood flow. Circulation 63:1259, 1981.
2. Schelbert, H. R., Phelps, M.E., Hoffman, E., et al.: Regional myocardial perfusion assessed with N-13 labeled ammonia and positron emission computerized axial tomography. Am. J. Cardiol. 43:209, 1979.
3. Schelbert, H.R.: Regional myocardial perfusion assessed with N-13 labeled ammonia and positron emission computerized axial tomography. Am. J. Cardiol. 45:39, 1980.
4. Schwaiger, M., Krivokapich, J., Ratib, O., et al.: Noninvasive quantification of coronary reserve by N-13 ammonia and positron emission tomography (PET). J. Am. Coll. Cardiol. 11:11A, 1988.
5. Schelbert, H.R., Wisenberg, G., Phelps, M.E., et al.: Non-invasive assessment of coronary stenoses by myocardial imaging during pharmacologic coronary vasodilation. VI. Detection of coronary artery disease in man with intravenous $13\text{-}NH_3$ and positron computed tomography. Am. J. Cardiol. 49:1197, 1982.
6. Selwyn, A.P., Allan, R.M., L'Abbate, A., et al.: Relation between regional myocardial uptake of Rb-82 and perfusion: Absolute reduction of cation uptake in ischemia. Am. J. Cardiol. 50:112, 1982.
7. Schwartz, R.S., Jackson, W.G., Celio, P.V., and Hickman, J.R.: Exercise thallium-201 scintigraphy for detecting coronary artery disease in asymptomatic young men. J. Am. Coll. Cardiol. 11:80A, 1988.
8. Shea, M.J., Wilson, R.A., deLandsheere, C.M., et al.: Use of short- and long-lived rubidium tracers for the study of transient ischemia. J. Nucl. Med. 28:989, 1987.
9. Sapirstein, L.A.: Fractionation of the cardiac output of rats with isotopic potassium. Circ. Res. 4:689, 1956.
10. Selwyn, A.P., Shea, M., Deanfield, J., et al.: The character of transient myocardial ischemia: Clinical studies and progress using positron emission tomography. Int. J. Card. Imag. 1:61, 1985.
11. Selwyn, A. P., Shea, M.J., Deanfield, J.E., et al.: Clinical problems in coronary disease are caused by wide variety of ischemic episodes that affect patients out of hospital. Am. J. Med. 79(3A):12, 1985.
12. Sobel, B.E., Bresnahan, G.F., Shell, W.E., and Yoder, R.D.: Estimation of infarct size in man and its relation to prognosis. Circulation 46:640, 1972.
13. Sobel, B.E., Geltman, E.M., Tiffenbrunn, A.J., et al.: Improvement of regional myocardial metabolism after coronary thrombolysis induced with tissue-type plasminogen activator or streptokinase. Circulation 69:983, 1984.
14. Sobel, B.E., Weiss, E.S., Welch, E.S., Welch, M.J., et al.: Detection of remote myocardial infarction in patients with positron emission transaxial tomography and intravenous C-11 palmitate. Circulation 55:853, 1977.
15. Schaper, W., Lewi, P., Flameng, W., and Gijpen, L.: Myocardial steal produced by coronary vasodilation in chronic coronary artery occlusion. Basic Res. Cardiol. 68:3, 1973.

T

1. Tamaki, N., Yonekura, Y., Senda, M., et al.: Myocardial positron computed tomography with N-13-ammonia at rest and during exercise. Eur. J. Nucl. Med. 11:246, 1985.
2. Tamaki, N., Yonekura, Y., Senda, M., et al.: Value and limitation of stress T1-201 tomography. Comparison with perfusion and metabolic imaging with positron tomography. Circulation 76(Suppl. IV):IV–4, 1987.
3. Tamaki, N., Yonekura, Y., Senda, M., et al.: Value and limitation of stress thallium-201 single photon emission computed tomography: Comparison with nitrogen-13 ammonia positron tomography. J. Nucl. Med. 29:1181, 1988.
4. Ter-Pogossian, M.M., Klein, M.S., Markham, J., et al.: Regional assessment of myocardial metabolic integrity in vivo by positron emission tomography with ^{11}C-labeled palmitate. Circulation 61:242, 1980.

V

1. Vogel, R., LeFree, M., Bates, E., et al.: Application of digital techniques to selective coronary arteriography: Use of myocardial contrast appearance time to measure coronary flow reserve. Am. Heart J. 107:153, 1984.
2. Van Train, K.F., Berman, D.S., Garcia, E.V., et al.: Quantitative analysis of stress thallium-201 myocardial scintigrams: A multicenter trial. J. Nucl. Med. 27:17, 1986.

W

1. Walsh, M.N., Bergmann, S.R., Baird, T.R., et al.: Improved myocardial perfusion after angioplasty delineated by positron emission tomography and $H2^{15}O$. Circulation 76:IV–401, 1987.
2. White, C.W., Wright, C.B., Doty, D.B., et al.: Does visual interpretation of the coronary arteriogram predict the physiologic importance of a coronary stenosis? N. Engl. J. Med. 310:819, 1984.
3. Wilson, R.F., Laughlin, D.E., Ackell, P.H., et al.: Transluminal, subselective measurement of coronary artery blood flow velocity and vasodilator reserve in man. Circulation 72:82, 1985.
4. Wisenberg, G., Schelbert, H.R., Hoffman, E.J., et al.: In vivo quantitation of regional myocardial blood flow by positron emission computed tomography. Circulation 63:1248, 1981.
5. Walsh, W.F., Harper, P.V., Resnekov, L., and Fill, H.: Noninvasive evaluation of regional myocardial perfusion in 112 patients using a mobile scintillation camera and intravenous nitrogen-13 labeled ammonia. Circulation 54:226, 1976.
6. Walsh, W.F., Fill, H.R., and Harper, P.V.: Nitrogen-13 labeled ammonia for myocardial imaging. Semin. Nucl. Med. 7:59, 1977.
7. Weiss, E.S., Ahmed, S.A., Welch, M.J., et al.: Quantification of infarction in cross-sections of canine myocardium in vitro with positron emission transaxial tomography and C-11 palmitate. Circulation 55:66, 1977.
8. Walsh, M.N., Bergmann, S.R., Steele, R.L., et al.: Delineation of impaired regional myocardial perfusion by positron emission tomography with $H_2{}^{15}O$. Circulation 78:612, 1988.

Y

1. Yano, Y., Cahoon, J.L., and Budinger, T.F.: A precision flow-controlled Rb-82 generator for bolus or constant-infusion studies of the heart and brain. J. Nucl. Med. 22:1006, 1981.
2. Yonekura, Y., Tamaki, N., Senda, M., et al. Detection of coronary artery disease with 13-N-ammonia and high resolution positron emission computed tomography. Am. Heart J. 113:645, 1987.

Z

1. Zir, L.M., Miller, S.W., Dinsmore R.E., et al.: Interobserver variability in coronary angiography. Circulation 53:627, 1976.
2. Zijlstra, F., Fioretti, P., Reiber, J.H.C., and Serruys, P.W.: Which cineangiographically assessed anatomic variable correlates best with functional measurements of stenosis severity? A comparison of quantitative analysis of the coronary cineangiogram with measured coronary flow reserve and exercise/redistribution thallium-201 scintigraphy. J. Am. Coll. Cardiol. 12:686, 1988.
3. Zierler, K.L.: Equations for measuring blood flow by external monitoring of radioisotopes. Circ. Res. 16:309, 1965.

Chapter 67

Evaluation of Myocardial Substrate Metabolism in Ischemic Heart Disease

RICHARD C. BRUNKEN, M.D. ▪ HEINRICH R. SCHELBERT, M.D.

ACUTE MYOCARDIAL ISCHEMIA 1191
Experimental Basis for Metabolic Studies 1191
Evaluation of Fatty Acid Metabolism with Carbon-11 Palmitate 1191
Evaluation of Oxidative Metabolism With Carbon-11 Acetate 1195
Evaluation of Glucose Metabolism with Fluorine-18 2-Fluoro 2-Deoxyglucose 1197
Synopsis 1198
Clinical Investigations with Tracers of Metabolism 1198
Studies with Carbon-11 Palmitate for Fatty Acid Metabolism 1198
Studies with Carbon-11 Acetate for Oxidative Metabolism 1199
Studies with Fluorine-18 2-Fluoro 2-Deoxyglucose for Alterations in Exogenous Glucose Utilization 1200
Synopsis 1203
ACUTE MYOCARDIAL INFARCTION AND REPERFUSION 1203
Experimental Basis for Metabolic Studies 1203
Evaluation of Fatty Acid Metabolism 1203
Evaluation of Oxidative Metabolism 1207
Evaluation of Glucose Metabolism 1209
Synopsis 1214
Clinical Investigations 1214
Metabolic Characterization of Acutely Infarcted Myocardium 1214
Relationship Between Electrocardiographic Changes and Metabolic Abnormalities 1217
Relationship Between Coronary Anatomy and Metabolic Findings 1218
Effects of Coronary Thrombolysis and Revascularization 1218
Synopsis 1219
METABOLIC ACTIVITY AS A CLINICAL INDICATOR OF TISSUE VIABILITY 1219
Effect of Revascularization on Hypoperfused, Metabolically Active Tissue 1222
Identification of Myocardial Viability 1222
Recovery of Blood Flow, Metabolism, and Contractile Function After Revascularization 1223
Synopsis 1225
Relationship Between Myocardial Metabolic Activity and Other Diagnostic Tests for Determination of Tissue Viability 1225
Electrocardiography 1225
Regional Myocardial Wall Motion 1227
Thallium-201 Redistribution Scintigraphy 1229
Synopsis 1231
Chronic Myocardial Ischemia and Infarction .. 1231
Chronic Myocardial Ischemia 1234
Chronic Myocardial Infarction 1234
Synopsis 1234
MYOCARDIAL METABOLIC IMAGING IN CLINICAL PRACTICE 1237
Indications for Metabolic Imaging 1237
Patient Care During Metabolic Imaging 1238
Standardization of Study Conditions 1239
Clinical Decision Making With Metabolic Imaging 1239
SUMMARY AND CONCLUSIONS 1240

Positron emission tomography with radiotracers of metabolic pathways enables evaluation and quantification of the fundamental biochemical abnormalities characteristic of myocardial ischemia in vivo. Assessment of both oxidative and anaerobic metabolism provides insights into the pathophysiology of myocardial ischemia and infarction and yields clinically useful information about the functional state of the myocardium. The tissue characterization provided by metabolic imaging with positron emission tomography predicts recovery from an ischemic insult more reliably than the assessment of blood flow alone and can be utilized to distinguish viable but functionally compromised tissue from the fibrosis of completed infarction. This chapter describes how positron emission tomography with tracers of blood flow and metabolism can demonstrate noninvasively the metabolic sequelae of human myocardial ischemia. It illustrates how metabolic imaging is used for disease characterization and further describes how this information contributes to the clinical decision-making process. The chapter begins with a description of the metabolic disturbances characteristic of acute myocardial ischemia, reviews the alterations in tissue metabolism observed in acute myocardial infarction, and proceeds to a summary of the biochemical perturbations characteristic of chronic coronary artery disease. It then compares the relative merits of metabolic imaging for the assess-

This work was supported in part by the Director of the Office of Energy Research, Office of Health and Environmental Research, Washington, D.C., by Grants #HL 29845 and #HL 33177 from the National Institutes of Health, Bethesda, Md., and by an Investigative Group Award from the Greater Los Angeles Affiliate of the American Heart Association, Los Angeles, Ca. Dr. Brunken is the recipient of a Clinical Investigator Award (#HL 02022–02) from the National Institutes of Health, Bethesda, Md.

ment of myocardial viability to those of routinely performed clinical tests. In each section, a review of observations in animal experimental studies precedes the description of the metabolic findings in human ischemic heart disease.

ACUTE MYOCARDIAL ISCHEMIA

Both the severity and the anatomic extent of the disturbances in myocardial metabolism resulting from an acute episode of ischemia depend upon the degree of blood flow reduction and the duration of the ischemic insult.[R1] Since experimental studies designed to assess the metabolic effects of acute ischemia frequently employ blood flow reductions of varying severity and duration, laboratory observations must be extrapolated with caution to acute human myocardial ischemia. However, because positron emission tomography is noninvasive, it is possible to utilize this technique to characterize and quantify the metabolic consequences of acute myocardial ischemia, both in experimental preparations and in patients with coronary artery disease.

Experimental Basis for Metabolic Studies

The myocardium utilizes a variety of substrates for energy production. Under normoxic conditions, it preferentially oxidizes free fatty acids over carbohydrates. Oxidation of free fatty acids accounts for about 60 to 70 percent of total myocardial oxygen consumption.[L1] Acute reductions in blood flow limit the availability of oxygen to the myocardium, thereby interfering with mitochondrial respiration and substrate oxidation.[L1, O1, O2] Ischemia not only depresses mitochrondrial β-oxidation of fatty acids but it also reduces uptake, cytosolic activation, and transmitochondrial transport of fatty acids.[L1] Because oxygen deprivation impairs fatty acid oxidation at several points in its biochemical pathway, acute ischemia may affect the tissue kinetics of a labeled fatty acid such as carbon-11 palmitate to a greater degree than the kinetics of carbon-11 acetate, a "pure" tracer of oxidative flux through the tricarboxylic acid cycle (see Chapters 4 and 65). As such, use of carbon-11 palmitate for metabolic imaging may prove more sensitive for detecting perturbations of intermediary metabolism in acute ischemia than carbon-11 acetate, even though the kinetics of the labeled fatty acid may reflect changes in regional oxidative substrate flux less directly than the kinetics of carbon-11 acetate.

Evaluation of Fatty Acid Metabolism with Carbon-11 Palmitate

In open-chest dog experiments, Lerch and associates analyzed the effects of 15 minutes of ischemia and hypoxia on the regional monoexponential myocardial clearance of carbon-11 palmitate.[L2] Myocardial ischemia was acutely induced in seven dogs by reducing blood flow in the left anterior descending coronary artery to 30 percent of normal. In a second group of seven animals, hypoxia was induced by perfusing the vessel with venous blood (PO_2 = 29.6 ± 2.4 mmHg) at a normal flow rate. Regional myocardial blood flow was determined from the washout rates of oxygen-15-labeled water. Regional myocardial tracer activity concentrations were measured with an external beta-probe. In the animals with myocardial hypoxia, blood flows in risk myocardium were unchanged from control values (1.16 ± 0.11 versus 1.43 ± 0.19 ml/min/g, P = NS), whereas blood flows in the ischemic group were reduced by an average of 64 percent (0.46 ± 0.09 versus 1.26 ± 0.23 ml/min/g, $P < 0.025$). Compared with control values, regional monoexponential carbon-11 palmitate clearance constants were reduced by 61 percent in the ischemia group (0.041 ± 0.013 versus 0.106 ± 0.014 min^{-1}, $P < 0.005$) and by 52 percent in the hypoxia group (0.047 ± 0.007 versus 0.098 ± 0.017 min^{-1}, $P < 0.02$). These data indicate that the impaired myocardial clearance of carbon-11 palmitate observed during oxygen deprivation reflects impaired fatty acid metabolism, rather than accumulation of label due to delayed washout of carbon-11-labeled metabolites.

Lerch and associates also employed serial positron emission tomographic imaging to determine monoexponential carbon-11 palmitate clearance rate constants in eight dogs with experimental stenoses of the circumflex coronary artery.[L3] In seven control dogs, positron tomographic imaging demonstrated homogeneous regional clearance of carbon-11 palmitate at rest (k = 0.060 ± 0.005 min^{-1}) and during more rapid heart rates induced by the administration of atropine (k = 0.070 ± 0.006 min^{-1}). Similar findings were observed in three animals with circumflex stenoses of less than 70 percent; carbon-11 clearance constants in risk myocardium did not differ significantly from those in normal myocardium, either at rest or with rapid atrial pacing. In contrast, five animals with greater than 70 percent circumflex stenoses had significantly lower carbon-11 palmitate clearance rate constants in the risk zone, both at rest (0.044 ± 0.011 versus 0.064 ± 0.011 min^{-1}, $P < 0.025$) and with rapid atrial pacing (0.044 ± 0.009 versus 0.073 ± 0.011 min^{-1}, $P < 0.025$). Thus sequential positron tomographic imaging with carbon-11 palmitate demonstrated impaired fatty acid oxidation in regions perfused by vessels with greater than 70 percent stenoses both at rest and with atrial pacing, reflecting inadequate myocardial delivery of oxygen under resting conditions and impaired tissue oxidative metabolic reserve.

Schön and colleagues also examined the effects of ischemia on the regional myocardial clearance of carbon-11 palmitate but injected the tracer directly into the coronary artery.[S1] They recorded the tissue carbon-11 time activity curves for a longer period of time in order to determine the effects of ischemia on the relationship between the rapid and slow clearance phases of the tissue clearance curve. Myocardial ischemia prolonged the half-time of the rapid clearance phase (from 3.5 to 10.3 min compared with 3.4 ± 0.7 min in normal myocardium[S2]). It is important to note that the relative size of the rapid clearance curve component declined in proportion to the decrease in oxygen consumption, whereas the ratio of the relative size of the slow-to-rapid clearance phase increased (Fig. 67–1). These observations indicate that the fraction of fatty acid that enters the endogenous lipid pool increases commensurate with the severity of ischemia, consistent with histopathologic reports demonstrating an increase in intracellular lipid content in acutely ischemic myocardium.[G1, S3, S4, V1]

The release of carbon-11 label from myocardium into coronary sinus effluent was also examined by these investigators.[S1] They noted that the rate of carbon-11 carbon dioxide release was directly proportional to myocardial oxygen consumption, decreasing as oxygen consumption declined. In addition, the fraction of carbon-11 label released from myocardium as carbon-11 carbon dioxide decreased as a function of oxygen consumption. Thus with more severe ischemia a disproportionately greater fraction of carbon-11 activity is released from myocardium in the form of nonmetabolized carbon-11 palmitate, an enhanced "back-diffusion" of label from tissue into the vascular space.

Subsequent studies by Fox and by Rosamond and their coworkers[F1, R2] confirmed the enhanced back-diffusion of nonmetabolized carbon-11 palmitate during ischemia. Fox and coworkers determined the myocardial extraction and clearance of carbon-11 palmitate in 21 open-chest dogs under normoxic, hypoxic (30 minutes), and ischemic (30 minutes) conditions.[F1] Following intracoronary tracer administration, myocardial tissue activity curves were monitored with a beta-probe, while efflux of nonmetabolized carbon-11 palmitate was determined by analysis of arterial and regional coronary venous blood. At baseline, 45.2 ± 3.8 percent of the initially extracted carbon-11 palmitate was oxidized during the first 20 minutes to carbon-11 carbon dioxide, while 6.2 ± 2.6 percent diffused back into the vascular space. During ischemia, however, when blood flow was decreased to 26 percent of normal, only 16.9 ± 9.8 percent of the extracted carbon-11 palmitate was recovered in the form of carbon-11 carbon dioxide ($P < 0.001$, compared with baseline), while the fraction of nonmetabolized carbon-11 palmitate increased to 15.6 ± 8.9 percent ($P < 0.05$). Virtually identical results were observed during myocardial hypoxia. Of the initially extracted carbon-11 palmitate, 15.1 ± 8.4 percent was released in the form of carbon-11 carbon dioxide, while 18.8 ± 11.7 percent

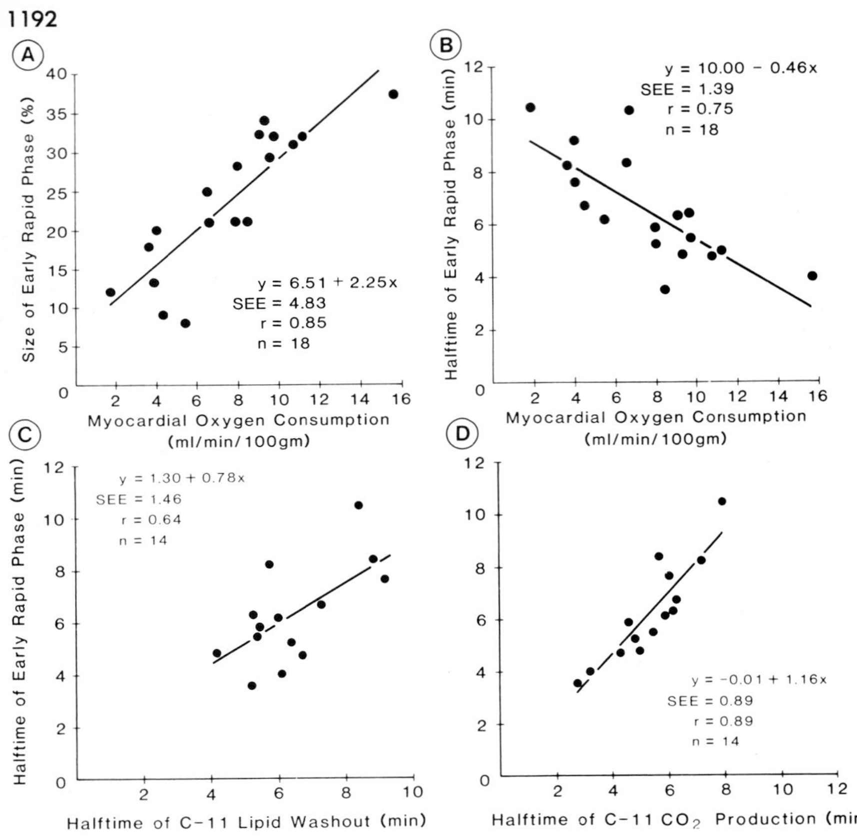

Figure 67–1. *Panel A,* Relationship between the size of the early rapid phase of the myocardial ^{11}C time activity curve and regional myocardial oxygen consumption in ischemic canine myocardium following the intra-arterial administration of ^{11}C-palmitate. *Panels B, C,* and *D:* Relationship between the half-times of the early rapid phase and regional myocardial oxygen consumption, half-time of ^{11}C-lipid washout, and half-time of ^{11}C-CO_2 production, respectively. (From Schön, H.R., Schelbert, H.R., Najafi, A., et al.: C-11 labeled palmitic acid for the noninvasive evaluation of regional myocardial fatty acid metabolism with positron computed tomography. II. Kinetics of C-11 palmitic acid in acutely ischemic myocardium. Am. Heart J. 103:548–561, 1982, with permission.)

diffused back into the vascular space. Thus, these observations indicate that back-diffusion of carbon-11 palmitate increases significantly during periods of hypoxia or ischemia and that this loss of nonmetabolized carbon-11 palmitate from myocardium might limit the value of the rapid clearance phase as an accurate quantitative measure of fatty acid oxidation.

Rosamond and associates performed studies in open-chest dogs subjected to 30 minutes of circumflex artery ischemia.[R2] They also observed an increase in the relative amount of nonmetabolized carbon-11 palmitate that diffused back into the vascular space in ischemic myocardium. Compared with 16.1 percent in normal myocardium, it increased to 44.4 percent in ischemic myocardium. Biochemical assays of tissue biopsies indicated that the relative fraction of the carbon-11 label incorporated into triglycerides, diglycerides, and nonesterified fatty acid progressively increased during the 30-minute period of ischemia. Deposition of carbon-11 label in the form of glycerides and phospholipids was significantly higher than in control myocardium.

To determine whether an acute increase in ventricular workload relative to oxygen delivery would similarly impair myocardial oxidative substrate metabolism, Schelbert and associates performed sequential carbon-11 palmitate positron tomographic imaging during rapid atrial pacing in nine open-chest dogs with partial occlusions of the left anterior descending artery (Fig. 67–2).[S5] With atrial pacing at 220 beats/min, there was no change in blood flow in risk myocardium (0.70 ± 0.22 versus 0.83 ± 0.37 ml/min/g, P = NS), whereas that in control myocardium rose from 0.83 ± 0.29 to 1.82 ± 0.14 ml/min/g ($P < 0.03$). During atrial pacing, the relative size of the early phase of the carbon-11 time-activity curve from myocardium in the ischemic risk zone was 45.5 percent smaller than that in normal myocardium. Conversely, the relative size of the slow phase was 35.7 percent higher than in normal tissue (Fig. 67–3). Furthermore, carbon-11 clearance half-times in ischemic myocardium were significantly longer than those of control myocardium (7.2 ± 2.4 versus 2.2 ± 0.5 min, $P < 0.05$), whereas peak myocardial carbon-11 palmitate uptake was linearly related to regional blood flow. In addition, the extraction fraction of carbon-11 palmitate was moderately but significantly lower in ischemic tissue than in control myocardium (0.38 ± 0.16 versus 0.47 ± 0.25, $P < 0.05$). Thus, these data indicate that acute demand-induced ischemia affects myocardial fatty acid metabolism in a manner similar to that of ischemia resulting from acute reductions in blood flow: there is a decline in the fraction of fatty acid directed into oxidative pathways, impaired oxidation of the fatty acid that enters oxidative pathways, and a greater incorporation of labeled fatty acid into the endogenous lipid pool.

The changes in fatty acid metabolism in ischemic myocardium identified with positron emission tomography and carbon-11 palmitate were correlated with ultrastructural abnormalities on electron microscopy by Schwaiger and colleagues.[S4] Regional myocardial ischemia was induced in closed-chest dogs by balloon occlusion of the left anterior descending artery. In nine animals, positron tomographic imaging with nitrogen-13 ammonia and carbon-11 palmitate was performed, while in an additional eleven animals the findings on electron microscopy were correlated with microsphere blood flow measurements. In this model of acute ischemia, the investigators identified a central ischemic zone and a second "border" zone surrounding the central ischemic zone (Fig. 67–4). The central ischemic zone was characterized by a marked reduction in blood flow (0.14 ± 0.14 ml/min/g) and depressed uptake (36.2 ± 11.4 percent) and delayed clearance (half-time = 45.5 ± 3.9 min) of carbon-11 palmitate. Changes characteristic of myocardial necrosis, such as cellular swelling and sarcolemmal bleb formation, widened I bands, glycogen depletion, and swollen and disrupted mitochondria containing amorphous matrix densities, were observed on electron microscopy (Fig. 67–5). In contrast, the border zone surrounding the central ischemic zone was characterized by a modest blood flow reduction (0.49 ± 0.18 ml/min/g), by mildly depressed uptake (80.0 ± 11.5 percent) and delayed clearance (half-time = 19.4 ± 8.1 min) of carbon-11 palmitate, and by an increase in intracellular small lipid droplets as the only morphologic abnormality on electron microscopy (Fig. 67–5). Thus, these investigators reported that functional abnormalities of fatty acid oxidation can be identified in ischemic myocardium without ultrastructural evidence of irreversible damage, indicating that disturbances in oxidative substrate metabolism can be detected and characterized on positron tomographic imaging with carbon-11 palmitate prior to the onset of irreversible cellular injury.

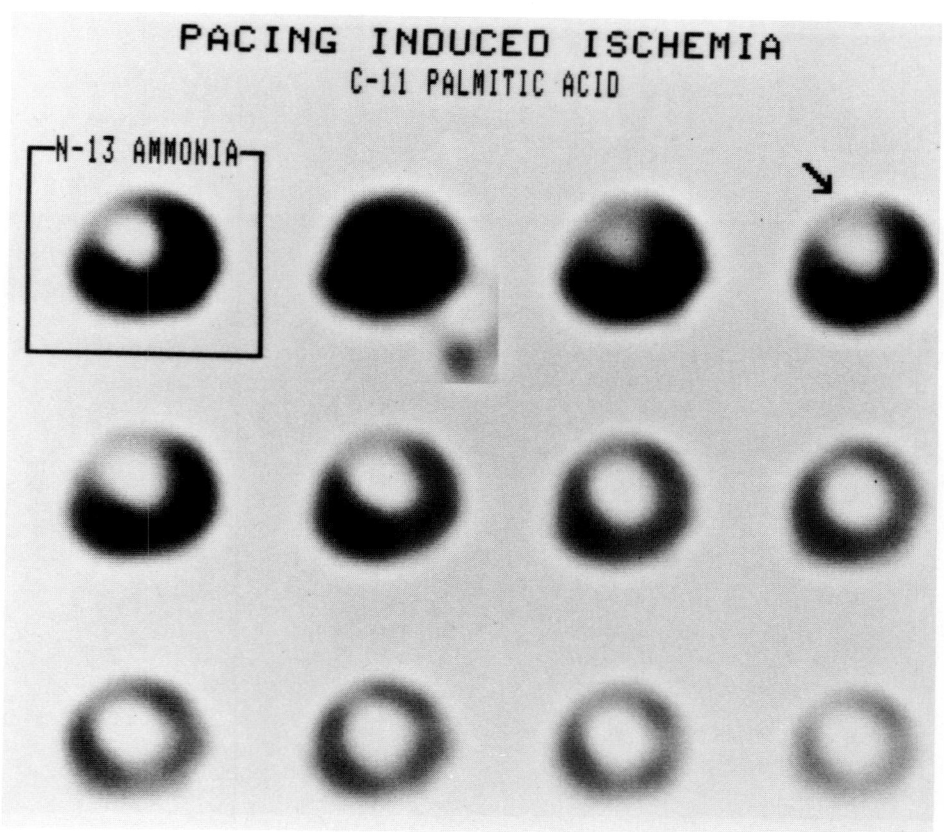

Figure 67–2. Serial cross-sectional positron emission tomographic images of the heart obtained following the intravenous administration of ^{11}C-palmitate during pacing-induced ischemia in a canine experiment. The relative distribution of regional blood flow during pacing is indicated by the [^{13}N]ammonia image in the upper left hand corner of the figure. Over the 32-minute ^{11}C-palmitate study, there is relatively homogeneous clearance of ^{11}C activity from the normally perfused lateral and inferior ventricular regions. In contrast, the decline in ^{11}C activity in the hypoperfused anterior region is slower than that of normal tissue (*arrow*), resulting in near normalization of relative myocardial ^{11}C activities on the latter images. (From Schelbert, H.R., Henze, E., Keen, R., et al.: C–11 palmitate for the noninvasive evaluation of regional myocardial fatty acid metabolism with positron computed tomography. IV. In vivo evaluation of acute demand induced ischemia in dogs. Am Heart J 106:736–750, 1983.)

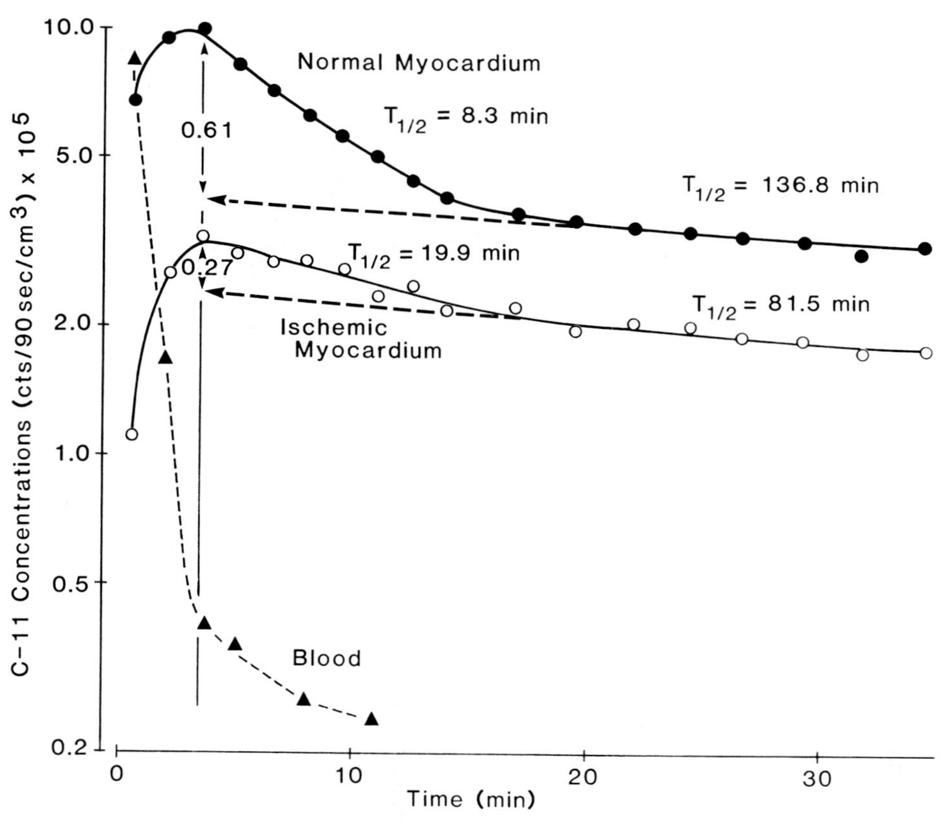

Figure 67–3. Myocardial ^{11}C time activity curves derived from regions of interest in normal and ischemic myocardium from the study illustrated in Figure 67–2. Maximal myocardial ^{11}C activity in both ischemic and normal myocardium reaches a maximum value at approximately 3.5 minutes. Clearance of the label from both ischemic and normal myocardium is biexponential. In ischemic myocardium, the relative size of the early portion of the time activity curve is smaller and the peak ^{11}C concentration is less than that in normal tissue. The half-time of the initial, early clearance of ^{11}C activity in ischemic myocardium is prolonged (19.9 versus 8.3 minutes), indicating impaired fatty acid oxidation. In contrast, the half-time of the second phase of the time activity curve is shorter than that of normal tissue (81.5 versus 136.8 minutes), indicating a more rapid entry of label into the endogenous lipid pool. (From Schelbert, H.R., Henze, E., Keen, R., et al.: C–11 palmitate for the noninvasive evaluation of regional myocardial fatty acid metabolism with positron computed tomography. IV. In vivo evaluation of acute demand-induced ischemia in dogs. Am. Heart. J. 106:736–750, 1983, with permission.)

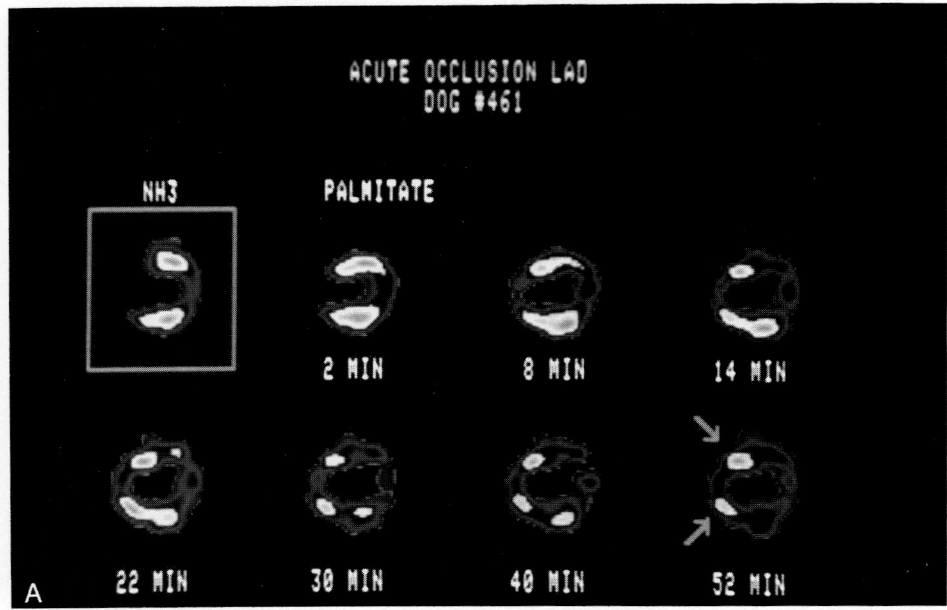

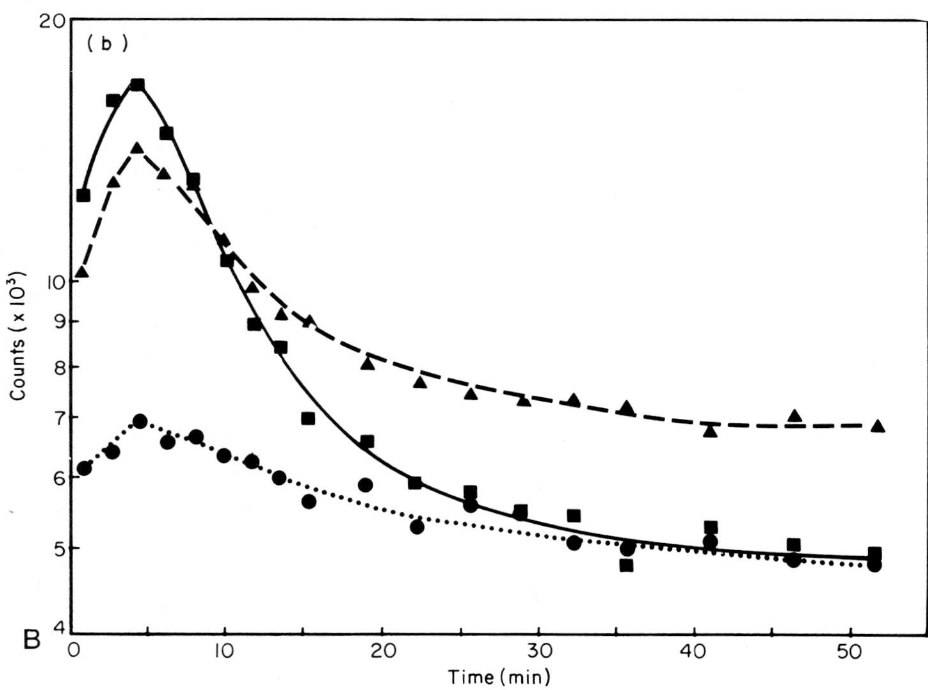

Figure 67–4. *Panel A*, Representative [^{13}N]-ammonia and serial ^{11}C-palmitate images in a canine preparation subjected to a balloon occlusion of the left anterior descending coronary artery. The [^{13}N]ammonia perfusion image (NH_3) demonstrates an anterior perfusion defect. On the serial ^{11}C-palmitate images there is impaired uptake and prolonged clearance of ^{11}C activity from the center and the border of the ischemic segment. The border zones are indicated by the arrows on the 52-minute image. *Panel B*, Myocardial ^{11}C time activity curves obtained from control (*square boxes*), ischemic (*circles*), and border regions (*triangles*). The central ischemic zone of necrosis is characterized by markedly decreased uptake and impaired clearance of ^{11}C activity, whereas normal myocardium reveals the typical biexponential clearance of ^{11}C activity with an early rapid phase and a late slow phase. In the border zone, uptake of the radiolabeled fatty acid is nearly as great as that in normal tissue, but the clearance of ^{11}C activity is prolonged and the relative amount of residual activity at the end of the initial rapid phase is increased. (From Schwaiger M., Fishbein, M.C., Block, M., et al.: Metabolic and ultrastructural abnormalities during ischemia in canine myocardium. Noninvasive assessment by positron emission tomography. J. Mol. Cell Cardiol. 19:259–269, 1987, with permission.)

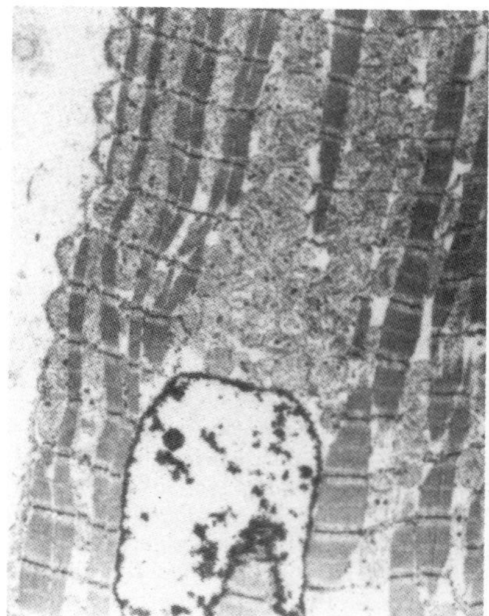
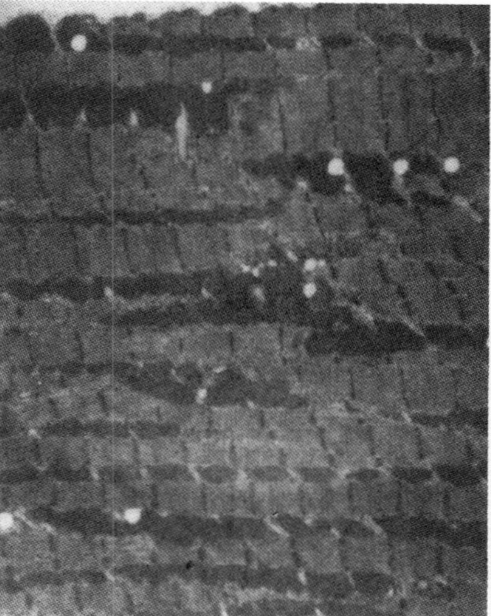
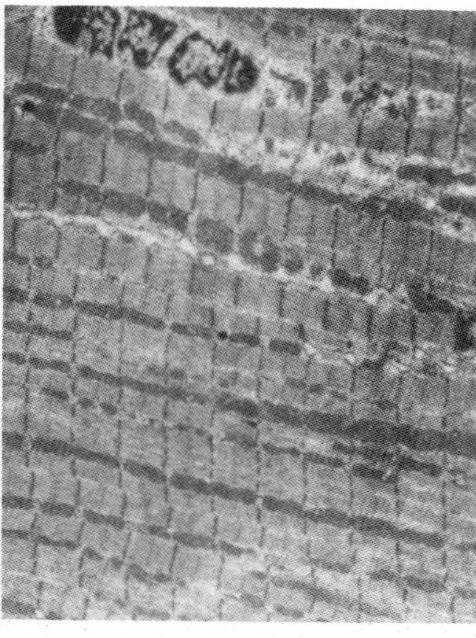

Figure 67–5. Typical ultrastructural findings in the central zone of necrosis (*left*), the peripheral border zone of ischemia (*middle*), and control myocardium (*right*) from the canine model of acute arterial occlusion employed for the studies in Figure 67–4. A sample from the central necrotic zone demonstrates mitochondrial matrix densities, swelling of the I bands, and chromatin clumping within the nucleus. The sample from the border zone shows normal mitochondria with lipid drop accumulation in close proximity to these organelles, along with maintained cellular glycogen stores. The electron microscopic sample from control myocardium demonstrates normal ultrastructure with no evidence for enhanced intracellular lipid accumulation. (From Schwaiger M., Fishbein, M.C., Block, M., et al.: Metabolic and ultrastructural abnormalities during ischemia in canine myocardium. Noninvasive assessment by positron emission tomography. J. Mol. Cell Cardiol. 19:259–269, 1987, with permission.)

In summary, serial positron tomographic imaging during acute ischemia in experimental animals demonstrates segmentally decreased uptake of carbon-11 palmitate and prolongation of the half-time of the rapid tissue clearance phase. The findings are consistent with a decrease in the relative amount of fatty acid entering oxidative metabolic pathways and with impaired metabolism of the substrate that does enter those aerobic pathways. Furthermore, the relative proportion of labeled fatty acid entering the endogenous lipid pool increases, and there is an increase in the relative amount of carbon-11 palmitate that diffuses back into the vascular space. The metabolic abnormalities in oxidative substrate metabolism identified with positron emission tomography and carbon-11 palmitate can occur in tissue without ultrastructural evidence of irreversible cellular damage, indicating the sensitivity of this imaging technique for detecting cellular dysfunction in acute ischemia. Finally, the increase in the fraction of carbon-11 palmitate that diffuses back from myocardium in nonmetabolized form may limit the accuracy of the clearance half-time as an index of fatty acid oxidation.

Evaluation of Oxidative Metabolism with Carbon-11 Acetate

Studies performed with carbon-14 acetate in isolated perfused hearts indicated a biexponential clearance pattern of this tracer from myocardium. The initial rapid clearance phase is linearly related to myocardial oxygen consumption.[B1, B2] In contrast to carbon-14 palmitate, the clearance of carbon-14 acetate is virtually independent of plasma substrate levels and thus affords quantitative assessment of myocardial oxidative metabolism independent of substrate availability and myocardial substrate selection (see also Chapter 65).

Brown and co-workers characterized the kinetics of carbon-14 acetate in studies performed in 37 isolated rabbit hearts.[B1] The steady-state extraction fraction of carbon-14 acetate averaged 63.4 ± 9.5 percent in control hearts, 94.9 ± 1.1 percent in ischemic hearts, and 54.8 ± 4.0 percent in hearts reperfused following 60 minutes of ischemia. Rates of efflux of carbon-14 carbon dioxide correlated closely with rates of oxygen consumption ($r = 0.97$, $P < 0.001$). Clearance half-times of carbon-14 carbon dioxide were 3.2 ± 0.9 minutes for control hearts, 15.0 ± 0.4 minutes for ischemic hearts, 9.3 ± 2.2 minutes for hypoxic hearts, and 3.1 ± 0.2 minutes for reperfused hearts. Thus, these findings indicate that the delayed clearance of carbon-14 carbon dioxide resulted from limited oxygen supply rather than from a flow-limited washout of carbon-14–labeled metabolites from tissue.

To determine whether back-diffusion of labeled acetate in ischemic hearts is as significant a problem as that for carbon-11 palmitate, these investigators analyzed the contribution of carbon-14 carbon dioxide to total radioactivity in the venous effluent. In control and reperfused hearts, 96.0 ± 1.1 percent of radioactivity in the venous effluent was in the form of carbon-14 carbon dioxide. This fraction decreased to 75.7 ± 7.2 percent of total venous radioactivity in ischemic hearts. The chemical species containing the label in venous effluent was determined using high-pressure liquid chromatography. In control hearts, 35 percent of non-CO_2 related carbon-14 activity was contributed by ketone bodies, primarily carbon-14-β-hydroxybutyrate and carbon-14 acetoacetate. In ischemic hearts, labeled ketone bodies accounted for 45 percent of non-carbon-14 carbon dioxide activity, while the remaining carbon-14 metabolites were largely labeled citrate, succinate, and lactate. These data suggest that back-diffusion of nonmetabolized carbon-14–labeled acetate does in fact occur and increases during ischemia. In addition, back-diffusion of labeled metabolites contributes to the overall clearance of carbon-14 activity from normal and ischemic myocardium.

The same investigators also co-injected carbon-11–labeled acetate with carbon-14–labeled acetate and compared the externally detected clearance of carbon-11 activity from myocardium with the release of carbon-14 activity in coronary sinus effluent in six control and four ischemic hearts. The rate constants of the rapid phase of the external clearance of carbon-11 acetate, k_1's, correlated significantly with the rate constants for efflux of total carbon-14 activity, carbon-14 carbon dioxide, as well as the rate of efflux of carbon-11 activity. In addition, rate constants for the carbon-11 acetate time activity curves correlated linearly with oxygen consumption measurements over a range of 0.01 to 0.12 O_2/min/g, indicating that the externally measured clearance of carbon-11 acetate is tightly coupled to oxygen consumption, even during states of severe myocardial ischemia or hypoxia. Other studies in isolated perfused hearts[B2] confirmed the linear relationship of the carbon-14 acetate clearance rate to myocardial oxygen consumption. Unlike the early observations, Buxton and associates noted that the tracer cleared from tissue in a biexponential rather than monoexponential fashion.[B2] Myocardial oxygen consumption in these experiments was reduced by induction of hypoxia or increased by the administration of phenylephrine. Despite alterations in tissue oxygen delivery and demand, and despite alteration of plasma substrate levels (2 mM lactate, 20 mM 3-hydroxybutyrate, or 0.1 mM palmitate), a good correlation was noted between k_1, the rate constant for the initial phase of carbon-

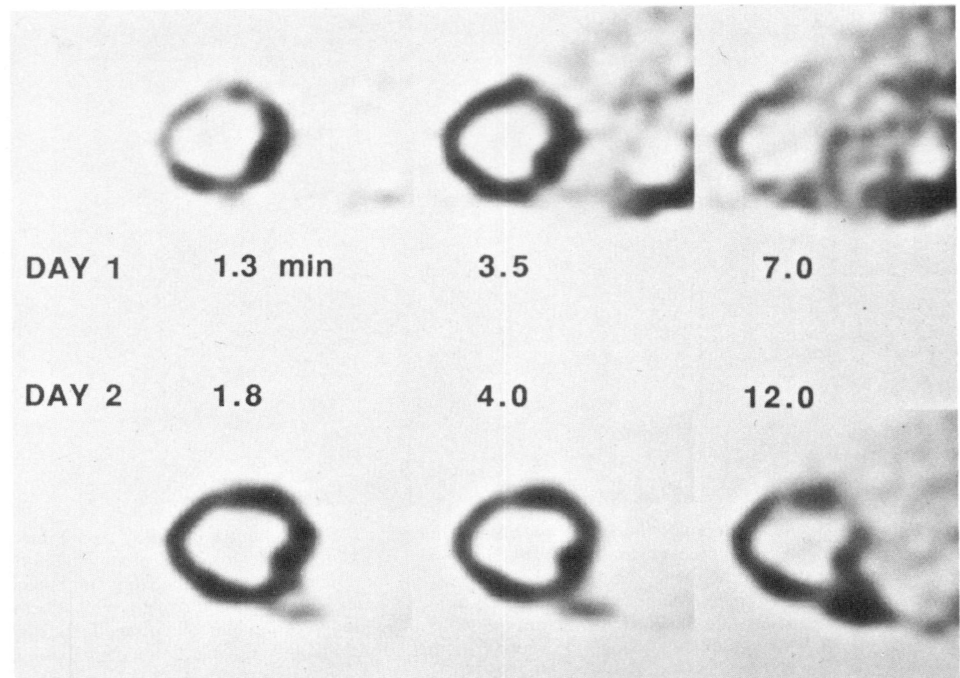

Figure 67–6. Cross-sectional dynamic transverse ^{11}C positron tomographic images of canine left ventricular myocardium following the intravenous administration of ^{11}C-acetate. The images on Day 1 were obtained 2 hours following release of a 20-minute balloon occlusion of the left anterior descending coronary artery. Delayed clearance of the radiolabel is noted in the anterior region of the ventricle. By Day 2, 24 hours after reperfusion, clearance of the ^{11}C label is homogeneous, indicating recovery from the acute ischemic insult. (From Buxton, D.B., Schwaiger, M., Vaghaiwalla, M.F., et al.: Regional abnormality of oxygen consumption in reperfused myocardium assessed with [1-^{11}C] acetate and positron emission tomography. Am. J. Cardiac Imaging 3:276–287, 1989, with permission.)

14 carbon dioxide clearance, and rates of myocardial oxygen consumption (r = 0.93). Unlike the report of Brown and associates,[B1] however, these investigators did not observe a statistically significant increase in back-diffusion of carbon-14 acetate during hypoxia and reported that more than 88 percent of carbon-14 activity in the venous effluent was released as carbon-14 carbon dioxide.

In subsequent studies in 12 intact dogs, Buxton and associates examined the utility of carbon-11 acetate for the noninvasive study of oxidative metabolism.[B3] The effect of varying myocardial workloads and substrate levels on the relationship between clearance rates of carbon-11 acetate and myocardial oxygen consumption was determined in 18 experiments. Cardiac workload was increased by infusion of norepinephrine or decreased by intramuscular administration of morphine sulfate. Substrate availability was varied by intravenous infusion of sodium lactate or by the administration of insulin and glucose. Myocardial consumption of oxygen, glucose, lactate, and free fatty acid was determined from arterial and coronary sinus sampling and the Fick technique. There was a linear relationship between myocardial oxygen consumption and microsphere blood flow measurements over a range of blood flows from 0.40 to 1.5 ml/min/g. Analysis of the dynamically acquired cross-sectional carbon-11 acetate images confirmed that the carbon-11 label cleared biexponentially from myocardium (Figs. 67–6 and 67–7). The rate constant for the initial rapid clearance phase, defined as k_1, was linearly related to oxygen consumption over a range of from 4.6 to 17.5 ml O_2/min/100 g. This relationship was independent of changes in plasma substrate availability. Rate constants for the second slow phase of acetate clearance, defined as k_2, however, were independent of myocardial oxygen consumption. The investigators postulated that this phase of the tissue clearance curve reflects incorporation of label into an endogenous amino acid pool or possibly a fatty acid pool.

The same workers further examined the homogeneity of carbon-11 acetate clearance constants from normal canine myocardium. Using dynamically acquired cross-sectional images, k_1's were approximately 7 percent lower in the interventricular septum than in the free wall of the left ventricle. This regional reduction in k_1's was correlated with a concomitant regional reduction in myocardial blood flow, as determined by microsphere measurements, and suggests a slightly lower rate of oxygen consumption in the interventricular septum compared with that in the left ventricular free wall.

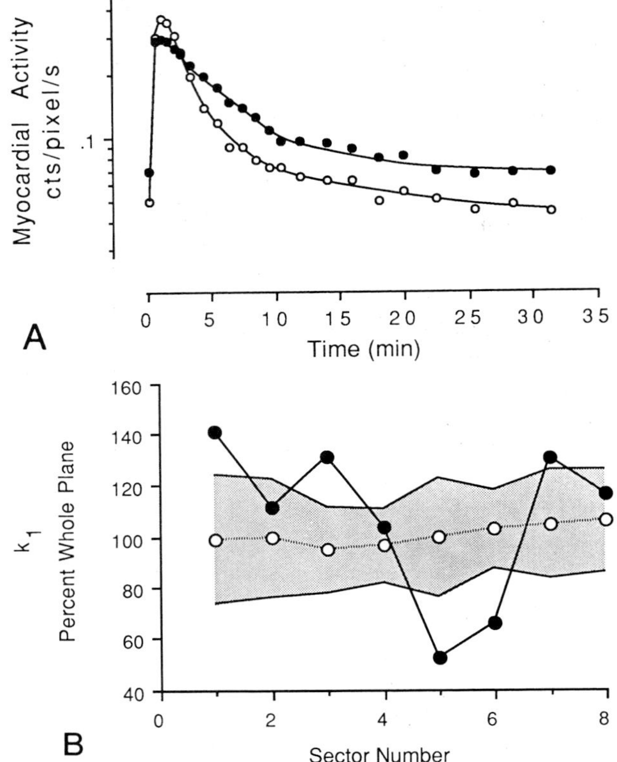

Figure 67–7. *Panel A,* Representative myocardial ^{11}C time activity curves in normal (*open circles*) and reperfused myocardium (*closed circles*). The curves were obtained from the Day 1 ^{11}C-acetate canine study illustrated in Figure 67–6 that was performed 2 hours after reperfusion. *Panel B,* Relative k_1's from an unrolled cross section of left ventricular myocardium. The data in solid circles represents that from a dog 2 hours post-reperfusion, whereas the open circles represent the means from 18 experiments in 12 control dogs. The ±2 standard deviation range is indicated for the control animals by the shaded area. In the reperfused myocardial region (Sectors 5 and 6), relative k_1's are depressed as compared with those in control animals. (From Buxton, D.B., Schwaiger, M., Vaghaiwalla, M.F., et al.: Regional abnormality of oxygen consumption in reperfused myocardium assessed with [1-^{11}C] acetate and positron emission tomography. Am. J. Cardiac Imaging 3:276–287, 1989, with permission.)

In summary, experimental studies have demonstrated that the myocardial clearance of radiolabeled acetate parallels regional oxygen consumption during acute myocardial ischemia. Because carbon-11 acetate is a "pure" tracer of tricarboxylic acid cycle flux, variations in plasma substrate levels affect its clearance from myocardium only slightly.[B2, B4, S6] Although back-diffusion of carbon-11 label from ischemic myocardium does occur with carbon-11 acetate, the relative amount of back-diffusion is quite small and does not seriously affect the quantitative determinations of regional myocardial oxygen consumption made with this tracer.

Evaluation of Glucose Metabolism with Fluorine-18 2-Fluoro 2-Deoxyglucose

Early laboratory studies indicated that utilization of exogenous glucose is accelerated in acutely ischemic myocardium.[B5, L1, M1, N1, O1, O2, V2] In patients with coronary artery disease, Most and associates noted that atrial pacing to the point of lactate production is associated with an increase in myocardial glucose extraction, confirming a similar augmentation in glucose utilization in acutely ischemic human myocardium.[M2] These observations implied that use of a radiolabeled marker of glucose metabolism, such as fluorine-18 2-fluoro 2-deoxyglucose, could prove useful in identifying and characterizing acutely ischemic myocardium with positron emission tomography.

Schelbert and associates induced acute ischemia by rapid atrial pacing in open-chest dogs with a partially occluded left anterior descending coronary artery.[S7] Following a control perfusion study with nitrogen-13 ammonia, a coronary constrictor positioned around the anterior descending artery was tightened sufficiently to abolish resting reactive hyperemia. The animals were then atrially paced at a rate of 200 beats/min for 11 minutes while a second nitrogen-13 ammonia perfusion study was performed. One hour following the nitrogen-13 ammonia pacing perfusion study, the animal was again paced at 200 beats/min while fluorine-18 2-fluoro 2-deoxyglucose was administered intravenously. After pacing for another 15 minutes, images of the regional myocardial fluorine-18 myocardial tracer concentrations were recorded. The externally recorded myocardial tracer concentrations were compared with regional blood flow measured by microspheres and with oxygen and glucose consumption determined by the Fick principle.

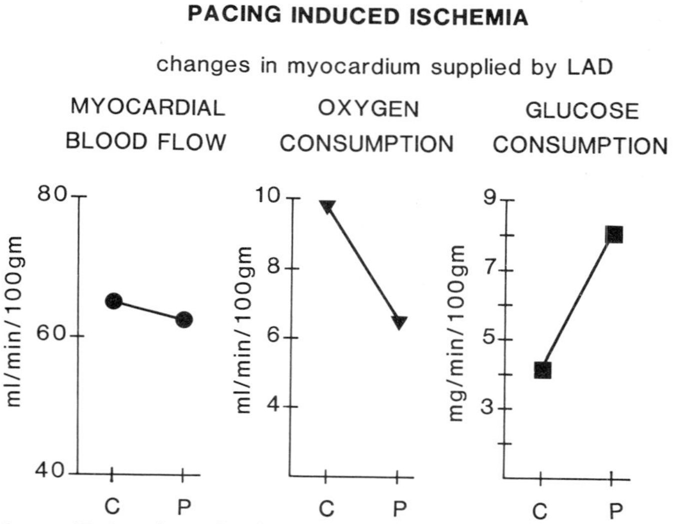

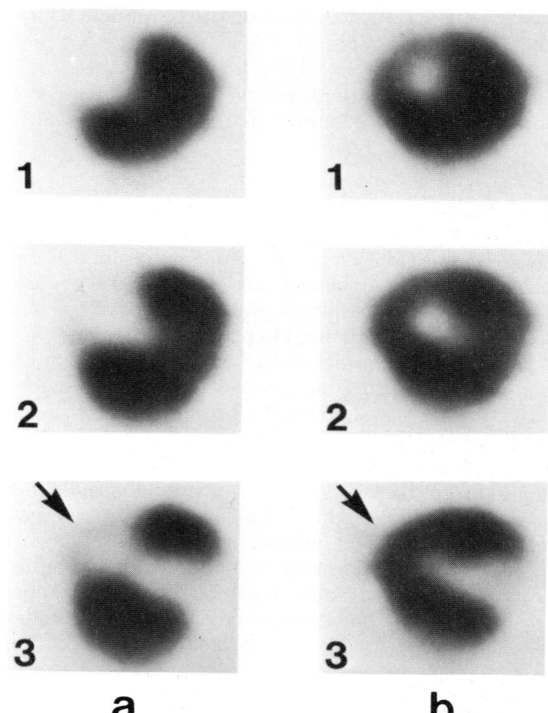

Figure 67–9. Representative cross-sectional positron emission tomographic images of relative blood flow ([^{13}N]ammonia, *Column a*) and exogenous glucose utilization ([18]F 2-fluoro 2-deoxyglucose, *Column b*) obtained during acute ischemia. Ischemia was induced by atrial pacing a canine preparation with a partially constricted left anterior descending artery. Level 1 is the most inferior cross-sectional level, and Level 3 is the most superior cross-sectional level. The [^{13}N]ammonia perfusion images demonstrate an anteroseptal perfusion defect (*arrow*.) The metabolic images obtained 45 minutes after the intravenous administration of [18]F 2-fluoro 2-deoxyglucose show preservation of exogenous glucose metabolism in the region of acute stress-induced myocardial ischemia (*arrow*). (From Schelbert H. R., Phelps, M.E., Selin, C., et al.: Regional myocardial ischemia assessed by [18]Fluoro 2-deoxyglucose and positron emission computed tomography. *In* Heiss, H.W. (ed.): Advances in Clinical Cardiology. Vol. I. Quantification of Myocardial Ischemia. Gerhard Witzstrock, New York, 1980, pp. 437–449, with permission.)

Figure 67–8. Relationship between changes in myocardial blood flow, oxygen consumption, and glucose consumption at rest (C) and with atrial pacing (P) in the vascular territory of a partially constricted left anterior descending coronary artery in a canine preparation. Changes in myocardial blood flow were assessed with the microsphere technique, whereas changes in oxygen and glucose consumption were derived from simultaneous arterial and interventricular coronary venous blood samples and application of the Fick technique. With atrial pacing, no significant change in myocardial blood flow is noted in risk myocardium and there is a decline in regional oxygen consumption. In contrast, glucose utilization increases nearly two-fold in the ischemic segment. (From Schelbert, H.R., Phelps, M.E., Selin, C., et al.: Regional myocardial ischemia assessed by [18]fluoro 2-deoxyglucose and positron emission computed tomography. *In* Heiss, H.W. (ed.): Advances in Clinical Cardiology. Vol. I. Quantification of Myocardial Ischemia. Gerhard Witzstrock, New York, 1980, pp. 437–449, with permission.)

With atrial pacing, mean myocardial blood flows in the risk zone were essentially unchanged (0.66 ml/min/g and 0.62 ml/min/g) and there was a decrease in regional oxygen consumption from 9.8 ml/min/100 g to 6.5 ml/min/100 g. However, regional glucose utilization increased from 4.2 to 8.1 ml/min/100 g (Fig. 67–8). Regional tissue concentrations of fluorine-18 2-fluoro 2-deoxyglucose were linearly related to regional myocardial blood flow for flows above 0.40 ml/min/g. For flows of 0.40 ml/min/g or less, however, tissue fluorine-18 2-fluoro 2-deoxyglucose concentrations exceeded those predicted by a simple linear relationship, indicating that the amount of substrate extracted per milliliter of blood delivered to tissue was accelerated in ischemic myocardium.

The enhancement of exogenous glucose utilization in ischemic tissue was readily appreciated on the positron emission tomographic images (Fig. 67–9). In the hypoperfused regions delineated on the nitrogen-13 ammonia studies, accelerated glucose utilization was identified by relative preservation of fluorine-18 2-fluoro 2-deoxyglucose uptake. This resulted in a visual "mismatch" between the nitrogen-13 ammonia perfusion defect and the uptake of fluorine-18 2-fluoro 2-deoxyglucose on the metabolic images. Thus, acute myocardial ischemia is associated with augmented uptake of glucose relative to blood flow, and this metabolic disturbance can be identified with positron emission tomography using fluorine-18 2-fluoro 2-deoxyglucose.

Synopsis

Determination of the metabolic disturbances induced by acute ischemia in experimental animal models forms the basis for application of positron emission tomography to the study of metabolism in ischemic human myocardium. In experimental studies, acute ischemia results in an impairment of the metabolic oxidative capacity of the tissue. On positron emission tomography with a "pure" tracer of mitochondrial oxidative substrate flux such as carbon-11 acetate, this impairment in aerobic metabolism is indicated by delayed segmental clearance of the radiolabel. Because the myocardial kinetics of carbon-11 acetate are virtually unaffected by varying arterial substrate levels and are less subject to errors due to back-diffusion of nonmetabolized carbon-11 acetate, determination of the carbon-11 acetate tissue clearance constant, k_1, is a reliable indirect means of assessing regional myocardial oxygen consumption. Impaired oxidation of free fatty acids in acute myocardial ischemia can be detected and quantified on positron emission tomography with carbon-11 palmitate. In ischemia, segmental uptake of carbon-11 palmitate is impaired, and there is prolongation of the half-time of the initial rapid tissue clearance phase. The proportion of labeled fatty acid that enters the endogenous lipid pool increases, and there is an increase in the relative amount of carbon-11 palmitate that "back-diffuses" into the vascular space. The disturbances in fatty acid metabolism in acutely ischemic myocardium detected on positron emission tomography can occur in tissue without ultrastructural evidence of irreversible cellular damage, indicating the sensitivity of this imaging technique for detecting cellular dysfunction. Under conditions of impaired tissue oxygen delivery, myocardial ATP production becomes increasingly dependent on anaerobic glycolytic pathways; this is reflected by augmented uptake of the glucose analog fluorine-18 2-fluoro 2-deoxyglucose in hypoperfused myocardial regions. It results in a visually detectable "mismatch" between tissue perfusion and exogenous glucose utilization on the positron tomographic images and forms the basis for the determination of metabolic viability in hypoperfused myocardial regions with positron emission tomography.

Clinical Investigations with Tracers of Metabolism

Initial clinical studies focused on the assessment of oxidative metabolism in human myocardium with carbon-11 palmitate. However, as evidence of the possible limitations of carbon-11 palmitate as a tracer of oxidative metabolism (as, for example, effects of substrate availability on its tissue kinetics[S8] and increased back-diffusion of tracer into the vascular space[F1, R2, S1]) was forthcoming from animal experiments, new investigations were undertaken with carbon-11 acetate as a more direct and "pure" tracer of tricarboxylic acid cycle activity and thus of oxidative metabolism in acute myocardial ischemia.

Studies with Carbon-11 Palmitate for Fatty Acid Metabolism

To assess the effects of acute ischemia on oxidative substrate metabolism in human myocardium, Grover-McKay and colleagues employed serial positron emission tomographic imaging with carbon-11 palmitate in 10 patients with exertional angina and significant (> 70 percent) coronary stenoses.[G2] Relative myocardial blood flow was first evaluated at rest with nitrogen-13 ammonia. Serial imaging with carbon-11 palmitate was then performed at rest (control) and again during atrial pacing at heart rates 10 percent lower than those provoking angina. Segmental wall motion was assessed with two-dimensional echocardiography at rest and during pacing.

Atrial pacing increased the mean heart rate of the subjects from 65 ± 12 beats/min to 102 ± 15 beats/min. Mean systolic and diastolic pressures remained constant (138 ± 21 versus 141 ± 23 mmHg and 83 ± 12 versus 80 ± 17 mmHg, respectively). Plasma levels of fatty acids (0.42 ± 0.26 versus 0.48 ± 0.11 mmol/L), triglycerides (242 ± 162 versus 311 ± 295 mg/dl), lactate (8.9 ± 2.9 versus 8.0 ± 2.2 mg/dl), and pyruvate (0.59 ± 0.25 versus 0.49 ± 0.22 mg/dl) did not differ significantly between the control and pacing studies, although there was a slight but statistically significant decrease in plasma glucose levels (99 ± 22 versus 92 ± 16 mg/dl). Thus increases in myocardial workload resulted primarily from increases in heart rate while the slight but statistically significant decline in plasma glucose levels during atrial pacing favored myocardial utilization of fatty acids.

The rest nitrogen-13 ammonia images revealed homogeneous myocardial blood flow in eight of the ten patients, whereas two patients with clinical histories of antecedent myocardial infarction had resting perfusion defects in the clinical infarct zone. The two patients with antecedent infarction had regional akinesis or dyskinesis at rest, which corresponded with the presence of Q waves on their electrocardiograms. With atrial pacing, five patients developed new regional akinesis or severe hypokinesis; three patients developed new hypokinesis, which was mild; and two patients had no apparent change in regional function. Visual analysis of the rest metabolic studies in the eight patients without prior myocardial infarction revealed homogeneous myocardial uptake and washout of carbon-11 palmitate. In the two patients with previous infarction, visual defects were apparent on both the early and late carbon-11 palmitate images, which corresponded to the defects noted on the nitrogen-13 ammonia perfusion studies. Half-times of the initial rapid phase of myocardial carbon-11 palmitate clearance were similar in both normal and risk myocardium (22.2 ± 5.2 versus 21.0 ± 5.4 min, P = NS), signifying that fatty acid oxidation was not impaired in the resting state (Fig. 67–10). The fraction of carbon-11 activity that was retained in myocardium and, conversely, the fraction of carbon-11 palmitate that became oxidized were virtually identical in risk and normal myocardium (51.8 ± 7.4 percent versus 54.0 ± 6.1 percent, P = NS).

With atrial pacing, the mean half-time of the rapid clearance phase decreased in both risk and normal myocardium, consistent with an increase in myocardial oxygen consumption and fatty acid oxidation as a result of the increased cardiac workload.[S2] Half-times in risk myocardium, however, were significantly longer than those in reference myocardium (15.6 ± 4.0 min versus 13.4 ± 2.5 min, $P < 0.01$), indicating an impaired oxidative metabolic reserve in the myocardial regions supplied by the vessels with significant coronary stenoses (Figs. 67–10 and 67–11). The fraction of carbon-11 activity that was retained in myocardium at the end of the initial rapid phase during pacing was significantly greater in the risk zones compared with reference myocardium (41.8 ± 10.9 percent versus 36.4 ± 9.0 percent, $P < 0.002$), implying that the flux of carbon-11 palmitate through oxidative pathways during pacing-induced ischemia was not commensurate with tissue demands as assessed by measurements in normal myocardium. For both the control and atrial pacing studies, tracer uptake in risk myocardium relative to reference myocardium remained unchanged (97.3 ± 14.3 percent at rest versus 97.9 ± 14.1 percent during pacing, P = NS).

When changes in myocardial clearance of carbon-11 palmitate were correlated with changes in regional function, the five patients who exhibited new akinesis or severe hypokinesis in the risk zones during atrial pacing also had a significant change in the percent difference in carbon-11 palmitate clearance half-times between risk myocardium and reference myocardium (−5.8 ± 13.2 percent at control versus 26.1 ± 30.6 percent during pacing, P = 0.01). In contrast, the percent difference in carbon-11 palmitate clearance half-times between risk and reference myocardium in the five patients exhibiting only mild hypokinesis or no change in function with pacing did not differ significantly between the control and pacing studies (−10.1 ± 18.2 percent versus 8.2 ± 11.2 percent, P = NS). Thus, regions with more severe deterioration of regional function during the stress of atrial pacing exhibited the greatest degree of impairment in myocardial

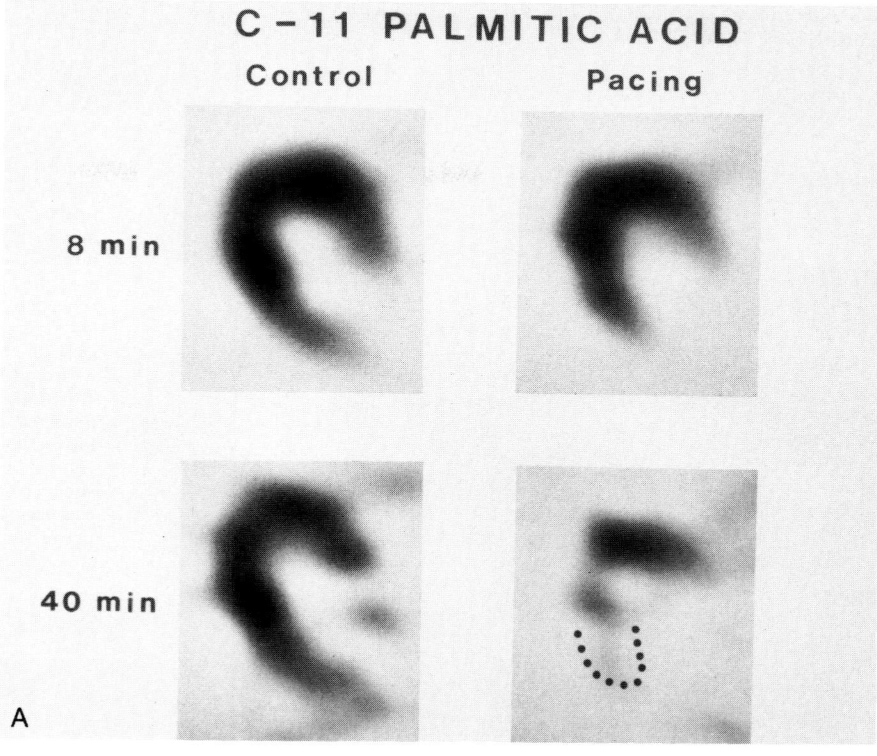

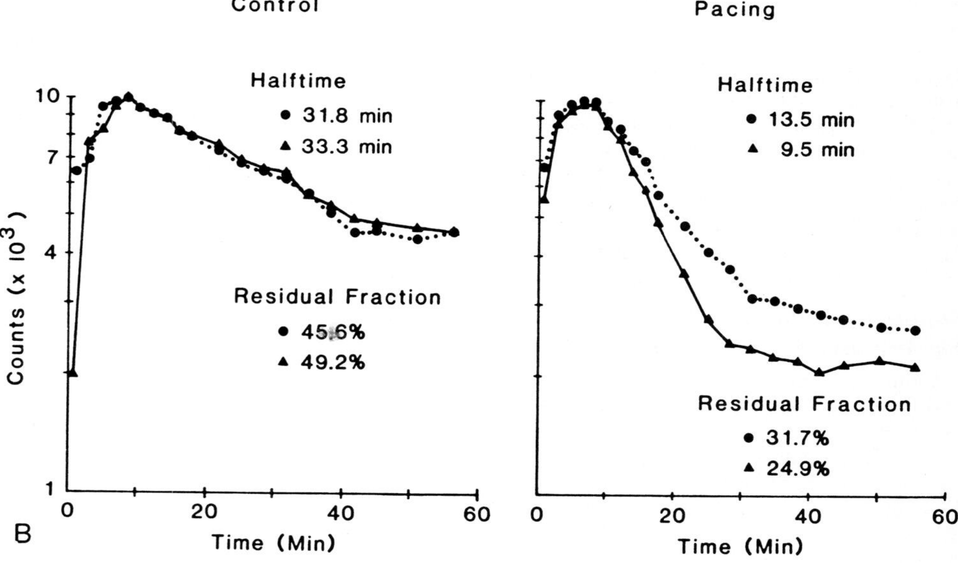

Figure 67–10. *Panel A*, Representative cross-sectional images of myocardial ^{11}C-palmitate activity in a patient with a proximal 90 percent stenosis of the left anterior descending coronary artery. The control images obtained in the resting state 8 and 40 minutes after the administration of the radiolabeled fatty acid are depicted in the column on the left, whereas images obtained at the corresponding time intervals during atrial pacing are displayed in the column on the right. Homogeneous uptake of the radiolabeled fatty acid is noted on the 8-minute images obtained both at control and during pacing. In the control resting state, there is uniform clearance of the labeled fatty acid from all myocardial regions, as indicated by a homogeneous distribution of the radiolabel on the delayed image at 40 minutes. In contrast, during atrial pacing there is rapid clearance of ^{11}C activity from the normally perfused lateral wall (*dotted region*) and an impairment in clearance of ^{11}C activity from the vascular territory of the anterior descending artery. *Panel B*, Representative myocardial ^{11}C time activity curves from the same patient at control and with atrial pacing. During the resting control study, uptake and clearance of ^{11}C activity in both the normal (*triangles*) and the anteroseptal regions (*circles*) are virtually identical. With atrial pacing, the ^{11}C clearance half-time is longer and the residual fraction is greater in the anteroseptal region, indicating impairment of free fatty acid oxidation during stress-induced myocardial ischemia and a relative increase in the amount of ^{11}C label entering the endogenous lipid pool. (From Grover-McKay, M., Schelbert, H.R., Schwaiger, M., et al.: Identification of impaired metabolic reserve by atrial pacing in patients with significant coronary artery disease. Circulation 74:281–292, 1986, by permission of the American Heart Association, Inc.)

oxidative reserve. Conversely, in regions without apparent stress-induced wall motion abnormalities, the changes in carbon-11 palmitate tissue kinetics tended to be attenuated, although not significantly when compared with control myocardium. This suggests that the ability to maintain systolic function in human myocardium may be coupled to the oxidative metabolic capacity of the tissue. Alternatively, normal regional function might have been maintained by a shift in local tissue metabolism to preferential utilization of glucose, a more oxygen-efficient substrate. However, further studies are required to confirm these possibilities.

Studies with Carbon-11 Acetate for Oxidative Metabolism

Early clinical studies demonstrated the feasibility of assessing overall myocardial oxidative metabolism with carbon-11 acetate in patients with coronary artery disease. In a preliminary report by Selwyn and co-workers, monoexponential carbon-11 acetate clearance constants were assessed in five patients with coronary artery disease and angina undergoing treadmill exercise.[89] Carbon-11 acetate was administered intravenously 1 to 2 minutes before the appearance of ischemic electrocardiographic changes. Although myocardial uptake of carbon-11 acetate was homogeneous on images obtained at 3 minutes, abnormal retention of activity was noted in ischemic regions on images obtained at 12 minutes. In this fashion, ischemic regions were positively labeled on the delayed carbon-11 acetate images. Compared with normal regions, clearance half-times were significantly longer (10.1 min versus 7.7 min, $P < 0.01$) and clearance constants were significantly lower (0.069 versus 0.090, $P < 0.01$) in ischemic regions. This initial report demonstrated that serial positron emission tomographic imaging with carbon-11 acetate could identify im-

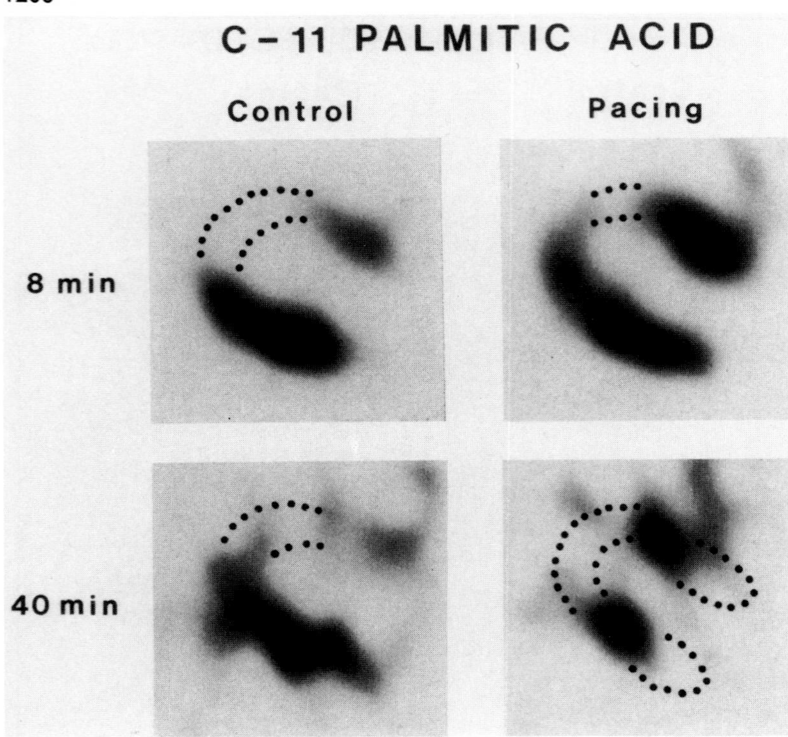

Figure 67–11. Representative ^{11}C-palmitate images from a patient with a 90 percent mid left anterior descending coronary artery stenosis and a history of prior myocardial infarction. On both the control and pacing images, defects are identified in the anterior region of the ventricle that are consistent with the patient's clinical history of prior infarction. On the study obtained during atrial pacing, impaired clearance of ^{11}C activity is noted in the peri-infarct zones as indicated by the persistence of activity in these areas on the 40-minute image. The ^{11}C-palmitate study thus identifies impaired oxidative metabolic reserve in the adjacent peri-infarct border zone. (From Grover-McKay, M., Schelbert, H.R., Schwaiger, M., et al.: Identification of impaired metabolic reserve by atrial pacing in patients with significant coronary artery disease. Circulation 74:281–292, 1986, with permission.)

paired myocardial oxidative metabolism in patients with angina at a workload insufficient to produce electrocardiographic signs of myocardial ischemia.

Similar findings were reported in another preliminary report by the same investigators.[A1] In five patients with coronary artery disease, serial carbon-11 acetate images were obtained at rest and then repeated during supine bicycle exercise. In normal myocardium, clearance constants were 0.065 ± 0.010 min^{-1} at rest and increased to 0.102 ± 0.009 min^{-1} with exercise. In contrast, regions with exercise-induced ischemia had clearance constants that remained depressed at 0.065 ± 0.011 min^{-1}. Again, these findings are consistent with a failure to increase oxidative substrate flux in response to increased demand.

Studies with Fluorine-18 2-Fluoro 2-Deoxyglucose for Alterations in Exogenous Glucose Utilization

Camici and colleagues employed positron emission tomography and fluorine-18 2-fluoro 2-deoxyglucose to examine the response of exogenous glucose utilization to acute exercise-induced ischemia in 12 patients with stable coronary artery disease.[C1] They compared the findings to those observed in 10 normal volunteers. Five of the twelve patients had evidence of prior transmural myocardial infarction and two had poor R wave progression in the anterior precordial leads on electrocardiography. None of the subjects had clinical histories of infarction in the 3 months prior to study. Regional myocardial blood flow and glucose metabolism were examined at rest with rubidium-82 and fluorine-18 2-fluoro 2-deoxyglucose in six patients and in five volunteers. Eight patients (including two with fluorine-18 2-fluoro 2-deoxyglucose studies at rest) and five volunteers had rubidium-82 studies at rest, during supine bicycle exercise, and immediately following exercise. Glucose metabolism in these eight patients was then evaluated after the patient's heart rate, blood pressure, and electrocardiogram had returned to baseline, and the exercise-induced rubidium-82 defect had resolved on the post-exercise perfusion images.

Both blood flow and glucose utilization were evaluated semiquantitatively by determining the fractional uptake of rubidium-82 (see Chapters 65 and 66) and of fluorine-18 2-fluoro 2-deoxyglucose. The latter was calculated by dividing the myocardial fluorine-18 activity concentrations at time t by the integral of the arterial fluorine-18 2-fluoro 2-deoxyglucose plasma concentration to time t.

At rest, the average myocardial fractional uptake of rubidium-82 in six regions of interest was similar in the patients and in the normal controls (0.44 ± 0.06 versus 0.47 ± 0.07). However, the range of regional rubidium-82 uptake (an indicator of the inhomogeneity in tracer uptake) was significantly greater in the patients than in the normal volunteers (0.14 ± 0.04 versus 0.06 ± 0.03, $P < 0.005$). When segments were classified according to exercise performance as ischemic or nonischemic, resting fractional uptake of rubidium-82 was similar in both the ischemic and nonischemic segments (0.41 ± 0.04 versus 0.45 ± 0.04, P = NS). In one patient with electrocardiographic criteria for an anterior infarction, resting regional rubidium-82 uptake was less than 2 standard deviations below normal in the clinical infarct zone.

The eight patients achieved a mean double product of 18,000 during supine bicycle exercise. Each experienced chest pain and exhibited electrocardiographic ST segment depression. At peak exercise, the average myocardial uptake of rubidium-82 in the patients was significantly lower than that in the normal subjects (0.52 ± 0.08 versus 0.65 ± 0.09, $P < 0.005$), while the range of myocardial rubidium-82 uptake in patients was again greater than that observed in the exercising normal volunteers (0.27 ± 0.09 versus 0.09 ± 0.03, $P < 0.001$). With exercise, rubidium-82 uptake increased significantly in the nonischemic segments in the patients (0.45 ± 0.04 versus 0.63 ± 0.07) but failed to increase in the ischemic segments (0.41 ± 0.04 versus 0.39 ± 0.04, P = NS). In five patients, regional rubidium-82 uptake actually decreased with exercise in myocardium supplied by diseased coronary arteries. This occurred in two patients with single-vessel disease and in the vascular territory supplied by the most severely diseased vessel in three patients with multivessel disease. Following exercise, fractional uptake of rubidium-82 in the ischemic segments persisted unchanged (0.42 ± 0.08; P = NS versus either baseline or exercise values), while uptake in the nonischemic segments returned to baseline levels (0.51 ± 0.09; $P < 0.02$ as compared with exercise, P = NS as compared with initial resting values).

The fractional uptake of fluorine-18 2-fluoro 2-deoxyglucose at rest in the patients with coronary artery disease did not differ from that in the normal subjects (0.11 ± 0.03 versus 0.07 ± 0.04, P = NS). Following exercise, uptake of fluorine-18 2-fluoro 2-deoxyglucose in the nonischemic segments was similar to that of normal subjects (0.33 ± 0.18 versus 0.35 ± 0.21). In contrast,

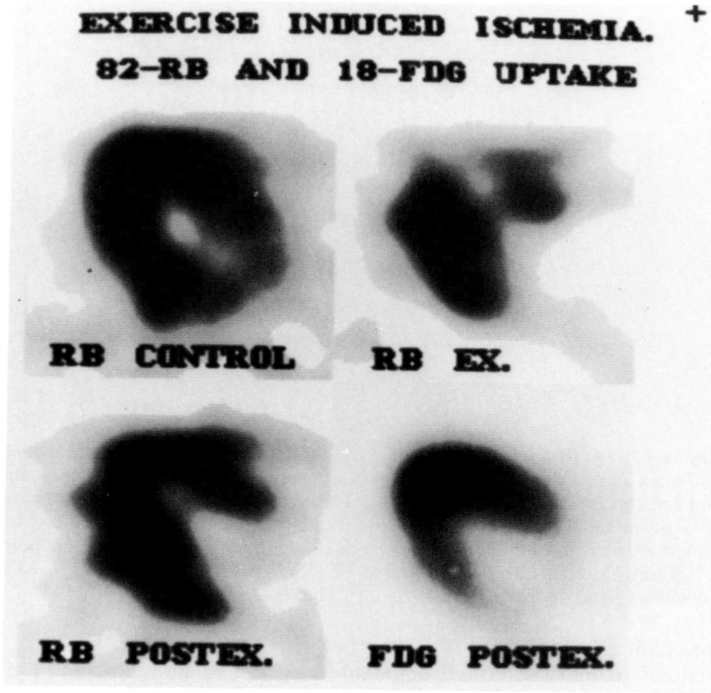

Figure 67–12. Representative ^{82}Rb perfusion and ^{18}F-2-fluoro 2-deoxyglucose (FDG) metabolic positron emission tomographic images in a patient with an 80 percent stenosis of the left anterior descending coronary artery. At rest (RB CONTROL), perfusion is homogeneous throughout all ventricular regions. With exercise (RB EX.), a stress-induced perfusion defect is identified in the anteroseptal region of the ventricle. On the post-exercise perfusion image (RB POSTEX.), obtained 6 minutes after termination of exercise, perfusion has normalized in the anteroseptal region. However, the glucose metabolic image (FDG POSTEX.) obtained 60 minutes later reveals prominent uptake of the glucose analog in the anteroseptal region (1.55 times higher than the lateral wall). Thus, the study with ^{18}F-2-fluoro 2-deoxyglucose demonstrates a persistently abnormal metabolic state in myocardium perfused by the diseased anterior descending artery despite the return of regional blood flow to normal levels. (From Camici, P., Araujo, L.I., Spinks, T., et al.: Increased uptake of ^{18}F-fluorodeoxyglucose in postischemic myocardium of patients with exercise-induced angina. Circulation 74: 81–88, 1986, with permission.)

ischemic segments exhibited significantly greater uptake of the glucose analog (0.47 ± 0.18, $P < 0.05$), compared with nonischemic regions (Fig. 67–12). Moreover, when compared with regional rubidium-82 uptake after exercise, uptake of fluorine-18 2-fluoro 2-deoxyglucose per unit of fractional rubidium-82 uptake in ischemic myocardium was 1.7 times higher than in normal segments, indicating that exogenous glucose utilization after exercise was augmented relative to flow in segments with stress-induced perfusion defects. Despite return of blood flow to resting levels, glucose metabolic imaging with positron emission tomography identified an abnormal postischemic state, suggesting delayed cellular recovery from the acute ischemic insult. The persistence of augmented glucose utilization after transient ischemia may be the metabolic expression of "stunned myocardium" as proposed by Braunwald and Kloner,[B6] in which myocardial contractile function remains depressed for some time after relief of ischemia.

To determine whether myocardial segments with stress-induced perfusion defects exhibit augmented utilization of glucose remote from the episodes of exercise-induced ischemia, Yonekura and colleagues performed rest and stress nitrogen-13 ammonia perfusion studies and remote (within 1 week) fluorine-18 2-fluoro 2-deoxyglucose glucose metabolic studies in 26 patients with angiographically confirmed coronary artery disease.[Y1] Of the 26 individuals studied, 6 had single-vessel disease, 12 had double-vessel disease, and 6 had triple-vessel disease, as defined by a luminal diameter narrowing of 75 percent or greater on coronary angiography. Two patients with stenoses of less than 75 percent were considered to have significant lesions because of clinically documented myocardial infarctions in the corresponding vascular territories.

The resting nitrogen-13 ammonia studies revealed flow defects in 26 (52 percent) of the vascular territories supplied by significantly stenosed coronary arteries. In 20 of these 26 territories, the electrocardiogram indicated evidence of antecedent infarction. The other six regions were perfused by vessels with 90 to 100 percent stenoses. In the two regions perfused by vessels with mild stenoses and electrocardiographic evidence of prior infarction, no resting perfusion abnormalities were identified on the nitrogen-13 ammonia images.

Supine bicycle exercise failed to alter the nitrogen-13 ammonia perfusion defects in 13 (50 percent) of the regions with resting abnormalities, whereas there was further deterioration of relative perfusion with exercise in the other 13 regions. In addition, 13 regions with normal perfusion at rest exhibited stress-induced nitrogen-13 ammonia perfusion defects, including the two regions perfused by vessels with mild stenoses and electrocardiographic evidence of prior infarction and one region perfused by a circumflex artery with a 50 percent stenosis.

Evaluation of regional myocardial glucose metabolism at rest revealed augmented exogenous glucose utilization in 12 of the 13 (92.3 percent) regions with resting flow defects that became more severe with exercise (Fig. 67–13); 6 of the 13 (46.2 percent) regions with only stress-induced perfusion defects also exhibited augmented exogenous glucose utilization. Therefore, the results of this investigation suggest that a significant proportion of myocardial regions with stress-induced defects or with stress-induced deterioration of a resting perfusion exhibit abnormally increased exogenous glucose utilization at rest. Of further interest was the observation that 4 of the 13 (31 percent) regions with resting perfusion defects with no change in perfusion with exercise also exhibited augmented uptake of fluorine-18 2-fluoro 2-deoxyglucose. This observation indicates that a fixed perfusion defect is not synonymous with the absence of metabolic tissue viability (see later section, Metabolic Activity as a Clinical Indicator of Tissue Viability).

Figure 67–13. See Color Plate 18.

The relationship between segmental stress-induced perfusion abnormalities and resting glucose metabolism was examined by Fudo and colleagues in 22 patients with prior anterior infarction.[F2] The mean interval from infarction to positron emission tomography was 20 weeks (range: 5 to 80 weeks). Of 21 patients with coronary arteriography, 8 had single-vessel disease, 5 had double-vessel disease, 5 had triple-vessel disease, and 2 had less than 75 percent diameter stenosis of the anterior descending coronary arteries.

The resting nitrogen-13 ammonia perfusion images exhibited defects corresponding to the clinical infarct region in 19 (86 percent) of the patients. Three patients with non-Q wave infarctions did not have a resting perfusion abnormality. With supine bicycle exercise, 16 of the 22 (73 percent) patients exhibited

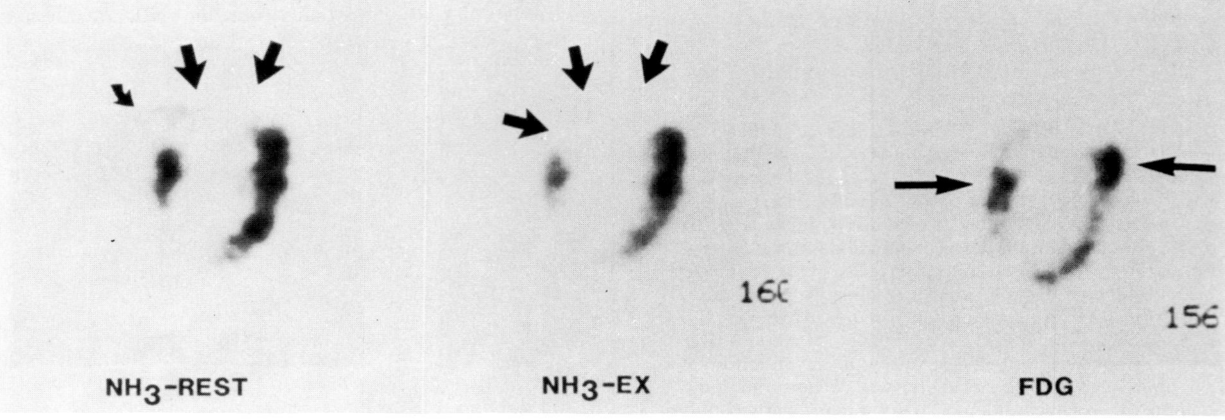

Figure 67–14. Rest (NH_3-REST) and stress (NH_3-EX) [^{13}N]ammonia perfusion and ^{18}F-2-fluoro 2-deoxyglucose metabolic (FDG) images from a 63-year-old man with a history of prior anterior infarction. The rest ^{13}N ammonia study demonstrates a perfusion defect involving the anteroseptal and anterolateral regions of the ventricle (*thick arrows*). With exercise, there is peripheral expansion of the resting perfusion defect (*thick arrows*). On the glucose metabolic study performed on a different day, there is enhanced uptake of ^{18}F-2-fluoro 2-deoxyglucose in the peripheral zones of perfusion defect expansion (*thin arrows*), indicating an abnormal postischemic metabolic state in the myocardium adjacent to the area of infarction. (From Fudo, T., Kambara, H., Hashimoto, T., et al.: F–18 deoxyglucose and stress N–13 ammonia positron emission tomography in anterior wall healed myocardial infarction. Am. J. Cardiol. 61:1191–1197, 1988).

peripheral expansion of a resting perfusion defect. Six of these sixteen patients exhibited augmented uptake of fluorine-18 2-fluoro 2-deoxyglucose in these peripheral zones on remote (within 1 week) metabolic imaging with positron emission tomography (Fig. 67–14), indicating that an altered myocardial metabolic state can be detected with positron emission tomography and fluorine-18 2-fluoro 2-deoxyglucose in the border zone in these patients with stress-induced expansion of their resting perfusion defects.

Of interest relative to these observations is the study of Thomassen and co-workers, in which low-dose intravenous glucose infusion had a beneficial effect on the pacing-induced anginal threshold in patients with coronary artery disease.[T1] These investigators assessed the time to the onset of angina and the extent of electrocardiographic ST segment depression during atrial pacing in nine patients with coronary artery disease, with and without intravenous glucose (350 mg/min). During atrial pacing, the administration of glucose significantly prolonged the time to the onset of angina (140 ± 24 versus 110 ± 24 seconds, $P < 0.05$) and decreased the extent of ST segment depression (0.9 ± 0.2 versus 1.8 ± 0.3 mm, $P < 0.01$). With glucose infusion, myocardial uptake of glucose increased by 100 percent while free fatty acid uptake fell by 50 percent. In addition, intravenous infusion of glucose prevented efflux of myocardial citrate during pacing, suggesting a glycogen-sparing effect. Thus, it is possible that the enhanced uptake of fluorine-18 2-fluoro 2-deoxyglucose in post-ischemic myocardium might represent cellular replenishment of glycogen stores that had become depleted during exercise-induced ischemia.

Araujo and associates recently examined regional myocardial perfusion and glucose metabolism in patients with unstable angina.[A2] The study population consisted of six normal volunteers, seven patients with chronic stable angina, and 22 patients with unstable angina. The diagnosis of unstable angina was based on a clinical history of a crescendo anginal pattern and the presence of electrocardiographic ST segment depression during chest pain. None of the individuals studied had evidence of recent infarction by serial plasma enzyme levels or by serial electrocardiography. Patients with stable angina were studied after discontinuing all medications for 48 hours. Patients with unstable angina were admitted to the coronary care unit and were treated with aspirin and, if necessary, sublingual nitrates. A 24-hour Holter monitor was performed immediately before positron emission tomography. Fractional myocardial uptake of rubidium-82 was calculated as described above, while an index of myocardial glucose utilization was obtained employing a modified Patlak graphical approach[P1] (see Chapter 65).

None of the patients with stable angina had chest pain or ST segment depression in the 24 hours prior to positron tomography. Of the 22 patients with unstable angina, 8 had angina with ST segment depression while 6 had angina without ST segment depression in the 24 hours prior to study. Five of these individuals had an episode of chest pain or ST segment depression within 2 hours of positron emission tomography.

Analysis of the positron emission tomographic images indicated similar mean fractional myocardial uptakes of rubidium-82 for patients with unstable angina (0.45 ± 0.07), normal volunteers (0.43 ± 0.09), and patients with stable angina (0.44 ± 0.06). In contrast, mean rates of myocardial glucose utilization were significantly higher in the patients with unstable angina (0.084 ± 0.047 μmol/ml/min) than in normals (0.012 ± 0.008 μmol/ml/min, $P < 0.001$) or in patients with stable angina (0.023 ± 0.32 μmol/ml/min, $P < 0.01$). It is important to note that the elevation in glucose utilization in the patients with unstable angina was diffuse rather than segmental in nature. The mean myocardial glucose utilization rate for patients with stable angina did not differ significantly from the mean rate for normals.

In order to assess differences in dietary state and in plasma substrate availability as possible explanations for their findings, the investigators determined plasma substrate levels and assessed rates of glucose utilization in skeletal muscle. Rates of glucose utilization in chest wall skeletal muscle were similar in the patients with unstable angina, in individuals with stable angina, and in the normal volunteers. Plasma glucose and insulin levels were similar in all three groups, indicating that differences in dietary state were unlikely to account for the observed differences in myocardial fluorine-18 2-fluoro 2-deoxyglucose uptake. Patients with chest pain or ST segment depression within 2 hours of positron emission tomography had myocardial glucose utilization rates that were similar to those of the patients without chest pain or ST segment depression immediately prior to imaging (0.085 ± 0.05 versus 0.078 ± 0.06 μmol/ml/min, P = NS), implying that there was no association between clinically identified episodes of myocardial ischemia and the metabolic findings on positron emission tomography.

Although the authors of this report postulated that the increased rates of myocardial glucose utilization observed in the patients with unstable angina might have reflected a prolonged metabolic derangement occurring as a result of multiple transient episodes of ischemia, it is unclear why a global increase in glucose myocardial utilization rates would be anticipated in patients with unstable angina, particularly in individuals with single-vessel disease. Because discrete regions of resting hypoperfusion were not identified on the rubidium-82 perfusion images, the investigators were unable to distinguish risk myocardium from normal myocardium. Thus, further studies of the metabolic abnormalities in individuals with unstable angina appear to be warranted, particularly in patients in whom a clearly defined risk zone can reliably be identified.

Synopsis

As predicted by animal experimental studies, both overall oxidative metabolism and fatty acid metabolism are depressed during acute ischemia in human myocardium. Both effects can be readily demonstrated as prolongation of the myocardial clearance rates of carbon-11 acetate and carbon-11 palmitate, respectively, in acutely ischemic myocardium. Studies with carbon-11 palmitate also demonstrate increased retention of carbon-11 activity in acutely ischemic myocardium, suggesting that a disproportionately greater fraction of the labeled fatty acid is deposited in the endogenous lipid pool. Other studies indicate that there is an increase in segmental glycolytic flux, as identified by a relative or absolute increase in fluorine-18 2-fluoro 2-deoxyglucose uptake on the positron tomographic metabolic images. An unexpected finding in these studies, however, was that increased glucose utilization may persist for some time after a single discrete ischemic event. This increase in glucose utilization may in fact represent a metabolic correlate to mechanical "stunning." From the available investigations, however, the length of time that such an abnormal metabolic state may persist is unknown. Although the observed increase in glucose utilization in normally perfused myocardial regions at rest suggests that such an abnormal metabolic state may exist for prolonged periods of time, the fact that the abnormal glucose uptake frequently occurs in regions with stress-induced perfusion defects raises the possibility that repeated episodes of acute ischemia alternating with "reperfusion" may result in a persistently abnormal metabolic state.

ACUTE MYOCARDIAL INFARCTION AND REPERFUSION

Acute myocardial infarction is a complex pathophysiologic process that typically begins with a disruption of myocardial blood flow, resulting in temporally and spatially inhomogeneous ischemia and cellular death.[R3, R4] A disruption of blood flow of sufficient severity and duration to cause cellular necrosis in one area of a vascular territory might also "stun," or produce transient myocardial mechanical dysfunction, in adjacent tissue.[B6, K1] In stunned tissue, myocardial blood flow is sufficient (either through collateral vessels or through "recanalization" of the occluded vessel) to maintain viability and prevent cellular death.[J1, R5] It is also possible that persistence or restoration of some degree of blood flow results in a state of myocardial "hibernation."

Because early coronary angiography in patients with acute myocardial infarction often reveals an occluded infarct artery,[D1] thrombolytic agents are being employed with increasing frequency in clinical practice in attempts to restore myocardial blood flow and limit myocardial infarct size. As such, assessment of the adequacy of reperfusion, whether occurring spontaneously[O3] or as a result of administration of thrombolytic agents,[G3, I1, K2, M3, N2, O4, S10, S11, V3, W1, W2] and determination of salvage of endangered myocardium in the clinical infarct zone are assuming increasingly important roles in clinical cardiology. Because it is difficult with routine tests to distinguish ischemically compromised tissue from that with irreversible injury early in the course of an infarction, the clinician may be unable to identify the patient with viable but jeopardized myocardium that could be salvaged by early intervention. Laboratory and clinical research efforts, therefore, have been directed at assessing the utility of metabolic imaging with positron emission tomography for identifying viable and therefore potentially salvageable tissue early in the course of an acute ischemic injury.

Experimental Basis for Metabolic Studies

Characterization of oxidative substrate metabolism in acutely injured tissue provides insights into the aerobic, energy-producing mitochondrial biochemical processes that are essential for recovery of mechanical function. It thus permits assessment of the beneficial or deleterious effects of restoration of blood flow. Although determination of the relative contributions of aerobic and anaerobic substrate metabolism to myocardial energy production in myocardium with ischemic injury is actively under investigation,[M4, S12] metabolic imaging with positron emission tomography is attractive because it offers noninvasive and quantitative assessment of regional tissue processes. In this way, both normal and ischemically injured tissue can be studied under identical neurohumoral and metabolic conditions. Observations made with these new techniques are likely to enhance our understanding of the pathophysiology of acute ischemic injury and reperfusion.

Evaluation of Fatty Acid Metabolism

One of the initial studies employing metabolic imaging with positron emission tomography to assess the severity of an acute ischemic injury was that of Bergmann and colleagues.[B7] These investigators sought to determine the beneficial effects of intracoronary thrombolysis on myocardial metabolism and the temporal dependence of these beneficial effects on the interval from coronary occlusion to reperfusion. A thrombus of the left anterior descending artery was induced in 23 closed-chest dogs by inserting a thrombogenic copper coil into the midportion of the vessel. Metabolic imaging with carbon-11 palmitate was performed 1 to 14 hours after coronary occlusion and was followed in 20 animals by intra-arterial administration of streptokinase. Three animals that did not receive streptokinase and three animals in which clot lysis could not be achieved served as controls; they had repeat imaging with carbon-11 palmitate between 1 and 6 hours following coronary occlusion. Clot lysis was achieved 1 to 2 hours after occlusion in 4 dogs, at 2 to 4 hours in 6 dogs, at 4 to 6 hours in 4 dogs, and at 12 to 14 hours in 3 dogs. Patency of the vessel was documented by repeat coronary angiography. A second carbon-11 palmitate study was then performed following successful lysis of the thrombus.

Prior to thrombolysis, each animal exhibited discrete defects in uptake of carbon-11 palmitate in the "infarct zone." In the control animals, no significant change in the extent and severity of the defect in carbon-11 palmitate uptake was noted on the second study. In the animals with successful thrombolysis, improvement in carbon-11 palmitate uptake on visual analysis depended highly on the duration of the arterial occlusion prior to reperfusion. Some of the visual carbon-11 palmitate defects did improve on the postreperfusion studies, primarily in the subepicardial regions and in the lateral borders of the initial defect. In general, longer intervals of arterial occlusion were associated with persistence of rather than improvement in the carbon-11 palmitate defects.

On quantitative analysis of carbon-11 palmitate defect size, animals with successful reperfusion within 4 hours of coronary occlusion had significant decreases in the percent of jeopardized myocardium on positron emission tomography (24.6 ± 3.8 percent versus 12.0 ± 2.3 percent for the 1- to 2-hour group and 25.7 ± 2.8 percent versus 20.3 ± 2.3 percent for the 2- to 4-hour group; $P < 0.01$ for both). In contrast, no significant change was noted in the animals in which reperfusion was achieved later than 4 hours after occlusion of the infarct vessel (24.7 ± 3.2 percent versus 21.6 ± 4.0 percent for the 4- to 6-hour group and 23.9 ± 3.1 percent versus 24.5 ± 3.7 percent for the 12- to 14-hour group; P = NS for both). Changes in the severity of the carbon-11 palmitate defects were similar. In animals with reperfusion less than 4 hours after coronary occlusion, there was a significant improvement in relative carbon-11 activity in the infarct zone (30.1 ± 2.6 percent versus 61.8 ± 4.6 percent for the 1- to 2-hour group and 39.1 ± 2.8 percent versus 55.6 ± 5.0 percent for the 2- to 4-hour group; $P < 0.01$ for both groups). In contrast, no significant improvement occurred in the animals with reperfusion later than 4 hours after coronary occlusion (28.2 ± 2.8 percent versus 37.6 ± 6.2 percent for the 4- to 6-hour group and 31.3 ± 3.9 percent versus 33.8 ± 1.6 percent for the 12- to 14-hour group; P = NS for both groups). Perhaps more importantly, these investigators noted that neither diminution in the size of the jeopardized zones nor increase in metabolic activity in these same regions could be successfully predicted from the electrocardiographic evolution of the infarction. Thus, these observations demonstrate that thrombolysis achieved less than 4 hours after coronary occlusion has a beneficial effect on myocardial uptake of carbon-11 palmitate in the infarct regions and that improvement in the carbon-11 palmitate metabolic images could not be successfully predicted by evolutionary changes on the electrocardiogram.

Schwaiger and colleagues compared the myocardial tissue kinetics of carbon-11 palmitate in reperfused myocardium with those in nonreperfused myocardium in an open-chest canine preparation.[S13] In six animals, the left anterior descending artery was permanently occluded by ligation of the vessel distal to the first diagonal branch. Following serial intra-arterial injections of carbon-11 palmitate, time activity curves were recorded in risk myocardium with a scintillation detector at baseline and 40, 110, and 200 minutes after coronary occlusion. Ten animals were subjected to a 20-minute occlusion of the vessel, followed by reperfusion. Serial time activity curves were recorded in risk myocardium in these animals in a similar fashion at control and 20, 90, and 180 minutes after release of the coronary artery ligature. The stability of the preparation and the reproducibility of the carbon-11 palmitate kinetic analyses were assessed by determination of serial time activity curves in six control animals.

In the six control animals, heart rate, blood pressure, and microsphere blood flow measurements were stable over the 300-minute study period. In the six animals with permanent occlusion of the left anterior descending artery, heart rate and blood pressure following ligature of the vessel did not differ significantly from control values, while blood flow decreased to 29.4 percent of control in the epicardium and 10.7 percent of control in the endocardium. In the ten animals with 20-minute arterial occlusions, heart rate and blood pressure did not differ significantly from control values throughout the study period. During coronary occlusion, blood flows in risk myocardium decreased to 30.1 percent of control values in the epicardium and 16.3 percent of control in the endocardium. Following reperfusion, however, both epicardial and endocardial blood flows returned to baseline values. In each group of animals, therefore, the cardiac workload (as estimated from the rate-pressure product) did not change over the course of the experiment. In addition, arterial levels of glucose, free fatty acids, and lactate remained constant except for a transient moderate increase in lactate concentrations in the early reperfusion period in the animals with the transient arterial occlusions. Thus, intergroup differences in the myocardial kinetics of carbon-11 palmitate could not be explained by differences in cardiac workload or by a variation in plasma substrate levels.

Analysis of myocardial carbon-11 palmitate kinetics in the six control dogs revealed that the initial capillary transit retention fraction and clearance half-times of carbon-11 palmitate, as well as the relative sizes of both the early and late phases of the myocardial carbon-11 time activity curves, remained constant over the 5-hour study interval. In the animals with permanent coronary artery occlusion, clearance half-times of carbon-11 palmitate were significantly longer (5.9 ± 1.9 min versus 3.7 ± 0.8 min, $P < 0.05$), and the relative sizes of the early rapid phase were markedly smaller (22.6 ± 4.9 percent versus 52.4 ± 9.4 percent, $P < 0.05$), indicating an impairment in fatty acid oxidation and a relative decrease in the amount of substrate entering oxidative pathways in the zone of ischemic injury. The observed changes in carbon-11 palmitate half-times and the relative sizes of the early rapid phase persisted throughout the study interval. In the animals subjected to transient arterial occlusions, clearance half-times of the rapid phase increased significantly after 20 minutes of reperfusion (7.1 ± 2.5 min versus 4.8 ± 1.1 min, $P < 0.05$) and remained prolonged even after 180 minutes of reperfusion (8.7 ± 2.4 min, $P < 0.05$ as compared with control). Although the relative size of the early rapid phase was significantly depressed after 20 minutes of reperfusion (39.6 ± 9.5 percent versus 57.7 ± 9.2 percent, $P < 0.05$ as compared with control values), the relative size of the rapid phase gradually recovered with time and was similar to control values by 180 minutes after reperfusion (49.6 ± 9.6 percent versus 57.7 ± 9.2 percent, P = NS).

Assessment of segmental shortening was performed with ultrasonic crystals in six of the animals with transient coronary occlusions. There was a significant deterioration in the percent fractional shortening (−2.6 ± 3.2 percent versus 15.1 ± 4.9 percent, $P < 0.05$) and a significant increase in the end diastolic length (12.8 ± 3.2 mm versus 14.1 ± 3.8 mm, $P < 0.05$) during coronary occlusion. At the end of the reperfusion period, however, both the percent fractional shortening and the end diastolic length did not differ significantly from control values (5.9 ± 3.7 percent and 13.4 ± 3.7 mm, respectively; P = NS for both as compared with control). In aggregate, these data indicate that improvement in the relative size of the early rapid phase paralleled functional recovery in the risk zone. Because carbon-11 palmitate clearance half-times in the early rapid phase did not improve with reperfusion (perhaps as a result of spatial and temporal inhomogeneity in the degree of ischemia or in the degree of back-diffusion of carbon-11 palmitate), the investigators suggested that the proportion of carbon-11 palmitate entering the endogenous lipid pool relative to that entering oxidative metabolic pathways might be a better index of metabolic recovery in reperfused myocardium.

Knabb and colleagues assessed the utility of positron emission tomography with oxygen-15 water and carbon-11 palmitate to predict recovery of myocardial oxidative metabolism in canine preparations in which a coronary thrombosis was induced by lodging a copper coil in the anterior descending artery.[K3] Four control animals were untreated, while six dogs received either intracoronary streptokinase or intravenous recombinant tissue-type plasminogen activator 2 hours after coronary occlusion. Reperfusion was confirmed in these animals by coronary angiography immediately following positron tomographic imaging, and persistence of vessel patency was documented by repeat angiography at 24 hours and at 4 weeks. Positron emission tomography was performed in all animals 90 minutes, 24 hours, and 4 weeks after angiographically documented occlusion of the anterior descending artery. In addition, positron emission tomography was performed 1 hour, 1 week, and 2 weeks following reperfusion in the dogs treated with thrombolytic agents. Thrombolytic therapy resulted in successful recanalization of the anterior descending artery within 45 minutes of the administration of the agent, and the recanalized vessels were patent in each animal on repeat angiography at 24 hours and at 4 weeks. In contrast, none of the animals in the control group had evidence of spontaneous reperfusion on follow-up coronary angiography.

During occlusion of the anterior descending coronary artery, blood flows in the risk zones in both the experimental and control groups were reduced to 15 ± 8 percent and 11 ± 7 percent of normal, respectively, as indicated by the oxygen-15 water studies. Following reperfusion, there was an early increase in blood flows in the risk zone of the thrombolysis group to 82 ± 25 percent ($P < 0.001$ as compared to occlusion), which was followed by a decline to 37 ± 16 percent at 24 hours ($P < 0.01$ as compared to reperfusion). Blood flow in the risk zones in the thrombolytic group increased again to 66 ± 11 percent at 1 week and remained unchanged at 4 weeks at 64 ± 18 percent. The pattern of reduction of flow with occlusion, restoration with reperfusion, decline at 24 hours, and gradual increase by 1 week was consistently observed in each of the six animals in the thrombolysis group. In the untreated animals, relative blood flows remained decreased at 13 ± 5 percent at 24 hours and increased significantly to 42 ± 16 percent at 4 weeks despite the presence of angiographically confirmed occlusion of the vessel, possibly as a result of the development of collateral blood flow. Thus in this canine model of 2-hour arterial occlusion followed by reperfusion, there was an initial improvement in risk myocardial blood flow after successful coronary thrombolysis. The initial improvement in perfusion was then followed by a decline in blood flow at 24 hours. Blood flow improved to 66 percent of normal at 1 week and remained depressed at this level on repeat study at 4 weeks. Perhaps more importantly, neither relative reductions in blood flow during occlusion in the risk zones nor those 1 hour after reperfusion correlated significantly with carbon-11 palmitate uptake at 4 weeks in the thrombolysis group. This suggests that early assessment of myocardial perfusion alone does not predict the extent of long-term recovery of myocardial fatty acid metabolism.

These investigators also correlated uptake of carbon-11 palmitate in risk myocardium at 4 weeks with uptake of the tracer early after thrombolysis. During coronary occlusion, uptake of carbon-11 palmitate in the risk zones was 32 ± 15 percent of normal in the thrombolysis group and 24 ± 14 percent in the control group. Upon reperfusion in the thrombolysis group, carbon-11 palmitate uptake transiently increased to 67 ± 22 percent in the risk zone ($P < 0.01$) but declined again to 36 ± 10 percent at 24 hours ($P < 0.02$ as compared with reperfusion; P = NS as compared with occlusion). By 1 week, carbon-11 palmitate uptake had increased to 64 ± 14 percent of normal, while over the next 3 weeks mean carbon-11 palmitate uptake declined to 45 ± 16 percent (attributed to a decline to 2 percent of normal in one animal). In the control animals, mean carbon-11 palmitate uptake remained depressed at 27 ± 9 percent at 24 hours and at 16 ± 12 percent at 4 weeks, indicating that tracer uptake remained depressed in this group despite the significant improvement in regional blood flow as determined by the oxygen-15 water studies. Thus, regional carbon-11 palmitate uptake appeared to recover more slowly and less consistently than myocardial perfusion. In contrast to assessment of myocardial perfusion, however, relative carbon-11 palmitate uptake 1 hour after reperfusion correlated significantly with carbon-11 palmitate activity at 4 weeks (r = 0.86, $P < 0.03$), implying that the extent of metabolic recovery following an acute infarction is more successfully predicted by early assessment of carbon-11 palmitate activity than assessment of myocardial perfusion. Unfortunately, these investigators did not compare the relative uptake of carbon-11 palmitate with histopathologic analyses of myocardium in the risk zone.

Schwaiger and associates assessed the temporal relationship between recovery of regional wall motion and myocardial metabolism in chronically instrumented dogs with reperfusion after a 3-hour balloon occlusion of the left anterior descending coronary artery.[S14] Before the ischemic insult, each of the animals underwent a baseline positron emission tomographic study with nitrogen-13 ammonia in order to ascertain that myocardial perfusion was homogeneous. Two to three days later, the left anterior descending coronary artery was occluded for 3 hours with a Fogarty catheter. Positron emission tomography with nitrogen-13 ammonia and carbon-11 palmitate was performed during occlusion of the vessel. After the intracoronary balloon was deflated, imaging with positron emission tomography and nitrogen-13 ammonia and carbon-11 palmitate was repeated (12 dogs). Serial positron emission tomographic studies were then performed at 24 hours (10 dogs), 1 week (8 dogs), and approximately 4 weeks (7 dogs), using nitrogen-13 ammonia, carbon-11 palmitate, and fluorine-18 2-fluoro 2-deoxyglucose. The imaging data were compared with regional microsphere blood flow measurements, segmental function as determined by ultrasonomicrometry, and with the histopathologic findings at the time of sacrifice at 4 weeks.

During occlusion, blood flows (Fig. 67–15) decreased to 24 ± 11 percent of control values (0.31 ± 0.15 versus 1.38 ± 0.52 ml/min/g, $P < 0.01$). Following reperfusion, blood flows increased to 78 ± 41 percent of control (1.01 ± 0.52 ml/min/g) at 2 hours and to 80 ± 51 percent of normal myocardium (1.02 ± 0.66 ml/min/g) at 24 hours. By 1 week, blood flows in risk myocardium no longer differed from those in normal myocardium (1.20 ± 0.65 versus 1.42 ± 0.35 ml/min/g at 1 week and 1.01 ± 0.69 versus 1.25 ± 0.37 ml/min/g at 4 weeks, respectively; P = NS for both).

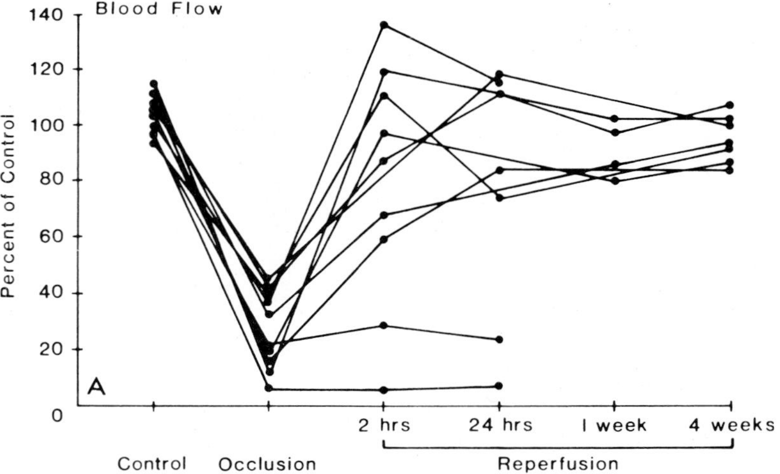

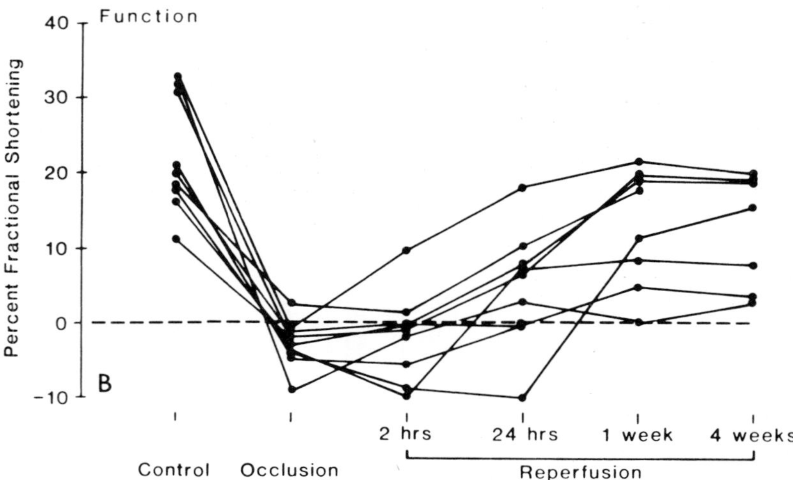

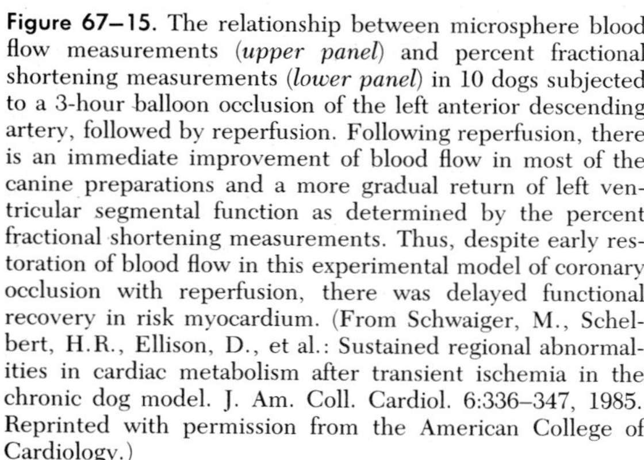

Figure 67–15. The relationship between microsphere blood flow measurements (*upper panel*) and percent fractional shortening measurements (*lower panel*) in 10 dogs subjected to a 3-hour balloon occlusion of the left anterior descending artery, followed by reperfusion. Following reperfusion, there is an immediate improvement of blood flow in most of the canine preparations and a more gradual return of left ventricular segmental function as determined by the percent fractional shortening measurements. Thus, despite early restoration of blood flow in this experimental model of coronary occlusion with reperfusion, there was delayed functional recovery in risk myocardium. (From Schwaiger, M., Schelbert, H.R., Ellison, D., et al.: Sustained regional abnormalities in cardiac metabolism after transient ischemia in the chronic dog model. J. Am. Coll. Cardiol. 6:336–347, 1985. Reprinted with permission from the American College of Cardiology.)

During occlusion, the percent systolic fractional shortening in risk myocardium (Fig. 67–15) decreased (−2.7 ± 3.7 percent versus 22.4 ± 8.5 percent, $P < 0.01$), while the end diastolic length increased (12.8 ± 2.7 versus 10.8 ± 2.4 mm, $P < 0.05$). Regional function remained abnormal 2 hours and 24 hours following reperfusion and recovered slowly over the ensuing 4 weeks. By 4 weeks, regional fractional shortening had returned to 56 percent of baseline values (12.6 ± 7.5 percent, $P < 0.05$), while end-diastolic length was normal (10.2 ± 1.8 mm, P = NS). Thus, despite normalization of blood flow by 1 week, regional function in risk myocardium improved only gradually over the 4 weeks following reperfusion. However, the researchers did observe a considerable variation in the degree of functional recovery among animals.

On positron emission tomography, relative nitrogen-13 ammonia activity decreased to 31.8 ± 10.6 percent of control values in the risk region during occlusion of the anterior descending artery. This was paralleled by a relative decrease in carbon-11 palmitate uptake to 36.0 ± 11 percent of normal values. Two hours following reperfusion, relative nitrogen-13 ammonia activity increased to 57 ± 18 percent of control values, and this was accompanied by an increase in carbon-11 palmitate uptake to 54 ± 26 percent of control values. By 4 weeks, both relative nitrogen-13 ammonia activity and carbon-11 palmitate activity in risk myocardium had returned to normal values (83 ± 21 percent and 76 ± 16 percent, respectively; P = NS for both). In general, ratios of nitrogen-13 ammonia activity in risk relative to control myocardium were paralleled by similar carbon-11 palmitate ratios (Fig. 67–16), indicating the dependence of initial carbon-11 palmitate uptake on myocardial blood flow.

Clearance half-times for carbon-11 palmitate were 36.0 ± 15.9 minutes in the ischemic segment during coronary occlusion, compared with 10.8 ± 3.6 minutes in control myocardium ($P < 0.05$). Two hours following reperfusion, carbon-11 clearance half-times increased further to 84.7 ± 102 minutes in the risk zone, compared with 15.1 ± 6.6 minutes in control myocardium ($P < 0.05$). Thus, despite an increase in myocardial blood flow and in the initial uptake of carbon-11 palmitate in acutely reperfused tissue, analysis of carbon-11 palmitate tissue kinetics demonstrated that oxidative substrate metabolism was even more profoundly impaired than during coronary occlusion. Similar findings were noted on the 24-hour studies. Uptake of carbon-11 palmitate was 56 ± 31 percent of control values, while clearance half-times of carbon-11 palmitate were markedly prolonged at 124.4 ± 149 minutes (Fig. 67–17). By 4 weeks, uptake of carbon-11 palmitate in risk myocardium did not differ significantly from that in control myocardium (76 ± 16 percent, P = NS), and clearance half-times of carbon-11 palmitate were no longer significantly prolonged (24.7 ± 9.9 versus 17.2 ± 4.1 minutes in normal myocardium, P = NS), indicating that fatty acid oxidation was no longer impaired in risk myocardium.

During occlusion of the artery, the percent of remaining carbon-11 activity in risk myocardium was 76.5 ± 13.5 percent, compared with 38.0 ± 8.5 percent in control regions ($P < 0.05$), implying that the relative proportion of labeled fatty acid entering nonoxidative metabolic pathways had increased in response to the ischemic insult. Similarly, the percent of remaining carbon-11 activity 2 hours following reperfusion was 82.8 ± 9.9 percent in ischemic regions, compared with 43.9 ± 11.9 percent in normal myocardium ($P < 0.05$). The percent of remaining carbon-11 activity remained abnormal relative to control myocardium until the 4-week study (see Fig. 67–15), indicating that the relative proportion of fatty acids entering nonoxidative pathways remained elevated for a prolonged period of time following the acute ischemic injury.

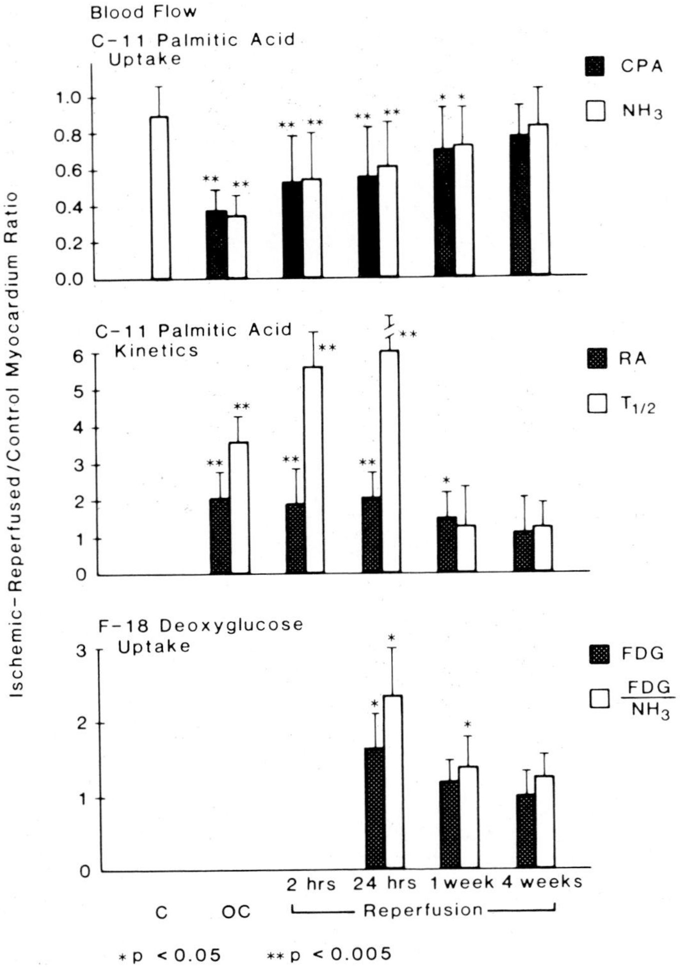

Figure 67–16. For the animal experiments illustrated in Figure 67–15, the relationship between myocardial metabolism and perfusion under control conditions (C), during a 3-hour balloon occlusion (OC) of the left anterior descending artery, and following reperfusion is shown. The top graph illustrates the uptake of ^{11}C-palmitic acid (CPA) and [^{13}N]ammonia (NH_3) in risk myocardium relative to control myocardium at each of the time points indicated. For each of the determinations, uptake of [^{13}N]ammonia is paralleled by that of ^{11}C palmitate, indicating the dependence of the early myocardial concentration of this tracer on blood flow. In the middle graph are displayed the clearance half-times (T½) of ^{11}C palmitate and residual ^{11}C activity (RA) at the corresponding times. During occlusion and for the first 24 hours thereafter, ^{11}C clearance half-times are markedly prolonged and there is an increase in residual myocardial ^{11}C activity. Thus, the ^{11}C-palmitate studies indicate impaired fatty acid oxidation and an increase in the relative proportion of label entering the endogenous lipid pool. At 1 week, ^{11}C clearance half-times do not differ significantly from those in normal myocardium, whereas the residual ^{11}C myocardial activity does not fully normalize until 4 weeks after reperfusion. The bottom graph displays the uptake of ^{18}F 2-fluoro 2-deoxyglucose and the ratio of ^{18}F 2-fluoro 2-deoxyglucose to [^{13}N]ammonia activity in risk myocardium relative to normal tissue. Uptake of ^{18}F 2-fluoro 2-deoxyglucose in risk myocardium is elevated relative to control values at 24 hours. Ratios of ^{18}F 2-fluoro 2-deoxyglucose to [^{13}N]ammonia activity are elevated at 1 week, normalizing only in the studies performed 4 weeks following reperfusion. Despite restoration of blood flow, sustained metabolic abnormalities in both fatty acid oxidation and glucose metabolism were identified with positron emission tomography in risk myocardium, paralleling the delayed recovery in segmental percent fractional shortening (Fig. 67–15). (From Schwaiger, M., Schelbert, H.R., Ellison, D., et al.: Sustained regional abnormalities in cardiac metabolism after transient ischemia in the chronic dog model. J. Am. Coll. Cardiol. 6:336–347, 1985. Reprinted with permission from the American College of Cardiology.)

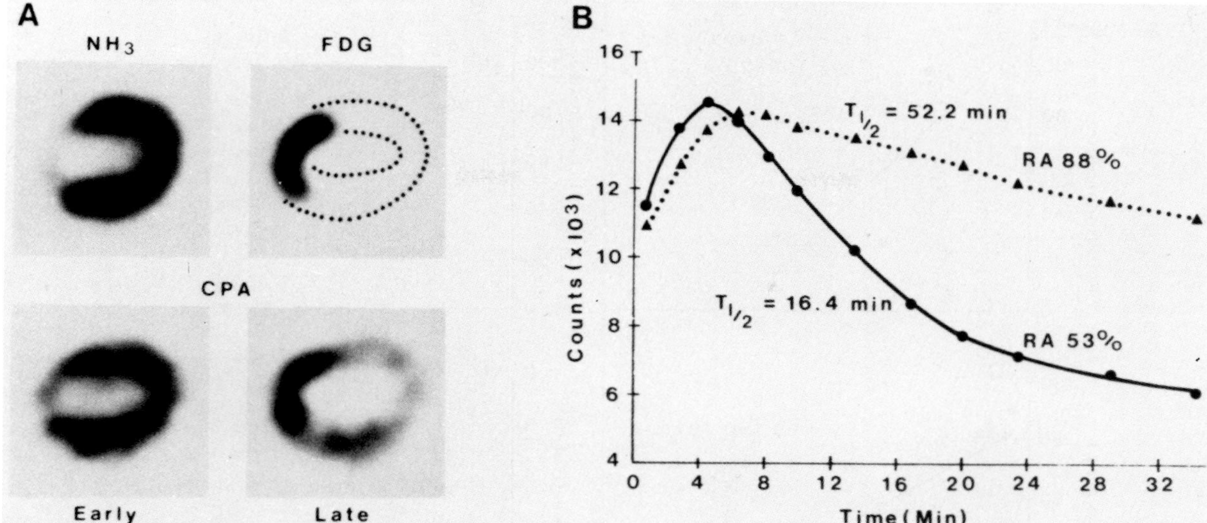

Figure 67–17. *Panel A*, Representative cross-sectional positron emission tomographic images in a canine model of acute ischemia with reperfusion. The images were obtained 24 hours after reperfusion following a 3-hour balloon occlusion of the left anterior descending artery. On the [^{13}N]ammonia (NH_3) perfusion image a defect is identified in the anterior region of the ventricle. On the ^{18}F 2-fluoro 2-deoxyglucose (FDG) metabolic image, there is augmented uptake of the labeled tracer of glucose metabolism in the hypoperfused anterior wall. The dots indicate normally perfused myocardium, which exhibits little uptake of the glucose analog owing to preferential utilization of free fatty acids in the fasting state. On the early ^{11}C-palmitate (CPA) image, there is an anterior defect that corresponds closely to the defect identified on the [^{13}N]ammonia perfusion image, indicating the dependency of the initial myocardial uptake of ^{11}C-palmitate on blood flow. On the late ^{11}C-palmitate image, there is retention of activity in the anterior region of the ventricle, indicating the delay in clearance of the radiolabel characteristic of impaired fatty acid metabolism. *Panel B*, Regional myocardial ^{11}C time activity curves from normal (*solid curve*) and reperfused (*dotted curve*) myocardium. As compared with normal myocardium, uptake of the labeled fatty acid is depressed and there is a slower clearance half-time (T½) and a higher residual activity (RA) at 20 minutes. The ^{11}C-palmitate study demonstrates impaired uptake and oxidation of the labeled fatty acid in reperfused myocardium and an increase in the relative proportion of label entering the endogenous lipid pool. Thus, the myocardium exhibits an abnormal metabolic state despite successful restoration of blood flow 24 hours prior to the study. (From Schwaiger, M., Schelbert, H.R., Ellison, D., et al.: Sustained regional abnormalities in cardiac metabolism after transient ischemia in the chronic dog model. J. Am. Coll. Cardiol. 6:336–347, 1985. Reprinted with permission from the American College of Cardiology.)

Analysis of myocardial fluorine-18 2-fluoro 2-deoxyglucose uptake on the 24-hour studies revealed that risk myocardium accumulated 1.49 ± 0.62 times more tracer than control myocardium (see Fig. 67–15). By 1 week, this relative uptake of fluorine-18 2-fluoro 2-deoxyglucose in risk myocardium had decreased to 1.2 ± 0.5 times that of control tissue (P = NS). However, when uptake of fluorine-18 2-fluoro 2-deoxyglucose was normalized for tracer delivery by dividing by nitrogen-13 ammonia counts, the highest measured ratios in risk myocardium relative to control tissue occurred at 24 hours (2.27 ± 1.4, $P < 0.05$), and these ratios remained abnormal even on the study at 1 week (1.6 ± 0.07, $P < 0.05$). By 4 weeks, ratios of fluorine-18 2-fluoro 2-deoxyglucose/nitrogen-13 ammonia counts had normalized in risk myocardium (1.22 ± 0.4, P = NS). In conjunction with the impairment in oxidative substrate metabolism demonstrated on the carbon-11 palmitate studies, the augmented uptake of fluorine-18 2-fluoro 2-deoxyglucose relative to blood flow is consistent with an accelerated rate of anaerobic glycolysis in the ischemically injured tissue.

When these workers correlated the histopathologic extent of tissue necrosis in individual animals with the relative degree of functional recovery in the risk myocardial segments, a statistically significant inverse linear relationship (Fig. 67–18) was identified (r = 0.79). Furthermore, uptake of both carbon-11 palmitate and nitrogen-13 ammonia (Fig. 67–18) 2 hours after reperfusion correlated closely with the extent of tissue necrosis on postmortem examination (r = 0.93 and r = 0.86, respectively). In contrast, uptake of fluorine-18 2-fluoro 2-deoxyglucose (Fig. 67–18) correlated only weakly with the amount of tissue necrosis (r = 0.52). Of the seven animals surviving to 4 weeks, three revealed virtually no recovery of function in the reperfused risk zone. Relative systolic fractional shortening averaged only 22 ± 11 percent of the preocclusion values. In these three animals the average percent necrosis was 37 ± 10 percent in the risk zones (Fig. 67–19). In the remaining four animals, regional function in risk myocardium improved to 90 ± 21 percent of control values. In these animals, the average percent necrosis was only 8 ± 3 percent (Fig. 67–20).

Thus, these observations imply that regional recovery of contractile function occurs gradually following an acute ischemic injury and indicate that improvement in function occurs in parallel with normalization of exogenous glucose utilization and recovery of oxidative metabolism. Characterization of the myocardium in the risk zone with positron emission tomography early in the course of the ischemic injury is helpful in predicting the eventual degree of recovery of regional function. Extensive tissue necrosis resulting from an acute ischemic injury is characterized on early positron emission tomographic imaging by markedly depressed blood flow, poor uptake, and prolonged myocardial clearance of carbon-11 palmitate and reduced fluorine-18 2-fluoro 2-deoxyglucose uptake. In contrast, viable but "stunned" myocardium is characterized by relative preservation of carbon-11 palmitate uptake and delayed tissue clearance of carbon-11 activity, and by enhanced utilization of fluorine-18 2-fluoro 2-deoxyglucose, indicating the utility of metabolic imaging with positron emission tomography early in the course of an ischemic injury for identifying viable but functionally impaired tissue in the clinical infarct zone.

Evaluation of Oxidative Metabolism

A preliminary report by Brown and associates compared the relative effects of an acute ischemic insult with reperfusion on the myocardial clearance of carbon-11 palmitate and carbon-11 acetate.[B8] As noted (Acute Myocardial Ischemia Experimental Studies: Oxidative Metabolism), a decrease in tissue oxygen delivery impairs myocardial fatty acid utilization at several loci, suggesting that the tissue clearance of a labeled fatty acid such as carbon-11 palmitate might be more severely affected by an acute ischemic insult than that of a "pure" tracer of oxidative flux like carbon-11 acetate. Thus, the purpose of the study of Brown and cohorts was to test the hypothesis that an acute ischemic injury might have a differential effect on the tissue clearance of

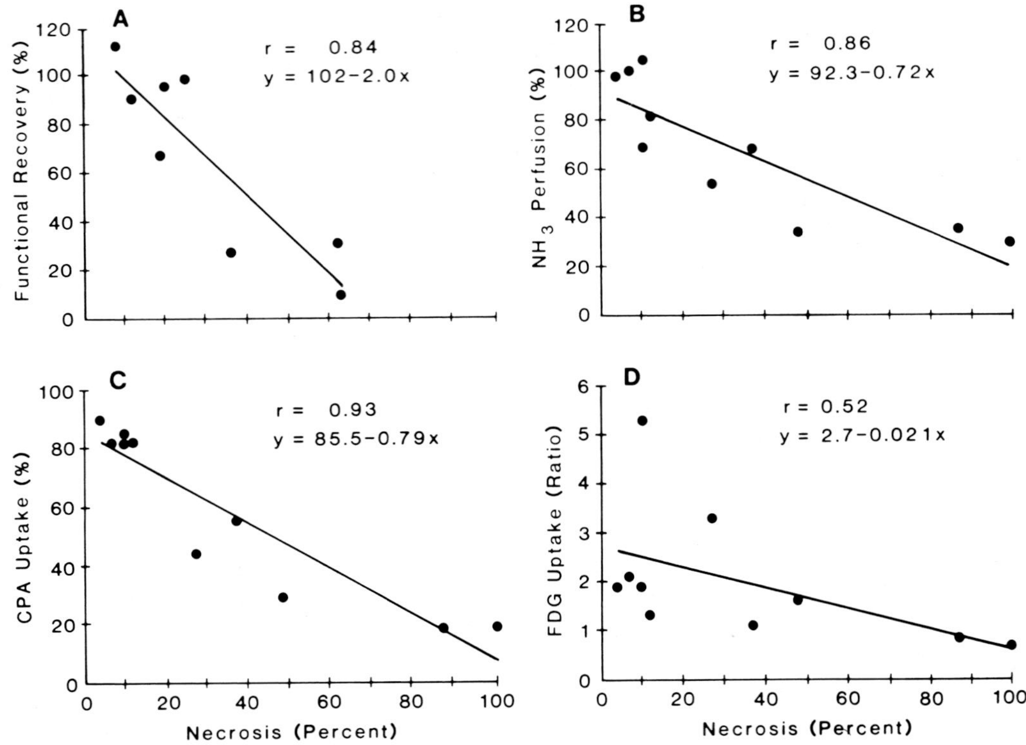

Figure 67–18. *Panel A,* Relationship between the extent of functional recovery and the histologic percent tissue necrosis in reperfused canine myocardium. *Panels B, C,* and *D,* Relationship between relative myocardial update of [^{13}N]ammonia (NH_3), ^{11}C-palmitic acid (CPA), and ^{18}F–2-fluoro 2-deoxyglucose (FDG) and percent tissue necrosis in reperfused canine myocardium. In this animal model, incorporating a 3-hour balloon occlusion of the left anterior descending artery followed by reperfusion, the extent of functional recovery was inversely related to the histologic percent of myocardial necrosis. Although there are strong and statistically significant inverse relationships between the myocardial update of [^{13}N]ammonia and the uptake of ^{11}C-palmitic acid and the percent tissue necrosis, the relationship between myocardial update of ^{18}F–2-fluoro 2-deoxyglucose and the percent myocardial necrosis is less pronounced. (From Schwaiger, M., Schelbert, H.R., Ellison, D., et al.: Sustained regional abnormalities in cardiac metabolism after transient ischemia in the chronic dog model. J. Am. Coll. Cardiol. 6:336–347, 1985. Reprinted with permission from the American College of Cardiology.)

carbon-11 palmitate, compared with that of carbon-11 acetate. In five dogs subjected to 1-hour occlusions of the anterior descending artery, the risk zone was delineated by imaging with oxygen-15 water during the period of occlusion. Following reperfusion, flow in the risk zone increased to 138 ± 47 percent that of normal tissue. Dynamic imaging with carbon-11 palmitate and carbon-11 acetate was then performed in random order. In normal myocardium, the initial carbon-11 clearance half-times for carbon-11 palmitate were 10.2 ± 7.3 minutes, while those for carbon-11 acetate were 4.4 ± 1.8 minutes. For risk myocardium, carbon-11 clearance half-times were 39.4 ± 23.9 minutes for carbon-11 palmitate (3.9 times that of normal myocardium) and 10.8 ± 2.9 minutes for carbon-11 acetate (2.4 times that of normal myocardium). Thus, while impaired oxidative substrate metabolism clearly could be identified with either tracer, the relative magnitude of the observed abnormality was nearly 63 percent greater on the carbon-11 palmitate study, consistent with previous reports indicating that acute ischemia may depress myocardial handling of fatty acids at several points in their metabolic pathway.[L1]

Buxton and colleagues used positron emission tomography to assess both aerobic and anaerobic metabolism in reperfused canine myocardium.[B9] Dynamic imaging with carbon-11 acetate and fluorine-18 2-fluoro 2-deoxyglucose was performed 2 and 24 hours following reperfusion in 11 closed-chest dogs subjected to a 20-minute balloon occlusion of the anterior descending artery. Regional function was determined simultaneously in ten animals with two-dimensional echocardiography. Following completion of the 24-hour studies, tissue slices were obtained for triphenyltetrazolium chloride (TTC) staining and for well counting.

For both the 2- and 24-hour imaging studies, heart rate (117 ± 32 versus 149 ± 30 beats/min, P = NS), systolic blood blood pressure (152 ± 13 versus 153 ± 31 mmHg, P = NS), and rate pressure product (18,452 ± 5773 versus 22,191 ± 2076 beats • mmHg/min, P = NS) were similar, indicating a comparable cardiac workload. Plasma glucose and lactate levels were similar for both the 2-hour and the 24-hour studies (5.4 ± 0.5 versus 5.5 ± 0.5 mM glucose and 1.0 ± 0.4 versus 0.7 ± 0.3 mM lactate; P = NS for both). However, free fatty acid levels were significantly higher at the time of the 24-hour study, compared with the 2-hour study (0.5 ± 0.3 versus 0.1 ± 0.1 mEq/L, $P < 0.001$), presumably as a result of prolonged fasting.

During coronary occlusion, blood flows in risk myocardium averaged 25 ± 24 percent of those in control myocardium ($P < 0.001$). By 24 hours, myocardial blood flow had increased to 86 ± 16 percent and no longer differed significantly from that in normal myocardium. With coronary occlusion, each of the animals exhibited an anterior wall motion abnormality ranging in severity from mild hypokinesis to akinesis. Following reperfusion, there was no immediate change in regional wall motion score in the risk zone, but by 24 hours the average wall motion score did not differ significantly from the mean baseline value. However, regional wall motion abnormalities were still present in six of the ten animals. On staining with triphenyltetrazolium chloride (TTC), none of the animals exhibited gross regions of myocardial infarction.

Dynamic imaging with positron emission tomography and carbon-11 acetate revealed the characteristic biexponential clearance of carbon-11 activity from both normal and reperfused myocardium. On the images obtained 2 hours following reperfusion, the initial uptake of carbon-11 acetate in reperfused sectors was 95 ± 5 percent of that in control sectors. When the clearance constant, k_1, in the risk sectors was normalized to the mean k_1 for control myocardium, it averaged 69 ± 15 percent ($P < 0.001$), indicating a marked impairment in oxidative metabolism in the reperfused tissue.

At 24 hours, uptake of carbon-11 acetate in the risk zone was 107 ± 16 percent of that in control myocardium (P = NS). In contrast, average tissue clearance rate constants in the risk zone

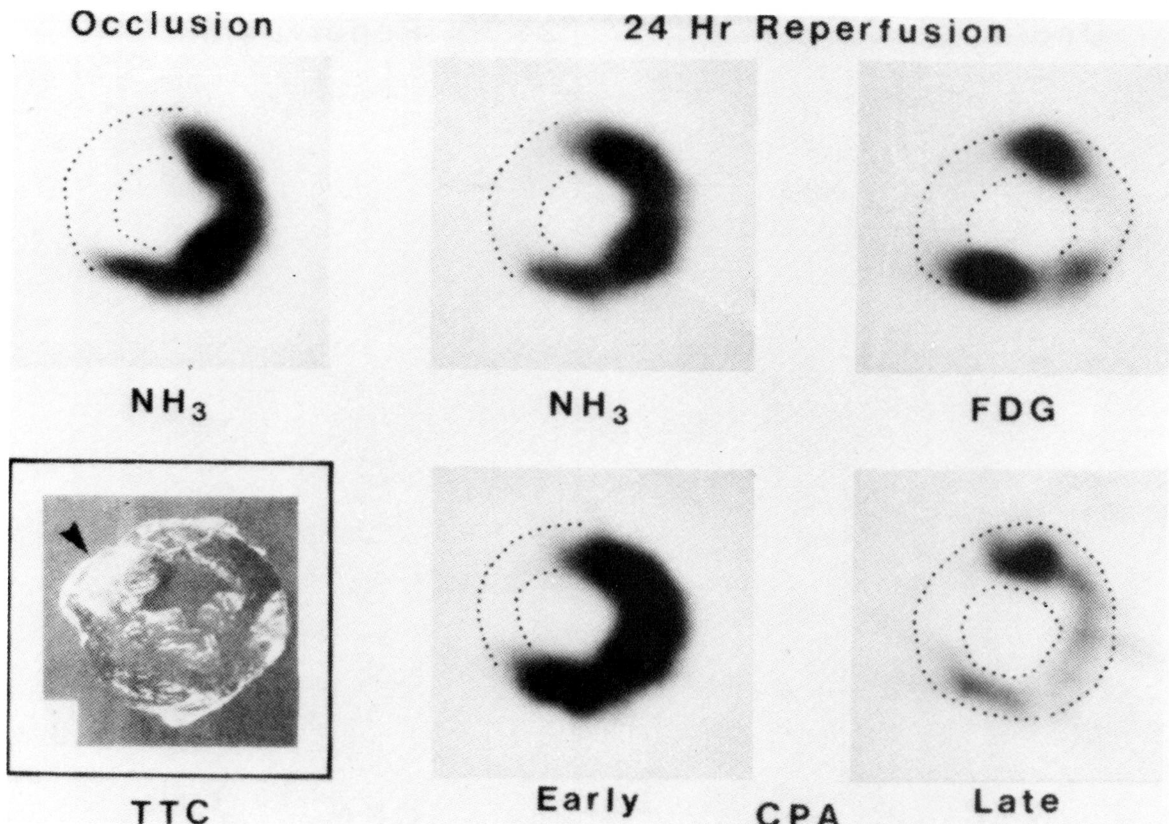

Figure 67–19. Representative positron emission tomographic images obtained 24 hours after release of a 3-hour balloon occlusion of the left anterior descending artery in a canine experiment. For comparison, the corresponding myocardial slice, which was stained with triphenyltetrazolium chloride (TTC) 4 weeks after the ischemic event, is displayed in the lower left-hand corner of the illustration. The [^{13}N]ammonia (NH_3) perfusion images obtained during occlusion and 24 hours after reperfusion demonstrate an extensive anterior perfusion defect. A similar defect is noted on the early ^{11}C-palmitate (CPA) image. The late (CPA) image demonstrates persistence of the anterior defect and abnormal retention of ^{11}C activity in the adjacent regions. The retention of ^{11}C activity in the adjacent regions indicates impaired fatty acid metabolism. In the corresponding glucose metabolic (FDG) images, a central anterior defect is again identified but, in addition, there is prominent uptake of the tracer in the peri-infarct areas. Positron emission tomography thus identifies a metabolic border zone of tissue with impaired fatty acid oxidation and enhanced glucose utilization surrounding the central area of necrosis. On histopathologic examination of the corresponding myocardial cross-sectional slice, there is a transmural infarction (*arrow*) in the anterior wall, with relative sparing of the peri-infarct regions demonstrating the abnormal metabolic state on positron emission tomography. (From Schwaiger, M., Schelbert, H.R., Ellison, D., et al.: Sustained regional abnormalities in cardiac metabolism after transient ischemia in the chronic dog model. J. Am. Coll. Cardiol. 6:336–347, 1985. Reprinted with permission from the American College of Cardiology.)

were 90 ± 17 percent of those in control myocardium (P = NS) and thus had improved significantly from those determined 2 hours following reperfusion ($P < 0.001$). In absolute terms, mean k_1 for reperfused sectors at 2 hours was 0.150 ± 0.039 min^{-1} and 0.225 ± 0.079 min^{-1} at 24 hours. Although the animals with the most severe wall motion abnormalities at 24 hours tended to have the most severe reductions in k_1 values, a statistically significant correlation was not demonstrated.

On the fluorine-18 2-fluoro 2-deoxyglucose glucose images there was no statistically significant difference in uptake of the glucose analog between risk and normal myocardium, either on the 2-hour or the 24-hour study. However, the myocardial response was heterogeneous. On the fluorine-18 2-fluoro 2-deoxyglucose images in three animals at 24 hours, the risk zone exhibited increased (greater than 2 standard deviations from the mean of control myocardium) uptake of fluorine-18 2-fluoro 2-deoxyglucose (Fig. 67–21), while uptake of the tracer was normal or even reduced in the remaining eight animals. When stratified according to the presence or absence of augmented uptake of fluorine-18 2-fluoro 2-deoxyglucose at 24 hours, the mean k_1 was significantly depressed in the animals with the augmented glucose metabolism (Fig. 67–22), consistent with an accelerated glycolytic flux in the myocardial regions, with impaired oxidative substrate metabolism. Furthermore, regional wall motion scores were significantly lower, both at 10 minutes and at 24 hours following reperfusion, in the animals with the augmented myocardial uptake of fluorine-18 2-fluoro 2-deoxyglucose. Thus, the results of this investigation indicate that regional oxygen consumption is impaired early (2 hours) following reperfusion after an acute ischemic insult and that failure of oxidative metabolism to recover with time is associated both with impaired regional function and with enhanced glucose utilization, consistent with an abnormal postischemic state.

Evaluation of Glucose Metabolism

Several of the experimental animal studies just described included the use of fluorine-18 2-fluoro 2-deoxyglucose and identified segmental increases in glucose utilization in reperfused, dysfunctional myocardium. Two recent experimental animal studies, published in preliminary form, indicated that with coronary occlusions of less than 30 minutes' duration, glucose utilization in acutely ischemic myocardium was normal or even elevated in myocardial regions with mild-to-moderate reductions in blood flow. For example, Russell and associates injected six dogs with fluorine-18 2-fluoro 2-deoxyglucose 5 minutes after coronary occlusion.[R6] Tissue samples obtained 30 minutes after coronary ligation revealed increased uptake of fluorine-18 2-fluoro 2-deoxyglucose in tissue samples, with flow decreased to as much as 60 to 80 percent of normal myocardium. Similar findings were reported by Kalff and colleagues, who observed that glucose utilization was maintained until flows decreased to 20 percent or less of that in normal myocardium.[K4]

The relationship between the severity of a blood flow reduction and tissue uptake of thallium-201, technetium-99m pyrophos-

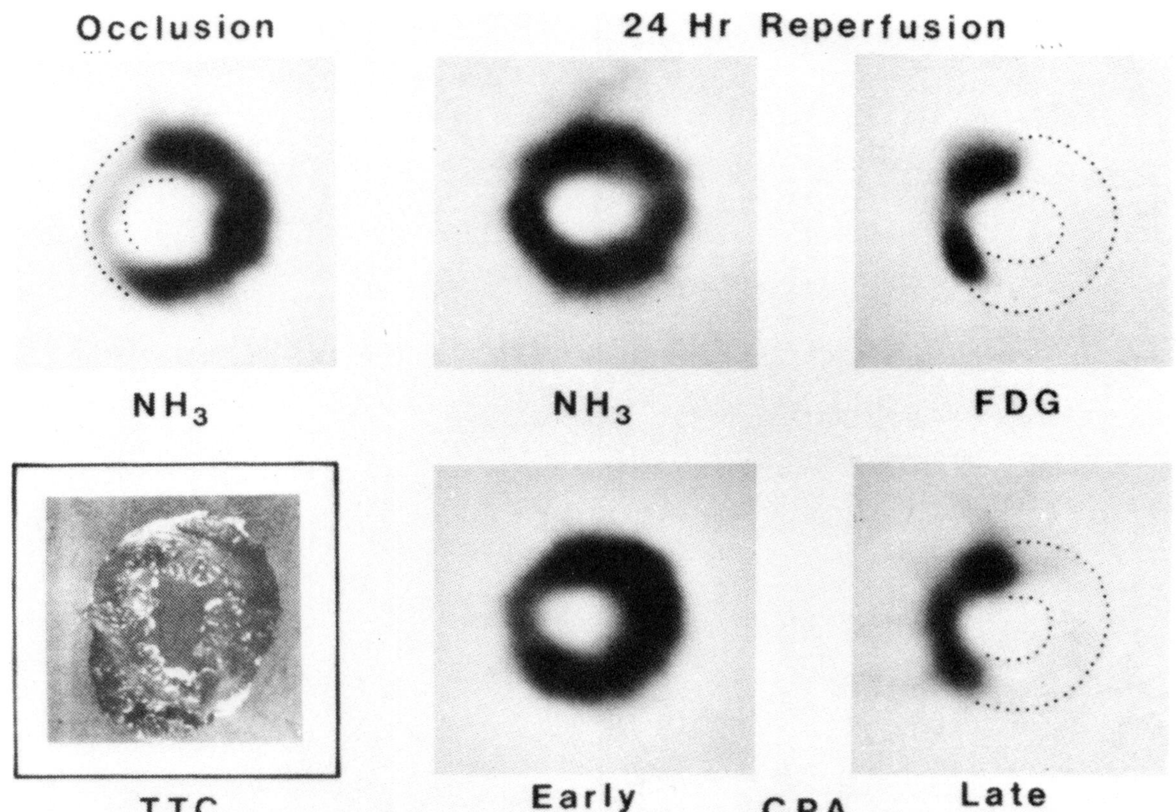

Figure 67–20. Representative positron emission tomographic images obtained 24 hours after a 3-hour occlusion of the left anterior descending artery in a second canine experiment. The [^{13}N]ammonia (NH_3) perfusion image during occlusion demonstrates an anterior perfusion defect. This has normalized on the perfusion study at 24 hours. The early ^{11}C-palmitate (CPA) image obtained 24 hours following reperfusion is similar to the NH_3 perfusion image. On the late CPA image, however, there is delayed clearance of the labeled fatty acid in the anterior wall, indicating impaired fatty acid oxidation. The ^{18}F–2-fluoro 2-deoxyglucose (FDG) image demonstrates augmented uptake of the tracer in this same region, illustrating an enhanced utilization of exogenous glucose. On triphenyltetrazolium chloride (TTC) stain of the corresponding cross-sectional myocardial slice 4 weeks later, there was no gross evidence of myocardial infarction. (From Schwaiger, M., Schelbert, H. R., Ellison, D., et al.: Sustained regional abnormalities in cardiac metabolism after transient ischemia in the chronic dog model. J. Am. Coll. Cardiol. 6:336–347, 1985. Reprinted with permission of the American College of Cardiology.)

phate, and fluorine-18 2-fluoro 2-deoxyglucose in reperfused canine myocardium was delineated in a study by Sochor and associates.[S15] In this investigation, seven dogs were subjected to a 3-hour balloon occlusion of the left anterior descending coronary artery. Segmental blood flow was determined with microspheres immediately before and at the end of the occlusion period. Twenty hours following reperfusion, fluorine-18 2-fluoro 2-deoxyglucose and technetium-99m pyrophosphate were simultaneously injected, and the arterial input function for both tracers was determined by rapid arterial blood sampling. Twenty-five minutes later, blood flow was measured, followed by the intravenous administration of thallium-201 with rapid arterial blood sampling for determination of the arterial input function. After sacrifice of the animals, myocardial cross sections were stained with triphenyltetrazolium chloride (TTC), and tissue samples were submitted for well counting.

During coronary occlusion, blood flows in the risk zones decreased to 42.5 percent that of control myocardium (32.9 ± 33.7 versus 77.4 ± 44.1 ml/min/100 g, $P < 0.01$). Twenty hours following reperfusion, blood flows in the risk segments remained 21.7 percent lower than flows in the control segments (70.2 ± 32.3 versus 89.7 ± 24.8 ml/min/100 g, $P < 0.05$). In reperfused myocardium, the net retention of thallium-201 was 24.5 percent lower than that of control myocardium (21.6 ± 12.2 percent versus 28.6 ± 10.0 percent, $P < 0.05$), paralleling the 21.7 percent reduction in blood flows. In contrast, the net tissue retention of technetium-99m pyrophosphate was 471 percent of that in control myocardium (3.72 ± 2.96 percent versus 0.79 ± 0.61 percent, $P < 0.05$). Furthermore, average rates of exogenous glucose utilization in reperfused myocardium were 293 percent higher than in control myocardium (4.4 ± 2.0 versus 1.5 ± 0.7 mg/min/100 g, $P < 0.01$). Thus, relative to myocardial blood flow, reperfused myocardium extracted 3.7 times more glucose per milliliter of blood flow than control myocardium (0.063 versus 0.017 mg/ml), indicating an accelerated glycolytic flux in the reperfused tissue 20 hours following restoration of blood flow.

When thallium-201 tissue concentrations were compared with microsphere blood flow measurements in risk myocardium, a linear relationship (r = 0.92) was observed, indicating that tissue thallium-201 concentrations paralleled reductions in blood flow. In contrast, tissue concentrations of fluorine-18 2-fluoro 2-deoxyglucose and technetium-99m pyrophosphate were not directly related to myocardial blood flow. Tissue technetium-99m pyrophosphate concentrations were highest in regions with blood flows 31 to 50 percent of control myocardium, with a mean ratio of activity in risk to control myocardium of 14.04 ± 2.66. For flows 30 percent of control or less, the ratio of activity in risk myocardium to control myocardium gradually declined, reaching 3.59 ± 1.71 in the regions with blood flows less than 15 percent of control. At higher blood flows, the ratio of activity in risk myocardium to control myocardium also decreased to 5.04 ± 4.02 for regions with blood flows greater than 70 percent of control myocardium.

In the case of fluorine-18 2-fluoro 2-deoxyglucose, highest tissue tracer concentrations were noted in the reperfused regions, with blood flows reduced by less than 30 percent relative to normal myocardium (ratio of risk to control myocardium = 1.75 ± 0.73). In risk regions with blood flows between 30 and 70 percent of control, tracer concentrations did not differ significantly from those in normal myocardium. In contrast, concentrations of fluorine-18 2-fluoro 2-deoxyglucose were significantly below those of normal myocardium in regions with blood flows

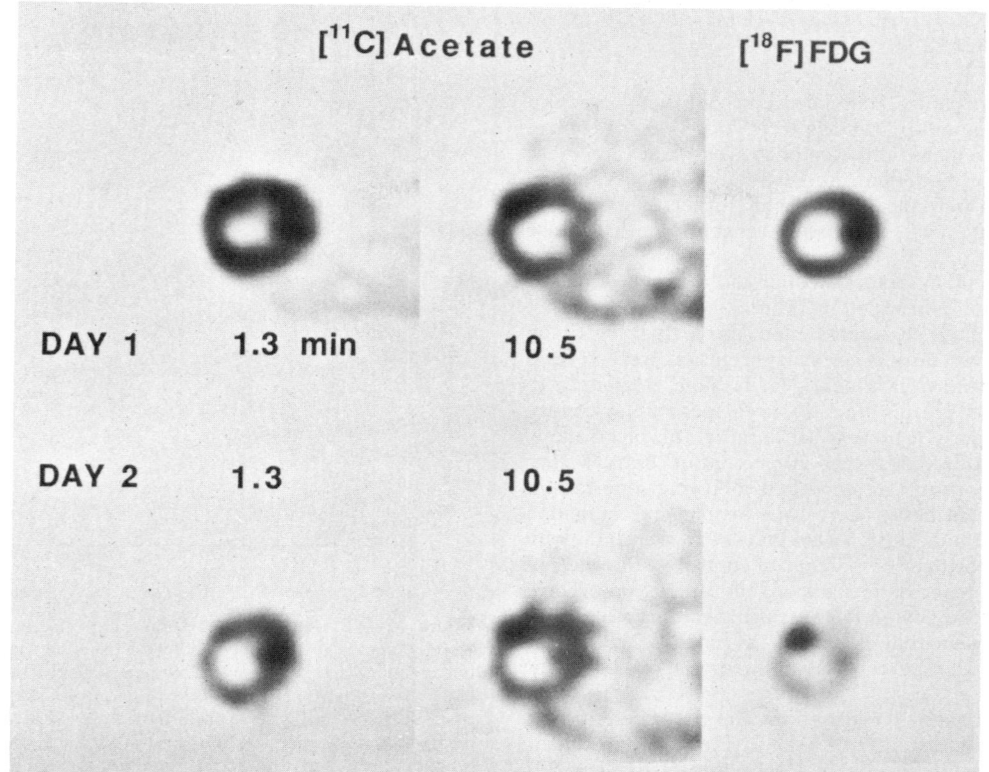

Figure 67–21. Representative cross-sectional ventricular images obtained in a canine preparation studied 3 and 24 hours after reperfusion following a 20-minute balloon occlusion of the left anterior descending artery. The early (1.3 minute) and late (10.5 minute) ^{11}C-acetate images obtained on Day 1 and Day 2 are displayed on the left, whereas the corresponding ^{18}F 2-fluoro 2-deoxyglucose images are displayed on the right. The early Day 1 acetate image shows slightly decreased uptake of ^{11}C-acetate in the territory of the anterior descending artery. Impaired oxidative substrate metabolism is also present in this region, as is indicated by the persistence of ^{11}C activity in the anterior ventricular region on the 10.5-minute image. Despite this impairment in oxidative substrate metabolism, there is preservation of ^{18}F 2-fluoro 2-deoxyglucose uptake on the 3-hour glucose metabolic image. When corrected for partial volume effect, the uptake of ^{18}F 2-fluoro 2-deoxyglucose was not statistically different from that in normal myocardium. At 24 hours, impaired uptake and clearance of ^{11}C-acetate are still present in the vascular territory of the anterior descending artery, indicating persistence of impaired oxidative substrate metabolism. In addition, there is a focal accumulation of ^{18}F 2-fluoro 2-deoxyglucose in the fasting state, indicating accelerated glycolytic metabolism in the reperfused myocardium. (From Buxton, D.B., Schwaiger, M., Vaghaiwalla, M.F., et al.: Regional abnormality of oxygen consumption in reperfused myocardium assessed with [1-^{11}C] acetate and positron emission tomography. Am. J. Cardiac Imaging 3:276–287, 1989, with permission.)

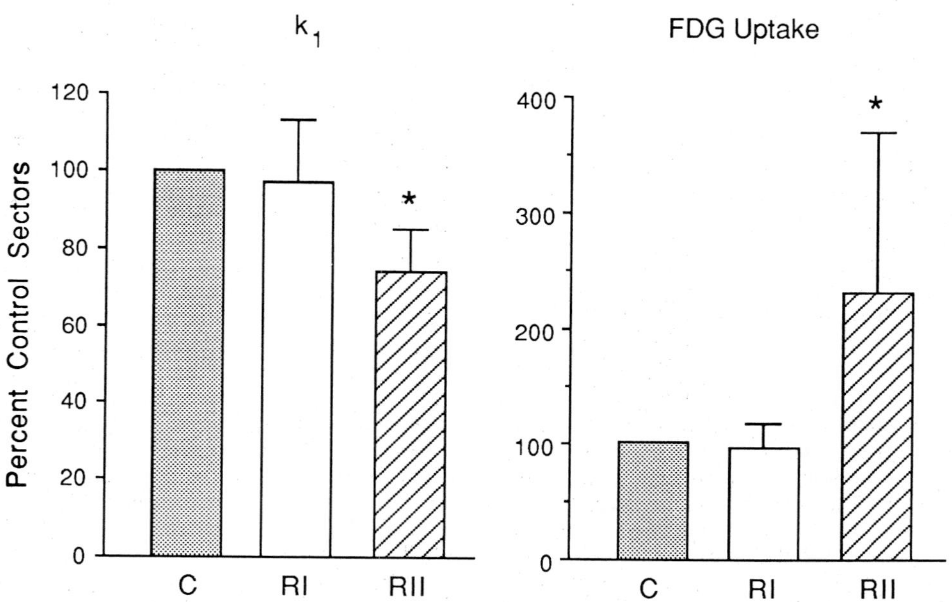

Figure 67–22. The relationship between ^{11}C-acetate clearance constants (k_1) and myocardial uptake of ^{18}F 2-fluoro 2-deoxyglucose (FDG Uptake) in dogs subjected to 20-minute balloon occlusions of the left anterior descending artery with subsequent reperfusion. The graphs display relative mean acetate clearance constant values (k_1) and relative uptake of FDG in control myocardium (C), in reperfused myocardium with normal uptake of the radiolabeled glucose tracer (RI), and in reperfused myocardium with increased uptake of FDG (RII). The measurements were obtained 24 hours after reperfusion, and the asterisk indicates $P<.02$ versus control values. When stratified according to the presence or absence of augmented uptake of FDG in the risk zone, segments with increased uptake of the labeled glucose analog had significantly poorer ^{11}C-acetate clearance constants. (From Buxton, D.B., Schwaiger, M., Vaghaiwalla, M.F., et al.: Regional abnormality of oxygen consumption in reperfused myocardium assessed with [1-^{11}C] acetate and positron emission tomography. Am. J. Cardiac Imaging 3:276–287, 1989, with permission.)

less than 30 percent of control (ratio of risk to control myocardium = 0.66 ± 0.42 for regions with flows 16 to 30 percent of control and 0.31 ± 0.23 for regions with blood flows less than 15 percent of control). Thus, for both fluorine-18 2-fluoro 2-deoxyglucose and technetium-99m pyrophosphate, factors other than myocardial blood flow influenced the tissue concentration of these tracers.

To elucidate these other factors, Sochor and colleagues further explored the relationship between myocardial blood flow, the net retention of each of these tracers, and the extent of tissue necrosis.[S15] Blood flows during coronary occlusion were related to reperfusion blood flows in a nonlinear fashion. Regions with occlusion blood flows greater than 20 to 40 percent of control myocardium had nearly complete restoration of blood flow, whereas regions with flows less than 20 percent of control values exhibited only partial return of blood flow following reperfusion. In addition, the percent tissue necrosis on histologic examination was inversely related to occlusion blood flows. Myocardium with occlusion flows greater than 60 percent of control values did not exhibit histologic evidence of necrosis on light microscopy. Thus, the severity of the blood flow reduction during coronary occlusion was related both to the extent of recovery of blood flow following reperfusion and to the percent tissue necrosis on histologic examination.

When these investigators correlated the net tissue retention of thallium-201 with the extent of tissue necrosis on histologic examination, they found that the net retention of thallium-201 declined as the percent of necrotic cells per tissue sample increased. For technetium-99m pyrophosphate, the net myocardial retention of the tracer was not correlated with the percent tissue necrosis. However, when the effects of varying blood flow were removed by calculation of the tissue retention fractions of technetium-99m pyrophosphate, there was a linear relationship (r = 0.93) between the logarithm of the retention fractions for this tracer and the percent tissue necrosis, indicating that the avidity of reperfused myocardium for this tracer increased in proportion to the degree of irreversible cell damage.

In control myocardium, absolute rates of exogenous glucose utilization calculated from uptake of fluorine-18 2-fluoro 2-deoxyglucose were linearly related to blood flow (glucose utilization rate = 0.078 + 0.33 · (blood flow), SEE = 1.19, r = 0.60). However, a linear relationship between blood flow and glucose utilization was not observed in reperfused myocardium. When these investigators compared ratios of absolute rates of glucose utilization in risk to control myocardium (to normalize for dietary state and myocardial workload), they found that this ratio was lowest in the tissue with the greatest percent tissue necrosis. As the percent of tissue necrosis in the samples decreased, the ratio of glucose utilization in risk to control myocardium precipitously increased, achieving its highest values in samples with less than 50 percent necrosis. Because the logarithm of the retention fraction of technetium-99m pyrophosphate was linearly related to the percent of histologic necrosis, ratios of glucose utilization rates in risk to control myocardium were plotted as a function of the logarithm of the retention fraction of technetium-99m pyrophosphate (Fig. 67–23). When displayed in this fashion, it becomes apparent that the highest relative rates of regional glucose utilization occurred in risk myocardium with lesser degrees of tissue injury and that relative glucose utilization rates approached unity as the the logarithm of the retention fraction of technetium-99m pyrophosphate approached values typical of normal myocardium. These data suggest that enhanced uptake of fluorine-18 2-fluoro 2-deoxyglucose distinguishes stunned myocardium with minimal tissue necrosis from tissue with extensive irreversible damage after an acute ischemic injury.

The study of Sochor and associates illustrates the utility of a multitracer approach for defining the presence and extent of reversibly and irreversibly injured tissue following an acute ischemic insult.[S15] In reperfused myocardium, uptake of thallium-201 reflects primarily blood flow, whereas the net tissue concentration of technetium-99m pyrophosphate is influenced both by blood flow and the amount of cellular necrosis. Perhaps more importantly, augmented uptake of fluorine-18 2-fluoro 2-deoxyglucose identifies ischemically compromised but viable tissue in the "infarct" zone.

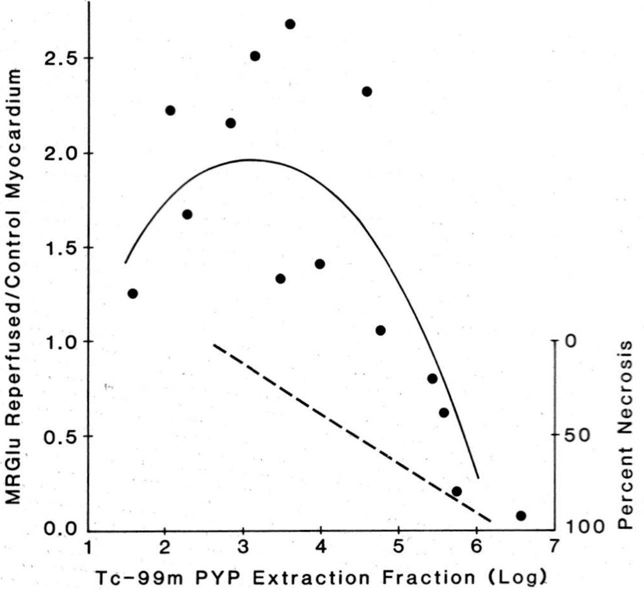

Figure 67–23. Data obtained from canine experiments in which dogs were subjected to a 3-hour balloon occlusion of the left anterior descending coronary artery, followed by reperfusion. On the left vertical axis, glucose consumption in reperfused myocardium relative to that in normal tissue is displayed, whereas, on the right vertical axis, the percent tissue necrosis is determined at the time of sacrifice. Both are displayed as a function of the logarithm of the retention fraction of ^{99m}Tc pyrophosphate. In these experiments, a close correlation was observed between the percent tissue necrosis and retention fractions of ^{99m}Tc pyrophosphate. In reperfused myocardium, rates of glucose utilization were increased in tissue with less severe degrees of histologic injury and were highest in tissue samples with less than 50 percent tissue necrosis. The broken line indicates the inverse of percent histologic tissue necrosis, whereas the solid line indicates the curvilinear fit of the glucose metabolic data, indicating an acceleration of glucose utilization in the myocardial segments with intermediate degrees of tissue necrosis due to an acute ischemic injury. (From Sochor, H., Schwaiger, M., Schelbert, H.R., et al.: Relationship between Tl–201, Tc–99m (Sn) pyrophosphate and F 18 2-deoxyglucose uptake in ischemically injured dog myocardium. Am. Heart J. 114:1066–1077, 1987, with permission.)

Melin and colleagues compared thallium-201 redistribution with myocardial uptake of fluorine-18 2-fluoro 2-deoxyglucose as an indicator of tissue viability in reperfused canine myocardium.[M5] Ten open-chest dogs were subjected to a 2-hour occlusion of the anterior descending artery. Twenty minutes prior to reperfusion, microsphere blood flow measurements were made, and thallium-201 was administered intravenously. Transmural myocardial biopsies were then obtained from risk and control myocardium, and the occlusion was released. Myocardial biopsies were repeated 2 hours following reperfusion, and repeat microsphere blood flow measurements were repeated 3 hours following reperfusion. Shortly after 3 hours of reperfusion, fluorine-18 2-fluoro 2-deoxyglucose was administered intravenously, and the arterial input function was obtained by rapid arterial sampling. Prior to sacrifice of the animals 4 hours after reperfusion, myocardial biopsies were again taken, and arterial and regional venous blood samples were obtained for measurement of oxygen content, glucose, lactate, and free fatty acids.

During coronary occlusion, myocardial blood flows fell to 41 ± 20 percent of normal in ischemic zones (myocardium exhibiting positive staining with triphenyltetrazolium chloride [TTC] within the vascular bed at risk), whereas regions with patchy necrosis had blood flows 18 ± 10 percent of normal, and necrotic regions (no staining with triphenyltetrazolium chloride) had blood flows

5 ± 4 percent of normal. Following reperfusion, blood flows in the ischemic regions increased to 84 ± 17 percent of normal, while flows in the regions with patchy necrosis increased to 94 ± 38 percent of normal and flows in the necrotic regions increased to 73 ± 65 percent of normal.

When these workers analyzed the myocardial thallium-201 time activity curves in the ischemic and nonischemic control regions, they found that the normalized thallium-201 activity in the control regions decreased from 100 percent prior to reperfusion to 59 ± 16 percent at 4 hours. Before reperfusion, relative thallium-201 activity in the ischemic regions was 28 ± 20 percent of normal values, and by 4 hours the relative activity had increased significantly to 47 ± 16 percent of control values. Although this was a significant improvement, relative thallium-201 activity in the ischemic regions remained significantly less than that in the normal regions ($P < 0.01$), suggesting that a perfusion defect might have been visually detectable had thallium-201 scintigraphy also been performed. Unfortunately, myocardial thallium-201 time activity curves were not provided for regions with patchy necrosis or regions with extensive necrosis. However, the investigators did report that the mean thallium-201 gradient 4 hours after reperfusion was 26 ± 13 percent between ischemic and normal myocardium, 48 ± 13 percent between the regions with patchy necrosis and normal myocardium, and 71 ± 26 percent between the necrotic regions and normal myocardium. Thus, the magnitude of the thallium-201 gradient between the affected region and normal tissue at 4 hours depended upon the degree of tissue necrosis.

When relative fluorine-18 activity was assessed in the risk zones, neither ischemic regions nor regions with patchy necrosis had values statistically different from those of normal myocardium (103 ± 37 percent and 97 ± 50 percent, respectively). In contrast, relative fluorine-18 activity in the necrotic regions was significantly reduced at 43 ± 26 percent ($P < 0.001$). Absolute rates of exogenous glucose utilization were not significantly different in ischemic regions (3.04 ± 1.92 mg/min/100 g) from rates in normal myocardium (3.85 ± 2.31 mg/min/100 g). Glucose utilization rates in regions with patchy necrosis (1.82 ± 1.02 mg/min/100 g) and necrotic regions (1.18 ± 0.74 mg/min/100 g) were significantly lower than rates in normal tissue. When glucose utilization rates were normalized to those in control myocardium to take into account varying cardiac workload and plasma substrate levels, only the necrotic regions had metabolic rates that were different from normal tissue (33 ± 25 percent, compared with 117 ± 68 percent for ischemic regions and 113 ± 72 percent for regions with patchy necrosis). These investigators did observe considerable heterogeneity in the measured metabolic rates, noting that three of nine dogs with ischemic tissue had a normalized transmural glucose metabolic rate of 150 percent, resulting in the rather large standard deviations in the measurements of these metabolic parameters.

When the arteriovenous differences in free fatty acids, lactate, and glucose were examined for all the reperfused regions in aggregate, reductions in the net myocardial uptake of both free fatty acids (22 ± 18 percent versus 41 ± 21 percent, $P < 0.001$) and lactate (7 ± 17 percent versus 29 ± 13 percent, $P < 0.01$) were observed. In contrast, glucose consumption rates in reperfused regions (6.29 ± 3.83 μmol/min/100 g) did not differ significantly from rates in normal myocardium (6.08 ± 6.4 μmol/min/100 g). Because oxygen consumption in the reperfused zones was significantly less than in normal myocardium (3.28 ± 2.26 versus 7.31 ± 2.23 ml/min/100 g, $P < 0.001$), the fact that glucose consumption was normal in these regions would imply that anaerobic glycolysis was occurring in at least a portion of the reperfused tissue.

The observations by Melin and co-workers indicate that thallium-201 redistribution and the presence of residual tissue glucose metabolic activity are both accurate indicators of myocardial viability in reperfused myocardium.[M5] From the data presented, it is not possible to determine whether assessment of tissue glucose metabolism might have identified additional tissue viability in regions with little or no thallium-201 redistribution. In reperfused myocardium, at least a portion of the observed consumption of glucose is via anaerobic pathways, consistent with an accelerated glycolytic flux in the postischemic state.

Schwaiger and colleagues utilized D-[6 carbon-14] glucose and L-[U carbon-13] lactate to determine the metabolic fate of exogenous glucose consumed by reperfused canine myocardium.[S12] On the first day of the study, 13 dogs were subjected to 3-hour balloon occlusions of the anterior descending artery, followed by reperfusion. Twenty-four hours later, these animals and four control animals were instrumented for determination of microsphere blood flows and for simultaneous arterial and regional venous blood sampling. Simultaneous infusions of D-[6 carbon-14] glucose (15 μCi/hr) and L-[U carbon-13] lactate (35 mg/hr) were begun in the 4 control dogs and in 9 of the 13 intervention dogs. After a 20- to 25-minute period of equilibration, arterial and regional venous sampling was performed to determine concentrations and specific activities of lactate and glucose and to determine carbon-14 carbon dioxide content. Four of the intervention animals underwent continuous infusion of L-[1 carbon-14] lactate acid to allow calculation of the rate of lactate oxidation in this preparation. At the end of the study the histologic extent and severity of the tissue injury were assessed on myocardial slices stained with triphenyltetrazolium chloride (TTC) while assessment of myocardial glycogen stores was performed on slices stained with periodic acid–Schiff (PAS) reagent.

On study 24 hours following reperfusion, blood flows in the reperfused myocardial regions were significantly less than those in normal tissue (66.8 ± 35.4 ml/min/100 g versus 87.2 ± 29.2 ml/min/100 g, $P < 0.01$). In the four control dogs, calculated chemical substrate extraction fractions were 62 percent for nonesterified fatty acids, 17 percent for lactate, and 65 percent for oxygen. In the intervention dogs, chemical extraction fractions calculated using venous samples from the anterior descending vein were significantly lower than those calculated with coronary sinus samples for nonesterified fatty acids (40 percent versus 48 percent, $P < 0.05$), lactate (2 percent versus 22 percent, $P < 0.05$), and oxygen (57 percent versus 66 percent, $P < 0.05$). These data suggest impaired regional oxidative substrate metabolism in risk myocardium.

Glucose uptake in the risk zones was significantly higher than that in normal myocardium in the control animals (0.40 ± 0.14 versus 0.15 ± 0.10 μmol/ml, extraction fractions of 9 percent and 2 percent, respectively, $P < 0.05$). In the four control dogs, 27 percent of the exogenous glucose extracted by the myocardium was oxidized to $^{14}CO_2$, while 6 percent was converted to lactate. Thus, in the control animals, 33 percent of extracted glucose entered glycolysis, while 67 percent entered a storage pool (glycogen). In contrast, in reperfused regions, 75 percent of exogenous glucose extracted by the myocardium entered glycolysis. Of this 75 percent, 32 percent was oxidized to $^{14}CO_2$ while 43 percent was converted to lactate. Lactate release from the risk zones was significantly higher than lactate release in control animals (0.37 ± 0.11 versus 0.08 ± 0.03 μmol/ml, $P < 0.05$). Thus, myocardium in the risk zones extracted greater amounts of exogenous glucose from the vascular space than normal tissue, and the proportion of extracted glucose entering anaerobic glycolysis in reperfused myocardium was significantly higher than that in control tissue.

On histopathologic examination, none of the control dogs exhibited tissue necrosis or regional depletion of cellular glycogen stores. In each of the intervention dogs, however, a central area of necrosis was identified that was smaller in anatomic extent than the zone of glycogen depletion. For all dogs, the average area of glycogen depletion in the risk zones (36.6 ± 19.2 percent) was significantly larger than the area of necrosis (17.4 ± 10.5 percent). Thus, this investigation would indicate that anaerobic glycolysis is accelerated in ischemically compromised tissue, and that this biochemically primitive means of energy production is important for maintaining cellular viability in reperfused myocardium. Because cellular glycogen stores are rapidly depleted during periods of diminished tissue oxygen delivery, augmented extraction of glucose from the vascular space is an important mechanism by which the myocyte provides substrate for the glycolytic processes operant in ischemically injured myocardium.

Synopsis

Myocardial infarction is a tissue injury characterized by both spatial and temporal inhomogeneity. Transient myocardial dysfunction due to ischemic stunning of adjacent viable myocardium may render early estimation of the actual extent of tissue necrosis difficult. In acute ischemic injury, assessment of myocardial metabolism with positron emission tomography predicts eventual recovery of regional function more successfully than assessment of myocardial perfusion alone, primarily by providing a better estimate of the amount of stunned myocardium relative to that which has undergone necrosis. Tissue that has been stunned by an acute reduction in blood flow exhibits an impairment in oxidative metabolism. The observed impairment in fatty acid metabolism is disproportionately greater than the impairment in overall oxidative metabolism, probably because ischemia interferes with the metabolism of fatty acids at several points in their biochemical pathway and not only with the process of mitochondrial oxidation. As a result of the impairment in oxidative metabolism, stunned myocardium resorts to more primitive anaerobic glycolytic pathways to maintain cellular viability. Because cellular glycogen stores are rapidly depleted during ischemia, accelerated extraction of glucose from the vascular space is an important means of maintaining substrate for the glycolytic processes operant in stunned myocardium. This augmented glycolytic flux is manifest on positron emission tomography by an enhanced uptake of fluorine-18 2-fluoro 2-deoxyglucose. Following restoration of blood flow by thrombolysis, recovery of segmental function in stunned myocardium seems to parallel recovery of the altered metabolic state.

Clinical Investigations

Relatively few clinical studies have employed positron emission tomography to assess myocardial oxidative metabolism in patients with acute myocardial infarction. As noted (Acute Myocardial Infarction Experimental Studies: Glucose Metabolism), experimental studies have indicated that viable but ischemically compromised tissue resorts to anaerobic glycolysis to sustain production of high-energy phosphate and thus to maintain cellular viability. Hence, most of the clinical studies of patients with acute myocardial infarction have focused on regional glucose metabolism in the clinical infarct zone. However, increasing interest in "purer" tracers of oxidative metabolism such as carbon-11 acetate, whose tissue kinetics are directly related to regional oxygen consumption, may prompt an in-depth look at the clinical utility of assessment of tissue oxidative substrate metabolism in patients with acute ischemic injury.

Metabolic Characterization of Acutely Infarcted Myocardium

Because laboratory studies suggested that myocardium that had been transiently stunned as a result of an ischemic insult retained the ability to metabolize glucose via glycolytic pathways, it seemed feasible that the noninvasive assessment of both myocardial perfusion and glucose metabolism in patients with acute myocardial infarction might prove clinically useful in distinguishing viable but functionally compromised tissue in the hypoperfused clinical infarct zone from areas with completed infarction. Furthermore, these studies suggested that acutely infarcted myocardium could be characterized more comprehensively with tracers of metabolism than with other parameters, such as segmental function, blood flow, or the resting electrocardiogram.

Marshall and colleagues utilized positron emission tomography with nitrogen-13 ammonia and fluorine-18 2-fluoro 2-deoxyglucose to assess relative myocardial perfusion and glucose metabolism in 15 patients in the subacute phase of myocardial infarction.[M6] Four electrocardiographically defined infarct regions were studied: anterior, septal, lateral, and inferoposterior. The study population included nine patients with postinfarction angina and six patients without postinfarction angina. The mean interval from the onset of chest pain to positron emission tomography was similar in both groups (2.2 ± 3.0 versus 3.7 ± 3.9 weeks, respectively; P = NS). Eleven patients had Q wave infarctions involving 13 electrocardiographic infarct regions, while four individuals had non-Q wave infarctions. In addition, two of the subjects had histories of remote Q wave infarctions. Thus, there were clinical histories of 19 infarctions (17 recent, 2 remote) in the patients studied.

On positron emission tomography, concordant decreases in myocardial perfusion and glucose utilization were noted on circumferential count profile analysis in 14 ventricular regions in 11 patients, consistent with completed infarction (Fig. 67–24). In contrast, myocardial uptake of fluorine-18 2-fluoro 2-deoxyglucose was preserved relative to that of nitrogen-13 ammonia in 11 regions in 10 patients (Fig. 67–24), indicating accelerated glucose metabolism relative to blood flow, and providing evidence for residual tissue metabolic viability. Of the 11 regions exhibiting the "metabolism-perfusion mismatch" of myocardial ischemia, 5 were in the vascular territory of the infarct artery, while three regions of ischemia were noted in the territories of remote coronary arteries. In one patient with left bundle branch block and lateral ischemia, it was not possible to correlate the metabolic findings with an electrocardiographic infarct region. One patient had ischemia both in the region of the acute infarction and in a remote vascular bed. Right ventricular ischemia was identified in two patients.

Eight of the ten patients with the metabolism-perfusion mismatch of myocardial ischemia had postinfarction angina at rest, whereas only one of the five patients without positron tomographic evidence of myocardial ischemia had postinfarction angina ($0.05 < P < 0.10$). In five patients who exhibited transient electrocardiographic ST-T changes with chest pain, the regions of ischemia identified with positron emission tomography correlated with the electrocardiographic regions demonstrating the ST-T changes. Thirteen of the patients had coronary angiography. In these, the metabolism-perfusion mismatch pattern of myocardial ischemia was associated with more extensive coronary disease (2.9 ± 0.4 versus 1.5 ± 0.6 coronary artery lesions, $P < 0.02$). Postmortem examination in two patients who died 10 days and 4 weeks after imaging confirmed the presence of significant amounts of viable tissue in the myocardial regions exhibiting the positron tomographic pattern of myocardial ischemia. Thus, these findings indicated that glucose metabolic imaging could identify viable tissue in some hypoperfused infarct regions in patients in the subacute stage of myocardial infarction and implied that positron emission tomography could prove useful for identifying viable tissue early in patients with acute infarction.

Schwaiger and associates subsequently assessed relative myocardial perfusion and exogenous glucose metabolism within 72 hours of the onset of chest pain in 13 patients presenting with acute myocardial infarction.[S16] Regional function was determined with two-dimensional echocardiography on the day of imaging and at 6.0 ± 4.6 weeks. All patients revealed electrocardiographic and/or serum enzymatic evidence of acute myocardial infarction. Twelve of the thirteen individuals evolved Q waves on the electrocardiogram, while one patient had left bundle branch block. The electrocardiographic site of the infarction was anterior in ten patients, inferior in one patient, posteroinferior in one patient, and undeterminable in the patient with left bundle branch block. In two patients there was electrocardiographic evidence of old inferior infarction. The peak creatine kinase serum level was 1384 ± 1640 U/L (normal = 20 to 120 U/L), and the peak serum level of the creatine kinase-MB isoenzyme was 39.9 ± 43.9 U/L (normal < 4 U/L).

Positron emission tomography was performed 54 ± 12 hours after the onset of chest pain. In the 13 patients, nitrogen-13 ammonia perfusion imaging identified 32 segments with diminished resting blood flow. In these hypoperfused segments, relative nitrogen-13 ammonia activity was 46 ± 13.9 percent of maximal myocardial nitrogen-13 ammonia activity. Regional myocardial perfusion was reduced in the anterior and apical segments

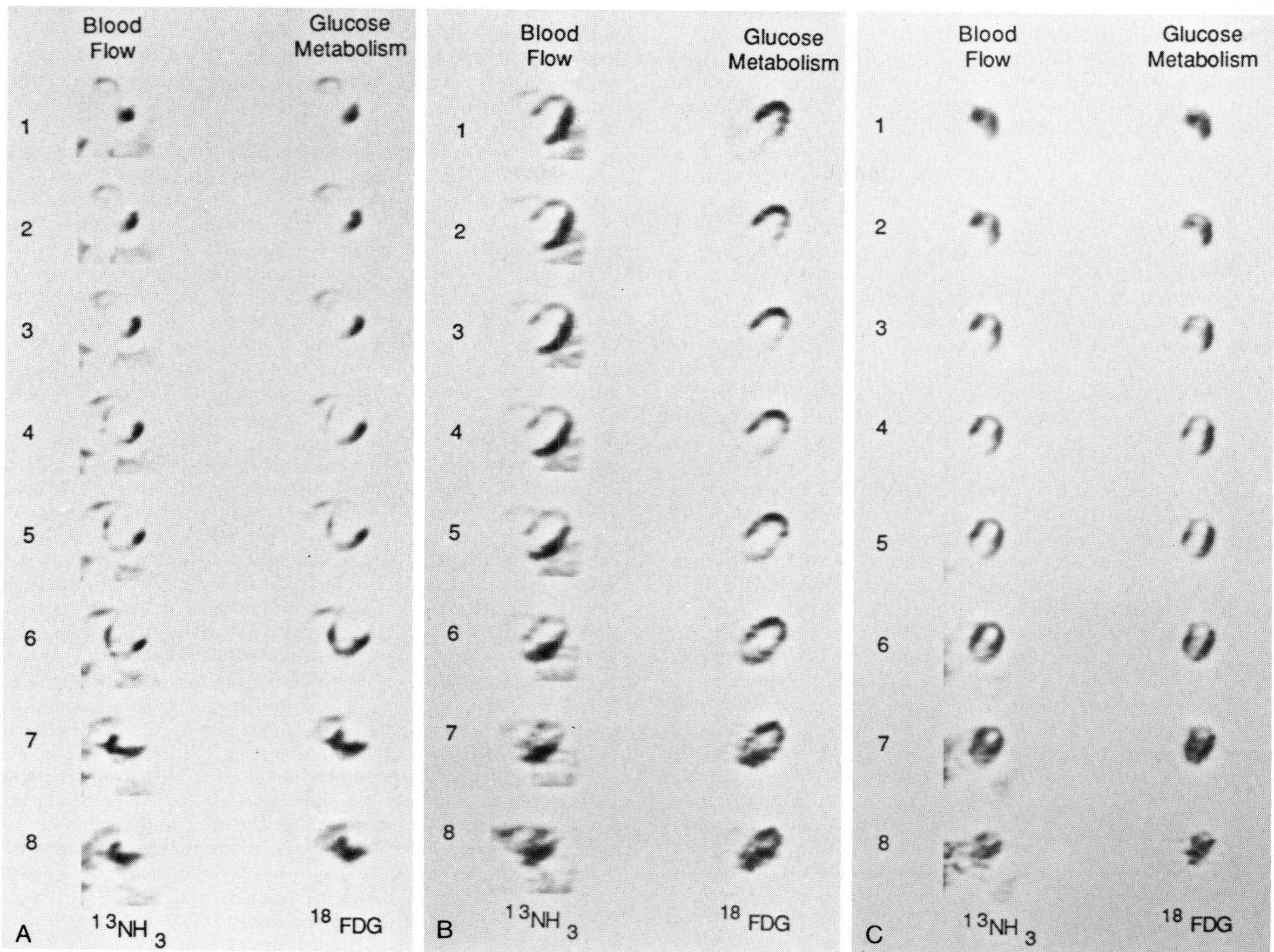

Figure 67–24. Representative [^{13}N]ammonia perfusion (NH_3) and ^{18}F 2-fluoro 2-deoxyglucose metabolic (^{18}FDG) images in three different patients with acute myocardial infarction. *Panel A,* Images from the study of a 52-year-old man with an uncomplicated acute anterolateral myocardial infarction. Matching defects in perfusion and glucose metabolism are noted in the anteroseptal and anteroapical regions of the ventricle, indicating completed infarction. *Panel B,* Representative images from a 76-year-old man with an acute anteroseptal infarction. On the [^{13}N]ammonia images, a large perfusion defect is identified in the anteroseptal and anteroapical regions of the ventricle. On the metabolic images, there is prominent uptake of the labeled glucose tracer, indicating metabolic viability in the hypoperfused infarct tissue. *Panel C,* Perfusion and glucose metabolic images from the study of a 71-year-old woman with an acute uncomplicated anteroseptal myocardial infarction. Only modest reductions in perfusion and glucose utilization are noted in the anteroapical region, indicating substantial residual myocardial viability in the clinical infarct zone.

in the ten patients with electrocardiographic anterior infarctions, whereas in the one patient with an acute inferior infarction, hypoperfusion was noted in the inferior and apical segments. The patient with a posteroinferior infarction exhibited a perfusion defect involving the inferior, apical, and lateral segments. In one of the two individuals with chronic inferior infarction, a perfusion defect was identified in the inferior wall.

On metabolic imaging with fluorine-18 2-fluoro 2-deoxyglucose, there were concordant decreases in exogenous glucose utilization in 16 (50 percent) of the hypoperfused regions, indicating an absence of metabolic tissue viability. In contrast, preserved glucose metabolism was identified in the remaining 16 (50 percent) hypoperfused segments, indicating residual tissue metabolic viability. Of the 13 patients, 9 (69.2 percent) had residual tissue glucose metabolism in hypoperfused ventricular segments, while concordant reductions in perfusion and glucose metabolism indicative of completed infarction were observed in 4 patients (30.8 percent). Each of the five patients who had postinfarction angina showed preservation of glucose metabolism in the hypoperfused infarct zone. In the segments with residual tissue metabolic viability, as identified with fluorine-18 2-fluoro 2-deoxyglucose, relative nitrogen-13 ammonia activity was not significantly different from that in the segments with a loss of metabolic viability (48.2 ± 15.9 percent versus 46.0 ± 7.4 percent of maximal myocardial nitrogen-13 ammonia activity, P = NS), indicating that assessment of myocardial perfusion alone could not have discriminated between the segments with and those without residual tissue metabolic viability on imaging with fluorine-18 2-fluoro 2-deoxyglucose.

Changes in segmental function were assessed by two independent observers who graded segmental wall motion in each of five myocardial segments according to the following scoring system: -1 = dyskinesia, 0 = akinesia, 1 = severe hypokinesia, 2 = mild hypokinesia, and 3 = normal function. On the day of positron emission tomography, there was no significant difference between the mean segmental wall motion score in segments with and those without preserved uptake of fluorine-18 2-fluoro 2-deoxyglucose (0.34 ± 0.84 versus 0.67 ± 0.83, P = NS), indicating that assessment of segmental wall motion could not have discriminated between segments with and those without metabolic evidence of viability. The mean left ventricular ejection fraction in patients with preserved glucose metabolism in the hypoperfused segments (44.4 ± 14.9 percent) did not differ significantly from that for the patients with the concordant reductions in flow and glucose metabolism (38.5 ± 4.4 percent, P = NS).

On follow-up assessment of segmental function in 12 patients at 6.0 ± 4.6 weeks, segments with a concordant reduction in perfusion and glucose metabolism exhibited no significant improvement in wall motion score (0.69 ± 0.99 versus 0.67 ± 0.83, P = NS), and the mean left ventricular ejection also did not change (38.8 ± 6.0 percent versus 38.5 ± 4.4 percent, P = NS). In contrast, the mean wall motion score improved significantly in the hypoperfused segments with metabolic activity on the early fluorine-18 2-fluoro 2-deoxyglucose images (1.12 ± 1.4 versus 0.34 ± 0.84, $P < 0.01$). Of the 16 hypoperfused segments with preserved fluorine-18 2-fluoro 2-deoxyglucose uptake, 8 showed improvement in segmental wall motion of at least one grade, while function remained unchanged in 6 segments and deteriorated in 2 segments. As a result, the mean left ventricular ejection fraction for these nine patients did not change significantly at 6 weeks (46.7 ± 12.9 percent versus 44.4 ± 14.9 percent, P = NS).

Assessment of both fatty acid metabolism and exogenous glucose utilization in the clinical infarct zone was performed in the case study reported by Brunken and co-workers.[B10] In this report of a 71-year-old woman admitted with an acute anteroseptal myocardial infarction, positron emission tomography with nitrogen-13 ammonia and fluorine-18 2-fluoro 2-deoxyglucose on the second hospital day revealed a prominent mismatch between regional perfusion and glucose utilization in the anteroseptal region of the ventricle (Fig. 67–25), indicating residual tissue viability in the clinical infarct zone. On subsequent study with carbon-11 palmitate, serial positron tomographic images demonstrated impaired tissue clearance of carbon-11 activity in the hypoperfused infarct zone, indicating impaired fatty acid oxidation in the myocardium with preserved exogenous glucose utilization.

Because the metabolic studies with positron emission tomography implied the presence of residual tissue viability in the infarct region, the patient underwent angioplasty of a long 80 percent stenosis of the anterior descending artery to salvage jeopardized myocardium. Unfortunately, the patient sustained a second infarction in the same region 3 days after the angioplasty (felt clinically to be due to plaque dissection with acute occlusion of the vessel), forcefully demonstrating that a significant amount of viable tissue did indeed remain in the clinical infarct zone following the initial ischemic insult. Thus, this initial case report suggested that the assessment of both glycolytic and oxidative substrate metabolism with positron emission tomography might prove clinically useful in characterizing the extent of ischemic tissue injury in patients with acute myocardial infarction.

Recent studies published in preliminary form have employed carbon-11 acetate to examine oxidative metabolism and its relationship to glucose utilization in acutely infarcted myocardium. Kalff and colleagues studied 14 patients within 4 ± 3 days of admission for an acute myocardial infarction.[K5] Carbon-11 acetate clearance rate constants, k_1's, were decreased in proportion to myocardial blood flow in the infarct territory. Compared with normal myocardium with average clearance half-times of 11.0 ± 3.3 min, half-times in infarct territories were longer, averaging 13.5 ± 1.5 minutes ($P < 0.05$). It is interesting that clearance half-times in normal myocardium were significantly shorter in the acute infarct patients than in a group of six normal volunteers, suggesting a compensatory increase in oxygen consumption in remote normal myocardium. Melin and associates also reported that reductions in carbon-11 acetate tissue clearance rates were proportional to the reductions in myocardial blood flow in infarct regions.[M7] These investigators noted that segmental tissue clearance rates of C-11 acetate in both groups were similarly depressed, when classified according to the presence or absence of preserved glucose metabolism.

Observations with metabolic imaging and positron emission tomography thus indicate that fluorine-18 2-fluoro 2-deoxyglucose can identify viable but compromised myocardium early after an acute myocardial infarction. Hypoperfused segments without

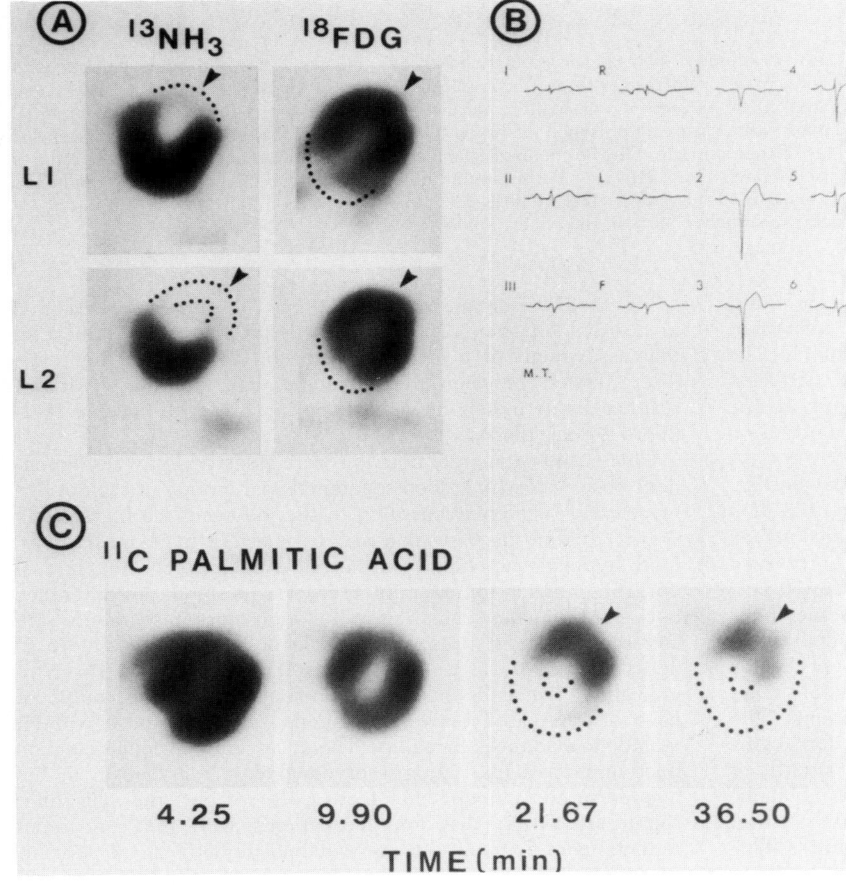

Figure 67–25. *Panel A*, Representative cross-sectional [^{13}N]ammonia ($^{13}NH_3$) perfusion and ^{18}F 2-fluoro 2-deoxyglucose (^{18}FDG) metabolic images from the study of a 71-year-old woman with a recent anteroseptal myocardial infarction. The images demonstrate an extensive mismatch between perfusion and glucose utilization in the clinical infarct zone, indicating residual tissue viability. *Panel B*, The patient's 12-lead electrocardiogram at the time of positron emission tomography. Q waves are present in V_1 and V_2 and there is a loss of R wave in the other anterior precordial leads. *Panel C*, Serial ^{11}C-palmitate images from the same patient. The ^{11}C palmitate study demonstrates impaired uptake and delayed clearance of ^{11}C activity in the zone of clinical infarction, indicating impaired fatty acid metabolism. (From Brunken, R.C., Schwaiger, M., and Schelbert, H.R.: PET detection of residual, viable tissue in acute MI. Applied Radiology 14:82–86, 1985, with permission.)

metabolic tissue viability on imaging with positron emission tomography and fluorine-18 2-fluoro 2-deoxyglucose uniformly fail to exhibit improvement in wall motion on delayed assessment of segmental function. Segments with diminished blood flow but with evidence of residual tissue glucose metabolism on study with positron emission tomography and fluorine-18 2-fluoro 2-deoxyglucose will have a variable functional outcome, if neither medical nor surgical intervention is performed to ensure salvage of ischemically compromised tissue (Fig. 67–26). Furthermore, rates of oxidative metabolism are invariably depressed in acutely infarcted myocardium. The degree of depression closely parallels the magnitude of the blood flow reduction and appears largely independent of simultaneously occurring rates of tissue glucose utilization.

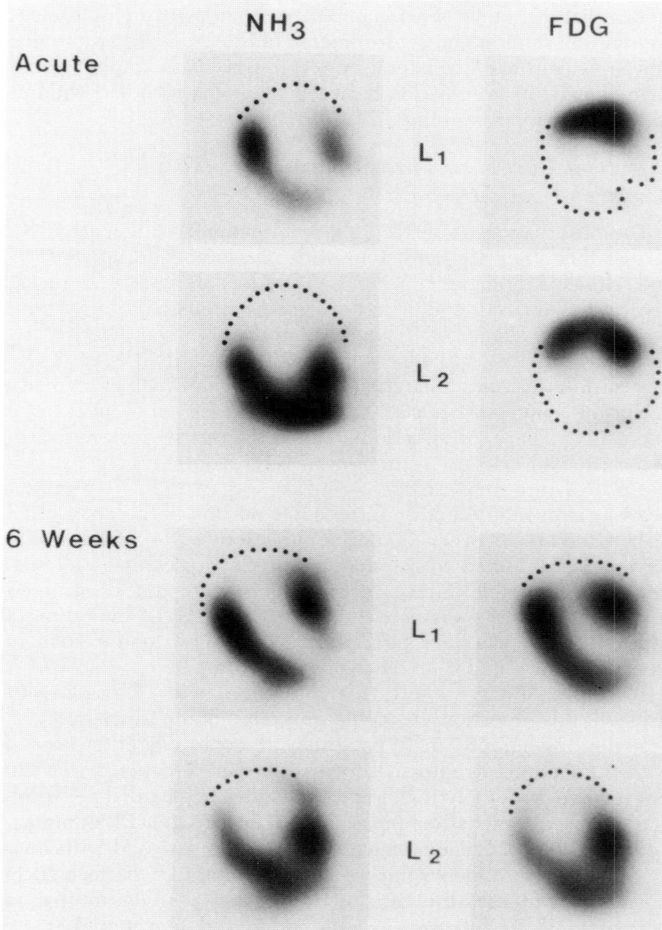

Figure 67–26. *Initial study*, Representative cross-sectional [^{13}N]ammonia (NH_3) perfusion and ^{18}F 2-fluoro 2-deoxyglucose (^{18}FDG) metabolic images obtained 48 hours after the onset of chest pain in a 71-year-old man with an acute anterior myocardial infarction. Coronary angiography revealed an 80 percent stenosis of the anterior descending coronary artery and a 50 percent stenosis of the circumflex artery. On the [^{13}N]ammonia perfusion images, there is an extensive anteroapical perfusion defect. The glucose metabolic study, performed in the fasting state, reveals enhanced uptake of the radiolabeled glucose analog in the zone of clinical infarction. *Study at 6 weeks*, Corresponding images obtained in the same patient 6 weeks after the patient's clinical myocardial infarction. In contrast to the initial study, there are concordant perfusion and glucose metabolic defects in the anteroapical region of the ventricle that are consistent with findings of completed myocardial infarction. In this patient, positron emission tomography performed early after infarction demonstrated evidence of residual metabolic viability in the clinical infarct zone. On the study at 6 weeks, however, the patient's infarct was complete. This suggests that interventional restoration of blood flow early after infarction might have salvaged viable but endangered myocardium in the clinical infarct region. (From Schwaiger, M., Brunken, R., Grover-McKay, M., et al.: Regional myocardial metabolism in patients with acute myocardial infarction assessed by positron emission tomography. J. Am. Coll. Cardiol. 8:800–808, 1986. Reprinted with permission from the American College of Cardiology.)

Relationship Between Electrocardiographic Changes and Metabolic Abnormalities

To assess the significance of electrocardiographic ST segment depression remote from the site of an acute ischemic injury, or "reciprocal" ST segment depression, Billadello and colleagues studied 20 patients with acute myocardial infarction, utilizing positron emission tomography and carbon-11 palmitate.[B11] In the 20 patients, there were 7 anterior and 13 inferior infarctions, as routinely defined electrocardiographically. Significant ST segment depression was defined by 0.1 mV or greater depression in at least two precordial (V_1 to V_6) or two inferior (II, III, aVF) leads. Total ST segment depression was defined as the sum of the ST segment depression in the anterior or inferior leads. Electrocardiograms were recorded at 3.4 ± 3.3 hours, and positron emission tomography was performed 9 ± 7 hours after the onset of chest pain. The mean interval between electrocardiography and positron emission tomography was 3 ± 3.2 hours. Imaging was repeated prior to hospital discharge at 14 ± 7 days. The patients were not treated with thrombolytic agents.

Of the seven patients with anterior infarction, none had reciprocal ST segment depression in the inferior leads. Each had defects in carbon-11 palmitate uptake limited to the septum and anterior and apical regions of the ventricle on the initial imaging studies. On delayed imaging at 14 ± 7 days, no new defects were identified. Each of the individuals with anterior infarction had angiographic evidence of significant (more than 50 percent reduction in luminal diameter) stenoses in the left anterior descending artery. Significant stenoses were also noted in the right coronary artery in one patient, and three had significant disease in the circumflex system. The mean left ventricular ejection fraction in this group was 0.45 ± 0.09, and assessment of regional function on contrast or radionuclide ventriculography revealed wall motion abnormalities limited to the anterior wall, septum, and apex.

Of the 13 patients with electrocardiographic inferior infarctions, 9 (69 percent) had ST depression in the anterior precordial leads. In each of the nine patients, positron emission tomography with carbon-11 palmitate revealed decreased accumulation of tracer in the inferior, posterior, apical, and posterolateral segments. In addition, accumulation of carbon-11 palmitate in the septal and anterior regions was reduced in three patients, corresponding to the anterior reciprocal ST segment changes noted on electrocardiography. At the time of hospital discharge, two of the three patients with the anterior carbon-11 palmitate defects showed improvement but not normalization of tracer uptake in the anterior and septal segments. This was observed despite normalization of the electrocardiographic anterior ST segment changes. In the third patient, there was no change in the diminished accumulation of carbon-11 palmitate in the anterior wall on delayed positron emission tomography. The three patients with the anterior carbon-11 palmitate defects each had multivessel coronary artery disease on coronary angiography. Of the six patients with reciprocal anterior ST segment depression and normal carbon-11 palmitate accumulation in the anterior and septal segments, two had stenoses only of the right coronary artery, one had stenoses of both the right and left anterior descending arteries, and two had severe three-vessel coronary artery disease. The remaining patient did not undergo cardiac catheterization. The three patients with abnormal uptake of carbon-11 palmitate had impaired wall motion in the anterior region, while the six patients with reciprocal ST changes and normal carbon-11 palmitate uptake had no anterior wall motion abnormalities. The mean left ventricular ejection fraction for these nine patients was 0.51 ± 0.12.

Of the four individuals with an acute inferior infarction without ST depression, none exhibited regional wall motion abnormalities in the anterior or septal regions of the ventricle. The mean left ventricular ejection fraction was 0.58 ± 0.17. Positron emission tomography revealed reduced uptake of carbon-11 palmitate in the inferoposterior region in each of the patients. In one individual with a nonhemodynamically significant (less than 50 percent) stenosis in the anterior descending artery, there was a small anterior region with decreased accumulation of carbon-11 palmitate. In this patient, the diminished accumulation of carbon-11 palmitate in the anterior region was no longer present at the time of hospital discharge, suggesting a transient depression of oxidative metabolism in this area of the ventricle.

Both the total inferior ST segment elevation (0.48 ± 0.35 versus 0.07 ± 0.19 mV, $P < 0.05$) and peak plasma MB creatine kinase levels (354 ± 134 versus 80 ± 34 IU/L, $P < 0.05$) in the patients with inferior infarction and reciprocal anterior ST segment changes were significantly larger than in the patients with inferior infarctions without reciprocal ST segment changes. In addition, the mean extent of metabolic compromise, the size of the defect on the carbon-11 palmitate images, was larger (58 ± 13 versus 33 ± 10 PET gram equivalents, $P < 0.02$). Thus, in this study, positron emission tomography with carbon-11 palmitate identified "ischemia at a distance" in one third of the patients with inferior infarctions and reciprocal anterior ST segment changes, and this ischemia was associated with impairment in regional wall motion.

Relationship Between Coronary Anatomy and Metabolic Findings

Schwaiger and associates examined the relationship between coronary anatomy and the metabolic findings in patients with an acute myocardial infarction.[S17] Positron emission tomography with nitrogen-13 ammonia and fluorine-18 2-fluoro 2-deoxyglucose was performed 5.1 (range: 2 to 14) days after the onset of chest pain in 15 patients with acute myocardial infarction. The physiologic and metabolic information derived from the imaging studies was then correlated with the anatomic information derived from coronary angiography.

Ten of the study patients had anterior infarctions and five had inferior infarctions. The plasma creatine kinase MB levels averaged 63.9 ± 38.1 U/L (normal: less than 4 U/L). The mean interval between positron emission tomography and coronary angiography was 4.4 ± 6.7 days. Segmental function was assessed in each of five ventricular segments within 24 hours of positron emission tomography in 14 patients using two-dimensional echocardiography (12 patients) or radionuclide ventriculography (2 patients).

Myocardial perfusion imaging with nitrogen-13 ammonia identified 37 hypoperfused left ventricular segments. In 20 (54.1 percent) of the segments, the decrease in relative perfusion was paralleled by a concordant decrease in exogenous glucose utilization on metabolic imaging with fluorine-18 2-fluoro 2-deoxyglucose, consistent with completed infarction. In contrast, 17 (45.9 percent) of the hypoperfused segments exhibited preserved uptake of fluorine-18 2-fluoro 2-deoxyglucose, consistent with metabolic tissue viability. On assessment of regional function, segments with preserved fluorine-18 2-fluoro 2-deoxyglucose uptake had wall motion scores as poor as those of the segments with matching perfusion and metabolic defects (0.79 ± 0.76 versus 0.52 ± 0.82, P = NS), signifying that assessment of segmental function could not discriminate between segments with and without tissue metabolic viability.

On coronary angiography at 8.4 ± 7.5 days, the infarct artery was occluded in eight patients and patent in seven patients. When segmental function was compared with coronary angiographic classification, segments in the distribution of patent arteries had wall motion scores as poor as those in the distribution of occluded arteries (0.68 ± 0.91 versus 0.60 ± 0.84, P = NS). Sixteen of the twenty (80 percent) infarct segments distal to an occluded artery exhibited matching defects on metabolic imaging, indicating completed infarction. Although significant collateral flow was noted on coronary angiography in seven of these segments, only two (28.6 percent) had preserved uptake of fluorine-18 2-fluoro 2-deoxyglucose, implying that the presence of visible collateral vessels on coronary angiography exerted no significant beneficial effect on tissue viability. The absence of such effect, however, may have also been related to the relatively small sample size. In contrast, 13 of the 17 (75.5 percent) hypoperfused infarct segments in the territory of a patent artery exhibited residual metabolic activity ($\chi^2 = 11.90$, $P < 0.001$).

Thus, this investigation in patients with acute myocardial infarction indicates a positive association between the presence of antegrade flow in the infarct artery and residual tissue metabolic activity. These observations are consistent with the hypothesis that anaerobic metabolism can be supported in acutely ischemic myocardium if some degree of residual blood flow exists for removal of inhibitory metabolites, such as hydrogen ion and lactate.[N1, R7] In addition, this study illustrates how metabolic imaging with positron emission tomography can provide new and clinically useful insights into the pathophysiology of acute human myocardial ischemia. For example, neither assessment of segmental wall motion nor determination of the presence or absence of visible coronary collaterals on coronary angiography would have allowed discrimination between segments with and without residual metabolic viability.

Effects of Coronary Thrombolysis and Revascularization

The observations described above in patients with acute myocardial infarction are consistent with previous experimental[R3, R4] and clinicopathologic[B12, F3, R8, S18, S19] studies demonstrating that myocardial infarction is a heterogeneous process. Reimer and Jennings have suggested that a "wavefront" of myocardial necrosis spreads from the subendocardial to the epicardial layer of the myocardium in acute infarction and that the duration of coronary occlusion is inversely related to the ultimate extent of myocardial necrosis.[R4] These observations imply that early restoration of myocardial blood flow, either occurring spontaneously[O3] or via the use of thrombolytic agents,[G3, I1, K2, M3, N2, O4, S11, V3, W1, W2] might prevent irreversible injury of the outer portion of the myocardial wall. Ultimate recovery of contractile function, therefore, would be inversely related to the amount of the myocardial wall sustaining irreversible injury relative to the amount of stunned myocardium in the vascular territory at risk. Thus, limitation of infarct size by early restoration of blood flow to the zone of ischemic injury might be clinically desirable.

In a preliminary report, DeLandsheere and colleagues addressed this question by comparing the findings on positron emission tomography in 16 patients with acute infarction treated with intravenous streptokinase with those in 10 patients who did not receive thrombolytic therapy.[D2] Relative myocardial perfusion was assessed with either potassium-38 or nitrogen-13 ammonia, while relative exogenous glucose uptake was assessed with fluorine-18 2-fluoro 2-deoxyglucose. Based on studies performed in normal volunteers, the ratio of fluorine-18 activity to that of potassium-38 or nitrogen-13 was considered elevated if it exceeded 1.41 (2 standard deviations above the mean for the normal volunteers). In the patients treated with intravenous streptokinase, the mean ratio of fluorine-18 counts to nitrogen-13 or potassium-38 counts was significantly greater than that in the patients not treated with thrombolytic therapy (2.44 ± 0.28 versus 1.42 ± 0.25, $P < 0.01$), suggesting a beneficial effect of streptokinase on myocardial metabolic viability in the clinical infarct zone.

In a subsequent report, these investigators detailed the results of positron emission tomography in 24 patients with acute anterior infarction who were treated with intravenous streptokinase.[D3] The mean peak plasma creatine kinase level was 2844 ± 1284 U/L, and the mean percent left anterior descending coronary artery stenosis on coronary angiography was 74.0 ± 23.3 percent. Myocardial blood flow was evaluated with nitrogen-13 ammonia or potassium-38, and myocardial glucose metabolism with fluorine-18 2-fluoro 2-deoxyglucose. The mean relative activity of the perfusion tracers in the territory of the left anterior descending coronary artery was decreased at 43.0 ± 20.0 percent. Fluorine-18 2-fluoro 2-deoxyglucose activity was 1.73 ± 0.75 (range: 1.0 to 3.88) times higher than that of the perfusion tracers. Glucose utilization was greater than 1.30 in 16 (66.7 percent) of the 24 patients. Thus, two thirds of the patients treated with streptokinase for acute anterior infarction had evidence of myocardial metabolic viability in the clinical infarct zone when studied with positron emission tomography. Because these investigators did not include an untreated control group of patients with acute infarction in this study, it is not possible to deduce the extent of the benefit, if any, derived from use of intravenous streptokinase in this particular investigation.

More recently, Henes and colleagues examined the recovery of myocardial blood flow and oxidative metabolism in eight patients with acute myocardial infarction following coronary thrombolysis.[H1] Positron emission tomography with oxygen-15 water and carbon-11 acetate was performed within 24 and 48 hours after thrombolysis and at hospital discharge. Myocardial blood flow in the "infarcted" but reperfused myocardium averaged 1.16 ± 0.6 ml/min/g of myocardium and remained unchanged at 48 hours and at hospital discharge. Regional myocardial oxygen consumption as estimated from the tissue clearance rate constants of carbon-11 acetate in reperfused myocardium was decreased at 24 hours to 43 ± 24 percent of that in normal myocardium. It significantly improved to 60 ± 15 percent at 48 hours and to 69 ± 19 percent at hospital discharge. The researchers noted that this gradual improvement in oxidative metabolism in the presence of normal blood flow sharply differed from findings in six patients without thrombolysis in whom both segmental blood flow and oxidative metabolism remained persistently depressed in the infarct regions on serial studies with positron emission tomography.

Brunken and Schelbert compared blood flow and glucose metabolism to scintigraphic evidence of irreversible tissue damage.[B13] They reported the case of a 64-year-old man with an acute anterior infarction who was treated with intravenous streptokinase within 3 hours of the onset of chest pain. Shortly after initiation of the streptokinase infusion the patient's chest pain resolved, and there were several brief episodes of ventricular tachycardia. Coronary angiography on the first hospital day revealed only a 60 percent stenosis of the left anterior descending artery, and the patient was treated medically. The peak creatine kinase plasma level was 1142 U/L (normal: 40 to 180 U/L), while the peak plasma creatine kinase MB level was 71.5 EU/L (normal: less than 3.5 EU/L). The initial electrocardiogram revealed a loss of anterior R waves, ST segment elevation in V_1 to V_5 and small Q waves in V_2 and V_3. On serial tracings, a Q wave infarction did not evolve but at 2 weeks the patient had persistent ST segment elevation and T wave inversion in V_2 to V_6 (Fig. 67–27). Echocardiography revealed severe anterior and apical hypokinesis, with an ejection fraction of 40 percent.

On infarct-avid scintigraphy with indium-111 antimyosin antibody fragments,[B14, J2, K6] prominent tracer uptake was noted in the septal, anterior, and apical regions of the ventricle, indicating acute myocardial necrosis (Fig. 67–27). Positron emission tomography with nitrogen-13 ammonia and fluorine-18 2-fluoro 2-deoxyglucose, performed on the fifth hospital day, revealed perfusion defects in the anterior, apical, and superior septal regions of the ventricle, which generally corresponded with the focal areas of uptake of indium-111 antimyosin uptake (Fig. 67–27). There was a concordant reduction in tracer activity in the apical region, consistent with irreversible tissue injury, but tracer uptake was preserved in the hypoperfused septal and anterior segments, indicating myocardial viability. Thus, the indium-111 antimyosin and glucose metabolic studies identified an admixture of necrotic and viable myocardium in the septal and anterior segments and a completed infarction at the ventricular apex.

The patient was discharged on medical therapy and did well over the ensuing 2 months. At that time, a repeat positron emission tomographic study revealed improved perfusion in the septal and anterior regions and a persistent apical defect (Fig. 67–27). On the metabolic images, exogenous glucose utilization had normalized in the septal and anterior segments, while the defect in the apical segment persisted. On stress echocardiography at 6 months, the patient's resting electrocardiogram was essentially normal (Fig. 67–27). With exercise to a heart rate of 153 beats/minute and a blood pressure of 180/80 mmHg, the T waves in the inferior leads became biphasic, and there were no ST segment changes to suggest exercise-induced ischemia. On the baseline echocardiogram the apex was akinetic to dyskinetic, and there was normal function in the remaining ventricular segments. The resting left ventricular ejection fraction was 58 percent, and it increased to 88 percent with exercise.

This case study illustrates the utility of glucose metabolic imaging for early myocardial tissue characterization in patients with an acute infarction. Despite identification of cellular necrosis with indium-111 antimyosin, positron emission tomography with fluorine-18 2-fluoro 2-deoxyglucose indicated that viable tissue persisted in the septal and anterior ventricular regions and suggested that thrombolysis had prevented transmural extension of the patient's infarction in these areas. Perhaps more importantly, early identification of tissue glucose metabolic activity predicted the delayed recovery of wall motion in the stunned myocardium in the septal and anterior segments. As quantitative determinations of myocardial blood flow, glucose utilization, and oxidative metabolism are now feasible with positron emission tomography, measurements of these physiologic parameters in patients with acute myocardial infarction should provide further insights into the pathophysiology of acute myocardial necrosis in humans and allow assessment of the beneficial (or deleterious) effects of medical or surgical interventions designed to salvage endangered myocardium.

Synopsis

Clinical studies of patients with acute myocardial infarction with positron emission tomography have demonstrated that myocardial infarction is an inhomogeneous process in humans as well as in the laboratory animal. Metabolic imaging reveals impaired fatty acid and overall oxidative substrate metabolism in the clinical infarct zone. Oxidative substrate flux in myocardium remote from the infarct region actually may be increased, perhaps as a result of the compensatory increase in regional myocardial work. On metabolic imaging with fluorine-18 2-fluoro 2-deoxyglucose, lack of residual tissue glucose metabolism in the hypoperfused infarct zone often presages a persistent depression in regional wall motion, suggesting completed infarction. In contrast, the presence of residual glucose metabolism in the zone of infarction is associated with a variable functional outcome, suggesting a metastable state with endangered but viable myocardium. Correlative studies with coronary angiography suggest that angiographically visible collateral vessels might not consistently exert a beneficial effect on myocardial metabolic viability in the clinical infarct region. However, residual antegrade blood flow through the infarct vessel does appear to exert a favorable effect on regional metabolic viability. Furthermore, several preliminary reports suggest that thrombolytic therapy beneficially affects the metabolic integrity of the infarct region.

METABOLIC ACTIVITY AS A CLINICAL INDICATOR OF TISSUE VIABILITY

Early patient studies with positron emission tomography clearly indicated that residual tissue glucose metabolism could be identified in hypoperfused human myocardium. However, the clinical implications of these observations remained uncertain. Although laboratory investigations indicated that exogenous glucose utilization was accelerated both in acutely ischemic tissue and in reperfused myocardium, and that the metabolic findings correlated with the histologic presence of significant amounts of viable myocytes, it was unclear whether these observations could be extrapolated to patients with ischemic heart disease, and further, whether they would affect patient care. In particular, it was unknown whether identification of tissue glucose metabolism in hypoperfused ventricular regions in individual subjects would indeed indicate that clinically significant amounts of viable tissue were present, and if so, whether the tissue characterization afforded by glucose metabolic imaging would provide additional information that could not be obtained with routinely performed clinical tests. Thus, clinical studies were undertaken to determine

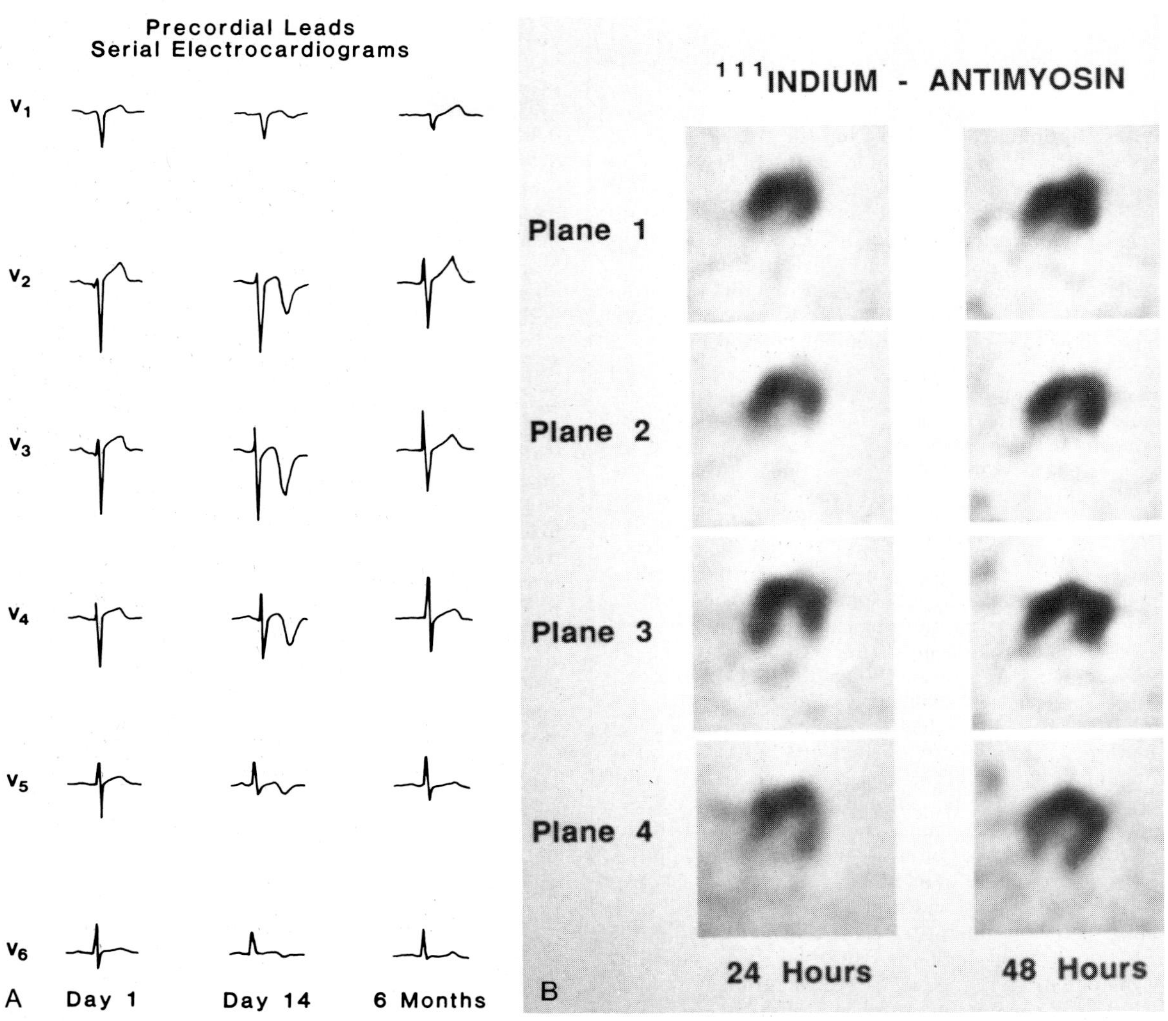

Figure 67–27. *Panel A,* Serial precordial electrocardiographic tracings obtained from a 64-year-old man with an acute anterior myocardial infarction who was treated with streptokinase. The initial set of tracings, obtained on the day of admission, demonstrate ST segment elevation in leads V_1 through V_5. On the second set of tracings, obtained 2 weeks following the onset of chest pain, there is persistent ST segment elevation and T wave inversion in leads V_2 through V_6. By 6 months, there is relatively normal R wave progression and only minor ST-T changes. Associated with the acute episode of chest pain was an elevation in the creatine kinase MB level to 71.5 EU/l (normal = 0.0 to 3.5). In light of the serial changes in enzymes, the clinical diagnosis of acute non-Q wave anterior myocardial infarction was established. *Panel B,* Representative single-photon emission tomographic indium-111 antimyosin images obtained 24 hours and 48 hours following the onset of chest pain in the patient whose electrocardiographic tracings are displayed in Panel A. In this display, the left ventricle points to the upper right-hand corner of the images. There is prominent uptake of the labeled antimyosin in the septum and anteroapical region of the ventricle, indicating an acute anteroseptal and anteroapical myocardial infarction.

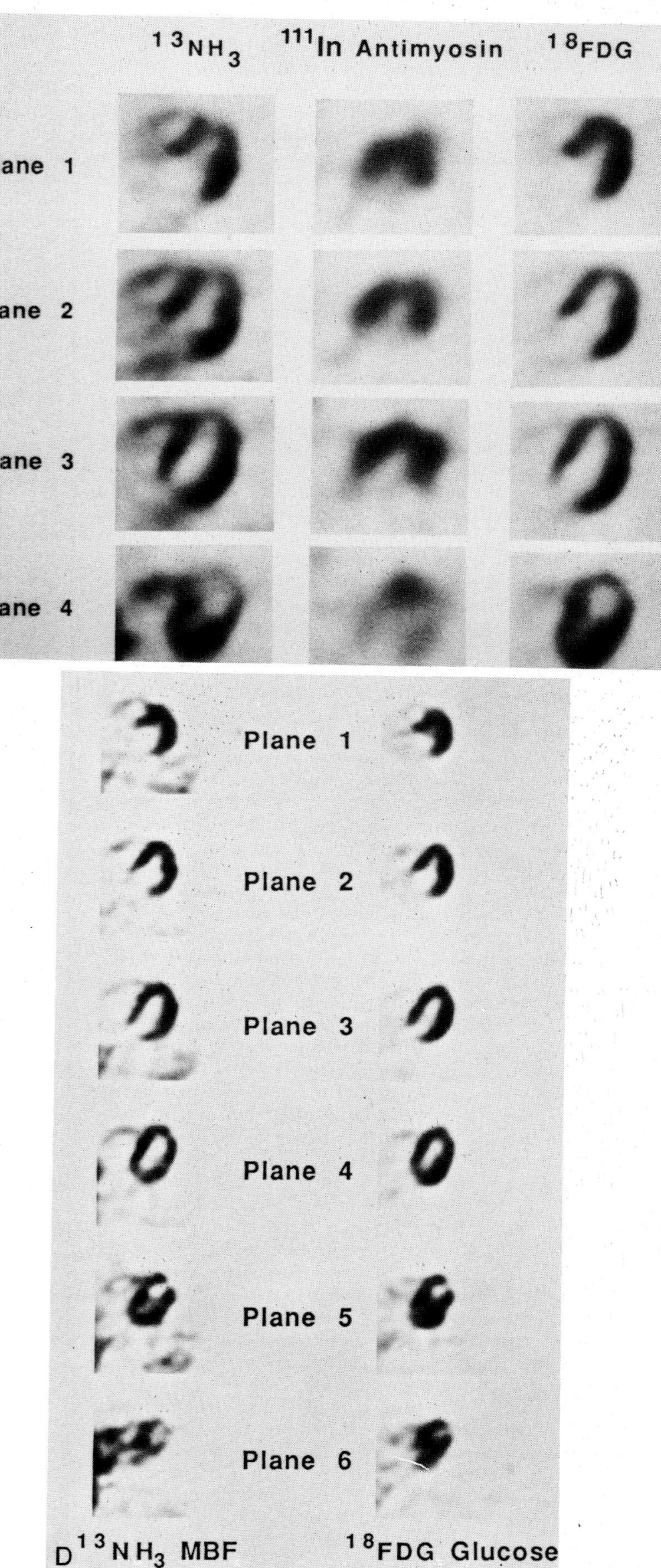

Figure 67–27. *Continued Panel C,* Corresponding [^{13}N]ammonia ($^{13}NH_3$) perfusion and ^{18}F-2-fluoro 2-deoxyglucose (^{18}FDG) metabolic images in the patient whose indium-111–antimyosin study is displayed in Panel B. On the [^{13}N]ammonia perfusion images, defects are present in the anteroseptal and anteroapical regions, which correspond to the areas with indium-111–antimyosin uptake. In the more superior aspect of the heart, glucose utilization is well preserved on the ^{18}F–2-fluoro 2-deoxyglucose metabolic images, indicating residual tissue viability. There is a small apical area that exhibits a concordant reduction in ^{18}F–2-fluoro 2-deoxyglucose uptake, which is consistent with completed infarction. *Panel D,* Repeat positron emission tomographic study in the same patient 8 weeks later. Concordant decreases in perfusion and glucose metabolism are noted in a small apical area of the ventricle, indicating completed infarction. Perfusion and glucose metabolism are essentially normal in the anterior segment and in the interventricular septum. The resting left ventricular ejection fraction increased from 40 to 58 percent, and segmental function in the septal and anterior segments improved from dyskinesia to normal. The apical segment remained akinetic to dyskinetic. Thus, positron emission tomography identified a large area of stunned myocardium, which was successfully salvaged by thrombolytic therapy, and correctly predicted the observed improvement in segmental wall motion. (From Brunken, R.C., and Schelbert, H.R.: Acute myocardial infarction: A case for metabolic imaging. The Leading Edge in Cardiology 3:1–11, 1989, with permission.)

whether metabolic imaging with positron emission tomography could identify viable tissue in patients with ischemic heart disease and further, to determine how the metabolic assessment of myocardial viability would compare with alternative tests routinely utilized in clinical practice.

Effect of Revascularization on Hypoperfused, Metabolically Active Tissue

Identification of Myocardial Viability

To test the hypothesis that the presence of myocardial glucose metabolism in hypoperfused ventricular regions is an accurate indicator of tissue viability, Tillisch and associates studied patients with resting wall motion abnormalities prior to elective coronary bypass surgery.[T2] The findings on positron emission tomography with nitrogen-13 ammonia and fluorine-18 2-fluoro 2-deoxyglucose prior to revascularization were compared with postoperative changes in segmental function. Because scar tissue is both avascular and metabolically inert, asynergic myocardial segments with concordant reductions in perfusion and glucose metabolism were not expected to exhibit improved function following revascularization. In contrast, segments with metabolically active tissue (either the metabolism-perfusion mismatch of myocardial ischemia or segments with a normal perfusion and metabolic pattern) were predicted to exhibit improved function once blood flow had been restored.

The study population consisted of 17 patients referred for coronary artery bypass surgery who had resting regional wall motion abnormalities identified on either contrast left ventriculography (4 patients) or radionuclide angiography (13 patients). Indications for coronary revascularization included double- or triple-vessel coronary artery disease, with an ejection fraction of less than 40 percent in 11 patients, persistent angina or a positive stress test at a low workload after myocardial infarction in 5 patients, and angina refractory to medical therapy in 1 patient. Sixteen of the seventeen patients had histories of antecedent myocardial infarction. Two patients had positron emission tomography within 2 weeks of an acute myocardial infarction, while the remaining fifteen were studied 8 weeks (range: 6 to 14 weeks) after myocardial infarction. Three experienced observers visually assessed segmental wall motion abnormalities on a grading scale of 0 (normal) to 4 (dyskinesia) in each of seven myocardial segments: apical, anteroseptal, anterolateral, anterobasal, lateral, posterior, and inferior. Following coronary artery bypass surgery, wall motion studies were performed within 3 weeks in 2 patients, at 6 to 10 weeks in 2 patients, and at 12 to 18 weeks in the remaining 13 patients. For the three observers, interobserver agreement on the directional change in segmental function (improvement, no change, or deterioration) was 98.8 percent.

Prior to coronary artery bypass surgery, 73 segments with resting wall motion abnormalities were identified in the 17 patients. After revascularization, improvement in the mean segmental score of at least one grade occurred in 9 of 21 (43 percent) mildly hypokinetic, 21 of 37 (57 percent) severely hypokinetic, and 6 of 14 (43 percent) akinetic segments. The only dyskinetic segment also exhibited improved function. There was no correlation between the severity of a wall motion abnormality prior to surgery and the extent of functional improvement on the postoperative studies. Of the segments with normal function before operation, two septal segments exhibited deterioration in function on the postoperative wall motion studies.

Of the 73 segments exhibiting resting wall motion abnormalities prior to revascularization, 67 were adequately revascularized at the time of coronary bypass surgery. Of 46 segments with preserved glucose metabolism, 41 were successfully revascularized. Of these 41 segments, 22 of 25 (88 percent) regions considered normal by circumferential profiles and 13 of 16 (81 percent) with the metabolism-perfusion mismatch of myocardial ischemia had improved wall motion postoperatively. The mean segmental wall motion score in these segments improved significantly on the delayed study (2.0 ± 0.08 versus 0.6 ± 0.6, $P < 0.05$). Furthermore, in the 11 patients with preserved glucose metabolism in three or more asynergic segments, the mean left ventricular ejection fraction increased significantly from 30 ± 11 percent to 45 ± 14 percent following coronary revascularization. This suggests that the patients with the largest amounts of jeopardized tissue derived the greatest benefit from revascularization, as determined by improvement in global left ventricular function. Three of the six segments with preserved glucose metabolism that did not exhibit improved function after revascularization were septal segments, in which determination of wall motion is complicated by the mechanical effects of the bypass operation itself.[R9]

The results in the segments with concordant reductions in perfusion and glucose metabolism were strikingly different. Of the 27 segments with concordant reductions in perfusion and glucose metabolism, 26 were adequately revascularized. Of these 26 segments, 24 (92 percent) had no improvement or further deterioration in wall motion following revascularization. In addition, the mean segmental wall motion score did not improve in these segments (2.4 ± 0.5 versus 2.6 ± 0.04, P = NS), implying that little functional benefit was derived by revascularizing these myocardial regions. Thus, this study demonstrated that metabolic imaging with positron emission tomography and fluorine-18 2-fluoro 2-deoxyglucose had an 85 percent positive predictive accuracy and a 92 percent negative predictive accuracy for identifying segments with functional improvement following coronary revascularization. Although the study was limited by the heterogeneity in the intervals from revascularization to postoperative determination of segmental function and by use of only a semiqualitative method to assess the anatomic extent of reversibly compromised tissue, it does indicate the utility of metabolic imaging for identifying viable but functionally compromised tissue that will benefit from restoration of blood flow.

Tamaki and associates confirmed these findings in 22 consecutive patients who were examined with nitrogen-13 ammonia and fluorine-18 2-fluoro 2-deoxyglucose and positron emission tomography within the 4 weeks prior to coronary artery bypass grafting.[T3] Segmental wall motion was evaluated with equilibrium radionuclide ventriculography and scored on visual inspection from 2 to −1, where 2 is normal, 1 hypokinetic, 0 akinetic and −1 dyskinetic. Wall motion was abnormal in 46 segments in 20 of the 22 patients. Positron emission tomography prior to surgery revealed concordantly reduced blood flow and glucose metabolism in 23 of the 46 segments with abnormal wall motion. Both blood flow and glucose uptake were normal in four segments, whereas blood flow was decreased and glucose uptake was elevated in 19 segments. Thus, abnormal wall motion was considered to be associated with ischemic but viable myocardium in 23 segments, whereas the remaining 23 segments were considered infarcted. When re-examined 5 to 7 weeks after surgery, wall motion had improved in 18 (78 percent) of the 23 segments with metabolic evidence of viability, but in only five (22 percent) of the other 23 segments with evidence of scar tissue on preoperative imaging. Thus, the findings by Tamaki and associates indicated a positive predictive accuracy of 78 percent and a negative predictive accuracy of 78 percent for improvement in segmental wall motion abnormalities following revascularization.

Although the study of Tamaki and associates[T3] was generally comparable to earlier findings, they reported a lower negative predictive accuracy of the "blood flow metabolism match." The value of only 78 percent, as compared with 92 percent by Tillisch and colleagues,[T2] may have resulted from two methodologic differences. First, Tamaki and his colleagues examined all patients in the fasted state. This resulted in low plasma insulin and glucose levels and high free fatty acid levels which suppressed fluorine-18 2-fluoro 2-deoxyglucose uptake in normal myocardium, and in which only ischemic but viable myocardium characteristically exhibited tracer uptake. In contrast, Tillisch and co-workers examined patients after glucose loading, resulting in fluorine-18 2-fluoro 2-deoxyglucose uptake in both ischemic and normal myocardium. Thus, the approach of Tamaki and associates detected even subtle increases in uptake of fluorine-18 2-fluoro 2-deoxyglucose, possibly owing to only small amounts of viable myocardium, which, if revascularized, may not have resulted in an improvement of segmental wall motion. Second, Tamaki and associates employed only visual inspection for their metabolic image analysis, whereas Tillisch and associates submitted both the nitrogen-13 ammonia perfusion and the fluorine-18 2-fluoro 2-deoxyglucose images to circumferential profile analysis of regional myocardial tracer activity concentrations. Viable myocardial regions were identified only if the discordance between blood flow and glucose utilization exceeded 2 standard deviations of a normal control population. It is therefore likely that the approach by Tamaki and associates is more sensitive for detecting myocardial viability, while the approach employed by Tillisch and associates is more specific for identifying myocardium that will exhibit improvement in contractile function if blood flow is restored.[T2, T3]

Recovery of Blood Flow, Metabolism, and Contractile Function After Revascularization

To assess both the temporal and quantitative relationships between recovery of myocardial perfusion, glucose metabolism, and segmental function following restoration of blood flow to ischemic myocardium, Nienaber and colleagues studied 11 patients with ischemic heart disease and resting segmental wall motion abnormalities undergoing percutaneous transluminal coronary angioplasty.[N3] Positron emission tomography with nitrogen-13 ammonia and fluorine-18 2-fluoro 2-deoxyglucose was performed 24 hours before and 48 hours and 2 months following coronary angioplasty. Segmental function was assessed with two-dimensional echocardiography.

Quantitative indices of abnormal wall motion were derived by multiplying visually assessed segmental wall motion scores by the percent of myocardium with abnormal function. Quantitative indices of abnormal perfusion were derived from the nitrogen-13 ammonia circumferential count profiles by multiplying the percent of visualized myocardium with abnormal perfusion by the severity of the deviation from normal laboratory values. In a similar fashion, quantitative indices of myocardial ischemia were calculated by multiplying the percent of visualized myocardium with an elevated nitrogen-13/fluorine-18 count difference by the severity of deviation from normal values. Changes in lesion geometry following coronary angioplasty were assessed with quantitative coronary angiography.

Coronary angioplasty improved coronary stenosis dimensions, as determined by a significant decrease in the percent area stenosis from 87.0 ± 13.5 percent to 54.0 ± 24.5 percent ($P < 0.05$) on quantitative coronary angiography. This was associated with a significant improvement in the mean nitrogen-13 ammonia perfusion defect score (Fig. 67–28) on the early postangioplasty positron emission tomography (115.9 ± 166.3 versus 31.2 ± 50.5, $P < 0.01$). However, despite the early improvement in resting myocardial perfusion, the mean echocardiographic wall motion score index did not improve significantly (108 ± 79 versus 97 ± 86, P = NS), indicating persistence of myocardial dysfunction despite improvement in blood flow.

Although there was improvement in the nitrogen-13 ammonia perfusion/fluorine-18 2-fluoro 2-deoxyglucose metabolism mismatch score (156 ± 175 versus 51 ± 33, $P < 0.05$) on positron emission tomography performed early after angioplasty, quantitative rates of myocardial glucose utilization obtained in eight of the patients revealed that ratios of values in risk myocardium relative to normal myocardium did not change significantly from the pre- to the early postangioplasty studies (1.68 ± 0.81 versus 1.24 ± 0.39, P = NS). This suggests that the early improvement in the nitrogen-13 ammonia perfusion/fluorine-18 2-fluoro 2-deoxyglucose metabolism mismatch score occurred primarily because of an improvement of perfusion rather than normalization of tissue glucose utilization.

On positron emission tomography two months following angioplasty, no further improvement in mean perfusion score was noted (31.2 ± 50.5 versus 24.2 ± 19.2, P = NS). However, there was further improvement in the nitrogen-13 ammonia perfusion/fluorine-18 2-fluoro 2-deoxyglucose metabolism mismatch score (51 ± 33 versus 15 ± 16, $P < 0.05$). In addition,

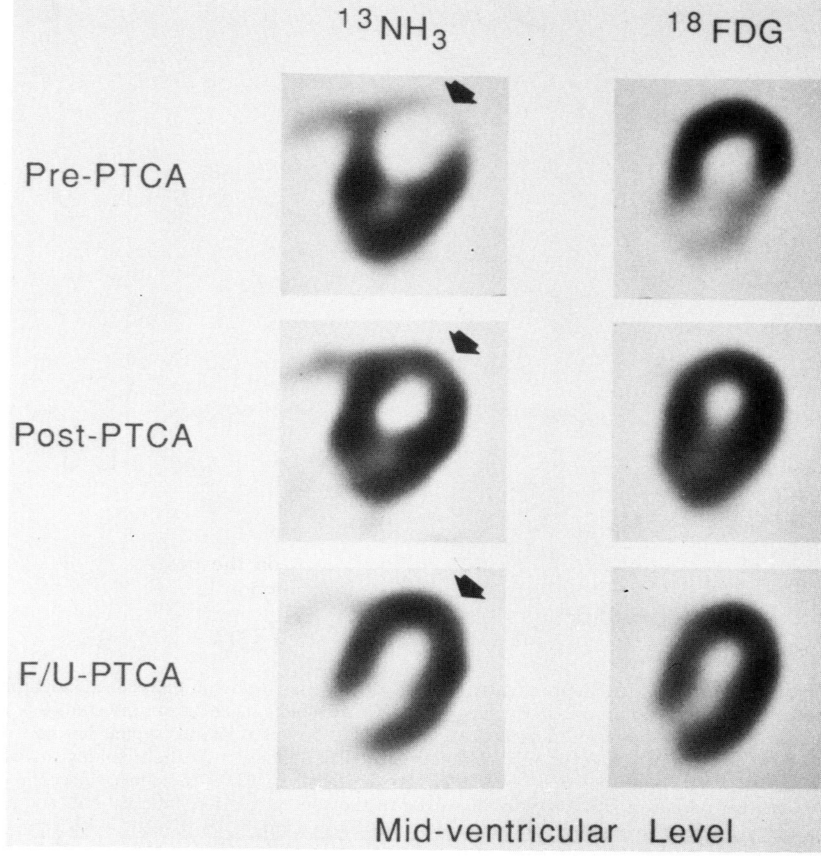

Figure 67–28. Sequential [^{13}N] ammonia perfusion ($^{13}NH_3$) and ^{18}F 2-fluoro 2-deoxyglucose (^{18}FDG) metabolic images in a patient just before (Pre-PTCA), early after (Post-PTCA), and 2 months (F/U-PTCA) following angioplasty of a proximal anterior left anterior descending coronary artery stenosis. The pre-PTCA positron emission tomographic study demonstrates an extensive metabolism perfusion mismatch in the anteroseptal and anteroapical regions of the ventricle. Early after successful angioplasty of the left anterior descending coronary lesion, there is considerable improvement in myocardial perfusion (*arrow*). However, glucose utilization remains enhanced relative to blood flow in the territory of the anterior descending coronary artery. By 2 months, both perfusion and glucose metabolism have normalized, indicating full recovery of tissue metabolism following successful restoration of blood flow by angioplasty of the culprit coronary lesion.

ratios of glucose utilization rates in risk myocardium relative to reference myocardium normalized (0.94 ± 0.37), suggesting that the late improvement in the nitrogen-13 ammonia perfusion/fluorine-18 2-fluoro 2-deoxyglucose metabolism mismatch score resulted primarily from a normalization of glucose metabolism in risk myocardium. A significant improvement in mean wall motion score was noted on the delayed studies at 2 months (56 ± 52, $P < 0.05$, compared with preangioplasty), and the quantitative extent of recovery of segmental function was linearly related to the preangioplasty mismatch score (change in wall motion score = 0.28 · preangioplasty mismatch score + 22, SEE = 27.9, r = 0.90, $P < 0.001$). Improvement in segmental function correlated only weakly with the preangioplasty perfusion score (r = 0.69), indicating that the tissue characterization afforded by concurrent perfusion and metabolic imaging more accurately predicts the ultimate degree of improvement in segmental function following restoration of blood flow than the assessment of myocardial perfusion alone.

Thus, full recovery of left ventricular function may be delayed following relief of chronic myocardial ischemia in humans. Improvement in tissue glucose metabolism appears to be paralleled by recovery of segmental function. Although there is a significant improvement in myocardial perfusion early after interventional restoration of blood flow, metabolic imaging with fluorine-18 2-fluoro 2-deoxyglucose identifies the persistence of an abnormal metabolic state. As demonstrated in animal experiments, this metabolic state is characterized by an accelerated rate of exogenous glucose utilization, which may reflect a period of cellular repair, necessary for return of full contractile function. Alternatively, it is also possible that the early persistence of enhanced regional glucose utilization reflects slow normalization of a chronic metabolic adaptive process to a persistent reduction in blood flow.[F4] For example, in the 22 patients studied by Tamaki and associates, repeat positron emission tomography performed 5 to 7 weeks after coronary artery bypass demonstrated persistently elevated myocardial uptake of fluorine-18 2-fluoro 2-deoxyglucose in 6 of the 19 (32 percent) segments with abnormal wall motion and enhanced glucose utilization prior to revascularization.[T3] Three of the six segments (50 percent) in which uptake of fluorine-18 2-fluoro 2-deoxyglucose remained elevated failed to exhibit improvement in wall motion. In contrast, wall motion invariably improved in the segments in which uptake of fluorine-18 2-fluoro 2-deoxyglucose had normalized. These data suggest that recovery of function in chronically ischemic human myocardium following restoration of blood flow may not be fully achieved until the abnormalities in tissue glucose metabolism have resolved.

The relationship between the severity of ischemic human myocardial dysfunction and the time course of recovery of left ventricular function after restoration of blood flow has not been well-defined. However, the case report of Luu and associates dramatically illustrates that recovery of left ventricular function may be quite prolonged following coronary artery revascularization in some patients with severe myocardial ischemia.[L4] Their patient, a 46-year-old man with ischemic cardiomyopathy (New York Heart Association Class IV), had an ejection fraction of 16 percent on resting radionuclide ventriculography. Although tomographic thallium-201 imaging revealed extensive and persistent perfusion defects, metabolic imaging with positron emission tomography uncovered significant viability in virtually all myo-

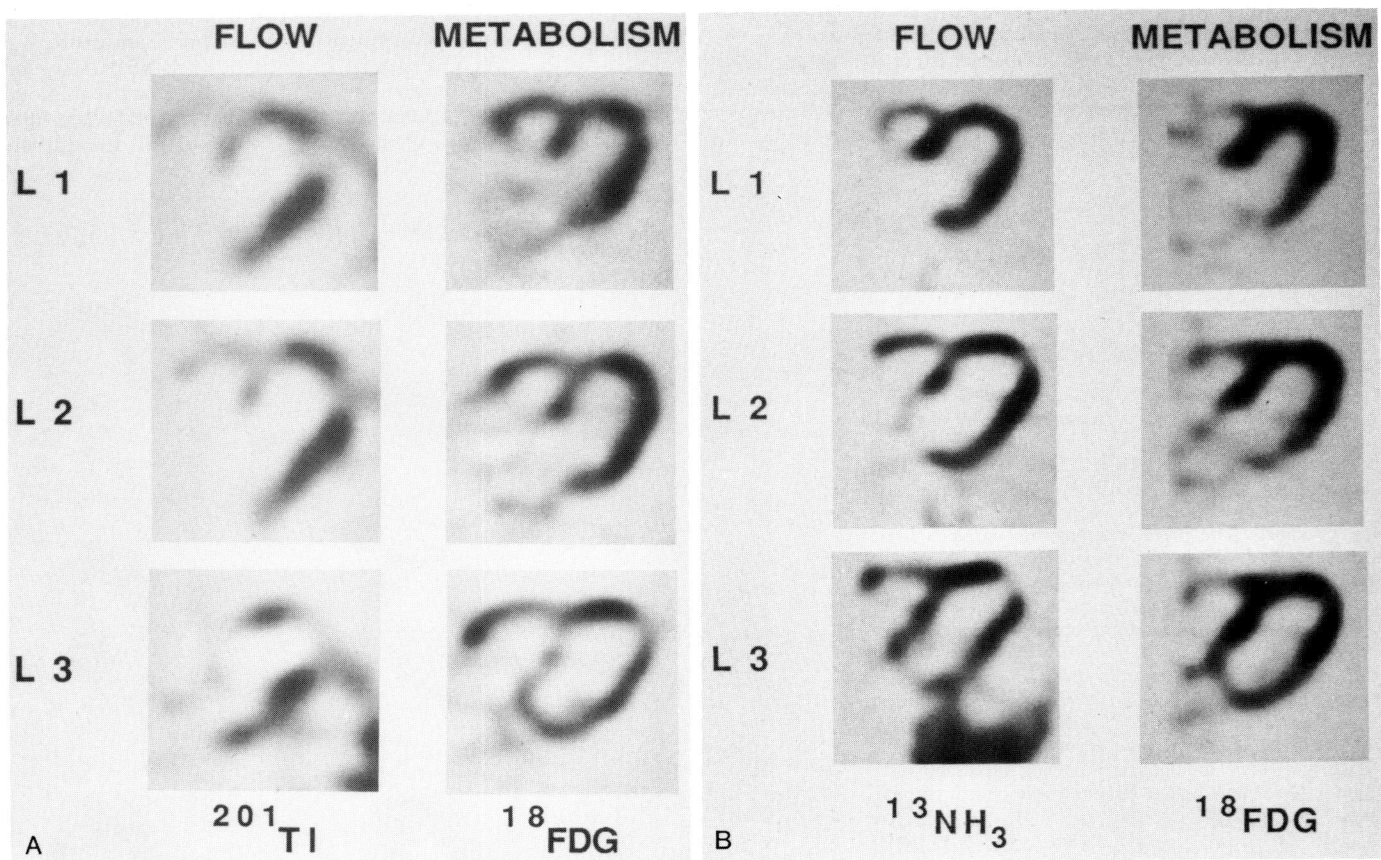

Figure 67–29. *Panel A*, Representative cross-sectional single-photon emission tomographic 24-hour redistribution thallium–201 images (^{201}Tl) and the corresponding ^{18}F 2-fluoro 2-deoxyglucose (^{18}FDG) metabolic images from the studies of a 45-year-old man with ischemic cardiomyopathy. On the ^{201}Tl images, extensive perfusion defects are identified in the anterolateral, septal, inferior, and inferolateral regions of the ventricle. In contrast, glucose metabolism is well preserved in the same ventricular regions, indicating residual myocardial viability. *Panel B*, Representative cross-sectional [^{13}N] ammonia ($^{13}NH_3$) perfusion and ^{18}F 2-fluoro 2-deoxyglucose (^{18}FDG) metabolic images in the same patient 2 months following coronary bypass surgery. Myocardial perfusion has markedly improved in the septal, inferior, inferolateral, and anteroapical regions of the ventricle. Although the resting left ventricular ejection fraction had increased from 16 percent to 26 percent at this point in time, ultimate recovery of ventricular function was not achieved until a full year after coronary bypass surgery (Table 67–1). (From Luu, M., Stevenson, L.W., Brunken, R.C., et al.: Delayed recovery of revascularized myocardium after referral for cardiac transplantation. Am. Heart. J. 119 (Part I):668–670, 1990, with permission.)

Table 67–1. LEFT VENTRICULAR FUNCTION FOLLOWING CABG IN A PATIENT WITH ISCHEMIC CARDIOMYOPATHY

	Echocardiography	LVEF (RNV)	
Date	*End Diastolic Dimension (mm)*	*Rest (%)*	*Exercise (%)*
Preoperative	66	16	15
One month	68	26	24
Six months	52	33	34
Twelve months	52	40	47

LVEF (RNV)—left ventricular ejection fraction (radionuclide ventriculography).

(From Luu, M., et al.: Delayed recovery of revascularized myocardium after referral for cardiac transplantation. Am. Heart J. 119(Part I):668, 1990, with permission.)

cardial segments (Fig. 67–29). The patient was referred for coronary revascularization rather than for heart transplantation. The patient's postoperative course was complicated by marked left ventricular failure requiring use of an intra-aortic balloon pump and the administration of vasopressors. Eventually, the patient's condition stabilized and he was discharged on medical therapy with little improvement in left ventricular function (Table 67–1). Over the ensuing three months the patient was admitted to the hospital on two separate occasions for treatment of congestive heart failure despite improvement on follow-up positron emission tomography (Fig. 67–29). On medical therapy, the patient's symptoms gradually improved to functional class II and he returned to work. On serial noninvasive testing, it was clear that left ventricular function had slowly improved over the 12 months after bypass surgery, indicating that the beneficial effects of restoration of blood flow to the chronically ischemic myocardium in this patient were not fully achieved for a considerable period of time. This case study suggests that recovery of contractile function after revascularization may require a considerable period of time and that therefore the beneficial effects of coronary revascularization on left ventricular function may be underestimated if assessment of function is performed too soon after restoration of blood flow.

Hashimoto and associates have suggested that some patients with depressed myocardial segmental uptake of fluorine-18 2-fluoro 2-deoxyglucose might also have residual tissue viability in the clinical infarct zone.[H2] They reported findings in two patients with chronic anterior infarction before and 4 and 8 months postangioplasty. In both cases, initially studied between 2 and 5 months after clinical myocardial infarction, marked decreases in both nitrogen-13 ammonia and fluorine-18 2-fluoro 2-deoxyglucose myocardial uptake were noted on the preangioplasty studies. At 4 and 8 months, both myocardial perfusion and glucose metabolism had improved. In one patient, wall motion in the anterior wall improved from akinesis to hypokinesis, but ventriculography was not repeated in the second patient.

Although the researchers suggested that the regions showing "PET infarction" might have been utilizing an alternative metabolic pathway for energy production and therefore exhibited only minimal uptake of fluorine-18 2-fluoro 2-deoxyglucose, another possible explanation is that myocardial uptake of fluorine-18 2-fluoro 2-deoxyglucose was underestimated because of technical factors. Since myocardial tracer uptake was assessed only visually, it is not possible to determine the myocardial extraction of fluorine-18 2-fluoro 2-deoxyglucose relative to that of nitrogen-13 ammonia. These case reports suggest that the myocardial tissue characterization in some patients might be enhanced by use of quantitative measurements of myocardial blood flow and glucose utilization rates, rather than reliance upon visual image analysis alone.

Synopsis

The reports of Tillisch,[T2] Tamaki,[T3] Nienaber,[N3] and their colleagues indicate that identification of residual tissue glucose metabolism in hypoperfused ventricular segments on metabolic imaging with positron emission tomography in patients with ischemic heart disease is a reliable marker of clinically important myocardial viability. Regional contractile function improves in metabolically active myocardial segments following interventional restoration of blood flow, and the ultimate degree of functional improvement is related to the anatomic extent and severity of the mismatch between perfusion and glucose metabolism on the preoperative positron emission tomographic images. The studies also suggest that recovery of both myocardial function and metabolism may be delayed following interventional restoration of blood flow.

Relationship Between Myocardial Metabolic Activity and Other Diagnostic Tests for Determination of Tissue Viability

Although identification of tissue glucose metabolism in clinical studies indicated the presence of ischemically compromised but viable tissue in patients with coronary artery disease, it remained to be determined whether the metabolic assessment of tissue viability with positron emission tomography provided unique information that could not be obtained with routine clinical tests. Accordingly, clinical studies in patients with chronic ischemic heart disease were performed to compare the tissue characterization afforded by positron emission tomography with that derived from routine clinical tests.

Electrocardiography

Although pathologic Q waves on the resting electrocardiogram have been attributed to "transmural" myocardial infarction,[C2, G4] careful clinicopathologic studies have shown that Q waves do not reliably distinguish transmural from subendocardial infarction.[D4, F3, R8, S18, S19] Both Durrer[D4] and Savage[S18] and their colleagues have reported that even small subendocardial infarctions may be associated with significant Q waves. In addition, chronic anterior Q waves have disappeared and associated regional ventricular dysfunction has improved following coronary revascularization,[C3, Z1] indicating that electrocardiographic Q waves and regional wall motion abnormalities are not always indicative of transmural scar formation.

Brunken and colleagues examined regional myocardial perfusion and glucose metabolism in 20 patients with 31 chronic electrocardiographic Q wave infarctions.[B15] All patients had clinical histories of one or more antecedent myocardial infarctions. The mean interval from the most recent clinical infarction to positron emission tomography was 20.6 months. Eight of the patients had triple-vessel disease, nine had double-vessel disease, one had single-vessel disease, and one patient with a well-documented clinical myocardial infarction had a 40 percent isolated stenosis of the left anterior descending artery. One patient did not have coronary angiography. Of the 20 patients, 10 (50 percent) had a history of congestive heart failure, and the mean left ventricular ejection fraction was depressed at 35.1 ± 12.1 percent. The mean interval between electrocardiography and positron emission tomography was 15.4 ± 20.1 days.

Each patient had persistent pathologic Q waves on serial electrocardiograms that were considered indicative of chronic myocardial infarction. Q waves were considered significant if greater than or equal to 0.04 second in duration or if deeper than one third of the following R wave. Four infarct regions were defined: septal, anterior, lateral, and inferior. Septal infarction was defined by pathologic Q waves in precordial leads V_1, V_2 ± V_3. Anterior infarction was diagnosed if the R wave in lead V_1 was preserved and if pathologic Q waves were present in any of the leads from V_2 to V_5. Lateral infarction was considered present when Q waves were noted in at least two of I, AVL, and V_6, while inferior infarction was identified by Q waves in at least two of the three inferior leads (II, III, AVF).

There were 31 Q wave regions in the 20 patients. Of these 31 regions, 11 were septal, 7 were anterior, 3 were lateral, and 10 were inferior. Only 10 of the 31 Q wave infarct regions (32 percent) exhibited the concordant reductions in perfusion and glucose metabolism indicative of completed infarction (Fig. 67–30). Six of the Q wave regions (20 percent) had the metabolism-perfusion mismatch of myocardial ischemia (Fig. 67–31). In 15 of

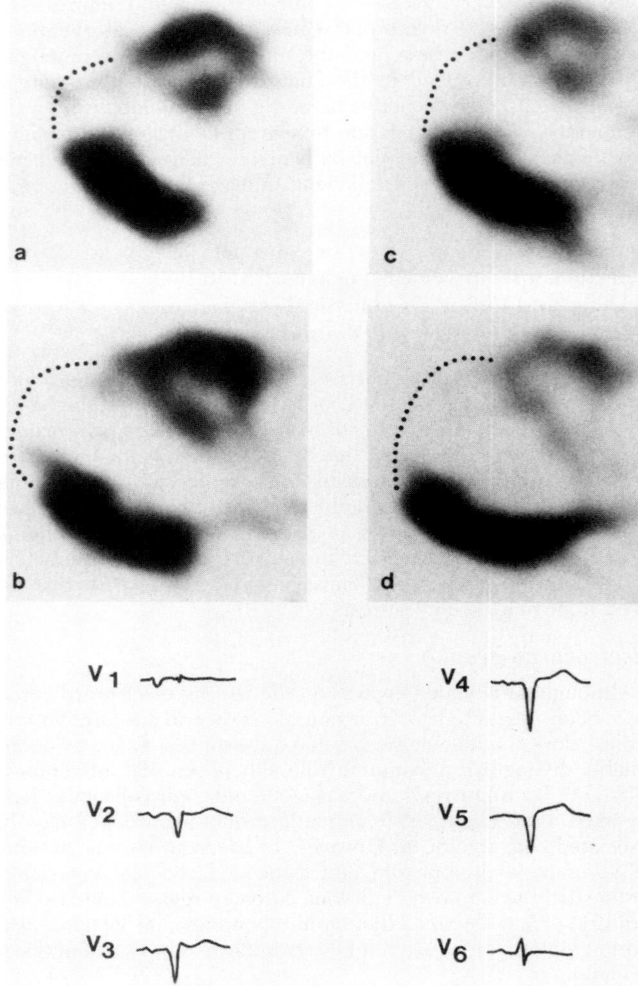

Figure 67–30. Representative [^{13}N] ammonia perfusion images (*panels a and b*) and ^{18}F 2-fluoro 2-deoxyglucose metabolic images (*panels c and d*) and the precordial electrocardiogram in a 68-year-old man with a history of myocardial infarction 5 months prior to study. On the electrocardiogram deep Q waves are noted in V_1 through V_5, in agreement with the concordant decreases in perfusion and glucose metabolism identified in the anteroapical and septal regions of the ventricle. The electrocardiogram and positron emission tomography both indicate completed myocardial infarction. (From Brunken, R., Tillisch, J., Schwaiger, M., et al.: Regional perfusion, glucose metabolism and wall motion in patients with chronic electrocardiographic Q-wave infarctions: Evidence for persistence of viable tissue in some infarct regions by positron emission tomography. Circulation 73:951–963, 1986, by permission of the American Heart Association, Inc.)

the Q wave infarct regions, regional tracer concentrations were within 2 standard deviations of established normal limits and therefore were considered normal (Fig. 67–32). Thus, positron emission tomography revealed metabolic evidence of tissue viability in 21 of 31 (68 percent) Q wave infarct regions.

Because previous investigations have shown an inexact relationship between the anatomic site of abnormal electrical activity and the surface electrocardiographic leads displaying Q waves[F5, G5, H3] a second analysis of the data was performed to avoid inadvertent bias in favor of positron emission tomography. In this analysis, Q wave regions were reassigned to maximize the agreement between the positron emission tomographic and the electrocardiographic "infarct regions." Even when this second analysis of the data was performed, the majority of myocardial Q wave infarct regions—15 of 28 Q wave regions (54 percent)—exhibited evidence of metabolic activity. No characteristic ST segment or T wave changes distinguished regions with metabolic criteria for ischemia from regions with criteria for completed infarction. T wave inversion and ST segment elevation and depression were noted with equal frequency in both groups. Thus, this report indicated that tissue viability could be identified with fluorine-18 2-fluoro 2-deoxyglucose and positron emission tomography in a significant proportion (54 percent) of electrocardiographic Q wave infarct regions, and that neither ST segment nor T wave changes were helpful in distinguishing hypoperfused regions with metabolic viability from regions with completed infarction.

Confirmation that glucose metabolic viability can be identified with metabolic imaging in regions with chronic myocardial infarction was provided in a subsequent report by Fudo and colleagues, who studied 22 patients with chronic anterior myocardial infarctions utilizing rest and stress nitrogen-13 ammonia

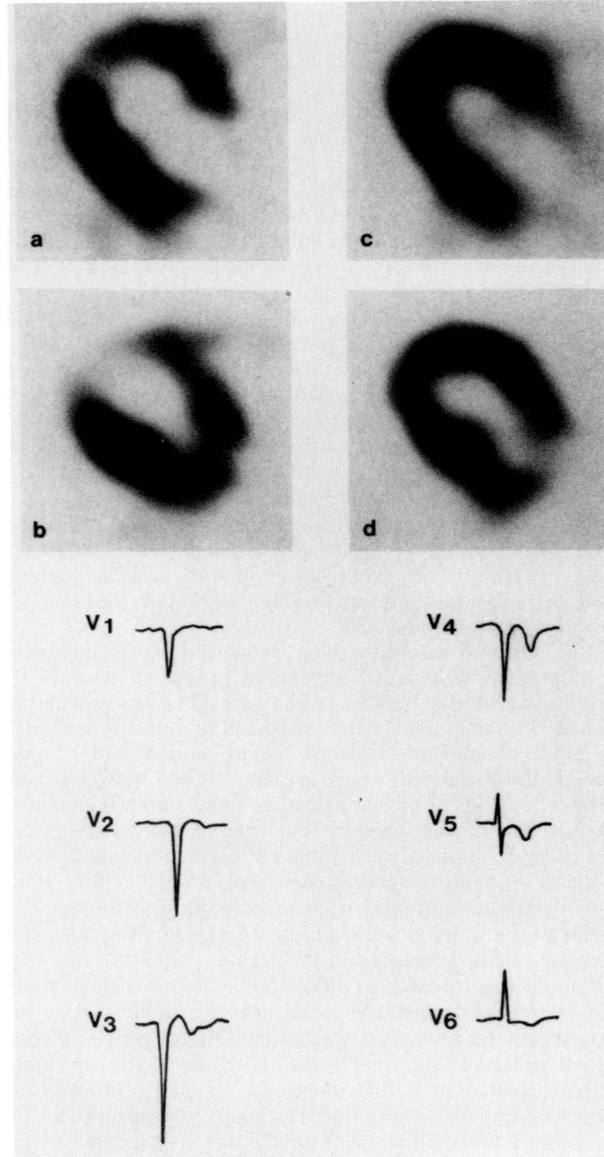

Figure 67–31. Precordial electrocardiogram and representative [^{13}N] ammonia perfusion images (*panels a and b*) and ^{18}F 2-fluoro 2-deoxyglucose metabolic images (*panels c and d*) in a 59-year-old man who sustained an anterior myocardial infarction 1 year prior to study. On the electrocardiogram pathologic Q waves are noted in V_1 through V_4. On the [^{13}N] ammonia perfusion images, defects are identified in the anterior and septal regions of the ventricle. In contrast, exogenous glucose utilization is well preserved in these hypoperfused ventricular regions, indicating the metabolism-perfusion mismatch of myocardial ischemia. (From Brunken, R., Tillisch, J., Schwaiger, M., et al.: Regional perfusion, glucose metabolism and wall motion in patients with chronic electrocardiographic Q-wave infarctions: Evidence for persistence of viable tissue in some infarct regions by positron emission tomography. Circulation 73:951–963, 1986, with permission.)

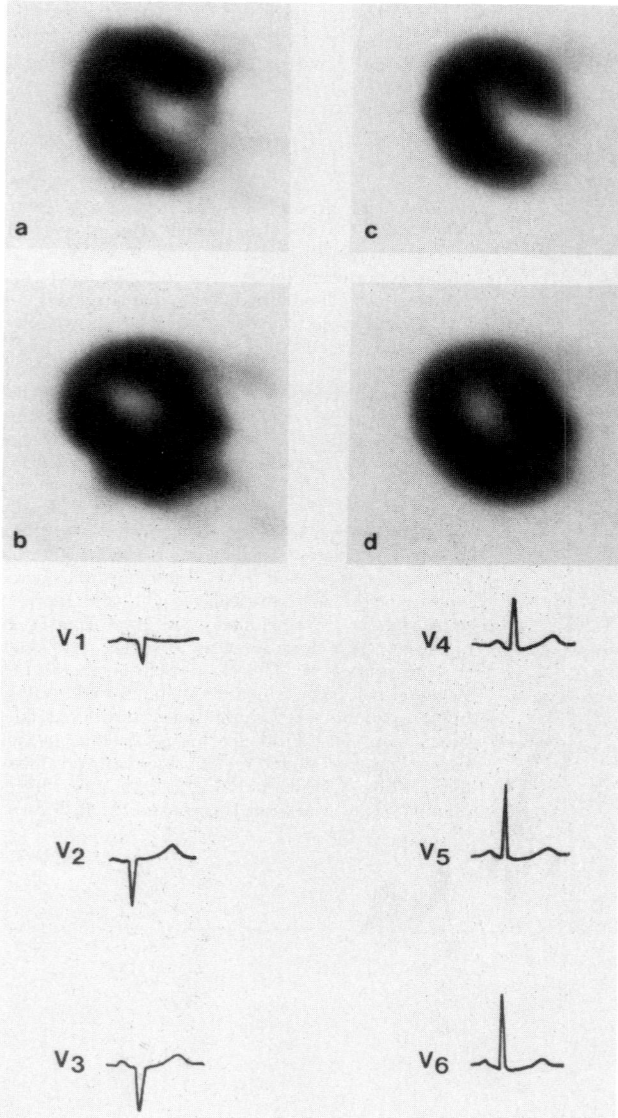

Figure 67–32. Representative [^{13}N] ammonia perfusion images (*panels a and b*) and ^{18}F 2-fluoro 2-deoxyglucose metabolic images (*panels c and d*) and precordial electrocardiogram of a 45-year-old woman with a well-documented anterior myocardial infarction 3 years prior to study. Although the electrocardiogram demonstrates pathologic Q waves in V_1 through V_3, regional perfusion and exogenous glucose utilization are within normal laboratory limits, indicating substantial tissue viability in the region with the electrocardiographic Q wave infarction. (From Brunken, R., Tillisch, J., Schwaiger, M., et al.: Regional perfusion, glucose metabolism and wall motion in patients with chronic electrocardiographic Q wave infarctions: Evidence for persistence of viable tissue in some infarct regions by positron emission tomography. Circulation 73:951–963, 1986, by permission of the American Heart Association, Inc.)

perfusion and remote (within 1 week) fluorine-18 2-fluoro 2-deoxyglucose metabolic imaging.[F2] The mean interval from anterior myocardial infarction to the positron emission tomographic study was 20 weeks. Although the myocardial infarctions were diagnosed by "electrocardiographic and enzymatic criteria," their report did not indicate the number of the patients with Q waves on the electrocardiogram. Twenty-one of the twenty-two patients had coronary angiography: eight patients had single-vessel disease of the left anterior descending artery, five had double-vessel disease, five had triple-vessel disease, and two had stenoses of the left anterior descending artery that were less than 70 percent.

When studied with positron emission tomography, 19 of the 22 patients (86 percent) had resting nitrogen-13 ammonia perfusion defects in the anterior wall. With exercise, 16 of the patients exhibited peripheral expansion of their resting perfusion defects, and 6 of these individuals had augmented uptake of fluorine-18 2-fluoro 2-deoxyglucose in these zones of peripheral perfusion defect expansion (see the section entitled Studies with Fluorine-18 2-Fluoro 2-Deoxyglucose for Alterations in Exogenous Glucose Utilization under the heading Acute Myocardial Ischemia). More importantly, 12 of the patients (54.5 percent) had diffuse uptake of fluorine-18 2-fluoro 2-deoxyglucose in the hypoperfused anterior regions, while an additional 2 patients (9.1 percent) without resting perfusion defects had elevated uptake of fluorine-18 2-fluoro 2-deoxyglucose in the electrocardiographic infarct region.

Hashimoto and associates compared the nitrogen-13 ammonia and fluorine-18 2-fluoro 2-deoxyglucose images in 11 patients with chronic non-Q wave infarctions with those obtained in 11 patients with chronic Q wave infarctions.[H4] The patient population consisted of 22 patients with documented anterior or lateral wall infarctions. Electrocardiographic Q wave infarction was defined by the presence of Q waves greater than or equal to 30 ms in duration in at least two adjacent electrocardiographic leads. Non-Q wave myocardial infarction was defined by a history of precordial chest pain of greater than 30 minutes' duration and elevation of MB creatine kinase levels on serial studies, along with significant evolution of ST segment or T wave changes or both on serial electrocardiograms. The mean interval from the most recent clinical infarction to positron emission tomography was 3.3 ± 2.6 months in the patients with the non-Q wave and 5.8 ± 6.7 months in patients with the Q wave infarctions (P = NS).

On the nitrogen-13 ammonia images, only 5 (45 percent) of the 11 patients with non-Q wave infarctions had resting perfusion defects. With exercise, 8 (73 percent) demonstrated a perfusion defect. In contrast, all 11 patients with Q wave myocardial infarction had perfusion defects, both on the resting and the stress studies. Of the 15 patients who had coronary angiography and resting perfusion defects, all had significant stenoses (greater than or equal to 90 percent) in the infarct-related artery. Four of the six patients without a resting perfusion defect had coronary stenoses of less than or equal to 50 percent in the infarct vessel. One patient with a 90 percent stenosis did not exhibit a perfusion defect, either at rest or with exercise, and this was attributed to the patient's use of a beta-blocker.

Of the 11 patients with Q wave myocardial infarction, 4 (36 percent) exhibited enhanced uptake of fluorine-18 2-fluoro 2-deoxyglucose in the hypoperfused infarct region. In contrast, 10 (91 percent) of the 11 patients with non-Q wave infarction had increased uptake of the labeled glucose tracer in the clinical infarct region ($P < 0.01$). Thus, while this study suggests that myocardial metabolic viability is observed more frequently in individuals with non-Q wave infarction than in those with Q wave infarction, it also confirms that a significant proportion (36 percent) of patients with chronic Q wave infarction will exhibit residual metabolic tissue viability on positron emission tomography with fluorine-18 2-fluoro 2-deoxyglucose.

The results of these clinical investigations are consistent with previous histologic studies demonstrating that myocardial infarction is an inhomogeneous process.[F3, S18, S19] In some patients an infarction may be nearly transmural in extent, whereas in other patients there may be only small amounts of subendocardial fibrosis. As noted, electrocardiographic Q waves reflect only abnormal electrical activation of the myocardium and do not establish etiology nor imply irreversibility of the underlying process (Fig. 67–33). Thus, glucose metabolic imaging with positron emission tomography provides an additional means of tissue characterization in patients with previous myocardial infarction, and the presence of chronic Q waves on the electrocardiogram does not preclude the existence of substantial amounts of viable tissue in the clinical infarct zone.

Regional Myocardial Wall Motion

Although assessment of segmental wall motion has been utilized to infer the presence or absence of viable myocardium in patients with ischemic heart disease, previous histopathologic studies have indicated that the severity of a resting wall motion abnormality is not always related to the extent of myocardial fibrosis.[C4, F6, I2, S20]

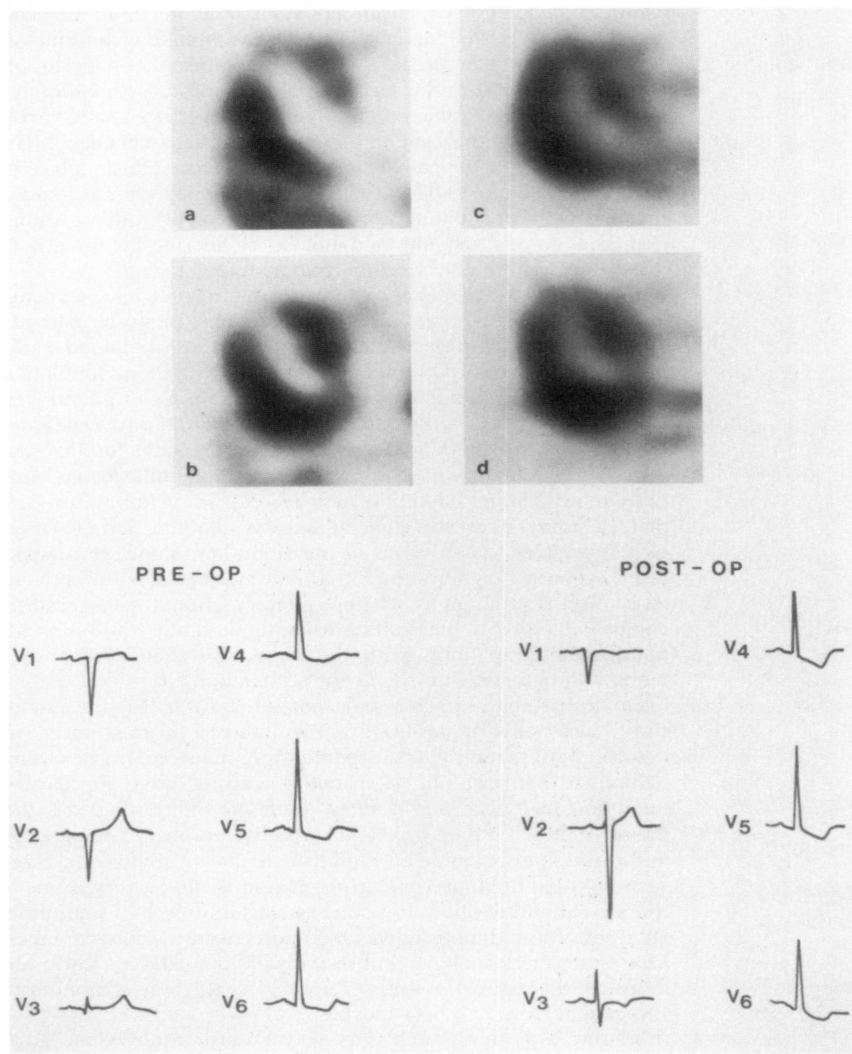

Figure 67–33. Precordial electrocardiograms obtained before (PRE-OP) and after (POST-OP) coronary bypass surgery along with representative preoperative [^{13}N] ammonia perfusion images (*panels a and b*) and ^{18}F 2-fluoro 2-deoxyglucose metabolic images (*panels c and d*) in a 73-year-old woman with a history of two remote myocardial infarctions and recurrent angina. The [^{13}N] ammonia perfusion images demonstrate an anteroapical perfusion defect. On the metabolic images there is preserved glucose metabolism in the hypoperfused region, indicating myocardial viability. On the preoperative electrocardiogram pathologic Q waves are noted in leads V_1 through V_3. Following coronary bypass surgery, the anterior Q waves are replaced by normal appearing R waves. Along with the electrocardiographic changes, the patient's left ventricular ejection fraction increased from 25 percent to 45 percent following coronary revascularization, and there was improvement in wall motion in the anteroapical region of the ventricle from akinesis to severe hypokinesis. (From Brunken, R., Tillisch, J., Schwaiger, M., et al.: Regional perfusion, glucose metabolism and wall motion in patients with chronic electrocardiographic Q wave infarctions: Evidence for persistence of viable tissue in some infarct regions by positron emission tomography. Circulation 73: 951–963, 1986, by permission of the American Heart Association, Inc.)

To determine whether analysis of regional wall motion might assist in distinguishing regions with and without metabolic activity, Brunken and colleagues assessed segmental wall motion in Q wave and non-Q wave regions considered normal, ischemic, and infarcted on positron emission tomography (see earlier section: Metabolism as a Clinical Indicator of Tissue Viability: Electrocardiography).[B15] Resting left ventricular wall motion abnormalities were assessed with gated radionuclide ventriculography in 14 patients, with two-dimensional echocardiography in 4 patients, and with contrast left ventriculography in 2 patients. The mean interval from the wall motion study to positron emission tomography was 20.5 ± 21.9 days. Regional wall motion was graded according to the following scale: normal = 0, mild hypokinesis = 1, severe hypokinesis = 2, akinesis = 3, and dyskinesis = 4. Three independent observers graded segmental wall motion, and their scores were averaged to give a mean regional wall motion score.

Regions with electrocardiographic Q waves that were considered normal on positron emission tomography had a mean wall motion score of 1.27 ± 0.85, whereas ischemic regions had a score of 2.17 ± 0.81, and infarcted regions had a score of 2.69 ± 0.59. The score for normal regions was significantly better than the score for ischemic regions ($P < 0.025$) or for infarcted regions ($P < 0.0005$). Perhaps more importantly, there was no significant difference between the scores for ischemic and infarcted regions, indicating that assessment of wall motion failed to distinguish between hypoperfused regions with and without metabolic evidence of tissue viability.

Analysis of wall motion in 52 non-Q wave regions yielded similar findings. Normal regions had a mean wall motion score of 1.02 ± 0.71, ischemic regions had a mean score of 1.82 ± 0.88 ($P < 0.05$ versus normal), and infarcted regions had a score of 2.00 ± 0.71 ($P < 0.01$ versus normal, P = NS versus ischemic regions). Thus, the findings in this study indicate that the assessment of regional wall motion cannot successfully discriminate between hypoperfused regions with and without metabolic viability as determined on metabolic imaging with positron emission tomography.

Fudo and colleagues also correlated the results of metabolic imaging with regional wall motion (see Metabolism as a Clinical Indicator of Tissue Viability: Electrocardiography) in their study of patients with chronic anterior myocardial infarctions.[F2] They grouped their patients according to regional function in the anterior wall. Group I consisted of eight patients with dyskinesis; in group II there were seven patients with anterior akinesis; in group III there were seven patients with anterior hypokinesis. Of the eight patients in group I, three (37.5 percent) exhibited diffuse uptake of fluorine-18 2-fluoro 2-deoxyglucose in the anterior dyskinetic region. Of the seven patients in group II, three (42.9 percent) exhibited uptake of the glucose metabolic tracer in the akinetic zone of infarction. In contrast, six of seven (85.7 percent) patients in group III had diffuse uptake of fluorine-18 2-fluoro 2-deoxyglucose in the hypokinetic anterior regions. Thus, while the results of this study indicate that the myocardial regions with chronic infarction and less severe impairment in wall motion have a better probability of exhibiting metabolic viability on study with positron emission tomography, a significant proportion of dyskinetic (37.5 percent) and akinetic (42.9 percent) clinical infarct regions manifest metabolic evidence of viability. The results also suggest that reliance upon the severity of a regional wall motion abnormality alone may seriously underestimate the extent of tissue viability in patients with ischemic heart disease.

These metabolic observations are consistent with previous clinicopathologic investigations indicating that myocardial infarction is a heterogeneous process and that the extent of myocardial fibrosis in patients with ischemic heart disease may vary considerably among individuals. For example, in the autopsy study of Ideker and colleagues, the measured percent fibrosis in hypokinetic segments ranged from 0 to 60 percent, in akinetic segments from 0 to 85 percent, and in dyskinetic segments from 5 to 85 percent.[12] In addition, these investigators also reported that some segments with normal wall motion displayed as much as 40 percent fibrosis on histologic examination. Comparable findings were reported by Stinson and Billingham, who correlated the results of transmural apical biopsies obtained at the time of coronary bypass surgery with regional function.[S20] Normal or only mild-to-moderate fibrosis was found in 81 percent (17 of 21) of hypokinetic regions, 47 percent (9 of 19) of akinetic regions, and 21 percent (3 of 14) of dyskinetic regions.

Further indirect evidence that there frequently is viable tissue in asynergeic ventricular regions comes from the functional outcome of these segments if they are revascularized. In individuals with stable angina, improvement or normalization of resting wall motion abnormalities occurs in 34 to 66 percent of segments following successful coronary bypass grafting,[B16, B17, C5, R10, S21, T4] including 29 percent of segments with previous infarction.[C5] In addition, both Cohen[C6] and Melchoir[M8] and their colleagues have reported that 83 percent and 65 percent, respectively, of patients with chronic ischemic left ventricular dysfunction will have improvement in regional function following angioplasty of the culprit vessel. Thus, assessment of segmental wall motion is not a reliable indicator of myocardial viability. The tissue characterization afforded by metabolic imaging with positron emission tomography is helpful in distinguishing asynergeic regions with extensive fibrosis from regions with viable but ischemically compromised tissue.

Thallium-201 Redistribution Scintigraphy

Thallium-201 redistribution scintigraphy has played an important clinical role in assessing myocardial viability.[B18, I3, I4, R11] Fixed thallium-201 defects usually have been attributed to completed infarction whereas resolution of defects on 4-hour delayed images has been associated with ischemic but viable tissue.[B19, P2, R11] Several clinical observations, however, suggest that thallium-201 redistribution scintigraphy might underestimate the extent of tissue viability in some patients. For example, Liu and associates noted that 12 of 16 (75 percent) myocardial segments with persistent defects on stress thallium-201 scintigraphy prior to angioplasty normalized on thallium-201 imaging after interventional restoration of blood flow.[L5] In a separate report, Gibson and group noted that 19 of 42 (45 percent) of myocardial segments with persistent defects on preoperative stress thallium-201 scintigraphy had normal thallium-201 uptake and normal washout kinetics after coronary revascularization.[G6] Thus, these reports indicate that some myocardial segments with fixed defects on thallium-201 scintigraphy might indeed harbor viable tissue.

To determine the metabolic viability of myocardial segments with persistent thallium-201 defects, Brunken and co-workers studied 12 consecutive patients with fixed defects on planar scintigraphy.[B20] Ten of the patients had a history of 14 prior myocardial infarctions. Eleven of the twelve patients had coronary angiography: seven had triple-vessel disease, two had double-vessel disease, and two had single-vessel disease. Of these 11 patients, 9 had one or more vessels with greater than 90 percent stenoses. The mean left ventricular ejection fraction was depressed at 32.1 ± 13.7 percent, and seven patients had congestive heart failure.

Planar thallium-201 images were assessed by three observers who independently graded myocardial thallium-201 uptake according to the following scale: 0 = normal, 1 = mild but definite defect, 2 = moderately severe defect, and 3 = complete defect (equal to background). Segmental scores on multiple views were averaged to give a mean value for each of seven anatomic segments: anterobasilar, anterolateral, apical, inferior, posterobasilar, anteroseptal, and lateral. A thallium-201 defect was defined by a mean segmental score of 0.66 or more—that is, at least two observers agreed that a defect was present on the initial images. Defects were considered fixed if the mean difference between the initial and redistribution scores was less than 0.5. Partial redistribution was defined by an improvement in the mean segmental score of 0.5 or more but failure to achieve a score of less than 0.33 on the redistribution study. A defect was considered completely reversible if the mean score on the redistribution study was less than 0.33—that is, at least two observers agreed that the defect had resolved on the delayed images.

Of the 51 segmental thallium-201 defects identified by the three observers, 36 were fixed, 11 were partially reversible, and 4 were completely reversible. Of the 36 segments with a fixed thallium-201 defect, only 15 (42 percent) exhibited the concordant defects in perfusion and glucose metabolism indicative of myocardial infarction on positron emission tomography. In contrast, the metabolism-perfusion mismatch of myocardial ischemia was present in 9 segments (25 percent), while 12 segments (33 percent) were normal on study with positron emission tomography. Thus, the majority of myocardial segments with a fixed thallium-201 defect (58 percent) exhibited evidence of myocardial metabolic viability on study with positron emission tomography.

Of the 11 segments with a partially reversible thallium-201 defect, 4 (36 percent) exhibited the concordant decreases in perfusion and glucose metabolism indicative of myocardial infarction. Four of the segments (36 percent) had the metabolism-perfusion mismatch of myocardial ischemia, while three segments (27 percent) were normal on positron emission tomography. Thus, residual tissue metabolic activity was detected in 64 percent of the segments with a partially reversible thallium-201 defect. Each of the four segments with completely reversible defects on thallium-201 scintigraphy was normal on positron emission tomography. In addition, positron emission tomography identified seven myocardial segments with resting perfusion defects that were not detected on planar thallium-201 imaging. Three of these segments exhibited positron tomographic criteria for myocardial infarction, whereas four segments exhibited the metabolism-perfusion mismatch of myocardial ischemia.

Nine of the twelve patients had one or more myocardial segments with the metabolism-perfusion mismatch of myocardial ischemia. In seven patients, ischemia was identified at sites remote from those of clinical infarction, or all the hypoperfused segments in a vascular territory exhibited positron tomographic ischemia. In only two patients, ischemia was identified adjacent to segments with completed myocardial infarction. Patients with metabolic criteria for myocardial ischemia were as likely to experience chest pain (five of nine versus two of three), to have triple-vessel coronary disease (six of nine versus one of two), or to require treatment for congestive heart failure (six of nine versus one of three) or ventricular ectopic activity (three of five versus two of five) as those without metabolic evidence for myocardial ischemia. The mean left ventricular ejection fraction was similarly depressed in patients with and without myocardial ischemia (32.0 ± 14.8 percent versus 32.3 ± 12.5 percent). Thus, none of the clinically available parameters reliably distinguished patients with positron tomographic criteria for myocardial ischemia from those with completed infarction on positron emission tomography. Perhaps more importantly, improvement or normalization of a thallium-201 defect on 4-hour redistribution images was not correlated with uptake of fluorine-18 2-fluoro 2-deoxyglucose (11 of 15 versus 21 of 26, P = NS), indicating that redistribution of thallium-201 was not associated statistically with myocardial viability in this patient population.

To assess both tissue glucose metabolism and regional wall motion in myocardial segments with persistent thallium-201 defects, Tamaki and associates correlated the findings on contrast left ventriculography and stress and 3-hour delayed single photon emission computed tomographic (SPECT) thallium-201 scintigraphy with positron emission tomography in 28 patients with remote myocardial infarction.[T5] The mean interval from the most recent infarction to study enrollment was 22 months (range: 2 to 108 months). Each patient underwent left ventriculography and coronary angiography within 4 weeks of the radionuclide studies. Regional function was graded on the contrast left ventriculograms by three observers who scored wall motion according to the following scale: 2 = normal, 1 = hypokinetic, 0 = akinetic, and −1 = dyskinetic. Differences in wall motion scores were resolved by mutual consensus.

Positron emission tomography with nitrogen-13 ammonia and fluorine-18 2-fluoro 2-deoxyglucose was performed within 2 weeks of thallium-201 scintigraphy. Quantitative analysis of thallium-201 uptake on the SPECT images and the nitrogen-13 ammonia images was performed with circumferential count profile analysis techniques, while thallium-201 defects in each of five myocardial segments were visually classified by three observers as fixed (no redistribution on delayed images) or transient (partial or complete redistribution on delayed images). The fluorine-18 2-fluoro 2-deoxyglucose images were interpreted by three observers who visually compared tracer uptake on the metabolic images with uptake of nitrogen-13 ammonia on the perfusion images. Segments with an increase in the uptake of the glucose analog were considered ischemic. In this investigation, the researchers analyzed only the segments "with thallium-201 perfusion defects in electrocardiographically defined infarcted areas" and excluded remote segments with perfusion defects from analysis. Thus a semiquantitative scoring system was not utilized to quantify the severity of the visually defined thallium-201 defects, nor were all myocardial segments with thallium-201 perfusion defects analyzed.

Each of the 28 patients had thallium-201 perfusion defects in the electrocardiographically defined infarct region. Transient thallium-201 defects were identified in at least one myocardial segment in 13 individuals, whereas persistent defects were identified in 15 individuals. In the 28 patients, 61 segmental thallium-201 defects were analyzed. Transient defects were present in 22 segments (36 percent) and persistent defects in 39 segments (64 percent). On positron emission tomography, myocardial glucose metabolism was preserved in 21 of the 22 segments with transient defects (95 percent) and 15 of the 39 segments with fixed defects (38 percent, $P < 0.001$). This study suggested, therefore, that redistribution of thallium-201 in a segmental defect was more frequently associated with preservation of myocardial glucose metabolism. In agreement with the findings of Brunken and colleagues, 40 percent of segments with fixed thallium-201 defects exhibited preservation of tissue glucose metabolism,[B20] again suggesting that analysis of relative myocardial perfusion underestimates the extent of tissue viability in a relatively large proportion of myocardial segments.

When Tamaki and co-workers assessed relative nitrogen-13 ammonia activity in the segments with the thallium-201 defects, segments with transient defects had less severe reductions in nitrogen-13 ammonia activity than the segments with fixed defects (−10 ± 4 percent versus − 19 ± 9 percent; $P< 0.05$).[T5] Of the segments with fixed defects, relative nitrogen-13 ammonia activity was less severely reduced when glucose metabolism was preserved, as compared with when glucose metabolism was absent (−13 ± 9 percent versus −23 ± 7 percent, $P< 0.005$).

Moreover, segmental wall motion was significantly better in segments with transient defects than in the segments with fixed thallium-201 defects (mean wall motion scores: 0.77 ± 0.60 versus 0.38 ± 0.74; $P < 0.05$). Also, segments with fixed thallium-201 defects but preserved glucose metabolic activity had significantly better wall motion scores than the segments without glucose metabolic activity (0.67 ± 0.70 versus 0.21 ± 0.71, $P < 0.05$). Thus, these data suggest that segments with persistent glucose metabolic activity have better wall motion (perhaps as a result of better preservation of blood flow) than segments with positron tomographic criteria for completed infarction. However, as indicated by the relatively large standard deviations of these measurements, considerable overlap occurred between each of the segmental classifications, so that assessment of relative perfusion and segmental wall motion in individual patients might prove clinically inadequate for distinguishing segments with completed infarction from segments with residual tissue viability, as assessed by metabolic imaging with positron emission tomography.

To determine whether positron emission tomography is superior to thallium-201 scintigraphy for detecting myocardial ischemia, the same investigators[T6] correlated the findings on stress and 3-hour delayed thallium-201 SPECT imaging with rest and exercise nitrogen-13 ammonia perfusion imaging and with fluorine-18 2-fluoro 2-deoxyglucose metabolic images. The study population consisted of 28 patients with angiographically confirmed coronary artery disease. Coronary stenoses of 50 percent or greater were considered hemodynamically significant. Positron emission tomography was performed within 2 weeks of thallium-201 SPECT imaging. After a rest perfusion study, an exercise nitrogen-13 ammonia perfusion study was performed, utilizing a supine bicycle ergometer. Metabolic imaging with fluorine-18 2-fluoro 2-deoxyglucose was performed within 1 week of the nitrogen-13 ammonia perfusion studies. Tracer uptake on both the thallium-201 SPECT images and the nitrogen-13 ammonia positron tomographic images was evaluated by circumferential count profile analysis techniques, as well as by visual analysis by three observers. Segments with a visual increase in the uptake of fluorine-18 2-fluoro 2-deoxyglucose relative to nitrogen-13 ammonia were considered ischemic. Observer differences were resolved by mutual consensus.

The sensitivity of stress and rest nitrogen-13 ammonia perfusion imaging for identifying significant coronary artery disease in the 28 patients was 80 percent (45 of the 56 vascular territories), compared with 79 percent for thallium-201 SPECT imaging (44 of 56 vascular territories). When analyzed according to vascular territory, similar sensitivities for detecting diseased vessels were noted for both thallium-201 SPECT scintigraphy and stress nitrogen-13 ammonia perfusion imaging (right coronary artery, 79 percent versus 80 percent; anterior descending artery, 88 percent versus 92 percent; circumflex artery, 62 percent versus 69 percent). The specificities for rest-stress nitrogen-13 ammonia perfusion imaging and thallium-201 SPECT imaging were also comparable (100 percent versus 96 percent, respectively).

When perfusion defects were classified as fixed, transient, or absent, there was a reasonable concordance between the nitrogen-13 ammonia perfusion studies and the thallium-201 SPECT studies, with an overall agreement of 72 percent (304 of 420 segments). In 47 segments (35 percent) with a fixed defect on thallium-201 SPECT scintigraphy, reversible (transient) defects were identified on nitrogen-13 ammonia perfusion imaging. In contrast, only 9 (11 percent) segments with persistent perfusion defects on positron emission tomography exhibited reversible (transient) defects on thallium-201 SPECT scintigraphy ($P < 0.001$). Thus, positron emission tomography identified reversible (transient) defects in 35 percent of the myocardial segments with fixed defects on thallium-201 SPECT scintigraphy, suggesting that the extent of myocardial viability might be underestimated by assessment of thallium-201 redistribution in some myocardial segments.

On metabolic imaging with fluorine-18 2-fluoro 2-deoxyglucose, residual metabolic activity was identified in 76 percent (87 of 115) of the myocardial segments with transient nitrogen-13 ammonia defects and 36 percent (30 of 82) of the segments with fixed nitrogen-13 ammonia perfusion defects. In addition, 2 percent (4 of 223) of the segments with normal nitrogen-13 ammonia perfusion studies exhibited augmented uptake of fluorine-18 2-fluoro 2-deoxyglucose in the fasting state, suggesting a postischemic state.

Similar findings were noted when comparison was made with the tomographic thallium-201 images. Augmented uptake of fluorine-18 2-fluoro 2-deoxyglucose was observed in 68 percent (52 of 77) of the myocardial segments with reversible and 41 percent (56 of 136) of the segments with fixed thallium-201 SPECT defects. In addition, 6 percent (13 of 207) of the segments normal on tomographic thallium-201 imaging exhibited augmented uptake of fluorine-18 2-fluoro 2-deoxyglucose. Thus, these studies illustrate the limitations of myocardial perfusion imaging for assessing tissue viability, indicating that underestimation of the extent of tissue viability (as determined by metabolic imaging with positron emission tomography and fluorine-18 2-fluoro 2-deoxyglucose) occurs in 36 to 41 percent of segments with fixed perfusion defects.

Brunken and colleagues compared thallium-201 SPECT scintigraphy with positron emission tomography in 26 patients (27 studies) with angiographically confirmed coronary artery disease.[B21] In the study population, 21 patients had a clinical history of 29 antecedent myocardial infarctions. The mean interval from coronary angiography to thallium-201 SPECT scintigraphy was 5.2 ± 6.8 weeks and to positron emission tomography, 5.3 ± 6.8 weeks. Two of the patients had left main coronary disease, seventeen had triple-vessel disease, five had double-vessel disease, and two had single-vessel disease. The mean left ventricular ejection fraction of the population was depressed at 32.3 ± 13.8 percent.

The mean interval between thallium-201 SPECT scintigraphy and positron emission tomography was 4.2 ± 4.8 days. Stress thallium-201 scintigraphy was performed in 20 patients, rest-redistribution thallium-201 scintigraphy in 5 patients, and dipyridamole thallium-201 scintigraphy in 1 patient. Three observers independently assessed thallium-201 uptake in each of the seven myocardial segments according to the following grading scale: 0 = normal, 1 = a definite but modest defect, 2 = a severe defect, and 3 = a complete defect (equal to background).

The three observers identified 152 segmental thallium-201 defects in the 27 patient studies. Ten segments with anterobasilar defects were not fully visualized on positron emission tomography and were therefore excluded from further analysis. Of the remaining 142 segmental thallium-201 defects, 101 were fixed, 31 were partially reversible, and 10 were completely reversible. Of the 101 segments with fixed defects, only 54 (53.4 percent) exhibited the concordant decreases in perfusion and glucose metabolism characteristic of completed infarction (Fig. 67–34). In contrast, myocardial ischemia was observed in 24 (23.8 percent) of the segments with fixed defects, indicating residual tissue metabolic viability (Fig. 67–35). Of the 31 segments with partially reversible defects, 11 (35.5 percent) exhibited metabolic criteria for myocardial infarction, whereas myocardial ischemia was observed in 9 (29 percent) of the segments. Thus, residual tissue metabolic viability was identified in 47 (46.5 percent) of the segments with fixed thallium-201 defects and 20 (64.5 percent) of the segments with partially reversible thallium-201 defects, again indicating that thallium-201 scintigraphy underestimates the extent of tissue viability in patients with ischemic heart disease.

Of the 10 segments with completely reversible defects, 5 (50 percent) were normal on positron emission tomography, while 5 (50 percent) exhibited the metabolism-perfusion mismatch of myocardial ischemia. Visual improvement in a persistent thallium-201 defect on redistribution imaging at 4 hours was not associated with the presence of glucose metabolic activity (20 of 31 partially reversible defects versus 47 of 101 fixed defects, $0.05 < P < 0.10$). Thus, apparent improvement in a persistent thallium-201 SPECT defect on redistribution images at 4 hours was not a reliable indicator of the presence or absence of tissue viability in this study population.

Because some have proposed that 3 or 4 hours is too short a time period for thallium-201 redistribution to occur in some individuals with tight coronary stenoses,[C7] delayed thallium-201 redistribution imaging at 24 hours has been advocated.[C7, H5, K7, Z2] For example, Kiat and co-workers reported that 74 of 122 (61 percent) persistent segmental thallium-201 defects on 4-hour delayed images exhibited further redistribution on repeat imaging at 18 to 72 hours.[K7] Similarly, Cloninger and colleagues noted that 13 of 28 (46.4 percent) patients with prior infarction and thallium-201 defects at 4 hours will exhibit further redistribution on delayed imaging at 24 hours.[C7] Thus, about half of myocardial segments with thallium-201 defects on 4-hour images will exhibit further redistribution on more delayed imaging.

In a preliminary report, Brunken and associates compared the results of 24-hour thallium-201 SPECT scintigraphy with the metabolic assessment of tissue viability by positron emission tomography in 14 patients with coronary artery disease.[B22] Uptake of thallium-201 was independently assessed by three observers in each of seven myocardial segments on the initial, 4-hour, and 24-hour SPECT images. The three observers identified 30 fixed, 31 partially reversible, and 10 completely reversible segmental thallium-201 defects. On positron emission tomography, only 14 (46.7 percent) of the segments with fixed defects and 12 (38.7 percent) of the segments with partially reversible defects exhibited criteria for completed infarction. Completed infarction was also identified in two (20 percent) of the segments with completely reversible thallium-201 defects, probably as a result of the superior spatial resolution of positron emission tomography. Thus, myocardial metabolic viability was identified in 53 percent of the segments with fixed defects, 61 percent of the segments with partially reversible defects, and 80 percent of the segments with completely reversible defects, indicating that a substantial proportion of myocardial segments with persistent defects on markedly delayed (24-hour) redistribution images will exhibit evidence of glucose metabolic activity, and hence tissue viability.

These comparative imaging studies demonstrate that a fixed thallium-201 perfusion defect, whether present on 4-hour images or on images acquired at later times, does not imply the absence of tissue viability. The metabolic studies with positron emission tomography corroborate the findings of Gibson[G6] and Liu[L5] and their colleagues, in which some myocardial segments with fixed thallium-201 defects normalized after revascularization. The metabolic images indicate why some myocardial segments with persistent thallium-201 defects may exhibit a normal perfusion pattern and normal thallium-201 washout kinetics following revascularization: viable tissue is present and is undetected on preoperative thallium-201 scintigraphy. In addition, the findings with positron emission tomography are in agreement with prior clinicopathologic studies,[B12] indicating that some myocardial regions with extensive thallium-201 perfusion defects contain only small amounts of myocardial fibrosis. Thus, thallium-201 scintigraphy may seriously underestimate the extent of residual tissue viability in some patients with ischemic heart disease, and metabolic imaging with fluorine-18 2-fluoro 2-deoxyglucose is helpful in identifying individuals with significant amounts of viable but jeopardized myocardium.

Synopsis

Identification of tissue glucose metabolism in hypoperfused ventricular regions with positron emission tomography and fluorine-18 2-fluoro 2-deoxyglucose indicates the presence of viable but jeopardized tissue in patients with coronary artery disease. The presence of glucose utilization in hypoperfused areas reliably predicts improvement in segmental function following revascularization and frequently identifies residual tissue viability when the electrocardiogram, assessment of wall motion, or thallium-201 scintigraphy indicates irreversible injury. Thus metabolic imaging with fluorine-18 2-fluoro 2-deoxyglucose provides unique information about tissue viability that cannot be obtained by the use of routinely employed clinical tests.

Chronic Myocardial Ischemia and Infarction

Left ventricular myocardial systolic dysfunction may result from a variety of causes, including ischemic heart disease, myocarditis, vasculitis, toxins such as doxorubicin, and idiopathic dilated cardiomyopathy. Often the initial aspect of the evaluation of patients with impaired systolic function is directed at distinguishing ischemic from nonischemic causes, for identifying patients with ischemic left ventricular dysfunction has therapeutic and prognostic ramifications.[F7, F8, H6, S22] Although noninvasive techniques such as radionuclide ventriculography, echocardiography, or thallium-201 scintigraphy occasionally may prove useful for identifying an ischemic etiology for the observed left ventricular dysfunction, often it is necessary to resort to invasive procedures, such as coronary angiography or myocardial biopsy or both, with their attendent risks,[D5, S23, W3] to delineate the cause of the left

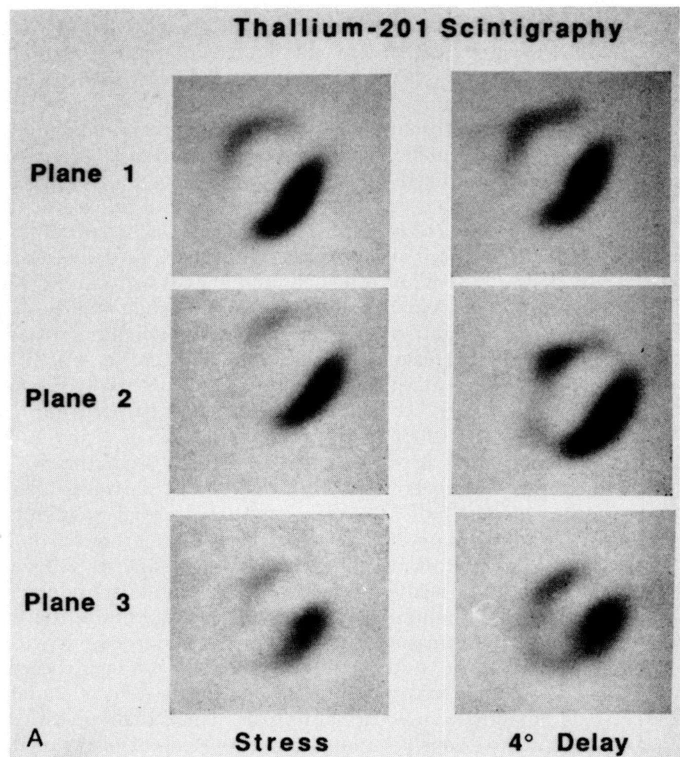

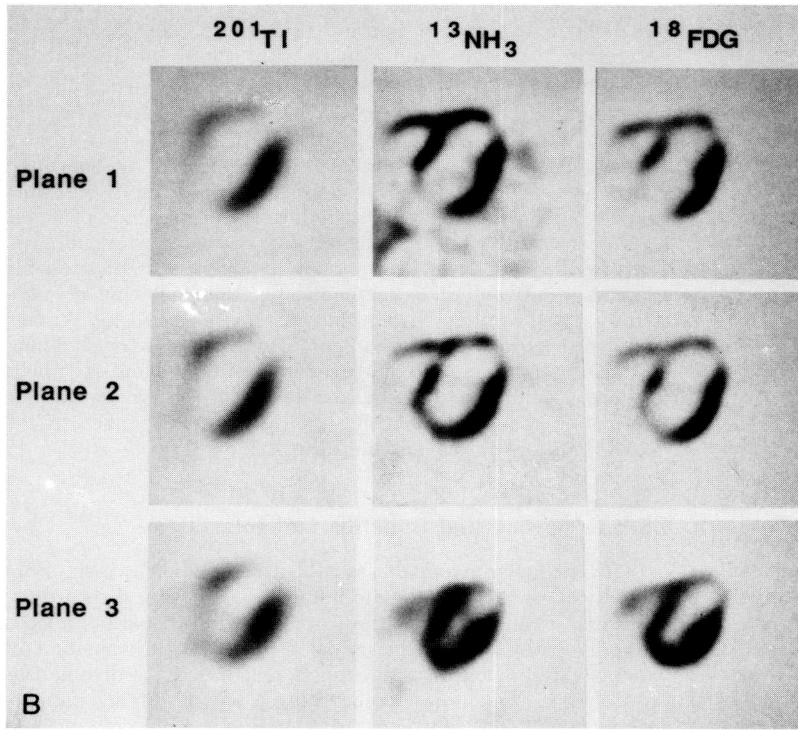

Figure 67–34. *Panel A,* Stress and 4-hour delayed single-photon emission tomographic thallium–201 (^{201}Tl) images from the study of a 62-year-old man with a history of previous myocardial infarction and triple-vessel coronary artery disease. The ^{201}Tl images demonstrate fixed defects in the anterior and apical regions of the ventricle and partially reversible anteroseptal and inferoseptal defects. *Panel B,* The corresponding [^{13}N] ammonia ($^{13}NH_3$) and ^{18}F 2-fluoro 2-deoxyglucose metabolic (^{18}FDG) images along with the 4-hour tomographic ^{201}Tl images. Concordant reductions in myocardial perfusion and glucose metabolism are identified in the anterior, apical, and anteroseptal segments, denoting completed myocardial infarction. In contrast, both perfusion and glucose metabolism are normal in the inferoseptal segment. (From Brunken, R. C., Kottou, S., Schwaiger, M., et al.: PET detection of viable tissue in myocardial segments with persistent defects at thallium–201 SPECT. Radiology 172:65–73, 1989, with permission.)

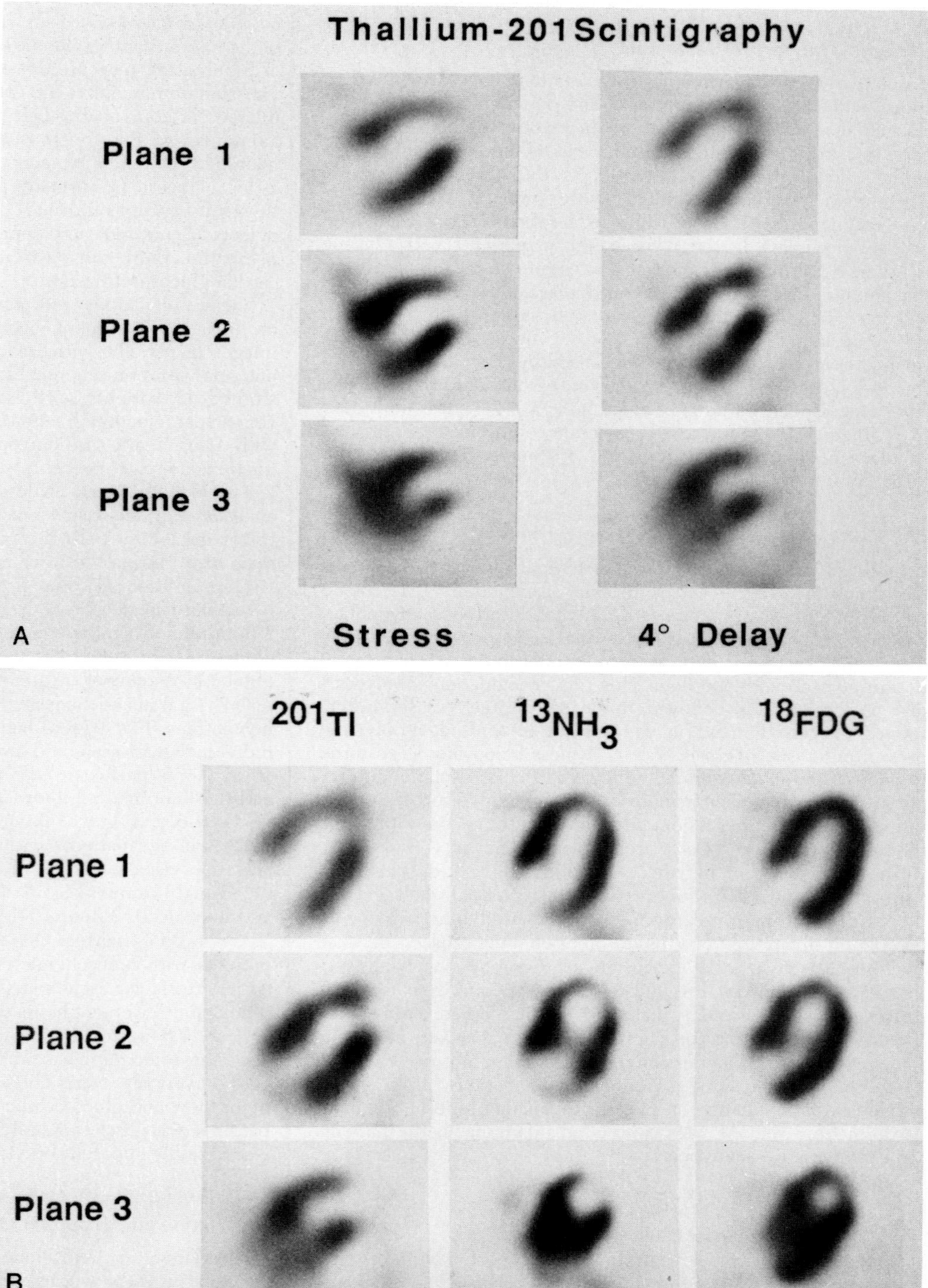

Figure 67–35. *Panel A,* Stress and 4-hour redistribution single photon emission tomographic thallium-201 (^{201}Tl) images in a 77-year-old woman with a history of prior myocardial infarction. On the tomographic cross-sectional thallium-201 images there is a fixed apical defect and partially reversible septal and anterior defects. *Panel B,* Four-hour tomographic ^{201}Tl images along with the corresponding ^{13}N ammonia ($^{13}NH_3$) perfusion images and ^{18}F 2-fluoro 2-deoxyglucose (^{18}FDG) metabolic images. Although perfusion defects similar to those noted on the ^{201}Tl study are identified on the ^{13}N ammonia perfusion images, there is preservation of glucose metabolism in the anterior and apical regions of the ventricle on the glucose metabolic images, indicating myocardial viability. (From Brunken, R. C., Kottou, S., Schwaiger, M., et al.: PET detection of viable tissue in myocardial segments with persistent defects at thallium-201 SPECT. Radiology 172:65–73, 1989, with permission.)

ventricular dysfunction. Thus, attention has been directed to the clinical utility of metabolic imaging with positron emission tomography for noninvasively distinguishing ischemic from other forms of left ventricular dysfunction, and for delineating the size and extent of chronically ischemic and infarcted ventricular regions in patients with left ventricular ischemic dysfunction.

Chronic Myocardial Ischemia

Relatively few experimental investigations have attempted to address the long-term functional and metabolic abnormalities associated with chronic reductions in myocardial blood flow. In part, this may be due to the difficulties inherent in devising an animal model that accurately reflects the chronic myocardial dysfunction observed in patients with coronary artery disease. The major impetus for further exploration of the metabolic changes occurring in the myocardium of patients with chronic ischemic heart disease is the fact that clinical studies demonstrate that some individuals with left ventricular contractile dysfunction will have improvement in regional wall motion following restoration of blood flow.[B16, B17, C5, R10, S21, T4] Because patients with reversible myocardial dysfunction caused by chronic ischemia are the ones most likely to benefit symptomatically and prognostically from successful restoration of blood flow,[B23, P3, P4, S21] it is important to distinguish individuals with ischemic compromise of left ventricular function from the patients with nonischemic causes for heart failure.

The Concept of Myocardial Hibernation

In 1985, Rahimtoola proposed that silent myocardial ischemia may result in sustained left ventricular dysfunction.[R12] He coined the term "hibernating myocardium" to describe a reversible, subacute, or chronic stage of myocardial ischemia in which resting contractile function is depressed in parallel to a sustained reduction in myocardial blood flow. This "down-regulation" of myocardial performance is believed to be self-protective, serving to reduce oxygen demand in the setting of limited supply and preventing tissue necrosis.[B24, K1, R13] Unless blood flow is restored to hibernating myocardium, the left ventricular dysfunction may persist indefinitely. The manner by which the myocardium enters into a state of hibernation and the length of time that the hibernating state can persist are, as yet, unknown.

The clinical problem, then, is to distinguish dysfunctional ventricular regions with hibernating (and potentially salvageable) myocardium from myocardium with impaired function due to completed infarction or due to nonischemic causes. Because thallium-201 myocardial perfusion scintigraphy has been suggested as a means of distinguishing nonischemic from ischemic causes of dilated cardiomyopathy,[B25, E1, I5] it seemed feasible that the tissue characterization afforded by perfusion and metabolic imaging with positron emission tomography might prove clinically useful in distinguishing ischemic cardiomyopathy from nonischemic cardiomyopathy, and for distinguishing hibernating myocardium from regions with completed infarction in the patients with ischemic cardiomyopathy.

Ischemic Versus Nonischemic Dilated Cardiomyopathy

Several investigators have preliminarily reported on the clinical utility of myocardial nitrogen-13 ammonia perfusion and fluorine-18 2-fluoro 2-deoxyglucose metabolic imaging for distinguishing ischemic cardiomyopathy from nonischemic cardiomyopathy. Fudo and associates utilized positron emission tomography with nitrogen-13 ammonia and fluorine-18 2-fluoro 2-deoxyglucose to study 18 patients with dilated cardiomyopathy and 20 patients with ischemic cardiomyopathy (left ventricular ejection fraction of 40 percent or less).[F9] In 19 (95 percent) of the patients with ischemic cardiomyopathy discrete perfusion defects were identified on the nitrogen-13 ammonia studies. In contrast, nitrogen-13 ammonia perfusion imaging revealed moderately inhomogeneous perfusion in the patients with dilated cardiomyopathy, and only three discrete perfusion defects were identified ($P < 0.01$).

On fluorine-18 2-fluoro 2-deoxyglucose metabolic imaging in the patients with ischemic cardiomyopathy, 14 individuals showed augmented uptake of glucose analog in hypoperfused regions, consistent with chronic myocardial ischemia. In five individuals, concordant reductions in uptake of fluorine-18 2-fluoro 2-deoxyglucose and nitrogen-13 ammonia were noted, consistent with completed infarction. Thus, a significant proportion (70 percent) of the patients with ischemic cardiomyopathy had discrete regions of hibernating myocardium on metabolic imaging with positron emission tomography. In contrast, 10 of the 18 patients with dilated cardiomyopathy had concordant *increases* in nitrogen-13 ammonia and fluorine-18 deoxyglucose uptake, whereas the remaining 8 patients had augmented uptake of fluorine-18 2-fluoro 2-deoxyglucose in normally perfused myocardial regions. Thus, these observations indicate that while discrete regional perfusion defects are not typically identified in patients with dilated cardiomyopathy, there can be tremendous regional variation in myocardial glucose utilization.

Vaghaiwalla Mody and colleagues also compared the findings on nitrogen-13 ammonia and fluorine-18 2-fluoro 2-deoxyglucose images in patients with ischemic cardiomyopathy with those in patients with nonischemic cardiomyopathy.[V4] These investigators studied 11 patients with ischemic cardiomyopathy (mean left ventricular ejection fraction, 23 ± 5 percent) and 10 patients with nonischemic cardiomyopathy (mean left ventricular ejection fraction, 18 ± 6 percent). The tomographic images were subjected to both visual analysis and circumferential count profile analysis. For the visual image analysis, three observers graded tracer uptake on both the perfusion and metabolic images on a scale of 0 (normal) to 3 (complete defect, equal to background). On circumferential count profile analysis, infarction was defined by concordant decreases in nitrogen-13 ammonia and fluorine-18 2-fluoro 2-deoxyglucose tracer concentrations, while ischemia was defined by preservation of fluorine-18 2-fluoro 2-deoxyglucose uptake in regions of resting hypoperfusion.

On visual image analysis, individuals with nonischemic cardiomyopathies (Fig. 67–36) had fewer defects per patient than the individuals with ischemic cardiomyopathy, on both the nitrogen-13 ammonia perfusion (2.7 ± 1.6 versus 5.0 ± 0.6, $P < 0.03$) and the fluorine-18 2-fluoro 2-deoxyglucose metabolic (2.8 ± 2.1 versus 4.6 ± 1.1, $P < 0.03$) studies. Not only were there fewer defects in the patients with nonischemic cardiomyopathies but also the visual severity of the defects was less for both the nitrogen-13 ammonia (1.0 ± 0.2 versus 1.8 ± 0.5, $P < 0.03$) and fluorine-18 2-fluoro 2-deoxyglucose (1.2 ± 0.7 versus 1.8 ± 0.4, $P < 0.03$) images. On circumferential count profile analysis, patients with nonischemic cardiomyopathy had fewer segments with criteria for ischemia (0.1 ± 0.3 versus 2.4 ± 1.4, $P < 0.001$) and fewer segments with criteria for completed infarction (0.4 ± 0.8 versus 2.5 ± 2.0, $P < 0.01$). Thus, the positron emission tomographic studies in the patients with nonischemic cardiomyopathy were characterized by fewer and less severe blood flow and glucose metabolic defects than the studies in the patients with ischemic cardiomyopathy, and these differences were readily apparent on visual inspection of the images.

Relationship Between Blood Flow and Metabolism in Chronically Hypoperfused Human Myocardium

The laboratory and clinical studies correlating tissue glucose metabolism with myocardial blood flow indicate that as myocardial blood flow decreases there is an increasing reliance upon exogenous glucose for energy production. However, if the degree of the blood flow reduction becomes too severe, then myocardial infarction ensues. Using dynamic positron emission tomography and appropriate tracer kinetic models for quantification of myocardial blood flow and rates of glucose utilization, Brunken and co-workers preliminarily reported on the relationship between myocardial blood flow and glucose utilization in chronically ischemic human myocardium.[B26]

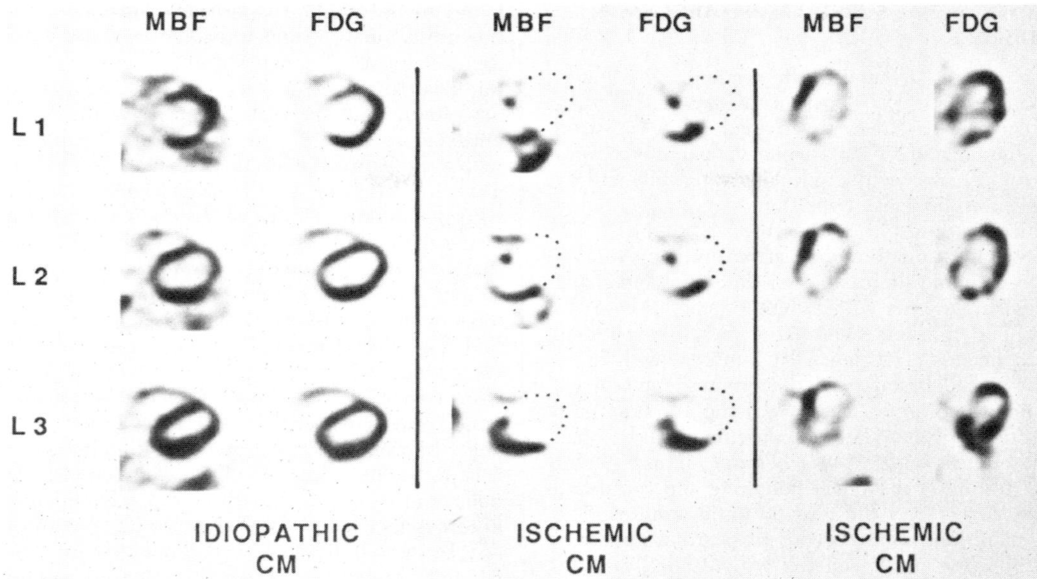

Figure 67–36. Positron emission tomographic images in three patients with dilated heart failure. In the *left panel* (IDIOPATHIC CM) are representative [^{13}N] ammonia (MBF) perfusion images and the corresponding ^{18}F 2-fluoro 2-deoxyglucose (^{18}FDG) metabolic images in a patient with idiopathic dilated cardiomyopathy. Both perfusion and glucose metabolism are homogeneous throughout the left ventricle. In the *center panel* (ISCHEMIC CM) are the images of a patient with ischemic cardiomyopathy. The [^{13}N] ammonia perfusion images (MBF) demonstrate extensive perfusion defects in the septal, lateral, anterior, and apical regions of the ventricle. These perfusion defects are matched on the ^{18}F 2-fluoro 2-deoxyglucose (^{18}FDG) metabolic images, indicating extensive antecedent myocardial infarction. In this patient, coronary revascularization would not be expected to improve left ventricular function. In contrast are images in the *right panel* (ISCHEMIC CM), from the study of a second patient with ischemic cardiomyopathy. On the [^{13}N] ammonia perfusion images (MBF) extensive perfusion defects are identified in the inferoseptal, lateral, and anteroapical regions of the ventricle. On the ^{18}F 2-fluoro 2-deoxyglucose (^{18}FDG) images, glucose metabolism is well preserved in these hypoperfused ventricular regions. In this patient with ischemic cardiomyopathy, positron emission tomography revealed extensive tissue viability that could be salvaged by coronary revascularization.

The study population consisted of 11 patients with ischemic cardiomyopathy. Quantitative myocardial blood measurements were calculated using a two-compartmental nitrogen-13 ammonia model,[S24] while absolute rates of glucose utilization were calculated using a modified Patlak graphical approach.[G8] In 50 myocardial segments, rates of glucose utilization ranged from 0.068 to 1.21 μmol/min/g, while blood flows ranged from 0.09 to 1.15 ml/min/g. When rates of glucose utilization were compared with myocardial blood flows, no clear relationship was noted. However, when rates of glucose utilization were divided by blood flows (to normalize for tracer delivery) and compared with blood flows, an inverse relationship was noted. For myocardial blood flows above about 0.45 ml/min/g, the amount of glucose extracted per milliliter of blood was relatively constant. At lower blood flows, however, the amount of glucose extracted per milliliter of blood increased, achieving a maximum of 2.2 μmol/ml at 0.12 ml/min/g of blood flow. Thus, these preliminary results of Brunken and colleagues are consistent with an accelerated glycolytic flux in moderately severe chronic human myocardial ischemia.[B26] However, no measurements were obtained at the very lowest range of blood flows, at which rates of glucose utilization would be expected to drop precipitously in regions with completed infarction.

In a preliminary communication, Brunken and colleagues have also reported on oxidative substrate metabolism in chronically hypoperfused human myocardium.[B27] In eight patients with angiographically confirmed coronary artery disease, dynamic positron tomographic imaging was performed with nitrogen-13 ammonia, carbon-11 acetate, and fluorine-18 2-fluoro 2-deoxyglucose. Segments with concordant decreases in both nitrogen-13 ammonia and fluorine-18 2-fluoro 2-deoxyglucose were classified as infarcted, whereas segments in which there was preservation of fluorine-18 2-fluoro 2-deoxyglucose uptake relative to that of nitrogen-13 ammonia were classified as ischemic. Estimates of the monoexponential clearance constants of carbon-11 acetate (k) were derived from myocardial time activity curves obtained from 16 regions in each image.

In the eight patients, 59 anatomic myocardial segments were studied. In the 33 segments classified as normal, k's for carbon-11 acetate averaged 0.072 ± 0.016 min^{-1}, and the ratio of k to the percent of peak nitrogen-13 ammonia activity was 0.081. In the 18 segments with myocardial ischemia, k's for carbon-11 acetate averaged 0.058 ± 0.010 min^{-1} ($P < 0.05$ versus normal), while ratios of k's to the percent of peak nitrogen-13 ammonia activity again averaged 0.81. In the eight segments with infarction, k's averaged 0.045 ± 0.019 min^{-1} ($P < 0.05$ versus ischemia), while ratios of k's relative to peak nitrogen-13 ammonia activity averaged 0.084. Thus, this preliminary report suggests that carbon-11 acetate clearance rate constants are depressed in proportion to the relative flow reduction in hypoperfused myocardial segments in patients with chronic ischemic heart disease, implying a constant extraction fraction for oxygen. In the hypoperfused segments with preservation of glucose metabolism, the intermediate reduction in the carbon-11 acetate clearance constants implies impaired oxidative substrate metabolism in the hypoperfused but metabolically viable tissue.

Chronic Myocardial Infarction

Initial experimental studies with positron emission tomography and carbon-11 palmitate indicated the ability of this technique to localize and quantify the extent of antecedent myocardial infarction. Weiss and colleagues induced myocardial infarction in canine preparations by ligating the left anterior descending artery distal to the first septal perforating artery.[W4] In six animals studied 48 hours after ligature of the artery, the relationship between myocardial creatine phosphokinase (CPK) depletion and carbon-14 palmitate accumulation was assessed. In six additional animals, myocardial infarct sizes determined by tomographic imaging with carbon-11 palmitate at 48 hours were correlated with depletion of myocardial creatine phosphokinase activity and with morphometric measurements of infarct size on postmortem examination. These investigators noted a linear relationship between the percent reduction in myocardial carbon-14 palmitate uptake and the percent depletion of myocardial creatine phosphokinase activity in 44 myocardial biopsy specimens obtained at 48 hours in the six animals. In addition, infarct sizes determined with positron emission tomography and carbon-11 palmitate were linearly related to morphologic infarct size and to the percent depletion of creatine phosphokinase activity. Thus, in this animal model, determinations of myocardial infarct size made with positron emission tomographic imaging with carbon-11 palmitate were linearly related to infarct sizes estimated morphologically and by myocardial creatine phosphokinase depletion.

In subsequent clinical studies from the same laboratory,[G9, S25, T7] imaging with carbon-11 palmitate and positron emission tomography was shown to be clinically feasible for detecting and sizing myocardial infarction in patients with ischemic heart disease. In a pilot study, Sobel and colleagues compared the cross-sectional carbon-11 palmitate images of 10 normal volunteers with those from 12 patients who had sustained a documented myocardial infarction 3 to 12 months prior to study.[S25] Of the 12 patients, 6 had anterior infarctions, 4 had lateral infarctions, and 2 had posteroinferior infarctions. Imaging was begun 3 minutes after intravenous administration of carbon-11 palmitate and continued at several transverse levels over the next 30 to 60 minutes. The normal volunteers exhibited homogeneous myocardial uptake of carbon-11 palmitate, whereas each of the patients had discrete defects in carbon-11 palmitate accumulation in regions corresponding to the electrocardiographic site of infarction.

Ter-Pogossian and associates prospectively compared the carbon-11 palmitate studies in 21 patients with documented myocardial infarction with those in 7 patients with suspected infarction in whom myocardial necrosis was subsequently excluded on the basis of serial electrocardiograms and plasma creatine kinase MB levels.[T7] Imaging with positron emission tomography was begun 3 minutes following the intravenous administration of carbon-11 palmitate. A set of 14 contiguous cross-sectional images of the heart was acquired. Blood pool imaging was then performed with carbon-11 carbon monoxide hemoglobin in the same planes. In addition to visual interpretation, carbon-11 palmitate images were quantitatively analyzed to assess the extent of myocardial injury. The total infarct volume was derived by summing the mass of myocardium with decreased carbon-11 palmitate uptake in each contiguous image plane according to the formula:

$$\text{infarct size (in PET g-Eq)} = \sum_{i=1}^{n} V_i \{ (100-a_i)/100 \} \times [1 \text{ g/cm}^3]$$

where the tomographic infarct size is expressed in PET gram-equivalents, V_i is the volume of infarction in plane_i (calculated by multiplying the total area of the carbon-11 palmitate defect by the plane thickness), a_i is the average background-corrected activity in the defect region, and the final term is an assumed myocardial specific density of 1 g/cm^3. The tomographic measurements of myocardial infarct size were then correlated with estimates of infarct size derived from analyses of plasma creatine kinase MB time activity curves[R14] and expressed in CK-gram equivalents.

None of the seven patients in whom myocardial infarction was excluded exhibited segmentally diminished uptake of carbon-11 palmitate. In contrast, each of the patients with documented clinical infarctions had clearly identifiable regions of diminished uptake of carbon-11 palmitate on transaxial, coronal, or sagittal images. The researchers noted that inferior and apical infarctions were less clearly visualized on transaxial tomographic images and implied that coronal or sagittal images were better for detecting inferior infarctions. The mean infarct size derived by positron emission tomography was 57.0 ± 32.3 PET g-equivalents, while the mean infarct size derived from creatine kinase MB time activity curves was 58.4 ± 49.3 CK g-equivalents (P = NS). When individual measurements of infarct size derived from the positron emission tomographic images were compared with those derived from plasma creatine kinase MB time activity curves, a linear relationship was observed (PET infarct size = 0.6 × enzymatic infarct size + 18, r = 0.92, $P < 0.001$). The reproducibility of the tomographic measurements of infarct size, as assessed by a second study in four patients 1 month later, was found to be within 10 percent. Thus, this study demonstrated the utility of positron emission tomography and carbon-11 palmitate for localizing and sizing infarctions in patients with ischemic heart disease.

Geltman and associates compared the findings on positron emission tomography using carbon-11 palmitate in 24 patients with non-Q wave infarctions with those in 22 patients with Q wave infarctions.[G9] Fourteen contiguous transverse planes were recorded and used for reconstruction of sagittal and coronal slices. Using the methods previously reported by Ter-Pogossian,[T7] quantitative measurements of infarct size were made. In each of the 22 patients with Q wave infarctions, regional defects with homogeneously reduced carbon-11 palmitate uptake were identified. The electrocardiographic and tomographic sites of infarction correlated well. The observed defects appeared confluent and were transmural in nature (Fig. 67–37). Of the 24 patients with non-Q wave myocardial infarctions, 23 (96 percent) had identifiable abnormalities of carbon-11 palmitate accumulation. In contrast to the patients with Q wave infarctions, carbon-11 palmitate defects in the patients with non-Q wave infarctions tended to be heterogeneous and often were not transmural in extent (Fig. 67–37). In some individuals, blood pool imaging with carbon-11 CO-labeled hemoglobin revealed a discrete space between the left ventricular cavity and myocardial accumulation of carbon-11

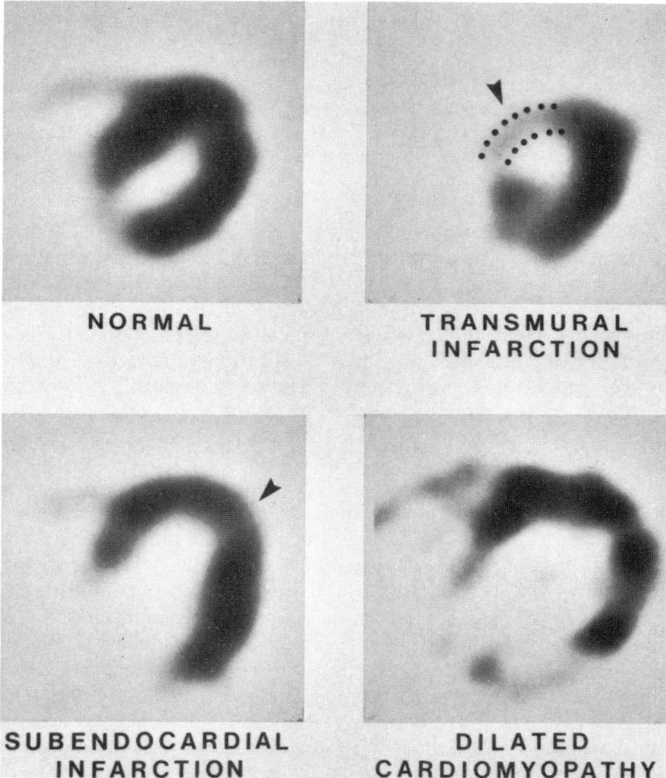

Figure 67–37. Representative ^{11}C palmitate images from a normal volunteer (NORMAL), a patient with transmural myocardial infarction (TRANSMURAL INFARCTION), a patient with subendocardial infarction (SUBENDOCARDIAL INFARCTION), and a patient with idiopathic dilated cardiomyopathy (DILATED CARDIOMYOPATHY). In the normal subject ^{11}C activity is generally uniform throughout the left ventricle. In the patient with transmural myocardial infarction a defect in ^{11}C activity is noted that encompasses the entire left ventricular myocardium (*arrow*). In contrast, the study in the patient with the subendocardial infarction demonstrates a modest focal reduction in ^{11}C activity (*arrow*) that does not involve the full thickness of the left ventricular myocardium. For comparison is the image from a patient with idiopathic dilated cardiomyopathy, demonstrating marked regional heterogeneity in ^{11}C myocardial activity. (From Schelbert, H.R., and Schwaiger, M.: PET studies of the heart. *In* Phelps, M.E., Mazziotta, J.C., and Schelbert, H.R. (eds.): Positron Emission Tomography and Autoradiography. Principles and Applications for the Brain and Heart. New York, Raven Press, 1986, pp. 581–661, with permission.)

palmitate, suggesting an interposed zone of metabolically inactive fibrosis. In addition, these investigators reported that mildly heterogeneous uptake of carbon-11 palmitate could be appreciated in "normal" adjacent myocardium by careful subtraction of background activity, implying mildly abnormal carbon-11 palmitate accumulation in the border zones of the non-Q wave infarctions. Patients with non-Q wave infarctions had significantly smaller infarct sizes than the patients with Q wave infarctions (19 ± 4 versus 50.4 ± 7.8 PET g-eq, $P < 0.01$). Relative carbon-11 activity in the zones of infarction was significantly higher (39 ± 1 percent versus 33 ± 1 percent, $P < 0.01$), implying less severe tissue fibrosis.

Planar rest thallium-201 images were obtained in 18 of the 24 patients with the non-Q wave infarctions. The sensitivity of thallium-201 scintigraphy for detecting non-Q wave myocardial infarction was significantly poorer than positron emission tomography with carbon-11 palmitate (61 percent versus 96 percent, $P < 0.05$), while both imaging techniques had similar specificities (90 percent versus 80 percent, P = NS).

Thus, positron emission tomography with carbon-11 palmitate accurately localized and sized antecedent infarctions. Q wave infarctions could be distinguished from non-Q wave infarctions by the more pronounced reduction in carbon-11 activity and apparent transmural extent of the metabolic defect. Although positron emission tomography imaging with carbon-11 palmitate appeared more sensitive for detecting non-Q wave myocardial infarction than planar thallium-201 scintigraphy, it is not certain that the same would have been observed had a tomographic thallium-201 imaging technique been utilized.[F10, K8]

Synopsis

Assessment of myocardial perfusion and glucose metabolism with positron emission tomography in patients with dilated heart failure is a reliable, noninvasive means of distinguishing ischemic cardiomyopathy from nonischemic cardiomyopathies. Patients with ischemic cardiomyopathy have larger and more severe perfusion and glucose metabolic defects on visual image analysis than do patients with nonischemic cardiomyopathies. On quantitative circumferential profile image analysis, patients with ischemic cardiomyopathy more frequently exhibit criteria for completed infarction or the metabolism-perfusion mismatch of chronic ischemia than do patients with other forms of dilated cardiomyopathy. Simultaneous perfusion and metabolic imaging with positron emission tomography enable not only discrimination between ischemic and nonischemic cardiomyopathies, but also permit evaluation of myocardial viability in patients who have ischemic cardiomyopathy.

Although reversible myocardial dysfunction is frequently observed in patients with chronic ischemic heart disease and can be identified readily utilizing positron tomographic imaging with fluorine-18 2-fluoro 2-deoxyglucose, the manner by which myocardium enters into the "hibernating state" and the length of time that the state of hibernation can persist are unknown. Preliminary reports suggest that oxidative substrate metabolism is depressed in proportion to the degree of blood flow reduction in human hibernating myocardium, and that the tissue resorts to anaerobic glycolysis under conditions of moderately severe blood flow reductions to maintain cellular viability. Further clinical studies employing quantitative measurements of blood flow and aerobic and anaerobic metabolic processes derived from positron emission tomography should increase our understanding of the relationship between blood flow and tissue metabolism in chronically hypoperfused human myocardium.

MYOCARDIAL METABOLIC IMAGING IN CLINICAL PRACTICE

Although assessment of myocardial metabolism with positron emission tomography provides clinically useful information about the state of the myocardium in patients with ischemic heart disease, it is important to attempt to define the role of this imaging technique in the practice of clinical cardiology. Although not all patients will benefit from metabolic imaging, in well-selected individuals the information derived from positron emission tomography will have a major impact on the patient's medical care. In this section, we identify the patients for whom metabolic imaging with positron emission tomography provides useful clinical information and discuss selected aspects of the care of the cardiac patient during myocardial metabolic imaging. Finally, we discuss how the information derived by positron emission tomography is incorporated into the clinical decision-making process for individual patient case management decisions.

Indications for Metabolic Imaging

In patients with ischemic heart disease, there are several clinical indications for myocardial glucose metabolic imaging. These include:

(1) *Detection and localization of stress-induced myocardial ischemia* in patients with chest pain in whom other physiologic stress tests are inconclusive, either for establishing the diagnosis or for localizing the ischemic region(s). An example of the utility of glucose metabolic imaging for detecting acute exercise-induced ischemia is illustrated in Figure 67–38.

(2) *Assessment of the physiologic significance and metabolic consequence of anatomically defined stenoses* in patients with known coronary artery disease by imaging with a perfusion tracer and fluorine-18 2-fluoro 2-deoxyglucose. In this way, both the blood flow reserve as well as the metabolic reserve of the vascular territory in question can be determined. In addition, it is possible to assess the myocardial response to interventions designed to augment blood flow to ischemic myocardial regions, such as coronary artery bypass surgery or coronary angioplasty.

(3) *Distinguishing myocardial regions with completed infarction from viable but ischemically compromised tissue* in patients with coronary artery disease and left ventricular dysfunction. This enables the clinician to determine more accurately the risk-benefit ratio of subjecting the patient to revascularization. Metabolic imaging is particularly helpful in patients in whom the electrocardiogram, assessment of regional wall motion, or thallium-201 scintigraphy would suggest completed infarction. As noted in the earlier section, Metabolism as an Indicator of Tissue Viability, these routine tests frequently underestimate the extent of salvageable tissue, compared with the tissue characterization afforded by metabolic imaging. Thus, some patients with the diagnosis of completed infarction on these routine tests actually might have significant amounts of viable tissue detected on metabolic imaging with fluorine-18 2-fluoro 2-deoxyglucose and therefore be reasonable candidates for coronary revascularization. On the other hand, positron emission tomography may confirm the presence of extensive infarction in some patients and therefore may influence the clinician to recommend medical therapy or cardiac transplantation rather than interventional revascularization.

(4) *Discrimination of ischemic from nonischemic forms of dilated cardiomyopathies* in patients with congestive heart failure of undetermined etiology. Although assessment of myocardial perfusion with thallium-201 might also distinguish between these two patient types, the advantage of simultaneous blood flow and glucose metabolic imaging is that it allows an independent, concurrent assessment of myocardial viability that may prove helpful in determining the need for invasive procedures such as coronary angiography.

(5) *Identification of residual myocardial viability and its extent in patients with acute ischemic injury.* Blood flow and glucose metabolic imaging in these patients provide the clinician with an estimate of the amount of viable but

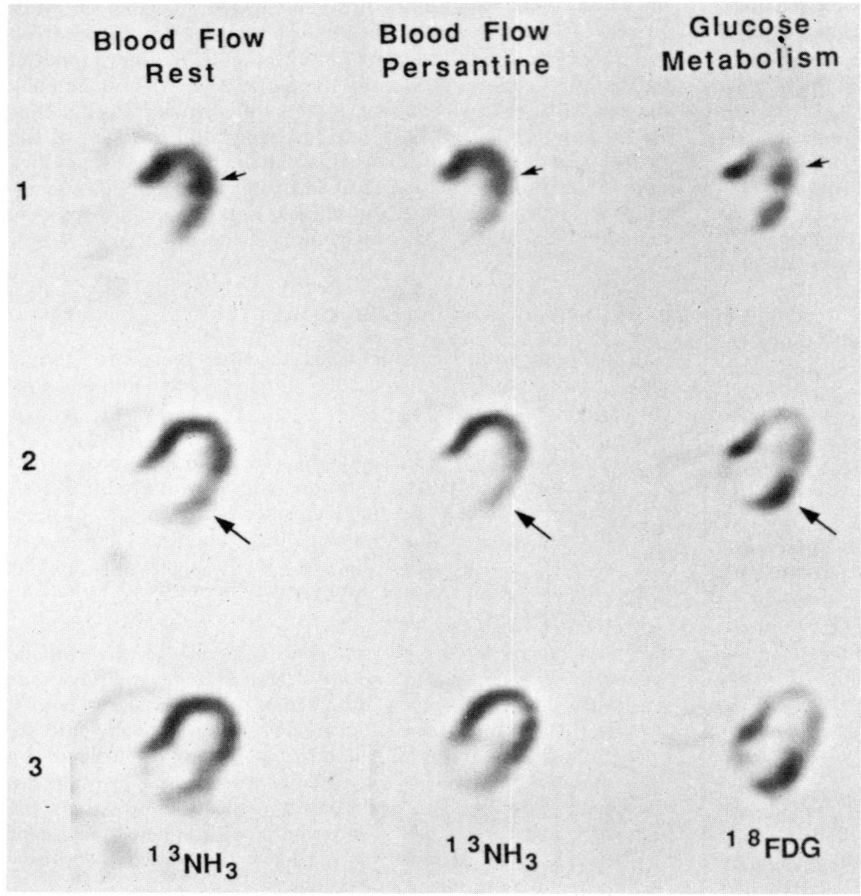

Figure 67–38. Rest and dipyridamole [^{13}N] ammonia ($^{13}NH_3$) perfusion images and the corresponding ^{18}F 2-fluoro 2-deoxyglucose (^{18}FDG) metabolic images in a patient with a history of previous bypass surgery and angina. With the administration of dipyridamole, subtle changes in relative myocardial blood flow are noted in the inferolateral region (*large arrows*) and in the anterior papillary muscle (*small arrows*). While striking differences in myocardial perfusion between the rest and dipyridamole [^{13}N] ammonia studies are not present, the ^{18}F 2-fluoro 2-deoxyglucose metabolic images demonstrate prominent uptake of the glucose analog in the inferolateral region and the anterior papillary muscle, indicative of acute myocardial ischemia. This study illustrates how metabolic imaging of acutely stunned myocardium with positron emission tomography can enhance the detection of stress-induced ischemia.

compromised tissue in the clinical infarct zone that will provide a rationale for instituting appropriate interventions designed to salvage endangered myocardium. In addition, positron emission tomography allows characterization of the state function of the myocardium remote from the zone of infarction. This is likely to be most helpful in the patient presenting with an acute ischemic injury who has a history of one or more previous infarctions, enabling the clinician to ascertain the extent of jeopardized tissue throughout the left ventricle.

As our understanding of the basic biochemistry of normal and ischemic myocardium in humans continues to grow and become more sophisticated, the list of clinical indications for positron emission tomography is likely to expand. For example, it may be possible to utilize quantitative blood flow and glucose utilization rates obtained with dynamic positron emission tomography to predict quantitatively both the extent and time course of recovery of regional and global left ventricular function in patients with ischemic left ventricular dysfunction following restoration of blood flow by coronary artery bypass surgery or by angioplasty. Thus, it is possible that metabolic imaging might prove useful in determining *quantitatively* the risk-benefit ratio of invasive interventions in individual patients with left ventricular dysfunction *prior* to intervention. In patients with chronic coronary artery disease, assessment of both oxidative and glycolytic metabolism, as well as quantitative regional measurements of blood flow, might prove more accurate for characterizing myocardial tissue, thereby improving the prognostic utility of myocardial perfusion imaging.[L6] As yet, the clinical indications for myocardial metabolic imaging have just begun to emerge and are likely to expand even farther as our understanding of the basic energy-producing processes in normal and diseased myocardium continues to grow.

Patient Care During Metabolic Imaging

By the very nature of the disease processes affecting the individual who is most likely to benefit from metabolic imaging, the patient with ischemic heart disease should be considered at risk for the development of complications during metabolic imaging. Although the information derived from metabolic imaging can contribute significantly to clinical decision making, the clinician should be aware that it may take 1 to 2 hours for a complete perfusion and metabolic study to be acquired. In some patients, therefore, it may be desirable to provide sedation prior to the positron emission tomographic study. During the imaging period, it is important that a physician knowledgeable in the care of patients with ischemic heart disease be present to assist in the monitoring of unstable patients and to treat promptly any complications occurring during imaging.

Stress or dipyridamole perfusion imaging to detect coronary artery disease may provoke acute myocardial ischemia. Myocardial ischemia is capable of precipitating life-threatening arrhythmias and cardiovascular collapse. In addition, dipyridamole may provoke acute respiratory failure in patients with bronchospastic pulmonary disease. In the patient with marked left ventricular failure, care must be taken to insure that exacerbation of cardiac dysfunction does not occur during imaging and that potentially lethal ventricular arrhythmias are adequately controlled. In addition, administration of intravenous fluids must be carefully regulated in order to avoid fluid overload and precipitation of acute pulmonary edema.

Because positron emission tomography is noninvasive, assessment of myocardial perfusion and metabolism in patients with acute myocardial infarction poses little additional risk to the individual beyond that engendered by the infarction itself. Whether in the intensive care unit or in the imaging suite, the key to the care of the patient with an acute infarction is careful monitoring by qualified personnel who are experienced and capable of handling the life-threatening sequelae of an acute ischemic injury. In some institutions, facilities for positron emission tomography are located next to the intensive care unit, thereby reducing the risks associated with transportation of the patient to an imaging facility. For patients undergoing positron emission tomography early in the course of an acute infarction, full electrocardiographic and hemodynamic monitoring capabilities should be available in the imaging suite. As in the intensive care unit, a crash cart with defibrillator and the drugs utilized to treat cardiac arrest should be readily available in case they are needed.

As with any procedure in medicine, the risks of performing the procedure must be balanced with the benefits derived by performing it. In our experience, almost any patient with a stable blood pressure and cardiac rhythm who is carefully monitored by a knowledgeable physician can derive the benefits of myocardial metabolic imaging.

Standardization of Study Conditions

Standardization of the patient's dietary state and monitoring of plasma substrate levels are important for performing metabolic imaging and, especially, for image interpretation. As outlined in Chapters 4 and 65, plasma substrate and insulin levels markedly influence myocardial substrate metabolism and selection of the primary fuel substrate. For example, the low insulin and glucose levels and the high free fatty acid levels in plasma characteristically present after periods of fasting result in preferential oxidation of free fatty acids by the myocardium and reduce exogenous glucose utilization. Thus, myocardial time activity curves derived from serial carbon-11 palmitate images typically exhibit a large relative size of the rapid clearance curve component and short clearance half-times. Conversely, glucose utilization is often low in the fasting state, resulting in nonvisualization of normal myocardium on the fluorine-18 2-fluoro 2-deoxyglucose studies. In contrast, in the postprandial state with higher insulin and glucose levels and lower free fatty acid plasma levels, the relative size of the rapid clearance curve component on the carbon-11 palmitate time activity curve declines, whereas fluorine-18 2-fluoro 2-deoxyglucose accumulation in normal myocardium markedly increases. Thus, the information contained on the metabolic images in normal myocardium depends upon the dietary state in a given patient.

In contrast, ischemically injured but viable myocardium appears to participate only incompletely in these metabolic responses to changes in plasma substrate levels. As determined in animal experiments,[V5] utilization of exogenous glucose in postischemic myocardium changes with plasma glucose levels. However, these changes are markedly attenuated. Glucose utilization and, thus, fluorine-18 2-fluoro 2-deoxyglucose uptake are lower in postischemic myocardium than in control myocardium during states of hyperglycemia, but higher than in control myocardium during euglycemic and low insulin states. Thus, compared with normal myocardium in humans, ischemically injured but viable myocardium characteristically will exhibit elevated fluorine-18 2-fluoro 2-deoxyglucose uptake in the fasted state, and normal or slightly reduced tracer uptake in the postprandial state. It is important to note, however, that fluorine-18 2-fluoro 2-deoxyglucose uptake is increased relative to segmental blood flow, forming the rationale for its utility in identifying myocardial viability.

Although the effects of dietary conditions and the influence of substrate levels on the myocardial metabolic images are the subjects of active investigation, patients in our laboratory are typically studied after an overnight fast and a standard oral glucose load (50 g) 1 hour prior to intravenous injection of fluorine-18 2-fluoro 2-deoxyglucose. This approach stimulates insulin secretion, lowers plasma free fatty acid levels, and characteristically results in good visualization of normal and ischemic myocardium. Circumferential profile analysis techniques are then applied to the cross-sectional perfusion and metabolic images and compared with a normal data base in order to define abnormalities of blood flow and exogenous glucose utilization.

Glucose metabolic studies in the fasted state characteristically result in "hot spot"images of ischemic tissue, in which only the regions with ischemic but viable myocardium are visualized as a focal area of increased fluorine-18 activity. As quantitative analytic techniques thus far have not been developed for these images, tissue metabolic activity is assessed visually. This approach appears to be highly sensitive for the detection of ischemic but viable myocardium. It is, however, relatively nonspecific for determining whether the amount of residual tissue viability will be sufficient for an improvement of contractile function if blood flow is restored by angioplasty or bypass surgery.

Standardization of study conditions may not always be possible. This is especially true for patients studied early after an acute myocardial infarction or those admitted with acute chest pain syndromes. In these situations, the myocardial blood flow images serve as a guide to lesion identification and characterization. Myocardial areas with normal perfusion but absent or low fluorine-18 2-fluoro 2-deoxyglucose uptake are considered normal. In contrast, abnormal myocardial areas are identified by segmental decreases in blood flow. Absence of fluorine-18 2-fluoro 2-deoxyglucose uptake in these hypoperfused segments is considered indicative of completed infarction, whereas increased uptake of fluorine-18 2-fluoro 2-deoxyglucose is considered indicative of ischemic but viable tissue.

Patients with coronary artery disease and diabetes mellitus pose a particular problem. Although systematic data are still lacking, observations in our laboratory suggest that fluorine-18 2-fluoro 2-deoxyglucose uptake may be poor in nonischemic myocardium in the diabetic patient. Because of slow tracer clearance from blood, fluorine-18 2-fluoro 2-deoxyglucose images often exhibit high blood pool activity. Delayed imaging or, as suggested by Besozzi (personal communication, October 1989), the administration of insulin may result in diagnostically acceptable myocardial images. It is interesting that ischemic but viable myocardium in the diabetic patient appears to utilize glucose and thus accumulates fluorine-18 2-fluoro 2-deoxyglucose. As a result, hypoperfused myocardial segments frequently exhibit increased fluorine-18 2-fluoro 2-deoxyglucose uptake well above blood pool activity. Because diabetes mellitus is frequently undiagnosed in coronary artery disease patients, we routinely determine plasma glucose levels in all patients prior to positron emission tomography. If plasma glucose levels exceed 150 mg/dl after an overnight fast, patients are not given an oral glucose load.

Clinical Decision Making with Metabolic Imaging

In patients with ischemic heart disease, clinical decisions are frequently based upon the cardiologist's estimate of the amount of viable but jeopardized tissue that could be salvaged by interventions designed to restore myocardial blood flow. In patients with coronary heart disease and symptoms predominantly of left ventricular dysfunction rather than angina, it may be especially difficult for the clinician to identify the individuals likely to benefit from coronary revascularization. Although individuals with depressed left ventricular function have the highest risk for both coronary bypass grafting[A3, K9, Z3] and coronary angioplasty, the patient with the largest amount of viable but dysfunctional myocardium is the one who will most benefit symptomatically and prognostically from coronary revascularization.[B23, P3, P4, S21, T2] Thus, distinguishing the individual with large amounts of viable tissue from the individual with extensive myocardial fibrosis is of paramount importance in the management of patients with ischemic heart disease and impaired left ventricular function. The individual with large amounts of hibernating myocardium might be a candidate for coronary revascularization, whereas the individual with extensive myocardial scar formation would be a candidate for medical therapy, or, in selected cases, for cardiac transplantation.

As noted earlier in Metabolism as a Clinical Indicator of Tissue Viability, identification of exogenous myocardial glucose utilization in hypoperfused ventricular regions accurately identifies viable tissue that will benefit functionally from restoration of myocardial blood flow. As such, positron emission tomography with fluorine-18 2-fluoro 2-deoxyglucose offers a unique means of assessing myocardial viability when routine clinical tests indicate completed infarction. From the comparative studies performed both in our laboratory and at other institutions, it is clear that the extent of residual myocardial viability is seriously underestimated by the electrocardiogram, assessment of regional function, and/or myocardial perfusion scintigraphy in some patients with ischemic heart disease. It is in these individuals that metabolic imaging with positron emission tomography is likely to have the largest clinical impact, reliably identifying viable myocardium when routine tests indicate completed infarction.

In the patient with acute ischemic injury, metabolic imaging with positron emission tomography identifies residual tissue viability in the clinical infarct zone, enabling the clinician to intervene, if deemed appropriate clinically, to restore blood flow to the zone of ischemic injury. Thus, a more conservative approach might be taken in patients with acute myocardial infarction with matching perfusion and glucose metabolic defects on positron emission tomography. In contrast, individuals with large metabolism-perfusion mismatches in the clinical infarct zone might be considered candidates for coronary angiography and perhaps angioplasty of the culprit lesion earlier, rather than later, in the course of the infarction, in an attempt to salvage viable but endangered tissue. As such, perfusion and metabolic imaging also can be utilized to assess the efficacy of interventions designed to restore blood flow or to reduce oxygen demand in the clinical infarct zone.

In the patient with congestive heart failure and dilated cardiomyopathy of undetermined etiology, positron emission tomography with a flow tracer and fluorine-18 2-fluoro 2-deoxyglucose might be considered prior to invasive diagnostic procedures. If a relatively homogeneous perfusion and glucose metabolic pattern is observed, then it is more likely that the etiology of the left ventricular dysfunction is nonischemic, and consideration might also be given to myocardial biopsy in addition to coronary angiography as a means of establishing the diagnosis. On the other hand, if large metabolism-perfusion mismatches are identified to indicate chronic left ventricular ischemia, then coronary angiography would appear warranted in most individuals in order to determine the suitability for coronary revascularization. On the other hand, if positron emission tomography identifies only large confluent areas of completed infarction, then revascularization would not likely be of clinical benefit, and medical management without coronary angiography might be proposed.

As positron emission tomography emerges into the clinical practice of cardiology, the role that metabolic imaging will assume in the decision-making process for patients with ischemic heart disease will continue to be defined and refined. A better understanding of the basic biochemical processes regulating myocardial energy production in both normal and ischemic tissue provides new and unique information that ultimately may enhance our care of the patient with ischemic heart disease and further reduce cardiac morbidity and mortality.

SUMMARY AND CONCLUSIONS

Positron emission tomography with tracers of blood flow and substrate metabolism allows the noninvasive determination of the metabolic consequences of acute and chronic ischemia in human myocardium. The observations made to date with this technique have provided new and unique insights into human coronary artery disease. These new insights have improved our understanding of the pathophysiology of human ischemic heart disease and have decisively contributed to patient care. Many of the past accomplishments are based upon semiquantitative analyses of normal and abnormal myocardial function. Use of quantitative analytic techniques for measurements of rates of blood flow and substrate utilization is likely to further enhance the characterization of the abnormal tissue metabolic processes resulting from myocardial ischemia. Further refinements, together with new insights that are both pathophysiologically and clinically important, are likely to be achieved as new tracers emerge and are applied to the study of human ischemic heart disease. Our challenge is to employ this newly derived knowledge in the most efficient manner in order to improve the detection of coronary artery disease and to reduce its human morbidity and mortality.

References

A

1. Allan, R.M., Pike, V.W., Maseri, A., and Selwyn, A.P.: Myocardial metabolism of ^{11}C-acetate: Experimental and patient studies. (Abstract.) Circulation 64(Suppl. IV):IV–75, 1981.
2. Araujo, L.I., Camici, P., Spinks, T., et al.: Abnormalities in myocardial metabolism in patients with unstable angina as assessed by positron emission tomography. Cardiovasc. Drugs Ther. 2:41, 1988.
3. Alderman, E.L., Fisher, L.D., Litwin, P., et al.: Results of coronary artery surgery in patients with poor left ventricular function (CASS). Circulation 68:785, 1983.

B

1. Brown, M., Marshall, D.R., Sobel, B.E., and Bergmann, S.R.: Delineation of myocardial oxygen utilization with carbon-11 labeled acetate. Circulation 76:687, 1987.
2. Buxton, D.B., Schwaiger, M., Nguyen, A., et al.: Radiolabeled acetate as a tracer of myocardial tricarboxylic acid cycle flux. Circ. Res. 63:628, 1988.
3. Buxton, D.B., Nienaber, C.A., Luxen, A., et al.: Noninvasive quantification of regional myocardial oxygen consumption in vivo with [1-^{11}C] acetate and dynamic positron emission tomography. Circulation 79:134, 1989.
4. Brown, M.A., Myears, D.W., and Bergmann, S.R.: Validity of estimates of myocardial oxidative metabolism with carbon-11 acetate and positron emission tomography despite altered patterns of substrate utilization. J. Nucl. Med. 30:187, 1989.
5. Brachfeld, N., and Scheuer, J.: Metabolism of glucose by the ischemic dog heart. Am. J. Physiol. 212:603, 1967.
6. Braunwald, E., and Kloner, R.A.: The stunned myocardium: Prolonged, postischemic ventricular dysfunction. Circulation 66:1146, 1982.
7. Bergmann, S.R., Lerch, R.A., Fox, K.A.A., et al.: Temporal dependence of beneficial effects of coronary thrombolysis characterized by positron tomography. Am. J. Med. 73:573, 1982.
8. Brown, M.A., Myears, D.W., Herrero, P., and Bergmann, S.R.: Disparity between oxidative and fatty acid metabolism in reperfused myocardium assessed with positron emission tomography. (Abstract.) Circulation 76(Suppl. IV):IV–4, 1987.
9. Buxton, D.B., Schwaiger, M., Vaghaiwalla Mody, F., et al.: Regional abnormality of oxygen consumption in reperfused myocardium assessed with [1-^{11}C] acetate and positron emission tomography. Am. J. Card. Imag. 3:276, 1989.
10. Brunken, R.C., Schwaiger, M., and Schelbert, H.R.: PET detection of residual, viable tissue in acute MI. Appl. Radiol. 14:82, 1985.
11. Billadello, J.J., Smith, J.L., Ludbrook, P.A., et al.: Implications of "reciprocal" ST segment depression associated with acute myocardial infarction identified by positron tomography. J. Am. Coll. Cardiol. 2:616, 1983.
12. Bulkley, B.H., Silverman, K., Weisfeldt, M.L., et al.: Pathologic basis of thallium-201 scintigraphic defects in patients with fatal myocardial injury. Circulation 60:785, 1979.
13. Brunken, R.C., and Schelbert, H.R.: Acute myocardial infarction: A case for metabolic imaging. Lead. Edge Cardiol. 3:1, 1989.
14. Berger, H., Lahiri, A., Leppo, J., et al.: Antimyosin imaging in patients with ischemic chest pain: Initial results of phase III multicenter trial. (Abstract.) J. Nucl. Med. 29:805, 1988.
15. Brunken, R., Tillisch, J., Schwaiger, M., et al.: Regional perfusion, glucose metabolism and wall motion in patients with chronic electrocardiographic Q wave infarctions: Evidence for persistence of viable tissue in some infarct regions by positron emission tomography. Circulation 73:951, 1986.
16. Bourassa, M.G., Lesperance, J., Campeau, L., and Saltiel, J.: Fate of left ventricular contraction abnormalities following aortocoronary venous grafts. Early and late postoperative modifications. Circulation 46:724, 1972.
17. Brundage, B.H., Massie, B.M., and Botvinick, E.H.: Improved regional ventricular function after successful surgical revascularization. J. Am. Coll. Cardiol. 3:902, 1984.
18. Berger, B.C., Watson, D.D., Burwell, L.R., et al.: Redistribution of thallium at rest in patients with stable and unstable angina and the effect of coronary artery bypass surgery. Circulation 60:1114, 1979.
19. Berman, D.S., Garcia, E.V., Maddahi, J., and Rozanski, A.: Thallium-201 myocardial perfusion scintigraphy: Redistribution. *In* Freeman, L.M. (ed.): Freeman and Johnson's Clinical Radionuclide Imaging. 3rd ed. Grune and Stratton, Orlando, Fla., 1984, pp. 481–482.
20. Brunken, R., Schwaiger, M., Grover-McKay, M., et al.: Positron emission tomography detects tissue metabolic activity in myocardial segments with persistent thallium perfusion defects. J. Am. Coll. Cardiol. 10:557, 1987.
21. Brunken, R.C., Kottou, S., Schwaiger, M., et al.: PET detection of viable tissue in myocardial segments with persistent defects at thallium-201 SPECT. Radiology 172:65, 1989.
22. Brunken, R.C., Mody, F.V., Hawkins, R.A., et al.: Positron tomography detects glucose metabolism in segments with 24-hour tomographic thallium defects. (Abstract.) Circulation 78(Suppl. II):II–91, 1988.
23. Bounous, E.P., Mark, D.B., Pollock, B.G., et al.: Surgical survival benefits for

coronary disease patients with left ventricular dysfunction. Circulation 78 (Suppl. I):I–151, 1988.
24. Braunwald, E., and Rutherford, J.D.: Reversible ischemic left ventricular dysfunction: Evidence for the "hibernating myocardium." (Editorial.) J. Am. Coll. Cardiol. 8:1467, 1986.
25. Bulkley, B.H., Hutchins, G.M., Bailey, I., et al.: Thallium-201 imaging and gated cardiac blood pool scans in patients with ischemic and idiopathic congestive cardiomyopathy. A clinical and pathologic study. Circulation 55:753, 1977.
26. Brunken, R.C., Vaghaiwalla Mody, F., Gambhir, S.S., et al.: Quantitative PET reveals accelerated glucose metabolism in ischemic human myocardium. (Abstract.) J. Nucl. Med. 30:867, 1989.
27. Brunken, R.C., Chan, S.Y., Armbrecht, J.J., et al.: ^{11}C-acetate kinetic analysis reveals impaired oxidative flux in hypoperfused human myocardium with maintained glucose metabolism. (Abstract.) Circulation 80 (Suppl. II):II–377, 1989.

C

1. Camici, P., Araujo, L.I., Spinks, T., et al.: Increased uptake of ^{18}F-fluorodeoxyglucose in postischemic myocardium of patients with exercise-induced angina. Circulation 74:81, 1986.
2. Chung, E.K.: Fundamentals of Electrocardiography. University Park Press, Baltimore, 1984, p. 83.
3. Conde, C.A., Meller, J., Espinoza, J., et al.: Disappearance of abnormal Q waves after aortocoronary bypass surgery. Am. J. Cardiol. 36:889, 1975.
4. Cabin, H.S., Soni Clubbs, K., Vita, N., and Zaret, B.L.: Regional dysfunction by equilibrium radionuclide angiography: A clinicopathologic study evaluating the relation of degree of dysfunction to the presence and extent of myocardial infarction. J. Am. Coll. Cardiol. 10:743, 1987.
5. Chatterjee, K., Swan, H.J.C., Parmley, W.W., et al.: Influence of direct myocardial revascularization on left ventricular asynergy and function in patients with coronary heart disease: With and without previous myocardial infarction. Circulation 47:276, 1973.
6. Cohen, M., Charney, R., Hershman, R., et al.: Reversal of chronic ischemic myocardial dysfunction after transluminal coronary angioplasty. J. Am. Coll. Cardiol. 12:1193, 1988.
7. Cloninger, K.G., DePuey, G., Garcia, E.V., et al.: Incomplete redistribution in delayed thallium-201 single photon emission computed (SPECT) images: An overestimation of myocardial scarring. J. Am. Coll. Cardiol. 12:955, 1988.

D

1. DeWood, M.A., Spores, J., Notske, R., et al.: Prevalence of total coronary occlusion during the early hours of transmural myocardial infarction. N. Engl. J. Med. 303:897, 1980.
2. DeLandsheere, C.M., Raets, D., Pierard, L.A., et al.: Fibrinolysis and viable myocardium after an acute infarction: A study of regional perfusion and glucose utilization with positron emission tomography. (Abstract.) Circulation 72 (Part II):II–393, 1985.
3. DeLandsheere, C.M., Raets, D., Pierard, L.A., et al.: Thrombolysis in anterior infarction: Effect on regional viability studied with positron emission tomography. (Abstract.) Circulation 76 (Suppl. IV):IV–5, 1987.
4. Durrer, D., Van Lier, A.A.W., and Buller, J.: Epicardial and intramural excitation in chronic myocardial infarction. Am. Heart J. 68:765, 1964.
5. Davis, K., Kennedy, J.W., Kemp, H.G., et al.: Complications of coronary arteriography from the collaborative study of coronary artery surgery [CASS]. Circulation 59:1105, 1979.

E

1. Eichhorn, E.J., Kosinski, E.J., Lewis, S.M., et al.: Usefulness of dipyridamole-thallium-201 perfusion scanning for distinguishing ischemic from nonischemic cardiomyopathy. Am. J. Cardiol. 62:945, 1988.

F

1. Fox, K.A.A., Abendschein, D.R., Ambos, H.D., et al.: Efflux of metabolized and nonmetabolized fatty acid from canine myocardium. Implications for quantifying myocardial metabolism tomographically. Circ. Res. 57:232, 1985.
2. Fudo, T., Kambara, H., Hashimoto, T., et al.: F–18 deoxyglucose and stress N–13 ammonia positron emission tomography in anterior wall healed myocardial infarction. Am. J. Cardiol. 61:1191, 1988.
3. Freifeld, A.G., Schuster, E.H., and Bulkley, B.: Nontransmural versus transmural myocardial infarction: A morphologic study. Am. J. Med. 75:423, 1983.
4. Fedele, F.A., Gewirtz, H., Capone, R.J., et al.: Metabolic response to prolonged reduction of myocardial blood flow distal to a severe coronary artery stenosis. Circulation 78:729, 1988.
5. Frank, E.: The image surface of a homogeneous torso. Am. Heart J. 47:757, 1954.
6. Flameng, W., Suy, R., Schwarz, F., et al.: Ultrastructural correlates of left ventricular contraction abnormalities in patients with chronic ischemic heart disease: Determinants of reversible segmental asynergy postrevascularization surgery. Am. Heart J. 102:846, 1981.
7. Franciosa, J.A., Wilen, M.W., Ziesche, S., and Cohn, J.: Survival in man with severe chronic left ventricular failure due to coronary heart disease or idiopathic dilated cardiomyopathy. Am. J. Cardiol. 51:831, 1983.
8. Fuster, V., Gersh, B.J., Giuliani, E.R., et al.: The natural history of idiopathic dilated cardiomyopathy. Am. J. Cardiol. 47:525, 1981.
9. Fudo, T., Kambara, H., Hayashi, M., et al.: Possible difference of metabolical condition in patients with dilated cardiomyopathy and severe coronary artery disease: Evaluation by positron emission tomography. (Abstract.) J. Am. Coll. Cardiol. 13:103A, 1989.
10. Fintel, D.J., Links, J.M., Brinker, J.A., et al.: Improved diagnostic performance of exercise thallium-201 single photon emission computed tomography over planar imaging in the diagnosis of coronary artery disease: A receiver operating characteristic analysis. J. Am. Coll. Cardiol. 13:600, 1989.

G

1. Goldstein, R.A., Klein, M.S., and Sobel, B.E.: Distribution of exogenous labeled palmitate in ischemic myocardium: Implications for positron emission tomography. *In* Vogel, J.H.K. (ed.): Advances in Cardiology. Vol. 27. S. Karger, Basel, 1980, pp. 71–82.
2. Grover-McKay, M., Schelbert, H.R., Schwaiger, M., et al.: Identification of impaired metabolic reserve by atrial pacing in patients with significant coronary artery disease. Circulation 74:281, 1986.
3. Guerci, A.D., Gerstenblith, G., Brinker, J.A., et al.: A randomized trial of intravenous tissue plasminogen activator for acute myocardial infarction with subsequent randomization to elective coronary angioplasty. N. Engl. J. Med. 317:1613, 1987.
4. Goldberger, A.L., and Goldberger, E.: Clinical Electrocardiography. 2nd ed. C.V. Mosby. St. Louis, 1981, p. 87.
5. Gardberg, M.: A simple geometric analysis of cardiac potentials as recorded at points close to the heart. Circulation 9:563, 1954.
6. Gibson, R.S., Watson, D.D., Taylor, G.J., et al.: Prospective assessment of regional myocardial perfusion before and after coronary revascularization surgery by quantitative thallium-201 scintigraphy. J. Am. Coll. Cardiol. 1:804, 1983.
7. Gutman, J., Berman, D.S., Freeman, M., et al.: Time to completed redistribution of thallium-201 in exercise myocardial scintigraphy: Relation to the degree of coronary artery stenosis. Am. Heart J. 106:989, 1983.
8. Gambhir, S.S., Schwaiger, M., Huang, S.C., et al.: Simple noninvasive quantification method for measuring glucose utilization in humans employing positron emission tomography and fluorine-18 deoxyglucose. J. Nucl. Med. 30:359, 1989.
9. Geltman, E.M., Biello, D., Welch, M.J., et al.: Characterization of nontransmural infarction by positron-emission tomography. Circulation 65:747, 1982.

H

1. Henes, C.G., Bergmann, S.R., Walch, M.N., and Geltman, E.M.: Recovery of myocardial perfusion and oxygen consumption after thrombolysis delineated with positron emission tomography (PET). (Abstract.) Circulation 80 (Suppl. II):II–312, 1989.
2. Hashimoto, T., Kambara, H., Fudo, T., et al.: Increased fluorine-18 deoxyglucose uptake after percutaneous transluminal coronary angioplasty in recently infarcted myocardium. Am. J. Cardiol. 63:743, 1989.
3. Horan, L.G., Flowers, N.C., and Johnson, J.C.: Significance of the diagnostic Q wave of myocardial infarction. Circulation 43:428, 1971.
4. Hashimoto, T., Kambara, H., Fudo, T., et al.: Non-Q wave versus Q wave myocardial infarction: Regional myocardial metabolism and blood flow assessed by positron emission tomography. J. Am. Coll. Cardiol. 12:88, 1988.
5. Hecht, H.S., Andreae, G., Myler, R.K, and Chin, H.: The role of 24 hour tomographic thallium-201 myocardial imaging in revascularization. (Abstract.) J. Nucl. Med. 29:769, 1988.
6. Hatle, L., Orjavik, O., and Storstein, O.: Chronic myocardial disease. Clinical picture related to long-term prognosis. Acta Med. Scand. 199:399, 1976.

I

1. ISAM Study Group: A prospective trial of intravenous streptokinase in acute myocardial infarction (I.S.A.M.). Mortality, morbidity and infarct size at 21 days. N. Engl. J. Med. 314:1465, 1986.
2. Ideker, R.E., Behar, V.S., Wagner, G.S., et al.: Evaluation of asynergy as an indicator of myocardial fibrosis. Circulation 57:715, 1978.
3. Iskandrian, A.S., Hakki, A.H., Kane, S.A., et al.: Rest and redistribution thallium-201 myocardial scintigraphy to predict improvement in left ventricular function after coronary arterial bypass grafting. Am. J. Cardiol. 51:1312, 1983.
4. Iskandrian, A.S., and Hakki, A.H.: Thallium-201 myocardial scintigraphy. Am. Heart J. 109:113, 1985.
5. Iskandrian, A.S., Hakki, A., and Kane, S.: Resting thallium-201 myocardial perfusion patterns in patients with severe left ventricular dysfunction: Differences between patients with primary cardiomyopathy, chronic coronary artery disease, or acute myocardial infarction. Am. Heart J. 111:760, 1986.

J

1. Jeremy, R.W., Hackworthy, R.A., Bautovich, G., et al.: Infarct artery perfusion and changes in left ventricular volume in the month after myocardial infarction. J. Am. Coll. Cardiol. 9:989, 1987.
2. Johnson, L., Seldin, D., Becker, L., et al.: Antimyosin imaging in acute transmural myocardial infarctions: Results of a multicenter clinical trial. J. Am. Coll. Cardiol. 13:27, 1989.

K

1. Kloner, R.A., and Przyklenk, K.: Altered myocardial states. The stunned and hibernating myocardium. Am. J. Med. 86(Suppl. 1A):14, 1989.
2. Kennedy, J.W., Martin, G.V., Davis, K.B., et al.: The Western Washington

intravenous streptokinase in acute myocardial infarction randomized trial. Circulation 77:345, 1988.
3. Knabb, R.M., Bergmann, S.R., Fox, K.A., and Sobel, B.E.: The temporal pattern of recovery of myocardial perfusion and metabolism delineated by positron emission tomography after coronary thrombolysis. J. Nucl. Med. 28:1563, 1987.
4. Kalff, V., Gallagher, K.P., Nguygen, N., et al.: Dissociation of glucose utilization and blood flow in canine myocardial ischemia. (Abstract.) Circulation 80(Suppl. II):II–638, 1989.
5. Kalff, V., Molina, E., Squicciarini, S., et al.: Regional C–11 acetate kinetics in patients with acute myocardial infarction as assessed by PET. (Abstract.) Circulation 80(Suppl. II):II–309, 1989.
6. Khaw, B., Yasuda, T., Gold, H., et al.: Acute myocardial infarct imaging with indium-111-labeled monoclonal antimyosin F_{ab}. J. Nucl. Med. 28:1671, 1987.
7. Kiat, H., Berman, D.S., Maddahi, J., et al.: Late reversibility of tomographic myocardial thallium-201 defects: An accurate marker of myocardial viability. J. Am. Coll. Cardiol. 12:1456, 1988.
8. Kiat, H., Berman, D.S., and Maddahi, J.: Comparison of planar and tomographic exercise thallium-201 imaging methods for the evaluation of coronary artery disease. (Editorial.) J. Am. Coll. Cardiol. 13:613, 1989.
9. Kennedy, J.W., Kaiser, G.C., Fisher, L.D., et al.: Clinical and angiographic predictors of operative mortality from the collaborative study in coronary artery surgery (CASS). Circulation 63:793, 1981.

L

1. Liedtke, A.J.: Alterations of carbohydrate and lipid metabolism in the acutely ischemic heart. Prog. Cardiovasc. Dis. 23:321, 1981.
2. Lerch, R.A., Bergmann, S.R., Ambos, H.D., et al.: Effect of flow-independent reduction of metabolism on regional myocardial clearance of ^{11}C-palmitate. Circulation 65:731, 1982.
3. Lerch, R.A., Ambos, H.D., Bergmann, S.R., et al.: Localization of viable, ischemic myocardium by positron-emission tomography with ^{11}C-palmitate. Circulation 64:689, 1981.
4. Luu, M., Stevenson, L.W., Brunken, R.C., et al.: Delayed recovery of revascularized myocardium after referral for cardiac transplantation. Am. Heart J. 119(Part I):668, 1990.
5. Liu, P., Kiess, M.C., Okada, R.D., et al.: The persistent defect on exercise thallium imaging and its fate after myocardial revascularization. Does it represent scar or ischemia? Am. Heart J. 110:996, 1985.
6. Ladenheim, M.L., Pollock, B.H., Rozanski, A., et al.: Extent and severity of myocardial hypoperfusion as predictors of prognosis in patients with suspected coronary artery disease. J. Am. Coll. Cardiol. 7:464, 1986.

M

1. Marshall, R.C., Nash, W.W., Shine, K.I., et al.: Glucose metabolism during ischemia due to excessive oxygen demand or altered coronary flow in the isolated arterially perfused rabbit septum. Circ. Res. 49:640, 1981.
2. Most, A.S., Gorlin, R., and Soeldner, J.S.: Glucose extraction by the human myocardium during pacing stress. Circulation 45:92, 1972.
3. Mathey, D.G., Sheehan, F.H., Schofer, J., and Dodge, H.T.: Time from onset of symptoms to thrombolytic therapy: A major determinant of myocardial salvage in patients with acute transmural infarction. J. Am. Coll. Cardiol. 6:S18, 1985.
4. Myears, D.W., Sobel, B.E., and Bergmann, S.R.: Substrate use in ischemic and reperfused canine myocardium: Quantitative considerations. Am. J. Physiol. 253 (Heart Circ. Physiol. 22): H107, 1987.
5. Melin, J.A., Wijns, W., Keyeux, A., et al.: Assessment of thallium-201 redistribution versus glucose uptake as predictors of viability after coronary occlusion and reperfusion. Circulation 77:927, 1988.
6. Marshall, R.C., Tillisch, J.H., Phelps, M.E., et al.: Identification and differentiation of resting myocardial ischemia and infarction in man with positron computed tomography, ^{18}F-labeled fluorodeoxyglucose and N–13 ammonia. Circulation 67:766, 1983.
7. Melin, J.A., Vanoverschelde, J.L., Bol, A., and Wijns, W.: Regional oxidative metabolism in patients with reperfused infarction: Relation to regional blood flow and glucose uptake. (Abstract.) Circulation 80 (Suppl. II):II–378, 1989.
8. Melchoir, J., Doriot, P.A., Chatelain, P., et al.: Improvement of left ventricular contraction and relaxation synchronism after recanalization of chronic total coronary occlusion by angioplasty. J. Am. Coll. Cardiol. 9:763, 1987.

N

1. Neely, J.R., Whitmer, J.T., and Rovetto, M.J.: Effect of coronary blood flow on glycolytic flux and intracellular pH in isolated rat hearts. Circ. Res. 37:733, 1975.
2. National Heart Foundation of Australia Coronary Thrombolysis Group: Coronary thrombolysis and myocardial salvage by tissue plasminogen activator given up to 4 hours after onset of myocardial infarction. Lancet 1:203, 1988.
3. Nienaber, C.A., Brunken, R.C., Sherman, C.T., et al.: Recovery of myocardial metabolism precedes functional improvement following relief of chronic myocardial ischemia by PTCA. (Abstract.) J. Nucl. Med. 30: 838, 1989.

O

1. Opie, L.H., Owen, P., and Riemersma, R.A.: Relative rates of oxidation of glucose and free fatty acids by ischaemic and nonischaemic myocardium after coronary artery ligation in the dog. Eur. J. Clin. Invest. 3:419, 1973.
2. Opie, L.H.: Effects of regional ischemia on metabolism of glucose and fatty acids. Circ. Res. 38(Suppl. I):I–52, 1976.
3. Ong, L., Reiser, P., Coromilas, J., et al.: Left ventricular function and rapid release of creatine kinase MB in acute myocardial infarction. Evidence for spontaneous reperfusion. N. Engl. J. Med. 309:1, 1983.
4. O'Rourke, M., Baron, D., Keogh, A., et al.: Limitation of myocardial infarction by early infusion of recombinant tissue-type plasminogen activator. Circulation 77:1311, 1988.

P

1. Patlak, C.S., Blasberg, R.G., and Fenstermacher, J.D.: Graphical evaluation of blood to brain transfer constants from multiple uptake data. J. Cereb. Blood. Flow Metabol. 3:1, 1983.
2. Pohost, G.M., Zir, L.M., Moore, R.H., et al.: Differentiation of transiently ischemic from infarcted myocardium by serial imaging after a single dose of thallium-201. Circulation 55:294, 1977.
3. Passamani, E., Davis, K.B., Gillespie, M.J., et al.: A randomized trial of coronary artery bypass surgery. Survival of patients with a low ejection fraction. N. Engl. J. Med. 312:1665, 1985.
4. Pibott, J.D., Kouchoukos, N.T., Oberman, A., and Cutter, G.R.: Late results of surgical and medical therapy for patients with coronary artery disease and depressed left ventricular function. J. Am. Coll. Cardiol. 5:1036, 1985.

R

1. Reimer, K.A., and Jennings, R.B.: Myocardial ischemia, hypoxia, and infarction: Cellular consequences of severe myocardial ischemia. *In* Fozzard, H.A., Haber, H., Jennings, R.B., et al. (eds.): The Heart and Cardiovascular System: Scientific Foundations. Vol. 2. Raven Press, New York, 1986, pp. 1148–1152.
2. Rosamond, T.L., Abendschein, D.R., Sobel, B.E., et al.: Metabolic fate of radiolabeled palmitate in ischemic canine myocardium: Implications for positron emission tomography. J. Nucl. Med. 28:1332, 1987.
3. Reimer, K.A., Lowe, J.E., Rasmussen, M.M., and Jennings, R.B.: The wavefront phenomenon of ischemic cell death. I. Myocardial infarct size vs. duration of coronary occlusion in dogs. Circulation 56:786, 1977.
4. Reimer, K.A., and Jennings, R.B.: The "wavefront phenomenon" of myocardial ischemic cell death. II. Transmural progression of necrosis within the framework of ischemic bed size (myocardium at risk) and collateral flow. Lab. Invest. 40:633, 1979.
5. Rogers, W.J., Hood, W.P., Mantle, J.A., et al.: Return of left ventricular function after reperfusion in patients with myocardial infarction: Importance of subtotal stenoses or intact collaterals. Circulation 69:338, 1984.
6. Russell, M., Coleman, E., Chu, A., and Cobb, F.R.: Relation of fluorodeoxyglucose uptake in ischemic myocardium to myocardial blood flow. (Abstract.) Circulation 80 (Suppl. II):II–638, 1989.
7. Rovetto, M.J., Whitmer, J.T., and Neely, J.R.: Comparison of the effects of anoxia and whole heart ischemia on carbohydrate utilization in isolated working hearts. Circ. Res. 32:699, 1973.
8. Raunio, H., Rissanen, V., Romppanen, T., et al.: Changes in the QRS complex and ST segment in transmural and subendocardial myocardial infarctions. A clinicopathologic study. Am. Heart J. 98:176, 1979.
9. Righetti, A., Crawford, M.H., O'Rourke, R., et al.: Interventricular septal motion and left ventricular function following coronary artery bypass surgery. Evaluation with echocardiography and radionuclide angiography. Am. J. Cardiol. 39:372, 1977.
10. Rankin, J.S., Newman, G.E., Muhlbaier, L.H., et al.: The effects of coronary revascularization on left ventricular function in ischemic heart disease. J. Thorac. Cardiovasc. Surg. 90: 818, 1985.
11. Rozanski, A., Berman, D.S., Gray, R., et al.: Use of thallium-201 redistribution scintigraphy in the preoperative differentiation of reversible and nonreversible myocardial asynergy. Circulation 64: 936, 1981.
12. Rahimtoola, S.H.: A perspective on the three large multicenter randomized clinical trials of coronary bypass surgery for chronic stable angina. Circulation 72: V–123, 1985.
13. Rahimtoola, S.H.: The hibernating myocardium. Am. Heart J. 117:211, 1989.
14. Roberts, R., Henry, P.D., and Sobel, B.E.: An improved basis for enzymatic estimation of infarct size. Circulation 52: 743, 1975.

S

1. Schön, H.R., Schelbert, H.R., Najafi, A., et al.: C-11 labeled palmitic acid for the noninvasive evaluation of regional myocardial fatty acid metabolism with positron-computed tomography. II. Kinetics of C–11 palmitic acid in acutely ischemic myocardium. Am. Heart J. 103:548, 1982.
2. Schön, H.R., Schelbert, H.R., Robinson, G., et al.: C-11 labeled palmitic acid for the noninvasive evaluation of regional myocardial fatty acid metabolism with positron-computed tomography. I. Kinetics of C-11 palmitic acid in normal myocardium. Am. Heart J. 103:532, 1982.
3. Scheuer, J., and Brachfeld, N.: Myocardial uptake and fractional distribution of palmitate-1-C^{14} by the ischemic dog heart. Metabolism 15:945, 1966.
4. Schwaiger, M., Fishbein, M.C., Block M., et al.: Metabolic and ultrastructural abnormalities during ischemia in canine myocardium: Noninvasive assessment by positron emission tomography. J. Mol. Cell. Cardiol. 19:259, 1987.
5. Schelbert, H.R., Henze, E., Keen, R., et al.: C–11 palmitate for the noninvasive evaluation of regional myocardial fatty acid metabolism with positron-computed tomography. IV. In vivo evaluation of acute demand-induced ischemia in dogs. Am. Heart J. 106:736, 1983.
6. Schwaiger, M., Hutchins, G.D., Bergin, P., et al.: Independence of C–11 acetate kinetics from dietary state in the human heart. (Abstract.) J. Nucl. Med. 30:837, 1989.

7. Schelbert, H.R., Phelps, M.E., Selin, C., et al.: Regional myocardial ischemia assessed by [18]Fluoro-2-deoxyglucose and positron emission computed tomography. *In* Heiss, H.W. (ed.): Advances in Clinical Cardiology. Vol. I. Quantification of Myocardial Ischemia. Gerhard Witzstrock, New York, 1980, pp. 437–449.
8. Schelbert, H.R., Henze, E., Schon, H.R., et al.: C–11 palmitate for the noninvasive evaluation of regional myocardial fatty acid metabolism with positron computed tomography. III. In vivo demonstration of the effects of substrate availability on myocardial metabolism. Am. Heart J. 105:492, 1983.
9. Selwyn, A.P., Allan, R.M., Pike, V., et al.: Positive labeling of ischemic myocardium: A new approach in patients with coronary disease. (Abstract.) Am. J. Cardiol. 47:481, 1981.
10. Sheehan, F.H.: Determinants of improved left ventricular function after thrombolytic therapy in acute myocardial infarction. J. Am. Coll. Cardiol. 9:937, 1987.
11. Sheehan, F.H., Braunwald, E., Conner, P., et al.: The effect of intravenous thrombolytic therapy on left ventricular function: A report on tissue type plasminogen activator and streptokinase from the Thrombolysis in Myocardial Infarction (TIMI Phase I) Trial. Circulation 75:817, 1987.
12. Schwaiger, M., Neese, R.A., Araujo, L., et al.: Sustained nonoxidative glucose utilization and depletion of glycogen in reperfused canine myocardium. J. Am. Coll. Cardiol. 13:745, 1989.
13. Schwaiger, M., Schelbert, H.R., Keen, R., et al.: Retention and clearance of C–11 palmitic acid in ischemic and reperfused canine myocardium. J. Am. Coll. Cardiol. 6:311, 1985.
14. Schwaiger, M., Schelbert, H.R., Ellison, D., et al.: Sustained regional abnormalities in cardiac metabolism after transient ischemia in the chronic dog model. J. Am. Coll. Cardiol. 6:336, 1985.
15. Sochor, H., Schwaiger, M., Schelbert, H.R., et al.: Relationship between Tl–201, Tc–99m (Sn) pyrophosphate and F–18 2-deoxyglucose uptake in ischemically injured dog myocardium. Am. Heart J. 114:1066, 1987.
16. Schwaiger, M., Brunken, R., Grover-McKay, M., et al.: Regional myocardial metabolism in patients with acute myocardial infarction assessed by positron emission tomography. J. Am. Coll. Cardiol. 8:800, 1986.
17. Schwaiger, M., Brunken, R.C., Krivokapich, J., et al.: Beneficial effect of residual anterograde flow on tissue viability as assessed by positron emission tomography in patients with myocardial infarction. Eur. Heart J. 8:981, 1987.
18. Savage, R.M., Wagner, G.S., Ideker, R.E., et al.: Correlation of postmortem anatomic findings with electrocardiographic changes in patients with myocardial infarction. Retrospective study of patients with typical anterior and posterior infarcts. Circulation 55:279, 1977.
19. Sullivan, W., Vlodaver, Z., Tuna, N., et al.: Correlation of electrocardiographic and pathologic findings in healed myocardial infarction. Am. J. Cardiol. 43:724, 1978.
20. Stinson, E.B., and Billingham, M.E.: Correlative study of regional left ventricular histology and contractile function. Am. J. Cardiol. 39:378, 1977.
21. Shearn, D.L., and Brent, B.N.: Coronary artery bypass surgery in patients with left ventricular dysfunction. Am. J. Med. 80:405, 1986.
22. Shugoli, G.I, Bowen, P.J., Moore, J.P., and Lenkin, M.L: Follow-up observations and prognosis in primary myocardial disease. Arch. Intern. Med. 129:67, 1972.
23. Schneiderman, J., Hager, W.D., and Gondos, B.: The endomyocardial biopsy. Ann. Clin. Lab. Sci. 16:134, 1986.
24. Smith, G.T., Huang, S.C., Nienaber, C.A., et al.: Noninvasive quantification of regional myocardial blood flow with N–13 ammonia and dynamic PET. (Abstract.) J. Nucl. Med. 29:940, 1988.
25. Sobel, B.E., Weiss E.S., Welch, M.J., et al.: Detection of remote myocardial infarction in patients with positron emission tomography and intravenous ^{11}C-palmitate. Circulation 55:853, 1977.

T

1. Thomassen, A., Nielsen, T.T., Bagger, J.P., and Henningsen, P.: Antianginal and cardiac metabolic effects of low-dose glucose infusion during pacing in patients with and without coronary artery disease. Am. Heart J. 118:25, 1989.
2. Tillisch, J., Brunken, R., Marshall, R., et al.: Reversibility of cardiac wall motion abnormalities predicted by positron tomography. N. Engl. J. Med. 314:884, 1986.
3. Tamaki, N., Yonekura, Y., Yamashita, K., et al.: Positron emission tomography using fluorine-18 deoxyglucose in evaluation of coronary artery bypass grafting. Am. J. Cardiol. 64:860, 1989.
4. Topol, E.J., Weiss, J.L., Guzman, P.A., et al.: Immediate improvement of dysfunctional myocardial segments after coronary revascularization: Detection by intraoperative transesophageal echocardiography. J. Am. Coll. Cardiol. 4:1123, 1984.
5. Tamaki, N., Yonekura, Y., Yamashita, K., et al.: Relation of left ventricular perfusion and wall motion with metabolic activity in persistent defects on thallium-201 tomography in healed myocardial infarction. Am. J. Cardiol. 62:202, 1988.
6. Tamaki, N., Yonekura, Y., Yamashita, K., et al.: SPECT thallium-201 tomography and positron tomography using N–13 ammonia and F–18 fluorodeoxyglucose in coronary heart disease. Am. J. Card. Imag. 3:3, 1989.
7. Ter-Pogossian, M.M., Klein, M.S., Markham, J., et al.: Regional assessment of myocardial metabolic integrity in vivo by positron-emission tomography with ^{11}C-palmitate. Circulation 61:242, 1980.

V

1. Van der Vusse, G.J., Roemen, T.H.M., Prinzen, F.W., et al.: Uptake and tissue content of fatty acids in dog myocardium under normoxic and ischemic conditions. Circ. Res. 50:538, 1982.
2. Vary, T.C., Reibel, D.K., and Neely, J.R.: Control of energy metabolism of heart muscle. Annu. Rev. Physiol. 43:419, 1981.
3. Van de Werf, F., Arnold, A.E.R., and the European Cooperative Study Group for Recombinant Tissue Type Plasminogen Activator: Intravenous tissue plasminogen activator and size of infarct, left ventricular function and survival in acute myocardial infarction. Br. Med. J. 297:1374, 1988.
4. Vaghaiwalla Mody, F., Brunken, R.C., Stevenson, L.W., et al.: Can positron tomography distinguish dilated from ischemic cardiomyopathy? (Abstract.) Circulation 78(Suppl. II):II–92, 1988.
5. Vaghaiwalla Mody, F., Buxton, D.B., Krivokapich, J., et al.: Attenuated response of glucose metabolism in reperfused canine myocardium to changes in substrate levels. J. Am. Coll. Cardiol. 15(Suppl. A):80A, 1990.

W

1. White, H.D., Norris, R.M., Brown, M.A., et al.: Effect of intravenous streptokinase on left ventricular function and early survival after acute myocardial infarction. N. Engl. J. Med. 317:850, 1987.
2. White, H.D., Rivers, J.T., Maslowski, A.H., et al.: Effect of intravenous streptokinase as compared with that of tissue plasminogen activator on left ventricular function after first myocardial infarction. N. Engl. J. Med. 320:817, 1989.
3. Wyman, R.M., Safian, R.D., Portway, V., et al.: Current complications of diagnostic and therapeutic catheterization. J. Am. Coll. Cardiol. 12:1400, 1988.
4. Weiss, E.S., Ahmed, S.A., Welch, M.J., et al.: Quantification of infarction in cross sections of canine myocardium *in vivo* with positron emission transaxial tomography and ^{11}C-palmitate. Circulation 55:66, 1977.

Y

1. Yonekura, Y., Tamaki, N., Kambara, H., et al.: Detection of metabolic alterations in ischemic myocardium by F–18 deoxyglucose uptake with positron emission tomography. Am. J. Card. Imag. 2:122, 1988.

Z

1. Zeft, H.J., Friedberg, H.D., King, J.F., et al.: Reappearance of anterior QRS forces after coronary bypass surgery: An electrovectorcardiographic study. Am. J. Cardiol. 36:163, 1975.
2. Ziessman, H.A., Sigler, C.J., Wells, T.M., et al.: Utility of delayed 24 hour redistribution on SPECT thallium-201 myocardial perfusion studies. (Abstract.) J. Nucl. Med. 29:769, 1988.
3. Zubiate, P., Kay, J.H., and Dunne, E.F.: Myocardial revascularization for patients with an ejection fraction of 0.2 or less—12 years' results. West. J. Med. 140:745, 1984.

Chapter 68

Metabolic Findings in Cardiomyopathies

EDWARD M. GELTMAN, M.D.

BIOCHEMISTRY OF MYOCARDIAL ENERGETICS 1244
SYSTEMIC METABOLIC ABNORMALITIES IN PATIENTS WITH CARDIOMYOPATHY 1246
DILATED CARDIOMYOPATHY: OBSERVATIONS ON POSITRON EMISSION TOMOGRAPHY .. 1247
DIFFERENTIATION OF ISCHEMIC FROM NONISCHEMIC DILATED CARDIOMYOPATHY 1247
Positron Emission Tomographic Imaging 1249
Comparison with Other Imaging Techniques .. 1251
HYPERTROPHIC CARDIOMYOPATHY 1251
Background 1251
Myocardial Metabolism in Hypertrophic Cardiomyopathy 1251
Findings on Positron Emission Tomography ... 1251
CARDIOMYOPATHIES ASSOCIATED WITH SYSTEMIC ILLNESSES 1252
Positron Emission Tomographic Imaging 1253
FUTURE DIRECTIONS 1253

The cardiomyopathies are a diverse group of syndromes characterized by primary or secondary abnormalities of the myocardium. In general, the diagnosis of cardiomyopathy is made after excluding congenital, valvular, and pericardial disease. Some investigators would also exclude patients with ischemic and hypertensive disease, although such patients are sometimes included in separate diagnostic categories, e.g., ischemic cardiomyopathy or hypertensive heart disease. The last-mentioned approach is employed in the discussion that follows.

The cardiomyopathies may be classified in either functional or etiologic terms. The functional classification separates patients into groups with dilated, restrictive, and hypertrophic physiologies. An etiologic classification is indicated in Table 68–1. The diversity of etiologies is great, and although the pathology and physiology of many cardiomyopathies have been well described, detailed metabolic studies are often lacking.

BIOCHEMISTRY OF MYOCARDIAL ENERGETICS

The myocardium has the ability to use multiple substrates to meet its metabolic needs (Fig. 68–1). Myocardial metabolism of fatty acids and carbohydrates has been well characterized in experimental animals and humans with invasive assessments of levels of substrates and metabolites in samples of arterial and coronary sinus blood, as well as with direct analysis of tissue. A more detailed discussion is included in Chapters 4 and 65. A few critical aspects of fatty acid and carbohydrate metabolism are discussed here. Under most physiologic conditions, the myocardium uses free fatty acids preferentially.[N1] After transport across the sarcolemma by transport proteins (a reversible process, allowing back diffusion),[F1] free fatty acids are activated to acetyl-CoA compounds and shuttled into the mitochondria for β-oxidation, or are incorporated into triglycerides or phospholipids. Retention of free fatty acid is decreased in myocardium during oxygen supply-demand imbalance whether due to epicardial coronary disease, microvascular disease, poor substrate diffusion (due to deposition in the interstitium of collagen, amyloid, mucopolysaccharide, or other substances), or to increased metabolic demand induced by increased wall stress caused by ventricular dilatation and increased preload and afterload.[R1, O1, S1]

The mitochondrial membrane is not freely permeable to high energy intermediates. Therefore, the carnitine shuttle mechanism is employed to transport free fatty acids into the mitochondria for β-oxidation.[B1, P1] Some of the cardiac metabolic effects of several diseases (including diabetes) may be mediated through alterations in levels of acyl carnitine and cytosolic free carnitine.[B2] In contrast, in ischemia, glycolysis leads to lactate production with decreased availability of pyruvate and decreased citric acid cycle flux. Subsequent decreases in free acetyl-CoA and decreased activity of thiokinase (due to increased lactate levels) lead to further decreases in citric acid cycle flux and decreased intracellular trapping of free fatty acids. Increased glycolytic flux increases cytosolic levels of α-glyceryl phosphate, facilitating the storage of free fatty acids.[O1] Although these abnormalities have been generally described in animal models of global or regional ischemia, they may well apply to many patients with dilated and hypertrophic cardiomyopathy. Patients with these syndromes may present with relative ischemia, either globally or of the subendocardium, due to poor myocardial perfusion secondary to increased wall stress, compressive forces, interstitial fibrosis, or microvascular disease.[C1, P2, O3] Similarly, they may experience increased metabolic demands due to increased circulating catecholamines and increased wall stress (both systolic and diastolic) owing to altered geometry and increased systemic vascular resistance secondary to neurohormonal activation.[P3, L1]

Uptake of glucose into myocytes is carrier mediated and not energy dependent.[N1] In the presence of insulin, this process is augmented.[P4] The degree to which insulin facilitates glucose uptake directly compared with indirect effects mediated by suppressed circulating free fatty acid levels is controversial.[N1, O1] Whether accomplished directly or indirectly, in intact animals and humans, increased levels of plasma glucose lead to augmented myocardial uptake and metabolism of glucose and decreased utilization of free fatty acids. In experimental animals, the rate of glycolysis increases acutely and markedly within 30 seconds after the induction of ischemia.[N1] The pyruvate generated by glycolysis is converted to lactate in ischemia, and its accumulation decreases pH, eventually slowing glycolysis if ischemia is profound and prolonged.[N1, O1, O2]

Defects in energy metabolism and transduction of metabolic events into myocardial contraction were thought to explain the basis of the mechanical defects observed in chronic congestive

Table 68–1. SELECTED CAUSES OF CARDIOMYOPATHY

1. Inflammatory
   a. Infective
      - Viral
      - Rickettsial
      - Bacterial
      - Mycobacterial
      - Spirochetal
      - Fungal
      - Parasitic
   b. Noninfective
      - Collagen diseases
      - Granulomatosis
      - Cardiac transplant rejection
2. Metabolic
   a. Nutritional
      - Thiamine deficiency
      - Kwashiorkor
      - Pellagra
   b. Endocrine
      - Acromegaly
      - Thyrotoxicosis
      - Myxedema
      - Cushing's disease
      - Pheochromocytoma
      - Diabetes mellitus
   c. Altered metabolism
      - Gout
      - Oxalosis
      - Porphyria
   d. Electrolyte imbalance
3. Toxic
   a. Alcohol
   b. Bleomycin
   c. Adriamycin
   d. Lead
   e. Cyclophosphamide
   f. Corticosteroids
   g. Cocaine
4. Infiltrative
   a. Amyloidosis
   b. Hemochromatosis
   c. Neoplastic
   d. Glycogen storage disorders
   e. Sarcoidosis
   f. Mucopolysaccharidosis
   g. Gaucher's disease
   h. Sphingolipidoses
5. Fibroplastic
   a. Endomyocardial fibrosis
   b. Endocardial fibroelastosis
   c. Loffler's fibroplastic endocarditis
   d. Becker's disease
   e. Carcinoid
6. Hematological
   a. Sickle cell anemia
   b. Polycythemia vera
   c. Leukemia
7. Hypersensitivity
   a. Methyldopa
   b. Penicillin
   c. Sulfonamides
   d. Tetracycline
   e. Giant cell myocarditis
8. Genetic
   a. Hypertrophic cardiomyopathy
      - With gradient
      - Without gradient
   b. Neuromuscular
      - Duchenne muscular dystrophy
      - Facioscapulohumeral muscular dystrophy
      - Limb-girdle dystrophy of Erb
      - Myotonia dystrophica
      - Friedreich's ataxia
9. Miscellaneous acquired
   a. Postpartum cardiomyopathy
   b. Obesity
10. Idiopathic
   a. Idiopathic dilated cardiomyopathy
   b. Idiopathic restrictive cardiomyopathy
   c. Idiopathic hypertrophic cardiomyopathy
11. Physical agents
   a. Heat stroke
   b. Hypothermia
   c. Radiation

Adapted from Wynne, J., and Braunwald, E.: The cardiomyopathies and myocarditides. *In* Braunwald, E. (ed.): Heart Disease. A Textbook of Cardiovascular Medicine. 3rd ed. W. B. Saunders Co., Philadelphia, 1988, p. 1411. (Reproduced with permission.)

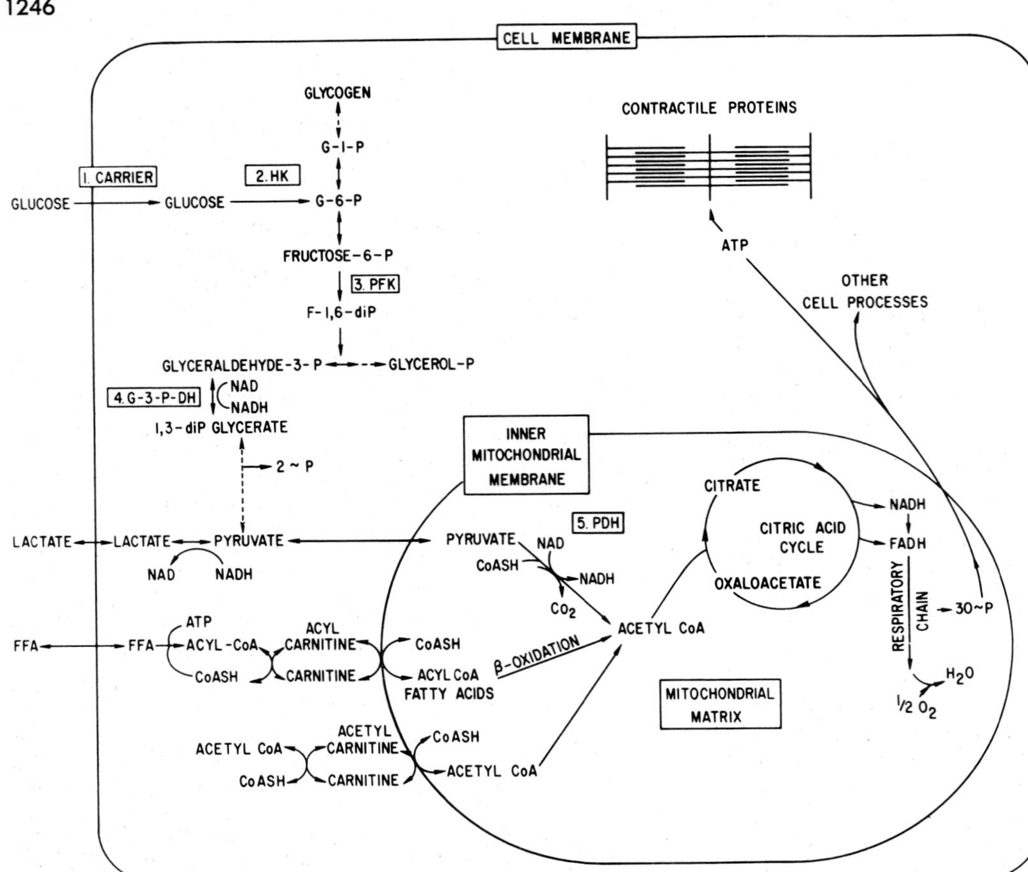

Figure 68–1. A schematic representation of the major pathways of metabolism of glucose, lactate, and free fatty acids, including glycolysis, the citric acid cycle, beta oxidation, and mitochondrial processes. (From Braunwald, E., Ross, J., and Sonnenblick, E. H. (eds.): Mechanisms of Contraction of the Normal and Failing Heart. 2nd ed. Little, Brown & Co., Boston, © 1976, p. 190, with permission.)

heart failure. The metabolic derangements observed in acute ischemia have been well described and delineated in Chapters 5 and 65. However, the processes involved in the slowly progressive syndrome of chronic congestive heart failure and the cardiomyopathies are less clearly defined. Although in some patients with symptoms of congestive heart failure, diastolic dysfunction predominates, in most patients with congestive heart failure, cardiac systolic mechanical reserve is diminished and there is a relative or absolute decrease in external cardiac work. In general (in the absence of acute ischemia due to obstructive coronary artery disease), the coronary circulation is exquisitely autoregulated. Even in patients or experimental animals with low-output congestive heart failure, total coronary blood flow and extraction of substrates (carbohydrates and free fatty acids) and oxygen (corrected for cardiac mass) remain within the normal range. There is close tracking between ventricular work, substrate utilization, and coronary perfusion.[B3, H1]

Defects in intermediary metabolism and respiration have been sought extensively in congestive heart failure. Clearly, in acute severe ischemia, adenosine triphosphate (ATP) production is limited, but in nonischemic chronic animal models of congestive heart failure and in humans, it is not clear whether or not there is a primary defect in mitochondrial function. Some investigators have shown defects in mitochondrial energy production in animal models of heart failure and in mitochondria obtained from hearts of patients with heart failure.[S2] In some animal models with hereditary cardiomyopathy (Syrian hamsters), severe depression of the ability to oxidize free fatty acids by the mitochondria has been demonstrated.[S3] Yet others have found close mitochondrial coupling and respiratory mitochondrial control with essentially normal myocardial mitochondrial function in papillary muscles from cats and humans with heart failure.[C2, S4] Since the mitochondrial abnormalities observed in some models of congestive heart failure are observed only late in the process, it seems likely that these abnormalities are not critical to the development of congestive heart failure. ATP and creatine phosphate depletion generally has not been found in experimental models of congestive heart failure or in patients, except in models with myocardial ischemia.[P5, C2] In contrast, there are abundant data indicating that there are abnormalities in the contractile proteins and myofibrillar ATPase activity associated with congestive heart failure.[A1, D1, G2, L2] Unfortunately, it appears that such defects are extremely difficult or impossible to evaluate noninvasively.

SYSTEMIC METABOLIC ABNORMALITIES IN PATIENTS WITH CARDIOMYOPATHY

With either systolic or diastolic dysfunction, there is activation of the renin-angiotensin-aldosterone system and the sympathetic nervous system.[P3] These processes result in increased levels of circulating angiotensin II and aldosterone but also result in induction and activation of local renin-angiotensin-aldosterone systems in specific tissue beds, including the heart.[D2] Similarly, systemic sympathetic activation is observed in patients with congestive heart failure with increased levels of circulating catecholamines and increased urinary excretion of catecholamine metabolites.[L1, H2] The heart is richly enervated with both sympathetic and parasympathetic efferent fibers providing direct cardiac regulation even in the absence of significant systemic sympathetic activation. In congestive heart failure, aortic coronary sinus sampling studies demonstrate excess catecholamine release into the coronary sinus during periods of myocardial stress and decompensation.[L1, H2, H3, K1]

Activation of the sympathetic nervous system and the renin-angiotensin-aldosterone system can have diverse effects on cardiac metabolism, depending on their effects on the coronary circulation, loading conditions, and direct cardiac inotropic stimulation. Increases in left ventricular preload and afterload and inotropic state induced by catecholamine stimulation in turn, induce increases in myocardial oxygen consumption with acceleration of the myocardial utilization of acetate and fatty acids as long as regional or global myocardial ischemia is not induced.[H4, B5] Conversely, high levels of exogenous catecholamines decrease myocardial glucose uptake in experimental animals.[M1]

DILATED CARDIOMYOPATHY: OBSERVATIONS ON POSITRON EMISSION TOMOGRAPHY

As indicated in Table 68–1, there are a considerable variety of etiologic processes that may lead to the development of a cardiomyopathy. The vast majority result in a dilated cardiomyopathy, including virtually all of those due to infectious processes, toxic agents, pregnancy and obesity, and metabolic and hematologic diseases. In most cases, there is a toxic or inflammatory process that destroys some myocytes, inducing scarring and the deposition of interstitial collagen. These processes increase the hemodynamic and metabolic burdens on the remaining viable myocytes while potentially impairing substrate delivery, particularly to the subendocardium, through fibrosis and increased left ventricular diastolic pressure with increased subendocardial wall stress. In most cases, no unique metabolic mechanism has been defined. In some dilated cardiomyopathies, the metabolic basis has been studied extensively (e.g., alcoholic cardiomyopathy[B5] and hereditary carnitine deficiency[T1, B2]) and specific derangements of intermediary metabolism defined, raising the hope that unique noninvasively detectable metabolic signatures may be defined for some types of dilated cardiomyopathy.

The dilated cardiomyopathies are the most prevalent form of cardiomyopathy and, accordingly, were the first to be studied with positron emission tomography (PET).[G3] Initial studies employed ^{11}C-palmitate imaged in the static mode employing a multi-slice PET device to define the spatial distribution of myocardial accumulation of fatty acids. Tomographic results in 17 patients with cardiomyopathies of different etiologies (three due to ethanol ingestion, two resulting from pregnancy and childbirth, two familial, one viral, and nine idiopathic) were compared with those of 13 normal subjects and 6 subjects with remote myocardial infarction. As expected, the tomographic images of patients with dilated cardiomyopathy demonstrated significant cardiac enlargement. Marked heterogeneity of the distribution of ^{11}C-palmitate was also observed throughout the hearts of patients with dilated cardiomyopathies (Fig. 68–2). Areas of avid accumulation of tracer were interspersed nearly randomly with zones of depressed accumulation. There was no consistent pattern to suggest a predilection for increased or decreased accumulation of ^{11}C-palmitate in any myocardial zone. Even when patients were grouped by etiologic diagnosis, no consistent patterns were detectable. Although the appearance was generally "moth-eaten," there were some small focal areas of moderately-to-markedly depressed accumulation of ^{11}C-palmitate.[G3]

Figure 68–2. See Color Plate 18.

The patterns observed in patients with dilated cardiomyopathy were distinctly different from those of normal subjects and patients with remote myocardial infarction. In normal subjects, accumulation of ^{11}C-palmitate was homogeneous with smooth transitions between zones of highest apparent activity and zones with lower activity. The slight variability observed in normal subjects was probably due to partial volume effects and spatial averaging in the ungated studies. Patients with remote myocardial infarction were found to have discrete zones of decreased accumulation of ^{11}C-palmitate, with homogeneous intense accumulation in remote normal zones. When analyzed quantitatively, patients with dilated cardiomyopathy demonstrated a significantly greater number of discrete zones of accumulation of ^{11}C-palmitate than either normal subjects or patients with myocardial infarction. The distribution of tracer was also altered in patients with dilated cardiomyopathy with a flatter frequency distribution curve, a lower mean myocardial radioactivity, and a higher proportion of the myocardium demonstrating low levels of accumulation of ^{11}C-palmitate when compared with normal subjects (Fig. 68–3).[G3] Alterations in regional accumulation of ^{11}C-palmitate could have been caused by regional decreases in uptake due to decreased delivery because of microvascular disease or fibrosis, decreased extraction induced by a primary metabolic derangement, a decreased amount of myocardium in zones replaced by fibrosis, or rapid clearance of ^{11}C-palmitate due to back diffusion of unaltered ^{11}C-palmitate or rapid metabolic clearance due to β-oxidation. Alternatively, local zones with avid accumulation of ^{11}C-palmitate could have decreased clearance due to diminished β-oxidation or increased storage of the tracer as triglycerides or phospholipids.

Although the left ventricular walls of patients with cardiomyopathy tend to be thinner and to demonstrate less systolic thickening than those of normal subjects, there was no correlation between the regional wall motion abnormalities and wall thickening and zones of regionally depressed accumulation of ^{11}C-palmitate. This suggests that regional tomographic abnormalities were not attributable primarily to partial volume effects.[G3]

There was also no clear association between myocardial metabolic abnormalities detected with tomography and abnormalities of myocardial perfusion detected with planar thallium-201 (^{201}Tl) scintigraphy. Among these patients, accumulation of ^{201}Tl in the myocardium was generally homogeneous except for mild apical thinning in two patients and focal defects in two additional patients, which correlated with tomographic metabolic abnormalities in only a single patient with idiopathic dilated cardiomyopathy.[G3]

Subsequent studies of patients with idiopathic dilated cardiomyopathy have employed dynamic analysis of the kinetics of ^{11}C-palmitate studied in the fasting and fed states.[S5, S6] In the fasting state, patients with cardiomyopathy incorporated a smaller percentage of administered ^{11}C-palmitate into the early rapidly turning over pool (presumably that pool undergoing β-oxidation) than did normal subjects, but did not demonstrate any alteration in the mean half-time of clearance of that early phase.[S5] In normal subjects, administration of glucose decreased the fraction of radioactivity entering the early rapidly turning over pool and decreased the rate of clearance of radioactivity from this pool. In patients with cardiomyopathy, the response was variable. Slightly more than half of the patients demonstrated a normal metabolic response to glucose administration. In contrast, more than 40 percent of patients with dilated cardiomyopathy demonstrated an aberrant pattern. In these patients, administration of glucose induced an increase in the fraction of radioactivity entering the early pool and markedly increased the rate of clearance from that pool (Fig. 68–4).[S5]

The spatial heterogeneity previously demonstrated with static studies was confirmed with dynamic studies as well.[S6] Patients with cardiomyopathy (predominantly dilated cardiomyopathy), when studied with ^{11}C-palmitate after the administration of glucose, demonstrated significantly greater regional variability in the clearance of ^{11}C-palmitate from myocardium than did normal subjects (Fig. 68–5). Similarly, there was a greater variability in the percentage of ^{11}C-palmitate taken up into the rapidly turning over pool by patients with dilated cardiomyopathy than by normal subjects.[S6] There was no clear association between the rates of clearance of ^{11}C-palmitate and the etiology of the cardiomyopathy, the changes in plasma substrate levels after the administration of glucose, or heart rate and blood pressure. There was a trend toward lower ejection fraction in patients who demonstrated an abnormal metabolic response to the administration of glucose.[S5] The metabolic basis for the abnormalities observed has not yet been defined, but it has been hypothesized that the pattern observed may be due to inhibition of citric acid cycle activity in the fasting state by augmented ketone body utilization (previously observed in some patients with congestive heart failure) that could be ameliorated by replenishment of Krebs cycle intermediates after glucose administration.[S5]

DIFFERENTIATION OF ISCHEMIC FROM NONISCHEMIC DILATED CARDIOMYOPATHY

It is often difficult or impossible to determine with a high degree of certainty whether a patient with congestive heart failure and an enlarged heart develops this syndrome because of exten-

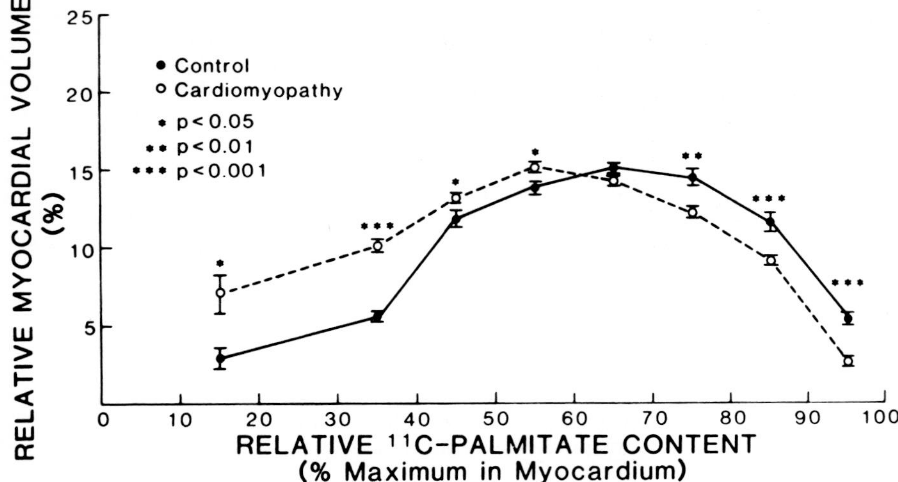

Figure 68–3. Frequency distribution of myocardial content of ^{11}C-palmitate calculated for a normal subject *(solid line)* and patients with cardiomyopathy *(broken line)*. Relative myocardial volume is plotted on the ordinate; myocardial content of ^{11}C-palmitate expressed as a percentage of maximal myocardial content of ^{11}C-palmitate is plotted on the abscissa. Data from the first 3 deciles were pooled and plotted at 15%. Data were calculated for each of the remaining 7 deciles and plotted at the midpoint of the decile. Brackets indicate standard error of the mean. (From Geltman, E. M., Smith, J. L., Beecher, D., et al.: Altered regional myocardial metabolism in congestive cardiomyopathy detected by positron tomography. Am. J. Med. 74:773–785, 1983, with permission.)

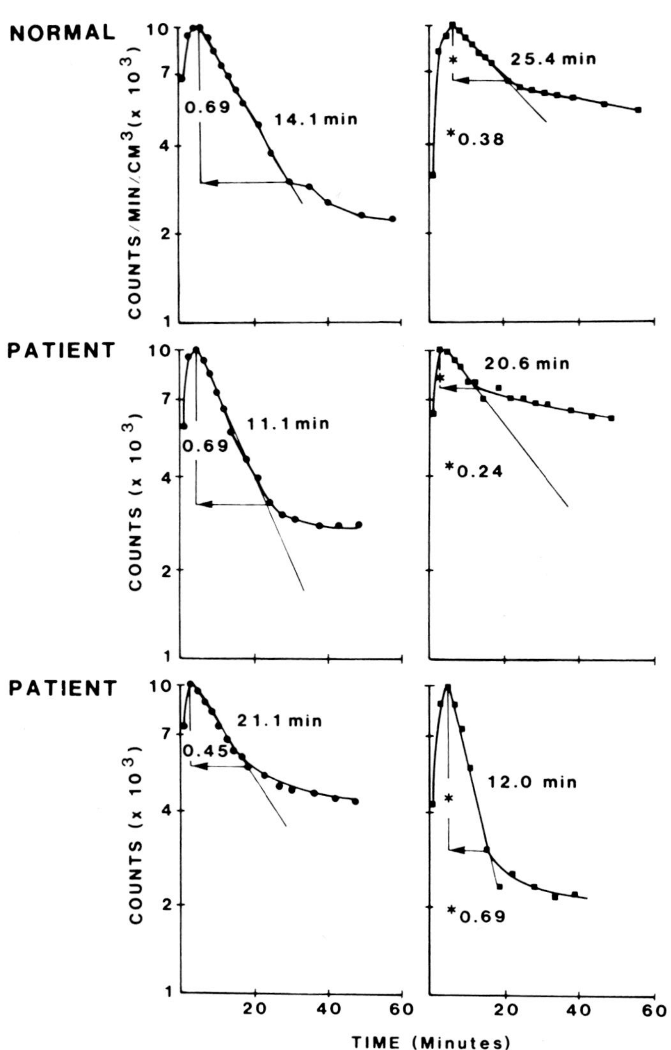

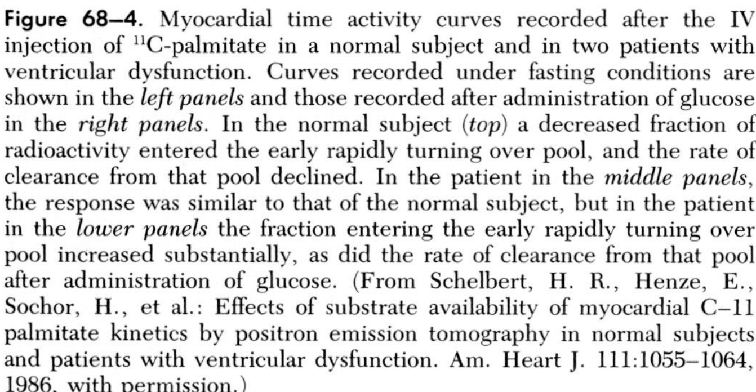

Figure 68–4. Myocardial time activity curves recorded after the IV injection of ^{11}C-palmitate in a normal subject and in two patients with ventricular dysfunction. Curves recorded under fasting conditions are shown in the *left panels* and those recorded after administration of glucose in the *right panels*. In the normal subject (*top*) a decreased fraction of radioactivity entered the early rapidly turning over pool, and the rate of clearance from that pool declined. In the patient in the *middle panels*, the response was similar to that of the normal subject, but in the patient in the *lower panels* the fraction entering the early rapidly turning over pool increased substantially, as did the rate of clearance from that pool after administration of glucose. (From Schelbert, H. R., Henze, E., Sochor, H., et al.: Effects of substrate availability of myocardial C-11 palmitate kinetics by positron emission tomography in normal subjects and patients with ventricular dysfunction. Am. Heart J. 111:1055–1064, 1986, with permission.)

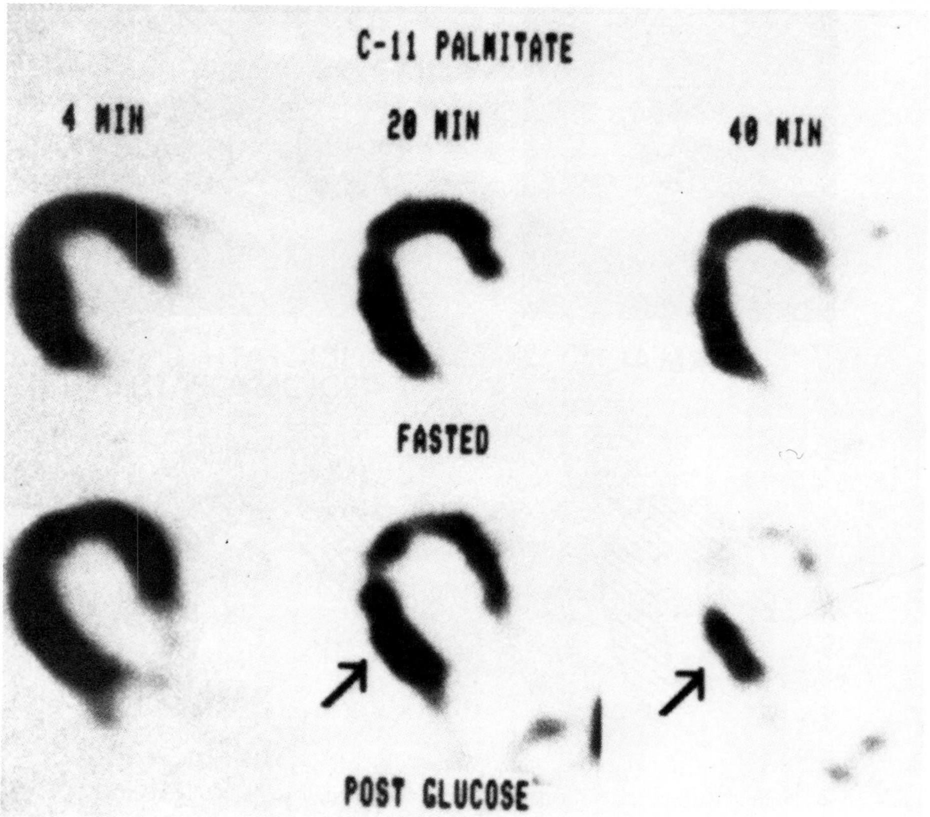

Figure 68–5. Serial tomographic images acquired after the IV administration of ^{11}C-palmitate in the fasting state (*top*) and after administration of glucose (*bottom*). In these images the top of each image represents the anterior, and the right of each image represents the patient's right. Evident in these images is substantial heterogeneity of accumulation of tracer, which is exaggerated after glucose administration. The clearance of radioactivity is rapid from the anterior and septal walls and markedly delayed in the posterolateral wall. (From Sochor, H., Schelbert, H. R., Schwaiger, M., et al.: Studies of fatty acid metabolism with positron emission tomography in patients with cardiomyopathy. Eur. J. Nucl. Med. 12(Suppl):S66–S69, 1986, with permission.)

sive coronary artery disease or a nonischemic dilated cardiomyopathy. When there is objective documentation of prior myocardial infarction, the diagnosis is made easily. However, in many other circumstances the distinction is difficult. Unfortunately, the electrocardiogram is insufficiently sensitive or specific to permit clear differentiation in many instances, since patients with myocardial infarction may not exhibit Q waves and since many patients with congestive cardiomyopathy may demonstrate on the electrocardiogram abnormalities suggestive of prior infarction. In many other instances, conduction abnormalities, such as left bundle branch block, preclude an electrocardiographic differentiation[E1, B7, B6, S7] Similarly, chest pain suggestive of ischemia may be encountered in several conditions in which the epicardial coronary arteries are normal. This syndrome has been observed in patients whose hearts are otherwise normal but whose microvasculature is abnormal, in patients with aortic insufficiency or stenosis, and in patients with nonischemic dilated cardiomyopathy.[P2, O3, C3] Patients presenting with idiopathic dilated cardiomyopathy and chest pain have been found to have normal coronary blood flow at rest but limited coronary flow reserve after dipyridamole infusion. In a group of 16 patients with idiopathic dilated cardiomyopathy, resting coronary flow assessed after the inhalation of argon gas averaged 78 ± 17 ml/100 gm/min at rest and increased to only 142 ± 38 with vasodilation. In contrast, coronary flow in normal subjects increased from 78 ± 9 to 301 ± 64 after dipyridamole infusion. Minimal coronary resistance (calculated after dipyridamole administration) correlated significantly with left ventricular end diastolic pressure and inversely with left ventricular ejection fraction.[O3]

Assessment of regional coronary perfusion with ^{201}Tl scintigraphy has demonstrated extensive zones of depressed uptake of thallium in patients with ischemic cardiomyopathy but only minimal apical thinning in patients with nonischemic cardiomyopathy, allowing some differentiation between patient groups.[B7] However, to detect an ischemic cardiomyopathy with this technique, a defect encompassing 40 percent of the circumference of the left ventricle was required, providing a relatively specific diagnostic technique but one with only modest sensitivity. Analysis of regional wall motion assessed echocardiographically or with radionuclide ventriculography has also been employed to attempt to differentiate patients with ischemic dilated cardiomyopathy from those with nonischemic dilated cardiomyopathy. Unfortunately, global hypokinesis is common in patients with ischemic cardiomyopathy, and some regional variability in the severity of wall motion abnormalities is commonly encountered in patients with nonischemic dilated cardiomyopathy, making accurate differentiation between these two entities difficult using traditional techniques.[E1, B6]

Positron Emission Tomographic Imaging

PET performed after IV administration of ^{11}C-palmitate has been used to differentiate patients with ischemic cardiomyopathy from those with nonischemic cardiomyopathy.[E1] PET revealed dramatic differences in the appearance of images acquired from patients with ischemic and nonischemic dilated cardiomyopathy. In a recent study, large defects encompassing more than 15 percent of the cross-sectional area of the left ventricle in transverse reconstructions were observed in 80 percent of patients with ischemic dilated cardiomyopathy but not in normal subjects or patients with nonischemic dilated cardiomyopathy. In general, patients with ischemic dilated cardiomyopathy had large zones of homogeneously depressed accumulation of ^{11}C-palmitate that contrasted sharply with the diffuse heterogeneity of accumulation of tracer observed in patients with idiopathic dilated cardiomyopathy (Fig. 68–6). This heterogeneity was exhibited as a greater number of discrete regions of radioactivity observed in patients with nonischemic cardiomyopathy compared with those with ischemic cardiomyopathy. Similarly, the frequency distribution of radioactivity per pixel was shifted toward lower values for patients with nonischemic dilated cardiomyopathy compared with those with ischemic disease. Among patients with ischemic dilated cardiomyopathy, those with diabetes mellitus demonstrated somewhat more tomographic heterogeneity than those without diabetes, which is in keeping with the more diffuse and

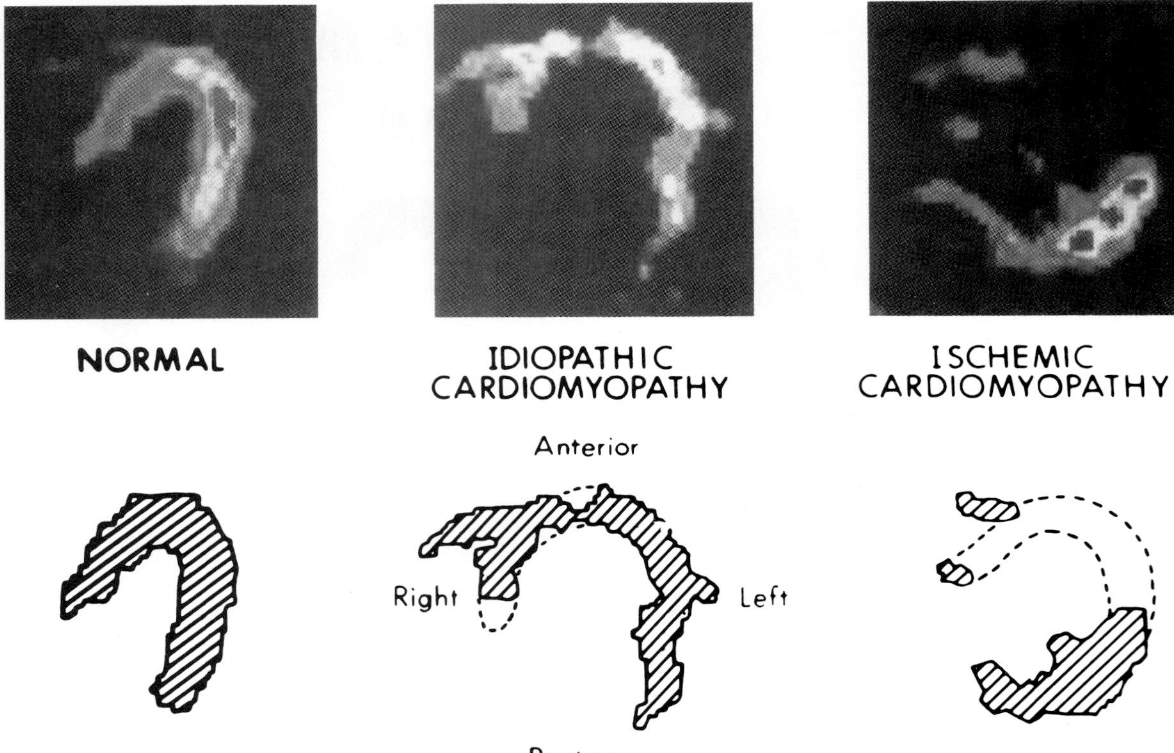

Figure 68–6. Representative midventricular tomograms acquired after the IV administration of ^{11}C-palmitate in a normal subject, in a patient with dilated cardiomyopathy, and in one with ischemic dilated cardiomyopathy. The orientation is the same as in Figure 68–2. Schematic representations are below each image with the expected myocardial borders indicated by the interrupted lines. In patients with ischemic cardiomyopathy, large zones of homogeneously depressed accumulation of ^{11}C-palmitate are noted. In contrast, in patients with dilated nonischemic cardiomyopathy, marked spatial heterogeneity is observed without large discrete zones of decreased accumulation of tracer. (From Eisenberg, J. D., Sobel, B. E., Geltman, E. M.: Differentiation of ischemic from nonischemic cardiomyopathy with positron emission tomography. Am. J. Cardiol. 59:1310–1414, 1987, with permission.)

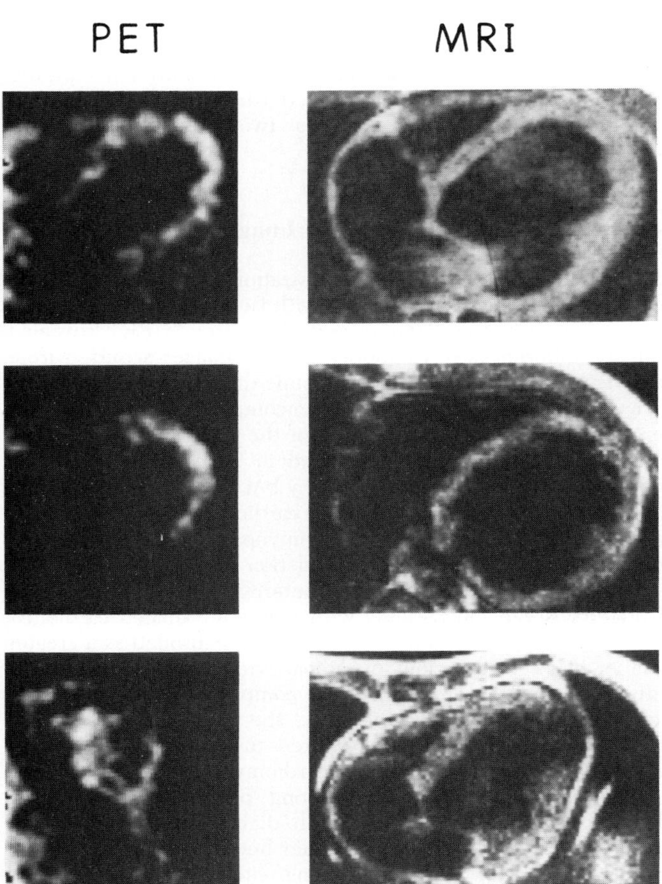

Figure 68–7. Transverse midventricular tomographic reconstructions acquired with positron emission tomography after the IV administration of ^{11}C-palmitate in the *left panels*, and in the same patients with proton magnetic resonance imaging employing spin-echo technique in the *right panels*. The diagnoses were sarcoidosis (*top*), idiopathic cardiomyopathy (*middle*), and ischemic cardiomyopathy (*bottom*). The two patients with nonischemic cardiomyopathy had diffuse spatial heterogeneity of metabolism reflected in the PET images. The patient with ischemic cardiomyopathy had a dense defect involving the anterior walls with an apparent transmural defect and an apparent nontransmural defect affecting the lateral wall. With MRI, the myocardial signal was essentially homogeneous for the patient in the *top panel;* there was fine speckling seen in the *middle panel*, but no regional wall thinning or apparent scarring to explain the PET imaging characteristics. Conversely, this metabolic heterogeneity observed on PET was not seen with MRI. The patient with ischemic cardiomyopathy demonstrated mild apical and anterolateral thinning indicated by the arrow, but the abnormality on MRI was subtle compared with the metabolic abnormality demonstrated by PET. (For further information, see Geltman, E. M., Eisenberg, J. D., Keim, S., et al.: Comparative magnetic resonance imaging and positron emission tomography in cardiomyopathy (abstr.). J. Am. Cardiol. 5:436, 1985, with permission.)

severe nature of the coronary disease typically encountered in patients with diabetes mellitus. Despite this increased heterogeneity, the tomographic patterns remained distinctly different from those of patients with nonischemic dilated cardiomyopathy.[E1]

Comparison with Other Imaging Techniques

Many imaging techniques have been employed for the evaluation of patients with dilated cardiomyopathy. In addition to echocardiography and ^{201}Tl scintigraphy (vida-supra), proton magnetic resonance imaging (MRI) and single-photon scintigraphy with iodinated fatty acids have been employed for the evaluation of patients with dilated cardiomyopathy.

Patients with dilated cardiomyopathy have been evaluated with proton MRI employing spin echo techniques for comparison with positron emission tomography performed after the IV administration of ^{11}C-palmitate.[G4] Although cardiac structure was well delineated with high spatial resolution with MRI, the metabolic heterogeneity observed with PET was not exhibited in MRI studies (Fig. 68–7). Ventricular dilatation, wall thinning, and other architectural details were observed with great clarity. However, within signals emanating from myocardial regions of interest, there were no significant differences between normal subjects and patients with dilated cardiomyopathy in signal intensity on ECG-gated spin-echo images (TE = 30 msec, or TE = 60 msec), in calculated T_2, or in the frequency distribution of signal intensity.[G4] Although some regional myocardial thinning could be observed with MRI in patients with ischemic dilated cardiomyopathy in zones of presumed infarction, the findings were often subtle and the technique did not differentiate between patients with ischemic cardiomyopathy and those with nonischemic cardiomyopathy as clearly as PET with ^{11}C-palmitate.

A number of fatty acid analogs have been synthesized and labeled with iodine-123 (^{123}I) for myocardial metabolic imaging (see Chapter 60). Several have been studied with either planar imaging or single-photon emission computed tomography in patients with dilated cardiomyopathy.[H5, U1, F2] In general, the spatial heterogeneity of accumulation observed with ^{11}C-palmitate in patients with dilated cardiomyopathy has been confirmed with the iodinated compounds. However, as observed with ^{11}C-palmitate, the spatial and kinetic abnormalities of fatty acid metabolism observed appeared relatively similar for patients with dilated cardiomyopathy of differing etiologies.[H5, U1] Although the patterns of clearance of the single-photon emitting tracers were distinctly different from those observed with normal subjects, the pattern of altered kinetics (prolongation or acceleration) observed in patients with cardiomyopathy depended on the specific compound tested.[H5, U1]

HYPERTROPHIC CARDIOMYOPATHY

Background

The hypertrophic cardiomyopathies comprise several syndromes exhibiting different pathologic findings, clinical presentations, and natural histories.[S8] All demonstrate significant left ventricular hypertrophy that may be generalized throughout the heart or predominate in the interventricular septum (particularly in the upper portion) or left ventricular apex (apical cardiomyopathy). Most are detected clinically because of abnormalities of diastolic function, characterized by pulmonary venous congestion with dyspnea. Despite signs and symptoms suggestive of left ventricular (LV) decompensation, systolic performance is generally well preserved or hyperdynamic.[S8] Paradoxically, limitation of forward output can occur if ventricular performance is supernormal, hypertrophy is severe, and geometry is altered sufficiently to induce LV outflow tract obstruction.

Hypertrophic cardiomyopathy may occur in either hereditary or sporadic patterns. There are numerous kindreds in which the disorder appears to be inherited as an autosomal dominant trait with variable penetrance. Up to one-third of cases of hypertrophic cardiomyopathy occur in a familial pattern with equal incidence in males and females,[M2] but many cases occur in a sporadic fashion. Because of the variability in patterns of inheritance, it has been postulated that the hereditary factor is the susceptibility to the development of hypertrophic cardiomyopathy, which could become manifest if an additional stimulus, such as hypertension or hyperthyroidism, is present.[S9]

It has also been postulated that hypertrophic cardiomyopathy may result from excessive responsiveness to sympathetic stimulation.[P6] Others have proposed that hyperthyroidism or increased responsiveness to thyroid hormone could induce or contribute to inappropriate cardiac hypertrophy.[S9] This concept is supported by the observation in experimental animals of the development of hypertrophic cardiomyopathy in the offspring of mothers made hyperthyroid during pregnancy.[O4] In many instances, hypertrophic cardiomyopathy only appears at an advanced age (about one-third of patients are over 60 years of age at presentation) and may represent an excessive hypertrophic response to hypertension.[M6, W1] Hypertrophic cardiomyopathy has also been described in patients with Friedreich's ataxia, although this group comprises a very small fraction of patients.[G5]

Myocardial Metabolism in Hypertrophic Cardiomyopathy

Coronary blood flow of patients with hypertrophic cardiomyopathy assessed with arterial-coronary sinus sampling techniques was normal or increased at rest, but was reduced when corrected for left ventricular mass.[P2] Myocardial oxygen consumption was normal or increased at rest and responded variably to pacing stress. Those with the highest myocardial oxygen consumption appeared to have the most extensive hypertrophy and demonstrated markedly reduced lactate extraction or lactate production with pacing, along with pacing-induced reductions in coronary blood flow or limited coronary flow reserve.[P2] When analysis was localized to the anterior circulation by selective catheterization of the great cardiac vein, a similar pattern was found, with increased total regional flow at rest but reduced coronary flow reserve with pacing.[C1, T2] Lactate balance was normal at rest, but lactate consumption decreased or converted to lactate production with pacing. Paradoxically, the arterial-coronary sinus oxygen difference narrowed rather than increased with pacing. Myocardial extraction of pyruvate appeared to parallel that of lactate, with decreased extraction of pyruvate demonstrated in patients who exhibited decreased extraction or production of lactate during cardiac pacing.[C1] Extraction of other substrates (beta hydroxybuterate, acetoacetate, free fatty acids, and glycerol) appeared normal at rest and with atrial pacing, and did not differ between patients with hypertrophic cardiomyopathies who did or did not develop ischemia during atrial pacing.[T2]

Initial invasive assessments of arterial-coronary sinus plasma levels of catecholamines in small numbers of patients have demonstrated only minor alterations.[H3] Recent studies have demonstrated substantial excesses of norepinephrine in great cardiac vein blood (compared with arterial blood).[B8] This appears to be due to diminished neuronal uptake of norepinephrine rather than excess release from sympathetic nerve endings. The percentage extraction of norepinephrine by patients with hypertrophic cardiomyopathy was unrelated to the severity of left ventricular obstruction, mean arterial pressure, coronary blood flow, or pulmonary artery occlusive pressure. In contrast, there were significant correlations between peak systolic left ventricular pressure and the arterial-coronary sinus differences in norepinephrine, arterial-coronary sinus production rate, and cardiac spillover rate of norepinephrine.[B8] These findings would suggest that the myocardium of patients with hypertrophic cardiomyopathy is exposed to more norepinephrine than normal subjects and that altered norepinephrine kinetics might play a role in the pathogenesis of hypertrophic cardiomyopathy.

Findings on Positron Emission Tomography

When patients with hypertrophic cardiomyopathy were studied at rest after a brief fast with PET and F-18-fluorodeoxyglucose

(^{18}FDG), ^{11}C-palmitate, and nitrogen-13–labeled ammonia ($^{13}NH_3$), a unique metabolic pattern was observed.[G6] Static images of relative perfusion ($^{13}NH_3$) demonstrated apparently homogeneous flow. When data were corrected for partial volume effects, regional perfusion in the septum was found to be mildly decreased. These data are concordant with invasive measurements of flow reported by others. Initial accumulation of ^{11}C-palmitate appeared homogeneous but was also mildly reduced in the septum when corrected for partial volume effects. However, the fraction extracted into the early rapidly turning over pool was similar in the septum and lateral walls, as was the half-time of clearance of ^{11}C-palmitate from both regions.[G6] The similarity of the extraction fraction and the clearance half-time of the early rapid phase suggests that regional ischemia at rest was not the cause of any decreased extraction of ^{11}C-palmitate. The decreased extraction in the septum relative to the lateral wall may merely reflect decreased delivery of tracer, since the diminished accumulation of ^{11}C-palmitate paralleled the reduction in accumulation of $^{13}NH_3$.

In contrast to the minor alterations in distribution of $^{13}NH_3$ and ^{11}C-palmitate, abnormalities of distribution of ^{18}FDG were marked.[G6] Adequate ^{18}FDG studies could not be obtained in the fasting state in all patients with hypertrophic cardiomyopathy due to high levels of circulating free fatty acids and suppressed uptake of glucose. However, in patients for whom data could be analyzed, accumulation of ^{18}FDG in the interventricular septum was suppressed with septum-to-lateral wall ratios of 0.83 ± 0.21 compared with 0.92 ± 0.07 in normal subjects (studied in the fed state). When data were corrected for partial volume effects, the differences were magnified. The septum-to-lateral wall ratio for ^{18}FDG after correction for partial volume effects was 0.55 ± 0.14. In some cases, the disparity between septum and lateral wall was dramatic (Fig. 68–8). The decreased ^{18}FDG accumulation in the septum was out of proportion to abnormalities in regional perfusion, as assessed with $^{13}NH_3$.[G6]

The explanation for the reduced ^{18}FDG accumulation in the septum is not clear. It appears unlikely that it is due to ischemia, since ^{11}C-palmitate kinetics were not altered substantially and perfusion was only mildly depressed. Septal ischemia would not be expected based on other studies of myocardial metabolism employing invasive techniques. Abnormal lactate extraction and production generally have not been observed at rest but only with atrial pacing, even when observations have been limited to the anterior circulation by catheterization of the great cardiac vein.

Altered catecholamine metabolism has been implicated as a possible mechanism for the observed metabolic inhomogeneity.[G6] In experimental animals, catecholamine infusion depressed myocardial uptake of ^{18}FDG in the absence of insulin, a process that was reversed by insulin administration.[M1] In the fasting state, insulin levels are low, and in patients with hypertrophic cardiomyopathy, norepinephrine kinetics are distinctly abnormal with increased exposure of myocardium to catecholamines. Although catecholamine kinetics have been studied in the great cardiac vein in patients with hypertrophic cardiomyopathy, no data are available to indicate that there are regional disparities in catecholamine kinetics between the septum or posterolateral walls in patients with hypertrophic cardiomyopathy.

The observed reduced accumulation of ^{18}FDG in the hypertrophic septum could also be an indication of decreased mechanical work and decreased oxygen requirements of the septum in patients with hypertrophic cardiomyopathy. Although the septum is thicker than the remaining cardiac walls, its thickening, a reflection of contractile function, is often substantially reduced in patients with hypertrophic cardiomyopathy, although septal thickening assessed echocardiographically was normal in many patients with hypertrophic cardiomyopathy studied with PET.[G6] Regional cardiac work in the septum might be decreased with a concomitant reduced myocardial oxygen demand in this region. Since the myocardium can use several substrates simultaneously,[M3] and since during fasting there was a relative abundance of free fatty acids, septal substrate requirements might have been met by fatty acids alone without the need for glucose utilization.

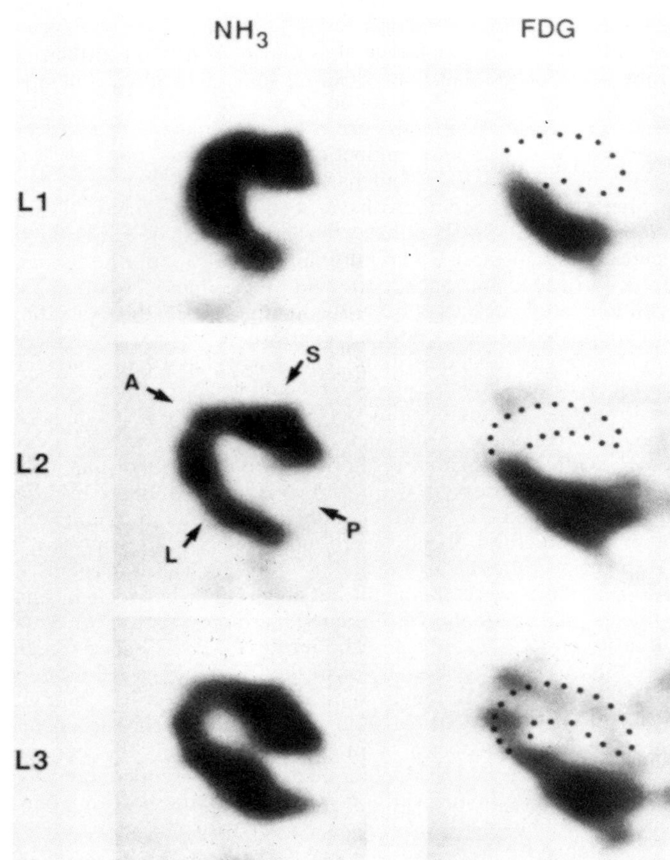

Figure 68–8. Transverse tomographic reconstructions acquired after the IV administration of ^{13}N ammonia ($^{13}NH_3$) (*left*) and ^{18}F-2-deoxyglucose (^{18}FDG) (*right*), acquired in the fasting state in a patient with hypertrophic cardiomyopathy. Three levels of the heart are shown; L-1 is the most basal and L-3 the most apical. The orientation is as in Figure 68–5. The distribution of $^{13}NH_3$ is relatively homogeneous, but there is markedly depressed accumulation of ^{18}FDG in the interventricular septum. The location of the septum is indicated by the dotted lines. (From Grover-McKay, M., Schwaiger, M., Krivokapich, J., et al.: Regional myocardial blood flow and metabolism at rest in mildly symptomatic patients with hypertrophic cardiomyopathy. J. Am. Coll. Cardiol. 13:317–324, 1989. Reprinted with permission from the American College of Cardiology.)

CARDIOMYOPATHIES ASSOCIATED WITH SYSTEMIC ILLNESSES

As indicated in Table 68–1, the diversity of causes of cardiomyopathy is great. Although the molecular basis of the underlying illness is understood for some (e.g., nutritional deficiency, endocrine disorders, glycogen storage diseases) and in others metabolic studies have been extensive (e.g., alcoholic heart disease, diabetes), few have been studied with PET. Duchenne muscular dystrophy is a prototype of a systemic metabolic disease that has been studied with PET.[P7]

Duchenne muscular dystrophy is an X-linked recessive disorder that affects approximately 3 of every 100,000 people within the United States.[B9] Up to one-third of cases occur in a nonfamilial pattern and are believed to arise from a spontaneous mutation.[B9] The disease usually becomes clinically apparent during the second year of life with a gait disturbance. Musculoskeletal abnormalities are progressive, with death occurring often due to pulmonary insufficiency in the second decade due to involvement of the diaphragm and the thoracic musculature. Cardiac involvement may be discovered relatively early owing to the detection of electrocardiographic abnormalities suggesting loss of electrically active tissue in the posterobasal region of the left ventricle.[S10] These abnormalities correlate closely with findings at postmortem in which fibrosis is found to be most extensive in the same location. Cardiac arrhythmias are prominent, including a variety of atrial arrhythmias and conduction disturbances. The illness is unique in several aspects but particularly in its predilection for involvement of a specific cardiac anatomic locus. Although many biochemical abnormalities have been defined, a specific pathogenetic mechanism has been elusive.[P8]

Positron Emission Tomographic Imaging

PET study of patients with Duchenne muscular dystrophy was performed in the fasting state after the IV administration of $^{13}NH_3$ for the assessment of perfusion and ^{18}FDG for the evaluation of regional uptake of glucose. Regional wall motion was assessed with gated blood pool imaging, and perfusion was assessed with planar ^{201}Tl scintigraphy. Abnormal regional wall motion was detected in only 20 percent of patients in the posterobasal, lateral, and/or inferolateral walls. Defects in the posterobasal or lateral walls, which were indicated by reduced accumulation of thallium, were detected in 27 percent of patients. Abnormalities were observed significantly more frequently with PET. Abnormalities of distribution of tracers were observed in 87 percent of patients with $^{13}NH_3$ and in 92 percent of patients who had a measurable accumulation of ^{18}FDG in the heart. Accumulation of $^{13}NH_3$ was decreased and accumulation of ^{18}FDG was increased in the posterobasal and lateral walls of the left ventricle, the zones of the left ventricle known to be most affected in this illness (Fig. 68–9). In patients with wall motion abnormalities and abnormalities seen on thallium scintigraphy, there was concordance between all techniques.[P7] Necropsy of a patient studied two years antemortem with PET demonstrated substantial fibrosis of the posterobasal and lateral walls of the left ventricle, with normal myocardium interspersed with areas of severe fibrosis. In addition, there were foci of fibrosis in remote, relatively normal portions of the left ventricle.[P7]

The biochemical explanation for the tomographic abnormalities remains speculative. The observed pattern of decreased accumulation of $^{13}NH_3$ and increased accumulation of ^{18}FDG in the posterobasal wall is typical of that observed in ischemic myocardium. However, there is no other evidence of ischemia in Duchenne muscular dystrophy. Specifically, coronary anatomy is normal in patients who are evaluated postmortem and there are generally no ECG abnormalities or symptoms to suggest ischemia. The decreased accumulation of $^{13}NH_3$ could be due to focal fibrosis, which decreases the number of myocytes capable of accumulating $^{13}NH_3$. Alternatively, the fibrosis could impair myocardial perfusion and diffusion, contributing to the reduced accumulation of this tracer. There could be islands of effectively ischemic cells (despite normal epicardial coronary arteries) due to the focal fibrosis interfering with local substrate delivery, leading to an increased accumulation of ^{18}FDG in residual viable myocardium. Alternatively, phosphorylation could be augmented because of abnormal adenylate cyclase or as a compensatory mechanism due to a primary defect in free fatty acid oxidation.[P7] Last, there could be a primary abnormality of membrane permeability, permitting increased diffusion of ^{18}FDG into myocytes.

Although there are a substantial number of additional systemic illnesses associated with dilated or hypertrophic cardiomyopathy, none have been studied with PET in a systematic fashion. In published studies, there are small groups with postpartum (n = 3) and alcoholic cardiomyopathy (n = 4), but in both conditions, the tomographic data acquired in the static mode after the administration of ^{11}C-palmitate were indistinguishable from the findings of other patients with dilated cardiomyopathy.[E1] A single patient with sarcoidosis and dilated cardiomyopathy has been included in a previously published series.[E1] In that patient, focal zones of reduced accumulation of ^{11}C-palmitate were observed in regions that were subsequently shown to represent confluent sarcoid granulomas and fibrosis when the patient was evaluated postmortem several months after tomography.

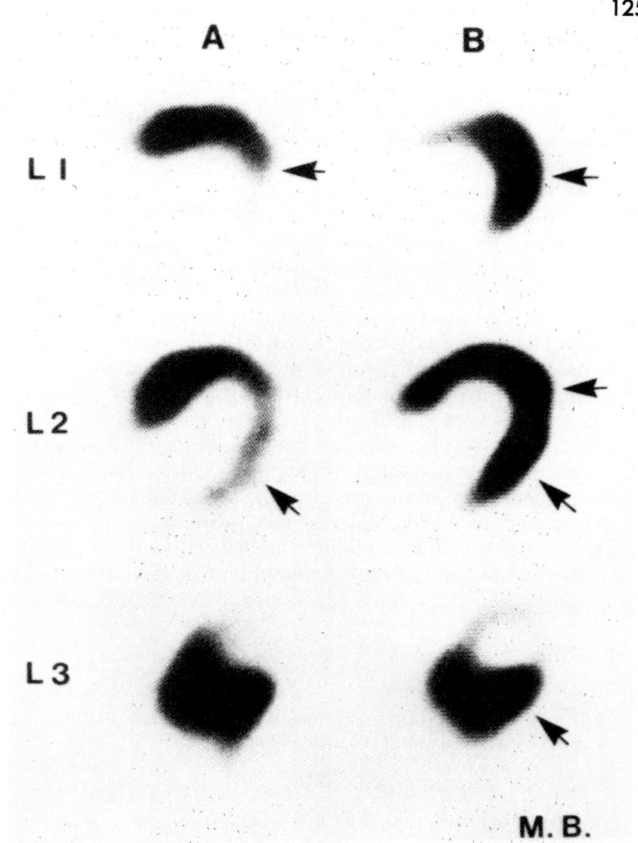

Figure 68–9. Regional accumulation of $^{13}NH_3$ (*Panel A*) and ^{18}FDG (*Panel B*) in three contiguous PET transverse reconstructions of the heart of a patient with Duchenne muscular dystrophy. The images at the top are most basal and the ones at the bottom most apical. There is regionally decreased accumulation of $^{13}NH_3$ in the posterolateral region in levels 1 and 2, with relative excess accumulation of ^{18}FDG in these same zones. This patient had a moderate posterolateral ^{201}Tl defect, posterolateral akinesis, and a left ventricular ejection fraction of 46%. (From Perloff, J. K., Henze, E., and Schelbert, H. R.: Alterations in regional myocardial metabolism, perfusion, and wall motion in Duchenne muscular dystrophy studied by radionuclide imaging. Circulation 69:33–42, 1984, by permission of the American Heart Association, Inc.)

FUTURE DIRECTIONS

Studies of patients with dilated or hypertrophic cardiomyopathy have provided a greater understanding of some of the abnormalities of myocardial perfusion and metabolism associated with these diverse illnesses, and have provided techniques for the differentiation of patients with ischemic and nonischemic dilated cardiomyopathy. Recently, several new radiopharmaceuticals have been developed that should add substantially to our diagnostic armamentarium. ^{11}C-acetate is such a compound (see Chapter 60). ^{11}C-acetate is avidly extracted by myocardium and subsequently enters the citric acid cycle. In studies in experimental animals, the clearance of radioactivity from the heart after administration of ^{11}C-acetate correlated closely with $^{11}CO_2$ production and myocardial oxygen consumption over a wide range of cardiac workloads.[B4, B11] The correlation between ^{11}C-acetate kinetics and myocardial oxygen consumption was not affected by circulating levels of free fatty acids or glucose.[B10, B11] In normal subjects, clearance of ^{11}C-acetate was homogeneous throughout the left ventricle and was augmented homogeneously by increased cardiac work induced by administration of catecholamines or dynamic exercise.[H4] There was a close correlation between accelerated clearance of ^{11}C-acetate and increased double-product, an indicator of myocardial oxygen consumption.[H4] The availability of this marker of oxidative metabolism should allow a more complete understanding of the metabolism of patients with cardiomyopathy in whom complex abnormalities of intermediary metabolism are expected. Thus, in a single patient, carbohydrate, fatty acid, and citric acid cycle flux can all be evaluated under similar conditions. As amino acids labeled with positron emitters become available, protein turnover may be evaluated as well.[H8]

The addition of markers of sympathetic nervous system activity such as ^{18}F-fluorometaraminol[M4] and ^{11}C-m-hydroxyephedrine[H7] may prove of great importance in furthering the understanding of many of the cardiomyopathies, particularly hypertrophic cardiomyopathy if they can be produced with sufficiently high specific activity to avoid inducing pharmacologic effects with the tracers.[M4] The availability of antimyosin FAB subunits,[M5] which may ultimately be labeled with positron emitters, should help in the assessment of inflammatory cardiomyopathies in which myocyte necrosis plays a significant part. Assessments of the relative roles of hypoperfusion and ischemia in the pathogenesis and clinical presentation of dilated and hypertrophic cardiomyopathies should be facilitated by the use of newly validated techniques for the assessment of myocardial perfusion with flow markers that are independent of the metabolic activity of the tissue, such as $H_2{}^{15}O$,[B12, H6, W2] and the recent development of selective markers of hypoxic myocardium, such as ^{18}F-misonidazole.[S11]

References

A

1. Alpert, N.R., and Gordon, M.S.: Myofibrillar adenosine triphosphate activity in congestive failure. Am. J. Physiol. 202:940, 1962.

B

1. Bremer, J.: Carnitine in intermediary metabolism. The metabolism of fatty acid esters of carnitine by mitochondria. J. Biol. Chem. 237:3628–3632, 1962.
2. Bremer, J., and Hokland, B.: Role of carnitine-dependent metabolic pathways in heart disease without primary ischemia. Z. Kardiol. 76 (Suppl. 5):9–13, 1987.
3. Bing, R.J.: Metabolic activity of intact heart. Am. J. Med. 30:679–691, 1961.
4. Brown, M., Marshall, D.R., Sobel, B.E., and Bergmann, S.R.: Delineation of myocardial oxygen utilization with carbon–11-labeled acetate. Circulation 76:687–696, 1987.
5. Bing, R.J.: Cardiac metabolism: Its contribution to alcoholic heart disease and myocardial failure. Circulation 58:965, 1978.
6. Boucher, C.A., Fallon, J.T., Johnson, R.A., and Yurchak, P.M.: Cardiomyopathic syndrome caused by coronary artery disease. III. Prospective clinicopathological study of its prevalence among patients with clinically unexplained chronic heart failure. Br. Heart J. 41:613–620, 1979.
7. Bulkley, B.H., Hutchins, G.M., Bailey, I., et al.: Thallium–201 imaging and gated cardiac blood pool scans in patients with ischemic and idiopathic congestive cardiomyopathy. A clinical and pathologic study. Circulation 55:753–760, 1977.
8. Brush, J.E., Jr., Eisenhofer, G., Garty, M., et al.: Cardiac norepinephrine kinetics in hypertrophic cardiomyopathy. Circulation 79:836–844, 1989.
9. Brooke, M.H.: A Clinician's View of Neuromuscular Diseases. Williams and Wilkins, Baltimore, 1979.
10. Brown, M.A., Myears, D.W., and Bergmann, S.R.: Validity of estimates of myocardial oxidative metabolism with carbon–11-acetate and positron emission tomography despite altered patterns of substrate utilization. J. Nucl. Med. 30:187–193, 1989.
11. Buxton, D.B., Schwaiger, M., Nguyen, A., et al.: Radiolabeled acetate as a tracer of myocardial tricarboxylic acid cycle flux. Circ. Res. 63:628–634, 1988.
12. Bergmann, S.R., Herrero, P., Markham, J., et al.: Noninvasive quantitation of myocardial blood flow in human subjects with oxygen–15 labeled water and positron emission tomography. J. Am. Coll. Cardiol., 14:639–652, 1989.

C

1. Cannon, R.O., III, Rosing, D.R., Maron, B.J., et al.: Myocardial ischemia in patients with hypertrophic cardiomyopathy: Contribution of inadequate vasodilator reserve and elevated left ventricular filling pressures. Circulation 71:234–243, 1985.
2. Chidsey, C.A., Weinbach, E.C., Pool, P.E., and Morrow, A.G.: Biochemical studies of energy production in the failing human heart. J. Clin. Invest. 45:40–50, 1966.
3. Cannon, R.O. III, Leon, M.B., Watson, R.M., et al.: Chest pain and "normal" coronary arteries—role of small coronary arteries. Am. J. Cardiol. 55:50B–60B, 1985.

D

1. Draper, M., Taylor, N., and Alpert, N.R.: Alteration in contractile protein in hypertrophied guinea pig hearts. *In* Alpert, N. (ed.): Cardiac Hypertrophy. Academic Press, New York, 1971, pp. 315–331.
2. Dzau, V.J.: Implications of local angiotensin production in cardiovascular physiology and pharmacology. Am. J. Cardiol. 59:59A–65A, 1987.

E

1. Eisenberg, J.D., Sobel, B.E., and Geltman, E.M.: Differentiation of ischemic from nonischemic cardiomyopathy with positron emission tomography. Am. J. Cardiol. 59:1310–1414, 1987.

F

1. Fox, K.A.A., Abendschein, D.R., Ambos, D., et al.: Efflux of metabolized and nonmetabolized fatty acid from canine myocardium. Circ. Res. 57:232–243, 1985.
2. Feinendegen, L.E., Vyska, K., Freundlieb, C., et al.: Noninvasive analysis of metabolic reactions in body tissues, the case of myocardial fatty acids. Eur. J. Nucl. Med. 6:191–200, 1981.

G

1. Graham, T.P., Jr., Ross, J., Jr., and Covell, J.W.: Myocardial oxygen consumption in acute experimental cardiac depression. Circ. Res. 21:123–138, 1967.
2. Gordon, M.S., and Brown, A.L.: Myofibrillar adenosine triphosphate activity of human heart tissue and congestive failure: Effects of ouabain and calcium. Circ. Res. 19:534, 1966.
3. Geltman, E.M., Smith, J.L., Beecher, D., et al.: Altered regional myocardial metabolism in congestive cardiomyopathy detected by positron tomography. Am. J. Med. 74:773–785, 1983.
4. Geltman, E.M., Eisenberg, J.D., Keim, S., et al.: Comparative magnetic resonance imaging and positron emission tomography in cardiomyopathy. J. Am. Cardiol. 5:436, 1985.
5. Gach, J.V., Andriange, M., and Franck, G.: Hypertrophic obstructive cardiomyopathy and Friedreich's ataxia. Am. J. Cardiol. 27:436, 1971.
6. Grover-McKay, M., Schwaiger, M., Krivokapich, J., et al.: Regional myocardial blood flow and metabolism at rest in mildly symptomatic patients with hypertrophic cardiomyopathy. J. Am. Coll. Cardiol. 13:317–324, 1989.

H

1. Henry, P.D., Eckberg, D., Gault, H.J., and Ross, J., Jr.: Depressed inotropic state and reduced myocardial oxygen consumption in the human heart. Am. J. Cardiol. 31:300–306, 1973.
2. Hasking, G.J., Esler, M.D., Jennings, G.L., et al.: Norepinephrine spillover to plasma in patients with congestive heart failure: Evidence of increased overall and cardiorenal sympathetic nervous activity. Circulation 73:615–621, 1986.
3. Haneda, T., Miura, Y., Miyazawa, K., et al.: Plasma norepinephrine concentration in the coronary sinus in cardiomyopathies. Cathet. Cardiovasc. Diagn. 4:399–405, 1978.
4. Henes, C.G., Bergmann, S.R., Walsh, M.N., et al.: Assessment of myocardial oxidative metabolic reserve with positron emission tomography and carbon–11-acetate. J. Nucl. Med. 30:1489–1499, 1989.
5. Höck, A., Freundlieb, C., Vyska, K., et al.: Myocardial imaging and metabolic studies with [17^{123}]iodoheptadecanoic acid in patients with idiopathic congestive cardiomyopathy. J. Nucl. Med. 24:22–28, 1983.
6. Herrero, P., Markham, J., Myears, D.W., et al.: Measurement of myocardial blood flow with positron emission tomography: Correction for count spillover and partial volume effects. Mathl. Comput. Modeling 11:807–812, 1988.
7. Haka, M.S., Rosenspire, K.C., Gildersleeve, D.L., et al.: Synthesis of [C–11]-m-hydroxyephedrine (HED) for neuronal cardiac imaging. (Abstract.) J. Nucl. Med. 30:783, 1989.
8. Henze, E., Schelbert, H.R., Barrio, J.R., et al.: Evaluation of myocardial metabolism with N–13 and C–11-labeled amino acids and positron computed tomography. J. Nucl. Med. 23:671–681, 1982.

K

1. Kawai, C., Yui, Y., Hoshino, T., et al.: Myocardial catecholamines in hypertrophic and dilated (congestive) cardiomyopathy: A biopsy study. J. Am. Coll. Cardiol. 2:834–840, 1983.

L

1. Levine, T.B., Francis, G.S., Goldsmith, S.R., et al.: Activity of the sympathetic nervous system and renin-angiotensin system assessed by plasma hormone levels and their relation to hemodynamic abnormalities in congestive heart failure. Am. J. Cardiol. 49:1659, 1982.
2. Luchi, R.J., Dritcher, E.M., and Thyrum, P.T.: Reduced cardiac myosin adenosine triphosphate activity in dogs with spontaneously occurring heart failure. Circ. Res. 24:5133, 1969.

M

1. Merhige, M.E., Ekas, R., Mossberg, K., et al.: Catecholamine stimulation, substrate competition, and myocardial glucose uptake in conscious dogs assessed with positron emission tomography. Circ. Res. 61(Suppl. II):II124–II129, 1987.
2. Maron, B.J., and Mulvihill, J.J.: The genetics of hypertrophic cardiomyopathy. Ann. Intern. Med. 105:610–613, 1986.
3. Myears, D.W., Sobel, B.E., and Bergmann, S.R.: Substrate use in ischemic and reperfused canine myocardium: Quantitative considerations. Am. J. Physiol. 253:H107–H114, 1987.
4. Mislanker, S.G., Gildersleeve, D.L., Wieland, D.M., et al.: 6-

[^{18}F]Fluorometaraminol: A radiotracer for in vivo mapping of adrenergic nerves of the heart. J. Med. Chem. 31:362–366, 1988.

5. Matsumori, A., Ohkusa, T., Matoba, Y., et al.: Myocardial uptake of antimyosin monoclonal antibody in a murine model of viral myocarditis. Circulation 79:400–405, 1989.
6. McKenna, W.J., and Kleinebenne, A.: Hypertrophic cardiomyopathy in the elderly. *In* Coodley, E.L. (ed.): Geriatric Heart Disease. PSG Publishing, Littleton, MA, 1985, pp. 260–268.

N

1. Neely, J.R., Rovetto, M.J., and Oram, J.F.: Myocardial utilization of carbohydrate and lipids. Prog. Cardiovasc. Dis. 15:289–329, 1972.

O

1. Opie, L.H.: Metabolism of the heart in health and disease. Part I. Am. Heart J. 76:685–698, 1968.
2. Opie, L.H.: Metabolism of the heart in health and disease. Part III. Am. Heart J. 77:383–410, 1969.
3. Opherk, D., Schwarz, F., Mall, G., et al.: Coronary dilatory capacity in idiopathic dilated cardiomyopathy: Analysis of 16 patients. Am. J. Cardiol. 51:1657–1662, 1983.
4. Olsen, E.G.J., Symons, C., and Hawkey, C.M.: The effect of triac and propranolol on the developing myocardium in rats. Br. Heart J. 40:1068, 1978.

P

1. Pande, S.V.: A mitochondrial carnitine acylcarnitine translocase system. Proc. Natl. Acad. Sci. USA 72:883–887, 1975.
2. Pasternac, A., Noble, J., Streulens, Y., et al.: Pathophysiology of chest pain in patients with cardiomyopathies and normal coronary arteries. Circulation 65:778–789, 1982.
3. Packer, M.: Neurohormonal interactions and adaptations in congestive heart failure. Circulation 77:721–730, 1988.
4. Post, R.L., Morgan, H.E., and Park, C.R.: Regulation of glucose uptake in muscle. III. The interaction of membrane transport and phosphorylation in the control of glucose uptake. J. Biol. Chem. 236:269–272, 1961.
5. Pool, P.E., Spann, J.F., Jr., Buiccino, R.A., et al.: Myocardial high energy phosphate stores in cardiac hypertrophy and heart failure. Circ. Res. 21:365–373, 1967.
6. Perloff, J.K.: Pathogenesis of hypertrophic cardiomyopathy: Hypothesis and speculation. Am. Heart J. 14:219, 1981.
7. Perloff, J.K., Henze, E., and Schelbert, H.R.: Alterations in regional myocardial metabolism, perfusion, and wall motion in Duchenne muscular dystrophy studied by radionuclide imaging. Circulation 69:33–42, 1984.
8. Perloff, J.K.: Cardiac involvement in heredofamilial neuroic diseases. Cardiovasc. Clin. 4:334–344, 1972.

R

1. Rose, C.P., and Goresky, C.A.: Constraints on the uptake of labeled palmitate by the heart. The barriers at the capillary and sarcolemmal surfaces and the control of intracellular sequestration. Circ. Res. 41:534–545, 1977.

S

1. Scheuer, J., and Brachfeld, N.: Myocardial uptake and fractional distribution of palmitate–1-C^{14} by the ischemic dog heart. Metabolism 15:945–954, 1966.
2. Schwartz, A., Sordahl, L.A., Entman, M.L., et al.: Abnormal biochemistry in myocardial failure. Am. J. Cardiol. 32:407–422, 1973.
3. Schwartz, A., Lindenmayer, G.E., and Harigaya, S.: Respiratory control and calcium transport in heart mitochondria from the cardiomyopathic Syrian hamster. Trans. NY Acad. Sci. 30 (Suppl. II):951–954, 1968.
4. Sobel, B.E., Spann, J.F., Jr., Pool, P.E., et al.: Normal oxidative phosphorylation in mitochondria from the failing heart. Circ. Res. 21:355–363, 1967.
5. Schelbert, H.R., Henze, E., Sochor, H., et al.: Effects of substrate availability on myocardial C–11 palmitate kinetics by positron emission tomography in normal subjects and patients with ventricular dysfunction. Am. Heart J. 111:1055–1064, 1986.
6. Sochor, H., Schelbert, H.R., Schwaiger, M., et al.: Studies of fatty acid metabolism with positron emission tomography in patients with cardiomyopathy. Eur. J. Nucl. Med. 12(Suppl.):S66–S69, 1986.
7. Schuster, E.H., and Bulkley, B.H.: Ischemic cardiomyopathy: A clinicopathologic study of fourteen patients. Am. Heart J. 100:506–512, 1980.
8. Shaver, J.A., Salerni, R., Curtiss, E.I., and Follansbee, W.P.: Clinical presentation and noninvasive evaluation of the patient with hypertrophic cardiomyopathy. Cardiovasc. Clin. 19:149–192, 1988.
9. Symons, C., Olsen, E.G.J., and Hawkey, C.: Association of hyperthyroidism with hypertrophic cardiomyopathy. *In* Sekiguchi, M., and Olsen, E.G.J. (eds.): Cardiomyopathy: Clinical, Pathological and Theoretical Aspects. University of Tokyo Press, Tokyo, 1980, pp. 369–373.
10. Slucka C: The electrocardiogram in Duchenne progressive muscular dystrophy. Circulation 38:933, 1968.
11. Shelton, M.E., Dence, C.S., Hwang, D.-R., et al.: Myocardial kinetics of fluorine–18 misonidazole: A marker of hypoxic myocardium. J. Nucl. Med. 30:351–358, 1989.

T

1. Tripp, M.E., Katcher, M.L., Peters, H.A., et al.: Systemic carnitine deficiency presenting as familial endocardial fibroelastosis. N. Engl. J. Med. 305:385–390, 1981.
2. Thompson, D.S., Naqvi, N., Juul, S.M., et al.: Effects of propranolol on myocardial oxygen consumption, substrate extraction, and haemodynamics in hypertrophic obstructive cardiomyopathy. Br. Heart J. 44:488–498, 1980.

U

1. Ugolini, V., Hansen, C.L., Kulkarni, V., et al.: Abnormal myocardial fatty acid metabolism in dilated cardiomyopathy detected by Iodine–123 phenylpentadecanoic acid and tomographic imaging. Am. J. Cardiol. 62:923–928, 1988.

W

1. Whiting, R.B., Powell, W.J., Dinsmore, R.E., and Sanders, C.A.: Idiopathic hypertrophic subaortic stenosis. N. Engl. J. Med. 285:196, 1971.
2. Walsh, M.N., Geltman, E.M., Steele, R.L., et al.: Delineation of impaired regional perfusion by positron emission tomography with $H_2{}^{15}O$. Circulation 78:612–620, 1988.

Chapter 69

Positron Emission Tomography: Evaluation of Cardiac Receptors

ANDRÉ SYROTA, M.D., Ph.D.

PRINCIPLES OF CARDIAC RECEPTOR IMAGING WITH POSITRON EMISSION TOMOGRAPHY 1256
COMPARISON OF IN VITRO AND IN VIVO RECEPTOR-BINDING TECHNIQUES 1257
In Vitro Binding Studies 1257
Saturation Experiments 1257
Kinetic Experiments 1258
Inhibition Experiments 1258
In Vivo Binding Studies 1258
Access of Ligand to Myocardium 1258
Interaction of Ligand Within the Myocardium 1259
Choice of Ligand 1259
CRITERIA FOR IDENTIFICATION OF LIGAND-RECEPTOR INTERACTION BY POSITRON EMISSION TOMOGRAPHY 1259
Main Criteria 1259
Saturability 1259
Stereoselectivity 1260
Correlation Between the Binding and a Biologic Effect 1260
Complementary Criteria 1260
IN VIVO RECEPTOR BINDING MODELS 1260
Kinetic Binding Studies 1261
Equilibrium Binding Studies 1262
CHARACTERIZATION OF CARDIAC ADRENERGIC RECEPTORS BY POSITRON EMISSION TOMOGRAPHY 1262
In Vivo Demonstration of β-Adrenergic Receptors 1262
Distribution and Subtypes of β-Adrenergic Receptors 1262
Positron Emission Tomographic Investigation of β-Adrenergic Receptors 1263
In Vivo Study of α-Adrenergic Receptors 1264
CHARACTERIZATION OF CARDIAC MUSCARINIC ACETYLCHOLINE RECEPTORS BY POSITRON EMISSION TOMOGRAPHY 1264
Distribution and Subtypes of Muscarinic Cholinergic Receptors 1264
Positron Emission Tomographic Investigation of Muscarinic Cholinergic Receptors 1265
CHARACTERIZATION OF THE PERIPHERAL-TYPE BENZODIAZEPINE RECEPTOR 1266
CLINICAL APPLICATIONS 1267
Functional and Pharmacologic Investigations 1267
Clinical Investigations 1267
Future Prospects 1267

Alterations of cardiac neurotransmitter receptors have been demonstrated in various heart diseases from samples collected mainly during surgery or autopsy. Positron emission tomography (PET) now allows us to obtain noninvasively quantitative determination of regional receptor density and affinity in humans. These measurements are based on the synthesis of a radioligand, usually a selective receptor antagonist labeled with a positron-emitting radioisotope such as carbon-11 (^{11}C). Mathematical compartmental models are fitted to time-activity curves obtained during saturation or displacement experiments in order to calculate the rate constants and the receptor density in meaningful regions of interest selected in the myocardium. Several receptor classes, such as β- and α-adrenergic, muscarinic cholinergic, and peripheral-type benzodiazepine, have thus been characterized in humans. PET can help to understand changes in receptor number that are associated with myocardial ischemia, heart failure, and cardiomyopathy as well as those changes associated with hormone dysfunctions or treatment with β-blocking agents.

PRINCIPLES OF CARDIAC RECEPTOR IMAGING WITH POSITRON EMISSION TOMOGRAPHY

Advances in basic cardiac physiology and cardiac pharmacology over the past two decades have shown that receptors in the heart are the major targets of many new drugs and neurotransmitters. Alterations in receptor molecules have also been demonstrated in various heart diseases.

Receptors form a class of intrinsic membrane proteins (or glycoproteins) defined by the high affinity and specificity with which they bind ligands. Implicit in the definition and naming of receptors (for example "β-adrenergic receptor") is the functional significance of their binding activity. Many receptors are associated directly or indirectly with membrane ion channels that open or close after a conformational change of the receptor induced by the binding of the neurotransmitter (e.g., norepinephrine) or of an agonist drug (isoproterenol) on the receptor specific site.

Changes in the number and/or the affinity of cardiac neurotransmitter receptors have been associated with myocardial ischemia and infarction, congestive heart failure, cardiomyopathy, and heart transplantation as well as diabetes or thyroid-induced heart muscle disease. These alterations of cardiac receptors have been demonstrated in vitro on membrane homogenates from samples collected mainly during surgery or postmortem examination. The disadvantage of these in vitro binding techniques is that receptors lose their natural environment and their relationships with the other components of the tissue. In vitro autoradiographic techniques in human tissue offer several advantages over homogenate binding techniques: an increase in sensitivity and the possibility of anatomic resolution allowing light microscopic mapping of relationships between the distribution of specific cell populations and neurotransmitter receptors. However, the evolution of receptor changes as the disease progresses or the effect of a drug cannot be analysed.

With the advent of PET, it is now possible to obtain noninvasively quantitative determination of regional biochemical processes in the heart.[B1]

The procedure involves several steps. The first one is the synthesis of radioligands labeled at sufficiently high specific activities with a positron-emitting isotope giving an externally detectable signal. The second step is the use of an imaging system that provides quantitative images of transverse sections of an organ with high sensitivity, good spatial resolution, and great accuracy (Fig. 69–1). The third step is the development of mathematical models that translate radioactive concentration values into physiologic binding parameters, such as receptor density and the equilibrium dissociation constant. This methodology is now applied clinically for studying the perfusion and the metabolism of the human heart in vivo under normal physiologic conditions and in disease states.[S1–S3] Since PET is an imaging technique that combines the advantages of quantitative autoradiography and of tomographic imaging by external detection, it has made possible both imaging and quantitative investigation of cardiac receptors. The feasibility of characterizing muscarinic acetylcholine receptors, β-adrenergic receptors, and α_1-adrenergic receptors has been shown in animals and in humans.[S4] The receptor PET technique is now beginning to be applied to clinical investigation.

Figure 69–1. See Color Plate 18.

In contrast to single-photon emission computed tomography (SPECT), PET gives the exact value of the radioactive concentration of a tracer in any pixel in the slice. It is then possible to select meaningful areas of interest in the septum or in the free wall of the left ventricle and to plot time-activity curves. Fitting these kinetic data to a mathematical model allows calculation of receptor density or drug affinity in any region of the myocardium. Furthermore, positron-emitting isotopes of natural elements have short half-lives (20 minutes for ^{11}C) and are produced at very high specific activity (400 to 1000 Ci/mmol) resulting in three advantages. First, drugs labeled by ^{11}C keep their pharmacologic properties contrary to analogs labeled by ^{123}I (unless they naturally contain iodine). Second, the injected amount of drug usually does not exceed 10 to 50 nanomoles, so that receptor occupancy by the tracer remains low. In addition, drugs that could have acute or chronic effects when administered at pharmacologic doses can be used in humans (e.g., β-blockers such as ^{11}C-practolol or ^{11}C-CGP 12 177). Third, for the same reason, the radiation burden is low although the amount of radioactivity injected is relatively high (10 to 20 mCi, 370 to 740 MBq). The reverse of the medal is the complexity and the cost of PET imaging. It is necessary to gather in the same facility a cyclotron to produce the positron emitter, a radiochemistry laboratory to synthesize the ^{11}C-labeled molecule in less than 40 minutes, and a positron tomograph to record the data. Table 69–1 shows a list of ligands labeled with ^{11}C or ^{18}F that have been synthesized for the investigation of cardiac receptors.[B2–B5, C1–C3, E1, M1, M15, M16] This chapter discusses those that have been most completely characterized. They include the muscarinic cholinergic receptor; β-adrenergic receptor; and peripheral-type benzodiazepine receptor.

COMPARISON OF IN VITRO AND IN VIVO RECEPTOR-BINDING TECHNIQUES

The main problem of in vitro and in vivo receptor studies is how to reduce data from receptor-binding experiments to parameters such as affinity constants, rate constants, and receptor densities. The in vivo analysis using PET is much more complicated than the in vitro analysis on tissue homogenates or on

Table 69–1. ^{11}C-LABELED LIGANDS FOR CARDIAC RECEPTOR STUDIES

Ligand		Class of Receptor
^{11}C MQNB	M1	muscarinic cholinergic
^{11}C TRB	M15	muscarinic cholinergic
^{11}C propranolol	B2	β-adrenergic
^{11}C practolol	B3	β-adrenergic
^{11}C pindolol	P1	β-adrenergic
^{11}C CGP 12177	B4	β-adrenergic
^{11}C prazosin	E1	α_1-adrenergic
^{11}C ketanserin	B5	serotonin S2
^{18}F setoperone	C1	serotonin S2
^{18}F ritanserin	C2	serotonin S2
^{11}C PK 11195	C3	peripheral-type benzodiazepine
^{18}F fluorometaraminol	M16	adrenergic neuronal mapping
^{11}C hydroxyephedrine	W9	adrenergic neuronal mapping

autoradiographic slices, but the basic principles are similar. It is thus necessary to briefly describe the main types of analyses that are used in vitro.[B6]

In Vitro Binding Studies

For the simple bimolecular association of a drug with its receptor in which the law of mass action is valid:

$$R + L + I \rightleftarrows RL + RI \qquad (1)$$

where R is the concentration of free (unoccupied) receptor, L is the concentration of free radioactive ligand, I is the concentration of unlabeled drug, and RL and RI are the concentrations of the receptor bound with each ligand. In most experiments, RL is the measured experimental variable; it represents the specific binding and not the total binding, specific plus nonspecific, observed experimentally. The total or added ligand concentration L_T is also known and is related to the free ligand concentration by:

$$L_T = L + RL \qquad (2)$$

Three basic types of experiments can be performed on a system following Equation 1 and are described in the following sections.

Saturation Experiments

Total radioligand concentration L_T is increased and RL determined at equilibrium in the absence of inhibitor (I = 0). Equation 1 becomes:

$$R + L \underset{k_{-1}}{\overset{k_{+1}}{\rightleftarrows}} RL \qquad (3)$$

where k_{+1} and k_{-1} are the association or forward rate constant and k_{-1} is the dissociation or reverse rate constant. The equilibrium dissociation constant K_D is defined as:

$$K_D = \frac{k_{-1}}{k_{+1}} = \frac{R \bullet L}{RL} \qquad (4)$$

The total receptor concentration R_T (often called B_{max}) must be the sum of the free and bound concentrations:

$$R_T = R + LR \qquad (5)$$

Combining Equations 2, 3, 4 and 5 gives at equilibrium:

$$RL = \frac{R_T \bullet L}{K_D + L} \qquad (6)$$

This equation describes a rectangular hyperbola and shows that at very high ligand concentrations ($L >> K_D$), all receptor sites are occupied and RL is not very different from R_T. This type of experiment gives also the value of K_D. It can be seen that when $L = K_D$, $RL = R_T/2$. The equilibrium dissociation constant is thus the concentration of ligand L that occupies half of the total receptors.

Kinetic Experiments

Bound ligand concentration RL is determined as a function of time, with L_T being held constant. Since the net rate at which RL is being formed is equal to the difference between the rate of formation of RL from R and L ($k_{+1} \cdot R \cdot L$) and the rate of dissociation of RL to give R and L ($k_{-1} \cdot RL$), one can write:

$$\frac{d\,RL}{dt} = k_{+1} \cdot R \cdot L - k_{-1} \cdot RL \tag{7}$$

The association rate constant k_{+1} is determined by measuring the amount of binding at various times after mixing the ligand with the tissue. The dissociation rate constant k_{-1} is easily obtained in experimental situations where the term $k_{+1} \cdot R \cdot L$ is essentially zero; that is, in conditions where rebinding of radioligand is prevented. This can be accomplished in two ways. In the first method, the reaction mixture is diluted by 50 fold or more so that L is reduced to nearly zero. In the second method, an excess of nonradioactive ligand is added so that all free binding sites become occupied by the added unlabeled ligand, then $R=0$. Under either of these experiments, Equation 7 reduces to:

$$\frac{d\,RL}{dt} = -k_{-1} \cdot RL \tag{8}$$

which, by integration, gives

$$RL = RL_o \cdot \exp(-k_{-1} \cdot t) \tag{9}$$

where RL_o is the concentration of bound ligand at $t=0$. One can notice that both methods must give the same value of k_{-1}.

Inhibition Experiments

The third basic type of experiment is the inhibition experiment, in which RL is measured as the concentration of an unlabeled drug (I) is increased and L_T is held constant. As can be seen from Equation 1, RI increases with increasing I, thus reducing RL because of a decrease in free binding sites R. This experiment is also referred to as a "competition study," since I is a competitive inhibitor. It is also commonly called the "displacement experiment," because the radioactive tracer seems to be displaced by the excess of unlabeled ligand. This term is, in fact, inappropriate, since the unlabeled drug only competes with the radioligand for the binding site and does not displace it. The term displacement is also widely used in PET studies. From Equation 1 one can demonstrate that:

$$RL = \frac{R_T \cdot L}{K_D(1 + I/K_i) + L} \tag{10}$$

where K_i is the inhibition constant, defined as $K_i = R \cdot I/RI$. The inhibition constant is related to the IC_{50}, the concentration of I giving 50 percent of the binding in the absence of I, by:

$$K_i = \frac{IC_{50}}{1 + L/K_D} \tag{11}$$

and one sees that $K_i = IC_{50}$ when $L = K_D$.

In Vivo Binding Studies

As applied to in vivo studies, the methods and the equations discussed previously remain valid but additional problems must be considered. Some methods have been adapted to PET studies, but the conditions of application of the equations must be carefully checked. Two kinds of problems can be defined. First, the radioactive ligand that is generally intravenously injected must reach its receptor sites within the studied organ without any modification. Second, the radioligand within the organ must interact with high affinity only with its specific receptor sites and must not bind either to other receptors or to nonspecific binding sites.

Access of Ligand to Myocardium

After intravenous injection, the radiotracer can bind to proteins or penetrate into red blood cells, thus reducing the amount of free ligand available for binding. Ligands such as peptides can be enzymatically degraded by circulating peptidases. Other molecules can be rapidly metabolized by the liver. About 90 percent of CGP 12177, a potent β-blocking agent, is metabolized five minutes after intravenous injection. After injection of ^{11}C-CGP 12177, most of the plasma radioactivity is due to ^{11}C-labeled metabolites, which do not bind to β-adrenoceptors. In addition, a time-dependent fraction of ^{11}C-CGP 12177 binds to red blood cells. The concentration of ^{11}C-CGP 12177 available for binding to receptors thus strongly differs from blood and plasma ^{11}C-radioactivities, but it can be calculated in each blood sample after centrifugation and thin-layer chromatography.

Another complication of in vivo studies is the presence of different serial barriers between the site of injection (a brachial vein in humans) and the receptor sites. These include the lungs, the capillary membrane, and the tissue itself. Lipophilic molecules are completely extracted during a single passage through the lung circulation. They can be metabolized by the pulmonary endothelial or epithelial cells before reaching the cardiac receptors. After intravenous injection, ^{11}C-propranolol showed a 90 to 100 percent lung uptake and the myocardium was never visualized during the 80 minutes of observation. ^{11}C-practolol is a thousand times more hydrophilic than ^{11}C-propranolol. It is not extracted by the lungs. Therefore, the myocardium is visualized a few minutes after injection. Pulmonary accumulation of drugs in patients may depend on the functional state of the pulmonary cells. The extraction by the lung of ^{11}C-labeled basic amines such as ^{11}C-propranolol is reduced in patients with chronic obstructive pulmonary disease; the tissue washout half-life is significantly greater in patients with active sarcoidosis (stage II) than in normal subjects.[P2]

The most puzzling situation was found when the myocardial serotonergic receptor was studied. Ketanserin, a potent antagonist of S-2 serotonergic receptors, was labeled with ^{11}C and intravenously injected in a group of normal volunteers. A large individual variation was observed: In some subjects, the myocardial concentration of ^{11}C-ketanserin was very high with low pulmonary uptake whereas the opposite was seen in others.[C4] Tobacco consumption accounted for this difference, since the radioactive ligand concentration in the lungs of smokers is linearly correlated to the amount of tobacco smoke absorption. The very high ^{11}C-ketanserin concentration seems to reflect the increasing cellularity (including alveolar macrophages that have serotonergic receptors on their membranes) induced by cigarette smoking.[C4] A low ligand concentration in the myocardium might thus be falsely attributed to a low receptor density when it is only the consequence of restricted access to receptor sites. In animals or humans, the amount of ligand that reaches the heart thus depends on its clearance from the lungs. The cardiac receptors cannot be visualized if the radioligand concentration in the lung decreases slowly compared with the physical half-life of the isotope.

The second barrier is the capillary barrier of the target organ. The problem is less severe in heart than in brain where the intercellular junctions are very tight. In contrast to the blood-brain barrier, the capillary membrane is permeable to small hydrophilic molecules. The biodistribution of the radiotracer is also important to consider; it may be extracted, trapped, or metabolized by other organs than the lungs and the heart. Many drugs are transformed into metabolites in the liver. Some of these metabolites are still labeled by the positron-emitting isotope but their physical and pharmacologic properties may have changed. Both the lipophilicity and the affinity of the metabolites may have been modified by several orders of magnitude. From these remarks one sees that Equation 1 must be modified into:

$$L_o + I_o \underset{k}{\overset{P}{\rightleftarrows}} L + I + R \underset{k_{-1}}{\overset{k_{+1}}{\rightleftarrows}} RL + RI \qquad (12)$$

where L_o is the concentration of unmetabolized labeled ligand and I_o is the concentration of inhibitor outside the "volume of reaction" of ligand with receptor. Parameters p and k are rate constants characterizing the transfer of ligand into and out of this volume of reaction. They may represent the exchange of ligand between plasma and tissue (for example through the blood-brain barrier)[F1, P3, W1, W2] or between blood and tissue on one hand and a smaller volume of reaction on the other hand that could correspond to the boundary layer in the vicinity of the membrane receptors.[S5] The limiting step for the exchange of tracer between blood and volume of reaction depends on several parameters; for example, the structure of the capillary membrane (continuous, fenestrated, discontinuous), the structure of the intercellular junctions (tight, leaky), the localization of the receptors (on endothelial cells, myocytes, or neuromuscular junctions), the chemicophysical properties of the labeled ligand, and of course, the functional integrity of the myocardium itself (normal, ischemic, denervated, cardiomyopathic).

Interaction of Ligand Within the Myocardium

Additional complexities are related to the removal process of the radioligand within the myocardium, such as uptake by different cells, enzymatic or chemical degradation, and intracellular trapping. A radioligand can also bind to different receptors or different receptor subtypes. The labeled ligand should ideally bind specifically to a single receptor type and even to a single receptor subtype, since subtypes of both α- and β-adrenergic receptors and of muscarinic cholinergic receptors exist.[H1, M2, S6] β-adrenergic receptors appear to exist as two subtypes, β_1 and β_2, with a predominance of β_1 over β_2 in the heart. It is well known that cardioselective β-blockers are generally hydrophilic, whereas nonselective β-blockers are generally lipophilic, although exceptions have been found. However, the affinity of the so-called cardioselective β-blockers is generally much lower than that of noncardioselective β-blockers.[W3]

PET detects the total radioactivity in the heart and, unlike in vitro studies, the distinction between specific binding and nonspecific binding is not immediate. In brain studies, one may subtract the radioactivity in the cerebellum from that in the striatum or in the cortex if receptors are known to be absent from the cerebellum.[W1] Such a correction is impossible in heart studies. Since nonspecific binding increases linearly with plasma ligand concentration whereas specific binding is perceived as a hyperbola, the ratio of specific to nonspecific binding can be increased by minimizing radiotracer plasma concentrations and maximizing specific radioactivity of the radioligand to detect enough radioactivity in the tissue. As a consequence, improving the affinity of a β-blocker by increasing its lipophilicity also leads to an increase in nonspecific binding. Intricate mechanisms thus interfere. The initial uptake of two tritiated antagonists of the muscarinic cholinergic receptor was compared in an isolated perfused rat heart preparation.[C5] The first, ^{3}H-QNB, a very potent antagonist, is a lipophilic molecule that is widely used in in vitro binding studies.[F2] The second, ^{3}H-MQNB, the methiodide salt of QNB, is a hydrophilic molecule that maintains a high affinity for the muscarinic acetylcholine receptor.[C1] After rapid injection in the perfusate, a high nonspecific uptake of ^{3}H-QNB was found contrasting with a 90 percent specific binding of ^{3}H-MQNB that could be inhibited by adding an excess of unlabeled MQNB or atropine in the perfusate.[C5] This example emphasizes the necessity of the search for new radioligands specially designed for in vivo studies. It also shows the need for preliminary in vitro studies on homogenates and on isolated organs and of pharmacokinetic studies on animals before trying to label a new ligand with a positron emitter.

Choice of Ligand

If the preliminary studies indicate that a ligand with high specificity and nanomolar binding affinity for receptor in vitro can reach its target (e.g., β_1-adrenergic receptors) in a few minutes in vivo without being highly extracted and metabolized by other tissues (particularly the lungs and the liver), one can try to label this ligand with ^{11}C since it is then possible to follow with PET the tissue kinetics of ^{11}C-labeled ligand for about 100 minutes. On the other hand, if the ligand reaches the myocardial receptors very slowly, it should be labeled with a positron-emitting isotope of a longer half-life, e.g., fluorine 18 (^{18}F) ($T_{1/2}$ = 1.8 hours), bromine 75 (^{75}Br) ($T_{1/2}$ = 1.7 hours) or bromine 76 (^{76}Br) ($T_{1/2}$ = 16.2 hours). Since ligand molecules do not generally contain a bromine or a fluorine atom, it is necessary to carefully study their binding properties in vitro; for example, the halogenation of QNB and MQNB lowers the tissue-to-blood and the specific-to-nonspecific binding ratios.

Although the 20-minute half-life of ^{11}C is a major advantage with regard to the fact that it entails minor radiation exposure of patients and minimal side effects, it adds to the complexity of the method because the ligand must be rapidly synthesized (in less than 40 minutes). Rapid labeling of the compound ideally can be accomplished by using a precursor of the ligand selected. By a single chemical reaction, the precursor may then be converted into the labeled molecule. The four labeled β-blocking agents, ^{11}C-propranolol,[B2] ^{11}C-practolol,[B3] ^{11}C-pindolol,[P1] and ^{11}C-CGP 12177,[B4] and the α_1-blocking agent, ^{11}C-prazosin,[E1] are obtained by using ^{11}C-phosgen as the labeled precursor.[L1] The muscarinic receptor antagonist ^{11}C-MQNB and the peripheral-type benzodiazepine receptor antagonist ^{11}C-PK 11195 are obtained by the reaction of ^{11}C-methyl iodide with QNB.[M1, C3] Two new ^{18}F-labeled antagonists of the serotonine S_2 receptor, ^{18}F-setoperone and ^{18}F-ritanserin, have been obtained by nucleophilic substitution.[C1, C2]

To summarize, in vivo characterization of cardiac receptors by PET requires high-affinity ligands displaying both a high specificity for a subtype of receptor and a low degree of nonspecific binding in vivo. Furthermore, the labeled ligand must rapidly reach the receptor within the myocardium in an unmetabolized state. The tissue-to-blood ratio must also be high to avoid having to correct for the circulating radioactivity. Also, side effects at saturating doses of ligand must be tolerable.

Although these requirements are difficult to fulfill, several ligands have already been found (Table 69–1). It is then necessary to demonstrate that the interaction of the ligand within the myocardium detected by PET corresponds to the interaction of a drug to a receptor and not to a specific binding site unrelated to a pharmacologic effect.

CRITERIA FOR IDENTIFICATION OF LIGAND-RECEPTOR INTERACTION BY POSITRON EMISSION TOMOGRAPHY

Receptor-mediated localization of a ligand in the myocardium must be validated in vivo by the same criteria as those for in vitro binding studies.[L2]

Main Criteria

Saturability

Saturability of the ligand-receptor complex can be demonstrated by two kinds of experiments. In the displacement experiments, an excess of cold agonist or antagonist is intravenously injected some time after injection of the labeled ligand. The radioactive concentration in the myocardium then rapidly decreases with time because of the competitive inhibition between the tracer and the excess of unlabeled ligand (Figs. 69–2 and 69–3).

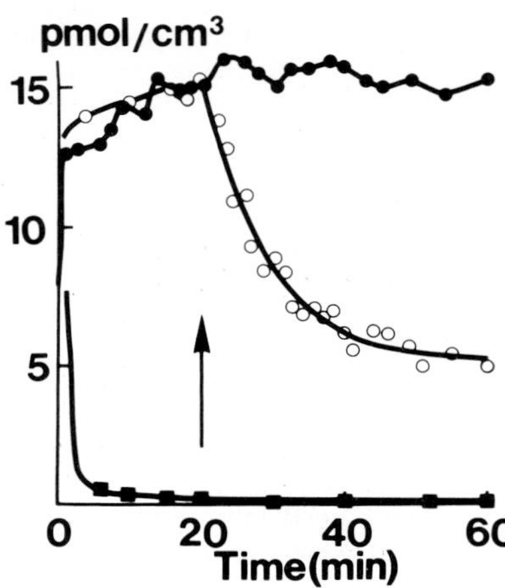

Figure 69–2. ^{11}C-MQNB radioactive concentration–vs.–time curves. After a bolus intravenous injection of 26 mCi of ^{11}C-MQNB at a high specific activity (639 Ci/mmol) in a normal subject, the tracer is rapidly cleared from the blood, and the MQNB concentration is around 0.1 pmol/cm^3 *(solid squares).* By contrast, the activity rises almost immediately in the ventricular septum *(solid circles)* and reaches a mean value around 15 pmol per cm^3 of tissue. In another subject *(open circles),* a similar dose of ^{11}C-MQNB was intravenously injected, but 20 minutes later *(arrow)* an additional intravenous injection of unlabeled atropine (18.7 nmol/kg) was performed. The injection of the competitive inhibitor results in a displacement of ^{11}C-MQNB from its binding sites *(open circles).* The displacement calculated 30 minutes after the injection of atropine is equal to 64%. (Adapted from Syrota, A., Comar, D., Paillotin, G., et al.: Muscarinic cholinergic receptor in the human heart evidenced under physiological conditions by positron emission tomography. Proc. Natl. Acad. Sci. USA 82:584–588, 1985.)

The receptor sites can also be blocked by an excess of unlabeled ligand injected prior to the radioligand. In this case, the tracer radioactive concentration in the tissue is lower than that measured in the absence of injection of the cold molecule (Fig. 69–4). Contrary to the saturation experiments described in in vitro studies, here the total amount of radioactivity L_T cannot be increased but the specific activity is decreased.

Stereoselectivity

Stereoselectivity is a powerful proof for receptor binding. If two stereoisomers are available, one with and the other without pharmacologic activity, the displacement must be obtained only with the active isomer. The stereospecificity of the binding of the muscarinic antagonist ^{11}C-MQNB was proved in this way: only the pharmacologically active isomer of benzetimide (dexetimide) could displace ^{11}C-MQNB, the inactive isomer (levetimide) being ineffective.[M1] These studies have the advantage of minimizing the effects of large amounts of cold ligand on blood flow, transport, and metabolism. However, selective effects of the active isomer on blood flow or metabolism cannot be totally excluded.

Correlation Between the Binding and a Biologic Effect

This criterion is essential for distinguishing between a displaceable binding site with no signal transmission and a receptor binding site that is related to physiologic responses. A correlation between receptor binding and biologic effect was shown with ^{11}C-pindolol, ^{11}C-CGP 12177, and ^{11}C-MQNB. The percentage of ^{11}C-MQNB or ^{11}C-CGP 12177 displaced by various amounts of unlabeled atropine or propranolol was proportional to the decrease or increase in heart rate (see Fig. 69–3).[D1, M1, S7]

Complementary Criteria

In addition to drug displacement (with agonist, antagonist, and stereoisomers) and correlation with pharmacologic activity, which are the most important and most decisive criteria, other criteria must be fulfilled. These are the specific regional distribution of the receptors and the high affinity of receptor sites for the radioligand. It must be noted that the receptors involved in neurotransmission have low affinity for the endogenous neurotransmitters, which, however, are released at high concentrations in the synaptic cleft.[C6] On the other hand, the antagonists of endogenous neurotransmitters behave like hormones; they bind with high affinity to receptors but their blood concentration is negligible. Therefore, better results are obtained with a labeled antagonist than with a labeled agonist; this was confirmed in vivo with PET, and all the ligands used to characterize cardiac receptors up to now are antagonists. Once all these criteria have been fulfilled, it becomes possible to develop a mathematical model that transforms values of radioactive concentrations measured in selected regions of interest of PET images into values of K_D and of receptor density.[D2]

IN VIVO RECEPTOR BINDING MODELS

Several models have recently been proposed as a framework for the analysis and quantification of ligand-receptor interactions investigated in vivo with PET.[F1, F3, P3, S5, W1, W2] The model commonly used is shown in Figure 69–5 and is described by Equation 12. As discussed earlier, two key features of in vivo experiments complicate the interpretation of receptor binding. First, the free ligand pool M_f, which is the product of free ligand concentration L by the volume of reaction V_R, cannot be measured directly. PET provides values of the total amount of ligand $M_T(t)$ (free and bound) in a region of interest of known volume:

$$M_T(t) = M_f(t) + M_b(t) \qquad (13)$$

with

$$M_f = V_R \cdot L \text{ and } M_b = V_R \cdot RL$$

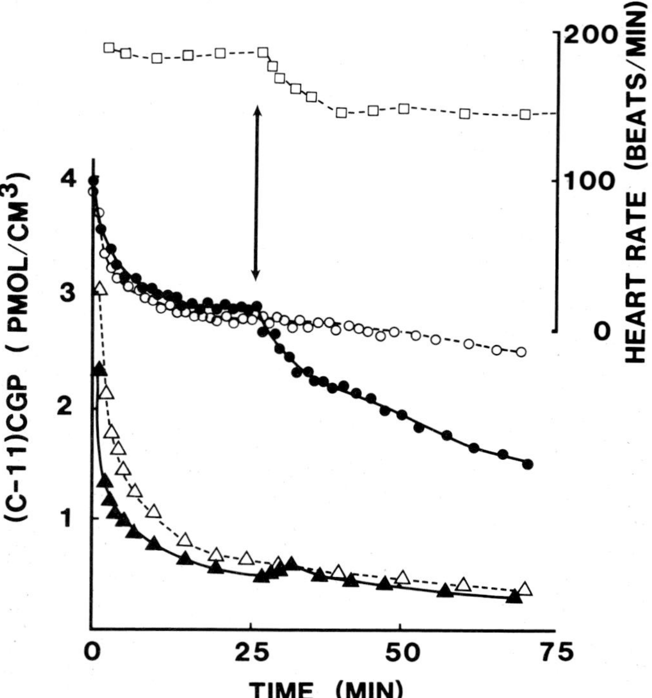

Figure 69–3. Control curve *(open circles)* and curve obtained after injection of an excess of unlabeled CGP 12177 (200 nmol) *(closed circles),* 25 minutes *(arrow)* after injection of a tracer dose of ^{11}C-CGP 12177 in a dog. Measurements were made from a region of interest selected from serial PET scans in the left ventricular myocardium. Concentration values are expressed as pmol/cm^3 of heart. The figure also shows the correlation between the decrease in heart rate *(open squares)* and the displacement of bound ligand *(closed circles).*

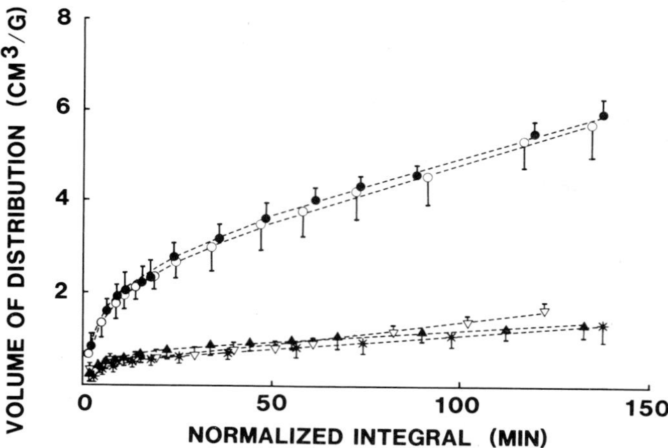

Figure 69–4. Volume of distribution (tissue/blood concentration ratio) of ^{11}C-CGP 12177 in dog myocardium as a function of the normalized time integral ($\int_0^t C[t]dt/C[T]$) in curarized control dogs (●), anesthetized control dogs (○), and in pre-saturation studies with unlabeled CGP 12177 (▽), pindolol (▲), and propranolol (*). In pre-saturation studies, 30 nmol/kg of unlabeled CGP, 400 nmol/kg of pindolol, or 2000 nmol/kg of propranolol were injected intravenously 10 min before ^{11}C-CGP 12177 injection. The heart rates at the time of radioligand injection in curarized dogs, anesthetized dogs, and dogs preloaded with unlabeled CGP, pindolol, and propranolol were 197±8, 129±28, 143±8, 153±8, and 113±15 (beats/min), respectively. The slope of the linear part of each curve was significantly lower in presaturation experiments with unlabeled CGP 12177, pindolol, and propranolol than in control studies. The slopes of the control curves obtained in curarized and anesthetized dogs were identical although the heart rate was much lower during anesthesia.

Second, this precursor pool changes with time independently of the concentration of free ligand in plasma because it depends on several variables: blood flow, capillary permeability, free receptor concentration, and affinity. Thus, in contrast to in vitro studies where L_0 is constant, in PET studies the plasma arterial concentration C_a and the free ligand pool M_f are a function of time. Two types of experimental approaches to the design of quantitative in vivo binding experiments have been proposed: the kinetic binding studies and the equilibrium binding studies.

Kinetic Binding Studies

The in vivo quantitation of binding sites is based on kinetic analysis of radioligand distribution in blood and tissue. A three-compartment model is usually employed (see Fig. 69–5). Tracer present in the myocardium is considered to exist in two major anatomic spaces: the intravascular (compartment 1) and the extravascular space (compartments 2 and 3). Tracer within the extravascular space may be further categorized as free (M_f) or specifically bound (M_b). A fourth compartment can be added if nonspecific binding of ligand to tissue cannot be neglected. The flux of free ligand that crosses the capillary barrier is equal to $p{\cdot}V_R{\cdot}C_a^*(t)$ where $C_a^*(t)$ is the blood radioactive concentration at time t, p an unknown rate constant (permeability), and V_R the volume of reaction (volume of water per unit volume of tissue).

The free radioactive ligand M_f^* can either bind directly to a free receptor site or escape with a rate constant, k. The binding probability depends on the rate constant (k_{+1}/V_R) and on the local concentration of available free receptors, which is equal to $[B'_{max} - M_b^*(t)]$ where B'_{max} is the unknown concentration of available receptor sites and $M_b^*(t)$ the bound ligand concentration. The rate constant for the dissociation of bound ligand is denoted by k_{-1}.

The differential equations describing tracer movement between the compartments in the model presented in Figure 69–5 are listed below:

$$\frac{dM_f^*(t)}{dt} = pV_R C_a^*(t) - kM_f^*(t) - \frac{k_{+1}}{V_R}[B'_{max} - M_b^*(t)]\,M_f^*(t) + k_{-1}M_b^*(t)$$
$$\frac{dM_b^*(t)}{dt} = \frac{k_{+1}}{V_R}[B'_{max} - M_b^*(t)]\,M_f^*(t) - k_{-1}M_b^*(t) \quad (14)$$

This model contains five parameters, the most important of which is the concentration of receptor sites available for ligand binding B'_{max} and the ratio of k_{-1} to k_{+1}, the equilibrium dissociation constant K_D. The model is nonlinear, but this is a great advantage because, first, it can be used whatever the amount of occupied receptors and, second, the receptor density B'_{max}, the association rate constant k_{+1}/V_R, and the dissociation rate constant k_{-1} can be identified separately. The model is identifiable in a no-noise case using a tracer pulse injection.[D2] However, fitting of noisy experimental data gave large parameter error estimates.[D2]

Most authors have used a simplified model assuming that the tracer occupies a negligible fraction of the available receptors[F3, M3, P3, W1] so that:

$$\frac{k_{+1}}{V_R}[B'_{max} - M_b^*(t)] \simeq \frac{k_{+1}}{V_R}B'_{max} = k_3 \quad (15)$$

The system of differential equations (14) becomes linear but neither the receptor density B'_{max} nor the equilibrium dissociation constant K_D can be separately measured with a single tracer injection. The rate constant k_3 gives only an indication of the binding potential that reflects the capacity of a given tissue to bind a labeled molecule.[M3, P3] The equations can be further simplified if it is assumed that the ligand binds irreversibly to receptor sites, i.e., if $k_{-1} = 0$. If both assumptions are made, a graphical method can then be used.[W1, W2]

These major simplifications have to be validated for each ligand-receptor interaction investigated, which has not been the case up to now. Therefore, we have investigated the possibility of improving parameter estimation by using a displacement experiment in which an excess of unlabeled ligand (J) is injected after a delay (t_D) following the injection of a trace amount of ^{11}C-labeled ligand (J*).[S5] This experimental protocol requires incorporation in the model of the kinetics of unlabeled ligand because it alters the local concentration of free receptor sites. The amounts of free unlabeled ligand and bound unlabeled ligand are denoted by $M_f(t)$ and $M_b(t)$, respectively.

Parameter identification requires knowledge of the blood time-activity curve $C_a^*(t)$, which is usually considered as a known and exact input function obtained from arterial blood samples. The arterial unlabeled ligand concentration $C_a(t)$ is assumed to be zero before the time of displacement t_D, and proportional to the arterial labeled ligand concentration measured at time $t - t_D$ when $t > t_D$, the proportionality factor being the ratio J/J*.

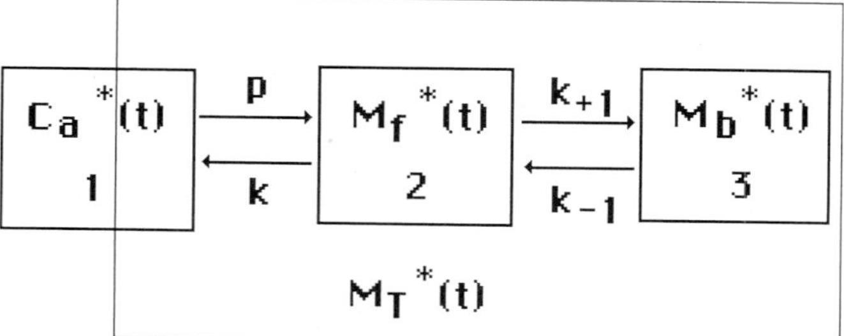

Figure 69–5. Compartmental model used in kinetic analysis of ligand binding to cardiac receptors. C_a* is the tracer concentration (corrected for metabolites) in arterial blood. M_f*, M_b*, and M_T* represent free, specifically bound, and total amount of tracer, respectively. The constants p and k are the transfer coefficients between blood and tissue. k_{+1} and k_{-1} are the association and dissociation rate constants, respectively.

Parameter identification and simulations of labeled and unlabeled ligand kinetics are performed using the following nonlinear differential equations:[D2, D7]

$$\frac{dM_f^*(t)}{dt} = pV_R\, C_a^*(t) - kM_f^*(t) - \frac{k_{+1}}{V_R}[B'_{max} - M_b^*(t) - M_b(t)]\, M_f^*(t) + k_{-1} M_b^*(t)$$

$$\frac{dM_b^*(t)}{dt} = \frac{k_{+1}}{V_R}[B'_{max} - M_b^*(t) - M_b(t)]\, M_f^*(t) - k_{-1} M_b^*(t) \tag{16}$$

$$\frac{dM_f(t)}{dt} = pV_R \frac{J}{J^*} C_a^*(t - t_D) - kM_f(t) - \frac{k_{+1}}{V_R}[B'_{max} - M_b^*(t) - M_b(t)]\, M_f(t) + k_{-1} M_b(t)$$

$$\frac{dM_b(t)}{dt} = \frac{k_{+1}}{V_R}[B'_{max} - M_b^*(t) - M_b(t)]\, M_f(t) - k_{-1} M_b(t)$$

where B'_{max}, $p{\cdot}V_R$, k, k_{+1}/V_R and k_{-1} are the unknown parameters. This model introduces no new parameter with regard to the first model described in Figure 69–5 and the result of the identifiability problem remains unchanged.

In PET studies, the experimental data acquired between time t_{i-1} and time t_i are given by the following integral relation:

$$M_T^*(t_i) = \frac{1}{t_i - t_{i-1}} \int_{t_{i-1}}^{t_i} (M_f^*(\pi) + M_b^*(\pi) + F_V C_a^*(\pi))dt \tag{17}$$

where F_V is a parameter representing the vascular fraction and identified at the same time as the model parameters.

Time-activity curves obtained from serial PET images recorded after intravenous injection of a tracer dose followed a few minutes later by an injection of an excess of the same unlabeled ligand were analyzed according to this model by using a nonlinear multiparameter least-squares curve-fitting procedure. The k_{+1}, k_{-1}, B'_{max} and K_D values were obtained using Equations 16 and 17 with small standard deviations.[D7] Such kinetic binding studies with displacement by cold ligand were used to measure B'_{max} and K_D for muscarinic acetylcholine receptor and β-adrenergic receptor in the dog and human heart, using ^{11}C-MQNB and ^{11}C-CGP 12177 as radiolabeled ligands.

Equilibrium Binding Studies

As an alternative to the single-dose, tracer-kinetic approach, B'_{max} and K_D have been measured by PET analysis of saturation kinetics performed at equilibrium.[F3] This assumption can be made if the ligand associates with and dissociates from receptors very rapidly because the duration of a PET study is limited by the short half-life of ^{11}C. At equilibrium, $dM_b^*/dt = 0$ and Equation 14 becomes:

$$M_b^* = \frac{B'_{max} \bullet M_f^*}{V_R K_D + M_F^*} \tag{18}$$

which is similar to Equation 6, commonly used in in vitro studies.

However, this methodology suffers several limitations. For measuring the ^{11}C-raclopride binding to dopaminergic D_2 receptor in the human brain, a series of five experiments was performed on each healthy subject.[F3] Bound ligand concentrations were measured at equilibrium and the five experimental data points, each obtained with different doses of ^{11}C-raclopride, were fitted to the hyperbola corresponding to Equation 18. The repetition of PET scans, if acceptable in volunteers, seems difficult to perform in clinical situations. Furthermore, the values of M_f^* must be known in order to calculate B'_{max} and K_D. When studying the D_2 receptor, one can consider that ^{11}C-raclopride binding in the cerebellum represents free ligand if nonspecific binding is not too large because it is known from in vitro studies that there are no dopaminergic receptors in the cerebellum. This approach is not applicable to the heart, where no such receptor regional distribution has ever been demonstrated.

CHARACTERIZATION OF CARDIAC ADRENERGIC RECEPTORS BY POSITRON EMISSION TOMOGRAPHY

Catecholamines, acting through α- and β-adrenergic receptors, modulate a variety of physiologic responses in the heart, the most important being an increase in the rate and force of cardiac contraction. Although the effects of sympathetic nervous stimulation on the heart have been investigated for many years, only more recently has it become possible to directly probe the receptors for catecholamines in the heart using in vitro radioligand-binding techniques.[M4, S6] Each of the two types of adrenergic receptors, α and β, can be classified into two subtypes termed α_1, α_2, and β_1, and β_2 using both pharmacologic and anatomic criteria.[M2, S6, S8] These receptor subtypes are coupled to G-proteins, which bind and hydrolyze the guanine nucleotide GTP. All of them have been purified and reconstituted with guanine nucleotide regulatory proteins in phospholipid vesicles, their functional regulation has been extensively studied, and the genes and/or cDNAs for the α_2−, β_1− and β_2− subtypes have been isolated and sequenced.[L3]

The adrenergic receptors are members of a large family. Recently cloned members of this family include human rhodopsin, the human color opsins, the α_2-adrenergic receptor in the hamster[D3] and human β_2-adrenergic receptor, the avian β-adrenergic receptor,[Y1] and the cerebral and cardiac muscarinic cholinergic receptors as well as two additional recently described muscarinic receptors.[B7, P4] Despite high similarities in amino acid sequences of the β_1- and β_2-receptor proteins (they are identical in 54 percent of their residues), the two receptors are products of different genes.

In Vivo Demonstration of β-Adrenergic Receptors

Distribution and Subtypes of β-Adrenergic Receptors

β-adrenergic receptor subtypes exhibit a characteristic tissue distribution. The β_1-adrenergic receptor appears to predominate in the heart whereas the β_2-adrenergic receptor predominates in the lung. However, both β_1- and β_2-adrenergic receptors are present in the mammalian heart. Basically, β_1-receptors exhibit equal affinity for both epinephrine and norepinephrine, whereas β_2-receptors exhibit a higher affinity for epinephrine than for norepinephrine.[M2] β_1-adrenergic receptors are the predominant β-adrenergic receptors in the human myocardium.[H2, S8] However, a relatively high proportion of β_2-receptors, up to 50 percent, has been found in the human heart, especially in the atria.[G2, H3, R1] The proportion of β_1- and β_2-adrenoceptors in the atrioventricular node of the rat heart is about 56 percent and 44 percent of the total binding capacity, respectively.[S9] It has been suggested that the β_2-receptors could be linked to the chronotropic changes, whereas the β_1-receptors could account for both inotropic and chronotropic responses.[M2] Controversies regarding the relative amount of β_1- and β_2-adrenoceptor subtypes could be attributable to differences in the preparative procedures, leading to varying degrees of endothelial contamination. Purified rat myocytes contain solely β_1-adrenoceptors.[B8] Following density gradient centrifugation of cardiac ventricular microsomes, β_1-adrenoceptors are associated with the peak corresponding to sarcolemmal membranes and β_2-adrenoceptors to the peak corresponding to endothelial cells.[F4] In guinea pig and rat ventricles, β_2-adrenoceptors would be primarily localized on the coronary endothelium, cardiomyocytes would contain only β_1-adrenoceptors.

Thus, coronary vessels also contain β-adrenoceptors. An inverse relationship between the density of β-receptors and the diameter of coronary vessels was determined with quantitative autoradiography.[M5] Incubation of slices of feline and dog heart with ^{125}I-iodocyanopindolol showed that β-receptor density was relatively low in the large epicardial conductance arteries, increased in the mural arteries, and was highest in the small resistance vessels, the coronary arterioles, where it was approximately 60 percent of the β-receptor density of nearby myocytes. Both β_1 and β_2 subtypes are present in large bovine coronary arteries,[V1] whereas small vessels would contain only β_2-adrenoceptors.[F4]

The most commonly used β-adrenergic ligands in in vitro binding studies, ^{3}H-dihydroalprenolol and ^{125}I-iodohydroxy-benzylpindolol, do not distinguish between β_1- and β_2-receptors. However, competition experiments can be performed.[S6] The nonselective radioligand is incubated with increasing concentrations of a β_1 subtype–selective antagonist, such as atenolol, practolol, metoprolol, or ICI 89406, or a β_2 subtype–selective agonist, such as zinterol, procaterol, or antagonist ICI 118151. Many antagonists, such as propranolol, alprenolol and pindolol, are nonselective. This strategy can be applied in vivo with PET. β_1-adrenergic antagonists appear to inhibit catecholamine action simply by occupying the β-adrenergic receptor and thus blocking the access of agonists to the receptor. Therefore, it is expected that agonists such as isoproterenol (a nonsubtype-selective agonist) or dobutamine (a β_1 subtype–selective agonist) would interact with a β-receptor in a different manner than that of antagonists since agonists promote physiologic changes and antagonists do not.[S6]

Positron Emission Tomography Investigation of β-Adrenergic Receptors

Four antagonists (propranolol, practolol, pindolol, and CGP 12 177) have been labeled with ^{11}C.[B2, B3, P1, B4] They differ in affinity, liposolubility and subtype-selectivity. It has been shown previously that ^{11}C-propranolol, a lipophilic nonselective antagonist could not be used for studying the β-adrenergic receptor with PET because it accumulates in the lungs after intravenous injection during the time of PET scanning. ^{11}C-practolol is a hydrophilic molecule that binds on homogenates to β_1-receptors. A few minutes after intravenous injection in humans, the heart is well visualized but the tracer concentration decreases rapidly with time, even when ^{11}C-practolol is injected at very high specific activity.[D1] The percentage of bound tracer that could be displaced by injection of an excess of unlabeled antagonist (practolol, propranolol, atenolol, pindolol) 20 minutes later was also low. Both results can be explained by the relatively low affinity of practolol (high K_D).

^{11}C-pindolol and ^{11}C-CGP 12177 have in common a high affinity (low K_D) and a low lipophilicity. ^{11}C-CGP 12177 presents the greatest advantages. It is a very potent hydrophilic β-blocker. It is usually considered to have no β-adrenoceptor subtype selectivity. However, a β_1-subtype–selectivity has recently been demonstrated on rat ventricular microsomes.[N1] The equilibrium dissociation constant K_D for β_1-adrenoceptors was 0.33 nmol, whereas the K_D for β_2-adrenoceptors was 0.90 nmol, suggesting a two- to threefold β_1-selectivity of ^{3}H-CGP 12177. This selectivity was identified by saturation binding in a tissue containing both β_1- and β_2-adrenoceptors under conditions in which subtype was blocked.[N1] The low β_1-selectivity of CGP 12177 cannot be detected in usual saturation binding studies because the two classes of binding sites must differ in their affinity by at least five- to sevenfold to be separately identified.[B9] It is therefore justified to consider that ^{11}C-CGP 12177 binds in vivo to a single class of myocardial β-adrenergic receptors.

Another interesting aspect of this ligand is its little nonspecific binding on membranes and little cellular uptake.[S10, S11] In addition, CGP 12177 does not bind to receptors that are removed from the plasma membrane and are internalized during short-term desensitization.[H4] Desensitization of adenylate cyclase is divided into two major categories. Homologous desensitization leads to sequestration of receptors away from the cell surface.[S12] These sequestered receptors can rapidly recycle to the cell surface or, with time, become down-regulated, being destroyed within the cell. In heterologous desensitization, receptor function is also regulated by phosphorylation by a β-adrenergic receptor kinase but receptors are neither sequestered nor down-regulated. Phosphorylation serves only to functionally uncouple the receptors; that is, to impair their interactions with the guanine nucleotide regulatory protein N_s.[S12] By using ^{3}H-CGP 12177, which is not taken up into intact cells, short-term homologous desensitization of β-adrenergic receptors was demonstrated in C6-glioma cells. Incubation of C6-cells with the agonist isoprenaline at 37°C for 15 to 20 minutes resulted in a 50 percent decrease in the number of binding sites of ^{3}H-CGP 12177, which paralleled the decrease in hormone-stimulated adenylate cyclase activity.[H4] Separation of the β-adrenergic receptors on a sucrose gradient showed that the loss of ^{3}H-CGP 12177 binding was related to a sequestration of receptors in a vesicular cell compartment that was accessible to the more hydrophobic antagonist ^{3}H-dihydroalprenolol but not to ^{3}H-CGP 12177. It must be noted that CGP 12177 also has a slight partial agonist effect. This hydrophilic β-adrenergic ligand that is not taken up by cells is, therefore, an ideal probe to specifically measure in vivo the cell surface receptors, i.e., the functionally active β-receptors.

A high myocardial uptake was measured after ^{11}C-pindolol or ^{11}C-CGP 12177 injection (Fig. 69–6), and a displacement of both bound tracers was obtained after injection of an excess of cold pindolol.[S7] Figure 69–3 shows a displacement of bound ^{11}C-CGP by an excess of cold CGP injected 25 minutes after the radiotracer. Saturation of the β-adrenergic receptor can also be demonstrated by a preinjection of an unlabeled β-blocker a few minutes before the injection of ^{11}C-CGP (see Fig. 69–4). The preinjection reduces the number of unoccupied receptor sites available for the binding of radiotracer. Therefore, compared with the control curve, the radioactive concentration measured in the ventricular myocardium is lower (see Fig. 69–4). Figure 69–3 also shows the correlation observed between the tracer displacement and the decrease in heart rate induced by the displacing agent. The validation of this important criterion is a strong indication that receptor sites, not only binding sites, are visualized.

Figure 69–6. See Color Plate 18.

Myocardial β-adrenergic receptor density has been found to differ among species: B_{max} = 152, 150, and 311 fmol/mg protein in rat, rabbit, and dog, respectively, using ^{3}H-DHA as ligand.[M6] β-Adrenoceptor density has been also measured in biopsies of the human left ventricle and found to vary between 30 fmol · mg^{-1} and 79 fmol · mg^{-1} using ^{125}I-cyanopindolol.[G2, H2, S8] β-Adrenergic receptor density has been measured in the ventricular myocardium of the dog by PET. From 39 measurements of CGP 12177 concentrations performed in different dogs after injection of various amounts of tracer (between 0.4 and 300 nmol/kg of weight), it was possible to calculate the receptor density by fitting experimental data close to equilibrium according to Equation 18. B'_{max} was found to be 113 pmol/g of tissue. The presence of β-adrenergic receptors in the ventricles of all studied species is consistent with the findings that sympathetic nerve fibers innervate all regions of the heart.[T1] In addition to the heterogeneity of binding sites with coexistence of about 50 percent of β_1- and 50 percent of β_2-adrenergic receptors in the human heart, there is a heterogeneous distribution of β-adrenoceptors in the heart. The density is greatest in the apex of the left ventricle in different species.[L4, W4] However, the norepinephrine distribution follows a gradient from base (maximum) to apex; areas of high tissue norepinephrine also represent regions rich in adrenergic supply and of high adrenergic activity.[P5] Therefore, discrepancies seem to exist between regional β-receptor density and reported catecholamine content or sympathetic innervation.[W4] These findings need further investigation in in vivo conditions in the human heart. Because of its larger size relative to that in most experimental animals, the human heart can be evaluated more conveniently and accurately with the high resolution PET systems, that are now available. The new positron-labeled false adrenergic transmitters, ^{18}F-fluorometaraminol and ^{11}C-hydroxyephedrine, could be markers for adrenergic nerves and could be used in the quantitative assessment of neuronal density in the human heart.[W8, W9]

Measurement of the association and dissociation rate constant values is based on the kinetic model shown on Figure 69–5. Quantification of receptors is based on accurate measurement of the arterial input function $C_a^*(t)$ in Equation 14. Very rapid sampling during the peak of activity following the injection of a ^{11}C-labeled tracer is now possible with the new time-of-flight PET systems capable of handling very high count rates concentrated within small regions. It is also possible to measure the ligand blood concentration in a ventricular region of interest without collecting arterial blood samples from a catheter inserted in the radial artery. The ^{11}C-blood radioactivity must then be transformed into ^{11}C-CGP 12177 plasma concentration. ^{11}C-CGP 12177 that has bound to red blood cells and the presence of metabolites in plasma have been determined in dog blood samples rapidly collected at various times from 0 to 60 minutes after injection. A fraction of ^{11}C-CGP 12177 binds to red blood cells; in addition, the ligand is rapidly metabolized. Identification of ^{11}C-labeled metabolites using over-pressure thin-layer chromatography (OPTLC) has shown that only about 10 percent of the ligand remains unchanged in plasma five minutes after intravenous injection. Thus, true ^{11}C-CGP 12177 input function differs strongly from the measured radioactive blood concentration. Preliminary results indicate that the best mathematical model that accounts for ^{11}C-CGP kinetics is the three-compartment model using the assumption of no dissociation of bound ligand ($k_{-1} = 0$). The association rate constant k_{+1} is 0.3 $nmol^{-1} \cdot min^{-1}$. In in vitro experiments at 37°C (98.6°F) with C6-glioma cell membranes and ^{3}H-CGP 12177, k_{+1} was 0.2 $nmol^{-1} \cdot min^{-1}$.[S10] In the same conditions, the k_{-1} value was 0.03 min^{-1} and the K_D was 0.2 nmol. A similar K_D value (0.3 nmol) was found in binding studies with intact cells.[S10] It is important to notice that the nonspecific binding has always been found to be low in these studies, probably because of the hydrophilic properties of CGP 12177.[P6, S10]

In Vivo Study of α-Adrenergic Receptors

α-Adrenergic receptors also have been classified into two subtypes, α_1 and α_2.[M2, M4, S6] The α_1-receptors are the classical postsynaptic α-receptors mediating smooth muscle contraction. α_2-Receptors are found in several locations, particularly on presynaptic nerve terminals, where they mediate feedback inhibition of norepinephrine release. The α_1- and α_2-receptors can be distinguished pharmacologically by their relative affinities for various agonists and antagonists. Yohimbine shows a high selectivity for α_2-adrenergic receptors, whereas prazosin demonstrates a 1,000- to 10,000-fold selectivity for α_1-adrenergic receptors. Much less information is available for α-adrenoreceptors than for β-adrenoreceptors.[M2]

Prazosin, a selective α_1-adrenergic blocker, was labeled with ^{11}C and injected into dogs.[E1] PET scans showed a high and homogeneous myocardial uptake with a much lower pulmonary uptake. However, the validation of criteria needed for the characterization of receptors could not be achieved probably because nonspecific binding was too high.

CHARACTERIZATION OF CARDIAC MUSCARINIC ACETYLCHOLINE RECEPTORS BY POSITRON EMISSION TOMOGRAPHY

Distribution and Subtypes of Muscarinic Cholinergic Receptors

The neurotransmitters acetylcholine and norepinephrine exert their chronotropic and inotropic effects on the heart by an opposite coupling of the cholinergic and β-adrenergic receptors to adenylate cyclase; β-adrenoceptors activate adenylate cyclase, whereas muscarinic cholinergic receptors inhibit it.[N2] The cholinergic receptor was historically the first receptor in which subtypes were clearly delineated. However, many classifications have been proposed.[H1] Currently, the accepted scheme is that muscarinic receptors exist in two subtypes. The M_1-subclass is defined as those receptors exhibiting a high affinity toward the antagonist pirenzepine, whereas the M_2-subclass is defined as those receptors exhibiting a low affinity toward pirenzepine.[H5] The high-affinity (M_1) sites are thought to be primarily located in the central nervous system, whereas the low-affinity (M_2) sites are thought to be mainly located on peripheral effector organs. Muscarinic receptors in the heart are thus considered to belong to the M_2 type. More recently, development of AF-DX 116, a new M_2-antagonist, has led to the suggestion that M_2-receptors may be subdivided further into two classes: one with high affinity for AF-DX 116 and one with low affinity.[G3, H6] Cardiac receptors have a high affinity for AF-DX 116 (M_2-subclass). Three subtypes of muscarinic receptors have thus now been proposed and are called M_1, M_2, and M_3. They can be differentiated on the basis of their affinity for pirenzepine, AF-DX 116, 4 DAMP, and dicyclomine.[D4] The existence of several subtypes of muscarinic receptors has been confirmed by cloning and sequencing DNA genes that code the receptor proteins.[B7, F5] The primary structure of a cardiac M_2-receptor from the porcine atria has recently been demonstrated.[P4] The amino acids sequence differs in neuronal M_1-receptor from porcine brain and in cardiac M_2-receptor, each receptor being clearly distinct mainly in the 5-6 loop of the cytoplasmic region.[F5, P4]

Attention must also be paid to vascular muscarinic receptors, because PET cannot localize acetylcholine receptors within the myocardium. Therefore, it is important to be able to characterize muscular and vascular receptors pharmacologically. Two different muscarinic effects have been demonstrated. Relaxation responses to cholinergic agonists are mediated by an action of acetylcholine on the endothelium to release a vasodilator substance: endothelium-dependent releasing factor (EDRF).[F6] The relaxation response to metacholine of rabbit ear artery has shown that the endothelial-dependent muscarinic receptors have a low affinity for the M_1-antagonist pirenzepine.[H7] However, these vascular receptors also have a low affinity for the cardioselective antagonist AF-DX 116. Other vessels respond to cholinergic agonists with a contractile response also mediated by muscarinic receptors.[O1] The bovine coronary artery displays both the endothelial-dependent relaxation response and the endothelial-independent contractile response involving vascular smooth muscle. Receptors mediating these effects have the same properties: they show low affinity for pirenzepine and AF-DX 116, and the putative M_1-selective agonist McN-A-343 produces no effect in either tissue.[D5] Thus, vascular muscarinic receptors appear to be distinct from myocardial receptors. They could belong in a same subclass of M_2-receptors; further studies are needed to determine whether or not they conform to the M_3-subclass. However, a new study suggests that porcine artery contains both M_1 and M_2 subtypes.[Y2] On the other hand, binding studies and functional assays also indicate heterogeneity for muscarinic receptors in the myocardium.[W5] Binding experiments with pirenzepine show that there is a population of muscarinic receptors in myocardium that could well be designated as M_1-receptors. Chick myocardium has a predominance of M_1-receptors in contrast to rat heart.[B10]

The most commonly used radiolabeled muscarinic antagonists, quinuclidinyl benzylate (^{3}H-QNB) and N-methylscopolamine (^{3}H-

NMS) appear to recognize identical populations of muscarinic receptors. The presence of a population of specific, saturable, high-affinity acetylcholine receptors in the mammalian heart was identified by the use of ^{3}H-QNB.[F2] The binding is saturable in vitro by increasing ligand concentration and is consistent with the mass action law for a single class of receptors. QNB does not differentiate between the M_1- and M_2-receptor subtypes. Competition curves for antagonists at the ^{3}H-QNB–labeled muscarinic sites are monophasic and are not affected by guanine nucleotides. In contrast, the competition curves for muscarinic agonists are biphasic, indicating the presence of high and low affinity states of the receptors.

When the same ligand was used to label intact cells instead of membrane preparations, a higher nonspecific binding prevented by methylamine suggested a trapping of the ligand within the cells, presumably into the lysosomes. The same results were found with ^{3}H-dexetimide.[G4] It has been very recently shown that ^{3}H-QNB labels significantly more sites than do two other hydrophilic muscarinic antagonists, ^{3}H-NMS and ^{3}H-MQNB (N-methyl QNB), the quaternary derivative of ^{3}H-QNB.[B11] It has been suggested that the subset of receptors detected only by ^{3}H-QNB are also muscarinic receptors, but that they probably do not participate in the physiologic responses, probably because they are sequestered in a hydrophobic compartment within the cell membrane.[B11]

It has been inferred from numerous functional studies that vascular muscarinic receptors mediating relaxation could be localized to endothelial cells. However, autoradiographic studies using either ^{3}H-QNB or ^{125}I-QNB demonstrated no binding sites over endothelial cells, whereas specific binding was seen over the smooth muscle cells.[S13] Furthermore, it has been observed that cultured endothelial cells do not have muscarinic binding sites.[P7]

Positron Emission Tomographic Investigation of Muscarinic Cholinergic Receptors

The studies reviewed earlier strengthen the rationale for the choice of labeling MQNB with ^{11}C to study the muscarinic acetylcholine receptor in vivo by PET.[M1] MQNB is a hydrophilic antagonist that is not extracted by the lungs and that displays a high affinity for the cholinergic receptors in rat heart homogenates: $K_D = 0.32$ nmol, $B_{max} = 228$ fmol/mg of protein.[S14] Analysis of in vitro kinetics of ^{3}H-MQNB binding gave a k_{+1} value of 2.73 $nmol^{-1} \cdot min^{-1}$ and a dissociation rate constant k_{-1} of 0.81 min^{-1}. All the criteria needed to characterize the muscarinic receptor were validated in the baboon and in the human with ^{11}C-MQNB. The ventricular septum and the left ventricle contained high concentrations of ^{11}C-MQNB, the radioactivity in the right ventricle was very low, and the atria were never visualized. Saturation experiments showed that the highest concentrations were found in the septum (98 pmol/g of heart) and in the left ventricle (89 pmol/g).[S14] It is reasonable to think that although the receptor concentration could be higher in atria than in ventricles,[F2] ventricle and septum contain a higher percentage of acetylcholine receptors than atria because of their greater weight.

The parasympathetic innervation of the heart is provided by efferent preganglionic parasympathetic neurons in the medulla oblongata, which project axons onto the heart where they synapse with efferent postganglionic parasympathetic neurons that innervate the heart. The perikarya of neurons in or on the heart have been considered to be primarily efferent postganglionic cholinergic parasympathetic neurons.[A1, B12] Muscarinic receptors have been identified on them by autoradiography.[H8] Although the existence of an abundant parasympathetic innervation of the atria is well known, that of the ventricles has been a subject of controversy. Both histologic and physiologic data were generally considered to indicate an absence of ventricular parasympathetic innervation, but in the past decade, numerous data, both chemical and physiological, have proved the existence of a direct parasympathetic innervation of the mammalian ventricle.[L5] Intraventricular parasympathetic ganglion cells are sparsely distributed in ventricular myocardium, if they exist at all.[N3, T1] However, it has been recently demonstrated that the primary vagal innervation of the canine ventricles is by way of postganglionic cholinergic axones whose cell bodies of origin are in the atria.[B12, T2] Long postganglionic axons cross the atrioventricular groove to innervate the ventricular myocardium. The ventricular muscarinic receptors seem to be localized in sarcolemma in dog;[M7] their precise role in the modulation of biochemical and electrophysiologic events at the cellular level remains a subject of considerable interest. Evidence of the presence of M_1- and M_2-receptors in the coronary vasculature of the dog has also been found recently. It has been suggested that M_1-muscarinic coronary receptors are responsible for the redistribution of blood flow to the subendocardium during cholinergic coronary vasodilatation, whereas both M_1- and M_2-receptors are involved in increasing myocardial perfusion.[P8] However, as discussed earlier, measurement of antagonist affinities indicates that the bovine coronary artery muscarinic receptors show low affinity for both pirenzepine and AF-DX 116, suggesting that they could be classified as M_3-receptors.[D5] Displacement studies with PET have been performed in dogs using various amounts of unlabeled pirenzepine and AF-DX 116. No displacement of bound ^{11}C-MQNB was observed after injection of pirenzepine (1 mg), whereas 25 percent of the radioactivity was displaced after injection of the same dose of AF-DX 116 (unpublished data). These in vivo results with PET suggest that M_1-receptors are not detectable in the adult dog heart.

Saturability of the binding was demonstrated by saturation experiments. After a bolus injection of ^{11}C-MQNB at a high-specific activity in a brachial vein in humans, the ^{11}C-MQNB blood concentration fell very rapidly to a negligible value a few minutes after intravenous injection (see Fig. 69–2). In contrast, the ^{11}C-MQNB concentration increased rapidly in the myocardium to reach a maximum in one to five minutes and then remained constant for 70 minutes. The rapid intravenous injection of unlabeled atropine led to a rapid decrease (lasting a few minutes) in the septal ^{11}C-MQNB concentration. The maximal percentage of ^{11}C-MQNB that could be displaced in dog was 94 percent. Atropine does not differentiate between muscarinic receptor subtypes of heart, brain, or glands,[G5] therefore, one can consider that less than 6 percent of ^{11}C-MQNB bound in the dog or human heart corresponds to nonspecific binding. This binding is stereospecific since dexetimide (the pharmacologically active isomer) but not levetimide can displace ^{11}C-MQNB from its binding site.[M1] A correlation between receptor occupancy and a physiologic effect also has been demonstrated;[S14] Figure 69–7 demonstrates a relationship between the percentage of MQNB found in 1 cm^3 of septum after rapid intravenous injection in 12

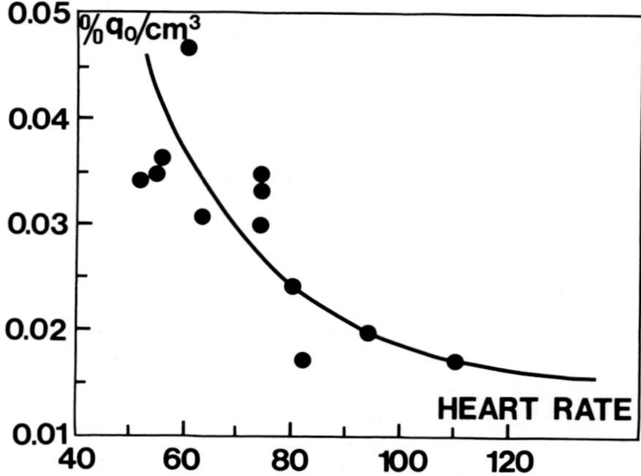

Figure 69–7. Dependence of ^{11}C-MQNB concentration in the ventricular septum on heart rate. In 12 individuals, the percentage of the injected dose present in 1 cm^3 of septum is plotted as a function of heart rate (expressed in beats per min) recorded at the time of ^{11}C-MQNB injection. The uptake of ^{11}C-MQNB is higher in subjects with lower heart rate at the time of injection.

subjects injected with comparable amounts of MQNB and the heart rate value recorded at the time of injection. For a given subject, the MQNB concentration in the ventricular septum was higher when the heart rate was lower. This result is apparently surprising, since muscarinic receptor function in the ventricle should be related to inotropic effects rather than to chronotropic effects. However, very recent results have shown that the ventricles primarily receive postganglionic cholinergic fibers from ganglion cells localized in the atria.[T2] The release of acetylcholine at parasympathetic nerve endings in the ventricles would thus depend on the activity of atrial cells mediating both the atrial chronotropic and the ventricular inotropic effects. A low frequency is related to a predominant vagal influence. The greater amount of ^{11}C-MQNB in the septum linked to vagal stimulation could be explained by an increase in either the number or the affinity of antagonist binding sites. In the physiologically active state, the agonist is released from the receptor in a low-affinity form, and more sites are available for ^{11}C-MQNB binding.[C6] The presence of two interconvertible forms of the muscarinic cholinergic receptor respectively favored by agonists and antagonists and displaying high-agonist/low-antagonist and low-agonist/high-antagonist affinities, respectively, has been demonstrated.[B13] According to this hypothesis, vagal stimulation would be characterized by a conversion to the low-agonist/high-antagonist affinity form of the muscarinic receptor. These findings suggest that PET allows the identification of the physiologically active conformation of the muscarinic receptor under sympathetic and parasympathetic physiologic control.[S14]

Binding characteristics of N-methyl scopolamine, atropine, pirenzepine, and AF-DX 116 have recently been measured in membranes of atria and ventricle from postmortem human tissue.[G5] The selectivity profiles of pirenzepine and AF-DX 116 previously described in rat tissues were confirmed in human tissues. The K_D values for ^{3}H-AF-DX 116 in atria and ventricle were 183 nmol and 174 nmol, respectively; it was much higher for ^{3}H-pirenzepine: 1021 nmol in atria and 760 nmol in ventricle. Rate constants and B_{max} values for ^{11}C-MQNB binding to cardiac muscarinic receptors have been calculated in six dogs using the three-compartment model described previously in displacement experiments with an excess of unlabeled MQNB.[D7] The association rate constant k_{+1} was 0.6 ± 0.1 nmol^{-1} · min^{-1}, the dissociation rate constant was 0.27 ± 0.03 min^{-1}, thus giving a K_D of 0.49 ± 0.14 nmol. The receptor density B_{max} was 42 ± 11 pmol per cm^3 of tissue. These values can be compared with those obtained in vitro in rat heart homogenates with ^{3}H-MQNB.[S14] The k_{+1}, k_{-1}, and K_D values were 2.73 nmol^{-1} · min^{-1}, 0.81 min^{-1}, and 0.3 nmol, respectively. The receptor density was 228 fmol/mg of protein. The dissociation rate constants for ^{3}H-QNB in intact chicken heart (0.33 min^{-1})[G6] and in embryonic chicken heart cell cultures (0.27 min^{-1})[G7] were also of the same order of magnitude as those measured in vivo with ^{11}C-MQNB and PET.

The receptor density calculated in each dog from the analysis of kinetic data (42 pmol/cm^3 of tissue) is also of the same order of magnitude as that previously obtained from saturation studies with ^{3}H-MQNB (98 pmol/cm^3 of tissue).[S14] In a recent study, analysis of ^{3}H-QNB saturation isotherms indicates B_{max} value of 9 pmol/g of wet weight of tissue in rat heart.[S15]

The advantage of using the kinetic model is that B_{max} can be obtained in a single experiment if a displacement of bound ^{11}C-MQNB by an excess of cold MQNB is performed 20 minutes later.[D7] In contrast, 34 separate experiments were needed to plot the ^{11}C-MQNB septal concentrations against the amount of MQNB injected.[S14]

It was found that ^{3}H-QNB bound to the muscarinic receptor by a two-step mechanism consistent with the formation of a low-affinity complex followed by conversion to a high-affinity complex.[G6, G7] These data can be explained by a fast-binding step followed by a slower isomerization of the receptor-antagonist complex.[J1] In displacement experiments, one should observe different dissociation rates, depending on the moment when the excess of unlabeled ligand is added. In three experiments performed in the same dog, the same amount of atropine was injected 5 minutes, 30 minutes, and 105 minutes after injection of a traced dose of ^{11}C-MQNB. The percentage of bound radioligand displaced was identical in all experiments, suggesting that no isomerization of the MQNB-muscarinic receptor complex occurs in vivo.[S14] A similar study performed in vitro with ^{3}H-QNB has been recently published.[E2] The QNB-complex dissociation reaction followed a mono-exponential kinetics if the ^{3}H-QNB-receptor complex had been incubated for a long time (more than one hour) before the excess of the nonradioactive ligand was added to displace the radioactive ligand from the complex. In contrast, the dissociation curve was bi-exponential with a rapid first slope if the displacement was started a few minutes after the complex formation.[E2] This discrepancy between our in vivo observations with PET and these in vitro data might be explained by an internalization or a trapping of the lipophilic ligand QNB.[G4] MQNB, the N-methyl quaternary salt of QNB, is highly hydrophilic and, like CGP 12177,[S11] would bind only to cell surface receptors.

CHARACTERIZATION OF THE PERIPHERAL-TYPE BENZODIAZEPINE RECEPTOR

Specific high-affinity benzodiazepine binding sites have been demonstrated in several peripheral organs including the heart.[D6, T3] The ligand specificity and affinity for the peripheral-type binding site is completely different from that of the central-type site.[T4] The demonstration of peripheral-type benzodiazepine binding sites was first made in vitro with ^{3}H-diazepam.[D6] New ligands that only bind to peripheral-type sites and not to the classical central type have been synthesized. RO 5-4864 and PK 11195 are almost inactive in binding inhibition of ^{3}H-diazepam on its sites in the brain but have a very high affinity for peripheral sites.[L6, L7] In vitro, the PK 11195 binding sites in rat cardiac membranes are specific, saturable with a K_D of 1.41 nmol and a B_{max} of 2250 pmol/g of protein.[L6, L7] PK 11195 was labeled with ^{11}C at very high specific activity[C3] and injected intravenously in dogs and humans. An initial uptake of ^{11}C-PK 11195 was seen in the lung, followed by a high uptake in the heart. Benzodiazepine binding sites were uniformly distributed.[C7] The amount of PK 11195 found in the heart was proportional to the quantity injected at values below 40 nmol/kg. Above 40 nmol/kg, however, the curve showed a plateau due to saturation of the benzodiazepine binding sites. This result agrees with the mathematical model of a ligand-receptor interaction studied in vivo.[S5] A similar curve was also obtained when studying the muscarinic acetylcholine receptor.[S14] From the PK 11195 concentration values, the number of benzodiazepine binding sites in the dog ventricular myocardium (B_{max}) was found to be around 6000 pmol/cm^3 of heart. Other criteria needed for identification of a ligand receptor interaction by PET were validated. Saturability was demonstrated by coinjection or displacement experiments with unlabeled PK 11195 and other ligands that compete for peripheral-type sites such as RO 5-4864 and diazepam. Ligands that only bind to sites resembling the brain, such as RO 15-1788 and clonazepam, were ineffective.[C7] The physiologic function of these receptors is still largely unknown. Recent studies have shown that PK 11195 binds to the mitochondrial outer membrane.[A2] In cardiac muscle and vascular smooth muscle, benzodiazepines have been shown to interfere with Ca^{++} movements. PK 11195 antagonizes the effects of several calcium channel blockers (diltiazem, nitrendipine, verapamil) and a calcium channel agonist (BAY K 8644) in a guinea pig papillary muscle preparation.[M8] It also inhibits arrythmias induced by ischemia and abnormalities after reperfusion in the dog heart.[M9] It has been recently shown that the peripheral-type benzodiazepine receptor antagonists RO 5-4864 and PK 11195 increase coronary flow in isolated retrograde perfused Langendorff rat heart preparations.[G8] A subpopulation of peripheral benzodiazepine receptors could also be associated with catecholaminergic neurons.[B14] Chemical sympathectomy increases B_{max} in the left ventricle (34 percent) one week after administration of 6-hydroxydopamine or reserpine. A PET study of these receptors in humans could thus be interesting in clinical situations.

CLINICAL APPLICATIONS

Functional and Pharmacologic Investigations

PET has only recently begun to be applied to the study of cardiac physiology and disease. It is the only technical method able to demonstrate the physiologic regulation of receptors. Receptors are dynamic entities regulated by a variety of pathophysiologic states.[M4] Treatment of cells or animals with agonists or antagonists influences the number of receptors. Agonist treatment leads to down-regulation (decrease in receptor density) and antagonist treatment leads to up-regulation. Prolonged exposure of tissue to catecholamines, acetylcholine, or carbamylcholine increases the number of β-adrenergic or muscarinic cholinergic receptors in the ventricular myocardium.[G9]

Changes in muscarinic cholinergic receptors with thyroid status have been observed in myocardial membranes of hypothyroid and hyperthyroid rats. Muscarinic receptor density was found to be increased by 58 percent in thyroidectomized rats and moderately decreased (20 percent) in rats injected with triodothyronine.[S16] In another study, a large increase in high-affinity binding sites (60 percent) and a decrease in low-affinity binding sites (30 percent) were seen in rats receiving PTU.[R2] In rats injected with L-thyroxine, there was a moderate decrease in both high-affinity binding sites (18 percent) and low-affinity binding sites (36 percent). An in vivo study using ^{11}C-MQNB and PET was performed in six patients with hypothyroidism and in six patients with hyperthyroidism.[S17] An increase in the number of high-affinity binding sites for acetylcholine was also found in patients with hypothyroidism, but no significant change was found in patients with hyperthyroidism,[S17] suggesting a direct effect of thyroid hormones on heart rate.[H9, K2, M10]

Many cardiovascular drugs influence synaptic mechanisms to elicit their therapeutic effects. They can influence neurotransmitter systems in several ways. They may interfere with synthesizing or degrading enzymes, alter the storage or release of the transmitter, or mimic or block the actions of neurotransmitters at receptor sites. The increased chronotropic sensitivity to isoproterenol in pigs is consequent to an up-regulation of β-adrenergic receptors in the right atrium.[H10] Treatment with β-blocking agents causes up-regulation of human myocardial β-receptor density. Among these agents, pindolol, a drug with intrinsic sympathomimetic activity, seems to favor up-regulation.[G10] Dysopyramide and quinidine exercise their anticholinergic effects by blocking cardiac muscarinic receptors in canine ventricular myocardium.[M11] Cocaine inhibits M_2 muscarinic cholinergic binding measured with ^{3}H-QNB in rat heart tissue and can act as an antimuscarinic agent, particularly at higher, toxic doses.[S15] Halothane decreases ^{11}C-CGP 12177 binding to dog myocardial tissue.[S18] In the future, measurement of in vivo receptor occupancy will allow us to predict extent and duration of effects of β-blockers. It will be possible to establish equivalently effective doses of β-blockers with different pharmacodynamic profiles in humans. In vitro studies with ^{3}H-CGP 12177 have proved the value of such studies in clinical pharmacology.[W6]

Clinical Investigations

PET could also be used to investigate changes in receptor number and affinity in cardiac diseases. Experimental studies have shown that coronary occlusion for 30 minutes to 1 hour is associated with an increase in the density of α- and β-adrenoceptors,[M12, M13, O2] whereas adenylate cyclase activity decreases progressively.[F7, V2] β-Adrenergic receptor density increases during relatively early stages of injury in metabolically impaired myocytes and decreases subsequently.[B15] This increase in receptors may account for the enhanced effects of catecholamines in the ischemic heart. The increased β-adrenoceptor density in moderately injured myocytes can be reversed on removal of the injurious agent and the restoration of the cellular ATP level.[M13] However, the mechanism mediating this up-regulation of receptors is unknown. Recent data provide evidence that β-adrenergic receptors of the heart may exist in several cellular environments, including the plasma membrane and an intracellular membrane location. During myocardial ischemia, β-adrenergic receptors could be redistributed from intracellular vesicles to sarcolemmal membranes.[M14] Since CGP 12177 recognizes cell surface β-adrenergic receptors and cannot be internalized unlike other lipophilic ligands,[H4] one may speculate that ^{11}C-CGP could be the ideal ligand to follow the receptor changes in patients with ischemic disease. There is no evidence of increased β-adrenergic receptor density after chronic canine myocardial infarction.[K3]

β_1- and β_2-receptor subtypes have been studied in congestive heart failure.[B16, B17, F8] Failing human ventricular myocardium shows a decrease in the β_1 proportion and an increase in the β_2 proportion owing to selective down-regulation of β_1-receptors.[B18, F9, V3] In dystrophic soleus muscle from CHF 147 dystrophic hamsters, the number of β-adrenergic receptors was elevated, suggesting that these receptors could be implicated in the pathogenesis of hamster cardiomyopathy.[W7] The number of β-receptors also increased twofold in an experimental animal model of cardiomyopathy.[R3] In patients with mitral valve disease, a significantly higher β-adrenoceptor density has been described in atrial than in ventricular myocardium. The relative proportions of β_1- and β_2- receptors were unchanged compared with normals, but the adenylate cyclase response to β-adrenergic agonists was higher in ventricular than in atrial tissue.[G11]

Cardiac β-receptor sensitivity to isoprenaline of the denervated donor heart has been compared with that of the innervated recipient heart.[H3] The observations are consistent with an increase in β-receptor density and probably no change in β-receptor affinity.[L8, Y3] Athletic training and diabetes reduce β-adrenergic receptor density. A decreased sensitivity of adenylate cyclase to isoproterenol stimulation is also observed after four weeks of experimentally induced diabetes.[A3]

Future Prospects

Binding of neurotransmitter to receptor is an essential step in synaptic transmission. The interaction between agonist and receptor leads to a cascade of molecular events via the second messenger system, culminating in the observed response. This series of molecular interactions has been shown to be altered in several cardiac diseases. However, there is also a complex sequence of events that takes place between the nerve terminal and the postsynaptic neuron or the cardiac muscle cell. It includes synthesis and release of neurotransmitter, binding to receptor, hydrolysis of neurotransmitter in the synaptic cleft, and reuptake of neurotransmitter. Several pathologic and therapeutic concepts in cardiology have been based on sympathetic neuroeffector mechanisms in the heart. A limitation in evaluating these concepts has been the inability to measure cardiac sympathetic function in vivo, especially the activity of the neuronal uptake process (uptake-1). A false adrenergic transmitter, metaraminol, has recently been labeled with ^{18}F for use in heart neuronal uptake determination by PET.[M16] ^{18}F-fluorometaraminol uptake is decreased following regional denervation of the dog heart.[W8] Postmortem measurements showed that norepinephrine and fluorometaraminol concentrations correlated closely over the entire dog heart. Another new molecule, ^{11}C-hydroxyephedrine, the N-methyl derivative of metaraminol, is also under investigation.[W9] In the near future, it should be possible to evaluate in vivo both adrenergic innervation and adrenergic receptors.

Thus, through a noninvasive method, PET is able to provide information not only on cardiac receptor density and affinity but also on the physiologically active form of the receptor under physiologic regulation in humans. It shows the interactions between drugs acting on the heart and myocardial receptors. One can, therefore, anticipate its value in the investigation of cardiac ischemia and cardiomyopathy in humans.

Acknowledgments

The author wishes to thank C. Crouzel and the cyclotron and chemistry staff, including K. Nakajima, M. Seto, B. Mazière, C. Loc'h, J. Delforge, B. Mazoyer, and the technicians, for their collaboration. The author is indebted to the skilled secretarial assistance of N. De Blecker for the preparation of the manuscript.

References

A

1. Ardell, J.L., and Randall, W.C.: Selective vagal innervation of sinoatrial and atrioventricular nodes in canine heart. Am. J. Physiol. (Heart Circ. Physiol. 20) 251:H764–H773, 1986.
2. Anholt, R.R.H., Pedersen, P.L., De Souza, E.B., and Snyder, S.H.: The peripheral-type benzodiazepine receptor. J. Biol. Chem. 261:576–583, 1986.
3. Atkins, F.L., Dowell, R.T., and Love, S.: β-Adrenergic receptors, adenylate cyclase activity, and cardiac dysfunction in the diabetic rat. J. Cardiovasc. Res. 7:66–70, 1985.

B

1. Bergman, S.R., Fox, K.A.A., Geltman, E.M., and Sobel, B.E.: Positron emission tomography of the heart. Progr. Cardiovasc. Dis. 28:165–194, 1985.
2. Berger, G., Mazière, M., Prenant, C., et al.: Synthesis of ^{11}C propranolol. J. Radioanal. Chem. 74:301–306, 1982.
3. Berger, G., Prenant, C., Sastre, J., et al.: Synthesis of a β-blocker for heart visualization: [^{11}C]practolol. Int. J. Appl. Radiat. Isot. 34:1556–1557, 1983.
4. Boullais, C., Crouzel, C., and Syrota, A.: Synthesis of 4-(3-t-butylamino-2-hydroxypropoxy)-benzimidazol-2(^{11}C)-one (CGP 12177). J. Label Compds. Radiopharm. 23:565–567, 1986.
5. Berridge, M., Comar, D., Crouzel, C., and Baron, J.C.: ^{11}C-labelled ketanserin, a selective serotonin S_2 antagonist. J. Label Compds. Radiopharm. 20:73–78, 1983.
6. Bennet, J.P., Jr.: Methods in binding studies. *In* Yamamura, H.I., Enna, S.J., and Kuhar, M.J. (eds.): Neurotransmitter Receptor Binding. Raven Press, New York, pp. 57–90, 1978.
7. Bonner, T.I., Buckley, N.J., Young, A.C., and Brann, M.R.: Identification of a family of muscarinic acetylcholine receptor genes. Science 237:527–532, 1987.
8. Buxton, I.L.O., and Brunton, L.L.:Direct analysis of β-adrenergic receptor subtypes on intact adult ventricular myocytes of the rat. Circ. Res. 56:126–132, 1985.
9. Burgisser, E.: Model testing in radioligand-receptor interaction by Monte Carlo simulations. J. Rec. Res. 3:261–281, 1983.
10. Brown, J.H., Goldstein, D., and Masters, S.H.: The putative M_1 muscarinic receptor does not regulate phosphoinositide hydrolysis: Studies with pirenzepine and McN A 343 in chick heart and astrocytoma cells. Mol. Pharmacol. 27:525–531, 1985.
11. Brown, J.H., and Goldstein, D.: Analysis of cardiac muscarinic receptors recognized selectively by nonquaternary but not by quaternary ligands. J. Pharmacol. Exp. Ther. 238:580–586, 1986.
12. Blomquist, T.M., Priola, D.V., and Romero, A.M.: Source of intrinsic innervation of canine ventricles: A functional study. Am. J. Physiol. (Heart Circ. Physiol. 21) 252:H638–H644, 1987.
13. Burgisser, E., De Lean, A., and Lefkowitz, R.J.: Reciprocal modulation of agonist and antagonist binding to muscarinic cholinergic receptor by guanine nucleotide. Proc. Natl. Acad. Sci. USA 79:1732–1736, 1985.
14. Basile, A.S., and Skolnik, P.: Tissue specific regulation of "peripheral-type" benzodiazepine receptor density after chemical sympathectomy. Life Sci. 42:273–283, 1988.
15. Buja, L.M., Muntz, K.H., Rosenbaum, T., et al.: Characterization of a potentially reversible increase in β-adrenergic receptors in isolated, neonatal rat cardial myocytes with impaired energy metabolism. Circ. Res. 57:640–645, 1985.
16. Bristow, M.R., Ginsburg, R., Minobe, W., et al.: Decreased catecholamine sensitivity and β-adrenergic receptor density in failing human heart. N. Engl. J. Med. 307:205–211, 1982.
17. Bristow, M.R., Kantrowitz, N.E., Ginsburg, R., and Fowler, M.B.: β-adrenergic function in heart muscle disease and heart failure. J. Mol. Cell Cardiol. S2:41–52, 1985.
18. Bristow, M.R., Ginsburg, R., Umans, V., et al.:β_1- and β_2-adrenergic receptor subpopulations in nonfailing and failing human ventricular myocardium: Coupling of both receptor subtypes to muscle contraction and selective β_1-receptor down-regulation in heart failure. Circ. Res. 59:297–309, 1986.

C

1. Crouzel, C., Venet, M., Irié, T., et al.: Labeling of a serotoninergic ligand with ^{18}F: [^{18}F]setoperone. J. Label Compds. Radiopharm. 25:403–414, 1988.
2. Crouzel, C., Venet, M., Sanz, G., and Denis, A.: Labelling of a new serotoninergic ligand: [^{18}F]ritanserine. J. Label Compds. Radiopharm. 25:827–832, 1988.
3. Camsonne, R., Crouzel, C., Comar, D., et al.: Synthesis of N-(^{11}C)methyl, N-(methyl-1 propyl), (chloro-2 phenyl)-1 isoquinoline carboxamide receptors. J. Label Compds. Radiopharm. 21:985–991, 1984.
4. Charbonneau, P., Syrota, A., Boullais, C., and Crouzel, C.: Serotonin receptors and lung phagocyte recruitment induced by cigarette smoking detected in vivo by positron emission tomography. J. Nucl. Med. 27:950, 1986.
5. Chaumet-Riffaud, Ph., Girault, M., and Syrota, A.: Characterization of muscarinic cholinergic receptors in the isolated perfused rat heart. J. Physiol. (London) 348:11P, 1984.
6. Changeux, J.P.: The acetylcholine receptor: An "allosteric" membrane protein. Harvey Lect. 75:85–254, 1981.
7. Charbonneau, P., Syrota, A., Crouzel, C., et al.: Peripheral-type benzodiazepine receptors in the living heart characterized by positron emission tomography. Circulation 73:476–483, 1986.

D

1. Dormont, D., Syrota, A., Berger, G., et al.: C-11 ligand binding to adrenergic and muscarinic receptors in the human heart studied in vivo by PET. J. Nucl. Med. 24:P20, 1983.
2. Delforge, J., Syrota, A., and Mazoyer, B.: Experimental design optimization: Theory and application to estimation of receptor model parameters using dynamic positron emission tomography. Phys. Med. Biol. 34:419–435, 1989.
3. Dixon, R.A.F., Kobilka, B.K., Strader, D.J., et al.: Cloning of the gene and cDNA for mammalian β-adrenergic receptor and homology with rhodopsine. Nature 321:75–79, 1986.
4. Doods, H.N., Mathy, M.-J., and Davidesko, D.: Selectivity of muscarinic antagonists in radioligand and in vivo experiments for the putative M_1, M_2 and M_3 receptors. J. Pharmacol. Exp. Ther. 242:257–262, 1987.
5. Duckles, S.P.: Vascular muscarinic receptors: Pharmacological characterization in the bovine coronary artery. J. Pharmacol. Exp. Ther. 246:929–934, 1988.
6. Davies, L.P., and Huston, V.: Peripheral benzodiazepine binding sites in heart and their interaction with dipyridamole. Eur. J. Pharmacol. 73:209–211, 1981.
7. Delforge, J., Janier, M., Syrota, A., et al.: Noninvasive quantification of muscarinic receptors in vivo with positron emission tomography in the dog heart. Circulation. (In press.)

E

1. Ehrin, E., Luthra, S.K., Crouzel, C., and Pike, V.W.: Preparation of carbon-11 labelled prazosin, a potent and selective α_1-adrenoceptor antagonist. J. Label Compds. Radiopharm. 25:177–183, 1988.
2. Eller, M., and Järv, J.: Two step isomerization of quinuclidinyl benzylate-muscarinic complex. Neurochem. Int. 12:285–289, 1988.

F

1. Frey, K.A., Hichwa, R.D., Ehrenkaufer, R.L.E., and Agranoff, B.W.: Quantitative in vivo receptor binding III: Tracer kinetic modeling of muscarinic cholinergic receptor binding. Proc. Natl. Acad. Sci. USA 82:6711–6715, 1985.
2. Fields, J.Z., Roeske, W.R., Morkin, E., and Yamamura, H.I.: Cardiac muscarinic cholinergic receptors. Biochemical identification and characterization. J. Biol. Chem. 253:3251–3258, 1978.
3. Farde, L., Hall, H., Ehrin, E., and Sedvall, G.: Quantitative analysis of D2 dopamine receptor binding in the living human brain by PET. Science 231:258–261, 1986.
4. Freissmuth, M., Hausleithner, V., Nees, S., et al.: Cardiac ventricular β_2-adrenoceptors in guinea pigs and rats are localized on the coronary endothelium. Arch. Pharmacol. 334:56–62, 1986.
5. Fukuda, K., Kubo, T., Akiba, I., et al.: Molecular distinction between muscarinic acetylcholine receptor subtypes. Nature 327:623–625, 1987.
6. Furchgott, R.F., and Zawadzki, J.V.: The obligatory role of endothelial cells in the relaxation of arterial smooth muscle by acetylcholine. Nature 288:373–376, 1980.
7. Freissmuth, M., Schütz, W., Weindlmayer-Göttel, et al.: Effects of ischemia on the canine myocardial β-adrenoceptor–linked adenylate cyclase system. J. Cardiovasc. Pharmacol. 10:568–574, 1987.
8. Fan, T.-HM., Liang, C.-S., Kawashima, S., and Banerjee, S.P.: Alterations in cardiac β-adrenoceptor responsiveness and adenylate cyclase system by congestive heart failure. Eur. J. Pharmacol. 140:123–132, 1987.
9. Fowler, M.B., Laser, J.A., Hopkins, D.L., et al.: Assessment of the β-adrenergic receptor pathway in the intact failing human heart: Progressive receptor down-regulation and subsensitivity to agonist response. Circulation 74:1290–1294, 1986.

G

1. Gibson, R.E., Eckelman, W.C., Vieras, F., and Reba, R.C.: The distribution of the muscarinic acetylcholine receptor antagonists, quinuclidinyl benzilate and quinuclidinyl benzilate methiodide (both tritiated) in rat, guinea pig and rabbit. J. Nucl. Med. 20:865–870, 1979.
2. Golf, S., Løvstad, R., and Hansson, V.: β-adrenoceptor density and relative number of β-adrenoceptor subtypes in biopsies from human right atrial, left ventricular, and right ventricular myocard. Cardiovasc. Res. 19:636–641, 1985.
3. Giachetti, A., Micheletti, R., and Montagna, E.: Cardioselective profile of AF-DX 116, a muscarinic M_2 receptor antagonist. Life Sci. 38:1663–1672, 1986.
4. Gossuin, A., Maloteaux, J.M., Trouet, A., and Laduron, P.: Differentiation between ligand trapping into intact cells and binding on muscarinic receptors. Biochim. Biophys. Acta 804:100–106, 1984.

5. Giraldo, E., Martos, F., Gomez, A., et al.: Characterization of muscarinic receptor subtypes in human tissues. Life Sci. 43:1507–1515, 1988.
6. Galper, J.B., Klein, W., and Catterall, W.A.: Muscarinic acetylcholine receptors in developing chicken heart. J. Biol. Chem. 252:8692–8699, 1977.
7. Galper, J.B., and Smith, T.W.: Properties of muscarinic acetylcholine receptors in heart cell cultures. Proc. Natl. Acad. Sci. USA 75:5831–5835, 1978.
8. Grupp, I.L., French, J.F., and Matlib, M.A.: Benzodiazepine RO 5-4864 increases coronary blood flow. Eur. J. Pharmacol. 134:143–147, 1987.
9. Galper, J.B., Dziekan, L.C., O'Hara, D.S., and Smith, T.W.: The biphasic response of muscarinic cholinergic receptors in culture heart cells to agonists. Effects on receptor number and affinity in intact cells and homogenates. J. Biol. Chem. 257:10344–10356, 1982.
10. Golf, S., and Hansson, V.: Effects of beta blocking agents on the density of beta adrenoceptors and adenylate cyclase response in human myocardium: Intrinsic sympathomimetic activity favours receptor regulation. Cardiovasc. Res. 20:637–644, 1986.
11. Golf, S., Andersen, D., and Hansson, V.: Beta adrenergic density and adenylate cyclase response in right atrial and left ventricular myocardium of patients with mitral valve disease. Cardiovasc. Res. 20:331–336, 1986.

H

1. Hirschowitz, B.I., Hammer, R., Giachetti, A., et al. (eds.): Subtypes of muscarinic receptors. Trends in Pharmacological Sciences, Suppl. Amsterdam, Elsevier, 1984.
2. Heitz, A., Schwartz, J., and Velly, J.: β-Adrenoceptors of the human myocardium: Determination of β_1 and β_2 subtypes by radioligand binding. Br. J. Pharmacol. 80:711–717, 1983.
3. Hedberg, A., Kempf, F., Jr., Josephson, M.E., and Molinoff, P.B.: Coexistence of beta-1 and beta-2 adrenergic receptors in the human heart: Effects of treatment with receptor antagonists or calcium entry blockers. J. Pharmacol. Exp. Ther. 234:561–568, 1985.
4. Hertel, C., Muller, P., Portenier, H., and Staehelin, M.: Determination of the desensitization of β-adrenergic receptors by [^{3}H]CGP-12 177. Biochem. J. 216:669–674, 1983.
5. Hammer, R., Berrie, C.P., Birdsall, N.J.M., et al.: Pirenzepine distinguishes between different subclasses of muscarinic receptors. Nature 283:90–92, 1980.
6. Hammer, R., Giraldo, E., Schiavi, G.B., et al.: Binding profile of a novel cardioselective muscarinic antagonist, AF-DX 116, to membranes of peripheral tissues and brain in the rat. Life Sci. 38:1653–1662, 1986.
7. Hynes, M.R., Banner, W., Jr., Yamamura, H.I., and Duckles, S.P.: Characterization of muscarinic receptors of the rabbit ear artery smooth muscle and endothelium. J. Pharmacol. Exp. Ther. 238:100–105, 1986.
8. Hassal, C.J.S., Buckley, N.J., and Burnstok, G.: Autoradiographic localization of muscarinic receptors on guinea pig intracardiac neurons and atrial myocytes in culture. Neurosci. Lett. 74:145–150, 1987.
9. Heimbach, D.M., and Crout, R.J.: Effect of atropine on the tachycardia of hyperthyroidism. Arch. Intern. Med. 129:430–432, 1972.
10. Hammond, H.K., White, F.C., Buxton, I.L.O., et al.: Increased myocardial β-receptors and adrenergic responses in hyperthyroid pigs. Am. J. Physiol. (Heart Circ. Physiol. 21) 252:H283–H290, 1987.

J

1. Järv, J., Hendlund, B., and Bartfai, T.: Isomerization of the muscarinic receptor-antagonist complex. J. Biol. Chem. 254:5595–5598, 1979.

K

1. Kloog, Y., Egozi, Y., and Sokolowsky, M.: Characterization of muscarinic acetylcholine receptors from mouse brain: Evidence for heterogeneity and isomerization. Mol. Pharmacol. 15:545–558, 1979.
2. Klein, I., and Levey, G.S.: New perspectives on thyroid hormone, cathecholamine, and the heart. Am. J. Med. 76:167–172, 1984.
3. Karliner, J.S., Stevens, M., Grattan, M., et al.: Beta-adrenergic receptor properties of canine myocardium: Effects of chronic myocardial infarction. J. Am. Coll. Cardiol. 8:349–356, 1986.

L

1. Landais, P., and Crouzel, C.: A new synthesis of carbon-11 labelled phosgene. Appl. Radiat. Isot. 38:297–300, 1987.
2. Laduron, P.M.: Criteria for receptor sites in binding studies. Biochem. Pharmacol. 33:833–839, 1984.
3. Lefkowitz, R.J., and Caron, M.G.: Adrenergic receptors. Models for the study of receptors coupled to guanine nucleotide regulatory proteins. J. Biol. Chem. 263:4993–4996, 1988.
4. Lathers, C.M., Levin, R.M., and Spivey, W.H.: Regional distribution of myocardial β-adrenoceptors in the cat. Eur. J. Pharmacol. 130:111–117, 1986.
5. Levy, M.N., and Martin, P.J.: Neural regulation of the heart beat. Ann. Rev. Physiol. 43:443–453, 1981.
6. Le Fur, G., Perrier, M.L., Vaucher, N., et al.: Peripheral benzodiazepine binding sites: Effect of PK 11195, 1-(2-chlorophenyl)-N-methyl-N-(1-methylpropyl)-3-isoquinolinecarboxamide. I. In vitro studies. Life Sci. 32:1839–1847, 1983.
7. Le Fur, G., Guilloux, F., Rufat, P., et al.: Peripheral benzodiazepine binding sites: Effect of PK 11195, 1-(2-chorophenyl)-N-methyl-N-(1-methyl-propyl)-3-isoquinolinecarboxamide. II. In vivo studies. Life Sci. 32:1849–1856, 1983.
8. Lurie, K.G., Bristow, M.R., and Reitz, B.A.: Increased β-adrenergic receptor density in an experimental model of cardiac transplantation. J. Thorac. Cardiovasc. Surg. 86:195–198, 1983.

M

1. Mazière, M., Comar, D., Godot, J.M., et al.: In vivo characterization of myocardium muscarinic receptors by positron emission tomography. Life Sci. 29:2391–2397, 1981.
2. Molinoff, P.B.: α- and β-adrenergic receptor subtypes properties, distribution and regulation. Drugs 28 (suppl 2):1–15, 1984.
3. Mintun, M.A., Raichle, M.E., Kilbourn, M.R., et al.: A quantitative model for the in vivo assessment of drug binding sites with positron emission tomography. Ann. Neurol. 15:217–227, 1984.
4. Motulsky, H.J., and Insel, P.A.: Adrenergic receptors in man. Direct identification, physiologic regulation, and clinical alterations. N. Engl. J. Med. 307:18–28, 1982.
5. Murphree, S.S., and Saffitz, J.E.: Delineation of β-adrenergic receptor subtypes in canine myocardium. Circ. Res. 63:117–125, 1988.
6. Mukherjee, A., Haghani, Z., Brady, J., et al.: Differences in myocardial α- and β-adrenergic receptor numbers in different species. Am. J. Physiol. (Heart Circ. Physiol. 14) 245:H957–H961, 1983.
7. Manalan, A.S., Werth, D.K., Jones, L.R., and Watanabe, A.M.: Enrichment, solubilization, and partial characterization of digitonin-solubilized muscarinic receptors derived from canine ventricular myocardium. Circ. Res. 52:664–676, 1983.
8. Mestre, M., Carriot, T., Belin, C., et al.: Electrophysiological and pharmacological evidence that peripheral type benzodiazepine receptors are coupled to calcium channels in the heart. Life Sci. 36:391–400, 1985.
9. Mestre, M., Bouetard, G., Uzan, A., et al.: PK 11195, an antagonist of peripheral benzodiazepine receptors, reduces ventricular arrythmias during myocardial ischemia and reperfusion in the dog. Eur. J. Pharmacol. 112:257–260, 1985.
10. McDevitt, D.G., Shanks, R.G., Hadden, D.R., et al.: The role of the thyroid in the control of heart rate. Lancet 1:998–1000, 1968.
11. Mirro, M.J., Manalan, A.S., Bailey, J.C., and Watanabe, A.M.: Anticholinergic effects of disopyramide and quinidine on guinea pig myocardium mediation by direct muscarinic receptor blockade. Circ. Res. 47:855–865, 1980.
12. Mukherjee, A., Wong, T.M., Buja, L.M., et al.: Beta adrenergic and muscarinic cholinergic receptors in canine myocardium: Effects of ischemia. J. Clin. Invest. 64:1423–1428, 1979.
13. Mukherjee, A., Bush, L.R., McCoy, K.E., et al.: Relationship between β-adrenergic receptor numbers and physiological responses during experimental canine myocardial ischemia. Circ. Res. 50:735–741, 1982.
14. Maisel, A.S., Motulsky, H.J., and Insel, P.A.: Externalization of β-adrenergic receptors promoted by myocardial ischemia. Science 230:183–186, 1985.
15. Mulholland, G.K., Schwaiger, M., Sherman, P.S., et al.: New positron labeled quaternized muscarinic ligand as potential PET imaging agent. Circulation 78:II598, 1988.
16. Mislankar, S.G., Gildersleeve, D.L., Wieland, D.M., et al.: 6-[^{18}F] fluorometaraminol: A radiotracer for in vivo mapping of adrenergic nerves of the heart. J. Med. Chem. 31:362–366, 1988.

N

1. Nanoff, C., Freissmuth, M., and Schütz, W.: The role of a low β_1-adrenoceptor selectivity of [^{3}H]CGP-12177 for resolving subtype-selectivity of competitive ligands. Arch. Pharmacol. 336:519–525, 1987.
2. Nathanson, N.M.: Molecular properties of the muscarinic acetylcholine receptor. Ann. Rev. Neurosci. 10:195–236, 1987.
3. Napolitano, L.M., Willman, V.L., Hanlon, C.R., and Cooper, T.: Intrinsic innervation of the heart. Am. J. Physiol. 208:455–458, 1965.

O

1. O'Rourke, S.T., and Vanhoutte, P.M.: Subtypes of muscarinic receptors on adrenergic nerves and vascular smooth muscle of the canine saphenous vein. J. Pharmacol. Exp. Ther. 241:64–67, 1987.
2. Ohyanagi, M., Matsumori, Y., and Iwasaki, T.: β-adrenergic receptors in ischemic and nonischemic canine myocardium: Relation to ventricular fibrillation and effects of pretreatment with propranolol and hexamethonium. J. Cardiovasc. Pharmacol. 11:107–114, 1988.

P

1. Prenant, C., Sastre, J., Crouzel, C., and Syrota, A.: Synthesis of ^{11}C-Pindolol. J. Label Compds. Radiopharm. 24:227–232, 1987.
2. Pascal, O., Syrota, A., Berger, G., et al.: Lung uptake of ^{11}C-imipramine and ^{11}C-propranolol in patients with sarcoidosis evaluated by positron emission tomography. *In* Marsac, J., and Chretien, J. (eds.): Sarcoidosis and Other Granulomatous Disorders. Pergamon Press, Paris, 1981, pp. 404–408.
3. Perlmutter, J.S., Larson, K.B., Raichle, M.E., et al.: Strategies for in vivo measurement of receptor binding using positron emission tomography. J. Cereb. Blood Flow Metab. 6:154–169, 1986.
4. Peralta, E.G., Winslow, J.W., Peterson, G.L., et al.: Primary structure and biochemical properties of an M_2 muscarinic receptor. Science 236:600–605, 1987.
5. Pierpont, G.L., DeMaster, E.G., and Cohn, J.N.: Regional differences in adrenergic function within the left ventricle. Am. J. Physiol. (Heart Circ. Physiol. 15) 246:H824–H829, 1984.

6. Porzig, H., Becker, C., and Reuter, H.: Competitive and noncompetitive interactions between specific ligands and beta-adrenoceptors in living cardiac cells. Arch. Pharmacol. 321:89–99, 1982.
7. Peach, M.J., Singer, H.A., and Loeba, L.: Mechanisms of endothelium-dependent vascular smooth muscle relaxation. Biochem. Pharmacol. 34:1867–1874, 1985.
8. Pelc, L.R., Gross, G.J., and Warltier, D.C.: Changes in regional myocardial perfusion by muscarinic receptor subtypes in dogs. Cardiovasc. Res. 20:482–489, 1986.

R

1. Robberecht, P., Delhaye, M., Taton, G., et al.: The human heart beta-adrenergic receptors. I. Heterogeneity of the binding sites: Presence of 50% beta$_1$- and 50% beta$_2$-adrenergic receptors. Mol. Pharmacol. 24:169–173, 1983.
2. Robberecht, P., Waelbroeck, M., Claeys, M., et al.: Rat cardiac muscarinic receptors. II. Influence of thyroid status and cardiac hypertrophy. Mol. Pharmacol. 21:589–593, 1982.
3. Raum, W.J., Laks, M.M., Garner, D., and Swerdloff, R.S.: β-adrenergic receptor and cyclic AMP alterations in the canine ventricular septum during long-term norepinephrine infusion: Implications for hypertrophic cardiomyopathy. Circulation 68:693–699, 1983.

S

1. Schelbert, H.R.: Positron-emission tomography: Assessment of myocardial blood flow and metabolism. Circulation 72:IV122–IV133, 1985.
2. Schwaiger, M., and Schelbert, H.R.: Assessment of tissue viability in ischemic heart disease by positron emission tomography. *In* Pohost, G.M., Higgins, C.B., Morganroth, J., et al. (eds.): New Concepts in Cardiac Imaging. Year Book Medical Publishing, Inc., Chicago, 1986, pp. 155–170.
3. Sobel, B.E.: Positron tomography and myocardial metabolism: An overview. Circulation 72:IV22–IV30, 1985.
4. Syrota, A.: In vivo study of receptors for neuromediators with PET. Int. J. Nucl. Med. Biol. 13:127–134, 1986.
5. Syrota, A., Paillotin, G., Davy, J.M., and Aumont, M.C.: Kinetics of in vivo binding of antagonist to muscarinic cholinergic receptor in the human heart studied by positron emission tomography. Life Sci. 35:937–945, 1984.
6. Stiles, G.L., and Lefkowitz, R.J.: Cardiac adrenergic receptors. Ann. Rev. Med. 35:149–164, 1984.
7. Seto, M., Syrota, A., Crouzel, C., et al.: Beta adrenergic receptors in the dog heart characterized by ^{11}C-CGP 12 177 and PET. J. Nucl. Med. 27:949, 1986.
8. Stiles, G.L., Taylor, S., and Lefkowitz, R.J.: Human cardiac beta-adrenergic receptors: Subtype heterogeneity delineated by direct ligand binding. Life Sci. 33:467–473, 1983.
9. Saito, K., Kurihara, M., Cruciani, R., et al.: Characterization of β_1- and β_2-adrenoceptor subtypes in the rat atrioventricular node by quantitative autoradiography. Circ. Res. 62:173–177, 1988.
10. Staehelin, M., Simons, P., Jaeggik, and Wigger, N.: CGP-12 177. A hydrophilic β-adrenergic receptor radioligand reveals high affinity binding of agonists to intact cells. J. Biol. Chem. 258:3496–3502, 1983.
11. Staehelin, M., and Hertel, C.: [^{3}H]CGP-12 177, a β-adrenergic ligand suitable for measuring cell surface receptors. J. Recept. Res. 3:35–43, 1983.
12. Sibley, D.R., and Lefkowitz, R.J.: β-adrenergic receptor-coupled adenylate cyclase. Biochemical mechanisms of regulation. Mol. Neurobiol. 1:121–154, 1987.
13. Stephenson, J.A., and Summers, R.J.: Autoradiographic analysis of receptors on vascular endothelium. Eur. J. Pharmacol. 134:35–43, 1987.
14. Syrota, A., Comar, D., Paillotin, G., et al.: Muscarinic cholinergic receptor in the human heart evidenced under physiological conditions by positron emission tomography. Proc. Natl. Acad. Sci. USA 82:584–588, 1985.
15. Sharkey, J., Ritz, M.C., Shenden, J.A., et al.: Cocaine inhibits muscarinic cholinergic receptors in heart and brain. J. Pharmacol. Exp. Ther. 246:1048–1052, 1988.
16. Sharma, V.K., and Banerjee, S.P.: Muscarinic cholinergic receptors in rat heart. Effects of thyroidectomy. J. Biol. Chem. 252:7444–7446, 1977.
17. Syrota, A., Le Guludec, D., Prenant, C., et al.: PET investigation of myocardial muscarinic acetylcholine receptor in patients with hyper- and hypothyroidism. J. Nucl. Med. 29:808, 1988.
18. Syrota, A., Marty, J., Seto, M., et al.: Halothane-induced decrease of ^{11}C-CGP 12177 binding to myocardial beta adrenergic receptor demonstrated by PET in the dog. J. Nucl. Med. 29:940, 1988.

T

1. Tcheng, K.T.: Innervation of the dog's heart. Am. Heart. J. 41:512–524, 1951.
2. Takahashi, N., Barber, M.J., and Zipes, D.P.: Efferent vagal innervation of canine ventricle. Ann. J. Physiol. (Heart Circ. Physiol. 17) 248:H89–H97, 1985.
3. Taniguchi, T., Wang, J.K.T., and Spector, S.: [^{3}H]Diazepam binding sites on rat heart and kidney. Biochem. Pharmacol. 31:589–590, 1982.
4. Trifiletti, R.R., Lo, M.M.S., and Snyder, S.H.: Kinetic differences between type I and type II benzodiazepine receptors. Mol. Pharmacol. 26:228–240, 1984.

V

1. Vatner, D.E., Knight, D.R., Homcy, C.J., et al.: Subtypes of β-adrenergic receptors in bovine coronary arteries. Circ. Res. 59:463–473, 1986.
2. Vatner, D.E., Knight, D.R., Shen, Y.T., et al.: One hour of myocardial ischemia in conscious dogs increases β-adrenergic receptors, but decreases adenylate cyclase activity. J. Mol. Cell Cardiol. 20:75–82, 1988.
3. Vatner, D.E., Vatner, S.F., Fujii, A.M., and Homcy, C.J.: Loss of high affinity cardiac beta adrenergic receptors in dogs with heart failure. J. Clin. Invest. 76:2259–2263, 1985.

W

1. Wong, D.F., Gjedde, A., and Wagner, H.N., Jr.: Quantification of neuroreceptors in the living human brain. I. Irreversible binding of ligands. J. Cerebr. Blood Flow Metab. 6:137–146, 1986.
2. Wong, D.F., Gjedde, A., Wagner, H.N., Jr., et al.: Quantification of neuroreceptors in the living human brain II. Inhibition studies of receptor density and affinity. J. Cerebr. Blood Flow Metab. 6:147–153, 1986.
3. Woods, P.B., and Robinson, M.L.: An investigation of the comparative liposolubilities of β-adrenoceptor blocking agents. J. Pharm. Pharmacol. 33:172–173, 1981.
4. Wei, J.-W., and Sulakhe, P.V.: Regional and subcellular distribution of β- and α-adrenergic receptors in the myocardium of different species. Gen. Pharmacol. 10:263–267, 1979.
5. Watson, M., Yamamura, H.I., and Roeske, W.R.: [^{3}H]pirenzepine and (-)-[^{3}H]quinuclidinyl benzilate binding to rat cerebral cortical and cardiac muscarinic cholinergic sites. I. Characterization and regulation of agonist binding to putative muscarinic subtypes. J. Pharmacol. Exp. Ther. 237:411–418, 1986.
6. Wellstein, A., Palm, D., Matthews, J.H., and Belz, G.G.: In vitro receptor occupancy allows to establish equieffective doses of β-blockers with different pharmacodynamic profiles in man. Investigations with propranolol and bufuralol. Meth. and Find. Exptl. Clin. Pharmacol. 7:645–651, 1985.
7. Watson-Wright, W.M., and Wilkinson, M.: β-adrenergic ([^{3}H]CGP-12177) receptors are elevated in slices of soleus muscle from CHF 147 dystrophic hamsters. Life Sci. 40:1171–1177, 1987.
8. Wieland, D.M., Rosenspire, K.C., Hutchins, G.D., and Schwaiger, M.: Validation of 6-[^{18}F]fluorometaraminol (FMR) for positron tomography. Circulation 78:II598, 1988.
9. Wieland, D.M., Hutchins, G.D., Rosenspire, K.C., et al.: [^{C}11]hydroxyephedrine (HED): a high specific activity alternative to 6-[^{18}F]fluorometaraminol (FMR) for heart neuronal imaging. J. Nucl. Med. 30:767–768, 1989.

Y

1. Yarden, Y., Rodriguez, H., Wong, S.K.-F., et al.: The avian β-adrenergic receptor: Primary structure and membrane topology. Proc. Natl. Acad. Sci. USA 83:6795–6799, 1986.
2. Yamada, S., Yamazawa, T., Harada, Y., et al.: Muscarinic receptor subtype in porcine coronary artery. Eur. J. Pharmacol. 150:373–376, 1988.
3. Yusuf, S., Theodoropoulos, S., Mathias, C.J., et al.: Increased sensitivity of the denervated transplanted human heart to isoprenaline both before and after β-adrenergic blockade. Circulation 75:696–704, 1987.

Glossary of NMR Terms

Aliasing—consequence of *sampling* in which any components of the signal that are at a higher *frequency* than the *Nyquist limit* is "folded" in the *spectrum* so that they appear to be at a lower frequency. In *Fourier transform imaging,* this can produce an apparent wrapping around to the opposite side of the image of a portion of the object that extends beyond the edge of the reconstructed region.

Angular frequency (ω)—*frequency* of oscillation or rotation (measured, e.g., in radians/second) commonly designated by the Greek letter ω:ω = 2πf, where f is frequency (e.g., in *hertz* (Hz)).

Angular momentum—a *vector* quantity given by the vector product of the momentum of a particle and its position vector. In the absence of external forces, the angular momentum remains constant, with the result that any rotating body tends to maintain the same axis of rotation. When a *torque* is applied to a rotating body in such a way as to change the direction of the rotation axis, the resulting change in angular momentum results in *precession.* Atomic nuclei possess an intrinsic angular momentum referred to as *spin,* measured in multiples of Planck's constant.

Annotation—a description of the factors used in creating an image should include the types and times of the *pulse sequence,* the number of signals averaged or added *(NSA),* the size of the reconstructed region, the size of the *acquisition matrix* in each direction, and the *slice thickness.*

Antenna—device to send or receive electromagnetic radiation. Electromagnetic radiation per se is not relevant to NMR, because it is the magnetic vector alone that couples the *spins* and the *coils,* and the term *coil* should be used instead.

Artifacts—false features in the image produced by the imaging process. The random fluctuation of intensity due to *noise* can be considered separately from artifacts.

B_o—a conventional symbol for the constant *magnetic (induction) field* in an *NMR* system. (Although historically used, H_o [units of *magnetic field* strength, ampere/meter] should be distinguished from the more appropriate B_o [units of magnetic induction, *telsa*].)

B_1—a conventional symbol for the *radiofrequency magnetic* induction field used in an MR system (another symbol historically used is H_1). It is useful to consider it as composed of two oppositely rotating *vectors,* usually in a plane transverse to B_o. *At the Larmor frequency,* the vector rotating in the same direction as the *precessing spins* interacts strongly with the spins.

Bandwidth—a general term referring to a range of *frequencies* (e.g., contained in a signal or passed by a signal processing system).

Baseline—a generally smooth background curve with respect to which either the *integrals* or peak heights of the *resonance spectral lines* in the *spectrum* are measured.

Bloch equations—phenomenologic "classical" equations of motion for the *macroscopic magnetization vector.* They include the effects of *precession* about the *magnetic field* (static and *RF*) and the *T1* and *T2 relaxation times.*

Boltzmann distribution—if a system of particles that are able to exchange energy in collisions is in thermal equilibrium, then the relative number *(population)* of particles, N_1 and N_2, in two particular *energy levels* with corresponding energies, E_1 and E_2, is given by

$$\frac{N_1}{N_2} = \exp\left[-(E_1 - E_2)/kT \right]$$

where k is Boltzmann's constant and T is absolute temperature. For example, in *NMR* of protons at room temperature in a *magnetic field* of 0.25 *tesla,* the difference in relative numbers of spins aligned with the magnetic field and against the field is about one part in a million; the small excess of nuclei in the lower energy state is the basis of the net *magnetization* and the *resonance* phenomenon.

Chemical shift (δ)—the change in the *Larmor frequency* of a given nucleus when bound in different sites in molecule, due to the magnetic shielding effects of the electron orbitals. Chemical shifts make possible the differentiation of different molecular compounds and different sites within the molecules in high-resolution NMR spectra. The amount of the shift is proportional to magnetic field strength and is usually specified in parts per million (ppm) of the resonance frequency relative to a standard. The actual frequency measured for a given *spectral line* may depend on environmental factors such as effects on the local magnetic field strength due to variations of *magnetic susceptibility.*

Chemical shift imaging—a magnetic resonance imaging technique that provides mapping of the regional distribution of intensity (images) of a restricted range of *chemical shifts,* corresponding to individual *spectral lines* or groups of lines.

Chemical shift reference—a compound with respect to whose *frequency* the chemical shifts of other compounds can be compared. The standard can either be internal or external to the sample. Because of the need for possible corrections due to differential magnetic *susceptibility* between an external standard and the sample being measured, the use of an internal standard is generally preferred.

C/N—see Contrast-to-noise ratio.

CNR—see Contrast-to-noise ratio.

Coil—single or multiple loops of wire (or other electrical conductor, such as tubing) designed either to produce a *magnetic field* from current flowing through the wire, or to detect a changing magnetic field by voltage induced in the wire.

Contrast—contrast can be defined as the relative difference of the signal intensities in two adjacent regions. In a general sense, we can consider image contrast, in which the strength of the image intensity in adjacent regions of the image is compared, or object contrast, in which the relative values of a parameter affecting the image (such as *spin density* or *relaxation time)* in corresponding adjacent regions of the object are compared. Relating image contrast to object contrast is more difficult in *MR imaging* than in conventional radiography, because there are more object parameters affecting the image and their relative contributions are very dependent on the particular imaging technique used. As in other kinds of imaging, image contrast in NMR also depends on region size, as reflected through the modulation transfer function (MTF) characteristics. The contrast between an object (e.g., lesion) and the background also depends on the

(From Glossary of MR Terms. 2nd ed. Reston, Virginia, American College of Radiology, 1986.)

particular choice of designated background (e.g., fat, muscle).

Contrast agent—substance administered to a subject being imaged in order to alter selectively the image intensity of a particular anatomic or functional region, typically by altering the *relaxation times.*)

Contrast-to-noise ratio—ratio of the absolute difference in intensities between two regions to the level of fluctuations in intensity due to *noise.*

Correlation time—the characteristic time between significant fluctuations in the local magnetic field experienced by a spin due to molecular motions. For values of the correlation time such that the magnetic field as a function of time has large *Fourier* components near the resonance frequency, the *T1 relaxation time* is shortened.

Cryostat—an apparatus for maintaining a constant low temperature (as by means of liquid helium). It requires vacuum chambers to help with thermal isolation.

dB/dt—the rate of change of the *magnetic field* (induction) with time. Because changing magnetic fields can induce electrical current, this is one area of potential concern for safety limits.

Decoupling—(1) specific irradiation designed to remove the *multiplet* structure in a particular *resonance* due to *spin-spin coupling* with other nuclei; (2) techniques used to avoid interactions between *coils,* such as separate transmitting and receiving coils.

Detector—portion of the *receiver* that demodulates the *RF MR signal* and converts it to a lower *frequency* signal. Most detectors now used are phase sensitive (e.g., *quadrature demodulator/detector*), and also give phase information about the RF signal.

Diamagnetic—a substance that slightly decreases a *magnetic field* when placed within it (its *magnetization* is oppositely directed to the magnetic field, i.e., with a small negative *magnetic susceptibility*).

Diffusion—the process by which molecules or other particles intermingle and migrate due to their random thermal motion. *NMR* provides a sensitive technique for measuring diffusion of some substances.

Dipole–dipole interaction—interaction between a spin and its neighbors due to their *magnetic dipole* moments. This is an important mechanism contributing to *relaxation times.* In solids and viscous liquids, this can result in broadening of the *spectral lines.*

Echo—see Spin echo.

Echo planar imaging—a technique of *planar imaging* in which a complete planar image is obtained from one *selective excitation pulse.* The *FID* is observed while periodically switching the *y-magnetic field gradient* field in the presence of a static *x-magnetic field gradient field.* The *Fourier transform* of the resulting *spin echo* train can be used to produce an image of the excited plane.

Echo time—see TE.

Eddy currents—electric currents induced in a conductor by a changing magnetic field or by motion of the conductor through a *magnetic field.* It represents one of the sources of concern about potential hazard to subjects in very high magnetic fields or rapidly varying *gradient* or main magnetic fields. It can be a practical problem in the *cryostat* of *superconducting magnets.*

Energy level—in a *magnetic field,* each *spin* can exist in one of a number of distinct states having different energies; this number is determined by the *spin quantum number.*

Excitation—putting energy into the *spin* system; if a net *transverse magnetization* is produced, an *MR signal* can be observed.

Faraday shield—electrical conductor interposed between *transmitter* and/or *receiver coil* and patient to block out electric fields.

Fast Fourier transform (FFT)—an efficient computational method of performing a *Fourier transform.*

Ferromagnetic—a substance, such as iron, that has a large positive *magnetic susceptibility.*

FID—see Free induction decay.

Field echo—see Gradient echo.

Field gradient—see Magnetic field gradient.

Filling factor—a measure of the geometrical relationship of the *RF coil* and the object being studied. It affects the efficiency of irradiating the object, and detecting *MR signals,* thereby affecting the *signal-to-noise ratio* and, ultimately, image quality. Achieving a high filling factor requires fitting the coil closely to the object, thus potentially decreasing patient comfort.

Flip angle—the amount of rotation of the *macroscopic magnetization vector* produced by an *RF pulse,* with respect to the direction of the static *magnetic field.*

Flow-related enhancement—*the increase in intensity that may be* seen for flowing blood or other liquids with some *MR imaging* techniques, due to the washout of *saturated* spins from the imaging region.

Fourier transform (FT)—a mathematical procedure to separate out the *frequency* components of a signal from its amplitudes as a function of time, or vice versa. The Fourier transform is used to generate the *spectrum* from the *FID* or *spin echo* in *pulse MR* techniques and is essential to most *MR imaging* techniques.

Free induction decay (FID)—if *transverse magnetization* of the spins is produced, e.g., by a 90-degree pulse, a transient *MR signal* will result that decays toward zero with a characteristic time constant *T2* (or *T2**); this decaying signal is the FID. In practice, the first part of the FID is not observable due to residual effects of the powerful exciting *RF pulse* on the electronics of the *receiver,* the *receiver dead time.*

Frequency (f)—the number of repetitions of a periodic process per unit time. For electromagnetic radiation, such as radio waves, the old unit, cycles per second (cps), has been replaced by the *SI* unit, *hertz,* abbreviated *Hz.* It is related to *angular frequency,* ω, by $f = \omega/2\pi$.

Frequency encoding—encoding the distribution of sources of *MR* signals along a direction by detecting the signal in the presence of a *magnetic field gradient* along that direction so that there is a corresponding gradient of *resonance frequencies* along that direction. In the absence of other position encoding, the Fourier transform of the resulting signal is a *projection profile* of the object.

G_x, G_y, G_z—conventional symbols for *magnetic field gradient.* Used with subscripts to denote spatial direction component of gradient, i.e., direction along which the field changes.

Gauss (G)—a unit of magnetic flux density in the older (CGS) system. The Earth's magnetic field is approximately one half gauss to one gauss, depending on a location. The currently preferred (SI) unit is the *tesla* (T) (1 T = 10,000 G).

Gradient—the amount and direction of the rate of change in space of some quantity, such as *magnetic field strength.* Also commonly used to refer to *magnetic field gradient.*

Gradient coils—current-carrying *coils* designed to produce a desired *magnetic field gradient* (so that the magnetic field is stronger in some locations than others). Proper design of the size and configuration of the coils is necessary to produce a controlled and uniform gradient.

Gradient echo—*spin echo* produced by reversing the direction of a *magnetic field gradient* or by applying balanced pulses of magnetic field gradient before and after a refocusing *RF pulse* so as to cancel out the position-dependent *phase* shifts that have accumulated due to the gradient. In the latter case, the gradient echo is generally adjusted to be coincident with the RF spin echo.

Gyromagnetic ratio (γ)—the ratio of the *magnetic moment* to the *angular momentum* of a particle. This is a constant for a given nucleus.

H_0—conventional symbol historically used for the constant *magnetic field* in an *MR system;* it is physically more correct to use B_o. A magnet provides a field strength, H; however, at a point in an object, the *spins* experience the *magnetic induction*, B.

H_1—conventional symbol historically used for the radiofrequency *magnetic field* in an *MR system;* it is physically more correct to use B_1. It is useful to consider it as composed of two oppositely rotating *vectors*. At the *Larmor frequency*, the vector rotating in the same direction as the *precessing spins* interacts strongly with the spins.

Hertz (Hz)—the standard *(SI)* unit of *frequency;* equal to the old unit cycles per second.

Homogeneity—uniformity. In *MR*, the homogeneity of the static *magnetic field* is an important criterion of the quality of the magnet. Homogeneity requirements for *MR imaging* are generally lower than the homogeneity requirements for NMR spectroscopy, but for most, imaging techniques must be maintained over a larger region.

I—see Nuclear spin number.

Image acquisition time—time required to carry out an *MR imaging* procedure comprising only the data acquisition time. The total image acquisition time is equal to the product of the repetition time, *TR*; the number of signals averaged, *NSA*; and the number of different signals (encoded for position) to be acquired for use in image reconstruction. The additional image reconstruction time also is important to determine how quickly the image can be viewed. In comparing *sequential plane imaging* and *volume imaging* techniques, the equivalent image acquisition time per slice must be considered, as well as the actual image acquisition time.

Inductance—measure of the magnetic coupling between two current carrying loops (mutual) reflecting their spatial relationship or of a loop (such as a *coil*) with itself (self). One of the principal determinants of the *resonance frequency* of an RF circuit.

Inhomogeneity—degree of lack of *homogeneity*, for example the fractional deviation of the local *magnetic field* from the average value of the field.

Interpulse times—times between successive *RF pulses* used in *pulse sequences*. Particularly important are the inversion time (TI) in *inversion recovery*, and the time between the *90-degree pulse* and the subsequent *180-degree pulse* to produce a *spin echo*, which is approximately one half the *spin echo time (TE)*. The time between repetitions of pulse sequences is the *repetition time (TR)*.

Inversion—a nonequilibrium state in which the *macroscopic magnetization vector* is oriented opposite to the *magnetic field*; usually produced by *adiabatic fast passage* or *180-degree RF pulses*.

Inversion-recovery (IR)—*pulse NMR* technique that can be incorporated into *MR imaging*, wherein the nuclear magnetization is inverted at a time on the order of *T1* before the regular imaging pulse-gradient sequences. The resulting partial *relaxation* of the spins in the different structures being imaged can be used to produce an image that depends strongly on T1. This may bring out differences in the appearance of structures with different T1 relaxation times. Note that this does *not* directly produce an image of T1. T1 in a given region can be calculated from the change in the *NMR signal* from the region due to the inversion pulse compared with the signal with no inversion pulse or an inversion pulse with a different inversion time (TI).

Kilohertz (kHz)—unit of *frequency*; equal to one thousand *hertz*.

Larmor equation—states that the *frequency* of precession of the nuclear *magnetic moment* is proportional to the *magnetic field*.

$$\omega_o = -\gamma B_o \quad \text{(radians per second)}$$

or

$$f_o = -\gamma B_o/2\pi \quad \text{(hertz)}$$

where ω_o or f_o is the frequency, γ is the *gyromagnetic ratio*, and B_o is the magnetic induction field. The negative sign indicates the direction of the rotation.

Larmor frequency (ω_o or f_o)—the *frequency* at which *magnetic resonance* can be excited; given by the *Larmor equation*. By varying the *magnetic* field across the body with a *magnetic field gradient*, the corresponding variation of the Larmor frequency can be used to encode position. For protons (hydrogen nuclei), the Larmor frequency is 42.58 MHz/tesla.

Lattice—by analogy to *NMR* in solids, the magnetic and thermal environment with which nuclei exchange energy in *longitudinal relaxation*.

Localization techniques—means of selecting a restricted region from which the signal is received. These can include the use of *surface coils*, with or without *magnetic field gradients*. Generally used to produce a *spectrum* from the desired region.

Longitudinal magnetization (M_z)—component of the *macroscopic magnetization vector* along the static *magnetic field*. Following excitation by *RF pulse*, M_z approaches its equilibrium value M_o, with a characteristic time constant *T1*.

Longitudinal relaxation—return of *longitudinal magnetization* to its equilibrium value after excitation; requires exchange of energy between the *nuclear spins* and the *lattice*.

Longitudinal relaxation time—see T1.

M—conventional symbol for *macroscopic magnetization vector*.

Mxy—see Transverse magnetization.

M_z—see Longitudinal magnetization.

M_o—equilibrium value of the *magnetization*; directed along the direction of the static *magnetic field*. Proportional to *spin* density, N.

Macroscopic magnetization vector—net *magnetic moment* per unit volume (a vector quantity) of a sample in a given region, considered as the integrated effect of all the individual microscopic nuclear magnetic moments. Most *MR* experiments actually deal with this.

Magnetic dipole—north and south magnetic poles separated by a finite distance. An electric current loop, including the effective current of a spinning nucleon or nucleus, can create an equivalent magnetic dipole.

Magnetic field (H)—the region surrounding a magnet (or current-carrying conductor) is endowed with certain properties. One is that a small magnet in such a region experiences a *torque* that tends to align it in a given direction. Magnetic field is a *vector* quantity; the direction of the field is defined as the direction that the north pole of the small magnet points when in equilibrium. A magnetic field produces a magnetizing force on a body within it. Although the dangers of large magnetic fields are largely hypothetical, this is an area of potential concern for safety limits.
Formerly, the forces experienced by moving charged particles, current-carrying wires, and small magnets in the vicinity of magnet are due to *magnetic induction* (B), which includes the effect of *magnetization*, whereas the magnetic field (H) is defined so as not to include magnetization. However, both B and H are often loosely used to denote magnetic fields.

Magnetic field gradient—a *magnetic field* that changes in strength in a certain given direction. Such fields are used in *NMR imaging* with *selective excitation* to select a region for imaging and also to encode the location of *NMR signals* received from the object being imaged. Measured (e.g.) in *teslas* per meter.

Magnetic induction (B)—also called magnetic flux density. The net magnetic effect from an externally applied *magnetic field* and the resulting *magnetization*. B is proportional to H($B = \mu H$), with the *SI* unit being the *tesla*.

Magnetic moment—a measure of the net magnetic properties of an object or particle. A nucleus with an intrinsic spin has an associated *magnetic dipole* moment, so that it interacts with the *magnetic field* (as if it were a tiny bar magnet).

Magnetic resonance (MR)—*resonance* phenomenon resulting in the absorption and/or emission of electromagnetic energy by nuclei or electrons in a static *magnetic field*, after excitation by a suitable *RF* magnetic field. The peak *resonance frequency* is proportional to the magnetic field, and is given by the *Larmor equation*. Only unpaired electrons or nuclei with a non-zero *spin* exhibit magnetic resonance.

Magnetic resonance imaging (MRI)—use of magnetic resonance to create images of objects such as the body. Currently, this primarily involves imaging the distribution of mobile hydrogen nuclei (protons) in the body. The image brightness depends jointly on the spin density (N(H)) and the relaxation times (T1 and T2), with their relative importance depending on the particular imaging technique and choice of interpulse times. Image brightness is also affected by any motion such as blood flow and respiration.

Magnetic shielding—means to confine the region of strong magnetic field surrounding a magnet; most commonly the use of material with high *permeability*.

Magnetic susceptibility (χ)—measure of the ability of a substance to become magnetized.

Magnetization—(see also Macroscopic magnetization vector—the magnetic polarization of a material produced by a magnetic field (magnetic moment per unit volume).

Megahertz (MHz)—unit of *frequency*, equal to one million *hertz*.

Multiple echo imaging—*spin echo imaging* using spin echoes acquired as a train. Typically a separate image is produced from each echo of the train.

Multiple slice imaging—variation of *sequential plane imaging* techniques that can be used with *selective excitation* techniques that do not affect adjacent slices. Adjacent slices are imaged while waiting for *relaxation of the first slice toward equilibrium, resulting in decreased image acquisition time* for the set of slices.

N(H)—see Spin density.

NEX—see NSA.

Noise—that component of the reconstructed image (or spectrum) due to random and unpredictable processes as opposed to the *signal* within the image itself that is due to predictable processes. Not to be confused with artifacts that are non-random errors in the image. It is commonly characterized by the standard deviation of signal intensity in the image of a uniform object (phantom) in the absence of *artifacts*. The measured noise may depend on the particular phantom used due to variable effects on the *Q* of the *receiver coil*.

NSA—number of signals averaged together to determine each distinct position-encoded signal to be used in image reconstruction.

Nuclear magnetic resonance (NMR)—the absorption of emission of electromagnetic energy by nuclei in a static *magnetic field*, afer *excitation* by a suitable *RF* magnetic field. The peak *resonance frequency* is proportional to the magnetic field, and is given by the *Larmor equation*. Only nuclei with a non-zero *spin* exhibit NMR.

Nuclear spin (see also Spin)—an intrinsic property of certain nuclei that gives them an associated characteristic *angular momentum* and *magnetic moment*.

Nuclear spin quantum number (I)—property of all nuclei related to the largest measurable component of the nuclear *angular momentum*. Non-zero values of nuclear angular momentum are quantized (fixed) as integral or half-integral multiples of ($h/2\pi$), where h is Planck's constant. The number of possible *energy levels* for a given nucleus in a fixed *magnetic field* is equal to $2I + 1$.

Nutation—a displacement of the axis of a spinning body away from the simple cone-shaped figure that would be traced by the axis during *precession*. In the *rotating frame of reference*, the nutation caused by an *RF pulse* appears as a simple precession, although the motion is more complex in the stationary frame of reference.

Orientation—a suggested standard orientation for the presentation of *NMR* images is (1) transverse: patient's right on the left side of the image, anterior or ventral on top; (2) coronal: patient's right to left side of image, superior or head to the top; (3) sagittal: patient's head to the top, anterior to the left side of image. R,L,S and A should be shown on the screen, as appropriate. In displaying sagittal images, it is helpful to indicate whether a slice is to the left or right of the midline.

Paramagnetic—a substance with a small but positive *magnetic susceptibility* (magnetizability). The addition of a small amount of paramagnetic substance may greatly reduce the *relaxation times* of water. Typical paramagnetic substances usually possess an unpaired electron and include atoms or ions of transition elements, rare earth elements, some metals, and some molecules including molecular oxygen and free radicals. Paramagnetic substances are considered promising for use as *contrast agents* in NMR imaging.

Partial saturation (PS)—*excitation* technique applying repeated *RF pulses* in times on the order of or shorter than *T1*. In *NMR imaging* systems, although it results in decreased signal amplitude, there is the possibility of generating images with increased *contrast* between regions with different relaxation times. It does *not* directly produce images of T1. The change in *NMR signal* from a region resulting from a change in the *interpulse time, TR*, can be used to calculate T1 for the region. Although partial saturation is also commonly referred to as *saturation recovery*, that term should properly be reserved for the particular case of partial saturation in which recovery after each *excitation* effectively takes place from true *saturation*.

Permeability (μ)—tendency of a substance to concentrate *magnetic field*, $\mu = B/H$.

Phantom—an artificial object of known dimensions and properties used to test aspects of an imaging machine.

Phase—in a periodic function (such as rotational or sinusoidal motion), the position relative to a particular part of the cycle.

Phase encoding—encoding the distribution of sources of *MR signals* along a direction in space with different phases by applying a pulsed *magnetic field gradient* along that direction prior to detection of the signal. In general, it is necessary to acquire a set of signals with a suitable set of different phase-encoding gradient pulses in order to reconstruct the distribution of the sources along the encoded direction.

Pixel—acronym for a picture element; the smallest discrete part of a digital image display. Note that the corresponding size of the pixel may be smaller than the actual spatial resolution.

Planar imaging—imaging technique in which an image of a plane is built up from signals received from the whole plane. See also Sequential plane imaging.

Precession—comparatively slow gyration of the axis of a spinning body so as to trace out a cone; caused by the application of a *torque* tending to change the direction of the rotation axis, and continuously directed at right angles to the plane of the torque. The *magnetic moment* of a nucleus with *spin* experiences such a torque when inclined at an angle to the *magnetic field*, resulting in precession at the *Larmor frequency*. A familiar example is the effect of gravity on the motion of a spinning top or gyroscope.

Probe—the portion of an *MR spectrometer* comprising the sample container and the *RF coils*, with some associated electronics. The RF coils may consist of separate *receiver* and *transmitter* coils in a *crossed-coil* configuration, or, alternatively, a single coil to perform both functions.

Pulse, 90 degrees ($\pi/2$ **pulse**)—*RF pulse* designed to rotate the *macroscopic magnetization vector* 90 degrees in space as referred to the *rotating frame of reference*, usually about an axis at right angles to the main *magnetic field*. If the *spins* are initially aligned with the magnetic field, this pulse will produce *transverse magnetization* and an *FID*.

Pulse, 180 degrees (π **pulse**)—*RF pulse* designed to rotate the *macroscopic magnetization vector* 180 degrees in space as referred to the *rotating frame of reference*, usually about an axis at right angles to the main *magnetic field*. If the *spins* are initially aligned with the magnetic field, this pulse will produce *inversion*.

Pulse length (width)—time duration of a pulse. For an *RF pulse* near the *Larmor frequency*, the longer the pulse length, the greater the angle of rotation of the *macroscopic magnetization vector* will be (greater than 180 degrees can bring it back toward its original orientation). For an RF pulse of a given shape as a function of time, the longer the pulse length, the narrower the equivalent range of frequencies in the pulse will be.

Pulse sequences—set of *RF* (and/or *gradient*) *magnetic field pulses* and time spacings between these pulses; used in conjunction with magnetic field gradients and *NMR signal* reception to produce NMR images. See also Interpulse times. A recommended shorthand designation of interpulse times used to generate a particular image is to list the repetition time *(TR)*, the echo time *(TE)* and, if using *inversion-recovery*, the inversion time, *TI*, with all times given in milliseconds. For example, 2500/30/1000 would indicate an inversion-recovery pulse sequence with TR of 2500 msec, TE of 30 msec, and TI of 1000 msec. If using multiple *spin echoes*, as in *CPMG*, the number of the spin echo used should be stated.

Quenching—loss of *superconductivity* of the current-carrying *coil* that may occur unexpectedly in a superconducting magnet. As the magnet becomes resistive, heat is released that can result in rapid evaporation of liquid helium in the *cryostat*. This may present a hazard if not properly planned for.

Radian—dimensionless unit of angular measure; 360 degrees = 2π radians.

Radiofrequency (RF)—wave *frequency* intermediate between auditory and infrared. The RF used in *NMR* studies is commonly in the *megahertz* (MHz) range. The RF used in *ESR* studies is commonly in the *gigahertz* (GHz) range. The principal effect of RF *magnetic fields* on the body is power deposition in the form of heating, mainly at the surface; this is a principal area of concern for safety limits.

Receiver—portion of the MR apparatus that detects and amplifies *RF signals* picked up by the *receiving coil*. Includes a preamplifier, amplifier, and *demodulator*.

Receiver dead time—time after exciting *RF pulse* during which *FID* is not detectable due to saturation of *receiver* electronics.

Relaxation rates—reciprocals of the *relaxation times*.

Relaxation times—after *excitation*, the *spins* tend to return to their equilibrium distribution, in which there is no *transverse magnetization* and the *longitudinal magnetization* is at its maximum value and oriented in the direction of the static *magnetic field*. It is observed that in the absence of applied *RF magnetic field*, the transverse magnetization decays toward zero with a characteristic time constant *T2*, and the longitudinal magnetization returns toward the equilibrium value M_o with a characteristic time constant *T1*.

Repetition time—see TR.

Rephasing gradient—*magnetic field gradient* applied for a brief period after a *selective excitation* pulse, in the opposite direction to the *gradient* used for the selective excitation. The result of the gradient reversal is a rephasing of the *spins* (which will have become out of *phase* with each other along the direction of the selection gradient), forming a *gradient echo* and improving the sensitivity of imaging after the selective excitation process.

Resonance—a large amplitude vibration in a mechanical or electrical system caused by a relatively small periodic stimulus with a *frequency* at or close to a natural frequency of the system; in *NMR* apparatus, resonance can refer to the NMR itself or to the tuning of the *RF* circuitry.

Resonance frequency—*frequency* at which *resonance* phenomenon occurs; given by the *Larmor equation* for *NMR*; determined by inductance and capacitance for *RF* circuits.

RF—see Radiofrequency.

Rotating frame of reference—a frame of reference (with corresponding coordinate systems) that is rotating about the axis of the static *magnetic field* B_0 (with respect to a stationary ["laboratory"] frame of reference) at a *frequency* equal to that of the applied *RF* magnetic field, B_1. Although B_1 is a rotating *vector*, it appears stationary in the rotating frame, leading to simpler mathematical formulations.

Saturation—a nonequilibrium state in *MR*, in which equal numbers of spins are aligned against and with the *magnetic field*, so that there is no net *magnetization*. Can be produced by repeatedly applying RF pulses at the *Larmor frequency* with interpulse times short compared with T1.

Saturation recovery (SR)—particular type of *partial saturation pulse sequence* in which the preceding pulses leave the *spins* in a state of *saturation*, so that recovery at the time of the next pulse has taken place from an initial condition of no *magnetization*.

Saturation transfer (or inversion transfer)—nuclei can retain their magnetic orientation through a chemical reaction. Thus, if *RF* radiation is supplied to the *spins* at a *frequency* corresponding to the *chemical shift* of the nuclei in one chemical state so as to produce *saturation* or *inversion*, and chemical reactions transform the nuclei into another chemical state with a different chemical shift in a shorter time compared with the *relaxation time*, the NMR *spectrum* may show the effects of the saturation or inversion on the corresponding, unirradiated, line in the spectrum. This technique can be used to study reaction kinetics of suitable molecules.

Scalar—a quantity having only magnitude.

Selective excitation—controlling the *frequency spectrum* of an irradiating *RF pulse* (via *tailoring*) while imposing a *magnetic field gradient* or *spins*, such that only a desired region has a suitable *resonant frequency* to be excited. Originally used to excite all but a desired region; now more commonly used to select only a desired region, such as a plane, for excitation.

Sensitive plane—technique of selecting a plane for *sequential plane imaging* by using an oscillating magnetic field *gradient* and filtering out the corresponding time dependent part of the *NMR signal*. The gradient used is at right angles to the desired plane and the magnitude of the oscillating magnetic field gradient is equal to zero only in the desired plane.

Sequence time—see TR.

Shift reagents—*paramagnetic* compounds designed to induce a shift in the *resonance frequency* of nuclei with which they interact. For example, many rare earths have been used as shift reagents for positive metal ions such as sodium and potassium.

Shimming—correction of *inhomogeneity* of the *magnetic field* produced by the main magnet of an *NMR* system due to imperfections in the magnet or to the presence of external *ferromagnetic* objects. May involve changing the configuration of the magnet or the addition of *shim coils (active shimming)* or small pieces of steel *(passive shimming)*.

Signal averaging—the averaging together of signals acquired under the same or similar conditions so as to suppress the effects of random variations or random artifacts. The number of signals averaged together can be abbreviated *NSA*.

Signal-to-noise ratio (SNR or S/N)—used to describe the relative contributions to a detected signal of the true signal and random superimposed signals *("noise")*. One common method to improve (increase) the SNR is to average several measurements of the signal on the expectation that random contributions will tend to cancel out. The SNR can also be improved by sampling larger volumes (with a corresponding loss of spatial resolution) or, within limits, by increasing the strength of the magnetic field used. The SNR depends on the electrical properties of the sample or patient being studied.

Slice—the effective physical extent of the "planar" region being imaged.

Slice thickness—the thickness of a *slice*. Because the *slice profile* may not be sharp edged, a criterion such as the distance between the points at half the sensitivity of the maximum *(FWHM)* or the equivalent rectangular width (the width of a rectangular slice profile with the same maximum height and same area) may be useful.

S/N—see Signal-to-noise ratio.

SNR—see Signal-to-noise ratio.

Spatial resolution—the smallest distance between two points in the object that can be distinguished as separate details in the image, generally indicated as a length or a number of black and white line pairs per mm. The specific criterion of resolution to be used depends on the type of test used (e.g., bar pattern or contrast-detail *phantom*). As the ability to separate or detect objects depends on their *contrast* and the noise, and the different *NMR* parameters of objects affect image contrast differently for different imaging techniques, care must be taken in comparing the results of resolution phantom tests of different machines and no single simple measure of resolution can be specified. The resolution may be anisotropic. The resolution may be larger than the size corresponding to the discrete image element *(pixel)*, although it cannot be smaller.

Spectral line—particular distinct *frequency* or narrow band of frequencies at which *resonance* occurs corresponding to a particular *chemical shift*.

Spectrometer—the portions of the *NMR* apparatus that actually produce the NMR phenomenon and acquire the signals, including the *magnet*, the *probe*, the *RF* circuitry, and the *gradient coils*. The spectrometer is controlled by the *computer* via the *interface* under the direction of the *software*.

Spectrum—an array of the *frequency components of the MR signal* according to frequency. Nuclei with different *resonant frequencies* show up as values at different corresponding frequencies in the spectrum. When resonances are relatively isolated, they appear as peaks or "lines" in the spectrum.

Spin—The intrinsic *angular momentum* of an elementary particle, or system of particles such as a nucleus, that is also responsible for the *magnetic moment;* or, a particle or nucleus possessing such a spin. The spins of nuclei have characteristic fixed values. Pairs of neutrons and protons align to cancel out their spins, so that nuclei with an odd number of neutrons and/or protons have a net non-zero rotational component characterized by an integer or half integer quantum *"nuclear spin number" (I)*.

Spin density (N)—the density of resonating *spins* in a given region; one of the principal determinants of the strength of the *NMR signal* from the region. The *SI* units would be moles/m^3. For water, there are about 1.1×10^5 moles of hydrogen per m^3, or .11 moles of hydrogen/cm^3. True spin density is *not* imaged directly, but must be calculated from signals received with different *interpulse times*.

Spin echo—reappearance of an *NMR signal* after the *FID* has apparently died away, as a result of the effective reversal of the dephasing of the spins (refocusing) by techniques such as specific *RF pulse sequences*, e.g., *Carr-Purcell sequence (RF spin echo)*, or pairs of *magnetic field gradient pulses (gradient echo)*, applied in times shorter than or on the order of *T2*. Unlike RF spin echoes, gradient echoes do not refocus phase differences due to *chemical shifts* or *inhomogeneities* of the *magnetic field*.

Spin-echo imaging—any of many *MR imaging* techniques in which the *spin echo* is used rather than the *FID*. Can be used to create images that depend strongly on *T2* if TE has a value on the order of a greater than T2 of the relevant image details. Note that spin echo imaging does *not* directly produce an image of T2 distribution. The spin echoes can be produced as a train of multiple echoes, e.g., using the *CPMG pulse sequence*.

Spin-lattice relaxation time—see T1.

Spin number, nuclear—see Nuclear spin number.

Spin-spin coupling—interaction between nuclei in the same molecule that results in a splitting of a single resonance line into two or more lines. For example, a ^{13}C nucleus with a directly bonded proton has two resonance frequencies corresponding to the two different orientations of the bonded proton.

Spin-spin relaxation time—see T2.

Spin tagging—nuclei will retain their magnetic orientation for a time on the order of *T1* even in the presence of motion. Thus, if the nuclei in a given region have their *spin* orientation changed, the altered spins will serve as a "tag" to trace the motion of any fluid that may have been in the tagged region for a time on the order of T1.

Spin-warp imaging—a form of *Fourier transform imaging* in which phase-encoding gradient pulses are applied for a constant duration but with varying amplitude. The spin warp method, as with other Fourier imaging techniques, is relatively tolerant of nonuniformities *(inhomogeneities)* in the *magnetic fields*.

Steady state free precession (SFP or SSFP)—method or *NMR excitation* in which strings of *RF pulses* are applied rapidly and repeatedly with interpulse intervals short compared with both *T1* and *T2*. Alternating the *phases* of the RF pulses by 180 degrees can be useful in obtaining maximal signal strength.

Superconductor—a substance whose electrical resistance essentially disappears at temperatures near absolute zero. A commonly used superconductor in *NMR imaging* system magnets is niobium-titanium, embedded in a copper matrix to help protect the superconductor from *quenching*.

Suppression—one of a number of techniques designed to minimize the contribution of a particular *spectral line* to the detected *signal*. Most commonly used to suppress the strong signal from water in order to detect other components.

Surface coil—*receiver coil* that does not surround the body and is placed close to the surface of the body. Used to restrict the region of the body contributing to the detected signal.

T_1 or T1 ("T-one")—spin-lattice or longitudinal *relaxation time;* the characteristic time constant for *spins* to tend to align themselves with the external *magnetic field*. Starting from zero *magnetization* in the z direction, the z magnetization will grow to 63 percent of its final maximum value in a time T1.

T_2 or T2 ("T-two")—spin-spin or transverse *relaxation time;* the *characteristic time constant for loss of phase* coherence among spins oriented at an angle to the static *magnetic field*, due to interactions between the spins, with resulting loss of *transverse magnetization* and *NMR signal*. Starting from a non-zero value of the magnetization in the xy plane, the xy magnetization will decay so that it loses 63 percent of its initial value in a time T2.

T2* ("T-two-star")—the observed time constant of the *FID* due to loss of *phase* coherence among spins oriented at an angle to the static *magnetic field*, commonly due to a combination of magnetic field *inhomogeneities*, ΔB, and *spin-spin transverse relaxation* with resultant more rapid loss in transverse magnetization and *NMR signal*. NMR signals can usually still be recovered as a spin echo in times less than or on the order of T2. $1/T2^* \cong 1/T2 + \Delta\omega/2$; $\Delta\omega = \gamma\Delta B$.

TE—echo time. Time between middle of 90-degree *pulse* and middle of *spin echo* production. For multiple echoes, use TE1, TE2. . . .

Tesla (T)—the preferred *(SI)* unit of magnetic flux density. One tesla is equal to 10,000 *gauss*, the older (CGS) unit.

Thermal equilibrium—a state in which all parts of a system are at the same effective temperature, in particular where the relative alignment of the *spins* with the *magnetic field* is determined solely by the thermal energy of the system (in which case the relative numbers of spins with different alignments is given by the *Boltzmann distribution*).

TI—inversion time. In *inversion recovery*, time between middle of *inverting (180-degree) RF pulse* and middle of the subsequent *exciting (90-degree)* pulse to detect amount of *longitudinal magnetization*.

TR—repetition time. The period of time between the beginning of a *pulse sequence* and the beginning of the succeeding (essentially identical) pulse sequence.

Transverse magnetization (M_{xy})—component of the *macroscopic magnetization vector* at right angles to the static *magnetic* *field* (B_o). *Precession* of the *transverse magnetization* at the *Larmor frequency* is responsible for the detectable *NMR signal.* In the absence of externally applied *RF magnetic field,* the transverse magnetization decays to zero with a characteristic time constant of *T2* or *T2**.

Tuning—process of adjusting the *resonant frequency,* e.g., of the *RF* circuit, to the desired value, e.g., the *Larmor frequency.* More generally, the process of adjusting the components of the *spectrometer* for optimal *NMR signal* strength.

Two-dimensional Fourier transform imaging (2DFT)—a form of *sequential plane imaging* using *Fourier transform imaging.*

Vector—a quantity having both magnitude and direction, frequently represented by an arrow whose legnth is proportional to the magnitude and with an arrowhead at one end to indicate the direction.

Volume imaging—imaging techniques in which *NMR signals* are gathered from the whole object volume to be imaged at once, with appropriate encoding *pulse RF and gradient sequences* to encode positions of the *spins.* Many *sequential plane imaging* techniques can be generalized to volume imaging, at least in principle. Advantages include potential improvement in *signal-to-noise ratio* by including signal from the whole volume at once; disadvantages include a bigger computational task for image reconstruction and longer *image acquisition times* (although the entire volume can be imaged from the one set of data). Also called simultaneous volume imaging.

Voxel—volume element; the element of three-dimensional space corresponding to a *pixel,* for a given slice thickness.

x—dimension in the stationary (laboratory) frame of reference in the plane orthogonal (at right angles) to the direction of the static *magnetic field* (B_o *or* H_o), z, and orthogonal to y, the other dimension in this plane.

x′—dimension in the *rotating frame of reference* in the plane at right angles to the direction of the *static magnetic field* (B_o *or* H_o), z; commonly defined to be the direction of the magnetic vector of the *exciting* RF field (B_1).

y—dimension in the stationary (laboratory) frame of reference in the plane orthogonal to the direction of the static *magnetic field* (B_o and H_o), z, and orthogonal to x, the other dimension in this place.

y′—dimension in the *rotating frame of reference* in the plane orthogonal (at right angles) to the direction of the static *magnetic field* (B_o *and* H_o), z, and orthogonal to the other dimension in the plane, x'.

z—dimension in the direction of the static *magnetic field* (B_o and H_o), in both the stationary and *rotating frames of reference.*

γ—see Gyromagnetic ratio.

δ—see Chemical shift.

μ—see Permeability.

τ—often used to denote different time delays between RF pulses. See Interpulse times.

χ—see Magnetic susceptibility.

ω—see Angular frequency.

ω_o—see Larmor frequency.

Index

Note: Numbers in *italics* refer to illustrations; numbers followed by (t) indicate tables.

Abscess, posterior ring, after endocarditis, transesophageal echocardiography of, 611
Absolute area stenosis, accuracy of, 237
Acetate, C-11–labeled, 1150, *1150*, 1151, *1151*
Acetoacetate, in lipid metabolism, 46, *48*
Acetoacetyl-CoA, in lipid metabolism, 46, *48*
Acetoacetyl-CoA thiolase, in lipid metabolism, 46, *48*
Acetrizoic acid, *164*, 165
Acetyl coenzyme A (acetyl-CoA), in myocardial metabolism, 39, *40*
Acetylcholine receptors, muscarinic, characterization of, positron emission tomography in, 1264–1266, *1265*
Acid(s), acetrizoic, *164*, 165
amino, labeling of, with carbon-11, 1152
with nitrogen-13, 1152
transport of, in protein synthesis, 50
diatrizoic, *164*, 165
ethylenediaminetetra-acetic, as chelating agent, 173
fatty, polyunsaturated, for hypercholesterolemia, 268
gadolinium diethylenetriamine pentaacetic. See *GdDTPA*.
iothalamic, *164*, 165
nicotinic, for hyperlipidemia, 267, 268, 268(t)
oleic, 1085
palmitic, 1085
Acidosis, intracellular, phosphorus magnetic resonance spectroscopy in, 848
Acoustic impedance, definition of, 539
Acoustic impedance mismatch, definition of, 539
Acoustic microscopy, 544
Acquired heart disease, chest roentgenography of, 103–108
Acquisition time, 737
ACTA scanner, 635
Activated partial thromboplastin time (APTT), in pulmonary embolism, 154
Activity spillover, in positron emission tomography, 1157, *1158*
Acyanosis, in congenital heart disease, with increased pulmonary blood flow, Doppler echocardiography in, 479–489
two-dimensional echocardiography in, 479–489
Acylcarnitine, in lipid metabolism, 45, *45*
Acyl-CoA, oxidation of, 46, *47*
transport of, into mitochondria, 45, 46, *46*
Acyl-CoA dehydrogenase, in lipid metabolism, 46, *47*
Acyl-CoA synthetase, in lipid metabolism, 44, *45*
ADAC system, 220, 221, 221(t)
Adenocarcinoma, metastatic, echocardiography of, 519, *520*
Adenosine, in maximal coronary dilation, 15, 16
Adenosine triphosphatase (ATPase), in myocardial metabolism, 39, *40*
Adenosine triphosphate (ATP), in cardiomyopathy, 932, 933, *933*
Adenosine triphosphate (ATP) *(Continued)*
hypertrophic, 971
in congestive heart failure, *973*
in myocardial ischemia, 970, *971*
in myocardial metabolism, 39, *40*
in normal myocardium, 969, *970*
phosphorus magnetic resonance spectroscopy of, 845, 847, *847*
utilization of, during exercise, 49
during ischemia, 50
during ischemic exercise, 972–974, *974*
"Adjacent nonischemic dyskinesis," 594
Admixture lesions, magnetic resonance imaging of, 892
Adrenergic cardiac receptors, characterization of, positron emission tomography in, 1262–1264
imaging of, 1138
Adriamycin, toxic effects of, phosphorus magnetic resonance spectroscopy of, 849
AF-DX 116, 1264
Afterload, in left ventricular function, 26
Age, influence of, on diastolic performance, 410, *411*
Alanine, in ischemia, 49
in myocardial metabolism, 42
Alanine aminotransferase, in myocardial metabolism, 42
Albumin, in sonicated contrast agents, 559
Albumin microspheres, positron-labeled, 1142, *1142*
Albunex, safety of, 559
Algorithm(s), analysis, in regional left ventricular function assessment, 382–388, *383–389*
for indicator dilution methods, of myocardial perfusion measurement, 691, *691*, 692
for systolic wall thickening analysis, 391, *391*
Aliasing, 370, *370*
definition of, 1271
in magnetic resonance imaging, 787, 788, *788*, *789*
Aliasing errors, 76, *76*
Allergy, to contrast agents, as pulmonary angiography contraindication, 149
for coronary angiography, 188, 189
Allograft, cardiac, rejection of, antimyosin imaging in, 1115, 1116, *1116*
gamma imaging in, 1114
phosphorus magnetic resonance spectroscopy in, 851
Alpha-adrenergic receptors, in vivo study of, positron emission tomography in, 1264
ALU (arithmetic logic unit), of digital image processor, 284
Amino acid(s), labeling of, with carbon-11, 1152
with nitrogen-13, 1152
transport of, in protein synthesis, 50
Aminoacyl-tRNA synthesis, 50
Amipaque, *164*
Ammonia, nitrogen-13. See *Nitrogen-13 ammonia*.
A-mode display, 356
Amplatz technique, of coronary angiography, 191, 192, *192*
Amplification, decibel values for, 351(t)
in echocardiography, 359, 360, *360*, *361*
Amplitude, loss of, factors in, 351
of nuclear magnetic resonance spectrum, 746
Amplitude-modulated pulse, 748, *749*
Amyloid heart disease, 457, *457*
Amyloidosis, cardiac, ultrasonic tissue characterization in, 551, *552*
Analog signal, in nuclear magnetic resonance, 737
Analog videotape, in archival storage, in digital angiography, 286
Analogs, fatty acid. See *Fatty acid analogs*.
Analog-to-digital conversion, 74
in densitometry, 291, 292
in nuclear magnetic resonance, 737
Analysis algorithms, in regional left ventricular function assessment, 382–388, *383–389*
ANALYZE software, 660, *660*
Anaphylactoid reaction, to angiographic contrast agents, 174–176
Anastomosis, coronary, graft–native vessel, evaluation of, high-frequency epicardial echocardiography in, 615–617, *626–629*
Anemia, in coronary reserve, 14
Aneurysm(s), apical, left ventricular thrombus with, echocardiography of, *523*
of aorta, ascending, magnetic resonance imaging of, 893, *893*
magnetic resonance imaging of, 874, *874*, *875*
roentgenographic evaluation of, *107*, 108
rupture of, ultrafast computed tomography of, 710, *711*
thoracic, ultrafast computed tomography of, 710–712, *711*
ultrafast computed tomography of, advantages of, 711, 712
disadvantages of, 711, 712
of arteries, imaging of, indium-111–labeled platelets in, 1127, 1128, *1128*
of interatrial septum, echocardiography of, 529, *530*
of left ventricle, 101, *103*
after myocardial infarction, 110, *116*, 600, *600*
cine magnetic resonance imaging of, *963*
of pulmonary artery, pulmonary angiography in, 156, 157, *158*
of sinus of Valsalva, magnetic resonance imaging of, 893
Rasmussen's, 157
ventricular function in, as predictor of survival, 138
Angina, as coronary angiography indication, 184
exertional, in atherosclerosis, 269, 270(t)
management of, equilibrium radionuclide angiography in, 1037
Angiocardiography, radionuclide. See *Radionuclide angiocardiography*.
Angiographic contrast agents, acute toxicity of, 166–168

Angiographic contrast agents *(Continued)*
anaphylactoid reaction to, 174–176
effects of, gastrointestinal, 176
hematologic, 176
noncardiovascular, 174–177
on blood vessels, 176, 177
on pulmonary function, 176
on renal function, 176
intravascular bolus injection of, 168
cardiac output after, 169, *171*
intravascular volume after, 168, *168*
systemic arterial pressure after, 169, *169*
systemic vascular resistance after, 168, *169*
ventricular filling pressure after, 169, *170, 171*
iodine concentration in, 165, 166, *166*, 167(t)
marketed in United States, 165, 166
pharmacologic effects of, 166–177, 167(t)
pharmacologic properties of, 167(t)
selection of, criteria for, 177–179, *178*, 178(t)
selective intracoronary injection of, 170–177
cardiac electrophysiology after, 171–174, *173, 174*
myocardial performance after, 170, 171, *171, 172*
systemic arterial pressure after, 170, 171, *171, 172*
Angiography, aortic root, in bypass graft assessment, 325, *325*
in coronary artery assessment, 312, 313
bypass graft, 193
cardiac. See *Cardiac angiography.*
coronary. See *Coronary angiography.*
digital. See *Digital angiography.*
direct, in bypass graft assessment, 325
in coronary artery assessment, 313
in valvular regurgitation, 67, 68, 68(t)
internal mammary artery, 193
intravenous, in bypass graft assessment, 324, 325
in coronary artery assessment, 312
magnetic resonance, 787, 881
of coronary flow reserve, image processing in, 247–249, *247, 248*, 248(t)
maximal hyperemic response in, 246
pulmonary. See *Pulmonary angiography.*
pulmonary vein wedge, 151
radionuclide. See *Radionuclide angiography.*
subtraction, digital. See *Digital subtraction angiography.*
vs. echocardiography, in ejection fraction measurement, 378(t)
in left ventricular volume measurement, 375, *376*, 378(t)
Angioplasty, as coronary angiography indication, 184
coronary, transluminal, percutaneous. See *Percutaneous transluminal coronary angioplasty (PTCA).*
coronary arterial stenosis before, digital analysis of, 317, 318, *318*
peripheral, imaging of, indium-111–labeled platelets in, 1127, 1128
Angiosarcoma, 512
echocardiography of, 518, *518, 519*
Angiovist, *164*, 165
intracoronary injection of, and ventricular fibrillation, 174
properties of, 166, 167(t)
Angle(s), Doppler, 61, 62, *62*
Ernst, 737
flip, definition of, 1272
in magnetic resonance spectroscopy, 844
Angle(s) *(Continued)*
steady-state longitudinal magnetization of, 756, *756*
of insonification, 544
phase, 740
Angle of incidence, 352
Angle of refraction, 352
Angular frequency, definition of, 1271
Angular momentum, definition of, 1271
Annotation, definition of, 1271
Annular array, in echocardiography, 355, *355*, 356
Annuloplasty, tricuspid, 441
Anomalous bands, echocardiography of, 529
Anomalous left coronary artery, thallium-201 scintigraphy of, 1066(t), 1067
Anomalous pulmonary venous connection, pulmonary angiography in, 159
Anoxia, metabolic consequences of, carbon magnetic resonance spectroscopy of, 853
Antenna, definition of, 1271
Anterior leaflet, cleft of, and mitral regurgitation, 435
Antibody(ies), antimyosin, immunoreactivity of, enzymatic fragmentation in, 1111, *1112*
radiolabeling of, 1110–1112, *1111, 1112*
in gamma imaging, of blood clots, 1118
monoclonal, in imaging, 1110–1120
Anticoagulation, for left ventricular thrombi, after myocardial infarction, 602
Antifibrin imaging, 1118
Antihistamines, in premedication, before coronary angiography, 189
for contrast agent allergy, 189
Antimyosin, adverse reactions to, 1117
monoclonal, preparation of, 1110, 1111, *1111*
uptake of, in myocardial infarction, 1112, *1112*
Antimyosin antibodies, immunoreactivity of, enzymatic fragmentation in, 1111, *1112*
radiolabeling of, 1110–1112, *1111, 1112*
Antimyosin antibody scintigraphy, in infarct size measurement, *136*
Antimyosin imaging, in cardiac allograft rejection, 1115, 1116, *1116*
in humans, 1114–1117, *1114–1118*
in myocardial infarction, 1114, 1115
in myocarditis, 1116, 1117, *1117, 1118*
principles of, 1110
vs. planar imaging, 1115
vs. single-photon emission computed tomography, 1115
Antiparallel orientation, 733
Aorta, abnormalities of, acquired, magnetic resonance imaging of, 871–876, *871–875*
congenital, magnetic resonance imaging of, 867–871, *868–871*
aneurysm of, magnetic resonance imaging of, 874, *874, 875*
roentgenographic evaluation of, *107*, 108
rupture of, ultrafast computed tomography of, 710, *711*
thoracic, ultrafast computed tomography of, 710–712, *711*
ultrafast computed tomography of, advantages of, 711, 712
disadvantages of, 711, 712
ascending, aneurysm of, magnetic resonance imaging of, 893, *893*
blood flow in, systolic acceleration of, 405
velocity of, magnetic resonance imaging of, 881, *882*
blood flow in, detection of, in aortic regurgitation, 427, *428*
Aorta *(Continued)*
cine magnetic resonance imaging of, 953, 954, *954*
coarctation of, cine magnetic resonance imaging of, 867, *869*
left ventricular outflow obstruction in, 491, *491, 492*
magnetic resonance imaging of, 867, *868, 869*, 893, *894*
ultrafast computed tomography of, 725, *727*
diameter of, measurement of, 489
disease of, chest roentgenography in, 107, *107*, 108
magnetic resonance imaging in, 893, *893, 894*
spin-echo imaging of, 953
Aortic arch, magnetic resonance imaging of, 893
right-sided, *94*
Aortic balloon valvuloplasty, 441, 442
Aortic dissection, cine magnetic resonance imaging in, 872, *873*
evaluation of, 953, 954
in bicuspid aortic valves, 420
magnetic resonance imaging in, 871–874, *871–874*
chemical shift artifacts in, 873, *874*
transesophageal echocardiography in, 609–611, *609*
two-dimensional echocardiography in, 426, *426*
ultrafast computed tomography in, 710, 711, *711, 712*
advantages of, 711, 712
disadvantages of, 711, 712
Aortic end-diastolic pressure, in valvular regurgitation, 68
Aortic insufficiency, equilibrium radionuclide angiography in, 1040, *1040, 1041*
exercise-induced left ventricular dysfunction in, 1041, *1041*
magnetic resonance imaging in, *899, 900*, 903
Aortic regurgitation, causes of, 425–427
cine magnetic resonance imaging in, 957, 958, *958–960*
contrast ventriculography in, 110, *115*
echocardiography in, 425–430, *426, 427*
Doppler, 427–430, *428, 429*
continuous-wave, 428, *429*, 430
in decision-making, 430
M-mode, 427, *427*
transesophageal, 425, 426
two-dimensional, 430
evaluation of, quantitative, 428–430
semiquantitative, 427–438
in Marfan's syndrome, 426, 427
left ventricular enlargement in, 101, *102*
left ventricular pressure-volume curve in, *140*
magnetic resonance imaging in, *901, 902*
premature mitral valve closure in, 68
radionuclide angiocardiography in, 1021
roentgenographic evaluation of, 104
severity of, color flow imaging of, 428
evaluation of, 67
pulsed-wave mapping of, 427
signal void in, 957, *958–960*
thoracic aortic blood flow in, 427, *428*
ultrafast computed tomography in, 679, *679*
valve repair for, intraoperative echocardiography during, 623, 624
valvular vegetations in, 425
Aortic root, angiography of, in bypass graft assessment, 325, *325*
in coronary artery assessment, 312, 313

Aortic root *(Continued)*
dilation of, cine magnetic resonance imaging of, 953, *954*
in aortic regurgitation, 426
size of, measurement of, magnetic resonance imaging in, 816, *816*
stroke volume of, calculation of, 58, *58*
Aortic stenosis, aortic valvular orifice area in, measurement of, 421
causes of, 419
cine magnetic resonance imaging in, 961, *961*
contrast ventriculography in, 110
diastolic left ventricular function in, 410
echocardiography in, 419–425, *420*
Doppler, 421–425, *422–425*
in decision-making, 425
two-dimensional, 420, *420*, 421
hemodynamic severity of, 421
left ventricular outflow obstruction in, 489, *490*
left ventricular pressure-volume curve in, *140*
magnetic resonance imaging in, 903, *905–909*
mean gradient in, Doppler echocardiographic measurement of, with catheterization, 421, *423*
modified Bernoulli equation in, 421
radionuclide angiocardiography in, 1021
senile, 419, 420
signal void in, 961, *961*
spin-echo imaging in, *909*
supravalvular, left ventricular outflow obstruction in, 491, *491*
magnetic resonance imaging in, 871, *871*, 893
transvalvular aortic velocity in, measurement of, 421
transvalvular pressure gradient in, measurement of, 421, *423*
valvular, subvalvular pressure gradients in, 60
Aortic stroke volume, in mitral regurgitation, 436
Aortic valve, area of, determination of, catheterization in, 421, *424*
continuity equation in, 421, *424*
bicuspid, aortic dissection in, 420
calcification of, 104
biplane transesophageal echocardiography of, *615*
calcification of, magnetic resonance imaging in, *905*, *906*
disease of, congenital, and aortic regurgitation, 426
rheumatic, 425
orifice area of, in aortic stenosis, 421
repair of, intraoperative echocardiography during, 623, 624, *624*
replacement of, equilibrium radionuclide angiography in, 1040, *1040*, *1041*
stenosis of, roentgenographic evaluation of, 104
Aortic valve gradient, underestimation of, by Doppler echocardiography, 425, *425*
Aortopulmonary window, magnetic resonance imaging of, 894
Apical wall motion, analysis of, 388–390
Appearance time, in coronary flow reserve measurement, *335*
in functional assessment, of coronary circulation, 334, *334–338*, 335
in hyperemia induction, 334, *334*
APTT (activated partial thromboplastin time), in pulmonary embolism, 154
Aquo-ion, relaxivity dispersion of, after chelation, *796*
Archival storage, in digital angiography, 286
analog videotape in, 286
cine film in, 286
digital optical disk in, 286
helical scan 8-mm magnetic tape in, 286
nine-track magnetic tape in, 286
Area-length method, of volume determination, 110, 111, *116*
Argon, in coronary blood flow measurement, 244
Arithmetic logic unit (ALU), of digital image processor, 284
Aromatic fatty acid analogs, 1088, 1089, *1089*
Array, annular, in echocardiography, 355, *355*, 356
linear, in electronic beam steering, 356, 357, *357*, *358*
phased, in electronic beam steering, 357, 358, *358*, *359*
orthogonal, in electronic beam steering, 359, *359*
Array processors, of digital images, 285
Arrhythmia(s), after intracoronary contrast agent injection, 187
coronary angiography and, 186, 186(t)
during exercise, equilibrium radionuclide angiography of, 1029
ventricular, as coronary angiography indication, 184
Arsenic, toxic effects of, phosphorus magnetic resonance spectroscopy of, 849
Arterial pressure, monitoring of, during coronary angiography, 190
systemic, effect on, of breath holding, 171, *172*
after intravascular bolus injection, of angiographic contrast agents, 169, *169*
after selective intracoronary injection, of angiographic contrast agents, 170, 171, *171*, *172*
Arteriography, coronary, in coronary artery disease diagnosis, vs. positron emission tomography, 1176, 1176(t), 1177, *1177*
quantitative. See *Quantitative coronary arteriography.*
digital subtraction, time-density analysis of, *331*
pulmonary, balloon occlusion, 150, 151
subjective vs. quantitative, 1174, 1175
Arteriovenous fistulae, pulmonary, pulmonary angiography in, 155, 156, *157*
Arteritis, Takayasu's, 156, *157*
magnetic resonance imaging in, 876
Artery(ies), aneurysms of, imaging of, indium-111–labeled platelets in, 1127, 1128
blood flow in, velocity of, 822(t)
coronary. See *Coronary artery(ies).*
dimensions of, densitometric validation studies of, 237, 238
nondensitometric validation studies of, 236, 237
great, transposition of, echocardiography in, 497, *497*, *506*, *507*
ultrafast computed tomography in, 722, *722*
injuries to, imaging of, indium-111–labeled platelets in, 1127, 1128
internal mammary, angiography of, 193
left anterior descending. See *Left anterior descending artery.*
pulmonary. See *Pulmonary artery.*
"roughness" of, measurement of, 227, *227*, 227(t)
stenotic, blood flow in, 215, *215*
Artifact(s), chemical shift, in magnetic resonance imaging, of aortic dissection, 873, *874*
Artifact(s) *(Continued)*
corduroy, 779, 788, *789*
definition of, 1271
echocardiography of, 528, 528(t), 529, *529–533*
flow, in magnetic resonance imaging, of aortic dissection, 872
from metal, in magnetic resonance imaging, 788, *790*
in fast computed tomography, in myocardial perfusion measurement, 695–698, *696–698*
in magnetic resonance imaging, of blood flow, 769–773, *772*, 785–787, 785(t)
suppression of, 773, 774
cardiac gating in, 773
phase compensation in, 774
saturation in, 773
prevention of, 791(t)
study of, 776
in x-ray computed tomography, 641
misregistration, in mask mode subtraction, 297, 298, *298*
moiré pattern of, 76, *77*
motion, cardiac, in magnetic resonance imaging, 781–783, 781(t), *782*
patient-related, in magnetic resonance imaging, 779–787, *781*
respiratory, in magnetic resonance imaging, 783, 783(t), 784
phase ghost, in magnetic resonance imaging, 786, *786*
phase-encoding, 865
pulsatile flow, in magnetic resonance imaging, 787
system-related, in magnetic resonance imaging, 787, 788, *788–791*
time-of-flight, *772*, 773
volume-averaging, in fast computed tomography, in myocardial perfusion measurement, 696
zipper, 788
Artifactual coarctation, 867
Ascending aorta, aneurysm of, magnetic resonance imaging of, 893, *893*
blood flow velocity in, magnetic resonance imaging of, 881, *882*
ASH (asymmetric septal hypertrophy), 450
Aspirin, with dipyridamole, for platelet deposition, on prosthetic grafts, 1130, *1131*
Asplenia, echocardiography in, 500, *505*
Asymmetric septal hypertrophy (ASH), 450
Asynchrony, measurement of, 140, 144
Atherosclerosis, angiographic intervention studies of, 267–270, 268(t), *269*, 270(t)
carotid, imaging of, indium-111–labeled platelets in, 1126, 1126(t)
coronary, high-frequency epicardial echocardiography in, 627, *630*
imaging of, indium-111–labeled platelets in, 1128
magnetic resonance imaging in, 881
progression of, 267–270
quantitative coronary angiography in, 267–270
radionuclide angiocardiography in, 1022
regression of, 267–270
ultrasonic tissue characterization in, 553, *553*
ATP. See *Adenosine triphosphate (ATP).*
ATPase (adenosine triphosphatase), in myocardial metabolism, 39, *40*
Atresia, congenital, of coronary arteries, 198
pulmonary. See *Pulmonary atresia.*
tricuspid. See *Tricuspid atresia.*
Atrial appendages, echocardiography of, 502, *504*

Atrial fibrillation, during exercise, equilibrium radionuclide angiography of, 1029
Atrial flutter, left atrial thrombi with, echocardiography of, 526, *527*
Atrial myxomas, ultrafast computed tomography of, 703, 704, *704*
imaging sequences in, 704
Atrial pacing, digital subtraction angiography with, 304–306, *305*
effects of, 304, *305*
in non-exercise stress echocardiography, 589
Atrial septal defect(s), *95*, *96*
blood flow in, pulmonary, 489
systemic, 489
echocardiography in, Doppler, *482*, 483
two-dimensional, *482*, 483
ostium primum as, 483, *487*
magnetic resonance imaging of, 888, *889*
ostium secundum as, *482*, 483
magnetic resonance imaging of, 888, *888*, *889*
pulmonary arterial hypertension in, 98, *99*
right ventricular volume overload with, 28
sinus venosus, ultrafast computed tomography of, 715, *716*
Atrial situs, ambiguus, echocardiography in, 500, *505*, *506*
determination of, 500
inversus, echocardiography in, 500, *505*, *506*
solitus, echocardiography in, 500, *507*, *508*
Atrioventricular canal, common, ultrafast computed tomography of, 717, *719*
Atrioventricular groove, 194
Atrioventricular septal defects, echocardiography in, Doppler, 487
two-dimensional, 486, 487, *487*, *488*
Atrioventricular sequence, in diastolic performance, 412, *413*
Atrioventricular valve(s), abnormalities of, ultrafast computed tomography of, 716, 717, *718*, *719*
disease of, magnetic resonance imaging of, 887
in atrioventricular defect, 487, *488*
incompetent, in restrictive cardiomyopathy, 458
Atrium(a), abnormalities of, ultrafast computed tomography of, 715, *716*
left. See *Left atrium(a)*.
right. See *Right atrium(a)*.
size of, echocardiography of, in dilated cardiomyopathy, 454
in restrictive cardiomyopathy, 457, *457*
Atropine, in premedication, before coronary angiography, 189
Attenuation, 351
correction for, in single-photon emission computed tomography, 987
decibel values for, 351(t)
definition of, 365
effect on, of ischemia, 545, *546*
in ultrasonic tissue characterization, 539
measurement of, in transmission, 540, *540*
Attenuation coefficient, 291, 351, 351(t), 540, *540*
collagen in, 543, *543*
in x-ray computed tomography, 640, 641
Autoregulation, of coronary blood flow, 243, *243*
regional aspects of, 9, 10, *10*
Averaging, respiratory, in magnetic resonance imaging, 783, 783(t), *784*
Axial resolution, determinants of, in echocardiography, 354
effect on, of pulse length, 353, *353*
Azimuthal resolution, 354. See also *Lateral resolution.*

B_0, 735
definition of, 1271
B_1, 735
definition of, 1271
B_1 field, in spectroscopy, 967, *968*
Background subtraction, in myocardial perfusion scintigraphy, 989
Back-projection, in single-photon emission computed tomography, 985, *985*, 986, *986*
Backscatter, cyclic variation in, 545, *545*, 546
after myocardial infarction, 548, *549*, *550*
after myocardial reperfusion, 546, *546*, 547
in dilated cardiomyopathy, 550, *551*
definition of, 539
integrated, 540, *541*
definition of, 539
in atherosclerosis, 553, *553*
ischemia effect on, 545, *546*
measurement of, in reflection, 540, *540*
point and blood, in cardiovascular Doppler physics, 367
Backscatter coefficient, collagen in, 543, *543*
definition of, 539
in infarction, 548, *548*
Backscatter imaging, integrated, 540, *540*, 541, *541*
real-time, 540, 541, *541*, *542*
Backscatter transfer function, 540, *541*
definition of, 539
Balloon occlusion pulmonary arteriography, 150, 151
Balloon valvuloplasty, aortic, 441, 442
mitral, 431, 441
Banding, pulmonary artery, magnetic resonance imaging of, 876–879, *878*
Bandwidth, definition of, 1271
of pulse, 748
receiver, 754
Baseline, definition of, 1271
BAY K 8644, 1266
Beam hardening, *636*, 637
in densitometry, 293
in fast computed tomography, in myocardial perfusion measurement, 696–698, *696–698*
Beam insertion, in echocardiography, instrumentation for, 353, *353*, 354
Beam thickness, 357
Benzodiazepine receptors, peripheral-type, characterization of, 1266, 1267
Bernoulli equation, 60, 61, *62*, 63
modified, in aortic stenosis, 421
in mitral regurgitation, 435
in mitral stenosis, 431
Beta oxidation, 1244–1246, *1246*
in fatty acid metabolism, 46, *47*
Beta-adrenergic receptors, distribution of, 1262, 1263
in vivo demonstration of, positron emission tomography in, 1263, 1264
subtypes of, 1262, 1263
Bicuspid aortic valve, calcification of, 104
Bicycle exercise, in equilibrium radionuclide angiography, 1028
in submaximal coronary dilation, 15
in systolic ventricular function, 407
left ventricular function during, evaluation of, ultrafast computed tomography in, 680
supine, Doppler echocardiography during, 578, *578*, *579*
Bicycle exercise *(Continued)*
two-dimensional echocardiography during, 576
upright, Doppler echocardiography during, 578, *578*, *579*
two-dimensional echocardiography during, 576, *576*
ventricular imaging during, 303, 304
Bifurcation, left anterior descending artery blood flow in, *327*
Bilinear interpolation, 81
Biochemical pathways, regulation of, 39
Bioenergetics, of substrates, in phosphorus magnetic resonance spectroscopy, 847, 848
Biomag 4125, *807*
Biplane analysis, interpretation of, 227
Biplane area-length volume model, 375
Bird's nest filter, for pulmonary embolism, 155
Blalock-Taussig shunt, magnetic resonance imaging of, 879, *880*
Bloch equation, definition of, 1271
Blood, "bright," 760
"dark," 760
effects on, of angiographic contrast agents, 176
Blood clots, gamma imaging of, with antibodies, 1118
Blood flow, coronary. See *Coronary blood flow*.
effects of, on magnetic resonance imaging, of great vessels, 864, 865, *866*, *867*
imaging of, techniques of, 774, *774*, 775
in aorta, detection of, in aortic regurgitation, 427, *428*
in congenital heart disease, ultrafast computed tomography of, 725–728, *728*
in hepatic vein, in tricuspid regurgitation, 438, *438*
in hypoperfused myocardium, 1234, 1235
in left anterior descending artery, before and after bifurcation, *327*
in myocardial acoustics, 544
in stenotic artery, 215, *215*
laminar, 59
effect of, on cine magnetic resonance imaging, 950, 951
magnetic resonance imaging of, 769–775
artifacts in, 769–773, *772*
suppression of, 773, 774
cardiac gating in, 773
phase compensation in, 774
saturation in, 773
excited spins in, washout of, 773
gradient-echo imaging effects in, 773
phase shifts in, 773
saturated spins in, washout of, 773
spin-echo imaging effects in, 773
measurement of, contrast echocardiography in, 563–565
electromagnetic flow probe in, *337*
pulsed-contrast injection method of, 328, *328*
techniques of, 774
time-of-flight, 774
myocardial, evaluation of, in cardiac disease, 1169–1189
measurement of, 1176(t)
positron emission tomography of, 1160–1163, *1161*, *1162*
analysis and interpretation of, 1172–1174, *1174*
circumferential profile analysis in, 1173, *1174*
equilibrium approach to, 1160
in therapeutic response evaluation, 1185–1187, *1186*

Blood flow *(Continued)*
quantification of, 1173
technique of, 1171, *1171–1173*, 1172
bolus, 1160, 1161, *1161*
tracers for, 1170, *1170*, 1170(t), 1171
kinetic models of, 1161–1163
positron-emitting tracers of, 1141–1144, 1141(t), *1142*
normal appearance of, in magnetic resonance imaging, 769–773, *770–772*
patterns of, in patent ductus arteriosus, *484*, 485, *485*, 486
physics of, 367, 368
flow profiles in, 367, 368, *368*
turbulence in, 368
viscosity in, 367, 368, *368*
pulmonary, calculation of, in left-to-right shunting, 487–489
in atrial septal defect, 489
in patent ductus arteriosus, 489
in ventricular septal defect, 489
increased, in congenital heart disease, two-dimensional echocardiography in, 479–489
with acyanosis, Doppler echocardiography in, 479–489
quantitation of, cine magnetic resonance imaging in, 965
magnetic resonance imaging in, 822–824, 822(t)
rate of, relationship of, to velocity, 58, 59, *59*
recovery of, after revascularization, 1223–1225, *1223*, *1224*, 1225(t)
regional, effect of, on iodo fatty acid analog uptake, 1092, 1093
systemic, calculation of, in left-to-right shunting, 487–489
in atrial septal defect, 489
in patent ductus arteriosus, 489
in ventricular septal defect, 489
systolic acceleration of, in ascending aorta, 405
turbulent, cine magnetic resonance imaging of, 950, 951, *951*, *952*
magnetic resonance imaging of, 769, *771*
Blood flow artifacts, in magnetic resonance imaging, 785–787, 785(t)
Blood flow–related enhancement, in magnetic resonance imaging, 785
Blood pressure, during exercise, 1020(t)
in valvular regurgitation, 68, *69*
Blood velocity, calculation of, in valve stenosis, Doppler equation in, 61, 62, *62*
phase shift in, 823, *823*
in arteries, 822(t)
in ascending aorta, magnetic resonance imaging of, 881, *882*
in left ventricular outflow tract, measurement of, 60
patterns of, in valvular regurgitation, 65–67, *65–67*
near stenotic valves, 59, 60, *60*, *61*
relationship of, to blood flow rate, 58, 59, *59*
to transvalvular pressure gradient, 60, 61, *62*
Blood vessels, effects on, of angiographic contrast agents, 176, 177
Blood volume, pulmonary, measurement of, equilibrium radionuclide angiography in, 1031
BMIPP, 1090
clearance rate of, 1090
fractional distribution of, 1090
in myocardial infarction, 1092
B-mode display, 356
B-mode images, real-time, formation of, 356–359
Boltzmann constant, 734
Boltzmann distribution, definition of, 1271
Border detection, in segmentation, 83
Bottom-up theory, of image perception, 88
Bradycardia, after intracoronary contrast agent injection, 187
Branch-chain fatty acid analogs, 1089, 1090
Breath holding, effect of, on systemic arterial pressure, 171, *172*
Bremsstrahlung beam, energy quality of, measurement of, 650, *654*
Bridging, coronary, 200
"Bright blood," 760
Bronchoconstriction, in pulmonary embolism, 153
Bronchogenic cysts, magnetic resonance imaging of, 940
Brown-Dodge method, of quantitative coronary angiography, 218, 219
Buffer, disk, 285
display, 285
Bulboventricular loop, echocardiography of, 500, *506*
Bull's eye plot, in myocardial perfusion quantification, 993, *993*
Bypass graft(s), angiography of, 193
assessment of, 324, 325
angiography in, aortic root, 325, *325*
direct, 325
intravenous, 324, 325
physiologic, 339, *343*
cine magnetic resonance imaging of, 963, 964, *964*
coronary artery, in ischemic cardiomyopathy, left ventricular function after, 1225, 1225(t)
flow rate in, determination of, ultrafast computed tomography in, 686
flow reserve in, determination of, ultrafast computed tomography in, 686
internal mammary artery, patency of, assessment of, ultrafast computed tomography in, 684, *684*
magnetic resonance imaging of, 874–876
patency of, determination of, computed tomography in, 682, 682(t)
ultrafast computed tomography in, 682–687
graft number in, 685, *685*
historical aspects of, 682, 682(t), *683*
interobserver variability in, 685
multicenter study of, 684, *684*, 685, *685*
pitfalls of, 685, *685*, 686
procedure for, 684
sensitivity and specificity of, 684, 684(t)
vs. other imaging techniques, 686
saphenous vein, patency of, assessment of, ultrafast computed tomography in, 684, *684*
stenotic, assessment of, ultrafast computed tomography in, 684, 685, *685*

C-11–labeled acetate, 1150, *1150*, 1151, *1151*
C-11–labeled ligands, for cardiac receptor studies, 1257, 1257(t)
C-11–labeled MQNB, 1152
C-11–labeled N-methyl quinuclidinyl benzylate, 1265, *1265*
C-11–labeled palmitate, 1145–1147, *1145–1148*
clearance of, 1147, *1147*
C-11–labeled palmitate *(Continued)*
in fatty acid metabolism, in myocardial ischemia, 1191–1195, *1192–1195*, 1198, 1199, *1199*, *1200*
in myocardial infarction, in detection, 1185, *1186*
in localization, 1235–1237, *1236*
myocardial tissue kinetics of, 1086, *1086*
vs. IPPA, 1089
C-11–labeled triphenylmethylphosphonium, 1153
Cadmium, toxic effects of, phosphorus magnetic resonance spectroscopy of, 849
Calcification, of aortic valve, bicuspid, 104
magnetic resonance imaging in, *905*, *906*
of mitral annulus, and mitral regurgitation, 435
pericardial, roentgenographic evaluation of, 106, *106*
Calcified cardiac structures, echocardiography of, 529, *533*
Calcium, deposition of, in damaged myocardial cells, 1077–1079, *1078*
Renografin-76 enrichment with, 171, *172*
Calcium antagonist, preangiographic administration of, 232, 233
Calibration, in quantitative coronary angiography, 224, *224*, 224(t), 225
of spatial measurements, in digital angiography, 290
Calipers, in quantitative coronary angiography, 218, *219*
Camera, digital, in radionuclide imaging, 980
gamma, in radionuclide angiocardiography, 1006, 1007
multicrystal, in radionuclide angiocardiography, *1009*
in radionuclide imaging, 980, 981
multiwire, in radionuclide imaging, 981, *981*
single-crystal, in radionuclide angiocardiography, *1009*
in radionuclide imaging, 978–980, 979, *980*
scintillation, 979, *979*, 980, *980*
video, in densitometry, 292
cAMP (cyclic adenosine monophosphate), in myocardial metabolism, 42
Carbohydrate metabolism, 39–44
glucose in, phosphorylation of, 39, 40, *41*
uptake of, 39, 40, *41*
glycogen metabolism in, 40–42, *41*
glycolysis in, 42, *43*
lactate metabolism in, 44
malate-aspartate shuttle in, 44, *45*
pyruvate dehydrogenase in, 42, *44*
pyruvate metabolism in, 42
Carbon, nucleus of, characteristics of, 842(t)
Carbon magnetic resonance spectroscopy, 851–854, *854*, *855*
Carbon spectroscopy, 975
Carbon-11, amino acid labeled with, 1152
Carbon-11 acetate, in oxidative metabolism, in myocardial ischemia, 1195–1197, *1196*, *1197*, 1199, 1200
Carcinoid syndrome, and pulmonary regurgitation, 440
and tricuspid regurgitation, 438
and tricuspid stenosis, 436, *437*
Carcinoma(s), embryonal, metastatic, echocardiography of, 520, *521*
lung, staging of, ultrafast computed tomography in, 712, *712*, 713
renal, metastatic, ultrafast computed tomography of, 404
renal cell, magnetic resonance imaging in, 881, *882*
Carcinosarcoma, pulmonary, 157

Cardiac allograft rejection, antimyosin imaging in, 1115, 1116, *1116*
gamma imaging in, 1114
phosphorus magnetic resonance spectroscopy in, 851
Cardiac amyloidosis, ultrasonic tissue characterization in, 551, *552*
Cardiac anatomy, analysis of, ultrafast computed tomography in, 715–725, *716–724*, *726*, *727*
Cardiac angiography, 109–148
applications of, 139–144
contrast agents for, selection of, 177–179, *178*, 178(t)
technique of, 109, 110
Cardiac catheterization, complications of, 186
outpatient, 206, 207
Cardiac chambers, flow to, differences in, 12, 13
Cardiac cycle, left ventricular function throughout, analysis of, 139–144, *139–143*
wall motion assessment throughout, 140–144, *141–143*
Cardiac drugs, effects of, measurement of, exercise Doppler echocardiography in, 578–580
Cardiac function, evaluation of, Doppler echocardiography in, 402–418
magnetic resonance imaging in, 819, *819–821*, 820
ultrafast computed tomography in, 669–681
global, assessment of, magnetic resonance imaging in, 819, *819*
segmental, assessment of, magnetic resonance imaging in, 819, 820
Cardiac hypertrophy, echocardiography of, 529, *533*
Cardiac imaging, effects on, of left ventricular function heterogeneity, 30
in anatomic assessment, 72–74
in functional assessment, 72–74
perceptual aspects of, 87–92
quantitative methods in, 72–86
Cardiac index, 122
Cardiac masses, chest roentgenography of, 106, *107*
echocardiographic evaluation of, 511–537
Cardiac motion, abnormalities of, in pericardial effusion, 464, *465*
Cardiac motion artifacts, in magnetic resonance imaging, 781–783, 781(t), *782*
prevention of, 791(t)
Cardiac output, 122
after intravascular bolus injection, of angiographic contrast agents, 169, *171*
Doppler, determination of, 403, 404
during exercise, 407, 1020(t)
measurement of, contrast echocardiography in, 568, *569*
magnetic resonance imaging in, 819, *819*
radionuclide angiocardiography in, 1014
ultrafast computed tomography in, 678, *678*
quantification of, 56–58
invasive standards for, 56, 57
velocity-based flow measurements in, 57, *57*, 58, *58*
Cardiac reserve, assessment of, stress ventriculography in, 135
Cardiac rhythm, in left ventricular function assessment, 34
Cardiac silhouette, heart size in, 99–103
left atrium enlargement on, *98–101*, 99, 100
left ventricle enlargement on, 100, 101, *102*, *103*
right atrium enlargement on, 101–103
Cardiac silhouette *(Continued)*
right ventricle enlargement on, 103, *103*
roentgenographic evaluation of, 98–103
lateral projection in, 99
posteroanterior projection in, 99
Cardiac situs, abnormal, magnetic resonance imaging in, 892
Cardiac structures, calcified, echocardiography of, 529, *533*
tissue of, ultrasonic characterization of. See *Ultrasonic tissue characterization.*
Cardiac tamponade, echocardiography in, 464–470, *466–471*
during pericardiocentesis, 470, *471*
effect of, on respiration, 469, *469*, *470*
pathophysiology of, 464, 465
pericardial effusion with, 708, *709*
postoperative, 466–468, *468*
Cardiac thrombi, imaging of, indium-111-labeled platelets in, 1124, *1124*, 1124(t), 1125, *1125*
Cardiac transplantation, as indication for coronary angiography, 184, *185*
spectroscopy in, 971, 972
Cardiac triggering. See also *Gating.*
in magnetic resonance imaging, 781–783, 781(t), *782*, *783*
Cardiac valves, evaluation of, ultrafast computed tomography in, 678, 679, *679*
Cardioactive drugs, hemodynamic effects of, 407
Cardiology, clinical, transesophageal echocardiography in, 605–617
Cardiomyopathy(ies), assessment of, magnetic resonance imaging in, 929–935
causes of, 1245(t)
chest roentgenography of, 105, 106
dilated. See *Dilated cardiomyopathy.*
Doppler left ventricular ejection velocity in, 405, *406*
echocardiography in, 449–459
equilibrium radionuclide angiography in, 1039, 1040
experimental, ultrasonic tissue characterization in, 551–553
hypertrophic. See *Hypertrophic cardiomyopathy.*
infiltrative, magnetic resonance imaging in, 933, 934, *934*
iodo fatty acid analogs in, 1093, *1093*, 1094
ischemic, left ventricular function in, after coronary artery bypass grafting, 1225, 1225(t)
myocardial metabolism in, 1244–1255
abnormalities of, 1246
magnetic resonance imaging of, 932, 933, *933*
obliterative, echocardiography in, 458
phosphorus magnetic resonance spectroscopy in, 848, 849
restrictive. See *Restrictive cardiomyopathy.*
ultrasonic tissue characterization in, 549–553, *551*, *552*
vs. constrictive pericarditis, ultrafast computed tomography in, 709
with systemic illnesses, 1252, 1253
Cardioplegic solutions, myocardial perfusion with, assessment of, contrast echocardiography in, 565–567
Cardiopulmonary bypass, echocardiography with, 622
Cardiothoracic (CT) ratio, 99
Cardiovascular tissue, ultrasonic characterization of, 538–556
Carnitine palmitoyltransferase, in lipid metabolism, 44
Carnitine shuttle, 45, 46, *46*
Carnitine translocase, in lipid metabolism, 44
Carotid atherosclerosis, imaging of, indium-111–labeled platelets in, 1126, 1126(t)
Carotid endarterectomy, imaging of, indium-111–labeled platelets in, 1127, *1127*
Carr-Purcell pulse sequence, *742*, 743
Carr-Purcell-Meiboom-Gill technique, 820
CASS (Coronary Artery Surgery Study), 213
Catecholamines, in glucose metabolism, 49
in myocardial metabolism, 49
in non-exercise stress echocardiography, 589
Catheter(ization), cardiac, complications of, 186
outpatient, 206, 207
Doppler echocardiography with, in aortic stenosis, in mean gradient measurement, 421, *423*
for quantitative coronary arteriography, selection of, 234, *235*
in aortic valve area determination, 421, *424*
in coronary angiography, brachial approach to, 190
femoral approach to, 190
transaxillary approach to, 190
in coronary stenosis measurement, 318
in pulmonary angiography, 150
in right ventricle, echocardiography of, 529, *530*
micrometric catheter measurement after, 234
pigtail, 109
with cardiomarker rings, 225
"Cavity obliteration," 110, *114*
Cell(s), alterations in, during experimental myocardial ischemia, 1074, *1076*
damaged, in myocardial infarcts, mitochondrial inclusions in, 1074–1077, *1076–1078*
function of, magnetic resonance spectroscopy of, 841–863
myocardial, damaged, calcium deposition in, 1077–1079, *1078*
Tc-99m-PPi deposition in, 1077–1079, *1078*
Centroid, 385, *386*
Cerebrovascular disease, imaging of, indium-111–labeled platelets in, 1126, 1126(t)
CFR. See *Coronary flow reserve (CFR).*
CGP 12177, 1152
CGR system, 220, 221, 221(t)
Chelation, in gadolinium potency, 804, *805*
in paramagnetic contrast agents, 795, 796, *796*
in relaxivity dispersion, 795, *796*
Chemical shift, 734
definition of, 1271
in magnetic resonance imaging, 777
of nuclei, 842(t)
Chemical shift imaging, definition of, 1271
Chemical shift reference, definition of, 1271
Chest, extracardiac abnormalities of, ultrafast computed tomography of, 703–713
Chest pain, as coronary angiography indication, 184
equilibrium radionuclide angiography in, in diagnosis, 1032–1034, 1032(t), *1033*
in prognosis, 1035–1037, *1036–1038*
Chest roentgenography, clinical aspects of, 93–108
interpretation in, 93–103
of acquired heart disease, 103–108
of aortic disease, 107, *107*, 108
of cardiac masses, 106, *107*
of cardiac silhouette, 98–103
of cardiomyopathy, 105, 106
of pericardial disease, 106
of pulmonary vasculature, 93–98
techniques of, 93

Chiari's network, echocardiography of, 512, *513*
Chirp-Z, 371, 372
Cholesterol, in atherosclerosis, 267–270, *269*
Cholesterol Lowering Atherosclerosis Study (CLAS), 270
Cholestyramine, for hyperlipidemia, 268, 268(t)
Cholinergic receptors, imaging of, 1138
  muscarinic, distribution of, 1264, 1265
    subtypes of, 1264, 1265
Chordae tendineae, ruptured, and mitral regurgitation, 433
Cimetidine, for contrast agent allergy, 189
Cine, flicker-free, in digital angiography, 287, 287(t)
Cine film, digitization of, cameras for, 219, 220(t)
    in quantitative coronary angiography, 219, 219(t), 220, *220*, 220(t)
  in archival storage, in digital angiography, 286
  in quantitative coronary angiography, 217, *217*, 218
  intravenous left ventriculography vs, 295–297
Cine frame, digitization of, variations in, 231, 232, 232(t)
  selection of, in quantitative coronary angiography, 241, 241(t), 242, 242(t)
Cine loop display, in digital angiography, 287
Cine magnetic resonance imaging, 783
  advantages of, 949, *950*
  effect on, of laminar blood flow, 950, 951
    of turbulent blood flow, 950, 951, *951*, *952*
  in aortic dissection, 872, *873*
  in blood flow quantitation, 965
  in cardiac chamber evaluation, 951–953, *953*
  in cardiac quantitation, 812, *814*
  in congenital heart disease, 962, *962*
  in coronary artery disease, 962–964, *963*, *964*
  in dilated cardiomyopathy, 931, *932*
  in hypertrophic cardiomyopathy, 931
  in valvular heart disease, 897, 898, *898*, 955–962, *957–961*
  limitations of, 949, 950
  multislice, 952
  of aortic coarctation, 867, *869*
  of great vessels, 953–955, *954–956*
  of intracardiac masses, 964, *964*, 965
  orthogonal, 952
  principles of, 948–966
    physical, 948, 949
  signal void in, 951, *951*, *952*
  technical implementation of, 949
Cineangiography, coronary. See *Coronary cineangiography.*
  digital subtraction, in coronary flow reserve measurement, 255, 256, *256*, *257*
    vs. intracoronary Doppler technique, 255, 256, *256–258*
  end-diastolic, in coronary blood flow measurement, 247, *247*
  in ejection fraction measurement, 379, *380*
  in end-diastolic volume measurement, *379*
  in end-systolic volume measurement, *379*
  intraventricular, vs digital angiography, 295–297, *296*, *297*
  of coronary circulation, 311
  vs. digital subtraction angiography, in coronary quantification, 319–322, *321–323*, 322(t), 323(t)
  x-ray gantry variability in, 240, 240(t)
Cineventriculogram, visual inspection of, 110, *111*
Circulation, coronary. See *Coronary circulation.*
  pulmonary, cine magnetic resonance imaging of, 954, 955, *955*, *956*
Circumferential profile, from tomographic slices, *992*, *993*
  generation of, in myocardial perfusion scintigraphy, 989, *989*, 990
  in positron emission tomography, of myocardial blood flow, 1173, *1174*
  of segmental wall motion, *999*
Circumflex coronary artery, anatomy of, 196
  collateral pathways to, 200
  left, atherosclerosis in, regression of, 270, 270(t)
  origin of, from right coronary artery, 198
    from right coronary sinus, 198
  reperfusion of, sodium imaging in, *835*, *836*
Citrate, in diabetes, 49
  in fasting, 49
Citrate synthetase, in tricarboxylic acid cycle, 47
Citric acid cycle, 1244–1246, *1246*
  carbon magnetic resonance spectroscopy of, 853
CIVICO III, 219, *220*
CIVICO IV, 219
CLAS (Cholesterol Lowering Atherosclerosis Study), 270
Cleft, of anterior leaflet, and mitral regurgitation, 435
Clofibrate, for hyperlipidemia, 267, 268, 268(t)
C/N, definition of, 1272
CNR, definition of, 1272
Coagulation, effects on, of angiographic contrast agents, 176
Coarctation, artifactual, 867
  of aorta, cine magnetic resonance imaging of, 867, *869*
    left ventricular outflow obstruction in, 491, *491*, *492*
    magnetic resonance imaging of, 867, *868*, *869*, 893, *894*
    ultrafast computed tomography of, 725, *727*
Coefficient, attenuation, 540, *540*
    collagen in, 543, *543*
  backscatter, collagen in, 543, *543*
    definition of, 539
    in infarction, 548, *548*
Coil, definition of, 1271
Cold pressor response, in non-exercise stress echocardiography, 589
Colestipol, for hyperlipidemia, 268, 268(t)
Collagen, in ultrasonic tissue characterization, 543, *543*, 544
Collateral circulation, coronary. See *Coronary collateral circulation.*
"Collateral steal," 18
Collimation, in radionuclide imaging, 980
  of x-ray beam, in computed tomography, 643
Color flow Doppler, instrumentation for, 371
  spectral analysis of, 372
Color flow imaging, in aortic regurgitation, 428
  in mitral regurgitation, 435
  in mitral stenosis, 431
  in patent ductus arteriosus, 486
  in pulmonary regurgitation, 440
  in tricuspid regurgitation, 438
  of left ventricular outflow obstruction, in hypertrophic cardiomyopathy, 451
  of ventricular septal defects, 481
Color flow mapping, of regurgitant jet, in mitral regurgitation, 622, 622(t)
Compensation, flow, 786
Compensatory hyperfunction, in infarcted myocardium, 33
Compression, gray scale, in digital imaging, 77, *78*
  in myocardial perfusion determination, 10
Computed tomography (CT), fast. See *Fast computed tomography.*
  gated, 644, 645, *645*
  half-value layer in, 650, *654*
  Hounsfield unit linearity in, 649, 650, 653(t), *654*
  in constrictive pericarditis, 943
  in indicator dilution methods, of myocardial perfusion measurement, 689–691, *690*, *692*
  in pericardial effusion, 941
  low-contrast resolution in, 648, 649, 650(t), *651*
  noise in, 649, 653(t)
  of bypass graft patency, 682, 682(t)
  radiation dosimetry in, 647, *647*, 648(t)
  slice thickness and contiguity in, 648, 648(t)
  spatial resolution in, 648, 649(t)
  stop-action, of moving organs, 645, *646*, *647*
  three-dimensional, dynamic, 643–665, *644*
    image analysis and display in, 659–665, *660–665*
  ultrafast. See *Ultrafast computed tomography.*
  uniformity in, 649, *652*, 652(t)
  with intravenous contrast agents, in myocardial perfusion measurement, 692–695, *693–695*
  x-ray, dynamic, instrumentation for, 634–668
      principles of, 634–668
    history of, 634, 635
    image quality in, 639–641
    scanner for, subsystems of, 641–643, *642*
Computed tomography dose index (CTDI), 647, *647*
Computer(s), host, in quantitative coronary angiography, 221, 221(t), 222, 222(t)
  of digital image processor, 285
  in x-ray computed tomography, 643
Computer languages, for quantitative coronary angiography, 222, 222(t)
Congenital heart disease, blood flow in, ultrafast computed tomography of, 725–728, *728*
  cine magnetic resonance imaging in, 962, *962*
  classification of, 887
  complex, echocardiographic approach to, 499–508, *500–508*
  echocardiography in, Doppler, 479–510
    intraoperative, 630, 631
    transesophageal, 612, *613*
    two-dimensional, 479–510
  magnetic resonance imaging in, 886–895
  radionuclide angiocardiography in, 1021
  right ventricular dimensions in, 394
  shunting in, ultrafast computed tomography of, 728, *728*
  surgical treatment of, 887
  ultrafast computed tomography in, 714–731
    clinical experience with, 714, 715
    technique of, 715
  ventricular volume and mass in, ultrafast computed tomography of, 728
  with acyanosis, and increased pulmonary blood flow, Doppler echocardiography in, 479–489
      two-dimensional echocardiography in, 479–489
    magnetic resonance imaging in, 887, 888

Congenital heart disease *(Continued)*
with cyanosis, and decreased pulmonary vascularity, Doppler echocardiography in, 492–496, *494–496*
two-dimensional echocardiography in, 492–496, *494–496*
and increased pulmonary vascularity, Doppler echocardiography in, 496–499
two-dimensional echocardiography in, 496–499, *497–499*
magnetic resonance imaging in, 887–892
with ventricular outflow obstruction, Doppler echocardiography in, 489–492
two-dimensional echocardiography in, 489–492
Congestive cardiomyopathy. See *Dilated cardiomyopathy.*
Congestive heart failure, ejection velocity in, after vasodilator therapy, 407
left ventricular dilatation in, 110, *113*
spectroscopy in, 972, *973*
thallium-201 scintigraphy in, 1066
Conotruncal defects, features of, 492
Conray, *164*, 165
Constrictive pericarditis, diagnosis of, 943, 944
echocardiography in, 470–475, *472–475*
Doppler, 473, *474*
M-mode, 470, *472*, *473*
two-dimensional, 470–475, *472*, *473*
filling dysfunction in, 473
mitral flow velocity in, 473, *474*, *475*
occult, 943
respiration in, 474, 475, *475*
ultrafast computed tomography in, 709, *709*
ventricular diastolic pressure in, 473, 474
vs. cardiomyopathy, ultrafast computed tomography in, 709
vs. restrictive cardiomyopathy, 943
Constructive interference, 352
Continuity equation, 58, 59, *59*
in aortic valve area determination, 421, *424*
in mitral stenosis, 433
Continuous loop display, in echocardiography, 363
Continuous wave echocardiography, of left ventricular outflow obstruction, in hypertrophic cardiomyopathy, 451, *451*
Continuous-wave Doppler echocardiography, in aortic regurgitation, 428, *429*, 430
in mitral stenosis, 431, *432*
in patent ductus arteriosus, *484*, 485, *485*
instrumentation for, 369
of left ventricular ejection, 403, *404*
spectral analysis of, 371, 372
Contour analysis, in quantitative coronary angiography, 225–227
Contour detection, in quantitative coronary angiography, 222–225
procedure for, minimal-cost, 223, *223*
Contractility, in left ventricular function, 26
Contraction, of left ventricle, analysis of, ultrafast computed tomography in, 674
regional, abnormalities of, detection of, 594–598, *595–597*, 597(t)
indices of, 594, *596*
studies of, nuclear magnetic resonance in, 923–925, *923*, *924*
Contrast, definition of, 1271, 1272
Contrast agent(s), administration of, electrocardiographically triggered injector in, in quantitative coronary arteriography, 234
intravenous, 296
computed tomography with, in myocardial perfusion measurement, 692–695, *693–695*
Contrast agent(s) *(Continued)*
left ventricular imaging with, 295–297, *296*, *297*
allergy to, as pulmonary angiography contraindication, 149
angiographic. See *Angiographic contrast agents.*
definition of, 1272
effect of, on ejection fraction, 119, 120, *120*
for contrast echocardiography, development of, 558–560, *559*
in myocardial perfusion quantification, 560
manually produced, 558
safety of, 559, 560
sonicated, 558, 559, *559*
for magnetic resonance imaging, 794–810, 794(t), 804(t)
relation of, to signal intensity, 798, 799
with sodium-23, 837
hyperosmolar, for maximal hyperemia, 338
in coronary angiography, effects of, 187–189, *188*
in left ventricular volume measurement, 119, 120, *120*
manganese-containing, in myocardial perfusion assessment, 824, *824*
nonionic, in indicator dilution methods, of myocardial perfusion measurement, 690, *690*
with iso-osmolality, in quantitative coronary arteriography, 233, 234, 234(t)
paramagnetic. See *Paramagnetic contrast agents.*
radiographic. See *Radiographic contrast agents.*
Contrast echocardiography, 557–574
cardiac applications of, 568–572, *569–572*
contrast agents for, development of, 558–560, *559*
safety of, 559, 560
during percutaneous transluminal coronary angioplasty, 568
in myocardial perfusion, 560–568, *566*, *567*
advantages of, 568
contrast agents for, 560
disadvantages of, 568
mathematical model for, 561–565, *563–565*
ultrasound equipment for, 560, *561*, *562*
myocardial, in coronary flow reserve assessment, 256, 257
Contrast input function, kinetics of, in myocardium, 699, 700, *700*
Contrast left ventriculography, qualitative assessment of, 110, *111–116*
quantitative analysis of, volume determination in, 110–124, *116*
in practice, 118–122, *119–121*
in theory, 110–118, *117*, *118*
parameters derived from, 122–124, *122–125*
Contrast nephropathy, 188
Contrast resolution, 76
in single-photon emission computed tomography, 985, *985*
in x-ray computed tomography, *640*
Contrast ventriculography, in aortic regurgitation, 110, *115*
in aortic stenosis, 110
in mitral regurgitation, 110, *114*
in mitral stenosis, 110
in mitral valve prolapse, 110, *115*
vs. equilibrium radionuclide angiography, 1029, 1029(t)
vs. two-dimensional echocardiography, 382
with electrocardiography, 118, *119*
Contrast washout analysis, in coronary flow reserve measurement, 330, 331, *332*, *333*
in functional assessment, of coronary circulation, 329–331, *330–333*
Contrast-detail curve, in x-ray computed tomography, *640*, 641
Contrast-to-noise ratio, definition of, 1272
in spin-echo imaging, 799
Contusion, myocardial, ultrasonic tissue characterization in, 553
Conversion, analog-to-digital, in densitometry, 291, 292
in nuclear magnetic resonance, 737
Convolution, in scatter and veiling glare correction, 292
Convolution method, 635
of projection reconstruction, in x-ray computed tomography, 638, *639*
Convolver, real-time, of digital image processor, 285
Coordinate system methods, of wall motion analysis, 127–129, *129*
Cor pulmonale, equilibrium radionuclide angiography in, 1042
"Corduroy artifact," 779, 788, *789*
Coronary anatomy, evaluation of, ultrafast computed tomography in, 680, *680*
Coronary and Left Ventricular Analysis System, 220
Coronary angiography, catheterization in, brachial approach to, 190
femoral approach to, 190
transaxillary approach to, 190
complications of, 185–187, 186(t)
avoidance of, 187
contraindications to, 184, 185
contrast media in, effects of, 187–189, *188*
data acquisition in, clinical aspects of, 182–210
development of, historic events in, 183
evaluation of, 201–206, *202–205*
implications of, 201–206, *202–205*
in unstable patient, 193
indications for, 183, 184, *185*
interpretation of, 201–206, *202–205*
interobserver variability in, 201
intraobserver variability in, 201
problems in, 213
traps to avoid in, 206
medication during, 190
patient preparation for, 189, 190
quantitative. See *Quantitative coronary angiography.*
techniques of, 190–193
Amplatz, 191, 192, *192*
Judkins, 191, *191*
percutaneous brachial, 193
Schoonmaker, 192, *192*
Sones, 190, 191, *191*
validity of, 200, 201
postmortem confirmation of, 200, 201
views in, adequate, importance of, 193, 194, *194*, *195*
angulated, benefits of, 194, *195*
caudocranial, 194, *194*
craniocaudal, 194, *194*
left anterior oblique, 193, 194
required number of, 214
right anterior oblique, 193, 194
Coronary anomalies, as coronary angiography indication, 184
Coronary arteriography, in coronary artery disease diagnosis, vs positron emission tomography, 1176, 1176(t), 1177, *1177*
quantitative. See *Quantitative coronary arteriography.*
Coronary artery(ies), anatomy of, normal, 194–196, *195*

Coronary artery(ies) *(Continued)*
assessment of, 312–324
aortic root angiography in, 312, 313
digital fluoroscopy in, 312
direct angiography in, 313
intravenous angiography in, 312
quantitative coronary arteriography in, 313–324, *313–323*, 315(t), 318(t), 322(t), 323(t)
roadmapping in, 313
videodensitometry in, with digital angiography, 324, 325(t)
circumflex. See *Circumflex coronary artery.*
congenital anomalies of, 196–199, *197*, 197(t), *198*
myocardial perfusion in, 197, 198
dimensions of, in coronary flow reserve, 249, *249*, 250, 250(t), *251*, 251(t)
dominant, 196
examination of, observer performance in, 91
fistulae of, 197, *197*
high origin of, 199
horseshoe, 199
left. See *Left coronary artery.*
magnetic resonance imaging of, 874–876
multiple ostia of, 199
occlusion of, and hypokinesis, 135, *136*, 137
temporary, acute myocardial infarct sizing after, Tc-99m-PPi in, 1083
right. See *Right coronary artery.*
single, 198, 199
stenosis of, functional effects of, 135
IPPA in, *1092*
thrombi of, imaging of, indium-111–labeled platelets in, 1124
ultrafast computed tomography of, 680, *680*
ultrasonography of, 602, 603, *603*, 625–630, *626*
visualization of, Dynamic Spatial Reconstructor in, *659*
Coronary artery bypass grafting, in ischemic cardiomyopathy, left ventricular function after, 1225, 1225(t)
Coronary artery disease, assessment of, physiologic, 339, *340–343*
chronic, iodo fatty acid analogs in, 1093, *1093*, 1094
exercise effect on, 1094
cine magnetic resonance imaging in, 962–964, *963*, *964*
coronary angiography in, 184
diagnosis of, exercise echocardiography in, 582–584, 583(t), *584*
two-dimensional, 582, 583
left ventricular ejection fraction in, during exercise, 585, *585*, 586, *586*
positron emission tomography in, 1174–1179, *1175*, 1176(t), *1177*
accuracy of, 1176–1178, 1176(t), *1177*
sensitivity/specificity analysis in, 1178
vs. coronary arteriography, 1176, 1176(t), 1177, *1177*
thallium-201 scanning in, 1023, 1058–1060, 1060(t)
wall motion analysis in, 583, 583(t), 584
echocardiography in, 594–604
applications of, 602, 603, *603*
effect of diet on, 1185
exercise echocardiography in, 580–584, *581*, *582*
IHDA uptake and clearance in, 1087, *1087*
localization of, positron emission tomography in, 1178
myocardial perfusion defects in, quantification of, 994, *995*
pretest probability of, 1032, 1032(t)
radionuclide angiocardiography in, 1021–1024, *1023*, *1024*
Coronary artery disease *(Continued)*
in risk stratification, 1022
severe, identification of, equilibrium radionuclide angiography in, 1034, 1034(t), *1035*
ventricular function in, 135–138
wall motion in, 144
Coronary Artery Surgery Study (CASS), 213
Coronary blood flow, autoregulation of, 243, *243*
measurement of, 244, 245
Doppler methods of, 245
end-diastolic cineangiography in, 247, *247*
first-pass distribution method of, 244
indicator-dilution principle in, 244
inert-substance washout method of, 244
thermodilution method of, 244
relation of, to coronary perfusion pressure, 244
Coronary bridging, 200
Coronary cineangiography, repeated, variability in, 238–241
long-term, 240, 240(t), 241
medium-term, 239, 240, 240(t)
overall, 238, 239
short-term, 239, 239(t)
Coronary circulation, assessment of, anatomic, 312–325
functional, 325–339
appearance time in, 334, *334–338*, 335
contrast washout analysis in, 329–331, *330–333*
density analysis in, 334, *334–338*, 335
impulse response analysis in, 331–334, *333*, *334*
indicator-dilution analysis in, 328, 329, *329*, *330*
transfer function analysis in, 331–334, *333*, *334*
transit-time analysis in, 325–328, *326–328*
cineangiography of, 311
collateral. See *Coronary collateral circulation.*
digital angiography of, 310–347
history of, 310–312, *311*
humoral control of, 11
neural activation effects on, 11
regulation of, endothelial relaxing factor in, 12
flow differences in, 12, 13
mechanisms in, 8
transmural perfusion in, 11, 12, *12*, *13*
Coronary collateral circulation, 16–18, 199, 200
contrast echocardiography of, 568
functional significance of, evaluation of, 1185–1187, *1186*
magnetic resonance imaging of, 894
mature, 17, *17*, 18
native, 16, 17, *17*
Coronary collateral steal, 1185, *1186*
Coronary dilation, intensive, in ventricular function, 27, 27(t)
Coronary dilators, maximal, 15, 16
submaximal, 15
Coronary disease, diagnosis of, angiographic vs. histologic, 201
diffuse, coronary stenosis in, 18
Coronary driving pressure, in autoregulation, 10
Coronary flow reserve (CFR), 13, *13*, 14, 243–259, *243*
after percutaneous transluminal coronary angioplasty, 255, *255*
angiography of, image processing in, 247–249, *247*, *248*, 248(t)
Coronary flow reserve (CFR) *(Continued)*
maximal hyperemic response in, 246
assessment of, absolute vs relative, 14
maximal hyperemia in, 338, *339*
myocardial contrast echocardiography in, 256, 257
density threshold in, 247, 248(t)
drug effects on, 14
hemodynamics of, 14
in coronary stenosis, 18, 19
limitation of, coronary obstructions in, 246
measurement of, 244, 245, 247–249, *247*, *248*, 248(t)
appearance time in, *335*
contrast washout analysis in, 330, 331, *332*, *333*
digital subtraction cineangiography in, 255, 256, *256*, *257*
Doppler probe in, 255, 256, *256*, *257*
electromagnetic flow probe in, *335*
myocardial densitometry in, 246
papaverine in, 246
time-density curve in, 329, *329*
variability in, 250–255
factors in, 258, 259
interobserver, 250, *252*
intraobserver, 250, *252*
long-term, 251, *254*
medium-term, 251, *252*, *253*
short-term, 251, *252*
videodensitometry in, 245
nonhemodynamic conditions in, 13, 14
prediction of, quantitative parameters in, 319
radiography of, 245–249, *246*
relationship of, to coronary artery dimensions, 249, *249*, 250, 250(t), *251*, 251(t)
to minimal luminal cross-sectional area, 249, *249*, 250, 250(t)
theoretic calculation of, 311, *311*
vs. myocardial perfusion reserve, 1176, 1176(t)
vs. stenosis flow reserve, 1175, 1176, 1176(t)
with exercise-induced radionuclide abnormalities, 339, *343*
Coronary infarction, 19
Coronary luminal area, 203, *204*
Coronary obstruction(s), description of, quantitative parameters in, 227, 227(t)
in coronary flow reserve limitation, 246
measurement of, long-term variability in, 240(t), 241
phantom studies of, 236, 237
physiologic significance of, 215, *215*, 216, *216*
quantitative analysis of, 217
severity of, determination of, 214, *214*, 215
symmetry measurements of, 226, *226*
Coronary occlusion, 19
Coronary perfusion pressure, relation of, to coronary blood flow, 244
Coronary reactive hyperemia, determination of, 243
Coronary revascularization, equilibrium radionuclide angiography of, 1037, 1038
Coronary sinus, dilated, vs pericardial effusion, 464
right, circumflex coronary artery originating from, 198
first septal perforator originating from, 199
left anterior descending artery originating from, 198
Coronary stenosis, 18, 18(t), 19
before angioplasty, digital analysis of, 317, 318, *318*
diffuse coronary disease in, 18

Coronary stenosis *(Continued)*
evaluation of, 307
hydraulic principles of, 18
in coronary flow reserve, 18, 19
measurement of, catheter in, 318
time-density curve in, 329, *330*
observer variability in, 18
Coronary thrombolysis, in myocardial infarction, effect of, on myocardial metabolism, 1218, 1219, *1220*, *1221*
Coronary vasodilation, effects of, on coronary vascular volume, 20
Coronary vasodilators, clinical use of, 15, *15*, 16
Correlation time, definition of, 1272
Cosine factor, in Doppler shift, 366, *366*, 367
Couch, in x-ray computed tomography, 641
CPI (technetium-99m carboxyisopropyl isonitrile), 1097, *1098*
CPT I, in lipid metabolism, 44, 45, *45*
CPT II, in lipid metabolism, 45, *45*
Creatine phosphokinase release, in infarct size measurement, *136*
Cross-plane resolution, 357
Cross-sectional area, geometric, measurement of, 315, 318(t)
videodensitometric, measured vs actual, linear regression analysis of, 315, *315*, *316*
Cryostat, definition of, 1272
Crystal-like spectrum, of sodium, 830
C-scan imaging, 359, *359*
CT (cardiothoracic) ratio, 99
CTDI (computed tomography dose index), 647, *647*
Currents, eddy, definition of, 1272
Cyanosis, in congenital heart disease, with decreased pulmonary vascularity, Doppler echocardiography in, 492–496, *494–496*
two-dimensional echocardiography in, 492–496, *494–496*
with increased pulmonary vascularity, Doppler echocardiography of, 496–499
two-dimensional echocardiography of, 496–499, *497–499*
Cyclic adenosine monophosphate (cAMP), in myocardial metabolism, 42
Cyst(s), bronchogenic, magnetic resonance imaging of, 940
pericardial, echocardiography of, 476
magnetic resonance imaging of, 940
ultrafast computed tomography of, 709, *710*
Cystic medial necrosis, of aorta, cine magnetic resonance imaging of, 953, *954*

Dacron grafts, platelet deposition in, drug effects on, 1130, 1131
thrombogeneity of, 1129, 1130
Damping, 353
"Dark blood," 760
Data analysis, standardization in, approaches to, 231, 232, 232(t)
dB/dt, definition of, 1272
Dechelation, of paramagnetic contrast agents, 796, 797, *797*
Deconvolution, analysis of, fast computed tomography in, 700
relaxation, in sodium magnetic resonance spectroscopy, 857, 858
Decoupling, definition of, 1272
Degradation, of protein, 52
Demerol-Phenergan-Thorazine, for sedation, in magnetic resonance imaging, 779
Densitometry, 290–293
Densitometry *(Continued)*
accuracy of, assessment of, 236
analog-to-digital conversion in, 291, 292
beam hardening in, 293
correction methods in, 291–293, *291–293*, 291(t)
density-time analysis in, 293
in percent area stenosis assessment, 229
in quantitative coronary angiography, 227–230, *228–230*
myocardial, in coronary flow reserve measurement, 246
scatter and veiling glare in, 292, *292*, 293, *293*
validation studies of, 230, 237, 238
in vivo, 237, 238
phantom, 237
repeated, variability in, 238
Density analysis, in functional assessment of coronary circulation, 334, *334–338*, 335
Density-time analysis, in densitometry, 293
Depth-Resolved Surface Coil Spectroscopy (DRESS), 968
Destructive interference, 352
Detector, definition of, 1272
in x-ray computed tomography, 641
Deuterium, nucleus of, characteristics of, 842(t)
Deuterium magnetic resonance spectroscopy, 858
Dextran-magnetite, in sodium imaging, 837
Dextro loop, 500, *508*
Dextrocardia, echocardiography in, *508*
DFT (discrete Fourier transform), 371, 372
Diabetes, diastolic left ventricular function in, 410
in protein turnover, 52
intracoronary contrast agent injection in, 188
myocardial metabolism in, 49
phosphorus magnetic resonance spectroscopy in, 848
thallium-201 scintigraphy in, 1066, 1066(t)
Diagnostic imaging, errors in, 87
Diamagnetic, definition of, 1272
Diastasis, heart rate effect on, 140, *142*
Diastole, diastolic pressure during, factors in, *34*
parameters for, measurement of, equilibrium radionuclide angiography in, 1031, 1032
phases of, 34, *35*
Diastolic function, in ischemia, detection of, 410
ventricular, 33–35
in restrictive cardiomyopathy, echocardiography of, 457, 458, *458*
left, in dilated cardiomyopathy, Doppler echocardiography of, 456
Diastolic orifice area, mean, 408
Diastolic performance, Doppler measures of, 410–413
"Diastolic pseudogating," 760
Diastolic stroke volume, transmitral, 408
Diatrizoate, bolus administration of, hemoglobin concentration after, *168*
effect of, on systemic arterial pressure, *169*
properties of, 166, 167(t)
sodium concentration of, 173
specifications of, 234(t)
Diatrizoic acid, *164*, 165
Diazepam, for sedation, in magnetic resonance imaging, 779
in premedication, before coronary angiography, 189
Diet, in coronary artery disease, 1185
Diffusion, definition of, 1272
Diffusion/perfusion imaging, in myocardial perfusion assessment, 823
Digital angiography, advantages of, 287, 287(t)
archival storage in, 286
analog videotape in, 286
cine film in, 286
digital optical disk in, 286
helical scan 8-mm magnetic tape in, 286
nine-track magnetic tape in, 286
edge detection in, 290, *290*
image enhancement in, 288, 289, *289*, 289(t)
spatial filtration in, 288, 289, *289*
image noise in, 282, 283
image workstations in, 286, 287
instrumentation for, 281–294
of coronary circulation, 310–347
history of, 310–312, *311*
on-line image storage in, 285, 285(t), 286
real-time digital magnetic disk in, 285, 286
solid-state memory in, 285
physical principles in, 281–294
pincushion distortion in, 290, *290*
pixels in, intensity of, 291, *291*
size of, 283, 283(t)
spatial measurements in, 289, 290
accuracy of, 290
calibration of, 290
video for, 283, *283*, 284
videodensitometry with, in coronary artery assessment, 324, 325(t)
in percutaneous transluminal coronary angioplasty, 324
vs. intraventricular cineangiography, 295–297, *296*, *297*
Digital camera, in radionuclide imaging, 980
Digital cardiac systems, on-line, in quantitative coronary angiography, 220, 221, 221(t)
Digital fluoroscopy, in coronary artery assessment, 312
Digital image(s), characteristics of, 74–77, *75–78*
display of, 77
processing of, 72–86
gray scale compression in, 77, *78*
image enhancement in, 77–82
filtering operations in, *81–83*, 82
geometric transformations in, 79–81
point operations in, 77, 78, *78–80*
segmentation in, 82, 83, *83*, *84*
storage of, 283, 283(t)
subtracted, 218
Digital image processor, 284, *284*, 285
arithmetic logic unit of, 284
array processors of, 285
hardware zoom of, 285
host computer of, 285
intensity transformation table of, 284
real-time convolver of, 285
Digital imaging, in left ventricular function assessment, during interventions, 303–308, *304–307*
principles of, 281–283, *282*, 283(t)
Digital optical disk, in archival storage, in digital angiography, 286
Digital scan conversion, in echocardiography, 360–363, *361*, *362*
Digital subtraction angiography, 287, 288
advantages of, 297–300, *298–300*, 298(t)
disadvantages of, 297–300, *298–300*, 298(t)
energy, 288
in ventricular function assessment, 295–309, *303*
temporal, 288
vs. cineangiography, in coronary quantification, 319–322, *321–323*, 322(t), 323(t)

Digital subtraction arteriography, time-density analysis of, *331*
Digital subtraction cineangiography, in coronary flow reserve measurement, 255, 256, *256*, *257*
vs. intracoronary Doppler technique, 255, 256, *256–258*
Digital subtraction videodensitometry, phantom studies of, 237
Digital-to-analog conversion, 77
Digitization, 74
bit depth in, 282
cine-frame, variations in, 231, 232, 232(t)
in quantitative coronary angiography, 217, *217*, 218
of cine film, cameras for, 219, 220(t)
in quantitative coronary angiography, 219, 219(t), 220, *220*, 220(t)
quantization in, 282
recursive, 231
sampling in, 282
scanning in, 282
Digitization noise, 282
Digitizing table, *x-y*, 120, 121, *121*
Dihydrolipoyl acetyltransferase, in myocardial metabolism, 42
Dihydrolipoyl dehydrogenase, in myocardial metabolism, 42
Dihydroxyacetone phosphate, in myocardial metabolism, 42, *43*
Dilated cardiomyopathy, atrial size in, echocardiography of, 454
contrast echocardiography in, 569, *571*
definition of, 449
differential diagnosis of, echocardiography in, 456
echocardiography in, 453–457, *454*
E-point–septal separation in, 454
functional assessment in, magnetic resonance imaging in, 931, 932, *932*
IHPA in, 1094
imaging of, 1251
ischemic vs nonischemic, 1234, *1235*, 1247–1251, *1250*
left ventricular function in, echocardiography of, 454
Doppler, 456
magnetic resonance imaging in, 931, 932
metabolism in, positron emission tomography of, 1247, *1248*, *1249*
metaiodobenzylguanidine uptake in, 1138
mitral valve function in, echocardiography of, 454–456
morphologic features of, magnetic resonance imaging of, 931
nonischemic, thallium-201 scintigraphy in, 1066, 1066(t)
prognosis in, echocardiography in, 456
pulmonary venous hypertension in, 95, *97*
roentgenographic evaluation of, 105
spectroscopy in, 970, 971
thrombi in, intracavitary, echocardiography of, 454, *455*
left ventricular, echocardiography of, 524, *524*, 525, *525*
tissue characterization in, magnetic resonance imaging in, 932
ultrasonic, 549–551, *551*
tricuspid valve function in, echocardiography of, 454–456
ventricular size in, echocardiography of, 453, 454
Diltiazem, effect of, on coronary flow reserve, 14
Diodrast, 163, *164*
Diphenhydramine, in premedication, before coronary angiography, 189
Dipole, magnetic, definition of, 1273
Dipole-dipole interaction, definition of, 1272
Dipyridamole, in acute myocardial ischemia detection, 912, 913
in exercise echocardiography, in coronary artery disease, 602
in maximal coronary dilation, 16
in non-exercise stress echocardiography, 589–591, 590(t)
with thallium-201 scintigraphy, 590
in thallium-201 scintigraphy, 1055, 1056, 1065, 1065(t), 1066
intravenous, for maximal hyperemia, 338, *339*
side effects of, 16
with aspirin, for platelet deposition, on prosthetic grafts, 1130, *1131*
Discrete Fourier transform (DFT), 371, 372
Disk buffer, 285
Dispersion, 759, *760*
Display, Doppler, 371, 372
from single-beam echocardiography system, 356
in positron emission tomography, of myocardial blood flow, 1172, *1172*, *1173*
in x-ray computed tomography, 643
of Dynamic Spatial Reconstructor, 656
shaded-surface, in three-dimensional computed tomography, 660, *664*
Display buffer, 285
Dissection, aortic. See *Aortic dissection.*
thoracic, ultrafast computed tomography of, 710, 711, *711*, *712*
Distal coronary perfusion pressure, in stenosis identification, 250, 251(t)
Distortion, pincushion, in digital angiography, 290, *290*
Diverticula, of pericardium, magnetic resonance imaging of, 940
DMIPP, 1090
clearance rate of, 1090
fractional distribution of, 1090
Dobutamine, in non-exercise stress echocardiography, 589
with ultrafast computed tomography, in left ventricular function evaluation, 679
Domain, frequency, 82
spatial, 82
Dominant coronary artery, 196
Doppler, color flow, spectral analysis of, 372
continuous-wave, in left ventricular ejection assessment, 403, *404*
spectral analysis of, 371, 372
display of, 371, 372
instrumentation for, 368–371
color flow, 371
continuous-wave, 369
pulsed, 369–371, *369*, *370*
physics of, 365–373
cardiovascular, frequency ambiguity in, 367
point and blood backscatter in, 367
reflection in, 367
principles of, 365–373
processing of, 371, 372
spectral analysis in, 371, 372, *372*
time-based, 371
pulsed, in left ventricular ejection assessment, 403, *404*
spectral analysis of, 371, 372, *372*
real-time two-dimensional, 371
Doppler angle, 61, 62, *62*
Doppler echocardiographic equation, 57, *57*, 58, *58*
Doppler echocardiography, continuous-wave, in aortic regurgitation, 428, *429*, 430
in mitral stenosis, 431, *432*
in patent ductus arteriosus, *484*, 485, *485*
during exercise, 577–580, *577–579*
Doppler echocardiography *(Continued)*
in cardiac drug effect measurement, 578–580
in ischemic heart disease, 586–588, *586*, *587*
vs thermodilution, in stroke volume measurement, 578, *579*
in aortic regurgitation, 427–430, *428*, *429*
in aortic stenosis, 421–425, *422–425*
in aortic valve gradient underestimation, 425, *425*
in assessment, of left ventricular ejection, 403–408, 403(t), *404–407*
during percutaneous transluminal coronary angioplasty, 407
of left ventricular filling, 408–413, 408(t), *409–413*
of left ventricular function, diastolic, 409, 410, *410*
during exercise, 580
in dilated cardiomyopathy, 456
of right ventricular ejection, 413–415
clinical applications of, 414, 415
of right ventricular filling, 415
of right ventricular systolic pressure, in tricuspid regurgitation, 438–440, *439*
of ventricular systolic function, after interventions, 407, *407*
at rest, 403–407, *406*
in atrial septal defects, *482*, 483
in atrioventricular septal defects, 487
in cardiac function evaluation, 402–418
in congenital heart disease, 479–510
with acyanosis, and increased pulmonary blood flow, 479–489
with cyanosis, and decreased pulmonary vascularity, 492–496, *494–496*
and increased pulmonary vascularity, 496–499
with ventricular outflow obstruction, 489–492
in constrictive pericarditis, 473, *474*
in hypertrophic cardiomyopathy, with cavity obliteration, 452, 453
with left ventricular outflow obstruction, 450, 451, *451*, *452*
with midventricular obstruction, 451, 452, *452*, *453*
in left ventricular outflow obstruction, 490–492, *490*, *492*
in mitral regurgitation, 435, 436
in mitral stenosis, 431–433, *432*
in patent ductus arteriosus, 483–486, *484–486*
in pulmonary valve disease, 440
in right ventricular outflow obstruction, 492
in tricuspid regurgitation, 438
in tricuspid stenosis, 436, *437*
in valvuloplasty, 441–443
in ventricular septal defects, 481–483, *481*
intraoperative, 618
of increased pulmonary arterial markings, 496–499
of increased pulmonary venous markings, 499
of left-to-right shunting, 487–489
of prosthetic valves, 441, *442*
of right-to-left shunting, at atrial level, 495, 496
at ventricular level, 492–495, *494*, *495*
vs. echocardiographic imaging, 402, 403
with catheterization, in mean gradient measurement, in aortic stenosis, 421, *423*
Doppler effect, 365–367
frequency shifts in, 365, 366, *366*
wave propagation in, 365

Doppler equation, in blood velocity calculation, 61, 62, *62*
Doppler measures, of diastolic performance, 410–413
age in, 410, *411*
atrioventricular sequence in, 412, *413*
heart rate in, 410, *412*
left atrial pressure in, 412, *413*
respiratory cycle in, 410, *411*
sampling size in, 410, *411*
ventricular, 408, 408(t)
of systolic performance, 407, 408
Doppler probe, in coronary flow reserve measurement, 255, 256, *256*, *257*
Doppler shift, cosine factor in, 366, *366*, 367
Doppler technique, intracoronary, vs digital subtraction cineangiography, 255, 256, *256–258*
Doppler transducers, 368, *368*, 369, *369*
Double aortic arch, magnetic resonance imaging of, 893
Double quantum filter, 831
Double quantum transition, 829
Double-outlet right ventricle, echocardiography in, 495, *495*
magnetic resonance imaging in, 891, *891*
ultrafast computed tomography in, *721*
Doxorubicin, toxicity of, diagnosis of, spectroscopy in, 970
monitoring of, equilibrium radionuclide angiography in, 1042
phosphorus magnetic resonance spectroscopy in, 849
DRESS (Depth-Resolved Surface Coil Spectroscopy), 968
Dressler's syndrome, 104, 942, 943, *943*
Drug(s), cardiac, effects of, exercise Doppler echocardiography of, 578–580
cardioactive, hemodynamic effects of, 407
effect of, on coronary vasodilator reserve, 14
on platelet deposition, on prosthetic grafts, 1130, 1131, *1131*
DSR. See *Dynamic Spatial Reconstructor (DSR).*
Dual-energy subtraction, 298(t), 299, *300*
Duchenne muscular dystrophy, cardiomyopathy with, 1252
positron emission tomography in, 1252, *1253*
thallium-201 scintigraphy in, 1066, 1066(t)
Dynamic mask subtraction, 299
Dynamic Spatial Reconstructor (DSR), 650–659, *654*, *655*
applications of, 657–659, *657–659*
imaging capabilities of, 656, *656*, 657, *657*
in image analysis, 656
scanner of, 652–656, *655*
Dyskinesia, relation of, to infarct size, 594, *595*
Dyskinesis, nonischemic, adjacent, 594
Dysplasia, congenital, of lungs, pulmonary angiography in, 157–159
Dyspnea, equilibrium radionuclide angiography in, 1042
Dysprosium, in sodium magnetic resonance spectroscopy, 857
Dysprosium bis-tripolyphosphate, in sodium magnetic resonance spectroscopy, 857
Dysprosium *o*-bis-(tripolyphosphatopropyloxy) benzene, in sodium magnetic resonance spectroscopy, 857
Dysprosium tetra(methylenephosphonate), in sodium magnetic resonance spectroscopy, 857
Dysprosium-DTPA, 824, *824*
Ebstein malformation, echocardiography in, 495, *496*
Ebstein's anomaly, and tricuspid regurgitation, 438
magnetic resonance imaging in, 891, *891*
of tricuspid valve, 105
ECG-gated mask subtraction, 298(t)
Echinococcosis, cardiac, 529
Echo, definition of, 1272
field, definition of, 1272
gradient, creation of, 747, *747*
definition of, 1272
granular, 367
spin, creation of, 747, *747*
definition of, 1276
Echo planar imaging, 757, *757*, 783, 883, *883*
definition of, 1272
in cardiac quantitation, 824, *824*
modulus blipped, 757, *757*
Echo time, *752*, 753
definition of, 1272
in magnetic resonance imaging, 778, *779*
Echocardiography, amplification in, 359, 360, *360*, *361*
axial resolution in, determinants of, 354
cardiopulmonary bypass with, 622
continuous loop display in, 363
continuous wave, of left ventricular outflow obstruction, in hypertrophic cardiomyopathy, 451, *451*
contrast. See *Contrast echocardiography.*
digital scan conversion in, 360–363, *360*, *361*
electronic beam steering in, linear array in, 356, 357, *357*, *358*
phased array in, 357, 358, *358*, *359*
orthogonal, 359, *359*
three-dimensional beam formation in, 359, *359*
epicardial, high-frequency, for graft–native vessel coronary anastomosis evaluation, 625–627, *626–629*
pathologic and physiologic correlations with, 627–630, *630*
imaging planes for, 618–620, *619*, *620*
esophageal, intraoperative, in coronary artery disease, 602
exercise. See *Exercise echocardiography.*
freeze-frames in, 363
history of, 348, 349
image formation in, 359, 360, *360*, *361*
in aortic regurgitation, 425–430, *426*, *427*
in decision-making, 430
in aortic stenosis, 419–425, *420*
in decision-making, 425
in assessment, of left ventricular ejection fraction, 377–379, 378(t), *380*
of left ventricular function, global, 374–381
regional, 381–391
of left ventricular mass, 380, 381, *381*
of left ventricular volume, 375–377, *376–379*, 378(t)
of right ventricular function, 391–398
regional, 396–398
in cardiac mass evaluation, 511–537
in cardiac tamponade, 464–470, *466–471*
in cardiomyopathy, 449–459
in complex congenital heart disease, 499–508, *500–508*
in constrictive pericarditis, 943
in coronary artery disease, 594–604
applications of, 602, 603, *603*
in dilated cardiomyopathy, 453–457, *454*
in differential diagnosis, 456
in prognosis, 456
in endomyocardial fibrosis, 458
in extracardiac mass evaluation, 511–537
Echocardiography *(Continued)*
in hypertrophic cardiomyopathy, 449–453, *450*
in mitral regurgitation, 433–436, *434*, *435*
in decision-making, 436
in mitral stenosis, 430–433, *431*
in decision-making, 433
in myocardial infarction, 594–604
in myocardial ischemia, 594–604
in obliterative cardiomyopathy, 458
in pericardial diseases, 460–478
in pericardial effusion, 941
in prosthetic regurgitation, 440, 441
in pulmonary regurgitation, 440
in pulmonary stenosis, 440
in pulmonary valve disease, 440
in restrictive cardiomyopathy, 457, 458
in tricuspid regurgitation, 437–440
in decision-making, 440
in tricuspid stenosis, 436, 437, *437*
in decision-making, 436, 437
in valvular heart disease, 419–448
in valvuloplasty, 441–443
instrumentation in, 348–364
for beam insertion, 353, *353*, 354
for electronic focusing, 355, *355*, 356
for lateral resolution, 354, *354*, 355, *355*
for pulse transmission, 353, *353*, 354
intraoperative, 618–633
during valvular surgery, 622–624
postpump, in mitral regurgitation, 623, *623*
M-mode. See *M-mode echocardiography.*
of artifacts, 528, 528(t), 529, *529–533*
of prosthetic stenosis, 440, 441
physics of, 348–364
postprocessing in, 363
preprocessing in, 363
quantitative, in right ventricular studies, 395(t)
reception in, 359, 360, *360*, *361*
single-beam, display from, 356
stress. See *Stress echocardiography.*
transesophageal. See *Transesophageal echocardiography.*
transgastric, 608
two-dimensional. See *Two-dimensional echocardiography.*
vs. angiography, in ejection fraction measurement, 378(t)
in left ventricular volume measurement, 375, *376*, 378(t)
vs. Doppler echocardiography, 402, 403
Ectopy, avoidance of, 118
Eddies, 59
Eddy currents, definition of, 1272
Edge detection, in digital angiography, 290, *290*
in quantitative coronary angiography, 223, *223*, 224
techniques for, accuracy of, 236
EDRF (endothelium-dependent releasing factor), 1264
EDTA (ethylenediaminetetra-acetic acid), as chelating agent, 173
Effusion, pericardial. See *Pericardial effusion.*
Effusive-constrictive pericarditis, 475, 943
eIF (eukaryotic initiation factors), in protein synthesis, 51, *51*, 52
Eisenmenger complex, 98, *99*
Eisenmenger's physiology, 892
Ejection, right ventricular, assessment of, Doppler echocardiography in, 413–415
clinical applications of, 414, 415
hemodynamics of, 414, *414*
Ejection fraction, 122, *122*
calculation of, cineangiography in, 379, *380*

Ejection fraction *(Continued)*
echocardiography vs. angiography in, 378(t)
exercise radionuclide angiography in, 585, *586*
in dilated cardiomyopathy, magnetic resonance imaging in, 931, *932*
magnetic resonance imaging in, 819, *819*
radionuclide angiography in, 379, *380*
radionuclide ventriculography in, 997, *997*, 998
two-dimensional echocardiography in, 379, *380*
during exercise, 1020(t)
relationship of, to metabolic equivalents, 1033, *1033*
effect on, of atrial pacing, 304, *305*
of contrast material, 119, 120, *120*
in chest pain prognosis, 1036, *1036*, *1037*
in global right ventricular function, 393–396, *393*, 395(t), *396*, *397*
left ventricular. See *Left ventricular ejection fraction.*
normal values for, 134(t)
regional, calculation of, radionuclide ventriculography in, 999, *999*, *1000*
normal limits of, 1001, 1002
right ventricular, 139
measurement of, equilibrium radionuclide angiography in, 1031
Ejection velocity, in heart failure, after vasodilator therapy, 407
systolic, Doppler, during percutaneous transluminal coronary angioplasty, 407
Elastance, of left ventricle, 140
Electrical alternans, 464
Electrical stimulation, in ventricular function evaluation, 27, 27(t)
Electrocardiographic gating, lead placement in, 781
Electrocardiographic triggering, 781, 781(t), *782*
Electrocardiography, after intracoronary contrast agent injection, 187, *188*
during coronary angiography, 190
exercise, vs. exercise echocardiography, 585
in acutely infarcted myocardium, 1217, 1218
vs. myocardial metabolic activity, in tissue viability determination, 1225–1227, *1226–1228*
with contrast ventriculography, 118, *119*
Electromagnetic flow probe, in blood flow measurement, *337*
in coronary flow reserve measurement, *335*
Electromotive force, 844
Electronic noise, 282
Electrons, unpaired, magnetic fields around, 795, *796*
Elongation factors, in protein synthesis, 52
Embolectomy, percutaneous, transvenous, 155
Embolism, pulmonary. See *Pulmonary embolism.*
Embolization, of left ventricular thrombi, 524
Embolization therapy, transcatheter, for arteriovenous fistulae, 156
Embryonal carcinoma, metastatic, echocardiography of, 520, *521*
EMI brain scanner, 635
Emission images, in positron emission tomography, of myocardial blood flow, 1171, 1172
Encoding, frequency, 746
definition of, 1272
phase, definition of, 1274
Endarterectomy, carotid, imaging of, indium-111–labeled platelets in, 1127, *1127*
End-diastole, contours of, tracing of, 120, *121*
hypertrophic cardiomyopathy at, 110, *114*
End-diastolic cineangiography, in coronary blood flow measurement, 247, *247*
End-diastolic mask mode subtraction, 299, *299*
End-diastolic pressure, aortic, in valvular regurgitation, 68
End-diastolic volume, 122
during exercise, 1020(t)
relationship of, to metabolic equivalents, 1033, *1033*
effect on, of atrial pacing, 304, *305*
left ventricular, 35
in Trendelenburg's position, 27
measurement of, equilibrium radionuclide angiography in, 1030, *1030*, 1031
measurement of, cineangiography in, *379*
two-dimensional echocardiography in, *379*
normal values for, 134(t)
uses for, 374
Endocardial motion, analysis of, 383, *383*
segmental, evaluation of, ultrafast computed tomography in, 673, *674*
Endocardial surface mapping, of ventricles, 388, *391*
Endocarditis, infectious, and aortic regurgitation, 425
and mitral regurgitation, 434
and tricuspid regurgitation, 437, 438
transesophageal echocardiography in, 611, *611*, 612
Endoluminal prostheses, efficacy of, 263–267
stent in, description of, 264, *264*, *265*
studies of, methods of, 264, *264*, *265*
use of, results of, 264–266, *265*, *266*, 266(t)
Endomyocardial fibroelastoma, and tricuspid stenosis, 436
Endomyocardial fibrosis, 449
and tricuspid stenosis, 436
echocardiography in, 458
Endothelial relaxing factor, in coronary circulation regulation, 12
Endothelium-dependent releasing factor (EDRF), 1264
End-systole, contours of, tracing of, 120
End-systolic pressure, relationship to, of left ventricular volume, 379, 380
End-systolic volume, 122
during exercise, 1020(t)
effect of atrial pacing on, 304, *305*
measurement of, cineangiography in, *379*
two-dimensional echocardiography in, *379*
normal values for, 134(t)
uses for, 374, 375
Energy, myocardial production of, 39, *40*
utilization of, compartmentation of, 50
Energy level, definition of, 1272
Energy subtraction, 288
Enhancement, flow-related, 865
definition of, 1272
in magnetic resonance imaging, 785
paradoxic, 760
Enoyl-CoA hydratase, in lipid metabolism, 46, *47*
Entry-slice phenomenon, 785
Envelope detection, 360
Enzyme(s), kinetics of, study of, phosphorus magnetic resonance spectroscopy in, 846, 847, *847*
Epicardial echocardiography, high-frequency, for graft–native vessel coronary anastomosis evaluation, 625–627, *626–629*
pathologic and physiologic correlations with, 627–630, *630*
Epicardial echocardiography *(Continued)*
imaging planes for, 618–620, *619*, *620*
transducer preparation for, 620
E-point–septal separation (EPSS), in dilated cardiomyopathy, 454
Equation(s), Bernoulli. See *Bernoulli equation.*
Bloch, definition of, 1271
continuity, in aortic valve area determination, 421, *424*
in mitral stenosis, 433
echocardiographic, Doppler, 57, *57*, 58, *58*
hemodynamic, for valvular heart disease quantification, 56–59
Larmor, definition of, 1273
Michaelis-Menten, 846
volume flow rate, 66
Equilibrium, thermal, definition of, 1276
Equilibrium binding, of cardiac receptors, 1262
Equilibrium magnetization, 735, *735*
Equilibrium radionuclide angiography, 1027–1046
after myocardial infarction, 1038, *1038*, 1039
after percutaneous transluminal coronary angioplasty, 1038
clinical applications of, 1032–1042
exercise equipment for, 1028
in cardiomyopathy, 1039, 1040
in patient management, 1037, 1038
in valvular heart disease, 1040, *1040*, 1041, *1041*
measurements from, 1029–1032, 1029(t), *1030*
of arrhythmias, during exercise, 1029
red blood cell labeling in, 1027, 1028
technical aspects of, 1027–1029, *1028*
vs. contrast ventriculography, 1029, 1029(t)
with single-photon emission computed tomography, 1032
Equipment, for contrast echocardiography, 560, *561*, *562*
Ernst angle, 737
Errors, in diagnostic imaging, 87
Erythrocytes, in ultrasound backscatter, 367
Esophageal echocardiography, intraoperative, in coronary artery disease, 602
Ethanol, spectrum of, 734, *735*
Ethylenediaminetetra-acetic acid (EDTA), as chelating agent, 173
Eukaryotic initiation factors (eIF), in protein synthesis, 51, *51*, 52
Eustachian valve, echocardiography of, 500, *501*, 511, *512*
Excitation, definition of, 1272
selective, 748
definition of, 1275
Excitation profile, 748, *749*
Excrescences, Lambl's, 529
Exercise, arrhythmias during, equilibrium radionuclide angiography of, 1029
bicycle, left ventricular function during, ultrafast computed tomography of, 680
ventricular imaging during, 303, 304
cardiac response to, 1020(t)
Doppler echocardiography during, 577–580, *577–579*
in cardiac drug effect measurement, 578–580
ejection fraction in, relationship of, to metabolic equivalents, 1033, *1033*
end-diastolic volume in, relationship of, to metabolic equivalents, 1033, *1033*
equilibrium radionuclide angiography during, 1028
exhaustive, in maximal coronary dilation, 15

Exercise *(Continued)*
in coronary artery disease, effect of, on iodo fatty acid analogs, 1094
increased, myocardial metabolism in, 49
IPPA uptake after, single-photon emission computed tomography of, 1093, *1093*, 1094
ischemic, spectroscopy in, 972–974, *974*
isometric, in ventricular function evaluation, 27, 27(t)
left ventricular ejection fraction during, in coronary artery disease diagnosis, 585, *585*, 586, *586*
radionuclide angiocardiography of, 1022, 1023, *1023*
left ventricular function in, Doppler echocardiography of, 580
M-mode echocardiography during, 575
peak ejection velocity during, in ischemic heart disease, 586, *586*, 587, *587*
positron emission tomography in, vs single-photon emission computed tomography, 1174, *1175*
radionuclide angiography during, in ejection fraction measurement, 585, *586*
reactive hyperemia during, *341*
stroke volume during, measurement of, Doppler echocardiography in, 578, *578*
vs. thermodilution, 578, *579*
supine, left ventricular hemodynamics during, 27
systolic ventricular function during, 407
thallium-201 scintigraphy during, 1053–1055, *1054–1056*
two-dimensional echocardiography during, 575–577, *576*
in coronary artery disease diagnosis, 582, 583
upright, left ventricular hemodynamics during, 27
Exercise echocardiography, clinical applications of, 580–589
Doppler, in ischemic heart disease, 586–588, *586*, *587*
in coronary artery disease, 602
in patient evaluation, after myocardial infarction, 588, *588*, 589(t)
vs. exercise electrocardiography, 585
vs. radionuclide angiography, 585, 586
vs. thallium-201 scintigraphy, 585, 586
Exercise electrocardiography, vs exercise echocardiography, 585
Exercise radionuclide angiography, limitations of, 1039
Exercise radionuclide ventriculography, in phase analysis, 1001, 1002
relationship of, to reactive hyperemia, *342*
External focusing, *354*, 355
Extracardial masses, echocardiographic evaluation of, 511–537
Extreme narrowing spectrum, of sodium, 830, *830*

FAD (flavin adenine dinucleotide), in myocardial metabolism, 39, *40*
Fan beam geometry, 637
Faraday shield, definition of, 1272
Faraday's induction law, 844
Fast computed tomography, half-value layer in, 650, *654*
Hounsfield unit linearity in, 649, 650, 653(t), *654*
in deconvolution analysis, 700
in measurement, of nonuniform myocardial perfusion, 700

Fast computed tomography *(Continued)*
of regional intramyocardial vascular volume, 698, 699, *699*
in myocardial contrast input function kinetics, 699, 700, *700*
in myocardial perfusion measurement, 688–702
imaging and reconstruction artifacts in, 695–698, *696–698*
low-contrast resolution in, 648, 649, 650(t), *651*, *652*
noise in, 649, 653(t)
radiation dosimetry in, 647, 648(t)
scanner for, 645–650, 689
slice thickness and contiguity in, 648, *648*, 648(t)
spatial resolution in, 648, *649*, 649(t), *650*
uniformity in, 649, 652(t), *653*
Fast exchange, two-state (FETS), 762, *762*
Fast Fourier transform, 371
definition of, 1272
Fast low-angle shot (FLASH) method, of magnetic resonance imaging, 756, 757
Fasting, myocardial metabolism in, 49
Fat pad, epicardial, vs pericardial effusion, 464
Fat protons, 760
Fatty acid analogs, aromatic, 1088, 1089, *1089*
branch-chain, 1089, 1090
comparison of, 1090
iodine-for-methyl, 1086–1088, *1087*, *1088*
iodo. See *Iodo fatty acid analogs.*
isoteric, 1090
Fatty acid binding protein, 44
Fatty acids, as myocardial fuel, 48
free, consumption of, during exercise, 49
in fasting, 49
metabolism of, 1244–1246, *1246*
level of, in reperfused myocardium, 50
metabolism of, 44–46, *45*
beta-oxidation in, 46, *47*
in myocardial infarction, 1203–1207, *1205–1210*
in myocardial ischemia, 50
C-11–labeled palmitate in, 1191–1195, *1192–1195*, 1198, 1199, *1199*, *1200*
myocardial, metabolism of, evaluation of, iodo fatty acid analogs in, 1086, 1087(t)
polyunsaturated, for hypercholesterolemia, 268
radioiodinated, myocardial imaging with, history of, 1085, 1086
Femoral vein, in pulmonary angiography, 150
Ferromagnetic, definition of, 1272
Ferromagnetic relaxing agents, 797, *797*, 798, *798*, 798(t)
FETS (fast exchange, two-state), 762, *762*
Fibrillation, after intracoronary contrast agent injection, 187
atrial, during exercise, equilibrium radionuclide angiography of, 1029
left atrial thrombi with, echocardiography of, 526, *527*
Fibroelastoma, endomyocardial, and tricuspid stenosis, 436
papillary, echocardiography of, 516, *516*
Fibroma, of left ventricle, echocardiography of, 516, *517*
ultrafast computed tomography of, 704
Fibrosarcoma, 512
pericardial, magnetic resonance imaging of, *945*
Fibrosing mediastinitis, cine magnetic resonance imaging in, 955, *956*
Fibrosis, endomyocardial, 449
and tricuspid stenosis, 436
echocardiography in, 458
Fick technique, errors in, 56, 57

Fick technique *(Continued)*
of quantifying cardiac output, 56, 57
FID. See *Free induction decay (FID).*
Field echo, definition of, 1272
Field gradient, definition of, 1272
magnetization of, in magnetic resonance imaging, 746, *746*, 747, *747*
Filling defects, intraluminal, in pulmonary embolism, *151–153*, 153
Filling dysfunction, in constrictive pericarditis, 473
Filling factor, definition of, 1272
Film, cine, in archival storage, in digital angiography, 286
Filter(s), double quantum, 831
frequency domain, 82, *83*
Ram-Lak, *639*
Shepp-Logan, *639*
Filtered back projection, in projection reconstruction, in x-ray computed tomography, 638, *639*
Filtering, in digital image processing, *81–83*, 82
in radionuclide angiocardiography, 1011, 1012
smoothing, in myocardial perfusion scintigraphy, 989
Filtration, spatial, in digital angiography, 288, 289, *289*
time domain, 288
First harmonic, 999
First septal perforator, origin of, from right coronary artery, 199
from right coronary sinus, 199
Fistula(e), arteriovenous, pulmonary, pulmonary angiography in, 155, 156, *157*
coronary artery, 197, *197*
Flail leaflets, detection of, transesophageal echocardiography in, 612, *612*
Flail porcine cusps, after endocarditis, transesophageal echocardiography of, 611
FLASH (fast low-angle shot) method, of magnetic resonance imaging, 756, 757
Flavin adenine dinucleotide (FAD), in myocardial metabolism, 39, *40*
Flip angle, definition of, 1272
in magnetic resonance spectroscopy, 844
steady-state longitudinal magnetization of, 756, *756*
Flow, regurgitant, 122, *122*, 123
Flow compensation (FR), 786
Flow mode, in ultrafast computed tomography, of atrial myxomas, 704
Flow profiles, in blood flow physics, 367, 368, *368*
laminar, 367
Flow reserve, coronary. See *Coronary flow reserve (CFR).*
in bypass grafts, ultrafast computed tomography of, 686
Flow velocity paradoxus, in cardiac tamponade, 469
Flow-related enhancement, 865
definition of, 1272
Fluorine, nucleus of, characteristics of, 842(t)
Fluorine magnetic resonance spectroscopy, 858
Fluorine-18 2–fluoro 2–deoxyglucose, in exogenous glucose utilization, in myocardial ischemia, 1200–1203, *1201*, *1202*
in glucose metabolism evaluation, in myocardial ischemia, 1197, *1197*, 1198
Fluorine-18 misonidazole, 1153
Fluorine-18–labeled 1–fluoro-2–deoxyglucose, in myocardial glucose metabolism, 1163, *1163*
Fluorine-18–labeled 2–fluoro-2–deoxyglucose, 1147–1150, *1149*, *1152*

Fluorine-18–labeled metaraminol, 1152
1–Fluoro-2–deoxyglucose, fluorine-18–labeled, in myocardial glucose metabolism, 1163, *1163*
2–Fluoro-2–deoxyglucose, fluorine-18–labeled, 1147–1150, *1149*, *1152*
Fluoroscopy, digital, in coronary artery assessment, 312
progressive scan, 287, 287(t)
"Focal attention," 88
Foreign bodies, echocardiography of, 529, *530*, *531*
"Forward mapping," 81
Forward stroke volume, in aortic regurgitation, 430
Fourier transform, 82, *82*
definition of, 1272
discrete, 371, 372
fast, 371
free induction decay in, 736, *736*, 737, *737*
three-dimensional, in magnetic resonance imaging, with sodium-23, 833, 834, *834–836*
two-dimensional, 752
Fourier transform imaging, two-dimensional, definition of, 1277
FR (flow compensation), 786
Fractionation principle, 1160
Frames, cine, selection of, in quantitative coronary angiography, 241, 241(t), 242, 242(t)
Fraunhofer zone, 354, *354*
Free fatty acids, consumption of, during exercise, 49
in fasting, 49
metabolism of, 1244–1246, *1246*
Free induction decay (FID), definition of, 1272
dependence of, on phase angle, 751, *751*
in Fourier transformation, 736, *736*, 737, *737*
in magnetic resonance imaging, 747
in magnetic resonance spectroscopy, interpretation of, 842, 843
in spin-warp imaging, 750–753, *751*
sodium imaging of, *836*, *837*
Freeze-frames, in echocardiography, 363
Frequency, ambiguity of, in cardiovascular Doppler physics, 367
angular, definition of, 1271
definition of, 365, 1272
fundamental, 999
Larmor, 733, 733(t), 734
definition of, 1273
in magnetic resonance imaging, 745
of sodium, 828
Nyquist, 753, 754
of precession, 733, *733*
pulse repetition, 369
resonance, 734
definition of, 1275
of magnetization, 748
spatial, 76
Frequency domain, 82
Frequency domain filters, 82, *83*
Frequency encoding, 746
definition of, 1272
"Frequency gradient," 778
Frequency shifts, in Doppler effect, 365, 366, *366*
Frequency-encoding gradient, 752
Fresnel zone, 354, *354*
Fructose-2, 6–biphosphate, in myocardial metabolism, 42, *43*
Fundamental frequency, 999
2G42D7, 1110
in cardiac allograft rejection imaging, 1114
in myocarditis, 1114
Gadolinium, in sodium magnetic resonance spectroscopy, 857
potency of, chelation in, 804, *805*
Gadolinium diethylenetriamine pentaacetic acid. See *GdDTPA*.
Gadolinium diethyltriamine pentamethylphosphonate (Gd-PMP), 806
Gamma imaging. See also *Antimyosin imaging*.
experimental, 1112–1114, *1112*, *1113*
in cardiac allograft rejection, 1114
in myocardial infarction, 1112, *1112*, 1113, *1113*
in myocarditis, 1114
of blood clots, antibodies in, 1118
triphenyltetrazolium chloride in, *1112*, 1113
Gantry, in x-ray computed tomography, 641, *642*
Gastrointestinal system, angiographic contrast agent effect on, 176
Gated blood pool imaging. See *Equilibrium radionuclide angiography*.
Gated computed tomography, 644, 645, *645*
Gated electrocardiography, in pericardial imaging, 937, 938
lead placement in, 781
Gating, in magnetic resonance imaging, of great vessels, 864, *865*
permutation, in pericardial imaging, 937, 938
retrospective, in magnetic resonance imaging, 783
Gauss, definition of, 1272
GdDTPA (gadolinium diethylenetriamine pentaacetic acid), effect of, on magnetic resonance imaging intensity, 799, *802*, *806*
in clinical studies, of ischemic myocardium, 925, 926, *926*
in detection, of acute myocardial ischemia, 911–913, *912*, *913*
in magnetic resonance imaging, with sodium-23, 837
in myocardial perfusion assessment, 823
in nuclear magnetic resonance imaging, in infarct size estimation, 921–923, 921(t), *922*, *923*
intravenous, plasma concentration after, 804, *804*
urinary excretion of, 804, 804(t)
whole body retention of, 804, 804(t)
relaxivity of, 804, 805, *805*
T1 effects of, 799, *801*, 801(t)
T2 effects of, 799, *801*, 801(t)
GdDTPA-albumin, 805, 806, *806*
GDP (guanosine diphosphate), in lipid metabolism, 46, *48*
Gd-PMP (gadolinium diethyltriamine pentaphosphonate), 806
Geometric diameter, measured vs actual, linear regression analysis of, 315, *315*, *316*
Geometric transformations, in digital image processing, 79–81
Geometry, fan beam, 637
parallel-beam, 637, *637*
G-frequency, 752
1, 4–a-Glucan branching enzyme, 41
Glucose, exogenous, utilization of, fluorine-18 2–fluoro 2–deoxyglucose in, in myocardial ischemia, 1200–1203, *1201*, *1202*
metabolism of, 1244–1246, *1246*
catecholamines in, 49
in myocardial infarction, 1209–1214, *1212*
in myocardial ischemia, 49
evaluation of, fluorine-18 2–fluoro 2–deoxyglucose in, 1197, *1197*, 1198
Glucose *(Continued)*
myocardial, measurement of, positron emission tomography in, 1163, *1163*, 1164, *1164*
phosphorylation of, in carbohydrate metabolism, 39, 40, *41*
transport of, insulin in, 39
uptake of, in carbohydrate metabolism, 39, 40, *41*
in reperfused myocardium, 50
Glucose-1–phosphate, in myocardial metabolism, 41
Glucose-6–phosphate, in fasting, 49
in myocardial metabolism, 40, 41, *41*
Glyceraldehyde-3–phosphate, in myocardial metabolism, 42, *43*
Glycogen, metabolism of, 40–42, *41*
carbon magnetic resonance spectroscopy of, 853
Glycogen phosphorylase, in myocardial metabolism, 41, *41*
Glycogen storage disease, in restrictive cardiomyopathy, 458
Glycogen synthetase, in myocardial metabolism, 41, 42
Glycolysis, 1244–1246, *1246*
in carbohydrate metabolism, 42, *43*
in diabetes, 49
in fasting, 49
in ischemia, 49
GMR (gradient moment reduction), 786
Gold-195, in radionuclide angiocardiography, 1010, 1010(t)
Gorlin equation, 63, 64
G-phase, 752, *752*, 753
Gradient(s), aortic valve, underestimation of, by Doppler echocardiography, 425, *425*
definition of, 1272
field, definition of, 1272
frequency, 778
frequency-encoding, 752
magnetic field, definition of, 1273
phase-encoding, 752
rephasing, definition of, 1275
Gradient coils, 745
definition of, 1272
Gradient echo, creation of, 747, *747*
definition of, 1272
Gradient moment nulling, in magnetic resonance imaging, 784, 786, *786*, 787, *787*
Gradient moment reduction (GMR), 786
Gradient reversal, temporal resolution in, in cine magnetic resonance imaging, 812
Gradient reversal pulse sequence, in magnetic resonance imaging, of great vessels, 864
Gradient-echo imaging, in magnetic resonance imaging, of blood flow, 773
Gradient-recalled acquisition in steady state (GRASS), 924, *924*
Graft(s), bypass. See *Bypass graft(s)*.
materials for, thrombogeneity of, 1129, 1130
prosthetic, platelet deposition on, 1129, *1131*, *1132*
drug effects on, 1130, 1131
Graft–native vessel coronary anastomosis, evaluation of, high-frequency epicardial echocardiography in, 625–627, *626–629*
"Granular echo," 367
GRASS (gradient-recalled acquisition in steady state), 924, *924*
Grating lobe, 357, *358*
Gray level, 541
echocardiographic, quantitation of, 542, 543
textures of, 541–543, *542*
in ischemia, 546, *547*
Gray level histogram, 78, *80*
Gray level run, 543

Gray level thresholds, in segmentation, 82, 83, *83*
Gray scale compression, in digital imaging, 77, *78*
Great arteries, transposition of, ultrafast computed tomography in, 722, *722*
Great vessels, anomalies of, magnetic resonance imaging of, 892–894, *893*, *894*
    ultrafast computed tomography of, 725, *726*, *727*
  cine magnetic resonance imaging of, 953–955, *954–956*
  magnetic resonance imaging of, blood flow effects on, 864, 865, *866*, *867*
    gating in, 864, *865*
    metallic prosthesis effects on, 865–867, *867*
    pulse sequences in, 864, *865*, *866*
      spin-echo, 864, *865*
    spin-phase effects on, 865, *866*
    time-of-flight effects on, 864, 865, *866*
  nuclear magnetic resonance of, 864–885
  transposition of, magnetic resonance imaging in, 876, *877*
GTP (guanosine triphosphate), in lipid metabolism, 46, *48*
Guanethidine, chemical structure for, *1135*
Guanosine diphosphate (GDP), in lipid metabolism, 46, *48*
Guanosine triphosphate (GTP), in lipid metabolism, 46, *48*
Gyromagnetic ratio, definition of, 1272
  of nuclei, in magnetic resonance imaging, 842(t)

H_0, definition of, 1272
H_1, definition of, 1273
Halcion, for sedation, in magnetic resonance imaging, 779
Halothane, toxic effects of, phosphorus magnetic resonance spectroscopy of, 849
Hanning filter, *986*
Hardware zoom, of digital image processor, 285
Harmonic, first, 999
  second, 999
  zero, 999
Heart, anatomy of, normal, 194–196, *195*
  cross-sectional images of, after nitrogen-13 ammonia administration, *1172*
  extracardiac masses adjacent to, 520, *522*, *523*
  extracardiac structures indenting, echocardiography of, 529, *531*
  gated computed tomography of, 644, 645, *645*
  innervation of, positron-emitting tracers of, 1141(t), 1152
  magnetic resonance imaging of, signal intensity in, 764, *764*
  normal variants of, 511, *511–513*, 512
  perfused, preparations of, phosphorus magnetic resonance spectroscopy of, 846–849
  quantitation of. See *Quantitation, cardiac.*
  shape of, complexities of, 25
    evaluation of, 73
  size of, in cardiac silhouette, 99–103
    measurement of, linear, magnetic resonance imaging in, 816, *816*, 816(t)
      magnetic resonance imaging in, 815–819
      volume, magnetic resonance imaging in, 816, 817, *817*
  structure of, evaluation of, ultrafast computed tomography in, 669–681
Heart *(Continued)*
  three-dimensional reconstruction of, 73, 73(t), 74, *74*
    shaded-surface displays in, 73, *74*
    wire-frame displays in, 73, *74*
  tissue characterization in, magnetic resonance imaging in, 820–822
      in infarct size measurement, 821, *821*, 822, *822*
      limitations of, 821
  translational motion of, correction for, 124, *127*
  wall thickness in, measurement of, magnetic resonance imaging in, 817–819
Heart chambers, size and function of, evaluation of, cine magnetic resonance imaging in, 951–953, *953*
Heart disease, acquired, chest roentgenography of, 103–108
  amyloid, 457, *457*
  congenital. See *Congenital heart disease.*
  evaluation of, perception in, 90, 91
  ischemic. See *Ischemic heart disease.*
  myocardial blood flow in, evaluation of, 1169–1189
  noncoronary, thallium-201 scintigraphy in, 1066, 1066(t), 1067
  skeletal muscle metabolism in, spectroscopy of, 972–974, *973*, *974*
  valvular. See *Valvular heart disease.*
Heart failure, ejection velocity in, after vasodilator therapy, 407
  vs. dilated cardiomyopathy, 456
Heart rate, after selective intracoronary injection, of angiographic contrast agents, 172, *173*
  calculation of, 118
  diastasis effect on, 140, *142*
  during exercise, 1020(t)
  in left ventricular function, 26, 34
  influence of, on diastolic performance, 410, *412*
Heart transplant, rejection of, magnetic resonance imaging in, 932
Helium, in coronary blood flow measurement, 244
Hemangioma, of left atrium, 516
Hematocrit, in myocardial acoustics, 544
Hemochromatosis, in restrictive cardiomyopathy, 458
Hemodynamic equations, for valvular heart disease quantification, 56–59
Hemodynamics, after intracoronary contrast agent injection, 187, 188
  in coronary vasodilator reserve, 14
  of left ventricle, exercise effects on, 27
  of right heart, in pulmonary embolism, 153
  of right ventricular ejection, 414, *414*
  of valvular lesions, 56–71
Hemoglobin, concentration of, after intravascular contrast agent bolus, 168, *168*
Hemorrhage, myocardial infarct with, magnetic resonance imaging of, 766, *767*
Heparin, for pulmonary embolism, 154
  in coronary angiography, 190
Hepatic vein, blood flow in, in tricuspid regurgitation, 438, *438*
Hernia, hiatal, echocardiography of, 529, *531*
Hertz, definition of, 1273
Hexabrix, properties of, 166, 167(t)
Hexadentate chelate, *796*
Hexokinase, in fasting, 49
Hexokinase reaction, 40
Hiatal hernia, echocardiography of, 529, *531*
Hibernation, myocardial, in myocardial ischemia, 1234
  in right ventricular function, 32
High-velocity signal loss, 864, *866*
High-velocity signal loss *(Continued)*
  in magnetic resonance imaging, 785
Histamine, effects of, on coronary circulation, 11
Histiocytoma, fibrous, malignant, 519, *519*
Histogram, gray level, 78, *80*
  R-R, 983, *984*
  time interval, 371
Histogram equalization, 78, *80*
Hodgkin's disease, mediastinal, echocardiography of, 520, *522*, *523*
Homogeneity, definition of, 1273
  of magnetic field, 744
Homogeneous spectrum, of sodium-23, 830, *830*, 831
Horseshoe coronary artery, 199
Host computer, of digital image processor, 285
Hounsfield unit, linearity of, in computed tomography, 649, 650, 653(t), *654*
    in fast computed tomography, 649, 650, 653(t), *654*
Huygens' principle, 352
Hybrid acquisition, 298(t)
Hydrogen, in coronary blood flow measurement, 244
Hydrolytic amylo-1, 6–glucosidase, in myocardial metabolism, 41
Hydrophone probe, 355
3–Hydroxyacyl-CoA dehydrogenase, in lipid metabolism, 46, *47*
3–Hydroxybutyrate, in lipid metabolism, 46, *48*
Hypaque, *164*, 165
Hypaque-76, intracoronary injection of, and ventricular fibrillation, 174
  properties of, 166, 167(t)
Hypercholesterolemia, polyunsaturated fatty acids for, 268
Hyperemia, induction of, appearance time in, 334, *334*
  maximal, in coronary flow reserve assessment, 338, *339*
  reactive. See *Reactive hyperemia.*
  time of arrival images in, *336*
Hyperkinesis, during myocardial infarction, 137, *137*
Hyperlipidemia, interventions for, 267, 268, 268(t)
Hyperosmolar contrast agents, for maximal hyperemia, 338
Hypertension, arterial, pulmonary, 98, *99*
    in atrial septal defect, 98, *99*
  chronic, autoregulation gain in, 10, *10*
  phosphorus magnetic resonance spectroscopy in, 848
  pulmonary, cine magnetic resonance imaging in, 954, 955, *956*
  thallium-201 scintigraphy in, 1066, 1066(t)
  venous, pulmonary. See *Pulmonary venous hypertension.*
Hypertrophic cardiomyopathy, 1251, 1252
  at end-diastole, 110, *114*
  cavitary size in, 450
  cavity obliteration in, echocardiography of, 452
    Doppler, 452, 453
  definition of, 449
  diastolic left ventricular function in, 410, 450
  echocardiography in, 449–453, *450*
  functional assessment of, magnetic resonance imaging in, 931
  intraventricular pressure gradients in, 450–453, *451–453*
  left ventricular contours in, *112*
  left ventricular outflow obstruction in, color flow imaging of, 451

Hypertrophic cardiomyopathy *(Continued)*
echocardiography of, 450, *451*
continuous wave, 451, *451*
Doppler, 450, 451, *451*, *452*
left ventricular systolic function in, 450
magnetic resonance imaging in, 929–931, *930*, *931*
metabolism in, 1251
positron emission tomography of, 1251, 1252, *1252*
midventricular obstruction in, echocardiography of, 451, 452, *452*, *453*
Doppler, 451, 452, *452*, *453*
mitral regurgitation in, echocardiography of, 453
morphologic features of, magnetic resonance imaging of, 929, *930*, *931*
muscular subaortic stenosis in, assessment of, 450, 451, *451*, *452*
roentgenographic evaluation of, 106
spectroscopy in, 971, *972*
surgery for, intraoperative echocardiography during, 624, *625*
systolic anterior motion in, 450, 451, *451*
thallium-201 scintigraphy in, 1066, 1066(t)
tissue characterization in, magnetic resonance imaging in, 931
ultrasonic, 551, *552*
Hypertrophy, cardiac, echocardiography of, 529, *533*
effect of, on myocardial perfusion, 19, *19*
in protein turnover regulation, 52
left ventricular, autoregulation gain in, 10, *10*
lipomatous, echocardiography of, 528, 529, *529*
reactive, in infarcted myocardium, 33
Hypokinesis, coronary artery occlusion and, 135, *136*, 137
Hypokinetic segment length, 129
Hypoplastic left heart syndrome, 489, 492, *493*
Hypoplastic right heart syndrome, echocardiography in, 496, *496*
Hypoxia, metabolic consequences of, carbon magnetic resonance spectroscopy of, 853
phosphorus magnetic resonance spectroscopy in, 848

IHDA, 1086–1088, *1087*, 1087(t)
in cardiomyopathy, 1094
in coronary artery disease, 1093
in myocardial infarction, 1091–1093, *1091*
intravenous, radiolabel fractional distribution after, 1088, *1088*
uptake and clearance of, *1089*, 1090
in coronary artery disease, 1087, *1087*
IHPA, 1086–1088, *1087*, 1087(t)
clearance rate of, 1090
in dilated cardiomyopathy, 1094
in myocardial infarction, 1091–1093
Image(s), analysis of, by Dynamic Spatial Reconstructor, 656
in positron emission tomography, 1157, *1157*, 1158, *1158*
in quantitative coronary arteriography, 231
three-dimensional computed tomography in, 659–665, *660–665*
B-mode, real-time, formation of, 356–359
cross-sectional, of heart, after nitrogen-13 ammonia administration, *1172*
digital, characteristics of, 74–77, *75–78*
storage of, 283, 283(t)
emission, in positron emission tomography, of myocardial blood flow, 1171, 1172

Image(s) *(Continued)*
formation of, in echocardiography, 359, 360, *360*, *361*
manipulation of, in digital angiography, 287
parametric flow ratio, *337*
perception of, theories of, 88
quality of, in x-ray computed tomography, 639–641
transmission, in positron emission tomography, of myocardial blood flow, 1171
Image acquisition, in iodo fatty acid imaging, 1091
in positron emission tomography, 1154–1157, *1154–1156*
in quantitative coronary angiography, 219, 220
in scintigraphy. See *Scintigraphy, image acquisition in.*
Image acquisition time, definition of, 1273
Image enhancement, in digital angiography, 288, 289, *289*, 289(t)
spatial filtration in, 288, 289, *289*
in digital image processing, 77–82
Image memory, 285
Image noise, in digital cardiac angiography, 282, 283
Image processing, in coronary flow reserve angiography, 247–249, *247*, *248*, 248(t)
quantitative, future directions of, 83–85, *84*
Image processors, in quantitative coronary angiography, 221, 221(t)
Image reconstruction, 634, 636
Image search, 88, 89
Image workstation, in digital angiography, 286, 287
Image-Selected in Vivo Spectroscopy (ISIS), 968, *968*
Imaging, antifibrin, 1118
antimyosin. See *Antimyosin imaging.*
backscatter, integrated, 540, *540*, 541, *541*
real-time, 540, *540*, 541, *541*
blood pool, gated. See *Equilibrium radionuclide angiography.*
chemical shift, definition of, 1271
color flow. See *Color flow imaging.*
C-scan, 359, *359*
diagnostic, errors in, 87
diffusion/perfusion, in myocardial perfusion assessment, 823
digital, in left ventricular function assessment, during interventions, 303–308, *304–307*
principles of, 281–283, *282*, 283(t)
echo, multiple, definition of, 1274
Fourier transform, two-dimensional, definition of, 1277
gamma. See *Gamma imaging.*
infarct avid, 1074–1084
iodo fatty acid. See *Iodo fatty acid imaging.*
metabolic, with single-photon-emitting tracers, 1085–1096
monoclonal antibody, 1110–1120
multiple slice, definition of, 1274
of blood flow, techniques of, 774, *774*, 775
of cardiac neurons, 1135–1139
of cardiac receptors, 1135–1139
of coronary arteries, ultrasonography in, 602, 603, *603*, 625–630, *626*
of left ventricle, 109, 110
contrast agents for, intravenous, 295–297, *296*
ventricular administration of, 297, *297*
of myocardial metabolism, in clinical practice, 1237–1240
of myocardial perfusion, thallium-201 in, 1047–1073
of pericardium, 937, 938
parametric, 299, *299*

Imaging *(Continued)*
planar. See *Planar imaging.*
radionuclide. See *Radionuclide imaging.*
rapid, in magnetic resonance imaging, 754–757, *755–757*
spectroscopic, 968, 969
spin-echo. See *Spin-echo imaging.*
spin-warp. See *Spin-warp imaging.*
time interval difference, 288
tomographic, 984–988
volume, definition of, 1277
x-ray, diagnostic, physics of, 162
Imaging chain, magnification in, correction of, 118, *118*
Imaging planes, for epicardial echocardiography, 618–620, *619*, *620*
for transesophageal echocardiography, 621, *621*
Imatron, 645
Imatron C-100 scanner, 669
Imipramine, administration of, metaiodobenzylguanidine uptake after, 1138
Impedance, 351, 351(t)
acoustic, definition of, 539
Impedance matching, 353, 354
Impulse conduction, after selective intracoronary injection, of angiographic contrast agents, 171–174, *173*
Impulse response analysis, in functional assessment, of coronary circulation, 331–334, *333*, *334*
Incidence, angle of, 352
Index, cardiac, 122
Indicator dilution curve, in radionuclide angiocardiography, 1012, *1012*, 1013
low-frequency, 1014, *1014*
Indicator dilution methods, of functional assessment, of coronary circulation, 328, 329, *329*, *330*
of myocardial perfusion measurement, algorithm for, 691, *691*, 692
application of, to computed tomography, 689–691, *690*, *692*
historical aspects of, 689
nonionic contrast agents in, 690, *690*
of quantifying cardiac output, 56, 57
Indium-111, in infarct avid imaging, 1083
Indium-111–labeled platelets, function of, 1122
imaging of, 1122–1124, *1123*
in cardiac thrombi imaging, 1124, *1124*, 1124(t), 1125, *1125*
in prosthesis imaging, 1129–1131, 1129(t), *1130*, *1131*
in pulmonary embolism imaging, 1128, 1129
in thrombosis imaging, 1121–1134
vascular, 1125–1128, 1126(t), *1127*, *1128*
venous, 1128, 1129
radiation dosimetry with, 1122
single-photon emission computed tomography of, 1122, 1123, *1123*
uptake of, quantification of, 1122–1124, *1123*
Induced electromotive force, 842
Inductance, definition of, 1273
Induction, magnetic, definition of, 1273
Infarct, apical, left ventricular thrombus with, echocardiography of, *524*
size of, measurement of, *136*
magnetic resonance imaging in, 821, *821*, 822, *822*
two-dimensional echocardiography in, 388, *390*
quantification of, single plane, 388, *390*
wall motion in, 388–391
relation of, to dyskinesia, 594, *595*
wall motion opposite, 137, *137*

Infarct avid imaging, 1074–1084
agents for, 1083
Infarcted myocardium, compensatory hyperfunction in, 33
in right ventricular function, 32, 33
infarct expansion in, 33
reactive hypertrophy in, 33
wall motion abnormalities in, 32
Infarction, acute, ultrasonic tissue characterization in, 545, 546, *546*, *547*
backscatter coefficient in, 548, *548*
chronic, ultrasonic tissue characterization in, 548, *549*, *550*
of right ventricle, paradoxic septal motion in, 396, 397(t)
regional wall motion abnormality in, 397
reperfused, detection of, nuclear magnetic resonance in, 918, 919, 919(t)
imaging of, nonproton nuclei in, 919
tissue property changes in, 918, 919, 919(t)
subacute, ultrasonic tissue characterization in, 548, *549*, *550*
systolic dysfunction in, 382
Infarct/risk relationship, 19
Inferior limbic band, echocardiography of, 500
Inferior vena cava filter, in pulmonary embolism, 155
Inferior vena caval plethora, in cardiac tamponade, 468
Infiltrative cardiomyopathy, magnetic resonance imaging in, 933, 934, *934*
Infundibular pulmonic stenosis, cine magnetic resonance imaging in, *962*
Infundibular septum, 479
Inhomogeneity, definition of, 1273
Inhomogeneous powder spectrum, of sodium-23, 830, *830*, 831
Inlet septum, 479
Innervation, cardiac, positron-emitting tracers of, 1141(t), 1152
Innominate vein, in aortic dissection, 872, *873*
Insonification, angle of, 544
Instrumentation, for digital angiography, 281–294
for Doppler, 368–371
for dynamic x-ray computed tomography, 634–668
for echocardiography, 348–364
for beam insertion, 353, *353*, 354
for lateral resolution, 354, *354*, 355, *355*
for pulse transmission, 353, *353*, 354
for radionuclide angiocardiography, 1006–1010, *1009*
for radionuclide imaging, 977–1005
for single-photon emission computed tomography, 1002
Insulin, in fasting, 49
in glucose transport, 39
in myocardial metabolism, 49
in protein turnover regulation, 52
Integrated backscatter, 540, *541*
definition of, 539
in atherosclerosis, 553, *553*
Integrated backscatter imaging, 540, *540*, 541, *541*
Intensity, in ultrasonography, 351
Intensity transformation table (ITT), of digital image processor, 284
Interatrial septum, aneurysm of, echocardiography of, 529, *530*
Interference, constructive, 352
destructive, 352
Interlace, in digital angiography, 284
Interleaved multislice mode, of magnetic resonance imaging, 754, *755*
Internal focusing, 354, *354*
Internal mammary artery, as bypass graft, ultrafast computed tomography of, 684, *684*
Internal mammary artery angiography, 193
Interpolation, bilinear, 81
nearest-neighbor, 81
Interpulse times, definition of, 1273
Interventricular septum, 194
measurement of, echocardiographic, 380, *381*
Intracardiac masses, cine magnetic resonance imaging of, 964, *964*, 965
ultrafast computed tomography of, 703–713
Intracardiac shunts, contrast echocardiography in, 568, 569
Intracardiac thrombi, ultrafast computed tomography of, 705–707, *705*, *706*
indications for, 706, *707*
Intracavitary thrombi, ultrafast computed tomography of, 706
Intraluminal filling defects, in pulmonary embolism, *151–153*, 153
Intramyocardial vascular volume, regional, measurement of, fast computed tomography in, 698, 699, *699*
Intravascular volume, after intravascular bolus injection, of angiographic contrast agents, 168, *168*
Intraventricular pressure gradients, in hypertrophic cardiomyopathy, 450–453, *451–453*
Inversion, definition of, 1273
Inversion pulse, 741
Inversion transfer, definition of, 1275
Inversion-recovery, definition of, 1273
Inversion-recovery sequence, in multipulse nuclear magnetic resonance, 740, *740*, 741, *741*
Iodide, clearance rate of, 1086–1088
Iodine, as radiographic contrast agent, 163, *163*
concentration of, in angiographic contrast agents, 165, 166, *166*, 167(t)
in left ventricular imaging, 296
Iodine ratio, 163
Iodine-123, in infarct avid imaging, 1083
Iodine-for-methyl fatty acid analogs, 1086–1088, *1087*, *1088*
Iodixanol, *164*, 165
Iodo fatty acid analogs, clearance of, in normal and diseased myocardium, 1089(t)
clinical experience with, 1091–1094, *1091–1093*
in cardiomyopathy, 1093, *1093*, 1094
in chronic coronary artery disease, 1093, *1093*, 1094
exercise effect on, 1094
in myocardial fatty acid metabolism, 1086, 1087(t)
tracer tissue kinetics of, 1086–1090, *1086–1089*, 1087(t), 1089(t)
uptake of, regional blood flow in, 1092, 1093
Iodo fatty acid imaging, analog for, 1090, 1091
background activity in, 1091
dietary conditions in, 1091
image acquisition in, 1091
planar vs. tomographic, 1091
technical aspects of, 1090, 1091
Iodo fatty acids, historical development of, 1085, 1086
16–[1–123] iodo hexadecanoic acid. See *IHDA.*
17–[1–123] iodo heptadecanoic acid. See *IHPA.*
Iodopyracet, 163, *164*
Iohexol, *164*, 165
properties of, 166, 167(t)
specifications of, 234(t)
Iopamidol, *164*, 165
effect of, on systemic arterial pressure, *169*
intracoronary injection of, and ventricular fibrillation, 174
effects of, *171*
properties of, 166, 167(t)
specifications of, 234(t)
Iopentol, 165
Iothalamate, intracoronary injection of, effects of, *171*
properties of, 166, 167(t)
Iothalamic acid, *164*, 165
Ioversol, *164*, 165
effect of, on systemic arterial pressure, *169*
properties of, 166, 167(t)
Ioxaglate, 165
bolus administration of, hemoglobin concentration after, *168*
intracoronary injection of, effects of, 170, *171*
properties of, 166, 167(t)
specifications of, 234(t)
IPPA, *1087*, 1088
clearance rates of, 1088, *1089*, 1089(t), 1090
fractional distribution of, 1088, *1089*, 1089(t)
in cardiomyopathy, 1094
in coronary artery disease, 1093
in coronary artery stenosis, *1092*
in myocardial infarction, 1092
uptake of, after exercise, single-photon emission computed tomography of, 1093, *1093*, 1094
vs. C-11–labeled palmitate, 1089
Iridium-191m, in radionuclide angiocardiography, 1010, 1010(t)
Ischemia, acute, ultrasonic tissue characterization in, 545, 546, *546*, *547*
diastolic function in, detection of, 410
effect of, on attenuation, 545, *546*
on backscatter, 545, *546*
gray level texture in, 546, *547*
in protein turnover regulation, 53
lactate changes after, proton magnetic resonance spectroscopy of, 854, *856*
myocardial. See *Myocardial ischemia.*
myocardial metabolism in, 49, 50
silent, detection of, positron emission tomography in, 1182, *1182–1184*, 1183
systolic dysfunction in, 382
transient, detection of, positron emission tomography in, 1182, *1182–1184*, 1183
in right ventricular function, 31
regional wall motion abnormalities in, 31
Ischemic cardiomyopathy, left ventricular function in, after coronary artery bypass grafting, 1225, 1225(t)
Ischemic exercise, spectroscopy in, 972–974, *974*
Ischemic heart disease, exercise echocardiography in, 580–584, *581*, *582*, 583(t), *584*
Doppler, 586–588, *586*, *587*
left ventricular function in, diastolic, 410
nuclear magnetic resonance imaging of, 923–925, *923*, *924*
myocardial substrate metabolism in, 1190–1243
nuclear magnetic resonance imaging in, 911–928
peak ejection velocity in, during exercise, 586, *586*, 587, *587*
roentgenographic evaluation of, 103, 104
thallium scintigraphy in, 587, *587*
ultrasonic tissue characterization in, 545–548, *546–550*
ISD (isosorbide dinitrate), preangiographic administration of, 233

ISIS (Image-Selected in Vivo Spectroscopy), 968, *968*
Isocenter, 745
Isochromat, 742, *742*
Isocitrate dehydrogenase, in tricarboxylic acid cycle, 47
Isometric exercise, in ventricular function evaluation, 27, 27(t)
Isonitriles, technetium-99m, 1053
imaging with, clinical application of, 1067, 1068
properties of, 1097–1100, *1098*, *1099*
Iso-osmolality, nonionic contrast agents with, in quantitative coronary arteriography, 233, 234, 234(t)
Isoproterenol, in non-exercise stress echocardiography, 589
Isosorbide dinitrate (ISD), preangiographic administration of, 233
Isoteric fatty acid analogs, 1090
Isovolumic relaxation, 409
right ventricular, 414
Isovolumic relaxation time, in cardiac tamponade, 469
Isovue, *164*
properties of, 166, 167(t)
ITT (intensity transformation table), of digital image processor, 284

Judgment calls, evaluation of, 90, *90*
faulty, 87
Judkins technique, of coronary angiography, 191, *191*

Kerley's lines, in pulmonary venous hypertension, *97*, 98
Kernel, pixel, 289
Ketone bodies, as myocardial fuel, 48
metabolism of, 46, *48*
Kilohertz, definition of, 1273
Kimray-Greenfield filter, for pulmonary embolism, 155, *156*
Kinetic binding, of cardiac receptors, 1261, *1261*

Lactate, concentration of, during exercise, 49
in ischemia, 49
proton magnetic resonance spectroscopy of, 854, *856*
metabolism of, 44, 1244–1246, *1246*
production of, during ischemic exercise, *974*
Lag, in digital angiography, 284
Lambert-Beer law, 228, 229, 635
Lambl's excrescences, 529
Laminar blood flow, 59
Languages, computer, for quantitative coronary angiography, 222, 222(t)
Laplace relationship, 123, 124
Larmor equation, definition of, 1273
Larmor frequency, 733, 733(t), 734
definition of, 1273
in magnetic resonance imaging, 745
of sodium, 828
Lateral resolution, determinants of, 354, *354*, 355, *355*
in echocardiography, instrumentation for, 354, *354*, 355, *355*
Lattice, definition of, 1273
Leads, placement of, in electrocardiographic gating, 781

Leaflet, anterior, cleft of, and mitral regurgitation, 435
Left anterior descending artery, atherosclerosis in, regression of, 270, 270(t)
blood flow in, before and after bifurcation, *327*
collateral pathways to, 199
lumen diameter of, effect of, on anterior wall motion, 307, *307*
origin of, from right coronary artery, 198
from right coronary sinus, 198
Left aortic arch, magnetic resonance imaging of, 893
Left atrial collapse, in cardiac tamponade, 466, *467*
Left atrial pressure, in diastolic performance, 412, *413*
in mitral regurgitation, 412, *413*
nitroglycerin effect on, 412, *413*
Left atrium(a), enlargement of, in mitral stenosis, 99, *101*
on cardiac silhouette, *98–101*, 99, 100
hemangioma of, 516
primary benign tumors of, echocardiography of, 512–516, *514–516*
thrombi of, echocardiography of, 525, 526, *526*, *527*
imaging of, indium-111–labeled platelets in, 1125
volume of, evaluation of, ultrafast computed tomography in, 678
Left bundle branch block, as pulmonary angiography contraindication, 149
thallium-201 scintigraphy in, 1066, 1066(t)
Left circumflex artery, atherosclerosis in, regression of, 270, 270(t)
Left coronary artery, anatomy of, 196
anomalous, thallium-201 scintigraphy in, 1066(t), 1067
origin of, from opposite coronary sinus, 198, *198*
from pulmonary artery, 197
Left heart, contrast echocardiography of, 569–572, *571*, *572*
Left pleural effusion, vs. pericardial effusion, 464, *465*
Left superior vena cava, persistent, echocardiography of, *503*, *504*
Left ventricle(s), abnormal wall motion in, causes of, 597(t)
anatomy and function of, 26, 73
aneurysm of, 101, *103*
after myocardial infarction, 110, *116*, 600, *600*
cine magnetic resonance imaging of, *963*
area of, calculation of, radionuclide angiocardiography in, 1016, *1017*
biplane transesophageal echocardiography of, 614, *614*
contours of, in hypertrophic cardiomyopathy, *112*
in mitral regurgitation, *112*
contraction of, analysis of, ultrafast computed tomography in, 674
indices of, *596*, 597(t)
elastance of, 140
enlargement of, autoregulation gain in, 10, *10*
gated spin-echo imaging in, *898*
in aortic regurgitation, 101, *102*
in congestive heart failure, 110, *113*
in Marfan's syndrome, *102*
on cardiac silhouette, 100, 101, *102*, *103*
evaluation of, cine magnetic resonance imaging in, 952, *953*
ultrafast computed tomography in, 671–676

Left ventricle(s) *(Continued)*
filling rate of, evaluation of, ultrafast computed tomography in, 675, *675*
hemodynamics of, exercise effects on, 27
imaging of, 109, 110
contrast agents for, intravenous, 295–297, *296*
ventricular administration of, 297, *297*
morphologic, echocardiography of, *508*
normal, shape of, 110, *111*, *112*
primary benign tumors of, echocardiography of, 516, *517*
psuedoaneurysm of, after myocardial infarction, 600, *601*
sectional performance of, ultrafast computed tomography of, 672, 673, *673*
segmental endocardial motion of, ultrafast computed tomography of, 673, *674*
segmental wall thickening in, ultrafast computed tomography of, 673, 674, *674*
size of, internal, measurement of, echocardiography in, 380, *381*
measurement of, magnetic resonance imaging in, 816, 816(t)
stroke volume of, determination of, 403, *405*
subendocardium of, autoregulation gain in, 9
subepicardium of, autoregulation gain in, 9
three-dimensional reconstruction of, ultrafast computed tomography in, 676, *676*
thrombi of, after myocardial infarction, 600, *601*, *602*
echocardiography of, 523–525, *523–526*
imaging of, indium-111–labeled platelets in, 1124, *1124*, 1125, *1125*
transmural perfusion of, 11, 12, *12*
Left ventricular diastolic collapse, in cardiac tamponade, 466–468, *468*
Left ventricular dysfunction, coronary angiography in, 184
exercise-induced, in aortic insufficiency, 1041, *1041*
in pulmonary venous hypertension, 95, 97, *98*
radionuclide angiocardiography in, 1022
Left ventricular ejection, assessment of, Doppler echocardiography in, 403–408, 403(t), *404–407*
Doppler, velocity of, in cardiomyopathy, 405, *406*
Left ventricular ejection fraction, calculation of, echocardiography in, 377–379, 378(t), *380*
equilibrium radionuclide angiography in, 1029, 1029(t)
technetium-99m agents in, *1106*
ultrafast computed tomography in, 671, *671*, 672, *673*
videodensitometry in, 300–302, *301–303*
during exercise, in coronary artery disease diagnosis, 584, 585, *585*, *586*
radionuclide angiocardiography of, 1022, 1023, *1023*
in dilated cardiomyopathy, 454
in hypertrophic cardiomyopathy, 450
in myocardial infarction, as predictor of survival, 138
Left ventricular end-diastolic pressure, after intravascular bolus injection, of angiographic contrast agents, 169, *170*, *171*
Left ventricular end-diastolic volume, measurement of, equilibrium radionuclide angiography in, 1030, *1030*, 1031
Left ventricular filling, assessment of, Doppler echocardiography in, 408–413, 408(t), *409–413*
diastolic, triphasic nature of, 34, 34(t), *35*

Left ventricular filling *(Continued)*
velocity of, in mitral prolapse, *412*
in mitral regurgitation, *412*
Left ventricular function, abnormal, 110
after coronary artery bypass grafting, in ischemic cardiomyopathy, 1225, 1225(t)
analysis of, throughout cardiac cycle, 139–144, *139–143*
assessment of, diagnostic, 135
digital imaging in, during interventions, 303–308, *304–307*
dobutamine in, with ultrafast computed tomography, 679, 680
determination of, intraoperative echocardiography in, 630
diastolic, assessment of, 34, 35
Doppler echocardiography in, 409, 410, *410*
ultrafast computed tomography in, 675, *675*, 676
factors in, 34, *34*
heterogeneity of, 34
in hypertrophic cardiomyopathy, 450
during exercise, bicycle, ultrafast computed tomography of, 680
Doppler echocardiography of, 580
effect on, of pressure overload, 124
of volume overload, 124
factors in, 26, 26(t), 27
global, assessment of, echocardiography in, 374–381
heterogeneity of, 30, *30*
cardiac imaging effects of, 30
impairment of, minimum coronary luminal diameter in, 306–308, *306*, *307*
in acute myocardial infarction, 135–137, *137*
as predictor of survival, 138
in aneurysms, as predictor of survival, 138
in dilated cardiomyopathy, echocardiography of, 454
Doppler, 456
in ischemic heart disease, assessment of, nuclear magnetic resonance in, 923–925, *923*, *924*
interventional studies of, ultrafast computed tomography in, 679, 680
regional, 28–30, *29*, 29(t)
assessment of, 29, 29(t)
analysis algorithms in, 382–388, *383–389*
echocardiography in, 381–391
ultrafast computed tomography in, 672–674, *673*, *674*
systolic, in hypertrophic cardiomyopathy, 450
Left ventricular mass, calculation of, 123, *123–125*, 124
echocardiography in, 380, 381, *381*
magnetic resonance imaging in, 818, *818*, *819*
ultrafast computed tomography in, 672, *672*, 672(t)
normal values for, 134–139, 134(t)
Left ventricular motion, complexities of, 25
components of, importance of, 25
during systole, 25
Left ventricular outflow tract, blood velocity in, 60
cross-sectional area of, calculation of, 58
obstruction of, Doppler echocardiography in, 490–492, *490*, *492*
in hypertrophic cardiomyopathy, color flow imaging of, 451
echocardiography of, 450, *451*
continuous wave, 451, *451*
Doppler, 450, 451, *451*, *452*
two-dimensional echocardiography in, 489–492, *490*, *491*
Left ventricular outflow tract *(Continued)*
vs. valvular stenosis, 420
Left ventricular output, measurement of, equilibrium radionuclide angiography in, 1031
Left ventricular performance, systolic, 35
Left ventricular pressure, systolic, in mitral regurgitation, 403, *405*
vs. left ventricular volume, 28, *28*
Left ventricular stress, 123, 124, *125*
Left ventricular volume, abnormality in, 110, *113*, *114*
calculation of, 110, 111, *116*, 300, 301
contrast material in, 119, 120, *120*
cube method of, 376
echocardiography in, 375–377, *376–379*, 378(t)
vs. angiography, 375, *376*, 378(t)
equilibrium radionuclide angiography in, 1030, *1030*, 1031
magnetic resonance imaging in, 816, 817, *817*
models for, 375, *375*, *376*
partial volume effects in, 815, 816
radionuclide angiocardiography in, 1016, *1016*
radionuclide ventriculography in, 997, 998
ultrafast computed tomography in, 671, *671*, 672
end-diastolic, 35
in Trendelenburg's position, 27
factors in, 26, 26(t), 27
normal values for, 134–139, 134(t)
relationship of, to end-systolic pressure, 379, 380
Left ventricular wall motion, assessment of, magnetic resonance imaging in, *821*
radionuclide angiocardiography in, 1017
quantitative analysis of, applications of, 134–139
parameter selection in, 138, 139
theoretical considerations in, 138
timing of, 138
regional, quantitative analysis of, 124–134, *126–134*
Left ventriculography, with intravenous contrast agents, vs. cine film, 295–297
Left-sided regurgitant lesions, evaluation of, 67
Left-to-right shunting, in patent ductus arteriosus, 483–486, *484*, *485*
quantitation of, Doppler echocardiography in, 487–489
radionuclide angiocardiography in, 1015, *1015*
Leiden Intervention Trial, 270, 270(t)
Lesion(s), admixture, magnetic resonance imaging in, 892
eccentric, Type I, 214
Type II, 214
geometric severity of, coronary angiographic assessment of, 214, 215, *215*
of pericardium, ultrafast computed tomography of, 709, *710*
regurgitant, cine magnetic resonance imaging of, 955–959, *957–961*
left-sided, evaluation of, 67
right-sided, evaluation of, 67
stenotic, cine magnetic resonance imaging of, 959–962, *961*
valvular, hemodynamics of, 56–71
vascular, pulmonary, pulmonary angiography for, 155–159
Level displays, 78, *80*
Levo loop, 500, *506*, *507*
Ligands, access of, to myocardium, 1258, 1259
Ligands *(Continued)*
C-11–labeled, for cardiac receptor studies, 1257, 1257(t)
cardiac receptor interaction with, positron emission tomography of, 1259, 1260, *1260*
choice of, 1259
interaction of, within myocardium, 1259
Limbic band, inferior, echocardiography of, 500
Line integral values, in x-ray computed tomography, 637
Linear array, in electronic beam steering, 356, 357, *357*, *358*
Linear magnetic field gradients, in magnetic resonance imaging, characteristics of, 744, 745, *745*
nuclear magnetic resonance projections in, 745, 746, *746*
production of, 744, 745
Linear systems theory, 331–334
Linear-array transducer, 357
Linearity, in digital angiography, 283, *283*, 284
Lipids, as myocardial fuel, 48
metabolism of, 44–46
Lipoma, ultrafast computed tomography of, 704
Lipomatous hypertrophy, echocardiography of, 528, 529, *529*
Localization techniques, definition of, 1273
Longitudinal magnetization, 738, *738*
definition of, 1273
steady-state, of flip angle, 756, *756*
Longitudinal relaxation, definition of, 1273
Longitudinal relaxation time, definition of, 1273
Lookup table, 77, 78, *78*, *79*
Low-contrast resolution, in computed tomography, 648, 649, 650(t), *651*
in fast computed tomography, 648, 649, 650(t), *651*, *652*
Lumen, of left anterior descending artery, diameter of, anterior wall motion effects of, 307, *307*
shapes of, 214
Lung(s), carcinoma of, staging of, ultrafast computed tomography in, 712, *712*, 713
congenital dysplasia of, pulmonary angiography in, 157–159
spindle cell sarcoma of, magnetic resonance imaging of, *944*
thallium-201 uptake by, 1051–1053, *1052*
Lung scan, radionuclide, before pulmonary angiography, 150
Lymphoma, extracardiac, echocardiography of, 520, *523*
metastatic, ultrafast computed tomography of, 404, *405*

M, definition of, 1273
precession of, 736, *736*, 739, *739*
M_0, 735, *735*
definition of, 1273
M_7, definition of, 1273
Macroautophagy, in protein synthesis, 52
Macroscopic magnetization vector, definition of, 1273
Magnetic dipole, definition of, 1273
Magnetic disk, digital, real-time, 285, 286
Magnetic field(s), around protons, 795, *796*
around unpaired electrons, 795, *796*
definition of, 1273
homogeneity of, 744
nucleus behavior in, 733, *733*, 734
Magnetic field gradient, definition of, 1273

Magnetic field gradient *(Continued)*
linear, in magnetic resonance imaging, characteristics of, 744, 745, *745*
nuclear magnetic resonance projections in, 745, 746, *746*
production of, 744, 745
Magnetic induction, definition of, 1273
Magnetic moment, 733
definition of, 1273
of nuclei, in magnetic resonance imaging, 842(t)
Magnetic resonance, definition of, 1273
phenomenology of, 759–761
Magnetic resonance angiography, 787, 881
Magnetic resonance imaging (MRI), artifacts in, blood flow, 785–787, 785(t)
engineering-related, 788, *791*
from metal, 788, *790*
local field inhomogeneity in, 788, *789*
motion, cardiac, 781–783, 781(t), *782*
prevention of, 791(t)
patient-related, 779–787, *781*
respiratory, 783, 783(t), 784
phase ghost, 786, *786*
prevention of, 791(t)
study of, 776
system-related, 787, 788, *788–791*
blood flow-related enhancement in, 785
cardiac, contrast agents for, 794–810, 794(t), 804(t)
cardiac triggering in, 781–783, 781(t), *782*, *783*
cine. See *Cine magnetic resonance imaging.*
definition of, 1274
echo planar, 783, 883, *883*
in cardiac quantitation, 824, *824*
field gradients in, magnetization of, 746, *746*, 747, *747*
flow phenomena in, 769–775
free induction decay in, 747
gradient moment nulling in, 784, 786, *786*, 787, *787*
high-speed, 783
high-velocity signal loss in, 785
image creation in, 776–779, *777*, 777(t)
data transfer in, 778, 779
scanning in, 777, 778, *779*, *780*
system tuning and preparation for, 777, *778*
image quality in, optimization of, 776–793
in anomalies of the great vessels, 892–894, *893*, *894*
in blood flow quantitation, 822–824, 822(t)
in cardiac quantitation, 811–827, *819–821*
in cardiomyopathy, 929–935
in congenital heart disease, 886–895
acyanotic, 887, 888
cyanotic, 887–892
in constrictive pericarditis, 943, 944
in dilated cardiomyopathy, 931, 932
in hypertrophic cardiomyopathy, 929–931, *930*, *931*
in infiltrative cardiomyopathy, 933, 934, *934*
in myocardial ischemia, 764–766, *764–767*, 764(t)
in early repair, 766, *767*
in late repair, 766
in reperfusion, 766, *766*
irreversible, 764–766, *765*
reversible, 764, *765*
in pericardial effusion, 941, 942
in pericardial thickening, 942
in restrictive cardiomyopathy, 933, 934, *934*
in systemic venous abnormalities, 879–881, *880–882*
in tissue characterization, 820–822
in valve stenosis, 903, *904–906*
Magnetic resonance imaging (MRI) *(Continued)*
in valvular disease, mechanisms of, 896, 897, *897*
in valvular regurgitancy, 898–903, *899–903*
linear magnetic field gradients in, 744–747
characteristics of, 744, 745, *745*
nuclear magnetic resonance projections in, 745, 746, *746*
production of, 744, 745
multislice imaging in, 754
of aorta, 867–876
of myocardial infarct, with hemorrhage, 766, *767*
of myocardial metabolism, in cardiomyopathy, 932, 933, *933*
of pericardium, gated, 938, 939, 939(t)
normal, 938, *938*, 939, 939(t)
of congenital anomalies, 940, 941
of neoplasms, 944, *944*, 945, *945*
postoperative, 944
phosphorus, of myocardial metabolism, in cardiomyopathy, 932, 933, *933*
principles of, 744–758
proton, in dilated cardiomyopathy, 1251
rapid imaging techniques in, 754–757, *755–757*
respiratory averaging in, 783, 783(t), *784*
respiratory triggering in, 783, 783(t), 784, *785*
retrospective gating in, 783
sedation in, 779–781
signal intensity in, GdDTPA in, 799, *801–803*, 801(t), *806*
in myocardial infarction, 913, 913(t), 914, *914–916*
in myocardium, in ischemic disease, 925, *925*
relation of, to contrast agent, 798, 799
slice selection in, 748, *748*, 749, *749*
sodium-23 in, 828–840, *833–837*
spatial presaturation in, 785, 786
spin-warp imaging in, concepts of, 750–752, *750*, *751*
practical aspects of, 752, *752*, 753, *753*
three-dimensional, in cardiac quantitation, 824, *824*
two-dimensional image formation in, 750–754
parameters for, 753, 754
Magnetic resonance sensitivity, of sodium-23, 831
Magnetic resonance spectra, of sodium-23, 830, *830*, 831
Magnetic resonance spectroscopy (MRS), carbon, 851–854, *854*, *855*
clinical uses of, 858, 859
definition of, 841–843, 842(t), *843*
deuterium, 858
fluorine, 858
in cardiac quantitation, 825, *825*
in vivo, data collection in, 844, 845
rationale for, 844
of cellular function, 841–863
of myocardial metabolism, 841–863
phosphorus. See *Phosphorus magnetic resonance spectroscopy.*
potassium, 856–858
proton, 854, *856*
sodium-23 in, 828–840. See also *Sodium magnetic resonance spectroscopy.*
surface coil for, 843, 844
Magnetic shielding, definition of, 1274
Magnetic susceptibility, definition of, 1274
Magnetic tape, 8-mm, in archival storage, in digital angiography, 286
nine-track, in archival storage, in digital angiography, 286
Magnetite, *807–809*
Magnetization, definition of, 1274
equilibrium, 735, *735*
longitudinal, 738, *738*
definition of, 1273
steady-state, of flip angle, 756, *756*
nonequilibrium, 736, *736*
of field gradients, in magnetic resonance imaging, 746, *746*, 747, *747*
off-resonance, 739, *739*
on-resonance, 738, *738*, 739, *739*
refocusing of, methods of, 747, *747*
resonance frequency of, 748
transverse, definition of, 1276
in magnetic resonance spectroscopy, 844
Magnetization transfer, 846, 847, *847*
Magnetization vector, macroscopic, definition of, 1273
Magnetogyric ratio, of nucleus, 733
Magnevist, 804, 805, 805(t)
Magnitude, definition of, 365
Malate dehydrogenase, in tricarboxylic acid cycle, 47
Malate-aspartate shuttle, in carbohydrate metabolism, 44, *45*
Malignancy, of pericardium, ultrafast computed tomography of, 709, *709*
Malrotation, of pulmonary artery, magnetic resonance imaging in, 876, *877*
Manganese chloride, in magnetic resonance imaging, 806
Manganese-containing contrast agents, in myocardial perfusion assessment, 824, *824*
Marfan's syndrome, aortic regurgitation in, 426, 427
left ventricular enlargement in, *102*
magnetic resonance imaging in, 867, *870*
Mask mode subtraction, 288, 298(t)
disadvantages of, 297–300
effects of, assessment of, 315, *317*
end-diastolic, 299, *299*
Mask operators, *81*, 82
Mass, of left ventricle, calculation of, 123, *123–125*, 124
echocardiography in, 380, 381, *381*
ultrafast computed tomography in, 672, *672*, 672(t)
normal values for, 134–139, 134(t)
of myocardium, estimation of, magnetic resonance imaging in, 817–819, *818*, *819*
of right ventricle, evaluation of, ultrafast computed tomography in, 677, *677*, 678
of ventricles, in congenital heart disease, ultrafast computed tomography of, 728
Mass(es), cardiac, transesophageal echocardiography in, *610*, 611
developmental, of pericardium, magnetic resonance imaging of, 940
echocardiographic evaluation of, 511–537
extracardiac, adjacent to heart, 520, *522*, *523*
intracardiac, assessment of, ultrafast computed tomography in, 703–713
cine magnetic resonance imaging of, 964, *964*, 965
ultrasonic tissue characterization in, 553
mediastinal, ultrafast computed tomography of, 712, *712*, 713
mimicking cardiac neoplasms, 528, 528(t), 529, *529–533*
MAST (motion artifact suppression technique), 786
Matrix size, in spatial resolution, *75*, 76
Mature collaterals, 17, *17*, 18
Maximal coronary dilators, 15, 16
Maximal hyperemic response, in coronary flow reserve angiography, 246

Maximal intensity image, 247, 248, *248*
MB-CK analysis, in acute myocardial infarct sizing, *1081*, *1082*
McN-A-343, 1264
Md-76, *164*, 165
  properties of, 166, 167(t)
Mean diastolic orifice area, 408
Mean gradient, in aortic stenosis, Doppler echocardiography in, with catheterization, 421, *423*
Mean mitral annular area, 408, *409*
Mean systolic gradient (MSG), 62, 63, *63*
Mean transit time, calculation of, contrast echocardiography in, 563–565, *564*
    radionuclide angiocardiography in, 1016
Mediastinitis, fibrosing, cine magnetic resonance imaging in, 955, *956*
Mediastinum, masses of, ultrafast computed tomography of, 712, *712*, 713
  tumors of, echocardiography of, 520, *522*, *523*
Medication, during coronary angiography, 190
Megahertz, definition of, 1274
Meglumine, 165
  in myocardial contrast echocardiography, 257
Melanoma, metastatic, ultrafast computed tomography of, 404
Membranous ventricular septum, 479, *480*, *481*
Memory, image, 285
  solid-state, in on-line image storage, in digital angiography, 285
Meridional wall stress, in dilated cardiomyopathy, magnetic resonance imaging of, 932
Mesothelioma, 512
  malignant, of pericardium, ultrafast computed tomography of, 709, *709*
Metabolic equivalents (METS), relationship of, to ejection fraction, in exercise, 1033, *1033*
    to end-diastolic volume, in exercise, 1033, *1033*
Metabolic imaging, with single-photon-emitting tracers, 1085–1096
Metabolism, as indicator, of myocardial tissue viability, 1219–1237
  carbohydrate. See *Carbohydrate metabolism.*
  disturbances of, after reperfusion, 50
  fatty acid, 44–46, *45*
    beta-oxidation in, 46, *47*
    C-11–labeled palmitate in, in myocardial ischemia, 50, 1191–1195, *1192–1195*, 1198, 1199, *1199*, *1200*
    free, 1244–1246, *1246*
    in ischemia, in myocardial infarction, 1203–1207, *1205–1210*
    myocardial, iodo fatty acid analogs in, 1086, 1087(t)
  glucose, 1244–1246, *1246*
    catecholamines in, 49
    in myocardial infarction, 1209–1214, *1212*
    in myocardial ischemia, 49
      fluorine-18 2–fluoro 2–deoxyglucose in, 1197, *1197*, 1198
  glycogen, 40–42, *41*
    carbon magnetic resonance spectroscopy of, 853
  in cardiomyopathy, 1244–1255
    abnormalities of, 1246
  in hypertrophic cardiomyopathy, 1251
    positron emission tomography of, 1251, 1252, *1252*
  in vivo, effect of, on relaxation dispersion, 797, *797*
  ketone, 46, *48*
  lactate, 44, 1244–1246, *1246*
Metabolism *(Continued)*
  lipid, 44–46
  myocardial. See *Myocardial metabolism.*
  skeletal muscle, in heart disease, spectroscopy of, 972–974, *973*, *974*
  sodium, abnormal, 856
  oxidative, in myocardial infarction, 1207–1209, *1211*
    in myocardial ischemia, carbon-11 acetate in, 1195–1197, *1196*, *1197*
  pyruvate, 42
  tracers of, in myocardial ischemia, 1198–1203
Metabolites, myocardial, quantification of, 843
Metaiodobenzylguanidine (MIBG), chemical structure for, *1136*
  myocardial uptake of, 1137, 1138
    after myocardial infarction, 1136, 1137
  neuronal localization of, experimental evidence for, 1135, 1136, *1137*
  radiolabeled, in sympathetic nerve assessment, 1135, *1136*
Metaraminol, fluorine-18–labeled, 1152
Metastasis(es), cardiac, echocardiography of, 519, 519(t), 520, *520*, *521*
  to pericardium, magnetic resonance imaging of, 944, *944*, 945, *945*
  ultrafast computed tomography of, 704, 705
Methionyl-tRNA, in protein synthesis, 50–52, *51*
Methylglucamine, 165
β-methyl-heptadecanoic acid, 1090
Methylprednisolone, for anaphylactoid reactions, 175, 176
Methysergide toxicity, and tricuspid stenosis, 436
Metrizamide, *164*, 165
  intracoronary injection of, effects of, *171*
METS (metabolic equivalents), relationship of, to ejection fraction, in exercise, 1033, *1033*
    to end-diastolic volume, in exercise, 1033, *1033*
MIBG. See *Metaiodobenzylguanidine (MIBG).*
Michaelis-Menten equation, 846
Microautophagy, in protein synthesis, 52
Microbubbles, in contrast echocardiography, 557, 558
    limitations of, 558
  in coronary artery disease diagnosis, 602
Microscopy, acoustic, 544
Microspheres, albumin, positron-labeled, 1142, *1142*
  radiolabeled, in transient ischemia, 31
Minimal diameter stenosis, regression analysis of, 321, *322*
Minimal luminal cross-sectional area, after percutaneous transluminal coronary angioplasty, with stent implantation, 266, *266*
  relationship of, to coronary flow reserve, 249, *249*, 250, 250(t)
Minimal stenosis diameter, measurement of, variability in, 315, 318(t)
Minimum coronary lumen diameter, correlation of, with left ventricular functional impairment, 306–308, *306*, *307*
Misonidazole, fluorine-18, 1153
Misregistration artifacts, in mask mode subtraction, 297, 298, *298*
Mitochondria, acyl coenzyme A transport to, 45, 46, *46*
Mitochondrial inclusions, of damaged myocardial infarct cells, 1074–1077, *1076–1078*
Mitral annular area, mean, 408, *409*
Mitral annulus, calcification of, and mitral regurgitation, 435
Mitral annulus *(Continued)*
  diameter of, measurement of, in mitral regurgitation, 436
Mitral balloon valvuloplasty, 431, 441
Mitral commissurotomy, open, for mitral stenosis, intraoperative echocardiography during, 624
Mitral flow velocity, in constrictive pericarditis, 473, *474*, *475*
Mitral insufficiency, equilibrium radionuclide angiography in, 1040
Mitral orifice area, measurement of, in mitral stenosis, 430, 431, *431*
Mitral prolapse, left ventricular filling velocity in, *412*
Mitral regurgitation, after myocardial infarction, *600*
  causes of, 433–435
  cine magnetic resonance imaging in, 951, *952*, 955–957, *957*
  contrast ventriculography in, 110, *114*
  echocardiography in, 433–436, *434*, *435*
    Doppler, 435, 436
    in decision-making, 436
    M-mode, 433, *433*
    two-dimensional, 433, *434*
  evaluation of, quantitative, 436
    semiquantitative, 435, 436
  in dilated cardiomyopathy, echocardiography of, 455
  in hypertrophic cardiomyopathy, echocardiography of, 453
  left atrial pressure in, 412, *413*
  left ventricle in, contours of, *112*
    filling velocity in, *412*
    pressure-volume curve in, *140*
    systolic pressure in, 403, *405*
  magnetic resonance imaging in, 898, *901*, *902*
  radionuclide angiocardiography in, 1021
  regurgitant jet in, color flow mapping of, 622, 622(t)
  rheumatic, 435
  roentgenographic evaluation of, 104, 105
  severity of, color flow imaging of, 435
    evaluation of, 67, 69
    pulsed-wave mapping of, 435
  signal void in, 955, *957*
  valve repair for, intraoperative echocardiography during, 622, 622(t), 623
      postpump, 623, *623*
Mitral stenosis, causes of, 430
  cine magnetic resonance imaging in, 962
  color flow imaging in, 431
  congenital, 430
  continuity equation in, 433
  contrast ventriculography in, 110
  echocardiography in, 430–433, *431*
    Doppler, 431–433, *432*
      continuous-wave, 431, *432*
    in decision-making, 433
    transesophageal, 430, 431
    two-dimensional, 430, 431
  left atrium enlargement in, 99, *101*
  left ventricular pressure-volume curve in, *140*
  open mitral commissurotomy for, intraoperative echocardiography during, 624
  pulmonary venous hypertension in, 95, *98*
  radionuclide angiocardiography in, 1021
  rheumatic, 430, *431*
  right ventricular pressure in, assessment of, 433
  roentgenographic evaluation of, 104
  severity of, clinical evaluation of, 64
  ultrafast computed tomography in, 679, *679*
Mitral stroke volume, in mitral regurgitation, 436

Mitral valve, area of, estimation of, 431, *432*
pressure half-time in, 431
overestimation of, *432*, 433
artificial, left atrial thrombi with, echocardiography of, 526, *526*
flail leaflet of, in mitral regurgitation, 433, 434
function of, in dilated cardiomyopathy, echocardiography of, 454–456
parachute, 430
premature closure of, in aortic regurgitation, 68
Mitral valve prolapse, and mitral regurgitation, 433, *434*
contrast ventriculography in, 110, *115*
M-mode display, 356
M-mode echocardiography, during exercise, 575
in aortic regurgitation, 427, *427*
in cardiac tamponade, 464–470, *466–471*
in constrictive pericarditis, 470, *472*, *473*
in mitral regurgitation, 433, *433*
in pericardial effusion, 460, *461*
in tricuspid regurgitation, 438
of left ventricular mass, 380, 381, *381*
of right ventricular function, 392
Mn-DPDP, 806
Mobin-Uddin filter, for pulmonary embolism, 155
Moderator band, echocardiography of, 511, *511*
Modified Bernoulli equation, in aortic stenosis, 421
in mitral regurgitation, 435
in mitral stenosis, 431
Modulus blipped echo-planar imaging, 757, *757*
Moiré pattern, 361, *361*
of artifacts, 76, *77*
Moment, magnetic, 733
definition of, 1273
of nuclei, in magnetic resonance imaging, 842(t)
Momentum, angular, definition of, 1271
Monitoring, in positron emission tomography, of myocardial blood flow, 1171
Monoclonal antibody imaging, 1110–1120
Monoclonal antimyosin, preparation of, 1110, 1111, *1111*
Motion, cardiac, abnormalities of, in pericardial effusion, 464, *465*
endocardial, analysis of, 383, *383*
segmental, evaluation of, ultrafast computed tomography in, 673, *674*
perception of, 88, *89*
periodic, 349, 350, *350*
translational, correction for, 124, *127*
Motion artifact suppression technique (MAST), 786
Motion artifacts, patient-related, in magnetic resonance imaging, 779–787, *781*
Movie mode, in ultrafast computed tomography, of atrial myxomas, 704
of intracardiac thrombi, 706
MPR. See *Myocardial perfusion reserve (MPR).*
MQNB, C-11–labeled, 1152
MRI. See *Magnetic resonance imaging (MRI).*
MRS. See *Magnetic resonance spectroscopy (MRS).*
MSG (mean systolic gradient), 62, 63, *63*
Multicrystal gamma camera, in radionuclide angiocardiography, *1009*
in radionuclide imaging, 980, 981
Multiple echo imaging, definition of, 1274
Multiple quantum filter technique, in intracellular vs. extracellular sodium-23 differentiation, 832, 833
Multiple quantum spectroscopy, 858
Multiple slice imaging, definition of, 1274
Multiple-gated single-photon emission computed tomography, 988, *988*
Multipulse nuclear magnetic resonance, 740–743
inversion-recovery sequence in, 740, *740*, 741, *741*
spin-echo sequence in, 741–743, *741*, *742*
Multislice spin echo, in cardiac quantitation, 812, *813*
multiphase, in cardiac quantitation, 812, *814*
Multiwire gamma camera, in radionuclide imaging, 981, *981*
Muscarinic acetylcholine receptors, characterization of, positron emission tomography in, 1264–1266, *1265*
Muscarinic cholinergic receptors, distribution of, 1264, 1265
subtypes of, 1264, 1265
Muscle(s), papillary, calcified, echocardiography of, 529, *533*
dysfunction of, and mitral regurgitation, 434
rupture of, after myocardial infarction, 599, *599*
vs. thrombi, on ultrafast computed tomography, 705
skeletal, metabolism of, in heart disease, spectroscopy of, 972–974, *973*, *974*
ventricular, fibers of, in myocardial acoustics, 544
Muscular dystrophy, Duchenne, cardiomyopathy with, 1252
positron emission tomography in, 1252, *1253*
thallium-201 scintigraphy in, 1066, 1066(t)
Muscular septum, 479
Muscular subaortic stenosis, in hypertrophic cardiomyopathy, assessment of, 450, 451, *451*, *452*
Mxy, definition of, 1273
Myocardial contrast echocardiography, in coronary flow reserve assessment, 256, 257
Myocardial contusion, ultrasonic tissue characterization in, 553
Myocardial densitometry, in coronary flow reserve measurement, 246
Myocardial fatty acids, metabolism of, iodo fatty acid analogs in, 1086, 1087(t)
Myocardial function, response of, to myocardial ischemia, 31
segmental, evaluation of, cine magnetic resonance imaging in, 963, *963*
Myocardial hibernation, in myocardial ischemia, 1234
Myocardial imaging, with radioiodinated fatty acids, history of, 1085, 1086
Myocardial infarct, acute, anatomy of, 1218
electrocardiographic changes in, 1217, 1218
metabolic characterization of, 1214–1217, *1215–1217*
sizing of, MB-CK analysis in, *1081*, *1082*
Tc-99m-PPi in, 1080–1083, *1081*
after temporary coronary artery occlusion, 1083
Tc-99m-PPi localization in, 1079, *1079*, *1080*
cells damaged by, mitochondrial inclusions in, 1074–1077, *1076–1078*
compensatory hyperfunction in, 33
GdDTPA in, in signal intensity, 799, *803*
in right ventricular function, 32, 33
infarct expansion in, 33
reactive hypertrophy in, 33
Myocardial infarct *(Continued)*
size of, estimation of, nuclear magnetic resonance in, 919–923, *920*, 921(t), *922*, *923*
with paramagnetic contrast agents, 921–923, 921(t), *922*, *923*
wall motion abnormalities in, 32
with hemorrhage, magnetic resonance imaging of, 766, *767*
Myocardial infarction, acute, detection of, nuclear magnetic resonance in, 913–918, *913–917*, 913(t), 917(t), 918(t)
left ventricular function in, 135–137, *137*
as predictor of survival, 138
magnetic resonance imaging in, signal intensity in, 913, 913(t), 914, *914–916*
substrate metabolism in, 1203–1219
antimyosin imaging in, 1114, *1114–1116*, 1115
complications of, *598–602*, 599–602
coronary angiography and, 186, 186(t)
detection of, Tc-99m-PPi in, 1080, *1081–1083*
echocardiography in, 594–604
equilibrium radionuclide angiography after, 1038, *1038*, 1039
functional recovery after, time course of, 137, 138
gamma imaging in, 1112, *1112*, 1113, *1113*
history of, as coronary angiography indication, 184
hyperkinesis during, 137, *137*
inferoposterior, acute, right ventricular dysfunction in, 397
iodo fatty acid analogs in, 1091–1093, *1091*, *1092*
left ventricular aneurysm after, 110, *116*
localization of, C-11–labeled palmitate in, 1235–1237, *1236*
positron emission tomography in, 1235–1237, *1236*
metabolic abnormalities in, 1231–1237
metaiodobenzylguanidine uptake after, 1136, 1137
myocardial relaxation times after, 914–918, *917*, 917–919(t)
patient evaluation after, exercise echocardiography in, 588, *588*, 589(t)
positron emission tomography in, 1183–1185, *1184–1186*
prognosis after, echocardiography in, 598, *598*, 599
systolic function after, assessment of, two-dimensional echocardiography in, 382
thallium-201 scintigraphy after, 1063, 1064, *1064*
therapeutic intervention for, evaluation of, 138
tissue viability after, identification of, 1222, 1223
ultrasonic backscatter in, 548, *549*, *550*
Myocardial ischemia, acute, detection of, nuclear magnetic resonance in, 911–913
with paramagnetic contrast agents, 911–913, *912*, *913*
myocardial metabolism in, 1191–1203
tissue property changes in, 911
chronic, metabolic abnormalities in, 1231–1237
clinical studies of, nuclear magnetic resonance imaging in, 925, *925*, 926, *926*, 926(t)
contrast echocardiography in, 567, 568
early repair of, magnetic resonance imaging in, 766, *767*
echocardiography in, 594–604

Myocardial ischemia *(Continued)*
experimental, cellular alterations in, 1074, *1076*
irreversible, 764–766, *765*
late repair of, 766
magnetic resonance imaging in, 764–766, *764–767*, 764(t)
myocardial function in, 31
myocardial hibernation in, 1234
myocyte ultrastructure in, 764, *765*, *766*
phosphorus magnetic resonance spectroscopy in, 848
reperfusion in, 766, *766*
reversible, 764, *765*
spectroscopy in, 970, *971*, *972*
Myocardial mass, estimation of, magnetic resonance imaging in, 817–819, *818*, *819*
Myocardial metabolism, 39–55
abnormalities of, in chronic ischemia, 1231–1237
after myocardial infarction, effect on, of coronary thrombolysis, 1218, 1219, *1220*, *1221*
of revascularization, 1218, 1219, *1220*, *1221*
and cardiac work, phosphorus magnetic resonance spectroscopy of, 846
catecholamines in, 49
imaging of, in clinical decision making, 1239, 1240
in clinical practice, 1237–1240
indications for, 1237, *1237*, 1238
patient care during, 1238, 1239
standardization of, 1239
in cardiomyopathy, magnetic resonance imaging of, 932, 933, *933*
in diabetes, 49
in fasting, 49
in hypoperfused myocardium, 1234, 1235
in ischemia, 49, 50
acute, 1191–1203
in reperfusion, 50
in vivo study of, phosphorus magnetic resonance spectroscopy in, 849–851, *850–854*
increased exercise in, 49
insulin in, 49
magnetic resonance spectroscopy of, 841–863
of glucose, measurement of, positron emission tomography in, 1163, *1163*, 1164, *1164*
of substrate, in ischemic heart disease, evaluation of, 1190–1243
positron-emitting tracers of, 1141(t), 1145–1152, *1145–1152*
regulators of, phosphorus magnetic resonance spectroscopy of, 845, 846
substrate of, evaluation of, 1151, 1152
vs. other diagnostic tests, in tissue viability determination, 1225–1231, *1226–1228*
Myocardial metabolites, quantification of, methods of, 843
Myocardial perfusion, absolute, measurement of, positron emission tomography in, 1179–1182, *1180–1182*
flow-dependent extraction in, 1180, *1180*
geometric limitations of, 1180
models for, 1180–1182, *1181*, *1182*
alteration of, coronary artery anomalies in, 197, 198
coronary anomalies not altering, 198, 199
defects of, in coronary artery disease, quantification of, 994, *995*
sizing of, 994
hypertrophy effect on, 19, *19*
imaging of, technetium-99m agents in, 1097–1109
Myocardial perfusion *(Continued)*
thallium-201 in, 1047–1073
measurement of, computed tomography in, with intravenous contrast agents, 692–695, *693–695*
fast computed tomography in, 688–702
beam hardening in, 696–698, *696–698*
imaging and reconstruction artifacts in, 695–698, *696–698*
photon scatter in, 696–698, *696–698*
theoretical considerations in, 689–692
indicator dilution methods of, algorithm for, 691, *691*, 692
application of, to computed tomography, 689–691, *690*, *692*
historical aspects of, 689
nonionic contrast agents in, 690, *690*
intraoperative echocardiography in, 630
nonuniformity of, assessment of, fast computed tomography in, 700
quantification of, contrast echocardiography in, 560–565
magnetic resonance imaging in, 823, 824, *824*
scintigraphy in, 989–996
planar methods of, 989–992, *989–991*
tomographic methods of, 992–995, *992*, *993*, *995*
studies of, contrast echocardiography in, 565–568, *566*, *567*
advantages of, 568
disadvantages of, 568
three-dimensional single-photon emission computed tomography of, 995, 996
Myocardial perfusion reserve (MPR), calculation of, positron emission tomography in, 1173, *1174*
percutaneous transluminal coronary angioplasty effect on, 1185, *1186*
vs. coronary flow reserve, 1176, 1176(t)
vs. stenosis flow reserve, 1179, *1179*
Myocardial revascularization, assessment of, thallium-201 scintigraphy in, 1064, *1065*
radionuclide angiocardiography in, 1024
Myocardial substrate interactions, 48–50
Myocardial tagging, magnetic resonance imaging in, 820, *820*
Myocarditis, antimyosin imaging in, 1116, 1117, *1117*, *1118*
gamma imaging in, 1114
thallium-201 scintigraphy in, 1066, 1066(t)
Myocardium, acoustic properties of, biologic determinants of, 543–545
blood flow in. See *Blood flow, myocardial.*
cells of, damaged, calcium deposition in, 1077–1079, *1078*
Tc-99m-PPi deposition in, 1077–1079, *1078*
contrast input function in, kinetics of, in fast computed tomography, 699, 700, *700*
damaged, Tc-99m-PPi concentration in, 1079, *1079*
diseased, iodo fatty acid analog clearance in, 1089(t)
energetics of, biochemistry of, 1244–1246, *1246*
energy production in, 39, *40*
fuel selection by, 48
heterogeneity of, 12, *13*
hibernating, right ventricular function in, 32
hypoperfused, blood flow and metabolism in, 1234, 1235
in ischemic disease, clinical studies of, nuclear magnetic resonance imaging in, 925, *925*, 926, *926*, 926(t)
ligand access to, 1258, 1259
Myocardium *(Continued)*
ligand interaction within, 1259
metaiodobenzylguanidine uptake in, 1137, 1138
normal, iodo fatty acid analog clearance in, 1089(t)
spectroscopy in, 969, *969*, 970, *970*
oxygen consumption in, 8, 9
performance of, after selective intracoronary injection, of angiographic contrast agents, 170, 171, *171*, *172*
radiolabel in, fractional distribution of, 1088, *1088*
reperfusion of, ultrasonic tissue characterization in, 546–548, *547*, *548*
respiratory control in, 47, 48
scatterers of, geometric attributes of, 544, *544*
stunned, 382, 597, 598
in right ventricular function, 31, 32
wall motion abnormalities in, 32
viability of, after infarction, identification of, 1222, 1223
assessment of, 135
Myocytes, in scattering, 545
ultrastructure of, in myocardial ischemia, 764, *765*, *766*
Myxoma(s), of atrium, left, echocardiography of, 512–516, *514*, *515*
right, echocardiography of, 516, 517, *517*, *518*
ultrafast computed tomography of, 703, 704, *704*
imaging sequences in, 704
transesophageal echocardiography in, *610*
ultrasonic tissue characterization in, 553

Native collaterals, 16, 17, *17*
Nearest-neighbor interpolation, 81
Necrosis, medial, cystic, of aorta, cine magnetic resonance imaging of, 954, *954*
Neighborhood, of pixels, 82
Neighborhood operations, 288, 289(t)
Nembutal, for sedation, in magnetic resonance imaging, 781
Neo-iopax, 163, *164*
Neoplasm(s), of pericardium, echocardiography of, 475
magnetic resonance imaging of, 944, *944*, 945, *945*
pulmonary angiography of, 157, *159*
Nephroma, metastatic, echocardiography of, 520, *521*
Nephropathy, contrast, 188
Nephrotoxicity, of contrast agents, for coronary angiography, 188
Nerve(s), activation of, effects of, on coronary circulation, 11
parasympathetic, in myocardial perfusion, 11
sympathetic, in myocardial perfusion, 10, 11
scintigraphic assessment of, 1135–1138, *1136*, *1137*
Neural activation, in ventricular function evaluation, 27, 27(t)
Neurons, cardiac, imaging of, 1135–1139
metaiodobenzylguanidine localization to, 1135, 1136, *1137*
Newtonian fluid, 367
NEX, definition of, 1274
N(H), definition of, 1274
Nicotinamide-adenine dinucleotide, in myocardial metabolism, 39, *40*
Nicotinic acid, for hyperlipidemia, 267, 268, 268(t)

Nifedipine, preangiographic administration of, 233, *233*
Nitrate, preangiographic administration of, 232, 233
Nitrogen-13, amino acid labeled with, 1152
Nitrogen-13 ammonia, *1142*, 1143, *1143*
  characteristics of, 1170(t)
  in myocardial blood flow evaluation, 1161, 1162, 1170
  in myocardial infarction detection, 1183
Nitroglycerin, effect of, on coronary flow reserve, 14
    on left atrial pressure, 412, *413*
  in coronary angiography, 190
  preangiographic administration of, 233
N-methyl quinuclidinyl benzylate, C-11–labeled, 1265, *1265*
N-methylscopolamine, 1264, 1265
NOE (nuclear Overhauser effect), 853
No-frequency-wrap, 788
Noise, definition of, 1274
  image, in digital cardiac angiography, 282, 283
  in computed tomography, 649, 653(t)
  in fast computed tomography, 649, 653(t)
Noncoronary heart disease, thallium-201 scintigraphy in, 1066, 1066(t), 1067
Nonequilibrium magnetization, 736, *736*
Non-exercise stress echocardiography, 589–591, 590(t)
Nonproton nuclei, in reperfused infarction imaging, 919
Nonselective pulse, 740
No-phase-wrap, 788
Norepinephrine, chemical structure for, *1135*
NSA, definition of, 1274
Nuclear magnetic resonance (NMR), definition of, 1274
  in detection, of acute myocardial infarction, 913–918, *913–917*, 913(t), 917(t), 918(t)
    of myocardial infarct size, 919–923, *920*, 921(t), *922*, *923*
    of reperfused infarction, 918, 919, 919(t)
  in ischemic heart disease, 911–928
    in clinical studies, 925, *925*, 926, *926*, 926(t)
    in left ventricular function assessment, 923–925, *923*, *924*
  in pericardial disease, 936–947
  in valvular disease, 896–910
  multipulse, 740–743
    inversion-recovery sequence in, 740, *740*, 741, *741*
    spin-echo sequence in, 741–743, *741*, *742*
  of great vessels, 864–885
  principles of, 732–743
  pulse Fourier transform, 735–740
    relaxation in, 737, 738, *738*
    rotating-frame concept in, 738–740, *738*, *739*
    signal averaging in, 737
    signal-to-noise ratio in, 737
    vectors in, 735, *735*, 736, *736*
  spectrum of, 734, 735, *735*
    amplitude of, 746
Nuclear magnetic resonance projections, in magnetic resonance imaging, 745, 746, *746*
Nuclear magnetic resonance spectroscopy, clinical applications of, 967–976
Nuclear Overhauser effect (NOE), 853
Nuclear relaxation, stimulated, requirements for, 761, 761(t)
Nuclear spin, 732, 733, 733(t)
  definition of, 1274
Nuclear spin quantum number, definition of, 1274
Nuclear stethoscope, 981
Nucleus(i), behavior of, in magnetic field, 733, *733*, 734
  in nuclear magnetic resonance, characteristics of, 842(t)
  magnetogyric ratio of, 733
  nonproton, in reperfused infarction imaging, 919
Nutation, definition of, 1274
Nyquist frequency, 753, 754
Nyquist sampling theorem, 76, 283, 370, 753

Obliterative cardiomyopathy, definition of, 449
  echocardiography in, 458
Occult constrictive pericarditis, 943
Off-resonance magnetization, 739, *739*
Oleic acid, 1085
Oligemia, pulmonary, magnetic resonance imaging in, 888–892, *890*, *891*
Omnipaque, *164*
  properties of, 166, 167(t)
O-mode scanning, 359
On-line digital cardiac systems, in quantitative coronary angiography, 220, 221, 221(t)
On-line image storage, in digital angiography, 285, 285(t), 286
    real-time digital magnetic disk in, 285, 286
    solid-state memory in, 285
On-resonance magnetization, 738, *738*, 739, *739*
Operating systems, for quantitative coronary angiography, 222, 222(t)
Optiray, *164*
  properties of, 166, 167(t)
Orientation, definition of, 1274
  in magnetic resonance imaging, in cardiac quantitation, 815, *815*
  of magnetic moment, 733
  parallel, 733
Orthogonal phased array, in electronic beam steering, 359, *359*
Orthogonality, triple, 322, *323*
Orthophosphate, in myocardial metabolism, 41
Osteogenic sarcoma, of sternum, magnetic resonance imaging of, *945*
Ostia, multiple, of coronary arteries, 199
Ostium primum atrial septal defect, 483, *487*
  magnetic resonance imaging of, 888, *889*
Ostium secundum atrial septal defect, *482*, 483
  magnetic resonance imaging of, 888, *888*, *889*
Ouabain, cardiac effects of, sodium magnetic resonance spectroscopy of, 857
Outlet septum, 479
Out-of-plane presaturation, 865
Outpatient cardiac catheterization, 206, 207
Output, cardiac. See *Cardiac output.*
Oxaloacetate, in myocardial metabolism, 42
Oxidation, beta, 1244–1246, *1246*
3-Oxoacid-CoA transferase, in lipid metabolism, 46, *48*
3-Oxoacyl-CoA thiolase, in lipid metabolism, 46, *47*
2-Oxoglutarate dehydrogenase, in tricarboxylic acid cycle, 47
Oxygen, consumption of, by myocardium, factors in, 8, 9
  metabolism of, carbon-11 acetate in, in myocardial ischemia, 1195–1197, *1196*, *1197*, 1199, 1200
    in myocardial infarction, 1207–1209, *1211*
Oxygen-15–labeled water, 1143
  characteristics of, 1170(t)
Oxygen-15–labeled water *(Continued)*
  in myocardial blood flow evaluation, 1162, *1162*, 1163, 1170

P-297, intracoronary injection of, effects of, *171*
Pacing, atrial, digital subtraction angiography with, 304–306, *305*
    effects of, 304, *305*
    in non-exercise stress echocardiography, 589
PACS (Picture Archiving and Communications Systems), 660
Pain, chest, coronary angiography in, 184
    diagnosis of, equilibrium radionuclide angiography in, 1032–1034, 1032(t), *1033*
    prognosis for, equilibrium radionuclide angiography in, 1035–1037, *1036–1038*
Palmitate, C-11–labeled. See *C-11–labeled palmitate.*
Palmitic acid, 1085
Papaverine, in coronary flow reserve measurement, 246
  in maximal coronary dilation, 15
  in myocardial contrast echocardiography, 257
  intracoronary, for maximal hyperemia, 338, *339*
Papillary fibroelastoma, echocardiography of, 516, *516*
Papillary muscle, calcified, echocardiography of, 529, *533*
  dysfunction of, and mitral regurgitation, 434
  rupture of, after myocardial infarction, 599, *599*
  vs. thrombi, on ultrafast computed tomography, 705
Parachute mitral valve, 430
"Paradoxic enhancement," 760
Paradoxic septal motion, in right ventricular infarction, 396, 397
Parallel orientation, 733
Parallel-beam geometry, 637, *637*
Paramagnetic, definition of, 1274
Paramagnetic contrast agents, blood pool, 805, 806, *806*
  cellular, 806, 807
  chelation in, 795, 796, *796*
  dechelation in, 796, 797, *797*
  extracellular, 804, *804*, 804(t), 805, *805*, 805(t)
  in myocardial perfusion assessment, 823
  in nuclear magnetic resonance imaging, in acute myocardial ischemia, 911–913, *912*, *913*
    in infarct size estimation, 921–923, 921(t), *922*, *923*
  in proton relaxation, *795*
  spin-echo pulse sequence interaction with, 799–808, *800–809*
Paramagnetic relaxing agents, 794–797, *795–797*
Paramagnetic shift reagents, in intracellular vs extracellular sodium-23 differentiation, 832
Parametric flow ratio images, *337*
Parametric imaging, 299, *299*
Parasympathetic nerves, in myocardial perfusion, 11
Paravalvular regurgitant leaks, after endocarditis, transesophageal echocardiography of, 611
Partial ileal bypass (PIB), for hyperlipidemia, 268, 268(t)

Partial saturation, definition of, 1274
Partial volume effect, in positron emission tomography, 1157, *1157*, *1158*
in ventricular volume measurement, 815, 816
Patency, of bypass graft. See *Bypass graft(s), patency of.*
Patent ductus arteriosus, *96*
blood flow in, patterns of, *484*, 485, *485*, 486
pulmonary, 489
systemic, 489
color flow imaging in, 486
echocardiography in, Doppler, 483–486, *484–486*
continuous-wave, *484*, 485, *485*
two-dimensional, 483, *484*
magnetic resonance imaging in, 876, *876*, 877, 894
Patient(s), asymptomatic, coronary artery disease in, positron emission tomography of, 1179
thallium-201 scintigraphy in, 1057, 1058, *1059*
care of, during myocardial metabolism imaging, 1238, 1239
evaluation of, after myocardial infarction, exercise echocardiography in, 588, *588*, 589(t)
before catheterization, 189
intensive care unit, transesophageal echocardiography in, 612
preparation of, for coronary angiography, 189, 190
unstable, coronary angiography in, 193
PCr. See *Phosphocreatine (PCr).*
Peak ejection velocity, during exercise, in ischemic heart disease, 586, *586*, 587, *587*
Peak instantaneous gradient, 62, *63*
Peak mitral regurgitant velocity, in mitral regurgitation, 435
Peak-to-peak gradient, 62, *63*
Pectus excavatum, echocardiography in, 529, *531*
Penetration, in ultrasonic tissue characterization, 539
Penn convention, 380, *381*
Pentobarbital, for sedation, in magnetic resonance imaging, 781
Pentose phosphate pathway, 40, *41*
Peptide chain initiation, in protein synthesis, 50–52, *51*
Peptides, elongation of, in protein synthesis, 52
termination of, in protein synthesis, 52
Percent area stenosis, accuracy of, 237
densitometric assessment of, 229
in reactive hyperemia, 318, *319*
measured vs. actual, linear regression analysis of, 315, *315*, *316*
Percent diameter narrowing, vs stenosis flow reserve, 1175, *1175*
Percent diameter stenosis, *202*, 203, *203*
coronary blood flow in, 216, *216*
in reactive hyperemia, 318, *319*, 339, *340*
in restenosis, after percutaneous transluminal coronary angioplasty, 260, *260–262*
interpolated, standard deviations in, 242(t)
limited value of, 215
measured vs. actual, linear regression analysis of, 315, *315*, *316*
measurement of, 218, *219*, 307
in quantitative coronary angiography, 225–227, *226*
regression analysis of, 321, *321*
visual interpretation of, interobserver variability in, 213
Perception, in heart disease evaluation, 90, 91
Perception *(Continued)*
of motion, 88, *89*
Perceptual aspects, of cardiac imaging, 87–92
Perceptual errors, strategies for, 89, 90
Percutaneous transluminal coronary angioplasty (PTCA), contrast echocardiography during, 568
coronary flow reserve after, 255, *255*
digital angiography vs videodensitometry in, 324
Doppler systolic ejection velocity during, 407
equilibrium radionuclide angiography after, 1038
functional result of, immediate, 251, *252*, *253*
long-term, 251, *254*
myocardial perfusion reserve after, 1185, *1186*
restenosis after, percent diameter stenosis in, 260, *260–262*
thallium-201 scintigraphy with, 1064, *1065*
with stent implantation, minimal luminal cross-sectional area after, 266, *266*
Percutaneous valvuloplasty, transesophageal echocardiography in, 612
Perfusion, absolute, vs tracer uptake, 1173
heterogeneity of, to myocardium, 12, *13*
myocardial. See *Myocardial perfusion.*
tissue, demonstration of, superparamagnetic agents for, 807, *807–809*, 808
transmural, regulation of, 11, 12, *12*, *13*
Perfusion pressure, coronary, distal, in stenosis identification, 250, 251(t)
relation of, to coronary blood flow, 244
Pericardial effusion, cardiac motion abnormalities in, 464, *465*
diagnosis of, 460, *461–463*, 941, 942
differential, 464, *465*
echocardiography in, 460–464, *461–465*
M-mode, 460, *461*
two-dimensional, 460, *463*
etiology of, 941(t)
fluid in, localization of, 460–463, *462*, *463*
quantitation of, 463, *464*
in restrictive cardiomyopathy, echocardiography of, 458
postoperative, 461, *463*
roentgenographic evaluation of, 106
second echo magnetic resonance signal intensity in, 942(t)
spin-echo imaging of, *903*
ultrafast computed tomography of, 708, *708*, *709*
with cardiac tamponade, 708, *709*
postoperative, 466–468, *468*
Pericardiocentesis, echocardiography during, in cardiac tamponade, 470, *471*
Pericarditis, constrictive. See *Constrictive pericarditis.*
echocardiography in, 475
effusive-constrictive, 475, 943
post-myocardial-infarction, 942, 943, *943*
Pericardium, absence of, congenital, ultrafast computed tomography in, 709
echocardiography in, 476
magnetic resonance imaging in, 940
anatomy of, 707, 708, *708*, 937
calcification of, roentgenographic evaluation of, 106, *106*
congenital anomalies of, magnetic resonance imaging in, 940, 941
cysts of, echocardiography of, 476
magnetic resonance imaging of, 940
ultrafast computed tomography of, 709, *710*
developmental masses of, magnetic resonance imaging of, 940
Pericardium *(Continued)*
diseases of, chest roentgenography in, 106
echocardiography in, 460–478
malignant, ultrafast computed tomography in, 709, *709*
neoplastic, echocardiography in, 475
nuclear magnetic resonance imaging in, 936–947
traumatic, echocardiography in, 476
diverticula of, magnetic resonance imaging of, 940
imaging of, 937, 938
lesions of, ultrafast computed tomography of, 709, *710*
magnetic resonance signal characteristics of, 939, 939(t), 940
metastases to, magnetic resonance imaging of, 944, *944*, 945, *945*
neoplasms of, magnetic resonance imaging of, 944, *944*, 945, *945*
normal, 938–940, *938*, 939(t)
echocardiographic appearance of, 460, *461*
magnetic resonance imaging of, 938, *938*, 939, 939(t)
gated, 938, 939, 939(t)
postoperative, magnetic resonance imaging of, 944
thickening of, magnetic resonance imaging of, 942
ultrafast computed tomography of, 708, 709
tumors of, benign, ultrafast computed tomography of, 709
ultrafast computed tomography of, 707–710
advantages of, 709, 710
disadvantages of, 709, 710
protocols for, 708
techniques of, 708
Periodic motion, 349, 350, *350*
Peripheral angioplasty, imaging of, indium-111–labeled platelets in, 1127, 1128
Permeability, definition of, 1274
Permutation gating, in pericardial imaging, 937, 938
Persistent left superior vena cava, magnetic resonance imaging of, 879, *880*
ultrafast computed tomography of, 716, *717*
PET. See *Positron emission tomography (PET).*
pH, intracellular, in cardiomyopathy, 932, 933, *933*
phosphorus magnetic resonance spectroscopy of, 845
Phantom, definition of, 1274
Phantom studies, of coronary obstruction, 236, 237
of digital subtraction videodensitometry, 237
Pharmacologic agents, in ventricular function evaluation, 27, 27(t)
Phase, definition of, 365, 1274
Phase analysis, radionuclide ventriculography in, 999–1001, *999–1001*
exercise, 1001, 1002
Phase angle, 740
free induction decay dependence on, 751, *751*
Phase cancellation effects, definition of, 539
Phase encoding, definition of, 1274
Phase ghost artifacts, in magnetic resonance imaging, 786, *786*
Phase shift, in blood flow velocity calculation, 823, *823*
Phased array, in electronic beam steering, 357, 358, *358*, *359*
orthogonal, in electronic beam steering, 359, *359*

Phase-encoding artifacts, 865
Phase-encoding gradients, 752
Phase-encoding time, 750
Phenylpropanolamine, administration of, metaiodobenzylguanidine uptake after, 1138
Philips DCI system, 220, 221, 221(t)
Phosphates, high-energy, phosphorus magnetic resonance spectroscopy of, 847
  inorganic, in cardiomyopathy, 932, 933, *933*
Phosphocreatine (PCr), in cardiomyopathy, 932, 933, *933*
  in congestive heart failure, *973*
  in hypertrophic cardiomyopathy, 971
  in myocardial ischemia, 970, *971*
  in myocardial metabolism, 39
  in normal myocardium, 969, *970*
  utilization of, in ischemic exercise, 972–974, *974*
Phosphodiesters, in hypertrophic cardiomyopathy, 971, *972*
  in normal myocardium, 969, *970*
Phosphofructokinase, activity of, in ischemia, 49
  in diabetes, 49
  in fasting, 49
  in myocardial metabolism, 42, *43*
Phosphoglucomutase, in myocardial metabolism, 41
Phospholipids, radioiodine-labeled, 1088, *1088*
Phosphomonoesters, in normal myocardium, 969
Phosphorus, nucleus of, characteristics of, 842(t)
Phosphorus magnetic resonance imaging, of myocardial metabolism, in cardiomyopathy, 932, 933, *933*
Phosphorus magnetic resonance spectroscopy, 845–851
  in allograft rejection, 851
  in cardiomyopathy, 848, 849
  in diabetes, 848
  in hypertension, 848
  in hypoxia, 848
  in intracellular acidosis, 848
  in myocardial ischemia, 848
  in perfused heart preparations, 846–849
  in study, of enzyme kinetics, 846, 847, *847*
    of high-energy phosphate changes, 847
    of in vivo myocardial metabolism, 849–851, *850–854*
    of myocardial metabolism regulation, 845, 846
    of substrate bioenergetics, 847, 848
  of toxic substances, 849
Phosphorus spectroscopy, 967
Phosphorylase kinase, in myocardial metabolism, 42
Phosphorylation, of glucose, in carbohydrate metabolism, 39, 40, *41*
  phosphorus magnetic resonance spectroscopy of, 845
Photon scatter, in fast computed tomography, in myocardial perfusion measurement, 696–698, *696–698*
Physics, of blood flow, 367, 368
    flow profiles in, 367, 368, *368*
    turbulence in, 368
    viscosity in, 367, 368, *368*
  of diagnostic x-ray imaging, 162
  of Doppler, 365–373
  of echocardiography, 348–364
  radiation, in x-ray computed tomography, 635–637, *636*
15-*p*-iodophenyl pentadecanoic acid. See *IPPA*.
15-(*p*-iodophenyl)-3, 3-dimethyl pentadecanoic acid (DMIPP), 1090
15-(*p*-iodophenyl)-3-R, S-methyl pentadecanoic acid. See *BMIPP*.
PIB (partial ileal bypass), for hyperlipidemia, 268, 268(t)
Picture Archiving and Communications Systems (PACS), 660
Piezoelectricity, in ultrasound generation, 350, *350*, 350(t)
Pigtail catheter, 109
Pincushion distortion, correction for, 118
  in digital angiography, 290, *290*
  in quantitative coronary angiography, 224
Pixel(s), 76
  definition of, 1274
  in digital angiography, intensity of, 291, *291*
  in magnetic resonance imaging, 754
  neighborhood of, 82
  size of, in digitized image, 222, 222(t), 283, 283(t)
PK 11195, 1266
Planar imaging, definition of, 1274
  echo, definition of, 1272
  in frame mode, 982–984, *982–984*
  in list mode, 984
    equilibrium studies of, 984
    first-pass studies of, 984
  Tc-sestamibi in, sensitivity of, *1103*, 1103(t)
    vs. thallium-201, 1105(t)
  thallium-201 in, sensitivity of, *1103*, 1103(t)
  vs. antimyosin imaging, 1115
  vs. single-photon emission computed tomography, 1090
Planck constant, 732
Plane, sensitive, definition of, 1275
Platelets, deposition of, on prosthetic grafts, 1129, *1131*, *1132*
    drug effects on, 1130, 1131
  indium-111–labeled. See *Indium-111–labeled platelets.*
  labeling of, 1121, 1122
Pleural effusion, left, vs pericardial effusion, 464, *465*
Point operations, 288, 289(t)
  in digital image processing, 77, 78, *78–80*
Point spread function (PSF), 292
Poiseuille resistance, after stenting, 266(t)
Polar coordinate profile, in myocardial perfusion quantification, 993, *993*
Polar scan line data, 360, *361*, *362*
Polycythemia, in coronary reserve, 14
Polysplenia, echocardiography in, 500, *506*
Polytetrafluoroethylene (PTFE) grafts, platelet deposition in, drug effects on, 1130, 1131
  thrombogeneity of, 1129, 1130
Polyunsaturated fatty acids, for hypercholesterolemia, 268
Pompe's disease, 934
Positioning, in positron emission tomography, of myocardial blood flow, 1171, *1171*
Positron emission tomography (PET), activity spillover in, 1157, *1158*
  image acquisition in, 1154–1157, *1154–1156*
  image analysis in, 1157, *1157*, 1158, *1158*
  in absolute myocardial perfusion measurement, 1179–1182, *1180–1182*
    flow-dependent extraction in, 1180, *1180*
    geometric limitations of, 1180
    models for, 1180–1182, *1181*, *1182*
  in coronary artery disease diagnosis, 1174–1179, *1175*, 1176(t), *1177*
    accuracy of, 1176–1178, 1176(t), *1177*
    in asymptomatic patients, 1179
    sensitivity/specificity analysis in, 1178
    vs. coronary arteriography, 1176, 1176(t), 1177, *1177*
  in Duchenne muscular dystrophy, 1252, *1253*
Positron emission tomography (PET) *(Continued)*
  in ligand-receptor interaction identification, 1259, 1260, *1260*
  in myocardial infarction, 1183–1185, *1184–1186*
    in localization, 1235–1237, *1236*
  in noninvasive measurement, of functional processes, 1159–1164, *1161–1164*
  in transient ischemia detection, 1182, *1182–1184*, 1183
  of cardiac receptors, adrenergic, 1262–1264
    evaluation of, 1256–1270
      clinical applications of, 1267
    muscarinic acetylcholine, 1264–1266, *1265*
  of ischemic vs. nonischemic cardiomyopathy, 1249–1251, *1250*
  of myocardial blood flow, 1160–1163, *1161*, *1162*, 1169–1189
    analysis and interpretation of, 1172–1174, *1174*
    circumferential profile analysis in, 1173, *1174*
    in therapeutic response evaluation, 1185–1187, *1186*
    quantification in, 1173
    technique of, 1171, *1171–1173*, 1172
    tracers for, 1170, *1170*, 1170(t), 1171
  of myocardial metabolism, in dilated cardiomyopathy, 1247, *1248*, *1249*
    in hypertrophic cardiomyopathy, 1251, 1252, *1252*
  of glucose, 1163, *1163*, 1164, *1164*
  partial volume effect in, 1157, *1157*, *1158*
  principles of, 1140–1168
    general, 1153, *1153*, 1154
  schematics of, 1153, *1153*
  tracers in, concentration of, 1157, *1157*, 1158, *1158*
    kinetics of, models of, 1158, 1159, *1159*
    uptake of, quantitative analysis of, 1179, *1179*
  vs. single-photon emission computed tomography, 1178, 1179
    during exercise, 1174, *1175*
  vs. thallium-201 scintigraphy, 1178, 1179
Positron-labeled albumin microspheres, 1142, *1142*
Positrons, decay of, detection of, 1153, *1153*
Posterior ring abscess, after endocarditis, transesophageal echocardiography of, 611
Posterior wall thickness, measurement of, echocardiographic, 380, *381*
Post-myocardial-infarction pericarditis, 942, 943, *943*
Postoperative pericardium, magnetic resonance imaging of, 944
Post-pericardiotomy syndrome, 942, 943
Postprocessing, in echocardiography, 363
Post-test probability, 1032
Potassium, nucleus of, characteristics of, 842(t)
Potassium magnetic resonance spectroscopy, 856–858
Precession, definition of, 1274
  free, steady state, definition of, 1276
  of frequency, 733, *733*
  of M, 739, *739*
Prednisone, for contrast agent allergy, 189
Preload, in left ventricular function, 26
Premedication, for coronary angiography, 189, 190
Preprocessing, in echocardiography, 363
Presaturation, out-of-plane, 865
  spatial, in magnetic resonance imaging, 785, 786
Pressure, right ventricular, in mitral stenosis, 433

Pressure gradient(s), intraventricular, in hypertrophic cardiomyopathy, 450–453, *451–453*
subvalvular, in valvular aortic stenosis, 60
transvalvular, in aortic stenosis, 421, *423*
in prosthetic stenosis, 441, *442*
in valvular regurgitation, 66, *66*, 68, *69*
measurement of, invasive standards for, 62, 63, *63*
quantification of, in valve stenosis, 60–63
relationship of, to blood velocity, 60, 61, *62*
Pressure half-time, in mitral valve area estimation, 431
in tricuspid valve area measurement, 436
Pressure overload, in left ventricular function, 124
Pressure-motion loop, *143*, 144
Pressure-volume loop, 28, *28*
end-systolic, 28, *28*
generation of, radionuclide angiocardiography in, 1018, *1018*
Pressure-volume relationship, in left ventricle, 139, 140, *140*
Pretest probability, 1032
of coronary artery disease, 1032, 1032(t)
Probability density function, 78
Probe, definition of, 1274
for magnetic resonance spectroscopy, 843, 844
for transesophageal echocardiography, 606, *606*
Progressive scan, 284
Progressive scan fluoroscopy, 287, 287(t)
Progressive systemic sclerosis, with scleroderma, thallium-201 scintigraphy in, 1066, 1066(t)
Projection(s), back, simple, 635
reconstruction from, in x-ray computed tomography, 637–639, *637–639*
Prolapse, mitral valve. See *Mitral valve prolapse.*
Promethazine, in premedication, before coronary angiography, 189
Propagation velocity, definition of, 365
in ultrasonic tissue characterization, 539
Propranolol, effects of, measurement of, exercise Doppler echocardiography in, 578–580
Prostacyclin, for platelet deposition, in prosthetic grafts, 1130
Prosthesis(es), endoluminal. See *Endoluminal prostheses.*
evaluation of, cine magnetic resonance imaging in, 962
imaging of, indium-111–labeled platelets in, 1129–1131, 1129(t), *1130*, *1131*
metallic, effect of, on magnetic resonance imaging, 865–867, *867*
Prosthetic grafts, platelet deposition on, 1129, *1131*, *1132*
drug effects on, 1130, 1131, *1131*
Prosthetic regurgitation, echocardiography in, 440, 441
Prosthetic stenosis, echocardiography in, 440, 441
two-dimensional, 440, 441
Prosthetic valve(s), Doppler echocardiography of, 441, *442*
evaluation of, transesophageal echocardiography in, 611
replacement of, intraoperative echocardiography during, 624
Protamine, in coronary angiography, 190
Protein, degradation of, 52
synthesis of, 50–52
amino acid transport in, 50
peptide chain initiation in, 50–52, *51*
Protein *(Continued)*
peptide elongation and termination in, 52
Protein turnover, 50–53
regulation of, 52, 53
diabetes in, 52
hypertrophy in, 52
insulin in, 52
ischemia in, 53
starvation in, 52
Proton(s), fat, 760
magnetic fields around, 795, *796*
nucleus of, characteristics of, 842(t)
of T1, in water, 759, 760
of T2, in water, 759, 760
water, 760
Proton magnetic resonance imaging, in dilated cardiomyopathy, 1251
Proton magnetic resonance spectroscopy, 854, *856*
Proton relaxation, 759, 760, *760*, 760(t)
biologic basis of, 759–768
effect on, of paramagnetic contrast agents, *795*
enhanced, 794–798
inherent, 794–798
measurement of, in vivo vs in vitro, 760, 761
mechanisms of, 761–763, 761(t), *762*, *763*
Proton spectroscopy, 974
Pseudoaneurysm, of left ventricle, after myocardial infarction, 600, *601*
Pseudogating, diastolic, 760
Pseudotruncus, *94*
PSF (point spread function), 292
PTCA. See *Percutaneous transluminal coronary angioplasty (PTCA).*
PTFE (polytetrafluoroethylene) grafts, platelet deposition in, drug effects on, 1130, 1131
thrombogeneity of, 1129, 1130
PTSM, 1144
Pulmonary angiography, 149–161
approach to, antecubital, 150
femoral vein, 150
catheterization in, 150
contraindications to, 149
in pulmonary embolism, 151–155
complications of, 154
interpretation of, *151–153*, 153
therapeutic maneuvers during, 154, *154*, 155, *156*
timing of, 152, 153
indications for, 149
of neoplasms, 157, *159*
of pulmonary vascular lesions, 155–159, *157*
pulmonary artery pressures during, 150
radionuclide lung scan before, 150
technique of, 149–151
Pulmonary arterial hypertension, 98, 99
in atrial septal defect, 98, *99*
Pulmonary arterial markings, increased, Doppler echocardiography of, 496–499
two-dimensional echocardiography of, 496–499, *497*, *498*
Pulmonary arteriography, balloon occlusion, 150, 151
Pulmonary arteriovenous fistulae, pulmonary angiography in, 155, 156, *157*
Pulmonary artery, abnormalities of, acquired, magnetic resonance imaging of, 876–879, *878–880*
congenital, magnetic resonance imaging of, *875–877*, 876
magnetic resonance imaging of, 894
ultrafast computed tomography of, 725, *726*
aneurysms of, pulmonary angiography of, 156, 157, *158*
Pulmonary artery *(Continued)*
banding of, magnetic resonance imaging of, 876–879, *878*
diameter of, measurement of, 489
left coronary artery origin from, 197
magnetic resonance imaging of, 876–879
occlusion of, after tetralogy of Fallot repair, magnetic resonance imaging of, 890, *891*
stenosis of, pulmonary angiography in, 156, *157*
thrombi of, ultrafast computed tomography of, 705–707, *707*
Pulmonary artery pressure, during pulmonary angiography, 150
in valvular regurgitation, 68
Pulmonary atresia, *96*
conduits in, magnetic resonance imaging of, 876–879, *879*
magnetic resonance imaging in, *875*, 876
ultrafast computed tomography in, *724*, 725
with intact ventricular septum, echocardiography in, 495, 496, *496*
with ventricular septal defect, echocardiography in, 494, *494*
Pulmonary blood volume, measurement of, equilibrium radionuclide angiography in, 1031
Pulmonary carcinosarcoma, 157
Pulmonary circulation, cine magnetic resonance imaging of, 954, 955, *955*, *956*
in congenital heart disease, with acyanosis, Doppler echocardiography of, 479–489
two-dimensional echocardiography of, 479–489
Pulmonary embolism, bronchoconstriction in, 153
cine magnetic resonance imaging in, 954, *955*
imaging of, indium-111–labeled platelets in, 1128, 1129
magnetic resonance imaging in, 876, *878*
pulmonary angiography in, 151–155
complications of, 154
interpretation of, *151–153*, 153
therapeutic maneuvers during, 154, *154*, 155, *156*
timing of, 152, 153
resolution rate of, 152
right atrial thrombi in, echocardiography of, 528, *529*
right heart hemodynamics in, 153
treatment of, 154, *154*, 155
ultrafast computed tomography in, 706, *707*
vasoconstriction in, 153
Pulmonary function, angiographic contrast agents in, 176
Pulmonary hypertension, as pulmonary angiography contraindication, 149
cine magnetic resonance imaging in, 954, 955, *956*
right ventricular ejection in, 414, *414*
Pulmonary oligemia, magnetic resonance imaging in, 888–892, *890*, *891*
Pulmonary regurgitation, causes of, 440
color flow imaging in, 440
echocardiography in, 440
pulsed-wave, 440
roentgenographic evaluation of, 105
Pulmonary sequestration, pulmonary angiography in, 157
Pulmonary slings, magnetic resonance imaging of, 893, 894
Pulmonary stenosis, causes of, 440
echocardiography in, 440, *507*
two-dimensional, 440
right ventricular enlargement in, 103, *103*
roentgenographic evaluation of, 105

Pulmonary stenosis *(Continued)*
subvalvular, in right ventricular outflow obstruction, 492, *494*
valvular, in right ventricular outflow obstruction, 492, *493*
Pulmonary valve disease, echocardiography in, 440
Doppler, 440
Pulmonary varix, pulmonary angiography in, 157
Pulmonary vascularity, in congenital heart disease with cyanosis, Doppler echocardiography in, 492–499, *494–496*
two-dimensional echocardiography in, 492–499, *494–499*
Pulmonary vasculature, lesions of, pulmonary angiography of, 155–159
normal anatomy of, 151
pulmonary flow in, decreased, 95, *96*
increased, 95, *95*, *96*
increased resistance to, 95–98, *97–99*
normal, 93–95, *94*
roentgenographic evaluation of, 93–98
Pulmonary vein wedge angiogram, 151
Pulmonary veins, drainage of, anomalous, pulmonary angiography in, 159
ultrafast computed tomography in, 716, *717*
evaluation of, cine magnetic resonance imaging in, 955
Pulmonary venous hypertension, 95, *97*, *98*
dilated cardiomyopathy in, 95, *97*, *98*
in mitral stenosis, 95, *98*
left ventricular dysfunction in, 95, *97*, *98*
Pulmonary venous markings, increased, Doppler echocardiography of, 499
two-dimensional echocardiography of, 499, *499*
Pulmonic regurgitation, cine magnetic resonance imaging in, 959, *962*
right ventricular ejection in, 414
severity of, evaluation of, 69
Pulmonic stenosis, infundibular, cine magnetic resonance imaging in, *962*
severity of, clinical evaluation of, 64
Pulse(s), amplitude-modulated, 748, *749*
bandwidth of, 748
90-degree, 736
definition of, 1274
180-degree, *740*, 741, *741*
definition of, 1274
inversion, 741
nonselective, 740
radiofrequency, in magnetic resonance spectroscopy, 842
selective, characteristics of, 749
read, 741
refocusing, 742
selective, 740
sinc, 748, *749*
transmission of, in echocardiography, instrumentation for, 353, *353*, 354
Pulse Fourier transform nuclear magnetic resonance, 735–740
relaxation in, 737, 738, *738*
rotating-frame concept in, 738–740, *738*, *739*
signal averaging in, 737
signal-to-noise ratio in, 737
vectors in, 735, *735*, 736, *736*
Pulse length, definition of, 1274
effect of, on axial resolution, 353, *353*
Pulse pressure, in valvular regurgitation, 68
Pulse repetition frequency, 369
Pulse sequences, definition of, 1275
in magnetic resonance imaging, of great vessels, 864, *865*, *866*
Pulse triggering, 781, 781(t), *782*
Pulsed Doppler, instrumentation for, 369–371, *369*, *370*
of left ventricular ejection, 403, *404*
spectral analysis of, 371, 372, *372*
Pulsed-wave echocardiography, in pulmonary regurgitation, 440
Pulsed-wave mapping, in aortic regurgitation, 427
in mitral regurgitation, 435
in tricuspid regurgitation, 438
Pulsus paradoxus, in cardiac tamponade, 465
Pyruvate, metabolism of, 42
Pyruvate decarboxylase, in myocardial metabolism, 42
Pyruvate dehydrogenase, in carbohydrate metabolism, 42, *44*
in diabetes, 49
in fasting, 49
in ischemia, 49
in tricarboxylic acid cycle, 47
Pyruvate dehydrogenase phosphatase, in myocardial metabolism, 42

Q-T interval, after selective intracoronary injection, of angiographic contrast agents, 173
Quadrature detection, 740
Quadrupolar interaction, sodium in, 829, *829*
Quality control, in quantitative coronary arteriography, 231–236
Quantification, in digital angiography, 287
of cardiac parameters, scintigraphy in, 988–1002
of myocardial blood flow, positron emission tomography in, 1173
of myocardial metabolites, methods of, 843
of myocardial perfusion defects, in coronary artery disease, 994, *995*
of radionuclide ventriculography, 996–1002
Quantitation, cardiac, magnetic resonance imaging in, 811–827
automated analysis of, 824
future of, 824, 825
general approach to, 811, 812
orientation of, 815, *815*
techniques of, 812–815, *812–814*
of blood flow, cine magnetic resonance imaging in, 965
magnetic resonance imaging in, 822–824, 822(t)
of myocardial perfusion, magnetic resonance imaging in, 823, 824, *824*
of shunting, radionuclide angiocardiography in, 1014, 1015, *1015*
of valvular regurgitation, magnetic resonance imaging in, 823, *823*
Quantitative coronary angiography, 211–280
applications of, 259–270
approaches to, 217–231, *217*
cine film, 217, *217*, 218
digital, 217, *217*, 218
biplane analysis in, 227
Brown-Dodge method of, 218, 219
calibration in, 224, 224(t), 225, *225*
calipers in, 218, *219*
cine film digitization in, 219, 219(t), 220, *220*, 220(t)
computer hardware and software in, 221, 221(t), 222, 222(t)
contour analysis in, 225–227
contour detection in, 222–225
densitometry in, 227–230, *228–230*
edge definition in, 223, *223*, 224
frame selection in, 241, 241(t), 242, 242(t)
image acquisition in, 219, 220
Quantitative coronary angiography *(Continued)*
on-line digital cardiac systems in, 220, 221, 221(t)
percent diameter stenosis measurement in, 225–227, *226*
pincushion distortion and correction in, 224
validation studies of, 236–242
computer analysis in, 238–241, 239(t), 240(t)
parameters describing, 236
Quantitative coronary arteriography, catheters for, selection of, 234, *235*
contrast media for, administration of, by electrocardiographically triggered injector, 234
nonionic, with iso-osmolality, 233, 234, 234(t)
data acquisition in, standardization of, 232–234, 232(t), *233*, 234(t)
image analysis in, 231
in coronary artery assessment, 313–324, *313–323*, 315(t), 318(t), 322(t), 323(t)
quality control in, 231–236
sources of error in, 322, 322(t), 323, 323(t)
vasodilators in, preangiographic administration of, 232, 233, *233*
Quantitative image processing, future directions of, 83–85, *84*
Quantization, in digitization, 282
Quantization errors, 76, *77*, 282
Quantum noise, 282
Quenching, definition of, 1275
Quinuclidinyl benzylate, 1264, 1265

R11D10, 1110
in cardiac allograft rejection imaging, 1114
Radian, definition of, 1275
Radiation, detection of, nonimaging devices for, 981, 982
principles of, 977, 978, *978*, *979*
Radiation dosimetry, in computed tomography, 647, *647*, 648(t)
in fast computed tomography, 647
Radiation physics, in x-ray computed tomography, 635–637, *636*
Radiofrequency, definition of, 1275
Radiofrequency data analysis, in ultrasonic tissue characterization, 540, *540*, 541, *541*
Radiofrequency field, 734
Radiofrequency pulse, in magnetic resonance spectroscopy, 842
selective, characteristics of, 749
Radiofrequency scan line, 360, *360*
Radiofrequency signal, in magnetic resonance spectroscopy, 844
Radiographic contrast agents, 162–181
actions of, cardiovascular, 167(t)
noncardiovascular, 167(t)
historical background of, 162–165, *163*, *164*
intravascular, performance criteria for, 162
Radiography, of coronary flow reserve, 245–249, *246*
Radiolabeled microspheres, in transient ischemia, 31
Radionuclide angiocardiography, 1006–1026
accuracy of, 1018
curve generation in, 1012–1014, *1012*, *1013*
data from, acquisition of, 1010, 1011, *1011*
curve, low-frequency, use of, 1014–1016, *1014*, *1015*
processing of, 1011–1018
filtering in, 1011, 1012
future of, 1024, 1025
history of, 1006, *1007*, *1008*
in congenital heart disease, 1021

Radionuclide angiocardiography *(Continued)*
in coronary artery disease, 1021–1024, *1023*, *1024*
in hemodynamic measurement, 1016–1018, *1016–1018*
in myocardial revascularization, 1024
in normal subjects, 1018–1021, *1019*, *1020*, 1020(t)
in valvular heart disease, 1021
instrumentation for, 1006–1010, *1009*
radiopharmaceuticals for, 1010, 1010(t)
reproducibility of, 1018, 1018(t)
Radionuclide angiography, equilibrium. See *Equilibrium radionuclide angiography.*
exercise, in ejection fraction measurement, 585, *586*
limitations of, 1039
in ejection fraction measurement, 379, *380*
vs. exercise echocardiography, 585, 586
Radionuclide imaging, artificial intelligence in, 1002
gamma camera in, multicrystal, 980, 981
single-crystal, 978–980, *979*, *980*
instrumentation for, 977–1005
of right ventricle, 303
physics of, 977–1005
Radionuclide lung scan, before pulmonary angiography, 150
Radionuclide ventriculography, exercise, in phase analysis, 1001, 1002
in reactive hyperemia, *342*
function calculations in, global, 997, *997*, 998
regional, 998–1002
image preprocessing in, 996
image processing in, 996, 997
background determination in, 996, 997
edge detection in, 997
left ventricular isolation in, 996
in phase analysis, 999–1001, *999–1001*
quantification of, 996–1002
Radiopharmaceuticals, for radionuclide angiocardiography, 1010, 1010(t)
RAM memory, 285
Ram-Lak filter, *639*
Ramp filter, 986, *986*
Range ambiguity, 370
Rasmussen's aneurysm, 157
Rastelli procedure, 892
1.5 Ratio ionic agents, 166
adverse reactions to, 177, *178*
anaphylactoid reaction to, 174–176
effects of, on renal function, 176
selection of, criteria for, 177–179
3.0 Ratio agents, effects of, on renal function, 176
3.0 Ratio ionic agents, 166
selection of, indications for, 178(t)
3.0 Ratio nonionic agents, 166
anaphylactoid reaction to, 174–176
selection of, criteria for, 177–179
Ray casting, in three-dimensional computed tomography, 663
Ray sums, in x-ray computed tomography, 637–639
Rayleigh scattering, 544
RC (respiratory compensation), 783
Reactive hyperemia, assessment of, 256, *257*, *258*
coronary, determination of, 243
relationship of, to exercise tests, *341*, *342*
to percent area stenosis, 318, *319*
to percent diameter stenosis, 318, *319*, 339, *340*
to stenotic segment area, 319, *319*, *320*
Reactive hypertrophy, in infarcted myocardium, 33
Read pulse, 741
Read-out time, 737
Reagants, shift, definition of, 1275
Real-time backscatter imaging, 540, 541, *541*, *542*
Real-time B-mode images, formation of, 356–359
Real-time convolver, of digital image processor, 285
Real-time digital magnetic disk, in on-line image storage, in digital angiography, 285, 286
"Real-time two-dimensional Doppler," 371
Receiver, definition of, 1275
Receiver bandwidth, 754
Receiver dead time, definition of, 1275
Receiver operating characteristic (ROC) analysis, 90, *90*
Reception, in echocardiography, 359, 360, *360*, *361*
Receptors, acetylcholine, muscarinic, characterization of, positron emission tomography in, 1264–1266, *1265*
alpha-adrenergic, in vivo study of, positron emission tomography in, 1264
benzodiazepine, peripheral-type, characterization of, 1266, 1267
beta-adrenergic, distribution of, 1262(t), 1263(t)
in vivo demonstration of, positron emission tomography in, 1263, 1264
subtypes of, 1262, 1263
cardiac, adrenergic, characterization of, positron emission tomography in, 1262–1264
binding of, in vivo models of, 1260–1262, *1261*
techniques of, 1257–1259
evaluation of, positron emission tomography in, 1256–1270
clinical applications of, 1267
imaging of, 1135–1139
ligand interaction with, positron emission tomography of, 1259, 1260, *1260*
positron-emitting tracers of, 1152
studies of, C-11–labeled ligands for, 1257, 1257(t)
cholinergic, muscarinic, distribution of, 1264, 1265
subtypes of, 1264, 1265
Recombinant human tissue-type plasminogen activator (rt-TPA), for pulmonary embolism, 155
Reconstruction, from projections, in x-ray computed tomography, 637–639, *637–639*
image, 634, 636
in single-photon emission computed tomography, 985, *985*, 986, *986*
filtering in, 986, *986*
three-dimensional, of left ventricle, ultrafast computed tomography in, 676, *676*
Reconstruction artifacts, in fast computed tomography, in myocardial perfusion measurement, 695–698, *696–698*
Recursive digitization, 231
Red blood cells, labeling of, in equilibrium radionuclide angiography, 1027, 1028
Reflection, backscatter in, measurement of, 540, *540*
in cardiovascular Doppler physics, 367
in ultrasound transmission, 351, 352, *352*
specular, 539
Reflection coefficient, 352
Refocusing, of magnetization, methods of, 747, *747*
Refocusing pulse, 742
Refraction, angle of, 352
in ultrasound transmission, 351, 352, *352*
Region growing, in segmentation, 83
Region of interest, wall motion measurement in, 132–134, *133*, *134*
Regional transfer function, assessment of, fast computed tomography in, 700
Region-partitioning, in segmentation, 83, *84*
Regurgitant flow, 122, *122*, 123
in mitral regurgitation, 436
Regurgitant fraction, 66, *66*, 67, *67*
in mitral regurgitation, 436
measurement of, equilibrium radionuclide angiography in, 1031
in aortic regurgitation, 430
Regurgitant lesions, cine magnetic resonance imaging of, 955–959, *957–961*
Regurgitant orifice, area of, cross-sectional, 66, *66*, 68, 69
measurement of, in aortic regurgitation, 430
transvalvular pressure gradient of, 66, *66*
Regurgitant stroke volume, in aortic regurgitation, 430
Regurgitant valves, comparison of, 69
Regurgitant velocity, mitral, peak, in mitral regurgitation, 435
Regurgitant volume, in aortic regurgitation, 430
in mitral regurgitation, 436
Regurgitation, left-sided, equilibrium radionuclide angiography in, 1040
mitral. See *Mitral regurgitation.*
prosthetic, echocardiography in, 440, 441
pulmonic. See *Pulmonic regurgitation.*
tricuspid. See *Tricuspid regurgitation.*
valvular, quantitation of, magnetic resonance imaging in, 823, *823*
Relative regional vascular volume, 247
Relaxation, in pulse Fourier transform nuclear magnetic resonance, 737, 738, *738*
longitudinal, definition of, 1273
nuclear, stimulated, requirements for, 761, 761(t)
proton. See *Proton relaxation.*
Relaxation deconvolution, in sodium magnetic resonance spectroscopy, 857, 858
Relaxation dispersion, in vivo metabolism in, 797, *797*
Relaxation rate, definition of, 1275
Relaxation time, calculation of, magnetic resonance imaging in, 820
definition of, 1275
isovolumic, in cardiac tamponade, 469
myocardial, changes in, after myocardial infarction, 914–918, *917*, 917–919(t)
in ischemic disease, 925, *925*
of sodium-23, 831, 832, 832(t)
of tissue, factors in, *763*
spin-lattice, 735, 753
definition of, 1276
spin-spin, 735–738, 753
definition of, 1276
T2, determination of, 820
Relaxing agents, ferromagnetic, 797, *797*, 798, *798*, 798(t)
paramagnetic, 794–797, *795–797*
superparamagnetic, 797, *797*, 798, *798*, 798(t)
Relaxivity, 794
of GdDTPA, 804, 805, *805*
Relaxivity dispersion, in chelation, 795, *796*
of aquoion, after chelation, *796*
Renal cell carcinoma, magnetic resonance imaging in, 881, *882*
metastatic, ultrafast computed tomography in, 404
Renal function, changes in, after intracoronary contrast agent injection, 188
effects on, of angiographic contrast agents, 176
Renografin, *164*, 165

Renografin-76, in contrast echocardiography, 558
intracoronary injection of, and ventricular fibrillation, 174
myocardial perfusion after, *566*
properties of, 166, 167(t)
with calcium enrichment, 171, *172*
Reperfusion, after thrombolytic therapy, technetium-99m isonitrile imaging in, 1068
in myocardial ischemia, magnetic resonance imaging in, 766, *766*
metabolic disturbances after, 50
of circumflex coronary artery, sodium imaging in, *835*, *836*
of infarction, imaging of, nonproton nuclei in, 919
nuclear magnetic resonance in, 918, 919, 919(t)
tissue property changes after, 918, 919, 919(t)
of myocardium, ultrasonic tissue characterization in, 546–548, *547*, *548*
substrate metabolism in, 1203–1219
Repetition time, definition of, 1275
in magnetic resonance imaging, 778, *779*
Rephasing gradient, definition of, 1275
Repolarization, after selective intracoronary injection, of angiographic contrast agents, 173, *174*
Resolution, aximuthal, 354
contrast, 76
in single-photon emission computed tomography, 985, *985*
in x-ray computed tomography, *640*
cross-plane, 357
lateral, determinants of, 354, *354*, 355, *355*
in echocardiography, instrumentation for, 354, *354*, 355, *355*
low-contrast, in computed tomography, 648, 649, 650(t), *651*
in fast computed tomography, 648, 649, 650(t), *651*, *652*
spatial. See *Spatial resolution.*
temporal. See *Temporal resolution.*
Resonance, definition of, 1275
magnetic, definition of, 1273
Resonance frequency, 734
definition of, 1275
of magnetization, 748
Resonance phenomenon, in nuclear magnetic resonance, 734, *734*, 735, *735*
Respiration, control of, in myocardium, 47, 48
in cardiac tamponade, 469, *469*, *470*
in constrictive pericarditis, 474, 475, *475*
Respiratory compensation (RC), 783
Respiratory cycle, in diastolic performance, 410, *411*
Respiratory maneuvers, in ventricular function evaluation, 27, 27(t)
Respiratory motion artifacts, in magnetic resonance imaging, 783, 783(t), 784
Respiratory triggering, in magnetic resonance imaging, 783, 783(t), 784, *785*
Respiratory-ordered phase-encoding (ROPE), 783
Respiratory-sorted phase-encoding (RSPE), 783
Restenosis, angiographic definition of, 259, 260, *260*, *261*
clinical studies of, methodologic considerations in, 263
incidence of, 260–262, 263(t), *264*
quantitative coronary angiography in, 259–263, *260–263*, 262(t)
risk factors for, 263
timing of, 262, 262(t), 263
videodensitometric analysis of, 263
Restrictive cardiomyopathy, atrial size in, echocardiography of, 457, *457*
atrioventricular valve incompetence in, echocardiography of, 458
conditions associated with, 458
echocardiography in, 457, 458
magnetic resonance imaging in, 933, 934, *934*
pericardial effusion in, echocardiography of, 458
roentgenographic evaluation of, 105, 106
spin-echo imaging in, 934, *934*
ultrasonic tissue characterization in, 551, *552*
ventricular function in, diastolic, echocardiography of, 457, 458, *458*
systolic, echocardiography of, 457
ventricular wall thickness in, echocardiography of, 457, *457*
vs. constrictive pericarditis, 943
Restrictive-infiltrative cardiomyopathy, definition of, 449
Retrospective gating, in magnetic resonance imaging, 783
Revascularization, blood flow recovery after, 1223–1225, *1223*, *1224*, 1225(t)
coronary, equilibrium radionuclide angiography of, 1037, 1038
in hypoperfused metabolically active tissue, 1222–1225, *1223*, *1224*, 1225(t)
in myocardial infarction, myocardial metabolism in, 1218, 1219, *1220*, *1221*
myocardial, radionuclide angiocardiography of, 1024
thallium-201 scintigraphy of, 1064, *1065*
Reverberation, 353
"Reverse mapping," 81
Reynolds number, 368
RF, definition of, 1275
Rhabdomyoma, 512
of left ventricle, echocardiography of, 516
of right ventricle, echocardiography of, 517, *518*
ultrafast computed tomography of, 704
Rhabdomyosarcoma, 512
Rheumatic disease, and mitral regurgitation, 435
and mitral stenosis, 430
and pulmonary regurgitation, 440
and tricuspid stenosis, 436
left atrial thrombi in, echocardiography of, 525, *526*
of aortic valve, 425
valvular, cine magnetic resonance imaging in, *960*
Right aortic arch, magnetic resonance imaging of, 893
Right atrium(a), collapse of, in cardiac tamponade, 466, *466*, *467*
enlargement of, on cardiac silhouette, 101–103
primary benign tumors of, echocardiography of, 516, 517, *517*, *518*
thrombi of, echocardiography of, 527, 528, *529*, *530*
volume of, evaluation of, ultrafast computed tomography in, 678
Right coronary artery, anatomy of, 196
atherosclerosis in, regression of, 270, 270(t)
circumflex coronary artery originating from, 198
collateral pathways to, 199, 200
first septal perforator originating from, 199
left anterior descending artery originating from, 198
origin of, from opposite coronary sinus, 198, *198*
"shepherd's crook" deformity of, 685, *687*
Right coronary sinus, circumflex coronary artery originating from, 198
Right heart, hemodynamics of, in pulmonary embolism, 153
studies of, contrast echocardiography in, 568, *570*
visualization of, Dynamic Spatial Reconstructor in, *657*
Right ventricle(s), anatomy of, 26
catheter in, echocardiography of, 529, *530*
dimensions of, assessment of, 392, *392*, 393
in congenital heart disease, 394
two-dimensional echocardiography of, 392, 393
double-outlet, echocardiography in, 495, *495*
magnetic resonance imaging in, 891, *891*
ultrafast computed tomography in, *721*
enlargement of, in pulmonary stenosis, 103, *103*
in right ventricular infarction, 396
on cardiac silhouette, 103, *103*
evaluation of, radionuclide angiocardiography in, 1018
ultrafast computed tomography in, 676–678
infarction of, paradoxic septal motion in, 396, 397
regional wall motion abnormality in, 397
right ventricular dilation in, 396
morphologic, echocardiography of, 500, *502*, *508*
primary benign tumors of, echocardiography of, 517, *518*
radionuclide imaging of, 303
studies of, echocardiographic, quantitative, 395(t)
thrombi of, echocardiography of, 527, *527*
wall motion in, in analysis of, 129, *130*
Right ventricular diastolic collapse, in cardiac tamponade, *464*, 466, *467*
Right ventricular diastolic pressure, in constrictive pericarditis, 473, 474
Right ventricular dysfunction, as pulmonary angiography contraindication, 149
in acute inferoposterior myocardial infarction, 397
Right ventricular ejection, assessment of, Doppler echocardiography in, 413–415
clinical applications of, 414, 415
hemodynamics of, 414, *414*
Right ventricular ejection fraction, 139
measurement of, equilibrium radionuclide angiography in, 1031
Right ventricular end-diastolic pressure, after intravascular bolus injection, of angiographic contrast agents, *170*
Right ventricular filling, assessment of, Doppler echocardiography in, 415
Right ventricular function, 26, 391–398
assessment of, digital subtraction angiography in, 302, 303, *303*
echocardiography in, 391–398
M-mode, 392
two-dimensional, 392
global, ejection fraction in, 393–396, *393*, 395(t), *396*, *397*
volumes in, 393–396, *393*, 395(t), *396*, *397*
modulation of, 28
regional, assessment of, echocardiography in, 396–398
Right ventricular mass, evaluation of, ultrafast computed tomography in, 677, *677*, 678
Right ventricular motion, complexities of, 25, 26
Right ventricular outflow tract, biplane transesophageal echocardiography of, *615*

Right ventricular outflow tract *(Continued)*
obstruction of, echocardiography in, Doppler, 492
two-dimensional, 492, *493*, *494*
Right ventricular pressure, in mitral stenosis, 433
systolic, in tricuspid regurgitation, Doppler echocardiography in, 438–440, *439*
Right ventricular volume, calculation of, Simpson's rule in, 393, *393*
ultrafast computed tomography in, 676, *676*, 677, *677*
modulation of, 28
Right ventricular volume overload, 392, *393*
with atrial septal defects, 28
Right ventriculography, 139
Right-sided aortic arch, *94*
Right-sided regurgitant lesions, evaluation of, 67
Right-to-left shunting, at atrial level, Doppler echocardiography of, 495, 496
two-dimensional echocardiography of, 495, 496, *496*
at ventricular level, Doppler echocardiography of, 492–495, *494*, *495*
two-dimensional echocardiography of, 492–495
in patent ductus arteriosus, 485, *485*, 486
quantitation of, radionuclide angiocardiography in, 1014, *1014*
Rigler's sign, 101
Ring-down time, 353, *353*
RO 5-4864, 1266
Roadmapping, in coronary artery assessment, 313
ROC (receiver operating characteristic) analysis, 90, *90*
ROPE (respiratory-ordered phase-encoding), 783
Rotating frame of reference, definition of, 1275
Rotating frame technique, of magnetic resonance imaging, with sodium-23, 836, 837, *837*
Rotating-frame concept, in pulse Fourier transform nuclear magnetic resonance, 738–740, *738*, *739*
Rotating-head transducer, 356
Rotational wall motion, 383, *384*
Rouleaux, 367
R-R histogram, 983, *984*
R-R interval, calculation of, 118
RSPE (respiratory-sorted phase-encoding), 783
rt-TPA (recombinant human tissue-type plasminogen activator), for pulmonary embolism, 155
Rubidium-81, 1152
Rubidium-82, 1144
characteristics of, 1170(t)
in myocardial blood flow evaluation, 1161, *1161*, 1162, *1162*, 1170, *1170*, 1171
in myocardial infarction detection, 1183
Rudimentary chambers, 500
Rule of 50 percent, 500
Run-length matrix, 543

Sampling, in digitization, 282
Saphenous vein, as bypass graft, assessment of, ultrafast computed tomography in, 684, *684*
Sarcoidosis, in restrictive cardiomyopathy, 458
Sarcoma, osteogenic, of sternum, magnetic resonance imaging of, *945*
spindle cell, of lung, magnetic resonance imaging of, *944*
Satisfaction of search, 89
Saturability, of ligand-receptor complex, 1259, 1260, *1260*
Saturation, definition of, 1275
partial, definition of, 1274
Saturation recovery, definition of, 1275
Saturation transfer, definition of, 1275
Scalar, definition of, 1275
Scan(ning), in digitization, 282
in image creation, in magnetic resonance imaging, 777, 778, *779*, *780*
lung, radionuclide, before pulmonary angiography, 150
O-mode, 359, *359*
progressive, 284
Scan conversion, digital, in echocardiography, 360–363, *361*, *362*
Scanner, ACTA, 635
brain, EMI, 635
for fast computed tomography, 645–650, *646*, *647*, 689
for x-ray computed tomography, subsystems of, 641–643, *642*
Imatron C-100, 669
of Dynamic Spatial Reconstructor, 652–656, *655*
Scatter, correction for, in single-photon emission computed tomography, 986, 987
in ultrasound transmission, 352, *352*, 353
photon, in fast computed tomography, in myocardial perfusion measurement, 696–698, *696–698*
Scatter and veiling glare (SVG), in densitometry, 292, *292*, 293, *293*
Scatterers, myocardial, geometric attributes of, 544, *544*
Scattering, definition of, 539
dynamic aspects of, 545, *545*
factors in, 543
Rayleigh, 544
specular, 544
Schoonmaker technique, of coronary angiography, 192, *192*
Scimitar syndrome, 159
Scinticor detector, *1009*
Scintigraphy, antimyosin antibody, in infarct size measurement, *136*
image acquisition in, 982–984
dynamic, 983, 984
first-pass, 983, 984
multiple-gated, 984
static, 982, *982–984*, 983
multiple-gated, 982, *982–984*, 983
non-gated, 982
in cardiac parameter quantification, 988–1002
in sympathetic nerve assessment, 1135–1138, *1136*, *1137*
thallium-201. See *Thallium-201 scintigraphy*.
Scintillation camera, 979, *979*, 980, *980*
Scintillation counter, 977, 978
Scleroderma, in restrictive cardiomyopathy, 458
progressive systemic sclerosis with, thallium-201 scintigraphy in, 1066, 1066(t)
Secobarbital, in premedication, before coronary angiography, 189
Second harmonic, 999
Sedation, in magnetic resonance imaging, 779–781
Segmental endocardial motion, ultrafast computed tomography of, 673, *674*
Segmental wall thickening, ultrafast computed tomography of, 673, 674, *674*
Segmentation, in digital image processing, 82, 83, *83*, *84*
Selectan, 163, *164*
Selective excitation, 748
definition of, 1275
Selective pulse, 740
Semilunar valves, abnormalities of, ultrafast computed tomography of, *724*, 725
disease of, magnetic resonance imaging of, 887
Sensitive plane, definition of, 1275
Sensitivity, magnetic resonance, of sodium-23, 831
of nuclei, in magnetic resonance imaging, 842(t)
Sensitometer, in densitometry, 229
Septum(a), interatrial, aneurysm of, echocardiography of, 529, *530*
interventricular, 194
motion of, paradoxic, in right ventricular infarction, 396, 397
ventricular, portions of, 479, *480*
Sequence repetition time, *752*, 753
Sequence time, definition of, 1275
Sequestration, pulmonary, pulmonary angiography in, 157
Serotonin, effects of, on coronary circulation, 11
SFR. See *Stenosis flow reserve (SFR)*.
Shaded-surface display, in three-dimensional computed tomography, 660, *664*
in three-dimensional heart reconstruction, 73, *74*
"Shadow phenomenon," 697
"Shepherd's crook" deformity, of right coronary artery, 685, *685*
Shepp-Logan filter, *639*
Shield, Faraday, definition of, 1272
Shift reagents, definition of, 1275
in sodium magnetic resonance spectroscopy, 856, 857, *857*
Shimming, 788
definition of, 1275
"Shock excitation," 353
Shunt(ing), assessment of, magnetic resonance imaging in, 822
radionuclide angiocardiography in, 1021
ultrafast computed tomography in, 678
Blalock-Taussig, magnetic resonance imaging of, 879, *880*
cine magnetic resonance imaging of, 962
congenital, magnetic resonance imaging of, 888, *888–890*
extracardiac, magnetic resonance imaging of, 894
in congenital heart disease, ultrafast computed tomography of, 728, *728*
intracardiac, contrast echocardiography in, 568, 569
left-to-right, in patent ductus arteriosus, 483–486, *484*, *485*
quantitation of, Doppler echocardiography in, 487–489
radionuclide angiocardiography in, 1015, *1015*
right-to-left, at atrial level, Doppler echocardiography of, 495, 496
two-dimensional echocardiography of, 495, 496, *496*
at ventricular level, Doppler echocardiography of, 492–495, *494*, *495*
two-dimensional echocardiography of, 492–495
in patent ductus arteriosus, 485, *485*, 486
quantitation of, radionuclide angiocardiography in, 1014, *1014*
surgical, evaluation of, ultrafast computed tomography in, 730, *730*
magnetic resonance imaging of, 894
systemic-to-pulmonary artery, magnetic resonance imaging of, 876–879, *880*

Side lobes, 355, *355*
with linear-array transducer, 357
Siemens Digitron III system, 220, 221, 221(t)
Siemens Polytron 1000 VR system, 220, 221, 221(t)
Signal, analog, in nuclear magnetic resonance, 737
high-velocity, loss of, 864, *866*
in magnetic resonance imaging, 785
intensity of, in cardiac magnetic resonance imaging, 764, *764*
Signal averaging, definition of, 1275
in pulse Fourier transform nuclear magnetic resonance, 737
Signal void, in aortic regurgitation, 957, *958–960*
in aortic stenosis, 961, *961*
in cine magnetic resonance imaging, 951, *951*, *952*
in mitral regurgitation, 955, *957*
in tricuspid regurgitation, 958, *960*
Signal-to-noise ratio, 283
definition of, 1275
in magnetic resonance spectroscopy, 844
in pulse Fourier transform nuclear magnetic resonance, 737
Simple back projection, 635
Simpson's rule, 73, 375–377, *376*, 388
in right ventricular volume calculation, 393, *393*
Simpson's rule technique, 816, 817
Sinc pulse, 748, *749*
Single quantum transition, 829
Single ventricle, cine magnetic resonance imaging in, *962*
echocardiography in, *500*, *501*
ultrafast computed tomography in, 722, *722*, *724*
Single-beam echocardiography, display from, 356
Single-crystal gamma camera, in radionuclide angiocardiography, *1009*
in radionuclide imaging, 978–980, *979*, *980*
Single-photon emission computed tomography (SPECT), 984–988, *985*
attenuation correction in, 987
back-projection in, 985, *985*
filtered, 985, 986, *986*
clinical interpretation of, factors in, 986–988
image reconstruction in, 985, *985*, 986, *986*
filtering in, 986, *986*
instrumentation for, 1002
IPPA uptake in, after exercise, 1093, *1093*, 1094
multiple-gated, 988, *988*
object size correction in, 987
of indium-111 labeled platelets, 1122, 1123, *1123*
patient motion correction in, 987
projection acquisition in, 985
scatter correction in, 986, 987
Tc-sestamibi in, sensitivity of, 1103(t), *1104*
vs. thallium-201, 1105(t)
technetium-99m in, vs thallium-201, 987, 988, *988*, 988(t)
thallium-201 in, 1057, 1065
sensitivity of, 1103(t), *1104*
three-dimensional, of myocardial perfusion, 995, 996
uniformity correction in, 987
vs. antimyosin imaging, 1115
vs. myocardial metabolic activity, in tissue viability determination, 1229–1231, *1232*, *1233*
vs. planar imaging, 1090
vs. positron emission tomography, 1178, 1179
during exercise, 1174, *1175*
Single-photon emission computed tomography (SPECT) *Continued*
with equilibrium radionuclide angiography, 1032
Single-photon-emitting tracers, metabolic imaging with, 1085–1096
Single-plane area-length volume model, 375
Sinus, coronary, dilated, vs pericardial effusion, 464
Sinus of Valsalva, aneurysm of, magnetic resonance imaging of, 893
Sinus septum, 479
Sinus venosus atrial septal defect, *482*, 483
ultrafast computed tomography of, 715, *716*
Skeletal muscle, metabolism of, in heart disease, spectroscopy of, 972–974, *973*, *974*
Slice, definition of, 1275
Slice thickness, definition of, 1275
Smoking, and silent ischemia, detection of, positron emission tomography in, 1182, *1183*
Smoothing filtering, in myocardial perfusion scintigraphy, 989
S/N, definition of, 1275
SNR, definition of, 1275
Sodium, concentration of, in diatrizoate, 173
Larmor frequency of, 828
metabolism of, abnormal, 856
nucleus of, characteristics of, 828, 829, *829*, 842(t)
physiologic properties of, 828
Sodium iodide, as radiographic contrast agent, 163
Sodium iodide thallium, in radiation detection, 977, 978, *978*
Sodium magnetic resonance spectroscopy, 856–858
multiple quantum, 858
relaxation deconvolution in, 857, 858
shift reagents in, 856, 857, *857*
Sodium pyrophosphate, 830
Sodium warfarin, for pulmonary embolism, 154
Sodium-23, characteristics of, 828, 829, *829*
in magnetic resonance imaging, 828–840, *833–837*
contrast agents in, 837
projection-reconstruction methods of, 833, *833*
rotating frame technique of, 836, 837, *837*
spin-echo pulse sequence in, 834, *834*, 835
surface coil techniques of, 835, 836, *836*, *837*
three-dimensional Fourier techniques of, 833, 834, *834–836*
in magnetic resonance spectroscopy, 828–840
intracellular, 831–833
vs. extracellular, determination of, multiple quantum filter techniques of, 832, 833
paramagnetic shift reagents in, 832
magnetic resonance sensitivity of, 831
magnetic resonance spectra of, 830, *830*, 831
relaxation times of, 831, 832, 832(t)
tissue, density of, 831
"invisibility" of, 831
Solid-state memory, in on-line image storage, in digital angiography, 285
Sones technique, of coronary angiography, 190, 191, *191*
Sonicated contrast agents, for contrast echocardiography, 558, 559, *559*
Sonomicrometers, in transient ischemia, 31
Sound amplitude, measurement of, in ultrasound transmission, 351, 351(t)
Spatial domain, 82
Spatial filtration, in digital angiography, 288, 289, *289*
Spatial frequency, 76
Spatial presaturation, in magnetic resonance imaging, 785, 786
"Spatial registration," 73
Spatial resolution, 76
definition of, 1276
in computed tomography, 648, 649(t)
fast, 648, *649*, 649(t), *650*
single-photon emission, 985, *985*
three-dimensional, 643, 644, *644*
x-ray, *640*, 641
relationship of, to matrix size, *75*, 76
to temporal resolution, 1008, *1009*
Speckle, acoustic, 353
definition of, 539
Spectral analysis, in Doppler processing, 371, 372, *372*
Spectral broadening, 369, *369*
Spectral line, definition of, 1276
Spectrometer, definition of, 1276
Spectroscopy, carbon, 975
clinical applications of, 967–976
imaging in, 968, 969
in cardiac transplantation, 971, 972
in clinical studies, methodology of, 967
in dilated cardiomyopathy, 970, 971
in hypertrophic cardiomyopathy, 971, *972*
in myocardial ischemia, 970, *971*, *972*
localization techniques in, 967–969, *968*, *969*
magnetic resonance. See *Magnetic resonance spectroscopy (MRS).*
multiple quantum, 858
of normal myocardium, 969, *969*, 970, *970*
of skeletal muscle metabolism, in heart disease, 972–974, *973*, *974*
phosphorus, 967
proton, 974
rotating frame technique in, 968, *968*
Spectrum(a), definition of, 1276
of ethanol, 734, *735*
of nuclear magnetic resonance, 734, 735, *735*
amplitude of, 746
of sodium-23, crystal-like, 830, *830*
extreme narrowing, 830, *830*
homogeneous, 830, *830*, 831
magnetic resonance, 830, *830*, 831
powder, inhomogeneous, 830, *830*, 831
Specular reflection, 539
Specular reflector, 351, 352, *352*
Specular scattering, 544
Spin, definition of, 1276
nuclear, 732, 733, 733(t)
definition of, 1274
in magnetic resonance imaging, 842(t)
tagged, washout of, 774, *774*
Spin angular momentum, 732
Spin density, definition of, 1276
Spin echo, creation of, 747, *747*
definition of, 1276
Spin echo pulse sequence, in magnetic resonance imaging, of great vessels, 864, *865*
Spin number, nuclear, definition of, 1276
Spin quantum number, 732
Spin states, 733, 734
Spin tagging, definition of, 1276
Spindle cell sarcoma, of lung, magnetic resonance imaging of, *944*
Spin-down orientation, 733
Spin-echo imaging, contrast-to-noise ratio in, 799
definition of, 1276
gated, in left ventricular hypertrophy, *898*
in aortic stenosis, *909*

Spin-echo imaging *(Continued)*
in hypertrophic cardiomyopathy, 929, *930*
in pericardial effusion, *903*
in restrictive cardiomyopathy, 934, *934*
in valvular disease, 896, 897, *897*
of aorta, 953
of aortic dissection, 871, *871*, *872*
of blood flow, 773
of chronic thrombi, 903, *903*
Spin-echo pulse sequence(s), hybrid, in sodium magnetic resonance imaging, 834
in magnetic resonance imaging, in cardiac quantitation, 812, *812*
with sodium-23, 834, *834*, 835
in multipulse nuclear magnetic resonance, 740, *740*, 741, *741*
interaction of, with paramagnetic contrast agents, 799–808, *800–809*
Spin-lattice relaxation time, 735, 753
definition of, 1276
Spin-phase effects, in magnetic resonance imaging, of great vessels, 865, *866*
Spin-spin coupling, definition of, 1276
Spin-spin relaxation time, 735–738, 753
definition of, 1276
Spin-up orientation, 733
Spin-warp imaging, concepts of, 750–752, *750*, *751*
definition of, 1276
practical aspects of, 752, *752*, 753, *753*
two-dimensional, 750, *750*
Split-and-merge techniques, in segmentation, 83, *84*
Standing wave pattern, 352
Starvation, in protein turnover regulation, 52
Steady state free precession, definition of, 1276
Stenosis, aortic. See *Aortic stenosis.*
aortic valve, roentgenographic evaluation of, 104
arterial, blood flow in, 215, *215*
bypass graft, ultrafast computed tomography of, 684, 685, *685*
coronary. See *Coronary stenosis.*
coronary artery, congenital, 198
severity of, in function, 135(t)
eccentricity of, 226
energy loss across, sources of, 215, *215*, *311*
identification of, distal coronary perfusion pressure in, 250, 251(t)
mitral. See *Mitral stenosis.*
percent diameter. See *Percent diameter stenosis.*
prosthetic, echocardiography in, 440, 441
pulmonary. See *Pulmonary stenosis.*
pulmonary artery, pulmonary angiography in, 156, *157*
pulmonic, infundibular, cine magnetic resonance imaging in, *962*
severity of, clinical evaluation of, 64
slit-like, with crescent shape, evaluation of, 228, *228*
tricuspid. See *Tricuspid stenosis.*
valvular. See *Valve stenosis.*
Stenosis flow reserve (SFR), 243
vs. coronary flow reserve, 1175, 1176, 1176(t)
vs. myocardial perfusion reserve, 1179, *1179*
vs. percent diameter narrowing, 1175, *1175*
Stenosis geometry, visual interpretation of, variability in, 213, *213*, 214
Stenotic lesions, cine magnetic resonance imaging of, 959–962, *961*
Stenotic segment area, in reactive hyperemia, 319, *319*, *320*
Stent(ing), implantation of, neointimal thickening after, 267
Stent(ing) *(Continued)*
percutaneous transluminal coronary angioplasty with, minimal luminal cross-sectional area after, 266, *266*
in endoluminal prostheses, description of, 264, *264*, *265*
results of, hemodynamic, 266(t)
morphologic, 266, 266(t), 267
Stereoselectivity, of ligand-receptor complex, 1259, 1260, *1260*
Sternum, osteogenic sarcoma of, magnetic resonance imaging of, *945*
Steroids, for contrast agent allergy, 189
Stethoscope, nuclear, 981
Streptokinase, assessment of, magnetic resonance imaging in, 925, 926, 926(t)
for pulmonary embolism, 155
Stress, and silent ischemia, detection of, positron emission tomography in, 1182, *1182*
imaging during, thallium-201 scintigraphy in, 1053–1057, *1054–1056*
in ventricular function evaluation, 27, 27(t)
left ventricular, 123, 124, *125*
Stress echocardiography, 575–593
non-exercise, 589–591, 590(t)
studies of, analysis of, 580
techniques of, 575–580
Stress ventriculography, in cardiac reserve assessment, 135
"Stroke distance," 403, *404*
Stroke volume, 122
aortic, in mitral regurgitation, 436
calculation of, magnetic resonance imaging in, 819, *819*
diastolic, transmitral, 408
Doppler, determination of, 403, 404
during exercise, measurement of, Doppler echocardiography in, 578, *578*
vs. thermodilution, 578, *579*
exercise-induced increase in, 407
in aortic regurgitation, forward, 430
regurgitant, 430
total, 430
in valvular regurgitation, 66
mitral, in mitral regurgitation, 436
of aortic root, calculation of, 58, *58*
of left ventricle, determination of, 403, *405*
ultrafast computed tomography in, 671, *671*
of right ventricle, evaluation of, ultrafast computed tomography in, *676*, 677, *677*
Stroke work, systolic, 139
Stunned myocardium, 597, 598
in right ventricular function, 31, 32
wall motion abnormalities in, 32
Subaortic stenosis, left ventricular outflow obstruction in, 490, *490*
muscular, in hypertrophic cardiomyopathy, 450, 451, *451*, *452*
Subendocardium, of left ventricle, autoregulation gain in, 9
Subepicardium, of left ventricle, autoregulation gain in, 9
Submaximal coronary dilators, 15
Substrates, bioenergetic effects of, in phosphorus magnetic resonance spectroscopy, 847, 848
Subtracted digital images, 218
Subtraction, energy, 288
mask mode, 288
temporal, 288
types of, 297–300, 298(t)
Subvalvular pulmonary stenosis, in right ventricular outflow obstruction, 492, *494*
Succinyl-CoA, in lipid metabolism, 46, *48*
Summation mask subtraction, 298(t), 299
Superconductor, definition of, 1276
Superior vena cava syndrome, magnetic resonance imaging in, 879–881, *881*
Superparamagnetic perfusion agents, 807, *807–809*, 808
Superparamagnetic relaxing agents, 797, *797*, 798, *798*, 798(t)
Suppression, definition of, 1276
Supravalvular aortic stenosis, left ventricular outflow obstruction in, 491, *491*
magnetic resonance imaging in, 871, *871*, 893
Surface coil, definition of, 1276
for magnetic resonance spectroscopy, 843, 844
Surface coil technique, in magnetic resonance imaging, with sodium-23, 835, 836, *836*, *837*
Susceptibility flowering, 788
Suture lines, surgical, echocardiography of, 529, *532*
SVG (scatter and veiling glare), in densitometry, 292, *292*, 293, *293*
Sympathetic nerves, in myocardial perfusion, 10, 11
scintigraphic assessment of, 1135–1138, *1136*, *1137*
Systemic arterial pressure, after intravascular bolus injection, of angiographic contrast agents, 169, *169*
after selective intracoronary injection, of angiographic contrast agents, 170, 171, *171*, *172*
during breath holding, 171, *172*
Systemic vascular resistance, after intravascular bolus injection, of angiographic contrast agents, 168, *169*
Systole, left ventricular motion during, 25
Systolic anterior motion, in hypertrophic cardiomyopathy, 450, 451, *451*
Systolic dysfunction, in infarction, 382
in ischemia, 382
Systolic ejection velocity, Doppler, during percutaneous transluminal coronary angioplasty, 407
Systolic function, after myocardial infarction, two-dimensional echocardiography of, 382
left ventricular, in dilated cardiomyopathy, Doppler echocardiography of, 456
ventricular, exercise effect on, 407
in restrictive cardiomyopathy, echocardiography of, 457
Systolic performance, Doppler indices of, 407, 408
left ventricular, 35
Systolic pressure, left ventricular, in mitral regurgitation, 403, *405*
right ventricular, in tricuspid regurgitation, Doppler echocardiography of, 438–440, *439*
Systolic stroke work, 139
Systolic velocity–time integral (VTI), 403, *404*
Systolic wall, thickening of, analysis of, 390, 391, *391*
algorithms for, 391, *391*
threshold phenomenon in, 390
vs. wall motion analysis, 390, 391, *391*

T1, 738, 896
definition of, 1276
estimation of, magnetic resonance imaging in, 820
GdDTPA effect on, 799, *801*, 801(t)
in acute myocardial infarction, 913, 913(t)
protons of, in water, 759, 760
T2, 738, 896
definition of, 1276

T2 *(Continued)*
GdDTPA effect on, 799, *801*, 801(t)
in acute myocardial infarction, 913, 913(t)
protons of, in water, 759, 760
T2 relaxation time, determination of, magnetic resonance imaging in, 820
Tachycardia, after intracoronary contrast agent injection, 187
in myocardial oxygen consumption, 9
Tagged spins, washout of, 774, *774*
Tagging, myocardial, magnetic resonance imaging in, 820, *820*
Takayasu's arteritis, 156, *157*
magnetic resonance imaging in, 876
Tantalum-178, in radionuclide angiocardiography, 1010, 1010(t)
TAPSE (tricuspid annular plane systolic excursion) index, 394
TBI (technetium-99m-t-butyl isonitrile), 1097, *1098*
Tc-99m-PPi, in damaged myocardium, concentration of, 1079, *1079*
deposition of, 1077–1079, *1078*
in acute myocardial infarct sizing, 1080–1083
after temporary coronary artery occlusion, 1083
in infarct avid imaging, 1074–1084, *1075*
in myocardial infarction, in detection, 1080, *1081–1083*
in localization, 1079, *1079*, *1080*
sensitivity of, 1080
Tc-sestamibi, 1097, *1098–1100*
clinical trials of, 1102–1107, 1102(t), *1103–1106*, 1103(t)
in left ventricular ejection fraction measurement, *1106*
in planar imaging, sensitivity of, *1103*, 1103(t)
vs. thallium-201, 1105(t)
in single-photon emission computed tomography, sensitivity of, 1103(t), *1104*
vs. thallium-201, 1105(t)
properties of, imaging, 1102(t)
physiologic, 1101, 1101(t)
uptake of, 1100, 1101(t)
Tc-teboroxime, 1100, *1100*, 1101
clinical trials of, 1107, *1107*, 1108
properties of, imaging, 1102(t)
physiologic, 1101, 1101(t)
uptake of, 1100, 1101(t)
vs. thallium-201, 1107, *1107*, 1108
TE, definition of, 1276
Technetium pyrophosphate imaging, in infarct size measurement, *136*
Technetium-99m, energy spectrum of, 978, *979*
in radionuclide angiocardiography, 1010, 1010(t)
vs. thallium-201, in single-photon emission computed tomography, 987, 988, *988*, 988(t)
Technetium-99m agents, in left ventricular ejection fraction measurement, *1106*
in myocardial perfusion imaging, 1097–1109
Technetium-99m BATO compounds, properties of, 1100, *1100*, 1101, 1101(t), 1102(t)
Technetium-99m carboxyisopropyl isonitrile, 1097, *1098*
Technetium-99m diethylene triamine pentaacetic acid, in left ventricular ejection fraction measurement, *1106*
Technetium-99m isonitriles, 1053
imaging with, clinical application of, 1067, 1068
properties of, 1097–1100, *1098*, *1099*
Technetium-99m methoxy-isobutyl isonitrile, 1097, *1098*
Technetium-99m pertechnetate, in left ventricular ejection fraction measurement, *1106*
Technetium-99m pyrophosphate, in myocardial infarction, 1113, *1113*
Technetium-99m-t-butyl isonitrile (TBI), 1097, *1098*
Tellurium, 1090
Temporal resolution, 76
in computed tomography, three-dimensional, 643, 644
ultrafast, 669
in gradient reversal, in cine magnetic resonance imaging, 812
spatial resolution relationship to, 1008, *1009*
Temporal subtraction, 288
Tendons, false, echocardiography of, 529, *530*
Teratoma, 512
of pericardium, magnetic resonance imaging of, 940
Tesla, definition of, 1276
Tethering, 382
Tetralogy of Fallot, echocardiography in, 494, *494*
magnetic resonance imaging in, 888–890, *890*, *891*
repair of, pulmonary artery occlusion after, magnetic resonance imaging of, 890, *891*
ultrafast computed tomography in, 719, *721*
Texture, of gray level, 541–543, *542*
in ischemia, 546, *547*
TGC (time gain compensation), 360, *360*
Thallium-201, in coronary artery disease, 1023, 1093
in myocardial infarction, 1091, *1091*
in myocardial perfusion imaging, 1047–1073
in planar imaging, sensitivity of, *1103*, 1103(t)
vs. Tc-sestamibi, 1105(t)
in single-photon emission computed tomography, 1057
sensitivity of, 1103(t), *1104*
vs. Tc-sestamibi, 1105(t)
vs. technetium-99m, 987, 988, *988*, 988(t)
persistent defects of, 1050, 1051, *1051*
redistribution of, delayed, 1048–1050, *1049*, *1050*
reverse, 1051
tissue tracer kinetics of, 1047–1053
uptake of, 1100, 1101(t)
by lung, 1051–1053, *1052*
kinetics of, 1047, 1048, *1048*
vs. Tc-teboroxime, 1107, *1107*, 1108
Thallium-201 scintigraphy, after myocardial infarction, 1063, 1064, *1064*
after thrombolytic therapy, 1064, 1065
applications of, clinical, 1057–1066, 1058(t)
prognostic, 1060–1063, *1061–1063*, 1061(t)
dipyridamole in, 1055, 1056, 1065, 1065(t), 1066
in non-exercise stress echocardiography, 590
history of, 1047
image analysis in, 1057
image display in, 1057
in asymptomatic patient, 1057, 1058, *1059*
in chest pain, 1058–1060, 1060(t)
in ischemic heart disease, 587, *587*
in myocardial revascularization assessment, 1064, *1065*
in noncoronary heart disease, 1066, 1066(t), 1067
in rest imaging, 1056, 1057
in single-photon emission computed tomography, 1065
in stress imaging, 1053–1057, *1054–1056*
Thallium-201 scintigraphy *(Continued)*
limitations of, 1067, 1067(t)
redistribution, vs. myocardial metabolic activity, in tissue viability determination, 1229–1231, *1232*, *1233*
vs. exercise echocardiography, 585, 586
vs. positron emission tomography, 1178, 1179
with percutaneous transluminal coronary angioplasty, 1064, *1065*
Thermal equilibrium, definition of, 1276
Thermodilution, during exercise, vs. Doppler echocardiography, in stroke volume measurement, 578, *579*
in coronary blood flow measurement, 244
Thoracic aortic aneurysm, ultrafast computed tomography of, 710–712, *711*
Thoracic dissection, ultrafast computed tomography of, 710, 711, *711*, *712*
Three-dimensional beam formation, in electronic beam steering, 359, *359*
Three-dimensional computed tomography, dynamic, 643–665, *644*
image analysis and display in, 659–665, *660–665*
Three-dimensional Fourier transform, in magnetic resonance imaging, with sodium-23, 833, 834, *834–836*
Three-dimensional magnetic resonance imaging, in cardiac quantitation, 824, *824*
Three-dimensional reconstruction, of heart, 73, 73(t), 74, *74*
shaded-surface displays in, 73, *74*
wire-frame displays in, 73, *74*
of left ventricle, ultrafast computed tomography in, 676, *676*
Three-dimensional single-photon emission computed tomography, in myocardial perfusion, 995, 996
Three-dimensional tomography, in myocardial perfusion quantification, 992–994, *992*, *993*
Threshold phenomenon, in systolic wall thickening analysis, 390
Thresholds, gray level, in segmentation, 82, 83, *83*
Thromboembolism, coronary angiography and, 186, 186(t)
Thrombogeneity, of graft materials, 1129, 1130
Thrombolysis, coronary, in myocardial infarction, myocardial metabolic effects of, 1218, 1219, *1220*, *1221*
Thrombolytic therapy, as coronary angiography indication, 184
for pulmonary embolism, 154, *154*
reperfusion after, technetium-99m isonitrile imaging in, 1068
thallium-201 scintigraphy after, 1064, 1065
Thrombosis, imaging of, indium-111–labeled platelets in, 1121–1134
venous, imaging of, indium-111–labeled platelets in, 1128, 1129
Thrombus(i), cardiac, imaging of, indium-111–labeled platelets in, 1124, *1124*, 1124(t), 1125, *1125*
chronic, spin-echo imaging of, 903, *903*
echocardiographic evaluation of, 520–528
intra-atrial, transesophageal echocardiography of, *610*, 611
intracardiac, echocardiography of, 520–528, *523–529*
ultrafast computed tomography of, 705–707, *705*, *706*
indications for, 706, *707*
scanning sequences in, 706
ultrasonic tissue characterization in, 553

Thrombus(i) *(Continued)*
intracavitary, detection of, ultrafast computed tomography in, 706
in dilated cardiomyopathy, echocardiography of, 454, *455*
of left ventricle, after myocardial infarction, 600, *601*, *602*
organization of, in chronic pulmonary embolism, 153
pulmonary artery, ultrafast computed tomography of, 705–707, *707*
vascular, imaging of, indium-111–labeled platelets in, 1125–1128, 1126(t), *1127*, *1128*
vs. papillary muscle, on ultrafast computed tomography, 705
TI, definition of, 1276
TID (time interval difference) imaging, 288
Time domain filtration, 288
Time gain compensation (TGC), 360, *360*
Time interval difference, 298(t)
Time interval difference (TID) imaging, 288
Time interval histogram, 371
Time of arrival images, in hyperemia, *336*
Time-density analysis, of digital subtraction arteriography, *331*
Time-density curve, in measurement, of coronary flow reserve, 329, *329*
of coronary stenosis, 329, *330*
Time-of-arrival mapping, 298(t)
Time-of-flight artifact, *772*, 773
Time-of-flight effects, in magnetic resonance imaging, of great vessels, 864, 865, *866*
Tissue, acoustically abnormal, 541, 542
hypoperfused and metabolically active, revascularization of, 1222–1225, *1223*, *1224*, 1225(t)
myocardial, viability of, determination of, myocardial metabolism in, 1219–1237, *1226–1228*
relaxation time of, factors in, *763*
in vivo, 760
ultrasonic characterization of. See *Ultrasonic tissue characterization.*
water in, in myocardial acoustics, 544
Tissue characterization, magnetic resonance imaging in, 820–822
in infarct size measurement, 821, *821*, 822, *822*
limitations of, 821
ultrasonic. See *Ultrasonic tissue characterization.*
Tomography, 984–988
computed. See *Computed tomography (CT).*
positron emission. See *Positron emission tomography (PET).*
three-dimensional, in myocardial perfusion quantification, 992–994, *992*, *993*
with scintigraphy, in myocardial perfusion quantification, 992–995, *992*, *993*, *995*
Top-down theory, of image perception, 88
Total anomalous pulmonary venous return, echocardiography in, 499, *499*
magnetic resonance imaging in, 892
Total stroke volume, in aortic regurgitation, 430
Toxicity, acute, of angiographic contrast agents, 166–168
doxorubicin, diagnosis of, spectroscopy in, 970
monitoring of, equilibrium radionuclide angiography in, 1042
methysergide, and tricuspid stenosis, 436
TR, definition of, 1276
Trabeculae, ventricular, echocardiography of, 529, *530*
Trabeculated septum, 479
Tracer(s), in positron emission tomography, concentration of, 1157, *1157*, 1158, *1158*
in myocardial blood flow evaluation, 1161–1163, 1170, *1170*, 1170(t), 1171
kinetics of, models of, 1158, 1159, *1159*
uptake of, quantitative analysis of, 1179, *1179*
of metabolism, in myocardial ischemia, clinical investigations with, 1198–1203
positron-emitting, 1141–1153, 1141(t)
of cardiac innervation, 1141(t), 1152
of myocardial blood flow, 1141–1145, 1141(t), *1142*, *1143*
of myocardial metabolism, 1141(t), 1145–1152, *1145–1152*
single-photon-emitting, metabolic imaging with, 1085–1096
uptake of, vs. absolute perfusion, 1173
Tracing, of endocardial contours, 120, *120*, *121*
Transcatheter embolization therapy, for arteriovenous fistulae, 156
Transducer(s), annular-array, focusing of, 355, *355*
design of, 353
Doppler, 368, *368*, 369, *369*
linear-array, 357
position of, in epicardial echocardiography, 618–620, *619*, *620*
aorta–pulmonary sulcus, 619, *619*, 620
aorta–superior vena cava, 620, *620*
parasternal equivalent, 619, *619*
subcostal equivalent, 620
preparation of, for epicardial echocardiography, 620
rotating-head, 356
single-crystal, focusing of, 354, *354*
wobbling, 356
Transesophageal echocardiography, ambulatory, indications for, 609–612, 609(t)
anatomic views in, 607, *607–609*, 608
biplane, 614–616, 614(t), 621, *621*
of aortic valve, *615*
of left ventricle, 614, *614*
of right ventricular outflow tract, *615*
complications of, 613
contraindications to, 613, 613(t)
future developments in, 614–616, *614*, 614(t), *615*
historical development of, 605, 605(t), 606
imaging planes for, 621, *621*
in aortic regurgitation, 425, 426
in clinical cardiology, 605–617
in left atrial thrombi, 526, *527*
in mitral regurgitation, 433, 434
in mitral stenosis, 430, 431
intraoperative, 620, 621
probes for, 606, *606*
safety of, 613, 614
technique of, 606, *606*, 606(t), 607
training for, 612, 613
Transfer, magnetization, 846, 847, *847*
Transfer function, 846
regional, assessment of, fast computed tomography in, 700
Transfer function analysis, in functional assessment, of coronary circulation, 331–334, *333*, *334*
Transgastric echocardiography, 608
Transient ischemia, in right ventricular function, 31
regional wall motion abnormalities in, 31
Transit times, calculation of, radionuclide angiocardiography in, *1014*, 1015
Transit velocity, 369
Transit-time analysis, in functional assessment, of coronary circulation, 325–328, *326–328*
Translational wall motion, 383, *384*
correction for, 124, *127*
Transmission, attenuation in, measurement of, 540, *540*
Transmission images, in positron emission tomography, of myocardial blood flow, 1171
"Transmit ghost," 788, *791*
Transmitral diastolic stroke volume, 408
Transplantation, cardiac, as coronary angiography indication, 184, *185*
spectroscopy in, 971, 972
Transposition, *96*
Transposition of great arteries, echocardiography of, 497, *497*, *506*, *507*
magnetic resonance imaging of, 876, *877*, 892, *892*
ultrafast computed tomography of, 722, *722*
Transvalvular aortic velocity, in aortic stenosis, 421
Transvalvular pressure gradient, in aortic stenosis, 421, *423*
in prosthetic stenosis, 441, *442*
Transvenous percutaneous embolectomy, 155
Transverse magnetization, definition of, 1276
in magnetic resonance spectroscopy, 844
Treadmill exercise, Doppler echocardiography during, 577, *577*
in submaximal coronary dilation, 15
systolic ventricular function during, 407
two-dimensional echocardiography during, 576, 577
Trendelenburg's position, end-diastolic left ventricular volume in, 27
Triazolam, for sedation, in magnetic resonance imaging, 779
Tricarboxylic acid cycle, 39, *40*, 46–48
during exercise, 49
in ischemia, 49
Tricuspid annular plane systolic excursion (TAPSE) index, 394
Tricuspid annuloplasty, 441
Tricuspid atresia, echocardiography in, 495, *495*
magnetic resonance imaging in, 890, 891, *891*
ultrafast computed tomography in, 717, *718*
Tricuspid regurgitation, causes of, 437, 438
cine magnetic resonance imaging in, 958, 959, *960*
echocardiography in, 437–440
Doppler, 438
in decision-making, 440
M-mode, 438
two-dimensional, 437, 438
hepatic vein blood flow in, 438, *438*
in dilated cardiomyopathy, echocardiography of, 455, 456
magnetic resonance imaging in, 903
right ventricular ejection in, 414
right ventricular systolic pressure in, estimation of, Doppler echocardiography in, 438–440, *439*
roentgenographic evaluation of, 105
severity of, color flow imaging in, 438
evaluation of, 69
pulsed-wave mapping of, 438
signal void in, 958, *960*
valve repair for, intraoperative echocardiography during, 624, 625
Tricuspid stenosis, causes of, 436
cine magnetic resonance imaging in, 962
echocardiography in, 436, 437, *437*
Doppler, 436, *437*
in decision-making, 436, 437
two-dimensional, 436
roentgenographic evaluation of, 105
severity of, clinical evaluation of, 64
Tricuspid valve, Ebstein's anomaly of, 105

Tricuspid valve *(Continued)*
function of, in dilated cardiomyopathy, echocardiography of, 454–456
prolapse of, 437
Triggering, cardiac. See also *Gating.*
in magnetic resonance imaging, 781–783, 781(t), *782, 783*
electrocardiographic, 781, 781(t), *782*
pulse, 781, 781(t), *782*
respiratory, in magnetic resonance imaging, 783, 783(t), 784, *785*
Triglycerides, in fasting, 49
in lipid metabolism, 44
radioiodine labeled, 1088, *1088*
Triphenylmethylphosphonium, C-11–labeled, 1153
Triphenyltetrazolium chloride (TTC), in gamma imaging, *1112*, 1113
"Triple orthogonality," 322, *323*, 324
Triple quantum transition, 829
Truncus arteriosus, echocardiography of, 497, 498, *498*
magnetic resonance imaging of, 894
TTC (triphenyltetrazolium chloride), in gamma imaging, *1112*, 1113
Tumor(s), benign, of pericardium, ultrafast computed tomography of, 709
cardiac, echocardiography of, 512–520
metastatic, echocardiography of, 519, 519(t), 520, *520, 521*
primary, benign, echocardiography of, 512–517, *514–518*
echocardiography of, 512–519, 512(t), *514–519*
malignant, echocardiography of, 517–519, *518, 519*
infradiaphragmatic, intracardiac extensions of, 704, 705, *705*
intracardiac, ultrafast computed tomography of, 703–705
metastatic, ultrafast computed tomography of, 704, 705
of mediastinum, echocardiography of, 520, *522, 523*
transesophageal echocardiography of, *610*, 611
Tuning, definition of, 1277
Turbulence, in blood flow physics, 368
Turbulent resistance, after stenting, 266(t)
"Twinkling" phenomenon, 12
Two-dimensional echocardiography, centerline method of, 387, *387*
during exercise, 575–577, *576*
in coronary artery disease diagnosis, 582, 583
in aortic dissection, 426, *426*
in aortic regurgitation, 430
in aortic stenosis, 420, *420*, 421
in atrial septal defects, *482*, 483
in atrioventricular septal defects, 486, 487, *487, 488*
in cardiac tamponade, 464–470, *466–471*
in congenital heart disease, 479–510
with acyanosis, and increased pulmonary flow, 479–489
with cyanosis, and decreased pulmonary vascularity, 492–496, *494–496*
and increased pulmonary vascularity, 496–499, *497–499*
with ventricular outflow obstruction, 489–492
in constrictive pericarditis, 470–475, *472, 473*
in ejection fraction measurement, 379, *380*
in end-diastolic volume measurement, *379*
in end-systolic volume measurement, *379*
in infarct size determination, 388, *390*
in left ventricular outflow obstruction, 489–492, *490, 491*

Two-dimensional echocardiography *(Continued)*
in mitral regurgitation, 433, *434*
in mitral stenosis, 430, 431
in patent ductus arteriosus, 483, *484*
in pericardial effusion, 460, *463*
in prosthetic stenosis, 440, 441
in pulmonary stenosis, 440
in systolic function assessment, after myocardial infarction, 382
in tricuspid regurgitation, 437, 438
in tricuspid stenosis, 436
in valvuloplasty, 441–443
in ventricular septal defects, 479–483, *480, 481*
intraoperative, 618
of increased pulmonary arterial markings, 496–499, *497, 498*
of increased pulmonary venous markings, 499, *499*
of right ventricle, in functional assessment, 392
in outflow obstruction, 492, *493, 494*
in size assessment, 392, 393
of right-to-left shunting, at atrial level, 495, 496, *496*
at ventricular level, 492–495
vs. contrast ventriculography, 382
vs. ultrafast computed tomography, in intracardiac thrombus detection, 706
Two-dimensional Fourier transform, 752
Two-dimensional Fourier transform imaging, definition of, 1277
Type I eccentric lesions, 214
Type II eccentric lesions, 214

UDPG (uridine diphosphate glucose), in myocardial metabolism, 40
Ultrafast computed tomography, advantages of, 669, 670
disadvantages of, 670, *670*, 671
in congenital heart disease, 714–731
clinical experience with, 714, 715
in postoperative evaluation, 728–730, 728(t), *729, 730*
technique of, 715
in evaluation, of bypass graft patency, 682–687
of cardiac anatomy, 715–725, *716–724, 726, 727*
of cardiac output, 678, *678*
of cardiac valves, 678, 679, *679*
of coronary anatomy, 680, *680*
of extracardiac abnormalities, 703–713
of intracardiac masses, 703–713
of left atrial volume, 678
of left ventricle, 671–676
of right atrial volume, 678
of right ventricular anatomy, 26, 676–678
of shunts, 678
of ventricular volume and mass, in congenital heart disease, 728
in interventional studies, of left ventricular function, 679, 680
in pulmonary emboli, 706, *707*
of blood flow, in congenital heart disease, 725–728, *728*
of intracardiac thrombi, 705–707, *705, 706*
of mediastinal masses, 712, *712*, 713
of pericardium, 707–710
of pulmonary artery thrombi, 705–707, *707*
of thoracic aortic aneurysms, 710–712, *711*
temporal resolution of, 669
vs. two-dimensional echocardiography, in intracardiac thrombus detection, 706
Ultrasonic contrast techniques, in coronary artery disease, 602

Ultrasonic tissue characterization, 538–556
approaches to, 540–543
basic concepts of, 539–543
definition of, 538
in atherosclerosis, 553, *553*
in cardiomyopathy, 549–553, *551, 552*
in coronary artery disease, 603
in intracardiac masses, 553
in ischemic heart disease, 545–548, *546–550*
in myocardial contusion, 553
measurement techniques in, 540–543, *540–542*
Ultrasonic wavelength, definition of, 539
Ultrasound, diagnostic, wavelengths in, 350(t)
generation of, piezoelectricity in, 350, *350*, 350(t)
in coronary artery imaging, 602, 603, *603*, 625–630, *626*
transmission of, 351–353
in imperfect medium, 351–353, 351(t)
reflection in, 351, 352, *352*
refraction in, 351, 352, *352*
scatter in, 352, *352*, 353
sound amplitude measurement in, 351, 351(t)
Undersampling, 76, *76*
Uniformity, in computed tomography, 649, *652*, 652(t)
in fast computed tomography, 649, 652(t), *653*
UPET (Urokinase Pulmonary Embolism Trial), 155
Uridine diphosphate glucose (UDPG), in myocardial metabolism, 40
Uridine triphosphate (UTP), in myocardial metabolism, 40
Urokinase, for pulmonary embolism, 155
Urokinase Pulmonary Embolism Trial (UPET), 155
Urokinase/Streptokinase Pulmonary Embolism Trial (USPET), 155
Urokon, *164*, 165
Uroselectan, 163, *164*
Uroselectan B, 163, *164*
USPET (Urokinase/Streptokinase Pulmonary Embolism Trial), 155
UTP (uridine triphosphate), in myocardial metabolism, 40

Vagal responses, coronary angiography and, 186
Validation studies, densitometric, in vivo, 237, 238
of arterial dimensions, 236, 237
phantom, 237
repeated, variability in, 238
nondensitometric, of arterial dimensions, 236, 237
of quantitative arteriography, in coronary artery assessment, 313–319, *315, 317*
of quantitative coronary angiography, 236–242
computer analysis in, 238–241, 239(t), 240(t)
results of, parameters describing, 236
Valium, for sedation, in magnetic resonance imaging, 779
Valve(s), abnormal motions of, in pericardial effusion, 464
aortic. See *Aortic valve.*
atrioventricular, abnormalities of, ultrafast computed tomography of, 716, 717, *718, 719*
disease of, magnetic resonance imaging of, 887

Valve(s) *(Continued)*
in atrioventricular defect, 487, *488*
cardiac, evaluation of, ultrafast computed tomography in, 678, 679, *679*
diseases of, cine magnetic resonance imaging in, 897, 898, *898*
magnetic resonance imaging in, mechanisms of, 896, 897, *897*
nuclear magnetic resonance in, 896–910
pulmonary, echocardiography in, 440
roentgenographic evaluation of, 104, 105
eustachian, echocardiography of, 500, *501*, 511, *512*
function of, after interventions, 440–443
evaluation of, physiologic basis for, 56–71
lesions of, hemodynamics of, 56–71
mitral. See *Mitral valve.*
prosthetic, Doppler echocardiography of, 441, *442*
evaluation of, transesophageal echocardiography in, 611
replacement of, intraoperative echocardiography during, 624
regurgitation of. See *Valvular regurgitation.*
semilunar, abnormalities of, ultrafast computed tomography of, *724*, 725
disease of, magnetic resonance imaging of, 887
tricuspid. See *Tricuspid valve.*
vegetations of, giant, echocardiography of, 529, *532*
in aortic regurgitation, 425
in mitral regurgitation, 434, *435*
Valve areas, 122, 123
Valve orifice velocity, measurement of, 60
Valve resistance, in valve stenosis, 64
Valve stenosis, 59–64
blood velocity in, calculation of, Doppler equation in, 61, 62, *62*
patterns of, 59, 60, *60*, *61*
clinical comparisons of, 64
flow-independent measurement of, 63, 64
magnetic resonance imaging in, 903, *904–906*
pressure gradients in, measurement of, invasive standards for, 62, 63, *63*
quantification of, 60–63
severity of, quantification of, 56
variable-orifice, 64, *65*
vs. left ventricular outflow obstruction, 420
Valvular aortic stenosis, subvalvular pressure gradients in, 60
Valvular heart disease, as coronary angiography indication, 184
cine magnetic resonance imaging in, 955–962, *957–961*
echocardiography in, 419–448
equilibrium radionuclide angiography in, 1040, *1040*, 1041, *1041*
native, 419–440
quantification of, hemodynamic equations for, 56–59
radionuclide angiocardiography in, 1021
rheumatic, cine magnetic resonance imaging in, *960*
Valvular pulmonary stenosis, in right ventricular outflow obstruction, 492, *493*
Valvular regurgitation, 64–69
blood velocity patterns in, 65–67, *65–67*
distal, 66, *66*, 67, *67*
proximal, 66, *66*
calculation of, radionuclide angiocardiography in, 1015
magnetic resonance imaging in, 898–903, *899–903*
quantification of, angiography in, 67, 68, 68(t)
Valvular regurgitation *(Continued)*
invasive standards for, 67, 68
magnetic resonance imaging in, 823, *823*
regurgitant fraction in, 66, *66*, 67, *67*
severity of, hemodynamic indicators of, 68, 69, *69*
transvalvular pressure gradients in, 66, *66*
Valvular surgery, intraoperative echocardiography during, 622–624
Valvuloplasty, aortic balloon, 441, 442
echocardiography in, 441–443
Doppler, 441–443
two-dimensional, 441–443
mitral balloon, 431, 441
percutaneous, transesophageal echocardiography in, 612
Variability, in wall motion analysis, 132, *132*
Variable-orifice stenotic valves, 64, *65*
Varix, pulmonary, pulmonary angiography in, 157
Vascoray, *164*
properties of, 166, 167(t)
Vascular lesions, pulmonary, pulmonary angiography for, 155–159
Vascular resistance, systemic, after intravascular bolus injection, of angiographic contrast agents, 168, *169*
Vascular ring, magnetic resonance imaging of, 867, *869*, *870*, 893, 894
Vascular thrombi, imaging of, indium-111–labeled platelets in, 1125–1128, 1126(t), *1127*, *1128*
Vasculature, pulmonary, normal anatomy of, 151
Vasoconstriction, in pulmonary embolism, 153
Vasodilation, coronary, effects of, on coronary vascular volume, 20
Vasodilator(s), coronary, clinical use of, 15, *15*, 16
in heart failure, ejection velocity after, 407
preangiographic administration of, in quantitative coronary arteriography, 232, 233, *233*
reserve of, 13, *13*, 14
Vasopressin, coronary circulatory effects of, 11
Vector(s), definition of, 1277
in pulse Fourier transform nuclear magnetic resonance, 735, *735*, 736, *736*
magnetization, macroscopic, definition of, 1273
Vegetations, ultrasonic tissue characterization of, 553
valvular, giant, echocardiography of, 529, *532*
in aortic regurgitation, 425
in mitral regurgitation, 434, *435*
Veiling glare, 291
scatter and, in densitometry, 292, *292*, 293, *293*
Vein(s), anomalies of, magnetic resonance imaging of, 894
hepatic, blood flow in, in tricuspid regurgitation, 438, *438*
innominate, in aortic dissection, 872, *873*
pulmonary, evaluation of, cine magnetic resonance imaging in, 955
saphenous, in bypass graft, ultrafast computed tomography of, 684, *684*
systemic, abnormalities of, magnetic resonance imaging of, 879–881, *880–882*
Velocity, aortic, transvalvular, in aortic stenosis, 421
flow, mitral, in constrictive pericarditis, 473, *474*
of blood flow, calculation of, phase shift in, 823, *823*
in arteries, 822(t)
Velocity *(Continued)*
in ascending aorta, magnetic resonance imaging of, 881, *882*
quantitation of, magnetic resonance imaging in, 823, *823*
of left ventricular ejection, 403
Doppler, in cardiomyopathy, 405, *406*
propagation, definition of, 365
regurgitant, mitral, peak, in mitral regurgitation, 435
transit, 369
Velocity-time envelope, 58, *58*
Vena cava, inferior, obstruction of, magnetic resonance imaging in, 881, *882*
superior, left, persistent, echocardiography of, *503*, *504*
magnetic resonance imaging of, 879, *880*
obstruction of, magnetic resonance imaging in, 879–881, *881*
ultrafast computed tomography of, 716, *717*
Vena caval plethora, inferior, in cardiac tamponade, 468
Vena contracta, 59, 60
Venous drainage, pulmonary, anomalous, ultrafast computed tomography in, 716, *717*
Venous return, abnormalities of, ultrafast computed tomography of, 715, 716, *717*
systemic, normal, *503*
Venous thrombosis, imaging of, indium-111–labeled platelets in, 1128, 1129
Ventricle(s), abnormalities of, ultrafast computed tomography of, 717–722, *720–724*
anteromedial translational motion of, analysis of, floating-axis system of, 385, *385*
endocardial surface mapping of, 388, *391*
imaging of, during bicycle exercise, 303, *304*
interdependence of, 28
left. See *Left ventricle(s).*
mass of, in congenital heart disease, ultrafast computed tomography of, 728
muscle fiber of, in myocardial acoustics, 544
right. See *Right ventricle(s).*
single, cine magnetic resonance imaging of, *962*
ultrafast computed tomography of, 722, *722*, *724*
size of, echocardiography of, in dilated cardiomyopathy, 453, 454
trabeculae of, echocardiography of, 529, *530*
volume of, in congenital heart disease, measurement of, ultrafast computed tomography in, 728
wall thickness in, in restrictive cardiomyopathy, echocardiography of, 457, *457*
whole, analysis of, integrative approaches to, 388, *391*
Ventricular arrhythmias, after intracoronary contrast agent injection, 187
as coronary angiography indication, 184
Ventricular diastolic pressure, in constrictive pericarditis, 473, 474
Ventricular fibrillation threshold, after selective intracoronary injection, of angiographic contrast agents, 173, 174, *174*, *175*
Ventricular filling pressure, after intravascular bolus injection, of angiographic contrast agents, 169, *170*, *171*
Ventricular function, assessment of, digital subtraction angiography in, 295–309
echocardiography in, 374–401
stress in, 27, 27(t)
diastolic, 33–35
assessment of, 301
determinants of, 24–38
Doppler measures of, 408, 408(t)

Ventricular function *(Continued)*
in restrictive cardiomyopathy, echocardiography of, 457, 458, *458*
in coronary artery disease, 135–138
pressure-volume measurements of, 27, 28, *28*
regional, modification of, pathologic states in, 31–33
normal, definition of, 382, 383
systolic, determinants of, 24–38
exercise effect on, 407
in restrictive cardiomyopathy, echocardiography of, 457
measurement of, Doppler echocardiography in, after interventions, 407, *407*
at rest, 403–407, *406*
Ventricular outflow, anomalies of, magnetic resonance imaging of, 887
obstruction of, in congenital heart disease, Doppler echocardiography in, 489–492
two-dimensional echocardiography in, 489–492
Ventricular septal defect, blood flow in, pulmonary, 489
systemic, 489
color flow imaging of, 481
echocardiography in, *507*
Doppler, 481–483, *481*
two-dimensional, 479–481, *480*, *481*
magnetic resonance imaging in, 888, *890*
pulmonary atresia with, echocardiography in, 494, *494*
ultrafast computed tomography in, 717, *720*
Ventricular septum, intact, pulmonary atresia with, echocardiography of, 495, 496, *496*
portions of, 479, *480*
rupture of, after myocardial infarction, *598*, 599, *599*
Ventriculography, contrast. See *Contrast ventriculography*.
radionuclide. See *Radionuclide ventriculography*.
right, 139
stress, in cardiac reserve assessment, 135
Verapamil, effects of, exercise Doppler echocardiography of, 578–580
Vessel cutoff, in pulmonary embolism, *151–153*, 153
Vessel midpoints, calculation of, 226
VEST, 981, 982
Video, for digital angiography, 283, *283*, 284
Video camera, in densitometry, 292
Videodensitometric cross-sectional area, measured vs. actual, linear regression analysis of, 315, *315*, *316*
Videodensitometry, 300–302
in coronary flow reserve measurement, 245
in coronary stenosis evaluation, 307
in left ventricular ejection fraction calculation, 300–302, *301–303*
in restenosis analysis, 263
limitations of, 324, 325(t)
with digital angiography, in coronary artery assessment, 324, 325(t)
in percutaneous transluminal coronary angioplasty, 324
Videotape, analog, in archival storage, in digital angiography, 286
Visceral situs, abnormal, magnetic resonance imaging of, 892
ultrafast computed tomography of, 715
Viscosity, in blood flow physics, 367, 368, *368*
Visual search, 88, 89
Volume, cardiac, measurement of, magnetic resonance imaging in, 816, 817, *817*
end-diastolic. See *End-diastolic volume*.
end-systolic. See *End-systolic volume*.

Volume *(Continued)*
in global right ventricular function, 393–396, *393*, 395(t), *396*, *397*
intramyocardial, measurement of, fast computed tomography in, 698, 699, *699*
intravascular, after intravascular bolus injection, of angiographic contrast agents, 168, *168*
of left atrium, evaluation of, ultrafast computed tomography in, 678
of left ventricle, calculation of, 300, 301
models for, 375, *375*, *376*
ultrafast computed tomography in, 671, *671*, 672
of right atrium, evaluation of, ultrafast computed tomography in, 678
of right ventricle, evaluation of, ultrafast computed tomography in, 676, *676*, 677, *677*
stroke. See *Stroke volume*.
ventricular, in congenital heart disease, measurement of, ultrafast computed tomography in, 728
Volume curve, left ventricular, 139, *139*
Volume determination, area-length method of, 110, 111, *116*
by contrast left ventriculography, 110–124, *116*
in practice, 118–122, *119–121*
in theory, 110–118, *117*, *118*
parameters derived from, 122–124, *122–125*
interobserver variability in, 118, *119*
Volume flow rate equation, 66
Volume imaging, definition of, 1277
Volume overload, left ventricular function in, 124
of right ventricle, 392, *393*
Volume rendering, in three-dimensional computed tomography, 660, 663, *664*, *665*
Volume-averaging artifacts, in fast computed tomography, in myocardial perfusion measurement, 696
Volumetric flow rate, calculation of, 403
Voxel, 76
definition of, 1277
VTI (systolic velocity-time integral), 403, *404*

Wall motion, abnormal, definition of, 131, 132
regional, in right ventricular infarction, 397
abnormal timing of, 110
analysis of, fixed-axis system of, 383–385, *384*, *386*
floating-axis system of, 383–385, *384*, *386*
in coronary artery disease diagnosis, 583, 583(t), 584
in right ventricle, 129, *130*
in theory, 124, *127*
methods of, 124–134, *128*
assumptions in, 127–129, *129*, *130*
selection of, 134
parameters in, 129–131, *131*
radial coordinate system in, 127, *129*
rectangular coordinate system in, 127, *129*
reference systems for, 383–386, *384–386*
reference-independent systems for, 387, 388
variability in, 132, *132*
vs. systolic wall thickening analysis, 390, 391, *391*
anterior, effect on, of left anterior descending lumen diameter, 307, *307*
apical, analysis of, 388–390

Wall motion *(Continued)*
assessment of, equilibrium radionuclide angiography in, 1028
magnetic resonance imaging in, 820, *821*
throughout cardiac cycle, 140–144, *141–143*
in coronary artery disease, 144
in infarct size quantification, 388–391
single plane, 388, *390*
in ischemic heart disease, analysis of, nuclear magnetic resonance in, 923
measurement of, exercise echocardiography in, 580, 581, *581*, *582*
in left ventricle, abnormal, causes of, 597(t)
assessment of, magnetic resonance imaging in, *821*
radionuclide angiocardiography in, 1017
quantitative analysis of, applications of, 134–139
parameter selection in, 138, 139
theoretical considerations in, 138
regional, quantitative analysis of, 124–134, *126–134*
timing of, 138
in myocardial infarction, as predictor of survival, 138
in normal subjects, standard deviation of, 127, *128*
measurements of, centerline method of, 124, *126*
in region of interest, 132–134, *133*, *134*
numbers of, 387
types of, 386, 387, *387*
opposite infarction site, 137, *137*
regional, measurement of, equilibrium radionuclide angiography in, 1029, 1029(t), 1030, *1030*
vs. myocardial metabolic activity, in tissue viability determination, 1227–1229
rotational, 383, *384*
sampling of, frequent, during cardiac cycle, 387, *388*, *389*
segmental, calculation of, radionuclide ventriculography in, 998, *998*, *999*
circumferential profile of, *999*
translational, 383, *384*
Wall motion score index, 598, *598*
Wall thickening, assessment of, magnetic resonance imaging in, 820, *821*
in dilated cardiomyopathy, magnetic resonance imaging of, 931, 932, *933*
in ischemic heart disease, nuclear magnetic resonance imaging of, 923–925, *924*
Wall thickness, normal values for, 134(t)
Warfarin, for left ventricular thrombi, 524
"Warping," 79
Washout, of tagged spins, 774, *774*
Washout rate profiles, generation of, in myocardial perfusion scintigraphy, 990, *990*
Water, in cardiac tissue, in myocardial acoustics, 544
measurement of, proton magnetic resonance spectroscopy in, 854
oxygen-15–labeled, 1143
characteristics of, 1170(t)
in myocardial blood flow evaluation, 1162, *1162*, 1163, 1170
protons of, 760
T1, 759, 760
T2, 759, 760
Wavelength, definition of, 365
in diagnostic ultrasound, 350(t)
ultrasonic, definition of, 539
Waves, 349, *349*, 350
mechanical, types of, 349, *349*
propagation of, in Doppler effect, 365

Window displays, 78, *80*
Windowing, 372
Wire-frame displays, in three-dimensional heart reconstruction, 73, *74*
Wobbling transducer, 356
Workstation, image, in digital angiography, 286, 287
Wraparound, in magnetic resonance imaging, 787, 788, *788*, *789*

Xenon-133, in coronary blood flow measurement, 244
X-ray computed tomography. See *Computed tomography, x-ray.*
X-ray gantry, geometry of, 232, *233*
  variability in, in cineangiography, 240, 240(t)
X-ray imaging, diagnostic, physics of, 162
X-ray system, setting of, on-line registration in, 232, *233*
X-ray tube, in x-ray computed tomography, 641, *642*
X-ray-cineangiographic acquisition system, block diagram of, 228, *229*
x-y digitizing table, 120, 121, *121*

Zero harmonic, 999
"Zipper" artifact, 788
Zoom, hardware, of digital image processor, 285